PRINCIPLES OF Surgery

Sixth Edition

NOTICE

Medicine is an ever-changing science. As new research and clinical experience broaden our knowledge, changes in treatment and drug therapy are required. The editors and the publisher of this work have checked with sources believed to be reliable in their efforts to provide information that is complete and generally in accord with the standards accepted at the time of publication. However, in view of the possibility of human error or changes in medical sciences, neither the editors nor the publisher nor any other party who has been involved in the preparation or publication of this work warrants that the information contained herein is in every respect accurate or complete, and they are not responsible for any errors or omissions or for the results obtained from use of such information. Readers are encouraged to confirm the information contained herein with other sources. For example and in particular, readers are advised to check the product information sheet included in the package of each drug they plan to administer to be certain that the information contained in this book is accurate and that changes have not been made in the recommended dose or in the contraindications for administration. This recommendation is of particular importance in connection with new or infrequently used drugs.

PRINCIPLES OF Surgery

Sixth Edition

Editor-in-Chief
SEYMOUR I. SCHWARTZ, M.D.
Professor and Chair
Department of Surgery
University of Rochester School of Medicine and Dentistry

Associate Editors
G. Tom Shires, M.D.
Professor and Chairman
Department of Surgery
Texas Tech University

Frank C. Spencer, M.D.
George David Stewart Professor and Chairman
Department of Surgery
New York University School of Medicine

With
Wendy Cowles Husser, M.A., M.P.A.
University of Rochester
School of Medicine and Dentistry

McGRAW-HILL, INC.
Health Professions Division
New York St. Louis San Francisco Auckland Bogotá Caracas Lisbon London Madrid
Mexico City Milan Montreal New Delhi Paris San Juan Singapore Sydney Tokyo Toronto

PRINCIPLES OF SURGERY

1 2 3 4 5 6 7 8 9 DOW DOW 9 8 7 6 5 4 3

ISBN 0-07-055928-7 {COMBO}
0-07-055929-5 {VOL 1}
0-07-055930-9 {VOL 2}
0-07-909967-X {SET}

This book was set in Times Roman by York Graphic Services, Inc. The editors were Michael J. Houston and Peter McCurdy. The production supervisor was Richard Ruzycka. The text was designed by Caliber and the cover by Ed Schultheis. Alexandra Nickerson Indexing Services prepared the index.
R. R. Donnelley and Sons was printer and binder.

This book is printed on acid-free paper.

The illustrations on the front cover were adapted from Georg Bartisch's *Augendienst* and Tagliacozzi's *De curtorum chirurgia*. The illustration on the back cover is from *An Explanation of the Fashion and Use of Three and Fifty Instruments of Chirurgery—Gathered out of Ambrosius Pareus*.

Library of Congress Cataloging-in-Publication Data
Principles of surgery / editor-in-chief, Seymour I. Schwartz ; associate editors, G. Tom Shires, Frank C. Spencer, with Wendy Cowles Husser. — 6th ed.
p. cm.
Includes bibliographical references and index.
ISBN 0-07-055928-7 (combo). — ISBN 0-07-055929-5 (v. 1). — ISBN 0-07-055930-9 (v. 2). — ISBN 0-07-909967-X (set)
1. Surgery. I. Schwartz, Seymour I., date
[DNLM: 1. Surgery. WO 100 P957 1994]
RD31.P88 1994
617—dc20
DNLM/DLC 93-28477
for Library of Congress CIP

To students of Surgery, at all levels, in their quest for knowledge

Contents

Contributors*

James T. Adams, M.D. *(33)*
Professor of Surgery
Department of Surgery
University of Rochester School of Medicine and Dentistry

R. Peter Altman, M.D. *(37)*
Professor of Surgery
Columbia University College of Physicians and Surgeons
Surgeon in Chief, Babies Hospital
Columbia Presbyterian Medical Center

Kathryn D. Anderson, M.D. *(37)*
Professor of Surgery
University of Southern California
Surgeon in Chief, Children's Hospital Los Angeles

Charles M. Balch, M.D. *(9)*
Professor and Head, Division of Surgery
Chairman, Department of General Surgery
University of Texas, MD Anderson Cancer Center

Elisa H. Birnbaum, M.D. *(26)*
Clinical Instructor in Surgery
Washington University School of Medicine
Jewish Hospital of St. Louis

Kirby I. Bland, M.D. *(14)*
Professor and Associate Chairman
Department of Surgery
University of Florida

Michael F. Boland, M.D. *(40)*
St. Luke's Hospital
Chesterfield, Missouri
Missouri Baptist Hospital, St. Louis

Timothy B. Boone, M.D., Ph.D. *(38)*
Assistant Professor of Urology
Baylor College of Medicine

Murray F. Brennan, M.D. *(9)*
Professor of Surgery
Cornell University Medical College
Memorial Sloan Kettering Cancer Center

*The numbers in parentheses following each contributor's name refer to the chapters written or co-written by that contributor.

Richard I. Burton, M.D. *(43)*
Professor and Chair
Department of Orthopaedics
University of Rochester School of Medicine and Dentistry

C. James Carrico, M.D. *(4)*
Professor and Chairman
University of Texas
Southwestern Medical School

Joseph M. Civetta, M.D. *(12)*
Professor of Surgery, Anesthesiology, Medicine, and Pathology
Chief, Division of Surgical Critical Care
University of Miami School of Medicine

I. Kelman Cohen, M.D. *(8)*
Professor and Chairman
Division of Plastic and Reconstructive Surgery
Medical College of Virginia of Virginia Commonwealth University

John J. Coleman III, M.D. *(15)*
Professor of Surgery
Chairman, Division of Plastic Surgery
Indiana University Medical Center

Stephen B. Colvin, M.D. *(17,18,19)*
Associate Professor of Surgery
Director, Cardiac Surgical Residency and Pediatric Cardiac Surgery
New York University School of Medicine

Robert E. Condon, M.D., M.S. *(32)*
Ausman Foundation Professor and Chairman
Department of Surgery
The Medical College of Wisconsin

Edward M. Copeland III, M.D. *(14)*
The Edward R. Woodward Professor and Chairman
Department of Surgery
University of Florida, Gainesville

William T. Couldwell, M.D. *(35)*
Assistant Professor of Surgery
Department of Neurologic Surgery
University of Southern California School of Medicine

Mary C. Crossland, B.S.N., R.N. *(8)*
Clinical Research Assistant
Division of Plastic and Reconstructive Surgery
Medical College of Virginia of Virginia Commonwealth University

Eric J. DeMaria, M.D. *(35)*
Assistant Professor of Surgery
Director of Trauma; Assistant Director Surgery/ Trauma ICU
Medical College of Virginia of Virginia Commonwealth University

Tom R. DeMeester, M.D. *(23)*
Professor and Chairman
Department of Surgery
University of Southern California School of Medicine

Robert F. Diegelmann, Ph.D. *(8)*
Professor of Surgery and Biochemistry
Division of Plastic and Reconstructive Surgery
Medical College of Virginia of Virginia Commonwealth University

Martin R. Eichelberger, M.D. *(37)*
Professor of Surgery
Department of Surgery
George Washington University

Patricia J. Eifel, M.D. *(9)*
Associate Professor
Department of Radiotherapy
University of Texas
MD Anderson Cancer Center

Jerome L. Finkelstein, M.D. *(7)*
Clinical Associate Professor of Surgery
Associate Director, Burn Center
Cornell University Medical College
New York Hospital–Cornell Medical Center

James W. Fleshman, M.D. *(26)*
Assistant Professor of Surgery
Washington University School of Medicine

Andrew H. Foster, M.D. *(1)*
Assistant Professor of Surgery
Division of Thoracic and Cardiovascular Surgery
Department of Surgery
University of Maryland Medical School

Irwin N. Frank, M.D. *(38)*
Professor of Urology
Department of Urology
University of Rochester School of Medicine and Dentistry

Robert D. Fry, M.D. *(26)*
Associate Professor of Surgery
Washington University School of Medicine
Program Director, Division of Colon and Rectal Surgery
Jewish Hospital of St. Louis

Aubrey C. Galloway, M.D. *(17,18,19)*
Associate Professor of Surgery
Director, Cardiac Surgical Research
New York University School of Medicine

Donald S. Gann, M.D. *(1,35)*
Professor and Executive Vice-Chairman
Department of Surgery
University of Maryland School of Medicine

Cleon W. Goodwin, M.D. *(7)*
Johnson and Johnson Distinguished Associate Professor of Surgery
Director, Burn Center
Cornell University Medical College
New York Hospital–Cornell Medical Center

Richard M. Green, M.D. *(20)*
Associate Professor of Surgery
Chief, Section of Vascular Surgery
University of Rochester School of Medicine and Dentistry

Lazar J. Greenfield, M.D. *(21)*
Frederick A. Coller Professor and Chairman
Department of Surgery
University of Michigan

Eugene A. Grossi, M.D. *(18)*
Assistant Professor of Surgery
New York University School of Medicine

Philip C. Guzzetta, Jr., M.D. *(37)*
Professor and Chairman
Division of Pediatric Surgery
University of Texas Southwestern Medical School

Julian T. Hoff, M.D. *(40)*
Professor of Surgery
Department of Surgery, Section of Neurosurgery
University of Michigan

Richard J. Howard, M.D. *(5)*
Professor of Surgery
Department of Surgery
University of Florida, Gainesville

Darryl T. Hiyama, M.D. *(11)*
Assistant Professor
Department of Surgery
University of California Los Angeles School of Medicine

Suzanne T. Ildstad, M.D. *(10)*
Assistant Professor of Surgery
Department of Surgery
University of Pittsburgh

Ronald C. Jones, M.D. *(6)*
Chief of Surgery
Baylor University Medical Center

M.J. Jurkiewicz, M.D. *(44)*
Professor of Surgery
Emory University School of Medicine

Edwin L. Kaplan, M.D. *(36)*
Professor of Surgery
Department of Surgery
The University of Chicago
Pritzker School of Medicine

Thomas C. King, M.D. *(16)*
Ferrer Professor of Surgery
Columbia Presbyterian Medical Center

Ira J. Kodner, M.D. *(26)*
Assistant Professor of Surgery
Washington University School of Medicine
Director, Division of Colon and Rectal Surgery
The Jewish Hospital of St. Louis

Stephen F. Lowry, M.D. *(2)*
Professor of Surgery
Department of Surgery
New York Hospital
Cornell Medical Center

John D. McConnell, M.D. *(38)*
Associate Professor of Urology
University of Texas Southwestern Medical School

David W. McFadden, M.D. *(22)*
Associate Professor of Surgery
Division of General Surgery
University of California Los Angeles
Chief, General Surgery, Sepulveda VA Medical Center

Michael R. Madden, M.D. *(7)*
Clinical Associate Professor of Surgery
Associate Director, Burn Center
Cornell University Medical College
New York Hospital
Cornell Medical Center

Stephen J. Mathes, M.D. *(13)*
Professor of Surgery
Head, Division of Plastic and Reconstructive Surgery
University of California San Francisco

Thomas A. Miller, M.D. *(24)*
Professor of Surgery
Department of Surgery
University of Texas Medical School at Houston

Frank G. Moody, M.D. *(24)*
Denton A. Cooley Professor and Chairman
Department of Surgery
University of Texas Medical School at Houston

Donald L. Morton, M.D. *(9)*
Emeritus Professor of Surgery
University of California Los Angeles School of Medicine

John S. Najarian, M.D. *(10)*
Jay Phillips Regents' Professor of Surgery
Director of Transplantation
Department of Surgery
University of Minnesota

Kurt D. Newman, M.D. *(37)*
Assistant Professor of Surgery
George Washington University

Kenneth Ouriel, M.D. *(20)*
Associate Professor
Department of Surgery
University of Rochester School of Medicine and Dentistry

Neal R. Pellis, Ph.D. *(9)*
Associate Professor of Surgery and Immunology
Department of General Surgery
University of Texas, MD Anderson Cancer Center

Malcolm O. Perry, M.D. *(6)*
Professor of Surgery
Department of Surgery
Texas Tech University Health Sciences Center

Jeffrey H. Peters, M.D. *(23)*
Assistant Professor of Surgery
University of Southern California School of Medicine
Chief, Division of General Surgery
University of Southern California University Hospital

Paul C. Peters, M.D. *(38)*
E. E. and Greer Garson Fogelson Distinguished Chair in Urology
Professor and Chairman, Division of Urology
University of Texas Southwestern Medical School

Glenn M. Preminger, M.D. *(38)*
Associate Professor of Urology
University of Texas Southwestern Medical School

Howard A. Reber, M.D. *(30)*
Professor of Surgery/Vice Chairman
Department of Surgery
University of California Los Angeles School of Medicine
Chief of Surgery, Sepulveda VA Medical Center

Keith Reemtsma, M.D. *(10)*
Valentine Mott and Johnson and Johnson Professor and Chairman
Department of Surgery
Columbia Presbyterian Medical Center

W. Bradford Rockwell, M.D. *(43)*
Assistant Professor of Surgery
Division of Plastic and Reconstructive Surgery
University of Utah School of Medicine

Robert E. Rogers, M.D. *(39)*
Professor of Obstetrics and Gynecology
Chief, Gynecology Division
Department of Obstetrics and Gynecology
Indiana University School of Medicine

Randy N. Rosier, M.D., Ph.D. *(41)*
Professor of Orthopaedics, Oncology, and Biophysics
Department of Orthopaedics
University of Rochester School of Medicine and Dentistry

Joel J. Roslyn, M.D. *(29)*
Alma Dea Morani Professor and Chairman
Department of Surgery
Medical College of Pennsylvania

Thomas M. Rouse, M.D. *(37)*
Director, Pediatric Trauma
Methodist Hospital of Indianapolis

Seymour I. Schwartz, M.D. *(3,27,28,31,42)*
Professor and Chair
Department of Surgery
University of Rochester School of Medicine and Dentistry

Jay J. Schnitzer, M.D. *(37)*
Instructor in Surgery
Harvard Medical School
Massachusetts General Hospital

G. Tom Shires, M.D. *(2,4,6)*
Professor and Chairman
Department of Surgery
Texas Tech University Health Sciences Center

G. Tom Shires III, M.D. *(2,4,6)*
Associate Professor
Department of Surgery
University of Texas
Southwestern Medical School

Marie F. Simard, M.D. *(35)*
Assistant Professor of Internal Medicine
Department of Internal Medicine
Division of Endocrinology
University of Southern California School of Medicine

Richard L. Simmons, M.D. *(10)*
George V. Foster Professor and Chair
Department of Surgery
University of Pittsburgh School of Medicine

Craig R. Smith, M.D. *(10,16)*
Associate Professor of Clinical Surgery
Columbia-Presbyterian Medical Center

Frank C. Spencer, M.D. *(17,18,19)*
George David Stewart Professor and Chairman
Department of Surgery
New York University School of Medicine

Mark R. Sultan, M.D. *(15)*
Assistant Professor of Surgery
Columbia-Presbyterian Medical Center

Gregory P. Sutton, M.D. *(39)*
Mary Fendrick Hulman Professor and Chief
Division of Gynecologic Oncology
Department of Obstetrics and Gynecology
Indiana University School of Medicine

Erwin R. Thal, M.D. *(6)*
Professor
Department of Surgery
University of Texas, Southwestern Medical School

James C. Thompson, M.D. *(25)*
John Woods Harris Professor and Chairman
Department of Surgery
University of Texas Medical Branch at Galveston

Courtney M. Townsend, Jr., M.D. *(25)*
Robertson-Poth Professor
Department of Surgery
University of Texas Medical Branch at Galveston

Albert J. Varon, M.D. *(12)*
Associate Professor of Clinical Anesthesiology, Surgery, and Medicine
Department of Anesthesiology
University of Miami School of Medicine

Alonzo P. Walker, M.D. *(32)*
Associate Professor of Surgery
Department of Surgery
The Medical College of Wisconsin

George E. Wantz, M.D. *(34)*
Clinical Professor of Surgery
Cornell University Medical College

Martin H. Weiss, M.D. *(35)*
Professor and Chairman
Department of Neurological Surgery
University of Southern California School of Medicine

Dietmar H. Wittmann, M.D., Ph.D. *(32)*
Associate Professor of Surgery
Department of Surgery
The Medical College of Wisconsin

Robert J. Wood, M.D. *(44)*
Assistant Professor of Surgery
Director, Emory University Center for Craniofacial and Pediatric Plastic Surgery
Emory University

David M. Young, M.D. *(13)*
Chief Resident
Division of Plastic and Reconstructive Surgery
University of California San Francisco

Michael J. Zinner, M.D. *(11,22,29)*
Professor and Chairman
Department of Surgery
University of California Los Angeles School of Medicine

Preface

The sixth edition of *Principles of Surgery* has special significance for the three editors, G. Tom Shires, Frank C. Spencer, and me. As we reflect on all that has ensued since the time we met as a group with David Hume, Richard C. Lillehei, and Edward Storer in the summer of 1966 and accepted the challenge from McGraw-Hill to create a new textbook of surgery, many thoughts enter our minds. The extraordinary explosion of scientific information and the advancement of the field of surgery are apparent. We have attempted to incorporate the advances in each of the editions.

The extent of change and update is readily manifest. In Basic Considerations, six of the twelve chapters have been completely revised by new authors. These are chapters on Surgical Infections, Burns, Wound Care and Wound Healing, Oncology, Surgical Complications, and Physiologic Monitoring. And many other chapters incorporate significant changes. In the Specific Considerations section, the chapters on Breast, Tumors of the Head and Neck, Peripheral Arterial Disease, Manifestations of Gastrointestinal Disease, Esophagus and Diaphragmatic Hernia, Colon, Rectum, and Anus, Gallbladder and Biliary Tract, Pancreas, Abdominal Wall Hernias, Pituitary, Urology, Gynecology, Neurosurgery, and Orthopaedics all represent new presentations by new authors. The application of minimally invasive procedures is considered in each of these chapters. New data leading to new concepts comprise the essence of each chapter, whether the chapter is a replacement or a revision.

The sixth edition is the most major revision we have produced; this is a deliberate effort on our part because we realize we have been privileged to participate in the education of an entire generation of medical students, surgical residents, and practitioners.

We are thankful to the many authors who over the years have contributed to the six editions of our book; it is the synthesis of their individual fields of expertise that has created a meaningful textbook. We are equally appreciative of our readership, both those readers who entrust their entrance into the arena of surgical education to us and those who have been loyal partners through several editions over the years.

ACKNOWLEDGMENTS

Associates who added significantly to the revised material for this 25 year anniversary edition are Aubrey C. Galloway, G. Tom Shires III, and Michael J. Zinner.

Throughout the production of the sixth edition, we have had the assistance of Amy Wilkin; the authors join us in an expression of gratitude for her commitment to the entire process.

Seymour I. Schwartz, M.D.

Preface to the First Edition

The raison d'être for a new textbook in a discipline which has been served by standard works for many years was the Editorial Board's initial conviction that a distinct need for a modern approach in the dissemination of surgical knowledge existed. As incoming chapters were reviewed, both the need and satisfaction became increasingly apparent and, at the completion, we felt a sense of excitement at having the opportunity to contribute to the education of modern and future students concerned with the care of surgical patients.

The recent explosion of factual knowledge has emphasized the need for a presentation which would provide the student an opportunity to assimilate pertinent facts in a logical fashion. This would then permit correlation, synthesis of concepts, and eventual extrapolation to specific situations. The physiologic bases for diseases are therefore emphasized and the manifestations and diagnostic studies are considered as a reflection of pathophysiology. Therapy then becomes logical in this schema and the necessity to regurgitate facts is minimized. In appreciation of the impact which Harrison's PRINCIPLES OF INTERNAL MEDICINE has had, the clinical manifestations of the disease processes are considered in detail for each area. Since the operative procedure represents the one element in the therapeutic armamentarium unique to the surgeon, the indications, important technical considerations, and complications receive appropriate emphasis. While we appreciate that a textbook cannot hope to incorporate an atlas of surgical procedures, we have provided the student a single book which will satisfy the sequential demands in the care and considerations of surgical patients.

The ultimate goal of the Editorial Board has been to collate a book which is deserving of the adjective "modern." We have therefore selected as authors dynamic and active contributors to their particular fields. The au courant concept is hopefully apparent throughout the entire work and is exemplified by appropriate emphasis on diseases of modern surgical interest, such as trauma, transplantation, and the recently appreciated importance of rehabilitation. Cardiovascular surgery is presented in keeping with the exponential strides recently achieved.

There are two major subdivisions to the text. In the first twelve chapters, subjects that transcend several organ systems are presented. The second portion of the book represents a consideration of specific organ systems and surgical specialties.

Throughout the text, the authors have addressed themselves to a sophisticated audience, regarding the medical student as a graduate student, incorporating material generally sought after by the surgeon in training and presenting information appropriate for the continuing education of the practicing surgeon. The need for a text such as we have envisioned is great and the goal admittedly high. It is our hope that this effort fulfills the expressed demands.

Seymour I. Schwartz, M.D.

PART I
BASIC CONSIDERATIONS

CHAPTER 1

Endocrine and Metabolic Responses to Injury

Donald S. Gann and Andrew H. Foster

INTRODUCTION

The response of the neuroendocrine system, the release of mediator substances, and the consequent alterations in cellular and intermediary metabolism, are tailored to the magnitude, duration, and nature of the injury. Although the precise interplay of neurohumoral and immunologic responses remains incompletely understood at this time, predictable patterns have been observed. Complete surgical care requires a thorough understanding of the injury response to distinguish those changes that are *physiologic,* and likely beneficial, from those that are deleterious or may indicate failure of homeostatic mechanisms. The ultimate recovery of the surgical patient hinges as much on appropriate and timely physiologic interventions in the intensive care unit as on an appropriately planned and expeditiously performed procedure in the operating room.

The technical achievements of the surgeon parallel advancements in device technology. Similarly, the improved resolution of laboratory techniques that are reexamining the neurohumoral responses to injury has sharpened the focus to include the characterization of bioactive substances to an astounding level of detail. The response to injury involves not only a complex interplay of substances between the hypothalamic-pituitary axis, autonomic nervous system (ANS), and classical hormone system, but also involves mediators that may have local and systemic actions, vascular endothelial cell products, and even the intracellular products of single cells.

The physiologic significance of recent experimental and clinical findings regarding mediators and other substances, and their potential interactions with established endocrine and neural responses are not fully understood at this time. Multiple, nested layers of stimulatory and inhibitory pathways are present, and undoubtedly all have important roles in fine control and modulation of homeostasis. These levels of complexity are difficult to translate to clinical situations. It seems inevitable that the next few years will see an evolving understanding of the relative importance of the neuroendocrine system, the immune system, and the vascular endothelium in the integration and modulation of the metabolic response to injury.

Cuthbertson and coworkers have described a useful framework for the metabolic response to injury in patients that temporally divides injury into the *ebb* and *flow* phases (Fig. 1-1). The ebb phase corresponds to the immediate consequence of injury that decreases the resting energy expenditure. In all injury there is some reduction in blood volume (e.g., hemorrhage), plasma volume (e.g., burn), and/or loss of effective circulating volume (e.g., third-space losses resulting from tissue trauma). These changes may produce cell sequestration or shock. Loss of vascular resistance is sensed by baroreceptors and stretch receptors and stimulates neural pathways via the sympathetic nervous system and activates catecholamine, arginine vasopressin (AVP), and angiotensin II release. The release of several hormones may be stimulated

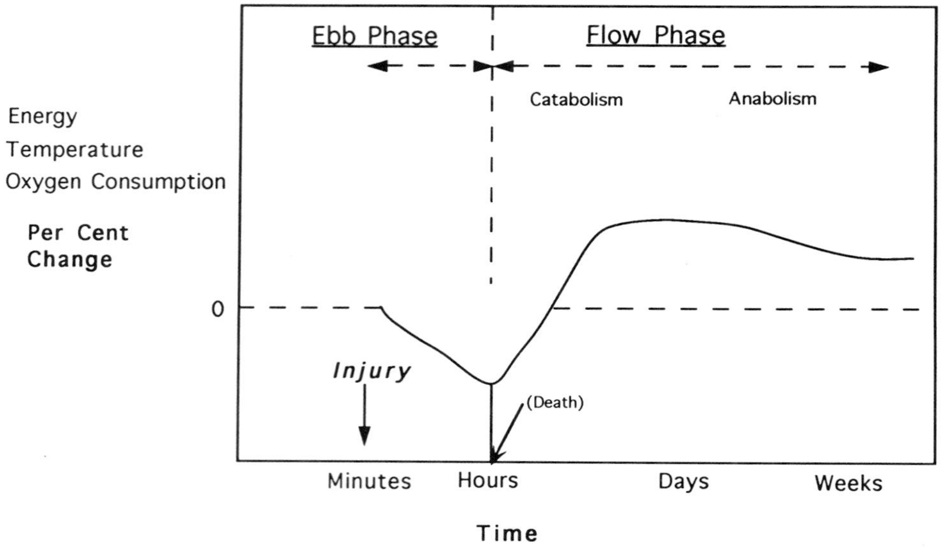

FIG. 1-1. The ebb and flow phases of the response to injury as described by Cuthbertson and later modified by Moore.

(Table 1-1). The flow phase corresponds to the period of compensation, with increases in metabolic rate, enzyme modulation directed to glucose production, and consequent restitution of blood volume, stimulation of the immune system, and production of hepatic acute phase reactants and intracellular heat shock proteins. Later, if compensatory systems prevail, energy expenditure diminishes and metabolism further shifts to anabolic pathways. Wound healing, capillary ingrowth, tissue remodeling, and functional recovery take place over a longer time period.

In this chapter, we have arbitrarily separated the response to injury into the following components: (1) stimuli, (2) neurohumoral response, (3) resultant alterations in metabolism, and (4) resultant alterations in fluid and electrolytes. The neurohumoral mediation of the injury response is further subdivided to describe the relevant responses of (1) the classical hormone system, (2) cytokines and other cell mediators, (3) endothelial cell products, and (4) the single cell.

STIMULI OF THE NEUROENDOCRINE REFLEX

The pattern of hormonal response to injury results from physiologic reflexes initiated by specific aspects of the injury itself. The stimuli are sensed by specialized peripheral and central receptors. These receptors transduce the stimulus into discrete neural afferent signals which are transmitted to the central nervous system (CNS) by specific pathways and are integrated with other signals, resulting in efferent output which modulates the release of numerous neuroendocrine substances that act to maintain homeostasis. The injury response is modulated by a number of factors such as patient age, nutritional status, concurrent illness, and medications.

In the absence of major hemorrhage, trauma, or sepsis, alterations in homeostasis are typically small and the response is directed at fine-tuning the internal milieu. In the presence of major injury, however, multiple and intense stimuli can initiate several reflexes and lead to the release of substances that appear directed to restoration of effective circulating volume and to delivery of critical energy substrates. When exaggerated, some of these responses may become deleterious.

Primary stimuli of neuroendocrine reflexes include alterations in (1) effective circulating volume, (2) oxygen, carbon dioxide, or hydrogen ion concentration, (3) pain, (4) emotional stimuli such as fear and anxiety, (5) energy substrates, (6) temperature, and (7) the wound.

Table 1-1
Neuroendocrine Response

Increased Release		*Decreased Release or Unchanged*
Epinephrine	Beta-endorphin	Insulin
Norepinephrine	Growth hormone	Estrogen
Dopamine	Prolactin	Testosterone
Glucagon	Somatostatin	Thyroxine
Renin	Eicosanoids	T_3
Angiotensin II	Histamine	TSH
AVP	Kinins	FSH
ACTH	Serotonin	LH
Cortisol	Interleukin-1	IGF
Aldosterone	TNF	

Effective Circulating Volume. Virtually all injuries are characterized by the loss of effective circulating volume. Causes include hemorrhage (trauma, ruptured aortic aneurysm), sequestration of plasma (acute pancreatitis, sepsis, burn), impaired circulation (cardiac failure, myocardial infarction, tamponade, pulmonary embolus), third-space formation (crush injury, surgical dissection, inflammation), or blood sequestration (sepsis, neurogenic collapse). Loss of effective circulating volume is sensed by high-pressure baroreceptors in the aorta, carotid arteries, and renal arteries, which are pressure-sensitive, and by low-pressure stretch receptors in the atria, which are sensitive to the changes in volume. Other arterial pressure receptors are located in the juxtaglomerular apparatus of the kidney that trigger the release of renin.

These afferent signals exert a tonic inhibition over the release of many hormones and the activities of the CNS and ANS (Fig. 1-2). Decreased effective circulating volume decreases baroreceptor and stretch receptor activities that act directly through central autonomic pathways to activate release of pituitary hormones such

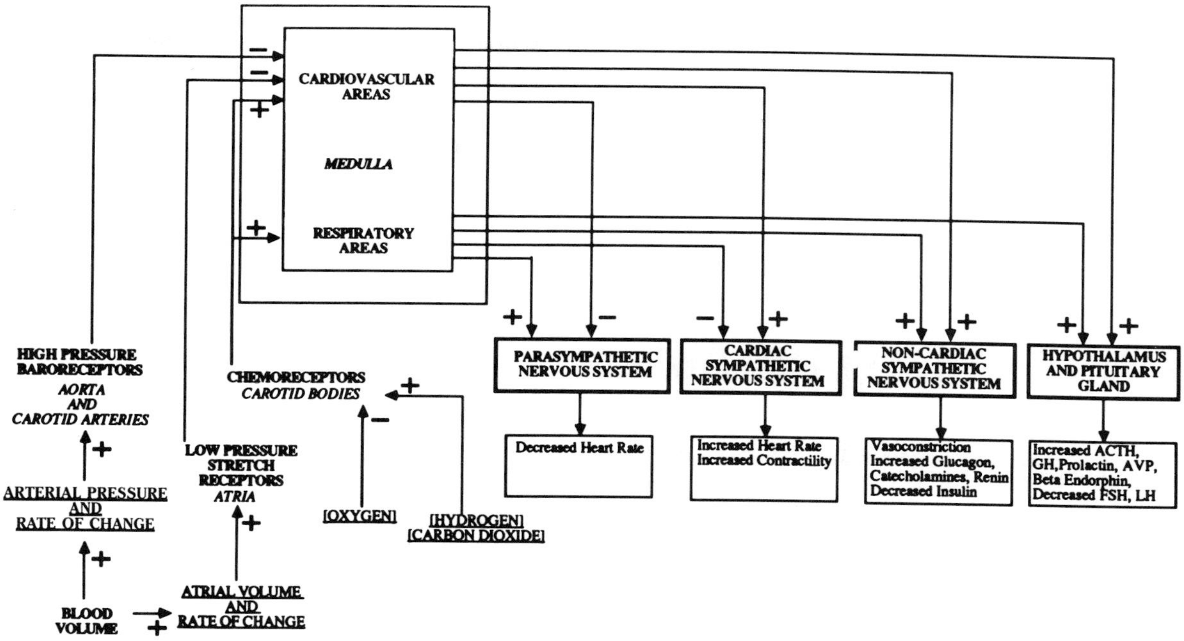

FIG. 1-2. Efferent limb of baroreceptor and chemoreceptor activation. Inactivation of baroreceptors or activation of chemoreceptors results in the stimulation of the hypothalamus and of the vascular component of the sympathetic nervous system.

as adrenocorticotropin (ACTH), vasopressin, growth hormone, and beta-endorphin and indirectly through the sympathetic nervous system to activate release of catecholamines, glucagon, and renin and to inhibit release of insulin for a given level of glucose. Decreases in the effective circulating volume that are sensed by high-pressure stretch receptors in the juxtaglomerular complexes of the kidney also may augment the secretion of renin and consequently promote angiotensin formation and aldosterone secretion. The decrease in baroreceptor and in stretch receptor discharge also stimulates the vascular component of the ANS. This causes peripheral vasoconstriction and increased cardiac contractility due to cardiac sympathetic stimulation and increased heart rate secondary to parasympathetic inhibition.

The neuroendocrine and autonomic responses initiated by a decrease in effective circulating volume are proportional to the magnitude of the volume loss. The neuroendocrine response to a 20 percent hemorrhage is greater than that observed following a 10 percent hemorrhage. Maximal neuroendocrine and cardiovascular responses occur when the effective circulating volume has been decreased by 30 to 40 percent. Further decreases in the effective circulating volume cannot be adequately handled by compensatory mechanisms, and shock follows.

Oxygen, Carbon Dioxide, and Hydrogen Ion. Changes in the concentration of oxygen, carbon dioxide, and hydrogen ions in the blood initiate cardiovascular, pulmonary, and neuroendocrine responses through the activation of peripheral chemoreceptors located in the carotid and the aortic bodies. Decreases in the concentration of oxygen or, to a lesser extent, increases in the concentrations of hydrogen ions and carbon dioxide are sensed by these receptors. Decreases in arterial blood flow or arterial oxygen tension increase chemoreceptor oxygen extraction, decrease venous P_{O_2}, and, through an unknown mechanism, activate the chemoreceptor which stimulates the hypothalamus and the vascular component of the sympathetic nervous system (Fig. 1-2). Chemoreceptor activation causes increased cardiac sympathetic nervous system activity and decreased parasympathetic nervous system activity, leading to increased heart rate and cardiac contractility. Chemoreceptor activation also stimulates the respiratory center causing increases in respiratory rate and stimulates release of ACTH and vasopressin. Hypovolemia may be accompanied by hyperventilation because the decrease in effective circulating volume and blood flow causes chemoreceptor stimulation. Furthermore, hypoxia may potentiate the hormonal reflex response to hypovolemia.

Pain. Pain acts as a stimulus to the neuroendocrine system via projections of peripheral nociceptive fibers to the CNS and consequent stimulation of the thalamus and the hypothalamus. Nociceptive stimuli do not activate the hormonal response unless neural pathways are intact. The response may be blunted or prevented by neural lesions, local anesthetics, or spinal cord lesions (Fig. 1-3).

Emotion. Emotional arousal, such as the perception or threat of injury, acts through the limbic system to projections to the hypothalamic and lower brainstem nuclei. These pathways, via the pituitary system, stimulate the secretion of AVP, ACTH, cortisol, and endogenous opiates and, via the ANS, the secretion of catecholamine and aldosterone.

Energy Substrates. Glucose is the primary substrate that activates neuroendocrine reflexes via receptors in the hypothalamic ventromedial nucleus. Peripheral receptors that have not yet been identified are also involved. Significant reduction in plasma glucose concentration stimulates the release of many hormones through central and autonomic pathways. These hormones include

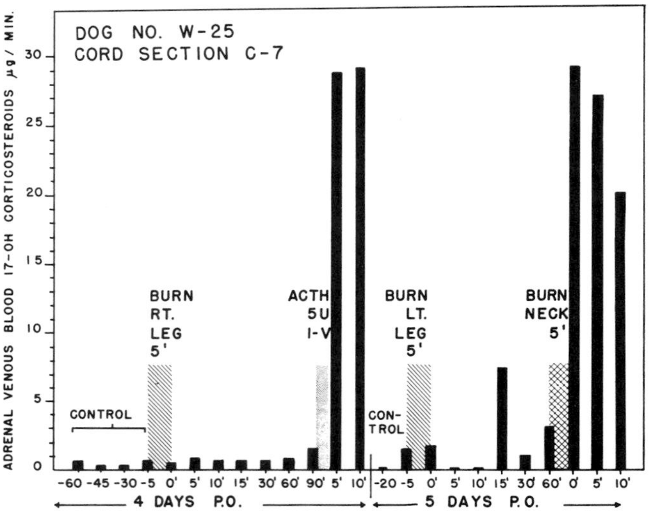

FIG. 1-3. Adrenocortical response to a burn following section of the cord at the level of C_7. A 5-min burn of the right leg, which was below the level of section, produced no increase in adrenocorticosteroid secretion over the control values. Five units of ACTH given intravenously produced an immediate and marked rise in adrenocortical output. With the dog under pentobarbital anesthesia, a burn of the left hindlimb produced no significant increase in adrenocorticosteroid output, but in marked contrast, a burn of the neck, which was above the level of cord section, produced an immediate and marked increase in adrenocortical secretion. (From: *Hume DM, Egdahl RH: Ann Surg 150:697, 1959, with permission.*)

ACTH, cortisol, growth hormone, beta-endorphin, AVP, and catecholamines. Glucagon release and insulin inhibition are mediated by ANS pathways and by direct pancreatic cell action.

Although changes in the concentrations of individual amino acids produce alterations in the secretion of various hormones, their potency varies from amino acid to amino acid, and the mechanisms by which they produce these alterations are not completely understood. In the beta islet cell, for example, arginine stimulates the secretion of both insulin and glucagon, possibly through production of nitric oxide, a free radical that has neurotransmitter properties, but leucine stimulates only the secretion of insulin. Cell surface receptors are implicated in this hormonal secretion because nonmetabolizable analogues of leucine and arginine are also effective stimuli.

The bioavailability of certain amino acids appears to be affected by the neurohumoral environment. For example, circulating glutamine is essential for maintenance of intestinal mucosal cell integrity. However, glutamine is not available to these cells during periods of sepsis and low flow but must be supplied enterally. Another example is observed in vascular endothelial cells, which release nitric oxide to act with endothelial cell relaxing factor to maintain normal local vascular tone, a process that is dependent on circulating L-arginine.

Temperature. Core temperature changes are sensed in the hypothalamic preoptic area and alter the secretion of hormones including ACTH, cortisol, AVP, growth hormone, aldosterone, thyroxine, and catecholamines. Temperature alterations are observed in a number of clinical situations such as hypovolemia with inadequate hepatic blood flow, starvation, sepsis with loss of peripheral vasomotor control, and burns with loss of thermal insulation. Induced moderate hypothermia, such as that employed during routine cardiopulmonary bypass, and profound hypothermia, such as that employed with total circulatory arrest and congenital heart repairs, are known to have far-reaching neuroendocrine and metabolic effects.

The Wound. Even sterile wounds activate inflammation and thereby involve systems directed to host defenses. The presence of inflammatory cells and activation of immunologic defense systems automatically implicates substances secreted by cells, such as the cytokines and other mediators, in the wound response. The magnitude of the wound has a direct relationship to the manifestations of the host response. The severity of injury has ramifications in the quantity of mediator substances which are released, since the spillover of some of these factors has been shown to cause systemic host effects that affect distant organs and neuroendocrine reflexes. Various substances, such as exotoxins, heat-labile proteins produced by gram-positive bacteria, and endotoxin, the lipopolysaccharide moiety of gram-negative bacteria cell walls, cause the release of mediator substances, such as interleukin 1 (IL-1) and tumor necrosis factor (TNF) from various cells and stimulate the release of hormones such as ACTH. As reviewed in a recent symposium by O'Dorisio and Panerai, many of these substances have complex and interrelated roles as messengers in the "neuroimmune axis."

NEUROHUMORAL MEDIATION OF THE INJURY RESPONSE

Integration of Stimuli and Modulation of Output

Classic experimental work has demonstrated that intact neural stimulus-signal transduction to the CNS is required for certain endocrine responses, such as that which mediates cortisol release through ACTH (Figs. 1-3 and 1-4). The ACTH response to operation is similarly absent in paraplegic patients with T_4-level spinal cord transection (Fig. 1-5). The response to nociceptive stimuli requires intact neural pathways. Anesthetic agents can initiate,

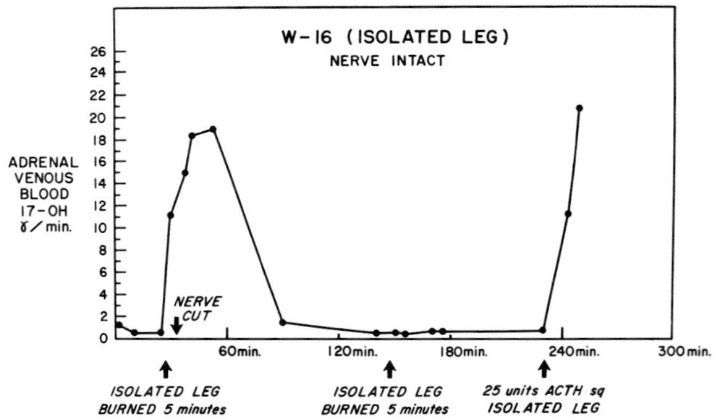

FIG. 1-4. The effect of limb denervation on ACTH secretion following trauma. The hind leg has been isolated so that it is attached to the body by only one artery, one vein, and one nerve. The burn of the isolated leg produces a marked and immediate response in adrenal venous corticosteroid secretion. During the height of this response the nerve was cut and the secretion dropped promptly to control values. A second burn of the leg now produced no adrenocortical response. ACTH injected subcutaneously into the isolated leg produced a prompt and marked increase in adrenocortical secretion. (From: *Hume DM et al: Surgery 52:174, 1962, with permission.*)

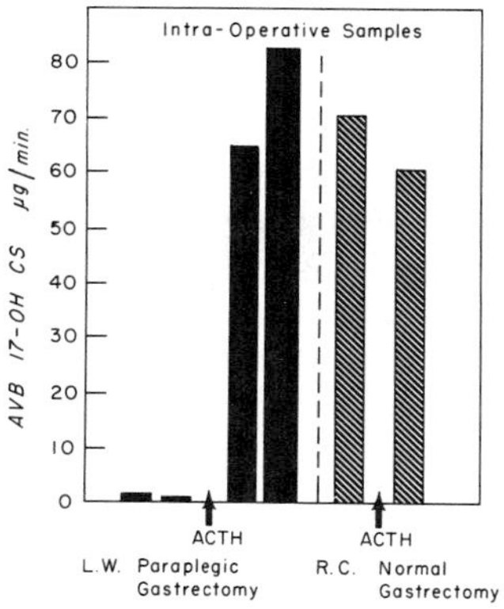

FIG. 1-5. Comparison of the adrenal venous blood content of 17-hydroxycorticosteroid (17-OHCS) in response to a gastric operation in a patient with spinal cord transection at T_4 and in a normal patient. The paraplegic patient fails to demonstrate an increase in 17-OHCS. This presumably results from the absence of ACTH production in response to surgery, since the ability of paraplegic patient's adrenal glands to respond to ACTH is demonstrated by the marked increase in 17-OHCS content of adrenal venous blood in response to intravenously administered ACTH. In contrast, the normal patient shows maximal secretion of 17-OHCS in response to the operation and no further increase is seen with intravenous ACTH. (From: *Hume DM et al: Surgery 52:174, 1962, with permission.*)

inhibit, or augment neuroendocrine reflexes and therefore must be considered as an additional factor in the injury response to operation.

The principal signals that initiate the neuroendocrine response to injury are those of hypovolemia and pain. The hormonal response is diffuse and stimulates the release of multiple hormones (Table 1-1). In each case, the prompt initiation of hormonal release depends on a reflex activated by afferent nerves. Although the reflex initiation of increased sympathetic activity may take place at the level of the medulla or spinal cord alone, it appears that even these reflexes require hypothalamic coordination similar to that observed in the control of the release of the anterior pituitary hormones. The precise pathways from afferent nerve endings to the hypothalamus have been studied in detail primarily for ACTH and to a lesser degree for AVP and catecholamines. Data for the control of other hormones, where they are available, seem analogous, and it is highly likely that the afferent pathways are shared to a considerable extent. The control of ACTH and AVP in response to the stimuli of hypovolemia and pain is an example of one neuroanatomic system by which humoral responses are integrated following injury (Fig. 1-6). Other nuclei in the hypothalamus play a central role in these reflexes by controlling the release of releasing factors, which in turn govern the secretion of various anterior pituitary hormones or ANS activity.

There is no clear overlap of function among the various hypothalamic nuclei. For example, the posterior hypothalamic area is involved in the control of ACTH and of descending sympathetic activities. The paraventricular nucleus is involved in the control of AVP, oxytocin, and ACTH. The ventromedial nucleus is involved in the control of growth hormone and ACTH. The arcuate nucleus controls gonadotropin releasing hormone. The supraoptic nucleus is active in the control of AVP and oxytocin. The suprachiasmatic nucleus appears to control the circadian rhythms of ACTH and gonadotropins. Hypothalamic control of the anterior pituitary is accomplished by the secretion of neurohormones into the capillary loops of the median eminence.

As a result of the similar pathways through which sensory inputs enter into the CNS, integration of afferent signals can result in modulation of efferent signals from the CNS. Consequently, the neuroendocrine response to a given stimulus is not an all-or-none phenomenon nor is it always the same. The response depends to a large extent on the nature, intensity, and duration of the stimulus; the presence of simultaneous and sequential stimuli; the status of

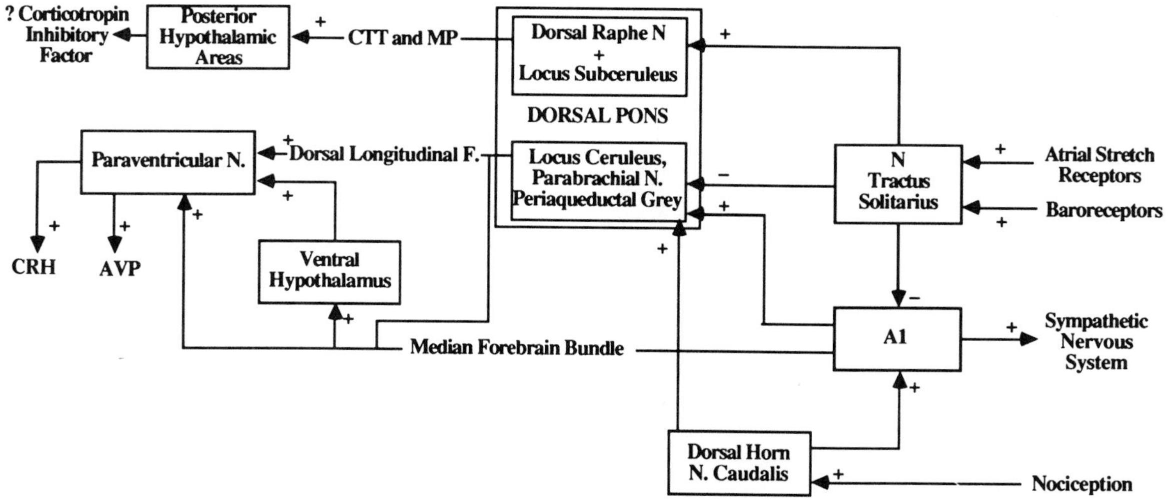

FIG. 1-6. Proposed neural organization of the ACTH and vasopressin (AVP) response to hypovolemia and nociception. Three principal areas of the hypothalamus receive signals from the pontine areas, projecting via the midbrain regions to modulate the release of vasopressin and of corticotropin releasing hormone (CRH) by the median eminence. Symbols: N, nucleus; F, fasciculus; CT, central tegmental tract; MP, mammillary peduncles; AVP, arginine vasopressin; Al, region of the caudal, ventrolateral medulla, which is the first possible site for interaction of pain and volume signals.

the receptor at the time of stimulation; and the time of day during which the stimulus occurs.

The dependence of the response to a stimulus on the intensity and duration of the stimulus, as well as the importance of CNS integration, is well described for cardiopulmonary reflexes and adrenomedullary secretion of catecholamines. Despite the potent activation of the sympathetic nervous system by small nonhypotensive hemorrhages, adrenomedullary secretion of catecholamines increases only slightly. Adrenal catecholamine secretion responds briskly to hypotensive hemorrhage in which both arterial and atrial receptors are activated, suggesting that high-pressure baroreceptors and low-pressure volume receptors both must be inactivated for adrenomedullary stimulation to be maximal. In addition to the intensity and the duration, the rate at which a stimulus is presented is also an important parameter in the modulation of efferent signals that are elicited by the stimulus. The neuroendocrine response of a traumatized individual with a ruptured spleen who loses 30 percent of blood volume in 1 h is considerably different from that observed in a patient with multiple long bone fractures who loses the same blood volume over 1 day.

The set point and the gain of baroreceptors may be altered by the convergence of other sensory inputs, such as viscerosomatic and somatosensory afferents, with baroreceptor inputs in the cardiovascular areas of the medulla. The responsiveness of baroreceptors themselves may be increased by the response they initiate, since baroreceptor responsiveness is increased by catecholamines, AVP, and angiotensin. Furthermore, the sensitivity of some end organs, such as the adrenal cortex, changes as a function of the time of day.

The stimuli accompanying injury, sepsis, and starvation rarely occur singly; in most situations, multiple stimuli are perceived simultaneously. The neuroendocrine response to injury is the summation of these stimuli and is often different from the response to any single stimulus alone (Fig. 1-7). For example, Egdahl and coworkers found hypothermic dogs responded with smaller increases in the secretions of ACTH, corticosteroids, and catecholamines than did normothermic dogs. Bereiter and coworkers demonstrated that the secretion of ACTH was greater to hemorrhage and noxious stimulation than either stimulus alone (Fig. 1-8). Experimental work has shown that the same 50 percent mortality observed after a 40 percent hemorrhage alone was observed after a 30 percent hemorrhage if combined with sciatic nerve stimulation.

In addition to multiple stimuli occurring simultaneously, it is not uncommon for multiple stimuli to occur sequentially as well. A patient involved in a motor vehicle accident may first experience pain from fractured ribs, then hypovolemia from a ruptured spleen, and then hypoxia from a slowly developing tension pneumothorax. According to classic endocrine feedback mechanisms, one might expect that the elevation of serum cortisol, for example, resulting from one set of stimuli would inhibit the release of ACTH by the second set, but the response may actually be potentiated by the second stimulus. Physiologic facilitation and potentiation for cortisol and catecholamines in response to sequential hemorrhages of the same magnitude and to sequential operations has

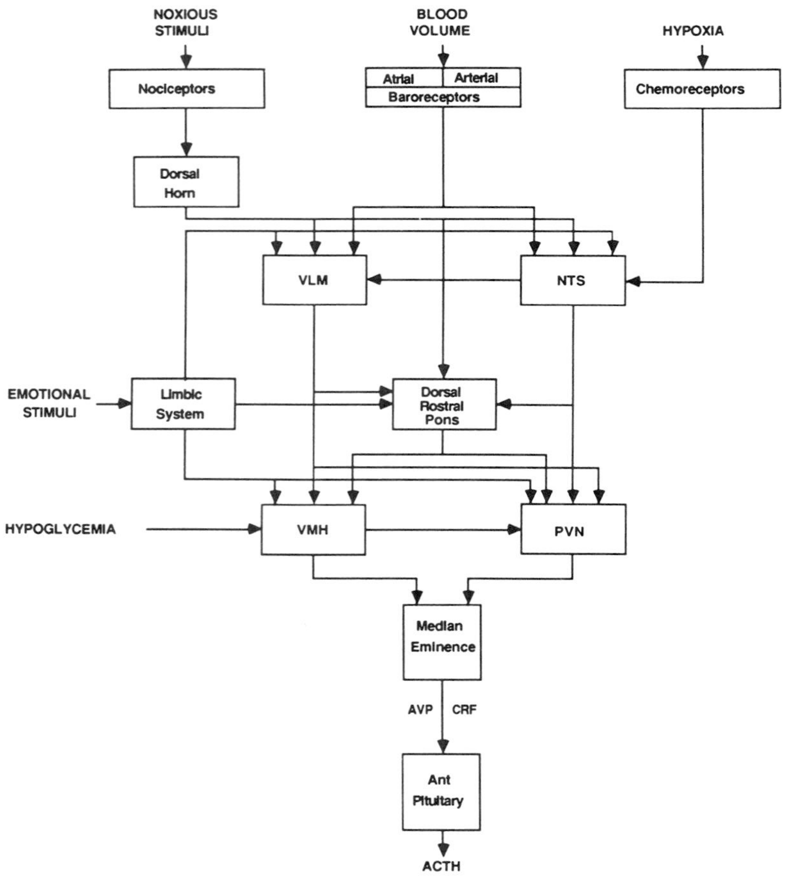

FIG. 1-7. Possible sites for the integration of the various stimuli elicited by injury are schematically represented. For example, noxious stimuli, hypovolemia, and hypoxia may first interact at NTS. Symbols: NTS, nucleus tractus solitarius; PVN, paraventricular nucleus; VLM, ventrolateral medulla; VMN, ventromedial hypothalamus (dorsomedial, arcuate, suprachlasmatic, periventricular, and premammillary nuclei). The dorsal rostral pons contains the loci ceruleus and subceruleus, the parabrachial nucleus, the perlaqueductal gray, and the dorsal raphe nucleus. Although this figure shows the release of ACTH, it is likely that other anterior pituitary hormones are controlled in a similar manner.

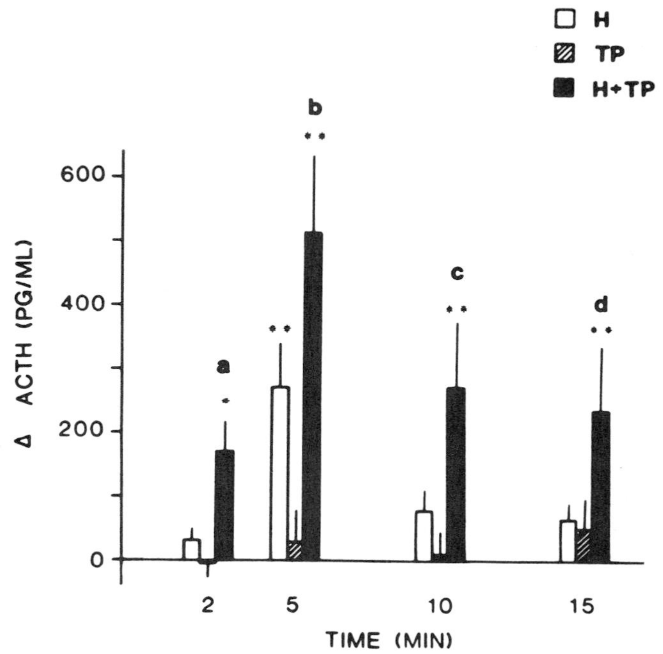

FIG. 1-8. Potentiation of the ACTH response to hemorrhage by nerve stimulation. H = hemorrhage, TP = tooth pulp, *= $p < 0.05$ vs. baseline, **= $p < 0.01$ vs. baseline. [Letters above each sample time point denote intragroup individual comparisons: $a = p < 0.05$ (H + TP vs. TP), $b = p < 0.01$ (H + TP vs. TP or H), $c = p < 0.05$ (H + TP vs. H), $d = p < 0.05$ (H + TP vs. TP or H).] At all time points, the response of ACTH to hemorrhage and tooth pulp stimulation was greater than the response to either hemorrhage or tooth pulp stimulation alone. (From: *Bereiter DA et al: Endocrinology 111:1127, 1982, with permission.*)

been demonstrated experimentally (Fig. 1-9). The neuroendocrine response to initial trauma, shock, or sepsis may modify the response to subsequent operation.

Efferent Output

Five arms to the efferent limb of the reflex neuroendocrine response to injury may be considered: (1) the autonomic response, (2) the hormonal response, (3) the local tissue response, (4) the vascular endothelial cell system response, and (5) the single cell response. The endocrine response may be divided into hormones whose secretion is primarily under hypothalamic-pituitary control (cortisol, thyroxine, growth hormone, and AVP) and hormones whose secretion is primarily under autonomic control (catecholamines, insulin, and glucagon). The release of cytokines and other mediators is related to the local tissue response, circulating toxins, and immunologic stimulation. Mediators may act systemically as well as locally. These substances have been shown to exert regulatory effects on each level of the ANS and CNS, on the classical hormone system, and on the vascular system and have known effects on intermediary metabolism and organ function as well. Recently, the vascular endothelial cell system has been considered as an endocrine organ in its own right because of the many potent substances that are elaborated by endothelial cells. Products of the *final* effector—the single cell—that are stimulated by injury will also be considered.

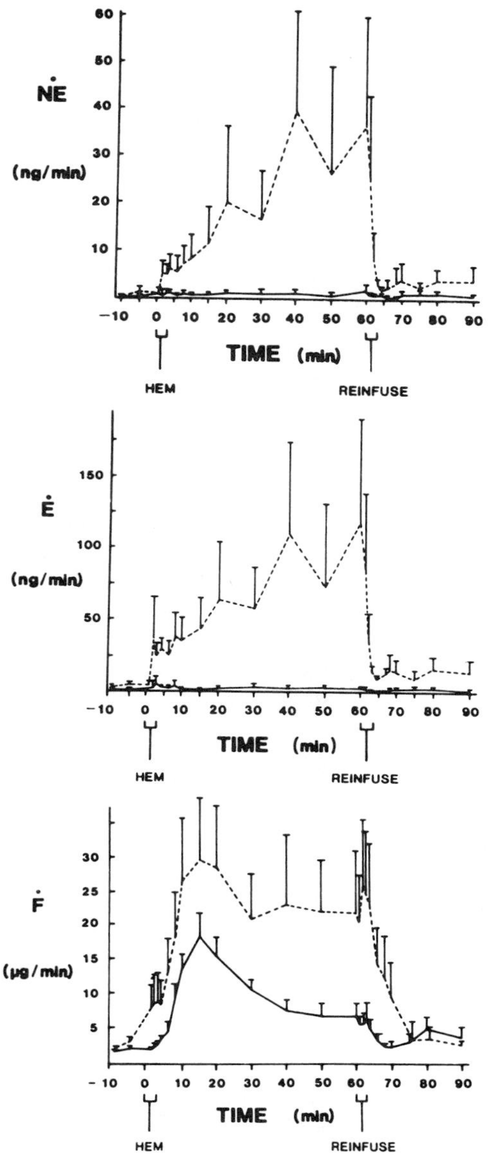

FIG. 1-9. Potentiation of the secretory rates of epinephrine (E), norepinephrine (NE), and cortisol (C) to a 6.5-mL/kg hemorrhage in dogs when a hemorrhage of the same magnitude was performed on the previous day. The pattern of response between E and NE is the same, but that for NE is at a lower absolute rate than that for E. Hemorrhages took place at 0 min; reinfusion occurred at 60 min. ________ = mean response on day 1; ________ = mean response on day 2. (From: *Lilly MP et al: Endocrinology 111:1917, 1982; 112:681, 1983, with permission.*)

Mechanisms of Hormone Action

Hormones may be broadly subdivided into groups based on chemical structure (Table 1-2). The chemical nature of these compounds determines the mechanism by which they exert their biologic effects. Receptors to these hormones are dynamic structures that may be found in varied tissue distribution and density, possess affinities that are modified by other compounds, and can be blocked by exogenous and endogenous substances.

Table 1-2
Chemical Classes of Some Hormones and Mediators

		Fatty Acid Derivatives	
Polypeptides	*Amino Acid Derivatives*	*Cholesterol*	*Arachidonic Acid*
Leutinizing hormone	Thyroxine	Cortisol	Prostaglandins
Insulin	Epinephrine	Testosterone	Leukotrienes
Glucagon	Norepinephrine	Aldosterone	
Vasopressin	Dopamine		
Interleukins	Serotonin		
TNF	Histamine		
Interferon	Thyroxine		
Endothelins			

The actions of hormones on cells require effector receptors that act through three major mechanisms for signal transduction (Fig. 1-10). Many hormone receptors and effectors have been characterized (Table 1-3). Some hormones, such as the peptides and amines, act through membrane-bound receptors coupled to guanine nucleotide-binding or G proteins and mediate changes in intracellular cyclic adenosine monophosphate (cAMP) or in calcium. These substances then act as second messengers to activate phosphorylases coupled to guanine triphosphate (GTP) hydrolysis (G protein action). G proteins coupled to adenylate cyclase increase cAMP. When G proteins are coupled to phospholipase C, the two principal active products are diacylglycerol (DAG) and inositol triphosphate (IP_3). DAG remains in the membrane where it activates protein kinase C, which in turn opens a membrane channel to allow calcium entry and, in some cells, may stimulate cell proliferation. IP_3 acts on the endoplasmic reticulum to release free calcium from the intracellular pool. The free calcium binds in turn to a calcium chelator, calmodulin, that activates a specific phosphorylase kinase. Calcium is utilized as a second messenger for stimulus-response coupling of many other key biologic processes including excitation-contraction coupling in muscle; excitation-secretion coupling at nerve endings and in exocrine and endocrine glands; maintenance of oxidative phosphorylation; activation of contractile and motile cell systems, such as microtubules and microfilaments; platelet activation; regulation of plasma membrane permeability; and tight gap junction and cell-to-cell communication. Insulin acts through tyrosine kinase.

Steroids and triiodothyronine (T_3) are examples of hormones that act primarily through cytosolic receptors (Fig. 1-11). Once bound to the receptor, the receptor-hormone complex is activated and translocated to the nucleus where the receptor-hormone complex binds to the nonhistone protein of nuclear chromatin, thereby modulating the transcription of genes into specific ribonucleic acid (RNA) that directs the synthesis of enzymatic, structural, and regulatory proteins. This explains the 1- to 2-h delay in onset of most of the primary steroid hormone actions.

In many cells, one of the principal by-products of hydrolysis of membrane phospholipid is arachidonic acid. As noted below, this substance is the principal precursor of prostaglandins and leukotrienes. The anti-inflammatory properties of cortisol are now be-

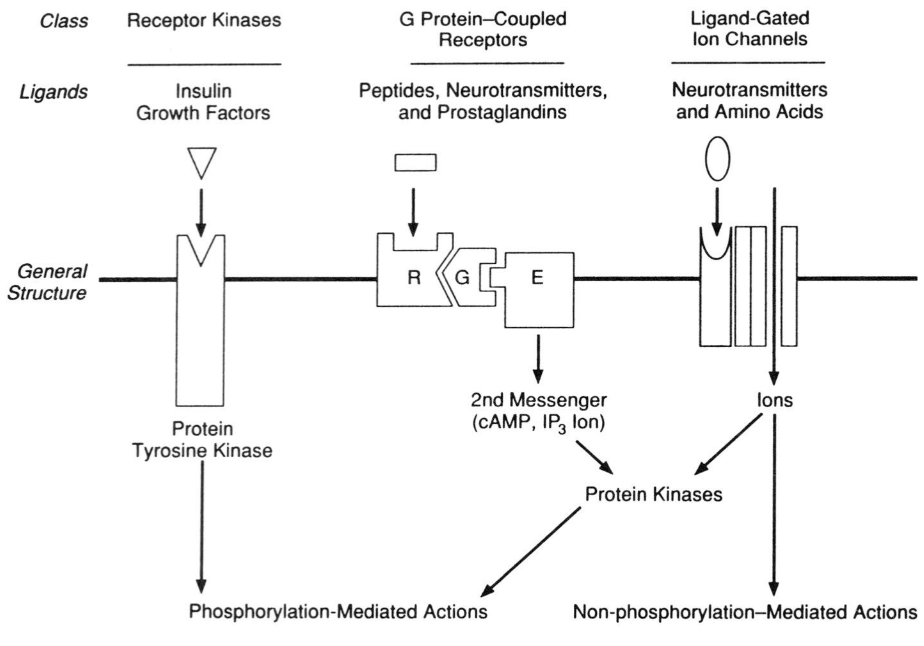

FIG. 1-10. Three major classes of membrane receptors exist for hormones and neurotransmitters. Many growth factors, including insulin, bind to cell surface receptors that act as protein tyrosine kinases stimulating the phosphorylation of proteins. A second class binds to receptors (R), coupled to separate effector (E) molecules by G proteins (G). Effectors may be enzymes that produce second messengers that in turn can activate distinct protein kinases. The third major class of receptors includes ligand-gated ion channels that may be coupled by G proteins. (From: *Habener JF: Genetic control of hormone formation, in Wilson JD, Foster DW: Williams Textbook of Endocrinology, 8th ed. Philadelphia, WB Saunders 1992, chap 4, with permission.)*

Table 1-3
Classification of Hormone Receptors and Effectors

Adenylate cyclase	
	Corticotropin
	Beta-adrenergic catecholamines
	Luteinizing hormone and human chorionic gonadotropin
	Follicle-stimulating hormone
	Glucagon
	Prostaglandins
	Parathyroid hormone
	TSH
	Alpha-adrenergic (inhibition)
	Somatostatin (inhibition)
Guanylate cyclase	
	Atrial peptide (AP, also called atrial natriuretic factor)
Receptor protein tyrosine kinases	
	Insulin
	Insulinlike growth factor (somatomedin-C)
	Epidermal growth factor
	Colony-stimulating factor 1
	Fibroblast growth factor
Phosphoinositol turnover and calcium flux	
	Acetylcholine receptor (muscarinic)
	Alpha-adrenergic catecholamines
	Angiotensin
	Luteinizing hormone releasing hormone
	Thyrotropin releasing hormone
	AVP
Ion channels	
	Acetylcholine receptor (nicotinic)
	Gamma-aminobutyric acid
Unknown effector system	
	Growth hormone
	Prolactin
	Erythropoietin
	Interleukins
	Nerve growth factor
	T-cell receptor

SOURCE: From Habener JF: Genetic control of hormone formation, in Wilson JD, Foster DW: *Williams Textbook of Endocrinology*, 8th ed. Philadelphia, WB Saunders, 1992, chap. 4, with permission.

lieved to result from its action to inhibit phospholipase A_2, thus limiting formation of prostaglandins and leukotrienes in certain tissues.

Hormone Systems

Hormones under Pituitary Control

CRH-ACTH-Cortisol. Hypothalamic, anterior pituitary, and adrenal cortical cells secrete corticotropin releasing hormone (CRH), ACTH, and cortisol, respectively. The latter hormone exerts proportionate direct effects on cells of the liver, skeletal muscle, and adipose tissue that establish metabolic availability of glucose during stress. Cortisol also has effects on cells of the immune system. The fine control of this neuroendocrine axis is achieved by feedback loop control, neural integration, and hormonal and mediator substance effects that act on each level of the system (Fig. 1-12).

CRH (formerly called corticotropin releasing factor, CRF) is synthesized primarily in the hypothalamic paraventricular nucleus in an area that overlaps with cells that secrete AVP (formerly called antidiuretic hormone, ADH), another potent corticotropin releasing factor (Fig. 1-13). CRH release into the hypophyseal portal venous system is stimulated by neurogenic hypothalamic input and is potentiated by angiotensin II. CRH release may also be stimulated by mediators such as IL-1, IL-6, and TNF via prostaglandins (Fig. 1-12).

ACTH is synthesized, stored, and released by chromophobe cells of the anterior pituitary as a fragment of a large molecule, proopiomelanocortin (POMC), that also contains gamma and beta lipotrophin, alpha melanocyte stimulating hormone (alpha MSH), and beta-endorphin. Pituitary ACTH release is stimulated by CRH and is potentiated by AVP, angiotensin II, and possibly oxytocin. Mediators such as IL-1 may stimulate ACTH release through noradrenergic or dopaminergic pathways which project to the hypothalamus. ACTH release is controlled by a short negative feedback loop and through cortisol action by a long feedback loop (Fig.

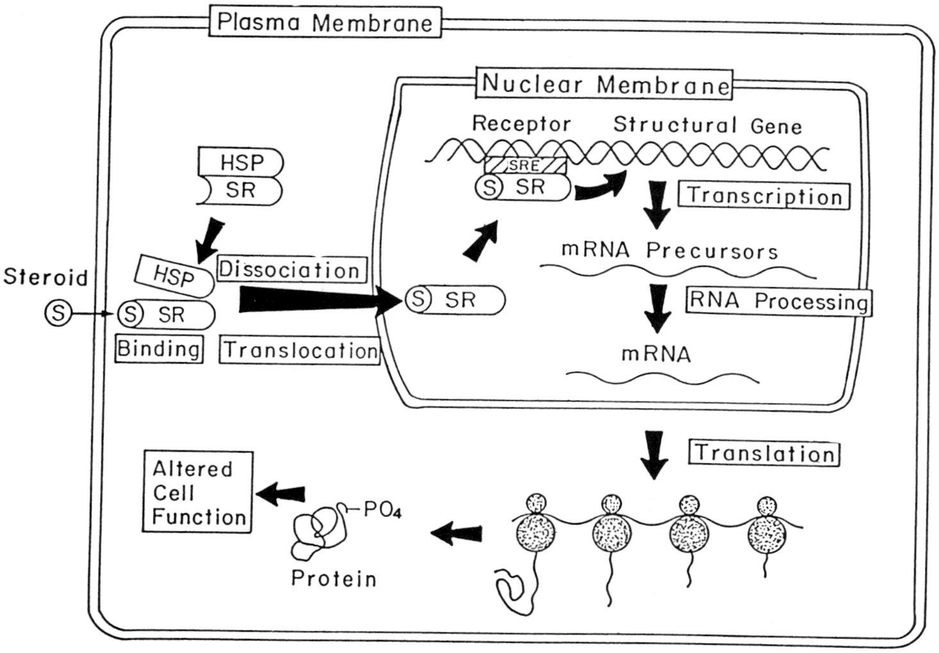

FIG. 1-11. Proposed model of steroid action. Steroid (S) readily diffuses across the plasma membrane and binds to a cytosolic receptor (SR). In the absence of steroid, the receptor resides in the cytoplasm as an inactive complex with heat-shock protein (HSP). Steroid binding causes HSP dissociation. The steroid-receptor complex is translocated to the nucleus, where it binds to a chromatin receptor consisting of the steroid receptor response DNA element (SRE), thereby activating the transcription of specific genes. RNA transcripts are translated into proteins that mediate changes in cell function. Alternative models in which steroid receptor resides in the nucleus have also been suggested. (From: *Habener JF: Genetic control of hormone formation, in Wilson JD, Foster DW: Williams Textbook of Endocrinology, 8th ed. Philadelphia, WB Saunders 1992, chap 2, with permission.*)

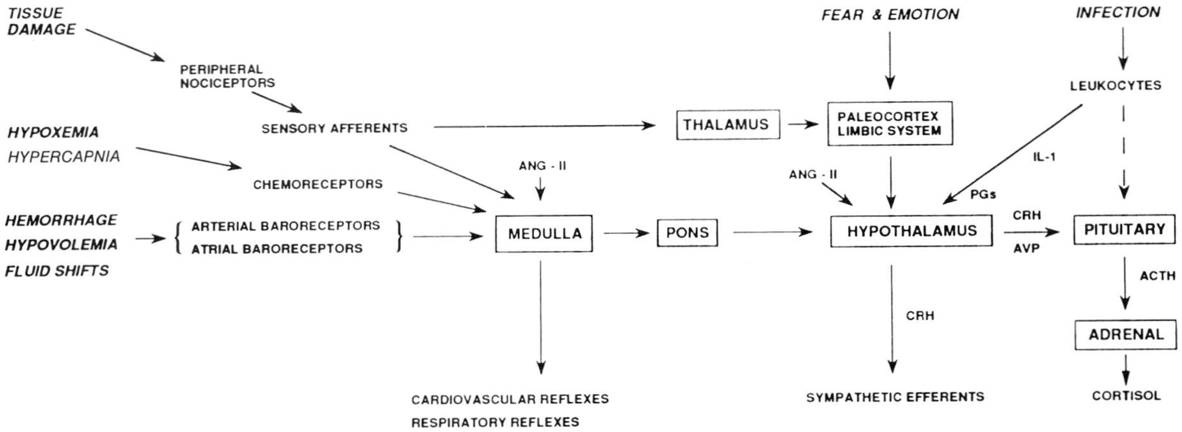

FIG. 1-12. Schematic diagram of the hypothelamic-pituitary-adrenal system showing major afferent inputs, neural pathways, and sites for modulation and for interaction. Abbreviations: ANG-II, angiotensin II; PGS, prostaglandins; IL-1, interleukin 1; CRH, corticotropin releasing hormone; AVP, arginine vasopressin; ACTH, adrenocorticotropin releasing hormone. (From: *Lilly MP, Gann DS: Arch Surg, in press, with permission.*)

1-14). The metabolic and systemic consequences of adrenal suppression secondary to exogenous corticosteroid administration are well known to the clinician.

Cortisol is synthesized, stored, and released from cells of the adrenal zona fasciculata. The release of cortisol is primarily controlled by ACTH binding to surface receptors and is mediated by changes in intracellular cAMP.

Most types of trauma are characterized by an increased secretion of CRH, ACTH, and cortisol that is positively correlated to the magnitude of the traumatic or thermal injury. The plasma concentration of cortisol, which loses its normal circadian rhythm, typically remains elevated for up to 4 weeks following thermal injury, for less than 1 week following soft tissue trauma, and for days following hemorrhage. In pure hypovolemia, the plasma cortisol concentration rapidly returns to normal when blood volume has been restored. Supervening infection prolongs the duration of the cortisol increase following injury. Persistent elevations of serum cortisol are associated with reduced survival.

Cortisol has widespread effects on the metabolism and utilization of glucose, amino acids, and fatty acids in hepatic and extrahepatic tissue. In the liver, cortisol inhibits the pentose phosphate shunt, the action of insulin, and several regulatory glycolytic enzymes. Through actions of ACTH and epinephrine, pyruvate dehydrogenase activity is reduced indirectly, and, as a consequence, the availability of pyruvate to be used for gluconeogenesis increases. Cortisol stimulates the activity and de novo synthesis of several regulatory gluconeogenic enzymes. Amino acid uptake and transaminase activities are also stimulated. Cortisol appears to exert an important role in maintaining, at least, euglycemia during stressful conditions by increasing the availability of gluconeogenic

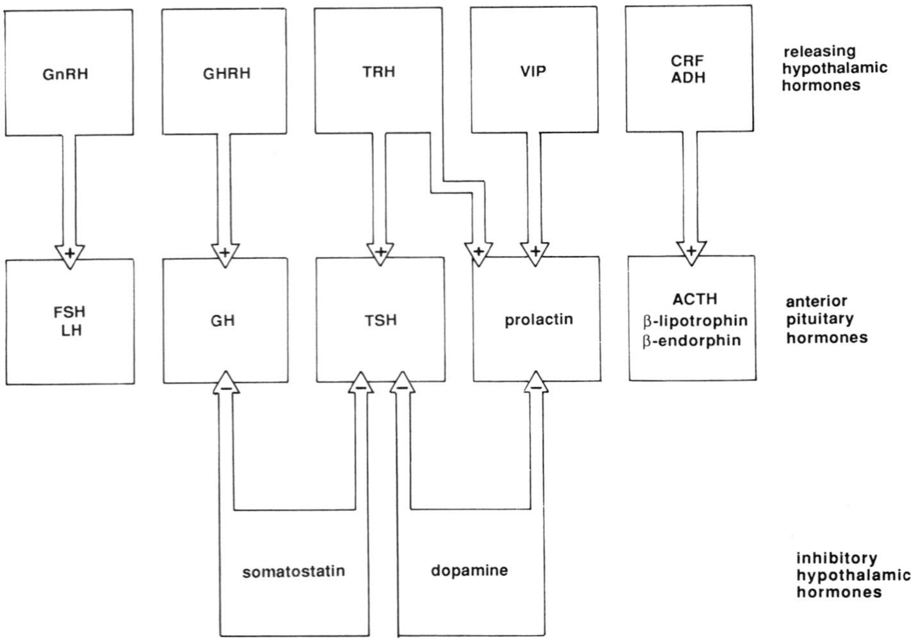

FIG. 1-13. Hormones produced in the anterior pituitary and the hypothalamic hormones that regulate their secretion. See text for abbreviations. (Adapted from: *Reichlin S: Neuroendocrine control of pituitary function, in Besser GM, Cudworth AG (eds): Clinical Endocrinology: An Illustrated Text. Philadelphia, JB Lippincott, 1987, with permission.*)

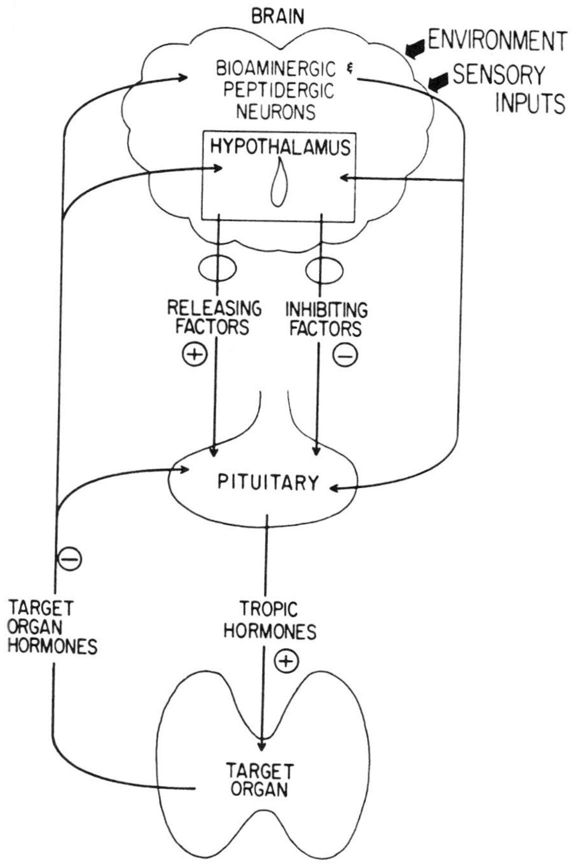

FIG. 1-14. Regulatory feedback loops of the hypothalamic-pituitary-target organ axis. (From: *Habener JF: Genetic control of hormone formation, in Wilson JD, Foster DW: Williams Textbook of Endocrinology, 8th ed. Philadelphia, WB Saunders 1992, chap 2, with permission.*)

substrates to the liver. Cortisol potentiates the hepatic actions of glucagon and epinephrine.

In skeletal muscle tissue, cortisol appears to lack direct gluconeogenic effects but does inhibit glucose uptake mediated by insulin. Cortisol inhibits amino acid uptake and stimulates amino acid release. The proteolytic effect of TNF in sepsis appears to be cortisol-dependent.

In adipose tissue, cortisol stimulates lipolysis and decreases glucose uptake. In addition, the action of other lipolytic hormones, including ACTH, growth hormone, glucagon, and epinephrine are potentiated. Plasma concentrations of free fatty acids and glycerol increase.

Corticosteroids administered in pharmacologic concentrations possess potent inhibitory effects on immunologic and inflammatory responses. Physiologic concentrations of circulating corticosteroids cause demargination and suppress leukocyte synthesis of IL-1, IL-2, gamma interferon, beta-endorphin, and various kinins and proteases associated with inflammatory responses. Cortisol inhibits phospholipase A_2, thereby limiting the production of prostaglandins and leukotrienes. Acting either directly or through inhibition of cytokine release, suppression of lymphocyte proliferation, of antibody formation, and of natural killer cell activity is also observed. Recent speculation that unchecked or excessive production of cytokines and/or other mediators may be important in the pathophysiology of the multiple organ failure syndrome suggests that endogenous corticosteroid interacts with these mediator substances to control or contain the immunologic defense response.

Death resulting from adrenal insufficiency in an injured patient is generally associated with hypoglycemia, hyponatremia, and hyperkalemia. The latter two findings result from the loss of the mineralocorticoid effect of sodium retention and kaliuresis due to aldosterone and, to a lesser extent, to cortisol. Hyponatremia in posttraumatic adrenal insufficiency is exaggerated by decreased free-water clearance from increased AVP secretion. Hypoglycemia arises because of the direct effects of cortisol on hepatic glucose production. It is noteworthy that, in the presence of injury or starvation, adrenalectomized human beings exhibit marked alterations in hepatic carbohydrate metabolism that result in rapid and fatal hypoglycemia. This appears to be, at least in part, the result of inability to store glycogen and carry out glucagon- and epinephrine-mediated gluconeogenesis in the absence of corticosteroid action.

The permissive action of cortisol was first proposed by Ingle to explain the finding that adrenalectomized animals given maintenance doses of corticosteroids showed some of the metabolic changes formerly ascribed to increased secretion of corticosteroids. He proposed that the primary role of cortisol in trauma was to permit or augment the action of other hormones. Hepatic gluconeogenesis stimulated by epinephrine or by glucagon is markedly enhanced in the presence of cortisol, lending support to this hypothesis (Fig. 1-15). Cortisol also has important direct actions following trauma. It has been shown experimentally, for example, that increased concentrations of cortisol are necessary to achieve complete blood volume restitution following hemorrhage (Fig. 1-16).

TRH-TSH-T_3/T_4. Hypothalamic thyrotropin releasing hormone (TRH) stimulates the release of thyroid stimulating hormone (TSH) which is synthesized, stored, and released by basophilic cells of the anterior pituitary. TSH stimulates the release of primarily thyroxine (T_4) from the thyroid gland which is converted to triiodothyroxine (T_3) in peripheral tissues. Both T_4 and T_3 bind to plasma proteins and thus exist in free and bound forms.

TRH is not limited to the hypothalamus, and, although it is not specific for the release of TSH, it does appear to be the primary agent responsible for pituitary TSH secretion. Administration of TRH during experimental hemorrhagic shock has been shown to be beneficial. The effect may occur via central pathways which modulate sympathoadrenal function. Hypothalamic TRH release is inhibited by T_3 and T_4. T_3 acts through a cytosolic receptor to bind to nuclear deoxyribonucleic acid (DNA) and mediate transcription. In consequence, a large number of enzymes and receptors are induced, with protean effects.

Thyroid hormones have numerous effects on cellular metabolism, growth, and differentiation. Among these are their ability to increase oxygen consumption, heat production, and the activities of the sympathetic nervous system. Thyroid hormones may also have profound metabolic effects when present in excess, which include increases in glucose oxidation, gluconeogenesis, glycogenolysis, proteolysis, lipolysis, and ketogenesis. Despite these actions, thyroid hormones do not appear to be important in the moment-to-moment regulation of plasma substrates, such as glucose.

In addition to TRH, the release of TSH is stimulated by estrogens and inhibited by T_3, corticosteroids, growth hormone, somatostatin, and by fasting. Pituitary TSH release is inhibited by T_3

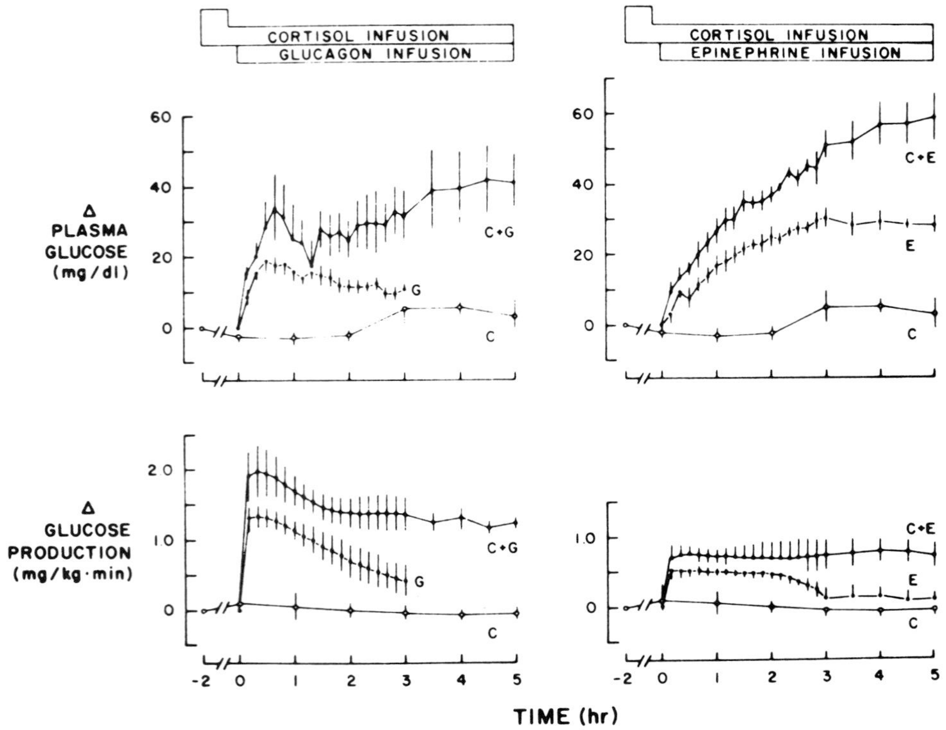

FIG. 1-15. The influence of cortisol (C) on the response of plasma glucose and glucose production to glucagon (G) or epinephrine (E). Cortisol, which by itself did not alter plasma glucose or glucose production, had the effect of increasing and more importantly prolonging the stimulatory effects of glucagon and epinephrine on glucose production. As a result, the effects of the combined hormone infusions on plasma glucose were more than additive. (From: *Eigler NJ et al: Clin Invest 63:114, 1979, with permission.*)

and T_4. Physiologically, T_3 is much more potent than T_4. Even though the plasma concentrations of free and total T_3 are frequently decreased after injury or surgery, TSH secretion is not increased. This results from rapid pituitary conversion of T_4 to T_3 and the fact that T_4 and T_3 become equipotent inhibitors of TSH secretion following injury. Reductions in serum TSH concentration have been observed in burn patients that are paradoxically associated with low serum concentrations of both free T_4 and free T_3. This situation is similar to the euthyroid sick syndrome observed in critically ill nonsurgical patients and may be the result of an impairment in hypothalamic or pituitary secretion or alterations in peripheral hormone binding.

Following injury, burns, and major operations the peripheral conversion of T_4 to T_3 is impaired, resulting in reduced circulating concentrations of both free and total T_3. In part, this is the result of a cortisol-mediated block of the conversion of T_4 to T_3 and of an increased conversion of T_4 to the biologically inactive molecule, reverse T_3. An increase in reverse T_3 is also characteristic of injury (Fig. 1-17). The plasma concentrations of total T_4 are frequently decreased after injury, but free T_4 concentrations usually remain

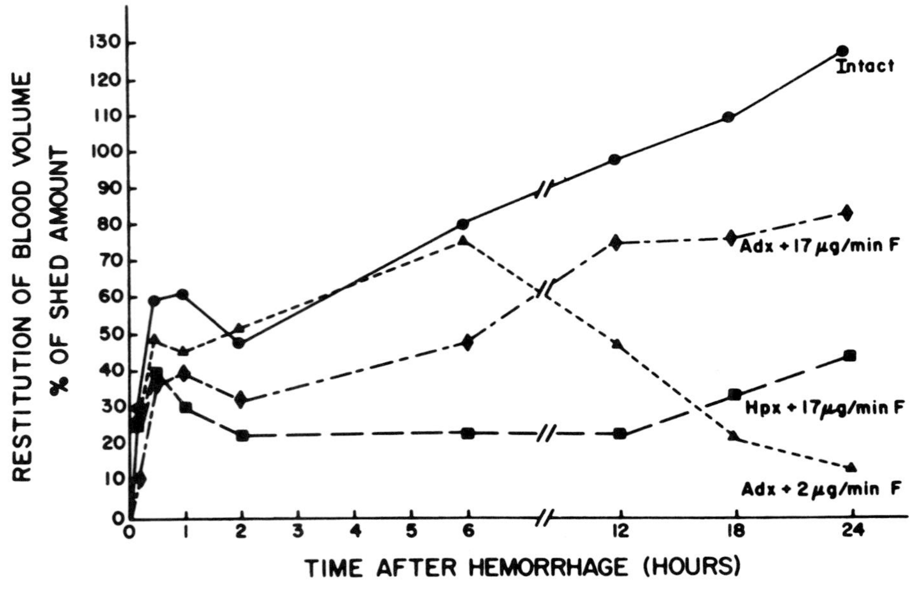

FIG. 1-16. Restitution of blood volume after 10 percent hemorrhage in four groups of splenectomized dogs: intact (●); adrenalectomized infused with cortisol at 2 μg/min (▲); adrenalectomized infused with cortisol at 2 μg/min prior to hemorrhage, then at 17 μg/min (◆); hypophysectomized infused with cortisol at 17 μg/min (■). The response of each group differed significantly from that of each other group ($p < 0.01$, analysis of variance). (From: *Gann et al: Recent Prog Horm Res 34:357, 1978, with permission.*)

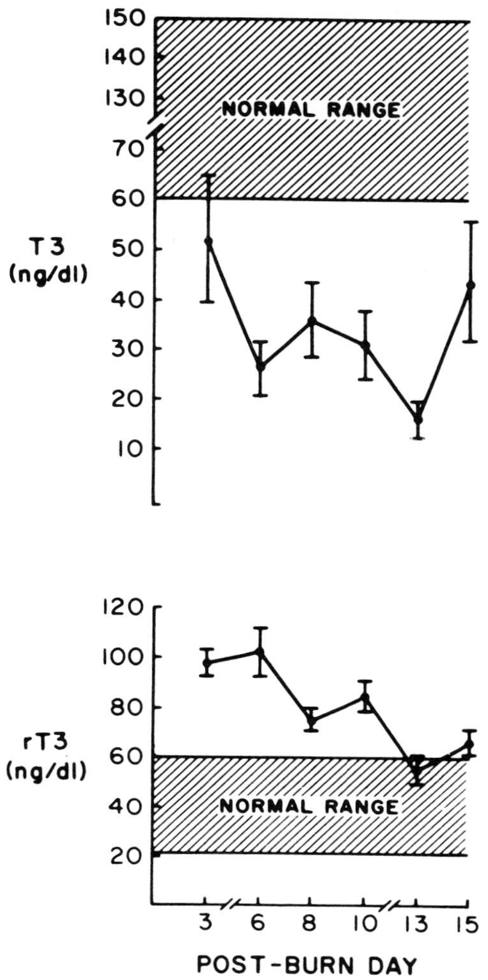

FIG. 1-17. Serum values (mean ± SEM) for T_3 and reverse T_3 in five male patients with a mean body surface area burn of 66.5 percent. Normal range represented by shaded area. T_3 values were decreased and reversed T_3 values were increased following thermal injury. (From: *Becker RA et al: J Trauma 20:713, 1980, with permission.*)

normal. Depressed concentrations of free T_4 appear to be an ominous clinical finding associated with death in traumatized, burned, and critically ill patients (Fig. 1-18).

Growth Hormone. The hypothalamus modulates the release of growth hormone (GH) through the stimulatory effect of growth hormone releasing hormone (GHRH) and the inhibitory effects of somatostatin. GHRH and somatostatin enter the circulation through the hypothalamohypophyseal portal system (Fig. 1-13). GH is synthesized, stored, and released from acidophilic cells of the anterior pituitary. GH effects are due to both direct action and the secondary release of insulinlike growth factors I and II (IGF-I and IGF-II), substances formerly called somatomedins. These growth factors are peptide hormones that are released by many cell types and act as endocrine, paracrine, and autocrine substances (Fig. 1-19).

Secretion of GH is governed by hypothalamic factors, autonomic stimulation, and hormonal and nonhormonal signals. Alpha-adrenergic stimulation, thyroxine, AVP, ACTH, alpha MSH, glucagon, testosterone, and estrogen stimulate GH release. Secretion of GH also occurs as a result of exercise, stress, reduction in effective circulating volume, fasting hypoglycemia, decreasing plasma fatty acid concentrations, and increasing concentrations of amino acids such as arginine. GH release is suppressed by hypothalamic release of somatostatin, beta-adrenergic stimulation, and cortisol. GH secretion is also inhibited by hyperglycemia and rising plasma fatty acid concentrations.

The primary metabolic actions of GH during stress are to promote protein synthesis and enhance breakdown of lipid and carbohydrate stores. The protein effects are primarily mediated by IGF-I which is released by hepatic and other target cells to cause suppression of proteolysis, increased amino acid uptake, and cellular proliferation in liver and skeletal muscle. GH increases plasma fatty acids and ketone bodies through direct stimulation of lipolysis and potentiation of catecholamine effects on adipose tissue and by stimulation of hepatic ketogenesis. GH release is also associated with decreased insulin levels. Consequently, plasma glucose is increased by inhibition of glucose transport in liver and skeletal muscle and by decreases in glucose oxidation.

Plasma concentrations of GH increase following injury, hemorrhage, operation, and anesthesia. Paradoxically, levels of IGF-I decrease after injury and correlate well with observed negative nitrogen balance. Malnutrition and fasting are also associated with marked decreases in IGF concentrations which are reversed with adequate protein and caloric intake. Recombinant IGF-I infusion attenuates nitrogen loss and improves intracellular glutamine during hypocaloric feedings in nonstressed human beings and may hold therapeutic promise following injury.

Gonadotrophins and Sex Hormones. Gonadotrophin releasing hormone (GnRH) is released from the hypothalamus to cause release of follicle-stimulating hormone (FSH) and luteinizing hormone (LH), which are synthesized, stored, and secreted by basophilic cells of the anterior pituitary. The release of these hormones is inhibited by CRF, prolactin, estrogen, progestins, and androgens.

The secretion of LH and FSH is suppressed after injury and during critical illness, an effect which may, in part, be related to CRF release. Following thermal injury, there appears to be an initial increase during the first day followed by prolonged decreased secretion.

In contrast to the increased release of ACTH and cortisol, estrogen and androgen concentrations decrease following injury. The mechanism for this may relate to reduced pituitary GnRH response or to altered release of FSH and LH. These changes account for the menstrual dysfunction and decreased libido that are observed after operation and injury. There is mounting evidence for potential links between the gonadal and the immune axis suggested by observations which include GnRH-induced decreases in immune function and IL-1 stimulation of GnRH release. Improved survival is observed when testosterone or conjugated estrogens are administered shortly before experimental shock.

Prolactin. Hypothalamic control of prolactin release is modulated by stimulatory (CRF, TRH, GHRH, serotonin, vasoactive intestinal peptide, and peptide histidine methionine) and inhibitory (dopamine, GnRH, and gonadotrophin-associated peptide) hormones and neuropeptides (Fig. 1-13). Prolactin is synthesized, stored, and released by acidophilic cells of the anterior pituitary gland. Unlike other anterior pituitary hormones, the predominant effect of the hypothalamus on prolactin secretion is one of tonic suppression.

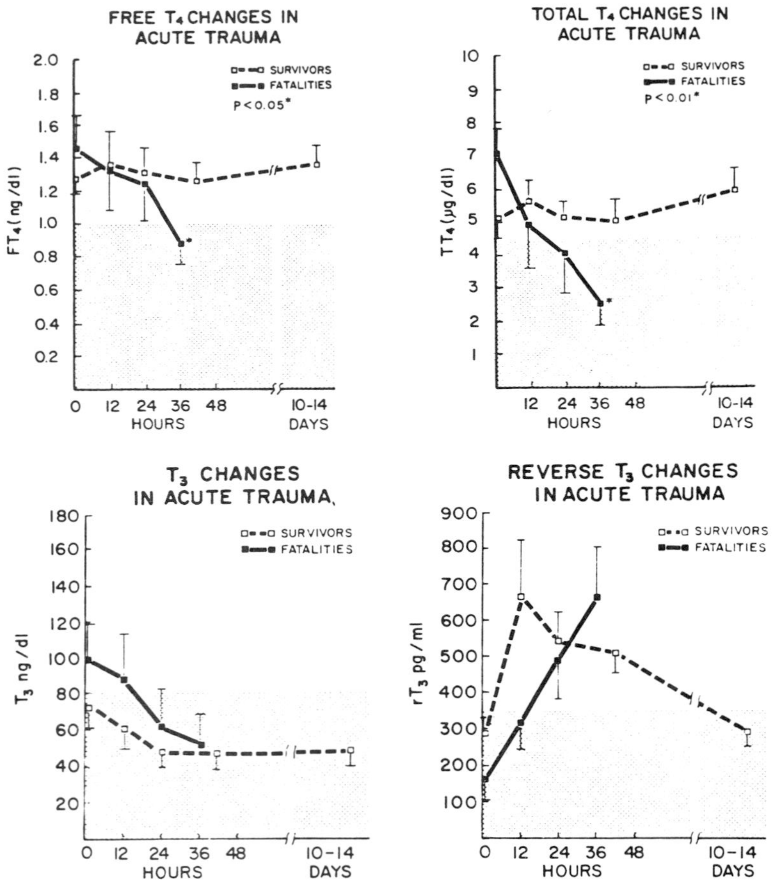

FIG. 1-18. Alterations in total T_4, free T_4, total T_3, and reverse T_3 in 19 acutely traumatized patients. Results are reported as mean ± SEM and statistically significant deviations are noted at matched time samples. Shaded regions denote subnormal levels of free T_4, total T_4, and total T_3 and normal range of reverse T_3. All patients had subnormal values of total T_3 and elevated values of reverse T_3 at some time point. Patients who died had subnormal values of total and free T_4, whereas survivors did not. (From: *Phillips RH et al: J Trauma 24:116, 1984, with permission.*)

Prolactin acts metabolically to promote increased nitrogen retention and to increase lipid mobilization. Fluid retentive effects on renal tubular cells have also been described.

Despite these functions, the physiologic importance of prolactin in human beings following injury is incompletely understood. Elevations in plasma prolactin have been documented in adults after trauma and operation and have correlated with the severity of injury. Decreases in prolactin concentrations have been observed in children and adolescents following thermal injury that are likely related to differences in CNS and reproductive system maturation. The increase in prolactin secretion that occurs following injury appears to be the result of direct stimulation, rather than a diminution of tonic dopaminergic prolactin inhibition. Prolactin has been shown to possess stimulatory effects on T-cell function.

Endogenous Opioids. The endogenous opioids derive from three precursors with multiple sites of origin (Table 1-4). Since pre-POMC contains the sequences for ACTH and beta-endorphin,

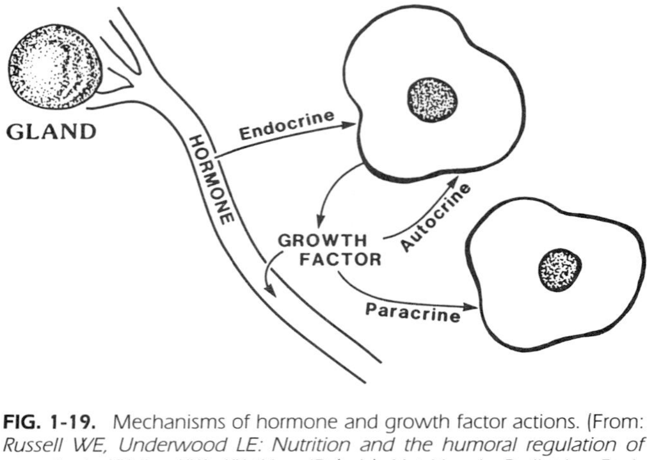

FIG. 1-19. Mechanisms of hormone and growth factor actions. (From: *Russell WE, Underwood LE: Nutrition and the humoral regulation of growth, in Walker WA, Watkins JB (eds): Nutrition in Pediatrics: Basic Science and Clinical Application. Boston, Little, Brown, 1985, pp 279–299, with permission.*)

Table 1-4
Precursors of Endogenous Opioids

Precursor	*Cleavage Products*
Pre-POMC	ACTH Beta-endorphin Alpha melanocyte stimulating hormone Gamma-endorphin Beta-lipotropin
Pre-proenkephalin-A	met-Enkephalin leu-Enkephalin
Pre-prodynorphin	Beta-endorphin Dynorphin

Pre-proopiomelanocortin (pre-POMC) is found primarily in the anterior pituitary. POMC gene expression has been found in monocytes, adrenal, lung, kidney, and gonadal tissues. Pre-proenkephalin-A is found in the brain, sympathetic ganglia, adrenal medulla, and gut. Pre-prodynorphin is found in brain, spinal cord, and gut.

both substances are cosecreted by the anterior pituitary. Gene expression for POMC has been detected in many human cell types.

Opioid compounds act at several receptors and few endogenous opioids have complete specificity for single receptor subtypes. In addition to analgesia, endogenous opioids have cardiovascular, metabolic, and immunologic actions. Beta-endorphin exerts a hypotensive effect mediated through a serotoninergic pathway. The enkephalins cause hypertension. The hyperglycemic effect of morphine and centrally administered beta-endorphin is well recognized. In addition, beta-endorphin, which does not appear to have any direct effect on glucose uptake in skeletal muscle or on hepatic glucose production, stimulates pancreatic glucagon and insulin release by the pancreas. Endogenous opioids may have an important central regulatory role in glucose metabolism, as suggested by the substantial increases in beta-endorphin caused by insulin-induced hypoglycemia. Opioid peptides are also known to possess immunologic suppressive effects.

Elevated endogenous opioid levels occur after major operation, sepsis, trauma, shock, and stress (Fig. 1-20). Clinical interest in opioid peptides resulted from the improved hemodynamics and survival observed after nalaxone administration in hemorrhagic, septic, and spinal shock. The precise humoral and immunologic role of opioids in the response to hemorrhage and sepsis remain active areas of investigation.

Arginine Vasopressin. AVP (formerly called antidiuretic hormone, ADH) is synthesized by cells of the supraoptic and paraventricular nuclei of the anterior hypothalamus and transported by axoplasmic flow to the posterior pituitary, where it is stored until neurally mediated release (Fig. 1-21). Release of AVP is modulated by neuroendocrine, afferent, and nonneuronal stimuli. The primary stimulus for AVP secretion is increased plasma osmolality, which is sensed by sodium-sensitive hypothalamic osmoreceptors and perhaps extracerebral osmoreceptors located in the liver or portal circulation. AVP release is enhanced by central and peripheral beta-adrenergic and angiotensin II stimulation, by agents such as opioids and anesthetics, and by a nonosmotic effect of elevated glucose concentrations. Pain also stimulates AVP release, while alpha-adrenergic agonists and atrial natriuretic peptide suppress AVP release. Changes in effective circulating volume stimulate AVP release through baroreceptors, left atrial stretch receptors, and chemoreceptors. Decreases of 10 percent in effective circulating volume, which is equivalent to that observed after changing from supine to upright position, result in a two- to threefold increase in plasma AVP.

The actions of AVP may be broadly classified as osmoregulatory, vasoactive, and metabolic. Osmoregulation occurs through the cAMP-mediated reabsorption of solute-free water in the renal distal tubules and collecting ducts. Vasoactive properties of AVP mediate peripheral vasoconstriction, especially in the splanchnic bed. AVP, on a molar basis, is more potent than glucagon in stimulation of hepatic glycogenolysis and gluconeogenesis and may have additional actions that lower concentrations of ketone bodies and nonesterified fatty acids.

Secretion of AVP is increased after a major operation, cardiopulmonary bypass, trauma, hemorrhage, sepsis, and burns (Fig. 1-22). The typical 5- to 7-day elevation of AVP that is observed

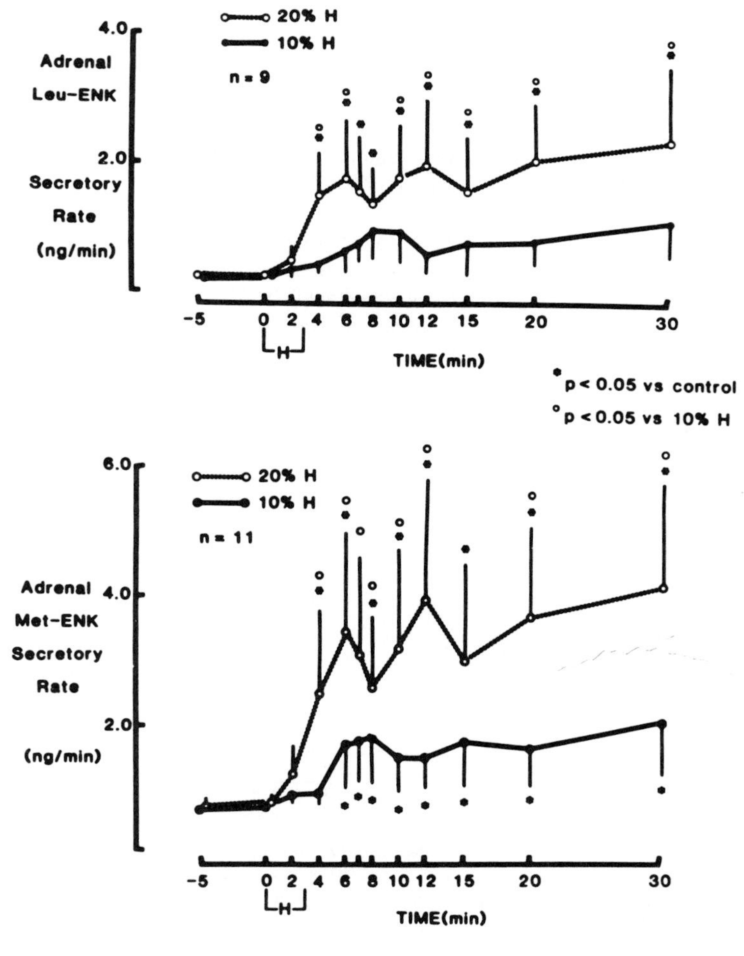

FIG. 1-20. Adrenomedullary secretion of methionine-enkephalin and leucine-enkephalin in dogs subjected to 10 or 20 percent hemorrhages. As shown, the secretion of met-enkephalin by the adrenal was always greater than that of leu-enkephalin, and although the ratio of secretory rates of met-enkephalin and leu-enkephalin varied from 2.8 to 4.9, it did not change in response to hemorrhage. (From: *Engeland WC, Dominique FB, Gann DS: Am J Physiol 251:R341, 1986, with permission.*)

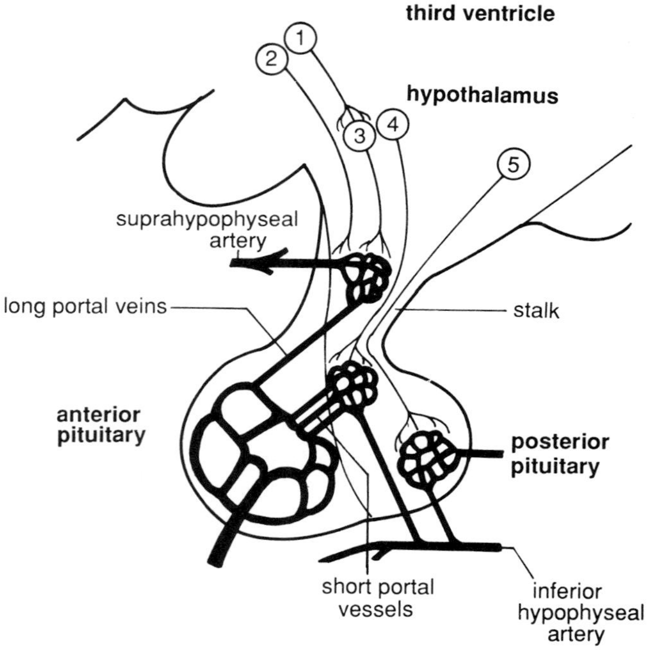

FIG. 1-21. Diagrammatic representation of the hypothalamopituitary regulatory system. The products of the posterior pituitary are synthesized in the supraoptic and paraventricular nuclei (5). Granules are transported by axoplasmic flow to the posterior pituitary and are released. The nuclei of the hypothalamus (1-4) produce hypothalamic factors which act on anterior pituitary cells to stimulate or inhibit hormone release. (From: *Reichlin S: Neuroendocrine control of pituitary function, in Besser GM, Cudworth AG (eds): Clinical Endocrinology: An Illustrated Text. Philadelphia, JB Lippincott, 1987, with permission.*)

after operation in the absence of abnormal osmolality or altered blood volume may be due to the stimulus of postoperative incisional pain. The immediate release of AVP that occurs following acute reductions in circulating volume is a complex event acting through afferents including baroreceptors, chemoreceptors, and left atrial receptors. AVP-mediated peripheral vasoconstriction in splanchnic vessels may decrease intestinal cell perfusion and play a role in the phenomenon of bacterial translocation in the gut. AVP-mediated hyperglycemia causes alterations in plasma osmolality that assist by Starling forces in restoration of effective circulating blood volume.

"Inappropriate" AVP secretion, also known as the syndrome of inappropriate antidiuretic hormone secretion (SIADH), is a term which was introduced in 1967 by Bartter and Schwartz to describe the excessive secretion of vasopressin that results in highly concentrated, low urinary output and profound dilutional hyponatremia. SIADH occurs after head injury and may occur after burns. The converse situation, in which there is an absence of vasopressin secretion from damage to the supraopticohypophyseal system (diabetes insipidus), is characterized by the production of large amounts of dilute urine with osmolality that is less than the elevated plasma osmolality. Since it frequently arises in comatose patients who cannot express thirst or regulate water intake, the continued excessive polyuria associated with diabetes insipidus leads to hypernatremia and eventually to hypotension if not treated with free water and exogenous vasopressin.

Hormones under Autonomic Control

Catecholamines. Norepinephrine (NE) is released from the axon terminals of sympathetic postganglionic neurons into the synaptic cleft. The rate of NE release correlates with sympathetic nervous system activity. NE in the cleft is metabolized by neuronal reuptake and nonneuronal mechanisms and appears to follow two-compartment kinetics as suggested by radiotracer studies using mathematical modeling techniques. Plasma NE levels represent spillover of NE from the synaptic cleft, which is the net result of NE production, clearance, and uptake processes. Plasma epinephrine (EPI) is secreted by the adrenal medulla primarily into the circulation to act hormonally at local and distant sites. The exact mechanisms involved in the adrenomedullary control of catecholamine secretion remain poorly understood.

Catecholamines exert metabolic, modulatory hormonal, and hemodynamic actions that differ according to target cell receptor type, receptor density, and circulating catecholamine concentration. EPI causes hepatic glycogenolysis, gluconeogenesis, lipolysis, and ketogenesis, increased lipolysis in adipose tissue, and inhibition of insulin-stimulated glucose uptake in skeletal muscle. EPI promotes stress-induced hyperglycemia by increasing hepatic glucose production and by decreasing peripheral glucose uptake.

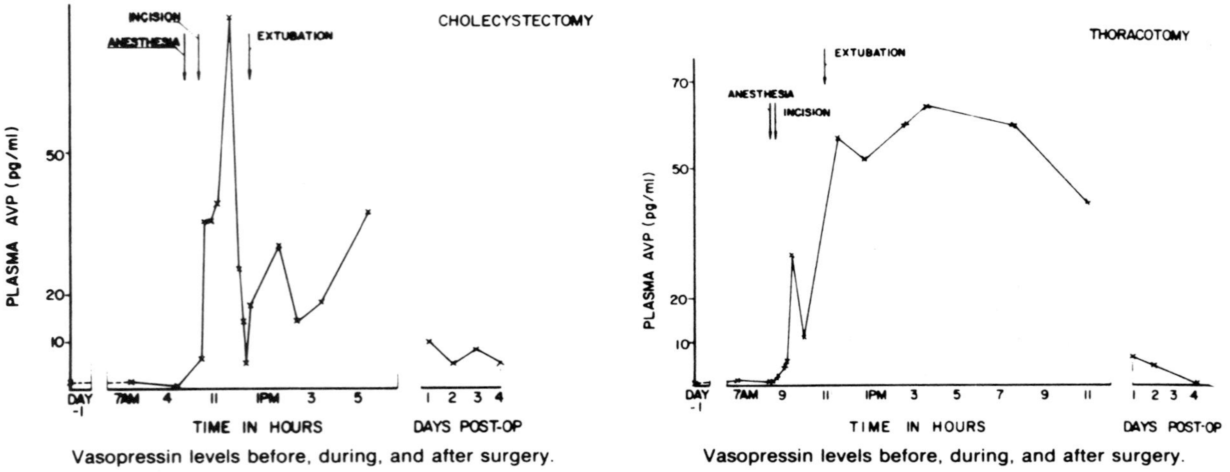

FIG. 1-22. Plasma vasopressin concentrations during cholecystectomy and thoracotomy. (From: *Haas M, Glick SM; Arch Surg 113:597, 1978, with permission.*)

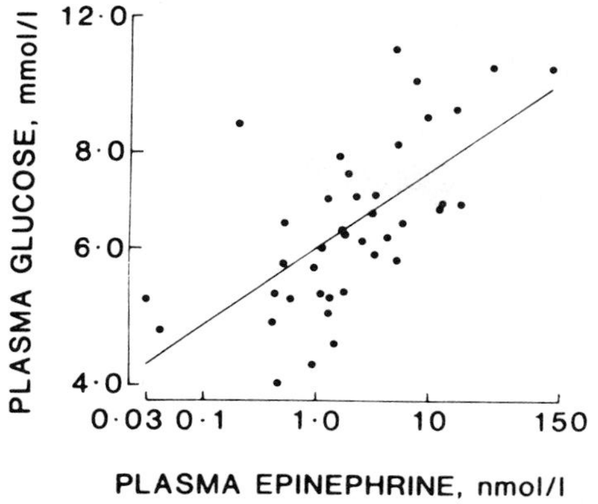

FIG. 1-23. The relationship between plasma concentrations of glucose and of epinephrine in 40 multiply injured patients. There was a positive correlation between plasma glucose and plasma epinephrine ($r = 0.64$, $p < 0.001$). (From: *Frayn KN, Little RA, Maycock PF: Circ Shock 16:299, 1985, with permission.*)

A positive correlation between plasma glucose and catecholamine concentrations is observed following injury (Fig. 1-23). Hormonal modulations produced by catecholamines include increased secretion of T_4 and T_3, renin, and parathyroid hormone and decreased secretion of aldosterone. Pancreatic catecholamine stimulation causes decreased insulin secretion and increased glucagon secretion. The hemodynamic effects of catecholamines are dependent on receptor subtype and dose.

Catecholamines increase immediately after injury and achieve peak concentrations approximately 24 to 48 h after injury, from which time they decrease to baseline. Despite different hormonal kinetics, plasma NE and EPI concentrations increase in parallel following injury. Numerous stimuli have been identified that lead to an increase in catecholamine secretion, and most are present following major injury including hypovolemia, hypoglycemia, hypoxemia, pain, and fear. Among these stimuli, plasma catecholamine concentrations following injury are best correlated with the volume of blood lost and are observed in patients after all forms of shock. The catecholamine response to operations involving cardiopulmonary bypass in neonates, for example, is blunted by administration of certain anesthetic agents, such as sufentanil, and is associated with improved outcome.

Aldosterone. Cells of the adrenal zona glomerulosa synthesize, store, and secrete the mineralocorticoid aldosterone in response to ACTH, angiotensin II, and elevations in serum potassium concentration. A pituitary glycoprotein, distinct from ACTH, called aldosterone stimulating factor (ASF) may also stimulate aldosterone release. ACTH is considerably more potent on a molar basis than angiotensin in stimulating aldosterone release. Tonic inhibition of aldosterone secretion is mediated through dopamine and through atrial natriuretic peptides through a pathway involved in aldosterone-mediated regulation of plasma sodium concentration and effective circulating volume.

The primary action of aldosterone is related to fluid and electrolyte metabolism. Aldosterone increases sodium and chloride reabsorption in the early distal convoluted tubule. Aldosterone also promotes sodium reabsorption and potassium secretion in the late distal convoluted tubules and early collecting ducts.

Following injury, ACTH and angiotensin increase and stimulate aldosterone release. ACTH mediates a short-duration release of aldosterone, which appears to be the most important stimulus to aldosterone secretion following injury. Aldosterone elevations, which persist well after ACTH has returned to normal, are also mediated through long-duration stress-induced increases in angiotensin II. Plasma aldosterone concentrations, like those of cortisol, lose normal diurnal circadian rhythm following injury. Aldosterone increases after anesthesia, injury, and major operation (Fig. 1-24). Highest aldosterone concentrations are noted in agonal or preterminal periods.

FIG. 1-24. Plasma aldosterone values in patients undergoing routine cholecystectomy. Patients who either had a conventional preoperative salt intake (LS) or a high salt intake (HS) both demonstrated an increase in plasma aldosterone secretion at the time of surgery. Only patients with a normal salt intake preoperatively demonstrated a persistent elevation in plasma aldosterone, whereas patients on a high salt diet demonstrated an immediate return to normal values in the postoperative period. (From: *Cochrane JPS: Br J Surg 65:774, 1978, with permission.*)

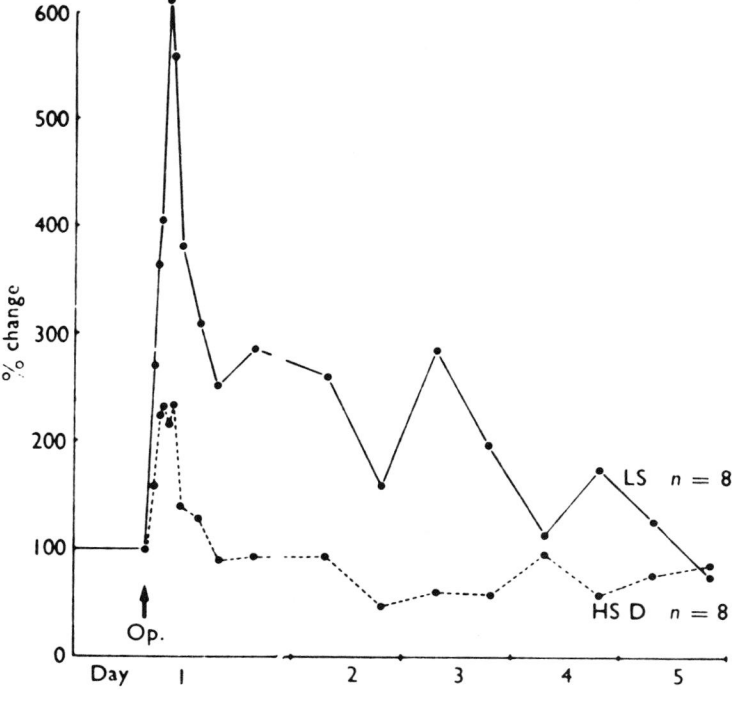

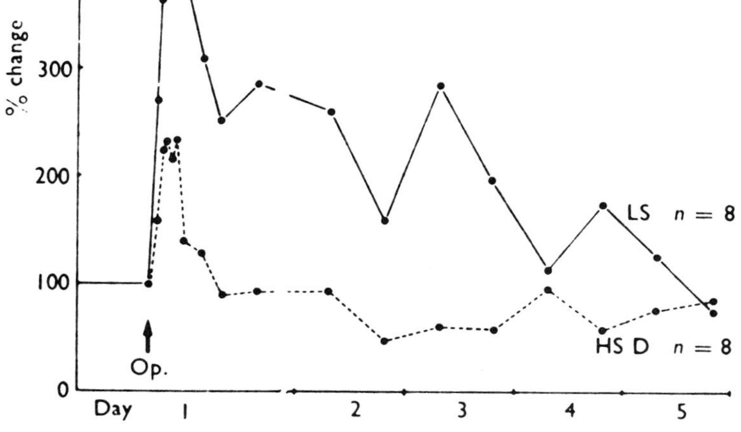

Renin-Angiotensin. Prorenin, the inactive form of renin, is found in the myoepithelial cells of the renal afferent arterioles. Proteolytic cleavage of prorenin and renin release are under the control of the juxtaglomerular neurogenic receptor, the juxtaglomerular cell, and the macula densa of the kidney. ACTH, AVP, glucagon, prostaglandins, potassium, magnesium, and calcium also influence renin secretion. Primary control of the renin system is through the neurogenic receptor of the juxtaglomerular apparatus which responds to beta-adrenergic stimulation by increasing renin release. The juxtaglomerular cell, acting as a stretch receptor, responds to a decrease in blood pressure with increased renin secretion. Increases in renin release are also stimulated when the macula densa receptor senses decreases in tubular chloride concentration in the distal nephron.

In the circulation, renin converts renin substrate or angiotensinogen, which is produced by the liver, into angiotensin I. Angiotensin I acts primarily as the precursor for the formation of angiotensin II, a process mediated in the pulmonary circulation by angiotensin converting enzyme.

Angiotensin II acts on the cardiovascular system, fluid and electrolyte balance, hormonal modulation, and metabolism. An extremely potent vasoconstrictor, it stimulates heart rate and myocardial contractility, and increases vascular permeability. Angiotensin II stimulates aldosterone synthesis and secretion, increases vasopressin secretion and participates in thirst regulation. Angiotensin II modulates hormonal actions by potentiating EPI release by the adrenal medulla, increasing CRF release, and increasing sympathetic neurotransmission. Metabolic actions include stimulation of hepatic glycogenolysis and gluconeogenesis.

Following injury, the normal circadian rhythm of renin is lost and sustained increases in renin activity are observed. Highest renin activity is noted in the agonal period. Renin secretion can be suppressed in the immediate postoperative period by salt and water loading (Fig. 1-25). Angiotensin II levels also increase immediately after injury.

Insulin. The synthesis, storage, and secretion of insulin by pancreatic beta islet cells are controlled by substrate concentrations, ANS activity, and hormone effects. Increases in glucose, amino acids, free fatty acids, and ketone bodies stimulate insulin secretion. Under normal physiologic conditions, the most important stimulus for insulin secretion is glucose. Neural and humoral mechanisms act during injury and stress to modulate the effect of glucose on insulin secretion. Sympathetic nervous system stimulation and EPI secretion inhibit insulin secretion in the presence of stress-induced hyperglycemia. Insulin secretion is further diminished by glucagon, somatostatin, gastrointestinal hormones, beta-endorphin, and IL-1, which act directly on beta islet cells, and by cortisol, estrogen, and progesterone, which interfere with peripheral actions of insulin.

Insulin, the primary anabolic hormone, promotes the storage of carbohydrate, protein, and lipid through its actions on the liver, fat, and skeletal muscle. Insulin acts on carbohydrate metabolism through the stimulation of membrane glucose transport into cells, the promotion of glycogenesis and glycolysis, and through the inhibition of hepatic gluconeogenesis. Lipid metabolism is affected by stimulation of lipid synthesis and inhibition of lipid degradation. Insulin acts on protein metabolism by promotion of protein synthesis, which is accomplished by increasing the transport of amino acids into the liver and other peripheral tissues and by inhibiting gluconeogenesis and amino acid oxidation.

Studies examining the plasma concentration of insulin following injury in human beings have noted a biphasic pattern of insulin release (Fig. 1-26). The first period, lasting only a few hours, is characterized by the suppression of insulin secretion, which is mediated by catecholamine release and sympathetic nervous system activity. This is followed by a period of normal to increased insulin secretion, which has been termed the phase of physiologic insulin resistance. Simple plasma insulin concentrations correlate poorly with injury. In this regard, the insulin/glucose ratio appears to be a better predictor of survival than either the plasma glucose or insulin concentrations.

Glucagon. Glucagon is synthesized, stored, and secreted by alpha islet cells of the pancreas. Glucagon release is modulated by substrate concentrations, ANS and CNS activity, and the effects of other hormones. The primary stimuli to glucagon secretion under normal conditions are plasma concentrations of glucose and amino acids and exercise. Glucose alters glucagon secretion in an inverse manner that appears to result primarily from direct action on the islet cell. Glucose ingestion has a greater effect on glucagon (and insulin) secretion than that observed following intravenously administered substrate. This may be a result of potentiating effects of gut hormones, differential portal blood substrate concentrations, or through the effects of central neural inputs activated by eating. Stimulation of the pancreas by the sympathetic nervous system stimulates alpha-adrenergic glucagon release. Beta-adrenergic or parasympathetic efferents inhibit glucagon release.

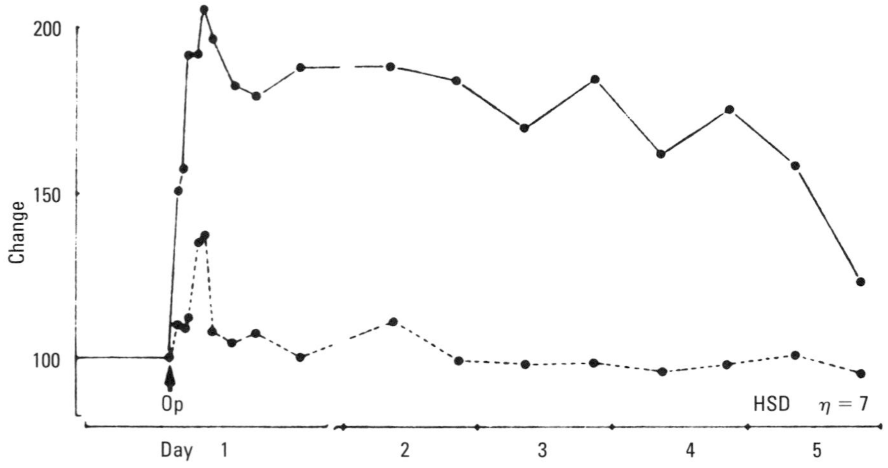

FIG. 1-25. Plasma renin activity in patients undergoing routine cholecystectomy. Patients who either had a conventional preoperative salt intake (LS) or a high salt intake (HS) both demonstrated an increase in plasma renin activity at the time of surgery. Only patients with a normal salt intake preoperatively demonstrated a persistent elevation in plasma renin activity whereas patients on a high salt diet demonstrated an immediate return to normal values in the postoperative period. (From: *Cochrane JPS: Br J Surg 65:744, 1978, with permission.*)

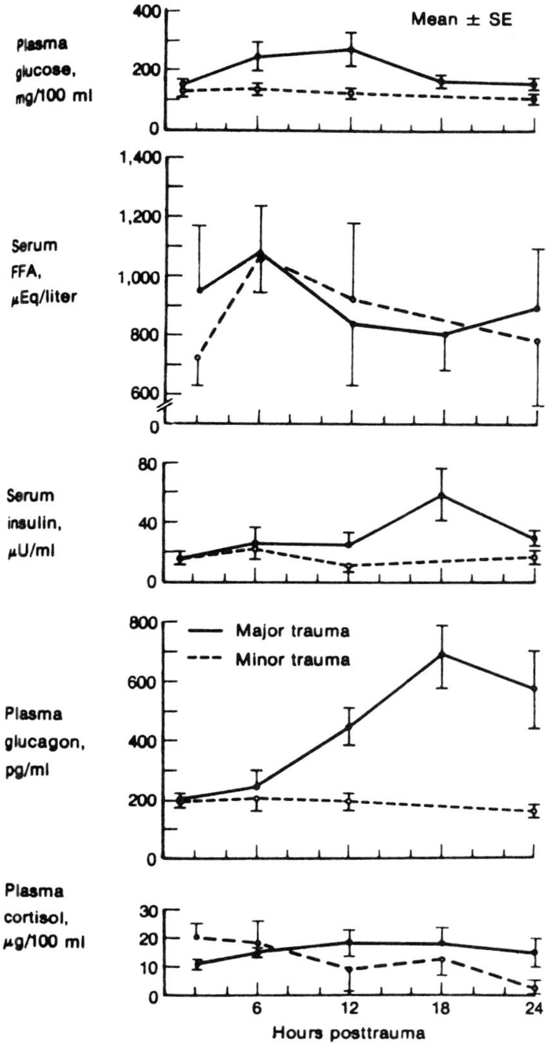

FIG. 1-26. Plasma concentrations of insulin, glucagon, cortisol, glucose, and free fatty acids in seven major and seven minor trauma patients observed over 24 h. The most significant findings were an early elevation of plasma glucose in association with a low-normal insulin concentration and a normal but gradually rising glucagon concentration that reached three times the normal value in 18 h. (From: *Meguid MM et al: Arch Surg 109:776, 1974, with permission.*)

Glucagon stimulates hepatic glycogenolysis and gluconeogenesis, which under basal conditions account for approximately 75 percent of the glucose produced by the liver. The presence of cortisol prolongs the duration and increases the peak effect of glucagon on hepatic carbohydrate metabolism. Glucagon also stimulates hepatic ketogenesis and lipolysis in adipose tissue.

Despite the increase in hepatic glucose production under normal circumstances, experimental work by McLeod and colleagues demonstrated that glucagon does not exert an important role in the immediate hyperglycemia that follows injury. Although an immediate increase in the plasma glucagon concentration that correlated with the plasma glucose concentration was noted following thermal injury, most studies of glucagon metabolism following nonthermal injury and hypovolemia find no increase in the plasma concentration of glucagon until 12 h after injury. During an operation there is an immediate decrease in the glucagon level, which returns to baseline 12 h later, increases above baseline 24 h later, and returns to normal by 3 days (Fig. 1-27). Despite the apparent difference between thermal and nonthermal injury, glucagon generally increases at some point in the immediate postinjury period after all forms of injury.

Somatostatin. Somatostatin, which is synthesized and secreted by pancreatic delta islet cells, central and peripheral neurons, and many other cells, is a potent inhibitor of GH, TSH, renin, insulin, and glucagon release. Infusion of somatostatin and other hormones in burn patients suggests complex interactions are involved in pancreatic islet cell function and carbohydrate homeostasis following thermal injury.

Insulinlike Growth Factors. The insulinlike growth factors, formerly referred to as the somatomedins, are a family of polypeptides that were originally isolated for their ability to stimulate proteoglycan synthesis in cartilage and DNA synthesis and cell replication in a variety of cell types. These growth factors (IGF-I and IGF-II) increase hepatic protein synthesis and glycogenesis, increase glucose uptake, oxidation and lipid synthesis in adipose tissue, and increase glucose uptake and protein synthesis in skeletal muscle. GH stimulation of protein synthesis is primarily mediated by IGF-I.

IGF-I concentration decreases after injury and correlates well with observed negative nitrogen balance. Preliminary studies of the effects of recombinant IGF-I infusion during hypocaloric feedings in nonstressed subjects suggest that nitrogen loss may be reduced by exogenous administration of this peptide.

Cytokines and Other Mediators

Emerging sophisticated cellular and molecular techniques of the last decade have led to the identification and preliminary understanding of factors released by activated cells that, on a very basic level, act as messengers in cellular communication (cytokines), at times spilling over into the circulation to function as hormones in response to hemorrhage, sepsis, inflammation, and other forms of injury. Among these mediators are the cytokines, eicosanoids, and endothelial cell factors. Mediator substances act locally as paracrine substances, as in the case of lymphokines acting on lymphocytes, and may also possess actions on distant cells or organs to function as hormones. Some factors that are stored within cells are released by the process of exocytosis from preformed intracellular packets; others exert their effects during the complex process of phagocytosis (Table 1-5). Mediators may be released as a consequence of cell death and exert their effects by diffusion. Other mediators are not carried within cells but circulate as inactive forms in plasma to exert their actions instantaneously by local activation processes; for example, the complement, coagulation, kinin, and angiotensin systems.

Cytokines are a newly discovered and as yet incompletely understood class of proteins that are stimulated by the host defense system and have paracrine, autocrine, and endocrine effects. The cytokines are bioactive in low concentrations (less than 10^{-11} mol/L) and are chiefly concerned with cell-to-cell communications. In some cases, the identification and naming of these compounds has been based on biologic function. This has led to redundancy in the naming of some compounds, since in many instances, multiple independent groups of researchers have focused on different actions of what prove to be identical compounds.

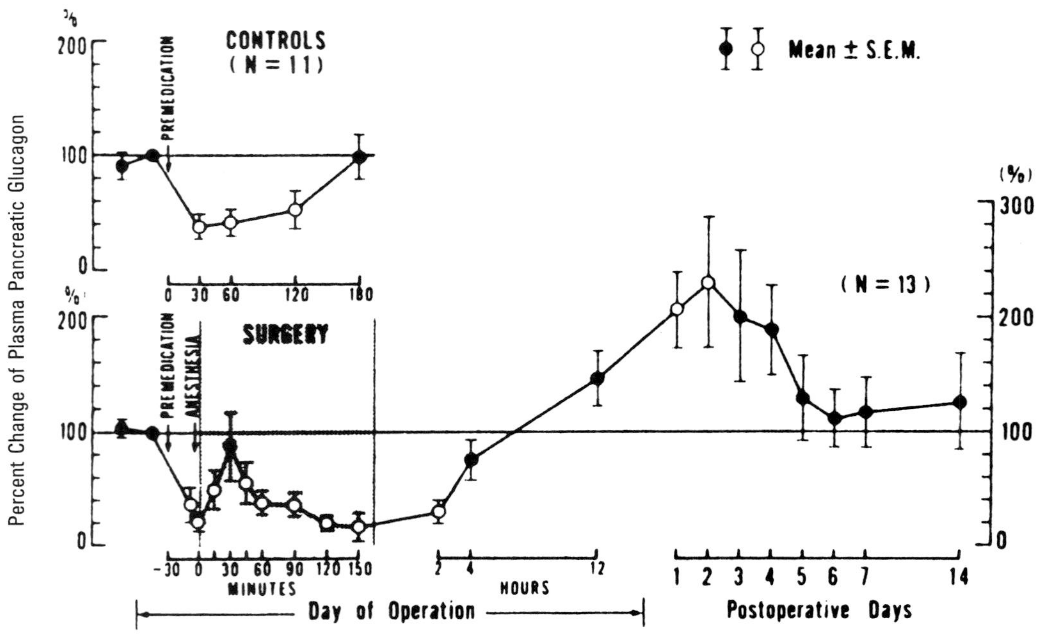

FIG. 1-27. Changes in plasma glucagon during and after elective surgery in 13 patients. Open circles represent significant differences when compared with the fasting value on the day of surgery. (From: *MIyata M, Yamamoto T, Nakao K: Horm Metab Res 8:239, 1976, with permission.*)

Interleukins. Some of the interleukins, such as IL-2, have effects that appear to be limited to the immunologic system and consequently are properly termed lymphokines. Others, such as IL-1, IL-3, and IL-6, have more diverse effects and are more properly termed cytokines.

Interleukin-1. The substance now known as interleukin-1 (IL-1) was first described in 1970 as a substance released from adherent accessory cells that augmented mixed lymphocyte responses in human beings and is responsible for the diverse biologic activities of lymphocyte-activating factor and endogenous pyrogen. IL-1 activity is now known to be mediated by two peptide molecules, termed IL-1 alpha and IL-1 beta. IL-1 beta is produced in 10-fold greater amounts than IL-1 alpha and has been thought to be the more physiologically relevant species. It appears that each IL-1 form has different mechanisms of action and bioactive states. Both species of IL-1 are translated in precursor form. IL-1 alpha has bioactivity as the precursor and is degraded rapidly to a smaller form that is principally membrane-bound. This cell-associated form may then induce killer cell cytotoxicity and other T-cell functions through cell contact without measurable release of further IL-1. The precursor form of IL-1 beta is not bioactive, and as much as 80 percent of this protein is retained in the cytosol after synthesis to be degraded to the active smaller species by tissue proteases when cell death and lysis occur. The nonbound IL-1 species have a circulating half-life of 6 min, are bound to the membrane receptor, internalized, and become associated with the nuclear chromosomes, possibly through a calcium-mediated process involving cAMP. Two classes of IL-1 receptors have been described with varied tissue distribution. An IL-1 specific inhibitor, termed IL-1 receptor antagonist (IL-1ra) has been described recently. It is produced by human monocytes, is found in urine, and blocks the binding of IL-1 to its cell surface receptors without agonist effects.

The stimulus to IL-1 release has been thought to include nearly all inflammatory, infectious, and immunologic processes. The bioassays that were used to determine the presence of IL-1 in the circulation may have been confounded by the presence and activity of other interleukins. The use of more specific radioimmunoassays and enzyme-linked immunosorbent assays (ELISAs) for detecting circulating IL-1 alpha and beta have failed to confirm the frequent appearance of IL-1 in clinical studies that had been observed using the original bioassays. The fact that IL-1 alpha has not been detected in the human circulation is consistent with the membrane-binding properties of this compound. Circulating IL-1 beta has been sporadically found in conditions of sepsis and in certain chronic disease states. IL-1 forms were not found in the circulation of human volunteers after intraveneous endotoxin, whereas other

Table 1-5
Cell-Derived Mediators

Macrophage or monocyte
Lysozyme, prostaglandins, leukotrienes, lipoprotein lipase, elastase, plasminogen activator, collagenase, arginase, fibronectin, complement, interleukin 1, tumor necrosis factor, interferon alpha and beta, angiogenesis factor
Neutrophil
Leukotriene B_4, elastase, acid hydrolases, lysozyme, hydroxyl radicals, prostaglandin E_2, cathepsin G, and collagenase
Mast cell
Histamine, proteases, heparin, eosinophil chemotactic factor-anaphylaxis, neutrophil chemotactic factor, prostaglandin D_2, leukotrienes C_4, D_4, E_4, PAF, tumor necrosis factor

SOURCE: From Yurt RW, Lowry SF: Role of the macrophage and endogenous mediators in multiple organ failure, in Deitch EA (ed): *Multiple Organ Failure*. New York, Thieme Medical Publishers, 1990, pp 60–66, with permission.

cytokines such as tumor necrosis factor (TNF), interferon (IFN), and IL-6 were readily detected.

The issue of whether IL-1 has a physiologic action at concentrations not detectable by currently available assays is not clearly settled at the present time. Many of the described actions of IL-1 under experimental conditions fall into the category of hormone effects, i.e., actions on distant organs or cells by IL-1 as a circulating cellular messenger, in addition to known paracrine and autocrine effects. However, many of these actions remain to be demonstrated in human beings.

The paracrine immunologic effects of IL-1 have been confirmed. IL-1 augments T-cell proliferation via enhanced IL-2 production and enhanced IL-2 receptor expression thereby acting as an immunologic adjuvant.

IL-1 acts on the CNS inducing fever by stimulating local release of prostaglandins in the anterior hyothalamus, inducing anorexia by direct action on the satiety center, lessening pain perception by increasing beta-endorphin release, and increasing the number of opiatelike receptors in the brain. IL-1 also increases the basal metabolic rate and increases oxygen consumption.

IL-1 acts with IL-6, TNF, and IFN to promote rapid synthesis of hepatic acute-phase proteins. In the modulating presence of cortisol, acute-phase proteins such as ceruloplasmin, fibrinogen, haptoglobin, C-reactive protein, complement factors, alpha 1 antitrypsin, and α_2-macroglobulin are induced and albumin synthesis is suppressed. The liver is stimulated to accumulate amino acids and zinc and iron from plasma pools. Copper is released and combines with ceruloplasmin to act in clearing oxygen-free radicals and donating copper to necessary enzyme systems such as lysyl oxidase which is essential for collagen cross-linkage. The acute-phase proteins alpha 1 antitrypsin and α_2-macroglobulin are protease inhibitors. C-reactive protein functions in bacterial opsonization, complement activation, and phagocytosis.

The energy and substrate demands for increased hepatic synthesis may also be in part modulated by actions of IL-1. The precise action of IL-1 on skeletal muscle metabolism remains unsettled, but it is clearly established that a breakdown fragment of IL-1 promotes skeletal muscle proteolysis, an effect which may require PGE_2. Recent work using infusions of IL-1 alpha in vivo has shown promotion of skeletal muscle proteolysis, whereas IL-1 induction in humans by injection of the inflammatory agent etiocholanolone has not been accompanied by changes in protein metabolism. It appears that IL-1 plays an important endocrine role in modulating protein metabolism to meet the demands of injury by inducing hepatic acute-phase protein synthesis and promoting breakdown of skeletal muscle to amino acids. The amino acids that are released appear to be used by the liver for energy as well as for protein synthesis since an appreciable amount of the amino acids released is oxidized. Other mediators, such as TNF, IFN, and PGE, also participate in this effect.

The metabolic effects of IL-1 may be related in part to central actions such as those on the hypothalamic-pituitary axis causing stimulation of CRF and ACTH. Blood levels of GH, alpha MSH, and prolactin are not markedly affected by IL-1, and catecholamines are increased only marginally. IL-1 may also act on pancreatic islet cells to stimulate insulin and glucagon secretion. Cytotoxic effects on insulin-producing beta cells for IL-1 and TNF have also been described. However, central noradrenergic pathways are stimulated by IL-1, and it may be that other (non–beta cell) central mechanisms also mediate the IL-1 effects on carbohydrate metabolism. Experimental work suggests that the effect of IL-1 on glucose metabolism, which is a mild hypoglycemic response, is related to a central alteration of the glucose set point, since IL-1 action appears to be independent of pancreatic endocrine cell function, peripheral insulin sensitivity, and serum glucose level.

Interleukin-2. IL-2 is a true lymphokine that, unlike the cytokines IL-1, IL-6, and TNF, appears to act predominantly as an immunostimulant. The substance was isolated originally as a T-cell growth factor and has been subsequently cloned and sequenced. Recombinant human IL-2 is a nonglycosylated protein molecule with a serum half-life of 6 to 10 min when administered intravenously. Antigen stimulation of lymphocytes triggers increased transcription of the genes for both IL-2 and IL-2 receptors. Use of IL-2 for generating lymphokine-activated killer (LAK) cells for the therapy of malignant disease is under investigation. Production of IL-2 has been impaired in patients following trauma and thermal injury.

Interleukin-6. Interleukin-6 (IL-6) is a family of glycoproteins known also by other names such as hepatocyte stimulatory factor, interferon $\beta 2$, and B-cell stimulatory factor 2. The primary biologic roles of IL-6 compounds appear to be enhancement of immune function and acting with IL-1 to promote synthesis of hepatic acute-phase proteins. IL-6 may also have central hormonal modulating effects, for example, causing prostaglandin-mediated CRF stimulation. IL-6 is rapidly released by a variety of cell types including monocytes, fibroblasts, and endothelial cells in response to bacterial products, viruses, and the cytokines IL-1 and TNF. IL-6 is detected in the human circulation within 60 min of intravenous endotoxin administration and is also stimulated following elective operation and thermal injury.

Tumor Necrosis Factor. TNF, or cachectin, is a cytokine protein that was originally isolated for its ability to produce cell death in certain tumors and to cause cachexia and hypertriglyceridemia during experimental infection. Human pro-TNF undergoes proteolysis to exist as dimer, trimer, or pentamer forms in solution. At least one intermediate species appears to be stable, bioactive, and cell-associated, with a circulating half-life of 14 to 18 min in human beings. A wide variety of cells produce TNF, including monocytes, pulmonary and peritoneal macrophages, Kupffer cells, mast cells, and endothelial cells, within minutes of stimulation. Complement activation products, particularly C5a, are involved in stimulation of TNF and IL-1.

TNF is believed to act synergistically with IL-1 to induce hypotension, tissue injury, and death in animals subjected to experimental sepsis and to cause the release of prostaglandin E_2 (PGE_2) neutrophil aggregation, thromboxane synthesis, and cytotoxicity for insulin-producing beta cells. TNF and IL-1 induce eicosanoids and platelet-activating factor (PAF). TNF also acts to suppress lipoprotein lipase activity in adipose cells and to cause a fall in transmembrane potential in skeletal muscle. TNF is not believed to have direct effects on proteolysis but has actions mediated by corticosteroids. Experimental work with IL-1 receptor antagonist suggests that TNF may mediate the early hypotension of sepsis and IL-1, or factors under the control of IL-1 may participate in later phases of sepsis-induced shock. Of interest, protein inhibitors of TNF activity have been found in the serum of patients with diseases such as sarcoidosis and tuberculosis, in the urine, and in malignant and benign pleural effusion fluid.

Although much of the initial cytokine research has focused on sepsis or endotoxemia, recent experimental work suggests that cytokines may play important roles in the response to loss of effective blood volume. In rats, infusion of monoclonal antibody to TNF before induction of hemorrhagic shock significantly ameliorated the TNF response and improved survival.

Interferon. Gamma interferon (IFN) is a glycoprotein released by stimulated T lymphocytes that activates macrophages to release IL-1 and TNF, increases monocyte IL-2 receptors, and inhibits viral replication. IFN reduces immunologic suppressor activity by inhibition of PGE_2 release. Elevated IFN levels have been observed in patients with pelvic inflammatory disease. Stimulation of cortisol has been observed after IFN infusions in cancer patients, but the mechanism is not fully understood.

Eicosanoids. The eicosanoids are a class of oxidation products of long-chain polyunsaturated fatty acids that are derived from arachidonic acid and are variously secreted by all nucleated cells except the lymphocyte. These substances include the prostaglandins, thromboxanes, leukotrienes, hydroxyeicosatetraenoic acids (HETEs), and lipoxins (Fig. 1-28). Esterified precursor fatty acids are released by acyl hydrolases, such as phospholipase A, to form arachidonic acid. Further intracellular metabolism to prostaglandins, thromboxane, and leukotrienes requires the enzymes cyclo-oxygenase, thromboxane synthetase, and lipoxygenase, respectively. Phospholipases are activated by many compounds such as epinephrine, angiotensin II, bradykinin, histamine, and thrombin. The activation of phospholipases can be inhibited by lipocortin, which is induced by cortisol.

Eicosanoids are not stored by cells but are synthesized de novo. Their effects depend on the nature of the stimulus and the nature of the producing cell type. For example, vascular endothelial cells convert arachidonic acid primarily to prostacyclin (PGI_2) via the enzyme prostacyclin synthetase which causes vasodilatation and inhibition of platelet aggregation. Platelets convert prostaglandin via thromboxane synthetase to thromboxane A_2 (TxA_2) which is a potent vasoconstrictor and promotes platelet aggregation. Macrophages, in contrast, synthesize a mixture of most of the cyclo-oxygenase and lipoxygenase products. Stimuli for eicosanoid synthesis include hypoxia, ischemia, tissue injury, pyrogen, endotoxin, NE, AVP, angiotensin II, bradykinin, serotonin, acetylcholine, and histamine. These stimuli result in the release of several prostaglandins whose structures depend on the tissue stimulated and not necessarily on the stimulus itself.

The biologic actions of eicosanoids depend on their effects on intracellular second messengers. Inhibitory effects of PGE compounds on AVP activity and hormone-stimulated lipolysis, for example, result from diminished expression of adenylate cyclase. PGE compounds mimic the effects of ACTH, TSH, and LH by stimulating intracellular cAMP. Thromboxane and leukotrienes have opposite effects from PGE compounds because they act by increasing intracellular free calcium via phosphatidylinositol transduction mechanisms.

The eicosanoids have widespread effects on systemic, pulmonary, and regional vasoregulation; on central and peripheral neurotransmission; on the local effects of hormones; and on immunologic function (Table 1-6). Leukotrienes are produced by a variety of cell types, including cells of the lung, connective tissue, smooth muscle, macrophages, mast cells, and monocytes. The slow-releasing substance of anaphylaxis has been found to be a mixture of these compounds. Leukotrienes are capable of increasing postcapillary leakage with 1000 times the potency of histamine and produce leukocyte adherence, bronchoconstriction, and vasoconstriction. Leukotrienes cause adhesion and chemotaxis and stimulate aggregation, enzyme release, and superoxide formation in neutrophils. Lipoxins are a newly isolated class of arachidonic acid metabolites that stimulate superoxide formation and degranulation of neutrophils. Prostaglandin administration causes stimulation of ACTH, GH, and prolactin in experimental models, whereas leukotrienes may induce LH release.

The prostaglandins are major components of the inflammatory response, whose importance is clearly demonstrated by the clinical resolution of inflammatory conditions such as bursitis, arthritis, and tenosynovitis with agents that block prostaglandin synthesis.

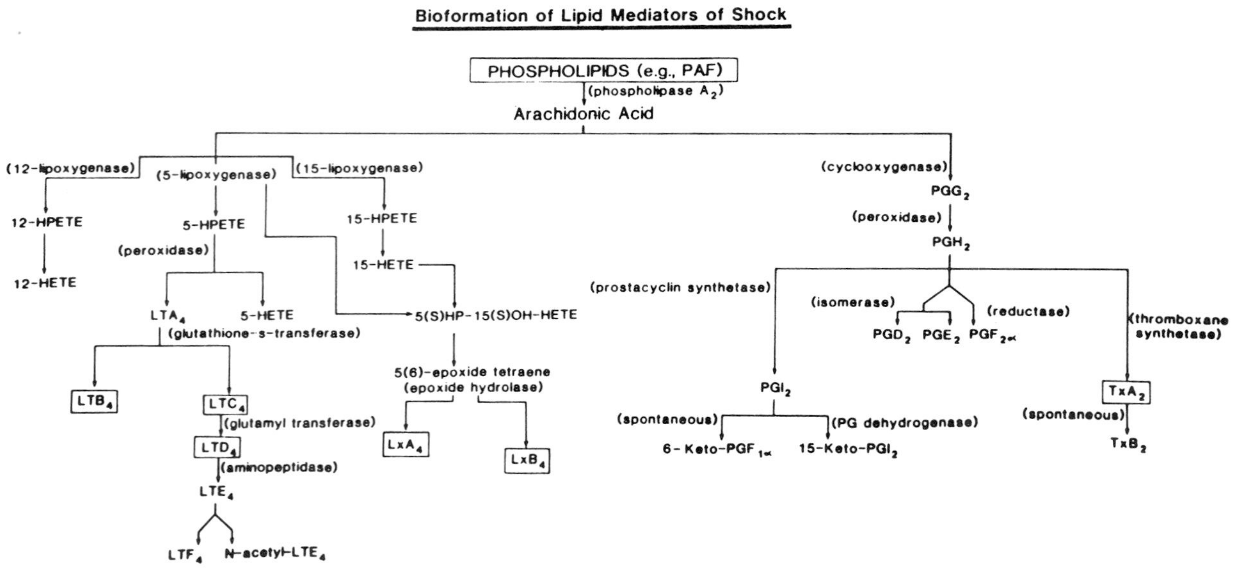

FIG. 1-28. The biosynthetic pathway of lipid mediators. Abbreviations: HP, hydroperoxide; LT, leukotriene; PG, prostaglandin; Tx, thromboxane; Lx, lipoxin. (From: *Lefer AM, et al: Circ Shock 27:3, 1989, with permission.*)

Table 1-6
Representative Pharmacologic Actions of Major Eicosanoids

Pharmacologic Action	*Eicosanoid Effectors*
Anterior pituitary peptide release	PGE_2, $PGF_{2\alpha}$
Bronchoconstriction	LTC_4, LTD_4, TxA_2, $PGF_{2\alpha}$
Bronchodilation	PGE_2, PGI_2
Chemotaxis	LTB_4
Gastrointestinal motility	PGE_2, $PGF_{2\alpha}$
Gastrointestinal cytoprotection	PGE_2, PGI_2, PGD_2
Lymphocyte proliferation	LTB_4
Inhibition of lymphocyte proliferation	PGI_2, PGE_2
Platelet aggregation and release reaction	TxA_2
Platelet inhibition	PGI_2, PGD_2
Renin release	PGI_2, PGE_2, PGD_2
Uterine contraction	PGE_2, $PGF_{2\alpha}$, TxA_2
Cervical ripening	PGE_2
Vasoconstriction	TxA_2, $PGF_{2\alpha}$, LTC_4, LTD_4
Vasodilation	PGI_2, PGE_2, PGD_2

SOURCE: From Myers A, Uotila P, et al: The eicosanoids: Prostaglandins, thromboxane, and leukotrienes, in DeGroot LJ: *Endocrinology*, 2d ed. Philadelphia, WB Saunders, 1989, chap. 150, with permission.

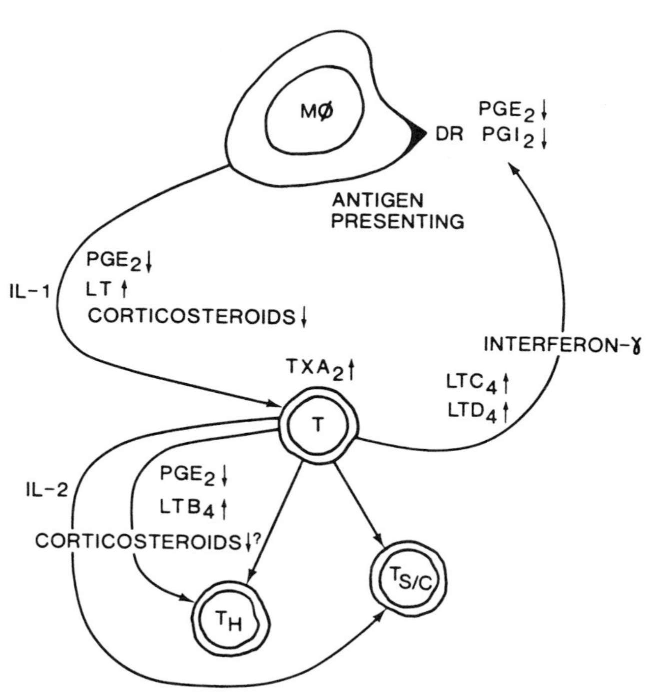

FIG. 1-29. Hypothetical model of eicosanoid modulation of lymphocyte-macrophage interaction. See text for abbreviations. (From: *Myers A, Uotila P, et al: The eicosanoids: Prostaglandin, thromboxane, and leukotrienes, in LJ DeGroot: Endocrinology, 2d ed. Philadelphia, WB Saunders 1989, chap 150, with permission.*)

The inflammatory response, which is characterized by increased vascular permeability, leukocyte migration, and vasodilation, is a group of cellular events that correspond to the classic clinical manifestations of rubor, dolor, tumor, and calor. Each of these symptoms and signs can result from the actions of eicosanoids. Plasma concentrations of eicosanoids are increased during hemorrhage, sepsis, endotoxemia, trauma, and thermal injury. The presence of these substances in increased concentrations has been implicated in adult respiratory distress syndrome (ARDS), pancreatitis, and renal failure. Some investigators believe, for example, that the primary event in ARDS is platelet aggregation and thromboxane release that produces pulmonary vasoconstriction, leukocyte trapping, oxygen-free radical release, and endothelial damage. This hypothesis is supported by the elevated ratio of TxB_2, the major metabolite of TxA_2, to 6-keto-$F_{1\alpha}$, the major metabolite of PGI_2, which is observed in patients with sepsis and ARDS compared to that observed in patients with sepsis alone.

Models for eicosanoid modulation of the immune response have been suggested (Fig. 1-29). Leukotrienes act indirectly by promoting IFN release from lymphocytes which stimulate DR antigen expression on macrophages. PGE_2 release is believed to inhibit IL-2 formation. Lipoxygenase products promote IL-1 formation. Recent studies suggest that increases in PGE_2 cause suppression of lymphocyte IL-2 production in burn patients.

Kallikreins-Kinins. Bradykinin in plasma and kallidin in tissues are produced through kininogen degradation by the serine protease kallikrein. Kallikrein exists in plasma as inactive prekallikrein (or Fletcher factor) that is activated by Hageman factor of the clotting system. Plasma kinins are rapidly broken down by kinase I and II. Kinase I, or anaphylatoxin inactivator, is a carboxypeptidase that degrades C3a, C4a, and C5a anaphylatoxins. Kinase II is a dipeptidase that is identical to angiotensin converting enzyme which converts angiotensin I to angiotensin II.

Bradykinin release is stimulated by hypoxia and ischemia. Increased kallikrein and bradykinin have been noted following hemorrhage, sepsis, endotoxemia, and tissue injury. These changes appear to correlate with severity of injury and survival.

The kinins are potent vasodilators that increase capillary permeability, produce edema, evoke pain, increase bronchial resistance, and enhance glucose clearance. It is postulated that bradykinin-induced increase in hepatic prostaglandins may inhibit gluconeogenesis through inhibition of glucagon-induced cAMP formation. Bradykinin infusions may increase nitrogen retention. Kinins have been implicated in the regulation of fluid and electrolytes by causing renal vasodilation, reduced renal blood flow, increased renin formation, and increased sodium and water retention when administered in pharmacologic doses.

Serotonin. Serotonin, or 5-hydroxytryptamine, is a neurotransmitter derived from tryptophan that is found in enterochromaffin cells of the intestine and in platelets. It is sometimes released in excessive quantities in patients with midgut embryonic types of carcinoid syndromes and can cause severe endocardial fibrosis. Serotonin stimulates vasoconstriction and bronchoconstriction, increases platelet aggregation, and stimulates myocardial heart rate and contractility. Serotonin is released at tissue injury, but its precise role following injury is incompletely understood.

Histamine. Histamine is synthesized from histidine and stored primarily in neurons, epidermis, gastric mucosa cells, mast cells, basophils, and platelets. Histamine release is stimulated by decreased intracellular cAMP and increased intracellular calcium. Histamine acts on two cell surface receptor subtypes. H_1 receptors mediate increased histamine precursor uptake, L-histidine, and stimulate bronchoconstriction, intestinal motility, and myocardial contractility. H_2 receptors inhibit histamine release and mediate changes in gastric secretion, heart rate, and immunologic function.

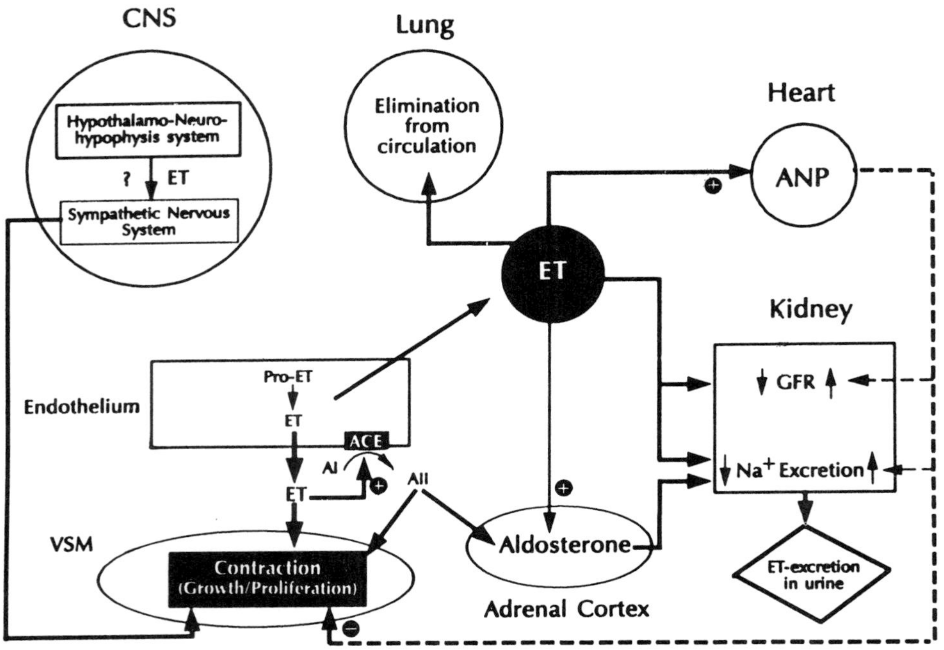

FIG. 1-30. Hypothetical integrated cardiovascular actions of endothelin (ET). By complex interactions with various endocrine systems, ET may indirectly modulate cardiovascular and renal function. Circulating ET (black circle) is removed by the lung and excreted by the kidney. Abbreviations: VSM, vascular smooth muscle; Pro-ET, precursors of ET; ACE, angiotensin-converting enzyme; AI, angiotensin I; AII, angiotensin II; ANP, atrial natriuretic peptide; GFR, glomerular filtration rate. (From: *Rubanyi GM, et al: FASEB 5:2717, 1991, with permission.*)

Both receptors cause local vasodilation and increased vascular permeability.

Elevated concentrations of histamine have been demonstrated after hemorrhagic shock, trauma, and thermal injury. Highest levels of histamine are associated with sepsis and endotoxemia and correlate with endotoxin-related decreases in arterial blood pressure and platelet count. Although histamine concentrations are inversely correlated with survival in septic shock, no significant correlation has been observed for patients with thermal injury. Histamine infusion causes hypotension, peripheral pooling of blood, increased capillary permeability, decreased venous return, and myocardial failure which are similar to changes that are frequently observed in shock and sepsis.

Endothelial Cell Mediators

The estimated aggregate weight of the endothelium in an adult is approximately 1.5 kg, stretching across a surface area of approximately 400 m^2. Substances elaborated by endothelial cells appear to have primarily local actions with extremely brief half-lives, suggesting primary paracrine roles. However, increases in plasma or urinary levels of some endothelial factors have been described in certain conditions, which suggests that pathophysiologic or systemic effects may occur. The endothelium may be considered to be an endocrine organ in its own right, responding to external stimuli by the production of paracrine hormones and growth factors that act on neighboring smooth muscle cells, monocytes, macrophages, fibroblasts, and organ-specific cells. Endothelial cell products may also modulate cardiovascular functions by acting on central cardiovascular, baroreceptor, and neuroeffector systems (Fig. 1-30). The primary action of endothelial-derived substances, however, is believed to be local vasomotor regulation and modulation of coagulation. Recent investigations also suggest that the endothelial cells act on immune function through elaboration of substances such as intercellular adhesion molecules, endothelial leukocyte adhesion molecules, and other molecules that promote platelet and lymphocyte binding, with secretion of cytokines such as IL-1, TNF, and IFN. The vascular system may thereby be considered an immunologic organ as well (Fig. 1-31).

Nitric Oxide. It has been known for some time that endothelial cells are required for the muscarinic receptor, vasodilatory action of acetylcholine, through the release of a substance termed endothelium-derived relaxing factor (EDRF). Only recently has it been appreciated that the effect of EDRF is due to the release of nitric oxide (NO). Endogenous NO, like the nitrovasodilatory drugs in clinical use, acts through the stimulation of the soluble guanylate cyclase. This enzyme forms cGMP which then activates cGMP-dependent protein kinases and leads ultimately to dephosphorylation of myosin light chains and muscle relaxation. NO formation is dependent on the presence of L-arginine and is released by many cell types in addition to endothelial cells, such as neutrophils, macrophages, cerebellar neurons, renal cells, and Kupffer

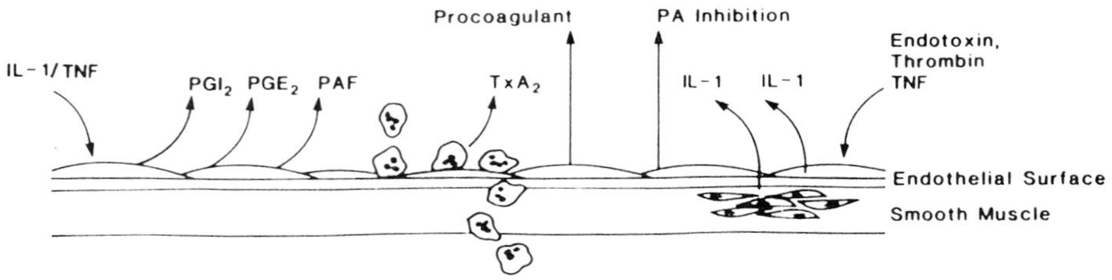

FIG. 1-31. Cytokine, IL-1, and TNF effects on vascular tissue. Abbreviation: PA, plasminogen activator; See text for others. (From: *Dinarello CA, et al: Adv Immunol 44:167, 1989, with permission.*)

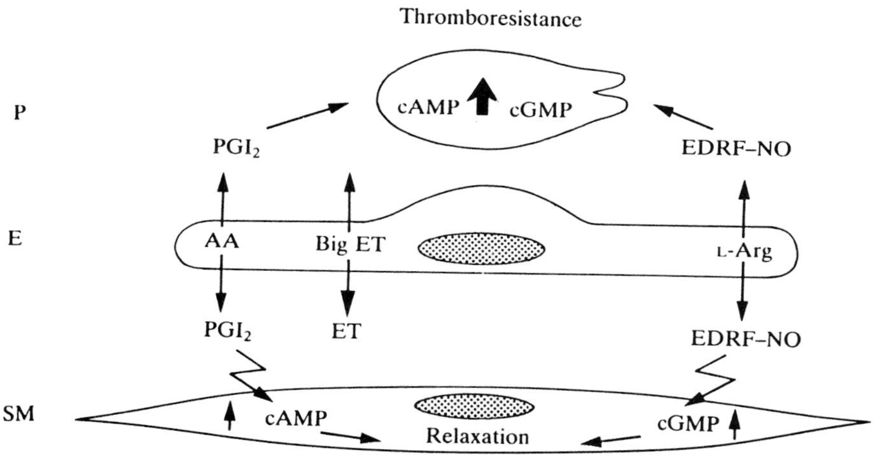

FIG. 1-32. Endothelial (E) cell mediators communicating with adjacent vascular smooth muscle cells (SM) and platelets (P). Prostacyclin (PGI_2) from arachidonic acid (AA) and endothelium-derived relaxing factor–nitric oxide (EDRF-NO) from L-arginine (L-arg) synergize by activating adenylate cyclase and guanylate cyclase, respectively, to cause SM relaxation and inhibition of platelet aggregation. Endothelin 1 (ET) is released from its precursor Big ET into the endothelial environment to cause vasoconstriction. (From: *Anggard EE, et al: J Endocrinol 127:373, 1990, with permission.*)

cells. There is evidence that blood vessels are dilated continuously by endothelial EDRF-NO, acting as a true paracrine compound with immediate inactivation by hemoglobin in the bloodstream, with synergistic vasodilatory actions by prostacyclin through adenylate cyclase (Fig. 1-32). The vasodilatory actions of these compounds appear to be countered by the potent endothelial cell products called endothelins which are described below.

NO causes vasodilation in human beings. Although the precise source of NO is not yet clearly established, a significant positive correlation between elevated serum concentration, the presence of endotoxin, and a clinical state of low vascular resistance has been observed in patients after trauma and during sepsis.

Other cells types, in addition to vascular endothelium, produce NO, including hepatocytes, Kupffer cells, macrophages, neutrophils, and cerebellar neurons, suggesting a wide spectrum of potential physiologic effects. NO also mediates protein synthesis in hepatocytes and electron transport in hepatocyte mitochondria.

Endothelins. In response to injury, vascular endothelial cells also elaborate endothelins (ET), a family of 21 amino acid peptides with potent vasoconstrictor properties, structurally related to the venom of the Israeli burrowing asp and to the gut peptide vasoactive intestinal contractor. The ETs originate from a large pre-propeptide from which a 38 amino acid peptide, big ET, is generated by proteolytic cleavage, and in turn is transformed to more active forms. Isopeptide ET forms have been found with different activities, tissue distributions, and receptors. ET-1 may be the most biologically active form. This form is the most potent vasoconstrictor known, being approximately 10 times more potent than angiotensin II. The mechanism of action of the ETs involves binding to G-protein–coupled receptors, activation of phospholipase with elevation of inositol triphosphate, diacylglycerol, eicosanoids, and calcium.

Increased serum levels of endothelin have been found to correlate with severity of injury in patients following major trauma and major operation and in patients during cardiogenic shock and sepsis. It is believed that the primary actions of ETs are paracrine, as the concentrations of circulating ETs (1 pg) are believed to be too low to exert systemic effects.

Factors affecting the release of ET are thrombin, catecholamines, and anoxia. ETs may be involved in counteracting basal levels of EDRF-NO and prostacyclins at the smooth muscle level of blood vessels to maintain physiologic tone (Fig. 1-32). These endothelial cells are also stimulated by mediators such as IL-1, TNF, and endotoxin (Fig. 1-31). Endothelin, NO, and substances such as endothelial leukocyte adhesion molecule-1 and oxygen-free radicals are produced and released by endothelium in the presence of cytokines such as IL-1, TNF, and endotoxins.

Other Endothelial Cell Factors. ***Prostaglandins.*** As discussed in the section on eicosanoids, endothelial cells synthesize predominantly prostacyclin and PGE_2 and only small amounts of TxA_2. These products act to promote vasodilatation and reduce platelet aggregation. The primary prostaglandin products of platelets, TxA_2 and 12-HETE, have opposite effects.

Platelet-Activating Factor. TNF, IL-1, AVP, and angiotensin II cause increased endothelial cell release of platelet activating factor (PAF), a phospholipid constituent of cell membranes, also known as acetyl glyceryl ether phosphorylcholine (AGEPc). Enhanced angiotensin II formation is facilitated by formation via endothelial-cell-membrane–bound angiotensin converting enzyme. Platelets in contact with PAF produce TxA_2 through the cyclo-oxygenase pathway to cause platelet aggregation and vasoconstriction (Fig. 1-28). PAF also mediates cytoskeletal changes in endothelial cells which increases barrier permeability to albumin. Among other potential actions, PAF is thought to be a possible mediator of hemodynamic and metabolic effects of endotoxin and has been isolated in the peritoneal fluid after experimental traumatic shock. Administration of specific PAF receptor antagonists has improved survival in experimental models of endotoxic, traumatic. and hemorrhagic shock. Experimental PAF infusion has altered glucose kinetics and suggests that PAF promotes release of glucagon and catecholamines.

Atrial Natriuretic Peptides. Atrial natriuretic peptides (ANP), or factors, are released by the CNS and by atrial tissue in response to changes in chamber distension. They are included here because the endocardium is a specialized endothelium. ANP are potent inhibitors of aldosterone secretion. They block perirenal tubular reabsorption of sodium, but their role in normal control of fluid and electrolyte balance remains controversial. ANP has been shown to be unaffected by coronary artery bypass operation but does change after atrial circulation is altered, as in certain congenital heart reconstructions. Similarly, fluid resuscitation does not appear to change plasma ANP concentrations. The role of ANP in postinjury responses is not yet clear.

Intracellular Mediators

Heat Shock Proteins. Originally named because of expression after heat stimulation, a group of intracellular proteins known as the heat shock proteins (HSPs) are induced following a variety of experimental stimuli including hypoxia, ether anesthesia, trauma, and hemorrhage. The HSPs are among the most highly conserved proteins in existence and are presumed to play an important role in protecting cells from the deleterious effects of stress. Current studies suggest that the HSPs interact with a variety of intracellular proteins and assist in their assembly, disassembly, stability, and intracellular transport (see Fig. 1-11 for example). The role of HSPs in the human cellular response to stress has not been defined. Experimental work has shown that HSP gene expression occurs in parallel with hypothalamic- pituitary axis activation and may be adrenal cortex–specific and also vascular cell–specific providing evidence for stress-induced interactions of the neurohumoral system and the molecular response to stress. This response may be ACTH-sensitive and age-dependent. Recent evidence suggests that HSP synthesis in shock may inhibit synthesis of hepatic acute-phase proteins. The full nature and significance of possible interactions between HSPs and other mediators of the injury response remains obscure.

Oxygen-free Radicals. The formation of short-lived highly reactive molecular oxygen species with an unpaired outer-orbit electron [oxygen-free radicals (OFR)] has been associated with damage to living tissues primarily by peroxidation of cell membrane unsaturated fatty acids. OFR species, such as the superoxide radical and hydroxyl radical and endogenous hydrogen peroxide that contribute to radical-mediated damage, are produced following ischemia and shock by activated granulocytes and by oxidases such as xanthine oxidase found in endothelium.

Various mechanisms are necessary and available for OFR protection. In the intracellular space, the enzyme superoxide dismutase (SOD) is present in high concentrations to react with the superoxide radical during the formation of hydrogen peroxide and oxygen. Catalase and glutathione peroxidase decompose hydrogen peroxide to water. In the extracellular space SOD-like activity is very low and has an affinity for endothelium. The fact that endothelium-derived relaxing factor is inactivated by superoxide anions may be important in the mechanisms of local blood flow regulation during and following ischemia and shock. Administration of substances known to inhibit OFR formation, such as allopurinol, which inhibits xanthine oxidase, or mannitol, which acts as a hydroxyl radical scavenger, have been shown experimentally and clinically to confer beneficial effects on organ preservation and overall survival. An intriguing recent observation found that allopurinol decreased bacterial translocation during experimental hemorrhagic shock.

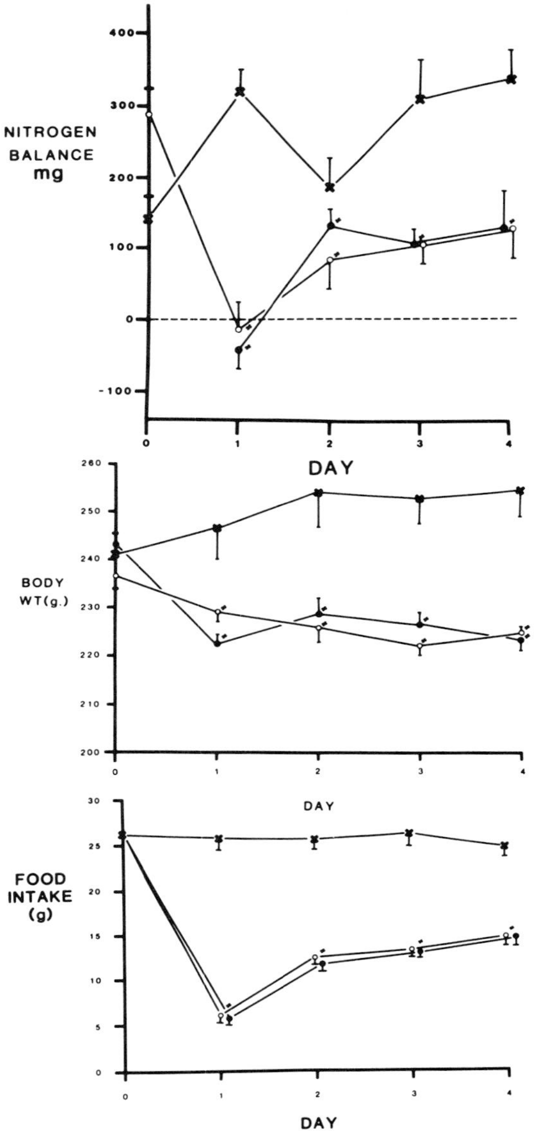

FIG. 1-33. Effect of wounding on food intake, nitrogen balance, and body weight. Food intake by wounded animals (●) was considerably less than that of animals allowed to eat ad libitum (×). When animals were pair-fed (○) to the reduced food intake of the wounded animals, negative nitrogen balance and weight loss were the same in these two groups. In contrast, there was a marked difference in nitrogen balance and body weight between wounded animals and animals allowed to eat ad libitum. (From: *Shearer JD et al: Am J Surg 147:456, 1984, with permission.*)

SUBSTRATE METABOLISM FOLLOWING INJURY

The metabolic response to injury is determined by the patient's baseline health and age, the nature and magnitude of the injury, the effects of injury-related starvation and immobilization, and the success of homeostatic systems in preventing further injury such as bacterial proliferation and sepsis during the phases of recovery. Early work suggested that the substrate metabolic changes observed after injury (negative nitrogen balance and weight loss, for example) could be accounted for by the fasting state (Fig. 1-33). It is now appreciated, however, that lipid, carbohydrate, and protein metabolism are altered by neurohumoral responses and by mediator-induced wound effects that are distinct from those observed in simple starvation. The metabolic response to fasting is a basic adaptive response that does have relevance to the posttraumatic state, since interruption of feeding usually accompanies injury.

Metabolism After Fasting

Substrate Metabolism. The average resting, 70-kg subject expends 1800 kcal/day of energy obtained from lipid, carbohydrate, and protein sources (Fig. 1-34). Obligate glycolytic cells,

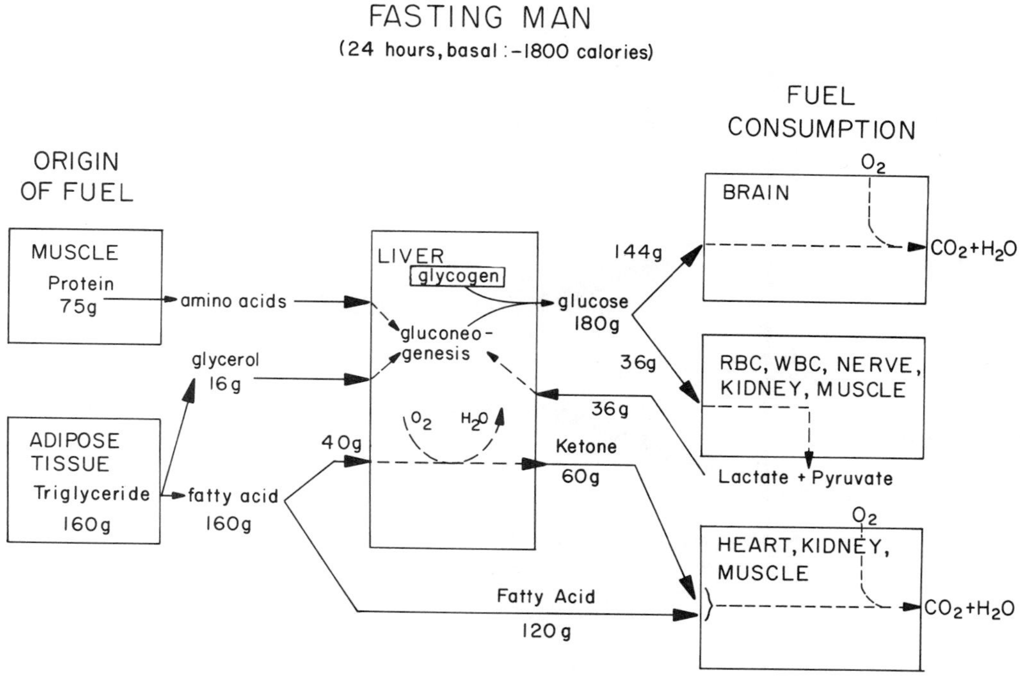

FIG. 1-34. Scheme of fuel utilization in a normal fasted man. The two primary sources are muscle protein and fat. The brain oxidizes glucose completely, the glycolyzers break down glucose by aerobic or anaerobic glycolysis into lactate and pyruvate, which are then remade in the liver into glucose, and the rest of the body burns fatty acids and ketones. (Adapted from: *Cahill GF: N Engl J Med 282:668, 1970, with permission.*)

such as neurons, leukocytes, and erythrocytes require 180 g/24 h of glucose for basal energy needs. In the absence of food, glucose must be supplied from preexisting body stores, which consist of 75 g of glucose stored as hepatic glycogen (Table 1-7). Skeletal muscle cannot directly release free glucose since it lacks the necessary enzyme glucose-6-phosphatase. The resulting reduction of circulating glucose during prolonged fasting serves as a primary stimulus to hormonal release that modulates gluconeogenesis and substrate substitution for those tissues that require glucose for energy (Fig. 1-35). Glucose concentration falls within 15 h of fasting, decreases insulin release, and increases secretion of glucagon, GH, catecholamines, AVP, and angiotensin II. Glucagon and EPI act through cAMP to promote glycogenolysis. Norepinephrine, AVP, and angiotensin II act through phosphatidylinositol and calcium and also promote glycogenolysis. Of all these hormones, AVP appears to be the most active on a molar basis. Cortisol and glucagon promote gluconeogenesis. Cortisol and EPI help to limit pyruvate utilization. The net effect of these actions is an apparent increase in glucose production. Reductions in the insulin/glucagon ratio correlate well with the alterations in hepatic glucose metabolism.

Sustained glucose production depends on presentation of amino acids, glycerol, and fatty acids to the liver (Figs. 1-36 and 1-37). The primary gluconeogenic precursors used by the liver and to a lesser extent by the kidney for gluconeogenesis are lactate, glycerol, and amino acids such as alanine and glutamine (Table 1-8).

Table 1-7
Glucose Available in Early and Late Starvation States in a 70-kg Man

Origin	*Early amount of glucose, g/24 h*	*Late amount of glucose, g/24 h*
New glucose (gluconeogenesis)		
Fat (glycerol)	16	18
Protein	43	12
Stores or recycled glucose		
Glycogen	85	0
Recycled glucose	36	50
Total	180	80

Table 1-8
Gluconeogenic Precursors

Gluconeogenesis	*Ketogenesis*	*Gluconeogenesis and Ketogenesis*
Alanine	Leucine*	Isoleucine*
Arginine*		Lysine*
Aspartic acid		Phenylalanine*
Asparagine		Tyrosine*
Cystine		Tryptophan*
Glutamic acid		
Glycine		
Histidine*		
Hydroxyproline		
Methionine*		
Proline		
Serine		
Threonine*		
Valine*		

*Essential amino acid.

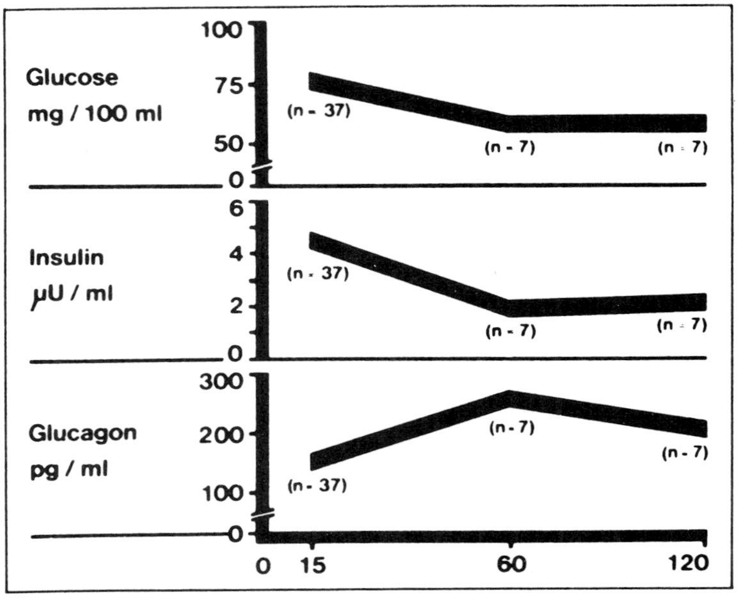

FIG. 1-35. The primary stimulus to the neuroendocrine response to fasting and starvation is hypoglycemia. Arterial concentrations of glucose, insulin, and glucagon after 15-, 60-, and 120-h of fasting are shown. (From: *Ahnefeld FW, Burri C, Dick W, Halmagyi M: Parenteral Nutrition. Heidelberg, Springer-Verlag, 1976, with permission.*)

Skeletal muscle releases lactate by breakdown of endogenous glycogen stores and by glycolysis of transported glucose. Lactate is also released by erythrocytes and white blood cells following aerobic glycolysis and release of newly formed lactate into the circulation. This lactate is reconverted to glucose in the liver by the Cori cycle (Fig. 1-38).

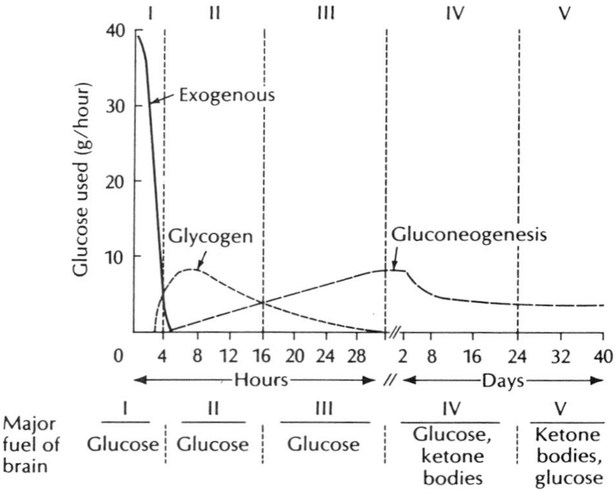

FIG. 1-36. The five phases of glucose homeostasis. This represents the origin of blood glucose in a 70-kg man who ingests 100 g of glucose and then fasts for 40 days. Phase I is the absorptive phase in which the 100 g of glucose enters the circulation by absorption from the gut. Phase II is the postabsorptive phase in which glucose is stored as glycogen in response to increased secretion of insulin and decreased secretion of glucagon. Phase III represents early starvation in which the fall in blood sugar leads to a decrease in insulin secretion and an increase in glucagon and catecholamine secretion. The latter results in an increase in gluconeogenesis and glycogenolysis. Phase IV is intermediary starvation in which hepatic glycogen stores have been depleted and the sole source of glucose is gluconeogenesis. Phase V represents prolonged starvation in which ketone bodies become the primary fuel, thereby resulting in a decrease in gluconeogenesis. (From: *Ruderman NB: Annu Rev Med 26:245, 1975, with permission.*)

The quantity of glucose made available from lactate from skeletal muscle is not sufficient to maintain glucose homeostasis. Consequently, approximately 75 g of protein are degraded daily during fasting and starvation to provide gluconeogenic amino acids to the liver (Table 1-9). Proteolysis, which results primarily from decreased insulin and increased cortisol, is associated with a rapid increase in the urinary nitrogen excretion from the normal 5 to 7 g/day to approximately 8 to 11 g during the first 2 to 4 days of fasting. Although the protein mobilized in starvation is derived primarily from skeletal muscle, the loss of protein from other organs is proportionately much greater (Fig. 1-39). In the liver, the synthesis of enzymes required for urea and serum protein synthesis are reduced. In the pancreas, the production of gastrointestinal hormones and enzymes is reduced and causes impaired exocrine function. In the gastrointestinal tract, digestive function is impaired by a reduction in the production of digestive enzymes and the regeneration of epithelial cells. For these reasons, starved patients often become paradoxically food-intolerant, as manifest by the development of diarrhea and malabsorption when small amounts of food or enteral feedings are given. The use of amino

Table 1-9
Fuel Composition of a Normal 70-kg Man

Fuel	*Weight, kg*	*Calories*
Tissues		
Fat (adipose triglyceride)	15	141,000
Protein (mainly muscle)	6	24,000
Glycogen (muscle)	0.150	600
Glycogen (liver)	0.075	300
Total		165,900
Circulating fuels		
Glucose (extracellular fluid)	0.020	80
Free fatty acids (plasma)	0.0003	3
Triglycerides (plasma)	0.003	30
Total		113

SOURCE: Adapted from Cahill GF, 1970.

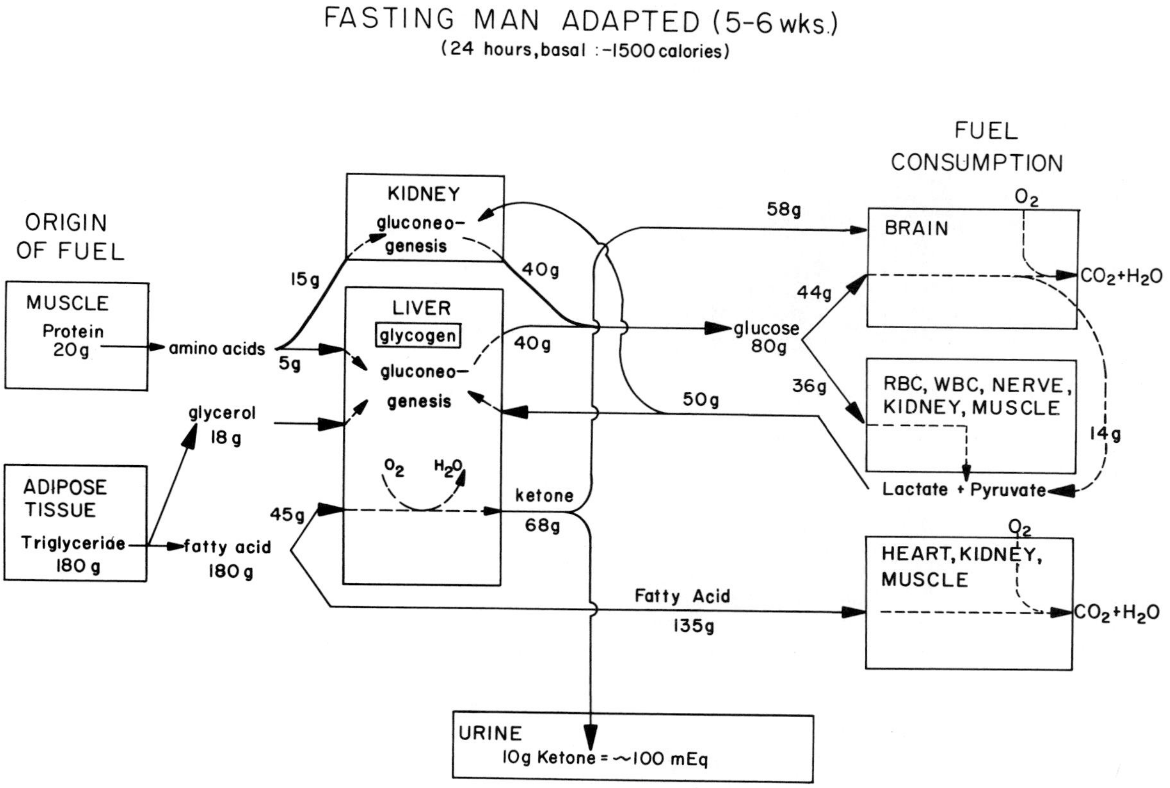

FIG. 1-37. Schema of fuel metabolism after 5 to 6 weeks of starvation. Liver glycogen sources are depleted, there is a diminished utilization of muscle protein, the brain is burning ketones, and gluconeogenesis from amino acids is taking place to a large extent in the kidney. (Adapted from: *Cahill GF: N Engl J Med 282:668, 1970, with permission.*)

FIG. 1-38. The Cori cycle (top) provides for the transfer of energy from the liver to the periphery. Glucose gives up energy to the periphery by anaerobic or aerobic glycolysis to lactate and pyruvate. The latter are then remade into glucose in the liver, utilizing energy derived from the metabolism of fatty acids. In the glucose to alanine cycle (bottom) described by Felig et al, glucose is metabolized to pyruvate in muscle; pyruvate is then converted to alanine, which is then transported to the liver, where it is remade into glucose.

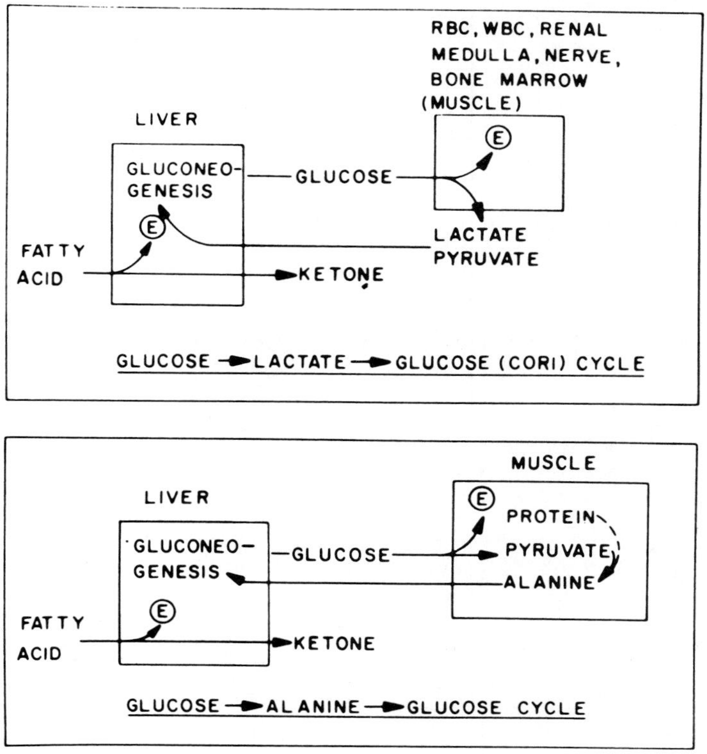

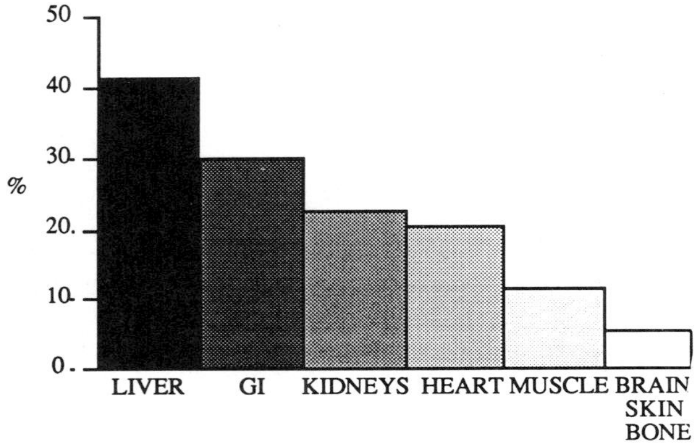

FIG. 1-39. The percentage of protein lost from various tissues during starvation. Although the greatest amount is derived from skeletal muscle, the tissue with the largest loss is the liver. (Modified from: *Addis T, Poo LJ, Lew W: J Biol Chem 115:111, 1936, with permission.*)

acids by the liver for gluconeogenesis creates a problem in handling the ammonia that is formed during the deamination of the amino acid, a necessary process before the carbon skeleton can be made available for gluconeogenesis. The renal excretion of ammonium ion becomes the primary route of elimination of alpha amino nitrogen during starvation because the normally active hepatic enzymes are diminished. Renal gluconeogenesis increases through metabolism of glutamine and glutamate which serve as the primary amino acids for amino group transport and gluconeogenesis in the kidney. The kidney may account for up to 45 percent of glucose production during late starvation.

The rapid proteolysis of body protein does not continue at the rate of 75 g/day for more than 5 to 6 days. Eventually, proteolysis diminishes to a nadir of 20 g/day which corresponds to the minimum urinary nitrogen excretion rate of approximately 2 to 4 g/day.

The reduction in proteolysis occurs as the CNS accommodates to ketones which substitute in part for glucose as an energy source. Although the brain can metabolize ketone bodies, transport systems at the blood-brain barrier limit ketone utilization and glucose is metabolized preferentially under normal conditions. During starvation, transport systems in the blood-brain barrier increase the rate of ketone body transport and metabolism of ketone bodies by the brain increases. Consequently, the amount of protein required for gluconeogenesis is significantly reduced (Fig. 1-37 and Table 1-7).

Energy requirements for gluconeogenesis and basal enzymatic and muscular function such as neural transmission and cardiac contraction can be met by the mobilization of approximately 160 g of triglycerides from adipose tissue in the form of free fatty acids and glycerol in a resting, fasting 70-kg subject (Fig. 1-40). Free fatty acid release is stimulated by a reduction in the serum insulin concentration and by an absolute or relative increase in the concentrations of glucagon, GH, EPI, and ACTH. The actions of these counterregulatory hormones require cortisol (permissive action) and other counterregulatory hormones. These endocrine alterations also stimulate ketogenesis. The free fatty acids and ketone bodies generated by the liver are used as a source of energy by nonglycolytic tissues such as the heart, kidney, muscle, and liver. As a consequence, the main source of energy in starvation is fat which provides up to 40 percent of the calories burned during starvation.

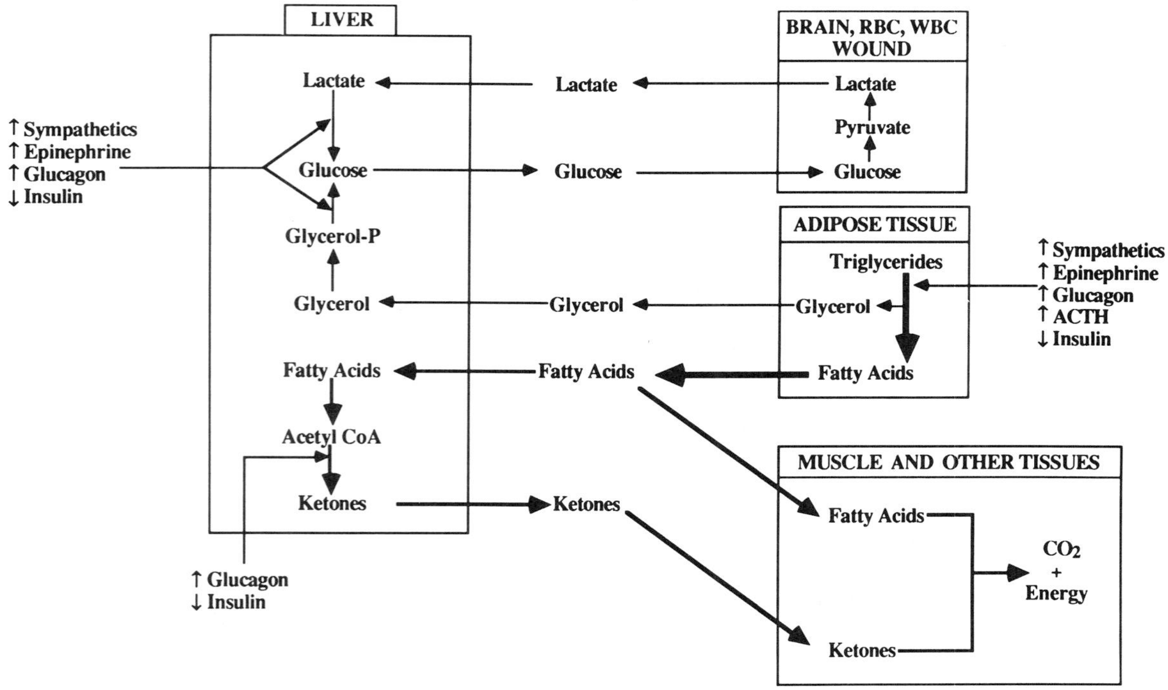

FIG. 1-40. Mobilization of fatty acids from adipose tissue during starvation provide fatty acids to various tissues that can be used for energy. In addition, fatty acids presented to the liver can be converted to ketone bodies for use throughout the body, and glycerol released during the degradation of triglycerides can be used by the liver to form new glucose. The primary hormones for lipolysis are catecholamines and for ketogenesis, glucagon.

Lipid metabolism during starvation decreases the overall amount of glucose that is required because fatty acid utilization occurs at a rate that is proportional to serum fatty acid concentration. Another important glucose sparing effect is that of ketone bodies which inhibit glucose uptake in most tissues by inhibition of pyruvate dehydrogenase. The utilization of fat as a main fuel source decreases the amount of mandatory glycolysis which therefore diminishes the requirements for gluconeogenesis and protein degradation.

Resting energy expenditure decreases by up to 31 percent during prolonged fasting. The classic studies by Benedict observed decreases in average energy expenditure from 1650 kcal/d in the first week to 1290 kcal/d in the third week of total starvation. This multifactorial reduction in resting energy expenditure is due in part to decreased sympathetic nervous system activity, metabolic activity of muscle and lean body cell mass, cardiac work, and body temperature.

The ability to utilize protein for gluconeogenesis and lipid for energy, the adaptation of the brain to utilize ketones, and the reduction of resting energy expenditure all work to permit survival during prolonged substrate shortages. Nonetheless, impairment and loss of important body functions does occur, and losses of 30 to 40 percent of the body weight are fatal.

Water and Electrolyte Metabolism. Major changes also occur in fluid and electrolyte metabolism during prolonged fasting. Initially, there is a loss of sodium, potassium, and water that accounts for the rapid and relatively large weight loss observed after fasting for short durations and the greater amount of weight lost early during the period of starvation as compared to later. The loss of sodium during this period is obligate and is related to the abrupt decrease in availability of carbohydrates, since small amounts of glucose will decrease the amount of sodium lost. Sodium loss gradually decreases from 150 to 250 meq/day to 1 to 15 meq/day as starvation persists. Alterations in sodium and water metabolism may also be the result of alterations in plasma membrane potential. Reductions in total body water and sodium are associated with reductions in the plasma volume. As a consequence, a starved patient tolerates hypovolemia poorly.

Metabolism After Injury

The altered metabolism that occurs following injury has been divided into two phases by Cuthbertson: the ebb and the flow phases (Fig. 1-1). The ebb phase, which occurs during the first several hours after injury, is characterized by normal or reduced energy expenditure, hyperglycemia, and the restoration of circulating volume and tissue perfusion. The flow phase, which occurs after tissue perfusion has been restored, is characterized by generalized hypermetabolism, negative nitrogen balance, hyperglycemia, and heat production. This phase may last from days to weeks, depending on the severity of the injury, previous health of the individual, and medical intervention. The early flow phase is catabolic, while the later flow phase has been termed by Moore as the anabolic phase. The catabolic phase continues even though volume deficits have been corrected, infection has been controlled, pain has been eliminated, and complete oxygenation has been restored. The late flow or anabolic phase is associated with a slow but progressive reaccumulation of protein followed by the reaccumulation of body fat. The duration of the anabolic phase is usually considerably longer than the catabolic portion of the flow phase since protein synthesis does not exceed 3 to 5 g/day.

Energy Balance. Injury of any type is associated with an increase in energy requirements. The energy expenditure of injured, septic, and burned individuals increases further and is associated with increases in oxygen consumption that vary directly with the severity of injury (Fig. 1-41) or burn surface area (Fig. 1-42). Fever alone increases metabolic rate by approximately 7 percent for each degree Fahrenheit of fever as noted by Dubois. Severe infections, however, such as peritonitis or intraabdominal abscesses are associated with an increase in resting energy expenditure of 20 to 75 percent, which is greater than that predicted by temperature elevation alone and is related to the inflammatory process itself. The most severe injury is a thermal burn, in which sustained increases in resting energy expenditure of greater than 100 percent have been noted. In large part, the increase in energy expenditure following injury results from the increased activity of the sympathetic nervous system and the increased circulating concentrations of catecholamines. The mechanism for this effect is not clear but may be related to catecholamine-induced increased cell membrane sodium permeability and the energy required for ion pump action to maintain normal transmembrane concentrations. The metabolic rate has been decreased by the administration of adrenergic blockers in severely burned patients. The action of IL-1 on the preoptic-anterior hypothalamic area causes fever and is blocked by circulating IL-1ra.

The increase in resting energy expenditure is also dependent on the patient size and environmental temperature. The largest increases in energy expenditure are observed in heavily muscled, well-nourished young men with large body cell mass, and the smallest increases are in elderly, poorly nourished women with small body cell mass. Normally, a linear relationship between body cell mass and resting energy expenditure is found.

The measurement of energy expenditure in critically ill patients can be performed by the reverse Fick equation or by the indirect calorimetry technique. The latter method, which measures simultaneous oxygen consumption and carbon dioxide production, can estimate the source of fuel by calculation of the respiratory quotient (ratio of carbon dioxide production to oxygen consumption). The respiratory quotient following injury and sepsis is usually 0.7 to 0.8, indicating primary utilization of fat.

Lipid Metabolism. Lipids are the primary source of energy following injury. Lipolysis is enhanced by the immediate elevations in ACTH, cortisol, catecholamines, glucagon, and GH; reduction in insulin; and increased sympathetic nervous system activity. Catecholamines are a chief stimulus to hormone-sensitive lipase. Both the sympathetic nervous system and circulating catecholamines are of paramount importance in the lipolytic response to stress. Recent investigations into the mechanism of catecholamine-induced posttraumatic lipolysis suggests that lipolysis may be increased by changes in adrenergic postreceptor (protein kinase hormone-sensitive lipase) response after elective operation. Other investigators have shown decreased basal and catecholamine-stimulated lipolysis during early intervals following severe trauma and emergency operation.

The net lipolysis observed during the ebb phase results in elevated plasma free fatty acids and glycerol despite increased metabolism of these substances. If the reduction in effective circulating volume is severe, as might be seen in severe hemorrhage or sepsis, an elevation in plasma free fatty acids may not occur. This may be due to altered delivery of hormones to peripheral adipose tissue or to alterations in catecholamine-mediated lipolysis. Increased re-esterification of fatty acids, such as that seen in the presence of

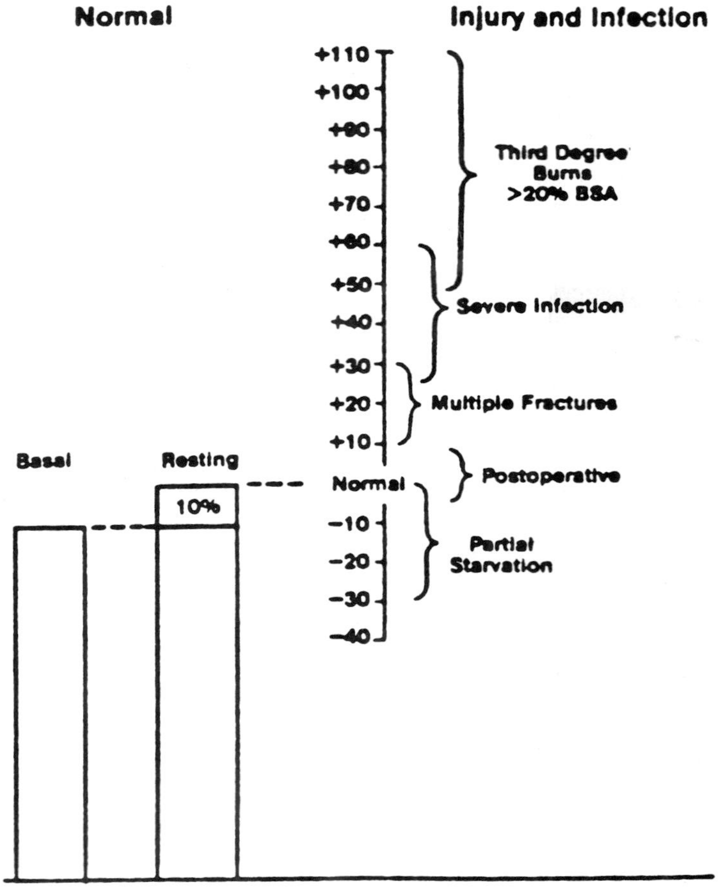

FIG. 1-41. Resting energy expenditure of adult patients during injury, stress, and starvation. The highest resting energy expenditures are seen following thermal injuries and severe infections. (From: *Kinney JM: The application of indirect calorimetry to clinical studies, in Assessment of Energy Metabolism in Health and Disease. Columbus, OH, Ross Laboratories, 1980, p 42, with permission.*)

high concentrations of lactate, may decrease net free fatty acid release. This explanation is supported by the observed rise in plasma glycerol noted after injury, which suggests that lipolysis is occurring, and by increased concentrations of lactate in studies in which there is no change in free fatty acid concentration. Acidosis, hyperglycemia and anesthetic agents also alter lipid mobilization after injury. For example, lipolysis is directly inhibited by pentobarbital anesthesia, and hemorrhage in the presence of pentobarbital usually results in a fall in the plasma free fatty acid and ketone body concentrations. Experimental hemorrhage using other anesthetic agents or in awake animals increases free fatty acid and ketone body concentrations.

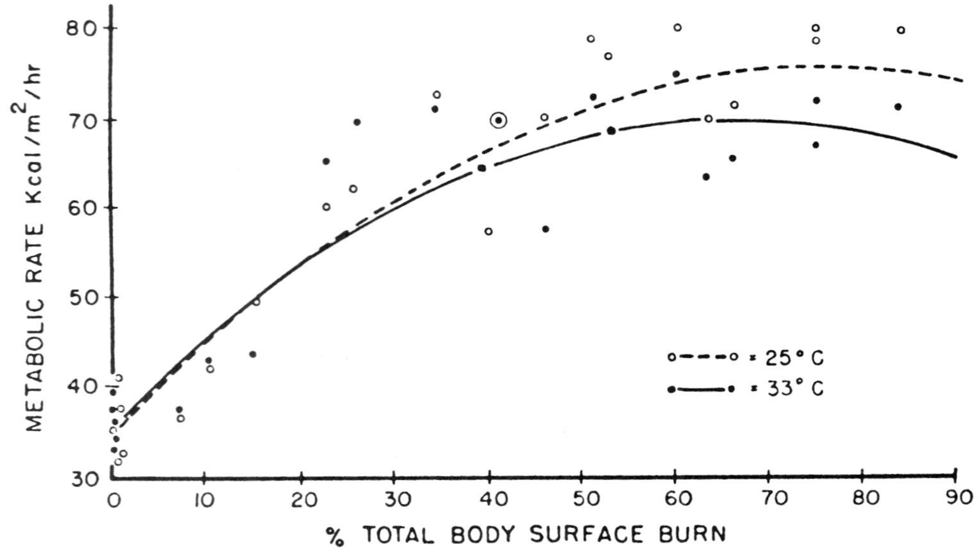

FIG. 1-42. Burned patients have a metabolic rate that correlates linearly with the size of the burn until massive thermal injuries are achieved, at which point the metabolic rate plateaus. This plateau suggests that patients with massive burns are at or near maximal rates of heat production. In addition, the increase in metabolic rate is secondary to endogenous heat production and not to a cold environment, since patients placed in a warm environment do not demonstrate a significant reduction in metabolic rate. (From: *Wilmore DW: Surg Clin North Am 56:999, 1976, with permission.*)

During the flow phase, net lipolysis continues despite increased insulin as reflected by increased concentrations and clearance of plasma free fatty acids. In the presence of oxygen, the released fatty acids can be oxidized by cardiac and skeletal muscle to produce energy. The plasma free fatty acid concentration is determined by the net balance of substrate appearance and clearance mechanisms. Therefore, even though an increase in the rate of appearance and oxidation of free fatty acids during sepsis and endotoxemia occurs, a rise in the plasma free fatty acid concentration is not always observed.

The precise role of fatty acids in inhibition of glycolysis following injury is controversial. Experimental evidence suggests that fatty acid–induced inhibition of glycolysis may be a major mechanism for reduced glycolysis during the flow phase after minor to moderate injury. This mechanism may not operate in severe injury, hemorrhage, or sepsis, conditions in which persistent glycolysis and net proteolysis are observed. Lipoprotein lipase, the endothelial cell membrane enzyme responsible for clearing plasma triglycerides, is suppressed in adipose tissue but not in muscle after trauma. In sepsis, however, this enzyme activity is suppressed in both muscle and adipose tissue. The roles of cytokines, such as TNF (which inhibit lipogenesis and decrease lipoprotein lipase activity), IL-1, and PGE_2, in fat metabolism are not fully understood.

Ketogenesis. The high concentrations of intracellular fatty acids and the elevated concentration of glucagon during the ebb and flow phases inhibit fatty acid synthesis. In hepatocytes, this also stimulates the transport of acylcoenzyme A (acyl-CoA) into the mitochondria for oxidation and ketogenesis. Ketogenesis is variable and correlates inversely with the severity of injury. In contrast to the situation in starvation, ketogenesis is decreased after major injury, severe shock, and sepsis and is suppressed by increases in insulin and other energy substrates, such as glucose, alanine, and lactate, and by increased uptake and oxidation of free fatty acids. After minor injury or mild infection, ketogenesis does increase but to a lesser extent than that seen during nonstressed starvation. Injuries that are associated with minor ketone body formation also appear to be associated with a small or absent increase in plasma free fatty acid concentrations. Interestingly, infusion of 3-hydroxybutyrate caused decreased release of alanine in patients after trauma. This suggests that the suppressive effect of ketone bodies on proteolysis during starvation may also be observed during posttraumatic protein metabolism when exogenous ketone body is supplied.

Carbohydrate Metabolism. Hyperglycemia was first reported following hemorrhage by Claude Bernard in 1853 and has subsequently been confirmed in different species following sepsis, trauma, and thermal injury. It occurs immediately after injury and persists into the flow phase.

The presence of hyperglycemia provides a ready source of energy to obligate tissues such as those of the CNS, the wound, and red blood cells, since these cells do not require insulin for glucose transport. As discussed in a subsequent section, the most homeostatically significant role of early hyperglycemia may be the resulting osmotically mediated transfer of fluids from cells to the interstitium which leads to blood volume restitution. Elevated concentrations of glucose may be necessary for leukocyte energy requirements within inflamed, wounded tissue with impaired vascular supply.

The following metabolic changes are substantially different from the situation observed in starvation. Increased hepatic gluconeogenesis and impaired peripheral glucose uptake result from increased secretion of catecholamines, cortisol, glucagon, GH, AVP, and angiotensin II and reduced secretion of insulin following injury. Hepatic glycogen is the primary source of glucose immediately after injury and appears to be mediated chiefly by catecholamines and cortisol. Glucose production during the flow phase results primarily from hepatic and renal gluconeogenesis mediated through glucagon and insulin using amino acids, lactate, pyruvate, and glycerol as substrates. IL-1 promotes release of both glucagon and insulin and alters carbohydrate metabolism through centrally mediated pathways. The systemic effects of mediators on carbohydrate metabolism during prolonged inflammation and/or sepsis are not fully understood, but their role in local wound metabolism is undoubtedly significant.

Insulin Resistance. Immediately after injury, the plasma insulin concentration is depressed in relation to the degree of hyperglycemia. This is due to a reduction in beta islet cell sensitivity to glucose which is mediated by catecholamines, cortisol, and the increased activity of the sympathetic nervous system. During the flow phase, insulin concentrations increase but hyperglycemia persists.

The persistent hyperglycemia is in part related to the delayed rate of assimilation of a glucose load, reflecting a resistance of normally insulin-sensitive tissues to insulin. This diabetes of injury, first noted by Drucker, may be important in mediating the shift of fluid from cells to the interstitium, discussed below. Accelerated gluconeogenesis has been demonstrated after injury utilizing radiotracer techniques. Glucose clearance, the ratio of glucose disposal to glucose concentration, is enhanced in injured patients and in those with sepsis. Studies using the insulin-clamp technique to assess whole-body insulin-dependent glucose disposal rates under steady-state conditions found significantly diminished maximal rates of glucose disposal and nearly twofold increases in insulin clearance rates in patients following injury. These observations suggest that a postreceptor, intracellular defect may be responsible for posttraumatic insulin resistance. Insulin-clamp studies of forearm glucose disposal and uptake in patients with multiple injuries suggest that skeletal muscle is a significant site of insulin resistance.

Possible mechanisms for inhibition of glucose oxidation include a reduction of skeletal muscle pyruvate dehydrogenase (PDH) activity in conditions of trauma and sepsis. This inhibition diminishes the rate at which pyruvate derived from glucose can be converted to acetyl-CoA and enter the tricarboxylic acid cycle (Fig. 1-43). This results in accumulation of pyruvate, alanine, and lactate which can be presented to the liver and promote gluconeogenesis. The decline in PDH activity may also contribute to the elevated lactate levels and acidosis which can occur in sepsis despite adequate tissue perfusion.

Increases in plasma glucose are proportional to the severity of injury and to some extent correlate with survival. The mortality rate of patients with sepsis and a normal glucose tolerance test was 10 percent but increased to 60 percent when abnormal glucose tolerance was observed.

Glucose Metabolism in Wounded Tissue. Glucose must be provided to the cells of wounded tissue. Glucose uptake and lactate production in wounded tissue are increased by up to 100 percent and are proportional to the circulating concentration of glucose present (Fig. 1-44). The increase in glucose uptake in

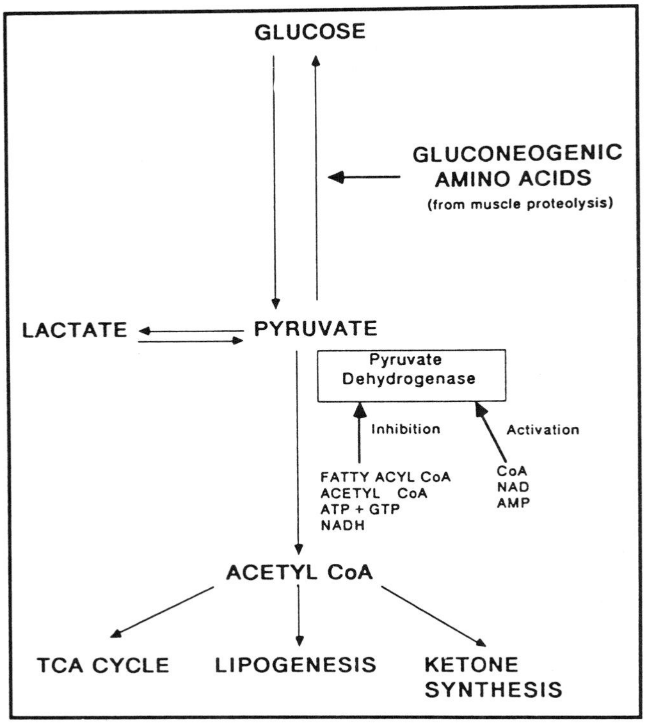

FIG. 1-43. Increased pyruvate dehydrogenase (PDH) activity results in the generation of acetyl-CoA for entry into the TCA cycle, lipogenesis, or ketone synthesis. Inhibition of PDH leads to the accumulation of lactate, pyruvate, and gluconeogenic amino acids, favoring gluconeogenesis. Septic inhibition of PDH leads to enhanced hepatic gluconeogenesis and depressed oxidation of substrates by peripheral tissues. Abbreviation: GTP, guanosine triphosphate. (From: *Kispert PH: Metabolic response to stress, in Simmons RL, Steed DL (eds): Basic Science Review for Surgeons. Philadelphia, WB Saunders, chap 7, p 121, 1992, with permission.*)

wounded tissue is associated with an increase in the activity of phosphofructokinase, a major rate-limiting enzyme in glycolysis. Despite the increase in glucose uptake and phosphofructokinase activity, wounded and burned tissues demonstrate decreased insulin sensitivity and fail to normally increase glucose uptake or glycogenesis in response to insulin (Fig. 1-45).

The accelerated glucose uptake in wounded and burned tissue correlates with the inflammatory cellular infiltrate and has accounted for as much as 70 percent of glucose uptake in experimental models. The inflammatory cells require glucose as an energy substrate. The white blood cells may also mediate an increase in glucose uptake by uninjured tissue through the release of mediators such as IL-1, TNF, and IFN.

Protein Metabolism. The intake of protein for a healthy young adult is approximately 80 to 120 g, or 13 to 20 g of nitrogen per day. Daily fecal and urinary excretion of nitrogen is 2 to 3 g and 13 to 20 g, respectively. Following injury, daily nitrogen excretion in the urine increases to 30 to 50 g as urea nitrogen and represents net proteolysis. Despite this significant draft on protein stores, only 20 percent is used for calories. The remainder is used by the liver and kidneys to produce glucose. These changes are mediated by increased secretion of cortisol, glucagon, and catecholamines and by decreased secretion and effect of insulin.

The increased excretion of urea following injury is also associated with the urinary loss of sulfur, phosphorus, potassium, magnesium, and creatinine, which indicates breakdown of intracellular compounds. Isotope dilution studies suggest that decreases in cell mass, not cell number, are responsible for these metabolites. The nitrogen/sulfur and nitrogen/potassium ratios suggest that skeletal muscle is the chief source of proteolysis. Radiolabeled amino acid incorporation studies and protein analyses confirm that skeletal muscle is depleted while visceral tissues, such as liver and kidney, are spared. The opposite situation is true during periods of nonstressed fasting.

In the setting of stable protein turnover rates, net protein loss takes place when increased breakdown, decreased synthesis, or a combination of these processes occurs. Available data on total body protein turnover suggest that after injury, the net changes in catabolism and synthesis depend on the severity of the injury. Elective operations and minor injury result in decreased protein synthesis and normal rates of protein breakdown. Severe trauma, burns, and sepsis are associated with increased protein turnover and greatly increased protein catabolism. Accelerated proteolysis and gluconeogenesis persist after major injury and during sepsis. The rise in urinary nitrogen and negative nitrogen balance begins shortly after injury, reaches a peak about the first week, and may continue for 3 to 7 weeks. The magnitude of nitrogen loss is also related to the age, sex, and physical condition of the patient. Young healthy males lose more protein in response to an injury than do women or the elderly, presumably because of smaller body cell mass in the latter two patient subsets.

Substrate cycling occurs between skeletal muscle, liver, and the wound (Fig. 1-46). Souba and colleagues have established the importance of the gut in substrate cycling with the liver (Fig. 1-47) and provide evidence for altered interactions after trauma and sepsis.

Amino Acid Metabolism. The amino acid composition of normal human beings differs according to tissue origin. Following trauma, the major source of amino acids is skeletal muscle which has different proportions of specific amino acids as protein and intracellular compounds compared to that of normal plasma (Fig. 1-48). The dynamics of specific amino acids following trauma are best understood for alanine and glutamine, the major carriers of nitrogen from skeletal muscle to visceral tissues. Immediately after injury there is little or no change in the total amino acid concentration, but increases are noted in alanine, cystine, taurine, and the aromatic amino acids. Although plasma amino acid concentrations in wounded animals are similar to those that occur in nonwounded pair-fed animals, the intracellular skeletal muscle concentrations of specific amino acids differ markedly between groups.

Increases in alanine as measured from extremity blood samples in traumatized individuals appear to be related to the overall extent of injury and whole body oxygen consumption rather than to the size of limb injury or local blood flow. Three- to fourfold increases in the splanchnic uptake of alanine, a major nitrogen transport compound from skeletal muscle to liver, has been demonstrated following injury (Fig. 1-47). Specific alterations in plasma amino acids are also time-related. Alanine concentrations, for example, increase early in the flow phase and later decrease.

The intracellular muscle concentrations and the muscle/plasma ratios of glutamine are reduced markedly in most studies of sepsis, wounding, and thermal injury. In general, the release of glutamine

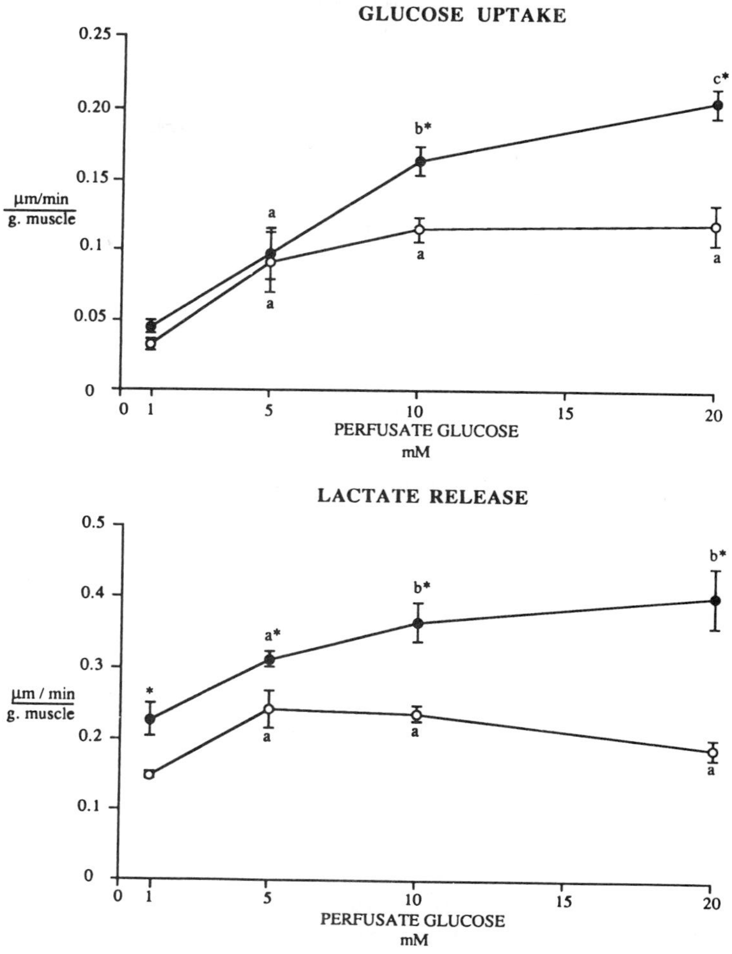

FIG. 1-44. Glucose uptake and lactate production by wounded (●) and nonwounded (○) hindlimbs of rats in response to increasing external glucose supply. Glucose uptake and lactate production by wounded hindlimbs increased as the concentration of external glucose increased. In contrast, glucose uptake and lactate production by nonwounded hindlimbs reached a plateau at an external glucose concentration of 5 mmol. $^*p < 0.05$ wounded vs. nonwounded; a. = $p < 0.05$ intragroup difference vs. 1 mmol; b. $= p < 0.05$ intragroup difference vs. 5 mmol; c. = $p < 0.05$ intragroup difference vs. 10 mmol. (From: *Amaral JF, Caldwell MD et al: Surgery 100:252, 1986, with permission.*)

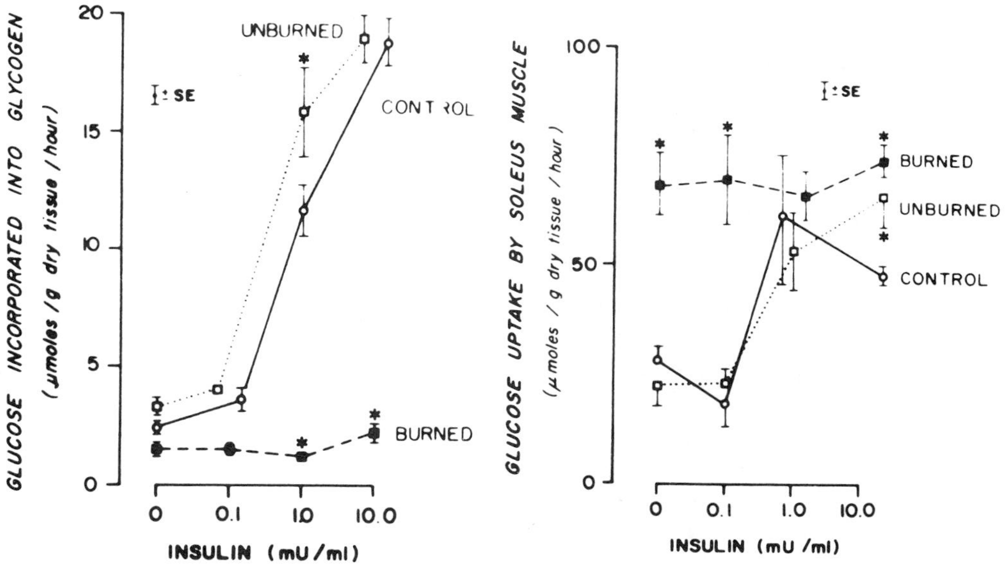

FIG. 1-45. Glucose uptake and glycogen synthesis by the soleus muscles from the burned and unburned limbs of rats 3 days after scald injury. Soleus muscles from the injured limb did not respond to insulin, whereas muscles from the uninjured limb responded to insulin in a dose-dependent fashion with an increase in glucose uptake and glycogen synthesis. (From: *Nelson KM, Turinsky J: J Surg Res 31:292, 1981, with permission.*)

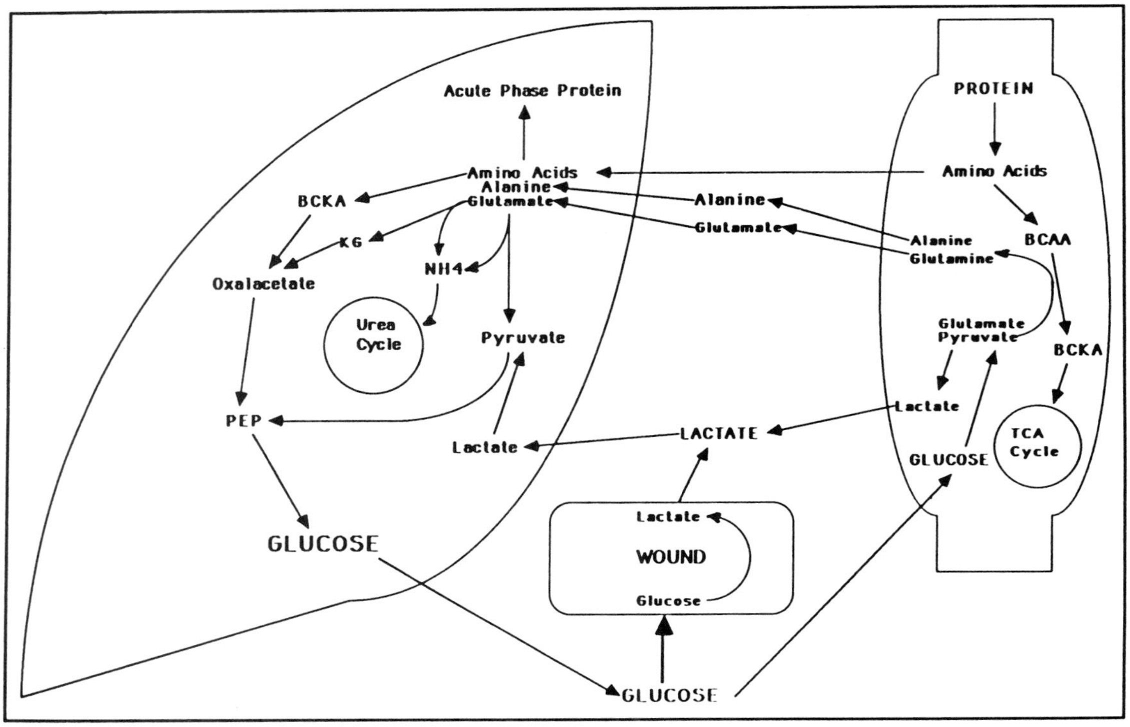

FIG. 1-46. Substrate cycling between the wound, liver, and skeletal muscle. Carbon skeletons from the muscle are used for hepatic gluconeogenesis. Abbreviations: BCAA, branched-chain amino acids; BCKA, branched-chain ketoacids; KG, α-ketoglutarate; NH_4, ammonium; PEP, phosphoenolpyruvate. (From: *Kispert PH: Metabolic response to stress, in Simmons RL, Steed DL (eds): Basic Science Review for Surgeons. Philadelphia, WB Saunders, 1992, chap 7, p 121, with permission.*)

is greater than can be predicted from its relative abundance in muscle tissue protein, indicating its synthesis in this tissue. Glutamine release from wounded and nonwounded muscle is not different, and if the release of glutamine is expressed as ratio to the phenylalanine released, there is a lower release rate in wounded tissue as compared to nonwounded tissue. Since phenylalanine is neither catabolized nor synthesized in muscle, a lower glutamine/phenylalanine ratio suggests that either the synthesis of glutamine in wounded tissue is reduced or the local catabolism in wounded muscle is increased.

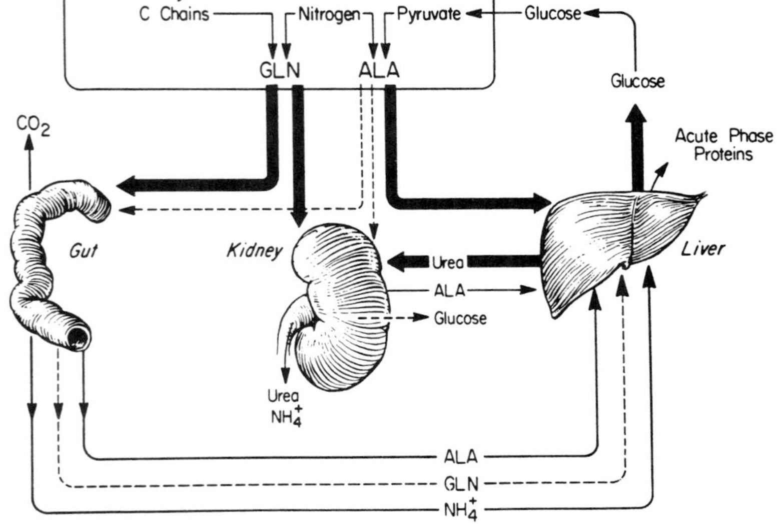

FIG. 1-47. In catabolic states, the net increase in skeletal muscle proteolysis results in efflux of primarily alanine and glutamine. The consumption of these amino acids by visceral organs results in the generation of urea and ammonia and loss of nitrogen. (From: *Souba WW, Smith RJ, Wilmore DW: JPEN 9:612, 1985, with permission.*)

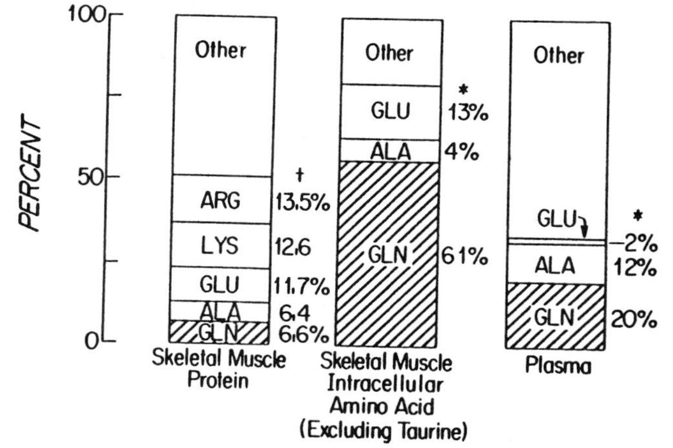

FIG. 1-48. Amino acid composition of a normal human being. Abbreviations: ARG, arginine; LYS, lysine; GLU, glutamate; ALA, alanine; GLN, glutamine. (From: *Souba WW: Adv Trauma 2:269, 1987, with permission.*)

Glutamine is a major energy source for lymphocytes, fibroblasts, and the gastrointestinal tract following injury. In the liver, periportal and perivenous hepatocytes metabolize glutamine differently (Fig. 1-49). In the small intestinal epithelial cell, glutamine is metabolized to carbon dioxide, alanine, citrulline, proline, and ammonia (Fig. 1-50).

Souba and colleagues have shown that glutamine is preferentially used as an energy source by the gut during catabolic states (Fig. 1-51). Failure to supply increased glutamine substrate requirements during these conditions has been implicated in the pathogenesis of bacterial translocation and the multiple organ failure syndrome. Glutamine may act as a conditional essential amino acid during periods of catabolism, since depletion of this substrate has pronounced negative effects on enterocytes and mucosal integrity and since administration of glutamine reverses these effects.

The role of other organs in amino acid homeostasis, in addition to the liver, muscle, and gastrointestinal tract, is under active investigation. The lung may be important in maintaining amino acid homeostasis in normal and septic states. Glutamine metabolism by pulmonary artery endothelial cells can be modulated by IL-1 and TNF.

The importance of circulating white blood cell and Kuppfer cell interactions with hepatocytes in protein metabolism is well known. IL-1, TNF, and to some extent IFN are known to stimulate proteolysis, some requiring cortisol and mediated in part through eicosanoids. IL-6 and IL-1 also stimulate production of hepatic acute-phase proteins and inhibit albumin synthesis by hepatocytes. Endothelial NO also inhibits hepatocyte albumin synthesis, thus increasing availability of amino acids for synthesis of acute-phase proteins.

Negative nitrogen balance can be reduced or eliminated by high-caloric nitrogen supplementation as with enteral or parenteral nutrition, with varying proportions and compositions of substrates. The loss of protein that occurs after injury is not entirely obligatory to the injury and is in part a manifestation of acute starvation and the increased need for gluconeogenetic precursors during periods of stress. Route of administration may also be important, as preliminary studies indicate that enteral glutamine has superior benefit compared to parenterally administered forms of glutamine. Other specific substrates such as arginine, ribonucleic acid, and polyunsaturated fatty acids may also hold future promise. Manipulation of the neurohumoral and the immunologic milieu after trauma through the use of growth factor infusions or monoclonal antibodies to cytokine mediators, for example, extend a limitless horizon to future therapy.

Wound Healing. It is particularly astounding that most wounds heal despite the presence of negative nitrogen balance, negative energy balance, and reduced tissue and plasma concentrations of zinc, thiamine, riboflavin, vitamin C, and vitamin A. Moore has termed this ability of wound healing to proceed in the presence and absence of abundant substrate supply the biologic priority of wound healing. Levenson has noted that "whereas the healing of a wound after injury appears satisfactory, it may be neither normal nor optimal." For example, there is a distinct delay in the healing of incisional wounds on burned animals when compared with incisional wounds on normal animals, and skin incisions on rodents with a fractured femur do not heal as well as skin incisions on rodents without a fractured femur. The biologic priority of wound healing does not mean that wound healing is normal in the severely injured patient.

The biologic priority of wound healing also does not mean that wound healing cannot be improved in severely injured patients. For example, large open wounds, such as burns, are associated with an inhibition of nitrogen anabolism of the host and may result in protein malnutrition and death if the substrate demands of the wounds are not met exogenously. Although it is not clear if the administration of protein improves wound healing per se, it has been shown to reduce negative nitrogen balance. Some investiga-

FIG. 1-49. Hepatocyte heterogeneity in the liver. Periportal hepatocytes contain glutaminase and urea cycle enzymes; the perivenous cells express glutamine synthetase. In the periportal cells, glutaminase is activated by ammonia and can therefore control flux through the urea cycle. Glutamine synthetase acts as a downstream scavenger by converting ammonia to glutamine and preventing ammonia intoxication. (From: *Souba WW: Annu Rev Nutr 11:285, 1991, with permission.*)

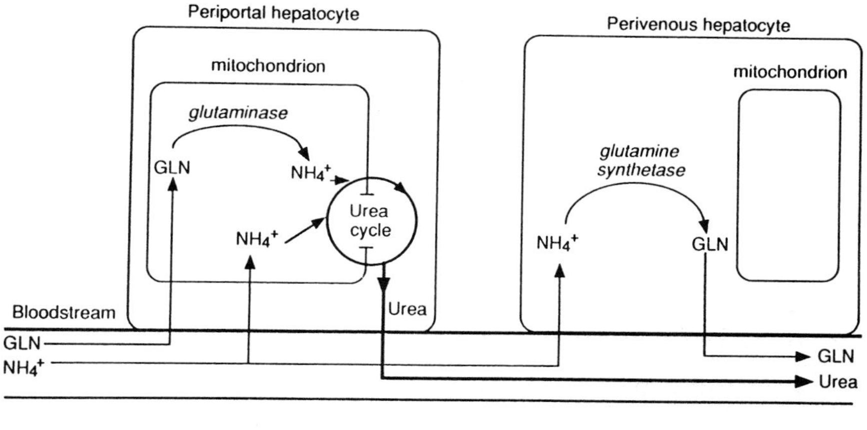

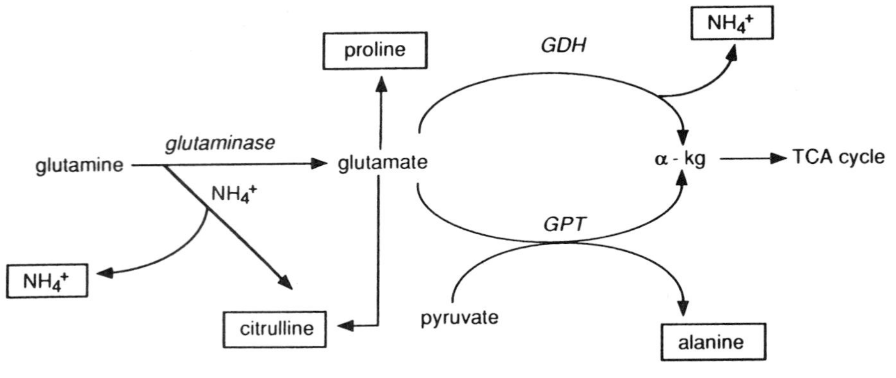

FIG. 1-50. Pathways of glutamine metabolism in the small intestinal epithelial cell. Glutamine is metabolized similarly whether it enters the enterocyte from the lumen or from the bloodstream. Two-thirds of the glutamine carbons are oxidized to carbon dioxide in the TCA cycle, while the glutamine nitrogens are released into the portal blood as ammonia, citrulline, alanine, and proline. The ammonia and alanine are extracted in large part by the liver. Citrulline is used by the kidneys for arginine biosynthesis. (From: *Souba WW: Annu Rev Nutr 11:285, 1991, with permission.*)

tors have also noted an improvement in wound healing with protein supplementation, but others have been unable to document any change.

Summary. Generalized catabolism, hyperglycemia, persistent gluconeogenesis, protein wasting, negative nitrogen balance, heat production, and loss of body mass are characteristic of all significant injuries. The degree of these metabolic alterations is directly related to the severity of injury, with the largest and most sustained changes being noted after sepsis and burns. Most of the energy required during the posttraumatic period is obtained from the oxidation of lipids; the net catabolism of 300 to 500 g of lean body cell mass per day is required as a source of amino acids for gluconeogenesis (Fig. 1-52). The persistence of the injury, particularly sepsis, through mechanisms that are unknown, but probably involve the cytokines, produces inhibition of the usual adaptive mechanisms that occur in starvation to reduce the amount of glucose needed per day. As a result, a highly catabolic state persists that in turn leads to protein wasting and malnutrition and ultimately to multiple-organ failure and death if the stimuli are not eliminated.

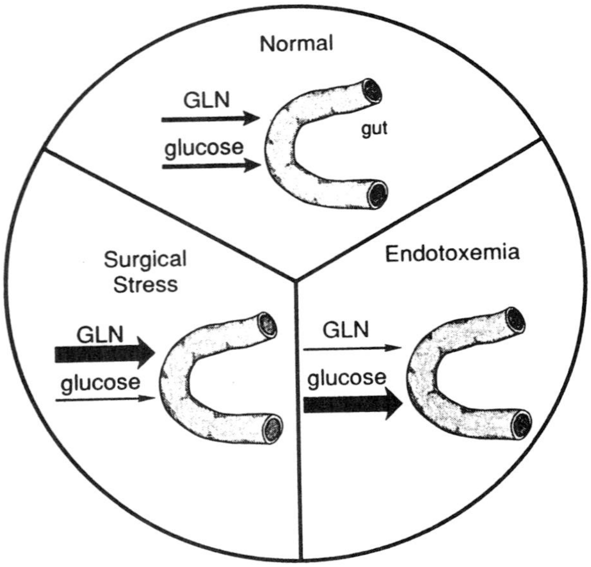

FIG. 1-51. Relative rates of consumption of glutamine and glucose by the gut in normal conditions, following operative stress, and during endotoxemia. (From: *Souba WW: Annu Rev Nutr 11:285, 1991, with permission.*)

ELECTROLYTE METABOLISM FOLLOWING INJURY

Almost all acute injuries are associated with changes in fluid and electrolyte metabolism, acid-base status, and renal function. In part, these alterations arise because patients do not usually have free access to water and electrolytes and frequently do not perceive thirst as a result of sedation, anesthesia, or head injury. A reduction in the effective circulating volume is characteristic of all injuries as a result of blood loss as in hemorrhage, of loss of vascular tone as in sepsis, of pump failure as in cardiac tamponade, of excessive unreplaced extrarenal losses as in diarrhea, of vomiting, of the drainage of fistulae, or of the sequestration of fluids.

The sequestration of fluids or third space is the result of an alteration in capillary permeability consequent to injury, ischemia, or inflammation. Since the fluid present in the third space has the same composition as the extracellular fluid (150 meq of sodium, 112 meq of chloride, 4.6 meq of potassium), one might think of this as an obligatory expansion of the total extracellular space. Although it is true that the total extracellular fluid space is expanded, the functional extracellular volume (that which can contribute to the maintenance of the effective circulating volume) is actually reduced because the fluid present in the third space is itself derived from the functional extracellular volume. Therefore, a liter of fluid trapped in the third space cannot be used, for example, during hemorrhage to replace the effective circulating volume lost. For this reason, the use of diuretics to mobilize fluid in an edematous postoperative patient who is not in congestive heart failure is pointless and potentially harmful, since it will result in a further reduction in the functional or exchangeable extracellular space and effective circulating volume but not in the volume of the third space. *Exchangeable* is not synonymous with *equilibrium* since the constituents of the third space are in dynamic equilibrium with those of the functional extracellular fluid volume. For example, fluid and electrolytes in a pleural effusion are in a constant state of recycling with the plasma, and antibiotics administered to a patient will enter the pleural effusion. The volume of the third space cannot be used to replace the volume of the functional extracellular space.

Blalock was the first to demonstrate that traumatic injury to an extremity resulted in the mobilization of fluid and electrolytes to an area of injury, thereby reducing the functional extracellular fluid volume. Even though the formation of the third space after nonthermal traumatic injury occurs immediately and is maximal by 5 to 6 h, the resolution of the third space is slower and may take longer than 10 days. Since the volume of the third space is directly proportional to the severity of injury, minor operative procedures, such as an appendectomy, are associated with considerably less

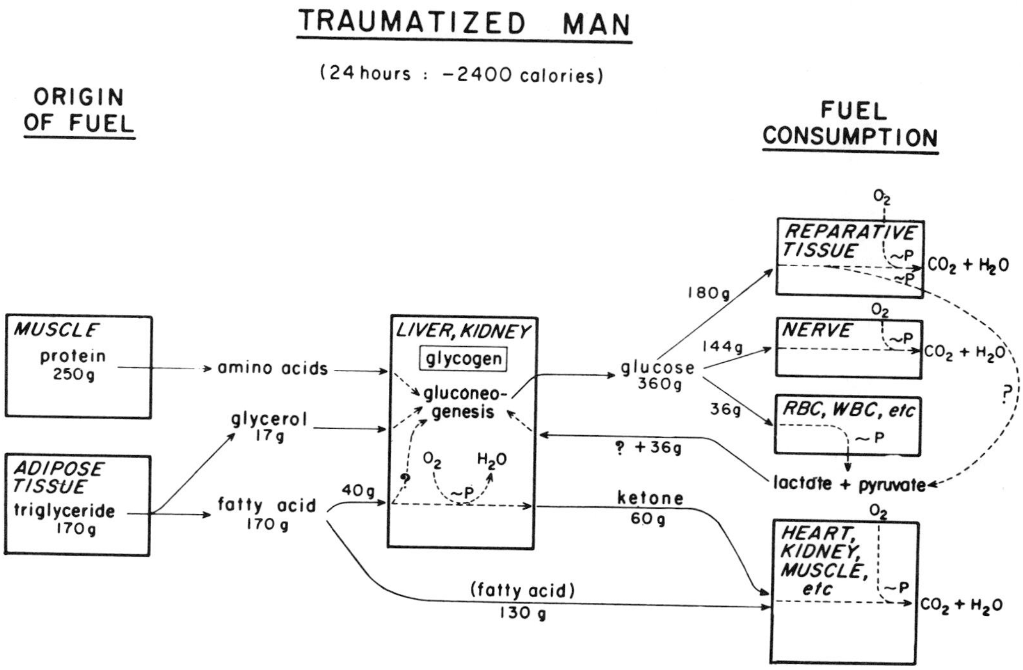

FIG. 1-52. Hypothetical scheme of rates of substrate flow in a traumatized individual excreting 40 g of nitrogen per day. Fat still provides the bulk of the calories. (From: *Cahill GF et al, in Fox CL Jr, Nahas GG (eds): Body Fluid Replacement in the Surgical Patient, New York, Grune and Stratton, 1970, p 286, with permission.*)

fluid sequestration than are major operative procedures such as an extensive retroperitoneal dissection. Similarly, minor traumatic injuries, such as an isolated simple limb fracture, are associated with less fluid sequestration than are those seen following major injuries, such as burns. If there is no intake of fluid into the functional extracellular space by either the oral or the intravenous route, the effective circulating volume will decline to a point at which hypotension ensues.

Hypovolemic shock is also associated with a reduction in the functional extracellular fluid volume in excess of the amount lost from the body by hemorrhage or by dehydration. Shires and colleagues have demonstrated that even though the return of shed blood alone after hemorrhage results in the return of the red blood cell mass and blood volume to normal, a deficit in the functional extracellular fluid volume persists. This deficit can be eliminated by the return of crystalloid solutions as well as shed blood. For this reason, patients who have sustained a major blood loss should receive blood or packed cells and crystalloid during their resuscitation. The site of this third-space formation appears to be the intracellular space as evidenced by a contraction of the intercellular space and an increase in the intracellular volume following hemorrhages of greater than 30 percent of the total blood volume and is thought to be the reason for the irreversible shock encountered in some patients. The mechanism for its formation remains unknown, but a protein that appears in the plasma of rats and dogs, and that can cause cell depolarization and increased intracellular water, has been found recently.

Major burns produce an alteration in the capillary permeability of the burned tissue that results in an exudation of plasma and an evaporative loss of water. There is also an increase in fluid flux across capillaries in nonburned tissue that appears to result from hypoproteinemia rather than from an alteration in capillary permeability. The formation of edema occurs primarily in the first 24 h with the greatest losses being incurred during the first 8 h. It is for this reason that thermally injured patients should receive 50 percent of their estimated fluid losses in the first 8 h. Colloid should be given on the second day to minimize edema formation in the nonburned tissue.

Sepsis produces a generalized capillary leak that again produces an increase in the total extracellular fluid volume but a decrease in the functional or exchangeable extracellular fluid volume. As sepsis persists, protein malnutrition produces hypoproteinemia, which in turn may increase the formation of edema. Therefore, the administration of colloid solutions during early sepsis when a capillary leak is present in the absence of hypoproteinemia may be unadvisable, since it may serve to further increase tissue edema. Once hypoproteinemia ensues, colloid administration may theoretically be helpful.

Any traumatic injury produces rapid changes in the functional extracellular fluid volume, effective circulating volume, extracellular osmolality, and electrolyte composition that result in the stimulation of the neuroendocrine system. In turn, the neuroendocrine response induces alterations in renal and circulatory function aimed at improving salt and water balance. Ultimately, the degree of impairment in fluid and electrolyte balance incurred following injury depends in part on the amount of functional extracellular volume lost, the ability of the neuroendocrine, renal, and circulatory systems to respond, the severity of the injury, the quality and quantity of fluid given, the age of the patient, preexisting illness, concurrent medications, and the anesthetic agents used.

Despite the potentially large number of variables noted, the overall response to the loss of effective circulating volume and electrolytes may be simplified as a coordinated physiologic effort to prevent further unnecessary losses of circulating volume and to replace the volume lost. The former involves the renal conservation of salt and water to minimize excretion and the latter involves the restoration of blood volume.

Renal Conservation of Salt and Water

The regulation of fluid and electrolytes by the kidney involves the formation of a large glomerular ultrafiltrate from which variable amounts of these substances are reabsorbed or into which they are secreted. The formation of tubular fluid at the glomerulus is dependent on the forces described in Starling's hypothesis of capillary equilibrium (Fig. 1-53). Thus, the quantity of filtrate formed is dependent on the renal perfusion pressure at the glomerulus. Under normal circumstances approximately 25 percent of the cardiac output is directed to the kidneys, resulting in the filtration of approximately 180 L of plasma water per day from the 1584 L of blood that pass through the kidneys. Although a reduction in the effective circulating volume and therefore in renal perfusion pressure should result in a reduction in the amount of glomerular ultrafiltrate that is formed, glomerular filtration remains unchanged despite a reduction in the renal perfusion pressure to 80 mmHg (Fig. 1-54). This occurs through the maintenance of renal blood flow, a process referred to as intrinsic autoregulation. The latter is thought to involve tubuloglomerular feedback in which individual nephrons sense their tubular fluid flow and alter the rate of glomerular filtration by changing the glomerular capillary pressure, primarily at the efferent arteriole. Decreases in tubular fluid flow lead

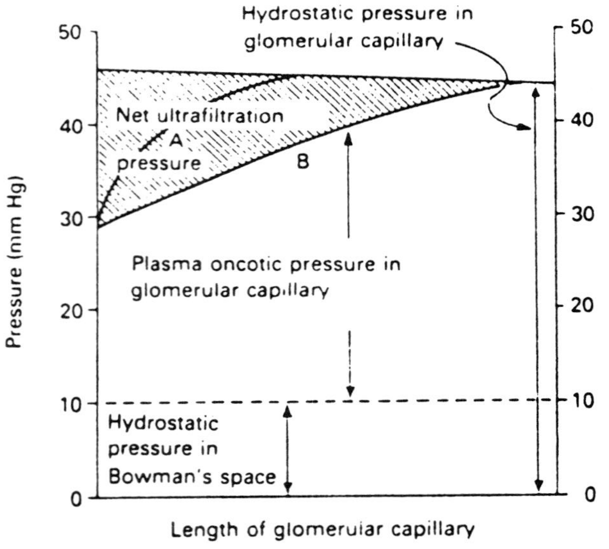

Balance of Mean Values

Hydrostatic pressure in glomerular capillary	45 mm Hg
Hydrostatic pressure in Bowman's space	10
Plasma oncotic pressure in glomerular capillary	27
Oncotic pressure of fluid in Bowman's space	0*
Net ultrafiltration pressure	8 mm Hg

FIG. 1-53. The Starling forces involved in the formation of the glomerular ultrafilitrate. Glomerular filtration pressure declines in the glomerular capillaries primarily as a result of a decrease in plasma oncotic pressure. In contrast, a decrease in the filtration pressure of extrarenal capillaries results primarily from a decrease in hydrostatic pressure. (From: *Valtin H: Renal Function: Mechanisms Preserving Fluid and Solute Balance in Health. Boston, Little, Brown, 1983, with permission.*)

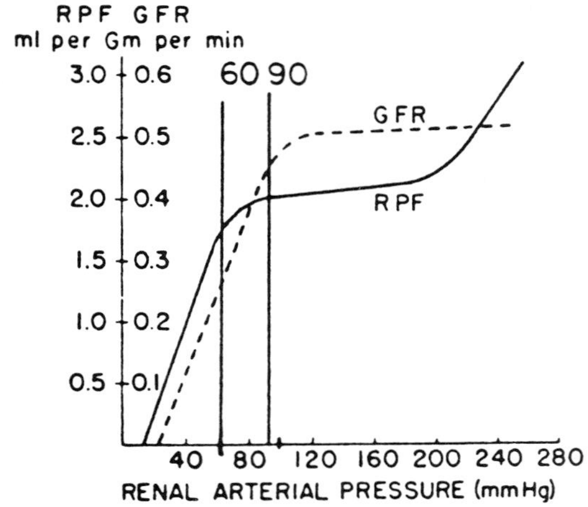

FIG. 1-54. Despite a reduction in renal arterial pressure to 90 mmHg, renal blood flow and glomerular filtration rate are maintained through intrinsic autoregulation. (From: *Powers RS: In Sabiston DC (ed): Davis-Christopher Textbook of Surgery, 12th ed. Philadelphia, Saunders, 1981, with permission.*)

to an increase in the efferent arteriolar resistance that, in turn, results in an increase in the fraction of peritubular blood that is filtered at the glomerulus. Thus, the rate of glomerular filtration is maintained.

An increase in the amount of blood filtered at the glomerulus relative to the amount that passes through it produces an increase in the oncotic pressure of the peritubular capillary blood perfusing the proximal tubule (Fig. 1-55). This results from the impermeability of the glomerular basement membranes to protein such that the glomerular filtrate is an ultrafiltrate of plasma. The increase in peritubular oncotic pressure, in turn, produces an increase in the net transfer of water, sodium, chloride, and bicarbonate from the proximal tubular filtrate to the peritubular blood. Sympathetic nervous system activity may directly increase the proximal tubular transport of sodium and suppress the release of cerebral natriuretic hormone and atrial natriuretic peptides.

The net result of these alterations is to decrease the delivery of sodium, chloride, and filtered fluid to the loop of Henle. Since the maintenance of the normal medullary osmotic gradient requires the adequate delivery of sodium and particularly of chloride to the long loops of Henle, a fall in medullary hyperosmolality frequently follows injury. A fall in medullary hyperosmolality may produce a defect in the ability of the kidneys to concentrate urine since the medullary gradient is essential to the renal countercurrent mechanism and the proper functioning of vasopressin. As a result, a larger amount of urine is necessary to eliminate the same amount of solute. This paradoxical increase in free-water clearance secondary to a defect in the inner medullary interstitial solute has been termed polyuric prerenal failure and has been implicated in the genesis of nonoliguric renal failure.

Concomitant with the increase in filtration fraction, there is a redistribution of blood flow from glomeruli of the superficial cortical nephrons to those in the juxtamedullary region that further increases sodium reabsorption. The ability of the juxtamedullary nephrons to further increase sodium reabsorption is related to the much longer loops of Henle they possess when compared with those in the superficial cortical area. The ability of the loops of Henle to reabsorb sodium is dependent on the presence of chlo-

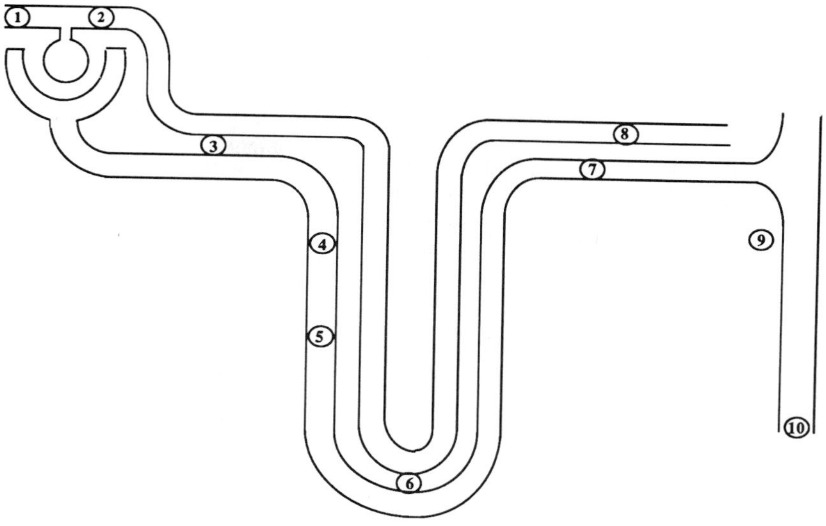

FIG. 1-55. Alterations in nephron function during injury. 1. Decreased renal perfusion pressure. 2. Increased efferent arteriolar resistance leading to a maintenance of GFR (autoregulation). 3. Increased peritubular capillary oncotic pressure from an increase in filtration of blood leads to increased proximal tubular reabsorption. 4. Shift from cortical nephrons to juxtamedullary nephrons. 5. Increased proximal reabsorption leads to decreased delivery of chloride to loop of Henle. 6. Diminished medullary gradient secondary to impaired sodium reabsorption. 7. Increased presentation of sodium to the distal tubules. 8. Increased exchange of sodium for hydrogen and potassium that is enhanced by aldosterone. 9. Increased free water reabsorption mediated by vasopressin that may be impaired by a fall in medullary osmotic gradient. 10. Kaliuresis, acid urine, and possibly loss of free water if action of vasopressin is impaired.

ride, since the reabsorption of sodium in the loops of Henle passively follows the active reabsorption of chloride. The increase in the filtration fraction consequent to a reduction in the renal perfusion pressure produces an increased movement of sodium and chloride to the peritubular fluid. As a result, the amount of chloride in the loop of Henle is low following injury and a large amount of sodium is delivered to the distal tubules. The increase in the distal delivery of sodium produces potassium wasting and metabolic alkalosis as sodium is reabsorbed and potassium and hydrogen ions secreted, a process that is augmented by the increased secretion of aldosterone that accompanies hypovolemia and injury. Conversely, if sodium delivery to the distal tubules is inadequate as a result of a marked decrease in glomerular filtration, potassium will not be excreted, even in the presence of aldosterone, and hyperkalemia and metabolic acidosis may ensue.

Sodium retention is a hallmark of injury that results in part from the increased secretion of aldosterone and other steroids. The amount of sodium retained depends more on the amount of sodium given than on the magnitude of injury. Sodium retention after injury cannot be explained solely on the basis of increased aldosterone and cortisol secretion since positive sodium balance persists well after the return of these hormones to normal concentrations (Fig. 1-56). Other factors that are known to contribute to positive sodium balance include an increase in the glomerular filtration fraction with an attendant increase in the proximal reabsorption of sodium and an increased blood flow to juxtamedullary nephrons.

Alkalosis. The increased delivery of sodium to the distal tubules is in part responsible for the metabolic alkalosis that commonly accompanies injury. Lyons and Moore have pointed out

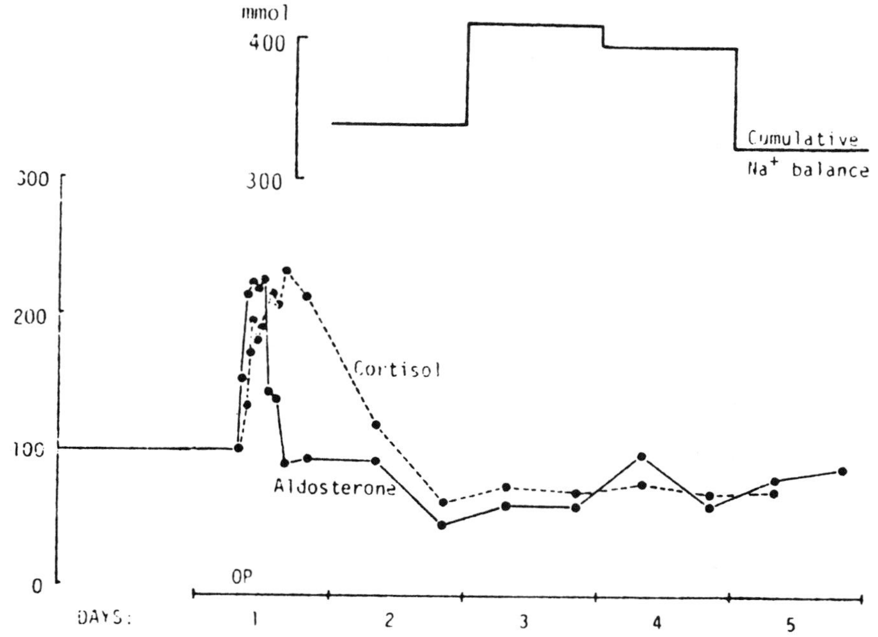

FIG. 1-56. Relationship of plasma aldosterone and plasma cortisol responses to postoperative sodium retention. The results are the median values for eight patients undergoing cholecystectomy at the start of day 1. All patients were in Na^+ and K^+ balance at the time of operation and the hormone changes are expressed as a percentage of the basal preoperative level. Intravenous intake was 259 mmol Na^+ on day 2, and 152 mmol Na^+ and 80 mmol K^+ on days 3 to 5, with a total of 3 L of water on each day. (From: *LeQuesne LP et al: Br Med Bull 41:212, 1985, with permission.*)

that the most common acid-base disturbance in patients who have not deteriorated to severe renal, circulatory, or pulmonary decompensation is either metabolic or respiratory alkalosis. In their study, 64 percent of the 105 surgical patients developed alkalosis in at least one determination in the postoperative period. It is important to prevent severe alkalosis in the surgical patient because of its potential hazards that include the production of tissue hypoxia through the effect of alkalosis on the oxygen-hemoglobin dissociation curve, hypokalemia, and alterations in vasomotor tone such as cerebral vasoconstriction.

Acidosis. The most common acid-base disturbance in severely injured patients or in those who deteriorated to severe renal circulatory or pulmonary decompensation is either metabolic acidosis or respiratory alkalosis. Foremost among the etiologies for acidosis following injury is shock. The metabolic acidosis that ensues is the result of tissue hypoperfusion and anaerobic metabolism. Metabolic acidosis may also occur in patients who have a respiratory alkalosis if hypoventilation occurs suddenly, since the rise in blood lactate that accompanies respiratory alkalosis will be unbuffered. Acidosis has profound effects on the cardiovascular system, producing a decrease in myocardial contractility, decreased response of the myocardium and peripheral vasculature to catecholamines, and a predisposition to arrhythmias.

Water Reabsorption. Injury and hypotension are also characterized by an increase in water reabsorption. In part, this is related to the increase in sodium reabsorption since the reabsorption of sodium is associated with the passive reabsorption of water. The increase in reabsorption is also the result of the stimulation of vasopressin secretion during hypotension and injury by osmotic and nonosmotic (baroreceptor) pathways. The increase in plasma AVP usually lasts 3 to 5 days after injury. Under most circumstances it results in water retention and oliguria unless specific preventive steps are taken. Postoperative oliguria was originally believed to be a normal accompaniment of injury that did no particular harm. Although it is well tolerated in most forms of mild to moderate surgical trauma, it is potentially harmful: first, it predisposes to acute tubular necrosis in severe trauma patients in whom hypovolemia and hypotension are apt to occur, and second, it sets the stage for the development of water intoxication (severe hyponatremia) if large volumes of non-solute-containing fluids are given to the patient before, during, or immediately after operation. The most common electrolyte abnormality observed following surgery and injury is hyponatremia as a result of the administration of hypotonic fluids under conditions that favor salt and water retention.

The action of AVP in effecting water retention requires the presence of an intact countercurrent mechanism in the loop of Henle. If the countercurrent mechanism is disrupted by a fall in medullary osmolality, the action of AVP is impaired, resulting in a defective urinary concentrating ability. Consequently, a normal or increased urine output in a hypotensive or injured patient does not necessarily reflect an adequate blood volume. In order to prevent a fall in the medullary gradient following injury, adequate tubular fluid flow must be ensured and maximal sodium reabsorption in the proximal nephron must be avoided. This is accomplished by the administration of liberal amounts of salt solutions such as Ringer's lactate or normal saline in the postoperative period. The administration of the solutions may result in marked positive sodium and solute balance and in edema as noted previously. During this period of increased AVP secretion the urine volume cannot be

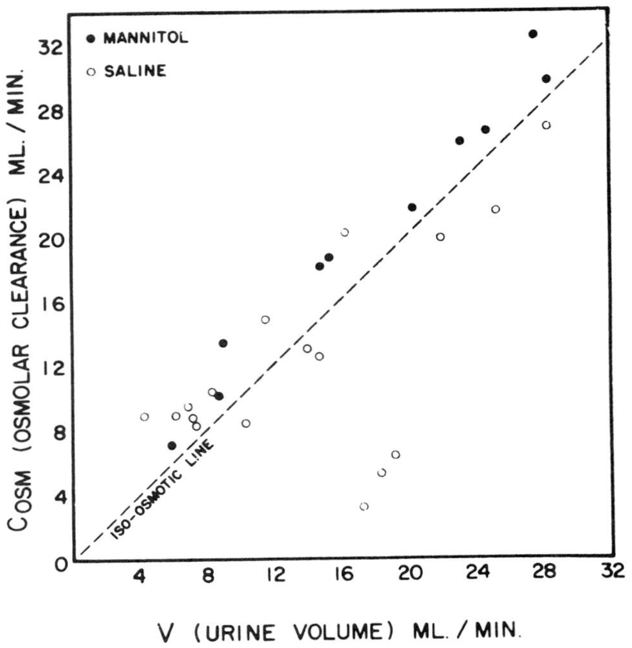

FIG. 1-57. Postoperative patients failed to excrete a water load when given 5% dextrose in water. These patients were then given either saline or mannitol. As shown, patients with high urine flow rates given saline were able to excrete free water whereas those with mannitol did not. This suggests that acute expansion of ECF volume in postoperative patients leads to suppression of the elevated AVP hormone activity normally seen during this period, and thus to excretion of hypotonic urine. (From: *Wright HK, Gann DS: Ann Surg 158:70, 1963, with permission.*)

increased by the administration of water alone. It is the solute load that determines urine volume, and free-water clearance will occur only when the extracellular fluid space has been expanded (Fig. 1-57). By increasing the solute load and the extracellular fluid volume, the urine output can be maintained. Although this may result in a "puffy" patient postoperatively, it will maximize the protection of renal function. The efficacy of treatment can be monitored by maintenance of urine output at 30 mL/h or greater.

The return of AVP secretion to normal is signaled by the brisk diuresis of free water and resolution of tissue edema that is seen in most surgical patients on the third to fifth postoperative days. This is the so-called fluid mobilization phase of injury. This period may take considerably longer in the presence of persistent hypovolemia, pain, hypoxia, or other stimuli to AVP release. The presence of a diminished urine output and hyponatremia several days after injury is not necessarily related to the inappropriate secretion of AVP (SIADH). The diagnosis of SIADH cannot be established until all possible stimuli to the secretion of AVP have been excluded.

Postoperative Patterns. The two patterns most commonly seen in the postoperative period are illustrated in Figs. 1-58 and 1-59. The first is that of a mild to moderate dilutional hyponatremia with hyperkalemia. This is primarily brought about by the secretion of vasopressin plus the overhydration of the patient with non-solute-containing fluids. The potassium level may be elevated, because potassium is lost from cells as a consequence of corticosteroid and starvation-induced catabolism. Other contributing factors include infusion of potassium-rich banked blood, reab-

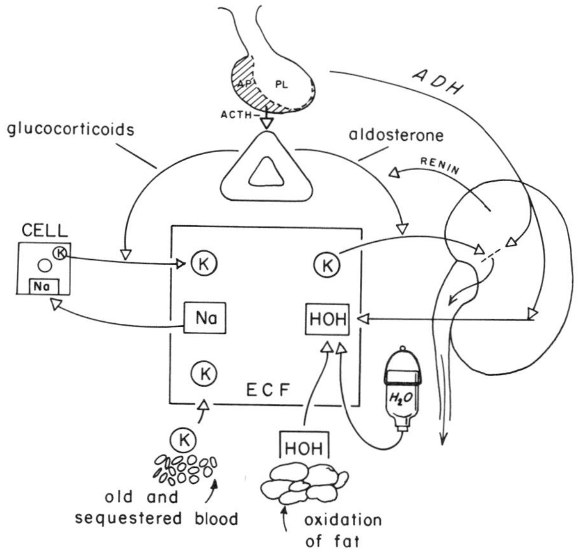

FIG. 1-58. Pattern of hyponatremia in the postoperative patient. Solute is diluted principally by excessive administration of water without salt. In addition, in severe trauma, sodium will move into cells in exchange for potassium. The hyperkalemia may be further aggravated by acidosis, by the action of cortisol, and by the breakdown of blood and may be opposed by the action of aldosterone.

sorption of blood from wound or peritoneum, and impaired potassium excretion due to diminished renal blood flow.

The hyponatremia and hyperkalemia are made much worse if the trauma is severe and prolonged or if the patient has had a chronic wasting illness before surgery. Other factors that can make the response worse include starvation, which as previously noted can itself produce hyponatremia through natriuresis; preexisting renal impairment, which predisposes to a further elevation of potassium level and depression of sodium level; cardiac disease with edema; preexisting hyponatremia; a pronounced shift of sodium into the cell with severe trauma; and episodes of hypotension, which further impair renal function. Consequently, cardiac patients may still need sodium replacement postoperatively, even though they may have an elevated total-body sodium and total-body water.

These changes can be prevented or minimized by the use of sodium chloride-containing solutions in the preoperative, intraoperative, and postoperative periods and by the replacement of third-space losses with normal saline. Potassium administration should be avoided unless the patient has unusual potassium losses or a declining serum potassium concentration.

The second pattern is one of hypokalemic alkalosis, classically seen in the patient with obstructing duodenal ulcer on continuous nasogastric suction or in the infant with hypertrophic pyloric stenosis with protracted vomiting. The alkalosis created by the loss of hydrogen ion from the stomach and the dehydration produced by the loss of water produces marked potassium losses in the urine since sodium reabsorption in the distal tubule must occur primarily in exchange for potassium rather than bicarbonate. The large quantities of chloride lost in gastric juice limit the ability of the kidney to reabsorb sodium proximally. As a result, a large amount of sodium is delivered to the distal tubules for reabsorption. Because of the large amount of sodium presented to the distal tubules and the increased secretion of aldosterone, patients with this condition usually have acid urine (paradoxical aciduria) from the exchange of hydrogen ion for sodium.

This condition is made worse by starvation, the intravenous administration of non-chloride-containing and non-potassium-containing solutions, the administration of proximal or loop diuretics, the administration of corticosteroids, the presence of diarrhea or a fistula, hyperventilation alkalosis, the preexistence of hypokalemia, and the administration of sodium bicarbonate. These changes can be eliminated by the administration of potassium chloride. Chloride is the most important of these two electrolytes, since without chloride the delivery of sodium to the distal tubules will remain increased and potassium and bicarbonate will continue to be wasted.

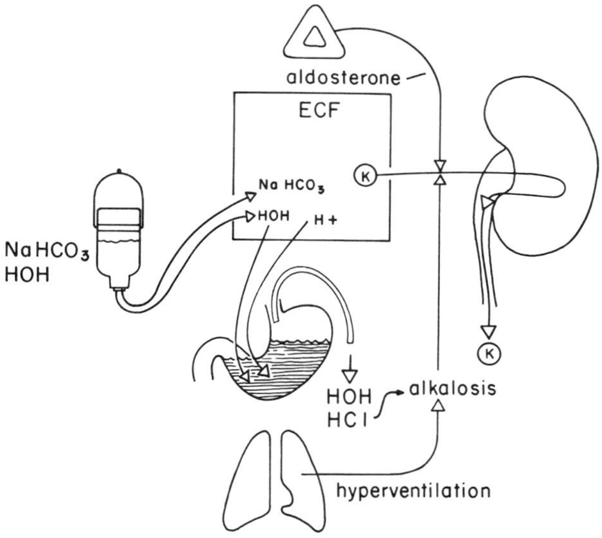

FIG. 1-59. Pattern of hypokalemic alkalosis in the postoperative patient. This is most commonly seen in patients who are alkalotic at the time of operation. The alkalosis produces an additional potassium loss in the urine. Hyperventilation increases the alkalosis and promotes further potassium loss. The administration of sodium bicarbonate, sometimes given in circumstances that are thought likely to be the result of acidosis, may further augment the alkalosis. These events then conspire to produce a severe hypokalemic alkalosis that, if renal function is maintained, may be made worse by the action of aldosterone in promoting potassium excretion.

Blood Volume Restitution

Despite the renal conservation of salt and water following injury, an increase in the functional extracellular fluid volume cannot occur even in the complete absence of renal excretion. In order for the functional extracellular fluid volume and effective circulating volume to return to normal following injury, the blood volume must be restored.

The restitution of blood volume can be accomplished by exogenous or endogenous fluids. The exogenous restitution of blood volume involves the administration of fluids. These fluids may be given intravenously, in which case the increase in blood volume is direct, or they may be given orally, in which case the increase in blood volume is indirectly mediated through intestinal absorption. The endogenous restitution of blood volume involves movement of fluids present in the interstitial fluid or cells to the effective circulating volume. This process may be thought of as occurring in two overlapping phases: the first involves the movement of essentially protein-free fluid from the interstitium to the plasma and the

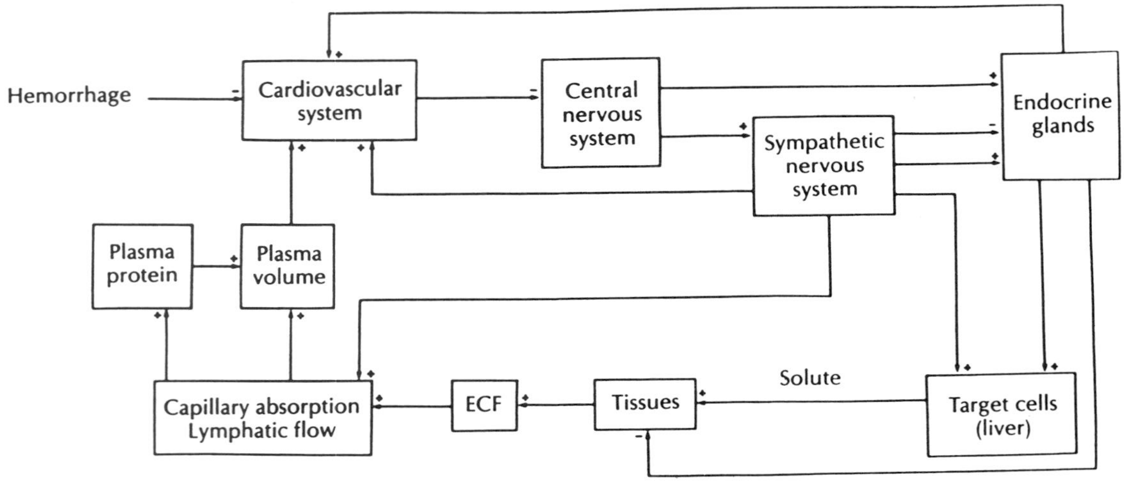

FIG. 1-60. Schematic representation of the restitution of blood volume. (From: *Gann DS, Amaral JF: The pathophysiology of trauma and shock, in Zuidema GD et al (eds): The Management of Trauma. Philadelphia, WB Saunders, 1985, with permission.*)

second involves the restitution of plasma protein that in turn mediates pari passu the movement of additional fluid, drawn osmotically from the cells, from the interstitium to the vascular space (Fig. 1-60).

A fall in capillary pressure mediates the net movement of protein-free fluid from the interstitium to the vascular space. The decrease in capillary pressure is initiated by hypotension and augmented by reflex sympathetic vasoconstriction. As capillary hydrostatic pressure decreases, the steady-state flux of fluid described in Starling's hypothesis of capillary equilibrium is changed. This results in the net movement of fluid into the capillary bed and in the restoration of approximately 20 to 50 percent of the blood volume lost. Because this fluid is protein-free, interstitial colloid oncotic pressure increases and interstitial hydrostatic pressure decreases, resulting in the establishment of a new steady state in which further net movement of fluid into the vascular space cannot occur.

The further movement of fluid and ultimately the complete restitution of blood volume depends on the movement of protein from the interstitium to the vascular space. The resultant increase in capillary oncotic pressure and decrease in interstitial oncotic pressure, in turn, mediates a shift of fluid from cells via the interstitial space to the capillary bed. The protein involved in this process is primarily in the form of albumin. This albumin must derive from the interstitium itself, since the restitution of blood volume is complete by 24 h, whereas albumin synthesis takes at least 48 h. The movement of albumin and protein from the interstitium to the capillary space may occur through either the lymphatics or the fenestrae of the capillary membrane. In order for either to be effective, interstitial pressure must increase. The latter can be accomplished through an increase in interstitial volume, since the compliance of the interstitium is fixed. The increase in interstitial volume cannot be derived from the plasma volume since it is already decreased. Water will move out of cells only down an osmotic gradient. Thus, an osmotic gradient between the intracellular and the extracellular space must exist in order for the interstitial volume to increase.

The movement of water from cells to the interstitium appears to be mediated by a hormonally induced increase in extracellular osmolality that was first described by Bergentz and Brief in experimental animals and later confirmed in human beings. The increase in serum osmolality occurs promptly after hemorrhage and correlates with the rate and degree of hemorrhage and the severity of the injury. An increase in cortisol is necessary but not sufficient to produce the increase in osmolality. An additional adrenal factor (probably catecholamines), a pituitary factor (probably AVP), and glucagon are required. The solute, derived primarily from the liver, includes glucose, phosphate, lactate, and pyruvate. Since these molecules are permeable to the capillary membrane but relatively impermeable to cell membranes, an osmotic gradient is established between interstitium and cells that moves fluid from the cells to the interstitium. The hydration of the interstitium either changes its colloidal state from gel to sol, or else opens up channels leading to the large capillary fenestrae. In either case, the capillary becomes permeable to albumin. The increase in interstitial volume results in an increase in interstitial pressure, thereby allowing protein to move through the capillary membrane and the lymphatics. The rise in osmolality also appears to contribute to the phase of transcapillary refill, since the increase in interstitial pressure requires the movement of water to the vascular space in order for the equilibrium between the interstitium and capillaries to be maintained (Fig. 1-61).

Nutritional status plays an important role in the hyperosmolality seen after hemorrhage. Fasted animals exhibit a lower degree of hyperglycemia and a slower rise in plasma osmolality than fed animals. As a result, the capacity for blood volume restitution is greater in animals who are fed than in those who are fasted. This difference presumably results from the depletion of hepatic glycogen stores during fasting, since the difference can be eliminated by the administration of glucose to the fasted animals.

One would predict that the higher the serum glucose, the more favorable the response. This is in marked contrast to the studies of combat victims by Carey and associates, in which a high glucose concentration correlated with high mortality. The production of solute after injury appears to be a function of the extent of the injury. In addition, it is important to recognize that the changes described result from an increase in the production of solute by the

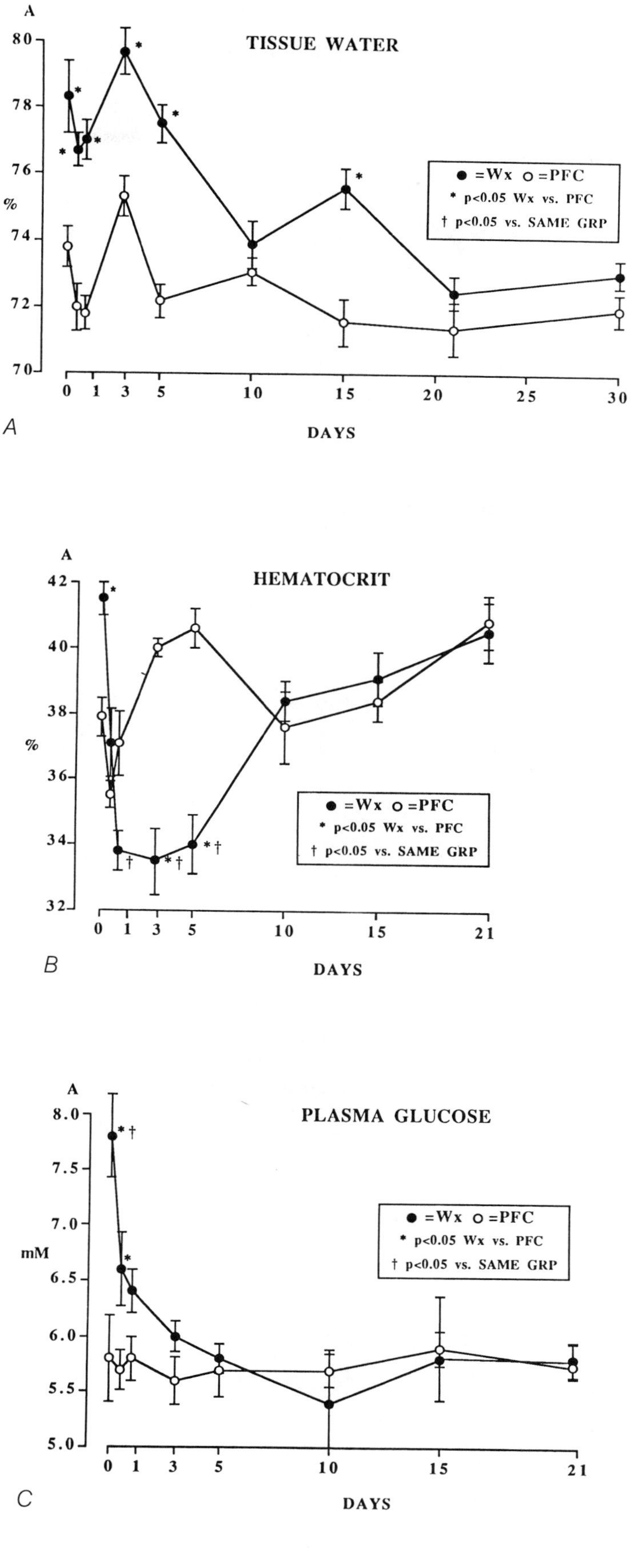

A

B

C

FIG. 1-61. Simultaneous, serial measurements in experimental and pair-fed control animals following hindlimb injury. The sequential changes in tissue water and hematocrit, in plasma concentrations of glucose, corticosterone, and catecholamines, and in insulin/glucagon ratios promote restitution of effective circulating blood volume. (From: *Amaral JF, Shearer JK, et al: J Trauma 28:1335, 1988, with permission.*)

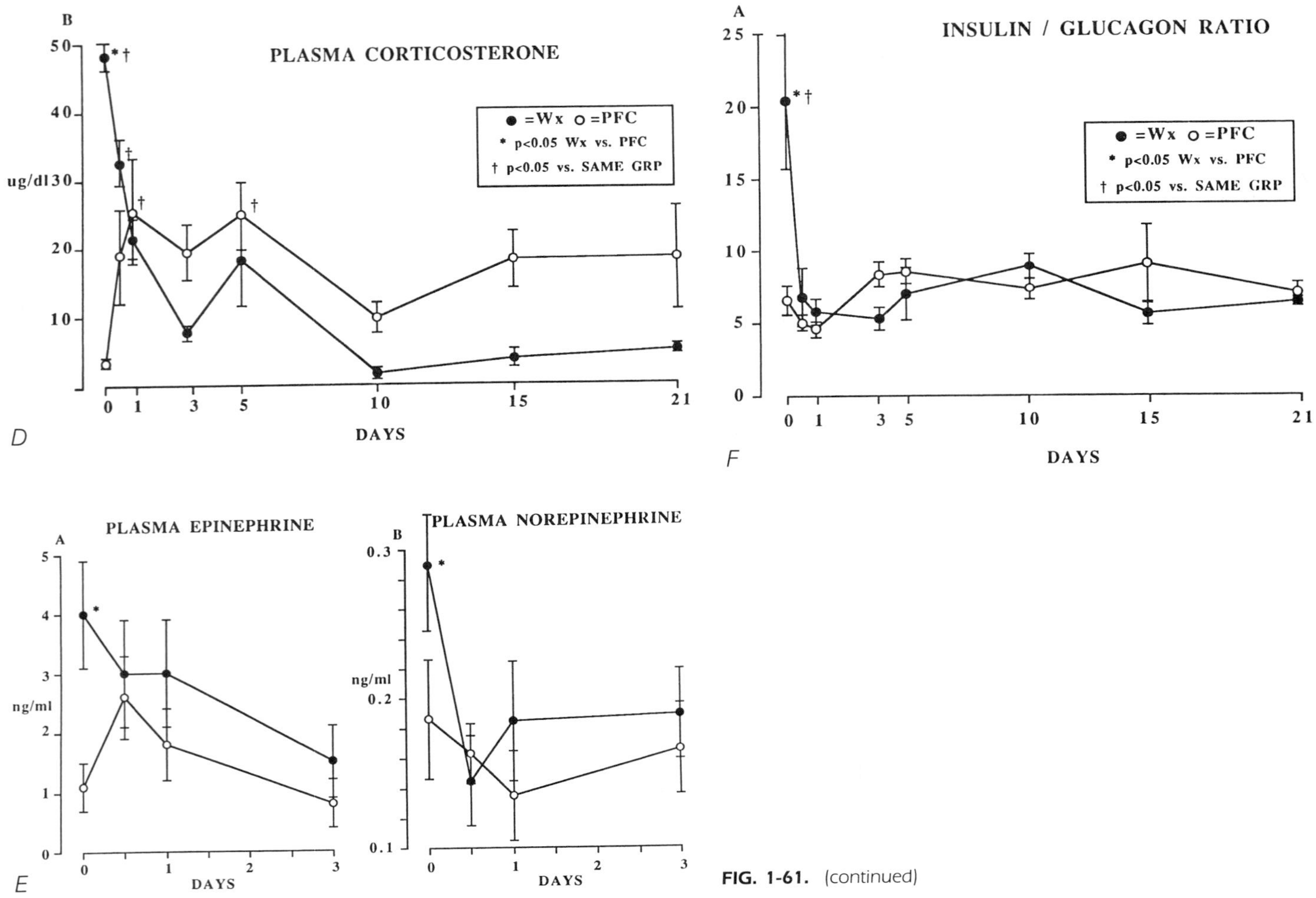

FIG. 1-61. (continued)

liver and its subsequent delivery to the interstitium bathing skeletal muscle. Given the same increase in solute production, changes in plasma solute concentrations will be smaller if muscle perfusion is adequate than if it is decreased by intense vasoconstriction. A very high increase in the serum glucose may be the result of inadequate tissue perfusion rather than of an accelerated rate of glucose production. In this setting, restitution would be significantly impaired and an increase in mortality would be expected. Although the second phase of blood volume restitution is present during all hemorrhages, the restitution in very large hemorrhages (>25 percent of the total blood volume) is no greater than that seen in small hemorrhages of 10 percent. This finding correlates with the appearance of a decrease in transmembrane potential, cell swelling, and eventually cell death.

Bibliography

Stimuli of the Neuroendocrine Reflex

Achtel RA, Downing SE: Ventricular responses to hypoxemia following chemoreceptor denervation and adrenalectomy. *Am Heart J* 84:377, 1972.

Baertschi AJ, Ward DG, Gann DS: Role of atrial receptors in the control of ACTH. *Am J Physiol* 231:692, 1976.

Bereiter DA, Plotsky PM, Gann DS: Tooth pulp stimulation potentiates the ACTH response to hemorrhage in cats. *Endocrinology* 111:1127, 1982.

Bereiter DA, Zaid AM, Gann DS: Adrenocorticotropin response to graded blood loss in the cat. *Am J Physiol* 247:E398, 1984.

Bereiter DA, Zaid AM, Gann DS: The effect of rate of hemorrhage on sympathoadrenal catecholamine release in the cat. *Am J Physiol* 250:E69, 1985.

Bereiter DA, Gann DS: Caudolateral areas of medulla-mediating release of ACTH in cats. *Am J Physiol* 251:R934, 1986.

Besedovsky HO, del Rey A: Immune-neuroendocrine circuits: Integrative role of cytokines. *Frontiers in Neuroendocrinology* 13:61, 1992.

Blalock JE: A molecular basis for bidirectional communication between the immune and neuroendocrine systems. *Physiol Rev* 69:1, 1989.

Blessing WW: Central neurotransmitter pathways for baroreceptor-initiated secretion of vasopressin. *NIPS* 1:90, 1986.

Brown AM: Receptors under pressure: an update on baroreceptors. *Circ Res* 46:1, 1980.

Claybaugh JR, Share L: Vasopressin, renin, and cardiovascular responses to continuous slow hemorrhage. *Am J Physiol* 224:519, 1973.

Egdahl RH: Pituitary-adrenal response following trauma to the isolated leg. *Surgery* 46:9, 1959.

Egdahl RH: The differential response of the adrenal cortex and medulla to bacterial endotoxin. *J Clin Invest* 38:1120, 1959.

Egdahl RH, Nelson DH, Hume DM: Adrenal cortical function in hypothermia. *Surg Gynecol Obstet* 101:15, 1955.

Engeland WC, Byrnes GJ, Gann DS: The pituitary adrenocortical response to hemorrhage depends on the time of day. *Endocrinology* 110:1856, 1982.

Gann DS, Cryer GL, Pirkle JC Jr: Physiological inhibition and facilitation of adrenocortical response to hemorrhage. *Am J Physiol* 232:R5, 1977.

Gann DS, Dallman MF, Engeland WC: Reflex control and modulation of ACTH and corticosteroids, in McCann SM (ed): *Endocrine Physiology,* III International Review of Physiology. Baltimore, University Park Press, 1981, vol 24, pp 157–199.

Gann DS, Berieter DA, et al: Neural interaction in control of adrenocorticotropin. *Fed Proc* 44:161, 1985.

Goldman WF, Saum WR: A direct excitatory action of catecholamines on rat aortic baroreceptors in vitro. *Circ Res* 55:18, 1984.

Grizzle WE, Dallman MF, et al: Inhibitory and facilitatory hypothalamic areas mediating ACTH release in the cat. *Endocrinology* 95:1450, 1974.

Hensel H: Neural processes in thermoregulation. *Physiol Rev* 53:948, 1973.

Heymans C, Neil E: *Reflexogenic Areas of the Cardiovascular System.* Boston, Little, Brown, 1958.

Holmes AE, Ledsome JR: Effect of norepinephrine and vasopressin on carotid sinus baroreceptor activity in the anesthetized rabbit. *Experientia* 40:825, 1984.

Hume DM, Bell CL, Bartter FC: Direct measurement of adrenal secretion during operative trauma and convalescence. *Surgery* 52:174, 1962.

Hume DM, Egdahl RH: The importance of the brain in the neuroendocrine response to injury. *Ann Surg* 150:697, 1959.

Lefcort AM, Ward DG, Gann DS: Electrolytic lesions of the dorsal rostral pons prevents adrenocorticotropin increases after hemorrhage. *Endocrinology* 114:2148, 1984.

Lilly MP, Engeland WC, Gann DS: Adrenomedullary responses to repeated hemorrhage in the anesthetized dog. *Endocrinology* 111:1917, 1982.

Lilly MP, Engeland WC, Gann DS: Responses of cortisol secretion to repeated hemorrhage in the anesthetized dog. *Endocrinology* 112:681, 1983.

Longnecker DE, McCoy S, Drucker WR: Anesthetic influence on response to hemorrhage in rats. *Circ Shock* 6:55, 1979.

McKinley MJ, McAllen RM, et al: Circumventricular organs: Neuroendocrine interfaces between the brain and the hemal milieu. *Frontiers in Neuroendocrinology* 11:91, 1990.

O'Berg B, White S: Circulatory effects of interruption and stimulation of cardiac vagal afferents. *Acta Physiol Scand* 80:383, 1970.

O'Dorisio MS, Panerai A (eds): Neuropeptides and immunopeptides: Messengers in a neuroimmune axis. *Ann N Y Acad Sci* 594:1, 1990.

Overman RR, Wang SG: The contributory role of the afferent nervous factor in experimental shock: Sublethal hemorrhage and sciatic nerve stimulation. *Am J Physiol* 148:289, 1947.

Quest JA, Gebber GL: Modulation of baroreceptor reflexes by somatic afferent nerve stimulation. *Am J Physiol* 222:1251, 1972.

Raff H, Shinsako J, Dallman MF: Surgery potentiates adrenocortical responses to hypoxia in dogs. *Proc Soc Exp Biol Med* 172:400, 1983.

Redding M, Mueller CB: Effect of ambient temperature upon responses to hypovolemic insult in the unanesthetized unrestrained albino rat. *Surgery* 64:110, 1968.

Wigger CJ: *Physiology of Shock.* New York, Commonwealth Fund, 1950.

Wood CE, Shinsako J, et al: Hormonal and hemodynamic responses to 15 mL/kg hemorrhage in conscious dogs: Responses to correlate to body temperature. *Proc Soc Exp Biol Med* 167:15, 1982.

Zimpfer M, Manders WT, et al: Pentobarbital alters compensatory neural and humoral mechanisms in response to hemorrhage. *Am J Physiol* 243:H713, 1982.

Mechanism of Hormone Action

Ali M, Vedeckis WV: The glucocorticoid receptor protein binds to transfer RNA. *Science* 235:467, 1987.

Cheung WY: Calmodulin. *Sci Am* 7:62, 1982.

Compton MM, Cidlowski JA: Vitamin B6 and glucocorticoid action. *Endocr Rev* 7:140, 1986.

Fain JN: Involvement of phosphatidylinositol breakdown in elevation of cytosol Ca^{++} by hormones and relationship to prostaglandin formation, in Kohn LD (ed): *Hormone Receptors.* New York, Wiley, 1982, vol 6, p 237.

Fain JN, Garcia-Sainz JA: Adrenergic regulation of adipocyte metabolism. *J Lipid Res* 24:945, 1983.

Farese RV: Phosphoinositide metabolism and hormone action. *Endocr Rev* 4:78, 1983.

Greengard P: Phosphorylated proteins as physiological effectors. *Science* 199:146, 1978.

Habener JF: Genetic control of hormone formation, in Wilson JD, Foster DF (eds): *Williams Textbook of Endocrinology,* 8th ed. Philadelphia, WB Saunders, chap 4, 1992.

Jensen EV: Interaction of steroid hormones with the nucleus. *Pharmacol Rev* 30:477, 1979.

Means AR, Lagace L, et al: Calmodulin as a mediator of hormone action and cell regulation. *J Cell Biochem* 20:317, 1982.

Motulsky JJ, Insel PA: Adrenergic receptors in man: Direct identification, physiologic regulations and clinical alterations. *N Engl J Med* 307:18, 1982.

Muldoon TG: Regulation of steroid hormone receptor activity. *Endocr Rev* 1:339, 1980.

O'Malley BW, Schrader WT: The receptors of steroid hormones. *Sci Am* 234:32, 1976.

Oppenheimer JH: Thyroid hormone action at the cellular level. *Science* 203:97, 1979.

Spiegel AM, Gierschik P, et al: Clinical implications of gaunine nucleotide binding proteins as receptor effector couplers. *N Engl J Med* 312:26, 1985.

Sterling K: Thyroid hormone action at the cell level. *N Engl J Med* 300:117, 173, 1979.

Hormone Systems

Aguilera G, Mendelsohn AO, Catt KJ: Dopaminergic regulation of aldosterone secretion, in Martini L, Ganong WF: *Frontiers in Neuroendocrinology.* New York, Raven, 1984, p 265.

Amir S, Berstein M: Endogenous opiates interact in stress-induced hyperglycemia in mice. *Physiol Behav* 28:575, 1982.

Anand KJS, Hickey PR: Halothane-morphine compared with high-dose sufentanil for anesthesia and postoperative analgesia in neonatal cardiac surgery. *N Engl J Med* 1:1, 1992.

Aono T et al: Influence of surgical stress under general anesthesia on serum gonadotropin levels. *J Clin Endocrinol Metab* 42:144, 1976.

Aun F, Medeiros-Neto GA, et al: The effect of major trauma on the pathways of thyroid hormone metabolism. *J Trauma* 23:104, 1983.

Averill DB, Scher AM, Feigl ED: Angiotensin causes vasoconstriction during hemorrhage in baroreceptor-denervated dogs. *Am J Physiol* 245:H667, 1983.

Baer PG, McGiff JC: Hormonal systems and renal hemodynamics. *Annu Rev Physiol* 42:589, 1980.

Barton RN: Neuroendocrine mobilization of body fuels after injury. *Br Med Bull* 41:218, 1985.

Bartter FC, Schwartz WB: The syndrome of inappropriate secretion of antidiuretic hormone. *Am J Med* 42:790, 1967.

Bauer WE, Vigar SNM, et al: Insulin response during hypovolemic shock. *Surgery* 66:80, 1969.

Baylis PH, Zepre RL, Robertson GL: Arginine vasopressin response to insulin-induced hypoglycemia in man. *J Clin Endocrinol Metab* 53:935, 1981.

Becker RA, Wilmore DW, et al: Free T4, free T3 and reverse T3 in critically ill, terminally injured patients. *J Trauma* 20:713, 1980.

Benedict CR, Grahame-Smith DG: Plasma noradrenaline and adrenaline concentrations and dopamine-B-hydroxylase activity in patients with shock due to septicaemia, trauma and hemorrhage. *Q J Med* 47:1, 1978.

Bernton EW, Long JB, Holaday JW: Opioids and neuropeptides; mechanisms in circulatory shock. *Fed Proc* 44:290, 1985.

Bie P: Osmoreceptors, vasopressin and control of renal water excretion. *Physiol Rev* 60:961, 1980.

Bonnet F, Harari A, et al: Suppression of antidiuretic hormone hypersecretion during surgery by extradural anaesthesia. *Br J Anaesth* 54:30, 1982.

Brizio-Molteni L, Molteni A, et al: Prolactin, corticotropin and gonadotropin concentrations following thermal injury in adults. *J Trauma* 24:1, 1984.

Buckingham J: Hypothalamic-pituitary responses to trauma. *Br Med Bull* 41:203, 1985.

Caldwell MD, Lacy WW, Exton JH: Effects of adrenalectomy on the amino acid and glucose metabolism of perfused rat hindlimbs. *J Biol Chem* 253:6837, 1978.

Carey LC, Lowery BD, Cloutier CT: Blood sugar and insulin response in human shock. *Ann Surg* 172:342, 1970.

Cartensen H, et al: Testosterone, luteinizing hormone and growth hormone in blood following surgical trauma. *Acta Chir Scand* 138:1, 1972.

Cerra FB: Nutrient modulation of inflammatory and immune function. *Am J Surg* 161:230, 1991.

Chaisson JL, Shikama H, et al: Inhibitory effect of epinephrine on insulin-stimulated glucose uptake by rat skeletal muscle. *J Clin Invest* 68:706, 1981.

Chan TM: The permissive effects of glucocorticoids on hepatic gluconeogenesis. *J Biol Chem* 259:7426, 1984.

Charters AC, O'Dell MWD, Thompson JC: Anterior pituitary function during surgical stress and convalescence. *J Clin Endocrinol Metab* 29:63, 1969.

Christiansen NJ, H:lsted J, et al: Effects of surgical stress and insulin on cardiovascular function and norepinephrine kinetics. *Am J Physiol* 247:E29, 1984.

Chwals WJ, Bistrian BR: Role of exogenous growth hormone and insulin-like growth factor-I in malnutrition and acute metabolic stress: A hypothesis. *Crit Care Med* 19:1317, 1991.

Cioffi WG Jr, Vaughan GM: Dissociation of blood volume and flow in regulation of salt and water balance in burn patients. *Ann Surg* 214:213, 1991.

Cobelli C, Toffolo G, Ferrannini E: A model of glucose kinetics and their control by insulin, compartmental and noncompartmental approaches. *Mathematical Biosciences* 72:291, 1984.

Cochrane JPS, Forsling ML, et al: Arginine vasopressin release following surgical operations. *Br J Surg* 68:209, 1981.

Cooper CE, Nelson DH: ACTH levels in plasma in preoperative and surgically stressed patients. *J Clin Invest* 41:1599, 1962.

Cowley AW, Quitlen EW, Skelton MM: Role of vasopressin in cardiovascular regulation. *Fed Proc* 42:3170, 1983.

Cryer, PE: Physiology and pathophysiology of the human sympathoadrenal neuroendocrine system. *N Engl J Med* 303:436, 1980.

Curtis T, Lefer A: Protective actions of naloxone in hemorrhagic shock. *Am J Physiol* 239:H416, 1980.

Daughaday WH: The adenohypophysis, in Williams RH: *Textbook of Endocrinology*. Philadelphia, WB Saunders, 1981, p 73.

Davies CL, Newman RJ, et al: The relationship between plasma catecholamines and severity of injury in man. *J Trauma* 24:99, 1984.

DeBold CR, Menefee JK, et al: Proopiomelanocorticotropin gene is expressed in many normal human tissues and in tumors not associated with ectopic adrenocorticotropin syndrome. *Mol Endocrinol* 2:862, 1989.

Deitch EA, Xo D, et al: Opioids modulate neutrophil lymphocyte function: Thermal injury alters plasma beta-endorphin levels. *Surgery* 104:41, 1988.

Edelman IS, Ismail-Beigi F: Thyroid thermogenesis and active sodium transport. *Recent Prog Horm Res* 30:235, 1974.

Eigler N, Sacca L, Sherwin RS: Synergistic interactions of physiologic increments of glucagon, epinephrine and cortisol in the dog. *J Clin Invest* 63:114, 1979.

Emerson TW: Participation of endogenous vasoactive agents in the pathogenesis of endotoxic shock. *Adv Exp Med Biol* 23:25, 1974.

Engeland WC, Bereiter DF, Gann DS: Sympathetic control of adrenal secretion after hemorrhage in awake dogs. *Am J Physiol* 251:R341, 1986.

Engeland WC, Demsher DP, et al: The adrenal medullary response to graded hemorrhage in awake dogs. *Endocrinology* 109:1539, 1981.

Engels FL, Fredricks J: Contribution to understanding of mechanism of permissive action of corticoids. *Proc Soc Exp Biol Med* 95:593, 1957.

Esler M, Jennings G, et al: Overflow of catecholamine neurotransmitters to the circulation: Source, fate and functions. *Physiol Rev* 70:963, 1990.

Feldman M, Kiser RS, et al: Beta-endorphin and the endocrine pancreas. *N Engl J Med* 308:350, 1983.

Felig P: The endocrine pancreas: Diabetes mellitus, in Felig P, Baxter JD, Broadus AE, Frohman LA (eds): *Endocrinology and Metabolism,* 2d ed. New York, McGraw-Hill, 1987, p 1043.

Felig P, Sherwin RS, et al: Hormonal interactions in the regulation of blood glucose. *Recent Prog Horm Res* 35:501, 1979.

Fisher JE, Hasselgren P-O: Cytokines and glucocorticoids in the regulation of the ''hepato-skeletal muscle axis'' in sepsis. *Am J Surg* 162:266, 1991.

Franchimont P: The regulation of follicle stimulating hormone and luteinizing hormone secretion in humans, in Martini L, Ganong WF (eds): *Frontiers in Neuroendocrinology*. New York, Oxford University Press, 1971, p 3331.

Fray JCS, Lush DJ, Valentine AND: Cellular mechanisms of renin secretion. *Fed Proc* 3250, 1983.

Frayn KN, Little RA, et al: The relationship of plasma catecholamines to acute metabolic and hormonal responses to injury in man. *Circ Shock* 16:229, 1985.

Frohman LA: CNS peptides and glucoregulation. *Annu Rev Physiol* 45:95, 1983.

Gann DS, Amaral JF: The pathophysiological response to injury, in Zuidema G, Rutherford R, Ballinger WF: *The Management of Trauma*. Philadelphia, WB Saunders, 1985, pp 35–100.

Gerich JE, Charles MA, et al: Regulation of pancreatic insulin and glucagon secretion. *Annu Rev Physiol* 38:353, 1976.

Grossman CJ: Regulation of the immune system by sex steroids. *Endocr Rev* 5:435, 1984.

Guillmen R, Vargo T, et al: β-Endorphin and adrenocorticotropin are secreted concomitantly by the pituitary gland. *Science* 197:1367, 1977.

Haberich FJ: Osmoreception in the portal circulation. *Fed Proc* 27:1137, 1968.

Halmagyi DFJ, Gillet DJ, et al: Blood glucose and serum insulin in reversible and irreversible post hemorrhagic shock. *J Trauma* 6:623, 1966.

Halmagyi DFJ, Neering IR, et al: Plasma glucagon in experimental post-hemorrhagic shock. *J Trauma* 9:320, 1969.

Halter JB, Pflug AE, et al: Mechanism of plasma catecholamine increases during surgical stress in man. *J Clin Endocrinol Metab* 45:936, 1977.

Harbour DV, Galin FS, et al: Role of leukocyte-derived pro-opiomelanocortin peptides in endotoxic shock. *Circ Shock* 35:181, 1991.

Hass M, Glock SM: Radioimmunoassayable plasma vasopressin associated with surgery. *Arch Surg* 113:597, 1978.

Hiebert JM, Kieler E, et al: Species differences in insulin secretion responses during hemorrhagic shock. *Surgery* 79:451, 1976.

Holaday JW, Black LE, Long JB: Neuropeptides in shock and trauma, in Gelhoed GW, Chernow B (eds): *Endocrine Aspects of Acute Illness*. London, Churchill Livingstone, 1985, p 257.

Horrobin DF: Prolactin as a regulator of fluid and electrolyte metabolism in mammals. *Fed Proc* 39:2567, 1980.

Ingenbleck Y: Thyroid function in non-thyroid illness, in De Vischer M (ed): *The Thyroid Gland*. New York, Raven, 1980.

Ippe E, Dobbs R, Unger RH: Morphine and beta endorphin influence the secretion of the endocrine pancreas. *Nature* 276:190, 1978.

Jackson I: Thyrotropin-releasing hormone. *N Engl J Med* 306:245, 1982.

Jahoor F, Herndon DN, et al: Role of insulin and glucagon in the response of glucose and alanine kinetics in burn-injured patients. *J Clin Invest* 78:807, 1986.

Kendler KS, Weitzman RE, Fisher DA: The effect of pain on plasma arginine vasopressin concentrations in man. *Clin Endocrinol* 8:89, 1978.

Kraus-Friedmann N: Hormonal regulation of hepatic gluconeogenesis. *Physiol Rev* 51:312, 1984.

Landgraf R, Landgraf-Leurs MMC: Prolactin: A diabetogenic hormone, *Diabetologia* 13:99, 1977.

Landsberg L, Young JB: Catecholamines and the adrenal medulla, in Wilson JD, Foster DW (eds): *Williams Textbook of Endocrinology,* 8th ed. Philadelphia, WB Saunders, 1992, p 621.

Lang RE, Bruckner UB, et al: Effect of hemorrhagic shock on the concomitant release of endorphin and enkephalin like peptides from the pituitary and adrenal gland in the dog, in Costa E, Trabucchi R (eds): *Regulatory Peptides: From Molecular Biology to Function*. New York, Raven, 1982.

Larsen PR: Thyroid-pituitary interaction. *N Engl J Med* 23:32, 1982.

Lautt WW, Dwan PD, Singh RR: Control of the hyperglycemic response to hemorrhage in cats. *Can J Physiol Pharmacol* 60:1630, 1982.

Lautt WW, Martens ES, Legare DJ: Insulin and glucagon response during hemorrhage induced hyperglycemia. *Can J Physiol Pharmacol* 60:1624, 1982.

Lefer AM: Significance of lipid mediators in shock states. *Circ Shock* 27:3, 1989.

Levy EM, McIntosh T, et al: Elevation of circulatory beta-endorphin levels with concomitant depression of immune parameters after traumatic injury. *J Trauma* 26:246, 1986.

Lilly MP, Gann DS: The hypothalamic-pituitary-adrenal-immune axis: A critical assessment. *Arch Surg* 127:1463, 1992.

Linares OA, Jacquez JA, et al: Norepinephrine metabolism in humans: Kinetic analysis and model. *J Clin Invest* 80:1332, 1987.

McIntosh TK, Faden AI: Thyrotropin-releasing hormone and circulatory shock. *Circ Shock* 18:241, 1986.

McLeod MK, Carlson DE, Gann DS: Hormonal responses associated with early hyperglycemia after graded hemorrhage in dogs. *Am J Physiol* 251:E597, 1986.

Marchetti B, Guarcello V, et al: Luteinizing hormone-releasing hormone agonist (LHRH-A) binds to lymphocytes and modulates the immune response, in Castagnetta L, Nenci I (eds): *Biology and Biochemistry of Normal and Cancer Cell Growth*. London, Harwood Academic Press, 1988, p 149.

Meguid MM, Brennan MF, et al: Hormone-substrate interrelationships following trauma. *Arch Surg* 109:776, 1974.

Merimer TJ, Zapf MJ, Froesch ER: Insulin-like growth factors in the fed and fasted states. *J Clin Endocrinol Metab* 55:999, 1982.

Miyata M, Yamomoto T, Nakao K: Suppression of glucagon secretion during surgery. *Horm Metab Res* 8:239, 1976.

Molteni A, Warphea RL, et al: Cicadian rhythms of serum aldosterone, cortisol and plasma renin activity in burn injuries. *Ann Clin Lab Sci* 9:518, 1979.

Morgan RJ, Martyn JAJ, et al: Water metabolism and antidiuretic hormone response following thermal injury. *J Trauma* 20:468, 1980.

Moss GS, Cerchio GM, et al: Serum insulin response in hemorrhagic shock in baboons. *Surgery* 68:34, 1970.

Munck A, Guyre PM, Holbrook NJ: Physiological functions of glucocorticoids in stress and their relation to pharmacological actions. *Endocr Rev* 5:25, 1984.

Nakao K, Nakai Y, et al: Substantial rise of plasma beta endorphin levels after insulin-induced hypoglycemia in human subjects. *J Clin Endocrinol Metab* 49:838, 1979.

Nelson DH: Corticosteroid-induced changes in phospholipid membranes as mediators of their action. *Endocr Rev* 1:180, 1980.

Newsome HH, Rose JC: The response of adrenocorticotrophic hormone and growth hormone to surgical stress. *J Clin Endocrinol Metab* 33:481, 1971.

Noel GL, Suh HK, et al: Human prolactin and growth hormone release during surgery and other conditions of stress. *J Clin Endocrinol Metab* 36:1255, 1973.

Novelli GP, Marsili M, Pieraccioli E: Anti-shock action of steroids other than cortisone. *Eur Surg Res* 5:169, 1973.

Ono N, Lumpkin MD, et al: Intrahypothalamic action of corticotropin-releasing factor to inhibit growth hormone and LH release in the rat. *Life Sci* 35:118, 1984.

Otsuki M, Dakoda M, Baba S: Influence of glucocorticoids on TRF-induced TSH response in man. *J Clin Endocrinol Metab* 36:945, 1973.

Parker RC, Baxter CR: Divergence in adrenal steroid secretory pattern after thermal injury in adult patients. *J Trauma* 25:508, 1985.

Parrillo JE, Fauci AS: Mechanisms of glucocorticoid action on immune processes. *Annu Rev Pharmacol Toxicol* 19:179, 1979.

Paterson SJ, Robson LE, Kosterlitz HW: Classification of opioid receptors. *Br J Med* 39:31, 1983.

Peach MJ: Renin-angiotensin system: Biochemistry and mechanisms of action. *Physiol Rev* 57:313, 1977.

Perdue JF: Chemistry structure and function of insulin-like growth factors and their receptors: A review. *Can J Biochem Cell Biol* 62:1237, 1984.

Pfeiffer A, Herz A: Endocrine action of opioids. *Horm Metab Res* 16:386, 1984.

Phillips LS, Vassilopoulou-Sellin R: Somatomedins. *N Engl J Med* 302:371, 1980.

Phillips RH, Valente WA, et al: Circulating thyroid hormone changes in acute trauma: Prognostic implications for clinical outcome. *J Trauma* 24:116, 1984.

Poole CJM, Carter DA, et al: Atrial natriuretic factor inhibits the stimulated in vivo and in vitro release of vasopressin and oxytocin in the rat. *J Endocrinol* 112:97, 1987.

Porte D Jr, Smith PH, Ensinck JW: Neurohumoral regulation of the pancreatic islet A and B cells. *Metabolism* 25:1453, 1976.

Raptis S, Dollinger HC, et al: Differences in insulin, growth hormone and pancreatic enzyme secretion after intravenous and intraduodenal administration of mixed amino acids in man. *N Engl J Med* 288:1199, 1973.

Rees M, Bowen JC, et al: Plasma beta endorphin immunoreactivity in dogs during anesthesia surgery, escherichia coli sepsis, and naloxone therapy. *Surgery* 93:386, 1983.

Reichlin S: Somatostatin. *N Engl J Med* 309:1495, 1983.

Rizza RA, Mandarino LJ, Gerich JE: Cortisol-induced insulin resistance in man: Impaired suppression of glucose production and stimulation of glucose utilization due to a postreceptor defect of insulin action. *J Clin Endocrinol Metab* 54:131, 1982.

Russell WE, Van Wyk JJ: Peptide growth factors, in Degroot LJ (ed): *Endocrinology,* 2d ed. Philadelphia, WB Saunders, chap 152, 1989, p 2504.

Samuelsson B: Prostaglandins and thromboxanes. *Recent Prog Horm Res* 34:239, 1978.

Sawchenko PE, Friedman MI: Sensory functions of the liver—a review. *Am J Physiol* 236:R5, 1979.

Schrier RW, Berl WT, Anderson RJ: Osmotic and non-osmotic control of vasopressin release. *Am J Physiol* 236:F321, 1979.

Share L: Control of plasma ADH titer in hemorrhage: Role of atrial and arterial receptors. *Am J Physiol* 215:1384, 1968.

Shavit Y, Lewis JW, et al: Opioid peptides mediate the suppressive effect of stress on natural killer cell cytotoxicity. *Science* 223:188, 1984.

Sherwin RS, Kramer KJ, et al: A model of the kinetics of insulin in man. *J Clin Invest* 53:1481, 1974.

Shirani KZ, Vaughan GM, et al: Inappropriate vasopressin secretion in burned patients. *J Trauma* 23:217, 1983.

Shirani KZ, Vaughan GM, et al: Reduced serum T4 and T3 and their altered transport binding after burn injury in rats. *J Trauma* 25:953, 1985.

Skillman JJ, Hedley-White J, Pallotta JA: Hormonal, fuel and respiratory relationships after acute blood loss in man. *Surg Forum* 21:23, 1970.

Skillman JJ, Lauler DP, et al: Hemorrhage in normal man: Effect on renin, cortisol, aldosterone, and urine composition. *Ann Surg* 166:865, 1967.

Sklar AH, Schrier RW: Central nervous system mediators of vasopressin release. *Physiol Rev* 63:1243, 1983.

Swerlick RA, Drucker NA, McCoy S: Insulin effectiveness in hypovolemic dogs. *J Trauma* 21:1013, 1981.

Thompson WA, Coyle SM, et al: The metabolic effects of continuous infusion of insulin-like growth factor (IGF-I) in parenterally fed men. *Surg Forum* 42:23, 1991.

Unger RH, Dobbs RE: Insulin, glucagon and somatostatin secretion in the regulation of metabolism. *Annu Rev Physiol* 40:307, 1978.

Vaughan GM, Becker RA, et al: Cortisol and corticotrophin in burned patients. *J Trauma* 22:263, 1982.

Vitek V, Lang DJ, Crowley RA: Admission serum insulin and glucose levels in 247 accident victims. *Clin Chim Acta* R95:93, 1979.

Vitek V, Shatney CH, et al: Thyroid hormone responses in hemorrhagic shock: Study in dogs and preliminary findings in humans. *Surgery* 93:768, 1983.

Wahl R, Grusseudorf M, et al: Changes of thyroid hormone concentrations after severe trauma and in hemorrhagic shock. *Eur Surg Res* 9 (suppl): 1, 1977.

Williams GH: Aldosterone, in Dunn MJ (ed): *Renal Endocrinology*. Baltimore, Williams and Wilkins, 1983, p 205.

Williamson DH: Regulation of ketone body metabolism and the effects of injury. *Acta Chir Scand* 22:9, 1981.

Wilmore DW, Long JM, et al: Catecholamines: Mediators of the hypermetabolic response to thermal injury. *Ann Surg* 180:653, 1974.

Wilmore DW, Mason AD, Pruitt BA: Insulin response to glucose in hypermetabolic burn patients. *Ann Surg* 183:314, 1976.

Wilmore WD, Moylan DA, et al: Hyperglucagonemia after burns. *Lancet* 1:73, 1974.

Wise L, Margraf HW, Ballinger WF: Adrenal cortical function in severe burns. *Arch Surg* 105:213, 1972.

Wolfe RR, Burk JF: Somatostatin infusion inhibits glucose production in burn patients. *Circ Shock* 9:521, 1982.

Wolfe RR, Herndon DN, et al: Effect of severe burn injury on substrate cycling by glucose and fatty acids. *N Engl J Med* 317:379, 1982.

Woloski BM, Smith EM, et al: Corticotropin releasing activity of monokines. *Science* 230:1035, 1985.

Woolfe PD, Hammill RW, et al: Transient hypogonadotropic hypogonadism caused by critical surgical illness. *J Clin Endocrinol Metab* 66:444, 1985.

Wright PD, Henderson K: Cellular glucose utilization during hemorrhagic shock in the pig. *Surgery* 77:322, 1975.

Wright PD, Johnston IDA: The effect of surgical operation on growth hormone levels in surgery. *Surgery* 77:479, 1975.

Cytokines and Other Mediators

Aasen AO, Smith-Erichsen N, et al: Plasma kallikrein-kinnin system in septicemia. *Arch Surg* 118:343, 1983.

Aggarwal BB, Kohr WJ, Hass PE, et al: Human tumor necrosis factor, production, purification and characterization. *J Biol Chem* 260:2345, 1985.

Arend WP, Joslin FG, et al: Effects of immune complexes on production by human monocytes of interleukin-1 or interleukin-1 inhibitor. *J Immunol* 134:3868, 1985.

Auron PE, Webb AC, et al: Nucleotide sequence of human monocyte interleukin 1 precursor cDNA. *Proc Natl Acad Sci USA* 81:7907, 1984.

Baracos V, Rodemann HP, et al: Stimulation of muscle protein degradation and prostaglandin E2 release by leukocyte pyrogen (interleukin-1). *N Engl J Med* 308:553, 1983.

Baughman RP, Lower EE: An inhibitor of tumor necrosis factor found in pleural effusions. *J Lab Clin Med* 118:326, 1991.

Baumann H, Isseroff H, et al: Phorbol ester modulates interleukin-6 and interleukin-1 regulates expression of acute phase plasma proteins in hepatoma cells. *J Biol Chem* 263:17390, 1988.

Berkenbosch F, De Goeij EC, et al: Neuroendocrine, sympathetic and metabolic responses induced by interleukin 1. *Neuroendocrinology* 50:570, 1989.

Berry HE, Collier JG, et al: The generation of kinins in the blood of dogs during hypotension due to hemorrhage. *Clin Sci* 39:349, 1970.

Besedovsky H, DelRey A, et al: Immunoregulatory feedback between interleukin-1 and glucocorticoid hormones. *Science* 233:652, 1986.

Besedovsky HO, Del Rey A: Metabolic and endocrine actions of interleukin-1. Effects on insulin-resistant animals. *Ann N Y Acad Sci* 594:214, 1990.

Beuschler HU, Fallon RJ, et al: Macrophage membrane interleukin 1 regulates the expression of acute phase proteins in human hepatoma Hep 3B cells. *J Immunol* 139:1896, 1987.

Beutler B, Cerami A: Cachectin and tumor necrosis factor as two sides of the same biological coin. *Nature* 320:584, 1986.

Beutler B, Cerami A: Cachectin: More than a tumor necrosis factor. *N Engl J Med* 316:379, 1987.

Beutler B, Mahoney J, et al: Purification of cachectin: A lipoprotein lipase-suppressing hormone secreted by endotoxin-induced RAW 264.7 cells. *J Exp Med* 161:984, 1985.

Bird TA, Saklatvala J: Studies on the fate of receptor bound ^{125}I-interleukin 1 beta in porcine synovial fibroblasts. *J Immunol* 139:92, 1987.

Blick M, Sherwin SA, et al: Phase I study of recombinant tumor necrosis factor in cancer patients. *Cancer Res* 47:286, 1987.

Brown JM, Grosso MA, et al: Cytokines, sepsis and the surgeon. *Surg Gynecol Obstet* 169:568, 1989.

Brown SL, Smith LR, et al: Interleukin 1 and interleukin 2 enhance proopiomelanocortin gene expression in pituitary cells. *J Immunol* 139:3181, 1987.

Caromona RH, Tsao RC, et al: The role of prostacyclin and thromboxane in sepsis and septic shock. *Arch Surg* 119:189, 1984.

Carswell EA, Old LJ, et al: An endotoxin-induced serum factor that causes necrosis of tumors. *Proc Natl Acad Sci USA* 72:3666, 1975.

Carter DB, Diebel MR Jr, et al: Purification, cloning, expression and biological characterization of an interleukin-1 receptor antagonist protein. *Nature (London)* 344:633, 1990.

Clowes GHA Jr, Hirsch E, et al: Survival from sepsis: The significance of altered protein metabolism regulated by proteolysis inducing factor, the circulating cleavage product of interleukin-1. *Ann Surg* 202:446, 1985.

Clowes GHA, George BC, et al: Muscle proteolysis induced by a circulating peptide in patients with sepsis or trauma. *N Engl J Med* 308:545, 1983.

Collort MA, Belin D, et al: Gamma interferon enhances macrophage transcription of the tumor necrosis factor/cachectin interleukin 1 and urokinase genes which are controlled by short lived repressors. *J Exp Med* 164:2113, 1986.

Dinarello CA, Clowes GHA Jr, et al: Cleavage of human interleukin-1: Isolation of a peptide fragment from plasma of febrile humans and activated monocytes. *J Immunol* 133:1332, 1984.

Dinarello CA, Savage N: Interleukin-1 and its receptor. *CRC Crit Rev Immunol* 9:1, 1989.

Dinarello CA: Interleukin-1 and its biologically related cytokines. *Adv Immunol* 44:153, 1989.

Doebber TW, Wu MS, et al: Platelet-activating factor involvement in endotoxin-induced hypotension in rats: Studies with PAF-receptor antagonist kadsurenone. *Biochem Biophys Res Commun* 127:799, 1985.

Dunn A: Systemic interleukin-1 administration stimulates hypothalamic norepinephrine metabolism paralleling the increased plasma corticosterone. *Life Sci* 43:429, 1988.

Engelmann H, Aderka D, et al: A tumor necrosis factor-binding protein purified to homogeneity from human urine protects cells from tumor necrosis factor toxicity. *J Biol Chem* 264:11974, 1989.

Fagarasan MO, Eskay R, et al: Interleukin 1 potentiates the secretion of beta endorphin induced by secretagogues in a mouse pituitary cell line (AtT-20). *Proc Natl Acad Sci USA* 86:2070, 1989.

Fernandez-Botran R: Soluble cytokine receptors: Their role in immunoregulation. *FASEB J* 5:2567, 1991.

Fletcher JR, Ramwell PW, et al: Prostaglandins and the hemodynamic course of endotoxin shock. *J Surg Res* 20:589, 1976.

Foley NM, McNicol MW, et al: Effect of serum from patients with sarcoidosis and tuberculosis on TNF-induced killing of murine cells. *Am Rev Respir Dis* 139:A58, 1989.

Fong Y, Moldawer LL, et al: Cachectin/TNF or IL-1 alpha induces cachexia with redistribution of body proteins. *Am J Physiol* 256:R659, 1989.

Fong Y, Moldawer LL, et al: Endotoxemia elicits increased circulating 2-IFN/IL-6 in man. *J Immunol* 142:2321 1989.

Fong Y, Moldawer LL, et al: The biological characteristics of cytokines and their implication in surgical injury. *Surg Gynecol Obstet* 170:363, 1990.

George DT, Abeles FB, et al: Effect of leukocyte endogenous mediators on endocrine pancreas secretory responses. *Am J Physiol* 233:E240, 1977.

Girardin E, Grau JM, et al: Tumor necrosis factor and interleukin-1 in the serum of children with severe infectious purpura. *N Engl J Med* 319:397, 1988.

Goetel EJ: Leukocyte recognition and metabolism of leukotrienes. *Fed Proc* 42:3128, 1983.

Goldberg AL, Kettlehut IC, et al: Activation of protein breakdown and prostaglandin E2 production in rat skeletal muscle in fever is signalled by a macrophage product distinct from interleukin 1 and other known cytokines. *J Clin Invest* 81:1378, 1988.

Grbic JT, Mannick JA, et al: The role of prostaglandin E2 in immune suppression following injury. *Ann Surg* 214:253, 1991.

Haberland GL: The role of kininogenases, kinin formation and kininogenase inhibition in post traumatic shock and related conditions. *Klin Vochenschr* 56:325, 1978.

Hartl WH, Herndon DN, et al: Kinin/prostaglandin system: Its therapeutic value in surgical stress. *Crit Care Med* 18:1167, 1990.

Jauch KW, Gunther B, et al: Improvement of impaired postoperative insulin action by bradykinin. *Biol Chem Hoppe Seyler* 367:27, 1986.

Jauch KW, Hartl WH, et al: Low-dose bradykinin infusion reduces endogenous glucose production in surgical patients. *Metabolism* 37:185, 1988.

Kaplan AP: Hageman factor-dependent pathways: Mechanisms of initiation and bradykinin formation. *Fed Proc* 42:3123, 1983.

Keogh C, Fong Y, et al: Identification of a novel tumor necrosis factor/cachectin from the livers of burned and infected rats. *Arch Surg* 125:79, 1990.

Kriegler M, Perez C, et al: A novel form of TNF/cachectin is a cell surface cytotoxic transmembrane protein: Ramifications for the complex physiology of TNF. *Cell* 53:45, 1988.

Kurt-Jones EA, Beller DI, et al: Identification of a membrane-associated interleukin-1 in macrophages. *Proc Natl Acad Sci USA* 82:1204, 1985.

Le J, Frederickson G, et al: Interleukin 2-dependent and interleukin 2-independent pathways of regulation of thymocyte function by interleukin 6. *Proc Natl Acad Sci USA* 85:8643, 1988.

Lefer AM: Eicosanoids as mediators of ischemia and shock. *Fed Proc* 44:275, 1985.

Lilly MP, Gann DS: The hypothalamo-pituitary-immune axis: A critical appraisal. *Arch Surg* 127:1463, 1992.

Lotz M, Jurik F, et al: B cell stimulating factor 2/interleukin 6 is a costimulant for human thymocytes and T lymphocytes. *J Exp Med* 167:1253, 1988.

Lumpin MD: The regulation of ACTH secretion by IL-1. *Science* 238:452, 1987.

March CJ, Mosley B, et al: Cloning, sequence and expression of two distinct human interleukin-1 complementary DNAs. *Nature* 315:641, 1985.

Matsuchima K, Taguchi M, et al: Intracellular localization of human monocyte associated interleukin 1 activity and release of biologically active IL-1 from monocytes by trypsin and plasmin. *J Immunol* 136:2883, 1986.

Maury CPJ, Salo E, et al: Circulating interleukin-1 beta in patients with Kawasaki disease. *N Engl J Med* 319:1670, 1988.

Mealy K, Van Lanschot JJB, et al: Are the catabolic effects of tumor necrosis factor mediated by glucocorticoids? *Arch Surg* 125:42, 1990.

Michie HR, Manogue KR, et al: Detection of circulating tumor necrosis factor after endotoxin administration. *N Engl J Med* 318:1481, 1988.

Moldawer LL, Svaninger G, et al: Interleukin 1 and tumor necrosis factor do not regulate protein balance in skeletal muscle. *Am J Physiol* 253:C766, 1987.

Myers A, Uotila P, et al: The eicosanoids: prostaglandins, thromboxane, and leukotrienes, in DeGroot LJ (ed): *Endocrinology,* 2d ed. Philadelphia, WB Saunders, 1989, p 2480.

Nagy S, Nagy A, et al: Histamine level changes in the plasma and tissues in hemorrhagic shock. *Circ Shock* 18:227, 1986.

Naitoh Y, Fukata J: Interleukin-6 stimulates the secretion of adrenocorticotropic hormone in conscious, freely-moving rats. *Biochem Biophys Res Commun* 155:1459, 1988.

Okubo A, Sone S, et al: Membrane-associated interleukin 1 alpha as a mediator of tumor cell killing by human blood monocytes fixed with paraformaldehyde. *Cancer Res* 49:265, 1989.

Okusawa S, Gelfand JA, et al: Interleukin-1 induces a shock-like state in rabbits. Synergism with tumor necrosis factor and the effect of cyclooxygenase inhibition. *J Clin Invest* 81:1162, 1988.

Okusawa S, Yancey KB, et al: C5a stimulates secretion of tumor necrosis factor from human mononuclear cells in vitro. *J Exp Med* 168:43, 1988.

Oomura Y: Chemical and neuronal control of feeding motivation. *Physiol Behav* 44:555, 1988.

Peetre C, Thysell H, et al: A tumor necrosis factor binding protein is present in human biological fluids. *Eur J Haematol* 41:414, 1988.

Pellicane JV, DeMaria EJ, et al: Tumor necrosis factor antibody (MOABTNF) improves survival following hemorrhagic shock in awake rats. Submitted to The Shock Society, 1992. In press.

Prieur AM, Jaufmann MT, et al: Specific interleukin-1 inhibitor in serum and urine of children with systemic juvenile chronic arthritis. *Lancet* 2:1240, 1987.

Ramadori G, Sipe JD, et al: Pretranslational modulation of acute phase hepatic protein synthesis by murine recombinant interleukin 1 (IL-1) and purified human IL-1. *J Exp Med* 162:930, 1985.

Regoli D, Barabe J: Pharmacology of bradykinin and related kinins. *Pharmacol Rev* 32:1, 1980.

Roberts LJ, Oates JA: Disorders of vasodilator hormones: the carcinoid syndrome and mastocytosis, in Wilson JD, Foster DW (eds): *Williams Textbook of Endocrinology,* 8th ed. Philadelphia, WB Saunders, 1992, chap 35.

Rodrick ML, Wood JJ, et al: Mechanisms of immunosuppression associated with severe nonthermal traumatic injuries in man: Production of interleukin 1 and 2. *J Clin Immunol* 6:310, 1986.

Sapolsky R, Rivier C, et al: Interleukin 1 stimulates the secretion of hypothalamic corticotropin-releasing factor. *Science* 238:522, 1987.

Seckinger P, Williamson K, et al: A urine inhibitor of interleukin 1 activity affects both interleukin alpha and beta but not tumor necrosis factor alpha. *J Immunol* 139:1541, 1987.

Shenkin A, Fraser WD, et al: The serum interleukin-6 response to elective surgery. *Lymphokine Res* 8:123, 1989.

Slotman GJ, Burchard KW, et al: Thromboxane and prostacyclin in clinical acute respiratory failure. *J Surg Res* 39:1, 1985.

Smedegard G, Cui L: Endotoxin-induced shock in the rat. A role for C5a. *Am J Pathol* 135:489, 1989.

Smith KA, Lachman LB, et al: The functional relationship of the interleukins. *J Exp Med* 151:1551, 1980.

Tracey KJ, Beutler B, et al: Shock and tissue injury induced by recombinant human cachectin. *Science* 234:470, 1986.

Tracey KJ, Lowry SF, et al: Cachectin/tumor necrosis factor mediates changes of skeletal muscle plasma membrane potential. *J Exp Med* 164:1368, 1986.

Tracey KJ, Lowry SF: The role of cytokine mediators in septic shock. *Adv Surg* 23:21, 1990.

Tracey KJ: Tumor necrosis factor (cachectin) in the biology of septic shock syndrome. *Circ Shock* 35:123, 1991.

Vilcek J, Gray PW, et al: Interferon gamma: A lymphokine for all seasons. *Lymphokine Res* 11:1, 1985.

Waage A, Brandtzaeg P: The complex pattern of cytokines in serum from patients with meningococcal septic shock. Association between interleukin 6, interleukin 1, and fatal outcome. *J Exp Med* 169:333, 1989.

Wakabayashi G, Gelfand JA, et al: Specific receptor antagonist for interleukin 1 prevents Escherichia coli-induced shock in rabbits. *FASEB J* 5:338, 1991.

Walter JS, Meyers P, et al: Microinjection of interleukin-1 into brain: Separation of sleep and fever responses. *Physiol Behav* 45:169, 1989.

Watters JM, Bessey PQ, et al: The induction of interleukin-1 in humans and its metabolic effects. *Surgery* 98:298, 1985.

Wicklmayr M, Dietze G, et al: Improvement of glucose assimilation and protein degradation by bradykinin in maturity onset diabetes and in surgical patients. *Adv Exp Med Biol* 12:569, 1979.

Wiedermann CJ: Interleukin-1 interaction with neuroregulatory systems: Selective enhancement by recombinant human and mouse interleukin-1 of in vitro opioid peptide receptor binding in rat brain. *J Neurosci Res* 22:172, 1989.

Woloski BM, Smith EM, et al: Corticotropin releasing activity of monokines. *Science* 230:1035, 1985.

Wood JJ, Rodrick ML, et al: Inadequate interleukin 2 production: A fundamental immunologic deficiency in patients with major burns. *Ann Surg* 200:31, 1984.

Endothelial Cell Mediators

Anggard EE: The endothelium—the body's largest endocrine gland? *J Endocrinol* 127:371, 1990.

Beveilacqua MP, et al: Endothelial leukocyte adhesion molecule 1: An inducible receptor for neutrophils related to complement regulatory proteins and lectins. *Science* 243:1160, 1989.

Billiar TR, Curran RD, et al: An L-arginine-dependent mechanism mediates Kupffer cell inhibition of hepatocyte protein synthesis *in vitro*. *J Exp Med* 170:1769, 1989.

Brigham KL, Meyrick B, et al: Antioxidants protect cultured bovine lung endothelial cells from injury from endotoxin. *J Appl Physiol* 63:840, 1987.

Bussolino E, Camussi G, et al: Human endothelial cells are targets for platelet-activating factor. I. Platelet-activating factor induces changes in cytoskeleton structures. *J Immunol* 139:2493, 1987.

Camussi G, Aglietta M, et al: The release of platelet-activating factor from human endothelial cells in culture. *J Immunol* 131:2397, 1983.

Cernacek P, Stewart DJ: Immunoreactive endothelin in human plasma: Marked elevation in patients in cardiogenic shock. *Biochem Biophys Res Commun* 161:562, 1989.

Cross JS, Gruber DP, et al: Hypertonic saline attenuates the hormonal response to injury. *Ann Surg* 209:684, 1989.

Curran RD, Billiar TR, et al: Multiple cytokines are required to induce hepatocyte nitric oxide production and inhibit total protein synthesis. *Ann Surg* 212:462, 1990.

Gala GJ, Lilly MP, et al: Interaction of sodium and volume in fluid resuscitation after hemorrhage. *J Trauma* 31:545, 1991.

Goetz KL, Wang BC, et al: Atrial stretch increases sodium excretion independently of release of atrial peptides. *Am J Physiol* 250:R946, 1986.

Hibbs JB Jr, Taintor R, et al: Nitric oxide: A cytotoxic activated macrophage effector molecule. *Biochem Biophys Res Commun* 156:87, 1988.

Hirata Y, Itoh K, et al: Plasma endothelin levels during surgery. *N Engl J Med* 321:1686, 1989.

Ignarro LJ, Buga GM, et al: Endothelium-derived relaxing factor. *Proc Natl Acad Sci USA* 84:9265, 1987.

Itoh K, Goseki N, et al: Intraoperative hemorrhage affects endothelin-1 concentrations. *Am J Gastroenterol* 86:118, 1991.

Kilbourn R, Belloni P: Endothelial cell production of nitrogen oxides in response to interferon gamma in combination with tumor necrosis factor, interleukin-1, or endotoxin. *J Natl Cancer Inst* 82:772, 1990.

Knowles RG, Palacios M, et al: Formation of nitric oxide from L-arginine in the central nervous system: A transduction mechanism for stimulation of the soluble guanylate cyclase. *Proc Natl Acad Sci USA* 86:5159, 1989.

Koller J, Mair P, et al: Endothelin and big endothelin concentrations in injured patients. *N Engl J Med* 325:1518, 1991.

Lang CH, Dobrescu C, et al: Platelet-activating factor-induced increases in glucose kinetics. *Am J Physiol* 254:E193, 1988.

Moncada S, Palmer RM, et al: Biosynthesis of nitric oxide from L-arginine. A pathway for the regulation of cell function and communication. *Biochem Pharmacol* 38:1709, 1989.

Naylor W: *Eur Pharmacol Sci* 11:96, 1990.

Ochoa JB, Udekwu AO, et al: Nitrogen oxide levels in patients after trauma and during sepsis. *Ann Surg* 214:621, 1991.

Palmer RMJ, Ferrife AG, et al: Nitric oxide release accounts for the biological activity of endothelium-derived relaxing factor. *Nature* 327:524, 1987.

Palombo JD, Blackburn GL, et al: Endothelial cell factors and response to injury. *Surg Gynecol Obstet* 173:505, 1991.

Pober JS, Cotran RS: Cytokines and endothelial cell biology. *Physiol Rev* 70:427, 1990.

Rubanyi GM, Botelho LHP: Endothelins. *FASEB J* 5:2713, 1991.

Ryan US (ed): *Endothelial Cells*. I–III. Boca Raton, CRC Press, 1988.

Saida K, Mitsui Y, Ishida N: A novel peptide, vasoactive intestinal contractor, of a new (endothelin) peptide family. *J Biol Chem* 264:14613, 1989.

Salvemini D, Korbut R, et al: Immediate release of a nitric oxide-like factor from bovine aortic endothelial cells by *Escherichia coli* lipopolysaccharide. *Proc Natl Acad Sci USA,* 87:2593, 1990.

Schmidt HHHW, Seifert R, et al: Formulation and release of nitric oxide from human neutrophils and HL-60 cells induced by a chemotactic peptide, platelet activating factor, and leukotriene B4. *FEBS Lett* 244:357, 1989.

Stewart JM, Gewitz MH, et al: The role of vasopressin and atrial natriuretic factor in postoperative fluid retention after the Fontan procedure. *J Thorac Cardiovasc Surg* 102:821, 1991.

Vallance P, Collier J, et al: Effects of endothelium-derived nitric oxide on peripheral arteriolar tone in man. *Lancet* II:997, 1989.

Vane JR, Anggard EE, et al: Regulatory functions of vascular endothelium. *N Engl J Med* 323:27, 1990.

Yanagisawa M, Kurihara H, et al: A novel potent vasoconstrictor peptide produced by vascular endothelial cells. *Nature* 332:411, 1988.

Intracellular Mediators

Blake MJ, Udelsman R, et al: Stress-induced heat shock protein 70 expression in adrenal cortex: An adrenocorticotropic hormone-sensitive, age-dependent response. *Proc Natl Acad Sci USA* 88:9873, 1991.

Carper SW, Duffy JJ, et al: Heat shock proteins in thermotolerance and other cellular processes. *Cancer Res* 47:5429, 1987.

Chirico WJ, Waters MG, et al: 70k heat shock related proteins stimulate protein translocation into microsomes. *Nature* 322:85, 1988.

Deitch EA, Bridges W, et al: Hemorrhagic shock, induced bacterial translocation is reduced by xanthine oxidase inhibition or inactivation. *Surgery* 104:191, 1988.

Haglund U, Gerdin B: Oxygen-free radicals and circulatory shock. *Circ Shock* 34:405, 1991.

Karlsson K, Marklund SL: Extracellular superoxide dismutase in the vascular system of mammals. *Biochem J* 255:223, 1988.

Lindquist S, Craig EA: The heat-shock proteins. *Annu Rev Genet* 22:631, 1988.

Morimoto RI, Tissieres A, et al: The stress response, function of the proteins, and perspectives, in Morimoto RI, Tissieres A, Georgopoulous EP, (eds): *Stress Proteins in Biology and Medicine*. Cold Spring Harbor, NY, Cold Spring Harbor Press, 1, 1990.

Rubanyi GM, Vanhoutte PM: Superoxide anions and hyperoxia inactivate endothelium-derived relaxing factor. *Am J Physiol* 250:H822, 1986.

Schoenige LO, Reilly P, et al: Heat shock gene expression excludes acute phase gene-expression following resuscitation from hemorrhagic shock. *Ann Surg* (In press.) 1993.

Udelsman R, Blake MJ, et al: Molecular response to surgical stress: Specific and simultaneous heat shock proteins induction in the adrenal cortex, aorta, and vena cava. *Surgery* 110:1125, 1991.

Vanhoutte PM, et al: Endothelial cell control of vascular function. *Hypertension* 13:658, 1989.

Substrate Metabolism Following Injury

Amaral JF, Shearer JD, et al: The temporal characteristics of the metabolic and endocrine response to trauma. *J Trauma* 28:1335, 1988.

Cuthbertson DP: The metabolic response to injury and its nutritional implications: Retrospect and prospect. *J Parenter Enter Nutr* 3:108, 1979.

Engels FL: The significance of the metabolic changes during shock. *Ann NY Acad Sci* 55:383, 1956.

Frayn KN: Substrate turnover after injury. *Br Med Bull* 41:232, 1985.

Moore FD, Brennan MF: Surgical injury: Body composition, protein metabolism and neuroendocrinology, in Ballanger WF, Collins JA, Drucker WR (eds): *Manual of Surgical Nutrition*. Philadelphia, WB Saunders, 1975, p 169.

Oppenheim W, Williamson D, Smith R: Early biochemical changes and severity of injury in man. *J Trauma* 20:135, 1980.

Siegel JH, Cerra FB, et al: Physiological and metabolic correlations in human sepsis. *Surgery* 86:163, 1979.

Stoner HB, Frayn KN, et al: The relationships between plasma substrates and hormones and the severity of injury in 277 recently injured patients. *Clin Sci* 56:563, 1979.

Stoner HB: Metabolism after trauma and sepsis. *Circ Shock* 19:75, 1986.

Turinsky J: Glucose metabolism in the region recovering from burn injury. *Endocrinology* 113:1370, 1983.

Volenec FJ, Clark GM, et al: Metabolic profiles of thermal trauma. *Ann Surg* 190:694, 1979.

Wilmore DW: Hormonal responses and their effect on metabolism. *Surg Clin North Am* 56:999, 1976.

Wilmore DW, Mason AD, et al: Insulin response to glucose in hypermetabolic burn patients. *Ann Surg* 183:314, 1976.

Metabolism after Fasting

Abbott NE, Anderson K: The effect of starvation, infection and injury on the metabolic processes and body composition. *Ann NY Acad Sci* 110:941, 1963.

Addis T, Poo LJ, Lew W: The quantities of protein lost by the various organs and tissues of the body during a fast. *J Biol Chem* 115:111, 1936.

Ahnefeld FW, Burri C, et al: *Parenteral Nutrition*. New York, Springer-Verlag, 1976.

Ashour B, Hansford RG: Effect of fatty acids and ketones on the activity of pyruvate dehydrogenase in skeletal muscle mitochondria. *Biochem J* 214:715, 1983.

Cahill GF: Starvation in man. *N Engl J Med* 282:668, 1970.

Cahill GF: Ketosis. *J Parenter Enterol Nutr* 5:281, 1981.

Carter WJ, Shakir KM, et al: Effect of thyroid hormone on the metabolic adaptation to fasting. *Metabolism* 24:1177, 1975.

Chaisson JL, Lilijenquist JE, et al: Gluconeogenesis from alanine in normal postabsorptive man: Intrahepatic stimulatory effect of glucagon. *Diabetes* 24:574, 1975.

Chopra IJ, Smith SR: Circulating thyroid hormones and thyrotropin in adult patients with protein caloric malnutrition. *J Clin Endocrinol Metab* 40:221, 1975.

Exton JH: Gluconeogenesis. *Metabolism* 21:945, 1972.

Felig P: The glucose-alanine cycle. *Metabolism* 22:17, 1973.

Hems DA, Whitton PD: Control of hepatic glycogenolysis. *Physiol Rev* 60:1, 1980.

Hers HG: The control of glycogen metabolism in the liver. *Annu Rev Biochem* 45:167, 1976.

Keys A, Brozek J, et al: *The Biology of Human Starvation*. University of Minnesota Press, 1950.

Korchak HM, Masoro EJ: Changes in the level of the fatty acids synthesizing enzymes during starvation. *Biochem Biophys Acta* 58:354, 1962.

Krebs HA: The metabolic fate of amino acids, in Munro HN, Allison JB (eds): *Mammalian Protein Metabolism*. New York, Academic, 1964, vol 1, p 125.

McGarry JD, Foser DW: Hormonal control of ketogenesis: Biochemical considerations. *Arch Intern Med* 137:495, 1977.

Mallette LE, Exton JH, Park CR: Control of gluconeogenesis from amino acids in the perfused rat liver. *J Biol Chem* 244:5713, 1969.

Masoro EJ: Lipids and lipid metabolism. *Annu Rev Physiol* 39:301, 1977.

Morgan HE, Earl DCN, et al: Regulation of protein synthesis in heart muscle. *J Biol Chem* 251:2151, 1971.

Munro HN, Crim MC: The proteins and amino acids, in Goodhart RS, Shils ME (eds): *Modern Nutrition in Health and Disease*. Philadelphia, Lea & Febiger, 1980, p 51.

Newsholme EA, Start C: *Regulation in Metabolism*. New York, Wiley, 1973.

Owen OE, Organ AP, et al: Brain metabolism during fasting. *J Clin Invest* 46:1589, 1967.

Palmblad J, et al: Effects of total energy withdrawal (fasting) on the level of growth hormone, thyrotropin, cortisol, adrenaline, noradrenaline, T4, T3 and rT3 in healthy males. *Acta Med Scand* 201:16, 1977.

Pozefsky T, Tancredi RG, et al: Effect of brief starvation on muscle amino acid metabolism in non-obese man. *J Clin Invest* 57:444, 1976.

Randle PJ, Newsholme EA, Garland PB: Regulation of glucose uptake by muscle: B. Effects of fatty acids, ketone bodies and pyruvate, and of alloxan-diabetes and starvation on the uptake and metabolic fate of glucose in rat heart and diaphragm muscles. *Biochem J* 93:652, 1964.

Sherwin RS, Hendler RG, Felig P: Effect of ketone infusion on amino acid and nitrogen metabolism in man. *J Clin Invest* 55:1382, 1975.

Energy Balance

Atkinson DE: The energy charge of the adenylate pool as a regulator parameter interaction with feedback modifiers. *Biochemistry* 7:4030, 1966.

Bartlett RH, Dechert RE, et al: Measurement of metabolism in multiple organ failure. *Surgery* 92:771, 1982.

Barton RN: The neuroendocrinology of physical injury. *Bailliere's Clin Endocrinol Metab* 1:355, 1987.

Benedict FG: *A Study of Prolonged Fasting*. Washington, DC, Carnegie Institute, 1915 (Publication No 203).

Chaudry IH, Sayeed MM, Baue AE: Depletion and restoration of tissue ATP in hemorrhagic shock. *Arch Surg* 108:208, 1974.

Chaudry IH, Wichterman KA, Baue AE: Effect of sepsis on tissue adenine nucleotide levels. *Surgery* 85:205, 1979.

Dubois EF: The mechanism of heat loss and temperature regulation, in Dubois EF (ed): *Lane Medical Lectures,* Stanford University Press, 1937.

Duke JH, Jorgensen SB, et al: Contribution of protein to caloric expenditure following injury. *Surgery* 68:168, 1970.

Giovanni I, Boldrini G, et al: Respiratory quotient and patterns of substrate utilization in human sepsis and trauma. *J Parenter Enterol Nutr* 7:226, 1983.

Hems DA, Brosnan JT: Effects of ischemia on content of metabolites in rat liver and kidney in vivo. *Biochem J* 120:105, 1970.

Horwitz BA: Role of active sodium transport in brown fat thermogenesis. *Isr J Med Sci* 12:1086, 1976.

Illner HP, Shires T: Membrane defect and energy status of rabbit skeletal muscle cells in sepsis and septic shock. *Arch Surg* 116:1302, 1981.

Im MJC, Hoopes JE: Energy metabolism in healing skin wounds. *J Surg Res* 10:459, 1970.

Kinney JM: Energy metabolism, in Fischer JE (ed): *Surgical Nutrition*. Boston, Little, Brown and Co., 1983, p 97.

Kinney JM, Lister J, Moore FD: Relationship of energy expenditure to total exchangeable potassium. *Ann NY Acad Sci* 110:722, 1963.

Kinney JM, Long CL, et al: Tissue composition of weight loss in surgical patients. I. Elective operations. *Ann Surg* 168:459, 1968.

Kinney JM, Morgan AP, et al: A method for gas exchange and expired radioactivity in acutely ill patients. *Metabolism* 13:205, 1964.

Kinney JM, Roe CF: Caloric equivalents of fever. Patterns of postoperative response. *Ann Surg* 156:610, 1962.

LePage GA: Biological energy transformations during shock as shown by tissue analysis. *Am J Physiol* 146:267, 1946.

Liaw KY, Askanazi J, et al: Effect of injury and sepsis on high energy phosphates in muscle and red cells. *J Trauma* 20:755, 1980.

Moore FD: Bodily changes during surgical convalescence. *Ann Surg* 137:289, 1953.

Moore FD: Energy and the maintenance of the body cell. *JPEN* 4:22, 1980.

Morris A, Henry W, et al: Macrophage interaction with skeletal muscle: a potential role of macrophages in determining the energy state of healing wounds. *J Trauma* 25:751, 985.

Nanni G, Siegel JH, et al: Increased lipid fuel dependence in the critically ill septic patient. *J Trauma* 24:14, 1983.

Pass LJ, Schloerb PR, et al: Liver adenosine triphosphate (ATP) in hypoxia and hemorrhagic shock. *J Trauma* 22:730, 1982.

Pruitt BA: Postburn hypermetabolism and nutrition in burn patients, in Ballinger WF, Collins JA, Drucker WR, Dudrick SJ, Zeppa R (eds): *Manual of Surgical Nutrition*. Philadelphia, WB Saunders, 1975, p 396.

Ryan NT: Metabolic adaptations for energy production during trauma and sepsis. *Surg Clin North Am* 56:1073, 1976.

Wilmore DW, Aulick LH, et al: Influence of the burn wound on local and systemic responses to injury. *Ann Surg* 186:444, 1977.

Wilmore DW, Long JM, et al: Catecholamines: Mediators of the hypermetabolic response to thermal injury. *Am Surg* 180:653, 1974.

Xin L, Blatteis CM: Blockade by interleukin-1 receptor antagonist of IL-1 beta induced neuronal activity in guinea pig preoptic area slices. *Brain Res* 569:348, 1992.

Lipid Metabolism

Allison SP, Hinton P, Chamberlain MJ: Intravenous glucose tolerance, insulin and free fatty acid levels in burn patients. *Lancet* 2:1118, 1968.

Bagby GJ, Corll CB, et al: Lipoprotein lipase suppressing mediator in serum of endotoxin-treated rats. *Am J Physiol* (Endocrinol Metab) 251:E470, 1986.

Bagby GJ, Corll CB, Martinez RR: Triglyceride and free fatty acid turnover in E. coli endotoxin treated rats. *Circ Shock* 16:76, 1985.

Beutler B, Cerami A: Recombinant interleukin-1 suppresses lipoprotein lipase in 3T3 cells. *J Immunol* 135:3969, 1985.

Birkhain RN, Long CL, et al: A comparison of the effects of skeletal trauma and surgery on the ketosis of starvation in man. *J Trauma* 513, 1981.

Forse RA, Leibel R, et al: Adrenergic control of adipocyte lipolysis in trauma and sepsis. *Ann Surg* 206:744, 1987.

Froholm BB: The effect of lactate in canine subcutaneous adipose tissue in situ. *Acta Physiol Scand* 81:110, 1971.

Galster AD, Bier DM, et al: Plasma palmitate turnover in subjects with thermal injury. *J Trauma* 24:938, 1984.

Hiraide A, Katayama M, et al: Effect of 3-hydroxybutyrate on posttraumatic metabolism in man. *Surgery* 109:176, 1991.

Jorgen N, Bjorn N, et al: Catecholamine regulation of adipocyte lipolysis after surgery. *Surgery* 109:488, 1991.

Kather H, Biger W, et al: Human fat cell lipolysis is primarily regulated by inhibitory modulators acting through distinct mechanisms. *J Clin Invest* 76:1559, 1985.

Kaufman RL, Matson CE, Beisel WR: Hypertriglyceridemia produced by endotoxin: Role of impaired triglyceride disposal mechanisms. *J Infect Dis* 133:548, 1976.

Kovach AGB, Russell S, et al: Blood flow, oxygen consumption and free fatty acid release in subcutaneous adipose tissue during hemorrhagic shock in control and phenoxybenzamine-treated dogs. *Circ Res* 26:733, 1970.

Nordenstrom J, Carpentier YA, et al: Free fatty acid mobilization and oxidation during total parenteral nutrition in trauma and infections. *Ann Surg* 198:725, 1983.

Rennie MJ, Holloszy JO: Inhibition of glucose uptake and glycogenolysis by availability of substrate in cell-oxygenated perfused skeletal muscle. *Biochem J* 168:161, 1977.

Robin AP, Nordenstrom J, et al: Influence of parenteral carbohydrate on fat oxidation in surgical patients. *Surgery* 195:608, 1984.

Smith R, Fuller DJ, et al: Initial effect of injury on ketone bodies and other blood metabolites. *Lancet* 1:1, 1975.

Wolfe RR, Shaw HF, Durkot MJ: Energy metabolism in trauma and sepsis: the role of fat, in Schumer W, Spitzer JJ, Marshall BE (eds): *Molecular and Cellular Aspects of Shock and Trauma*. New York, AR Liss, 1983, p 89.

Carbohydrate Metabolism

Amaral JF, Shearer JD, et al: Can lactate be used as a fuel by wounded tissue? *Surgery* 100:252, 1986.

Amaral JF, Shearer JD, et al: The effect of endotoxin on glucose metabolism in skeletal muscle requires the presence of plasma. *Arch Surg* 124:727, 1989.

Askanazi J, Elwyn DH, et al: Respiratory distress secondary to a high carbohydrate load. *Surgery* 86:596, 1980.

Bessey PQ, Brooks DC, et al: Epinephrine acutely mediates skeletal muscle insulin resistance. *Surgery* 94:172, 1983.

Black PR, Brooks DC, et al: Mechanisms of insulin resistance following injury. *Ann Surg* 196:420, 1982.

Caldwell MD, Shearer J, et al: Evidence for aerobic glycolysis in λ-carrageenan wounded skeletal muscle. *J Surg Res* 37:63, 1984.

Cannon WB: *The Wisdom of the Body*. New York, W.W. Norton, 1939.

Clark EJ, Rossiter R: Carbohydrate metabolism after burning. *Q J Exp Physiol* 32:279, 1944.

Cryer PE, White NH, Santiago JV: The relevance of glucose counterregulatory systems to patients with insulin-dependent diabetes mellitus. *Endocr Rev* 7:131, 1986.

Dahn M, Bouwnard DG, et al: The sepsis-glucose intolerance riddle: A hormonal explanation. *Surgery* 86:423, 1977.

Drucker WR, Dekieweit JC: Glucose uptake by diaphragms from rats subjected to hemorrhagic shock. *Am J Physiol* 206:317, 1964.

Drucker WR, Gallie BL, et al: The effect of persisting hypovolemic shock on pancreatic output of insulin, in Kovach AGB, Stoner HB, Spitzer JJ (eds): *Neurohumoral and Metabolic Response to Injury*. New York, Plenum, 1978, pp 187-198.

Forster J, Morris AS, et al: Glucose uptake and flux through phosphofructokinase in wounded rat skeletal muscle. *Am J Physiol* 256:E788, 1989.

Hagg SA, Taylor SI, et al: Glucose metabolism in perfused skeletal muscle. *Biochem J* 158:203, 1976.

Halmagyi DFJ, Irving MH, Varga D: Effect of adrenergic blockade on the metabolic response to hemorrhagic shock. *J Appl Physiol* 25:384, 1968.

Hiebert JM, Celik Z, et al: Insulin response to hemorrhagic shock in the intact and adrenalectomized primate. *Am J Surg* 125:501, 1973.

Hinton P, Allison SP, et al: Insulin and glucose to reduce catabolic response to injury in burned patients. *Lancet* 1:767, 1971.

Hunt TK, Conolly WB, et al: Anaerobic metabolism and wound healing: An hypothesis for the initiation and cessation of collagen synthesis in wounds. *Am J Surg* 135:328, 1978.

Jordan GL, Fischer EP, Lefiak EA: Glucose metabolism and traumatic shock in human. *Ann Surg* 175:685, 1972.

Kahn CR: Insulin resistance, insulin insensitivity and insulin unresponsiveness: A necessary definition. *Metabolism* 27:1893, 1973.

Kenney PR, Allen-Rowlands CF, et al: Glucose and osmolality as predictors of injury severity. *J Trauma* 23:712, 1983.

Kispert PH: Metabolic response to stress, in Simmons RL, Steed DL (eds): *Basic Science Review for Surgeons*. Philadelphia, WB Saunders, 1992, p 109.

Long CL, Spencer JL, et al: Carbohydrate metabolism in men: Effect of elective operations and major injury. *J Appl Physiol* 31:110, 1971.

Morris AS, Shearer J, Caldwell MD: The role of the cellular infiltrate on glucose metabolism in wounded tissue. *Surg Forum* 36:95, 1985.

Nelson KM, Turinsky J: Local effect of burn on skeletal muscle insulin responsiveness. *J Surg Res* 31:288, 1981.

Pekala P, Kawakami M, et al: Studies of insulin resistance in adipocytes induced by a macrophage mediator. *J Exp Med* 157:1360, 1983.

Randle PJ, Garland PB, et al: Interactions of metabolism and the physiological role of insulin. *Recent Prog Horm Res* 22:1, 1966.

Romanosky AJ, Bagby GJ, et al: Increased muscle glucose uptake and lactate release after endotoxin administration. *Am J Physiol* 239:E391, 1980.

Ryan NT, George BC, et al: Chronic tissue insulin resistance following hemorrhagic shock. *Ann Surg* 80:402, 1974.

Shangraw RE, Turinsky J: Local response of muscle to burns: Relationship of glycolysis and amino acid release. *JPEN* 5:193, 1981.

Stoner HB: Studies on the mechanism of shock: The quantitative aspects of glycogen metabolism after limb ischemia in the rat. *Br J Exp Pathol* 39:635, 1958.

Vary TC, Siegel JH, et al: Effect of sepsis on activity of pyruvate dehydrogenase complex in skeletal muscle and liver. *Am J Physiol* 250:E634, 1986.

Vary TC, Siegel JH, et al: Regulation of glucose metabolism by altered pyruvate dehydrogenase activity in sepsis. *JPEN* 10:351, 1986.

Wolfe RR, Durkot MJ, et al: Glucose metabolism in severely burned patients. *Metabolism* 28:1031, 1979.

Protein Metabolism

Albina JE, Henry W, et al: Glutamine metabolism in rat skeletal muscle wounded with λ-carregeenan. *Am J Physiol* 250:E24, 1986.

Albina JE, Shearer JD, et al: Amino acid metabolism following λ-carrageenan injury to rat skeletal muscle. *Am J Physiol* 250:E24, 1986.

Andrews RP, Morgan HC, Jhrkiewitz MJ: Relationship of dietary protein to the healing of experimental burns. *Surg Forum* 6:72, 1955.

Ardawi MSM, Newsholme EA: Glutamine metabolism in lymphoid tissue, in Haussinger D, Sies H (eds): *Glutamine Metabolism in Mammalian Tissues*. New York, Springer-Verlag, 1984, p 235.

Askanazi I, Carpentier YA, et al: Muscle and plasma amino acids following injury: Influence of intercurrent infection. *Ann Surg* 192:78, 1980.

Askanazi S, Elwyn DH, et al: Muscle and plasma amino acids after injury: The role of inactivity. *Ann Surg* 188:797, 1978.

Aulick LH, Wilmore DH: Increased peripheral amino acid release following burn injury. *Surgery* 85:560, 1979.

Bilmazer C, et al: Quantitative contribution by skeletal muscle to elevated ratio of whole-body protein breakdown in burned children as measured by 3-MEH output. *Metabolism* 27:671, 1978.

Birkhain RH, et al: Effects of major skeletal trauma on whole body protein turnover in man measured by {14C}leucine. *Surgery* 888:294, 1980.

Calloway DH, Grossman MI, et al: Effect of previous level of protein feeding on wound healing and on metabolic response to injury. *Surgery* 37:935, 1955.

Calwell FT Jr: Metabolic responses to thermal trauma. II: Nutritional studies with rats at two environmental temperatures. *Ann Surg* 155:119, 1962.

Chassin JL, McDougall HA, et al: The effect of adrenalectomy on wound healing in normal and in stressed rats. *Proc Soc Exp Biol Med* 86:466, 1954.

Clowes G, Randall H, Cha C: Amino acid and energy metabolism in septic and traumatized patients. *J Parenter Enterol Nutr* 4:195, 1980.

Crane CW, et al: Protein turnover in patients before and after elective orthopedic operations. *Br J Surg* 64:129, 1977.

Crowley CV, Seifter E, et al: Effects of environmental temperature and femoral fracture on wound healing in rats. *J Trauma* 17:436, 1977.

Curran RD, Ferrari FK, et al: Nitric oxide and nitric oxide-generating compounds inhibit hepatocyte protein synthesis. *FASEB J* 5:2085, 1991.

Cuthbertson DP: Observations on the disturbances of metabolism by injury to the limbs. *Q J Med* 1:233, 1932.

Cuthbertson DP, Tilstone WJ: Effects of environmental temperature on the closure of full thickness skin wounds in the rat. *Q J Exp Physiol* 52:249, 1967.

Dale G, et al: The effect of surgical operation on venous plasma free amino acids. *Surgery* 81:295, 1977.

Elwyn DH, Parikh HC, et al: Inter-organ transport of amino acids in hemorrhagic shock. *Am J Phys* 231:377, 1976.

Engels FL, Winton MG, Long CNH: Biochemical studies on shock. I. The metabolism of amino acids and carbohydrates during hemorrhagic shock in the rat. *J Exp Med* 77:397, 1942.

Frawley JP, Artz CP, Howard JM: Muscle metabolism and catabolism in combat casualties. *Arch Surg* 71:612, 1955.

Freund HR, Ryan JA, Fischer JE: Amino acid derangements in patients with sepsis: Treatment with branched chain amino acid rich infusions. *Ann Surg* 188:423, 1978.

Furst P, Bergstrom S, Chao L: Influence of amino acid sulphur on nitrogen and amino acid metabolism in severe trauma. *Acta Chir Scand Suppl* 494:136, 1979.

Howard JE, Bingham RS Jr, Mason RE: Studies on convalescence: In nitrogen and mineral balances during starvation and graduated feeding in healthy young males at bed rest. *Trans Assoc Am Physicians* 59:242, 1946.

Keller GA, West MA, et al: Multiple systems organ failure: Modulation of hepatocyte protein synthesis by endotoxin activated Kuppfer cells. *Ann Surg* 201:87, 1985.

Kien CL, et al: Increased rates of whole body protein synthesis and breakdown in children recovering from burns. *Ann Surg* 187:383, 1978.

Kinney JM, Elwyn DH: Protein metabolism and injury. *Annu Rev Nutr* 3:433, 1983.

Kline DL: The effect of hemorrhage on the plasma amino acid nitrogen of the dog. *Am J Physiol* 146:654, 1946.

LaBrosse EH, Beech JA, et al: Plasma amino acids in normal humans and patients with shock. *Surg Gynecol Obstet* 125:516, 1967.

Levenson SJ, Howard J, Rosen J: Studies of the plasma amino acids and amino conjugates in patients with several battle wounds. *Surg Gynecol Obstet* 101:35, 1955.

Levenson SM, Green RW, et al: Ascorbic acid, riboflavin, thiamine, and nicotinic acid in relation to severe injury, hemorrhage and infection in the human. *Ann Surg* 124:840, 1946.

Levenson SM, Pirani CL, et al: The effect of thermal burns on wound healing. *Surg Gynecol Obstet* 99:74, 1954.

Levenson SM, Seifter E, Van Winkle W: Nutrition, in Hunt TK, Dunphy JE (eds): *Fundamentals of Wound Management*. New York, Appleton Century Croft, 1979, p 286.

Long CL, Schiller WR, et al: Muscle protein catabolism in the septic patient as measured by 3-methylhistidine exertion. *Am J Clin Nutr* 30:1349, 1977.

Lund CL, Levenson SM, et al: Ascorbic acid, thiamine, riboflavin and nicotinic acid in relation to acute burns in man. *Arch Surg* 55:557, 1947.

McCoy S, Case SA, et al: Determinants of blood amino acid concentration after hemorrhage. *Ann Surg* 43:787, 1977.

Miller JDB, Bistran BR, Blackburn GL: Failure of postoperative infection to increase nitrogen excretion in patients maintained on peripheral amino acids. *Am J Clin Nutr* 30:1523, 1977.

Moore RN, Goodrum KJ, Berry LJ: Mediation of an endotoxic effect by macrophages. *J Reticuloendothel Soc* 17:187, 1976.

Odessey R, Khairallah EA, Goldberg AL: Origin and probable significance of alanine production by skeletal muscle. *J Biol Chem* 249:7623, 1974.

O'Donnell TF, Clowes GHA, et al: Proteolysis associated with a deficit of peripheral energy fuel substrates in septic man. *Surgery* 80:192, 1976.

O'Keefe SJD, Sender PM, James WPT: Catabolic loss of body nitrogen in response to surgery. *Lancet* 2:1035, 1974.

Plumley DA, Austgen TR, et al: Role of the lungs in maintaining amino acid homeostasis. *JPEN* 14:569, 1990.

Plumley DA, Souba WW, et al: Accelerated lung amino acid release in hyperdynamic septic surgical patients. *Arch Surg* 125:57, 1990.

Ruderman NB, Berger M: The formation of glutamine and alanine in skeletal muscle. *J Biol Chem* 249:5500, 1974.

Russell JA, Long CH, Engel FL: Biochemical studies of shock: The role of peripheral tissues on the metabolism of protein and carbohydrate during hemorrhagic shock in the rat. *J Exp Med* 79:1, 1944.

Shearer J, Morris A, et al: Effect of starvation on the local and systemic metabolic effects of the λ-carrageenan wound. *Am J Surg* 147:456, 1984.

Shizgal HM, Milne CA, Spainer HA: The effect of nitrogen-sparing intravenously administered fluids on postoperative body composition. *Surgery* 86:60, 1979.

Souba WW: Glutamine: A key substrate for the splanchnic bed. *Annu Rev Nutr* 11:285, 1991.

Souba WW: The metabolic role of the gut in the systematic response to injury. *Adv Trauma* 2:269, 1987.

Souba WW, Salloum RM, et al: Cytokine modulation of glutamine transport by pulmonary artery endothelial cells. *Surgery* 110:295, 1991.

Souba WW, Wilmore DW: Postoperative alteration of arteriovenous exchange of amino acids across the gastrointestinal tract. *Surgery* 94:342, 1983.

Stein TP, Leskin MJ, et al: Changes in protein synthesis after trauma: Importance of nutrition. *Am J Physiol* 233:E348, 1976.

West MA, Keller GA, et al: Mechanism of hepatic insufficiency in septic multiple system organ failure. *Surg Forum* 35:44, 1984.

Williamson MB, McCarthy TH, Fromm HJ: Relation of protein nutrition to the healing of experimental wounds. *Proc Soc Exp Biol Med* 77:302, 1957.

Williamson OH, et al: Muscle-protein catabolism after injury in man, as measured by urinary excretion of 3-methyl histidine. *Clin Sci Mol Med* 52:527, 1977.

Wilmore DM, Goodwin CW, et al: Effect of injury and infection on visceral metabolism and circulation. *Ann Surg* 192:491, 1980.

Woolfe LIU: Arterial plasma amino acids in patients with serious postoperative infections and in patients with major fractures. *Surgery* 79:283, 1976.

Electrolyte Metabolism Following Injury

Andersson B: Regulation of body fluids. *Annu Rev Physiol* 39:185, 1977.

Arturson G: Microvascular permeability to macromolecules in thermal injury. *Acta Physiol Scand* 463:111, 1979.

Baxter CR, Shires T: Physiological response to crystalloid resuscitation of severe burns. *Ann NY Acad Sci* 150:874, 1968.

Blalock A: Experimental shock: The cause of low blood pressure caused by muscle injury. *Arch Surg* 20:959, 1930.

Demling RH, Kramer G, Harms B: Role of thermal injury-induced hypoproteinemia on fluid flux and protein permeability in burned and unburned tissue. *Surgery* 95:136, 1984.

Elder JM, Miles AA: The action of the lethal toxins of gas gangrene clostridia on capillary permeability. *J Pathol* 74:133, 1957.

Harms B, Bodai B, et al: Microvascular fluid and protein flux in pulmonary and systemic circulations after thermal injury. *Microvas Res* 23:77, 1982.

Shires GT, Carrico CJ, Cannizaro PC (eds): *Shock. Modern Problems in Clinical Surgery.* Philadelphia, WB Saunders, 1973.

Shires GT III, Peitzman AB, et al: Change in red blood cell transmembrane potential in hemorrhagic shock. *Surg Forum* 32:5, 1981.

Shires T, Williams J, Brown L: Acute changes in extracellular fluids associated with major surgical procedures. *Ann Surg* 154:803, 1961.

Tom WW, Villalba M, et al: Fluorophotometric evaluation of capillary permeability in gram negative-shock. *Arch Surg* 118:636, 1983.

Renal Conservation of Salt and Water

Anderson RJ, Gordon JA, et al: Renal concentration defect following nonoliguric acute renal failure in the rat. *Kidney Int* 21:583, 1979.

Anderson RJ, Linas SL, et al: Nonoliguric renal failure. *N Engl J Med* 296:1134, 1977.

Cantin M, Genest J: The heart and atrial natriuretic factor. *Endocr Rev* 6:1, 1985.

Cochrane JPS: The aldosterone response to surgery and the relationship of this response to postoperative sodium retention. *Br J Surg* 65:744, 1978.

Gill JR Jr, Casper AGT: Effect of renal alpha-adrenergic stimulation on proximal sodium resorption. *Am J Physiol* 223:1201, 1972.

Gill JR Jr, Caspter AGT: Role of sympathetic nervous system in the renal response to hemorrhage. *J Clin Invest* 48:915, 1969.

Hall JE, Guvton AC, Cowley AW Jr: Control of glomerular filtration rate by renin-angiotensin system. *Am J Physiol* 232:F215, 1979.

Itskovitz HD, McGriff JC: Hormonal regulation of renal circulation. *Circ Res* 34/35(suppl I):165, 1974.

Johnson MD, Park CS, Malrin RL: Antidiuretic hormone and the distribution of renal cortical blood flow. *Am J Physiol* 232:F111, 1977.

LeQuesne LP, Cochrane JPS, Fieldman NR: Fluid and electrolyte disturbances after trauma: the role of adrenocortical and pituitary hormones. *Br Med Bull* 41:212, 1985.

Lyons JH, Moore FD: Postraumatic alkalosis: Incidence and pathophysiology of alkalosis in surgery. *Surgery* 60:93, 1966.

Miller PD, Krebs RA, et al: Polyuric prerenal failure. *Arch Intern Med* 140:907, 1980.

Navar AG: Renal autoregulation; perspectives from whole kidney and single nephron studies. *Am J Physiol* 234:F357, 1978.

Navar LG, Ploth DW, Bell PD: Distal tubular feedback control of renal hemodynamics and autoregulation. *Annu Rev Physiol* 42:557, 1980.

Schrier RW: Effects of adrenergic nervous system and catecholamines on systemic and renal hemodynamics, sodium and water excretion and renin secretion. *Kidney Int* 6:291, 1974.

Stein JH, Boonjaren S, et al: Mechanism of the redistribution of renal cortical blood flow during hemorrhagic hypotension in the dog. *J Clin Invest* 52:3, 1973.

Valtin H: *Renal Function: Mechanisms Preserving Fluid and Solute Balance in Health,* 2d ed. Boston, Little, Brown and Company, 1983.

Blood Volume Restitution

Bergentz SE, Brief DD: The effect of pH and osmolality on the production of canine hemorrhagic shock. *Surgery* 58:412, 1965.

Boyd DR, Mansberger AR: Serum water and osmolal changes in hemorrhagic shock. *Am Surg* 34:744, 1968.

Brooks DK, Williams WG, et al: Osmolar and electrolyte changes in hemorrhagic shock. *Lancet* 1:521, 1963.

Byrnes GJ, Pirkle JC Jr, Gann DS: Cardiovascular stabilization after hemorrhage depends upon restitution of blood volume. *J Trauma* 18:623, 1978.

Casley-Smith JR: The functioning and interrelationships of blood capillaries and lymphatics. *Experientia* 32:1, 1976.

Chien S: Role of the sympathetic nervous system in hemorrhage. *Physiol Rev* 47:214, 1967.

Cope O, Litwin SB: Contribution of the lymphatic system to the replenishment of plasma volume following a hemorrhage. *Ann Surg* 156:655, 1962.

Drucker WR, Chadwick CDJ, Gann DS: Transcapillary refill in hemorrhage and shock. *Arch Surg* 116:1344, 1981.

Evans JA, Darlington DN, et al: A circulating factor(s) mediates cell depolarization in hemorrhagic shock. *Ann Surg* 213:549, 1991.

Friedman SG, Pearce FJ, Drucker WR: The role of blood glucose in the defense of plasma volume during hemorrhage. *J Trauma* 22:86, 1982.

Gann DS: Endocrine control of plasma protein and volume. *Surg Clin North Am* 56:1135, 1976.

Gann DS, Carlson DE, et al: Impaired restitution of blood volume after large hemorrhage. *J Trauma* 21:598, 1981.

Gann DS, Carlson DE, et al: Role of solute in the early restitution of blood volume after hemorrhage. *Surgery* 94:439, 1983.

Haddy FJ, Scott JB, Molnar JJ: Mechanisms of volume replacement and vascular constriction following hemorrhage. *Am J Physiol* 208:169, 1965.

Jarhult J, Lundvall J, et al: Osmolar control of plasma volume during hemorrhagic hypotension. *Acta Physiol Scand* 85:142, 1972.

Kenney PR, Allen-Rowlands CF, Gann DS: Glucose and osmolality as predictors of injury severity. *J Trauma* 23:712, 1983.

Leaf A, Cotran R: *Renal Pathophysiology*. New York, Oxford University Press, 1976.

Menguy R, Master YF: Influence of hyperglycemia on survival after hemorrhagic shock. *Adv Shock Res* 1:43, 1979.

Pirkle JC Jr, Gann DS: Expansion of interstitial fluid is required for full restoration of blood volume. *J Trauma* 16:937, 1977.

Pitts RF: *Physiology of the Body Fluids,* 3d ed. Chicago, Yearbook Medical Publishers, 1974.

Quiros G, Ware J: Modification of cardiovascular responses to hemorrhage by induced hyperosmolality in the rat. *Acta Physiol Scand* 117:391, 1983.

Ware J, Ljanquist O, et al: Osmolar changes in hemorrhage. The effect of an altered nutritional status. *Acta Chir Scand* 148:8, 1982.

Weil M, Afifi AA: Experimental and clinical studies on lactate and pyruvate as indicators of the severity of acute circulatory failure. *Circulation* XLI:989, 1970.

Wright FS, Briggs JP: Feedback control of glomerular blood flow, pressure and filtration rate. *Physiol Rev* 59:958, 1979.

Wright HK, Gann DS: A defect in urinary concentrating ability during postoperative anti-diuresis. *Surgery Gynecol Obstet* 121:47, 1965.

Wright HK, Gann DS: Correction of defect in free water excretion in postoperative patients by extracellular fluid volume expansion. *Ann Surg* 158:70, 1963.

CHAPTER 2

Fluid, Electrolyte, and Nutritional Management of the Surgical Patient

G. Tom Shires, G. Tom Shires III, and Stephen F. Lowry

ANATOMY OF BODY FLUIDS

One of the most critical aspects of patient care is management of the body composition of fluid and electrolytes. Most diseases, many injuries, and even operative trauma impose a great impact on the physiology of fluid and electrolytes within the body. These changes often exceed those brought about by acute lack of alimentation. Therefore, a thorough understanding of the metabolism of salt, water, and electrolytes and of certain metabolic responses is essential to the care of surgical patients.

The anatomy of body fluids and the physiologic principles that maintain normal fluid and electrolytes will be defined. In addition, a classification of derangements will be outlined to allow an organized therapeutic approach.

A prerequisite to the understanding of fluid and electrolyte management is knowledge of the extent and composition of the various body fluid compartments. Early attempts to define these compartments were relatively accurate, but a more precise definition has been obtained by many investigators through the use of isotope tracer techniques. The wide range of normal values is a function of body size, weight, and sex, but these compartments are relatively constant in the individual patient in the normal steady state. The figures used in this section, therefore, are approximate and presented as a percentage of body weight.

Total Body Water

Water constitutes between 50 and 70 percent of total body weight. Using deuterium oxide or tritiated water for measurement of total

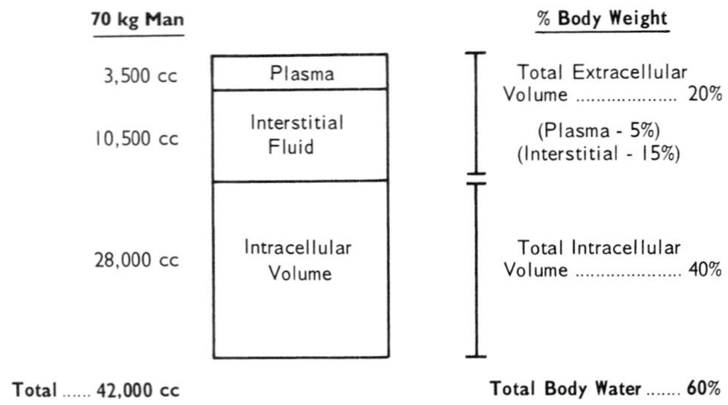

FIG. 2-1. Functional compartments of body fluids.

body water, the average normal value for young adult males is 60 percent of body weight and 50 percent for young adult females. A normal variation of ±15 percent applies to both groups. The actual figure for each healthy individual is remarkably constant and is a function of several variables, including lean body mass and age. Since fat contains little water, the lean individual has a greater proportion of water to total body weight than the obese person. The lower percentage of total body water in females correlates well with a relatively large amount of subcutaneous adipose tissue and small muscle mass. Moore et al. have shown that total body water, as a percentage of total body weight, decreases steadily and significantly with age to a low of 52 and 47 percent in males and females, respectively. Conversely, the highest proportion of total body water to body weight is found in newborn infants, with a maximum of 75 to 80 percent. During the first several months following birth there is a gradual "physiologic" loss of body water as infants adjust to their environment. At 1 year of age, the total body water averages approximately 65 percent of the body weight and remains relatively constant throughout the remainder of infancy and childhood.

The water of the body is divided into three functional compartments (Fig. 2-1). The fluid within the body's diverse cell population represents between 30 and 40 percent of the body weight. The extracellular water represents 20 percent of the body weight and is divided between the intravascular fluid, or plasma (5 percent of body weight), and the interstitial, or extravascular, extracellular fluid (15 percent of body weight).

Intracellular Fluid

Measurement of intracellular fluid is determined indirectly by subtraction of the measured extracellular fluid from the measured total body water. The intracellular water is between 30 and 40 percent of the body weight, with the largest proportion in the skeletal muscle mass. Because of the smaller muscle mass in the female, the percentage of intracellular water is lower than in the male.

The chemical composition of the intracellular fluid is shown in Fig. 2-2, with potassium and magnesium the principal cations, and phosphates and proteins the principal anions. This is an approximation, since so few data concerning the intracellular fluid are available.

Extracellular Fluid

The total extracellular fluid volume represents approximately 20 percent of the body weight. The extracellular fluid compartment

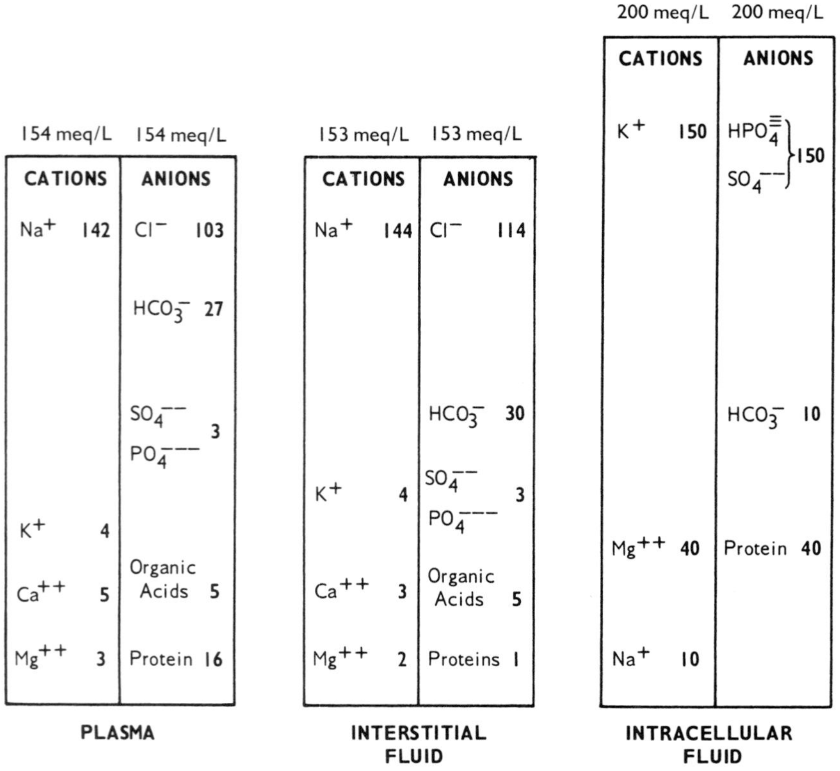

FIG. 2-2. Chemical composition of body fluid compartments.

has two major subdivisions. The plasma volume comprises approximately 5 percent of the body weight in the normal adult. The interstitial, or extravascular, extracellular fluid volume comprises approximately 15 percent of the body weight.

The interstitial fluid is further complicated by having a rapidly equilibrating functional component, as well as several more slowly equilibrating nonfunctioning components. The nonfunctioning components include connective tissue water as well as water that has been termed *transcellular,* which includes cerebrospinal and joint fluids. This nonfunctional component normally represents only 10 percent of the interstitial fluid volume (1 to 2 percent of body weight) and is not to be confused with the *relatively* nonfunctional extracellular fluid, often called a "third space," found in burns and soft tissue injuries.

The normal constituents of the extracellular fluid are shown in Fig. 2-2, with sodium the principal cation, and chloride and bicarbonate the principal anions. There are minor differences in ionic composition between the plasma and interstitial fluid that are primarily due to the difference in protein concentration. Because of the higher protein content (organic anions) of the plasma, the total concentration of cations is higher and the concentration of inorganic anions somewhat lower than in the interstitial fluid, as explained by the Gibbs-Donnan equilibrium equation (i.e., the product of the concentrations of any pair of diffusible cations and anions on one side of a semipermeable membrane will equal the product of the same pair of ions on the other side). For practical consideration, however, they may be considered equal. The total concentration of intracellular ions exceeds that of the extracellular compartment and would seem to violate the concept of osmolar equilibrium between the two compartments. This apparent discrepancy is due to the fact that the concentration of ions is expressed in milliequivalents (meq) without regard to osmotic activity. In addition, some of the intracellular cations probably exist in undissociated form.

Osmotic Pressure

The physiologic and chemical activity of electrolytes depend on (1) the *number of particles* present per unit volume [moles or millimoles (mmol) per liter], (2) the *number of electric charges* per unit volume (equivalents or milliequivalents per liter), and (3) the *number of osmotically active particles* or ions per unit volume [osmoles or milliosmoles (mO) per liter]. The use of the terms *grams* or *milligrams per 100 milliliters* expresses the weight of the electrolytes per unit volume but does not allow a physiologic comparison of the solutes in a solution.

A mole of a substance is the molecular weight of that substance in grams, and a millimole is that figure expressed in milligrams. For example, a mole of sodium chloride is 58 g (Na–23, Cl–35), and a millimole is 58 mg. The expression, however, gives no direct information as to the number of osmotically active ions in solution or the electric charges that they carry.

The electrolytes of the body fluids then may be expressed in terms of chemical combining activity, or "equivalents." An equivalent of an ion is its atomic weight expressed in grams divided by the valence, whereas 1 meq of an ion is that figure expressed in milligrams. In the case of univalent ions, 1 meq is the same as a millimole. In the case of divalent ions, such as calcium or magnesium, 1 mmol equals 2 meq. The importance of this expression is that 1 meq of any substance will combine chemically with 1 meq of any other substance; in any given solution, the number of milliequivalents of cations present is balanced by precisely the same number of milliequivalents of anions.

When the osmotic pressure of a solution is considered, it is more descriptive to employ the terms osmole and milliosmole. These terms refer to the actual number of osmotically active particles present in solution but are not dependent on the chemical combining capacities of the substances. Thus, a millimole of sodium chloride, which dissociates nearly completely into sodium and chloride, contributes 2 mO, and 1 mmol of sodium sulfate (Na_2SO_4), which dissociates into three particles, contributes 3 mO. One millimole of an un-ionized substance such as glucose is equal to 1 mO of the substance.

The differences in ionic composition between intracellular and extracellular fluid are maintained by the semipermeable cell membrane. The total number of osmotically active particles is 290 to 310 mO in each compartment. Although the total osmotic pressure of a fluid is the sum of the partial pressures contributed by each of the solutes in that fluid, the *effective* osmotic pressure is dependent on those substances that fail to pass through the pores of the semipermeable membrane. The dissolved proteins in the plasma, therefore, are primarily responsible for effective osmotic pressure between the plasma and the interstitial fluid compartments. This is frequently referred to as the *colloid oncotic pressure*. The effective osmotic pressure between the extracellular and intracellular fluid compartments would be contributed to by any substance that does not traverse the cell membranes freely. Thus, while sodium as the principal cation of the extracellular fluid contributes a major portion of the osmotic pressure, other substances that fail to penetrate the cell membrane freely, such as glucose, also increase the effective osmotic pressure.

Because the cell membranes are completely permeable to water, the effective osmotic pressures in the two compartments are considered to be equal. Any condition that alters the effective osmotic pressure in either compartment will result in redistribution of water between the compartments. Thus, an increase in effective osmotic pressure in the extracellular fluid, which would occur most frequently as a result of increased sodium concentration, would cause a net transfer of water from the intracellular to the extracellular fluid compartment. This transfer of water would continue until the effective osmotic pressures in the two compartments were equal. Conversely, a decrease in the sodium concentration in the extracellular fluid will cause a transfer of water from the extracellular to the intracellular fluid compartment. Depletion of the extracellular fluid volume without a change in the concentration of ions will not result in transfer of free water from the intracellular space.

Thus, the intracellular fluid shares in losses that involve a change in concentration or composition of the extracellular fluid but shares only slowly in changes involving loss of isotonic volume alone. For practical consideration, most losses and gains of body fluid are directly from the extracellular compartment.

NORMAL EXCHANGE OF FLUID AND ELECTROLYTES

Knowledge of the basic principles governing both the internal and external exchanges of water and salt is mandatory for care of the patient undergoing major operative surgery. The stable internal fluid environment, which is maintained by the kidneys, brain, lungs, skin, and gastrointestinal tract, may be compromised by severe surgical stress or direct damage to any of these organs.

Table 2-1
Water Exchange (60- to 80-kg Man)

Routes	*Average Daily Volume, mL*	*Minimal, mL*	*Maximal, mL*
H_2O gain:			
Sensible:			
Oral fluids	800–1500	0	1500/h
Solid foods	500–700	0	1500
Insensible:			
Water of oxidation	250	125	800
Water of solution	0	0	500
H_2O loss:			
Sensible:			
Urine	800–1500	300	1400/h (diabetes insipidus)
Intestinal	0–250	0	2500/h
Sweat	0	0	4000/h
Insensible:			
Lungs and skin	600	600	1500

Water Exchange

The normal individual consumes an average of 2000 to 2500 mL water/day; approximately 1500 mL water is taken by mouth, and the rest is extracted from solid food, either from the contents of the food or as the product of oxidation (Table 2-1). The daily water losses include 250 mL in stools, 800 to 1500 mL as urine, and approximately 600 mL as insensible loss. A patient deprived of all external access to water must still excrete a minimum of 500 to 800 mL urine/day in order to excrete the products of catabolism, in addition to the mandatory insensible loss through the skin and lungs.

Insensible loss of water occurs through the skin (75 percent) and the lungs (25 percent) and is increased by hypermetabolism, hyperventilation, and fever. The insensible water loss through the skin is not from evaporation of water from sweat glands but from water vapor formed within the body and lost through the skin. With excessive heat production (or excessive environmental heat), the capacity for insensible loss through the skin is exceeded, and sweating occurs. These losses may, but seldom do, exceed 250 mL/day per degree of fever. An unhumidified tracheostomy with hyperventilation increases the loss through the lungs and results in a total insensible loss up to 1.5 L/day.

A frequently overlooked source of gain is the water of solution, which is the water that holds carbohydrates and proteins in solution in the cell. Normally, gain of water from this source is zero, but after 4 to 5 days without food intake, the postoperative patient may begin to gain significant quantities of water (up to 500 mL daily) from excessive cellular catabolism.

Salt Gain and Losses

In the normal individual, the salt intake per day varies between 50 and 90 meq (3 and 5 g) as sodium chloride (Table 2-2). Balance is maintained primarily by the normal kidneys that excrete the excess salt. Under conditions of reduced intake or extrarenal losses, the normal kidney can reduce sodium excretion to less than 1 meq/day within 24 h after restriction. In the patient with salt-wasting kidneys, however, the loss may exceed 200 meq/L of urine. Sweat represents a hypotonic loss of fluids with an average sodium concentration of 15 meq/L in the acclimatized patient. In the unacclimatized individual, the sodium concentration in sweat may be 60 meq/L or more. Insensible fluid lost from the skin and lungs, by definition, is pure water. For practical considerations, then, normal losses may be relatively free of salt in the healthy individual with normal renal function.

Table 2-2
Sodium (Salt) Exchange (60- to 80-kg Man)

Sodium Exchange	*Average*	*Minimal*	*Maximal*
Sodium gain:			
Diet	50–90 meq/day	0	75–100 meq/h oral
Sodium loss:			
Skin (sweat)	10–60 meq/day*	0	300 meq/h
Urine	10–80 meq/day	<1 meq/day†	110–200 meq/L‡
Intestines	0–20 meq/day	0	300 meq/h

*Depending on the degree of acclimatization of the individual.
†With normal renal function.
‡With renal salt wasting.

The volume and composition of various types of gastrointestinal secretions are shown in Table 2-3. Gastrointestinal losses are usually isotonic or slightly hypotonic, although there is considerable variation in the composition. These should be replaced by an essentially isotonic salt solution. It is also important to reiterate that distributional or sequestration losses of extracellular fluid at any point in the operative or postoperative course also represent isotonic losses of salt and water.

CLASSIFICATION OF BODY FLUID CHANGES

The disorders in fluid balance may be classified in three general categories: disturbances of (1) volume, (2) concentration, and (3) composition. Of primary importance is the concept that although these disturbances are interrelated, each is a separate entity.

If an isotonic salt solution is added to or lost from the body fluids, only the *volume* of the extracellular fluid is changed. The acute loss of an isotonic extracellular solution, such as intestinal juice, is followed by a significant decrease in the extracellular fluid volume and little, if any, change in the intracellular fluid volume. Fluid will not be transferred from the intracellular space to refill the depleted extracellular space as long as the osmolarity remains the same in the two compartments.

If water alone is added to or lost from the extracellular fluid, the *concentration* of osmotically active particles will change. Sodium ions account for 90 percent of the osmotically active particles in the extracellular fluid and generally reflect the tonicity of body fluid compartments. If the extracellular fluid is depleted of sodium, water will pass into the intracellular space until osmolarity is again equal in the two compartments.

The concentration of most other ions within the extracellular fluid compartment can be altered without significant change in the total number of osmotically active particles, thus producing only a *compositional* change. For instance, a rise of the serum potassium concentration from 4 to 8 meq/L would have a significant effect on the myocardium, but it would not significantly change the effec-

Table 2-3
Composition of Gastrointestinal Secretions

Type of Secretion	*Volume (mL/24 h)*	*Na (meq/L)*	*K (meq/L)*	*Cl (meq/L)*	*HCO_3 (meq/L)*
Salivary	1500 (500–2000)	10 (2–10)	26 (20–30)	10 (8–18)	30
Stomach	1500 (100–4000)	60 (9–116)	10 (0–32)	130 (8–154)	
Duodenum	(100–2000)	140	5	80	
Ileum	3000 (100–9000)	140 (80–150)	5 (2–8)	104 (43–137)	30
Colon		60	30	40	
Pancreas	(100–800)	140 (113–185)	5 (3–7)	75 (54–95)	115
Bile	(50–800)	145 (131–164)	5 (3–12)	100 (89–180)	35

tive osmotic pressure of the extracellular fluid compartment. Normally functioning kidneys minimize these changes considerably, particularly if the addition or loss of solute or water is gradual.

An internal loss of extracellular fluid into a nonfunctional space, such as the sequestration of isotonic fluid in a burn, peritonitis, ascites, or muscle trauma, is termed a *distributional* change. This transfer or functional loss of extracellular fluid internally may be extracellular (e.g., peritonitis) or intracellular (e.g., hemorrhagic shock) or both (e.g., major burns). In any event, all distributional shifts or losses result in a contraction of the *functional* extracellular fluid space.

Volume Changes

Volume deficit or excess is usually diagnosed by clinical examination of the patient. There are no readily available laboratory tests of benefit in the acute phase except measurement of the plasma volume. Direct measurement of the extracellular fluid volume using radioisotopic tracers is feasible only in a research setting. There are several laboratory tests, however, that indirectly reflect changes in extracellular fluid volume. The blood urea nitrogen (BUN) level rises with an extracellular fluid deficit of sufficient magnitude to reduce glomerular filtration. The serum creatinine may not increase proportionally in young people with healthy kidneys, and this discrepancy is often used as one test to differentiate prerenal and renal azotemia. The concentration of formed elements in the blood, such as the hematocrit, increases with an extracellular fluid deficit and decreases with an extracellular fluid excess. The concentration of serum sodium is *not* related to the volume status of extracellular fluid; a severe volume deficit may exist with a normal, low, or high serum level.

Volume Deficit. Extracellular fluid volume deficit is the most common fluid disorder in the surgical patient. The loss of fluid is not water alone, but water and electrolytes in approximately the same proportion as they exist in normal extracellular fluid. The most common disorders leading to an extracellular fluid volume deficit include losses of gastrointestinal fluids due to vomiting, nasogastric suction, diarrhea, and fistular drainage. Other common causes include sequestration of fluid in soft tissue injuries and infections, intraabdominal and retroperitoneal inflammatory processes, peritonitis, intestinal obstruction, and burns. The signs and symptoms of this state are easily recognized and are listed in Table 2-4. The central nervous system and cardiovascular signs occur early with acute rapid losses, whereas tissue signs may be absent until the deficit has existed for at least 24 h. The central nervous system signs are similar to barbiturate intoxication and may be missed if the volume deficit is mild. The cardiovascular signs are secondary to a decrease in plasma volume and may be associated with varying degrees of hypotension in the patient with a severe extracellular fluid volume deficit. Skin turgor may be difficult to assess in the elderly patient or in the patient with recent weight loss and is not diagnostic in the absence of other confirmatory signs. The body temperature tends to vary with the environmental temperature. In a cool room, the patient may be slightly hypothermic and the febrile response to illness may be suppressed. This occurs frequently and can be very misleading during clinical evaluation of the septic patient. After partial correction of the volume deficit, the temperature will generally rise to the appropriate level. Severe volume depletion depresses all body systems and interferes with the clinical evaluation of a patient. For example, a volume-depleted patient with severe sepsis from peritonitis may have a normal temperature and white blood cell count, complain of little pain, and have unimpressive findings on abdominal examination. The clinical picture may change dramatically, however, as the extracellular fluid volume is restored.

Oliguria is secondary to renal hypoperfusion (prerenal axotemia) and occasionally may be difficult to distinguish from oliguria caused by intrinsic renal disease (renal azotemia). In addition to the patient's history and examination of urinary sediment, the tests of urinary function listed in Table 2-5 may be beneficial. Some of these tests are of limited value in the differential diagnosis of oliguria in elderly patients because of the diminished ability to concentrate urine generally associated with aging.

Volume Excess. Extracellular fluid volume excess may be generally iatrogenic or secondary to renal insufficiency, cirrhosis, or congestive heart failure. Both the plasma and interstitial fluid volumes are increased. In the healthy young adult, the signs are generally those of circulatory overload, manifested primarily in the pulmonary circulation, and of excessive fluid in other tissue (Table 2-4). In the elderly patient, congestive heart failure with pulmonary edema may develop quickly with a moderate volume excess.

Table 2-4
Extracellular Fluid Volume

	Deficit		*Excess*	
Type of Sign	*Moderate*	*Severe*	*Moderate*	*Severe*
Central nervous system	Sleepiness Apathy Slow responses Anorexia Cessation of usual activity	Decreased tension reflexes Anesthesia distal extremities Stupor Coma	None	None
Gastrointestinal	Progressive decrease in food consumption	Nausea, vomiting Refusal to eat Silent ileus and distention	At operation: Edema of stomach, colon, lesser and greater omenta, and small bowel mesentery	
Cardiovascular	Orthostatic hypotension Tachycardia Collapsed veins Collapsing pulse	Cutaneous lividity Hypotension Distant heart sounds Cold extremities Absent peripheral pulses	Elevated venous pressure Distention of peripheral veins Increased cardiac output Loud heart sounds Functional murmurs Bounding pulse High pulse pressure Increased pulmonary 2d sound Gallop	Pulmonary edema
Tissue	Soft, small tongue with longitudinal wrinkling Decreased skin turgor	Atonic muscles Sunken eyes	Subcutaneous pitting edema Basilar rales	Anasarca Moist rales Vomiting Diarrhea
Metabolic	Mild decrease temperature, 97–99°R	Marked decrease temperature, 95–98°R	None	None

Concentration Changes

Sodium is primarily responsible for the osmolarity of the extracellular fluid space: determination of the serum concentration of sodium generally indicates the tonicity of body fluids. Hyponatremia and hypernatremia can be diagnosed on clinical grounds (Table 2-6), but signs and symptoms are not generally present until the changes are severe. Clinical signs of hyponatremia or hypernatremia tend to occur early and with greater severity if the rate of change in extracellular sodium concentration is very rapid. Changes in concentration should be noted early by laboratory tests and corrected promptly.

Hyponatremia. Acute symptomatic hyponatremia (sodium less than 130 meq/L) clinically is characterized by central nervous system signs of increased intracranial pressure and tissue signs of excessive intracellular water. The hypertension is probably induced by the rise in intracranial pressure, since the blood pressure generally returns to normal with the administration of hypertonic solutions of sodium salts. Of importance with severe hyponatremia is the relatively rapid development of oliguric renal failure, which may not be reversible if therapy is delayed.

Many chronic hyponatremic states are asymptomatic until the serum sodium level falls below 120 meq/L. One important exception is the patient with increased cerebrospinal fluid pressure, after closed head injury, in whom mild hyponatremia may be fatal, because of the progressive increase in intracellular water as the extracellular fluid osmolarity falls.

Table 2-5
Oliguria

	Prerenal	*Renal*
Urine osmolality (mO/kgH_2O)	>500	<350
Urine sodium (meq/L)	<20	>40
BUN/serum creatinine	>15	<10
Urine/plasma urea	>8	<3
Urine/plasma creatinine	>40	<20

SOURCE: Adapted from: Miller TR, et al: *Ann Intern Med* 89:47, 1978.

Hypernatremia. Central nervous system and tissue signs characterize acute symptomatic hypernatremia. This is the only state in which dry, sticky mucous membranes are characteristic. This sign does not occur with pure extracellular fluid volume deficit alone and may be misleading in the patient who breathes through the mouth. Body temperature is generally elevated and may approach a lethal level, as in the patient with heatstroke.

While volume changes occur frequently without a change in serum sodium, the reverse is not true. The disease states that cause a significant acute alteration in the serum sodium frequently produce a concomitant change in the extracellular fluid volume.

Mixed Volume and Concentration Abnormalities

Mixed volume and concentration abnormalities may develop as a consequence of the disease state or occasionally may result from inappropriate parenteral fluid therapy. Moyer noted that the clinical picture associated with a combination of fluid abnormalities will tend to be an algebraic composite of the signs and symptoms of each state. Like signs produced by both abnormalities will be

Table 2-6
Acute Changes in Osmolar Concentration

Type of Signs	*Hyponatremia (Water Intoxication)*		*Hypernatremia (Water Deficit)*	
Central nervous system	Moderate: Muscle twitching; Hyperactive tendon reflexes; Increased intracranial pressure (compensated phase)	Severe: Convulsions; Loss of reflexes; Increased intracranial pressure (decompensated) phase)	Moderate: Restlessness; Weakness	Severe: Delirium; Maniacal behavior
Cardiovascular	Changes in blood pressure and pulse secondary to increased intracranial pressure		Tachycardia; Hypotension (if severe)	
Tissue	Salivation, lacrimation, watery diarrhea; "Fingerprinting" of skin (sign of intracellular volume excess)		Decreased saliva and tears; Dry and sticky mucous membranes; Red, swollen tongue; Skin flushed	
Renal	Oliguria progressing to anuria		Oliguria	
Metabolic	None		Fever	

additive, and opposing signs will tend to nullify one another. For example, the tendency for the body temperature to fall with an extracellular volume deficit may be counteracted by the tendency for it to rise with severe hypernatremia.

One of the more common mixed abnormalities is an extracellular fluid deficit and hyponatremia. This state is readily produced in the patient who continues to drink water while losing large volumes of gastrointestinal fluids. It may also occur in the postoperative period when gastrointestinal losses are replaced with inadequate volumes of only 5% dextrose in water or a hypotonic sodium solution. An extracellular volume deficit accompanied by hypernatremia may be produced by the loss of a large amount of hypotonic salt solution, such as sweat, in the absence of fluid intake.

The prolonged administration of excessive quantities of sodium salts with restricted water intake may result in an extracellular volume excess and hypernatremia. This may also occur when pure water losses (such as insensible loss of water from the skin and lungs) are replaced with sodium-containing solutions only. Similarly, the excessive administration of water or hypotonic salt solutions to the patient with oliguric renal failure may rapidly produce an extracellular volume excess and hyponatremia.

Normally functioning kidneys may minimize these changes to some extent and compensate for many of the imprecise replacements associated with parenteral fluid administration. In contrast, the patient in anuric or oliguric renal failure is particularly prone to develop these mixed volume and osmolar concentration abnormalities. Fluid and electrolyte management in these patients, therefore, must be precise. Unfortunately, the fact that a patient with normal kidneys who develops a significant volume deficit may be in a state of "functional" renal failure is often not appreciated. As the volume deficit progresses, the glomerular filtration rate falls precipitously, and the kidneys' unique functions for maintaining fluid homeostasis are lost. These changes may occur with only a mild volume deficit in the elderly patient with borderline renal function. In these elderly patients, the blood urea nitrogen level may rise higher than 100 mg/dL in response to the fluid deficit with a concomitant rise in the serum creatinine level. Fortunately, these changes are usually reversible with early and adequate correction of the extracellular fluid volume deficit.

Composition Changes

Compositional abnormalities of importance include changes in acid-base balance and concentration changes of potassium, calcium, and magnesium.

Acid-Base Balance

The pH (the negative logarithm of the hydrogen ion concentration) of the body fluids is normally maintained within narrow limits in spite of the large load of acid produced endogenously as a by-product of body metabolism. The acids are neutralized efficiently by several buffer systems and subsequently excreted by the lungs and kidneys.

The important buffers include proteins and phosphates, which play a primary role in maintaining intracellular pH, and the bicarbonate-carbonic acid system, which operates principally in the extracellular fluid space. The proteins and hemoglobin have only minor influence in the extracellular fluid space, but the latter is of prime significance as an intracellular buffer in the red cell.

A buffer system consists of a weak acid or base and the salt of that acid or base. The buffering effect is the result of the formation of an amount of weak acid or base equivalent to the amount of strong acid or base added to the system. The resultant change in pH is considerably less than if the substance were added to water alone. Thus, inorganic acids (e.g., hydrochloric, sulfuric, phosphoric) and organic acids (e.g., lactic, pyruvic, keto acids) combine with base bicarbonate producing the sodium salt of the acid and carbonic acid:

$$HCl + NaHCO_3 \longrightarrow NaCl + H_2CO_3$$

The carbonic acid formed is then excreted via the lungs as CO_2. The inorganic acid anions are excreted by the kidneys with hydrogen or as ammonium salts. The organic acid anions generally are metabolized as the underlying disorder is corrected, although some renal excretion may occur with high levels.

The functions of the buffer systems are expressed in the Henderson-Hasselbalch equation, which defines the pH in terms of the ratio of the salt and acid. The pH of the extracellular fluid is defined primarily by the ratio of the amount of base bicarbonate (majority as sodium bicarbonate) to the amount of carbonic acid (related to the CO_2 content of alveolar air) present in the blood:

$$\text{pH} = pK + \log \frac{\text{BHCO}_3}{\text{H}_2\text{CO}_3} = \frac{27 \text{ meq/L}}{1.33 \text{ meq/L}} = \frac{20}{1} = 7.4$$

pK represents the dissociation constant of carbonic acid in the presence of base bicarbonate and by measurement is 6.1. At a body pH of 7.4, the ratio must be 20:1, as depicted. From a chemical standpoint, this is an inefficient buffer system, but the unusual property of CO_2 to behave as an acid or change to a neutral gas subsequently excreted by the lungs makes it quite efficient biologically.

As long as the 20:1 ratio is maintained, regardless of the absolute values, the pH will remain at 7.4. When an acid is added to the system, the concentration of bicarbonate (the numerator in the Henderson-Hasselbalch equation) will decrease. Ventilation will immediately increase to eliminate larger quantities of CO_2 with a subsequent decrease in the carbonic acid (the denominator in the Henderson-Hasselbalch equation) until the 20:1 ratio is reestablished. Slower, more complete compensation is effected by the kidneys with increased excretion of acid salts and retention of bicarbonate. The reverse will occur if an alkali is added to the system. Respiratory acidosis and alkalosis are produced by disturbances of ventilation, with an increase or decrease in the denominator and a resultant change of the 20:1 ratio. Compensation is primarily renal, with a retention of bicarbonate and increased excretion of acid salts in respiratory acidosis and the reverse process in respiratory alkalosis.

The four types of acid-base disturbances are listed in Table 2-7. Use of the CO_2 combining power (approximates the plasma bicarbonate) or CO_2 content (includes bicarbonate, carbonic acid, and dissolved CO_2) and knowledge of the patient's disease may allow an accurate diagnosis in the uncomplicated case. Use of the serum CO_2 content or CO_2 combining power alone is generally inadequate as an index of acid-base balance. This test principally reflects the level of plasma bicarbonate, since dissolved CO_2 and carbonic acid contribute no more than a few millimoles under most circumstances. In the acute phase, therefore, respiratory acidosis or alkalosis may exist without any change in the serum CO_2 content; determinations of the pH and P_{CO_2} from a freshly drawn arterial blood sample are necessary for diagnosis.

Unfortunately, more complex acid-base disturbances are frequently encountered. Combinations of respiratory and metabolic changes occur and may represent compensation for the initial acid-base disturbance or may indicate two or more coexisting primary disorders (Table 2-8).

As previously noted, a knowledge of the pH, bicarbonate concentration, and P_{CO_2} will allow an accurate diagnosis of most acid-base disturbances. However, the clinical interpretation of these measurements is associated with some inherent problems. Although the arterial P_{CO_2} is considered an accurate index of primary respiratory disturbances, changes in the level may represent compensation for a primary metabolic alteration. Thus, a depressed P_{CO_2} (below 40 mmHg) is characteristic of respiratory alkalosis but also represents the normal compensatory response to a metabolic acidosis. Similarly, the level of plasma bicarbonate cannot

Table 2-7
Acidosis-Alkalosis

Type of Acid-Base Disorder	*Defect*	*Common Causes*	$\frac{BHCO_3}{H_2CO_3} = \frac{20}{1}$	*Compensation*
Respiratory acidosis	Retention of CO_2 (Decreased alveolar ventilation)	Depression of respiratory center—morphine, CNS injury Pulmonary disease—emphysema, pneumonia	↑ Denominator Ratio less than 20:1	Renal Retention of bicarbonate, excretion of acid salts, increased ammonia formation Chloride shift into red cells
Respiratory alkalosis	Excessive loss of CO_2 (increased alveolar ventilation)	Hyperventilation: Emotional, severe pain, assisted ventilation, encephalitis	↓ Denominator Ratio greater than 20:1	Renal Excretion of bicarbonate, retention of acid salts, decreased ammonia formation
Metabolic acidosis	Retention of fixed acids or Loss of base bicarbonate	Diabetes, azotemia, lactic acid accumulation, starvation Diarrhea, small bowel fistulae	↓ Numerator Ratio less than 20:1	Pulmonary (rapid) Increase rate and depth of breathing Renal (slow) As in respiratory acidosis
Metabolic alkalosis	Loss of fixed acids Gain of base bicarbonate Potassium depletion	Vomiting or gastric suction with pyloric obstruction Excessive intake of bicarbonate Diuretics	↑ Numerator Ratio greater than 20:1	Pulmonary (rapid) Decrease rate and depth of breathing Renal (slow) As in respiratory alkalosis

Table 2-8
Respiratory and Metabolic Components of Acid-Base Disorders

	Acute (Uncompensated)			Chronic (Partially Compensated)		
Type of Acid-Base Disorder	*pH*	P_{CO_2} *(Respiratory Component)*	*Plasma* HCO_3^-* *(Metabolic Component)*	*pH*	P_{CO_2} *(Respiratory Component)*	*Plasma* HCO_3^-* *(Metabolic Component)*
Respiratory acidosis	↓↓	↑↑	N	↓	↑↑	↑
Respiratory alkalosis	↑↑	↓↓	N	↑	↓↓	↓
Metabolic acidosis	↓↓	N	↓↓	↓	↓	↓
Metabolic alkalosis	↑↑	N	↑↑	↑	↑?	↑

*Measured as standard bicarbonate, whole blood buffer base, CO_2 content, or CO_2 combining power. The *base excess value* is positive when the standard bicarbonate is above normal and negative when the standard bicarbonate is below normal.

be regarded exclusively as an index of metabolic disturbances. An elevated plasma bicarbonate level may indicate a primary metabolic alkalosis or a compensatory response to chronic respiratory acidosis. Astrup and colleagues proposed the use of the standard bicarbonate and base excess values. Base excess (or deficit) directly expresses, in meq/L, the amount of fixed base (or acid) added to each liter of blood. This defines the *metabolic* component of acid-base disorders.

One useful approach to defining pure, combined, or compensated disturbances relates measured changes in P_{CO_2} and pH to calculated changes that would be expected from pure etiologies. Within reasonable physiologic ranges, a 10-torr change in P_{CO_2} yields a 0.08 change in pH from the normal values of P_{CO_2} (40 torr) and pH (7.4).

Respiratory Acidosis. This condition is associated with retention of CO_2 secondary to decreased alveolar ventilation. The more common causes are listed in Table 2-7. Initially, the arterial P_{CO_2} is elevated (usually above 50 mmHg), and the serum bicarbonate concentration (measured as CO_2 content) is normal. In the chronic form, the P_{CO_2} remains elevated, and the bicarbonate concentration rises as renal compensation occurs.

This problem may be particularly serious in the patient with chronic pulmonary disease in whom preexisting respiratory acidosis may be accentuated in the postoperative period. A number of conditions resulting in inadequate ventilation (e.g., airway obstruction, atelectasis, pneumonia, pleural effusion, pain from an upper abdominal incision, or abdominal distention limiting diaphragmatic excursion) may exist singly or in combination to produce respiratory acidosis. Although restlessness, hypertension, and tachycardia in the immediate postoperative period may be due to pain, similar signs indicate inadequate ventilation with hypercapnia. The use of narcotics in this situation will compound the problem by depressing respiration.

Management involves prompt correction of the pulmonary defect, when feasible, and measures to ensure adequate ventilation. Endotracheal intubation and mechanical ventilation are occasionally necessary to achieve this objective. Strict attention to tracheobronchial hygiene during the postoperative period is an important preventive measure in all patients, particularly those with chronic pulmonary disease. Encouraging deep breathing and coughing, using humidified air to prevent inspissation of secretions, and avoiding oversedation are all indicated.

Respiratory Alkalosis. Respiratory alkalosis is a more common problem in the surgical patient than previously recognized. Hyperventilation due to apprehension, pain, hypoxia, central nervous system injury, and assisted ventilation are all common causes. Any of these conditions may cause a rapid decrease in the arterial P_{CO_2} and increase in serum pH. The serum bicarbonate concentration is normal in the acute phase but falls with compensation if the condition persists.

The majority of patients who require ventilatory support in the postoperative period will develop varying degrees of respiratory alkalosis. This may be inadvertent, due to improper use of the mechanical respirator, or it may occur during attempts to raise the P_{O_2} in a hypoxic patient. Proper management of the patient on a mechanical ventilator requires frequent measurements of blood gases and appropriate corrections of the ventilatory pattern when indicated. The arterial P_{CO_2} should not be allowed to fall below 30 mmHg, as serious complications may occur, particularly in the presence of a complicating hypokalemia or metabolic alkalosis. Generally, the P_{CO_2} can be maintained at an acceptable level by proper adjustments of the ventilatory rate and volume.

The dangers of a severe respiratory alkalosis are those related to potassium depletion and include the development of ventricular arrhythmias and fibrillation, particularly in patients who are digitalized or have preexisting hypokalemia. Other complications include a shift of the oxyhemoglobin dissociation curve to the left, which limits the ability of hemoglobin to unload oxygen at the tissue level except at low tissue oxygen tensions, and the development of tetany and convulsions if the level of ionized calcium is significantly depressed. The development of hypokalemia may be quite sudden and is related to entry of potassium ions into the cells in exchange for hydrogen and an excessive urinary potassium loss in exchange for sodium. Severe and persistent respiratory alkalosis is often difficult to correct and may be associated with a poor prognosis because of the underlying cause of hyperventilation. Treatment is primarily directed toward preventing the condition by the proper use of mechanical ventilation and correcting preexisting potassium deficits.

Metabolic Acidosis. Metabolic acidosis results from the retention or gain of fixed acids (diabetic ketoacidosis, lactic acidosis, azotemia) or the loss of base bicarbonate (diarrhea, small bowel fistula, renal insufficiency with inability to resorb bicarbonate). The excess of hydrogen ion results in lower pH and serum bicarbonate concentration. The initial compensation is pulmonary, with an increase of the rate and depth of breathing and depression of the arterial P_{CO_2}.

Renal damage may interfere with the important role of the kidneys in the regulation of acid-base balance. The kidneys serve a vital function in this regard through the excretion of nitrogenous waste products and acid metabolites and the resorption of bicarbonates. If renal damage occurs and these functions are lost, metabolic acidosis develops rapidly and may be difficult to control.

With normal kidneys, metabolic acidosis may develop when the capacity of the kidneys for handling a large chloride is exceeded. This is particularly common in patients who have excessive losses of alkaline gastrointestinal fluids (biliary, pancreatic, small bowel secretions) and are maintained on parenteral fluids for an extended period of time. Continued replacement of these losses with fluids having an inappropriate chloride-bicarbonate ratio, such as isotonic sodium chloride solution, will not correct the pH change; the use of a balanced salt solution, such as lactated Ringer's, is indicated. Anion gap has become a useful tool in the management of acid-base disorders. This value can be determined routinely when evaluating serum electrolytes. The gap is calculated from the sum of serum chloride and bicarbonate subtracted from the serum sodium concentration. The normal value is 10 to 15 meq/L. The anion gap is a laboratory anomaly, since routine clinical laboratory tests measure the cations sodium and potassium and the anions chloride and bicarbonate. The unmeasured anions that account for the "gap" are sulfate and phosphate plus lactate and other organic anions. If the acidosis is due to loss of bicarbonate (e.g., diarrhea) or gain of a chloride acid (e.g., administration of ammonium chloride), the anion gap will be normal. Conversely, if the acidosis is due to increased production of an organic acid (e.g., lactic acid in circulatory shock) or the retention of sulfuric or phosphoric acid (e.g., renal failure), the concentration of unmeasured anions (anion gap) will be increased.

Conditions associated with an elevated anion gap are listed in Table 2-9. The most common cause of an elevated anion gap is shock or inadequate tissue perfusion from any number of causes, resulting in accumulation of large quantities of lactic acid. Diabetic ketoacidosis, starvation, and ethanol intoxication cause elevation of the anion gap by the formation of ketoacids; renal failure and uremia cause such elevation by the retention of sulfuric and phosphoric acids. Poisoning by methanol, ethylene glycol, and aspirin produce increased anion gaps by elevation of their organic acid counterparts (formic, oxalic, and salicylic acids). In a patient with an elevated anion gap, therefore, one or more of these causes should be considered.

One of the most common causes of severe metabolic acidosis in surgical patients is acute circulatory failure with accumulation of lactic acid. This is a reflection of tissue hypoxia due to inadequate perfusion, although it is only one of the manifestations of cellular dysfunction. Acute hemorrhagic shock may result in a rapid and profound drop in the pH, and attempts to raise the blood pressure with vasopressors will simply compound the problem by further compromising tissue perfusion. Similarly, attempts to correct the acidosis by the infusion of large quantities of sodium bicarbonate without restoration of flow are futile. Following restoration of adequate tissue perfusion by proper volume replacement, the lactic acid is quickly metabolized and the pH returned to normal. The use of lactated Ringer's solution to replace the extracellular fluid deficit incurred with hemorrhagic shock concomitant with administration of whole blood does not accentuate the lactic acidosis. Instead, there is a rapid decrease in the serum lactate and return of pH toward normal, which is not the case when whole blood alone is used (Table 2-9).

Table 2-9
Causes of Metabolic Acidosis

Causes	*Mechanisms*
Normal anion gap:	
Diarrhea, small bowel fistula, uterosigmoidostomy	Loss of HCO_3
Proximal renal tubular acidosis	Decreased tubular reabsorption of HCO_3
Distal renal tubular acidosis	Decreased acid excretion
Acid administration (NH_4Cl, HCl)	Increased acid load
"Dilutional" acidosis	Volume expansion with HCO_3^- free fluids
Elevated anion gap:	
Shock (inadequate perfusion)	Increased lactic acid
Diabetes, starvation, alcohol intoxication	Increased keto acids
Uremia	Retention of sulfuric and phosphoric acids
Ingestion of methanol, ethylene glycol, aspirin	Conversion to formic, oxalic, and salicylic acids

The indiscriminate use of sodium bicarbonate during the resuscitation of patients in hypovolemic shock is discouraged for several reasons. A mild metabolic alkalosis is a common finding following resuscitation, in part due to the alkalinizing effects of blood transfusions and the administration of lactated Ringer's solution. After infusion (and partial restoration of hepatic blood flow), the citrate contained in the transfused blood and the lactate in lactated Ringer's solution are metabolized and bicarbonate is formed. The organic acidosis (lactic acid) that developed during the shock episode is rapidly cleared once adequate tissue perfusion is restored. Lactic acid production ceases, the hydrogen ion load is buffered and excreted via the lungs as CO_2, and the organic anion, lactate, is metabolized to bicarbonate by the liver. If excessive quantities of sodium bicarbonate are administered simultaneously, severe metabolic alkalosis can result. An alkaline pH may be highly undesirable in this situation, particularly in patients with hypoxia or low fixed cardiac outputs, because it shifts the oxyhemoglobin dissociation curve to the left. Other factors that tend to shift the oxygen dissociation curve to the left in this situation include the depressed level of erythrocyte 2,3-diphosphoglycerate in the transfused blood and the development of hypothermia. If the curve shifts far enough to the left, significant interference with oxygen unloading at the tissue level may occur.

The treatment of metabolic acidosis, therefore, should be directed toward correction of the underlying disorder when possible. Bicarbonate therapy properly may be reserved for the treatment of severe metabolic acidosis, particularly following cardiac arrest, when partial correction of the pH may be essential to restore myocardial function. Recent studies indicate that the acidosis accompanying cardiac arrest is well compensated for a significant period of time if the patient is well ventilated and not previously acidotic. In addition, the administration of bicarbonate in the usual recommended doses may induce an acute and severe hypernatremia and hyperosmolarity. Thus bicarbonate should be used judiciously during cardiac arrest, the initial dose of bicarbonate not exceeding 50 mL of 7.5% solution (45 meq $NaHCO_3$ containing 90 mO) and the decision for additional doses being based on measurements of pH and P_{CO_2} when possible.

Similarly, pH correction of more protracted states of metabolic acidosis may be indicated but should be accomplished slowly. Frequent measurements of serum electrolytes and blood pH are the best guides to therapy, since a satisfactory formula to estimate the amount of alkali needed has not been devised.

Metabolic Alkalosis. Metabolic alkalosis results from the loss of fixed acids or the gain of bicarbonate and is aggravated by any preexisting potassium depletion. Both the pH and plasma bicarbonate concentration are elevated. Compensation for metabolic alkalosis is primarily by renal mechanisms, since respiratory compensation is generally small and cannot be detected in most patients. Rarely, hypercapnia may represent a compensatory response to metabolic alkalosis in patients without chronic pulmonary disease. When this is suspected, rapid reduction in P_{CO_2} by mechanical ventilation should be avoided. Rather, the P_{CO_2} will fall as the metabolic alkalosis is corrected.

The majority of patients with metabolic alkalosis have some degree of hypokalemia, due in part to influx of potassium ions into the cells, as hydrogen ions efflux into the serum. The dangers of metabolic alkalosis are the same as discussed with respiratory alkalosis.

A problem commonly encountered in the surgical patient is hypochloremic, hypokalemic metabolic alkalosis resulting from persistent vomiting or gastric suction in the patient with pyloric obstruction. Unlike vomiting with an open pylorus involving a combined loss of gastric, pancreatic, biliary, and intestinal secretions, this entity results in loss of fluid with high chloride and hydrogen ion concentrations in relation to sodium. Initially, the urinary excretion of bicarbonate increases to compensate for the alkalosis. This increase in urinary bicarbonate excretion results from net hydrogen ion resorption by the renal tubular cells, with accompanying potassium ion excretion. As the volume deficit progresses, aldosterone-mediated sodium resorption is accompanied by potassium excretion. The resulting hypokalemia leads to excretion of hydrogen ion in place of potassium ion by this mechanism, producing paradoxic aciduria. The net result is a self-perpetuating alkalosis with hypokalemia. Proper management includes replacement of the extracellular fluid volume deficit with isotonic sodium chloride solution in addition to replacement of potassium. Volume repletion should be started and a good urine output obtained before potassium is administered.

Rarely, severe hypokalemic metabolic alkalosis in a patient with pyloric outlet obstruction may be refractory to standard therapy. This occurs most often in patients who also have severe hypochloremia and several liters of nasogastric drainage daily. In the past, the infusion of ammonium chloride or arginine hydrochloride was the usual method for increasing the level of nonvolatile acids. However, infusion of the first may produce ammonia toxicity, and the latter solution is no longer available commercially. Recently, the use of 0.1 *N* to 0.2 *N* hydrochloric acid has been shown to be safe and effective therapy for correction of severe, resistant metabolic alkalosis. The infusion should be administered over a 6- to 24-h period, with measurements of pH, P_{CO_2}, and serum electrolytes every 4 h. Generally, 1 or 2 L of solution over a period of 24 h is sufficient, although one should not hesitate to infuse additional hydrochloric acid when the need is based on appropriate clinical and laboratory evidence. Temporary control of the alkalosis with this method is usually successful, but the underlying cause should be controlled as soon as possible.

Potassium Abnormalities

The normal dietary intake of potassium is approximately 50 to 100 meq daily, and in the absence of hypokalemia, the majority of this is excreted in the urine. Ninety-eight percent of the potassium in the body is located within the intracellular compartment at a concentration of approximately 150 meq/L, and it is the major cation of intracellular water. Although the total extracellular potassium in a 70-kg male would approximate only 63 meq (4.5 meq/L × 14 L), this small amount is critical to cardiac and neuromuscular function. In addition, the turnover rate in the extracellular fluid compartment may be extremely rapid.

The intracellular and extracellular distribution of potassium is influenced by many factors. Significant quantities of intracellular potassium are released into the extracellular space in response to severe injury or surgical stress, acidosis, and the catabolic state. A significant rise in serum potassium may occur in these states in the presence of oliguric or anuric renal failure, but dangerous hyperkalemia (greater than 6 meq/L) is rarely encountered if renal function is normal. After severe trauma, however, normal or excessive urinary volumes may not reflect the ability of the kidney to clear solutes or to excrete potassium. (See the section High-Output Renal Failure.)

Hyperkalemia. The signs of a significant hyperkalemia are limited to the cardiovascular and gastrointestinal systems. The gastrointestinal symptoms include nausea, vomiting, intermittent intestinal colic, and diarrhea. The cardiovascular signs are apparent on the electrocardiogram initially, with high peaked T waves, widened QRS complex, and depressed ST segments. Disappearance of T waves, heart block, and diastolic cardiac arrest may develop with increasing levels of potassium.

Treatment of hyperkalemia consists of immediate measures to reduce the serum potassium level, withholding of exogenous potassium, and correction of the underlying cause if possible. Temporary suppression of the myocardial effects of a sudden rapid rise of potassium level can be accomplished by the intravenous administration of 1 g of 10% calcium gluconate under ECG monitoring. Serum potassium levels may be transiently decreased by administration of bicarbonate and glucose with insulin (45 meq $NaHCO_3$ in 1000 mL/D_{10}W with 20 units regular insulin), both of which promote cellular uptake of potassium. However, the definitive treatment of hyperkalemia requires either the enteral administration of cation exchange resins (kayexalate) or dialysis.

Hypokalemia. The more common problem in the surgical patient is hypokalemia, which may occur as a result of (1) excessive renal excretion, (2) movement of potassium into cells, (3) prolonged administration of potassium-free parenteral fluids with continued obligatory renal loss of potassium (20 meq/day or more), (4) total parenteral hyperalimentation with inadequate potassium replacement, and (5) loss in gastrointestinal secretions.

Potassium plays an important role in the regulation of acid-base balance. Increased renal excretion occurs with both respiratory and metabolic alkalosis. Potassium is in competition with hydrogen ion for renal tubular excretion in exchange for sodium ion. Thus, in alkalosis, the increased potassium ion excretion in exchange for sodium ion permits hydrogen ion conservation. Hypokalemia itself may produce a metabolic alkalosis, since an increase in excretion of hydrogen ions occurs when the concentration of potassium in the tubular cell is low. In addition, movement of hydrogen ions into the cells as a consequence of potassium loss is partly responsible for the alkalosis. In metabolic acidosis the reverse process occurs, and the excess hydrogen ion exchanges for sodium with retention of greater amounts of potassium.

Renal tubular excretion of potassium ion is increased when large quantities of sodium are available for excretion. The more sodium ion available for resorption, the more potassium is exchanged for it in the lumen. Potassium requirements for prolonged or massive isotonic fluid volume replacement are increased, probably on this basis.

The renal excretion of potassium may be small when compared with the amount of potassium that may be lost in gastrointestinal secretions. The amount per liter in various types of gastrointestinal fluids is shown in Table 2-3. Although the average potassium concentration of some of these fluids is relatively low, significant hypokalemia will result if potassium-free fluids are used for replacement.

Hypokalemia also may be a serious problem in the patient maintained on intravenous nutrition. Large quantities of supplemental potassium generally are necessary to restore depleted intracellular stores and to meet the requirements for tissue synthesis during the anabolic phase.

In summary, most of the factors that tend to influence potassium metabolism result in excess excretion, and a tendency toward hypokalemia occurs frequently in the surgical patient except when shock or acidosis interferes with the normal renal handling of potassium.

The signs of potassium deficit are related to failure of normal contractility of skeletal, smooth, and cardiac muscle and include weakness that may progress to flaccid paralysis, diminished to absent tendon reflexes, and paralytic ileus. Sensitivity to digitalis with cardiac arrhythmias and electrocardiographic signs of low voltage, flattening of T waves, and depression of ST segments are characteristic. Signs of potassium deficit may be masked by those of a severe extracellular fluid volume deficit. Repletion of the volume deficit may further aggravate the situation by lowering the serum potassium level secondary to dilution.

The treatment of hypokalemia involves, first, prevention of this state. In the replacement of gastrointestinal fluids, it is safe to replace the upper limits of loss, since an excess is readily handled by the patient with normal renal function. No more than 40 meq should be added to a liter of intravenous fluid, and the rate of administration should not exceed 40 meq/h unless the electrocardiogram is being monitored. In the absence of specific indications, potassium should not be given to the oliguric patient or during the first 24 h following severe surgical stress or trauma.

Calcium Abnormalities

The majority of the 1000 to 1200 g of body calcium in the average-sized adult is found in the bone in the form of phosphate and carbonate. Normal daily intake of calcium is between 1 and 3 g. Most of this is excreted via the gastrointestinal tract, and 200 mg or less is excreted in the urine daily. The normal serum level is between 8.5 and 10.5 mg/dL, and approximately half of this is not ionized and is bound to plasma protein. An additional nonionized fraction (5 percent) is bound to other substances in the plasma and interstitial fluid, whereas the remaining 45 percent is the ionized portion that is responsible for neuromuscular stability. Determination of the plasma protein level, therefore, is essential for proper analysis of the serum calcium level. The ratio of ionized to nonionized calcium is also related to the pH; acidosis causes an increase in the ionized fraction, whereas alkalosis causes a decrease.

Disturbances of calcium metabolism generally are not a problem in the uncomplicated postoperative patient, with the exception of skeletal loss during prolonged immobilization. Routine administration of calcium to the surgical patient, therefore, is not needed in the absence of specific indications.

Hypocalcemia. The symptoms of hypocalcemia may be seen at serum levels less than 8 mg/dL and include numbness and tingling of the circumoral region and the tips of the fingers and toes. The signs are of neuromuscular origin and include hyperactive tendon reflexes, positive Chvostek's sign, muscle and abdominal cramps, tetany with carpopedal spasm, convulsions (with severe deficit), and prolongation of the Q-T interval on the electrocardiogram.

The common causes include acute pancreatitis, massive soft tissue infections (necrotizing fasciitis), acute and chronic renal failure, pancreatic and small intestinal fistulas, and hypoparathyroidism. Transient hypocalcemia is a frequent occurrence in the hyperparathyroid patient following removal of a parathyroid adenoma, owing to atrophy of the remaining glands and avid bone uptake. Asymptomatic hypocalcemia may occur with hypoproteinemia (normal ionized fraction), whereas symptoms may appear with a normal serum calcium level in a patient with severe alkalosis. The latter is due to a decrease in the physiologically active or ionized fraction of total serum calcium. Calcium levels also may fall with a severe depletion of magnesium.

Treatment is directed toward correction of the underlying cause with concomitant repletion of the deficit. Acute symptoms may be relieved by the intravenous administration of calcium gluconate or calcium chloride. Calcium lactate may be given orally, with or without supplemental vitamin D, in the patient requiring prolonged replacement. The routine administration of calcium during massive transfusions of blood remains controversial and reflects a paucity of studies where calcium *ion* levels are measured. In the majority of studies, calcium ion concentrations have been estimated from measured *total* serum calcium levels. Presently, available data indicate that the majority of patients receiving blood transfusions do not require calcium supplementation. The binding of ionized calcium by citrate is generally compensated for by the mobilization of calcium from body stores. For patients receiving blood as rapidly as 500 mL every 5 to 10 min, however, calcium administration is recommended. An appropriate dose, from the data of Moore, is 0.2 g of calcium chloride (2 mL of 10% calcium chloride solution), administered intravenously in a separate line, for every 500 mL of blood transfused. To avoid dangerous levels of hypercalcemia, this dose of calcium is recommended only while blood is being transfused at the rate noted above. Additionally, the total dose of calcium generally should not exceed 3 g unless there is objective evidence of hypocalcemia. Larger doses are rarely indicated since there is some mobilization of calcium and citrate breakdown with release of calcium ion even with shock and inadequate peripheral perfusion. During massive transfusions, some attempt should be made to monitor the calcium level. A rough approximation of calcium ion concentration can be obtained by monitoring the Q-T interval on the ECG, although techniques for the rapid measurement of calcium ion concentration are now available.

Hypercalcemia. The symptoms of hypercalcemia are rather vague and of gastrointestinal, renal, musculoskeletal, and central nervous system origin. The early manifestations of hypercalcemia include easy fatigue, lassitude, weakness of varying degree, anorexia, nausea, vomiting, and weight loss. With higher serum calcium levels, lassitude gives way to somnambulism, stupor, and finally coma. Other symptoms include severe headaches, pains in the back and extremities, thirst, polydipsia, and polyuria. The critical level for serum calcium is greater than 15 mg/dL, and unless treatment is instituted promptly, the symptoms may rapidly progress to death. The two major causes of hypercalcemia are hyperparathyroidism and cancer with bony metastasis. The latter is most frequently seen in the patient with metastatic breast cancer who is receiving estrogen therapy.

A serum calcium concentration of 15 mg/dL or higher requires emergency treatment. Most patients have an extracellular fluid volume deficit due to the effects of hypercalcemia (vomiting, polyuria), and vigorous volume repletion with salt solutions lowers the calcium level by dilution and increased urinary calcium excretion. Rapid correction of the associated extracellular fluid volume deficit will immediately lower the serum calcium level by dilution and by increased renal clearance that may be augmented by furosemide administration.

Oral or intravenous inorganic phosphates effectively lower serum calcium by inhibiting bone resorption and forming calcium-phosphate complexes that are deposited in soft tissues and bone. Intravenous use may cause an abrupt fall in calcium, however, and tetany, hypotension, and acute renal failure have been reported with this form of therapy. If used, intravenous phosphorus should be given slowly over a period of approximately 12 h once daily for no more than 2 or 3 days. Inorganic phosphates are contraindicated in patients with hyperphosphatemia or renal failure. Intravenous sodium sulfate will also lower serum calcium by increasing urinary excretion of this ion. It is less effective than phosphate salts, however, and is probably no more effective than normal saline.

Corticosteroids decrease resorption of calcium from bone and reduce the intestinal absorption of vitamin D. They have been found useful in treating hypercalcemic patients with sarcoidosis, myelomas, lymphomas, and leukemias, although the reduction in serum calcium may not be apparent for 1 or 2 weeks. Mithramycin, a cytotoxic drug, effectively lowers serum calcium in 24 to 48 h by direct action on the bones. The drug is relatively safe in the small doses used, and the calcium level may remain normal for several days to weeks following a single dose. Calcitonin induces a moderate decrease in serum calcium, but the effect is diminished with repeated administration. The definitive treatment of acute hypercalcemic crisis in patients with hyperparathyroidism is immediate surgery.

Treatment of hypercalcemia in the patient with metastatic cancer is primarily that of prevention. The serum calcium level is checked frequently; if it is elevated, the patient is placed on a low-calcium diet, and measures to ensure adequate hydration are instituted.

Magnesium Abnormalities

The total body content of magnesium in the average adult is approximately 2000 meq, about half of which is incorporated in bone and only slowly exchangeable. The distribution of magnesium is similar to that of potassium, the major portion being intracellular. Serum magnesium concentration normally ranges between 1.5 and 2.5 meq/L. The normal dietary intake of magnesium is approximately 20 meq (240 mg) daily. The larger part is excreted in the feces, and the remainder in the urine. The kidneys show a remarkable ability to conserve magnesium; on a magnesium-free diet, renal excretion of this ion may be less than 1 meq/day.

Magnesium Deficiency. Magnesium deficiency is known to occur with starvation, malabsorption syndromes, protracted losses of gastrointestinal fluid, and prolonged intravenous fluid therapy with magnesium-free solutions, and during total parenteral nutrition when inadequate quantities of magnesium have been added to the solutions. Other causes include acute pancreatitis, treatment of diabetic ketoacidosis, primary aldosteronism, chronic alcoholism, amphotericin B therapy, and a protracted course following thermal injury.

The magnesium ion is essential for proper function of most enzyme systems, and depletion is characterized by neuromuscular and central nervous system hyperactivity. The signs and symptoms are quite similar to those of calcium deficiency, including hyperactive tendon reflexes, muscle tremors, and tetany with a positive Chvostek sign. Progression to delirium and convulsions may occur with a severe deficit. A concomitant calcium deficiency occasionally is noted and will be refractory to treatment in the absence of magnesium repletion.

The diagnosis of magnesium deficiency depends on an awareness of the syndrome and clinical recognition of the symptoms. Laboratory confirmation is available but not reliable, as the syndrome may exist in the presence of a normal serum magnesium level. The possibility of magnesium deficiency should always be considered in the surgical patient who exhibits disturbed neuromuscular or cerebral activity in the postoperative period. This is particularly important in patients who have had protracted dysfunction of the gastrointestinal tract with long-term maintenance on parenteral fluids and in patients on parenteral hyperalimentation. Routine magnesium is always indicated in the management of these patients.

Treatment of magnesium deficiency is by the parenteral administration of magnesium sulfate or magnesium chloride solution. If renal function is normal, as much as 2 meq of magnesium/kg of body weight can be administered daily by the intravenous or intramuscular route in the face of severe depletion. The intravenous route is preferable for the initial treatment of a severe symptomatic deficit. The solution is prepared by the addition of 80 meq of magnesium sulfate (20 mL of 50% solution containing 4 meq/mL magnesium) to a liter of intravenous fluid and is administered over a 4-h period. If the patient is not symptomatic, the infusion should be given over a longer period of time. The possibility of acute magnesium toxicity should be kept in mind when giving this ion intravenously. When large doses are given, the heart rate, blood pressure, respiration, and ECG should be monitored closely for signs of magnesium toxicity, which could lead to cardiac arrest. It is advisable to have calcium chloride or calcium gluconate available to counteract any adverse effects of a rapidly rising serum magnesium level.

Partial or complete relief of symptoms may follow this infusion as a result of increased concentration of magnesium ion in the extracellular fluid compartment, although continued replacement over a 1- to 3-week period is necessary to replenish the intracellular compartment. For this purpose and for the asymptomatic patient who may have significant magnesium depletion, 10 to 20 meq of 50% magnesium sulfate solution may be given daily by the intramuscular route, in intravenous fluids, or orally as magnesium oxide (800 mg). When intramuscular magnesium sulfate is used, it should be given in divided doses or at multiple sites, since the intramuscular injection of this salt is painful. After complete repletion of intracellular magnesium and in the absence of abnormal loss, balance may be maintained by the administration of as little as 4 meq of magnesium ion daily. The amount of magnesium supplementation required for patients on parenteral hyperalimentation varies but approximates 12 to 24 meq daily for the average patient.

Magnesium ion should not be given to the oliguric patient or in the presence of severe volume deficit unless actual magnesium depletion is demonstrated. If given to a patient with renal insufficiency, considerably smaller dosages are used, and the patient is carefully observed for signs or symptoms of toxicity.

Magnesium Excess. Symptomatic hypermagnesemia, although rare, is most commonly seen with severe renal insufficiency. Retention and accumulation of magnesium may occur in any patient with impaired glomerular or renal tubular function, and the presence of acidosis may rapidly compound the situation. Serum magnesium levels tend to parallel changes in potassium concentration in these cases. In patients on ordinary dietary intakes of magnesium, increased serum concentrations of the ion do not occur until the glomerular filtration rate falls below 30 mL/min. Magnesium-containing antacids and laxatives (milk of magnesia, epsom salts, Gelusil, Maalox) are commonly administered in quantities sufficient to produce toxic serum levels of magnesium where impaired renal function is present. Other conditions that may be associated with symptomatic hypermagnesemia include early thermal injury, massive trauma or surgical stress, severe extracellular volume deficit, and severe acidosis.

The early signs and symptoms include lethargy and weakness with progressive loss of deep tendon reflexes. Interference with cardiac conduction occurs with increasing levels of magnesium and changes in the ECG (increased P-R interval, widened QRS complex, and elevated T waves) resemble those seen with hyperkalemia. Somnolence leading to coma and muscular paralysis occur in the later stages, and death is usually caused by respiratory or cardiac arrest.

Treatment consists of immediate measures to lower the serum magnesium level by correcting coexisting acidosis, replenishing preexisting extracellular volume deficit, and withholding exogenous magnesium. Acute symptoms may be temporarily controlled by the slow intravenous administration of 5 to 10 meq of calcium chloride or calcium gluconate. If elevated levels or symptoms persist, peritoneal dialysis or hemodialysis is indicated.

FLUID AND ELECTROLYTE THERAPY

Parenteral Solutions

There are many electrolyte solutions of varied compositions that are available for parenteral administration (Table 2-10). Several of the more commonly used solutions are discussed below. Choice of a particular fluid depends on the volume status of the patient and the type of concentration or compositional abnormality present.

A cost-effective extracellular "mimic" of isotonic salt solution for replacing gastrointestinal losses and extracellular fluid volume deficits, in the absence of gross abnormalities of concentration and composition, is lactated Ringer's solution. This solution is physiologic and contains 130 meq of sodium balanced by 109 meq of chloride and 28 meq of lactate. Lactate is used instead of bicarbonate, since the former is more stable in intravenous fluids during storage. The lactate is readily converted to bicarbonate by the liver following infusion. Concern about the ability of the liver to metabolize lactate is unwarranted even when infusing large quantities of lactated Ringer's solution to patients in hemorrhagic shock. This fluid has minimal effects on normal body fluid composition and pH even when infused in large quantities. There are other balanced salt solutions available, some with sodium acetate or bicarbonate instead of lactate; all are considered interchangeable.

Isotonic sodium chloride contains 154 meq of sodium and 154 meq of chloride per liter. The high concentration of chloride above the normal serum concentration of 103 meq/L imposes on the kidneys an appreciable load of excess chloride that cannot be rapidly excreted. Thus, a dilutional acidosis may develop by reducing base bicarbonate relative to carbonic acid. This solution is ideal, however, for the initial correction of an extracellular fluid volume deficit in the presence of hyponatremia, hypochloremia, and metabolic alkalosis. In a similar situation with moderate metabolic acidosis, M/6 sodium lactate (167 meq/L each of sodium and lactate) may be given.

For maintenance fluid in the postoperative period, 0.45% sodium chloride in 5% dextrose solution is often used to provide free water for insensible losses and some sodium for renal adjustment of serum concentration. With added potassium, this is a reasonable solution to use for maintenance requirements in an uncomplicated patient requiring only a short period of parenteral fluids.

Preoperative Fluid Therapy

Preoperative evaluation and correction of existing fluid disorders is an integral part of surgical care. An orderly approach to these problems requires an understanding of the common fluid disturbances associated with surgical illness and adherence to a few simple guidelines.

The analysis of a particular fluid disorder may be facilitated by categorizing the abnormalities into volume, concentration, and compositional changes. Although some disease states produce characteristic changes in fluid balance, much confusion may be avoided by regarding each disturbance as a separate entity. There are no shortcuts; close observation of the patient and frequent reevaluation of the clinical situation is the most rewarding approach. For example, volume changes cannot be accurately predicted from a knowledge of the level of serum sodium, since an extracellular fluid volume deficit or excess may exist with a normal, low, or

Table 2-10
Composition of Parenteral Fluids (Electrolyte Content, meq/L)

	Cations				*Anions*		
Solutions	*Na*	*K*	*Ca*	*Mg*	*Cl*	*HCO_3*	*Osmolality, mO*
Extracellular fluid	142	4	5	3	103	27	280–310
Lactated Ringer's	130	4	3	—	109	28*	273
0.9% sodium chloride	154	—	—	—	154	—	308
D_5 45% sodium chloride	77	—	—	—	77	—	407
D_5W	—	—	—	—	—	—	253
M/6 sodium lactate	167	—	—	—	—	167*	334
3% sodium chloride	513	—	—	—	513	—	1026

*Present in solution as lactate that is converted to bicarbonate.

high sodium concentration. Similarly, any of the four primary acid-base disturbances may be associated with any combination of volume and concentration abnormalities.

Correction of Volume Changes

Changes in the volume of extracellular fluid are the most frequent and important abnormalities encountered in the surgical patient. Depletion of the extracellular fluid compartment without changes in concentration or composition is a common problem. The diagnosis of volume changes is made almost entirely on clinical grounds. The signs that will be present in an individual patient depend not only on the relative or absolute quantity of extracellular fluid that has been lost but also on the rapidity with which it is lost and the presence or absence of signs of associated disease.

Volume deficits in the surgical patient may result from external loss of fluids or from an internal redistribution of extracellular fluid into a nonfunctional compartment. Generally, it involves a combination of the two, but the internal redistribution is frequently overlooked.

The phenomenon of internal redistribution or translocation of extracellular fluid is peculiar to many surgical diseases; in the individual patient, the loss may be quite large. Although the concept of a ''third space'' is not new, it is generally considered only in relation to patients with massive ascites, burns, or crush injuries. Of more importance, however, is the third-space loss into the peritoneum, the bowel wall, and other tissues with inflammatory lesions of the intraabdominal organs. The magnitude of these losses may not be fully appreciated without realization of the fact that the peritoneum alone has approximately 1 m^2 of surface area. A slight increase in thickness from sequestration of fluid, which would not be appreciated on casual observation, may result in a functional loss of several liters of fluid. Swelling of the bowel wall and mesentery and secretion of fluid into the lumen of the bowel will cause even larger losses. Similar deficits may occur with massive infection of the subcutaneous tissues (necrotizing fasciitis) or with severe crush injury.

These ''parasitic'' losses remain a part of the extracellular fluid space and may be measured as a slowly equilibrating volume. The term *nonfunctional* is used because the fluid is no longer able to participate in the normal functions of the extracellular compartment and may just as well have been lost externally. Any transfer of intracellular fluid to the extracellular compartment for replenishment of the loss is insignificant in the acute phase. The patient with ascites may have an enormous total extracellular fluid volume although the functional component is severely depleted. The same is true of extensive inflammatory or obstructive lesions of the gastrointestinal tract, although the loss is not as obvious. These losses will evoke the signs and symptoms of an extracellular fluid volume deficit with or without the concomitant external loss of fluids.

Exact quantification of these deficits is impossible and, at the present time, probably unnecessary. The defect can be estimated on the basis of the severity of the clinical signs. A mild deficit represents a loss of approximately 4 percent of body weight, a moderate loss is 6 to 8 percent of body weight, and a severe deficit is approximately 10 percent of body weight. It is important to reemphasize the fact that cardiovascular signs predominate when there is acute rapid loss of fluid from the extracellular fluid compartment with few or no tissue signs. In addition to the estimated deficit, fluids lost during the period of treatment must be replaced.

Immediately following diagnosis of a volume deficit, prompt fluid replacement with a balanced salt solution should be started. Continuing therapy is tailored to the response of the patient, based on frequent clinical examination. Reliance on a formula or single clinical sign to determine adequacy of resuscitation is fraught with danger. Rather, reversal of the signs of the volume deficit, combined with stabilization of the blood pressure and pulse, and an hourly urine volume of 30 to 50 mL are used as general guidelines. An adequate hourly urine output, although usually a reliable index of volume replacement, may be totally misleading. The excessive administration of glucose (over 50 g in a 2- to 3-h period) may result in osmotic diuresis, while an osmotic agent such as mannitol tends to produce urine at the expense of the vascular volume. Patients with chronic renal disease or incipient acute renal damage from shock and injury also may have inappropriately high urinary volumes. In addition, the rapid administration of salt solutions may transiently expand the intravascular volume, increase the glomerular filtration rate, and result in an immediate outpouring of urine, although the total extracellular fluid space remains quite depleted.

The choice of the proper fluid for replacement depends on the existence of concomitant concentration or compositional abnormalities. With pure extracellular fluid volume loss or when only minimal concentration or compositional abnormalities are present, the use of a balanced salt solution, such as lactated Ringer's, is desirable.

Rate of Fluid Administration. This varies considerably, depending on the severity and type of fluid disturbance, the presence of continuing losses, and the cardiac status. In general, the most severe volume deficits may be safely replaced initially with isotonic solutions at rates up to 2000 mL/h, reducing the rate as the fluid status improves. Constant observation by a physician is mandatory when the administration exceeds 1000 mL/h. At these rates, a significant portion may be lost as urinary output owing to a transient overexpansion of the plasma volume.

In elderly patients, associated cardiovascular disorders do not preclude correction of existing volume deficits, but they do require slower, more careful correction with constant monitoring of the cardiopulmonary system. If urinary output is not promptly restored, this may require measurements of central filling pressures and cardiac output to prevent ongoing renal injury from overcautious volume restoration.

Correction of Concentration Changes

If severe *symptomatic* hyponatremia or hypernatremia complicates the volume loss, prompt correction of the concentration abnormality to the extent that symptoms are relieved is necessary. Volume replenishment should be accomplished with slower correction of the remaining concentration abnormality. For immediate correction of severe hyponatremia, 5% sodium chloride solution or molar sodium lactate solution is used, depending on the patient's acid-base status. In any case, the sodium deficit can be estimated by multiplying the decrease in serum sodium concentration below normal (in milliequivalents per liter) by the liters of total body water. Initially, up to one-half of the calculated amount of sodium may be administered slowly, followed by clinical and chemical reevaluation of the patient before any additional infusion of sodium salts.

Note that this estimate is based on total body water, since the effective osmotic pressure in the extracellular compartment cannot be increased without increasing this function proportionately in the intracellular compartment. Although absolute reliance on any formula is undesirable, proper use of this estimate will allow a safe quantitative approximation of the sodium deficit. Generally, only a portion of the total deficit is replaced initially to relieve acute symptoms. Further correction is facilitated when renal function is restored by correction of the volume deficit. If the total calculated deficit were given rapidly, severe hypervolemia might occur particularly in patients with limited cardiac reserve. In practice, the infusion of small, successive increments of hypertonic saline solution with frequent evaluation of the clinical response and serum sodium concentration is recommended.

In the treatment of moderate hyponatremia with an associated volume deficit, volume replacement can be started immediately with concomitant correction of the serum sodium deficit. Isotonic sodium chloride solution (normal saline) is used initially in the presence of metabolic alkalosis, whereas M/6 sodium lactate (167 meq/L each of sodium and lactate) is used to correct an associated acidosis. Only a few liters of these solutions may be necessary to correct the serum sodium concentration; the remainder of the volume deficit may be replaced with lactated Ringer's solution.

Treatment of hyponatremia associated with volume excess is by restriction of water. In the presence of severe symptomatic hyponatremia, a small amount of hypertonic salt solution may be infused cautiously to alleviate symptoms. As this will cause additional volume expansion, it is contraindicated in patients with limited cardiac reserve; peritoneal dialysis or hemodialysis is preferred in this situation.

For the correction of severe, symptomatic hypernatremia with an associated volume deficit, 5% dextrose in water may be infused slowly until symptoms are relieved. If the extracellular osmolarity is reduced too rapidly, however, convulsions and coma may result. For this reason, correction of hypernatremia concomitant with repletion of the volume deficit by half-strength sodium chloride or half-strength lactated Ringer's solution is safer in most cases. In the absence of a significant volume deficit, water should be administered cautiously since dangerous hypervolemia may result; constant observation and frequent determinations of the serum sodium concentration are indicated. The problem is somewhat simplified once a sufficient quantity of fluid has been given to permit renal excretion of the solute load.

Composition and Miscellaneous Considerations

Correction of existing potassium deficits should be started *after* an adequate urine output is obtained, particularly in the patient with metabolic alkalosis since this may be secondary to or aggravated by potassium depletion. Calcium and magnesium rarely are needed during preoperative resuscitation but should be given as indicated, particularly to patients with massive subcutaneous infections, acute pancreatitis, or chronic starvation.

Fluid abnormalities also must be suspected in the patient for whom an elective procedure is planned. Chronic illnesses frequently are associated with extracellular fluid volume deficits, and concentration and compositional changes are not uncommon. Correction of anemia and recognition of the fact that a concentrated blood volume may exist in the chronically debilitated patient is of obvious importance. The hematocrit increases approximately 3 percent after the infusion of one unit of packed cells into the adult of average size. The increase may be significantly greater in the patient with a contracted intravascular volume, indicating the need for concurrent volume replacement. Of additional importance is the prevention of volume depletion during the preoperative period. Prolonged periods of fluid restriction in preparation for various diagnostic procedures, the use of cathartics and enemas for preparation of the bowel, and osmotic diuresis from contrast agents may cause a significant acute loss of extracellular fluid. Prompt recognition and treatment of these losses before surgery is necessary to prevent complications during the operative period.

Of additional importance is the prevention of volume depletion during the preoperative period. Prolonged periods of fluid restriction in preparation for various diagnostic procedures, and the use of cathartics and enemas for preparation of the bowel may cause a significant acute loss of extracellular fluid. Prompt recognition and treatment of these losses is necessary to prevent complications during the operative period.

Intraoperative Fluid Management

If preoperative replacement of extracellular fluid volume has been incomplete, hypotension may develop promptly with the induction of anesthesia. This can be quite insidious, as the ability of the awake patient to compensate for mild volume deficit is revealed only when the compensatory mechanisms are abolished with anesthesia. This problem is prevented by maintaining base-line requirements and replacing abnormal losses of fluids and electrolytes by intravenous infusions in the preoperative period.

In addition to blood losses during operation, there appears to be extracellular fluid losses during major operative procedures. Some of these, including edema from extensive dissection, collections within the lumen and wall of the small bowel, and accumulations of fluid in the peritoneal cavity, are clinically discernible and well recognized. They generally are felt to represent distributional shifts, in that the functional volume of extracellular fluid is reduced but not externally lost from the body. These functional losses are often referred to as "parasitic losses, third space edema, or sequestration" of extracellular fluid. Another source of extracellular fluid loss during major operative trauma is the wound itself. This is a relatively smaller loss and very difficult to quantify except in extensive and major operative procedures.

At the beginning of this century, surgeons became aware that many changes occurred in urinary output, blood volume, and fluid and electrolyte composition during and after surgery. Assessment of these changes, however, awaited the development of analytic techniques and their application to patient studies. In the following 25 years, saline solutions in varying combinations were given to patients undergoing operation, often in excessive amounts. Work in the late 1930s and early 1940s by Moyer and by many others indicated that during and after operative procedures, saline and water solutions should be withheld entirely, because most of the fluid administered was retained.

The possibility existed that the operative and postoperative retention of salt and water administered in relatively small amounts might simply be physiologic retention to replace a deficit of salt and water incurred by the operative procedure. Subsequent studies have revealed that functional extracellular fluid decreases with major abdominal operations, largely as sequestered loss into the operative site. This extracellular fluid volume deficit can be replaced during the operative procedure. These data have led to the conclusion that the need for an extracellular "mimic" in the form of balanced salt solution now can be clinically estimated. Intraoperative correction of the volume deficit with salt solution markedly reduces postoperative oliguria, but is not intended to substitute for blood replacement. Rather, it is felt to be a physiologic supplement, or adjunct, to replace sequestered losses.

Thus, the pendulum has swung from indiscriminate use of salt solutions in the first quarter of this century to almost total withholding of fluid and electrolytes from surgical patients in the second quarter of the century; indications at present are that proper management lies somewhere between these two extremes. Some guidelines are necessary for the intraoperative administration of saline solutions as a "mimic" for the sequestered extracellular fluid. Because this varies from an almost imperceptible minimum to a high of approximately 3 L during an uncomplicated procedure, quantification is extremely difficult with the presently available means of measuring functional extracellular fluid. Consequently, no accurate formula for intraoperative fluid administration can yet be derived. Some arbitrary but clinically useful guidelines are the following: (1) Blood should be replaced to maintain an acceptable red blood cell mass irrespective of any additional fluid and electrolyte therapy. (2) The replacement of extracellular fluid should begin during the operative procedure. (3) Balanced salt solution needed during operation is approximately 0.5 to 1 L/h, but only to a maximum of 2 to 3 L during a 4-h major abdominal procedure, unless there are other measurable losses.

Using a similar fluid regimen, Thompson and associates reported experiences in a series of 670 patients undergoing major aortoiliac reconstructive procedures. In this group of patients, the average amount of Ringer's lactate solution administered was 3555 mL, giving an average intraoperative replacement of salt solution of 677 mL/h of operative procedure. In the last 6 years of this study there were only two deaths in 298 operations, an operative mortality of 0.67 percent. Among the entire 670 patients, only two patients died of renal failure, an incidence of 0.3 percent. No patient died of pulmonary insufficiency. This extremely low incidence of renal failure, even in the presence of extensive operative trauma, is similar to the authors' data for major abdominal operative procedures.

Data by Virgilio and others have indicated that in the previously healthy surgical patient, the addition of albumin to intraoperative blood and extracellular fluid replacement is not only unnecessary but potentially harmful. More recent data by Shires with operative measurements of cardiac function and extravascular lung water indicate optimal function with replacement of blood and an extracellular "mimic" without the addition of extra albumin.

In summary, the addition of crystalloid fluid resuscitation, in appropriate volume, to blood replacement in the last quarter century has markedly improved the ability to maintain intraoperative homeostasis and avoid organ injury associated with inadequate volume replacement.

Postoperative Fluid Management

Immediate Postoperative Period

Orders for postoperative fluids are not written until the patient is in the recovery room and the fluid status has been assessed. Evaluation at this point should include a review of preoperative fluid status, the amount of fluid loss and gain during operation, and clinical examination of the patient with assessment of the vital signs and urinary output. Initial fluid orders are written to correct any *existing* deficit, followed by maintenance fluids for the remainder of the day. For the patient with complications who has received or lost large amounts of fluid, it is frequently difficult to estimate the fluid requirements for the ensuing 24 h. In this situation, intravenous fluids are ordered 1 L at a time and the patient is checked frequently until the situation is clarified. Proper replacement of fluids during this relatively short period will facilitate subsequent fluid management.

Immediately after operation, extracellular fluid volume depletion may occur as a result of continued losses of fluid at the site of injury or operative trauma—for example, into the wall or lumen of the small intestine. Several liters of extracellular fluid may be slowly deposited in such areas within a few hours or more during the first day or so from the time of the injury. Unrecognized deficits of extracellular fluid volume during the early postoperative period are manifest primarily as circulatory instability. The signs of volume deficiency in other organ systems may be delayed for several hours with this type of fluid loss. Postoperative hypotension and tachycardia require prompt investigation, followed by appropriate therapy. The generally accepted adequate blood pressure of 90/60 and a pulse of less than 120 in postoperative patients may not be sufficient to prevent renal ischemia unless, in addition to lack of signs of shock, urine flow is adequate. Evaluation of the level of consciousness, pupillary size, airway patency, breathing patterns, pulse rate and volume, skin warmth, color, body temperature, and a 30- to 50-mL hourly urine output, combined with critical review of the operative procedure and the operative fluid management, usually is recommended. Since operative trauma frequently involves loss or transfer of significant quantities of whole blood, plasma, or extracellular fluid that can be only grossly estimated, circulatory instability is most commonly caused by underestimated initial losses or insidious, concealed continued losses. Operative blood loss is usually estimated by the operating surgeon to be 15 to 40 percent less than the isotopically measured blood loss from that patient. For a patient with circulatory instability, further volume replacement of an additional 1000 mL isotonic salt solution, while determining whether continuing losses or other causes are present, often resolves the problem.

It is unnecessary and probably unwise to administer potassium during the first 24 h postoperatively, unless a definite potassium deficit exists. This is particularly important for the patient subjected to prolonged operative trauma involving one or more episodes of hypotension and for the posttraumatic patient with hemorrhagic hypotension. Oliguric renal failure or the more insidious high-output renal failure may develop, and the administration of even a small quantity of potassium may be quite detrimental.

Later Postoperative Period

The problem of volume management during the postoperative convalescent phase is one of accurate measurement and replacement of all losses. In the otherwise healthy individual, this involves the replacement of measured sensible losses, which are generally of gastrointestinal origin, and the estimation and replacement of insensible losses.

The insensible loss is usually relatively constant and will average 600 mL/day. This may be increased by hypermetabolism, hyperventilation, and fever to a maximum of approximately 1500 mL/day. The estimated insensible loss is replaced with 5% dextrose in water. This loss may be partially offset by an insensible gain of water from excessive tissue catabolism in the complicated postoperative patient, particularly if associated with oliguric renal failure.

Approximately 1 L of fluid should be given to replace that volume of urine required to excrete the catabolic end products of metabolism (800 to 1000 mL/day). In the individual with normal renal function, this may be given as 5% dextrose in water, since the kidneys are able to conserve sodium with excretion of less than 1 meq daily. It is probably unnecessary to stress the kidneys to this degree, however, and a small amount of salt solution may be given in addition to water to cover urinary loss. In the elderly patient with salt-losing kidneys or in patients with head injuries, an insidious hyponatremia may develop if urinary losses are replaced with water. Urinary sodium in these circumstances may exceed 100 meq/L and result in a daily loss of significant amounts of sodium. Measurement of urinary sodium will facilitate accurate replacement.

Urine volume is not replaced on a milliliter-for-milliliter basis. A urinary output of 2000 to 3000 mL on a given day may simply represent diuresis of fluids given during surgery or may represent excessive fluid administration. If these large losses are completely replaced, the urine output will progressively increase, and this may logically progress to a unique situation resembling diabetes insipidus with urinary outputs in excess of 10 L/day.

Sensible losses, by definition, can be measured or, as in the case of sweating, the amount can be estimated. Gastrointestinal losses are usually isotonic or slightly hypotonic, and they are replaced with an essentially isotonic salt solution. When the estimated loss is slightly above or below isotonicity, appropriate corrections can be made in the daily water administration, while isotonic salt solutions are used to replace these losses volume for volume. Sweating is not usually a problem except with the febrile patient in whom losses may, but seldom do, exceed 250 mL/day per degree of fever. Excessive sweating may, in addition, represent a considerable loss of sodium in the unacclimatized individual.

Determination of serum electrolyte levels is generally unnecessary in the patient with an uncomplicated postoperative course maintained on parenteral fluids for 2 to 3 days. A more prolonged period of parenteral replacement or one complicated by excessive fluid losses requires frequent determinations of the serum sodium, potassium, and chloride levels, and carbon dioxide combining power. Adjustments then can be made with intravenous fluids of appropriate composition.

Daily maintenance fluid should be administered at a steady rate as the losses are incurred. If given over a shorter period of time, renal excretion of the excess salt and water may occur while the normal losses continue over the full 24-h period. For the same reason, fluids of different composition are alternated, and additives to intravenous fluids (e.g., potassium chloride and antibiotics) are evenly distributed in the total volume of fluid given.

In summary, daily fluid orders should begin with an assessment of the patient's volume status and a check for possible concentration of compositional disorders as reflected by proper laboratory determinations. All measured and insensible losses are replaced with fluids of appropriate composition, allowing for any preexisting deficit or excess. The amount of potassium replacement is 40 meq daily for renal excretion of potassium in addition to approximately 20 meq/L for replacement of gastrointestinal losses. Inadequate replacement may prolong the usual postoperative ileus and contribute to the insidious development of a resistant metabolic alkalosis. Calcium and magnesium are replaced when needed, as previously discussed.

Special Considerations in the Postoperative Patient

Volume Excesses. The administration of isotonic salt solutions in excess of volume losses (external or internal) may result in overexpansion of the extracellular fluid space. The otherwise normal person in a postoperative state tolerates an acute overexpansion extremely well. Excesses administered over a period of several days, however, will soon exceed the kidney's ability to excrete sodium. Therefore, it is important to determine as accurately as possible from intake and output records and serum sodium concentrations the actual needs of the patient managed over several postoperative days. Attention to the signs and symptoms of overload usually prevents this fluid abnormality. It arises most frequently with attempts to meet excessive volume losses that are not measurable, such as those occurring from incompletely controlled fistula drainage.

The earliest sign is a weight gain during the catabolic period, when the patient should be losing ¼ to ½ lb/day. Heavy eyelids, hoarseness, or dyspnea on exertion may rapidly appear. Circulatory and pulmonary signs of overload appear late and represent a rather massive overload. Peripheral edema may be a sign, but it does not necessarily indicate volume excess. In the absence of additional evidence for volume overload, other causes for peripheral edema should be considered. Overexpansion of the *total* extracellular fluid may coexist with *depletion* of the functional extracellular fluid compartment, along with decreased effective circulating plasma volume.

Hyponatremia. Significant postoperative alterations in serum sodium concentration are infrequent if the fluid resuscitation during operation has included adequate volumes of isotonic salt solutions. The kidneys retain the ability to excrete moderate excesses of salt water administered in the early postoperative period if functional extracellular fluid has been adequately replaced during the operative or immediate postoperative period. Previous studies of sodium balance have revealed that patients do excrete sodium after the functional deficit incurred by the shift of extracellular fluid has been replaced. Wright and Gann have demonstrated normal capacity to excrete water postoperatively when isotonic salt solutions are administered before a challenge with a water load. Thus, the commonly described hyponatremia associated with surgical procedures and traumatic injury is prevented by the replacement of extracellular fluid deficits. The daily maintenance of normal osmolarity is simplified by the replacement of observable losses of known sodium content.

Hyponatremia may easily occur when water is given to replace losses of sodium-containing fluids or when water administration consistently exceeds water losses. The latter may occur with oliguria or in association with decreased water loss through the skin and lungs, intracellular shifts of sodium, or the cellular release of excessive amounts of endogenous water. Severe or refractory hyponatremia, however, is difficult to produce if renal function remains normal.

In the presence of hyperglycemia, determination of the glucose concentration is necessary to evaluate the significance of a depressed serum sodium level. Since glucose does not enter cells by passive diffusion, it exerts an osmotic force in the extracellular compartment. This contribution to osmotic pressure is normally small, but with an elevated glucose concentration, the increased osmotic pressure causes the transfer of cellular water into the extracellular compartment, resulting in a dilutional hyponatremia. Hyponatremia may therefore be observed when the total effective osmotic pressure in the extracellular compartment is normal or even above normal. Each 100 mg/dL rise in the blood glucose above normal results in a decrease in the serum sodium concentration of approximately 1.6 to 3 meq/L.

Endogenous Water Release. The patient maintained on intravenous fluids without adequate caloric intake will, between the fifth and tenth days, gain significant quantities of water (maximum, 500 mL/day) from excessive cellular catabolism, thus decreasing the quantity of exogenous water required per day.

Intracellular Shifts. Systemic bacterial sepsis is often accompanied by a precipitous drop in serum sodium concentration. This sudden change is poorly understood but usually accompanies loss of extracellular fluid as either interstitial or intracellular sequestrations. This can be treated by withholding free water, restoring extracellular fluid volume, and initiating treatment of the sepsis.

Hypernatremia. Hypernatremia (serum sodium concentration above 150 meq/L), although uncommon, is a dangerous abnormality. In contradistinction to decreased serum sodium concentration, hypernatremia is easily produced when renal function is normal. The extracellular fluid hyperosmolarity results in a shift of intracellular water from within the cell to the extracellular fluid compartment; in this situation, a high serum sodium level may indicate a significant deficit of total body water. In surgical patients hypernatremia arises most often from excessive or unexpected water losses, although it may result from use of salt-containing solutions to replace water losses. Classification of water losses may be helpful in preventing and treating this abnormality.

Excessive Extrarenal Water Losses. With increased metabolism from any cause, but particularly associated with fever, the water loss through evaporation of sweat may reach several liters daily. Patients with tracheostomy in dry environments can (with high minute volumes) lose as much as 1 to 1.5 L of water/day by this route. Increased water evaporation from a granulating surface is of significant magnitude in the thermally injured patient, and losses may be as great as 3 to 5 L/day.

Increased Renal Water Losses. Extremely large volumes of solute-poor urine may result from hypoxic damage to the distal tubules and collecting ducts or loss of antidiuretic hormone stimulation from damage to the central nervous system. In both instances, facultative water resorption is impaired. The former occurs in high-output renal failure; in our experience, this is the most common type of renal failure following severe injury or operative trauma. The latter occurs with extensive head injuries accompanied by temporary diabetes insipidus.

Solute Loading. High protein intake may produce an increased osmotic load of urea, which necessitates the excretion of large volumes of water. Hypernatremia, azotemia, and extracellular fluid volume deficits follow. In general, these can be prevented by an intake of 7 mL of water/g of dietary protein.

Excessive glucose administration results in the need for a large volume of water for excretion. Osmotic diuretics such as mannitol and urea also result in the obligatory excretion of a large volume of water as well as increasing urinary sodium losses. In addition, isotonic salt solutions, if used to replace pure water losses, rapidly produce hypernatremia.

High-Output Renal Failure. Acute renal insufficiency following trauma or surgical stress is a highly lethal complication. The diagnosis is based on persistent oliguria and chemical evidence of uremia after stabilization of the circulation. The clinical course is characterized by oliguria lasting from several days to several weeks, followed by a progressive rise in daily urine volume until both the excretory and concentrating functions of the kidney are gradually restored.

Uremia, occurring without a period of oliguria and accompanied by a daily urine volume greater than 1000 to 1500 mL/day, is a more frequent but less well recognized entity. Clinical experience and laboratory experiments suggest the high-output renal failure represents the renal response to a less severe or modified episode of renal injury than that required to produce classic oliguric renal failure. It is a milder form of renal insufficiency and its presence, by serial measurement of blood urea nitrogen and serum electrolytes, permits intelligent chemical and fluid volume management with a much greater latitude because of the daily urine volume excretion. Normal extracellular fluid volume and normal serum sodium concentration, therefore, are quite easily maintained when accurate daily outputs of each are obtained and replaced accordingly. The sodium-containing fluids may be administered as lactate to control the mild metabolic acidosis that occurs. Severe acidosis may develop if isotonic losses from the gastrointestinal tract or renal excretion of sodium are replaced with sodium chloride.

The chief danger of high-output renal failure is the failure to recognize its existence because of normal output. The inappropriate administration of intravenous potassium in this setting may result in hyperkalemia. Good urinary output and gastrointestinal involvement requiring suction usually indicate the need for daily potassium replacement. With this type of renal failure, however, potassium intoxication may be produced. As little as 20 meq of potassium chloride given intravenously may rapidly produce myocardial potassium intoxication requiring exchange resin or hemodialysis treatment.

The typical course of high-output renal failure begins without a period of oliguria. The daily urine volumes are normal or greater than normal, often reaching levels of 3 to 5 L/day while blood urea nitrogen is increasing. An attempt to decrease urine output by water restriction rapidly results in hypernatremia without a change in urine volume. On the average, urea nitrogen continues to increase for 8 to 12 days before a downward trend occurs. The blood urine urea ratio is about 1:10 until a decrease occurs in the blood urea concentration.

Functionally, the lesion is characterized by a glomerular filtration rate of less than 20 percent of normal and complete resistance to vasopressin for 1 to 3 weeks after the blood urea nitrogen has declined. During the next 6 to 8 weeks, the glomerular filtration rate gradually rises, and the response to vasopressin becomes normal.

NUTRITION IN THE SURGICAL PATIENT

The majority of patients undergoing elective surgical operations withstand the brief period of catabolism and starvation without noticeable difficulty. Maintaining an adequate nutritional regimen may be of critical importance in managing seriously ill surgical patients with preexisting weight loss and depleted energy reserves. Between these two extremes are patients for whom nutritional support is not essential for life but may serve to shorten the postoperative recovery phase and minimize the number of complications. Not infrequently a patient may become ill or even die from complications secondary to starvation rather than the underlying disorder. Therefore, it is essential that the surgeon have a sound grasp of the fundamental metabolic changes associated with surgery, trauma, and sepsis and an awareness of the methods available to reverse or ameliorate these events. A detailed discussion of the neuroendocrine and metabolic response to injury has been presented in Chap. 1.

Body Fuel Reserves

The body must mobilize appropriate nutrients from fuel reserves in order to withstand the necessary periods of partial or complete starvation and to meet the additional requirements imposed by surgery, trauma, or sepsis. The extent and availability of these reserves may be of critical importance for successful recovery from an illness. Available information concerning body fuel composition and the rate of fuel comsumption in human beings has been reviewed by Cahill and is summarized below.

Carbohydrates, proteins, and fats are the three sources of fuel in human beings. Their relative contributions by both weight and caloric potential are illustrated in Fig. 2-3. Carbohydrate stores, primarily in the form of liver and muscle glycogen, are relatively small and could supply basal caloric requirements for less than 1 day. This relatively small quantity, however, is absolutely essential in the emergency situation for the production of high-energy phosphates during anaerobic metabolism. Although glucose yields approximately 4 kcal/g, its storage as glycogen requires the addition of 1 or 2 g of intracellular water and electrolytes. Therefore, it yields only 1 or 2 kcal/g of wet weight.

Protein represents a considerably larger source of fuel, but, as emphasized by Cahill, every molecule of protein in the body has a specific purpose, such as an enzyme, a structural component, or a contractile protein in muscle. Thus, any protein loss represents loss of an essential function. Additionally, the amount of total body protein is relatively fixed in the normal healthy individual, and any additional protein is metabolized, the excess calories being stored as fat. Protein, like glycogen, represents an inefficient energy source relative to its wet weight, since it exists in an aqueous environment.

In contrast to glycogen and protein, fat is stored in a relatively anhydrous state. By weight, then, it is a relatively rich source of

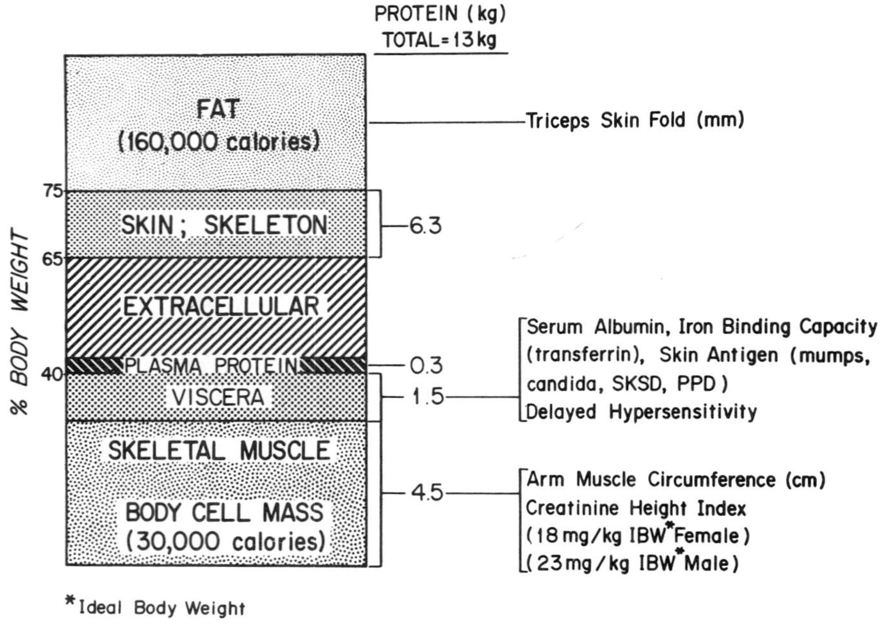

FIG. 2-3. Body fuel composition, exclusive of glycogen (900 kcal), in a normal individual. Nutritional assessment techniques corresponding to components of body composition. (From: *Blackburn GL, Bothe A Jr: Cancer Bulletin 30:90, 1978, with permission.*)

energy, supplying approximately 9 kcal/g. Most of the fat in the body serves as a readily available energy source; the few areas where fat serves a specific function (e.g., mechanical fat pads) are the last to be mobilized during starvation.

In summary, protein and fat are the only major sources of fuel. Total protein mass is relatively fixed in amount, and caloric excess or deficiency is met by an increase or decrease in the body's fat mass. Fat depots serve as sources of energy, protein stores represent *potential* sources of energy but only through the loss of some important function, and the small stores of carbohydrates are generally protected except for emergency use during anaerobic glycolysis.

Starvation

During the first several days of complete starvation, caloric needs are supplied by body fat and proteins: the small glycogen reserve is largely spared. Previous studies have shown an obligatory loss of approximately 10 to 15 g of nitrogen daily in the urine during this period, indicating the utilization of approximately 60 to 90 g of protein (each gram of nitrogen represents approximately 6.25 g of muscle protein). The majority of this protein, which is largely derived from skeletal muscle, is converted to glucose in the liver by the process of gluconeogenesis; most of this endogenously produced glucose is used by the brain. The remainder is used by certain tissues such as red blood cells and leukocytes which convert the glucose to lactate and pyruvate. These are returned to the liver and resynthesized into glucose (the Cori cycle). This obligatory nitrogen loss, then, reflects the use of amino acids derived from muscle protein for gluconeogenesis to supply glucose to the brain. No patient, however, should be allowed to starve completely. The administration of at least 100 g of glucose will obviate most of this gluconeogenesis and reduce the nitrogen loss by at least one-half—the well-known "protein-sparing effect" described by Gamble. Available evidence from Cahill indicates that this protein-sparing effect is regulated by insulin, which is released when exogenous glucose is infused for use by the brain. The slightly elevated insulin level reduces amino acid release from the muscle, amino acid extraction by the liver, and gluconeogenesis. In the diabetic with an absolute or relative lack of insulin, the infusion of glucose does not inhibit gluconeogenesis, and muscle breakdown to amino acids continues unabated. The liver derives its energy by oxidizing fatty acids to ketones, and the remainder of the body utilizes both fatty acids and ketones to meet caloric requirements. Generally a small quantity of the ketones is excreted into the urine.

If complete starvation continues for more than a few days, the obligatory nitrogen loss progressively decreases, as the brain begins to use fat as its fuel source. Unlike other body tissues, however, the brain cannot utilize free fatty acids, since they do not cross the blood-brain barrier. Instead, use of keto acids that are produced by the liver and readily cross the blood-brain barrier gradually displaces the use of glucose by the brain. After prolonged starvation, the net effect of this adaptation to ketone utilization is a protein-sparing effect with reduction of urinary nitrogen excretion to approximately 4 g/day. This 4 g of nitrogen represents approximately 25 g of protein, or about 100 g of lean wet muscle. Thus, the normal individual with an average supply of fat and muscle may survive total starvation for several months. Insulin again may be the signal for the reduction in muscle catabolism and gluconeogenesis (coincident with the increased use of keto acids by the brain), according to Cahill. However, changes in the blood level of alanine, which is quantitatively one of the more important amino acids, may also play a role. A fall in the blood level of this amino acid appears to decrease gluconeogenesis and glucose production by the liver.

Surgery, Trauma, Sepsis

In contrast to the whole-body and tissue-specific energy and protein conservation response exhibited during unstressed starvation, the injured patient manifests variable, but obligatory, increases in energy expenditure and nitrogen excretion (Fig. 2-4, Table 2-11). While the extent and duration of this response to injury are modified by a variety of factors, including the adequacy of resuscitation, infection, and medication, the inability to down-regulate body energy expenditure and nitrogen losses may rapidly deplete both labile and functional energy stores. The postinjury metabolic environment precludes the efficient oxidation of fat and ketone production, thereby promoting the continued erosion of protein pools. This enhanced net protein catabolic process, if unchecked by effective disease-specific therapy and allowed to progress for an extended period without nutritional intervention, eventuates in critical organ failure.

The sequence of metabolic and endocrine events occasioned by surgery, trauma, or sepsis may be divided into several phases. The magnitude of the changes and the duration of each phase vary considerably and are directly related to the severity of the injury.

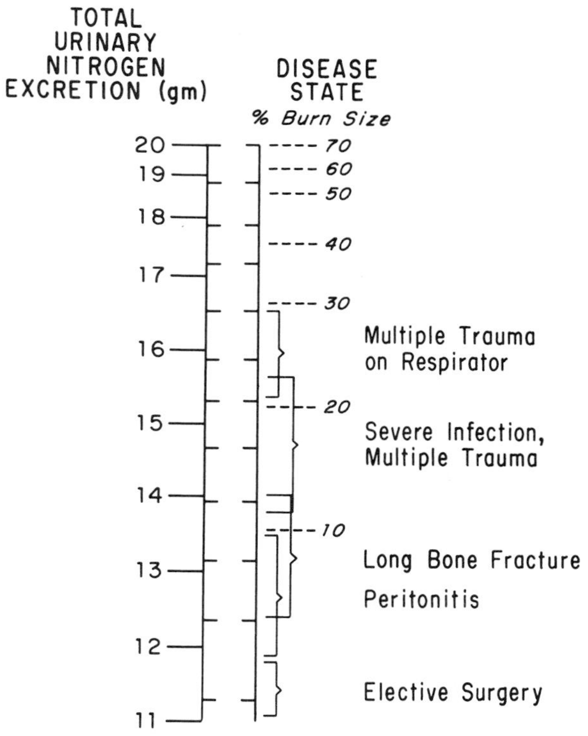

FIG. 2-4. The *minimum* anticipated daily urinary nitrogen excretion of adult patients in relation to the injury stimulus. These losses may be modulated by a number of variables including the age and nutritional status of the patient. (Adapted from: *Grant JP: Handbook of Total Parenteral Nutrition, Philadelphia, WB Saunders, 1980, with permission.*)

Table 2-11
Correlation of Increased Energy Expenditure and Urinary Nitrogen Excretion After Injury and Illness

	% Increase Above Basal Energy Expenditure	*Daily Urinary N Excretion per kg*
Normal	—	0.09
Elective, major surgery	24	0.21
Skeletal trauma	32	0.32
Blunt trauma	37	0.32
Head trauma/steroids	61	0.34
Sepsis	79	0.37
40% thermal injury	132	0.37

SOURCE: Adapted from Long CL, et al: *J Parenter Enterol Nutr* 3:452, 1979.

Catabolic Phase. This phase has also been termed the *adrenergic-corticoid phase* since it corresponds to the period during which changes induced by adrenergic and adrenal corticoid hormones are most striking. Immediately after surgery or trauma, there is a sudden increase in metabolic demands and urinary excretion of nitrogen beyond the levels associated with simple starvation. Patients generally cannot eat, cannot lower their metabolic rate, and cannot effectively alter the source of endogenous fuels to spare protein utilization. This is in distinct contrast to events in the normal individual subjected to prolonged starvation, where most body tissues use fat as their main source of fuel, thereby sparing protein. Trauma apparently results in an obligatory and excessive mobilization of protein in an attempt to provide skeletons for gluconeogenesis, acute phase, and wound repair proteins. The administration of moderate amounts of glucose to these individuals produces little or no change in the rate of protein catabolism, although recent evidence using isotopic determinations of protein kinetics suggests that provision of sufficient nonprotein calories in combination with amino acids does reduce the rate of body protein breakdown.

Glucose turnover is increased, while Cori cycle activity is stimulated and three-carbon intermediates are converted back to glucose in the liver by pyruvate carboxylase and phosphoenolpyruvate carboxylase. Increased synthesis of these two enzymes occurs in the presence of elevated levels of glucagon, glucocorticoids, and catecholamines and low concentration of insulin—the hormonal environment present during the catabolic phase of injury. Lipolysis also is stimulated by this hormonal milieu, and an obligatory oxidation of fatty acids is evident.

Efforts directed at interruption of afferent neurogenic stimuli by extradural anesthesia have met with partial success in attenuating some of these abnormalities of energy substrate turnover. The impact of such therapy on nitrogen loss has been far less dramatic, suggesting that circulating or tissue paracrine factors other than classical neuroendocrine hormones are of major importance in early postinjury metabolic responses. Recent evidence would suggest that a class of macrophage and lymphocyte-produced peptides (cytokines), some of which, such as cachectin/tumor necrosis factor and interleukin-1, are already known to enhance hepatic acute-phase protein mRNA and tissue glucose transporter protein production, are likely participants in the derangements of catabolic phase responses. The extent of the negative nitrogen balance in these patients varies considerably and is largely related to the magnitude of the injury.

Early Anabolic Phase. Depending on the severity of injury, the body turns from a catabolic to an anabolic phase. This may occur within 3 to 8 days after uncomplicated elective surgery or after weeks in patients with extensive cross-sectional tissue injury, sepsis, or ungrafted thermal injury. This turning point, also known as the *corticoid-withdrawal phase,* is characterized by a sharp decline in nitrogen excretion and restoration of appropriate potassium-nitrogen balance. Generally, this transition period lasts no more than a day or two and coincides with diuresis of retained free water. Renewed interest in oral nutrition and the patient's immediate environment promotes greater muscular activity.

The early anabolic phase may last from a few weeks to a few months depending on the capacity to ingest adequate nutrition and the extent to which erosion of protein stores has occurred. Nitrogen balance is positive, indicating synthesis of proteins, and there is a rapid and progressive gain in weight and muscular strength. Positive nitrogen balance reaches a maximum of approximately 4 g/day, which represents the synthesis of approximately 25 g of protein and the gain of over 100 g of lean body mass/day. The total amount of nitrogen gain will ultimately equal the amount lost during the catabolic phase, although the rate of gain will be much slower than the rate of initial loss.

Late Anabolic Phase. The final period of convalescence or the late anabolic phase may last from several weeks to several months after a severe injury. This phase is associated with the gradual restoration of adipose stores as the previously positive nitrogen balance declines toward normal. Weight gain is much slower during this phase because of the higher caloric content of fat and can be realized only if intake is in excess of caloric expenditure. In most individuals, the phase ends with a gradual return to the previously normal body weight. The patient who is partially immobilized during this period of time, however, may exhibit a marked gain in weight due to decreased energy expenditure.

Assessment and Requirements

Nutritional homeotasis presupposes that proper timing and administration of nutrients will impact favorably on the outcome of therapy. Muller has reported a randomized, prospective trial documenting a significant reduction of postoperative morbidity and mortality following intravenous nutritional support. Similar reductions in the complication rate following nutritional support have been observed by other groups in a variety of surgical and traumatic illnesses. Reports that up to 50 percent of selected surgical populations may manifest evidence of protein-calorie malnutrition underscores the importance of identifying patients at increased risk from nutritional morbidity.

Nutritional assessment is undertaken to determine the severity of nutrient deficiencies or excess and to aid in predicting nutritional requirements (Fig. 2-3). Important information is obtained by determining the presence of weight loss and of chronic illnesses or dietary habits that influence the quantity and quality of food intake. Social habits predisposing to malnutrition and the use of medications that may influence food intake or utilization should also be investigated. Physical examination seeks to assess loss of muscle and adipose tissues, organ dysfunction, and subtle change in skin, hair, or neuromuscular function reflecting a frank or impending nutritional deficiency. Anthropometric data (weight change, skin fold thickness, and arm circumference muscle area) and biochemical determinations (creatinine excretion, albumin, and transferrin) may be used to substantiate the historical and

Table 2-12
Elemental Requirements for Depleted Adult Subjects

Element	*Daily Infusion, per kg**
N	0.4 g
PO_4^{2-}	0.018 g
K^+	0.65 meq
Na^+	0.74 meq
Cl^-	0.56 meq
Ca^{2+}	0.13 meq

*Requirements listed are based on kilogram of ideal body weight; appropriate adjustment to current body weight may be necessary.

SOURCE: Adapted from Rudman D, et al: *J Clin Invest* 55:94, 1975.

physical findings. It is imprecise to rely on any single or fixed combination of the above findings to accurately assess nutritional status or morbidity. Appreciation for the stresses and natural history of the disease process, in combination with nutritional assessment, remains the basis for identifying patients in acute or anticipated need of nutritional support.

Balance studies have documented the basal requirements for nonstressed, depleted patients who are undergoing nutritional support (Table 2-12). These guidelines must be considered in relation to goals for gradual repletion of a malnourished patient or for maintenance of lean tissue stores in an otherwise well-nourished subject.

The above basal requirements are inadequate for patients who have undergone major surgery or who have suffered severe trauma or sepsis. The exact caloric and nitrogen requirements necessary to maintain an individual in balance after severe injury are dependent on the extent of injury, the source and route of administered nutrients, and, to some extent, the degree of antecedent malnutrition.

A fundamental goal of nutritional support is to meet the energy requirements for metabolic processes, core temperature maintenance, and tissue repair. Failure to provide adequate nonprotein energy sources will lead to dissolution of lean tissue stores. The requirement for energy may be measured by indirect calorimetry or estimated from urinary nitrogen excretion which is proportional to resting energy expenditure (REE) (Table 2-11). Basal energy expenditure (BEE) may also be estimated by the equations of Harris and Benedict:

$$\text{BEE (men)} = 66.47 + 13.75\ (W) + 5.0\ (H) - 6.76\ (A)\ \text{kcal/day}$$

$$\text{BEE (women)} = 655.1 + 9.56\ (W) + 1.85\ (H) - 4.68\ (A)\ \text{kcal/dal}$$

where W = weight, kg
H = height, cm
A = age, years

These equations are suitable for estimating energy requirements in 80 percent of hospitalized patients. A suitable correction for the degree of operative or traumatic stress may then be applied as in Table 2-11 to determine the resting energy expenditure. Nonprotein calories are supplied in excess of energy expenditure because the utilization of exogenous nutrients is decreased and energy substrate demands are increased after traumatic or septic insult. Appropriate nonprotein caloric needs are 1.2 to 1.5 times REE during enteral nutrition and 1.5 to 2.0 times REE during intravenous nutrition.

The second objective of nutritional support is to meet the substrate requirements for protein synthesis. Maintenance of protein synthesis is dependent on many factors, including the nature and degree of insult, the source and amount of exogenous protein, and prior nutritional status. As a consequence, no single nutritional formulation is appropriate for all patients. An appropriate calorie-nitrogen ratio (150 to 200 : 1) should be maintained, although recent evidence suggests that increased protein intake (and a lower ratio) may be efficient in selected hypermetabolic patients. In the absence of severe renal or hepatic dysfunction precluding the use of standard nutritional regimens, approximately 0.25 to 0.35 g of nitrogen/kg of body weight should be provided daily.

Amino acid formulations designed to improve protein kinetics in the posttraumatic or organ failure setting are under investigation. Solutions enriched in branched-chain amino acids are being used to preserve or enhance muscle protein synthesis. Branched-chain amino acids are also used in combination with reduced aromatic amino acid concentrations to alleviate encephalopathy secondary to hepatocellular dysfunction. Formulations designed to improve nitrogen utilization by providing intact or keto analogues of essential amino acids have gained wide acceptance in the management of acute renal failure.

The requirements for vitamins and essential trace minerals usually can be easily met in the average patient with an uncomplicated postoperative course, and vitamins usually are not given in the absence of preoperative deficiencies. Patients maintained on elemental diets or parenteral hyperalimentation require complete vitamin and mineral supplementation. The commercial defined-formula enteral diets contain varying amounts of essential minerals and vitamins (Tables 2-13 and 2-14). It is necessary to ensure that adequate replacement is available in the diet or by supplementation. Numerous commercial vitamin preparations are available for intravenous or intramuscular use, although most do not contain vitamin K and some do not contain vitamin B_{12} or folic acid. Supplemental trace minerals may now be given intravenously by commercial preparations. Essential fatty acid supplementation may also be necessary, especially in patients with depletion of adipose stores. Patients receiving intravenous feeding will require all the above micronutrients to prevent evolution of deficiencies.

Indications and Methods for Nutritional Support

The selection of patients who require partial or complete nutritional support has become increasingly important. The ability to provide complete nutritional support in the starving patient and to counteract the nitrogen losses in catabolic states with elemental diets or parenteral hyperalimentation represents a substantial contribution. The need for nutritional support should be assessed during the preoperative and postoperative course of all but the most routine cases. The majority of surgical patients, however, do *not* require special nutritional regimens. The reasonably well-nourished and otherwise healthy individual who undergoes an uncomplicated major surgical procedure has sufficient body fuel reserves to withstand the catabolic insult and partial starvation for at least 1 week. Adequate quantities of parenteral fluids with appropriate electrolyte composition and a minimum of 100 g of glucose daily to minimize protein catabolism will be all that is necessary in most patients. Assuming that the patient has a relatively uncomplicated postoperative course and resumes normal oral intake at the end of this period, defined-formula diets or parenteral hyperalimentation

Table 2-13
Caseinates and Whole Protein Formulas*

Formula	*Criti-care HN§*	*Ensure*	*Ensure HN*	*Ensure Plus*	*Ensure plus HN*	*Entri-ton*	*Iso-tein HN*	*Isocal*	*Isocal HCN*	*Magna-cal*	*Nutri-Aid*	*Osmo-lite*	*Osmo-lite HN*	*Preci-sion Iso-tonic*	*Preci-sion HN*	*Preci-sion LR*	*Renu*	*Susta-cal*	*Susta-cal HC*	*Trauma-Cal*	*Trava-sorb MCT*
NP, kcal/mL†	0.85	0.86	0.88	1.28	1.25	0.86	0.93	0.92	1.70	1.72	0.94	0.91	0.88	0.84	0.87	0.99	0.87	0.76	1.26	1.17	1.45
Nitrogen, g/L	6.00	5.92	7.10	8.80	10.0	5.60	10.8	5.44	12.0	11.2	6.29	5.92	7.10	4.64	7.04	4.16	5.60	9.60	9.76	13.20	5.92
Osmolality, mO/kg	650	450	470	600	650	300	300	300	740	590	350	300	310	300	557	525	330	625	650	550	312
Na, meq/L	27	32	40	46	50	61	27	23	34	43	33	23	40	34	42	30	21	40	36	52	32
K, meq/L	33	32	40	48	46	61	27	33	35	32	33	27	40	24	23	22	32	52	38	36	32
Cl, meq/L	30	30	40	46	45	56	27	30	34	26	30	23	40	28	33	31	18	44	36	45	30
Ca, meq/L	26	26	37	32	52	50	28	31	33	50	27	26	37	32	17	29	25	50	42	38	26
P, mmol/L	17	17	24	20	33	32	18	17	21	32	18	17	24	20	11	18	16	29	27	24	17
Mg, meq/L	17	17	25	26	34	33	19	17	22	33	17	17	25	21	11	19	16	31	28	17	17
Zn, mg/L	10	16	17	24	16	15	8.5	10	20	15	16	16	17	10	5	9	10	14	13	15	16
Cu, mg/L	1	1	1.5	1.6	1	2	1.1	1	2	2	1.1	1	1.5	1	0.7	1	2	2	2	1.5	1
Vitamins, 1/RDA/day‡	1.9	1.9	1.4	1.6	1.0	2.0	1.6	2.0	1.5	1.0	2.0	1.9	1.4	1.6	2.9	1.8	2.0	1.1	1.8	2.0	2.0

*Lactose-free.

†NP = nonprotein kilocalories per milliliters of solution.

‡Volume in liters needed to meet the U.S. RDA per day.

§This formula also contains synthetic amino acids.

SOURCE: Adapted from Legaspi A, Lowry SF: Agents affecting nutrition and homeostasis, in *Manual of Drug Therapy*. New York, Raven Press, 1985.

Table 2-14
Elemental and Peptide Diets*

Formula	*Vivonex*	*Vivonex HN*	*Vivonex TEN*	*Vital*	*Travasorb STD*	*Travasorb HN*
NP, kcal/mL†	0.92	0.82	0.85	0.83	0.88	0.82
Nitrogen, g/L	3.36	6.72	6.08	6.72	4.80	7.20
Osmolality, mO/kg	550	810	630	460	560	560
Na, meq/L	20	23	20	16	40	40
K, meq/L	30	30	20	30	30	30
Cl, meq/L	20	23	23	19	42	38
Ca, meq/L	28	16	25	33	25	25
P, mmol/L	18	10	49	21	16	16
Mg, meq/L	18	10	17	22	16	16
Zn, mg/L	8	5	10	10	7.5	7.5
Cu, mg/L	1	0.7	1	1.3	1	1
Vitamins (1/RDA/day)‡	1.8	3.0	2.0	1.5	2.0	2.0

*Lactose-free.

†NP = nonprotein kilocalories per milliliter of solution.

‡Volume in liters needed to meet the U.S. RDA per day.

SOURCE: Adapted from Legaspi A, Lowry SF: Agents affecting nutrition and homeostasis, in *Manual of Drug Therapy*. New York, Raven Press, 1985.

are probably unnecessary and inadvisable because of the associated risks. During the early anabolic phase, the patient must be provided with an adequate caloric intake of proper composition to meet the energy needs of the body and allow protein synthesis. A high calorie-nitrogen ratio (optimal ratio approximately 150 kcal/g nitrogen) and an adequate supply of vitamins and minerals are necessary for maximum anabolism during this period.

In contrast to this group, there are populations of surgical patients for whom an adequate nutritional regimen may be of critical importance for a successful outcome. These categories include preoperative patients who are chronically debilitated from their diseases or malnutrition and patients who have suffered trauma, sepsis, or surgical complications and cannot maintain an adequate caloric intake.

Specialized nutritional support can be given by enteral, enteral plus peripheral vein, and by central venous routes. The enteral route should be initially considered because it is simple, economical, and usually well tolerated in most patients. Nasopharyngeal, gastrostomy, and jejunostomy tube feedings may be considered for alimentation in patients who have a relatively normal gastrointestinal tract but cannot or will not eat. Elemental diets may be administered by similar routes when bulk and fat-free nutrients requiring minimal digestion are indicated. Finally, parenteral alimentation may be used for supplementation in the patient with limited oral intake or, more commonly, for complete nutritional management in the absence of oral intake. Recent data demonstrate that parenteral feeding potentially enhances the magnitude of both macroendocrine (stress hormones) and microendocrine (cytokine) mediator responses to an antigenic challenge, such as endotoxin (Fig. 2-5). While the mechanisms for such an amplification of counter-regulatory hormone and inflammatory cytokine levels in parenterally fed subjects remains to be fully elucidated, a loss of intestinal barrier function permitting acute or chronic host exposure to luminal toxins likely exerts a significant influence in this process.

Despite the failure to document clinical differences between the enteral and parenteral feeding routes with respect to the utilization of exogenous nutrients, the gastrointestinal tract serves a number of synthetic and immunologic functions that bear consideration in the design of nutritional support regimens. Toward this end, a number of approaches for preserving gastrointestinal mucosal integrity and gut mass, including luminal stimulation by digestible or nondigestible substrates, as well as infusion of critical intestinal fuel sources such as glutamine, are currently undergoing clinical trials.

The patient's ability to tolerate and absorb enteral feedings is determined by the rate of infusion, the osmolality, and the chemical nature of the product. Enteral feedings are often begun at a rate of 30 to 50 mL/h and are increased by 10 to 25 mL/h a day until the optimal volume is delivered. After full volume is attained, the concentration of the solution is increased slowly to the desired strength. If esophageal or gastric feedings are given, residual gastric volume should be monitored to reduce the risk of a major aspiration episode. If abdominal cramping or diarrhea occurs, the rate of administration or the concentration of the solution should be decreased. All feeding tubes should be thoroughly irrigated clear of solutions if feedings are interrupted or medications are given by this route.

Nasoenteric Tube Feeding

The development of mercury-weighted silastic feeding tubes has improved the ability to provide safe and effective enteral nutrition. Use of such tubes represents a safer alternative to the practice of nasoesophageal or gastric feeding by large-bore red rubber or plastic tubes. Exceptions to this rule include patients with head and neck malignancies who will tolerate a blenderized diet that cannot easily be administered by smaller diameter tubes.

Nasoesophageal or gastric feedings should be used only in alert patients. The foremost contraindication for nasoesophageal or gastric tube feeding is unconsciousness or lack of protective laryngeal reflexes, which may result in life-threatening pulmonary complications due to aspiration. Even with a tracheostomy, it is inadvisable to feed mentally obtunded patients via such route, since feedings often can be recovered from tracheostomy suction, indicating continued aspiration of gastric contents. Pharyngeal tube feedings

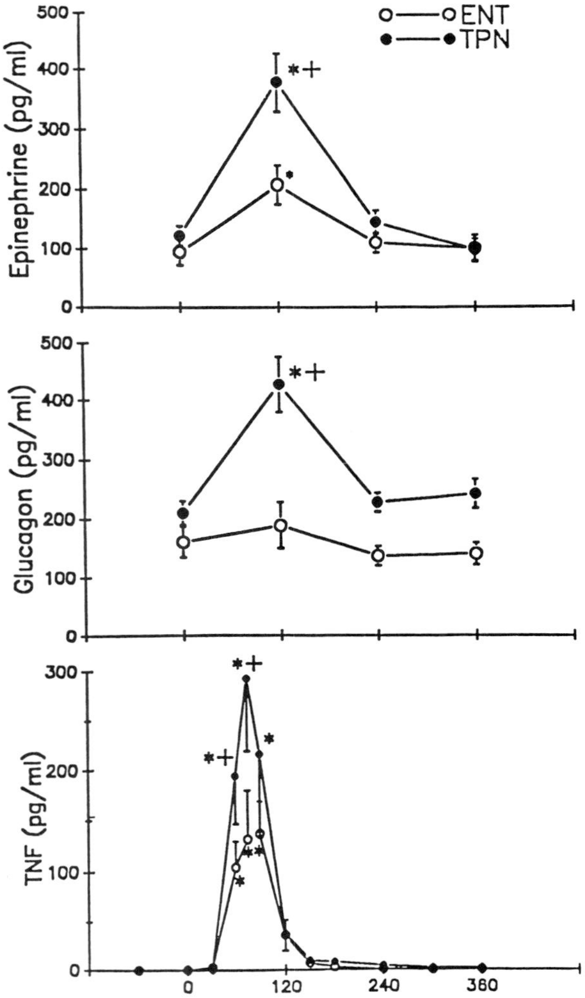

FIG. 2-5. Hormonal and tumor necrosis factor (TNF) levels in response to endotoxin in normal subjects. Epinephrine, glucagon, and TNF levels in arterial blood before ($t = 0$) and after intravenous endotoxin administration. Subjects were studied 12 h after the cessation of 7 days of enteral feedings (ENT) or total parenteral nutrition (TPN). (Adapted from: *Fong and Lowry: Cytokines and the cellular response to injury and infection, in Care of the Surgical Patient. New York, Scientific American, 1990.*)

may be indicated for patients with oropharyngeal tumor; irritation may be prevented by inserting the tube into the pyriform sinus.

The nasojejunal tube may allow feeding beyond dysfunctional gastric stomas and high gastrointestinal fistulas. In such cases, it may be possible to maintain nutrition without a jejunostomy tube until stomal dysfunction relents or the fistula heals. Such tubes may be positioned in the upper small intestine by positioning the patient in a manner that promotes passage of the mercury-weighted tube into the desired intestinal segment. If this technique proves unsuccessful, placement may be effected by fluoroscopic guidance or by an experienced endoscopist. Proper position of the tube must be confirmed radiographically (with water-soluble opaque medium if necessary).

Whenever dietary preparations are administered into the gastrointestinal tract via tubes, it is advisable to employ bedside infusion pumps to ensure a constant rate of delivery over each 24-h period. The utilization of such pumps decreases the incidence of gastrointestinal side effects induced by too rapid delivery of hyperosmolar solutions, while at the same time allowing safer administration of larger daily volumes of nutrients, since gastric distention is minimized. Investigation is required for all abdominal complaints in such patients in view of reports of intussusception around feeding tubes placed more distally in the small intestine.

Gastrostomy Tube Feeding

The administration of blended food through a gastrostomy tube is a good method for feeding patients with a variety of chronic gastrointestinal lesions arising at or above the cardioesophageal junction. However, gastrostomy tube feedings are contraindicated for mentally obtunded patients with inadequate laryngeal reflexes. This feeding method should be used only in alert patients or in patients with total obstruction of the distal esophagus.

Generally, gastrostomies of the Stamm (serosa-lined, temporary) or modified Glassman (mucosa-lined, permanent) type are constructed. Percutaneous endoscopic gastrostomies (PEG) have proved to be a safe and effective method for pursuing enteral nutritional support. The feeding mixture may be ordinarily prepared food converted by a blender into a semiliquid. Hyperosmolarity of the feeding formula is not generally a problem as long as the pylorus is intact.

Jejunostomy Tube Feeding

Jejunostomy tube feedings are generally required for patients in whom nasoesophageal or gastrostomy tube feedings are contraindicated, e.g., comatose patients or patients with high gastrointestinal fistulas or obstructions, or in whom a nasojejunal feeding tube cannot be placed. The jejunostomy may be of the Roux en Y (permanent) or the Witzel (temporary) type. The latter is constructed by inserting a #18 French rubber catheter into the proximal jejunum approximately 12 in. distal to the ligament of Treitz. The wall of the jejunum is inverted over the tube for about 3 cm as it emerges from the bowel to create a serosa-lined tunnel that allows rapid sealing of the jejunal opening when the tube is removed. An alternative procedure is the placement of a smaller-bore polyethylene or silastic catheter. The tube is brought out through a stab wound in the left upper quadrant of the abdomen. The jejunum is sutured to the anterior abdominal wall at the point of tube entry to seal it from the peritoneal cavity.

Alternate methods that have gained wide acceptance include the needle catheter jejunostomy that is available in commercial kit form or may be constructed using subclavian catheter materials. In selected instances, jejunostomies may be placed endoscopically or converted from PEG catheters.

If the jejunostomy tube is inadvertently removed, blind attempts at reinsertion are contraindicated. If discovered within a few hours, the tube may be reinserted under fluoroscopic control to be sure it is in the bowel before feedings are resumed. The patient is observed for signs of peritonitis for 12 to 18 h after feedings are restarted. If there is any doubt about the position of the tube, it should be replaced surgically.

Feedings are safely begun 12 to 18 h after jejunostomy construction, even though peristalsis is not audible. Jejunostomy tube feedings are usually initiated with one of the many commercially available defined formula diets (Tables 2-13 and 2-14). Such formulas, when provided by continuous infusion, are usually well tolerated.

With proper care, about 85 percent of jejunostomy patients tolerate their feedings. Diarrhea is usually controlled if the concentration and volume of formula are temporarily reduced. Failing this, feeding is halted for a day, then resumed from the beginning of the feeding regimen, progressing somewhat more slowly than before. If mild diarrhea or cramping persists, a pulverized Lomotil tablet or 8 to 10 drops of tincture of belladonna may be given through the tube 30 min before formula infusion. At times it may be necessary to give 5 mL paregoric 15 to 30 min before the formula to control cramping and diarrhea, but this should be employed sparingly and for as short a period as possible. In many cases, symptoms are relieved if the rate and volume of infusion are reduced and cold formula avoided. Failing control of diarrhea by the above means, or as an alternative method to opiates, the periodic administration of bulk-forming agents (Metamucil) may be helpful.

If the patient with a jejunostomy has a proximal bowel or biliary fistula draining more than 300 mL daily for prolonged periods, the fistular drainage may be collected by sump suction, cooled in an ice basin at bedside, and promptly refed in small increments throughout the day. To avoid jejunal overloading, the fistular fluid is refed between formula feedings. It is not advisable to refeed aspirated gastric juice, for this may cause jejunal irritation and profuse diarrhea. If the fistular drainage is profuse, it is usually not possible to refeed more than 2 L/day, and fluid and electrolyte losses must be replaced by appropriate intravenous supplements. Additional water may be given with the feedings or administered between the feedings as indicated. Occasionally, an elemental diet, as discussed below, may be indicated when other jejunostomy formulas are not tolerated.

Elemental Diets

Commercial production of nutritionally complete liquid diets, derived in purified form either from natural foods or from foods prepared synthetically, has been given such designations as chemically defined or elemental diets.

Clinical experience with chemically formulated bulk-free elemental diets has been encouraging. These diets may be used for complete nutritional support or as dietary supplements for patients who are unable to eat or digest enough food to meet their energy requirements. They may be preferable to high-caloric parenteral feedings for patients who have at least part of the small bowel available for the absorption of simple sugars and amino acids. Elemental diets have been found useful for patients with depleted protein reserves secondary to gastrointestinal tract disease, such as ulcerative or granulomatous colitis and malabsorption syndrome, and for patients with only partial function of the gastrointestinal tract, such as the short bowel syndrome or gastric or small bowel fistulas with feeding distal to the fistula. The diets also have been used during preoperative bowel preparation.

As commercially prepared, these diets also contain base-line electrolytes, water- and fat-soluble vitamins (except vitamin K), and trace minerals. They contain no bulk and therefore produce a minimum of residue. Products such as Carnation Instant Breakfast and Meritene contain intact protein derived from milk products, eggs, or both and are designed for oral consumption in lactose tolerant patients. Other preparations contain intact protein from semipurified isolates of milk, soybean, or egg (Table 2-13). These do not contain lactose and are more readily tolerated in such lactase-deficiency states as gastroenteritis, intestinal resection, radiation, or genetic predisposition. Finally, there are several products whose protein content is either partially hydrolyzed or completely hydrolyzed to amino acids or dipeptides (Table 2-14). When digestion and absorption are normal, there appears to be little therapeutic advantage to the use of crystalline amino acid formulas. A listing of the basic constituents for several commercial preparations, as well as the volume necessary to achieve minimal daily requirements, is given in Table 2-13.

Special products designed for use in the presence of organ dysfunction are also available (Table 2-15). Amin-Aid provides essential amino acids and histidine with minimal electrolytes, vitamins, or bulk, but does yield 2 kcal/mL for use in the setting of renal failure. Hepatic Aid, which may be used in the presence of severe liver insufficiency, is enriched with branched-chain amino acids and is deficient in aromatic, ringed amino acids.

Fat may contribute less than 1 or as much as 47 percent of the calories in these commercial formulas. Most contain long-chain fats as corn oil, soy oil, or safflower oil. Some include medium-chain triglycerides, such as Precision-LR and Vital. Despite the high caloric density of fat, it does not increase the osmolality of the formula. When significant maldigestion or malabsorption is present, a diet low in fat or one supplemented with medium-chain triglycerides may be useful.

Specific products are limited in their overall clinical usefulness by virtue of the fixed content of nutrients. In recent years, there has been a trend in preparing enteral diets in modular form, where certain critical items, such as sodium, potassium, and fat, can be modified in concentration as dictated by clinical circumstances.

The amount of elemental diet required to maintain weight and nitrogen balance varies with the individual patient. In severe catabolic states the standard diet often fails to achieve positive nitrogen balance. Careful attention to water and electrolyte balance is mandatory, particularly when large quantities of fluid are being lost through fistulas or other routes. Additional sodium and potassium may be added to the mixture (not to exceed a total of 100 meq), although they should be given in intravenous fluids when larger quantities are needed. Water may be added to the mixture in the face of excessive pure water losses.

Complications include nausea, vomiting, and diarrhea which develop because of the high osmolarity of the diets. This generally can be controlled by decreasing the rate and or concentration of the mixture. Hypertonic nonketotic coma may occur in the presence of excessive water losses or if the diets are administered at concentrations above those recommended. Hyperglycemia and glycosuria may occur in any severely ill patient, particularly latent diabetics, and insulin may be indicated.

Parenteral Alimentation

Dudrick et al. have demonstrated the clinical practicality of providing complete nutritional needs for an extended period of time using high-caloric parenteral feedings. Parenteral alimentation involves the continuous infusion of a hyperosmolar solution containing carbohydrates, proteins, fat, and other necessary nutrients through an indwelling catheter inserted into the superior vena cava. In order to obtain the maximum benefit, the ratio of calories to nitrogen must be adequate (at least 100 to 150 kcal/g nitrogen) and the two materials must be infused simultaneously. When the sources of calories and nitrogen are given at different times, there is a significant decrease in nitrogen utilization. These nutrients can be given in quantities considerably greater than the basic caloric and nitrogen requirements, and this method has proved to be highly successful in achieving growth and development, positive nitrogen balance, and weight gain in a variety of clinical situations.

Table 2-15
Specialized Formulations for Enteral Nutrition During Organ Failure*

Formula	*Amin-Aid*	*Hepatic Aid*	*Travasorb Hepatic*	*Travasorb Renal*	*TraumAid*	*Stresstein*
NP, kcal/mL†	1.88	1.47	0.98	1.26	0.83	0.93
Nitrogen, g/L	2.35	6.47	4.4	4.4	7.58	11.2
Osmolality, mO/kg	1095	1150	690	590	675	910
EAA, g/L‡	18.6	22.15	20.0	13.8	26.2	89.6
BCAA, g/L§	7.5	15.3	14.5	6.67	15.0	61.6
Protein, g/L	19.4	42.6	29.0	23.0	43.0	70.0
Na, meq/L	<15	<15	19	0	23	28
K, meq/L	<6	<6	29	0	30	28
Cl, meq/L	0	0	19	0	23	29
Ca, meq/L	0	0	19	0	20	25
P, mmol/L	0	0	16	0	13	16
Mg, meq/L	0	0	15	0	11	17
Zn, mg/L	0	0	6.6	0	6.7	7.5
Cu, mg/L	0	0	0.8	0	0.7	1.0
Vitamins (1/RDA/day)‖	—	—	2.1	—	3.0	2.0

*Lactose-free.

†NP = nonprotein kilocalories per milliliter of solution.

‡Essential amino acids, branched-chain amino acids included.

§Branched-chain amino acids only; leucine, isoleucine, and valine.

‖Volume in liters needed to meet the U.S. RDA per day.

SOURCE: Adapted from Legaspi A, Lowry SF: Agents affecting nutrition and homeostasis, in *Manual of Drug Therapy*. New York, Raven Press, 1985.

Indications for the Use of Intravenous Hyperalimentation. It is often difficult to demonstrate that parenteral feeding significantly alters the clinical course or outcome in most nonsurgical patient populations. Recently reported clinical trials and meta-analysis of parenteral feeding in the perioperative period have, however, suggested that preoperative nutritional support may benefit some surgical patients, particularly those with extensive malnutrition. By contrast, definitive evidence of benefit accruing to use of nutritional support in the postoperative setting is lacking. The routine use of this technology in the critical care environment has yet to be adequately assessed and, as a consequence, is currently more intuitively utilized. The evidence underlying the application of parenteral nutrition in situations of surgical relevance was reviewed before the formulation of clinical practice guidelines published by a recent Georgetown University panel. The principal indications for parenteral alimentation are found in seriously ill patients suffering from malnutrition, sepsis, or surgical or accidental trauma when use of the gastrointestinal tract for feedings is not possible. It has been used in many instances either where it is not needed or where use of the gastrointestinal tract is more appropriate. In some instances, intravenous nutrition may be used to supplement inadequate oral intake. The safe and successful use of this regimen requires proper selection of patients with specific nutritional needs, experience with the technique, and an awareness of the associated complications. The fundamental goals are to provide sufficient calories and nitrogen substrate to promote tissue repair and to maintain the integrity or growth of the lean tissue mass. Listed below are situations where parenteral nutrition has been used in an effort to achieve these goals.

1. Newborn infants with catastrophic gastrointestinal anomalies, such as tracheoesophageal fistula, gastroschisis, omphalocele, or massive intestinal atresia
2. Infants who fail to thrive nonspecifically or secondarily to gastrointestinal insufficiency associated with the short bowel syndrome, malabsorption, enzyme deficiency, meconium ileus, or idiopathic diarrhea
3. Adult patients with short bowel syndrome secondary to massive small bowel resection or enteroenteric, enterocolic, enterovesical, or enterocutaneous fistulas
4. Patients with high alimentary tract obstructions without vascular compromise, secondary to achalasia, stricture, or neoplasia of the esophagus; gastric carcinoma; or pyloric obstruction
5. Surgical patients with prolonged paralytic ileus following major operations, multiple injuries, or blunt or open abdominal trauma, or patients with reflex ileus complicating various medical diseases
6. Patients with normal bowel length but with malabsorption secondary to sprue, hypoproteinemia, enzyme or pancreatic insufficiency, regional enteritis, or ulcerative colitis
7. Adult patients with functional gastrointestinal disorders such as esophageal dyskinesia following cerebral vascular accident, idiopathic diarrhea, psychogenic vomiting, or anorexia nervosa
8. Patients who cannot ingest food or who regurgitate and aspirate oral or tube feedings because of depressed or obtunded sensorium following severe metabolic derangements, neurologic disorders, intracranial surgery, or central nervous system trauma
9. Patients with excessive metabolic requirements secondary to severe trauma, such as extensive full-thickness burns, major fractures, or soft tissue injuries
10. Patients with granulomatous colitis, ulcerative colitis, and tuberculous enteritis, in which major portions of the absorptive mucosa are diseased
11. Paraplegics, quadriplegics, or debilitated patients with indolent decubitus ulcers in the pelvic areas, particularly when soilage and fecal contamination are a problem
12. Patients with malignancy, with or without cachexia, in whom malnutrition might jeopardize successful delivery of a therapeutic option
13. Patients with potentially reversible acute renal failure, in whom marked catabolism results in the liberation of intracellular anions and

cations, inducing hyperkalemia, hypermagnesemia, and hyperphosphatemia

Conditions *contraindicating* hyperalimentation include the following:

1. Lack of a specific goal for patient management, or where instead of extending a meaningful life, inevitable dying is prolonged
2. Periods of cardiovascular instability or severe metabolic derangement requiring control or correction before attempting hypertonic intravenous feeding
3. Feasible gastrointestinal tract feeding; in the vast majority of instances, this is the best route by which to provide nutrition
4. Patients in good nutritional status, in whom only short-term parenteral nutrition support is required or anticipated
5. Infants with less than 8 cm of small bowel, since virtually all have been unable to adapt sufficiently despite prolonged periods of parenteral nutrition
6. Patients who are irreversibly decerebrate or otherwise dehumanized

Insertion of Central Venous Infusion Catheter. The successful use of intravenous hyperalimentation generally depends upon the proper placement and management of the central venous feeding catheter. A 16-gauge, 8- or 12-in. radiopaque catheter is introduced percutaneously through the subclavian or internal jugular vein and threaded into the superior vena cava. Although the technique for subclavian vein puncture (Fig. 2-6) has been quite popular, the internal jugular approach may be used (Fig. 2-7).

For insertion of the intravenous catheter through the subclavian vein, the patient is placed supine in a 15° head-down position with a small pad placed between the shoulder blades to allow the shoulders to drop posteriorly. This allows expansion of the subclavian vein and easier penetration. The skin is scrubbed with ether or acetone to defat the surface and then with an iodophor compound. Drapes are carefully placed, and *scrupulous* aseptic precautions are observed. Local anesthetic is infiltrated into the skin, subcutaneous tissue, and periosteum at the inferior border of the midpoint of the clavicle. A 2-in.-long, 14-gauge needle attached to a small syringe is inserted, beveled down through the wheal, and advanced toward the tip of the operator's finger, which is pressed well into the patient's suprasternal notch. The needle should hug the inferior clavicular surface and go over the first rib into the subclavian vein. With slight negative pressure applied to the syringe, entrance into the vein will be noted by the appearance of blood. The needle is advanced a few millimeters further to be sure that it is entirely within the lumen of the vein. The patient is asked to perform a Valsalva maneuver, or the thumb is held over the

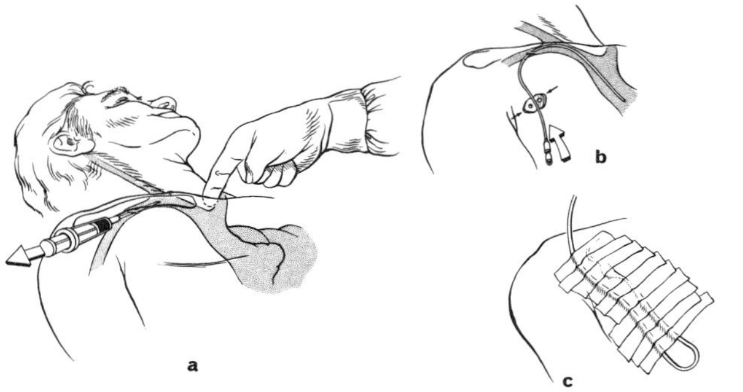

FIG. 2-6. Use of the subclavian vein for insertion of central venous catheter.

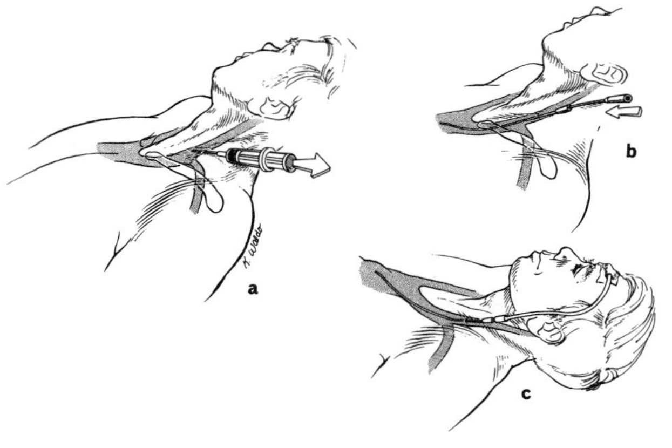

FIG. 2-7. Use of internal jugular vein for insertion of central venous catheter.

needle hub as the syringe is removed to avoid air embolism. A 16-gauge, 8- or 12-in. radiopaque catheter is then introduced through the needle and threaded into the superior vena cava. The needle is then withdrawn from the patient, and a small plastic splint is fitted over the junction of the catheter and needle to prevent catheter severance by the needle. The catheter is connected to a sterile intravenous administration tubing, and a slow infusion is begun while the catheter is sewn to the skin with a small synthetic suture. Antibiotic ointment is applied around the entrance of the catheter into the skin, and an occlusive dressing is applied over it including the junction of the intravenous tubing with the catheter. A chest film is immediately obtained to confirm the position of the radiopaque catheter in the vena cava and to check for a possible pneumothorax.

Every 2 or 3 days, the intravenous tubing is changed at the catheter entry site, the catheter site is scrubbed as for an operative procedure, and antibiotic ointment and a new occlusive dressing are applied. In general, withdrawal or administration of blood through the catheter or the use of the catheter for central venous pressure measurements should be avoided, since the risk of contamination and catheter occlusion are significantly increased.

The use of the internal jugular approach has also been quite satisfactory, especially for the pediatric age group. It is probably unwise, unless absolutely necessary, to place catheters into the inferior vena cava from the lower extremities because of the greater likelihood of sepsis and thromboembolic phenomena. Additionally, cutdown catheter insertions into the cephalic or basilic veins have not proved satisfactory.

Preparation and Administration of Solutions. The basic solution contains a final concentration of 20 to 25% dextrose and 3 to 5% crystalline amino acids. The solutions are usually prepared in the pharmacy from commercially available kits containing the component solutions and transfer apparatus. Preparation in the pharmacy under laminar flow reduces the incidence of bacterial contamination of the solution. Proper preparation with suitable quality control is absolutely essential to avoid septic complications.

Since the formulation of commercially available alimentation solutions varies considerably with regard to amino acid and electrolyte concentration, it is imperative that the physician become thoroughly familiar with the levels of the components within the

Table 2-16
Dextrose–Amino Acid Formulas Delivered via a Central Line

	Aminosyn			*Freamine III*		*Novamine*		*Travasol*	
Formula	*10%*	*8.5%*	*7%*	*10%*	*8.5%*	*11.4%*	*8.5%*	*10%*	*8.5%*
Osmolality, mO/L	1000	850	700	950	810	1049	785	1000	1322
Total AA, g/100 mL*	9.86	8.53	6.97	9.70	8.25	11.41	8.50	10.00	8.50
Total EAA, g/100 mL†	4.70	4.06	3.32	4.63	3.94	5.11	3.80	4.05	3.34
PE, g/L‡	100	85	70	96	82	113	84	103	89
N§	15.7	13.4	11.0	15.3	13.0	18.0	13.4	16.5	14.3

Vitamins are usually supplemented with a multiple vitamin preparation containing: vitamin A, 10,000 units; ergocalciferol, 1000 units; vitamin E, 5 units; thiamine HCl, 50 mg; riboflavin, 10 mg; pyridoxine HCl, 15 mg; niacinamide, 100 mg; dexpanthenal, 25 mg; ascorbic acid, 500 mg.

*Total AA = total amino acids.

†Total EAA = total essential amino acids.

‡PE = protein equivalent.

§N = nitrogen.

SOURCE: Adapted from Legaspi A, Lowry SF: Agents affecting nutrition and homeostasis, in *Manual of Drug Therapy*. New York, Raven Press, 1985.

solution utilized (Table 2-16). Only in this manner may additives, in the form of additional electrolytes, be rationally planned to meet specific metabolic needs of the patient. One should recognize that the recommended concentrations of electrolytes are only estimates and that actual requirements may vary considerably (Table 2-12) between individual patients, dependent on routes of fluid and electrolyte loss, renal function, metabolic rate, cardiac function, and the underlying disease state.

Intravenous vitamin preparations should be added as recommended in Table 2-12. In addition, phytonadione (vitamin K_1) 10 mg and folic acid 5 mg should be administered intramuscularly once a week, since these are unstable in the hyperalimentation solution. Cyanocobalamin (vitamin B_{12}) 1 mg is given by intramuscular injection once a month. Intramuscular administration of iron may be required for patients with iron deficiency anemia although adequate mobilization of iron stores may occur once the patient is anabolic. During prolonged fat-free parenteral nutrition essential fatty acid deficiency may become clinically apparent, manifested by a dry, scaly dermatitis and loss of hair. The syndrome may be prevented by periodic infusion of a fat emulsion at a rate equal to 4 to 5% of total calories. Essential trace minerals may be required after prolonged total parenteral nutrition and may be supplied by direct addition of commercial preparations to dextrose amino acid solutions. The most frequent presentation of trace mineral deficiencies is the eczamatoid rash developing both diffusely and at intertriginous areas in zinc-deficient patients. Other rare trace mineral deficiencies include a microcytic anemia associated with copper deficiency and glucose intolerance presumably related to chromium deficiency. The latter complications are seldom seen except in patients receiving parenteral nutrition for extended periods of time. The daily administration of commercially available trace mineral supplements will obviate most such problems.

Depending on fluid and nitrogen tolerance, parenteral nutrition solutions can generally be increased over 2 to 3 days to achieve the desired infusion rate. Insulin may be supplemented as necessary to ensure glucose tolerance. Wolfe and Elwyn have demonstrated that maximum efficiency of glucose utilization occurs at an infusion rate of 7 mg/(kg · min). Dextrose infusions above this level result in increased fat synthesis and provide no additional suppression of amino acid gluconeogenesis.

Rarely, additional intravenous fluids and electrolytes may be necessary with continued abnormal large losses of fluids. The patient should be carefully monitored for development of electrolyte, volume, acid-base, and septic complications. Vital signs and urinary output are regularly observed, and the patient should be weighed daily. Frequent adjustments of the volume and composition of the solutions are necessary during the course of therapy. Electrolytes are drawn daily until stable and every 2 or 3 days thereafter, and the hemogram, blood urea nitrogen, liver functions, phosphate, and magnesium are determined at least weekly.

The urine sugar level is checked every 6 h and blood sugar concentration at least once daily during the first few days of the infusion and at frequent intervals thereafter. Relative glucose intolerance may occur following initiation of parenteral alimentation. Insulin may be supplemented as necessary to improve carbohydrate tolerance. The response of blood glucose to exogenous insulin is evaluated by frequent capillary blood determinations, rather than reliance upon glycosuria. If the blood sugar levels remain elevated or glycosuria persists, the dextrose concentration may be decreased, the infusion rate slowed, or regular insulin added to each bottle. The rise in blood glucose concentration observed after initiating an intravenous alimentation program may be temporary, as the normal pancreas increases its output of insulin in response to the continuous carbohydrate infusion. In patients with diabetes mellitus, additional crystalline or human insulin may be required.

The administration of adequate amounts of potassium is essential to achieve positive nitrogen balance and replace depleted intracellular stores. In addition, a significant shift of potassium ion from the extracellular to the intracellular space may take place because of the large glucose infusion, with resultant hypokalemia, metabolic alkalosis, and poor glucose utilization. In some cases as much as 240 meq of potassium ion daily may be required. Hypokalemia may cause glycosuria, which would be treated with potassium, not insulin. Thus, before giving insulin, the serum potassium level must be checked to avoid compounding the hypokalemia.

By virtue of the stress response following major trauma, sepsis, or burns, some patients may remain extremely insulin resistant.

Patients with insulin-dependent diabetes mellitus may exhibit wide fluctuations in blood glucose during parenteral nutrition. Partial replacement of lipid emulsions for dextrose calories may alleviate these problems in selected patients.

Fat Emulsions. Lipid emulsions derived from soybean or safflower oils are widely used as an adjunctive nutrient to prevent the development of essential fatty acid deficiency. Recent attention has also focused on their use as a major energy source in parenteral alimentation. Fat emulsion, dextrose, and amino acid combinations appear equally effective to carbohydrate and amino acid solutions in the repletion of nonstressed patients. The efficiency of fat as a caloric source in the traumatized, hypermetabolic patient is not well documented. There appears to be a theoretical advantage to the utilization of lipid emulsions in some septic and trauma patients where nonsuppressible fat oxidation and increased norepinephrine excretion accompany glucose infusion. Patients with abnormal fat transport or metabolism, lipoid nephrosis, coagulopathy, or serious pulmonary disease should not receive fat emulsions. Most investigators advise limitation of administered fat emulsions to between 2.0 and 2.5 g/kg of body weight per day.

Special Formulations. Numerous studies have documented the safety of parenteral alimentation in patients with renal failure. For this purpose, special formulations of essential amino acids may be indicated. Selection of the appropriate calorie and nitrogen concentrations must be judged by fluid tolerance, associated illnesses, and the frequency of dialysis. Appropriate use of dialysis is additive to nutritional support in improving survival of these patients. Solutions for patients with acute, oliguric renal failure contain a final dextrose concentration of 40 to 45% and only essential L-amino acids. In patients with nonoliguric renal failure, it may be possible to use both essential and nonessential amino acids to further promote protein synthesis.

Solutions designed for patients with hepatic failure contain increased levels of branched-chain amino acids and decreased concentrations of aromatic amino acids. Such solutions appear to improve encephalopathy but may not improve survival, which is dictated by the underlying hepatic pathology. Patients with moderate hepatic reserve and alcoholic hepatitis may also be treated with standard parenteral formulas to control encephalopathy and ascites.

Cachexia related to severe cardiac disease may be judiciously treated with highly concentrated dextrose and amino acid formulas that are low in sodium content.

Complications. Problems may arise either in the placement and maintenance of venous access or in the formulation and delivery of parenteral solutions. One of the more common and serious complications associated with long-term parenteral feeding is sepsis secondary to contamination of the central venous catheter. Contamination of solutions should be considered but is rare when proper pharmacy protocols have been followed. This problem occurs more frequently in patients with systemic sepsis and in many cases is due to hematogenous seeding of the catheter with bacteria. Usually, it is due to failure to observe strict aseptic precautions during preparation and administration of the solutions. One of the earliest signs of systemic sepsis may be the sudden development of glucose intolerance (with or without temperature increase) in a patient who previously has been maintained on parenteral alimentation without difficulty. When this occurs or if fever develops without obvious cause, a diligent search for a potential septic forcus is indicated. Other causes of fever should also be investigated. If fever persists, the infusion catheter should be removed and cultured. Some centers are now replacing catheters considered at low risk for infection over a J-wire. Should evidence of infection persist over 24 to 48 h without a definable source, the catheter should be replaced in the opposite subclavian vein or into one of the internal jugular veins and the infusion restarted. It may be advisable to wait a short period of time before reinserting the catheter, especially if bacteremia or hemodynamic instability are present.

Other complications related to catheter placement include the development of pneumothorax, hemothorax, or hydrothorax; subclavian artery injury; cardiac arrhythmias if the catheter is placed into the atrium or the ventricle; air embolism or catheter embolism; and, rarely, cardiac perforation with tamponade. Clinically evident thrombophlebitis or thrombosis of the superior vena cava has been rare, but radiographically proved thrombophlebitis has been noted in up to 25 percent of selected patients. All these complications may be avoided by strict adherence to the techniques previously outlined.

Although there is a trend for increased utilization of multiple lumen catheters for purposes of infusion therapy and monitoring critically ill patients, the risks, particularly of sepsis and of venous thrombosis, attending the prolonged use of such catheters may be increased. Efforts should be directed at replacing these catheters with standard single lumen intravenous feeding catheters at the earliest possible time. The acute nutritional management of surgical patients seldom requires the use of permanently implanted catheters (Fig. 2-8). Use of these catheters should be restricted to those nonseptic or high-risk patients requiring prolonged periods of nutritional and/or fluid therapy or for selected patients requiring frequent blood sampling.

Hyperosmolar nonketotic hyperglycemia may develop with normal rates of infusion in patients with impaired glucose toler-

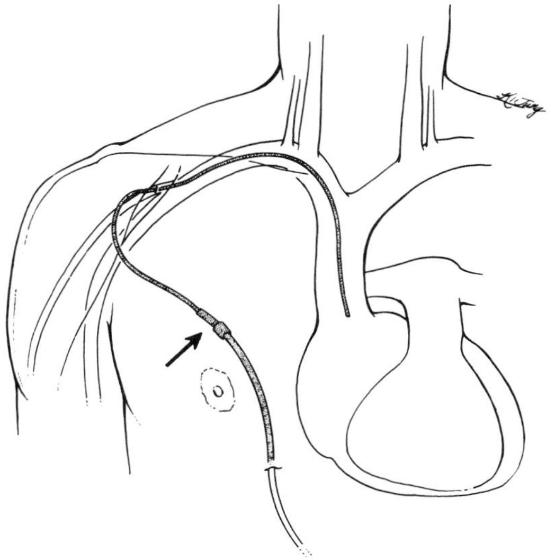

FIG. 2-8. A silastic catheter of the Hickman of Broviac type may be placed by percutaneous means into the superior vena cava or, as shown, by a venotomy in the cephalic, external, or internal jugular veins. The dacron cuff (arrow) may be positioned closer to the skin exit site than is demonstrated above. (Modified from: *Hickman RO et al: Surg Gynecol Obstet 148:871, 1979, with permission.*)

ance or in any patient if the hypertonic solutions are administered too rapidly. This is a particularly common complication in latent diabetics and in patients following severe surgical stress or trauma. Treatment of the condition consists of volume replacement with correction of electrolyte abnormalities and the administration of insulin. This particularly serious complication can be avoided with careful attention to daily fluid balance and frequent determinations of urine and blood sugar levels and serum electrolyte content.

A number of volume, concentration, and compositional abnormalities may also develop, but these are largely avoided by careful attention to the details of patient management. This is particularly important for elderly patients and for patients with significant cardiovascular, renal, or hepatic disorders. Increasing experience has emphasized the importance of not ''overfeeding'' the parenterally nourished patient. This is particularly true of the depleted patient in whom excess calorie infusion may result in carbon dioxide retention and respiratory insufficiency. In addition, excess feeding has also been related to the development of hepatic steatosis or marked glycogen deposition in selected patients. Mild abnormalities of serum transaminases, alkaline phosphatase, and bilirubin may occur in many parenterally nourished patients. Failure of the tests to plateau or return toward normal over 7 to 14 days should suggest another etiology.

Home Parenteral Nutrition

Patients who do not require a hospital environment for management of their primary disease, yet cannot tolerate adequate enteral or oral feeding, *may* be candidates for home parenteral nutrition. Silastic catheters placed in the superior vena cava by the cephalic or internal jugular vein and tunneled over the chest wall to exit near the sternum have proved effective for this purpose (Fig. 2-8). Alternatives to this technique include the placement of subcutaneous infusion ports, which in preliminary trials have proved to be effective for long-term intravenous nutritional support. An absolute catheter-related infection rate of 0.3 per year per patient may be anticipated.

While home parenteral nutrition is generally more cost-effective than similar inpatient methods, criteria for selection of patients must be more stringent than those listed above for hospitalized patients. Patients with terminal illnesses, lack of self-care ability, or lack of a supportive home environment are *not* candidates for this method. The majority of patients will suffer from inflammatory bowel disease, motility disorders, or ischemic bowel infarction and resection.

An extended period of inpatient training is necesary to acquaint the patient and family with appropriate methods of solution preparation and delivery. This is best done in a multidisciplinary setting where professionals are thoroughly familiar with the acute and chronic complications of home parenteral nutrition. All patients on home parenteral nutrition should be placed on the registry maintained by Howard at the Oley Foundation (Albany Medical College). This will allow continued refinements in the clinical and technical management of these patients.

Bibliography

Fluid and Electrolyte Therapy

Abouna GM, Veazey PR, Terry DB: Intravenous infusion of hydrochloric acid for treatment for severe metabolic alkalosis. *Surgery* 75:194, 1974.

Anderson OS, Engel K: A new acid-based nomogram: An improved method for the calculation of the relevant blood acid-base data. *Scand J Clin Lab Invest* 12:177, 1960.

Astrup P, Jorgensen K, Andersen OS, et al: The acid-based metabolism: A new approach. *Lancet* 1:1035, 1960.

Bartlett WC: Acute hyperparathyroid crisis. *Am J Surg* 114:796, 1967.

Baxter CR, Zedlitz WH, Shires GT: High-output acute renal failure complicating acute traumatic injury. *J Trauma* 4:467, 1964.

Bear RA, Dyck RF: Clinical approach to the diagnosis of acid-base disorders. *Can Med Assoc J* 120:172, 1979.

Bishop RL, Weisfeldt ML: Sodium bicarbonate administration during cardiac arrest: Effect on arterial pH, pCO_2 and osmolality. *JAMA* 235:506, 1976

Brenner BM, Rector FC (eds): *The Kidney,* 3d ed. Philadelphia, WB Saunders, 1987.

Canizaro PC: Oxygen transport in shock, in Shires GT (ed): *Shock and Related Problems*. New York, Churchill Livingstone, 1984, pp 95–110.

Canizaro PC, Prager MD, Shires GT: The infusion of Ringer's lactate solution during shock. *Am J Surg* 122:494, 1971.

Christensen MS, Brodersen P, et al: Cerebral apoplexy (stroke) treated with or without prolonged artificial hyperventilation. II. Cerebrospinal fluid acid-base balance and intracranial pressure. *Stroke* 4:620, 1973.

Collins JA: Problems associated with the massive transfusion of stored blood. *Surgery* 75:274, 1974.

Collins JA, Murawski K, Shafer WA (eds): *Massive Transfusion in Surgery and Trauma*. New York, Alan R. Liss, 1982.

Cooper N, Brazier JR, et al: Myocardial depression following citrated blood transfusion. *Arch Surg* 107:756, 1973.

Dudrick SJ, et al: General principles and techniques of intravenous hyperalimentation, in Cowan GSM, Schutz WL (eds): *Intravenous Hyperalimentation,* Philadelphia, Lea & Febiger, 1972.

Elias EG, Evans JT: Hypercalcemic crisis in neoplastic disease: Management with mithramycin. *Surgery* 71:631, 1972.

Guyton AC, Taylor AE, Granger HJ: *Circulatory Physiology. II. Dynamics and Control of the Body Fluids*. Philadelphia, WB Saunders, 1975.

Harken AH, Gabel RA, et al: Hydrochloric acid in the correction of metabolic acidosis. *Arch Surg* 110:819, 1975.

Henzel JH, DeWeese MS, Ridenhour C: Significance of magnesium and zinc metabolism in the surgical patient. I. Magnesium. *Arch Surg* 95:974, 1967.

Jenkins MT, Beck GP: Differential diagnosis of hypotension occuring during anesthesia and surgery. *Clin Anesthesiol* 3:106, 1963.

Kassirer J, Berkman P, et al: The critical role of chloride in the correction of hypokalemic alkalosis in man. *Am J Med* 38:172, 1965.

Katz MA: Hyperglycemia induced hyponatremia. Calculations of expected serum sodium depression. *N Engl J Med* 289:843, 1973.

Lassen NA: Control of cerebral circulation in health and disease. *Circ Res* 34:749, 1974.

Laurens R, Karp BI: Pontine and extrapontine myelinolysis following rapid correction of hyponatremia. *Lancet* 1:1439, 1988.

Mattar JA, Weil MH, Shubin H, et al: Cardiac arrest in the critically ill. II. Hyperosmolal states following cardiac arrest. *Am J Med* 56:162, 1974.

Maxwell MH, Kleeman CR, Narins RG (eds): *Clinical Disorders of Fluid and Electrolyte Metabolism,* 5th ed. New York, McGraw-Hill, 1994.

McClelland RN, Shires GT, et al: Balanced salt solution in the treatment of hemorrhagic shock studies in dogs. *JAMA* 199:830, 1967.

Mellemgaard K, Astrup P: The quantitative determination of surplus amounts of acid or base in the human body. *Scand J Clin Lab Invest* 12:187,1960.

Mengoli LR: Experts from the history of postoperative fluid therapy. *Am J Surg* 121:311, 1971.

Miller TR, Anderson RJ, et al: Urinary diagnostic indices in acute renal failure. *Ann Intern Med* 89:47, 1978.

Moncrief JA, Mason AD: Water vapor loss in the burned patient. *Surg Forum* 13:38, 1962.

Moore FD, Olesen KH, McMurrey JD, et al: *Body Cell Mass and Its Supporting Environment: Body Composition in Health and Disease*. Philadelphia, WB Saunders, 1963.

Pitts RF: Acid-base regulation by the kidneys. *Am J Med* 9:356, 1950.

Randall RE Jr, Cohen MD, et al: Hypermagnesemia in renal failure: Etiology and toxic manifestations. *Ann Intern Med* 61:73, 1964.

Roberts JP, Roberts JD, Skinner C, et al: Extracellular fluid deficit following operation and its correction with Ringer's lactate; a reassessment. *Ann Surg* 202:1, 1985.

Schwartz WB, Relman AS: A critique of the parameters used in the evaluation of acid-base disorders. *N Engl J Med* 268:1382, 1963.

Shires GT, Cunningham JN, et al: Alterations in cellular membrane function during hemorrhagic shock in primates. *Ann Surg* 176:288, 1972.

Shires GT, Holman V: Dilutional acidosis. *Ann Intern Med* 28:551, 1948.

Shires GT, Jackson DE: Postoperative salt tolerance. *Arch Surg* 84:703, 1962.

Shires GT, Williams J, Brown F: Acute changes in extracellular fluids associated with major surgical procedures. *Ann Surg* 154:803, 1961.

Shires GT III, Peitzman AB, et al: Response of extravascular lung water to intraoperative fluids. *Ann Surg* 197:515, 1983.

Singer RB, Hastings AB: An improved clinical method for the estimation of disturbances of the acid-base balance of human blood. *Medicine* 27:223, 1948.

Sporn N, Lancestremere RG, Papper S: Differential diagnosis of oliguria in aged patients. *N Engl J Med* 267:130, 1962.

Thompson JE, Vollman RW, et al: Prevention of hypotensive and renal complications of aortic surgery using balanced salt solution: Thirteen year experience with 670 cases. *Ann Surg* 167:767, 1968.

Tuller MA, Mehdi F: Compensatory hypoventilation and hypercapnia in primary metabolic alkalosis. *Am J Med* 50:281, 1971.

Vanatta JD, Fogelman MJ: *Moyer's Fluid Balance,* 3d ed. Chicago, Year Book Medical Publishers, 1982.

Virgilio RW, Rice CL, et al: Crystalloid vs. colloid resuscitation: Is one better? *Surgery* 85:129, 1979.

Williams DB, Lyons JH: Treatment of severe metabolic alkalosis with intravenous infusion of hydrochloric acid. *Surg Gynecol Obstet* 150:315, 1980.

Wilson RF, Sibbold WJ: Approach to acid-base problems in the critically ill and injured. *J Am Coll Emerg Physicians* 5:515, 1976.

Wright HK, Gann DS: Correction of defect in free water excretion in postoperative patients by extracellular fluid volume expansion. *Ann Surg* 158:70, 1963.

Nutrition

Alexander JW, MacMillan BG, et al: Beneficial effects of aggressive protein feeding in severely burned children. *Ann Surg* 192:505, 1980.

Askanazi J, Rosenbaum SH, et al: Respiratory changes induced by the large glucose loads of total parenteral nutrition. *JAMA* 243:1444, 1980.

Baker JP, Detsky AS, et al: Randomized trial of total parenteral nutrition in critically ill patients: Metabolic effects of varying glucose-lipid ratios as the energy source. *Gastroenterology* 87:53, 1984.

Bessey PQ, Watters JM, et al: Combined hormonal infusion simulates the metabolic response to injury. *Ann Surg* 200:264, 1984.

Cahill GF Jr: Starvation in man. *N Engl J Med* 282:668, 1970.

Cerra FB: Hypermetabolism, organ failure, and metabolic support. *Surgery* 101:1, 1987.

Cerra FB, McPherson JP, et al: Enteral nutrition does not prevent multiple organ failure syndrome (MOFS) after sepsis. *Surgery* 104:727, 1988.

Clague MB, Keir MJ, et al: The effects of nutrition and trauma on whole-body protein metabolism in man. *Clin Sci* 65:165, 1983.

Cuthbertson DP: The disturbance of metabolism produced by bony and non-bony injury, with notes on certain abnormal conditions of bone. *Biochem J* 24:1244, 1930.

Dahn MS, Lange P, et al: Splanchnic and total body oxygen consumption differences in septic and injured patients. *Surgery* 101:69, 1987.

Dudrick SJ, Wilmore DW, et al: Long-term parenteral nutrition with growth, development, and positive nitrogen balance. *Surgery* 64:134, 1968.

Fong Y, Marano MA, et al: Total parenteral nutrition and bowel rest modify the metabolic response to endotoxin in man. *Ann Surg* 210:449, 1989.

Heymsfield SB, Bethel RA, et al: Enteral hyperalimentation: An alternative to central venous hyperalimentation. *Ann Intern Med* 90:63, 1979.

Hook E, Jacox AK, et al: Evaluating total parenteral nutrition: Core statement of the technology assessment and practice guidelines forum. *Nutrition* 6:474, 1990.

Klein S, Simes J, Blackburn GL: Total parenteral nutrition and cancer clinical trials. *Cancer* 58:1378, 1986.

Lindmark L, Bennegard K, et al: Resting energy expenditure in malnourished patients with and without cancer. *Gastroenterology* 87:402, 1984.

Lowry SF: Host metabolic response to injury, in Shires GT, Davis JM (eds): *Host Defenses Advance in Trauma and Surgery*. New York, Raven Press, 1986.

Lowry SF: The route of feeding influences injury responses. *J Trauma* 30:510, 1990.

Mirtallo JM, Schneider PJ, et al: A comparison of essential and general amino acid infusions on the nutritional support of patients with compromised renal function. *J Parenter Enterol Nutr* 6:109, 1982.

Moore FA, Moore EE, et al: TEN versus TPN following major abdominal trauma-reduced septic morbidity. *J Trauma* 29:916, 1989.

Mullen JL, Buzby GP, et al: Reduction of operative morbidity and mortality by combined preoperative and postoperative nutritional support. *Ann Surg* 192:604, 1980.

Muller JM, Dienst C, et al: Pre-operative parenteral feeding in patients with gastrointestinal carcinoma. *Lancet* 1:68, 1982.

Twomey PL, Patching SC: Cost-effectiveness of nutritional support. *J Parenter Enterol Nutr* 9:3, 1985.

Veterans Affairs total parenteral nutrition cooperative study group: Perioperative total parenteral nutrition in surgical patients. *N Engl J Med* 325:525, 1991.

CHAPTER 3

Hemostasis, Surgical Bleeding, and Transfusion

Seymour I. Schwartz

BIOLOGY OF HEMOSTASIS

Hemostasis is a complex process that prevents or terminates blood loss from a disrupted intravascular space, provides a fibrin network for tissue repair, and, ultimately, removes the fibrin when it is no longer needed. Endothelial cells functionally act to prevent clotting. They interfere with platelet recruitment by inactivating adenosine diphosphate (ADP). They provide an environment in which thrombin is also inactivated by complexing with antithrombin III. Endothelial cells release thrombomodulin that downmodulates the coagulation process (Fig. 3-1). Four major physiologic events participate, both in sequence and interdependently, in the hemostatic process. Vascular constriction, platelet plug formation, fibrin formation, and fibrinolysis occur in that general order, but the products of each of these four processes are interrelated in such a fashion that there is a continuum and multiple reinforcements (Fig. 3-2).

Vascular Constriction

Vasoconstriction is the initial vascular response to injury even at the capillary level. It is dependent upon local contraction of smooth muscle that has a reflex response to various stimuli. The initial vascular constriction occurs prior to platelet adherence at the site of injury. Adherence of endothelial cells to adjacent endothelial cells may be sufficient to cause cessation of blood loss from the intravascular space. Vasoconstriction is subsequently linked to

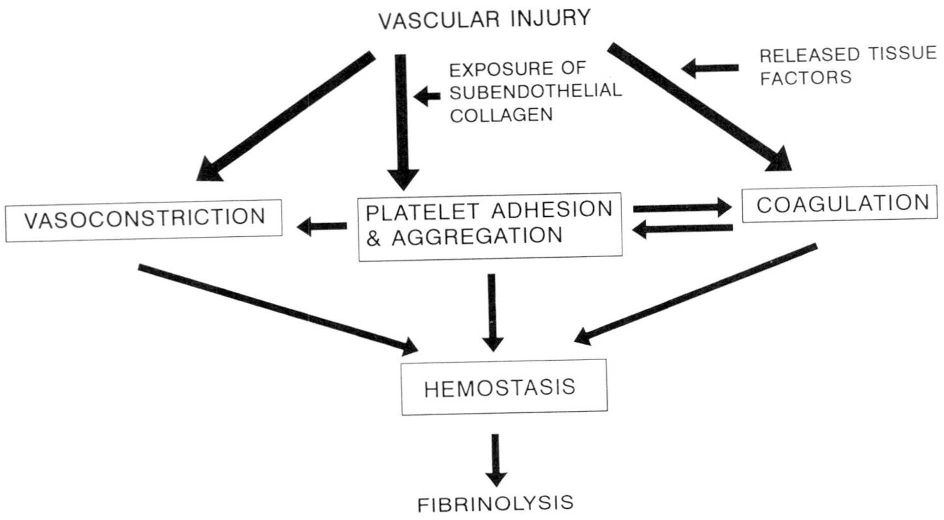

FIG. 3-1. Simplified view of the process involved in hemostasis.

platelet plug and fibrin formation. Thromboxane A_2 (TXA_2), which results from the release of arachidonic acid from platelet membranes during aggregation, is a powerful vasoconstrictor. By contrast, prostacycline, which is also secreted during the platelet release reaction, is a potent vasodilator. Serotonin, 5-hydroxytryptamine (5-HT), released during platelet aggregation, is another vasoconstrictor, but it has been shown that when platelets have been depleted of serotonin in vivo, constriction is not inhibited. Bradykinin and fibrinopeptides in the coagulation schema are also capable of contracting smooth muscle. Some patients with mild bleeding disorders and a prolonged bleeding time have, as their only abnormality, capillary loops that fail to constrict in response to injury.

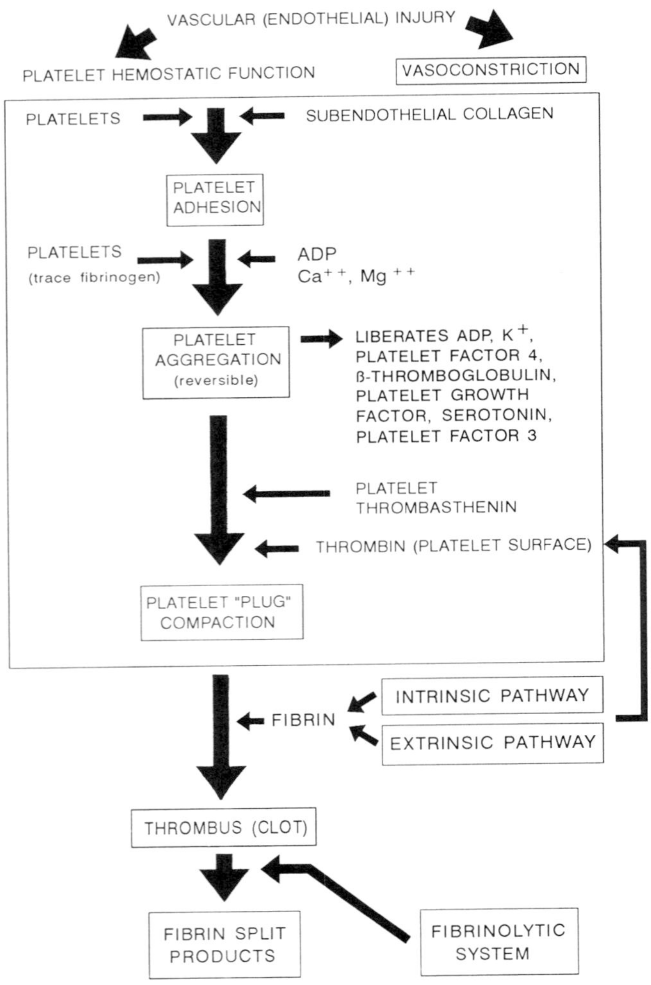

FIG. 3-2. Schematic representation of hemostasis.

A lateral incision in a small artery may remain open because of physical forces, while complete transection of a similarly sized vessel contracts to the extent that bleeding may cease spontaneously. The vascular response factor should also include the contribution of pressure provided by surrounding tissues. Bleeding from a small venule ruptured by trauma, in the thigh of an athlete, may be negligible because of the compressive effect of surrounding muscle. In the same individual, bleeding from a similar vessel in the nasal mucosa may be significant. When there is low perivascular pressure, as seen in patients with muscle atrophy accompanying aging, in patients on prolonged steroid therapy, and in patients with the Ehlers-Danlos syndrome, bleeding tends to be more persistent.

Platelet Function

Platelets are 2-μm diameter fragments of megakaryocytes and number 200,000 to 400,000/mm^3 in circulating blood with a life span of 7 to 9 days. They play an integral role in hemostasis along two pathways. Platelets, which normally do not adhere to each other or to the normal vessel wall, form a plug that stops bleeding when vascular disruption occurs. Injury to the intima exposes subendothelial collagen to which platelets adhere within 15 s of the traumatic event. This requires von Willebrand factor (vWF), a protein that is lacking in patients with von Willebrand's disease. The platelets then expand and develop pseudopodal processes and also initiate a release reaction that recruits other platelets from the circulating blood. As a consequence, a loose platelet aggregate forms, sealing the disrupted blood vessel. The aggregation up to this point is reversible and is not associated with secretion. This process is known as *primary hemostasis*. The administration of heparin does not interfere with this reaction, and that fact explains why hemostasis can occur in the heparinized patient. ADP and serotonin are principal mediators in this process of adhesion and aggregation. Various prostaglandins have opposing activities.

Arachidonic acid, released from platelet membranes, is converted by cyclooxygenase to prostaglandin G_2 (PGG_2) and PGH_2, which, in turn, are converted to TXA_2, a potent platelet aggregator and vasoconstrictor. By contrast, PGI_2 (prostacyclin) and PGE_2 inhibit aggregation and act as vasodilators.

ADP, released from damaged tissues and platelets, plus platelet factor 4 and trace thrombin on the platelet surface in the face of Ca^{2+} and Mg^{2+}, stimulate a platelet release reaction by which the content of the platelet and its granules is discharged. Fibrinogen is required for this process. During this process, platelet factor 4, β-thromboglobulin, platelet-derived growth factor, ADP, serotonin, and calcium are introduced into the plasma. The release reaction results in compaction of the platelets and the formation of an "amorphous" plug, which is no longer reversible. This process is inhibited by cyclic adenosine monophosphate (cAMP). As a consequence of the release reaction, platelet factor 3 is made available and contributes phospholipid to several stages of the coagulation cascade.

The lipoprotein surface provided by platelets catalyzes reactions that are involved in the conversion of prothrombin (factor II) into thrombin (Fig. 3-3). Platelet factor 3 is involved in the reaction by which activated factor IX (IXa), factor VIII, and calcium activate factor X. It is also involved in the reaction by which Xa, factor V, and Ca^{2+} activate factor II. Platelets may also play a role in the initial activation of factors XI and XII. Platelet factor 4 and β-thromboglobulin are also made available during the release reaction, and they may inhibit the activity of heparin and modify fibrin formation. The platelets also play a role in the fibrinolytic process by releasing an inhibitor of plasminogen activation.

Coagulation

Coagulation is the process by which prothrombin is converted into the proteolytic enzyme thrombin, which, in turn, cleaves the fibrinogen molecule to form insoluble fibrin in order to stabilize and add to the platelet plug. Coagulation consists of a series of zymogen activation stages in which circulating proenzymes are converted in sequence to activated proteases (Fig. 3-4). The traditional concept of the clotting system evolved from test tube analysis and follows two pathways. The two pathways are the *intrinsic* pathway, which involves components normally present in blood, and the *extrinsic* pathway that is initiated by the tissue lipoprotein (Fig. 3-5). In the intrinsic pathway factor XII is activated by binding to subendothelial collagen. Prekallikrein and high molecular weight kinogen amplify this contact phase. Activated factor XII (XIIa) proteolytically cleaves factor XI and also prekallikrein to form XIa and kallikrein. In the presence of Ca^{2+}, XIa activates factor IX (IXa). This, in turn, complexes with factor VIII, which can be activated to a more potent form by thrombin, and, in the presence of Ca^{2+} and the phospholipid platelet factor 3, activates factor X. In the extrinsic pathway, the tissue phospholipid, thromboplastin, reacts with factor VII and Ca^{2+} to activate factor X.

Activated factor X (Xa), produced by the two pathways, proteolyzes prothrombin (factor II) to form thrombin. The effects of thrombin are limited to the area of endothelial disruption by several processes. The escape of thrombin into the circulation is prevented from complexing with antithrombin locally by the binding of the thrombin to thrombomodulin on the endothelium, creating a complex that cannot cleave fibrinogen and also activating protein C, which, in turn, inactivates factors V and VIII. Additionally, circulating thrombin is inactivated by plasma protease inhibitors. This process is accelerated by factor V, tissue lipoproteins, platelet surface phospholipids, and Ca^{2+}. Thrombin activates the fibrin stabilizing factor (XIII) and cleaves fibrinopeptides A and B from fibrinogen (factor I) to form fibrin, a monomer that is cross-linked with XIIIa, to form a stable clot (Fig. 3-6).

All the coagulation factors except thromboplastin, Ca^{2+}, and most of factor VIII are synthesized in the liver. Factors II, VII, IX, and X require vitamin K for their production (Table 3-1).

Fibrinolysis

Fibrinolysis is a natural process directed at maintaining the patency of blood vessels by lysis of fibrin deposits. Also involved in the maintenance of vascular patency is circulating antithrombin III (ATIII) which neutralizes the action of thrombin and other proteases in the coagulation cascade.

Fibrinolysis is initiated at the same time as the clotting mechanism under the influence of circulating kinases, tissue activators,

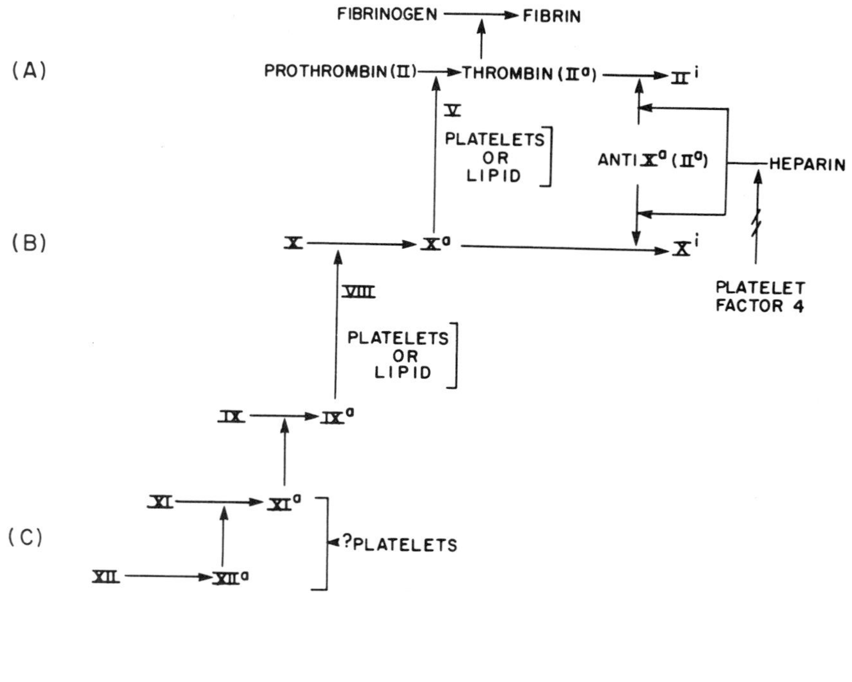

FIG. 3-3. Role of platelets in coagulation. Platelets or phospholipid accelerate reactions *A* and *B*. In addition, the role of platelets may be more complex in reaction *B* and may serve to protect factor X_a from inactivation by plasma inhibitors. Platelets may also play a part in activating the contact system *C*. Platelet factor 4 is the heparin-neutralizing substance (i = inactivated clotting factor). (From: *Weiss HJ: 1975, with permission.*)

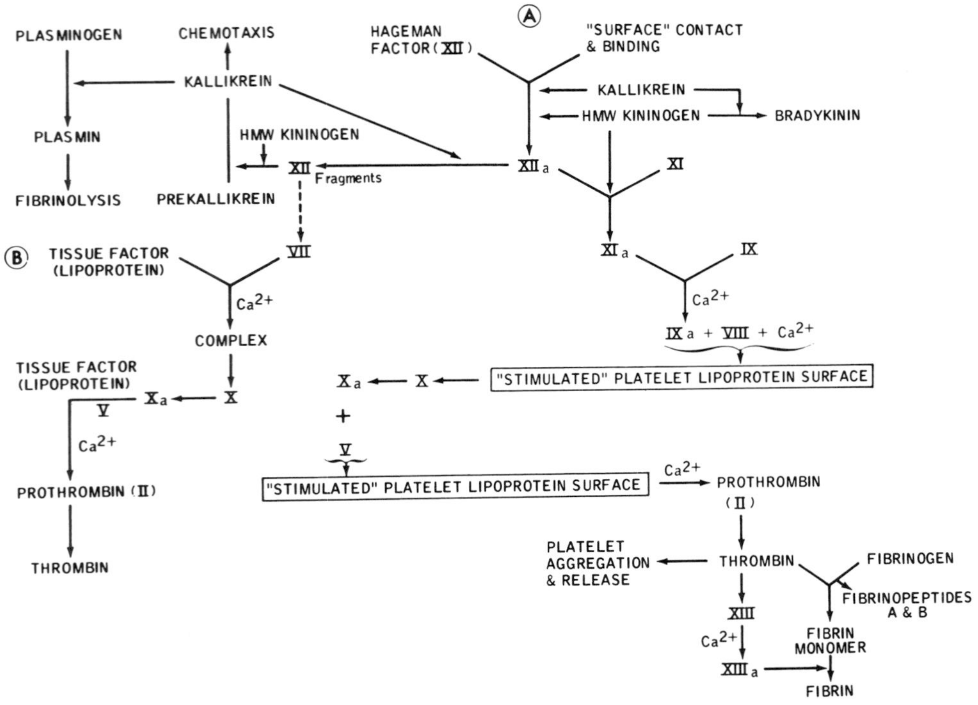

FIG. 3-4. Outline of the intrinsic (*A*) and extrinsic (*B*) pathways of fibrin formation.

and kallikrein present in many organs including venous endothelium. Fibrinolysis is dependent on the enzyme, plasmin, which is derived from a precursor plasma protein (plasminogen) (Fig. 3-7). Plasminogen levels are known to rise as a consequence of exercise, venous occlusion, and anoxia. Plasminogen activation is also initiated by the activation of factor XII. The plasminogen is preferentially absorbed on fibrin deposits. The enzyme plasmin lyses fibrin and acts on other coagulant proteins, including fibrinogen, factor V, and factor VIII, as well. The smaller fragments of polypeptide products of fibrin that are produced interfere with normal platelet aggregation; the larger fragments are incorporated into the clot in lieu of normal fibrin monomers and result in an unstable clot. Human blood also contains an anti-plasmin that inhibits plasminogen activation, and platelets are believed to possess anti-fibrinolytic activity.

CONGENITAL HEMOSTATIC DEFECTS

Inheritance

The modes of inheritance of hemostatic disorders, with only rare exceptions, are three in type: (1) autosomal dominant, (2) autosomal recessive, and (3) sex-linked recessive. The most common hemostatic disorder transmitted by the autosomal dominant mode is von Willebrand's disease. Hereditary hemorrhagic telangiectasia and factor XI deficiency also appear to be transmitted in this fashion.

Occasionally, in a pedigree with an autosomal dominant gene, an *apparently* normal person may transmit disease to his or her child. The parent clearly carried the gene, which clinically expressed no defect.

In inherited hemostatic disorders, the difference in clinical expression between dominant and recessive genes is a graded one rather than an ''all-or-none'' phenomenon. The heterozygous individual with an autosomal recessive trait may have a measurable deficiency of the factor governed by that gene, but no clinical disease. In order to demonstrate clinical expression of disease, the individual must be homozygous. This appears to be the case, for example, in factor X deficiency. Other hemostatic disorders probably inherited in this mode are factor V, factor VII, and factor I deficiencies.

Sex-linked recessive inheritance governs true hemophilia (factor VIII deficiency) and factor IX deficiency (Christmas disease).

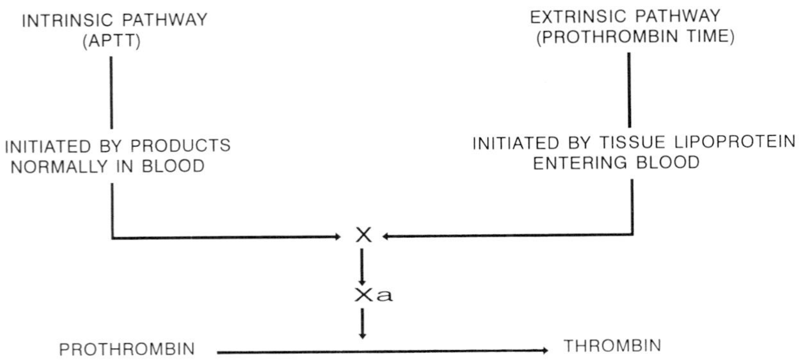

FIG. 3-5. Pathways of blood coagulation.

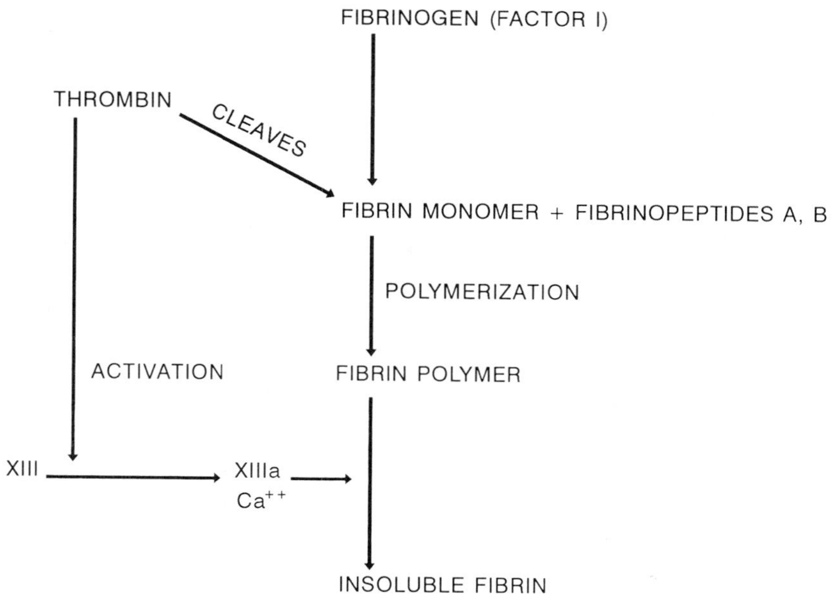

FIG. 3-6. Formation of fibrin.

The genes for these diseases are recessive in expression and are carried on the female (X) chromosome. When paired with the normal X chromosome (the female carrier state), clinical disease is not present. When the affected X chromosome is paired with the normal male (Y) chromosome, clinical disease is expressed.

Platelet Deficiencies

The most common congenital platelet deficiency is an abnormality seen in *von Willebrand's disease* (see material below). In this disorder, the von Willebrand factor (vWF), which is missing, has been shown to be required for platelet adhesion to subendothelial collagen. Also, unlike platelets of normal patients that aggregate in vitro when ristocetin is added, platelets from patients with von Willebrand's disease fail to aggregate with the addition of ristocetin. Another inherited disorder affecting platelets is the rare *Bernard-Soulier syndrome*. Patients with Bernard-Soulier syndrome have normal levels of vWF and the addition of that factor does not affect aggregation of platelets in the presence of ristocetin. In Bernard-Soulier syndrome, the platelet membrane receptor for vWF, a portion of the glycoprotein I complex, is missing.

Glanzmann's thrombasthenia is a rare congenital disorder in which platelets fail to aggregate in the presence of ADP and mediation of factors involved in clot retention is impaired also. Patients with *congenital afibrinogenemia* also have impairment of platelet aggregation because fibrinogen is required for this process to occur. Patients with congenital afibrinogenemia have disturbed platelet function, manifested by a prolonged bleeding time correctable by fibrinogen administration.

Congenital disorders of platelet secretion include *storage pool disease,* in which the platelets lack the storage capability of ADP required for aggregation. The Hermansky-Pudlak syndrome (occulocutaneous albinism, ceroidlike deposits in macrophages, and bleeding diathesis) is classified in this category. Congenital *primary release defects* have also been described and are responsible for prolonged bleeding time.

Table 3-1
Nomenclature of Coagulation Factors

Factor I	Fibrinogen
Factor II	Prothrombin
Factor III	Thromboplastin (tissue or platelet factors)
Factor IV	Calcium
Factor V	Proaccelerin
Factor VI	(Same as factor V)
Factor VII	Proconvertin
Factor VIII	Antihemophilic factor
Factor IX	Plasma thromboplastin component (Christmas factor)
Factor X	Stuart-Prower factor
Factor XI	Plasma thromboplastin antecedent (PTA)
Factor XII	Hageman factor
Factor XIII	Fibrin stabilizing factor (Laki-Lorand)

Congenital Defects of Coagulation Factors

Factor VIII Deficiency (Classical Hemophilia)

Classical hemophilia (hemophilia A) is a disease of males. The failure to synthesize normal factor VIII activity is inherited as a

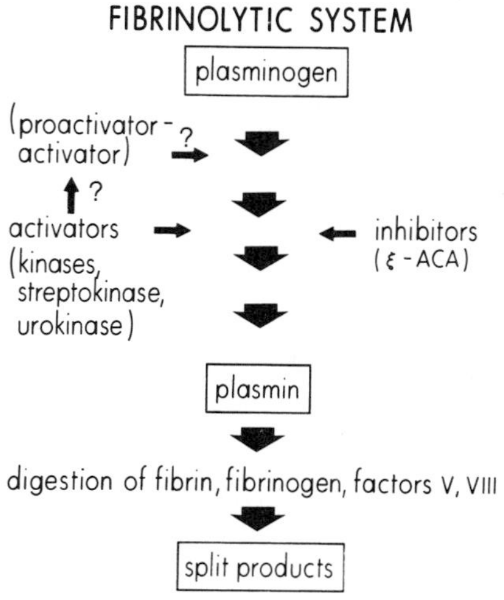

FIG. 3-7. Fibrinolyt . system.

sex-linked recessive trait. Spontaneous mutations account for almost 20 percent of cases. The incidence of the disease is approximately 1:10,000 to 1:15,000 population, and the clinical manifestations can be extremely variable. The accuracy for detecting the carrier state now approaches 90 percent.

Clinical Manifestations. Characteristically, the severity of clinical manifestations is related to the degree of deficiency of factor VIII. Spontaneous bleeding and severe complications are the rule when virtually no factor VIII can be detected in the plasma. When plasma factor VIII concentrations are in the range of 5 percent of normal, the patient may have no spontaneous bleeding yet may bleed severely with trauma or surgical treatment. Patients with levels greater than 5 percent of normal (greater than 0.05 units/mL) are considered mild hemophiliacs. Patients whose factor VIII levels fall between 1 and 5 percent of normal are considered moderately severe hemophiliacs. Typically, members of the same pedigree with true hemophilia will have approximately the same degree of clinical manifestations.

While the severely affected patient may bleed during early infancy, significant bleeding typically is noted first when the child is a toddler. At that time, in addition to the classic bleeding into joints, epistaxis and hematuria may be noted. Bleeding that is life-threatening may follow injury to the tongue or frenulum. Tracheal compression and retropharyngeal bleeding may follow tonsillar infection. Intracranial bleeding, associated with trauma in half the cases, accounts for 25 percent of deaths. Vascular and neural compromise may occur in relation to pressure secondary to bleeding into a soft tissue closed space. Equinus contracture deformity may be seen in severely hemophilic patients secondary to bleeding into the calf. Volkmann's contracture of the forearm and flexion contractures of the knees and elbows are also disabling sequelae of deep soft tissue bleeding.

Hemarthrosis is the most characteristic orthopaedic problem. Bleeding into the joint may cause few symptoms until distention of the joint capsule occurs. A large hemarthrosis generally is manifested by a tender, swollen, warm, and painful joint. Muscle spasm and pain around the joint arise from involvement of periarticular structures. These signs may mimic infection. The same orthopaedic problems are noted in association with severe factor IX deficiency (Christmas disease).

Retroperitoneal bleeding may follow lifting of a heavy object or strenuous exercise. Signs of posterior peritoneal irritation and spasm of the iliopsoas suggest the diagnosis. Hypovolemic shock may occur, since the amount of blood loss that can take place in this setting is enormous. The clinical manifestations of intramural intestinal hematoma are nausea and vomiting, crampy abdominal pain, and signs of peritoneal irritation mimic those of appendicitis. Fever and leukocytosis may be noted. Radiographs of the abdomen may fail to reveal an abnormality or may display a modest amount of ileus. Upper gastrointestinal examination may demonstrate a uniform thickening of mucosal folds which has been described as a "picket fence" or "stack of coins" appearance (Fig. 3-8). Intramural hematomas of the intestine occur with other hemostatic disorders and, therefore, should be considered when any patient with a hemostatic problem presents with findings suggesting an acute intraabdominal process.

Treatment. ***Replacement Therapy.*** The plasma concentration of factor VIII necessary for maintenance of hemostatic integrity is normally quite small. Patients with as little as 2 to 3 percent of factor VIII activity usually do not bleed spontaneously. Once serious bleeding begins, however, a much higher level of factor VIII activity, probably approaching 30 percent, is necessary to achieve hemostasis.

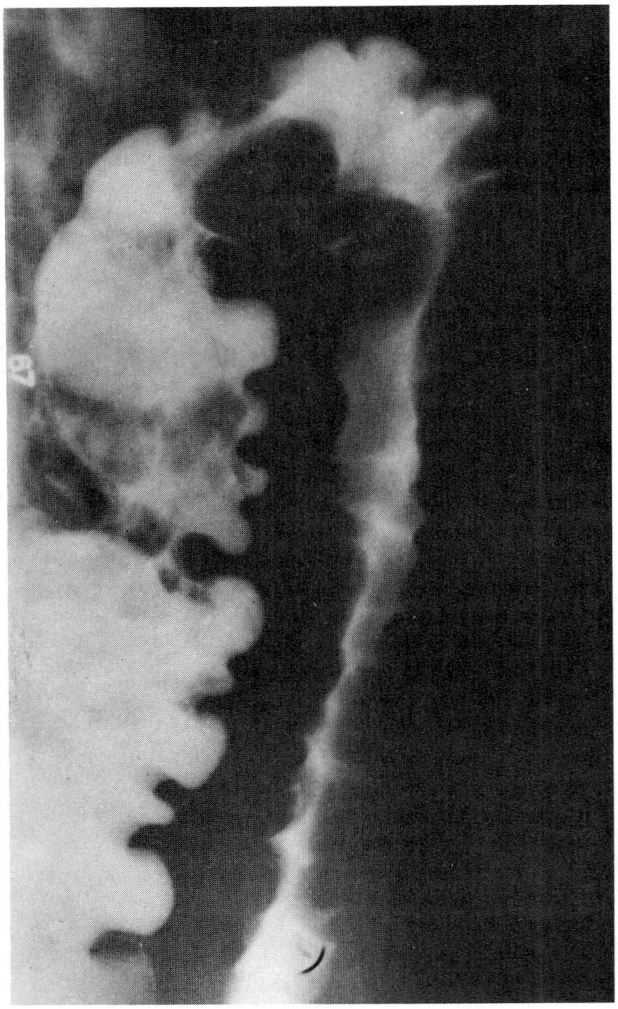

FIG. 3-8. Radiograph of patient with hemophilia. Note thickening of mucosal folds indicative of an intramural hematoma.

The half-life of factor VIII is 8 to 12 h. Following administration of a given dose of factor VIII, approximately one-half of the initial posttransfusion activity disappears from the plasma in 4 h. This early disappearance is thought to be due, in large part, to diffusion from the intravascular space. The period of equilibration can extend for as long as 8 h, at which time only about one-quarter of the initial level remains in the circulating blood. From that time on, the slope of disappearance is less steep. Twenty-four hours after a given dose, no more than 7 to 8 percent of administered factor VIII activity remains within the circulation.

One unit of factor VIII activity is considered that amount present in 1 mL of normal plasma. Actually, fresh frozen plasma contains 0.60 unit/mL. Theoretically, in a patient with 0 percent activity, to achieve an initial posttransfusion level of 60 percent of normal, using fresh plasma, a volume of plasma equal to 60 percent of the patient's estimated plasma volume would have to be administered. Table 3-2 shows approximate levels of factor VIII required for hemostasis in different lesions. The minimum hemo-

Table 3-2
Principles of Substitution Therapy in Surgery in Patients with Severe Bleeding Disorders

	Day of Operation				*Day 2–7 Postoperatively*			*Day 8 Postoperatively*		
	Dosage				*Dosage*			*Dosage*		
Type of Operation and Disease	*Desirable Level of (%)*	*Initial Units/kg*	*Maintenance Units/kg BW**	*Interval (h)*	*Desirable Level of (%)*	*Maintenance Units/kg BW*	*Interval (h)*	*Desirable Level of (%)*	*Maintenance Units/kg BW*	*Interval (h)*
Hemophilia A	VII:C	VIII:C			VIII:C			VIII:C		
Major surgery	50–150	50–60	25–30	4–6	40–60	20–40	4–8	15–25	10–25	12–24
Minor surgery	40–50	25–40	20–30	4–8	30–50	15–20	6–12			
Hemophilia B	IX:C	IX:C			IX:C			IX:C		
Major surgery	50–150	60–70	30–40	8–12	40–60	30–40	12–24	15–25	10–20	24–48
Minor surgery	40–50	25–40	20–30	8–12	30–50	15–20	24			
von Willebrand's disease	VIII:C	VIII:C			VIII:C			VIII:C		
Major surgery	50–70 BT† < 5 min	30–40	30–40	4–5	> 40 BT < 10 min	10–20	12	20–40	5–10	24–48
	VIII:C				VIII:C					
Minor surgery	20–50 BT < 5 min	10–20	10–20	4–5	> 40 BT < 10 min	5–10	12			

*Body weight.

†Bleeding time according to Duke.

SOURCE: Nilsson IM, Larsson SA, Bergentz SE, 1987, with permission.

static level of factor VIII for mild hemorrhages is 30 percent; for joint and muscle bleeding and major hemorrhages, it is 50 percent. For major surgery and life-threatening bleeding, levels of 80 to 100 percent should be reached preoperatively and maintained above 30 percent for 2 weeks. Remembering the loss from the circulation, one-half the initial dose would need to be supplied every 12 h. The use of fresh plasma in such a circumstance would require a volume that is excessive. Factor VIII concentrates now available circumvent this problem. Cryoprecipitate concentrates of factor VIII can be regarded as containing 9.6 units/mL. The amount of material to be given can be computed from the formula

$$\frac{\text{Patient's weight (kg)} \times \text{desired rise of factor VIII (\% average normal)}}{\text{Total units of factor VIII in dose}} = R$$

where R is a factor that is fairly constant for any given type of material and represents the rise of factor VIII obtained in the patient's plasma for every unit of transfused factor VIII per kilogram of the patient's body weight. Half that amount is subsequently administered every 4 to 6 h to maintain a safe level. There is now a variety of factor VIII concentrates available. Regardless of the preparation employed, continued laboratory assessment of circulating factor VIII level is an important element in the control of these patients. Wet-frozen cryoprecipitate is preferred for replacement in patients with mild hemophilia since the risk of hepatitis is less than it is with factor VIII concentrates. The latter are preferred for major replacement problems. In mild hemophilia A and in mild von Willebrand's disease, DDAVP (1-desamino-8-D-arginine vasopressin), a synthetic derivative of vasopressin, has been used to effect a dose-dependent increase of all factor VIII activities and to effect release of plasminogen activator. Patients undergoing orthopaedic or neurosurgical procedures should also receive a fibrinolytic inhibitor.

Following major surgical treatment of the hemophiliac, transfusion replacement of factor VIII should be continued for at least 10 days. Wounds should be well healed and all drains removed before termination of therapy. If sutures remain, transfusion should be reinstituted prior to their removal. Many recent reports document the safety of major surgical procedures in hemophilic patients receiving replacement therapy. But in one large series, the incidence of postoperative hemorrhage did not improve over a 16-year period despite a threefold increase in dosage of factor VIII, suggesting that circulating factor VIII levels are not the sole determinant of bleeding in these patients.

The virus of homologous serum hepatitis is transmitted by the various concentrates of plasma. Other complications of replacement therapy include the appearance of inhibitors of factor VIII, which may arise in the hemophiliacs who have had transfusion. These inhibitors have been characterized as antibodies of the γG variety. They tend to diminish in several weeks if further transfusion is not employed. Laboratory search for these factors should be carried out in every hemophilic patient who is considered a candidate for elective surgical treatment, as their presence complicates transfusion management. Paradoxical bleeding may occur in patients transfused to an appropriate factor VIII level due to the development of abnormal platelet function.

Adjunctive Management. Treatment of soft tissue bleeding is directed at the prevention of airway obstruction and vascular and neural damage. These are accomplished best by the administration of sufficient factor VIII. Bed rest and cold packs can be of some assistance. In general, results of fasciotomy to relieve pressure have varied from disappointing to disastrous. The occasional development of large cysts has resulted in sufficient deformity and disability to require amputation.

The primary treatment of hemophilic hemarthrosis is directed at maintaining full range of motion and minimal destruction of the cartilage. Aspiration of blood from the hemophilic joint is not uniformly endorsed, and when regarded as necessary, it should be considered a major surgical event. Elevation of factor VIII level by transfusion is necessary. The procedure should be carried out in the operating room under strict sterile precautions. In most instances, aspiration is not required, and the combination of factor VIII replacement and local cold packing proves sufficient. Physiotherapy plays a critical role and should consist of *active* exercises, since the patient is unlikely to move the extremity to a point where bleeding will recur. Passive exercises often result in recurrence of bleeding. The reader is referred to the review by Curtiss for details of orthopaedic management.

The management of intramural intestinal hematoma and retroperitoneal bleeding is predicated on appropriate transfusion therapy and avoidance of surgical treatment. Even when a relatively minor procedure, such as tracheostomy, is performed, the plasma level of factor VIII should be raised above 25 to 30 percent. Since dental hygiene usually is poor in hemophilic patients, dental and oral surgical treatment frequently are necessary.

Factor IX Deficiency (Christmas Disease)

Factor IX deficiency clinically is indistinguishable from factor VIII deficiency and also has an X-linked recessive mode of inheritance. These two entities were considered a single disease until 1952, when their unique deficiencies were documented. Factor IX deficiency accounts for 20 percent of hemophiliacs. Christmas disease, like classical hemophilia, can occur in severe, moderate, or mild forms according to the level of factor IX activity in the plasma. The severe form has a factor IX level of less than 1 percent: one-half of the patients belong to this group.

Treatment. Most patients with severe factor IX deficiency require substitution therapy on a regular basis. All patients require substitution therapy whenever minor or major surgery is performed. Currently, therapy is generally based on the administration of factor IX concentrates. Initially the rate of disappearance of factor IX from the circulation is more rapid than that of factor VIII; subsequently factor IX, with a half-life of 18 to 40 h, has a slower disappearance rate. Konyne, which contains 10 to 60 units of factor IX/mL, has produced good results, but thromboembolic complications have been reported. More recently, the preparations have had other activated clotting factors removed, and the incidence of thromboembolic complications has decreased. During severe hemorrhage, treatment should be directed at achieving plasma factor IX levels of 20 to 50 percent of normal for the first 3 to 5 days, and then maintaining the plasma level at 10 to 20 percent of normal for approximately 10 days. The usual daily dose is 30 to 50 μm/kg of body weight, followed by 20 μm/kg of body weight/24 h. When an operation is required, the plasma level of approximately 50 to 70 percent of normal should be achieved. Sixty microns per kilogram of body weight every 24 h is recommended during the operation and the first postoperative day, followed by 30 to 40 μm/kg every 24 h for the next 2 to 3 days, and 20 μm/kg every 24 h for the remainder of the week. In all instances, the levels should be monitored by laboratory determinations. The development of antibodies against factor IX represents a serious complication that is difficult to deal with. This occurs in about 10 percent of patients with Christmas disease. These patients are managed by withholding all infusion therapy with blood or plasma. High doses of factor IX concentrates combined with cyclophosphamide have been effective.

von Willebrand's Disease

von Willebrand's disease occurs as commonly as true hemophilia. The increasing recognition of this disease is related to more reliable factor VIII assays. This hereditary disorder of hemostasis is usually transmitted as an autosomally dominant trait but recessive inheritance may occur. The disease is characterized by a diminution of the level of factor VIII:C (procoagulant) activity that corrects the clotting abnormality in hemophilia A plasma. The reduction of factor VIII:C activity usually is not as great as that seen in classical hemophilia. Also unlike classical hemophilia, where factor VIII:C activity remains constant, in the patient with von Willebrand's disease variation in the level of circulating factor VIII:C activity may be noted. Characteristically, these patients also have a prolonged bleeding time, but this is less constant than the factor VIII:C reduction. A given patient may have an abnormal bleeding time on one occasion and a normal bleeding time on another. The level of factor VIII-related antigen (factor VIII:Ag) is disproportionately lower than that of factor VIII:C, and ristocetin fails to cause platelet aggregation in about 70 percent of patients with the disease. The vast majority of patients has a prolonged activated partial thromboplastin time (aPTT).

Clinical Manifestations. The manifestations of bleeding usually are mild and often overlooked until trauma or the stress of surgical treatment makes them apparent. A careful clinical history is, therefore, of great importance in these patients. Spontaneous manifestations often are limited to bleeding into the skin or mild mucous membrane bleeding. Epistaxis and menorrhagia have been relatively common in our personal experience. Serious bleeding following dental extractions and tonsillectomy also are not uncommon. Fatal bleeding from the gastrointestinal tract has been described.

Treatment. Treatment is directed at correcting the bleeding time and factor VIII R:vWF (the von Willebrand factor). Only cryoprecipitate is reliably effective. Lyophilized concentrates of factor VIII:C lack the required factor VIII R:vWF. Newer factor VIII concentrates have a full complement of vWF. Ten to forty units per kilogram of cryoprecipitate are administered every 12 h to correct the bleeding time. Replacement therapy should be begun 1 day before a surgical procedure. Aspirin *must* be avoided for 10 days before an elective operation. Duration of treatment should be the same as that described for the patient with classical hemophilia. Intravenous high-dose γ-globulin has successfully treated an acquired type of von Willebrand's disease associated with myeloproliferative disorders, leukemias, and lymphomas.

An analogue of the antidiuretic hormone DDAVP (stimate, 1-desamino-8-D-arginine vasopressin) administered intravenously temporarily (for 1 to 2 h) increases vWF:Ag, ristocetin cofactor, and VIII:C and shortens the bleeding time. DDAVP may induce thrombocytopenia and release tissue plasminogen activator.

Rare Deficiencies of Coagulation Factors

Factor XI [plasma thromboplastin antecedent (PTA)] deficiency (Rosenthal's syndrome) is a mild disorder occurring mainly in patients of Jewish ancestry. Patients may undergo major procedures without significant bleeding. Fresh frozen plasma is therapeutic. *Factor V (proaccelerin) deficiency (parahemophilia)* is extremely rare; significant bleeding usually occurs in homozygotes. Excessive bleeding is characteristically associated with factor levels lower than 1 percent of normal. Administration of fresh frozen plasma to raise the level to 25 percent of normal is sufficient. *Factor VII (proconvertin) deficiency* also is associated with excessive operative bleeding in homozygous patients. Administration of banked plasma to raise the factor level above 10 percent of normal provides adequate hemostasis. *Factor X (Stuart-Prower) deficiency* is associated with both amyloidosis and familial carotid body tumors. Frozen or normal plasma is therapeutic. *Factor II (prothrombin) deficiency* is extremely rare and can be corrected with plasma infusion to achieve levels greater than the percent of normal.

Although the prothrombin time will detect factor VII deficiency, it cannot be used as a guide to therapy because it remains abnormal when adequate levels of factor VII are achieved. Patients with factor VII deficiency have normal PTT and thrombin time. Specific assays can define any of these deficiencies. Vitamin K therapy is ineffective in raising levels of factors II, V, VII, X, and XI.

When the transfusion programs outlined above for deficiency of the prothrombin group of factors (factors II, V, VII, and X) are employed, the one-stage prothrombin time does not return to normal. Rather, a one-stage prothrombin time slightly less than twice the control value is achieved. This is sufficient to result in normal hemostasis. Of the four "prothrombin" factors, only factor V must be provided as fresh or freshly frozen plasma. Stored plasma is equally effective as therapy for factors II, VII, and X.

Inherited Fibrinogen Abnormalities

Included in this category are patients with congenital afibrinogenemia, hypofibrinogenemia, and dysfibrinogenemia. Fewer than 200 cases of afibrinogenemia have been reported. This disorder is ascribed to an autosomal, recessive mode of inheritance. The affected individuals are presumably homozygous for the trait. Bleeding time may be markedly prolonged in some patients because fibrinogen is required for platelet aggregation. Conventional methods for measuring fibrinogen in the plasma give a zero value, but immunologic techniques may detect trace amounts of a fibrinogen-like protein. Patients have an indefinitely prolonged whole blood coagulation time, which can be corrected by the addition of fibrinogen. The deficiency, however, usually is less a clinical problem than is classical hemophilia. Bleeding usually begins early in life, and bleeding from the umbilical cord is a characteristic symptom. Bleeding may follow operations, dental extraction, and trauma, but the most feared complication is intracranial bleeding following minor injury to the head.

Less profound inherited deficiencies of fibrinogen have been observed and categorized as congenital hypofibrinogenemia. Two groups of hypofibrinogenemic patients have been differentiated: those with fibrinogen values below 50 mg/dL and those with higher levels. The clinical manifestations depend on the fibrinogen concentration. Another congenital disorder is dysfibrinogenemia, in which there are structural defects in the fibrinogen molecule. Both the hypofibrinogenemia and the dysfibrinogenemia have a dominant mode of inheritance. Dysfibrinogenemic patients are frequently asymptomatic but may have moderate or severe bleeding associated with an operation. They have a propensity for thromboembolic disorders and have a higher incidence of wound dehiscence following operative intervention. The thrombin clotting time is diagnostic for this general category of abnormalities, but definition of the precise abnormality requires a series of complex laboratory studies.

Treatment. Although the hemostatically optimal level of fibrinogen is not known, a level greater than 100 mg/dL is generally required during an operation. The patient's fibrinogen level should be raised above this prior to the procedure. Substitution therapy may be affected by the infusion of fresh frozen plasma or cryoprecipitate. In order to achieve a fibrinogen level near 100 mg/dL for 24 h, an initial dose of 20 to 25 mg fibrinogen/kg of body weight should be administered, followed by one-third the initial amount given on a daily basis throughout the postoperative period. But appropriate corrections must be based on actual fibrinogen measurements. Normal fibrinogen concentration should be maintained until wound healing is shown to be adequate.

Congenital Factor XIII Deficiency

This rare disorder is manifest by umbilical bleeding in the newborn and slow wound healing following an operation. In general, most of the bleeding manifestations are mild, but intracranial bleeding may result as a consequence of minor trauma. The mode of inheritance is an autosomal recessive trait. Immunologic assays have demonstrated deficiency of the protein. Therapy is accomplished with fresh frozen plasma, cryoprecipitate, or factor XIII concentrates. With major bleeding, or accompanying surgical intervention, the desired concentration of the recipient's plasma is 0.3 to 0.5 μm/mL. With minor bleeding or as prophylaxis, a level greater than 0.05 μm/mL is all that is required.

ACQUIRED HEMOSTATIC DEFECTS

Platelet Abnormalities

Thrombocytopenia is the most common abnormality of hemostasis that results in bleeding in the surgical patient. The patient may have a reduced platelet count due to a variety of disease processes such as idiopathic thrombocytopenic purpura, thrombotic thrombocytopenic purpura, and systemic lupus erythematosus, or secondary hypersplenism and splenomegaly of sarcoid, Gaucher's disease, lymphoma, and portal hypertension. In these circumstances the marrow usually demonstrates normal or increased number of megakaryocytes. By contrast, when thrombocytopenia occurs in patients with leukemia or uremia, and in those patients on cytotoxic therapy, there is generally a reduced number of megakaryocytes in the marrow.

Thrombocytopenia may occur acutely as the result of massive blood loss followed by replacement with stored blood. Exchange of one blood volume (11 units in a 75-kg man) decreases the platelet count from approximately 250,000/mm^3 to approximately 80,000/mm^3. Thrombocytopenia may be induced acutely by the administration of heparin and may be associated with thrombohemorrhagic complications. This situation, which is thought to have an immunologic basis, has been reported in 0.6 percent of patients receiving heparin. The lowest platelet counts occur after 4 to 15 days of treatment in patients given heparin for the first time and after 2 to 9 days in those given subsequent courses.

Thrombocytopenia is often accompanied by impaired platelet function. Impaired aggregation following the addition of ADP has been demonstrated in patients receiving a blood transfusion of more than 10 units. Uremia may be associated with increased bleeding time and an impaired aggregation, which can be corrected by hemodialysis or peritoneal dialysis. Defective aggregation and platelet secretion can occur in patients with thrombocythemia, polycythemia vera, or myelofibrosis. A variety of drugs interferes with platelet function. These include: aspirin, indomethacin, ibuprofen, dipyridamole, phenothiazides, penicillins, chelating agents, lidocaine, and cocaine.

The presence and extent of thrombocytopenia can be defined rapidly by a platelet count. In general, 60,000 platelets/mm^3 are adequate for normal hemostasis, but if there is associated platelet dysfunction, there may be a poor circulation between the platelet count and the extent of bleeding. The template bleeding time is the most reliable in vivo test of platelet function.

When thrombocytopenia is present in a patient in whom an elective operation is entertained, it is managed based on the extent of the reduction of platelet count and the etiology. A count greater than 50,000/mm^3 requires no specific therapy. If thrombocytopenia is due to acute alcoholism, drug effect, or viral infection, the platelet level will return to near normal within 1 to 3 weeks. Occasionally, severe thrombocytopenia may be secondary to vitamin B_{12} or to folic acid deficiency, in which case it is associated with a megaloblastic bone marrow. This condition generally occurs 2 to 3 years after total gastrectomy or in association with severe intestinal malabsorption. In either case, supplying the appropriate nutrient will correct the thrombocytopenia in 2 to 3 days.

If the patient has idiopathic thrombocytopenia or lupus erythematosus, and a platelet count less than 50,000/mm^3, an attempt to raise the platelet count with steroid therapy or plasmapheresis may prove successful (see Chap. 31). The administration of platelet transfusions in these patients with the spleen in place is generally ineffective. The administration of γ-globulin may temporarily increase the platelet count. Splenectomy alone should not be performed to correct the thrombocytopenia associated with splenomegaly secondary to portal hypertension.

Prophylactic platelet administration as a routine accompaniment to massive blood transfusion is not required or indicated to prevent a hemostatic defect. Platelet packs are administered preoperatively to rapidly increase the platelet count in surgical patients with thrombocytopenia due to marrow depression or in association with massive bleeding and replacement with banked blood. Special platelet transfusion sets are used to reduce the loss of platelets due to adherence. One unit of platelet concentrate contains approximately 5.5×10^{10} platelets and would be expected to increase the circulating platelet count by about 10×10^9/L in the average 70-kg person. Thus, a transfusion of 4 to 8 pool platelet concentrates should raise the count by 40 to 80×10^9/L and should provide adequate hemostasis, as documented by bleeding time and control of the hemorrhagic manifestations. Fever, infection, hepatosplenomegaly, and the presence of antiplatelet alloantibodies decrease the effectiveness of platelet transfusions. In patients refractory to standard platelet transfusions, the use of human lymphocyte antigen (HLA)–compatible platelets coupled with special processors has proved effective. Platelet aggregometry has been applied to screening for potential donors.

Acquired Hypofibrinogenemia

Defibrination Syndrome

The largest proportion of patients with fibrinogen-related problems of surgical concern are in this group. The fibrinogen deficiency rarely is an isolated defect because thrombocytopenia and factors II, V, VII, VIII, and X deficiencies of variable severity usually accompany this state.

The majority of patients with acquired hypofibrinogenemia suffer from intravascular coagulation, more properly known as *defibrination syndrome* or *consumptive coagulopathy,* and it is to this group of patients that the term *disseminated intravascular coagulation* (DIC) has been applied. Systemic bleeding, however, dominates the clinical manifestations; thrombi are rarely found at autopsy. The syndrome, now recognized with increasing frequency, is caused by the introduction of thromboplastic materials into the circulation. Because this material is found in most tissues, many disease processes may activate the coagulation system. The hemorrhagic disasters of the perinatal period, e.g., retained dead fetus, premature separation of the placenta, and amniotic fluid embolus, primarily are due to this pathophysiologic mechanism. The hemorrhagic state following hemolytic transfusion reaction is also related to this process. Defibrination has been observed as a complication of extracorporeal circulation, head trauma, disseminated carcinoma, lymphomas, thrombotic thrombocytopenia, rickettsial infection, snakebite, burns, and shock from any cause. Release of thromboplastic material has long been a recognized complication of gram-negative sepsis and has been attributed to the effects of circulating endotoxin on platelets. Septicemia due to gram-positive organisms may also be associated with DIC.

The differentiation of DIC with secondary protective fibrinolysis from primary fibrinolytic states can be extremely difficult because the thrombin time (TT) is prolonged in both cases, as is the prothrombin time (PT) and partial thromboplastin time (PTT). There is no laboratory test to confirm or exclude the diagnosis. The combination of a low platelet count, a positive plasma protamine test indicating the presence of fibrin monomer-fibrinogen complexes in the plasma, and reduced fibrinogen accompanied by increased fibrin degradation products viewed in the context of the patient's underlying disease is highly suggestive of the diagnosis. The fibrinogen level is generally below 100 mg/dL when there is significant diffuse bleeding.

Treatment. The most important facets of treatment are relieving the patient's causative, primary medical or surgical problem and maintaining adequate capillary flow. The use of intravenous fluids to maintain volume and, at times, vasodilators to open the arterioles is indicated. If blood flow deficiency is related to the inability of a damaged heart to pump, the use of drugs such as digitalis or isoproterenol may be indicated. Viscosity may be affected by an increased hematocrit, and, therefore, a plasma expander may be beneficial.

If there is active bleeding, hemostatic factors should be replaced with fresh frozen plasma, which is usually sufficient to correct the hypofibrinogenemia; cryoprecipitate, which also provides fibrinogen (250 mg/10 mL); and platelet concentrates. There is little evidence that this replacement therapy will "fuel the fire" and accelerate the pathophysiologic process. Most studies show that heparin is not helpful in acute forms of DIC, but the drug is indicated for purpura fulminans or venous thromboembolism. Fibrinolytic inhibitors such as ϵ-aminocaproic acid (EACA) may be used to block the accumulation of degradation products but are dangerous if the thrombotic process is still active. They should not be used without prior effective antithrombotic treatment with heparin.

Fibrinolysis

The acquired hypofibrinogenemic state in the surgical patient also can be due to pathologic fibrinolysis. This may occur in patients with metastatic prostatic carcinoma, shock, sepsis, hypoxia, neoplasia, cirrhosis, and portal hypertension and in those patients on extracorporeal bypass.

The pathogenesis of this bleeding disorder is complex. Secondary to shock or hypoxia, a release of excessive plasminogen activator into the circulation occurs. This is thought to consist of endogenous kinases which can be released from vascular endothelium and other tissues. Pharmacologic activation of plasminogen also occurs with pyrogens, epinephrine, nicotinic acid, and acetylcholine. Electric shock and pneumoencephalography have also been reported to cause activation. Patients with cirrhosis and portal hypertension have a diminished ability to clear normal amounts of plasminogen activator from the blood.

In addition to the reduction in levels of plasma fibrinogen, diminution of factors V and VIII also occurs, since they also serve as substrates for the enzyme plasmin. Thrombocytopenia is not an accompaniment of the purely fibrinolytic state. Polymerization of fibrin monomers, a step in normal fibrin formation, is interfered with by the proteolytic residue of fibrinogen and fibrin. The fibrin and fibrinogen breakdown products usually disappear from the circulation in a matter of hours. The whole blood clot lysis time defines increased fibrinolytic activity if a non-anticoagulated blood sample lyses in a test tube in less than 8 h. A euglobulin lysis time of 20 min or less provides a more rapid assessment.

Treatment. The successful treatment of the underlying disorder usually is followed by rapid spontaneous recovery, since the severity of fibrinolytic bleeding is dependent upon the concentration of breakdown products in the circulation. EACA, which is a synthetic amino acid, interferes with fibrinolysis by inhibiting plasminogen activation. The drug may be administered intravenously or orally. An initial dose of 5 g for the average-sized adult is followed by another 1 g every 1 to 2 h until the hemorrhagic state subsides. Treatment rarely is required for more than 2 or 3 days. Just as the administration of EACA in a patient with consumptive coagulopathy is potentially dangerous, the administration of heparin in the patient who has a primary pathologic fibrinolysis is fraught with danger. Thus, fine clinical judgment and reliable laboratories are needed to avoid therapeutic complications. Restraint in definitive treatment of both fibrinolysis and consumptive coagulopathy is recommended, while measures designed to reverse the shock and stabilize the patient are emphasized.

Myeloproliferative Diseases

The polycythemic patient, particularly with marked thrombocytosis, is a major surgical risk. Operations should be considered only for the most grave surgical emergency. If possible, the operation should be deferred until medical management has effected normal blood volume, hematocrit, and platelet count. Spontaneous thrombosis is a complication of polycythemia vera and can be explained, in part, by increased blood viscosity, increased platelet count, and increased tendency toward stasis. Paradoxically, a significant tendency toward spontaneous hemorrhage is noted in these patients also.

Myeloid metaplasia frequently represents part of the natural history of polycythemia vera. Approximately 50 percent of patients with myeloid metaplasia are postpolycythemic. There is evidence suggesting qualitative platelet abnormalities in these patients. Abnormalities in platelet factor 3 release and in platelet aggregation with ADP have been demonstrated.

Treatment. Thrombocytosis can be reduced by the careful administration of alkylating agents such as busulfan or chlorambucil. Elective surgical procedures should be delayed weeks to months following institution of treatment. Ideally the hematocrit should be kept below 48 percent and the platelet count less than 400,000/mm^3. Before operation, a thorough laboratory examination of hemostatic function should be conducted. When an emergency procedure is required, the erythremic and thrombocytotic states should be reduced by phlebotomy and replacement of the blood removed with Ringer's lactate. The operation, at all times, must be performed fastidiously.

Other Diseases

Illnesses resulting in severe impairment of hepatic function may limit synthesis of plasma factors essential to normal coagulation. The patient with advanced cirrhosis may be lacking in factors of the prothrombin complex (II, V, VII, X), as well as factor XIII. In addition, there may be increased fibrinolysis due to failure of the liver to clear plasminogen activators.

Other diseases, such as macroglobulinemia, may be associated with the abnormal production of proteins that coat the platelets and interfere with their function. Multiple myeloma and the disorders associated with the excess production of cryoglobulins may also bind certain blood-clotting factors.

Anticoagulation and Bleeding

Spontaneous bleeding may be a complication of anticoagulant therapy with either heparin or the coumarin and indanedione derivatives. The incidence of bleeding complications related to heparin is reduced with a continuous infusion technique, regulating the PTT between 60 to 100 s (control: 30 to 35). An exaggerated response to oral anticoagulants may occur if dietary vitamin K is inadequate. The anticoagulant effect of coumarin is consistently reduced in patients receiving barbiturates, and increased coumarin requirements have also been documented in patients taking contraceptives, other estrogen-containing compounds, corticosteroids, and ACTH. Therefore, reduced anticoagulant dosage should be instituted following discontinuance of any of these drugs. Medications known to increase the effect of oral anticoagulants include phenylbutazone, the cholesterol-lowering agent clofibrate, anabolic steroids (norethandrolone), D-thyroxine, glucagon, quinidine, and a variety of antibiotics.

Unexplained bleeding in medical and paramedical personnel occasionally is due to surreptitious anticoagulation. The onset of hematuria or melena in the patient receiving anticoagulants should be investigated, since it has been shown that anticoagulants may unmask underlying tumors. Patients with bleeding secondary to anticoagulation may present only with epistaxis, gastrointestinal hemorrhage, or hematuria. Physical examination, however, almost always reveals other signs of bleeding such as ecchymoses, petechiae, or hematoma. Bleeding secondary to anticoagulation is not an uncommon cause of rectus sheath hematoma, simulating appendicitis, and intramural intestinal or retroperitoneal hematoma.

Surgical intervention may prove necessary in patients receiving anticoagulant therapy. Increasing experience suggests that surgical treatment can be undertaken without discontinuing the anticoagulant program. The risk of thrombotic complications reportedly is increased when anticoagulant therapy is discontinued suddenly. If so, this may not be related to what has been called the "rebound phenomenon" but may represent an event in a patient who has an underlying thrombotic tendency. When the clotting time is less than 25 min in the heparinized patient or when the prothrombin time is greater than 20 percent of normal in a patient on coumarin, reversal of anticoagulant therapy may not be necessary. Meticulous surgical technique is mandatory, and the patient must be observed closely.

Certain surgical procedures should not be performed in the face of anticoagulation. In sites where even minor bleeding can cause great morbidity, e.g., the central nervous system and the eye, anticoagulants should be discontinued and, if necessary, reversed. Because of the added problem of local fibrinolysis, prostatic surgical treatment should not be carried out in a patient on anticoagulants. Procedures requiring blind needle introduction should be avoided. Deaths have been reported following sympathetic block for peripheral vascular disease in patients receiving anticoagulation.

Emergency operation occasionally is necessary in patients who have been heparinized as treatment for deep venous thrombosis. The first step in managing these patients is discontinuation of heparin; this may be sufficient if the operation can be delayed for several hours. For more rapid reversal, 1 mg of protamine sulfate for every 100 units of heparin most recently administered is immediately effective. For each hour that has elapsed since the last heparin dose, the amount of protamine should be halved. The formation of both extrinsic and intrinsic prothrombinase can be retarded, prolonging the one-stage PT test and the PTT test. Some patients exhibit the phenomenon of "heparin rebound" following apparently adequate heparin neutralization with protamine. Prolongation of the clotting time again recurs after adequate postoperative antagonism of the heparin. This can contribute to postoperative bleeding. In our experience, this is the major cause of "unexplained" postoperative bleeding following cardiac and vascular surgical procedures. Activation of fibrinolysis and thrombocytopenia may also contribute to this problem.

Bleeding infrequently is related to hypoprothrombinemia if the prothrombin concentration is greater than 15 percent. In the elective surgical patient receiving coumarin therapy sufficient to effect anticoagulation, the drug can be discontinued several days prior to operation, and the prothrombin concentration then checked. A level greater than 50 percent is considered safe. If emergency surgical treatment is required, parenteral injection of vitamin K can be used. Since the reversal effect may take 6 h, transfusion of whole blood or, preferably, freshly frozen plasma may be required. Parenteral administration of vitamin K also is indicated in elective surgical treatment of patients with biliary obstruction, malabsorption, and hypoprothrombinemia. The drug should result in a normal PT. By contrast, if the hypoprothrombinemia is related to hepatocellular dysfunction, vitamin K therapy is ineffective and should not be prolonged over a week if no response is noted. Vitamin K is an oxidant, and one must be aware that patients with red cell enzyme deficiencies may sustain hemolysis following its administration.

Cardiopulmonary Bypass

Overheparinization, heparin rebound, inadequate protamine neutralization, protamine excess, and thrombocytopenia have all been indicted as causes of excessive bleeding in patients undergoing cardiopulmonary bypass. DIC is difficult to document in most patients. The predisposing factors that seem to be associated with excessive bleeding are prolonged perfusion times, prior use of oral anticoagulants, cyanotic heart disease, hypothermia, and prior use of antiplatelet drugs. It is currently believed that the two factors most important in triggering excessive bleeding associated with cardiopulmonary bypass are excessive fibrinolysis and platelet functional defects, with the latter the more important element.

The laboratory evaluation of patients with bleeding should include PT, PTT, complete blood count (CBC) and platelet count, examination of the peripheral blood smear, and measurement of fibrin degradation products. Heparin assay can indicate the heparin level; plasminogen and plasmin assays are also available.

The management of cardiopulmonary bypass hemorrhage should include the empiric administration of 6 to 8 units of platelet concentrates as rapidly as possible. If hyperheparinemia is believed to be the major factor, 25 percent of the calculated dose of protamine should be administered and repeated every 30 to 60 min until the bleeding ceases. If there is laboratory evidence of excess fibrinolysis, EACA should be given at an initial dose of 5 to 10 g followed by 1 to 2 g/h until bleeding ceases. EACA may be associated with ventricular arrythmia, hypotension, and hypokalemia.

TESTS OF HEMOSTASIS AND BLOOD COAGULATION (TABLE 3-3)

The most important assessment of hemostasis is a careful history and physical examination. Only the history can indicate whether the patient has a hemorrhagic diathesis. Rather than asking a patient if he or she is a "bleeder," specific questions should be asked. These should include queries to determine if there was untoward bleeding during a major surgical procedure, or if there was *any* bleeding after a minor operation such as tonsillectomy, circumcision, or dental extraction, or if spontaneous bleeding was ever experienced. If there is a suggestion of bleeding diathesis, the age of onset and family history is helpful to determine whether a hereditary or acquired defect should be investigated. Questions should uncover a history of exposure to toxic agents, oral anticoagulants, and drugs that might interfere with hemostasis. Aspirin and ibuprofen are two of the more common medications in this category. A history of a recent regimen of broad spectrum antibiotics should alert the physician to the possibility of a deficiency of vitamin K-dependent clotting factors. Patients with malignancy may have a variety of abnormalities, such as compensated intravascular coagulation, and increased circulating fibrin complexes. Complex hemostatic disorders may accompany liver and renal failure.

Platelet Count. Because thrombocytopenia is the most common abnormality of hemostasis in the surgical patient, determination of the level of circulating platelets is a critical screening test. Direct enumeration of blood platelets can be accomplished quite accurately. *Spontaneous* bleeding only rarely can be related to thrombocytopenia with platelet counts greater than 40,000/mm^3. Platelet counts of 60,000 to 70,000/mm^3 usually are sufficient to provide adequate hemostasis following trauma or surgical procedures if other hemostatic factors are normal. An abnormal count should be confirmed by inspection of the blood smear.

When an area where the red blood cells display their customary central pallor and where few of the red blood cells overlap one

Table 3-3
Screening Tests in Adults, Healthy Term Infants, and Premature Infants

	Adults	*Term Infants*	*Premature Infants (32–35 Weeks' Gestation)*
Platelet count (10^3/cm)*	300±50	259±35	239±50
Bleeding time (min)*	4±1.5	4±1.5	4±1.5
Prothrombin time (PT) (s)*	12–14	13–17	18
Partial thromboplastin time (PTT) (s)*	45	71	100
Thrombin time (TT) (s)*	10	14	14
Fibrinogen (mg/dL)†	200–350	117–225	—

*Values published by Hathaway and Bonnar.

†Values obtained in this laboratory.

Values for infants 35 to 39 weeks' gestation lie between those of term and 32- to 35-week infants. Values for older children (>3 months) are the same as those for adults.

SOURCE: Karpatkin M, 1980, with permission.

another is examined, 15 to 20 platelets per oil immersion field should be noted. If the blood is not anticoagulated before the smear is prepared, as many as half of these may be in clumps of three or four platelets. A well-stained blood smear that fails to display more than three or four platelets in at least every other oil immersion field can be considered significantly thrombocytopenic. In this situation, the patient's platelet count generally is less than 75,000/mm^3. Blood smears which must be searched because platelets appear in only every four or five oil immersion fields usually represent platelet counts of fewer than 40,000/mm^3. If cover slip smears have been prepared, the cover slips always should be mounted as matched pairs. Platelets occasionally stick to one of the cover slips, and examination of both will obviate a false impression of thrombocytopenia. Lightly stained blood smears may appear thrombocytopenic in that the platelets are not prominent enough to attract the examiner's attention.

Inspection of the blood smear has the other obvious advantage of permitting the examiner to identify additional pathologic features which may have meaning in the care of the patient. The presence of nucleated red blood cells or abnormal white cells can provide information important to the diagnosis. The presence of giant platelets or large fragments of megakaryocyte cytoplasm will also alert the examiner to possible pathologic platelet function.

Bleeding Time. This assesses both the interaction between platelets and a damaged blood vessel and the formation of the platelet plug. Bleeding time may be abnormal in thrombocytopenia, qualitative platelet disorders, von Willebrand's disease, and also in some patients with factor V deficiency, or hypofibrinogenemia. Aspirin ingested within 1 week will affect the results. The tests can be performed by a variety of techniques that do not have the same normal times or the same degree of accuracy. The Duke bleeding time, performed by incising the most dependent portion of the earlobe and measuring the time lapse until the bleeding ceases, normally should not exceed 3½ min. The Ivy method is performed on the forearm after a blood pressure cuff has been inflated to 40 mmHg. It has an upper limit of normal of 5 min. The Mielke template technique, a modification of the Ivy method, provides more accurate results but may leave a scar.

Other Tests of Platelet Function. Platelet aggregation can be assessed with a variety of induction agents to uncover specific abnormalities. The results may be affected by venipuncture, blood pH, temperature, duration of storage, and the equipment itself. The degree of abnormality detected by the test does not correlate with the extent of untoward bleeding. Aspirin is the most common cause of platelet aggregation abnormality. Failure of platelets to aggregate with the addition of arachidonate defines an aspirin effect. The failure of platelets to aggregate with ADP, epinephrine, and collagen is characteristic of Glanzmann's thrombasthenia. Abnormal platelet aggregation with ristocetin occurs in von Willebrand's disease and in Bernard-Soulier syndrome.

The ability of the platelets to liberate platelet factor 3 (phospholipid), essential in tiny amounts at several stages of the blood-clotting process (see Fig. 3-3), also can be measured. Impairment of platelet factor 3 release has been reported in conditions described as *thrombocytopathia*. This defect can represent a primary disease entity, but similar impairment has been described as a secondary phenomenon in uremia and liver disease. The inability of the platelet to make platelet factor 3 available for the clotting process may be a part of a more fundamental surface membrane abnormality. The ability of ADP, epinephrine, collagen, and arachidonic acid to liberate serotonin β-thromboglobulin, or platelet factor 4 can be measured.

Prothrombin Time. This test measures the speed of the events described earlier as the extrinsic pathway of blood coagulation. A tissue source of procoagulant (thromboplastin), a lipoprotein, is added with calcium to an aliquot of citrated plasma and the clotting time determined. The laboratory should establish a normal dilution curve and normal values daily. The PT will be prolonged in the presence of even minute amounts of heparin. The presence of heparin, by its antithrombin action, will artificially prolong the clotting time of the mixture so that it appears that the prothrombin complex is low. Accordingly, an accurate prothrombin determination cannot be carried out in a patient receiving anticoagulation treatment with heparin until the heparin has disappeared from the plasma. This should be at least 5 h following the last intravenous dose. The amount of heparin used to maintain patency of an intravenous line is usually insufficient to alter the PT.

The use of tissue procoagulants in the test eliminates the roles of factors VIII, IX, XI, XII, and platelets. Properly done, the test will detect deficiencies of factors II, V, VII, X, and fibrinogen.

The one-stage PT is the preferred method of controlling anticoagulation with the coumarin and indanedione drugs.

Partial Thromboplastin Time. The PTT is a screening test for the intrinsic clotting pathway. The in vitro clotting system now is sensitive to factors VIII, IX, XI, and XII, as well as the factors normally detected by the one-stage PT. The range of normal with this test varies with the product used. The patient's plasma must be compared with a normal control.

The PTT, when used in conjunction with the one-stage PT, can help to place a clotting defect in the first or second stage of the clotting process. If the PTT is prolonged and the one-stage PT is normal, factors VIII, IX, XI, or XII may be deficient. If the PTT is normal and the one-stage PT is prolonged, a single or multiple deficiency of factors II, V, VII, or X or of fibrinogen may be present. The PTT is also abnormal in the presence of circulating anticoagulants or during heparin administration. It may be prolonged when heparin is used to maintain the patency of an intravenous line. The sensitivity of the test is such that only extremely mild cases of factor VIII or IX deficiency may be missed.

Thrombin Time. This test is of value in detecting qualitative abnormalities in fibrinogen and in detecting circulating anticoagulants and inhibitors of fibrin polymerization. The clotting time of the patient's plasma is measured following the addition of a standard amount of thrombin to a fixed volume of plasma. Controls of normal plasma must be run in parallel. Failure of the clot to form, in the absence of circulating inhibitors such as heparin or the fibrinolytic degradation products of fibrin and fibrinogen, is consistent with severe diminution of fibrinogen, usually well below 100 mg/dL. It is also prolonged when fibrinolysis is taking place.

Other Tests of Coagulation. The fibrinogen level can be determined by clotting time measurements or gravimetrically. Specific assays of coagulation factors are performed by measuring clotting time of plasma congenitally lacking in one of these factors. Relatively simple tests permit identification of circulating anticoagulants. The simplest of these are based on the retardation of clotting of normal recalcified plasma by varying mixtures of the test plasma. The sensitivity of such tests usually can be increased by incubating the test plasma with the normal plasma for 30 min at body temperature prior to recalcification. Detection of factor XIII deficiency requires a special test.

Tests of Fibrinolysis. Fibrin degradation products (FDP) can be measured by immunologic methods. Normally, dissolution of a recently formed blood clot will not occur for 48 h or more. When fibrinolysis is a significant factor in hemostatic failure, dissolution of the whole blood clot is observed in 2 h or less. The test has the disadvantage of being time-consuming in a circumstance where time may be of the essence. In addition, a false impression of increased fibrinolytic activity may be gained from clots formed in patients with high hematocrits or in thrombocytopenia, where red cells may fall away from the clot. The euglobulin clot lysis time and dilute whole blood or plasma clot lysis time are more sensitive indices and permit more rapid evaluation of fibrinolysis.

The *thromboelastogram* is a graphic representation of clotting. The record obtained provides information about the clotting time, the speed of fibrin polymerization, and the strength and tendency toward dissolution of the clot.

EVALUATION OF THE SURGICAL PATIENT AS A HEMOSTATIC RISK

Preoperative Evaluation of Hemostasis

The patient's history provides meaningful clues for the presence of a bleeding tendency. It is reasonable to use a questionnaire on which the patient indicates: (1) prolonged bleeding or swelling after biting the lip or tongue, (2) bruises without apparent injury, (3) prolonged bleeding after dental extraction, (4) excessive menstrual bleeding, (5) bleeding problems associated with major and minor operations, (6) medical problems receiving a physician's attention within the past 5 years, (7) medications including aspirin or remedies for headache taken within the past 10 days, and (8) a relative with a bleeding problem. Rapaport indicates that, based on the answers to these questions, one of the following conclusions can be reached: (1) hemostasis is apparently normal, (2) the history contains insufficient tests of hemostasis, or (3) there is a possibility or likelihood of a defect. He also proposes that this information, coupled with an appreciation of the planned operation, can be used to establish four levels of concern to determine the extent of preoperative testing.

In Level I, the history is negative and the procedure contemplated is relatively minor, e.g., breast biopsy or hernia repair: no screening tests are recommended. In Level II, the history is negative, screening tests may have been performed in the past, and a major operation is planned, but the procedure is usually not attended by significant bleeding: a platelet count and blood smear and PTT are recommended to detect thrombocytopenia, a circulating anticoagulant, or intravascular coagulation. Level III pertains to the patient whose history is suggestive of defective hemostasis and also to the patient who is to undergo an operative procedure in which hemostasis may be impaired, for example, operating using pump oxygenation or cell savers, or procedures in which a large, raw surface is anticipated. Level III also pertains to situations, such as intracranial operations, in which minimal postoperative bleeding could be injurious. In this level, a platelet count and bleeding time test should be performed to assess platelet function; a PT and PTT should be used to assess coagulation, and the fibrin clot should be incubated to screen for abnormal fibrinolysis. Level IV pertains to patients who present with a history highly suggestive of a hemostatic defect. A hematologist should be consulted, and, in addition to the tests prescribed for Level III patients, the bleeding time test should be repeated in 4 h following the ingestion of 600 mg of aspirin, provided that the operation is scheduled to take place 10 or more days after this study. In the case of an emergency procedure, platelet aggregation tests using ADP, collagen, epinephrine, and ristocetin should be performed, and a TT is indicated to detect dysfibrinogenemia or a circulating, weak, heparin-like anticoagulant. Patients with liver disease, renal failure, obstructive jaundice, and the possibility of a disseminated malignancy should have a platelet count, PT, and PTT performed preoperatively.

Evaluation of Excessive Intraoperative or Postoperative Bleeding

Excessive bleeding during or shortly after a surgical procedure may be due to one or more of the following factors: (1) ineffective local hemostasis, (2) complications of blood transfusion, (3) a previously undetected hemostatic defect, (4) consumptive coagulopathy and/or fibrinolysis. Excessive bleeding from the field of the procedure, unassociated with bleeding from other sites, e.g., central venous pressure or intravenous line or tracheostomy, usually suggests inadequate mechanical hemostasis rather than a defect in the biologic process. An exception to this rule applies to operations on the prostate, pancreas, and liver because operative trauma may stimulate local plasminogen activation and lead to increased fibrinolysis on the raw surface. In this circumstance 24 to 48 h interruption of plasminogen activation by the administration of EACA may prove effective.

Although one may be reasonably certain on clinical grounds that surgical bleeding is related to local problems, laboratory investigation must be confirmatory. Prompt examination should be made of the blood smear to determine the number of platelets, and an actual platelet count should be done if the smear is equivocal. A PTT, one-stage PT, and a TT all can be determined within minutes. Correct interpretation of the results should confirm the clinical impression or identify the problem.

As pointed out previously, massive blood transfusion is a well-documented cause of thrombocytopenia. Although most patients who receive 10 units or more of banked blood within a period of 24 h will be measurably thrombocytopenic, this is usually *not* associated with hemostatic failure. Therefore, prophylactic administration of platelets is not indicated, but if there is evidence of diffuse bleeding, 8 to 10 packs of fresh platelet concentrates should be given empirically, because no clear association has been documented between the platelet count, bleeding time, and the occurrence of profuse bleeding.

Another cause of hemostatic failure related to the administration of blood is a hemolytic transfusion reaction. The first hint of a transfusion reaction in an anesthetized patient may be diffuse bleeding in an operative field that had previously been dry. The pathogenesis of this bleeding is thought to be related to the release of ADP from hemolyzed red cells, resulting in diffuse platelet aggregation, following which the platelet clumps are swept out of the circulation. Release of procoagulants may result in progression of the clotting mechanism and intravascular defibrination. In addition, the fibrinolytic mechanism may be triggered.

Transfusion purpura is an uncommon cause of thrombocytopenia and associated bleeding following transfusion. In this circumstance, the donor platelets are of the uncommon Pl^{A1} group. These platelets sensitize the recipient, who makes antibody to the foreign platelet antigen. The foreign platelet antigen does not completely disappear from the recipient circulation but seems to attach to the recipient's own platelets. The antibody, which attains a sufficient titer within 6 or 7 days following the sensitizing transfusion, then destroys the recipient's own platelets. The resultant thrombocytopenia and bleeding may continue for several weeks. This uncommon cause of thrombocytopenia should be considered if bleeding follows transfusion by 5 or 6 days. Platelet transfusions are of little help in the management of this syndrome, since the new donor platelets usually are subject to the binding of antigen and damage from the antibody. Corticosteroids may be of some help in reducing the bleeding tendency. Posttransfusion purpura is self-limited, and the passage of several weeks inevitably leads to subsidence of the problem.

DIC and disseminated fibrinolysis occur intraoperatively or postoperatively when control mechanisms fail to restrain the hemostatic process to the area of tissue damage. Either process can cause diffuse bleeding and can be caused by trauma, incompatible transfused blood, sepsis, necrotic tissue, fat emboli, retained products of conception, toxemia of pregnancy, large aneurysms, and liver diseases. It is important to distinguish between the two processes or the dominant element causing intraoperative or postoperative bleeding. No single test can confirm or exclude the diagnosis or distinguish between the two disorders. The combination of thrombocytopenia, defined by smear or platelet count, positive plasma protamine test for fibrin monomers, a low fibrinogen level, and an elevated FDP provides strong indications for DIC. The euglobulin lysis time provides a method of detecting diffuse fibrinolysis.

Diffuse intraoperative and postoperative bleeding is a complication of biliary tract surgery in cirrhotic patients. This has been related to portal hypertension and coagulopathy associated with chronic liver disease. The tests used to distinguish DIC from fibrinolysis pertain. The therapeutic approach includes the intravenous administration of vasopressin to effect a temporary reduction in portal hypertension, and EACA to correct the increased fibrinolysis.

At times, an operation performed in a patient with sepsis is attended by continued bleeding. Severe hemorrhagic disorders due to thrombocytopenia have occurred consequent to gram-negative sepsis. The pathogenesis of endotoxin-induced thrombocytopenia has been studied in detail, and it has been suggested that a labile factor, possibly factor V, is necessary for this interaction. Defibrination and hemostatic failure also may occur with meningococcemia, *Clostridium welchii* sepsis, and staphylococcal sepsis. Hemolysis appears to be one mechanism in sepsis leading to defibrination. Evaluation of these patients includes platelet count, PT, PTT, and TT.

LOCAL HEMOSTASIS

Surgical bleeding, even when alarmingly excessive, is usually caused by ineffective local hemostasis. The goal of local hemostasis is to prevent the flow of blood from incised or transected blood vessels. This may be accomplished by interrupting the flow of blood to the involved area or by direct closure of the blood vessel wall defect. The techniques may be classified as mechanical, thermal, or chemical.

Mechanical Procedures

The oldest mechanical device to effect closure of a bleeding point or to prevent blood from entering the area of disruption is digital pressure. When pressure is applied to an artery proximal to an area of bleeding, profuse bleeding is reduced, permitting more definitive action. The Pringle maneuver of occluding the hepatic artery in the hepatoduodenal ligament as a method of controlling bleeding from a transected cystic artery or from the surface of the liver is a classic example. Direct digital pressure over a bleeding site, such as a lateral rent in the inferior vena cava, is also effective. The finger has the advantage of being the least traumatic vascular hemostat. All clamps, including the so-called atraumatic vascular clamps, do result in damage to the intimal wall of the blood vessel. The obvious disadvantage of digital pressure is that it cannot be used permanently.

The hemostat also represents a temporary mechanical device to stem bleeding. In smaller and noncritical vessels, the trauma and adjacent tissue necrosis associated with the application of a hemostat are of little consequence. These minor disadvantages are outweighed by the mechanical advantage that the instrument offers to subsequent ligation. When bleeding occurs from a vessel that should be preserved, relatively atraumatic hemostats should be employed to limit the extent of intimal damage and subsequent thrombosis.

In general, a ligature replaces the hemostat as a permanent method of effecting hemostasis in a single vessel. When a vessel is transected, a simple ligature usually is sufficient. For large arteries with pulsation and longitudinal motion, transfixion suture to prevent slipping is indicated. When the bleeding site is from a lateral defect in the blood vessel wall, suture ligatures are required. The adventitia and media constitute the major holding forces within the walls of large vessels, and therefore multiple fine sutures are preferable to fewer larger sutures.

Historically, Aulus Cornelius Celsus devised the use of ligatures in the first century A.D. Because of the strong influence of Galen, who was inclined to cautery, this method did not gain popularity. Paré, in 1552, rediscovered the principle of ligature. In 1800, Physick used absorbable sutures of buckskin and parchment. In 1858, Simpson introduced the wire suture, and in 1881 Lister employed chromic catgut. Halsted, in the early 1900s, emphasized the importance of incorporating as little tissue as possible in the suture and indicated the advantages of silk. In 1911, Cushing reported on the use of silver clips to effect hemostasis in delicate vessels in critical areas. A wide variety of staples made of different metals, relatively inert in tissue, has been used.

All sutures represent foreign material, and their selection is based on the characteristics of the material and the state of the wound. Nonabsorbable sutures, such as silk, polyethylene, and wire, evoke less tissue reaction than absorbable materials, such as catgut, polyglycolic acid (Dexon), and polygalactin (Vicryl). The latter are preferable, however, in the face of overt infection. The presence of nonabsorbable material in an infected wound can lead to extrusion or sinus tract formation. Wire is the least reactive of the nonabsorbable sutures but the most difficult to handle. Monofilament wire and coated sutures have an advantage over multifilament sutures in the presence of infection. The latter tend to fragment and permit sinus formation due to the interstices.

Diffuse bleeding from multiple transected vessels may be controlled by mechanical techniques which employ pressure directly over the bleeding area, pressure at a distance, or generalized pressure. These techniques are based on the premise that as pressure and flow are decreased in the area of vascular disruption, a clot will occur. As a standard procedure of military surgeons in the seventeenth century, pressure at a distance was effected by application of tourniquets and other pressure devices at pressure points proximal to bleeding sites. Now it is generally felt that direct pressure is preferable and is not attended by the danger of tissue necrosis associated with prolonged use of tourniquets. Gravitational suits have been used to create generalized pressure and temporarily decrease bleeding from ruptured major intraabdominal vessels.

Direct pressure applied by means of packs affords the best method of controlling diffuse bleeding from large areas. Rarely is it necessary to leave a pack at the bleeding site and remove it at a second sitting. If this is done, several days should elapse before removal, and the possibility of recurrent bleeding should be anticipated. The question as to whether hot wet packs or cold wet packs should be applied has been investigated. Unless the heat is so great as to denature protein, it may actually increase bleeding, whereas cold packs promote hemostasis by inducing vascular spasm and increasing endothelial adhesiveness. Bleeding from cut bone may be controlled by packing beeswax in the area. This material effects pressure and is relatively nonirritative to the body.

Thermal Agents

Galen's favoring of cautery influenced medicine for 1500 years, until the teachings of Paré were appreciated. The use of cautery was revitalized in 1928, when Cushing and Bovie applied this technique for effecting hemostasis of delicate vessels in recessed areas, such as the brain. Heat achieves hemostasis by denaturation of protein, which results in coagulation of large areas of tissue. With actual cautery, heat is transmitted from the instrument by conduction directly to the tissue; with electrocautery, heating occurs by induction from an alternating-current source.

When electrocautery is employed, the amplitude setting should be high enough to produce prompt coagulation but not so high as to set up an arc between the tissue and the cautery tip. This avoids burns outside the operative field and prevents exit of current through electrocardiographic leads or other monitoring devices. A negative plate should be placed beneath the patient whenever cautery is employed to avoid severe skin burns. The advantage of cautery is that it saves time; its disadvantage is that more tissue is necrosed than with precise ligature. Certain anesthetic agents cannot be used with electrocautery because of the hazard of explosion.

A direct current can also result in electrical hemostasis. Since the protein moieties and cellular elements of blood have a negative surface charge, they are attracted to the positive pole, where a thrombus is formed. Direct currents in the 20- to 100-mA range have been applied to control diffuse bleeding from large serous surfaces. High-power argon gas has been applied successfully to the control of bleeding from superficial erosions.

At the other end of the thermal spectrum, cooling has been applied to control bleeding, particularly from the mucosa of the esophagus and stomach. Generalized hypothermia is of little avail, since, in order to reduce the blood flow to visceral organs, the systemic temperature must be brought down to the level of 35°C. At this point shivering and ventricular fibrillation may be encountered. Thrombocytopenia may also be a consequence of generalized cooling. Direct cooling with iced saline is effective and acts by increasing the local intravascular hematocrit and decreasing blood flow by vasoconstriction.

Extreme cooling, i.e., cryogenic surgery, has been applicable particularly in gynecology and neurosurgery. Temperatures ranging between −20 to −180°C are used, and freezing occurs around the tip of the cannula within 5 s. At temperatures of −20°C or below, the tissue, capillaries, small arterioles, and venules undergo cryogenic necrosis. This is caused by dehydration and denaturation of lipid molecules. The muscular walls of large arteries are an exception. Although the major arteries and blood may be frozen solid, the blood contained in these vessels does not clot. When thawing occurs, normal circulation is resumed.

Chemical Agents

Chemical agents vary in their hemostatic action. Some are vasoconstrictive, while others have coagulant properties. Still others are relatively inert but possess hygroscopic properties which increase their bulk and aid in plugging disrupted blood vessels.

Epinephrine, applied topically, induces vasoconstriction, but extensive application can result in considerable absorption and systemic effects. The drug generally is used on oozing sites in mucosal areas, during tonsillectomy, for example.

Historically, skeletal muscle was one of the first materials with locally hemostatic properties to be employed, its use having been introduced by Cushing in 1911. Shortly thereafter, hemostatic fibrin was manufactured. The properties required for local hemostatic materials include handling ease, rapid absorption, nonirritation, and hemostatic action independent of the general clotting mechanism. The most widely used of the commercially available materials are gelatin foam (Gelfoam), oxidized cellulose (Oxycel), oxidized regenerated cellulose (Surgicel), and micronized collagen (Avitene). All these materials act, in part, by transmitting pressure against the wound surface, and the interstices provide a scaffold on which the clot can organize (Table 3-4).

Gelfoam is made from animal skin gelatin which has been denatured. In itself, Gelfoam has no intrinsic hemostatic action, but it can be used in combination with topical thrombin, for which it serves as an absorbable carrier. Its main hemostatic activity is related to the contact between blood and the large surface area of the sponge and to the pressure exerted by the weight of the sponge and absorbed blood. Prior to application of Gelfoam, the sponge should be moistened in saline or thrombin solution, and all the air should be removed from the interstices.

Oxycel and Surgicel are altered cellulose materials capable of reacting chemically with blood and producing a sticky mass which functions as an artificial clot. These substances are relatively inert and are removed by liquefaction in 1 week to 1 month. They should be dry when they are applied. Like Gelfoam, these materials are nontoxic and relatively nonirritating but are somewhat detrimental to wound healing and require phagocytosis to be removed. Surgicel has been shown to have an antibacterial effect. Microcrystalline collagen has been shown to be as effective as other materials as a topical hemostatic agent where a large surface is oozing.

Fibrin glue is commercially available in Europe and Canada but not in the United States, because of the potential of disease transmission when fibrinogen is obtained from pooled plasma. Single-donor fibrinogen can be mixed with bovine thrombin to make the sealant. The glue is particularly effective in controlling surface bleeding from the liver and spleen.

TRANSFUSION

Background

In 1967, the tercentennial anniversary of the transfusion of blood into human beings was celebrated. In June of 1667, Jean-Baptiste Denis and a surgeon, Emmerez, transfused blood from a sheep into a 15-year-old boy who had been bled many times as treatment for fever. The patient apparently improved, and a successful experience was reported simultaneously in another patient. Because of two subsequent deaths associated with transfusion from animals to humans, criminal charges were brought against Denis. In April of 1668, further transfusions in humans were forbidden unless approved by the Faculty of Medicine in Paris. It was not until the nineteenth century that human blood was recognized as the only appropriate replacement. In 1900, Landsteiner and his associates introduced the concept of blood grouping and identified the major A, B, and O groups. In 1939, the Rh group was recognized. The introduction of various preservative solutions, such as acid citrate dextrose (ACD), citrate-phosphate-dextrose (CPD), and citrate-phosphate-double-dextrose adenine (CP2D-A), and newer additive solutions have extended the shelf life of blood up to 42 days.

Preservation of blood and its constituents has been achieved by freezing, and emphasis has been placed on the use of plasma expanders and component therapy.

Characteristics of Blood and Replacement Therapy

Blood

Blood has been described as a vehicular organ that perfuses all other organs. It provides transportation of oxygen to satisfy the body's metabolic demands and removes the by-product carbon dioxide. Blood also transports chemical nutriments for, and waste products from, metabolic activity. Homeostatic governors, including hormones, coagulation factors, and antibodies, are carried to and from appropriate sites within the fluid portion of the blood. Red blood cells, with their oxygen-carrying capacity; white blood cells, which function in body defense processes; and platelets, which contribute to the hemostatic process, comprise the formed elements.

Replacement Therapy

Banked Whole Blood. This is now rarely indicated and rarely available. With the new preservatives, the shelf life has been extended to 40 ± 5 days. At least 70 percent of the transfused erythrocytes remain in the circulation for 24 h posttransfusion and are viable. The changes in the red cell that occur during storage include reduction of intracellular ATP and 2,3 diphosphoglycerate (2,3 DPG) which alters the curve of oxygen disassociation from hemoglobin, decreasing oxygen transport function. Banked blood is a poor source of platelets, because platelets lose their ability to survive transfusion after 24 h of storage. Among the clotting factors, II, VII, IX, and XI are stable in banked blood. Within 21 days of storage, the pH decreases from 7 to 6.68, and the lactic acid increases from 20 to 150 mg/dL. The potassium concentration rises steadily to 32 meq and the ammonia concentration rises from 50 to 680 mg at the end of 21 days for CPD whole blood. The hemolysis that occurs during storage is insignificant.

Typing and Cross Matching. In selecting blood for transfusion, serologic compatibility is established routinely for the recipients' and donors' A, B, O, and Rh groups. Cross matching between the donors' red cells and recipients' sera (the "major" cross match) is performed. As a rule, Rh-negative recipients should be transfused only with Rh-negative blood. Since this group represents 15 percent of the donor population, the supply may be limited. If the recipient is an elderly male who has not been transfused previously, the transfusion of Rh-positive blood is reasonable if Rh-negative blood is unavailable. Anti-Rh antibodies form within several weeks of transfusion. If further transfusions are needed within a few days, more Rh-positive blood can be used. Rh-positive blood should not be transfused to Rh-negative females who are capable of childbearing. Administration of hyperimmune anti-Rh globulin to Rh-negative women shortly before or after childbirth largely eliminates Rh disease in subsequent offspring.

A variety of cell-serum interactions may be detected by careful cross matching. Incompatibility may be due to the fact that either the donor or recipient has been wrongly grouped.

In the patient who is receiving repeated transfusions, serum drawn not more than 72 h prior to cross matching should be utilized for matching with cells of the donor. Emergency blood transfusion can be performed with type O blood. O-negative and type-specific red blood cells are equally safe for emergency transfusion.

Table 3-4
Topical Absorbable Hemostatic Agents

	Oxidized Cellulose	*Collagen*	*Thrombin*	*Gelatin Sponge*
Material	Oxidized gauze (OG) Oxidized regenerated cellulose knit (ORC)	Purified bovine Collagen sponge Microfibrillar Powder Web Nonwoven web	Protein of bovine origin; powder	Purified gelatin
Time to hemostasis	Average 2–8 min.	Average 1–5 min.	Concentration-dependent Usually less than 1 min.	Not specified on label
Absorption time	OG = 3–4 weeks ORC = 1–2 weeks	Approximately 8–12 weeks	Absorbed immediately	4–6 weeks
Handling characteristics	Conforms well Easy to wrap Packs easily Good suture base	Sponges: Easy to apply & remove Conforms wet or dry Hold suture Microfibrillar: Packs well Difficult to apply and remove Sticks to gloves and instruments	May be used as: Powder Liquid With gelatin sponge Requires preparation and/or special storage	Friable sponge, may be used wet or dry Conforms only if pre-moistened Poor suture base
Special features	ORC—Bactericidal	Sponges: Good wet integrity	Fast acting	

Problems are associated with the administration of 4 or more units of O-negative blood because there is a significant increase in the risk of a hemolytic reaction.

In patients with malignant lymphoma and leukemia, cryoglobulins may be present, and the blood should be administered through a blood warmer. If these antibodies are present in high titer, hypothermia may be contraindicated.

In patients with thalassemia who have been multiply-transfused and, more particularly, with acquired hemolytic anemia, typing and cross matching may be difficult, and sufficient time should be allotted during the preoperative period to accumulate blood that may be required during the operation. Cross matching should always be carried out prior to the administration of dextran, since dextran interferes with the typing procedure.

Because banked blood may be stored for 40 ± 5 days, the use of autologous predeposit transfusion is growing. In otherwise healthy, nonanemic patients, up to 5 to 6 units of blood may be collected for use in elective surgical procedures. Patients may donate blood if the hemoglobin level exceeds 11 g/dL or if the hematocrit is greater than 34 percent. The first procurement is performed 40 days before the planned operation and the last one, 3 days before the procedure. Donations can be scheduled at intervals of 4 to 5 days. Recombinant human erythropoietin (rHmEPO) accelerates generation of red cells and will allow for more frequent harvest for elective operative procedures.

Fresh Whole Blood. This term refers to blood that is administered within 24 h of its donation. It is rarely indicated. Due to time requirements to test for infectious disease, fresh blood is only available untested. One unit of platelet concentrate has more viable platelets than 1 unit of fresh whole blood, which is also an inadequate source of factor VIII.

Packed Red Cells and Frozen Red Cells. Packed red cells is the product of choice for most clinical situations. Concentrated suspensions of cells can be prepared by removing most of the supernatant plasma following centrifugation. The preparation reduces but does not eliminate reaction caused by plasma components. It also reduces the amount of sodium, potassium, lactic acid, and citrate administered. Essentially it provides oxygen-carrying capacity.

Frozen red cells are not available for use in emergencies. They are often used for patients who have been previously sensitized because they have been selected for lack of certain antigens. The red cell viability is improved, and the ATP and 2,3-DPG concentrations are maintained.

Leukocyte Poor Washed Cells. These are prepared by aspirating the buffy coat and supernatant plasma and passing them through a specific white-cell filter. The red cells then are washed with sterile isotonic solution. This should be done only for patients with demonstrated hypersensitivity to either leukocytes or platelets (buffy coat reactions). Usually this syndrome is manifest by fever, chilly sensations, and urticaria due to plasma proteins in the absence of hemolysis.

Platelet Concentrates. The indications for platelet transfusion are as follows: thrombocytopenia due to massive blood loss and replacement with platelet-poor products, thrombocytopenia due to inadequate production, and qualitative platelet disorders. The preparations should be used within 120 h of blood donation. One unit of platelet concentrates has a volume of approximately 50 mL. Platelet preparations may transmit infectious diseases and account for allergic reactions similar to those due to whole blood. When treating thrombocytopenic bleeding or preparing some thrombocytopenic patients for surgery, it is advisable to elevate the platelet levels to the range of 50,000 to 100,000/mm^3 to provide continued protection. The development of isoimmunity remains one of the most important factors limiting usefulness of platelet transfusion. Isoantibodies are demonstrable in about 5 percent of patients after 1 to 10 transfusions, in 20 percent after 10 to 20 transfusions, and in 80 percent after more than 100 transfusions. The use of HLA-compatible platelets addresses this problem.

Frozen Plasma and Volume Expanders. Frozen plasma prepared from freshly donated blood or fresh plasma is necessary to provide factors V and VIII. The other plasma clotting factors are present in banked preparations. The risk of infectious disease is the same whether fresh frozen plasma or whole blood/red cells is administered. Ringer's lactate or buffered saline solution, administered in amounts two to three times the estimated blood loss, is effective and is associated with fewer complications. Dextran or a combination of Ringer's lactate solution and normal human serum albumin are preferred for rapid plasma expansion. Commercially available dextran preparations probably should not be administered in amounts exceeding 1 L/day, since prolongation of bleeding time and hemorrhage can occur. Low-molecular-weight dextran, i.e., molecular weight of 30,000 to 40,000, has achieved recent popularity because it possesses a higher colloidal pressure than plasma and effects some reversal of erythrocyte agglutination.

Concentrates. *Antihemophilic concentrates* are prepared from plasma and are available for the treatment of factor VIII deficiency. Some of these concentrates are twenty to thirty times as potent as an equal volume of fresh frozen plasma. The simplest factor VIII concentrate is the plasma cryoprecipitate. *Albumin* also has been concentrated, so 25 g may be administered and provide the osmotic equivalent of 500 mL of plasma. The advantage of albumin is that it is a hepatitis-free product.

Indications for Replacement of Blood or Its Elements

Improvement in Oxygen-Carrying Capacity. This is primarily a function of the red cell. When anemia can be treated by specific therapy, such as erythropoietin, transfusion should be withheld. Acute anemias, such as hemolytic anemia, are more disabling physiologically than chronic anemia, since most patients with chronic anemia have undergone an adjustment to the situation. In pregnancy, there is a moderate drop in hematrocrit, and transfusions are not indicated to correct the physiologic anemia of pregnancy prior to surgical treatment. The correction of chronic anemia prior to surgical treatment, though often performed, is difficult to justify. In a 1988 National Institutes of Health Concensus Report, the dictum was challenged that a hemoglobin value of less than 10 g/dL or a hematocrit of less than 30 percent indicates a need for a preoperative red cell transfusion. It is suggested that cardiac output does not increase significantly in healthy individuals until the hemoglobin value decreases to approximately 7 g/dL. Patients with chronic anemia and a hemoglobin value less than 7 g/dL in whom significant bleeding intraoperatively is not anticipated do not require a transfusion preoperatively. There is no correlation between anemia and dehiscence or severity of postoperative infection.

Blood volume may be replaced with dextran solution or Ringer's lactate solution with a reduction of the hemoglobin to levels below 10 g and little demonstrable change in the effects of a reduction in oxygen-carrying capacity or the capacity to remove metabolic gaseous by-products. A stroma-free hemoglobin solution has been shown to have the ability to carry and exchange oxygen. Also, a whole blood substitute, Fluosol-DA, has been proposed as a solution with oxygen-handling capabilities.

Volume Replacement. The most common indication for blood transfusion in surgical patients is the replenishment of the circulating blood volume. It is difficult to evaluate the volume deficit accurately.

Values for "normal blood volume" are variable, and the techniques of measurement are relatively inaccurate when there is a rapidly changing situation, such as hemorrhage. Chronically ill and elderly patients may have a diminution of blood volume. In patients with cardiac decompensation, the blood volume may be greater than normal. Many patients with chronically reduced blood volume are well accommodated to that volume.

Measurement of hemoglobin or hematocrit is also used to interpret blood loss. This measurement is misleading in the face of acute blood loss, since the hematocrit may be normal in spite of a severely contracted blood volume. It has been shown that, after a healthy adult male lost approximately 1000 mL of blood rapidly, the venous hematocrit fell only 3 percent during the first hour, 5 percent at 24 h, 6 percent at 48 h, and 8 percent at 72 h, thus indicating the time required for the body to restore blood volume.

Both the amount and the rate of bleeding are factors in the development of the signs and symptoms of blood loss. A healthy person can lose 500 mL in 15 min with only minor effects on the circulation and little change in blood pressure or pulse. Loss of 15 to 30 percent of blood volume (class II hemorrhage) is associated with tachycardia and decreased pulse pressure. Loss of 30 to 40 percent (class III hemorrhage) generally results in tachycardia, tachypnea, hypotension, oliguria, and changes in mental status.

Loss of blood may be evaluated in the operating room by estimating the amount of blood in the wound and on the drapes and by weighing sponges. The loss determined by weighing sponges is only about 70 percent of true loss. In patients who have normal preoperative blood values, blood loss up to 20 percent of total blood volume (TBV) is replaced with crystalloid solutions. Blood loss up to 50 percent TBV is replaced with crystalloids and red blood cell concentrates. Blood loss above 50 percent TBV is replaced with crystalloids, red blood cells, and albumin or plasma. Continued bleeding above 50 percent TBV should receive the same components and fresh frozen plasma. If electrolyte solutions are used to replace blood volume, an amount three to four times the lost volume is required because of immediate diffusion into the interstitial space.

Replacement of Clotting Factors. Transfusion of platelets and/or proteins contributing to coagulation may be indicated in specific patients either prior to or during operation (Table 3-5). In the treatment of certain hemorrhagic conditions, it is to be appreciated that the clotting defects may be multiple. Efficacy of fresh frozen plasma in the management of coagulopathy in patients with liver disease and in patients receiving large amounts of volume replacement for acute blood loss is not well defined. There are insufficient data to specify criteria for transfusion of fresh frozen plasma. The initial volume of fresh frozen plasma needed for an effect on coagulation ranges between 600 to 2000 mL administered in 1 to 2 h. The rigid use of the PT and PTT to anticipate the effect of fresh frozen plasma is not justified.

Specific Indications

Massive Transfusion. The term *massive transfusion* implies a single transfusion greater than 2500 mL, or 5000 mL transfused over a period of 24 h. The approximate percentages of *original* blood volume remaining after varying degrees of hemorrhage

Table 3-5
Replacement of Clotting Factors

Factors	*Normal Level*	*Life Span in Vivo (½ Life)*	*Fate During Coagulation*	*Level Required for Safe Hemostasis*	*Stability in ACD Bank Blood (4°)*	*Ideal Agent for Replacing Deficit*
I (fibrinogen)	200–400 mg/100 mL	72 h	Consumed	60–100 mg/100 mL	Very stable	Bank blood; concentrated fibrinogen
II (prothrombin)	20 mg/100 mL (100%)	72 h	Consumed	15–20%	Stable	Bank blood; concentrated preparation
V (proaccelerin, accelerator globulin labile factor)	100%	36 h	Consumed	5–20%	Labile (40% at 1 week)	Frozen fresh plasma; blood under 7 days
VII [proconvertin, serum prothrombin conversion accelerator (SPCA) stable factor]	100%	5 h	Survives	5–30%	Stable	Bank blood; concentrated preparation
VIII [antihemophilic factor (AHF), antihemophilic globulin (AHG)]	100% (50–150)	6–12 h	Consumed	30%	Labile (20–40% at 1 week)	Fresh frozen plasma; concentrated AHF; cryoprecipitate
IX [Christmas factor, plasma thromboplastin component (PTC)]	100%	24 h	Survives	20–30%	Stable	Fresh frozen plasma; bank blood concentrated preparation
X (Stuart-Prower factor)	100%	40 h	Survives	15–20%	Stable	Bank blood; concentrated preparation
XI [plasma thromboplasma antecedent (PTA)]	100%	Probably 40–80 h	Survives	10%	Probably stable	Bank blood
XII (Hageman factor)	100%	Unknown	Survives	Deficit produces no bleeding tendency	Stable	Replacement not required
XIII [fibrinase, fibrin-stabilizing factor (FSF)]	100%	4–7 days	Survives	Probably less than 1%	Stable	Bank blood
Platelets	150,000–400,000/mm^3	8–11 days	Consumed	60,000–100,000/mm^3	Very labile (40% at 20 h; 0 at 48 h)	Fresh blood or plasma; fresh platelet concentrate (not frozen plasma)

SOURCE: Salzman EW: Hemorrhagic disorders, in Kinney JM, Egdahl RH, Zuidema GD (eds): *Manual of Preoperative and Postoperative Care*. Philadelphia, WB Saunders, 1971, p 157, with permission.

and transfusion are shown in Table 3-6. A variety of problems may attend the use of massive transfusion. Circulatory overload or DIC may occur. Dilutional thrombocytopenia, impaired platelet function, and deficiencies of factors V, VIII, and XI may occur. Routine alkalinization is not advisable, since this could have an adverse effect on the oxyhemoglobin dissociation curve and presents an additional sodium load to a compromised patient. The increased potassium content of multiple units of stored blood does not provide clinical effects unless the patient is severely oliguric.

Citrate toxicity may be associated with massive transfusion, particularly in young children and patients with severe hypotension or liver disease. This is related to an excessive binding of ionized calcium and is usually corrected by spontaneous mobilization of calcium from bone. The physiologic consequences of citrate toxicity rarely have a significant effect. The function of hemoglobin is altered by storage in that the concentration of 2,3-DPG falls to a negligible level by the third week. This results in an increased affinity of the red blood cells for oxygen and a less efficient oxygen delivery system. In itself, reduction of 2,3-DPG may not have a significant effect, but when combined with acute anemia it may be an important factor.

When large transfusions are administered, a heat exchanger may be used to warm the blood, since hypothermia may cause a decrease in cardiac rate and output and a reduction in the blood pH. Warming the blood decreases significantly the frequency of intraoperative cardiac arrest.

The use of blood from many donors increases the possibility of hemolytic transfusion reaction due to incompatibility. This can be reduced by screening each potential donor in the pool and eliminating those who show possible incompatibility. Paradoxically, patients who survive a massive transfusion do not have a high probability of developing isoantibodies subsequently, and the risk is no greater than that from a single transfusion. The risk of infectious disease increases progressively with each succeeding unit. When administering massive transfusions, the pH, blood gases, and potassium should be measured regularly. Acidosis and abnormalities should be corrected. If diffuse bleeding occurs, coagula-

Table 3-6
Percentage of Original Blood Volume Remaining in a Patient with a 5-L Blood Volume Transfused with 500-mL Units

	Magnitude of Hemorrhage and Transfusion		
*Situation**	*1 Blood Volume (10 Units)*	*2 Blood Volumes (20 Units)*	*3 Blood Volumes (30 Units)*
Best	37	14	5
Usual	25–30	10	2–4
Worst	18	3	0.4

*The "best" situation requires simultaneous and equal replacement during hemorrhage; the "worst" situation means initial loss of one-half blood volume not replaced until the hemorrhage has stopped.

SOURCE: After Collins, 1976.

tion screening tests and platelet counts should be performed, and deficits corrected with frozen plasma and platelet concentrates.

Methods of Administering Blood

Routine Administration. The rate of transfusion depends upon the patient's status. Usually, 5 mL/min is administered for 1 min, following which 10 to 20 mL/min may be administered to complete routine transfusion. When marked oligemia is being treated, the first 500 mL may be given within 10 min, and the second 500 mL may be given equally rapidly in most cases. Cold blood may be used for this amount, but when larger amounts are administered, warm blood is desirable. As much as 1500 mL/min can be administered through two 7.5 French catheters.

When large transfusions are administered, it is important not to overload the circulation, and the use of central venous pressure monitoring is particularly pertinent. There is no practical advantage in the use of intraarterial transfusion over the intravenous route in the treatment of oligemia. It has been shown that coronary flow and systemic arterial pressure respond as rapidly and to the same extent whether the blood is administered intravenously or intraarterially.

Other Methods. Blood may be instilled intraperitoneally or into the medullary cavity of the sternum and long bones. Intrasternal and intramedullary transfusion may be painful, and the rate of administration is limited. Approximately 90 percent of red cells injected intraperitoneally enter the circulation, but uptake is not complete for at least a week, and therefore the method is not suitable when immediate transfusion is required.

Intraoperative autotransfusion has become increasingly popular; it is a potentially life-saving adjunct to the management of trauma and is useful in elective operations in which multiple transfusions are likely to be required. Approximately 250 mL of blood can be retrieved, washed, and returned to the patient over a 5- to 6-min period. Another approach to anticipated intraoperative large blood losses is hemodilution. At the onset of the procedure, red cells are removed while the intravascular volume is maintained with crystalloid or colloid. The reduced blood viscosity improves microcirculatory profusion. The removed blood can then be retransfused during the operation to replace lost blood or be reinfused near the completion of the procedure.

Complications

Hemolytic Reactions. The incidence of nonfatal hemolytic transfusion reactions is approximately 1 per 6000 units of blood administered. Fatal hemolytic transfusion reactions occur once in every 100,000 units administered. Hemolytic reactions due to incompatibility of A, B, O, and Rh groups or many other independent systems may result from errors in the laboratory of a clerical or technical nature or the administration of the wrong blood at the time of transfusion. Hemolytic reactions are characterized by intravascular destruction of red blood cells and consequent hemoglobinemia and hemoglobinuria. Circulating haptoglobin is capable of binding 100 mg of hemoglobin/dL of plasma, and the complex is cleared by the reticuloendothelial system. When the binding capacity is exceeded, free hemoglobin circulates, and the heme is released and combines with albumin to form methemalbumin. This is detected by a positive Schumm's test. When free hemoglobin exceeds 25 mg/dL of plasma, some is excreted in the urine, but in most subjects hemoglobinuria occurs when the total plasma level exceeds 150 mg/dL. The renal lesions that may occur consist of tubular necrosis and precipitation of hemoglobin within the tubules. Red cell stromal lipid is liberated, and this may initiate a disseminated intravascular coagulation. But DIC is more likely initiated by antibody-antigen complexes activating factor XII end complement, leading to activation of the coagulation cascade. The kallikrein-bradykinin system may be activated and affect the circulatory system. Minor incompatibilities may occur, causing hemolysis within the reticuloendothelial system manifested by fever, a mild decrease in hemoglobin, and an increase in bilirubin. If the recipient has a low antibody titer at the time of transfusion, reaction may be delayed for several days.

Clinical Manifestations. There is an increased hazard in patients with a previous transfusion reaction. If the patient is awake, the most common symptoms are the sensation of heat and pain along the vein into which the blood is being transfused, flushing of the face, pain in the lumbar region, and constricting pain in the chest. The patient may experience chills, fever, and respiratory distress, hypotension, and tachycardia from amounts as small as 50 mL. In patients who are anesthetized and undergoing operation, the two signs which may call attention are abnormal bleeding and continued hypotension despite adequate replacement. The mortality and morbidity resulting from hemolytic reactions is high if the patient receives a full unit of incompatible blood. Acute hemorrhagic diatheses occur in 8 to 30 percent of patients. There is a sudden fall in the platelet count, an increase in fibrinolytic activity, and consumption of coagulation factors, especially V and VIII, due to disseminated intravascular clotting.

Rudowski reported the following incidences of clinical manifestations in a large series with hemolytic posttransfusion reactions: oliguria, 58 percent; hemoglobinuria, 56 percent; arterial hypotension, 50 percent; jaundice, 40 percent; nausea and vomiting, 30 percent; flank pain, 25 percent; cyanosis and hypothermia, 22 percent; dyspnea, 20 percent; chills, 18 percent; diffuse bleeding, 16 percent; neurologic signs, 10 percent; and allergic reaction, 6 percent. The laboratory criteria are hemoglobinuria with a concentration of free hemoglobin over 5 mg/dL, a serum haptoglobin level below 50 mg/dL, and serologic criteria to show antigen incompatibility of the donor and recipient blood. The simplest clinical diagnostic test is insertion of a bladder catheter and evaluation of the color and volume of the excreted urine, since hemoglobinuria and oliguria are the most characteristic signs. A positive Coombs' test indicating transfused cells coated with patient antibody also provides evidence.

Treatment. If a transfusion reaction is suspected, the transfusion should be stopped immediately, and a sample of the recipient's blood should be drawn and sent along with the suspected unit to the blood bank for comparison with the pretransfusion samples. The serum bilirubin should be determined in the recipient. Each gram of hemoglobin is converted to about 40 mg of bilirubin. The hemolytic reaction is characterized by an increase in the indirect reacting fraction.

A Foley catheter should be inserted and the hourly urine output recorded. Since renal toxicity is affected by the rate of urinary excretion and the pH and since alkalinizing the urine prevents precipitation of hemoglobin within the tubules, attempts are made to initiate diuresis and alkalinize the urine. This can be accomplished with mannitol or furosemide plus 45 meq of bicarbonate. If marked oliguria or anuria occurs, the fluid intake and potassium intake are restricted, and the patient is treated as a case of renal shutdown. In some instances, dialysis is required. Following recovery from oliguria or anuria, diuresis is often copious and may be associated with significant losses of potassium and sodium that require replacement.

Febrile and Allergic Reactions. These are relatively frequent, occurring in about 1 percent of transfusions. Reactions are usually mild and are manifested by urticaria and fever and occur within 60 to 90 min of the start of transfusion. In rare instances, the reaction may be severe enough to cause anaphylactic shock. Allergic reactions are caused by transfusion of antibodies from hypersensitive donors or the transfusion of antigens to which the recipient is hypersensitive. Reactions may occur following the administration of whole blood, packed red cells, plasma, and antihemophilic factor. Treatment consists of antihistamines, epinephrine, and steroids, depending on the severity of the reaction. Repeated reactions can be prevented by use of leukocyte-depleted or washed red cells.

Bacterial Sepsis. Bacterial contamination of infused blood is rare and may be acquired either from the contents of the container or the skin of the donor. Gram-negative organisms, especially coliform and *Pseudomonas* species, which are capable of growth at 4°C, are the most common cause. Clinical manifestations include fever, chills, abdominal cramps, vomiting, and diarrhea. There may be hemorrhagic manifestations and increased bleeding if the patient is undergoing surgical treatment. In some instances, bacterial toxins can produce profound shock. If the diagnosis is suspected, the transfusion should be discontinued and the blood cultured. Emergency treatment includes adrenergic blocking agents, oxygen, antibiotics, and, in some cases, judicious transfusion.

Embolism. Although air embolism has been reported as a complication of intravenous transfusion, healthy animals tolerate large amounts of air injected intravenously at a rapid rate. It has been suggested that the normal adult generally will tolerate an embolism of 200 mL of air. Smaller amounts, however, can cause alarming signs and may be fatal. Manifestations of venous air embolism include a rise in venous pressure and cyanosis, a "mill wheel" murmur heard over the precordium, hypotension, tachycardia, and syncope. Death usually is related to primary respiratory failure. Treatment consists of placing the patient on the left side in a head-down position with the feet up. Arterial air embolism is manifested by dizziness and fainting, loss of consciousness, and convulsions. Air may be visible in the retinal arteries, and bubbles of air may flow from transected vessels.

Plastic tubes used for transfusion have also embolized after they have broken off within the vein. Plastic tubes have passed into the right atrium and the pulmonary artery, resulting in death. Embolized catheters have been removed successfully.

Thrombophlebitis. Prolonged infusions into peripheral veins using either needles, cannulae, or plastic tubes are associated with superficial venous thrombosis. Intravenous infusions which last more than 8 h are more likely to be followed by thrombophlebitis. There is an increased incidence in the lower limb as compared to upper limb infusions. Treatment consists of discontinuation of the infusion and local compressing. Embolism from superficial thrombophlebitis of this nature is extremely rare.

Overtransfusion and Pulmonary Edema. Overloading the circulation is an avoidable complication. It may occur with rapid infusion of blood, plasma expanders, and other fluids, particularly in patients with heart disease. In order to prevent this complication, the central venous pressure should be monitored in these patients and whenever large amounts of fluid are administered.

Circulatory overloading is manifested by a rise in the venous pressure, dyspnea, and cough. Rales generally can be heard at the bases of the lungs. Treatment consists of stopping the infusion, placing the patient in a sitting position, and, occasionally, venous section for removal of blood.

Although acute pulmonary edema occurs more frequently following large transfusions, it has been reported in patients receiving small transfusions. A syndrome which can be confused with pulmonary edema consists of postoperative hypoxia seen in patients who have undergone cardiac surgical treatment and extracorporeal bypass procedures. A damaging factor apparently is carried by the perfusing blood, and immature plasma cells are found in the interalveolar tissue. The lesion represents an immune response to blood. The incidence is reduced by employing the hemodilution technique of pump priming.

Transmission of Disease. Malaria, Chagas' disease, brucellosis, and syphilis are among the diseases that can be transmitted by blood transfusion. Syphilis has been reported following the transfusion of platelets. The storage temperature used for all other blood components (4°C or lower) kills the spirochete. The incubation period ranges from 4 weeks to 4 months. The first manifestation is the skin rash of secondary syphilis. Cure is readily achieved with brief penicillin therapy. Malaria can be transmitted by all blood components, including platelets, fresh frozen plasma, and frozen or deglycerolized red cells. The species most commonly implicated is *Plasmodium malariae*. The incubation period ranges between 8 to 100 days; the initial clinical manifestation is shaking chill and spiking fever. Cytomegalovirus (CMV) infection, causing a syndrome resembling infectious mononucleosis, was commonly observed following open heart surgery when large amounts of heparinized blood were used to prime the pump. The most significant morbidity and mortality occurs following transfusion of CMV-infected blood in low-birthweight infants born of mothers who were CMV antibody negative.

Posttransfusion viral hepatitis remains the most common fatal complication of blood transfusion. It is estimated that for every case of icteric posttransfusion viral hepatitis there are four anicteric cases, many of which are asymptomatic. Hepatitis is caused either by hepatitis B virus, or the non-A, non-B viruses, including C. The incubation period of the former is up to 6 months, the latter's may be as short as 2 weeks. Serologic markers for hepatitis B surface antigen (HB_sAg) and hepatitis C are available, and collecting agencies are required to test all units of blood for these antigens. The risk of hepatitis transmission per unit of blood is 0.035 percent.

The clinical manifestations of hepatitis include lethargy and anorexia as part of anicteric disease, icterus, and chronic liver disease. HB_sAg persists in about 35 percent of patients who develop serum hepatitis of type B. There is no risk from human serum albumin and other plasma protein fractions.

Immune serum globulin is effective in preventing type A hepatitis but is inconsistent in regard to type B. Accidental self-inoculation with material that is definitely known to contain HB_sAg, or transfusion of blood which is HB_sAg-positive, constitutes an indication for immediate use of human specific immunoglobulin (HSI) anti-HB_sAg. The presently recommended dose is 0.5 IgG given as an intramuscular injection. A vaccine has been developed against

HB_sAg, and it is recommended that all surgeons undergo vaccination.

The risk of AIDS following blood transfusion has been estimated to be one case per 225,000 patients transfused and blood collecting agencies have taken measures to preclude donors in high-risk groups and to apply screening techniques. Blood donors are *not* at risk.

Bibliography

General

Colman RW, Hirsh J, Marder VJ, Salzman EW (eds): *Hemostasis and Thrombosis: Basic Principles and Clinical Practice,* 2d ed. Philadelphia, Lippincott, 1987.

Ratnoff OD, Forbes CD (eds): *Disorders of Hemostasis*. Philadelphia, WB Saunders, 1991.

Rudowski WJ (ed): *Disorders of Hemostasis in Surgery*. Hanover, NH, The University Press of New England, 1977.

Biology of Hemostasis

Jackson CM, Nemerson Y: Blood coagulation. *Annu Rev Biochem* 49:765, 1980.

Marcus AJ: The role of lipids in platelet function: With particular reference to the arachidonic acid pathway. *J Lipid Res* 19:793, 1978.

Rodman NF: The morphologic basis of platelet function, in Brinkhous KM, Shermer RW, Mostofi FK (eds): *The Platelet*. Baltimore, Williams & Wilkins, 1971.

Shattil AJ, Bennett JS: Platelets and their membranes in hemostasis: Physiology and pathophysiology. *Ann Intern Med* 94:108, 1980.

Weiss HJ: Platelet physiology and abnormalities of platelet function. *N Engl J Med* 293:531, 1975.

Weiss HJ: Platelet physiology and abnormalities of platelet function. *N Engl J Med* 293:580, 1975.

Congenital Hemostatic Defects

Brown B, Steed DL, et al: General surgery in adult hemophiliacs. *Surgery* 99:154, 1986.

Curtiss PH Jr: Orthopedic management of patients with hereditary disorders of blood coagulation. *Mod Treat* 5:84, 1968.

Kasper CK, Bowlen AL, et al: Hematologic management of hemophilia A for surgery. *JAMA* 253:1279, 1985.

Nilsson IM, Larsson SA, Bergentz S-E: The use of blood components in the treatment of congenital coagulation disorders. *World J Surg* 11:14, 1987.

Rudowski WJ: Major surgery in haemophilia. *Annu Rev Coll Surg Engl* 63:111, 1981.

Acquired Hemostatic Defects

Bell WR: Disseminated intravascular coagulation. *Johns Hopkins Med J* 146:289, 1980.

Bennett B, Towler HMA: Haemostatic response to trauma. *Br Med Bull* 41:274, 1985.

Bick RL: Disseminated intravascular coagulation and related syndromes: A clinical review. *Semin Thromb Hemost* 14:299, 1988.

Feinstein DI: Treatment of disseminated intravascular coagulation. *Semin Thromb Hemost* 14:351, 1988.

Hoak JC, Koepke JA: Platelet transfusions. *Clin Haematol* 5:69, 1976.

Schwartz SI: Myeloproliferative disorders. *Ann Surg* 182:464, 1975.

Schwartz SI, Hoepp LM, Sachs S: Splenectomy for thrombocytopenia. *Surgery* 88:497, 1980.

Silver D, Kapsch DN, Tsoi EKM: Heparin-induced thrombocytopenia, thrombosis, and hemorrhage. *Ann Surg* 198:301, 1983.

Slichter SJ: Identification and management of defects in platelet hemostasis in massively transfused patients. *Prog Clin Biol Res* 108:225, 1982.

Tests of Hemostasis and Blood Coagulation

Bowie EJ, Owen CA Jr: The significance of abnormal preoperative hemostatic tests. *Prog Hemost Thromb* 5:179, 1980.

Karpatkin M: Screening tests in hemostasis. *Pediatr Clin North Am* 27:831, 1980.

Rapaport SI: Preoperative hemostatic evaluation: Which tests, if any? *Blood* 61:229, 1983.

Reid WO, Henry RL, et al: Hemostasis: The balance concept of procoagulant and inhibitor systems and use of the serial thrombin time (STT). *Medical Hypotheses* 15:169, 1984.

Local Hemostasis

Abbott W, Austen WG: The effectiveness and mechanism of collagen-induced topical hemostasis. *Surgery* 78:723, 1975.

Cushing H: The control of bleeding in operations for brain tumor. *Ann Surg* 54:1, 1911.

Evans BE: Local hemostatic agents (and techniques). *Scand J Haematol* 33 (suppl 40):417, 1984.

Jenkins HP, Clarke JS: Gelatin sponge: A new hemostatic substance. *Arch Surg* 51:253, 1945.

Matthew TL, Spotnitz WD, et al: Four year's experience with fibrin sealant in thoracic and cardiovascular surgery. *Ann Thorac Surg* 50:40, 1990.

Silverstein FE, Auth DC, et al: High power argon laser treatment via standard endoscope. I. A preliminary study of efficacy in control of experimental erosive bleeding. *Gastroenterology* 71:558, 1976.

Willman VL, Hanlon CR: The influence of temperature on surface bleeding: Favorable effects of local hypothermia. *Ann Surg* 143:660, 1956.

Transfusion

Allen JB, Allen FB: The minimum acceptable level of hemoglobin. *Int Anesthesiol Clin* 20:1, 1982.

Busch MP, Eble BE, et al: Evaluation of screened blood donations for human immunodeficiency virus type 1 infection by culture and DNA amplification of pooled cells. *N Engl J Med* 325:1, 1991.

Caceres E, Whittembury G: Evaluation of blood losses during surgical operations: Comparison of the gravimetric method with the blood volume determination. *Surgery* 45:681, 1959.

Carson JL, Poses RM, et al: Severity of anaemia and operative mortality and morbidity. *Lancet* 1:727, 1988.

Collins JA: Massive blood transfusions, in *Clinics in Hematology*. Philadelphia, WB Saunders, 1976.

Council on Scientific Affairs: Autologous blood transfusions. *JAMA* 256:2378, 1986.

Glover JL, Broadie TA: Intraoperative autotransfusion. *World J Surg* 11:60, 1987.

Ham JM: Transfusion reactions, in Condon RE, DeCosse JJ (eds): *Surgical Care*. Philadelphia, Lea & Febiger, 1980, chap 12, pp 178–186.

Harrigan C, Lucas CE, et al: Serial changes in primary hemostasis after massive transfusion. *Surgery* 98:836, 1985.

Hoff HE, Guillemin R: The tercentenary of transfusion in man. *Cardiovasc Res Cent Bull* 6:47, 1967.

Hogman CF, Bagge L, Thoren L: The use of blood components in surgical transfusion therapy. *World J Surg* 11:2, 1987.

Katz R, Rodriguez J, Ward R: Posttransfusion hepatitis: Effect of modified gamma-globulin added to blood in vitro. *N Engl J Med* 285:925, 1971.

Keeling MM, Gray LA, et al: Intraoperative autotransfusion: Experience in 725 consecutive cases. *Ann Surg* 197:536, 1983.

Krevans JR, Jackson DP: Hemorrhagic disorder following massive whole blood transfusions. *JAMA* 159:171, 1955.

Krugman S, Giles JP, Hammond J: Viral hepatitis, type B (MS-2 strain): Prevention with specific hepatitis B immune serum globulin. *JAMA* 218:1665, 1971.

Maloney JV Jr, Smythe CMcC, et al: Intra-arterial and intravenous transfusion. *Surg Gynecol Obstet* 97:529, 1953.

Messmer KFW: Hemodilution. *Surg Clin North Am* 55:659, 1975.

Messmer KFW: Acceptable hematocrit levels in surgical patients. *World J Surg* 11:41, 1987.

Mitsuno T, Ohyanagai H, Naito R: Clinical studies of a perfluorochemical whole blood substitute (Fluosol-DA). *Ann Surg* 195:60, 1982.

Perioperative Red Cell Transfusion: National Institutes of Health Consensus Development Conference Statement, vol. 7, no. 4, June 27–29, 1988. US Dept. of Health and Human Services, Bethesda, MD.

Peterman T: Transfusion-associated acquired immunodeficiency syndrome. *World J Surg* 11:38, 1987.

Reed RL, Ciavarella D, et al: Prophylactic platelet administration during massive transfusion. *Ann Surg* 203:40, 1986.

Rizza CR: Coagulation factor therapy. *Clin Haematol* 5:113, 1976.

Shah DM, Prichard MN, et al: Increased cardiac output and oxygen transport after intraoperative isovolemic hemodilution: A study in patients with peripheral vascular disease. *Arch Surg* 115:597, 1980.

Snyder EL (ed): *Blood Transfusion Therapy: A Physician's Handbook.* Arlington, VA, American Association of Blood Banks, 1983.

Wallace J: Blood transfusion and transmissible disease. *Clin Haematol* 5:183, 1976.

CHAPTER 4

Shock

G. Tom Shires III, G. Tom Shires, and C. James Carrico

DEFINITION

Shock is a pathophysiologic condition clinically recognized as a state of inadequate tissue perfusion. Obtaining a more exact yet succinct scientific definition of the shock state has become increasingly difficult as the complexities of the biochemical and physiologic alterations become better defined by modern investigation. Shock was recognized as a ''rude unhinging of the machinery of life'' by the elder Gross in 1872. The futility of the early treatment of this condition was emphasized by Warren's description in 1895 as ''a momentary pause in the act of death.'' The term shock was most often applied to the clinical setting of arterial hypotension following external blood loss or trauma. Blalock's recognition that ''shock is a peripheral circulatory failure, resulting from a discrepancy in the size of the vascular bed and the volume of the intravascular fluid,'' in 1940, acknowledged the components of the heart, the vessels, and circulating volume in maintaining homeostasis. In 1942, Wiggers offered the following definition: Shock ''is a syndrome resulting from a depression of many functions but in which reduction of the effective circulating blood volume is of basic importance and in which impairment of the circulation steadily progresses until it eventuates into a state of irreversible circulatory failure.''

The etiologic classification offered by Blalock in 1934 is still a useful outline for a modern definition. Blalock suggested four categories: (1) hematogenic, (2) neurogenic, (3) vasogenic, and (4) cardiogenic. It is now clear that shock is a systemic disorder that disrupts vital organ function as the end result of a variety of causes. While hemorrhagic or traumatic shock is characterized by global hypoperfusion, septic shock may be associated with hyperdynamic circulation yet result in a maldistribution of regional or intraorgan blood flow. Consequently, Cerra's recent description of shock as a ''disordered response of organisms to an inappropriate balance of substrate supply and demand at a cellular level'' may more accurately reflect the unifying functional abnormality at the metabolic level.

CIRCULATORY HOMEOSTASIS

Preload. The majority of the blood volume at rest is contained within the venous system. The effect of the return of this venous blood to the heart produces ventricular end-diastolic wall tension, a major determinant of cardiac output. Gravitational shifts in blood volume distribution are rapidly compensated for by active and passive alterations in venous capacity. The thin-walled systemic veins are highly compliant. As arteriolar inflow increases, the venous pressure rises and venous capacitance passively increases. With decreased arteriolar inflow, active contraction of the venous smooth muscle cells and passive elastic recoil combine to increase return of blood flow to the heart, maintaining adequate ventricular filling and supporting cardiac output.

In the normal heart, most changes in cardiac output are a reflection of alterations in preload. Changes in position, intrathoracic pressure, intrapericardial pressure, and circulating blood volume produce major changes in cardiac output. Different venous beds play different roles in regulating preload. Veins in the skeletal muscles show a minor response to sympathetic stimulation and respond more to external factors, predominantly the balance between gravitational forces and the muscle pump. Increases in sympathetic outflow to the splanchnic vascular bed produce a rapid and dramatic reduction in the splanchnic blood volume which normally contains about 20 percent of the total blood volume. Exercise and the response of central baroreceptors during hemorrhage reflexly decrease the splanchnic capacitance following these stimuli of sympathetic outflow. Cutaneous noradrenergic nerves respond to hypothalamic control and alter venous tone of the skin to promote thermal regulation during resting heat stress, exercise demands, and the febrile response.

The normal circulating blood volume is maintained within narrow limits by balancing salt and water intake with external losses by the ability of the kidney to respond to alterations in hemodynamics and the hormonal effects of renin, angiotensin, and antidiuretic hormone. The summation of these relatively slow responses, which maintain adequate preload by altering the circulating blood volume, are overshadowed in the acute setting by the changes in venous tone, systemic vascular resistance, and intrathoracic pressure as outlined above. In addition, the net effect of preload on the ventricle also responds to the cardiac determinants of ventricular function, including coordinated atrial contraction, which augments ventricular diastolic filling, and tachycardia, which drops the effect of preload on the ventricle by compromising diastolic filling time.

Ventricular Contraction. The Frank-Starling phenomenon describes the varying force of ventricular contraction as a function of its preload. The changes in force development are explained by the ultrastructural property of the myocardium, which generates a force of contraction dependent on initial muscle length. A variety of disease states, including myocardial injury, valve dysfunction, and cardiac hypertrophy, may alter the mechanical performance of the heart. Experimental studies in burn, septic, hemorrhagic, and traumatic shock have documented deteriorating intrinsic cardiac function during these injury states. While the mechanisms of these alterations in myocardial performance are unclear, their effect on the evaluation and management of global perfusion in clinical shock may be assessed by Swan-Ganz catheterization which measures preload indirectly as end-diastolic pressure, thermodilution cardiac output, and estimations of calculated vascular resistance.

Afterload. Afterload is the force acting to resist myocardial work during contraction. Arterial pressure is the major component of afterload that influences the ejection fraction. This vascular resistance is primarily determined by precapillary smooth muscle sphincters in conjunction with other rheologic factors such as blood viscosity. If afterload increases, stroke volume can be maintained in the presence of an increase in preload. Unlike the normal heart, which can maintain stroke volume in the face of increased vascular resistance by increasing preload, the decreased effective circulating volume in shock states prevents this compensatory maintenance of cardiac output. This imbalance of preload-afterload effects overwhelms the normal increase in inotropic state produced by increased sympathetic nerve activity in the heart and by increased circulating catecholamines released by the stress response.

PATHOPHYSIOLOGY OF HYPOVOLEMIC SHOCK

Hypovolemic shock results from a decrease in the circulating or effective intravascular volume. Consequently, most of the signs of clinical shock are characteristic of peripheral hypoperfusion and increased adrenergic activity. Initially, young, healthy patients appear anxious and exhibit restlessness. This behavior gives way to apathy and lethargy following initiation of treatment. Frank coma rarely results from blood loss alone and is most often a sign of concomitant direct brain injury or is coincident with complete cardiovascular collapse.

As intravascular volume is lost, an increase in peripheral vascular resistance occurs to defend the blood pressure in compensation for falling cardiac output. Differential increases in peripheral resistance in regional arteriolar beds, particularly the skin, gut, and kidney, will further defend pressure at the cost of further decreasing organ flow. The pale, cool skin noted on exam and the blanching of the bowel with decreased pulses in the mesentery are gross signs seen at the bedside and at laparotomy.

A decrease in circulating blood volume also results in tachycardia in response to decreased stroke volume from inadequate preload. The tachycardic response depends on the rate of blood loss and the position of the patient, as orthostatic testing may unmask cardiovascular instability with tachycardia and hypotension in a patient who appears stable when examined in the supine position. Significant orthostasis reflects a decrement in circulating blood volume approaching 30 percent in young patients.

Organ Responses

The baroreceptor reflex, mediated through high-pressure stretch receptors in the aorta and carotid, produces the increased sympathetic nervous system activation that leads to an increase in myocardial contractility initially, before decreased coronary perfusion or other mediators of a negative inotropic state appear later in established shock. Myocardial perfusion may be further impaired by leukotrienes and platelet activating factor released in trauma, while direct myocardial depression may result from cachectin/tumor necrosis factor (TNF) or other circulating factors, perhaps as a result of intestinal hypoperfusion.

The compensatory splanchnic vasoconstriction in defense of falling preload and central blood pressure may play some role in the eventual progression to multiple organ system failure in the resuscitated patient. Although gross dysfunction in the absorptive mechanism or frank ischemic necrosis is unusual in the patient who initially survives resuscitation from profound hypovolemia, gut barrier dysfunction, in terms of translocation of bacteria and endotoxin from the lumen into the systemic lymphatic or venous circulation, might play a role in the acquired immune dysfunction resulting in septic death a few weeks later. The liver also participates in the splanchnic redistribution of blood flow, as portal blood flow is the major component of hepatic perfusion. Although clinically significant "shock liver" or ischemic hepatic necrosis is unusual, the liver plays a central role in the compensatory metabolic responses mediated by epinephrine, norepinephrine, glucagon, and cortisol. Hepatic dysfunction is a frequent component of multiple organ system failure in patients who survive initial therapy.

Renal responses to hypovolemic shock are dramatic. Not only is total renal blood flow decreased, but also intrarenal distribution of blood flow shifts from the cortex to the medulla. Renal renin secretion, mediated directly by renal sympathetic innervation, begins the cascade of angiotensin conversion to angiotensin II. This potent systemic arteriolar vasoconstrictor also stimulates renal prostaglandin production, the release of aldosterone and antidiuretic hormone. The net effect is to decrease glomerular filtration rate and increase tubular reabsorption of salt and water in an attempt to replace the circulating intravascular volume deficits.

Extracellular Fluid Response

Although the most common form of hypovolemic shock results from external blood loss, internal redistribution of the extracellular fluid from the intravascular to the extravascular space can also result in a decrease in effective circulating blood volume. This nonhemorrhagic hypovolemia occurs in a variety of surgical illness, including burns, bowel obstruction, peritonitis, pancreatitis, and crush injuries. Methodology that measures the total body red cell mass with ^{51}Cr-tagged red blood cells, a total body plasma volume with ^{125}I-tagged human serum albumin, and total body extracellular fluid with ^{35}S-tagged sodium sulfate allowed insight into this redistribution phenomenon in shock in both injured human and animal models. An initial loss of circulating intravascular volume decreases capillary hydrostatic pressure. Starling forces predict the increased transcapillary influx of extracellular fluid from the interstitial to the intravascular space following subcritical hemorrhage of less than 10 percent of the blood volume.

Using the same animal model, identical measurement of the body fluid compartments following 25, 35, 45, or over 50 percent of circulating blood volume, which produced hypotension, resulted in a disproportionate reduction in the functional extracellular fluid volume above the measured loss from red blood cells and plasma. This 18 to 26 percent reduction is presumed to be a change in internal redistribution of extracellular fluid, out of the interstitial fluid space, in response to hemorrhagic shock. Although total anatomic extracellular fluid may be normal, the reduction in the early equilibrating extracellular fluid available for transcapillary or transcellular flux, as measured by this isotope equilibration technique, persists in the absence of volume resuscitation.

Animals treated by reinfusion of whole blood had restoration of the measured deficiencies in red cell mass and plasma volume, while the deficiency in extracellular fluid volume persisted. The additional infusion of 10 mg/kg of plasma following return of shed blood also failed to restore the functional extracellular fluid volume. However, dogs treated with an extracellular mimic such as a balanced salt solution, plus shed blood, exhibited a return of the functional extracellular fluid volumes to control levels. This was associated with a dramatic reduction in mortality from 80 percent following blood replacement alone to 30 percent following lactated Ringer's resuscitation of the functional extracellular fluid volume (Fig. 4-1).

When volume distribution curves are obtained following prolonged shock, there is a reduction in the total or anatomic extracellular fluid space when compared with preshock volumes. If the shock is not of sufficient duration to produce a reduction in both functional and total extracellular fluid, the early reduction may be only in the functional extracellular fluid. If volume restitution occurs with prompt therapy, no long-term reduction in extracellular fluid volume may be measured (Fig. 4-2). Because the magnitude of the loss of extracellular fluid cannot be fully explained by Starling forces producing transcapillary refill, and no external losses occur, the isotonic movement of interstitial water and sodium into the proportionally much larger cell mass represents the most likely mechanism for this additional measured reduction in extracellular fluid volume (Fig. 4-3).

In summary, reduction in extracellular fluid in reversible hemorrhagic shock can consistently be shown (1) with extracellular fluid markers that enter cells slowly or not at all in the shock state when (2) reinjection of the extracellular fluid markers is utilized in the shock state, (3) extracellular fluid markers or tracers are allowed sufficient time for equilibration, (4) shock measurements

FIG. 4-1. Acute hemorrhagic shock: survival study.

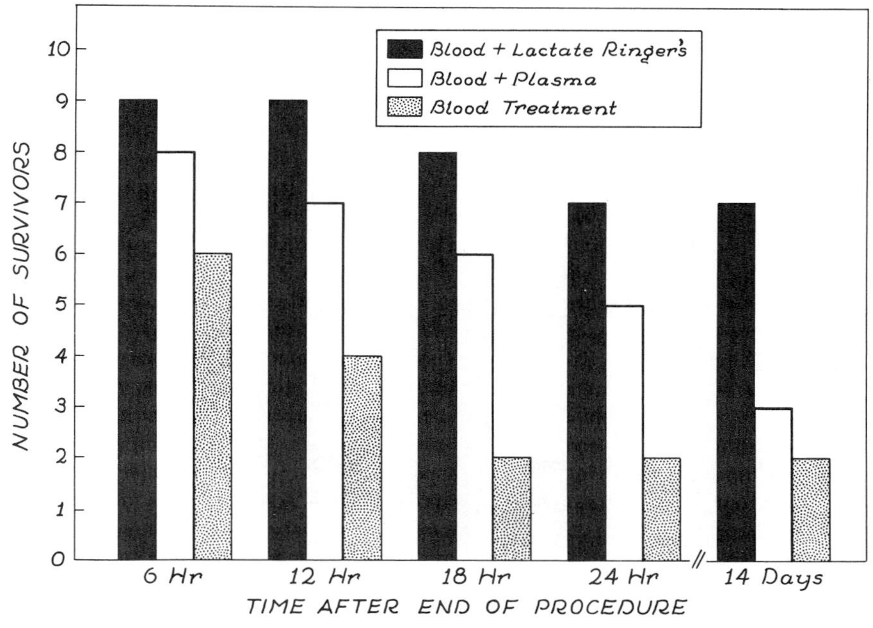

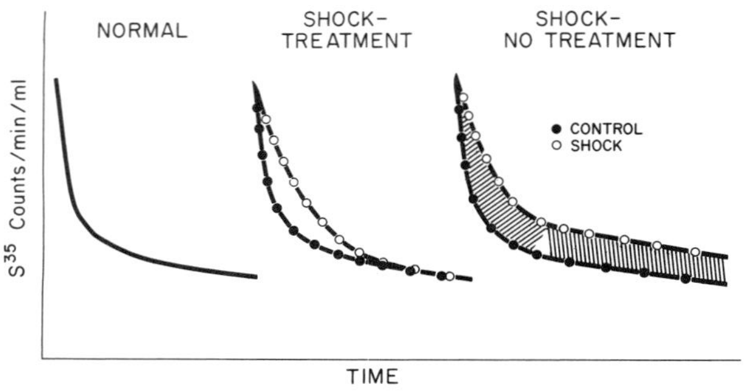

FIG. 4-2. Radiosulfate equilibration curve: semilogarithmic plot, summary model.

are obtained while hemorrhagic shock is sustained, and (5) the shock preparation is sufficiently severe and is maintained until there is a change in cellular membrane transport.

Cellular Responses

Studies of ion transport across the cell membrane were undertaken in order to determine the possibility of intracellular swelling in skeletal muscle in response to hemorrhagic shock. Using a Ling-Gerard ultramicroelectrode with glass tip diameter of less than 1 μm, intracellular transmembrane potential recordings were made. The electrode was modified to record intracellular transmembrane potentials in vivo before, during, and after shock.

Skeletal muscle measurements in acute hemorrhagic shock demonstrate a consistent and sustained fall in the normally negative intracellular transmembrane potential. This may represent a reduction in efficiency of the sodium pump induced by tissue hypoxia; it is present only during shock-producing hypotension. Additional studies in splenectomized dogs showed that changes in variables such as pH, P_{CO_2}, and bicarbonate do not influence the transmembrane potential in shock. Even with progressive metabolic acidosis and its subsequent correction, the potential still follows the blood pressure and shock state.

Combining the ultramicroelectrode measurement of transmembrane potential with direct aspiration of skeletal muscle interstitial fluid found that as blood pressure fell and transmembrane potential was reduced, plasma potassium rose slowly during the shock period. The directly aspirated interstitial fluid potassium during the same period of time rose to a height of more than 15 meq/L of interstitial fluid. The potassium, moving out of skeletal muscle cells, was being sequestered in the interstitium as sodium chloride and water moved into muscle cells. This functional correlate of inadequate ion movement out of the interstitial fluid emphasized the importance of the extracellular environment to substrate transport in shock.

The resting potential difference (PD) is generally agreed to depend on an energy-dependent $Na^+ - K^+$ transport mechanism. The specific energy substrate of this membrane-bound complex is adenosine triphosphate (ATP).

Depletion of ATP in skeletal muscle, liver, and kidney in a hemorrhagic shock model in rats led to the proposal that the cellular dysfunction observed in hemorrhagic shock was secondary to inadequate energy stores. Subsequent studies reported markedly improved survival rates after hemorrhagic shock in animals that were administered ATP-$MgCl_2$.

Subsequent studies indicate that skeletal muscle ATP levels were maintained during prolonged hemorrhagic shock (Fig. 4-4).

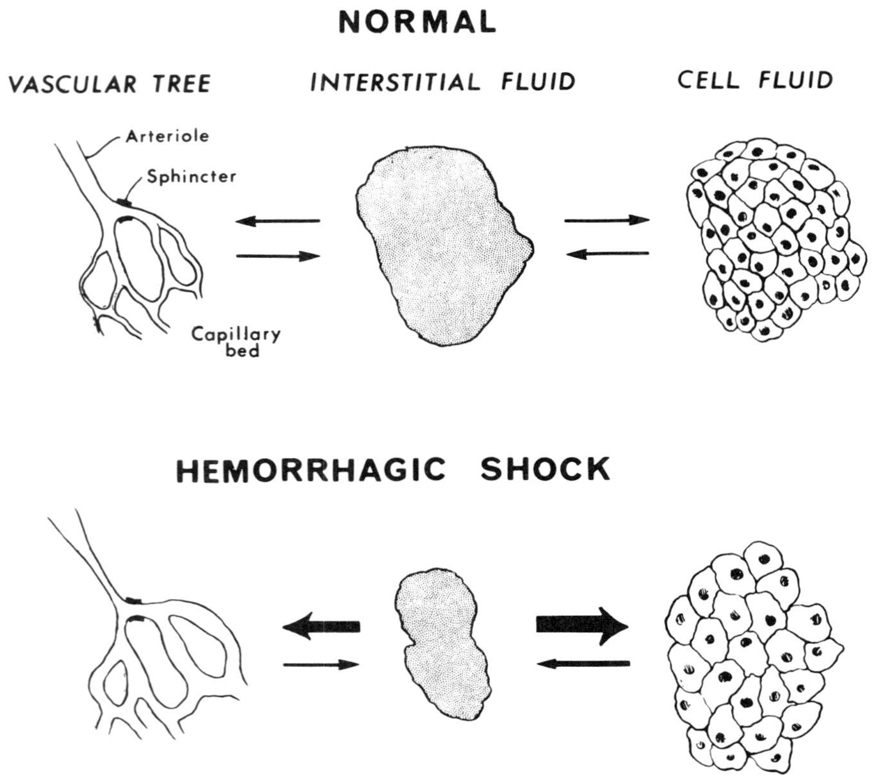

FIG. 4-3. Interstitial fluid response to hemorrhagic shock.

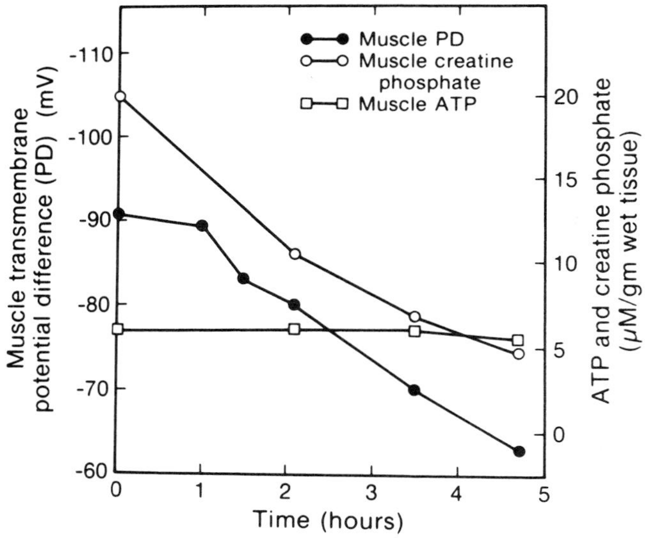

FIG. 4-4. A significant decline in skeletal muscle transmembrane potential difference (PD) and muscle creatine phosphate content occurred by 2.1 h into the shock period. Final creatine phosphate content was 25 percent of the control value. Muscle adenosine triphosphate (ATP) stores were maintained throughout the shock period. (From: *Peitzman AB, Corbett WA, et al: Surg Gynecol Obstet 161:420, 1985, with permission.*)

Depletion of liver ATP or skeletal muscle creatine phosphate was not prevented by administration of intravenous ATP-$MgCl_2$. Cellular dysfunction in liver and muscle, indicated by depolarization of PD, was not ameliorated by infusion of ATP-$MgCl_2$. Thus, late changes in cell energy contents appear to be the result of failing cellular function, rather than the primary cause of membrane failure in shock.

The present data suggest that skeletal muscle cells may be a principal site of fluid and electrolyte sequestration after severe, prolonged hemorrhagic shock. The exact mechanism for the production of electrolyte changes as well as for the notable diminution in extracellular fluid that occurs after hemorrhagic shock is not known. It appears that the changes may well represent a reduction in the efficiency of an active ionic pump mechanism or a selective increase in muscle cell membrane permeability to sodium, or both.

With a reset membrane potential, extracellular fluid electrolyte concentrations are unchanged. Consequently, from the Nernst equation, intracellular Cl^- must rise from 3.5 to 10 meq and intracellular Na^+ from 10 to 22 meq. Transposition of these data to the previously cited measurements in hemorrhagic shock is illustrated (Fig. 4-5). This model shows that only a 6 percent isotonic swelling of muscle cells will explain the major reduction in extracellular fluid measured in hemorrhagic shock.

In summary, the cellular response to hypovolemic hypotension is characterized by a consistent change in active transport of ions. Evidence obtained in vivo indicates that sodium and water enter muscle cells, with resultant loss of cellular potassium to the extracellular fluid. The interstitial fluid holds the extruded potassium. Depletion of cellular ATP below rate-limiting concentrations for ion transport does not appear to be a primary event. Replenishment of the depleted extracellular fluid counteracts these changes at the cellular level and is an important feature of therapy in patients with hypovolemic shock.

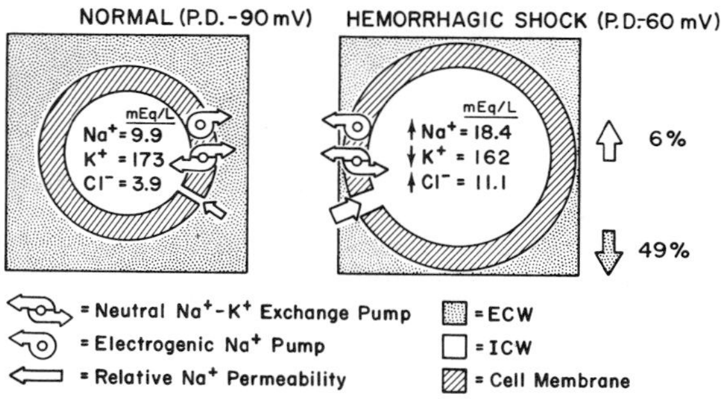

FIG. 4-5. Theoretic transport mechanisms responsible for alterations in potential difference (PD) and fluid-electrolyte distribution in hemorrhagic shock.

Pulmonary Responses

With advances in the management of hemorrhagic shock and support of circulatory and renal function in injured patients, 1 to 2 percent of significantly injured patients (with previously normal lungs) develop acute respiratory failure in the postinjury period. Initially this lung injury was thought to be specifically related to the shock state and its resuscitation. This was implied by such names as "shock lung" and "traumatic wet lung," which have been applied to acute respiratory insufficiency following injury. It is now recognized that there are many similarities in the pathophysiology and clinical presentation of acute lung injury following a variety of insults. This has resulted in the realization that the lung has a limited number of ways of reacting to injury and that several different causes of acute diffuse lung injury result in a similar pathophysiologic response. The common denominator of this response appears to be damage at the alveolar-capillary interface, with resulting leakage of proteinaceous fluid from the intravascular space into the interstitium and subsequently into alveolar spaces.

Clinical Presentation. This injury with its resulting interstitial (and alveolar) edema produces a clinical picture ranging in severity from mild pulmonary dysfunction to progressive pulmonary failure. It differs from "classic" pulmonary failure in that the patients *are usually hypocarbic* rather than hypercarbic. The severe form has been labeled *adult respiratory distress* syndrome (ARDS) and is characterized by

1. Hypoxemia, which is relatively unresponsive to elevations of inspired oxygen concentration (indicating ventilation perfusion imbalance and shunting).
2. Decreased pulmonary compliance (progressively increased airway pressure required to achieve adequate tidal volume).
3. Chest x-ray changes, which are characteristically minimal in the early stages; with progression of the syndrome interstitial edema and diffuse bilateral infiltrates appear that may progress to widespread areas of consolidation.
4. Pulmonary edema unrelated to cardiogenic causes or increased hydrostatic pressure should be ruled out. This is generally done by the measurement of filling pressures.

The clinical criteria are summarized in Table 4-1.

Four clinical stages were described. The first is quite subtle and is characterized by spontaneous hyperventilation with hypocarbia, diminished pulmonary compliance, and respiratory alkalosis. If the process continues, the patient progresses to the second stage,

Table 4-1
Clinical Criteria for Postinjury Pulmonary Insufficiency (ARDS)

Major

A. Hypoxemia (unresponsive)
B. Stiff lung (low compliance)
C. ↓ Resting volume (functional residual capacity)
D. X-ray (diffuse interstitial pattern)
E. ↑ Dead space ventilation

Minor

A. ↑ Cardiac output
B. Hyperventilation
C. R/O cardiogenic pulmonary edema

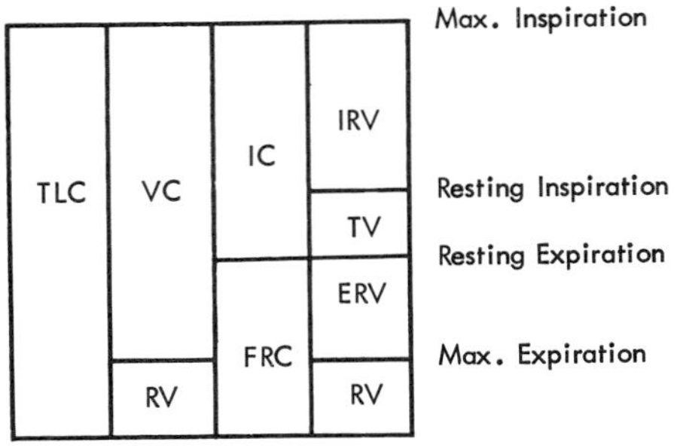

FIG. 4-6. Lung volumes and capacities: TLC, total lung capacity; VC, vital capacity; IC, inspiratory capacity; FRC, functional residual capacity; RV, residual volume; ERV, expiratory reserve volume; TV, tidal volume; IRV, inspiratory reserve volume.

during which respiratory problems become more apparent. Persistent hyperventilation (with hypocarbia), progressive hypoxemia, decreased compliance, and an increase in pulmonary shunt fraction indicate that further pulmonary deterioration is occurring. Changes in chest roentgenograms are characteristically subtle during the early stages. As the syndrome advances to stage three (progressive pulmonary insufficiency) and stage four (terminal hypoxia with cardiac asystole), interstitial edema and diffuse infiltrates are observed on the roentgenograms, while gas exchange and pulmonary mechanics progressively deteriorate.

While these initial clinical descriptions are useful, several qualifying points are important. First, the early changes are nonspecific. Similar findings result from a variety of causes (e.g., early pneumonia, atelectasis, pulmonary edema). Second, the progression can be rapid and the stages are not clearly distinguishable. Studies of the incidence of ARDS have shown that >75 percent of patients developing ''full-blown'' ARDS do so within 24 h of the inciting cause and that 95 percent do so within 72 h. In these studies the diagnosis of ARDS required the following:

1. $Pa_{O_2} \leq 75$ mmHg while receiving $FI_{O_2} \geq 0.5$
2. Diffuse pulmonary infiltrates
3. Pulmonary artery wedge pressure ≤18 mmHg
4. No alternate explanation for the above

Third, with currently available pulmonary support, progression to ''stage four'' is rare. While the mortality *associated with* ARDS remains high, death is rarely the result of respiratory failure alone.

Pathophysiology. A review of basic terminology is shown in Table 4-2. The prominent derangements in pulmonary function associated with ARDS are (1) hypoxia that is unresponsive to increased inspired oxygen concentrations, (2) decreased pulmonary compliance (compliance defined as the amount of volume increase in the lungs obtained by a given increase in pressure), which clinically appears as ''stiff lungs,'' and (3) a fall in resting lung volume, specifically a fall in the functional residual capacity. The functional residual capacity, as shown in Fig. 4-6, is the amount of air remaining in the lungs after a normal expiration.

The traditional causes of hypoxia (decreased arterial P_{O_2}) are shown in Table 4-3. It is unlikely that hypoventilation is responsible for the hypoxia in this syndrome. Hypoventilation significant enough to produce hypoxia is associated with a rise in the P_{CO_2}. These patients, however, have an abnormally low P_{CO_2}.

Although diffusion defects can theoretically result from interstitial edema, they rarely cause clinical hypoxia and should respond to the administration of 100% oxygen. Diffusion defects alone appear to be unlikely causes of the clinical syndrome.

Ventilation/perfusion inequalities can explain the hypoxia seen in these patients, and shunting represents the ultimate ventilation/perfusion abnormality. Normally, there is autoregulation of ventilation and perfusion within the lung so that a balance exists between ventilation and perfusion of alveolar groups. When a group of alveoli become nonventilated or have decreased ventilation, compensatory mechanisms bring about a reflex decrease in blood supply to these alveoli. This, in its extreme, results in no ventilation and no perfusion to these alveolar units; thus no abnormality in terms of dead space ventilation or shunting occurs. The effects of loss of this normal balance or loss of compensatory mechanisms are shown in Fig. 4-7. On the left, alterations in blood flow are demonstrated. It can be seen that progressive decrease in blood flow with continued ventilation affects primarily carbon dioxide elimination. This can be defined as high ventilation/perfusion ratio and is usually detected by increases in dead space ventilation. Such changes do not result in hypoxia. On the right side of Fig. 4-7 is shown the effect of reduction in ventilation while perfusion is maintained. It can be seen that progressive lowering of ventilation can result in hypoxia until the ultimate reduction, i.e., nonventilation, occurs. In theory, as long as any ventilation of the

Table 4-2
Basic Terminology and Symbols

$\overline{V}_{O_2}$	Oxygen consumption
Q_T	Cardiac output
V_D/V_T	Physiologic dead space ventilation as fraction of tidal volume
Q_s/Q_t	Physiologic shunt as fraction of total cardiac output
AaD_{O_2}	Alveolar arterial gradient—oxygen
FI_{O_2}	Fraction of inspired O_2
$\dot{V}/\dot{Q}$	Ratio of ventilation to perfusion
Pa_{O_2}	Partial pressure, arterial, oxygen

Table 4-3
Causes of Hypoxemia

1. Hypoventilation
2. Diffusion defects
3. V/Q abnormalities
4. Shunting

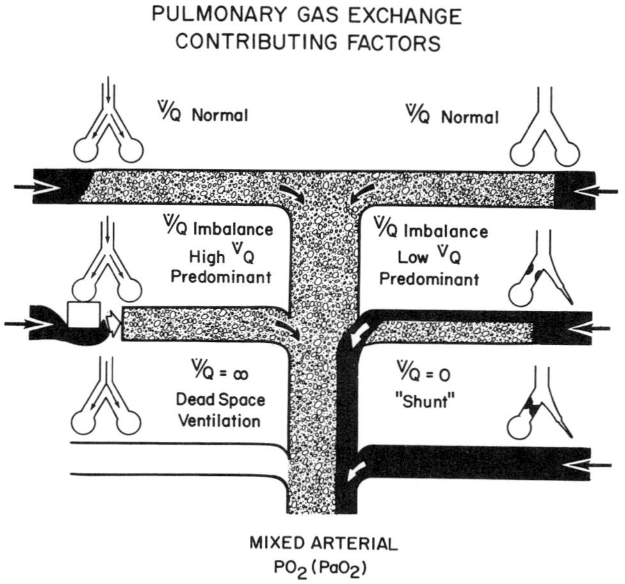

FIG. 4-7. Diagrammatic representation of ventilation/perfusion ratio (V/Q) abnormalities.

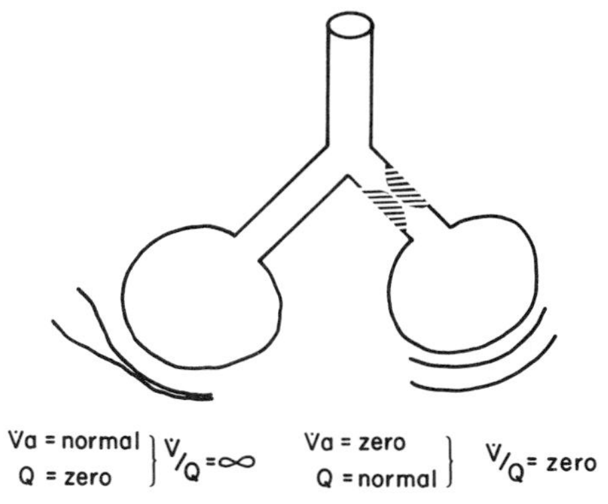

FIG. 4-9. Diagrammatic representation of mismatched ventilation and perfusion.

alveolus occurs, the hypoxia should be responsive to oxygen. This, then, is generally referred to as a ventilation/perfusion abnormality characterized by a low V/Q ratio. When alveolar collapse or nonventilation occurs, the hypoxia secondary to this is no longer responsive to oxygen; this is defined as a shunt.

Causes of pulmonary shunting are shown in Fig. 4-8. Shunting normally takes place, to the extent of about 3 percent of the cardiac output, through both intrapulmonary and extrapulmonary routes. Although pathologic shunts occur from extrapulmonary causes, intrapulmonary shunting appears to be the problem in ARDS. Basically, there is perfusion of alveoli that are collapsed or for other reasons cannot be ventilated. The alveoli, for example, may be filled with secretions, exudate, blood, or edema.

Whatever the basic cause, the clinical picture of ARDS appears to result from a distortion of the normal ventilation/perfusion balance. This concept is shown in Fig. 4-9. In some areas of the lung there is perfusion with poor ventilation; in other areas there is ventilation of nonperfused alveoli. This combination of abnormalities will produce decreased resting lung volume (functional residual capacity, or FRC), shunting, and increased dead space ventilation.

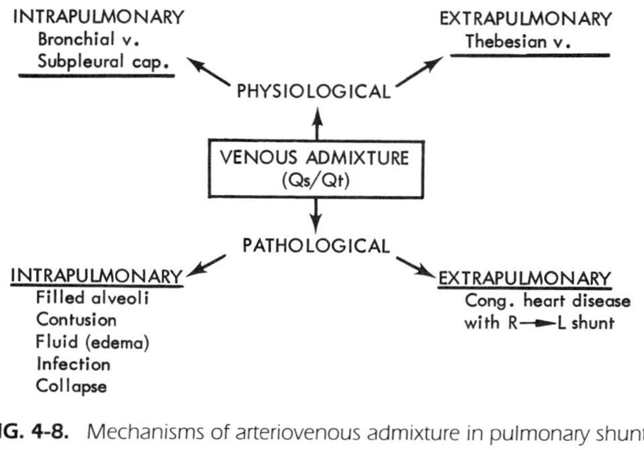

FIG. 4-8. Mechanisms of arteriovenous admixture in pulmonary shunting.

The common denominator producing the abnormalities in ventilation and perfusion and other abnormalities seen in ARDS is thought to be injury to the pulmonary capillary endothelium or alveolar epithelium. Injury to the capillary endothelium results in loss of integrity of the membrane, with increased permeability to albumin. The consequent leak of protein-rich fluid leads to *interstitial pulmonary edema* and decreased pulmonary compliance. With continued leakage, the alveolar units become fluid-filled and hypoxia (shunting) ensues. Thus the entire clinical picture of ventilation of poorly perfused segments (capillary injury), decreased compliance (interstitial edema), perfusion of poorly ventilated segments, and loss of lung volume (partially and completely fluid-filled alveoli) appears to result from capillary injury with a "capillary leak."

Etiology. A variety of factors have been suggested as capable of producing ARDS (Table 4-4). Several of these are specific to, or frequently present in the trauma patient. Some of these have been clearly shown to predispose patients to the development of ARDS as shown in Table 4-5. The definition of these factors and possible mechanism of production are discussed below.

Blood-Borne Injury. Among individual conditions, *sepsis syndrome* is the most frequent single precipitant of ARDS. Sepsis syndrome has been defined as evidence of a significant inflammatory state (temperature ≤35°C or ≥39°C, white blood cell count <2000 or >12,000 cells/mm^3, positive blood cultures, or source of infection) accompanied by a deleterious systemic effect (unexplained arterial hypotension with systolic blood pressure <90 mmHg for greater than 2 h, systemic vascular resistance less than 800 dyne · s/cm^5, or unexplained metabolic acidosis).

The risk of ARDS after bacteremia alone, on the other hand, is relatively low, increasing markedly if bacteremia is accompanied by a deleterious systemic response such as hypotension or thrombocytopenia. While sepsis can serve as an example of factors that produce ARDS as a result of blood-borne injury, the precise mechanism by which this occurs has not yet been elucidated. Some propose that the injury is a direct result of bacterial products on the capillary endothelium. Others present evidence for extensive injury resulting from products of activated leukocytes or platelets. Whatever the precise mechanisms, it is becoming clearer that the end result of this blood-borne injury is massive disruption of the capillary endothelium and alveolar epithelium. The end result is

Table 4-4
Disorders Associated with (Causing) Adult Respiratory Distress Syndrome

Blood-Borne or Vascular Source of Injury	
Trauma (soft tissue or skeletal)*	Drug overdoses:
Sepsis*	Heroin, methadone, ethchlorvynol, acetylsalicylic acid, propoxyphene
Fat embolism	Drug idiosyncratic reaction
Pancreatitis	Thrombotic thrombocytopenic purpura
Shock	Leukemia
Multiple transfusions:	Venous air embolism
Microemboli	Head injury
Leukoagglutinin reaction	Paraquat
Disseminated intravascular coagulation	Cardiopulmonary bypass/hemodialysis
Surface burns	
Miliary tuberculosis	
Inhalation or Airway Source	***Direct or Physical Source***
Aspiration of gastric contents*	Lung contusion
Diffuse infectious pneumonia:* viral, mycoplasma, Legionnaires', pneumocystis	Radiation
Near-drowning*	High altitude
Irritant gas inhalation: NO_2, Cl_2, SO_2, NH_3	Hanging
Smoke inhalation	Reexpansion
O_2 toxicity	

*Common cause of ARDS.

loss of selectivity of the endothelium for albumin, interstitial edema, and eventual alveolar flooding, all producing the clinical picture of ARDS.

Other predisposing factors for ARDS probably operate in a similar fashion. These include: massive soft tissue and skeletal trauma (with microemboli as a possible circulating agent); multiple blood transfusions (with particulate or activated humoral agents causing capillary injury); fat embolism; disseminated intervascular coagulation; and activation (or lack of metabolism) of other circulating agents as might occur in pancreatic injury, pancreatitis, and massive hepatic injury.

The role of hypotension (shock) alone as a precipitating factor continues to be questioned. It appears probable that the presence of severe hypotension may augment injury from other causes but that hypotension alone is rarely the sole cause.

Inhalation or Airway Injury. Aspiration of gastric contents is among the most common causes of ARDS in several series. The clinical picture and roentgenographic findings that we now call ARDS were described by Mendelson in a classic paper in which he also presented animal studies on the pathophysiology of lung injury, stressing the role of acid pH. As in sepsis, the precise mechanism remains under investigation. Although a pH of 2.5 or less was originally suggested as being necessary to produce lung injury in human beings, data now exist that suggest that aspiration of substances with pHs greater than 2.5 can also produce this clinical picture. Despite the need to further define the mechanism, there is little question that aspiration of large amounts of gastric contents is a cause of ARDS. In addition, aspiration can serve as an example of other airway sources of injury. These include near-drowning, inhalation of toxic products (from burning wood, plastic, or chemical agents), oxygen toxicity, and diffuse infectious pneumonias.

Direct or Physical Lung Injury. Thoracic trauma with lung contusion is a well-established cause of ARDS. ARDS can occur as a result of bilateral lung contusion due to chest trauma or blast injury. Lung contusion is usually localized and unilateral. Even a localized contusion can produce significant intrapulmonary shunting. The severe ARDS picture associated with pulmonary contusions is more likely if the thoracic trauma is bilateral, although a

Table 4-5
Incidence of ARDS After Predisposing Clinical Conditions

	Single Condition Present			*Multiple Conditions Present*		
Clinical Condition	*Number*	*Number with ARDS*	*Incidence, %*	*Number**	*Number with ARDS*	*Incidence, %*
Sepsis syndrome	46	18	39	21	8	38
Aspiration	64	8	13	20	8	40
Multiple transfusions	31	8	26	37	12	32
Lung contusion	57	6	11	40	17	43
Multiple fractures	34	3	9	32	10	31
Near-drowning	5	2	40	6	4	67
Total	237	45	19	69	30	43

*Number with given condition as one of multiple risk conditions.

severe unilateral blast injury can also result in ARDS involving both lungs. It has been suggested that significant increases in intrathoracic pressure occur with thoracic or abdominal injuries that produce much more extensive damage than initially appreciated on roentgenogram. There is little doubt that whatever the mechanism, "pulmonary contusions" are a predisposing factor in this devastating clinical picture. It is important to recognize that this may not require extensive chest wall trauma. This is particularly true in children with their compliant chest walls.

Type and Amount of Resuscitative Fluid. The role of resuscitative fluids and the questions of the benefits of colloid versus crystalloid solutions have been a major area of controversy. Much of this concern has been based on concepts of fluid exchange in the normal lung. This information is described mathematically in the following formula: $Q_f = K_w[(P_c - P_i) - \sigma_s(\pi_c - \pi_i)]$. A description of the symbols is as follows:

Q_f = net exchange of fluid across membrane
K_w = filtration coefficient of water
P_c = capillary hydrostatic pressure
P_i = interstitial hydrostatic pressure
σ_s = reflection coefficient of solute (factor by which ideal osmotic pressure is reduced owing to membrane permeability to solute; range of σ is 0 to 1.0)
π_c = capillary osmotic pressure
π_i = interstitial osmotic pressure

This concept is represented diagrammatically in Fig. 4-10.

If the pulmonary vasculature is normal, a fall in serum oncotic pressure renders the lungs more susceptible to pulmonary edema.

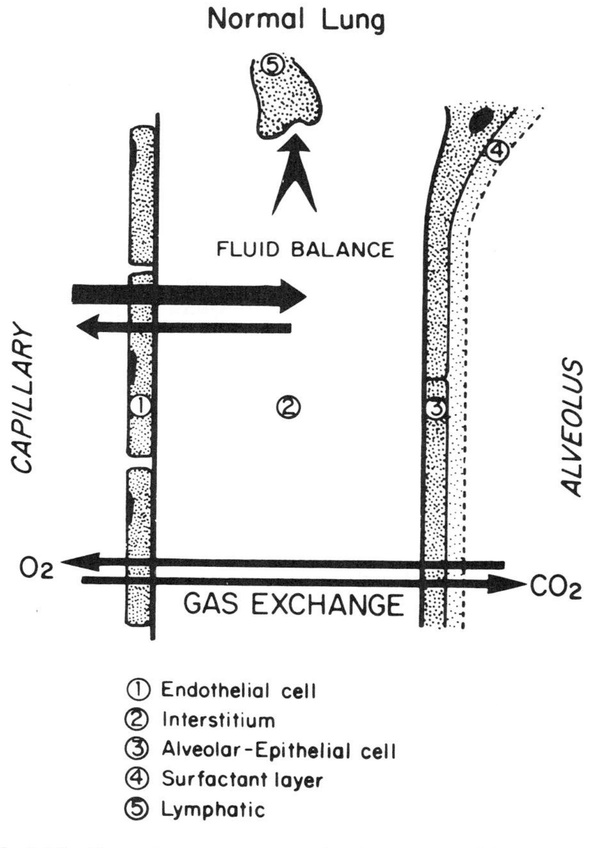

FIG. 4-10. Dynamic processes occurring in the normal lung.

Some authors reason that if crystalloid solutions are used in resuscitation, a fall in oncotic pressure might occur and cause or compound a pulmonary abnormality. If this were the case, the administration of colloid might be beneficial to the patient. The crucial flaw in the reasoning hinges on the word "normal." Whether the injury leading to ARDS is to the endothelium or to the alveolar epithelium, the selectivity of the capillary for albumin and other large molecules is lost or impaired. Thus, the potential benefit of solutions containing high–molecular-weight compounds and the potential detriment of reasonable amounts of electrolyte-containing solutions become a nonissue.

Diagnosis. Criteria for the diagnosis of ARDS have been previously outlined. It is generally agreed that if one waits until patients meet these criteria, any opportunity for preventive or early therapeutic measures is lost. The general approach to these patients is to attempt to identify high-risk patients, place them in an intensive care area, and carefully observe them for signs of ARDS. Particular emphasis is placed on changes in oxygenation, changes in respiratory rate or arterial P_{CO_2}, and changes in lung mechanics.

Assessment of the adequacy of pulmonary function should begin immediately after injury in those patients at risk for developing ARDS. Endotracheal tubes inserted for airway control during surgery should sometimes be left in place until high-risk patients can be evaluated. In many such patients an additional 4 to 6 h of intubation postoperatively will be sufficient to allow the physician to detect the presence of early ARDS. Extubation should be considered when adequate lung function has been demonstrated (described below). If several days of intubation are contemplated, a nasotracheal tube may be substituted for the orotracheal tube in the operating room. This will allow for greater patient comfort and acceptance.

A prerequisite for optimal lung function is normal cardiovascular status. Hemodynamic monitoring, therefore, should be instituted routinely. This includes recording of heart rate, arterial pressure, electrocardiogram, central venous pressure, and pulmonary artery pressure if indicated. Serial body weight, intake and output balance, bacteriologic studies, coagulation profile, and chest x-rays are important data.

Monitoring of pulmonary function can be conveniently divided into three general areas: evaluation of oxygenation, ventilation, and lung-thorax mechanics. Table 4-6 details the most easily obtained tests and includes "normal" values. As a general principle, isolated determinations are not as valuable as serial measurements obtained at regular intervals. Hypoxemia is often detected in patients who appear to be doing well clinically.

The effective compliance (C_{eff}) may be valuable as an assessment of the ease of distensibility of the lung and thoracic cage. This derived value is obtained by dividing the VT by the peak airway pressure. C_{eff} indicates the "stiffness" of the lungs, i.e., how difficult they are to ventilate (low C_{eff} means increased stiffness). A decreased C_{eff} may indicate increased extravascular lung water, airway constriction, or increased chest wall resistance (impaired bellows activity). Low values are usually found in patients with ARDS.

An adequate assessment of pulmonary function can be achieved by serial measurement of arterial blood gases, tidal volume, minute ventilation, and effective compliance. Several other monitoring indices have been advocated. The work of breathing is almost always increased in ARDS. This value is a measure of the mechanical cost of achieving adequate ventilation. The major dis-

Table 4-6
Assessment of Pulmonary Function

Function	*Acceptable*	*Consider Institution of Therapy**
Oxygenation:		
Partial pressure oxygen arterial blood	$Pa_{O_2} > 90$ mm on 40% FI_{O_2}	<90 mmHg on 40% FI_{O_2} or decreasing
Partial pressure oxygen arterial blood to fraction inspired oxygen ratio (Pa_{O_2}/FI_{O_2})	$Pa_{O_2}/FI_{O_2} > 250$	<250 or decreasing
Alveolar-arterial oxygen gradient (breathing 100% O_2 for 10 to 15 min)	50–200 mmHg	>200 mmHg or increasing
Ventilation:		
Partial pressure carbon dioxide arterial blood	35–40 mmHg	30 or decreasing
Minute volume	<12 L/min	Increasing
Mechanics:		
Rate	12–25/min	25 or increasing
Effective compliance	50 cm^3/cmH_2O	50 or decreasing

*Trends over a period of time are useful in marginal situations.

advantage of this test is that the measurement and interpretation is difficult in the critically ill patient.

Table 4-6 is intended as a guide for identifying patients who require increased attention. Careful investigation for causes of pulmonary deterioration (pneumothorax, fluid excess, lobar atelectasis, etc.) is indicated, and more extensive monitoring may be required before instituting therapy for ARDS.

Management. ***Support of Pulmonary Function (Support of Oxygenation, and CO_2 Elimination).*** The most common indication for beginning ventilatory therapy is hypoxemia. Initial management should be to increase the FI_{O_2}, both as a diagnostic test and to temporarily relieve hypoxemia, if the Pa_{O_2} is less than 65 mmHg. For effective therapy, control of the airway must be achieved. The most rapid and reliable way to do this is the insertion of an endotracheal or nasotracheal tube. Mechanical ventilation may then be applied. Since a defect in the matching of ventilation to perfusion is present, therapy is directed at maintaining ventilation to marginally ventilated alveoli and recruiting collapsed or partially occluded alveoli. This will directly increase the FRC of the lungs.

Technique. The volume ventilator is the device most often chosen for the treatment of ARDS. The initial tidal volume setting may be 10 to 15 mL/kg body weight at a rate of 12 to 14 breaths per minute, with an inspiration:expiration ratio of 1:2. The ventilator is adjusted so that the patient can "trigger" additional ventilator breaths. This can be described as assisted mechanical ventilation (AMV). An FI_{O_2} of 0.4 should be applied initially and blood-gas determinations used to indicate the efficacy of this treatment. Humidification of the inspired air via a heated nebulizer is essential.

Blood gases are checked within 10 to 20 min of beginning respiratory treatment to determine the patient's response. If hypoxemia persists on 40 percent oxygen, increasing the VT still further may be warranted in an effort to increase the FRC. The effect of this maneuver is best assessed by following serial compliance changes. If the C_{eff} is improving, benefit from increased VT may be expected. If C_{eff} decreases with an increase in VT, too much volume is being given to the patient. Lower tidal volume ventilation will then be required to minimize the risk of complications of ventilatory therapy. The compliance curve is shaped somewhat like the Starling curve of cardiac function, i.e., a plateau is reached, after which any increase in volume is achieved only at the expense of a marked increase in airway pressure.

Alternative methods of mechanical ventilatory support are available. One that is being used more frequently is intermittent mandatory ventilation (IMV). This is a technique of mechanical ventilation that allows the patient to breathe spontaneously and at the same time to receive periodic support from the ventilator.

Acceptable levels of Pa_{O_2} are between 65 and 80 mmHg. If this cannot be achieved with the treatment outlined above, there are two alternatives: manipulation of FI_{O_2} or more vigorous support of lung volume.

The FI_{O_2} may be increased to higher levels. Since pulmonary shunting is caused by continued perfusion of nonventilated alveoli, simply increasing the concentration of oxygen will have no significant effect on the shunt. In addition, washout of nitrogen from poorly ventilated alveoli will make them more susceptible to collapse, thus converting low V/Q areas to areas of shunt resulting in more atelectasis. Although there is still controversy over the role of O_2 toxicity in the genesis of ARDS, the literature clearly indicates that prolonged use of high O_2 concentrations can produce a clinical picture similar to ARDS. A concentration of more than 50% O_2 is required to produce deleterious effects in patients with normal lungs, depending on the amount of time alveolar hyperoxia is maintained. The higher the O_2 concentrations, the less the time required to produce damage. Therefore every effort should be made to limit the FI_{O_2} to less than 0.5.

Since manipulation of the FI_{O_2} is of short-term benefit, the second alternative is to recruit collapsed or partially collapsed alveoli with some modification of ventilatory therapy. This can be done by applying continuous positive end-expiratory pressure (PEEP) to the airway. PEEP may be achieved by either inserting an airflow resistance during expiration or using a ventilator with an end-expiratory plateau of positive pressure. Providing positive pressure throughout the respiratory cycle prevents alveolar and small airway collapse and may recruit lung units that were previously collapsed. The beneficial effects of this modality are (1) increased FRC, compliance, and Pa_{O_2}; (2) increased V/Q ratio (when initially low); and (3) decreased pulmonary shunting.

Technique of PEEP. The commonly used volume ventilators have the capability of instituting PEEP without modifying the equipment. Although there is some controversy about the absolute level required, incremental increases in pressure are advocated. The usual beginning level is 5 cmH_2O of PEEP. Cardiorespiratory function is monitored after 10 to 15 min to assess the effects. If no beneficial effect is noted, further increases in PEEP follow in increments of 3 to 5 cmH_2O pressure. There may be variable response to PEEP. While some patients respond with an immediate increase in Pa_{O_2}, others may not show improvement for $\frac{1}{2}$ to 1 h or longer. Therefore, absence of immediate response should not be interpreted as an absolute failure of PEEP.

Complications of PEEP. Cardiac output can be decreased secondary to an increase in intrathoracic pressure and decreased venous return. This is usually significant only when the intravascular volume is decreased. Therefore, fluids should be given to assure a normal volume status before beginning PEEP therapy. Monitoring of the pulmonary wedge pressure is valuable in the assessment of volume before and during the administration of PEEP. Cardiac output can also be measured to assure normal values.

Excessive pressure applied to the terminal airways can overdistend and rupture normal alveoli, leading to pneumothorax. This complication of PEEP is uncommon below 20 cmH_2O pressure.

Close attention to the effective compliance can prevent excessive airway and alveolar pressure being applied during PEEP therapy. PEEP is most beneficial when FRC is low initially. In patients with a high FRC from preexisting lung disease (chronic obstructive pulmonary disease), any level of PEEP may be detrimental. This can be determined only by closely monitoring the patient's response to treatment.

Control of Pa_{CO_2}. Hyperventilation is a common problem in patients who are being artificially ventilated. Hypocarbia has been shown to be deleterious to the cerebral circulation (vasoconstriction) and the pulmonary circulation. Therefore, ventilatory therapy should be set to maintain normal levels of Pa_{CO_2}. With high tidal volume ventilation, a compensatory decrease in respiratory rate is necessary to maintain a normal Pa_{CO_2}. Increasing the inspired concentration of CO_2 or adding dead space have both been advocated as methods of increasing the Pa_{CO_2} but are rarely effective in patients with ARDS. Effective control of the Pa_{CO_2} requires heavy sedation or muscle relaxation and control of the patient's respiration. Decrease of the Pa_{CO_2} below 30 is an indication for instituting respiratory control.

Oxygen-Carrying Capacity of Blood. Although the Pa_{O_2} can be increased by higher levels of $F_{I_{O_2}}$, it is the red blood cell that carries almost all the O_2 to the tissues. One unit of packed red cells carries more O_2 than plasma exposed to pure O_2 at hyperbaric pressure. Therefore, a hemoglobin (Hgb) concentration mean 12 g/dL is optimal. Attention should also be given to the acid-base status of the patient. Both acidosis and alkalosis produce shifts of the Hgb-O_2 dissociation curve that can affect the ability of Hgb to off-load O_2 at the tissue level.

Fluid Management. Fluid therapy can arbitrarily be divided into two phases when one is dealing with the acutely traumatized or critically ill patient. In the initial phase, or resuscitation phase, careful control of fluid administration is important but may be difficult. Later, in the maintenance phase of fluid therapy, careful regulation of intake and output can be accomplished more easily. In both phases, the ideal would be the complete normalization of pulmonary vascular pressure. This can best be accomplished by invasive monitoring of pulmonary artery and central venous pressures. To avoid the complications of hydrostatic edema with resultant pulmonary dysfunction, continued monitoring of these parameters in acutely ill patients is essential. The values of these hemodynamic indices can guide the minute-by-minute volume replacement in the resuscitation phase and the hourly rates in the maintenance phase.

The type of fluid used for resuscitation and maintenance therapy is controversial. The two most common asanguinous fluids are isotonic balanced salt solutions and solutions containing albumin (colloid). Proponents of colloid therapy have stressed the physiologic principle of maintaining colloid osmotic pressure of the plasma (π_c) in the prevention of interstitial edema. Others have argued that little or no change occurs in plasma oncotic pressure despite large volumes of balanced salt solutions. It is reasonable to assume that if the pulmonary membranes are injured the effect of oncotic pressure will be reduced.

Randomized trials of crystalloid versus colloid therapy in acutely ill patients have been conducted. Lowe and associates reported no difference with regard to survival, incidence of pulmonary failure, or postresuscitation pulmonary function. Similarly, Virgilio and colleagues demonstrated the greater ease with which isotonic fluid therapy can be managed, despite its large volumes, as opposed to colloid therapy. On the other hand, others have suggested that the use of colloid solutions enhances the function of the myocardium and oxygen transport in patients with high cardiac indexes, whereas crystalloid tends to worsen pulmonary gas exchange.

Detrimental effects of albumin treatment have been proposed. It has been demonstrated that albumin in the first several days of resuscitation has a negative inotropic effect and promotes fluid retention by limiting salt and water excretion. This same group has also suggested that albumin therapy may alter blood coagulation. Other investigators demonstrated an increased extravasation of albumin in the lungs after resuscitation with colloid solutions. This extravascular albumin may adversely affect fluid and protein movement in the lung.

In considering the conflict in the literature regarding the pros and cons of colloid therapy (albumin solutions), several points should be emphasized. Clinical and experimental studies generally find balanced salt solutions satisfactory for volume replacement. A second point is that massive volumes of isotonic salt solutions are necessary before severe changes in plasma osmotic pressure occur. Third, the changes that occur in colloid osmotic pressure may not be of importance in the injured lung because of the increased permeability of protein at the membrane level. Also, the cost of albumin-containing solutions can be up to fifty times that of balanced salt solutions.

Based on the above, our approach is to treat the acutely ill or traumatized patient with blood and/or isotonic salt solutions, depending on the clinical status. Pulmonary vascular pressures are closely monitored to prevent the sequelae of overzealous therapy or hypovolemia.

Diuretics. Administration of diuretics has been proposed as a method for indirectly decreasing the amount of interstitial edema. Reports claiming a therapeutic role for diuretics in treating ARDS are not conclusive. Our practice is to give small doses of furosemide *when hemodynamic studies indicate that fluid overload has occurred,* e.g., an elevated pulmonary artery wedge pressure. No attempt is made to ''dry out'' the patient by the long-term administration of diuretics. There is no solid evidence to suggest that lowering fluid volumes below normal will decrease the leak from injured capillaries. Such decreases in volume may have serious deleterious effects.

Corticosteroids and Anti-inflammatory Agents. There is no conclusive proof that pharmacologic doses of steroid should be part of the specific therapy of the ARDS syndrome. Data do exist to indicate that steroids may be effective in treating pulmonary fat embolism and in selected patients with extensive acute fibrosis. Therefore, we reserve steroid therapy for these clinical entities. Similarly, the use of other antiinflammatory agents is unproved and should be confined to carefully constructed experimental trials.

Antibiotics. Prophylactic use of broad-spectrum antibiotics has no place in the primary therapy of ARDS. Indiscriminate use of these agents can allow the emergence of resistant strains of bacteria that are very difficult to treat. Many patients will already have been given antibiotics because of certain types of injury. Specific antibiotics are used to treat pulmonary sepsis. Their choice is determined by serial cultures of the sputum.

Ancillary Pulmonary Care. Patients treated in the intensive care unit tend to be bound to the bed by numerous tubes, wires, and catheters. Change in position then becomes a difficult problem. It has been shown, however, that significant improvement in oxygenation can result from frequent position changes. Maintenance of one position is likely to compound pulmonary abnormalities.

Routine pulmonary toilet, suctioning with sterile technique, and attempts to prevent pulmonary infection are very important. These must all be done on a routine basis.

Additional Ventilatory Support. Additional modifications of ventilatory therapy are available for patients with unique problems and those who do not respond to conventional methods. These include *pressure support,* which is useful in overcoming airway resistance; *selective lung ventilation,* which may be useful in patients with nonuniform disease; *high frequency (JET) ventilation,* which may be useful in patients with bronchopleural fistulae; and *reverse inspiratory/expiratory ratio ventilation,* which may be effective in selected patients who fail to respond to conventional ventilatory support.

Prevention. Early application of PEEP in high-risk patients could reduce the incidence of ARDS. This concept has been challenged. We prospectively randomized 92 patients meeting entry criteria for ARDS risk factors to receive mechanical ventilation either without PEEP (control) or with 8 cm water PEEP (early PEEP). These therapies were continued for 72 h unless (1) ARDS developed or (2) the Pa_{O_2} was greater than 140 ($FI_{O_2} = 0.5$) at 24 h and continued so following PEEP removal. This group included 65 trauma patients. The groups were comparable for age, severity of injury, number and types of ARDS risk factors, and additional oxygenation. The incidence of atelectasis, pneumonia, and barotrauma was the same in both groups as was mortality. Thus, we were unable to demonstrate any effect of early application of 8 cm of PEEP to high-risk patients on the incidence of ARDS. While there may be valid reasons for intubation and early mechanical support of injured patients, the probability that such treatment will significantly decrease the incidence of true ARDS is low. This is compatible with the concept that a physical injury to the alveolar capillary interface has occurred. The impact of ventilatory support on the long-term progress of the disease remains debatable.

Table 4-7
Early and Late Mortality in ARDS Patients by Immediate Cause of Death

	Early Deaths (≤72 h)	*Late Deaths (>72 h)*
Sepsis	3*	8
Respiratory	1	4†
Cardiac	1	5‡
Neurologic	3	4
Other	2	1

*Sepsis present prior to ARDS.
†All four with sepsis as a contributory cause.
‡Three with sepsis as a contributory cause.

Outcome. Despite advances in ventilatory support and fluid management, the mortality associated with ARDS remains high. Most centers report mortalities of 50 percent or greater in patients who sustain rigidly defined ARDS. The causes of death, however, are rarely respiratory failure (Table 4-7). Most of the early deaths (less than 72 h) are related to the underlying illness or injury. In contrast, sepsis is directly responsible for 38 percent of the late (greater than 72 h) ARDS deaths and is a contributing factor in 76 percent. This supports the intuitive impression that long-term survival in surgical patients with ARDS frequently depends on identification and elimination of the septic focus.

Alterations in Oxygen Transport

Cell hypoxia and eventually cell death may result from the complex changes induced by shock. In the past, attention was directed primarily toward the factors affecting oxygen transport capability, including the concentration and partial pressure of oxygen in the inspired air, alveolar ventilation, ventilation/perfusion relationships, cardiac output, blood volume, and hemoglobin concentration. The demonstration that the level of organic phosphates in the red blood cell has a significant effect on the position of the oxygen/hemoglobin dissociation curve has served to focus attention on the processes responsible for release of oxygen at the tissue level.

Oxygen Transport

The oxygen transport system consists of several component processes that function collectively to extract oxygen from inspired air and deliver it at a partial pressure sufficient to allow rapid diffusion from blood into the body cells. Each of the component processes has its own internal controls, and failure of any one may be compensated for by adjustments in the remainder of the system. The functions of the oxygen transport system are summarized in the following formula:

$$\text{Oxygen consumption} = \text{arteriovenous oxygen difference} \times \frac{\text{cardiac output (L/min)}}{100}$$

The amount of oxygen in whole blood includes that bound to hemoglobin (1.38 mL O_2/g of hemoglobin) and a small amount dissolved in plasma (0.003 mL/mm of oxygen tension). The oxygen content of arterial (Ca_{O_2}) and venous blood (Cv_{O_2}) are calculated by the formula

$$\text{Oxygen content} = (1.38 \times Hb_{conc} \times Hb_{sat}) + (0.003 \times P_{O_2})$$

Consider a person with a hemoglobin of 15 g/dL, an arterial oxygen tension of 100 mmHg, a venous oxygen tension of 40 mmHg, arterial and venous hemoglobin saturations of 97 and 75 percent, respectively, and a cardiac output of 6 L/min. Substituting these values in the formulas above, arterial oxygen content is 20.4 vol%, venous oxygen content is 15.6 vol%, arteriovenous oxygen difference is 4.8 vol%, and oxygen consumption is 288 mL/min.

Changes in any one of these factors are of variable significance regarding oxygen delivery. For instance, pulmonary gas exchange with 20 percent inspired oxygen concentration (FI_{O_2}) normally produces an arterial oxygen tension (Pa_{O_2}) of approximately 100 mmHg, slightly less than average alveolar oxygen tension. Increasing the FI_{O_2} to 100 percent would raise Pa_{O_2} to approximately 650 mmHg. This would increase the amount of dissolved oxygen in the plasma from 0.3 to 2.0 vol% but would only increase the hemoglobin saturation from 97 to 100 percent. By contrast, even moderate changes in hemoglobin concentration or cardiac output have a strong influence on oxygen transport capability. A hemoglobin concentration of 10 g/dL (instead of 15) in the example above would reduce the oxygen-carrying capacity of the blood by one-third (Ca_{O_2} = 13.7 vol%). Coupled with a fall in cardiac output from 6 to 3 L/min, assuming that other variables remain unchanged, oxygen consumption theoretically would fall from 288 to 96 mL/min. This is a not infrequent clinical occurrence, although oxygen consumption would be maintained at a higher level by adjustments in other parts of the system (e.g., increase of arteriovenous oxygen difference).

Therapy designed to improve tissue oxygenation, therefore, includes an evaluation of all factors affecting the oxygen transport system. Adjustment of inspired oxygen concentration and efforts to improve alveolar ventilation are of obvious importance; however, therapeutic attempts to maintain a normal hemoglobin concentration and cardiac output deserve special attention.

Oxygen/Hemoglobin Dissociation Curve

The oxyhemoglobin dissociation curve describes hemoglobin affinity for oxygen, and its unusual sigmoid shape reflects the phenomenon of heme-heme interaction. Each of four heme groups in the hemoglobin molecule reacts with oxygen in a prescribed order, and uptake of an oxygen molecule by one heme group facilitates the oxygenation of the next heme group. The sigmoid configuration of this curve is particularly suitable for the uptake, transport, and subsequent release of oxygen. Since the upper portion of the dissociation curve is relatively flat, oxygen loading by hemoglobin may remain relatively normal despite wide variations in the alveolar oxygen tension. As oxygenated blood traverses the peripheral capillary, however, P_{O_2} drops from approximately 100 to 40 mmHg, hemoglobin saturation falls from 97 to 75 percent, and the blood releases just over 22 percent of its oxygen load (Fig. 4-11). Since P_{O_2} values at the peripheral capillary level fall on the steep portion of the curve, significant changes in oxygen release are produced by only small alterations in oxygen tension.

The position of the oxyhemoglobin dissociation curve along the horizontal axis is characteristically termed the P_{50} value. This reflects the oxygen tension necessary to saturate 50 percent of the

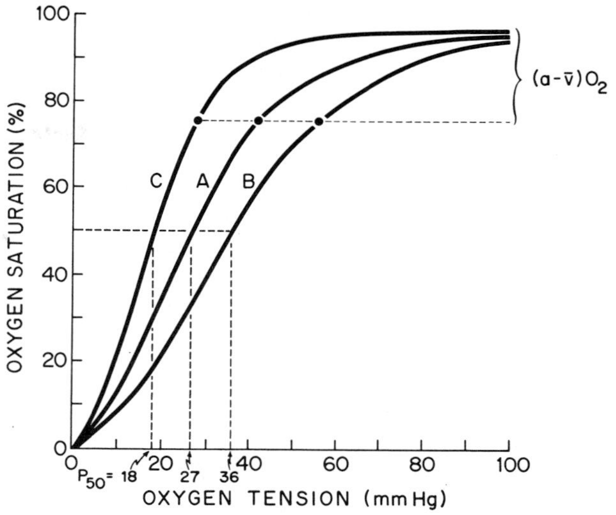

FIG. 4-11. Oxygen-hemoglobin dissociation curves in *(A)* normal, *(B)* rightward-shifted, and *(C)* leftward-shifted positions. The P_{50} value denotes the position of the curve along the horizontal axis and represents the oxygen tension (in mmHg) necessary to saturate 50 percent of available hemoglobin with oxygen. Note that as the curve moves toward the left, the arteriovenous oxygen difference, $(a-\bar{v})\ O_2$, can be maintained only by decreasing venous oxygen tension. (Adapted from: *Shappell SD, Lenfant CJM: Anesthesiology 37:127, 1972, with permission.*)

hemoglobin with oxygen; the normal value is approximately 27 mmHg.

The importance of positional changes of the curve is also related to its sigmoid shape. Within limits, rightward or leftward shifts have little effect on arterial oxygen saturation if Pa_{O_2} is above 80 mmHg. At the peripheral capillary level, however, even small shifts of the curve may be important. A rightward shift of the dissociation curve (P_{50} above 27 mmHg) indicates decreased hemoglobin affinity for oxygen, while a leftward shift (P_{50} below 27 mmHg) is associated with an increase of hemoglobin/oxygen affinity. Compared with the normally positioned curve, more oxygen is released at any given P_{O_2} with a rightward-shifted curve and less is released with a leftward-shifted curve. Therefore, if arterial and venous oxygen tensions remain constant, arteriovenous oxygen difference increases with a rightward shift of the curve and decreases with a leftward shift (Fig. 4-12).

Changes in position of the oxygen/hemoglobin dissociation curve are significant in at least two respects. The transfer of oxygen from the blood to the sites of intracellular utilization is directly related to the oxygen pressure differential. A rightward shift of the curve is theoretically advantageous, since an equivalent amount of oxygen is released at a higher P_{O_2} than with a leftward-positioned curve. (Note that in curve *B* of Fig. 4-11, half of the oxygen would be released at a P_{O_2} of 36 mmHg; in curve *C*, less than 10 percent of the oxygen would be released at the same P_{O_2}.) The ability to maintain or enlarge the arteriovenous oxygen difference is dependent to some extent on the position of the curve. Normally, arterial hemoglobin saturation is near the upper limit and cannot be increased appreciably. Any enlargement of the arteriovenous oxygen difference necessitates reduction in venous hemoglobin saturation and venous oxygen tension Pv_{O_2}. As the curve moves to the left, maintenance of any given arteriovenous oxygen difference requires a progressive decrease in Pv_{O_2}. The fall in Pv_{O_2} is finally limited by the fact that a certain partial pressure is necessary for

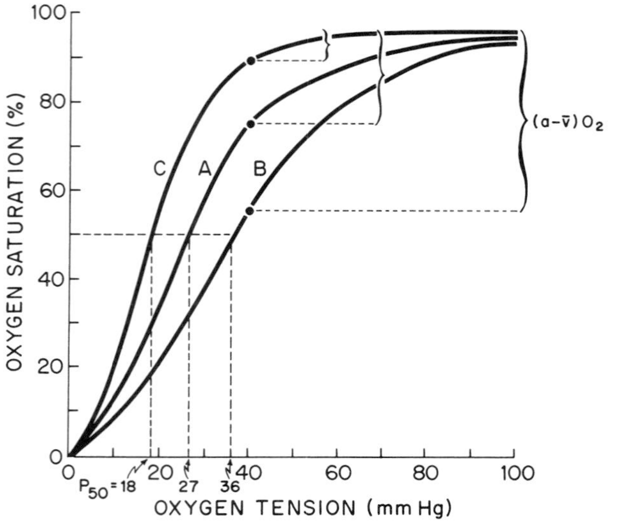

FIG. 4-12. Oxygen-hemoglobin dissociation curves similar to those in Fig. 4-11. Note that if arterial and venous oxygen tensions remain constant, arteriovenous oxygen difference decreases as the curve moves toward the left.

Table 4-8
Factors that Alter Hemoglobin/Oxygen Affinity

Increase P_{50}	*Decrease P_{50}*
By direct effect:	By direct effect:
Increased $[H^+]$	Decreased $[H^+]$
temperature	temperature
P_{CO_2}	P_{CO_2}
DPG, ATP	DPG, ATP
Hb conc	Hb conc
Ionic strength	Ionic strength
Abnormal hemoglobin	Abnormal hemoglobin
Aldosterone	Carboxyhemoglobin
	Methemoglobin
By increasing DPG:	By decreasing DPG:
Decreased $[H^+]$	Increased $[H^+]$
Thyroid hormone	Decreased thyroid hormone
Pyruvate kinase deficiency	Hexokinase deficiency
Increased inorganic phosphate	Decreased inorganic phosphate
Cortisol	
Cell age (young)	Cell age (old)

SOURCE: Adapted from Shappell SD, Lenfant CJM: Adaptive, genetic and iatrogenic alterations of the oxyhemoglobin dissociation curve. *Anesthesiology* 37:127, 1971.

transfer of oxygen from the blood to the tissue cell. That level of oxygen pressure below which diffusion may be theoretically impaired and cellular function disturbed has been termed the "critical P_{O_2}."

Available data concerning the critical P_{O_2} are limited but suggest that it varies in individual organ systems and may depend on the level of activity of the tissues. Opitz and Schneider showed that oxygen uptake by the brain is impaired when venous oxygen tension falls below 20 to 25 mmHg, while Berne and associates indicated loss of myocardial function at oxygen tensions between 10 and 12 mmHg. With a leftward movement of the curve, therefore, maintaining or enlarging the arteriovenous oxygen difference is theoretically limited as the Pv_{O_2} approaches this critical level. Tissue oxygen delivery may be sustained in this instance by other mechanisms, principally by increasing cardiac output.

During hypovolemic shock, cardiac output is low and relatively fixed. Normally, enlargement of arteriovenous oxygen difference will partially compensate for the diminished blood flow; however, the response may be totally inadequate with a leftward shift of the dissociation curve. Continued survival and maintenance of essential organ function may be obtained only by shunting blood from tissues that tolerate a limited period of severe hypoxia (skin, skeletal muscle) to organs that require high oxygen flow rates (brain, heart).

Factors Influencing the Position of the Oxygen/Hemoglobin Dissociation Curve

Attempts to ensure a normal or rightward-positioned dissociation curve may be essential during treatment of patients with low-flow states. Factors affecting the position of the curve have been summarized by Shappell and Lenfant and are outlined in Table 4-8. The main in vivo influences include changes in pH, temperature, partial pressure of carbon dioxide, and level of red blood cell organic phosphates. Changes in hydrogen ion concentration and temperature have predictable and instantaneous effects on the position of the curve, while P_{CO_2} exerts its influence both by changing pH and by a pH-independent effect.

The position of the dissociation curve is also influenced by interaction of hemoglobin with organic phosphates in the red blood cell. Both ATP and 2,3-diphosphoglycerate (DPG) bind to hemoglobin and lower the affinity of hemoglobin for oxygen, i.e., shift the dissociation curve to the right. In a quantitative sense, DPG is the more important of the two phosphates and exerts an additional influence in the intact red blood cell by lowering intracellular pH via Donnan equilibrium. Significant concentrations of DPG are found only in the red blood cell, and DPG is present in a concentration approximately equimolar with that of hemoglobin. DPG is a product of erythrocyte glycolysis, formed via a branch of the Embden-Myerhof pathway by conversion of 1,3-DPG to 2,3-DPG, catalyzed by diphosphoglycerate mutase.

Erythrocyte DPG undergoes considerable changes in response to several stimuli, with parallel changes in the position of the dissociation curve. Hypoxia increases erythrocyte DPG in conditions such as exercise, anemia, exposure to high altitude, cardiac failure, and various pulmonary diseases. The concomitant rightward shifts of the dissociation curve are thought to represent significant compensatory responses, allowing release of more oxygen at a higher P_{O_2}.

The regulation of DPG synthesis is complex and as yet not fully clarified. Although numerous factors influence the level of DPG (Table 4-8), the principal *mechanism* for increasing or decreasing its concentration appears to be related to the level of hydrogen ions in the red cell. DPG concentration increases as the red blood cell pH rises and decreases as the pH falls. These changes are due, in part, to the differential effects of pH on the activity of two red cell enzymes, DPG mutase and phosphatase. For instance, alkalosis stimulates DPG synthesis by increasing DPG-mutase activity and reducing the breakdown of DPG by DPG-phosphatase. The rise in red cell pH may be secondary to elevation of whole blood pH or, as in hypoxic states, a relative increase in the amount of deoxyhemoglobin. The pH also influences DPG binding to hemoglobin and may affect other enzymes in the glycolytic cycle. The net effect of pH changes on DPG concentration, therefore, probably represents a combination of these (and other unknown) influences. It should be noted that the pH-induced changes in DPG concentration tend to counteract the direct pH effects on the curve via the Bohr effect. Therefore, the immediate rightward shift of the curve secondary to acute acidosis is eventually offset by a pH-induced reduction in DPG concentration.

DPG synthesis is also responsive to hormonal influences and the level of inorganic phosphate. The phosphate level is directly related to DPG concentration, and maintenance of a normal inorganic phosphate level during intravenous hyperalimentation is necessary to prevent a reduction in the level of erythrocyte 2,3-DPG. Thyroid hormone acts directly to increase DPG synthesis, a fact that probably explains the elevated levels of this compound in hyperthyroid patients. Cortisol and aldosterone both shift the dissociation curve to the right, thereby decreasing hemoglobin/oxygen affinity. The effects of cortisol are probably secondary to direct stimulation of DPG synthesis. Hemoglobin/oxygen affinity also increases as the erythrocyte ages, presumably owing to a decreasing DPG concentration.

Blood Transfusions, Erythrocyte DPG, and Oxygen Delivery

The acceptability for transfusion of blood that has been stored in ACD (acid citrate dextrose) solution for up to 3 weeks is based on survival of at least 70 percent of the cells in the recipient's circulation. During this 3-week period, however, there is a rapid decline in erythrocyte DPG and a progressive increase in hemoglobin/oxygen affinity. Following transfusion, several hours are required for the DPG levels to return to normal. These findings suggest that oxygen delivery may be impaired after the administration of large quantities of stored blood and have led to a reevaluation of transfusion practices.

Several studies in both experimental animals and human beings have failed to show significant impairment of tissue oxygenation with markedly reduced levels of erythrocyte DPG and leftward shifts of the oxygen dissociation curve. Similar findings were noted in our study of 45 injured patients who received more than 5 units of whole blood stored in ACD solution during resuscitation and the subsequent operative procedure. Erythrocyte DPG levels were below normal in a majority of these patients and correlated well with the amount and storage time of the transfused blood. There were no consistent correlations, however, between DPG concentration and the measured parameters of oxygen delivery. This lack of correlation may be explained by two observations. First, the position of the dissociation curve cannot be reliably predicted from a knowledge of the DPG concentration alone. DPG represents only one of several factors that affect the curve, and the final P_{50} represents a composite of these influences. Normal or elevated P_{50} values noted in several patients with low DPG concentrations were probably due to other factors (e.g., pH and temperature) that tended to counteract the influence of DPG. A second observation is the lack of a consistent relationship between the P_{50} value and oxygen consumption. The majority of patients with leftward shifts of the dissociation curve had reasonably normal arteriovenous oxygen difference and oxygen consumption. Additionally, several of the patients with narrowed arteriovenous oxygen differences maintained oxygen delivery simply by increasing the cardiac output.

These findings do not imply that the position of the dissociation curve and the factors that influence it are unimportant. They do suggest that a person with reasonably intact cardiovascular and

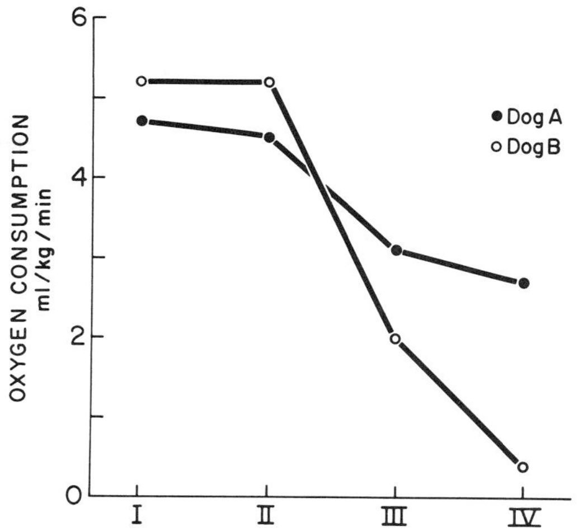

FIG. 4-13. Effects of hemorrhagic shock and sodium bicarbonate infusion on oxygen consumption after exchange transfusion with fresh blood (dog *A*) and DPG-depleted blood (dog *B*). I, Control period; II, after exchange transfusion (DPG concentration 6.20 μM/mL RBC in dog *B*); III, after induction of hypotension; IV, continued hypotension and sodium bicarbonate infusion.

pulmonary systems is able to tolerate rather significant leftward shifts of the oxygen dissociation curve. The consequences may be quite different, however, in a patient with limited compensatory mechanisms and in some therapeutic regimens followed without understanding of their effects on the position of the curve. An example of this is shown in Fig. 4-13. Despite the sharp reduction in cardiac output following hemorrhage to a mean blood pressure of 50 mmHg, the control dog with a normal P_{50} value was able to maintain normal oxygen delivery by increasing the arteriovenous oxygen difference from 4.5 to 10.6 mL. By contrast the DPG-depleted dog was unable to expand the arteriovenous oxygen difference sufficiently (P_{50} value 15 mmHg). The problem was compounded by attempts to correct pH to normal by infusion of sodium bicarbonate solution. The dissociation curve moved farther to the left (P_{50} value 8 mmHg), the hemoglobin concentration fell secondary to hemodilution, and oxygen consumption fell to near zero. Although extreme, the experimental conditions are not unlike those that may be found in the clinical setting.

In summary, available evidence suggests that changes in hemoglobin/oxygen affinity, as reflected by the position of the oxygen dissociation curve, may be important in several circumstances. The elevated DPG concentrations and rightward shifts of the dissociation curve observed in hypoxic states (pulmonary disease, cardiac failure, anemia, exposure to high altitude, and so on) probably represent compensatory responses that facilitate oxygen unloading in the tissue capillaries. Oxygenation can be maintained in these instances by other mechanisms (e.g., increasing cardiac output) but at greater expense to body economy.

Leftward shifts of the dissociation curve observed following transfusions of stored blood, acute alkalosis, hypothermia, and so forth are, at best, undesirable phenomena and can significantly impair oxygen unloading. Although leftward shifts are tolerated in many circumstances, maintenance of a normally positioned dissociation curve may be of singular importance in patients with hypoxia, anemia, or hypotension when compensatory responses are limited.

Therapeutic Implications

Obtaining a sufficient quantity of fresh blood for resuscitation of patients in hemorrhagic shock is difficult, and attempts are being made to find a suitable storage medium that will maintain the levels of organic phosphates (DPG, ATP) in red blood cells. In addition to DPG, maintenance of a sufficiently high ATP level is essential to maintain a flexible and highly deformable red cell membrane. The biconcave disc shape of a normal red blood cell is transformed toward a nondeformable spherocyte during storage. This loss of deformability hinders passage through the microcirculation and increases susceptibility of the cell to destruction. Although both DPG and ATP levels rapidly return to normal within 6 to 24 h, restoration may be delayed in the critically ill and massively transfused patient who is least able to tolerate increased microvascular resistance to flow and depression of tissue oxygenation.

When large quantities of blood are administered, particularly in critically ill patients, some attention should be paid to the storage age of each unit of blood. If a significant portion of the blood administered has been stored for more than 7 to 10 days, every attempt should be made to obtain fresh blood for additional transfusion requirements. In our experience the institution of these simple changes, including conversion to CPDA-1 storage media, has been rewarding. The large reductions in DPG and P_{50} noted in the past are rarely seen today, even after massive transfusions.

Other factors that influence the position of the dissociation curve (Table 4-8) may also be important in the individual patient. For instance, the induction of respiratory alkalosis can produce an abrupt increase in hemoglobin/oxygen affinity. This is a common occurrence during operations and in patients requiring ventilatory assistance in the postoperative period; coupled with other factors that limit oxygen transport, the capacity to maintain tissue oxygenation may be sharply reduced. Similarly, the sudden correction of an acidosis, whether metabolic or respiratory, may have undesirable effects. In this regard the indiscriminate use of sodium bicarbonate during resuscitation of patients in hypovolemic shock is discouraged. The presence of a mild metabolic alkalosis is a common finding after resuscitation, owing in part to the alkalinizing effects of blood transfusions and the administration of lactated Ringer's solution. After infusion (and partial restoration of hepatic blood flow), the citrate and lactate contained in transfused blood and the lactate in lactated Ringer's solution are metabolized and bicarbonate is formed. If excessive quantities of sodium bicarbonate are administered simultaneously, a severe metabolic alkalosis may result. The alkaline pH may be highly undesirable, particularly in patients with hypoxia or low fixed cardiac output. Combined with other factors incident to blood replacement that increase hemoglobin/oxygen affinity (low DPG concentration and hypothermia), significant interference with oxygen unloading at the cellular level may occur.

The immediate and direct pH influences on the curve (via the Bohr effect) are eventually offset by reciprocal changes in DPG concentration. There is, however, a lag period of approximately 4 h before any change in DPG concentration is noted, and the final level is not reached until 48 h after induction of acidosis or alkalosis. The fact that the effects of sudden large changes in pH may persist for several hours should be considered during therapy. Correction of a metabolic acidosis, therefore, is properly directed toward correction of the underlying disorder. Bicarbonate therapy may be reversed for the treatment of severe metabolic acidosis, particularly following cardiac arrest, when *partial* correction of pH is essential to restore myocardial function. Similarly, pH correction in more protracted states of metabolic acidosis may be indicated but should be accomplished slowly.

Lowering body temperature also causes a leftward shift of the dissociation curve and an increase in hemoglobin/oxygen affinity, but any interference in oxygen delivery may be countered effectively by the hypothermia-induced reduction in metabolic requirements.

Rightward shifts of the curve are usually desirable and, unless extreme, rarely interfere with oxygen uptake in the lungs. Rightward shifts generally occur as a compensatory response to hypoxia, regardless of the cause. Nevertheless, in patients with severe arterial desaturation (exposure to high altitude, cogestive failure, right-to-left cardiac shunts), any potential benefit from shifting the curve farther to the right may be offset by interference with oxygen loading.

Techniques for constructing an oxygen dissociation curve are time-consuming and not readily available in most hospitals. For this reason we have developed a rapid, though less precise, method for estimating the position of the curve (the P_{50} value). Since the shape and slope of the curve do not change appreciably with changes in position, determination of a single point of the steep part of the slope should allow a rough estimate of the entire curve. To obviate the use of a tonometer, a single sample of venous blood is drawn anaerobically and the P_{O_2} and oxygen saturation are measured. (An arterial sample is unsuitable, since the values fall on the upper flat portion of the curve.) An estimated P_{50} value may then be obtained using the Severinghaus slide rule or a nomogram as depicted in Fig. 4-14. The nomogram represents a computer plot of a family of O_2 dissociation curves, using the

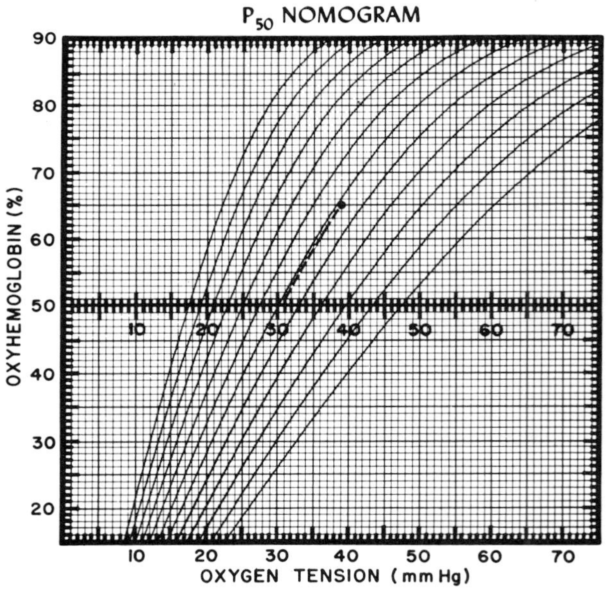

FIG. 4-14. Nomogram for estimation of P_{50} value (position of the oxygen-hemoglobin dissociation curve). The point on the nomogram corresponding to the measured P_{O_2} and saturation of a sample of venous blood is traced to the line representing 50 percent oxygen saturation. This intersection represents the estimated P_{50} (normal value approximately 27 mmHg). In the example shown, the venous blood sample P_{O_2} is 39 mmHg, the oxygen saturation 65 percent, and the P_{50} value 31 mmHg (a rightward-positioned dissociation curve).

correction factor for pH as suggested by Severinghaus. The point on the nomogram corresponding to the measured P_{O_2} and saturation values is found and traced to the line representing 50 percent oxygen saturation. This intersect represents the estimated P_{50}; the normal value is approximately 27 mmHg. A P_{50} above this level represents a rightward shift of the oxygen dissociation curve, while a lower value represents a leftward shift.

Estimates of P_{50} have become routine in our care of critically ill patients. Combining this with measurements of both arterial and venous blood gases, a considerable amount of information may be obtained about the state of oxygenation and oxygen transport capability.

THERAPY OF SHOCK

Hypovolemic Shock

Therapy depends on detection of the causative mechanisms and provision of support to the patient. Initial care of the injured patient should follow the guidelines from the advanced trauma life support procedures of the American College of Surgeons Committee on Trauma. In a patient who has undergone trauma, more than one causative factor may be operating. Once the diagnosis of shock has been made and supportive therapy begun, a diligent search can be made for the causative factor or factors. Recognition of deficits of total body water and electrolytes is usually subtle, and correction requires specific therapy with crystalloid solutions. Reductions in the extracellular fluid volume (plasma and interstitial fluids) primarily, as in burns, peritonitis, and some forms of crush injury, are more easily recognized. Specific therapy should be started with electrolyte solutions and rarely may require the use of plasma or some source of protein. External blood loss should be corrected immediately with appropriate fluid therapy.

Fluid Resuscitation

Extracellular Fluid Replacement. When patients are admitted to the emergency room in hemorrhagic shock, at least two large-gauge catheters are inserted into appropriate veins and an infusion of lactated Ringer's solution is begun immediately. At the same time, blood is drawn for typing and cross matching. The lactated Ringer's solution is run at a rapid rate so that in a period of 45 min between 1000 and 2000 mL of lactated Ringer's solution is given intravenously.

The procedure is a highly effective therapeutic trial to determine the preexisting amount of blood loss or the presence of continuing blood loss. It is often observed that blood pressure will return to normal, become stable, and remain so in patients with initially severe hypotension after infusion of 1 or 2 L of a balanced salt solution. When such a response is correlated with measurements of red blood cell mass, plasma volume, and extracellular fluid volume, the preexisting blood loss is shown to be relatively minimal. If blood loss has been minimal and hemorrhage is not continuing, hemorrhagic hypotension can be alleviated simply by the infusion of a balanced salt solution.

If blood loss has been severe or hemorrhage is continuing, the elevation of blood pressure and decrease in pulse rate that occur with rapid intravenous infusion of lactated Ringer's solution is usually transient. When this occurs, blood that has been accurately typed and cross-matched is available and can be given immediately. Consequently, the initial use of the balanced salt solution allows time for accurate typing and cross matching.

In view of the disparate reduction in the extravascular, extracellular fluid as demonstrated in animals and human beings, it is felt that even though blood is needed, as it is in the majority of patients admitted in hemorrhagic hypovolemia, alleviation of the reduction in functional extracellular fluid is desirable.

Lactated Ringer's solution as initial therapy, both from the standpoint of a therapeutic trial and as a therapeutic adjunct, is a procedure that has been found to be effective. This is understandable, since lactated Ringer's solution is isotonic, essentially free from side reactions, and virtually harmless from the standpoint of aggravation of other fluid and electrolyte imbalances that may be present.

Further, it appears that the use of a balanced salt solution in this fashion significantly reduces the requirement of whole blood in the patient with hemorrhagic hypotension. This is true not only from the standpoint of proper hemoglobin and hemoconcentrations following therapy, but also from the standpoint of prevention of, or recovery from, renal failure.

A concern that Ringer's lactate solution may aggravate the existing lactate acidosis when used to treat patients in shock has been expressed by several investigators, but previous studies in both experimental animals and patients do not support this view. The use of blood plus Ringer's lactate solution to treat hemorrhagic shock in experimental animals and in patients results in a more rapid return to normal of lactate, excess lactate, and pH than does treatment with return of shed blood alone.

Blood Transfusions. Blood transfusions have been discussed above under Blood Transfusions, Erythrocyte DPG, and Oxygen Delivery.

Albumin Solutions. In the absence of whole blood, many substances have been proposed as transient substitutes for the combination of red blood cells and plasma available in whole blood. The most popular and commonly used substitute has been human plasma. Historically, in some circumstances, e.g., battlefield conditions, plasma has been a highly serviceable substitute. Currently, there appears to be little justification for the addition of albumin to balanced salt solutions for volume resuscitation in hypovolemic shock.

The primary hypothetical advantage of albumin resuscitation concerns the transient increase in intravascular colloid oncotic pressure. It had been felt that this might protect the lung from interstitial edema. However, an excellent review by Civetta points out that the lung does not function according to classic Starling forces. There is a rapid albumin flux across the normal pulmonary capillary membrane, and lung lymphatics rapidly clear the interstitium. Substantial evidence from our laboratory and others has failed to show increases in lung water induced by hemorrhagic shock, crystalloid resuscitation, or the hypooncotic state.

Albumin infusion does transiently produce a greater increase in intravascular volume, per unit volume administered, than Ringer's lactate. The administered albumin rapidly disperses to the extravascular space. Practical and potential disadvantages of colloid administration include postresuscitation hypertension, increased intravascular volume at the expense of necessary interstitial fluid resuscitation, depression of circulating immunoglobulins, and suppression of albumin synthesis. Although clinical and experimental evidence supports the safety and efficacy of both colloid and crystalloid solutions, when titrated to measured physiologic end points, a recent meta-analysis of several clinical studies also concluded that trauma patients should receive crystalloid resuscitation.

Hypertonic Saline Solutions. Clinical and experimental studies have shown that hypertonic saline is an effective fluid for initial resuscitation. Similar to burn studies in previous decades, the primary measurable change is a decrease in free water load compared to balanced salt solutions, when subjects were resuscitated to similar hemodynamic end points. As noted in burn patients, the serum electrolytes require continuous monitoring to prevent hypernatremia and hyperosmolar coma, particularly if other resuscitation fluids cannot be given promptly following the initial infusion of hypertonic saline. Current clinical data do not show an improvement in survival in patients initially given small volumes of 7.5% sodium chloride in 6% dextran 70, when followed by standard resuscitation in a state-of-the-art trauma care environment. Hypertonic saline resuscitation in uncontrolled hemorrhagic shock appears to increase bleeding from the splanchnic bed by peripheral vasodilatation in the face of increased arterial blood pressure. Nevertheless, these solutions may find some role, probably in the prehospital setting, when reliable access for large-volume resuscitation or skilled personnel are unavailable, as it may be given by interosseous infusion. The greatest potential benefit of hypertonic resuscitation may be in patients with head injury and hypovolemic shock.

Artificial Blood Substitutes. The consequences of the human immunodeficiency virus and the unavoidable risks of transfusion complications have renewed an interest in synthetic oxygen-carrying blood substitutes. Perfluorochemical compounds have the ability to deliver dissolved gases into the circulation when emulsified. The Japanese have successfully used Perfluorodecalin (Fluorosol-DA) in treatment of chronic anemia. This solution has found limited use in this country because of its short shelf life and potential toxicities, including complement and coagulation activation and reticuloendothelial system depression. It is quite expensive and requires a long preparation time, further limiting its use in the therapy of hemorrhagic shock.

Early preparations of free hemoglobin from outdated banked human blood initially had significant side effects from retained erythrocyte stroma, including allergic reactions, renal failure, coagulopathy, and immunodepression. Highly purified, stroma-free hemoglobin (SFH) has minimized these side effects and allowed early clinical trials. SFH has excellent oxygen-carrying capacity and does not require the potentially toxic inspired oxygen concentrations associated with the perfluorochemicals. The limited availability of human sources may eventually be overcome by ongoing development of bovine SFH, which would allow more practical and widespread applications in the future. Currently, there are no appropriate substitutes for red blood cell transfusion to improve the oxygen-carrying capacity in shock patients.

Artificial Plasma Substitutes. Artificial colloid solutions have been devised to replace human albumin for plasma expansion. Hydroxyethyl starch (hetastarch), an amylopectin, and dextran, a polysaccharide, are the most commonly employed. Both are reasonably safe and inexpensive drugs, although both hetastarch and dextran have been associated with rare anaphylactoid reactions and ill-defined transient coagulopathies. A concern of reticuloendothelial depression during blood clearance of these unphysiologic compounds has also been raised. These solutions have colloidal properties and physiologic impact that are similar to albumin. The concerns regarding the administration of albumin solutions to unstable patients in shock also argue against the use of these artificial colloid solutions in this setting.

The partial pressure of oxygen in the arterial blood (Pa_{O_2}) is the hallmark of adequacy of oxygenation. This must be considered in the light of the inspired oxygen concentration (FI_{O_2}). A simple means of establishing a measurable relationship between Pa_{O_2} and FI_{O_2} is their ratio (Pa_{O_2}/FI_{O_2}). Ratios between 250 and 500 are considered adequate, while a value of less than 250 is definitely abnormal. This ratio provides the clinician with a gross estimate of the efficacy of oxygenation at the bedside during rapid changes in therapy. It appears to be most reliable when the FI_{O_2} is between 0.3 and 0.7. Of the classical causes of hypoxemia (hypoventilation, diffusion defects, ventilation/perfusion abnormalities, and pulmonary shunt), only the intrapulmonary shunt should affect this index if the patient is breathing pure oxygen. In contrast, the AaD_{O_2} is affected by cardiac output, O_2 consumption, the position of the hemoglobin/O_2 dissociation curve, and the magnitude of the pulmonary shunt. In particular, as the FI_{O_2} varies, the AaD_{O_2} varies widely. This greatly limits its value as an initial screening test.

The adequacy of ventilation is measured by the arterial partial pressure of carbon dioxide (Pa_{CO_2}). By definition, hypoventilation occurs when the Pa_{CO_2} is elevated. Postinjury pulmonary failure is usually associated with hypocapnia (hyperventilation). Therefore, the patient with a decrease in both Pa_{CO_2} and Pa_{O_2} probably has ARDS. Tidal volume (VT)—the amount of air breathed during one respiratory cycle—is another indication of the adequacy of ventilation. VT multiplied by the respiratory rate is called the *minute ventilation*. This value is easily derived but by itself is only a rough guide to adequate ventilation. In many postinjury patients, high minute ventilations are recorded. This may be a compensatory response or an indicator of a pathologic condition.

Vasopressors. In the past the use of drugs that cause vasoconstriction in hypovolemic shock had been popular because blood pressure in human beings can usually be elevated by these agents. The objective in treating hypovolemic shock, however, is to increase tissue perfusion. Vasopressors raise blood pressure by increasing peripheral vascular resistance and decreasing tissue perfusion. Therefore, the injurious effects of shock may be aggravated.

In 1923, Cannon condemned the use of vasopressors on this physiologic basis: "Damming the blood in the arterial portion of the circulation, when the organism is suffering primarily from a diminished quantity of blood flow, obviously does not improve the volume flow in the capillaries." Recent studies have more clearly defined the hazards of using vasopressors in hypovolemic shock, including evidence that the administration of vasopressors during hypovolemia reduces the already depleted plasma volume.

It is doubtful that the use of vasopressors in the treatment of uncomplicated hypovolemic shock is ever warranted. Their use in place of adequate volume resuscitation, administered by any necessary means, is particularly condemned as their deleterious effects will be magnified in the patient who is still hypovolemic. More complex clinical situations with a component of cardiogenic shock may well require chronotropic or vasoactive drug support as outlined under therapy for cardiogenic shock.

Vasodilators. Despite the theoretic attractiveness of directly reversing the reflex vasoconstriction during hemorrhagic shock, the use of vasodilators has not proven clinically useful. The tightly controlled animal preparations that appear to support its use in graded hemorrhage are not mimicked in the clinical arena.

Another vasoactive compound, ATP-$MgCl_2$ improves survival in a lethal shock model in animals when combined with fluid resuscitation. Because the highly polar ATP molecule cannot cross the intact cell membrane and is rapidly degraded in circulation, its effect may be due to restoration of local flow by a vasodilatory effect rather than to augmentation of intracellular high-energy charge. As with other compounds with vasodilatory properties, ATP-$MgCl_2$ infusion results in further hemodynamic instability in the hypovolemic patient, further limiting its potential value in clinical application.

Positioning. Most first-aid courses teach that the patient in shock should be placed in the head-down position. Although it is true that some forms of shock, particularly neurogenic shock, will respond to the head-down position, the effect of posture on the cerebral circulation in the face of true hypovolemia has not been defined. Frequently the patient with multiple trauma has sustained other injuries, within both the abdomen and the chest, so that the routine use of the Trendelenburg, or head-down, position may interfere with respiratory exchange far more than when the patient is left supine. The beneficial effect of the head-down position is probably the result of transient autotransfusion of pooled blood in the capacity or venous side of the peripheral circulation. This beneficial effect can be obtained easily by elevating both legs while maintaining the trunk and the remainder of the patient in the supine position. This is probably the preferable position for the treatment of hypovolemic shock.

Mast Garment. There has been enthusiasm for the in-the-field application of military antishock trousers, the MAST garment. When applied to the extremities with modest pressures, the garment functions well as a splint and may control some venous bleeding. When applied at high pressures, the resultant increase in total peripheral resistance may elevate the systemic pressure while decreasing cardiac output and peripheral perfusion. In addition, inflation of the abdominal bolster may compress the inferior vena cava, impairing venous return to the heart by further increasing the venous resistance. Several reports of reperfusion injury with compartment syndromes in uninjured limbs have appeared. The MAST device may be of value when used strictly as a temporizing device or rarely as specific treatment of bleeding pelvic fractures. Its use must not delay the immediate repletion of intravascular and extravascular volume by fluid therapy or interfere with rapid transport of the injured patient.

Pulmonary Support. In the past, most writings on the treatment of hypovolemic shock stated that breathing high oxygen concentrations is probably of little value during a period of hypotension. These conclusions were based on the concept that the principal defect is in volume flow to tissues and decreased cardiac output. The oxygen saturation in the majority of patients with uncomplicated hypovolemic shock is generally normal, and the small increase in dissolved oxygen in the blood contributed by raising the P_{O_2} above this level is insignificant, particularly in the face of a markedly decreased cardiac output. This concept continues to be valid in terms of improvement of the shock state or tissue oxygenation itself. Nevertheless, in the small but significant group of patients in hypovolemic shock in whom the oxygen saturation is not normal, the *initial* use of increased oxygen concentrations may be extremely important, since the fall in cardiac output accompanying hemorrhagic shock has been shown to compound existing defects in oxygenation. This can occur in patients with preexisting defects, such as chronic obstructive lung disease. More frequently problems in oxygenation arise directly from the patient's injury and may include a coexisting pneumothorax, pulmonary contusion, aspiration of gastric contents or blood, or airway obstruction. Thus, although oxygen is not routinely administered to patients in shock, if any doubt exists as to the possibility of one of these circumstances or as to the adequacy of oxygenation of arterial blood, the initial administration of oxygen until the injuries to the patient have been diligently assessed is certainly justified. If oxygen is to be administered to patients under these circumstances, it should be delivered through loose-fitting face masks designed for this purpose. If controlled airway is indicated for other reasons, an endotracheal tube is ideal. The use of nasal catheters, particularly those passed into the nasopharynx, is avoided because of potential complications of pharyngeal lacerations and gastric distention. Gastric rupture has been recorded secondary to such a catheter being inadvertently placed in the esophagus.

Antibiotics. Antibiotics were used in the treatment of hypovolemic shock for many years and were thought to exert a protective mechanism against the ravages of hypovolemia. Subsequent data fail to support this hypothesis. The use of antibiotics in patients who have open or potentially contaminated wounds, however, continues to be sound practice, when combined with good surgical debridement and care. Consequently, the use of wide-spectrum antibiotics is advisable as a preventive measure in the severely injured patient. Cefoxitin, 2 g I.V., has proved to be a safe and effective single agent in multiorgan abdominal injuries.

Analgesics. Treatment of pain in the patient with hypovolemic shock is rarely a problem from the standpoint of shock itself. If, however, the causative injury produces severe pain, as in fracture, peritonitis, injury to the chest wall, and the like, control of pain becomes mandatory. Generally, when the patient is moved to the emergency facility where physicians and care are available, simple supportive measures (administration of intravenous fluids, passing of catheters) will give reassurance. The need for analgesics is greatly reduced, since the need to allay fear and anxiety is decreased. If, however, the patient continues to have severe pain, the observations made by Henry K. Beecher in World War II become extremely pertinent. Many battle casualties received morphine or other narcotic agents by subcutaneous administration soon after wounding. Since these analgesics did not enter the circulation immediately, the pain continued and the patient ultimately received several doses that were poorly absorbed. Once effective therapy was begun for shock, the doses previously administered were absorbed and profound sedation resulted. As a result, the recommendation was made that small doses of narcotics be given *intravenously* for the management of pain in the patient with shock.

Steroids. Adrenocorticoid depletion was commonly regarded as a contributory factor in shock after it was learned that the presence of hypovolemic shock could in itself deplete the adrenal cortex of adrenocortical steroids. Subsequent studies, however, have shown that adrenocortical steroid production is stimulated maximally by the presence of hypovolemic shock. Steroid depletion with hypovolemic shock may possibly occur in the elderly patient or in patients who have specific adrenocortical diseases such as incipient Addison's disease, postadrenalectomy patients, or patients who have had adrenal suppression with exogenous adrenocortical steroids. In these specific instances the intravenous administration of hydrocortisone is desirable. In the trauma patient with hypovolemic shock, administration of adrenocorticoids is not indicated. The use of steroids in more complicated unresponsive shock states, particularly when septic shock is suspected, remains controversial.

Monitoring. Continuous bedside monitoring of circulatory efficacy, including assessment of the heart rate, arterial blood pressure, urinary output, and peripheral perfusion remains the cornerstone for resuscitation. Adequate resuscitation is indicated when adequate cerebral function and urinary output are restored. In the patient with multiple injuries, central venous pressure (CVP) monitoring is useful. Although left ventricular overload can occur while right ventricular function and CVP remain normal, this is not often the case in the absence of myocardial injury. Changes over time in the CVP with fluid infusion do indicate the ability of the myocardium to pump the volume presented to it. A normal to depressed CVP that does not rise with rapid administration of crystalloid fluid usually indicates continuing hypovolemia. The presence of an elevated CVP or its rapid rise in response to fluid administration is indicative of impairment of the pumping mechanism. Although this usually represents primary myocardial deficiency and should be treated as outlined under cardiogenic shock, a mechanical obstruction to venous return with cardiac tamponade or mediastinal compression by intrapleural air or blood must be immediately addressed in the injured patient. The use of a balloon-tipped Swan-Ganz catheter allows measurement of pulmonary artery and pulmonary wedge pressures, in addition to thermodilution cardiac output determinations. The early use of the Swan-Ganz catheter is rarely necessary in the initial emergency department resuscitation from hemorrhagic shock.

At some point, hemorrhagic shock becomes refractory to the above therapies and is irreversible. Complete vascular collapse with hypotension unresponsive to volume or drug intervention eventually leads to lethal central nervous system and cardiac dysfunction. Irreversibility is difficult to define but has been related to the duration and volume of hemorrhage, the age and preexisting cardiovascular fitness of the patient, and the coexistence of massive trauma with multiple direct organ derangement. Before the conclusion that refractory shock has occurred, the multiple causes of failure to respond to therapy should be resolved. These include continuing unsuspected blood loss into the chest or abdomen, inadequate volume replacement, multisystem trauma with occult thoracic injuries including cardiac tamponade and hemopneumothorax, and acute myocardial insufficiency from direct injury or secondary to prolonged coronary hypoperfusion.

Cardiogenic Shock

This form of shock occurs when the heart is unable to generate sufficient cardiac output to maintain adequate tissue perfusion. Unlike hypovolemic shock, cardiogenic shock is manifest by hypotension in the face of adequate intravascular volume. Cardiogenic shock that is unresponsive to the measures outlined below carries significant mortality and morbidity, particularly when associated with myocardial infarction and the secondary end-organ injuries of pulmonary edema, oliguric renal failure, and coma.

Pathophysiology. Myocardial failure may result from a variety of diseases, including valvular heart disease, cardiomyopathy, and direct myocardial contusion. Acute myocardial infarction is the most frequent cause of cardiogenic shock, which is often fatal when 40 percent of the left ventricular mass has been lost. Papillary muscle dysfunction, ischemic ventricular septal defects, massive left ventricular infarction, and arrhythmias are complications of acute myocardial infarction that may lead to cardiogenic shock.

The initial compensatory response to diminished myocardial contraction is tachycardia that attempts to maintain cardiac output, despite a decreased left ventricular ejection fraction, at the expense of increasing myocardial oxygen consumption. As cardiac index falls below 2 L/min/m^2 hypotension produces reflex sympathetic vasoconstriction. This attempt to maintain central pressure by increasing peripheral vascular resistance leads to decreasing organ perfusion. An increase in afterload further impairs left ventricular function and increases myocardial work. The combination of increased myocardial oxygen demand, hypotension, and shortened diastole amplifies the mismatch between coronary arterial oxygen delivery and myocardial oxygen demand, extending the zone of infarction in the patient who does not receive prompt intervention.

Treatment. Although the goal of medical management of cardiogenic shock has been to enhance ventricular performance and improve global perfusion, the traditional management with inotropic drugs and fluids continues to yield a high mortality of 80 to 90 percent. The techniques that maximize ventricular performance paradoxically increase myocardial oxygen demand at a time when therapy to limit infarct size and salvage reversibly ischemic myocardium should include minimizing myocardial demand and attempting to provide early reperfusion. Nevertheless, initial therapy includes optimizing ventricular preload by manipulating filling pressure, decreasing afterload in the patient with adequate systolic pressure, correction of arrhythmias, and improving contractility to sustain vital organ perfusion.

Monitoring and Volume Management. Supplemental oxygen, pain relief and sedation, and continuous electrocardiographic monitoring should be initiated early. A Foley catheter is inserted for monitoring urine output. Cutaneous oximetry and automated arterial blood pressure cuff measurements can be used in place of an intraarterial catheter for continuous arterial pressure monitoring and blood gas determinations. Placement of a Swan-Ganz catheter, with measurement of cardiac output and pulmonary artery wedge pressure, is crucial to therapeutic decision making in these critically ill patients. Cardiogenic shock with low cardiac output and arterial hypotension can occur in some patients with normal to slightly elevated pulmonary artery wedge pressures. A small increase in left ventricular filling pressure by volume infusion may maximize cardiac output by the Frank-Starling mechanism. It should be stressed that, although hemodynamic measurements suggest myocardial insufficiency, mechanical obstruction such as cardiac tamponade in the injured patient or pulmonary embolism in the postoperative patient may be present. Although these diagnoses must be made largely on clinical grounds in the emergency setting, volume infusion is usually of some benefit while echocardiography, pericardiocentesis, or thoracentesis are quickly performed. Constant vigilance is required during volume challenge in this setting, as increased filling pressures may lead to further myocardial ischemia and acute pulmonary edema. If any pulmonary complications evolve, early intubation and mechanical ventilation will both decrease the myocardial oxygen demand as a consequence of increased work of breathing and correct arterial hypoxemia which may further impair cardiac performance.

Inotropic Agents. The beta$_1$-adrenergic receptors of the myocardium respond to exogenous sympathomimetic drugs by increasing contractility and improving cardiac output. These effects are at the cost of increasing myocardial oxygen demand in the setting of already compromised myocardial perfusion. Nevertheless, intravenous infusion of dopamine may promptly reverse life-threatening hypotension and restore mean arterial pressure to about 80 mmHg. The dopaminergic effects of splanchnic, coronary, and renal vasodilatation at low (2 to 5 μg/kg/min) doses are augmented by adrenergic-mediated increases in contractility and heart rate as dosages rise to 5 to 8 μg/kg/min. At higher doses, alpha-adrenergic receptor effects predominate, and central arterial pressure can increase while coronary artery constriction further decreases coronary blood flow. Dopamine also causes a variable increase in heart rate and can precipitate other arrhythmias, emphasizing the need to titrate the lowest acceptable dose. Dobutamine, a synthetic catecholamine with predominantly inotropic effect, appears to be less arrhythmogenic and may redistribute cardiac output to the coronary circulation. Studies appear to favor dobutamine over dopamine for treating cardiogenic shock following cardiopulmonary bypass or myocardial infarction. Digitalis remains a controversial drug in acute pump failure. Although very useful in the treatment of supraventricular arrhythmias, digitalis increases myocardial oxygen consumption and probably adds very little hemodynamic benefit relative to therapy with sympathomimetic agents.

Vasodilator Agents. Some patients with low cardiac output and high filling pressures have near-normal arterial blood pressure in the setting of profoundly decreased perfusion by clinical assessment. In this circumstance, systolic ventricular wall stress is high, and reducing afterload should increase cardiac output and decrease myocardial work. An agent such as sodium nitroprusside should be used with extreme caution in hypotensive patients because redistribution of an already depressed cardiac output away from the coronary and cerebral circulation can occur, and any decrease in systemic diastolic pressure would further depress coronary perfusion pressures.

Mechanical Support. As the role of early reperfusion strategies, including thrombolysis, percutaneous transluminal coronary angioplasty, and emergency bypass, evolves, mechanical therapy can temporarily support the failing myocardium until these modalities may be undertaken or some myocardial recovery occurs. Despite significant associated morbidity, successful mechanical cardiac support will maintain organ perfusion while decreasing myocardial oxygen demand by unloading the left ventricle and reducing myocardial work. The intraaortic balloon pulsation device has been most widely used. It can be inserted at the bedside and fulfills the criteria of elevating diastolic blood pressure, which increases pulmonary perfusion while decreasing myocardial work, by increasing cardiac output distal to the ventricle. It is unclear whether this device improves long-term survival, but it clearly does support the failing myocardium while recovery or other interventions proceed. Those patients who had surgically correctable problems following acute myocardial infarction appear to fare better than patients who were not operative candidates following temporary mechanical support.

Left heart bypass by left atrium to femoral artery circulatory bypass and temporary implantation of left ventricular assist devices may be even more effective in assuming cardiac work. These techniques have been usually limited to patients with cardiogenic shock following cardiac surgery, as operative placement is required. The role of all these techniques may broaden if ongoing studies support improved survival from early revascularization by thrombolytic therapy, coronary angioplasty, and emergency surgery.

Arrhythmias. Rapid ventricular rates can depress cardiac output to shock levels. Ventricular end-diastolic pressure decreases due to shortened filling time, and ventricular relaxation is incomplete by the end of the abbreviated diastolic period. Cardiac output falls because impaired stroke volume cannot be compensated for by the rapid heart rate. Digoxin is the drug of choice for atrial fibrillation or atrial flutter. However, electrical cardioversion should be promptly undertaken for tachycardia that produces hypotension and hypoperfusion. Resistant sinus tachycardia, while well tolerated by the normal heart, may produce a low flow state in the diseased heart. Verapamil has been useful in treating tachyarrhythmias of atrial origin, while propranolol will slow sinus tachycardia. Beta blockade can further decrease cardiac output in this setting, and a careful search for the cause of the sinus tachycardia, including fever, hypovolemia, and drug effect, should be evaluated. Immediate nonsynchronized direct current electrical shock is mandatory treatment for ventricular fibrillation or ventricular flutter that has caused cardiogenic shock with loss of consciousness. Ventricular fibrillation rarely converts spontaneously, and the rapid development of cardiovascular collapse that follows demands prompt therapy. In the patient with acute myocardial injury, premature ventricular complexes may lead to ventricular tachyarrhythmias. Intravenous lidocaine is generally the initial treatment and is also given following cardioversion to prevent recurrent ventricular fibrillation. Bretylium tosylate has been useful in treating life-threatening ventricular tachyarrhythmias that have not responded to lidocaine or class 1A agents such as procainamide.

Low cardiac output with ventricular rates less than 70 beats/min may occur in patients with impaired cardiac performance. Stroke volume cannot increase to compensate for the pathologic bradycardia. Electrical pacing of the heart at a rate of 80 to 100 beats/min can restore sufficient cardiac output, whether the underlying mechanism is sinus bradycardia, atrial fibrillation with slow ventricular rate as in digitalis toxicity, or atrioventricular disassociation.

Neurogenic Shock

Neurogenic shock, or, by the older classification, "primary shock," is that form of shock which follows serious interference with the balance of vasodilator and vasoconstrictor influences to both arterioles and venules. This is the shock that is seen with clinical syncope, as with sudden exposure to unpleasant events such as the sight of blood, the hearing of bad tidings, or even the sudden onset of pain. Similarly, neurogenic shock is often observed with serious paralysis of vasomotor influences, as in high spinal anesthesia or injury to the spinal cord. The reflex interruption of nerve impulses also occurs with acute gastric dilatation.

The clinical picture of neurogenic shock is quite different from that classically seen in hypovolemic shock. While the blood pressure may be extremely low, the pulse rate is usually slower than normal and is accompanied by dry, warm, and even flushed skin. Measurements made during neurogenic shock indicate a reduction in cardiac output, but this is accompanied by a decrease in resistance of arteriolar vessels as well as a decrease in the venous tone. Consequently there appears to be a normovolemic state with a greatly increased reservoir capacity in both arterioles and venules, thereby inducing a decreased venous return to the right side of the heart and subsequently a reduction in cardiac output.

If neurogenic shock is not corrected, a reduction of blood flow to the kidneys and damage to the brain result, and subsequently all the ravages of hypovolemic shock appear. Treatment of neurogenic shock is usually obvious. Gastric dilatation can be rapidly treated with nasogastric suction. Shock in high spinal anesthesia can be treated effectively with fluid administration and a vasopressor such as ephedrine or phenylephrine (Neo-Synephrine). These drugs will increase cardiac output, restore venous tone, and elevate systemic blood pressure by arteriolar constriction. With the milder forms of neurogenic shock, such as fainting, simply removing the patient from the stimulus, relieving the pain, and elevating the legs will be adequate therapy while the vasoconstrictor nerves regain the ability to maintain normal arteriolar and venous resistance.

There is rarely need for hemodynamic measurement in this usually self-limited form of hypotension. The exception to this occurs when this form of shock results from injury, as with spinal cord transection from trauma. In this instance there may be significant loss of blood and extracellular fluid into the area of injury surrounding the cord and vertebral column. Considerable confusion can arise as to the relative need for fluid replacement, as opposed to the need for vasopressor drugs, under these circumstances. Similarly, if surgical intervention for any reason becomes necessary, hemodynamic measurements may be of great value in the management of these patients. In uncomplicated neurogenic shock, central venous pressure should be slightly low, with a near-normal cardiac output. If hypovolemia ensues, central venous pressure decreases, as does cardiac output. Thus, careful monitoring of central venous pressure may be necessary. Fluid administration without vasopressors in this form of hypotension may produce a gradually rising arterial pressure and cardiac output without elevation of central venous pressure, by gradually "filling" the expanded vascular pool; therefore, caution must be utilized during fluid administration.

In management of these patients balancing the two forms of therapy, slight volume overexpansion is much less deleterious than excessive vasopressor administration. The latter decreases organ perfusion in the presence of inadequate fluid replacement, particularly in the body proximal to the cord injury. Balance can best be obtained by maintaining a normal central venous pressure that rises slightly with rapid fluid administration (thus ensuring adequate volume) and using a vasopressor such as phenylephrine judiciously to support arterial pressure.

Septic Shock

Sepsis, the sepsis syndrome, and septic shock define the continuum of human response to infection. Although any agent capable of producing infection, including viruses, parasites, and fungi, may result in septic shock, the most frequent etiologic organisms in the antibiotic era are gram-negative and occasionally gram-positive bacteria. The initial infectious process now appears to only be a stimulus for a series of host responses that may culminate in death even in the absence of infection at the time of death. Over the past few decades, the incidence of gram-negative sepsis has risen dramatically, from fewer than 100 reported cases in the early 1920s to an estimate of 400,000 cases per year. Of those, approximately 100,000 episodes of septic shock are treated annually in the United States. Even in the most recent series, overall mortality exceeds 30 percent, with mortality greater than 80 percent in complicated cases with associated multiple organ system failure.

Gram-negative organisms supplanted gram-positive organisms as the predominant etiology of septic shock following the widespread application of effective antibiotics for gram-positive infections. Despite increasingly powerful gram-negative antibiotics, the incidence of gram-negative sepsis continues to rise. Proposed causes for this increasing incidence include a developing reservoir of resistent and virulent organisms, concentration of infected patients in critical care settings, more extensive operations in elderly and poor-risk patients, initial salvage of the severely injured, and a growing population of patients immunosuppressed by organ transplant protocols, radiotherapy, and chemotherapy.

The most common source of gram-negative infection is the genitourinary system. This frequently follows instrumentation of the urinary tract, which is performed at some point in up to one-third of hospitalized patients. The second most frequent site of origin is the respiratory system, followed by the alimentary system, including the biliary tract. Increasing and prolonged use of indwelling catheters for monitoring and hyperalimentation is responsible for many bloodstream infections. The early and aggressive use of appropriate antibiotic therapy, in addition to other treatments outlined below, plays a crucial role in favorable outcome. Patients with a surgically correctable focus of infection have a more favorable prognosis.

Clinical Manifestations. Gram-negative infections are frequently heralded by the onset of chills and temperature elevations above 38°C (101°F). In the setting of clinical evidence for infection, the patient may rapidly progress to evidence of altered organ function, most often renal and pulmonary in nature. The above clinical picture plus the development of hypotension completes the picture of septic shock. Unlike most other forms of shock, the patient who is normovolemic has hypotension despite an increased cardiac output and a reasonable filling pressure. The peripheral resistance is low and produces the paradoxical "warm shock" with pink, dry extremities. The high cardiac output is often associated with a decrease in oxygen utilization and a narrowed arteriovenous oxygen difference.

In a patient who is initially hypovolemic or persists in the shock state, a hypodynamic pattern emerges characterized by a falling cardiac output, low central pressures, and increased peripheral resistance with more typical cold, pale extremities consistent with global hypoperfusion. If early, volume replacement will frequently increase cardiac output and produce a hyperdynamic circulation, while the patient later in shock will be unresponsive to volume replacement and have a low cardiac output with increasing metabolic acidosis.

Concomitant laboratory tests usually show an elevation in the white blood cell count, but leukopenia may be present in immunosuppressed and debilitated patients or those with overwhelming white cell consumption from sepsis. Thrombocytopenia may be an early indicator of gram-negative sepsis, particularly in pediatric and burn patients. Mild hypoxia with compensatory hyperventilation and respiratory alkalosis are common early findings, despite clinical or radiological evidence of intrinsic pulmonary disease. Although the onset of hypotension may be coincident with these clinical signs of infection, a patient can have relatively subtle findings of hyperventilation, respiratory alkalosis, and altered sensorium for a prolonged period before shock ensues.

Pathophysiology. Septic shock is the end result of numerous complex interactions between exogenous and endogenous mediators and host responses to these stimuli. The wide individual variation in human and experimental studies regarding septic shock and response to various interventions emphasizes this intricate and poorly understood pathogenesis. Necessary host responses to local injury and infection form the local defenses against progression to systemic illness. When the ability to contain local infection is overwhelmed, systemic illness may result from the inappropriate systemic effects of these mediators.

At the organ level, cardiovascular response to systemic infection, in the absence of hypovolemia, is the development of a hyperdynamic state. A number of vasoregulatory mediators combine to produce a net decrease in systemic vascular resistance. This is quite distinct from the increased vascular resistance seen in response to hypoperfusion in other forms of shock. As cardiac index increases, the arterial-venous oxygen difference narrows. An apparent defect in peripheral oxygen extraction was originally ascribed to pathologic arteriovenous shunting. However, microvascular blood flow in many capillary beds does not appear to be altered in septic shock. In addition, neither cellular hypoxia nor any defects in the energy-producing metabolic pathways have been documented by recent studies using in vivo nuclear magnetic resonance spectroscopy. Despite increased cardiac index and decreased oxygen extraction, no direct evidence for cellular hypoxia was detected.

Although patients with hyperdynamic septic shock have an increased cardiac output, detailed studies in both patients and animals report a depression in myocardial function. The long-postulated myocardial depressant factor, although poorly characterized biochemically, appears to be a reasonable explanation for documented decreases in left ventricular ejection fraction despite acceptable filling pressures. The pathophysiologic mechanisms that produce organ dysfunction in the septic state, prior to the onset of hypotension, are compounded by the development of refractory hypotension, with tissue ischemia probably contributing a component of cell death in end-stage hypodynamic septic shock.

Mediators of Septic Shock. By the end of the nineteenth century, toxic properties of bacteria and their cellular components were recognized. The term *endotoxin* was first applied by Pfeiffer to cell wall extracts from killed cholera bacteria. The physiologic effects of endotoxin were eventually attributed to the lipopolysaccharide outer membrane common to gram-negative bacteria. The inner core in lipid A regions appears to mediate the inflammatory responses following administration of endotoxin. By the 1950s, the important interaction between white cells and the host response to infection was described. The interaction between lipopolysaccharides and the recipient host produces complex interacting cascades with a spectrum of physiologic effects.

A central and proximal mediator of the host response to bacteremia and endotoxin administration is cachectin/tumor necrosis factor (TNF), a 17 KD cytokine released from activated macrophages. Following purification and sequencing of this protein by Beutler and Cerami, early studies documented cellular defects identical to those seen from intravenous bacterial administration. Monoclonal antibodies to human cachectin/TNF completely protected against the development of septic shock following challenge with a lethal dose of intravenous *Escherichia coli* in baboons. Other laboratories confirmed anticachectin antibody protection from lethal shock in endotoxin models as well.

TNF administration produces renal, gastrointestinal, and pulmonary pathology characteristic of human septic shock. Hypermetabolism, lactic acidosis, pulmonary hypertension, and increased capillary permeability also result from TNF administration. TNF produces chemical and cellular alterations by several mechanisms, including the direct cytotoxicity to endothelial cells and indirectly by stimulating neutrophil adherence and the generation of toxic oxygen metabolites. TNF also induces the production of interleukin-1 (IL-1) by monocytes and endothelial cells, which can act synergistically to augment the above effects.

IL-1 is also capable of producing hypotension and pathologic organ changes similar to TNF and endotoxin administration. Although IL-1 administration alone does not result in a shock state, it markedly potentiates the lethal effects of TNF in mice. IL-1 can have a major role in promoting the cellular effects of TNF.

Several other cytokines have been identified in the serum of patients with septic shock, and in animal models of bacteremia and endotoxemia, including interleukin-6, interleukin-8, granulocyte-monocyte colony-stimulating factor, and macrophage inflammatory proteins 1 and 2. The role of these and other recently isolated cytokines in the pathogenesis of human septic shock remains to be demonstrated.

Arachidonic acid metabolites, both via the cyclooxygenase and the lipoxygenase pathways, play a role in mediating septic shock responses. Leukotriene B_4 markedly increases endothelial permeability and is chemotactic for neutrophils. One of the many TNF-cytokine interactions recently demonstrated included the enhancement of leukotriene D_4 generation from neutrophils by TNF. Specific 5′-lipoxygenase inhibition will also diminish the systemic responses to endotoxin in rats. Inhibition of the cyclooxygenase pathway will likewise diminish the toxic effect of TNF infusion with concomitant depression of circulating PGE_2. Although these complex interactions require further investigation, it appears that TNF may both amplify the cellular effects and augment the production of eicosinoids, further amplifying the systemic response to endotoxin.

Platelet activating factor (PAF) is a phospholipid product of leukocytes and endothelial cells that has been implicated in the development of septic shock. PAF administration produces a shock state in a variety of experimental models. It appears to have numerous interactions with the organ effects of TNF and endotoxin, including pathologic alterations in the gut, kidney, and lung. Like the leukotrienes, enhanced PAF synthesis and release is also induced by TNF administration.

Complement activation occurs during septic shock. Many of the endothelial and neutrophil effects noted in sepsis are mimicked by complement breakdown products. TNF appears to augment the response to complement activation by the induction of neutrophil complement receptors.

The Gut in Sepsis. A resurgent interest in the role of the gut during trauma and sepsis has come about due to the recent recognition that the gut is metabolically active in stress states. The route of feeding alters metabolic and cytokine responses and may influence neutrophil and macrophage function in humans. Impairment of the normal gut barrier function may contribute to postinjury hypermetabolism and ultimately sepsis syndrome and septic shock by allowing bacteria or endotoxin to translocate from the lumen to the lymphatics, blood, and organs. Although experimental evidence in humans is scant at this time, numerous injury models in rats suggest that bacterial translocation-related phenomena may be due to amplified cytokine responses. The bowel lumen is a primary reservoir for gram-negative bacteria and the source of inoculum for aspiration pneumonia. Despite results of early clinical trials, the role of whole gut decontamination in injured patients awaits a better understanding of the pathophysiology.

Treatment. The only effective way to reduce mortality in septic shock is by prompt recognition and treatment of the associated infection before the onset of shock. Once shock occurs, the control of infection by early surgical debridement or drainage and use of appropriate antibiotics represents *definitive* therapy. Other recommended measures, including fluid replacement and the use of vasoactive drugs, represent *adjunctive* forms of therapy and are useful to prepare the patient before surgical intervention or to support the patient until the infectious process is controlled.

As soon as gram-negative sepsis and shock are apparent, a prompt and thorough search for the source of infection is made while instituting other supportive measures. Because of the multiple complicating factors that may accompany endotoxemia, the patient is best treated in an intensive care unit. Careful monitoring of direct arterial pressure, central venous pressure, pulmonary artery and pulmonary wedge pressures measured via a Swan-Ganz catheter, urine output, and arterial and central venous blood gases may be essential for proper management.

If the infectious process is amenable to drainage, operation is performed as soon as possible after initial stabilization of the patient's condition. In some cases surgical debridement or drainage of the infection must be accomplished for the patient to respond. These procedures can be performed under local or general anesthesia. For example, a patient with ascending cholangitis and shock secondary to sepsis may respond temporarily to supportive treatment. Improvement may be short-lived, however, unless timely drainage of the biliary tract is instituted. Prompt surgical drainage is of central importance in determining survival in patients with septic shock. Several reports have shown marked improvement in survival in septic shock patients with infectious foci amenable to surgical drainage. Other factors influencing prognosis include the severity of underlying illnesses, prompt treatment with appropriate antibiotics, and the development of other organ complications, particularly ARDS and renal failure.

Antibiotic Therapy. The use of specific antibiotics based on appropriate cultures and sensitivity tests is desirable when possible. The results may not be available for several days, but useful information may be gained from previous wound and blood cultures obtained during an earlier phase of the septic process and Gram stain of appropriate material. Antibiotics must often be chosen, however, on the basis of the suspected organisms and their previous sensitivity patterns. Properly directed empiric therapy is crucial, as appropriate antibiotic coverage, defined as the use of an antibiotic with in vitro activity against the recovered organism, has repeatedly been shown to influence survival in these patients.

Until the recent development of extended-spectrum penicillins, third-generation cephalosporins, and carbapenems, the need for multiple antibiotics, usually including an aminoglycoside, was widely accepted. Most double antibiotic regimens had the theoretical advantages of a broadened spectrum, potential synergy, and prevention of emerging bacterial resistance during therapy. The presumed focus of infection and the potential for nosocomial infection with resistant organisms unique to the admitting hospital also influence the choice of antibiotic regimens. Until the mid 1980s, most multiple-drug regimens for septic shock in medical patients used an aminoglycoside and either third-generation cephalosporins or antipseudomonal penicillins. Surgical infections, most often of intraabdominal origin, should be treated with an agent with good activity against *Bacteroides,* and consideration should be given to coverage against enterococcus in immunoimpaired patients. Most recent randomized prospect trials have focused on neutropenic patients in whom impaired host defenses should magnify the weakness of the antibiotics chosen. Most studies support the use of ceftazidime or imipenem-cilastatin as acceptable single agents. The standard antibiotic combinations have undergone more rigorous evaluation than newer monotherapies, particularly in the presence of *Pseudomonas aeruginosa* bacteremia. Monotherapy more often requires early modification of treatment. Because shock is an added risk factor for aminoglycoside-induced nephrotoxicity, many current regimens attempt to avoid aminoglycosides and use double beta-lactam combinations.

Fluid Replacement. Prompt correction of preexisting fluid deficits is essential. A majority of patients will incur fluid losses from the disease processes that initiate sepsis and shock. "Third space losses," with massive sequestration of plasma and extracellular fluid, are characteristic of many surgical conditions, including peritonitis, burns, strangulation obstruction of the bowel, and extensive soft tissue infections.

The type of fluid used will vary, although most "third space losses" are properly replaced with a balanced salt solution such as Ringer's lactate. Any deficits in red blood cell mass should be corrected by the administration of packed cells in order to maintain optimal oxygen-carrying capacity of the blood. Large quantities of replacement fluids are often needed in order to maintain an effective circulating volume. A fine balance exists between the need for volume replacement and the harmful effects that fluid overload with increased pulmonary capillary wedge pressure may have on lungs already injured by the septic process.

Insertion of a Swan-Ganz catheter for measurements of *both* pulmonary artery and pulmonary capillary wedge pressure, the latter a reflection of left ventricular end-diastolic pressure, is necessary. This is particularly true in patients on mechanical ventilation and positive end-expiratory pressure. Many patients will respond favorably to fluid administration combined with prompt control of the infection with a rise in blood pressure, an increase in urine output, warming of the extremities, and clearing of the sensorium. In these instances no additional therapy may be indicated.

Steroids. High-dose steroids appear to reduce the release of lysozymal enzymes, exert a modest inotropic effect on the heart, and produce mild peripheral vasodilatation. Early animal studies showed improved survival, particularly when given as pretreatment. Several large well-controlled prospective, randomized clinical trials have shown that even early administration of high-dose corticosteroids improves neither survival nor the shock state in septic patients. Steroids were significantly detrimental in patients with evolving ARDS or renal insufficiency. Consequently, pharmacologic doses of steroids are not indicated in the treatment of septic shock. Documented or suspected adrenal insufficiency, however, should be promptly addressed by physiologic replacement doses during this period of profound stress.

Pharmacologic Support. Although fluid resuscitation remains the initial therapy for hypotension in sepsis, it is frequently necessary to administer drugs with inotropic or vasopressor activity. Dopamine and dobutamine are the initial inotropic agents usually used. As discussed above in cardiogenic shock, dopamine has some vasopressor activity at higher doses that may be required in the volume-loaded patient with persistent profound hypotension. Augmentation of the impaired myocardial performance in septic shock appears to be a reasonable goal. Dobutamine will often increase cardiac input with less tachycardia and arrhythmia than dopamine. The beta-adrenergic vasodilatation from dobutamine infusion may not be tolerated by these hypotensive patients. Vasodilator drugs have been shown to improve cardiac output and oxygen delivery in normotensive septic patients. Their use in septic shock is limited by low systemic pressure or decreased cardiac filling pressures. More potent vasopressors, despite their obvious detrimental effect on peripheral perfusion, may be transiently unavoidable in patients who have persistent life-threatening hypotension, despite optimum fluid and dopamine infusions. Norepinephrine is a potent alpha receptor agonist that is usually effective in raising pressure in patients who have failed the above support. Its balance of beneficial and adverse effects is controversial. Epinephrine, a catecholamine with potent alpha- and beta-adrenergic activity, may support the blood pressure in patients who do not respond to norepinephrine. Polypharmacy is frequently ineffective and may be harmful in these patients with complex cardiovascular alterations. Their use is primarily for transient support, while primary definitive therapy with antibiotics and drainage of surgical infection are being instituted.

Manipulations of Humoral Responses. Given the obviously complex and as yet ill-defined interactions among a large number of mediators, therapy directed at any single agent will probably be ineffective. Carefully tailored multidrug therapy may eventually allow modulation of the deleterious systemic effects of the necessary host responses to injury and infection.

Initial trials of steroids, fibronectin, and naloxone were disappointing. More specific immunotherapy using monoclonal IgM antibodies to core lipopolysaccharide have been completed. Only small subsets of patients from each study showed statistical benefit. The HA-1A improved survival and organ function in the presence of gram-negative bacteremia with or without shock. The E-5 trial was of benefit in patients with gram-negative bacteremia only in the absence of shock. None of the antibodies directed to lipid A or other epitopes of the core lipopolysaccharide are established therapeutic modalities.

The naturally occuring IL-1 receptor antagonist has been manufactured by recombinant technology. Because IL-1 RA has shown benefit in several animal models, a large-scale clinical trial is under way to assess its use in human sepsis. Monoclonal antibodies to TNF are also available and undergoing clinical assessment. The persistent significant morbidity and mortality from sepsis, despite powerful antibiotic therapy, prompt surgery, and carefully titrated fluid and drug support suggests that the future for improved therapeutic results lies in these exciting new treatments in the next decade.

Bibliography

Pathophysiology of Hypovolemic Shock

Blalock A: *Principles of Surgical Care, Shock and Other Problems*. St Louis, CV Mosby, 1940.

Braunwald E, Sonnenblick EH, et al: Mechanisms of cardiac contraction and relaxation, in Braunwald E (ed): *Heart Disease: A Textbook of Cardiovascular Medicine*. Philadelphia, WB Saunders, 1992, p 351.

Canizaro PC, Prager MD, Shires GT: The infusion of Ringer's lactate solution during shock. *Am J Surg* 122:494, 1971.

Dahn MS, Lange P, et al: Hepatic blood flow and splanchnic oxygen consumption measurements in clinical sepsis. *Surgery* 107:295, 1990.

Davis JM, Stevens JM, et al: Neutrophil laboratory activity in severe hemorrhage shock. *Circ Shock* 10:199, 1983.

Gross SG: *A System of Surgery: Pathological, Diagnostic, Therapeutic and Operative*. Philadelphia, Lea & Febiger, 1872.

Holcroft JW: Impairment of venous return in hemorrhage shock. *Surg Clin North Am* 62:25, 1982.

Horton JW: Hemorrhagic shock depresses myocardial contractile function in the guinea pig. *Circ Shock* 28:23, 1989.

Hotchkiss RS, Karl IE: Reevaluation of the role of cellular hypoxia and bioenergetic failure in sepsis. *JAMA* 267(11):1503, 1992.

Hotchkiss RS, Song SK, et al: Sepsis does not impair tricarboxylic acid cycle in the heart. *Am J Phys* 260(1, part 1):C50-7, 1991.

Natanson C, Danner RL, et al: Role of endotoxemia in cardiovascular dysfunction and mortality: *Escherichia coli* and *Staphylococcus aureus* challenges in a canine model of human septic shock. *J Clin Invest* 83:243, 1989.

Parrillo JE: The cardiovascular pathophysiology of sepsis. *Annu Rev Med* 40:469, 1989.

Porter JM, Sussman MS, et al: Splanchnic vasospasm in circulatory shock, in Marston A, Bulkley GB, Fiddian-Green RG, Haglund UH (eds): *Splanchnic Ischemia and Multiple Organ Failure*. London, Edward Arnold, 1989, p 73.

Rush BF Jr, Redan JA, et al: Does the bacteremia observed in hemorrhagic shock have clinical significance? A study in germ-free animals. *Ann Surg* 210:342, 1989.

Shenkin HS, et al: On the diagnosis of hemorrhage in man: A study of volunteers bled large amounts. *Am J Med Sci* 208:421, 1944.

Suffredini AF, Fromm RE, et al: The cardiovascular response of normal humans to the administration of endotoxin. *N Engl J Med* 321:280, 1989.

Wiggers CJ: Present status of shock problem. *Physiol Rev* 22:74, 1942.

Extracellular Fluid Response

Campion DS, et al: The effect of hemorrhagic shock on transmembrane potential. *Surgery* 66:1051, 1969.

Chiao JJ, Minei JP, et al: In vivo myocyte sodium activity and concentration during hemorrhagic shock. *Am J Phys* R684, 1990.

Cunningham JN Jr, Shires GT, Wagner Y: Cellular transport defects in hemorrhagic shock. *Surgery* 70:215, 1971.

Illner HP, Shires GT: The effect of hemorrhagic shock on potassium transport in skeletal muscle. *Surg Gynecol Obstet* 150:17, 1980.

Lucas CE, Ledgerwood AM, et al: Colloid oncotic pressure and body water dynamics in septic and injured patients. *J Trauma* 31(7):927, 1991.

Middleton ES, Mathews R, Shires GT: Radiosulphate as a measure of the extracellular fluid in acute hemorrhagic shock. *Ann Surg* 170:174, 1969.

Roberts JP, Roberts JD, et al: Extracellular fluid deficit following operation and its correction with Ringer's lactate. *Ann Surg* 202:1, 1985.

Shires GT, et al: Alterations in cellular membrane function during hemorrhagic shock in primates. *Ann Surg* 176:288,1972.

Shires GT, Brown FT, Canizaro PC: *Shock*. Philadelphia, WB Saunders, 1973, chap 4.

Wilde WS: The chloride equilibrium in muscle. *Am J Physiol* 143:666, 1945.

Pulmonary Responses

Baldwin RE, Rice CL, et al: Adult respiratory distress syndrome, in Shields TW (ed): *General Thoracic Surgery*. Philadelphia, Lea & Febiger, 1989, pp 474–482.

Bell RC, Coalson JJ, et al: Multiple organ system failure and infection in adult respiratory distress syndrome. *Ann Intern Med* 99:293, 1983.

Clauss RH, et al: Effects of changing body position upon improved ventilation-perfusion relationships. *Circulation* 38(suppl II-37):214, 1968.

Dahn MS, Lucas CE, et al: Negative inotropic effects of albumin resuscitation for shock. *Surgery* 86:235, 1979.

Fowler AA, Hamman RF, et al: Adult respiratory distress syndrome: Risk with common predispositions. *Ann Intern Med* 98:593, 1983.

Froese AB, Bryan AC: High frequency ventilation. *Am Rev Resp Dis* 136:1363, 1987.

Lucas CE, Ledgerwood AM, Higgins RF: Impaired salt and water excretion after albumin resuscitation for hypovolemic shock. *Surgery* 86:544, 1979.

MacIntyre NR: New forms of mechanical ventilation in the adult. *Clin Chest Med* 9(1):47, 1988.

Maunder RJ, Hudson LD: Pharmacologic strategies for treating the adult respiratory distress syndrome. *Respir Care* 35:241, 1990.

Montgomery AB, Stager MA, et al: Causes of mortality associated with the adult respiratory distress syndrome. *Am Rev Respir Dis* 132:485, 1985.

Pepe PE, Hudson LD, et al: Early application of positive end-expiratory pressure in patients at risk for the adult respiratory distress syndrome. *N Engl J Med* 311:281, 1984.

Sinanan M, Maier RV, Carrico CJ: Laparotomy for intraabdominal sepsis in ICU patients: Indications and outcome. *Arch Surg* 119:652, 1984.

Alterations in Oxygen Transport

Bellingham AJ, Detter JC, Lenfant C: Regulatory mechanisms of hemoglobin oxygen affinity in acidosis and alkalosis. *J Clin Invest* 50:700, 1971.

Canizaro, PC: Oxygen transport in shock, in Shires GT (ed): *Shock and Related Problems, Clinical Surgery International*. New York, Churchill Livingstone, 1984, vol 9, pp 127–147.

Consensus Conference: Perioperative red blood cell transfusion. *JAMA* 260:2700, 1988.

Feola M, Gonzalez HF, et al: Development of a bovine stroma free hemoglobin solution as a blood substitute. *Surg Gynecol Obstet* 157:399, 1983.

Gould SA, Rosen AL, et al: Fluosol-DA as a red cell substitute in acute anemia. *N Engl J Med* 314(26):1653, 1986.

Gould SA, Sehgal LR, et al: The efficacy of polymerized pyridoxylated hemoglobin solution as an O_2 carrier. *Ann Surg* 211:394, 1990.

Hoyt DB, Greenburg AG, et al: Resuscitation with fluosol-DA 20%-tolerance to sepsis. *J Trauma* 26:8, 713, 1986.

Levine EA, Rosen AL, et al: Treatment of acute postoperative anemia with recombinant human erythropoietin. *J Trauma* 19:1134, 1989.

Lucas CE, Ledgerwood AM, Huggins RF: Impaired salt and water excretion after albumin resuscitation for hypovolemic shock. *Surgery* 86:544, 1979.

Samsel RW, Schumacker PT, et al: Oxygen delivery to tissues. *European Respiratory Journal* 4(10):1258, 1991.

Tremper KK, Friedman AE, et al: The preoperative treatment of severely anemic patients with a perfluorochemical oxygen-transport fluid, Fluosol-DA. *N Engl J Med* 307:277, 1982.

Woodson RD, Wranne B, Detter JC: Effect of increased blood oxygen affinity on work performance in rats. *J Clin Invest* 52:2717, 1973.

Therapy of Shock

Beecher HK: Preparation of battle casualties for surgery. *Ann Surg* 121:769, 1945.

Chavez-Negreta A, Majluf CS, et al: Treatment of hemorrhagic shock with intraosseous or intravenous infusion of hypertonic saline dextran solution. *Eur Surg Res* 23(2):123, 1991.

Civetta JM: A new look at the Starling equation. *Crit Care Med* 7(3):84, 1979.

Claussen MS, Landercasper J, et al: Acute adrenal insufficiency presenting as shock after trauma and surgery: Three cases and review of literature. *J Trauma* 32(1):94, 1992.

Hackford AW, Talley FP, et al: Prospective study comparing imipenem-cilastatin with clindamycin and gentamicin for the treatment of serious surgical infections. *Arch Surg* 123:322, 1988.

Hagman CF, Bagge L, Thoren L: The use of blood components in surgical transfusion therapy. *World J Surg* 11:2, 1987.

Isom OW: Cardiogenic shock, in Shires GT (ed): *Fluids, Electrolytes, and Acid Bases*. New York, Churchill-Livingstone, 1988, p 133.

Lee L, Bates ER, et al: Percutaneous transluminal coronary angioplasty improves survival in acute myocardial infarction complicated by cardiogenic shock. *Circulation* 76:1345, 1988.

Lucas CE, Ledgerwood AM, et al: Impaired pulmonary function after albumin resuscitation from shock. *J Trauma* 20:446, 1980.

Mattox KL, Bickell W, et al: Prospective MAST study in 911 patients. *J Trauma* 29(8):1104, 1989.

Nasraway SA, Rackow EC, et al: Inotropic response to digoxin and dopamine in patients with severe sepsis, cardiac failure, and systemic hypoperfusion. *Chest* 95:612, 1989.

Pizzo PA, Hathorne JW, et al: A randomized trial comparing ceftazidime alone with combination antibiotic therapy in cancer patients with fever and neutropenia. *N Engl J Med* 315:552, 1986.

Vassar MJ, Perry CA, et al: Analysis of potential risks associated with 7.5% sodium chloride resuscitation of traumatic shock. *Arch Surg* 125(10):1309, 1990.

Velanovich V: Crystalloid versus colloid fluid resuscitation: A meta-analysis of mortality. *Surgery* 105:65, 1989.

The Veterans Administration Systemic Sepsis Cooperative Study Group. Effect of high-dose glucocorticoid therapy on mortality in patients with clinical signs of systemic sepsis. *N Engl J Med* 317:659, 1987.

Humoral Mediators

Abraham E, Freitas AA: Hemorrhage produces abnormalities in lymphocyte function and lymphokine generation. *J Immunol* 142:899, 1989.

Berger M, Wetzler EM, et al: Tumor necrosis factor is the major monocyte product that increases complement receptor expression on mature human neutrophils. *Blood* 71:151, 1988.

Bitterman H, Smith BA, et al: Beneficial actions of antagonism of peptide leukotrienes in hemorrhagic shock. *Circ Shock* 24:159, 1988.

Cohn SM, Fink MP, et al: LY171883, a leukotriene D.E. receptor antagonist, preserves mesenteric perfusion and ameliorates intestinal intramucosal acidosis in porcine endotoxic shock. *J Surg Res* 49:37, 1990.

Dinarello CA: The proinflammatory cytokines interleukin-1 and tumor necrosis factor and treatment of the septic shock syndrome. *J Infect Dis* 163(6):1177, 1991.

Haglund U: The splanchnic organs as the source of toxic mediators in shock. *Progress in Clinical and Biological Research* 264:135, 1988.

Hesse DG, Tracey KJ, et al: Cytokine appearance in human endotoxemia and primate bacteremia. *Surg Gynecol Obstet* 166:147, 1988.

Lefer AM: Significance of lipid mediators in shock states. *Circ Shock* 27:3, 1989.

Minei JP, Fantini GA, et al: Endotoxin infusion in human volunteers: Assessment of the early cellular membrane response. *Surg Forum* 38:102, 1987.

Minei JP, Shires GT III, et al: Platelet activating factor antagonist CV-3988 prevents hepatocellular membrane dysfunction during live *E. coli* bacteremia. *Surg Forum* 39:24, 1988.

Natanson C, Eichenholz PW, et al: Endotoxin and tumor necrosis factor challenges in dogs stimulates the cardiovascular profile of human septic shock. *J Exp Med* 169:823, 1989.

Rothstein JL, Schreiber H: Synergy between necrosis factor and bacterial products causes hemorrhagic necrosis and lethal shock in normal mice. *Proc Natl Acad Sci (USA)* 85:607, 1988.

Rush BF Jr, Sori AJ, et al: Endotoxemia and bacteremia during hemorrhagic shock. The link between trauma and sepsis? *Ann Surg* 207(5):549, 1988.

Sun X, Hsueh W: Bowel necrosis induced by tumor necrosis factor in rats is mediated by platelet-activating factor. *J Clin Invest* 81:1328, 1988.

Tracey KJ, Fong Y, et al: Anti-cachectin TNF monoclonal antibodies prevent septic shock during lethal bacteremia. *Nature* 330:662, 1987.

Tracey KJ: Tumor necrosis factor (cachectin) in the biology of septic shock syndrome. *Circ Shock* 35(2):123, 1991.

Wolpe SD, Cerami A: Macrophage inflammatory proteins 1 and 2: Members of a novel superfamily of cytokines. *FASEB J* 3:2565, 1989.

CHAPTER 5

Surgical Infections

Richard J. Howard

HISTORICAL BACKGROUND

Infection is encountered by all surgeons, who, by the nature of their craft, invariably impair the first lines of host defenses—the cutaneous or mucosal barrier—between environmental microbes and the host's internal milieu. The entrance of microbes into host tissues is the initial requirement for infection. Preventing microbial penetration, reducing the microbial inoculum, and treating established infection have been important developments in reducing the mortality associated with surgery.

For most of surgical history, death from infection was the expected result, although it was not until the end of the nineteenth century that bacterial cause of surgical infection was appreciated. Death from infection was so common after compound fracture or fracture due to a gunshot wound that amputation was the standard treatment. Before antiseptic practices were instituted, mortality rates for amputation in times of war, 1745 to 1865, were between 25 to 90 percent. Mortality rates for amputation in civilian practice during the same period ranged between 5 to 50 percent.

The introduction of anesthesia by Long in 1842, and by Morton in 1846, increased the scope of surgery by permitting operations on body cavities and allowing surgeons to operate more slowly and deliberately so that death from blood loss was diminished. Infection still remained a great problem. Erysipelas, hospital gangrene (a term popularized during the Civil War describing a necrotizing infection presumably due to *Streptococcus*), and tetanus continued to plague surgeons and their patients. Many surgeons realized that a more favorable prognosis was associated with an infection that developed ''laudable pus,'' rather than a more serious infection that was not associated with purulence. Surgeons still did not yet understand the cause of infection.

Joseph Lister (1827–1912) made one of the great contributions to surgery by demonstrating that antisepsis could prevent infection and, as a consequence, compound fractures did not have to be treated by amputation. In March 1865, he began placing pure carbolic acid into wounds. Later he reduced the concentration to 10.5

and 2.5%. In 1867, he published his initial articles reporting that compound fractures healed without infection when wounds were treated with carbolic acid.

Wound antisepsis was not new with Lister. More than 20 articles appeared in British medical publications between 1859 and 1865 describing antiseptic treatment of wounds. Numerous agents had been placed in wounds since ancient times in an attempt to foster healing and prevent death. These agents included resins such as turpentine, pitch and tar, balsams and balms, myrrh and frankincense, honey, alcohol, glycerin, mercuric chloride, silver nitrate, iodine, hypochlorites, creosote, ferric chloride, zinc chloride, and carbolic acid. In 1871, Lister began to use a carbolic acid spray to reduce contamination of the operating room atmosphere, a practice he abandoned in 1887.

The "antiseptic principle" or "Listerian method" emphasized antiseptic treatment of wounds after the operation. Although initially resisted by many surgeons (more by British surgeons than surgeons on the continent), they were gradually adopted.

Even late in the nineteenth century aseptic surgery was not practiced. Surgeons washed their hands after, but seldom before, operations. When asked what was new in surgery in 1882, Ernst Bergmann said, "today we wash our hands before an operation." Gloves were not worn routinely until the early part of the twentieth century. Only gradually and with much opposition was aseptic surgery adopted. Sterilization of instruments, first by chemicals and then by steam, came into practice in the 1880s and 1890s. Hand washing and wearing of masks, caps, gowns, and gloves were also introduced about this time.

William S. Halstead introduced rubber gloves for his scrub nurse (and future Mrs. Halstead) Caroline Hampton because the corrosive sublimate (HgCl) used to sterilize instruments irritated her skin. Halstead's student Joseph Bloodgood introduced their routine use by the entire operating team.

The introduction of antibiotics was a major step in the treatment of infections. Although the discovery of penicillin was first reported by Alexander Fleming in 1928, the drug was not used clinically until administration by Howard Florey in the 1940s. It was rapidly introduced in general clinical medicine and followed by streptomycin and numerous other antibiotics. Antibiotics, it was hoped, would eliminate the risk of infection as a surgical complication and would enable established infections to be easily cured. Such, however, has not been the case. Wound infection and other postoperative infections continue to be a problem even though prophylactic antibiotics have reduced the risk. The bacteria causing wound infection have changed. With more elective abdominal surgery the cause of wound infection has changed from gram-positive cocci to gram-negative enteric bacteria. The wide use of antibiotics has even led to the emergence of strains of antibiotic-resistant bacteria. The nature of postoperative infection has also changed because of the many patients being operated on who have compromised host defenses (debilitated, elderly, cancer patients) or who are given drugs that inhibit host defenses (cancer chemotherapy agents, drugs to prevent organ transplant rejection).

It was also hoped that antibiotics would allow for the cure of most infections even without operation. While the introduction of antibiotic therapy was a giant step in the treatment of nonsurgical infections, it made a much smaller impact in the treatment of surgical infections. The mortality rate of acute appendicitis was approximately 50 percent in the latter part of the nineteenth century. The recognition in the 1890s that a person with acute appendicitis required an immediate operation led to a dramatic decrease in mortality rate in the early part of the twentieth century. Until that time surgeons believed that waiting a few days would allow the intestines to isolate the appendix, after which an abscess could be safely drained. The availability of intravenous fluid therapy and blood transfusion led to another decrease in mortality rate in the early part of the twentieth century. By the time penicillin became available, the mortality rate of acute appendicitis was only 5 percent. Continuing improvement in anesthesia, surgical technique, and postoperative care have also contributed to the decline in mortality—as has antibiotic therapy.

Although antibiotic therapy was a monumental advance in the treatment of infections, for patients with surgical infection it constitutes only one part of treatment. Surgical infections virtually always require an operative procedure for a successful outcome. In the future, continued improvement in the treatment outcome of surgical infection is more likely to stem from such factors as earlier and better means of diagnosis, improved patient care, and therapy directed against bacterial products or host response modifiers, rather than from improvements in antimicrobial therapy.

GENERAL CONSIDERATIONS

Surgical infections can conveniently be defined as infections that require operative treatment or result from operative treatment. Infections that require operative treatment include (1) necrotizing soft tissue infections; (2) body cavity infections such as peritonitis, suppurative pericarditis, and empyema; (3) confined tissue, organ, and joint infection such as abscess and septic arthritis; and (4) prosthetic device–associated infections.

Infections that result from operative treatment include wound infection, postoperative abscess, postoperative (tertiary) peritonitis, other postoperative body cavity infections, other hospital-acquired infections among which are pneumonias, urinary tract infection, and vascular catheter-related infection. Immunocompromised patients are subject to viral and fungal infections that seldom cause infection in the normal host.

Principles of Therapy

The patient's own host defenses and antibiotic therapy are adequate to overcome most infections. Nonoperative treatments can assist recovery from some infections. Chest physiotherapy is useful in patients with pneumonia—especially for those with thickened secretions. Increasing fluid intake and thus increasing urine flow is helpful in patients with urinary tract infections. Immobilization and elevation can relieve pain and reduce swelling of an extremity involved with cellulitis or lymphangitis.

Operative treatment is generally required in situations where host defenses cannot function properly or where there is continuing contamination with microorganisms: infected fluid collections must be drained, infected necrotic tissue must be debrided, and infected foreign bodies must be removed. Fluid collections such as abscesses must be drained because phagocytic cells cannot function properly with the low oxygen tension usually present. Antibiotics penetrate abscesses poorly. Since most bacteria are not actively dividing and antibiotics work best on actively dividing bacteria, they are not very effective against bacteria in abscesses. Similarly, necrotic tissue and foreign bodies inhibit the proper functioning of host defenses.

Defects in the gastrointestinal tract provide a continuing source of bacteria that rapidly overwhelms host defenses. Operation is required to correct this continuing source by closing the defect in the gastrointestinal tract or bringing it to the outside as an ileostomy or colostomy.

Determinants of Infection

The development of a surgical infection depends on several factors: (1) microbial pathogenicity, (2) host defenses, (3) the local environment, and (4) surgical technique (for postoperative infection).

Microbial Pathogenicity. Microbial pathogenicity is really a balance between host defenses and microbial virulence. Some microbes that have virtually no ability to cause infection in the normal host can cause lethal infection in an individual with severely compromised defenses.

Many bacteria *(S. pneumoniae, Klebsiella pneumoniae, S. pyogenes, Staphylococcus aureus, Salmonella typhi)* and fungi *(Histoplasma capsulatum, Candida albicans, Cryptococcus neoformans)* have thick capsules that make them resistant to phagocytosis (see section on Surgical Microbiology below). Other microbes *(Mycobacterium tuberculosis, Aspergillus flavus,* and *Toxoplasma gondii)* resist intracellular killing after they have been phagocytosed when lysosomes containing enzymes that digest microbes do not fuse with the phagosome. Other microbes successfully resist digestion by lysosomal enzymes.

Some bacteria can elaborate toxins, many of which are enzymes that injure or kill cells or promote spread within tissues. Exotoxins play an important role in the pathogenicity of *Clostridium, Staph. aureus,* and *Strep. pyogenes*. Other bacteria *(C. tetani, C. botulinum)* elaborate neurotoxins that alter normal neural transmission.

Endotoxins are lipopolysaccharide-protein complexes that are normal constituents of the cell wall of gram-negative bacteria. These molecules activate many biologic pathways including the complement and coagulation systems and cause release of interleukins and other biologic mediators from macrophages, release of hormones, and alteration in metabolism.

Host Defenses. Local host defenses are important in preventing microbial invasion into the tissues. Systemic host defenses are needed to rid the tissues of microbes once invasion has occurred.

Local Host Defenses. Tissues are protected from microbial invasion by a layer of epithelium. The epithelium of the skin is multilayered, and the superficial layers are keratinized. The epithelium also is multilayered in the nasopharynx, oral cavity, esophagus, and genitourinary tract. At other sites (the tracheobronchial tree, gastrointestinal tract, and eye) a single layer of epithelium protects the underlying tissues. Each site also provides a local environment that is not conducive to microbial attachment and growth. Among these local environmental features are lack of moisture (skin), flushing action of tears and urine, cilia (trachea, bronchia), and peristalsis, mucus, pH (gastrointestinal tract), and local immunity (IgA).

Systemic Host Defenses. A complex system of defense mechanisms exists throughout the body that can inactivate and kill microbial agents. These host defenses consist of phagocytic cells, the immune system, and molecular cascades such as the complement system, the coagulation system, and the kinin system. Phagocytic cells that can ingest and kill microbes include polymorphonuclear leukocytes (PMNs) and tissue macrophages (monocytes in the blood). Through a complex set of interactions of microbes with complement and other activation molecules, PMNs adhere to vascular endothelium; migrate across the endothelium and move in the direction of the microbes (chemotaxis); attach to the microbes, a process that may involve immunoglobulins or other opsonins; and phagocytose the microbes. Finally, lysosomes containing a variety of enzymes fuse with the phagosome, and the microbe is rapidly digested. The initiation of this process and its attendant chemical, cellular, and physiologic changes results in inflammation.

Macrophages are phagocytic cells found throughout the body tissues: in liver (Küpffer cells), spleen, lymphoid tissue, lung (alveolar microphages), brain (glial cells), connective tissue (histiocytes), pleura, and peritoneum. Macrophages can also move toward microbes in response to chemotactic agents and phagocytose and kill them. In addition, macrophages are important in initiating the immune response and can elaborate cytokines, tissue necrosis factor, interferon, and other biologically active molecules. Humoral and cellular immunity are important systemic host defense mechanisms for many microbial agents. The complement system, clotting system, kinin system, leukotrienes and other biologically active molecules are also activated by microbial agents and play an important role in mediating host defenses.

Host defenses are altered in individuals at either end of the age spectrum, malnourished individuals, trauma patients, postoperative patients, burn patients, patients with malignant neoplasms, patients receiving cancer chemotherapeutic agents or immunosuppressive drugs to prevent rejection of organ transplants, and patients taking steroids or other agents that have immunosuppressive effects.

Local Environmental Factors. Local factors may permit an infection to occur in a person with minimal microbial contamination and with otherwise adequate host defenses. These environmental factors inhibit systemic host defenses from being fully effective. A traumatic wound that normally would heal without infection has a greatly increased likelihood of becoming infected if the trauma has resulted in devitalization of tissue or if foreign bodies have become deposited in the wound. Phagocytic cells do not function as effectively in the presence of devitalized tissue or foreign bodies. A suture can reduce the number of *S. aureus* required to produce a subcutaneous infection by a factor of 100,000. Fluid collections and edema also increase the likelihood of infection because they inhibit phagocytosis.

Peripheral vascular disease contributes to soft tissue infection by preventing blood and the systemic host defenses it contains (phagocytic cells, immune globulins) from reaching the site of microbial contamination. Shock also decreases the amount of blood that reaches these sites.

All the above environmental considerations can prevent phagocytic cells from functioning efficiently by lowering tissue P_{O_2}. The lowered P_{O_2} inhibits function of phagocytic cells and promotes the growth of anaerobes.

Surgical Technique. Surgical technique is an important determinant of postoperative wound infection and other postoperative infections. Gentle handling of tissues, removing of devitalized tissues, not using the cautery excessively, not performing intestinal anastomoses under tension or when there is any question of inadequate blood supply, removing blood and other potential adjuvants that can promote growth of microbes, and appropriate use (and avoiding inappropriate use) of drains are some of the ways surgeons can decrease the likelihood of postoperative infection.

TYPES OF SURGICAL INFECTIONS

Soft Tissue Infections

Infection of the soft tissues (Table 5-1), skin, subcutaneous fat, fascia, and muscle, usually can be treated by antibiotics unless an abscess is present or tissue necrosis is present.

Cellulitis and Lymphangitis

Cellulitis is a spreading infection of the skin and subcutaneous tissues. There may or may not be evidence of injury to the skin. It is characterized by local pain and tenderness, edema, and erythema. Usually the border between infected and uninvolved skin is indistinct with the region of erythema gradually fading into normal appearing skin. Erysipelas is characterized by intense erythema with a sharp line of demarcation between involved and uninvolved skin and is caused by *S. pyogenes* Lancefield group A (beta-hemolytic streptococci). Cellulitis may be accompanied by systemic manifestations such as fever, chills, malaise, and toxicity.

Cellulitis may be due to numerous bacteria in addition to *S. pyogenes* such as *S. aureus, S. pneumoniae,* other streptococci, *Haemophilus influenzae,* and aerobic and anaerobic gram-negative bacteria. Lymphangitis is inflammation of the lymphatic channels in the subcutaneous tissues and presents as visible red streaks. Bacteria may reach the lymph nodes and cause lymphadenitis.

Cellulitis and lymphangitis can be treated by antibiotics alone. Local care includes immobilization and elevation to reduce pain and swelling. Failure to achieve prompt clinical response should suggest that suppuration has occurred and that surgical drainage is required.

Other skin infections that can be treated by local cleansing and local or systemic antibiotics include impetigo *(S. aureus),* erysipeloid *(Erysipelothrix insidiosa (rhusiopathiae),* folliculitis, and furunculosis.

Some microbial factors that cause granulomatous infections produce ulcers, nodules, sinuses, or infiltrated plaques. Biopsy with culture and histologic examination of tissue with special stains may be required for such lesions. Mycobacterial and fungal infections can manifest themselves in this way.

Soft Tissue Abscess

Surgical treatment is usually required if the soft tissue infection results in abscess or tissue necrosis. Furuncles and carbuncles (boils), breast abscess, and perirectal abscess require surgical incision and drainage and usually antibiotic therapy. A *carbuncle* is a subcutaneous abscess usually formed by a confluent infection of multiple contiguous hair follicles. They are most frequently found on the back of the neck and on the upper back. The most common cause is *S. aureus*. Overlying erythema may lead to the mistaken diagnosis of cellulitis, but the presence of a fluctuant mass usually leads to the correct diagnosis. A *felon* is a purulent collection in the distal phalanx of the fingers that causes intense pain and pressure in that compartment. Swelling may be minimal because of the fibrous bands between the skin and bone. Treatment requires incision and drainage. *Breast abscess* is usually caused by *S. aureus* but can be due to gram-negative bacteria as well. It frequently occurs in nursing mothers. Treatment consists of incision and drainage and antibiotics (see Chap. 14). *Perirectal abscess* begins as an infection of one of the crypt glands that then extends into the perirectal space and may present subcutaneously near the anus. It is caused by aerobic and anaerobic gram-negative bacteria that are normal residents of the colon. Incision and drainage and antibiotic

Table 5-1
Skin and Soft Tissue Infections

Type of Infection	*Etiologic Agents*
Pyogenic bacterial infections	
Cellulitis	*S. aureus,* group A streptococcus, various other bacteria
Lymphangitis	*S. aureus,* group A streptococcus, various other bacteria
Impetigo	*S. aureus,* group A streptococcus
Ecthyma	*S. aureus,* group A streptococcus, *P. aeruginosa*
Erysipelas	Group A streptococcus
Erysipeloid	*E. insidiosa*
Erythrasma	*C. minutissimum*
Hidradenitis suppurativa	*S. aureus*
Folliculitis	*S. aureus, Candida,* gram-negative bacteria
Furuncles and carbuncles	*S. aureus*
Paronychia	*S. aureus,* group A streptococcus, *Candida, P. aeruginosa*
Nodular and ulceronodular infections	
Bacterial	*S. aureus,* group A streptococcus, *Treponema pallidum,* mycobacteria Granuloma inguinale, Lymphogranuloma venereum, various other bacteria
Fungal	*Candida,* mycetoma (90% due to *Nocardia brasiliensis,* but other fungi also) chromoblastomycosis, histoplasmosis, (*Histoplasma capsulatum*), cryptococcosis (*Cryptococcus neoformans*), blastomycosis (*Blastomyces dermatidis*), coccidioidomycosis (*Coccidioides immitus*), sporotrichosis (*Sporotrichum schenekii*), phycomycosis (due to fungi of the genera *Mucor, Rhizopus,* and *Absidia*), aspergillosis (*Aspergillus fumigatus* ano, rarely, other species of *Aspergillus*)
Viral	Warts (*papilloma virus*), molluscum contagiosum (caused by a pox virus, specific one not determined)
Necrotizing soft tissue infections	
Bacterial	*Clostridium, Streptococcus,* microaerophilic streptococcus plus *S. aureus,* mixed anaerobic and aerobic bacteria, *P. aeruginosa, S. aureus,* marine *Vibrio*
Fungal	*Rhizopus, Mucor, Absidia*
Secondary infections complicating previous lesions	
Human and animal bites	*S. aureus,* streptococci, *Bacteroides, Pasteurella multocida*
Diabetic food infections	*S. aureus,* multiple anaerobic and aerobic bacteria (an average of 5.8 species per specimen)
Burns	*S. aureus,* streptococci, *P. aeruginosa, Candida,* various other bacteria, *Aspergillus*
Pilonidal and sebaceous cysts	*S. aureus,* various anaerobic and aerobic bacteria
Chronic ulcers (varicose, decubitus)	Various aerobic and anaerobic bacteria
Cutaneous involvement in blood-borne infections	
Bacterial	*Neisseria meningitidis, P. aeruginosa, S. aureus*
Fungal	*Candida, Cryptococcus*

therapy are the appropriate initial treatment. Up to 50 percent of perirectal abscesses may result in a fistula communicating with the anal crypt and may require later treatment. The fistula may be difficult to identify because of the intense inflammation of the abscess, and it is usually best to drain the abscess rather than risk making a passage into the anus looking for a fistula where none may have existed previously (see Chap. 26).

Necrotizing Soft Tissue Infections

Soft tissue infections that result in tissue necrosis are less common than other forms of soft tissue infections but are more serious because of their propensity for extensive destruction of tissues and high mortality rate. The nomenclature for necrotizing soft tissue infection is confusing. It is based both on tissues affected and causative organism. Names such as necrotizing fasciitis, streptococcal gangrene, gas gangrene, bacterial synergistic gangrene, clostridial myonecrosis, and Fournier's gangrene are commonly used. Attempts to differentiate these infections clinically are based on predisposing conditions, presence of pain, toxicity, fever, presence of crepitus, appearance of the skin and subcutaneous tissues, and whether or not bullae are present. Such classifications and clinical appearances are of little help in the initial treatment of these infections. Bacteria seldom respect anatomic barriers and thus necrotizing fasciitis is rarely limited to fascia and myonecrosis is rarely limited to muscle.

Most necrotizing soft tissue infections are caused by mixed aerobic and anaerobic gram-negative and gram-positive bacteria. *Clostridium* species, of which *C. perfringens, C. novyi,* and *C. septicum* are the most common, cause the most dramatic infections with rapid progression, early toxicity, and high mortality rate. The term *gas gangrene* has been used to indicate clostridial infection. But the presence of gas in tissue simply means that anaerobic bacterial metabolism has produced insoluble gases such as hydrogen, nitrogen, and methane. Both facultative and obligate anaerobes are capable of such metabolic activity. Gas in tissues is much more likely not to be due to *Clostridium* species. *Streptococcus pyogenes* can also cause extensive tissue necrosis. It seems to have been a more common cause of these infections in the early part of this century than currently. Halophilic marine *Vibrio* species are uncommon causes of rapidly progressive necrotizing soft tissue infections, especially in individuals with liver disease. Fungi can also cause necrotizing cutaneous and subcutaneous infection, but these infections progress much more slowly than do bacterial infections.

Necrotizing soft tissue infections must be recognized early and treated promptly. Diagnosis is not difficult when skin necrosis or bullae are present, but the clinical findings can be subtle before extensive necrosis has occurred. The overlying skin may appear to be normal or involved only with cellulitis. Early mental confusion, toxicity, and failure to respond to nonoperative therapy may be the earliest clues to the presence of a necrotizing infection. The presence of cutaneous necrosis, bullae, or crepitus strongly suggests a necrotizing infection and surgical exploration is warranted.

Surgical treatment requires debridement of all necrotic tissue. Computed tomography is a sensitive method of detecting soft tissue gas and may allow a better understanding of the extent of tissue necrosis. All necrotic tissue must be removed. Amputation may be required for myonecrosis of the extremities. It may be difficult to evaluate fully the extent of necrosis at the initial operation, or viable tissue may become necrotic after the initial debridement. Therefore, the wound must be inspected daily with adequate (usually general) anesthesia either in the operating room or intensive care unit until the surgeon can be sure there is no further necrosis. Extensive debridement, which can leave the patient with large tissue defects and extensive wounds, may be required. The goal of treatment is to remove all necrotic tissue and worry about reconstruction later. Initially, broad-spectrum antibiotics including penicillin should be administered. A Gram stain of the tissue and fluid should be done to look for gram-positive rods *(Clostridium)* or cocci *(Streptococcus).*

The use of hyperbaric oxygen to treat necrotizing soft tissue infections is controversial. Patients are placed in a chamber at three times atmospheric pressure absolute. Hyperbaric oxygen inhibits production of alpha toxin by *Clostridium.* Proponents of hyperbaric oxygen claim it makes the patient less toxic and diminishes the amount of tissue requiring excision. Although hyperbaric oxygen can decrease mortality due to *Clostridium* in experimental animals, there are no controlled clinical trials of hyperbaric oxygen in humans. Even proponents, however, admit hyperbaric oxygen does not improve outcome for patients with necrotizing soft tissue infections caused by nonclostridial organisms. Hyperbaric oxygen should not be used before surgical debridement. If adequate debridement is carried out, the patient usually rapidly improves and hyperbaric oxygen is usually not required. Since clostridial infections account for only a small number of necrotizing soft tissue infections, the number of patients who can benefit from this form of therapy is small.

Hyperbaric oxygen therapy has possible complications. Barotrauma can cause injury to the middle ear if the eustachian tube is blocked, trauma to a sinus, pneumothorax, and air embolism. Oxygen toxicity can cause neurotoxicity resulting in reduced seizure threshold and pulmonary toxicity if treatment is prolonged. A feeling of claustrophobia by the patient and reversible visual changes are other potential problems associated with hyperbaric oxygen therapy.

Tetanus

Tetanus is caused by *C. tetani,* a large gram-positive spore-forming bacillus. In recent years the number of cases in the United States has decreased sharply from over 450 in 1955 to fewer than 100 in 1975, and currently there are approximately 50 cases of tetanus reported per year.

Clostridium tetani is usually acquired by implantation of the organisms into tissues by means of breaks in the mucosal or skin barriers. Although it is frequently said that tetanus occurs in dirty, necrotic, and uncared-for wounds, the majority of cases in the United States appear after punctures, lacerations, and abrasions. Tetanus can appear after surgical wounds, injections, and in patients who have no apparent injury at all. Organisms proliferate at the site of inoculation and have virtually no capacity for causing an invasive infection. Clinical tetanus is as much an intoxication as an infection.

Clostridium tetani elaborates two toxins, tetanospasmin and tetanolysin. Tetanospasmin acts on the anterior horn cells of the spinal cord and on the brainstem. It blocks inhibitor synapses at these sites, leading to muscle spasms and hyperreflexia. These physiologic effects are similar to those of strychnine poisoning. Tetanolysin is cardiotoxic and causes hemolysis, but it is not thought to be of major clinical importance.

The median incubation period for both fatal and nonfatal cases is 7 to 8 days. Tetanus usually appears in generalized form but occasionally appears as localized tetanus with increased muscle tone and spasms confined to muscles near the wound and without systemic signs. Neonatal tetanus is recognized as difficulty in sucking beginning at 3 to 10 days of age and progressing to generalized tetanus.

In generalized tetanus, some patients have symptoms of restlessness and headache. In others, the first symptoms are muscle spasms with vague discomfort in the neck, lumbar region, and jaws. Spasm of the pharyngeal muscles makes swallowing difficult. A stiff neck is one of the early signs. Progressively, other muscle groups become involved until the spasms become generalized. Orthotonos, opisthotonos, and emprosthotonos can develop. Generalized toxic convulsions are frequent, exhausting, and unpredictable. Any slight external stimulus (a breeze, sudden movement, noise, or light) and internal stimuli (cough, swallow, distended bladder) may trigger generalized convulsions. These convulsions may involve the laryngeal and respiratory muscles and result in fatal acute asphyxia.

Throughout these spasms, which can be extremely painful and even cause fractures, the patient remains mentally alert. The pulse is elevated and there is profuse perspiration. Fever may or may not be present.

Diagnosis of tetanus is based on the clinical picture associated with no prior history of immunization. Although laboratory studies may show an elevated white blood cell count, they are not helpful in making the diagnosis. The demonstration of gram-positive organisms in the wound does not establish the diagnosis of tetanus; failure to demonstrate that the bacillus is in the wound does not eliminate the diagnosis. Consequently, the differential diagnosis can be difficult in early tetanus. Even with adequate treatment, the mortality rate can exceed 50 percent.

Treatment. Patients with clinical tetanus require exquisite nursing care to avoid complications. Initially therapy consists of administration of tetanus immune globulin (TIG), 500 to 10,000 units, as soon as the diagnosis is made. The exact effective dosage of TIG has not been established. Routine laboratory tests should be obtained and the patients should be monitored. Nursing care must be provided constantly in an intensive care unit setting. Formerly these patients were cared for in quiet rooms that provided a minimum of stimulation. Currently most are treated in an intensive care unit on a respirator with paralytic drugs given to prevent muscle spasms.

Mild cases can be treated with sedation, but most physicians administer muscle relaxants. Adequate doses of analgesics are required because of the pain associated with muscle spasms. Detailed attention must be given to caring for a paralyzed individual who is on a respirator. Adequate nutrition must be provided. Laxatives are generally indicated so that gastrointestinal elimination can be facilitated. A urinary catheter should be provided. The patient will require eye protection to prevent desiccation. Because the patient is paralyzed, pressure sores can occur rapidly, and these must be prevented with appropriate skin protection, hygiene, and cushions. Patients may require tracheostomy if they become dependent on a respirator for a prolonged period of time. X-ray studies are used to monitor the development of fractures. Pulmonary emboli can be a problem in patients who have minimal movement. Cardiac exhaustion and circulatory disruption can occur from sympathetic overstimulation. Hyperbaric oxygen is not recommended because it is ineffective. Oxygen has no effect on the toxemia.

The wound must be treated to remove as much of the *C. tetani* and nonviolable tissue as possible. Debridement of all necrotic tissue should be done. Penicillin G should be administered to treat any bacteria that remain behind, but antibiotics are no substitute for good wound care.

Table 5-2
Summary of Immunization Practices Advisory Committee Recommendations for Tetanus Prophylaxis in Routine Wound Management

History of Adsorbed Tetanus Toxoid (Doses)	*Clean Minor Wounds*		*All Other Wounds*[a]	
	Td[b]	*TIG*	*Td*[b]	*TIG*
Unknown or < 3 doses	Yes	No	Yes	Yes
≥ 3 doses[c]	No[d]	No	No[e]	No

[a]Such as, but not limited to, wounds contaminated with dirt, feces, soil, or saliva; puncture wounds; avulsions; and wounds resulting from missiles, crushing, burns, or frostbite.

[b]For children < 7 years of age, diphtheria, pertussis, and tetanus (DPT) immunization is used [or diphtheria and tetanus (DT) if pertussis vaccine is contraindicated]. For persons ≥ 7 years of age, Td is preferred to tetanus toxoid alone.

[c]If only three doses of fluid toxoid have been received, a fourth dose of toxoid, preferably an adsorbed toxoid, should be given.

[d]Yes, if > 10 years since last dose.

[e]Yes, if > 5 years since last dose.

Td = tetanus-diphtheria toxoid.

TIG = tetanus immune globulin.

SOURCE: Reproduced from Centers for Disease Control: Tetanus—United States, 1987 and 1988. *MMWR* 39:37, 1990.

Prevention. Active immunization with tetanus toxoid (TD) is a safe and effective way of preventing tetanus (Table 5-2). Unfortunately many children in the United States are not adequately vaccinated; immunization is also inadequate in many developing countries.

One month after the diagnosis of tetanus is made, the patient should be begun on tetanus toxoid immunization. The dose of tetanus toxin mediated during an infection is so small that immunization does not occur.

Body Cavity Infections

Peritonitis and Intraabdominal Abscess

Primary peritonitis is caused by a single organism and occurs most commonly in young children and in adults with ascites or with renal failure that is being treated by peritoneal dialysis. Primary peritonitis can be treated with antibiotics and other medical measures.

Secondary bacterial peritonitis is usually due to a defect in the gastrointestinal tract and requires operative intervention. The goals of surgery are to control the source of contamination, remove bacteria and adjuvant materials from the peritoneal cavity, and prevent postoperative abscess or recurrent peritonitis. Antibiotic therapy that is effective against aerobic and anaerobic enteric bacteria has an important role in treating patients with secondary bacterial peritonitis, but it should never delay or replace operative intervention.

Percutaneous or operative drainage along with antibiotic therapy is necessary for the treatment of intraabdominal abscesses. The etiology, clinical presentation, diagnosis, and treatment of peritonitis and intraabdominal abscess are discussed in Chap. 32.

Empyema

Empyema (Chap. 16) is usually due to pneumonia. Other causes are pulmonary infarct, septic emboli to the lung, tracheal or bronchial fistula, esophageal perforation, leaking esophageal anastomosis, hepatic abscess, subphrenic abscess, trauma, leaking bronchial closure, infected hemothorax, and paravertebral abscess.

Empyema may be encapsulated and localized or may involve the entire pleural cavity. Initially the fluid in the chest is thin, but with increasing numbers of PMNs and fibrin deposition the fluid becomes thicker and the visceral and parietal peritoneum adhere to each other.

The clinical manifestations of empyema initially resemble those of pneumonia, with pleuritic chest pain and fever. But unresponsiveness to antibiotic therapy may suggest the diagnosis. Chronic empyema can be manifested by dyspnea, fatigue, anemia, debility, and clubbing of the fingers.

Treatment of empyema is aimed at evacuation of the empyema contents and restoration of normal pulmonary function by expansion of the lung. Most empyemas can be treated by tube thoracostomy, especially in early empyema when the fluid is thin, and antibiotic therapy. The course of the disease is followed by the patient's clinical response and chest roentgenograms. The tube may be converted to open drainage after 2 to 3 weeks when the visceral and parietal pleurae have become adherent and the lung will not collapse.

Open drainage should be used if there are multiple pus pockets, if the pus is very thick, or if it is inadequately drained by tube thoracostomy. In special cases a decortication procedure may be necessary to reexpand the lung or if a bronchopleural fistula is present, a thoracoplasty may be required.

Other Closed-Space Infections

Purulence in closed spaces usually requires drainage and antibiotic therapy. If the diagnosis of septic arthritis is made promptly, antibiotic therapy alone may be sufficient to treat the infection. If the diagnosis is delayed, surgical treatment is required to preserve joint function and to eradicate the infection.

Suppurative pericarditis generally requires operative intervention. Although antibiotic therapy alone may be able to treat some early infections, operative therapy is usually required once suppuration has occurred.

Prosthetic Device–Associated Infections

Infections in prosthetic devices, such as cardiac valves, pacemakers, vascular grafts, and artificial joints, are associated with great morbidity, defeat of the goals of the operation, and too frequently end with the death of the patient. Although intensive antibiotic therapy alone can occasionally cure the infection, frequently the infection can be eradicated only by complete removal of all foreign material and antibiotic therapy. Replacement of cardiac valves with a new porcine or homograft valve and antibiotic therapy has met with some success. Vascular grafts have occasionally been salvaged without graft removal by treatment with debridement, povidone-iodine–soaked dressings, and antibiotic therapy as long as the suture line is not infected. Infected prosthetic joints and pacemakers have occasionally been salvaged by antibiotic irrigation of the joint or pacemaker. Usually infected prosthetic devices require complete removal.

Hospital-Acquired (Nosocomial) Infections

Hospital-acquired infections are infections that develop within a hospital or are acquired within a hospital. These infections are costly in terms of the suffering and death they can cause and from the cost of increased hospital stay, time lost from work, and legal liability. Each year in the United States there are an estimated 2,000,000 hospital-acquired infections that result in 150,000 deaths. Hospital-acquired infections add 1.5 days to the hospital stay of patients who develop lymphangitis, 14.8 days for patients with septicemia, and 16.6 days for patients who have infection at multiple sites. The total yearly cost of these infections is estimated at several billion dollars.

The Centers for Disease Control examines hospital-acquired infections through the National Nosocomial Infections Surveillance Study (Table 5-3). Infection rates are greatest on the surgical service, 44.3 per 1000 discharges. On surgical services urinary tract infections are the most common, followed by wound infection, lower respiratory infection, bacteremia, and cutaneous infections. Vascular catheter-related infections are frequently classified under bacteremia or cutaneous infection.

Wound Infections

Classification. For many years wounds have been classified according to the theoretical number of bacteria that contaminate wounds into clean, clean-contaminated, contaminated, and dirty (Table 5-4). Wound infection rates in large series are approximately 1.5 to 3.9 percent for clean wounds, 3.0 to 4.0 percent for clean-contaminated wounds, and approximately 8.5 percent for contaminated wounds. Dirty wounds generally are left open, but wound infection rates for dirty wounds of 28 and 40 percent have been reported (Table 5-5).

Wound infections encompass infections that occur above the fascia (superficial wound infection) and those that occur below the fascia (deep wound infection). Some authors have proposed more inclusive terms of surgical field or surgical site infection that would include all operative sites potentially exposed to bacteria. These more inclusive terms would include superficial and deep wound infections and infections that do not occur in direct proximity to the surgical incision (e.g., postoperative intraabdominal abscess).

Definition of Surgical Wound Infection. An incisional (superficial) wound infection must meet the following criteria: Infection occurs at an incision site within 30 days after operation and involves skin or subcutaneous tissue above the fascial layer and any of the following:

1. There is purulent drainage from incision or drain located above fascial layer.
2. Organism is isolated from culture of fluid aseptically obtained from wound closed primarily.
3. Wound is opened deliberately by surgeon, unless wound is culture-negative.

Deep surgical wound infection must meet the following criteria: Infection occurs at operative site within 30 days after operation if no prosthesis was permanently placed or within 1 year if an implant was placed, and infection involves tissues or spaces at or beneath the fascial layer and any of the following:

1. Wound spontaneously dehisces or is opened deliberately by surgeon when patient has fever (>38°C) and/or localized pain or tenderness, unless wound is culture-negative.

Table 5-3
Hospital-Wide Surveillance Component, Medians of Hospital Overall and Site-Specific Infection Rates, by Service

		Median Rates				
Service	*No. Hospitals*[a]	*Overall*	*Bloodstream Infection*	*Surgical Wound Infection*	*Urinary Tract Infection*	*Pneumonia*
Medicine	86	3.5	0.3		1.7	0.6
Oncology	63	5.1	1.0		1.6	0.6
Burn/trauma	20	14.9	1.4	1.1	4.5	3.1
Cardiac surgery	45	9.8	0.8	2.5	2.1	1.8
Dental	37	0.0	0.0	0.0	0.0	0.0
ENT[b]	72	1.1	0.0	0.3	0.0	0.2
General surgery	89	6.4	0.4	1.9	1.5	1.1
Urology	81	2.1	0.1	0.4	0.7	0.2
Neurosurgery	72	6.4	0.2	0.7	2.9	1.1
Ophthalmology	58	0.0	0.0	0.0	0.0	0.0
Orthopedics	88	3.9	0.1	0.8	1.9	0.3
Plastic surgery	53	2.0	0.0	0.8	0.4	0.0
Obstetrics	72	0.9	0.0		0.2	0.0
Gynecology	82	2.4	0.0		1.0	0.1
Pediatrics	74	0.4	0.0		0.0	0.0
High-risk nursery	44	14.0	3.9		0.3	1.4
Well-baby nursery	71	0.4	0.1		0.0	0.0

[a]For each service, the number of nosocomial infections per 100 discharges was calculated. Only those hospitals who reported at least 50 discharges were included. Because the distributions of all these rates were positively skewed, the median, which is a better measure of central tendency than the mean, is shown.

[b]Ear, nose, throat.

SOURCE: Reproduced from Centers for Disease Control: Nosocomial infection rates for interhospital comparison: Limitations and possible solutions. *Infect Control Hosp Epidemiol* 12:609, 1991, with permission.

Table 5-4
Classification of Operative Wounds in Relation to Contamination and Increasing Risk of Infection

Clean
- Elective, primarily closed, and undrained
- Nontraumatic, uninfected
- No inflammation encountered
- No break in asepsis
- Respiratory, alimentary, genitourinary, or oropharyngeal tracts not entered

Clean-contaminated
- Alimentary, respiratory, or genitourinary tracts entered under controlled conditions and without unusual contamination
- Appendectomy
- Oropharynx entered
- Vagina entered
- Genitourinary tract entered in absence of culture-positive urine
- Biliary tract entered in absence of infected bile
- Minor break in technique
- Mechanical drainage

Contaminated
- Open, fresh traumatic wounds
- Gross spillage from gastrointestinal tract
- Entrance of genitourinary or biliary tracts in presence of infected urine or bile
- Major break in technique
- Incisions in which acute nonpurulent inflammation is present

Dirty and Infected
- Traumatic wound with retained devitalized tissue, foreign bodies, fecal contamination, or delayed treatment, or from a dirty source
- Perforated viscus encountered
- Acute bacterial inflammation with pus encountered during operation

SOURCE: Reproduced from Altemeier WA, Burke JF, Pruitt BA Jr, Sandusky WR (eds): in *Manual on Control of Infection in Surgical Patients,* 2d ed. Philadelphia, Lippincott, 1984, p 28, with permission.

Table 5-5
Surgical Wound Infection Rates[a] Among 84,691 Operations by Traditional Wound Classification and NNIS Risk Index[b]

	Risk Category					
Wound Class	*0*	*1*	*2*	*3*	*(G)*[c]	*All Operations*
Clean	1.0	2.3	5.4	—	(0.47)	2.1
Clean-contaminated	2.1	4.0	9.5	—	(0.40)	3.3
Contaminated	—	3.4	6.8	13.2	(0.44)	6.4
Dirty	—	3.1	8.1	12.8	(0.43)	7.1
All operations	1.5	2.9	6.8	13.0		

[a]Number of surgical wound infections per 100 operations.

[b]The National Nosocomial Infection Survey surgical wound infection risk index includes the following elements: the patient's wound class was contaminated or dirty; the patient was assigned an American Society of Anesthesiology score of 3, 4, or 5 by the anesthesiologist prior to the operation; and the procedure lasted longer than the 75th percentile of the duration of surgery for the various operative procedures reported. A patient's risk score (range 0–3) was determined by adding the number of these risk factors present.

[c]Goodman-Kruskal correlation coefficient.

SOURCE: Reproduced from Centers for Disease Control: Nosocomial infection rates for interhospital comparison: Limitations and possible solutions. *Infect Control Hosp Epidemiol* 12:609, 1991, with permission.

2. An abscess or other evidence of infection directly under the incision is seen on direct examination, during operation, or by histopathologic examination.
3. Surgeon diagnoses infection.

Bacteria can gain entrance to the wound from endogenous or exogenous sources. Virtually all infections in clean-contaminated and contaminated wounds and also in the majority of clean wounds are due to endogenous bacteria present on the skin or mucosal surfaces.

Prophylaxis

Operating Room Environment. Air-handling systems are designed to reduce the number of airborne microbes. Filtration of air can reduce the number of dust particles to which microbes can adsorb. Operating room air should have a positive pressure with respect to air in the corridors so that unfiltered air does not enter the operating room. Special laminar flow systems with high-efficiency particulate air (HEPA) filters are frequently used when prosthetic joints are implanted to reduce the likelihood of airborne contamination. Reducing the number of people in the operating room and limiting talking are also advocated by some surgeons to reduce the number of airborne microbes.

Instruments and Drapes. Properly sterilized instruments should never be a source of infection. If drapes become wet, bacteria can move from underneath the drapes to the surgical field by capillary movement, i.e., "moist bacterial strikethrough." These bacteria theoretically can then enter the wound and cause a wound infection. Disposable drapes with plastic liners and cloth drapes with tighter weaves are designed to minimize bacterial strikethrough. It is difficult to establish if one type of drape is associated with fewer wound infections. The choice of drapes should be based on other considerations such as cost and ecologic effects.

Adhesive plastic drapes do not lower the incidence of wound infection. Cruse found that using adhesive plastic drapes in addition to routine draping was associated with an increased wound infection of 2.3 percent (214 of 9252) compared to 1.5 percent (405 of 26,303) when plastic drapes were not used.

Skin bacteria may actually proliferate under the warm, moist environment provided by the plastic drape, and these bacteria may enter the wound when the edges of the plastic drape lift off the wound margins as so frequently happens. Plastic drapes can be helpful, however, in isolating potential sources of contamination such as ostomies or fistulae near the incision.

Hand Washing. Hand washing with soap and an antiseptic agent should accomplish removal of dirt and desquamated skin and reduction of the number of microbes on the skin. Although tradition calls for scrubbing for 10 min and using two brushes, washing for 5 min and using one brush accomplishes equal reduction in skin bacterial counts. In practice, many surgeons scrub for a shorter time, especially after the first operation when, presumably, most dirt and desquamated skin should have already been removed.

Hexachlorophene, povidone-iodine, and chlorhexidine are the most commonly used disinfectants for hand washing. Hexachlorophene has the disadvantage of acting slowly. It should be used daily to achieve maximal reduction of skin bacteria. It has been replaced in some hospitals because of its slow action and because it can be absorbed through the skin. Both povidone-iodine and chlorhexidine result in prompt reduction of skin microbes.

Gloves. Gloves are usually made of latex and should fit snugly over the fingers and hands and over the cuff of the surgical gown. Thirty percent of gloves have defects in them by the end of the operation. Surgeons are potentially exposed to infectious agents harbored by their patients when blood enters through these holes and gets onto their skin. Glove perforations are more likely to occur with long operations, operations for trauma, and when patient blood loss is great.

Other Barriers. Caps prevent hair and skin scales (and adherent bacteria) from falling into the patient's wound, masks prevent droplets produced during speaking or coughing from entering the patient's wound, and gowns prevent desquamated skin and other particles from entering the patient's wound. There are no data that demonstrate unequivocally that wearing these barriers lowers the wound infection rate. Two recent studies found that when surgeons did not wear masks, the wound infection rate was not increased. In one study surgeons did not wear masks for a 6-month period and compared wound infection rates for the same 6-month period for the preceding 5 years. The wound infection rate actually fell to 1.8 percent from 5.7 percent. In another study more than 3000 patients were randomized to be operated on by surgeons wearing masks or not wearing masks. There was no difference in wound infection rate. But these barriers should still be worn if for no other reason than to prevent blood of the patient from coming in contact with the operating room team.

Preoperative Stay. Patients who have longer preoperative hospitalizations are more likely to develop postoperative wound infections. These patients may acquire more virulent or antibiotic-resistant hospital bacteria. Since patients who are more ill and whose host defenses may be compromised are the ones likely to have long preoperative hospital stays, it is not surprising that they are more likely to develop wound infections.

Preoperative Shower. A preoperative shower with an antiseptic soap such as chlorhexidine or povidone-iodine can reduce the resident skin bacteria especially in those patients who may have increased skin bacteria such as hospitalized patients or obese patients with large, moist intertriginous areas. Cruse reported that infection rate fell to 1.3 percent for patients taking a preoperative shower with soap containing hexachlorophene from 2.1 percent if they took a shower with ordinary soap and 2.3 percent if the patient did not shower. But another study of 5536 patients found no reduction in wound infection rates in patients who had a preoperative shower with 4% chlorhexidine detergent.

Remote Infections. Remote infections can triple the rate of wound infection. Elective operations should generally be delayed until the infection has been eliminated. Areas of dermatitis are generally moist, and bacterial growth at these sites increases dramatically. Elective operations should be delayed until the dermatitis is treated, especially if the skin incision is near or through such regions.

Hair Removal. Shaving, clipping, and depilatory agents have been used to remove hair. Shaving remains the most commonly used method of hair removal. But nicks and cuts caused by shaving are sites where bacteria can proliferate.

If shaving is done the night before operation, there is ample time for bacterial proliferation in any nicks or cuts, and the wound infection rate is higher than when shaving is done in the operating room immediately before operation. When hair is removed by clipping with an electric clipper, the wound infection rate can be reduced further.

Skin Preparation. Degerming of the operative site usually entails washing the operative site with a germicidal soap solution for 5 to 10 min followed by painting the site with an antimicrobial solution such as tincture of iodine, of chlorhexidine, or povidone-iodine. Painting the operation site with an alcohol solution of povidone-iodine, which can be accomplished in less than 1 min, is as effective as a 5-min scrub with povidone-iodine followed by painting with povidone-iodine solution.

Reduction of Colonic Bacteria. There are approximately 10^{10} to 10^{11} bacteria per gram of feces. Colon procedures thus potentially expose the wound to numerous bacteria. Colonic bacteria can be greatly reduced by cleansing the colon of feces. A variety of enemas or cathartics such as magnesium citrate solution or electrolyte solutions in polyethylene glycol can be used. These agents should be used before all elective colon surgery. Oral antibiotics can further reduce the number of colonic bacteria. A combination of neomycin and erythromycin base is used most commonly, but other antibiotics are equally effective.

Improving Host Defenses. Malnutrition should be corrected to restore the patient's resistance to infection to normal. Obesity should be corrected since it is associated with an increased rate of wound infection. Weight reduction also lowers the risk of pulmonary complications. Abnormal physiologic states that result from cirrhosis, uremia, and diabetes should be corrected as far as possible. Patients with pulmonary disease should have therapy before elective surgery to have their pulmonary status optimized. Patients who smoke should cease smoking before the operation. Since smoking inhibits ciliary movement, people who smoke might not be able to clear tracheal secretions as well as nonsmokers.

Surgical Technique. Every surgical incision injures tissues. Bacteria contaminate the wounds of virtually all clean-contaminated and contaminated procedures and, probably, most clean operations as well. The surgeon's goal should be to make the local wound environment as unfavorable to the growth of these bacteria as possible.

The incision should be made in a manner to injure as little tissue as possible and to prevent the accumulation of agents that facilitate bacterial growth or that inhibit host defenses such as devitalized tissue, foreign bodies, blood, and serum. The initial skin incision should be made with a scalpel through the entire skin layer. The subcutaneous fat should then be divided with a single incision down to the fascia. It may not be possible to do so in obese patients, but the fewest passes of the scalpel should be used. It is important to begin each new pass of the scalpel in the depths of the wound so that tissue is not devitalized. Some surgeons prefer to use the laser or electrocautery for the incision. These techniques may result in less bleeding but can cause more tissue destruction. There are no well-controlled studies showing that one technique results in fewer wound infections than another.

The surgeon should be fastidious in assuring there is no bleeding before closure. Blood in the incision provides a good environment for bacterial growth. The surgeon should not rely on drains to remove blood. It is more likely to clot and form a hematoma rather than be removed by a drain.

The wound edges can become desiccated leading to increased tissue necrosis at the wound margins. Desiccation should be prevented by placing moist laparotomy pads over the edges of the wound and keeping them wet. Some surgeons place antibiotics in the irrigant. There is no solid evidence that local antibiotics lessen the likelihood of infection. When the wound is closed, there is a potential space where a seroma can collect. There are no well-controlled studies that provide data on whether subcutaneous sutures affect the risk of wound infection.

If the surgeon is concerned about the possibility of a wound seroma such as might occur in the subcutaneous tissue of an extremely obese individual, a closed suction drain should be used. Penrose drains should not be used because bacteria can actually enter the wound through the drain tract. Penrose drains lead to a higher wound infection rate than not using a drain.

All devitalized tissue and foreign bodies should be removed from traumatic wounds. Irrigation with saline can facilitate removing small particles, especially if the irrigation is performed with the saline under pressure. When complete removal of devitalized tissue and foreign bodies cannot be assured or if the wound is heavily contaminated with bacteria, it can be left open and closed secondarily. If the wound is left open, saline-soaked gauze should be placed in the depths of the wound to keep the edges apart. There are no well-controlled studies that demonstrate that using antibiotic solutions inhibits infection or improves healing.

Prophylactic Antibiotics. Antibiotic administration can reduce the incidence of postoperative wound infection in patients having selected operations. There are certain principles that guide antibiotic prophylaxis (Table 5-6). Prophylactic antibiotic therapy directed against the bacteria likely to contaminate the wound should be selected (Table 5-7). For clean operations for which antibiotic prophylaxis is appropriate, *S. aureus, S. epidermidis,* and gram-negative enteric bacteria are the most likely bacteria to cause wound infections. Gram-negative enteric bacteria are the most likely causes of wound infection following gastroduodenal and biliary tract procedures, colorectal surgery, appendectomy, and gynecologic surgery.

The antibiotics should generally be given intravenously 30 to 60 min before operation so that adequate blood and tissue levels are present at the time the skin incision is made. The antibiotic dose should be repeated if the operation lasts longer than 4 h or twice the half-life of the antibiotic or if blood loss has been great. Prophylactic antibiotics should not be continued beyond the day of operation. The most commonly violated principle is giving the antibiotic longer than actually needed, which not only increases costs but also increases the likelihood of promoting antibiotic resistance among hospital strains of bacteria.

Table 5-6
Principles of Antibiotic Prophylaxis

Choose an antibiotic effective against the pathogens most likely to be encountered
Choose an antibiotic with low toxicity
Administer a single, fully therapeutic dose intravenously 30 to 60 minutes preoperatively
Administer a second dose of antibiotic if the operation lasts longer than 4 h or twice the half-life of the antibiotic
Give two to three doses postoperatively. There is no need to extend administration beyond 24 h
Use of antibiotics is appropriate when infection is frequent or when consequences of infection would be unusually severe

Table 5-7
Prevention of Wound Infection and Sepsis in Surgical Patients

Nature of Operation	*Likely Pathogens*	*Recommended Drugs*	*Adult Dosage Before Surgery*[a]
Clean			
Cardiac			
Prosthetic valve, coronary artery bypass, and other open-heart surgery	*S. epidermidis, S. aureus, Corynebacterium,* enteric gram-negative bacilli	cefazolin *or* vancomycin[b]	1 g IV 1 g IV
Vascular			
Arterial surgery involving the abdominal aorta, a prosthesis, or a groin incision	*S. aureus, S. epidermidis,* enteric gram-negative bacilli	cefazolin *or* vancomycin[b]	1 g IV 1 g IV
Lower extremity amputation or ischemia	*S. aureus, S. epidermidis,* enteric gram-negative bacilli, clostridia	cefazolin *or* vancomycin[b]	1 g IV 1 g IV
Neurosurgery			
Craniotomy	*S. aureus, S. epidermidis*	cefazolin *or* vancomycin[b]	1 g IV 1 g IV
Orthopaedic			
Total joint replacement, internal fixation of fractures	*S. aureus, S. epidermidis*	cefazolin *or* vancomycin[b]	1 g IV 1 g IV
Ocular	*S. aureus, S. epidermidis,* streptococci, enteric gram-negative bacilli, *Pseudomonas*	gentamicin *or* tobramycin *or* neomycin-gramicidin-polymyxin B cefazolin	Multiple drops topically over 2 to 24 h 100 mg subconjunctivally at end of procedure
Clean-Contaminated			
Head and neck			
Entering oral cavity or pharynx	*S. aureus,* streptococci, oral anaerobes	cefazolin *or* clindamycin	1 g IV 600 mg IV
Gastroduodenal	Enteric gram-negative bacilli, gram-positive cocci	*High risk, gastric bypass,* or *percutaneous endoscopic gastrostomy only:* cefazolin	1 g IV
Biliary tract	Enteric gram-negative bacilli, enterococci, clostridia	*High risk only:* cefazolin	1 g IV
Colorectal	Enteric gram-negative bacilli, anaerobes	*Oral:* neomycin + erythromycin base[c] *Parenteral:* cefoxitin *or* cefotetan	 1 g IV
Appendectomy	Enteric gram-negative bacilli, anaerobes	cefoxitin *or* cefotetan	1 g IV
Vaginal or abdominal hysterectomy	Enteric gram-negative bacilli, anaerobes, Group B streptococci, enterococci	cefazolin	1 g IV
Cesarean section	Same as for hysterectomy	*High risk only:* cefazolin	1 g IV after cord clamping
Abortion[d]	Same as for hysterectomy	aqueous penicillin G *or* doxycycline	1 million units IV 300 mg by mouth[d]
Dirty[e]			
Ruptured viscus	Enteric gram-negative bacilli, anaerobes, enterococci	cefoxitin *or* cefotetan either ± gentamicin *or* clindamycin + gentamicin	1 g IV q6h 1 g IV q12h 1.5 mg/kg IV q8h 600 mg IV q6h 1.5 mg/kg IV q8h
Traumatic wound[f]	*S. aureus,* Group A streptococci, clostridia	cefazolin	1 g IV q8h

[a]Parenteral prophylactic antimicrobials for clean and clean-contaminated surgery can be given as a single intravenous dose just before the operation. Cefazolin can also be given intramuscularly. For prolonged operations, additional intraoperative doses should be given every 4 to 8 h (q4–8 h) for the duration of the procedure.

[b]For hospitals in which methicillin-resistant *S. aureus* and *S. epidermidis* frequently cause wound infection, or for patients allergic to penicillins or cephalosporins. Rapid IV administration may cause hypotension, which could be especially dangerous during induction of anesthesia.

[c]After appropriate diet and catharsis, 1 g of each at 1 P.M., 2 P.M., and 11 P.M., the day before the operation. An alternative is oral lavage solution (Golytely, and others—*Med Lett* 27:39, 1985) from 1 P.M. to 6 P.M. (4–6 h) until rectal effluent is clear, followed by neomycin 2 g and metronidazole 2 g orally at 7 P.M. and 11 P.M. (Wolff BG, et al: *Arch Surg,* 1234:895, 1988).

[d]Aqueous penicillin G or doxycycline is recommended for first-trimester abortion in patients considered at high risk for pelvic infection, including those with previous pelvic inflammatory disease, previous gonorrhea, or multiple sex partners. The dosage of doxycycline should be divided into 100 mg 1 h before the abortion and 200 mg ½ h after. For mid-trimester abortion, cefazolin, 1 g IV, is recommended.

[e]For "dirty" surgery, therapy should usually be continued for 5 to 10 days.

[f]For bite wounds, in which likely pathogens may also include oral anaerobes, *Eikenella corrodens* (human), and *Pasteurella multocida* (dog and cat) (DJ Weber and AR Hansen, *Infect Dis Clin North Am,* 5:663, Sept 1991), some *Medical Letter* consultants recommend use of amoxicillin-clavulanic acid (*Augmentin*) or ampicillin-sulbactam (*Unasyn*).

SOURCE: Reproduced from Antimicrobial prophylaxis in surgery. *Med Lett* 34:5, 1992, with permission.

Cephalosporins are the most commonly used antibiotics for prophylaxis because of their broad antibacterial spectrum that provides activity against the gram-positive pyogenic cocci, gram-negative enteric bacteria, and anaerobic bacteria (some cephalosporins) and because of their low toxicity. But despite their safety profile, allergic reactions can occur with these antibiotics, so they should not be used indiscriminately. Cefazolin, a first-generation cephalosporin, is an effective antibiotic prophylaxis for indicated clean, gastroduodenal, biliary tract, head and neck operations, and for traumatic wounds. Vancomycin can be substituted in hospitals where methicillin-resistant *S. aureus* or *S. epidermidis* is a problem and in patients who are allergic to penicillins or cephalosporins. For colorectal procedures oral neomycin plus erythromycin base and/or cefoxitin or cefotetan provide effective coverage.

First- or second-generation cephalosporins provide effective prophylaxis for gynecologic surgery and cesarean section. Third-generation cephalosporins are no more effective than first- or second-generation agents and are more expensive. Many other antibiotic classes also provide effective prophylaxis, but none has gained the popularity of the cephalosporins.

Indications. Prophylactic antibiotics are indicated in patients where bacterial contamination of the wound is likely or in patients having clean operations in which a prosthetic device is placed where infection could lead to disastrous results such as an infected cardiac valve, vascular graft, or artificial joint. Bacterial contamination is likely in traumatic wounds, when the intestinal tract has been entered as a result of trauma, in elective operations on the intestine or colon, in gastroduodenal operations in which the patient has increased gastric flora, in high-risk biliary tract operations, and in gynecologic operations.

The bacteria in the stomach are increased in patients who have gastric outlet obstruction, decreased gastric acidity (achlorhydria, antacid or H_2 blocker therapy, gastric cancer), and normal or high acidity if bleeding has occurred. High-risk biliary tract operations include the presence of jaundice, bile duct obstruction, stones in the common bile duct reoperative biliary tract operation, acute cholecystitis, and patient's age greater than 70 years.

Infection Surveillance. An infection surveillance program can help to reduce the rate of wound infections and is required by the Joint Commission on Accreditation of Health Organizations. Large studies have shown the usefulness of regular wound surveillance. The introduction of a good wound surveillance program lowered the wound infection rate of more than 20,000 wounds to 1.9 percent from 4.9 percent over a 5-year period.

Other Hospital-Acquired Infections

Urinary Tract Infection. Urinary tract infection accounts for 40 percent of hospital-acquired infections. Two-thirds of patients with hospital-acquired urinary tract infection have had operation on the lower urinary tract, instrumentation of the bladder, or catheterization. Because of the large number of patients who fit one of these categories there are an estimated 400,000 urinary tract infections per year in hospitalized patients. Catheter-associated urinary infections cause bacteremia in 2 to 4 percent of patients and are associated with a case fatality rate three times as high as nonbacteriuric patients.

Bacteriuria occurs in 1 to 5 percent of patients after a single short-term catheterization. The risk of infection is higher in pregnant patients, elderly, or debilitated patients and in patients with urologic abnormalities. The risk of bacteriuria in patients with long-term indwelling catheters is approximately 5 to 10 percent for each day the catheter is in place. Therefore, urinary catheters should be placed only when necessary and should be removed as soon as possible. If prolonged urinary tract catheterization is required as in comatose patients, incontinent men, or spine-injured patients, suprapubic or condom catheters can be used to reduce the risk of infection.

Appropriate catheter insertion after careful cleansing of the urethral meatus and postinsertion care of the catheter can reduce the risk of infection. Irrigation of the catheter (i.e., to remove blood clots) should only be done by trained individuals.

Lower Respiratory Tract Infection. Lower respiratory infections are the third most common hospital-acquired infection according to the National Nosocomial Infections Study. Anesthesia, operations on the head and neck, and postoperative endotracheal intubation interfere with the normal protective cough reflex and may permit aspiration of contaminated material. Pain associated with thoracic or upper abdominal operations and trauma interferes with coughing and deep breathing which promotes collection of material in the tracheobronchial tree and atelectasis which predispose to infection. Pulmonary edema or adult respiratory distress syndrome resulting from injudicious use of intravenous fluids, cardiac failure, trauma, sepsis, renal failure, or inhalation of hot gases by burn patients also predispose to pulmonary infection. Fluid that accumulates in alveoli inhibits the phagocytic capacity of pulmonary macrophages.

Hospitalized patients may have gram-negative bacteria as part of their oral flora. These bacteria may be aspirated into the lungs during the postoperative period. Tracheostomies and respiratory care devices also predispose to entry of bacteria into the lower respiratory tract.

The most common causes of lower respiratory tract infection in hospitalized patients are *S. aureus, Pseudomonas aeruginosa, Klebsiella* sp., *Escherichia coli,* and *Enterobacter* sp. These bacteria, especially if they occur in the intensive care unit setting, may be resistant to commonly used antibiotics. Pulmonary infections in hospitalized patients are frequently not associated with sputum production, and culture of sputum specimens may not reflect the cause of pneumonia. Specially tipped swabs can be introduced into the lungs through a flexible bronchoscope, but even culturing by this method is not infallible.

Lower respiratory tract infections are common in intubated patients in intensive care units, occurring in as many as 20 to 25 percent of patients with a mortality rate of 50 percent. Many of these pneumonias are attributed to low levels of aspiration. Oropharyngeal decontamination using topical nonabsorbable antibiotics or antiseptics can reduce tracheobronchial contamination by gram-negative bacteria and pneumonia in these patients.

Vascular Catheter-Related Infection. Vascular catheter-related infections have increased greatly with the increased use of central vascular catheters that are left in place for prolonged periods in patients with compromised host defenses. It is estimated that 20 million hospitalized patients each year undergo vascular catheterization of some sort. An estimated 20,000 to 50,000 cases of hospital-acquired bacteremia per year are secondary to vascular catheters. Central venous catheters have a higher infection rate than do peripheral venous catheters, and polyethylene catheters have a higher infection rate than Silastic catheters. The most common source of catheter sepsis is believed to be microorganisms at the skin exit site that follow the catheter into the vein rather than originating from a distant site that colonizes the catheter via the bloodstream.

The skin is the most common source of organisms causing catheter-related infection. *S. aureus* and *S. epidermidis* causing catheter infections usually originate from the skin. Most yeast vascular-access infections result from hematogenous dissemination from another site. Gram-negative enteric bacteria also may infect catheters by a hematogenous route.

The duration of catheterization, the number of catheter manipulations, inexperience of the inserter, violations of aseptic technique, and use of multilumen catheters are all associated with an increased risk of infection. Transparent plastic dressings increase the risk of infection two- to fourfold compared with traditional gauze dressings. Having teams designated for catheter insertion and maintenance can reduce the risk of catheter infection. Skin preparation with chlorhexidine gluconate and use of topical antibiotics can also reduce the risk of infection. There are no data proving that practices such as changing catheters at intervals over guide wires, changing infusion tubing every 24 to 48 h, and using in-line filters reduce the risk of infection.

Finding bacteria on culture of the catheter tip does not establish if it was infected, since the bacteria may have come from the blood that inevitably contaminates catheter tips. Some investigators have attempted to do semi-quantitative cultures of catheter tips by rolling them on solid culture plates, flushing sterile broth through the catheter, or subjecting them to sonication to remove adherent organisms before quantitative culture. If there is unequivocal purulent discharge around the catheter insertion site, the diagnosis of vascular-access infection can be made without a positive catheter culture.

Any evidence of phlebitis, cellulitis, or suspicion of septic complications due to intravenous cannulas should lead to prompt removal of the cannulas. Because many central venous catheters are used in compromised hosts who are prone to fever, these catheters generally should not be removed because of fever alone until other potential sources of fever have been eliminated. Most surgeons remove central venous catheters that are suspected of being infected and replace them after 24 to 48 h.

Catheter infections due to *S. epidermidis* can occasionally be treated with antibiotics alone or by removal of the catheter. If antibiotics are used, a short course (3 to 7 days) is recommended. Vascular-access infections due to *S. aureus* always require antibiotic therapy. The controversy in the treatment of catheter infections due to *S. aureus* is in the duration of antibiotic therapy with most experts recommending a 2- to 3-week course. Vascular-access infections caused by yeasts should always be treated by catheter removal and amphotericin B if cultures remain positive following removal or if there is infection elsewhere.

SURGICAL MICROBIOLOGY

Surgical infections are usually caused by bacteria, but fungal and viral infections can also occur, especially as postoperative infections in immunocompromised hosts. Most bacterial infections are due to organisms that are part of the patient's endogenous flora—bacteria that are normal residents of the skin or gastrointestinal tract.

Bacteria

Bacteria can be classified according to staining characteristics with Gram stain (positive or negative), shape (cocci, rods, spirals), and sensitivity to oxygen (aerobic, facultative, anaerobic), or according to a combination of these characteristics. Gram-positive cocci, gram-negative aerobic and facultative rods, and anaerobic bacteria are three groups into which most bacteria causing surgical infections can be placed.

Gram-Positive Cocci

Staphylococcus and some *Streptococcus* species are the gram-positive cocci (often referred to as pyogenic cocci) of interest to surgeons because of their ability to cause primary surgical infections and postoperative infections.

The genus *Staphylococcus* is comprised of facultatively anaerobic gram-positive cocci that are found on moist areas of the body, anterior nares, and mucous membranes. In addition, these bacteria can be found on the body surface of many species of mammals and birds, in the air and dust of occupied buildings, and in milk, food, and sewage.

Staphylococcus aureus is the most common pathogen isolated from wound infections. A major factor in its pathogenicity is coagulase production, although the mechanism whereby coagulase production increases virulence is not known. In addition to coagulase production, a variety of other cell surface components and extracellular products are related to its pathogenicity.

Cell wall peptidoglycan inhibits edema production and migration of leukocytes, allowing bacteria to proliferate in tissues. Capsules inhibit opsonization and thus phagocytosis. The ability of some strains to produce a loosely surface-associated exopolysaccharide or glycocalyx (slime) is associated with virulence, probably by permitting the bacteria to resist phagocytosis and adhere to prosthetic materials.

Other extracellular products also contribute to the pathogenicity of *S. aureus*. An enterotoxin is responsible for food poisoning. Epidermolytic toxin can cause a variety of skin lesions. The most characteristic are diffuse exfoliative bullae seen in children with the scalded skin syndrome. Another exotoxin, TSS toxin-1, is responsible for toxic shock syndrome. Other extracellular products make *S. aureus* resistant to H_2O_2-mediated intracellular killing (catalase) and cause cell death (leukocidin, alpha toxin, beta toxin).

Staphylococcus epidermidis, a member of the flora of the skin and mucous membranes, for many years was thought to be a commensal. Although not as pathogenic as *S. aureus, S. epidermidis* causes infection in the presence of foreign bodies such as plastic catheters, ventricular shunts, and prosthetic heart valves and joints. *Staphylococcus aureus* and *S. epidermidis* are important surgical pathogens. *S. aureus* is a major cause of wound infection. It can cause infection of skin and soft tissues and abscesses of these and other structures. Bacteremia can lead to infection of heart valves and other deep structures such as bone, kidney, and brain.

Surgically important members of the genus *Streptococcus* include *S. pyogenes, S. pneumoniae,* and the viridans group which includes *S. mutans, S. mitior, S. salivarius, S. sanguis,* and *S. mulleri*. Streptococci are classified according to Lancefield classification (based on cell surface antigens) and ability to cause hemolysis on blood agar: alpha-hemolysis, a zone of green discoloration around colonies containing intact red blood cells; beta-hemolysis, complete clearing of the area around colonies and destruction of red blood cells; and gamma-hemolysis, no hemolysis. *S. pyogenes* is Lancefield group A and beta-hemolytic. Group A streptococci have cell surface components and extracellular products that inhibit host defenses or promote spread of the bacterium. The cell surface M protein and the capsule help streptococci resist phagocytosis. Hyaluronidase and streptokinase promote the spread of infection. Streptolysin O and streptolysin S are hemolysins. Streptococcal proteinase may be responsible for tissue invasion. Pyogenic exotoxins share many properties with endotoxins from gram negative bacteria.

Group A streptococci can cause infection of almost any organ, although the skin, subcutaneous tissues, and pharynx are by far the most frequently affected sites. *S. pyogenes* can cause pharyngitis giving rise to scarlet fever and rheumatic fever. Erysipelas is streptococcal cellulitis and lymphangitis and is a spreading infection with sharp, irregular, red borders. Erythrogenic toxin produced by the streptococci is responsible for the intense cutaneous erythema but is not found in all streptococcal infections.

Streptococci are important pathogens because of their ability to cause postoperative infections including cellulitis wound infection, endocarditis, urinary tract infection, and bacteremia. These bacteria can also cause primary necrotizing soft tissue infections and abscesses. In some hospitals streptococci other than group A streptococci are the principal streptococcal pathogens. *S. pyogenes* is currently an uncommon cause of necrotizing soft tissue infections. In the early part of this century and in the nineteenth century, streptococci were believed to be the most common cause of necrotizing soft tissue infection.

Enterococcus faecalis, E. faecium, and *E. durans* were formerly members of the genus *Streptococcus,* but recently a separate genus was recognized. They are part of the normal flora of the gastrointestinal tract and the vagina. They are commonly found in patients with peritoneal and pelvic infections as part of the mixed flora typical of these infections. Whether they are true pathogens is controversial. Enterococcal bacteremia has a poor prognosis in combination with intraabdominal or pelvic infection and is found most often in patients who have been hospitalized for a long time.

Aerobic and Facultatively Anaerobic Gram-negative Bacilli

During the last 40 to 50 years gram-negative bacilli, frequently in association with anaerobic bacteria, have replaced the gram-positive cocci as the cause of most surgical infections other than wound infection. There are numerous gram-negative rods that can cause human disease, but relatively few are of surgical significance. Their cell walls have common chemical constituents, most prominent of which is lipopolysaccharide or endotoxin which is responsible for most of the biologic effects of these bacteria. Some genera also have capsules. Most are members of the family Enterobacteriaceae, which are inhabitants of the gastrointestinal tract. The genera *Escherichia, Klebsiella, Proteus, Enterobacter, Serratia,* and *Providencia* frequently can be cultured from patients with intraabdominal and pelvic peritonitis and abscess, postoperative wound infection, pneumonia, and urinary tract infection.

The family Vibrionaceae includes *Vibrio* among its genera. Some *Vibrio* species are found in marine water and can cause bacteremia and necrotizing soft tissue infections in susceptible hosts, usually those with hepatic disease. They can be found in seafood and can cause bacteremia and death if the uncooked seafood is ingested.

The family Pseudomonadaceae is composed of obligate aerobes that lack the ability to ferment sugars as do members of the Enterobacteriaceae. *Pseudomonas aeruginosa* is the species responsible for most surgical infections. They cause infections similar to those of gram-negative enteric bacteria in association with gastrointestinal disease, pneumonia, urinary tract infection, and burns. They are frequently found in immunologically compromised patients, especially if they have been hospitalized for some time. They cause necrotizing infections, especially pneumonia and vasculitis. Ecthyma gangrenosum is the cutaneous manifestation of necrotizing vasculitis due to *Pseudomonas* bacteremia and is characterized by small, round necrotic skin lesions. Because of its resistance to single antibiotic therapy, *Pseudomonas* infections are frequently treated with a combination of two antibiotics.

Anaerobic Bacteria

Anaerobic bacteria require reduced oxygen tension for growth. They are found predominantly in the mouth, vagina, and gastrointestinal tract where they greatly outnumber the aerobic bacteria. Anaerobic bacteria, which are pathogenic, can tolerate an initial exposure of up to 3% oxygen. Virtually all anaerobic infections arise endogenously. A low oxidation-reduction potential is common to all anaerobic infection. Vascular disease, epinephrine injection, cold, shock, edema, trauma, operation, foreign bodies, malignancy, and gas production by microorganisms can lower the oxidation-reduction potential and predispose to infection with these organisms.

Most infections with anaerobic bacteria are mixed with facultative or aerobic bacteria. Aerobic or facultative bacteria make conditions favorable for anaerobic bacteria by using up available oxygen and lowering oxidation-reduction potential. The aerobic bacteria may also supply a growth factor necessary for another organism or may interfere with local or systemic host resistance.

Anaerobes such as the *Bacteroides fragilis* group have an endotoxin that differs chemically from the endotoxin of the enteric facultative or aerobic gram-negative bacilli and exhibits poor biologic activity. The cell wall of anaerobic bacteria is important in abscess formation.

The genus *Clostridium* is the most virulent of all anaerobes. *Clostridium* is widely distributed in soil and nature and can be cultured from the stool. *Clostridium* can cause necrotizing soft tissue. Clostridia produce exotoxins that can be shown to have biologic effects in cell culture, in animals. Their precise role in clinical disease is unclear. Exotoxins produced by these bacteria are responsible for most of the local and systemic manifestations. *C. perfringens, C. septicum,* and *C. novyi,* which can cause necrotizing infections, produce toxins that can destroy cell membranes and lyse red blood cells, collagenase, hyaluronidase, and other enzyme toxins that enhance spread of the infection throughout the tissues.

Clostridium perfringens and *C. difficile* both produce an enterotoxin. *C. difficile* causes pseudomembranous colitis and occurs in patients on antimicrobial therapy. It produces a cytotoxin that is cytopathic for almost all tissue culture cell lines. *C. tetani* and *C. botulinum* produce neurotoxins that cause muscle spasms and paralysis, respectively.

In the colon, the ratio of anaerobic bacteria to aerobic bacteria is between 300:1 and 1000:1. The most common pathogens in the colon are members of the genera *Bacteroides, Fusobacterium,* and *Peptostreptococcus.* Of these, *Bacteroides* is the most commonly cultured genus in patients with intraabdominal infections. The *Bacteroides fragilis* group, composed of *B. fragilis, B. thetaiotaomicron, B. distasonis, B. ovatus,* and *B. vulgatus,* accounts for most infections with this genus. Colonic anaerobes virtually never cause infections by themselves but only as part of a mixed flora often with facultative enteric gram-negative bacilli.

Fungi

Together with algae and protozoa, fungi are classified as protists, the most primitive eukaryotic organism. They grow as single-celled organisms, yeasts, or as long, branching filaments known as hyphae. Their cell wall shows little similarity to bacteria, but they have much in common with mammalian cells. Because of this and other structural and biochemical similarities to mammalian cells, they are not sensitive to antibacterial agents, and many antifungal agents are toxic to human cells.

Fungi can be grouped as primary pathogens, which can cause disease in individuals with intact host defenses, and opportunists, which cause disease in patients with compromised host defenses. Among the primary pathogens are *Histoplasma, Coccidioides,* and *Blastomyces*. *Candida, Cryptococcus, Aspergillus,* and the phycomycetes (*Mucor* and *Rhizopus*) cause most of the opportunistic infections.

In surgical patients opportunists cause most infections. *Candida albicans* and other *Candida* species are by far the most common. They cause infections in patients being treated with broad-spectrum antibiotics and in those receiving steroids and other immunosuppressive agents, in malnourished patients, in patients with malignant neoplasms, and in other compromised hosts. In these patients they can cause vascular catheter-related infections, bacteremia, intraabdominal infection, pneumonia, and urinary tract infection. These infections can be treated by stopping antibiotics, correcting host defenses, and therapy with amphotericin B or one of the azole antifungal agents.

Viruses

Viruses are distinguished by their small size, by their being obligate intracellular parasites, and by their having either ribonucleic acid (RNA) or deoxyribonucleic acid (DNA) but not both. Members of the herpes virus family, especially cytomegalovirus (CMV), herpes simplex virus, varicella-zoster virus, and Epstein-Barr virus can cause infections in recipients of organ transplants and other immunosuppressed patients.

CMV causes most viral infections in organ transplant recipients. In these patients CMV can cause ulcerative lesions of the gastrointestinal tract leading to bleeding or perforation for which operations might be required. Epstein-Barr virus is implicated as the cause of a polyclonal B-cell lymphoma in transplant recipients.

Hepatitis B virus, hepatitis C virus, and human immunodeficiency virus (HIV) are of importance to surgeons because of the possibility that they can become infected from patient exposure and that patients can potentially be infected from physicians who harbor these viruses. Hepatitis B prophylaxis is available should a health care worker sustain a percutaneous or permucosal exposure (Table 5-8).

Human Immunodeficiency Virus

An apparently new disease was first reported in December 1981, with the description of opportunist infections and Kaposi's sarcoma occurring in homosexual men. These men also had a profound depletion of T lymphocytes. Human immunodeficiency virus (HIV), the cause of acquired immunodeficiency syndrome (AIDS), was isolated in 1983. Since 1983, more than 200,000 individuals in the United States have developed AIDS.

HIV is a retrovirus of the lentivirus family. It is an RNA virus with a cylindrical core containing RNA, the RNA-dependent DNA polymerase (reverse transcriptase), and core proteins. The core is surrounded by a viral envelope derived from cells of the host nuclear membrane. A glycoprotein (GP-120) on the envelope has an affinity for the CD4 receptor on T lymphocytes. After binding of the GP-120 to the CD4 receptor on T-helper/inducer cells, the virus is internalized and uncoated. The reverse transcriptase synthesizes DNA complementary to viral RNA. This DNA is incorporated into the host genome leading to a lifelong infection.

Infected CD4-positive cells are not able to carry out their normal immune functions, which leads to opportunist infections in the

Table 5-8
Recommendations for Hepatitis B Prophylaxis After Percutaneous or Permucosal Exposure

HB Vaccination Status of Exposed Person	*HB_sAg Status of Source of Exposure*		
	HB_sAg-Positive	*HB_sAg-Negative*	*Untested or Unknown*
Unvaccinated	Give single doses of HBIG Initiate HB vaccine series	Initiate HB vaccine series	Initiate HB vaccine series
Previously vaccinated Known responder	Test exposed person for anti-HB_s. If anti-HB_s levels are adequate,* no treatment is needed; if they are inadequate, give an HB vaccine booster dose	No treated is needed	No treatment is needed
Known nonresponder	Give two doses of HBIG or one dose of HBIG plus one dose of HB vaccine	No treatment is needed	If source is at high risk for HB infection, consider proceeding as if it had been demonstrated to be HB_sAg-positive
Response unknown	Test exposed person for anti-HB_s. If anti-HB_s levels are adequate,* no treatment is needed; if they are inadequate, give one dose of HBIG plus an HB vaccine booster dose	No treatment is needed	Test exposed person for anti-HB_s. If anti-HB_s levels are adequate,* no treatment is needed; if they are inadequate, give an HB vaccine booster dose

*An adequate anti-HB_s level is $\geq$ 10 mU/mL, which is approximately equivalent to 10 sample ratio units (SRU) on radioimmunoassay or positive result on enzyme immunoassay.

HBIG = hepatitis B immune globulin; HB = hepatitis B

SOURCE: From Centers for Disease Control: Recommendations for protection against viral hepatitis. *MMWR* 34:313, 1985.

host and the development of Kaposi's sarcoma. The development of opportunist infections and tumors (Kaposi's sarcoma and lymphomas) is accompanied by a decrease in the number of T cells to less than 200/mm^3. There has recently been a move to define AIDS as all patients infected with HIV who have a CD4 count less than 200 cells/mm^3.

Epidemiology. The Centers for Disease Control (CDC) estimates that between 390,000 and 480,000 cases of AIDS will have been diagnosed in the United States by the end of 1993. Between 285,000 and 340,000 of these patients will have died. The CDC does not collect data on the number of individuals infected with HIV but estimates that for every person with AIDS there are approximately eight individuals with HIV infection who have not yet developed clinical AIDS. There are approximately 1,000,000 people infected with HIV in the United States. Approximately 8,000,000 to 10,000,000 people are infected with HIV worldwide.

HIV has been isolated from blood, semen, saliva, tears, vaginal secretions, alveolar fluid, cerebrospinal fluid, breast milk, synovial fluid, and amniotic fluid. Only blood and blood products, semen, vaginal secretions, and breast milk have been linked to transmission.

Groups at highest risk for HIV infection are (1) homosexual and bisexual men, (2) intravenous drug abusers, (3) persons with hemophilia or other coagulation disorders, (4) heterosexual contacts with the individuals in the three previous categories, and (5) children born to HIV-positive mothers. Recipients of transfusions of blood and blood products from HIV-positive donors have approximately a 95 percent chance of developing HIV infection, and over 4500 cases of transfusion-acquired AIDS have been reported to the CDC. This number could eventually reach 12,000 because of HIV-positive transfusion recipients who are thought to exist but who have not yet developed AIDS. Since testing blood donors for evidence of HIV became mandatory in 1985, transfusion-acquired HIV infection has been virtually eliminated.

HIV seroprevalence varies greatly depending on the specific population studied, the location of the population, sex, race and ethnic origin, and year of study. The lowest HIV seropositive rates are found among blood donors (0.0041 percent for repeat female donors, 0.0189 percent for repeat male donors) and are highest among hemophiliacs (50 to 100 percent positive), intravenous drug users (20 to 60 percent positive), homosexual and bisexual men (30 to 60 percent positive).

Relatively few seroprevalence studies have been done among hospital or emergency room patients. Seroprevalence rates differ greatly depending on the type of hospital studied ranging from 0.24 percent among 26,275 patients in the CDC sentinel hospital study to 9.1 percent at St. Paul-Ramsey Medical Center. One can expect that hospital type, location, and specific hospital population will greatly affect HIV-seropositivity rates. According to a later sentinel hospital study of 89,547 blood specimens from hospitalized patients conducted by the CDC, the overall seropositivity was 1.3 percent, but the HIV-seropositive rate of individual hospitals ranged from 0.1 to 7.8 percent.

Serologic Events. Patients infected with HIV develop viremia accompanied by a generalized lymphadenopathy, fever, and malaise. Approximately 6 to 12 weeks after infection antibody to HIV develops. During this time the viral titer in blood decreases markedly from 10^4/mL to 10 to 100/mL. A low level of virus persists until the patient develops AIDS approximately 7 to 9 years after infection. When AIDS develops, the virus titer rapidly increases to a level of 10^4/mL. Since serologic testing examines antibody to HIV, it is seldom positive before 12 weeks after infection. During this early period ("the window") it is possible for patients to have circulating virus and be potentially infectious to those around them and yet test negative for HIV.

Surgery in HIV-Infected Individuals. While surgeons do not primarily care for individuals with HIV infection and AIDS, patients with this infection may require operation for unrelated reasons, for diagnosis of an infection, and for treatment of surgical complications of AIDS. Patients with HIV infection and AIDS generally do not require any extra preoperative preparation because of their infection. Malnutrition associated with HIV infection may require correction of the undernourished state if time permits. Perioperative antimicrobial therapy is given for the same indications as patients without HIV infections. These patients generally do not have difficulty with wound healing and do not have a higher rate of wound infections or other postoperative hospital-acquired infections. The use of drains and open wounds requires extra cautions to avoid contamination with HIV-infected blood and other body fluids.

Patients with HIV infection and AIDS may require surgery for problems related to their viral illness or to other infectious or neoplastic causes. These problems include (1) peritonitis due to bowel perforation which occurs as a result of CMV infection; (2) gastrointestinal obstruction due to Kaposi's sarcoma or lymphoma of the gastrointestinal tract; (3) gastrointestinal hemorrhage due to CMV, lymphoma, or Kaposi's sarcoma; and (4) intraabdominal or retroperitoneal infections by mycobacteria and other opportunistic organisms.

HIV and AIDS in Health Care Workers. Over 7250 health care workers with AIDS have been reported to the CDC. There may be more than 50,000 health care workers infected with HIV based on an estimate of eight persons infected with HIV for every patient with AIDS.

Health care workers with AIDS comprise approximately 5 percent of the total number of patients with AIDS in the United States. Approximately 5.7 percent of the labor force in the United States is comprised of health care workers. Most health care workers with AIDS are homosexual or bisexual men (Table 5-9). Significantly fewer, however, are intravenous drug abusers. A large

Table 5-9
Comparison of Health Care Workers and Non-Health Care Workers with AIDS by Transmission Category

Transmission Category	*Health Care Workers, %*	*Non-Health Care Workers, %*
Male homosexual or bisexual contact	71.8	61.1*
Heterosexual intravenous drug user	6.6	21.1*
Male homosexual or bisexual contact and intravenous drug user	7.4	7.0
Heterosexual contact	5.3	4.5
Recipient of blood or blood product	3.0	3.3
Other	$<$1.0	0.0
Undetermined	5.9	2.9*

*$p < 0.001$.

SOURCE: Howard RJ (ed): *Infections Risks in Surgery*, Norwalk, CT, Appleton & Lange, 1991, p 66, with permission.

"undetermined" category accounts for 5.9 percent of health care workers with AIDS. On further examination, one-half of these patients can be classified under one of the other risk factors, one-fourth are dead or refused to be interviewed, and the remaining one-fourth are still being investigated.

As of October 1, 1992, 96 health care workers have developed HIV infection as a result of exposure to blood from HIV-infected patients. Thirty-one of the 96 health care workers had the patient-acquired infection confirmed by being seronegative at the time of exposure and becoming seropositive after exposure. Six of these 31 health care workers have developed AIDS. Sixty-five health care workers did not have a blood specimen obtained at the time of exposure, but other risk factors were excluded. Most of these 96 individuals are nurses or technicians. Two are surgeons. Not all health care workers with occupationally acquired HIV infection may be included in the CDC data set.

Risk of HIV Seroconversion in Health Care Workers. Fourteen prospective studies have examined the actual risk of health care workers becoming infected with HIV after sustaining a percutaneous exposure to blood or blood-containing body fluids from patients with HIV infection. Six (0.29 percent per exposure) of 1948 health care workers who sustained 2042 percutaneous exposures seroconverted to HIV. On the other hand, none of 668 health care workers in 12 reports who sustained a total of 1051 mucous membrane exposures to blood or blood-containing body fluids from HIV-infected patients seroconverted.

Surgeons are frequently exposed to patient's blood and other body fluids, but until recently there were no studies documenting the actual risk of blood exposure to operating room personnel. Most exposures are to the skin and can be decreased by wearing two pairs of gloves and face shields. Survey studies place the percutaneous injury rate high with injuries occurring in 5.6 percent of operations and with 86 percent of surgeons reporting one percutaneous injury per year. None of these studies attempted to assess the risk of transmission of HIV or hepatitis or the amount of blood transferred to operating room personnel during percutaneous injury.

Prevention of Blood-borne Infections in Health Care Workers. Beginning in 1983, the CDC began issuing guidelines designed to minimize the risk of transmission of HIV in the health care setting. In 1987, the CDC issued new guidelines, which have come to be called "universal precautions" (Table 5-10). These guidelines have been updated and extended but not substantially altered. They are applicable to clinical and laboratory staffs, emergency service personnel, and to health care workers performing invasive procedures as well as to those who are not included in direct patient care (e.g., housekeeping personnel, kitchen staff, and laundry workers). Although universal precautions were issued to reduce the transmission of HIV in health care settings, they are also appropriate for reducing the transmission of other blood-borne viruses including hepatitis B (HBV); non-A, non-B hepatitis; and hepatitis C (HCV).

The intent of the CDC guidelines is that all patients should be regarded as potentially harboring blood-borne pathogens, because the medical history, physical examination, and laboratory testing cannot identify all patients infected with HIV or other blood-borne pathogens and because in emergencies there may be no time for testing patients for various pathogens. Since all patients should be treated alike (as if they potentially have a blood-borne infection), there is no need for testing patients because it will not alter health care worker behavior.

Table 5-10
Guidelines to Prevent Transmission of HIV

Universal Precautions

1. All health care workers should use appropriate barrier precautions routinely to prevent skin and mucous membrane exposure when contact with blood or other body fluids of any patient is anticipated. Gloves should be worn for touching blood and body fluids, mucous membranes, or nonintact skin of all patients; for handling items or surfaces soiled with blood or body fluids; and for performing venipuncture and other vascular-access procedures. Gloves should be changed after contact with each patient. During procedures that are likely to generate aerosolized droplets of blood or other body fluids, masks and protective eyewear or face shields should be worn to prevent exposure of mucous membranes of the mouth, nose, and eyes. Gowns or aprons should be worn during procedures that are likely to generate splashes of blood or other body fluids.
2. Hands and other skin surfaces should be washed immediately and thoroughly if contaminated with blood or other body fluids. Hands should be washed immediately after gloves are removed.
3. All health care workers should take precautions to prevent injuries caused by needles, scalpels, and other sharp instruments or devices during procedures; when cleaning used instruments; during disposal of used needles; and when handling sharp instruments after procedures. To prevent needlestick injuries, needles should not be recapped, purposely bent or broken by hand, removed from disposable syringes, or otherwise manipulated by hand. After they are used, disposable syringes and needles, scalpel blades, and other sharp items should be placed in puncture-resistant containers for disposal; the puncture-resistant containers should be located as close as practical to the area of use. Large-bore reusable needles should be placed in a puncture-resistant container for transport to the reprocessing area.
4. Although saliva has not been implicated in HIV transmission, to minimize the need for emergency mouth-to-mouth resuscitation, mouth-pieces, resuscitation bags, or other ventilation devices should be available for use in areas in which the need for resuscitation is predictable.
5. Health care workers who have exudative lesions or weeping dermatitis should refrain from all direct patient care and from handling patient care equipment until condition resolves.
6. Pregnant health care workers are not known to be at greater risk for contracting HIV infection than health care workers who are not pregnant; however, if a health care worker acquires HIV infection during pregnancy, the infant is at risk for infection resulting from perinatal transmission. Because of this risk, pregnant health care workers should be especially familiar with and strictly adhere to precautions to minimize the risk of HIV transmission.

Additional Precautions for Invasive Procedures

1. All health care workers who participate in invasive procedures must use appropriate barrier precautions routinely to prevent skin and mucous membrane contact with blood and other body fluids of all patients. Gloves and surgical masks must be worn for all invasive procedures. Protective eyewear or face shields should be worn for procedures that commonly result in the generation of aerosolized droplets, splashing of blood or other body fluids, or the generation of bone chips. Gowns or aprons made of materials that provide an effective barrier should be worn during invasive procedures that are likely to result in the splashing of blood or other body fluids. All health care workers who perform or assist in vaginal or cesarean deliveries should wear gloves and gowns when handling the placenta or the infant until blood and amniotic fluid have been removed from the infant's skin and should wear gloves during postdelivery care of the umbilical cord.
2. If a glove is torn or a needlestick or other injury occurs, the glove should be removed and a new glove used as promptly as patient safety permits; the needle or instrument involved in the incident should also be removed from the sterile field.

SOURCE: Centers for Disease Control: Recommendations for prevention of HIV transmission in health-care settings. *MMWR* 36(2S):1S, 1987.

Compliance with universal precautions has been examined in the emergency room and hospital environment. Compliance with universal precautions was only 18 percent in a large inner-city hospital emergency room, and it fell to 5 percent if the patient was bleeding from an external injury. The rates of noncompliance with universal precautions are reported to be 74 percent in the surgical intensive care unit and 34 percent on the surgical wards. The noncompliance rate fell to 43 percent in the intensive care unit after an educational program about universal precautions, but it did not change on the surgical wards. On the other hand, Wong and associates found the frequency of use of barrier precautions increased from 54 to 73 percent and blood exposures decreased after universal precautions were put into effect. In the 1990s, it is unacceptable not to use universal precautions.

Testing Patients for Blood-borne Pathogens. Ever since serologic testing for antibodies to HIV became available in 1985, there has been heated discussion among physicians, medical ethicists, and lay groups about the effectiveness, ethics, and social consequences of testing patients (Table 5-11). Surgeons have generally favored patient testing so that they could take special precautions with HIV-positive patients. Some surgeons have developed special protocols for the operating room believing universal precautions to be insufficient for that high-risk environment. Others have argued against testing.

The CDC does not recommend routine HIV testing of all patients. HIV testing of patients is recommended for management of health care workers who sustain parenteral or mucous membrane exposure to blood or other body fluids from a patient, for patient diagnosis and management, and for counseling associated with efforts to prevent and control HIV transmission in the community.

If hospitals, physicians, or other health care agencies choose to perform HIV testing, the CDC advocates certain principles: (1) obtain consent for testing, (2) inform patients of results and provide counseling for seropositive patients, (3) ensure confidentiality, (4) ensure that seropositive patients will not receive compromised care, and (5) prospectively evaluate the efficacy of the program in reducing the incidence of exposure of health care workers to blood or other body fluids of patients who are infected with HIV. Most states have laws regulating testing of patients for HIV. Many of these laws require written informed consent of the patient with pretest and posttest counseling for both HIV-positive and HIV-negative patients.

Management of Health Care Workers Exposed to Patients' Blood and Other Body Fluids. The CDC and others have issued recommendations for the management of health care workers exposed to patient blood and other body fluids. Hospitals, physicians' offices, and other employers of health care workers should establish a systematic approach for managing adverse exposures that is consistent with CDC and Department of Labor guidelines and state laws. The Department of Labor and CDC have published detailed employer responsibilities in protecting workers from acquisition of blood-borne diseases in the workplace. Employers should develop standard operating procedures for all activities having the potential for exposure and should provide an initial and periodic workers education program.

The CDC recommends that if an exposure occurs, a blood sample should be drawn after consent is obtained from the individual from whom the exposure occurred and tested for hepatitis B surface antigen (HBsAg) and antibody to HIV. Local laws regarding consent for testing source individuals should be followed. Policies should be available for testing source individuals when consent cannot be obtained (e.g., an unconscious patient). Pretest counseling, posttest counseling, and referral for treatment, if appropriate, of the source individual should be provided.

HIV Postexposure Management. If a health care worker is exposed percutaneously or by a splash to the eye or mucous membrane from a patient who has HIV infection, AIDS, or who refuses to be tested, the worker should be counseled regarding the risk of infection and be evaluated clinically and serologically for evidence of HIV infection as soon as possible after the exposure. The worker should be advised to report and seek medical evaluation for any acute febrile illness that occurs within 12 weeks after exposure. Following the initial test at the time of exposure, seronegative workers should be retested 6 weeks, 12 weeks, and 6 months

Table 5-11
Arguments for and Against Testing of Patients for Blood-Borne Pathogens, Especially HIV

For	*Against*
1. Physicians have a right to know of infections patients may have	1. Confidentiality of test results cannot be maintained
2. Knowing will allow physicians to take proper precautions	2. Informed consent is unlikely to be obtained
3. Valuable epidemiologic data can be collected	3. Psychological and social consequences of being found to be seropositive can be devastating
4. Treatment of infected patients can be instituted	4. Insurance may be impossible to obtain for seropositive patients
5. Others at risk (e.g., sexual partners, needle sharers) can be warned or appropriate precautions can be taken	5. A seronegative patient does not assure the physician the patient cannot transmit disease because it takes from 2 weeks to 6 months, and even longer in some cases to develop HIV antibodies
6. Universal precautions and additional appropriate precautions—especially in the operating room—are too cumbersome and impractical to be taken for every patient. Knowing who harbors disease would allow intense, focused precautions to be taken for individuals most at risk of spreading infections	6. There are some false-positive tests for HIV and false-negative tests for HIV
7. While universal precautions are to be taken for all patients, additional precautions are taken for patients known to be HIV-, HBsAg-, or HCV-positive	7. Seropositive patients will likely be denied medical and dental care
8. No matter how much a surgeon says only universal precautions alone are sufficient, his or her behavior is likely to be different when operating on seropositive patients, i.e., he or she is likely to take additional care, move more slowly and deliberately	8. For low-prevalence populations the cost of screening and confirmatory tests is great for every positive test result
9. HIV testing is currently so reliable that false-positive tests are extremely unlikely	9. If the health care worker adheres to universal precautions, there is no need for testing because it will not change behavior
	10. At least one study has shown that knowing a person is seropositive does not affect the rate of percutaneous blood exposure
	11. A false sense of security may be instilled in caring for seronegative patients who may still transmit HIV and other blood-borne pathogens

after exposure to determine whether transmission has occurred. During this period the worker should refrain from blood or semen donation and should use appropriate protection during sexual intercourse. If the source individual is found to be seronegative, baseline testing of the exposed worker with follow-up 12 weeks later may be performed if desired or recommended by the health care provider.

Zidovudine (AZT) is used to treat patients with HIV infection and has been proposed as chemoprophylaxis to prevent occupational infection in health care workers. There are no data that indicate prophylactic AZT therapy can prevent HIV infection in humans, although AZT given immediately after exposure can alter the course of animal retroviral (not HIV) infection. There are no clear indications for AZT prophylaxis, but some institutions recommend it for employees sustaining massive exposures (e.g., injections or transfusions of HIV-containing blood), endorse it for serious parenteral exposures (e.g., deep needlesticks), and have it available but do not recommend it for less severe exposure. The final decision is left to the employee following counseling about the toxicity and applicable data. AZT should be given within 24 h, preferably as soon as possible, after exposure. If the HIV status of the source patient is unknown, AZT therapy can be begun until test results are available. A dilemma arises when the source individual refuses to be tested.

AZT prophylaxis protocols generally advise administering 200 mg AZT every 4 h for 28 to 42 days. Some protocols skip the 4 A.M. dose. Since an adverse exposure can occur anytime, AZT should be available 24 hours a day.

Transmission of Blood-borne Pathogens From Health Care Workers to Patients. Blood-borne pathogens can also be transmitted from health care workers to patients. HIV, HBV, and non-A, non-B hepatitis (HCV) can potentially be transmitted from surgeons to patient during invasive procedures when they sustain a percutaneous injury with a needle or sharp instrument which then recontacts the patient. Only HBV has been demonstrated to be transmitted from physicians to patients. One dentist has transmitted HIV to five patients. There are no other reports of transmission of HIV from a health care worker to a patient. There are four reports following patients of surgeons with AIDS. None of 767 serologically tested patients developed HIV infection as a result of being cared for by HIV-infected surgeons. None of more than 1000 patients of another surgeon who died of AIDS developed HIV infection, but there is as yet no published report. More than 9000 patients cared for by more than 75 health care workers with AIDS have been followed, and no cases of transmission by health care worker to patient were reported. Approximately 60 of the 9000 patients were HIV-positive, but they were positive before being cared for by the health care worker, had other risk factors, or transmission from the health care worker was excluded.

Management of the HIV- or HB_sAG-Positive Health Care Worker. The report of a dentist passing HIV to his patients sparked considerable discussion in the scientific and popular press about the HIV-positive health care worker, especially surgeons and dentists since they were most likely to participate in invasive procedures. The CDC first issued guidelines for the management of HIV-infected personnel in 1985. It subsequently issued guidelines for management of HIV-infected health care workers who participate in invasive procedures. In its early guidelines the CDC recommended that health care personnel who are otherwise fit for duty and who do not participate in invasive procedures be allowed to perform their regular duties. In its subsequent guidelines the CDC recommended that HIV-infected personnel who do participate in invasive procedures be evaluated on a case-by-case basis. These recommendations were consolidated in 1987 with the suggestion that whether health care workers could perform their regular duties be decided on an individual basis.

Following the report of transmission of HIV by a dentist, the CDC issued a subsequent set of recommendations. Defining "exposure-prone" procedures has met with resistance from the medical community. These recommendations do not require testing of health care workers for HIV or HBV but suggest that they should be tested voluntarily. Health care workers who are infected with HIV or HBV should not perform exposure-prone procedures unless they have sought counsel from an expert panel, and their patients should be informed of their seropositivity. The recommendations specify the composition of the panel but provide no guidelines for the panel on which to base their decisions.

ANTIMICROBIAL THERAPY

The use of antimicrobials in treating surgical infections does not differ fundamentally from antimicrobial usage in general medicine. The same basic considerations apply in treating all infections. One difference, however, is that antimicrobial therapy is only an adjunct in treating surgical infection; operative treatment (or percutaneous radiologic drainage of infected material) is the main method of therapy. The goal of antimicrobial therapy is to prevent or treat infection by reducing or eliminating pathogenic organisms until the host's own defenses can get rid of the last pathogens.

The basic considerations in antimicrobial therapy are efficacy, toxicity, and cost. Effectiveness is the most important consideration in choosing antimicrobial therapy. Effective antimicrobial agents must be active against the pathogens causing the infection and must be able to reach the site of infection in adequate concentrations.

All antibiotics have potential toxicity. Toxic effects may be idiosyncratic such as allergy or the rare instance of bone marrow aplasia caused by chloramphenicol or result in damage to tissues and organs as renal or ototoxicity seen with the aminoglycosides or amphotericin B. Antimicrobial agents also exert selective pressures on the microbial ecology of the hospital that lead to resistant microbes, a problem that can occur especially in intensive care unit settings.

Cost is the final consideration in the selection of antimicrobial agents. Determining antimicrobial costs includes more than just the cost of the drug. Drug administration charges, nursing time, intravenous fluid and lines, and monitoring costs must also be added to drug costs. The increased hospital time that occurs when an inexpensive but also less effective agent is used should also be included in costs. Obviously an inexpensive agent that is not effective or that causes more toxicity ultimately becomes a more expensive antimicrobial.

Distribution of Antimicrobial Agents

Successful treatment of localized infections with systemic antimicrobial agents requires that an adequate concentration of drug be delivered to the site of infection. Ideally the tissue concentration of antibiotics should exceed the minimum inhibitory concentration. Tissue penetration depends in part on protein binding of antibiotics. Only the unbound form of antibiotics will pass through the capillary wall or act to inhibit bacterial growth. Therapeutic outcome, on the other hand, appears uncorrelated with protein affinity, presumably because protein binding is easily reversible. Lipid solubility of antibiotics is also an important factor in tissue penetration. It determines the ability of antibiotics to pass through membranes by nonionic diffusion or into wounds, bone, cerebrospinal fluid, the eye, endolymph of the ear, vegetations of bacterial endocarditis, and abscesses.

Blood. Rapidity of excretion and protein binding are two main determinants of blood concentration of antimicrobial agents. Protein binding affects the rapidity of excretion. Antibiotics that are highly protein bound are not excreted as rapidly as those with a low binding affinity and thus have longer half-lives. Therefore, highly protein bound antibiotics generally do not have to be given as frequently as those with low protein binding. Efficacy of penicillins, cephalosporins, and other antibiotics that affect bacterial cell wall synthesis depends on the time during which serum levels are above the minimum inhibitory concentrations rather than a peak serum concentration. Efficacy of aminoglycosides, on the other hand, is related to achieving peak serum concentrations that are four to eight times the minimum inhibitory concentration. Monitoring of serum aminoglycoside concentrations is usually necessary to ensure that these concentrations have been achieved; patients more commonly have subtherapeutic levels rather than toxic levels. On the other hand, some antimicrobial agents such as nitrofurantoin and norfloxacin are excreted so rapidly in the urine that they never achieve blood (or tissue) levels sufficient to achieve effective antibacterial concentrations. They do, however, reach high urinary concentrations and are effective agents for treating urinary tract infections.

Urine. Most commonly used antibiotics (sulfonamides, penicillins, cephalosporins, aminoglycosides, tetracyclines, quinolones, azoles) are excreted principally in the urine and achieve high urinary concentrations—up to 50 to 200 times their serum concentration. Notable exceptions are erythromycin and chloramphenicol. Since concentrating ability is severely compromised in patients with renal disease, infections of the urinary tract are more difficult to treat in these patients. The pH of urine can be changed to facilitate antibiotic activity. For instance aminoglycosides are more active in an alkaline medium, whereas other urinary antibacterial agents [tetracyclines, nitrofurantoin, methenamine (Mandelamine)] are more active in an acidic environment. Fortunately, the antimicrobials most commonly used to treat urinary tract infections have antimicrobial activity across a broad pH range.

Bile. Besides urine, only bile regularly has concentrations of antibiotics higher than found in serum. The biliary concentrations of many of the penicillins especially nafcillin, piperacillin, mezlocillin, and azlocillin; cephalosporins especially cefazolin, cefamandole, ceforanide, cefoxitin, cefoperazone, and cefadroxil; tetracyclines; and clindamycin frequently are several times their serum contractions. Nafcillin and rifampin achieve biliary concentrations 20 to 100 times that of serum. Aminoglycoside antibiotics enter bile less well, especially in the presence of liver disease. Their biliary concentrations are usually lower than serum levels.

Interstitial Fluid and Tissue. High, prolonged serum concentration and low protein binding favor diffusion of antibiotics from serum into extravascular tissues. Absolute tissue levels may not accurately reflect the therapeutic potential of the antibiotic, however, because the agent may be tightly bound to tissue and thus be unavailable for binding to bacteria.

Abscesses. There are few data of clinical relevance concerning the distribution of antibiotics into abscesses. The generalization that no antibiotics penetrate abscesses is not true. While the penicillins, cephalosporins, and some other antibiotics penetrate mature abscesses poorly, others such as metronidazole, chloramphenicol, and clindamycin can achieve inhibitory concentrations in abscesses.

A separate problem is whether, after penetration, an antibiotic can retain its antimicrobial efficacy under the conditions that exist in an abscess. The acidic pH, low redox potential, and the large numbers of microbial and tissue products that can bind antibiotics all serve to reduce antimicrobial efficacy. Multiple types of bacteria within an abscess make it more likely that one type will inactivate an agent effective against it or another bacteria. The lack of efficacy of penicillins and cephalosporins in treating most abscesses may be due to high concentrations of beta lactamases that accumulate there. Metronidazole and clindamycin can both enter abscesses and retain antibacterial activity in such environments. But these antibiotics are not effective against the aerobic gram-negative bacteria that are usually present together with the anaerobic bacteria against which they are effective, so the abscess usually persists.

An additional reason that antibiotics alone are seldom effective in treating abscesses is that antibiotics are most effective against actively metabolizing, rapidly dividing bacteria. Conditions in abscesses are usually unfavorable for such active metabolic activity, so the antibiotic is not able to enter and be active against the bacteria.

For all these reasons antibiotics alone should not be relied on to treat most abscesses. Despite occasional reports of success with such treatment, drainage remains the mainstay of abscess treatment.

Use of Antibiotics in Surgery

Prophylactic Antibiotics. Antibiotics are frequently administered prophylactically to patients undergoing operation to prevent wound infection where the likelihood of infection is high (when the tissues have been exposed to bacteria such as occurs during colon surgery) or where the consequences of infection are great even though the risk of infection is low (when a prosthetic device is implanted). The use of prophylactic antibiotics to prevent wound infection have been discussed in the section on wound infection. Antibiotic prophylaxis should also be administered to many patients with previously placed prosthetic devices such as cardiac valves who are having operations or dental procedures.

Therapeutic Use of Antibiotics. Many infections can be successfully treated with oral antibiotics on an outpatient basis. Severe surgical infections should be treated with intravenous antibiotics. Initial antibiotic therapy is usually empiric since it should be postponed until microbiologic studies are complete (Table 5-12). Antibiotic therapy should generally be initiated before cultures are obtained in patients with peritonitis, abscesses, and necrotizing soft tissue infections. Since cultures are usually obtained promptly during operative procedures or when percutaneous drainage has been performed, it is unlikely that prior antibiotic therapy will affect culture results for most surgical infections.

Empiric Therapy. Rational empiric antibiotic therapy requires familiarity with the microbes most likely to cause infection at the involved site and antibiotic susceptibility patterns in the hospital or unit (e.g., intensive care unit). Intraabdominal surgical infections

Table 5-12
Antimicrobial Drugs of Choice

Infecting Organism	*Drug of Choice*	*Alternative Drugs*
Gram-Positive Cocci		
Enterococcus		
Endocarditis[1] or other severe infection	Penicillin G or ampicillin with gentamicin	Vancomycin with gentamicin
Uncomplicated urinary tract infection[2]	Ampicillin or amoxicillin	Norfloxacin;[3] ciprofloxacin;[3] nitrofurantoin
S. aureus or *epidermidis**		
Non-penicillinase-producing	Penicillin G or V[4]	A cephalosporin;[5,6] vancomycin; imipenem; clindamycin; ciprofloxacin[3]
Penicillinase-producing	A penicillinase-resistant penicillin[7]	A cephalosporin;[5,6] vancomycin; amoxicillin-clavulanic acid; ticarcillin-clavulanic acid; ampicillin-sulbactam; impenem; clindamycin; ciprofloxacin[3]
Methicillin-resistant[8]	Vancomycin, with or without gentamicin and/or rifampin	Trimethoprim-sulfamethoxazole; ciprofloxacin[3]
S. pyogenes Groups C and G	Penicillin G or V[4]	An erythromycin;[9] a (Group A) and cephalosporin;[5,6] vancomycin; clindamycin
Streptococcus, Group B	Penicillin G or ampicillin	A cephalosporin;[5,6] vancomycin; an erythromycin
Streptococcus, viridans group[1]	Penicillin G with or without gentamicin	A cephalosporin;[5,6] vancomycin
S. bovis[1]	Penicillin G	A cephalosporin;[5,6] vancomycin
Streptococcus, anaerobic or *Peptostreptococcus*	Penicillin G	Clindamycin; a cephalosporin;[5,6] vancomycin
S. pneumoniae[10,*] (pneumococcus)	Penicillin G or V[4]	An erythromycin;[9] a cephalosporin;[5,6] chloramphenicol;[11] vancomycin
Gram-Negative Cocci		
*N. gonorrhoeae** (gonococcus)	Ceftriaxone[5]	Spectinomycin; ciprofloxacin;[3] penicillin G; amoxicillin with probenecid; cefoxitin;[5] trimethoprim-sulfamethoxazole chloramphenicol[11]
Gram-Positive Bacilli		
C. perfringens[13]	Penicillin G	Chloramphenicol;[11] metronidazole; clindamycin; a tetracycline[12]
C. tetani[14]	Penicillin G	A tetracycline[12]
C. difficile	Vancomycin	Metronidazole; bacitracin
Listeria monocytogenes	Ampicillin with or without gentamicin	Trimethoprim-sulfamethoxazole
Enteric Gram-Negative Bacilli		
*Bacteroides**		
Oropharyngeal strains	Penicillin G[15]	Clindamycin; cefoxitin;[5] metronidazole; chloramphenicol;[11] cefotetan[5]
Gastrointestinal strains[16]	Metronidazole	Clindamycin; cefoxitin;[5] chloramphenicol;[11] mezlocillin, ticarcillin, or piperacillin; imipenem; ticarcillin-clavulanic acid; ampicillin-sulbactam; cefotetan[5]
*Campylobacter jejuni**	Ciprofloxacin[3] or erythromycin	A tetracycline;[12] gentamicin
*Enterobacter**	Cefotaxime,[5,17] ceftizoxime,[5,17] or ceftriaxone[5,17]	Gentamicin, tobramycin, or amikacin; imipenem;[17] carbenicillin,[18] ticarcillin,[18] mezlocillin,[18] piperacillin,[18] or azlocillin;[18] aztreonam;[17] ceftazidime;[5,17] trimethoprim-sulfamethoxazole; ciprofloxacin;[3] norfloxacin;[3,19] chloramphenicol[11]
Escherichia coli[20,*]	A cephalosporin[5,6,17]	Ampicillin[21] with or without gentamicin, tobramycin, or amikacin; carbenicillin,[18] ticarcillin,[18] mezlocillin,[18] piperacillin,[18] or azlocillin;[18] gentamicin, tobramycin, or amikacin; amoxicillin-clavulanic acid;[17] ticarcillin-clavulanic acid;[18] ampicillin-sulbactam;[17] trimethoprim-sulfamethoxazole; imipenem;[17] a tetracycline;[12] ciprofloxacin;[3] norfloxacin;[3,14] chloramphenicol[11]
Klebsiella pneumoniae[20,*]	A cephalosporin[5,6,17]	Gentamicin, tobramycin, or amikacin; amoxicillin-clavulanic acid;[17] ticarcillin-clavulanic acid;[18] ampicillin-sulbactam;[17] trimethoprim-sulfamethoxazole; imipenem;[17] aztreonam;[17] a tetracycline;[12] ciprofloxacin;[3] norfloxacin;[3,23] chloramphenicol;[11] mezlocillin[24] or piperacillin[23]

Table 5-12
Antimicrobial Drugs of Choice ***(cont.)***

Infecting Organism	*Drug of Choice*	*Alternative Drugs*
Enteric Gram-Negative Bacilli (cont.)		
Proteus mirabilis[20,]*	Ampicillin[22]	A cephalosporin;[5,6,17] carbenicillin,[18] ticarcillin,[18] mezlocillin,[18] piperacillin,[18] or azlocillin;[18] gentamicin, tobramycin, or amikacin; trimethoprim-sulfamethoxazole; imipenem;[17] aztreonam;[17] ciprofloxacin;[3] norfloxacin;[3,19] chloramphenicol[11]
*Proteus,** indole-positive (including *Providencia rettgeri, Morganella morganii,* and *Proteus vulgaris*)	cefotaxime,[5,17] ceftizoxime,[5,17] or ceftriaxone[5,17]	Gentamicin, tobramycin, or amikacin; carbenicillin,[18] ticarcillin,[18] mezlocillin,[18] piperacillin,[18] or azlocillin;[18] amoxicillin-clavulanic acid;[17] ticarcillin-clavulanic acid;[18] ampicillin-sulbactam;[17] imipenem;[17] aztreonam;[17] ceftazidime;[5,17] trimethoprim-sulfamethoxazole; a tetracycline;[12] ciprofloxacin;[3] norfloxacin;[3,19] chloramphenicol[11]
*Providencia stuartii**	Cefotaxime,[5,17] ceftizoxime,[5,17] or ceftriaxone[5,17]	Imipenem;[17] ticarcillin-clavulanic acid;[18] gentamicin, tobramycin, or amikacin; carbenicillin,[18] ticarcillin,[18] mezlocillin,[18] piperacillin,[18] or azlocillin;[18] aztreonam;[17] ceftazidime;[5,17] trimethoprim-sulfamethoxazole; ciprofloxacin;[3] norfloxacin;[3,19] chloramphenicol[11]
*Serratia**	Cefotaxime,[5,23] ceftizoxime,[5,23] ceftriaxone[5,23]	Gentamicin or amikacin; or imipenem;[23] aztreonam;[23] ceftazidime;[23] trimethoprim-sulfamethoxazole; carbenicillin,[23] ticarcillin,[24] mezlocillin,[24] piperacillin,[24] or azlocillin;[24] ciprofloxacin;[3] norfloxacin[3,19]
Other Gram-Negative Bacilli		
*Acinetobacter**	Imipenem[17]	Tobramycin, gentamicin, or amikacin; carbenicillin,[18] ticarcillin,[18] mezlocillin,[18] piperacillin,[18] or azlocillin;[18] trimethoprim-sulfamethoxazole; minocycline;[12] doxycycline[12]
*Aeromonas**	Trimethoprim-sulfamethoxazole	Gentamicin or tobramycin; imipenem; a tetracycline[12]
*Eikenella corrodens**	Ampicillin	An erythromycin; a tetracycline;[12] amoxicillin-clavulanic acid; ampicillin sulbactam
*Fusobacterium**	Penicillin G	Metronidazole; clindamycin; chloramphenicol[11]
*P. aeruginosa**		
Urinary tract infection	Carbenicillin or ticarcillin	Piperacillin, mezlocillin, or azlocillin; ceftazidime;[5] imipenem; aztreonam; gentamicin; tobramycin; amikacin; norfloxacin;[3] ciprofloxacin[3]
Other infections	Carbenicillin, ticarcillin, mezlocillin, piperacillin, or azlocillin plus tobramycin, gentamicin, or amikacin[25]	Tobramycin, gentamicin, or amikacin with ceftazidime,[5] imipenem, or aztreonam; ciprofloxacin[3]
P. cepacia	Trimethoprim-sulfamethoxazole	Chloramphenicol;[11] ceftazidime;[5] imipenem
Vibrio vulnificus	A tetracycline[12]	Penicillin G
*Xanthomonas maltophilia** (*P. maltophilia*)	Trimethoprim-sulfamethoxazole	Minocycline;[2] ceftazidime;[5] ciprofloxacin[3]
Acid-Fast Bacilli		
Mycobacterium tuberculosis	Isoniazid with rifampin[26] with or without pyrazinamide	Ethambutol; streptomycin;[11] cycloserine;[11] ethionamide;[11] kanamycin;[11] capreomycin[11]
Mycobacterium kansasii	Isoniazid with rifampin with or without ethambutol or streptomycin[11]	Ethionamide;[11] cycloserine[11]
Mycobacterium avium complex[27]	Rifampin with ethambutol, ciprofloxacin,[3] and clofazimine with or without amikacin[11]	Ethionamide;[11] cycloserine;[11] rifabutin (ansamycin)[28]; imipenem
Mycobacterium fortuitum complex	Amikacin[11] and doxycycline[12]	Cefoxitin;[5] rifampin; and erythromycin; a sulfonamide
Mycobacterium marinum (balnei)[29]	Minocycline[12]	Trimethoprim-sulfamethoxazole; rifampin; cycloserine[11]
Mycobacterium leprae (leprosy)	Dapsone with rifampin with or without clofazimine	Ethionamide;[11] protionamide[28]
Actinomycetes		
Actinomyces israelii (actinomycesis)	Penicillin G	A tetracycline[12]
Chlamydia pneumoniae (TWAR strain)	A tetracycline[12]	An erythromycin

Table 5-12
Antimicrobial Drugs of Choice *(cont.)*

Infecting Organism	*Drug of Choice*	*Alternative Drugs*
Actinomycetes (cont.)		
Nocardia	A sulfonamide	Trimethoprim-sulfamethoxazole; amikacin; minocycline;[12] trisulfapyrimidines with minocycline,[12] ampicillin, or erythromycin; cycloserine[11]
Spirochetes		
Treponema pallidum	Penicillin G[4]	A tetracycline;[12] ceftriaxone[5]
Fungi		
Candidiasis (deep-seated)	Amphotericin B (± flucytosine)	Fluconazole
Histoplasa capsultum	Ketoconazole	Intraconazole
Cryptococcus neoformans	Amphotericin B (+ flucytosine)	
Other deep-seated mycoses	Amphotericin B (+ flucytosine ?)	
Coccidioides immitis	Amphotericin B (IV + intrathecal)	Fluconazole, intraconazole
Other deep-seated mycoses	Amphotericin B or ketoconazole	Fluconazole, intraconazole
Blastomyces dermatitidis	Ketoconazole	Amphotericin B, intraconazole
Aspergillus	Amphotericin B (+ flucytosine ?)	Intraconazole
Sporothrix schenckii		
Lymphocutaneous	Potassium iodide	Intraconazole, fluconazole
Deep-seated	Amphotericin B	Ketoconazole, intraconazole
Pseudallescheria boydii	Miconazole	Amphotericin B
Mucormycosis	Amphotericin B	
Viruses		
Cytomegalovirus	Ganciclovir	Foscarnet
Hepatitis B or C virus	Alfa-2a or alfa-2b interferon	
Herpes simplex virus		
Genital	Acyclovir	Vidarabine, foscarnet
Encephalitis	Acyclovir	Vidarabine
Disseminated, adult	Acyclovir	Vidarabine; foscarnet
Human immunodeficiency virus	Zidovudine	Dideoxyinosine
Varicella-zoster virus	Acyclovir	Vidarabine

*Resistance may be a problem; susceptibility tests should be performed.

[1]In endocarditis, disk sensitivity testing does not provide adequate information; dilution tests for susceptibility should be used to assess bactericidal as well as inhibitory end points. Peak bactericidal activity of the serum against the patient's own organism should be present at a serum dilution of at least 1:8.

[2]Routine antimicrobial susceptibility tests may be misleading. Because of high urine concentrations, ampicillin may be effective in urinary tract infections even when the organism is reported to be "resistant."

[3]Not recommended for children.

[4]Penicillin V is preferred for oral treatment of infections caused by non-penicillinase-producing staphylococci and other gram-positive cocci. For initial therapy of severe infections, penicillin G, administered parenterally, is the first choice. For somewhat longer action in less severe infections due to Group A streptococci, pneumococci, or *Treponema pallidum,* procaine penicillin G, an intramuscular formulation, is given once or twice daily. Benzathine penicillin G, a slowly absorbed intramuscular preparation, is usually given in a single monthly injection for prophylaxis of rheumatic fever, once for treatment of Group A streptococcal pharyngitis, and once or more for treatment of syphilis.

[5]The cephalosporins have been used as alternatives to penicillins in patients allergic to penicillins, but such patients may also have allergic reactions to cephalosporins.

[6]For parenteral treatment of staphylococcal or non-enterococcal streptococcal infections, a first-generation cephalosporin such as cephalothin, cephapirin, cephradine, or cefazolin can be used; for staphylococcal endocarditis, some *Medical Letter* consultants prefer cephalothin or cephapirin. For oral therapy, cephalexin or cephradine can be used. The second-generation cephalosporins cefamandole, cefuroxime axetil, cefonicid, ceforanide, cefotetan, and cefoxitin are more active than the first-generation drugs against gram-negative bacteria. Cefuroxime and cefamandole are active against ampicillin-resistant strains of *H. influenzae,* but cefamandole has been associated with prothrombin deficiency and occasional bleeding. Cefoxitin and cefotetan are active against *B. fragilis.* The third-generation cephalosporins cefotaxime, cefoperazone, ceftizoxime, ceftriaxone, and ceftazidime have greater activity than the second-generation drugs against enteric gram-negative bacilli. Cefixime is an oral cephalosporin with more activity than second-generation cephalosporins against facultative gram-negative bacilli but has no useful activity against staphylococci, anaerobes, or *P. aeruginosa* (*Med Lett,* 31:73, 1989). With the exception of cefoperazone (which can also cause bleeding) and ceftazidime, the activity of all currently available cephalosporins against *P. aeruginosa* is poor or inconsistent (GR Donowitz, GL Mandell: *N Engl J Med,* 318:490, 1988).

[7]For oral use against penicillinase-producing staphylococci, cloxacillin or dicloxacillin is preferred; for severe infections a parenteral formulation of methicillin, nafcillin, or oxacillin should be used. Neither ampicillin, amoxicillin, amdinocillin, bacampicillin, cyclacillin, hetacillin, carbenicillin, ticarcillin, mezlocillin, azlocillin, nor piperacillin is effective against penicillinase-producing staphylococci. However, the combinations of clavulanic acid with amoxicillin or ticarcillin and of sulbactam with ampicillin are active against these organisms.

[8]Occasional strains of coagulase-positive staphylococci and many strains of coagulase-negative staphylococci are resistant to penicillinase-resistant penicillins; these strains are also resistant to cephalosporins and to imipenem.

[9]Occasional strains of Group A streptococci and pneumococci may be resistant to erythromycins.

[10]In patients allergic to penicillin, an erythromycin is preferred for respiratory infections and chloramphenicol is recommended for meningitis. Rare strains of *S. pneumoniae* may be relatively resistant or resistant to penicillin; these strains are susceptible to vancomycin.

[11]Because of the frequency of serious adverse effects, this drug should be used only for severe infections when less hazardous drugs are ineffective.

[12]Tetracyclines are generally not recommended for pregnant women or children less than 8 years old.

[13]Debridement is primary. Large doses of penicillin G are required. Hyperbaric oxygen therapy may be a useful adjunct to surgical debridement in management of the spreading, necrotic type.

Table 5-12 (continued)

[14]For prophylaxis, a tetanus toxoid booster and, for some patients, tetanus immune globulin (human) are required.

[15]The proportion of penicillin-resistant *Bacteroides* sp. from the oropharynx has been increasing recently; for patients seriously ill with infections that may be due to these organisms, or when response to penicillin is delayed, clindamycin is preferred.

[16]When infection is in the central nervous system, either intravenous metronidazole or chloramphenicol is recommended.

[17]In severely ill patients, some *Medical Letter* consultants would add gentamicin, tobramycin, or amikacin.

[18]In severely ill patients, some *Medical Letter* consultants would add gentamicin, tobramycin, or amikacin (but see footnote 25).

[19]Indicated for treatment of urinary tract infections only.

[20]For acute, uncomplicated urinary tract infection, before the infecting organism is known, the drug of first choice is one of the soluble sulfonamides, such as sulfisoxazole, or (for *E. coli* or *Proteus mirabilis*) ampicillin or amoxicillin or (for *Klebsiella*) a cephalosporin. Trimethoprim or trimethoprim-sulfamethoxazole is also useful for treatment of urinary infections caused by susceptible organisms.

[21]In some areas, a fairly high percentage of *E. coli* strains may be resistant to ampicillin.

[22]Large doses (6 g or more daily) are usually necessary for systemic infections. In severely ill patients, some *Medical Letter* consultants would add gentamicin, tobramycin, or amikacin.

[23]In severely ill patients, some *Medical Letter* consultants would add gentamicin or amikacin.

[24]In severely ill patients, some *Medical Letter* consultants would add gentamicin or amikacin (but see footnote 25).

[25]Neither gentamicin, tobramyicn, netilmicin, or amikacin should be mixed in the same bottle with carbenicillin, ticarcillin, mezlocillin, piperacillin, or azlocillin for intravenous administration. In high concentrations or in patients with renal failure, carbenicillin or ticarcillin may inactivate the aminoglycosides.

[26]Rifampin should be used concurrently with other drugs to prevent emergence of resistance. It is always included in treatment regimens for isoniazid-resistant organisms and is generally used together with isoniazid in the treatment of cavitary and far-advanced pulmonary tuberculosis as well as for extrapulmonary tuberculosis.

[27]The first-choice combination is currently under study in patients with AIDS.

[28]An investigational drug in the United States.

[29]Most infections are self-limited without drug treatment.

SOURCE: Adapted from: The choice of antimicrobial drugs. *Med Lett* 32:41, 1990, with permission.

are virtually always caused by mixed gram-negative and gram-positive aerobic and anaerobic bacteria. Initial antibiotic therapy should provide broad-spectrum activity against these bacteria.

Most necrotizing soft tissue infections, especially those originating after an intraabdominal operation or occurring below the waist, are also due to a mixed bacterial flora, and broad-spectrum empiric therapy should be initiated. Because clostridia or streptococci can also cause these infections, penicillin G should generally be included. Once Gram stain and culture results are available, antibiotic therapy can be modified.

Prosthetic device infections usually progress much more slowly than intraabdominal or necrotizing soft tissue infections. Gram-positive cocci, especially *S. aureus* and *S. epidermidis*, play a prominent role in these infections, but they can also be caused by gram-negative bacteria.

Numerous single and combination antimicrobials are available for initial and imperative therapy. The Surgical Infection Society (SIS) has made recommendations for antimicrobials that can be used for empiric therapy of intraabdominal infections. They recommend against using drugs such as cefazolin and other first-generation cephalosporins, penicillin, cloxacillin and other antistaphylococcal penicillins, ampicillin, erythromycin, and vancomycin because these drugs do not provide adequate coverage for both aerobic and anaerobic organisms.

Metronidazole and clindamycin should not be used as single agents because they lack activity against aerobic enteric organisms. Other antibiotics, such as aminoglycosides, aztreonam, cefuroxime, cefonicid, cefamandole, ceforanide, cefotetan, cefotaxime, ceftizoxime, cefoperazone, ceftriaxone, ceftazidime, and polymyxin should not be used alone because of the inadequate coverage of anaerobic gram-negative bacilli. Because of inadequate clinical data documenting efficacy and concerns about resistance, the SIS also recommends against using as single agents for empiric therapy antibiotics such as piperacillin, mezlocillin, azlocillin, ticarcillin, and carbenicillin despite their relative safety in broad in vitro antibacterial activity. Chloramphenicol has an appropriate in vitro spectrum of activity but is not acceptable because it produces serious side effects.

Acceptable agents for community-acquired intraabdominal infections include cefoxitin, cefotetan, cefmetazole, and ticarcillin/clavulanic acid. However, these antibiotics should not be used for patients whose abdominal infection develops in the hospital after previous antibiotic therapy. For these infections and serious intraabdominal infections imipenem-cilastatin (Primaxin) should be used. Combination therapy such as metronidazole or clindamycin plus an aminoglycoside or an antianaerobic antibacterial agent plus a third-generation cephalosporin or clindamycin plus a monobactam is acceptable. Cost consideration and toxicity consideration make one of these recommendations preferable to another. The combination of an antianaerobic antibiotic plus an aminoglycoside plus penicillin or ampicillin is recommended only if enterococcal infection is suspected based on Gram stain or thought to be clinically relevant (e.g., associated with enterococcus bacteremia). Community-acquired intraabdominal infections are seldom associated with serious enterococcus infections.

Definitive Therapy. Antimicrobial therapy may have to be altered when the results of Gram stain and culture insensitivity data are available (Table 5-13). For instance, if only gram-positive organisms are seen in patients with soft tissue infections, broad-spectrum antimicrobial coverage can generally be stopped and only antibiotics that provide coverage for these gram-positive bacteria continued. Sensitivity data may determine that one of the antibiotics currently being used is not active against one of the bacteria isolated. In this case antimicrobial therapy should be altered. In addition, change to a less toxic or less costly antimicrobial agent may be possible once laboratory results are available.

Infections originating in the intensive care unit are frequently due to antibiotic-resistant bacteria. This is especially true for hospital-acquired *S. aureus* which is frequently resistant to methicillin. For hospital-acquired staphylococcal infections vancomycin should generally be initiated if methicillin-resistant *S. aureus* is a problem in the hospital until definitive sensitivity is available. If

Table 5-13
Intravenous Antimicrobials Commonly Used in Surgery

Class of Agent	*Specific Agent*	*Trade Name*	*Usual Total Daily Dose*	*Interval, h*	*Dose Adjustment for Renal Failure*	*Effect of Hemo-Dialysis*
Penicillins						
Natural penicillins	Penicillin G	Numerous manufacturers	1.2–24 million units	2–6	Minor	Yes
Penicillinase-resistant penicillins	Methicillin	Staphcillin	4–12 g	4–6	Minor	Yes
	Nafcillin	Unipen, Nafcil, Naftopen, Nallpin	4–12 g	4–6	Minor	No
	Oxacillin	Prostaphlin, Bactocil, others	4–12 g	4–6	Minor	No
Extended spectrum penicillins						
Aminopenicillin	Ampicillin	Polycillin, Omnipen, Principen, others	2–12 g	2–6	Minor	Yes
Antipseudomonal penicillins	Carbenicillin	Geopen	400–500 mg/kg	4–6	Major	Yes
	Ticarcillin	Ticar	200–300 mg/kg	4–6	Major	Yes
	Azlocillin	Azlin	200–300 mg/kg	4–6	Minor	Yes
	Piperacillin	Pipracil	200–300 mg/kg	4–6	Minor	Yes
Penicillins with beta lactamase inhibitors	Ampicillin-sulbactam	Unasyn	6–12 g	6	Minor	Yes
	Ticarcillin-clavulanate	Timentin	200–300 mg/kg	4–6	Major	Yes
Cephalosporins						
First-generation cephalosporins	Cephazolin	Ancef, Kefzol	2–6 g	6–8	Major	Yes
	Cephalothin	Keflin	2–12 g	4–6	Minor	Yes
	Cephapirin	Cephadyl	2–12 g	4–6	Minor	Yes
	Cephradine	Anspor, Velosef	2–8 g	4–6	Major	Yes
Second-generation cephalosporins	Cefamandole	Mandol	1.5–12 g	4–8	Minor	Yes
	Cefmetazole	Zefazone	6–8 g	6–12	Major	Yes
	Cefonicid	Monocid	0.5–2 g	24	Major	No
	Ceforanide	Precef	1–2 g	12	Major	Yes
	Cefotetan	Cefotan	2–4 g	12	Major	Yes
	Cefoxitin	Mefoxin	6–8 g	4–8	Major	Yes
	Cefuroxime	Zinacef, Kefurox	2.25–8 g	6–8	Major	Yes
Third-generation cephalosporins	Moxalactam	Moxam	4–12 g	8–12	Major	Yes
	Cefotaxime	Claforan	2–12 g	4–8	Minor	Yes
	Ceftizoxime	Cefizox	2–12 g	6–12	Major	Yes
	Ceftriaxone	Rocephin	1–4 g	12–24	No	Yes
Third-generation cephalosporins with antipseudomonal activity	Cefoperazone	Cefobid	2–12 g	6–12	No	No
	Ceftazidime	Fortaz, Tazidime, Tazicef	2–6 g	8–12	Major	Yes
Carbapenems	Imipenem-cilastatin	Primaxin	2–4 g	6–8	Major	Yes
Monobactams	Aztreonam	Azactam	6–8 g	6–8	Minor	Yes
Aminoglycosides	Amikacin	Amikin	15 mg/kg	6–8	Major	Yes
	Gentamicin	Garamycin	3–5 mg/kg	8	Major	Yes
	Netilimicin	Netromycin	4–6.5 mg/kg	8–12	Major	Yes
	Tobramycin	Nebcin	3–5 mg/kg	8	Major	Yes
Fluoroquinolones	Ciprofloxacin	Cipro	800 mg	12	Minor	Yes
Tetracyclines	Tetracycline	Achromycin	0.5–2 g	6–12	Major	No data
	Minocycline	Minocin	100 mg	12	Minor	No
Macrolids	Erythromycin	E-mycin, Erythrocin	2–4 g	6	No	No
Miscellaneous antibacterial agents	Clindamycin	Cleocin	600–1200 mg	6–12	No	No
	Metronidazole	Flagyl	15 mg/kg loading dose then 30 mg/kg/day	6	Minor	Yes
	Chloramphenicol	Chloromycetin	50 mg/kg	6	Minor	No
	Vancomycin	Vancocin	2 g	6–12	Major	No
Antifungal Agents						
Polyenes	Amphotericin B	Fungizone	0.5–1.5 mg/kg (slow infusion)	24	Major	No
Azoles	Fluconazole	Diflucan	400 mg first day then 200 mg	24	Major	Yes
	Ketoconazole (oral only)	Nizoral	By infusion 200 mg	24	No	No
	Intraconazole (oral only)	Sporanox	200 mg	24	No	No
Antimetabolite	Flucytosine (oral only)	Ancobon	150 mg/kg		Major	Yes
Antiviral Agents	Vidarabine	Vira-A	10–15 mg/kg (infuse over 12–24 h)	24	Minor	Yes
	Acyclovir	Zovirax	5–10 mg/kg (1 h infusion)	8	Minor	Yes
	Ganciclovir	Cytovene	10 mg/kg	12	Major (infusion)	Yes
	Foscarnet	Foscavir	180 mg/kg (infusion)	8	Major	

the *S. aureus* is sensitive to penicillin G or methicillin, these agents should be used because they are more effective and the cost is substantially less than vancomycin. Two drugs are generally used to treat *P. aeruginosa* infections, an antipseudomonas beta lactam drug such as mezlocillin, or ceftazidime in combination with an aminoglycoside, in an attempt to prevent development of resistance and to take advantage of possible synergism.

Drug Administration

Route. For seriously ill surgical patients the antimicrobial agent should be administered intravenously to assure adequate serum levels. Seriously ill patients whose gastrointestinal tract is not functioning properly and who have problems maintaining blood pressure have inconsistent absorption when antibiotics are given by other routes. If patients need prolonged antimicrobial therapy once they have begun to recover, other routes can possibly be used or the patient can be given long-term intravenous antimicrobial agents as an outpatient.

Recommendations provided by the manufacturer in the package insert should be used as guidelines for appropriate doses of antimicrobial agents. In general, there is a wide margin between therapeutic and toxic concentrations with drugs such as the penicillins and cephalosporins. Other agents such as aminoglycosides have a much narrower margin between therapeutic and toxic levels. For these antibiotics the calculated dose in adults is based on lean body weight. For children, antibody dosing is frequently based on surface area.

Duration. There are few data defining the appropriate duration of antibiotic treatment. Most surgical infections can be treated effectively with 5 to 7 days of antibiotic therapy. As long as the patient is making clinical progress, gastrointestinal function has returned in patients with peritonitis, and the patient's temperature and white blood cell count are normal, it is generally safe to stop antibiotics. If clinical improvement is not evident within 4 to 5 days of operation and fever or leukocytosis persist after more than 5 days of therapy, a reason for the apparent treatment failure should be sought.

Treatment Failure. Although failure of a bacterial infection to respond to a particular antibiotic is commonly regarded as evidence that the wrong antibiotic was selected, other factors are usually responsible. Patients with intraabdominal infections who remain febrile or have persistent leukocytosis usually have recurrent (tertiary) peritonitis or an intraabdominal abscess that requires drainage. Patients with necrotizing soft tissue infections may have persistent infections. Other causes of fever and infection, such as pneumonia, urinary tract infection, vascular catheter-related infections, drug fever, and thrombophlebitis, should be investigated.

Finally, the antibiotic may be inappropriate. It may be the wrong antibiotic, or it may have been given in an inadequate dose or by an inappropriate route. The bacteria may not be susceptible to the antibiotic at the concentration achievable at the site of infection, or the site may have become superinfected by another bacterium not sensitive to the antibiotic.

Drug Toxicity. Normally antibiotics are excreted primarily by the kidneys and accumulate in the serum of patients with impaired renal function. Therefore, with many antibiotics it is necessary to reduce the dose or to increase the interval between doses in patients with renal failure (there are many schedules that detail how to estimate dosages of antibiotics strongly excreted by the kidneys, but none of them is perfect). Toxic drugs such as the aminoglycosides should either not be used in patients with renal failure or impaired renal function, or if used, their serum or plasma concentration levels must be obtained frequently to verify that toxic levels are not being reached.

The general approach to antibiotic usage in patients with renal failure is to give a first dose of 80 to 100 percent of the usual amount and then to estimate the timing and the amount of the second dose according to various schedules based on the normal half-life of the antibiotic.

Immunotherapy of Infection

Antibodies to bacterial products and to mediators of sepsis are new (and extremely costly) therapeutic modalities that are currently being evaluated. The Food and Drug Administration has approved one antibody (HA-1A) for treatment of patients with gram-negative bacteremia. HA-1A is a human monoclonal IgM antibody to the lipid A domain of endotoxin. In a controlled clinical trial HA-1A resulted in fewer (30 percent) deaths than in recipients of placebo (49 percent). For patients with gram-negative bacteremia and shock, recipients of HA-1A had a mortality of 33 percent compared to 57 percent for placebo recipients. No benefit was seen in patients who were clinically septic but did not have documented gram-negative bacteremia. E5, a murine monoclonal IgM antibody to endotoxin, also reduced mortality (11 percent of patients with gram-negative sepsis who were not in shock compared to 23 percent of placebo-treated patients).

Bibliography

Selected Readings

Bennett JV, Brachman P (eds): *Nosocomial Infections*. Boston, New York, Little, Brown and Co., 1986.

Howard RJ (ed): *Infectious Risks in Surgery*. Norwalk, CT, Appleton & Lange, 1991.

Howard RJ (ed): Surgical infections. *Surg Clin North Am* 68:1, 1988.

Howard RJ, Simmons RL (eds): *Surgical Infectious Diseases,* 2nd ed. Norwalk, CT, Appleton & Lange, 1988.

Historical Background

Earle AS: The germ theory in America: Antisepsis and asepsis (1867–1900). *Surgery* 65:508, 1969.

Wangensteen OH, Wangensteen SD: Military surgeons and surgery, old and new: An instructive chapter in management of contaminated wounds. *Surgery* 62:1102, 1967.

Wangensteen OH, Wangensteen SD, Klinger CF: Some pre-Listerian and post-Listerian antiseptic wound practices and the emergence of asepsis. *Surg Gynecol Obstet* 137:677, 1973.

General Considerations

Brown JM, Grosso MA, Harken AH: Cytokines, sepsis and the surgeon. *Surg Gynecol Obstet* 169:568, 1989.

Ganz T, Selsted ME, et al.: Neutrophils and host defense. *Ann Intern Med* 109:127, 1988.

Howard RJ: Host defense against infection. *Curr Probl Surg* 17:267, 1980.

Lubran MM: Bacterial toxins. *Ann Clin Lab Sci* 18:58, 1988.

Mims CA: *The Pathogenesis of Infectious Disease,* 2d ed. New York, Grune & Stratton, 1982, p 13.

Smith H: Microbial surfaces in relation to pathogenicity. *Bacteriol Rev* 41:475, 1977.

Tracey KJ, Lowry SF: The role of cytokine mediators in septic shock. *Adv Surg* 23:21, 1990.

Volankis JE: The complement system. *Survey of Immunology Research* 3:202, 1984.

Westphal O, Jann K, Himmelspach K: Chemistry and immunochemistry of bacterial lipopolysaccharides as cell wall antigens and endotoxins. *Progress in Allergy* 33:9, 1983.

Types of Surgical Infections

Skin and Soft Tissue Infections

Ahrenholz DH: Necrotizing soft-tissue infections. *Surg Clin North Am* 68:199, 1988.

Barzilai A, Zaaroor M, Toledano C: Necrotizing fasciitis: Early awareness and principles of treatment. *Isr J Med Sci* 21:127, 1985.

Dellinger EP: Severe necrotizing soft tissue infections: Multiple disease entities requiring a common approach. *JAMA* 246:1717, 1981.

Freischlag JA, Ajalat G, Busuttil RW: Treatment of necrotizing soft tissue infections: The need for a new approach. *Am J Surg* 149:751, 1985.

Furste W, Lobe TE, Botros NN: Gangrenous soft tissue infections. *Infectection and Surgery* 4:837, 1985.

Gleckman RA, Czachor JS: Managing diabetes-related infections in the elderly. *Geriatrics* 44:37, 1989.

Gozal D, Ziser A, et al.: Necrotizing fasciitis. *Arch Surg* 121:233, 1986.

Kingston D, Seal DV: Current hypotheses on synergistic microbial gangrene. *Br J Surg* 77:260, 1990.

Llera JL, Levy RC: Treatment of cutaneous abscess: A double-blind clinical study. *Ann Emerg Med* 14:15, 1985.

Mbonu OO, Nwako FA: Synergistic bacterial gangrene and allied lesions: A unified etiological theory. *Int Surg* 68:122, 1984.

Sudarsky LA, Laschinger JC, et al.: Improved results from a standardized approach in treating patients with necrotizing fasciitis. *Ann Surg* 206:661, 1987.

Ward RG, Walsh MS: Necrotizing fasciitis: 10 years experience in a district general hospital. *Br J Surg* 78:488, 1991.

Tetanus

Bleck TP: Tetanus: Pathophysiology, management and prophylaxis. *Dis Mon* 37:545, 1991.

Centers for Disease Control: Tetanus—United States, 1982–1984. *MMWR* 39:602, 1985.

Roos KL: Tetanus. *Semin Neurol* 11:206, 1991.

Peritonitis and Intraabdominal Abscess

Bunt TJ: Urgent relaparotomy: The high-risk no-choice operation. *Surgery* 98:555, 1985.

Dellinger EP, Wertz ME, et al.: Surgical infection stratification system for intra-abdominal infection: Multicenter. *Arch Surg* 120:21, 1985.

Hau T, Ahrenholz DH, Simmons RL: Secondary bacterial peritonitis: The biologic basis of treatment. *Curr Probl Surg* 16:1, 1979.

Hau T, Haaga JR, Aeder MI: Pathophysiology, diagnosis, and treatment of abdominal abscess. *Curr Probl Surg* 21:1, 1984.

Lennard ES, Dellinger EP, et al.: Implications of leukocytosis and fever at conclusion of antibiotic therapy for intra-abdominal sepsis. *Ann Surg* 195:19, 1982.

Olson MM, Allen MO: Nosocomial abscess. Results of an eight year prospective study of 32,284 operations. *Arch Surg* 124:356, 1989.

Shuck JM: Newer concepts in intra-abdominal infection. *Am Surg* 51:304, 1985.

Other Closed Space Infections

Esterhai JL Jr, Gelb I: Adult septic arthritis. *Orthop Clin North Am* 22:503, 1991.

Gainor BJ: Septic arthritis: Common pitfalls. *Orthop Rev* 18:555, 1989.

Hanssen AD: Surgical treatment of septic arthritis and infected prostheses. *Curr Opin Rheumatol* 2:154, 1990.

Ho G Jr: Bacterial arthritis. *Curr Opin Rheumatol* 3:603, 1991.

Schurman DJ, Smith RL: Surgical approach to the management of septic arthritis. *Orthop Rev* 16:241, 1987.

Prosthetic Device–Associated Infections

Dougherty SH: Pathobiology of infection in prosthetic devices. *Rev Infect Dis* 10:1102, 1988.

Sugarman B, Young EJ: Infections associated with prosthetic devices and magnitude of the problem. *Infect Dis Clin North Am* 3:189, 1989.

Young EJ, Sugarman B: Infections in prosthetic devices. *Surg Clin North Am* 68:167, 1988.

Hospital-Acquired Infections

Bozzetti F, Terno G, et al.: Prevention and treatment of central venous catheter sepsis by exchange via a guidewire. A prospective controlled trial. *Ann Surg* 198:48, 1983.

Carlisle EJ, Blake P, et al.: Septicemia in long-term jugular hemodialysis catheters; eradicating infection by changing the catheter over a guidewire. *Int J Artif Organs* 14:150, 1991.

Centers for Disease Control: Nosocomial infection rates for inter-hospital comparison: Limitations and possible solutions. *Infect Control Hosp Epidemiol* 12:609, 1991.

Craig CP: Infection surveillance for ambulatory surgery patients: An overview. *QRB* 9:107, 1983.

Craven DE, Steger KA, Barber TW: Preventing nosocomial pneumonia: State of the art and perspectives for the 1990s. *Am J Med* 91:44S, 1991.

Fabry J, Meynet R, et al.: Cost of nosocomial infections: Analysis of 512 digestive surgery patients. *World J Surg* 6:362, 1982.

Garner JS, Jarvis WR, et al.: CDC definitions for nosocomial infections. *Am J Infect Control* 16:128, 1988.

Gross PA: Epidemiology of hospital-acquired pneumonia. *Semin Respir Infect* 2:2, 1987.

Haley RW, Culver DH, et al.: Identifying patients at high risk of surgical wound infections: A simple multivariate index of patient susceptibility and wound contamination. *Am J Epidemiol* 121:206, 1985.

Haley RW, Culver DH, et al.: The efficacy of infection surveillance and control programs in preventing nosocomial infection in US hospitals. *Am J Epidemiol* 121:182, 1985.

Hampton AA, Sheretz RJ: Vascular-access infections in hospitalized patients. *Surg Clin North Am* 68:57, 1988.

Jarvis WR, White JW, et al.: Nosocomial infection surveillance, 1983. *MMWR-CDC Surveillance Summaries* 33:9SS, 1984.

Martone WJ, Garner JS (eds): Proceedings of the third decennial international conference on nosocomial infections. *Am J Med* 91(3B):1S, 1991.

Platt R, Murdock B, et al.: Reduction of mortality associated with nosocomial urinary tract infection. *Lancet* 1:893, 1983.

Press OW, Ramsey PG, et al.: Hickman catheter infections in patients with malignancies. *Medicine* 63:189, 1984.

Septimus EJ: Nosocomial bacterial pneumonias. *Semin Respir Infect* 4:245, 1989.

Shinozaki T, Deane RS, et al.: Bacterial contamination of arterial lines. A prospective study. *JAMA* 249:223, 1983.

Stamm WE: Catheter-associated urinary tract infections: Epidemiology, pathogenesis, and prevention. *Am J Med* 91:65S, 1991.

Stamm WE: Guidelines for prevention of catheter-associated urinary tract infections. *Ann Intern Med* 82:386, 1975.

Tager IB, Ginsberg MD, et al.: An epidemiological study of the risks associated with peripheral intravenous catheters. *Am J Epidemiol* 118:839, 1983.

Weinstein RA: Epidemiology and control of nosocomial infections in adult intensive care units. *Am J Med* 91:179S, 1991.

Wound Infections

Brown RB, Bradley S, et al.: Surgical wound infections documented after hospital discharge. *Am J Infect Control* 15:54, 1987.

Burns JJ, Dippe SE: Postoperative wound infections detected during hospitalization and after discharge in a community hospital. *Am J Infect Control* 10:60, 1982.

Condon RE, Haley RW, et al.: Does infection control, control infection? *Arch Surg* 123:250, 1988.
Condon RE, Schulte WJ, et al.: Effectiveness of a surgical wound surveillance program. *Arch Surg* 118:303, 1983.
Cruse PJE, Foord R: The epidemiology of wound infection: A 10 year prospective study of 62,939 wounds. *Surg Clin North Am* 60:27, 1980.
Culver DH, Horan TC, et al.: Surgical wound infection rate by wound class, operative procedure and patient risk index. *Am J Med* 91(3B):158S, 1991.
Garibaldi RA, Cushing D, Lerer T: Risk factors for postoperative infection. *Am J Med* 91(3B):158S, 1991.
Gil-Egea MJ, Pi-Sunyer MT, et al.: Surgical wound infections: Prospective study of 4,468 clean wounds. *Infect Control* 8:277, 1987.
Haley RW, Culver DH, et al.: Identifying patients at high risk of surgical wound infections: A simple multivariate index of patient susceptibility and wound contamination. *Am J Epidemiol* 121:206, 1985.
Nichols RL: Surgical wound infection. *Am J Med* 91:54S, 1991.
Olson M, O'Connor M, Schwartz ML: Surgical wound infections: A 5-year prospective study of 20,193 wounds at the Minneapolis VA Medical Center. *Ann Surg* 199:253, 1984.
Olson MM, Lee JT Jr: Continuous, 10-year wound infection surveillance: Results, advantages and unanswered questions. *Arch Surg* 125:794, 1990.
Orr NW: Is a mask necessary in the operating theatre? *Ann R Coll Surg Engl* 63:390, 1981.
Penin GB, Ehrenkranz NJ: Priorities for surveillance and cost-effective control of postoperative infection. *Arch Surg* 123:1305, 1988.
Seaman M, Lammers R: Inability of patients to self-diagnose wound infections. *J Emerg Med* 9:215, 1991.
Tunevall TG: Postoperative wound infections and surgical face masks: A controlled study. *World J Surg* 15:383, 1991.

Surgical Microbiology

Ahrenholz DH, Simmons RL: Mixed and synergistic infections, in Howard RJ, Simmons RL (eds): *Surgical Infectious Diseases,* 2d ed. Norwalk, CT, Appleton & Lange, 1991, chap. 2, p 87.
Altemeier WA, Culbertson WR, et al.: Intra-abdominal abscess. *Am J Surg* 125:70, 1973.
Bennion RS, Thompson JE, et al.: Gangrenous and perforated appendicitis with peritonitis: Treatment and bacteriology. *Clin Ther* 12(suppl C): 31, 1990.
Brook I: A 12 year study of aerobic and anaerobic bacteria in intra-abdominal and post-surgical abdominal wound infection. *Surg Gynecol Obstet* 196:387, 1989.
Finegold SM, George WL, Mulligan ME: Anaerobic infections. *Dis Mon* 31:1, 1985.
Gialdroni-Grassi G: Infections by gram-positive bacteria: An overview. *J Antimicrob Chemother* 21(suppl C):1, 1988.
Howard RJ: Viruses, in Howard RJ, Simmons RL (eds): *Surgical Infectious Diseases,* 2nd ed. Norwalk, CT, Appleton & Lange, 1991, chap. 1, p 115.
Martin WJ, Young LS: Enteric gram-negative bacteria and pseudomonades, in Howard RJ, Simmons RL (eds): *Surgical Infectious Diseases,* 2d ed. Norwalk, CT, Appleton & Lange, 1991, p 35.
Peterson PK: The pyogenic cocci, in Howard RJ, Simmons RL (eds): *Surgical Infectious Diseases,* 2d ed. Norwalk, CT, Appleton & Lange, 1991, p 23.

Human Immunodeficiency Virus

Armstrong FP, Miner JC, et al.: Investigation of health care workers with symptomatic human immunodeficiency virus infection: An epidemiologic approach. *Mil Med* 152:414, 1987.
Barone JE, Gingold BS, et al.: Abdominal pain in patients with acquired immune deficiency syndrome. *Ann Surg* 204(6):619, 1986.
Buehrer JL, Weber DJ, et al.: Wound infection rates after invasive procedures in HIV-1 seropositive versus HIV-1 seronegative hemophiliacs. *Ann Surg* 211(4):492, 1990.
Centers for Disease Control: Recommendations for prevention of HIV transmission in health-care settings. *MMWR* 36(2S):1S, 1987.
Centers for Disease Control: Recommendations for preventing transmission of human immunodeficiency virus and hepatitis B virus to patients during exposure-prone invasive procedures. *MMWR* 40(RR-8):1, 1991.
Centers for Disease Control: The HIV/AIDS epidemic: The first 10 years. *MMWR* 40:357, 1991.
Charache P, Cameron JL, et al.: Prevalence of infection with human immunodeficiency virus in elective surgery patients. *Ann Surg* 214:562, 1991.
Gerberding JL, Littell C, et al.: Risk of exposure of surgical personnel to patients' blood during surgery at San Francisco General Hospital. *N Engl J Med* 322:1788, 1990.
Henderson DK, Fahey BJ, et al.: Risk of occupational transmission of human immunodeficiency virus type 1 (HIV) associated with clinical exposure: A prospective evaluation. *Ann Intern Med* 113:740, 1990.
Henderson DK, Gerberding JL: Prophylactic idovudine after occupational exposure to the human immunodeficiency virus: An interim analysis. *J Infect Dis* 160:321, 1989.
LaRaja RD, Rotherenberg RE, et al.: The incidence of intra-abdominal surgery in acquired immunodeficiency syndrome: A statistical review of 904 patients. *Surgery* 105:175, 1989.
Mishu B, Schaffner W, et al.: A surgeon with AIDS: Lack of evidence of transmission to patients. *JAMA* 264:467, 1990.
Panlilio AL, Foy DR, et al.: Blood contact during surgical procedures. *JAMA* 265:1533, 1991.
Popjoy SL, Fry DE: Blood contact and exposure in the operating room. *Surg Gynecol Obstet* 172:480, 1991.
Porter JD, Cruickshank JG, et al.: Management of patients treated by surgeon with HIV infection. *Lancet* 335:113, 1990. Letter.
Quebbeman EJ, Telford GL, et al.: Risk of blood contamination and injury to operating room personnel. *Ann Surg* 214:614, 1991.
Sacks JJ: Correspondence: AIDS in a surgeon. *N Engl J Med* 313(16):1017, 1985.
St. Louis ME, Rauch KJ, et al.: Seroprevalence rates of human immunodeficiency virus infection at sentinel hospital in the United States. The Sentinel Hospital Surveillance Group. *N Engl J Med* 323:213, 1990.
Vetto JT, Robinson GL, et al: Surgery for non-Hodgkin's lymphoma of the gastrointestinal tract associated with human immunodeficiency (HIV) virus. *Surg Res Commun* 6:79, 1989.
Wilson SE, Robinson G, et al.: Acquired immune deficiency syndrome (AIDS): Indications for abdominal surgery, pathology, and outcome. *Ann Surg* 210(4):428, 1989.
Wong ES, Stotka JL, et al.: Are universal precautions effective in reducing the number of occupational exposures among health care workers? A prospective study of physicians on a medical service. *JAMA* 265:1123, 1991.

Antibiotics

Antimicrobial prophylaxis in surgery. *Med Lett* 34:5, 1992.
Balfour HH Jr, Chace BA, et al.: A randomized, placebo-controlled trial of oral acyclovir for the prevention of cytomegalovirus disease in recipients of renal allografts. *N Engl J Med* 320:1381, 1989.
Balfour HH Jr: Management of cytomegalovirus disease with antiviral drugs. *Rev Infect Dis* 12(suppl 7):S849, 1990.
Bernstein JM, Erk SD: Choice of antibiotics, pharmacokinetics, and dose adjustments in acute and chronic renal failure. *Med Clin North Am* 74:1059, 1990.
Bohnen JMA, Solomkin JS, et al.: Guidelines for clinical care: Anti-infective agents for intra-abdominal infection. A Surgical Infection Society Policy Statement. *Arch Surg* 127:83, 1992.
Greenman RL, Schein RM, et al.: A controlled trial of E5 murine monoclonal IgM antibody to endotoxin in the treatment of gram-negative sepsis. *JAMA* 266:1097, 1991.
Kaiser AB: Antimicrobial prophylaxis in surgery. *N Engl J Med* 315:1129, 1986.
Karam GH, Sanders CV, Aldrige KE: Role of newer antimicrobial agents

in the treatment of mixed aerobic and anaerobic infections. *Surg Gynecol Obstet* 172(suppl):57, 1991.

Platt R, Kaiser AB (eds): International symposium on perioperative antibiotic prophylaxis. *Rev Infect Dis* 13:S779, 1991.

Segret J, Levin S: The role of prophylactic antibiotics in the prevention of prosthetic device infections. *Infect Dis Clin North Am* 3:357, 1989.

Solomkin JS, Dellinger EP, et al.: Results of a multicenter trial comparing inipenam/cilistatin to tobramycin/clindamycin for intra-abdominal infections. *Ann Surg* 212:581, 1990.

Solomkin JS, Meakins JL Jr, et al.: Antibiotic trials in intra-abdominal infections. A critical evaluation of study design and outcome reporting. *Ann Surg* 200:29, 1983.

Terrel CL, Huges CE: Antifungal agents used for deep-seated mycotic infections. *Mayo Clin Proc* 67:69, 1992.

Terrell CL (ed): Symposium on antimicrobial agents. Parts I-IV. *Mayo Clin Proc* 66:930, 1047, 1152, 1249; 1991.

Ziegler EJ, Fisher CJ Jr, et al.: Treatment of gram-negative bacteremia and septic shock with HA-1A human monoclonal antibody against endotoxin. A randomized, double-blind, placebo-controlled trial. *N Engl J Med* 324:429, 1991.

CHAPTER 6

Trauma

G. Tom Shires, Erwin R. Thal, Ronald C. Jones, G. Tom Shires III,
and Malcolm O. Perry

GENERAL CONSIDERATIONS

The magnitude of the problem of trauma in the United States is probably not adequately appreciated. In this country trauma is the leading cause of death in the first four decades of life. It ranks overall as the fourth leading cause of death in the United States today; if arteriosclerosis is considered as a single entity, trauma is the third leading cause of death. Over 140,000 deaths occur each year from accidents. Automobile accidents alone kill more Americans annually than were lost during the entire Korean conflict. Unlike many serious disease entities in the United States, the incidence of and mortality from injuries is increasing each year.

Injury is the leading cause of physician contacts and leads to over 140 million bed days of annual disability. The Centers for Disease Control found that over 4 million years of future worklife are lost each year to injury versus 2.1 million to heart disease and 1.7 million to cancer.

Initial Resuscitation of the Severely Injured Patient

The patient with multiple injuries is best managed by one physician. When the responsibility is divided, evaluation of the patient's overall problems may be lacking and complications may not be recognized for several hours.

Priority by Injury

There are three categories of patients, according to immediacy of injury. The first group includes injuries that interfere with vital physiologic function and therefore immediately threaten life, such as obstruction of an airway or bleeding from a gunshot wound. The primary treatment is to establish an airway and control the bleeding. This type of patient may require surgical treatment for massive internal bleeding within 5 to 10 min following arrival in the emergency room. The operating room should be alerted when the patient is admitted to the emergency room, and no time is wasted in getting the patient into "operative" condition. Often the control of hemorrhage is dependent on a rapid thoracotomy or laparotomy to occlude injured major vessels.

A second group of patients are those with injuries that offer no immediate threat to life. These include patients who have received gunshot wounds, stab wounds, or blunt trauma to the chest and abdomen but whose vital signs are stable. The majority of injured patients are in this category. Although they will require surgical procedures within 1 to 2 h, there is time for additional information to be obtained. Blood for typing and cross matching is drawn, and blood is made available if there is any possibility that the patient will require surgical intervention. If vital signs are stable, x-rays may be obtained to determine the course of the missile and the extent of possible associated injuries, such as fractures. Cystography and pyelography may be performed to assess hematuria. Since patients with penetrating and blunt abdominal injuries may develop shock at any moment, a physician must be in constant attendance during all evaluations. Patients who suddenly develop shock are immediately taken to the operating room without additional diagnostic procedures.

The third group of patients are those whose injuries produce occult damage. This group is composed primarily of patients who have sustained blunt trauma to the abdomen that may or may not require surgical intervention and in whom the exact nature of the injury is not apparent. These patients usually have time for extensive laboratory studies, x-rays, and more complete physical examination. Surgical intervention in this group may be delayed hours or days.

Patients who are severely injured are admitted to the emergency room in a trauma area equipped for emergency resuscitation. This room should contain such items as intravenous fluids, overhead operating-room light, oxygen, cardiac monitor and defibrillator, and a portable carriage that is suitable for an operating-room table in an emergency situation. A cabinet should be in the room containing equipment for endotracheal intubation, tracheostomy tray, closed drainage tray, venous section tray, central venous catheters, closed-chest drainage tubes, intravenous fluids with tubing, needles, and equipment for paracentesis, and pericardiocentesis and peritoneal lavage catheters. The cabinet shelf should have clearly visible labels under each tray or set of instruments. These trays and instruments should be kept in this trauma room and not in central supply, as a waiting period of even 5 min may prove fatal.

Adequate Airway. The first and most important emergency measure in the management of the severely injured patient is to establish an effective airway. A cabinet should be available at the head of the emergency room carriage in which a laryngoscope and cuffed endotracheal tubes of various sizes are available. Endotracheal intubation is the most rapid method of obtaining an adequate airway. Once an airway is established, a means of positive-pressure breathing such as an Ambu bag or anesthesia machine should be available, and a cuffed endotracheal tube is desirable, so that positive-pressure breathing may be accomplished if needed in the resuscitation or in the administration of anesthesia. Either wall suction or a portable suction machine must be available in the trauma room to remove pulmonary secretions, foreign bodies, and frequently, blood from the upper respiratory tract. In the presence of suspected cervical spine injuries, when an endotracheal tube cannot be readily inserted, a cricothyroidotomy or tracheostomy may be required.

Shock and Hemorrhage. Shock is usually controlled while the patient's airway is being addressed by another person. Internal hemorrhage will require immediate surgical intervention. Hypovolemic shock is best prevented or controlled by starting intravenous infusions in at least two extremities, using 18-gauge or larger catheters. A balanced salt solution such as Ringer's lactate solution is usually started until blood is available. Blood for typing and cross matching is drawn at the time the intravenous fluid is started, and the balanced salt solution is given in addition to the blood. Shock resulting from a blood loss of 750 mL can usually be corrected by rapid administration of 2 L of Ringer's lactate solution over a 15- to 20-min period. Blood loss in excess of 750 mL usually requires the administration of whole blood in addition to balanced salt solution. Often, 2 L of balanced salt solution will replace the volume and correct hypotension so that no blood is necessary, reducing the possibility of blood transfusion reaction. When a patient initially responds to 1 to 2 L of balanced salt solution, as evidenced by a normal blood pressure and decrease in pulse rate, but subsequently becomes hypotensive, blood administration usually is indicated. By this time, type-specific blood usually is available and often cross-matched, which reduces the chances for a transfusion reaction. Should a patient not respond to the rapid administration of 2 L of balanced salt solution, uncross-matched, type O, Rh-negative blood is administered without hesitation. The development of the rapid infusion system with counter current warming has been a significant improvement in the treatment of shock. Warming obviates interference with platelet function by hypothermia.

External bleeding is best controlled by direct finger pressure on the bleeding wound or vessel. Tourniquets are of little benefit in the control of major arterial bleeding and often injurious if they occlude collateral circulation. A frequent mistake is the placement of a tourniquet on an extremity tight enough to obstruct venous return but loose enough not to inhibit arterial flow; this only increases the blood loss and edema. The danger of tissue loss from tourniquet use is always present.

Superficial vessels may be ligated if they are readily seen; however, wounds are not probed in a blind attempt to place a hemostat on a vessel. As soon as bleeding is controlled, the wound is covered with a sterile dressing, and the patient is taken to the operating room, where the wound is more adequately visualized and proper instruments are available. The needless probing of wounds in the emergency room may lead to severe infection, which can be avoided by proper exploration including adequate irrigation and sterile surgical technique in the operating room.

Neurologic Evaluation. After an adequate airway has been obtained and hemorrhage has been controlled, a gross neurologic evaluation of the patient is undertaken. Motor function in the four extremities should be verified. A progressing neurologic deficit following injury to the spinal cord may indicate the necessity for an emergency laminectomy. Decompression of a hematoma may result in return of function. Thoracoabdominal injuries usually take precedence over orthopaedic or neurologic injury.

Chest Injuries. Airway obstruction may be due to mucus, fragments of bone from facial fractures, dirt and debris, and, commonly, broken teeth or dentures. If the patient does not ventilate normally after an endotracheal tube is inserted, or a tracheostomy has been performed, several injuries should be considered. These include pneumothorax, hemothorax, cardiac tamponade, flail chest, and ruptured bronchus.

Pneumothorax. If a pneumothorax is questionable, an 18-gauge needle may be inserted into the chest in the anterior axillary line and aspiration done to reveal the presence of air. An initial chest x-ray is preferable, but often severe respiratory distress precludes time for x-ray confirmation. Tension pneumothorax with mediastinal shift is suggested by displacement of the trachea to the opposite side. Auscultation of the chest may reveal decreased breath sounds. The patient with a pneumothorax is treated with closed-chest drainage. As there is little danger from the insertion of a chest tube in the absence of a pneumothorax, an anterior chest tube should be inserted if there is doubt.

Hemothorax. Diagnosis of hemothorax is similar to that of pneumothorax. If the patient on the emergency-room cart is in distress, a needle may be inserted in the eighth interspace in the posterior axillary line and aspiration done to reveal a hemothorax. This is best drained with both anterior and posterior chest tubes. The anterior chest tube is placed in the second interspace in the midclavicular line and the posterior chest tube is placed in the eighth interspace in the posterior axillary line in the region between the midaxillary and posterior axillary line. Chest tubes are of large caliber so that adequate drainage may be maintained. Thoracotomy may be indicated, depending on the rate of bleeding or the presence of intrathoracic clots.

Cardiac Tamponade. During initial observation, an unsuspected cardiac tamponade may develop secondary to blunt or penetrating trauma. This is often not present on arrival in the emergency room but may develop after 1 to 2 h of observation. The clinical signs pathognomonic for cardiac tamponade are increased venous pressure, decreased pulse pressure, particularly with a paradoxical pulse and with or without cyanosis, and decreased heart sounds. The diagnosis may be subtle until the subsequent development of hypotension. Emergency treatment includes aspiration of the pericardial sac with an 18-gauge needle through the xiphocostal angle. Decompression of as little as 20 mL of aspirated blood may make a remarkable difference in the patient's vital signs. The high incidence of false-positive and false-negative findings with pericardiocentesis has led to the use of subxiphoid pericardial window in some centers. Depending on the cause of cardiac tamponade, immediate thoracotomy is usually required to repair the cardiac wound. When a patient arrives at the emergency room in shock without evidence of blood loss, this diagnosis should be suspected.

Flail Chest. Paradoxical chest wall motion from major blunt trauma has historically been managed by endotracheal intubation and mechanical ventilation or operative stabilization of the rib fractures. This approach has been replaced by ventilatory management based on the physiologic derangement of the associated lung injury. Although this requires the careful assessment of arterial blood gases and clinical parameters of pulmonary function combined with vigorous pulmonary toilet, it allows many patients to overcome the morbidity associated with prolonged intubation and ventilation.

Ruptured Bronchus. After rupture of a bronchus, respiratory distress, hemoptysis, cyanosis, and a massive air leak with both mediastinal and subcutaneous emphysema and/or tension pneumothorax may be observed. Often the diagnosis is not obvious. There is a close relationship between fractures of the first and second ribs and rupture of a bronchus. If extrapleural hematoma is noted, special views of the first ribs are indicated. A ruptured bronchus is treated initially with closed-chest drainage. If this does not effectively keep the lung expanded, bronchoscopy and open thoracotomy with repair of the bronchus is indicated.

Open Chest Wounds. The patient with a chest injury resulting in a sucking chest wound is best managed by immediately covering the open wound with whatever material is available, such as a large vaseline gauze bandage or a thin sheet of plastic wrap. This prevents further shifting of the mediastinum and allows ventilation of the opposite lung. Chest tubes are usually inserted before operation, and immediate surgical intervention is indicated.

Ruptured Thoracic Aorta. The diagnosis may be suspected from chest x-ray showing a widened mediastinum and confirmed by arteriography. Immediate operation usually is indicated.

Penetrating Wounds of the Abdominal Wall. All penetrating injuries to the abdominal wall are explored locally in the emergency room to determine if the peritoneal cavity is penetrated. Exploration is usually accomplished by extending the stab wound and determining its depth. In the event that the extent of penetration cannot be determined or if the stab wound violates the peritoneal cavity, the abdominal cavity is explored. The mortality and morbidity from a negative abdominal exploration is negligible, but failure to discover such injuries as colon or liver injury for several hours may allow peritonitis and other complications to develop. All gunshot wounds of the abdomen should be explored whether penetration is evident or not. Shock waves from nonpenetrating gunshot wounds of the abdominal wall can easily transect bowel or lacerate the liver or spleen without entering the abdominal cavity. Most gunshot wounds that enter the peritoneal cavity damage a vessel, organ, or hollow viscus.

The Unconscious Patient. Patients with closed head injuries who are unconscious must have an airway established immediately. Hypotension rarely results from a closed head injury but is almost always caused by blood loss, usually in the thorax or abdomen. The absence of blood does not rule out an intraabdominal or thoracic injury. Extreme care should be used in moving unconscious patients until injuries of the spine have been ruled out.

Immediate Nonoperative Surgical Care

Hematuria. A Foley catheter is routinely inserted, particularly following blunt trauma to the abdomen, to determine the presence of hematuria and to follow the urinary output during and immediately following the surgical procedure. Gross hematuria is evidence of urinary tract injury resulting from contusion, laceration, or rupture. If the patient's vital signs are stable and hematuria is present, a combined cystogram and intravenous pyelogram should be done. A single 15-min film is usually adequate to determine kidney function and extravasation from the bladder, ureter, or kidneys. Failure to demonstrate extravasation does not rule out the possibility of a ruptured bladder or kidney. Should a nephrectomy be required during a laparotomy, functioning of the kidney on the opposite side should be proved. It is useless to attempt to visualize the kidneys by intravenous pyelogram when the patient is hypotensive. X-rays are delayed until the patient has been resuscitated and bleeding has been controlled in the operating room. If time is not available preoperatively for an intravenous pyelogram, a cassette may be placed under the patient prior to the start of surgical procedures and a pyelogram or renal arteriogram obtained intraoperatively.

Fractures. Fractures of the extremities are best managed immediately with splints for the extremities. Immobilization may prevent additional nerve and blood vessel injury and conversion of a closed fracture to an open one. The presence or absence of pulses in the fractured extremities should be noted on initial examination. Intravenous infusions should not be started in an injured extremity. Massive thoracoabdominal bleeding takes precedence over fractures, unless there is an accompanying arterial injury of such magnitude that there is danger of loss of limb. In such instances, it is often necessary to have two surgical teams working simultaneously.

Unstable pelvic ring fractures are best treated by early stabilization. The immediate application of external pelvic fixation not only allows early mobilization and pain relief but also may be lifesaving by controlling bleeding into the fracture hematoma.

Arterial Injuries. Any penetrating injury in the region of a major blood vessel or nerve deserves evaluation by arteriography. On initial examination, 18 percent of subsequently proved arterial injuries are noted to have a normal pulse distal to the arterial injury, and one-third of the patients have a palpable but diminished distal pulse. Vessel exploration in the region of the neck should be done under endotracheal anesthesia and may require resection of a portion of the clavicle for adequate visualization. Early recognition of an arterial injury is the most important factor in preserving a viable extremity or functioning distal organ.

Diagnosis and Management of Unapparent Injury

Blunt trauma to the abdomen may produce severe intraperitoneal or retroperitoneal injury with minimal physical findings. Bowel sounds may not be lost for several hours, and evidence of retroperitoneal or intraabdominal injury may not become apparent for as long as 18 h.

An abdominal diagnostic peritoneal lavage may be performed early in the observation period in patients with injuries from blunt trauma to the abdomen who have equivocal physical findings or altered consciousness. A 95 percent diagnostic accuracy is associated with a positive lavage tap. A negative abdominal tap does not rule out intraabdominal injury and should be followed by peritoneal lavage or CT scan. Patients with signs of peritoneal irritation require exploratory laparotomy even in the absence of a positive peritoneal lavage.

Radiographs. These are taken when a patient's vital signs remain stable but are omitted for patients in severe shock. X-rays of the chest and abdomen are routinely performed to rule out foreign bodies such as knife blades within the depths of the wound. Patients sustaining gunshot wounds should have x-rays when possible in an attempt to trace the course of the missile. Patients sustaining blunt trauma often require multiple x-rays to rule out obscure fractures of the vertebral spine and retroperitoneal injuries. X-rays of extremities will be of value in determining whether or not the missile struck bone, fractured bone, or passed near vital structures. Cervical spine x-rays are obtained in all unconscious patients, or patients who could not demonstrate upper extremity deficits.

Nasogastric Intubation. A Levin tube is routinely inserted in most severely injured patients; exceptions include those patients with penetrating neck wounds, complex facial injuries, or suspected cervical spine fractures. Passage of the tube may provoke vomiting and empty the stomach of large particles, preventing subsequent aspiration during anesthesia. Esophageal or gastric injury from penetrating or blunt trauma may be diagnosed by finding bright red blood in the Levin tube drainage. Gastric intubation prevents gastric dilation during tracheal intubation and aids in the prevention of postoperative distention of the small bowel.

Prophylactic Antibiotics. Antibiotics are administered preoperatively to all patients sustaining penetrating wounds of the abdomen, beginning as soon as possible after the injured patient arrives in the emergency room. They may be discontinued if exploratory laparotomy is negative. Considerable experimental evidence indicates that prophylactic antibiotics in trauma are of benefit if administered within the first 3 h following injury. Retrospective reviews of patients who sustained penetrating abdominal injuries show that there is a decrease in the incidence of infections in those patients who received antibiotics preoperatively or intraoperatively as opposed to those who received antibiotics in the immediate postoperative period or therapeutically. Prospective studies indicate coverage should be against both aerobes and anaerobes.

Tetanus Prophylaxis. Following injury, immunized patients are administered a tetanus toxoid booster. In unimmunized patients the wound is debrided, and 250 units of tetanus human immune globulin is administered. Patients who were previously immunized but are now taking steroids, immunosuppressive therapy, or chemotherapy or who have had extensive irradiation should receive human immune globulin, since they may not have normal antibody response. Severely contaminated wounds should be left open or converted to open wounds when feasible.

PRINCIPLES IN THE MANAGEMENT OF WOUNDS

Primary Wound Management

The most important single factor in the management of contaminated wounds is adequate debridement. This old surgical principle frequently has been forgotten since the advent of antibiotics. All tissue that is dead, has a poor blood supply, or is heavily contaminated should be removed if at all possible. This is particularly true of subcutaneous fat and muscle. Skin with impaired blood supply should be removed initially because of its tendency to become infected. Granulation tissue formation and later grafting procedures are preferable. Following sharp debridement and hemostasis, the wound is irrigated with copious quantities of saline solution, depending on the area and degree of soft tissue injury and contamination. That the incidence of wound infection is inversely proportional to the amount of irrigation and debridement at the time of injury has been demonstrated by Singleton and by Peterson and confirmed clinically many times.

Local Care of Wounds

Glass or sharp instruments usually carry a minimal amount of foreign material into a wound and cause a minimal amount of tissue trauma. X-rays should be taken of any area in which the depth of the wound cannot clearly be seen. It is not uncommon for the deep portion of a stab wound to contain the tip of a knife blade or other foreign body. Stab wounds of soft tissues are explored in the emergency room with the gloved finger or under local anesthesia by extending the length of the laceration to determine the direction and extent of the wound and to rule out any major vessel, nerve, or organ injury. The wound is then irrigated with copious amounts of saline solution. If the wound doesn't penetrate the peritoneal cavity, a small soft-rubber Penrose drain is inserted and the wound is left open for drainage. The drain is removed in 24 h.

Gunshot wounds are debrided externally and left open for drainage. Suturing these wounds leaves a closed contaminated space, and the infection can easily spread to surrounding soft tissue structures. Deep lacerations involving the extremity with damage to major vessels and tendons and massive muscle injury are managed by controlling major vessel bleeding and immediately wrapping the wound in sterile dressings. An x-ray is taken, if indicated, but a severe laceration is not explored until the patient is in the operating room. This procedure prevents undue contamination of the wound in the emergency room before the patient is adequately prepared. Minor lacerations can be managed in the emergency room.

Fascia usually can be approximated, and, depending on the type of wound, the skin and subcutaneous tissue may or may not be closed initially. These wounds are often left open and have delayed primary closure in 3 to 5 days. Damaged muscle due to gunshot wounds is debrided, hemostasis is obtained, and the wound is irrigated as outlined above. The wounds are packed open and closed with delayed closure. All patients with such wounds receive antibiotics and tetanus toxoid.

Antibacterial soaps or detergent materials are not used to irrigate wounds when muscle, tendon, or blood vessels are visible. Severe chemical irritation to these structures may occur, with resultant structure impairment and delayed wound healing.

Many factors, such as the number and virulence of organisms, blood supply of tissue, host resistance, shock, adequacy of surgical debridement, tissue tension, dead space, hemostasis, age, and associated diseases, are responsible for infection. Viable bacteria can be demonstrated in many surgical wounds at the time of closure; however, few incisions become infected.

Cosmetic appearance is a secondary consideration; the primary aim is to avoid infection and cover vital structures. No attempt at plastic repair is made at the initial closure of a potentially contaminated wound. Jagged edges of skin with poor blood supply are trimmed, and any resulting unpleasant scar can be cared for at a later date when no infection is present. Most lacerations, regardless of location, will never need revision if they meet the criteria previously outlined for the primary closure.

Puncture Wounds. The most frequent puncture injury is that caused by a rusty nail in the foot. The patient is administered antibiotics both to prevent secondary infection and to aid in the prevention of tetanus, since this wound is not completely open to the air. Puncture wounds are debrided conservatively if they involve only the skin and subcutaneous tissue. Human tetanus immune globulin is given (250 mg) to the unimmunized patient. Debridement with conversion to an open wound and the administration of antibiotics and tetanus toxoid, whether or not the patient has been previously immunized, is also performed.

Power Mower Injuries. Injuries resulting from the use of power mowers have increased in recent years. These include injuries from flying objects thrown from the power mower and from the mower itself to the hands and feet, particularly the fingers and toes. Treatment has consisted of covering exposed bones with muscle and leaving the entire wound open. These injuries almost uniformly become infected if an attempt is made to close the wound primarily. Patients are treated with systemic antibiotics and tetanus prophylaxis, and the wounds are packed with fine-mesh gauze. Skin grafting and reconstructive procedures should be delayed.

Emergency Laparotomy

Incisions. A midline incision is regularly used for exploratory laparotomy in patients with abdominal trauma and does not endanger the abdominal muscle, blood supply, or nerve supply, or damage aponeuroses. Minimal ligatures are used on bleeders that are contained in small bits of tissue, as each extra ligature is a foreign body and enhances the chance of a wound infection. Tissues should be kept moistened and gently handled. Surgical technique governs the development of wound infection as significantly as any single factor.

Suture. Number 0-Prolene is the suture material of choice for closing the uncomplicated midline abdominal incision, particularly in operations for traumatic lesions. It has not been the cause of draining sinuses following postoperative wound infections. Suture placement is probably the most important factor in the prevention of wound dehiscence. Sutures should not be placed at equal distances from the edge of the fascia, as they will fall in the same group of fibers; should one suture tear the fascia longitudinally, the tear may extend from suture to suture until dehiscence occurs. Sutures should be staggered or placed at varying intervals from the edge of the fascia. With such a closure, there should be no fear in having a patient cough vigorously for adequate postoperative pulmonary care. An occasional patient with minimal subcutaneous tissue will complain of pain in the incision when the suture is under a pressure point such as a belt. These sutures are easily removed under local anesthesia.

Simple interrupted suture is used to close the fascia and peritoneum in a single layer. This is felt to be superior to the figure-of-eight suture, because less tissue is gathered and the suture can be placed faster, thus reducing anesthesia time. Interrupted sutures are used instead of running sutures because a break in the suture material will not loosen the entire incision. Regardless of the type of suture or method of placement, the fascia should be loosely approximated and not strangulated. Tightening fascial sutures may lead to necrosis with the suture subsequently cutting through the tissue. Retention sutures have not been regularly used. Routine antibiotic irrigation of the wound for the prevention of infection has not been necessary.

Through-and-Through Closure. Several local and systemic factors noted at the time of the original operation may make through-and-through closure the procedure of choice (Fig. 6-1). This uses adjustable bridges and large braided nonabsorbable suture or German silver wire swaged on a large cutting needle. The

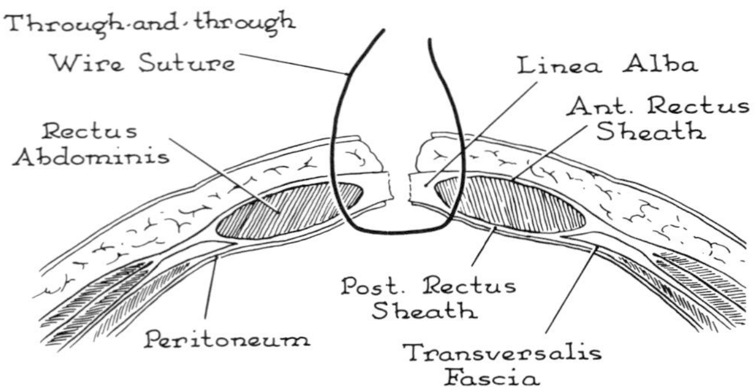

FIG. 6-1. Through-and-through wire closure. (From: *Shires GT: Care of the Trauma Patient. New York, McGraw-Hill, 1966, p 37, with permission.*)

bridges prevent cutting of skin by the wire and allow for swelling that occurs in the first 24 to 48 h postoperatively. The bridges can be adjusted to compensate for swelling of tissues. Wounds massively contaminated from shotgun wadding and fecal material, in patients with steroids, or associated with massive infection and peritonitis are best handled with through-and-through closure. Often a single patient may have several indications for this type of closure such as chronic pulmonary disease, obesity, and/or chronic debilitating disease. Occasionally through-and-through closure is used at the end of a lengthy operation with a long incision to shorten anesthesia time if the patient is not tolerating the procedure well. This type of closure is routinely used in the patient requiring reoperation in the early postoperative period because of gastrointestinal bleeding or intestinal obstruction. The sutures are left in place for 3 weeks. This measure has proved to be sure, safe, timesaving, and often lifesaving.

Infection. Infection and severe abdominal distention are frequently mentioned as causative factors in dehiscence. Wound infection may be prevented in the markedly contaminated abdomen by leaving the skin and subcutaneous tissue open down to the fascia for delayed primary closure. This method is frequently used in long operations or with excessive contamination such as from feces. Abdominal wounds frequently harbor coliform organisms if bowel injury has been sustained. These wounds are packed open with fine-mesh gauze, changed daily for debridement, and either closed at 5 days or allowed to granulate until closure. This procedure will usually result in an excellent scar.

Drains. Subcutaneous drains will not substitute for good hemostasis. Failure to obtain hemostasis will give rise to a hematoma which is an excellent culture medium for an already contaminated wound. Drains from the abdominal cavity are usually brought out through a separate stab wound and by the most direct route. This is especially true for some liver and pancreatic injuries. Drainage of the free peritoneal cavity is not attempted.

Antibiotics

Following hemorrhage and closed head injury, sepsis is the next most common cause of death in patients who sustain abdominal trauma, and it is a leading cause of postoperative morbidity. Up to one-fourth of trauma patients admitted to hospitals develop a nosocomial infection, and patients requiring 5 days or more in the ICU have a 60 percent infection rate. Infection following penetrating abdominal trauma usually results from endogenous organisms introduced by perforation of the gastrointestinal tract. The bacterial population of the large bowel is 10^{11} to 10^{12} bacterial count/gram of stool, and anaerobes outnumber aerobes by 1000 to 10,000. The most common aerobe is *Escherichia coli,* and the most common anaerobe is *Bacteroides fragilis.*

The incidence of infection after gunshot wounds is 2 or 3 times greater than after stab wounds. Antibiotics are started as soon as possible after injury. Jones evaluated 257 patients sustaining penetrating abdominal trauma at Parkland Memorial Hospital in Dallas and found that cefoxitin was statistically more effective than cefamandole and comparable with a combined regimen of clindamycin and tobramycin. Cefoxitin was also an effective agent in serious infections such as bacteremia, intraabdominal abscess, and severe operative soft tissue infections. Infections are more common in patients who have been hypotensive preoperatively or intraoperatively than in normotensive patients. Several other studies have confirmed that single-agent antimicrobial therapy is as effective as combination therapy. Antibiotics must be active against *B. fragilis* and other anaerobes in addition to gram-positive and gram-negative bacteria. Not only has single-agent cefoxitin (2 g every 6 h) been demonstrated to prevent infection following abdominal trauma but also Timentin (3 g every 4 h), mezlocillin (4 g every 6 h), and combination therapy such as ticarcillin (3 g every 4 h), tobramycin (1.5 mg/kg every 8 h) or clindamycin (600 mg every 6 h), and Gentamicin (1.5 mg/kg every 8 h). Routine administration of an aminoglycoside is unnecessary following penetrating abdominal trauma and may contribute to renal failure. Alternatives to aminoglycoside antibiotics are aztreonam and third-generation cephalosporins such as ceftazidime.

Risk factors for development of infection following trauma include older age, massive transfusion, shock, and multiple injured organs. The appropriate duration of preventive antibiotic treatment is unknown. For gastrointestinal injury, between 2 and 5 days is adequate. Patients without gastrointestinal injury and without massive soft tissue destruction can probably have antibiotics discontinued after 24 h, but additional studies are needed to clearly define the proper interval of antibiotic administration.

Intraabdominal abscess formation is a frequent complication particularly following gunshot wounds to the abdomen. Colon injury is a predictor of increased incidence of bacteremia and intraabdominal abscess formation. Of patients with intraabdominal abscess, more than one-third have associated bacteremia. Clinical findings include temperature elevation from 102 to 105°F and white blood cell count from 20,000 to 50,000. The mortality for intraabdominal abscess remains at 15 to 20 percent.

Patients who develop bacteremia following abdominal trauma often have an associated colon injury and 75 percent are associated with gunshot wounds. Antibiotics effective in the management of bacteremia and intraabdominal abscess include imipenem (Primaxin), a carbapenem, which has the broadest antimicrobial activity of an antibiotic, is relatively nontoxic, and is active against both aerobes and anaerobes. Others include ticarcillin-clavulanic acid (Timentin), ampicillin-sulbactum (Unasyn), piperacillin, cefoxitin, cefotetan, and semi-synthetic penicillins. Early diagnosis of intraabdominal abscess is usually made by CT scan. Mortality from intraabdominal abscess has been reduced using this diagnostic technique. With proper patient selection, percutaneous drainage of intraabdominal abscess can be accomplished.

Failure to debride nonviable tissue results in infection and antibiotic failure. Surgical technique and appropriate surgical judgment is just as important as proper antibiotic selection.

BITES AND STINGS OF ANIMALS AND INSECTS

Rabies

In 1950, approximately 5000 cases of rabies were reported among dogs and 18 were reported in humans. In comparison, only 160 cases of rabies in dogs were reported in 1989. In 1991, there were three patients in the United States who died from rabies. Wild animals, therefore, now constitute the most important potential source of infection for both humans and domestic animals in the United States; however, the many possible exposures that result from frequent contact between domestic dogs and humans continue to be the basis of most antirabies treatment.

Approximately 10,000 patients receive postexposure prophylaxis for rabies annually. Rabies among wild animals, especially skunks, foxes, raccoons, and bats, account for greater than 85 percent of cases. Any mammalian animal may carry rabies. Rodents are almost never found to be infected with rabies and have not been known to cause rabies among humans in the United States. Woodchucks accounted for 70 percent of rabies among rodents reported to the CDC. In all cases involving rodents, the state or local health department should be consulted before a decision is made to initiate postexposure antirabies prophylaxis. Many of the cases of human rabies reported in the past 10 years have resulted from exposure outside the United States. The dog remains the major species with rabies and the major source of rabies among humans in the rest of the world.

Diagnosis. Circumstances surrounding the attack frequently furnish vital information as to whether or not vaccine is indicated. Most domestic animal bites are provoked attacks; if this history is obtained, rabies vaccine can usually be withheld if the animal appears healthy. Children are frequently bitten while attempting to separate fighting animals or while teasing or accidentally hurting the animal. Bites during attempts to feed or handle an apparently healthy animal are generally regarded as provoked. Postexposure prophylaxis combining local wound treatment, passive immunization, and vaccination is over 90 percent effective when appropriately applied. An unprovoked attack by a domestic animal is more likely than a provoked attack to indicate that the animal is rabid. A fully vaccinated dog or cat is unlikely to become infected with rabies, although rare cases have been reported.

Extent and Location of the Bite. Any penetration of the skin by teeth constitutes a bite exposure. Bites to the face and hands carry the highest risk, but the site of the bite should not influence the decision to begin treatment. Nonbites include scratches, abrasions, open wounds, or mucous membranes contaminated with saliva. If the material containing the virus is dry, the virus can be considered noninfectious. Other contact by itself, such as petting a rabid animal and contact with the blood, urine, or feces of a rabid animal, does not constitute an exposure and is not an indication for prophylaxis.

Management of Biting Animals. Most animal bites sustained by human beings are caused by dogs and cats, and in most instances it is possible to observe the biting animal for the development of rabies. Domestic animals that bite a person should be captured and observed for symptoms of rabies for 10 days. If none develop, the animals may be assumed to be nonrabid. If the animals dies or is killed, the head is sent promptly to a public health laboratory for examination. The tissue requires refrigeration, but not freezing, and transportation to the laboratory following death of the animal must be rapid. Clinical signs of rabies in wild animals cannot be interpreted reliably; therefore, any wild animal that bites or scratches a person should be killed at once (without unnecessary damage to the head) and the brain examined for evidence of rabies. Travelers to Asia, Africa, and Central and South America should be aware that greater than 50 percent of the rabies cases among humans in the United States result from exposure to dogs outside the United States (Table 6-1).

Postexposure Prophylaxis. It is generally accepted that the incubation period for rabies in human beings ranges from 10 days to 1 year, most cases occurring 20 to 90 days from exposure. In cases of exposure of the head, neck, or upper extremities, the incubation period is potentially less than 30 days. Local care of the

Table 6-1
Rabies Postexposure Prophylaxis Guide, United States, 1991

Animal Type	*Evaluation and Disposition of Animal*	*Postexposure Prophylaxis Recommendations*
Dogs and cats	Healthy and available for 10 days observation	Should not begin prophylaxis unless animal develops symptoms of rabies*
	Rabid or suspected rabid	Immediate vaccination
	Unknown (escaped)	Consult public health officials
Skunks, raccoons, bats, foxes, and most other carnivores; woodchucks	Regarded as rabid unless geographic area is known to be free of rabies or until animal proven negative by laboratory tests†	Immediate vaccination
Livestock, rodents, and lagomorphs (rabbits and hares)	Consider individually	Consult public health officials. Bites of squirrels, hamsters, guinea pigs, gerbils, chipmunks, rats, mice, other rodents, rabbits, and hares almost never require antirabies treatment

*During the 10-day holding period, begin treatment with HRIG and HDCV or RVA at first sign of rabies in a dog or cat that has bitten someone. The symptomatic animal should be killed immediately and tested.

†The animals should be killed and tested as soon as possible. Holding for observation is not recommended. Discontinue vaccine if immunofluorescence test results of the animal are negative.

SOURCE: Rabies Prevention—United States 1991. *Morbidity and Mortality Weekly Report,* vol 40. March 22, 1991.

animal bite should consist of thorough irrigation, cleansing with a soap solution, and debridement. Administration of tetanus toxoid and an antibiotic might be indicated.

Postexposure prophylaxis in addition to local wound treatment consists of both human rabies immune globulin (HRIG) (Imogam® Rabies) and vaccine. There are two rabies vaccines currently available in the United States. Human diploid cell rabies vaccine (HDCV) or rabies vaccine adsorbed (RVA) (Imovax®). Either is administered in conjunction with HRIG at the beginning of postexposure therapy. A regimen of five 1-mL doses of HDCV or RVA is given intramuscularly. The first dose of the five-dose course is given as soon as possible after exposure. Additional doses are given on days 3, 7, 14, and 28 after the first vaccination. For adults, the vaccine is always administered intramuscularly in the deltoid area. For children, the anterolateral aspect of the thigh is also acceptable. The gluteal area should never be used for HDCV or RVA injections since administration in this area results in lower neutralizing antibody titers.

Postexposure antirabies vaccinations should always include administration of both passive antibody and vaccine, with the exception of persons who have previously received complete vaccination regimens with a cell culture vaccine, or person who have been vaccinated with other types of vaccines and have had documented rabies antibody titers. These persons should receive only vaccine. Because the antibody response after the recommended postexposure vaccination regimen has been satisfactory, routine postvaccination serologic testing is not recommended, unless the patient is known to be immunosuppressed. The state health department may be contacted for recommendations on this matter.

HRIG is administered only once to provide immediate antibodies until the patient responds to the vaccine by actively producing antibodies. If HRIG was not given when vaccination was begun, it can be given through the seventh day after administration of the first dose of vaccine. Beyond the seventh day, HRIG is not indicated since an antibody response to cell culture vaccine is presumed to have occurred. The recommended dosage of HRIG is 20 IU/kg. This formula is applicable for all age groups, including children. If anatomically feasible, up to one-half the dose of HRIG should be thoroughly infiltrated in the area around the wound, and the rest should be administered intramuscularly in the gluteal area. HRIG should never be administered in the same syringe or into the same anatomic site as vaccine. Because HRIG may partially suppress active production of antibody, no more than the recommended dose should be given (Table 6-2).

Side Reaction to Vaccine. Local reaction such as pain, erythema, and swelling or itching at the injection site has been reported in 30 to 75 percent of recipients. Headache, nausea, abdominal pain, muscle aches, and dizziness have been reported from 5 to 40 percent of recipients. Cases of neurologic illness resembling Guillain-Barré syndrome that resolved have been reported. Local pain and low-grade fever may follow injections of HRIG. There is no evidence that hepatitis B virus, human immunodeficiency virus, or other viruses have ever been transmitted by commercially available HRIG in the United States.

Precautions and Contraindications. Corticosteroids can interfere with the development of active immunity after vaccination and may predispose the patient to rabies. When rabies postexposure prophylaxis is administered to persons receiving steroids or other immunosuppressive therapy, it is especially important that a serum sample to be tested for rabies antibody to ensure that an acceptable antibody response has developed.

Because of the potential consequences of inadequately treated rabies exposure, and because there is not indication that fetal abnormalities have been associated with rabies vaccination, pregnancy is not considered a contraindication to postexposure prophylaxis.

Manifestations and Treatment of Disease. Symptoms of rabies include a 2- to 4-day prodromal period in which the patient reaches the excited stage. Paresthesia in the region of the

Table 6-2
Rabies Postexposure Prophylaxis Schedule, United States, 1991

Vaccination Status	*Treatment*	*Regimen**
Not previously vaccinated	Local wound cleansing	All postexposure treatment should begin with immediate thorough cleansing of all wounds with soap and water
	HRIG	20 IU/kg body weight. If anatomically feasible, up to one-half the dose should be infiltrated around the wound(s) and the rest should be administered IM in the gluteal area. HRIG should not be administered in the same syringe or into the same anatomic site as vaccine. Because HRIG may partially suppress active production of antibody, no more than the recommended dose should be given
	Vaccine	HDCV or RVA, 1.0 mL, IM (deltoid area†) one each on days 0, 3, 7, 14, and 28
Previously vaccinated§	Local wound cleansing	All postexposure treatment should begin with immediate thorough cleansing of all wounds with soap and water
	HRIG	HRIG should not be administered
	Vaccine	HDCV or RVA, 1.0 mL, IM (deltoid area†), one each on days 0 and 3

*These regimens are applicable for all age groups, including children.

†The deltoid area is the only acceptable site of vaccination for adults and older children. For younger children, the outer aspect of the thigh may be used. Vaccine should never be administered in the gluteal area.

§Any person with a history of preexposure vaccination with HDCV or RVA, prior postexposure prophylaxis with HDCV or RVA, or previous vaccination with any other type of rabies vaccine and a documented history of antibody response to the prior vaccination.

SOURCE: Rabies Prevention—United States 1991. *Morbidity and Mortality Weekly Report*, vol 40. March 22, 1991.

bite is an important early symptom. Other symptoms include headaches, vertigo, stiff neck, malaise, lethargy, and severe pulmonary symptoms including wheezing, hyperventilation, and dyspnea. The patient may have spasm of the throat muscles with dysphagia. The outstanding clinical symptom of rabies is related to swallowing. Drooling, maniacal behavior, and convulsions ensue and are followed by coma, paralysis and death. Intensive respiratory supportive care might be beneficial. This can include tracheostomy. Dilantin can be used for seizures.

Snakebites

Incidence. In North America all the poisonous snakes of medical importance are members of the family Crotalidae, or pit vipers, with the exception of the coral snake, of the Elapidae family. The pit vipers include the rattlesnake, cottonmouth, moccasin, and copperhead. Approximately 8000 persons are bitten each year by poisonous snakes with over 98 percent of bites occurring on the extremities. Rattlesnakes are responsible for approximately 70 percent of all deaths due to snakebites, while death from the bite of a copperhead is extremely rare.

Poisonous versus Nonpoisonous Snakes. Pit vipers are named for the characteristic pit, a heat-sensitive organ, that is located between the eye and the nostril on each side of the head. As a rule, these snakes may be identified by their elliptical pupils, as opposed to the round pupil of harmless snakes. Nonpoisonous snakes do not have pits. However, the coral snake does have a round pupil and lacks the facial pit. Pit vipers have two well-developed fangs that protrude from the maxillae, whereas nonpoisonous snakes have rows of teeth without fangs. Pit vipers also may be identified by turning the snake's belly upward and noting the single row of subcaudal plates (Fig. 6-2). The coral snake is a brightly colored small snake with red, yellow, and black rings. This color combination occurs also in nonpoisonous snakes, but the alternating colors are different. Only the coral snake has a red ring next to a yellow ring; when red touches yellow, it is a coral snake. The nose of the coral snake is black.

The venoms of poisonous snakes consist of enzymatic, complex proteins that affect all soft tissues. Venoms have been shown to have neurotoxic, hemorrhagic, thrombogenic, hemolytic, cytotoxic, antifibrin, and anticoagulant effects. Most venoms contain hyaluronidase, which enhances the rapid spread of venom by way of the superficial lymphatics. There may be considerable variation in the venom effect. Either neurotoxic features such as muscle cramping, fasciculation, weakness, and respiratory paralysis or hemolytic characteristics may predominate depending on the snake.

Clinical Manifestations. Pain from the bite of a poisonous snake is excruciating and probably the symptom that most easily differentiates poisonous from nonpoisonous snakebites. Poisonous snakes characteristically produce one or two fang marks, whereas nonpoisonous snakes may produce rows of punctures. Hypotension, weakness, sweating and chills, dizziness, nausea, and vomiting are other systemic symptoms. Local signs and symptoms may include swelling, tenderness, pain, and ecchymosis and may appear within minutes at the site of the venom injection. If no edema or pain is present within 30 min following injury, the pit viper probably did not inject any venom. Swelling may continue to increase for 24 h. Hemorrhagic vesiculations, bullae, and petechiae may appear between 8 and 36 h, with thrombosis of superficial vessels and eventual sloughing of tissues. Systemic symptoms include paresthesias and muscle fasciculations. Muscle fasciculations are most common following a rattlesnake bite and often are in the perioral region. Fasciculations almost never follow a copperhead bite and rarely follow a cottonmouth bite. They are often seen in the face muscles and over the neck, back, and the involved extremity and can occur within 10 min.

Rattlesnakes. The venom produces deleterious changes in the blood cells, defects in blood coagulation, injuries to the intimal linings of vessels, damage to the heart muscles, alterations in respiration, and, to a lesser extent, changes in neuromuscular conduction. Pulmonary edema is common in severe poisoning, and hemorrhage into the lungs, kidneys, heart, and peritoneum may occur. Hematemesis, melena, changes in salivation, and muscle

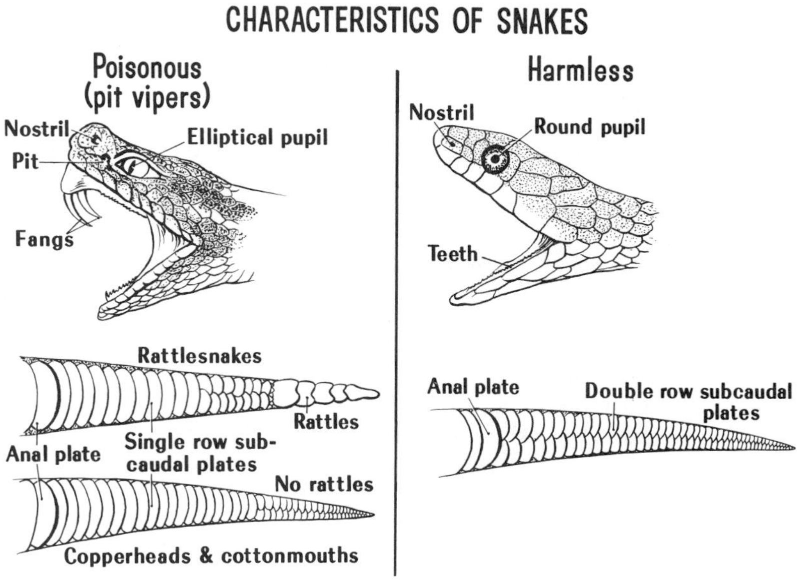

FIG. 6-2. Characteristics of poisonous and nonpoisonous snakes. (From: *Parrish HM: Texas State J Med 60:592, 1964, with permission.*)

fasciculations may be seen. Urinalysis may reveal hematuria, glycosuria, and proteinuria. Red blood cells and platelets can decrease, and bleeding and clotting times are usually prolonged.

Coral Snakes. The coral snake contributes to only 3 percent of all bites and 1.5 percent of all deaths from poisonous snakes. Bites by the coral snake occasionally provoke blurred vision, ptosis, drowsiness, increased salivation, and sweating. The patient may notice paresthesia about the mouth and throat, sometimes slurring of speech and nausea and vomiting. Pain is not a constant complaint nor is edema a constant finding. Thus coral snake venom causes more extensive changes in the nervous system, but death may occur from cardiovascular collapse.

Laboratory Evaluation. Blood should be immediately drawn for typing and cross matching because hemolysis may later make this difficult. Since hemolysis and injury to kidneys and liver may occur, it is important to follow alterations in clotting mechanism, renal and liver function, as well as electrolyte status.

Management. ***Tourniquet.*** Application of a tourniquet, incision, and suction are appropriate if used within 1 h from the time of the bite. The snake injects venom into the subcutaneous tissue, and this is absorbed by the lymphatics. As almost none of the venom is absorbed through the blood stream, the tourniquet is applied loosely to obstruct only venous and lymphatic flow. The index finger should be easily inserted beneath the tourniquet after its application. The distal pulse is checked and should be palpable after tourniquet application. The tourniquet is not released once applied and may be left in place during the 30 min that suction is being applied. The tourniquet may be removed (1) as soon as an intravenous infusion is started, (2) when antivenin is ready for administration, and (3) if the patient is not in shock.

Incision and Suction. Incision and suction for 30 min may be of benefit if accomplished within 30 min after snakebite. The incision should be longitudinal and not cruciate. When two fang marks are seen, the depth of the venom injection is generally considered to be one-third of the distance between the fang marks. Severe bites may result in envenomations deep to the fascia, and surgical exploration may be indicated. Incisions made proximal to the bite are contraindicated.

Excision. The average snakebite does not require surgical excision. This procedure is reserved for the most severe envenomations. Snyder and Knowles showed that wide excision of the entire area around the snakebite within 1 h from the time of injection can remove most of the venom. Excision of the fang marks including skin and subcutaneous tissue should be considered in severe bites and in patients known to be allergic to horse serum who are seen within 1 h following the bite. Most fatalities from snakebites do not occur for 6 to 48 h following the bite, giving time to institute other first aid measures.

Systemic Treatment. The most important treatment for a snakebite is antivenin, although many patients will not require it. Copperhead venom rarely necessitates antivenin. Most snakebite fatalities in the United States during the past 20 years have involved either delay in obtaining treatment, no antivenin treatment, or inadequate dosage. Because antivenin contains horse serum, before its administration skin testing is required. Epinephrine 1/1000 in a syringe should be available before antivenin is given.

Because the rattlesnake, cottonmouth, moccasin, and copperhead belong to the same biologic family, their bites can be treated by the same antivenin (antivenin Crotalidae polyvalent). The coral snakebite is rare, and the antivenin is different from that for the pit vipers. A North American coral snake (*Micrurus fulvius*) antivenin has been developed. It effectively treats *Micrurus* coral snakebites but is not effective in treating bites of *Micruroides,* the genus native to Arizona and New Mexico. Coral snake antivenin can be obtained from many state health departments.

Information concerning identification of a snake or the proper antivenin frequently can be obtained from the nearest zoo herpetarium. A major problem with bites by exotic poisonous snakes is the choice and availability of suitable antiserum. Physicians confronted with this situation may obtain advice from the local poison control center or the Antivenin Index Center of the Oklahoma Poison Information Center, Oklahoma City, Oklahoma (405-271-5454).

Antivenin should be withheld until a physician can determine if it is indicated. Approximately 30 percent of all poisonous snakebites in the United States result in no envenomation. The indication for antivenin is governed by the degree of envenomation.

Grade O—no envenomation. One or more fang marks, minimal pain, less than 1 in of surrounding edema and erythema at 12 h, no systemic involvement.

Grade I—minimal envenomation. Fang marks, moderate to severe pain, 1 to 5 in of surrounding edema and erythema in the first 12 h after bite, systemic involvement usually not present.

Grade II—moderate envenomation. Fang marks; severe pain; 6 to 12 in of surrounding edema and erythema in the first 12 h after bite; possible systemic involvement including nausea, vomiting, giddiness, shock, or neurotoxic symptoms.

Grade III—severe envenomation. Fang marks, severe pain, more than 12 in of surrounding edema and erythema in first 12 h after bite, grade II symptoms of systemic involvement usually present and may include generalized petechiae and ecchymosis.

Grade IV—very severe envenomation. Systemic involvement is always present, and symptoms may include renal failure, blood-tinged secretions, coma, and death; local edema may extend beyond the involved extremity to the ipsilateral trunk.

With frequent observations using this classification, the severity of the bite will be found to increase with time, and thus change in grade is observed. Most bites will have reached a final staging within 12 h. Antivenin usually is not required for grades 0 or I envenomation. Grade II may require 3 or 4 ampules, and grade III usually requires 5 to 15 ampules. If symptoms increase, several ampules may be required during the first 2 h. The smaller the patient, the relatively larger the required dose of antivenin. Proper dosage can be estimated by observing the clinical signs and symptoms. If systemic manifestations are severe, antivenin should be given rapidly, by intravenous drip, in large doses. The injection of antivenin locally around the bite is not advised, as massive edema usually occurs in that area. Absorption from this area is poor, and additional antivenin fluid will further decrease perfusion and perhaps increase tissue anoxia.

If antivenin is indicated, three to five vials are given by intravenous drip in 500 mL of normal saline solution or 5% glucose solution. If severe systemic symptoms are already present, six to eight vials are added. The dose of intravenously administered antivenin can be more easily titrated with response to treatment, and the amount administered is based on improvement in signs and symptoms, not on weight of the patient. Antivenin is administered until severe local or systemic symptoms improve. When it is obvious that antivenin therapy will be instituted, the tourniquet should be left in place until antivenin is started.

If too much time has elapsed for excision to be effective and the patient is allergic to horse serum, a slow infusion of 1 ampule of antivenin in 250 mL of 5% glucose solution may be given in a

90-min period with constant monitoring of the blood pressure and electrocardiogram depending on the seriousness of the bite. This is accomplished in an active emergency department or an intensive care unit. If an immediate reaction occurs, the antivenin is stopped, and a vasopressor and epinephrine may be required.

The incidence of serum sickness is directly related to the volume of horse serum injected. Of patients receiving 100 to 200 mL of horse serum, 85 percent will have some degree of sensitivity within 8 to 12 days following injection.

Intravenous fluids are frequently required to replace the decreased extracellular fluid volume resulting from edema formation. Fascial planes may become very tense with obstruction of venous and later arterial flow, requiring fasciotomy. Adequate antivenin treatment usually makes surgical intervention unnecessary. These patients may need blood, since anemia can develop from the hematologic effects. As afibrinogenemia has been reported, fibrinogen may be required. Vitamin K may also be required. Bleeding and clotting abnormalities are treated with antivenin in addition to blood components. Antibiotics are started immediately to prevent secondary infection, and tetanus toxoid is administered. The most common species of organisms isolated from rattlesnake venom are *P. aeruginosa, Proteus* sp., *Clostridium* sp., and *B. fragilis*.

Stinging Insects and Animals

Hymenoptera

The most important insects that produce serious and possibly fatal anaphylactic reactions are the arthropods of the order Hymenoptera. This group includes the honeybee, bumblebee, wasp, yellow and black hornet, and the fire ant. The venom of these stinging insects is just as potent as that of snakes and causes more deaths in the United States yearly than are caused by snakebites.

Insects of the Hymenoptera group, except the bee, retain their stinger and are in a position to sting repeatedly, each time injecting some portion of the venom sac contents. The worker honeybee sinks its barbed sting into the skin and it cannot be withdrawn. As the bee attempts to escape, it is disemboweled. The stinger with the bowel, muscles, and venom sac attached is left behind. The muscles controlling the venom sac, although separated from the bee, rhythmically contract for as long as 20 min driving the stinger deeper and deeper into the skin and continuing to inject venom.

Clinical Manifestations. Symptoms consist of one or more of the following: localized pain, swelling, generalized erythema, a feeling of intense heat throughout the body, headache, blurred vision, injected conjunctivae, swollen and tender joints, itching, apprehension, urticaria, petechial hemorrhages of skin and mucous membranes, dizziness, weakness, sweating, severe nausea, abdominal cramps, dyspnea, constriction of the chest, asthma, angioneurotic edema, vascular collapse, and possible death from anaphylaxis. Fatal cases may manifest glottal and laryngeal edema, pulmonary and cerebral edema, visceral congestion, meningeal hyperemia, and intraventricular hemorrhage. Death apparently results from a combination of shock, respiratory failure, and central nervous system changes. Most deaths from insect stings occur within 15 to 30 min.

Treatment. Early application of a tourniquet may prevent rapid spread of the venom. Affected persons should be taught to remove the venom sac if present, being careful not to squeeze the sac. It may be necessary for some patients to carry an emergency kit, which is commercially available. Patients should be taught to give themselves an epinephrine injection. Patients having severe reactions should first receive 0.3 to 0.5 mL of a 1:1000 solution of epinephrine intravenously.

Stingrays

Approximately 750 persons each year are stung by stingrays. As the spine, which is curved and has serrated edges, enters the flesh, the sheath surrounding the spine ruptures, and venom is released. As the spine is withdrawn, fragments of the sheath may remain in the wound. The wound edges are often jagged and bleed freely. Pain is usually immediate and severe, increasing to maximum intensity in 1 to 2 h and lasting for 12 to 48 h. This consists of copious irrigation with water to wash out any toxin and fragments of the spine's integumentary sheath. Russell noted that the venom is inactivated when exposed to heat. Therefore, the area of the bite should be placed in water as hot as the patient can stand without injury for 30 min to 1 h. After soaking, the wound may be further debrided and treated appropriately. Patients treated in this manner were shown to have rapid and uncomplicated healing of the wound. Patients not treated with heat had tissue necrosis with prolonged drainage and chronically infected wounds.

Portuguese Man-of-War

Following a severe sting there may be almost immediate severe nausea, gastric cramping, constriction and tightness of throat and chest with severe muscle spasm. There is intense burning pain with weakness and perhaps respiratory distress. The most important emergency treatment is to inactivate the nematocysts immediately, to prevent their continuous firing of toxins. This is accomplished by application of a substance of high alcohol content, such as rubbing alcohol, followed by application of a drying agent, such as flour, baking soda, talc, or shaving cream. The tentacles may then be removed by shaving. Alkaline agents, such as baking soda, are then applied in order to neutralize the toxins, which are acidic. Demerol and Benadryl may dramatically relieve the pain and symptoms. Aerosol corticosteroid-analgesic balm is helpful.

Spider Bites

Black Widow Spider

The most common biting spider in the United States is the black widow (*Latrodectus mactans*) (Fig. 6-3). The female spider

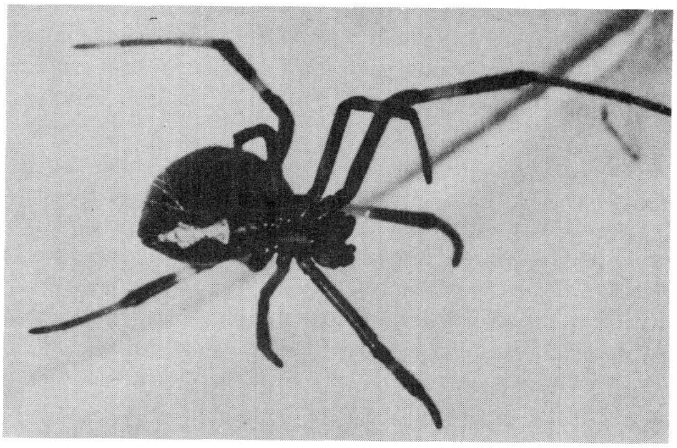

FIG. 6-3. Abdominal view of a female black widow spider showing the hourglass marking. (From: *Paton BC: Surg Clin North Am 43:537, 1963, with permission.*)

has a reddish orange hourglass on its ventral surface. *Latrodectus* venom is primarily neurotoxic in action and appears to center on the spinal cord. Following a bite by the black widow spider, the majority of patients experience pain within 30 min and a small wheal with an area of erythema appears. Nausea and vomiting occur in approximately one-third of patients, headache in one-fourth, and dyspnea may develop. The time of onset of symptoms following the bite is from 30 min to 6 h. The severe symptoms last from 24 to 48 h. Generalized muscle spasm is the most prominent physical finding. Cramping muscle spams occur in the thighs, lumbar region, abdomen, or thorax. Priapism and ejaculation have been reported. Most patients recover within 24 h.

Treatment. Treatment consists of narcotics for the relief of pain and a muscle relaxant for relief of spasm. Either methocarbamol (Robaxin) or 10 mL of a 10% solution of calcium gluconate relieves symptoms. It is believed that calcium acts by depressing the threshold for depolarization at the neuromuscular junctions. Calcium gluconate may give instant relief of muscular pain and methocarbamol can be administered intravenously, 10 mL over a 5-min period with a second ampule started in a saline solution drip. Although *Latrodectus mactans* antivenin is available, it is rarely required. The manufacturer recommends its use for patients younger than 16 years or older than 60 years and for patients with underlying cardiovascular diseases. The antivenin is prepared from horse serum and is administered intramuscularly after appropriate skin tests. Hospitalization may be required for the young, elderly, and patients with significant chronic diseases or with severe signs and symptoms of envenomation.

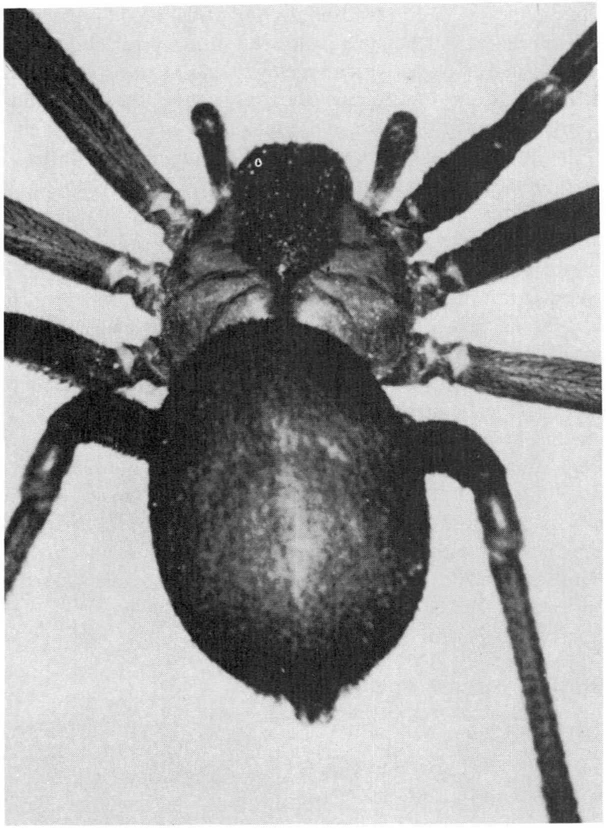

FIG. 6-4. The distinguishing mark of the *Loxosceles reclusa* is the darker violin-shaped band over the dorsal cephalothorax. (From: *Dillaha CJ, Jansen GT, et al: JAMA 188:33, 1964, with permission.*)

North American Loxoscelism

The distinguishing mark of the *Loxosceles reclusa* is the darker violin-shaped band over the dorsal cephalothorax (Fig. 6-4). The spider is native to the south central United States. The body ranges from 7 mm to 1.2 cm and including the legs ranges from 2 to 3 cm.

Clinical Manifestations. The initial bite may go unnoticed or be accompanied by a mild stinging sensation. Pain may recur 6 to 8 h afterward. A mild envenomation is associated with local urticaria and erythema which usually resolves spontaneously. More severe bites results in progression to necrosis and sloughing of skin with residual ulcer formation. A generalized macular and erythematous rash may appear in 12 to 24 h. Erythema develops, with bleb or blister formation surrounded by an irregular area of ischemia. A zone of hemorrhage and induration and a surrounding halo of erythema may develop peripherally. The central ischemia turns dark, an eschar forms by the seventh day, and by the fourteenth day the area sloughs, leaving an open ulcer. Approximately 3 weeks is required for the lesion to heal. The pain may be out of proportion for the size of the area involved. The progression from blue to black gives the bite a necrotic appearance, and the more severe ones develop within a few hours to 2 days. Systemically, the patient may have fever, nausea, vomiting, weakness, arthralgia, malaise, and even petechiae. The two principal systemic effects, hemolysis and thrombocytopenia, have been responsible for deaths. Hemoglobinemia, hemoglobinuria, leukocytosis, and proteinuria may also occur, and there may be eventual renal failure. *Loxosceles* venom is chiefly cytotoxic in action. Laboratory studies are obtained in patients with severe envenomation including prothrombin time, partial thromboplastin time (PTT), platelet count, and urinalysis. The pathophysiology of the bite is that intravascular coagulation and the formation of microthrombi within the capillary occur, leading to capillary occlusion, hemorrhage, and necrosis.

Treatment. Treatment is conservative, because of the difficulty in predicting the severity of the bite. Various treatments have been advocated in addition to early excision including corticosteroids, heparin, regitine, dextran, and infusion, but clinical studies have failed to identify the benefit of these agents. The dose for steroids has varied from 30 to 80 mg of methylprednisolone daily tapered over a period of several days. Rees has reported a leukocyte inhibitor, dapsone, used in leprosy, to be effective in reducing inflammation at the site of the brown recluse venom injection. Treatment was with dapsone 100 mg daily for 14 days before surgical excision, if required. The incidence of scarring and deformity was much less in the dapsone-treated group than with observation and subsequent surgical excision. However, there are significant side effects associated with dapsone treatment including dose-dependent hemolytic anemia, methemoglobinemia, and rash. Whether or not dapsone improves morbidity following brown spider bites awaits further clinical evaluation. Conservative therapy seems to be the preferred treatment. Excision of the necrotic area with skin grafting may be required at a later date.

PENETRATING WOUNDS OF THE NECK AND THORACIC INLET

Although penetrating injuries of the neck are uncommon in civilian surgical practice, the concentration of deep vital structures makes any cutaneous wound a potentially serious injury. Life-threatening consequences of unrepaired injuries of the larynx, trachea, pharynx, esophagus, and blood vessels of the neck and thoracic inlet mandate early diagnosis and operative correction. There is general agreement that penetrating wounds with overt evidence of deep injuries require urgent operations. A difference of opinion exists regarding the necessity for operative exploration of patients without evidence of such injuries. Numerous reports document similar results in patients treated by routine operative explorations and those observed, with or without adjunctive diagnostic studies, and operated on for positive tests or evolving clinical findings.

General Considerations

Before World War II, the treatment of penetrating wounds of the neck was largely nonsurgical unless major bleeding or deep injuries were obvious. Reported mortality rates were 18 percent of 188 cases in the Spanish-American War and 11 percent of 594 cases in World War I. During World War II the mortality rate fell to 7 percent, probably because of a variety of factors, including earlier tracheostomy, more frequent and expedient surgical exploration, antibiotics, and improvements in surgical and anesthetic techniques.

Since 1960, numerous civilian series have been reported and mortality rates approximate 5 percent. Most deaths are due to spinal cord and blood vessel injuries, although tracheal and esophageal wounds account for some. Fogelman and Stewart pointed out that the mortality rate for their cases that were promptly explored was 6 percent, whereas for those in which surgical intervention was omitted or postponed the mortality rate was 35 percent.

Mandatory (Routine) Exploration. Based on the improved results of operative care of penetrating neck injuries, the policy evolved in many major trauma centers of "treating the platysma like the peritoneum" and exploring virtually all neck wounds that penetrated the platysma. In 1967, Jones and associates reviewed 274 penetrating neck wounds treated in this manner at Parkland Memorial Hospital. There were 11 deaths, for a mortality rate of 3.6 percent. Of the fatalities, four were due to complications from spinal cord injuries, three from massive hemorrhage, and the remainder from cerebral complications of vascular or laryngotracheal injuries. Of the 274 cases, 103 (38 percent) explorations were negative, i.e., with no hematoma, no significant bleeding, and no damage to any named structure in the neck, although the tract of the injury frequently was within millimeters of vital structures. In the negative explorations there were no deaths and the only complication was a superficial wound infection that cleared promptly with drainage. These patients usually were discharged within 72 h to clinic follow-up if there were no associated injuries. Similar results have been documented more recently in the series reported by Saletta and associates and by Roon and Christensen. These three series represent 700 patients, 327 (47 percent) of whom had major structural injuries. Thirty-one (4.4 percent) of these patients with important injuries were considered preoperatively to be "clinically negative." Most of these silent injuries were not life-threatening, but many patients with serious injuries had soft signs indicating their presence.

Selective Exploration. Because of the frequency of negative explorations resulting from the policy of mandatory exploration, a number of trauma centers have begun the selective management of penetrating neck injuries. Patients with overt signs of vascular or visceral injuries are promptly operated on and those with "clinically negative" penetrating wounds are monitored by repeated physical examinations, with or without radiographic and endoscopic diagnostic procedures. Reports summarizing the results of selective management of more than 1200 patients with penetrating neck trauma have been published since 1983. About half the patients in most series underwent explorations because of clinical or radiographic evidence of deep injuries, and the rate of negative explorations was in the range of 20 to 30 percent. Subsequent explorations were infrequently required and minimal morbidity occurred in observed patients. No significant differences in mortality or morbidity were demonstrated between series managed by mandatory or selective exploration, including the randomized single-institution study by Golueke. Variable cost saving may result from a selective management policy, depending on the extent to which diagnostic studies are used.

Clinical evidence of an underlying vascular or visceral injury mandates operative exploration in any patient with penetrating cervical trauma. Acute symptoms and signs suggesting cervical vascular injuries include arterial bleeding, hematoma, diminished distal pulsation, bruit, unexplained shock, and cerebral changes indicative of an ischemic or embolic event. Findings suggesting aerodigestive tract injuries include stridor, dysphonia, aphonia, hemoptysis, hematemesis, dysphagia, odynophagia, and subcutaneous emphysema. Most laryngotracheal injuries acutely cause symptoms and physical findings, while vascular and pharyngoesophageal injuries are more often initially occult.

In hemodynamically stable and "clinically negative" patients with penetrating neck trauma, careful examination of the wound is an important aspect of estimating the potential for morbid injuries. If the extent of the injury is not apparent, the wound is very gently probed with a small hemostat, only to the depth of the platysma muscle. If the platysma has been penetrated, the probing is discontinued. Neck wounds should not be probed beneath the platysma muscle because hemostasis may be disrupted. A valid appraisal of the likelihood of deep injury requires knowledge of the anatomic relationships of the visceral and vascular structures of the neck. Wounds in the posterior triangle are less often associated with serious visceral and vascular injuries than those in the anterior and lateral aspects of the neck. Directly anterior wounds infrequently injure the esophagus without an intervening tracheal injury that is usually manifest by subcutaneous emphysema or air escaping from the wound. Plain films of the neck may be useful diagnostically by demonstrating subfascial air or, in the case of missile wounds, may assist in defining the trajectory by revealing a retained bullet or metallic fragments in bone.

Because a penetrating wound may be the only sign indicating the presence of a major vascular injury, arteriography has become an important modality in the management of neck injuries. In the management of trauma patients, arteriography is used mainly for one of three norms: (1) to exclude the need for operation in a patient who has no indication for surgery, (2) to define a vascular wound not detectable by other means, and (3) to plan the repair of a major vascular injury. Duplex ultrasonography can be helpful in concert with other diagnostic methods in the detection and evaluation of vascular wounds. In patients who have no clinical features of vascular injury, these adjunctive noninvasive techniques assist in determining whether or not arteriograms are needed. These studies may be useful in precisely defining the site of an arterial injury, as well as for the purpose of confirming arterial integrity. Monson's division of the neck into three zones is useful in considering the arteriographic evaluation of penetrating neck trauma (Fig. 6-5): Zone I—below a horizontal line 1 cm above the claviculomanubrial junction or inferior to the cricoid cartilage; Zone II—between Zone I and the angle of the mandible; and Zone III—between the angle of the mandible and the base of the skull. Zones II and III are considered the neck proper, and Zone I is the base of the neck or thoracic inlet.

Arteriography has been used extensively and successfully to exclude arterial injuries in the selective management of cervical trauma. Many authors recommend its routine use in stable patients with overt signs of arterial injury, especially in Zones I and III because of the potential technical problems with exposure and vascular control in these regions. This will be considered more thoroughly in the section on specific injuries.

The possibility of underlying pharyngoesophageal injury has remained a problem in the management of "clinically negative" penetrating neck trauma. Important laryngotracheal injuries are essentially always overt, arterial injuries can be accurately diagnosed arteriographically, and occult venous injuries are unlikely to have much morbid potential. The validity of nonoperative exclusion of pharyngoesophageal injuries has not been thoroughly addressed.

In an attempt to resolve this issue, 118 patients with penetrating neck trauma in Zones II or III were prospectively studied. Essentially all patients had cervical arteriography, barium esophagrams, and flexible and rigid endoscopies, followed by operative neck explorations. Esophageal injuries were found at exploration in 10 patients; barium swallows and rigid esophagoscopies detected the injuries in eight of the nine patients so studied. Flexible endoscopy was inaccurate, yielding falsely negative results in five of the eight patients with esophageal perforations having this examination. Of 108 patients in whom esophageal injuries were operatively excluded, false-positive studies occurred in none of the 103 patients having barium swallows, one of the 98 patients having flexible esophagoscopies, and five of the 107 patients undergoing rigid endoscopies. The patient with a falsely negative barium swallow had a positive rigid endoscopy, and the esophogram demonstrated the injury in the single patient with a negative rigid endoscopic

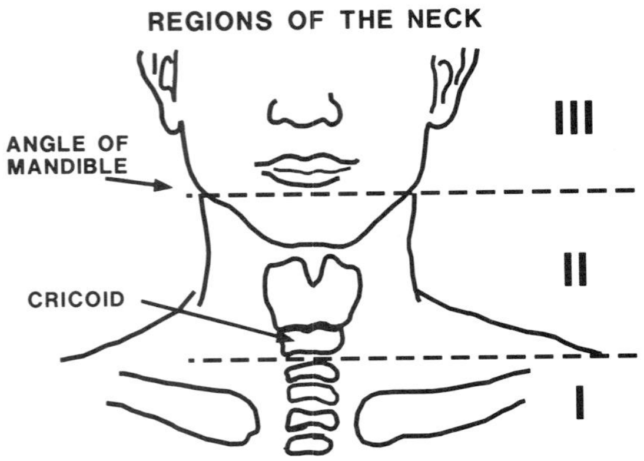

FIG. 6-5. Arbitrary division of the cervical region into three zones. Management of penetrating wounds of the neck is based on the area involved. (From: *Monson DO et al: 1969, with permission.*)

examination. Therefore, all patients with esophageal injuries had at least one positive study preoperatively. The sensitivity (ability of a test to detect an injury if present) for barium swallow and rigid esophagoscopy was 89 percent. The specificity (ability of a test to exclude an injury if absent) was 100 and 95 percent for barium swallow and rigid esophagoscopy, respectively.

Summary. Patients with clinical findings of vascular or visceral injuries are operatively explored in the operating room under general anesthesia. Patients with altered sensoriums in whom appropriate information, examinations, and diagnostic studies are impossible are also explored. Based on the above data, our current recommendations for stable patients with penetrating injuries in Zones II and III, without clinical evidence of vascular or aerodigestive tract injuries, include biplane four-vessel cervical angiography, barium esophagography in two projections with cineradiography, and rigid esophagoscopy. If arteriography reveals an injury requiring operation, no further studies are performed and the patient is operatively explored. If arteriography is negative, barium esophagography is performed. If esophagography is normal, important injury is considered unlikely and the patient is admitted for observation. If esophagography is positive, operative exploration is recommended, preceded by rigid esophagoscopy under general anesthesia. If esophagoscopy is negative, the judgment regarding proceeding with operative exploration is based on the certainty of the abnormality seen on esophagram. If any of the aforementioned studies cannot be adequately completed or are equivocal, operative exploration is recommended. Patients with injuries in Zone I are more liberally explored, despite the absence of objective clinical findings, because the site of injury is less amenable to observation, unexpected bleeding is difficult to control nonoperatively, and the validity of arteriographic exclusion is questionable.

Success with selective management of penetrating neck trauma requires surgeons and radiologists experienced in evaluating such injuries and the 24-h availability of precise radiologic studies. In addition, the necessary commitment of time and personnel for careful and repeated patient observation is substantially greater than is required for a cervical exploration. Routine exploration probably remains the safest approach to the management of penetrating neck injuries for surgeons working in hospitals caring for a limited number of traumatized patients.

The cost of observation without radiologic studies is clearly less than for an operative procedure and a brief postoperative stay. The expense of several radiologic studies makes the cost of the two modes of treatment more similar. Additional expenses mount related to the number of patients requiring operative procedures after the diagnostic studies. It seems that the total expense of a policy of mandatory exploration is likely to be at least equal to if not less than for selective management.

Treatment. ***Initial Evaluation and Management.*** On admission to the emergency room, all patients with neck injuries are immediately evaluated regarding their systemic condition, i.e., airway patency and adequacy of ventilation, blood pressure, pulse, and mental state. Peripheral signs of shock such as sweating, cold skin, and collapsed veins should be recorded. If there is external bleeding, pressure is applied for temporary hemostasis. Adequate ventilation may require endotracheal intubation in obtunded patients or tracheostomy if a laryngotracheal injury or a cervical hematoma has caused upper airway obstruction.

One or two large-bore intravenous cannulas are inserted in peripheral veins and an infusion of Ringer's lactate solution is started while blood is drawn for typing and cross matching. If shock is present, the fluid is given rapidly; if there is no evidence of blood loss, the intravenous solutions are kept going by slow drip. When indicated, whole blood is administered as soon as it is available. Usually the salt solution will temporarily reverse the shock state until cross-matched blood is available. If shock is severe and is not improved promptly by the Ringer's lactate solution, type O, Rh-negative low-titer unmatched blood is infused rapidly until matched blood is available. Plasma has also been used but has no advantage over salt solutions; i.e., both are quite helpful temporarily, although neither is a substitute for whole blood.

Tube thoracostomy is often necessary for intrathoracic bleeding or pneumothorax from the commonly associated pulmonary injuries. If there is no clinical evidence of pneumothorax or hemothorax and the patient's condition is stable, an upright chest film is obtained with a physician in constant attendance. No attempt is made to pass a nasogastric tube in the emergency room because of the danger of recurrent hemorrhage as a result of coughing or gagging.

The major initial risk is airway compromise for patients with injuries of the neck proper and exsanguinating hemorrhage for those with penetrating trauma entering the mediastinum. The clinical presentation of patients with superior mediastinal vascular injuries varies from innocuous-appearing cutaneous wounds to terminal hemorrhagic shock. Hemostasis may be transient and spontaneously break down, or it may be disrupted by changes in intravascular or intrathoracic pressure. Acute hemorrhage from these injuries can sometimes be controlled by external pressure, but occasionally control requires an anterolateral thoracotomy in the emergency room. The innominate and right subclavian vessels can be controlled through a right thoracotomy and the left subclavian artery controlled through a left chest incision.

Special x-ray studies such as contrast esophagography and arteriography may be useful but are considered only in hemodynamically stable patients. An upper neck wound whose course extends above the angle of the mandible (Zone III) often presents dangerous intraoperative problems. Arteriographic definition of the site and extent of arterial injury may importantly alter operative plans. Internal carotid injuries near the base of the skull are difficult to expose and cephalad control may be essentially impossible. Initial extracranial-intracranial arterial bypass (EC-IC) is a reasonable consideration in patients with such injuries. Operative control of midneck carotid wounds (between the mandible and the level of the cricoid cartilage—Zone II) is usually simple and arteriographic definition is less important. Vertebral artery injuries that may otherwise go undetected may be demonstrated if arteriography is performed on patients with injuries in this region.

Preoperative arteriography is frequently helpful in evaluating patients with potential arterial injuries of the neck and thoracic inlet, but it should not be used to obviate the need for operative exploration in patients with intrathoracic bleeding, and arteriograms should be considered only in stable patients.

The frequent absence of overt signs of vascular trauma and the minimal morbidity imposed by operative exploration was documented by Flint and associates. Thirty-two percent of these patients had no diagnostic signs of vascular injuries. Even innominate and subclavian vessel wounds had no overt manifestations in 29 percent of these patients with such injuries. Most of the injuries in these patients were adequately managed with cervical or transverse clavicular incisions, and very few of those without overt injury manifestations required thoracic incisions.

Anesthesia. Exploration is performed under general anesthesia, using an orotracheal airway with an inflatable cuff. The anesthetic agent varies considerably according to the specific problem, necessity for rapid induction, circulatory status, and preexisting disease.

Anesthetic induction requires attention to different problems in patients with superior mediastinal injuries as compared with those with wounds of the neck proper. Intubation while awake is preferred in patients with wounds of the neck proper because difficulties imposed by cervical hematomas or upper airway edema may delay adequate oxygenation in paralyzed patients. In these wounds, disruption of existing hemostasis by retching or struggling with intubation is usually amenable to control by external pressure.

On the other hand, intubation in patients with superior mediastinal wounds may produce major hemorrhage that cannot be controlled by local pressure. These patients less often have structural alterations of the upper airway, and intubation can more safely follow the infusion of muscle relaxants. Because gastric decompression is omitted to avoid sudden alterations in intrathoracic pressure, precautions are necessary in the technique of induction to minimize the aspiration risk. In either instance, preinduction preparation for emergency tracheostomy is essential.

The chest is again examined just before induction, because pneumothorax may develop slowly following a neck wound, appearing an hour or longer after an initially negative chest x-ray. Wounds in the base of the neck following a downward path may cause minimal apical pulmonary injuries so that a pneumothorax is not apparent initially and may not be manifest until after the patient is intubated. This should be kept in mind as a cause for hypotension or hypoxia during anesthesia.

Technique of Operation. Patient positioning and preparation of the sterile field require foresight concerning operative exposure and the need for venous autografts. The supine position with some cervical extension is used. The prepared operative field includes the neck, chest, anterior shoulders, and a separate site for harvesting saphenous vein.

The incision is planned to allow full exposure of the tract of injury. Proximal and distal control of the major blood vessels must also be considered in the length and position of the incision. Incisions commonly used are the oblique incision along the anterior border of the sternocleidomastoid muscle, the horizontal clavicular incision with resection of the medial portion of the clavicle, median sternotomy, and anterolateral thoracotomy. A collar incision is occasionally useful for bilateral injuries or those primarily involving the larynx or proximal trachea.

The tract of injury is followed to its depth, with systematic examination of each adjacent structure. Blast injury, especially from high-velocity missiles, may not be immediately apparent and requires careful evaluation. If injuries to the major blood vessels are suspected, tapes are passed around the vessels proximal and distal to the point of suspected injury before local clots are removed. Injured structures are repaired as outlined in the following paragraphs and muscles are anatomically approximated.

Most soft tissue neck wounds are drained for 24 to 48 h using Penrose drains or Silastic suction catheters to prevent the accumulation of blood and serum. If the pharynx or esophagus is injured, drainage is continued for 4 to 8 days. In the case of a massive gunshot wound, such as close-range shotgun injury, the wound is left open initially and, if possible, a delayed primary closure is performed 3 to 4 days later.

Specific Injuries

Vascular Injuries. Clinical problems posed by acute vascular injuries are best considered by dividing the discussion into injuries of the neck proper (Zones II and III) and those of the base of the neck or thoracic inlet (Zone I). Cerebral ischemia and tracheal compression from contained bleeding are the major concerns with injuries of the middle and upper neck. External hemorrhage can usually be controlled by pressure, and the diagnosis is signaled by an adjacent penetrating wound, a bruit, or a neurologic deficit. The major problems of vascular injuries of the thoracic inlet are exsanguinating hemorrhage, early diagnosis, and operative exposure. Operative techniques of vessel repair are straightforward and infrequently pose important management problems. Although the specific vessel injured is sometimes defined by preoperative arteriography, the surgical management of potential vascular injuries must often proceed without this information.

Cervical Blood Vessels. Major vascular injuries in this region include the common carotid artery and its extracranial branches, the vertebral artery, and the internal jugular vein. Special attention is directed to preoperative neurologic evaluation because cerebral infarction may affect the intraoperative decision regarding flow restoration. Transient hypotension may exaggerate cerebral ischemia, but it does not appear to have a predictably deleterious effect on eventual neurologic status. Rapid fluid volume restitution and restoration of normal blood pressure is important for physiologic reasons and also allows a more accurate evaluation of the neurologic consequences of the injury. Thal and associates described the relationship between preoperative neurologic status, vascular procedure, and results in patients with carotid injuries. It was concluded that vascular reconstruction was advisable in patients with mild deficits and in those with severe deficits in whom prograde flow was present preoperatively. Ligation was recommended in patients with severe neurologic deficits and no preoperative prograde flow. Ligation may occasionally be appropriate for patients with neurologic deficits and persistent prograde flow in whom thrombus exists in the cephalad vessel. If thrombectomy cannot be performed without risk of cerebral embolization, ligation may be the best choice.

Arterial reconstruction, if feasible, is recommended in essentially all neurologically intact patients. The only exception is the patient with obstructed prograde flow and intraluminal thrombus in the cephalad vessel. If reconstruction risks cerebral embolization, ligation is suggested.

Controversy continues regarding the therapeutic implications of preoperative neurologic deficits. Recent reviews by Unger and associates and by Liekweg and Greenfield support the recommendation that injured carotid arteries should be reconstructed, if technically feasible, in all except comatose patients with prograde flow. In these authors' opinion, flow should also be restored in patients without prograde flow, except those with severe or rapidly progressing deficits and seriously depressed sensoriums.

Operative Technique. Before the induction of anesthesia, preparations are made for the performance of emergency tracheostomy in the event of intubation difficulties. Stability of the cervical spine should be confirmed before intubation, particularly in high-velocity missile trauma. If an internal carotid injury near the base of the skull has been demonstrated arteriographically, exposure may be difficult and an additional 1 to 2 cm can be obtained by subluxation of the jaw. The mandible is pulled inferiorly and anteriorly and held in place with dental wires.

Patients with potential or proved carotid injuries should be handled with consideration given to the tenuous hemostasis provided by soft tissue tamponade and the likelihood of intraluminal thrombus. A vigorous antiseptic scrub may dislodge a clot and cause either bleeding or embolization. Preparation of the operative field preferably includes the shoulder and anterior chest in case further exposure is required, as well as a site for harvesting a venous autograft.

Incision extensions that may be necessary are described with vascular injuries of the thoracic inlet. Shunts are rarely needed for repairs of common carotid injuries if the cephalad clamp does not occlude communication between the external and internal carotid arteries. Adequate collateral flow from the external carotid is easily verified by momentarily releasing the cephalad clamp. Following proximal and distal occlusion, with or without an intraluminal shunt, repair is carried out by standard vascular techniques. Injuries of the internal jugular vein are primarily repaired if this can be readily accomplished by lateral venorrhaphy, patch venoplasty, or end-to-end anastomosis. Unilateral ligation is well tolerated and the use of interposition grafts to restore venous continuity is not justified.

The common use of preoperative arteriography in recent years has uncovered an increasing number of vertebral artery injuries. Acute complications of vertebral artery injury are rare, but massive hemorrhage may be lethal. An AV fistula is the most common late complication, usually diagnosed months or years after injury. The incidence of these sequelae is unknown. Meier and associates described a series of 13 patients with acute vertebral artery trauma. During this time period 54 carotid injuries were treated, yielding a comparative incidence of about 20 percent for vertebral artery injuries.

A review of forty-one patients with penetrating vertebral artery injuries revealed that five of these patients were in shock on arrival but no patient presented with or developed neurologic signs attributable to the vertebral-basilar system. Three-quarters of the patients had no clinical findings of arterial injuries other than the penetrating wound or a stable hematoma. The remaining patients had expanding hematomas and four had overt arterial hemorrhage. The diagnosis was made arteriographically in 35 patients and during urgent operative explorations in the remainder. Proximal and distal vertebral artery ligations were performed in 28 patients; 13 had only proximal ligations and two were treated nonoperatively. Several complications developed in the patients having only proximal ligations, and the authors recommend both proximal and distal ligations when feasible. Reid and Weigelt recommended ligation of injured vertebral arteries in all patients with normal contralateral arteries if no spinal cord branches arise from the injured vessels but state that nonoperative management may be reasonable in asymptomatic patients with arteriographically minimal injuries. The site of proximal ligation is immediately distal to the subclavian origin of the vertebral artery. The site of distal ligation depends on the location of injury and can be performed as high as the C1-C2 interspace, when the artery is free of the bony canal.

Base of the Neck (Thoracic Inlet). Thoracic inlet injuries may involve the innominate, the subclavian, and the proximal common carotid arteries and adjacent veins. Anatomic characteristics make the diagnosis of injured vessels difficult and impede rapid hemostasis and operative exposure for vascular control and repair. Exsanguinating hemorrhage is the predominant risk; bleeding may not be easily recognized because of free decompression into the pleural spaces. Abundant collateral blood supply generally protects against cerebral or upper extremity ischemia but also disguises the injury by maintaining distal perfusion and exaggerates blood loss during operative exposure.

Rapid resuscitation, liberal surgical exploration, and a thorough knowledge of the operative approach are the necessary ingredients of success. Indications to consider early surgical exploration are listed in Table 6-3. Diagnostic errors and subsequent inappropriately conservative management rarely occur with overt signs of major vascular injury. Unfortunately, many of these injuries appear innocuous at the time of presentation, and a high index of suspicion is necessary. In this circumstance platysmal penetration and proximity of the wound to a major vascular structure are used as indications for surgical exploration. As previously discussed, arteriography to modify the principle of proximity and penetration exploration remains controversial. It may prove useful if immediately available, but valuable time should not be wasted with studies if objective evidence of major vascular injury exists.

Important factors in the management of these injuries are emphasized by the series of Flint and associates. During an 11-year period, 146 patients with 206 injuries of major vascular structures at the base of the neck were treated. Arterial injuries accounted for 49 percent, including 36 injuries to the subclavian artery, 29 to the common carotid, and 7 to the innominate artery. Of the 74 venous injuries, there were 31 to the subclavian vein, 32 to the internal jugular, and 11 to the innominate vein. Signs and symptoms of major vascular injury were equivocal in many patients and totally absent in 32 percent of the patients. These patients were explored on the basis of platysmal penetration and the proximity of the wound to a major vascular structure. The overall mortality was 7.8 percent and was generally related to the magnitude of associated injuries or the extent of blood loss before operation. Thirteen percent of the patients with arterial trauma died, compared with 3 percent of those with venous injuries. Early and liberal surgical exploration with emphasis on adequate exposure resulted in low mortality and morbidity rates in this large series.

Operative Technique. Vessel exposure and control of hemorrhage are the major problems in the operative management of thoracic inlet injuries. The inaccuracy of preoperative wound localization and the wide exposure often required for vascular control make a flexible operative approach essential. A variety of incisions may be needed, often involving the mobilization of overlying bony structures, as illustrated in Fig. 6-6. The initial incision may not provide adequate exposure and may require extension or another separate incision. The supine position and a wide operative field including the entire neck, chest, and upper arms offers the most operative flexibility.

Table 6-3
Findings Suggesting Major Vascular Injury

Obvious or direct evidence of injury:
1. Circulatory instability
2. Excessive external bleeding
3. A large or progressing hematoma
4. Distal pulse deficit
5. Neurologic deficit involving nerves anatomically adjacent to major vascular structures
6. Massive or continued intrathoracic bleeding
7. Ischemia

Indirect evidence indicating injury:
1. A wound above the clavicle or manubrium that penetrates the platysma muscle
2. Thoracic wounds whose trajectory traverses the superior mediastinum or thoracic inlet
3. Mediastinal widening demonstrated radiographically

The approaches used to expose these injuries are the oblique cervical and horizontal clavicular incisions, median sternotomy, left anterolateral thoracotomy, and a musculoskeletal chest wall flap (see Fig. 6-6). The right oblique cervical incision generally is adequate to expose the entire right common carotid artery. The horizontal clavicular incision with subperiosteal resection of the medial half of the clavicle adequately exposes the right subclavian vessels. Extension to a median sternotomy is necessary to expose the innominate artery. The distal left common carotid artery is easily exposed through a left oblique neck incision, but the proximal vessel requires a sternal extension. The distal left subclavian artery can be reached through a horizontal clavicular incision, but its proximal portion requires a sternotomy or, more appropriately, a left anterolateral thoracotomy. A musculoskeletal flap, or ''trapdoor,'' may be used to expose the proximal left carotid and the entire left subclavian arteries and the left innominate vein. This is formed by combining horizontal clavicular, superior median sternotomy, and anterolateral thoracotomy incisions. Most base-of-the-neck injuries can be exposed through the oblique cervical and/or horizontal clavicular incisions. The vascular repair seldom is difficult and most often can be accomplished by lateral arteriorrhaphy or end-to-end anastomosis. When graft interposition is required, autogenous material is preferred.

In unstable patients with suspected major mediastinal injuries, especially in the presence of large or continuing intrathoracic bleeding, initial thoracic incisions are advisable. This usually implies a median sternotomy, but if the wound is on the left and a

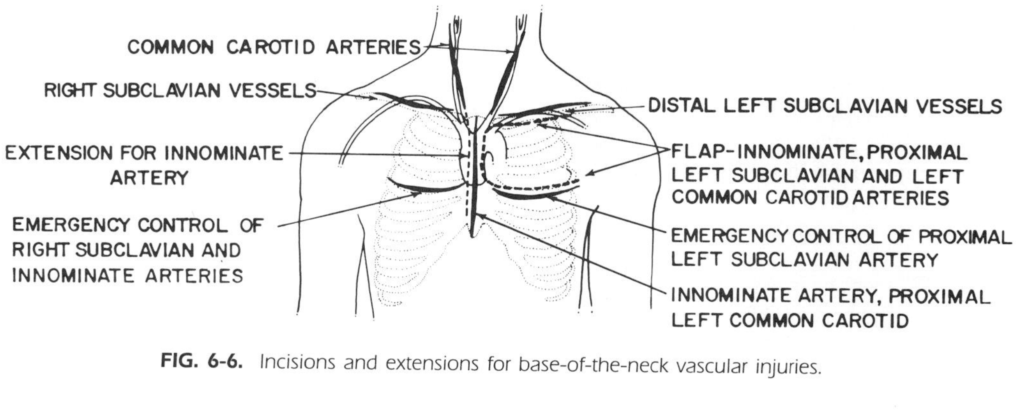

FIG. 6-6. Incisions and extensions for base-of-the-neck vascular injuries.

proximal left subclavian injury is suspected, an anterolateral thoracotomy is performed. Anterolateral thoracotomy is performed on the side of injury in patients with massive intrathoracic bleeding if sternal splitting instruments are not immediately available.

Oblique cervical and horizontal clavicular incisions often provide adequate exposure in stable patients with cervical, periclavicular, or supramanubrial wounds without evidence of deep mediastinal penetration or intrathoracic hemorrhage. A wide operative field is essential, however, and extension to a thoracic incision is made without hesitation.

The oblique cervical incision provides adequate exposure for most cervical wounds without evidence of mediastinal penetration. Lateral extension with resection of the medial half of the clavicle is sometimes necessary for additional exposure. Using this extension, satisfactory access was obtained in more than 90 percent of patients with common carotid and internal jugular injuries. If difficulty with proximal exposure is encountered during the dissection of either common carotid artery, a midsternal extension is made.

The horizontal clavicular incision is initially used in stable patients with periclavicular or supramanubrial wounds and suspected mediastinal penetration but without notable intrathoracic bleeding. Eighty-seven percent of subclavian vein injuries, 75 percent of innominate vein injuries, and 60 percent of subclavian artery injuries were successfully repaired by Flint and associates using this incision.

If possible, complete proximal and distal vascular control should precede dissection into the immediate area of suspected injury and the tamponading hematoma. If exposure is inadequate during the dissection of either proximal common carotid artery or the right subclavian artery, a midsternal extension should be made without hesitation. If proximal exposure is inadequate during the transclavicular dissection of the left subclavian artery, a left anterolateral thoracotomy is performed and, if additional exposure is required, midsternal extension forms a musculoskeletal flap.

The repair of the vascular injury, once isolated, seldom presents a major problem and can usually be accomplished by lateral arteriorrhaphy or end-to-end anastomosis. When graft interposition is required, autogenous material is preferred. The use of shunts or extracorporeal circulation to maintain cerebral flow should be considered if flow is reduced in more than one of the vessels supplying the brain. Vascular reconstruction is desirable, but because of the rich collateral circulation, single arterial ligations can usually be safely performed, especially when survival depends on early completion of the operation. Measurement of "stump" pressures may be helpful in predicting the consequences of major arterial ligations. Venous ligation usually results in minimal morbidity and may be indicated when optimal repair is not possible, although both innominate veins should not be ligated.

Larynx and Trachea. The signs and symptoms of laryngeal and tracheal injuries include respiratory distress, hoarseness, hemoptysis, and subcutaneous emphysema. Essentially all penetrating laryngotracheal injuries are clinically obvious and this fact may be useful in predicting the course of a missile. Subcutaneous air is not diagnostic of such an injury since air may enter through the skin wound or be due to an injury of the esophagus, bronchus, or lung.

Whenever laryngeal or tracheal injury produces difficulty breathing in the emergency room, a tracheostomy is performed before transfer of the patient to the operating suite. If the patient is hoarse or the wound is near the thyroid or larynx, laryngoscopy is performed preoperatively, when feasible, to evaluate the larynx and function of the recurrent laryngeal nerves. Direct laryngoscopy, using a small-diameter flexible endoscope, is more often successful and less cumbersome than indirect laryngoscopy in the acutely traumatized patient.

Tracheal wounds are usually obvious during operative exploration, but if the injury cannot be identified, the endotracheal tube cuff should be deflated to increase intratracheal pressure and enhance the air leak. Clean lacerations of the trachea or larynx are closed using synthetic absorbable suture such as Dexon or Vicryl. These materials result in less frequent problems with chronic granulation tissue postoperatively. If a tracheostomy is not performed, an endotracheal tube may be indicated for several days postoperatively to ensure an adequate airway.

A tracheostomy may be required instead of or in addition to primary repair, depending on the site and size of the defect and the magnitude of associated injuries. Patients with laryngeal injuries should have normal anatomy reconstructed as accurately as possible to lessen subsequent airway and speech difficulties. If a tracheostomy is required, it is maintained until healing is complete and laryngeal or tracheal edema has subsided, usually in 4 to 8 days.

Pharynx and Esophagus. The clinical findings suggesting pharyngeal or esophageal injury are hematemesis, dysphagia, and subcutaneous emphysema. Carefully performed barium esophagography with cineradiography in two projections may be used to exclude esophageal injury in the asymptomatic patient with platysmal penetration. False-negative examinations occasionally occur, and all patients are closely observed in the hospital and without oral intake for at least 24 h. Pharyngoesophageal injuries are notoriously silent, and a high index of suspicion and a liberal attitude regarding operative exploration result in the lowest incidence of missed esophageal perforations.

After adequate debridement, injuries of the pharynx and esophagus usually may be primarily repaired using an inner layer of absorbable suture such as Vicryl or Dexon and an outer layer of silk, cotton, or Prolene. If a small esophageal injury is suspected but cannot be demonstrated during exploration, an anesthetic mask may be applied to the nose and mouth and positive pressure exerted while the wound is filled with saline solution. Bubbles may disclose the point of injury. It is vital to drain all such wounds, because infections and salivary leaks are potential complications. If there is massive loss of esophageal tissue, as with a close-range shotgun blast, it may be necessary to perform a cutaneous esophagostomy for feeding purposes and a cutaneous pharyngostomy for salivary drainage. A secondary reconstruction will be required after initial healing is complete. A small plastic nasogastric tube is used for feeding for 8 to 10 days following major esophageal injuries, unless a gastrostomy is deemed preferable.

Nerve Injuries. A preoperative neurologic examination is performed, whenever possible, to identify injured nerves. The brachial plexus, deep cervical plexus, phrenic nerves, and the cranial nerves are systematically tested. The vagus and recurrent laryngeal nerves can be evaluated by examining the vocal cords. A hypoglossal or spinal accessory nerve injury is particularly easy to miss unless a preoperative neurologic examination is performed. An associated head injury or alcoholic intoxication often impedes an adequate neurologic examination. Whenever possible, severed or lacerated nerves are debrided and repaired primarily using interrupted fine silk sutures on the perineurium.

Salivary Glands. The diagnosis of salivary gland injury is usually made during operative exploration but, if suspected preoperatively, may be made with sialography. Debridement, hemostasis, and simple drainage provide effective treatment. In the absence of ductal obstruction, a salivary fistula rarely occurs after injury to the gland substance.

When the major duct is injured, it may be repaired with fine silk over a ureteral catheter stent. The catheter should be removed after repair is completed. When repair is not feasible because of the patient's condition or for some other compelling reason, the duct may be ligated and the gland allowed to atrophy, or the duct may be reimplanted in the mucosa at a later time. If a salivary fistula does occur postoperatively and fails to close spontaneously, irradiation usually arrests salivary flow, but it is not advisable in children or young adults.

Miscellaneous Injuries. Thyroid injuries require only debridement of devitalized tissue, hemostasis, and adequate drainage. The thoracic duct may be injured with wounds near the left innominate-jugular venous bifurcation. Repair of the duct is not feasible because of its friability, but simple ligation is adequate. The duct may divide immediately before entering the vein or there may be tributaries from the head and arm and multiple ligations may be required for lymphostasis. The area should be thoroughly dried and inspected before closing, because a large collection of lymph may occur postoperatively from even a small leak. If lymph does accumulate, incision and drainage with the application of a bulky pressure dressing for a few days will usually effect closure of the lymphatic fistula. Injured right thoracic ducts, though less frequent, are treated similarly.

ABDOMINAL TRAUMA

The incidence of abdominal trauma continues to increase. Each year about 3.5 million persons in the United States are injured in automobile accidents, and many of these injuries involve the abdominal contents. Mortality rates are generally higher in patients sustaining blunt trauma than in those with penetrating wounds. Although newer and better diagnostic techniques such as computed tomography are now available, blunt trauma still presents a difficult challenge to the clinician. The spleen, liver, kidneys, and bowel are the most frequently injured abdominal organs (Table 6-4).

Early diagnosis facilitates optimal management. Initial evaluation serves as a baseline but is frequently difficult because of the masking of abdominal injury by other associated injuries. Often the patient is unconscious because of alcoholism, drug abuse, shock, or associated head injury. Chest trauma, orthopaedic problems, and retroperitoneal injuries may further complicate the diagnostic process. Another misleading factor in diagnosis, often not recognized, is that relatively trivial injuries may rupture abdominal viscera. The index of suspicion must be high, even in cases of supposedly minor abdominal trauma, if diagnostic errors are to be avoided.

Table 6-4
Frequency of Injury in Abdominal Trauma

Viscera Injured	*Frequency, %*
Spleen	26.2
Kidneys	24.2
Intestines	16.2
Liver	15.6
Abdominal wall	3.6
Retroperitoneal hematoma	2.7
Mesentery	2.5
Pancreas	1.4
Diaphragm	1.1

Clinical Manifestations. The evaluation of the patient with blunt abdominal trauma begins with a careful history and physical examination. Knowing the mechanism of injury is essential in discerning the likelihood of abdominal injury. Information about the patient and the accident scene can be obtained from the paramedics, witnesses, family, police, and the patient as well. Factors such as rapid deceleration, impaling forces, and seat belt restraints make abdominal viscera prone to injury. Physical examination in the alert patient remains the most reliable predictor of injury, yet this will be misleading as either a false-positive or false-negative examination in 10 to 20 percent of patients. The entire patient must be examined as well as the abdomen because of the high incidence of associated trauma. Fitzgerald and associates reported extraabdominal injuries were present in 97 percent of patients with abdominal injuries who were dead on arrival at the hospital and in 70 percent of those admitted alive. In spite of the explosion of diagnostic technology, if the diagnosis is unclear, one must depend on repeated physical examinations done at frequent intervals by the same examiner. One cannot overemphasize the importance of the bedside clinical evaluation in determining which patients will benefit from operative management of their injuries.

Abdominal pain and tenderness when present are very reliable findings. Abdominal rigidity, and/or involuntary guarding, are indicative of intraperitoneal injury, and even when present alone, warrant exploratory celiotomy without further diagnostic procedures. It is important to note that blood in the peritoneal cavity may or may not cause irritation; hence hemoperitoneum may or may not produce significant physical findings. Patients with an altered state of consciousness resulting from closed head injuries, alcoholism, or drug abuse also may demonstrate evidence of abdominal discomfort. Injuries to organs in the retroperitoneal space such as pancreas, duodenum, kidney, and blood vessels, by virtue of their anatomic location, frequently do not produce signs of peritoneal irritation such as rebound tenderness, referred pain, and abdominal wall rigidity.

Newer diagnostic studies and better imaging techniques such as computed tomography have increased the clinician's ability to rapidly identify abdominal injuries. These studies have significantly helped to reduce the number of negative celiotomies. In a small number of cases it will be difficult to determine the extent of injury and occasional negative procedures will be performed. It is still preferable to perform a negative celiotomy on occasion with virtually no mortality and very little morbidity than to suffer the consequences of a missed injury.

In patients with blunt abdominal trauma, determinations of alterations in blood pressure are often useful. A valuable sign of continuing intraabdominal hemorrhage is transient elevation of the blood pressure to normal levels for a few minutes followed by return to hypotensive levels with the rapid infusion of 500 to 1000 mL of Ringer's lactate solution. Patients who are hypotensive from minimal blood loss or from neurogenic shock usually do not behave in this manner. The Ringer's lactate solution generally is infused over a period of 15 to 20 min while other measures, such as blood typing and cross matching, are being carried out. Postural hypotension, when the patient assumes the erect position, is another useful sign of continuing intraabdominal bleeding. Often subtle signs of hemorrhage such as mild to moderate tachycardia, tachypnea, narrowing of the pulse pressure, and cool skin temperature will be early manifestations of intraabdominal hemorrhage. Blood loss in the range of 30 to 40 percent of the blood volume will be necessary to produce sustained marked hypotension with a systolic blood pressure consistently below 60 to 70 mmHg.

Diagnostic Procedures. Whereas history and physical examination remain the most reliable diagnostic modalities, other diagnostic aids will frequently confirm clinical suspicions. In general, laboratory determinations do not offer much help in the young, previously healthy traumatized patient.

Sudden acute blood loss may not be adequately reflected by early hemograms; hence, a normal hemoglobin and hematocrit shortly after injury may be misleading. Serum glucose and creatinine determinations may be helpful in elderly patients suspected of having diabetes or renal insufficiency. Whereas serum electrolytes are rarely abnormal, the serum potassium level is extremely important if operation is contemplated. Unrecognized hypokalemia may lead to disastrous consequences. A serum amylase level, when elevated, is a relatively reliable predictor of intraabdominal injury although not always an indication for operative intervention. In addition to being elevated with pancreatic injury, abnormal amylase levels are also seen in injuries to the duodenum and upper small bowel. Leakage of the amylase-containing fluid is rapidly absorbed into the blood from the peritoneal cavity.

Serum isoenzyme amylase analysis has been advocated by some authors to be more specific than total amylase for pancreatic injury; however, other reports refute this hypothesis.

Studies of urinary sediment are useful, since hematuria may indicate injury to the genitourinary tract. Studies indicate that dipstick urinalysis is very accurate in determining hematuria in addition to being very cost-effective. If the patient with abdominal injury cannot void, catheterization should be done to obtain urine for examination. Catheterization is contraindicated before obtaining an urethrogram, if there is a scrotal hematoma, perineal hematoma, blood at the tip of the male meatus, or a high-riding or floating prostate on rectal examination. In these instances injury to the urethra is suspected and additional damage may be done if a catheter is blindly inserted.

Levin tubes should be inserted as soon as possible in all patients sustaining blunt abdominal trauma. The stomach contents are aspirated and the aspirate is examined for the presence of blood. In addition, a Levin tube provides decompression of the stomach, prevents gastric dilatation, and prevents aspiration with the induction of anesthesia. The instillation of 30 to 60 mL of an antacid in the Levin tube will neutralize the stomach contents and further minimize the ravages of aspiration, should it occur.

Blood-gas determinations should be obtained in all multiply injured patients and, in particular, those patients with a history of chronic pulmonary disease, chest injuries, or possible aspiration.

Radiologic Findings. For patients who have sustained severe abdominal injury and in whom other clinical signs obviously point to such injury, radiography, for diagnosis, may dangerously delay surgical intervention. For some patients with stable vital signs and questionable diagnoses of intraabdominal injury, x-ray studies may occasionally be helpful. When a patient is suspected of having intraabdominal injuries, upright films of the chest should be made, in addition to supine films of the abdomen. Occasionally additional information may be obtained from lateral and left lateral decubitus films. The skeletal system is surveyed for fractures or dislocations. Examination of the soft tissues may give information about changes in size, shape, or position of many viscera. Pneumoperitoneum may be diagnosed with the patient in the erect or lateral decubitus positions. Indirect evidence of solid viscera rupture with secondary hemorrhage may be presumed by an increase in density in the region, by displacement of neighboring viscera, or by accumulation of fluid between the gas shadows of bowel loops. If a gastric, duodenal, or upper jejunal rupture is suspected, the appearance of pneumoperitoneum may be facilitated by injecting 750 to 1000 mL of air into the nasogastric tube, after which the patient sits in a semierect position for 10 min before an upright chest film or left lateral decubitus film of the abdomen is made. Films should also be made before the air injection for purposes of comparison if the patient's condition permits. Abdominal films are obtained if the patient has sustained penetrating trauma. It is important to document the location of missiles or the presence of retained fragments.

Examination of the upper gastrointestinal tract by contrast radiography using a water-soluble opaque medium may identify an injury of the stomach, duodenum, or upper small bowel. Contrast material is always used in conjunction with computed tomography. The use of barium mixtures for this is dangerous, since a severe peritoneal reaction may be caused by barium if it leaks through a gastrointestinal perforation. This is especially true if there is fecal contamination in the peritoneal cavity from a concomitant colon injury.

Intravenous pyelograms are performed less frequently than in the past. A single-shot urogram may provide useful information as a screening procedure in a patient who is being taken to the operating room urgently. It may establish the nature of the injury, but more importantly it will determine if both kidneys are functioning before surgical intervention in case an injured kidney must be removed. If arteriography or CT scan is contemplated, the intravenous pyelogram and cystogram can be obtained at the conclusion of the angiogram, thereby eliminating one study and conserving time. If necessary, intravenous pyelograms may be done during the surgical procedure to determine the presence of a functional kidney on one side before removing the other kidney.

Cystograms using a minimum of 300 mL of contrast material to adequately distend the bladder may also be useful for diagnosing bladder injury or perforation from blunt abdominal trauma, but normal cystograms do not necessarily rule out bladder injury.

Computed Tomography. The CT scan will provide excellent images of intraabdominal viscera. Resolution is excellent for solid organs such as the liver and spleen as seen in Fig. 6-7. Whereas lavage is unreliable for retroperitoneal injuries, the CT scan has a distinct advantage in this area. Pancreatic injuries are frequently identified with clarity; however, several reports of missed pancreatic injuries including complete transections have been noted.

Hollow organs are harder to evaluate unless contrast material is used. This is recommended and given both orally and intravenously. Some authors have used rectal contrast to identify colon injuries. Intravenous contrast will permit assessment of the genitourinary system and possibly obviate the need for an intravenous pyelogram.

Fluid collections, usually blood, may be seen surrounding organs or in dependent places such as the pelvis (Fig. 6-8). Con-

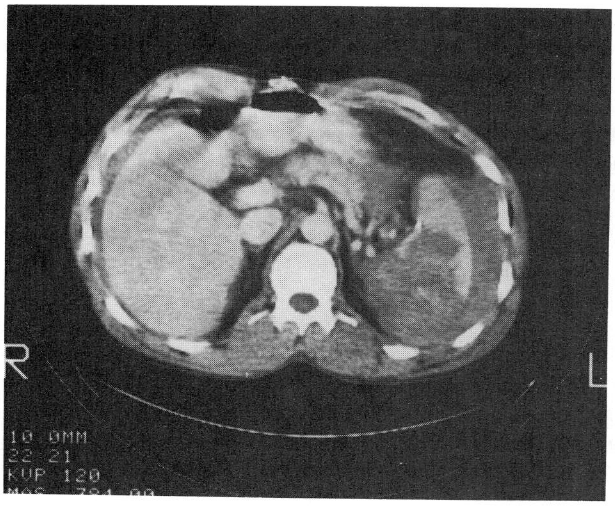

FIG. 6-7. Markedly disrupted spleen with blood seen surrounding the splenic remnant.

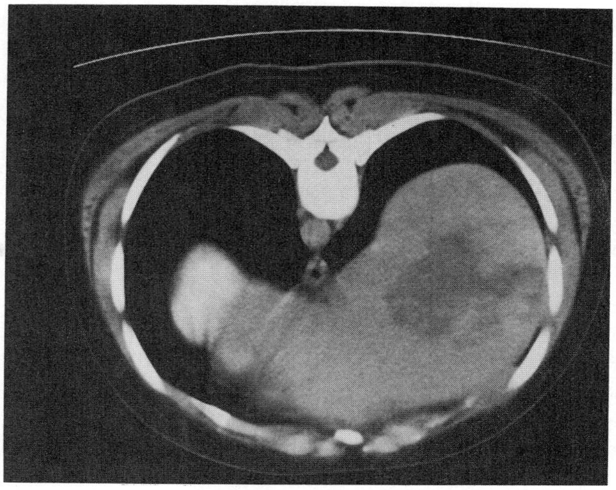

FIG. 6-9. Patient fell two stories. Large intraparenchymal hematoma seen in right lobe of liver.

tained hematomas can be seen within solid organs that would be missed with lavage if there is no free blood in the peritoneal cavity (Fig. 6-9).

Unstable patients are not candidates for computed tomography. The length of the procedure will vary according to whether contrast is used, experience with the technology, and the availability of the scanner. Again, valuable time should not be wasted if hemodynamic stability is in question.

Reports are very enthusiastic, but caution must be given to the fact that significant injuries have been missed with CT scans. The incidence of false negatives is 7 to 10 percent, and hence continued clinical evaluation is essential for optimal care in spite of a negative procedure.

The emergence of the CT scan has led to consideration of nonoperative management of some selected injuries. Repeated CT scans or sonography have been used to follow the progress of patients who are operated on.

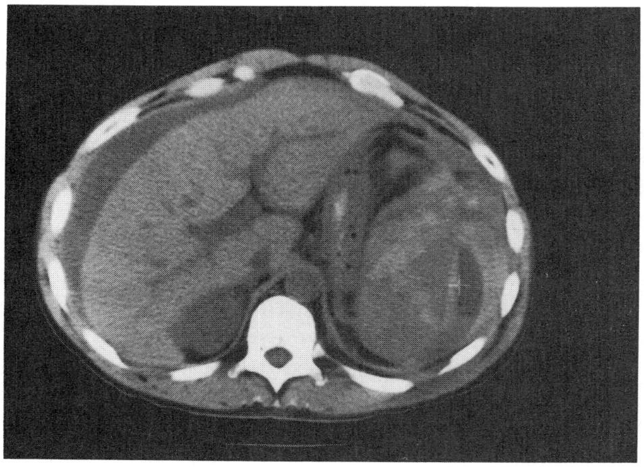

FIG. 6-8. Large spleen with inhomogeneous density representing blood in and around the spleen. Small fluid level seen within the spleen. Free fluid (blood) in the abdomen and surrounding liver. There are areas of high density (clotted blood) within lower-density fluid.

Arteriography. Selective arteriography is another available study occasionally used in diagnosis of blunt abdominal trauma. Selective catheterization of the celiac, mesenteric, or renal vessels may be performed. A film taken several minutes after injection can be used as an excretory urogram.

Arteriography is useful in assessing renal artery injury and is routinely used if a kidney is not promptly visualized with intravenous pyelography or CT scan. Intimal tears, aortic occlusion, and traumatic aneurysms are often seen in conjunction with seat belt injuries and are occasionally associated with serious lumbosacral trauma.

When continued pelvic bleeding occurs with extension into the retroperitoneal space secondary to pelvic fractures, arteriography may be beneficial in localizing the site of bleeding. Additionally, vasospastic agents or hemostatic agents such as autologous clot may be embolized to control bleeding. Again, it must be emphasized that time should not be wasted on adjunctive procedures when surgical intervention is indicated.

Peritoneal Lavage. Canizaro and associates described the use of intraperitoneal saline infusions in animals. Root and associates first described the technique of peritoneal lavage in human beings in 1965 and subsequently reported a series of 304 patients with a 96 percent accuracy. Numerous reviews of this procedure have proved peritoneal lavage to be a safe and reliable adjunctive procedure for evaluating patients with blunt abdominal trauma. The indications for this technique are patients with closed head injuries, altered consciousness, spinal cord injuries, equivocal abdominal findings, and negative needle paracentesis. It is not recommended for patients with gunshot wounds to the lower chest or abdomen, stab wounds to the back, previous abdominal procedures, presence of dilated bowel, late pregnancy, or positive needle paracentesis.

Several techniques have been described. The Lazarus-Nelson approach utilizes a small Teflon catheter inserted over a previously placed flexible guide wire. The technique popularized by Perry selects a point in the lower midline below the umbilicus approximately one-third of the distance between that and the pubic symphysis. After decompression of the urinary bladder and the stomach by the use of a Levin tube, the skin is cleansed and prepared with an iodinated antiseptic solution. A wheal is raised with 1%

lidocaine with epinephrine and the skin incised with a #11 scalpel. At this point a standard peritoneal dialysis catheter can be inserted, and the trocar advanced carefully until it just penetrates the peritoneum (Fig. 6-10). An alternative and perhaps safer method is to incise the abdominal wall to the peritoneum and insert the trocar under direct vision. Once the peritoneum is penetrated, the trocar is removed and the dialysis catheter advanced toward the pelvis. A syringe is then attached to the catheter and the peritoneal cavity is aspirated.

Nonclotting blood will often be aspirated through the larger catheter in spite of a negative needle paracentesis. If no blood is aspirated, a liter of balanced salt solution (Ringer's lactate) is rapidly infused into the peritoneal cavity over 5 to 10 min. For children and small adults 10 to 15 mL/kg is used. The patient is then turned from side to side in order to further mix the blood and fluid. If other injuries such as pelvic or long bone fractures are present, this step is eliminated.

The empty intravenous-fluid bottle is lowered and the fluid siphoned out of the peritoneal cavity. A sample is sent to the laboratory for quantitative analysis. In addition to obtaining red cell and white cell counts, it is important to determine the presence or absence of amylase, bile, or bacteria. Greater than 100,000 RBC/mm^3, 500 WBC/mm^3, or detection of bile, bacteria, food fibers, or amylase in excess of normal serum values is considered a positive study. Controversy exists regarding the number of red cells that constitute a positive study. Most authors agree with 100,000 for blunt trauma but figures as low as 1000 have been reported for penetrating trauma.

It must be emphasized that peritoneal lavage is very inaccurate in predicting retroperitoneal injuries. Unless the posterior peritoneum has been torn or considerable time has elapsed between the injury and lavage, most pancreatic injuries are not detected. The same is true for duodenal, urologic, and major vessel injuries that are retroperitoneal. Diaphragmatic injuries likewise are rarely detected by peritoneal lavage. Complications, although very rare (1 to 2 percent), occur frequently enough that lavage is not recommended for every patient suspected of abdominal injury. A negative lavage, however, may spare the patient an exploratory celiotomy. The role of peritoneal lavage is now being reassessed and its use redefined since the emergence of computed tomography. There clearly is a place for both diagnostic tests.

Other Procedures. Sonography has been used in the evaluation of blunt abdominal injury but is not nearly as accurate as computed tomography. The recent surge of interest in laparoscopy has not escaped the trauma patient. Early studies are beginning to emerge indicating a select group of patients may benefit from this procedure. This would include those patients thought to have penetrating injuries who have no other indication for operation. The absence of penetration coupled with a pristine abdomen may obviate the need for operation. On the other hand, numerous injuries have been missed on laparoscopy and found at celiotomy. These include ureteral injuries, pancreatic transections, liver, colon, and diaphragmatic injuries.

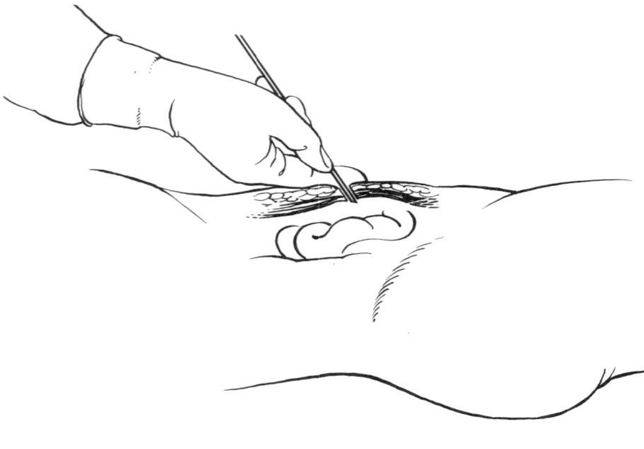

FIG. 6-10. Insertion of catheter for peritoneal lavage in the lower midline below the umbilicus.

Penetrating Trauma

Stab Wounds

Diagnosis of penetrating injuries of the abdomen does not usually present the difficult problem often posed by blunt abdominal trauma. Three methods of management have evolved: (1) routine exploration of all patients with abdominal stab wounds, (2) selective management, or (3) exploration following demonstration of peritoneal cavity and/or visceral injury.

Before 1960 there was little controversy, since essentially all surgeons agreed that penetrating trauma to the abdomen required exploratory celiotomy to rule out visceral injury. This agreement was first challenged by Shaftan in 1960, who recommended exploratory celiotomy only for patients with physical evidence of injury due to penetrating abdominal trauma and observation in the hospital for those without evidence of visceral injury. The major controversy now revolves around the following issues, which assume paramount importance: (1) How reliable are the various diagnostic criteria for visceral injury? (2) What is the effect of delayed celiotomy on the complication and mortality rate in patients who have no clinical manifestations of visceral injury after penetrating trauma, but who subsequently develop such manifestations? (3) Does negative celiotomy cause significant morbidity and mortality?

Some clinicians favor mandatory celiotomy for all patients who have sustained penetrating abdominal trauma. This point of view was supported by Bull and Mathewson, who found that 23 percent of 78 patients with significant intraabdominal injury confirmed at celiotomy and due to penetrating abdominal wounds had had no physical signs preoperatively. In contrast, 18 percent of 100 patients with possible penetrating injuries in whom the peritoneal cavity was not entered did have physical findings suggestive of visceral injury.

In spite of the fact that there is virtually no mortality associated with a negative celiotomy, most series report postoperative complications in the range of 10 to 20 percent. A review of 247 patients with negative celiotomies revealed a 2 percent incidence of small bowel obstruction. Seventy-five percent of the patients had an average follow-up of 57 months. Because of the high incidence of negative celiotomy following routine exploration, most trauma centers have abandoned this approach.

Selective management of abdominal stab wounds is recommended by many authors. Following clinical assessment, the decision to perform exploratory celiotomy is based on the following factors: (1) physical signs of peritoneal injury; (2) unexplained shock; (3) loss of bowel sounds; (4) evisceration of omentum or a viscus; (5) evidence of blood in the stomach, bladder, or rectum; and (6) evidence of visceral injury such as pneumoperitoneum or visceral displacement on x-ray films. Occasionally, other diagnostic studies are used, including intravenous pyelography, cystography, arteriography, peritoneal lavage, or computed tomography

(CT). In the absence of any indication of visceral injury, these patients are admitted to the hospital for a 24- to 48-h period of observation and are reevaluated frequently, preferably by the same observer. If the patient's condition deteriorates or changes significantly, exploratory celiotomy is performed.

Local exploration can provide useful information. The abdominal wall is prepared with an antiseptic agent. Using local anesthesia, the wound is opened sufficiently to visualize the complete course and depth of the tract. Often with adequate light, instruments, assistance, and exposure, it is obvious that a wound thought to have penetrated the peritoneal cavity is actually superficial and limited to the abdominal wall. These patients are managed by simple wound care and outpatient follow-up if other injuries do not require hospitalization.

Local wound exploration must involve more than simple instrument probing to determine penetration. Blind probing may be misleading, since a tortuous wound tract may allow passage of the probe for only a short distance, creating a false impression of nonpenetration. If the end of the tract cannot be visualized or the peritoneum is penetrated, local exploration is considered positive. This technique is equally useful for stab wounds of the back, although the thickness of the paraspinous muscles may prevent visualization of the end of the wound tract. Frequently, innocuous small stab wounds of the back significantly damage such retroperitoneal structures as the inferior vena cava, ureter, pancreas, or duodenum. A review of over 300 abdominal stab wounds by the authors indicated that nearly 20 percent of the patients could be discharged from the emergency room without hospital admission based on a negative local exploration that clearly demonstrated the end of the tract.

The abdominal viscera are at risk to injury with stab wounds of the lower chest as well as the abdomen. Figure 6-11 indicates the diaphragmatic excursion with maximal inspiration and expiration and clearly demonstrates elevation of the diaphragm as high as the fourth to fifth intercostal space anteriorly. Wounds at or below this level are therefore evaluated for abdominal injury as well.

If the stab wound to the chest is located below the fifth intercostal space and medial to the anterior axillary line and there is no obvious indication for operation, peritoneal lavage is performed. If lavage is negative, the patient is admitted to the hospital and observed for 24 to 48 h. If lavage is positive, operation is performed.

Patients with stab wounds of the abdomen located medial to the anterior axillary line are evaluated clinically. If there is no indication for operation, local exploration is performed. If the end of the tract is not visualized or the peritoneum has been penetrated but the abdominal physical findings are considered negative, lavage is similarly performed. Since lavage is unpredictable in determining retroperitoneal injuries, this method of management is limited to lower chest and abdominal wounds that are located between the two anterior axillary lines. Whereas these wounds have previously been treated by routine celiotomy, a review of 123 patients treated in this manner successfully reduced the incidence of negative celiotomies from 25.6 to 4.1 percent; 70 percent of the patients in this series were spared operative procedures, while 2.3 percent of the 88 patients initially observed were subsequently operated on but did not suffer any ill effects from delayed surgical treatment.

Patients with posterior wounds lateral to the anterior axillary line are not lavaged because of this method's unreliability with retroperitoneal injuries. In many centers these wounds are treated according to the criteria for selective management; other institutions recommend operative intervention to rule out visceral injury. Local exploration in this area may be beneficial. If the wound tracks anteriorly, peritoneal lavage may be performed. If the wound tracks posteriorly, computed tomography with contrast has been found to be extremely reliable with a sensitivity of 88 percent.

Since lower chest wounds may penetrate the diaphragm, it is important to evacuate air and blood from the pleural space with chest tubes before celiotomy. Although a pneumothorax may not be indicated by x-ray or physical examination, prophylactic insertion of an anterior chest tube will decrease the danger of a tension pneumothorax developing during induction of anesthesia and subsequent abdominal exploration. If a chest tube is not inserted, attention should be turned to the diaphragm shortly after entering the abdomen and the anesthesiologist should be alerted to watch for pulmonary problems.

Gunshot Wounds

The incidence of visceral injury in patients with abdominal gunshot wounds is at least 90 percent, as compared with 30 to 40 percent in patients with abdominal stab wounds. There is an eight-

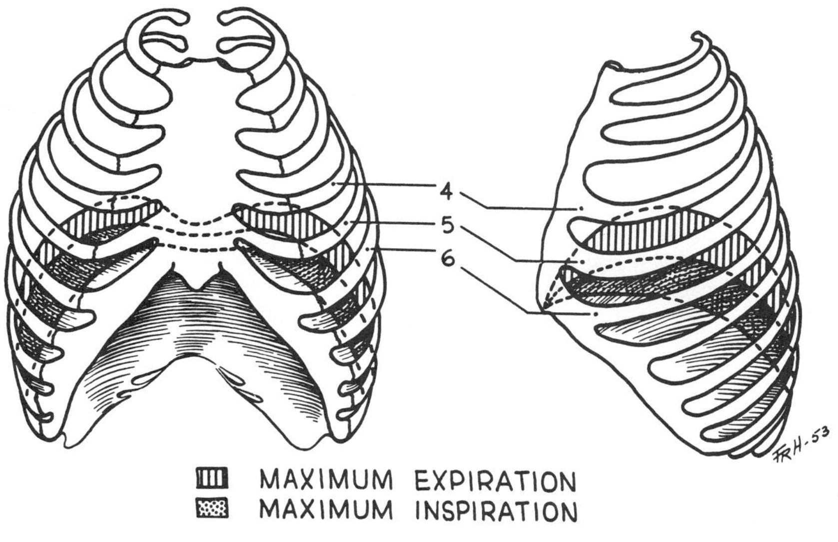

FIG. 6-11. Maximum diaphragmatic respiratory excursion. (From: *Shefts LM: Surg Clin North Am 38:1577, 1958, with permission.*)

fold to tenfold difference in mortality rates associated with gunshot wounds when compared with stab wounds.

It is not possible to predict the path of a missile by merely observing the entrance and exit wounds or connecting a line between an entrance wound and the appearance of a bullet on the x-ray film. These missiles may bounce, tumble, ricochet, and embolize.

Extraperitoneal gunshot wounds may produce intraabdominal injury by blast effect. In a report by Edwards and Gaspard, 14 percent of 35 patients sustaining gunshot wounds to the abdomen without penetration of the peritoneal cavity sustained at least one visceral injury.

Any bullet passing in proximity to the peritoneal cavity requires exploratory celiotomy. This includes all wounds of the lower chest and abdomen, flank, and back. Approximately 25 percent of lower chest wounds will produce intraabdominal injury. Celiotomy is recommended for patients with entrance wounds below the fifth intercostal space. If the patient's condition permits, anterior-posterior and lateral films of the abdomen should be made to locate the missile. Selective management, the use of radiopaque material, local exploration, or peritoneal lavage are not recommended for patients sustaining gunshot wounds in proximity to the abdomen. A review of 59 gunshot wound patients all of whom were taken to the operating room in spite of a negative physical examination and negative periotoneal lavage had a 25 percent incidence of visceral injury. Injuries not detected by either modality included the colon, diaphragm, kidney, pancreas, and aorta.

Once the diagnosis of intraabdominal injury is established and resuscitation is instituted, the abdomen is explored. A long midline incision is preferred for the following reasons: (1) It may be made much more rapidly than other incisions, a matter of vital importance when attempting rapid control of exsanguinating hemorrhage. (2) It gives wide access to all parts of the abdomen, which transverse incisions do not. (3) It may be readily extended into either side of the thorax or continued superiorly as a median sternotomy in case of combined thoracoabdominal injury or when better abdominal exposure is required. (4) It may be rapidly closed, which is of great importance in decreasing the anesthesia and operative time in gravely injured patients.

Management of Patients with Exsanguinating Abdominal Hemorrhage. With improvement of prehospital care, more patients are arriving at the hospital in extremis. Frequently this condition is due to massive intraabdominal hemorrhage that is refractory to standard resuscitative measures. Some authors have advocated performing preliminary left thoracotomy and temporary thoracic aortic occlusion before opening the abdomen in patients with massive hemoperitoneum, tense abdominal distention, and persistent hypotension. Bleeding can usually be controlled through the abdomen. Control of life-threatening hemorrhage from the aorta or its branches can be obtained by placing a vascular clamp on the supraceliac aorta. The exposure is through the gastrohepatic ligament, with blunt separation of the diaphragmatic crura crossing the aorta at the hiatus. The aorta is not encircled but simply clamped in an anterior-posterior plane while precise identification and control of the injuries is obtained. This maneuver is preferred where feasible and carries less morbidity than a thoracoabdominal incision and clamping of the decending thoracic aorta. The descending thoracic aorta is quickly and bluntly dissected circumferentially and occluded by a straight vascular clamp just above the diaphragm. Although this procedure may have occasional applicability, caution is expressed because it requires opening another major cavity, it increases afterload on the heart, the blood supply to the spinal cord may be interrupted, renal circulation is diminished, and it is ineffective in controlling major venous bleeding.

Once the abdomen is opened, the aortic clamp can be slowly released following stabilization of the patient, and proximal control gained at a lower level. A medium or large Richardson retractor may be used to obtain rapid temporary occlusion of the abdominal aorta just below the diaphragm. The lesser curvature of the stomach is pulled inferiorly, and the flat surface of the retractor blade is compressed firmly against the abdominal aorta, thus occluding it against the vertebra just beneath the diaphragm.

With effective control of massive hemorrhage, resuscitation can be successfully completed, ensuring continuous perfusion to the heart and brain and minimizing the possibility of sudden cardiac arrest.

Stomach

Injuries to the stomach from blunt trauma are infrequent, perhaps because of a relative lack of fixation of the stomach and its protected position; but penetrating injuries of the stomach from gunshot wounds occur frequently.

Diagnosis. The diagnosis of gastric injury is generally suspected from the course of the penetrating object, and, at times, additional suspicion of gastric injury arises from the presence of bloody fluid aspirated from the Levin tube. Generally, wounds of the anterior stomach wall are easily seen at celiotomy. Because of the possibility of missing posterior stomach wall wounds, it is important in all cases of proved or possible gastric injury to open the lesser sac through the gastrocolic omentum. This permits the entire posterior aspect of the stomach to be searched for injury. The points of attachment of the greater and lesser omenta on the greater and lesser curvatures of the stomach, respectively, should also be carefully inspected. If a hematoma is noted at the mesenteric attachment, it should be evacuated and the stomach wall at that site carefully inspected for injury.

Treatment. Gastric wounds are repaired by first placing a continuous locked 2-0 suture through all layers of the gastric wall. This hemostatic stitch is very important to control extensive bleeding that may occur from the rich submucosal network of blood vessels in the stomach. After this inner layer closure, an outer inverting row of interrupted nonabsorbable mattress sutures of the Lembert or Halsted type is placed. The outer row of sutures provides adequate approximation of the stomach wall, seals off readily, and prevents leaks. These sutures in the outer layer should not be through-and-through, as is the first row of sutures, but should extend through the seromuscular coat and the submucosal layer of the stomach. Wounds of the stomach are not drained externally, since they are unlikely to leak, as duodenal wounds may. It is very important to irrigate the peritoneal cavity, with special attention to the subhepatic and subphrenic spaces and the lesser sac, so that all food particles and gastric juice spilled into these areas are removed.

After operation for a gastric wound, nasogastric tube suction should be maintained for several days until active peristalsis resumes and the danger of postoperative gastric dilatation passes. The gastric aspirate should be observed for excessive bleeding, which may occur if the hemostatic suture line is inadequate. If bleeding is brisk or persists, the patient should be immediately reexplored to control the gastric bleeding point. After peristalsis resumes, gastric aspiration is discontinued and the patient is initially started on clear liquids and rapidly advanced to a normal diet.

Complications. Complications that may develop after stomach injury are hemorrhage from, or leakage of, the suture line and development of subhepatic, subphrenic, or lesser sac abscesses secondary to spilling of contaminated gastric contents. Development of such abscesses is suspected after gastric wounds in patients who fail to do well postoperatively and who have unexplainable fever for more than a few days. If contamination seems heavy, the skin and subcutaneous tissue should be left open until the wound appears clean.

Duodenum

Injuries to the duodenum and small bowel comprise about one-quarter of blunt and penetrating abdominal trauma. Mortality rates for duodenal injuries have steadily decreased and are directly proportional to the number and severity of associated injuries as well as the time between injury and treatment. Lucas and Ledgerwood reported a mortality rate of 40 percent in patients who were not operated on in the first 24 h after injury, in contrast to a mortality of only 11 percent among those operated on within less than 24 h. The improving mortality rate among patients with duodenal injuries is indicated by four series of duodenal wounds reported since 1978. The total number of patients in these series was 677 and the mortality rates ranged from 10.5 to 14 percent. The mortality rate for simple stab wounds involving only the duodenum should be significantly less than 5 percent, while the mortality for severe blunt trauma or shotgun wounds to the duodenum ranges from about 35 to more than 50 percent, especially when such trauma is combined with serious pancreatic injuries.

Diagnosis. The diagnosis of blunt trauma to the duodenum and small bowel is considerably more difficult than that of penetrating trauma to these organs. With duodenal or small bowel trauma, all the characteristic signs of injury to abdominal viscera may be minimal or absent for several reasons: (1) The injury of the duodenum following blunt trauma is frequently retroperitoneal, so that duodenal contents leak into the retroperitoneal area rather than into the free periotoneal cavity. (2) Duodenal and small bowel fluid may cause minimal contamination and may not lead to early signs of bacterial peritonitis. This is not true of injuries of the intraperitoneal duodenum, in which duodenal fluid freely flows into the peritoneal cavity. The highly alkaline pH of this fluid causes immediate chemical irritation of the peritoneum and physical signs of such irritation.

Injuries of the duodenum or upper small bowel should be suspected in any patient who receives a blow to the upper abdomen or lower chest, such as from a steering wheel. Testicular pain should raise suspicion of retroperitoneal duodenal rupture. Also, pain referred to the shoulders, chest, and back may be associated with perforation of the duodenum and small intestine.

Several diagnostic aids may be helpful in determining rupture of the duodenum or small bowel. Plain radiographs of the abdomen are helpful and may be diagnostic, but absence of free intraperitoneal air does not rule out bowel perforation. Retroperitoneal rupture of the duodenum is not often diagnosed by x-ray. The diagnosis may be based on detection of a large accumulation of air about the right kidney or along the psoas muscle margins. The accuracy of radiographic studies may also be increased by giving the patient a water-soluble radiopaque contrast medium orally and making abdominal x-ray films to detect leakage of the medium from the duodenum or small bowel. Such diagnostic procedures are unnecessary if other clinical signs indicate the need for exploratory celiotomy.

When a celiotomy is done for suspected intraabdominal injury, duodenal lesions are often missed, especially retroperitoneal lesions of the third or fourth portions. This is due to superficial observation, inadequate exposure, and lack of persistence on the part of the surgeon. Duodenal perforations have been missed initially in 33 to 50 percent of the various reported series of retroperitoneal duodenal injuries. To avoid overlooking duodenal trauma and contributing to the high mortality from duodenal wounds, it is important to inspect the entire duodenum during abdominal exploration. This is especially true if a retroperitoneal hematoma is noted near the duodenum or if there is crepitation or bile-stained fluid along the lateral margins of the duodenum retroperitoneally. Additional signs that require careful exploration of the duodenum and the retroduodenal area include: elevation of the posterior peritoneum with glassy-appearing edema; petechiae or fat necrosis over the ascending and transverse colon or mesocolon; retroperitoneal phlegmon; hematoma over the head of the pancreas extending into the base of the mesocolon; fat necrosis of the retroperitoneal tissues; and/or discoloration of retroperitoneal tissues—dark from hemorrhage, grayish from suppuration, or yellowish from bile.

If these signs are noted or if the duodenum is contused, it should be widely mobilized by the Kocher maneuver, incising the peritoneum along its lateral margin, so that the duodenum can be completely mobilized along with the head of the pancreas. Thus, small areas of perforation in the retroperitoneal aspect of the duodenum may be identified. Often retroperitoneal wounds of the duodenum that were missed at initial exploration are not recognized until several days later when bile-stained fluid drains from the abdominal wound of a patient who has continued to do poorly postoperatively.

The third and fourth portions of the duodenum may be exposed by mobilizing the cecum, right colon, hepatic flexure of the colon, and mesenteries of these organs up to and including the ligament of Treitz, carrying the dissection of the mesocolon along the attachment at the root of the small bowel mesentery.

Treatment. Treatment of duodenal perforation itself depends more on the size of the perforation than on any other single factor. In general, an attempt is made to close the duodenal perforation if this can be done without decreasing the lumen of the duodenum. This closure is carried out with a continuous locking 3-0 suture through all layers of the duodenal wall followed by an outer layer of nonabsorbable interrupted mattress sutures in the seromuscular layer of the duodenum. If the perforation is so large that simple closure will cause a stricture of the duodenum, consideration should be given to (1) complete division of the duodenum and an end-to-end anastomosis or (2) division of the duodenum, closure of both ends, and a gastroenterostomy.

If the region of the ampulla is involved in a duodenal injury, the common bile duct should be identified by insertion of a T tube, since reimplantation of the common duct sometimes may be necessary. Approximately 75 to 80 percent of all duodenal injuries can be closed by debridement of the wound edges and simple suture. For the other 20 to 25 percent, one of the reparative proce-

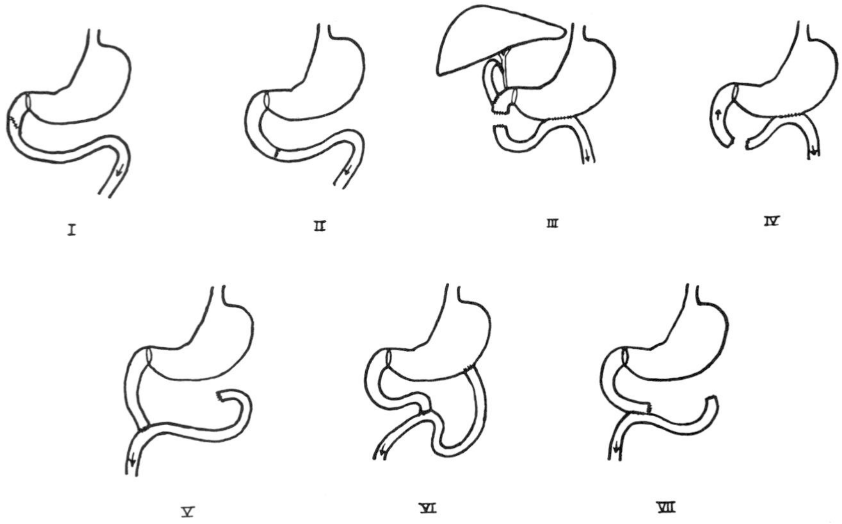

FIG. 6-12. Diagrammatic representation of various operative procedures in a series of cases. I, Simple closure; II, end-to-end duodenoduodenostomy; III and IV, closure of both ends of duodenum and gastroenterostomy; V, closure of distal duodenum and duodenojejunostomy; VI, duodenojejunostomy and gastroduodenostomy; VII, resection of fourth part of duodenum and duodenojejunostomy. (From: *Cleveland HC, Waddell WR: Surg Clin North Am 43:413, 1963, with permission.*)

dures such as a seromuscular patch using a loop of small intestine or suturing the open end of a Roux limb to the defect can be used (Fig. 6-12). Rarely, a pancreaticoduodenectomy may be necessary to manage extensive devitalizing trauma to the duodenum and periampullar region, especially when such injuries are combined with severe pancreatic trauma and it is difficult to control bleeding.

Severe injuries of the duodenum or combined severe injuries of the pancreas and duodenum may be treated by a Berne duodenal "diverticulization" procedure instead of by pancreatoduodenal resection unless the destruction and devitalization of the pancreas and duodenum is too extensive. This operation is illustrated in Fig. 6-13. This operation consists of diversion of the alimentary stream away from the injured duodenum and pancreatic head. This is achieved by removing the gastric antrum, closing the duodenal stump, and performing a Billroth II gastrojejunostomy and vagotomy. The duodenal laceration is closed with interrupted monofilament nonabsorbable sutures, and the duodenum is decompressed with a tube duodenostomy to reduce the possibility of disruption of the duodenal suture line from increased pressure within the duodenal stump. The tube duodenostomy is performed by inserting a #12 or #14 French straight rubber catheter into the lateral duodenal wall through a stab wound, securing the tube with a pursestring suture. The area of the combined pancreatic and duodenal injuries is then extensively drained with several large Penrose drains and a soft suction drain. Closed suction drains may be preferable to Penrose drains if the area of tissue destruction is not too extensive. The biliary tract is drained by inserting a T tube into the common duct or by performing a tube cholecystostomy. In 1974, Berne and associates reported the use of this operation in the treatment of 50 patients with severe pancreatic and duodenal injuries with a mortality rate of only 16 percent, which is gratifyingly low for patients with such grave injuries. Even though duodenal and pancreatic fistulae may develop in patients undergoing the Berne duodenal diverticulization procedure, these lesions are generally well tolerated since they are, in effect, end rather than lateral fistulae because the gastric contents are diverted from the duodenum and pancreas. In the experience reported by Berne and associates, there were seven duodenal fistulae and five pancreatic fistulae among their 50 patients, but all closed spontaneously.

An alternative method for diverting the gastric contents from severe duodenal injuries was reported by Vaughan and associates. This procedure consists of repair of the duodenal wound, followed by a gastrotomy on the greater curvature of the antrum of the stomach in a site selected for gastrojejunostomy. Through this opening, the pylorus is closed with absorbable sutures. Gastrojejunostomy, side-to-side, is then accomplished (Fig. 6-14). These surgeons used this procedure in 75 patients selected from 175 consecutive patients who had duodenal trauma. The mortality was 19 percent and the rate of fistula formation was 5 percent among the patients treated by pyloric exclusion and gastrojejunostomy. Two of the three patients who developed duodenal fistulae after pyloric exclusion had spontaneous closure of the fistula, and the remaining patient required surgical closure. Vaughan and associates note that in other series of duodenal injuries the rate of lateral duodenal fistula formation has ranged between 6 and 14 percent regardless of the type of closure. Kelly and associates have performed the same type of pyloric exclusion with gastrojejunostomy but have used staples instead of sutures as employed by Vaughan and associates to close the pylorus.

Prevention of Duodenal Fistulization after Duodenal Trauma. Some surgeons suggest that duodenal fistulas can be prevented by prolonged decompression of the duodenum after clo-

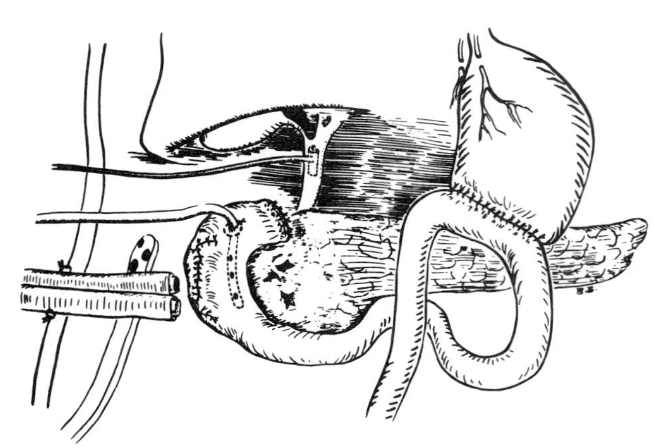

FIG. 6-13. The essential components of duodenal diverticulization including gastric antrectomy, tube duodenostomy, gastrojejunostomy, and drainage of the biliary tract may be advisable. (From: *Berne CJ, Donovan AJ, et al: Am J Surg 127:503, 1974, with permission.*)

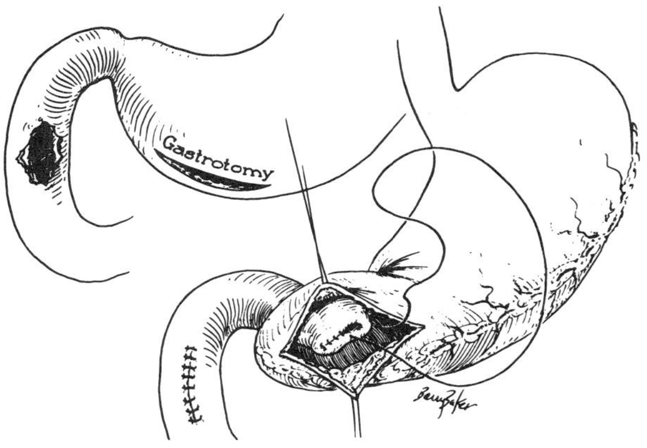

FIG. 6-14. Duodenal injury and method of excluding the pylorus. (From: *Vaughan GD, Frazier OH, et al: Am J Surg 134:785, 1977, with permission.*)

sure of the wound. This may be especially indicated in more severe injuries of the duodenum and can be accomplished in several ways. Snyder and associates performed duodenal tube decompression in 53 percent of the 190 of their patients with duodenal injuries who had duodenorrhaphies. In this series, duodenal fistulae developed in 9 percent and caused death in 4 percent of those who had duodenal decompression. Stone and Fabian reported a series of 321 patients with duodenal wounds and the last 237 were all managed with duodenal decompression via a gastrostomy tube and twin jejunostomy tubes (one passing retrograde into the duodenum). Only one duodenal fistula (0.5 percent) occurred in 210 surviving patients. In contrast, failure to decompress the duodenum was associated with an 8 percent leak rate. Thus, tube decompression of the duodenum is a reasonable and probably effective adjunct in the management of selected duodenal injuries.

Reliance on an abdominal drain in the management of duodenal trauma has varied considerably, although several reports suggest that routine drainage of the duodenal suture line may favor fistula formation. A secure closure in the absence of a pancreatic injury does not require drainage. If drainage is used, closed suction is preferred.

Postoperative Care. After repair of duodenal injuries, decompression with a nasogastric or gastrostomy tube is usually continued until bowel function returns. If a fistula forms, gastroduodenal decompression should be continued for prolonged periods and a sump drain should be inserted into the drain site for continuous active suction of the fistulous tract. This is done to prevent the spread of duodenal fluid throughout the peritoneal cavity and to aid in the calculation and replacement of fluid and electrolyte losses from the fistula. Meticulous nutritional support is important when fistulae occur. This can be accomplished by using jejunostomy tubes distal to the fistula, which may have been inserted at the initial operation. If enteral feedings are not reasonable, it may be necessary to support the patient with intravenous hyperalimentation. Occasionally, a fistula does not close with nonoperative therapy. In such cases, when a reasonable trial of conservative treatment has been made and the patient is in optimal condition for reoperation, the abdomen is opened and completely explored to rule out distal bowel obstruction that may be causing the fistula to persist. The fistula is exposed at its origin from the duodenum, and a Roux en Y defunctionalized limb of proximal jejunum is brought up to the fistula and anastomosed to it. This anastomosis may use either the end or the side (after closing the end of the jejunal limb) of the defunctionalized jejunum. This procedure permanently diverts the fistula drainage internally and is very effective.

Intramural Hematoma

Intramural hematoma of the duodenum is usually due to blunt abdominal trauma, including child abuse, which causes rupture of intramural duodenal blood vessels with formation of a dark, sausage-shaped mass in the submucosal layer of the duodenal wall. The hematoma may cause partial or complete duodenal obstruction, but the obstruction is usually partial. The patient has signs of a high small bowel obstruction, with nausea and vomiting associated with upper abdominal pain and tenderness, and sometimes a suggestion of a right upper quadrant mass on palpation of the abdomen. Plain films of the abdomen may show an ill-defined right upper quadrant mass and obliteration of the right psoas shadow. Felson and Levin have shown that an upper gastrointestinal tract series is generally diagnostic, showing dilation of the duodenal lumen with the appearance of a "coiled spring" in the second and third portions of the duodenum due to the crowding of the valvulae conniventes by the hematoma. The serum amylase level may be elevated. An intramural duodenal hematoma may also occur spontaneously in patients on anticoagulants.

Most infants and children with intramural duodenal hematomas can successfully be treated without surgical intervention. Nonsurgical treatment of these patients consists of cessation of oral intake, nasogastric suction, and intravenous replacement of fluids and electrolytes.

Small Bowel

Injuries to the small bowel are more common than injuries to the duodenum or colon. Eighty percent of bowel injuries occur between the duodenojejunal junction and the terminal ileum, with approximately 10 percent each in the duodenum and the large intestine. The usual mechanism of small bowel injury from blunt trauma is crushing of the small bowel against the vertebral column. Rupture of the small bowel is also caused by shearing and tearing forces applied to the abdomen, and rarely by sudden elevation of the intraluminal pressure of the bowel with bursting from such sudden high pressure.

In exploring the abdomen for injuries to the small bowel, it is important to inspect minutely the entire circumference of the small bowel and its attached mesentery from the ligament of Treitz to the ileocecal valve. The bowel may be completely transected in one or more places in blunt trauma with or without severe injury to the mesentery and its blood supply; at times, the mesentery may be torn from a segment of bowel, thus depriving the bowel of its blood supply. Penetrating trauma to the small bowel from a gunshot wound or stab wound is common.

Treatment. Small, single perforations of the small bowel may be closed safely with a single layer of interrupted nonabsorbable mattress sutures that include and invert the seromuscular and submucosal coats of the bowel. A hemostatic stitch, as required for stomach wounds, is not necessary for small bowel injuries, because the small bowel does not tend to continue bleeding from the submucosal plexus, as does the stomach. However, individual bleeders should be ligated with fine suture material. Two advantages of a single-layer closure are the rapidity of performance, which is important in patients in precarious condition after multiple trauma, and the reduced likelihood of compromising the bowel lumen.

Two small perforations of the bowel that are very close together may often be repaired by converting the wounds into one and closing the resulting defect as a single linear wound. This type of repair does not constrict the lumen of the bowel as much as two separate lines of suture placed close together and is more secure. Multiple perforations of the small bowel may occur after injury from shotgun pellets. Each one of these injuries should be carefully sought out and closed with interrupted rows of nonabsorbable sutures.

Long linear lacerations of the small bowel lumen also should be closed with a single row of nonabsorbable sutures after ligating any persistent bleeders with small nonabsorbable sutures. Longitudinal lacerations may be closed in a longitudinal direction or transversely according to the Heineke-Mikulicz principle.

Small bowel injuries produced by high-velocity missiles cause severe contusions of tissue surrounding the actual perforation. Because the contusion is a site of potential tissue necrosis and bowel leakage caused by thrombosis of vessels in the area of blast injury, it should be debrided. The debridement should extend into viable bowel where active bleeding is obtained. If the wound is too large or is long and longitudinal, the bowel may not be adequately closed without compromising the lumen, and the damaged segment should be resected. If there are multiple wounds in a short segment of bowel, it is much safer and easier to resect the injured segment than to attempt to suture each of the closely spaced wounds. Perforations or lacerations to the mesenteric border, unless they are quite small, are difficult to repair and frequently are associated with vascular impairment. They also should be managed by resection of the involved bowel if an adequate closure cannot be obtained without impairment of the blood supply. Following transection the bowel should be reanastomosed after debriding contused and damaged areas on either side of the wound back to normal intestine that has a good blood supply. Careful attention should be given to leaving uninjured mesentery adjacent to the suture line of the reanastomosis.

Extensive segments of bowel may be avulsed from the mesentery, so that the bowel loses its blood supply. All the necrotic or potentially necrotic bowel and injured mesentery must be resected and an end-to-end anastomosis made between uninjured bowel attached to uninjured mesentery.

Contusions of the small bowel should be assumed to be larger than is apparent. Such injuries are dangerous, since they may lead to subsequent necrosis and perforation. Contusions up to 1 cm in diameter may be turned in with a row of fine nonabsorbable mattress sutures. Larger contusions should be resected.

Temporary control of bowel spillage can be quickly obtained by stapling either the perforation or both ends of a transection while attention is directed toward managing more serious problems. After stabilization has been accomplished, the bowel can be repaired more leisurely as described above. Postoperative care of patients with wounds of the small bowel includes maintenance of nasogastric suction and low oral intake until adequate bowel activity returns. Leakage from suture lines and intestinal obstruction rarely occur if small bowel wounds are properly managed.

Colon

The morbidity and mortality from acute injuries to the colon and rectum have been significantly reduced by an aggressive surgical approach. This has been largely influenced by the experiences of military surgeons during World War II, the Korean conflict, and the Vietnam War.

In World War II, an impressive improvement in the mortality from wounds of the colon was noted. This was due to several factors including improved methods of triage and transportation, effective replacement of blood and fluid, and early surgical intervention combined with ancillary use of antibiotics.

The mortality rate for wounds of the colon of 37 percent in World War II was reduced to approximately 15 percent during the action in Korea. The majority of military surgeons treating acute injuries of the colon tended to exteriorize the wound as an artificial anus to prevent further soilage of the peritoneal cavity. This approach to these particular wounds was duly carried over into civilian practice and reflected in the subsequent reduction in mortality and morbidity. In the later phase of the Korean conflict, however, some modification of the aggressive technique was noted in that small, primary wounds treated early were handled by primary closure without exteriorization.

Acute wounds of the colon that occur in a civilian environment exhibit features that may modify the indications for exteriorization of the wound. The types of injury usually noted in a military situation resulted from either high-velocity missiles or fragmentation missiles in which there was massive destruction of tissue and usually gross soilage of the peritoneal cavity. In the civilian environment, the wounds more often are caused by low-velocity missiles and usually are unassociated with massive destruction of surrounding organs and tissue. The time from wounding to initial treatment in the civilian situation is generally somewhat less than that noted during military conflict. Similarly, associated injuries occurring in civilian accidents do not tend to be so numerous or so massive as those in a military environment, and this has a definite influence on morbidity and mortality.

Etiology. Acute injuries of the colon and rectum can be divided into penetrating wounds and wounds resulting from blunt trauma. Acts of violence constitute an important source of injuries to the colon, and these are generally penetrating injuries caused by guns or knives or, on rarer occasions, blunt abdominal trauma. Wounds of the rectum, particularly, may be the result of instrumentation during the process of sigmoidoscopy, the administration of enemas, or sexual behavior. There may also be perforations of the colorectum by foreign bodies that pass through the alimentary canal into the colon. Inadvertent penetration of the colon or rectum may occur during difficult operations; this is especially true of pelvic operations for neoplastic or severe inflammatory disease. Falls resulting in impalement on sharp objects may produce wounds of the rectum. Automobile accidents and other forms of blunt trauma may also produce acute injuries to the colon and rectum.

Diagnosis. A systematic diagnostic approach to problems of abdominal trauma is necessary, but specific examinations of the colon and rectum may be necessary to delineate an injury. This is particularly pertinent in those instances in which instrumentation is the cause of suspected perforation. Rectal examination and sigmoidoscopy should occupy a prominent place in the examination of these patients. Diagnostic abdominal x-ray studies should be used to determine if there is a perforation with leakage of air into the free peritoneal cavity. Anteroposterior and lateral decubitus views are particularly helpful in these instances. Contrast studies of the colon should be used rarely and cautiously in view of the high morbidity and mortality associated with leakage of barium and feces into the free peritoneal cavity. Aqueous opaque media, such as Gastrografin, are preferable when penetration of the colon is suspected. If colon injuries are suspected in a patient having a CT scan, rectal contrast material in addition to standard IV and oral contrast material could help identify these injuries.

Treatment. The management principles of patients with abdominal trauma apply to those patients who have acute injuries of the colon. It is important that the time from wounding to definitive operation be as short as possible, and aggressive replacement of fluid and blood losses should be undertaken at once. Patients with penetrating abdominal trauma or suspected colon or rectal injury should have a broad-spectrum antibiotic with aerobic and anaerobic coverage begun before surgery.

A thorough and complete exploration of all abdominal viscera is made, for the morbidity and mortality vary directly with the number of associated injuries. Bleeding should be controlled as rapidly as possible and immediate efforts made to reduce peritoneal soilage from any penetrating wound of an abdominal viscus. The specific care of the wound of the colon should be approached by noting the anatomic differences between the intraperitoneal and extraperitoneal large intestine. Particular attention must be paid to the type of wound, its location, the amount of tissue destruction, the presence of associated injuries, and the time from wounding to definitive care.

Small primary wounds located on the antimesenteric border that are seen quite early, in which there is minimal tissue destruction, and minimal or no peritoneal soiling including those of the left colon, in the absence of associated injuries of other abdominal viscera, may often be adequately managed by a primary two-layer closure.

The mucosa is approximated with a running lock suture of 3-0 absorbable suture and the seromuscular layers are closed with interrupted permanent sutures using the Lembert technique. High-velocity missile wounds associated with shock, large fecal contamination, and significant associated injuries should rarely if ever be closed primarily. Tissue destruction in these cases is often excessive and may not be readily apparent.

A less well-accepted modification of primary closure in which the repaired colon wound is exteriorized and then returned to the abdominal cavity, usually about 10 to 14 days later, has been reported but is seldom used. If the repaired colon wound fails to heal after exteriorization, it is converted to a colostomy and managed in the usual manner.

Flint and associates classified colon injuries into three grades. The classification has been used to determine the type of repair that is most appropriate. It includes: Grade 1—isolated colonic injuries with minimal fecal contamination, no shock and minimal delay (these injuries are most suitable for primary repair). Grade 2—through and through perforation, lacerations, moderate contamination, and associated injuries. Grade 3—severe tissue loss, devascularization of the colon, heavy contamination, prolonged hypotension, or significant delay in treatment (these wounds should routinely be managed by exteriorization as a colostomy, by primary repair and a proximal colostomy, resection and colostomy with mucous fistula, or a Hartmann closure of the distal colonic segment).

Burch and associates reported a series of 727 patients with colon injuries. Primary repair was accomplished in 52 percent, the majority of which were simple closure. Seventy-eight percent of right colon injuries, 62 percent of transverse colon injuries, and 32 percent of left colon injuries were closed primarily. The late mortality rate (>48 h) was 1.2 percent for primary repair compared with 9.2 percent for patients treated with a colostomy. It should be noted that more seriously injured patients had a colostomy, hence the higher mortality rate, but with careful selection primary repair can be safely accomplished.

Acute injuries of the intraperitoneal colon resulting from high-velocity missiles that are associated with extensive destruction of tissues or that are large and ragged in nature and are located near or involve the mesenteric border should not be closed primarily. If located in the ascending, transverse, or descending colon, the wound may be exteriorized as a colostomy. Similarly, if the time from wounding to definitive care is relatively long, allowing seeding of the peritoneal cavity with a large number of bacteria, some type of colostomy should be performed either as a wound exteriorization or as a proximal diverting colostomy. Primary closure of the distal wounds is then permissible. Although a loop colostomy may be done for expediency, a completely diverting double-barrel colostomy is favored. It is preferable to open the loop colostomy immediately, usually with the cautery in order to secure early, complete fecal diversion. This is performed in the operating room after all the wounds are closed and dressed. When there are associated massive injuries to other viscera, although the colon wound itself might fulfill the indications for primary closure, a colostomy is indicated. In some instances, there may be massive injury of the cecum or of the ileocecal area, in which case it will be necessary to resect the injured bowel and do an ileotransverse colostomy.

Enthusiasm for primary repair in part has been predicated on a feeling that there is an excessive morbidity associated with colostomy closure. Thal and Yeary reported their experience with 137 patients who had colostomy closures following trauma. The morbidity in their series was 10.2 percent, including wound infection 5.1 percent, bowel obstruction 2.9 percent, and fistula formation 1.5 percent. There was no mortality in their series. They concluded that the morbidity following colostomy closure was low enough so as not to be a factor in the consideration of primary repair versus colostomy as an initial operative procedure.

Wounds of the right colon and cecum that do not produce extensive destruction of the large bowel and are not associated with massive soilage or serious injuries to other viscera may often be managed by primary closure and appendicostomy. In these instances, after debridement and careful closure of the laceration of the cecum, tube appendicostomy is performed to decompress this segment. Seromuscular sutures are placed about the base of the appendix and secured to the lateral parietal peritoneum in order to prevent intraperitoneal leakage about the area of the tube insertion. By this technique, suitable decompression of the cecum and right colon may be obtained, and removal of the tube appendicostomy permits the vent to close spontaneously.

The extraperitoneal perforations of the rectum must be evaluated under the same principles used for colon injuries within the peritoneal cavity. If clean lacerations with minimal spillage are seen early, primary bowel repair may be indicated if the wound is accessible. Presacral drains should then be inserted. Associated perineal wounds should be debrided and, if grossly contaminated, left open. If debridement is adequate and these wounds are clean, they may be closed with drainage. Any damage to the anal sphincter may be repaired at this time. When a perineal wound is present but not penetrating the colon, it should be debrided widely and if not grossly contaminated then may be closed with drainage. Where there is no perineal wound but there is significant tissue destruction about the extraperitoneal rectum, presacral drainage should be instituted.

For all injuries of the rectum, complete diversion of the fecal stream is mandatory and can be accomplished by constructing a proximal double-barrel colostomy. Even in those instances where the rectal wound has been closed and diverting colostomy performed, presacral drainage is necessary.

Drainage of the retrorectal area is extremely important. This can be established by making a curvilinear incision in the posterior perianal area, incising the anococcygeal ligament, and bluntly dissecting into the presacral space. Two Penrose drains will usually suffice, but with extensive injuries, it may be necessary to utilize sump drainage for a few days.

Lavenson and Cohen, on the basis of their experience in the Vietnam conflict, strongly recommended removal of all feces from the distal rectum. This is accomplished by irrigating copious amounts of saline solution through the defunctionalized segment until the return is clear. They report a significant decrease in mortality and complication rates when utilizing this technique. Military injuries are generally associated with higher-velocity missiles and cause more fecal contamination and blast injury to surrounding pelvic tissue. In civilian injuries, distal irrigation might not be as important, as evidenced by Trunkey and Shires, who report a lower morbidity and mortality rate in their series, in which distal irrigation was not used but adequate drainage and diversion were used.

Serious perineal injuries are treated in a similar manner. Even in the absence of rectal injury, sepsis can be avoided by early fecal diversion. Failure to recognize this potential problem may lead to extensive soft tissue infections extending from the knee to the axilla, with potential involvement of the anterior and posterior abdominal wall.

Early closure of the colostomy is indicated in patients who have completely recovered and have no distal colon injury. It is desirable to close the simple colostomy in 2 or 3 weeks. Before closure, both limbs of the colon should be visualized radiographically to assure that no lesion persists. Mechanical and bacterial cleansing of the colon is effected preoperatively.

Liver

Injury to the liver is suspected in all patients with penetrating or blunt trauma that involves the lower chest and upper abdomen. Among patients with penetrating abdominal trauma, the liver is second only to the small bowel as the organ most commonly injured; among those with blunt trauma, the liver is second only to the spleen as the most commonly injured organ. About 80 percent of liver injuries occur as a result of penetrating trauma from stab wounds or gunshot wounds; only 15 to 20 percent occur from blunt trauma. In recent years, the incidence of stab wounds has diminished while the incidence of gunshot wounds, especially those caused by higher-velocity and larger-caliber missiles, and blunt trauma has increased. These changes in the types of liver injuries, the more rapid transport of patients with hepatic trauma to treatment facilities, and better resuscitation methods have caused an increase in the severity of liver injuries that are likely to confront the surgeon.

Early exploration, prompt resuscitation, antibiotics, and proper choice of surgical treatment, have led to increased survival rates. The average overall mortality rate of patients with hepatic trauma is about 10 to 15 percent. This rate is directly related to the severity of the liver injury and the presence of associated visceral trauma. The mortality rate of stab wounds to the liver without associated organ injury is only about 1 percent. When significant liver trauma is associated with injuries of more than five other intraabdominal organs, or when major hepatic resection is required to control the bleeding, the mortality rate rises to about 45 to 50 percent.

Liver injuries run the spectrum from minor capsular tears to shattered stellate fractures. The American Association for the Surgery of Trauma through its Organ Injury Scaling Committee has devised the following classification system that will facilitate comparing similar injuries and help determine appropriate therapy depending on injury severity (Table 6-5).

Treatment. After initial resuscitation and diagnostic maneuvers, patients with suspected hepatic injuries are rapidly moved to the operating room. The entire abdomen and chest are "prepped" and draped, and a long upper midline abdominal incision is made. Sources of bleeding from the liver and abdomen are quickly appraised, and temporary control of the bleeding is obtained by manual compression or packs placed over the bleeding sites and by temporary occlusion of appropriate major vessels. Digital compression of the hepatic artery and portal vein to occlude temporarily the blood flow to the liver (the Pringle maneuver) may control or slow hepatic hemorrhage in some patients, but more often it is necessary to combine the Pringle maneuver with compression packs placed over the liver injury to control hemorrhage effectively. There is general agreement that, in the normothermic liver, blood flow to the liver can be completely occluded with safety for at least 60 min and probably longer without causing any hepatocellular damage. If it is necessary to occlude the hepatic blood supply for more than 60 min, the vascular occlusion can be briefly interrupted to allow short periods of uninterrupted hepatic blood flow.

Table 6-5
Liver Injury Scale

	Grade	*Injury Description*
I.	Hematoma	Subcapsular, nonexpanding, <10% surface area
	Laceration	Capsular tear, nonbleeding, with <1-cm-deep parenchymal disruption
II.	Hematoma	Subcapsular, nonexpanding, hematoma 10–50%; intraparenchymal nonexpanding <2 cm in diameter
	Laceration	<3 cm parenchymal depth, <10 cm in length
III.	Hematoma	Subcapsular, >50% of surface area or expanding; ruptured subcapsular hematoma with active bleeding; intraparenchymal hematoma >2 cm
	Laceration	>3 cm parenchymal depth
IV.	Hematoma	Ruptured central hematoma
	Laceration	Parenchymal destruction involving 25–75% of hepatic lobe
V.	Laceration	Parenchymal destruction >75% of hepatic lobe
	Vascular	Juxtahepatic venous injuries (retrohepatic cava/major hepatic veins)
VI.	Vascular	Hepatic avulsion

Definitive treatment of liver injuries may be accomplished by drainage alone, suture or hemostatic maneuvers and drainage, or variations of hepatic resection or resectional debridement.

Drainage Alone. Hepatic hemorrhage ceases spontaneously by the time the abdomen is opened or stops soon after compression of the bleeding site in about half of patients with liver injuries. In such patients, the only treatment necessary is adequate drainage of the injury. Suturing of nonbleeding liver injuries is unnecessary. This is emphasized by Trunkey, Shires, McClelland and by Lucas and Ledgerwood who reported no rebleeding among several hundred patients with liver injuries that stopped bleeding spontaneously or soon after temporary pack compression. Suturing of nonbleeding liver wounds may cause bleeding and needlessly traumatizes hepatic tissue.

In the past, all liver injuries were drained externally. Many injuries, especially those not requiring sutures or debridement, are no longer drained. Adequate drainage of the perihepatic space in patients with liver injuries greatly reduces the formation of infected collections of bile, blood, and tissue fluid in the subphrenic and subhepatic spaces. It is preferable to bring suction drains out through small stab wounds in the abdominal wall that are separate from the Penrose drains if both types are used. In large patients with more extensive liver wounds, it may be preferable to resect the lateral half or two-thirds of the right twelfth rib to achieve more effective gravity drainage. The Penrose drains are left in place 5 to 10 days, thereafter being slowly removed over a 3-day period. Only at this time is a firm, fibrinous tract formed about the drains that ensures adequate external drainage of the material that accumulates in the abdomen after the drain is removed. Suction drains generally should remain in place until drainage is less than 25 to 30 mL of fluid daily.

Suture, Hemostatic Techniques, and Drainage. Hemostasis should be achieved by direct ligation of the bleeding vessel. Definitive hemostasis of persistently bleeding liver injuries usually can be achieved by liver sutures. Simple interrupted sutures are placed 2 cm from the wound margins, using 2-0 or 0 chromic sutures swaged onto a 2-in. blunt-tipped "liver needle." This allows gentle but firm approximation of the wound edges, thereby stopping most bleeding that originates from the outer 2 cm of the liver parenchyma immediately beneath the hepatic capsule. Passage of the suture through buttressing material such as Surgicel, Gelfoam, or omentum is seldom needed if the sutures are placed 2 cm from the margin of the injury and tied gently. If a bolster is needed, it is preferable to use a vascularized pedicle of omentum instead of foreign material.

Microcrystalline collagen powder (Avitene) may be used in selected patients to control bleeding from minor liver wounds. Unlike other material such as Gelfoam, Avitene can be left in liver wounds without inciting significant foreign body reaction. The argon coagulator effectively stops minor bleeding from the raw parenchymal surface as does fibrin glue.

The use of liver sutures to obtain hemostasis from both the entrance and exit sites of long gunshot tracts in the liver is controversial. Lucas and Ledgerwood state that this technique was successfully used in several of their patients who otherwise would have required extensive surgery. Placement of the liver sutures at both ends of the bullet tract stops bleeding arising from the subcapsular area, which is the usual source. During their 5-year prospective review, Lucas and Ledgerwood found that only one patient developed an intrahepatic abscess following use of this technique, and no patients developed hemobilia after closure of both ends of a long gunshot tract. They noted that continued bleeding that persists after closure of both ends of a tract is usually identified at the initial operation by blood oozing between the liver sutures or by an increase in the size of the liver within 10 min after placement of the sutures. If there is persistent bleeding from the tract, hemostasis is best achieved by opening the tract and individually ligating the bleeding vessels.

Ligation of an appropriate major branch of the hepatic artery (i.e., the right or left branch) while reported in the past is now rarely advocated. Lucas and Ledgerwood did not find ligation of major branches of the hepatic artery to be effective in arresting hemorrhage, possibly because some of these patients were bleeding from major venous injuries. It is suggested that the right or left hepatic artery should not be ligated if a simple temporary compression pack or suturing of a bleeding injury controls the hemorrhage.

The unrealistic expectation that hepatic artery ligation would control venous bleeding undoubtedly can lead to late recognition of hepatic and portal vein injuries in patients who continue to bleed after hepatic artery ligation. If bleeding recurs after the pack is removed, the porta is occluded temporarily with a vascular clamp. If hemorrhage continues after the Pringle maneuver, the wound is repacked and a search is made for hepatic venous injury. When porta compression controls hemorrhage, the laceration is gently explored for specific bleeding sites amenable to suture ligation. After this, devitalized liver tissue is debrided and the area is drained.

Resection. Resectional debridement or limited wedge resection is recommended to control bleeding from ragged liver injuries that may be caused by shotgun wounds, high-velocity rifle wounds, and severe blunt injuries. Limited resectional debridement of shattered liver tissue usually achieves hemostasis from such injuries effectively and safely. The margins of resectional debridement should be 2 or 3 cm beyond the point of injury, and bleeding during debridement is controlled by digital parenchymal compression and/or temporary occlusion of the inflow of blood to the liver at the porta hepatis. The liver parenchyma is separated bluntly by finger fracture, a suction tip, or a scalpel handle. Vessels and bile ducts are secured by individual suture ligation or by metal hemoclips as these structures are encountered. It is not necessary to oppose the margins of the resection with interrupted liver sutures if bleeding from the resected surface is controlled. If such hemostasis is not achieved, the omental pack referred to above can be used.

Anatomic hepatic lobectomy to control bleeding, especially from the right lobe, is preferably reserved for patients in whom (1) hepatic suturing is unsuccessful; (2) resectional debridement or hepatotomy with intraparenchymal hemostasis is precluded by the anatomic location of the injury; (3) occlusion of the hepatic artery fails to control hemorrhage. Although resectional debridement or sublobar hepatic resection may be required in about 4 or 5 percent of all patients with liver injuries, no more than 2 or 3 percent require anatomic, lobar resection to control hemorrhage. Most of the few patients with liver injuries who require major hepatic lobectomies to control bleeding have massive, shattering injuries to the major hepatic veins at or near the junction with the vena cava (Fig. 6-15). If it becomes apparent that major lobar resection is necessary, the hepatic bleeding is temporarily controlled by manual compression of packs placed over the liver wound and by a Pringle maneuver while the midline abdominal incision is extended by performing a median sternotomy.

A median sternotomy is much more quickly and easily made and closed than a right thoracoabdominal incision, causes considerably less diaphragmatic injury, provides much easier access to

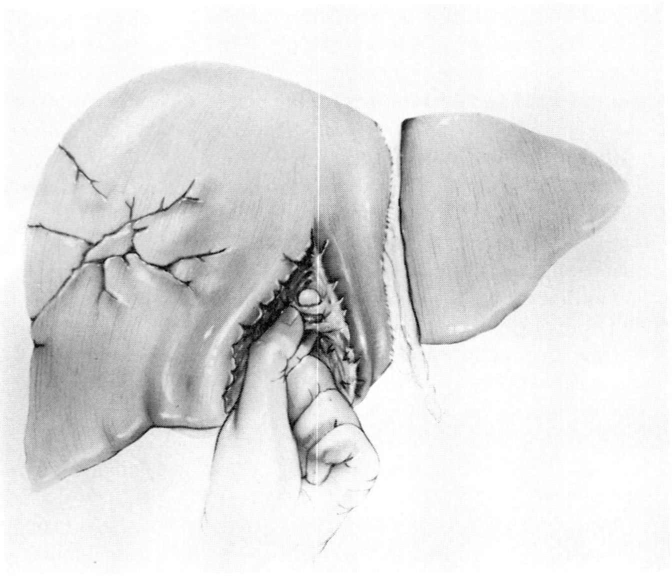

FIG. 6-15. Typical liver injury requiring hepatic resection.

the vena cava and hepatic veins, permits easier insertion of a retrohepatic vena caval shunt if this is required, and causes less postoperative pain and pulmonary morbidity than a right thoracoabdominal incision.

After wide exposure is obtained by the median sternotomy extension of the midline abdominal incision, Rumel tourniquets are placed about the vena cava superior and inferior to the liver. The superior tape is placed about the vena cava superior to the central tendon of the diaphragm after this portion of the vena cava is exposed by opening the pericardium. These tapes permit temporary occlusion of the vena cava for insertion of an intracaval shunt if vascular isolation of the liver is required during hepatic lobectomy because of major retrohepatic vena cava or major hepatic vein injury near where these veins enter the vena cava. The hepatic artery, portal vein, and bile ducts supplying the lobe to be resected are then suture-ligated and divided. After this, hepatic resection can be done by dividing Glisson's capsule with a cautery along the line appropriate for the lobe being removed. The lobe is removed by fracturing through the liver substance along the line of resection with the thumb and forefinger or with the top of an abdominal suction tube from which the guard has been removed. As the blood vessels and bile ducts are encountered within the liver, they are isolated by passing a right-angle clamp around them and are then ligated and divided. After the larger vessels and ducts are suture-ligated, the smaller ones are secured with metal hemoclips. No attempt is made to secure the hepatic veins at their junction with the retrohepatic vena cava before beginning the resection; instead, it is much easier and safer to isolate and suture-ligate or oversew the appropriate major hepatic veins as they are encountered posteriorly during the liver resection. The resection begins anteriorly and progresses posteriorly toward the right or left side of the vena cava, keeping to the right or left of the middle hepatic vein (depending on whether a right or left lobectomy is being done). The middle hepatic vein demarcates the right from the left lobe of the liver and passes in a line from the middle of the gallbladder bed posteriorly to the midportion of the retrohepatic vena cava. The hepatic veins and other large vascular structures must be oversewn, since simple ligatures on these large structures often slip off and cause catastrophic bleeding.

Vascular Isolation. Vascular isolation may be required in a highly selective group of patients with liver injuries. This technique allows the surgeon to control bleeding from and to repair retrohepatic vena caval or major hepatic venous injuries. Vascular isolation of the liver is attained by using one of two techniques. The first of these techniques uses occlusive vascular clamps placed across the aorta just below the diaphragm, on the porta hepatis, and across the inferior vena cava above and below the liver. This technique may be associated with cardiac dysrhythmias and renal insufficiency. The second technique for obtaining vascular isolation of the liver was first described and reported by Schrock and associates and further successful experience with this reported by Yellin and associates. When this technique is used, retrohepatic vena caval and hepatic venous isolation is attained by inserting a #36 endotracheal tube with an inflatable balloon near the caudal end via the right atrial appendage of the heart. The tube is then passed down the retrohepatic cava and shunts blood around the liver from the lower portion of the body to the right heart. Control of vascular inflow to the liver is obtained by placing a Rumel tourniquet or vascular clamp on the porta hepatis. The introduction of the intracaval shunt via the right atrial appendage is most expeditiously done through a median sternotomy. Also, it is suggested that three equidistant "guy" sutures should be placed in the right atrial wall somewhat outside the atrial purse-string suture before making the atrial opening in the center of the purse-string suture to insert the shunt tube. These "guy" sutures are then spread apart and held up by assistants as the atrium is opened; this greatly facilitates insertion of the shunt by stabilization of the atrial wall. Defore and associates reported survival of 7 of 15 patients with major vena caval or hepatic vein injuries following vascular isolation and introduction of an intracaval shunt as described. Nevertheless, this technique is difficult and somewhat dangerous to perform and should be used only when it is certain that the vena caval and/or hepatic vein injuries are severe enough that bleeding can be controlled in no other way. In the latter instance, the shunt may be lifesaving. It is also emphasized that the results with the shunt probably can be improved if it is used promptly as soon as it becomes apparent that no other method will achieve hemostasis. In some experiences reporting poor results with the shunt, its use may have been delayed too long and the massive transfusions required in the interim may have led to an intractable coagulopathy. In reviewing 60 patients from several institutions in whom the shunt was used, Walt found a survival rate of 20 percent and very probably most of these patients would not have survived without the shunt.

Another method for controlling hemorrhage from the retrohepatic vena cava or major hepatic veins has been described by the authors. If the major venous laceration is in such a position in the suprahepatic vena cava or the extrahepatic portion of the hepatic veins, a Foley catheter may be quickly inserted into the exposed laceration. The balloon of the Foley catheter is then inflated and gently pulled up against the wall of the vena cava or hepatic vein to occlude the laceration, arrest the hemorrhage, and thus permit repair of the venous laceration with relatively good exposure and little blood loss.

Packing. In some patients with severe injuries, hemostasis may not be possible. Massive bleeding can be temporarily controlled by compression packing with laparotomy packs while the anesthesiologist resuscitates the patient with blood and crystalloids. Only after the patient is stabilized should the packs be gently removed. If massive blood loss ensues, the patient becomes hypothermic, or acidemia (pH 7.2 to 7.3) occurs, one should quickly make the decision to tightly pack the liver and return the patient to the intensive care unit. Once the patient has been stabilized, the patient is returned to the operating room where the pack is carefully removed. This is generally done within 36 to 72 h after the initial procedure. If necessary, the injury can be debrided; however, in most cases, bleeding does not recur and little more than removing the packs and irrigation is needed.

Packing is a valuable adjunct for controlling hepatic hemorrhage in highly selected patients and should be performed early (less than 10 units blood replacement). If indicated, appropriate use of this packing technique will often preclude massive transfusions and subsequent fatal coagulopathy problems. Placing a steridrape between the liver surface and the pack has been recommended. This technical point will facilitate removal of the pack without disturbing the hemostasis or clot formation that has been achieved at the injury site.

Subcapsular Hematoma. The treatment of subcapsular hematomas of the liver is somewhat controversial. Left alone, these may (1) resolve spontaneously, (2) expand and burst with delayed intraperitoneal bleeding, (3) cause a hepatic abscess, or (4) decompress into the biliary tree and cause hematobilia. The risk of inducing massive hemorrhage, at times uncontrollable, accompanies attempts at incision and evacuation.

Richie and Fonkalsrud reported a series of subcapsular hematoma patients who were treated nonoperatively. They emphasized that severe bleeding may result in some patients in whom hematomas of the liver are unroofed, and they further noted that since some hematomas are centrally located within the liver, they often do not lend themselves to resection or control by hepatic artery ligation.

With the advent of computed tomography, nonoperative management of liver injuries, especially subcapsular or intraparenchymal hematomas, has become quite popular. The CT scan allows one to accurately assess the severity of the liver injury. It is possible to quantify the amount of intraabdominal blood in the pelvis as well as the amount of blood surrounding the liver.

In patients with grade I, II, and some grade III injuries, nonoperative management is preferable so long as there are no other indications for operative therapy, such as hemodynamic instability, signs of peritonitis, or other associated injuries. Depending on the mechanism and severity of injury, these patients are followed with serial CT scans or sonography at varying intervals. Little agreement exists as to how often one should scan the patient and for what length of time activity should be restricted following discharge from the hospital. Although it is not necessary to limit activity until complete resolution occurs, one needs to be certain that healing has occurred, as indicated by a significant reduction of the hematoma in follow-up studies. Patients who are managed nonoperatively must be reliable and readily available for close follow-up care.

Emergency hepatic arteriography for patients in stable condition with probable subcapsular or intrahepatic hematomas due to blunt trauma may be used on rare occasions. An advantage of hepatic arteriography in some stable patients with intrahepatic hematomas is that this technique can be used therapeutically as well as diagnostically. If a site of arterial hemorrhage is visualized arteriographically, the hemorrhage may be controlled nonoperatively and atraumatically by embolizing several 2-mm^2 pieces of Gelfoam through the hepatic arterial catheter. These emboli obstruct the bleeding site and prevent further bleeding.

Hematobilia. Hematobilia is caused by arterial hemorrhage into the biliary tract after liver trauma; classically it presents with a triad of findings consisting of upper or lower gastrointestinal hemorrhage, obstructing jaundice, and colicky abdominal pain. In the past, the standard treatment for this condition consisted of hepatic resection or hepatotomy with direct exposure and suture ligation of the bleeding artery. Such treatment is often associated with considerable blood loss and high operative mortality and morbidity. There are now several reports of successful management of traumatic hematobilia by ligation of the hepatic arteries supplying the involved lobe of the liver. Hepatic arterial embolization also has been effective therapy.

Complications. Major nonfatal complications occur in approximately 20 percent of patients with liver injuries. Since the thorax is involved in many hepatic injuries, there is a high incidence of pulmonary complications. Also, the incidence of intraabdominal and perihepatic abscesses ranges from 4.5 to 20 percent. The probability of such abscess formation increases with more complex injuries of the liver and with the presence of associated colon injuries.

Patients with major lobar resections may be expected to have some postoperative bilirubin elevation, probably secondary to transient biliary obstruction by blood clots and temporary hepatic insufficiency (due to shock, loss of hepatic mass, operative trauma, and occasionally, postoperative sepsis). Hyperbilirubinemia usually disappears within about 3 weeks, with no further surgical treatment required for the relief of jaundice. Liver function studies generally show hepatic impairment but usually return to normal after several weeks. Glucose metabolism is altered after resection, and in the early postoperative period it may be necessary to give the patient supplemental glucose solutions. Studies indicate that survival is possible with only 20 percent of the normal hepatic mass, and that within several months most of the resected hepatic tissue is replaced by hepatic regeneration.

Well-controlled prospective studies, support the position that effective biliary decompression is not achieved by the T tube and that drainage of the common duct may increase the incidence of complications in patients with hepatic trauma, especially those due to infection and bile duct obstruction (i.e., jaundice, cholangitis, and bile duct stricture). T-tube drainage of the uninjured bile duct associated with hepatic injuries is no longer advocated.

Gallbladder

Although perforations of the gallbladder due to blunt trauma are very unusual, penetrating abdominal trauma frequently causes gallbladder injuries. Penetrating or avulsion injuries of the gallbladder are best managed by cholecystectomy, but in unstable patients with other severe injuries, when, in the surgeon's judgment, cholecystectomy is inadvisable, a tube cholecystostomy should be done, with placement of drains around the gallbladder and the subhepatic space. In general, simple suture of a gallbladder perforation is not recommended because of the probability of bile leakage. After about 4 weeks, if a patient who has had a tube cholecystostomy is doing well, a cholangiogram is performed through the cholecystostomy tube, and if this shows that the gallbladder and biliary ducts are normal, with free flow of contrast material into the duodenum, the cholecystostomy tube can be removed. Routine cholecystectomy after removal of the cholecystostomy tube in patients who have sustained gallbladder trauma is unnecessary, but it is probably advisable to perform an oral cholecystogram or sonogram several months after injury to determine the status of the gallbladder.

Extrahepatic Biliary Tree

Penetrating Injuries

The diagnosis of penetrating injuries of the extrahepatic biliary tree usually presents no problem as compared with the diagnosis of blunt trauma of the biliary tree, which may be difficult unless intraabdominal hemorrhage occurs. When the hepatic artery and portal vein are involved, the mortality rate is inordinately high because of massive hemorrhage that may be virtually impossible to control before irreversible hypoxic damage occurs to the brain and myocardium.

While opening the abdomen, blood and bile seen issuing from the subhepatic region indicate possible injury to the biliary tree. At times, the amount of bile, blood, or contusion may be minimal, and the gallbladder, cystic duct, and hepatoduodenal structures must be carefully inspected to evaluate the significance of any subserosal hematoma or bile staining. If the patient has survived to be surgically explored, generally no massive bleeding from the subhepatic region will be noted initially. Many times in obtaining exposure of the hepatoduodenal ligament structures, clots that have formed and tamponaded major bleeding sites may be dislodged, with recurrence of vigorous bleeding from the portal vein, hepatic artery, or their branches, which are frequently injured when the bile ducts are injured.

The hemorrhage can be controlled by placing the fingers in the foramen of Winslow and compressing the hepatoduodenal ligament (the Pringle maneuver). After removing the free blood and obtaining good exposure while maintaining finger tamponade as above, more definitive control of the hemorrhage may be obtained by placing vascular or rubbershod clamps across all the structures in the hepatoduodenal ligament. One clamp should be placed as far distal as possible on the hepatoduodenal ligament, and this maneuver is aided by dividing the lateral serosal reflection of the duodenum and reflecting the duodenum and head of the pancreas medially. Another clamp is then placed on the hepatoduodenal ligament through the foramen of Winslow as near the liver hilus as possible.

After hemorrhage is controlled, the serosa of the hepatoduodenal ligament at the site of the hematoma formation is incised, and the disruption of the portal vein or hepatic artery is visualized by rapidly dissecting out these structures. When the defects in the major vessels are located, repair is carried out with 5-0 arterial sutures using the general principles and techniques of vascular surgery.

Busuttil and associates stated that the most important factor in determining how to manage the bile duct injury is whether or not the duct is completely or incompletely transected. From their experience, complete transection almost always ends with stricture if the duct is primarily repaired end-to-end but has a favorable outcome if some type of duct-enteric anastomosis is done. These findings were reported by Belzer some years ago when he showed that an incomplete ductal injury could be successfully repaired by duct anastomosis or patch (vein or gallbladder graft); however, a complete division, when mobilized for primary anastomosis or patch, almost always ends in stricture. Also, Longmire recommended duct-enteric anastomosis as the best method for the early treatment of injuries to the extrahepatic bile ducts.

Busuttil and his colleagues further state that if the duct has been perforated or incompletely divided, primary repair can be successfully performed. There seems to be no definitive evidence that the presence or absence of a T-tube stent makes any difference in the rate of success in these cases. However, Busuttil and associates believe that a T-tube stent should not be used if the duct is of small caliber.

If the patient is in poor condition and cannot tolerate a prolonged procedure for definitive repair of the bile duct, then the defects of the biliary duct may be repaired by simple bridging with a T tube fixed in place with a suture at either end of the ductal defect; secondary repair can then be done as soon as the patient can tolerate it. If possible, however, definitive repair should be done, since recurrent strictures are more likely after the more difficult secondary repairs of the bile ducts.

If the gallbladder and cystic duct are intact, the biliary-enteric bypass to repair a ductal injury also may be done between the gallbladder and jejunum with ligation of the distal and proximal limbs of the damaged common duct. Also, it may be more expedient at times to use a simple loop of jejunum instead of a Roux en Y limb to perform the bypass procedure.

Blunt Trauma

Blunt trauma to the biliary tree deserves separate discussion, not because the surgical management differs, but because of its relative rarity and difficulty of diagnosis. The usual mechanism of closed injury to the extrahepatic biliary tree is a shearing force applied to the common duct.

When blunt trauma to the biliary tree is severe enough to result in a free flow of bile into the peritoneal cavity, the characteristic picture of bile peritonitis occurs. The usual history involves a crushing injury to the right upper quadrant, the epigastrium, or the lower part of the chest, which results in severe pain and may be followed by shock. Bile or nonclotting blood may be found on peritoneal tap or lavage.

Shock is usually secondary to the marked outpouring of extracellular fluid into the peritoneal cavity due to the chemical irritation of the peritoneum by bile. The initial chemical peritonitis caused by bile may be followed shortly after by bacterial peritonitis. If biliary leakage is minimal, shock may be of relatively short duration or may be absent, and abdominal signs initially may be slight. This may be followed by the recovery and well-being of the patient, which may last for periods up to 5 or 10 days. The onset of jaundice on about the third day is a fairly constant sign. The appearance of clay-colored stools and the presence of bile in the urine may be noticed from the second to the fifth day after injury of the duct.

A gradual increase in abdominal size may occur during the first 10 days that may be unattended by the usual signs of peritonitis in patients with bile duct rupture. This increasing abdominal girth is accompanied by progressive signs of extracellular fluid volume deficit and by evidence of infection manifest by fever and leukocytosis. In the reported cases of transection of the common duct, the site of transection was uniformly in the retroduodenal area of the superior margin of the pancreas. This serves to emphasize the importance of extensive medial reflection of the duodenum to explore the retroperitoneal duodenum as well as the distal common duct and pancreas in patients undergoing celiotomy for blunt abdominal trauma.

In reviewing the surgical treatment of the 34 patients reported to have blunt injuries of the common bile duct, Carmichael noted that simple drainage is unwise because of the high mortality and high stricture rate associated with this method of treatment. Carmichael advocated choledochoduodenostomy when the distal duct is unsuitable for primary repair or is missing. Of eight choledochoduodenostomies in his review, all did well except one, who required a cholecystojejunostomy to reestablish bile flow. No duodenal fistulae occurred. Choledochojejunostomy with or without a Roux en Y jejunal limb was done in six patients, and all of these did well. Carmichael concluded that the most successful procedures in reconstruction of the avulsed common bile duct are Roux en Y choledochojejunostomy or choledochoduodenostomy. Choledochojejunostomy offers a better exposure if a future operation is required, a tension-free anastomosis, and a technically easier mucosa-to-mucosa anastomosis. Also, this procedure avoids the lateral duodenal fistula that may occur after choledochoduodenostomy.

The postoperative therapy of biliary tract injuries, in which bile peritonitis is an important complicating feature, should include adequate replacement of extracellular fluid volume deficits, which may require intravenous infusion of several liters of balanced salt solutions in 24 h. These solutions should be given as soon as possible preoperatively and continued throughout the surgical procedure and postoperatively to avoid extracellular fluid volume deficit. Broad-spectrum antibiotics should be given before the surgical procedure and continued during the operation and postoperatively until the chances of sepsis diminish.

The overall mortality in the collected series of common duct injuries reported by Carmichael was 35 percent; however, the mortality from biliary tract injuries probably should be below 5 to 10 percent if they are discovered early and treated appropriately.

Portal Vein

Approximately 90 percent of portal vein injuries occur because of penetrating trauma. They are frequently associated with other visceral injuries, most commonly to the inferior vena cava, liver, pancreas, and stomach. Mattox and associates reported a survival rate of 50 percent in their series of 22 patients with portal vein injuries. Lateral venorrhaphy, if possible, is the preferred method of treatment. Mattox suggests performing a portacaval or mesocaval shunt as an alternative treatment of portal vein injury if suture repair is impossible and the patient's general condition is stable. In contrast, Fish reported that four of five patients who had portacaval shunts for portal vein reconstruction after trauma developed hepatic decompensation or encephalopathy, whereas those complications were not observed in patients undergoing portal vein ligation.

The insertion of an autogenous vein graft to bridge the defect in the portal vein (using the left common iliac vein, left renal vein, or a paneled saphenous vein graft) may be preferable to a portacaval shunt if the patient's condition is stable and the proximal and distal ends of the injured vein are suitable for the insertion of a graft. This procedure should prevent portal hypertension or hepatic deterioration that may occur if the vein is ligated. If associated injuries are severe, ligation of the portal vein may make it possible to save the patient. Even though portal vein ligation may cause portal hypertension, interruption of the vein is compatible with patient's survival in about 80 percent of the cases. It should be emphasized that in those with associated hepatic arterial injuries, a good repair of the hepatic artery must be achieved before accepting treatment of portal vein injuries by ligation. Because of obstruction to portal outflow, acute splanchnic hypervolemia develops simultaneously with peripheral hypovolemia. Patients have died of such splanchnic pooling after portal vein ligation. Since this problem has been appreciated, these patients have been followed closely with either central venous or pulmonary artery pressure measurements to maintain a functionally normal peripheral blood volume. This may require overtransfusions of a volume of blood almost equal to the patient's own normal blood volume.

Pancreas

Travers described the first pancreatic injury in England in 1827. This was an intoxicated woman who was struck by a stagecoach wheel. Autopsy revealed a complete transection of the pancreas. Approximately 70 percent of pancreatic injuries result from penetrating injuries and 30 percent from blunt injuries. The overall mortality is approximately 20 percent but is usually due to associated injuries. Pancreatic trauma is associated with a high morbidity but less than 3 percent of patients actually die of the pancreatic injury. Early mortality is due to associated hemorrhage or severe head injury, whereas mortality after 48 h is usually secondary to sepsis often in association with a colon injury. Although it is rare for a patient sustaining penetrating abdominal trauma to have an isolated pancreatic injury, approximately 20 percent of patients sustaining blunt pancreatic trauma have an isolated pancreatic injury.

Diagnosis. Diagnosis of pancreatic injuries is based on a complete history, including the mechanism of injury, thorough physical examination, serum amylase level, and most important is adequate visualization of the pancreas at surgical exploration. Following isolated blunt pancreatic trauma, symptoms are often mild and loss of bowel sounds, tenderness, guarding, or spasm may not be present for several hours.

The role of CT in the preoperative evaluation of pancreatic injury remains to be defined. CT may demonstrate pancreatic edema following pancreatic contusion. However, some patients thought to have focal or diffuse enlargement have been found to have a normal pancreas at surgery. The majority of false-positive diagnoses is due to unopacified bowel loops adjacent to the pancreas that may be mistaken for focal pancreatic swelling. Peripancreatic hematoma from trauma to the spleen and left kidney are other causes for diagnostic errors. In small series, up to 20 percent of acute pancreatic injuries were missed. Because of the time required and the expense of this procedure, it is not indicated as a routine diagnostic study. In a stable patient with a positive CT scan an endoscopic retrograde cholangiopancreatogram (ERCP) may be performed to document ductal injury.

ERCP is rarely used in an emergency since the patient requires surgery for other organ injuries and the pancreas can be evaluated intraoperatively by direct inspection. On rare occasion, if an extensive resection or pancreaticoduodenectomy is anticipated, ductal injury may be proven. ERCP may be of benefit in the patient following blunt trauma in which there has been a delay of several hours to days in diagnosis. An ERCP may confirm or deny a suspected pancreatic injury identified on CT scan.

Serum Amylase. A preoperative elevation of the serum amylase level in the absence of peritoneal signs is not used as an indication for exploratory laparotomy. Many patients have been found to have an elevated serum amylase level but negative abdominal findings. These patients are closely observed for evidence of peritonitis or until the amylase level returns to normal. An elevation of the amylase level on peritoneal lavage fluid is more often associated with small bowel injury than pancreatic injury. Between 15 and 30 percent of patients sustaining penetrating abdominal trauma have a preoperative elevation of the serum amylase. Only 50 to 65 percent of patients have an elevation of amylase preoperatively following blunt trauma even with complete transection of the pancreas. Approximately one-third of patients with hyperamylasemia do not have significant pancreatic trauma. Although the serum amylase level may be elevated following blunt trauma, it is not cost-effective to measure it routinely for penetrating abdominal trauma.

Surgical Exploration. The duodenum is completely mobilized using a Kocher maneuver. The gastrocolic omentum is divided and the lesser sac is entered and the entire pancreas is visualized. A peripancreatic or capsular hematoma is considered presumptive evidence of pancreatic injury and should be explored. Over 60 percent of patients sustaining penetrating trauma to the pancreas have an associated retroperitoneal injury. It is important to identify any major pancreatic duct injury in order that appropriate treatment may be given. Before an extensive resection, pancreatic duct violation is usually determined. Pancreatography through an injured duodenum may be performed although the uninjured duodenum is rarely opened. Untreated disruption of the pancreatic duct has been the main source of morbidity associated with pancreatic injury. When profuse bleeding occurs from the pancreatic area, the pancreas is mobilized and the superior mesenteric and splenic vessels, the aorta, and vena cava are inspected, since they may be the source of severe hemorrhage. A needle cholangiogram is performed if there is question of injury to the common bile duct.

Associated Injuries. Following penetrating pancreatic trauma, the most common associated injuries are to the liver, stomach, and colon, whereas injuries to the liver and spleen are most often associated with blunt pancreatic trauma. The 25 percent incidence of associated colon injuries in patients with penetrating trauma greatly enhances the chance of intraabdominal abscess which occurs in 25 percent of patients with a combined pancreatic and colon injury. Approximately 20 percent of penetrating pancreatic injuries also have duodenal injuries. Major retroperitoneal artery and vein injuries occur in over 40 percent of patients sustaining pancreatic trauma and account for a high mortality rate.

Classification of Pancreatic Trauma. One classification of pancreatic trauma is according to anatomic severity. Grade I is partial thickness lesion in the duodenum and injury to the pancreas without ductal involvement. Grade II is a full-thickness injury to the duodenum and pancreas without ductal involvement. Grade III is ductal injury in the body or tail of the pancreas, whereas a grade IV is ductal injury in the head of the pancreas with greater than 75 percent circumferential injury of the duodenum or common bile duct. A grade V injury is a massive devascularizing injury to the pancreatic head and adjacent duodenum.

Management. Approximately 75 percent of patients sustaining pancreatic injury are managed with external drainage. Closed drainage is implemented in an effort to decrease the incidence of drain tract and intraabdominal abscess formation rather than the combination of Penrose and Sump drains. Nevertheless, intraabdominal abscess formation continues to be a significant problem particularly when there is associated colon injury. The drains are left in place for 10 days. Patients have been observed to have minimal pancreatic drainage for up to 1 week and then have a significant increase in drainage. All pancreatic injuries including contusions are drained since there may be unrecognized injury. Failure to drain may lead to complications such as pseudocysts and pancreatic abscesses (Table 6-6). Following drainage alone in 342 patients, only 10 fistulae and two pseudocysts developed. In only 2 to 3 percent of patients who died can the pancreatic injury be confirmed as contributing to the cause of death, usually in association with sepsis and other organ injuries. Postoperative hemorrhagic pancreatitis is responsible for some deaths.

The majority of gunshot wounds to the head of the pancreas may be treated with drainage alone, unless it is obvious that additional operative procedures must be performed. Mortality for a penetrating injury to the head of the pancreas is approximately 30 percent and is related to hemorrhage or trauma to other organs.

Complete transection usually follows blunt trauma secondary to an automobile accident. Presumably, there is external force pressing the pancreas across the vertebral column and transecting it at the neck directly over the superior mesenteric vessels. The usual treatment for this injury is distal pancreatectomy. Patients without associated injury, who are stable, may have a Roux en Y anastomosis to the distal pancreas if greater than 80 percent (12 cm) of the pancreas is to be resected. Attempts to reanastomose a transected pancreatic duct are difficult and may give rise

Table 6-6
Pancreatic Trauma Method of Management, $N = 450$

	Pt	*Fistula*	*Pseudo-cyst*	*Lesser Sac Abscess*	*Death*	*Death 48 h hem. or CNS*
Drainage alone	342	10	2	14	40	(15)
Distal pancreatectomy	48	2		4	3	(1)
Distal pancreatectomy and Roux en y	23			1	5	(1)
Pancreaticoduodenectomy	8				3	(1)
Diverticulization	5	1			1	
Roux en y to injury	11			2	1	
Roux en y both ends	7			1	2	
Roux en y to head-common duct	1					
Uncinate resection	1					
No drainage	4				1	

to a pseudocyst or pancreatic fistula. Distal pancreatectomy is indicated for injuries to the left of the superior mesenteric vessels. Pancreaticojejunostomy is usually not indicated when there is associated colonic contamination.

Distal Pancreatectomy. The most effective method of treating pancreatic injury with obvious disruption of the pancreatic duct in the body or tail of the gland is distal pancreatectomy. When performing a distal pancreatectomy to prevent unnecessary blood loss, sutures are placed in the superior and inferior borders of the pancreas approximately 2 cm from the edge. If the patient is unstable, rapid division and ligation of the splenic vessels and splenectomy may be preferable to attempting to salvage the spleen, particularly if it is also injured. The transected duct of Wirsung in the remaining proximal gland is ligated with a transfixion suture of fine monofilament. The cut surface of the transected proximal pancreas is oversewn with interrupted, interlocking mattress sutures. A large stapler may be used to transect the pancreas. If the pancreatic duct can be identified, it is ligated.

In the unstable patient, even with suspected ductal injury, drainage is always a method of management. The pancreas is drained with closed suction drainage. Most patients sustaining a stab or gunshot wound to the pancreas do not require surgical resection. Only about 10 to 15 percent of patients require distal pancreatectomy. A conservative approach in the absence of proven ductal injury results in a low mortality. Complications and mortality increase in patients undergoing distal resection. The trend is currently toward conservative management of the pancreatic injury. Routinely performing a distal pancreatectomy for all penetrating injuries to the body and tail of the pancreas, significantly prolongs the operative time and contributes to additional hemorrhage and hypothermia. This in turn increases the incidence of coagulopathy. Approximately 25 percent of patients undergoing a distal pancreatectomy develop an intraabdominal abscess. In a multicenter study, intraabdominal abscess formation occurred in one-third of patients following distal pancreatectomy. In one large review of over 1400 patients, it was determined that approximately 25 percent of patients underwent distal pancreatectomy with a mortality of 14 percent.

The incidence of fistula and abscess formation appears to be the same whether the pancreas is stapled or sutured followed resection. If pancreatic ductal injury is doubtful, simple drainage is performed. In an unstable patient with questionable ductal injury, drainage is the treatment of choice.

Roux en Y Pancreaticojejunostomy. In 1971, Jones and Shires described placing a Roux en Y anastomosis to both ends of the transected pancreas. This was performed in an effort to prevent pancreatic insufficiency, diabetes mellitus, and pancreatic fistula. The procedure was used only in patients who would have required 80 percent or more of the pancreas to be resected. If pancreatic salvage is attempted, a more simple procedure described by Letton is a Roux en Y anastomosis to the proximal end of the distal pancreas (Fig. 6-16). Transections of lesser magnitude are treated by distal pancreatectomy. The Roux en Y anastomosis is accomplished using permanent sutures placed approximately 1 cm apart in a single-layer anastomosis. The consistency of the pancreas must be suitable for suturing.

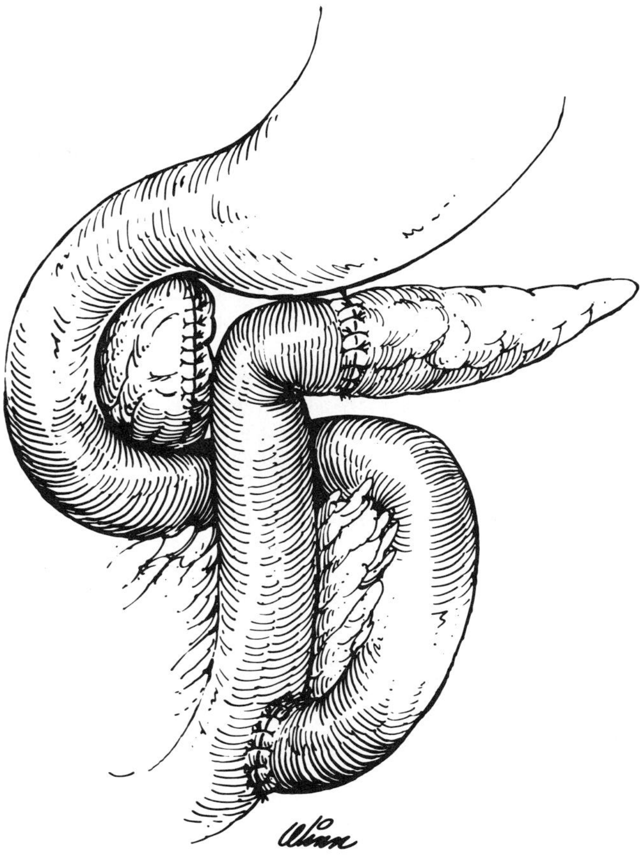

FIG. 6-16. Technique of Roux en Y anastomosis to the transected body of the pancreas.

Management of Pancreaticoduodenal Injuries. Approximately 20 percent of penetrating pancreatic injuries are associated with duodenal trauma, but less than 10 percent of blunt injuries have associated duodenal injury. The mortality for combined pancreaticoduodenal trauma is 20 percent, mostly from associated injuries. These injuries are usually managed by structure of the duodenum and drainage of the pancreas. A duodenostomy tube may be inserted, but it is difficult to demonstrate that this decreases morbidity or mortality. Duodenal fistula following duodenostomy tube insertion is approximately the same as in those patients treated with pyloric exclusion. Simple through-and-through injuries to the duodenum and pancreas are managed by suture of the duodenum and drainage.

Pyloric Exclusion. Vaughan and associates described pyloric exclusion as a simple method of managing combined pancreaticoduodenal injuries. A recent update of their series reports a 7 percent duodenal fistula rate. Pyloric exclusion consists of repair or resection and reanastomosis of the duodenum, a gastrotomy with oversew of the pylorus from inside using permanent suture material or a stapling device followed by a gastroenterostomy. The division is temporary, and the pylorus is usually open in 3 weeks in over 90 percent of the patients. An occasional marginal ulcer may develop.

Diverticularization. Berne and associates described performing a gastric resection, vagotomy, gastroenterostomy, duodenostomy, choledochostomy and suction drainage for patients with combined pancreaticoduodenal injuries. Criteria for selection of patients to undergo the diverticularization procedure have not been well described.

Pancreaticoduodenectomy. A recent review describing over 150 pancreaticoduodenectomies performed for penetrating trauma and blunt trauma demonstrated a mortality of 30 percent. Indications for pancreaticoduodenectomy include combined pancreaticoduodenal injuries in which the duodenum cannot be repaired or is nonviable or there is uncontrollable hemorrhage from the pancreas. Before performing a pancreaticoduodenectomy, the presence of a pancreatic ductal injury should be verified. A needle cholangiogram may occasionally demonstrate the pancreatic duct. The overall condition of the patient and associated injuries must be assessed before submitting the patient to several hours of surgery. Only 2 percent of patients require pancreaticoduodenectomy for management of their injury. In addition to fistula formation and abscesses, marginal ulceration with upper gastrointestinal hemorrhage has occurred following pancreaticoduodenectomy.

Complication. Mortality and morbidity from pancreatic trauma may be associated with pancreatic fistula, pancreatitis, pseudocysts, intraabdominal abscess, and pancreatic insufficiency.

Fistula. The incidence of pancreatic fistula varies with the definition of duration of the fistula and volume of drainage. Fistulae may develop following penetrating injuries or simple contusion. The fistulae almost always close spontaneously and very rarely require reoperation. The fistula may contribute, however, to sepsis and eventual death. Total parenteral nutrition in association with somatostatin has been shown to decrease the number of days of fistula drainage as well as to decrease the volume. The serum amylase level may be elevated while the fistula is present, probably because of transperitoneal absorption.

Pseudocyst. A pancreatic pseudocyst is a false cyst, the wall of which is inflammatory fibrous tissue that does not contain epithelium and is made of those structures surrounding the pancreas in the retroperitoneum. Diagnosis of pancreatic pseudocyst is by sonography or CT. Pancreatic pseudocyst is now a rare complication following pancreatic trauma if the pancreas has been managed appropriately at the time of initial injury. The preferred method of treatment is internal drainage, by either cyst gastrostomy or Roux en Y cyst jejunostomy. The Roux-en-Y limb is at least 45 cm.

Hemorrhagic Pancreatitis. Bleeding from the drain tract in the postoperative period may represent hemorrhagic pancreatitis with erosion of a ligated retroperitoneal vessel. This herald hemorrhage is an indication for exploration and control of the bleeding vessel, appropriate debridement, and additional drainage.

Pancreatic Insufficiency and Diabetes. Several reports have noted pancreatic insufficiency and diabetes as complications if over 80 percent of the pancreas was resected. Rarely with a proximal transection of the pancreas, in a stable patient and in the absence of splenic injury, an internal Roux en Y drainage to the distal pancreas should be considered to preserve pancreatic function.

Sepsis. Intraabdominal sepsis is a common complication following multiple abdominal trauma and is the second most common cause of death. Abscess formation occurs in 25 to 30 percent of patients who have a pancreatic injury and is often in association with a colon injury. Over three-fourths of patients who develop an intraabdominal abscess have had an associated gastrointestinal tract injury. The location of an intraabdominal abscess in the right or left subdiaphragmatic region is predictable in most patients depending on whether they have had an associated spleen or liver injury. Sepsis relates to hemorrhagic shock in that one-third of patients who are hypotensive develop an infection whereas in patients who never developed hypotension, only 15 percent developed infection. The serum amylase is not consistently elevated in patients with a pancreatic or lesser sac abscess. Some abscesses may be drained percutaneously, while others will require open drainage. Antibiotic therapy consists of an agent active against both aerobes and anaerobes since many of these abscesses follow a colon injury.

Mortality. The overall mortality for pancreatic trauma is approximately 20 percent for penetrating injuries and 15 percent for blunt trauma. Recognition of pancreatic injury at the time of initial surgical exploration is the key to decreasing the morbidity and mortality of pancreatic trauma. There are several reasons why the pancreatic injury appears not to be the cause of death. The mortality for isolated pancreatic injury is less than 1 percent. Patients developing shock following injury have a 40 percent mortality in association with pancreatic trauma, whereas the normotensive patient with pancreatic injury has less than a 5 percent mortality. The mortality due to the pancreatic injury in the multiply injured patient is less than 3 percent.

Spleen

The spleen is the abdominal organ most frequently injured by blunt trauma: such injuries to the spleen represent approximately one-quarter of all blunt injuries of the abdominal viscera. The spleen also is often injured by penetrating abdominal trauma and is frequently associated with blunt and penetrating thoracoabdominal injuries.

Diagnosis. The diagnosis of splenic injury is usually easily made with penetrating trauma but is often more difficult in patients sustaining blunt trauma. The clinical manifestations are the systemic symptoms and signs of hemorrhage and local evidence of peritoneal irritation in the region of the spleen. Approximately 30 to 40 percent of patients with splenic injury present with a systolic blood pressure below 100 mmHg. But many patients with splenic trauma may develop hypotension and tachycardia when assuming the sitting position.

A history of injury, which may be seemingly slight, followed by abdominal pain, predominantly in the left upper quadrant; left shoulder pain; and syncope is very significant. Often the left shoulder pain, or Kehr's sign, occurs only when the patient is in a supine or head-down position. This is caused by irritation of the inferior surface of the left side of the diaphragm by free blood or blood clots. Elevation of the foot of the bed or pressure in the left subcostal region may occasionally reproduce pain at the top of the left shoulder. Ballance's sign, which refers to fixed dullness to percussion in the left flank and dullness in the right flank that disappears on change of position of the patient, thus indicating large quantities of clot in the perisplenic region and free blood in the remainder of the peritoneal cavity, may be helpful in establishing the diagnosis. Whereas a decreased or falling hematocrit, leukocytosis of more than 15,000, x-ray findings such as fractures of the left lower ribs, gastric displacement, loss of splenic outline, and splinting or elevation of the left diaphragm are useful diagnostic findings, they are frequently absent.

Abdominal paracentesis, although seldom used, and diagnostic peritoneal lavage are extremely helpful in establishing the diagnosis in doubtful cases, especially in patients who have an altered state of consciousness. In patients with splenic trauma the incidence of false-negative diagnostic peritoneal lavage is reported, in repeated series, to be less than 1 percent.

Computerized tomography is now the preferable procedure in both pediatric and adult patients. It is an accurate, simple way to diagnose subcapsular hematomas and more extensive transcapsular lacerations. As with liver injuries, one can evaluate the degree of splenic injury and use this study to determine if the patient would be best served by operative or nonoperative therapy. Although extremely accurate, the CT scan may, on occasion, be falsely negative, thereby requiring close clinical evaluation for optimal patient care.

Delayed rupture of the spleen was first described by Baudet in 1902, and the asymptomatic interval between abdominal injury and rupture of the spleen is known as the latent period of Baudet. It was postulated that bleeding appeared several days after injury because (1) a subcapsular splenic hematoma gradually increased in size until it caused a delayed rupture of the splenic capsule and intraperitoneal hemorrhage or (2) there was initial bleeding from a splenic laceration that ceased spontaneously but began again in several days or weeks when the perisplenic hematoma became dislodged. This concept has been challenged by Olsen and Polley and by Benjamin and associates. These authors report a rate of delayed rupture of the spleen of less than 1 percent in over 600 patients. They suggest that delayed splenic rupture is an unusual occurrence and that the 15 percent incidence reported in older papers actually represents a delay in diagnosis rather than a delayed rupture in those patients.

Treatment. King and Shumacker in 1952 reported that all five patients under 6 months who had splenectomies developed meningitis or overwhelming septicemia. Two of these five patients died. This observation stimulated further investigation followed by considerable confusion and contradictory remarks into the relationship between splenectomy and what was later termed overwhelming postsplenectomy infection (OPSI). This syndrome is characterized by an abrupt onset of overwhelming sepsis, massive bacteremia, usually pneumococcal, followed by early death.

Eraklis and Filler reported a mortality rate of 0.8 percent in 342 patients under age 16 who had splenectomy for trauma. Singer reviewed 23 series from the literature including 2795 patients. The risk of sepsis was 1.45 percent in the 688 patients (300 adults) who had splenectomy for trauma. Only four of these patients died for a mortality rate of 0.58 percent. This has been compared with the general population where a death rate due to sepsis is estimated at 0.01 percent. This comparison is not accurate as the two groups are dissimilar by virtue of the fact the former group have all sustained some type of trauma and undergone an operative procedure that is not accounted for in the control group.

O'Neal and McDonald reported a mortality rate of 2.7 percent in a series of 356 adult patients. There were no fatalities in the 115 patients with splenectomy for trauma. All the deaths in the series occurred in patients whose spleen was removed in conjunction with other nontraumatic elective procedures or patients with proved malignancies.

Stimulated by these and many other reports describing the immunologic abnormalities and pathophysiology of the overwhelming sepsis syndrome, a more conservative approach has evolved concerning the management of splenic trauma. Similar to liver injuries, a classification system for splenic trauma has been developed by the Organ Injury Scaling Committee of the American Association for the Surgery of Trauma (Table 6-7). Most grade I and II injuries can be managed nonoperatively or by splenic salvage procedures. Selected guide III injuries may be salvaged as well. Nonoperative therapy in the pediatric age group has been the preferred method of management for many years. The same principles now seem applicable to adult trauma patients, but to a lesser degree. Shackford and Molin compared 13 series from the literature and found 12.7 percent of adult patients were managed nonoperatively. Thirty-one percent failed observation and subsequently required operation for hemorrhage. Seventy-five percent of the spleens in the total group of 237 patients were salvaged. These figures compare favorably to the pediatric population. Two hundred and eight patients compared from six series had a splenic salvage rate of 81 percent. Only 11 percent of this group failed nonoperative management. By comparison, 70 percent of the pediatric patients were initially observed, whereas only 12 percent of adult patients were selected for nonoperative management.

In assessing the patient with multiple trauma, one cannot assume the spleen is the only injured organ; hence other injuries may be missed in as many as 30 percent of patients. Nonoperative therapy requires a prolonged hospitalization that is generally accomplished in an intensive care unit. Other drawbacks include a prolonged convalescence, increased hospital cost, and risk and complications associated with repeated blood transfusions, such as delayed autoimmune disease.

Table 6-7
Splenic Injury Scale

*Grade**		*Injury Description*
I.	Hematoma	Subcapsular, nonexpanding, <10% surface area
	Laceration	Capsular tear, nonbleeding, <1 cm parenchymal depth
II.	Hematoma	Subcapsular, nonexpanding, 10–50% surface area; intraparenchymal, nonexpanding <2 cm in diameter
	Laceration	Capsular tear, active bleeding, 1–3 cm parenchymal depth that does not involve a trabecular vessel
III.	Hematoma	Subcapsular, >50% surface area or expanding; ruptured subcapsular hematoma with active bleeding; intraparenchymal hematoma, <2 cm or expanding
	Laceration	>3 cm parenchymal depth or involving trabecular vessels
IV.	Hematoma	Ruptured intraparenchymal hematoma with active bleeding
	Laceration	Laceration involving segmental or hilar vessel producing major devascularization (>25% of spleen)
V.	Laceration	Completely shattered spleen
	Vascular	Hilar vascular injury that devascularizes spleen

*Advance one grade for multiple injuries to the same organ. Based on most accurate assessment at autopsy, laparotomy, or radiologic study.

Based on an extensive review of the literature, Luna and Dellinger concluded that the 1 to 2 percent incidence figures for postsplenectomy infection represented a 10- to 20-fold overestimation of the true incidence. These authors quoted a 60 percent success rate in three series of nonoperative observation in adults who were initially stable without evidence of blood loss. Ninety-three percent of the patients who failed nonoperative management required a splenectomy, suggesting that splenic salvage rates were not improved by nonoperative observation when the initial injury was felt to be relatively minor.

Luna and associates further stated it has been estimated that 35 to 40 percent of patients who are successfully observed will require a blood transfusion that averages 40 to 50 percent of their blood volume. Although symptoms may occur in only 50 percent of patients with non-A non-B hepatitis and only 20 percent become icteric, it is estimated that the per-unit risk for a single-unit transfusion may approach 3 percent. The posttransfusion hepatitis death rate per unit of blood transfused is 0.14 percent.

Proper management of patients with splenic injuries is still controversial, and continued reevaluation of data is necessary. It is possible that failure of nonoperative therapy frequently results in splenectomy rather than splenorraphy (the preferable procedure) and the increased incidence of blood transfusion with its attendant disease transmission problems may outweigh any theoretic advantages of avoiding surgery. Luna and Dellinger also concluded that in adults 0.26 percent of the observed patients die (0.17 percent for pediatric patients) compared with 0.06 percent for those operated on initially.

A more rational approach to the problem is splenic preservation in carefully selected patients at the time of operation. The procedures include (1) no therapy for nonbleeding capsular lacerations, (2) application of microfibrillar collagen or other hemostatic agents to minor lacerations with minimal bleeding, (3) suture repair of more extensive injuries, (4) partial splenectomy for splenic injuries that do not involve the hilus. Contraindications to splenic salvage procedures as recommended by Traub and Perry include (1) patient instability secondary to major associated injuries, (2) splenic avulsion or extensive fragmentation, (3) extensive hilar vascular injury, (4) failure to attain splenic hemostasis. Relative contraindications include significant peritoneal contamination from concomitant bowel injury and rupture of a diseased spleen.

Increasing experimental data and clinical evidence indicate that an intact spleen is required to produce important opsonic antibodies that are necessary for optimal function of the macrophage system and production of immunoglobulins. Sepsis is a rather frequent occurrence following splenectomy for certain hematologic disorders, many of which have diffuse reticuloendothelial abnormalities. Many of these patients, however, receive various forms of therapy that alter immunity and response to infection. Splenectomy is still a safe procedure and the indicated procedure of choice in many patients.

Operative Technique (See Chap. 31). Most authors do not recommend drainage of the splenic bed after elective splenectomy; it is used still in selected trauma cases, however. The incidence of drain tract infections and subphrenic abscess has been reported to be as high as 25 to 50 percent when drains were used, in contrast to 5 to 12 percent when drains were not employed. Many of these infections, however, were related to the presence of associated injuries, usually in the gastrointestinal tract, or to the immunologic defects often present in patients requiring splenectomies for conditions other than trauma, and not to the drains per se. The routine use of drains following splenectomy for trauma is supported by the series reported by Naylor, Cohn, and Shires. These authors reported an incidence of subphrenic abscess of only 3.4 percent in 408 patients undergoing splenectomy for trauma. Among the 72 patients who had splenectomy for trauma involving the spleen alone, there were no subphrenic abscesses and an incidence of drain tract infection of only 1.3 percent. Thus, while it cannot be proved that drainage of the splenic bed after splenectomy for trauma reduces the incidence of subphrenic collections, it is most probable that drainage in such cases does not increase the incidence of subphrenic abscess. Also in those instances of splenic injury in which there is any question of associated pancreatic or gastric trauma, drainage of the splenic bed may prevent complications that could arise if such unrecognized injuries were not drained. Even those authors who incriminate the usage of splenic bed drains report no higher incidence of subphrenic abscess or other infections if the drains are removed before the sixth postsplenectomy day.

Another area of controversy is the issue of prophylactic antibiotics in the postsplenectomized patient, particularly in the pediatric age group. Most authors advocate prophylactic penicillin therapy until at least age 5 years, but it has been recommended that protection be extended into the teenage years, and isolated reports suggest indefinite protection. The use of long-term antibiotics is not without untoward effects, such as drug sensitivity, bacterial resistance, and suppression of natural immunologic defenses. Patient compliance over a long period of time is very poor. Patients who have undergone splenectomy are advised to contact their physician at the first sign of any febrile illness.

Pneumococcal vaccination is recommended following splenectomy. This should protect against 80 to 85 percent of the pneumococcal strains leading to sepsis. It must be stressed, however, that although pneumococcus is the most prevalent offending organism, the syndrome can be caused by other organisms such as meningococcus and *Haemophilus influenzae*. Currently there are no recommendations for a second or booster dose of pneumococcal vaccine. Asplenic patients should be considered immunocompromised, receive close follow-up, and be instructed about the potential risks of the asplenic state.

Mortality. Factors contributing to mortality following splenic injury include (1) associated injury, (2) mechanism of injury, (3) presence of shock on admission to hospital, and (4) advanced age. Naylor and associates reported an overall mortality rate of 11.2 percent in their series of 408 patients, which compares favorably with that in other reports.

Retroperitoneal Hematoma

The most common cause of retroperitoneal hemorrhage is pelvic fracture, which accounts for about 60 percent of all traumatic retroperitoneal hematomas. The diagnosis of retroperitoneal hematoma is most difficult following blunt, nonpenetrating trauma to the abdomen, and should be suspected in any patient following trauma who has signs and symptoms of hemorrhagic shock but no obvious source of hemorrhage. Hemorrhage within the retroperitoneal area may be massive and may exceed 2000 mL of blood. Experimental data have shown that as much as 4000 mL of fluid can extravasate into the retroperitoneal space under pressure.

Diagnosis. Abdominal pain occurs in approximately 60 percent of patients, and back pain in about 25 percent. The abdominal pain is usually vague and generalized but is occasionally localized over the hematoma. Local or generalized tenderness is present in about two-thirds of the patients, and shock occurs in approximately 40 percent. Occasionally, a tender mass is palpable through the abdomen or in the flanks, and in some cases, rectal examination will reveal a boggy mass anterior or posterior to the rectum. Dullness to percussion over the flanks or the abdomen that does not vary with changing positions of the patient has been recorded in some instances. At times, discoloration of the flanks from retroperitoneal hemorrhage has been noted after the lapse of a few hours (Grey Turner's sign). Progressive decreases in the hemoglobin and hematocrit is a consistent finding, and hematuria is found in 80 percent of patients.

If a large pelvic hematoma is suspected, special care should be taken when performing lavage so as not to inadvertently enter the hematoma, which may cause significant and difficult-to-control hemorrhage. A supraumbilical open lavage is suggested in these cases.

Radiography can be helpful in establishing the diagnosis. Approximately two-thirds of the patients with peritoneal hematoma have had fractures of the pelvis, and other x-ray findings have included obliteration of the psoas shadow in 30 percent, abdominal mass in 5 percent, and paralytic ileus in 8 percent. Also, displaced bowel-gas shadows and fractured vertebrae have been noted. CT scan and, occasionally, arteriography may be helpful in establishing the diagnosis of retroperitoneal injury. In the patient whose condition is deteriorating, however, immediate exploration is performed without obtaining such studies, in order to attempt rapid control of progressive bleeding. Many retroperitoneal hematomas from pelvic fractures will tamponade themselves within a short time, and the patient's condition will remain stable. The use of the pneumatic antishock garment, external fixators, and occasionally arteriography with embolization will often control or temporize pelvic bleeding until definitive care can be rendered.

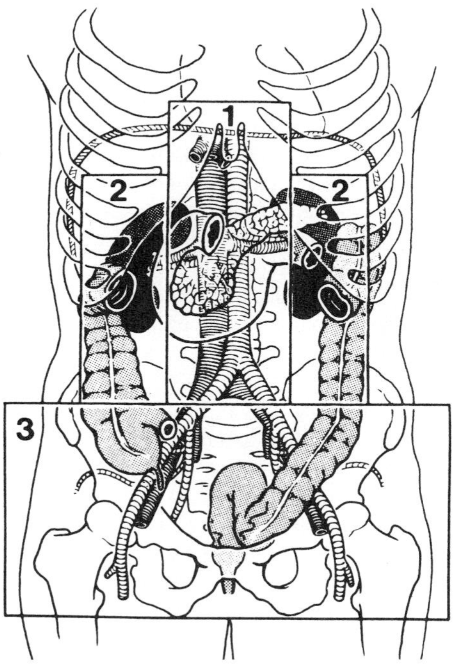

FIG. 6-17. Retroperitoneal classification. Zone 1 = central-medial retroperitoneal hematomas. Zone 2 = flank retroperitoneal hematomas. Zone 3 = pelvic retroperitoneal hematomas. [From: *Sheldon GF: Retroperitoneal hematoma, in Blaisdell WF, Trunkey DD (eds): Abdominal Trauma. New York, Thieme-Stratton, 1982, p 281, with permission.*]

Treatment. One of the most frequently debated areas of abdominal surgery is that of the proper management of retroperitoneal injuries. The major controversy centers around the question of whether to open and explore retroperitoneal hematomas depending on the anatomic location. The retroperitoneum has been divided into three areas in an attempt to clarify the various problems encountered (Fig. 6-17). Area 1 is the upper central area and extends from the diaphragmatic hiatus to the sacral promontory. Area 2 consists of the right and left flank, and area 3 consists of the pelvis.

The decision to open the hematoma is dependent on several considerations. These include the wounding mechanism, the location, and the intraoperative evaluation of the size of the hematoma. There is general agreement that all penetrating injuries should be explored as well as all hematomas in the central medial area from the hiatus to the sacrum (area 1).

When retroperitoneal vascular injuries are suspected, proximal control is essential before entering the hematoma. Suprarenal aortic injuries are controlled by approaching the aorta from the lateral aspect. This is accomplished by reflecting the left colon, kidney, spleen, and pancreas toward the midline and applying a vascular clamp above and below the injury. Infrarenal aortic injuries are best approached through the root of the mesentery with the transverse colon retracted superiorly and the small bowel packed off to the right. Iliac artery and vena cava injuries can be exposed and controlled by approaching them from the right side. Mobilization of the right colon may facilitate this exposure.

If uncontrollable hemorrhage occurs, pressure can be applied immediately above and below the area of injury. An assistant's hand or retractor applied just below the crus of the diaphragm will occasionally be helpful. Preoperative thoracotomy to cross-clamp the aorta is not recommended unless the injury is located at the diaphragm and it is the only way to obtain proximal control.

Injuries located in the flanks (area 2) are frequently individualized. The most common injury in this area is the kidney, renovascular pedicle, and posterior colon. Once again, penetrating injuries in this area should be explored. Patients with blunt trauma are often managed selectively. If the evaluation of the kidney has been unremarkable, including an arteriogram, and the hematoma is lateral or contained in Gerota's fascia and not expanding, many authors recommend nonexploration. If, however, the hematoma is expanding or large and the preoperative evaluation is incomplete or inconclusive, it is best to investigate this area of potential injury. Before opening Gerota's fascia, it is extremely important to gain control of the renal artery and vein so that if massive hemorrhage is encountered the surgeon will be in a position to control it. If there is any question of a hematoma around the large bowel, it must be completely explored.

Large retroperitoneal hematomas that are located deep in the pelvis (area 3) and associated with pelvis fractures are best not explored. It is important to be certain there is no injury to the distal aorta, iliac vessels, or takeoff of the internal iliac vessels. If major vessels are not explored at the time that hematomas occur near them, major and sometimes fatal postoperative bleeding may occur. Present-day vascular surgical techniques obviate the fear of incurring massive hemorrhage as a contraindication to exploring retroperitoneal hematomas.

Ligation of one or both hypogastric arteries, popular in the past, may control persistent bleeding in the pelvic retroperitoneal space but in general is ineffective. Certainly it is preferable to locate a single vessel that is bleeding and either ligate or repair it. Selective arteriography, either intraoperatively or in the x-ray department, and infusion of vasospastic drugs or the embolization of autologous clots or hemostatic agents may be beneficial in controlling this type of hemorrhage. On rare occasions it may be necessary to pack the pelvis with large lap packs for 24 to 48 h in order to achieve hemostasis.

Inferior Vena Cava

Inferior vena caval injuries associated with penetrating abdominal wounds are being seen with increasing frequency. It has been reported that 1 in every 50 gunshot wounds and 1 in every 300 knife wounds of the abdomen will injure the vena cava. These are serious injuries: one-third of the patients die before reaching the hospital, and up to half the remaining persons will die during hospitalization. Most deaths occur from bleeding because of the inherent difficulties in controlling injuries of large veins, but significant wounds of other structures, especially in the retroperitoneum, are common and often adversely affect therapeutic efforts.

Etiology and Distribution. Most injuries of the inferior vena cava are caused by gunshot wounds, but stab wounds or blunt trauma may also be involved (Table 6-8). Simple penetrating wounds produced by knives and low-velocity missiles are less lethal than those wounds caused by shotguns, high-velocity bullets, and especially blunt trauma. Widespread serious damage to other structures, particularly liver and major arteries and veins, are likely to result from shotgun wounds and blunt trauma to the abdomen and lower part of the chest.

The infrarenal vena cava is most susceptible and most often injured (Table 6-9). The level of injury is a major determinant of survival, and injuries of the suprarenal, intrahepatic vena cava are extremely dangerous, especially when accompanied by wounds of hepatic and renal veins. Difficulties in exposure and control are invariably encountered, and adjunctive measures are often necessary.

Diagnosis. Injuries of the inferior vena cava should be considered in all cases of penetrating wounds of the abdomen and lower part of the chest. Because of the vagaries of the trajectory of bullets, innocent-appearing small-caliber wounds may produce serious damage to retroperitoneal structures, without intraabdominal organ injury. Patients who have suffered stab wounds of the back or lower part of the chest may also harbor unsuspected caval injuries.

Table 6-8
Causes of Inferior Vena Caval Injuries

	Total	*Died*	*Mortality, %*
Bullet	69	23	33
Shotgun	8	6	75
Stab	12	2	17
Blunt	12	11	92
Total	101	42	42

Table 6-9
Location of Inferior Vena Caval Injury

	Total	*Died*	*Mortality, %*
Above renal veins	19	11	58
At renal vein level	21	13	62
Below renal veins	47	14	30
Bifurcation	14	4	29

One of the major determinants of survival of these patients is the presence of hemorrhagic shock on admission. This is often a clue that despite the absence of identifying physical findings, major vascular injuries are present. Hemoperitoneum, hemothorax, subcutaneous blood staining from retroperitoneal bleeding, and evidence of distal vena caval obstruction may be helpful in diagnosis.

Except for direct venous studies with contrast media, radiographic examination is rarely specific. Routine x-ray studies, including anteroposterior and lateral films of the chest and abdomen, are useful and are recommended, but it is usually best not to delay surgery for elaborate studies if firm indications for exploration exist.

Treatment. Associated injuries are common and are a major factor in survival of these patients (Table 6-10). Before exploration, resuscitation and attention to other problems often are important. An adequate airway must be obtained, volume and blood deficits repaired, and fractures stabilized. Vena caval injuries that require clamping may reduce the effectiveness of using lower-extremity veins for fluid administration, and at least one large-bore catheter should be placed into the upper-extremity venous system. This line is best reserved for blood and fluid administration and should not be used for primary anesthetic manipulations.

Thoracotomy may be required, especially in patients with suprarenal caval injuries. If transatrial intracaval shunts are needed, a median sternotomy offers good exposure for this maneuver as well as for control of associated hepatic injuries.

Abdominal exploration is performed through a midline incision that can be extended as required, and median sternotomy can be added if necessary. Rapid abdominal exploration will usually expose major injuries and establish priorities of repair. It is usually wise to control the bleeding, pause, and complete volume and blood restoration before definitive repairs are begun. Attempts to complete bowel repairs while bleeding persists from other injuries often extend the hypotensive episode and increase blood loss.

Centrally located retroperitoneal hematomas above the pelvis often harbor significant injuries, and usually are explored. Damage to other retroperitoneal structures is common (79 percent) and not always evident without formal exploration. The size or stability of the hematoma does not offer reliable evidence as to the presence or absence of significant injuries. Continued bleeding

Table 6-10
Injuries Associated with Inferior Vena Caval Injury

Aorta, iliac artery	13	Kidney	21
Major splanchnic vessel	26	Pancreas	18
Renal artery or vein	20	Spleen	10
Liver	46	Colon	27
Duodenum	27	Other	21

from the vena caval injury, however, is ominous. Patients actively bleeding at the time of operation have a very high mortality rate, especially if the vena caval injury is at or above the renal arteries and veins (Table 6-11).

Initial control of bleeding can usually be obtained with pressure and packs. Occasionally temporary occlusion of the abdominal aorta at the diaphragmatic hiatus is useful in reducing blood loss from high caval injuries. Exposure of the inferior vena cava is obtained by reflecting medially the right colon, duodenum, and pancreas. Direct tamponade, manually or with sponge sticks, is usually effective in controlling bleeding. Simple lacerations or punctures are most common, but transections, avulsion, or multiple lacerations may be encountered, and control may be very difficult in the last group.

Simple lacerations can be controlled with gentle digital pressure and sutured by simply passing the needle under the occluding finger. In some cases the edge of the wound can be held gently in apposition with vascular forceps or blunt Allis clamps while repair is effected. Balloon catheter tamponade has also been used for control of these wounds. Partial occlusion with vascular clamps is a useful technique and can be instituted after the initial use of other maneuvers (Fig. 6-18). These simple tangential wounds usually can be repaired without injury to lumbar veins, but occasionally ligation of gonadal and lumbar tributaries is required (Fig. 6-19).

Transections may be repaired by end-to-end vascular surgical techniques after mobilizing the vena cava. If there are multiple caval wounds requiring complicated repairs, or if repair poses an undue risk in a patient with multiple injuries, infrarenal ligation is preferable. In most cases construction of venous grafts is not required, and the time and effort necessary to perform these repairs may increase the operative morbidity and mortality.

Wounds at or above the renal veins are difficult to expose and repair. If bleeding from behind the liver is encountered and is not easily identified as coming from a laceration of the anterior cava wall below the caudate lobe, an intracaval shunt may be needed. The liver can be rotated medially after division of supporting ligaments, and if intrahepatic vena cava or combined hepatic vein lacerations are present, the shunt can be inserted as described by Schrock et al. The transatrial approach is easier than inserting the shunt from the intrarenal vena cava and is very useful in managing these extremely dangerous wounds. A large chest tube (34 to 38 F tube) with a proximal side hole is inserted through the atrial appendage, and the tip is placed near the orifices of the renal veins. Umbilical tapes encircling the inferior vena cava within the pericardium and above the renal veins secure the catheter. The side hole in the catheter is placed at a level to permit the return of blood via the tube into the right atrium. This shunt, occasionally combined with temporary occlusion of the portal triad, will usually allow sufficient control of bleeding to effect repairs. This technique is rarely required.

Table 6-11
Relationship of Bleeding and Mortality from Inferior Vena Caval Injuries

	Total	*Died*	*Mortality, %*
Active bleeding	41	32	78
Tamponade	57	9	16
Not specified	3	0	0

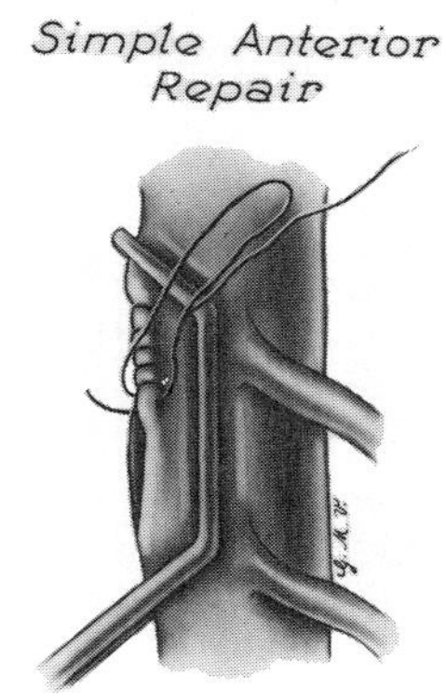

FIG. 6-18. Repair of anterior laceration of the inferior vena cava. Note the use of a partially occlusive clamp.

Unlike injuries of the infrarenal cava, most wounds above the renal veins should be repaired. Ligation of the inferior vena cava at this level produces serious complications. Some survivors have been reported, and those were usually in operations uncomplicated by hypotension, shock, or multiple injuries.

Those vascular procedures used in other areas are effective in repairing the suprarenal vena cava. Simple venorrhaphy often may suffice, but patch graft angioplasty or anastomosis may be needed (Fig. 6-20). If graft interposition is required, autogenous venous grafts obtained from the infrarenal cava or iliac vein are preferred (Fig. 6-21). Concomitant repair of hepatic vein injuries can be effected, but in some cases ligation may be preferable.

These repairs can usually be completed within 30 min, a period of ischemia well tolerated by the normothermic liver. Regional hypothermia may be induced with iced saline solution by irrigation techniques, thus conferring further protection of the liver during more prolonged ischemia.

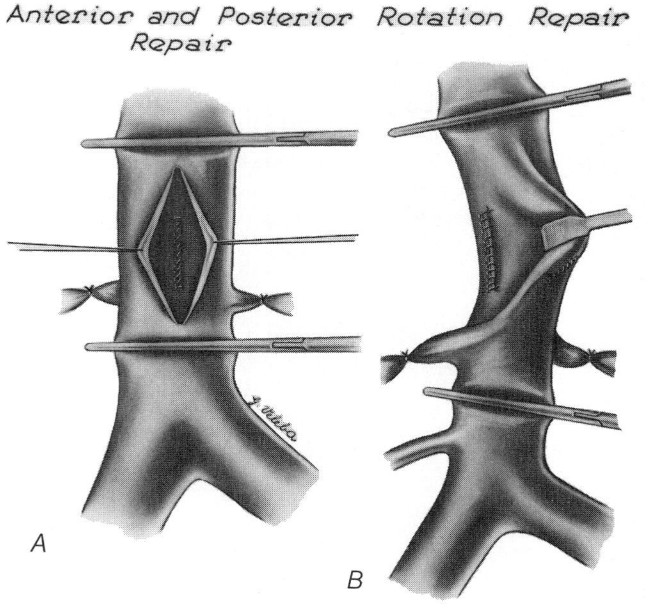

FIG. 6-19. Repair of through-and-through injury to the inferior vena cava. *A.* Anterior laceration is enlarged to permit closure of the posterior wall from within the lumen. *B.* Rotation of the posteroinferior vena cava.

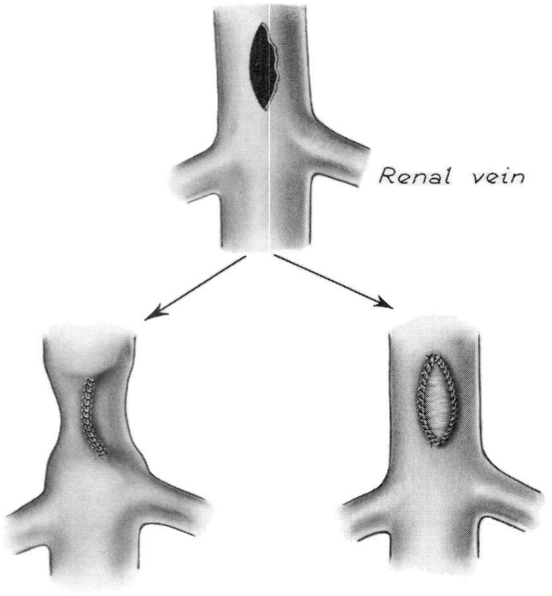

FIG. 6-20. Repair of the inferior vena cava using a patch graft to prevent stenosis.

Complications. In patients with isolated wounds of the inferior vena cava, repair is usually effective and complications are few. In these patients, ileofemoral venous thrombosis and pulmonary embolus have been encountered. Pancreatitis has also been encountered, and recurrent retroperitoneal bleeding might occur.

The mortality in patients with isolated inferior vena caval injuries was 11 percent in one series, but 67 percent of the patients with one or more major vessel injuries died. All the patients with inferior vena caval wounds at or above the renal veins had significant associated injuries, usually liver and bowel, occasionally pancreas, stomach, and lung. The mortality is high in this group of patients, especially if the inferior vena cava is actively bleeding at surgery.

Female Reproductive Organs

Injuries to the female reproductive organs are infrequently seen following either blunt or penetrating trauma to the abdomen. Except for sexual assault, injury to the female reproductive system in the nonpregnant patient is extremely uncommon. Rupture of the pregnant uterus due to blunt trauma is rare but has occurred in a number of instances. The major threat to the fetus in blunt trauma is placental abruption, which if complete, will result in fetal demise. Of blunt and penetrating wounds to the female reproductive tract, 90 percent involve the uterine corpus and 10 percent involve the remaining adnexa.

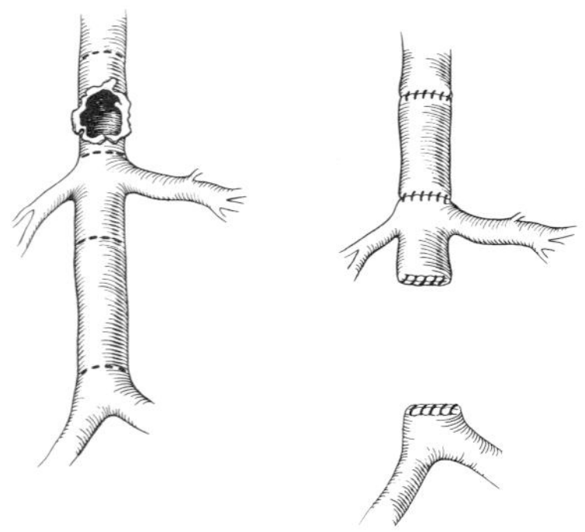

FIG. 6-21. Interposition of an excised segment of the infrarenal inferior vena cava to establish continuity of the suprarenal inferior vena cava.

In the past, serious questions have been raised about the efficacy of pregnant patients wearing seat belts in automobiles. Crosby has shown rather conclusively that more maternal and fetal lives have been saved by the use of lap belts, with or without shoulder harnesses, than by not using them.

The diagnostic evaluation of the pregnant patient sustaining traumatic injury should be undertaken with careful consideration for radiation exposure. Many procedures can be condensed to give maximum information with minimal exposure. On the contrary, no necessary procedure should be withheld because of a known or suspected pregnancy.

The most common cause of fetal death in automobile accidents is maternal death; therefore, important diagnostic and therapeutic measures designed to save the mother should be performed. In general, intrauterine exposure to diagnostic radiation is not an indication to terminate a pregnancy.

Pregnant patients sustaining penetrating trauma are managed the same as nonpregnant patients. It may be difficult to perform lavage in the late second and third trimester for stab wounds, but patients sustaining gunshot wounds should be formally explored in the operating room. In spite of the fact the gravid uterus may afford considerable protection to abdominal viscera, these organs are still at risk.

Treatment. The signs and symptoms from a ruptured pregnant uterus are those of abrupt and massive intraperitoneal hemorrhage. Associated with these findings are generalized abdominal pain and tenderness, abdominal distention, ileus, and the absence of fetal heart sounds and movements. If the patient arrives at the hospital alive (which is not often the case), immediate blood volume and extracellular fluid replacement must be instituted through several large-bore intravenous catheters, preferably placed in the upper extremities, since there may be an interference with venous return from lower extremities of those patients. Urgent celiotomy is necessary to control hemorrhage, even though the patient may still be in shock at the time. Probably the only anesthesia that will be required is assisted respiration with 100% oxygen administered through an endotracheal tube. Other agents may be added if and when shock abates. The treatment of choice is evacuation of the uterus, closure of the disruption with large chromic catgut sutures, and thorough peritoneal toilet with removal of all blood and foreign tissue.

Wounds of the uterus and adnexa are repaired by figure-of-eight chromic catgut sutures without drainage in most instances, although in occasional patients hysterectomy is indicated, as in injury of the lower uterine segment and major uterine vessels caused by high-velocity missiles. In these instances, hysterectomy is preferable to an attempted suture repair, since repair may cause stenosis of the cervical canal with resultant hematometra and dystocia. Also, hysterectomy for lower-uterine-segment injuries is indicated to obtain proper control of bleeding vessels and to help rule out uretheral injury at the point where the ureter and uterine artery are in juxtaposition.

It is best to leave the vaginal cuff partially open following hysterectomy for trauma, because of the likelihood of vaginal cuff or cul-de-sac abscess formation, especially if there is appreciable blast injury or concomitant colon injury. If abscesses occur and the vaginal cuff has been left open, it is usually a relatively simple matter to drain the abscess with a finger inserted through the vagina into the open cuff. If gross fecal contamination is present from colon injury, the cuff should be left open and a Penrose drain led out of the vagina from the cul-de-sac.

If massive uncontrollable or recurrent bleeding occurs following trauma to the female pelvic organs, it may be rapidly and adequately controlled by bilateral in-continuity ligations of the hypogastric arteries with nonabsorbable suture material. This will not often be required but should be borne in mind as a very helpful and possibly lifesaving procedure.

Following injury to the pregnant uterus, the incidence of fetal loss is quite high. Instances have been reported in which penetrating uterine injury during pregnancy has been repaired with ensuing normal delivery. One report found that over 80 percent of patients with uterine injuries during pregnancy delivered subsequently per vagina with no difficulty. Of the patients followed after uterine injury, all who were of childbearing age subsequently were able to conceive children. If a dying pregnant patient presents with a live fetus, rapid cesarean section will occasionally salvage the baby. Conversely, a pregnant patient may present in a neurologically devastated state late in her pregnancy. A viable fetus may be delivered if the mother is kept alive by mechanical means for a period of time to allow further intrauterine development of the infant. These situations require difficult moral and ethical decisions.

By far the majority of pregnant patients with uterine injuries will abort shortly after the injury, frequently requiring curettage to control bleeding after spontaneous abortion. Others will require elective emptying of the uterine contents at the time of celiotomy in order to secure adequate hemostasis and uterine repair.

Abdominal Wall

Injury to the abdominal wall without peritoneal injury is often difficult to diagnose. Muscular guarding and rigidity are frequently present, and it may be impossible to rule out intraabdominal injury from a hematoma of the abdominal wall. Such hematomas are usually due to rupture of the rectus abdominis or the epigastric artery by direct trauma or severe muscular exertion. The epigastric artery may also be injured by penetrating trauma, resulting in a hemoperitoneum. The patient may become hypotensive from such an injury because of the severe intraperitoneal bleeding that sometimes occurs.

The mass from the rectus abdominis hematoma is below the umbilicus in over 80 percent of the cases. To distinguish this mass from intraperitoneal masses, patients should be requested to raise their heads against resistance; the mass should disappear if it is intraperitoneal and remain the same if it is in the abdominal wall. This sign is not completely reliable, and if adjunctive diagnostic aids such as paracentesis and lavage are equivocal, then abdominal celiotomy should be performed.

On occasion missile injuries will appear to be limited to the abdominal wall. Depending on the bullet caliber, distance at which it was shot, and body habitus blast effect may injure hollow and solid abdominal viscera without actual penetration of the peritoneum. Local wound exploration, peritoneal lavage, and computed tomography are unreliable in these cases. As stated above, these patients are best treated by celiotomy.

Bibliography

General Considerations

Shires GT: *Principles of Trauma Care*. New York, McGraw-Hill, 1985.

Principles in Wound Management and Antibiotics

Alexander JW, Kaplan JZ, Altemeier WA: Role of suture materials in the development of wound infection. *Ann Surg* 165:192, 1967.

Bartlett JG: The normal flora, in Condon RE, Gorbach SL (eds): *Surgical Infections, Selective Antibiotic Therapy*. Baltimore, Williams & Wilkins, 1981, pp 4–5.

Caplan ES, Hoyt N: Infection surveillance and control in the severely traumatized patient. *Am J Med* 70:638, 1981.

Condie JP, Ferguson DJ: Experimental wound infections: Contamination versus surgical technique. *Surgery* 50:367, 1961.

Dunphy JE, Jackson DS: Practical applications of experimental studies in the care of the primarily closed wound. *Am J Surg* 104:273, 1962.

Fabian TC, Boldreghini SJ: Antibiotics in penetrating abdominal trauma. Comparison of ticarcillin plus clavulanic acid with gentamicin plus clindamycin. *Am J Med* (suppl 5B):157, 1985.

Francke EL, Neu HC: Postsplenectomy infection. *Surg Clin North Am* 61:135, 1981.

Gentry LO, Feliciano DV, et al: Perioperative antibiotic therapy for penetrating injuries to the abdomen. *Ann Surg* 200:561, 1984.

Gorbach SL: Intestinal microflora. *Gastroenterology* 60:1110, 1971.

Gorbach SL, Nahas L, et al: Studies of intestinal microflora. I. Effects of diet, age, and periodic sampling on numbers of fecal micro-organisms in man. *Gastroenterology* 53:845, 1967.

Grover FL, Richardson JD, et al: Prophylactic antibiotics in the treatment of penetrating chest wounds. *J Thoracic Cardiovasc Surg* 74:538, 1977.

Hofstetter SR: A prospective comparison of two regimens of prophylactic antibiotics in abdominal trauma: Cefoxitin versus triple drug. *J Trauma* 24(4):307, 1984.

Jones RC: Management of pancreatic trauma. *Ann Surg* 187:555, 1978.

Jones RC: New Directions in Antimicrobial Therapy. Infections in Trauma—A Symposium. St. James, Barbados, Stuart Pharmaceuticals, 1983, p 17.

Jones RC, Thal ER, et al: Evaluation of antibiotic therapy following penetrating abdominal trauma. *Ann Surg* 201:576, 1985.

Jones RC: Newer antibiotics for the surgeon. *Am J Surg* 152:577, 1986.

LoCurto JJ, Tischler CD, et al: Tube thoracostomy and trauma—antibiotics or not? *J Trauma* 26:1067, 1986.

Malangoni MA, Dillon LD, et al: Factors influencing the risk of early and late serious infections in adults after splenectomy for trauma. *Surgery* 96:775, 1984.

Mandel AK: Prophylactic antibiotics and no antibiotics compared in penetrating chest trauma. *J Trauma* 25(7):639, 1985.

Mann LS, Spinazzola AJ, et al: Disruption of abdominal wounds. *JAMA* 180:99, 1962.

Nichols RL, Smith JW, Klein DB: Risk of infection after penetrating abdominal trauma. *N Engl J Med* 311:1065, 1984.

Onderdonk AD, Bartlett JG, Louie T: Microbial synergy in experimental abdominal abscess. *Infect Immun* 13:22, 1976.

Oreskovitch MD, Dellinger EP, Lennard S: Duration of preventive antibiotic administration for penetrating abdominal trauma. *Arch Surg* 117:200, 1982.

Schimpff SC, Miller RM, et al: Infection in the severely traumatized patient. *Ann Surg* 179:353, 1974.

Thorngate S, Ferguson DJ: Effect of tension on healing of aponeurotic wounds. *Surgery* 44:619, 1958.

Wagner DH: Errors in the choice of abdominal wall incisions and in their closure. *Surg Clin North Am* 38:175, 1958.

Bites and Stings of Animals and Insects

Auer AI, Hershey FB: Surgery for necrotic bites of the brown spider. *Arch Surg* 108:612, 1974.

Berger RS, Addelstein GH, Anderson PC: Intravascular coagulation: The cause of necrotic arachnoidism. *Invest Dermatol* 61:142, 1973.

Bernstein B, Erhlich F: Brown recluse spider bites. *J Emerg Med* 4:457, 1986.

Bitseff EL, Garoni WJ, et al: The management of stingray injuries of the extremities. *South Med J* 63:417, 1970.

Christopher DG, Rodning CB: *Crotalidae* envenomation. *South Med J* 79:159, 1986.

Dillaha CJ, Jansen GT, et al: North American loxoscelism. *JAMA* 188:33, 1964.

Emergency Department Management of Poisonous Snake Bites, American College of Surgeons Committee on Trauma, February 1981.

Fardon DW, Wingo CW, et al: The treatment of brown spider bites. *Plast Reconstr Surg* 40:482, 1967.

Fishbein DB, Bernard KW, Miller KD: Early kinetics of the antibody response after booster immunizations after human diploid cell vaccine. *Am J Trop Med Hyg* 35:663, 1986.

Golden DBK, Langlois J, et al: Treatment failures with whole-body extract therapy of insect sting allergy. *JAMA* 246(21):2460, 1981.

Goldstein EJC, Citron DM, et al: Bacteriology of rattlesnake venom and implications for therapy. *J Infect Dis* 140(5):818, 1979.

Huang TT, Blackwell SJ, Lewis SR: Tissue necrosis in snakebite. *Tex Med* 77:53, 1981.

Huang TT, Lynch JB, et al: The use of excisional therapy in the management of snakebite. *Ann Surg* 179:598, 1974.

Hunt KJ, Valentine MD, et al: A controlled trial of immunotherapy in insect hypersensitivity. *N Engl J Med* 299:157, 1978.

Levine MI: Insect stings. *JAMA* 217:964, 1971.

Marr JJ: Portuguese man-of-war envenomization. *JAMA* 199:115, 1967.

Marteic Z: Lactrodectism: Variations in clinical manifestations produced by *Lactrodectus* species of spiders. *Toxicon* 21:457, 1983.

Parrish HM: Incidence of treated snakebites in the United States. *Public Health Rept (US)* 31:269,1966.

Parrish HM, Carr CA: Bites by copperheads in the United States. *JAMA* 201:927, 1967.

Rabies Prevention—United States, 1991. *Morbidity and Mortality Weekly Report,* vol. 40. R.R.-3 March 22, 1991.

Rees R, Shack RB, Withers E: Management of brown recluse spider bites. *Plast Reconstr Surg* 68:768, 1981.

Rees RS, Altenbern DP, et al: Brown recluse spider bites: A comparison of early surgical excision vs. dapsone and delayed surgical excision. *Ann Surg* 202:659, 1985.

Reisman RE, Arbesman CE, Lazell M: Clinical and immunological studies of venom immunotherapy. *Clin Allergy* 9:167, 1979.

Roberts RS: Csenscsitz TA, Heard CW: Upper extremity compartment syndromes following pit viper envenomation. *Clin Orthop* 193:184, 1985.

Russell FE: *Snake Venom Poisoning*. Philadelphia, Lippincott, 1980.

Russell FE, Carlson RW, et al: Snake venom poisoning in the United States—Experiences with 550 cases. *JAMA* 233:341, 1975.

Schwartz HJ, Lockey RF, et al: A multicenter study on skin test reactivity of human volunteers to venom as compared to whole-body hymenoptera antigens. *J Allergy Clin Immunol* 67:81, 1981.

Sprenger TR, Bailey WJ: Snakebite treatment in the United States—Review. *Int J Dermatol* 25:479, 1986.

Strauss MB, Orris WL: Injuries to divers by marine animals: A simplified approach to recognition and management. *Milit Med* February 1974.

Timms PK, Gibbons RB: Lactrodectism—Effects of the black widow spider bites. *West J Med* 144:315, 1986.

Van Mierop LHS: Poisonous snakebite: A review. II. Symptomatology and treatment. *J Fla Med Assoc* 63(3):201, 1976.

Van Mierop LHS, Kitchesn CS: Defibrination syndrome following bites by the eastern diamondback rattlesnake. *J Fla Med Assoc* 67:31, 1980.

Wasserman GS, Anderson PC: Loxoscelism and necrotic arachnoidism. *J Toxicol Clin Toxicol* 21:451, 1984.

Penetrating Wounds of the Neck and Thoracic Inlet

Ayuyao AM, Kaledzi YL, et al: Penetrating neck wounds: Mandatory versus selective exploration. *Ann Surg* 202:563, 1985.

Dunbar LL, Adkins RB, Waterhouse G: Penetrating injuries to the neck: Selective management. *Am Surg* 50:198, 1984.

Flint LM, Snyder WH, et al: Management of major vascular injuries in the base of the neck: An 11-year experience with 146 cases. *Arch Surg* 106:407, 1973.

Fogelman MJ, Stewart RD: Penetrating wounds of the neck. *Am J Surg* 91:581, 1956.

Gewertz BL, Samson DS, et al: Management of penetrating injuries of the internal carotid artery at the base of the skull utilizing extracranial-intracranial bypass. *J Trauma* 20:365, 1980.

Golueke PJ, Goldstein AS, et al: Routine versus selective exploration of penetrating neck injuries: A randomized prospective study. *J Trauma* 24:1010, 1984.

Graham JM, Feliciano DV, et al: Management of subclavian vascular injuries. *J Trauma* 20:537, 1980.

Hiatt JR, Busuttil RW, Wilson SE: Impact of routine arteriography on management of penetrating neck injuries. *J Vasc Surg* 1:860, 1984.

Jones RF, Terrell JC, Salyer KE: Penetrating wounds of the neck: An analysis of 274 cases. *J Trauma* 7:228, 1967.

Jurkovich GJ, Zingarelli W, et al: Penetrating neck trauma: Diagnostic studies in the asymptomatic patient. *J Trauma* 25:819, 1985.

Larson DL, Cohn AM: Management of acute laryngeal injury: A critical review. *J Trauma* 16:858, 1976.

Liekweg WG, Greenfield LJ: Management of penetrating carotid artery injury. *Ann Surg* 188:587, 1978.

Meier DE, Brink BE, Fry WJ: Vertebral artery trauma: Acute recognition and treatment. *Arch Surg* 116:236, 1981.

Metzdorff MT, Lowe DK: Operation or observation for penetrating neck wounds? A retrospective analysis. *Am J Surg* 147:646, 1984.

Monson DO, Saletta JD, Freeark RJ: Carotid-vertebral trauma. *J Trauma* 9:987, 1969.

Narrod JA, Moore EE: Selective management of penetrating neck injuries. *Arch Surg* 119:574, 1984.

Noyes LD, McSwain NE Jr, Markowitz IP: Panendoscopy with arteriography versus mandatory exploration of penetrating wounds of the neck. *Ann Surg* 204:21, 1986.

Obeid FN, Haddad GS, et al: A critical reappraisal of a mandatory exploration policy for penetrating wounds of the neck. *Surg Gynecol Obstet* 160:517, 1985.

Ordog GJ, Albin D, et al: 110 bullet wounds to the neck. *J Trauma* 25:238, 1985.

Prakashchandra MR, Bhatti MFK, et al: Penetrating injuries of the neck: Criteria for exploration. *J Trauma* 23:47, 1983.

Reid JDS, Weigelt JA: Forty-three cases of vertebral artery trauma. Presented at the 47th Annual Meeting of The American Association for the Surgery of Trauma, Montreal, Quebec, Canada, September 1987.

Roon AJ, Christensen N: Evaluation and treatment of penetrating cervical injuries. *J Trauma* 19:391, 1979.

Rosoff L Sr, White EJ: Perforation of the esophagus. *Am J Surg* 128:207, 1974.

Saletta JD, Lowe RJ, et al: Penetrating trauma of the neck. *J Trauma* 16:579, 1976.

Snyder WH III, Thal ER, et al: The validity of normal arteriography in penetrating trauma. *Arch Surg* 113:424, 1978.

Symbas PN, Hatcher CR Jr, Boehm GAW: Acute penetrating tracheal trauma. *Ann Thorac Surg* 22:473, 1976.

Thal ER, Snyder WH III, et al: Management of carotid artery injuries. *Surgery* 76:955, 1974.

Thomas AN, Goodman PC, Roon AJ: Role of angiography in cervicothoracic trauma. *J Thorac Cardiovasc Surg* 76:633, 1978.

Unger WS, Tucker WS Jr, et al: Carotid arterial trauma. *Surgery* 87:477, 1980.

Weigelt JA, Thal ER, et al: Diagnosis of penetrating cervical esophageal injuries. Presented at the 39th Annual Meeting of the Southwestern Surgical Congress, San Diego, California, April 1987.

Abdominal Trauma

Arajarvi E, Santavirta S, Tolonen J: Abdominal injuries sustained in severe traffic accidents by seatbelt wearers. *J Trauma* 27:393, 1987.

Arango A, Baxter CR, Shires GT: Surgical management of traumatic injuries of the right colon; 20 years civilian experience. *Arch Surg* 114:703, 1979.

Backwinkel K: Rupture of the rectus abdominis muscle. *Arch Surg* 90:35, 1965.

Balasegaram M: Surgical management of pancreatic trauma. *Curr Prob Surg* 16(12):1, 1979.

Bass EM, Crosier JH: Percutaneous control of posttraumatic hepatic hemorrhage by gelfoam embolization. *J Trauma* 17(1):61, 1977.

Baudet quoted by Terry JH, Self MM, Howard JM: A discussion of injuries of the spleen. *Surgery* 40:615, 1956.

Beal SL, Spisso JM: The risk of splenorrhaphy. *Arch Surg* 123:1158, 1988.

Beal SL, Ward RE: Successful atrial caval shunting in the management of retrohepatic venous injuries. *Am J Surg* 158:409, 1989.

Beall AC, Bricker DL, et al: Surgical considerations in the management of civilian colon injuries. *Ann Surg* 173:971, 1971.

Bender JS, Geller ER, Wilson RF: Intra-abdominal sepsis following liver trauma. *J Trauma* 29:1140, 1989.

Benjamin CI, Engrav LH, Perry JF Jr: Delayed rupture or delayed diagnosis of rupture of the spleen. *Surg Gynecol Obstet* 142:171, 1976.

Berne CJ, Donovan AJ, et al: Duodenal ''diverticulization'' for duodenal and pancreatic injury. *Am J Surg* 127:503, 1974.

Berni GA, Bandyk DF, et al: Role of intraoperative pancreatography in patients with injury to the pancreas. *Am J Surg* 143:602, 1982.

Buechter KJ, Zeppa R, Gomez G: The use of segmental anatomy for an operative classification of liver injuries. *Ann Surg* 211:669, 1990.

Bull JC Jr, Mathewson C Jr: Exploratory laparotomy in patients with penetrating wounds of the abdomen. *Am J Surg* 116:223, 1968.

Buntain WC, Gould HR, Maull KI: Predictability of splenic salvage by computed tomography. *J Trauma* 28:24, 1988.

Buntain WL, Lynn HB: Splenorrhaphy: Changing concepts for the traumatized spleen. *Surgery* 86:784, 1977.

Burch JM, Brock JC, et al: The injured colon. *Surgery* 203(6):701, 1986.

Burch JM, Feliciano DV, Mattox KL: The atriocaval shunt. *Ann Surg* 207:555, 1988.

Busuttil RW, Kitahama A, et al: Management of injuries to the porta hepatis. *Ann Surg* 191(5):641, 1980.

Canizaro PC, Fitts CT, Sawyer RB: Diagnostic abdominal paracentesis: A proposed adjunctive measure. *US Army Surg Res Unit Annl Rept* June 1964.

Carmichael DH: Avulsion of the common bile duct by blunt trauma. *South Med J* 72(2):166, 1980.

Cerise EJ, Scully JH Jr: Blunt trauma to the small intestine. *J Trauma* 10(1):46, 1970.

Cheatham JE Jr, Smith EI, et al: Nonoperative management of subcapsular hematomas of the liver. *Am J Surg* 140:851, 1980.

Cobb LM, Vinocur CD, et al: Intestinal perforation due to blunt trauma in children in an era of increased nonoperative treatment. *J Trauma* 26(5):461, 1986.

Cogbill TH, Moore EE, et al: Distal pancreatectomy for trauma: A multicenter experience. *J Trauma* 31:1600, 1991.

Cogbill TH, Moore EE, et al: Nonoperative management of blunt splenic trauma: A multicenter experience. *J Trauma* 29:1312, 1989.

Cook A, Levine BA, et al: Traditional treatment of colon injuries. *Arch Surg* 119:591, 1984.

Cook DE, Walsh JW, et al: Upper abdominal trauma: Pitfalls in CT diagnosis. *Radiology* 159:65, 1986.

Cox EF, Flancbaum L, et al: Blunt trauma to the liver: Analysis of management and mortality in 323 consecutive patients. *Ann Surg* 207:126, 1988.

Crosby W: Safety of lap belt restraints for pregnant victims of automobile collisions. *N Engl J Med* 248:632, 1971.

Crosby W: Committee on medical aspects of automobile safety belts during pregnancy. *JAMA* 221:20, 1972.

Dang CV, Peter ET, et al: Trauma of the colon. Early drop-back of exteriorized repair. *Arch Surg* 117:652, 1982.

Dauterive AH, Flancbaum L, Cox EF: Blunt intestinal trauma. A modern-day review. *Ann Surg* 201(2):198, 1985.

Dawes LG, Aprahamian C, et al: The risk of infection after colon injury. *Surgery* 100(4):796, 1986.

Defore WW Jr, Mattox KL, et al: Management of 1,590 consecutive cases of liver trauma. *Arch Surg* 111:493, 1976.

Delva E, Camus Y, et al: Vascular occlusions for liver resections operative management and tolerance to hepatic ischemia: 142 cases. *Ann Surg* 209:211, 1989.

Dickerman JD: Bacterial infection and the asplenic host: A review. *J Trauma* 16(8):662, 1976.

Dickerman JD: Splenectomy and sepsis: A warning. *Pediatrics* 63:938, 1979.

Dixon JA, Miller F, McCloskey D: Anatomy and techniques in segmental splenectomy. *Surg Gynecol Obstet* 150:516, 1980.

Donohue JH, Crass RA, Trunkey DD: The management of duodenal and other small intestinal trauma. *World J Surg* 9(6):904, 1985.

Douglas GJ, Simpson JS: The conservative management of splenic trauma. *J Pediatr Surg* 6:565, 1971.

Dudrick SJ, Wilmore DW, et al: Spontaneous closure of traumatic pancreatoduodenal fistulas with total intravenous nutrition. *J Trauma* 10(7):542, 1970.

Duke JH, Jones RC, Shires GT: Management of injuries to the inferior vena cava. *Am J Surg* 110:759, 1965.

Durham R: Management of gastric injuries. *Surg Clin North Am* 70:517, 1990.

Edwards J, Gaspard DJ: Visceral injury due to extraperitoneal gunshot wounds. *Arch Surg* 108:865, 1974.

Ein SH, Shandling B, Simpson JS: Nonoperative management of traumatized spleen in children: How and why. *J Pediatr Surg* 13:117, 1978.

Elmore JR, Clark DE, et al: Selective nonoperative management of blunt splenic trauma in adults. *Arch Surg* 124:581, 1989.

Eraklis AJ, Filler RM: Splenectomy in childhood: A review of 1413 cases. *J Pediatr Surg* 4:382, 1972.

Fabian TC, Mangiante EC, et al: A prospective study of 91 patients undergoing both computed tomography and peritoneal lavage following blunt abdominal trauma. *J Trauma* 26(7):602, 1986.

Farnell MB, Spencer MP, et al: Nonoperative management of blunt hepatic trauma in adults. *Surgery* 104:748, 1988.

Federle MP, Richard AC, et al: Computed tomography in blunt abdominal trauma. *Arch Surg* 117:645, 1982.

Feliciano DV: Management of traumatic retroperitoneal hematoma. *Ann Surg* 211:109, 1990.

Feliciano DV, Jordan GL, et al: Management of 1000 consecutive cases of hepatic trauma (1979–1984). *Ann Surg* 204(4):438, 1986.

Feliciano DV, Martin TD, Cruse PA: Management of combined pancreatoduodenal injuries. *Ann Surg* 205:673, 1987.

Feliciano DV, Mattox KL, Jordan GL Jr: Intra-abdominal packing for control of hepatic hemorrhage: A reappraisal. *J Trauma* 21(4):285, 1981.

Feliciano DV, Mattox KL, et al: Packing for control of hepatic hemorrhage. *J Trauma* 26(8):738, 1986.

Fischer RP, Beverlin BC, et al: Diagnostic peritoneal lavage: Fourteen years and 2586 patients later. *Am J Surg* 136:701, 1978.

Fish JC: Reconstruction of the portal vein: Case reports and literature review. *Am Surg* 32:472, 1966.

Flint LM, Vitale GC, et al: The injured colon. Relationships of management to complications. *Ann Surg* 193:619, 1981.

Flint LM Jr, McCoy M, et al: Duodenal injury. Analysis of common misconceptions in diagnosis and treatment. *Ann Surg* 191:697, 1980.

Flint LM, Polk HC Jr: Selective hepatic artery ligation: Limitations and failures. *J Trauma* 19(5):319, 1979.

Forde KA, Ganepola AP: Is mandatory exploration for penetrating abdominal trauma extinct? The morbidity and mortality of negative exploration in a large municipal hospital. *J Trauma* 14(9):764, 1974.

Fullen WD, McDonough JJ, et al: Sternal splitting approach for major hepatic or retrohepatic vena cava injury. *J Trauma* 14(11):903, 1974.

Fullen WD, Selle JG, et al: Intramural duodenal hematoma. *Ann Surg* 179:549, 1974.

Geis WP, Schulz KA, et al: The fate of unruptured intrahepatic hematomas. *Surgery* 90(4):689, 1981.

Gentilello LM, Cortes V: Whipple procedure for trauma: Is duct ligation a safe alternative to pancreatico jejunostomy? *J Trauma* 31:661, 1991.

George SM Jr, Fabian TC, Mangiante ED: Colon trauma: Further support for primary repair. *Am J Surg* 156:16, 1988.

George SM Jr, Fabian TC, et al: Primary repair of colon wounds. *Ann Surg* 209:728, 1989.

Giuliano A: Is splenic salvage safe in the traumatized patient? *Arch Surg* 116:651, 1981.

Glancy KE. Review of pancreatic trauma. *West J Med* 151:45, 1989.

Graham JM, Mattox KL, et al: Traumatic injuries of the inferior vena cava. *Arch Surg* 113:413, 1978.

Green JB, Shackford SR, et al: Late septic complications in adults following splenectomy for trauma: A prospective analysis in 144 patients. *J Trauma* 26(11):999, 1986.

Heimansohn DA, Canal DF, McCarthy MC: The role of pancreaticoduodenectomy in the management of traumatic injuries to the pancreas and duodenum. *Am Surg* 56:511, 1990.

Heimbach DM, Ferguson GS, Harley JD: Treatment of traumatic hemobilia with angiographic embolization. *J Trauma* 18(3):221, 1978.

Holgerson LO, Bishop HC: Nonoperative treatment of duodenal hematoma. *J Pediatr Surg* 12:11, 1976.

Ivatury RR, Nallathambi M, et al: Liver packing for uncontrolled hemorrhage. *J Trauma* 26(8):744, 1986.

Ivatury RR, Nallathambi M, et al: Penetrating pancreatic injuries: Analysis of 103 consecutive cases. *Am Surg* 56:90, 1990.

Izant RJ, Drucker WR: Duodenal obstruction due to intramural hematoma in children. *J Trauma* 4:797, 1964.

Jackson GL, Thal ER: Management of stabwounds of the back and flank. *J Trauma* 19(9):660, 1979.

Jeffrey RB, Federle MP, Goodman PC: CT of splenic trauma. *Radiology* 141:729, 1981.

Jeffrey RB Jr, Federle MP, Crass RA: Computed tomography of pancreatic trauma. *Radiology* 147:491, 1983.

Jones RC: Management of pancreatic trauma. *Ann Surg* 187(5):555, May 1978.

Jones RC: Management of pancreatic trauma. *Am J Surg* 150:698, 1985.

Jones RC, McClelland RN, et al: Difficult closures of the duodenal stump. *Arch Surg* 94:696, 1967.

Jones RC, Thal ER, et al: Evaluation of antibiotic therapy following penetrating abdominal trauma. *Ann Surg* 120(5):576, 1985.

Jordan GL: Injury to the pancreas and duodenum, in Mattox K, Moore E, Feliciano D (eds): *Trauma*. East Norwalk, Conn, Appleton & Lange, 1988, chap 33, p 473.

Jurkovich GJ, Carrico CJ: Pancreatic trauma. *Surg Clin North Am* 70:575, 1990.

Jurkovich GJ, Greiser WB, et al: Hypothermia in trauma victims: An ominous predictor of survival. *J Trauma* 27:1019, 1987.

Kelly G, Norton L, et al: The continuing challenge of duodenal injuries. *J Trauma* 18(3):160, 1978.

King H, Shumacker HB Jr: Splenic studies: I. Susceptibility to infection after splenectomy performed in infancy. *Ann Surg* 136:239, 1952.

Kobold EE, Thal AP: A simple method for the management of experimental wounds of the duodenum. *Surg Gynecol Obstet* 116:340, 1963.

Kudsk KA, Sheldon GF, Lim RC Jr: Atrial-caval shunting (ACS) after trauma. *J Trauma* 22(2):81, 1982.

Lambeth W, Rubin BR: Nonoperative management of intrahepatic hemorrhage and hematoma following blunt trauma. *Surg Gynecol Obstet* 148:507, 1979.

Lavenson GS, Cohen A: Management of rectal injuries. *Am J Surg* 122:226, 1971.

Ledgerwood AM, Kazmers M, Lucas CE: The role of thoracic aortic occlusion for massive hemoperitoneum. *J Trauma* 16(8):610, 1976.

Levison MA, Peterson SR, et al: Duodenal trauma: Experience of a trauma center. *J Trauma* 24:475, 1984.

Lim RC, Glickman MG, Hunt TK: Angiography in patients with blunt trauma to the chest and abdomen. *Surg Clin North Am* 52(3):551, 1972.

Longmire WP: Early management of injury to the extrahepatic biliary tract. *JAMA* 195:623, 1966.

Longo WE, Baker CC, et al: Nonoperative management of adult blunt splenic trauma. *Ann Surg* 210:626, 1989.

Lou Sister MA, Johnson AP, et al: Exteriorized repair in the management of colon injuries. *Arch Surg* 116:926, 1981.

Lucas CE: What is the role of biliary drainage in liver trauma? *Am J Surg* 120:509, 1970.

Lucas CE, Ledgerwood AM: Factors influencing outcome after blunt duodenal injury. *J Trauma* 15(10):839, 1975.

Lucas CE, Walt AJ: Analysis of randomized biliary drainage for liver trauma in 189 patients. *J Trauma* 12(11):925, 1972.

Lucas CE, Canizaro PC, Shires GT: Repair of hepatic venous intrahepatic vena caval, and portal venous injuries, in Madding GF, Kennedy PA: *Trauma to the Liver,* 2d ed. Philadelphia, Saunders, 1971, chap 10, p 146.

Luna G, Dellinger EP: Nonoperative observation therapy for splenic injuries. *Am J Surg* 153:462, 1987.

Luna GK, Maier RV, et al: Incidence and effect of hypothermia in seriously injured patients. *J Trauma* 27:1014, 1987.

McClelland RN, Shires T: Management of liver trauma in 259 consecutive patients. *Ann Surg* 161:248, 1965.

McClelland RN, Shires T, Poulos E: Hepatic resection for massive trauma. *J Trauma* 4:282, 1964.

McInnis WD, Aust JB, et al: Traumatic injuries of the duodenum: A comparison of 1° closure and the jejunal patch. *J Trauma* 15(10):847, 1975.

McLelland BA, Hanna SS, et al: Analysis of peritoneal lavage parameters in blunt abdominal trauma. *J Trauma* 25(5):393, 1985.

Mahon PA, Sutton JE Jr: Nonoperative management of adult splenic injury due to blunt trauma: A warning. *Am J Surg* 149:716, 1985.

Malangoni MA, Cue JI, et al: Evaluation of splenic injury by computed tomography and its impact on treatment. *Ann Surg* 211:592, 1990.

Malangoni MA, Levine AW, et al: Management of injury to the spleen in adults. Results of early operation and observation. *Ann Surg* 200(6):702, 1984.

Mansour MA, Moore JB, Moore EE: Conservative management of combined pancreatoduodenal injuries. *Am J Surg* 158:531, 1989.

Martin TD, Feliciano DV, et al: Severe duodenal injuries. Treatment with pyloric exclusion and gastrojejunostomy. *Arch Surg* 118(17):631, 1983.

Mattox KL, Espada R, Beall AC Jr: Traumatic injury to the portal vein. *Ann Surg* 181:519, 1975.

Miller DR: Median sternotomy extension of abdominal incision for hepatic lobectomy. *Ann Surg* 175:193, 1972.

Moore EE, Shackford SR, et al: Organ injury scaling: Spleen, liver, and kidney. *J Trauma* 29:1664, 1989.

Moore FA, Moore EE, et al: Risk of splenic salvage after trauma. *Am J Surg* 148:800, 1984.

Moretz JA III, Campbell DP, et al: Significance of serum amylase level in evaluating pancreatic trauma. *Am J Surg* 130:739, 1975.

Morgenstern L: Microcrystalline collagen used in experimental splenic injury: A new surface hemostatic agent. *Arch Surg* 109:44, 1974.

Morgenstern L, Shapiro SJ: Techniques of splenic conservation. *Arch Surg* 114:449, 1979.

Morton JR, Jordan GL: Traumatic duodenal injuries: Review of 131 cases. *J Trauma* 8(2):127, 1968.

Mucha P Jr, Daly RC, Farnell MB: Selective management of blunt splenic trauma. *J Trauma* 26(11):970, 1986.

Nallathambi MN, Ivatury RR, et al: Nonoperative management versus early operation for blunt splenic trauma in adults. *Surg Gynecol Obstet* 166:252, 1988.

Nance FC, Cohn I Jr: Surgical judgment in the management of stab wounds of the abdomen: A retrospective and prospective analysis based on a study of 600 stabbed patients. *Ann Surg* 170:569, 1969.

Nance FC, Wennar MH, et al: Surgical judgment in the management of penetrating wounds of the abdomen: Experience with 2212 patients. *Ann Surg* 179:639, 1974.

Naylor R, Coln D, Shires GT: Morbidity and mortality from injuries to the spleen. *J Trauma* 14(9):773, 1974.

Nichols RL, Smith JW, et al: Risk of infection after penetrating abdominal trauma. *N Engl J Med* 311(17):1065, 1984.

Noyes LD, Doyle DJ, McSwain NE: Septic complications associated with the use of peritoneal drains in liver trauma. *J Trauma* 28:337, 1988.

Oakes DD: Splenic trauma. *Curr Probl Surg* 17:342, 1981.

O'Brien JA, Coustan DR, et al: Prepartum diagnosis of traumatic fetal-maternal hemorrhage. *Am J Perinatol* 2:214, 1985.

Olsen WR, Redman HC, Hildreth DH: Quantitative peritoneal lavage in blunt abdominal trauma. *Arch Surg* 104:536, 1972.

O'Neal BJ, McDonald JC: The risk of sepsis in the asplenic adult. *Ann Surg* 194:775, 1981.

Oreskovich MR, Carrico CJ: Stab wounds of the anterior abdomen. Analysis of management plan using local wound exploration and quantitative peritoneal lavage. *Ann Surg* 198(4):411, 1983.

Pachter HL, Pennington R, et al: Simplified distal pancreatectomy with the auto suture stapler: Preliminary clinical observations. *Surgery* 85:166, 1979.

Pachter HL, Spencer FC: Recent concepts in the treatment of hepatic trauma. Facts and fallacies. *Ann Surg* 190(4):423, 1979.

Pachter HL, Spencer FC, et al: The management of juxtahepatic venous injuries without an atriocaval shunt: Preliminary clinical observations. *Surgery* 99(5):569, 1986.

Parvin S, Smith DE, et al: Effectiveness of peritoneal lavage in blunt abdominal trauma. *Ann Surg* 181:255, 1975.

Peitzman AB, Makaroun MS, et al: Prospective study of computed tomography in initial management of blunt abdominal trauma, *J Trauma* 26(7):585, 1986.

Perlberger RR: Control of hemobilia by angiographic embolization. *AJR* 128:672, 1977.

Perry JF Jr, DeMeules JE, Root HD: Diagnostic peritoneal lavage in blunt abdominal trauma. *Surg Gynecol Obstet* 131:742, 1970.

Perry MO: *The Management of Acute Vascular Injuries*. Baltimore, Williams & Wilkins, 1981, p 105.

Perry MO, Thal ER, Shires GT: Management of arterial injuries. *Ann Surg* 173:403, 1971.

Phillips T, Sclafani SJA, et al: Use of the contrast-enhanced CT enema in the management of penetrating trauma to the flank and back. *J Trauma* 26:593, 1986.

Pickhardt B, Moore EE, et al: Operative splenic salvage in adults: A decade perspective. *J Trauma* 29:1386, 1989.

Prinz RA, Pickleman J, Hoffman JP: Treatment of pancreatic cutaneous fistulas with a somatostatin analog. *Am J Surg* 155:36, 1988.

Quast DC, Jordan GL: Traumatic wounds of the female reproductive organs. *J Trauma* 4:839, 1964.

Reinhardt GF, Hubay CA: Surgical management of traumatic hemobilia. *Am J Surg* 121:328, 1971.

Richie JP, Fonkalsrud EW: Subcapsular hematoma of the liver. *Arch Surg* 104:781, 1972.

Root HD, Hauser CW, et al: Diagnostic peritoneal lavage. *Surgery* 57:633, 1965.

Rosoff L, Cohen JL, et al: Injuries of the spleen. *Surg Clin North Am* 52(3):667, 1972.

Rozycki GS: Trauma in pregnancy, in Moore EE (ed): *Early Care of the Injured Patient*. Philadelphia, BC Decker, 1990, chap 16, p 182.

Rydell WB Jr: Complete transection of the common bile duct due to blunt abdominal trauma. *Arch Surg* 100:724, 1970.

Saifi J, Fortune JB, et al: Benefits of intra-abdominal pack placement for the management of nonmechanical hemorrhage. *Arch Surg* 125:199, 1990.

Schrock T, Blaisdell FW, Mathewson C: Management of blunt trauma to the liver and hepatic veins. *Arch Surg* 96:698, 1968.

Schrock T, Christensen N: Management of perforating injuries of the colon. *Surg Gynecol Obstet* 135:65, 1972.

Shackford SR, Molin M: Management of splenic injuries. *Surg Clin North Am* 70:595, 1990.

Shackford SR, Sise MJ, et al: Evaluation of splenorrhaphy: A grading system for splenic trauma. *J Trauma* 21(7):538, 1981.

Shaftan GW: Indications for operation in abdominal trauma. *Am J Surg* 99:657, 1960.

Shannon FL, Moore EE: Primary repair of the colon: When is it a safe alternative? *Surgery* 98(4):851, 1985.

Sheldon GF, Cohn L, Blaisdell W: Surgical treatment of pancreatic trauma. *J Trauma* 10:795, 1970.

Sheldon GF, Lim RC Jr, et al: *Ann Surg* 202(5):539, 1985.

Singer DB: Postsplenectomy sepsis, in Rosenberg HS, Bolande RP (eds): *Perspectives in Pediatric Pathology*. Chicago, Year Book Medical, 1973, vol 1, p 285.

Smiley K, Perry MO: Balloon catheter tamponade of major vascular wounds. *Am J Surg* 121:326, 1971.

Snyder WH III, Weigelt JA, et al: The surgical management of duodenal trauma. *Arch Surg* 115:422, 1980.

Soderstrom CA, Maekawa K, et al: Gallbladder injuries resulting from blunt abdominal trauma. An experience and review. *Ann Surg* 193(1):60, 1981.

Stain SC, Yellin AE, Donovan AJ: Hepatic trauma. *Arch Surg* 123:1251, 1988.

Starzl TE, Kaupp HA, et al: Penetrating injuries of the inferior vena cava. *Surg Clin North Am* 43:387, 1963.

Stevens SL, Maull KI: Small bowel injuries. *Surg Clin North Am* 70:541, 1990.

Stone HH, Fabian TC: Management of duodenal wounds. *J Trauma* 19(5):334, 1979.

Stone HH, Lamb JM: Use of pedicled omentum as an autogenous pack for control of hemorrhage in major injuries of the liver. *Surg Gynecol Obstet* 141:92, 1975.

Stone A, Sugawa C, et al: The role of endoscopic retrograde pancreatography (ERP) in blunt abdominal trauma. *Am Surg* 56:715, 1990.

Strate RG, Grieco JC: Blunt injury to the colon and rectum. *J Trauma* 23(5):384, 1983.

Strauch GO: Preservation of splenic function in adults and children with injured spleens. *Am J Surg* 137:478, 1979.

Sturmer FC, Wilt KE: Complete division of the common duct from external blunt trauma. *Am J Surg* 105:781, 1963.

Taxier M, Sivak MV, et al: Endoscopic retrograde pancreatography in the evaluation of trauma to the pancreas. *Surg Gynecol Obstet* 150:65, 1980.

Thal ER: Evaluation of peritoneal lavage and local exploration in lower chest and abdominal stabwounds. *J Trauma* 17:642, 1977.

Thal ER: Peritoneal lavage. Reliability of RBC count in patients with stab wounds to the chest. *Arch Surg* 119:579, 1984.

Thal ER, May RA, Beesinger D: Peritoneal lavage: Its unreliability in gunshot wounds of the lower chest and abdomen. *Arch Surg* 115:430, 1980.

Thal ER, Shires GT: Peritoneal lavage in blunt abdominal trauma. *Am J Surg* 125:64, 1973.

Thal ER, Yeary EC: Morbidity of colostomy closure following colon trauma. *J Trauma* 20(4):287, 1980.

Thompson JS, Moore EE, Moore JB: Comparison of penetrating injuries of the right and left colon. *Ann Surg* 193:414, 1981.

Traub AC, Perry JF: Splenic preservation following splenic trauma. *J Trauma* 22(6):496, 1982.

Trunkey D, Hays RJ, Shires GT: Management of rectal trauma. *J Trauma* 13(5):411, 1973.

Trunkey D, Shires GT, McClelland RN: Management of liver trauma in 811 consecutive patients. *Ann Surg* 179(5):522, 1974.

Tuggle D, Huber PJ Jr: Management of rectal trauma. *Am J Surg* 148:806, 1984.

Turpin I, State D, Schwartz A: Injuries to the inferior vena cava and their management. *Am J Surg* 134:25, 1977.

Van Stiegmann G, Moore EE, Moore GE: Failure of spleen repair. *J Trauma* 19:698, 1979.

Vaughan GD III, Frazier OH, et al: The use of pyloric exclusion in the management of severe duodenal injuries. *Am J Surg* 134:785, 1977.

Weichert RF III, Hewitt RL, Drapanas T: Blunt injuries to intrahepatic vena cava and hepatic veins with survival. *Am J Surg* 121:322, 1971.

Weinstein ME, Govin GG, Rice CL: Splenorrhaphy for splenic trauma. *J Trauma* 19:692, 1979.

Wilder JR, Lotfi MW, Jurani P: Comparative study of mandatory and selective surgical intervention in stab wounds of the abdomen. *Surgery* 69:546, 1971.

Wisner DH, Wold RL, Frey CF: Diagnosis and treatment of pancreatic injuries. *Arch Surg* 125:1109, 1990.

Woolley MM, Mahour GH, Sloan T: Duodenal hematoma in infancy and childhood. Changing etiology and changing treatment. *Am J Surg* 136:8, 1978.

Yajko RD, Seydel F, Trimble C: Rupture of the stomach from blunt abdominal trauma. *J Trauma* 15(3):177, 1975.

Yellin AE, Chaffee CB, Donovan AJ: Vascular isolation in treatment of juxtahepatic venous injuries. *Arch Surg* 102:566, 1971.

Yasugi H, Mizumoto R, et al: Changes in carbohydrate metabolism and endocrine function of remnant pancreas after major pancreatic resection. *Am J Surg* 132:577, 1976.

Yasugi H, Rosoff L Sr: Pancreatoduodenectomy for combined pancreatoduodenal injuries. *Arch Surg* 110:1177, 1975.

CHAPTER 7

Burns

Cleon W. Goodwin, Jerome L. Finkelstein, and Michael R. Madden

Thermal burns and related injuries continue to be a major cause of death and disability in the United States. The introduction of the burn center concept in 1945 by the United States Army heralded a rapid improvement in survival and a reduction of morbidity of burned patients and provided the basis for regional specialty treatment centers in other disciplines. The surgical critical care of the thermally injured patient is provided by an interactive multidisciplinary team, which has proved to be the most efficient and effective and least expensive method of treating major burn injury. Burn injury, however, is a chronic disease, of which the initial hospitalization may be only a small part of total treatment. Burned patients often require years of supervised rehabilitation, reconstructive surgery, and psychosocial support. Omission of any step along the road to full recovery can result in wasted resources and a lost patient. Burn centers are best equipped to provide long-term support services, either on-site or at satellite facilities, for patients with smaller burns who do not require in-patient care. In a 2-year experience in the care of 12,623 cases of burn injury, only 1094 (8.8 percent) required hospitalization. The remainder were treated on an outpatient basis. The clinical scope of burn care encompasses fluid and electrolyte physiology, surgical infection, nutritional maintenance, cardiopulmonary support, and wound care, none of which can be treated as separate entities without an understanding of the entire disease process. As such, treatment of extensive thermal injury is essentially an exercise in surgical critical care and requires the full-time commitment of individuals skilled in all facets of burn therapy.

EPIDEMIOLOGY

In the United States, over two million civilians each year seek medical care for burn injury. Five hundred thousand individuals are treated in emergency rooms, and approximately 74,000 patients are hospitalized (275 to 300/million population). Over 20,000 patients (80 to 100/million) are burned so severely that they require admission to a specialized burn treatment center. Twelve thousand burn victims die of their injuries. Military burn casualties range from 18 percent of wounds in the Falkland Islands conflict to many thousands when nuclear munitions are used.

Demographics. Burn injuries have unique age and sex distributions. The largest group of burned patients are children under 6 years of age (Fig. 7-1). Within their age range the overwhelming majority are less than 2 years old. During adolescence, the incidence of thermal injuries falls, although burn injury is the fourth

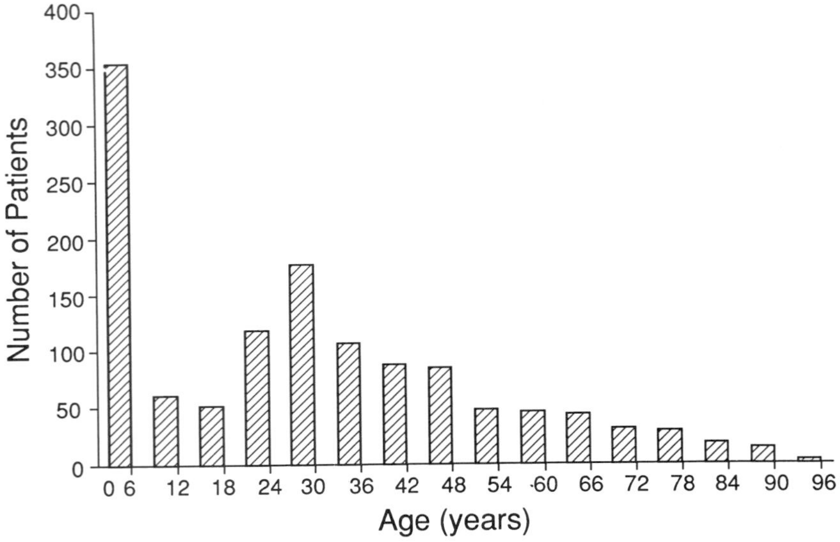

FIG. 7-1 The age distribution of 1264 patients admitted to the Shires Burn Center at the New York Hospital-Cornell Medical Center in 1991. Small children and patients with occupational injuries comprise the largest populations in most urban burn centers.

most common cause of accidental death in this age group. Occupational burn injuries produce a secondary peak incidence at 25 to 35 years of age before a gradual decline with advancing age. The significant aspect about the number of elderly burned patients is that they do occur and are admitted to specialized burn facilities for care. Moreover, in recent years, survival with return to preinjury status has improved faster than for the general burn population.

Males dominate the incidence of burn injury except for the elderly. This is thought to be related to the predominance of males working in heavy industry and increased risk-taking behavior in males compared to females. Equalization of gender incidence of burn injury occurs primarily because women outlive men by a large margin over 70 years of age. The reason for male predominance in infants and small children is not known.

Burn injury preferentially involves less socioeconomically advantaged citizens. A number of epidemiologic studies demonstrate strong associations between calculated burn rate and socioeconomic variables. Per capita income, percentage of persons below the poverty level, percentage of residences built before 1940, proportion of adults with 16 years or more of education, and percentage of persons moving from a prior residence in the same county were strongly associated with hospitalized burn injuries in New England counties. In New York State, the nonwhite population is involved with serious burns nearly three times more often than the white population (66 per million versus 23 per million). The relationship between mean family income is strong and linear: for every $1000 decrease in family income, the burn rate increases 4.9 burns per 10,000 person years. The use of portable, open-flame heating equipment, faulty heating and electrical systems, crowded living conditions, and the absence of smoke detectors are responsible for many burns. Although a large percentage of hospitalized burn patients abuse illicit drugs and alcohol, it is not known if these habits promote thermal injury. Mechanisms of thermal injury in these patients included questionably accidental burns related to acute intoxication and self-injury due to psychosis or depression. Also, although households with alcohol drinkers are at higher risk for burn injury, such households tend to have higher smoking levels.

Etiology. The etiology of burns varies to some degree with the location of the burn center. Centers in suburban locations or near petroleum-based industries tend to treat more flame-related injuries, whereas urban burn centers see a larger proportion of scald injuries. In our urban burn center in a densely populated, highly mobile metropolitan area, scalding is the most common mechanism of thermal injury (Table 7-1). This is of particular importance, since most scald burns potentially are preventable. Electrical injuries either are occupationally related or are accidental contacts with the high-voltage rail of mass transit subways. Undoubtedly, smoking-related fires and burns are proportionately greater than represented here since many structure fires almost certainly were ignited by cigarettes but not reported. A small but constant number of burn injuries occur in health care facilities, particularly in those dedicated primarily to the care of the elderly and mentally ill. Steam burns almost universally occur in people who work with the production and distribution of superheated steam.

Pediatric Burns. Over 80 percent of burns to children under 5 years of age are scald burns. Generally, tap water burns are more severe and extensive than other scald burns (spills from containers). Scald burns often occur when inadequately supervised infants or young children are put in bathtubs in which the water is exces-

Table 7-1
Etiology of Thermal Injuries (%)

Scalds	37
Structure fires	18
Flammable liquids/gases	15
Electrical	7
Smoking related	6
Open flames	6
Contact burns	5
Vehicle fires	2
Fireworks/explosives	2
Chemical	1
Miscellaneous	1

Based on 9833 admissions to Shires Burn Center at the New York Hospital-Cornell Medical Center, 1977 to 1991.

sively hot and the children are unable to remove themselves. While some states regulate hot water temperature in multiple occupancy housing, this preventive measure is not universal. In some series, the most common activities leading to burn injury are food preparation and food consumption. Further, the skin of young children is thinner than that of older children and adults and is more susceptible to injury. Skin grafting is required in up to 40 percent of hospitalized children, and long-term hypertrophic scarring occurs in more than half of burned children and is more severe than in older individuals. Burn injury, especially in skin-grafted children, causes a profound growth arrest during the first postburn year, and this growth delay is not recovered for at least 3 years following injury. Most pediatric burns occur in a residential setting. Almost all fireworks burns occur in children.

Finally, child abuse may be present as a thermal injury. Of the 222 reported cases of child abuse from the New York Hospital in 1989, 73 (33 percent) sustained burns because of intentional abuse or neglect. These 73 children represented approximately one-quarter of the pediatric admissions under 6 years of age. Only a minority of the abused children demonstrated the typical physical findings of an immersion scald. Such findings include scald burns of the feet, posterior legs, buttocks, and hands. Contact burns caused by cigarettes account for many inflicted injuries, but scalding is the most common mechanism. The most accurate indications of abuse were derived from extensive discussions with guardians and on-site evaluations by social workers and child-protection personnel. Factors predisposing to child abuse include teen-aged parents, mental deficits in either the child or abuser, unwed motherhood, a single-parent household, and low socioeconomic status.

DELIVERY OF BURN CARE

Prehospital Triage. First-responder care for burn patients includes that needed by any injured patient as well as that which is burn specific. The burning process should be stopped as rapidly as possible by extinguishing the flames, diluting and washing away offending chemicals, or removing the patient from contact with an electric current. The rescuer must take every precaution to avoid becoming part of the circuit when trying to break contact between a patient and a source of electricity. Cardiopulmonary resuscitation should be instituted as indicated and is most often necessary in patients who have sustained high-voltage electric injury. Subsequent ventilatory support is dependent on both the patient's general condition and pulmonary status. If the patient was burned in a closed space, some degree of carbon-monoxide poisoning should be assumed, and 100 percent oxygen should be administered by a tight-fitting nonrebreathing face mask. If the patient has impaired ventilatory exchange because of obtundation or some other reason, an endotracheal tube should be placed and mechanical ventilatory support provided.

The burn wounds should be covered with a clean sheet or dressing to prevent further contamination of the wound surface and to reduce the pain in areas of partial-thickness burn. The patient should then be covered with a clean blanket to conserve body heat and minimize the risk of hypothermia. If the patient's hemodynamic status will permit, burned extremities should be elevated.

Following the described field resuscitation, patients with moderate and major burn injuries should be promptly transported to a hospital for definitive care. If the patient has only burns, and transport to the hospital will require no more than 30 to 34 minutes, intravenous fluids need not be started in the field. If transportation to a definitive treatment facility will require more than 45 min, or if the patient has experienced blood loss caused by associated mechanical injuries, a physiologic saline solution should be administered through as large a cannula as can be readily inserted into a peripheral vein. Transportation should not be delayed by prolonged unsuccessful efforts to establish intavenous access.

The use of room temperature water soaks will rapidly reduce the pain present in small areas of partial-thickness burns and may also reduce the extent of tissue damage in those patients in whom such treatment can be initiated within 10 to 15 min of the time of injury. If more time has elapsed, radiative loss of heat and heat transfer by the circulation at the periphery of the burn will have returned tissue temperature to essentially normal levels, and tissue injury will be little influenced by such treatment. Cold soaks and ice packs should not be used.

Admission Criteria. The determinants of burn patient disposition include the extent and depth of the injury, the location of the burns, the age of the patient, the agent of injury, presence of associated mechanical trauma, and preexisting diseases. Guidelines mandating burn unit/burn center hospitalization are outlined in Table 7-2. These criteria expand on those of the American Burn Association and reflect particular social and medical needs of urban populations. Patients with lesser injuries can be cared for in other hospital facilities or as outpatients, depending on the extent of the burn and the patient's response to the injury. Several other diseases, such as toxic epidermal necrolysis and other causes of massive cutaneous injury, closely resemble thermal injury and require the same resources and expertise. Optimal care is provided for patients with such injuries at burn centers or burn units.

Table 7-2
Guidelines for Burn Unit/Center Hospitalization

1. Second-degree burns—15% TBSA
2. Third-degree burns—5% TBSA (such burns will require surgical excision and closure)
3. Burns of the face, feet, hands, and perineum
4. Electrical injuries
5. Inhalation injury, including smoke inhalation and carbon monoxide poisoning
6. Chemical burns (such burns require prolonged irrigation, are deeply invasive, and usually are third-degree burns)
7. Burned patients with associated injuries, including fractures and major blunt and penetrating trauma
8. Any burn in patients under the age of 10 years and over the age of 50 years
9. Burns in patients with concomitant serious medical diseases (e.g., diabetes mellitus, chronic alcoholism, cirrhosis, heart disease, acquired immunodeficiency syndrome)
10. All children suspected of being victims of child abuse or neglect
11. Infected burns originally treated on an outpatient basis
12. Small third-degree burns best treated with early excision and grafting
13. Smaller burns in patients not able to care for the burn, which if left unattended, pose a significant potential for development of burn infection: (a) drug abusers; (b) mentally ill; (c) homeless; (d) patients hospitalized at other institutions who experience a serious burn; (e) unreliable home environment for small children
14. Acute massive skin loss syndromes requiring burn center quality of care (e.g., Stevens-Johnson syndrome/toxic epidermal necrolysis, large traumatic degloving injuries)

TBSA, total body surface area

Minor burns should be cleansed with a surgical detergent disinfectant, debrided, and allowed to dry. The use of occlusive dressings is optional and depends on the location of the burn and the patient's desires. If dressings are used, they should be changed every 3 days and the wound inspected. If healing is progressing satisfactorily, a dressing is reapplied, but if infection develops, the patient should be admitted to the hospital and the wound treated with a topical chemotherapeutic agent and systemic antibiotics.

Burn Patient Transfer. The transfer of a burn patient must be coordinated between the referring and receiving physicians. The physicians involved should review the resuscitative care received by the patient (i.e., fluids infused, medications given, pertinent laboratory values, and the patient's current hemodynamic and pulmonary status) to assess patient stability and optimize patient safety during transfer. Needed alterations in treatment should be identified by the burn center physician and recommendations made for treatment alteration before patient movement. In general, burn patients best tolerate transfer as soon as resuscitative therapy has achieved hemodynamic and pulmonary stability. If there is any question about the adequacy of resuscitation, transfer should be delayed until such concerns have been addressed.

Continuity and safety of burn patient transfer are optimized if a physician can accompany the patient during the transfer. If such escort is not possible, an appropriately trained and credentialed nurse or emergency medical technician should accompany the patient. Ground transportation, rotary-wing aircraft, and fixed-wing aircraft can all be used for the transfer of burn patients, depending on the distance involved. Pretransfer stability is particularly important in patients who are to be transferred by helicopters, where limited space, poor lighting, noise, and vibration make anything but the simplest of monitoring procedures difficult. The physician who is directing the aeromedical transfer team should assess the patient to be transferred while still in the referring hospital and make any necessary adjustments in treatment at that time. Contraindications to burn patient movement are most frequently encountered when aeromedical transfer is considered later in the postburn course and consist of pneumonia, congestive heart failure, cardiac arrhythmias, active gastrointestinal hemorrhage, and systemic sepsis. Such problems should be addressed and the underlying process brought under control before transfer requiring more than 30 to 60 min is undertaken. All pertinent records or copies thereof should accompany the patient.

UTILIZATION OF RESOURCES

Service standards for specialized burn facilities have been established by a number of accreditation agencies at the local, state, and national levels. Individual standards require unit organization and integration with other units in the supporting institution, delineated responsibilities of the staff according to special patient-care needs, education, policies and procedures for patient care, and guidelines for facility design and equipment. Required personnel reflect the true interdisciplinary composition of a full-service burn center, the major emphasis being on continuous individualized burn care (Table 7-3). In addition, physician consultative services from all major clinical departments must be readily available at all times.

The costs of burn center care have proved to be relatively elusive to define. One problem has been the diversity of recognized burn treatment facilities, which range from four-bed units to centers with more than 40 beds. It is likely that burn facilities begin to approach economic efficiency at the size of an 8- to 10-bed unit, given the multidisciplinary personnel needed for burn care. Smaller facilities often experience great difficulty in routinely keeping these expensive beds filled and the dedicated staff intact.

Table 7-3
Burn Center Staffing Requirements

Director
Associate Director(s)
Fellow(s)
Residents: two for every 15 patients (total physicians)
Nurses: one for every two ICU patients
Clinical nurse instructor
Occupational therapists: one for every 10 patients
Physical therapists: one for every seven patients
Social workers: full-time assignment to burn center
Nutritionists
Respiratory therapists: 24 h/day, 7 days/week

SOURCE: Modified from standards of Burn Advisory Committee, New York City Emergency Medical Services, 1991.

The New York Hospital Burn Center is an example of an urban burn care facility serving the population of the greater New York City metropolitan area. It consists of a 24-bed intensive care unit (ICU) floor and a 22-bed step-down area. Census ranges from 35 to 75 patients, with a mean inpatient population of approximately 50 patients. The ICU is configured so that when the patients require complex monitoring and nursing care they are located in one half of the ICU, and as they recover they are gradually moved toward the other half as their conditions improve. Although the latter beds are less densely equipped, all are configured to provide full ICU-level support. The step-down floor is also staffed as described in Table 7-3 and is engineered so that it can act as a primary burn ICU in the event of a mass casualty incident. In this way, bed occupancy can be maintained while resources and staff are distributed in the most efficient manner. Activity of nursing care is extremely high for massively burned patients and may require one nurse assigned to each critically ill patient. The proportion of patient days requiring category 3 and 4 nursing intensity (on a four-part nursing intensity scale) was more than 93 percent for extensively burned patients. Both of the categories entail one-on-one staffing assignments. Validated nursing workload management systems must be used when staffing a burn center. The usual activity-based methods fail to capture the total acuity and personnel required to treat patients with large burns.

The adequacy of reimbursement in the long term determines whether or not a burn center can survive. Reimbursement based on the patient's diagnosis is the major prospective payment system used by funding agencies. Diagnosis-related groups (DRGs) were developed in the 1970s initially as a tool for utilization review. Hospitalized patients were classified according to patterns of care received, lengths of stay, and use of services. The original 383 DRGs recognized only the presence or absence of a secondary diagnosis and did not recognize the variable severity of an illness within broad disease categories. Additional DRGs have been added during the last decade, and the current number exceeds 800.

Each DRG is assigned a case mix index (CMI), which is a weighted average service intensity multiplier that theoretically reflects relative resource consumption associated with each DRG. The higher the index, the more seriously ill the patient is, and the greater are the hospital revenues. Each DRG is characterized by an expected length of stay (LOS) based on statistical evaluation of that disease complex in the past. Long-stay outliers occur when actual LOS exceeds the expected LOS of the patient's DRG by 20 days or 1.94 standard deviations, whichever is less. Cost outliers are derived in the same manner based on the reimbursement rate for each DRG.

There are six burn categories, ranging from DRG 456 to the more recent DRG 472, which was added in October 1986 (Table 7-4). In addition, four additional DRGs are frequently used for patients with inhalation injury, with or without cutaneous burns. The burn DRGs are based only on extent of burn injury and the occurrence of a surgical procedure. A nonextensive burn can be as large as 49 percent total body surface area (TBSA) if it is all second degree, and an extensive burn can be as small as 20 percent TBSA if it is all third degree. Debridement that uses surgical excision qualifies for inclusion into DRG 459, whereas hydrotherapy or enzymatic debridement for wound care is not classified as an operative procedure. Furthermore, a number of procedures performed in appropriately equipped and staffed burn centers qualify as operating room procedures. These procedures include tracheostomy, escharotomy, and fasciotomy. Together, the combinations of burn extent and operative status result in 279 burn-related ICD-9-CM codes (International Classification of Disease, Version 9, Clinical Manual).

We assessed the ability of the five burn DRGs to explain the variation in resource consumption of 400 evaluable burned patients admitted in 1983. The cost data, not charges, were evaluated by an analysis of variance to assay degree of variation within each DRG and by a reduced-form model relating resource consumption to clincial and nonclinical factors. The burn DRGs explained only 17 percent of the variation of resource consumption, which is lower than other DRGs or competing classification methods. The impact of future modifications of health care reimbursement is not known, but the unique needs of regional specialty care centers will have to be recognized if the facilities are to remain financially viable.

MORTALITY AND OUTCOME

Survival of burn injury is related most strongly to age, burn size, and the presence or absence of inhalation injury. Because of the many variables, including associated injury, chronic diseases, postburn time of admission, and events surrounding the injury, raw mortality is of little value and often is misleading when trying to assess treatment outcome. A technique of data transformation (probit or logit transformations) is necessary to transform the sigmoid dose-response relationship between burn size and mortality to a straight line relationship to generate an error term that will permit comparisons of outcome. To determine burn-specific mortality, a previously healthy population without preexisting morbidity and admitted within hours of injury should constitute the study population for outcome assessment. Even then, it is doubtful that burn center outcomes can be accurately compared among institutions with these data. More sophisticated statistical techniques, such as logistic regression or analysis of covariance procedures, can evaluate the multiple effects of many variables and provide better data for comparisons of burn centers and the effects of multiple comorbid factors. Complications that occur during hospitalization should not be considered in such data analysis. Changing trends, such as the increasing tendency to admit more superficial burns, may require replotting of burn size several weeks after injury to offset any attendant improvement in survival.

The conventional statistic for assessment and comparison of burn-patient mortality is the LA_{50} (the extent of burn that is associated with death in 50 percent of the patients having burns of that extent). Probit analysis of 37,000 patients in 1980 from the National Burn Information Exchange Data Collection Program demonstrates an overall LA_{50} of 71.2 percent for burn patients aged 5 to 34 years. Most studies indicate that children under age four have a significantly higher mortality rate than older children and young adults. Part of this higher mortality in the very young may reflect relative unfamiliarity with pediatric clinical care techniques. Recent developments in biomedical technology may produce a major improvement in survival in the next few years.

Table 7-4
DRGs Associated with Thermal Injury

456—Burn patient transferred to another acute care facility
457—Extensive burns without OR procedures
458—Nonextensive burns with skin grafts
459—Nonextensive burns with wound debridement or other OR procedures
460—Nonextensive burns without OR procedures
472—Extensive burn with OR procedures

Inhalation Injury

101—Other respiratory system diagnosis
474—Respiratory system diagnosis with tracheostomy (Medicare)
475—Respiratory system diagnosis with ventilatory support
736—Tracheostomy other than for mouth, larynx, or pharynx disorder (non-Medicare)

DRGs, diagnosis-related groups; OR, operating room

PATIENT ASSESSMENT

History. Obtaining a thorough history is one of the most important and often most difficult tasks in the care of burned patients. Patient care and outcome assessment is highly dependent on many factors, and this information may require several days to accumulate. Consumer product safety, liability, reimbursement, and discharge planning vitally depend on accurate documentation of preinjury status and of the events surrounding the injury. Emergency medical personnel, fire officers, and emergency department staff are excellent sources at the time of admission. Social workers and family physicians or clinics are effective in obtaining information about chronic illnesses and functional capacity.

Date, time, and geographic location of the injury are essential for instituting initial treatment. Any treatment required at the scene, especially if the patient was unconscious or in cardiopulmonary arrest, should be documented. While cardiac arrest is poorly tolerated in older adults, children found in cardiac arrest and resuscitated at the scene of a fire have a reasonable chance of survival. The cause and circumstances of the burn provide information about the potential for associated injuries or intoxications. An explosion or jump from upper floors often is accompanied by major fractures. The possibility of drug abuse, including alcohol, should be investigated. Preexisting chronic diseases, including coronary artery disease, diabetes mellitus, chronic lung disease, cerebrovascular disease, and acquired immunodeficiency syndrome (AIDS), adversely affect outcome and should be documented. Certain medications cannot be safely interrupted, and therefore should be identified (phenytoin, insulin, antidepressants, antihypertensives, including beta-blocking agents, digitalis, and others). The possibility of child abuse should be considered when treating any burned child. Burns in some adults are the results of criminal assaults, and information about the injury should be obtained and recorded with the recognition that the medical record will be used in a court of law. All entries to the medical chart should be timed, dated, and legibly signed by the recorder.

Estimation of Burn Severity. The extent, or TBSA, burned determines fluid requirements, drug doses, and outcome (mortality and disability). Initial triage to the appropriate level of medical care is determined primarily by the extent of injury. Burn size can be estimated conveniently and with reasonable accuracy by the "rule of nines" (Table 7-5). Using this artifice, specific body parts represent 9 percent TBSA or multiples thereof. In patients with massive burns it is easier to use this method to estimate the proportion of unburned skin. For small burns, the area defined by the patient's hand represents approximately 1 percent of the body surface.

Once the burned patient reaches the facility for definitive care, burn diagrams are used to determine more accurately the extent of burn injury (Fig. 7-2). This is best carried out immediately following the initial wound debridement. Standing alongside the patient, the exact location of the burn is drawn on the body diagram; in addition, areas of second-degree burn should be identified separately from third-degree burn when possible. Great care must be taken in diagramming accurate locations of the burn, since many treatments and legal decisions often are based on this initial documentation. Extent of injury is more important than depth for directing care during the first few days after admission. Burn depth becomes important later when evaluating the patient for surgical procedures and long-term rehabilitative care. It is often useful to reestimate burn extent and depth after several weeks to develop a more accurate record of injury and any needed surgical procedures. Serial photographic records are extremely helpful but are expensive to provide.

The proper approach to the burn wound is dictated by both the extent and depth of injury (Table 7-6). *First-degree* burns involving primarily the epidermis most commonly result from prolonged exposure to ultraviolet light or very brief exposure to heat. These burns usually are physiologically unimportant and, therefore, are not considered when calculating the TBSA burned. Occasionally, visitors to tropical climates underestimate their susceptibility to sunburn and sustain severe near total body exposure. These unfortunate individuals may require a brief hospitalization for fluid replacement and pain control. These burns appear pink or light red, and are dry, without blisters; they usually heal within 2 to 3 days. Symptomatic treatment with cool compresses to alleviate pain is the best treatment.

BURN ESTIMATE AND DIAGRAM

AGE vs. AREA

Area	Birth 1 yr.	1–4 yr.	5–9 yr.	10–14 yr.	15 yr.	Adult	2°	3°	Total	Donor Areas
Head	19	17	13	11	9	7				
Neck	2	2	2	2	2	2				
Ant. Trunk	13	13	13	13	13	13				
Post. Trunk	13	13	13	13	13	13				
R. Buttock	2½	2½	2½	2½	2½	2½				
L. Buttock	2½	2½	2½	2½	2½	2½				
Genitalia	1	1	1	1	1	1				
R.U. Arm	4	4	4	4	4	4				
L.U. Arm	4	4	4	4	4	4				
R.L. Arm	3	3	3	3	3	3				
L.L. Arm	3	3	3	3	3	3				
R. Hand	2½	2½	2½	2½	2½	2½				
L. Hand	2½	2½	2½	2½	2½	2½				
R. Thigh	5½	6½	8	8½	9	9½				
L. Thigh	5½	6½	8	8½	9	9½				
R. Leg	5	5	5½	6	6½	7				
L. Leg	5	5	5½	6	6½	7				
R. Foot	3½	3½	3½	3½	3½	3½				
L. Foot	3½	3½	3½	3½	3½	3½				
						TOTAL				

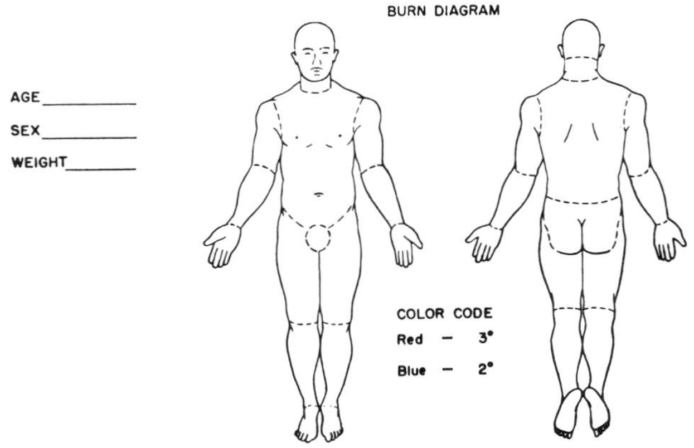

FIG. 7-2. Burn diagram for documenting extent and depth of burn. The most important concept of such diagrams is its provision for changing proportions of body surface area with increasing age. Clinical data for the burn diagram are most accurately obtained immediately after the admission wound debridement.

Burn wounds that involve the epidermis and dermis are referred to as *partial-thickness*, or *second-degree*, wounds; they in turn can be divided into three subtypes: superficial, deep, and indeterminate. Superficial partial-thickness burns affect the epidermis and the superficial level of the dermis and are easily recognized by their moist, pink appearance, characteristic bullae formation, and exquisite sensitivity to stimuli (even a current of air) (Fig. 7-3). They are produced by brief contact with hot liquids or flashes of flame. These wounds heal spontaneously within 2 weeks from the time of injury. The skin remains quite elastic in superficial second-degree burns and underlying tissues can swell massively with only a modest increase in tissue pressure beneath the burn. Extremities with circumferential superficial second-degree burns rarely, if ever, require decompression by escharotomy (see below). If vascular perfusion below such burns is compromised, other causes of injury, such as a fracture, should be sought.

Table 7-5
"Rule of Nines" for Calculating Percentage of Body Burned (% TBSA)

	Child	*Adult*
Head/neck	18	9
Arm	9	9
Anterior trunk	18	18
Posterior trunk	18	18
Leg (groin to toe)	14	18

TBSA, total body surface area

Table 7-6
Diagnosis of Burn Wound Depth

	Second-Degree Burns		
First-Degree Burns	*Superficial*	*Deep Dermal*	*Third-Degree Burns*
Cause			
Sun Minor flash	Hot liquids Flashes of flame Brief exposure to dilute chemicals	Hot liquids Flashes of flame Prolonged exposure to dilute chemicals	Flame Immersion scalds High voltage electricity Exposure to concentrated chemicals Contact with hot objects
Color			
Pink	Pink to bright red	Dark red or mottled yellow-white	Pearly white or charred Translucent and parchment-like
Surface			
Dry or small blisters	Variably sized, usually large bullae Copious exudate	Smaller bullae, often ruptured Slightly moist	Dry with adherent nonviable epidermis Thrombosed vessels may be visible
Sensation			
Painful	Painful	Decreased pinprick sensation Intact deep pressure sensation	Anesthetic Deep pressure sensation
Texture			
Soft with minimal edema and later superficial exfoliation	Thickened by edema but pliable	Moderate edema with decreased elasticity	Inelastic and leathery
Healing			
2 to 3 days	5 to 21 days	3 weeks	None—grafting required

Deep partial-thickness wounds are defined as those wounds that take longer than 3 weeks to heal; this prolonged healing often results in hypertrophic scar formation. Deep dermal burns are caused by immersion in hot liquids and by flame, are characteristically bright red or yellow-white, have a slightly moist surface, and show decreased sensitivity to stimuli (pinprick). Skin with these burns is less elastic than that sustaining more superficial burns. If optimal healing is not achieved with conventional daily wound management, improved results can be attained with split-thickness skin grafts. It is difficult on admission to reliably assess some deep burn wounds, which either could heal spontaneously or require a skin graft. These indeterminate wounds must be observed over a 10-day to 2-week period by an experienced burn surgeon to predict accurately whether excision and skin grafting would prove superior to the natural healing process. A variety of techniques to determine burn depth have been used, including fluorescein and indocyanine green fluorometry, laser Doppler flowmetry, thermography, ultrasonography, nuclear magnetic resonance imaging, and light reflectance; however, until further refinements of these techniques occur, clinical observation remains the most accurate method for determining the need for grafting.

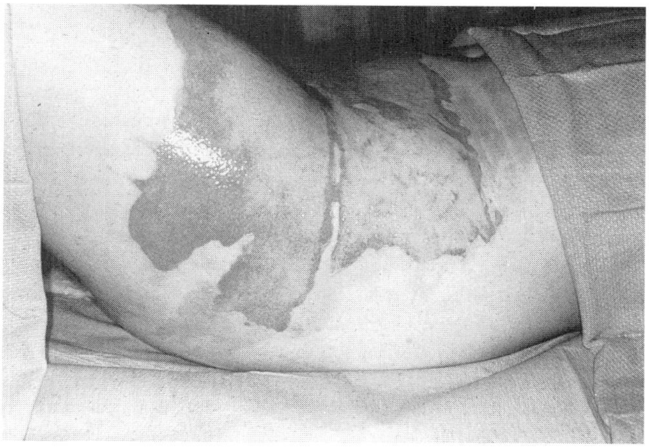

FIG. 7-3. Second-degree burn on the abdomen and left thigh. This burn demonstrates the characteristic moist appearance of a partial-thickness burn. It is bright pink on the lower thigh and becomes more pale and less moist as it extends onto the abdomen, indicating a deeper second-degree burn.

Full-thickness, or *third-degree*, burns generally are readily recognized. They are caused by exposure to concentrated chemicals or high-voltage electricity, and prolonged contact with flames and hot objects. They may appear pearly white, charred, or parchmentlike, and thrombosed veins may be seen through the devitalized tissue, referred to as *eschar* (Fig. 7-4). They are characteristically dry and insensate. Third-degree burned skin is inelastic, and the occurrence of such burns in a strategic location can cause rapid physiologic compromise as edema accumulates and tissue pressure rises. Such burns may require escharotomies (see below).

The evaluation of burns in small children (less than 4 years of age) differs significantly from that of older children and adults. The head represents a much greater proportion of the surface area. More importantly, the visual appearance of the burn can be misleading to those accustomed to treating adults. Burns that appear to be more superficial in adults are much deeper in small children. On admission, third-degree burns in these children characteristi-

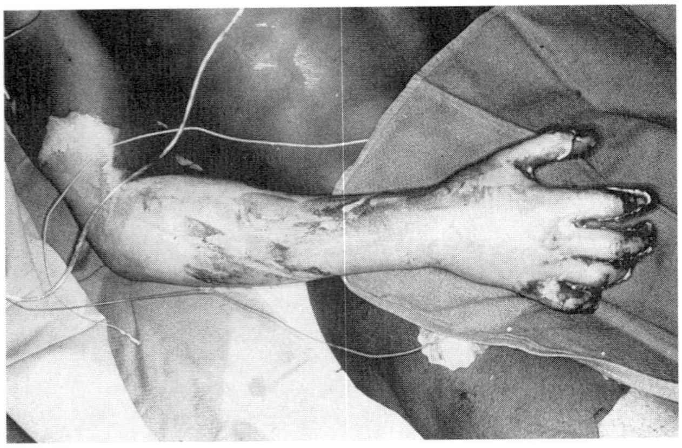

FIG. 7-4. Third-degree, or full-thickness, burn of the right arm. The surface of the burn is ivory-colored, dry, and insensate. Dark patches represent incinerated epidermis firmly adherent to underlying eschar. Burns with this appearance typically penetrate into, but not through, the underlying subcutaneous tissue.

cally have a rich red color, and typical white or parched burns are almost never seen (Fig. 7-5). These red burns often are classified initially as second-degree burns. Only over the succeeding 4 or 5 days do these burns assume a more classic full-thickness appearance. At this time, parents become quite disturbed when informed that a skin graft will be necessary.

Physical Examination. A burned patient is a trauma patient and evaluation can be carried out safely and expeditiously by following the format of the Advanced Trauma Life Support guidelines of the American College of Surgeons. The most common cause of early instability in burned patients is severe inhalation injury producing massive upper airway damage with pending obstruction or near lethal carbon monoxide poisoning. If treatment was not already instituted in the field, the primary survey should identify quickly these difficulties. A thorough secondary survey will detect associated injuries. Particularly important is an early and thorough neurologic examination, with emphasis on mental status. Overlooked neurologic deficits present on admission may be attributed to a misadventure in the hospital when finally documented at a later date. Changing neurologic status may indicate a closed head injury. Baseline vital signs and assessment of peripheral pulses allow interpretation of subsequent alterations, particularly in patients with circumferential extremity burns. A thorough abdominal examination should be carried out before the patient receives analgesics and sedatives. The detection of turbulent airflow in the upper airway, hoarseness, and wheezing indicates inhalation injury, and clinical progresison of these findings may require endotracheal intubation. Small children should have a thorough ear, nose, and throat evaluation since approximately one-third of children admitted to a burn treatment facility have preexisting otitis media or other upper respiratory tract infection. All patients should have a rectal examination.

Laboratory Studies. Complete blood count, electrolytes, and standard biochemistry profile should be obtained immediately upon arrival to the receiving treatment facility. Disease processes that significantly affect survival, such as cirrhosis, hepatitis, and gastrointestinal malignancy, may be detected. Blood gases and carboxyhemoglobin concentration should be measured promptly since oxygen administration can obscure the initial severity of carbon monoxide poisoning. When available, cyanide levels should be measured in patients at risk for inhalation injury. A drug screen, including alcohol, facilitates assessment of the patient's mental status and can anticipate the development of withdrawal symptoms later in the hospital course. A chest radiograph should be obtained for all patients: blast overpressure, attempts at central venous cannulation, and rib fractures may cause pneumothorax or hemothorax. Radiographs of the entire spine, long bones, and pelvis should be obtained for patients with electrical contact injury or sustaining blunt trauma in association with the burn injury.

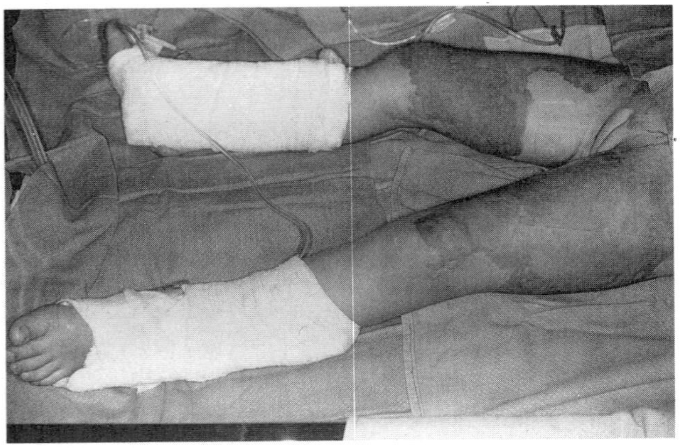

FIG. 7-5. Third-degree burns of legs in a small child shortly after injury. Although the burn was bright red in appearance, it has a violaceous hue and is dry. This appearance is characteristic of acute full-thickness burns in children less than 2 years of age. Over the next 72 h, such burns assume the more typical ashen appearance of a full-thickness injury.

FLUID RESUSCITATION

Physiology of Resuscitation. Cutaneous thermal injury manifests as coagulation necrosis with microvascular thrombosis in areas of deepest damage. The surrounding tissue usually is less extensively burned, with ill-defined zones of stasis and hyperemia. These areas of incomplete necrosis are characterized by potentially salvageable tissue that is perfused by a microcirculation that is damaged. This loss of capillary integrity allows loss of fluid from the intravascular compartment and subsequent edema formation. If patients with a large thermal injury do not receive prompt and appropriate fluid resuscitation, burn shock ensues and the injured but viable portions of the burn proceed to complete necrosis. In addition to direct physical damage to the microvasculature, kinins, prostanoids, histamine, and oxygen radicals appear to play important roles in determining the severity of tissue injury. Ibuprofen preserves dermal vasculature and decreases early postburn edema. Blockade of histamine H_2 receptors in animal studies substantially ameliorates fluid loss and edema formation after burn injury.

Edema formation is most extensive in the damaged but still viable portions of the burn wound. In the classic model of the burn wound, this area would correspond to the zone of stasis. Fluid is also lost into remote uninjured tissues, albeit at a much slower rate and lesser volume. Fluid resuscitation greatly accentuates edema formation in both burned and unburned tissue. Edema is not inherently detrimental; once resolved, no significant permanent damage remains. Edema in critical locations, such as around the upper airway or beneath full-thickness eschar encircling the extremities or the chest, however, can pose potentially dangerous situations. The fluid lost from the intravascular space closely resembles plasma in both protein and electrolyte content, and these losses are proportional to the size of injury. Baxter and Shires have demonstrated that sodium losses are approximately 0.5 to 0.6 meq/kg body weight/percent body surface burned. A resuscitation regimen must include large doses of sodium as well as fluid volume to replace intravascular losses acutely.

Red blood cells are proportionately retained in the circulation. Whereas hemolysis of as much of 40 percent of the red cell mass occurs in some extensive flame burns, only 10 percent of red cells are damaged in most patients. Acute hemolysis is caused by direct thermal damage to red cells. Burn-induced complement activation and subsequent oxygen radical production by neutrophils increase osmotic fragility of red blood cells and sustained hemolysis for several days following thermal injury. During the first 24 h following injury, hemoconcentration rapidly develops, and hematocrit values as high as 70 percent are relatively common in young, previously healthy patients. Viscosity rises as the circulating hematocrit increases, but potential detrimental effects of hyperviscosity have not been demonstrated in burned patients.

The increase in capillary permeability leads to a fall in intravascular volume and cardiac output. Although systemic arterial pressure often is initially maintained near normal, continued contraction of the intravascular volume leads to hypotension, further depression of cardiac output, decreased peripheral perfusion, and tissue acidosis as hypovolemic burn shock becomes established. Loss of intravascular fluid is too rapid and too massive in burns exceeding 20 to 25 percent of the body surface to allow partial correction of fluid deficits by the shift of fluid from the intracellular space. Initially, the increased capillary permeability results in an obligatory net plasma volume loss. As intravascular pressure falls and extravascular tissue pressure rises, the rate of plasma loss into injured tissues decreases in patients not receiving fluid resuscitation. During the second 24 h postburn, capillary permeability returns to normal, with a small net increase in intravascular plasma volume. Exogenous colloid administered at this time will remain in the circulation in a normal fashion.

Replacement of fluid sequestered in burned tissues is the cornerstone of treating and preventing burn shock. With institution of adequate crystalloid resuscitation, cardiac output begins to rise and usually returns to normal by 18 to 24 h postinjury. At the same time, however, plasma volume and blood volume continue to fall for another 12 to 24 h before intravascular volume begins to rise. By this time, cardiac output has increased to supranormal levels, reflecting the onset of postburn hypermetabolism. However, blood volume deficits persist for as long as 2 weeks following large burn injuries. Such data emphasize the superiority of cardiac output measurements over blood volume determinations as a guide to resuscitation. The response of systemic arterial pressure is variable. Whereas the patient initially may demonstrate pronounced hypotension while severely hypovolemic, blood pressure often remains in the low to low-normal range after adequate resuscitation has begun and cardiac output has stabilized. Accurate peripheral arterial pressures are difficult to measure in edematous burned extremities. Experimental studies have shown that the kidney is the most poorly perfused organ following thermal injury. With resuscitation, renal blood flow returns to normal only after restoration of perfusion to other visceral organs. As such, adequate renal perfusion implies adequate flow to other organs. Although it does not precisely reflect total renal blood flow, urinary output is the most readily accessible index by which to monitor resuscitation.

The initial persistence of reduced cardiac output after apparently adequate fluid therapy, as evidenced by an appropriate pulse rate and restoration of both arterial blood pressure and urinary output, has been attributed to the presence of circulating myocardial depressant factors, which possibly originate from the burn wound. Horton and coworkers demonstrated in isolated, coronary-perfused guinea pig hearts that burn injury resulted in decreased left ventricular contractility and a shift of ventricular function curves downward and to the right. This dysfunction was more pronounced in hearts from aged animals and was not totally reversed by fluid resuscitation. This persistent postburn myocardial depression was not identified by Cioffi and colleagues in a similar model when animals received resuscitation synchronous with the thermal injury: timely resuscitation totally reversed contraction and relaxation abnormalities after burn injury. Such studies emphasize the importance of early intervention. Similar studies using noninvasive M-mode echocardiographic assessment of cardiac function, cardiac output, indices of left ventricular volume, and myocardial contractility parallel Cioffi's experimental findings. Cardiac index fell by 12 h postinjury and returned to normal only by the end of the second postburn day. The cardiac index changes were paralleled by similar reductions in left-ventricular volumes, indicating that the reduced cardiac outputs were related to intravascular volume deficits. Ejection fractions were normal at all time points, and mean velocity of left-ventricular internal fiber shortening was significantly elevated at all time intervals, indicating a hypercontractile state. These findings implicate intravascular volume deficits as the cause of decreased cardiac output after thermal injury and demonstrate that physiologically relevant myocardial depression is not an inherent aspect of burn injury.

Choice of Resuscitation Fluid. Although the effectiveness of sodium-containing fluid in the treatment of hypovolemia was recognized early in the twentieth century, large-volume crystalloid resuscitation is a relatively recent development. Because of the similarity of wound fluid to plasma, balanced electrolyte solutions closely approximating plasma electrolyte concentrations have emerged as effective resuscitation fluids for the treatment of shock syndromes. Baxter adopted lactated Ringer's solution as an inexpensive, readily available extracellular fluid mimic and successfully resuscitated severely burned patients without the complications of fluid overload and electrolyte derangements. Lactated Ringer's solution is slightly hypotonic with respect to sodium (130 meq/L), providing some free water, as advocated by the earlier Evans and Brooke formulas.

Earlier resuscitation formulas included colloid products, and such solutions remain popular in many burn treatment facilities. Baxter demonstrated that plasma volume changes are independent of plasma colloid content in the first 24 h postburn, and therefore colloid-containing fluid resuscitation is of little benefit during this time interval. A major concern with administering colloid at this time is its rapid loss into the extravascular space. At best, colloid would seem ineffective and may be deleterious by promoting edema formation by subtraction effect with accumulation of colloid in physiologically critical tissues such as the lung. During the second 24 h following thermal injury, colloid is retained in the plasma compartment and exerts a positive effect on the restoration of blood volume.

The relative merits of colloid and crystalloid solutions for initial resuscitation of the burned patient were evaluated in a randomized controlled trial (Table 7-7). The colloid-containing solutions clearly were more effective in restoring intravascular volume and cardiac index to normal levels by the end of the first 24 h postinjury. While the patients receiving colloid-containing fluid required significantly less volume for adequate resuscitation during this time than did the patients receiving crystalloid-only solutions, by the end of the second postburn day, there were no differences between the two treatment groups in terms of fluid administered, cardiac output, left-ventricular contractility, and intravascular volume.

The potential advantages of colloid-containing resuscitation solutions appeared to be more than offset by the deleterious effects of colloid on the lungs. Whereas both crystalloid and colloid solutions were equally effective in maintaining hemodynamic stability during the first postburn week, extravascular lung water increased significantly above normal in patients resuscitated with colloid-containing fluids (Fig. 7-6). Furthermore, later pulmonary complications and mortality were higher in the colloid-treated patients. Therefore, colloid administration should be avoided in most burned patients until capillary integrity is restored and administered colloid is retained in the plasma compartment. A few patients who require fluid resuscitation greatly in excess of predicted needs but who remain severely hypotensive and have marginal urinary output may benefit from albumin infusions during the latter part of the first 24 h following burn injury.

Table 7-7
Left-Ventricular Indices During Postburn Resuscitation

Time Period (h)	*Treatment*	*Cardiac Index**	*End Diastolic Volume Index†*	*Stroke Index‡*
0–12	Colloid	3.05	42	32
	Crystalloid	3.11	43	34
12–24	Colloid	4.67	56	40
	Crystalloid	2.75	36	27
24–48	Colloid	4.42	52	39
	Crystalloid	4.03	51	37

*Normal = 3.40 L/min/m^2
†Normal = 60 mL/m^2
‡Normal = 44 mL/cycle/m^2

Hypertonic saline solutions have been used successfully to resuscitate extensively burned patients. The most commonly utilized solution contains 250 meq sodium per liter. The major advantage of hypertonic sodium solutions is the smaller volume required for adequate resuscitation during the first 24 h postburn. During this time, edema formation is less than that associated with isotonic resuscitation, and patients with encircling third-degree burns may require escharotomy less frequently. Although this reduced volume of resuscitation may be advantageous in patients with inhalation injury, improved outcome has never been demonstrated. Urine output is well supported by hypertonic fluids, but cardiac output is lower than that in comparable patients receiving lactated Ringer's solution. Hypertonic solutions may not restore intravascular volume and organ perfusion effectively; preservation of urinary output in part may be a direct effect of the large sodium load. Hypertonic saline resuscitation is limited by the development of hypernatremia. Sodium concentrations exceeding 165 meq/L

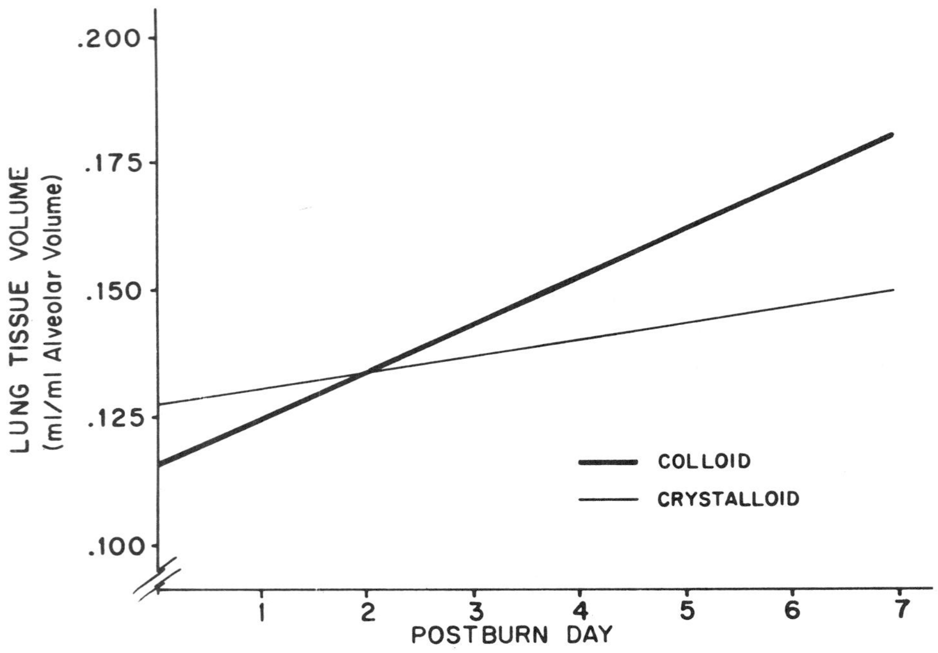

FIG. 7-6. Effect of resuscitation fluid composition on lung water. While lung water, measured as lung tissue volume, remained unchanged over the 7 days in severely burned patients receiving lactated Ringer's solution, lung water in patients receiving lactated Ringer's/2.5% albumin colloid solution progressively increased.

cause acute renal failure, and a rising serum sodium concentration dictates discontinuance of hypertonic resuscitation and institution of isotonic or even hypotonic fluids. At the end of 72 h postburn, the sodium dose and total volume of isotonic and hypertonic resuscitations are similar. Hypertonic saline resuscitation works best in centers that utilize silver nitrate-soaked dressings for topical antimicrobial therapy: large amounts of sodium are rapidly lost into the dressings and significant hypernatremia occurs less frequently.

Resuscitation in the First 24 Hours. Fluid requirements during the first 24 h postburn are directly related to the size of the patient (body weight) and the magnitude of the injury (% TBSA). Lactated Ringer's solution is the most commonly used electrolyte solution in burn resuscitation. The resuscitation regimen used at the New York Hospital incorporates modifications of the Parkland and Brooke formulas (Table 7-8). The New York Hospital formula calculates fluid requirements as 4 mL/kg body weight/% TBSA burned. Small children require additional fluid during this time to obtain adequate resuscitation. Children weighing up to 30 kg receive added maintenance fluid and are given a lactated Ringer's solution.

Although burned patients tend to require a greater proportion of fluid during the first 24 h, this uneven requirement becomes more balanced the sooner resuscitation is instituted after injury. Thus, initial infusion rates can be calculated simply by dividing the predicted first day volume by 24 h. It is critical to recognize that resuscitation formulas serve only as a planning tool for initiating resuscitation. Once fluid resuscitation begins, all subsequent therapy is based on the patient's physiologic response to the infusion during the previous hour. It is a mistake to write fluid orders for the entire 24-h period; rather, the rate of resuscitation must be assessed at least hourly and must be based on criteria for the adequacy of resuscitation (see below). The fluid should be infused at a constant rate and any changes titrated in a deliberate fashion. Bolus fluid administration, although occasionally necessary early in treatment, is detrimental because proportionately more fluid is lost from the intravascular compartment into the injured tissues.

In adults and older children, the resuscitation fluid administered during the first 24 h after injury generally should not contain dextrose. With the large fluid volumes commonly required by extensively burned patients, 5 percent dextrose concentrations in the lactated Ringer's solution would deliver massive doses of dextrose. Before the recognition of the adverse effects of these large dextrose doses, burn patients were believed to be susceptible to an unusual syndrome called *burn stress pseudodiabetes*, which was characterized by hyperglycemia, glycosuria, polyuria, and difficulty with resuscitation. An exception to avoidance of dextrose administration is the very young burned child, who characteristically has reduced liver glycogen stores. Without dextrose supplementation during resuscitation, hypoglycemia is not uncommon in pediatric burn patients. In such patients, serum glucose concentrations should be monitored frequently and glucose supplemented as indicated.

Resuscitation in the Second 24 Hours. Fluid management undergoes substantial alterations during the second 24 h postburn. The plasma protein estimated to have been lost into the burn wound during the first 24 h is replaced at this time (see Table 7-8). The increase in microvascular endothelial permeability of the previous day has reversed, and administered colloid is now retained in the intravascular compartment. Colloid is replaced as plasma or a plasma-equivalent solution. Such solutions contain isotonic saline, and this additional sodium dose is essential for the success of most crystalloid resuscitations. While fresh-frozen plasma has enjoyed much popularity as a colloid replacement, it has been replaced by various pasteurized protein fractions because of the infectious potential of the former. The colloid should be given early on the second postburn day, usually within 4 to 8 hours. The major fluid component of resuscitation during the second postburn day is sufficient water to provide an adequate urine output and replacement of increasing evaporative and other insensible water losses. The latter can be voluminous and is essentially free of sodium. Most patients do well with infusion of 5 percent dextrose in water or in 0.2 percent sodium chloride. Because small children are more susceptible to hyponatremia, they tend to require more sodium at this time than do adults. Frequent measurements of serum sodium guide the optimal fluid composition. Fluid infusion rates during the second 24 h are instituted at approximately one-half of the last hour's rate of lactated Ringer's solution and then adjusted up or down depending on the overall response. If urinary output requires a steady increase in fluid administration, lactated Ringer's solution should be used.

Table 7-8
New York Hospital Method for Estimating Resuscitation Fluid Requirements for Burned Patients

	Adults	*Children**
First 24 h postburn	Lactated Ringer's solution 4 mL/kg/% burn	Lactated Ringer's solution 4 mL/kg/% burn *plus* First 10 kg–100 mL/kg Second 10 kg–50 mL/kg Third 10 kg–20 mL/kg
Second 24 h postburn	D5/W *plus* Colloid-containing fluid† 0.5 mL/kg/% burn	D5/0.45% saline *plus* Colloid-containing fluid† 0.5 mL/kg/% burn

*Children under 30-kg body weight

†Administered as plasma equivalent (e.g., 5% albumin in 0.9% sodium chloride solution)

Monitoring Resuscitation. Urinary output is the most readily accessible and efficacious monitor of the adequacy of resuscitation (Table 7-9). Restoration of renal perfusion occurs only after flow in other organs has been restored, and an adequate urine output implies hemodynamic stability. Desirable urinary volumes are 40 to 60 mL/h in adults and 1 mL/kg body weight/h in children weighing up to 30 kg. Larger resuscitation volumes producing greater urinary outputs do not improve oxygen consumption or other indices of organ function.

The major exceptions to these guidelines are in patients with direct electrical injury and myoglobinuria. Free myoglobin is toxic to the renal tubules and can cause acute tubular necrosis and anuria. The therapeutic goal in these patients is to increase urinary output to wash out this toxic pigment quickly. If the urine in electrically injured patients is pink, red, or brown, intravenous infusion rates are increased to raise urine output to 100 to 150 mL/h. As the pigment disappears from the urine, the fluid infusion rate is reduced and urine output is allowed to decrease to 40 to 60 mL/h. If the urine is darkly pigmented, increased infusion rates may not raise the urinary output successfully. In these patients, sodium bicarbonate is administered to alkalinize the urine to a pH greater than 5.6 and increase the solubility of myoglobin. Forty-five milliequivalents of bicarbonate may be added to each liter of lactated Ringer's solution. In addition, mannitol is given to promote diuresis. Twenty-five grams is given immediately to adults and 12.5 g is added to each liter of resuscitation fluid. Urine output in these conditions, however, becomes a poor guide to resuscitation, and additional methods of monitoring may be required.

Heart rate, blood pH, and systemic blood pressure are relatively nonspecific indicators of perfusion, and their accuracy in reflecting the state of the resuscitation effort is variable. Heart rate is the most reliable of these indicators. Shortly after thermal injury, heart rate in adults rises to between 110 and 130 beats/min, and this sinus tachycardia persists for as long as the burn wound remains open. Slower heart rates may be seen in well-trained athletes with small burns and in the elderly. In this latter group, the inability to sustain this mild tachycardia is associated with a markedly higher mortality rate. Heart rates higher than 130 beats/min almost always reflect significant hypovolemia and are accompanied by oliguria. Volume loading in such patients reduces abnormally elevated heart rates more quickly than it increases urinary output. This is an extremely useful observation, since fluid infusion volumes can be reduced earlier, avoiding excessive tissue edema and overshoot of urinary output. Proportionately higher heart rates are seen in children, but they too demonstrate these responses to intravascular volume changes.

Although arterial blood pH is a relatively nonspecific indicator of blood flow, a normal pH usually reflects adequate tissue perfusion. A moderately low pH (7.2 to 7.3) is fairly common in the early stages of resuscitation but nearly always rises to normal as the fluid infusion continues. Administration of sodium bicarbonate rarely is required, but, for those patients in whom faster correction of the acidemia is believed necessary, the addition of 45 mEq of sodium bicarbonate to each liter of lactated Ringer's solution provides effective treatment. Arterial blood pH below 7.2 reflects prolonged shock and is seen almost entirely in patients who fail to respond to fluid therapy.

Arterial blood pressure may be low, normal, or elevated; hypertension is frequently seen in small children. Mild hypotension in the presence of an otherwise stable patient with adequate urine output is well tolerated and does not require treatment. There probably is an arterial pressure below which autoregulation in certain organ functions (e.g., kidney, brain) fails; therefore, arterial systolic blood pressure below 80 to 85 mmHg in most situations should be supported. Blood pressure is difficult to measure in burned and edematous extremities, and treatment directed specifically at the control of arterial pressure, whether it be abnormally low or high, should be guided by invasive monitoring.

If the burned patient fails to respond to predicted fluid volumes, direct monitoring of vascular pressures is indicated (Table 7-10). A useful guideline for instituting invasive monitoring is a fluid requirement exceeding 150 to 200 percent of burn formula calculations (i.e., greater than 6 to 8 mL/kg/% TBSA burned). Pulmonary capillary wedge pressure is the most useful measure of intravascular volume capacity and of the ability to infuse additional fluid. Inadequate resuscitation can be supplemented to a pulmonary wedge pressure of 18 to 20 mmHg in most individuals. Cardiac output, determined by the same catheter, is a valuable guide to pharmacologic intervention. When using inotropic drugs to support cardiac output, one must be aware of the natural time course of cardiac output changes following burn injury. Therapy should be directed to supporting cardiac output at or just above the level required for that point in time.

Causes of Resuscitation Failure. Delayed resuscitation prolongs tissue ischemia, promotes tissue acidosis, and generates toxic products that impair capillary membrane integrity and increase permeability; such conditions lead to total necrosis of potentially salvageable tissue and an increased probability of mortality. Most instances of delayed resuscitation occur when the extent of injury is underestimated or not recognized at all, and involve primarily children and the elderly. Occasionally, patients living in remote locations are difficult to transport to a burn center in a timely manner and the onset of effective resuscitation measures may be delayed.

Electrical injuries require more fluid than would be estimated by the extent of cutaneous burn alone, for two reasons. First, substantial quantities of thermally injured tissues may lie beneath the skin and escape consideration in fluid calculations. In many cases, only small entrance and exit burns may be visible, while all inter-

Table 7-9
Major Indicators of Effective Intravascular Volume

Urinary output
Pulmonary capillary wedge pressure
Cardiac output
Blood pH
Systemic blood pressure

Table 7-10
Indications for Intravascular Monitoring

Carbon monoxide poisoning
Delayed resuscitation
Extremes of age
Inhalation injury (severe)
High positive end-expiratory pressure
History of cirrhosis/alcoholism
Massive burns
Severe electrical injury
Pre-existing cardiac disease
Pre-existing renal failure

vening muscle, nerves, and vessels may be destroyed. The associated third-space loss may be enormous, with a consequent requirement for large volumes of resuscitation fluid. Second, as described earlier, additional fluid is needed to initiate diuresis to excrete hemochromagens released from damaged muscle.

Inhalation injury is the most common major associated injury in burned patients. As with electrical injury, the major cause for the additional fluid requirement in inhalation injury is the additional tissue injury in the lungs. Concomitant inhalation injury increases fluid requirements in burned patients by 40 to 50 percent. Attempts to restrict fluid administration and to maintain intentional hypovolemia result only in underresuscitation of the patient, with all its adverse consequences and accentuation of pulmonary edema.

Escharotomy is often necessary in patients with third-degree burns encircling an extremity. Escharotomy allows the underlying tissue to expand, producing a larger volume into which edema fluid can accumulate. Following escharotomy, a previously stable patient responding well to intravenous resuscitation may suddenly become oliguric and more tachycardiac. These indices of hypovolemia should be expected following escharotomy and mandate an increase in the fluid infusion rate.

Carbon monoxide poisoning produces cardiac failure. Cardiac dysfunction may continue long after carboxyhemoglobin levels have fallen to zero. Such patients respond poorly to fluid and to pharmacologic support of cardiac function. Larger volumes of fluid are often required in such patients to obtain adequate tissue perfusion.

Few studies are available in burned patients with acute drug and alcohol intoxication, but experience in burn centers with large drug-abusing patient populations indicates that these patients require more fluid and higher filling pressures than do nonabusing patients with burns of equivalent sizes. Both primary cardiac dysfunction and increased capillary permeability appear to be involved.

Coronary artery disease and advanced age are associated with cardiac dysfunction similar to that encountered in patients with carbon monoxide intoxication or drug abuse. Alcoholic cardiomyopathy may compound the toxicity of acute ethanol intoxication. The hemodynamic response is similar for all forms of cardiac dysfunction: additional fluid is required to increase filling pressures in an attempt to augment cardiac output.

Adjuncts to Resuscitation. Thermal injury is the quintessential disease of massive third-space fluid loss. As described previously, most of the physiologic instability during the first 48 h postburn is due to hypovolemia and the essential element of therapy is volume replacement. Before any other mode of therapy is instituted to treat burned patients in shock, adequate replacement of intravascular volume must be confirmed by direct measurement. If the patient remains oliguric and in shock after volume is replaced to a pulmonary wedge pressure of 18 to 20 mmHg, further expansion of intravascular volume is unlikely to produce any additional beneficial effect and pharmacologic therapy should be utilized.

Low-dose dopamine (2 to 3 μg/kg/min) has the unique effect of increasing urinary output in many patients. Even in this dose range, cardiac output may increase modestly. If urinary output increases to desired levels, usually no further medication is necessary, and resuscitation can proceed according to the usual guidelines. Doses of dopamine can be increased in patients whose systemic vascular resistance (SVR) is decreased, but a low SVR is unusual during the resuscitation phase of burn injury. Only after the onset of postburn hypermetabolism does SVR drop to very low levels. Dopamine may increase pulmonary artery pressures in acutely burned patients who usually already have moderate pulmonary hypertension. Doses of dopamine greater than 5 to 10 μg/kg/min do not improve right-ventricular function in burned patients and may accentuate pulmonary congestion.

Unlike dopamine, dobutamine decreases preload and afterload and relieves pulmonary congestion while increasing cardiac output. If inotropic support is needed after low-dose dopamine fails to improve urinary output, dobutamine is the agent of choice at the present time. The goal of inotropic support is to restore a low cardiac output to the normal or slightly above-normal level appropriate for that time on the postinjury cardiac output curve.

Digitalis for inotropic support should be avoided. When used in conjunction with dopamine, dobutamine, and other adrenergic drugs, no additional inotropic effect occurs. Furthermore, digoxin (the most commonly used form) is relatively long-acting and is difficult to counteract if acute toxicity develops. Elderly patients taking digitalis before injury usually require reinstitution of the drug when weaned from the infusible inotropes. Digitalis is a very effective drug for most supraventricular tachyarrhythmias in burned patients. Such arrhythmias should not be pharmacologically decreased below 110 beats/min in most adult burn patients unless the patient has angina or electrocardiographic rate-related ST-T segment depression. Certain supraventricular arrhythmias should be treated first with adenosine. Vasodilators may be helpful in the occasional burn patient with increased afterload and SVR. Short-acting agents that can be easily titrated are safest. Nitroprusside is especially convenient to use, although tachyphylaxis develops after several days. Nitroglycerin is another valuable agent for the temporary control of hypertension due to volume shifts during resuscitation, particularly for patients with ischemic heart disease. Intravenous nicardipine is equally effective and better maintains cardiac output.

Beta-adrenergic blocking agents and calcium channel blockers such as verapamil decrease cardiac output and blunt the hypermetabolic response to injury. These actions are deleterious in burned patients. Beta-blockers should be used only in patients who have been taking such drugs chronically; sudden withdrawal of beta-blockers is associated with rebound tachycardia and an increased incidence of sudden death. Verapamil may be useful for temporarily slowing a supraventricular tachycardia so that an accurate diagnosis can be made. The tachycardia is then treated with a more specific agent. As stated earlier, excessive sinus tachycardia in a burned patient almost always requires more fluid infusion, not pharmacologic agents. Vasoconstrictors generally have no role in the treatment of burn shock.

Diuretics almost never are indicated during resuscitation; oliguria is assumed to reflect hypovolemia until proved otherwise. Only after wedge pressure and cardiac output are optimized is a diuretic indicated for reduced urinary output. Elderly patients on chronic diuretic therapy may require a diuretic but, even in these patients, volume replacement and inotropic support (including low-dose dopamine) should be tried first. Small doses of a loop diuretic (furosemide 10 to 40 mg intravenously) generally are sufficient.

Intravascular Access. Reliable intravascular access is a critical concern. At least one large (16-gauge) intravenous cannula should be inserted, and two reliable routes of access are often necessary. The selection of a peripheral vein or a central vein depends on the operator's skill with venous cannulation and the potential need to measure cardiac filling pressures. If the latter is likely in a patient in whom a large fluid requirement is anticipated, the introducer sheath for the pulmonary artery catheter should be inserted as soon after injury as possible. Later in the resuscitation period, when the patient has become massively edematous, normal anatomic landmarks are unidentifiable, and insertion of the introducer at this time is comparably difficult and dangerous. An introducer has a large diameter and provides ideal vascular access for high-volume flow rates. A multiple-lumen catheter can be inserted into the introducer sheath if several incompatible drugs or infusions are needed. The subclavian and internal jugular veins are the safest locations for central access. Both inspiratory and expiratory chest radiographs should be obtained to confirm proper cannula placement and to verify the absence of a pneumothorax. The femoral vein may also be used for large-bore venous access. Cutdowns are virtually never necessary and cause major infectious morbidity and even mortality later in the postburn course. High-volume flow rates through the saphenous vein can use massive leg edema and dangerously high compartment pressures. Veins accessed by cutdowns become unusable for access at a later time and are the most common cause of suppurative thrombophlebitis. Steel needles or short cannulas may dislodge from the vein as edema accumulates; therefore, longer catheters should be used for all access.

The same considerations apply for arterial monitoring catheters. Short 20-gauge cannulas may be used (in adults) for dorsalis pedis, posterior tibial, and radial artery cannulas. Longer catheters should be used for femoral and axillary artery access. The brachial artery should not be used for arterial access because risk of limb loss with the use of this site is high. It makes little difference whether a cannula is inserted through burned or unburned skin. With a rigidly enforced schedule of changing such cannulas every 72 h, infectious complications are minimized and are similar for burned and unburned insertion sites. Proportionately smaller catheters are used for pediatric patients.

Fluid Management After 48 Hours. After 48 h, burned patients begin to demonstrate the physiologic changes associated with the postinjury hypermetabolic response, which reaches its peak approximately 1 week after injury and persists until the burn wound is closed. Cardiac output approximately doubles in patients with burns covering more than 40 percent TBSA. Minute ventilation increases, with a similar elevation of oxygen consumption and carbon dioxide production. Thermal injury to skin destroys its ability to retain water vapor, and evaporative water loss through the burn can be enormous. Evaporative water loss can be estimated by calculating (25 + % TBSA burned) × m^2 body surface area/h or 2.1 to 3 mL/kg body weight/% TBSA burned. Mobilization of edema and urinary output increase at this time, and diuresis may be sizable as the renal solute load produced by hypercatabolic processes increases. Failure to mobilize edema fluid at this time is an accurate predictor of mortality.

Fluid management during the postresuscitation phase is guided by urinary output, careful control of weight loss, and maintenance of serum sodium in the normal range. Burned patients maintain a positive sodium and water balance for up to 2 weeks following injury (Table 7-11), therefore, sodium-free or low-sodium solutions should be used following completion of the resuscitation phase. As with resuscitation, a minimum urine output of 40 to 60 mL/h is necessary. Higher volumes of urine may not be related to fluid balance but instead may reflect an obligatory diuresis in response to large solute concentrations in the urine or to increased levels of atrial natriuretic peptide. Fluid administration is titrated to allow a slow but progressive loss of weight so that the patient returns to preinjury weight by postburn day seven to ten. A faster weight loss is associated with hypernatremia and usually arises from the underestimation of evaporative water loss (Table 7-12). If weight loss is delayed, hyponatremia develops. Hyponatremia is the most common cause of convulsions after burn injury and is particularly dangerous in small children (Fig. 7-7). Severe cerebral edema may require treatment with hypertonic saline solutions. In the absence of neurologic symptoms, most patients respond to restriction of free water intake.

Urinary potassium losses in the postresuscitation period average 50 to 200 meq daily and may be as high as 600 meq daily. Replacement is easily managed by monitoring serum and urine concentrations. Red cell loss is progressive, and most adults require two to three units each week to maintain a hematocrit greater than 30 percent. Recombinant human erythropoietin may reduce the need for blood transfusion.

MAINTENANCE OF PERIPHERAL CIRCULATION

Following thermal injury, fluid accumulates in damaged tissue, and edema soon becomes clinically apparent. Edema formation is accelerated by the large fluid volumes required for adequate resuscitation. Skin with full-thickness destruction will not expand as fluid accumulates beneath the unyielding eschar. If an extremity is encircled by a full-thickness burn, increasing edema formation progressively elevates tissue pressure until blood flow ceases. Is-

Table 7-11
Retention of Fluid and Sodium Administered During Resuscitation of Eight Extensively Burned Patients*

	Exchangeable Sodium Mass (Percentage of Predicted)	*Extracellular Fluid Volume (Increase Above Predicted)*
Fifth postburn day	145%	153%
Twelfth postburn day	121%	128%

*Mean burn size: 47.6% TBSA

SOURCE: From: Pruitt, 1979, with permission.

Table 7-12
Causes of Hypernatremia in Burn Patients

Cause	*Number of Patients*
Inadequate replacement of insensible water loss	31
Sepsis	16
Osmotic diuresis associated with diabetes mellitus or hypermetabolism	2
Defect in osmotic regulation (diabetes insipidus)	2
Total patients with hypernatremia	51*

*10.9% of 468 admissions

SOURCE: From: Warden, et al., 1973, with permission.

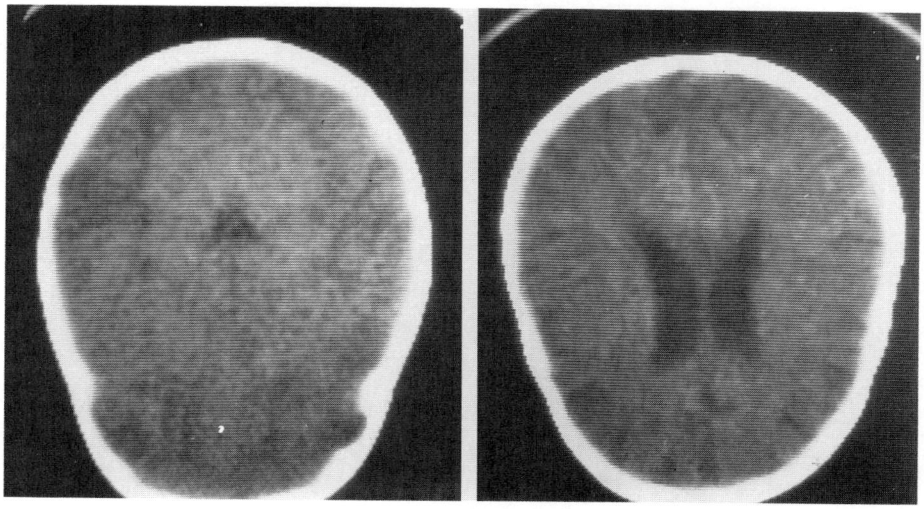

FIG. 7-7. Computed tomography scans of a burned child. Hyponatremia and neurologic symptoms were associated with cerebral edema *(left)*. With correction of hyponatremia, the patient's neurologic abnormalities and cerebral edema resolved *(right)*.

chemia and loss of that limb may occur if adequate circulation is not restored. Distal cyanosis, delayed capillary refill, deep pain, and neurologic deficits suggest vascular compromise but are relatively nonspecific signs in a severely burned extremity. Swelling and coolness of unburned skin distal to the burn are common but are not indications for surgical intervention.

Use of the Doppler ultrasonic flow probe greatly increases the accuracy of perfusion assessment and has reduced the need for escharotomy by as much as 50 percent. The posterior tibial and dorsalis pedis pulses in the lower extremities and the palmar arch pulses in the upper extremities should be assessed hourly. Disappearance of the Doppler signal or a progressive reduction of its intensity indicates vascular compromise and the need for decompression.

Burned extremities should be elevated immediately following injury and actively exercised for 5 min each hour. Such conservative measures will maintain adequate peripheral circulation in many patients with circumferential full-thickness extremity burns. If such measures fail, escharotomy is indicated. The eschar of involved extremities is incised along the midmedial and midlateral lines down to and just through the subdermal fascial attachments (Fig. 7-8). Inadvertent extension into the subcutaneous tissue results in copious bleeding and should be avoided (Fig. 7-9). This procedure is carried out at the bedside and requires no anesthesia since eschar is insensate. Pulses may not be restored in some patients with deep thermal burns or additional trauma below the level of the investing fascia. Fasciotomy is indicated in these patients, and usually should be carried out in the operating room after the patient is hemodynamically stabilized. Thoracic escharotomy may be necessary in a rare patient whose chest wall activity is restricted by an encircling deep third-degree burn. Escharotomy incisions should be covered with a topical antimicrobial agent. Excessive bleeding can be controlled by packing the escharotomy incision with gauze and temporarily wrapping the extremity with elastic bandages. After 2 to 3 h, these dressings can be removed.

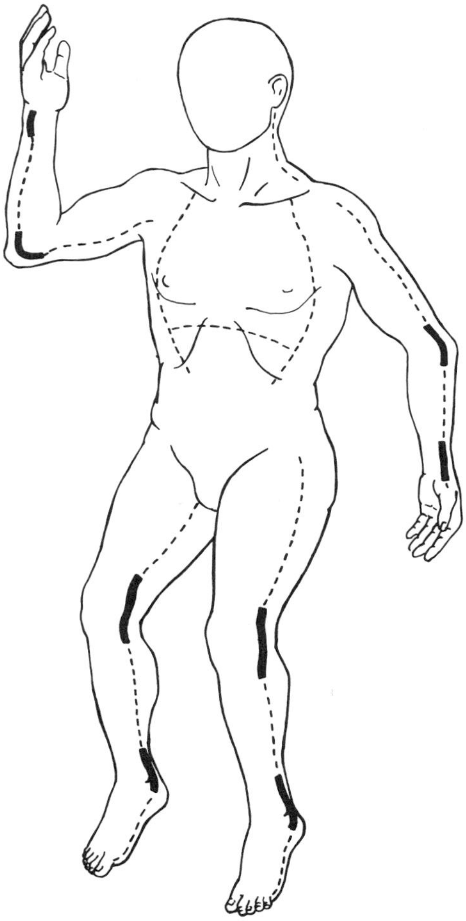

FIG. 7-8. Locations for escharotomy incisions. These incisions are placed along the midmedial and midlateral lines of the extremities. The skin is especially tight along major joints, and decompression at these sites must be complete. Chest and neck escharotomies rarely are needed.

OTHER SUPPORT MEASURES

Nasogastric Intubation. Ileus usually develops soon after injury in children with burns over 15 percent TBSA and in adults with burns over 20 percent TBSA. A nasogastric tube should be

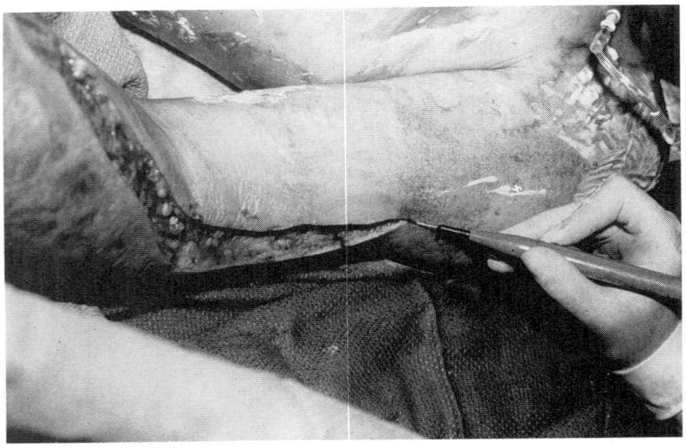

FIG. 7-9. The escharotomy incision extends through all cutaneous attachments just into the underlying subcutaneous tissue. Deeper incisions into the subcutaneous fat produce copious bleeding and do not further release the tight esochar. Electrocautery is especially useful for this procedure.

inserted until ileus resolves. Nasogastric intubation is particularly important for patients who require aeromedical evacuation. Decreasing ambient atmospheric pressure with increasing cabin altitude accentuates gastric dilatation and the risk of aspiration. Resolution of ileus is indicated by passage of flatus or stool. Bowel sounds may be present in the presence of gastric and colon ileus and are not reliable signs of adequate return of gastrointestinal function. Ileus is more severe and prolonged in patients with larger burns.

Pain Control. Burned patients are extremely sensitive to analgesics during the resuscitative phases. Small doses given frequently are safer than a single large dose. Burn treatment facilities should adopt a restricted number of narcotic agents and become familiar with their actions. The use of multiple agents leads to poor pain control and promotes treatment errors with these dangerous drugs. Morphine sulfate is an effective and cost-efficient agent. Immediately following injury, opioid analgesic potency is increased, sharing many of the features of stress-induced analgesia. Adults should be treated with 2 to 5 mg morphine in titrated doses each hour; children may require up to 0.1 mg/kg/h.

All drugs should be given intravenously during the resuscitative phase. Narcotics injected into the muscle or subcutaneous tissue in hypovolemic patients are not readily absorbed and accumulate with multiple doses until peripheral perfusion is reestablished. At that time, the multiple doses are rapidly absorbed into the circulation and profound and often fatal cardiovascular collapse occurs. Later in the postburn course, larger doses will be necessary to moderate burn-associated pain, and continuous infusion of morphine is especially effective. Supplemental doses are usually required for debridement procedures. Self-administration of nitrous oxide is also a useful adjunct during debridement procedures, as is ketamine administered in subanesthetic doses. Total elimination of pain in burned patients is not possible short of general anesthesia. All of these drugs compromise respiratory function and should be given only under the direct supervision by personnel skilled in airway control and respiratory support. The concomitant use of benzodiazepines, hypnosis, and psychological support promotes pain tolerance in burned patients and reduces narcotic requirements. During the convalescent phase, a regularly scheduled dose of an oral analgesic, such as methadone, produces more effective pain relief than unscheduled ''prn'' doses.

Antibiotics and Tetanus Prophylaxis. Prophylactic antibiotics are not used for in-hospital care of burned patients. Such use is associated with the emergence of organisms resistant to multiple antibiotics. Daily inspection of the burn will detect cellulitis surrounding the burn wound in its earliest stages and antibiotic therapy can be instituted safely at that time. Approximately 1 week following thermal injury, a 1- to 2-cm border of erythema often surrounds the margins of the burn; this erythema is usually caused by tissue reaction to wound breakdown products and does not represent bacterial infection. More diffuse erythema, especially if accompanied by edema with a peau d'orange appearance usually is due to gram-positive bacterial cellulitis and should be treated with appropriate antibiotics. Small burns in outpatients may be treated prophylactically with penicillin or a substitute antibiotic if the patient is allergic to penicillin. Before wound excision, antibiotics reflecting the resident bacterial population in the eschar are given on call to the operating room; these antibiotics are not strictly prophylactic since wound manipulation is associated with bacteremia in a large proportion of burned patients. Tetanus prophylaxis is based on the patient's prior immunization status and should proceed according to the guidelines established by the American College of Surgeons. If the patient's immunization status is unknown, both the toxoid and human immune globulin should be administered.

INHALATION INJURY

Pathophysiology. Cutaneous burns cause alterations of pulmonary physiology even in the absence of inhalation injury. Large volumes of fluid resuscitation necessary for the treatment of burn shock undoubtedly cause a modest increase in interstitial lung water. In humans without inhalation injury, abnormalities of pulmonary function and gas exchange are difficult to detect and probably have minimal clinical impact. In experimental models of thermal injury, cutaneous burns activate the complement system, which in turn initiates C5a-related chemotactic activity in the serum, transient neutropenia, sequestration of neutrophils in the pulmonary capillaries, and ultimately hydroxyl radical generation by the entrapped neutrophils. This sequence of events leads to increased pulmonary vascular permeability and morphologic changes indicative of endothelial damage and tissue edema and hemorrhage. Prostanoids and other mediators also participate in this response. The resulting decreased dynamic compliance appears to be due to mediator-induced bronchoconstriction; extravascular lung water does not increase significantly.

The occurrence of inhalation injury produces dramatic pathologic and physiologic effects in the lung. The extent of injury is related to the composition of inhaled gases, size of particulates, duration of toxicant exposure, and quantity of concomitant fluid administration. Short-term exposure to carbon monoxide produces no histologic changes. Aldehydes, particularly acrolein, cause pulmonary edema and large-airway injury. Other organic and inorganic acids, common combustible by-products of burning household goods, also produce airway and parenchymal injury. Particulates less than 0.05 μm in diameter are deposited in the terminal bronchioles and pulmonary parenchyma and in combination with combustion by-products provoke extensive damage.

Accumulation of edema and deterioration of lung function usually do not occur immediately but appear after several days following exposure. Lung edema is peribronchiolar and appears to be derived from the systemic, and not the pulmonary, circulation. In animal experiments bronchial artery ligation delays the onset and reduces the magnitude of edema formation. Many studies have shown that the microvascular permeability of the bronchial circulation is extremely sensitive to inflammation and that inhalation injury causes selective vasodilation of the entire airway systemic vasculature.

Histologically, inhalation injury produces edema, progressive necrotizing tracheobronchitis with pseudomembrane formation, and airway obstruction. This is accompanied by congestion, alveolar edema, atelectasis, and bronchopneumonia. Tissue repair of lung injury begins approximately 1 week following smoke inhalation. The reparative phase usually restores normal features to lung tissue but occasionally produces squamous metaplasia, intraalveolar fibrosis, and severe bronchiectasis. These latter events can severely compromise airway patency and pulmonary function.

Clinical Implications. The respiratory tract injury produced by smoke or toxic gas inhalation presents a major challenge to the burn center. Inhalation injury in the absence of cutaneous burns can be life-threatening and require long-term critical care unit resources. Combined cutaneous and pulmonary burns result in an extremely high fatality rate. In some large clinical series, the added presence of inhalation injury increases mortality tenfold when compared to equivalent-sized burns with no inhalation injury. Inhalation injury in burned patients is associated with a three- to fourfold prolongation in hospitalization, especially among the elderly, by increasing the incidence of pneumonia and accompanying mortality. In addition to age and burn size, the presence or absence of inhalation injury is the strongest predictor of outcome at the time of admission.

Up to one-third of hospitalized burn patients in large series have inhalation injury. It most often occurs in patients who have sustained their burns in an enclosed space. High concentrations of carbon monoxide and the toxic products of incomplete combustion are concentrated in such an environment, increasing the chances of pulmonary exposure and damage. Patients who have decreased mentation (from head trauma, alcohol or drug abuse) or who are comatose at the scene have prolonged exposure to smoke and suffer severe inhalation injury. Children tend to hide under beds and in closets during a house fire and often are difficult to locate and remove from the fire scene. Inhalation injury happens less frequently in open spaces, but may occur after explosions with noxious gases forced down the airway by the blast overpressure.

Carbon Monoxide Poisoning. Inhalation injury occurs in three basic forms alone or in combination: carbon monoxide poisoning, upper airway injury, and lower airway injury. Carbon monoxide is the major cause of hypoxia in fire-related deaths in urban environments. Eighty percent of deaths due to smoke inhalation result from carbon monoxide intoxication and asphyxia. Carbon monoxide is a colorless, odorless, and tasteless gas with an affinity for hemoglobin that is more than 200 times that for oxygen. It reduces the oxygen delivery capacity of blood, and causes a leftward shift of the oxyhemoglobin dissociation curve. Both of these effects reduce oxygen availability and cause hypoxia. Although carbon monoxide binds avidly to mitochondrial and cytoplasmic heme proteins and blocks electron transport in in vitro preparations, the role of this mechanism as a causative factor for toxic clinical manifestations has never been demonstrated. In unique animal model systems in which the blood has been replaced by perfluorocarbons, carbon monoxide exposure that would have been lethal in blood-perfused animals was well tolerated when perfused with oxygen-containing artificial blood. This study strongly suggests that the major mechanism for carbon monoxide toxicity is the impairment of oxygen delivery and not any cytotoxic action on heme-containing proteins.

The important clinical manifestations of severe carbon monoxide poisoning are related to the central nervous system and the heart. Mental obtundation roughly corresponds with the carboxyhemoglobin levels. Carboxyhemoglobin concentrations in excess of 60 percent usually are associated with coma and death. Many other medical conditions, however, can cause this degree of neurologic dysfunction, and carbon monoxide poisoning must be quantified by spectrophotometry before therapy is instituted (Table 7-13). Carbon monoxide concentrations should be measured in all victims of a fire environment.

Low carbon monoxide levels do not mean that inhalation injury in this environment has not occurred, and such patients require further airway evaluation. With prolonged carbon monoxide exposure, myocardial depression may be profound and unresponsive to fluid replacement and inotropic agents. Cardiac output remains low and is often followed by shock, acidosis, and death. The cherry-red skin color said to be characteristic of carbon monoxide poisoning is almost never observed in burn patients. A normal arterial partial pressure of oxygen (P_{O_2}) is not helpful because arterial oxygen tension may be quite high in the presence of dangerously low oxygen content of carbon monoxide-saturated hemoglobin. Optimal treatment of carbon monoxide poisoning consists of 100 percent oxygen administered either by a tight-fitting mask if the patient is conscious or by endotracheal intubation and mechanical ventilation if the patient is unconscious. The relative efficiencies of enriched oxygen environments are listed in Table 7-14. The role of hyperbaric oxygen in the treatment of carbon monoxide poisoning remains unclear. Its efficacy in accelerating carbon monoxide elimination is unquestioned; however, its superiority to 100 percent oxygen breathing for mitigating long-term neurologic

Table 7-13
Common Conditions Clinically Similar to Carbon Monoxide Intoxication in Burned Patients

Drug overdose
Alcohol intoxication
Uncontrolled diabetes
Insulin overdose
Acute head injury
Postictal state
Acute central nervous system infection
Acute psychotic reaction
Hypovolemic or septic shock

Table 7-14
The Effect of Increasing Oxygen Administration on Carbon Monoxide Elimination

O_2 Pressure (atm)	$T_{1/2}$ (Min)
0.21	240
1.0	40
3.0	25

sequelae and maintaining survival has never been demonstrated in controlled clinical trials. Hyperbaric oxygen, if immediately available, appears to be a reasonable choice for solitary carbon monoxide poisoning in the absence of other life-threatening diseases or injuries. The difficult logistics of using the chamber for burned patients usually outweighs the potential benefits because concurrent care of the burn and other associated injuries take priority in triage. Patients with thermal injuries and potential carbon monoxide poisoning should undergo initial assessment in a burn center. After stabilization, the triage of appropriate patients to the hyperbaric chamber then can be arranged.

Neuropsychiatric sequelae may persist in up to 10 percent of carbon monoxide-exposed patients. Several weeks after exposure, some patients develop a syndrome characterized by mental deterioration, urinary incontinence, and disturbance of gait. Computed tomography of the brain demonstrates bilateral areas of decreased density in the globus pallidus. Plum points out that this syndrome is not unique to carbon monoxide poisoning and that it is seen following other severe anoxic episodes in which the initial coma lasted more than 24 h. These neurologic symptoms do not respond to hyperbaric oxygen, whether it is administered for the initial hypoxic episode or for the relapse.

Upper Airway Burns. Burns of the upper airway include those involving the nasal cavity, pharynx, larynx, glottis, trachea, and larger bronchi (Table 7-15). Direct heat injury to the upper airway is rare because the heat-carrying capacity of dry air is quite low, and the heated air is rapidly cooled to body temperature as it passes through the nasopharyngeal area and upper airway. The heat capacity of steam is 4000 times that of dry air, and steam inhalation can cause direct thermal injury down to the alveoli. Reflex closure of the glottis occurs rapidly and prevents prolonged exposure. Nevertheless, steam inhalation usually is rapidly fatal, with death ensuing within 24 h. In the majority of cases of inhalation injury, injury results from chemical injury to the mucosal surfaces by the inhaled gases. The common products of incomplete combustion include cyanides, aldehydes, and hydrocarbons.

The presence of facial burns alerts the surgeon to the possibility of inhalation injury. Other signs and symptoms that corroborate the diagnosis include hoarseness, stridor, bronchorrhea, wheezing, carbonaceous sputum, singed nasal hair, and singed eyebrows. Diagnostic procedures should be carried out to define the extent of injury and to facilitate treatment. Fiberoptic bronchoscopy is readily available and the most reliable modality for the diagnosis and management of inhalation injury. In patients with potential obstruction of the upper airway, bronchoscopy is performed with the bronchoscope threaded through an endotracheal tube to ensure accurate and prompt placement of the endotracheal tube if severe supraglottic injury is observed (Fig. 7-10). Bronchoscopy should be carried out only after fluid resuscitation has begun and hypovolemia has been corrected. Bronchoscopy during the shock phase often leads to cardiac arrest and can lead to false-negative diagnosis in the damaged but unperfused bronchial mucosa.

Positive findings of injury viewed through the bronchoscope can be divided into mucosal and extramucosal lesions. Abnormalities of the mucosa include edema, erythema, blebs, and mucosal slough. Carbonaceous debris and bronchorrhea constitute extramucosal findings. Mild injury to the upper airways is accompanied commonly by some edema but no compromise of airway patency. Serial examinations may be necessary. If progressive edema is detected, nasotracheal intubation over the bronchoscope is performed. Mild injury of the upper airway usually requires the administration of warm, humidified oxygen and serial evaluation by the same observer. More severe injury can be managed temporarily in some patients with racemic epinephrine (0.5 mL in 2 mL normal saline administered by nebulizer every 4 h). Signs of advancing obstruction of the airway, especially in patients with large fluid requirements, mandate intubation. Maximal edema peaks 24 to 48 h after the initial insult, and the endotracheal tube is not removed until after the third postburn day and resolution of edema. Direct visualization of the patient's pharynx and larynx is performed with the bronchoscope prior to extubation to ascertain edema reduction.

Lower Airway Burns. Approximately 85 percent of patients with bronchoscopic evidence of injury to the large airways will have clinically important pulmonary parenchymal injury. Injury to the lower airway involves primarily the terminal bronchioles and alveoli (Fig. 7-11). In the absence of complication, the pulmonary parenchymal injury will heal in 7 to 10 days (see Table 7-15). These injuries result from the distal propagation of the products of incomplete combustion at the time of the fire. The structural lining cells are physically damaged and commonly slough, with obstruction of the small airways. In the alveoli, the immediately adjacent vascular endothelial cells may be injured and permit loss of intravascular fluid.

The primary complications are pneumonia, atelectasis, and pulmonary edema. Typically these complications are not clinically evident until some 4 to 7 days after the injury. Once this occurs, the subsequent mortality is approximately 60 percent. Xenon 133 ventilation-perfusion scans can be performed in patients suspected of inhalation injury. Unequal lung field radiation density and/or retention of radiolabeled gas in the lung field greater than 90 s

Table 7-15
Characteristics of the Three Major Presentations of Inhalation Injury

Injury	*Time of Onset*	*Duration*	*Complications*	*Therapy*
Supraglottic	0–24 h	48–72 h	Airway obstruction	Tracheal intubation
Upper airway	0–24 h	2–7 days	Airway debris; secondary infection with tracheobronchitis	Airway access & toilet with suctioning
Lower airway	4–7 days	Weeks	Pulmonary edema; bronchopneumonia	Mechanical ventilatory assistance

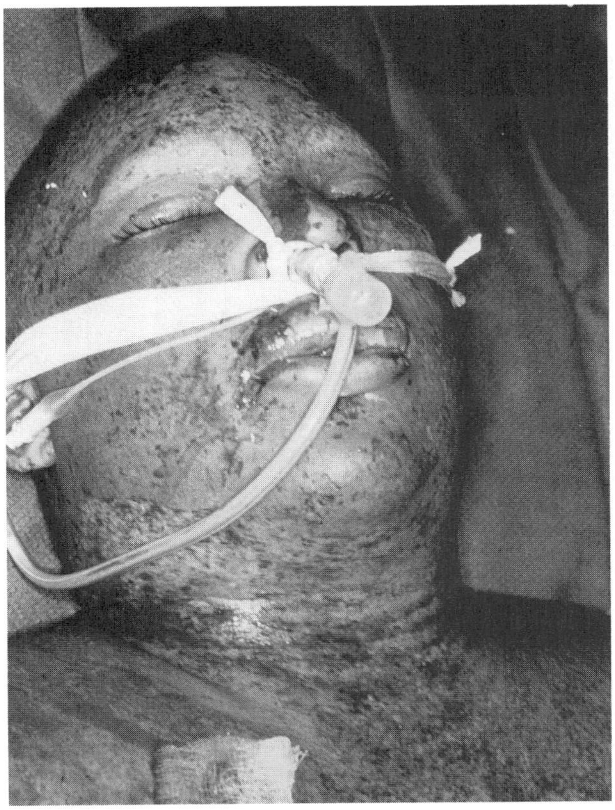

FIG. 7-10. Nasotracheal intubation during bronchoscopy in a patient with severe facial burns and upper airway injury. The tube is secured with cloth tapes that are tied around the patient's head. The use of adhesive tape in such patients is to be condemned, because the moist burn, denuding skin, and topical antimicrobial agent prevent long-term adherence of adhesives to burns, and accidental extubation in such a patient would likely be fatal.

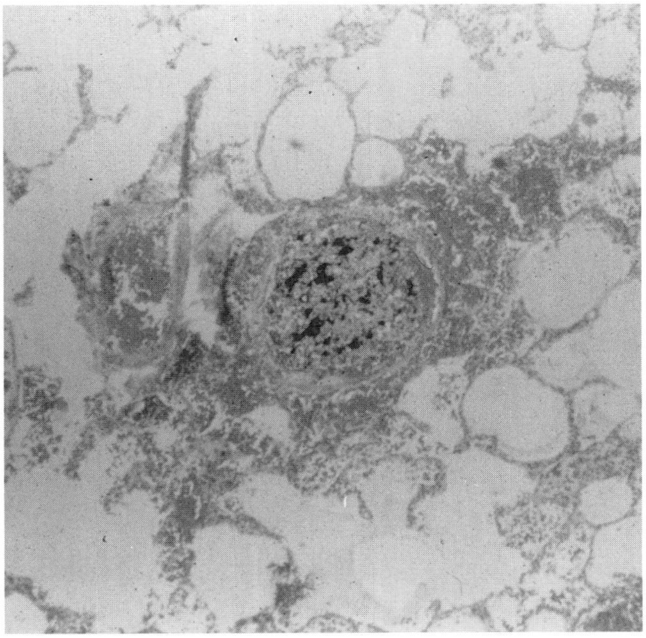

FIG. 7-11. Necrotic debris occluding a respiratory bronchiole in a patient with smoke inhalation and pulmonary parenchymal injury. The distal alveolar ducts and sacs are obstructed and eventually develop edema and infection. This inhalation injury is easily detected by xenon[133] ventilation-perfusion scintigraphy.

following peripheral vein injection of 10 mC of radiolabeled xenon constitutes a positive scan. This method has an accuracy of more than 9C percent and, when combined with fiberoptic bronchoscopy, has a diagnostic accuracy of more than 96 percent. It requires movement of severely ill patients to specialized nuclear medicine facilities.

Chest radiographs and arterial P_{O_2} often are usually normal on admission. Patients with parenchymal inhalation injury first demonstrate abnormalities on the chest film approximately 4 days following burn injury (Fig. 7-12). A P_{O_2} less than 60 mmHg on room air, or a P_{O_2} less than 300 mmHg on a fraction of inspired oxygen (F_{IO_2}) of 100 percent is a reliable indicator of inhalation injury, with an accuracy of 86 percent.

The treatment of patients with parenchymal inhalation injury is largely symptomatic. Patients without respiratory failure or airway obstruction are treated with frequent suctioning, incentive spirometry, and humidified, oxygen-enriched air. Prophylactic antibiotics, either aerosolized or systemic, are of no value and may result in the emergence of resistant organisms and subsequent infection. Similarly, the prophylactic administration of steroids has no effect on the course of inhalation injury and increases infectious complications. Inspissated exudates causing acute obstruction of the airway require emergent removal with a flexible or rigid bronchoscope. Once pneumonia develops, antibiotic treatment is based on sputum verification of infection and isolation of the offending organism. Surveillance respiratory cultures are valuable in allowing proper selection of antibiotics while awaiting definitive results of culture.

Acute respiratory failure is common in patients with inhalation injury, especially if the patient develops pneumonia. Mechanical ventilatory support in the adult is indicated by the following criteria of acute respiratory failure: respiratory rate greater than 40/min, an arterial oxygen tension less than 60 mmHg on an F_{IO_2} greater than 0.4, and an arterial partial pressure of carbon dioxide (P_{CO_2}) greater than 50 mmHg. Respiratory distress is a clinical diagnosis, and its appearance before the above criteria occur mandates ventilatory support in some patients. High-frequency percussive ventilation has demonstrated the ability to provide adequate oxygenation at lower inspired oxygen concentrations and lower peak and mean airway pressures and to produce better clearance of endobronchial secretions than conventional ventilation. Patients who respond to mechanical ventilation with positive end-expiratory pressure can be weaned from the ventilator during the second week after the burn if weaning parameters are met. If pulmonary infection supervenes in ventilated patients, a prolonged course of sepsis and respiratory failure is certain and the endotracheal tube should be replaced by tracheostomy in patients requiring intubation for longer than 1 to 2 weeks. Following extubation or decannulation, follow-up fiberoptic bronchoscopy to detect any persistent airway injury should be carried out routinely in most patients in whom the duration of intubation exceeds 10 days. Tracheal stenosis and granuloma formation are the most common lesions and sudden airway occlusion can occur if the compromised airway is not recognized.

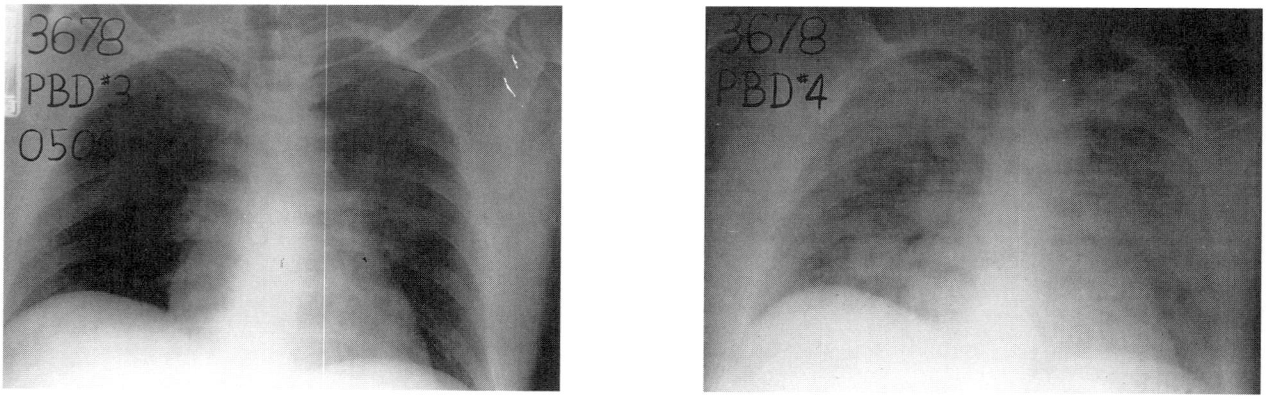

FIG. 7-12. Serial chest radiographs in a patient with inhalation injury documented on the day of admission by xenon[133] photoscintigraphy. Characteristically, the chest radiograph remained normal through the third postburn day (left). On the fourth postburn day, at a time when the patient was mobilizing wound edema fluid and losing weight, the chest radiograph demonstrated florid pulmonary edema (right). This patient later died of acute respiratory failure and bronchopneumonia.

WOUND CARE

Initial Debridement. Following stabilization of the airway and institution of fluid resuscitation, care of the burn wound begins. Except in chemical injuries, where prompt irrigation should be instituted as soon as possible, the burn wound in the newly admitted patient requires a relatively low priority for care. Initial wound debridement is best carried out in a specially designed wound treatment facility (''the tank room''). Such facilities should be capable of maintaining a warm environment and providing permanently mounted electronic monitoring facilities. Immersion in large tubs now is rarely employed; this form of therapy leads to large fluid shifts and acute electrolyte derangements, and hemodynamic decompensation in these immersion tubs is common. Custom-designed mobile stretchers, which can be individually sterilized and placed beneath longitudinal showers and heat shields, provide safe and convenient means to wash and debride the burn wound.

Although bullae may be left intact in outpatients with small burns, all bullae in hospitalized burned patients should be collapsed and debrided. Adherent tissue is sharply excised. Gentle scrubbing is effective for removing very fragile necrotic tissue, but total debridement of all nonviable tissue can be carried out over several days (Fig. 7-13). Once the initial debridement is completed, the burn diagram is filled out. The extent and depth of injured tissue is best evaluated at this time; earlier burn assessment, such as that in the emergency department, invariably leads to underestimation of burn severity. The burn wound should be bathed in an antibacterial detergent: chlorhexidine is the most effective agent for cleansing and decontaminating the burn wound. No resistance by colonizing bacteria has developed to chlorhexidine, nor has cross-resistance between this detergent and silver sulfadiazine developed. Chlorhexidine can damage the eyes, and great care must be taken to avoid ocular exposure. Finally, a topical antimicrobial burn cream is applied to the wound. This is most easily accomplished by spreading the cream by hand wearing ster-

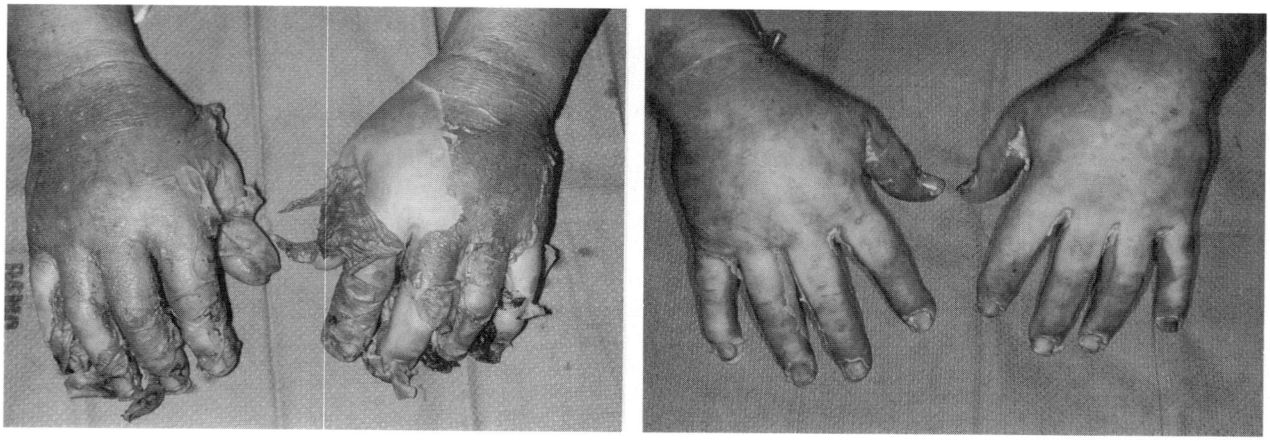

FIG. 7-13. Deep second-degree burns of the dorsal surface of the hands. Before debridement, necrotic tissue is loosely adherent to the underlying eschar or has spontaneously sloughed (left). Sharp debridement extends laterally to the unburned palmar margins, where the external skin layer becomes tightly adherent to underlying dermis. The pinkish-white color of the burns is indicative of a very deep dermal burn that will benefit from early excision and grafting (right).

ile gloves. Tongue blades are useful for applying burn cream to small areas.

Daily Care. The unhealed burn wound should be debrided and cleansed at least twice daily. The necrotic material removed at this time is the nonviable cheese-like surface of the burn. Only tissue that is spontaneously separating should be removed; attempts to remove adherent debris will cause further injury to partial-thickness burns and retard epithelialization. Occasionally, beneath a very thick full-thickness burn, subeschar collections of purulent material accumulate and require surgical unroofing to prevent invasive infection. This twice-daily wound care schedule allows the alternating use of several topical chemotherapeutic agents.

The wounds of all burned patients should be examined at least once daily, and more often if systemic signs of sepsis are present. Any prominent change in the appearance of the burn wound suggests infection (Fig. 7-14). Dark brown or violaceous discoloration of the wound and hemorrhage into the subeschar tissue are the most common signs of burn wound infection (although these signs most often prove to represent noninfectious lesions) (Table 7-16). The peripheral hemorrhagic infarcts of ecthyma gangrenosum are specific for *Pseudomonas* wound infection. Crusted serrations of the burn wound margin indicate viral infection. Biopsy is required for diagnosis (see below).

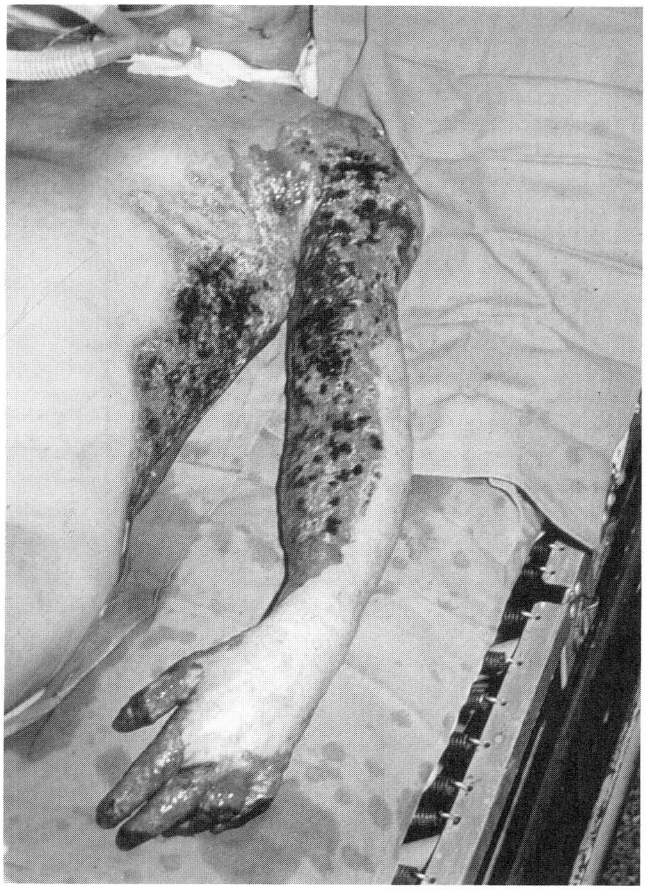

FIG. 7-14. Focal invasion by *Aspergillus* species in a chronic burn wound. This fungus produces sharply demarcated lesions, an appearance relatively unique for this organism. A burn wound biopsy should be placed through one of these nodules and adjacent unburned skin.

Burn Wound Infection. Thermal injury causes coagulation necrosis of the epidermis and of varying levels of the dermis and subcutaneous tissue. Potentially salvageable skin may undergo full-thickness necrosis if poor tissue perfusion or bacterial infection supervenes. Meticulous patient care can limit the extent of tissue loss. Once necrosis occurs, the wound is essentially avascular, which prevents effective delivery of systemic antibiotics if infection occurs. Damage to the cutaneous barrier allows bacterial penetration into viable tissue and subsequent infection.

The pattern of burn wound infection has changed over the past several decades and may be related to the proliferation of broad-spectrum antibiotics. Before the availability of penicillin, streptococci and staphylococci were the predominant organisms. By the late 1950s, gram-negative bacteria, primarily *Pseudomonas* species, emerged as the dominant organisms causing fatal wound infections in burned patients.

In general, all wounds become contaminated soon after injury with either the patient's endogenous flora or with the resident organisms in the treatment facility. Microbial species colonize the surface of the wound and may penetrate the avascular eschar. This event is without clinical significance. Bacterial proliferation may occur beneath the eschar at the viable-nonviable interface, leading to subeschar suppuration and separation of the eschar. In a few patients, microorganisms may breach this barrier and invade the underlying viable tissue, producing systemic sepsis. The burn wound is a potential portal for bacterial entry into the blood, and *P. aeruginosa* produces the prototypical lesion of invasive burn wound sepsis.

The essential pathologic feature of burn wound sepsis is invasion by the organism into viable tissue. The organisms then spread to the perivascular structures and directly invade the vessel wall, causing a capillaritis with subsequent vascular occlusion. Hemorrhagic necrosis of the surrounding tissue follows, and later the organisms gain entry into the bloodstream to produce metastatic lesions. In unburned tissue, metastatic *P. aeruginosa* results in ecthyma gangrenosum. Depending on the infecting agent, other histologic presentations may occur.

Any organism capable of invading tissue can produce burn wound sepsis. The predominant organism causing wound infection varies with each burn treatment facility. These facilities experience cyclical variations in the pattern of major offending organisms. Burn wound infection could be focal, multifocal, or generalized. Clinically, the likelihood of septicemia appears to increase as the area of burn wound involvement increases. Septicemia caused by an infected burn wound is less frequent in patients with focal

Table 7-16
Clinical Signs of Burn Wound Infection

Conversion of second-degree burn to full-thickness necrosis
Focal dark-brown or black discoloration of wound
Degeneration of wound with "neoeschar" formation
Unexpectedly rapid eschar separation
Hemorrhagic discoloration of subeschar fat
Erythematous or violaceous edematous wound margin
Metastatic septic lesions in unburned tissue (ecthyma gangrenosum)
Crusted serrations of wound margin
Green pigment in subcutaneous fat

invasion and multifocal invasion involving less than 20 percent TBSA. Generalized burn wound invasion is considered to be present when the infection involves areas exceeding 20 percent TBSA and is associated with a high frequency of septicemia.

Since the introduction of effective topical chemotherapy, fungal burn wound infection has increased and primarily involves highly invasive *Phycomycetes* and *Aspergillus* species. *Candida*, while frequently colonizing the wound surface, has little invasive potential and rarely causes burn wound sepsis. Viral infection, usually with herpes virus, affects partial-thickness wounds and is of clinical significance only when causing visceral lesions.

Monitoring Wound Infection. Certain groups of patients—children and those with burns larger than 30 percent TBSA or with multisystem organ failure—are more likely to develop invasive infection of the burn wound. The definitive diagnosis of burn wound infection can be made only by wound biopsy. Quantitative surface swab cultures are inaccurate and misleading. The wound should be prepared by mechanical cleansing. Antibacterial solutions and organic solvents should not be used, since these agents may destroy bacteria in the biopsy sample, producing a false-negative result. The biopsy should be sufficiently large so that portions can be evaluated by histologic and microbiologic methods. A wedge-shaped specimen must include not only the lesion-bearing eschar but also underlying or adjacent viable tissue in order to confirm the presence of microbial invasion (Figs. 7-15 and 7-16). Half of the specimen is placed in 10 percent formalin and subsequently processed by rapid frozen and fixed techniques. Bacteria are identified by Gram stain or hematoxylin-eosin stain and fungi by periodic acid-Schiff stain. Such processing can be completed in less than 3 to 4 h. The findings are graded on the basis of microbial involvement (Table 7-17), with the single most important sign of burn wound infection being the presence of microbial organisms in unburned viable tissue (Fig. 7-17). The remainder of the biopsy sample is sent to the microbiology laboratory for quantitative culture and for antimicrobial sensitivities. The

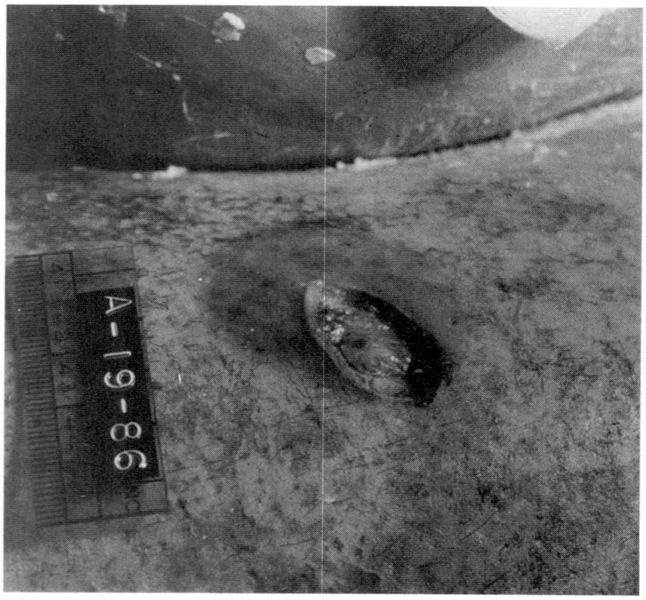

FIG. 7-15. Wedge-shaped defect produced by biopsy through an area of wound discoloration. The depth of the biopsy extends down to viable subcutaneous tissue.

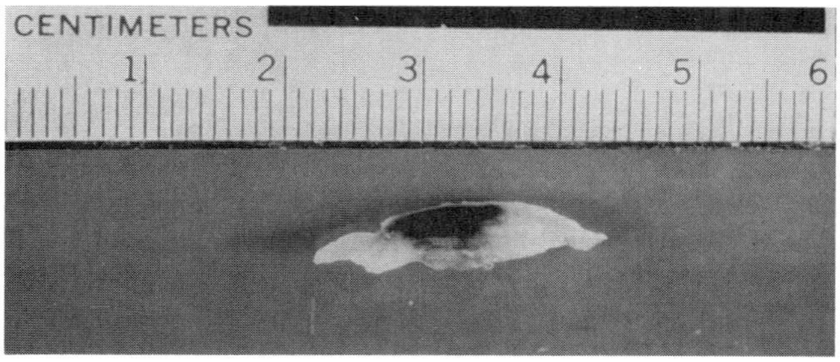

FIG. 7-16. Biopsy specimen of appropriate size for both histologic and microbiologic examination. This specimen should be bisected vertically through the middle of the dark zone and each position sent for appropriate evaluation.

recovery of more than 10^5 organisms per gram of tissue is highly suggestive of, but not diagnostic of, burn wound infection. Inappropriate selection of biopsy site in separated eschar and failure to include viable tissue may suggest infection when none exists. Similarly, lower counts may accompany histologically confirmed invasion and associated septicemia. When biopsy histology is not available, bacterial density greater than 10^5 organisms per gram of tissue with a concomitant positive blood culture with the same organism is a relatively reliable indicator of wound sepsis.

Topical Antimicrobial Chemotherapy. Before the introduction of effective topical antimicrobial agents, up to 60 percent of deaths in specialized burn treatment facilities were caused by burn wound sepsis. Each of the three agents with proven effectiveness has a wide spectrum of activity, is applied topically to the burn wound (Fig. 7-18), and has its own unique advantage and disadvantages (Table 7-18). All appear to be equally effective in controlling burn wound infection when applied early before heavy colonization has occurred. Only mafenide acetate is able to penetrate the eschar, and it is the only agent capable of suppressing dense bacterial proliferation beneath the eschar surface. Mafenide is especially effective against clostridia. The main disadvantage of mafenide acetate is its strong carbonic anhydrase inhibition, which

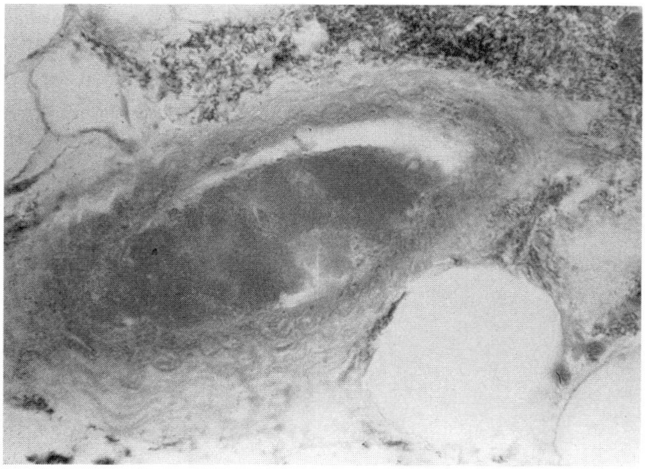

FIG. 7-17. Histologic appearance of bacterial burn wound invasion. Darkly staining gram-negative bacteria are invading viable subcutaneous fat and partially encompass a thrombosed blood vessel. Blood-borne spread of infection and focal ischemic necrosis promote rapid progression of burn wound sepsis and hemodynamic collapse.

Table 7-17
Histologic Indicators of Burn Wound Infection

Microorganisms in unburned tissue
Hemorrhage in unburned tissue
Marked inflammatory reaction in adjacent viable tissue
Small-vessel thrombosis or ischemic necrosis of unburned tissue
Perineural and intralymphatic migration of organisms
Vasculitis with perivascular "cuffing" of organisms
Intracellular viral inclusions

interferes with renal buffering mechanisms. Bicarbonate is wasted, chloride is retained, and the resulting hyperchloremia is compensated for by an increase in ventilation and subsequent respiratory alkalosis.

The primary disadvantages of silver sulfadiazine are its lack of eschar penetration and the development of bacterial resistance to its antibacterial actions. If bacterial density in the wound increases while silver sulfadiazine is being used, the agent must be discontinued and mafenide acetate, which can penetrate the eschar, substituted. Of greater concern is the increasing development of gram-negative bacterial resistance to this agent. The mode of resistance in some facilities is a transferable, multiple antibiotic-resistant plasmid with selective sulfonamide resistance. The use of silver sulfadiazine in these situations can lead to the selection of organisms that are resistant to all clinically available antibiotics.

Silver nitrate must be used soon after injury, before bacteria have proliferated on the wound. Although gram-positive organisms are slightly less susceptible to silver nitrate, true resistance does not develop. Its most serious disadvantages are the associated electrolyte imbalances, which are common, and methemoglobinemia formation, which is unusual. Methemoglobin may form in patients whose burns are colonized by nitrate-reducing bacteria. A two-log increase in bacterial density of surveillance biopsies dictates a change in topical agent. Cerium nitrate in a small number of clinical studies has been shown to be an effective topical antimicrobial drug and currently is undergoing clinical evaluation. No

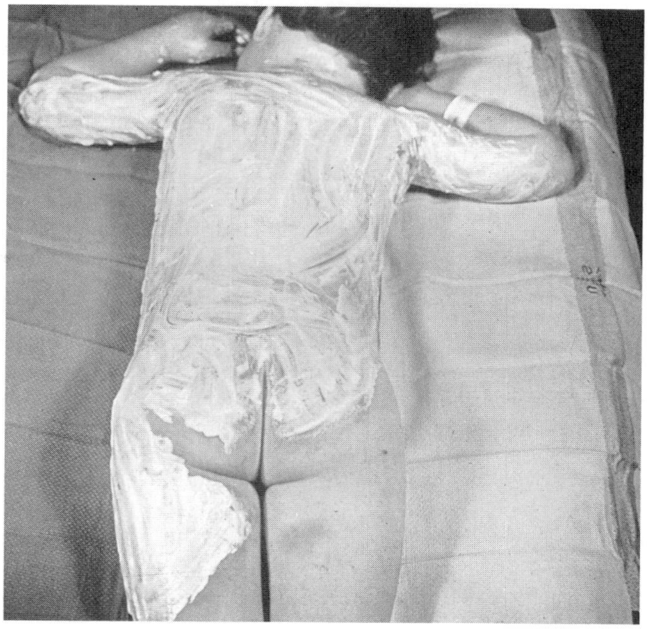

FIG. 7-18. Topical application of an antimicrobial agent to the surface of a burn. This cream is easily applied by the gloved hand from that patient's container. A thin layer of nonadherent synthetic "bridal veil" dressing placed over the burn cream prevents active patients from inadvertently removing the topical agent.

Table 7-18
Topical Antimicrobial Agents for Burn Wound Care

	Silver Nitrate	*Mafenide Acetate*	*Silver Sulfadiazine*
Active component	0.5% in aqueous solution	11.1% in water miscible base	1.0% in water miscible base
Spectrum of antibacterial activity	Gram-negative—good Gram-positive—good Yeast—good	Gram-negative—good Gram-positive—good Yeast—poor	Gram-negative—variable Gram-positive—good Yeast—good
Method of wound care	Occlusive dressings	Exposure	Exposure or single-layer dressings
Advantages	Painless No hypersensitivity reaction No gram-negative resistance Dressings reduce evaporative heat loss Greater effectiveness against yeasts	Penetrates eschar Wound appearance readily monitored Joint motion unrestricted No gram-negative resistance	Painless Wound appearance readily monitored when exposure method used Easily applied Joint motion unrestricted when exposure method used Greater effectiveness against yeasts
Disadvantages	Deficits of sodium, potassium, calcium, and chloride No eschar penetration Limitation of joint motion by dressings Methemoglobinemia—rare Argyria—rare Staining of environment and equipment	Painful on partial-thickness burns Susceptibility to acidosis as a result of carbonic anhydrase inhibition Hypersensitivity reactions in 7% of patients	Neutropenia and thrombocytopenia Hypersensitivity—infrequent Limited eschar penetration

other agents have demonstrated clinical efficacy in clinical trials of topical chemoprophylaxis of burn wounds.

Subeschar Clysis and Surgery. Although topical chemotherapeutic agents have significantly reduced the incidence of burn wound sepsis (Table 7-19), this complication continues to be an important major cause of mortality in patients with large burns. Once generalized burn wound sepsis has developed, the probability of survival is less than 10 percent. Subeschar infusion of antibiotics has been proposed to prevent or treat wound invasion in burn wounds that escape topical chemotherapeutic control. This therapeutic modality has been systemically examined in an established animal model of burn wound infection and subsequently in burned patients. In a strain of *P. aeruginosa* that predictably produces lethal burn wound sepsis, a range of antibiotics and routes of administration were evaluated. This organism was selected because *pseudomonal* wound infection remains a major wound-related source of sepsis. The organisms were sensitive by standard tube dilution techniques to carbenicillin, colistimethate, gentamicin, and neomycin. Only the semisynthetic penicillins, represented in this study by carbenicillin, when injected beneath the infected eschar, resulted in universal survival. The introduction of carbenicillin by the subeschar and subcutaneous routes appears to provide a depot from which sustained blood levels are maintained. The effectiveness of subeschar clysis was demonstrated in a clinical series of 19 consecutive patients who developed burn wound infection over a 2-year period. All patients had histologically proven burn wound invasion and were subsequently treated with subeschar clysis of carbenicillin. Five of 19 patients (26 percent) survived and were discharged from the hospital. Five additional patients died later without evidence of residual burn wound infection. Altogether, subeschar clysis eradicated burn wound invasion in 53 percent of treated patients.

Subeschar clysis is best used as adjunctive therapy in preparation of patients for eschar excision or as primary treatment for patients who are too unstable hemodynamically to tolerate surgical intervention. Once the diagnosis of bacterial burn wound invasion is confirmed, topical therapy is changed to mafenide acetate, which is capable of penetrating into underlying viable tissue. Appropriate systemic antibiotics are instituted, usually an aminoglycoside for control of gram-negative bacteria and an antibiotic effective against gram-positive bacteria. The invaded burn wound is treated directly by subeschar clysis of a semisynthetic penicillin, usually piperacillin. Even when mycotic burn wound invasion has occurred, subeschar clysis can be used since mixed mycotic/bacterial wound infection occurs in a proportion of these patients. Although focal infection may be totally eradicated by these interventions, excision of the infected wound is the definitive therapy of burn wound invasion. If localized infection is treated only by antimicrobial agents, the successful eradication of the invaded focus must be verified by biopsy and histologic examination. Generalized wound involvement in stable patients should be treated by surgical excision. The excised wound should be covered immediately with biologic dressings.

Table 7-19
Burn Wound Sepsis as a Cause of Death

	Autopsies Performed	*Autopsy Diagnosis of Burn Wound Sepsis No. (%)*
No topical chemotherapy	167	100 (60)
Topical chemotherapy	394	109 (28)

SOURCE: From: U.S. Army Institute of Surgical Research.

WOUND CLOSURE

Surgical Excision. Excision of the burn wound is indicated for full-thickness wounds and deep partial-thickness wounds, particularly in functionally important locations. Expedient closure of full-thickness wounds decreases the risk of infection, reduces pain, and allows aggressive and effective physical therapy, which results in a better functional recovery. Excision can be initiated once the patient has stabilized, resuscitation is complete, and fluid mobilization is in progress, 3 to 5 days after injury. Total excision of a large burn in a single procedure is associated with massive blood loss with no apparent advantage. The removal of burn eschar in order to avoid invasive burn wound infection is appealing; however, conclusive evidence of improved mortality rates with early excision has not been demonstrated in any population of burned patients.

The two most common techniques of early escharotomy include tangential excision and fascial excision. Tangential excision involves sequentially excising the eschar down to bleeding, viable tissue using a guarded dermatome. The excision is completed when viable dermis or healthy subcutaneous tissue is encountered. Intraoperative hemorrhage may be profuse with this procedure, and the amount of surface area excised is usually limited by this factor. We limit the extent of each surgical excision to 20 percent of the TBSA, blood loss equivalent to the patient's blood volume, or 2 h of operative time, unless the burn wound is invaded. Blood loss can be reduced with the use of tourniquets with extremity burns, and a healthy wound bed is demonstrated by the presence of moist, white dermis or bright yellow fat in the subdermal tissues.

Particularly deep wounds that involve the underlying fat may require fascial excision, especially if the wound is infected. Fascial excision is carried out using an electrocautery and tourniquet to limit the blood loss. Loss of body contour is inevitable with fascial excision, and this technique should be avoided when possible. After excision and hemostasis, split-thickness skin grafts are harvested using any of a variety of dermatomes. Donor skin thickness ranges from .010 to .012 inch and these grafts can be expanded using a Tanner-Vanderput mesh apparatus when large surface areas require coverage or when wound drainage is expected to be large. When adequate skin is available, sheet grafts may be used to achieve an improved appearance in cosmetically important areas. The grafts are secured into position using staples on the periphery, and adjacent grafts are joined with small vascular clips. The use of these clips avoids separation of adjacent grafts, which can result in hypertrophic scar formation at the site of separation.

If autograft is limited, the graft may be meshed $1\frac{1}{2}$ to 1, 2 to 1, 3 to 1, or 6 to 1, depending on the needs of the particular patient. When 3 to 1 or 6 to 1 autografts are required, the autografts are covered with $1\frac{1}{2}$ to 1 meshed homograft to protect the interstices until epithelialization has been achieved. The homograft subsequently sloughs when the autograft underneath has healed. If all available skin has been used, homograft can be applied to excised areas until previously used donor sites have healed and can be reharvested. This process usually requires 2 to 3 weeks before reharvesting can occur.

Biologic Wound Coverings. In large burns, closure of the wound is limited by available autograft, and biologic dressings are acceptable substitutes. Biologic dressings limit the growth and proliferation of bacteria present on the wound surface, prevent wound desiccation, and reduce evaporative water and heat loss from the wound. They also decrease exudative protein and red blood cell loss from the wound surface, mitigate wound pain, facilitate joint motion, and promote tissue angiogenesis.

Cadaver homograft (also called *allograft*), which will develop a blood supply from the underlying wound bed, is the most frequently used and effective biologic dressing and remains the "gold standard" when autograft is not available. All cadaver skin must be screened for transmissible diseases. Homograft can be used fresh or after cryopreservation for indefinite periods of time. Amnion is an alternative biologic dressing that can be obtained from the delivery room and is relatively inexpensive. It too must be screened for transmissible diseases. It promotes angiogenesis and improves patient comfort but now is rarely used. Cutaneous xenografts are available from a variety of species, and most commonly, porcine material is used in either fresh-frozen or lyophilized preparations. Xenograft is not as effective as allograft in reducing bacterial contamination. Capillary ingrowth does not occur with xenografts; rather, it is held in place by plasmatic circulation, but progressively degenerates and needs to be replaced. These biologic dressings can also be used as a test material to determine the readiness of a burn wound for autografting and as debriding dressings to prepare clean wounds.

Skin Substitutes. Skin substitutes were developed to surmount the limitations of biologic dressings, which include possible disease transmission, complex storage requirements, finite shelf life, and supply and demand. These substitutes can be categorized as epidermal, dermal, or a combination of the two.

Epidermal-Derived Tissue. Advances in tissue culture techniques over the past 20 years have enabled researchers to grow confluent sheets of epidermis in vitro suitable for grafting. In 1981, O'Conner et al. reported the successful use of autologous epithelial graft grown over a period of 3 weeks and applied to two burn patients. These grafts were reported to provide adequate coverage of full-thickness wounds without the need for underlying dermis. Several institutions since that time have had a limited experience using cultured autografts, with a "take" rate varying from 0 to 85 percent. The use of autologous epidermal sheets has also been limited by the obligatory waiting period of 3 weeks for growth of sufficient material. This prolonged wait delays timely surgery in patients with major burn injury. Long-range durability of these grafts due to the lack of anchoring fibrils and hemidesmisomes resulted in subsequent separation of the epidermal-dermal junction and severe scarring in many patients. Advantages of this technique over the use of widely meshed autograft have not been clearly established.

In a parallel effort, investigators have transplanted cultured allogeneic epidermis using cadaver keratinocytes. This approach offers several advantages over an autologous system, including the ready availability of cultured grafts and avoidance of the obligatory 3-week waiting period. In addition, successful cryopreservation can make allogeneic epidermis available to other institutions without extensive tissue culture facilities. The epidermal cells grown according to this method stimulated the proliferation of allogeneic T lymphocytes in vitro and did not express histocompatibility transplantation antigens. Deep partial-thickness wounds, which traditionally are autografted, heal in an accelerated fashion when covered with cultured allogeneic grafts. The transplanted allogeneic cells fail to adhere on full-thickness wounds. Using DNA fingerprinting techniques allogeneic grafts were shown not to persist on partial-thickness wounds, but rather are replaced by the patient's own skin cells. The clinical observation of improved healing with these grafts on partial-thickness wounds appears unrelated to the "take" of the transplanted cells on the wound and the beneficial effect may be related to the presence of growth factors in the culture system. Further studies are necessary in order to determine the clinical role for these grafts.

Dermal Substitutes. A dermal sheet matrix comprised of a collagen matrix enriched with chondroitin-6-sulfate and a Silastic epidermal analogue has been used as a bilaminate skin substitute. When granulation tissue ingrowth has produced adequate vascularization of the dermal analogue of that skin substitute, the Silastic membrane is removed and the wound closed by direct application of a thin split-thickness skin graft to the underlying vascularized collagen dermal analogue. The exogenous collagen apparently is replaced by host tissue. It was used in a prospective randomized trial in 149 patients, with an 80 percent "take" rate as compared to 95 percent "take" rate with autograft. In the majority of the cases, the dermal matrix covered by thin autograft was as effective as the wounds covered with traditional autograft of .010 to .012 inch thickness. This material is not currently available for further evaluation or clinical use.

A biodegradable matrix composed of polyglycolic acid populated with cultured human fibroblasts also has been evaluated. Both layers are allowed to be incorporated into the wound bed and subsequent epithelialization of the interstices occurs over the viable dermal structure. Others have used allograft cadaver skin after having removed the epidermal layer; the dermal remnant on the wound serves as a recipient layer for cultured keratinocytes or thin autograft. Since the dermal layer is relatively nonimmunogenic, it appears to persist. Clinical experience with the use of dermal equivalents has been limited and further study is necessary to determine its beneficial effects. The goal of burn wound care is completion of wound coverage with a combination dressing of epithelium and dermis in order to prevent scar contracture.

Donor Sites. Donor sites are surgically created, superficial partial-thickness wounds that usually heal within 2 weeks of procurement. Donor site dressings that create a moist environment result in optimal healing. Expedient rates of healing and decreased pain associated with these dressings occurs without any evidence of clinical infection. In addition, the exudates collected from beneath these dressings stimulate the proliferation of epidermal cells in culture when examined by multiparameter flow cytometric analysis.

One occlusive dressing is a bilaminate membrane consisting of an outer layer of silicone rubber bonded to a fine-knit, flexible, nylon fabric, is semipermeable, and allows water vapor to escape from the wound surface. It appears to work best on the scalp and back, where continuous pressure can be applied. The specific dressing used must be tailored to the anatomic location of the donor site. Occlusive dressings with adhesive margins require a 1-½inch border around the donor site to secure the dressing and they result in fluid accumulation underneath the dressing. When a border is unavailable due to adjacent burns or when leakage of fluid causes patient discomfort, other dressings must be chosen. A large variety of these dressings achieve comparable results by similarly creating a moist environment.

Growth Factors. Growth factors are being investigated actively as potential accelerants for wound healing. Epidermal growth factor has been reported to increase the epithelialization of human graft donor sites; however, when these results are compared to occluded donor sites, there does not appear to be any advantage in healing time. Growth factors have been shown to be present within the exudate of wound fluid beneath occlusive dressings, which may represent a potential mechanism for the increased rate of healing observed with these dressings. Human growth hormones administered systemically to burned children also appear to increase healing of donor sites and to shorten hospital stay. Further studies with proper controls are required to evaluate the topical and systemic use of growth factors on the healing of partial-thickness wounds.

Special Burns. ***Eye Lids.*** Burns to the eyelid can result in contraction and ectropion formation, which results in exposure of the cornea. Release of the ectropion and application of skin grafts are necessary to avoid the consequences of the exposed cornea. The ectropion can result from either extrinsic or intrinsic causes. Extrinsic causes such as facial and neck burn scar contractures are corrected first if present. If there is burn injury to the eyelid with associated contracture then lid release is carried out. Initially the eye surface is protected by Bell's phenomenon, in which the globe spontaneously rotates upward and behind the shortened lid when the patient sleeps.

Operative correction of the ectropion is indicated when conjunctivitis, keratitis, or corneal ulceration develops. The lid must be overcorrected to anticipate the inevitable graft contraction that can lead to subsequent reexposure of the cornea. Therefore, upper and lower lids are not released at the same time to facilitate overcorrection. The release should extend beyond the medial and lateral canthi. Full-thickness grafts obtained from the posterior auricular area minimize subsequent contraction. Secretions from eyes with corneal defects should be cultured. Ophthalmic ointment containing an antibiotic active against both gram-positive and gram-negative species, including *Pseudomonas*, is applied until corneal injury has healed.

Scalp. Full-thickness burns of the scalp that extend down to the periosteum can be treated with split-thickness grafts as long as the periosteum is viable. Deeper injuries destroying the periosteum require debridement of the outer table of the calvarium. Granulation tissue is rapidly produced from the diploe, which are subsequently skin grafted. After maturation of the wounds, tissue expanders can be used effectively to remove healed areas of alopecia with expansion of full-thickness scalp and enclosure of the previously covered wound. Rotation of full-thickness flaps also can be used to cover denuded and exposed bone.

Facial Burns. Deep wounds of the face require grafting, and usually this is carried out approximately 10 days after injury, when it is clear that deep wounds are present and will result in hypertrophic scar formation or complete skin loss. Skin grafts are placed as aesthetic units when possible (Figs. 7-19 and 7-20). Grafts to the face are best staged with excision and homograft application applied during the first stage and definitive autograft during the second stage. The homograft tests the recipient site for adequate take and avoids loss of subsequent autograft, which can be devastating on the face. Split-thickness skin grafts are successfully used for the forehead, but thick sheet grafts provide superior results over the cheeks. Flaps generally are not used on the face because of the inherent lack of facial expression and the obscuring of the angles and contours of the face. Split-thickness skin grafts for the forehead are harvested from the scalp or supraclavicular areas to obtain the best color match. Alternatively, skin from the neck enlarged with tissue expanders can be used to cover burns of the cheeks. A Uvex mask is molded in the operating room and used postoperatively when the grafts are secure in order to retard hypertrophic scar formation.

Hand Burns. Deep burns to the hands can result in shortening of the collateral ligaments and when combined with proximal interphalangeal flexion, wrist flexion, and distal interphalangeal flexion, classic claw deformity occurs. This deformity must be counteracted by splinting the hand in the anticlaw position using thermoplastic material. The proximal interphalangeal joints are kept straight and the metacarpophalangeal joints flexed. Rapid coverage of the wound with skin can lead to early rehabilitation

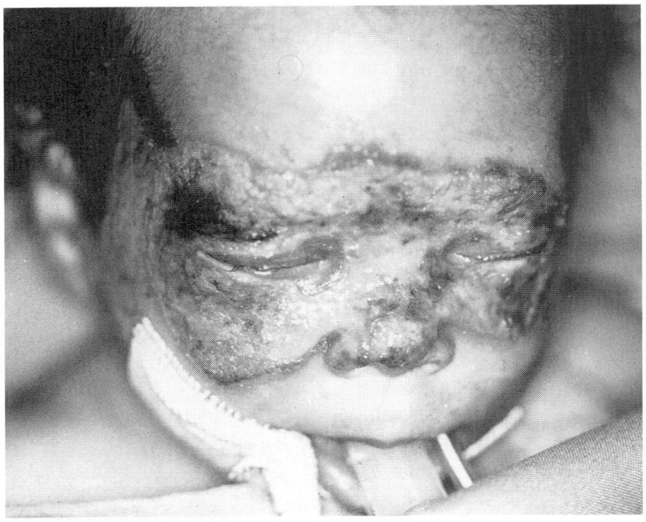

FIG. 7-19. Two-month-old child who rolled onto a radiator. This third-degree burn spared the eyelid margins, an important consideration for planning surgical intervention.

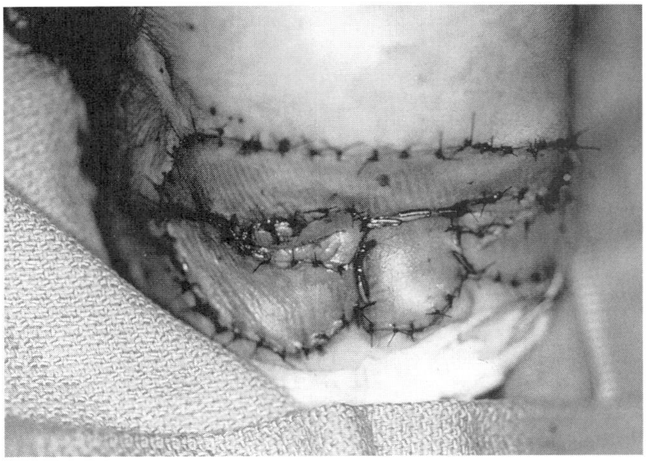

FIG. 7-20. Same child as in Fig. 7-19 following burn excision and thick split-thickness skin grafting. Where possible, the sheet grafts were placed as aesthetic units.

(Fig. 7-21). Split-thickness skin grafts are used for the dorsum of the hand; however, full-thickness grafts may be necessary for palmar burns, which are relatively unusual.

METABOLISM

The metabolic response to major thermal injury is manifested as a biphasic response, as originally described by Cuthbertson for other forms of trauma. The *ebb* phase begins immediately following the burn injury and is characterized by hypotension, decreased intravascular volume, decreased total-body blood flow, poor tissue perfusion, and generalized hemodynamic instability. Although loss of intravascular volume into the injured tissues can explain the majority of this initial response, neurohumoral mechanisms play an important role in burn injury, since the initial fall in cardiac output is extremely rapid, and occurs before major loss of intravascular volume. As described above, histamine, activated complement factors, oxidants, and prostanoids appear to be the major mediators of this phase of the injury response. Metabolic expenditure measured at this time documents a general hypometabolic state, with a decrease in total-body oxygen consumption below normal levels.

Following successful resuscitation, the patient enters the *flow* phase of the physiologic response to trauma. This response is related to the severity of injury but may be altered by intervening infection. In the burned patient, cardiac output is restored to normal between the first and second postburn days and rises between the fifth and tenth postburn days to a plateau approximately two to two and one-half times that of the resting state for uninjured individuals. The concomitant hypermetabolic response is characterized by a large increase in metabolic expenditure, erosion of body mass, abnormal substrate utilization, increased heat elimination, and weight loss.

Hypermetabolism. In parallel with the increase in total-body blood flow, metabolic rate begins to rise during the flow phase and plateaus at levels of two to two and one-half times that for the uninjured individual. The magnitude of this response is proportional to the size of thermal injury and increases in a linear fashion with increasing burn size. The increased metabolic expenditure remains relatively constant over the next few weeks until the burn wound either spontaneously heals or is closed by skin grafting. Although early excision of the burn wound prevents the hypermetabolic response in animal models, excision of the burn and wound closure in patients at any time postburn does not alter the natural course of the metabolic response to injury. The patient remains hypermetabolic for as long as wound healing continues, and subsurface remodeling and contraction after wound closure presents clinically as a hyperemic, immature wound. Studies indicate that the increased metabolic rate persists as long as the wound is hyperemic and immature and only declines to normal values when the wound is fully mature and blanched. Thus, increased nutritional support must be continued even after closure of the wound surface.

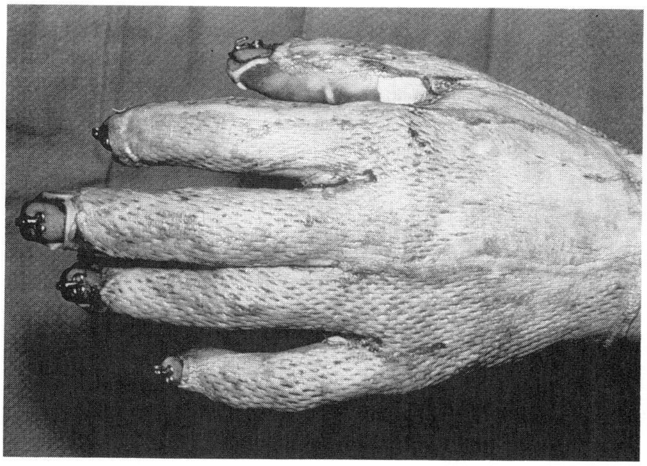

FIG. 7-21. Meshed split-thickness skin grafting of a dorsal hand burn. The fingernail hooks are attached with an epoxy glue and are used to maintain dynamic finger traction while the hand is splinted. The use of sheet grafts in patients with ample donor sites avoids the tiny permanent scars of the mesh pattern, but subgraft fluid accumulations remain undrained.

Erosion of Body Mass. Nitrogen loss increases following thermal injury, and 80 to 90 percent of nitrogen appears in the urine as urea, which may exceed 40 g/day in alimented patients with severe burns. The amount of nitrogen excreted in the urine is directly proportional to the metabolic rate of the patient. Skin losses of nitrogen through the burn wound may account for 20 to 25 percent of total daily nitrogen losses.

Over a wide range of metabolic responses varying from that of normal subjects to those of severely burned patients, body protein contributes a constant 15 to 20 percent of energy required to meet metabolic needs. Measurement of whole-body protein turnover in burned patients indicates that although protein breakdown proceeds at accelerated rates, protein synthesis also occurs, albeit at slower rates. Alterations in nitrogen economy in regional organ beds are reflected by changes in nitrogen transfer as amino acids. Following severe burns, peripheral amino acids, principally alanine and glutamine, are released in increased quantities into the circulation. Alanine appears to act as a carrier of nitrogen from muscle to liver and is derived from the transamination of pyruvate by branched-chain amino acids. Skeletal muscle is a primary source of nitrogen loss in the urine, and muscle proteolysis is reflected by the increased excretion of creatinine and 3-methylhistidine. Glutamine is a major precursor for renal ammoniogenesis.

This increased nitrogen exertion in the unalimented patient is paralleled by a decrease in lean body mass and weight loss. Whereas weight loss is only minimal in patients with a small burn, approximately 5 percent of body weight for a 10 percent burn, for patients with massive burns it can be enormous. In burns exceeding 40 percent of body surface, weight losses exceeding 30 percent of preinjury weight can occur with the first few weeks following injury if nutritional support is not provided.

Circulatory Changes. As noted earlier, cardiac output and oxygen utilization in the hypermetabolic patient nearly double. The proportional rise in cardiac output is slightly larger than the increase in oxygen consumption, and as a result, the difference between arterial and mixed venous oxygen concentrations moderately narrows in the stable, noninfected burned patient. Regional blood flow to the visceral organs generally increases, but this increase is proportional to the overall elevated blood flow, and the fractional oxygen extraction by the liver, kidneys, and other abdominal viscera remains approximately unchanged. Also, the fraction of oxygen consumed by each organ maintains approximately the same proportion as before injury. Muscle and neural tissue do not appear to participate in this response. Muscle blood flow and muscle oxygen consumption remain unchanged following severe thermal injury. This response is quite unexpected, since muscle mass has an important role in substrate homeostasis in the thermally injured patient. Similarly, blood flow and oxygen utilization by the brain, and presumably other neural tissue, are not affected by the presence of the burn.

The burn wound elicits an entirely different response. Blood flow to the wound increases massively, exceeding by over ten times the blood flow to an equivalent area of uninjured skin. Further, the wound itself utilizes little or no oxygen for its metabolic processes and appears to be essentially an anaerobic organ. Large amounts of glucose are consumed by the wound and comparable amounts of lactate and pyruvate are produced. Thus, the wound preferentially utilizes anaerobic glycolytic pathways, which are inefficient for energy production, and the increased blood flow to the wound appears to be necessary to provide adequate glucose substrate for the energy requirements of wound healing. The wound vasculature appears to respond only to hydraulic forces. It appears to be denervated, with a loss of both neurogenic vasoconstrictor tone and active reflex vasoconstriction.

Thus, during clinical episodes of hypovolemia and reduced cardiac output, blood flow to the wound passively decreases, predisposing the healing wound to infection and necrosis of poorly perfused tissues. This increase in blood flow without a concomitant increase in oxygen extraction is most likely responsible for the systemic narrowing of arterial to mixed venous oxygen content difference. Technically, the wound acts as a localized shunt, but in this case, the decreased oxygen extraction does not reflect derangement of organ distribution of blood flow and substrate utilization. Conversely, normalization of the difference between arterial and mixed venous oxygen content in the burned patient often may be a premonitory sign of an impending low flow state and patient decompensation.

Altered Thermoregulation. With the onset of postburn hypermetabolism, heat production is elevated, and burned patients commonly exhibit elevated core and skin temperatures and higher core to skin heat transfer coefficients. Central thermoregulation appears to be altered in burned patients, with an upward shift of the temperature of maximal comfort and least metabolic expenditure. For burned patients, this zone of thermal neutrality appears to be between 31° and 33°C and these patients seem to be internally warm and not externally cold. Attempts to modulate the hypermetabolic response by externally heating thermally injured patients above temperatures of thermal neutrality do not decrease the metabolic rate. Inadvertent cooling of the burned patient, such as by failure to maintain an adequate environmental temperature, however, will increase metabolic rate substantially in those patients capable of this added physiologic stress (Fig. 7-22). However, for those patients already at the limits of their physiologic reserve, this added cold stress may precipitate cardiovascular collapse and death.

Evaporation of 1 mL water requires approximately 0.580 kcal heat. Since thermal injury abolishes the water vapor barrier of skin, evaporative water loss through the burn wound has been suggested as the etiology of the hypermetabolic response. Coverage of the burn wound with water-impermeable dressings under environmentally controlled conditions reduces evaporative water loss but produces only a modest reduction in metabolic rate. Although animal studies indicate that caloric intake increases metabolic response over that expected from the specific dynamic action of nutrients, such findings have not been demonstrated in burned patients. Only a small fraction of the hypermetabolic response can be ascribed to the endogenous specific dynamic action of accelerated protein breakdown. The Q_{10} of hyperpyrexia accounts for only a modest fraction of postburn hypermetabolism, and the augmented heat production following injury is a consequence of an elevated metabolic state, not of increased thermoregulatory drives.

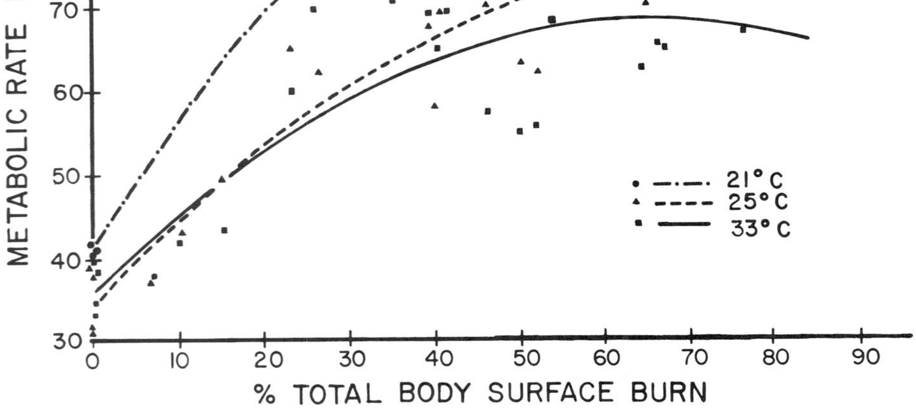

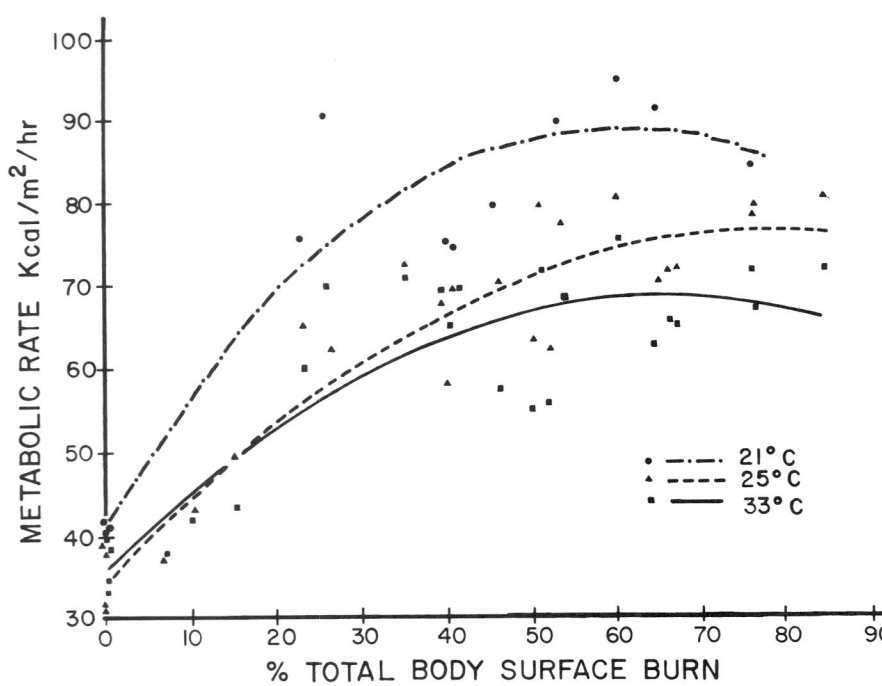

FIG. 7-22. The effect of environmental cooling on energy expenditure of burned patients. Metabolic rate is minimized at room temperatures at or above thermal neutrality for burned patients (31°C). Environmental cooling, such as by inappropriate use of room air conditioning, increases metabolic rate and physiologic stress and can precipitate unexpected decompensation.

Neuroendocrine-Mediator Response. The catecholamines appear to be the major endocrine mediators of the hypermetabolic response in the thermally injured patient. Catecholamine excretion correlates in a curvilinear fashion with the size of burn and with metabolic rate. Pharmacologic blockade of beta, but not alpha, receptors substantially diminishes the intensity of postburn hypermetabolism, including the increases in metabolic rate, respiratory rate, minute ventilation, and concentrations of free fatty acid. Conversely, infusion of beta receptor agonists produces a response that partially mimics postinjury hypermetabolism. Full beta receptor blockade, as verified by isoproterenol infusion, abolishes only a portion of the hypermetabolism, suggesting that other hormonal mediators are involved.

Although increased levels of thyroid hormones can produce hypermetabolism, such as occurs in hyperthyroid patients, these humoral agents are not elevated in patients with large burns. In burned patients, total thyronine (T3) and thyroxine (T4) concentrations are reduced, and reverse T3 concentrations are elevated. As such, thermal injury is another in the list of nonthyroidal illnesses that result in suppression of thyroid hormone. Free T3 and T4 concentrations fall to the lower range of normal or are slightly depressed in stable burned patients, and these moderate reductions in concentrations appear to be related to a burn-induced circulating inhibitor of the binding of T3 and T4 to transport proteins. Concentrations of free T3 and T4 fall markedly when burned patients become septic. That adequate thyroid function may be necessary to facilitate physiologic adaptation by severely burned patients to postinjury metabolic demands is demonstrated by the apparent relationship between plasma levels of T_3, T_4, and catecholamines.

Burn injury alters adrenal activity by abolishing the normal diurnal variations in glucocorticoid concentrations, but these hormones do not appear to influence metabolic activity directly and play only a permissive role with the cathecholamines. Adrenocorticotropic hormone (ACTH) does not correlate with burn size, and although cortisol does correlate with metabolic rate and postburn day, there is no connection between cortisol and thermogenesis. Glucagon concentrations are directly related to metabolic rate and cortisol concentrations and may also modulate resting metabolism by its anti-insulin effects.

Recent studies implicate several cytokines in the physiologic response to injury. During healing, the wound is populated by inflammatory cells, particularly monocytes and macrophages, which are important to the tissue repair process. Interleukins -1 (IL-1) and -6 (IL-6), tumor necrosis factor, and probably gamma interferon appear to be the dominant cytokines involved in both promoting wound healing and amplifying the hypermetabolic response. The cytokines individually increase oxygen consumption, cardiac output, heat production, and body temperature, while markedly reducing systemic vascular response. This response does not reflect sepsis; it continues unabated in the absence of bacteria in the wound and selective gut decontamination. Further, circulating levels of IL-1 and IL-6 are increased in stressed germ-free animals when compared to infected endotoxemic animals. Misinterpreting the hypermetabolic response to injury as infection, or even microbe, related leads to inadequate support or intentional mitigation of this altered physiologic state, often with increased morbidity and mortality.

NUTRITIONAL SUPPORT

Since the nutritional effects of the hypermetabolic response manifest primarily as exaggerated energy expenditure and massive nitrogen loss, nutritional support should be directed primarily toward provision of calories to match energy expenditure and of nitrogen to replace or support body protein stores.

Nutrient Selection. ***Carbohydrate.*** Carbohydrate, primarily in the form of glucose, appears to be the best source of nonprotein calories in the thermally injured patient. Certain tissues, including the burn wound, neural tissues, and the formed elements of the blood, utilize glucose in an obligatory fashion. Provision of glucose to these tissues occurs at the expense of lean body mass if adequate nutrition is not provided. In the unalimented state, the major sources of three carbon precursors for new glucose production by the liver are the wound and skeletal muscle. As described earlier, the wound utilizes glucose by anaerobic glycolytic pathways, producing large amounts of lactate as an end product. The wound meets its high glucose requirements by high glucose delivery rates, which are made possible by the enhanced circulation to the wound.

In the liver, lactate is extracted and utilized for new glucose production by the Cori cycle. Concomitantly, alanine, glutamine, and other glycogenic amino acids also contribute to increased gluconeogenesis. Increased ureagenesis, with urea ultimately derived from body protein stores, parallels the rise in hepatic glucose output. Peripheral amino acids and wound lactate account for approximately one-half to two-thirds of new glucose produced by the liver. The mild hyperglycemia characteristically observed in hypermetabolic burned patients is a consequence of accelerated glucose flow arising from increased hepatic glucose production, not from decreased peripheral utilization.

Since glucose that is obtained by gluconeogenic pathways is ultimately derived from protein stores, depletion of body protein during periods of starvation leads to energy deficits and malfunctioning of glucose-dependent energetic processes at the cellular level. Active transport mechanisms responsible for maintaining transmembrane ionic gradients in erythrocytes are deranged in catabolic, thermally injured patients. The abnormal sodium and potassium gradients in red cells can be reversed by providing these injured patients with high caloric levels of carbohydrate as glucose. Hepatic clearance of indocyanine green, an energy-dependent active transport process, is decreased in severely injured patients when energy normally supplied as glucose is replaced by an isocaloric glucose-free source. Glucose-insulin solutions correct the "sick cell syndrome" in burned patients, who exhibit a prompt natriuresis and nonosmotic diuresis when metabolic requirements are met by glucose.

Estimation of Calorie Requirements. The cornerstone of energy maintenance is the provision of calories as carbohydrates. A number of methods are available for estimating caloric requirements. Based on a comparison of percentage weight change with daily caloric consumption for adult patients with a wide range of burn sizes, ideal daily caloric intake can be calculated by the following formula: 25 kcal/kg body weight + 40 kcal/% TBSA burned. More frequently used is the Harris-Benedict equation, which predicts basal energy expenditure; a multiple of this equation is used to estimate energy needs in burned patients. Daily caloric intake for patients with extensive burns may be estimated quite conveniently as 2000 to 2200 kcal/m^2 TBSA burned. In those few patients with difficult nutritional management problems, indirect calorimetry can be measured at the bedside. Measured energy expenditure by this method is increased by an activity factor, usually 25 percent of resting expenditure for most burned patients.

Nitrogen. The combination of glucose with nitrogen-containing nutrients improves nitrogen balance and allows more calories to be utilized for the restoration of nitrogen balance than would be the case if either nutrient group were used alone. Energy and protein thus cooperatively contribute to this improvement in protein economy. Following injury, the individual effects of glucose and amino acids on nitrogen equilibrium appear to operate by at least two different mechanisms. Amino acid administration promotes synthesis of visceral and muscle protein without affecting the rate of protein breakdown. Glucose retards whole-body protein breakdown and decreases the total amino acid pool but exerts little effect on protein synthesis. Both mechanisms improve nitrogen balance, and both glucose and nitrogen should be components of the nutritional regiment for the severely burned catabolic patient.

The unique importance of glutamine as a fuel source has been recently recognized. The gastrointestinal tract uses glutamine as a respiratory energy source and disposes of the majority of glutamine as ammonia, urea, and citrulline. The alanine generated from glutamine in the intestine and kidney is used for gluconeocentesis. During critical illness, circulating concentrations of glutamine fall, and supplemental glutamine is required to meet gastrointestinal energy requirements. While glutamine can be supplied easily by the enteral route, parenteral preparations are not routinely available.

Fat. The role of fat as a source of nonprotein calories is dependent on the extent of injury and the associated hypermetabolic response. When hypercaloric diets that do not contain nitrogen are administered, carbohydrate is more effective in sparing body protein than is fat when each calorie source is used alone. The reduction in nitrogen excretion by parenteral fat emulsions is accounted for solely by the glycerol content of the fat emulsions. In patients with small burns and a moderate rise in metabolic expenditure, fat and carbohydrates, when combined with protein, produce equal improvements in nitrogen balance. Such is not the case, however, in patients with large thermal injuries. In these severely hypermetabolic patients receiving constant doses of amino acid, carbohydrate decreases nitrogen exertion, but equal caloric doses of fat (as lipid emulsions) fail to exert a similar effect. In contrast to the response of starved-adapted patients, the signals that increase skeletal muscle proteolysis and gluconeogenesis in hypermetabolic burned patients override the ability to adapt to starvation by causing ketosis, decreasing nitrogen excretion, reducing energy expenditure, and utilizing lipid substrate.

Thus, fat appears to be a poor calorie source for the maintenance of nitrogen equilibrium and lean body mass in hypermetabolic patients with large burns. Patients with only moderate elevations of metabolic rate can utilize lipid calories more efficiently; however, such individuals rarely require parenteral nutrition, and most table foods and defined formula diets contain all necessary fat nutrients.

When fat is omitted from enteral and parenteral solutions, essential fatty acid deficiency may develop after prolonged nutritional therapy. Patients with this deficiency have dermatitis, hemolytic anemia, thrombocytopenia, impaired wound healing, loss of hair, and early death. Although no precise requirement is known, 2 to 4 percent of daily energy requirements should consist of linoleic acid. This can be accomplished easily by weekly administration of 1 L lipid emulsion to patients receiving parenteral support and by the addition of safflower oil to the enteral solution of patients receiving nutrition by this route. Recently, diets containing fish oils (eicosapentanoic acid) have been shown in experimental models of thermal injury to produce less weight loss, better preservation of skeletal muscle mass, and lower resting metabolic expenditure. Small trials in burned patients appear to confirm these initial findings.

Vitamins and Minerals. Vitamin requirements in critically ill, hypermetabolic burned patients remain poorly defined. The fat-soluble vitamins (A, D, E, and K) are stored in fat depots and are slowly depleted during prolonged feeding of solutions that do not contain any vitamin formulations. The water-soluble vitamins (B-complex and C) are not stored in appreciable amounts and are depleted rapidly. Care must be taken to ensure that all vitamins are supplemented. The dosage guidelines recommended by the National Advisory Group/American Medical Association (NAG/AMA) are reasonable for burned patients unless symptoms of deficiency occur. Ascorbic acid plays an essential role in wound repair and plasma levels are frequently depressed in burned patients. Therefore, it seems prudent to supplement the NAG/AMA formulation with 250 to 500 mg vitamin C daily. Larger doses may cause diarrhea and formation of renal stones and will interfere with laboratory studies. Excessive doses of vitamins A and D produce toxic symptoms, and monitoring of serum levels is misleading when the concentrations of the vitamin carrier proteins are decreased, as commonly occurs in critically ill patients.

Mineral balance plays an important role in the administration of nutrients and their utilization for metabolic processes. Frequent determinations of serum sodium, potassium, chloride, calcium, magnesium, and phosphorus are the best clinical guides to electrolyte replacement. Less is known about trace metal requirements following thermal injury. Zinc is an important cofactor in wound repair, and zinc deficiency has been documented in burned patients. Following injury in an animal model, zinc and other trace metals seem necessary for nitrogen retention, but these metals may only reflect nitrogen balance and have little direct implication. Periodic measurements of zinc, copper, manganese, and chromium provide the best guidelines for replacement dosages. Trace elements are present in varying concentrations as contaminants in amino acid parenteral solutions.

Administration of Nutrition. The goal of nutritional support in the severely burned patient is energy and nitrogen balance. These nutritional requirements can be calculated by the methods described earlier, and in most cases their successful utilization will meet energy expenditure and preserve lean body mass. Hypocaloric feedings result in continued loss of lean body mass and should not be used except during episodes of patient deterioration, when fluid, glucose, and osmolar tolerance are reduced. Supranormal caloric feedings often can be successfully administered to burned patients, but such a regimen does not improve nitrogen balance and promotes a number of associated complications. Most thermally injured patients are healthy before the time of injury, and a repletion nutrition program is not required. As these burned patients become stable, gain wound coverage, and return to normal activities, metabolic needs decrease, and diets that previously met only maintenance requirements now provide a positive balance of nitrogen and energy. At this time, such supranormal diets may be tolerated safely and allow the patient to restore lost fat and lean body mass. Attempts to meet the predicted nutritional requirements of severely burned patients during the period of resuscitation and hemodynamic instability usually are unsuccessful. Resuscitation is carried out by glucose-free balanced electrolyte solutions. The infusion of glucose at this time results in marked hyperglycemia. Ileus develops soon after injury and precludes the use of the gastrointestinal tract for either resuscitation or feeding. After 48 to 72 h, tissue fluid begins to be reabsorbed and nutritional support can begin.

Whenever possible, nutrients should be administered by the gastrointestinal route; parenteral nutrition should be reserved only for those patients with an inoperative gut. In patients with smaller burns (less than 30 percent TBSA) and no other complicating diseases, the gastrointestinal tract returns to functional status quickly following burn injury, within 24 to 72 h. When evidence of gut function, such as the passage of stool or flatus, is present, enteral feedings (either orally or by tube) can be instituted and quickly advanced to full requirements. Certain thermally injured patients, particularly those with massive burns (greater than 30 percent TBSA), the elderly, and those with inhalation injury or complicating diseases, experience a prolonged period of paralytic ileus following thermal injury, and bowel activity may not return until second postburn week. If gastrointestinal function has not returned in such a patient, parenteral feedings should be instituted within 3 to 5 days postburn. Administration of nutrients through the gastrointestinal tract may be only partially successful in some patients, and enteral intake can be supplemented by parenteral infusion.

Enteral feeding offers a number of advantages over parenteral feeding. Enteral nutrients appear to maintain the integrity of the gastrointestinal tract and reduce the incidence of bacterial translocation from the gut. An oral diet preserves gut mucosal mass and maintains digestive enzyme content, whereas parenteral feeding results in decreased mucosal cell turnover. Other studies have verified that oral feeding stimulates the gut to elaborate trophic hormones, particularly gastrin. Enteral calories initiate greater insulin release when compared with parenteral nutrition, and insulin appears to promote anabolism. A number of clinical studies have shown that institution of enteral feeding immediately after admission is both feasible and beneficial. This feeding technique blunts the intensity of the hypercatabolic response and more effectively maintains preinjury weight. Associated findings are decreased circulating concentrations of the counterregulatory hormones. This method was most successful in patients with small burns and usually failed in patients with large burns and inhalation injury.

Total parenteral nutrition should be instituted when the gastrointestinal tract proves inadequate to supply calories. Prolonged postresuscitation ileus, overuse of narcotics, and constipation are frequent causes of failure of successful enteral alimentation. Sepsis, which may occur at any time during hospitalization, is associated with ileus and severe glucose intolerance, and such symptoms initially may be the only evidence of this complication. Previously tolerated feedings often must be discontinued while hyperglycemia is being controlled and the patient is being resuscitated. Ileus commonly persists, and nutrition is reinstituted by the parenteral route, often requiring large doses of insulin. Late complications involving the gastrointestinal tract may preclude use of the gut and require parenteral alimentation to meet nutritional goals.

Ancillary Nutritional Support Measures. Metabolic expenditure can be minimized by blunting a variety of stressful stimuli. Thermally injured patients, particularly children, have difficulty maintaining body temperature in cold environments. Because of the apparent change in the hypothalamic set point of thermal neutrality, burned patients require higher ambient temperatures for comfort. The temperature of thermoneutrality is approximately 31°C, four degrees higher than that of normal subjects. Warming burned patients to this level decreases the metabolic rate and corresponding energy requirements (see Fig. 7-22). Thermal blankets, radiation reflectors, and heat lamps may be required to maintain the patient's temperature above 37°C.

Pain accompanies wound manipulation and other patient-care procedures. Such pain accentuates metabolic expenditure, and controlled administration of narcotics will reduce metabolic rate in such patients. Adequate analgesia and sedation should be provided so that patients will have periods of uninterrupted rest. Hypovolemia, dehydration, and sepsis are potent stimuli of catecholamine secretion and appropriate volume replacement and antibiotic administration should be utilized as indicated. Systemic infection accentuates erosion of body mass, and additional calories must be supplied to maintain nitrogen balance at the same level obtained before infection.

Human growth hormone increases nitrogen retention when administered with adequate calories in nitrogen. Improved nitrogen balance is reflected by increased retention of potassium, phosphorus, and amino acid. The actions of exogenous growth hormone appear to be mediated by the effects of increased insulin secretion on carbohydrate metabolism. Lack of activity promotes muscle wasting and atrophy. Vigorous physical therapy promotes preservation of muscle bulk, and supervised activity must be provided on a daily basis to all patients requiring prolonged hospitalization. Skeletal traction and air fluidized beds encourage immobility and loss of lean body mass; simple isometric exercises usually can be carried out by these patients. Wound care and expeditious wound closure are the most effective measures for limiting the injury and its metabolic sequelae.

Nutritional Assessment. Assessment of nutritional adequacy in thermally injured patients uses fairly straightforward indices, namely, daily weight, calorie count, and nitrogen balance determinations. Once the burned patient has mobilized edema fluid from the wound during the first postburn week, daily weight is the single most effective index of nutritional balance. Although body weight must be interpreted in the context of daily fluid balance, a progressive gain in body weight usually indicates a positive energy balance and an increase in body mass. Conversely, a steady loss of body weight indicates loss of body mass, particularly from tissue protein stores. Calorie counts furnish quantitative data for verifying energy and nitrogen balance. All burn centers should have the full-time services of clinical and research dieticians. Food on trays must be carefully weighed before and after presentation to the patients, and all parenteral fluid infusions must be assessed in terms of their caloric and nitrogen content. Measurements of nitrogen balance are relatively difficult to perform in burned patients, since a large percentage of nitrogen loss occurs through the burn wound. Such studies, however, are quite helpful in identifying the occasional patient who continues to lose body mass in spite of apparently adequate caloric support. The use of standard anthropometric methods are unreliable and are of no value in patients with massive burns. The various skinfold thickness indices often are meaningless since the areas to be assessed are often covered by thick eschar and underlying wound edema. Indices based on standard measurements of height and weight obviously cannot be applied to burned patients with multiple extremity amputations. Various indices of immunologic status and visceral protein pool may be markedly abnormal, but none has been demonstrated to accurately predict specific nutritional deficiencies or patient outcome.

INFECTION AND IMMUNITY

Infection remains the most frequent cause of death in burned patients (Fig. 7-23). Thermal injury causes severe immunosuppression, which is related to the size of the burn wound. Although a direct relation between specific immune defects and infection has yet to be established, it is likely that this global immunosuppression predisposes the burned patient to infection. Sepsis occurs when the balance of interactions between host and opportunistic organisms is altered unfavorably. Such factors as the creation of new portals of entry, altered host defenses, and exposure to potentially pathogenic and opportunistic organisms are important determinants of sepsis in burned patients.

Immunologic Alterations. Circulating phagocytes, principally neutrophils and macrophages, demonstrate major alterations in function following thermal injury. Decreased granulocyte chemotaxis correlates in a linear fashion with burn size. While neutrophil phagocytosis remains normal, intracellular killing of both gram-positive and gram-negative bacteria is decreased. This bactericidal defect is related to elevation of intracellular 3′:5′-cyclic adenosine monophosphate and is mediated by increased prostaglandin E_1 in neutrophils from burned subjects. After an initial decrease, bone marrow and splenic production of granulocytes and macrophages increases after burn injury. This increased production presumably is necessary to maintain increased demands for these myeloid cells placed on the host as a consequence of the initial response to injury. Once burned, removal of the wound does not alter the marrow or splenic response. Supervening infection is associated with a decline in colony stimulating factor and decreased proliferation of granulocyte-macrophage stem cells. The end result is leukopenia. Lactoferrin, a known inhibitor of colony stimulating factor, appears to mediate this process.

The complement system acts as an important nonspecific mediator of host defense, and burn injury is associated with abnormal activation of both the alternative and classic complement pathways. Activation of the alternative complement pathway appears to be dominant following thermal injury and is associated with increased neutrophil aggregating activity in plasma, neutrophil aggregates in the lung, and increased pulmonary vascular permeability. Neutrophil adhesion to microvascular endothelium can be inhibited by monoclonal antibodies directed against the leukocyte CD18 adhesion complex or its endothelial ligand, intercellular adhesion molecule (ICAM-1). This inhibition mitigates the increase in microvascular permeability and burn wound progression. Tissue damage also can activate the intrinsic coagulation and fibrinolytic system, which in turn leads to complement activation.

Defects in specific immunity are most profound in cell-mediated responses, which are under the control of T lymphocytes. Although initial clinical studies indicated that burn injury was associated with greater reduction of helper T cells than suppressor T cells and was predictive of septic death, later studies demonstrated that burn injury alone did not alter T-cell populations, and that selective depletion of helper T lymphocytes and a decrease in the ratio of helper to suppressor T cells occurred only after the advent of infection. This discrepancy was shown to be caused by contamination of the lymphocyte population by immature nonlymphoid cells, primarily granulocytes. After thermal injury, T-cell activation increases spontaneously and after interleukin-2 (IL-2) stimulation; concurrently, B-cell activation was significantly reduced. The number of T and B lymphocytes, however, remained unchanged in these burned patients. T-cell proliferative function is depressed in burned patients and is associated with an increase in serum factors that inhibit IL-2-mediated T-cell functions. Increased circulating soluble, cell-free IL-2 receptors explain, in part, the inhibited IL-2 response and do not appear to be a direct result of endotoxin exposure.

Predictors of Infection. Since most morbidity and mortality in severely burned patients is related to infection, reliable predictors of those patients who are about to become infected would allow more timely intervention with anti-infective agents and potentially improved outcome. In addition, many aspects of the hypermetabolic response of uninfected burned patients are similar to those of infected and septic patients without large inflammatory wound surfaces. Extent of burn injury is one of the major demographic predictors of outcome. Incidence of infection and sepsis rises as burn size increases. In burns involving less than a 10 to 20 percent TBSA, life-threatening infection in otherwise healthy burned patients almost never occurs. Children appear to be more susceptible to systemic infection for a given burn size. The presence of inhalation injury correlates highly with infection and mortality, and patients with severe inhalation injury and no burn may have a fatal outcome. A large study of 5882 burned patients indicated significantly increased mortality in patients with gram-

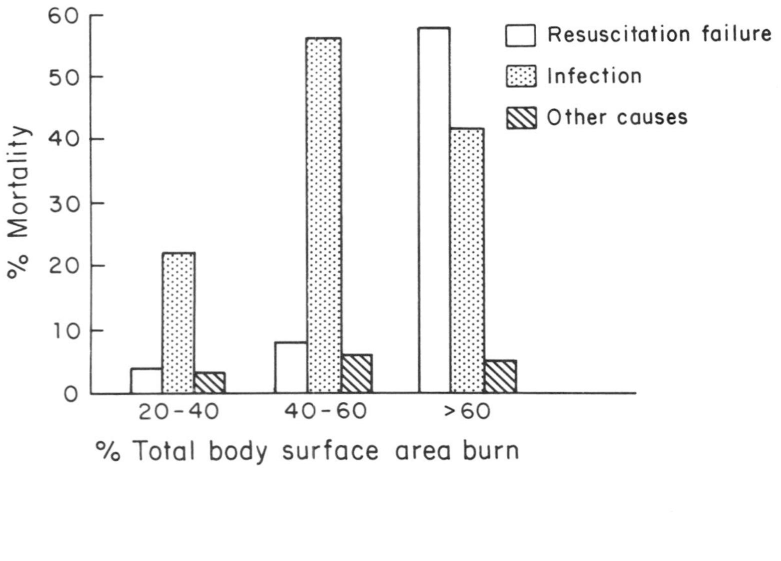

FIG. 7-23. Infection is the primary cause of death in burned patients, including patients with massive burns who survive the resuscitation phase. Patients dying of resuscitation failure were most often elderly, had sustained severe carbon monoxide poisoning, or had debilitating chronic diseases.

negative bacteremia, an equivocal increase in patients with blood cultures positive for yeastlike organisms, and no increase attributable to gram-positive bacteremia. Methicillin resistance in *Staphylococcus aureus* does not increase the probability of mortality, at least when these gram-positive infections are treated with vancomycin. This observation questions the economic value of infection control resources devoted to this group of patients. Epidemiologic studies of burned patients have demonstrated a relationship between the number of transfusions received and infectious morbidity that was independent of age and burn size, but no significant relationship between the number of transfusions and mortality.

The search for a laboratory study that could facilitate the early diagnosis of infection has led to intense examination of postinjury alterations of hormones, acute-phase proteins, and fluorescent substances in the blood and plasma of burned patients. Most of these laboratory alterations were nonspecific and could not distinguish between inflammation and infection. One of these fluorescent substances, identified as neopterin by thermospray mass spectrometry, has been shown to correlate strongly with episodes of bacteremia. Monitoring of serum concentrations may allow early identification of bacteremia before systemic mediator activation and sepsis occurs.

Clinical Manifestations of Sepsis. Many of the physiologic criteria commonly claimed to reflect sepsis are noninfectious manifestations of postinjury hypermetabolism. Hyperthermia, tachycardia, increased ventilation, and high cardiac output are present routinely in otherwise healthy patients with large burns. The added effect of sepsis may accentuate this nonspecific physiologic response in patients with small burns but often causes a suppression of these hypermetabolic responses in patients with large burns. Thus, a reduction of cardiac output to normal may represent a low-output syndrome in a septic burned patient. Certain systemic responses, however, are highly suggestive of infection and sepsis.

Body temperature in patients is dependent in part on environmental conditions. Hyperthermia (39°C or greater) occasionally represents a febrile response to infection, particularly in children. Episodic elevations, however, in temperatures are common in uninfected burned patients. Nevertheless, this diagnosis is one of exclusion, and an infection workup is required for most of these patients. Hypothermia, on the other hand, commonly indicates sepsis, usually due to gram-negative organisms. Leukocytosis also is nonspecific; while large burn wounds remain open, moderate elevations of the leukocyte count are common. Leukocyte counts above 16,000 to 18,000/mm^3 usually reflect gram-positive infection, while leukopenia (below 5000 to 6000/mm^3) indicates gram-negative infection and impending sepsis. While thrombocytopenia is caused by a number of factors, including infection and sepsis, normal to high platelet counts almost always occur in burned patients who are stable with no imminent likelihood of sepsis.

Other potential systemic manifestations are more nonspecific. Decreasing mental status can be caused by excessive sedation, histamine receptor blocking agents, and cerebrovascular disease. Hyperglycemia may be due to irregular administration of high-calorie nutrition solutions or hypokalemia. Increased fluid requirements, hypotension, and oliguria may be related to underreplacement of evaporative water loss or unrecognized diarrhea. The most important observation is the temporal relationship of these physiologic events. The precipitant onset of hyperglycemia, fall in blood pressure (even when modest), and decreased urinary output should suggest the possibility that the patient is beginning to become unstable. If these findings are associated with the development of hypothermia, leukopenia, and a falling platelet count, the patient is likely developing sepsis, and a rapid infection evaluation and antibiotic administration should be instituted.

Infectious Complications. With the introduction of topical antimicrobial chemotherapy, the most common location of lethal infection has shifted from the burn wound to the respiratory tract. Awareness of the variety of infections commonly encountered in burned patients allows an orderly evaluation of the potentially septic patient and reduces the possibility that an otherwise unusual infection will be overlooked (Table 7-20).

Pneumonia. With prolonged survival in critical care units as a result of modern patient support techniques, the respiratory tract has become the most common locus of infection. Bronchopneumonia has replaced hematogenous pneumonia as the most common form of pulmonary infection in burned patients. The decrease in the incidence of invasive burn wound infection has greatly reduced the occurrence of hematogenous pneumonia. Hematogenous pneumonia represents systemic dissemination of microorganisms from a remote locus of infection. The sudden appearance of a solitary ''cannonball'' pulmonary infiltrate is indicative of hematogenous pneumonia and should prompt a search for the primary source of infection (Fig. 7-24). The more common sources of hematogenous infection include the infected burn wound, suppurative thrombophlebitis, and infection from a perforated viscus. Inhalation injury greatly increases the incidence of pneumonia, and the use of artificial airways provides a portal of entry for nosocomial organisms always indigenous in a critical care unit.

The diagnosis of pneumonia is confirmed by the presence of characteristic chest radiograph patterns and the presence of the offending organism and inflammatory cells in the sputum. Following inhalation injury, early infiltrates usually represent chemical pneumonitis and not infectious pneumonia. Although this damaged lung tissue may become infected, subsequently, the use of prophylactic antibiotics only selects resistant organisms, does not alter the incidence of pneumonia and should not be used. Colonization of the upper airway of patients requiring intubation and mechanical ventilation should not be confused with respiratory tract infection. Bacterial tracheobronchitis, which can cause life-threatening sepsis, may be difficult to distinguish from airway colonization, even with protected brush specimens and appropriate staining techniques, and antimicrobial therapy may be instigated by relatively nonspecific signs of sepsis.

Table 7-20
Infections in Burned Patients

Invasive burn wound sepsis
Pneumonia—airborne or hematogenous
Septic thrombophlebitis
Endocarditis
Urinary tract infection—cystitis, pyelonephritis, renal abscess, prostatitis
Intraabdominal sepsis—perforated Curling's ulcer, acalculous cholecystitis, necrotizing enterocolitis, pancreatitis
Parotitis
Sinusitis
Generalized sepsis—usually arising from other infections listed in this table

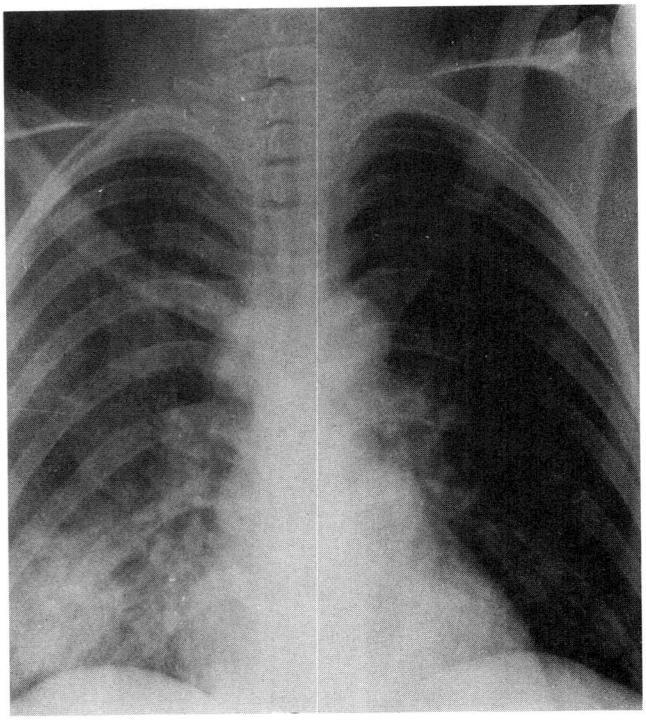

FIG. 7-24. Chest radiograph demonstrating a solitary infiltrate typical of early hematogenous pneumonia. Such discrete patterns represent a septic embolus from a distant site to the lung. In this instance, the source was septic thrombophlebitis in an extremity.

Suppurative Thrombophlebitis. Suppurative thrombophlebitis is a major source of sepsis, occurring in up to 5 percent of patients with major burns. It is associated with the use of intravenous catheters, especially if inserted by cutdown techniques, and its incidence increases with prolonged duration of vein cannulation. The nidus of infection is usually located in the vein at the site of the catheter tip, which produces endothelial injury and formation of a fibrin clot. The fibrin mesh subsequently is seeded during bacteremias that may occur throughout the patient's hospital course.

Over half of the infected patients demonstrate no local signs or symptoms, and unexplained sepsis or the appearance of hematogenous pneumonia should prompt inspection of all previously cannulated veins. The vein suspected of harboring infection initially is examined by opening any previous cutdown incisions. The venotomy is exposed, all ligatures are removed, and the vein lumen is opened. If free flow of blood occurs, the vein is probably free of infection, and the search for the septic source must be directed elsewhere. Identification of pus in the vein confirms the diagnosis. If no free backbleeding occurs, the vein must be explored more proximally until backbleeding is obtained (Fig. 7-25).

Once the diagnosis of suppurative thrombophlebitis is confirmed, the vein is ligated at its proximal extent to prevent seeding during the operative manipulation, and excision of the infected vein completes the treatment. Because skip areas of infection frequently occur along the course of an infected vein, all involved vein and its tributaries are excised up to an uninvolved major branch point. To minimize this complication, catheters should be placed percutaneously in high-flow veins, and insertion sites should be changed every 48 to 72 h.

In the absence of a concurrent bacteremia, cannulas may be changed once over a guidewire. The next change should be placed through a new site. If the patient is bacteremic, the new catheter is placed in a new location. Occasionally, arterial cannulas cause local vascular infection. The cannulas should be removed promptly and replaced elsewhere. Arterial cannula infection may progress to a rapidly expanding aneurysm at the site of vessel puncture. Most occur in the radial artery and are treated by ligation of the aneurysm. This complication can be minimized by reducing the frequency of arterial puncture and rotating arterial lines to all available vessels, including the dorsalis pedis and axillary arteries.

Bacterial Endocarditis. Endocarditis occasionally is a cause of occult sepsis in burned patients, and its incidence continues to

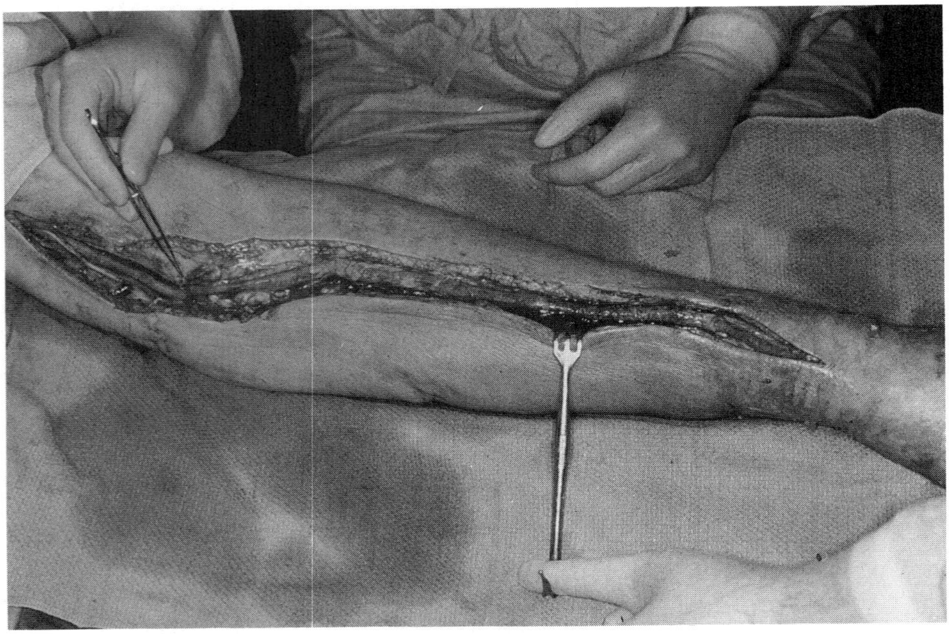

FIG. 7-25. Excision of a pus-filled vein that had been previously cannulated for fluid administration. Suppurative thrombophlebitis requires total excision of the involved vein up to the point of free backflow of blood from the axillary vein (left).

rise with the increasing use of intravascular catheters for hemodynamic monitoring. Endocarditis is suspected in patients with positive blood cultures and no other identifiable source of bacteremia. Such patients should be examined repeatedly by biplanar transthoracic and transesophageal echocardiography until the source of septicemia is identified. Most lesions are found on the right side of the heart, and over 85 percent of cases occur in patients who have had central venous or pulmonary artery catheters in the right atrium or through the right ventricle. Cannulation-induced injury probably is initiated by endothelial fibrin deposition and secondary seeding by bacteria from distant foci. Once the diagnosis of bacterial endocarditis is confirmed, systemic antibiotic therapy using agents to which the isolated organism is sensitive should be instituted and continued for at least 4 weeks. Echocardiography and blood cultures should be repeated after the patient has completed antibiotic therapy. Prompt angiography and valve replacement may be indicated in those patients who develop cardiac failure or multiple septic emboli.

Urinary Tract Infections. Most patients with large burns (greater than 20 percent TBSA) require indwelling urinary catheter to guide fluid resuscitation. Aseptic technique of insertion and catheter care, the use of closed drainage systems, and the removal of the catheter at the earliest clinically indicated time are effective measures for preventing urinary tract infections. With increasing duration of catheter placement, the likelihood of obtaining positive urine cultures rises, so that after 7 to 10 days, most patients will have positive urine cultures. Causative organisms usually reflect the flora of the burn wound.

In the absence of an inflammatory response (negative urinalysis), the majority of positive urine cultures do not require antimicrobial treatment. Pyuria (greater than 10 white blood cells/high-power field) with positive urine cultures usually requires treatment with systemic antibiotics. Occasionally in a patient with occult sepsis, treatment of bacteriuria may be indicated in the absence of pyuria, but workup for pyelonephritis, although relatively rare in burned patients, should be initiated. Pyelonephritis occurs either as an ascending infection from concurrent cystitis or by way of hematogenous spread of infection. Hematogenous infections may result in renal abscesses. Candiduria in the absence of signs of systemic infection often can be treated with bladder irrigations with amphotericin B. Burns of the penis usually do not require bladder catheter drainage unless they are severe. In such cases, a suprapubic cystostomy usually is preferred. Prolonged catheter drainage may lead to prostatic or periurethral abscesses.

Chondritis of the Ear. The pinna of the ear is composed almost entirely of cartilage with minimal blood supply and is vulnerable to infection. One-third of burn injuries involve the face, neck, and ears, and in older reports chondritis has occurred in 5 to 25 percent of patients with burned ears. The infection arises most frequently between the second and fifth week after injury and is commonly associated with organisms such as *Pseudomonas, Staphylococcus,* and *Candida* species. Pressure on the burned ear is a major factor leading to the development of chondritis. The diagnosis is based on swelling, erythema, warmth, and exquisite tenderness elicited on palpation (Fig. 7-26). The ear protrudes from the head because of the increased auriculocephalic angle and is easily distinguishable from the uninvolved ear.

Severe cases of chondritis require bivalving of the ear in the longitudinal plane with debridement of all infected cartilage and placement of a gauze wick to separate the soft tissue halves. This procedure results in a severe cosmetic deformity: the ear loses its cartilaginous support and the surrounding soft tissue collapses. Burned ears are placed in mafenide acetate as a topical agent because it diffuses through the eschar and attains effective tissue levels in the underlying soft tissue and cartilage. However, mafenide acetate also can cause auricular pseudochondritis in those patients allergic to this drug. This simulated chondritis is actually allergic edema of the involved partial-thickness burn of the ear. The use of systemic antibiotics generally is ineffective because of the poor blood supply to the auricular cartilage. Pressure on the ear is avoided by the use of foam donuts on the head and by restricting the use of pillows. The premature separation of eschar exposes viable cartilage that then may become desiccated and susceptible to bacterial colonization and infection. If this should occur, the exposed cartilage should be covered with a biologic dressing.

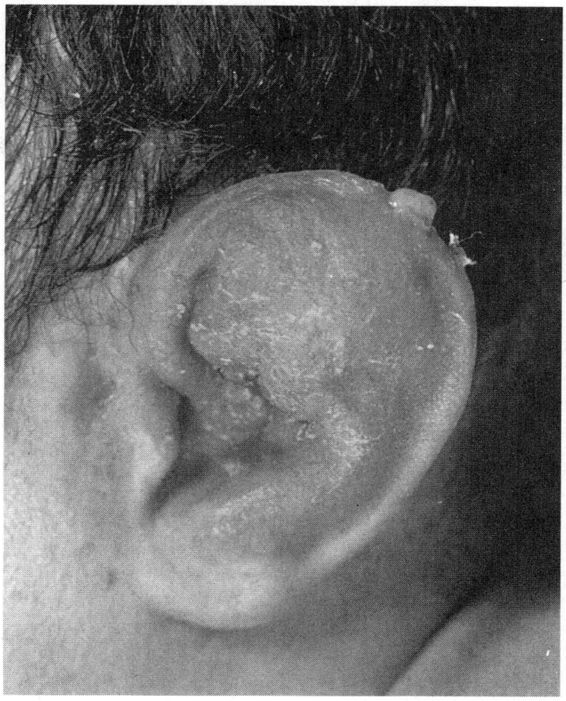

FIG. 7-26. Bacterial chondritis of the pinna of the ear. Most of the cartilaginous contour is obscured by purulent fluid beneath the burned skin. This infection is treated by bivalving the ear through the plane of its outer margins.

Other Infections. Intraabdominal infections may be a cause of occult infection. Several burn-associated complications of the gastrointestinal tract (Curling's ulcer, acalculous cholecystitis, colitis) can lead to perforation of a viscus and subsequent peritonitis or abscess formation. Acute appendicitis can occur in severely burned patients. All of these intraabdominal conditions are extremely difficult to detect in critically ill burned patients. Burn injury often is accompanied by ileus requiring nasogastric decompression. Obtundation produced by injury or sedation may mask symptoms and makes examination of the abdomen unreliable. Burn injury to the abdominal wall and tissue edema further complicate abdominal evaluation.

Herpetic infections may occur in the burn wound, primarily in healing second-degree burns of the face. Where possible, biopsy of the herpetic lesion will demonstrate the characteristic intranuclear inclusion bodies. Herpetic infections of the upper gastrointestinal tract, liver, and lungs, although rare, can lead to perforation and systemic viremia. Treatment requires the use of systemic viral agents, such as acyclovir. Chicken pox lesions most commonly appear in partial-thickness wounds, including donor sites, and may cause conversion of these wounds to full-thickness injuries. Tetanus is rare, as are other clostridial infections. Tetanus prophylaxis and timely surgical extirpation of necrotic tissue, especially muscle, will prevent clostridial sepsis in nearly all patients.

Infection Surveillance. Patients with burns more than 2 to 3 days old who have been treated in other medical institutions should have the burn wound biopsied on admission to the burn center. This biopsy will provide valuable information about wound bacterial density and about the nosocomial organisms imported with the patient. On occasion, this allows identification of the index case for a subsequent epidemic that may occur in the receiving institution. Two to three times a week following admission surveillance cultures of sputum, urine, wound (by biopsy), blood, and stool (if diarrhea is present) should be obtained from all patients with major burns. Except for blood cultures, positive cultures do not necessarily indicate infection but reflect the likely organism responsible if infection is present. The distinction between colonization and true tissue infection can only be made in conjunction with clinical or laboratory evidence of a tissue response to infection. Thus, a Gram stain must accompany all respiratory tract cultures, as should a urinalysis with a urine culture. Organisms colonizing the burn wound early in the postburn course often are the agents causing later life-threatening infections during hospitalization. As such, diagnosis and the selection of appropriate antibiotic therapy is facilitated by reviewing surveillance cultures and sensitivity data on newly septic patients. Surveillance data provide an overall picture of the organisms present in the burn center and, by timely detection, help prevent potentially dangerous epidemics.

Work-up of Suspected Infection. Most infections will be apparent in burned patients. Burn wound evaluation is described above. Chest radiographs to verify central venous catheter position also will detect new infiltrates or effusions. Routine urinalysis may suggest pyelonephritis, a relatively rare infection in burned patients; renal sonography is an accurated bedside procedure for confirming this diagnosis in patients too critically ill to be moved from the burn center. The long-term use of nasogastric and endotracheal tubes suggests the possibility of parotitis and paranasal sinusitis. Prostatic and scrotal abscesses are not unusual in males with indwelling bladder catheters; routine rectal examination provides much useful information on a patient's physical status. Lumbar puncture should be carried out more readily in children with suspected sepsis. Adoption of a planned protocol for evaluating sepsis in burned patients will avoid overlooking inapparent infection (Table 7-21).

Treatment of Infection. The treatment of burn wound sepsis is discussed above. The definitive therapy of the infected burn is expeditious excision of the wound. Many of the other infections commonly encountered in burned patients require surgical intervention and emphasize the essential nature of burn injury as primarily one of surgical infectious disease and critical care. Most acquired infections in hospitalized burned patients involve the organisms that originally colonized the burn wound.

Table 7-21
Work-up of Occult Sepsis

Primary
Cultures of blood, sputum, urine
Wound biopsy
Culture of stool (if diarrhea present) and titers for *C. difficile*
Chest radiograph
Gram stains of urine, sputum
Secondary
Evaluation/exploration of previously cannulated vessels
Lumbar puncture (especially in children)
Echocardiography
Renal sonogram
Radiographs of paranasal sinuses
Other (as indicated by clinical examination and initial diagnostic studies)
Abdominal sonogram and computed tomography
Computed tomography of head
Viral titers

Antibiotics. The number and types of antibiotics used in a burn center should be restricted (Table 7-22), and the criteria for documenting infection should be well defined. In general, an infection caused by an identified organism is treated by a single antibiotic. No controlled trails in burned patients have demonstrated any improvement in survival by the routine use of antibiotic combinations to treat serious infection. Under certain circumstances, multiple antibiotics may be indicated. A bacteremia that persists in the face of documented therapeutic levels of the antibiotic to which the organism has been shown to be sensitive should be treated by an additional susceptibility-proven agent. Some infections are associated with several predominant microbes with different sensitivity patterns and will require an antibiotic for each organism. Suspected sepsis before the isolation of responsible organisms can be isolated requires the use of suitable agents for gram-positive and gram-negative organisms. Patient and burn center microbial surveillance data are extremely useful for choosing effective coverage. Anaerobic infection almost never occurs in burned patients, but the use of an antibiotic effective against anaerobic organisms may be indicated in the rare patient with severe muscle necrosis or intraabdominal infection.

The indiscriminate use of multiple agents promotes overgrowth of *Candida* species, enterococci, and multiple antibiotic-resistant organisms, both in the patient and in the burn center. The current problem of increasing staphylococcal and enterococcal resistance to vancomycin emphasizes the importance of using the least com-

Table 7-22
Antibiotic Use in the Treatment of Burn-Associated Infection

Presumed sepsis
Gram-positive and gram-negative antibiotic based on patient surveillance cultures and unit epidemiology
Documented infection
One antibiotic per dominant organism
Exceptions, requiring additional coverage
Anaerobes
Persistent bacteremia with therapeutic levels

plex (and cheapest) antibiotic shown to be effective against the organism. Therapy generally is continued 10 to 14 days for most infections.

Numerous studies have demonstrated altered pharmacokinetics of antibiotics in burned patients resulting in lowered serum drug levels when the usual recommended dosage is employed. In many cases such dosages are subtherapeutic in the burned patient, especially among antibiotics that are predominately excreted renally. Serum levels should be monitored frequently and early in the course of therapy. Inappropriate peak levels should prompt alteration in the dosage, while inadequate trough levels should prompt shortening of the dosage interval. The presence of renal insufficiency should not be considered a contraindication to the use of any drug in the case of life-threatening sepsis in the burned patient, but the toxic effects can be avoided or minimized by the use of serum level monitoring.

Immunomodulators. The use of immunomodulators to prevent or to treat infection in burned patients has a long history marked by virtually complete failure. At the present time, a number of somatic and myelopoietic growth factors are undergoing evaluation. Human growth hormone has been shown to improve burn wound healing and by inference to reduce infectious complications. Recombinant human granulocyte colony stimulating factor improves survival times in experimental models of *Pseudomonas* burn wound sepsis. Although this agent increased leukocyte count and neutrophil oxidative function in humans, it had no effect in early trials on morbidity and mortality. Although monoclonal antibodies against the lipid A component of endotoxin have produced marginal improvements in survival of patients with gram-negative bacteremia and shock, these biologics have yet to be evaluated in burned patients. It is likely that in the near future, monoclonal antibodies to cytokines and their receptors will prove to be effective for treating patients with life-threatening infections.

Infection Control in the Burn Center. Patients with major burns should be treated in single rooms isolated from other patients. Significant reductions in infectious events and mortality have been associated with the conversion from multiple-patient to single-patient enclosures. The rooms should be ventilated with nonrecirculating ultrafiltration air exchange systems. The single rooms should be closed periodically for decontamination and repainting. Universal precaution barrier techniques now are required by government regulation. Although the effectiveness of these techniques has not been proved, they probably help to decrease cross-contamination and to remind the burn center staff to wash their hands. Hand washing is the single most effective means of preventing nosocomial infection, and separate sinks in each patient room are mandatory if hand washing is to be effective. Shared common sinks serve only to promote cross-contamination. Chlorhexidine gluconate appears to be the most effective cleaning agent for reducing nosocomial infections in critical care units.

The flow of patients and burn-care personnel should be directed away from the critical-care unit to the convalescent floor. Patients and staff on step-down units should not return to visit friends and relatives who still have critical burn injuries. As described above, the convalescent patients are the major reservoirs for life-threatening nosocomial infections. Only patients experiencing unexpected physiologic instability should be transferred back to the burn critical care area. Cohorting burned patients into separate geographic sections of the hospital, although proven effective in controlling burn-center epidemics, is too expensive and impractical in most medical centers, where it is not economically feasible to leave large blocks of beds continually unoccupied.

COMPLICATIONS

Gastrointestinal Complications. The gastrointestinal tract is one of the major target organs of the physiologic response to massive thermal injury. Gastrointestinal complications associated with large burns include stress ulceration of the stomach and duodenum (Curling's ulcer), acalculous cholecystitis, acute pancreatitis, superior mesenteric artery syndrome, nonocclusive ischemic enterocolitis, and hepatic dysfunction.

Curling's Ulcer. Stress ulceration of the stomach and duodenum, or Curling's ulcer, presents as a spectrum of lesions in the stomach and duodenum, and the clinical course of this complication is strongly influenced by preventive measures. Serial endoscopic examinations have shown that 85 percent of patients with burns exceeding 35 percent of TBSA demonstrate superficial mucosal disease with 72 h of injury (Fig. 7-27). In the absence of prophylactic measures, this mucosal disease heals in the majority (80 percent) of patients within 1 week. The disease progresses in approximately 20 percent of patients to frank gastric and duodenal ulcers, which first become evident 96 h after injury. With current preventive measures, these lesions heal following successful resuscitation and initiation of enteral feeding. The presence of gastric acid is required for the progression of the early erosions to more extensive ulcers, but the concentrations of acid and gastrin most often are within the normal range in patients with active ulceration.

Controlled randomized trials of antacids and placebo have demonstrated definitively the beneficial effects of continuous gastric acid neutralization in preventing upper gastrointestinal hemorrhage and perforation of stress ulcers. Until the burn wound is healed, 30 mL antacid is administered each hour through the naso-

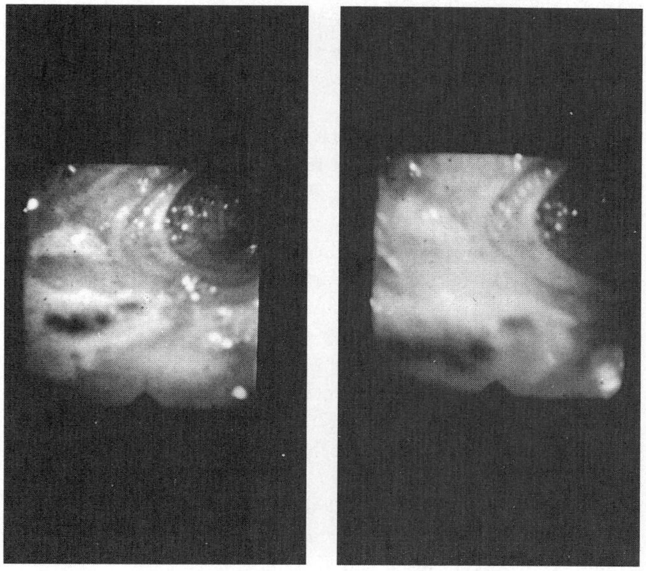

FIG. 7-27. Superficial prepyloric gastric erosions in a recently admitted burned patient. Nasogastric irrigation was clear, although it was guaiac positive. These lesions characteristically heal with antacid prophylaxis and enteral feeding.

gastric tube to maintain the gastric pH above 5. The dosage can be increased if gastric acidity persists below this level. Cimetidine is equally effective in preventing Curling's ulcers, and in patients who cannot tolerate antacids, histamine H_2 blockers are an acceptable alternative to antacids. Thrombocytopenia and severe alterations in mental status are associated with the use of cimetidine therapy in burned patients and may be confused with the clinical presentation of sepsis. Recent clinical trials suggest that early enteral feeding may be as effective as antacids and histamine H_2 antagonists. In the rare patient who requires surgery for severe hemorrhage or perforation of Curling's ulcer, vagotomy and gastric resection has produced the best immediate and long-term survival. Curling's ulcers are often multiple and are found simultaneously in the stomach and duodenum. The entire stomach and duodenum must be inspected through a wide gastrotomy incision. A perforated Curling's ulcer with subsequent abscess formation occasionally causes occult sepsis.

Superior Mesenteric Artery Syndrome. Superior mesenteric artery syndrome may develop in burned patients who experience marked weight loss. The superior mesenteric artery obstructs the transverse portion of the duodenum, and enteral alimentation becomes impossible. Gastric decompression and intravenous nutrition have reduced the need for operative intervention.

Acute Pancreatitis. Acute pancreatitis may occur in patients with extensive burns, with an incidence as high as 35 percent in those requiring treatment in a critical-care unit. Abdominal pain is often absent, and pancreatitis is suggested by increasing fluid requirements and the new onset of hyperglycemia. Measurement of amylase excretion rates appears to be the most sensitive laboratory diagnostic study. Treatment is directed toward general supportive measures, nasogastric drainage, and parenteral nutrition.

Acute Acalculous Cholecystitis. Acute acalculous cholecystitis in burned patients occurs under two distinct clinical circumstances. In one form, the gallbladder is infected by hematogenous seeding from a primary source in the septic patient, usually from the invaded burn wound. The other presentation occurs in critically ill patients who have developed marked dehydration, ileus, or pancreatitis. Almost all of these latter patients are hypernatremic and hyperosmolar, and sepsis usually is not the initiating event. The gallbladder and bile in the latter presentation are often sterile.

Physical examination may be difficult in the burned patient, who often is obtunded and has painful abdominal burn wounds. Jaundice and complaints of abdominal pain in critically ill patients suggest acalculous cholecystitis, and such patients should be evaluated by ultrasonography and computed tomography. Increased gallbladder wall thickness, sloughing mucosa, and intraluminal gas in the gallbladder suggest acute acalculous cholecystitis. Cholescintigraphy is of little value in these critically ill patients. Nonvisualization of the gallbladder occurs in nearly all seriously ill burned patients, and subsequent laparotomy has confirmed the high false-positive rate of this study.

Once the diagnosis is made, cholecystectomy is indicated to avoid rupture of the gallbladder. Tube cholecystostomy occasionally is used in unstable, critically ill patients and can be carried out at the bedside, if necessary. Because this diagnosis is difficult to make preoperatively in critically ill patients, laparoscopic evaluation of the gallbladder may be useful for planning therapy.

Nonocclusive Ischemic Enterocolitis. Nonocclusive ischemic enterocolitis is being recognized increasingly in severely burned patients with multisystem organ failure. The lesion is located in the distal small bowel and colon, and it clinically and histologically resembles the lesions of Curling's ulcer in the upper gastrointestinal tract. The lesions bleed and perforate less often, but if the patient recovers, healing of the bowel often occurs with stricture formation. Patients who develop this complication should be put at bowel rest and nourished intravenously. Pseudoobstruction of the colon may be a clinical variant of this entity; it occurs in 1 percent of young, thermally injured patients and is more frequent in elderly populations as early survival increases. Proctoscopy and barium enema examinations should be carried out to confirm the absence of mechanical obstruction. Decompression of distended colon by colonoscopy generally is unsuccessful, and in patients with an enlarged cecum, laparotomy and cecostomy may be necessary to avoid infarction and perforation of the colon. Nonocclusive ischemic enterocolitis may represent the anatomic basis of bacterial translocation.

Myocardial Infarction. Myocardial infarction in burned patients occurs almost exclusively in the elderly population. In some urban burn centers, young cocaine users develop acute myocardial infarction soon after admission. Infarction usually occurs toward the end of the first week after burn, when the hypermetabolic response reaches its peak. The demands for greatly elevated cardiac output at this time appears to exceed the ability of the diseased heart to meet its own perfusion and metabolic demands, and infarction occurs. All patients with large burns should be monitored electrocardiographically. If an infarct pattern or an arrhythmia develops, infarction should be confirmed by the serial measurement of cardiac enzymes and electrocardiograms.

Associated cardiac failure is treated with inotropic agents as needed to maintain total-body perfusion appropriate for the time course of that patient's injury. Short-acting infusible drugs, such as dopamine, dobutamine, or amrinone, are preferable to long-acting drugs, such as digitalis. Increased afterload is treated with intravenous nitroprusside or nitroglycerin. Adequate intravascular volume must be maintained to meet the perfusion requirements of the wound and visceral organs. Unless the patient has been so treated before injury, beta-adrenergic blocking agents should not be used to treat cardiac disease in burned patients; such agents blunt the rise in total-body blood flow after burn injury. The inability to increase cardiac output during the hypermetabolic phase of injury results in a relative low-output syndrome and almost universal mortality.

ELECTRICAL INJURIES

Each year in the United States, more than 1000 deaths result from electrical and lightning injuries. These injuries, however, are relatively uncommon events, comprising about 5 percent of admissions to most burn units. In adults, electrical burns are commonly occupational hazards, particularly with electrical utility workers. More recently, many have been related to installation of home radio and television antennas and unsafe operation of electrical appliances. In urban environments, electric-powered mass transit conduits are one of the most common sources of such injuries. Household appliances and unprotected electric sockets cause most electrical injuries in children. Lightning injury affects all age groups, especially in rural areas.

Pathophysiology. Electrical injury manifests in a variety of forms, ranging from cardiopulmonary arrest and minimal tissue damage to devastating electrocution and vaporization of major body parts. Tissue damage is a direct consequence of thermal injury generated by the flow of alternating or direct current. Alternating current is more dangerous because it can produce tonic muscle contractions and the victim may be unable to release the source of electricity. Further, cardiac arrest and coma frequently accompany electrocution with alternating current, and these events are most likely to occur at current frequencies of 50 to 60 cycles/s. As frequency increases above 60 cycles/s, tissue damage and risk of cardiac arrest decrease. Tissue damage caused by line voltages less than 1000 volts arbitrarily is designated as low-voltage injury. High-tension electrical injury is caused by line voltages above 1000 volts.

Electricity causes injury by four mechanisms: direct contact, conduction, arc, and secondary ignition. Low-voltage electrical sources produce direct injury at the point of contact. Skin and subcutaneous tissue are involved most commonly, although occasionally muscle and bone beneath the cutaneous burn may be damaged. High-voltage current not only causes direct injury at the point of contact but also damages tissues that conduct the electricity through the body. Arc burns occur without actual contact of the body surface with the source of electricity. Very high voltages are required to produce this charge transfer, and when arcing occurs, extremely high temperatures are produced. The duration of the arc is brief, and the "flash" injury produced is usually limited to the body surface. A variant of arc injury occurs when electrical current being conducted along a body part flashes directly to an adjacent body part; such injuries are frequently observed in the axilla and other flexion creases where surface moisture tends to accumulate. Burns occur when the electrical source ignites clothing and other flammable materials. Very deep flame burns may occur, especially if the patient is also unconscious. The victim may not be able to verify whether direct contact has occurred, and patient evaluation and management personnel must assume that diverse multisystem effects of electrical injury may be present.

Tissue damage associated with electrical injury occurs when electrical energy is converted to thermal energy. The resulting injury is a thermal burn that produces physiologic responses similar to those caused by other mechanisms of thermal injury. Skin represents the initial barrier to current flow and is an effective insulator to deeper tissues. After electrical contact and the onset of current flow, the skin undergoes coagulation necrosis and desiccation. With low-voltage injuries, the charred skin at the point of contact terminates current flow and limits the extent of injury. The skin surrounding the contact point may sustain an arc burn as the increase in skin resistance terminates current flow. At high voltages (over 1000 volts), skin resistance initially is overcome, and current flow through deep tissues in the body is unimpeded. Except for bone, these internal tissues act as a volume conductor, offering little resistance to flow. Current flow is terminated when the tissue at the point of electrical contact desiccates and resistance increases markedly (Fig. 7-28). At this point, electrical arcing frequently occurs. The charred tissue then acts as an electrical insulator. No further tissue damage is possible.

Deep tissue damage is related to the density and duration of current flow through these tissues. Heat production and, hence, thermal injury depend on the density of current flow. In body parts with small cross-sectional areas, such as an extremity, current density is high, and tissue destruction is severe. In regions of the body with large cross-sectional areas, such as the trunk, current density is reduced, and deep injuries are unusual. Surface tissues

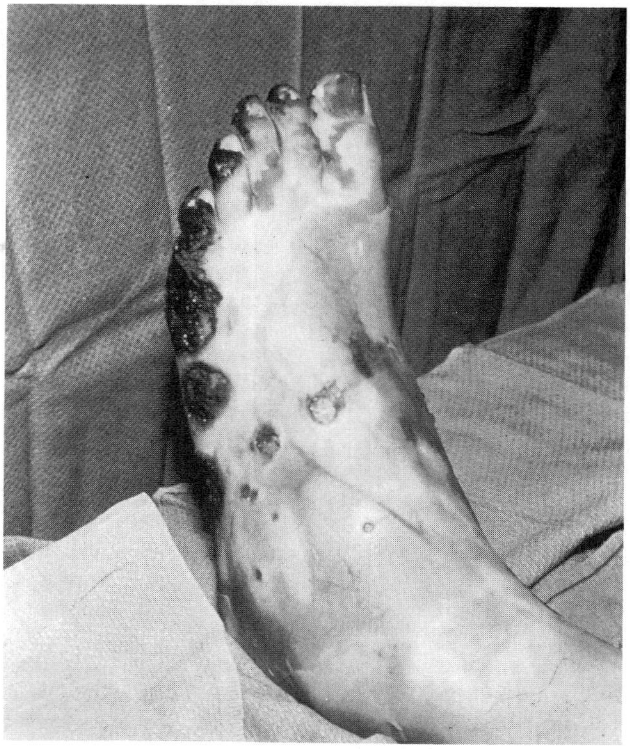

FIG. 7-28. Electrical injury involving the foot. Exit and entry contact points demonstrate areas of severe desiccation and tissue loss. The charred skin presents a high-resistance barrier to further current flow, and the electrical circuit terminates. The extreme depth of this burn is illustrated by the coagulated subcutaneous vessels on the dorsum of the foot. At surgical exploration, all muscle compartments in the lower leg were nonviable.

cool faster than deep tissues. Because bone has high resistance to current flow, it heats to higher temperatures than does surrounding soft tissue. As a result, the most severely heat-damaged soft tissues are usually muscle and nerves directly adjacent to the bone, a position almost impervious to clinical detection. The most severe cutaneous and deep injuries are adjacent to contact sites, and damage decreases with increasing distance from contact points. The hallmark of electrical injury is the likelihood of extensive deep tissue damage far out of proportion to the visible cutaneous burn.

Clinical Manifestations. The characteristics of electric injury frequently necessitate modification of the treatment used for patients with conventional thermal injury. Cardiopulmonary arrest frequently occurs in patients who have sustained high-voltage electric injuries and must be treated promptly by cardiopulmonary resuscitation. Cardiac arrhythmias may also occur during and even after resuscitation. Patients who have sustained a cardiac arrest should undergo continuous electrocardiographic monitoring for at least 48 h beyond the last evidence of arrhythmia. This can be accomplished safely by telemetry on the burn center step-down unit if no other major injuries are present.

The risk of acute renal failure is relatively high in patients with electric injury. Renal failure occurs as a result of underestimation of fluid needs and the liberation of myoglobin from injured muscle. Unless a brisk urinary output is maintained, myoglobin will precipitate in renal tubules and cause acute tubular necrosis. Extensive tissue destruction may also cause release of potassium, and the resulting hyperkalemia may reach sufficient levels to interfere with cardiac function. Edema of tissues beneath the muscle fascia of a limb injured by high-voltage electricity may impair nutrient blood flow to those deep tissues and blood flow to distal unburned tissue, necessitating a fasciotomy to reduce the tissue pressure within the muscle compartment and restore circulation. Electric injury on occasion has caused intestinal perforation, pancreatic necrosis, gallbladder necrosis, and hepatic injury.

Deficits of peripheral nerve, spinal cord, cerebellar, and cerebral function may present immediately following injury or may be delayed in onset. A thorough neurologic examination should be performed on admission and at scheduled intervals thereafter to identify and record any neurologic deficit. Following direct nerve injury return of function is uncommon, but resolution of early functional deficits of nerves not directly injured is common. Sensory nerves appear to be less sensitive to current injury than motor nerves. Late-appearing functional deficits of nerves far removed from the points of contact may be part of a polyneuritic syndrome. Immediate spinal cord deficits resulting from direct axonal damage are more commonly transient than are later-appearing spinal cord deficits, and present as quadriplegia, hemiplegia, transverse myelitis, or ascending paralysis.

Moderate to large blood vessels subjected to high-voltage electric current may be the site of delayed hemorrhage. Hemorrhage from such vessels seems to occur only when wound debridement has been inadequate or a vessel exposed by debridement has undergone exposure-related desiccation and necrosis following debridement. An arteritis initiated at the time of electrical injury leads eventually to thrombosis of the smaller nutrient vessels and subsequent tissue necrosis.

Compression fractures of vertebral bodies may be produced by the tetanic contractions of the paraspinus muscles, and long-bone fractures may be caused by falls occurring at the time of the injury. Appropriate radiographic studies should be obtained at the time of admission to identify such fractures.

Management. As with any other tissue injury, fluid loss into damaged tissue is one of the major physiologic derangements after electrical burns. Intravascular volume deficits are replaced with lactated Ringer's solution sufficient to maintain a urinary output of 50 to 75 mL/h. If the patient has grossly visible myoglobinuria, urinary output should be increased to 100 to 150 mL/h by raising the fluid infusion rate. The increased urine production facilitates dilution of myoglobin and its washout from renal tubules. If myoglobinuria is severe or urinary output remains low in spite of an increased rate of fluid administration, 12.5 g mannitol is added to each liter of lactated Ringer's solution. The addition of sodium bicarbonate to the resuscitation solution alkalinizes the urine and increases the solubility of myoglobin.

Wound care involves treatment of both cutaneous and deep soft tissue injuries. Immediately after electrical injury, second- and third-degree cutaneous wounds are debrided, cleansed, and placed in topical antimicrobial burn creams. Mafenide acetate is preferred for electrical injuries because of its superior ability to penetrate injured tissue deeply and its unique anticlostridial spectrum. Tetanus prophylaxis is brought up to date. Prophylactic antibiotics have not been shown to decrease episodes of infection and are not used. Extremity muscle compartment pressures are monitored by physical palpation and by Doppler ultrasonography of major arterial pulses. If the extremity has been injured by a circumferential third-degree burn, and arterial flow becomes compromised, escharotomy is carried out. If the compartment symptom persists, fasciotomy involving all major compartments is performed. Since blood loss may be difficult to control, fasciotomy usually should be carried out in an operating room. While timely fasciotomy may allow preservation of nutrient blood flow to potentially viable tissue, it is likely that the ultimate extent of tissue damage is determined at the time of electrical injury and that progression of tissue loss seldom occurs.

Dead tissue promotes infection, which may be life threatening, and definitive therapy of the electrical burn must be directed toward the timely removal of necrotic tissue. At the present time, the amputation of electrically injured extremities is not routine. The availability of several diagnostic tools may allow definition of viable and nonviable tissue in wounds whose surface appearance may not reflect deeper injuries. Technetium 99m pyrophosphate scintigraphy is the most common diagnostic technique employed for evaluation of injured extremities and may provide useful results within the first 24 h. Normal isotopic uptake reflects normal perfusion, while totally nonviable tissue exhibits no uptake. Areas of potentially reversible injury demonstrate increased isotope uptake, and serial scanning may be useful in determining the need for debridement. In extremities with intact flow of the major arteries, arteriography may be helpful. Truncation of flow to nutrient muscle branches indicates irreversible injury. Ultimately, the viability of deep tissue is determined most accurately by serial surgical exploration of the injured extremity.

The timing of surgical intervention and the extent of debridement are determined by the stability of the patient and the nature of the injury. Generally, initial exploration and debridement may commence at the end of the resuscitation phase, within 24 to 48 h of injury. Distal portions of electrocuted extremities that are desiccated and mummified should be amputated. More proximally, it may be impossible to determine grossly the extent of deep tissue injury. These areas should be explored thoroughly, utilizing fasciotomy incisions if previously placed. All muscle groups should be inspected, especially those adjacent to bone. Only obviously necrotic tissue is removed, and every attempt should be made to salvage viable tissue. This approach requires daily wound examination and sequential operative debridements until all necrotic tissue is removed. Intervening complications, such as intractable hyperkalemia, severe myoglobinuria, or infection, may force abandonment of this sequential approach and require urgent amputation. It is rarely advisable to proceed to early closure following amputation, and definitive closure of the debrided wound is carried out only when all necrotic tissue has been removed. Similarly, excision or grafting of full-thickness cutaneous burns may be delayed until this time. Long-term care requires multidisciplinary rehabilitation and prosthetics services.

Associated Complications. Patients sustaining electrical injuries may develop a number of apparently unrelated late complications that develop from a few months to several years after injury. As with cutaneous burns, more than half of electrically injured patients develop posttraumatic stress disorders, especially if a body part has been lost. Associated psychiatric symptoms respond well to psychotherapy and medication. Contractures require extensive rehabilitation care and reconstructive surgery. Cholelithiasis occurs with increased frequency in patients who have sustained electrical burns. Cataracts are particularly troublesome and occur in up to 6 percent of electrically injured patients. The physical examination carried out on the admission of such patients should include a careful ophthalmologic evaluation to identify preexisting cataracts. Although vision loss may be extensive, surgical correction is highly effective.

Small children may sustain house current electric burns of the mouth as a consequence of sucking on electrical outlets or chewing a live extension cord (Fig. 7-29). The burn often involves the oral commissure and characteristically has the appearance of an avascular full-thickness burn. The high frequency of bleeding from the labial artery justifies initial in-hospital care of these patients. Because early surgical excision usually accentuates the long-term cosmetic lip deformity, all such injuries are treated with periodic debridement of only grossly nonviable tissue until primary healing is complete. What initially appeared to be a severe lesion heals with a lesser cosmetic defect. Following spontaneous closure, elective repair of any significant microstomia can be carried out.

Lightning Injury. Lightning injury is a relatively unusual form of electrical injury but is seen with rising frequency with the increase in outdoor leisure activities. Almost as many human lightning strikes occur to individuals inside dwellings. Most of the latter injuries occur to persons near windows, particularly those adjacent to plumbing in bathrooms or kitchens. The electrical energy produced by lightning typically is extremely high amperage of very short duration, and the thermal injuries produced resemble other forms of electrical injury. Most lightning strike victims sustain immediate cardiopulmonary arrest as a result of apnea caused by electrical paralysis of the brainstem respiratory center. The cutaneous injury is unique in its serpiginous and arborizing pattern of usually second-degree burn (Fig. 7-30). Cardiac abnormalities in survivors are frequent and consist of persistent arrhythmias and infarction patterns. Neurologic injuries manifest primarily as isolated and multiple peripheral nerve injuries. Tympanic membrane rupture is common and may be associated with hearing loss. Cataracts associated with lightning injuries were first reported in 1722. Treatment follows the general guidelines for electrical injury.

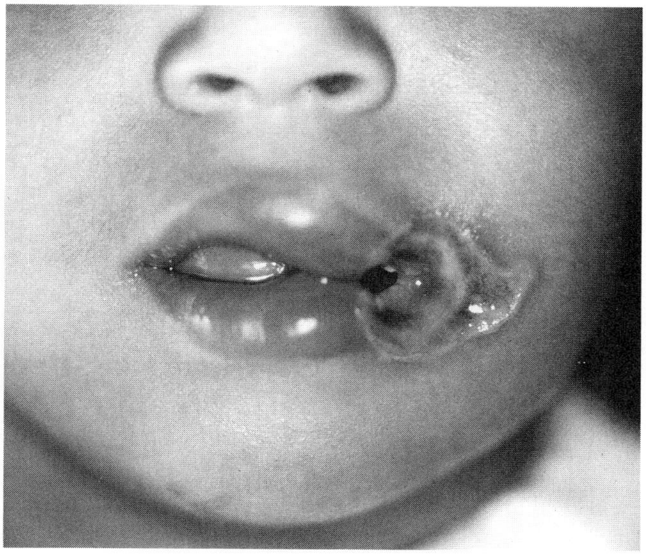

FIG. 7-29. Electrical injury of the oral commissure of a small child. This accident occurred as the child was chewing on the electrical cord of a household appliance. As the eschar of such burns spontaneously separates, a branch of the labial artery in this location often will rupture with massive hemorrhage.

CHEMICAL INJURIES

Chemical burns are produced by the thermal injury released during the reaction of strong acids or strong bases with viable tissue. Further, this destruction continues for as long as these chemicals remain in contact with tissue. Other toxic chemicals cause injury by desiccating tissue and allowing subsequent absorption through the burn with systemic toxicity. Immediate removal of these toxic agents is mandatory to limit further damage and toxicity, and first-responder personnel and other health-care workers are subject to chemical injury during this process. The incidence of chemical burns is rapidly increasing, and many of these injuries are the subject of expensive litigation. Chemical burns display discoloration of the skin that suggests a superficial burn, but most often the entire depth of skin and even the subcutaneous tissue are nonviable. With few exceptions, immediate irrigation with large quantities of water or saline commonly is the single most effective means of preventing tissue damage.

General Principles. The first priority of the treatment of chemical burns is rapid termination of the burning process. All clothing, including shoes and socks, should be promptly removed. With the exception of a few liquid chemicals and dry powders, all affected body areas should be irrigated immediately with large quantities of water or saline. The washing will remove or dilute the chemical agents and prevent further skin damage and absorption. The duration of continual irrigation depends on the nature of the burn. For ordinary acids, it is necessary to wash for at least 30 to 60 min; in burns with alkali, washing for hours is required. In burns of the head and face, cleansing of the eyes, nose, ears, and oral cavity demands special attention, and the eyes, in particular, should be washed first. Although dilution of many chemicals generates heat, the continuous administration of large quantities of irrigation should keep damaged tissues below the temperature of injury. Dry alkali powders should be brushed away carefully before copious irrigation is instituted. In almost no circumstance should specific neutralizing solutions be used; the heat of neutralization often is substantial and can cause additional thermal destruction.

Following irrigation, wound care is similar to that of other burns. Gentle debridement should be carried out. Initially, the appearance of the chemical burn appears deceptively benign and superficial. Only after several days does the extent of the destruction become evident, and recognition of the evolution of wound appearance is necessary to avoid misinforming the patient. Topical antimicrobial agents are applied to the burn, and if the burn is extensive, fluid resuscitation is instituted. Some agents cause systemic toxicities that must be treated as they present. Aerosolization of caustic chemicals can cause severe inhalation injury. Full-thickness chemical burns are excised and grafted in a timely fashion. Often underlying structures such as tendon or bone are involved, and several procedures by a multidisciplinary team may be necessary.

Acid Burns. A strong acid generally has a pH below 2.0 and causes coagulation necrosis of tissue. As such, its destructive effect is limited by the barrier of coagulated tissue, and irrigation is required for a short period of time. With certain exceptions, acid

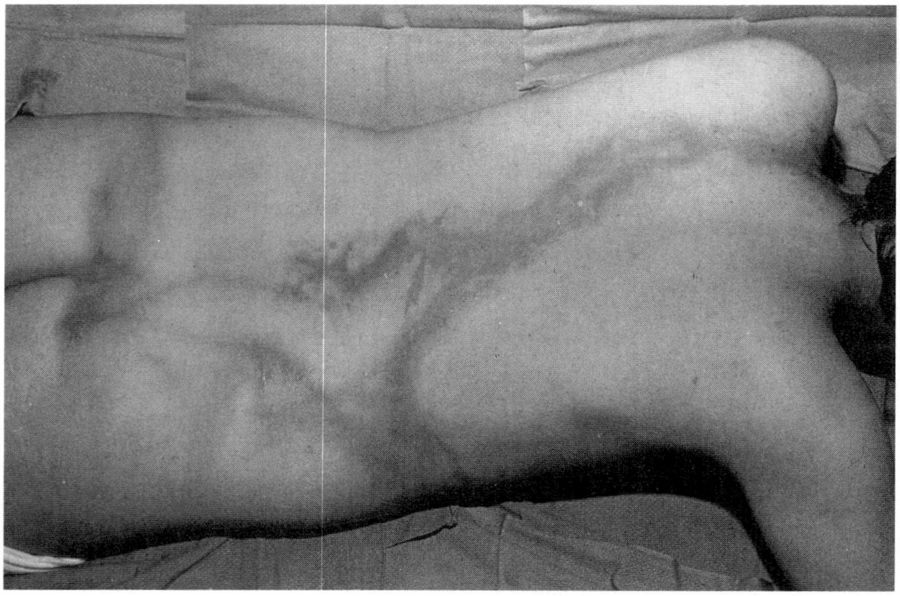

FIG. 7-30. Lightning injury in a young man. The splashed-on, serpentine pattern is characteristic for such injuries. Extensive deep tissue damage is unusual.

chemical burns are less destructive than alkali burns. The coagulated protein of the burn eschar has a characteristic appearance for many of the acids, and these distinctions may aid diagnosis. As with all caustic chemicals, increasing duration of contact accentuates the depth of injury. If the eschar is dark, has a leathery texture, and is desiccated, the chemical burn is likely a full-thickness injury.

Nitric Acid. Nitric acid is usually used as an industrial agent. It is highly corrosive and produces a yellow eschar. Nitric acid burns should be copiously irrigated.

Hydrochloric Acid. Hydrochloric acid is also an industrial chemical. The eschar it produces is white or grayish-brown. Its burns should be irrigated.

Sulfuric Acid. Sulfuric acid is a strong dehydrating agent. It produces a dry black or brown eschar and commonly extends through the skin into the subcutaneous tissue. Furthermore, sulfuric acid may form an indolent erosive surface and, because this acid produces considerable heat during tissue burning, causes severe pain. Concentrated sulfuric acid will produce intense heat when in contact with water and the amount of water used in washing must be copious to dilute the sulfuric acid and to disperse the heat produced. Chlorosulfonic acid is dissociated into sulfuric acid and hydrochloric acid when it comes into contact with water; it causes more severe burns than ordinary strong acids.

Hydrofluoric Acid. Hydrofluoric acid is a highly corrosive acid that produces toxicity by two distinct mechanisms. The hydrogen ions produce protein coagulation and tissue destruction in much the same manner as the other strong acids. In addition the free fluoride ion causes liquefaction and penetrates deeply to form salts with calcium and magnesium. This progressive tissue destruction is accompanied by intense deep pain and edema. Underlying tendons and bone may be damaged by direct contact with this agent. The subungual nail bed appears to be particularly susceptible to injury, leading to onycholysis and permanent nail deformities. Life-threatening hypocalcemia may develop following extensive contact with hydrofluoric acid.

Administration of calcium gluconate to the body area with the hydrofluoric acid burn is the most effective treatment for both relieving the burn-associated pain and terminating the invasive tissue destruction. Calcium reacts with hydrofluoric acid to form inactive calcium fluoride. The most effective route of calcium administration is uncertain. While local injection of calcium gluconate into the injured tissue is widely practiced, extremity burns appear to be best treated by regional intravenous perfusion of diluted (2 percent) calcium gluconate using the Bier tourniquet technique. Hydrofluoric acid burns on the torso are amenable only to local infiltration. Persistent hypocalcemia requires systemic administration of calcium gluconate.

Oxalic Acid. Oxalic acid may combine with calcium to cause devitalization of cell cytoplasm. Following contact with oxalic acid, the skin and mucosa will show white, indolent erosions. Besides immediate washing with running water, calcium gluconate should be injected locally and intravenously. Hypocalcemia may appear if oxalic acid burns extending over a considerable surface are not treated in time.

Phenol. Phenol, or carbolic acid, and its derivatives are highly corrosive acid alcohols that cause extensive coagulation necrosis. Light gray or light brown eschar may be formed following contact of the skin with phenol, and the skin becomes firm and thickened. The wound surface is dry, has well-defined margins, and demonstrates minimal swelling. Pain and numbness may be felt locally. Because of its high lipid solubility, phenol penetrates deeply into adjacent tissues. Phenol is sparsely soluble in water, and irrigation with water may promote tissue invasion. Therefore, flushing with water is not recommended unless a high-volume source is available. Phenol is most soluble in polyethylglycol; a 50% solution of polyethylene glycol in water is recommended since a high concentration causes a significant exothermic reaction. The burn is thoroughly rinsed until the smell of phenol on the wound surface disappears completely. The polyethylene glycol should be removed from the skin by copious water irrigation because it too can cause systemic toxicity following absorption through the burn wound.

Systemic absorption of phenol may cause central nervous system depression, hypothermia, intravascular hemolysis, acute tubular necrosis, pulmonary edema, and cardiovascular collapse.

While phenol is not a common household agent, its derivative cresol is used in several cleaning products. While industrial concentrations of cresol are required to produce deep cutaneous burns, systemic absorption of more dilute preparations will produce all of the toxic effects of phenol. Affected patients are best treated with hemodialysis and standard burn wound care.

Formic Acid. Formic acid is an organic acid used in agriculture and industry and can cause full-thickness chemical burns and systemic toxicity. Absorption of formic acid will cause acidosis, hemolysis, and hemoglobinuria. Copious water lavage is effective in removing surface accumulations. Acidosis and the presence of hemochromagens in the urine are treated as described above. Hemodialysis may be helpful in reversing severe systemic toxicity.

Alkali Burns. A strong alkali has a pH of 11.5 or greater and causes liquefaction necrosis. Because a barrier of coagulated protein never forms, alkali burns are much more invasive and require prolonged periods of water irrigation (up to 12 h). Dry powdered lime first should be brushed away before instituting irrigation. A strong alkali can dissolve protein and collagen, forming alkaline protein compounds; it can also saponify fat and causes cellular dehydration of the tissues. The heat produced during saponification will cause further necrosis of the deeper tissues. Consequently, the depth of burn in the early stage is often underestimated, and when reestimated at later stages the surface area of a third-degree burn often is found to be greater than originally estimated. Edema is marked during the shock stage of an alkali burn, with extensive loss of fluids and hypovolemia. Such burns are prone to infection and wound sepsis.

Nearly all of the strong alkalis are hydroxides of sodium, potassium, and other metals. Ammonia is an irritative gas and also belongs to the category of strong alkalis. Ammonia water is the aqueous solution of ammonia, ammonium hydroxide. It is alkaline, with ammonia forming approximately 20 percent of its content. Prolonged contact with mucosa or skin will produce severe burns. When ammonia is in contact with water in the airway mucosa, it leads to the local formation of ammonium hydroxide, which can cause liquefaction necrosis with edema and mucosal slough. Ammonia causes death by laryngospasm and asphyxia.

Burns caused by lime are usually deep second or third degree, and the wound surface appears rather dry or desiccated. In the management of such burns, the lime powder must first be wiped clean; washing with a large amount of running water then may be carried out. This will prevent aggravation of the burn by the heat produced by the contact of lime with water.

Other Chemicals Burns. ***White Phosphorus.*** White phosphorus is a commonly used incendiary in military munitions and fireworks and in agricultural products (fertilizers). When exposed to air, white phosphorus spontaneously oxidizes to phosphorus pentoxide, which will hydrolyze in water to form potentially caustic phosphoric acid. Upon spontaneous oxidation, the phosphorus ignites with a yellow flame and produces a dense white smoke with a characteristic garlic smell. Besides the direct thermal injury produced by the burning phosphorus particles, clothing often ignites and produces an even longer burn. Because of the explosive nature of the spontaneous ignition, phosphorus particles often are deeply embedded below the skin. Phosphorus ignition is prevented by eliminating the presence of oxygen. This is best accomplished by covering the wound with water or saline-soaked dressings. White phosphorus melts at 44°C and the oily liquid readily spreads to clothing and may be difficult to detect. Imbedded particles are best removed in the operating room and the retrieved particles must be placed in water to prevent ignition and injury to the surgical staff. A Wood's lamp is helpful in identifying phosphorus particles, which fluoresce under ultraviolet light.

Copper sulfate solutions have been used extensively to neutralize and identify phosphorus particles. Copper sulfate forms black cupric phosphide granules, which prevent further oxidation. However, copper sulfate solutions, particularly in concentrations greater than 1%, are systemically absorbed and produce acute nausea, vomiting, renal and hepatic failure, and massive hemolysis. These solutions are now rarely used. Phosphorus may be absorbed through the burn wound and produce cardiac arrhythmias. Patients should be monitored with continuous electrocardiography and with frequent determinations of serum electrolytes.

Hydrocarbons. Gasoline burns occur most commonly in patients in motor vehicle accidents but also arise from criminal assaults. Subsequent ignition produces typical flame burns. Patients sustaining such burns require significantly greater fluid resuscitations and have more prolonged and complicated clinical courses. Gasoline and other hydrocarbons also can produce burns without ignition. Dousing or immersion with prolonged exposure will produce partial- or even full-thickness burns. These solvents are cytotoxic and promote dissolution of tissue lipids, causing cutaneous injury. Systemic absorption of hydrocarbons, both through the skin and the respiratory tract, can cause chemical pneumonitis and bronchitis, glomerulonephritis, hepatitis, and cardiac instability. Tetraethyl lead in gasoline can be absorbed through the skin and cause symptomatic lead poisoning. Blood and urine lead levels should be monitored, and the lead poisoning syndrome should be treated with chelating agents (dimercaprol, ethylene diaminetetraacetic acid, and penicillamine).

Tar. Tar is the residue after fractional distillation of petroleum. There are four kinds of tar: coal tar, petroleum tar, oil-shale tar, and natural tar. Coal tar contains the greatest amount of volatile substances and causes the most marked tissue damage; petroleum tar and oil-shale tar contain the least amount of volatile substances and cause less chemical damage; and natural tar does not contain any volatile substance and is not directly harmful to human skin. Depending on its temperature, hot tar causes direct thermal cutaneous injury. The severity of the burn is compounded in proportion to the volatile hydrocarbon content of the tar. Immediate cooling of the hot tar to body temperature is the most important aspect of treatment. Burns caused by hot liquid tar avidly stick to the skin and any attempt to remove the tar at this time will accentuate the cutaneous injury. Removal of the tar should be delayed until the resuscitation phase is completed. The best method of removal is to apply a petroleum-based ointment to solubilize the tar and facilitate removal. Over several days the tar will begin to loosen and detach. Second- and third-degree burns are evident with equal frequency once the tar is removed.

Cement. Wet cement will cause a chemical burn. Cement is a mixture of calcium silicates, alumina, and iron oxide. The pH of cement usually exceeds 12 because of the presence of calcium oxide and, in the presence of water, of sodium, potassium, and calcium hydroxides. Such injuries often are not recognized until many hours after initial contact.

Magnesium. Burns caused by magnesium are unusual. Magnesium may penetrate into the deep-lying tissues if it is not removed promptly from the skin. It reacts with the tissue fluids in the subcutaneous tissue to form magnesium oxide and liberates hydrogen, causing local formation of emphysematous lesions and massive necrosis simulating gas gangrene. The ulcers formed by the magnesium are small initially but they gradually enlarge several weeks later. Some ulcers are undermined with irregular bases; red granulomatous nodules may appear, and the ulcers heal slowly. After a magnesium burn, the wound surface should be tangentially excised to remove the magnesium together with the necrotic tissue, thus preventing delayed healing of the wound surface. If magnesium is absorbed through the skin or inhaled, respiratory symptoms, nausea, vomiting, chills, or high fever may occur.

Ocular Injuries. Immediate and copious lavage of chemically injured eyes with water or saline is essential to retain vision and minimize damage to the globe and surrounding structures. Initial irrigation can be started by everting the eyelids and dripping normal saline through intravenous tubing directly onto the globe. Extended irrigation is necessary in patients with injuries caused by strong alkalis, and a contact lens with an irrigating side arm facilitates lavage. A local anesthetic should be instilled to prevent blepharospasm, and a cycloplegic agent in combination with a miotic agent is administered to reduce the effects of iritis. Surveillance cultures dictate the choice of ophthalmic antibiotics. The subconjunctival injection of autologous serum, the local application of edetic acid or cysteine, and mucosal grafts have been recommended to reduce scar formation, but such interventions have had only limited success. Symblepharon adhesions should be lysed before dense scarring forms between the globe and the eyelid. An injured eye should not be patched. Xerophthalmia is treated with tear solutions and a bandage lens. Alkali injuries often cause devastating scar formations in the cornea and deeper ocular structures, and globe perforation is not uncommon. Corneal transplants have been generally unsuccessful in restoring vision. Chemical eyelid burns often lead to the formation of ectropions with exposure of the globe; subsequent desiccation leads to corneal perforation and collapse of the globe, necessitating enucleation. Tarsorrhaphies can be used to maintain eyelid coverage, but symblepharons often become unavoidable.

LONG-TERM CARE

Rehabilitation. ***Inpatient Therapy.*** Maintaining function and preventing the complications of prolonged immobility are the specific goals of the rehabilitative treatment of burn patients. Daily assessment of the patient's range of motion, ambulating ability, and functional status is necessary to determine the effectiveness of ongoing treatment plans and to make modifications as needed for new deficits. These assessments begin on the day of admission for all burn patients. The location of the burn in relation to the joint axis determines what movement will be limited as the burn heals. In most extremity burns, the position of maximal comfort promotes the formation of scar contractures. Because compliance is a major factor in a successful rehabilitation program, the burn therapist must work closely with the entire burn team in developing the patient's trust, understanding, and confidence. Our burn team includes not only physical and occupational therapists, but also a play therapist who engages children in physical activities in an environment in which they often are not aware of the therapeutic nature of the active exercises they are performing. This facility commonly enables children to achieve full range of motion independently. Passive exercises must be used with great caution, since overzealous ranging may lead to tendon disruption, muscle tears, heterotopic ossification, and traumatic release of scar contractures.

Physical therapy begins on the day of admission. Burned extremities are elevated and actively exercised to minimize edema and reduce the need for escharotomy. Stable patients initially are placed in chairs and then begin ambulation as tolerated. Injudicious use of analgesics and antianxiety drugs impede a successful mobilization program, and great skill is required to find the optimal doses of these drugs. When out of bed, burned legs are wrapped with disposable compression bandages to prevent venous stasis and edema. Even when in bed, nearly all burned extremities develop varying degrees of edema. Active exercises maintain muscle mass and strength. Passive exercises are employed most commonly in debilitated and mentally obtunded patients, and therapists must be careful not to exceed the limits of tissue extensibility. Continuous passive motion devices and dynamic splinting increase function in such patients and do not require the continual presence of the rehabilitation therapists. Objective measurements of joint stiffness can be quantified by piston-drive displacement transducers, and these devices provide useful documentation of patient progress.

Burn contractures are unlike other types of contractures. Burn scars commonly envelop the entire circumference of single joints, and the scar may involve multiple joints. Contraction may pull a joint in one direction and an adjacent joint in the opposite direction (Fig. 7-31). A classic example is boutonnière deformity of the fifth finger. Therefore, the entire burn scar must be uniformly stretched, and complex splints or even multiple joint pin fixation often is required. Positioning of body parts in the antideformity posture best prevents wound contracture. Splints also are used for

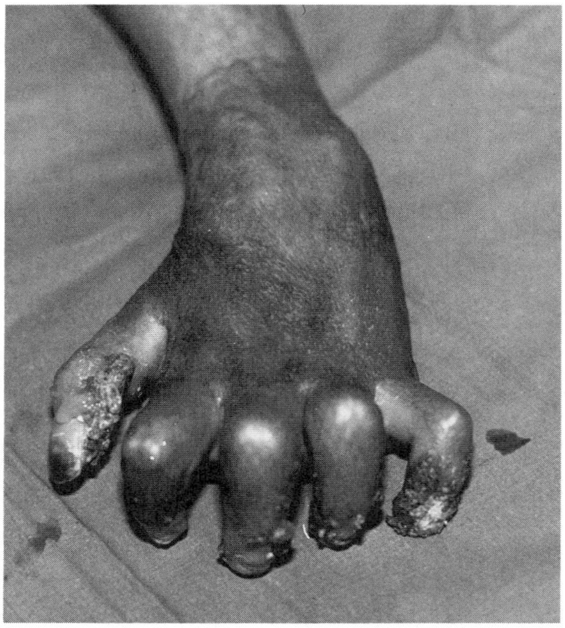

FIG. 7-31. Scar hypertrophy and contraction of a grafted deep third-degree burn of the hand. With tendon and joint capsule damage, timely splinting and joint fixation is necessary to prevent the development of a functionally useless claw.

immobilizing freshly grafted extremities to prevent inadvertent shearing of the new autograft.

Hypertrophic scarring is one of the most troublesome sequelae of cutaneous burns. All second- and third-degree burns produce permanent scarring. Some scars in healed second-degree burns are barely noticeable, while deeper burns, even when grafted, may develop bulky scar. Certain individuals are prone to severe hypertrophic scar formation. Scar hypertrophy can be retarded by the use of custom-fitted pressure garments over healed scars. Specially fitted inserts may be necessary to apply pressure to concave areas of skin. All individuals whose burns do not heal by the second postburn week should be treated with pressure devices, first with a generic tubular elastic stocking and later, after the surface of the burn scar stabilizes, with custom-made compression garments. Adults usually wear these garments for 3 to 6 months, while small children require up to 4 years of compression therapy before scar maturation occurs.

Outpatient Therapy. Many functional deficits persist after discharge. The burn center outpatient facility must provide the structure for frequent and continuous follow-up for as long as 10 years. For many patients, the burn center outpatient facility provides their only access to primary care. Pressure garments require regular refitting. At this time, patients are able to use complex physical training devices and special techniques for reducing contractures, and some require daily visits to the rehabilitation department. Outpatients are evaluated 1 week after discharge, and the intervals between the following visits are gradually lengthened, depending on individual patient needs. As burn scars mature, permanent residual deficits or deformities may be amenable to reconstructive surgical correction. Usually, multiple small operations are employed, and total corrective surgery may extend over 10 years. Patients develop follicular infection in the burn wound several months after injury. These plugged follicles usually disappear once hair erupts through the overlying epithelium. Severe itching and vague but intense neuritic pain are long lasting and are poorly responsive to antipruritic medications and analgesics. Printed explanations of burn care and detailed treatment procedures are effective in allaying anxiety and ameliorating patient discomfort.

Psychological Support. Burned patients display a variety of psychological responses to their injury, including anxiety, depression, denial, withdrawal, and regression. Withdrawal and regression are especially common in children, who may refuse to participate and cooperate with their care. Play therapy provides a forum for interaction between children who are often injured by similar mechanisms and may suffer the same cosmetic deformities or functional deficits. The rapport provided by the team of play therapists, physical and occupational therapists, burn nurses, and physicians promotes compliance among the patients and encourages the proper use of pressure garments and assistive devices.

Nearly half of older children and adults develop the posttraumatic stress disorder following thermal injury. The disorder is characterized by recurrent and intrusive recollections of the initial injury, avoidance of circumstances that invoke memories of the event, loss of interest in daily activities, feelings of isolation, hyperalertness, memory impairment, and sleep disturbances. Noncompliance with burn therapy is a serious outward manifestation of the patient's attempt to avoid recollections of the traumatic event. The individual's psychological state following the burn injury predicts the likelihood of occurrence of posttraumatic stress disorder. The presence of symptoms of the posttraumatic stress disorder during the acute hospitalization correlates with psychological impairment during convalescence. The severity of injury is not related to the symptoms. Both short- and long-term psychotherapeutic support frequently is necessary in burned patients, and a full-time psychiatrist is an essential member of the burn team. Burned patients rarely seek treatment for psychological problems and the burn staff must actively evaluate this potential need. The frequency of this disorder increases with length of follow-up.

Family support groups convene on a weekly basis and are instrumental in enabling the burn team to present an update on the patient's progress, to address specific short- and long-term goals of burn management, to respond to questions pertaining to current treatment plans, and to allay anxieties and fears voiced by family members regarding their expectations for the patient's eventual convalescence. This type of psychosocial support system plays a critical role in the comprehensive care of the burn patient, not only during the inpatient stay but also throughout outpatient follow-up, which continues for years postinjury.

Reconstructive Problems. ***Hypertrophic Scar and Keloid Formation.*** Burn scar hypertrophy typically develops in deeper partial-thickness injuries and third-degree burns that are allowed to heal primarily. Hypertrophy of grafted areas of excised burn wound occurs less frequently and is dependent, in part, on the time from injury to excision, on the involved anatomic part, and on the particular surgical technique employed (see Fig. 7-31). Tangential excision of the burn wound was introduced by Janzekovic to obtain a better cosmetic and functional result. With tangential excision, necrotic tissue of a partial-thickness burn is removed in successive layers until a base of partially viable dermis is reached; in most circumstances, the wound is then immediately grafted. Depending on the depth of the burn wound, sequential excision extends to varying levels of the skin and subcutaneous tissue until all nonviable tissue is removed. Sequential excision, therefore, encompasses tangential excision, but goes beyond it to include the complete excision of necrotic full-thickness injuries. Delayed tangential excision is more likely to result in residual scar hypertrophy in grafted burn wound.

Because only a few epithelial elements, sweat glands, and hair follicles remain viable in deep partial-thickness burns, healing takes place from these remnants over a period of 3 to 6 weeks. The resulting scar epithelium is of poor quality and is prone to form hypertrophic scar. Although both exhibit excessive collagen production, hypertrophic scar should be distinguished from a keloid. A keloid overgrows the original dimensions of the initial injury (Fig. 7-32). Hypertrophic scar develops in the bed of the injured tissue and is confined to its original anatomic boundaries. Hypertrophic scars frequently will flatten with time and pressure, whereas keloids often do not respond. As described above, burn scar hypertrophy is most commonly treated with a constant application of pressure on healed wounds by elastic garments. Although long-term controlled trials have not clearly demonstrated permanent beneficial effects from compression therapy, compression garments quickly reduce the mass of hypertrophic immature scars and provide patients with tangible evidence of the benefits of conscientious follow-up after injury. The mechanism by which constant compression application reduces scar mass is not well defined. It can cause profound changes in the partially occluded microvasculature of hypertrophic scars. The pressure then leads to focal degeneration of selected cells because of anoxia following microvascular occlusion. Electron microscopy has demonstrated

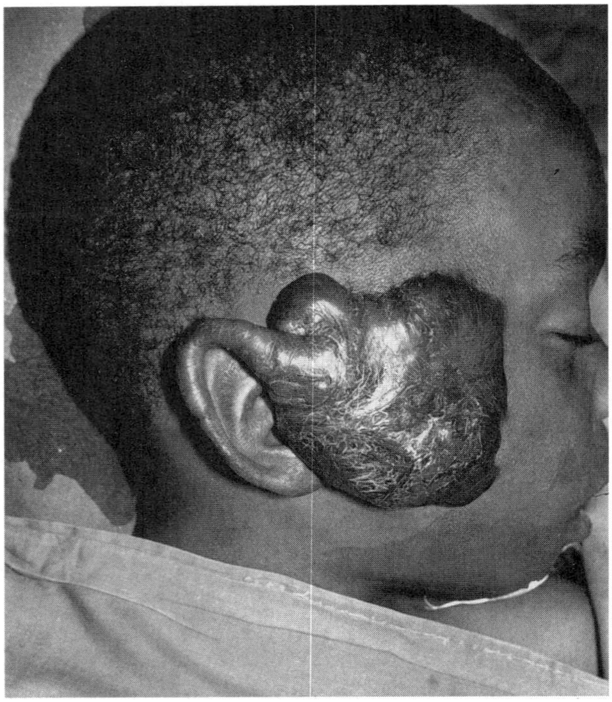

FIG. 7-32. Large keloid arising from a small burn just anterior to the tragus of the ear. Reconstructive surgery is necessary to reduce the bulk of this keloid, although the long-term appearance may be only modestly improved.

that fibroblasts in pressure-treated wounds are more linearly organized and collagen is manufactured in a more organized fashion.

Other forms of therapy for hypertrophic scarring include radiotherapy, cryotherapy, and reexcision and wound closure. Radiotherapy in doses of 1500 to 2000 rads has been used with varying results. Radiation probably produces an inhibitory effect on both fibroplasia and capillary budding. Cryotherapy is now rarely used. It is associated with depigmentation and increased melanocyte sensitivity to subsequent cold exposure. The most successful approach to residual hypertrophic burn scars is initial pressure therapy until the wound matures, followed by subsequent excision and application of skin grafts. Tissue expansion has been used to expand normal skin and replace the excised hypertrophic scar or keloid. Complication rates with tissue expansion are as high as 40 percent and include infection, implant extrusion, and device rupture. Such complications usually require removal of the original implant, treatment of any infection, and replacement.

Because of their marked propensity to recur, keloids are much more difficult to treat. Therapy has included excision of the keloid and primary closure, which is effective for linearly oriented keloids with a narrow base; however, excessive wound tension leads to recurrence. Broad-based keloids may be removed flush with the surrounding skin and a split-thickness skin graft placed over the base of the keloid to prevent it from recurring. Unfortunately, excision alone has a recurrence rate of greater than 50 percent. Intralesional injection of corticosteroids has been advocated as a means to reduce the bulk of keloid and hypertrophic scar mass. This therapeutic modality may be used in combination with excision or split-thickness skin grafting. Triamcinolone is the most commonly used steroid and is believed to act by decreasing collagen synthesis and increasing collagen degradation through its effect on the collagen inhibitors, alpha-2 macroglobulin and alpha-1 antitrypsin. When steroid injection is used in conjunction with surgery, keloids should be injected for at least 1 month prior to the operation. Some surgeons inject triamcinolone in the base of the wound and along its edges during the surgical procedure. Postoperatively, the patient receives injections monthly until the wound matures. The major side-effects of intralesional injection of steroids are hypopigmentation and atrophy of the skin surrounding the keloid.

Many burns heal with loss of pigmentation, and burn scar hypopigmentation and surface irregularity can be significantly improved by dermabrasion and thin split-thickness grafting. Adequate pigmentation and flat surfaces are obtained in most patients. Tissue expanders are particularly effective for treating burn scar alopecia. Approximately 20 percent of patients treated in burn facilities are readmitted for reconstructive procedures. The most common areas of reconstruction involve the hand and wrist (most common), arm and forearm, face, and neck. Improved inpatient burn treatment and scar management are reducing the need for subsequent reconstructive surgery.

Marjolin's Ulcer. Chronic ulceration of old burn scars was noted by Marjolin to lead frequently to malignant degeneration (Fig. 7-33). The most common lesion is squamous cell carcinoma, although basal cell carcinomas occasionally occur (Fig. 7-34). Rare tumors, including malignant fibrous histiocytoma, sarcoma, and neurotropic malignant melanoma, also have been described. Therefore, it is critical to suspect malignant degeneration in any patient who exhibits chronic breakdown of a healed burn wound scar. Although such lesions typically appear decades after the

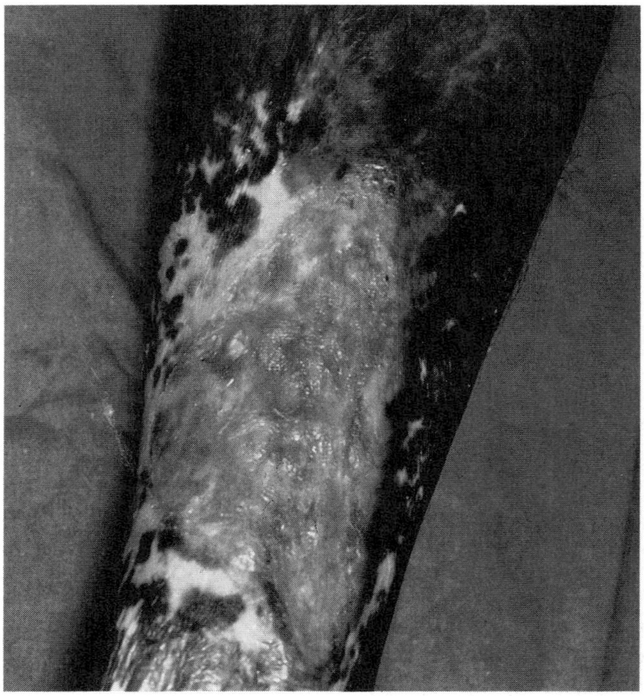

FIG. 7-33. Chronically unstable scar in a 20-year-old burn. Biopsy of this scar confirmed the presence of malignant changes in this Marjolin's ulcer. The patient underwent wide excision of all chronically irritated skin and thick split-thickness skin grafting.

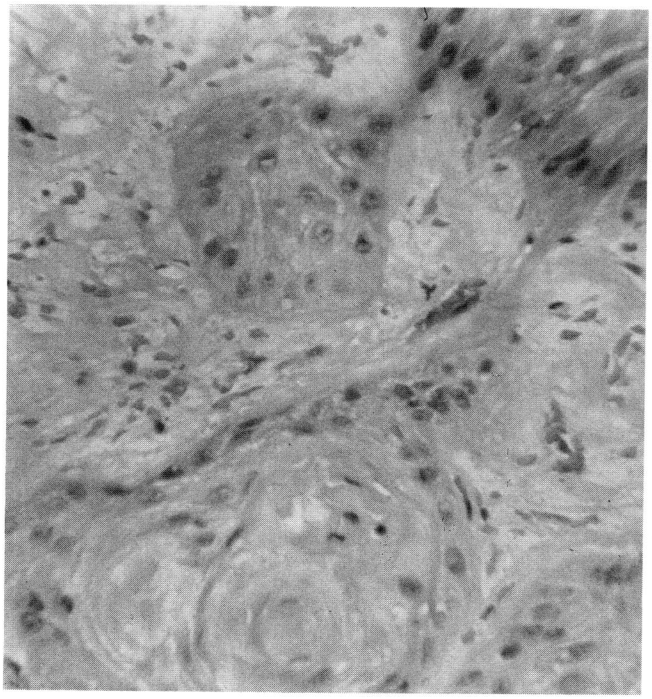

FIG. 7-34. Squamous cell carcinoma in Marjolin's ulcer. Nests of epithelial cells characteristic of this lesion are evident on histologic examination.

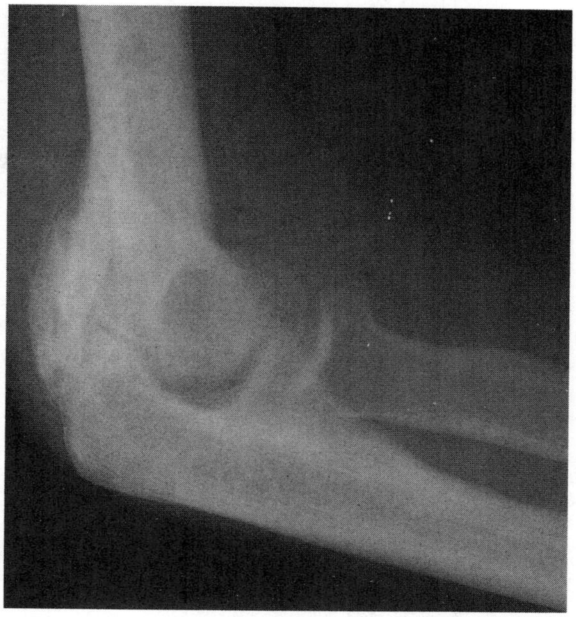

FIG. 7-35. Heterotopic ossification of the elbow. Pain on flexion and restriction of motion prompted radiographic examination. The calcification is located in the muscle and soft tissue around the joint but seldom directly affects the tendons.

original injury, burn scar carcinoma may be encountered within the first year. A biopsy of chronic wound ulcers with histologic confirmation of malignancy dictates wide excision. In the absence of cancer, most unstable burn scars should be excised and resurfaced. Burn scar carcinomas may metastasize aggressively; however, prophylactic regional node dissection has not improved mortality. Approximately 30 percent of burn scar carcinomas occur in the head and neck, and adjuvant radiotherapy for these lesions improves survival. Very deep dermal burns that have not healed by the third or fourth postburn week occasionally develop nodules in the burn wound bed. When these wounds are excised and grafted, the pathologic diagnosis of the surgical specimen is often confused. Usually these nodules represent pseudoepitheliomatous hyperplasia or keratoacanthomas; on occasion, these lesions are erroneously interpreted as carcinoma or lymphoma.

Heterotopic Ossification. Heterotopic ossification occurs in up to 13 percent of burned patients. Although this complication may develop in patients with partial-thickness burns and around extremities not involved with the injury, it most commonly involves patients with full-thickness burns greater than 20 percent TBSA and adjacent to the involved joint 1 to 3 months after injury. The elbow is the most commonly affected joint (Fig. 7-35). The diagnosis usually is made by the physical or occupational therapist, who discovers increased pain and decreased range of motion of the involved joints (Fig. 7-36). Limitation of physical activity usually precedes radiographic evidence of calcification, which is located in the muscle and surrounding soft tissue of the joint. Although the mechanism causing heterotopic ossification is not known, aggressive physical therapy with bleeding into the soft tissue has been incriminated. Prolonged immobilization of a joint encompassed by a burn also appears to promote heterotopic ossification. Restricted activity promotes mobilization of body calcium stores and may lead to deposition of calcium in the soft tissues. Treatment remains controversial. Some suggest surgical removal of all ossified soft tissue, but others recommend supervised rehabilitation therapy and allowing reabsorption of ossified tissue.

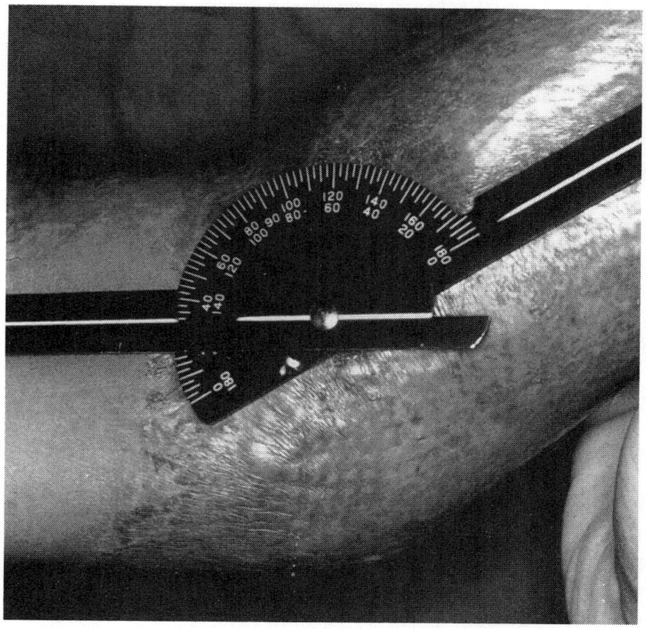

FIG. 7-36. Reduced range of motion in a patient with heterotopic ossification. Although the patient had been burned and grafted over the antecubital fossa, graft contracture did not cause the reduced range of motion.

Fractures. Up to 10 percent of burned patients have associated fractures. Until recently, fractures were treated conservatively, ranging from casting to splinting and traction to external fixation. Placement of internal hardware was thought to promote infection at the site of the appliance. More recently, internal fixation has been shown not to increase the risk of infection. In applicable situations, early reduction and internal fixation of fractures can be carried out safely in most burned patients.

Fractures in patients with large burns are treated with splints or traction until resuscitation is complete. Operative repair preferably is performed within 48 to 72 h of burn injury. Burn wounds adjacent to fracture sites are usually excised and autografted at the time of internal fixation. If internal fixation is not possible, external fixation is used, which permits access to the burn wound and provides effective practical stability of the injury.

Bibliography

General

Artz CP, Moncrief JA, Pruitt BA: *Burns: A Team Approach*. Philadelphia, WB Saunders, 1979.

Clark WB, Fromm BS: Burn mortality: Experience at a regional burn unit. *Acta Chir Scand* (suppl 537), 1987.

Haponik EF, Munster AM: *Respiratory Injury: Smoke Inhalation and Burns*. New York, McGraw-Hill, 1990.

Proceedings of the NIH Conference: Advances in understanding trauma and burn injury. *J Trauma* (suppl) 12, 1990.

Wachtel TL, Kahn V, Frank HA: *Current Topics in Burn Care*. Rockville, MD, Aspen, 1983.

Wilmore DW, Brennan MF, Harken AH, Holcroft JW, Meakins JL (eds): *American College of Surgeons Care of the Surgical Patient*. New York, Scientific American, 1993.

Epidemiology

Amy BW, McManus WF, et al: Lightning injury with survival in five patients. *JAMA* 253:243, 1985.

Baker SP, O'Neill B, Karpf RS: *The Injury Fact Book*. Lexington, MA, Lexington Books, 1984, p. 139.

Ballard JE, Koepsell TD, Rivara F: Association of smoking and alcohol drinking with residential fire injuries. *Am J Epidemiol* 135:26, 1992.

Bowden ML, Grant ST, et al: The elderly, disabled and handicapped adult burned through abuse and neglect. *Burns* 14:447, 1988.

Clark WR, Lerner D: Regional burn survey: Two years of hospitalized burns in central New York. *J Trauma* 18:524, 1978.

Deitch EA, Staats M: Child abuse through burning. *J Burn Care Rehabil* 3:89, 1982.

Erikson EJ, Merrell SW, et al: Differences in mortality from thermal injury between pediatric and adult patients. *J Pediat Surg* 26:821, 1991.

Finkelstein JL, Schwartz SB, et al: Pediatric burns: An overview. *Pediatr Clin North Am* 39:1145, 1992.

Graiteer PL, Sniezek JE: Hospitalization due to tap water scalds, 1978–1985. *MMWR* 37:35, 1987.

Kawakami M, Switzer BR, et al: Immune suppression after acute ethanol ingestion and thermal injury. *J Surg Res* 51:210, 1991.

Kobayashi JM: Fireworks-related injuries—Washington. *MMWR* 32:285, 1983.

Lenoski EF, Hunter KA: Specific patterns of inflicted burn injuries. *J Trauma* 17:842, 1977.

Locke JA, Rossignol AM, Burke JF: Socio-economic factors and the incidence of hospitalized burn injuries in New England counties, USA. *Burns* 16:273, 1990.

Mierley MC, Baker SP: Fatal house fires in an urban population. *JAMA* 249:1466, 1983.

Moir GC, Shakespeare V, Shakespeare PG: Audit of thermally injured children under 5 years of age. *Burns* 17:406, 1991.

Mozingo DW, Smith AA, et al: Chemical burns. *J Trauma* 28:642, 1988.

National Safety Council Accident Facts, 1981 Edition. Chicago, National Safety Council, 1981.

O'Neill JA, Meacham WF, et al: Patterns of injury in the battered child syndrome. *J Trauma* 13:332, 1973.

Perrotta DM, Boender J, et al: Occupational electrocution—Texas 1981–1985. *MMWR* 36:725, 1987.

Pruitt BA Jr: Forces and factors influencing trauma care: 1983 AAST Presidential Address. *J Trauma* 24:463, 1984.

Pruitt BA Jr: The universal trauma model. *Bull Am Coll Surg* 70 (No. 10):2, 1985.

Pruitt BA Jr, Mason AD Jr, Goodwin CW: Epidemiology of burn injury and demography of burn care facilities. *Probl Gen Surg* 7:235, 1990.

Purdue GF, Hunt JL, Prescott PE: Child abuse by burning: An index of suspicion. *J Trauma* 28:221, 1988.

Runyon CW, Gerken EA: Epidemiology and prevention of adolescent injury: A review and research agenda. *JAMA* 262:2273, 1989.

Showers J, Garrison KM: Burn abuse: A four-year study. *J Trauma* 28:1581, 1988.

Sorenson B: Management of burns occurring as mass casualties after nuclear explosion. *Burns* 6:33, 1979.

Spitz MC: Severe burns as a consequence of seizures in patients with epilepsy. *Epilepsia* 33:103, 1992.

Swenson JR, Dimsdale JE, et al: Drug and alcohol abuse in patients with acute burn injuries. *J Psychosomat Med* 3:287, 1991.

Trier H, Spaabaek J: The nursing home patient, a burn-prone person: An epidemiological study. *Burns* 13:484, 1987.

Delivery of Burn Care

American Burn Association, Appendix B. Guidelines for service standards and severity classifications in the treatment of thermal injury. Cincinnati, American Burn Association, 1983.

Bull JP, Squire JR: A study of mortality in a burns unit: Standards for the evaluation of alternative methods of treatment. *Ann Surg* 130:160, 1949.

Burn Care Resources in North America, 1991–1992. Cincinnati, American Burn Association, 1991.

Curreri PW, Luterman A, et al: Burn injury: Analysis of survival and hospitalization time for 937 patients. *Ann Surg* 192:472, 1980.

Halebian PH, Madden MR, et al: Improved burn center survival of patients with toxic epidermal necrolysis managed without corticosteroids. *Ann Surg* 204:503, 1986.

Herndon DN, LeMaster J, et al: The quality of life after major thermal injury in children: An analysis of 12 survivors with greater than 80% total body, 70% third-degree burns. *J Trauma* 26:609, 1986.

Jones WG, Halebian P, et al: Drug-induced toxic epidermal necrolysis in children. *J Pediatr Surg* 24:167, 1989.

Krob MJ, D'Amica FJ, Ross DL: Do trauma scores accurately predict outcomes for patients with burns? *J Burn Care Rehabil* 12:560, 1991.

Molter NC: Workload management systems for nurses: Application to the burn unit. *J Burn Care Rehabil* 11:267, 1990.

Peterson VM, Murphy JR, et al: Identification of novel prognostic indicators in burned patients. *J Trauma* 28:632, 1988.

Piccolo NS, Piccolo-Lobo MS, Piccolo-Daher MTJ: Two years in burn care, an analysis of 12423 cases. *Burns* 17:490, 1991.

Pre-Hospital Advanced Burn Life Support Course. Lincoln, Nebraska Burn Institute, 1991.

Pruitt BA Jr: Burn treatment for the unburned. *JAMA* 257:2207, 1987.

Pruitt BA Jr: Improvement in burn care. *JAMA* 244:2090, 1980.

Pruitt BA Jr, Tumbusch WT, et al: Mortality in 1100 consecutive burns treated at a burn unit. *Ann Surg* 159:396, 1964.

Reese JM, Dimick AR: The cost of burn care and the federal government's response in the 1990's. *Clin Plast Surg* 3:561, 1992.

Shirani KZ, Pruitt BA Jr, Mason AD Jr: The influence of inhalation injury and pneumonia on burn mortality. *Ann Surg* 205:82, 1987.

Smith DJ Jr, Robson MC, et al: DRG-driven change in burn wound management: A success story. *Plast Reconstr Surg* 82:710, 1988.

Thorpe, KE, Kim JO, Goodwin CW: Variation in resource consumption within burn DRGs. *Proc Am Burn Assoc* 18:116, 1986.

Treat RC, Sirinek KR, et al: Air evacuation of thermally injured patients: Principles of treatment and results. *J Trauma* 20:275, 1980.

Wasserman D, Schlotterer M: Survival rates of patients hospitalized in French burn units during 1985. *Burns* 15:261, 1989.

Zawackie BE, Azen SP, et al: Multifactorial probit analysis of mortality in burned patients. *Ann Surg* 189:1, 1979.

Zoch G, Schemper M, et al: Comparison of prognostic indices for burns and assessment of their accuracy. *Burns* 18:370, 1992.

Resuscitation

Arturson G: Microvascular permeability to macromolecules in thermal injury. *Acta Physiol Scand* (suppl) 463:111, 1979.

Asch MJ, Mersol PM, et al: Regional blood flow in the burned anesthetized dog. *Surg Forum* 22:55, 1971.

Aulick LH, Goodwin CW, et al: Visceral blood flow following thermal injury. *Ann Surg* 193:112, 1985.

Baxter CR: Fluid volume and electrolyte changes in the early postburn period. *Clin Plast Surg* 1:693, 1974.

Baxter CR, Shires GT: Physiological response to crystalloid resuscitation of severe burns. *Ann N Y Acad Sci* 150:874, 1968.

Blalock A: Trauma to the intestine: The importance of the local loss of fluid in the production of low blood pressure. *Arch Surg* 22:314, 1931.

Boshkov LK, Tredget EE, Janowska-Wieczorek A: Recombinant human erythropoietin for a Jehovah's Witness with anemia of thermal injury. *Am J Hematol* 37:53, 1991.

Bowser B, Caldwell FT: The effects of resuscitation with hypertonic vs hypotonic vs colloid on wound and urine fluid and electrolyte losses in severely burned children. *J Trauma* 23:916, 1983.

Cioffi WG, DeMeules JE, Gamelli RL: The effects of burn injury and fluid resuscitation on cardiac function in vitro. *J Trauma* 26:638, 1986.

Cioffi WG, Vaughn GM, et al: Dissociation of blood volume and flow in regulation of salt and water balance. *Ann Surg* 214:213, 1991.

Clark WR, Neimen GF, et al: Effects of crystalloid on lung fluid balance after smoke inhalation. *Ann Surg* 208:56, 1988.

Cope O, Moore FD: The redistribution of body water in the fluid therapy of the burned patient. *Ann Surg* 126:1013, 1947.

Demling RH, Lalonde C: Topical ibuprofen decreases early postburn edema. *Surgery* 102:857, 1987.

Dries DJ, Waxman K: Adequate resuscitation of burn patients may not be measured by urine output and vital signs. *Crit Care Med* 19:327, 1991.

Dyess DL, Ardell JL, et al: Effects of hypertonic saline and dextran 70 to resuscitation on microvascular permeability after burn. *Am J Physiol* 262:H1832, 1992.

Ehrlich HP: Anti-inflammatory drugs in the vascular response to burn injury. *J Trauma* 24:311, 1984.

Fallner B, Reven S, et al: Hypertension in children with burns. *J Trauma* 18:213, 1978.

Goodwin CW, Dorethy J, et al: Randomized trial of efficacy of crystalloid and colloid resuscitation on hemodynamic response and lung water following thermal injury. *Ann Surg* 197:520, 1983.

Goodwin CW, Long JM, et al: Paradoxical effect of hyperoncotic albumin in acutely burned children. *J Trauma* 21:63, 1981.

Graves TA, Cioffi WG Jr, et al: Fluid resuscitation of infants and children with massive thermal injury. *J Trauma* 28:1656, 1988.

Herndon DN, Barrow RE, et al: Extravascular lung water changes following smoke inhalation and massive burn injury. *Surgery* 102:341, 1987.

Herndon DN, Traber DL, Traber LD: The effect of resuscitation on inhalation injury. *Surgery* 100:248, 1986.

Hatherhill JR, Till GO, et al: Thermal injury, intravascular hemolysis, and toxic oxygen products. *J Clin Invest* 78:629, 1986.

Horton JW, Baxter CR, White DJ: Differences in cardiac responses to resuscitation from burn shock. *Surg Gynecol Obstet* 168:201, 1989.

Kaufman TM, Horton JW: Burn induced alterations in cardiac B-adrenergic receptors. *Am J Physiol* 262:H1585, 1992.

Kowal-Vern A, Gamelli RL, et al: The effect of burn wound size on hemostasis: a correlation of the hemostatic changes to the clinical state. *J Trauma* 33:50, 1992.

Kuwagata Y, Sugimoto H, et al: Left ventricular performance in patients with thermal injury or multiple trauma. A clinical study with echocardiography. *J Trauma* 32:158, 1992.

Lund CC, Browder MC: The estimation of burns. *Surg Gynecol Obstet* 79:352, 1944.

Monafo WW, Halverson JD, et al: The role of concentrated sodium solutions in the resuscitation of patients with severe burns. *Surgery* 95:129, 1984.

Morehouse JD, Goodwin CW, et al: Resuscitation of the thermally injured patient. *Crit Care Clin* 8:355, 1992.

Moylan JA, Mason AD Jr, et al: Postburn shock: A critical evaluation of resuscitation. *J Trauma* 13:354, 1973.

Navar PD, Saffle JR, Warden GD: Effect of inhalation injury on fluid resuscitation requirements after thermal injury. *Am J Surg* 150:716, 1985.

O'Brien R, Murdoch J, et al: The effect of albumin or crystalloid resuscitation on bacterial translocation and endotoxin absorption flowing experimental burn injury. *J Surg Res* 52:161, 1992.

O'Neill JA: Fluid resuscitation in the burned child. *J Pediatr Surg* 17:604, 1982.

Pruitt BA Jr: The effectiveness of fluid resuscitation. *J Trauma* 19:868, 1979.

Pruitt BA Jr, Mason AD Jr, Moncrief JA: Hemodynamic changes in the early postburn patient: The influence of fluid administration and of a vasodilator (hydralazine). *J Trauma* 11:36, 1971.

Raker JW, Rovit RL: The acute red blood cell destruction following severe thermal trauma in dogs. *Surg Gynecol Obstet* 98:169, 1954.

Shimazaki S, Yoshioka T, et al: Body fluid changes during hypertonic lactated saline solution therapy for burn shock. *J Trauma* 17:38, 1977.

Shirani KZ, Vaughn GM, et al: Inappropriate vasopressin secretion (SIADH) in burned patients. *J Trauma* 23:217, 1983.

Till GO, Hatherill JR, et al: Lipid peroxidation and acute lung injury after thermal trauma to skin: Evidence of a role for hydroxyl radical. *Am J Pathol* 119:376, 1985.

Tokay R, Zeigler ST, et al: Effects of hypertonic saline dextran resuscitation on oxygen delivery, oxygen consumption, and lipid peroxidation after burn injury. *J Trauma* 32:704, 1992.

Topley E, Jackson DM, et al: Assessment of red cell loss in the first two days after severe burns. *Ann Surg* 155:581, 1962.

Tranbaugh RF, Lewis FR, et al: Lung water changes after thermal injury: The effects of crystalloid resuscitation and sepsis. *Ann Surg* 192:479, 1980.

Warden GD, Wilmore DW, et al: Hypernatremic state in hypermetabolic burn patients. *Arch Surg* 106:420, 1973.

Yurt RW, Pruitt BA Jr: Base line and postthermal injury plasma histamine in rats. *J Appl Physiol* 60:1782, 1986.

Inhalation Injury

Agee RN, Long JM III, et al: Use of ^{133}xenon in early diagnosis of inhalation injury. *J Trauma* 16:218, 1976.

Basadre JO, Sugi K, et al: The effect of leukocyte depletion on smoke inhalation injury in sheep. *Surgery* 104:208, 1988.

Cioffi WG Jr, Graves TA, et al: High frequency percussive ventilation in patients with inhalation injury. *J Trauma* 29:350, 1989.

Cioffi WG Jr, Rue LW III, et al: Prophylactic use of high-frequency percussive ventilation in patients with inhalation injury. *Ann Surg* 213:575, 1991.

Goodwin CW Jr, Pruitt BA Jr: Underestimation of thermal lung water volume in high cardiac output patients. *Surgery* 92:401, 1982.

Hales CA, Barkin P, et al: Bronchial artery ligation modifies pulmonary edema after exposure to smoke with acrolein. *J Appl Physiol* 67:1001, 1989.

Hubbard GB, Langlinais PC, et al: The morphology of smoke inhalation in sheep. *J Trauma* 31:1477, 1991.

Hunt JL, Agee RN, Pruitt BA Jr: Fiberoptic bronchoscopy in acute inhalation injury. *J Trauma* 15:641, 1975.

Jin LJ, Lalonde C, Demling RH: Lung dysfunction after thermal injury in relation to prostanoid and oxygen radical release. *J Appl Physiol* 61:103, 1986.

Jones WG, Madden MR, et al: Tracheostomies in burn patients. *Ann Surg* 209:471, 1989.

Kleinerman J: Respiratory tract pathology in patients with severe burns. *Hum Pathol* 21:1212, 1990.

Kramer GC, Herndon DN, et al: Effects of inhalation injury on airway blood flow and edema formation. *J Burn Care Rehabil* 10:45, 1989.

Levine BA, Petroff PA, et al: Prospective trials of dexamethasone and aerosolized gentamicin in the burned patient. *J Trauma* 18:188, 1978.

Linares HA, Herndon DN, Traber D: Sequence of morphologic events in experimental smoke inhalation. *J Burn Care Rehabil* 10:27, 1989.

Lund T, Goodwin CW, et al: Upper airway sequelae in burn patients requiring endotracheal intubation or tracheostomy. *Ann Surg* 201:324, 1985.

Madden MR, Finkelstein JL, Goodwin CW: Respiratory care of the burn patient. *Clin Plast Surg* 13:29, 1986.

Moylan JA, Adib K, Burnbaum M: Fiberoptic bronchoscopy following thermal injury. *Surg Gynecol Obstet* 140:541, 1975.

Naraizzi LR: Computerized tomographic correlate of carbon monoxide poisoning. *Arch Neurol* 36:38, 1979.

Pierce EC II, Bensky WH, et al: A registry for carbon monoxide poisoning in New York City. *Clin Toxicol* 26:419, 1988.

Plum F, Posner J, Raymond RN: Delayed neurological deterioration after anoxia. *Arch Intern Med* 110:18, 1976.

Prien T, Traber LD, et al: Pulmonary edema with smoke inhalation, undetected by indicator dilution technique. *J Appl Physiol* 63:907, 1987.

Prien T, Traber DL, et al: Early effects of inhalation injury on lung mechanics and pulmonary perfusion. *Intensive Care Med* 14:25, 1988.

Pruitt BA Jr, Cioffi WG, et al: Evaluation and management of patients with inhalation injury. *J Trauma* 30:563, 1990.

Shimazu T, Ikeuchi H, et al: Smoke inhalation injury and the effect of carbon monoxide in the sheep model. *J Trauma* 30:170, 1990.

Stewart RD: The effect of carbon monoxide on humans. *Ann Rev Pharmacol* 15:409, 1975.

Thompson PB, Herndon DN, et al: Effect on mortality of inhalation injury. *J Trauma* 26:163, 1986.

Tredget EE, Shankowsky HA, et al: The role of inhalation injury in burn trauma: A Canadian experience. *Ann Surg* 212:720, 1990.

Welch GW, Lull RJ, et al: The use of steroids in inhalation injury. *Surg Gynecol Obstet* 145:539, 1977.

Zikria BA, Budd DC, et al: What is clinical smoke poisoning? *Ann Surg* 181:151, 1976.

Burn Wound Care

Chu CS, McManus AT, et al: Multiple harvestings from deep partial-thickness scald wounds healed under the influence of weak direct current. *J Trauma* 30:1044, 1990.

Compton CC, Gill JM, et al: Skin regenerated from cultured epithelial autografts on full-thickness burn wounds from 6 days to 5 years after grafting: A light, electron microscopic and immunohistochemical study. *Lab Invest* 60:600, 1989.

Demling RH, Katz A, et al: The immediate effect of burn wound excision on pulmonary function in sheep: The role of prostanoids, oxygen radicals, and chemoattractants. *Surgery* 101:44, 1987.

Goodwin CW, Maguire MS, et al: Prospective study of burn wound excision of the hands. *J Trauma* 23:510, 1983.

Goodwin CW, McManus WF, et al: Management of abdominal wounds in thermally injured patients. *J Trauma* 22:92, 1982.

Green H, Kehinde O, Thomas J: Growth of cultured human epidermal cells into multiple epithelia suitable for grafting. *Proc Natl Acad Sci* 76:5665, 1979.

Green HA, Bua D, et al: Burn depth estimation using indocyanine green fluorescence. *Arch Dermatol* 128:43, 1992.

Janzekovic Z: A new concept in the immediate early excision and grafting of burns. *J Trauma* 10:1103, 1990.

Ketchum LD, Cohen IK, et al: Hypertrophic scars and keloids. *Plast Reconstr Surg* 53:448, 1974.

Kischer CW, Shelton MR: Microvasculature and hypertrophic scars and the effect of pressure. *J Trauma* 19:757, 1979.

Kischer CW, Shelton MR, et al: Hypertrophic scars and keloids: A review of new concepts concerning their origin. *Scan Electron Microsc* 4:1699, 1982.

Levine BA, Sirinek KR, Pruitt BA Jr: Wound excision to fascia in burn patients. *Arch Surg* 113:403, 1978.

Madden MR, Finkelstein JL, et al: Grafting of cultured allogeneic epidermis on second and third degree burn wounds on 26 patients. *J Trauma* 26:955, 1986.

Madden MR, Nolan E, et al: Comparison of an occlusive and a semi-occlusive dressing and the effect of the wound exudate upon keratinocyte proliferation. *J Trauma* 29:924, 1989.

Marano MA, Madden MR, et al: Early excision in burn therapy: Selection, technique, results. *Adv Trauma Crit Care* 6:73, 1991.

McManus WF, Mason AD Jr, Pruitt BA Jr: Excision of the burn wound in patients with large burns. *Arch Surg* 124:718, 1989.

Munster AM, Weiner SH, Spense RJ: Cultured epidermis for the coverage of massive burn wounds. *Ann Surg* 211:676, 1990.

Perry AW, Goodwin CW, et al: Use of vascular clips to approximate skin grafts. *J Burn Care Rehabil* 9:490, 1988.

Shuck JM, Pruitt BA Jr, et al: Homograft skin for wound coverage: A study in versatility. *Arch Surg* 98:472, 1969.

Teepe RGC, Koebrugge EJ, et al: Fresh versus cryopreserved cultured allografts for the treatment of chronic skin ulcers. *Br J Dermatol* 122:81, 1990.

Woodley DT, Briggaman RK, et al: Characterization of ''neo-dermis'' formation beneath cultured epidermal autograft transplanted on muscle fascia. *J Invest Dermatol* 95:20, 1990.

Metabolism and Nutrition

Alexander JW, Saito H, et al: The importance of lipid type in the diet after burn injury. *Ann Surg* 204:1, 1986.

Aulick LH, Baze WB, et al: Control of blood flow in large surface wound. *Ann Surg* 191:249, 1980.

Aulick LH, Wilmore DW, et al: Muscle blood flow following thermal injury. *Ann Surg* 188:778, 1978.

Aulick LH, Goodwin CW, et al: Visceral blood flow following thermal injury. *Ann Surg* 193:112, 1981.

Aulick LH, Wilmore DW: Increased peripheral amino acid release following burn injury. *Surgery* 85:560, 1979.

Aulick, LH, Wilmore DW, et al: Depressed reflex vasomotor control of the burn wound. *Cardiovasc Res* 16:113, 1982.

Becker RA, Vaughn GM, et al: Hypermetabolic low triiodothyronine syndrome of burn injury. *Crit Care Med* 10:870, 1982.

Becker RA, Wilmore DW, et al: Free T_4, free T_3 and reverse-T_3 in critically ill, thermally injured patients. *J Trauma* 20:713, 1980.

Brown RO, Buonpane EA, et al: Comparison of modified amino acids and standard amino acids in parenteral nutrition support of thermally injured patients. *Crit Care Med* 18:1096, 1990.

Carlson DE, Cioffi WG Jr, et al: Evaluation of serum visceral protein levels as indicators of nitrogen balance in thermally injured patients. *JPEN* 15:440, 1991.

Carlson DE, Cioffi WG Jr, et al: Resting energy expenditure in patients with thermal injuries. *Surg Gynecol Obstet* 174:270, 1992.

Chiarelli A, Enzi G, et al: Very early nutrition supplementation in burned patients. *Am J Clin Nutr* 51:1035, 1990.

Curreri PW, Wilmore DW, et al: Intracellular cation alterations following major trauma: Effect of supranormal caloric intake. *J Trauma* 11:390, 1971.

Cuthbertson DP, Tilstone WJ: Metabolism during the postinjury period, in

Advances in Clinical Chemistry. Vol. 12. New York, Academic Press, 1969.

Demling RH, Frye E, Read T: Effect of sequential early burn wound excision and closure on postburn oxygen consumption. *Crit Care Med* 19:861, 1991.

Demling RH, Lalonde C, et al: Comparison of the postburn hyperdynamic state and changes in lung function (effect of wound bacterial content). *Surgery* 100:828, 1986.

Enzi G, Casadei A, et al: Metabolic and hormonal effects of early nutritional supplementation after surgery in burn patients. *Crit Care Med* 18:719, 1990.

Fleming RYD, Rutan RL, et al: Effect of recombinant human growth hormone on catabolic hormones and free fatty acids following thermal injury. *J Trauma* 32:698, 1992.

Goodwin CW, Mason AD Jr, Pruitt BA Jr: Increased mitochondrial oxygen consumption in the hypermetabolic injured rat. *Surg Forum* 33:1, 1982.

Goodwin CW, Wilmore DW: Surgery and burns, in Paige DM (ed): *Manual of Clinical Nutrition*. St. Louis, CV Mosby, 1988, p. 372.

Goodwin CW Jr: Metabolism and nutrition in the thermally injured patient. *Crit Care Clin* 1:97, 1985.

Goran MI, Peters EJ, et al: Total energy expenditure in burned children using the doubly labeled water techniques. *Am J Physiol* 259:E576, 1990.

Gore DC, Honeycutt D, et al: Effect of exogenous growth hormone on whole-body and isolated-limb protein kinetics in burned patients. *Arch Surg* 126:38, 1990.

Gore DC, Honeycutt D, et al: Propranolol diminishes extremity blood flow in burned patients. *Ann Surg* 213:568, 1991.

Jaksic T, Wagner D, et al: Proline metabolism in adult male burned patients and healthy control subjects. *Am J Clin Nutr* 54:408, 1991.

Lalonde C, Demling RH, Goad ME: Tissue inflammation without bacteria produces increased oxygen consumption and distant organ lipid peroxidation. *Surgery* 104:49, 1988.

Lalonde C, Demling RH: The effect of complete burn wound excision and closure on postburn oxygen consumption. *Surgery* 102:862, 1987.

Long JM, Wilmore DW, et al: Effect of carbohydrate and fat intake in nitrogen excretion during total intravenous feeding. *Ann Surg* 185:417, 1977.

McDougal WS, Heimburger S, et al: The effect of exogenous substrate on hepatic metabolism and membrane transport during endotoxemia. *Surgery* 84:55, 1978.

McDougal WS, Wilmore DW, Pruitt BA Jr: Glucose-dependent hepatic membrane transport in nonbacteremic and bacteremic thermally injured patients. *J Surg Res* 22:697, 1977.

Martensson J, Goodwin CW, Blake R: Mitochondrial glutathione in hypermetabolic rats following burn injury and thyroid hormone administration: Evidence of a selective effect on brain glutathione by burn injury. *Metabolism* 41:273, 1992.

Newsome TW, Mason AD Jr, Pruitt BA Jr: Weight loss following thermal injury. *Ann Surg* 178:215, 1973.

Plymate SR, Vaughn GM, et al: Central hypogonadism in burned men. *Hormone Res* 27:152, 1987.

Saito H, Trochi O, et al: The effect of route of nutrient administration on the nutritional state, catabolic hormone secretion, and gut mucosal integrity after burn injury. *JPEN* 11:1, 1987.

Souba WW, Smith RJ, Wilmore DW: Glutamine metabolism by the intestinal tract. *JPEN* 9:608, 1985.

Strome DR, Newman JJ, et al: Mechanisms of reduced lipolytic response in rat adipocytes following thermal injury. *Surg Forum* 34:103, 1983.

Taylor JW, Hander EW, et al: The effect of central nervous system narcosis on the sympathetic response to stress. *J Surg Res* 20:313, 1976.

Vaughn GM, Becker RA, et al: Nonthyroidal control of metabolism after burn injury: Possible role of glucagon. *Metabolism* 34:637, 1985.

Vaughn GM, Mason AD Jr, et al: Alterations of mental status and thyroid hormones after thermal injury. *J Clin Endocrinol Metab* 60:1221, 1985.

Vaughn GM, Becker RA, et al: Visceral blood flow following thermal injury. *Ann Surg* 193:112, 1981.

Wallace BH, Caldwell FT, Cone JB: Ibuprofen lowers body temperature and metabolic rate of humans with burn injury. *J Trauma* 32:154, 1992.

Wilmore DW: Catabolic illness: Strategies for enhancing recovery. *N Engl J Med* 325:695, 1991.

Wilmore DW, Goodwin CW, et al: Effect of injury and infection on visceral metabolism and circulation. *Ann Surg* 192:491, 1980.

Wilmore DW, Long JM, et al: Catecholamines: Mediator of the hypermetabolic response to thermal injury. *Ann Surg* 180:653, 1974.

Wilmore DW, Mason AD Jr, et al: Effect of ambient temperature on heat production and heat loss in burn patients. *J Appl Physiol* 38:593, 1975.

Wilmore DW, Mason AD Jr, Pruitt BA Jr: Insulin response to glucose in hypermetabolic burn patient. *Ann Surg* 183:314, 1976.

Infection and Immunology

Amy BW, McManus WF, Pruitt BA Jr: Tetanus following a major thermal injury. *J Trauma* 25:654, 1984.

Baskin TW, Rosenthal A, Pruitt BA Jr: Acute bacterial endocarditis: A silent source of sepsis in the burned patient. *Ann Surg* 184:618, 1976.

Becker WK, Cioffi WG Jr, et al: Fungal burn wound infection: A 10 year experience. *Arch Surg* 126:44, 1991.

Bjornson AB, Knippenberg RW, Bjornson HS: Bactericidal defect of neutrophils in a guinea pig model of thermal injury is related to elevation of intracellular cyclic 3′-, 5′- adenosine monophosphate. *J Immunol* 143:2609, 1989.

Bowers BL, Purdue GF, Hunt JL: Paranasal sinusitis in burn patients following nasotracheal intubation. *Arch Surg* 126:1411, 1991.

Bruck HM, Nash G, et al: Opportunistic fungal infection in the burn wound with phycomycetes and aspergillus: A clinical pathological review. *Arch Surg* 102:476, 1971.

Burleson DG, Mason AD Jr, Pruitt AD Jr: Lymphoid subpopulation changes after thermal injury with infection in an experimental model. *Ann Surg* 207:208, 1988.

Burleson DG, Johnson A, et al: Identification of neopterin as a potential indicator of infection in burned patients. *Proc Soc Exp Biol Med* 199:305, 1992.

Cioffi WG Jr, Burleson DG, et al: Effects of granulocyte-macrophage colony-stimulating factor in burn patients. *Arch Surg* 126:74, 1991.

Deitch EA, Berg RD: Endotoxin but not malnutrition promotes bacterial translocation of the gut flora in burned mice. *J Trauma* 27:161, 1987.

Desai MH, Rutan R, et al: *Candida* infection with and without nystatin prophylaxis. *Arch Surg* 127:159, 1992.

Doebbeling BN, Stanley GL, et al: Comparative efficacy of alternative hand-washing agents in reducing nosocomial infections in intensive care units. *N Engl J Med* 327:88, 1992.

Eldad A, Neuman A, et al: Silver sulfadiazine-induced hemolytic anaemia in a glucose-6-phosphate dehydrogenase deficient burn patient. *Burns* 17:430, 1991.

Foley FD, Greenwald KA, et al: Herpes virus infection in burn patients. *N Engl J Med* 282:652, 1970.

Gamelli RL, Hebert JC, Foster RS Jr: Effect of burn injury on granulocyte and macrophage production. *J Trauma* 25:615, 1985.

Gelfand JA, Donelan M, et al: Alternative complement pathway activation increases mortality in a model of burn injury in mice. *J Clin Invest* 70:1170, 1982.

Gough DB, Jordan A, et al: Suppressor T-cell levels are unreliable indicators of the impaired response following thermal injuries. *J Trauma* 32:677, 1992.

Graves TA, Cioffi WG, et al: Relationship of transfusion and infections in a burn population. *J Trauma* 29:948, 1989.

Kagan RJ, Naraqi S, et al: Herpes simplex virus and cytomegalovirus infections in burned patients. *J Trauma* 25:40, 1985.

Kim SH, Hubbard GB, et al: Frozen section technique to evaluate early burn wound biopsy: Comparison with the rapid section technique. *J Trauma* 25:1134, 1985.

McManus AT, Kim SH, et al: Comparison of quantitative microbiology and histopathology in divided burn wound biopsy specimens. *Arch Surg* 122:74, 1987.

McManus AT, Mason AD Jr, et al: What's in a name? Is methicillin-resistant *Staphylococcus aureus* just another *S. aureus* when treated with vancomycin? *Arch Surg* 124:1456, 1989.

McManus AT, Moody EE, Mason AD: Bacterial motility: A component in experimental *Pseudomonas aeruginosa* burn wound sepsis. *Burns* 6:235, 1979.

McManus AT, Denton CL, Mason AD Jr: Mechanisms of in vitro sensitivity to sulfadiazine silver. *Arch Surg* 118:161, 1983.

McManus AT, Denton CL, Mason AD Jr: Topical chlorhexidine diphosphanilate (WP-973) in burn wound sepsis. *Arch Surg* 119:206, 1984.

McManus WF, Mason AD Jr, Pruitt BA Jr: Subeschar antibiotic infusion in the treatment of burn wound infection. *J Trauma* 20:1021, 1980.

Mason AD Jr, McManus AT, Pruitt BA Jr: Association of burn mortality and bacteremia: A 25 year review. *Arch Surg* 121:1027, 1986.

Michie HR, Manoque KR, et al: Role of circulating tumor necrosis factor after endotoxin administration. *N Engl J Med* 318:1481, 1988.

Mileski W, Borgstrom D, et al: Inhibition of leukocyte-endothelial adherence following thermal injury. *J Surg Res* 52:334, 1992.

Mills DC II, Roberts LW, et al: Suppurative chondritis: Its incidence, prevention, and treatment in burn patients. *Plast Reconstr Surg* 82:267, 1988.

Mooney DP, Gamelli RL, et al: Recombinant human granulocyte colony-stimulating factor and *Pseudomonas* burn wound sepsis. *Arch Surg* 123:1353, 1988.

Peterson VM, Ambruso DR, et al: Inhibition of colony-stimulating factor (CSF) production by postburn serum: Negative feedback inhibition mediated by lactoferrin. *J Trauma* 28:1001, 1988.

Pruitt BA Jr, McManus WF, et al: Diagnosis and treatment of cannula-related intravenous sepsis in burn patients. *Ann Surg* 191:546, 1980.

Pruitt BA Jr: Host-opportunist interactions in surgical infection. *Arch Surg* 121:13, 1986.

Pruitt BA Jr: Biopsy diagnosis of surgical infections. *N Engl J Med* 310:1737, 1984.

Pruitt BA Jr, McManus AT: Opportunistic infections in severely burned patients. *Am J Med* 80:146, 1984.

Pruitt BA Jr, Foley FD: The use of biopsies in burn patient care. *Surgery* 73:887, 1973.

Pruitt BA Jr: Phycomycotic infections. *Probl Gen Surg* 4:664, 1984.

Pruitt BA Jr, DiVincenti FC, et al: The occurrence and significance of pneumonia and other pulmonary complications in burn patients: Comparison of conventional and topical treatment. *J Trauma* 10:519, 1970.

Pruitt BA Jr, Erickson DR, Morris A: Progressive pulmonary insufficiency and other pulmonary complications of thermal injury. *J Trauma* 15:369, 1975.

Sasaki TM, Panke TW, et al: The relationship of central venous and pulmonary artery catheter position to acute right-sided endocarditis in severe thermal injury. *J Trauma* 19:740, 1979.

Sasaki TM, Welch GW, et al: Burn wound manipulation-induced bacteremia. *J Trauma* 19:46, 1979.

Schluter B, Konig W, et al: Differential regulation of T- and B-lymphocyte activation in severely burned patients. *J Trauma* 31:239, 1991.

Shirani KZ, McManus AT, et al: Effects of environment on infection in burn patients. *Arch Surg* 121:31, 1986.

Smith DJ, Thompson PD: Changing flora in burn and trauma units: Historical perspective—experience in the United States. *J Burn Care Rehabil* 13:276, 1992.

Till GO, Guilds LS, et al: Role of xanthine oxidase in thermal injury of skin. *Am J Pathol* 135:195, 1989.

Wann AT, Conyers RAJ, et al: Determination of silver in blood, urine and tissues of volunteers and burn patients. *Clin Chem* 37:1683, 1991.

Wasserman D, Schlotterer M, et al: Use of topically applied silver-sulfadiazine plus cerium nitrate in major burns. *Burns* 15:257, 1989.

Waymack JP: Antibiotics and the postburn hypermetabolic response. *J Trauma* 30:530, 1990.

Winchurch RA, Thupari JN, Munster AM: Endotoxemia in burn patients: Level of circulating endotoxins related to burn size. *Surgery* 102:808, 1987.

Wolff SM: Monoclonal antibodies and the treatment of gram-negative bacteremia and shock. *N Engl J Med* 324:486, 1991.

Xiao GX, Chopra RK, et al: Altered expression of lymphocyte I1-2 receptors in burned patients. *J Trauma* 28:1669, 1988.

Yurt RW, Pruitt BA Jr: Decreased wound neutrophils and indiscrete margination in the pathogenesis of wound infection. *Surgery* 98:191, 1985.

Yurt RW, McManus AT, et al: Increased susceptibility to infection related to extent of burn injury. *Arch Surg* 119:183, 1984.

Electrical Injury

Baker MD, Chiaviello C: Household electrical injuries in children. *Am J Dis Child* 143:59, 1989.

Bizhko IP, Slesarenko SV: Operative treatment of deep burns of the scalp and skull. *Burns* 18:220, 1992.

Chandra NC, Sui CO, et al: Clinical predictors of myocardial image after high voltage electrical injury. *Crit Care Med* 18:193, 1990.

Chang LY, Yang JY: The role of bone scans in electrical burns. *Burns* 17:250, 1991.

Comer RW, Fitchie JG, et al: Oral trauma. Emergency care of lacerations, fractures and burns. *Postgrad Med* 85:34, 1989.

Critchley M: Neurological effects of lightning and electricity. *Lancet* 1:68, 1934.

Daniel RK, Ballard PA, et al: High-voltage electrical injury: Acute pathophysiology. *J Hand Surg (Am)* 13:44, 1988.

Gilbert TB, Shaffer M, et al: Electrical shock by dislodged spark gap in bipolar electrosurgical device. *Anesth Analg* 73:355, 1991.

Goodwin CW: Electrical injury, in Wyngaarden JB, Smith LH Jr, Bennett JC (eds): *Cecil Textbook of Medicine*. Philadelphia, WB Saunders, 1992, p. 2356.

Grube BJ, Heimbach DM: Neurologic consequences of electrical burns. *J Trauma* 30:25, 1990.

Housinger TA, Green L, et al: A prospective study of myocardial damage in electrical injuries. *J Trauma* 25:122, 1985.

Hunt JL, McManus WF, et al: Vascular lesions in acute electric injuries. *J Trauma* 14:461, 1974.

Hunt JL, Mason AD Jr, et al: The pathophysiology of acute electric injury. *J Trauma* 16:335, 1976.

Imai K, Inoue T, et al: Reconstruction of two separated electrical burn ulcers. *Ann Plast Surg* 27:146, 1991.

Murphy P, Herbert K: Burns from electric fire-guards. *Burns* 18:243, 1992.

Rosenberg DB: Neurologic sequelae of minor electric burns. *Arch Phys Med Rehabil* 70:914, 1989.

Rosenberg DB, Nelson M: Rehabilitation concerns in electrical burn patients: A review of the literature. *J Trauma* 28:808, 1988.

Schein RM, Kett DH, et al: Pulmonary edema associated with electrical injury. *Chest* 97:1248, 1990.

Strachan D, McCombe AW, et al: The long-term results of electric fire hand burns in children. *Br J Plast Surg* 42:468, 1989.

Chemical Injuries

Berone GJ, Brennan JT: Glomerulonephritis associated with hydro-carbon solvents: Mediated by antiglomerular basement membrane antibody. *Arch Environ Health* 25:365, 1972.

Bowen TE Jr, Whelan TJ Jr, Nelson TG: Sudden death after phosphorus burns: Experimental observations on hypocalcemia, hyperphosphatemia, and electrocardiographic abnormalities following production of a standard white phosphorus burn. *Ann Surg* 174:779, 1971.

Bruns DE, Herold DA, et al: Polyethylene glycol intoxication in burn patients. *Burns* 9:49, 1982.

Divatia JV, Upadhye SM, et al: Fiberoptic intubation in cicatricial membranes of the pharynx. *Anesthesia* 47, 1992.

Hankins CL, Hackett ME, Vaoma G: An analysis of resuscitative requirements of petrol (gasoline) burns. *Burns* 18:141, 1992.

Hansbrough JF, Zapata-Sirvent R, et al: Hydrocarbon contact injuries. *J Trauma* 25:250, 1985.

Haores JC, Rumack BH, et al: Methemoglobinemia resulting from absorption of nitrates. *JAMA* 242:2869, 1979.

Henry JA, Hla KK: Intravenous regional calcium gluconate perfusion for hydrofluoric acid burns. *Clin Toxicol* 30:203, 1992.

Lin CH, Yang JY: Chemical burn with cresol intoxication and multiple organ failure. *Burns* 18:162, 1992.

Mozengo DW, Smith AA, et al: Chemical burns. *J Trauma* 28:642, 1988.

Ohji M, Ohmi G, et al: Goblet cell density in thermal and chemical injuries. *Arch Ophthalmol* 105:1686, 1987.

Pardoe R, Minami RT, et al: Phenol burns. *Burns* 3:29, 1977.

Sellars SL, Spence RA: Chemical burns of the oesophagus. *J Occup Med* 32:726, 1990.

Simpson LA, Cruse CW: Gasoline immersion injury. *Plast Reconstr Surg* 67:54, 1981.

Upfal M, Doyle C: Medical management of hydrofluoric acid exposure. *J Occup Med* 32:726, 1990.

Rehabilitation and Reconstructive Surgery

Apfeberg D, Lash H: The use of epidermis over keloid as an autograft after resection of the keloid. *J Dermatol Surg* 2:402, 1976.

Babu M, Diegelmann R, Olwer N: Fibronectin is overproduced by keloid fibroblasts during abnormal wound healing. *Mol Cell Biol* 9:1642, 1989.

Bernstein L, Jacobsberg L, et al: Detection of alcoholism among burn patients. *Hosp Community Psychiatry* 43:255, 1992.

Boyd BM, Roberts WW, Miller GR: Periarticular ossification following burns. *South Med J* 52:1048, 1959.

Buhrer DP, Huang TT, et al: Treatment of burn alopecia with tissue expanders in children. *Plast Reconstr Surg* 81:512, 1988.

Ceilley RI, Babu A: The combined use of cryosurgery and intralesional injections of suspensions of fluorinated adrenal corticosteroids for reducing keloids and hypertrophic scars. *J Dermatol Surg Oncol* 5:54, 1979.

Cella DF, Perry SW, et al: Stress and coping in relatives of burn patients: A longitudinal study. *Hosp Community Psychiatry* 39:159, 1988.

Cella DF, Perry SW, et al: Depression and stress responses in parents of burned children. *J Pediatr Psychol* 13:87, 1988.

Da Matta A: Reconstruction of postburn sequelae with expanded flaps. *Burns* 15:407, 1989.

Dossett AB, Hunt JL, et al: Early orthopedic intervention in burn patients with major fractures. *J Trauma* 31:888, 1991.

Elledge ES, Smith AA, et al: Heterotopic bone formation in burned patients. *J Trauma* 28:684, 1988.

Erol OO, Atabay K: The treatment of burn scar hypopigmentation and surface irregularity by dermabrasion and thin skin grafting. *Plast Reconstr Surg* 85:754, 1990.

Evans EB: Orthopedic measures in the treatment of severe burns. *J Bone Joint Surg* 48B:643, 1966.

Evans EB: Heterotopic bone formation in thermal burns. *Clin Orthop* 263:94, 1991.

Helm PA: Burn rehabilitation: Dimensions of the problem. *Clin Plast Surg* 19:512, 1988.

Hoffman S: Radiotherapy for keloids? *Ann Plast Surg* 9:265, 1982.

Luster SH, Patterson PE, et al: An evaluation device for quantifying joint stiffness in the burned hand. *J Burn Care Rehab* 11:312, 1990.

Maguire HC: Treatment of keloids with triamcinolone acetonide injected intralesionally. *JAMA* 192:325, 1968.

Munster AM, Bruck HB, et al: Heterotopic ossification following burns: A prospective study. *J Trauma* 12:1071, 1973.

Perry S, Difede J, et al: Predictors of posttraumatic stress disorder after burn injury. *Am J Psychiatry* 149:931, 1992.

Perry SW, Cella DF, et al: Pain perception vs pain response in burn patients. *Am J Nursing* 87:698, 1987.

Zellweger G, Kunzi W: Tissue expanders in reconstruction of burn sequelae. *Ann Plast Surg* 26:380, 1991.

Complications and Special Problems

Canter TG, Korek JS: Central nervous system reactions to histamine-2 receptor blockers. *Ann Intern Med* 114:1027, 1991.

Cheng DH, Slogoff S, Allen GW: Ketamine-induced stress ulcers in the rat. *Anesthesiology* 40:531, 1974.

Czaja AJ, McAlhany JD, Pruitt BA Jr: Acute gastroduodenal disease after thermal injury: An endoscopic evaluation of incidence and natural history. *N Engl J Med* 291:925, 1974.

Czaja AJ, McAlhany JC, Pruitt BA Jr: Acute duodenitis and duodenal ulceration after burn: Clinical and pathologic characteristics. *JAMA* 232:621, 1975.

Dowling JA, Foley FD, Moncrief JA: Chondritis of the burned ear. *Plast Reconstr Surg* 42:115, 1968.

Gargon TJ, Mitchell L, Plaus W: Burn scar sarcoma. *Ann Plast Surg* 20:477, 1988.

Giblin T, Pickrell L, et al: Malignant degeneration of burn scars: Marjolin's ulcer. *Ann Surg* 162:291, 1965.

Hendricks WM: Sudden appearance of multiple keratoacanthomas three weeks after thermal burns. *J Dermatol* 47:410, 1991.

Lee JY, Kapadia SB, et al: Neurotropic malignant melanoma occurrence in a stable burn scar. *J Cutan Pathol* 19:145, 1992.

Lesher TJ, Sirinek KR, Pruitt BA Jr: Superior mesenteric artery syndrome in thermally injured patients. *J Trauma* 19:567, 1979.

Lesher TJ, Teegarden DK, Pruitt BA Jr: Acute pseudo-obstruction of the colon in thermally injured patients. *Dis Colon Rectum* 21:618, 1978.

Levine BA, Sirinek KR, et al: Effect of cimetidine on gastric secretory function during stress. *J Surg Res* 24:178, 1978.

Levine BA, Sirinek KR, Pruitt BA Jr: Cimetidine protects against stress-induced gastric injury augmented by mucosal barrier breakers. *Am J Surg* 137:328, 1979.

McElwee HP, Sirinek KR, Levine BA: Cimetidine affords protection equal to antacids in prevention of stress ulceration following thermal injury. *Surgery* 86:620, 1979.

Mossberg DA, Crane RT, et al: Burn scar carcinoma of the head and neck. *Arch Otolaryngol Head Neck Surg* 114:1038, 1988.

Munster AM, Goodwin MN, Pruitt BA Jr: Acalculous cholecystitis in burned patients. *Am J Surg* 122:591, 1971.

Newsome TW, Asch MJ, et al: Gastrin levels following thermal injury. *Arch Surg* 107:622, 1973.

Perry AW, Gotlieb LH, et al: Mafenide induced "pseudochondritis." *J Burn Care Rehabil* 9:145, 1988.

Pruitt BA Jr, Goodwin CW: Stress ulcer disease in the burned patient. *World J Surg* 5:209, 1981.

Pruitt BA Jr, Dowling JA, Moncrief JA: Escharotomy in early burn care. *Arch Surg* 96:502, 1968.

Purdue GF, Hunt JL: Chondritis of the burned ear: A preventable condition. *Am J Surg* 152:257, 1986.

Rosenthal A, Czaja AJ, Pruitt BA Jr: Gastrin levels and gastric acidity in the pathogenesis of acute gastroduodenal disease after burns. *Surg Gynecol Obstet* 144:232, 1977.

Rossignol AM, Locke JA, Burke JF: Paediatric burn injuries in New England, USA. *Burns* 16:41, 1990.

Rutan RL, Herndon DN: Growth delay in postburn pediatric patients. *Arch Surg* 125:392, 1990.

Silbert BS, Lipkowski AW, et al: Enhanced potency of receptor-selective opioids after acute burn injury. *Anesth Analg* 73:427, 1991.

Slogoff S, Allan GW, et al: Clinical experience with subanesthetic ketamine. *Anesth Analg* 53:354, 1974.

Stromberg BV, Klingman R, Schluter WW: Basal cell burn carcinoma. *Ann Plast Surg* 24:186, 1990.

CHAPTER 8

Wound Care and Wound Healing

I. Kelman Cohen, Robert F. Diegelmann, and Mary C. Crossland

INTRODUCTION

Wound healing has been described throughout recorded history. Empirically, the ancients recognized that foreign bodies and dead tissue must be removed from wounds. They knew that cleanliness prevented infection and pus required drainage. Wound elixirs such as honey decreased wound suppuration (hypertonic glucose is bactericidal) and fresh open wounds could be closed primarily using hairs, cloth, or insect jaws. Later Paré realized that surgical destruction of tissue was harmful. Lister, Semmelweis, Ehrlich, Fleming, and Florey realized, with increasing sophistication, that bacteria were pathogens. Control of bacteria by asepsis, antiseptics, and antimicrobials heralded a new era in wound management.

Antibiotics, understanding fluid and blood replacement, and control of pain were the major contributions to wound management during the first 25 years of the twentieth century. During the past two decades, wound care has made more advances than over the past two thousand years. This is because of five major factors: (1) the biologic mechanisms of repair are now being defined on an anatomic, a biochemical, and a molecular level; (2) the social and financial devastation of chronic wounds is finally being appreciated by health care providers and federal health care funding agencies; (3) the medical-industrial complex can envision profit in the discovery of more efficacious modalities for wound care and, hence, is supporting wound healing research; (4) the development of new pharmacologic agents through the breakthroughs in molecular biology will enhance the healing of both acute and chronic wounds; and (5) reconstructive surgical techniques have changed drastically in the past two decades with the advent of muscular and musculocutaneous flaps as well as microvascular free-tissue transfers. The advances of the previous decades are only a prelude to the changes in wound care and management that will occur in the next two decades.

Unlike those creatures low on the phylogenetic scale that heal by *regeneration,* humans heal by the rather involved mechanisms of inflammation, matrix deposition, and scar remodeling. Ultimately, science should be able to alter human wound healing to more of a regenerative phenomenon. This is the Nirvana of the wound healer!

GENERAL CONSIDERATIONS

Wound healing is a vague term that often confuses and diverts the clinician from focusing on a specific diagnosis. It is only by defining the specific biologic processes of a particular wound or wound problem that one can formulate a rational approach to therapy. Therefore, the reader must first have a very clear definition of the *mechanisms* of wound healing and how they contribute to various *types of wound closure*.

Types of Wound Closure

Primary closure approximates the disrupted tissue by sutures, staples, or tapes. With time, the synthesis, deposition, and cross-linking of collagen provide the tissue with strength and integrity and are of primary importance in this type of repair (Fig. 8-1).

In *delayed primary closure,* approximation is delayed until several days after the wound has been created (Fig. 8-2). Delay in closure is indicated to prevent infection in those wounds where there is significant bacterial contamination, foreign bodies, or extensive tissue trauma. During the period that the wound remains open, moist, sterile saline dressings should be changed at least twice a day to optimize the wound for closure. The use of peroxide and iodophores in these open wounds should be avoided because these solutions destroy the host's tissues as well as bacteria. In the open wound being prepared for delayed primary closure, angiogenesis proceeds to provide enhanced blood supply and needed oxygen. Leukocytes are attracted to destroy and remove bacteria, and the phases of healing progress to improve the wound environment for soft tissue closure. Wound tensile strength following delayed primary closure becomes the same as the primarily closed wound with time. *Spontaneous closure,* or *''secondary'' wound closure,* occurs when the margins of the open wound move together by the biologic process of contraction (Fig. 8-3). A striking example is the lower extremity amputation stump which, if left open, will heal as the margins contract toward one another. Failure of spontaneous open wound closure results in a chronic wound.

Partial-thickness wounds heal by the process of epithelization. This occurs first by migration and then mitosis of epithelial cells (Fig. 8-4). Venous stasis ulcers appear to heal without clinical evidence of contraction. This has been confirmed by studies where tattooed margins in venous stasis ulcers did not move inward as the wound healed. Therefore, these open wounds are healing by a process other than contraction. The process appears to be epithelization with the induction of neodermis.

Mechanisms Involved in Wound Healing

Three very separate biologic mechanisms are involved in all healing processes; however, there are significant differences in the contribution of each mechanism depending on the type of wound. *Epithelization* is the process whereby keratinocytes migrate and then divide to resurface partial-thickness loss of skin or mucosa. Examples include partial-thickness skin graft donor sites, abrasions, blisters, and both first- and second-degree burns. *Contraction* is the process whereby there is spontaneous closure of full-thickness skin wounds or constriction of tubular organs such as the common bile duct or esophagus after injury. *Connective tissue matrix deposition* is the process whereby fibroblasts are recruited to the site of injury and produce a new connective tissue matrix. This process is of major importance in primary wound closure, be it skin, tendon, or intestinal anastomosis. The cross-linked collagen in the connective tissue provides the strength and integrity to all tissues.

Phases of Healing

The healing of an acute, primarily closed wound or a wound created by any mechanism, be it trauma, chemical, friction, heat, or cold, usually follows a predictable pattern under *normal circumstances*. Chronic dermal wounds (such as pressure, diabetic, and venous stasis ulcers) or chronic parenchymal injury (such as subacute chronic hepatic fibrosis) will not be considered in this discussion. Under *normal* conditions, the phases of healing are divided into four specific events. Although they are described in a sequential fashion, they really consist of an overlapping symphony of complex interactions. There is not a ''lag phase'' in the healing process. This is a misnomer propagated by several generations of authors. From the moment of injury, healing is an active, dynamic process.

Coagulation. Injury causes hemorrhage from damaged vessels and lymphatics (Fig. 8-5). Vasoconstriction occurs almost immediately as a result of release of catecholamines. Various other vasoactive compounds such as bradykinin, serotonin, and histamine are released from tissue mast cells. They initiate the process of diapedesis, a passage of intravascular cells into the extravascular space within the wound area. Platelets derived from the hemorrhage form a hemostatic clot.

The platelets release clotting factors to produce fibrin, which is both hemostatic and forms a mesh for the further migration of inflammatory cells and fibroblasts. Fibrin is produced from fibrinogen, which is activated by thrombin derived from its precursor prothrombin in the presence of thromboplastin. If the fibrin mesh is eliminated, ultimate wound strength is diminished.

Platelets are also extremely important because they are the first cells to produce several essential cytokines which modulate most of the subsequent wound healing events. The subject of cytokines will be discussed in detail later in this chapter.

Inflammation. The inflammatory phase is characterized by the sequential migration of leukocytes into the wound. Within 24 hours the wound is predominated by polymorphonuclear leukocytes followed by a preponderance of macrophages (Fig. 8-6). Although it is well known that inflammatory cells regulate connective tissue matrix repair, the messengers of regulation are now being defined. These are the various cytokines which in the past have been termed ''growth factors.''

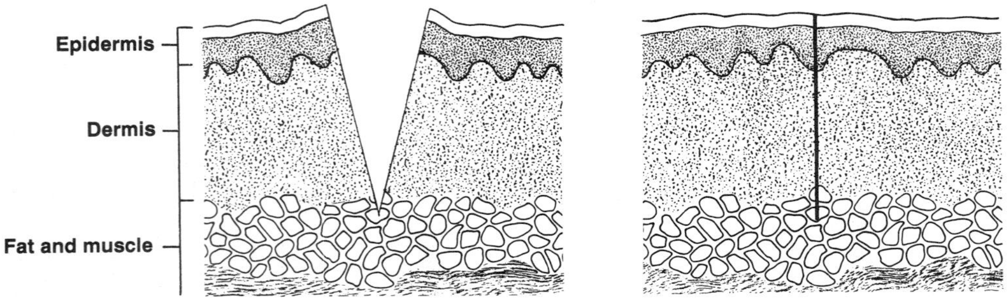

FIG. 8-1. Primary closure. The wound margins are pulled together with sutures, staples, or adhesive tapes. (Modified from: Cohen IK, Diegelmann RF: Wound healing, in Greenfield LJ, et al, (eds): Surgery, Scientific Principles and Practice, Chap 3. Philadelphia, JB Lippincott, 1993, with permission.)

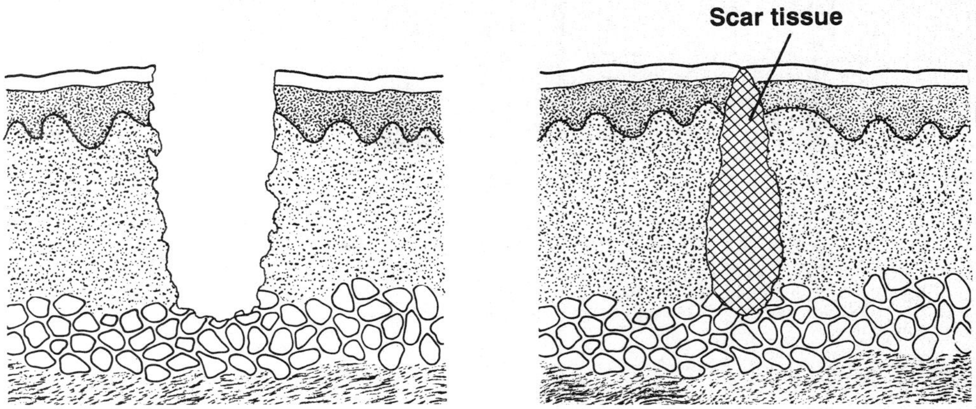

FIG. 8-2. Delayed primary closure. The wound is allowed to remain open for several days to ensure all contamination is removed before it is closed. The wound then undergoes primary healing with deposition of scar tissue in the center of the wound. (Modified from: Cohen IK, Diegelmann RF: Wound healing, in Greenfield LJ, et al, (eds): Surgery, Scientific Principles and Practice, Chap 3. Philadelphia, JB Lippincott, 1993, with permission.)

Fibroplasia. During the phase of fibroplasia the healing events most important to the surgeon occur. Fibroplasia increases wound strength; hence tissue integrity is restored (Fig. 8-7). Within 10 hours after injury, there is evidence of increased wound collagen synthesis. By day 5 to 7, collagen synthesis has peaked and then declines gradually. In addition, there is significant production of ground substance within the matrix and proliferation of blood vessels.

Remodeling. The wound is an "up-regulated" process until "remodeling" (Fig. 8-8). At that point, acute and chronic inflammatory cells diminish gradually, angiogenesis ceases, and fibroplasia ends. The equilibrium between collagen synthesis and collagen degradation is gradually restored. Normally, a fibrous repair is imperfect, but functional and not excessive. The complex interactions and associations of the various processes that take place during normal dermal wound healing are summarized in Fig. 8-9.

Cytokines

Cytokines provide all the communications for cell-cell interactions and are the most exciting wound healing breakthrough of the decade (Table 8-1). Their potential clinical use is just beginning to unfold. These cytokines may have important pharmacologic roles in the many areas of clinical management of wound healing. For example, cytokines appear to play roles in the regulation of fibrosis, the healing of chronic wounds and skin grafts, vascularization, the enhancement of bone and tendon strength after repair, and perhaps even in the control of malignancy.

Cytokines are really "wound hormones" (Fig. 8-10). They may be *endocrine,* like somatomedin or insulinlike growth factor (IGF-1), when they are secreted by one cell then circulate in the bloodstream to reach a distant target cell (see Fig. 8-10). Others are *paracrine,* produced by one cell and affecting an adjacent target cell; examples include transforming growth factor beta (TGF-β) and platelet-derived growth factor (PDGF). *Autocrine* factors are secreted by a cell and then act on receptors on the same cell. Finally, *intracrine* factors are produced by a cell and remain active in the same cell.

Cytokines in Wound Healing. Cytokines may be either *competence factors*—i.e., they get the cell into G_1 phase, such as PDGF—or *progression factors,* such as IGF-1, and act to promote the cell through the proliferation cycle. In addition to cell division, cytokines stimulate cells to migrate to the wound site and to produce specific components needed for matrix repair (Fig. 8-11). These include proteins, enzymes, proteoglycans, and attachment glycoproteins. The cytokine nomenclature is complex and somewhat confusing. Some factors such as PDGF (platelet-derived growth factor) derive their name from the cell of origin. Others are named for their action—e.g., EGF (epithelial growth factor)—whereas others derive their name for their first reported action, e.g., TGF-β (transforming growth factor). Several of these

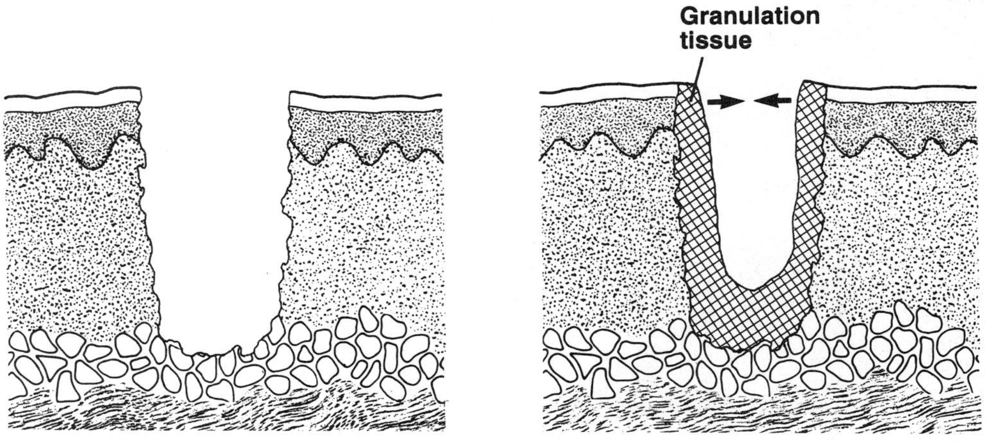

FIG. 8-3. Spontaneous or "secondary" wound closure. The open wound is not closed by external means, and it heals by contraction with some deposition of scar tissue. (Modified from: Cohen IK, Diegelmann RF: Wound healing, in Greenfield LJ, et al, (eds): Surgery, Scientific Principles and Practice, Chap 3. Philadelphia, JB Lippincott, 1993, with permission.)

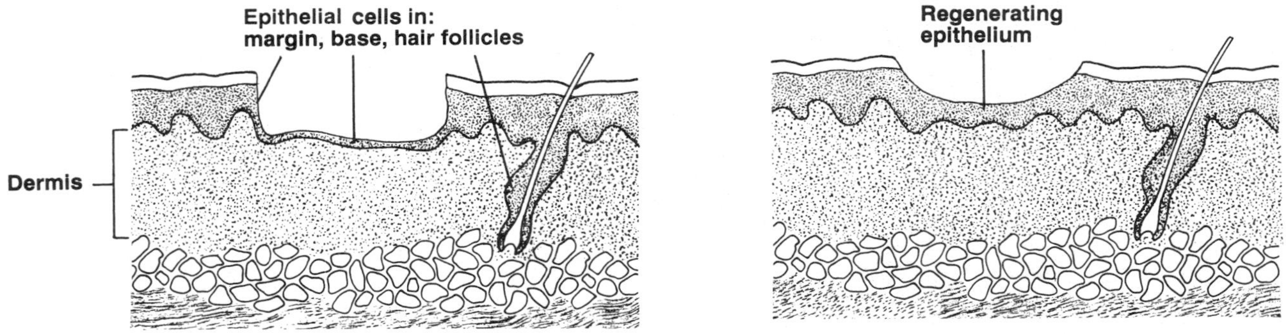

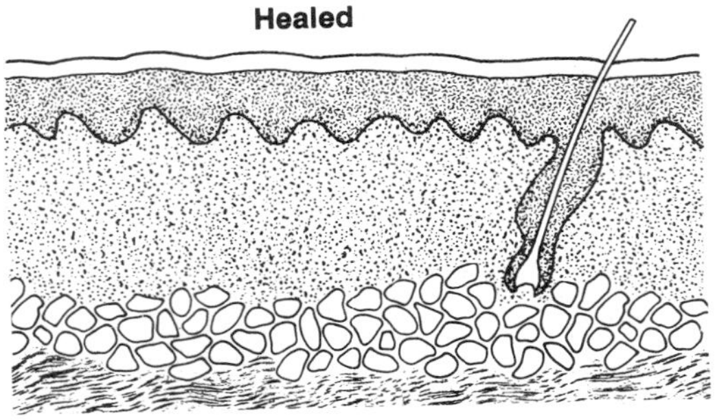

FIG. 8-4. Partial-thickness healing. Superficial wounds heal mainly by replacement of the epithelial layer. (Modified from: Cohen IK, Diegelmann RF: Wound healing, in Greenfield LJ, et al, (eds): Surgery, Scientific Principles and Practice, Chap 3. Philadelphia, JB Lippincott, 1993, with permission.)

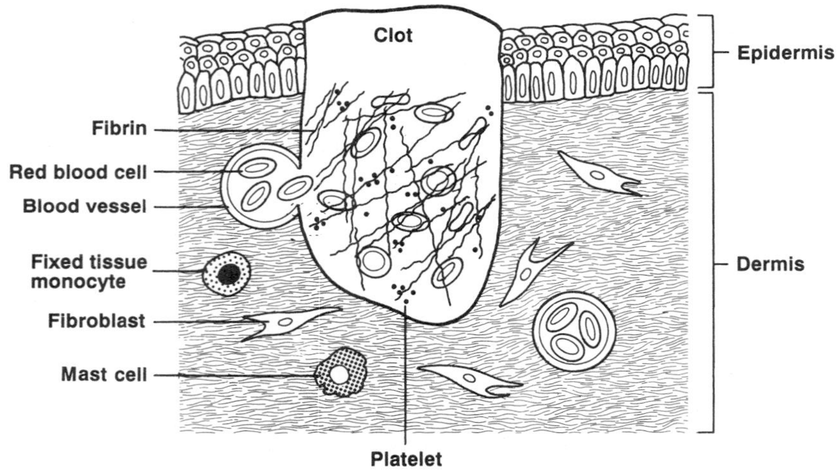

FIG. 8-5. At the initial time of tissue disruption, platelets release coagulation factors and cytokines to initiate the healing process. (Modified from: Cohen IK, Diegelmann RF: Wound healing, in Greenfield LJ, et al, (eds): Surgery, Scientific Principles and Practice, Chap 3. Philadelphia, JB Lippincott, 1993, with permission.)

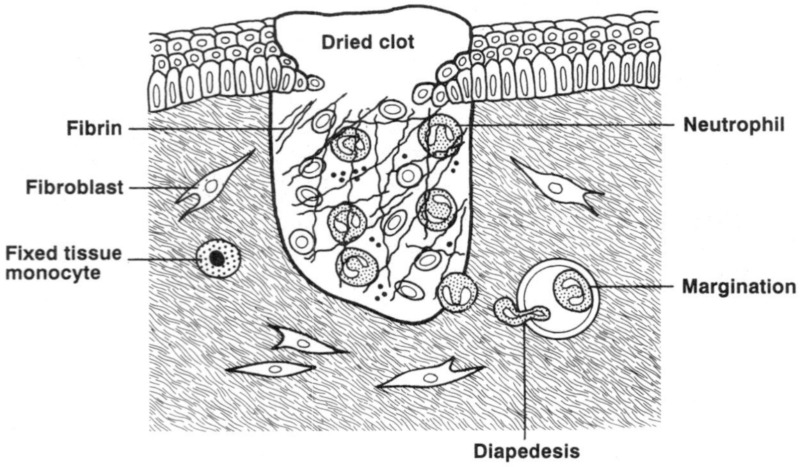

FIG. 8-6. Within the first day following tissue injury, neutrophils attach to surrounding vessel walls (margination) and then move through the vessel walls (diapedesis) to migrate (chemotaxis) to the wound site. (Modified from: Cohen IK, Diegelmann RF: Wound healing, in Greenfield LJ, et al, (eds): Surgery, Scientific Principles and Practice, Chap 3. Philadelphia, JB Lippincott, 1993, with permission.)

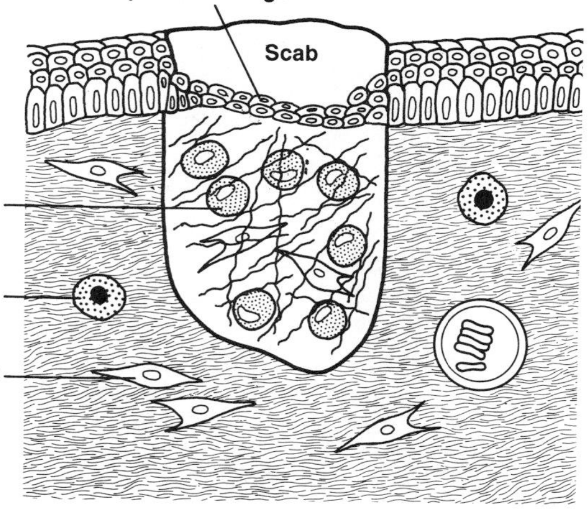

FIG. 8-7. The fibroplasia phase is characterized by movement of wound macrophages into the site of injury, which in turn attract fibroblasts. The fibroblasts then repair the site by producing new connective tissue matrix. (Modified from: Cohen IK, Diegelmann RF: Wound healing, in Greenfield LJ, et al, (eds): Surgery, Scientific Principles and Practice, Chap 3. Philadelphia, JB Lippincott, 1993, with permission.)

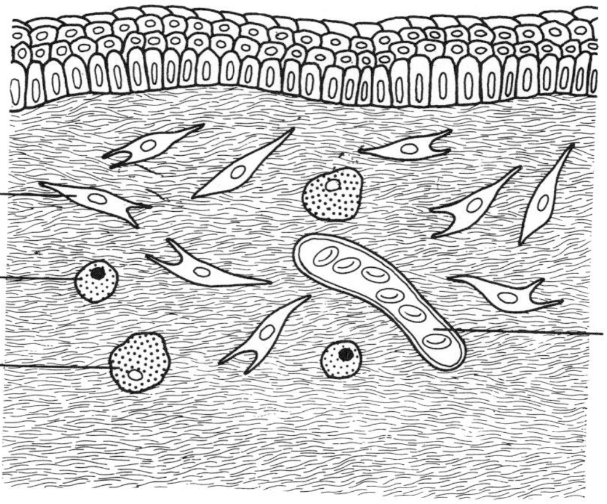

FIG. 8-8. The remodeling phase is characterized by an equilibrium between collagen synthesis and collagen degradation in an effort to reestablish the connective tissue matrix that was destroyed by the tissue injury. (Modified from: Cohen IK, Diegelmann RF: Wound healing, in Greenfield LJ, et al, (eds): Surgery, Scientific Principles and Practice, Chap 3. Philadelphia, JB Lippincott, 1993, with permission.)

Table 8-1
Cytokines That Affect Wound Healing

Cytokine	*Symbol*	*Source*	*Functions*
Platelet-derived growth factor	PDGF	Platelets, macrophages, endothelial cells, and smooth muscle cells	Fibroblast proliferation, chemotaxis, and collagen metabolism; chemotaxis and activation of neutrophils, macrophages; angiogenesis
Transforming growth factor β	TGF-β	Platelets, neutrophils, lymphocytes, macrophages, and many other tissues and cells	Fibroblast proliferation, chemotaxis, collagen metabolism, indirect angiogenesis, and action of other growth factors
Epidermal growth factor	EGF	Platelets, saliva, urine, milk, and plasma	Stimulates epithelial cell and fibroblast proliferation and granulation tissue formation
Transforming growth factor α	TGF-α	Activated macrophages, platelets, keratinocytes, and many tissues	Similar to EGF functions
Interleukins	IL-1 etc	Macrophages, lymphocytes, and many other tissues and cells	Fibroblast proliferation, collagenase, neutrophil chemotaxis
Tumor necrosis factor	TNF	Macrophages, mast cells, and T lymphocytes	Fibroblast proliferation
Fibroblast growth factors	FGF	Brain, pituitary, macrophages, and many other tissues and cells	Fibroblast and epithelial cell proliferation; stimulates matrix deposition, wound contraction and angiogenesis
Keratinocyte growth factors	KGF	Fibroblasts	Epithelial cell proliferation
Insulinlike growth factor-1	IGF-1	Liver, plasma, and fibroblasts	Stimulates synthesis of sulfated proteoglycans, collagen, and fibroblast proliferation
Human growth hormone	huGH	Pituitary and thus plasma	Anabolism, stimulates IGF-1
Interferons	IFN	Lymphocytes and fibroblasts	Inhibition of fibroblast proliferation and collagen synthesis

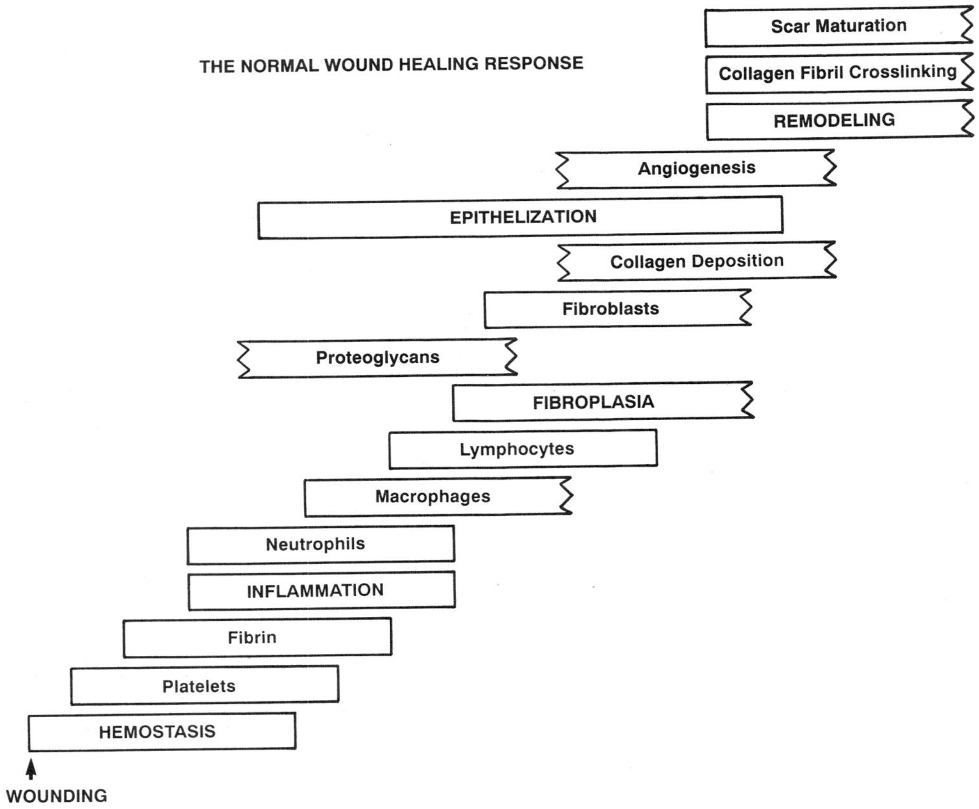

FIG. 8-9. Sequence of events in wound healing. (Modified from: *Mast BA: The skin, in Cohen IK, Diegelmann RF, Lindblad WJ (eds): Wound Healing: Biochemical and Clinical Aspects, Chap 22. Philadelphia, Saunders, 1992, with permission.*)

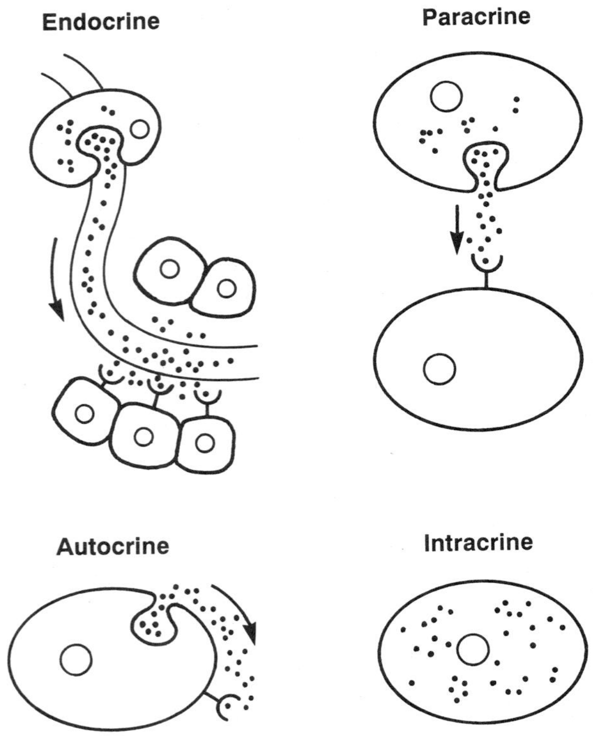

FIG. 8-10. Cell signaling by cytokines.

cytokines are of major importance in wound healing processes (see Table 8-1).

PDGF is one of several platelet-derived growth factors and initiates many wound healing events. Moreover, it stimulates production of several other wound cytokines. PDGF functions include chemotaxis for fibroblasts and macrophages as well as smooth muscle cells.

TGF-β is produced by platelets and a host of other cells, including fibroblasts and macrophages. This important cytokine increases collagen synthesis by specifically enhancing matrix gene expression and by inhibiting collagenase production and activity. As a result, there is a significant stimulation of collagen deposition mediated by TGF-β. Therefore, this cytokine appears to be essential for normal healing, and an excessive amount of TGF-β may be extremely important in the pathophysiology of fibrotic states such as hypertrophic scar and keloid.

There is a family of TGF betas, and the specific isoforms may have diverse activities during wound healing. If TGF-β1 is neutralized by specific antibodies, then the healing of linear incisions is scarless! These exciting animal studies suggest that control of healing by alteration of the cytokine environment may be possible.

The FGF family is another group of cytokines which bind to heparin and heparinlike glycosoaminoglycans. Basic FGF is a potent angiogenic factor and causes increased epithelial cell migration and hastens wound contraction.

EGF-stimulated epithelial migration and mitosis have been reported to hasten reepithelization of burn wound donor sites. However, a study in a group of healthy, nonsmoking, medical students

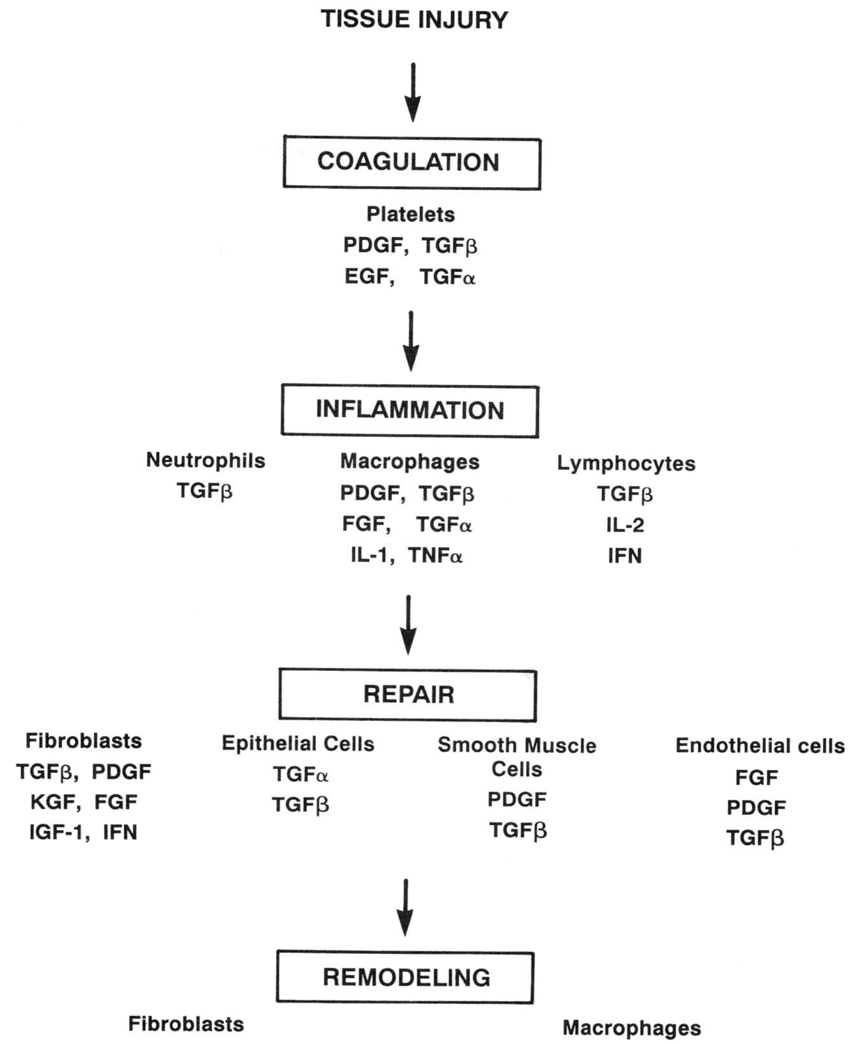

FIG. 8-11. Cytokines released by cells involved in tissue repair.

with split-thickness donor sites failed to reveal a difference between EGF treatment and controls. Recent data suggest that EGF activity may be inhibited by wound proteases, and inhibition of these proteases may allow EGF to function. EGF and the closely related compound TGF-α continue to have clinical promise as wound healing agents. As summarized in Table 8-1, there are several other cytokines from a variety of cell and tissue sources which probably have key roles in the complex process of wound healing. Much of the basic information about these factors has been obtained by animal and cell culture studies where single compounds were analyzed. Obviously in vivo, they interact in complex associations.

Extracellular Matrix Metabolism

The extracellular matrix is a complex structure where a number of cell types and components interact (Fig. 8-12). Collagen is the major component of the extracellular matrix of all soft tissues, tendons, ligaments, and bone. There are at least 13 distinct forms of collagen that have been characterized, and the first 5 major forms are described in Table 8-2. In addition to collagen, glycosaminoglycans, proteoglycans, fibronectin, laminin, and elastin are also present. The role of these components in normal connective tissue and during wound repair is summarized in Table 8-3.

Synthesis. There are several major points where collagen synthesis is regulated (Fig. 8-13). One is at the transcription step, where the amount of mRNA for the specific collagen is controlled. Once synthesized, the mRNA undergoes extensive modifications before it is ready to be translated. The next point of control is at the translational step, where the actual synthesis occurs on ribosomes on the rough endoplasmic reticulum.

Collagen is composed of three polypeptide chains, and each chain is formed in a very orderly sequence with a high frequency of glycine-proline-x (Fig. 8-14). Collagen is unique because it contains the amino acid hydroxyproline. Hydroxyproline, however, is not incorporated as such into the collagen chain, but hydroxylation occurs to specific prolines as synthesis occurs. This step is extremely important because failure to hydroxylate proline produces an unstable collagen molecule which is degraded rapidly in the intracellular or extracellular environment. This key hydroxylation step requires several cofactors and cosubstrates. A lack of ascorbic acid or oxygen will compromise collagen production and result in insufficient wound strength.

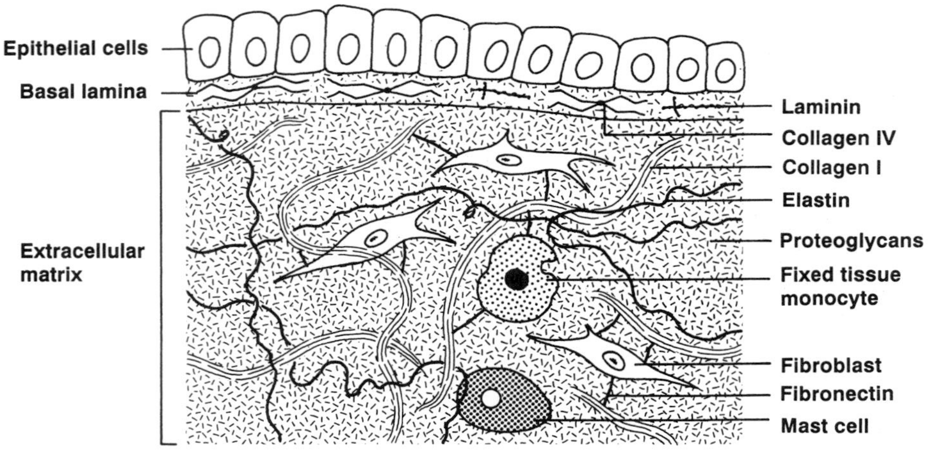

FIG. 8-12. Extracellular matrix.

Table 8-2
The Five Major Collagen Types

Type	*Chains*	*Major molecular form*	*Distribution*	*Function*
I	$\alpha 1(I)$ $\alpha 2(I)$	$[\alpha 1(I)]_2\alpha 2(I)$	All connective tissues except hyaline cartilage and basement membranes	Formation of supporting connective tissues
II	$\alpha 1(II)$	$[\alpha 1(II)]_3$	Cartilagelike tissues	Shock absorption and joint mobility
III	$\alpha 1(III)$	$[\alpha 1(III)]_3$	Distensible connective tissues, e.g., blood vessels; increased in fetal skin	Formation of small fibrous elements
IV	$\alpha 1(IV)$ $\alpha 2(IV)$ $\alpha 3(IV)$ $\alpha 4(IV)$ $\alpha 5(IV)$	$[\alpha 1(IV)]_2\alpha 2(IV)$	Basement membranes and basal lamina in skin	Formation of meshlike scaffold for filtration
V	$\alpha 1(V)$ $\alpha 2(V)$ $\alpha 3(V)$	$[\alpha 1(V)]_2\alpha 2(V)$	Essentially all tissues	Similar to Type III collagen and cytoskeleton around cells

Table 8-3
Components of the Extracellular Matrix and Their Function

Component	*Structure*	*Function*
Collagen	Triple helical glycoprotein molecules rich in proline, hydroxyproline, and glycine	Strength, support and structure for all tissues and organs
Elastin	Stretchable hydrophobic protein interacting with glycosylated microfibrils	Allows tissues and structures to expand and contract
Fibronectin	Specialized adhesive glycoprotein	Mediates cell-matrix adhesion
Laminin	Large, complex adhesive glycoprotein	Binds cells to Type IV collagen and heparan sulfate
Proteoglycans	Heterogeneous, long glycosaminoglycan chains covalently linked to a core protein	Moisture stores, shock absorption, sequestration of cytokines
Hyaluronic acid	A very large, specialized, nonsulfated glycosaminoglycan	Provides a fluid environment for cell movement and differentiation and binds to cytokines

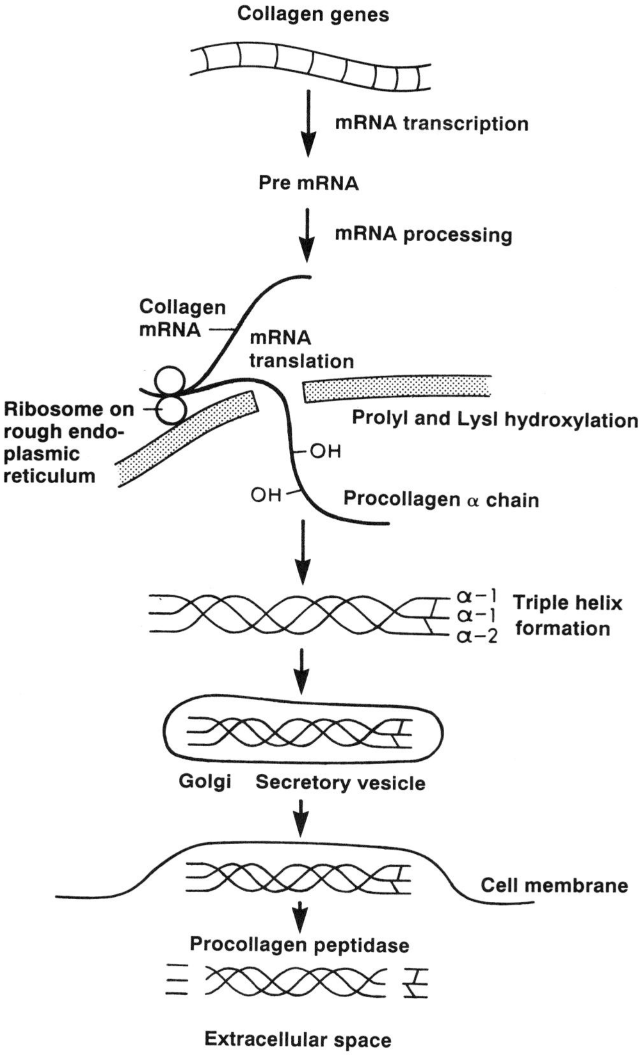

FIG. 8-13. Pathway of collagen synthesis. Each collagen alpha chain is encoded on a specific gene. After transcription, the pre-mRNA is processed to a functional mRNA. The procollagen α chains are synthesized on membrane-bound ribosomes. The α chains then interact to form the triple-helix molecule. The molecule is packaged into secretory vesicles where it is moved to the cell membrane for secretion. At the surface of the cell, the procollagen extension peptides are removed by procollagen peptidases. (Modified from: Cohen IK, Diegelmann RF: Wound healing, in Greenfield LJ, et al, (eds): Surgery, Scientific Principles and Practice, Chap 3. Philadelphia, JB Lippincott, 1993, with permission.)

As the collagen molecules are assembled, they are glycosylated by the addition of galactose and glucose to specific hydroxylysine residues and then the three chains are stabilized to one another by hydrogen bonds. Moreover, at the amino and carboxyl terminal ends of the molecule are extra pieces termed ''extension peptides'' (see Fig. 8-14). The carboxyl extension peptides ''register'' and hold the molecule in position as it is shipped extracellularly via microtubules in the cytoplasm.

Collagen is different from all other proteins because it undergoes several modifications once it has reached the extracellular environment. Here, collagen cross-linking occurs to form fibrils and fibers of collagen. The enzyme responsible for this step, lysyl oxidase, requires copper and can be inhibited by collagen cross-link inhibitors such as beta-aminopropionitrile (BAPN) and D-penicillamine. These collagen cross-link inhibitors have been used in animals and to a limited degree in humans in an attempt to prevent excessive collagen deposition and subsequent adhesions and fibrosis. The results have been modest.

Degradation. For normal wound healing, collagen must be degraded as well as produced. The breakdown of collagen is initiated by very specific enzymes termed *mammalian collagenases,* made by a variety of cells including inflammatory cells, fibroblasts, and epithelial cells. They initiate degradation of the collagen molecule by splitting it into specific three-quarter and one-quarter fragments termed the TC_A and TC_B fragments. After this initial split, other nonspecific proteases can further degrade the pieces into peptides and eventually amino acids. Collagenase exists in a nonactive or zymogen form that must be activated by other proteases such as plasmin. Once the collagenase is activated, it can be inhibited by complexing with the plasma and tissue protein alpha-2 macroglobulin.

Ground Substance. The exact role of ground substance or proteoglycans and glycosaminoglycans in wound healing remains unclear. Recent evidence suggests that ground substance has more importance in the healing process than recognized previously. Proteoglycans are composed of glycosaminoglycan subunits attached by covalent bonds to a protein core. They form a ''bottle brush''-like structure and, as macromolecules, occupy significant space in the extracellular matrix. They function as molecular ''shock absorbers'' in combination with cartilage, provide for moisture storage, and also sequester cytokines. Some evidence suggests that following tissue injury, when ground substances are degraded, the bound cytokines are released to provide initial signals to facilitate the repair process. One specific glycosaminoglycan, hyaluronic acid, is most unusual because it is not sulfated and not bound to protein. It has a very high molecular weight and provides a fluid

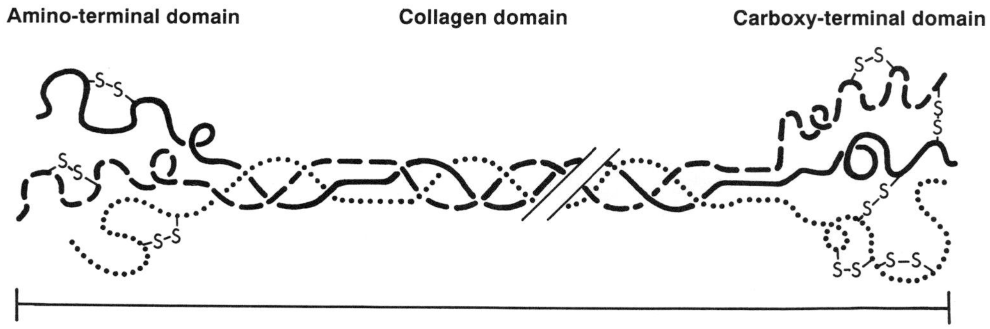

FIG. 8-14. Structure of Type I procollagen molecule. When first synthesized, the collagen molecule contains extension peptides at both amino- and carboxy-terminal ends. The basic molecule is composed of three α chains in a helical complex. (Modified from: Cohen IK, Diegelmann RF: Wound healing, in Greenfield LJ, et al, (eds): Surgery, Scientific Principles and Practice, Chap 3. Philadelphia, JB Lippincott, 1993, with permission.)

environment, thus facilitating rapid cell movement and cell differentiation. Hyaluronic acid has an early and transient appearance soon after injury in the adult and has a much longer persistence in fetal skin and fetal wounds.

Genetic Disorders. Molecular biology has provided new data on wound healing since the last edition of this text. Most exciting is information on a host of genetically controlled defects of collagen and glycosaminoglycan metabolism that result in both subtle and lethal diseases of connective tissue. There are probably hundreds of variants awaiting characterization and chromosomal identification. All of these genetic defects in connective tissue metabolism result in a poor wound healing response.

Osteogenesis Imperfecta. Osteogenesis imperfecta (OI) is a congenital form of osteopenia due mainly to mutations in the genes for Type I collagen. There are four types of OI. These range from mild to lethal manifestations (Table 8-4). Patients with OI present a unique problem to the surgeon because of (1) the increased propensity of the bones to break under minimal stress, (2) dermal thinning, and (3) increased bruisability. Scarring is usually normal in these patients, and the skin has normal extensibility.

Patients affected severely with OI may have difficulty with diaphoresis, which is not only unpleasant but coupled with fasting before surgery may lead to dehydration and fever. The administration of parenteral fluids preoperatively may circumvent these problems. Children with OI also have a higher incidence of hernias, especially umbilical and inguinal. These can be corrected successfully with surgery.

Table 8-4
Osteogenesis Imperfecta

Type	*Inheritance*	*Clinical features*
I	Dominant	Mild bone fragility, blue sclera
II	New dominant	Lethal, shortening and fragility of long bones
III	Dominant recessive	Severe, progressively deforming, early loss of ambulation
IV	Autosomal dominant	Mild to moderate bone fragility

Ehlers-Danlos Syndrome. Ehlers-Danlos syndrome is a genetically, biochemically, and clinically distinct group of collagen disorders characterized mainly by joint laxity, skin hyperextensibility and fragility, poor wound healing, and vascular rupture. At least ten types of this disorder have been distinguished. The enzyme or biochemical deficiency is known only for a few of the types. Each type presents a distinct challenge to the surgeon. These challenges encompass vascular complications such as AV fistulas, true and false aneurysms, varicose veins, bleeding ulcers, arterial rupture, and defective platelet adhesion. Invasive procedures in these patients such as angiography and surgery carry a very high morbidity and mortality. Rupture or dissection of a major artery may occur spontaneously in Ehlers-Danlos patients after minor trauma or with angiographic manipulation. Due to connective tissue weakness, adolescent males are at an increased risk with normal growth and development as well as with the increased stresses of physical activities common in this age group. Due to connective tissue weakness, adolescent females are at a higher risk with the hormonal changes of menstruation. The types of Ehlers-Danlos syndrome are summarized in Table 8-5.

Marfan's Syndrome. Marfan patients are characterized by tall stature, arachnodactyly, lax ligaments, myopia, scoliosis, pectus excavatum and often dissecting aneurysms of the root and ascend-

Table 8-5
Ehlers-Danlos Syndrome

Type	*Inheritance*	*Clinical features*	*Biochemical defect*
I	AD	Soft, hyperextensible skin; easy bruising; thin, atrophic scars; hypermobile joints; varicose veins; prematurity of affected newborns	Not known
II	AD	Similar to Type I but less severe	Not known
III	AD	Soft skin; large and small joint hypermobiity	Not known
IV	AD	Thin, translucent skin with visible veins; easy bruising; absence of skin and joint extensibility; arterial, bowel, and uterine rupture	Abnormal Type III collagen
V	XLR	Similar to Type II	Not known
VI	AR	Soft, muscle hypotonia; scoliosis; joint laxity; hyperextensible skin	Lysyl hydroxylase deficiency
VII	AD	Congenital hip dislocation; severe joint hypermobility; soft skin with normal scarring	Abnormal Type I collagen
VIII	AD	Generalized periodontitis; soft hyper-extensible skin	Not known
IX	XLR	Soft, extensible, lax skin; bladder diverticula and rupture; short arms, limited pronation and supination; broad clavicles; occipital horns	Lysyl oxidase defect
X	AR	Similar to Type II with abnormal clotting studies	Possible defect in fibronectin

SOURCE: Modified from Phillips C, Wenstrup RJ: Biosynthetic and genetic disorders of collagen, Chap 9, in Cohen IK, Diegelmann RF, Lindblad WJ (eds): *Wound Healing: Biochemical and Clinical Aspects*. Philadelphia, Saunders, 1992.

ing portions of the aorta. Some of these patients have defects in collagen structure, and some have abnormal fibrillin in their elastin. Spontaneous rupture of the aorta can cause sudden death if not suspected early. All these diseases may make surgery more difficult and wound healing more complicated.

Epidermolysis Bullosa. Epidermolysis bullosa is characterized by blistering and ulcerations. It is thought to be due to excessive production of collagenase by fibroblasts. The basic defect is one of tissue adhesion within the epidermis, basement membrane, and/or dermis, resulting in tissue separation and blistering of skin with minimal trauma. The majority of these ulcers will heal spontaneously through contraction, but in the more severe forms the epithelium cannot regenerate adequately, and chronic inflammation and scarring ensue. This genetic disease creates a challenge for the surgeon in several realms. Alimentary tract surgery exhibits poor healing impaired by stenosis and strictures in many cases. Dermal incisions and tissue injury must have meticulous skin care to limit the amount and severity of blistering in the traumatized tissue.

Clinical Importance. Patients with these genetic disorders provide a unique challenge for the surgeon. Because of the relatively rare occurrences of these genetic defects, any one surgeon may see no more than one or two cases within a lifetime. Despite this low exposure rate, it behooves the surgeon to be aware of the physical and clinical signs of these diseases so that disaster during surgery can be avoided. A thorough history and physical, with emphasis on the family history, may alert the unsuspecting surgeon to a potential problem, which can then be successfully overcome. At times, preoperative diagnosis is impossible.

Control of extracellular matrix metabolism is one of the most important challenges in health management and far beyond the confines of surgery. Diseases characterized by excessive or inadequate matrix deposition are among the leading causes of morbidity and mortality in man. Excessive collagen deposition of keloid, hypertrophic scar on the skin is quite analogous to the disease processes that result in hepatic fibrosis, intestinal strictures, retroperitoneal fibrosis, and tendon adhesions; these topics will be discussed in detail in a later section of this chapter. Inadequate or poor-quality matrix production may be secondary to a variety of causes, such as malnourishment, various drugs that inhibit cell proliferation and protein synthesis, and the genetic disorders just described. These may lead to infection, wound dehiscence, multiple fractures, and bowel leak, which are but a few examples of the consequences of altered connective tissue metabolism characteristic of genetic defects.

Wound Contraction

Contraction is one of the most powerful mechanical forces in the body. Controversy still exists regarding the exact biologic mechanisms of the process. Surgeons have always found the process of wound contraction both an ally and a foe. Even the ancients knew that open skin wounds healed if kept clean and protected with a dressing. During the healing process, the skin margins move in until they meet one another to provide a healed wound.

In the Civil War, more extremity amputations were performed than at any other time in the history of man. The wounds were left open because of the recognition that closure would usually lead to sepsis and death. Although healing often took months, very large dinner-plate-sized above-the-knee amputation sites would heal with a sturdy stump for a weight-bearing prosthesis. Similarly, hidradenitis suppurativa in the groin region, which can be very difficult to heal, is often managed best by total excision of all involved skin in the groin and perianal area and then allowing the wound margins to come together spontaneously until the wound is healed. In both instances, contraction is the ally of the surgeon, allowing closure without added morbidity.

However, in many instances, *contraction* (the normal, active biologic process) results in a *contracture,* a fixed deformity which is an aesthetic and functional disability to the patient. Most dramatic are contractures of skin and hollow organs. Loss of skin, secondary to either burn injury or trauma, may result in a contracture as the skin edges are drawn together to fill a defect. In addition, if there is no other skin present, a contracture will result. This is especially true over flexor joint surfaces such as the neck (Fig. 8-15) or volar surfaces of digits. But the process is not limited to the skin. Any type of injury to hollow organs such as the esophagus or common bile duct may trigger the contractile process resulting in a contracture, which mechanically blocks the function of the hollow organ.

Mechanism. The earliest observations in this century on contraction were made by Carrel. He noted that open animal skin wounds healed by a process wherein the wound margins would remain open for a few days, a ''lag phase,'' followed by a rapid rate of closure. There were and still remain questions as to whether the cells responsible for these powerful forces of tissue movement are located within the central granulation tissue of the wound or at the wound margins (picture-frame theory).

In the early 1970s, researchers noted the presence of fibroblast-like cells in contracting open skin wounds which had smooth muscle components in the cytoplasm as well as fibroblast characteristics. They termed these cells *myofibroblasts.* When strips of open wound granulation tissue were placed in a water bath, they contracted in the presence of smooth muscle agonists and relaxed in the presence of smooth muscle antagonists. Furthermore, myofibroblasts have been identified in a number of contracted human tissues such as Dupuytren's contracture, burn contractures, and contractures of capsules around silicone breast implants. These cells are at their peak during and following the process of contraction.

Others state that the myofibroblast is present only after contraction has been completed. They postulate that the extracellular matrix may be as important as the cell type within the contracting tissue. The work that supports this hypothesis is based on experiments done in vitro in a tissue culture system of a collagen gel lattice. Perhaps the varying evidence points to a contribution of both elements, i.e., contracting cell acting upon a matrix more susceptible to contraction.

All attempts to use pharmacologic agents to control contraction of wounds have failed. For example, some investigators attempted to inhibit open wound contraction with smooth muscle inhibitors such as Trocinate, which was successful only as long as the agent was present on the wound surface. Splinting a wound open will not prevent contracture. As soon as the splint is removed, the powerful biologic forces of the process place the wound margins in just the position they would be had the splint not been placed.

Clinical Approaches. In the surgical correction of contractures, there are several helpful clinical principles. Before surgery, it should be determined whether the scar is mature or immature. Mature scar is soft and pliable whereas immature scar may be stiff,

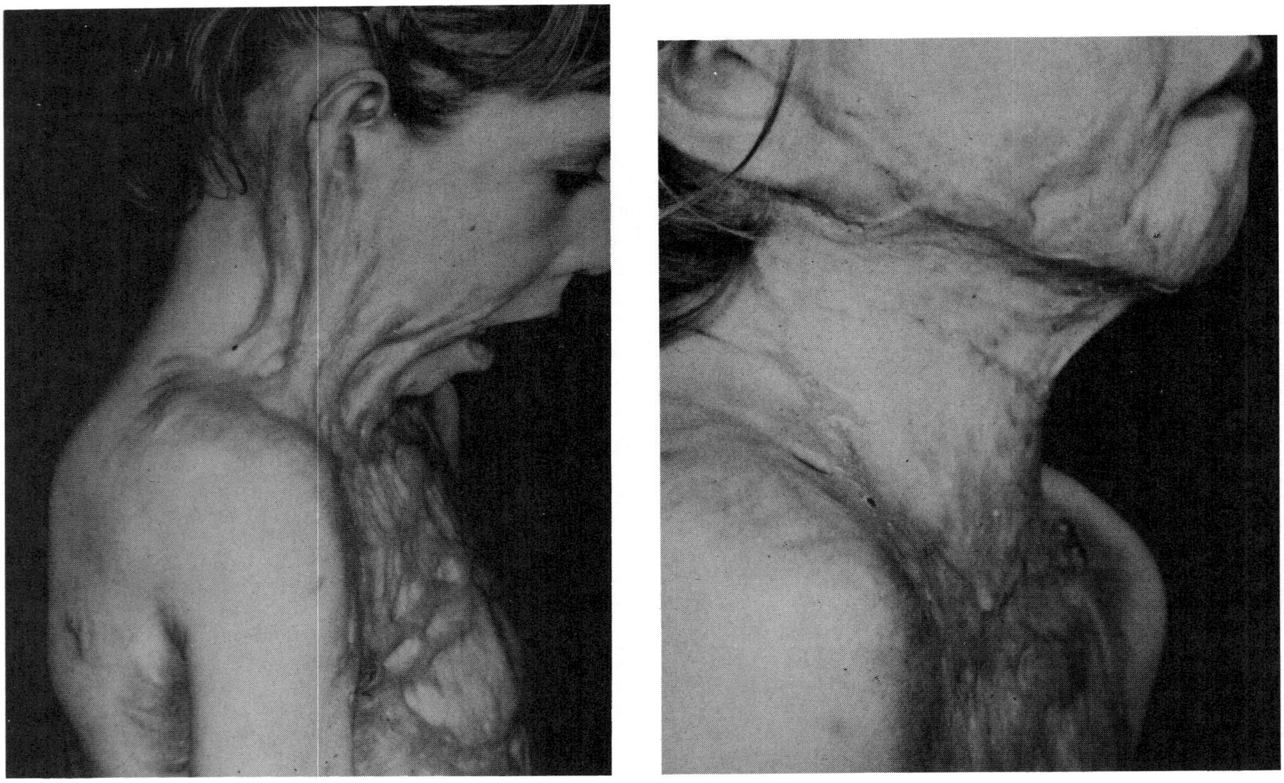

A B

FIG. 8-15. *A.* Severe contracture produced by full-thickness skin loss in burn wound of neck and face. Note ectropion of lower lip. *B.* Release of contracture in same patient shown in Fig. 8-15*A*. Contracture was released by excising scar tissue and resurfacing the defect with several split-thickness skin grafts. Note absence of wrinkling of graft and restoration of cervical profile. Facial scars ultimately excised and resurfaced.

indurated, hypertrophic, and even tender. Immature scar still has inflammatory cell components and residual myofibroblasts which will tend to facilitate contracture of the bed under any skin graft that may be used to correct the deformity. In many cases, it is preferable to correct the defect by placement of a *flap* which contains both skin and subcutaneous tissue and in some cases muscle. Because a flap is made of composite tissue, and supplies the defect with all of the components of soft tissue, contraction is rare.

If one corrects a mature contracture, a skin graft may be used to fill the defect. For reasons unknown, the open wound contracts less after placement of a full-thickness graft than after a partial-thickness graft (Fig. 8-16). It is not a matter of graft thickness, but a matter of *full* or *partial*. In both instances, it is advisable to splint the repaired wound in a fully open position. This may be required for several months. It appears that splinting is required until all myofibroblasts and inflammation are gone from the wound. The time required for splinting is highly variable and must rely on ''clinical judgment'' rather than science.

Epithelization

All surfaces exposed to the external environment are covered by epithelial cells. Skin is an example of epithelization but mechanisms of epithelial repair are similar throughout the body. The outer layer of skin, the epidermis, is composed of a multilayered stratified squamous epithelium that protects the body from fluid loss, bacterial invasion, electromagnetic radiation, and general trauma. Normally, the epidermal thickness is maintained at a constant level. Cells in the basal layer of the epidermis divide and migrate superficially and mature in the process. They become anuclear and die as they reach the surface and slough or desquamate, by which time they are really mere acellular masses of keratin. Although the term *keratinocyte* is used often interchangeably with the term *epithelial cell,* the epithelium is composed of several types of cells. The majority are keratinocytes but the epithelium also contains other types such as Langerhans cells, which are involved in immunologic responses.

The collagen-rich dermis, and not the epidermis, provides all the strength attributed to skin. The epidermis, however, provides the barrier that protects the internal milieux of the host from the external environment. The basement membrane of the basal lamina provides structural support for the epidermis and attaches epidermis to dermis (see Fig. 8-12). It is a thin glycoprotein-rich layer with complex layering and structures. A true adult-type wound healing response with classic inflammatory changes only occurs once the basal layer has been violated.

Mechanisms. Partial-thickness wounds heal by the process of epithelization (see Fig. 8-4). There are two major phenomena in the process of epithelization: migration and mitosis.

After epithelial destruction, a blood clot is formed; it dries and forms a scab on the exposed dermis. This response protects the dermis. Epithelial cell migration then begins the reparative process

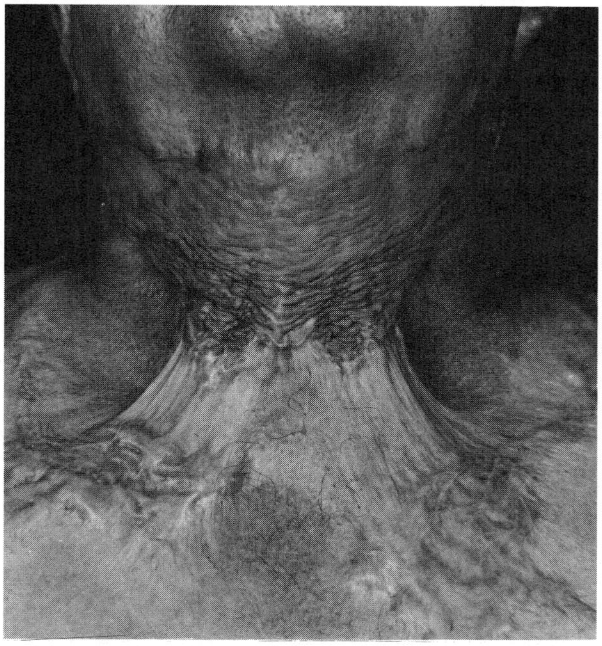

FIG. 8-16. Appearance of partial-thickness skin graft applied to granulating wound while undergoing contraction. Note wrinkled appearance of graft and effect of continued contraction on surrounding skin.

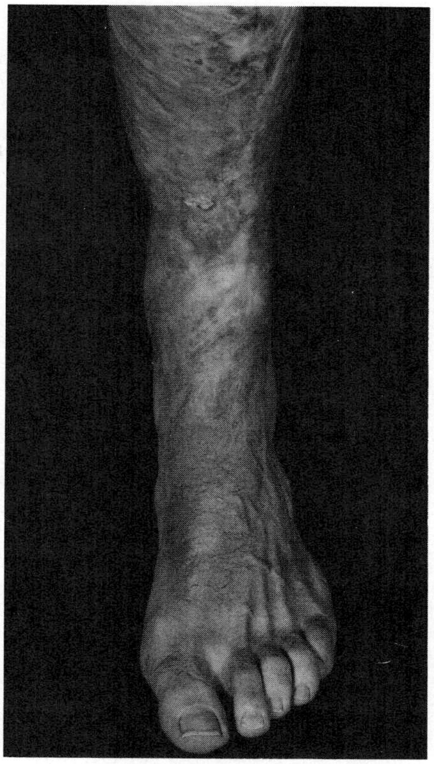

FIG. 8-17. Third-degree burn of lower leg following healing by epithelization. Absence of dermis accounts for shiny appearance and relative fragility of the suffface.

and is independent of epithelial mitosis. Migration of cells is the dominant process in epithelization. Under experimental conditions, blocking cell mitosis has no significant effect on cell migration or closure of the wound. These migrating cells are derived from the margins of the wound and from hair follicles and sebaceous glands within the dermal base of the wound (see Fig. 8-4). The more superficial the wound, the more rapid the process of reepithelization. Very superficial wounds, such as minor burns and abrasions, that do not penetrate the basal membrane heal by regeneration. Deeper dermal burn wounds that penetrate the basement membrane may heal by epithelization also, but the process requires a longer time. In addition, the result is often unsatisfactory because the inflammatory or healing response is initiated once the basement membrane is violated (Fig. 8-17).

Regardless of the type of injury, the basal layer of epithelium and the epithelium in the deeper hair follicles and sweat glands is where migration is initiated (see Fig. 8-4). One can observe these cells as they change morphologically. They flatten out and send out cytoplasmic projections which extend into the surrounding tissue (Fig. 8-18). These cells also lose their attachments to their neighboring basal cells and begin to migrate, with the leading cells phagocytizing debris and blazing a path for those keratinocytes migrating behind them. The epithelial cells do not migrate as single cells but in a sheet of cells. Some researchers have proposed that the keratinocyte sheets pile up at the leading edge and that cells tumble over the top in leap-frog fashion by a process called *epiboly*. A few days after migration begins, these migrating cells pause to divide.

Some of the biochemical mechanisms of these processes have been clarified. The blood and tissue fluids contain both fibronectin and vitronectin—both of which support epithelial cell migration. Moreover, several growth factors stimulate keratinocyte migration and mitosis. These include bFGF, PDGF, TGF-α and EGF. By contrast, TGF-β inhibits epidermal cell proliferation but stimulates motility. Although the mechanical aspects of epidermal cell motility are not defined clearly, it is known that these cells contain a cytoskeleton and move by an actin-myosin contractile system. Once the surface is covered, the epithelial cells revert to their normal phenotypic behavior, with intercellular and basement membrane attachments. This reversion to a normal state may be a key to understanding epithelial cancer (Fig. 8-19).

The movement of epithelial sheets is most important in healing of partial-thickness wounds. Clinically, this process is enhanced by keeping the surface moist rather than dry. Nature's scab may be satisfactory, but appropriate nonadherent dressings that will keep the wound moist are of vital importance and can enhance significantly the process of epithelization (see section on Wound Dressings). Growth factors will also be used in the near future to accelerate these processes. In addition, agents that enhance the detachment of cells and enhancement of the epibolic mechanisms will be added to the therapeutic regimen.

Nutrition

Inadequate nutrition devastates the healing process. If caloric protein intake stops for a mere 24 hours, collagen synthesis ceases. Inadequate nutrition inhibits the immune response, and opsonization of bacteria is ineffective. Several dietary insufficiencies have been described.

Ascorbic acid is essential for man, and its lack is the most common cause of wound healing deficiency. The diseased state associated with a lack of vitamin C (ascorbic acid) is known as *scurvy*. Historians have recounted how old scars in sailors would

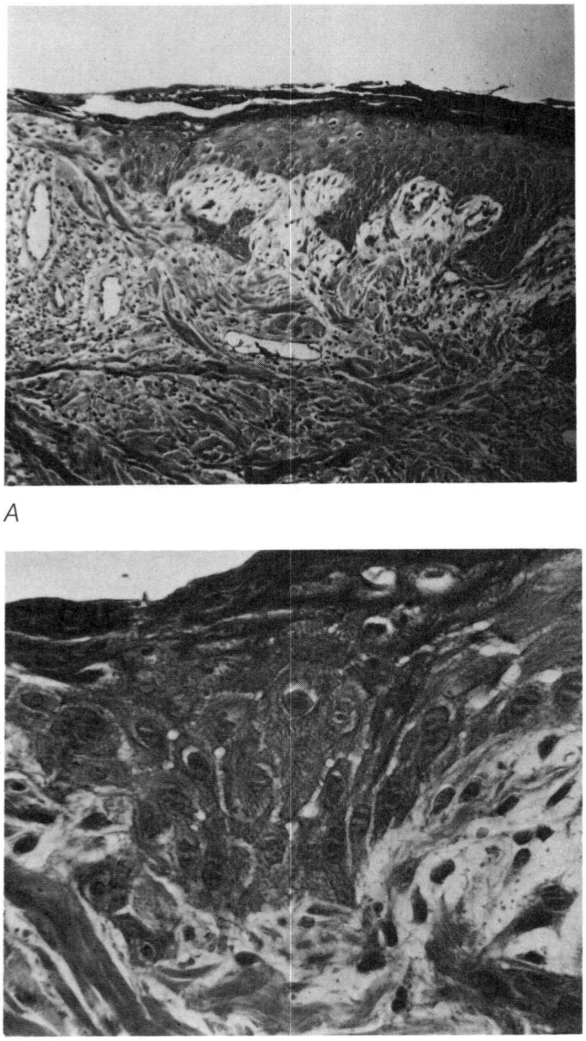

A

B

FIG. 8-18. *A.* Low-power view of epithelium advancing over granulating surface in a human wound. Note decreased thickness of advancing margin. *B.* High-power view of advancing epithelium in granulating human wound. Note dedifferentiation of cells, deep migratory activity suggesting subsurface metabolic activity at epithelial-mesenchymal tissue interface, and absence of visible mitotic activity.

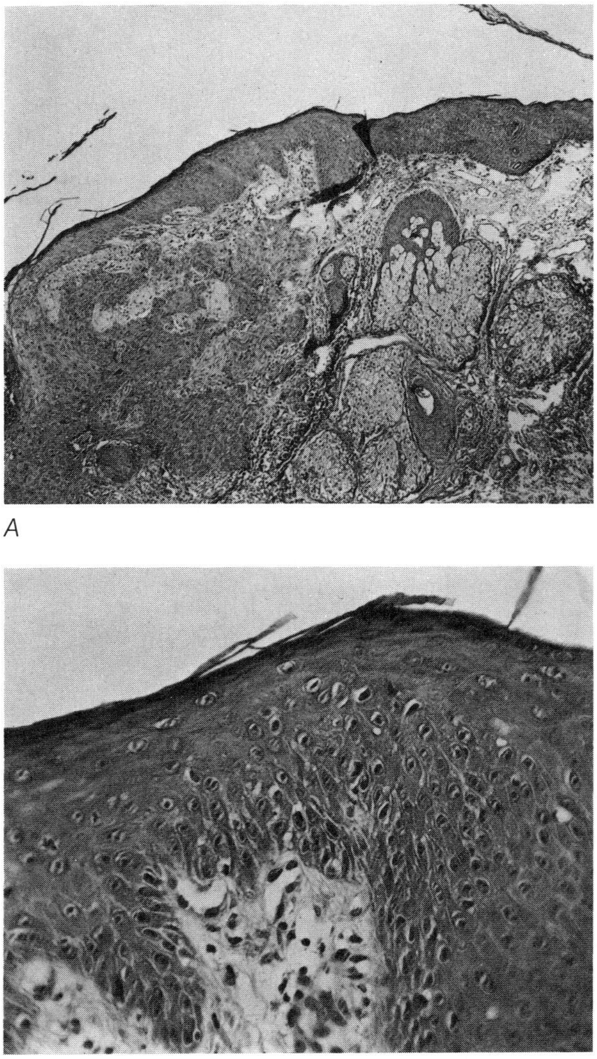

A

B

FIG. 8-19. *A.* Low-power view of epidermoid carcinoma of skin. Note accumulation of cells producing increased thickness of epithelium without purposeful migratory activity. *B.* High-power view of epidermoid carcinoma. Note numerous mitotic figures.

spontaneously open years after healing when the sailors were at sea for many months and without fresh fruits which contain large quantities of ascorbate. Long before biochemical analysis for ascorbate was available, the British admiralty recognized that scurvy could be avoided if all ships carried adequate supplies of ascorbate-containing fruits—hence the term ''Limey'' became affixed to British throughout the world.

The biochemical function of vitamin C is well known, and secondary functions relating to collagen gene expression have also been described. As mentioned in the discussion of collagen metabolism, ascorbate is a cofactor in the hydroxylation of proline to form the amino acid hydroxyproline during the synthesis of collagen. Ascorbate is essential for the addition of molecular oxygen to form the hydroxyl group of hydroxyproline. In humans, thermally unstable collagen is produced if ascorbate is not in sufficient dietary supply. Therefore, old healed wounds tend to disrupt preferentially compared with the normal surrounding skin for two reasons: First, the scar is never as strong as surrounding skin. Second, there is more collagenase activity in normal scar than in normal skin. Hence, in the scorbutic patient, scar breaks down before there is breakdown of the normal skin. The problem is of more than mere historic and biochemical interest. Ascorbate deficiency is found commonly after major trauma and is more common than generally realized in some of the malnourished members of lower socioeconomic classes in the United States. The mechanism of acute ascorbate deficiency after major trauma is not clear. There may be rapid sequestration of ascorbate in organs, or there may be renal loss, degradation, or lower absorption of this vitamin. Aggressive replacement of vitamin C should be undertaken immediately after major trauma to prevent would healing complications.

Up to a gram of vitamin C per day has been recommended in severely traumatized patients.

The trace metal iron is needed for prolyl hydroxylation. The minerals calcium and magnesium are required for collagenase activity and protein synthesis in general. All the essential amino acids required for protein synthesis are needed for wound healing. Supplementation of the diet with increased levels of arginine enhances the wound healing response. An adequate oxygen supply is essential; some speculate that many chronic wound healing problems and perhaps impaired wound healing following trauma can be treated effectively by increasing tissue oxygenation.

Immunosuppression

Several groups of patients are immunosuppressed. Interestingly, only a small number of these patients actually manifest clinical wound healing problems. Acquired immunodeficiency disease is manifested by myriad signs and symptoms. A direct relationship between the leukocyte defect and healing per se, however, has not been reported. The wound complications found in AIDS patients are secondary to other manifestations of the disease. For example, various skin lesions such as Kaposi's sarcoma or infected traumatic wounds do occur. Chronic wounds in these patients should undergo the same therapy as any other chronic wound (see section on Chronic Wounds later in this chapter).

Chemotherapeutic drugs inhibit healing. It is often unclear if the clinical wound healing problems are caused by the drugs or by the malignant tumor. Malignancies deplete nutrients as well as inhibiting wound healing directly. In animal models, chemotherapeutic agents have been demonstrated to be very harmful to healing. Various growth factors such as PDGF and TGF-β are able to prevent the harmful effects of these drugs on collagen metabolism.

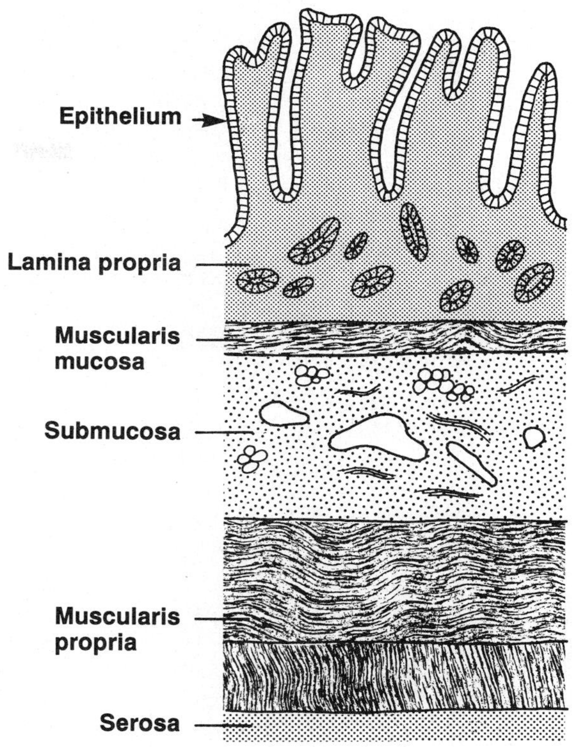

FIG. 8-20. Schematic representation of the multiple tissue layers in the gastrointestinal tract wall. (Modified from: *Graham MF, Blomquist P, Zederfeldt B: The alimentary canal, in Cohen IK, Diegelmann, RF, Lindblad WJ (eds): Wound Healing: Biochemical and Clinical Aspects, Chap 27. Philadelphia, Saunders, 1992.*)

SPECIFIC WOUND HEALING PROBLEMS

Gastrointestinal Tract

Little is known about the healing of the gastrointestinal tract when compared with skin and other organ systems. It has been observed that bowel anastomotic tensile strength develops more rapidly than skin tensile strength. The chronic wounds of bowel are classified as inflammatory bowel diseases. Gastric ulcers are not merely a matter of ischemia and erosion, and duodenal ulcers are not merely a matter of excessive acid and mucosal erosion. Crohn's disease and other forms of inflammatory bowel disease remain as much of an enigma as diabetic leg ulcers or hepatic fibrosis.

Anatomy. The gastrointestinal tract is divided into several distinct layers (Fig. 8-20). The inner mucosal layer is for absorption, and the outer muscularis mucosae layer functions for motility. They are wrapped in a strong serosal layer which is an extension of the peritoneum.

The mucosal epithelium is only one cell thick and renews itself about every 8 days. Beneath the epithelium is a basement membrane composed of Type IV collagen similar to the basement membrane of skin. Beneath this is the lamina propria, which is made up of collagen Types I, III, and V and elastin with an array of specialized cell types including various inflammatory cells. The outermost layer of the mucosa is a very thin layer of smooth muscle, the muscularis mucosae, which contributes to gut motility.

The submucosa separates the mucosa from the muscularis propria and appears to attach these two important layers to one another. It is composed of several collagen types in a ratio similar to that found in human aorta.

The muscularis propria is densely packed smooth muscle with a predominance of Types I and III collagen and a small amount of Type V. This collagen serves as an intramuscular tendon, or the source of strength through which a force can be transmitted through the smooth muscle cells. This is supported by the fact that hypertrophy of the muscularis propria also increases the collagen content of the muscle.

Injury and Repair. Healing of the gastrointestinal tract is similar to that of skin, in that penetration of the basement membrane marks the difference between total restoration of the tissue and the normal healing process by inflammation and fibrous matrix deposition (Fig. 8-21). The stomach is subjected continuously to hydrochloric acid and pepsin under normal conditions. When this combination is excessive, it can overcome the gastric mucosa's resistance to autodigestion and lead to penetration of the basement membrane and ulcer formation. Drugs such as aspirin and hydrocortisone or chemotherapeutic agents can enhance this damage. Short-term exposure to these agents can cause mucosal necrosis and detachment, but as long as the basal lamina is intact, the epithelial cells will migrate over the surface to repair the defect without any evidence of inflammatory cell activation. If the process is severe enough to permeate the basal lamina, into the lamina propria, then the inflammatory process is initiated. Once the lesion penetrates the mucosa, it is called an ulcer and healing is slower.

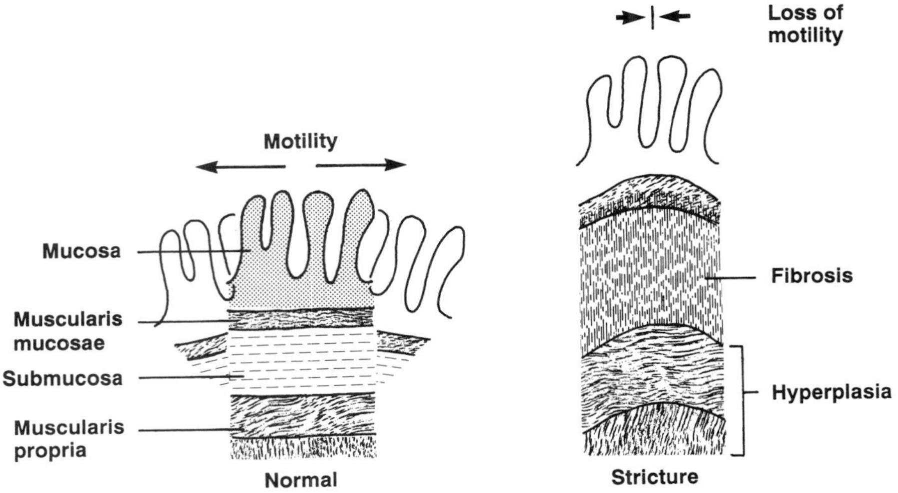

FIG. 8-21. The normal compliant relationship between mucosa and muscularis propria is lost when the submucosa becomes fibrotic. (Modified from: *Graham MF, Blomquist, P, Zederfeldt B: The alimentary canal, in Cohen IK, Diegelmann RF, Lindblad WJ (eds): Wound Healing: Biochemical and Clinical Aspects, Chap 27. Philadelphia, Saunders, 1992.*)

The distinction is of biologic and clinical importance, because ulcers always heal with some evidence of scarring (Fig. 8-22).

Crohn's disease is a chronic idiopathic inflammatory bowel disease that affects the terminal ileum and cecum most frequently but can involve any part of the gastrointestinal tract. It is characterized by inflammation in the submucosa rather than mucosa and often extends from mucosa to serosa, hence the term *transmural*. Inflammation leads to collagen deposition and contraction which cause stricture and symptoms of intestinal obstruction. Biochemically there is increased collagen Type I and V content in the involved bowel compared with normal. This is in contrast to ulcerative colitis where the bowel tends to have thinning of its matrix and to perforate rather than get thicker and develop strictures. The healing process of ulcerative colitis is much different from that of Crohn's disease. In ulcerative colitis, the inflammation is confined to the mucosa and does not extend into the submucosa.

Human intestinal smooth muscle cells isolated from normal human jejunum have been used to clarify further the pathogenesis of bowel healing. Demonstrating their differences when compared with normal skin, the bowel cells in vitro produce twice the collagen as skin fibroblasts. Moreover, TGF-β enhances collagen synthesis by intestinal smooth muscle cells. Although corticosteroids inhibit collagen production by dermal fibroblasts, they are not effective in down-regulating collagen synthesis by human intestinal smooth muscle cells.

Radiation injury is commonly seen in the alimentary tract and terminates in extensive and progressive submucosal, muscularis, and serosal fibrosis with striking hyalinization of the accumulated collagen. Resection is required in some patients but is hazardous because bowel anastomosis in radiated tissue is associated with anastomotic leak and fistula formation.

Lye ingestion is a common cause of esophageal tissue injury. The mucosa is penetrated and hence fibrosis and stricture occur. Although parenteral corticosteroids have proven to be efficacious in animals, there has never been a well-controlled study in man.

Healing in the Gastrointestinal Tract. The same basic process of repair occurs with anastomotic healing in the gastrointestinal tract as occurs in skin. The same factors that inhibit development of tensile strength in skin do the same in the gastrointestinal tract. But the gastrointestinal tract is a unique tubular structure; it is closed with sutures or staple devices and must then rely on the anastomosis to provide bowel integrity until the anastomosis has developed sufficient tensile strength to prevent disruption. The major complications of intestinal anastomoses are anastomotic leakage and actual bowel wall disruption. These are associated with a significant morbidity and mortality. Although clinical complications of anastomotic leak occur in 2 to 18 percent of patients, up to 50 percent of anastomotic sites leak early, as demonstrated by contrast radiographic studies.

Eventually, the submucosa provides the major strength in anastomotic closures because it contains the majority of the fibrous connective tissue, which is mainly collagen. It is during the early period following anastomosis that leak occurs. During this time, the sutures or staples, and not the connective tissue matrix, hold the anastomosis together. However, most studies have focused on collagen metabolism. During the first few days following anastomosis, there is significant turnover of collagen not only at the anastomotic site but in the adjacent bowel wall. Reduction in collagen content extends a significant distance from the actual anastomotic site. Although most studies of anastomosis and anastomotic leak have centered around the strength of the closure (i.e., sutures followed by collagen deposition and cross-linking), much of the problem with anastomotic leakage may be related to the early absence of a new mucosal lining. Intestinal content can pass through the bowel wall which lacks a mucosal scar.

Skin

More wound healing data comes from skin than from any other organ system. Most of the information gained from the study of skin in animal models and in humans can be applied to the process of tissue repair in all other organ systems.

Keloids and Hypertrophic Scars. Keloids and hypertrophic scars are both abnormal healing processes that occur after injury from trauma or surgery. However, they are different both clinically and biochemically. Hypertrophic scars remain within the boundaries of the original wound and almost always regress over a period of time (Fig. 8-23). By contrast, keloids extend beyond the boundaries of the original wound and usually do not regress (Fig. 8-24); they usually recur after excision unless additional therapy is given.

Under normal conditions there is an equilibrium between collagen synthesis and collagen degradation in skin and normal scar.

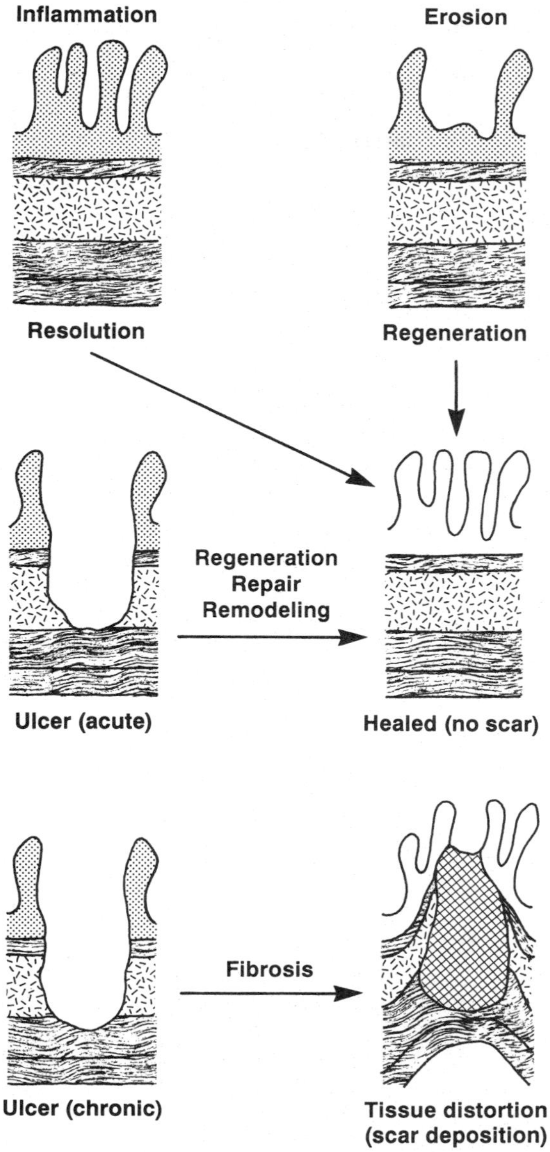

FIG. 8-22. Pattern of gastrointestinal repair depends on the depth of mucosal inflammation. (Modified from: *Graham MF, Blomquist P, Zederfeldt B: The alimentary canal, in Cohen IK, Diegelmann RF, Lindblad WJ (eds): Wound Healing: Biochemical and Clinical Aspects, Chap 27, Philadelphia, Saunders, 1992.*)

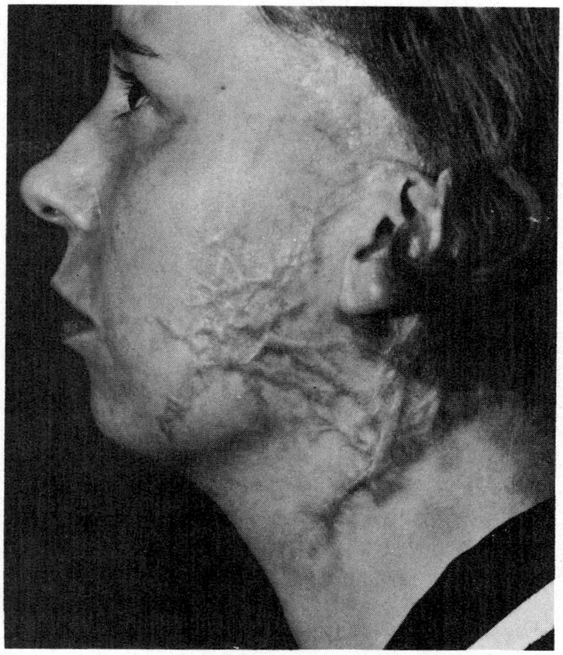

A

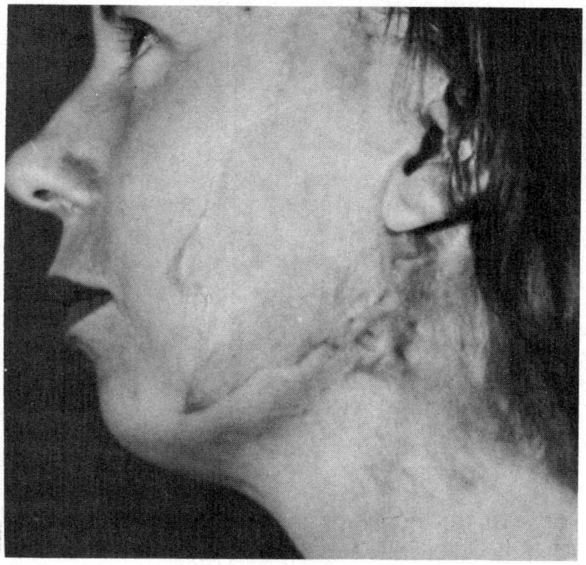

B

FIG. 8-23. *A.* Hypertrophic scar produced by deep second-degree burn. Although a significant amount of full-thickness skin has not been lost, overproduction of collagen has produced an unsightly scar. *B.* Patient shown in Fig. 8-23*A* following excision of facial portion of scar and application of a thick split-thickness skin graft. Cervical portion of scar resurfaced later. A single graft covering facial and cervical areas would obliterate submandibular groove. Note that scar at junction of graft and skin is most prominent near angle of mouth, where motion and tension are unavoidable. Although different in texture, hue, and thickness from normal skin, the graft provides a smooth surface over which cosmetics can be applied more effectively than over previous scar.

By contrast, both keloids and hypertrophic scars are characterized histologically by an overabundant deposition of collagen. The rate of collagen synthesis in keloid tissue, however, is significantly greater than in hypertrophic scar. The keloid tissue contains more soluble collagen and has a greater water content. Fibroblasts isolated from keloids continue to produce more collagen, through up to 40 passages in cell culture, than hypertrophic scars or normal skin. The equilibrium may be disrupted further by the collagenase inhibitor α_2-macroglobulin, which is abundant in keloid and hypertrophic scar tissue. Both increased collagen synthesis and decreased degradation seem responsible for the increased collagen deposition in keloid and even hypertrophic scar. Molecular biologic studies applied to these earlier findings seem to confirm the

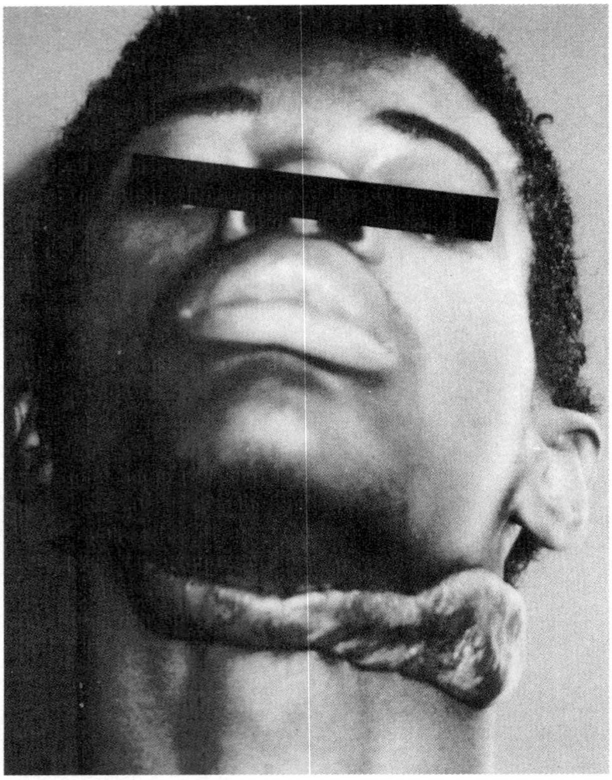

FIG. 8-24. Recurrent keloid on the neck of a seventeen-year-old man that had been revised several times. (From: *Murray JC, Pinnell SR: Keloids and excessive dermal scarring, in Cohen IK, Diegelmann RF, Lindblad WJ (eds): Wound Healing: Biochemical and Clinical Aspects, Chap 30. Philadelphia, Saunders, 1992.*)

routine biochemistry. There is increased messenger RNA for Type I collagen, which suggests that these lesions result from abnormal regulation of collagen production at the level of transcription.

Growth factors may be very important in the regulation of these lesions. Early data suggest that cultured keloid cells produce increased amounts of cytokines compared with normal skin fibroblasts and that keloids may contain increased concentrations of TGF-β. Neutralizing antibodies to TGF-β placed in primary guinea pig wounds at the time of closure resulted in scarless healing. These observations suggest that inhibition of TGF-β may make a significant contribution in the clinical control of keloids and hypertrophic scars.

At present, the clinical treatment of keloids and hypertrophic scars is not optimal. Surgical excision should be done only after careful consideration. Hypertrophic scar will regress usually without operation. Keloid tends to return after excision. There may, however, be clear indications for surgery in either group of patients. In some patients, keloid is very disfiguring, and this alone may be reason enough to excise the lesion. Excision may be used for debulking so that pharmacologic agents may be used to control the abnormal scar. In other patients excision is indicated to improve function. All patients must be aware of the high risk of recurrence and the importance of careful follow-up.

As in any disease process that is not understood clearly, there are many treatments that have been advocated for keloids and hypertrophic scars. Perhaps the most popular and effective is the intralesional injection of triamcinolone, which is a long-lasting 9-alpha-fluorocorticosteroid. Such treatment will make the lesion softer and often smaller, and may be the only treatment required for small lesions. Moreover, such treatment will often relieve the burning, itching, and pain associated with keloids and hypertrophic scars. If these somatic symptoms are the patient's complaints, then corticosteroids may be all that is required regardless of the size or appearance of the lesion. The authors recommend 40 mg/mL of triamcinolone, never using more than 2 mL every 6 to 8 weeks in adults to avoid any systemic effects. Complications include local atrophy of skin and subcutaneous tissue, which may be severe. Telangiectasia may appear locally, and there may be depigmentation in dark-skinned patients. Pregnant women should never be so treated because of the remote possibility that a birth deformity may be related to the use of corticosteroids. We do not recommend the use of a "Dermojet" to deliver triamcinolone through the epidermis to the keloid in the underlying dermis. Triamcinolone may be used in conjunction with surgery. Some inject triamcinolone into the wound margins at the time of closure after excision, whereas others begin treatment at various times after operation. The newer "supersteroids" such as Temovate may be effective, topically.

Keloids are known to contain a significant number of mast cells and have increased histamine content as compared with normal skin or scar. As a result, these patients often suffer severe itching. An oral antihistamine is often helpful to control this symptom. Drug therapy has included retinoic acid applied topically and Retin-A cream which give symptomatic relief and tend to make the lesions softer. Several other topical devices have been used to treat both these lesions including a sponge, steroid-impregnated tape, and silicone sheets. There are no valid data that any of these methods are efficacious. Radiation therapy is mentioned only to be condemned. There have been no long-term follow-ups reported, and the late development of skin cancer after radiation constitutes a potential hazard.

Factitious Wounds. Factitious lesions are much more common than one would expect. The surgeon should always be on the alert for factitious diseases of a surgical nature. Beware of any patient who has had multiple surgical procedures, especially patients with some relationship to the health care field. When examining patients, note the pattern of scars, accessibility to self-mutilation, "la belle indifférence." Confrontation will often lead to the patient leaving—never to return. Both diagnosis and treatment are extremely difficult.

Marjolin's Ulcer. Any nonhealing wound in an area of previous trauma may represent squamous cell carcinoma termed Marjolin's ulcer. These virulent malignancies arise from old areas of trauma. Although the causation may be multifactorial, they appear to arise because the dense scar of the lesion does not allow normal immunologic surveillance of the area by the host. Therefore, the host cannot destroy the malignant transformation within a burn scar.

Tendon

Tendons link muscle to bone and thereby allow muscular force to exert motion. They are composed mainly of Type I collagen, with a significant amount of proteoglycan which arranges and regulates the size of the collagen fibrils. If fetal muscle development is prevented, tendons do not develop. When tendons cross the concavity of a joint such as finger or wrist, they pass under fibrous structures called pulleys. Specialized cells located in the pulleys and elsewhere lubricate the tendons. In the areas where tendons are compressed, they receive blood supply from vincula.

There are some unique factors in tendon healing. The flexor tendons within fibrous flexor sheaths of the digits present the surgeon with a unique healing problem so challenging that some termed the area ''no-man's-land''; surgical results in this area were poor. This is because healing must occur in the sutured ends of the tendon as well as in the sheath itself. Both are collagenous structures. When they heal together as a unit rather than separately, tendon function is lost because gliding is impeded by the scar between tendon and sheath. Empirically, surgeons have learned to make ''no-man's-land'' into ''some-man's-land'' by using meticulous technique and early mobilization. A major contribution to the functional healing of tendon within a fibrous flexor sheath has been the revelation that the segmental blood supply to tendon through the vincula is extremely important in promoting healing with less-restricting scar.

There is excellent experimental and clinical work to show that early motion provides the stress forces to lengthen scar. Motion cannot prevent collagen deposition but it can lengthen the scar and allow enough motion for functional gliding of tendon. Motion may also enhance lubrication from synovial fluid.

Several experimental methods to enhance tendon healing include electrical stimulation, nonsteroidal anti-inflammatory agents, and growth factors, but there is no evidence of effectiveness. Experimentally, pharmacologic agents have been used in an attempt to reduce tendon adhesions. Hyaluronic acid holds some promise. The use of proline analogues has not been successful. β-Aminopropionitrile was used successfully in humans undergoing flexor tendon grafting, but side effects led to termination of the study.

Bone

Fracture repair combines physical, biochemical, and biomechanical factors in a process that often leads to scarless healing. After fracture, the dead material is removed and hematoma resorbs. Revascularization occurs and granulation tissue bridges the defect. Within a few days, connective tissue (''soft callus'') is found both externally and internally along the marrow cavity of the bone. This material is a fibrocartilaginous splint for early healing. Soft callus is mineralized as cartilage and is replaced by osteoid or bony material to form hard callus over the next few months. This provides fracture stabilization. Remodeling begins as the cortical callus is replaced with compact bone (Fig. 8-25). Over a period that may even take years, the bone is reshaped by the forces transmitted through the bone (''Wolfe's law''). Osteoconductive and osteoinductive factors are extremely important in bone healing. Osteoinductive factors such as bone morphogenic protein (BMP) and osteogenic protein-1 (OP-1), both members of the TGF-β family of cytokines, activate local cells to accelerate the healing process of bone. Various other cytokines such as PDGF, TGF-β, bFGF are but a few that will probably have use in the clinical control of fracture healing. Oxygen tension and electrical forces are also important. Electrical field stimulation has proven to be clinically efficacious—especially in delayed nonunion.

Chronic Wounds

Chronic wounds remain one of the most costly unsolved problems in health care. It is estimated that approximately 15 percent of diabetics develop skin ulcers, which result in about 60,000 amputations per year. The range of medical costs has been estimated at

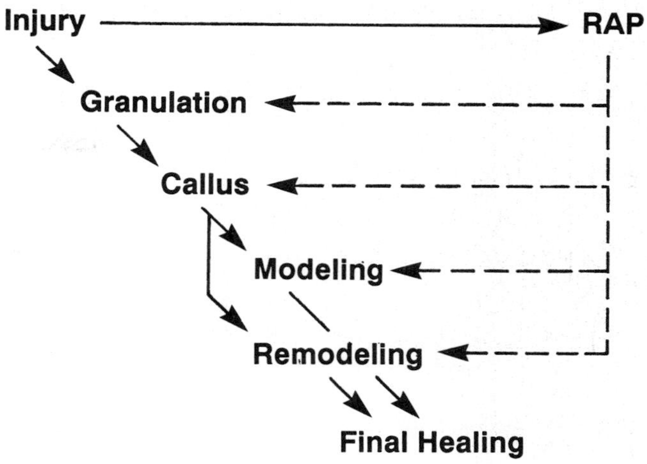

FIG. 8-25. Diagrammatic representation of the relationship of the regional acceleratory phenomenon (RAP) with bone healing processes. (From: *Frost HM: The biology of fracture healing. Clin Orthop Rel Res 248:288, 1989.*)

$24,000 to $36,000 per patient, and the overall cost of diabetic ulcers, including loss of productivity, could be as high as $20 billion per year. In addition, there are about 175,000 to 250,000 spinal cord injury patients in the United States and approximately 7000 to 10,000 new patients per year. Approximately 25 to 85 percent develop pressure ulcers, and cost estimates range from $14,000 to $25,000 per patient for medical, surgical, and nursing care. If the elderly nursing home population is added in with the spinal cord injury population, then the figure for the care of all pressure ulcers is also very significant. The care of venous stasis ulcers is also very costly.

Acute versus Chronic Wounds. There are significant differences between acute and chronic wounds. An *acute wound* usually occurs in a normal, healthy person and is either closed primarily or allowed to close by ''secondary intention.'' Most injuries to whole organs or tissues can be considered acute wounds. For example, liver insulted with a viral infection or a chemical toxin is a ''wounded'' tissue, but this type of wound in the liver usually resolves completely without any evidence of hepatic fibrosis and undergoes tissue regeneration. It is only the occasional patient in whom the hepatic injury results in a chronic wound with subsequent fibrosis which can even lead to hepatic failure.

A *chronic wound* is one that fails to heal because of some underlying pathologic condition. For example, pressure ulcers, diabetic ulcers, and venous stasis ulcers are chronic wounds. These complex wounds will not heal until the underlying cause is corrected. Curiously, many of these chronic wounds heal to a point and then there is an arrest of the healing process. The exact factors that cause this phenomenon remain unknown. With proper clinical management, most chronic wound healing problems are resolved and healing occurs, but recurrence is common.

Chronic Wound Healing Mechanisms. Sometimes, the basic biologic mechanism of healing chronic wounds is contraction, which reduces the area of the wound. Usually, minimal epithelization is required to heal chronic wounds, and the result is often cosmetically and functionally acceptable. There are exceptions to the predominance of contraction. Epithelization may be more important than was thought. For example, venous stasis ulcers do not heal by contraction. If the margins of these ulcers are tattooed and then the wound heals, one observes that the tattoo marks are still in their peripheral location. It would appear that epithelial cells cover the wound and that these cells lead to the induction of a neodermis. This is supported by the evidence that cultured epithelial cells applied to a granulating wound bed will induce new dermis formation.

Chronic Wound Care. Most chronic wounds of various causes will heal by secondary intention only if the underlying mechanical causative factors are treated first. For example, compression stocking or bandages must be used to relieve venous hypertension in order for venous stasis ulcers to heal. Conversely, pressure must be eliminated over the pressure sore. Special pressure-relieving beds and other devices have been designed for this purpose. Diabetes must be controlled to ensure healing of diabetic ulcers.

The objective of the management of chronic wounds healing by secondary intention is to create optimal conditions for healing by contraction and epithelization or to prepare the wound bed for flaps or skin grafting. Cleaning of the wound should remove microorganisms, necrotic tissue, and foreign bodies and simultaneously not injure surrounding healthy tissue. The wound itself must not come into contact with agents that harm the wound bed. Disinfectants not only destroy microorganisms but also the healthy tissue in the wound. Strong cleansers such as hydrogen peroxide and iodophores can hinder the wound healing process. In some cases irrigation of the wound with normal, sterile saline is helpful. Although power spray and jet lavage of chronic wounds are widely used, they are often ineffective in removing debris and may even force bacteria deeper into granulating tissue, and the process may injure the new cells. For some patients, whirlpool may be helpful in debridement with lower leg ulcers or with extensive burns. The whirlpool environment is comfortable, and the moving water carries off dead tissue. Care must be taken to prevent infection between patients by strict hygienic control of whirlpools. Debridement with a knife—so-called sharp debridement—may be the best method for wound cleaning when feasible.

Another method for debridement and cleaning of the wound is the use of wet to dry gauze. In addition to cleaning the wound, wet gauze provides a moist environment. Bacteria and proteinaceous material are wicked into the interstices of the gauze as drying occurs. This is especially helpful in treating deep wounds because the gauze dressing can be packed into the deepest recesses of the wound. This moist environment enhances granulation tissue growth. There are a wide variety of wound dressings that may be used to serve this protective function (see section on Wound Dressings).

In addition to dressings, several aspects of general patient care are important. Sometimes it is necessary to assist the patient's immune system by means of systemic or topical antibiotics to prevent or control infection and sepsis. This is especially important in large burns, where both systemic and topical antibiotics are used, since systemic antibiotics generally do not penetrate granulation tissue. There are also a number of extrinsic factors that can impair chronic wounds from healing. As outlined in a previous section of this chapter, patients with genetic disorders of collagen metabolism usually have associated problems of wound healing. Inadequate vitamin C, low tissue P_{O_2} and poor nutrition in general can also impair the healing of chronic wounds. Other extrinsic factors associated with delayed healing of chronic wounds include old age, uremia, jaundice, diabetes, glucocorticoid steroids, distant malignancies, and any pharmacologic agent that interferes with protein synthesis.

WOUND DRESSINGS

During the past decade, dressings for both acute and chronic wounds have changed dramatically. As new principles of wound care have evolved, many new dressings have become available. The clinician must match the characteristics of the dressing to the type of wound being treated.

Primarily closed wounds are often covered for a few days with a sterile dressing to protect the wound from bacterial invasion until the margins have formed an epithelial seal. In addition, the dressing serves to absorb fluid that may leak out of the wound. In some cases, the dressing is of psychologic benefit, as the patient and family are spared the vision of the wound. Early removal of dressings from primarily closed wounds allows the care team to be alerted to signs of infection, necrosis, and/or wound separation.

Semiocclusive Dressing. Semiocclusive dressings provide a moist environment which enhances the reepithelization of partial-thickness wounds. There can be relative control of the water and gases transmitted through these dressings. If a semiocclusive dressing is applied early to a partial-thickness wound, scab formation is avoided. Not only can scab formation damage the underlying dermis, the removal of the scab may be painful, cause bleeding, and damage the new epithelium. Semiocclusive film dressings are commonly used to provide a moist environment for reepithelization but have a tendency to collect fluid and trap wound exudate which may cause the dressing to leak and require frequent changing. The combining of a calcium alginate and a film dressing can both provide a moist wound environment and assist with the absorption in these highly secreting wounds.

The classification, composition, indications, and functions of dressings are summarized in Table 8-6. Occlusive/semiocclusive dressings may further exacerbate infection when covering areas where the bacterial count is greater than 1×10^5 organisms per gram of tissue. This risk may be reduced by first controlling the wound bacterial count with topical antimicrobial and/or systemic antibodies. In addition, several of the hydrogels can be used effectively with antibiotic creams. These hydrogels accelerate the rate of penetration of the antibiotic into the granulation tissue.

If dressings are used to debride, it is important that a slower and more gentle process is used when tendons are exposed. This can be accomplished with several of the hydrogels. When eschar tissue is present, a hydrocolloid may be more appropriate than a hydrogel dressing. This type of debridement occurs through autolysis. The hydrocolloid traps the wound exudate and creates a moist environment that softens and lifts or causes proteolytic digestion of the eschar.

Wounds with a large amount of exudate require dressing with a greater capacity to absorb. When dressings do not adequately absorb, the healthy tissue around the wound may become macerated. The use of a skin protectant around the wound may alleviate this problem. There has been concern that hydrocolloids leave pectin base in wounds which form granuloma. There are, however, several nonpectin-based hydrocolloids that address this problem and also absorb wound secretions.

MECHANICAL WOUND CLOSURE

The materials used for wound closure are much less important than the techniques of closure. Basically, sutures may be classified as

Table 8-6
Wound Dressings

Classification	*Compositions*	*Indications*	*Functions*	*Examples*
Films	Semiocclusive (semipermeable). Polyurethane or copolyester.	Acute. Partial- or full-thickness wounds with minimal exudate. Nondraining primarily closed wounds.	Mimic skin performance. Water vapor permeable. Water/bacterial impermeable. Retention dressing for gels. Provides moist environment.	Op-site, Bioclusive, Tegaderm, Blisterfilm, Visulin
Hydrocolloids	Contain hydrophil colloidal particles (quar, karaya, gelatic, carboxymethyl cellulose) in an adhesive mass (usually polyisobutylene).	Acute or chronic partial- or full-thickness wounds. Stage I to IV pressure ulcers.	Absorbs fluid. Debrides soft necrotic tissue by autolysis. Protects wounds. Good adhesiveness without adherence to wound. Encourages granulation. Promotes reepithelization. Protects wounds from trauma.	Cutinova Hydro, Duoderm, Comfeel. Restore, Intrasite, Ultec, J & J ulcer dressing
Hydrogels	Contain 80–99% water. Cross-linked polymer such as polyethyleneoxide, polyvinyl pyrollidone or acrylamide.	Acute or chronic partial-thickness wound with minimal exudate.	Creates moist environment. Usually requires secondary dressing. Low absorbency. Debrides minimally. Decreases pain. Does not adhere to wound.	Vigilon, Geliperm, Elastogel, Intrasite Gel, Span Gel
Foams	Either hydrophilic or hydrophobic. Nonocclusive. Usually polyurethane or gel film coated. High absorbency.	Acute or chronic partial-thickness wounds that are highly secreting and require mechanical debriding.	Debrides. High absorbency rates. Water vapor permeable.	Cutinova Plus, Lyofoam, Allevyn
Impregnates	Fine mesh gauze impregnated with either moisturizing, antibacterial or bacteriocidal compounds. Nonadherent.	Acute or chronic partial-thickness wounds with minimal to moderate exudate.	Does not adhere to wound. Promotes reepithelization. May contain antibacterial or bactericidal agents. Requires secondary dressing.	Aquaphor-gauze, Adaptic, Biobrane, Scarlet red
Absorptive powders and pastes	Consist of starch, copolymers or colloidal, hydrophillic particles. Can absorb up to 100 times their weight.	Chronic full-thickness wounds with large amounts of exudate.	High absorbency. Debrides necrotic and fibrous material from wound.	Granulat, Debrisan wound cleansing paste, Bard absorptive dressing, Duoderm granules
Calcium alginate	Nonwoven composite of fibers from calcium alginate, a celluloselike polysaccharide.	Full- or partial-thickness wounds with high exudate.	Highly absorbent. Dressing material becomes a gel to facilitate moist healing. Requires secondary dressing.	Sorbsan, Kaltostat

absorbable or *nonabsorbable*. The absorbable are synthetic such as polyglycolic acid or biologic such as ''catgut'' which is plain or chromium-treated. Traditional teaching is that absorbable sutures are buried and, as they absorb, will not be a nidus for late infection. Nonabsorbable sutures are used on the skin because they are less reactive and allegedly provide a better-appearing scar. These dogma make little sense in the schema of healing. Although it is true that gut sutures are more reactive than polyglycolic acid, which is more reactive than nylon, the argument that tissue reactivity to particular sutures is of significance in the healing process has never been validated. Nonabsorbable sutures may be used in subcutaneous tissue as well as fascia or for organ repair. By contrast, absorbable sutures are often used on the skin in infants and children. For example, 6-0 plain gut sutures placed in the skin do not require removal in a child, thus avoiding the major trauma of suture removal. Similarly, absorbable sutures are used commonly for closure of hand wounds—even in adults.

The most important fact about sutures is that any woven suture is more prone to infection than a smooth suture because bacteria can become entrapped in the interstices of a woven suture and not be destroyed by the normal host responses, thus leading to bacterial propagation and infection. Therefore, woven suture material should not be used in closure of contaminated wounds.

A few suture materials deserve special comment. The nonabsorbable polypropylene is extremely smooth and, therefore, the best material to use when creating a subcuticular pull-out suture. The absorbable polyglycolic dermal suture (PDS) is best for areas where long-term tensile strength is required. Although stainless steel sutures are still used, they should be banned in the operating room because they often cut through gloves and create an environment where the surgical team may be more susceptible to pathogens such as hepatitis or AIDS virus.

Staples. Although these devices have revolutionized repair of organ parenchyma and anastomosis of various hollow organs, they must be used with discretion on the skin. Well-designed staples applied properly are excellent for everting the skin margins appropriately. Staples must be removed within a few days if one is to avoid permanent skin marks.

Adhesive Strips. In certain types of wounds, adhesive tape strips can be used. For example, once dermal sutures are in place, tapes may be substituted for surface skin sutures as long as the wound edges are well approximated. In addition, the strips can be very helpful to support the wound margins after early removal of skin sutures. The tape strips are simple and clean, and many small lacerations can be closed painlessly using strips without the need for local anesthetics.

FETAL WOUND HEALING

During the past decade, there has been a logarithmic increase in interest in fetal surgery and fetal wound healing. Animal fetal surgery has led to repair of life-threatening conditions in human fetuses without maternal mortality. Fetal surgery will become routine in future decades. It is imperative that the mechanisms of fetal tissue repair are appreciated if human fetal surgical repairs are to be performed optimally. An even more important reason to study fetal healing is to dissect out the mechanisms that make fetal repair so dramatically different from adult healing. Understanding fetal healing should allow for major advances in our treatment of the adult healing problems of scar, contraction, and wound disruption.

There is little evidence of an inflammatory response during fetal healing. An inflammatory response, however, can be induced by the addition of living or dead bacteria, removal of hyaluronic acid from the connective tissue matrix, or a variety of cytokines including TGF-β, PDGF, and EGF. Rather than collagen, the major component of the wound matrix is the glycosaminoglycan hyaluronic acid.

Primarily closed skin wounds in a third-trimester rabbit cannot be detected on routine histology or by electron microscopy. There are no inflammation and no evidence of excessive collagen deposition. There are no architectural abnormalities of the matrix. Collagen synthesis measured daily after wounding is significantly greater in fetal wounds than in normal fetal skin. In addition, there is an astonishing gain in the tensile strength of the closed fetal skin wound by 5 days, in marked contrast to the adult who gains little strength in this time period. These data lead to the inescapable conclusion that there must be a very rapid turnover and remodeling of collagen during fetal repair.

Third-trimester open fetal rabbit wounds do not contract, in contrast to second-trimester fetal sheep wounds, which do contract. There is no evidence of myofibroblasts in the noncontracting fetal rabbit wounds. If the wound is sealed from the amniotic fluid environment by a silicone patch, the wound will close by either contraction or regeneration. There is reasonable evidence that amniotic fluid may inhibit fetal wound contraction, but the mechanisms and component(s) remain unclear. The content of the matrix of the open fetal wound is mainly hyaluronic acid, and this may be an important factor in the contractile process in both adult and fetus. There is promise that adult wound contraction can be controlled by the data obtained from the noncontracting fetal wound.

Bibliography

General

Clark RAF, Henson PM: *The Molecular and Cellular Biology of Wound Repair*. New York, Plenum Press, 1988.

Cohen IK, Diegelmann RF, Lindblad WJ (eds): *Wound Healing: Biochemical and Clinical Aspects*. Philadelphia, Saunders, 1992.

Kang AH, Nimmi ME (eds): *Collagen: Vol. 5, Pathobiochemistry*. Boca Raton, FL, CRC Press, 1992.

Nimmi ME (ed): *Collagen: Vol. 1, Biochemistry*. Boca Raton, FL, CRC Press, 1988.

Videos: "The Principles of Wound Healing," "Secondary Wound Closure," "Partial Thickness Healing," and "Treatment of Primary Healing Wounds." These four videos are available from the Wound Healing Center, Box 117, Richmond, VA 23298-0117.

Collagen Metabolism

Bauer EA, Striklin GP, et al: Collagenase, in Goldsmith, LA (ed): *Biochemistry and Physiology of the Skin,* Chap 18. Oxford, Oxford University Press, 1983, pp 411–432.

Cohen IK: Can collagen metabolism be controlled: theoretical considerations. *J Trauma* 25:410, 1985.

Gay S, Miller EJ: *Collagen in the Physiology and Pathology of Connective Tissue*. Stuttgart-New York, Fischer, 1978, p 75.

Haukipuro K, Melkko J, et al: Connective tissue response to major surgery and postoperative infection. *Eur J Clin Invest* 22(5):333, 1992.

Hering TM, Marchant RE, Anderson JM: Type V collagen during granulation tissue development. *Exp Mol Pathol* 39:219, 1983.

Miller EJ: The structure of fibril-forming collagens. *Ann NY Acad Sci* 406:1, 1985.

Nerlich AG, Poschl E, et al: Biosynthesis of collagen and its control, in Kuhn K, Krieg T (eds): *Connective Tissue: Biological and Clinical Aspects*. Basel, Karger, 1986, pp 70–90.

Nimni ME: Collagen: structure, function, and metabolism in normal and fibrotic tissues. *Semin Arthritis Rheum* 13:1, 1983.

Prockop DJ, Kivirikko KI, et al: The biosynthesis of collagen and its disorders. *N Engl J Med* 301:13, 77, 1979.

Uitto J, Murray LW, et al: Biochemistry of collagen in disease. *Ann Intern Med* 105:740, 1986.

Weiss JB, Ayad S: *Cell Biology of Extracellular Matrix,* 2nd ed, Hay ED (ed). New York, Plenum Press, 1981.

Weiss JB, Ayad S: An introduction to collagen, in Weiss JB, Jayson MIV (eds): *Collagen in Health and Disease,* Chap 1. Edinburgh, Churchill Livingstone, 1982, pp 1–17.

Cytokines and Wound Healing

Glaser BM, Michels RG, et al: Transforming growth factor-β_2 for the treatment of full-thickness macular holes: a prospective randomized study. *Ophthalmology* 99:1162, 1992.

Granstein RD, Flotte TJ, Amento EP: Interferons and collagen production. *J Invest Dermatol* 95:755, 1990.

Grotendorst GR, Martin GR, et al: Stimulation of granulation tissue formation by platelet-derived growth factor in normal and diabetic rats. *J Clin Invest* 76:2323, 1985.

Lynch SE, Colvin RB, Antoniades HN: Growth factors in wound healing: single and synergistic effects on partial thickness porcine skin wounds. *J Clin Invest* 84:640, 1989.

McGrath MH: Peptide growth factors and wound healing. *Clin Plast Surg* 17(3):421, 1990.

Nathan C, Sporn M: Cytokines in context. *J Cell Biol* 113(5):981, 1991.

Peltonen J, Kahari L, et al: Evaluation of transforming browth factor β and type I procollagen gene expression in fibrotic skin diseases by in situ hybridization. *J Invest Dermatol* 94(3):365, 1990.

Pierce GF, Mustoe TA, et al: Transforming growth factor β reverses the glucocorticoid-induced wound healing deficit in rats: possible regulation in macrophages by platelet-derived growth factor. *Proc Natl Acad Sci USA* 86:2229, 1989.

Roberts AB, Flanders KC, et al: Transforming growth factor β: biochemistry and roles in embryogenesis, tissue repair and remodeling, and carcinogenesis. *Recent Prog Horm Res* 44:157, 1988.

Roberts AB, Sporn MB, et al: Transforming growth factor type beta: rapid induction of fibrosis and angiogenesis in vivo and collagen formation in vitro. *Proc Natl Acad Sci USA* 83:4167, 1986.

Robson MC, Phillips LG, et al: Platelet-derived growth factor BB for the treatment of chronic pressure ulcers. *Lancet* 339:23, 1992.

Shah M, Foreman DM, Ferguson MWJ: Control of scarring in adult wounds by neutralising antibodies to transforming growth factor beta (TGFβ). *Lancet* 339:213, 1992.

Sporn MB, Roberts AB: Peptide growth factors and inflammation, tissue repair, and cancer. *J Clin Invest* 78:329, 1986.

Sporn MB, Roberts AB, et al: Transforming growth factor-beta: biological function and chemical structure. *Science* 233:532, 1986.

Wahl SM, Hunt OA, et al: Transforming growth-factor type-beta induces monocyte chemotaxis and growth factor production. *Proc Natl Acad Sci USA* 84:5788, 1987.

Proteoglycan Glycoconjugates

Comper WD (ed): *Heparin and Related Polysaccharides: Structural and Functional Properties*. New York, Gordon and Breach, 1981.

Dorfman A: Proteoglycan biosynthesis, in Hay ED (ed): *Cell Biology of the Extracellular Matrix*. New York, Plenum Press, 1981, pp 115–138.

Lindahl U, Hook M: Glycosaminoglycans and their binding to biological macromolecules. *Ann Rev Biochem* 47:385, 1978.

Roden L: Structure and metabolism of connective tissue proteoglycans, in Lennarz WJ (ed): *The Biochemistry of Glycoproteins and Proteoglycans*. New York, Plenum Press, 1980, pp 267–371.

Silbert JE: Structure and metabolism of proteoglycans and glycosaminoglycans. *J Invest Dermatol* 79:31S, 1982.

Weigel PH, Fuller GM, LeBoeuf RD: A model for the role of hyaluronic acid and fibrin in the early events during the inflammatory response and wound healing. *J Theor Biol* 119:219, 1986.

Genetic Defects in Connective Tissue Metabolism

Bauer EA, Gedde-Dahl T, Eizen AZ: The role of human skin collagenase in epidermolysis bullosa. *J Invest Dermatol* 68:119, 1977.

Hollister DW, Lee B, et al: Linkage of Marfan syndrome and a phenotypically related disorder of two different fibrillin genes. *Nature* 352:330, 1991.

Kashiwagi H, Riddle JM, et al: Functional and ultrastructural abnormalities of platelets in Ehlers-Danlos syndrome. *Ann Intern Med* 63:249, 1965.

Krieg T, Hume A, et al: Molecular defects of collagen metabolism in the Ehlers-Danlos syndrome. *Int Soc Trop Dermatol* 20:415, 1981.

Marini JC: Osteogenesis imperfecta: comprehensive management. *Adv Pediatr* 35:391, 1988.

McKusick VA: The defect in Marfan syndrome. *Nature* 352:279, 1991.

Sillence DD, Senn AS, Danks DM: Genetic heterogeneity in osteogenesis imperfection. *J Med Genet* 16:101, 1979.

Wenstrup RJ, Willing MC, et al: Distinct biochemical phenotypes predict clinical severity in nonlethal variants of osteogenesis imperfecta. *Am J Hum Genet* 46:975, 1990.

Wesley JR, Mahour GH, Woolley MM: Multiple surgical problems in two patients with Ehlers-Danlos syndrome. *Surgery* 87:319, 1980.

Wound Contraction

Abercrombie M, Flint MH, James DW: Wound contraction in relation to collagen formation in scorbutic guinea pigs. *J Embryol Exp Morphol* 4:167, 1956.

Billingham RE, Russell PS: Studies on wound healing with special reference to the phenomenon of contracture in experimental wounds in rabbits' skin. *Ann Surg* 144:961, 1956.

Craven JL: Wound contraction in lathyritic rats. *Arch Pathol* 89:526, 1970.

Cronin TD: The use of molded splint to prevent contracture after split skin grafting on the neck. *Plast Reconstr Surg* 27:7, 1961.

Ehrlich HP: The modulation of contraction of fibroblast populated collagen lattices by types I, II, and III collagen. *Tissue Cell* 20:47, 1988.

Ehrlich HP, Wylver DP: Fibroblast contraction of collagen lattices in vitro: inhibition by chronic inflammatory cell mediators *J Cell Physiol* 116:345, 1983.

Gabbinai G, Ryan GB, Majno G: Presence of modified fibroblasts in granulation tissue and possible role of wound contraction. *Experientia* 27:549, 1971.

Madden JW, Morton D Jr, Peacock EE Jr: Contraction of experimental wounds. I. Inhibiting wound contraction by using a topical smooth muscle antagonist. *Surgery* 76:8, 1974.

McGrath M: Healing of the open wound, in Rudolph, R (ed): *Problems in Aesthetic Surgery. Biological Causes and Clinical Solutions*. St Louis, CV Mosby, 1986, pp 13–48.

McGrath MH, Simon RH: Wound geometry and the kinetics of wound contraction. *Plast Reconstr Surg* 72:66, 1983.

Peacock EE Jr: Pharmacological control of surgical scar tissue. *Am Surg* 44:693, 1978.

Robee D (ed): *Soft and Hard Tissue Repair: Biological and Clinical Aspects*. New York, Praeger Press, 1984.

Rudolph R: The effect of skin graft preparation on wound contraction. *Surg Gynecol Obstet* 142:49, 1976.

Rudolph R: Inhibition of myofibroblasts by skin graft. *Plast Reconstr Surg* 63:473, 1979.

Rudolph R: Location of the force of wound contraction. *Surg Gynecol Obstet* 148:547, 1979.

Rudolph R: Contraction and the control of contraction. *World J Surg* 4:279, 1980.

Rudolph R, Guber S, Woodward M: The life cycle of the myofibroblast. *Surg Gynecol Obstet* 145:389, 1977.

Rudolph R, Utley J, Woodward M: Contractile fibroblasts (myofibroblasts) in a painful pacemaker pocket. *Ann Thorac Surg* 31:373, 1981.

Van Winkle W Jr: Wound contraction. *Surg Gynecol Obstet* 125:131, 1967.

Watts GT, Grillo HC, Gross J: Studies in wound healing. II. The role of granulation tissue in contraction. *Ann Surg* 148:153, 1958.

Epithelization

Clark RAF, Winn HJ, et al: Fibronectin beneath re-epithelialization epidermis in vivo: Sources and significance. *J Invest Dermatol* 80(suppl):26S, 1983.

Donaldson DJ, Mahan JT: Keratinocyte migration and the extracellular matrix. *J Invest Dermatol* 90:623, 1988.

Fine J-D: The skin basement membrane zone. *Adv Dermatol* 2:283, 1987.

Mertz PM, Davis SC, et al: Pulsed rhEGF treatment increased epithelialization of partial thickness wounds. *J Invest Dermatol* 90:588a, 1988.

Nanney L-B: Epidermal and dermal effects of epidermal growth factor during wound repair. *J Invest Dermatol* 94(5):624, 1990.

Poh-Fitzpatrick MB: Skin care of the healed burned patient. *Clin Plast Surg* 19(3):745, 1992.

Stenn KS: Coepibolin, the activity of human serum that enhances the cell spreading properties of epibolin, associates with albumin. *J Invest Dermatol* 89:59, 1987.

Stenn KS, Bhawan J: The normal histology of skin, in Farmer ER, Hood AF (eds): *Dermatopathology*. East Norwalk, CT, Appleton-Century-Crofts, 1990, pp 3–29.

Stenn KS, Madri JA, et al: Multiple mechanisms of disassociated epidermal cell spreading. *J Cell Biol* 96:63, 1983.

Stenn KS, Milstone LM: Epidermal cell confluence and implications for a two step mechanism of wound closure. *J Invest Dermatol* 83:445, 1984.

Winter GD: Epidermal regeneration studied in the domestic pig, in Maibach HI, Rovee DT (eds): *Epidermal Wound Healing*. Chicago, Year Book, 1972, pp 71–112.

Woodley DT, Kalabec T, et al: Adult human keratinocytes migrating over nonviable dermal collagen produce collagenolytic enzymes that degrade Type I and Type IV collagen. *J Invest Dermatol* 86:418, 1986.

Woodley DT, O'Keefe EJ, Prunieras M: Cutaneous wound healing: a model for cell-matrix interactions. *J Am Dermatol* 12:420, 1985.

Wright N, Alison M: *The Biology of Epithelial Cell Populations,* Vol I. Oxford, Clarendon Press, 1984, pp 283–345.

Nutrition

Albina JE, Mills CD, et al: Arginine metabolism in wounds. *Am J Physiol* 254:E459, 1988.

Breslow R: Nutritional status and dietary intake of patients with pressure ulcers: review of research literature 1943 to 1989. *Decubitus* 4:16, 1991.

Daly JM, Lieberman MD, et al: Enteral nutrition with supplemental arginine, RNA, and omega-3 fatty acids in patients after operation: immunologic, metabolic, and clinical outcome. *Surgery* 112(1):56, 1992.

Dvlewski DF, Froman DM: Vitamin C supplementation in the patient with burns and renal failure. *J Burn Care Rehabil* 13(3):378, 1992.

Ehrlichman RJ, Seckel BR, et al: Common complications of wound healing. Prevention and management. *Surg Clin North Am* 71(6):1323, 1991.

Falcone PA, Caldwell MD: Wound metabolism. *Clin Plast Surg* 17:443, 1990.

Hadley SA, Fitzsimmons L: Nutrition and wound healing. *Top Clin Nutr* 5:72, 1990.

Harju E, Huttunen J, Yla-Herttual AS: Clinical and metabolic effects and wound healing metabolism in controlled total parenteral nutrition with high vs. low nitrogen content for seven days after abdominoperineal rectum resection for carcinoma. *Chir Ital* 42(506):151, 1990.

Orgill D, Demlilng RH: Current concepts and approaches to wound healing. *Crit Care Med* 16:899, 1988.

Winkler MF, Mandrym MK: Nutrition and wound healing. *Supp Line* 1-4, 1992.

Young ME: Malnutrition and wound healing. *Heart Lung* 17:60, 1988.

Zaloga GP, Bortenschlager L, et al: Immediate postoperative enteral feeding decreases weight loss and improves wound healing after abdominal surgery in rats. *Crit Care Med* 20(1):115, 1992.

Crohn's Disease

Graham MF: Collagen production by the intestinal smooth muscle cell in response to inflammation: wound healing in the gut, in Snape WJ, Collins SM (eds): *Effects of Immune Cells and Inflammation on Smooth Muscle and Enteric Nerves.* Boca Raton, FL, CRC Press, 1991, pp 119–126.

Graham MF: Stricture formation: pathophysiologic and therapeutic concepts, in MacDermott R, et al (eds): *Inflammatory Bowel Disease.* New York, Elsevier, 1991.

Graham MF, Bryson GR, Diegelmann RF: Transforming growth factor-β_1 selectively augments collagen production by human intestinal smooth muscle cells. *Gastroenterology* 99:447, 1990.

Graham MF, Diegelmann RF, et al: Collagen content and types in the intestinal strictures of Crohn's disease. *Gastroenterology* 94:257, 1988.

Graham MF, Drucker DEM, et al: Collagen synthesis by human intestinal smooth muscle cells in culture. *Gastroenterology* 90:400, 1987.

Hypertrophic Scars and Keloids

Cohen IK, McCoy BJ: The biology and control of surface over-healing. *World J Surg* 4:289, 1980.

Crockett DJ: Regional keloid susceptibility. *Br J Plast Surg* 17:245, 1964.

Diegelmann RF, Cohen IK, McCoy BJ: Growth kinetics and collagen synthesis of normal skin, normal scar, and keloid fibroblasts in vitro. *J Cell Physiol* 98:341, 1979.

Griffith BH, Monroe CW, McKinney P: A follow-up study on the treatment of keloids with triamcinolone acetonide. *Plast Reconstr Surg* 46:145, 1970.

Kamin AJ: The etiology of keloids: a review of the literature and a new hypothesis. *S Afr Med J* 38:913, 1964.

Ketchum LD, Cohen IK, Masters FW: Hypertrophic scars and keloids: a collective review. *Plast Reconstr Surg* 53:140, 1974.

Ketchum LD, Smith J, et al: Treatment of hypertrophic scars, keloids, and scar contracture by triamcinolone acetonide. *Plast Reconstr Surg* 38:209, 1966.

Macguire HC: Treatment of keloids with triamcinolone acetonide injected intralesionally. *JAMA* 192:325, 1965.

Minkowitz F: Regression of massive keloid following partial excision and postoperative intralesional administration of triamcinolone. *Br J Plast Surg* 20:432, 1967.

Murray JC, Pollock SV, Pinnell SR: Keloids: a review. *Clin J Am Acad Dermatol* 4(4):461, 1981.

Oluwasanmi JO: Keloids in the African. *Clin Plast Surg* 1:179, 1974.

Omo-Dare P: Genetic studies on keloids. *J Natl Med Assoc* 67:428, 1975.

Peacock EE, Madden JW, Trier WC: Biologic basis for the treatment of keloids and hypertrophic scars. *South Med J* 63:755, 1970.

Rockwell WB, Cohen IK, Ehrlich HP: Keloids and hypertrophic scars: a comprehensive review. *Plast Reconstr Surg* 84(5):827, 1989.

Chronic Wounds

Allman RM, Laprade CA, et al: Pressure sores among hospitalized patients. *Ann Intern Med* 105:337, 1986.

Allman RM, Walker JM, et al: Air-fluidized beds or conventional therapy for pressure sores. *Ann Intern Med* 107:641, 1987.

Alvarez O, Rozint J, Wiseman D: Moist environment for healing: matching the dressing to the wound. *Wounds* 1:35, 1989.

Barnett A, Berkowitz RL, Vistnes LM: Comparison of synthetic adhesive moisture vapor permeable and fine mesh gauze dressings for split thickness skin graft donor sites. *Am J Surg* 145:379, 1983.

Bryant RA (ed): *Acute and Chronic Wounds.* St Louis, Mosby Yearbook, 1992.

Cuzzell J: The new RYB color code. *Am J Nurs* 88:1342, 1988.

Falanga V, Eaglstein WH, et al: Topical use of human recombinant epidermal growth factor (h-EGF) in venous ulcers. *J Dermatol Surg Oncol* 18(7):604, 1992.

Hinman CD, Maibach HI: Effect of air exposure and occlusion on experimental human skin wounds. *Nature* 200:377, 1973.

Jones PL, Millman A: Wound healing and the aged patient. *Nurs Clin North Am* 25:2634, 1990.

Kemp MG, Keithley JK, et al: Factors that contribute to pressure sores in surgical patients. *Res Nurs Health* 13:2934, 1990.

Kindwall EP, Gottlieb LJ, Larson DL: Hyperbaric oxygen therapy in plastic surgery: a review article. *Plast Reconstr Surg* 88(5):898, 1991.

Maklebust J: Pressure ulcers: etiology and prevention. *Nurs Clin North Am* 22:359, 1987.

National Pressure Ulcer Advisory Panel: Pressure ulcers prevalence, cost and risk assessment consensus development conference statement. *Decubitus* 2(2):24, 1989.

Robinson CE, Coghlan JK, Jackson G: Decubitus ulcers in paraplegics: financial implications. *Can J Public Health* 69:199, 1978.

Rudolph R, Noe JM: *Chronic Problem Wounds.* Boston, Little, Brown & Co, 1983.

US Department of Health and Human Services: *Pressure Ulcers in Adults: Prediction and Prevention.* AHCPR Publication No. 92-0047, Rockville, MD, 1992.

Wound Dressings

Alvarez OM, Mertz PM, Eaglstein WH: The effect of occlusive dressings on collagen synthesis in superficial wounds. *J Surg Res* 35:142, 1983.

Alvarez O, Rozint J, Wiseman D: Moist environment for healing: matching the dressing to the wound. *Wounds* 1:35, 1989.

Barnett A, Berkowitz RL, Vistnes LM: Comparison of synthetic adhesive

moisture vapor permeable and fine mesh gauze dressings for split thickness skin graft donor sites. *Am J Surg* 145:379, 1983.
Bryant RA: *Acute and Chronic Wounds*. St Louis, Mosby Yearbook, 1992.
Cuzzell J: The new RYB color code. *Am J Nurs* 88:1342, 1988.
Eaglstein WH, Mertz PM, Falanga V: Occlusive dressings. *Am Fam Physician* 35:211, 1987.
Eisinger M, Kraft ER, Fortner JG: Wound coverage by epidermal cells grown in vitro, in Hunt TK, Heppenstall RB, et al (eds): *Soft and Hard Tissue Repair: Biological and Clinical Aspects*. New York, Praeger, 1984, pp 293–310.
Falanga V: Occlusive wound dressings. *Arch Dermatol* 124:872, 1988.
Hinman CD, Maibach HI: Effect of air exposure and occlusion on experimental human skin wounds. *Nature* 200:377, 1963.
James JH, Watson AC: The use of Opsite, a vapor permeable dressing, on skin graft donor sites. *Br J Plast Surg* 28:107, 1975.
Katz S, McGiley K, Leyden JJ: Semipermeable occlusive dressings: effects on growth of pathogenic bacteria and reepithelization of superficial wounds. *Arch Dermatol* 122:58, 1986.
Kiuirikho KI, Myllyla R: Post-translational enzymes in the biosynthesis of collagen: intracellular enzymes. *Methods Enzymol* 82A:245, 1982.
Magee C, Havry BB, et al: A rapid technique for quantitating wound bacterial count. *Am J Surg* 133:760, 1977.
Martinez J, Burns C: Wound management. *Curr Concepts Wound Care* Summer:9–16, 1987.
Mertz PM, Eaglstein WH: The effect of a semiocclusive dressing on the microbial population in superficial wounds. *Arch Surg* 119:287, 1984.
Mertz PM, Marshall DA, Eaglstein WH: Occlusive wound dressings to prevent bacterial invasion and wound infection. *J Am Acad Dermatol* 12:662, 1985.
Rovee DT, Kurowsky CA, Labun J: Local wound environment and epidermal healing. *Arch Dermatol* 106:330, 1972.
Sirvio LM, Grussing DM; The effect of gas permeability of film dressings on wound healing. *J Invest Dermatol* 93:528, 1989.
Thomas S, Loveless P: Moisture vapour permeability of hydrocolloid dressings. *Pharm J* 241:806, 1988.
Thomas S, Loveless P, Hay NP: Comparative review of the properties of six semipermeable film dressings. *Pharm J* 240:785, 1988.
Varghese MC, Balin AK, et al: Local environment of chronic wounds under synthetic dressings. *Arch Dermatol* 122:52, 1986.
Winter GD: Healing of skin wounds and the influence of dressings on the repair process, in Harkiss KJ (ed): *Surgical Dressings and Wound Healing*. London, Crosby Lockwood, 1971, pp 46–60.
Winter GD, Scales JT: Effect of air drying and dressings on the surface of a wound. *Nature* 197:91, 1963.

Mechanical Wound Closure

deHoll D, Rodeheaver G, et al: Potentiation of infection by suture closure of dead space. *Am J Surg* 127:716, 1974.
Edlich RF, Becker DG, et al: Scientific basis for selecting staple and tape skin closures. *Clin Plast Surg* 17:571, 1990.
Edlich RF, Panek PH, et al: Physical and chemical configuration of sutures in the development of surgical infection. *Ann Surg* 177:679, 1973.
Edlich RF, Rodeheaver GT, Thacker JG: Technical factors in the prevention of infections, in Simmons RL, Howard RJ (eds): *Surgical Infectious Diseases*. New York, Appleton-Century-Crofts, 1982, p 449.
Frazza EJ, Schmitt EE: A new absorbable suture. *J Biomed Mater Res* 1:43, 1971.
Harrison I, Williams DF, Cuschieri A: The effect of metal clips on the tensile properties of healing skin wounds. *Br J Surg* 62:945, 1975.
Jewell ML, Sato R, Rahija R: A comparison of wound healing in wounds closed with staples versus skin sutures. *Contemp Surg* 22:29, 1983.
Johnson A, Rodeheaver GR, et al: Automatic disposable stapling devices for wound closure. *Ann Emerg Med* 10:631, 1981.
Laufman H, Rubel T: Synthetic absorbable sutures. *Surg Gynecol Obstet* 145:597, 1977.
Myers MB, Cherry G, Heinburger S: Augmentation of wound tensile strength by early removal of sutures. *Am J Surg* 117:338, 1969.
Nordstrom REA, Nordstrom RM: Absorbable versus nonabsorbable sutures to prevent postoperative stretching of wound area. *Plast Reconstr Surg* 78:186, 1986.
Postlethwait RW: Long-term comparative study of nonabsorbable sutures. *Ann Surg* 171:892, 1970.
Rodeheaver GT, Halverson JM, Edlich RF: Mechanical performance of wound closure tapes. *Ann Emerg Med* 12:203, 1983.
Rodeheaver GT, Thacker JG, Edlich RF: Mechanical performance of polyglycolic acid and polyglactin 910 synthetic absorbable sutures. *Surg Gynecol Obstet* 153:835, 1981.
Rodeheaver GT, Thacker JG, et al: Knotting and handling characteristics of coated synthetic absorbable sutures. *J Surg Res* 35:525, 1983.
Salthouse TN, Williams JA, Willigan DA: Relationship of cellular enzyme activity to catgut and collagen suture absorption. *Surg Gynecol Obstet* 129:691, 1969.
Silloway KA, Morgan RF, et al: Arcuate staple: its influence on pain of staple penetration and removal. *Am J Surg* 150:612, 1985.
Stillman RM, Marino CA, Seligman SJ: Skin staples in potentially contaminated wounds. *Arch Surg* 119:821, 1984.
Tera H, Aberg C: Tensile strength of twelve types of knot employed in surgery, using different suture materials. *Acta Chir Scand* 142:1, 1976.
Thacker JG, Rodeheaver GT, et al: Mechanical performance of sutures in surgery. *Am J Surg* 133:713, 1977.

Fetal Wound Healing

DePalma RL, Krummel TM, et al: Characterization and quantitation of wound matrix in the fetal rabbit. *Matrix* 9:224, 1989.
Krummel TM, Ehrlich HP, et al: In vitro and in vivo analysis of the inability of fetal rabbit wounds to contract. *Wound Repair and Regeneration* 1:1993 (in press).
Longaker MT, Adzick NS: The biology of fetal wound healing: a review. *Plast Reconstr Surg* 87:788, 1991.
Longaker MT, Chiu ES, et al: Studies in fetal wound healing. V: Prolonged presence of hyaluronic acid characterizes fetal wound fluid. *Ann Surg* 213:292, 1991.
Longaker MT, Golbus MS, et al: Maternal outcome after open fetal surgery: a review of the first 17 human cases. *JAMA* 265:737, 1991.
Mast BA, Diegelmann RF, et al: Scarless wound healing in the mammalian fetus. *Surg Gynecol Obstet* 174:441, 1992.
Mast BA, Haynes JH, et al: In vivo degradation of fetal wound hyaluronic acid results in increased fibroplasia, collagen deposition, and neovascularization. *Plast Reconstr Surg* 89(3):503, 1992.
Siebert JW, Burd AR, et al: Fetal wound healing: a biochemical study of scarless healing. *Plast Reconstr Surg* 85:495, 1990.

Acknowledgment

The authors wish to thank Cary Klett, M.D., for her helpful contribution to the section on genetic defects in connective tissue metabolism.

CHAPTER 9

Oncology

Charles M. Balch, Neal R. Pellis, Donald L. Morton, Patricia J. Eifel, and Murray F. Brennan

INTRODUCTION

Cancer is indiscriminant of age, ethnic and racial origins, and socioeconomic strata and continues to be one of the most prevalent diseases of the latter twentieth century. Effective treatment of cancer is limited by our present understanding of the causes of (1) cell transformation, (2) the reasons host defense mechanisms fail to eliminate errant cells, and (3) the long latent period (i.e., many years) from initiation to clinical detection. Treatment in the past decade has expanded from surgery alone playing the major role to the adoption of a multidisciplinary approach for many cancer patients. Treatments now involve combinations of surgery, radiation therapy, chemotherapy, hormonal therapy, and biologic therapy directed against visible tumor. Technological advances propel investigations toward an understanding of the causes and consequences of malignant changes at the tissue, cellular, genomic, and molecular levels. This new knowledge is only beginning to translate into clinical successes.

In the era of clinical specialization and subspecialization, it is apparent that cancer management requires a multimodality approach and understanding. Indeed, most cancer patients, now and in the future, will receive two or more modalities of cancer treatment as their standard care. The surgeon, medical oncologist, radiation oncologist, radiologist, immunologist, and pathologist have become clinical partners. For the surgeon to continue as a meaningful partner on a cancer care team, he or she must know the indications, risks, and benefits of all cancer treatments and how to coordinate them in the right combination and sequence in an individual cancer patient. A second partnership is now developing between the laboratory investigator and clinician, bringing questions and investigations of tumor biology into the clinic. As reports of flow cytometry, cell-receptor expression, genetic analysis, and serum tumor markers now routinely appear in medical records of patients, clinicians increasingly incorporate these laboratory parameters into clinical decisions and treatment planning.

Participation in multimodality patient care conferences now requires at least a working knowledge of each specialty's perspective, tools, and limitations. The surgeon has traditionally been responsible for coordinating cancer care and has generally provided the entry point into the cancer care system by making the diagnosis and providing the first treatment. Advances in technology, as well as the increasing effectiveness of radiation and systemic therapy, however, have brought new treatment options to the care of the surgical patient with cancer.

EPIDEMIOLOGY AND ETIOLOGY

Epidemiology

The distribution of cancer within the human species is the product of multifactorial influences. Genetic predispositions may include race, ethnicity, or simply skin color. While geographic influences may include environmental factors, such as incident sunlight, chemical exposure, endemic etiologic agents, and domestic confinement, dietary considerations determined by the available food resources are also a factor. As travel, cultural exchange, emigration, and communication continue to advance, the geographic boundaries of various forms of cancer have become less well defined and genetic influences may become more apparent.

Geographic Patterns. Although a genetic predisposition exists for some cancers, most available information favors environmental variation as the major contributor to the disparate geographic incidences of different cancer types. In many cases, the high incidence of a specific cancer in a particular region or country is linked to a specific causative agent. Chewing a mixture of betel nut, tobacco, and lime in regions of India has resulted in a high incidence of oropharyngeal tumors. The high incidence of gastric carcinoma in Japan is putatively linked to a diet of smoked and highly salted foods, and food contaminated with aflatoxin. The high incidence of hepatocellular carcinoma in parts of Africa and Asia is presumed to be associated with the frequency of hepatitis B infections in these regions. Geographic differences in the incidence of several other common solid tumors are less clearly explained. Breast and colon carcinoma are common in North America, but rare in Africa and Asia. Although carcinomas of the stomach, esophagus, and cervix are more common in developed countries, they are relatively infrequent in North America. Tobacco-smoking regions display increases in several solid tumors, not the least of which are most types of lung cancer. Regions of industrial use of asbestos have a greater frequency of mesothelioma as well as other tumors. Europeans living in subtropical and equatorial zones are at increased risk of skin cancer, particularly melanoma.

Cancer Statistics. The incidence of cancer is rising in nearly all populations. Estimates of overall cancer incidence by site and gender in the United States were recently reported by the National Cancer Institute's Surveillance, Epidemiology and End Results (SEER) program (Fig. 9-1). Lung, colorectal, and prostate carcinoma in decreasing order account for most cancer in men. Breast carcinoma accounts for 29 percent of all cancer in women, followed by colorectal, lung, and uterine carcinoma. There are substantial variations in cancer incidence at different sites within ethnic and racial subpopulations in the United States (Table 9-1). Environmental factors are at least partially responsible, since after a few decades immigrant populations develop cancer risks that approach those of the indigenous population. For example, Japanese immigrants to Hawaii have an increased risk of developing cancer compared with Japanese in their native country (Fig. 9-2).

Analysis of age-adjusted mortality from cancer at selected sites for men and women from 1930 to 1986 (Fig. 9-3) provides an analysis of clinically useful trends. For both sexes, the dramatic

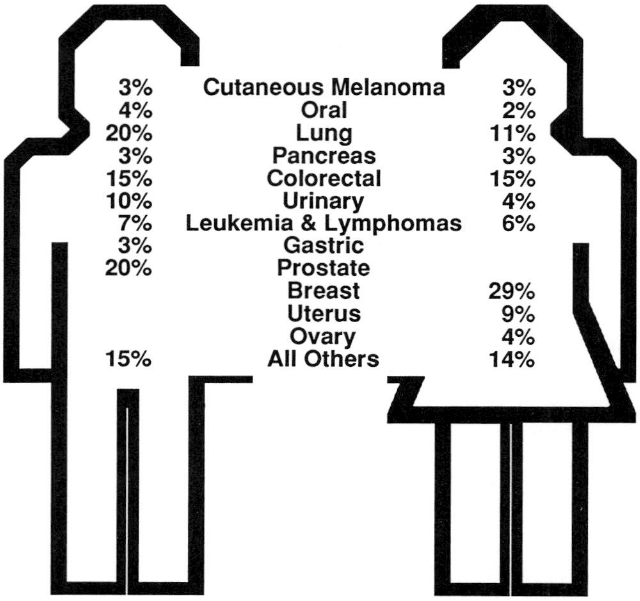

FIG. 9-1. Cancer distribution in human beings by gender and site. *(Adapted from SEER, 1987.)*

Table 9-1
Annual Age-Adjusted Incidence Rates per 100,000 for Selected Cancer Sites by Ethnic Group, 1975–1985, U.S. Males

	Whites	*Blacks*	*Hispanics*	*Native Americans*
All sites	404	490	266	185
Bladder	11	15	11	4
Brain, other nervous system	7	4	5	3
Colon	40	41	18	8
Esophagus	5	18	3	2
Gallbladder	1	1	2	9
Hodgkin's disease	4	3	3	1
(Non)-Hodgkin's lymphoma	13	9	7	5
Kidney	10	10	9	9
Larynx	9	12	4	1
Leukemia	14	11	8	6
Lip	4	0	3	0
Liver	1	1	2	9
Lung and bronchus	82	120	32	14
Melanoma and skin	10	1	2	2
Multiple myeloma	5	10	3	3
Nasopharynx	1	1	1	1
Other biliary	2	1	2	3
Other oral cavity, pharynx	12	21	5	2
Pancreas	11	17	12	9
Prostate	77	123	72	46
Rectum	20	15	12	5
Stomach	12	21	21	26
Testis	4	1	3	2
Thyroid	2	1	3	2
All others	28	31	22	19

SOURCE: Adapted from SEER program data.

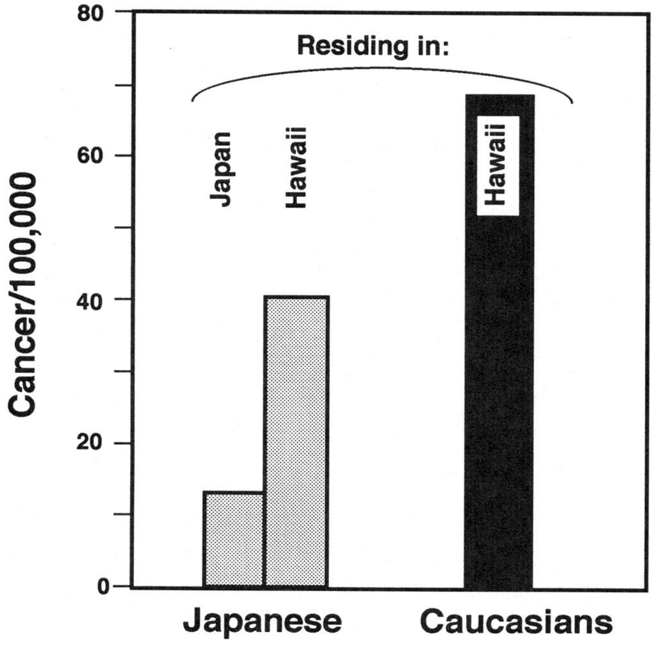

FIG. 9-2. Influence of geographic location on the frequency of cancer in an immigrant population.

increases in the death rates observed for lung carcinoma are attributed to increased cigarette smoking. From 1973 to 1987, there was a 15 percent increase in incidence of all cancers (Fig. 9-4). Cutaneous melanoma had the greatest increase, 83 percent, with non-Hodgkin's lymphoma and prostate carcinoma following at increases of approximately 50 percent. The scientific bases of the increases are unknown. By contrast, carcinoma of the cervix declined 36 percent, as did endometrial carcinoma and gastric carcinoma. Reduction in cervical carcinoma is due to the early detection and treatment of cervical dysplasia resulting from the widespread use of routine cervial cytologic screening (Pap smear). In summary, most cancers are rising in frequency. Although no singular influence predominates as causal in the increase, longer life expectancy, emotional stress, and environmental deterioration are significant.

Cancer is second to heart disease as the most common cause of death in the United States, accounting for 22 percent of all deaths. The fairly steep decline in mortality from gastric cancer in both sexes reflects a genuine decrease in incidence, since routine endoscopic screening has not gained acceptance in the United States, and current therapeutic intervention has had little impact on survival. From 1973 to 1987, overall cancer mortality has increased 13 percent in persons age 65 and older, with an increase for all ages of 5.4 percent. The few cancers that are highly sensitive to chemotherapy show the greatest decrease in mortality. From 1973

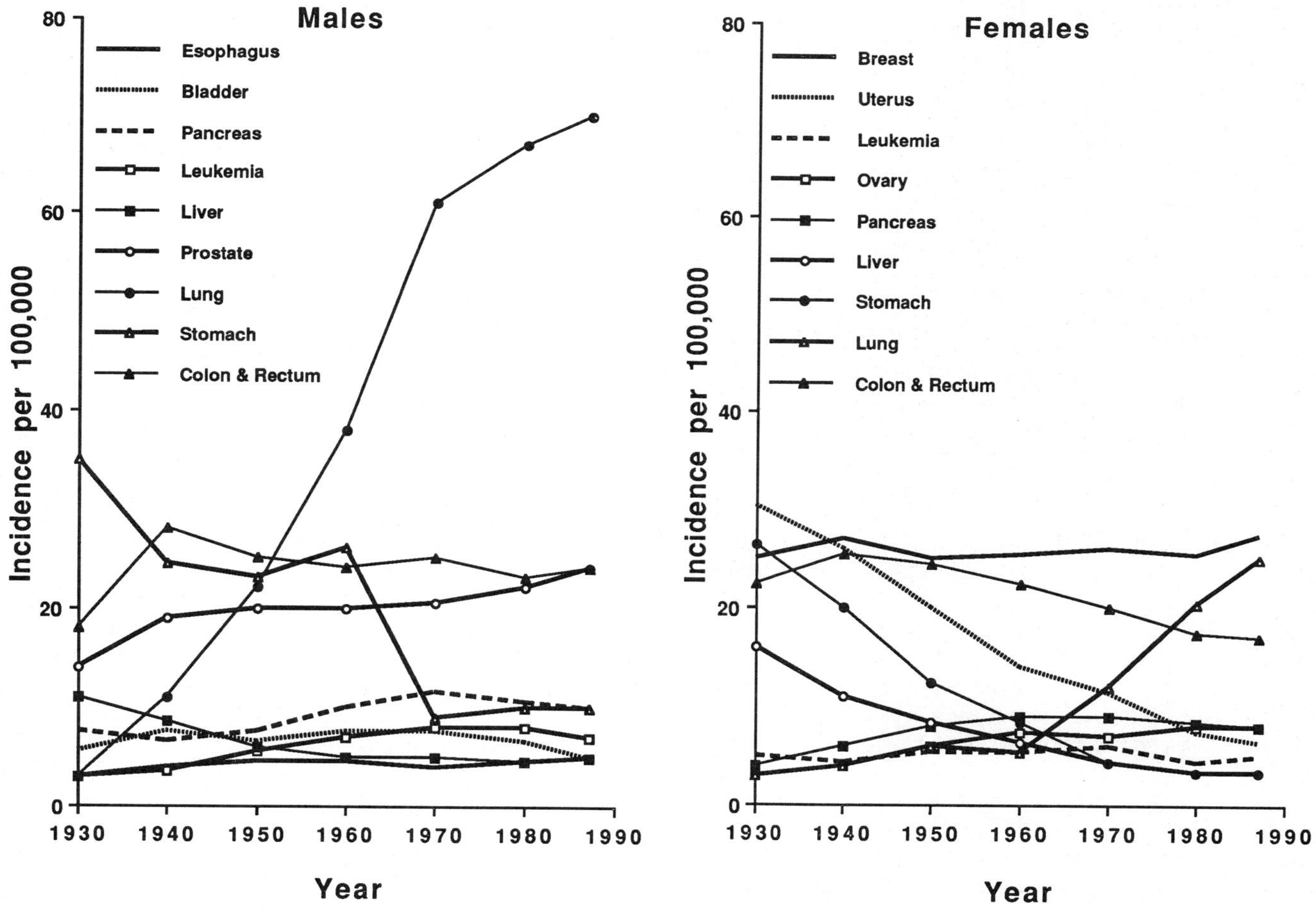

FIG. 9-3. Changing trends in the incidence of major cancers from 1930 to 1987.

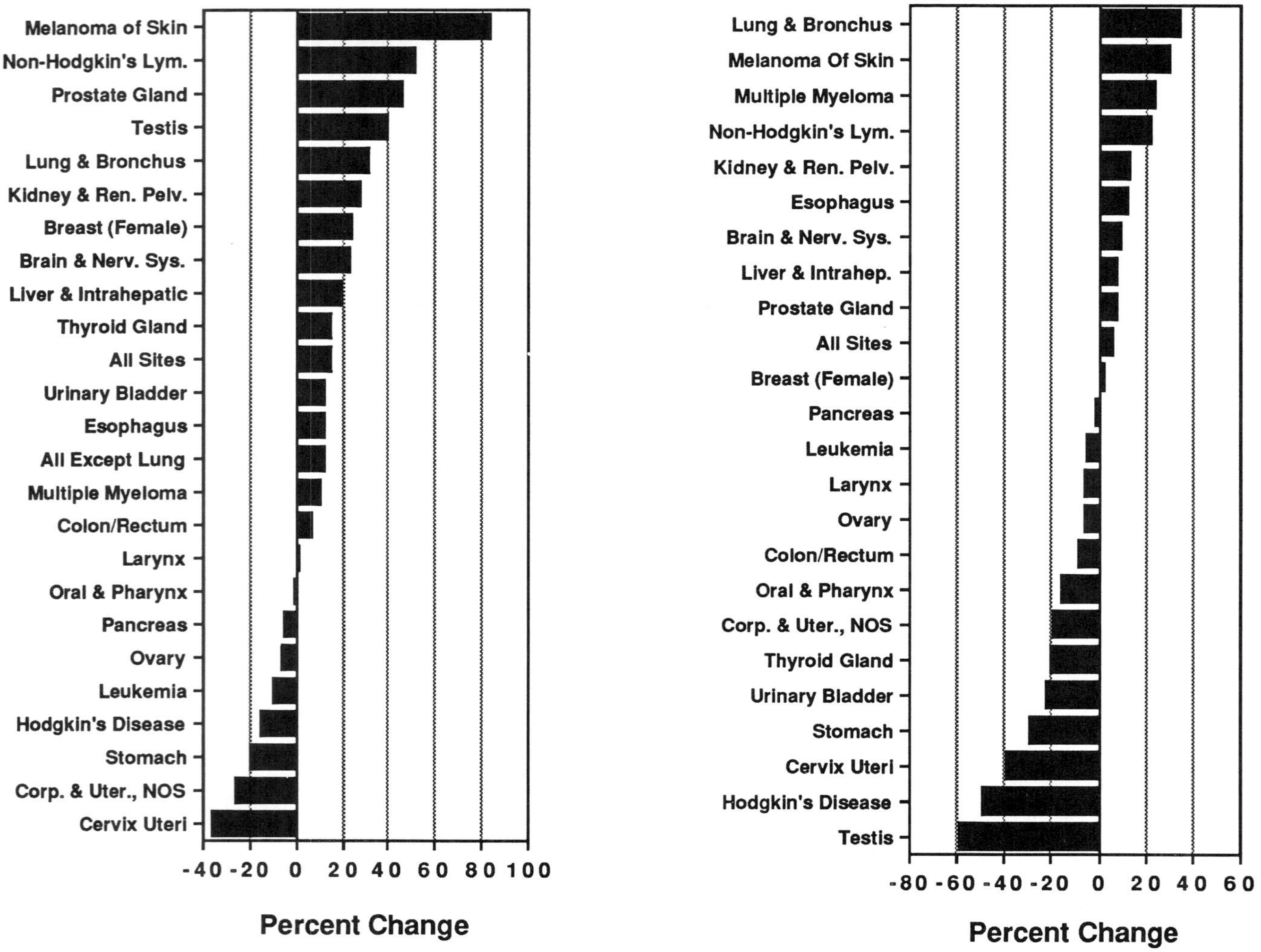

FIG. 9-4. Percent change in the incidence of cancers *(left panel)* and in mortality due to cancers *(right panel)* during the period 1973 to 1987.

to 1987, cancer mortality from testicular carcinoma and Hodgkin's disease has been reduced by 60 percent and 50 percent, respectively (see Fig. 9-4).

Because cancer continues to be a major cause of loss of life and productivity worldwide, the need to emphasize education, regular health evaluations, and screening is compelling. Emphasis on detection of premalignant lesions or early malignancies in geographic regions with a high cancer incidence may result in genetic identification of populations at high risk. The goals of investigations in tumor biology include identification of cancer causation, markers for early detection, mechanisms of cellular transformation and tumor cell growth regulation, and alterations of host-tumor immune interactions, as well as the development of novel and complementary therapeutic strategies.

Etiology

In conjunction with the epidemiologic findings, there is an intense effort under way to identify the specific agents that induce neoplastic outgrowth from normal tissue (Table 9-2). Generally neoplastic transformation is induced by an organism or mutagenic chemical, or by radiation, however, there are exceptions that are less well defined by experimental animal models. Much of our understanding of the biology of carcinogenesis is rooted in animal models and in vitro systems. The following reviews the immunobiology and molecular genetics of chemical- and virus-induced tumors.

Carcinogenesis

Physical Carcinogenesis. Tumor induction by physical agents occurs by essentially two mechanisms: (1) induction of cell proliferation over an extended period of time, which increases the opportunity for events leading to transformation, and (2) exposure to physical agents that induce damage or changes in the fidelity of DNA replication. The former has been demonstrated in experimental models, involving implantation of essentially nondegradable objects such as urethane film. Clinically, oral prostheses, orthopaedic prostheses, and, less frequently, self-induced chronic irritation have been observed to induce neoplasia in human beings. A second mechanism of physical carcinogenesis is exposure to ionizing radiations or ultraviolet light. In either setting, the result is progressive neoplasia that in animals is usually immunogenic and displays highly polymorphic tumor-associated antigens. In

Table 9-2
Agents that Induce Tumor in Human Beings

Type of Carcinogen	*Agent*	*Example*
Physical	Foreign body, ultraviolet light, gamma- and x-radiation	Asbestos, sunlight, occupational exposure
Chemical	Organics	Polycyclic hydrocarbons, fossil fuel combustion products
	Inorganics	Heavy metals, residue from smelting, fuel combustion
Viral	DNA RNA	Epstein-Barr, herpes, retroviurses

human beings, the biology of these neoplasms is forthcoming.

Foreign-Body Response. In human beings, it is difficult to attribute the induction of a neoplasm solely to the presence of a foreign body. Foreign bodies may act as cocarcinogens or promoters, or, alternatively, may produce a chronic irritation that exposes tissue to carcinogenesis by otherwise subtumorigenic doses of environmental agents. Alternatively, the foreign body-induced irritation may promote only cellular proliferation, thereby increasing the possibility for errors in DNA replication that may lead to neoplastic transformation. The increased risk for skin cancer in patients with burns or chemically induced irritations, such as that following ingestion of potassium hydroxide, provides an example of the close link between tumorigenesis and the induction of cell proliferation. Cellular accumulation and proliferation associated with chronic inflammatory conditions may contribute to the carcinogenicity of other agents or may increase the probability for genetic changes resulting in neoplastic transformation. An example may be the increased cancer risk in inflammatory bowel disease.

Response to foreign bodies often involves inflammation. This process results in the accumulation of infiltrating cells, which elaborates factors that may affect other cells in situ. Such processes are fundamental to tumors resulting from introduction of foreign, ostensibly inert, material. In some instances, removal of the foreign body results in tumor regression.

Exposure to asbestos fibers and/or dust markedly increases the risk for neoplastic disease. Among the inorganic carcinogens, asbestos is unusual in its induction of otherwise rare mesotheliomas. In addition to lung cancers, workers exposed to asebestos have increased incidences of bladder carcinoma, gastrointestinal tract neoplasms, and laryngeal and esophageal tumors. Clinical and experimental model investigations reveal that asbestos may act as a primary carcinogen or as a cocarcinogen. Thus, individuals who smoke tobacco and are exposed to asbestos fibers increase their risk beyond the sum of individual susceptibilities.

The role of multiple agents in the induction of tumors has been demonstrated in animal models. The ability to identify exposure to each agent and subsequent irritation can demonstrate the relative contribution of each. Brief exposure of animals to subcarcinogenic doses of croton oil followed by chronic (daily) abrasion with a wire brush induces tumors, many of which are fibrosarcomas. These observations strongly suggest that in the multistage process of tumorigenesis, the chronic irritation may fulfill one or more of the critical steps necessary to induce a tumor.

Ionizing Radiation. When administered in experimental animals, alpha-, gamma-, and x-radiation, as well as ultraviolet light, induce tumors. Exposure of experimental animals to gamma or x-rays results in the induction of leukemia, lymphomas, and thymomas, and, to a lesser extent, brain and visceral tumors. Ultraviolet light is biologically significant in the 280- to 320-nm (UV-B) range. UV-C (less than 280 nm) does not penetrate the ozone, and UV-A (more than 320 nm) is substantially less carcinogenic. Ultraviolet light induces skin tumors (primarily sarcomas) and occasionally squamous cell carcinomas or melanomas in rodents. The mechanism of carcinogenesis usually involves chromosomal changes, induction of DNA adducts, mutations, altered DNA methylation, and activation of oncogenes. In the presence of oncogenic viruses, whether exogenous or endogenous, radiation may accelerate tumor induction. In addition to the direct effects on the tissue that lead to transformation, radiation is a potent immunosuppressive, thereby decreasing a potentially important tumor surveillance mechanism. Both gamma- and x-rays directly and indirectly affect viability and function of lymphocytes. By contrast, ultraviolet light induces immunosuppression indirectly, possibly through release of biologically active substances from cells in the skin.

In human beings, results of exposure and dose are time related. Gamma- and x-radiation may occur in carcinogenic doses as a consequence of occupational exposure, usually with significant impact upon lymphogenesis. Resulting leukemias are progressive and lethal. Ultraviolet light from the UV-B range may be responsible for induction or promotion of a number of human skin tumors, including basal cell carcinoma, squamous cell carcinoma, and malignant melanoma, especially in fair-skinned individuals, whose skin tends to sunburn rather than suntan. Basal and squamous cell carcinomas are found with greater prevalence on sun-exposed skin of older individuals, especially those who have had a chronic exposure to sunlight, such as fishermen and construction workers. A role for UV-B light in melanoma may be in its promotion rather than its induction. All other conditions (genetic, skin pigmentation, exposure to carcinogen) met, ultraviolet light may contribute an essential step, whether it be immunosuppression, damage to skin cells such as keratinocytes and Langerhans cells, or induction of cellular changes that eventuate as tumor (Fig. 9-5). There is evidence from experimental models to support all three possibilities.

Chemical Carcinogenesis. Exposure to chemicals in the environment increases the risk for nearly all cancers. Designation of specific chemicals as carcinogens is based on two broad criteria: (1) documented induction of neoplasms in human beings or exper-

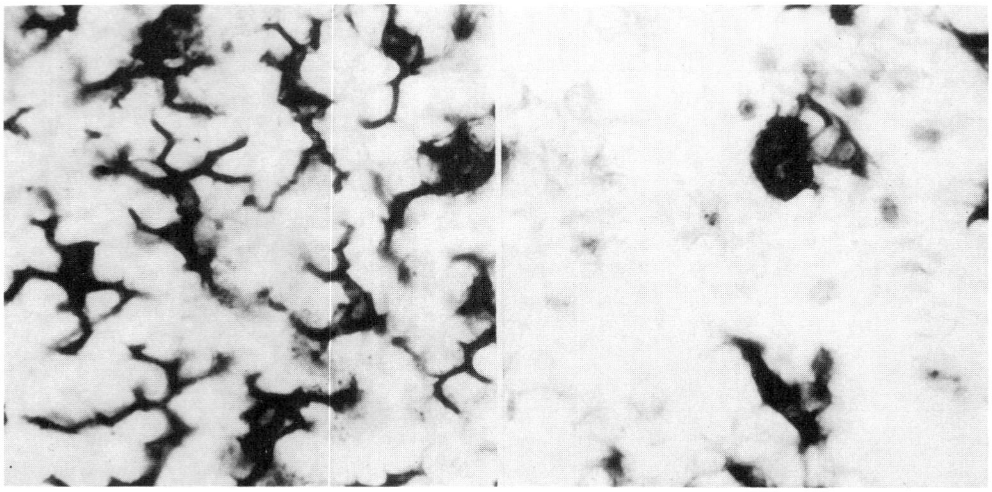

FIG. 9-5. Effect of UV-B light on Langerhans cells in human skin. This individual was exposed to one minimum erythema dose of UV-B. Twenty-four hours later punch biopsies were obtained from normal *(left panel)* and exposed skin *(right panel)*, sectioned, stained for ATPase, and compared for presence of Langerhans cells. *(Courtesy of Dr. Margaret L. Kripke.)*

imental animals and (2) evidence of mutagenic potential. Mutagenicity is an important, but possibly not a necessary, characteristic of carcinogenic chemicals. Carcinogenesis may occur as a result of external contact with, or, alternatively, ingestion or inhalation of the agent. The spectrum of responses and tumors that arise from chemical carcinogenesis is wide. Often the nature of the resulting neoplasm is determined by the route of introduction and by the tissues that accumulate the carcinogens. Chemical carcinogens may be organic or inorganic and the nature of the carcinogen has significant impact on the resultant neoplastic disease. A hallmark of chemical carcinogenesis is polymorphic tumor antigen specificity. Each tumor induced by a chemical carcinogen results in a unique immunologic specificity (Fig. 9-6).

Organic Carcinogens. Organic carcinogens, such as the polycyclic hydrocarbons and nitrosamines, induce a wide variety of neoplasms. Polycyclic hydrocarbons must undergo chemical transformation by host tissues to an ''active'' carcinogen to induce a neoplasm. Combustion products, such as benzo[a]pyrene, are believed etiologic of a variety of visceral cancers. In animals, these agents have been used to induce soft tissue and visceral tumors after relatively short exposures. In the experimental setting, the latent period (the time from exposure to the development of a tumor) for most organic carcinogens is often inversely related to carcinogen dose. The experimental tumors are immunogenic and they seldom metastasize. In human beings, many tumors arise slowly, are poorly antigenic, and occur when primaries are small, suggesting that they are the result of prolonged exposure to low doses of carcinogens.

The relation of rodent carcinogenesis to tumorigenesis in human beings has been the subject of protracted controversy. The significance of a single bolus dose of carcinogen into an otherwise healthy host probably does not reflect the natural history of most human cancers. Nevertheless, the rodent models have enabled identification of potential carcinogens, as well as elucidation of some of the basic mechanisms by which organic carcinogens induce cancer. The organic carcinogens have provided the models for investigation of the immunobiology of tumors in rodents. An interesting and challenging aspect of chemical carcinogenesis is illustrated in the highly polymorphic tumor antigen specificity demonstrated in transplantation tests (see Fig. 9-6).

Inorganic Carcinogens. Inorganic carcinogens are often heavy-metal residues from fossil fuel combustion or industrial pro-

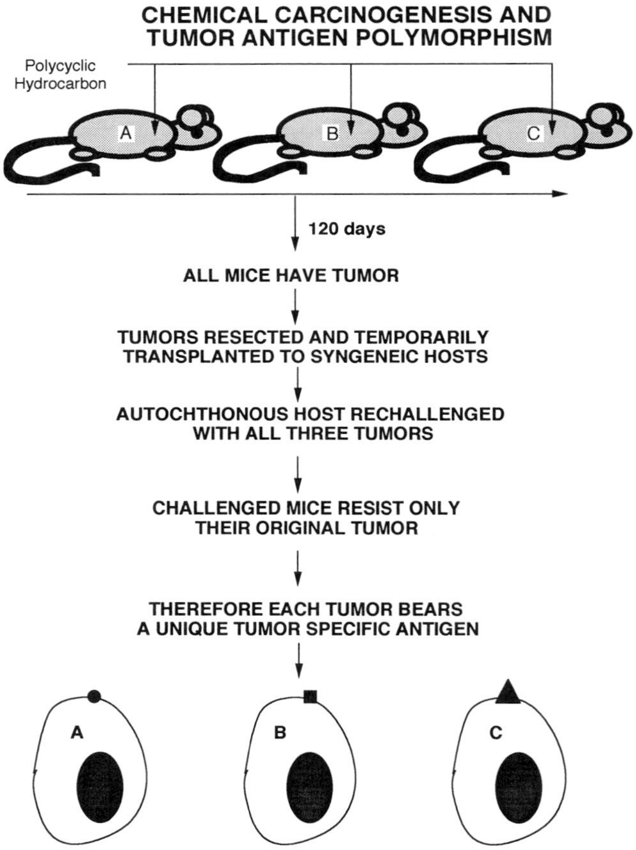

FIG. 9-6. Chemical carcinogenesis in mice. Intramuscular or subcutaneous administration of carcinogens such as 3-methylcholanthrene results in tumors in nearly all hosts within several months. Tumors are transplantable in syngeneic hosts and are subsequently used for investigations. Detailed are the immunization and challenge protocols that reveal the antigenic polymorphism of chemical carcinogenesis.

cesses such as smelting. In human beings, tumors are induced in the respiratory and urogenital systems. In human beings and rodents, compounds of nickel, cadmium, chromium, arsenic, and possibly lead induce a wide variety of neoplasms. Of the inorganic carcinogens, nickel is the most widely investigated. Insoluble forms such as sulfides and subsulfides of nickel are more carcinogenic. Exposure to the inorganic carcinogens is often occupational. Frequently the exposure is chronic and in subtoxic doses. Nickel-smelting products induce nasopharyngeal carcinomas. In rodents, administration of insoluble nickel into the subcutis results in sarcomas. Intraocular injection induces sarcomas, carcinomas, and even melanomas. Metal carcinogens induce DNA adducts and DNA-protein crosslinks that then decrease the fidelity of DNA replication. It is hypothesized that the DNA changes increase the probability for transformation.

The biologic aspects of the host-tumor relationship in tumors induced by inorganic carcinogens are unknown. Nevertheless, experimental tumors are immunogenic and in many respects indistinguishable from their histologically identical counterparts induced by organic carcinogenesis.

Viruses. Induction of tumors by infectious agents was a long-disputed concept in the early part of this century. Today it is unequivocal that both RNA and DNA viruses induce tumors in animals from amphibians to primates. It is only in recent years that this conviction has included human beings. Oncogenic RNA viruses are subdivided into acute-acting types and chronic types. Acute-acting types induce sarcomas, leukemias, and lymphoid tumors in experimental animals. Chronic types induce leukemias and mammary tumors in animals and include human T-lymphotrophic viruses. The RNA viruses and the mechanisms of transformation of cells are discussed in a subsequent section. Oncogenesis by RNA virus results in the appearance of tumor-associated antigens on the surface of tumor cells. A subset of the antigens may be shared among tumors induced by several different oncogenic viruses, whereas other tumor-associated antigens are unique to the individual oncogenic virus. All tumors induced by a single virus share the same virus-induced tumor antigens (Fig. 9-7). In addition to the cell-surface antigens, there are antigens expressed in the cytoplasm and in the nucleus.

Three groups of DNA viruses have oncogenic strains. The papova viruses, including the papilloma, polyoma, and SV40 viruses, induce tumors in animals. Two others, JC and BK, were isolated from human tumors. The second group is made up of adenoviruses, and the third comprises the herpes group. Adenoviruses were isolated from a variety of animal tumors; most of these are tumorigenic in newborn animals. An example of the herpes group is the Epstein-Barr virus (EBV), which has been implicated in the etiology of Burkitt's lymphoma and nasopharyngeal carcinoma. There is an accumulating body of evidence to suggest that DNA viruses, as well as RNA viruses, also may participate in the initiation and promotion phases of human tumorigenesis.

Evidence for EBV etiology in Burkitt's lymphoma includes the following observations:

1. Patients have higher titers of antibodies against the tumor-associated antigens and virus-determined antigens than unaffected individuals from the same family or age group.
2. Tumor cells have at least one copy of the viral DNA integrated into the host cell genome.
3. EBV transforms human cells in vitro.
4. EBV induces tumors after inoculation into subhuman primates.

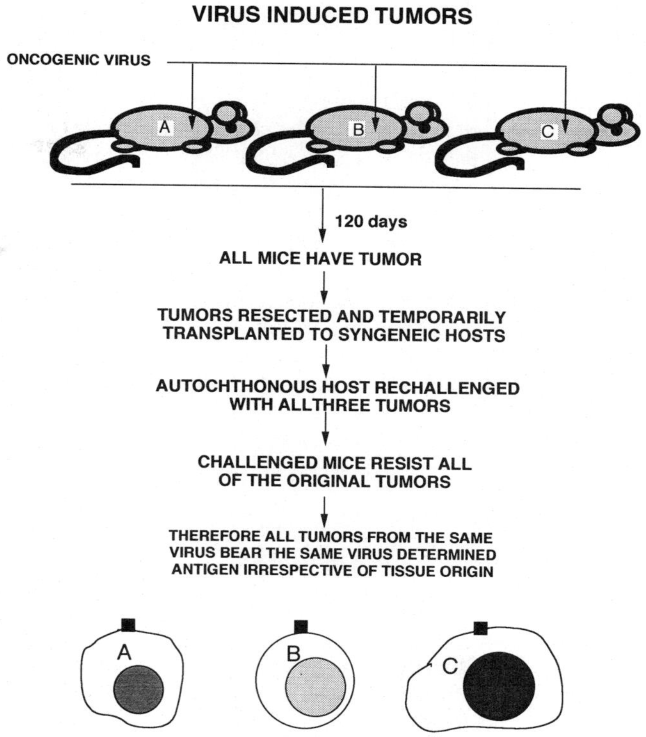

FIG. 9-7. Induction of tumors in mice with oncogenic viruses. Using a protocol similar to that in Figure 9-6 illustrates there is antigenic similarity among tumors induced by a single virus strain. DNA virus tumors display virus-specific antigenic signature while groups of RNA viruses may induce shared antigen.

The World Health Organization has indicated that previous and continued exposure to EBV results in high titers of antibody to the virus capsid antigen and a 30-fold increase in risk compared to control populations. Tumor induction does not occur by exposure to virus alone. EBV is worldwide, but the tumor incidence is restricted to Africa and New Guinea. Thus, there is a possibility for climate-related cofactors or participating organisms endemic to these regions. These factors no doubt are superimposed on a background of some unknown host genetic factors.

Herpes simplex virus-2 (HSV-2) is the etiologic agent of genital herpes. Infected women with early sexual activity and a large number of sexual partners have significantly increased risk for cervical carcinoma. Women with invasive carcinoma have antibodies to HSV-2, and about 40 percent of cervical biopsies with severe dysplasia or carcinoma display HSV-2-specific DNA-binding protein. A similar relationship has been established for human papova virus (HPV). The DNA of HPV16 and HPV18 have been demonstrated in cervical carcinoma biopsies. Indeed, factors in addition to mere infection with HSV-2 or HPV are necessary to result in transformation and tumorigenesis.

Immunodeficiency. The role of the immune system in the prevention of neoplastic disease has been the subject of extensive debate. Clinical observations and results from animal models are inconsistent. Immunodeficient individuals or immunosuppressed transplant recipients are at greater risk for neoplastic disease, frequently tumors of the lymphoreticular system. Only selected nonlymphoid tissues exhibit increased incidence of neoplasia.

In experiments with carcinogen-induced murine models, loss of T lymphocytes does not significantly affect carcinogenesis but does diminish host response to transplantable tumors. Analysis of the immune cellular participants in the surveillance against neoplastic progression reveals that in the normal host, several lymphoid cell compartments participate in the prevention of, and destruction of, aberrant cells. Proposed mechanisms include T, B, and NK lymphocytes as well as macrophages cytotoxic to transformed cells. Unlike chemical carcinogenesis, compromising cellular immunity significantly increases animal susceptibility to viral oncogenesis. Thus, the precise role of host immunity in tumor surveillance, whether in human beings or in animals, is yet to be elucidated. Present evidence suggests that the immune system is important in preventing the clinical emergence of cancer and that specific components of host immunity may be activated in the treatment of residual disease after surgery.

BIOLOGY OF NEOPLASTIC DISEASE

Cell Biology of Transformation

Histology of Abnormal Cell Growth. Neoplastic cells proliferate more rapidly than adjacent normal tissue and fail to respond to signals that regulate the rate of cell division. This proliferation results in an abnormal mass—a *tumor*, or *neoplasm*. Malignant status is determined by the clinical behavior of a neoplasm, and not exclusively by the presence of abnormal growth. Malignancy is characterized by uncontrollable growth and/or dissemination. *Cancer* is a general term used to describe malignant neoplasia with a substantial probability for local recurrence and/or dissemination to organ systems, thus resulting in death. The progression of the cell to frank malignancy is histologically characterized in a series of "plasias" (Fig. 9-8).

Hyperplasia is an increase in cell number demonstrable in both normal and neoplastic tissues. Rapid basal growth rates are normal for bone marrow, intestinal crypt epithelium, and skin. Following injury, the local growth rate increases over baseline in the normal response of wound healing. As wound closure is achieved cell division returns to that of the adjacent tissue. Liver regeneration after hepatic injury or hepatectomy induces a dramatic hyperplastic response manifest as increased cell numbers and size, and a hypertrophy of the tissue. Colonic hyperplastic polyps are frequently observed, and appear to be potential precancers in the evolution of colonic malignancy. In breast ductal epithelium, florid, but not mild, hyperplasia is associated with a 1.5- to 2-fold increased risk of subsequent breast carcinoma (see Fig. 9-8).

Metaplasia is reversible transformation of one mature cell type to another, such as when the replacing mature cell type is present in tissue or in areas of tissue where it is not normally found. The possible basis of this poorly understood transformation may be a redirection of stem cell differentiation or, alternatively, the dedifferentiation of fully mature differentiated cells. The most extensively investigated is the epithelial metaplasia secondary to chronic inflammation. In chronic gastroesophageal reflux, the normal distal esophageal squamous cell mucosa exhibits metaplasia to a "gastric-type" columnar epithelium.

Dysplasia describes epithelial tissues containing altered cell size, shape, and organization. Stratification of dysplasia as mild, moderate, or severe is based on the degree of cellular dedifferentiation. Although frequently the cause of dysplasia is unknown, it is presumed secondary to chronic inflammation or exposure to environmental toxins or irritants. The gastrointestinal tract, respiratory tree, urinary bladder, cervix, vagina, breast, and skin all have foci of dysplasia. Morphologically, nuclear polymorphism and hyperchromatism are present, often accompanied by total loss of cellular and epithelial polarity. Mitoses are more frequent in the afflicted areas than in the surrounding normal epithelium. There is no penetration of abnormal cells through the epithelial basement membrane (see Fig. 9-8). Carcinoma in situ demonstrates all of these changes. Despite the association of dysplasia with synchronous or metachronous invasive carcinoma, not all dysplastic tissue progresses to carcinoma. Many tissues may demonstrate a "field effect," with multiple, patchy areas of dysplasia. In some tissues the extent of dysplasia is subject to hormonal control. Thus, clinicians advocate close visual, radiologic, and endoscopic surveillance, and consideration of prophylactic resection of all tissue at risk.

Gompertzian Progression. Biologic growth occurs according to a mathematical relationship with time. In the early stages growth is clearly exponential, with a high growth fraction and very short volume doubling times (Fig. 9-9). As time passes, the doubling time lengthens and the growth fraction decreases. The general slope of this curve can therefore be expressed mathematically as an exponentially decreasing function. The specific equation describing this relationship was originally derived by the eighteenth century mathematician Gompertz; thus, biologic growth that conforms to this pattern is referred to as *gompertzian growth*. Evidence that not only normal cell growth but neoplastic cell growth follows a gompertzian pattern is increasing. Many different animal tumors conform to a gompertzian growth curve, and human myelomas follow a gompertzian growth pattern as well. The duration of a neoplastic disease and its relationship to current detection methods is exemplified in the progression of mammary tumors (Fig. 9-10), which undergo numerous changes and persist in the environment of host regulatory mechanisms for many years before becoming clinically apparent.

Angiogenesis. Propagation of the tumor mass requires neovascularization. Much of our understanding of this process emerges from the work of Folkman, who in pioneering the investigation of tumor angiogenesis determined that the production of angiogenesis factors stimulates endothelial cells to form new vessels. Endothelial cells in the vicinity or angiogenic stimuli undertake several different morphologies based on their distance from the originating vessel. In response to angiogenic induction, endothelial cells migrate, propagate, and mature as their leading front approaches the tumor zone (Fig. 9-11).

Progression to malignancy disturbs host homeostatic mechanisms, as characterized by (1) unresponsiveness to normal growth regulators, (2) invasive phenotype, and (3) evasion of immune-mediated tumor destruction. Our understanding of these changes relies on the advances in basic research of the molecular biology of tumor initiation, progression, and metastasis.

Molecular Biology and Oncogenes

Oncogenesis occurs in three distinct stages: (1) initiation, (2) promotion, and (3) progression. In each stage occur a series of changes in molecular mechanisms (growth factors and their receptors, signal transduction molecules, oncogenes, and "antioncogenes") governing normal cellular differentiation and growth. Accumulation of a critical number of perturbations in the regulatory circuit results in malignant transformation.

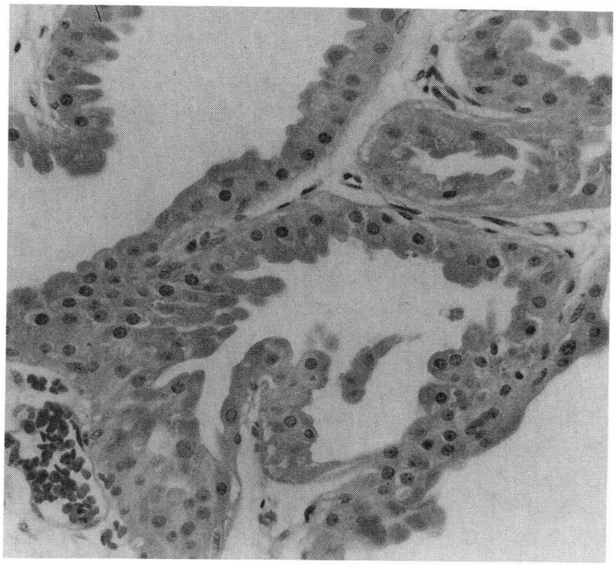

A

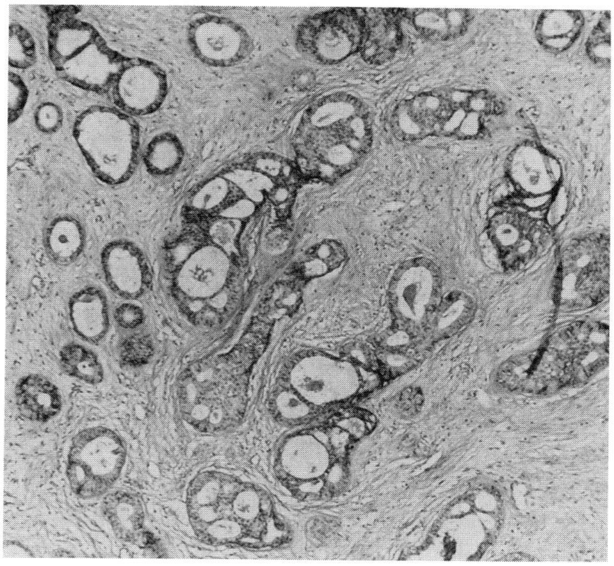

B

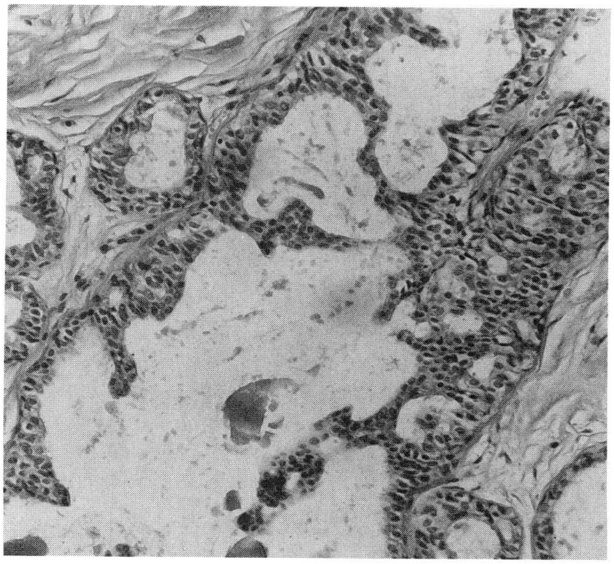

C

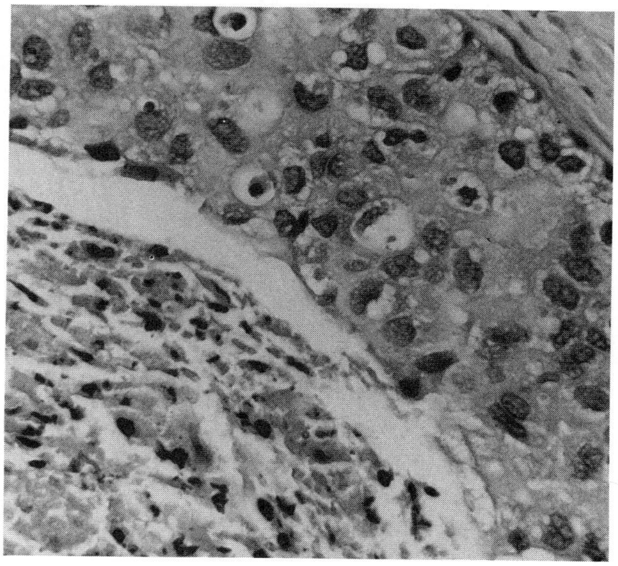

D

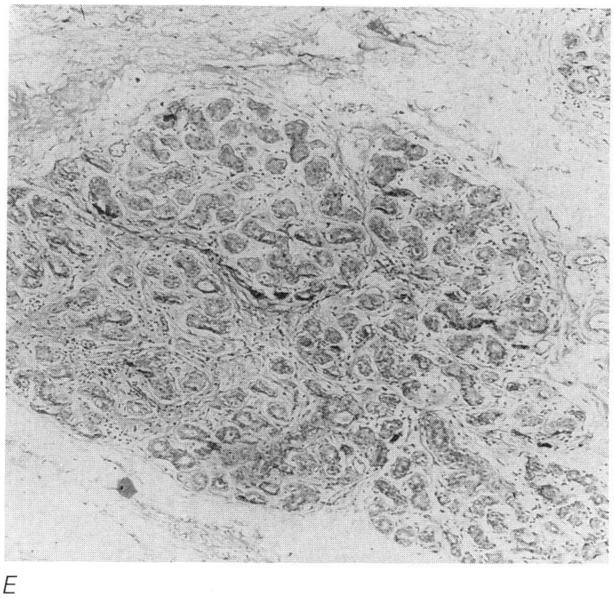

E

FIG. 9-8. Spectrum of "plasias" in breast ductal epithelium. *A.* Normal ductal epithelium displaying a single layer of cuboidal cells. *B.* Apocrine metaplasia, in which cuboidal cells are replaced by eosinophilic columnar cells (increased magnification). *C.* Mild hyperplasia characterized by three or four layers of cuboidal cells with uniform nuclei. *D.* Dysplasia or atypical hyperplasia, with more than one cell layer, nuclei of more than one size, and frank chromasia, and a cribriform pattern. *E.* Neoplasia displaying a ductal carcinoma in situ (DCIS), with intraductal calcifications and cellular replacement of the ductal lumen. *(Courtesy of Dr. Nour Sneige, M.D. Anderson Cancer Center.)*

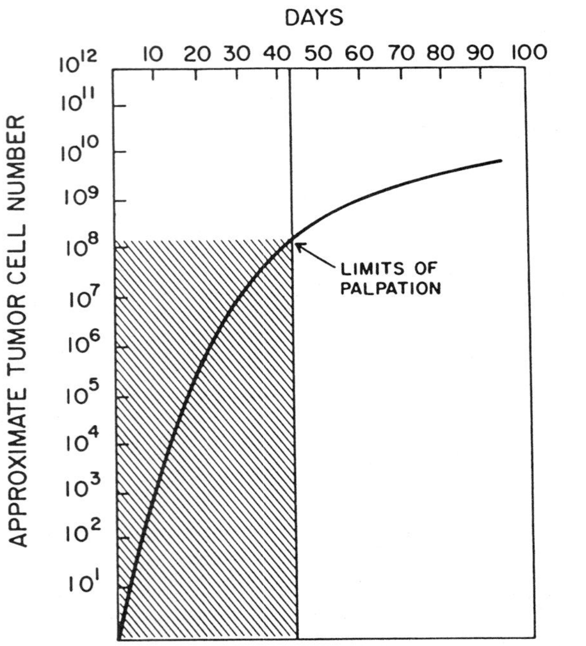

RELATIVE GROWTH RATE	RAPID	SLOW
TUMOR SIZE	MICROSCOPIC	MACROSCOPIC
CLINICALLY DETECTABLE	NO	YES
DRUG AND RADIATION THERAPY	MORE SENSITIVE	LESS SENSITIVE
SURGICAL TREATMENT	NO	YES

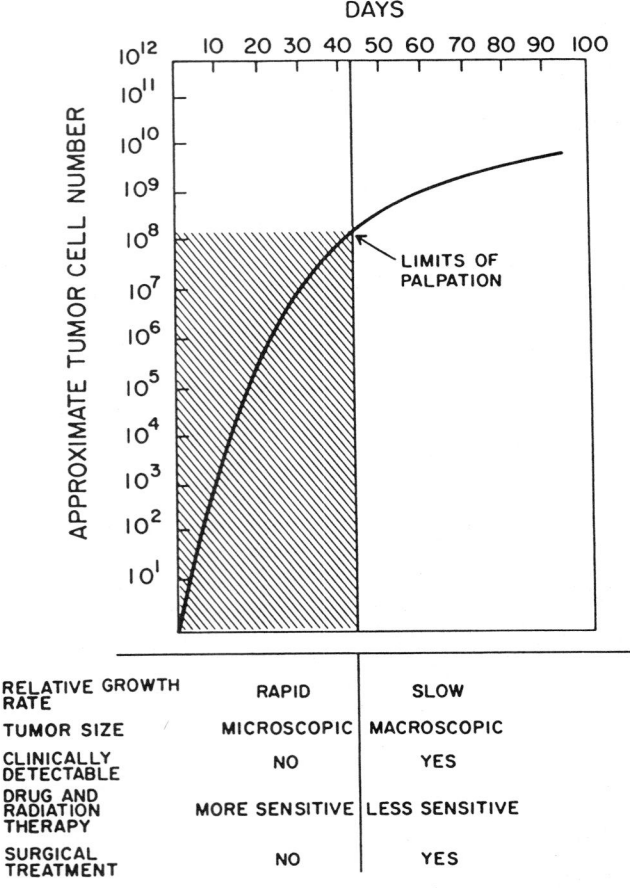

FIG. 9-9. Tumor growth-curve–based propagation of a chemically induced tumor in mice. The gompertzian mathematical relationship illustrates that tumor cells grow exponentially at a rate that is simultaneously decreasing exponentially with time. The limit of palpation is 1 mm diameter in mice or 10^8 cells. This limit may be an order of magnitude higher in human breast cancer. *(Adapted from Skipper, 1971.)*

Tumor Viruses. The discovery of tumor viruses, postulated more than 25 years ago, set the stage for elucidation of retroviral oncogenes. Molecular analysis of viral oncogenesis laid the foundation for establishing the relationship of oncogenes to tumorigenesis and the role of specific genes in neoplastic transformation. Viruses are packaged genetic information, either in the form of DNA or RNA, protected by a structural protein coat. In nonlytic infections, viruses may insert their genetic material into host cells and induce changes morphologically consistent with neoplastic transformation (Fig. 9-12).

There are six families of DNA tumor viruses. Virus DNA is either replicated epigenetically or incorporated into the host cell genome and subsequently replicated. Among DNA viruses, hepatitis B virus is strongly associated with the development of hepatocellular carcinoma, and more than 80 percent of cervical carcinomas evidence papilloma virus infection. Tumor-inducing RNA viruses are retroviruses that introduce a DNA copy into the host genome. Evidence that RNA retroviruses induce human tumors is provided in only a few instances, while in rodent leukemias and adenocarcinomas and in avian leukemias and sarcomas there is a substantial body of evidence supporting retroviral etiology in cancer.

The molecular basis of oncogenesis by DNA viruses has been difficult to elucidate, largely because of the involvement of viral genes in the expression and replication of viral DNA without integration into the host genome. Second, many DNA viruses lyse the host cell, causing release of the progeny virus. In vitro models of SV40 and polyoma virus indicate that DNA viruses may regulate host cell transcription and create a state of continued proliferation without completion of the normal lytic cycle.

RNA retroviruses were first isolated in 1911 from chicken sarcoma by Rous. Their discovery provided the foundation for research and led to our present understanding of oncogenes and their precursors, proto-oncogenes. After infection, the retroviral RNA is transcribed into a double-stranded DNA by the viral enzyme reverse transcriptase. Retroviral DNA is then integrated into the host chromosomal DNA, forming a DNA provirus. The viral DNA

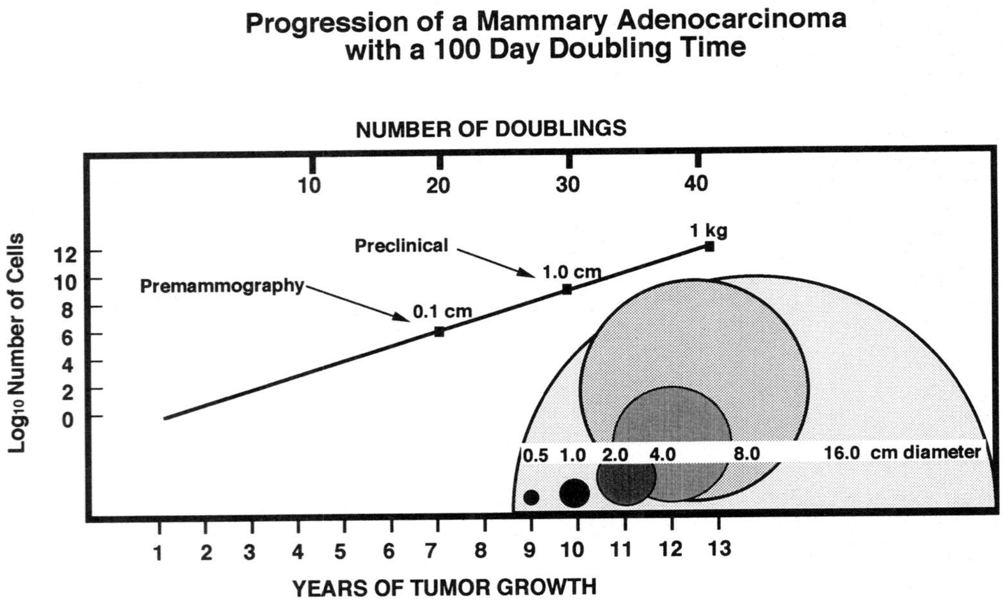

FIG. 9-10. Proposed progression of mammary cancer in human beings using some aspects of the gompertzian relationship.

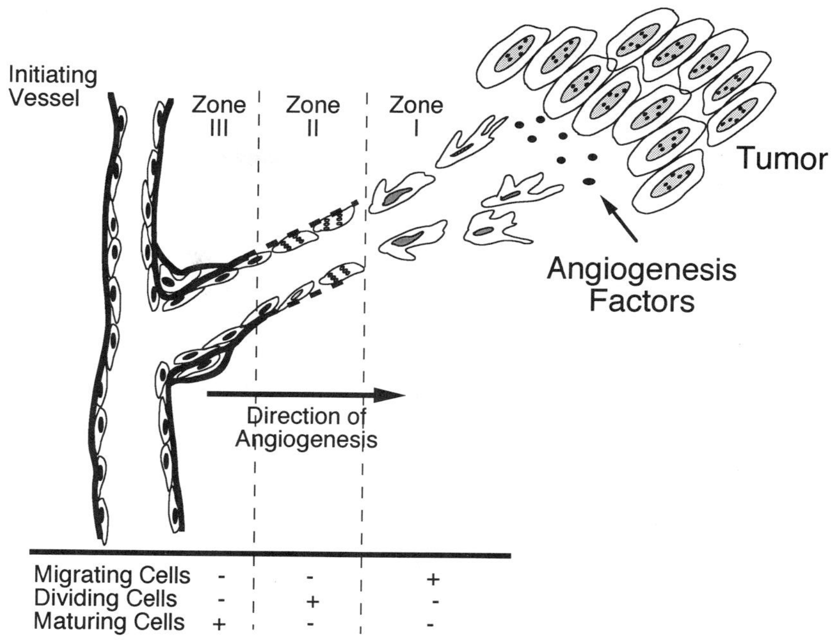

FIG. 9-11. Model of neovascularization as it occurs in the vicinity of a progressing neoplasm. Endothelial cells respond to angiogenic factors, some of which may originate at the tumor, by forming a new vessel from a nearby "parent" vessel. The leading edge zone I has a number of migrating endothelial cells, while the next level is composed of proliferating cells. In zone III, the cells nearest the initiating vessel are maturing and morphologically resemble vascular endothelium. *(Adapted from Folkman, 1984.)*

is transcribed by host cell RNA polymerase into RNA copies of the viral genome and mRNA. The mRNA is then translated into proteins for assembly of viral progeny. New virus particles are then released by budding from the plasma membrane without cell lysis or death.

Oncogenic retroviruses neoplastically transform cells in vitro and induce tumors in animals. Rous sarcoma virus contains the *src* gene, which encodes a membrane-associated enzyme responsible for phosphorylation of cellular proteins. Oncogenic retroviruses have at least one gene not involved in viral replication but that participates in transformation. The oncogenes are designated by three-letter names often related to the tumors induced or the source cell line. The products of oncogenes differ in their cellular location, function, and proposed mechanism for transformation. In all retroviruses, the oncogenes are an integral part of the viral genome, not involved in replication, but essential for the malignant potential of the virus.

Viral Oncogenes. Retroviral oncogenes originate from normal cell genes called *proto-oncogenes*. The genes are incorporated or transduced into the viral genome during recombination events between the virus and host DNA. During this transduction process, the normal genes may undergo rearrangement or mutation. Oncogenes isolated from viruses are designated with the letter "v" (e.g., v-*src*), and when isolated from the host DNA bear the letter "c" (e.g., c-*fos*).

Identification of cellular oncogenes by gene transfer experiments advanced our understanding of the molecular basis of cancer. DNA isolated from human tumors and transferred to recipient cells induced transformation. The cellular oncogenes were identified as forms of the normal proto-oncogenes altered by point mutations or DNA rearrangements. Additionally, some cellular oncogenes are homologous to the viral oncogenes found in retroviruses. For example, v-*mos* and c-*mos* sequences differ at only 25 positions out of 1157 nucleotides, and the corresponding proteins differ by only 11 amino acids.

Oncogenes in Human Neoplasms. There is increasing support for the hypothesis that human tumors arise consequent to cellular oncogene activation. Normally, many proto-oncogenes are expressed during periods of proliferation, development, and differentiation, suggesting their key regulatory role in growth. Abnormal proto-oncogene expression, function, or activation may induce the deregulated proliferation and dedifferentiation characteristic of the neoplastic state.

Members of the gene family designated "*ras*" are frequently activated oncogenes in solid human tumors. *Ras*-gene products are plasma membrane proteins capable of binding GTP. These G-binding proteins are involved in intracellular signal transduction. Point mutations resulting in single amino acid substitutions in the *ras*-protein change a normal protein into one with transforming activity.

Oncogene activation may be manifest as a chromosomal translocation. A well-known example is the Philadelphia chromosome of chronic myelogenous leukemia. The proto-oncogene c-*abl* is translocated from chromosome 9 to the *bcr* locus on chromosome 22. Transcription of the new *bcr*/*abl* locus results in the formation of a fusion protein with enhanced tyrosine kinase activity and transforming capabilities (Fig. 9-13). Burkitt's lymphoma is characterized by the translocation of c-*myc* from chromosome 8 to chromosome 2, 14, or 22. It becomes positioned near highly transcribed genes involved in immunoglobulin production, resulting in a deregulation of c-*myc* expression.

Changes in Gene Expression. In other tumors, an oncogene may be amplified based on an increased number of gene copies per cell, which in turn results in an increased level of gene expression. Amplification of N-*myc* has been found to correlate with prognosis in patients with neuroblastoma. Patients with N-*myc* amplification, even in early stages, had much more aggressive tumors. Clinically, the result was a higher incidence of tumor recurrence, progression, and resistance to chemotherapy. These are examples of what future analyses on other tumors may pro-

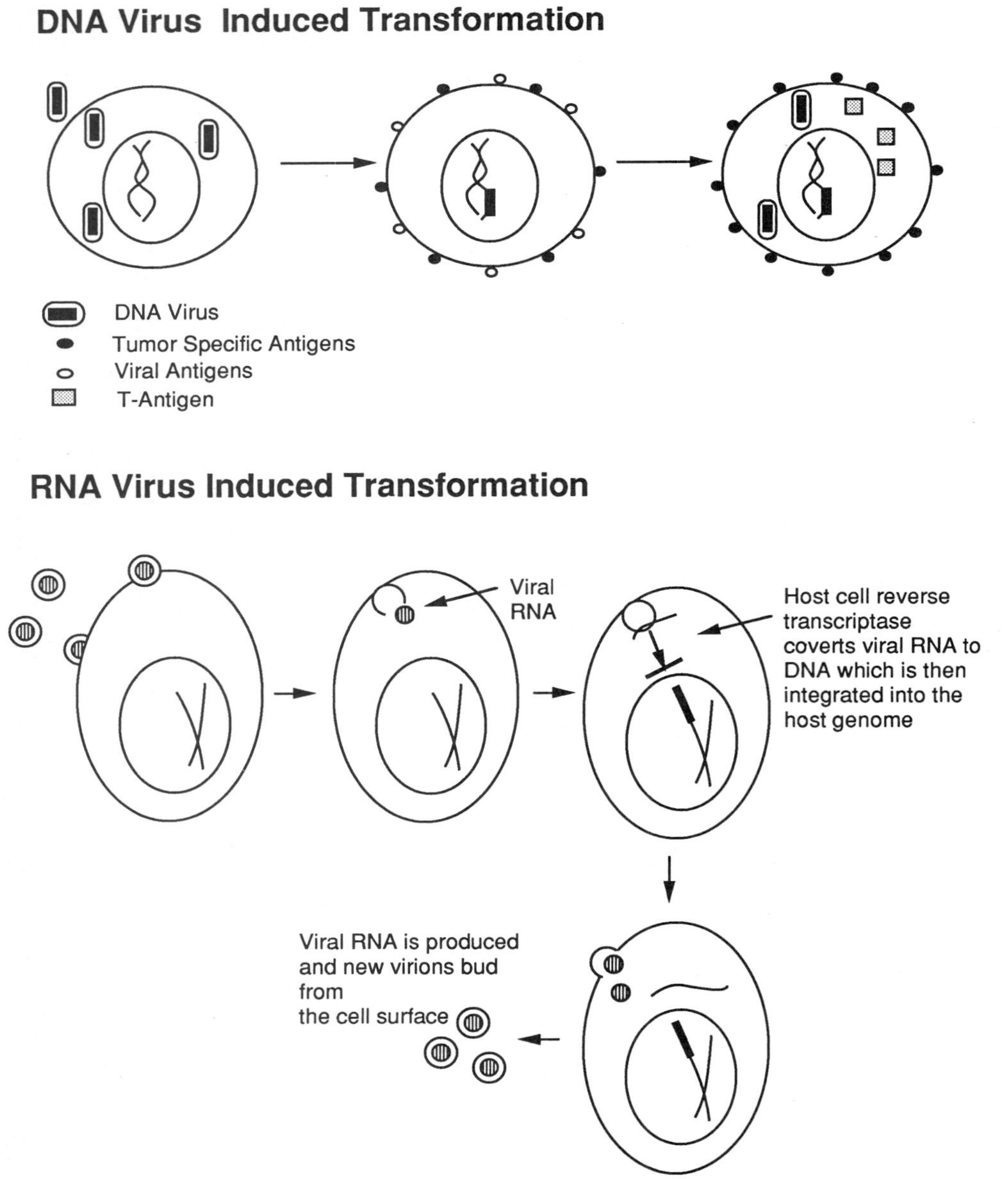

FIG. 9-12. Transformation of cells by oncogenic DNA viruses and RNA retroviruses.

vide. A partial list of oncogenes and their mechanisms of activation is provided in Table 9-3.

Investigation of inherited tumors suggests a loss of specific chromosomal regions may play a permissive role in the development of a neoplasia. Usually the losses involve only one of the two parental chromosomes present in normal cells where the lost genes encode potential growth inhibitory signals. The tumor-suppressor genes, or *antioncogenes*, are often described as acting "recessively" at the cellular level. This refers to the ability of the cell to maintain the normal phenotype in the presence of one normal parental gene or wild-type allele. A second genetic event or mutation in the normal allele results in transformation to the cancerous phenotype. Table 9-4 lists several tumor-suppressor genes or chromosomal losses found in human neoplasms.

Classification of Oncogenes. Despite the ever-increasing number of oncogenes identified, many of these genes are classified according to the function of their protein products. The groupings are based on the action of the oncogene protein in the membrane, cytoplasm, or nucleus. For example, the gene products may function as abnormal growth-stimulating factors in the extracellular compartment or as abnormal growth-factor receptors (GFR) on the cell surface. Alternatively, the oncogenes may control levels of critical second messengers in various signal-transduction pathways. The oncogenes also act within the nucleus as regulators of transcription. Table 9-5 lists some of the known oncogenes, classified according to presumed action and associated neoplasms.

Growth Factors and Receptors. One of the most intriguing aspects emerging from oncogene research is the relationship between oncogenes, peptide growth factors, and their receptors. The first correlation between an oncogene and a normal cellular protein was demonstrated when the amino acid sequence of

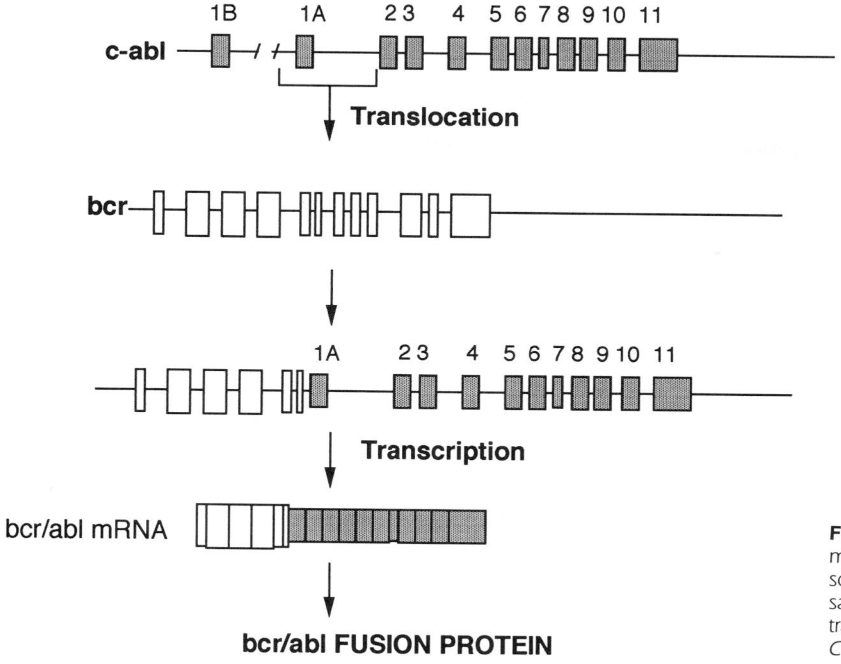

FIG. 9-13. Activation of *c-abl* by translocation into the middle of the *bcr* promoter. Following translocation transcription proceeds through *abl,* resulting in a fused message containing all but the 1A exon. The message is then translated into a *bcr/abl* fusion protein. *(Adapted from Cooper, 1990.)*

the *sis* oncogene product displayed significant homology to the beta chain of platelet-derived growth factor (PDGF), a major growth factor isolated from platelets, used by fibroblasts in culture, and presumed to support the growth of several mesenchymal tissues. The suggestion is that transformation results from the production of extracellular mitogenic peptides, and is the basis of the autocrine stimulation model. In the autocrine model, the cell produces a growth factor to which it responds by cell proliferation (Fig. 9-14).

The oncogenes *int*-2, *hst*, and *fgf*-5 encode proteins related to fibroblastic growth factor (FGF). Growth factors implicated in transformation are listed in Table 9-6. Autocrine stimulation by growth factors is dependent on the presence of GFR on the cell surface. In some neoplasms, oncogenes may be responsible for altered GFR expression. An increase in the numbers of receptors may have a similar effect as an increase in levels of the growth factor. Indeed, tumors with extremely high numbers of receptors for epidermal growth factor (EGF) have been described in head and neck squamous cell carcinomas, colon tumors, and breast cancers. In breast cancer, EGF receptor status has been correlated with early recurrence and a decrease in disease-free survival.

GFR consist of three distinct domains: (1) an amino-terminal, extracellular, ligand-binding domain, (2) a hydrophobic transmembrane domain, and (3) a tyrosine kinase carboxyl-terminus on the cytoplasmic side of the membrane. The tyrosine kinase domain phosphorylates groups of proteins that act as important second messengers (Fig. 9-15).

The ligand-binding domain is deleted in the *erb* B oncogene (EGFB-like) product (Fig. 9-16). The truncated receptor is constitutively active and is able to generate a mitogenic signal in the absence of EGF binding.

Several other receptors encoded by oncogenes (*kit, ros, met, ret,* and *trk*) demonstrate deletions of the ligand-binding domains. Thus, oncogenes encode proteins that may function in an autocrine manner to stimulate cell proliferation. Oncogenes may also result in the expression of altered GFR with abnormal signal transduction

Table 9-3
Human Neoplasms and Associated Oncogene Activation

Neoplasm	*Oncogene*	*Activation Mechanism*
Chronic myelogenous leukemia	*abl*	Translocation
Acute lymphocytic leukemia		
Follicular B-cell lymphoma	*bcl*-2	Translocation
Breast and ovarian carcinoma	*erb*B-2	Amplification
Burkitt's lymphoma	c-*myc*	Translocation
Breast and lung carcinoma		Amplification
Lung carcinoma	L-*myc*	Amplification
Neuroblastoma	N-*myc*	Amplification
Lung carcinoma		Amplification
Colon and pancreatic carcinoma	K-*ras*	Point mutation
Acute myeloid and lymphoid leukemias	N-*ras*	Point mutation

Table 9-4
Tumor Suppressor Gene Loss in Human Cancers

Tumor Suppressor Gene or Chromosome	*Neoplasm*
Chromosome 1	Neuroblastoma
Chromosome 3	Lung and renal cell carcinoma
Chromosome 5	Colon carcinoma
Chromosome 11	Wilms' tumor, hepatoblastoma, adrenal carcinoma, rhabdomyosarcoma, bladder, and breast carcinoma
Chromosome 13 (Rb)	Retinoblastoma, osteosarcoma, breast, bladder, and small cell lung carcinoma
Chromosome 17 (p53)	Lung and colon carcinoma
Chromosome 18	Colon carcinoma
Chromosome 22	Acoustic neuroma, meningioma

SOURCE: Adapted from *Cooper GM: Oncogenes. Boston, Jones & Bartlett, 1990.*

activity. Growth factors may also exert effects through the activation of certain proto-oncogenes.

Second Messengers. Most oncogenes encode proteins associated with the inner surface of the cell membrane and transmit signals from GFR on the cell surface to cytoplasmic messengers signaling cell proliferation. The *src* and *ras* families of oncogenes are representative proteins involved in signal transduction. The *src* family has tyrosine kinase activity, while the *ras* proteins bind guanine nucleotides (GDP and GTP). Phosphorylation of tyrosine residues is a key regulatory mechanism in enzyme activity. Tyrosine kinases include members of the *src* family, *abl* and *fps* oncogenes. The physiologic stimuli responsible for activation of the nonreceptor kinases are not clearly defined yet. Thus their roles in signal transduction pathways are not as well described as those of the receptor kinases. There is evidence, however, that control of nonreceptor tyrosine kinase activity plays a key role in multiple cellular processes involving cellular metabolism, cytoskeletal integrity, and cellular proliferation.

Tyrosine kinases, such as the *src* protein, may themselves be regulated by phosphorylation. The activity of the *src* gene product, pp60c-*src* (a 60-kD phosphoprotein), is elevated in colon adeno-

Table 9-5
Categories of Oncogenes and Their Associated Neoplasms

Oncogene Product	*Oncogene*	*Normal Homologue*	*Neoplasm*
Growth factors	*sis*	PDGF	
	int-2	PGF	Breast carcinoma
Transmembrane growth factor receptors	*erb*B	EGF receptor	
	neu		Breast carcinoma
	fms	M-CSF receptor	
	ros, *kit*		
Membrane-associated tyrosine kinases	*abl*		Chronic myelogenous leukemia, acute lymphocytic leukemia, acute myelogenous leukemia
	src		
	fcs, *fps*		
Membrane-associated guanine nucleotide binding proteins	K-, N-, and H-*ras*		Colorectal, lung, prostate carcinoma
Cytoplasmic serine-threonine kinases	*raf*/*mil*		
	mos		
Cytoplasmic hormone receptors	*erb*A	Thyroid hormone receptor	
Nuclear factors	c-*myc*		Burkitt's lymphoma
	N-*myc*		Neuroblastoma
	L-*myc*		Small cell lung carcinoma
	N-*myc fos*		
	jun		
	myb, *ets*, *ski*		
Antioncogenes	Rb		Retinoblastoma
Others	*bcl*-2		Non-Hodgkin's lymphomas
	bcl-1		
	int-1		Breast carcinoma

PDGF, platelet-derived growth factor; FGF, fibroblast growth factor; EGF, epidermal growth factor; and M-CSF, mononuclear cell colony-stimulating factor.

SOURCE: Adapted from *Ducker BJ, Mamon HV, Roberts U: Oncogenes. Growth factors and signal transduction.* N Engl J Med *321:1383, 1989.*

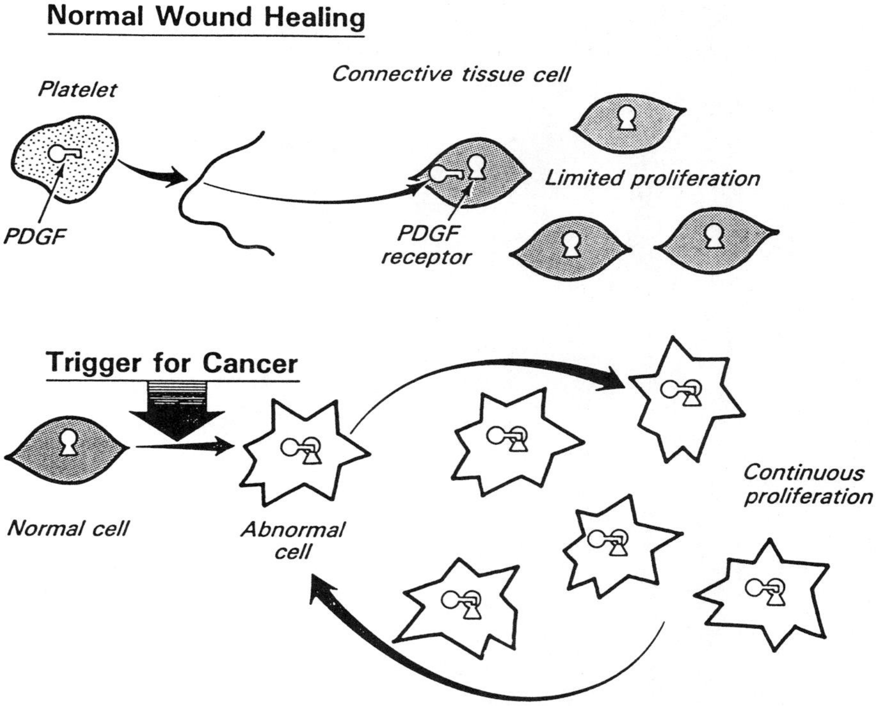

FIG. 9-14. The *sis* oncogene is similar to the gene that produces PDGF. During the normal wound-healing process PDGF induces limited proliferation of connective tissue as a part of the repair process. Transformation induces alteration in the expression of this gene, resulting in continuous proliferation. (From: *DeVita VT, Hellman S, Rosenberg SA (eds): Important Advances in Oncology. Philadelphia, JB Lippincott, 1985, with permission.*)

Table 9-6
Growth Factors Involved in Transformation

Growth Factor	*Source*	*Target Tissue*	*Biologic Activity*
Insulin Family			
Insulin	Beta-islet cells of pancreas	Liver, adipose, muscle	Supports growth, modulates metabolism of lipids, amino acids, and sugars
IGF-1 and IGF-11	Human plasma	Liver, adipose, muscle, cartilage, fibroblasts	Insulin-like metabolic effects; mitogens; stimulate incorporation of sulfate into cartilage proteoglycans
EGF Family			
EGF	Mouse submaxillary gland, human urine	Epidermal cells, fibroblasts, epithelial cells	Mitogen, promotes keratinization, inhibits gastric acid secretion
TGF-alpha	Transformed cells	Identical to EGF	Identical to EGF
PDGF Family			
Dimers of A and B chains	Alpha-granules, platelets	Fibroblasts, smooth muscle cells, glial cells	Supports growth of various mesenchymal cells, chemotactic agent
TGF-Beta Family			
TGF-beta-1 and -2	Alpha-granules, platelets	All cell types	Often inhibits growth, augments matrix accumulation, chemotactic
MIS	Testis	Mullerian duct	Inhibits growth of cells derived from the mullerian duct
FGF Family			
alpha-FGF beta-FGF	Brain Pituitary	All cell types	Mitogenic for cells of mesodermal and neuroectodermal origin
Bombesin Family			
Bombesin Gastrin-releasing peptide	Frog skin Porcine gut	Many epithelial and mesenchymal cells	Mitogenic for gastrointestinal, respiratory tract, and 3T3 cells

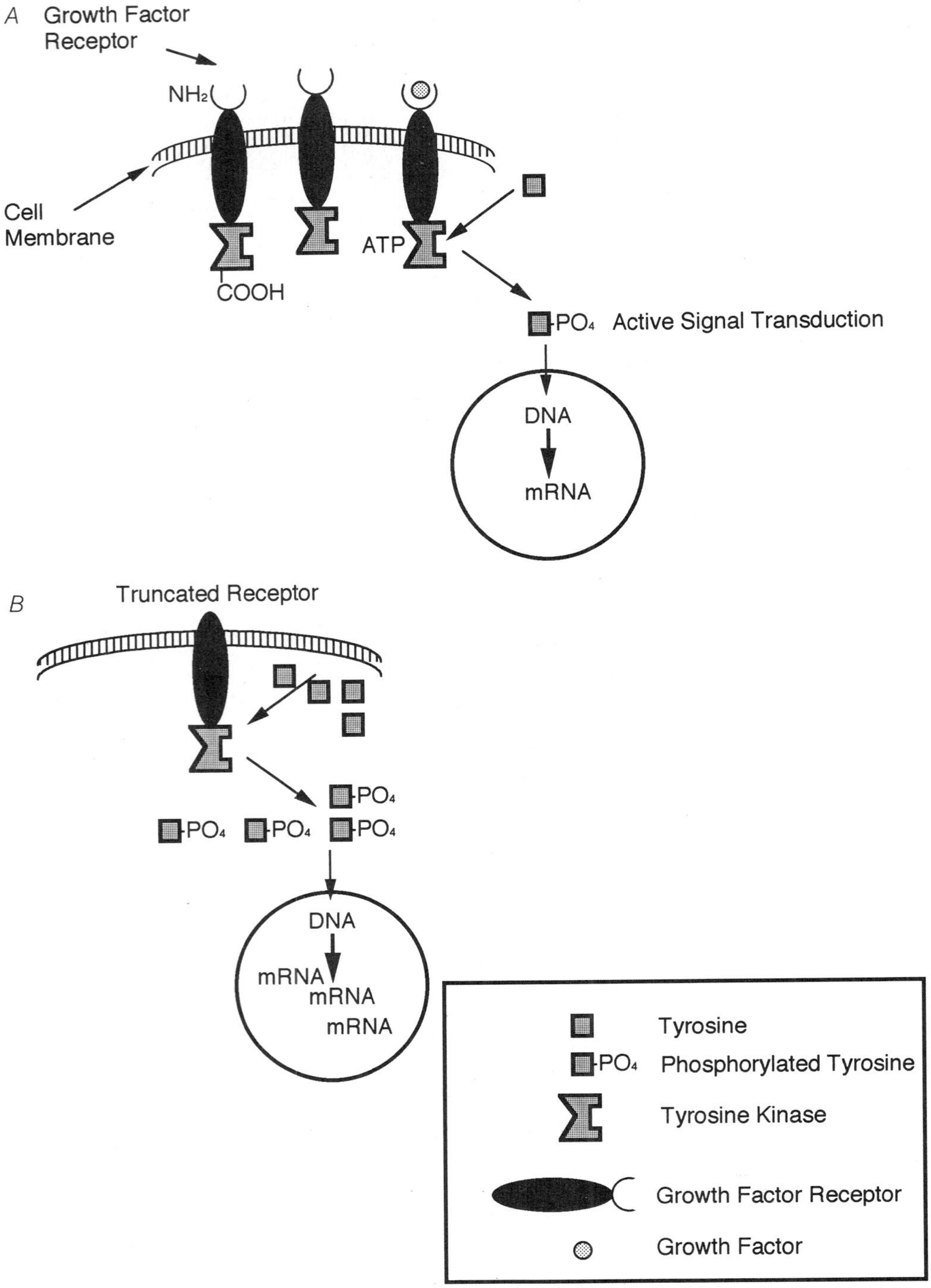

FIG. 9-15. Signal transduction initiated by GFR binding of ligand (*A*) and following mutation of the GFR. The extracellular domain binds ligand and the signal is transmitted through the transmembrane anchor to the cytoplasmic domain containing the tyrosine kinase domain. The activated tyrosine kinase phosphorylates tyrosine residues of proteins that regulate gene expression. In the mutated version (*B*) the signal is constitutively transduced.

carcinomas relative to normal colon epithelial cells. In a normal cell, the phosphorylation of an enzyme is a transient, regulatory event. In the oncoprotein, the enzyme may be constitutively activated, resulting in the unregulated transfer of phosphate to tyrosine residues on targeted proteins. The targets or effector proteins send abnormal or uncontrolled mitogenic signals to the cell nucleus. Characterization of these molecular messengers will help clarify signal transduction pathways. Ultimately, secondary messengers may serve as targets for specific chemotherapeutic inhibitors of tyrosine kinase function.

G-Protein Binding of GTP. Stimulation of a cell surface receptor induces exchange of GDP for GTP and the G protein is then converted to an activated configuration. While in the active state, secondary messengers are generated in specific signal transduction pathways such as the phosphatidylinositol and protein kinase C systems.

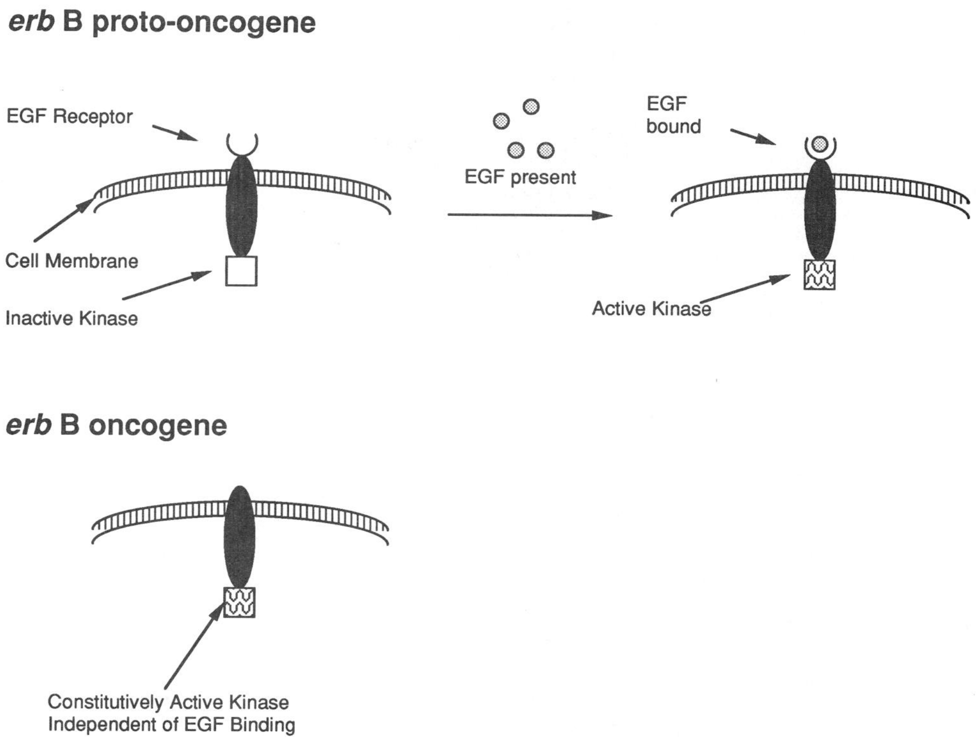

FIG. 9-16. The *erb* B proto-oncogene and the *erb* B oncogene. The *erb* B proto-oncogene is the EGF receptor complex with the intracellular tyrosine kinase domain. Binding of EGF to the extracellular domain activates the kinase. The *erb* B oncogene product is missing the extracellular domain.

Hormonal activation of adenylate cyclase is an example of such a system. Binding of activated G proteins may phosphorylate and activate phospholipase-C, which splits phosphatidylinositol 4,5-biphosphate into inositol triphosphate (ITP3) and diacylglycerol (DAG). ITP3 stimulates release of calcium from intracellular stores and DAG activates the protein kinase C (PKC) system in conjunction with released Ca^{++}.

Thus, the abnormal expression or activation of the receptors or any of the molecules within the signal system may be responsible for transformation of the cell. An example of this concept is the characteristic point mutations of the *ras* gene, which result in a constitutively activated protein. Mutations at position 12, 13, or 61 within the *ras* gene will result in proteins capable of increasing the rate of GDP/GTP exchange or decreasing hydrolysis of GTP and conversion of the enzyme to its inactive state. The PKC system is thus receiving continual proliferative signals ultimately leading to cell transformation. Altered or abnormal expression of a normal proto-oncogene results in the production of an oncoprotein with transforming potential.

Nucleus Changes. Many proto-oncogenes function normally as integrated members of precise signal transduction pathways. Malignant transformation must ultimately involve abnormal mitogenic signals transmitted to the cell nucleus and the subsequent loss of the normal gene expression. Therefore, some oncogenes encode proteins that are localized to the nucleus.

"Nuclear oncogenes" have a variety of activities, all of which function within the nucleus (Table 9-7). Some of the nuclear oncogenes, such as c-*fos*, c-*jun*, and c-*myb*, are transcriptional regulatory molecules. Other nuclear oncogenes, such as c-*myc* and n-*myc*, may control cell cycle. For example, the c-*erb* A protein is a thyroid hormone receptor that serves as a negative regulator of thyroid-induced cell proliferation. The c-*fos* and c-*jun* oncogene products are components of a transcriptional activator termed AP-1. Binding of the *fos* and *jun* proteins forms a heterodimer with enhanced DNA-binding affinity. The basic regions of this heterodimer bind to an AP-1 target site on the DNA. The ultimate result is increased transcription of the AP-1 target genes. The c-*erb* A oncoprotein has lost the ability to bind thyroid hormone. The oncoprotein is thus functioning as a constitutive, hormone-independent repressor of thyroid hormone inducible genes. This loss of normal function leads to increased transforming potential (Fig. 9-17). The *myc* family of nuclear oncogenes are activated in a wide variety of human malignancies. Oncoproteins from c-*myc* may stimulate cells to progress from G1 into S-phase (DNA synthesis), resulting in persistent cellular proliferation.

Coordination of Oncogene Changes. In the normally regulated cell, binding of extracellular ligands by specific cell membrane receptors is transmitted as a mitogenic signal to the cell nucleus, leading to increased transcription of target genes, DNA synthesis, and cell proliferation. It has been demonstrated that many of the proto-oncogenes are linked and act in a cooperative fashion involving signal transduction. For example, binding of PDGF to its receptor on fibroblasts results in increased transcription of the c-*myc* gene (see Fig. 9-14). Examples of binding of specific growth factors and activation of the receptor with subsequent changes in activity or expression of linked proto-oncogene products have been demonstrated in several systems. Activation of PDGF and EGF receptor tyrosine kinases result in increased activation of the phosphatidyl-inositol and protein kinase C systems. Similarly, PDGF binding may result in tyrosine phosphorylation of the c-*raf* kinase with subsequent increase in its enzyme activity. Growth factor stimulation may also regulate the transcription of

Table 9-7
Nuclear Oncogene Products

Proto-oncogene	*Protein Molecular Weight (in kD)*
Thyroid Hormone Receptor (*erb*)	52
Myc Family	
c-*myc*	64
L-*myc*	66
N-*myc*	64
Transcription Factor AP-1 Components	
c-*jun*	47
jun-B	40
jun-D	40
c-*fos*	62
fra-1	38
fos-B	45
Other Nuclear Oncogenes	
myb	75
ets-1	51
ets-2	56
ski	60
rel	68

nuclear oncogenes such as c-*fos* and c-*jun*. These in turn function as important regulators of the mitogenic signals originating from growth factor binding.

It is unlikely that a single genetic event leads to complete malignant transformation. Rather, the capabilities for extended proliferation, invasion of adjacent tissues, and metastasis are probably acquired as a sequence of genetic events. Multiple changes in the elaborate biochemical regulation issue from abnormal expression or activation of several cooperating oncogenes. The gradual acquisition of these molecular changes may involve target sites at any of the various classes of oncogenes described herein. While the oncogenes are viewed to be positive signals leading to transformation, another distinct class of genes are negative regulators of cell proliferation. These genes are growth suppressor genes, recessive oncogenes, antioncogenes, or tumor-suppressor genes. Loss of suppressor genes facilitates tumor development. Tumor suppressor genes may function as governors of growth and proliferative signals, and actually suppress malignant transformation. Evidence of tumor suppressor genes is derived from several investigations. Karyotype analysis reveals that certain malignancies have characteristic losses of specific chromosomes, while chromosomal banding demonstrates deletion of particular chromosomal bands in other diploid cancers. More detailed information regarding the existence of tumor-suppressor genes developed from cell hybridization experiments, the study of familial cancers, and the loss of heterozygosity in tumors. Fusion between malignant and normal cells yielded hybrids that were nontumorigenic unless specific chromosomes were lost from the hybrids. Tumorigenicity was

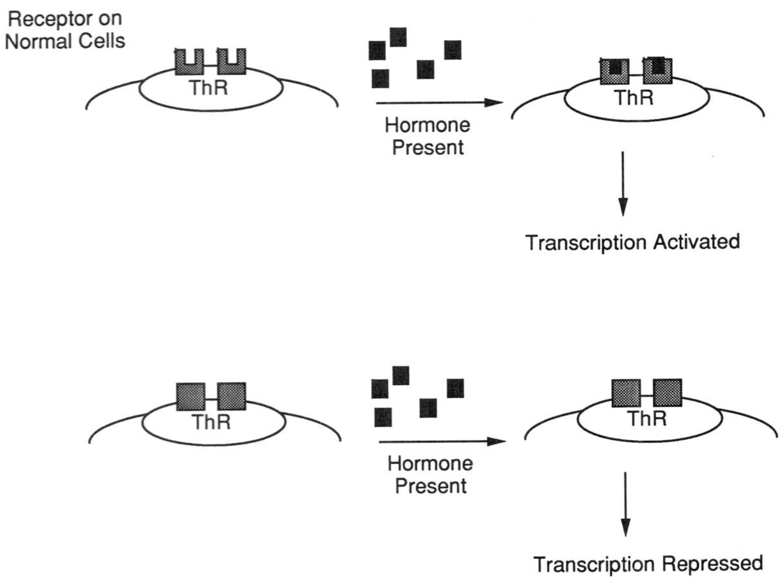

FIG. 9-17. The *erb* A oncogene and the thyroid hormone receptor.

suppressed in the hybrids by the addition of genetic material that was absent in the original malignant cell.

Retinoblastoma Gene. The genetic changes that are fundamental to the cancer process suggest potential congenital patterns of expression. Genetic analysis of families with hereditary and sporadic retinoblastomas provides evidence for the role of tumor-suppressor genes in human tumors. In inherited retinoblastomas, an abnormal Rb gene is transmitted to 50 percent of offspring. In the presence of a normal allele tumors do not develop and the abnormal germ-line mutation behaves in a recessive fashion. However, a second mutation of the normal allele (somatic cell mutation) may occur in a retinal cell, leading to the development of the tumor. Thus, loss of both parental alleles of the suppressor gene results in malignant transformation of the retinal cell. In sporadic retinoblastomas, development of a tumor requires two somatic mutations (Fig. 9-18). In either case, the result is the loss of any normal allele capable of inhibiting tumor formation. The genetic loss in retinoblastomas involves deletion of chromosome 13 band q14. Using the technique of restriction-fragment-length polymorphism (RFLP), tumor-suppressor genes may be identified through the loss of heterozygosity of the allele in question or a specific marker associated with that allele. *Heterozygosity* refers to the presence of two different alleles for a given gene. RFLP allows the identification of these different alleles based on differences in the restriction sites of DNA digesting enzymes. Following treatment with the restriction endonucleases, the DNA can be hybridized with a polymorphic gene probe.

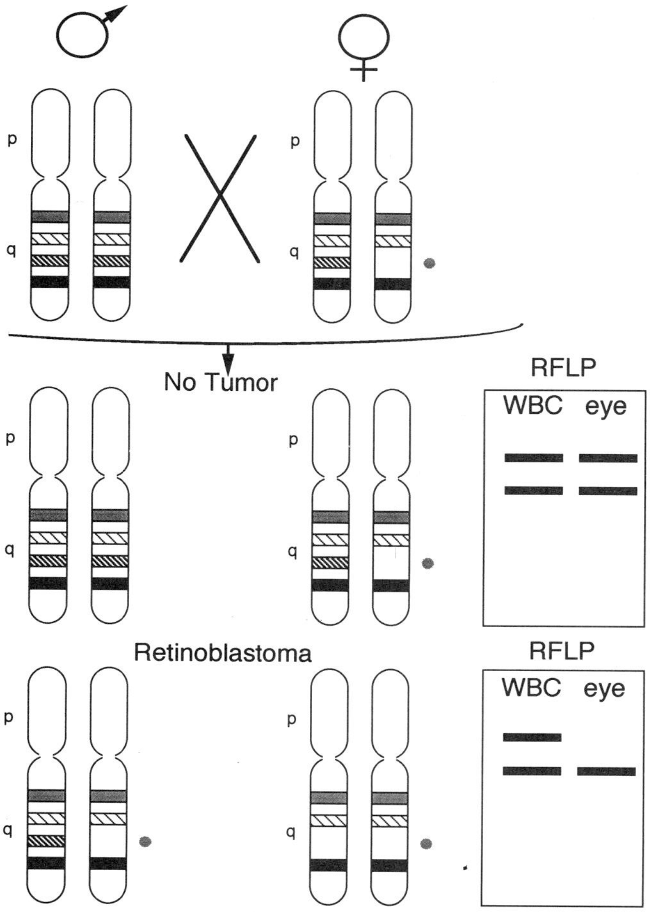

FIG. 9-18. Retinoblastoma is associated with a deletion in the 14th band in the long arm of chromosome 13. When heterozygous for the deletion there may be no tumor. However, if loss occurs in the other chromosome in cells of the eye, retinoblastoma develops. Analysis of the DNA from blood cells and cells from the eye of offspring (using RFLP) reveals the homozygous deletion in the eye while the heterozygous peripheral white blood cells give a normal phenotype.

p53. The p53 gene, named for the protein it encodes and located on chromosome 17q12, is a suppressor gene associated with carcinoma of the breast, lung, and colon, and osteosarcomas. Other possible suppressor genes are thought to exist based on the frequency and consistency of specific chromosomal deletions and rearrangements in certain neoplasms. Table 9-4 lists representative tumor-suppressor genes and the associated neoplasms.

The mechanism of action of the proteins encoded by these genes is being examined. In general, these gene products may act in a coordinated, balanced fashion to regulate the actions of the dominantly transforming genes. The proteins p53 and p105-Rb are nuclear phosphoproteins that are probably transcriptional regulators. The tumor-suppressor gene involved in type 1 neurofibromatosis (NF1) encodes a protein that may regulate several *ras* proteins. It is highly unlikely that any of the dominant oncogenes or recessive tumor-suppressor genes would function in any mutually exclusive fashion. Rather, these genes are likely to function in a precise, coordinated biochemical circuit of elaborate checks and balances.

Colorectal Cancer. Colorectal tumors appear to arise from a mutational activation of dominant oncogenes coupled with the mutational inactivation of tumor-suppressor genes. Mutations in at least four to five genes are required for full malignant transformation. It is the total accumulation of changes rather than the sequence of the accumulation that is important. Finally, the mutant tumor-suppressor genes may predispose to further genetic changes even when present in the heterozygous state. Metastatic potential is unrelated to the acquisition of other, as yet unknown, alterations. The future holds promise that revelations of molecular biology will become useful in the care of the cancer patient. Application of this knowledge may prove beneficial in terms of diagnosis, prognosis, and treatment, as identification of allelic deletions in the Rb gene can be used in screening to detect high-risk individuals. Deletions of chromosome 5 have been identified in individuals with the hereditary familial polyposis syndrome.

Prognostic Indicators. The use of oncogenes as prognostic indicators is also continuing to evolve. For example, amplification of the HER-a/*neu* gene in breast cancer is associated with both an increased frequency of lymph node metastasis and a decreased disease-free survival. Similarly, amplification of N-*myc* in neuroblastomas is predictive of rapid disease progression and unresponsiveness to chemotherapy.

Potential Therapeutic Strategies. The final challenge is development of molecular antineoplastic therapy that addresses specific genetic lesions that enable cell proliferation. A reasonable approach may involve targeting the protein products of oncogenes. Exceptional specificity may be gained by developing unique tyrosine kinase inhibitors or the use of monoclonal antibodies against overexpressed growth factor receptors.

Heritable Influences

Many factors contribute to the initiation and progression of cancer. Some are inherited characteristics that may be magnified by cultural influences. Ethnic influences less frequently confer the neoplasm than increase the risk for specific cancers. In this section, the examples presented illustrate the diversity of influences that may increase the incidence of tumors in specific populations.

Familial Breast Cancer. The family medical history provides an important aspect to patient evaluation in breast cancer. Investigations of family histories in breast cancer patients reveal increased risks for breast cancer and also increased predisposition to other neoplasms in first-degree relatives (Fig. 9-19). In familial breast cancer there is (1) earlier age of onset, (2) frequent bilateral disease, (3) genetic heterogeneity, and (4) vertical transmission, suggesting autosomal dominance. Ten to 15 percent of breast cancer cases have familial aggregation but fewer meet all the criteria for familial breast cancer. There are no accepted histologic or cytogenetic markers that identify familial tendency in breast cancer. Proto-oncogene polymorphisms such as those observed in c-Ha-*ras* offer no molecular genetic discriminators. Potential differences are only suggested in isolated reports of mammary tumor-associated antigens. There is no conclusive association of familial breast cancers with hormone dependency. There may be as much as a twofold higher incidence of blood group B in familial versus sporadic cancer in some studies. Familial arrays may include males with breast cancer. More often, familial analysis reveals increased risk for a group of cancers such as colon, ovarian, esophageal, and stomach carcinomas, and to a lesser extent, sarcoma, lung tumors, and adrenocortical carcinomas. Heritable characteristics that modify risks may be better identified as the molecular genetic analysis of cancers progresses.

Dysplastic Nevus. Familial melanomas are an uncommon occurrence. At three major centers between 4 and 10 percent of melanoma patients have a history of melanoma in first-degree relatives. Despite the frequency of association, there are no known genetic markers for malignant melanoma. There is an autosomal dominant hereditary occurrence of melanoma originally termed B-K mole syndrome and now called dysplastic nevus syndrome (Fig. 9-20). Patients typically have between 10 and 100 pigmented lesions usually larger than the junctional and compound nevi of childhood. Patients with familial melanoma frequently display immunologic abnormalities. Dysplastic nevi occur most frequently on the back and, less commonly, below the waist. The dysplasia is probably preneoplastic stage. Dysplastic nevus is indistinguishable

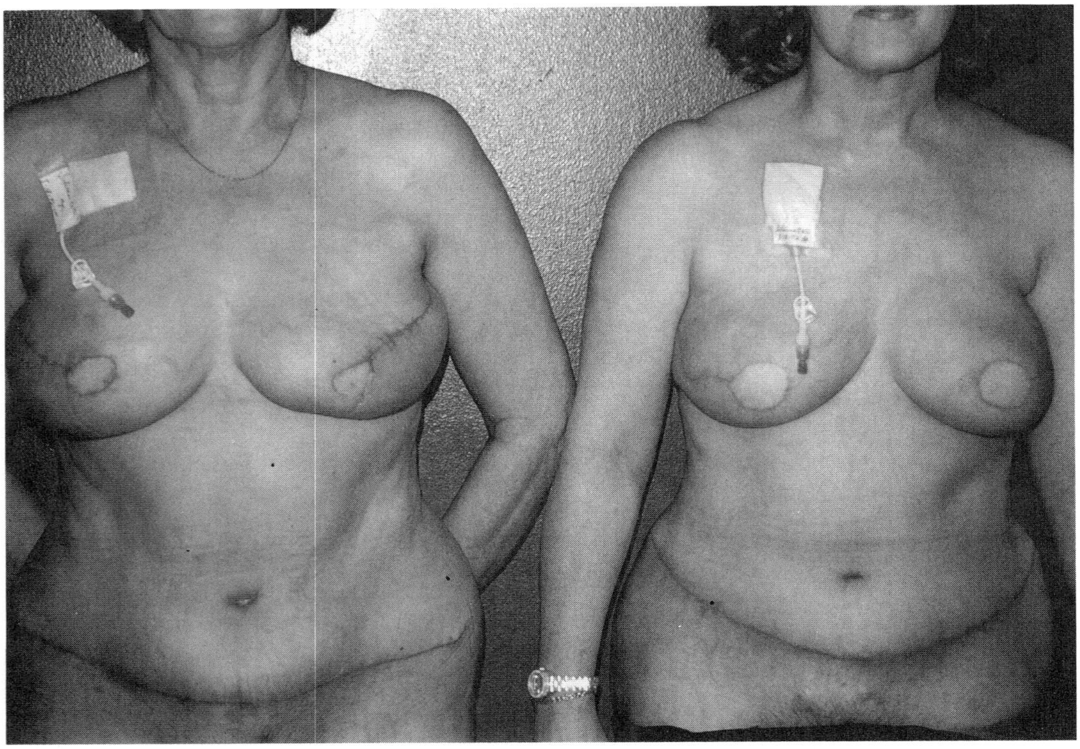

FIG. 9-19. An example of multidisciplinary breast cancer treatment. Two sisters were simultaneously diagnosed with a left breast cancer. Their mother had bilateral breast cancer and all other females in the family for two generations had breast cancer. Both patients chose to have a left modified radical mastectomy (as a cancer treatment) and a right total mastectomy (as cancer prevention) with immediate TRAM (transverse rectus abdominus musculocutaneous) flap breast reconstruction (as cancer rehabilitation). Both patients had metastasis to the lymph nodes and will receive postoperative adjuvant chemotherapy using doxorubicin, 5-FU, and cyclophosphamide. The photograph shows both women 3 weeks after surgery. A nipple reconstruction will be scheduled later. A left subclavian catheter has been inserted to facilitate a 6-month course of chemotherapy. Both tumors were strongly positive for expression of estrogen receptors, so both patients will receive adjuvant tamoxifen chemotherapy.

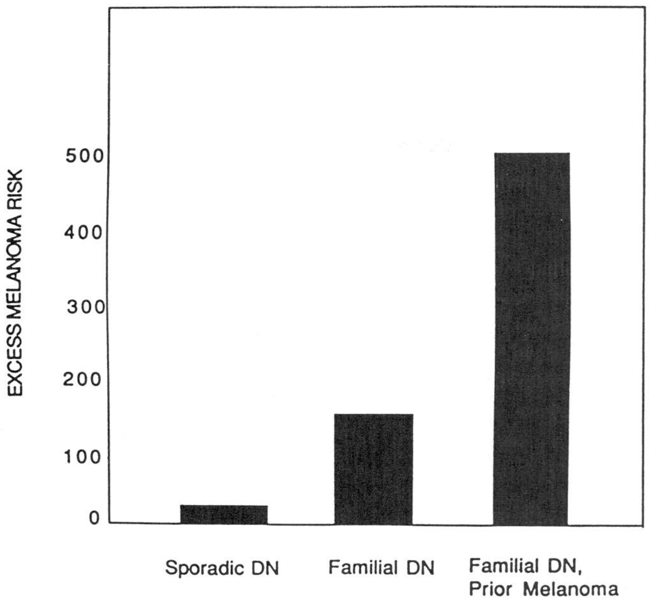

FIG. 9-20. Dysplastic nevus (DN) syndrome. Excess melanoma risk (relative to the general population) in persons with dysplastic nevi varies, depending on family history and personal history of melanoma.

from melanoma in situ upon gross examination of a single lesion. Presumably, 40 percent of melanoma in situ began as dysplastic nevus. Patients with dysplastic nevus syndrome and a family history of melanoma have a greater risk of developing melanoma (50 percent or more by age 60).

Multiple Endocrine Neoplasias. There are at least three different autosomal dominant familial cancer syndromes that result in one of the multiple endocrine neoplasias (MEN). Type I (Wermer's syndrome) presents with tumors of the anterior pituitary, parathyroids, and pancreatic islets. Occasionally, symptoms include tumor or hyperfunction of the adrenal glands. Cytogenetic analysis suggests that an allelic loss in 11q12-11q13 occurs in both the sporadic and familial form of MEN I. Other studies report loss on both 11p and 11q. There may be linkage to the *int*-2 oncogene. MEN I patients have a "basic fibroblast growth factor-like" activity in their serum, while serum from normal individuals is devoid of such activity. More than 50 percent of patients with MEN I display multiple adenomas in two or more different glands, and 20 percent have three or more glands involved. Hyperparathyroidism, pituitary adenomas, hypersecretion of gastrin, insulin, or other pancreatic hormones, and adrenocortical hyperfunction are common characteristics. MEN I may include schwannomas, multiple cutaneous lipomas, thymomas, and bronchial or small intestinal carcinoids.

MEN II patients are subdivided into subgroups IIa and IIb. Both subgroups display medullary thyroid carcinoma (MTC) and pheochromocytomas. MEN IIa also includes parathyroid hyperplasia. MEN IIb includes mucosal neuromas, ganglioneuromatosis of the gastrointestinal tract, and a Marfan-like habitus. MEN IIa is associated with losses in chromosomes 1 and 10 with the break for the deletion demonstrated at 1p32. Genotyping with a panel RFLP probes identified marker D10Z1, a pericentromeric region of chromosome 10 in MTC in both MEN IIa and IIb. These results suggest possible loss of a tumor-suppressor gene and allelic mutations in the same locus in the two different familial cancer syndromes. RFLP analysis may be useful in identifying patients at risk for MEN II.

Lynch Syndrome. Familial cancer trends are also manifest in colorectal cancers. The most widely investigated familial cancer of the colon is the heredity nonpolyposis colorectal cancer (HNPCC) syndrome. HPNCC syndrome is divided into two main categories: (1) hereditary site-specific colon cancer, or Lynch syndrome I, and (2) colorectal cancer in association with other forms of cancer, or Lynch syndrome II. The main characteristics of Lynch syndrome I are autosomal dominant heredity, no associated polyposis, the vulnerable site being the right colon in patients with two or more close relatives with cancer, multiple colon cancers, and long survival. In Lynch syndrome II, many of the characteristics are the same as Lynch syndrome I with the added burden of increased risk for endometrial, ovarian, stomach, and urinary tract tumors. In addition to these, Lynch syndrome II patients are at greater risk for recurrence of all types. The HPNCC group comprises nearly 5 percent of all colorectal cancers (in some centers as high as 15 to 20 percent). At present, there are no discriminating immunologic or biochemical markers that facilitate identification of Lynch syndrome, as well as no marker to distinguish syndrome I from II. Control of this form of colorectal cancer in current and future generations of families will be facilitated by computer registries and clinical surveillance of the high-risk group.

Tumor Progression and Metastasis

In the process of changing from normal to neoplastic, cells undergo numerous changes that result in unregulated growth. Cells cease to respond to the growth regulatory networks within the tissue system. Concomitantly, their requirements for growth factors diminish, and tumor cells may begin to synthesize their own growth factors or induce surrounding host cells to do so. Figure 9-21 illustrates the theoretical stages in the progression of cells to-

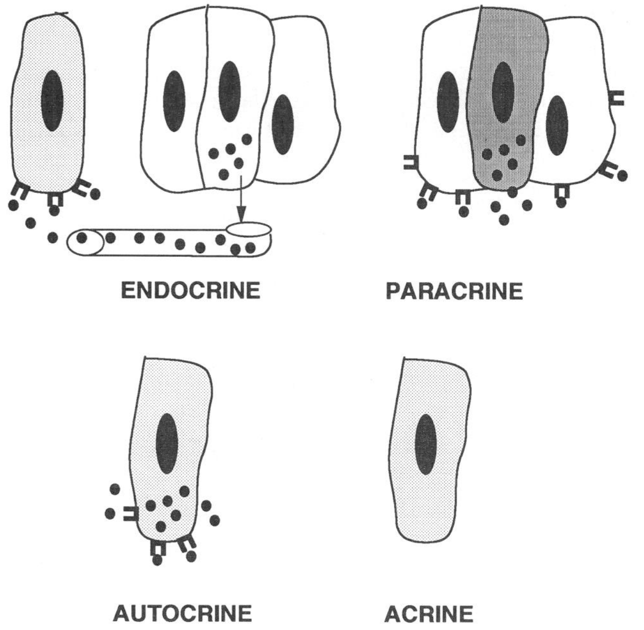

FIG. 9-21. Spectrum of growth factor dependence in tumorigenesis.

ward growth factor independence. Growth factors provided by adjacent normal cells are considered paracrine, while those provided by the tumor are autocrine. Potentially tumors may become growth factor independent, or acrine.

Other aspects of progression are discussed in the oncogene section, while growth properties of tumor masses are presented in the section on chemotherapy.

Theoretical Bases for Metastasis. Metastasis is the active or passive dissemination of disease from the site of origin to a distant site or organ. In cancer, the primary site undergoes changes that enable tumor cells to enter the microcirculation (intravasation), thereafter increasing the possibility for seeding distal sites (Fig. 9-22). Vascularization of the tumor provides the initial opportunity for entry into the circulation. As tumor cells traverse the vasculature, microemboli may trap cells in capillary beds of organs, thus enabling adherence to the vessel wall, followed by extravasation and establishment in the stroma (Fig. 9-23). The biologic basis of each of these stages remains to be determined, but as our understanding of this complex process emerges, we are presented with more possibilities for therapeutic intervention.

As tumors progress, they occupy space within the normal tissue. As progression ensues, cells depart the initiating mass and metastasize to distal sites. The metastasis process involves enzymes, adhesion molecules, growth factors, and the ability of distal organ sites to support tumor growth. Although there are numerous factors involved in the process of progression, several critical stages are well characterized in model systems. It is essential that the tumor cells survive and compete physiologically in the host and effectively evade the immune response (Fig. 9-24). The means by which tumors disseminate has been the subject of a century of controversy. Nevertheless, there are four theories for the mechanism by which tumor cells metastasize (Fig. 9-25). Although there is no single universally applicable theory for the mechanism of metastasis, each of the following includes the characteristics of (1) tumor heterogeneity, (2) cell surface receptors, (3) matrix degrading enzymes, (4) and cell–cell interactions. In the *random theory* advanced by Ewing, any cell within the primary tumor has the capacity to metastasize at any time during neoplastic progression. In this theory, metastasis is governed by lodgement of tumor cells in various compartments. The random theory conveniently explains regional spread of disease to lymph nodes and occasionally the blood-borne spread to the first organ with a complex microvascular bed. The *selection theory* espouses that only certain cells within the primary tumor achieve the capacity to dislodge and metastasize. The ''selected'' cells possess the capacity to course the vascular and lymphatic channels to access different organ sites. Malignant tumors are heterogeneous for this property, and the metastatic clones are selected during the multistep process of formation of metastases. Selection also occurs at the target organ site. Those cells capable of propagating at the site will do so, and those that cannot may degenerate. In the *metastatic compartment theory*, every cell in the primary tumor has the inherent capacity to be metastatic. Conversion to metastatic phenotype is determined by the tumor microenvironment. Finally, the *dynamic equilibrium theory* proposes that cells continually change from metastatic to nonmetastatic and back at a rate of 10^5 to 10^6 cells per generation toward metastatic phenotype and 10^{-2} to 10^{-6} cells per generation back to a nonmetastatic state. At the metastatic site, the cells then return to a more nonmetastatic posture. There are animal models as well as clinical data to support each of these theories.

Random Theory. In recent years, with the emergence of understanding the complex array of the molecules, genes, and signals involved in the process of cell growth, the random theory has received greater support. There are tumor cells that may spread to random secondary sites based on mechanical factors, such as the formation of blood-borne multicell emboli that randomly lodge in the microcirculation, usually in the first capillary bed encountered. This is especially apparent in regional lymph node metastasis, wherein the draining nodes are the most common site for metastatic deposits. About 50 percent of the attempts to in vivo select for more metastatic variant cells failed to demonstrate more metastatic cells in the secondary deposits. In opposition to this concept there are some tumor cells that spread to particular secondary sites (for example, melanoma metastases to brain and bowel, breast cancer metastases to bone and adrenal glands). Using genetically marked cells (drug resistance, chromosome markers, isozymes, RFLP patterns), secondary tumors are shown to contain unique cells or sets of cells. Cloning primary tumor cell populations yields some metastatic and some nonmetastatic cells.

Selection Theory. Specific histologic types of neoplasms have a remarkable proclivity for metastasis to selected organ sites (Table 9-8). There is a longstanding wealth of clinical evidence to support the concept that organ sites may provide unique milieu to

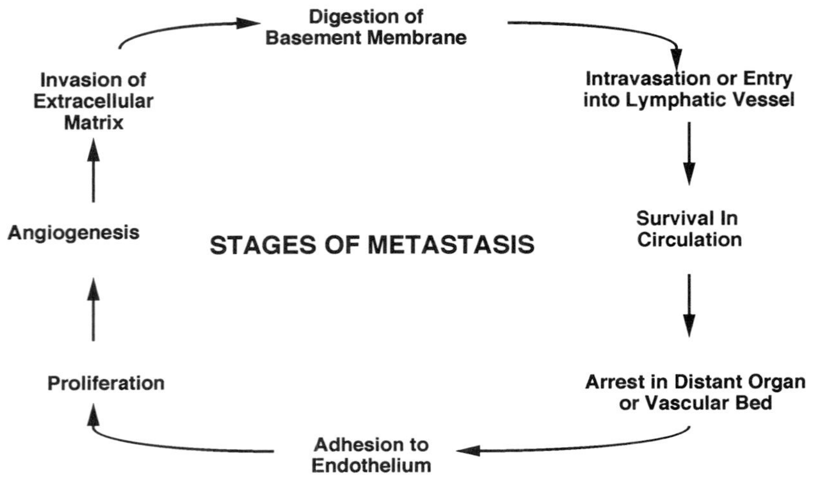

FIG. 9-22. Progression of events that occur in the establishment of metastatic growth.

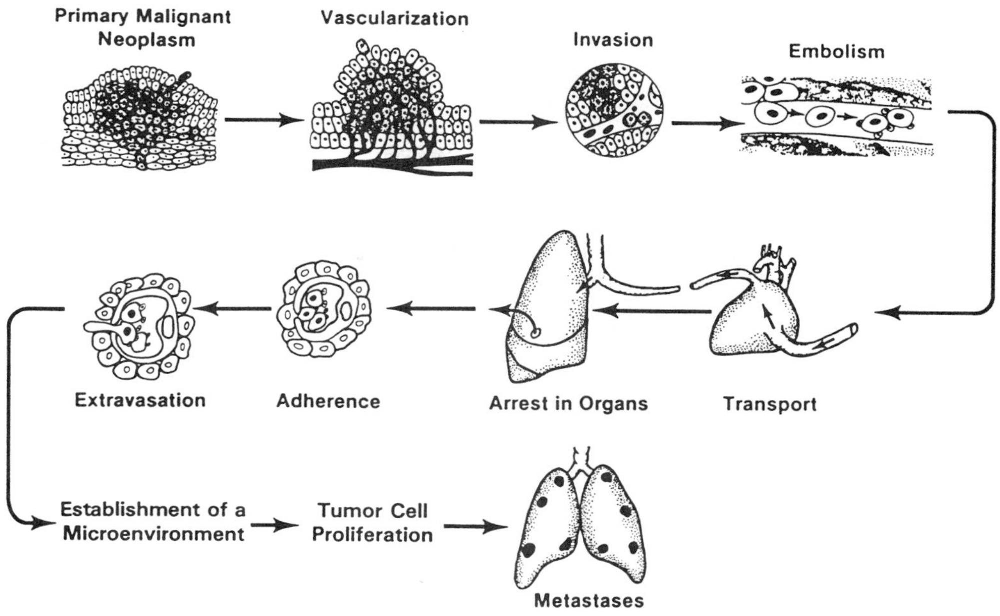

FIG. 9-23. Critical stages in the biology of metastasis. At each stage there are biochemical events that involve specific cell surface structures, and intracellular and extracellular events.

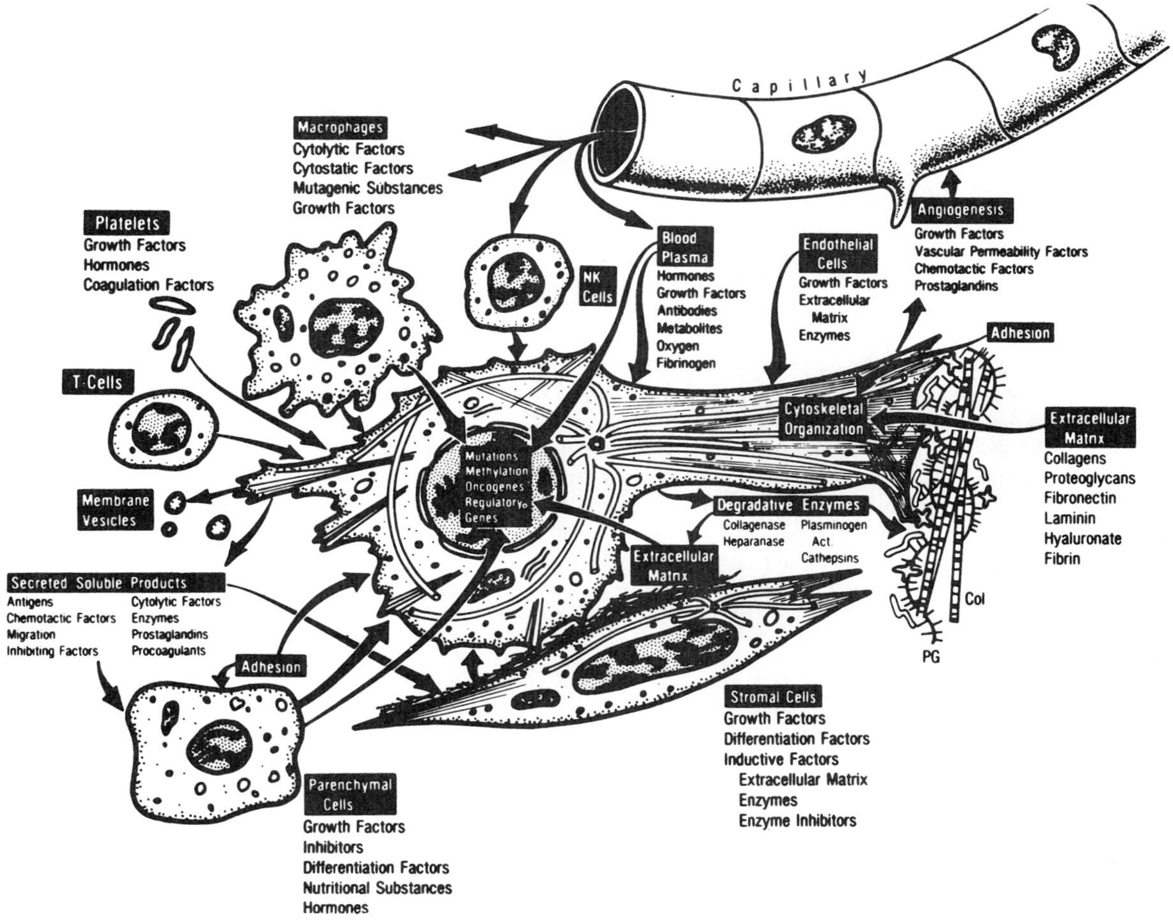

FIG. 9-24. Components of host-tumor relationships. The complexity and diversity of cells that interact with the tumor are depicted. These include immune effective cells, stromal cells, vascular cells. Products of these cells are combined as host defense mechanisms to contain or eliminate tumor at the metastatic site. Numerous biochemical interactions are involved in the progression and metastasis of tumors. The tumor relies on growth factors, cytokines, enzymes, matrix, and adhesion molecules as it proceeds through the stages progressing to disseminated growth. *(Courtesy of Dr. Garth L. Nicolson.)*

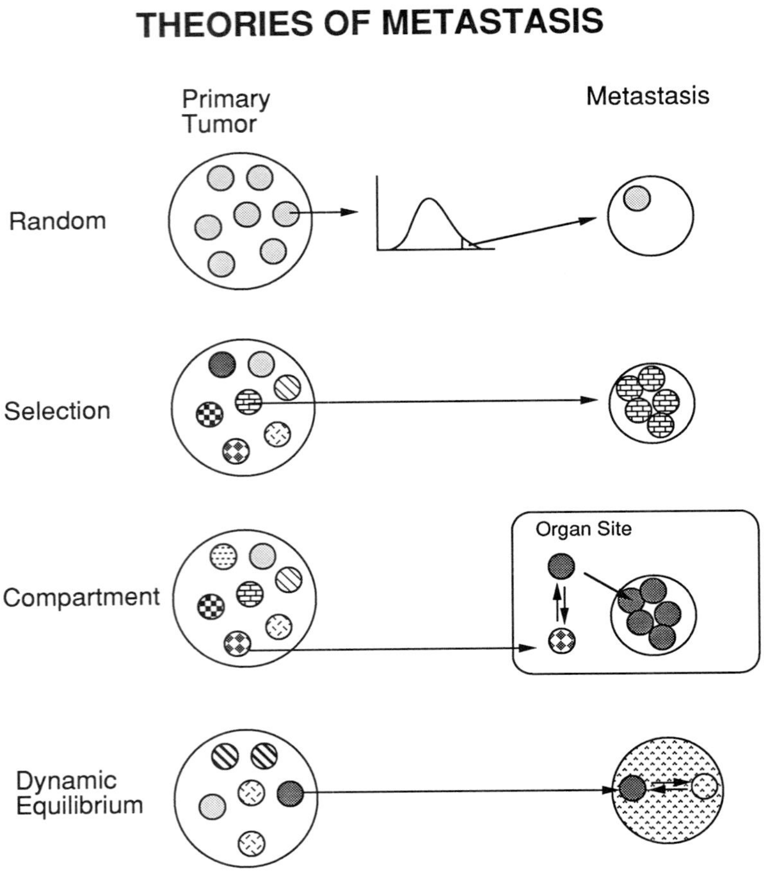

FIG. 9-25. Metastasis may occur by any of four theoretical mechanisms. The basis of metastasis.

support the growth of errant tumor cells. Experiments conducted in vivo in animal models revealed that cell populations can be selected for variants that metastasize to particular sites by sequential isolation of the metastatic cells and reinoculation into sygeneic hosts. In vitro, selection of heterogeneous low or nonmetastatic cells for properties that are associated with metastasis can yield rare variants that are metastatic. As may be shown by using genetically marked cells (drug resistance, chromosome markers, isozymes, RFLP patterns) secondary tumors contain unique cells or sets of cells. Again, this concept is not universally applicable.

Table 9-8
Site Predilection of Blood-Borne Metastases

Type of Primary Tumor	*Most Frequent Site of Distant Metastases*
Bladder carcinoma	Lung, bone
Breast cancer	Bone, liver, lung
Colorectal carcinoma	Liver, peritoneal surfaces, ovary
Renal carcinoma	Lung, liver, bone
Lung cancer	Liver, bone, brain
Melanoma (cutaneous)	Skin/subcutaneous, lung, liver
Melanoma (ocular)	Liver
Prostatic carcinoma	Bone
Sarcomas (bone, soft tissue)	Lung
Testicular carcinoma	Lung
Thyroid adenocarcinoma	Bone, lung
Uterus	Peritoneum, omentum, liver

Some tumors spread randomly to secondary sites. In vivo sequential selection for enrichment of metastatic variant cells was only successful in about one-half of the models. Indeed, there are occasions when in vivo selections led to fewer metastatic cell subpopulations.

Metastatic Compartment Theory. In support of this theory, some tumor cells change their phenotypic properties as dictated by organ site or when in contact with normal cells or other tumor cells. These changes can be reversible and may occur at a rate too rapid to be explained by host selection. On the other hand, tumor cell clones in some instances appear to be relatively stable in their metastatic properties and are not affected by the presence of other cell types. This theory predicts that cells from metastases should be no more metastatic than cells from primary tumors. In about one-half of the experimental models, however, analysis of metastatic foci revealed greater frequency of metastatic clones. Using genetically marked cells, it can be shown that secondary tumors contain unique cells or sets of cells, which would not be expected by the metastatic compartment theory.

Dynamic Equilibrium Theory. The metastatic potential of a cell is relatively unstable but is inherited for at least a short time period. In time, the cell population will reach an equilibrium, with the continuous generation of metastatic and nonmetastatic cells at definable rates. Phenotypic drift in numerous properties of tumor cells does occur in many cell populations. In opposition to this theory, the metastatic properties of some tumor cell clones appear to be relatively stable and do not undergo phenotypic drift. This theory erroneously predicts that with time cells from metastases should be no more metastatic than cells from first-degree tumors.

In addition, the fact that secondary tumor sites contain unique cells or sets of cells does not support the dynamic equilibrium theory.

Obviously the metastatic process must involve elements of more than one of the above theories. It is perhaps best explained by various combinations of these theories, depending on the system examined.

Invasion. The malignant potential of a tumor is related to its ability to dissociate and seed other sites. Distribution of tumor cells from the primary site of tumorigenesis may occur by direct spread, wherein the leading front of tumor margin advances into another tissue, vessel, or cavity. Invasion and infiltration into host tissues surrounding the primary tumor eventuate in penetration of blood vessels, lymph vessels, or both, providing access for widespread dispersion. The mechanisms responsible for invasion of local host tissues are biochemical and, less frequently, mechanical. Mechanical pressure as a result of neoplastic proliferation may force encroaching projections of tumor cells along lines of least resistance. Pressure atrophy is independent of the rate of tumor proliferation. Not all invasive tumors grow rapidly; some highly invasive tumors have very slow growth rates.

Intrinsic cell motility may play a role in tumor cell invasion, and there is experimental evidence to suggest that some tumors produce autocrine motility factors. The association between increased cell motility and tumorigenic potential is being investigated using the rates of migration of tumor cells and homologous normal cells determined in vitro. As yet no direct proof of an association has been revealed. Tumor cells possess the organelles necessary for active locomotion and can form cellular cytoplasmic processes, indicative of motility, during the invasive process. On the other hand, inhibition of cell motility prevents invasion in some in vitro models. For example, treatment of tumor cells with cytoskeleton-disrupting agents before introduction into experimental animals alters metastatic patterns. In summary, the role of cell motility as a single factor in tumor invasion is poorly substantiated. Therefore it is considered one of a number of conditions that must be accommodated before tumor cells can successfully invade distant tissues.

In addition to cellular movement, the production and activation of specific enzymes, hydrolases, and collagenases is critical to tumor invasion. Histologic examination of tissues obtained from sites of tumor invasion displays variation in the degree of tissue damage. Many human and animal malignant neoplasms have higher levels of lytic enzyme activity than benign tumors or corresponding normal tissues. Evidence for the involvement of tissue-degradative enzymes in neoplastic invasion is convincing. Lysosomal catheptic activities are elevated within some tumor tissues, and increased production of cathepsin B in breast carcinomas compared with that in normal or benign tissue has been observed; therefore, there may be a critical role for this enzyme in the expression of the aggressive malignant phenotype. Enhanced production and secretion of the serine protease plasminogen activator is associated with the neoplastic transformation.

Invasion of normal tissues, the intercellular matrix, and vascular basement membranes by metastatic cells requires the active participation of hydrolytic enzymes (see Fig. 9-24). Connective tissue proteins are classified into four major groups: collagen, elastin, glycoproteins, and proteoglycans. The distribution of each protein differs among different tissues. The constituents of the extracellular matrix are stabilized and organized by interactions among the tissue proteins, and the stability is easily disordered by degradative enzymes released from tumor cells.

Both intravasation and extravasation are pivotal in hematogenous, systemic metastasis. In either instance, the tumor cells are confronted with a barrier significantly composed of type IV collagen. Therefore, it is consistent that there is a strong correlation between the ability of murine tumor cells to produce spontaneous metastases and increased levels of collagenase IV. Tumor cells that invade blood vessels or leave capillaries of distant organs in which they have been lodged must penetrate the basement membrane (Fig. 9-26). Dissolution of the basement membrane, suggestive of enzymatic action, has been observed in areas adjacent to arrested tumor cells. Type IV collagen is a major structural protein of basement membranes between parenchymal cells and the connective tissue on which cells rest. Type IV collagen is chemically and genetically distinct from cartilage collagen type II and stromal collagen types I and III.

The collagenase prepared from metastatic murine tumor cells preferentially digests this basement membrane collagen. Cells recovered from the venous effluent of a murine fibrosarcoma, potentially the invasive population, have been observed to solubilize basement membrane collagen to a significantly greater extent than cells from the parent population. It appears that metastatic tumor cells exhibit a preferential attachment to type IV collagen substrates. Since tumor cells can lodge selectively in areas of endothelial damage, the possession of high levels of collagenase type IV may be fundamental to invasion and metastasis.

Lymphatic-Hematogenous Spread. Clinical observations suggest that carcinomas spread by the lymphatic route and mesenchymal tumors spread by means of the bloodstream. Experimental models contradict this notion, however. Disseminating tumor cells may pass from one system to another. The two systems are inseparable, and the division into lymphatic spread and hematogenous spread is arbitrary and only useful for academic discussion.

Lymphatic Access to Distant Tissue. The process of infiltration and expansion into host tissues results in the penetration of small lymphatic vessels by tumor cells. Tumor cell emboli in the vessels are responsible for initiation of lymphatic metastases. Tumor emboli may be trapped in the first lymph node encountered, or they may traverse lymph nodes or even bypass them to form distant nodal metastases (the "skip" metastasis). Although this phenomenon was recognized in the late 1800s, its implications for treatment were frequently ignored in the development of surgical approaches.

The view that the lymphatics are the primary route for spread of carcinomas is an oversimplification of the process. Of prime importance is the role that lymph nodes, in particular, may play in the control or regulation of metastatic spread. Lymph nodes in the area of a primary neoplasm are often enlarged and clinically palpable, signifying hyperplasia of lymph node follicles accompanied by proliferation of reticulum cells and sinus endothelium and/or growth of tumor cells.

Lymph nodes are immunologically responsive in patients with neoplasms. Tumor presence stimulates the activation, proliferation, and release of immunocompetent cells in the lymphoreticular system. The reaction commences in the regional lymph nodes and later proceeds to distant nodes and the spleen. Proliferative changes in the regional nodes often precede the spread and subsequent growth of tumor emboli within them. Initial entrapment and growth of lymphatic-borne tumor emboli usually occur in the subcapsular sinus of the lymph node. Additional emboli may be released from the sinus, or the tumor may grow toward the hilar region and the efferent channels. Thus, a significant proportion of the host immune response to disseminated tumor growth occurs

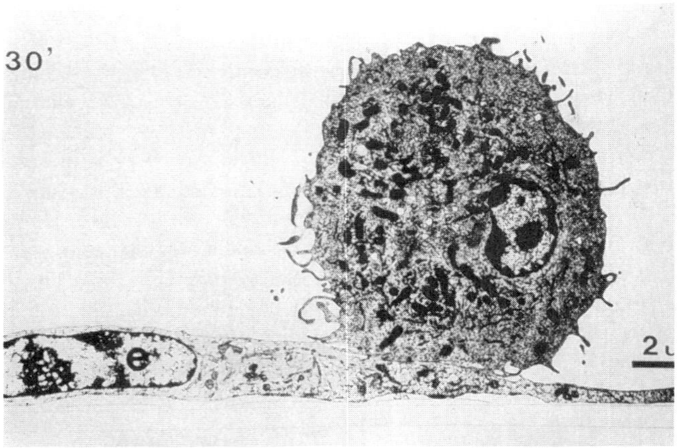

A

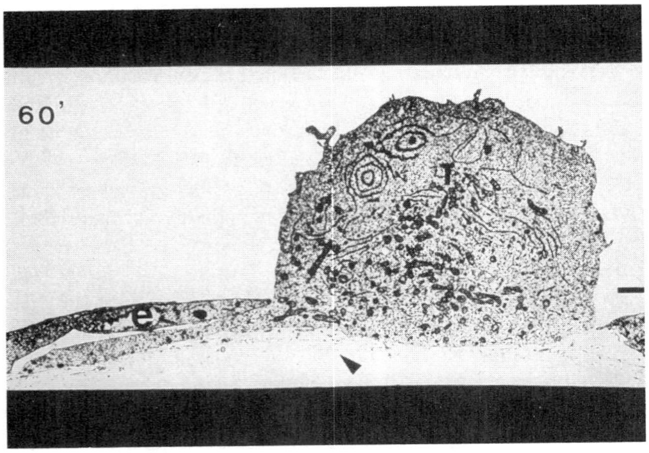

B

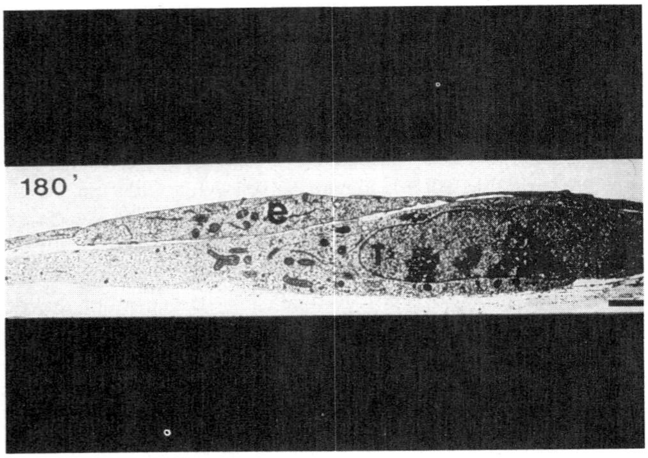

C

FIG. 9-26. Transmission electron micrograph of the invasion of basement membrane in vitro by a tumor cell mass. *A.* By 30 minutes incubation there is frank attachment to the endothelial layer. At 60 (*B*) and 180 (*C*) minutes there is obvious invasion of the endothelium and an establishment of the neoplastic cells in the model endothelium.

through interactions with the immune cells in the peripheral lymphatic network.

Barrier Function of Lymph Nodes. It is hypothesized that lymph nodes serve as a temporary "filter" for metastatic tumor cells. While lymph nodes (of normal animals) can be an effective, though temporary, barrier to tumor spread, they also may serve as a repository for immunoselected, resistant tumor cells. In experimental animals, administration of carcinoma cells directly into the afferent popliteal lymphatics of rabbits, followed by removal of lymph nodes 1 to 42 days after injection, revealed that only 2 of 30 animals developed distant metastases. Thus, there is evidence for a lymph node role as a temporary barrier to tumor spread. By contrast, another experimental study with radiolabeled tumor cells from rats showed that most cells that reached the lymph node rapidly entered the efferent lymphatics and then the bloodstream. Furthermore, tumor cells may cross from lymphatics to the vasculature and even return to the lymphatics. Most of the experimental animal systems used to investigate this strongly suggest that normal nonreactive lymph nodes are subjected to a sudden influx of a large number of tumor cells. This model may not be at all analogous to the regional nodes in the early stages of cancer spread in human beings, wherein tumor depositions to the regional nodes occur.

Filtration capacity of lymph nodes is influenced in several ways. Tumor growth, acute or chronic inflammatory reactions, and fibrosis resulting from local x-radiation may reduce the efficiency of filtration. Another consideration is that the properties of tumor cells per se, rather than the filtration capacity of the lymph node, determine whether neoplastic cells are trapped and destroyed.

The role of the regional lymphatics in neoplasia in general and in metastasis in particular is as controversial as it is important. Unquestionably, the regional nodes may be involved immunologically in the host response to a neoplasm. The importance of the regional nodes in the initiation of systemic immunity has been investigated in a series of models, which permits a focused approach. First, adoptive transfer of regional lymphatic cells by the intraperitoneal administration of regional node cells of tumor-bearing animals has been shown to induce tumor allograft immunity in normal animals. Furthermore, skin allografts lacking lymphatic connections were found to be tolerated only until restoration of the lymphatic system occurs. Finally, construction of skin pedicles in guinea pigs lacking afferent lymphatics led to indefinite retention of skin allografts. These observations have served as a touchstone for the use of immunotherapy in the treatment of cancer. There are, however, substantial differences in the quality and quantity of immune response to tumors and to allografts. In similar models, tumor allografts were rejected, although skin allografts remained viable.

Twenty years ago, Crile challenged the classic concept of en bloc resection of primary tumors of the breast and their regional lymphatics. He advocated simple mastectomy, or local tumor excision and preservation of the regional nodes. The retention of the nodes free of metastatic cells was hypothesized to be important in maintaining a high level of systemic tumor immunity to aid in the prevention of growth of disseminated micrometastases. Subsequent clinical trials by Fisher et al. comparing simple and radical mastectomy showed no improvement in survival rates despite an increased incidence of axillary lymph node metastasis in the patients who underwent simple mastectomy. While the presence of lymph node metastases is a harbinger of distant metastases in many patients, their removal does not protect against subsequent relapse, either because the mode of spread (lymphatic versus hematogenous) is a random event, or because metastases had begun to spread beyond the regional lymph nodes prior to clinical detection of the original cancer.

Studies in mice reveal that the regional lymphatics may be important for the initiation of immunity against a transplantable syngeneic tumor. The effect, however, is dependent on the immunogenicity of the tumor. Immunogenicity is based on the ability of the tumor to induce complete protection against transplant challenge in genetically identical hosts. In weakly immunogenic tumors, regional nodes were important in the initiation of systemic immunity, but strongly immunogenic tumors induced systemic immunity independent of their presence.

The contradictory findings on the role of regional lymph nodes in controlling cancer metastasis are consistent with our knowledge of the heterogeneity of tumor cells, metastases, antigens, and the host model. Different tumor models, and especially differences in experimental conditions, influence the relative biologic behavior of tumor cells. Therefore one may question the biologic relevance and accuracy of some animal models for human cutaneous melanoma. In cutaneous melanoma, there is extensive involvement of local and regional lymphatics. By contrast, human ocular melanoma or mucosal melanoma show early metastasis to visceral organs, and not lymph node metastases. Clearly, then, different animal tumor models (for melanoma) must be applied carefully to the individual types in the spectrum of human melanoma. Restricted adaptation of biologic principles from animal models applies not only within one tumor, but also across histologic barriers. An animal model using lymphosarcoma cells may have little relevance to human clinical cancer metastasis of solid tumors.

Hematogenous Metastasis. Widespread tumor cell dissemination is a consequence of the penetration of blood vessels, lymphatics, or both. Cells of malignant neoplasms frequently penetrate thin-walled capillaries, but rarely invade the elastin fiber-rich arteries or arteriolar walls. This resistance to invasion is not necessarily mediated by mechanical strength alone. Connective tissues possess protease inhibitors that may block the enzyme-dependent process of invasion. Malignant tumors do not produce their own blood vessels, but induce the ingrowth of new capillaries from host tissue by releasing tumor angiogenesis factor. Neovascularization of the tumor may result in vessels that are qualitatively different from "normal" vessels. The penetration of the new vascular channels may be aided by defective endothelium and increased permeability.

Once in the blood vessels, tumor cells may be passively carried away or, alternatively, adhere and grow at the penetration site. Subsequently, the latter may result in release of tumor emboli into the circulation. The accumulation of tumor emboli correlates with the development of tumor vascularization. Since most cells released into the bloodstream are eliminated rapidly, the mere presence of tumor cells in the circulation does not constitute metastasis. The rate of tumor cell release from an implanted murine fibrosarcoma is related mathematically to the development of pulmonary metastases. Although most tumor cells are destroyed within the bloodstream, it appears that the greater the number of cells released by a primary tumor, the greater the probability that some cells will survive to form metastases. The number of tumor emboli in the circulation correlates well with the size and clinical duration of the primary tumor. The development of necrotic and hemorrhagic areas within large tumors facilitates metastasis by providing easy access to the circulation.

The rapid death of most circulating tumor cells is probably due to the traumatic nature of blood turbulence (shear stress), but the isolated nature of the emboli allows for interaction with a variety of blood components. Tumor cells either aggregate with each other (homotypic aggregation) or with host cells (heterotypic aggregation), such as platelets and lymphocytes. Formation of multicellular emboli affords a survival advantage to the tumor cells in the circulation. In an experimental model, the number of pulmonary metastases formed after intravenous injection of tumor cells is related to the size of tumor emboli. Although the relationship may be the consequence of enhanced trapping of larger emboli in the microcirculation, it may also be due to the protective effect of an outer layer of cells. Metastases may result from undamaged "central" cells protected from the hostile circulatory environment by peripheral tumor or host cells in the embolus.

Tumor cell entrapment in the capillary bed of distant organs is a necessary prelude to secondary tumor growth. Although the morphologic aspects of tumor cell arrest are studied extensively, relatively little is known about the dynamics of the process. Exposure of the capillary basement membrane is a result of the normal and continuous physiologic process of endothelial cell-shredding and may allow adhesion of tumor emboli. Platelet adherence to damaged areas (naked basement membrane) followed by degranulation causes further retraction of endothelial cells and augments attachment of tumor emboli or platelet-tumor cell emboli. Fibrin deposits around an arrested tumor embolus are frequently observed. The role of fibrin in tumor cell arrest and metastasis is uncertain. Theoretically, a protective coat of fibrin around the tumor embolus shields the neoplastic cells from the attacks of host immunocytes or blood turbulence. Increased coagulation is commonly observed in patients with cancer and may be related to the increase in thromboplastin found in tumors. Some neoplasms produce large quantities of procoagulant-A, which directly activates factor X in the clotting process. A reduced rate of blood flow then leads to increased trapping of circulating tumor cells and survival of already trapped cells. The use of anticoagulants in the treatment or control of metastasis is based on the consideration of the above observations. A major limitation of this approach is the increased risk of hemorrhage and hematoma formation in anticoagulated patients undergoing major surgery.

Extravasation of arrested tumor cells is presumed to occur by mechanisms comparable to those that control intravasation. Tumor cells grow and destroy the arresting vessel as a prelude to attaining an extravascular position, or follow white blood cells through the vascular wall. To grow in the organ parenchyma, the metastases must develop a vascular network and evade the host immune system. When the metastases have attained a certain size, they may give rise to additional metastases, the so-called metastasis of metastases. Thus, in a short time, a small primary tumor may initiate multiple sites of affliction, each with the capacity to cycle the process of invasion of the vasculature and subsequent seeding of other organ sites.

Heterogeneity. In neoplasia, heterogeneity is carried to its largest exponent. Heterogeneity is introduced at the level of etiology. The differences due to histology, anatomic location, and ploidy all impact by multiplying the possibilities for heterogeneity.

Recently, it has been demonstrated that a vast heterogeneity exists in a single neoplasm. Diversity is manifest in (1) malignant potential, that is, the ability to produce tumors in syngeneic hosts (animals) or upon transplantation into immunologically deficient tumors (human tumor specimens); (2) quantitative expression of cell surface histocompatibility, as well as other antigens; and (3) different antigenic specificities expressed by cells within a tumor, or different specificities expressed between primary and metastatic cells. The following discussion addresses the aspects of heterogeneity that impact upon the biology of metastasis.

To produce a clinically apparent metastasis, malignant tumor cells must complete a sequence of potentially lethal interactions with host homeostatic mechanisms, not the least of which is avoidance of recognition and destruction by host defense. Failure to complete any step in the metastatic program results in elimination of the errant tumor cells. The complexity of the pathogenesis of metastasis explains, in part, why the process is deemed inefficient. For example, the presence of tumor cells in the circulation does not predict that metastasis will occur, because most tumor cells that enter the blood stream are rapidly destroyed. By 24 hours after entry into the circulation, less than 1 percent of radiolabeled tumor cells are still viable, and furthermore, less than 0.1 percent of tumor cells introduced into the circulation survive to produce metastases. The 0.1 percent of circulating cells responsible for the development of metastases either survived by random chance or are selected for survival and growth from preexistent subpopulations of cells. Do all cells growing in a primary neoplasm produce metastases, or only specific and unique cells by virtue of properties that enable the potentially destructive stepwise sojourn from the primary tumor to metastatic sites?

At the time of diagnosis, many human and animal neoplasms are composed of numerous subpopulations of cells with distinctly different biologic properties. Cells isolated from individual neoplasms differ in morphology, karyotype, growth rate, antigenicity-immunogenicity, cell surface receptors for lectins, hormone receptors, response to therapies, and potential for invasion and metastasis. Indeed, during the last decade, the concept that neoplasms are heterogeneous and contain multiple subpopulations of cells with different biologic properties has gained wide consensus. Almost a century ago, Paget analyzed autopsies of a large number of patients with breast cancer and concluded that the nonrandom pattern of metastasis was not due to chance, but rather to the environment provided by target organs (''soil''). Metastases developed only when the ''seed and soil'' were matched. A present definition of the ''seed and soil'' hypothesis could consist of three important principles. First, the process of metastasis may not be random. Second, neoplasms are not uniform entities but contain cells exhibiting heterogeneous metastatic capabilities. Third, the outcome of metastasis depends on the properties of both tumor cells and host factors, and the balance of these contributions varies among tumors arising in different tissues, and even among tumors of similar histologic origin in different patients.

The specificity with which metastatic tumor cells display a predilection for selected target organs suggests a molecular recognition system whereby tumor cells are able to specifically bind to target tissues to establish the mechanism of residence. Cell surface molecules, some of which may be integrins or ligands of integrins, may assign organ specificity to the metastatic phenotype. The study of these molecules will elucidate the mechanisms of organ/tissue predilection in metastasis and also afford a biologic basis for novel strategies to prevent establishment of metastases.

Cellular Diversity in Neoplasia. Cells with a spectrum of metastatic potential may be isolated from parent tumor lines (animals) or surgically excised primary tumors (human beings). The majority of cells do not evidence metastatic behavior.

Assessment of metastatic potential in human tumors is now performed in vivo in congenitally athymic nu/nu (nude) mice. These animals have severely impaired cell-mediated immunity and are therefore incapable of rejecting foreign tissue transplants. These animals afford an in vivo setting in which to assess malignant potential and metastatic proclivity. Recently, several human tumor lines and primary tumor displayed subpopulations of cells with widely differing metastatic properties.

The difference in metastatic propensities among tumor cells of an individual neoplasm is no longer controversial. Three aspects of the extensive cellular heterogeneity are investigated in tumor biology laboratories: (1) when do variants appear? (2) what is the origin of the diversity, and (3) what regulates variant expression? As answers to these questions emerge, they may help surgeons in making decisions critical to the timing and sequence of multimodality treatments for primary tumors and metastases.

The first question seeks a fundamental aspect of carcinogenesis irrespective of unicellular or multicellular origin; most tumors are heterogeneous and contain subpopulations of cells with differing biologic behavior. Tumors may arise as the result of a rare event, somatic mutation, wherein the origin is presumed unicellular. Indeed, substantial evidence from studies using a marker immunoglobulin or glucose 6-phosphate dehydrogenase (G6PD) in women with X-chromosome inactivation mosaicism suggests that chronic myelogenous leukemia, Burkitt's lymphoma, and multiple myeloma arise from a single cell. In contrast, hereditary trichoepithelioma and colon carcinoma are presumed to be of multicellular origin. Some of the most widely investigated animal model tumors, such as chemically induced murine fibrosarcomas, are also multicellular in origin.

Cellular diversity is consistent with neoplasms that are multicellular in origin. Such tumors are probably populated by the progeny of several transformed cells. In chemically induced sarcomas, cells obtained from different areas of the tumor differed in their growth rate, susceptibility to cytotoxic drugs, and antigenicity. Tumors that are unicellular in origin are not uniform. The evidence that diversity is continually generated is substantial.

Foulds suggested that tumors undergo a series of changes as part of the natural history of the disease. For example, tumors initially diagnosed as benign over a period of many months or even years assume a malignant phenotype. Nowell suggested that acquired genetic variability within developing clones of tumors, coupled with host selection pressures, results in new clonal sublines of increased growth autonomy or malignancy.

In four different experimental tumor models, highly metastatic cells were less phenotypically stable than their nonmetastatic counterparts isolated from the same single neoplasm. The rapid generation of diversity is presumed the product of increased genetic instability. Highly metastatic clones exhibit a higher rate of spontaneous mutation than the cells from poorly metastatic lines. These results are in accord with the hypothesis that tumor progression occurs as a result of acquired genetic alterations. Additional evidence that genetic mechanisms are responsible for tumor progression is from experiments using mutagens such as nitrosoguanidine or ultraviolet radiation. Treatment of tumor cell populations with mutagens induces variants with (1) increased tumorigenicity, (2) increased metastatic capacities, (3) decreased tumorigenic potential, and (4) increased immunogenicity. The more metastatic a tumor cell population is, the greater the likelihood that the constituent cells will undergo spontaneous mutations that result in rapid phenotypic diversification and increased opportunities for escape from various therapeutic modalities. Diversification may be further exaggerated by the mutagenic action of many of the cytotoxic antineoplastic drugs used in therapy.

Tumors of unicellular origin may exhibit metastatic heterogeneity very early in development. This conclusion is based upon the in vivo behavior of murine fibroblasts transformed by an oncogenic virus. Six colonies of murine embryo fibroblasts, each derived from a single cell, were infected in vivo with murine sarcoma virus and then propagated as pedigree cell lines. Intravenous injection of viable cells from each clone resulted in marked differences among the clones with regard to colonization of the lung. Because the parent cell population was derived from a single transformed cell, the differences resulted from rapid phenotypic diversification. Similarly, when the clones from two colonies (one of high and one of low experimental metastatic capacity) are subcloned and evaluated in the same manner, both clones exhibited a pattern of metastatic heterogeneity. As indicated earlier, the more metastatic tumors display greater heterogeneity. The clone with higher metastatic capacity exhibited a greater degree of variability than the clone with lower metastatic capacity. Thus, despite its single-cell origin, diversification occurred during the 6 weeks following the subcloning, to yield cells with different metastatic properties. Thus, generation of metastatic heterogeneity in neoplasms does not require a prolonged latent period.

Cells within the tumor mass are not autonomous units but are regulated by the proximity of other neoplastic cells. Different subpopulations of mammary tumor cells affect the growth patterns and chemosensitivity of other groups of cells (paracrine). Similar regulatory control may exist for the metastatic phenotype of different cells within a mixed tumor. Data from models and clinical observation provide evidence that different subpopulations of tumor cells stabilize their relative proportions and thereby impose an equilibrium on the combined population. Removal of the stabilizing effect, by isolating clones or by applying a strong selection pressure such as chemotherapy, leads to rapid diversification in the resurgent populations. Although the nature of these stabilizing influences and their mode of action are not yet understood, their very existence argues against randomness in tumor development. Rather, the "society" of tumor cells imposes regulatory constraints upon its individual members to maintain cellular diversity and its concomitant benefits for tumor survival. Certainly, this phenomenon, irrespective of its underlying mechanisms, further complicates attempts to understand the process of tumor progression toward malignancy.

Heterogeneity in Metastases. The origin of heterogeneity in metastases may occur as a consequence of primary tumor diversification. Pathologists have long recognized that primary tumors are made up of zones of morphologically distinct cells. Recent studies demonstrated that these zonal differences are not restricted to morphology, but include many other characteristics. Repeated passage of small tumor fragments rapidly imposes an artificial uniformity on tumor cell populations that is absent when larger, more representative populations are used. It is conceivable that embolic aggregates may arise from a single one of these zones and thus exhibit a degree of uniformity for specific characteristics even as resultant metastases. The same situation may arise when the embolus originates from an area of zonal junctions containing populations with varying phenotypes, and then selective cell death leads to the survival of only one cell. Alternatively, many or all of the cells forming such a mixed embolus may survive to act as the progenitors of metastatic tumors, in which case the generation of diversity, as in some primary tumors, is then a consequence of the multicellular origin of the neoplasm. Metastases may have a unicellular or a multicellular origin. To determine whether individual metastases are clonal and whether different metastases can be produced by different progenitor cells, tumor cells were x-irradiated to induce random chromosome breaks and rearrangements to serve as markers. If a metastasis were derived from a single cell, all the chromosome spreads examined within an individual metastasis would exhibit the same karyotype. By contrast, if metastases were formed from more than one progenitor cell, its constituent cells would exhibit different chromosomal arrangements, assuming, of course, that the different cells involved carried distinguishable karyotypic markers. The cellular composition of 21 individual metastases was analyzed after cultivation of cells from individual lesions. In 11 of 21 lesions, unique karyotypic patterns of abnormal, marker chromosomes were found, suggesting that each metastasis originated from a single progenitor cell. This experiment cannot resolve, however, whether metastases arose as a consequence of individual cells surviving in the bloodstream or whether homogeneous clumps (i.e., a multicellular embolus of cells with the same chromosome marker) survived in the circulation, but it does establish that many metastases do originate from single cells. The finding that different metastases are populated exclusively by cells with different chromosome markers indicates that different metastases originate from different progenitor cells.

These results from experiments in animal models using clones bearing identifiable biochemical markers demonstrated not only that the majority of metastases are of clonal origin, but also subsequently variant clones with diverse phenotypes rapidly formed to generate significant cellular diversity within individual metastases.

Collectively, these observations indicate that different metastases arise from different progenitor cells and account for the well-documented differences in the behavior of individual metastases in the same patient, including differences in response to therapy (i.e., interlesional heterogeneity). However, within individual metastases of proven clonal origin, heterogeneity can develop rapidly to create significant intralesional heterogeneity.

Metastatic Patterns. Metastasizing tumors have predilection for selected organ sites. In human beings, colon tumors frequently metastasize to the liver, renal cell carcinoma to the lung, melanoma to the lung and brain, and prostate cancer to the bone. Several hypotheses have been advanced to explain the selectivity observed in human as well as animal tumors. Indeed, specific organs may elaborate essential growth factors that enable tumors to proliferate. In human beings, evidence is emerging to suggest that bone marrow produces growth factors that facilitate propagation of prostatic cancer cells. In mice, implantation of mammary tumors into the mammary fat pad results in better tumor propagation than at other sites. Selection of cell lines from metastatic primary tumors results in enrichment of the cell population that metastasizes to a selected organ (e.g., the lung). Subcutaneous administration of the selected line results in an accumulation of tumor colonies in the lung. Specificity is illustrated in the same protocol, where ectopically transplanted lung tissue is also invaded by the lung-selected line. In addition to the optimum environment provided by selected organs, sites of metastases may be determined by interaction between tumor cell surface adhesion molecules (Table 9-9) or ligands of adhesion molecules. Adhesion molecules mediate many cell-cell and cell-matrix interactions. Metastatic melanoma cells express more VLA-4 than nonmetastatic cells, suggesting that this adhesion receptor may have some role in determining the endothelium that may be a site for interaction with the VLA-4 ligand, V-CAM. It is difficult to ascribe the adhesion molecule expression on tumor cells as an index of metastatic behavior or site of metastasis. Metastasis is a multistage process in which tumor cells acquire greater and greater autonomy with regard to growth factor requirements. Concurrently, the array of cell surface adhesion receptors or ligands may change thereby determining sites of metastasis.

No doubt metastasis is a complex process with no universally applicable mechanism. The only unifying concept is the dissemination of neoplastic disease to other sites and the challenge they present to the surgeon in the quest for successful eradication of residual disease. Knowledge of the biologic and biochemical events that induce, sustain, and disseminate neoplastic disease provides us with the basis for the development of new therapeutic strategies. The therapies may then address multiple targets within the tumor biology, thereby maximizing our chances for success.

CLINICAL MANIFESTATIONS

The clinical presentation of cancer is varied and inconstant. Cancer may appear as an asymptomatic lesion too small to be seen without magnification or special studies, such as mammography. It may appear as an asymptomatic lump, or the patient may complain of symptoms that are subsequently found to be caused by an underlying malignancy. Often, symptoms are nonspecific and may resemble those of nonmalignant diseases.

The clinical abnormalities produced by advancing neoplastic diseases are grouped into two categories, those abnormalities that stem directly from the presence of a tumor mass and those physiologic derangements that are produced indirectly. By teaching patients the key symptoms of cancer that require medical evaluation, earlier diagnosis and treatment may be achieved (Table 9-10).

Table 9-10
Cancer's Seven Warning Signals

Change in bowel or bladder habits
A sore that does not heal
Unusual bleeding or discharge
Thickening or lump in breast or elsewhere
Indigestion or difficulty in swallowing
Obvious change in wart or mole
Nagging cough or hoarseness

SOURCE: Adapted from the American Cancer Society.

The onset and latency period of the neoplastic state is difficult to establish in human cancers. As previously discussed, it may take as long as 5 to 8 years from the onset of an established cancer until clinically detectable disease (i.e., with a tumor of at least one billion cells comprising 1 mL in volume) evolves. Therefore, the use of the word *early* in describing a cancer may lead to confusion. To avoid this, we will use the terms *early* and *late* in relation to the clinical stage of a neoplasm rather than to indicate its duration in the body. When viewed in this manner, the curable cancer may have been present for years before its diagnosis and therapy. The term *early* usually refers to a neoplasm that can be effectively treated. These neoplasms are small rather than large, do not extend into essential organs, and have not metastasized. Some lesions that have been present for years still may be early stage, whereas other lesions with more rapid growth rates may be late stage even if present for only a few months.

The seven danger signals of cancer, as formulated by the American Cancer Society, are listed in Table 9-10. These may be helpful in the ongoing effort to educate people and increase the frequency of early diagnosis for certain major tumors. The more common patterns of clinical presentation, and some of the more common syndromes related to cancer, are discussed in detail in the paragraphs that follow. Symptoms of cancer result from inexorable growth, so there is a typical tempo or pattern of symptoms that increase in intensity, duration, and frequency.

Table 9-9
Adhesion Molecules, Cell Expression, and Ligands

Adhesion group	*Molecule*	*Ligand*	*Distribution*
Selectins	L-selectin	Carbohydrates	
Integrin supergene family	LFA-1	ICAM-1, -2	All leukocytes
	Mac-1	Fibrinogen, iC3b, LPS	Neutrophils, lymphocytes, some monocytes
	gp150/95	iC3b	Granulocytes, monocytes
	Vitronectin receptor	Vitronectin	
	Platelet IIb/IIIa	Vitronectin, fibrinogen, thromboplastin	
	VLA-1	Laminin (type I collagen)	
	VLA-2	Type I collagen (laminin)	
	VLA-3	Fibronectin (laminin and collagen)	
	VLA-4	V-CAM and fibronectin	Lymphocytes, melanoma calls
	VLA-5	Fibronectin	
	VLA-6	Laminin	
Immunoglobulin supergene family	LFA-3	CD2 (LFA-2)	
	ICAM-1	LDA-1	
	VCAM-1	VLA-4	Endothelium
	PECAM	?	
	Carcinoembryonic antigen	?	

Signs of Expansile Growth. The signs attributable to the expansile growth of a tumor depend on its location. When the neoplasm is either on or near the surface of the body, it may present simply as a visible or palpable mass. In the gastrointestinal, biliary, respiratory, and urinary tracts, signs are frequently related to obstruction. Examples are vomiting, jaundice, cough, and urinary retention. Within the central nervous system, expansile growth may cause pain, paralysis, or sensory loss.

Expansile growth of a tumor may also result in destruction of host tissues. Examples are pathologic fractures, hepatic insufficiency, and Addison's disease.

Signs of Infiltrative Growth. Pain, numbness, and paralysis may result when tumor infiltrates nerves. Frequently, signs of nerve invasion are also signs of incurability. Examples are lumbosacral plexus pain in cancer of the cervix and rectum, dorsal and lumbar spine pain in cancer of the pancreas, and the shoulder and arm pain and palsy when carcinoma of the lung infiltrates the brachial plexus. Other signs of infiltration, generally denoting incurability, are thickening of the uterine ligaments in cancer of the cervix and fixation to the chest wall in breast cancer.

Signs of Tumor Necrosis. Tumors may become necrotic, ulcerate, and bleed. Fatigue and weakness may be the only symptoms in cancer of the stomach or right colon, because the tumor ulceration and bleeding have resulted in anemia. If a tumor becomes ulcerated and infected, the signs and symptoms of inflammation will include edema, pain, tenderness, and fever. The inflammation caused by cecal cancer can mimic the clinical symptoms of acute appendicitis or cholecystitis. Therefore, response of such inflammation to antibiotics or the healing of an ulcer does *not* necessarily indicate a nonneoplastic lesion.

Tumor necrosis at any site may produce fever, leukocytosis, elevation of the erythrocyte sedimentation rate, anorexia, and malaise. Such necrosis constitutes one of the causes of the *fever of unknown origin*. Keller and Williams, in studies of 46 patients with unexplained fever, found that in 19 who underwent exploratory laparotomy the cause of the fever was intra-abdominal malignant disease.

Diagnosis of Nodal Metastases. Lymph nodes containing metastatic melanoma are generally more firm and rubbery, and are nontender compared with inflammatory nodes, which are usually softer, more resilient, and tender. For benign causes of adenopathy, there usually is evidence of infection or injury in the drainage region. It should be emphasized that some normal regional nodes are palpable in thin people, and others may merely have benign ''shotty'' nodes that have persisted for months or years.

Any adenopathy suspected of harboring metastatic disease should be investigated. If the index of suspicion for metastatic disease is low, the patient may be followed with frequent examination until a diagnosis can be made. If the examination is equivocal or close follow-up is not possible, either fine-needle or open biopsy may be warranted.

Unknown Primary Tumors Presenting as Metastases. Usually the site of origin of a metastasis is known. The initial presentation of a tumor, however, may be at a distance from its origin. The primary neoplasm giving rise to the metastasis may have regressed completely and may never be detected in some neoplasms, such as malignant melanoma and carcinomas of the oropharynx. Surgical resection of the metastatic lesions may result in long-term cure without the site of the primary ever being detected.

The most frequent sites of presentation of metastatic neoplasms are the cervical and supraclavicular lymph nodes, lungs, liver, bones, and brain. The most common metastatic sites for unknown primary neoplasms are listed in Table 9-11.

Systemic Manifestations of Malignant Disease. Tumors may have a variety of remote and systemic effects that contribute to morbidity. Cancer patients frequently develop unusual symptoms and physiologic derangements that cannot be attributed to the mechanical presence of primary or metastatic disease, or to physiologic changes resulting from hormones normally secreted by the tissue of origin.

Some symptoms, such as the cachexia of carcinomatosis, may result from competition between the tumor and the host for basic components of the same metabolic pool. The pathogenesis of many of these disorders is unknown, however. Some of these nonmetastatic, systemic manifestations of malignant tumors are thought to result from (1) the ectopic production of known hormones; (2) the secretion of unidentified, physiologically active substances that do not resemble known hormones but that have hormone-like effects; (3) autoimmune phenomena, in which the host is sensitized to an antigen from the tumor; and/or (4) toxic substances secreted from the tumor.

The systemic clinical manifestations of malignant disease and the neoplasms with which they are associated are presented in Table 9-12. Sometimes palliative surgery is indicated to treat these systemic manifestations (e.g., resection of metastases that are producing hormones that induce hypercalcemia or hypoglycemia).

DIAGNOSIS AND STAGING

Diagnosis

Diagnosis of cancer should proceed in an orderly fashion: careful history, thorough physical examination with examination of the blood and urine, and investigation of suspicious findings by appropriate radiologic examinations and radioisotope scans.

Table 9-11
Unknown Primary Tumors Presenting as Metastases

Site of metastasis	*Primary neoplasm*
Lymph nodes:	
Cervical nodes	Nasopharynx, pharnyx, oral cavity, thyroid, larynx, lymphomas
Supraclavicular nodes	Bronchus, breast, stomach, esophagus, pancreas, colon, testis, ovary, cervix
Axillary nodes	Breast, melanoma, lymphoma
Inguinal nodes	Genitalia, anus, melanoma
Skin and subcutaneous tissues	Melanoma, breast, bronchus, stomach, kidney
Lung	Breast, colon, kidney, stomach, testis, melanoma, thyroid, sarcomas
Liver	Stomach, colon, breast, pancreas, bronchus
Ovary	Colon, stomach
Bones	Breast, bronchus, prostate, thyroid
Central nervous system	Breast, bronchus, kidney, colon
Serous cavities	Bronchus, breast, ovary, lymphoma
Gastrointestinal tract	Melanoma

Table 9-12
Systemic Manifestations of Malignant Disease

Clinical Manifestations	*Associated Neoplasms*	*Clinical Manifestations*	*Associated Neoplasms*
Cutaneous			
Acanthosis nigricans	Cancer of stomach, lung, and breast	Hormonal and metabolic effects of nonendocrine tumors	
Dermatomyositis	Cancer of stomach, breast, lung, and ovary	Hypoglycemia (mechanism unknown)	Retroperitoneal or mediastinal mesenchymal tumors, hepatic tumors
Erythema multiforme, exfoliative dermatitis, bullous pemphigoid	Allergic response to a variety of neoplasms, lymphoma, myeloma		
Peutz-Jeghers syndrome	Intestinal polyposis	Cushing's syndrome (increased ACTH)	Cancer of the lung, malignant thymoma, pancreatic cancer
Hematologic		Hypercalcemia (increased PTH, vitamin D-like substances or bone destruction)	Cancer of lung, kidney, breast, uterus, sarcomas, hemopoietic neoplasms
Abdominal red cell mass			
Erythrocytosis (increased erythropoietin)	Renal cell carcinoma, hepatoma, uterine myoma, cerebellar tumors, pheochromocytoma	Hyponatremia (increased ADH)	Cancer of lung, intracranial tumors
Anemia		Hyperthyroidism (increased)	Choriocarcinoma (TSH) testicular embryonal carcinoma
Myelophthisic	All tumors		
Hypoproliferative	Thymoma, renal cell carcinoma	Precocious puberty and/or gynecomastia (increased gonadotropin)	Hepatoma, lung, adrenal cancer, testicular tumors
Hemolytic	Hemopoietic neoplasm	Zollinger-Ellison syndrome (increased gastrin secretion)	Pancreatic nonbeta islet cell adenomas
Miscellaneous causes (infection, bleeding, radiation effects, uremia, etc.)		Elevated liver enzymes	Renal cell carcinoma
Abnormal leukocyte or platelet mass	Miscellaneous neoplasms	Anorexia and weight loss	Most neoplasms
		Hyperuricemia	Hemopoietic neoplasms
Leukemoid reactions	Hemopoietic neoplasms, lung, pancreas	Atypical carcinoid syndrome	Pancreatic duct, islet cell gastric, thyroid, and oat cell cancer of lung
Leukopenia			
Thrombocytosis		Nonmetastatic neuromuscular multifocal leukoencephalopathy	Hemopoietic neoplasms
Coagulation and bleeding disorder			
Disseminated intravascular coagulation	Mucin-secreting adenocarcinoma	Subacute cerebellar degeneration	Multiple neoplasms, especially of lung, ovary, and breast
Vascular			

A *history* of any of the warning signs listed in Table 9-10 should prompt a search for cancer.

Physical examination includes a thorough search of the entire skin surface for squamous cell and basal cell carcinomas, indurated lesions, ulcers, suspicious or irritated nevi, nodules, and other signs of malignant disease. Lymph nodes should be palpated for enlargement. Breasts should be carefully examined. All body orifices should be examined. A Pap smear from the cervix should be obtained at a biannual pelvic examination. Rectal examination should include proctoscopic examination of patients who have hemorrhoids or rectal symptoms. The oropharynx should be examined, with special attention to the floor of the mouth. Indirect laryngoscopy should be performed if the patient is hoarse, has a neck mass, or is suspected of having an intrathoracic neoplasm or cancer of the thyroid gland.

Laboratory examination should include a complete blood cell count, urinalysis, examination of stool for occult blood, and chest x-ray. Other tests should be ordered where indicated by symptoms. Before operating on a patient for cure or palliation, a metastatic workup should be done, directed by symptoms and the most likely site of metastases. Prior to extensive disfiguring or disabling procedures, tomograms of the lungs, bone marrow biopsy, scalene node biopsy, isotope scans, or arteriography may be useful in determining whether the neoplasm is still localized. Cytologic examination should be performed if a pleural effusion or ascites is present.

Diagnosis of solid tumors rests on locating and performing a biopsy of the lesion. This goal is most easily fulfilled when the tumor is near the body surface or involves one of the orifices of the body that can be examined with appropriate visual instruments, such as a bronchoscope, proctoscope, or cystoscope. Carcinomas of the breast, tongue, or rectum can be seen or palpated, and a portion can be excised for definitive diagnosis.

The most difficult cancers to diagnose, and unfortunately the most lethal ones, occur in the internal organs. Space-occupying lesions in the internal organs may grow quite large before causing symptoms. Techniques that may be useful in localizing such lesions include barium examinations of the gastrointestinal tract; examination of the bronchial tree by endoscopy; selective arteriography of major vessels supplying internal organs; radiographic examination using radioisotopes and radiopaque dyes that concentrate in various organs such as the liver, gallbladder, kidney, and lymph nodes; and ultrasonography and abdominal computer-assisted tomography (CT), which is rapidly becoming the most useful investigative technique for intra-abdominal tumors). Exploratory surgery is often required to confirm the diagnosis and obtain biopsy.

Screening and Detection

All physicians should participate actively in cancer screening and early detection programs. Successful screening programs must have both a cost-effective method for detecting early cancers and a targeted group of individuals at high enough risk to justify its application. Early detection of cancer not only has the potential to improve cure rates but in many instances enables the surgeon to limit the extent of surgery.

In the future, the surgeon will become increasingly involved in prevention of cancer by identifying high-risk patients and intervening to diminish their risks. The surgeon can clarify how simple changes in life-style, such as quitting smoking to prevent lung cancer and decreasing sunlight exposure for fair-skinned individuals at risk for melanoma, can effect prevention. Pharmacologic measures to modulate those conditions that predispose an individual to cancer are also becoming a reality. An excellent example of this chemopreventive approach is a recent study demonstrating a significant decrease in the incidence of severe oral leukoplakia in subjects using 13-cis-retinoic acid.

The list of cancers, the treatment and prognosis of which can be improved by early detection, grows longer each year. Today it is estimated that more than 18,000 lives would be saved each year if women older than age 40 would undergo screening mammography according to American Cancer Society guidelines. Once a cancer is detected in its early stages, the surgeon has a number of treatment options. Most melanomas are now detected early and treated by relatively narrow excision; furthermore, the cure rate has doubled to 80 percent or greater during the 1970s and 1980s. The national mortality rate from cervical carcinoma has declined dramatically since the advent of the Pap test, which allows for treatment of precursor lesions or early cancers, often without hysterectomy. Individuals with small rectal cancers are another group with a high probability for cure (greater than 80 percent) for whom local excision of the carcinoma might be considered; in this case, local excision replaces abdominal and perineal resection of the rectum. Even patients with lung cancer have a 50 percent 5-year survival rate and generally have less lung tissue removed if the tumor is detected early.

Screening programs should cover especially those who have an inherited susceptibility to cancer. Among these are individuals with a family history of breast cancer, colon cancer, and medullary thyroid cancer, and those with predisposing conditions such as dysplastic nevus syndrome and polyposis of the colon.

Any given individual stands approximately 1 chance in 4 of developing cancer during his or her lifetime. Therefore, in screening 1000 persons for an entire life span, we will find cancer in 250 of them. Since a person can harbor more than one primary cancer and a second lesion will develop with increasing frequency as the number of people who have survived the first one increases, we might count on a very crude estimate of 350 cancers in our population of 1000. Since we expect people to live an average of 72 years, we must carry out 72,000 annual examinations to discover 350 cancers, or less than 5 cancers per 1000 examinations. By directing our research to the middle and late adult years when the incidence is highest, we might conceivably double the yield to 10 per 1000. Thus, the chances of detecting cancer in a given annual examination are no more than 1 in 100 even under the most optimal circumstances.

Biopsy

It is imperative that microscopic proof of malignant disease be obtained prior to institution of treatment, since significant morbidity and mortality may result from all forms of cancer therapy. The specific type of antitumor therapy will depend on the histologic type of tumor, which must be established by biopsy. Significant errors have been made when biopsies were not obtained (radical mastectomies for fat necrosis and radiation therapy for renal cysts, for example).

Even when biopsy reports from another hospital are available, the slides of the previous biopsy must be obtained and reviewed prior to the institution of therapy. This is essential because, not infrequently and particularly in rare neoplasms, an erroneous interpretation may have been made. *Definitive therapy cannot be planned rationally without knowing the nature of the neoplastic lesion.*

Three methods for biopsy of suspicious tissue are commonly used. They are the *needle*, the *incisional*, and the *excisional*, or open, biopsy; each has its advantages and disadvantages. Regardless of the method used, the pathologic interpretation of the tumor mass can be valid only if a representative section of tumor is obtained. A problem of "sampling error" can occur with the needle and the incisional biopsies when only a small portion of the total tumor mass is submitted for pathologic examination.

Needle biopsy is the simplest method and may be used for biopsy of subcutaneous masses, muscular masses, and some internal organs, such as liver, kidney, and pancreas. Furthermore, this method is inexpensive and causes minimal disturbance of the surrounding tissue. The danger of implanting tumor cells in a needle track during aspiration biopsy is extremely small and can be avoided if the location of the needle track is such that it can be excised easily at the time of the definitive surgical procedure. Needle biopsy may be disadvantageous when the specimen is quite small and not representative of the total tumor, or the needle may miss the space-occupying lesion. Hence, a needle or aspiration biopsy does require experience to interpret. A negative report for malignant disease is always viewed with skepticism and should be followed by incisional or excisional biopsy if there is any doubt.

Some centers have used fine-needle aspiration cytology. In this procedure, a fine needle is inserted into the tumor, and strands of single cells are obtained for cytologic diagnosis. This procedure is extremely useful for a number of tumors but requires considerable skill to interpret and should only be done by an experienced pathologist.

Incisional biopsy involves removal of only a portion of a tumor mass for pathologic examination. An incisional biopsy may be performed using a scalpel or a core biopsy punch. It is best performed so that, if tumor cells are spilled at the time of biopsy, the incisional wound can be encompassed and totally excised at the time of the definitive surgical procedure. Incisional biopsy includes removal of portions of tumor with forceps during endoscopic examination of the bronchus, esophagus, rectum, and bladder. Incisional biopsy is indicated for deeper subcutaneous or muscular tumor masses when needle biopsy fails to establish a diagnosis.

The incisional biopsy is also used when a tumor is so large that total local excision would prejudice any subsequent adequate, wide locally curative resection because of the wide tissue planes that are necessarily exposed by biopsy. It may also be performed for larger tumors around the face or digits, where preservation of tissue is particularly important to preserve function or cosmesis. Such biopsy should take a deep section of tumor, as well as a margin of normal tissues, if possible. Incisional biopsy does suffer from the same hazard as the needle biopsy in that the removed portion may not be representative of all the involved tissue; hence, a negative biopsy does not preclude the presence of cancer in the remaining mass. Another theoretical objection to the incisional method is the possibility that the surgeon may seed cancer cells into the operative wound or that exposed open lymphatics may transport the cells to distant sites. Despite these dangers, one must keep in mind that definitive surgical procedures cannot be planned rationally without knowing the nature of the neoplastic lesion.

Excisional biopsy is total local removal of the tumor mass. This is used for small, discrete masses, 2 to 3 cm in diameter, when local removal will not interfere with the wider excision required for permanent local control. A major advantage of an excisional biopsy is that it gives the entire lesion to the pathologist. This method is contraindicated in large tumor masses because, again, the biopsy procedure may scatter tumor cells throughout a large biopsy incision that must be widely and totally encompassed by subsequent definitive surgical procedures. Therefore, excisional biopsy is usually contraindicated for skeletal and soft tissue sarcomas, although it is ideally suitable for superficial squamous or basal cell carcinomas and malignant melanomas.

A narrow margin (i.e., several millimeters) of normal-appearing tissue is removed with tumor mass. A wider margin is generally not indicated because the biopsy as a diagnostic procedure may be insufficient treatment for a malignant tumor but excessive for a benign one. Surgeons should always mark the excisional biopsy margins with sutures so that if removal is incomplete, they will know where tumor margin was positive should further excision be indicated.

Biopsy incisions should be closed with meticulous hemostasis, since it may be possible for a collecting hematoma to extend tumor cell contamination by widespread infiltration of tissue planes. Contaminated instruments, gloves, gowns, and drapes should be discarded and replaced with noncontaminated substitutes when the definitive procedure is to follow immediately after the biopsy procedure.

The excisional method is principally used for polypoid lesions of the colon, for thyroid and breast nodules, for small skin lesions, and when the pathologist cannot make a definitive diagnosis from tissue removed by incisional biopsy. An unbiopsied lump is surgically removed when the suspicious character of the lesion, the need for its removal whatever the diagnosis, and the nonmutilating nature of the operation make such an approach reasonably definitive. Examples of such procedures include hemithyroidectomy for thyroid nodules, partial colectomy for lesions at any point beyond the reach of the sigmoidoscope, and a right colectomy for a cecal mass that might be inflammatory or neoplastic.

Lymph nodes should be carefully selected for biopsy. Cervical lymph nodes should not be biopsied until a careful search for a primary tumor has been made. Indirect laryngoscopy, pharyngoscopy, esophagoscopy, bronchoscopy, and thyroid scan may be included in the workup. Enlargement of the upper cervical nodes is usually due to metastases from laryngeal, oropharyngeal, and nasopharyngeal neoplasms. Supraclavicular nodes are more frequently enlarged from metastases originating in the thoracic or abdominal cavity.

The specimen may be prepared for pathologic examination by either frozen or permanent sections. Frozen sections are made immediately, and pathologic diagnosis can be obtained within 10 to 20 minutes. Although frozen sections may be as adequate as permanent sections for diagnosis of some neoplasms, most pathologists would prefer to make a definitive diagnosis in questionable cases on permanent sections. In circumstances when pathology might be difficult to interpret, a thin slice of the tumor mass should be fixed in a glutaraldehyde solution so that it can be processed for electron microscopy if the light microscopic evaluation of the tissue is not definitive. If the tumor mass might be a lymphoma, the freshly biopsied specimen should be examined for lymphoid cell-surface marker expression. Although permanent sections or special stains require 1 to 2 days for processing, it is usually best to have a definite diagnosis before discussing the therapeutic options. Therefore, frozen sections are used when the diagnosis is required at the time of major surgery and when it is in the patient's best interests to have the definitive resectional surgery carried out at that time.

Occasionally, an exploratory thoracotomy or laparotomy will be necessary to obtain tissue for microscopic examination and confirmation of diagnosis. These procedures are being replaced by thoracoscopy and laparoscopy. As a general rule, regardless of the clinical picture, the neoplastic nature of the disease process must be confirmed by frozen section examination prior to closure of the wound. This is critical because the permanent sections may fail to confirm the neoplastic nature of the pathologic process, and the patient will have experienced the morbidity of operation without obtaining a diagnosis.

Exfoliative cytology constitutes one possible method for the early diagnosis of certain types of neoplasms. This technique is based on the fact that cancer cells are shed from the surfaces of neoplasms arising in epithelial-lined body cavities and orifices, such as the vagina, bronchus, and stomach. These cells can be collected, stained, and recognized as malignant because of their individual morphologic changes.

Staging

The extent of the patient's tumor as determined by clinical evaluation at the time of initial presentation is called the *clinical stage*. In addition to making an exact histologic diagnosis of cancer, it is essential that the clinical stage of the disease be determined prior to making a decision regarding therapy. This is especially important when the patient initially presents for treatment, but also it is often desirable to repeat some of the diagnostic procedures periodically during the patient's course in order to assess his or her true status. The recognized importance of this staging has led to a variety of international and national attempts to standardize the staging of the patient with cancer. The staging system published by the American Joint Committee on Cancer is now accepted as the standard criteria for cancer staging (Table 9-13). Stage I usually indicates a small neoplasm confined to its primary site of origin. Stage II is for larger tumors or metastases to the regional lymph nodes, while stages III and IV indicate regional or distant metastatic spread.

Cancer staging uses the TNM system, which focuses on the extent of tumor in terms of the primary tumor (T), presence or absence of node metastases (N), and the presence or absence of distant metastases (M). The system was developed following careful analysis of the results of treatment in patients with various constellations of clinical findings. It was found that patients with larger tumors did less well than those with smaller tumors; hence, the separation of various stages on the basis of tumor size. For different tumors size criteria vary, but in this system decreasing prognosis is indicated by increasing numbers after the T, such as T1, T2, T3, or T4 for lesions of increasing sizes. The presence or absence of regional spread is usually indicated by variations in the secondary category, under N for nodes. The absence of nodal metastasis is designated as N0; the presence of nodal metastasis is N1;

Table 9-13
TNM Classification of Patients

Tumor	
T0	No evidence of primary tumor
Tis	Carcinoma in situ
T1,T2,T3,T4	Progressive increase in tumor size or involvement
Nodes	
N0	No evidence of regional node involvement
N1,N2,N3,N4	Increasing degrees of demonstrable abnormality of regiona lymph nodes
Metastasis	
M0	No evidence of distant metastasis
M1	Distant metastasis present
Histopathology	(Histopathology refers to the histologic type of cancer.)
Grade (G)	
GX	Grade cannot be assessed
G1	Well-differentiated
G2	Moderately well-differentiated
G3–G4	Poorly to very poorly differentiated; use whichever indicator is most appropriate (term or G+ number).

for more extensive nodal involvement, additional numbers may be used. Finally, distant metastases are indicated by adding a subscript 1 following M for metastases, or a subscript 0 for their absence. Thus, a small lesion that has neither spread to regional nodes nor metastasized would be designated as a T1N0M0 lesion. A lesion that was larger and involved regional nodes but without distant metastases might be identified as a T2N1M0 lesion. A larger neoplasm with both regional and distant metastases would be designated a T3N1M1 lesion. For some tumor types such as soft tissue sarcoma, a G for grade of malignancy is added. High-grade tumors are more anaplastic and tend to metastasize sooner.

The American Joint Committee on Cancer recognizes several types of cancer staging schemas. The clinical-diagnostic staging (cTNM) represents the extent of disease prior to first definitive treatment. Postsurgical resection-pathologic staging (pTNM) provides additional information after operation, and is especially useful in planning adjuvant therapy for many types of tumors. Other staging types include surgical-evaluative staging (sTNM), usually used for tumors that cannot be resected, retreatment staging (rTNM), usually used after a disease-free interval, and autopsy staging (aTNM).

The importance of accurate staging when designating a therapeutic program for a patient with cancer cannot be overemphasized. It is an important consideration when comparing the results of therapy in different centers, and as therapeutic methods for cancer improve, it is only by careful staging that new forms of therapy can be appropriately evaluated. For example, only accurate staging can identify patients, such as those with stage II breast cancer, whose more advanced disease is still potentially curable by adjuvant therapy. These patients probably have subclinical metastases at the time of operation.

The present staging methods cannot characterize subclinical microscopic metastatic lesions. Many patients who are treated for apparently localized cancers already have disseminated metastases. For example, about one-half of those patients who have cancer of the breast and who undergo various types of mastectomy have subclinical distant metastasis at the time of the operation. However, this problem can be approached by assigning prognostic risk factors for undetected metastatic diseases to a clinical stage.

Posttreatment Screening and Surveillance

After treatment for the initial presentation of cancer, patients are followed periodically to detect recurrences. Surveillance and follow-up for distant metastatic disease should be tempered by the patient's initial stage of disease. For patients with early cancer, a judicious metastatic workup should be performed at regular intervals. Natural history studies have demonstrated that about 75 percent of recurrences will occur within the first 2 years, and 95 percent within the first 5 years. However, some patients are at continuing risk for developing a distant metastatic disease even 10 years after treatment and beyond.

Metastatic breast cancer can occur anywhere in the body. However, there are specific patterns of recurrence, especially for first recurrences, that should be taken into account that will direct a more selective metastatic evaluation. For example, the liver is the most common site of relapse for colorectal cancer, bone for breast cancer, the lung for extremity sarcomas, and the skin and subcutaneous tissue for melanomas. In our practice, we perform a metastatic survey at 3- to 4-month intervals during the first 2 years, at 6-month intervals to the fifth year, and yearly thereafter. In general, this evaluation consists of a history and physical examination, chest x-ray, and serum liver enzyme level determination, particularly alkaline phosphatase. A metastatic bone scan can be performed on an optional basis for early disease at the second and fifth year in those patients at risk. It is useful to have a baseline bone scan performed before or after surgery, especially for patients with stage II or III breast cancer, because they are at higher risk of developing bone metastasis, compared with patients with stage I breast cancer. Currently, available tumor markers, such as carcinoembryonic antigen, CA125, and other markers, are not sufficiently sensitive or cost effective to justify being used for routine screening.

TREATMENT

Surgery and radiation therapy today represent the most successful means of dealing with cancer as long as it remains localized to the primary site and regional lymph nodes. Since these forms of therapy exert their effect locally, neither can be considered curative once the disease has metastasized beyond the local region, although both methods of therapy may be useful as palliative treatment. Chemotherapy, hormone therapy, and immunotherapy, unlike surgery and radiation therapy, represent systemic forms of treatment effective against tumor cells already metastatic to distant organ sites. These systemic therapeutic modalities offer a greater chance of curing patients with a minimal number of tumor cells than those with clinically evident disease. Thus, though surgery and radiation therapy cannot be curative unless the tumor is confined locally or regionally, they can decrease the patient's tumor burden so that chemotherapy, hormone therapy, or immunotherapy may become more effective. During the past several years, enough evidence has accumulated to suggest that treatment combining surgery, radiation therapy, chemotherapy, hormone therapy, and, possibly, immunotherapy will significantly improve cure rates above those achieved with any single therapeutic modality.

Just as oncology should be approached as a unique field of study, so cancer should be regarded as a single but complex disease requiring a multidisciplinary approach. The practice of assigning certain types of neoplasms to surgery, radiation therapy, or medicine with a further division into various anatomically oriented specialties should be discontinued.

Goals of Therapy: Cure or Palliation. Once the diagnosis of malignant disease has been made and the extent of disease determined, a decision must be made about the goal of the therapy. *Is the patient curable?* This is the foremost question that must be answered before the physician recommends aggressive therapy with its attendant complications. The goals of therapy vary with the extent of the cancer. If the cancer is localized without evidence of spread, the goal is to eradicate the cancer and cure the patient. When the cancer is spread beyond local cure, the goal is to control the patient's symptoms and to maintain maximum activity for the longest possible period of time. Palliation should be measured in terms of useful life.

Patients are generally judged as incurable if they have distant metastases or evidence of extensive local infiltration of adjacent organs or structures. The most common criterion for incurability is distant metastasis. Some patients, however, are potentially curable even if they have distant metastases. For example, patients with solitary pulmonary metastases may be curable by resection, and even those with widespread metastases who have choriocarcinoma may be curable with chemotherapy. Histologic proof of distant metastases should be obtained before the patient is assessed as incurable. Occasionally, an exploratory celiotomy, thoracotomy, or laparoscopy/thoracoscopy may be necessary to determine the nature of equivocal lesions in the lungs or liver. In some situations (e.g., multiple pulmonary metastases) the clinical situation may point so overwhelmingly to distant metastases that the patient may safely be considered incurable without biopsy.

Local extension may be a criterion of incurability. For each anatomic site, there are certain local criteria that place the patient unequivocally in an incurable status, while others imply a poor prognosis but are not absolutely indicative of incurability. In equivocal situations after extensive studies have failed to demonstrate metastatic or incurable local extension, the patient deserves the benefit of doubt and should be treated for cure.

Choice of Therapy. Radiation therapy and chemotherapy are the most frequently used therapeutic modalities in the fight against cancer. Each may play a role in both curative and palliative therapy. Biologic therapy is a new modality that has a limited role in cancer therapy at the present time, but one that may become increasingly useful in the future. In choosing therapy, a variety of factors must be considered regardless of whether the aim is cure or palliation. The natural history of the disease and the results obtained from each type of therapy must be known prior to choosing a modality or combination of modalities.

The patient's general condition and the presence of any coexisting disease must be considered in planning therapy. Surgery may be contraindicated in a patient who has recently experienced a myocardial infarction. A patient with pre-existing diabetes will be much more susceptible to the toxic effects of hormonal therapy with corticosteroids. Renal disease may increase the toxicity of some of the chemotherapeutic drugs, such as methotrexate. In addition, any evidence of infection or bleeding in a patient may make any form of cancer therapy dangerous, requiring vigorous treatment prior to the initiation of definitive therapy.

The psychologic makeup of the patient and the patient's life situation must be considered. A patient who is unable to accept the realities of a given treatment should be offered an alternative approach when possible. This is particularly true of any surgical procedures that significantly alter appearance or that involve change of organ function requiring the patient's daily care, such as colostomy. Experimental forms of therapy, such as intra-arterial infusion of drugs, should also be avoided in some patients. Obviously, a patient who is going to be unwilling to tolerate the inconvenience of an intra-arterial catheter and who might remove it without medical approval should not undergo such treatment.

Multimodality Cancer Therapy and Clinical Decision-Making

Determining the most appropriate treatment plan for a cancer patient is one of the most difficult decision-making processes in clinical medicine. The biologic presentations are varied, the treatment options are many, and the patient's differing perception of "quality of life" all have to be incorporated into the decision-making process.

This section is intended to provide a framework for decision-making involving the management of cancer patients, including the coordination of the overall care of the patient, not only for surgical treatment, but also for the coordination of a multidisciplinary care involving two, three, or even four different modalities of cancer treatment. An example is the algorithm of breast cancer decisions shown in Figure 9-27.

Why should the surgeon be involved in the broader issues of oncology management? In the past, there have been very few treatment options available and surgical treatment was the mainstay of breast cancer management. The surgeon made the diagnosis and provided the first (and usually the only) treatment. In recent years, however, decision-making regarding cancer treatment for many types of cancer have undergone fundamental changes. For example, it has evolved to a point where multidisciplinary cancer care is the standard of treatment for most breast and colon cancer patients.

If the surgeon is to retain the primary coordinating role in cancer management, then he or she must fully understand all aspects of oncology management and know how to deploy them in individual patients. This includes knowledge about the indications, risks, and benefits of various cancer surgery options, adjuvant chemotherapy, hormonal therapy, radiation therapy, and the importance of reconstructive surgery. The proper treatment for an individual patient depends on planning the right combination and sequence of treatments in an individual situation that take into account the patient's physical, emotional, psychological, and rehabilitation needs. An example of this approach is shown in Figure 9-19.

Principles of Cancer Decision-Making

The decision-making process that leads to a treatment plan requires the integration of information from four areas: (1) natural history of the disease by histological type, (2) clinical staging, (3) goals of treatment, and (4) indications and risks for each treatment (or combination of treatments) based on results of clinical trials.

Natural History. Clinical decision-making for cancer patients requires knowledge about the natural history of the disease as a starting point. For example, there are four components of breast cancer that must be taken into account in treatment planning: (1) the primary breast cancer itself, (2) multicentric (or multifocal) cancer elsewhere in the breast, (3) axillary nodal metasta-

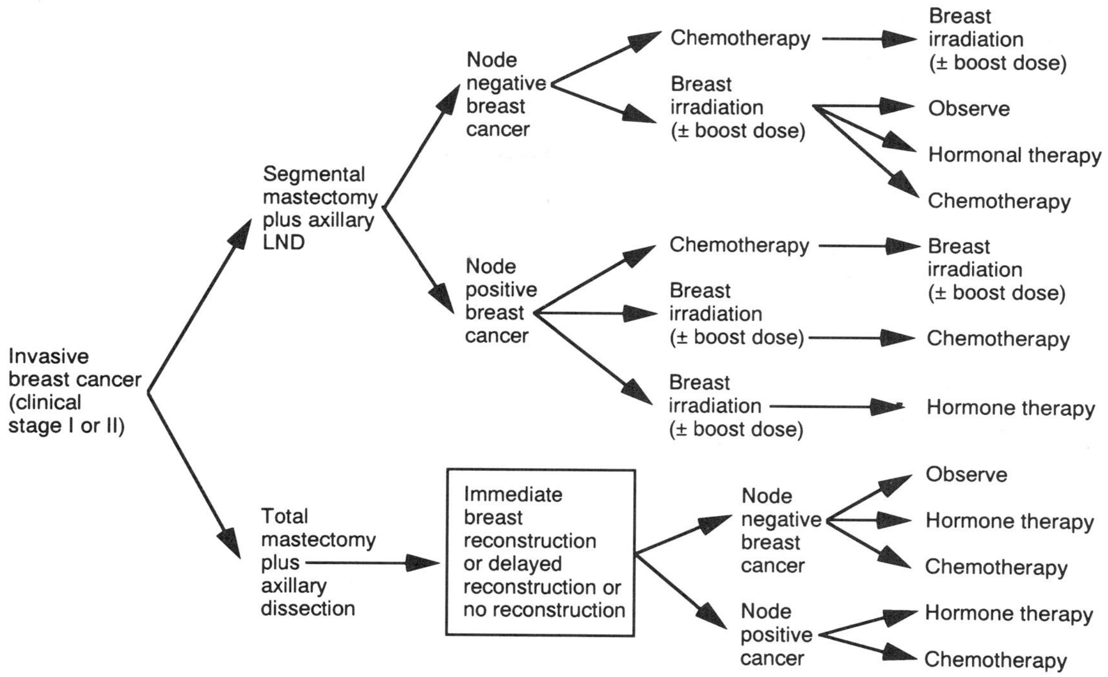

FIG. 9-27. An algorithm depicting treatment options for early-stage breast cancer. The first-level treatment decisions involve options for local/regional treatment. The basic choice here is between breast conservation surgery plus irradiation or modified radical mastectomy with the option of breast reconstructive surgery. A second level of decision is made postoperatively regarding the deployment of adjuvant chemotherapy or hormonal therapy.

ses, and (4) distant microscopic metastases. The presence of ductal carcinoma in situ is a marker in individuals who might develop invasive breast cancer in the *ipsilateral* breast, while lobular carcinoma in situ is a marker of patients who are at high risk for developing invasive breast cancer in *either* breast. A mastectomy or breast irradiation would adequately treat the first condition but not the second. Cystosarcoma phyloides, invasive tubular carcinoma, and small in situ ductal carcinomas do not metastasize to the axillary lymph nodes, so an operation to remove these glands is unnecessary. The patient's genetic background may also affect the biology of the disease. Thus, patients with breast cancer family syndrome have a high risk for developing bilateral breast cancer compared to those with sporadic (nonfamilial) breast cancer.

Staging and Prognosis. The stage of cancer and knowledge about prognostic factors that predict the risk of metastases are both important to delineate before embarking on treatment decisions. Despite the fact that many cancer patients have microscopic metastatic disease at the time of the initial presentation, our ability to detect metastases with currently available tests is low. A metastatic workup for most early cancers (i.e., stages I and II) consists of a history and physical examination, chest x-ray, and liver function enzymes as a starting point. CT scans of the brain, chest, and abdomen are not indicated in the absence of the signs or symptoms suggestive of metastatic cancer based on the preliminary screening test described above.

The tumor size and nodal status are still the primary parameters for clinical staging. However, the surgeon must take into account the risk of microscopic metastatic disease based on prognostic factors. For example, a woman with a stage I melanoma located on her leg has a 10 percent risk or less of having microscopic metastatases, while a man with a stage I scalp melanoma has a 60 percent risk or greater of harboring occult metastases. Estimating the risk of microscopic distant metastases in a patient with node-negative breast cancer based on histologic grade, tumor size, hormone receptor expression, and flow cytometry data is important for recommending adjuvant systemic chemotherapy or hormonal therapy. There is no single prognostic factor that helps in these decisions, and the surgeon must take into account the net effect of combinations of prognostic features of the tumor.

Goals of Treatment. There are six potential goals for surgical treatment of breast cancer:

1. Cure
2. Local disease control
3. Staging
4. Cosmetic result
5. Rehabilitation
6. Prevention

Each of these goals must be taken into account when arriving at a final treatment plan. In many circumstances, variations in surgical treatment will not influence ultimate survival outcome. Nevertheless, the type of surgery used (alone or in combination with radiation therapy) may affect the other goals of cancer treatment described above. For example, a limited axillary dissection may result in understaging of the cancer (which may in turn influence subsequent decisions regarding adjuvant systemic therapy) and also expose the patient to the risk of having a subsequent operation for axillary recurrences in the future. Performing a modified radical mastectomy without discussing the option of breast reconstructive surgery with the patient is simply not good rehabilitation for most breast cancer patients.

Risk/Benefit Ratio. Each component of cancer treatment has its own indications, risks, and benefits. When used in combinations, these treatments may have additive or cumulative effects. For example, arm edema increases significantly after a complete axillary dissection and axillary irradiation. When planning surgical excision of a melanoma, the margins of excision are critically important. If too narrow, the risk of a local recurrence increases, and is associated with a high mortality from metastases. If the margins are too wide, the patient may be severely disfigured.

Adjuvant chemotherapy is being deployed increasingly, even preoperatively in some patients. The use of adjuvant chemotherapy has proved beneficial in some circumstances but not in others. For example, adjuvant chemotherapy may increase survival rates for node-positive patients with breast cancer and colon cancer, but not for most patients with node-negative cancers of the breast or colon. Adjuvant therapy has no proven benefit for any subgroup of surgically treated melanoma patients. Some adjuvant chemotherapy regimens can entail serious morbidity and even mortality. The surgeon must understand the deployment of systemic therapy in sufficient detail in order to counsel with the patient and to decide when to consult with the medical oncologist.

It should be clear from this brief discussion that modern cancer management often requires a team of surgeons and physicians, each of whom bring a perspective and treatment benefit to the cancer patient. The surgeon should be an effective partner in this team and be able to coordinate the overall care of the breast cancer patient after consulting with radiation oncologists, medical oncologists and reconstructive surgeons.

Curative Treatment. The primary goal of cancer surgery is to excise the offending cancer (at the primary site, at multicentric sites, and in the axillary lymph nodes) so that the cancer cells at these sites will not be a continuing source of metastases to other organs. Clearly, surgical excision for early forms of cancer, such as early breast cancer detected by mammography, is curative in the majority of patients. On the other hand, patients with more biologically aggressive or later-stage cancers already have a high risk of harboring distant microscopic metastases that will override the curative effects of surgery as a local or regional treatment.

Local Disease Control. Another important goal of cancer surgery is to prevent residual tumor cells from arising at a later time as a clinical recurrence because they were not excised at the first operation. This is a valid goal of surgical treatment, even when the probability for cure is low. The value of surgical treatment has sometimes not been fully appreciated because it is difficult to prove that the details of surgical approaches have a measurable impact on survival rates. However, a surgical procedure that leaves the patient with a risk of 10 to 15 percent or greater that a subsequent major operation under general anesthesia will be required is simply not adequate surgical treatment. This is true even if the salvage surgery for such patients does not impact on their overall cure rates. For example, leaving a positive or close surgical margin around a primary breast cancer would result in a 20 percent failure rate within the breast and the subsequent need for mastectomy under general anesthesia, which is not acceptable surgical treatment for achieving local disease control.

Cancer Staging. Documenting the presence or absence of the primary tumor, multicentric disease, and nodal metastasis is a vitally important part of the breast cancer operation. For example, a more complete axillary lymph node dissection (i.e., levels I and II) is appropriate for staging as well as local disease control, because the nodal status will influence subsequent decisions regarding adjuvant systemic therapy. Even if radiation therapy can achieve local disease control of axillary metastasis, it negates important staging information regarding the presence or absence of lymph node metastasis.

Cancer Rehabilitation. An important, but often underemphasized, goal of cancer management is the rehabilitation of the patient back to his or her previous status as closely as possible, from a physical, emotional, social, and employment perspective. It is insufficient to treat the cancer without addressing the individual rehabilitation needs of the patient. For example, in a woman with breast cancer, the goals of rehabilitation entail (1) a minimal trauma scar and swelling of the tissues of the chest and arm, (2) return of strength and mobility in the shoulder after axillary lymphadenectomy, and (3) restoration of contour and symmetry of the breast to an extent necessary for the patient to resume as normal a life-style as possible. For some women, an external prosthesis is satisfactory, while others significantly benefit from breast reconstructive surgery. Patients with extremity sarcomas may be considered candidates for limb salvage surgery or prosthesis use to maximize function (Fig. 9-28).

Cancer Prevention. In some circumstances, surgical removal of tissue as in mastectomy (unilateral or bilateral) may be justified solely on the basis of cancer prevention. Such a circumstance usually involves a patient who is at very high risk for harboring occult multifocal breast cancer at the time of diagnosis, or who is at high risk for subsequently developing cancer later during her lifetime. For example, a contralateral mastectomy might be used as a form of cancer prevention in a breast cancer patient who is at high risk for subsequently developing cancer in her other breast. The presence of lobular carcinoma in situ breast cancer and breast cancer family syndrome are two circumstances in which a contralateral mastectomy may be justified as a form of cancer prevention. There

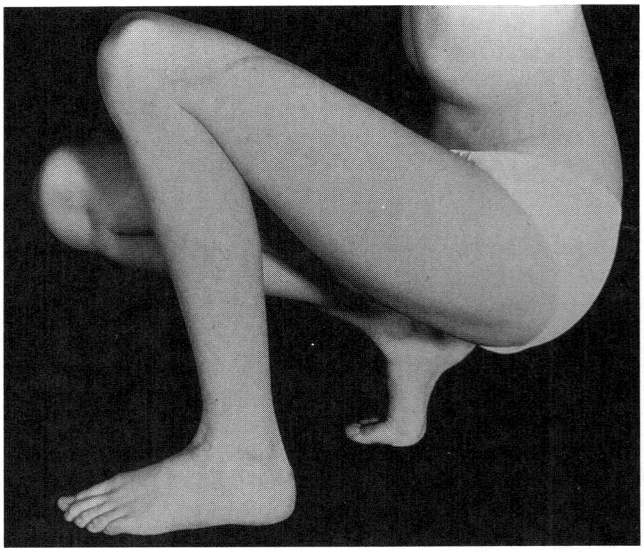

FIG. 9-28. This patient with an osteogenic sarcoma in the distal left femur underwent preoperative chemotherapy and resection of the affected distal femur followed by implantation of a total knee prosthesis. The figure illustrates the degree of mobility that can be achieved with this limb salvage approach.

is also preliminary evidence to suggest that the administration of tamoxifen as a form of chemoprevention might be effective, but this must be confirmed with a prospective clinical trial, which is now ongoing.

Counseling with Patients. On the average, it will take 20 to 30 minutes of physician time to adequately inform the cancer patient about treatment options and to arrive at a decision about the most appropriate treatment in an individual patient. Most patients expect to understand and participate in the decision-making process, however, many are confused because of conflicting input from family, friends, and even other physicians. Anxiety and uncertainty about the life-threatening nature of cancer and the prospects of physical disfigurement contribute to a negative, emotional overtone that makes it difficult for some patients to comprehend the issues about treatment options and how to provide his or her own enlightened input into the decision-making process. Empathetic listening by the physician and a clear but comprehensive discussion about treatment options is essential. The use of patient education materials (both written and videotaped) and counseling by nurses or physician-assistants all help to streamline the decision-making process and to ensure that the patient is more comfortable and informed about the treatment plan.

Management of Primary Cancers and Regional Metastases

Surgical Therapy

Surgical treatment represents the most frequently used and the most successful single method of cancer therapy currently available. More patients are cured of cancer by surgery than by any other therapeutic modality. However, only about one-half of cancer patients are cured by surgery alone, since surgical therapy, with few exceptions, is curative only in those patients in whom the disease is localized to the primary site and regional nodes.

The surgical procedure is designed to remove the primary neoplasms and the contiguous routes of spread (lymphatics and regional lymph nodes), with the goal of removing every cancer cell serving as a source of metastasis, to cure the patient or to control the disease locally even when the probability of cure is low. Decreasing tumor burden by removing the primary tumor and any regional metastases might alter the host-tumor balance to favor the patient with minimal residual metastases.

Advances in surgical techniques, anesthesia, and supportive care (blood transfusions, antibiotics, and fluid and electrolyte management) have permitted the development of more radical and extensive operative procedures. These advances have resulted in significant improvements in the local control rates for certain human neoplasms.

Preoperative Preparation. Many malignant tumors seem to have a toxic effect on the patient disproportionate to the size of the lesion, and often the patient's physical condition is relatively poor. The patient may have a poor nutritional status because of interference with normal alimentary function, as with cancers of the oropharynx, esophagus, and intestinal tract. Pain may contribute to anorexia and severe electrolyte disorder. Anemia, vitamin deficiencies, and defects in the coagulation mechanisms must be corrected before an operation can be safely performed.

Every effort should be made to correct nutritional deficiencies, restore depleted blood volume, and correct hypoproteinemia before an extensive surgical procedure (e.g., total parenteral nutrition can be used to prepare the malnourished patient for a major operation); otherwise the risk of operative morbidity or death will be excessive.

Once the decision has been made to proceed with surgical therapy, the procedure should be planned carefully. It is essential to realize that the best, and often the only, opportunity for cure is at the time of the first operation. If the neoplasm is incompletely excised at that time, the violation of tissue planes, lymphatics, and blood vessels will allow tumor cell seeding throughout the wound. In addition, any recurrence may be difficult to separate from the inflammatory reaction and scarring of the first operation, which can distort tissue planes to a point where tumor margins are indistinct. Therefore, enucleation or incomplete excision of a tumor mass is never indicated as a therapeutic measure.

Types of Cancer Operations. ***Local Resection.*** Wide local resection, in which an adequate margin of normal tissue is removed with the tumor mass, may be adequate treatment for certain low-grade neoplasms that do not metastasize to regional nodes or widely infiltrate adjacent tissues. Basal cell carcinomas, thin melanomas (i.e., less than 1.0 mm), and mixed tumors of the parotid gland are examples of such neoplasms. It is essential that at least some normal tissue surrounding the tumor be excised in order to prevent local recurrence.

Radical Local Resection. Some neoplasms may spread widely by infiltration into adjacent tissues. This is especially true of soft tissue sarcomas and esophageal and gastric carcinomas. For this reason, it is necessary to remove a wide margin of normal tissue with the neoplasm in these cases. The wide normal-tissue margin between the line of excision and the tumor mass also acts as a protective barrier against tumor cell spill into the severed lymphatics and vessels. The greater the width of normal tissues between the plane of dissection and the tumor, the greater likelihood of a complete local excision.

If the tumor was previously explored but not removed or if an incisional biopsy was performed, it is extremely important that a segment of skin and the underlying muscles, fat, and fascia be removed far beyond the limits of the original incision, because tumor cells may have been implanted in the incision at the time of this initial operation.

Malignant neoplasms are not well encapsulated. A pseudocapsule composed of a compression zone of neoplastic cells may surround the tumor. This apparent encapsulation offers a great temptation for simple enucleation, because the tumor may be dislodged from its bed so easily. This temptation must be resisted. The surgeon must cut through normal tissue at all times and should never disrupt the neoplasm during its removal. Dissection should proceed with meticulous care to avoid tumor cell spill. It is important for the surgeon to remember to resect as far as possible from the gross extent of the tumor on all sides, including the deep aspect. Skin, subcutaneous fat, and some muscles may have to be sacrificed, but usually this causes little functional loss. Involvement of major vessels, nerves, joints, or bones may require sacrifice of these structures and even amputation in order to obtain a curative result. During the surgical procedure, the extent of operation should be determined by concern not only for cure, but also for functional integrity.

Radical Resection with en bloc Excision of Lymphatics. Since many neoplasms commonly metastasize by way of the lymphatics, operations have been designed to remove the primary neoplasm and the regional lymph nodes draining that area in continuity with all the intervening tissues. Conditions are best for this type of operation when the collecting nodes of the lymphatic channels draining the neoplasm lie adjacent to the primary site or when there is a single avenue of lymphatic drainage that can be removed without sacrificing vital structures. It is important to avoid cutting across involved lymphatic channels because such action may increase the possibility of local disease recurrence.

It is generally agreed that such en bloc regional lymph node dissections should be performed in patients having clinical involvement of lymph nodes by metastatic tumor. The modified radical mastectomy and radical total gastrectomy are two examples of en bloc dissections. In many cases, the tumor has already spread beyond the regional nodes, and the likelihood of cure following such procedures may be quite low. En bloc removal of the involved nodes offers the only chance for cure and provides significant palliation and local control.

The high rate of local cancer recurrence following surgical resection when lymph nodes are grossly involved and the high error rate when palpation is used to assess the extent of the involvement have led to routine dissection of regional nodes close to the primary tumor even though they are not clinically involved. Microscopic examination of the excised lymph nodes in these patients who have no clinical evidence of palpable enlargement reveals evidence of tumor spread in 20 to 40 percent of carcinomas and melanomas. A higher 5-year survival rate has been reported for patients showing microscopic involvement of lymph nodes when compared to that of patients in whom lymph node involvement was clinically recognizable.

Recently some surgeons have challenged the concept of elective, or prophylactic, lymph node dissection in cases where the regional nodes are not obviously involved, because it is not clear whether cure rates are improved if the nodes are removed before they are palpable. In many types of cancer the foreknowledge of tumor in regional nodes does affect the staging of the patient and can alter the treatment modality. For example, patients with breast cancer who have metastases to regional nodes may benefit considerably from adjuvant chemotherapy, as may some patients with deep melanomas. Furthermore, a comparison of experimental results from one institution with another depends on accurate staging of each patient at the time of the initiation of therapy. For these reasons, the decision to recommend a prophylactic lymph node dissection must be based on the likelihood of benefit to the patient. The argument against lymphadenectomy because it diminishes the host's immune system has not been proved by experimental studies, and should not be a consideration when planning therapy.

Extensive Surgical Procedures. Some slow-growing primary tumors may reach enormous size and may locally infiltrate widely without the development of distant metastases. Supraradical operative procedures can be undertaken for these extensive, nearly inoperable tumors, with cure of occasional patients. Although surgical care, anesthesia, blood replacement, and physiologic monitoring are much improved over the past, these operations should not be undertaken except by experienced surgeons who can select those patients most likely to benefit. Furthermore, these extensive surgical procedures sometimes offer a chance for a cure that is not possible by other means, and are justified in selected situations when extensive laboratory work-up shows no evidence of distant metastases. The surgeon, however, must be willing to accept the responsibility for the postoperative emotional rehabilitation of the patient before undertaking such extensive procedures as pelvic exenteration, hemipelvectomy, forequarter amputation, or radical operations for head and neck carcinomas.

Pelvic exenteration is a well-conceived operation capable of curing patients with radiation-treated recurrent cancer of the cervix and certain well-differentiated and locally extensive adenocarcinomas of the rectum. This operation removes the pelvic organs (bladder, uterus, and rectum) and all soft tissues within the pelvis. Bowel function is restored with colostomy. Urinary tract drainage is established by anastomosis of ureters into a segment of bowel (ileum or sigmoid colon). The 5-year relapse-free survival after pelvic exenteration is 25 percent.

Hemipelvectomy (resection of the lower extremity and iliac bone) can sometimes be curative for skeletal sarcomas limited to the head of the femur or acetabulum or to one-half of the pelvic structures, and in some slowly growing soft tissue sarcomas of the upper thigh and buttock that recur locally but metastasize slowly. Forequarter amputation (resection of the upper extremity and scapula) can offer similar results when the neoplasm is limited to the bones of the scapula and upper humerus or to the soft tissues of the shoulder girdle.

Lymphadenectomy. There are some general principles common to lymph node dissection at various anatomic sites, particularly the neck, axilla, and groin (Fig. 9-29).

1. The surgeon must thoroughly understand the anatomy of the lymph nodes in each area of the body and should incorporate all the draining nodes at risk into the surgical specimen. With regard to lymphatic anatomy and its implications for cancer, the treatise by Haagensen and colleagues is particularly enlightening. Morton and colleagues have recently described an interesting and potentially useful approach to identify the primary draining lymph nodes that might contain metastatic melanoma. This intraoperative lymphatic mapping technique, which uses vital blue dyes, may provide a staging procedure to accurately identify patients with clinically occult metastases for whom a therapeutic lymphadenectomy would be beneficial.
2. The goals of a lymph node dissection must be clearly defined. They include any one or a combination of the following: (1) curative intent, (2) local disease control (i.e., palliation), or (3) staging. Each type of regional lymph node dissection has its own set of acceptable risks for different patients based on such variables as age and general health. For example, some patients with bulky nodal metastases may be cured by surgical excision; therefore, it is imperative for the surgeon to perform a thorough operation. A palliative lymph node dissection may be indicated in patients with large, symptomatic metastases even if other distant metastases are present. In such a setting, removal of the nodal metastases may be beneficial as long as the distant metastases are not an immediate threat to life. Staging to determine whether metastatic disease is present in the lymph nodes will assume increased importance as adjuvant chemotherapy, hormonal therapy, or immunotherapy is used for patients with nodal metastases.
3. An incomplete lymph node dissection is generally not acceptable except when the goals of surgery are strictly palliative. When the intent is curative surgery, such as with melanoma, a complete lymphadenectomy is vital, especially when there are no other effective modalities of regional therapy. The majority of patients with nodal metastases have at least one additional involved node elsewhere in the regional nodal basin. For example, melanoma patients having a biopsy or partial lymphadenectomy for metastatic disease have significantly lower survival rates compared with those who have a complete lymphadenectomy. On the other hand, a partial axillary dissection (levels I and II) is satisfactory for breast cancer where the goals are staging and local disease control.
4. The incision providing access to the underlying regional nodes should be correctly placed to minimize the risk of dividing lymphatic vessels that could contain malignant cells.
5. For dissections of lymph nodes in the neck, axilla, or groin, use of closed-suction catheter drains is important because they evacuate blood and serum and keep the tissues in apposition, minimizing the risk of

A

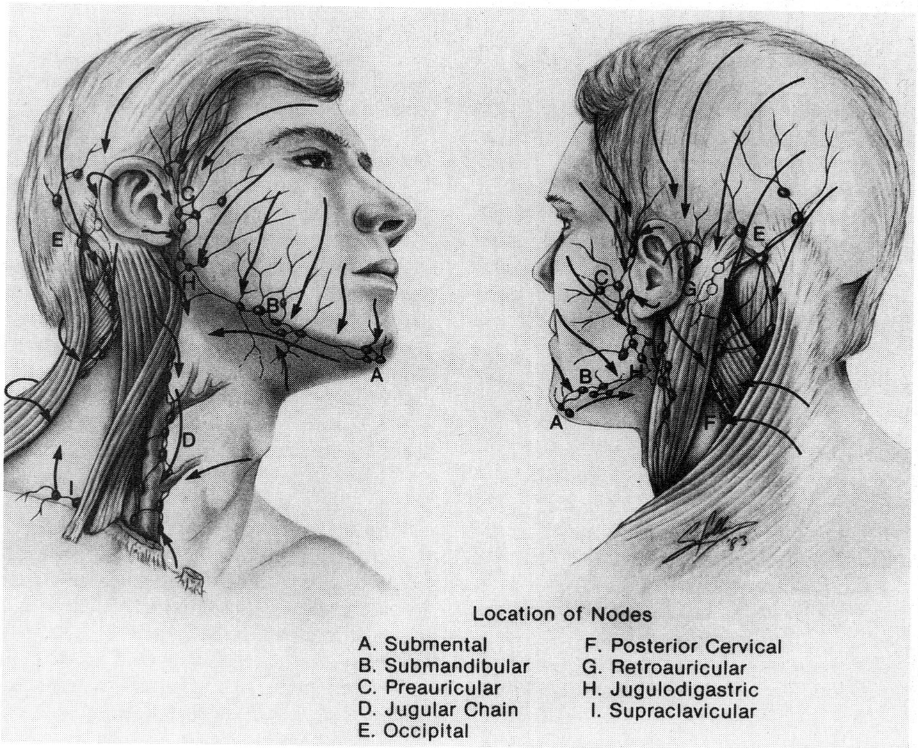

B

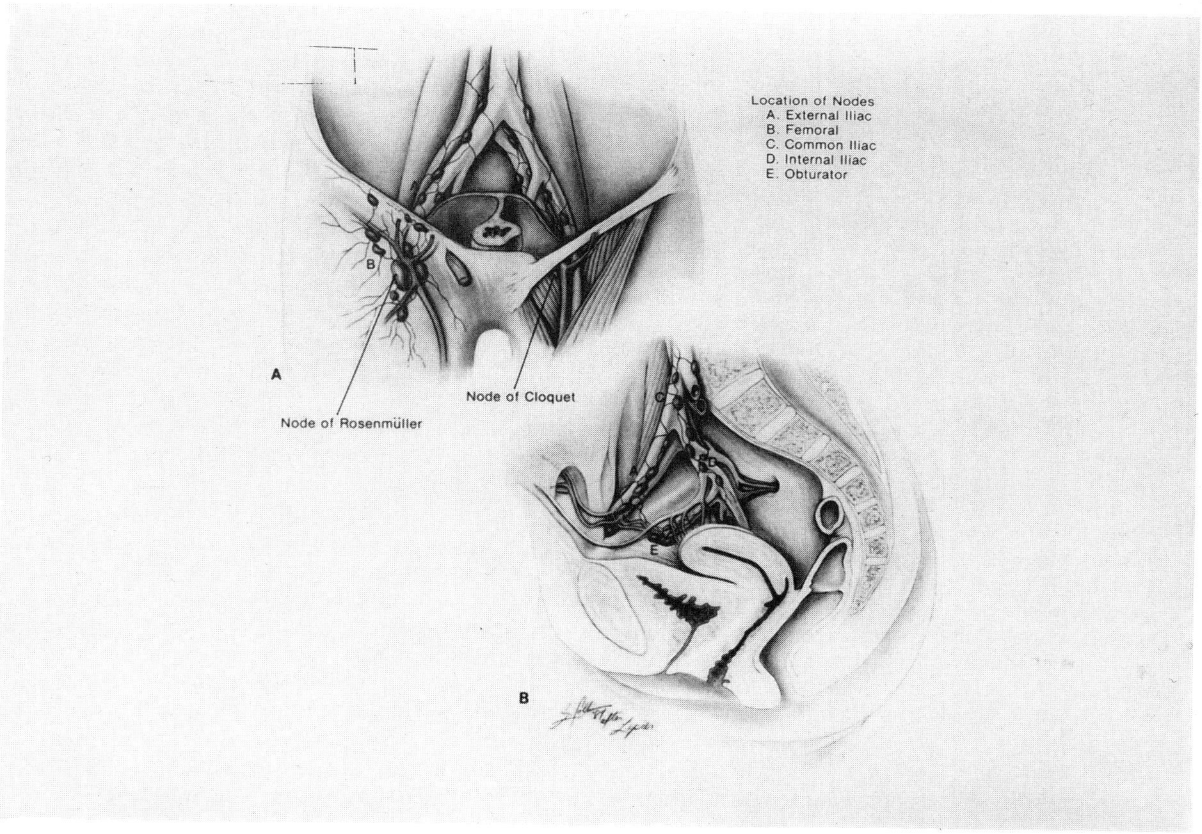

FIG. 9-29. Understanding the lymphatic drainage patterns for many forms of superficially located cancer is important for treating cancers, such as those involving skin, breast, and head and neck. *A*. Location of cervical and supraclavicular lymph nodes along with their drainage patterns from various sites of the head and neck. *B*. Location of lymph nodes in the groin involving the femoral lymph nodes, iliac, and obturator lymph nodes. The node of Rosenmüller is commonly involved with metastatic melanoma in the femoral triangle; the node of Cloquet is a transitional lymph node between the femoral and the iliac lymph node chain that often is sampled to identify patients at risk for iliac metastases. *C*. The three levels of axillary lymph nodes. The lower axillary lymph nodes (level I) are lateral to the pectoralis minor muscle; level II lymph nodes lie behind the muscle, while the apical lymph nodes (level II) are medial to the pectoralis minor muscle. A level I and II lymph node dissection is appropriate in the treatment of breast cancer, while resection of all three levels is necessary for curative operations involving melanoma.

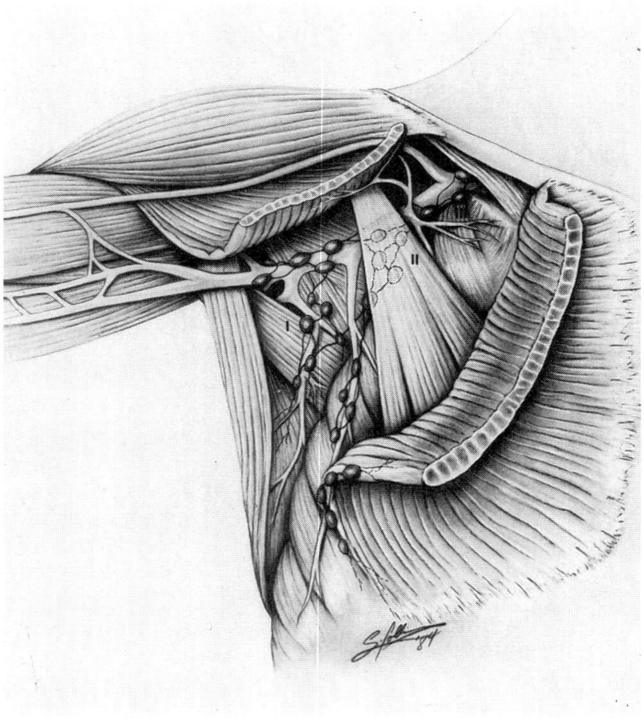

C

FIG. 9-29. Cont.

seroma formation. We use one or two large catheters inserted percutaneously through the lower flap and placed in a dependent part of the wound. There are no objective data on the best time to remove these devices. The incidence of seroma formation increases if they are removed too early, and the incidence of wound infection increases if they are kept in too long (especially longer than 10 days). Based on empirical evidence, we recommend that the catheters be removed when the drainage is less than 40 mL per 24 hours or 8 days after surgery, whichever comes first.

6. The use of prophylactic antibiotics is controversial. The incidence of wound infection is highest after a groin dissection and lowest after a neck dissection. Staphylococci and streptococci are the most common organisms isolated from these wound infections. The use of prophylactic antibiotics is probably justified on an empirical basis for groin and axillary lymphadenectomies, but such a practice must be confirmed with controlled clinical trials.
7. In patients with bulky nodal metastases, especially with invasion and fixation into surrounding tissues, such as in the axilla for metastatic breast cancer and in the neck for metastatic melanoma, the risk of regional recurrence is high (greater than 20 percent). Based on data from prospective clinical trials, adjuvant radiotherapy might be considered in such circumstances to improve regional disease control.

Radiation Therapy

The effectiveness of radiation therapy, like surgical therapy, must be assessed by comparing the frequency of local and regional tumor control to the frequency of treatment-induced morbidity. Ionizing radiation is effective in management of a wide variety of malignant tumors and is part of the treatment of 50 to 60 percent of patients with cancer. Maximizing radiation therapy requires that the radiation oncologist be directly involved in the selection of patients and in the evaluation of these patients before, during, and after treatment.

With radiation, tumors can be destroyed while anatomy is preserved. Often function and cosmesis can also be preserved if the anatomy is intact before treatment. Concurrent medical problems have less influence on radiation than on surgical or chemotherapy, although treatment-related sequelae may be more frequent or more severe in patients with certain systemic illnesses such as diabetes or collagen vascular disease.

The differential effect of radiation on tumors and normal tissues results in a favorable therapeutic ratio in most clinical situations. Radiation can, however, have immediate and delayed side effects on normal tissues. The incidence and severity of late sequelae, which may progress over many years, are highly dependent on treatment technique. The type of equipment used, field arrangement, accuracy of tumor localization and field placement, treatment schedule, and expertise of the treating physician all influence the quality of outcome. The appearance of late sequelae today may be the unfortunate consequence of treatment techniques long abandoned. Thus, the selection of radiation therapy should be based on the results of treatment with modern techniques.

Physical Basis. Ionizing radiations are characterized by their capacity to ionize (and excite) atoms and molecules in an absorber such as tissue. Electromagnetic radiations can be produced artificially in kilovoltage radiation therapy units and linear accelerators by impinging energetic electrons on a target (e.g., tungsten). The energy of the resulting x-rays is related to the energy of the accelerated electrons as they reach the target material. Electromagnetic radiations of characteristic energy (gamma-rays) are also produced by the radioactive decay of naturally occurring radioisotopes (e.g., radium 226) or artificially produced isotopes (e.g., cobalt 60). According to quantum physics, x-rays and gamma-rays can also be represented as particles called *photons*. Removal of the target in a linear accelerator results in an emitted beam of high-energy electrons that have different absorption characteristics from photons and are very useful in the treatment of relatively superficial malignancies. Other types of particulate radiations (e.g., protons, neutrons, pi mesons, and helium ions) are produced by very powerful linear accelerators, or *cyclotrons*, and have been used therapeutically, primarily in investigative settings. Because the basic physical mechanisms of action of all ionizing radiations are the same, the different effects observed with equal physical doses result from differences in spatial or temporal distributions.

For decades, doses at the point of interest, such as the tumor or spinal cord, were grossly extrapolated from skin reactions or doses measured in air (the roentgen). Currently, clinical specification of radiation doses are derived from direct measurements of absorbed doses within the patient (using thermoluminescent dosimeters) or from doses calculated within a tissue phantom that simulates the human being. Phantom measurements are adapted for precise clinical application through the use of computer programs. Recent technological advances have made it possible to correct for tissue inhomogeneities (air cavities and bone) within the treatment volume using CT-based treatment planning.

Until 1980, absorbed radiation doses were quantified in rads, with 1 rad equal to 0.01 joule per kilogram of the absorber. According to the 1980 recommendations of the International Commission on Radiological Units, doses should be quantified in Gray (Gy) units, with 1 Gy = 100 rad = 1 joule per kilogram of the absorber, and 1 cGy = 1 rad.

The availability of modern radiation therapy was initially facilitated by widespread distribution of cobalt 60 teletherapy units, dating to 1949, and the later versatile 4- to 6-MeV linear accelerators. Linear accelerators that produce a range of photon and electron energies between 4 and 25 MeV are available and are useful in a wide variety of clinical situations. Modern equipment provides deeply penetrating beams, short treatment times, isocentric patient setups, improved skin sparing, decreased bone absorption (compared with kilovoltage units), and sharp beam margins with less side scatter than cobalt 60 units.

In some clinical situations, brachytherapy, or the direct placement of radioactive sources within tissue, may permit delivery of tumor doses higher than those achievable with external beam radiation therapy. Because the dose delivered falls off in a manner proportional to the square of the distance from the source, very high doses can be delivered to tissues immediately adjacent to the implant with relative sparing of surrounding normal tissues. A variety of artificially produced radioisotopes, including Iridium 192, Cesium 137, and Iodine 125, are used in the treatment of cancers of the breast, prostate, brain, lung, head and neck, gynecologic organs, soft tissues, and eye. These brachytherapy techniques have led the radiation oncologist into the operating room and into closer cooperation with many surgeons.

Biologic Basis. The development of the clinical radiation therapy practice has often been based on empirical observation. Studies of radiation biology have provided a scientific basis for these observations, have guided investigative programs, and are providing a basis for future studies.

Modern cellular radiobiology dates to the development of tumor cell culture by Puck and Marcus in the mid-1950s. Mammalian cell dose-survival curves quantitatively correlate reproductive cell death with total radiation dose. The inherent radiosensitivity of most normal and transformed mammalian cells are remarkably similar, with doses of 110 to 240 cGy consistently reducing reproductive cell survival to 37 percent (D_0 dose). Therefore, differences in the rapidity and completeness of response of human tumors and normal tissues must be based on other factors, such as the capacity to repair sublethal damage, tissue oxygenation, cell cycle time and distribution, and repopulation.

Radiosensitivity should not be confused with radioresponsiveness and radiocurability. *Radiosensitivity* is the measure of susceptibility of cells to injury by ionizing radiation. This injury may cause reproductive cell death by interrupting the cells' capacity to replicate indefinitely. Radiation can also kill cells by interfering with critical cell functions unassociated with cell replication (''interphase death''). The latter has been shown to be an important mechanism of radiation-induced cell death in lymphocytes and in normal salivary gland.

Radiocurability refers to the ability of radiation to permanently control a tumor, allowing survival of the host. Tumor type, size, site, and extent have a greater influence on radiocurability than cellular radiosensitivity. *Radioresponsiveness*, or the rapidity of a tumor's response to radiation, may not correlate well with radiocurability. Whereas, epidermoid carcinomas of the oral cavity, larynx, skin, and cervix and adenocarcinomas of the breast, cervix, and prostate may be radiocurable despite relatively slow responses to radiation, undifferentiated carcinomas often respond rapidly to radiation treatment but are usually not cured because of widespread tumor dissemination. However, differences in radioresponsiveness of tumors of a specific type and site may correlate with local tumor control.

The ability of cells to accumulate and repair sublethal injury varies widely. Generally, normal tissues have a greater capacity to repair injury than tumor cells. Fractionation, or the division of a radiation dose into multiple smaller doses, allows recovery of this damage between radiation fractions. Laboratory and clinical studies indicate that an interfraction interval of at least 4 to 6 hours is necessary to permit maximal repair of sublethal injury. Because of their greater repair capacity, slowly dividing normal tissues are usually spared more than tumor cells by the use of relatively small fraction sizes. However, rapidly dividing stem cell populations such as bone marrow and mucosal surfaces have less capacity for repair. The use of small doses per fraction improves the therapeutic ratio by reducing the late normal tissue effects of radiation more than the tumor effects. Although some protraction of treatment is necessary to permit repopulation of acutely responding normal stem cell populations and avoid intolerable acute normal tissue effects, treatment protraction also permits repopulation of tumor cells and should not be excessive. Empirical evidence suggests that daily fractions of approximately 2 Gy optimize the balance between these effects. Recently, clinicians have been investigating the use of altered, hyperfractionated schedules that use two or three small fractions per day in an effort to further decrease late normal tissue complications without increasing the overall duration of treatment.

For similar reasons, cell killing can be modified by changes of the dose rate. To achieve tolerable individual treatment durations, external beam radiation therapy is usually delivered at a dose rate of 2 to 5 Gy/min. As the dose rate decreases, cell killing per unit of dose decreases. Low dose rates (i.e., less than 10 cGy/min) may favor repair in normal tissues. This effect is exploited clinically to improve normal tissue tolerance (particularly of the lung) in total-body irradiation and to allow delivery of very large total doses with low dose rate interstitial and intracavitary brachytherapy techniques.

Radiation-induced cell killing can be modified in other ways. Because molecular oxygen must be present for maximal cell killing by ionizing radiation, tumor cellular hypoxia can decrease the effectiveness of radiation therapy by as much as a factor of 3. This ''oxygen effect'' may explain the postirradiation persistence of tumor cells when there is necrosis or fibrosis.

The intrinsic radiosensitivity of cells can be increased by altering the target DNA, such as by replacing thymidine with halogenated pyrimidine analogues (BUdR, IUdR) during cell replication. Cell killing can be increased by inhibiting postirradiation repair processes. For example, the repair of DNA strand breaks can be inhibited by actinomycin D and doxorubicin and by heat (42° to 45°C). Unfortunately, current methods of altering the target DNA and inhibiting postirradiation repair are not selective for tumor cells and, consequently, may not improve the therapeutic ratio.

Clinical Basis. Like surgery and chemotherapy, radiation therapy has definite and relative indications and contraindications. Table 9-14 is a partial list of tumors that are treated with radiation.

Irradiation may be the only anticipated treatment or may be combined with surgery and/or chemotherapy. The intent of treatment may be curative or palliative. In some clinical situations, surgery and radiation provide comparable rates of local tumor control with qualitatively different side effects. In such cases the choice of treatment can be made only by a patient who has been carefully informed by a surgeon and radiation oncologist. Whenever curative treatment of malignancy is being considered, it is important that all the specialists (medical, surgical, and radiation oncologists) be involved before initiation of any form of therapy. Previous surgical and chemotherapeutic management can signifi-

Table 9-14
Indications for Radiation Therapy

Before or after conservative surgery permitting organ preservation:
Early carcinomas of the larynx, pharynx, oral cavity
Carcinoma of the breast
Soft tissue sarcomas
Ewing's sarcoma
Carcinoma of the vulva, vagina
Anal carcinoma
Early carcinomas of the distal rectum
Prostate cancer
Early carcinoma of the bladder
Skin cancer (e.g., of the eyelid, nose, ear)
Retinoblastoma, ocular melanoma (diagnosed clinically)
Radiation therapy alone or with chemotherapy:
Hodgkin's disease
Selected localized non-Hodgkin's lymphomas
Carcinoma of the cervix
Nasopharyngeal carcinoma
Brain tumors
Before or after radical surgery in selected patients with tumor exhibiting high-risk features:
Breast carcinoma
Locoregionally advanced carcinomas of the head and neck
Lung cancer
Carcinoma of the cervix following radical hysterectomy
Carcinoma of the endometrium
Adenocarcinoma of the rectosigmoid
Brain tumors
Indications for emergency palliative radiation:
Spinal cord compression
Superior vena caval syndrome
Airway obstruction
Cranial nerve compression

cantly influence the therapeutic ratio of subsequent radiation therapy. Furthermore, close cooperation from the beginning of therapy can often improve treatment outcome significantly. For example, careful marking of the margins of a tumor during surgery can help the radiation oncologist define a more accurate target volume and decrease the morbidity of therapy. Awkward placement of a surgical incision can dramatically increase the volume, complexity, and morbidity of subsequent irradiation. In some cases, the radiation oncologist can obtain valuable information by observing the operative field.

Decisions about the utility of radiation therapy are based on tumor-related factors (type, site, extent, typical natural history) and host factors (general condition, local and regional tissues status). A definitive tissue diagnosis should be obtained before treatment in almost all cases to avoid inappropriately morbid treatment of benign conditions that mimic malignancy. On rare occasions when biopsy poses an unreasonable risk to the patient (e.g., tumors of the brainstem and optic tract), treatment may be initiated on the basis of strong radiologic diagnostic evidence. The introduction of CT and magnetic resonance imaging (MRI) should reduce unfortunate diagnostic errors in these situations.

Histologic tumor type and grade may be useful pretherapeutic predictors of biologic behavior and radiocurability. The potential for local and regional tumor control, however, is more closely related to tumor size and the primary site. In most cases, radiation dose is limited by the tolerance of surrounding normal tissues. In general, the probability of controlling a tumor with a tolerable dose of radiation is inversely proportional to its size and the number of proliferating clonogens that must be eliminated. While surgical tumor debulking procedures that leave gross residual disease are sometimes necessary to relieve tumor-related symptoms, they usually reduce the number of clonogens by less than one log, may increase tumor hypoxia, may decrease the tolerance of adjacent normal tissues, and rarely improve radiocurability. Large tumors are more likely to have spread regionally, sometimes requiring treatment of a larger volume with a consequent reduction of normal tissue tolerance.

The primary tumor site predicts biologic behavior and dictates which normal tissues will be affected by treatment. For example, small tumors of the glottic larynx rarely spread to regional nodes, and more than 90 percent of such tumors are cured with moderate doses of radiation to a small local field. By contrast, similar-sized tumors originating a few millimeters away in the supraglottic larynx have a richer lymphatic supply, have a much greater likelihood of regional spread, and often require treatment with relatively large fields encompassing the regional lymph nodes. Even fairly large tumors of the cervix can be controlled locally with minimal risk of serious morbidity because of the high radiation tolerance of the uterus and vagina and the opportunity to deliver high doses with intracavitary therapy. Carcinomas of similar size in the upper abdomen are rarely controllable with radiation therapy alone because surrounding normal tissues such as liver, kidney, bowel, and spinal cord limit the deliverable doses of external beam radiotherapy. Intraoperative radiotherapy (the delivery of external beam radiotherapy directly to a tumor exposed during an operation) is currently being investigated as a possible means of increasing the radiation dose that can be delivered in such situations.

After initial evaluation of the patient, the objective of radiation therapy must be defined. If the cancer is curable, a prolonged treatment course and a moderate risk of serious treatment-related morbidity are often accepted in an effort to overcome life-threatening disease. If the objective is palliation of bothersome cancer-related symptoms, treatment must be designed to minimize morbidity and inconvenience and maximize symptom relief.

Radiation treatment planning and delivery have become increasingly sophisticated. The radiation oncologist must begin by defining a target volume. This involves careful synthesis of information from the patient's medical history, physical examination, radiologic studies, operative description, and pathology reports. Knowledge about the characteristic natural history of the disease, anatomic routes of spread, and possible interactions among radiation and surgery, chemotherapy, and intercurrent disease must all be included in the determination. Armed with this information, the radiation oncologist must design a therapeutic approach that will maximize the chance of tumor control and minimize the risk of treatment-related morbidity. In most cases, the primary tumor and adjacent volume at risk for regional spread are graphically displayed and incorporated in a planned treatment volume.

The best method of delivery of radiation is selected from a range of options, including multiple beams of photons or electrons, sometimes augmented by interstitial or intracavitary applications. Various types of beam shaping devices may be used to alter depth dose distributions and to shape the radiation field. The dosimetry data are incorporated in computer-assisted programs that allow rapid, accurate calculations of the desired options. The chosen treatment fields are then simulated on the patient using a specialized machine built to the geometric specifications of the treatment machine but fitted with a diagnostic x-ray head and fluoroscope. The patient may be fitted with immobilization devices to improve the reproducibility of treatment. Marks on the patient's skin make it possible to reproduce the simulated fields during treatment. With careful immobilization and field localization, repetitive treatment delivery can be accurate to within a few millimeters. Modern treatment planning and delivery require close cooperation between multiple health professionals, including medical physicists, dosimetrists, radiation therapy technologists, radiation therapy nurses, and radiation oncologists.

Different sites in the same patient may be treated with different doses according to risk and the amount of tumor involvement. A relatively large volume, including the primary tumor and surrounding areas at risk for harboring microscopic disease, may be treated to a moderate dose. The primary tumor, grossly involved lymph nodes, or positive surgical margins may then be "boosted" to a higher dose either with smaller external beam fields or with brachytherapy.

Radiation therapy alone is curative in many clinical situations. Aggressive local or local and regional treatment yields high cure rates in many types of head and neck cancer, gynecologic malignancies, anal cancer, prostate cancer, Hodgkin's disease, and other neoplasms.

In other cases, radiation is used in combination with surgery or chemotherapy. Such multidisciplinary approaches require continuous cooperation between all the physicians and health professionals involved. Radiation and surgery may be directed to the same site, as when resection of a cancer of the hypopharynx is followed by irradiation, or when irradiation of a soft tissue sarcoma in an extremity is followed by surgery. The use of combined treatment may permit less morbid treatment than would be necessary with either modality alone. Local tumor excision plus radiation therapy is now commonly used as an equal alternative to mastectomy in the treatment of breast cancer. Treatment of soft tissue sarcomas with wide local excision and preoperative or postoperative irradiation achieves local control rates comparable to amputation but with preservation of the limb. In some cases, radiation and surgical treatment are directed to different sites, as when orchiectomy is followed by irradiation of the retroperitoneal lymph nodes, or when a neck dissection follows interstitial irradiation of a cancer of the oral tongue.

The expectations and indications of combined treatment are not always clear. Postoperative radiation has been demonstrated to improve local and regional control rates in many postsurgical situations. Because patients with unfavorable clinical or histologic features are usually selected for postoperative therapy, retrospective comparisons between patients who received radiation alone or combined therapy usually do not compare similar groups of patients and do not answer important questions about the influence of postoperative treatment on survival. Even when the survival benefit of postoperative radiation is uncertain, treatment may be indicated to prevent morbid local recurrence.

When surgery and radiation therapy are directed to the same site, the interval between their use depends on a range of factors. Moderate-dose irradiation of a soft tissue sarcoma may be followed by resection in 10 to 14 days, while rectosigmoid resection should be delayed 4 to 6 weeks after pelvic irradiation to allow for regression of edema and hyperemia. Most postoperative radiation therapy is delivered with relatively high doses directed to sites at high risk for persistent tumor. The optimal timing of postoperative radiotherapy depends on the type of surgical procedure, patient recovery, wound healing, and tumor characteristics, and should be decided by the surgeon and radiotherapist in concert. Unnecessary delays should be avoided since they may allow time for tumor regrowth and decrease the efficacy of radiotherapy.

Such planned combined treatment is usually much more effective than the use of one method to rescue the failure of the other. In these circumstances, the effectiveness of the second method is often reduced. Fibrosis, loss of tissue planes, and decreased vascularity that can occur many months after an aggressive course of radiation therapy increase the incidence of major surgical complications. Irradiation of a tumor regrowing in tissues altered by surgery is likely to be ineffective because of decreased vascularity and increased tumor volume and to be more morbid because of surgical sequelae such as abdominal adhesions that fix segments of bowel within the high-dose volume.

When the goal of treatment is palliation, the treatment dose and schedule are chosen to achieve symptom relief as quickly as possible with little or no treatment-related morbidity. Because the dose is usually not pushed to normal tissue tolerance and the patient is not expected to survive to experience late effects of radiation, relatively large daily fractions may be used to shorten the overall treatment time. Treatment is given only to relieve symptoms or occasionally to prevent imminent problems (e.g., to prevent fracture in tumorous weight-bearing bones). Occasionally, aggressive radiotherapeutic treatment of hematogenous metastases may be indicated, particularly if the lesion is solitary and presents after a long disease-free interval.

Even when seemingly indicated, radiation therapy may be inappropriate because of host factors. Debilitated or disoriented patients may not tolerate daily treatment. Local tissue changes induced by comorbid disease may cause the risk of curative treatment to outweigh the chance of benefit.

Any effective anticancer therapy may produce undesirable and, occasionally, dangerous side effects. The incidence and severity of late complications has decreased with modern radiotherapy techniques, but in many situations, efforts to eliminate a small-to-moderate risk of major complications by reducing the radiotherapy dose will result in an even greater increase in tumor recurrences.

Acute radiation-induced side effects may be distressing but can usually be managed conservatively and are almost always self-limited. The nature of these effects, summarized in Table 9-15, depends on the tissues included within the treatment volume.

The clinically important late sequelae of radiation therapy may not be apparent until months or even years after completion of treatment. The risk of late complications can usually be minimized (but not eliminated) by careful technique. Although curative, high-dose radiotherapy necessarily attends a risk of major late complications, this should be viewed in the same context as other, sometimes unavoidable, sequelae of curative cancer treatment (e.g., colostomy for abdominal perineal resection or amputation for sarcoma).

On rare occasions, ionizing radiation can induce second malignancies in treated patients. Clinical studies, however, have demonstrated that this risk is small. In studies of more than 2000 patients with head and neck cancer and 2000 patients with cancer of the breast, no increase in the incidence of second cancers could be demonstrated in patients treated with radiotherapy. The increased incidence of leukemia in patients treated for Hodgkin's disease correlated most strongly with exposure to alkylating agents, although many of the patients also received radiation therapy. A very slight increase in the incidence of myelogenous leukemias (observed:expected = 1.4) was noted in 29,493 patients observed for 60,000 person-years after radiation for cervical carcinoma.

Table 9-15
Local Effects of Radiation

Organ	*Acute Changes*	*Chronic Changes*
Skin	Erythema, wet or dry desquamation, epilation	Telangectasia, subcutaneous fibrosis, ulceration
Gastrointestinal tract	Nausea, diarrhea, edema, ulceration, hepatitis	Stricture, ulceration, perforation, hematochezia
Kidney		Nephropathy, renal insufficiency
Bladder	Dysuria	Hematuria, ulceration, perforation
Gonads	Sterility	Atrophy, ovarian failure
Hemopoietic tissue	Lymphopenia, neutropenia, thrombocytopenia	Pancytopenia
Bone	Epiphyseal growth arrest	Necrosis
Lung	Pneumonitis	Pulmonary fibrosis
Heart		Pericarditis, vascular damage
Upper aerodigestive tract	Mucositis, xerostomia, anosmia, dysgeusia	Xerostomia, dental caries
Eye	Conjunctivitis	Cataract, keratitis, optic nerve atrophy
Nervous system	Cerebral edema	Necrosis, myelitis

Management of Cancer at Distant Sites

Clinical Evaluation and Screening for Distant Metastases

The clinician must evaluate the patient for the presence and extent of metastases before instituting treatment. The diagnostic evaluation should be suitably comprehensive but cost-effective. In the absence of symptoms or signs of metastases, a minimal number of laboratory and radiologic tests should be ordered because their costs are an additional burden to the patient and his or her family, and the diagnostic yield is often small. Rather than order a battery of expensive tests, the physician should first perform an initial screening appraisal, with a more extensive metastatic survey pursued on a more selective basis, depending on the presence of signs and symptoms of disease in a particular area. Such an approach has been described using algorithms. Guidelines for metastatic evaluation at specific sites are listed in Table 9-16.

The goals of treatment (cure versus palliation) are important factors in determining the extent of metastatic evaluation to be performed. In general, laboratory tests, except for screening, should not be ordered unless a positive result would lead to a change in the treatment plan. Other factors, such as cost and availability, are involved as well. Knowledge of prognostic factors and the natural history of the disease will help to determine whether the

Table 9-16
Tests for Evaluating Metastatic Cancer

Metastatic Site	*Symptoms*	*Initial Studies*	*Confirmatory Studies (If Necessary)*
Lung	Usually none (may have some dyspnea, cough or hemoptysis)	Chest x-ray film	CT scan or tomograms
Liver	Weight loss, anorexia, abdominal pain, fever	↑ AP ↑ LDH Px; Liver mass, ascites	Liver ultrasound scan Abdominal CT scan, needle biopsy
Skin, SQ	New nodule	Px	Biopsy
Gastro-intestinal tract	Anemia, hematemesis, melena, obstruction, abdominal pain	Px Stool guaiac	Gastrointestinal endoscopy, UGI with small bowel follow through, barium enema
Brain	Change in affect, headache, numbness, motor weakness	Hx and Px	Brain MRI scan CT scan
Bone	Localized pain, fracture	↑ AP	Bone scan Bone x-ray film
Kidneys, bladder	Hematuria	Urinalysis	Intravenous pyelogram, cystoscopy

Abbreviations: SQ, subcutaneous tissue; Hx, medical history; Px, physical examination; AP, alkaline phosphatase; LDH, lactic dehydrogenase; UGI, upper gastrointestinal series.

probability of detecting metastases warrants a more or less comprehensive metastatic evaluation. These same principles are also important postoperatively in determining how long to follow the patient, the frequency of follow-up visits, and the types of screening tests to be used.

History and Physical Examination. A complete history and physician examination are the most important parts of the initial metastatic evaluation. A hallmark of metastatic disease is a symptom complex that progresses in either intensity or frequency. A careful history and physical examination are the most sensitive, specific, and cost-effective means of evaluating possible metastatic disease short of a biopsy.

Laboratory and Radiological Tests. The chest x-ray should be used routinely for screening purposes. Whole-lung tomograms or CT scans of the chest are useful for evaluating suspected pulmonary, pleural, or mediastinal metastases. In general, serum liver function tests, including lactic dehydrogenase level, are important screening tools for metastatic disease. An isolated elevation of the serum alkaline phosphatase or lactic dehydrogenase level is presumptive evidence of metastatic disease. For patients who, on the basis of physical examination or abnormal liver chemistries, have suspected intra-abdominal metastases, a CT or ultrasound (US) scan of the abdomen should be obtained if possible.

Bone, brain, and liver radioisotope scans have been used as screening tests for metastatic disease. Numerous studies have now shown, however, that these scans are not indicated for routine screening of occult metastatic disease because their diagnostic yield is low, except for those cancers which frequently relapse first in the bone, such as breast cancer and prostate cancer. A bone scan is the most sensitive test for skeletal metastatic disease, but a careful history and directed radiographs are necessary to ensure that areas of uptake do not represent areas of old trauma or inflammation.

Pathologic Tests. The definitive diagnosis of metastatic disease is made by biopsy. An excisional or needle biopsy is relatively easy to perform when the suspected metastasis is superficially located. More deeply situated lesions may also be approached with a thin-needle biopsy. In many circumstances, however, the clinical diagnosis is sufficient when made by radiologic studies, especially if metastases involve more than one site at the same time and the abnormality was absent on previous studies.

Cytologic examination of urine, sputum, or cerebrospinal, peritoneal, or pleural fluid, as well as bone marrow examination, also may yield a diagnosis of metastatic disease, especially when there are specific symptoms referable to these areas. A common problem in the diagnosis of metastatic cancer is distinguishing a metastatic lesion from a primary anaplastic or undifferentiated carcinoma or lymphoma, as, for instance, when an anaplastic lung lesion appears in a patient who had a primary anaplastic or undifferentiated carcinoma or lymphoma. When an anaplastic lung lesion appears in a patient who had a primary melanoma removed 5 years previously and is a very heavy cigarette smoker, should this be diagnosed as a metastatic melanoma or a lung carcinoma? Electron microscopy and immunostaining with antibodies of cytologic specimens and tissue specimens can be crucial in aiding the pathologist in the diagnosis.

Screening for Metastases. The frequency of examination may vary among patients according to their risk of metastases, but our practice is to evaluate the patient every 3 to 4 months for the first 2 years, at 6-month intervals to the fifth year, and then at least once a year indefinitely. Patients with very early cancer (e.g., melanomas less than 1.0 mm) might be followed at 6-month to 12-month intervals from the beginning whereas those with high risk for metastases should be followed at 2-month to 3-month intervals during the first 2 years after initial surgery.

Because a large proportion of recurrences are detected by the patients themselves, it is advocated that high-risk patients be briefed on the possible symptoms they may develop and urged to seek immediate medical attention should such symptoms manifest themselves. Annual review of all patients is recommended for an indefinite period to detect both additional primary melanomas and late recurrences.

Treatment of Advanced Cancer: General Principles

The clinical source of systemic metastases can vary widely among patients. Cure is usually not a realistic aim in such cases, so the treatment must reflect a carefully considered judgment that will preserve the quality of life while attempting to prolong it. Even though advanced cancer cannot usually be cured, debilitating symptoms can often be relieved or prevented. Experimental therapies are often considered for these patients.

The treatment of a patient with advanced cancer depends on several factors, including the sites and numbers of metastases, their rate of growth, types of and responses to previous treatment, and the age, overall condition, and desires of the patient. For example, a vigorous treatment might be appropriate for a slowly growing solitary metastasis, but only symptomatic treatment or none at all might be used in a debilitated patient with multiple metastases in whom prior treatment has failed.

In general, the number of organs or tissues containing metastases is the most significant factor predicting survival in patients with distant metastases. For example, the median survival is 7 months for melanoma patients with metastasis to one site, 4 months for those with metastases to two sites, and only 2 months for those with metastatic disease at three or more sites. The locations of the metastases are also important. Sites associated with relatively favorable outcomes for melanoma and breast cancer include (in approximately descending order) the skin, subcutaneous tissue, distant lymph nodes, bone, and lung. Unfavorable outcomes are associated with metastases to the liver and brain. Metastases in favorable sites are associated with long-term survival (i.e., 2 to 5 years) in a small but measurable proportion of patients. If the patient has received previous therapy, such as chemotherapy or surgery for a systemic metastasis, the survival is likely to be shorter. Patients in a debilitated state are less likely to withstand vigorous treatments than those who are not suffering the constitutional symptoms of metastatic disease. The patient's desires regarding treatment after he or she has received counseling about the therapies' benefits and risks should be strongly considered when choosing among alternative forms of palliative treatment.

Defining Goals and Benefits of Treatment. Balancing the goals of treatment with its risks and benefits is especially important and should be incorporated into the overall assessment of each patient and his or her treatment plan. The goals of treatment are relief of symptoms and prolongation of life. Treatment directed at relieving symptoms is generally worthwhile, especially when the anticipated benefit from relieving symptoms exceeds the toxic effects and risk of morbidity from the treatment itself. In addition, the effectiveness of the treatment can be monitored by both subjective and objective assessment of the symptoms caused by the metastases.

The second goal, to prolong life, has not been achieved in most patients with advanced cancer. One exception is in the surgical removal of solitary metastases from skin and subcutaneous tissues or visceral sites such as the lung or brain (Fig. 9-30). Surgical excision of solitary metastases of melanoma in visceral organs can lead to survival of more than 5 years in 5 to 20 percent of patients (Table 9-17). Chemotherapy, biologic therapy, and radiation therapy have not been shown to directly influence survival in any but a few circumstances.

Each treatment has its own set of risks, and the physician using these treatments should thoroughly understand these potential risks as they apply to each patient. Experimental treatments are an option for most patients who are first diagnosed with distant metastases. Patients who have a good performance status (who are able to care for themselves and have no debilitating symptoms from their disease), good cardiac and pulmonary function, and adequate white blood cell and platelet counts are usually candidates for clinical trials. Available effective methods for relief of symptomatic disease should be considered first.

Patient Counseling. In general, the patient should know about his or her situation and should participate in deciding among treatment alternatives. One of the greatest causes of anxiety is uncertainty; therefore, patients should be counseled about their situations so that they may be able to cope with their disease more realistically and arrange their personal lives accordingly. However, some patients are unable to cope if a completely honest approach is adopted. Nevertheless, some discussion is warranted because it is difficult to initiate treatment without explaining the reasons for it. If the physician and patient do not communicate with one another honestly and openly, the patient may lose trust in the physician and may not accept subsequent treatment recommendations.

When counseling patients and their families, the physician must be not only sympathetic and realistic but also hopeful about the results of treatment. Patients need hope, and even in grim situations treatment can achieve certain measurable goals, if only the relief of symptoms. In other words, the physician should continue treating the patient even when it is no longer possible to treat the cancer. The approach taken for each patient depends on that person's prognosis, physical condition, and emotional stability.

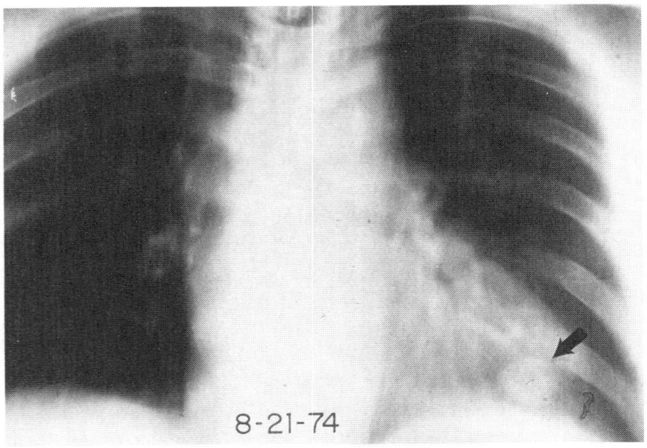

FIG. 9-30. Chest tomogram of a solitary pulmonary metastasis in a 47-year-old man diagnosed in 1974. There was no other evidence of metastatic disease and the lesion was surgically resected. The patient was free of melanoma 16 years later.

Occasional Treatment Modalities. Multiple treatment modalities are available for patients with metastatic disease. These therapies, along with their indications and risks, are listed in Table 9-18. The choice of treatment should take into account the potential toxicity, requirements for hospitalization, frequency of treatments, and median time necessary to attain antitumor response.

No Treatment. The option of providing no treatment is an important one to consider, especially for asymptomatic patients, those who are terminally ill, or those who are very old. There are circumstances in which, for an asymptomatic patient with slowly growing tumors in some sites, such as the lung, the physician may elect to observe the lesions. Quality of life is maintained in this instance and treatment can be instituted when there is further progression, evidenced by increasing size or number of metastases, or when the patient develops symptoms. Another circumstance concerns patients who are terminally ill or at an extreme age, where the risk/benefit ratio is small. The decision to forgo treatment can be difficult, and is often best made with the patient after he or she has received the counsel and assistance of relatives or medical or nursing advisers. Naturally, a patient should not be denied treatment when there is a reasonable expectation that the treatment will be successful and the risks of toxic effects are acceptable.

Surgical Resection of Metastases. Although logic would suggest that once a neoplasm has metastasized to a distant site it should no longer be curable by surgical resection, removal of metastatic lesions in the lung, liver, or brain has occasionally produced a clinical cure. Therefore, in selected patients with slowly growing neoplasms, resections of the metastatic lesions may be indicated, especially if the metastasis is solitary. Prior to undertaking resection, an extensive laboratory workup should rule out metastatic spread to other body areas. To avoid an early relapse, patients should be selected for surgery carefully. Sometimes, several weeks or months of observation provide relevant information about the rate of tumor growth and the possibility of metastases emerging at other sites. Surgery should only be used in cases of accessible lesions and in cases in which the patient can undergo surgery safely.

Palliative Surgery. Surgical procedures are sometimes indicated to relieve symptoms, to reduce the severity of the patient's illness, or to prolong a useful, comfortable life without attempting to cure the patient. Such an operation is justified to relieve pain, hemorrhage, obstruction, or infection when it can be done without great discomfort to the patient, and when it improves the quality of life even if it does not prolong it. Surgery that only prolongs a miserable existence certainly does not benefit the patient.

Some examples of palliative surgical procedures are (1) colostomy, enteroenterostomy, or gastrojejunostomy to relieve obstruction; (2) chordotomy to control pain; (3) cystectomy for infected, bleeding tumors of the bladder; (4) amputation for painful infected tumors in the extremities; (5) simple mastectomy for carcinoma of the breast, even in the presence of distant metastases, when the primary tumor is infected, large, ulcerated, and locally resectable; and (6) colon resection in the presence of hepatic metastases.

The decision to use palliative surgery depends on the site of the disease and the duration of anticipated survival. If the patient's life

Table 9-17
Median Survival in Months of Patients After Complete Surgical Resection of Distant Metastases From Melanoma

Metastatic Site	*M.D. Anderson Hospital*	*Memorial Hospital*	*University of Alabama Hospitals*	*Roswell Park Memorial Institute*
Skin, subcutaneous	23 (64)*	25 (12)	17 (13)	31 (25)
Lung	16 (26)	19 (17)	9 (17)	9 (13)
Brain	15 (16)	7.5 (5)	8 (17)	5 (4)
Gastrointestinal (excluding liver)	18 (9)	15 (12)	8 (5)	8 (3)
2-Year survival rate	15%	21%	16%	31%

*Number of patients with metastases at that site is given in parentheses.

SOURCE: *Balch CM, Houghton A, Milton GW, Sober A, Soong SJ (eds): Cutaneous Melanoma, 2d ed. Philadelphia, JB Lippincott, 1992, with permission.*

Table 9-18
Treatment Options for Systemic Metastatic Disease

Treatment Option	*General Indications*	*Possible Risks*	*Comment*
Chemotherapy	Systemic disease (especially multisystem) Symptomatic lesions	Vomiting, diarrhea, marrow depression, infection, organ toxicity	Low activity for most single agents
Biologic therapy	Systemic disease Symptomatic lesions	Fever, fatigue, liver toxicity	Investigational treatment Low activity, but some durable responses
Surgery	Superficial lesions Solitary brain lesion Symptomatic visceral lesions Occasional solitary lung lesion	Anesthesia, infection, hemorrhage	Best for isolated lesions, especially symptomatic, low-risk patients
Radiation therapy	Superficial lesions Brain lesions Bone lesions	Normal tissue injury	Dose fraction may be important, especially for melanoma
Hyperthermia	Large superficial lesions	Normal tissue injury	An experimental treatment

is likely to be measured in weeks, the surgical ablation of a metastasis is not justified, whereas longer anticipated survival may render excision of gross disease worthwhile. Each case must be considered on its own merit.

Radiation Therapy for Distant Metastases. Irradiation has a role in the treatment of patients with advanced cancer, particularly those with symptomatic lesions.

Radiation is used as palliative treatment for patients with bone or brain metastases and for symptomatic lesions located in the skin, subcutaneous tissues, or lymph nodes (Fig. 9-31). Radiation therapy using high-energy beams relieves the pain of bone metastases, often within 1 week. Cranial (whole-brain) and spinal cord irradiation is used for central nervous system metastases. Irradiation from high-energy proton beams using a linear accelerator can also effectively treat superficially located metastases in the skin or soft tissues.

Chemotherapy

Modern use of chemotherapy began in the 1940s with the administration of hormonal therapy using androgens and estrogens, and the use of the alkylating agent, nitrogen mustard (Fig. 9-32). There are now over 30 drugs in common clinical use and well over 100 involved in investigational studies. Throughout the 1950s, chemotherapy was given on empirical grounds, using doses and scheduling previously found to be successful in antimicrobial therapy. Daily oral administration of fixed drugs was generally used. Although responses were occasionally seen, clinical relapse was universal. In the early 1960s, Skipper founded the principles still used in designing chemotherapeutic trials:

1. A single cancer cell could grow into a lethal tumor mass.
2. Tumors follow gompertzian growth kinetics in vivo, with a slowing of tumor doubling time with increasing tumor burden in the later stages of tumor growth.
3. Most chemotherapeutic agents exhibit log cell kill kinetics, with the same increment of log cell kill seen with subsequent doses.
4. An inverse relationship exists between tumor burden and curability by chemotherapeutic agents.

The comparison of antimicrobial therapy for bacterial infections and chemotherapy for malignant disease has major limitations. Bacterial infection results from a bolus exposure of bacteria introduced into an immunocompetent host capable of easily recognizing bacterial antigens as foreign. Antimicrobial therapy will kill

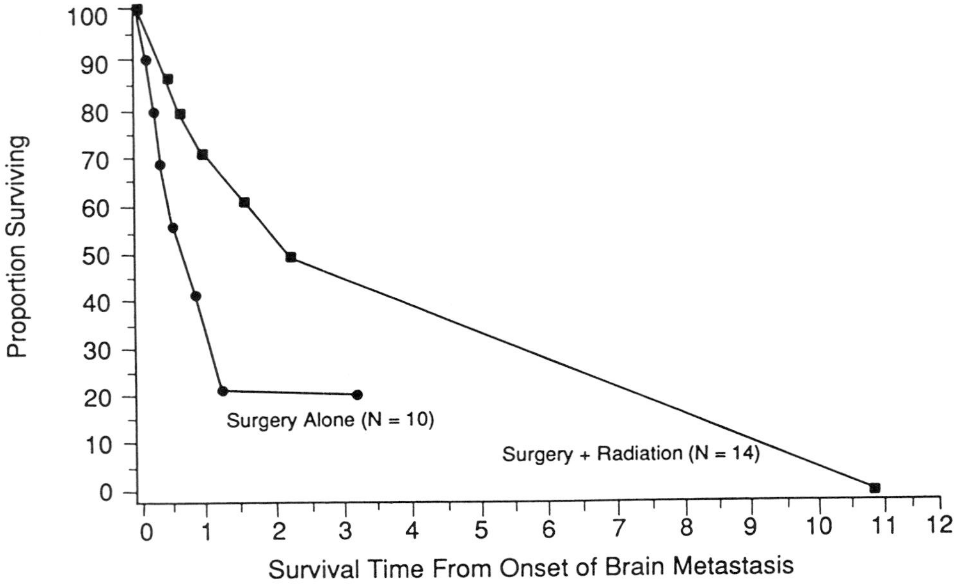

FIG. 9-31. Retrospective analysis of 24 patients with solitary brain metastases treated by surgical excision. Patients receiving postoperative cranial irradiation had apparently better survival (P = 0.07) than those not treated with irradiation. Survival time shown in months.

bacteria or arrest bacterial proliferation until host antibodies and immune effector cells expand to eliminate remaining viable bacteria. Tumors arise from normal cells through mutational events that uncommonly lead to significant cell-surface alterations. Even after significant cell kill by chemotherapy, the host may not recognize the remaining viable tumor cells as foreign, allowing regrowth of tumors.

Pharmacologic manipulation of tumors employs the systemic or regional delivery of diffusible agents to destroy or arrest tumor cells capable of proliferation. Unfortunately, currently available drugs are not selective in the exclusive destruction of tumor cells. All dividing and some quiescent cells are affected. Since most agents act on one or more stages of cell cycle, cells and tissues with the highest growth fraction will be most greatly affected. The

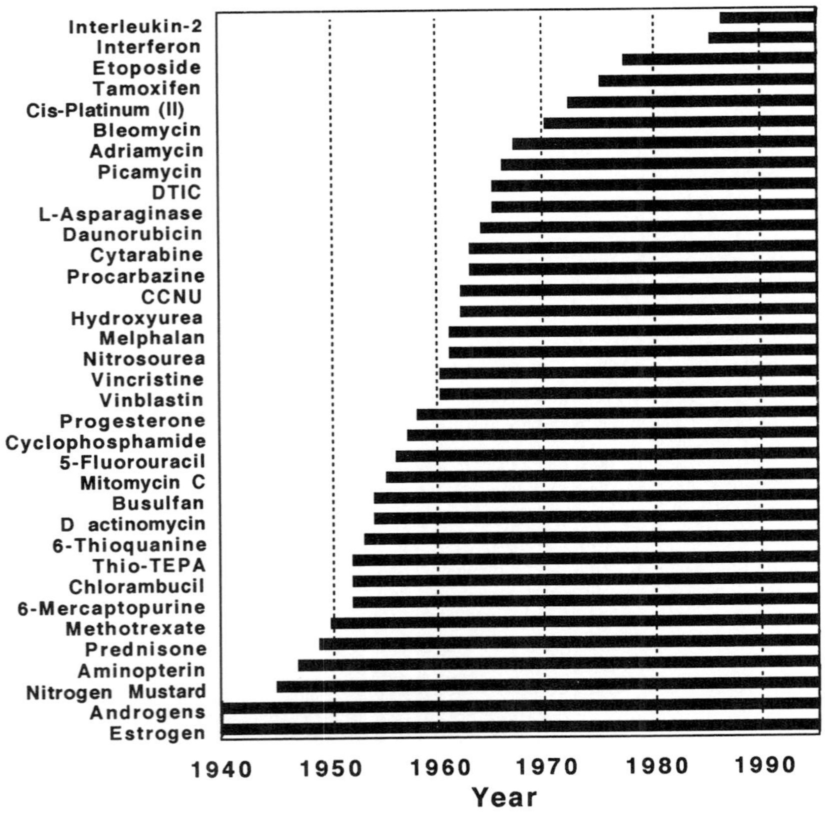

FIG. 9-32. Historical perspective for the use of therapeutic agents in the treatment of cancer. While the development of chemotherapeutic agents continues, there is a recent emergence of biologic treatments. *(Adapted from Krakoff IH: Cancer chemotherapeutic agents. Ca 37:93–15, 1987.)*

practical administration of chemotherapy considers a dynamic balance of maximal tumor cell kill with minimal and acceptable toxicity to normal host tissues.

The primary target of chemotherapeutic drugs is the tumor stem cell. Complete destruction of all tumor stem cells is essential to effect a cure. Skipper's pioneering studies with L1210 murine leukemia, which has a 100 percent growth fraction, fostered the concept of log tumor killing (Fig. 9-33). If a single dose of drug reduces the tumor cell number by 99 percent (a 2-log kill), then subsequent identical drug doses will decrease tumor cell number by the same log decrements. A 1-cm tumor contains approximately 10^9 cells and even a 99.999 percent cell kill (a 5-log kill) will result in 10^4 viable tumor cells and will fail to cure the tumor. This model established the principle of the inverse relationship between tumor burden and curability. It is therefore not surprising that the so-called clinical complete response, defined as disappearance of all measurable disease, usually results in recurrent disease, since several million viable, but undetectable, proliferating cells may still be present in one or more sites.

As previously discussed, most human tumors do not undergo exponential growth in vivo, but demonstrate a slowing of growth with progressive tumor size. The growth fraction peaks well before clinical detection, thus smaller volume disease is presumed to be more responsive to drugs active against proliferating cells, and provides the rationale for treatment in a postoperative or adjuvant setting.

The initial use of chemotherapy was to attempt to cure for macrometastatic disease. Although treatment of gross metastatic disease remains a dominant application of chemotherapy since no other modality is effective, it is known that even after dramatic clinical responses, cures are rare and currently limited to some pediatric malignancies, hematologic malignancies, Hodgkin's and some non-Hodgkin's lymphomas, testicular neoplasms, and choriocarcinoma. Equal attention is now being directed toward preoperative chemotherapy and postoperative treatment for presumed micrometastatic disease.

Resistance to Chemotherapeutic Drugs. The concept of tumor cell log kill presumes that all cell subpopulations within a tumor are chemosensitive. It is known that clinical drug resistance is responsible for the majority of chemotherapy treatment failures. Resistant subpopulations of cells may exist de novo within tumors or may arise by spontaneous or induced mutations. In animal models, Goldie and Coldman have demonstrated spontaneous mutation rates from 10^{-4} to 10^{-7}, conferring chemoresistance to a variety of chemotherapeutic drugs (Fig. 9-34). These rates are assumed, but not known, to be similar for human tumors. It is likely that a time interval exists during the natural growth of a tumor from single-cell neoplastic transformation to a tumor burden of approximately ten thousand to ten million cells where no chemoresistant cells have emerged. This interval may be several years for many solid tumors. Above this mass, the likelihood for the emergence of one or more chemoresistant clones increases exponentially with subsequent tumor growth. This concept re-emphasizes the importance of chemotherapy delivery at the earliest recognized stage of tumor growth and in clinical situations in which the risk for subclinical disease is high to achieve the greatest likelihood of cure.

Elucidation of the mechanisms involved in drug resistance has revealed a complex picture. There appear to be several different general mechanisms for different classes of chemotherapeutic agents (Table 9-19). Often tumors are found to be resistant to several agents that may be structurally unrelated. This "multidrug resistance" (mdr) may also occur by several different mechanisms. An mdr gene has recently been identified and its protein product, P-glycoprotein, has been found to cause the efflux of several different drugs from the intracellular space of target host cells in vitro. Drugs affected by overexpression of the mdr gene include several natural product agents such as the anthracycline doxorubicin, the vinca alkaloids vinblastine and vincristine, actinomycin D, and the epidophyllotoxins, such as etoposide (VP-16). High levels of P-glycoprotein are found in normal cells lining luminal spaces of the gastrointestinal tract, liver, and kidney, where the normal function of this gene product is presumed to include an active efflux of environmental toxins from the body. This efflux pump can be blocked in vitro by calcium channel blockers such as verapamil, which is currently undergoing clinical study. Other mechanisms of mdr include alterations in drug-conjugating enzymes such as glutathione S-transferase, alterations in components of the cytochrome P-450 enzyme complex such as aryl hydrocarbon hydroxylase, or alterations in drug transport enzymes such as glucuronyl transferase. Another mechanism of mdr may involve allosteric alterations in DNA, through interference with activity of topoisomerase II, an enzyme responsible for maintaining DNA's secondary and tertiary structure.

Overcoming clinical drug resistance is a major area of laboratory investigation. Molecular probes are being developed to iden-

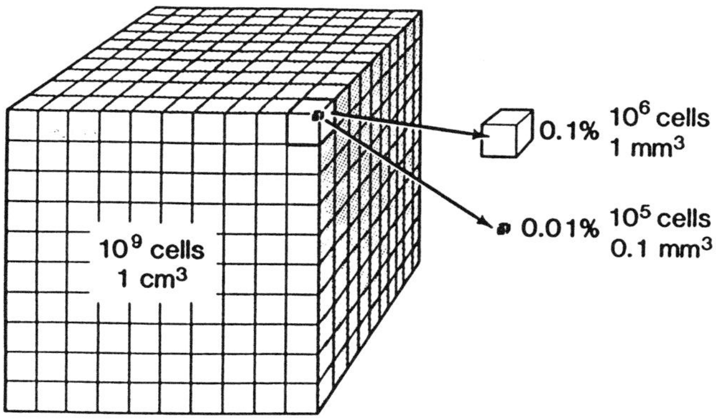

FIG. 9-33. In a mass containing 10^9 tumor cells, destruction of 99.9 percent of the cells leaves 10^6 viable cells capable of regrowth or metastasis. The surviving cells may then propagate as a resistant population.

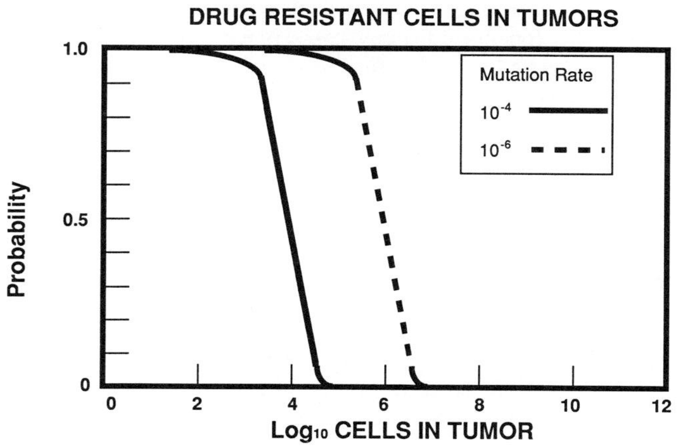

FIG. 9-34. Influence of mutation rate on drug resistance frequency.

Table 9-19
Mechanisms of Drug Resistance

Mechanism	*Drug*
Multidrug resistance	Vinca alkaloids Antitumor antibiotics Etoposide
Transport defect	Methotrexate Melphalan Nitrogen mustard Cytosine arabinoside
Poor activation	Cytosine arabinoside 5-Azacytidine 5-Fluorouracil 6-Thioguanine 6-Mercaptopurine Methotrexate Doxorubicin
Drug activation	Cytosine arabinoside Alkylating agents 6-Thioguanine 6-Mercaptopurine
Improved DNA repair	Alkylating agents Antitumor antibiotics Cisplatin
Gene amplification	Methotrexate 2-Deoxycoformycin 5-Fluorouracil
Alternate pathways	Methotrexate 5-Fluorouracil
Altered pools of competing substrate	Cytosine arabinoside 5-Fluorouracil
Target alterations	Vincristine Methotrexate 5-Fluorouracil Hydroxyurea Steroids

SOURCE: Adapted from *DeVita VT: Principles of chemotherapy, in. DeVita VT, Hellman S, Rosenber SA, (eds): Cancer: Principles and Practice of Oncology, 3rd ed. Philadelphia, JB Lippincott, 1989.*

tify additional genes involved in mdr. Antibodies against P-glycoprotein are already available and are under investigation for both diagnostic and potential therapeutic use.

Classification of Chemotherapeutic Drugs. In consideration of preoperative therapy, the surgeon should know the effects of drugs on normal tissues in order to predict changes in a patient's general medical status prior to surgery and to know the optimal timing of surgery relative to the recovery of bone marrow stem cells and the effects on wound healing. The surgeon also has the best perspective on the safe timing and tolerance of planned postoperative therapy with respect to wound healing and rehabilitation. An awareness of chemotherapeutic side effects or complications peculiar to specific drugs is also essential in order to recognize potential problems requiring prompt surgical intervention (Table 9-20).

Anticancer drugs may kill tumor cells, but the majority act by preventing cell division and thus cell proliferation. Most drugs act through effects on one or more components of the cell cycle. The classification of anticancer drugs as non-cell cycle-specific, cell cycle-specific, or phase-specific is a relative rather than an absolute description of the effects on the cell cycle. DNA synthesis can be prevented by blocking the availability of purine and pyrimidine nucleotide precursors. DNA may be damaged by crosslinking with unstable alkyl groups. DNA transcription can be prevented by direct binding of drug to DNA. Mitosis can be arrested through binding of tubulin and prevention of mitotic spindle formation. Drug combinations are often based on the complementary effects of phase-specific agents on rapidly dividing cells and the effects of non-cell cycle-specific agents on dividing and nondividing cells.

Alkylating Agents. Alkylating agents are non-cell cycle-specific agents whose mechanism of action involves contribution of an unstable alkyl group to cross-link nucleic acids (primarily DNA). The major effect is on cells in G1 or mitosis, but there may also be cytotoxic effects with high doses on cells in G0. Alkylating agents have demonstrated antitumor activity in the treatment of Hodgkin's and non-Hodgkin's lymphoma, leukemias, multiple myeloma, and carcinomas of the breast, endometrium, testis, and lung. Cyclophosphamide and cisplatin (CDDP) are commonly used in a variety of solid tumors. Dacarbazine (DTIC) and ifosfamide have documented antitumor activity against soft tissue sarcomas and other neoplasms.

Nitrosoureas represent a subgroup of alkylating agents with increased lipid solubility and thus, better central nervous system penetration. An additional mechanism of action may include carbamoylation, affecting both DNA and RNA. They do not exhibit cross-resistance with other alkylating agents. One recently described clinical concern is the rare, but important, late appearance of secondary malignancies (especially leukemias) several years after therapy with nitrosoureas (see Table 9-20).

Antimetabolites. These agents interfere with DNA and RNA synthesis and are thus phase-specific for the synthesis phase of the cell cycle. An exception is 5-fluorouracil (5-FU), which is both phase-specific and cell cycle-specific (Fig. 9-35). These drugs are most active in rapidly proliferating tumors such as the hematologic malignancies, but also have wide applicability in many solid tumors, especially breast cancer and gastrointestinal malignancies. These drugs may include structural analogues of metabolites essential in normal growth and proliferation that become incorporated as a false message, such as the pyrimidine analogue cytarabine (Ara-C). Other actions include reversible or irreversible binding to key or rate-limiting enzymes in the synthesis pathways, such as the relatively irreversible binding of methotrexate to the enzyme dihydrofolate reductase (DHFR) (Fig. 9-36). Leucovorin (folinic acid or citrovorum factor) is the most stable form of folic

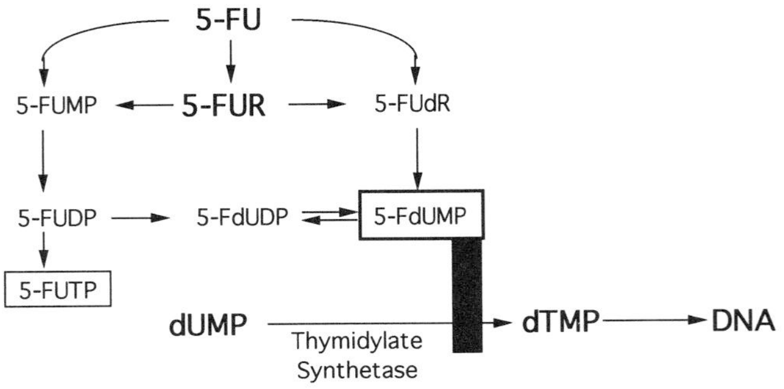

FIG. 9-35. Mechanism of the antimitotic 5-FU in the inhibition of tumor cell division.

Table 9-20
Toxicities of Common Chemotherapeutic Agents

Agent	*Route of Administration*	*Major Toxicity*	*Toxicity of Surgical Interest*
Alkylating Agents			
		General: myelosuppression, n/v, renal, hepatic, gonadal dysfunction, leukemia, cataracts	
Busulfan	P.O.	Myelosuppression, pulmonary fibrosis, gonadal dysfunction	Severe thrombocytopenia, gynecomastia
Chlorambucil	P.O.	Myelosuppression, gonadal dysfunction, leukemia	
Cisplatin (CDDP)	I.V.	Renal, severe n/v, ototoxicity, neurotoxicity, anaphylaxis, nausea, vomiting, alopecia	Hypomagnesemia, Raynaud's local vesicant
Dacarbazine (DTIC)	I.V., I.A.	Severe n/v, flu-like syndrome, myelosuppression	Diarrhea, hepatic vein thrombosis, local vesicant
Ifosfamide	I.V.	Myelosuppression, renal, acute cystitis, hepatic, alopecia, confusion	Hemorrhage, cystitis, ADH effect, local vesicant
Mechlorethamine hydrochloride (N2 mustard)	I.V., intracavitary	Severe n/v, myelosuppression, neurotoxicity, maculopapular rash	Strong local vesicant
Melphalan (L-PAM)	P.O., I.V., I.A.	Prolonged myelosuppression	
Nitrosoureas			
Carmustine (BCNU)	I.V.	N/v, hepatic, renal, pulmonary fibrosis, leukemia	Delayed leukopenia, thrombocytopenia
Lomustine (CCNU)	P.O.	Marked myelosuppression, renal, pulmonary fibrosis, leukemia	Delayed leukopenia, thrombocytopenia
Antimetabolites			
Pyrimidine analogues			
Cytarabine (Ara-C)	I.V., S.Q.	Myelosuppression, cholestasis, mucositis, pericarditis, paraparesis	Ischemic bowel, pulmonary edema
5-Fluorouracil (5-FU)	I.V., I.A.	Myelosuppression, n/v, mucositis, cerebellar dysfunction, dermatitis	Diarrhea, endotoxic shock, hepatic (I.A. route)
Floxuridine (FudR)	I.A.	N/v, myelosuppression (mild)	Diarrhea, severe gastritis, biliary sclerosis
purine analogues			
6-Mercaptopurine	P.O.	Myelosuppression, cholestasis, rash	Ileus, cumulative hepatic toxicity
folate antagonists			
methotrexate (leucovorin)	P.O. I.V., intrathecal	Myelosuppression, n/v, renal, pneumonitis, stomatitis, alopecia	Diarrhea, hemorrhagic enteritis, progressive hepatic fibrosis
Plant Alkaloids			
Etoposide (VP-16)	I.V., P.O.	Myelosuppression, n/v, alopecia	Bronchospasm, hypotension, ileus
Vinblastine	I.V.	Myelosuppression, n/v (mild), peripheral neuropathy (<vincristine)	Abdominal pain, ileus, Raynaud's local vesicant
Vincristine	I.V.	Neuropathy (peripheral and CNS), myelosuppression (mild), alopecia	Ileus, ADH effect, local vesicant
Antibiotics			
Bleomycin	I.V., I.M., S.Q., I.A., intracavitary	Fever, pulmonary fibrosis, dermatitis, anaphylaxis, myelosuppression (mild), alopecia, mucositis	Fever, Raynaud's
Dactinomycin (actinomycin D)	I.V.	N/v (severe), myelosuppression, mucositis, alopecia, dermatitis	Diarrhea, local vesicant
Doxorubicin	I.V.	Myelosuppression, cardiomyopathy, n/v, alopecia, mucositis, ECG changes	CHF secondary to cardiomyopathy, ECG changes, local vesicant
Mitomycin (mitomycin C)	I.V., I.A., intracavitary	Myelosuppression, n/v, malaise, pulmonary fibrosis, hemolytic anemia	Prolonged myelosuppression, local vesicant
Miscellaneous			
Leucovorin (folinic acid, chlorovorum factor)	P.O., I.V., I.M.	Augments with 5-FU, recues with methotrexate; anaphylaxis, worsens B-12 deficiency	
Levamisole	P.O.	Transient granulocytopenia, n/v, dermatitis, headache, nervousness	Ileus, abdominal pain, fever
Mitotane	P.O.	N/v, lethargy, depression, dermatitis, adrenal insufficiency	Diarrhea, hypotension, hemorrhagic cystitis
Tamoxifen	P.O.	Thrombocytopenia or leukopenia, tumor "flare," cataracts	Carcinoma

Abbreviations: P.O., oral; I.V., intravenous; I.A., intra-arterial; S.Q., subcutaneous; I.M., intramuscular; n/v, nausea/vomiting; CHF, congestive heart failure; ADH, antidiuretic hormone; CNS, central nervous system.

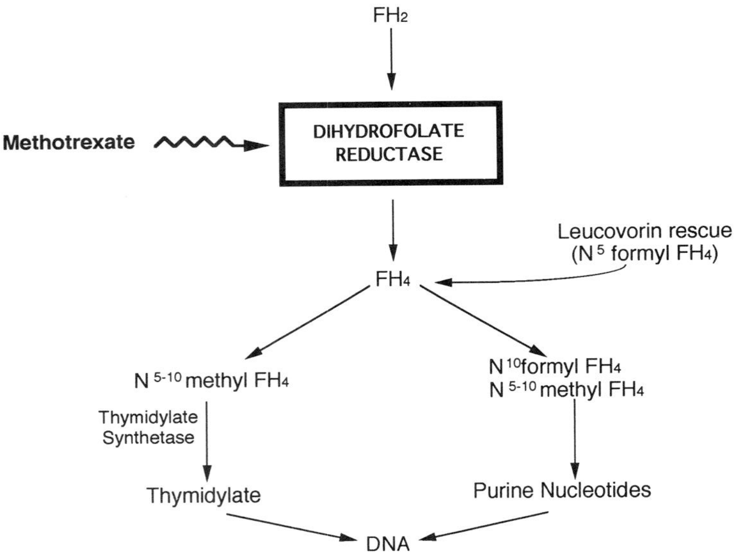

FIG. 9-36. Mechanism of the antimetabolic activity of folic acid antagonists.

acid and may be given to replenish the intracellular folate pool. It may be administered after high-dose methotrexate to "rescue" normal tissues by repleting folate and bypassing the block at DHFR. If given in combination with 5-FU, leucovorin potentiates the antitumor effect of 5-FU by stabilizing the covalent bond of 5-FdUMP (the active metabolite of 5-FU) to the enzyme thymidylate synthase.

Plant Alkaloids. Derivatives of the periwinkle plant include the vinca alkaloids vinblastine, vincristine, and vindesine. All three act as inhibitors of mitosis by binding microtubules and causing arrest in metaphase. The vinca alkaloids have demonstrated antitumor activity against Hodgkin's and non-Hodgkin's lymphomas, acute leukemias, breast, testicular, head and neck, renal, and cervical carcinomas, and other solid tumors. Although these three compounds share a similar chemical structure, there is a wide spectrum of clinical activity and toxicity (see Table 9-20).

Derivatives of the mandrake plant, the epidophyllotoxins etoposide (VP-16) and teniposide (VM-26), may act through inhibition of nucleoside transport and incorporation into DNA and RNA. These drugs show phase-specific activity for cells in G2 and late S phase. Clinical activity has been seen against lymphomas, leukemias, lung, bladder, prostate, and testicular carcinomas, hepatomas, and other solid tumors.

The plant alkaloids are prominent targets for the P-glycoprotein product of the mdr gene, resulting in clinical drug resistance.

Antibiotics. A wide spectrum of antitumor drugs have been isolated from microorganisms. These drugs are generally considered non-cell cycle-specific agents and appear to interfere with the synthesis and/or function of nucleic acids. Doxorubicin, bleomycin, mitomycin C, and dactinomycin are examples with wide current clinical applications.

Doxorubicin was derived from *Streptomyces* species and has demonstrated activity against many solid tumors, such as soft tissue sarcomas and carcinomas of the breast, lung, esophagus, stomach, liver, bladder, prostate, head and neck, testis, and endometrium, among others. The mechanism of action appears to involve intercalation into DNA with triggering of topoisomerase II-mediated DNA cleavage to alter the tertiary structure of DNA. A close analogue, daunomycin, has shown antitumor activity against acute lymphoblastic and myeloblastic leukemia.

Bleomycin was also derived from a *Streptomyces* species and causes single- and double-strand breaks in DNA (but not RNA). Antitumor activity has been shown against a variety of squamous cell carcinomas, lymphomas, testicular and lung carcinomas, malignant melanoma, soft tissue sarcomas, and mycosis fungoides.

Mitomycin C is a non-cell cycle-specific antitumor antibiotic that acts as an alkylating agent to cross-link DNA and inhibit DNA and RNA synthesis. Antitumor activity has been demonstrated against many gastrointestinal malignancies, as well as breast, lung, cervix, and bladder carcinomas.

Dactinomycin (actinomycin D) is an antitumor antibiotic derived from a *Streptomyces* species that prevents DNA and RNA synthesis by binding to the deoxyguanosine moieties of DNA. Single-stranded DNA breaks have also been demonstrated. Antitumor activity has been shown against malignant melanoma, testicular tumors, choriocarcinoma, Wilms' tumor, neuroblastoma, retinoblastoma, and several sarcomas.

Miscellaneous. Tamoxifen citrate is a nonsteroidal antiestrogen with cytostatic effects mediated through competitive inhibition of the estrogen receptor and several other emerging nonestrogen receptor pathways. Tamoxifen has a clearly documented role in the therapy of hormone-dependent tumors of the breast and prostate. Recent large studies have demonstrated antitumor activity against hormone receptor-negative breast carcinoma and possible protection against contralateral and recurrent breast carcinoma. In addition, some beneficial claims have been made regarding the possible prevention of osteoporosis and atherosclerotic heart disease through an estrogen receptor effect. Although the estrogen receptor-mediated mechanisms of tamoxifen have become more complex and confusing, the clinical applications have expanded secondary to the apparent benefits and the relatively low toxicity of outpatient oral therapy (see Table 9-20).

Levamisole is an antihelminthic drug recently used as an antitumor agent because of reported immunorestorative activity for functionally impaired macrophages and T-lymphocytes. Two large randomized, prospective trials have shown a survival benefit with levamisole combined with 5-FU in the adjuvant treatment of modified Dukes' C adenocarcinoma of the colon. Concomitant with confirmation of this finding, levamisole treatment is being extended to rectal carcinoma in combination with other agents.

Basis of Drug Selection. New drug development has rapidly evolved over the last 20 years from the identification of antitumor activity through clinical serendipity to the selection of agents through deliberate manipulations of the chemical structure of organic compounds predicted to inhibit antitumor activity by computer analysis. National and public demands to urgently find and market antitumor agents has increased funding for new drug development. The National Cancer Institute (NCI) has developed a steeply tapering pyramid for new drug testing prior to general availability to clinicians, with an emphasis on short-term and long-term safety.

Concomitant with new drug development, the NCI has the goal of doubling patient entry into national clinical trials between 1988 and 1992. There are limitations to the interpretation and relevance of in vitro drug assays and in vivo xenograft studies using chemotherapeutic drugs. Well-designed human, controlled, clinical trials represent the "gold standard" for the advancement of drug and multimodality therapy.

Phase I clinical trials are designed to determine the maximal tolerated dose (MTD) of drug, drug toxicity, and schedule for use in phase II trials. Patient eligibility is usually limited to patients with advanced disease for whom standard treatments have failed. Schema frequently include three patients at each escalating dose until toxicity is observed. Patients are informed that the likelihood for a major clinical response is small, but responses are monitored and documented.

Phase II clinical trials attempt to estimate the response rate of specific tumor types to a particular drug. Fifteen to 25 patients with a specific tumor type are initially entered. If no responses are seen, the study is usually terminated. Phase II trials may or may not randomize patients. Patients with a good performance status and a minimum of previous treatment are preferred to allow the highest probability of showing a favorable effect. Response to the drug must be measurable to allow quantitative assessment. Phase II trials assess the activity but not the efficacy of a particular drug. A minimal response rate of 20 percent is generally required to proceed to phase III trials.

Phase III trials determine whether a drug with known activity contributes significantly to the treatment of a disease. A comparative study with new treatment versus standard treatment(s) is used to determine the efficacy of the new treatment. The standard treatment may consist of no treatment or other chemotherapeutic agents. Large numbers of patients, long regular patient follow-up, and extensive resources are usually required. It is critical that different treatment groups are comparable in every way, including stratification for known or suspected prognostic variables such as sex, age, and tumor stage, among others. A randomized, controlled trial does not use historical controls and assigns comparable patients to randomly receive only one treatment modality, or arm. The study design may contain multiple treatment arms, but requires increasing numbers of patients as treatment arms are added to allow statistically valid comparisons between treatment groups. Patient eligibility and entry, the timing and method of randomization, and the endpoints to evaluate response and toxicity should be determined prior to the start of the study. The endpoint of many phase III trials is overall survival, but disease-free survival, tumor response rates, and palliation of symptoms are other common study endpoints. Phase III trials often require multi-institutional participation to accrue sufficient numbers of comparable patients over a reasonable period of time. Intra- and interinstitutional quality control is required to reach valid conclusions.

Dose and Timing of Chemotherapy. To achieve maximal tumor cell kill, the goal of chemotherapy is to give the highest tolerated dose over the shortest possible time. The dosage of drug or drugs to be administered is based on the MTD derived from phase I and II studies and must be tailored to a patient's performance status, medical illness, or organ dysfunction.

Drug dosing was traditionally described in milligrams per kilogram (mg/kg). The current and more reliable standard of drug dosing is in terms of body surface area, described as milligrams per meter squared (mg/m^2). Many nomograms are readily available to convert mg/kg to mg/m^2. A simple and relatively accurate conversion is calculated by multiplying the mg/kg dose by 40 to yield the mg/m^2 dose. Alterations are often made for patients whose actual weight varies widely from their ideal weight, as in obese patients or patients with large volumes of "third-spaced" fluid collections, such as pleural effusions, ascites, or edema. Although no universally accepted formula exists for these patients, knowledge of the pharmacology and volume of distribution of different drugs provides a rational basis for dose alterations.

The interval for repeated drug dosing is dependent on toxicity patterns to normal tissues. For most chemotherapeutic agents with bone marrow toxicity, leukopenia and thrombocytopenia become evident on a complete blood count by day 9 or 10 and reach a nadir between days 14 and 18. Recovery is usually beginning by day 21 and is approximately 90 percent complete by day 28. This provides the rationale for a 28-day course or cycle of marrow suppressive agents. Bone marrow recovery time may be delayed in onset or prolonged secondary to previous chemotherapy, radiation therapy to marrow-producing bone, or inherent toxicities of a few specific drugs (see Table 9-20).

The interval required to assure the safe recovery of bone marrow production or other dose-limiting toxicities may also allow recovery and repopulation of remaining tumor cells. The administration of drug combinations was begun to overcome the problems of single-drug toxicity and existing or emergent drug-resistant cell populations.

Combination Therapy and Dose Intensification. The Goldie-Coldman hypothesis predicts that chemoresistant cell populations are present at the time tumor is clinically apparent. Single-agent therapy has only produced cures in choriocarcinoma and Burkitt's lymphoma. Combination chemotherapy is an attempt to provide antitumor therapy to all resistant cell populations at the earliest possible time, without increasing the toxicity to normal tissues.

With rate exceptions, only drugs known to be effective as single agents against a particular tumor are considered for combination therapy. Drugs from different classes are often selected with cell cycle and non-cell cycle specificity to affect dividing and quiescent tumor subpopulations. Careful selection of drugs with non-overlapping toxicities is essential to avoid life-threatening injury to normal tissues. If such combinations require lowering of individual drug doses to avoid excess toxicity, the reduced antitumor activity, as suggested by suboptimal dose intensification, outweighs the potential benefit of the drug combination.

The concept of dose intensification has been promoted by Hyrniuk et al. to allow comparisons of the relative effectiveness of each drug used in combination therapy and to optimize drug dose delivery during a course of combination chemotherapy. Relative dose intensity (RDI) is the proportion of drug delivered per unit of time (usually 1 week) relative to an arbitrary standard dose of that drug over the same interval. For example, during a 28-day cycle of combination therapy, if one chooses a cyclophosphamide standard dose (as in the Cooper CMFVP breast cancer regimen) given as 80 mg/m^2/day by continuous infusion (a dose intensity of 560 mg/m^2/week) and compares a test regimen consisting of 100 mg/m^2/day given only on days 1 to 14 (a dose intensity of 350 mg/m^2/week), the RDI of the test regimen is 350/560 = 0.62. The test dose of cyclophosphamide is higher during the first half of the 28-day course, but the overall total dose per course is less than in the standard dose.

The importance of optimizing dose intensification has been well documented in laboratory animal models bearing curable tumors, in which as little as a 20 percent decrease in dose intensity of an effective drug can result in a 50 percent decrease in cure rate. Comparisons of dose intensity in combination drug trials for breast, ovarian, and colon carcinomas, and lymphomas have demonstrated a strong correlation between dose intensity and response rates.

Induction Chemotherapy. The term *induction chemotherapy* best describes the use of chemotherapy as the sole form of treatment for advanced disease. The usual clinical situation is the presence of multiple sites of metastatic disease, where local-regional treatment by surgery and radiation would not address the systemic disease, which is the primary determinant of clinical outcome. If a patient progresses or fails to respond to induction chemotherapy, a change to other agents or combinations, or *salvage therapy,* is considered.

Adjuvant Chemotherapy. *Adjuvant chemotherapy* describes the use of regional or systemic therapy after local-regional tumor elimination by surgery or radiation therapy. All adjuvant therapy is the treatment of presumed micrometastatic disease. This treatment is usually limited to those patient groups known through historical controls to be at moderate-to-high risk for local or distant recurrence. Since there is no tumor visible at the time of treatment, response can only be evaluated over time through observed rather than expected recurrence rates, disease-free survival, and overall survival.

Although the choice of agents for adjuvant chemotherapy is based on response rates seen with advanced disease of the same histologic type, the correlation of sensitivity between micrometastatic disease and established bulky metastatic disease is often inferred and not absolutely known. A limited but intensive duration of therapy is usually employed since any benefit against microscopic disease is likely to occur during the first few courses as long as adequate cytotoxic doses are given. Few studies show any added benefit to ''maintenance'' adjuvant chemotherapy.

Chemotherapy as Initial Treatment. The use of chemotherapy in a multimodality treatment strategy for localized disease is known as *primary* or *neoadjuvant chemotherapy*. There is an increasing use of primary chemotherapy for a variety of solid tumors, such as breast, gastrointestinal, and pediatric carcinomas, extremity sarcomas, and localized lymphomas, among others (Fig. 9-37).

There are several theoretical advantages to primary chemotherapy. First, large or locally advanced tumors may be downstaged to allow a safer resection and spare surrounding normal tissues, as in breast conservation surgery, anal sphincter preservation with mid-to-low rectal tumors, and limb preservation with extremity sarcomas. Second, tumor responsiveness to chemotherapy can often be determined within one to three initial courses while grossly or radiologically visible tumor is still present, and can be used to clinically guide postoperative chemotherapy. Those tumors with an initial complete or major partial response will be continued on the same agents postoperatively. Tumors not responding or progressing with primary chemotherapy would either not be subjected to postoperative chemotherapy or would be treated by alternative chemotherapeutic agents. A third potential advantage is immediate

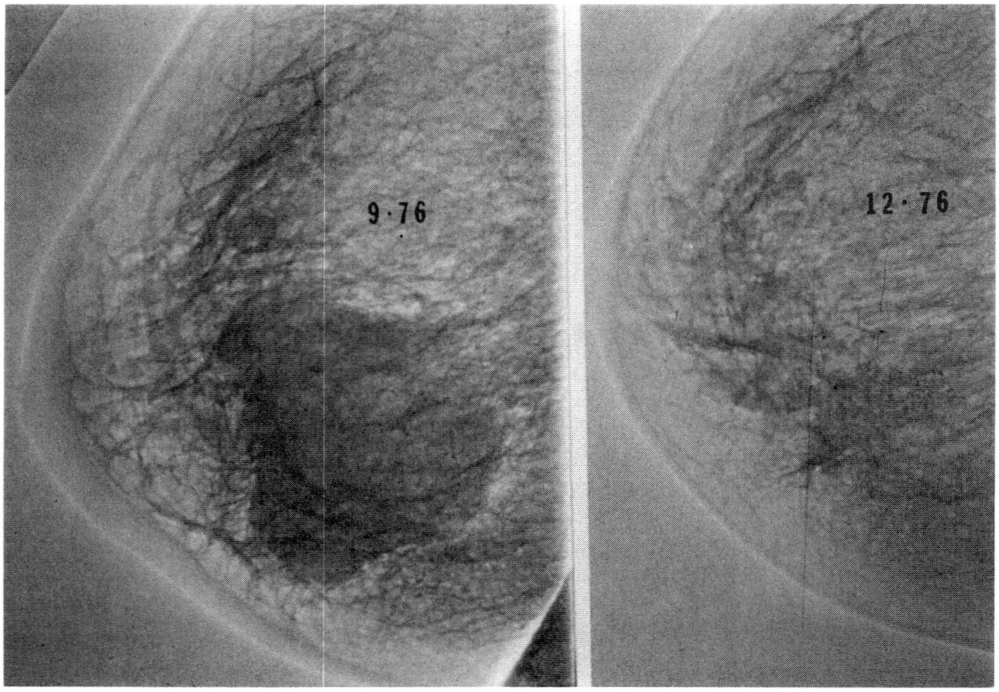

FIG. 9-37. A striking example of preoperative chemotherapy in a patient with locally advanced (stage III) breast cancer. *Left panel.* A pretreatment mammogram showing a large tumor occupying the lower half of the breast. *Right panel.* Three months later there is a complete response to the doxorubicin-based chemotherapy regimen, as measured by physical examination and mammography. However, after mastectomy, pathological examination showed viable tumor cells at a microscopic level. The patient subsequently received postoperative chemotherapy and radiotherapy as part of a multimodality treatment approach used at the M.D. Anderson Cancer Center for stage III breast cancer.

treatment of possible micrometastatic disease instead of delaying systemic therapy until completion of a several-week course of radiotherapy or until full recovery from resection of the primary tumor.

Potential disadvantages of primary chemotherapy include a delay in local-regional management of tumor if there is no response or progressive disease. Second, tumors that progress on primary therapy may preclude a safe resection or lead to sacrifice of additional normal surrounding structures to obtain adequate resection margins. Third, a positive chemotherapeutic tissue effect may confuse the pathologic staging of resected tissues, complicating future treatment decisions and prognosis.

Drug Delivery Strategies. Intravenous administration is the most common route of chemotherapeutic drug delivery. One or more drugs are given to deliver uniform doses of drug to all capillary beds and end organs with known or presumed metastatic disease. Other common routes of delivery include regional arterial chemotherapy and intraperitoneal chemotherapy. Less common applications include intravesical bladder therapy, topical therapy of skin tumors, intrathecal therapy for meningeal disease, and intrapleural drug instillation for malignant pleural effusions.

Regional Chemotherapy. Intraperitoneal chemotherapy has been used in abdominal neoplasms that demonstrate abdominal carcinomatosis or malignant ascites as a dominant pattern of metastatic spread, such as ovarian, colorectal, pancreatic, and gastric carcinomas, retroperitoneal sarcomas, pseudomyxoma peritonei, and abdominal mesotheliomas. Although results from clinical trials with intraperitoneal chemotherapy for macrometastatic disease have been disappointing, systemic therapy is rarely effective, thus providing the impetus for its use as an adjuvant treatment to control micrometastatic disease in patients at high risk for this pattern of failure. Positive peritoneal cytology obtained by washings at the time of laparotomy or laparoscopy represents an ideal clinical setting for intraperitoneal chemotherapy in view of the high risk of clinically significant peritoneal failure at the time of lowest detectable peritoneal disease. A role for preoperative intraperitoneal chemotherapy has not been defined.

It is known that fluid in the abdominal cavity will primarily diffuse through serosal surfaces and into the portal circulation draining to the liver. A small amount of fluid drains via lymphatics that empty through pores in the diaphragm. The depth and rate of diffusion of several chemotherapeutic drugs through peritoneal serosa and into peritoneal tumor implants has been established in animal models and is dependent on size, lipid solubility, and charge. The larger the molecule, a low lipid content, and the presence of a positive or negative charge will all decrease the rate of peritoneal surface absorption and thus increase the time of exposure of drug to peritoneal surfaces.

The rationale for intraperitoneal chemotherapy is to gain a therapeutic advantage by delivering relatively high-dose drug to the serosal surfaces of the peritoneal cavity with low plasma and other tissue levels. Several conditions should be present to consider this route of drug delivery: (1) peritoneal metastasis and/or liver metastasis should be a dominant pattern of failure; (2) the drug should have known tumoricidal activity against the tumors; (3) the drug should have a low peritoneal permeability to maximize the duration of peritoneal drug exposure; and (4) there should be rapid plasma clearance of drug.

There are several technical considerations in the delivery of intraperitoneal chemotherapy. The use of soft, indwelling peritoneal catheters connected to a subcutaneous access port has greatly diminished the risk of catheter-related infections. It is important that drug concentration be distributed equally throughout the peritoneal cavity, both to optimize drug exposure to tumor and to prevent sequestering of high drug concentrations in focal fluid loculations. Equal drug distribution requires the absence of adhesions, necessitating the administration of therapy perioperatively and a duration of therapy limited to days. Additionally, studies of peritoneal cavity fluid distribution after transperitoneal catheter infusion using soluble water-soluble contrast or radionuclides have demonstrated the need for instillation of 1 to 2 liters of crystalloid to assure equal distribution.

Although intraperitoneal chemotherapy has been investigated for several years in the treatment of minimal residual disease in ovarian carcinoma, an overall survival advantage has been difficult to demonstrate because of the lack of randomized, controlled clinical trials. The efficacy of this therapy in other intra-abdominal, abdominal, and pelvic malignancies is under investigation.

Regional arterial drug therapy to specific organ sites has been used for several primary and metastatic solid tumors, including head and neck carcinomas, primary and recurrent gastrointestinal and pelvic malignancies, extremity sarcomas, in-transit metastatic melanoma, and primary or metastatic hepatic tumors.

Limb perfusion in extremity melanoma employs vascular isolation of an affected extremity through external iliac or axillary arterial and venous cannulation and placement of a proximal limb tourniquet to minimize systemic drug leakage. A high concentration of drug with or without limb hyperthermia can then be perfused over approximately 1 hour and extracted via an extracorporeal dialysate pump oxygenator before re-establishment of normal limb perfusion. The maximal drug dosage becomes limited by limb tissue toxicity and not by systemic drug levels, but is accompanied by the considerable additional morbidity associated with operative limb vascular access and compromised wound healing.

Chemoembolization, used in the treatment of primary hepatomas or neuroendocrine tumors metastatic to the liver, employs delivery of drug-impregnated pellets or sponge spheroids that temporarily or permanently occlude end-arteries selectively supplying tumor-bearing liver, thus slowing tumor blood flow and increasing the time of drug exposure to the tumor. The same decrease in flow has been accomplished with internal or external, surgically placed, temporary hepatic artery occlusion catheters, which can be manipulated to cause tumor ischemia after hepatic arterial infusion of drug.

The high tissue extraction of some drugs by hepatic parenchyma has also been exploited. The fluoropyrimidines demonstrate high hepatic extraction, with removal of more than 90 percent of floxuridine (FUdR) and 75 to 85 percent of 5-FU on a single pass after hepatic artery bolus infection. Clinical trials using hepatic arterial FUdR have demonstrated that biliary sclerosis (that appears to be irreversible) and elevation of hepatic enzymes represent the dose-limiting toxicities seen with hepatic intra-arterial FUdR administration.

Drugs such as doxorubicin and mitomycin C that have some demonstrated tumoricidal activity against primary hepatomas and metastatic colon carcinoma may also be given by hepatic arterial infusion. However, systemic toxicity becomes dose-limiting, since the hepatic extraction of these drugs is approximately 25 percent and 12 percent, respectively. Attempts to increase the extracorporeal extraction of these and other drugs from the venous effluent of the liver and other regional infusion sites is under investigation using regional venous filtration techniques.

Measuring the Response to Chemotherapy. Established guidelines are available to evaluate clinical response to chemotherapy for visible, palpable, or radiologically measurable tumors. A partial response is most commonly defined as a 50 percent or greater reduction in summed measurable tumor mass. Each tumor mass is measured as the product of the two greatest perpendicular diameters. A partial response is occasionally subdivided into minor responses (less than 50 percent size reduction) and major responses (greater than 50 percent size reduction, but less than a complete response). This subdivision is clinically insignificant since only a complete response has the potential for cure. A complete response requires total disappearance of tumor on physical examination and radiologic studies for at least 4 weeks. Tumor progression is defined as a greater than 50 percent increase in summed measurable tumor mass. Stable disease indicates no change in tumor mass, size reduction less than a partial response, or any increase in size less than progression.

An absence of change in tumor size does not always indicate a lack of tumor response. Many large tumors may undergo necrosis, fibrosis, or granuloma formation with marked destruction of viable tumor cells, but minimal or no change in size. The increasing use of preoperative or primary chemotherapy has enabled histologic evaluation of pretreated tumor and normal tissue. There are currently no universally accepted guidelines to evaluate biologic tumor response other than gross estimates of the percentage of visibly unaffected tumor cells identified through histologic examination of sectioned tumor.

Adjuvant chemotherapy is, by definition, the treatment of presumed micrometastases. Since no tumor is detectable, physical measurement of response to therapy cannot be performed. The end points become time to relapse, relapse-free or disease-free survival, and overall survival, compared to matched historical or concurrent untreated control patients.

The many possible clinical responses to chemotherapy require measurement of disease over a prolonged length of time. The most common clinical course of a drug-sensitive tumor that undergoes a complete response to therapy is early relapse. A concept frequently overlooked by clinicians and one difficult for patients to understand is that success in curing malignant disease is won or lost when the disease is clinically undetectable. There is often patient or physician hesitancy to continue courses of toxic chemotherapy when the tumor appears to have disappeared, or to start adjuvant treatment when a clinically aggressive tumor appears to have been completely resected.

Side Effects and Toxicity. Some degree of drug toxicity during the administration of chemotherapy is not only expected but is often desirable as it indicates a cellular damage response to the agent or agents. With rare exceptions, the maximal tolerated dose (MTD) of most chemotherapeutic agents is sought to achieve the highest tumor cell kill. Therefore, close attention to normal tissue injury is essential to optimize the risk/benefit ratio and assure that the treatment is not worse than the disease.

Patterns of organ toxicity have been well described for the different classes of drugs. The degree of toxicity is dependent on concentration of drug(s), time of exposure, and the host response to drug. Anticipated drug toxicity is based on the nonspecific damage caused by most chemotherapeutic agents to rapidly proliferating normal tissues such as bone marrow stem cells, gastrointestinal crypt lining cells, and hair follicles. Even within the same class of drugs, differential organ injury may be seen. There may also be rare idiosyncratic systemic drug reactions within any drug category that cause unexpected, and occasionally life-threatening toxicity.

Objective and subjective measurements of toxicity are serially recorded to allow the delivery of maximal tumoricidal drug doses with minimal and reversible injury to normal tissues. Several grading scales have been formulated to quantitate and follow toxicity with subsequent courses of drug therapy. The Eastern Cooperative Oncology Group (ECOG) and other groups or centers have developed scales that attempt to standardize toxicity criteria for measurement and reporting in clinical trials. The severity of signs, symptoms, and alterations in laboratory tests are graded for all major organ systems. Grade 0 denotes no toxicity and grade 4 usually denotes life-threatening toxicity. The duration, chronicity, and reversibility of toxicity are also important. Clinical trials often have provisions for dose reduction or cessation of drug therapy for toxicity greater than grade 2 or 3, depending on the organ system affected. Surgical consultation of a patient receiving chemotherapy is one of the most challenging situations requiring thoughtful surgical judgment. The neutropenic patient with idiopathic sepsis, abdominal pain, perirectal pain, or soft tissue infection requires frequent and careful examination and knowledge of the expected leukocyte nadir and recovery time.

Quality of Life. The overall use of chemotherapeutic agents to treat solid tumors is rapidly increasing. Patients with advanced disease will often respond transiently or not at all to even intensive multiagent therapy. Since the median survival of these patients is measured in months, the toxicity and duration of therapy must be carefully weighed against any expected or likely increase in survival to maximize the quality of life.

Attempts to measure quality of life require subjective analyses of pre-and posttreatment patient performance status and symptoms over time. The subjective nature of this analysis is difficult to quantitate and requires a repeated and reproducible written record of graded symptoms and alterations in life-style. The disease interval to maximize is the *time without symptoms* (from persistent or progressive disease) *or toxicity,* called the TWiST score. If a marginal increase in overall survival results in a shortened TWiST interval during prolonged course of toxic chemotherapy, then any antitumor benefits of that therapy will not translate into an improved quality of that patient's remaining life.

An informed and interested patient can be a vital and equal partner in the decision to pursue chemotherapy. The clinician's role is to know the experience with chemotherapy, describe the therapeutic options, toxicity, and expected benefits, encourage the partnership of those patients eager to take a prominent role in guided clinical decisions, and remove the burden of decision-making from patients unable or unwilling to participate in these difficult decisions. Clinician adaptability is essential to maintain the trusting patient/physician relationship necessary for completion of a prolonged chemotherapy program.

Biologic Therapy

The rationale of biologic therapies for human cancer is to augment host immunity and intensify a tumor rejection response. Immunobiologic therapy is usually administered in combination with other agents or surgical procedures. Biologic therapy also includes novel and experimental therapies involving the incorporation of specific gene sequences that increase cytokine synthesis, regulate tumor cell division, and augment immune-mediated tumor rejection. Gene therapy may involve the transfection of drug sensitivity, lymphokine, or tumor suppressor genes. Transfected materials may be promoter sequences, the entire sequence for a specific product, or an antisense sequence to confound macromolecular synthesis of a specific product.

Immunology of Neoplastic Disease. ***Absence or Impairment of Immune Function.*** Immunodeficiency in human beings is associated with an increase in the incidence of specific neoplasms. Frequently, these are tumors of the immune system or skin, and some epithelial tumors caused by viruses. Seldom is there a significant increase in the risk for common tumors such as breast cancer and colon carcinoma. Many immunodeficiencies do not significantly affect the function of macrophages and NK lymphocyte populations, which have critical roles in the surveillance against neoplastic disease. Therefore, given the vast redundancy in the capacity of the immune system it is difficult to ascribe a singular mechanism within the immune system that is charged with surveillance against neoplastic disease. The consensus from experimental models and from clinical experience is that the immune system is critical in preventing the outgrowth of transformed cancer cells at metastatic sites.

Tumors That Evoke Adaptive and Native Immune Responses. Implicit in the ability of the immune system to recognize neoplastic cells is the existence of tumor-associated antigens that can initiate an immune response in the autochthonous host. In animal models there is convincing evidence that tumors express tumor antigens that evoke protective immunity to transplantation with lethal numbers of syngeneic tumor cells. Depending on the etiology of the neoplasms, antigenic specificities may be exquisitely unique (as in chemically induced neoplasms of mice) or shared among all tumors of a common etiology (virus induced).

Evidence that human tumors are immunogenic in the autochthonous host is growing despite several decades of controversy. In melanoma as well as ovarian carcinoma and in squamous cell carcinoma of the head and neck, analysis of the T-cell-mediated responses in peripheral blood and tumor infiltrates reveals substantial numbers of clones that possess antigen-specific receptors for biochemical structures expressed on the surface of tumor cells. Immunity to tumors may be manifest as production of specific antibody and the activation of specific T-lymphocytes that are cytotoxic to in vitro propagated tumor and that secrete lymphokines when stimulated by tumor antigen. With these initial findings there was an expansion of investigative protocols addressing the potentiation of tumor immune responses in cancer patients by targeting the T-cell population.

From laboratory experimentation and clinical observation, it is known that many tumors induce immune responses in their hosts and that the immune effector mechanisms are thwarted locally and systemically by (1) the insufficient nature of the effector mechanism, (2) activation of immunoregulatory networks that suppress tumor rejection, and (3) actions or products of the tumor that interfere with the rejection process. No single possibility has universal application, but as our understanding of the host immune response to autologous tumor antigens in various neoplastic diseases improves, the strategies for biologic approaches to treatment will improve vastly.

In most experiences, induction of antitumor antibody affords little protection. In the rodent models immunity to solid tumors cannot be transferred to normal syngeneic hosts using serum or purified antibody preparations. By contrast, T lymphocytes play a critical role in the rejection of solid tumors in these models. In addition to the adoptive specific immunity afforded by T lymphocytes, the native NK lymphocytes of the large granular lymphocyte (LGL) series are capable of lysing a wide variety of tumor and virus infected cells without the use of antigen-specific receptors and recognition of the major histocompatibility complex (MHC).

The use of biologic agents that shift the host immune response toward rejection of the growing neoplasm is a clinical strategy that continues to increase in use with our knowledge of the molecular mechanisms. The immune system has the capacity to distinguish neoplastic from normal cells through differential expression of an array of tumor-associated antigens. Theoretically the immune system may be activated or reactivated to specifically attack and destroy tumor leaving normal tissue largely unaffected. Present strategies using immunology employ a variety of biologic agents in conjunction with antibodies and immune cells. Table 9-21 summarizes the modalities of immunotherapy, and Table 9-22 summarizes some of the source materials used in the design of biologic therapies that employ immunologic agents. It is intended that biologic therapy will serve as an adjunct in the treatment of cancer wherein it may serve to augment the treatments initiated as surgery, radiation, or chemotherapy.

Rapidly emerging advances in the basic mechanisms of cell-mediated immunity provide new strategies for biologic therapy based on the prospect that the host immune system may be manipulated either in vivo and ex vivo to reject neoplastic outgrowth. Molecular biology and cell cloning enable investigation of a new

Table 9-21
Immunotherapy Strategies

Therapeutic Strategy	*Agent*	*Desired Biologic Effect*
Active specific	Vaccine	Induction of tumor-specific immunity
Passive specific	Immune lymphocytes or antibody	Establish tumor immunity
Active nonspecific	BCG and other immunologic adjuvants	Activate macrophages Promote specific immunity
Passive nonspecific	LAK cells	Establish a large population of nonspecific cytolytic lymphocytes in the host

Table 9-22
Source Materials for Biologic Therapy of Neoplastic Disease

Agent	*Description*
LAK cells	Peripheral blood lymphocytes activated by incubation with IL 2. Usually large granular lymphocytes of the NK lineage. Antigen independent lysis of tumor cells with little or no effect on normal tissue. Used in adoptive transfer protocols.
TIL	Tumor infiltrating lymphocytes that have been propagated ex vivo in the presence of tumor antigen and IL-2. Often are T-lymphocytes. May also be NK. Used in adoptive transfer protocols.
Genetically modified immune cells	Immune cells transfected with genes that modulate lytic activity or homing patterns.
Allogeneic vaccine	Vaccine preparation composed of tumor cells obtained from several different donors. Tumor cells inactivated by irradiation ex vivo.
Autologous vaccine	Vaccine prepared from the patient's own tumor. Tumor cells inactivated by irradiation.
Oncolysate vaccine	Prepared by infecting and lysing tumor cells with a nononcogenic virus such as vaccinia.
Recombinant vaccines	Incorporation of the gene encoding a tumor associated antigen into an immunogenic, nononcogenic virus.
Monoclonal antibody	Antibodies to tumor-associated antigens that can mediate lysis through complement or by facilitation of lysis by Fc-receptor bearing cells. Additionally, labeled antibody may be used in imaging.
Immunoconjugate	Antibodies to tumor-associated antigens may be conjugated to cytotoxic drugs and thereby facilitate targeting of drug to the tumor while maintaining subtoxic levels systemically
Antisense sequences	Prevention of translation of molecules that down-regulate host immunity to tumor may be achievable by ex vivo or in vivo delivery of potently regulatory antisense DNA.

level of the biology of host-tumor relationships and for development of biologic agents to administer to cancer patients. Early clinical trials in patients treated with prototypic strategies suggest a long future for biotherapy. Considering the vast possibilities in biologic and molecular genetic approaches to the modulation of host immunity, the present clinical trial battery constitutes only a small fraction of the potential options.

Previous immunologic investigations in cancer patients addressed antibody levels and cytotoxic lymphocytes from human blood. Demonstration of antibodies against human cancers is occurring more frequently as detection assays become more sensitive and specific. As suggested by animal models, the majority of antibodies in human peripheral blood are not protective even though some may be directed against tumor-associated antigens. Therefore a major effort has been launched to elucidate the role of various lymphocyte populations in human tumor immunity. Figure 9-38 shows the major lymphocyte populations and their associated cell surface markers (cluster designate, CD) and biologic activities. The majority of peripheral blood lymphocytes, whether T cells or NK cells, have low and sometimes undetectable cytotoxicity against autologous tumor cell targets. Clinical studies of pretherapy and postsurgery patients suggest that the peripheral blood NK cells consistently lyse human tumors, but the extent of cytotoxicity usually does not correlate with the stage of disease nor the prognosis. Possibly measurement of immune effector mechanisms in the peripheral compartment is not an appropriate indicator for assessment of the tumor immunity at the site of neoplastic outgrowth.

Important new information emerged with investigations of the nature and function of lymphocytes emigrating directly into human cancers (tumor-infiltrating lymphocytes, TIL). Functional analysis of TIL in melanoma and renal cell carcinoma resulted in a two-compartment model of host immune response, in which (1) the host immune defense in the vascular compartment is primarily concerned with antibodies, and, more importantly, NK cells that destroy tumors in transit within the circulatory system, and (2) the tissue level at which cytotoxic T lymphocytes and macrophages are the primary effector cells responsible for an immune rejection response. No doubt the critical aspects of host-tumor interaction should take place at the site of the tumor. It is at this level that the defect in host immunity is most apparent. The profound immunologic shortfall of TIL extracted from a human melanoma is illustrated in Figure 9-39. Herein, freshly isolated TIL do not recognize nor bind to adjacent autologous tumor cells, two critical aspects of cytotoxic effector function. In addition, the TIL respond poorly to antigenic stimulus, polyclonal activators, and cytokines when compared to peripheral blood lymphocytes. On the other hand, the absence of effector function in TIL is overcome ex vivo by long-term (2 to 6 weeks) incubation of TIL with interleukin-2 (IL-2) and tumor-associated antigen, which often restores the proliferative potential, cytokine synthesis, and cytotoxic capacity.

Clinical investigations identified several populations of human TIL cytotoxic T lymphocytes recovered from melanoma and renal cell carcinoma that differ based on their response to tumor and tumor-associated antigen (Fig. 9-40). Thus, there is likely an extraordinary diversity in effector cell type and function among different human cancers. Important differences are evident in comparison of the populations of TIL that marginate into melanoma and renal cell carcinoma. Melanoma TIL frequently are cytotoxic T lymphocytes that proliferate in the presence of IL-2 and antigens. Ex vivo propagated melanoma TIL kill only autologous cells by recognition of either self (histocompatibility antigens) or individually specific melanoma antigens (see discussion of carcinogen-induced murine tumors). In contrast, TIL from human renal

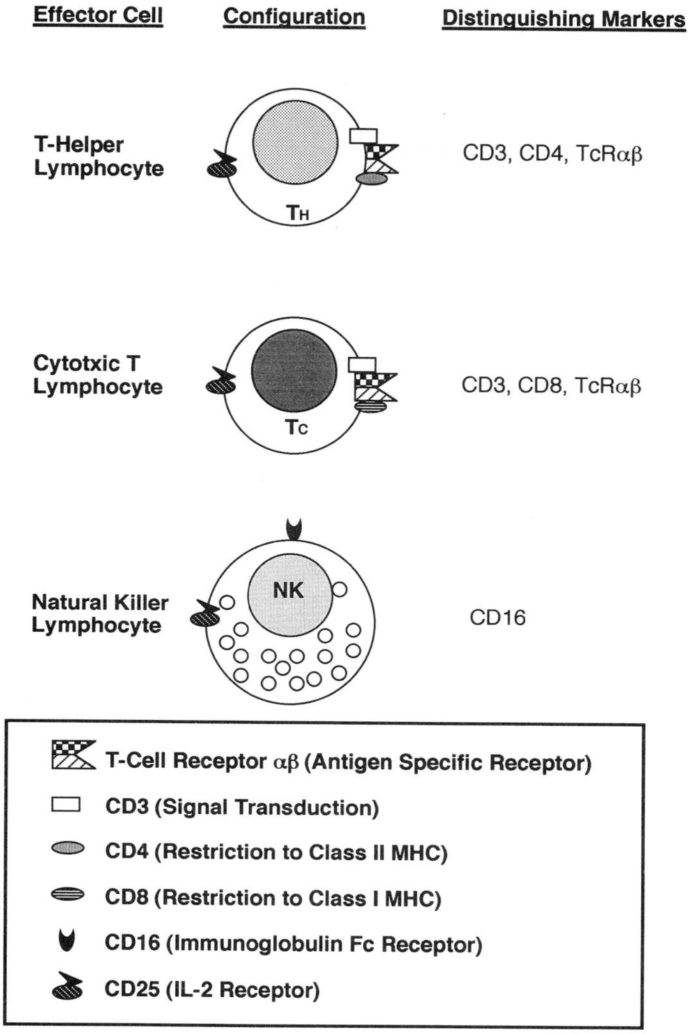

FIG. 9-38. Effector cells that may be propagated from the TIL populations. Bulk cultures of TIL from several different neoplasms result in a predominating population from one or more of the illustrated phenotypes. In unselected populations of cultured TIL the phenotypic expression of cell surface markers (CD) has strong correlation with immune function. In cloned populations of lymphocytes the phenotype and function may not coincide.

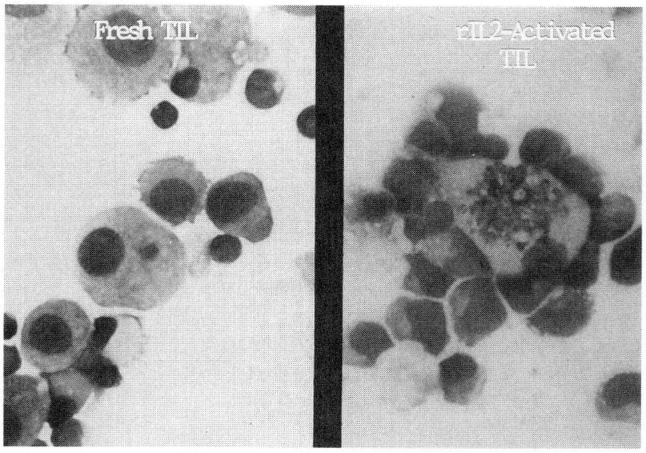

FIG. 9-39. Comparison of fresh TIL isolates with TIL cultured in the presence of IL-2 and tumor antigen. A critical step in immune-mediated destruction of tumor cells is recognition (the binding of effector cell to the target). Fresh TIL *(left panel)* evidence little if any target cell recognition, while cultured TIL *(right panel)* bind to the tumor in substantial numbers.

cell carcinomas have the capacity to kill both autologous and allogeneic human cancer cells after IL-2 activation. Initially it was concluded that the unrestricted cytotoxicity of renal cell carcinoma by TIL was due solely to predominance of NK cells known to lyse a vast array of allogeneic targets. Phenotypic analysis of TIL separated by fluorescence-activated cell sorter (FACS), however, revealed an ''anomalous'' T cell that was cytotoxic in vitro for both autologous and allogeneic targets. The novel modality of T-cell-mediated tumor lysis in the absence of MHC compatibility may suggest in renal cell carcinoma the possibility of producing antitumor T cells from allogeneic donors. Thus, there is substantial diversity in tumor infiltrates. Part of the diversity is due to the multilevel redundancy in immune effectors and part is determined by the target tissue or the host organ of the tumor.

The function of human TIL does not necessarily correlate with the phenotypic (CD) marker expression ascribed to T and NK cells. CD3 is the cell surface marker for nearly all the T lymphocytes in the peripheral compartment. $CD3^+CD4^+$ lymphocytes are frequently associated with helper function, whereas $CD3^+CD8^+$ T lymphocytes have cytotoxic or suppressor cell function. Experiments performed in our laboratory using cloned human TIL showed no correlation between the CD4 or CD8 expression and

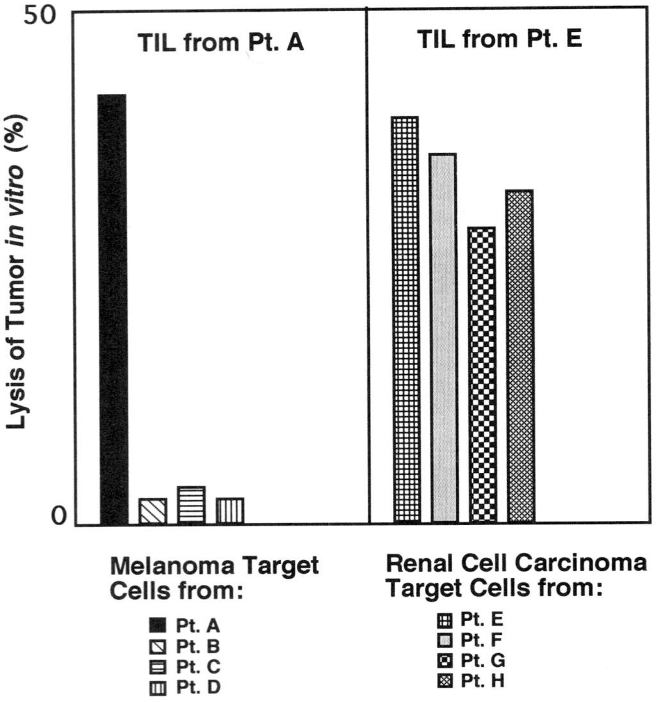

FIG. 9-40. Difference in the effector cell populations propagated from the TIL of melanoma and renal cell carcinoma. The TIL from melanoma lyse only the autologous tumor cells and not melanoma cells from other patients. Melanoma cytotoxic TIL are frequently antigen-specific T lymphocytes. In contrast, propagated TIL from renal cell carcinoma (RCC) lyse RCC cells from many patients. The TIL from RCC may be MHC-unrestricted T lymphocytes or NK lymphocytes.

the functional capacity of cloned $CD3^+$ T cells. Thus, $CD4^+$ cells, otherwise known as TH lymphocytes, enigmatically possess cytotoxic capabilities, while $CD8^+$ cells produce different cytokines such as IL-2 and IL-4, functions usually ascribed to $CD4^+$ helper cells.

In summary, analysis of the TIL in two human neoplasms has revealed (1) overwhelming impairment of lymphocyte function at the tumor site; (2) a strategy for reinstating immune function ex vivo; (3) potential diversity of the nature and function of TIL from histologically different tumors; and (4) in TIL, that phenotypic expression may not correlate with function of T lymphocytes. Therapy strategies will address the unique aspects of each TIL population to maximize host immune function, reversing the unbalanced equilibrium that promotes the progressive neoplasm.

Scientific Basis of Biologic Therapy. The major premise of biologic therapy is that (1) cancer progression results from failure of the host immune defenses to recognize and reject the tumor; and (2) biologic agents, either alone or in combination, augment the immune response and thereby elicit a rejection response that will reverse the imbalance in host-tumor relationships by blunting tumor progression. There are a variety of biologic therapy agents presently available for clinical trials (Table 9-23). The objective in the clinical trials is to stimulate function of effector cells, including T lymphocytes, NK cells and cytotoxic macrophages, and B lymphocytes (i.e., antibodies). The choice of agents depends on many variables. Most important are the lymphocyte populations sought for augmentation. Thus, therapy may invoke vaccines, cytokines, drugs, and adoptively transferred lymphocytes.

Vaccines. Immunization of cancer patients against tumor-associated antigens has been attempted during the past decade. Some vaccines may elicit an antibody response against tumor-associated agents, but evocation of T-cell-mediated immunity as reflected in the peripheral compartment has been difficult. More-

Table 9-23
Biologic Agents in Clinical Trials

Agent	*Immune Function*	*Anticipated Effect in Cancer Patients*
IL-2	Activation of NK-lymphocyte cell growth factor	Proliferation of antitumor cytotoxic T cells
IL-3	Promotes growth of myeloid cells	Stimulation of hematopoietic stem cells
IL-4	Growth factor for B and T lymphocytes	Improve survival of T cells
TNF	Lyses transformed cells	Direct cytotoxicity of lymphomas and sarcomas
IFN-gamma	Activation of macrophage and NK cells	Promotion of nonspecific immunity
IFN-alpha	Increased expression of histocompatibility antigens	Increase target susceptibility
MTP-PE	Activates macrophages	Adjuvant for tumor-associated antigens and activation of phagocytic cells
Tumor vaccines	Induction of tumor-specific immunity	Activation of specific cytotoxic lymphocytes and antibodies
Monoclonal antibody	Passive immunization	Mediate tumor destruction. As a conjugate, delivery of cytotoxic drugs
Cellular therapy	Adoptive transfer of tumor immunity	Cell-mediated tumor rejection
Extracorporeal immunoabsorption	Removal of suppressor factors from blood	Augmentation of cell-mediated tumor immunity

over, it is much more difficult to demonstrate an individual immune response from peripheral blood in patients who have received tumor immunizations, probably owing to their compromised immune function.

One approach is to combine the tumor cells with a strong antigen such as a nonpathogenic virus in the form an oncolysate. In experimental models, the addition of virus antigens to tumor promotes an associative immune recognition that affords stronger host immunity to tumor-associated antigens. The use of the nononcogenic viruses available as attenuated vaccines enables rapid adaptation to therapy in human beings. For example, many investigators have used polyvalent allogeneic oncolysates using different cultured melanoma cell lines that display most of the previously identified melanoma-associated antigens. Clinical studies demonstrated that more than 70 percent of patients were immunized, as evidenced by a new serum antibody against tumor-associated antigens. The toxicity was minimal, and there were improved survival rates in the phase II study as compared to computer-matched historical controls. Randomized prospective, multi-institutional studies are being conducted.

Alternatively, other vaccine protocols are currently undergoing clinical trials for melanoma, colon carcinoma, renal cell carcinoma, and ovarian carcinoma. These strategies include the use of (1) autologous tumor cell vaccines, (2) subcellular fractions, and (3) isolated or synthetic tumor antigens. Each modality offers the prospect of vaccine preparations that activate tumor-specific immunity with emphasis on activation of cell-mediated immunity or a protective antitumor antibody.

Recombinant Cytokines. Advances in molecular biology have enabled the development of pure forms of a variety of interleukins and interferons and their administration in pharmacologic doses to a population of cancer patients sufficient to assess their efficacy (Table 9-24). These interferons comprise three different families, each with peculiar mechanisms of action. Moreover, a pure product has become available in unlimited quantities in multiple laboratories at a cost that permits extensive clinical trials. Subsequently, similar technology has provided several of the interleukins for clinical trials.

The availability of recombinant pure cytokines enabled clinical trials that (1) address specific biologic questions, (2) provide interpretable analyses, and (3) offer a potentially more effective form of treatment. A composite of early trials with nonrecombinant interferon in patients with advanced melanoma demonstrated a major response rate of only 4 percent. In comparison, several years later, trials using recombinant alpha-interferon (rIFN-α) for metastatic melanoma showed a major response rate of about 23 percent (range 14 to 28 percent). IL-2, the T-cell growth factor, induces a major response, particularly in patients with metastatic melanoma and metastatic renal cell carcinoma, but not with breast cancer, colon cancer, or lymphoma. Some responses are quite dramatic, including significant regression in major organs such as liver and lung. The intravenous administration of the cytokines is not without significant toxicity, however, and it is clear that they trigger a cascade of effects that results in other lymphocyte activities as well as the direct effects of IL-2 on other tissues. Some of the side effects are similar to those seen with septic shock.

Table 9-24
Cytokines

Cytokine	*Source*	*Activity*
IL-1	Monocytes, macrophages, dendritic cells, NK cells, astrocytes, keratinocytes	Induces lymphokine release from T cells, growth of fibroblasts and synovial cells, PGE release, fever
IL-2	Activated T cells	Induces cytotoxic activity, growth of activated T, NK, B, and LAK cells, and lymphokine production
IL-3	Activated T cells, lectin-stimulated PBL	Stimulates the growth of multipotential stem cells
IL-4	Activated T cells	B-cell stimulating factor (BSF), also stimulates T, B cells, and macrophages
IL-5	T cells	Induces differentiation of eosinophils
IL-6	Monocytes, fibroblasts, some tumors	Induces Class I HLA expression on fibroblasts, and production of acute phase proteins by hepatocytes
IL-7	T cells	Stimulates T-cell proliferation, promotes expansion of B-cell populations
IL-8	Activated T cells	Activation of granulocytes, induction of chemotactic response
IL-9	T-helper cells	Mitogen for TH subpopulations, promotes growth of mast cells
IL-10	T-helper cells	Suppresses cytokine production in other TH populations producing IL-2 and IFN
IFN-gamma	T cells	Activates macrophages, Tc, Tdth, and NK cells, increases MHC expression
GM-CSF	Activated T cells	Mitogenic for many cells, activates macrophages and granulocytes, promotes T-cell proliferation
TNF	Macrophages, T cells	Antitumor activity, mitogenic for many lymphoid cells

Adoptive Cellular Therapy. The concept of adoptive cellular therapy as a treatment strategy awaited the ability to propagate large numbers (over 10^{11}) of lymphocytes in vitro. The initial strategy used ex vivo prepared lymphokine-activated killer (LAK) cells in combination with high doses of IL-2. The LAK cells were prepared from peripheral blood lymphocytes. Although major response rates of 18 to 20 percent were seen, it was not clear whether the major contributor to the response was the IL-2 or LAK cells. Subsequent studies suggest that IL-2 and not LAK cells may be the major contributor to the responses. Some evidence suggests that LAK cells may be more important in renal cell carcinoma than in melanoma. Subsequently the methodology was developed for isolating TIL from human melanoma and renal cell carcinoma, and following proliferation ex vivo in the presence of IL-2, the TIL were returned to the patients and IL-2 therapy administered concurrently. In preliminary studies, response rates of up to 40 percent were obtained. Thus, unlike LAK cells, the TIL may have an important role in the therapy of local and regional disease, while LAK cells may remain useful in treatment of hematogenous dissemination and some renal cell carcinomas.

Combined Therapy Using Biologic Agents. Combination biologic therapy is now in clinical trials for treatment of most major human cancers. The multiagent concept is plausible because (1) multiple immune abnormalities are likely to occur in cancer patients; (2) there is heterogeneity in immune response (nature of lymphocytes, role of antibody, presence of macrophages) relative to the site of the metastases; and (3) combinations of agents with different mechanisms of action are more likely to augment individual aspects of immune response additively or synergistically in a diverse population of cancer patients. For example, combinations of IL-2 plus IFN-α elicits a higher rate and more durable response time for metastatic melanoma than either cytokine alone. Combinations of tumor antigen, lymphokines, and cyclophosphamides are intended to activate tumor-specific immunity, promote effector T-cell proliferation, and down-regulate suppressor T cells.

Immunotherapy is a logical adjunct for the treatment of subclinical microscopic disease following definitive cancer surgery, radiation therapy, or chemotherapy, for the following reasons: (1) patients who have only small foci of cancer cells remaining after destruction of the major tumor bulk are the most likely to benefit from immunotherapy, because the tumor mass that must be destroyed is smallest at that time; (2) the specificity of the immune response provides a possible therapeutic tool that has selectivity for small numbers of cancer cells not possible with any other therapeutic modality; (3) patients with disease in earlier stages are more likely to respond to immunotherapeutic maneuvers, since the cancer patient's general immune competence is greatest when the disease is localized and is often impaired after metastasis; and (4) immunotherapy should complement rather than interfere with currently available methods of cancer therapy. Because both irradiation and chemotherapy are immunosuppressive, the use of immunotherapy in combination with these therapeutic modalities must be carefully controlled.

Numerous attempts at immunotherapy of cancer have been undertaken since the turn of the century. Although an occasional striking regression was obtained, in most cases the results were neither impressive nor consistent, and interest in this treatment modality declined until recently. With the availability of large quantities of purified biologic response modifiers (such as IL-1 and -2, interferon, tumor necrosis factor) made possible by recombinant DNA technology, a patient's immune defenses may be dramatically manipulated in a number of ways.

New Approaches to Delivery. Concern over the toxicity of intravenously administered cytokines has promoted development of methods to target cytokines and thereby reduce systemic effects. Cytokines are administered aggressively and frequently because of their short half-life in the blood. In addition, cytokines are not always distributed to all areas of the body and often do not traverse the blood-brain barrier. An innovative approach is incorporation of interferon and adjuvants into liposomes, thus directing the cytokine to a specific host cell population. In animal models, liposomes are ingested by macrophages. Degradation of the "packaged" therapy results in intracellular release of adjuvants such as muramyl tripeptides (MTP-PE) and the interferon, which then activate macrophages to become cytotoxic against cancers, both in vitro and in vivo. A randomized study in dog osteogenic sarcoma showed significantly greater response and survival rates in animals that received the MTP-PE liposomes as compared with those that received empty liposomes. This novel approach has been extended to human studies, beginning with a pilot study of patients with osteogenic sarcoma and melanoma.

Neoadjuvant Biologic Therapy. Administration of agents preoperatively in patients with measurable and surgically resectable metastatic disease thus affords the advantages of determining clinical response in a measurable tumor, comparing pathologic response to clinical response, and examining the in vivo effects of biologics on host-tumor relationships. Several current clinical trials are being conducted at the M.D. Anderson Cancer Center in which patients receive a preoperative course of IL-2 plus IFN-α or MTP-PE liposomes for a 3- to 4-week period of time. Measurable tumors are then resected and a postoperative decision to continue the therapy is made based on demonstrated immunologic activity as measured by pathologic and immunologic assessment of the surgical specimen.

Adoptive Immunotherapy. In adoptive immunotherapy, immune lymphoid cells are transferred to a recipient to mediate tumor destruction. In many experimental murine tumors, in vivo transfer of lymphocytes from an immune mouse to a tumor-bearing mouse can cause dramatic tumor regression. These immune lymphocytes are tumor-antigen-specific, display major histocompatibility complex restriction, and have classical T-cell markers; thus, they are classic cytolytic T lymphocytes. In these animal models, it is necessary to use large numbers of cells from immunized, syngeneic (generally identical) donor mice. This effective immunotherapeutic modality is, unfortunately, technically impractical in human beings.

Rosenberg and colleagues have pioneered the study of adoptive immunotherapy using LAK cells. LAK cells are cytolytic lymphocytes that are generated in the presence of IL-2. Treatment of human lymphocytes from almost any source (peripheral blood, lymph nodes, spleen, thymus, bone marrow) results in the creation of cytolytic cells capable of killing a wide range of fresh and cultured human cancer cells but not normal cells. The biochemical nature of this tumor-specific recognition and killing is not fully defined. Human LAK cells do not have T-cell markers and are not MHC- or antigen-specific in their killing. A similar strategy was used to obtain activated T cells from TIL populations to be propagated ex vivo and then reinfused into the autologous patient with metastatic disease.

Extensive animal experiments demonstrate the ability of systemically administered LAK cells and IL-2 to cause dramatic regression of many different types of primary and metastatic tumors. Clinical trials using autologous LAK cells (obtained by repeated leukopheresis and in vitro IL-2 expansion) and systemically administered IL-2 have resulted in clear, objective responses in some patients with bulky metastatic cancer. Administration of high doses of IL-2 alone have some clinical efficacy but considerable toxicity. Even greater toxicity is seen with combined administration of LAK cells and IL-2 and includes fluid retention and renal dysfunction. Nevertheless, these impressive studies, in patients with large tumor burdens, are an exciting glimpse of the potential of properly manipulated immune systems.

Nonspecific Immunotherapy. The theoretical basis for nonspecific immunotherapy depends on the observation that certain substances, such as mixed bacterial toxins and fractions of the tubercle bacillus, have the ability to nonspecifically enhance host resistance to most viral, fungal, and bacterial agents. Although the exact mechanism is unknown, these agents do appear to stimulate immune response to a wide variety of antigens, including tumor antigens.

Historically, a type of nonspecific immunotherapy was described by Coley at the turn of the century in one of the first reports of a tumor regression possibly induced by immunogenic means. Coley's interest in the possible value of such therapy was stimulated when he observed a recurrent inoperable sarcoma of the neck regress completely for 7 years after the patient had had attacks of erysipelas. This observation led to the development of Coley's toxins, a mixture of killed bacterial vaccines. Coley injected this admixture directly into tumor lesions or gave it intravenously. Some impressive regressions of tumors and long-term cures resulted from these agents. Because the responses were inconsistent, Coley's toxins never received widespread use, and interest in them died out.

Interest in a similar nonspecific immunotherapy was revived more than 20 years ago using attenuated bovine tuberculosis bacillus (bacille Calmette-Guerin, BCG). Some tumor regressions were observed but consistent responses in any one treatment group were difficult to achieve. There are several possible mechanisms to explain tumor regression following BCG injection; both specific and nonspecific immune reactions were probably involved. The tumor cells may be killed as "innocent bystanders" during the delayed cutaneous hypersensitivity reaction that occurs when lymphocytes and macrophages attack BCG dispersed throughout the tumor nodule. This is supported by the observation that the intratumor injection of BCG works only in patients who can be sensitized to BCG, as shown by their delayed cutaneous hypersensitivity reaction to purified protein derivative.

In addition to the nonspecific effect, a specific immune response to melanoma-associated tumor antigens also occurs in some patients because an associated rising titer of antimelanoma antibody is observed following BCG immunotherapy. Sequential biopsies of tumor nodules following BCG inoculation reveal that the regression of these nodules is associated with granulomatous infiltration of lymphocytes, monocytes, and fibroblasts surrounding and infiltrating the melanoma cells. Furthermore, the regression of melanoma nodules not injected with BCG is accompanied by the appearance of lymphocyte infiltrates within the regressing melanoma tumor nodules. The specific antitumor effect may result from more lymphocytes and macrophages coming into contact with the tumor cells and promoting antigen presentation. Conversely, it may work via the effector limb of the immune response by bringing greater numbers of both stimulated and unstimulated lymphocytes to the tumor.

Examples of other nonspecific agents include *Corynebacterium parvum, Bordatella pertussus,* MTP-PE, methanol-extractable residue of BCG, bacterial endotoxins, and polynucleotides. Another form of nonspecific immunotherapy involves the use of agents capable of restoring depressed immune responses. Several agents have been proposed in such a context, including thymic hormones such as thymosin and the antihelminthic drug levamisole.

The rational application of immunotherapy to human cancer will depend, to a large extent, on a better knowledge of tumor-associated antigens in human neoplasms and methods for increasing the immune response against these agents. Specificity for cancer cells cannot be achieved by other known therapeutic means, but the potency of immunotherapy is limited. Expectations of dramatic benefits from immunotherapy for malignant disease have been high; however, the results of many clinical trials have fallen short of these expectations. The theoretical advantages of a specific systemic antitumor adjuvant with minimal toxicity continues to make immunotherapy a promising avenue of future investigation. At the present time, its use should be limited to cancer facilities, where the effects of this form of treatment can be scientifically evaluated.

Passive Immunotherapy. In passive immunotherapy, tumor-specific antiserum is used systemically in an effort to suppress tumor. This approach is fraught with a number of theoretical and practical problems. Passive immunotherapy, for a number of reasons, is only effective in suppressing small numbers of tumor cells and must work in concert with host effectors (complement, macrophages, K cells, etc.) to effect a cytotoxic action on target cells. Moreover, only antibodies of certain classes and subclasses can interact effectively with certain cellular effectors. Most of the better characterized human tumor-specific antisera are murine monoclonal antibodies that, because of their antigenicity, have limited applications in human beings.

Immunotoxins. Immunotoxins are tumor-specific antibodies to which are attached toxic molecules. This intuitively appealing concept, first proposed by Ehrlich one century ago, uses the antibody molecule to preferentially localize anticancer agents in the vicinity of tumors. It obviates the need for the host to supply effector cells or complement to mediate tumor destruction. Monoclonal antibodies are preferred to heterologous antiserum since they permit the use of homogeneous, purified antibodies of defined specificity. A wide range of toxic molecules has been tested in vitro and includes radioactive isotopes, traditional cancer drugs, and plant and bacterial toxins. Recombinant DNA technology now permits the creation of hybrid or chimeric immunotoxin molecules in which the Fc fragment of the immunoglobulin molecule has been replaced by a polypeptide toxin sequence. Immunotoxins are currently undergoing clinical trials, although their overall therapeutic efficiency in clinical oncology is unproved.

Gene Therapy. The ability to clone genes introduces a new era of biologic therapy that will have an impact on human clinical trials in ensuing years. An example is the elegant studies by Hellstrom and colleagues, in which a cloned gene for one of the major human melanoma tumor-associated antigens (p97) was introduced into the genome of a vaccinia virus. The virus then expressed both immunogenic viral antigens plus the more weakly immunogenic human melanoma antigens on the surface. This reagent will be tested in human studies in the near future. A novel approach is transfection of human TIL with genes for producing cytokines such as tumor-necrosing factor. The ability to transfect cytokine genes into human TIL has been demonstrated and proposals exist that seek to use adoptive cellular therapy with genetically transfected cells capable of producing high concentrations of tumor-necrosing factor or other lymphokines at the tumor site. One of the practical aspects of this approach is the prospect of achieving accumulation of cytokine at the tumor site while sparing the vascular compartment of the otherwise deleterious effects of high-dose, systemic cytokine.

A modest survey of the recent findings in the molecular genetics and biology of the human immune system reveals a vast warehouse of new strategies for treatment of neoplastic disease. As our knowledge base accumulates, the previous concerns about (1) the existence of human tumor antigens, (2) the impaired immunity in cancer patients, and (3) the harnessing of naturally occurring endogenous immunoregulators are rapidly dissipating.

Management of Distant Metastases at Specific Sites

Lung, Pleura, and Mediastinum. Two of the most common initial sites of metastasis are the lungs and pleura. Nearly all patients with disseminated cancer will develop metastases in the chest prior to death. These lesions are evaluated by chest x-ray as the screening test (preoperatively and during follow-up), with suspicious intrathoracic metastases evaluated by tomograms, CT scans, or bronchoscopy.

For screening purposes, a standard chest x-ray is sufficiently sensitive and cost-effective to be used for screening in all cancer patients. The yield of the more expensive pulmonary tomograms or CT scans is too low and the cost too high to be justified when the chest x-ray is normal. Moreover, the false-positive rate of CT scans or tomograms can be as high as 15 percent. Even in patients with distant metastases (stage IV), they are not indicated unless the presence of pulmonary metastases would alter the treatment plan or a better definition of lesions is required for entry into a research protocol.

Definitive evaluation of suspicious metastases begins when one or more lesions are seen on the chest x-ray. Hilar and mediastinal adenopathy frequently accompany pulmonary metastases. Whole-lung tomograms or CT scans of the chest are of value in evaluating suspicious chest lesions or in determining whether the metastatic disease seen on the chest x-ray is also present elsewhere in the chest. Both tomograms and CT scans have advantages and disadvantages in evaluating thoracic metastases from melanoma. Basically, tomograms can detect lesions as small as 6 mm in diameter, while CT scans can identify lesions down to 3 mm, although the increased sensitivity is offset by decreased specificity. Which of these is utilized by the clinician will often depend on available facilities, the cost of the test, and the skills of the radiologist involved. It also must take into account the need to detect metastases as small as 3 mm when making an individual patient treatment decision.

Pulmonary metastases are generally asymptomatic. Sooner or later, however, they may cause one or more of the following symptoms: persistent cough, hemoptysis, shortness of breath, or chest pain. An irritating, dry, and unproductive cough may progress to hemoptysis.

Bronchoscopy with biopsy may be considered in patients when the diagnosis of the pulmonary lesion (e.g., metastatic disease, fungal disease, benign tumor, or bronchogenic carcinoma) is in doubt, especially when symptoms suggest bronchial involvement (e.g., a productive cough or a centrally placed or cavitary lesion). A scalene lymph node biopsy is indicated for palpable nodes. Mediastinoscopy is indicated if mediastinal nodes that are accessible through the instrument are present on the chest x-ray, tomogram, or CT scan. Thoracentesis or pleural biopsies may be helpful when evaluating effusions. Thin-needle biopsy of a pulmonary lesion under CT scan guidance may be useful in selected instances to establish the histologic diagnosis. If the diagnosis remains in doubt, an exploratory thoracotomy may be necessary, especially for a solitary lesion, because some patients will have potentially curable primary lung cancer.

The treatment approach is determined by the location and number of thoracic metastases. Surgical resection of pulmonary metastases appears to benefit a small number of highly selected patients. In most series, the median survival was 17 months, with a 5-year survival rate of 20 to 25 percent. Some patients live more than 10 years. In fact, resection of a solitary pulmonary metastasis provides a higher rate of 5-year survival than resection of primary bronchogenic carcinoma of the lung. Resection of pulmonary metastases may be indicated even when more than one metastatic lesion is present. Our experience has shown that sarcoma patients with tumor doubling times greater than 40 days received significant palliation from pulmonary resection and remained free of disease for as long as 5 years. In contrast, patients with tumor doubling times of less than 20 days did not significantly benefit from resection of their metastatic lesions.

Criteria for resection should include an absence of metastases at other sites, control of the primary tumor, and the potential for complete resection. CT scans should be obtained preoperatively because the number of lesions demonstrated by tomography is often greater than that shown by chest x-ray.

Lung parenchyma should be conserved during resection. Fortunately, most metastases occur just below the pleura, and a wedge of tissue removed by segmental resection suffices. Several techniques have proved useful for these resections, including stapling, electrocautery, and laser surgery. Lobectomy is rarely needed, and pneumonectomy is usually not indicated.

Patients who are ineligible for surgery, such as those with multiple slow-growing tumors, might be monitored but receive no treatment at all while they are asymptomatic. If the pulmonary metastases progress rapidly, especially if multiple visceral metastases exist at other sites or if the patient has disease symptoms, chemotherapy should be given.

Pleural effusions are generally associated with a short survival time. If patients are symptomatic, they can treated by thoracentesis or by tube thoracostomy and chemical pleurodesis.

Liver, Biliary Tract, and Spleen. Hepatic metastases can occur in most patients with metastatic disease, especially those with abdominal and breast cancer. There are no reliable and accurate tests for detecting liver metastases at an early stage of their evolution. Thus, it is generally not worthwhile to order tests other than serum liver chemistries for screening purposes unless there are signs or symptoms suggesting metastatic liver disease. Hepatic metastases are usually not detected by radiologic tests until they are large (more than 2 cm in diameter) and multiple. The prognosis of these patients is poor (i.e., a median survival of 2 to 4 months) and treatment options few.

A radiologic assessment of the liver may be warranted to evaluate the patient's overall status when deciding treatment options for metastases at some other site. Screening tests for liver metastases should consist only of a history and physical examination and serum liver chemistries. These are sufficiently accurate and the most cost-effective of all available tests. The patterns of abnormal liver chemistries that suggest liver metastases are an elevated lactic dehydrogenase and/or alkaline phosphatase level in the presence of normal or only slightly elevated serum glutamic-oxaloacetic transaminase or bilirubin level. An elevated lactic dehydrogenase level is a clinically useful and relatively specific indicator for metastatic melanoma.

Symptoms and physical signs of early liver metastases are uncommon. The patient may experience decreased appetite with loss of weight followed within weeks by general lassitude and debility. The loss of appetite may precede a clinically palpable liver by a month or more. On the other hand, the patient may have an easily palpable liver and feel perfectly well. As the disease in the liver progresses, distressing nausea, vomiting, or even spiking night sweats and fever may develop.

When liver metastases are suspected, the confirmatory radiologic tests to be considered are the (1) US scan, (2) CT scan, (3) radionuclide liver scan, and (4) hepatic arteriogram. The tests to be used depend on availability and cost at individual hospitals, the interpretive skills of the radiologist, and the generation of equipment used, which is especially important in regard to CT scanners and US units. Most comparative studies have found that the abdominal CT scans are more accurate and reliable than US and radionuclide liver scans for evaluation of liver masses.

The role of angiography in evaluating suspected metastases in the abdomen and retroperitoneum is generally limited to the few instances in which the differential diagnosis cannot be resolved by noninvasive techniques and in which the information gained would be an essential part of the treatment decision. It is also important when hepatic resection is contemplated.

It is usually not necessary to confirm the diagnosis of liver metastases by biopsy. In the few instances in which the confirmed diagnosis is essential to treatment decisions, a needle biopsy can be performed percutaneously, by laparoscopy, or at the time of laparotomy.

For most types of liver metastases, surgical excision is not beneficial and chemotherapy is the treatment of choice. Some patients with isolated liver metastases from colorectal cancers may benefit from surgical resection. Those patients with a solitary metastasis, or metastases located in one lobe, are often successfully treated with resection. Approximately 25 percent of these patients will survive for 5 years. However, fewer than 5 percent with colon cancer metastatic to the liver are candidates for this type of treatment. Most patients with colorectal cancer have diffuse disease and are best treated with systemic or intra-arterial chemotherapy.

Brain and Spinal Cord. Many cancers, particularly melanoma and lung cancer, metastasize to the brain, a common cause of death.

Headache and mental deficits are the most common symptoms of brain metastasis. Headache resulting from brain metastasis characteristically begins as a mild morning headache. As the condition progresses and the intracranial pressure increases, the headache will persist longer into the day and become more severe. It is usually generalized, although it may be slightly worse in the frontal or occipital region and may be associated with visual changes. Seizures are uncommon.

The most common physical sign of brain metastases is a focal neurologic defect. The presence of papilledema is a helpful sign, but its absence is not useful diagnostically.

The best tests for diagnosing intracerebral metastases are MRI and CT with contrast enhancement. MRI, a technique that depends on the intrinsic paramagnetic properties of biologic tissue, is generally the preferred test to detect and stage brain and spinal metastases. MRI can detect tumors that cannot be visualized by CT scans. MRI has an advantage, particularly for lesions at the base of the skull and posterior fossa, because only a weak signal is generated from the adjacent bone. Furthermore, MRI scans appear to have an increased tissue sensitivity, including a better ability to distinguish hemorrhage from tumor, as compared with CT scans.

The accuracy and sensitivity of these scans make it unnecessary in most cases to perform either a radionuclide brain scan or electroencephalogram, unless there are some equivocal findings that warrant these complementary studies. A carotid arteriogram may be indicated to rule out possible vascular abnormalities. A spinal tap to diagnose meningeal involvement is occasionally necessary (after a CT scan) for a patient who has a cranial nerve palsy, bladder dysfunction, or nonlocalizing or bilateral neurologic signs and symptoms.

The mainstay of initial treatment is corticosteroids, the most effective of which is dexamethasone (up to 100 mg/day). Dexamethasone reduces edema around the tumor and helps relieve symptoms in the majority of patients, at least temporarily. The steroid dose should be tapered over 2 to 4 weeks as tolerated and the therapy stopped after definitive treatment unless the patient's symptoms intensify during steroid withdrawal. Steroids often do not help patients with rapid neurologic deterioration because this condition is usually owing to intracerebral hemorrhage around the metastasis. Chemotherapy is not usually effective for brain metastasis, although responses do occur occasionally.

Surgical excision followed by cranial irradiation is the treatment of choice in the case of a solitary, surgically accessible metastasis. Tumor excision by means of a craniotomy is relatively safe; it alleviates symptoms in most patients and prevents further neurologic damage in patients with demonstrable metastases. The treatment may even be considered in some patients who have disease at other sites plus symptomatic brain metastases, since their estimated life span can exceed 3 months and their neurologic status usually improves.

No study has directly proved whether surgery, radiation, or a combination of the two provides the most effective palliation for solitary metastases in the brain. Patients treated with irradiation alone, however, do not survive long-term. Thus, although the overall results and the quality of life obtained through these treatment approaches are probably similar, the occasional dramatic prolongation of life brought about by surgery renders it the somewhat superior treatment in cases of solitary metastases. Radiotherapy is preferred when the lesions are numerous or are located in an area that precludes a safe operation.

Bone. Bone metastases are commonly observed in patients with advanced breast or prostate cancer, but occur infrequently in patients with gastrointestinal cancers. Bone metastases are medullary in location and destructive in nature. They are generally osteolytic in appearance on radiography and provoke little if any bone formation. Some patients with prostate cancer have bone metastases that are osteoblastic. Axial metastases account for up to 80 percent of bony lesions, being most common in the spine and rib. When bony lesions involve the vertebral body, there are often compression fractures, which may lead to neurologic symptoms such as radicular back pain, paresthesia or paresis of the legs, and urinary retention. Only about 10 percent of lytic lesions occur in weight-bearing bones, but these could result in pathologic fractures.

Bone metastases are most frequently diagnosed in symptomatic patients, although occasionally they are seen incidentally on radiographs (e.g., rib metastases on routine chest x-ray) or a bone scan prompted by an elevated serum alkaline phosphatase level in the absence of liver metastases. The pain from bony metastases is typically nocturnal at first, becoming persistent, progressive, and localized. It is boring in nature and can be quite severe in intensity.

These metastases are imaged radiographically or scintigraphically. The radionuclide bone scan has clearly established itself over radiographic skeletal surveys as the initial test for evaluating suspected bone metastases. It has remarkable sensitivity, which is reported to be 50 to 80 percent greater than radiographs alone, allows detection of skeletal lesions far earlier than their appearance on skeletal x-ray films. However, scan abnormalities are nonspecific and must be correlated with radiographic study and patient history (for fractures, trauma, arthritis, etc.) to distinguish between benign and malignant causes. It may be necessary to perform a bone biopsy to establish the diagnosis in some situations before instituting treatment.

The treatment of bone metastases depends on (1) the degree of symptoms, (2) the location and magnitude of the lesions, and (3) the patient's life expectancy. The goals of therapy are to relieve pain, maximize ambulation, and minimize medical care. In general, patients without symptoms should be monitored to assess the progression of their lesions but should receive no major treatment unless they become symptomatic.

Symptomatic metastases most frequently involve non-weight-bearing bones, particularly the spine and ribs. In these cases, irradiation of the lesions usually provides relief. The radiation fields should generally be restricted to those lesions responsible for the symptoms. Symptomatic bone lesions only occasionally respond to systemic chemotherapy, but bone metastases from breast cancer may respond quite well to hormonal therapy in some patients.

Symptomatic metastases in weight-bearing bones (e.g., the femur) require special consideration. If the lesion is large, and especially if there is evidence of cortical destruction, prophylactic stabilization and irradiation are sometimes used when the patient's expected life span is at least 2 months. Stabilization includes operative metallic bone fixation (e.g., with intramedullary rods), joint replacement, repair with methyl methacrylate, or external braces or a cast. Radiotherapy is generally given postoperatively.

Alternatively, the lesion might be treated with radiation alone, in which case the patient must be monitored closely for evidence of pathologic fracture. Unless the risk of surgery is high or the patient's expected life span is short, pathologic fracture of a weight-bearing bone should be stabilized, maximizing the patient's quality of life and decreasing hospital or nursing home costs.

Patients in whom fractures of the vertebrae have compressed the spinal cord require prompt treatment to avert paralysis. The treatment may require both decompressive laminectomy and postoperative irradiation, or irradiation alone, depending on the extent of the disease and the patient's overall medical condition.

Skin, Subcutaneous Tissues, and Distant Lymph Nodes. These are the most common sites of distant metastases. Metastases here are often the first sign of hematogenous spread. Skin and subcutaneous metastases are generally 0.5 to 2.0 cm in diameter and are readily detectable by physical examination. Distant lymph node metastases can occur in any area. The more superficial nodal metastases are easily diagnosed by physical examination. Those within the thorax can usually be detected on chest x-ray, with CT scans or tomograms used as confirmatory tests, whereas abdominal nodal metastases are generally detected by CT or US scans. These lesions are generally treated, especially when symptomatic and isolated, by surgical excision (if superficially located) or radiation therapy. They might also be treated with chemotherapy or hormone therapy, especially when there are multiple lesions or simultaneous visceral metastases.

Gastrointestinal Tract. Some cancers, particularly melanoma, can metastasize to the gastrointestinal tract. Metastases to the gastrointestinal tract usually occur in multiple sites simultaneously.

Early involvement of the gastrointestinal tract usually causes vague and subtle symptoms, so it is necessary to suspect intestinal metastases in patients with persistent, nonspecific complaints such as epigastric distress, nausea, anorexia, or weight loss, which occur in a large number of patients. Only occasionally do some acute and potentially catastrophic symptoms occur. The most common clinical manifestations are due to (1) chronic bleeding, with anemia, anorexia, and weight loss; (2) obstruction of the small bowel, with abdominal pain, nausea, and vomiting; or (3) acute bleeding, with hematemesis or melena. Metastases in the gastrointestinal tract are difficult to detect by radiologic studies, so their routine use is not indicated for screening purposes.

Chronic bleeding is a common symptomatic manifestation of gastrointestinal metastases. In anemic patients, the bleeding can be treated with repeated blood transfusions. Chemotherapy can be considered for patients with multiple gastrointestinal lesions, whereas surgical excision should be considered for gastrointestinal metastases, provided that the patient's condition is good and no other visceral metastases exist.

Surgery is recommended for most patients who have acute complications of obstruction, massive bleeding, or perforation. These conditions cannot be treated in any other way, and the only alternative is to allow the patient to die. The final decision depends on the patient's overall clinical condition, but symptoms can be successfully alleviated in most cases, and survival after surgical excision of the offending metastases averages 4 to 8 months.

Psychologic Management and Rehabilitation

The physician can ease the cancer patient's fear of the disease by free and open communication. Psychologic support and education are necessary in order for the patient to deal with any disability that may result from therapy. Examples include training in the care of a stoma following curative surgery for colonic and rectal cancer and referral to lay groups associated with the American Cancer Society for counseling the anxious patient with an altered body image resulting from mastectomy.

Despite the prognostic factors discussed previously, it is still impossible to predict the exact course of any malignant tumor. Patients with the most grim prognoses are occasionally cured by aggressive therapy, and spontaneous regressions are sometimes observed even in patients with metastases. In contrast, some patients with apparently localized disease may be dead of disseminated cancer in a few months. This uncertainty about the future is one of the most difficult adjustments faced by cancer patients and their families. Most reassuring in this regard is to emphasize that for each month that passes following successful treatment of the primary neoplasm, the chances for cure improve. This is particularly correct for tumors such as squamous cell carcinoma of the lung or oropharynx. Although other, more slowly growing neoplasms, such as carcinoma of the breast and malignant melanoma, may recur after disease-free intervals of 10 to 20 years, the chances of recurrence also decrease with time. Recognition that cancer is a chronic disease is an important aspect of management. Long-term, consistent follow-up provides opportunities for reassurance and usually can ensure detection of recurrence at an early stage.

Some patients do not want to know about their illness for fear of having their suspicions verified. A patient should never be lied to, even if requested by the family. In general, gentle and optimistic truth is best. Untruths often create barriers between patients and their families that can lead to psychologic isolation of patients who are unable to discuss their fears and anxieties with those they need most.

With the patient for whom primary cancer therapy has failed, one of the most difficult problems faced by the physician is ''What should the patient be told?'' Most oncologists who deal exclusively with cancer patients agree that the incurable patient also must be told the truth as gently and optimistically as possible. Hope and reassurance as to the physician's continuing concern are best sustained by continuing active treatment until it is certain that the patient can no longer benefit. Realistic and consistent support is actually more important to the patient and family at this stage of the disease than earlier. There is increasing evidence that patients tolerate the process of dying much better when cared for in this manner.

Some incurable patients are unable to accept the realities of the situation. In this case, it is essential that a responsible family member be informed. The duration of the incurable patient's life is so uncertain that predictions should be avoided. If, as frequently happens, the relatives insist on some estimate, a combined minimum-maximum prognosis, such as from 6 months to 2 years, will help the family accept this uncertainty.

The basic aim in caring for the patient with advanced cancer is to prolong useful life, but not useless suffering. The patient should be permitted to die with dignity when active therapy can no longer be of benefit.

Bibliography

General References

Balch CM, Houghton A, Milton GW, Sober A, Soong S-J (eds): *Cutaneous Melanoma* (2d ed). Philadelphia, JB Lippincott, 1992.

Balch CM, Houghton AN: Diagnosis of metastatic melanoma at distant sites, in Balch CM, Houghton AN, Milton GW, Sober A, Soong S-J (eds): *Cutaneous Melanoma* (2d ed). Philadelphia, JB Lippincott, 1992, p. 439.

Bitran JD, Golumb HM, Little AG, Weichselbaum RR (eds): *Lung Cancer—A Comprehensive Treatise*. Orlando, Grune & Stratton, 1988.

Bland KI: *The Breast: Comprehensive Management of Benign and Malignant Diseases*. Philadelphia, WB Saunders, 1991.

DeVita VT, Hellman S, Rosenberg SA (eds): *Cancer: Principles and Practice of Oncology* (4th ed). Philadelphia, JB Lippincott, 1993.

DiSaia PJ, Creasman WT (eds): *Clinical Gynecologic Oncology* (3rd ed). St. Louis, CV Mosby, 1989.

Economou SG, Witt TR, Deziel DJ, Saclarides TJ, Staren ED, Bines SD (eds): *Adjuncts to Cancer Surgery*. Philadelphia, Lea & Febiger, 1991.

Eilber FR, Nizze A, Morton DL: Sequential evaluation of general immune competence in cancer patients: correlation with clinical course. *Cancer* 35:660, 1975.

Frykberg ER, Bland KI, Copeland EM: The detection and treatment of early breast cancer. *Adv Surg* 23:119, 1990.

Haskell CM (ed): *Cancer Treatment* (2d ed). Philadelphia, WB Saunders, 1985.

Hays DM (ed): *Pediatric Surgical Oncology—The Principles and Practices of the Pediatric Surgical Specialities*. Orlando, Grune & Stratton, 1986.

Hellmann K, Carter SK (eds): *Fundamentals of Cancer Chemotherapy*. New York, McGraw-Hill, 1987.

Houghton AN, Balch CM: Treatment for advanced melanoma, in Balch CM, Houghton AN, Milton GW, Sober A, Soong S-J (eds): *Cutaneous Melanoma* (2d ed). Philadelphia, JB Lippincott, 1992, p. 213.

Larson DL, Ballantyne AJ, Guillamondegui OM (eds): *Cancers in the Neck—Evaluation and Treatment*. New York, Macmillan, 1986.

McKenna RJ, Murphy GP (eds): *Fundamentals of Surgical Oncology*. New York, Macmillan, 1986.

Moosa AR, Schimpff SC, Robson MC (eds): *Comprehensive Textbook of Oncology* (2d ed), vol. 1. Baltimore, Williams & Wilkins, 1991.

Morton DL, Eilber FR, Sondak VK, Economou JS (eds): *The Soft Tissue Sarcomas*. Orlando, Grune & Stratton, 1987.

Pitot HC (ed): *Fundamentals of Oncology* (3rd ed). New York, Marcel Dekker, 1986.

Rosenberg SA: Gene therapy of cancer. *Important Adv Oncol* p. 17, 1992.

Roth JA, Ruckdeschel JC, Weisenburger TH (eds): *Thoracic Oncology*. Philadelphia, WB Saunders, 1989.

Sclafani LM, Brennan MF: Nutritional support in the cancer patient, in Fischer JE (ed): *Total Parenteral Nutrition* (2d ed): Boston, Little, Brown, 1991, p. 323.

Shiu MH, Brennan MR (eds): *Surgical Management of Soft Tissue Sarcoma*. Philadelphia, Lea & Febiger, 1989.

Staren ED, Szeluga DJ, Doolas A: Hyperalimentation of the cancer patient, in SG Economou, Witt, TR, Deziel DJ, Saclarides TJ, Staren ED, Bines SD (eds): *Adjuncts to Cancer Surgery*. Philadelphia, Lea & Febiger, 1991, p. 631.

Storm FK (ed): *Hyperthermia in Cancer Therapy*. Chicago, Year Book Medical Publishers, 1985.

Yeatman TM, Weber RS, Balch CM: The contemporary management of skin cancers, in Copeland EM, Howard RJ, Warshaw AL, Levine BA, Sugerman H (eds): *Current Practice of Surgery,* 1993 (in press).

Epidemiology and Etiology

American Cancer Society: *Cancer Facts and Figures*. New York, 1987.

Barbocid M: Human oncogenes, in De Vita VY, Hellmen S, Rosenberg SA (eds): *Important Advances in Oncology*. Philadelphia, JB Lippincott, 1986, p. 3.

Barratt RW, Tatum EL: Carcinogenic mutagens. *Ann NY Acad Sci* 71:1072, 1958.

Boice JD Jr, Fraumeni JF Jr (eds): *Radiation Carcinogenesis: Epidemiology and Biological Significance*. New York, Raven, 1984.

Boyland E: The history and future of chemical carcinogenesis. *Br Med Bull* 36:5, 1980.

Campisi J, Fingert HJ, Pardee AB: Basic biology and biochemistry of cancer, in Knapp RC, Berkowitz RS (eds): *Gynecologic Oncology,* chap 2. New York, Macmillan, 1984.

Doll R: The epidemiology of cancer. *Cancer* 45:2475, 1980.
Elson LE, Betts TE: Death rates from cancer of the respiratory and oral tracts in different countries in relation to the types of tobacco smoked. *Eur J Cancer* 17:109, 1981.
Garfinkel MA: Cancer mortality in nonsmokers: Prospective study by the American Cancer Society. *J Natl Cancer Inst* 65:1169, 1981.
Gatti RA, Good RA: Occurrence of malignancy in immunodeficiency diseases: A literature review. *Cancer* 28:89, 1971.
Heuper WC: Environmental cancer, in Homburger F (ed): *The Physiopathology of Cancer*. New York, Harper & Row, 1959, p. 91.
Kindt TJ, Robinson MA: Major histocompatibility complex antigens, in Paul WE (ed): *Fundamental Immunology*. New York, Raven, 1984, p. 347.
Land H, Parada LF, Weinberg RA: Cellular oncogenes and multistep carcinogenesis. *Science* 222:771, 1983.
Lee Y-T (Margaret): Cancer statistics of Chinese versus Americans. *J Surg Oncol* 27:355, 1981.
Locke FB, King H: Cancer mortality risk among Japanese in the United States. *J Natl Cancer Inst* 65:1149, 1980.
Minz B, Fleischman RA: Teratocarcinomas and other neoplasms as developmental defects in gene expression. *Adv Cancer Res* 34:211, 1981.
Prehn RT: Specific isoantigenicities among chemically induced tumors. *Ann NY Acad Sci* 101:107, 1962.
Seeger RG, Brodeur GM, et al: Association of multiple copies of the V-*myc* oncogene with rapid progression of neuroblastomas. *N Engl J Med* 313:1111, 1985.
Slaga TJ: Mechanisms of chemical carcinogenesis, in Moosa AR, Schimpff SC, Robson MC (eds): *Comprehensive Textbook of Oncology* (2d ed), vol. 1. Baltimore, Williams & Wilkins, 1991.
Storer JB: Radiation carcinogenesis, in Becker FF (ed): *Cancer: A Comprehensive Treatise*. (2d ed), vol. 1. Plenum, New York, 1982, p. 629.
VanBeveren C, Vermal M: Homology among oncogenes. *Curr Top Microbiol Immunol* 123:73, 1986.
Varmus HE: The discovery of cellular oncogenes and their role in neoplasia. *Cancer* 55:2324, 1985.
Waterfield MD, Scrace GT, et al: Platelet-derived growth factor is structurally related to the putative transforming protein p28 in sarcoma virus. *Nature* 304:35, 1983.
Wigle DT, Mae Y, et al: Relative importance of smoking as a risk factor for selected cancers. *Can J Publ Health* 71:269, 1980.

Biology of Neoplastic Disease

Abbas AK, Lichtman AH, Pober JS (eds): *Cellular and Molecular Immunology*. Philadelphia, WB Saunders, 1991.
Albers B, Bray D, et al: *The Molecular Biology of the Cell*. New York, Garland, 1983.
Arbeit JM: Molecules, cancer, and the surgeon. *Ann Surg* 212:3, 1990.
Bishop JM: Cellular oncogenes and retroviruses. *Ann Rev Biochem* 52:301, 1983.
Bishop JM: Retroviruses and cancer genes. *Cancer* 55:2329, 1985.
Bishop JM: The molecular genetics of cancer. *Science* 235:305, 1987.
Bishop JM: Molecular themes in oncogenesis. *Cell* 64:235. 1991.
Bister K, Jansen HW: Oncogenes in retroviruses and cells; biochemistry and molecular genetics. *Adv Cancer Res* 47:99, 1986.
Black PH: Shedding from the cell surface of normal and cancer cells. *Adv Cancer Res* 32:75, 1980.
Brown JM, Harken AH, Sharefkin JB: Recombinant DNA and surgery. *Ann Surg* 212:178, 1990.
Cantley LC, Auger KR, et al: Oncogenes and signal transduction. *Cell* 64:281, 1991.
Cooper GM: *Oncogenes*. Boston, Jones and Bartlett, 1990.
Cross M, Dexter TM: Growth factors in development, transformation, and tumorigenesis. *Cell* 64:271, 1991.
Doyle LA: Interrelationships between growth factors and oncogenes, in Moosa AR, Schimpff SC, Robson MC (eds): *Comprehensive Textbook of Oncology* (2d ed), vol. 1. Baltimore, Williams & Wilkins, 1991, p. 63.
Ducker BJ, Mamon HJ, Roberts M: Oncogenes, growth factors and signal transduction. *N Engl J Med* 321:1383, 1989.
Fearon ER, Vogelstein B: A genetic model for colorectal tumorigenesis. *Cell* 61:759, 1990.
Fidler IJ, Hart IR: Biological diversity in metastatic neoplasms: Origins and implications. *Science* 217:998, 1982.
Fidler IJ, Price JE: The influence of organ microenvironment on the development of cancer metastases, in Larson DL, Ballantyne AJ, Guillamondegui OM (eds): *Cancer in the Neck—Evaluation and Treatment*. New York, Macmillan, 1986, p. 23.
Fidler IJ, Balch CM: The biology of cancer metastasis and implications for therapy, in Ravitch MM, Stelchen FM (eds): *Current Problems in Surgery*, vol. 24. Chicago, Year Book Medical Publishers, 1987, p. 3.
Folkman J: Tumor angiogenesis. *Adv Cancer Res* 43:175, 1985.
Folkman J, Li W, Casey R: Inflammation and angiogenesis, in Melchers F (ed): *Progress in Immunology*. Heidelberg, Springer-Verlag, 1989, p. 61.
Folkman J: The role of angiogenesis in tumor growth. *Semin Cancer Biol* 3:65, 1992.
Folkman J, Ingber D: Inhibition of angiogenesis. *Semin Cancer Biol* 3:89, 1992.
Foulds L: *Neoplastic Development*, vol. 1. London Academic Press, 1969; vol. 2. London Academic Press, 1975.
Grimm EA, Ramsey KM, et al: Lymphokine-activated killer cell phenomenon. II. Precursor phenotype is serologically distinct from peripheral T lymphocytes, memory cytotoxic thymus-derived lymphocytes, and natural killer cells. *J Exp Med* 157:884, 1983.
Hamburger AW: Cell transformation, in Moosa AR, Schimpff SC, Robson MC (eds): *Comprehensive Textbook of Oncology* (2d ed), vol. 1. Baltimore, Williams & Wilkins, 1991, p. 22.
Hunter T: Cooperation between oncogenes. *Cell* 64:249, 1991.
Liotta LA, Steeg PS, Stetler-Stevenson WG: Cancer metastasis and angiogenesis: an imbalance of positive and negative regulation. *Cell* 64:327, 1991.
Male D, Champion B, Cooke A: *Advanced Immunology*. Philadelphia, JB Lippincott, 1987.
Marshall CJ: Tumor suppressor genes. *Cell* 64:313, 1991.
Needleman SW: Retroviral and cellular oncogenes, in Moosa AR, Schimpff SC, Robson MC (eds): *Comprehensive Textbook of Oncology* (2d ed), vol. 1. Baltimore, Williams & Wilkins, 1991, p. 55.
Nicolson GL: Properties of metastatic tumor cells and the generation of tumor phenotypic diversity, in Larson DL, Ballantyne AJ, Guillamondegui OM (eds): *Cancer in the Neck—Evaluation and Treatment*. New York, Macmillan, 1986, p. 3.
Nicolson GL: Oncogenes, genetic instability, and evolution of the metastatic phenotype. *Adv Viral Oncol* 6:143, 1987.
Nicolson GL: Molecular mechanisms of cancer metastasis: Tumor and host properties and the role of oncogenes and suppressor genes. *Curr Opin Oncol* 3:75, 1991.
Nowell PC: The clonal evolution of tumor cell populations. *Science* 194:23, 1976.
Pellis N, Balch CM, et al: Tumor biology, in Greenfield LJ, Mulholland MW, Oldham KT, Zelenock GB (eds): *Surgery: Scientific Principles and Practice*. Philadelphia, JB Lippincott, 1992, p. 407.
Pitot HC: The natural history of neoplastic development: The relation of experimental models to human cancer. *Cancer* 49:1206, 1982.
Prehn RT, Main JM: Immunity to methylcholanthrene-induced sarcomas. *J Natl Cancer Inst* 18:769, 1957.
Southam CM, Brunschwig W, et al: The effect of leukocytes on transplantability of human cancer. *Cancer* 19:1743, 1966.
Stutman O: The immunological surveillance hypothesis, in Herberman RB (ed): *Basic and Clinical Tumor Immunology*. Boston, Martinus Nijhoff, 1983, p. 1.
Weinberg RA: A molecular basis for cancer. *Sci Am* 249:126, 1983.

Cancer Diagnosis, Staging, and Pathology

American Joint Committee on Cancer. *Manual for Staging of Cancer* (3rd ed). Philadelphia, JB Lippincott, 1988.

Archie JT, Witt TR: Peritoneoscopy for biopsy, staging, and therapy of intra-abdominal tumors, in Economou SG, Witt TR, Deziel DJ, Saclarides TJ, Staren ED, Bines SD (eds): *Adjuncts to Cancer Surgery*. Philadelphia, Lea & Febiger, 1991, p. 195.

Batsakis JG, Medina JE: Pathological evaluation of neck dissection lymph nodes: A status report, in Larson DL, Ballantyne AJ, Guillamondegui OM (eds): *Cancer in the Neck—Evaluation and Treatment*. New York, Macmillan, 1986, p. 33.

Bland KI, McCoy DM, et al: Application of magnetic resonance imaging and computerized tomography as an adjunct to the surgical management of soft tissue sarcomas. *Ann Surg* 205:473, 1987.

Bloom HJG, Richardson WW, Harries EJ: Natural history of untreated breast cancer (1805–1933): Comparison of untreated and treated cases according to histological grade of malignancy. *Br Med J* 2:213, 1962.

Cohn SL, Robinson, et al: Tumor markers and phenotyping techniques, in Economou SG, Witt TR, Deziel DJ, Saclarides TJ, Staren ED, Bines SD (eds): *Adjuncts to Cancer Surgery*. Philadelphia, Lea & Febiger, 1991, p. 207.

Collins VP, Loeffler RK, Tivey H: Observations on growth rates of human tumors. *Am J Roentgenol Radium Ther Nucl Med* 76:988, 1956.

Commission on Clinical Oncology of the Union Internationale Contre Cancrum: *TNM Classification of Malignant Tumors*. Geneva, International Clinics Against Cancer, 1968.

Doyle LA, Aisner J: Clinical presentation of lung cancer, in Roth JA, Ruckdeschel JC, Weisenburger TH (eds): *Thoracic Oncology*. Philadelphia, WB Saunders, 1989, p. 52.

Everson TC: Spontaneous regression of cancer. *Ann NY Acad Sci* 114:721, 1964.

Garland LH, Coulson W, Wollin E: The rate of growth and apparent duration of untreated primary bronchial carcinoma. *Cancer* 16:694, 1963.

Gold P, Freeman SO: Specific carcinoembryonic antigens of the human digestive system. *J Exp Med* 122:467, 1965.

Jones SE: Importance of staging in Hodgkin's disease. *Semin Oncol* 7:126, 1980.

LeVeen EG, LeVeen HH: Peritoneovenous shunt in the treatment of malignant ascites, in Economou SG, Witt TR, Deziel DJ, Saclarides TJ, Staren ED, Bines SD (eds): *Adjuncts to Cancer Surgery*. Philadelphia, Lea & Febiger, 1991, p. 339.

Putman JB Jr, Roth JA: Prognostic indicators in patients with pulmonary metastases. *Semin Surg Oncol* 6:291, 1990.

Russell WO, Cohen J, et al: A clinical and pathological staging system for soft tissue sarcomas. *Cancer* 40:1562, 1977.

Turner DA, Fruin ME: Magnetic resonance imaging in cancer, in Economou SG, Witt TR, Deziel DJ, Saclarides TJ, Staren ED, Bines SD (eds): *Adjuncts to Cancer Surgery*. Philadelphia, Lea & Febiger, 1991, p. 95.

Wang RC, Goepfert H, et al: Squamous cell carcinoma metastatic to the neck from an unknown primary site, in Larson DL, Ballantyne AJ, Guillamondegui OM (eds): *Cancer in the Neck—Evaluation and Treatment*. New York, Macmillan, 1986, p. 183.

Williams PA: A productive history and physical examination in the prevention and early detection of cancer. *Cancer* 47:1146, 1981.

Williams ST, Beart RW Jr: Staging of colorectal cancer. *Semin Surg Oncol* 8:83, 1992.

Cancer Surgery

Ames F, Balch CM: Management of local and regional recurrence after mastectomy or breast-conserving treatment, in Cady B, Bland KL (eds): *The Surgical Clinics of North America*. Philadelphia, WB Saunders, 1990, p. 1115.

Ames FC, Balch CM, McCarthy WH: Axillary lymph node dissection, in Balch CM, Houghton AN, Milton GW, Sober A, Soong S-J (eds): *Cutaneous Melanoma* (2d ed). Philadelphia, JB Lippincott, 1992, p. 384.

Austgen TR, Souba WW, Bland KI: Reoperation for colorectal carcinoma. *Surg Clin North Am* 71:175, 1991.

Balch CM: Surgical oncology in the 21st century. *Arch Surg* 127:1272, 1992.

Brennan MF: Surgical management of peripancreatic cancer, in Karakousis CP, Copeland EM III, Bland KI (eds): *Atlas of Surgical Oncology*. Philadelphia, WB Saunders, (in press).

DeMeester TR, Albertucci M: Surgical therapy, in Bitran JD, Golumb HM, Little AG, Weichselbaum RR (eds): *Lung Cancer–A Comprehensive Treatise*. Orlando, Grune & Stratton, 1988, p. 135.

Edwards MJ, Balch CM: Surgical aspects of lymphoma, in Tompkins RK, Balch CM, Cameron JL, et al (eds): *Advances in Surgery*. 22:225, Chicago, Yearbook Medical Publishers, 1989.

Haagensen CD, Feind CR, Herter FP, et al: *The Lymphatics in Cancer*. Philadelphia, WB Saunders 1972.

Holmes EC: Adjuvant treatment in resected lung cancer. *Semin Surg Oncol* 6:255, 1990.

McCormack P: Surgical resection of pulmonary metastases. *Semin Surg Oncol* 6:297, 1990.

Pollock RE, Kroll SS, Balch CM: Surgical procedures for advanced local and regional malignancy of the breast, in Bland K, Copeland E (eds): *The Breast*. Philadelphia, WB Saunders, 1990, p. 948.

Pommier R, Woltering EA: Follow-up of patients after primary colorectal cancer resection. *Semin Surg Oncol* 7:133, 1991.

Roh M, Balch CM, et al: *Atlas of Advanced Oncologic Surgery*. Philadelphia, Gower, 1990.

Sherry RMN, Pass HI, et al: Surgical resection of metastatic renal cell carcinoma and melanoma after response to interleukin-2-based immunotherapy. *Cancer* 69:1850, 1992.

Sondak VK, Economou JS, Eilber FR: Soft tissue sarcomas of the extremity and retroperitoneum: Advances in management. *Adv Surg* 24:333, 1991.

Williard WC, Hajdu SI, et al: Comparison of amputation with limb-sparing operations for adult soft tissue sarcoma of the extremity. *Ann Surg* 215:269, 1992.

Yeatman TJ, Bland KI: The basis for surgical decisions in the management of in situ breast cancer. *Compr Ther* 16:12, 1990.

Radiation Oncology

Fletcher GH: Radiation therapy of cancers of the head and neck, in McKenna RJ, Murphy GP (eds): *Fundamentals of Surgical Oncology*. New York, Macmillan, 1986, p. 258.

Fu KK: Biological basis for the interaction of chemotherapeutic agents and radiation therapy. *Cancer* 55:2123, 1985.

Gunderson LL, Rich TA, Tepper JE: Radiation therapy of gastrointestinal cancer, in McKenna RJ, Murphy GP (eds): *Fundamentals of Surgical Oncology*. New York, Macmillan, 1986, p. 282.

Hall EJ: Radiation biology. *Cancer* 55:2051, 1985.

Hellman S: Principles of radiation therapy, in DeVita VT Jr, Hellman S, Rosenberg SA (eds): *Cancer: Principles and Practice of Oncology*. Philadelphia, JB Lippincott, 1989.

Johnson R: Introduction to radiation oncology, in McKenna RJ, Murphy GP (eds): *Fundamentals of Surgical Oncology*. New York, Macmillan, 1986, p. 255.

Kaplan HS: Historic milestones in radiobiology and radiation therapy. *Semin Oncol* 6:479, 1979.

Little AG: Principles of radiation oncology, in Bitran JD, Golumb HM, Little AG, Weichselbaum RR (eds): *Lung Cancer—A Comprehensive Treatise*. Orlando, Grune & Stratton, 1988, p. 55.

Montague ED, Fletcher GH: Radiation therapy of breast cancer, in McKenna RJ, Murphy GP (eds): *Fundamentals of Surgical Oncology*. New York, Macmillan, 1986, p. 268.

Peters, LJ: Basic principles of radiobiology in head and neck oncology, in Larson DL, Ballantyne AJ, Guillamondegui OM (eds): *Cancer in the Neck—Evaluation and Treatment*. New York, Macmillan, 1986, p. 75.

Chemotherapy

Calabresi P, Schein PS, Rosenberg SA: *Medical Oncology: Basic Principles and Clinical Management of Cancer*. New York, Macmillan, 1985.

Chabner BA: The oncologic end game (Karnofsky Memorial Lecture). *J Clin Oncol* 4:625, 1986.

Chabner BA, Collins JM (eds): *Cancer Chemotherapy: Principles and Practice*. Philadelphia, JB Lippincott, 1990.

Creaven PJ: Pharmacologic principles of cancer chemotherapy, in McKenna RJ, Murphy GP (eds): *Fundamentals of Surgical Oncology*. New York, Macmillan, 1986, p. 233.

Crown J, Norton L: Adjuvant systemic therapy for early breast cancer. *Semin Surg Oncol* 7:271, 1991.

Einhorn LH: Testicular cancer as a model for a curable neoplasm: The Richard and Hinda Rosenthal Foundation Award Lecture. *Cancer Res* 41:3275, 1981.

Erlichman C: Potential applications of therapeutic drug monitoring in treatment of neoplastic disease by antineoplastic agents. *Clin Biochem* 19:101, 1986.

Pazdur R: Adjuvant chemotherapy of tumors of the gastrointestinal tract, in Economou SG, Witt TR, Deziel DJ, Saclarides TJ, Staren ED, Bines SD (eds): *Adjuncts to Cancer Surgery*. Philadelphia, Lea & Febiger, 1991, p. 467.

Schabel FM Jr: The use of tumor growth kinetics in planning ''curative'' chemotherapy of advanced solid tumors. *Cancer Res* 29:2384, 1969.

Schnipper LE: Clinical implications of tumor-cell heterogeneity. *N Engl J Med* 314:1423, 1986.

Tannock IF: Experimental chemotherapy and concepts related to the cell cycle. *Int J Radiat Biol* 49:335, 1986.

Multimodality Therapy

Balch CM, Singletary SE: Clinical decision making in early breast cancer. *Ann Surg* 217:207, 1993.

Bitran JD, Golomb HM, et al: The multimodality approach to lung cancer, in Bitran JD, Golumb HM, Little AG, Weichselbaum RR (eds): *Lung Cancer—A Comprehensive Treatise*. Orlando, Grune & Stratton, 1988, p. 3.

Brennan MF, Casper ES, et al: The role of multimodality therapy in soft-tissue sarcoma. *Ann Surg* 214:328, 1991.

Rosen G, Murphy ML, et al: Chemotherapy, enbloc resection and prosthetic bone replacement in the treatment of osteogenic sarcoma. *Cancer* 37:1, 1976.

Suit HD, Todoroki T: Rationale for combining surgery and radiation therapy. *Cancer* 55:2246, 1985.

Suit HD, Todoroki T: Rationale for the laboratory and clinical basis for combining radiation and surgery in the treatment of primary malignant disease, in McKenna RJ, Murphy GP (eds): *Fundamentals of Surgical Oncology*. New York, Macmillan, 1986, p. 329.

Rehabilitation and Psychological Management

Fink DJ: Cancer rehabilitation, in McKenna RJ, Murphy GP (eds): *Fundamentals of Surgical Oncology*. New York, Macmillan, 1986, p. 345.

McGuire DB, Yarbro CH (eds): *Cancer Pain Management*. Orlando, Grune & Stratton, 1987.

Osoba D (ed): *Effect of Cancer on Quality of Life*. Boca Raton, CRC Press, 1991.

Penn RD: Neurosurgical techniques for pain control in cancer patients, in Economou SG, Witt TR, Deziel DJ, Saclarides TJ, Staren ED, Bines SD (eds): *Adjuncts to Cancer Surgery*. Philadelphia, Lea & Febiger, 1991, p. 622.

Biologic Therapy

Balch CM, Pellis N: Clinical immunology and biological therapy of human cancer, in Najarian JS (moderator): *Proceedings from the 1990 Surgical Research and Education Symposium*. Chicago, American College of Surgeons, 1991, p. 13.

Coley WB: The treatment of malignant tumors by repeated inoculation of erysipelas, with a report of original cases. *Am J Med Sci* 105:487, 1893.

Culver K, Cornetta K, et al: Lymphocytes as cellular vehicles for gene therapy in mouse and man. *Proc Natl Acad Sci USA* 88:3155, 1991.

Economou JS, Staren ED: Immune modulators in the treatment of cancer, in Economou SG, Witt TR, Deziel DJ, Saclarides TJ, Staren ED, Bines SD (eds): *Adjuncts to Cancer Surgery*. Philadelphia, Lea & Febiger, 1991, p. 575.

Irie RF, Morton DC: Regression of cutaneous metastatic melanoma by intralesional injection with human monoclonal antibody to ganglioside GD2. *Proc Natl Acad Sci USA* 83:8694, 1986.

Golub SH, D'Amore P, et al: Systemic administration of human leukocyte interferon to melanoma patients. II. Cellular events associated with changes in NK cytotoxicity. *J Natl Cancer Inst* 68:711, 1982.

Lotze MT, Matory YL, et al: Clinical effects and toxicity of interleukin-2 in patients with cancer. *Cancer* 58:2764, 1986.

Morton DL: Changing concepts of cancer surgery: Surgery as immunotherapy. *Am J Surg* 135:367, 1978.

Morton DL, Foshag LJ, et al: Active specific immunotherapy in malignant melanoma. *Semin Surg Oncol* 5:420, 1989.

Rosenberg SA, Lotze MT, et al: Observations on the systemic administration of autologous lymphokine-activated killer cells and recombinant interleukin-2 to patients with metastatic cancer. *N Engl J Med* 313:1485, 1985.

Rosenberg SA: *Biologic Therapy of Cancer*. Philadelphia, JB Lippincott, 1991.

Rosenberg SA: Karnofsky Memorial Lecture. The immunotherapy and gene therapy of cancer. *J Clin Oncol* 10:180, 1992.

Wong JH, Irie RF, Morton DL: Human monoclonal antibodies: Prospects for the therapy of cancer. *Semin Surg Oncol* 5:448, 1989.

CHAPTER 10

Transplantation

Richard L. Simmons, Suzanne T. Ildstad, Craig R. Smith, Keith Reemtsma, and John S. Najarian

Human beings do not burst like balloons—they fall apart, piece by piece. Clinical organ transplantation is designed to replace the exhausted parts as they fall. Because the immunologic barrier of allograft rejection stands in the way of attaining chimerism between host and graft, immunologists and surgeons have been working together since World War II to circumvent the rejection reaction.

Transplantation of solid organs and even cells for treatment of end-organ failure and genetic and metabolic diseases is one of the greatest success stories in surgery and immunobiology for this century. After Alexis Carrel described the technique for vascular anastomoses, the transplantation of primarily vascularized solid organs became technically possible. Rejection occurred in all grafts except those between identical twins, leading to recognition that individuals possess unique heritable differences in tissue histocompatibility antigens. The development of histocompatibility typing followed.

The recognition that anticancer agents (i.e., irradiation, alkylating agents) prolonged graft survival through nonspecific suppression of the immune system to prevent graft rejection allowed transplantation of tissues and organs between genetically different individuals to proceed. In 40 short years, transplantation of hearts, lungs, livers, kidneys, pancreas, small intestine, and even cellular grafts are now clinically accepted therapeutic approaches for a wide variety of disease states. Transplantation has been so successful that the supply of grafts for transplantation has become increasingly limited.

The first part of this chapter discusses the immunobiology of the allograft, the rejection reaction, and the means for achieving immunosuppression. The current and incipient clinical applications of these biologic principles and techniques to the human patient are discussed in the second section. The combination of immunobiology with clinical transplantation has benefitted both fields greatly. As the mechanisms of graft rejection and acceptance become increasingly understood, further advances in the field can be anticipated.

IMMUNOBIOLOGY OF THE ALLOGRAFT

In general, the greater the genetic difference between the graft and the recipient, the more vigorous that rejection response. Tissue or organ grafts between individuals of the same species (*allografts*, or *homografts*) are rejected with a vigor proportional to the degree of the genetic disparity between the individuals. Grafts between individuals of different species (*xenografts*, or *heterografts*) are rejected even more rapidly. Grafts between identical twins (*isografts, isogenic grafts*, or *syngenic grafts*) or from individuals to themselves (*autografts*) survive indefinitely after the vascular supply has been reestablished.

Allografts normally survive the transplant operation as well as isografts. If the recipient has not previously encountered the antigens present on the donor graft, the allograft is not morphologically or physiologically distinguishable from the isograft in the early posttransplant period—the rejection process normally takes several days. Medawar first noted that skin grafts between unrelated rabbits appeared normal until the fourth or fifth day. At that time inflammation appeared within the graft bed in the form of a dense leukocyte infiltrate that led to necrosis of the entire graft by about the tenth day. He further demonstrated that the rejection process is the result of immunologic mechanisms. Whereas the "first-set rejection" took place in 10 or 11 days, a second graft from the same rabbit resulted in an accelerated "second-set rejection." The process of first-set and second-set rejection of an allogenic graft takes place whether or not the graft is *orthotopic* (a graft placed in the anatomic position normally occupied by such tissue) or *heterotopic* (placed in other than the original location). The reaction is immunologically specific for the antigens involved, and the second-act rejections occur only when the recipient has been sensitized to antigens shared with the first graft.

Transplantation (Histocompatibility) Antigens

The rejection of an allograft is elicited by foreign histocompatibility antigens on the cell surfaces of the grafted tissue. Many antigens can serve as histocompatibility antigens. For example, the ABO blood group antigens will elicit rapid graft rejection in hosts with natural isoantibody. Similarly, xenografts between distant species are rejected rapidly because tissue incompatibilities are so profound between most species that circulating preformed antibodies may exist in the serum of the recipient of the graft. Alloantigenic incompatibilities between members of a species vary, however, and strong antigens can lead to graft rejection within 8 days, while weaker differences will permit graft survival of well over 100 days.

The Immunogenetics of Histocompatibility

The strongest of the transplantation antigens is the expression of a single chromosomal region called the *major histocompatibility complex* (MHC) (Fig. 10-1). The MHC is a large gene complex that controls traits which influence the entire immune response. In humans the MHC is located on chromosome 6. All mammals have

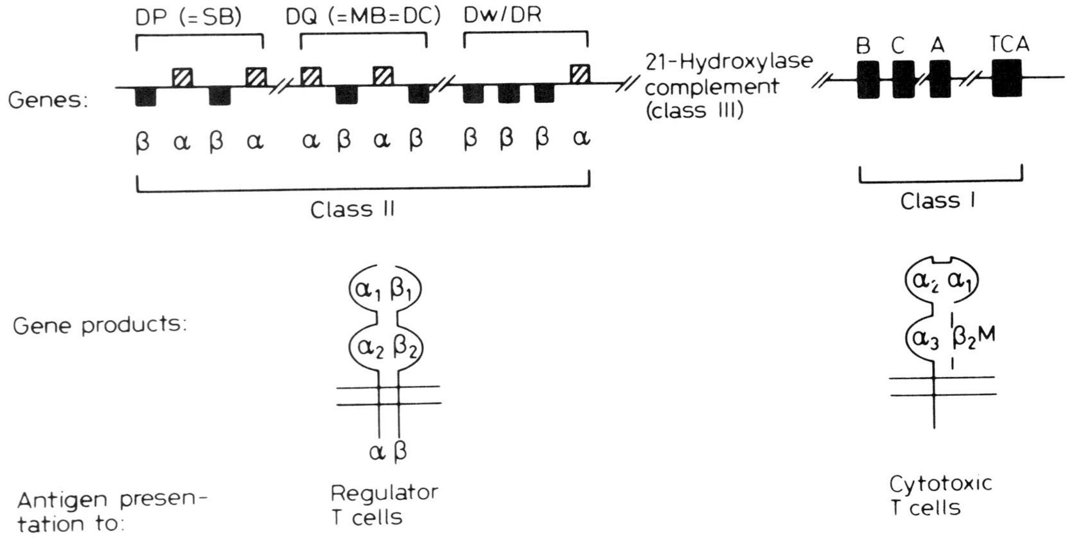

FIG. 10-1. Gene map of chromosome 6 in human beings. This segment of the chromosome between the locus coding for the enzyme glyoxylase (GLO) and HLA-A is usually referred to as the HLA complex. The loci of HLA can be divided into two classes: Class I loci include HLA-A, HLA-B, and HLA-C, whereas the Class II loci include HLA-DR, HLA-DP, and HLA-DQ. Gene products of the Class I molecules are glycoproteins consisting of a heavy chain that penetrates the cell membrane. The heavy chain is folded into three immunoglobulinlike domains (α_1, α_2, and α_3). A β_2-microglobulin unit completes the structure. The Class II antigens consist of two polypeptide chains, both of which penetrate the cell membrane. The extracellular part of each chain is folded into two domains. The domains adjacent to the cell membrane are homologous with the α_3 and β_2M domains of the Class I molecules and the constant domain of the immunoglobulin molecule. (From: *deVries RRP, Van Rood JJ [eds]: Immunobiology of HLA Class I and Class II Molecules. Basel, Switzerland, Karger, 1985, with permission.*)

a similar MHC, but the nomenclature varies among species. In humans, the gene products of the MHC were first investigated on leukocytes and were named *human leukocyte antigens* (HLA).

The presence of HLA antigens on a cell surface can be detected in one of two ways. The serologic method uses antigen-specific antisera, which binds to cells carrying the antigen. A second method measures the proliferation of host lymphocytes in response to histocompatibility antigens on the cells of potential graft donors. The MHC antigens that can best trigger the proliferation of allogenic lymphocytes were designated *Class II molecules*. The antigens that trigger allogenic lymphocyte proliferation poorly were designated *Class I molecules*. Both Class I and Class II molecules can now be detected by specific antisera. The Class I molecules are expressions of those portions of the MHC supergene called HLA-A, HLA-B, and HLA-C. The Class II molecules are expressions of HLA-D, DR, DQ, and DW/DR subloci. Because of the genetic diversity in the human race, not all histocompatibility antigens have been identified.

The MHC genes have been classically divided into three classes: Class I, Class II, and Class III. Only Class I and Class II molecules have a major influence in transplantation. Although Class I and Class II determinants were once thought of as *antigens*, they are now known to play a critical role in T-cell and B-cell activation, in addition to providing histocompatibility recognition.

HLA Class I molecules can be detected on the cell surfaces of almost all nucleated cells. In contrast HLA Class II molecules are found only on cells of the immune system—macrophages, dendritic cells, B cells, and activated T cells. Resting T lymphocytes do not express Class II molecules. Both Class I and Class II molecules are each composed of two polypeptide chains with variable and constant regions similar to those seen in immunoglobulin structure. The polymorphism is expressed in the variable regions of each molecule distant from the cell membrane. The constant portion of molecule is closest to the cell membrane and shows considerable homology between Class I and Class II molecules. This fact suggests that a common evolutionary origin exists between these three molecules (see Fig. 10-1). The Class I genes encode cell surface transplantation antigens which serve as the primary targets for cytotoxic T lymphocytes in graft rejection.

The Class I heavy chains (37–45 KDa) are highly polymorphic and are noncovalently associated on the cell surface with the β_2-microglobulin light chain (β_2M), which is remarkably conserved. Class I expression cannot occur in the absence of β_2M. The three-dimensional structure of a number of the Class I molecules has now been characterized (Fig. 10-2). Class I molecules are integral membrane proteins which function in the presentation of transplantation antigens to T cells. They are developmentally regulated and are not detectable until the midsomite stage of embryogenesis. Although they are expressed on almost all cells of the adult, the level of expression varies from tissue to tissue. Expression is greatest in lymphoid cells.

The *interferons* (IFN-α, IFN-β, IFN-γ) induce increased expression of Class I molecules in a wide variety of cell types through binding to a specific cell surface receptor. IFN-α and IFN-β are produced by fibroblasts while IFN-γ is produced by T lymphocytes.

The *Class II genes*, also known as the immune response genes, encode the genetic material for the immune response. They control the immune response to many antigens and also encode a number of antigens that are expressed on lymphocytes. Class II gene products are the primary targets for helper T lymphocytes. The Class II loci in humans include HLA-DR, DQ, and DP. Class II antigenic

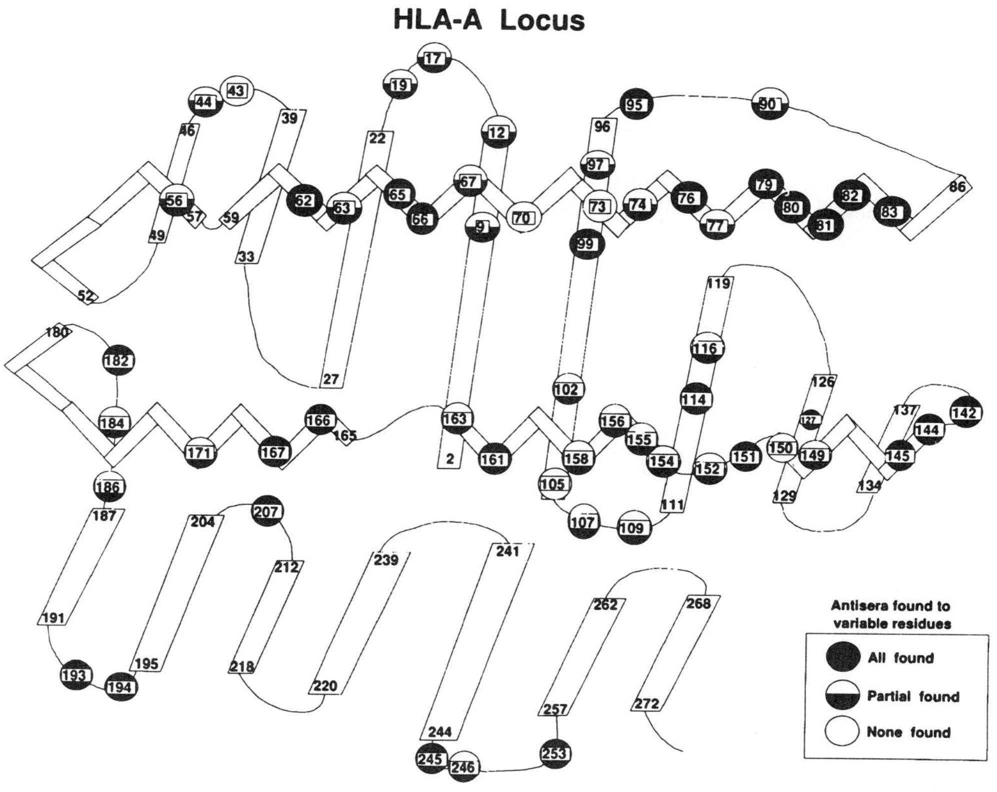

FIG. 10-2. 3-dimensional structure of HLA-A locus. Antisera or monoclonal antibodies are available to a number of variable residues to allow more precise typing. A change in only one amino acid is sufficient to change the antigenicity. Similar information is known for the HLA-B locus as well. (From: *Terasaki PI [ed]: Clinical Transplants 1990. Los Angeles, UCLA Tissue Typing Laboratory, 1991, p 525, with permission.*)

expression is normally limited to cells of bone marrow stem cell origin, although expression of Class II on other tissues may be induced by inflammatory cytokines like IFN-α; thus during the inflammatory response that accompanies rejection, both Class I and Class II antigen expression occurs in cells that normally do not express these molecules.

Minor transplantation antigens are expressions of genes located on other chromosomes, and they elicit a weaker rejection response. However, an isolated minor antigen disparity can have a major impact on the outcome of a transplanted organ. Grafts between HLA (MHC)-identical siblings will reject if chronic immunosuppression is not utilized after transplantation of a solid organ because of the presence of these minor transplantation antigens. Only identical twins accept grafts from each other without need for immunosuppression.

The HLA antigens have formed the basis for transplantation tissue typing for many years. Because of extreme polymorphism, only rarely do two unrelated individuals share all the antigens expressed. Relatives, on the other hand, often share some antigens because each person inherits one chromosome and, hence, one set of HLA antigens from each parent (Fig. 10-3), and because all the HLA antigens are expressed (codominant) on the cell surface.

The MHC subloci have been found to be closely linked but separable, and therefore genetic crossover between them, though unusual, can occur. As shown in Fig. 10-3, the parental HLA-A, -B, and -D pairs are usually inherited together, and the antigens originating from one chromosome are called *HLA haplotypes*. Almost always the haplotype the child receives from each parent corresponds to the haplotype of one of the parental chromosomes. When crossover occurs during meiosis, however, the child receives a recombinant haplotype from a parent. (In the example shown, recombination occurred between A and B antigens. Recombination can occur between B and D also.)

Detection of the A, B, and D alleles for tissue typing requires banks of monospecific antisera. Typing was thought to be clinically useful because it seemed clear that survival of transplanted organs between family members correlated with the closeness of the HLA antigen match. The clinical results of organ transplantation have not, however, clearly demonstrated the importance of HLA-A and -B identity in organ transplantation between unrelated (cadaver) donor-recipient pairs, especially with the availability of improved immunosuppressive agents.

Normal Role for the MHC. The functions of histocompatibility antigens are not toally understood, but they do not exist merely to thwart the efforts of transplant surgeons. They are critical to the recognition phenomena during cell-cell interactions within the same organism. Both MHC Class I and Class II molecules are membrane glycoproteins that serve to bind and display on the surface of cells peptide antigens. The peptides are the products of digestion of proteins processed by antigen-presenting accessory cells like dendritic cells and macrophages. Thus, antigens are always presented in the context of "self" MHC molecules, and the recognition of the foreign peptide-self MHC molecule complex by the antigen-specific receptor on the T lymphocytes leads to the T-cell proliferation and the cascade of cellular immune responses. It is likely that foreign MHC molecules are presented as peptide fragments by host MHC molecules on the surface of host antigen-presenting cells.

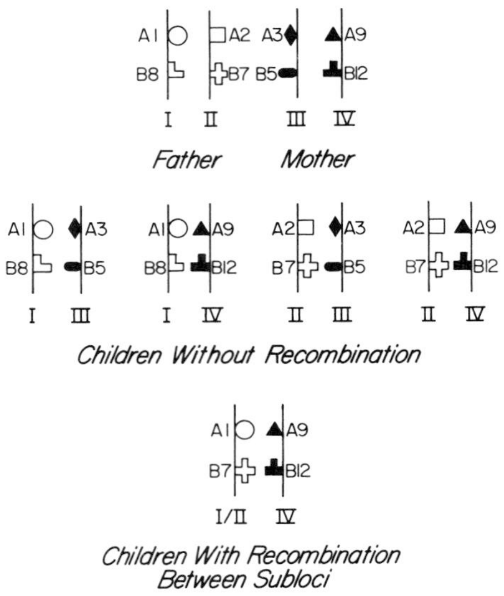

FIG. 10-3. Hypothetical examples of inheritance of serologically detectable HLA antigens of the A and B series. Four offspring of mating between parents with chromosomes labeled I-II and III–IV are shown, as well as one possible result of recombination within the HLA region and subsequent inheritance. The parental chromosomes are usually transmitted intact, and the offspring receive one chromosome containing an A and B pair from each parent. Occasionally, however, crossover occurs and the child receives a recombinant antigen pair from a parent. For simplicity, genes coding for the C and D series of antigens within the HLA complex are not shown. See Fig. 10-1 for the presumed location of the genes within the HLA complex.

Histocompatibility Matching

It is obvious that, other things being equal, the less antigenic the graft, the less the host will react against it. In human transplantation, when the donor and recipient are identical twins, there is no antigenic difference, and the tissues are accepted. When the donor and recipient are siblings or when a parent donor is used for offspring, there is a greater statistical likelihood of antigen sharing between donor and recipient than when a cadaver or other unrelated donor is used.

Several methods have been developed for the purpose of demonstrating antigenic similarities between donor and recipient prior to transplantation, so that donor and recipient pairs that are relatively histocompatible may be selected.

The best current method is called *serologic* or *leukocyte typing*. HLA antigens on circulating lymphocytes can be detected with antisera derived originally from multiply transfused patients or from women with multiple pregnancies. Some of the antisera recognize groups of antigens, and others recognize single antigens (*monospecific antisera*). Using the patient's leukocytes and a group of standard antisera, it is thus possible to characterize most of the strong HLA antigens in both donor and host. Table 10-1 demonstrates typical results from a typing panel. Only HLA antigens can be routinely determined in this way. Weaker histocompatibility antigens at other loci have not been detected by serologic techniques in human beings.

Histocompatibility typing is useful in determining the best match between donor and recipient when family donors are utilized. Siblings who share all HLA antigens are the best possible

Table 10-1
Lymphocyte Antigen Typing Report of Theoretical Family*

		HLA-A Locus											*HLA-DR Locus*									
Family Member	*ABO*	*A1*	*A2*	*A3*	*A9*	*A10*	*A11*	*A28*	*Aw19*	*Aw34*	*Aw36*	*Aw43*	*DR1*	*DR2*	*DR3*	*DR4*	*DR5*	*DRw6*	*DR7*	*DRw8*	*DRw9*	*DRw10*
Father AB	A	+	−	+	−	−	−	−	−	−	−	−	−	−	+	+	−	−	−	−	−	−
Mother CD	A	−	+	−	−	−	−	+	−	−	−	−	+	−	−	−	−	−	+	−	−	−
Son AC (patient)	O	+	−	−	−	−	−	+	−	−	−	−	+	−	+	−	−	−	−	−	−	−
Son AD	A	+	+	−	−	−	−	−	−	−	−	−	−	−	+	−	−	−	+	−	−	−
Daughter BC	O	−	−	+	−	−	−	+	−	−	−	−	+	−	−	+	−	−	−	−	−	−
Daughter BD	A	−	+	+	−	−	−	−	−	−	−	−	−	−	−	+	−	−	+	−	−	−
Daughter AC	O	+	−	−	−	−	−	+	−	−	−	−	+	−	+	−	−	−	−	−	−	−

		HLB-B Locus																		
Family Member	*ABO*	*B5*	*B7*	*B8*	*B12*	*B13*	*B14*	*B15*	*Bw16*	*B17*	*B18*	*Bw21*	*Bw22*	*B27*	*Bw35*	*B37*	*B40*	*Bw41*	*Bw42*	*Bw47*
Father AB	A	−	−	+	−	−	−	−	−	−	−	−	−	−	+	−	−	−	−	−
Mother CD	A	−	−	−	−	−	−	−	−	−	+	−	−	+	−	−	−	−	−	−
Son AC (patient)	O	−	−	+	−	−	−	−	−	−	−	−	−	+	−	−	−	−	−	−
Son AD	A	−	−	+	−	−	−	−	−	−	+	−	−	−	−	−	−	−	−	−
Daughter BC	O	−	−	−	−	−	−	−	−	−	−	−	−	+	+	−	−	−	−	−
Daughter BD	A	−	−	−	−	−	−	−	−	−	+	−	−	−	+	−	−	−	−	−
Daughter AC	O	−	−	+	−	−	−	−	−	−	−	−	−	+	−	−	−	−	−	−

*The specifications for the A, B, C, and DR loci are those currently used at the University of Minnesota.

Son AC is the prospective transplant recipient. Daughter AC is a perfect match for all four antigens; she shares the inheritance of both HLA haplotypes and is the ideal donor. Both parents, son AD, and daughter BC share only one haplotype with the potential recipient and are theoretically not as good donors. Daughter BD shares no HLA haplotypes with the recipient and is the poorest donor in the family.

More important than the HLA type are the ABO blood types. The father, mother, son AD, and daughter BD *cannot* donate, because they are all blood group A and the recipient is blood group O and possesses anti-A antibodies in his serum.

donor-recipient pair. But several points about histocompatibility matching deserve emphasis:

1. Recipients receiving grafts, even from donors who are HLA identical matches with them, will still reject the graft (although more slowly) unless immunosuppressive drugs are utilized. Only an identical twin is truly a perfect match.
2. Even with poor histocompatibility matches between relatives, the results are frequently good, which probably indicates it is sometimes possible to suppress even great degrees of antigenic incompatibility.
3. Even with a good histocompatibility match, the graft may fail if the host has performed antibodies against a donor's tissue. These antibodies can be recognized if recipient serum is allowed to react with donor lymphocytes in a cytotoxicity test. This test, called *cross matching*, should be performed with fresh serum as a final test of compatibility prior to transplant. Preformed cytotoxic antibodies to donor tissue cannot be detected by the usual typing procedure itself.
4. The presence of ABO isohemagglutinins will lead to the prompt rejection of tissue bearing incompatible blood group substances for most solid organ grafts.
5. Despite the results of tissue typing, a related donor has generally produced better transplant results than an unrelated (cadaver) donor.
6. Tissue typing for unrelated cadaver donors has not been successful, with one exception: HLA identity of all detectable antigens correlates with a higher incidence of graft success. But such identity is rare.

Mixed Lymphocyte Culture (MLC). The other method capable of detecting degrees of histocompatibility between donor and recipient is the MLC test, which detects differences principally at the Class II locus. This is referred to as *functional typing*. Lymphocytes of the recipient are mixed with lymphocytes of the donor in tissue culture. If significant antigenic differences exist between the two, they will respond by proliferation, with transformation into blast cells, DNA synthesis, and mitosis. The incorporation of tritiated thymidine into DNA can be quantified to assess the degree of stimulation. As the test was originally devised, it was a two-way test—cells of the donor were capable of reacting against cells of the recipient and vice versa. In order to isolate the response of the recipient cells to the donor antigens, the donor lymphocytes can be inactivated by irradiation. The test is not useful as a screening test for cadaver organ transplantation but retains usefulness in related bone-marrow transplantation.

The Immune Apparatus

The immune response to the histocompatibility antigens on the cells of transplanted organs triggers the rejection reaction. At birth, human beings are already immunologically competent and have undergone a complex developmental process. It is now agreed that there is a single pluripotent hemopoietic stem cell, found in the extraembryonic yolk sac. The daughter stem cells migrate to various centers for further differentiation.

Ontogeny of the Immune Response. The cellular components of the immune system are all derived from a *pluripotent bone marrow stem cell*, which produces at least 12 cell lineages, including B cells, T cells, natural killer (NK) cells, neutrophils, platelets, macrophages, eosinophils, basophils, erythrocytes, mast cells, glial cells, and dendritic cells (Fig. 10-4). Production of the lineages by the stem cell is under direct regulation by *cytokines*, including *colony-stimulating factors*, which induce differentiation and proliferation of bone marrow stem cell progeny. The pluripotent stem cell, however, itself never matures, and must therefore be regulated in a different fashion from the progenitor cells produced by it. The critical cytokines which influence lineage maturation at the early stages include *stem cell factor* (SCF), IL-3, GM-CSF (granulocyte-macrophage–colony-stimulating factor), IL-1, and erythropoietin. Clinical use of two of these factors (GM-CSF and erythropoietin) has had significant impact. The administration of GM-CSF to patients rendered neutropenic from chemotherapy and following bone marrow transplantation has markedly reduced the incidence of infection. Similarly, patients with anemia secondary to renal failure who receive erythropoietin rarely require transfusion. The potential application of these factors for treatment of organ disease states is promising.

The first immature cell lines to be established are the *lymphoid* and *myeloid* (see Fig. 10-4). The lymphoid progenitor cells migrate to the thymus (T cells) or bursal equivalent (B cells) to differentiate into mature T and B lymphocytes. The thymus and bone marrow are, therefore, considered *primary lymphoid organs*. The peripheral lymphoid tissues (spleen, peripheral lymph node and various tissues including skin) populated by the mature T and B lymphocytes are termed the *secondary lymphoid* tissues. Two major cell types of lymphoid lineage play a major role in transplant rejection: B lymphocytes and T lymphocytes. The B cells produce a *humoral* or *antibody* response to antigen, while T cells are responsible for cell-mediated functions of the immune system. Two main subsets of T-cells exist. CD8+ mature T cells mediate *effector functions* such as direct cytotoxic attack to produce graft rejection, while CD4+ T cells play an *immunoregulatory (helper)* role through secretion of cytokines which exert a paracrine effect to up- or down-regulate nearly all aspects of immune response.

Both the thymus and the bursa (or its equivalent) are responsible for the further development of the peripheral lymphoid tissues, i.e., spleen, lymph nodes, Peyer's patches. Certain areas of the lymph node are dependent on the functional presence of the thymus and the bursa (Figs. 10-5 and 10-6). The paracortical regions between the cortical germinal centers and the medulla are dependent on the thymus, while the germinal centers themselves and the medullary cord lymphoid tissue are under the developmental control of the bursal equivalent. Therefore, thymectomy early in the neonatal period or congenital thymic deficiency results in failure of development of the paracortical regions of the lymph nodes. In chickens, bursectomy leads to failure of development of germinal centers and medullary cord lymphoid tissues.

T lymphocytes are *the* specifically reactive cell in graft rejection. T cells represent the immunocompetent cell population responsible for the development of cellular rather than humoral immunity. T-cell responses include delayed hypersensitivity reactions, antiviral activity, and many of the early reactions responsible for allograft rejection.

The *B cells* descend from stem cells in the bone marrow and become responsible for the manufacture of circulating immunoglobulins and thus for humoral immunity (see Fig. 10-4). The B

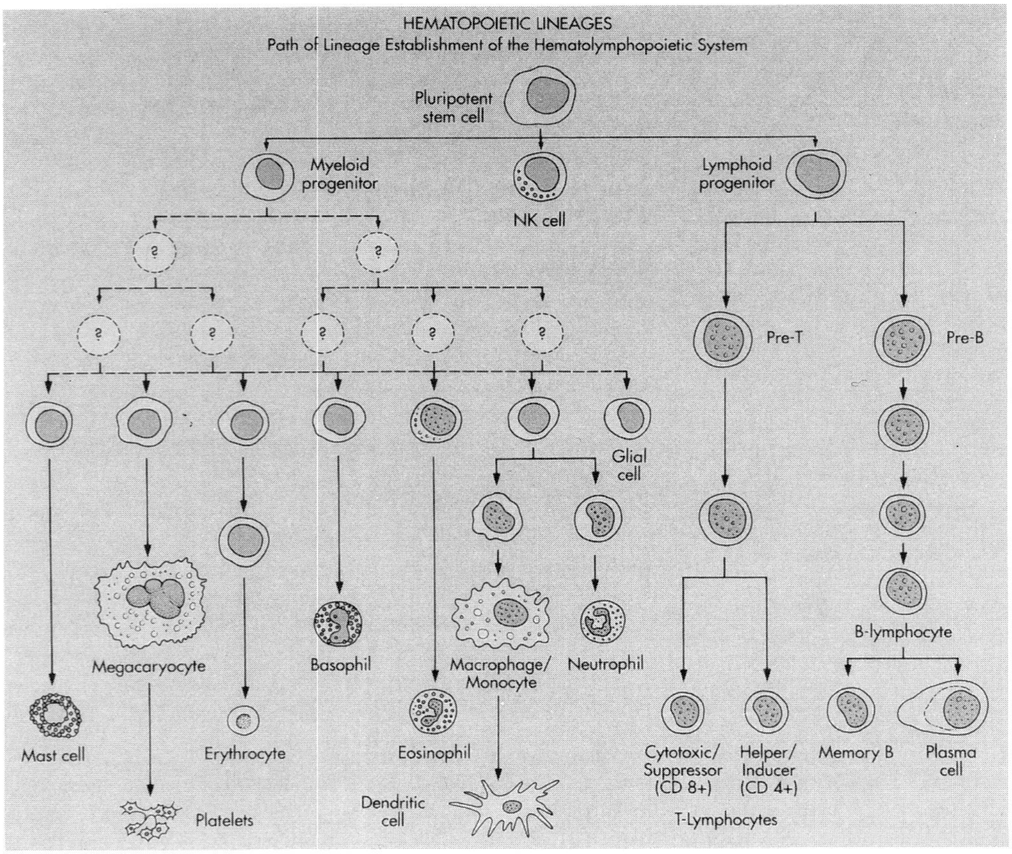

FIG. 10-4. Components of the immune system. A pluripotent bone marrow stem cell produces all components of the immune response, including megakaryocytes, red blood cells, lymphocytes, neutrophils, eosinophils, macrophages and other antigen-presenting cells, and glial cells of the brain. (From: *Starzl TE, Shapiro R, Simmons RL [eds]: Atlas of Organ Transplantation. New York, Gower Medical Publishing, 1992, p 1.3, with permission.*)

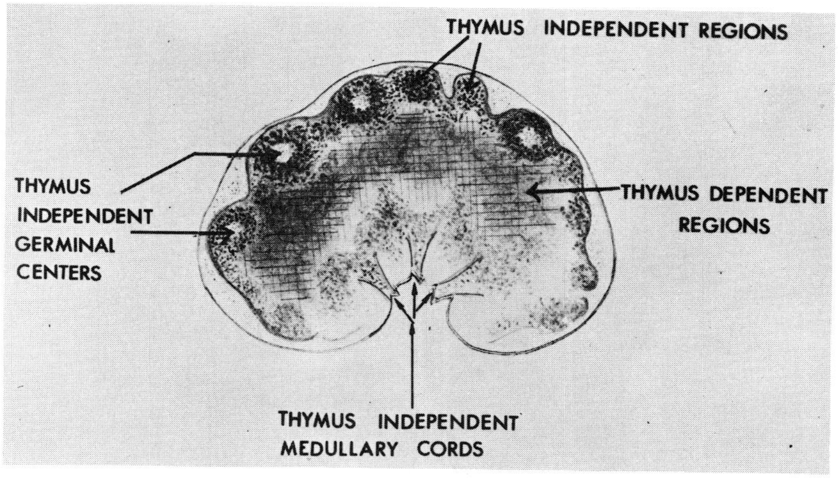

FIG. 10-5. The thymus-dependent and thymus-independent areas are illustrated in this schematic representation of a lymph node. (From: *Good RA, Finstad J: Structure and development of the immune system, in Najarian JS, Simmons RL [eds]: Transplantation. Philadelphia, Lea & Febiger, 1972, p 26, with permission.*)

cells appear to be relatively sessile, but their end products, immunoglobulin antibodies, can interact with foreign antigens at distant sites. The T cells responsible for cell-mediated immunity are of necessity more peripatetic and must migrate to the periphery in order to neutralize foreign antigens.

The lymphoid system is the seat of the body's immunologic response, and the small mature lymphocytes and the plasma cells are the immunocompetent cells. Once the lymphocytes (T or B cells) have migrated to the peripheral lymphoid tissue, they are fully immunocompetent. They exist in a resting state, ready to respond to any invading antigen to which they are specifically reactive. It is likely that Burnet's clonal selection theory holds true—i.e., a state of preparedness for a certain antigen or group of related antigens exists within a lymphoid cell so that it is only capable of responding to a narrow range of genetically determined antigenic specificities. For this reason only a small percentage of the lymphocytes in the body will respond to any one specific antigen.

Lymphocytes: The Specifically Reactive Cell in Rejection. Precursor T lymphocytes are produced by the pluripotent bone marrow stem cell through progenitors which differentiate into pre-T cells. The precursor T cells then migrate to the *thymus* and mature there through a series of genetically dictated events that result in acquisition of specific cell-surface receptors. All T lymphocytes express on their cell membrane a specific *T-cell receptor (TCR)*, which is the antigen binding site, and associated transmembrane proteins (CD3), which together constitute the *T-cell receptor complex*. Foreign antigens bind to the binding groove of the T-cell receptor and activate the immune response through transmembrane signaling via CD3 (Fig. 10-7).

The T-cell receptor complex is acquired in the thymus in a series of maturational steps. At the same time, immature T cells acquire *subset* or *differentiation* receptors called *cluster of differentiation (CD) antigens*, the best known of which are CD4 and CD8. With the recognition that CD antigens expressed on the cell surface denote specific function, a new nomenclature evolved which would allow general application of the same terminology to all species. T-lymphocyte cellular subsets are now designated by cellular function. The most frequently encountered CD antigens for each cellular type are listed in Table 10-2. These CD antigens determine function: the CD8+ *cytotoxic/suppressor* group lyses target cells and kills cells infected with virus and the CD4+ T cells serve an *immunoregulatory cell (helper/inducer)* role which medi-

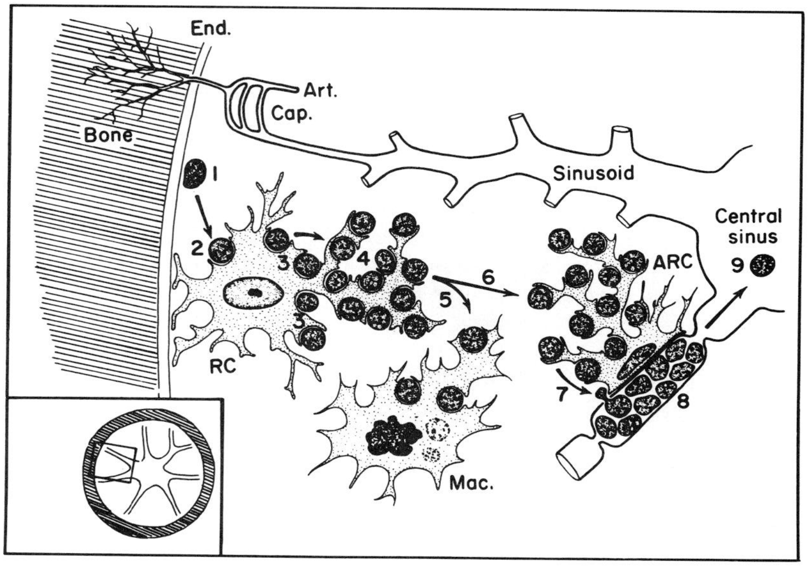

FIG. 10-6. The bone marrow is now believed to be the bursal equivalent in vertebrates lacking a bursa. Precursor B lymphocytes are believed to follow the numbered sequence while proliferating and differentiating. RC: reticular cell; ARC: adventitial reticular cell; Mac.: macrophage; End.: endosteum; Art.: artery; Cap.: capillary. (From: *Gallagher RB, Osmond DG: To B, or not to B: that is the question. Immunol Today 12:2, 1991, with permission.*)

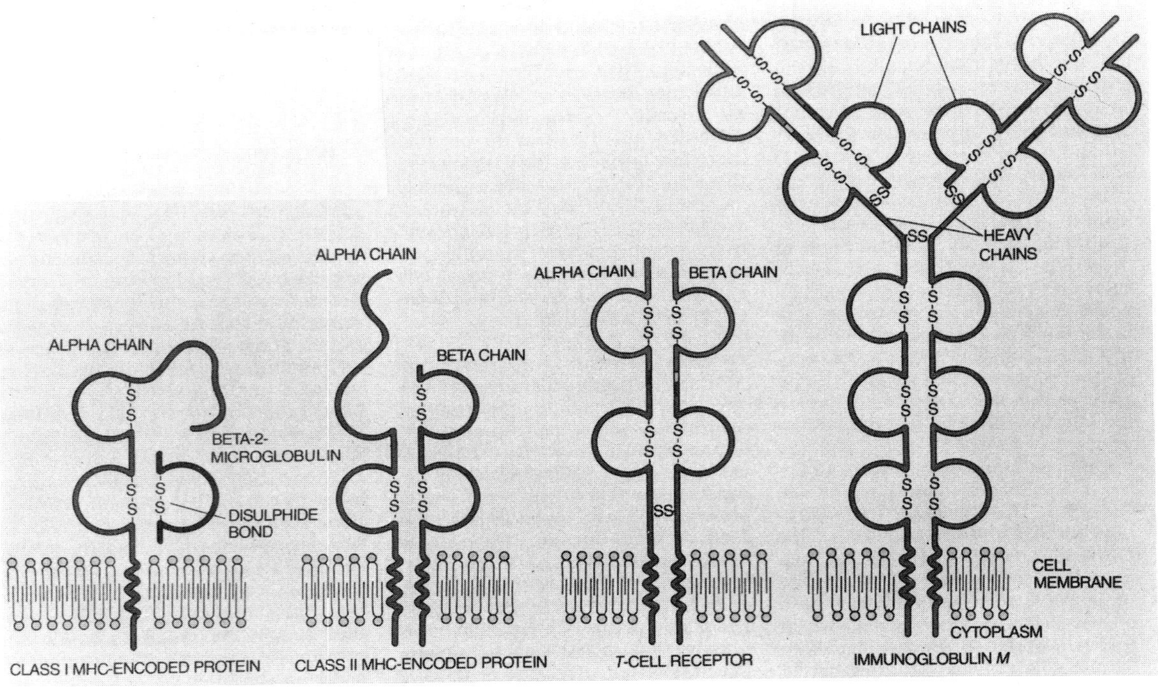

FIG. 10-7. Homology between HLA antigens and antigen binding molecules on the surfaces of lymphocytes. The molecular structures are similar and the molecules share similar amino acid sequences. (From: *Mannack P, Kappler J: The T cell and its receptor. Sci Am 254:36, 1986, with permission.*)

ates interactions of T cells, B cells, macrophages, and other cells through *cytokine* production. Functionally mature T lymphocytes then emerge from the thymus to populate the peripheral lymphoid tissues. Once mature, they cannot reenter the thymus.

T-Cell Receptor. The role of the immune system in maintaining health is critically dependent on recognition of foreign antigen by T-cell antigen receptors (TCR). These TCRs must be able to specifically recognize foreign antigen and yet be unreactive against *self antigens*. The ability to discriminate between self and nonself is learned within the thymus.

The T-cell receptor is a heterodimer composed of two polypeptide chains referred to as the alpha (α) and beta (β) chains which are linked by disulfide bonds (Fig. 10-8). δ-T cells are functionally distinct T cells that mature extrathymically. They tend to be concentrated in the skin and in mucosal tissues that interface directly with the outside world. In all T-cell receptors, each chain has a *variable region* that confers antigen specificity plus a *constant region*.

A great deal is known about the composition of T-cell receptor complex and how binding specificity is conferred. The T-cell receptor (TCR) is a cell surface complex consisting of a 90 kDa alpha-beta ($\alpha\beta$) heterodimer. It is associated with three invariant polypeptides collectively referred to as the T-cell receptor complex (CD3). This is remarkably constant for all species characterized.

Immunologic Events in Allograft Rejection

Induction of Immunity

Lymphocytes. Mature lymphocytes appear to sit in a state of immunologic readiness. Resting lymphocytes react to antigen that binds to its receptor by proliferation, differentiation, maturation, and the production of molecules (antibodies, protein markers on the cell surface, lymphokines) that can react with the antigen and recruit other mediators of the immune response. After proliferation some of these cells have a life span of many years so that a much larger pool of antigen-reactive cells (memory cells) remains. Such cells also may be capable of a more rapid response.

The Afferent Arc. The small lymphocyte that recognizes the immunogenic determinants must translate that recognition into an immunologic response. The first phase of the immunologic response has been called the afferent arc. It involves the grafting process itself, the release of the immunogenic histocompatibility antigens from the graft, the processing and recognition of the immunogens, and the stimulation of the responsive lymphoid cell population. After organ allografting, this process takes place both within the graft and in those lymphoid depots that receive antigenic stimuli.

The immunogens of a grafted organ, being surface components of the cell membrane, are readily available to the recipient's T lymphocytes that percolate through the transplanted organ. In order for the lymphocyte to become sensitized, however, an accessory *antigen-presenting cell* (APC) cell of the monocyte-macrophage lineage is necessary. In the case of protein antigens, the macrophage efficiently traps an antigen, processes it, and presents it in a form more easily recognized by the T-cell receptor. For this to occur, the responding lymphocyte and the macrophage must share identical Class II molecules on their cell surfaces. The Class II of the APC provides a *costimulatory* signal which is essential for the activation of the T lymphocyte as well as for IL-1 production by the macrophage. This is strong evidence for the importance of self-recognition of cooperating cells in the immune response.

The accessory cell has a second function as well, namely, to provide a second signal by means of a secreted cytokine molecule

Table 10-2
Representative Cell Surface Cluster of Differentiation (CD) Markers

CD Antigen	Ligand (target)	Distribution	Chromosome Number
T-Cell-Associated			
CD1	—	Thymocytes; dendritic cells	Ig22-g23
CD2 (CFA-2)	LFA-3	T cells; NK cells	—
CD3	—	T cells	11g23
CD4	Class II (MHC)	Helper T cells	12pter-p12
CD5	—	T cells; activated B cells	11g12-13
CD8	Class I (MHC)	T cells; NK cells	2p12
B-Cell-Associated			
CD20	—	B lineage cells	12g12-13
CD10	—	CALLA; pre-B cells; some mature B cells	3
CD19	—	B cells	12g12-13
CD76	—	Mature B cells; some T cells	12g12-13
Myeloid-Cell-Associated			
CD11a (LFA-1)	ICAM-1	Leukocytes	16p11-p13
CD11b	iC36 fibrinogen	Granulocytes; monocytes; NK cells; T cells	16p11-p13
CDw12	—	Myeloid cells (monocytes; granulocytes)	—
NK-Cell-Associated			
CD16a	Fc receptor	NK cells; granulocytes; some T cells	1
CD57	—	NK cells; some T cells	11
Activation-Associated Antigens			
CD58 (LFA-3)	CD2	All leukocytes (broadly expressed)	1
CD56	CD56	Isoform of N-CAM; NK cells; T cell subsets	11g23

SOURCE: Adapted from: Clark EA, Lanier LL. Report from Vienna: in search of all surface molecules expressed on human leukocytes. *J Clin Immunol* 9:266, 1989.

that enhances T-cell responses in its immediate vicinity. The most important cytokine in the activation of T-cell responses is called interleukin-1 (IL-1). Like all cytokines, interleukin-1 has many other functions, including mediating the production of fever and metabolic change during inflammatory responses.

Within the microenvironment of the immune cellular response, however, IL-1 has well-defined functions. In cooperation with antigen binding by the T cell, IL-1 fosters the appearance of receptors for a second lymphokine on the cell surface of the antigen-reactive T cell, namely, IL-2 receptors (IL-2R). Interleukin-2 (IL-2) is simultaneously secreted by antigen-responsive CD4+ helper T cells. Interaction of IL-2 with its receptor allows the cell to proliferate and mature (Fig. 10-9). IL-2R are not expressed on the surface of resting T cells. With T-cell activation as in the rejection response, however, they appear at the cell surface. The production of IL-2 by helper T cells exerts an *autocrine* feedback on the same cell and *paracrine* effect to activate other T cells in the local microenvironment, thus amplifying the immune response.

Cell-Cell Interactions. During graft rejection, antigen-responsive clones of lymphocytes do not act alone. They not only require accessory cells plus interleukin, they also interact with other lymphocytes. Extensive lymphocyte-lymphocyte interaction is needed for the development of maximum lymphocyte proliferative and cytotoxic activity. The cooperation occurs both between T and B cells and between defined subpopulations of T cells.

The requirement for cooperation between T and B cells was established by showing that neither cell population alone could mount an immune response to certain antigens, whereas mixtures of the two cell types resulted in the production of high levels of antibody. The CD4+ T-cell subset contains the ''helper'' T cells (T_H) that secrete cytokines soon after antigen stimulation. An-

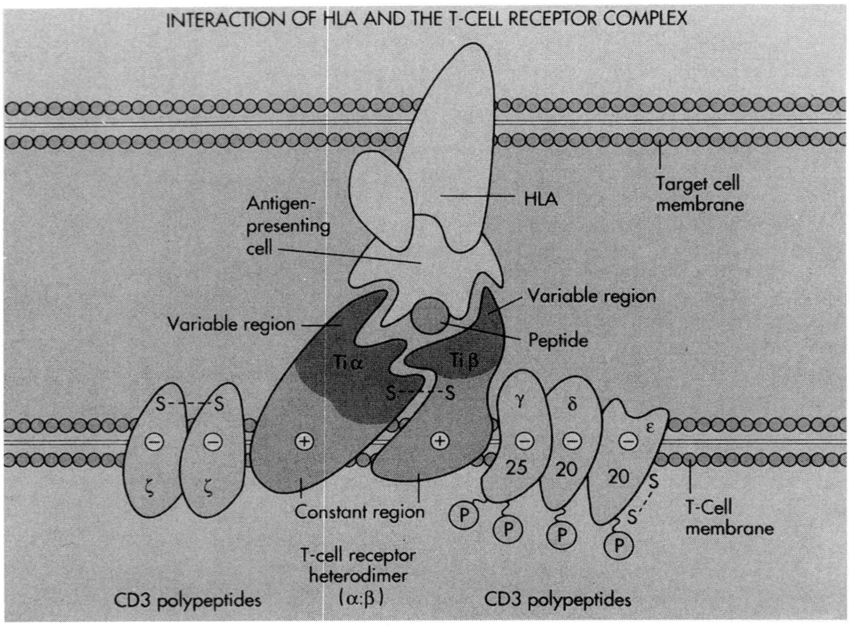

FIG. 10-8. The α and β polypeptide chains of the T-cell receptor form a heterodimer linked by a disulfide bond (S-S) and anchored in the T-cell membrane. The heterodimer recognizes and binds to peptide associated with an HLA molecule on the surface of a presenting cell. The nonpolymorphic CD3 polypeptides (designated γ, δ, ϵ, and ξ) are assembled together with the T-cell antigen receptor and are probably involved in signal transduction. P denotes phosphorylation site. (From: *Starzl TE, Shapiro R, Simmons RL [eds]: Atlas of Organ Transplantation. New York, Gower Medical Publishing, 1992, p 1.9, with permission.*)

tigen-stimulated B cells require T-helper cytokines in order to proliferate, mature, and produce antibody. Just as T_H cytokines are necessary for B-cell antibody response, these cytokines are needed for the development of lymphocyte-mediated cytotoxicity by cytotoxic CD8+ T cells. Once mature, these CD8+ cells recognize antigen in the donor cells, and kill them directly. Thus, graft destruction can be accomplished either by antibody from B cells or by direct cytotoxicity by cytotoxic T cells. The maturation of both

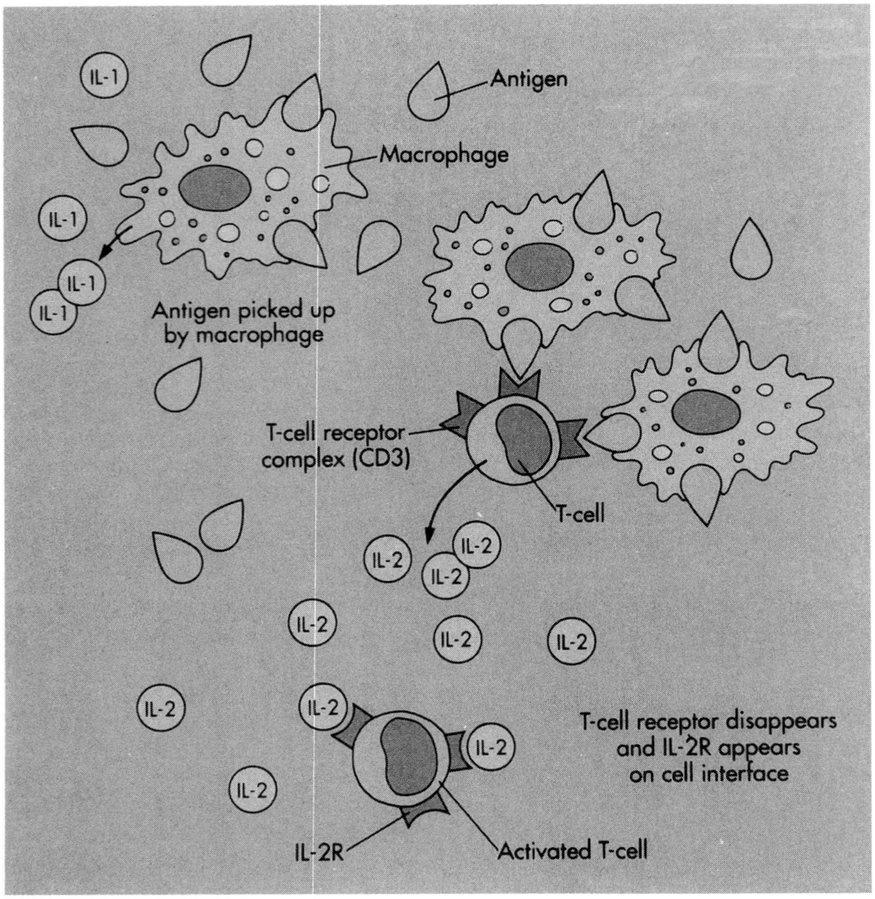

FIG. 10-9. Steps in T-cell activation. T-cell activation occurs through the T-cell receptor complex, IL-2, and the IL-2 receptor (IL-2R). Resting T cells express CD3 but not the IL-2 receptor. When T-cell receptors are stimulated by antigen (Ag) plus MHC gene products, they manufacture IL-2 receptors (IL-2R), which appear at the cell surface. Simultaneously, IL-2 secreted by these cells binds to the new IL-2R to stimulate proliferation and differentiation. At the same time, macrophages (M) which present antigen to the T cell are stimulated to produce IL-1. When the antigenic stimulus is no longer present, the number of IL-2R decreases and the T-cell CD3 receptor complex is again reexpressed on the cell surface. In this way, a feedback control mechanism is maintained. (From: *Starzl TE, Shapiro R, Simmons RL [eds]: Atlas of Organ Transplantation. New York, Gower Medical Publishing, 1992, p 1.8, with permission.*)

effector cell populations requires antigen-presenting cells and T_H cells.

There is evidence that yet another T-cell subgroup can inhibit either the development of antibody-producing B cells or the generation of T_H cells. These regulatory lymphocytes have been called suppressor T (T_S) cells. They are also believed to reside among the CD8+ subset of T lymphocytes.

The elucidation of these interactions has occupied many cellular immunologists during the past 20 years. Convincing experimental demonstration of lymphocyte-lymphocyte interaction required the various cells to be identified and separated from the bulk populations of lymphocytes in vitro. This was facilitated by the discovery of distinct antigenic proteins on the surfaces of the various subsets of lymphocytes. Antibodies to these surface marker proteins could then be used to deplete or enrich the bulk populations of a specific cell type and thereby clarify the function of each cell type. Table 10-2 lists some of the functional lymphocyte subtypes, the markers they possess, and their *ligands* (what they bind to).

Once the lymphocyte subpopulations were identified, the mechanisms of their interaction could be elucidated. Most interactions seem to involve the manufacture and release of soluble substances (*cytokines*) by stimulated cells that trigger responder cells that bear receptors for these cytokines. Table 10-3 lists some of the cytokines that have been studied and their putative function.

The most powerful of the cytokines secreted by activated T_H cells is called interleukin-2. CD8+ cytotoxic T cells cannot secrete interleukin-2, but they require it to proliferate and mature. The interaction of the antigen-responsive T_H cell with the antigen plus interleukin-1 permits it to secrete interleukin-2, which acts on both helper and cytotoxic T cells to permit expansion of the antigen-sensitive clones. A second set of cytokines that act on antigen-stimulated B cells is necessary for B-cell expansion (see Table 10-3).

Most evidence supports the idea that B lymphoid differentiation to antibody-producing cells is accompanied by cellular proliferation. When the B cell proliferates, morphologic differentiation accompanies the proliferation, and the result is a plasma cell busily engaged in making specific antibody. Conversion from a transformed cell to a plasma cell is seen within a few days of grafting, in both organ allografts and the lymphoid tissue stimulated by these transplants.

The situation for T cells responding to Class I and Class II alloantigens during allograft rejection has proved to be a fascinat-

Table 10-3
Biologic Activities of Some Cytokines

Cytokine	*Secreting Cells*	*Activities*
Interleukin-1	Monocytic cells; T & B cells; NK cells; fibroblasts; endothelial cells; neutrophils; smooth muscle cells	Proliferation of T & B cells; endothelial cell activation; fever, inflammation; increases liver protein synthesis
Interleukin-2	Activated T cells	T-cell growth factor; cytotoxic T-cell generation; B-cell proliferation/differentiation; growth of NK & LAK cells
Interleukin-4	T cells; mast cells; bone marrow stromal cells	B-cell activation/differentiation; T & mast cell growth factor
Interleukin-6	Activated T cells; macrophages; fibroblasts; endothelial cells	B-cell proliferation/differentiation; T-cell activation; fever, inflammation; increases liver acute phase protein synthesis
Interleukin-8	Monocytes; fibroblasts; endothelial cells; synoviocytes; keratinocytes; chondrocytes; antigen-activated T cells	Neutrophil migration & degranulation; T & basophil chemotactic protective effect from neutrophil-mediated damage
Interleukin-10 (CSIF)	T helper 2 cells	Suppress cytokine production by Th1 cells; growth costimulator for thymocytes; suppress antigen presentation by macrophages; growth costimulator for mast cells; B cell viability enhancement; thymocyte costimulator
Granulocyte-macrophage-CSF (GM-CSF)	Activated T cells; macrophages; fibroblasts; thymic epithelium; endothelial cells	Promotes neutrophils, eosinophil, & macrophage bone marrow colonies; activates mature granulocytes; promotes growth and differentiation of bone marrow progenitors
Granulocyte-CSF (G-CSF)	Macrophages; endothelial cells; fibroblasts; T cells	Promotes neutrophil lineage maturation; chemoattractant for monocytes and endothelial cells
Interferon gamma (IFNγ)	T cells NK cells	Induces Class II (DR) expression; activates macrophages and endothelial cells; augments or inhibits other lymphokine activities; augments NK activity; potent antiviral activity
Interferon alpha,beta (IFNα,β)	T & B cells; fibroblasts; macrophages; endothelial & epithelial cells	Inhibits cell growth; exerts antiviral activity; induces Class I & Class II antigen expression; augments NK activity; has fever-inducing & antiproliferative properties; increases CTL generation; inhibits tumor cell growth
Tumor necrosis factor alpha,beta (TNFα,β)	T cells; macrophages; NK cells	Major inflammatory mediator; tumoricidal activity; B-cell growth/differentiation; procoagulant activity; inhibition of lipoprotein lipase; enhances T-cell function; macrophage & neutrophil activation; fever

ing variation on the standard immunologic response. Class II alloantigens stimulate CD4+ T_H cells preferentially and Class I alloantigens stimulate CD8+ cytotoxic T cells preferentially. After proliferation under the influence of interleukin-2 from helper cells responding to Class II antigens, T cytotoxic cells mature into cells that interact with cells bearing Class I antigens. Such an interaction leads to donor cell death. The CD4+ and CD8+ T-cell precursors respond to different alloantigens within the closely linked HLA complex, and different T-cell types appear to accomplish differentiation and proliferation. Differentiation requires proliferation, but quite unexpectedly they occur in different cells.

Expression of Immunity: Graft Destruction

Specifically sensitized cytotoxic T cells are present within most rejecting allografts and are capable of inflicting damage. Alloantigenically stimulated T_H cells are there as well, and can secrete cytokines (see Table 10-3) capable of mediating delayed hypersensitivity reactions. But specifically sensitized cells are in the minority, and it is likely that a small number of specifically sensitized lymphoid cells initiate a rejection reaction but that the completion of reaction also requires many nonsensitized cells recruited by cytokines that amplify the immune response. Polymorphonuclear leukocytes (PMNs), eosinophils, plasma cells, and unsensitized mononuclear cells are all part of the rejection process. Of course, antibody can initiate graft destruction in the relative absence of a cellular reaction under appropriate circumstances.

In Vitro Lysis of Target Cells by Cytotoxic Lymphocytes. The specifically sensitized lymphoid cells that collect at the site of an allograft have long been known to damage the donor tissues directly in the absence of humoral antibody or complement. Direct contact between the sensitized lymphocyte and the target cell appears to be important. Reports have begun to characterize the model for delivery of a lethal hit by cytotoxic T lymphocyte (Fig. 10-10). Large granules are present in the cytoplasm of activated *cytotoxic T lymphocytes* and *NK cells*. While granule-independent killing can occur, most cytotoxic T-cell activity is believed to be due to *granule exocytosis*. *Perforin* and serine esterases are located within the granule substructures. *Perforin* is a pore-forming protein (70 kDa) which is homologous in part to the complement component C9. When the cytotoxic T cell binds to the antigen on the target cell membrane, perforin undergoes a conformational change which enables it to insert into the lipid bilayer and polymerize to form tubular transmembrane pores. The final result is a unidirectional granule exocytosis with destruction of target cell.

Cytokines: Effector Molecules Released by Activated Lymphocytes. The release of cytotoxic factors by lymphocytes infiltrating an allograft would be the most direct way to damage foreign cells, but probably not the most efficient. Specifically sensitized T cells release a number of cytokines that serve to activate and enlist macrophages, polymorphonuclear leukocytes (PMNs), lymphocytes, etc., so that the initial cellular response is amplified (see Table 10-3). In effect, cytokines are a way for the cellular components of the immune response to communicate with each other. They primarily act in an *autocrine* fashion to affect the same cell type that produced them, or work in a *paracrine* fashion to stimulate cells of other types in the local vicinity. They rarely exert a systemic (*endocrine*) effect except in disease states and are usually not detectable in serum.

Cytokines play a critical role in rejection of transplanted tissue. The response of a cell to a given cytokine is influenced by the local concentration of the cytokine, the cell type, and other cytokines to which it has been exposed. Binding of the cytokine to a cell surface receptor results in transmembrane signal transduction, which results in increased cellular RNA and protein synthesis, and ultimately altered cell behavior. Cytokines function in a number of ways to (1) induce each other, (2) modulate cell surface receptors, and (3) modify the immune response by additive or antagonistic interactions on cell function. All cytokines have more than one effect and may be stimulatory for some cell types yet inhibitory for

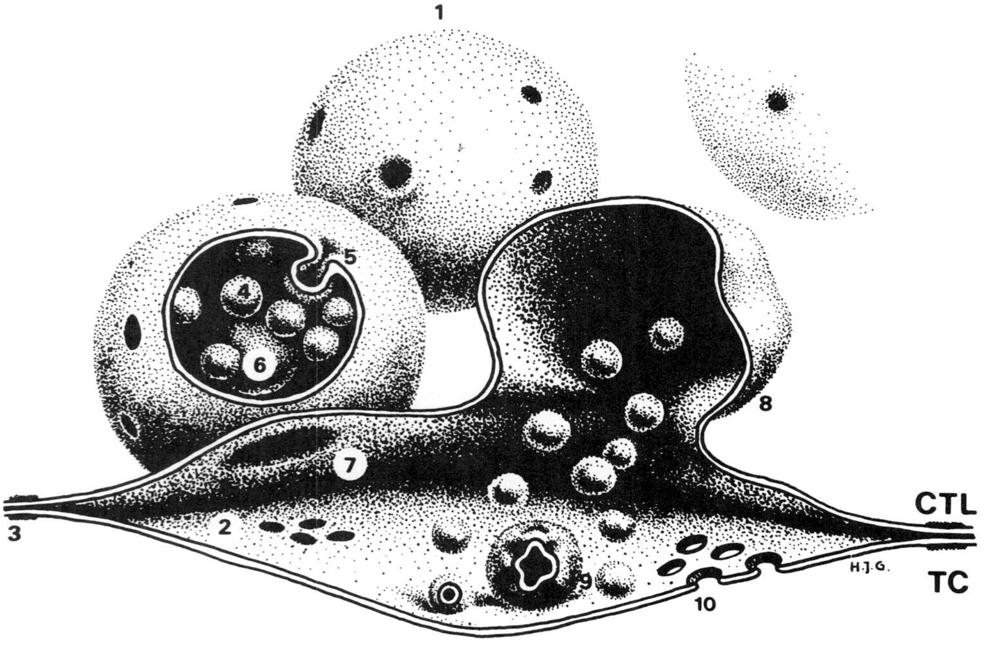

FIG. 10-10. Three-dimensional illustration of lethal hit delivery. The upper part of the drawing represents the CTL (cytotoxic T lymphocyte) and shows the cytotoxic granules (1) and the plasma membrane area lining the intercellular cleft (2) between CTL and TC (target cell). This cleft is bordered by special membrane interactions (3). One opened granule is shown to contain internal vesicles (4), which form by budding from the granule outer membrane (5) and a dense core (6). This granule is in the process of fusing with the CTL plasma membrane (7). Another granule (8) has already done so and has released its contents into the cleft. The vesicles and dense core interact (9) with the TC membrane, which, as a result of perforin action, contains pores (10). (From: *Peters PJ, Geuze HJ, van der Donk HA, Borst J: A new model for lethal hit delivery by cytotoxic T lymphocytes. Immunol Today 11:30, 1990, with permission.*)

others. Each cytokine generally reacts specifically with its own *receptor*, which means that diversity of cytokines is paralleled by receptor diversity.

Cytokines: The Soluble Immune Cell Regulators. *Interleukins* or *cytokines* are a group of soluble hormonelike glycoproteins that function as immune cell regulators. They play a pivotal role in the immune response, are participants in a number of disease processes, and have been used therapeutically. They were previously named based on the cell of origin. *Lymphokines* are produced by lymphocytes and *monokines* by macrophages. At the present time, newly discovered cytokines are called *interleukins*. All cytokines exert more than one effect and may be inhibitory for some cells and stimulatory for others. Although they are small glycoproteins (< 80 kDa), they are very potent, generally acting at picomolar concentrations. They bind to specific cell surface receptors to exert their influence (see Table 10-3). Most cytokines are not secreted constitutively but instead are produced in response to various stimuli. The induction of cytokine secretion by lymphocytes may require antigen stimulation, but secretion of macrophage-derived cytokines (IL-1, IL-6, TNFα) is dependent on other stimuli such as endotoxin virus or other cytokines. In vivo, cytokines do not act alone but in combination with other cytokines and stimuli.

Because of the profound biologic effects of these hormonelike glycoproteins and their potency, it is not surprising that their activities are tightly regulated. Regulation of cytokine secretion occurs at the following levels: (1) regulation of *cytokine secretion itself*; (2) regulation of *cytokine receptor expression*; (3) cross-regulation of the activity of *one cytokine by other cytokines*; and (4) regulation by *soluble cytokine-binding factors* and/or inhibitors.

Macrophages are very active participants in graft rejection; their role does not end with antigen processing. They are highly secretory cells. The best known product is IL-1, which is pivotal to lymphocyte activation.

Interleukin-1. Interleukin-1 (IL-1) is produced by activated macrophages as well as T and B lymphocytes, NK cells, skin keratinocytes, brain astrocytes, epithelial cells, and vascular endothelial cells. Production of IL-1 by APC requires, for the most part, binding of T_H cells to the antigen/MHC complex on the APC. The IL-1 produced, in turn, acts in an autocrine fashion to stimulate the APCs and as an activation factor for T cells. The effects of IL-1 are broad, including fever, the release of hepatic acute-phase proteins, the release of neutrophils, ACTH, cortisol, and insulin. Effects on endothelial cells result in increased leukocyte adherence, prostaglandin release, and hypotension. IL-1 is cytotoxic for tumor cells and insulin-producing beta cells.

Tumor Necrosis Factor (TNF). Tumor necrosis factor shares many of the acute-phase response properties with IL-1. It is produced by activated macrophages but appears to have no direct effect on lymphocyte activation. It acts synergistically with IL-1 to mediate a variety of acute-phase changes including tumor necrosis, hypotension, and inflammatory reactions. The vascular endothelium and several endocrine organs are the primary targets for TNF.

Other cytokines function to activate the macrophage. Macrophages resemble lymphocytes in that they have resting and activated states. In the latter phase, the cytoplasm has the appearance of great activity, both morphologically and enzymatically. Phagocytosis, pinocytosis, and bacteriostatic and tumoricidal activities are increased. The levels of many intracellular enzymes, including the digestive enzymes found in lysosomes, are markedly elevated. Macrophages found at the site of graft rejection appear to be in the activated state and thus better able to participate in tissue destruction.

Role of Antibody in Allograft Rejection. Circulating antibody is not an obligatory participant in the rejection of solid tissue allografts. In fact, the inability to make immunoglobulin does not preclude graft rejection. There is now no doubt, however, that rejection can be mediated by alloantibodies—especially the rejection of vascularized organ allografts.

Humoral antibody provides only the recognition portion of graft rejection. Unlike cell-mediated immunity, where the recognition system is intimately associated with the destruction of the target, humoral antibody must activate other systems in order to effect cell death.

Although antibodies bind to allografts, such binding is of no consequence by itself, and the antibody would probably be cleared during the course of normal cell membrane repair. The combination of antibody with the antigen produces an active complex, which triggers a number of nonspecific effector pathways (Fig. 10-11). Each effector pathway typically consists of a sequential activation of enzymes that attract and hold active cells, produce vascular permeability, release enzymes capable of degrading cell surfaces and other proteins, release factors causing smooth muscle contraction, and precipitate the formation of fibrin clots.

The immunologic response, therefore, has evolved as both efficient and discriminatory. Relatively few specifically differentiated cells can produce molecules that will perform the recognition function. Since few cells are committed to each antigen, many more antigens can be discriminated. The antibodies in turn initiate a relatively general effector mechanism that can destroy the graft.

The Complement System. The most important of the several effector molecular cascade systems triggered by antigen binding by antibody is the complement system. The combination of antibody (of IgG_1, IgG_2, IgG_3, or IgM classes) with antigen changes the conformation of the antibody molecule. Included in this change is the activation of a site on the constant (Fc) end of the antibody molecule, which then triggers the complement pathway. The alternate (properdin) pathway can be set off by the immunologically nonspecific serum proteins of the properdin system reacting with sugar structures found on bacterial surfaces and conceivably mammalian cells; its role in graft rejection, however, is unknown. The components of both pathways are circulating protein molecules that, when activated, react in a sequential fashion. At present, the system is known to be made up of a number of distinct molecules that are capable of interacting with one another, with antibody, and with cell membranes. Once activated they can act enzymatically on the next molecule in the sequence, which serves as the inactive substrate. Components C6 and C9 are nonenzymatic and bind to the previous components, resulting in conformational and activity changes.

Most of the biologically significant activities of the complement system arise during activation of the last six reacting complement components, C3 and C5 through C9 (Fig. 10-12). The two parallel but entirely independent initial pathways—the classic and the alternate pathways—both lead to activation of the terminal, biologically important portion of the sequence, involving the reactions of C5 through C9. The terminal portion of the complement

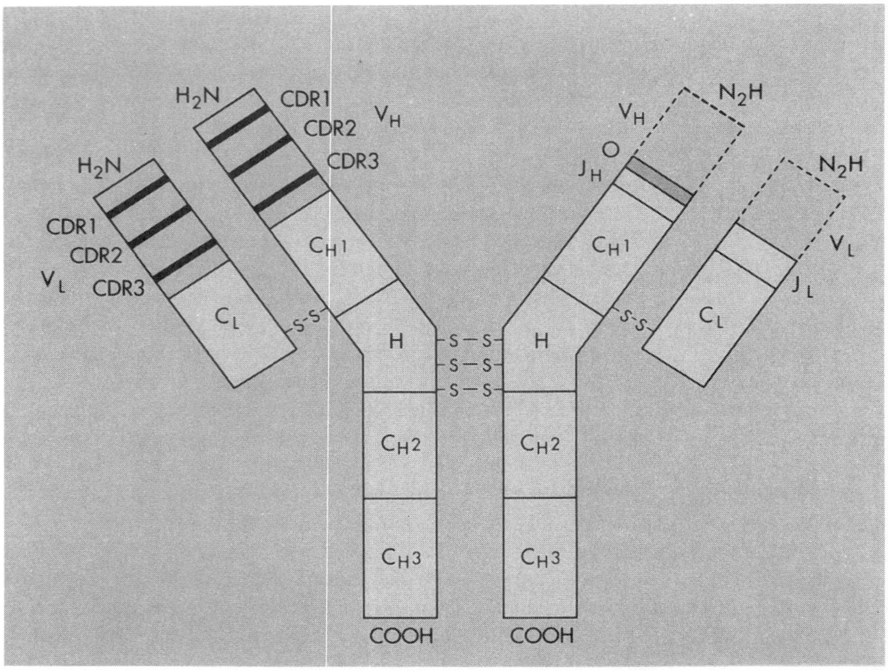

FIG. 10-11. Typical subunit of an Ig molecule, composed of two identical heavy chains and two identical light chains linked by disulfide bridges. Variable regions are indicated on the right subunit; CDR (complementarity-determining region) sequences are indicated on the left subunit. CH_{1-3} refer to heavy chain constant regions; C_L denotes constant region, light chain; V_L variable region, light chain; V_H variable region, heavy chain; H, hinge region. (From: *Starzl TE, Shapiro R, Simmons RL [eds]: Atlas of Organ Transplantation. New York, Gower Medical Publishing, 1992, p 1.14, with permission.*)

sequence may also be directly activated by certain noncomplement serum and cellular enzymes without participation of the early reaction factors. For example, fibrinolytic enzymes in plasma and certain lysosomal enzymes will activate the C3 and C5 stages.

The classic complement pathway (see Fig. 10-12) appears to be the most important for immune reactions. Three biologic consequences of complement activation are most important in transplantation rejection.

1. Complement has been shown to be capable of mediating lytic destruction of many kinds of cells to which antibodies have bound. The active components are in the C8 and C9 complexes, but the mechanism of lysis is not clear; perhaps enzymatic activity of the complex damages the membrane directly.
2. Many kinds of cells possess receptors for the C3b or C4b (activated) components, including B lymphocytes, neutrophils, monocytes, and macrophages. If C3b or C4b attach to a damaged cell they may act as opsonins, bringing the target cells in contact with the phagocytic macrophages and monocytes or exposing the surface antigens of these cells to B lymphocytes.
3. Many of the complement cleavage products have biologic actions of their own. For example, C4a and C2b act as kinins. C3a has chemotactic activity for polymorphonuclear leukocytes, causes the release of histamine from mast cells (anaphylatoxin activity), has a kinin activity, and causes immune adherence. C5a is a very potent chemotactic factor, stimulates histamine release from mast cells, and attracts neutrophils and liberates lysosomes from them.

Therefore, complement activation releases kinins that increase vascular permeability, leading to edema; attracts polymorphonuclear leukocytes that release other vasoactive compounds and lysosomal enzymes; encourages phagocytosis of damaged tissue; releases lysosomal enzymes from macrophages; opsonizes cells; binds cells to damaged cell surfaces (immune adherence); and leads to cell death.

An important biologic characteristic of the complement system as well as the other cascade systems discussed in this section is that they are capable of self-amplification. Thus, in one study 450 C4 molecules were found fixed to each sensitized sheep red blood cell, but each erythrocyte had approximately 100,000 C3 components on its surface. In addition, the C3 components were distributed over the cell membrane surface, rather than confined to the site of the antigen-antibody combination, thus enlarging the area of effect. Although this step produces the greatest numerical amplification, other steps in the complement pathway also expand the number of active molecules.

The Clotting System. Theoretically the deposition of fibrin in the allografted organ may arise in two ways. The first, the so-called *extrinsic pathway* of thrombin formation, requires tissue thromboplastin to initiate the sequence of events. The release of this cellular substance may follow damage to the endothelial cell membranes either by antibody and complement or through the direct cytotoxic effect of lymphocytes. The activation of complement through C3 would also promote the adherence of platelets, which, in turn, would stimulate platelet retraction and release of platelet phospholipids. These phospholipids have been shown to promote clotting.

The second method of inducing clot formation, the *intrinsic pathway*, has the potential to be activated directly by immunologic reaction. In the intrinsic pathway, Hageman factor (factor XII) begins a sequence that proceeds through factors XI, IX, VII, and V to the activation of prothrombin factor to form thrombin with the eventual polymerization of fibrin. Antigen-antibody complexes will activate Hageman factor to trigger this cascade and produce clotting in vitro in the absence of platelets. Thus, an entry into the intrinsic pathway is present within the interactions of antigens and antibodies (Fig. 10-13).

As the reaction proceeds and tissue damage is produced, tissue thromboplastin is released, collagen fibers are exposed, and clotting is facilitated. It is now generally hypothesized that the pro-

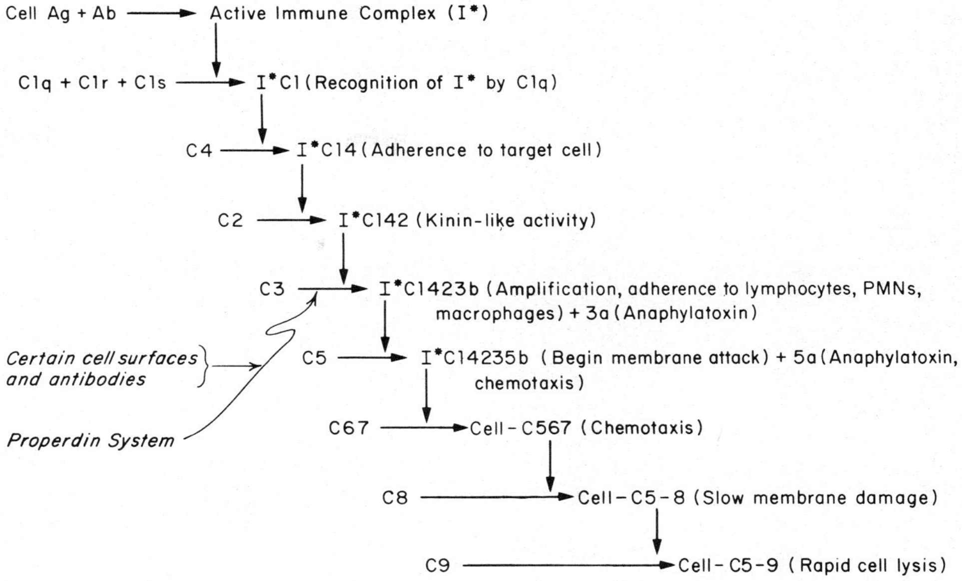

FIG. 10-12. The complement pathways and the biologic activity released at each step. The classic pathway begins with a specific antigen-antibody reaction. The properdin pathway is triggered by a more nonspecific interaction between cell surfaces and the molecules that make up the properdin systems. Both pathways, however, converge at the C3 step, where most of the biologic activity associated with complement activation begins. Amplification also occurs at several steps, but it is greatest at C3. The subsequent steps lead to the molecular condensation on the target cell surface, which ultimately results in membrane damage and lysis. There are several other important consequences of complement activation. The presence of these molecules on the target cell surface makes them adherent to other cells. Macrophages, platelets, polymorphonuclear leukocytes, and lymphocytes adhere and increase the damage to the graft cells. The steps through C5 are largely enzymatic in nature; the C3 and C5 components, for example, are split during activation, releasing chemotactic and vasoactive (anaphylatoxin) molecules. Attachment of the C5b molecule to the cell begins the condensation ending in membrane damage; this seems to occur away from the immune complex. Interaction of the C6,C7 components results, additionally, in the release of another chemotactic factor. The activation of the complement pathway, therefore, contributes to many of the features seen in allograft rejection—cellular infiltrates, adherent PMNs and platelets, thrombosed vessels, interstitial edema, and cellular damage.

FIG. 10-13. The coagulation cascade system. Fibrin and two vasoactive peptides are the final products of the cascade. The two modes of activation of the system are diagramed. Factor XII (Hageman factor) can be activated by immune complexes initiating the intrinsic pathway. Tissue damage (presumably produced by immunologic damage) could precipitate the extrinsic system. In both systems, the factors shown, with the probable exceptions of V and VIII, are enzymes. Activation of the pathways involves the sequential conversions of these enzymes to active forms (represented by XII*a*, XI*a*, etc.). (From: *Najarian JS, Foker JE: Allograft rejection: II. The expression of immunity: the efferent arc, in Najarian JS, Simmons RL [eds]: Transplantation. Philadelphia, Lea & Febiger, 1972, p 94, with permission.*)

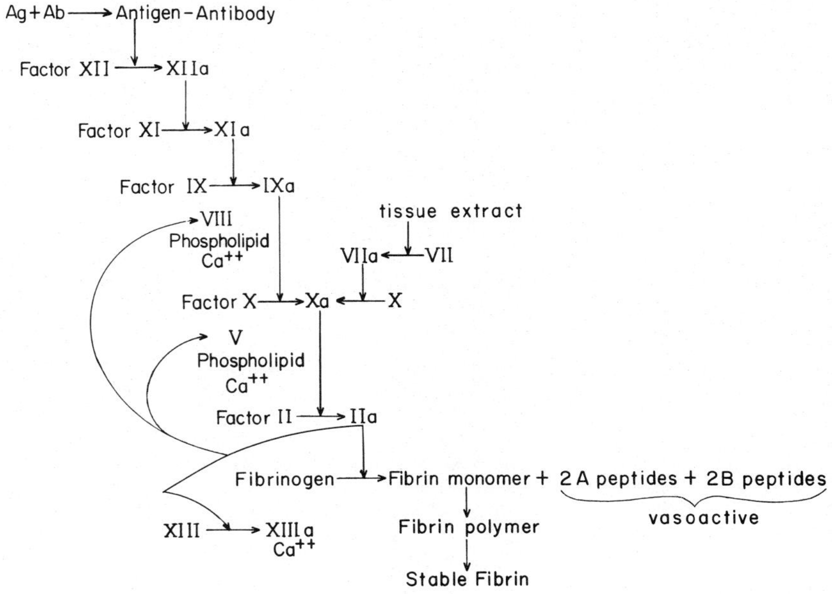

gressive obliterative vascular reaction of a chronically rejecting allograft is a by-product of fibrin laid down along endothelium that has been damaged by immune mechanisms.

The Kinin System. The kinin, or kallikrein, system is initiated by activation of coagulation factor XII, leading eventually to the formation of kallikrein, which acts on kininogen, an α-globulin substrate in the plasma, and results in bradykinin. Bradykinin is one of the kinins, a group of active peptides that are rather rapidly inactivated, after formation, by kininases present in plasma. The kinins possess a variety of biologic activities, including chemotaxis of PMNs, smooth muscle contraction, dilatation of peripheral arterioles, and increase of capillary permeability. The involvement of the kinin system in graft rejection is likely but is as yet unproved.

Interrelationships of the Molecular Cascade Systems (Fig. 10-14). Antigen-antibody complexes activate complement and Hageman factor. Hageman factor in turn produces clotting, activates plasmin, and perhaps directly activates complement. Plasmin in turn can activate C3 to produce, among other effects, chemotactic factors, immune adherence, and opsonization. Activation of Hageman factor also leads to kinin production. Activation of the complement system produces aggregation of platelets and, consequently, initiation of the clotting mechanism. Thrombin formation, in turn, stimulates the production of plasmin from plasminogen. Prostaglandin activity is released following complement activation, and may contribute to vascular permeability, although the significance of this in allograft rejection remains unclear.

Not only are the activators of these systems interrelated, but also the inhibitors are intertwined. The C1 esterase inhibitor also decreases the activity of the kinin and plasmin systems. Neither activation nor inhibition of one system can occur without affecting the other pathways.

The complexity of the allograft reaction is just beginning to be understood. Not only does it involve a variety of recognition molecules (antibodies) and presumably a similar variety of specifically sensitized cells; there is much recent evidence that unsensitized

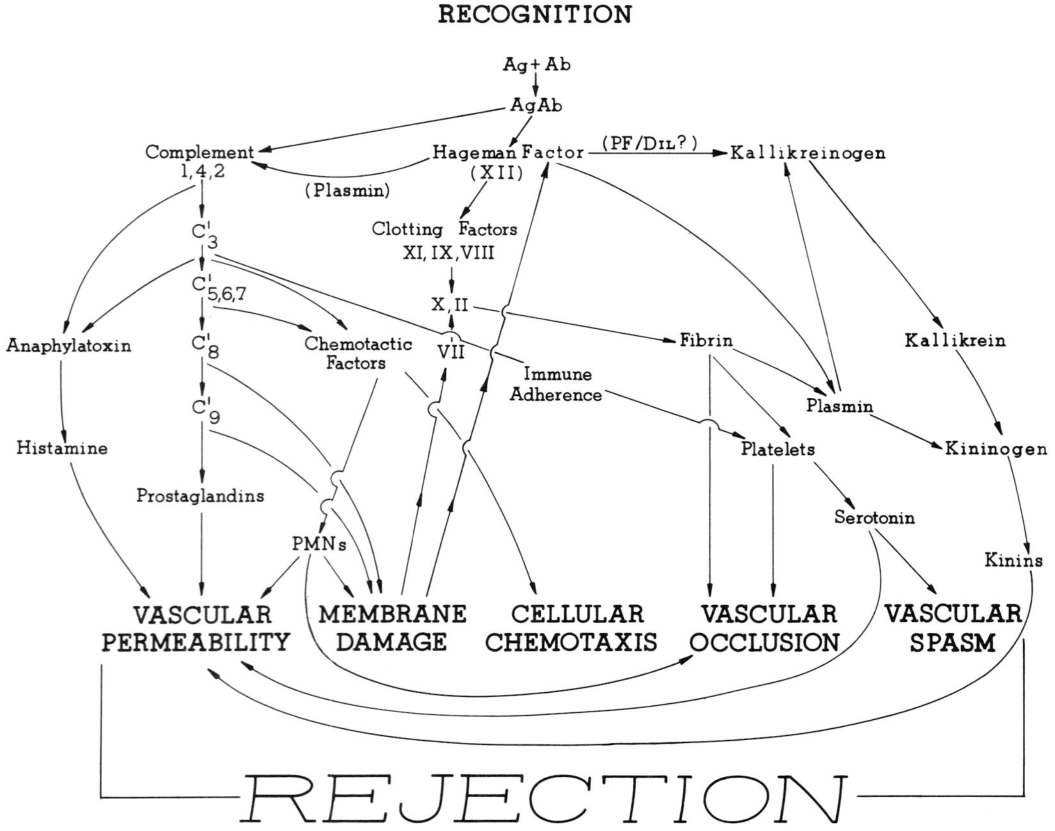

FIG. 10-14. Integration of the humoral amplification system in graft rejection. This diagram suggests the complexity of allograft rejection. The three main cascade pathways—complement, clotting, and kinin—generate many active molecules, including the kinins, chemotactic factors, anaphylatoxins, histamine, and serotonin. These molecules, together with platelets and polymorphonuclear leukocytes (PMNs), produce the destructive effects on the graft. The most prominent consequences include increased vascular permeability (edema), spasm, and occlusion, as well as cell and basement membrane damage and cellular chemotaxis (infiltration). It is clear that these systems do not operate singly but tend to activate each other. Not shown are the many interlocking inhibitory factors that keep these systems in check once they are activated. (From: *Najarian JS, Foker JE: Allograft rejection: II. The expression of immunity: the efferent arc, in Najarian JS, Simmons RL [eds]: Transplantation. Philadelphia, Lea & Febiger, 1972, p 94, with permission.*)

lymphocytes can be specifically directed and actively lyse target allogenic cells by a coating with antibody. In addition, the main force of the reaction may be produced by a bewildering array of amplifying chain reactions that include both molecular amplification schemes and cellular amplifiers. The activation of complement, the clotting system, kinin formation, and the stimulation of PMN, macrophages, and platelet assault produce a variety of damage to the transplanted organ. Included are occlusive phenomena within the graft vessels, induced permeability of these same vessels with interstitial edema accumulation, disruption of cellular basement membranes, and the infiltration of the graft with a profusion of cell types (see Fig. 10-14).

An Integrated View of the Rejection of Organ Allografts. Rejection morphology has two main components: The first component is the host response, and it is composed of effector cells and molecules, both immunologically specific and nonspecific. In rapid rejections these constitute most, if not all, of the pathologic picture, so that the speed of the reaction virtually precludes response by the organ cells. The second component becomes prominent only with longer survival of the transplanted organ and encompasses morphologic alterations peculiar to the injured organ.

A predictable series of events ensues when an unsensitized patient is allografted. The first visible change is a perivascular infiltration of round cells (Fig. 10-15). The accumulation of cells is not significant for several hours after transplantation but can reach considerable numbers within 48 h. The original enclaves around small vessels spread, and the interstitial space is further infiltrated. A potpourri of cells accumulates: cells resembling small lymphocytes are seen, as well as large transformed lymphocytes with basophilic cytoplasm. Large histiocytes or macrophages are just beginning to arrive in numbers. Plasma cells are still relatively scarce; as a terminal product of cellular differentiation, they may require several cell divisions before they appear in the organ (Fig. 10-16).

Antibody and complement are deposited in the area of the capillaries, and some of the infiltrating lymphoid cells are producing immunoglobulins by the third day. Recognition molecules (antibody) as well as sensitized cells are therefore present early in the allograft reaction.

Sensitized lymphoid cells, on recognizing the foreign tissue, release several mediators of inflammation and cell damage. The release of cytotoxic factors directly injures membranes of adjacent cells. Mitogenic products stimulate division of lymphoid cells, perhaps expanding the immunocompetent population. Activated, phagocytic macrophages are effectively concentrated in the area by migration inhibitory factor, other chemotactic factors, and cytokines produced by the activated cells. In addition, vascular permeability agents are released.

Meanwhile, complement is fixed, thereby producing chemotactic factors, anaphylatoxins, and finally cellular damage when the terminal components are activated. Capillary permeability is increased by anaphylatoxins from the complement chain and probably by kinins. Interstitial edema becomes prominent. At the same time there are several additional inducements to cellular infiltration. The complement cascade generates molecules that produce immune adherence and others that have chemotactic activity. Damaged cells release additional compounds that contribute to infiltration by PMNs as well as other cells. PMNs in turn release vasoactive amines (including histamine or serotonin, depending on the species) and additional vascular permeability-promoting factors. The PMNs squeeze through the enlarged endothelial cell junctions and release proteolytic cathepsins D and E, causing basement membrane damage.

Fibrin and α-macroglobulins, whose contribution is not understood, are deposited by 7 days. During this time, lymphoid cells have continued to accumulate and, joined by significant numbers of plasma cells and PMNs, obscure the normal architecture. The

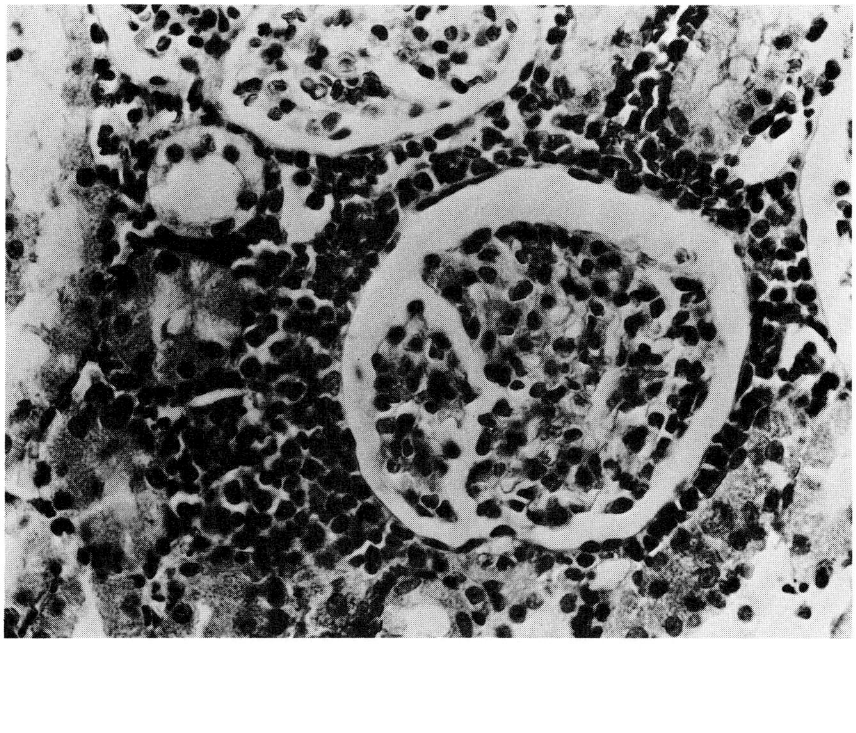

FIG. 10-15. Canine renal allograft 48 h after transplantation into unmodified recipient. Round cell infiltration, usually the first overt sign of host activity against the allograft, is apparent within 6 to 12 h after transplantation. By 48 h the number of invading cells is substantial. The original perivascular infiltrate has surrounded a glomerulus and adjacent tubules. (From: *Foker JE, Najarian JS: Allograft rejection: III. The pathobiology of organ rejection, in Najarian JS, Simmons RL [eds]: Transplantation. Philadelphia, Lea & Febiger, 1972, p 122, with permission.*)

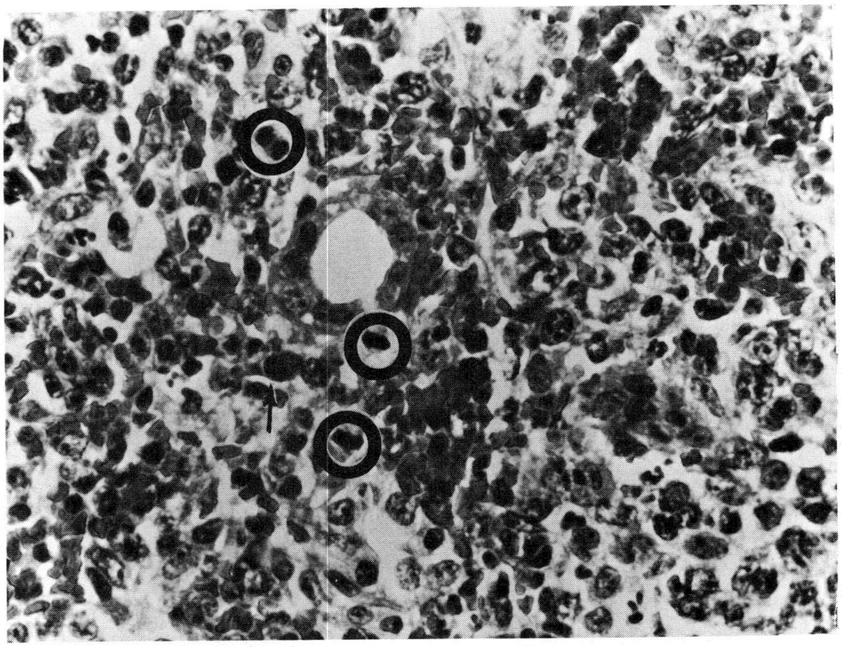

FIG. 10-16. Canine renal allograft 4 days after transplantation into an unmodified recipient. Invading cells all but obscure the architecture of the kidney. Numerous mitoses *(circles)* can be found, and this cellular proliferation may be producing immunologically competent cells within the graft. A plasma cell *(arrow)* is present, but most of the cells resemble lymphocytes and macrophages. (From: *Foker JE, Najarian JS: Allograft rejection: III. The pathobiology of organ rejection, in Najarian JS, Simmons RL [eds]: Transplantation. Philadelphia, Lea & Febiger, 1972, p 122, with permission.*)

round cell population presumably contains many macrophages and other immunologic nonspecific cells at this point. Increasingly frequent mitoses may indicate the production of immunocompetent cells within the graft.

The small vessels become plugged with fibrin and platelets, diminishing the perfusion and preventing function. In this relatively rapid sequence of events, the organ has little chance to respond, and the pathologic process is dominated by the host effector pathways.

Obviously, rejection modified by immunosuppressive agents is not a distinct morphologic classification. The morphologic features associated with this more chronic rejection become dominated by the response of the organ tissue itself. Here the normal response of tissue to injury predominates in the pathologic picture. A good deal of endothelial cell damage occurs in the allograft, and the responses of cellular repair, hypertrophy and hyperplasia, follow.

Endothelial cell damage also elicits repair processes called, for convenience, *accelerated atherosclerosis*. Aggregations of platelets within the intimal layer are resolved, and the dissolution of the thrombi is accompanied by the infiltration of macrophages and foam cells. The result is a thickened intimal layer with the loss of smooth endothelial lining and the presence of vacuolated cells. The lumen narrows as a result. Narrowing of the vessel lumen is also a consequence of the medial thickening. Studies using nonimmunologic disease models have shown that most of the cells proliferating in response to the stimulus of injury are smooth muscle cells. A reasonable extrapolation is that hyperplasia of these cells produces much of the luminal narrowing in the allograft (Fig. 10-17).

Although the exposed position of the endothelial cells and the striking proliferation of the smooth muscle cells argue for their being an important target of the immune reaction, there is evidence that the basement and elastic membranes of the vessel absorb a major portion of immune-mediated damage. Either immune complexes or antibodies to the vascular basement membrane activate complement and attract polymorphonuclear cells. These nonspecific effector cells release at least four protein factors that increase the permeability of the vessel and in addition produce cathepsins D and E, which digest basement membranes. The PMNs are active in reaching the basement membrane and will lift the endothelial cells to gain this access.

Platelets may be of greater significance than PMNs in mediating damage. Immune complexes (which activate complement) will result in platelet adherence and the release of vasoactive substances. Platelet aggregation leads to the release of histamine, serotonin, and other capillary permeability factors that expose more basement membrane; the exposed collagen fibers of the basement membrane further enhance platelet aggregation. Platelets and PMNs drawn to these sites release cathepsins, elastases, and phosphatases that increase destruction and attract other nonspecific cellular effectors including macrophages.

The myocardial cell is the characteristic cell of the heart, the tubular cell of the kidney, the acinar and islet cell of the pancreas, etc. The differentiation and function of these cells demand an ample oxygen supply, and if destroyed, they cannot be replaced by further cellular division. Therefore, compromise of respiration by vascular endothelial and medial hypertrophy, intravascular aggregations of platelets, and interstitial accumulations of edema and mononuclear cells will have predictable consequences for these cells. They will atrophy, and death may be followed by replacement fibrosis (Fig. 10-18).

The interstitial area concomitantly increases in size. The interstitial area, however, has much activity in its own right. Repair of immunologic damage stimulates many fibroblastic cells to proliferate, and it attracts macrophages. The persisting immunogenic capacity of the allograft is indicated by the inevitable presence of infiltrating plasma cells and lymphoid cells.

It is impossible to determine what proportions of these effects result from ischemia produced by vascular occlusion, interstitial

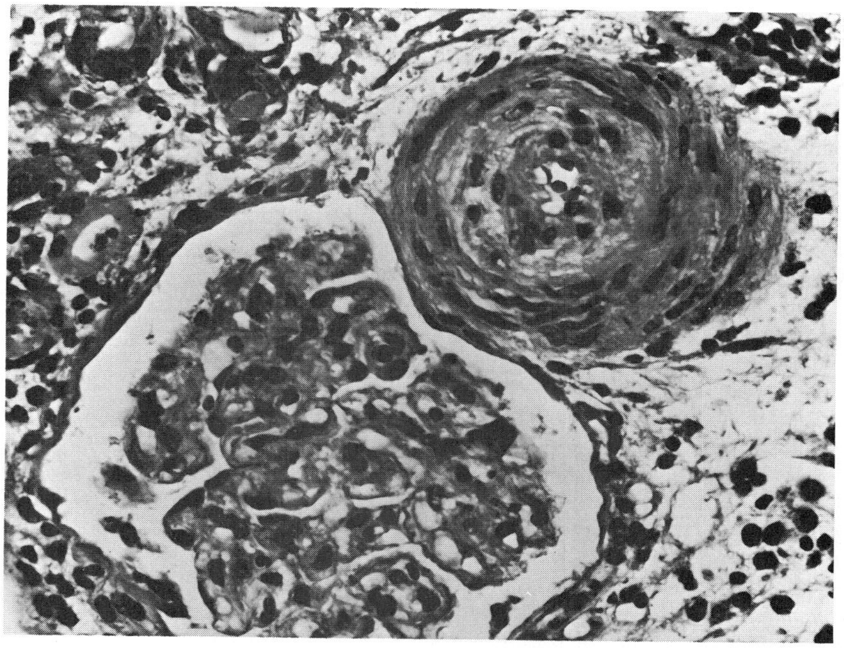

FIG. 10-17. A rejected human allograft removed 18 months posttransplant. The lumen of the arteriole has all but disappeared as a consequence of hyperplasia of the cells of the vessel. Most of the thickening of the wall is probably due to proliferation of smooth muscle cells with spindle-shaped nuclei. Endothelial cells, with rounder nuclei, almost fill the lumen. (From: *Foker JE, Najarian JS: Allograft rejection: III. The pathobiology of organ rejection, in Najarian JS, Simmons RL [eds]: Transplantation. Philadelphia, Lea & Febiger, 1972, p 122, with permission.*)

edema, or cellular infiltrates. Similarly, the contribution made by the direct cytotoxic action of specific and nonspecific effector cells and molecules is unknown.

PREVENTING GRAFT REJECTION

Clinical Immunosuppression

The development of immunosuppressive agents has revolutionized the field of transplantation. The clinical use of these agents has made transplantation of solid organs and cellular grafts an accepted therapy for end-organ failure. For the most part, if these agents are discontinued, graft rejection will occur. The only exception to this rule is for recipients of bone marrow stem cells, who become specifically tolerant to the graft donor after acceptance of the graft. Historically, as the mechanisms responsible for graft rejection became increasingly understood, it has been possible to design more specific antirejection drugs.

Theoretically, there are a number of methods by which the allograft rejection response can be suppressed, including (1) de-

FIG. 10-18. Extensive damage to the small artery in a human renal allograft removed 14 months posttransplant is apparent. The elastic membranes are badly frayed, and the elastica interna has been destroyed entirely along half the circumference of the vessel. The intimal layer shows extensive disruption and loss of cells. The cells remaining are often vacuolated. The lumen is narrowed by tissue from several origins: proliferation of smooth muscle cells in the media, endothelial cell swelling and hyperplasia, and the presence of an organized thrombus. The adventitial area shows damage and edema formation. Note also that severe tubular atrophy and interstitial fibrosis are present. (From: *Foker JE, Najarian JS: Allograft rejection: III. The pathobiology of organ rejection, in Najarian JS, Simmons RL [eds]: Transplantation. Philadelphia, Lea & Febiger, 1972, p 122, with permission.*)

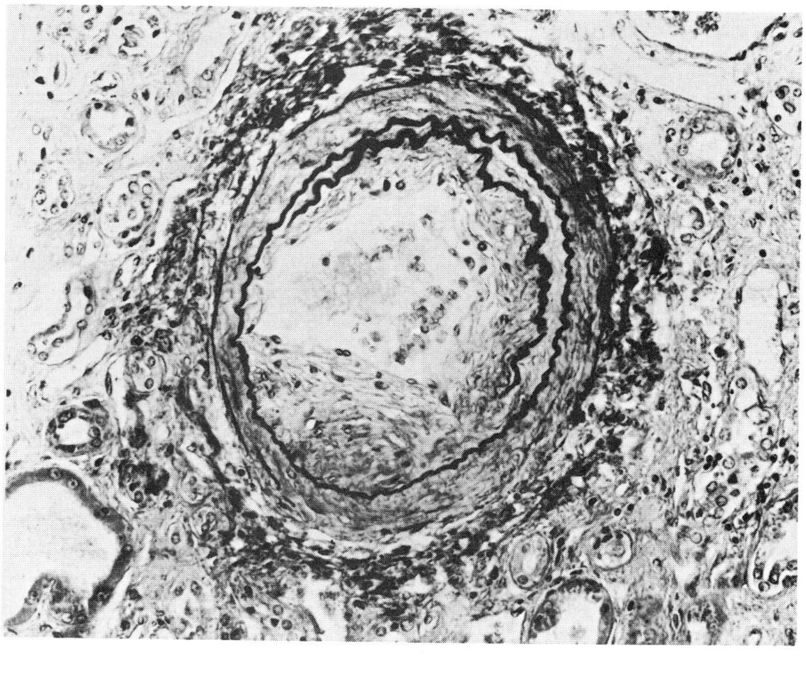

stroying the immunocompetent cells before transplantation, (2) making the antigen unrecognizable or even toxic to the reactive lymphocyte clones, (3) interfering with antigen processing by the recipient cells, (4) inhibiting lymphocyte transformation and proliferation, (5) limiting lymphocyte differentiation into killer or antibody-synthesizing cells, (6) activating sufficient numbers of suppressor lymphocytes, (7) inhibiting destruction of graft cells by killer lymphocytes, (8) interfering with the combination of immunoglobulins with target antigens, (9) preventing tissue damage by the nonspecific cells or antigen-antibody complexes, or (10) inducing true specific immunologic tolerance of the graft antigens.

In practice, a clinically useful immunosuppressive agent largely depends on either the destruction of the immunocompetent cells or inhibiting the differentiation and proliferation of these cells. Inducing specific immune tolerance before grafting has been successful only in bone marrow transplantation. Inhibiting sensitized cells and antibodies after they have been produced is only transiently effective in slowing graft damage. To be most effective, immunosuppression must be present at the time of transplantation, or even before.

A number of methods have been used to prevent graft rejection. Clinically, most of the agents in use are directed at T_H lymphocyte responses. They act in a nonspecific fashion to inhibit T-lymphocyte activation and proliferation. Historically, single agents were initially used in an attempt to control graft rejection. The first agents used included *irradiation*, which was fraught with morbidity and mortality, and *corticosteroids*, which were not sufficient to control rejection even at very high doses. The introduction of *multimodal therapy*, using a combination of agents which may act additively or synergistically via different mechanisms, has been found to allow maximum immunosuppression with a minimum of side effects, since lower doses of each agent are required. Figure 10-19 lists some points of action of frequently used agents with respect to the cell cycle. At the present time, all immunosuppressive agents in use function through nonspecific suppression of the immune system. Table 10-4A lists some of the most frequently used immunosuppressive agents.

Antiproliferative Agents

Most traditional immunosuppressive agents act to impair the proliferation of lymphocytes. Such agents include the antimetabolites, alkylating agents, toxic antibiotics, and x-ray. They inhibit the full expression of the immune response by preventing the differentiation and division of the immunocompetent lymphocyte after it encounters the antigen. All of them, however, fall into one of two broad mechanistic categories. Either they structurally resemble needed metabolites or they combine with certain cellular components, such as DNA, and thereby interfere with cell function.

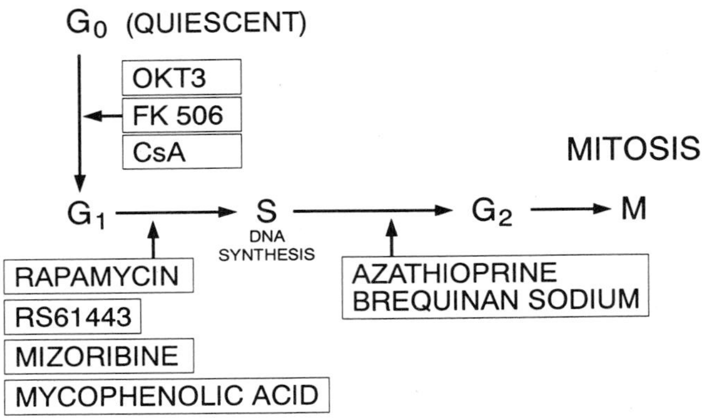

FIG. 10-19. Point in cell cycle at which some commonly utilized immunosuppressive agents function.

The former group, the antimetabolites, have a structural similarity to cell metabolites and either inhibit enzymes of that metabolic pathway or are incorporated during synthesis to produce faulty molecules. The antimetabolites include purine, pyrimidine, and folic acid analogues, which are most effective against proliferating and differentiating cells. They are given at the time of transplantation when the immunocompetent cells are first stimulated, and then for the life of the graft to interfere with the continuing stimulus to the immune system.

Alkylating agents and certain antibiotics include those compounds that combine with DNA and other cellular components. Although these agents would be useful in the pretransplant period to reduce the number of effective immunocompetent cells in the recipients, and thereafter to prevent proliferation, they are so toxic that their use has been limited to bone marrow transplantation and as occasional substitutes for azathioprine.

Purine Analogues. The purine analogue azathioprine (AZ) (Imuran) has been the most widely used immunosuppressive drug

Table 10-4A
Common Immunosuppressive Agents: Classification and Mechanism of Action

Classification	*Agent*	*Mechanism of Action*
Antimetabolite	Azathioprine	Purine analogue; interference with DNA synthesis
Lymphocyte depletion compound	Antilymphocyte globulin (ALG)	Sera directed against mature T lymphocytes
Lymphocyte depletion compound	Steroids	Produce a decrease in total T lymphocytes
T-cell-directed immunotherapy	Cyclosporine	Inhibits T-cell activation and maturation
T-cell-directed immunotherapy	FK506	Macrolide antibiotic which inhibits T-cell activation and maturation
T-cell-directed immunotherapy	Rapamycin	Macrolide antibiotic inhibits T-cell activation and maturation as well as inhibiting activity of activated T cells
Monoclonal antibody	OKT3	Binds to CD3 portion of T-cell receptor complex

in clinical organ transplantation. Azathioprine is 6-mercaptopurine (6-MP) plus a side chain to protect the labile sulfhydryl group. In the liver, the side chain is split off to form the active compound, 6-MP. The mechanism of action would seem to be similar for these two compounds; however, azathioprine seems to enjoy the advantage of slightly lower toxicity.

Full metabolic activity occurs in the cell with the addition of ribose 5-phosphate from phosphoribosyl pyrophosphate to form 6-MP ribonucleotide. The structural resemblance of this molecule to inosine monophosphate is obvious, and 6-MP ribonucleotide inhibits the enzymes that begin to convert inosine nucleotide to adenosine and guanosine monophosphate (Fig. 10-20). In addition, the presence of 6-MP ribonucleotides slows the entire purine biosynthetic pathway by fraudulent feedback inhibition of an early step. The steric similarity to either adenosine or guanine nucleotides is not great enough to allow significant incorporation into DNA or RNA and synthesis of faulty molecules. The result of inhibiting these several enzymes, however, is to block the synthesis of cellular RNA, DNA, certain cofactors, and other active nucleotides.

The toxicity of azathioprine results from the same mechanisms. Its primary toxic effect is bone marrow suppression, leading to leukopenia. Liver toxicity can also result, possibly because of the high rate of RNA synthesis by these cells. The mechanism is unclear, however, because hepatic dysfunction does not seem to be dose-related. Fortunately, both of these toxic effects are relatively mild and readily reversible.

Although pyrimidine analogues have been studied extensively as immunosuppressants in the laboratory, only brequinan shows clinical promise.

Folic Acid Antagonists. The folic acid antagonists, aminopterin and methotrexate, inhibit the enzyme dihydrofolate reductase and prevent the conversion of folic acid to tetrahydrofolic acid. This step is necessary for the synthesis of DNA, RNA, and certain coenzymes; again, proliferating cell systems are most affected.

Some of the toxicity of aminopterin and methotrexate can be abrogated by the administration of folinic acid some hours or even days after the use of the antagonist. Nevertheless, the ratio of immunosuppression to toxicity has not justified their use in clinical kidney transplantation. The immune reactions that accompany bone marrow transplantation are more difficult to control, and methotrexate has been used to both prevent and reverse the severe graft-versus-host (GVH) reactions that occur. It is now used clinically in bone marrow transplantation only if cyclosporine or FK506 as GVH-prophylaxis is contraindicated.

Alkylating Agents. The alkylating agents have highly reactive rings as part of the molecular structure. These unstable rings have electron-seeking points that combine with electron-rich nucleophilic groups such as the tertiary nitrogens in purines and pyrimidines, or with —NH_2, —COOH, —SH, and —PO_3H_2 groups on a variety of molecules. The high-energy rings of alkylating agents break and combine with these constituents to form stable covalent bonds. Obviously, many cell components have such groups, including DNA, RNA, and the enzymatic and structural proteins. Alkylation of DNA is probably the most detrimental. If the DNA strands are not repaired, chromosomal replication will be faulty in proliferating cells. Both DNA and RNA can be alkylated at several points, but a common site appears to be N-7 of the guanine ring (Fig. 10-21). Mispairing of DNA during replication may result from the presence of the alkylating agent itself, the clipping out of the alkylated guanine residue, or the cleavage of an alkylated guanine ring. Also chain breaks and cross-linkages frequently interfere with chain replication.

Since the damage to DNA can be repaired, these effects are apparently time-dependent. Consequently, the administration of alkylating agents just before and during stimulation by the antigen would most interfere with the ability of the immunocompetent cells to respond to that antigen. Continued use of the alkylating agents would also muffle the proliferative response of these cells in the face of a persistent stimulus. There are differences, however, in the response of T and B cells. The B cell seems to be more susceptible to cyclophosphamide than the T cell. This drug is a potent inhibitor of antibody formation, but its effect on skin or kidney rejection is much less spectacular. The reason for this apparent difference is unknown.

The usefulness of alkylating agents, which include nitrogen mustard, phenylalanine mustard, busulfan, and cyclophosphamide, is limited by their toxicity. Even so, cyclophosphamide has been used with good results in renal transplantation when liver toxicity prohibited the use of azathioprine. Cyclophosphamide is frequently used in clinical bone marrow transplantation, where it potentiates the effects of radiation and enhances the disruption of DNA. When cyclophosphamide is used, lower doses of radiation are required to deplete the recipient bone marrow population and provide space for donor cells. When leukemia is the indication for bone marrow transplantation, cyclophosphamide will aid in the destruction of these cells.

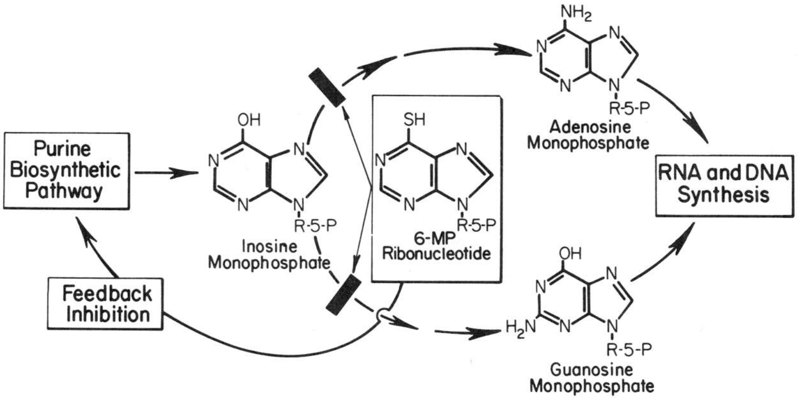

FIG. 10-20. Mechanism of antimetabolite action. 6-Mercaptopurine (6-MP) ribonucleotide resembles inosine monophosphate in its steric configuration. It thereby competes with inosine in its transformation into adenosine monophosphate and guanosine monophosphate and their subsequent incorporation into RNA and DNA. In addition, 6-MP inhibits the purine biosynthetic pathway, since it resembles a product of that biosynthetic pathway (feedback inhibition). (From: *Simmons RL, Foker JE, Najarian JS: Principles of immunosuppression, in Sabiston DC Jr [ed]: Davis-Christopher Textbook of Surgery. Philadelphia, Saunders, 1972, p 471, with permission.*)

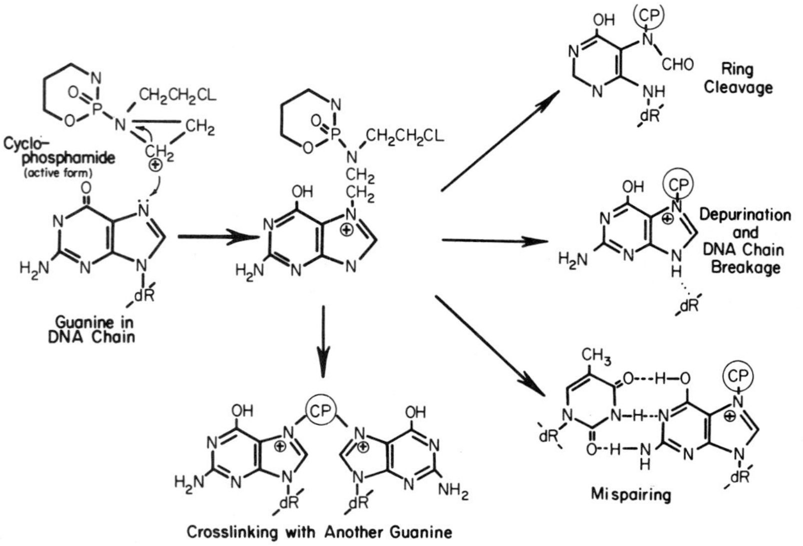

FIG. 10-21. Mechanism of action of the alkylating agent cyclophosphamide (CP). CP binds to the guanine molecule within the DNA chain. The guanine-CP complex leads to further damage to the DNA molecule. Four examples of the damage to DNA are shown. (From: *Simmons RL, Foker JE, Najarian JS: Principles of immunosuppression, in Sabiston DC Jr [ed]: Davis-Christopher Textbook of Surgery. Philadelphia, Saunders, 1972, p 471, with permission.*)

Toxicity is high, however, and predictable reactions occur, principally to rapidly replicating cell populations. Stomatitis, nausea, vomiting, diarrhea, skin rash, anemia, and alopecia are all common reactions. The more specific effects of cyclophosphamide administration are prompt fluid retention, occasionally severe hemorrhagic cystitis, and cardiac toxicity. The cardiac and edema problems suggest that even nonreplicating cell populations are adversely affected by this drug.

Cyclosporine. The discovery of cyclosporine in 1972 initiated a new era for the field of transplantation. The use of cyclosporine made liver and heart transplantation clinically feasible. It provided a more precise form of T-cell-specific immunotherapy to control graft rejection. It is now one of the most frequently used immunosuppressive agents. The use of cyclosporine in combination with modest doses of prednisone and/or azathioprine provides superior control of graft rejection with fewer side effects.

Cyclosporine is a completely new class of immunosuppressive agent. It is a cyclic peptide produced by a fungus (Fig. 10-22). Many of its suppressive effects are T-cell-specific. Cyclosporine inhibits activation of resting T lymphocytes, resulting in an inhibition of IL-2 production. However, once T lymphocytes have been activated, cyclosporine is *not* effective for suppression of the immune response (Fig. 10-23).

Cyclosporine is insoluble in aqueous solutions. Absorption from the gastrointestinal tract is slow and incomplete. Excretion of cyclosporine is primarily through the bile, and there is a well-documented enterohepatic cycle. Adverse effects of cyclosporine include hirsutism, neurotoxicities, hyperkalemia, nephrotoxicity, and hepatotoxicity. The most frequent toxic effects are nephrotoxicity, hypertension, and tremors.

A number of clinical trials for transplantation of kidneys, livers, lungs, hearts, and small bowel have demonstrated that cyclosporine provides potent immunosuppression without the myelosuppression associated with antimetabolite use.

FK506. FK506 is a *macrolide antibiotic* which, like cyclosporine, is produced by a fungus. The immunosuppressive potency of FK506 is at least 500 times greater than that for cyclosporine A. It is composed of hydroxy groups, carbonyl groups, and an amide group and is virtually insoluble in water (Fig. 10-24). FK506, like cyclosporine, inhibits cell activation but it does not prevent function of previously activated T lymphocytes. Its mechanism of action results in inhibition of interleukin-2 (IL-2) production. Although it inhibits the production of IL-3 and IFN-γ, it does not suppress hematopoiesis. In humans, FK506 treatment inhibits the appearance of IL-2 receptors on activated T lymphocytes. However, once T cells have been activated, FK506 has no effect. In clinical trials for liver, lung, cardiac, renal, small intestine, and pancreatic islet allografts, preliminary data indicate that it is at least as effective as cyclosporine in preventing graft rejection. Most important, it appears to be steroid-sparing, allowing a fairly rapid tapering of corticosteroids. Although FK506 is a potent immunosuppressive agent in preventing allograft rejection, it has not been effective in prevention of rejection in xenogenic (cross-species) combinations. Two primary drug toxicities have been observed in preliminary clinical trials: (1) anorexia and weight loss; and (2) nephrotoxicity secondary to vascular changes involving fibrinoid necrosis of the small arteries and arterioles. These effects appear to be dose-related.

FK506 has played a critical role in characterizing the mechanisms of intracellular *signal transduction*, the process by which *extracellular* molecules bind to a cell surface receptor or intramembrane receptor to influence *intracellular* events at the gene level. Signal transduction occurs in at least two steps: (1) a signal is transmitted from a cell surface or intramembrane receptor across the cell membrane and is (2) subsequently transmitted across the cytoplasm to regulate gene expression. Two categories of *immunophilins*, receptors in the cytoplasm of T cells, have been described to date: *cyclophilins* (bind cyclosporine) and *FK binding proteins (FKBP)*.

Binding of FK506 to FKBP in the cytoplasm of T lymphocytes results in the production of an *FKBP-FK506 complex*, which interferes with a Ca^{+2}-dependent signaling mechanism via an intermediary intracytoplasmic enzyme, *calcineurin*. The next step(s) in intracellular signal transduction that influence activation or suppression of the genes that control the immune response are yet to be defined. Characterization of the ligand (target, i.e., FK506)–

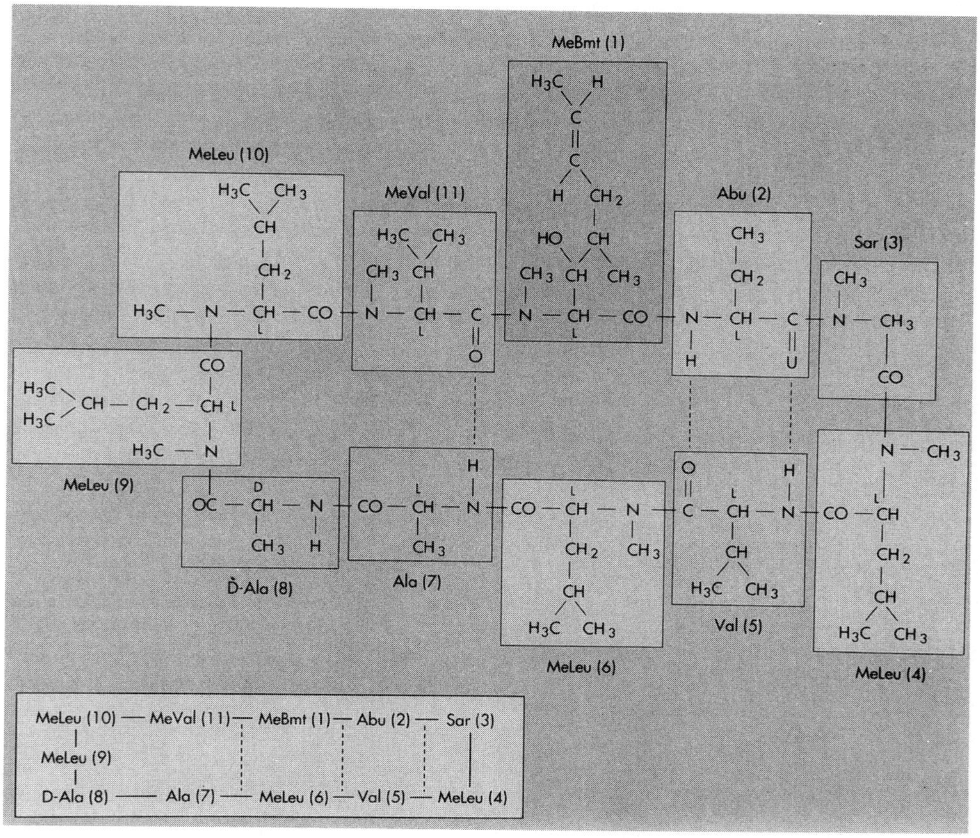

FIG. 10-22. Atomic structure *(top)* and alignment of amino acids *(bottom)* of cyclosporine. The unique structure at position 1 is MeBmt, a novel β-hydroxy, unsaturated, 9-carbon amino acid ((4R)-4-[(E)-2-butenyl)]-4,N-dimethyl-L-threonine). Abu denotes α-aminobutyric acid; Sar, sarcosine; MeLeu, N-methyl-L-leucine; Val, valine; Ala, L-alanine; D-Ala, alanine; and MeVal, N-methyl-L-valine. (From: *Starzl TE, Shapiro R, Simmons RL [eds]: Atlas of Organ Transplantation. New York, Gower Medical Publishing, 1992, p 1.24, with permission.*)

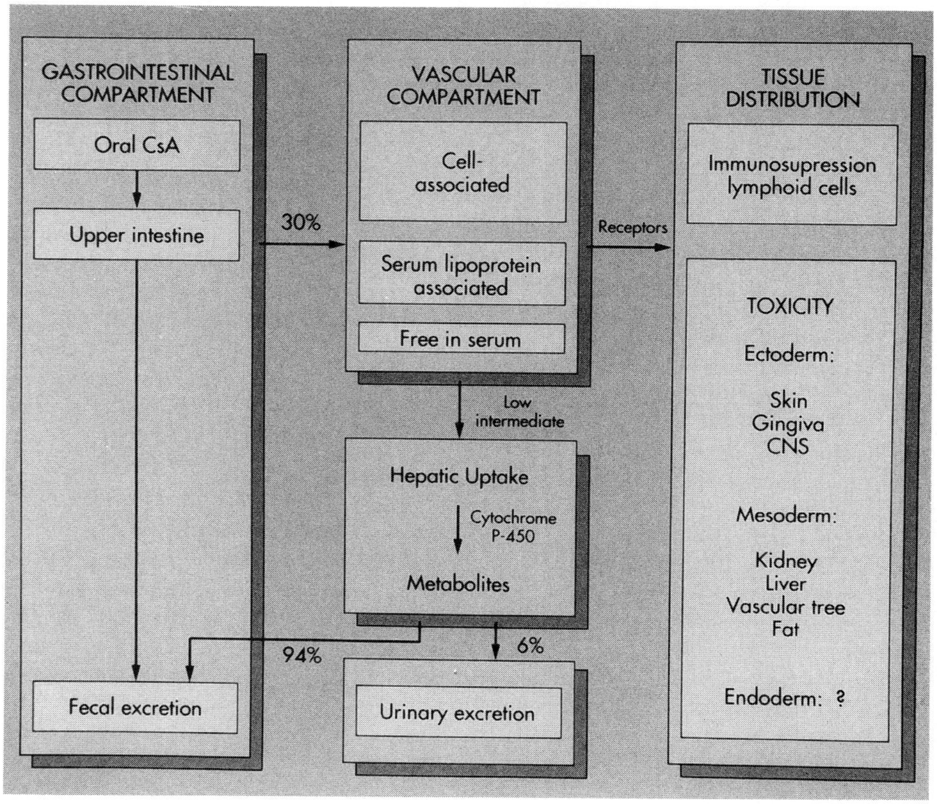

FIG. 10-23. Disposition of cyclosporine (CsA). The drug is absorbed from the gastrointestinal tract into the vascular compartment, where the major drug fraction becomes cell-associated, and the largest serum fraction binds to lipoproteins, with only a small "free" fraction. The tissue distribution of the drug causes immunosuppression of lymphoid cells, on the one hand, and toxicity to ectodermal and mesodermal structures, on the other. After the drug is taken up by the liver, it is metabolized by the cytochrome P-450 system, producing metabolites that are primarily excreted in the bile and to a small extent in the urine. CNS denotes central nevous system. (From: *Starzl TE, Shapiro R, Simmons RL [eds]: Atlas of Organ Transplantation. New York, Gower Medical Publishing, 1992, p 1.26, with permission.*)

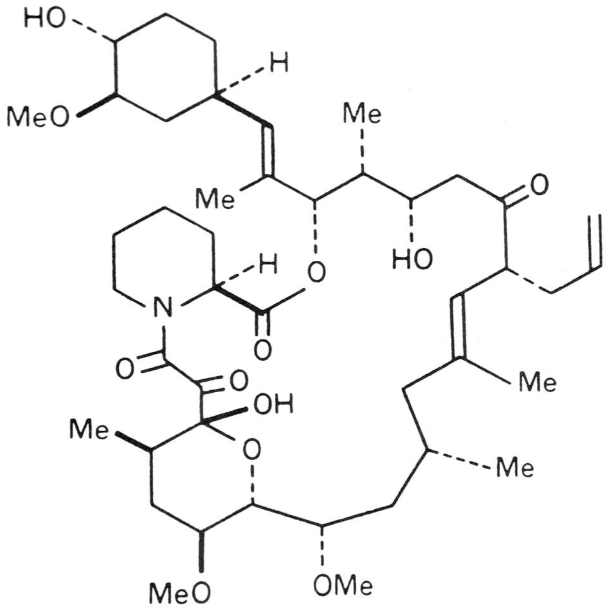

FIG. 10-24. Chemical structure of FK506. (From *Ochiai T: A novel immunosuppressive agent: FK506. Transplant Immunol Lett 7:4, 1990, with permission.*)

receptor (i.e., FKBP) interaction might allow even more focused approaches for immunotherapy to prevent rejection.

Rapamycin (RAPA), like FK506, is a macrolide antibiotic. Its structure resembles that of FK506. In vitro, RAPA is a potent inhibitor of T-cell and B-cell proliferation. Most important, it has virtually no effect on IL-2 production. Instead, it strongly inhibits IL-4 and IL-2 driven T-cell proliferation. Specifically, it blocks the ability of the IL-2 receptor to induce signal transduction. In blocking studies, RAPA was antagonized by FK506 but not by cyclosporine, which is not surprising in view of the fact that they bind to the same immunophilin receptor (FKBP). This critical difference has further elucidated the mechanisms of *intracellular signal transduction* (Fig. 10-25). It is currently believed that binding of RAPA to FKBP results in an *immunophilin-drug complex* which is different in configuration from the FK506-FKBP complex. Therefore, a different signal is transmitted through the cellular cytoplasm, this time in a *calcium-independent* fashion. Therefore, FK506 and rapamycin, although structurally similar, are very different in their activity.

Like FK506, RAPA inhibits Ca^{+2}-dependent T- and B-cell division. However, rapamycin also inhibits Ca^{+2}-independent T- and B-cell division, cell proliferation induced by IL-2 and IL-4, and gamma-interferon (IFN-γ) production induced by IL-1. FK506 has no effect on any of these elements of the immune response in vitro.

Initial studies of RAPA and FK506 indicated that they were antagonistic if used in excess. However, used in combination in *low doses*, RAPA and FK506 are synergistic in their immunosuppressive function rather than antagonistic. Since only a low concentration of drug is required to produce the immunosuppressive effects, combination therapy may have significant clinical application.

Immunosuppression by Lymphocyte Depletion

Adrenal Corticosteroids. Adrenal corticosteroids have played a major historical role in clinical transplantation. Despite uncertainty about their mechanism of action, steroids are still often necessary for successful human organ transplantation and are commonly used to produce immunosuppression in other types of patients.

Many effects of steroids are known (Fig. 10-26). The problem is deciding which are primary and which are secondary actions. Steroids cross the cell membrane and bind to specific receptors in the cytoplasm of most cells, lymphocytes included. The steroid-receptor complex then enters the nucleus and interacts with DNA in an unknown way. In lymphocytes, DNA, RNA, and protein synthesis is inhibited, as is glucose and amino acid transport. At a sufficient dosage, lymphocyte degeneration and lysis occur. Cytolysis can readily be produced in vivo, and T cells appear to be most susceptible. The primary antilymphocyte action of steroids may be to deplete small lymphocytes before they are activated by antigen. Steroids also suppress most of the accessory functions of macrophages, including the ability to secrete interleukin-1.

The functional effects of steroids are predictable, and all T-cell responses are depressed. Paradoxically, the steroid-resistant thymocytes that remain after an injection of steroids have increased activity, but the net immunologic capability of the treated animal is reduced.

Although B-cell activity and antibody production are relatively unaffected by steroids, many other cell types that participate in graft rejection are damaged. Both macrophage and neutrophil chemotaxis and phagocytosis are inhibited. The accumulation of neutrophils, macrophages, and monocytes at sites of immune and inflammatory activity is reduced. Steroids also increase the membrane stability of digestive lysosomal particles in these cells, which reduces their inflammatory activity. Inflammation is so intertwined with any substantial immune reaction that the various effects are inseparable. The variety of immunologic activities that steroids will suppress means that their effectiveness against the rejection reaction is probably the sum of many influences. Steroids alone cannot prevent clinical allograft rejection, but, together with other compounds, they are potent in both preventing and reversing rejection reactions.

Steroid toxicity of some degree is frequent and commonly includes a cushingoid appearance. Other characteristic problems from steroid therapy are hypertension; weight gain; peptic ulcers and gastrointestinal bleeding; euphoric personality changes; cataract formation; hyperglycemia, which may progress to steroid diabetes; and osteoporosis with avascular necrosis of bone. The appearance and severity of these complications vary considerably, but all too frequently they are life-threatening or disabling. Clinical transplantation will be improved tremendously when more specific means of immunosuppression are developed and present steroid dosages can be reduced.

Antilymphocyte Globulin (ALG). A variety of antibody preparations designed to react with immunoresponsive lymphocytes are available. The first agent applied was ALG, a polyclonal serum. Subsequently, monoclonal antibodies have also become available (Table 10-4B). They are designed to prevent and to treat graft rejection.

Heterologous polyclonal antilymphocyte globulins (ALG) are produced when thoracic duct, peripheral blood, lymph node, thy-

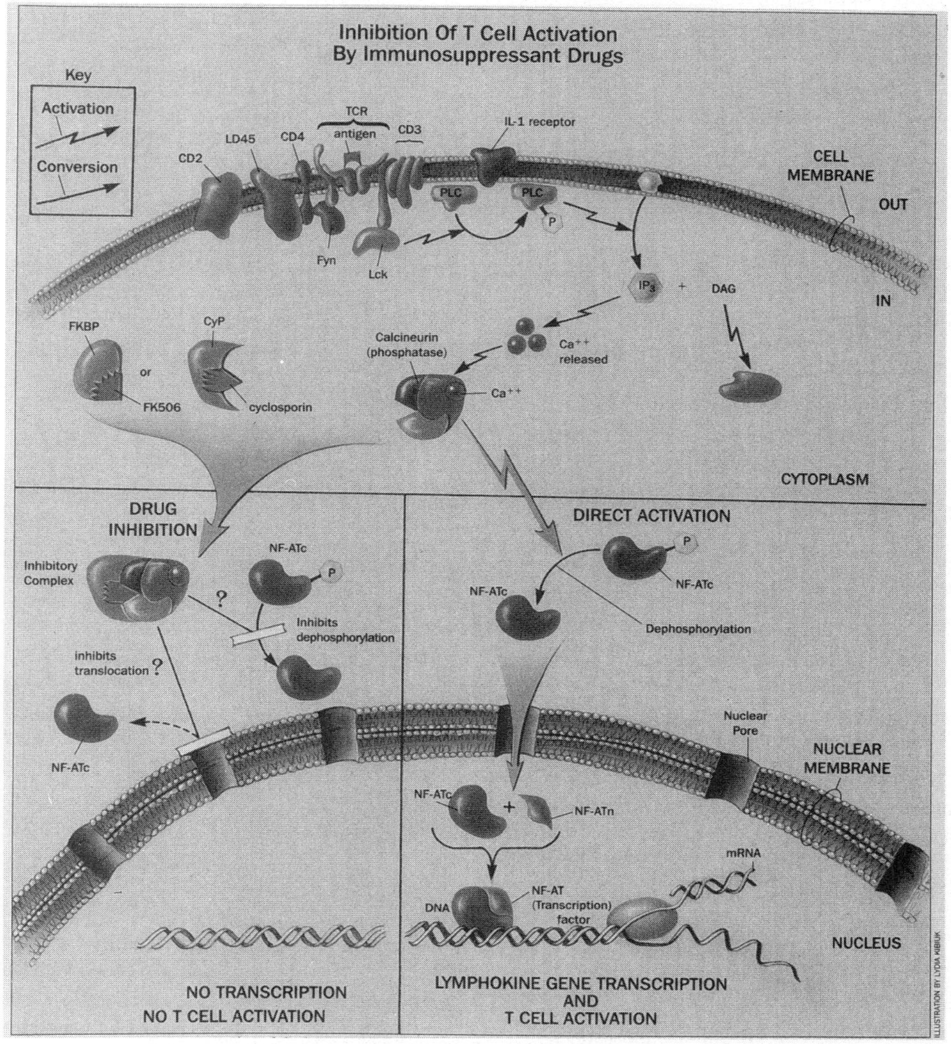

FIG. 10-25. Proposed model of inhibitory action of the immunosuppressant drugs FK506 and cyclosporine A on T-cell activation. Binding of antigen to the T-cell receptor complex (TCR) stimulates at least one tyrosine kinase, such as Lck or Fyn, shown here. The kinase phosphorylates phospholipase C (PLC), which triggers breakdown of phosphatidyl inositol 4,5-biphosphate (PIP_2) to inositol 1,4,5-triphosphate (IP_3) and diacylglycerol (DAG). DAG activates protein kinase C, and IP_3 triggers the intracellular release of calcium ions. Calcium activates the phosphatase calcineurin which dephosphorylates the cytoplasmic component of nuclear factor of activated t cells (NF-ATc), which facilitates its translocation into the nucleus. NF-ATc combines with its nuclear cofactor, NF-ATn, to form an activated transcription factor that activates RNA polymerase (POL) and regulates the transcription of genes encoding interleukin-2 (IL-2) and other lymphokines and cytokines needed for T-cell activation. T-cell activation is blocked *(left panel)* when immunosuppressant drugs FK506 or cyclosporine bind to their receptor proteins, FKBP and cyclophilin (CyP). Both drug-receptor complexes can inhibit calcineurin, which blocks nuclear translocation of NF-ATc, either by inhibiting phosphate removal or by other mechanisms that prevent entry into the nucleus. (From: *Touchette N: Immune suppressants signal surprises in T cell activation. J NIH Res 3(9):71, 1991, with permission.*)

mus, or spleen lymphocytes are injected into animals of a different species. Cell membranes or cultured lymphocytes serve equally well to provide the antigenic stimulation. The addition of adjuvants, usually Freund's complete adjuvant, is used to enhance the immunogenicity of the foreign lymphocytes and produce sera that are consistently more immunosuppressive. The rabbit and the horse are commonly used to produce antisera for clinical transplantation.

The antibodies produced in this crude way are polyclonal and therefore reactive with a number of different epitopes on the many subsets of lymphocytes injected. As a consequence, the immunosuppressive effect is the net result of the destruction of many lymphocyte subsets.

The action of heterologous polyclonal ALG seems to be directed mainly against the T cell. ALG therefore interferes most with the cell-mediated reactions—allograft rejection, tuberculin sensitivity, and the graft-versus-host reaction. ALG can abolish preexisting delayed hypersensitivity reactions, and larger doses will prolong the survival of some xenografts. ALG has a definite, but lesser, effect on the production of antibodies to T-cell-dependent antigens.

Although these preparations, purified and administered intravenously, have been widely used in clinical transplantation with beneficial results in both the prevention and treatment of organ allograft rejection, monoclonal reagents with more predictable reactivity are now available. In work for which they were awarded the Nobel Prize, Kohler and Milstein developed a simple technique to produce unlimited quantities of specific *monoclonal antibodies* (1975). This technology has revolutionized the field of immunology. The application of monoclonal antibodies has had a profound impact on understanding the biology of transplantation, the immune response, and rejection.

The technology for monoclonal antibody production is simple yet elegant. While normal B cells cannot be grown in long-term culture, B-cell tumors, called *myelomas*, reproduce indefinitely. Fusion of a single normal antibody-forming B cell with a non-antibody-producing myeloma cell results in production of a single immortal monoclonal antibody-producing hybrid of the two cells called a *hybridoma*. Because an individual B cell produces only one antibody, potentially unlimited types of monoclonal antibodies can be produced, depending on which B-cell clones are activated by a specific immunizing antigen.

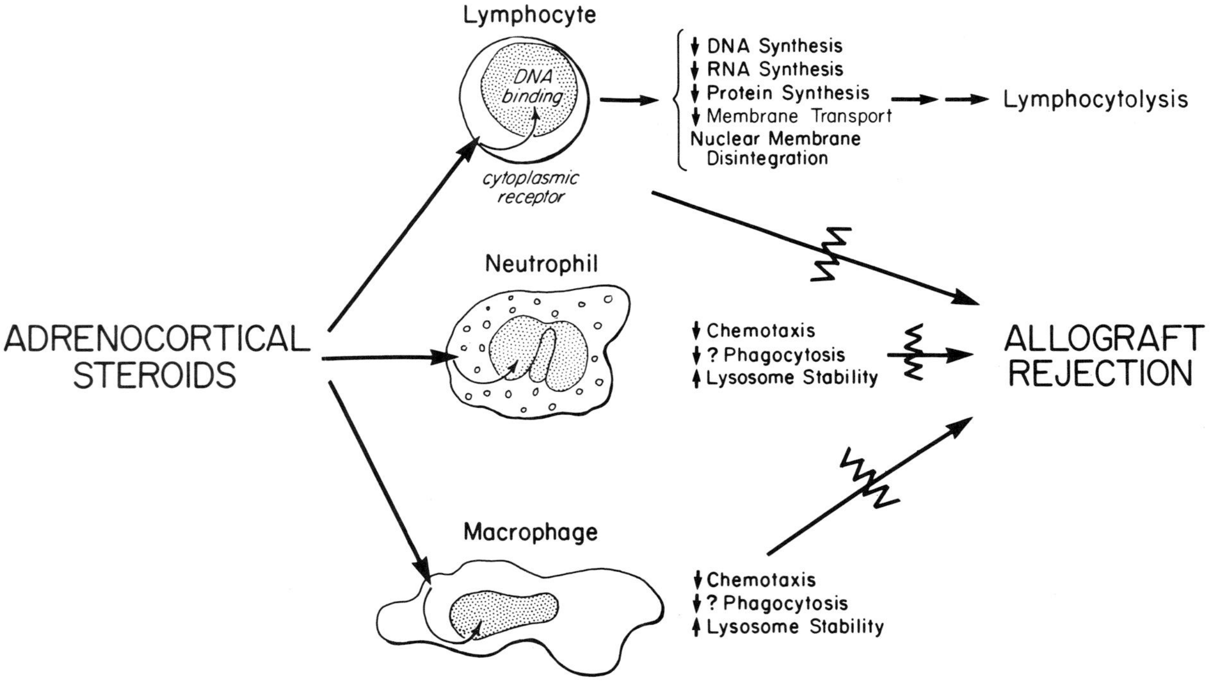

FIG. 10-26. Adrenocortical steroids play an important role in clinical allograft immunosuppression. Many apparent sites of action have been located experimentally. These compounds bind to cytoplasmic receptors, and this complex combines with DNA. How this relates to the many functional consequences of steroids presented in this diagram is unclear. In the complex clinical transplantation setting it is not possible to determine if the primary suppression of lymphocytes is more important than the anti-inflammatory effects on neutrophils and macrophages in the suppression of allograft rejection reactions. This suppression of interleukin-1 production by macrophages is probably a most important mechanism.

Monoclonal antibodies have been used clinically to control rejection and to monitor changes in lymphocyte subpopulations during immunosuppressive therapy. Table 10-4B lists some of the monoclonal antibodies available for clinical use. OKT3 is the prototype. OKT3 is an anti-CD3 monoclonal antibody that binds to the T-cell receptor complex (CD3) present on all mature T cells. Because the CD3 receptor to which OKT3 binds is the signaling portion of the T-cell receptor complex, lymphocyte function is inhibited. Anti-CD4 is also in use in clinical trials.

Table 10-4B
Representative Monoclonal Antibodies

CD Class	*Monoclonal Antibody*	*Target Cell*
CD3	OKT3	All T cells (both $\alpha\beta$-TCR and $\gamma\delta$-TCR positive)
CD4	OKT4, Leu3a	Helper and inducer T cells (Class II)
CD5	Leu1	T cells, activated B cells
CD8	OKT8, Leu2	Suppressor and cytotoxic T cells (Class I)
CD14	LeuM3	Monocytes (granulocytes)
CD16	Leu11[a]	NK cells, granulocytes, macrophages
CD19	Leu12, B4	B cells
CD20	Leu16	B cells
CD34	My10	Hematopoietic stem cells
CD39	G28-8	B cells, macrophages

The toxicity of any heterologous antibody prepared against human tissue depends in part on its cross reactivity with other tissue antigens, and the ability of the patient to make antibodies against the protein itself. Polyclonal ALG can produce anemia and thrombocytopenia despite prior absorption with human platelets and red cell stroma. Monoclonal antibodies have few cross reactions, but fever, chills, nausea, diarrhea, and aseptic meningitis are frequently seen during the intravenous administration of the first few doses. All heterologous globulins can elicit allergic reactions against themselves. These are generally mild and infrequent, but monoclonal antibodies are strongly antigenic so that they are less effective after 1 or 2 weeks of use due to the formation of antibodies directed against the monoclonal antibodies. Polyclonal antibody preparations seem to be repeatedly effective.

Radiation. Radiation was probably the first agent used to produce immunosuppression. Ionizing radiation (x-rays, alpha rays, beta rays) affects both cellular proteins and nucleic acids. Despite the fact that relatively small doses of irradiation may disrupt the secondary protein structure formed by hydrogen bonding and the tertiary conformation that results, biologically significant alterations of protein function seem to require very high doses. Consequently, most of the immunosuppressive effects of x-radiation are caused by changes produced in nucleic acids. DNA is particularly vulnerable, and therefore so is cellular replication. The most important of the several modes of damage is the production of scattered breaks in the deoxyribose-phosphate backbone of DNA (Fig. 10-27). Disruption of either the carbon-carbon bonds

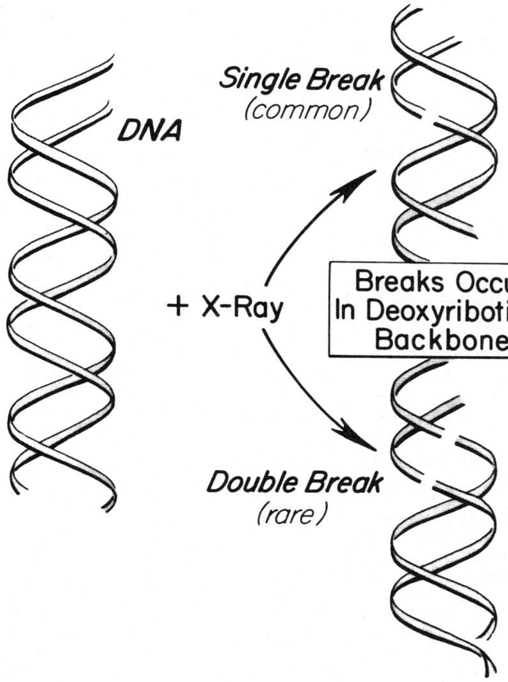

FIG. 10-27. X-ray-induced damage of DNA molecule. Irradiation frequently induces single breaks in the deoxyribotide backbone of the DNA double helix. More rarely, irradiation induces double breaks within the backbone. (From: *Simmons RL, Foker JE, Najarian JS: Principles of immunosuppression, in Sabiston DC Jr [ed]: Davis-Christopher Textbook of Surgery. Philadelphia, Saunders, 1972, p 471, with permission.*)

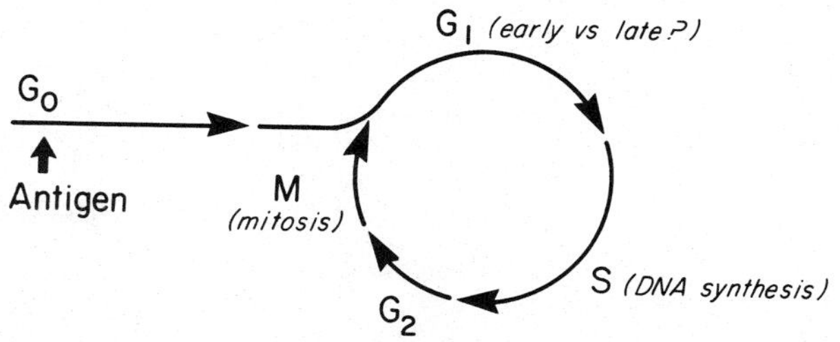

FIG. 10-28. The phases of the cell cycle. Following stimulation by an antigen, or other type of mitogen, small lymphocytes are activated. They are converted from the resting G_0 phase to the active G_1 phase. The G_1 phase lasts 10 h or longer before DNA synthesis (S phase) begins. The S phase lasts about 10 h and is followed by a short (2 to 4 h) G_2 phase before mitosis (M phase). M phase is relatively brief, usually less than 2 to 3 h, after which the cells are returned to the G_1 phase. The susceptibility of the cell to the immunosuppressive agents used in transplantation varies with the phase of the cycle. Periods of most intense nucleic acid synthesis, particularly S phase, are most vulnerable to the antimetabolites. As discussed in the text, the resting G_0 lymphocyte is also susceptible to several of the clinically used immunosuppressive agents. (From: *Foker JE, Simmons RL, Najarian JS: Principles of immunosuppression, in Sabiston DC Jr [ed]: Davis-Christopher Textbook of Surgery. Philadelphia, Saunders, 1977, p 509, with permission.*)

of the deoxyribotides or the bonds involving the phosphate groups produces breaks in one of the DNA strands. Occasionally both strands are broken at the same point. Other sites of damage, such as the bases themselves, are even less frequent.

Repair mechanisms exist to mend the breaks, but insufficient time may be available in the dividing cell. Therefore, the effectiveness of radiation is dependent on the phase of the cell cycle in which the cell is found (Fig. 10-28). Cells in the M or G_2 phase are most sensitive to irradiation. Presumably, DNA breaks that occur during these phases cannot be repaired quickly enough, and the synthetic events and precise apportionment of cellular components that occur during mitosis may become scrambled. Conversely, the early G_1 phase and the latter part of the S phase are the most resistant portions of the cell cycle. Although irradiation is, in general, most effective just prior to or during mitosis, lymphocytes are a special case. For reasons that are not known, these cells are also sensitive in their resting, or G_0, phase.

The effect of irradiation on the immune response depends greatly on its timing with relation to antigen exposure. When an antigen is given soon after irradiation, the immune response will be inhibited because there is insufficient time for the immunocompetent cell population to recover before the antigen is encountered. If radiation is given during the time of maximal proliferation of the immunocompetent population to an antigen (soon after antigen administration), the immune response will be strongly inhibited. On the other hand, if antigenic stimulation is delayed long enough for the precursor cells to recover from the radiation, there will even be a slight augmentation of the response. Radiation is ineffective if given long after the antigen, when a mature population of effector cells has been formed.

Total body irradiation has limited use in clinical transplantation because the toxicity is too great. Fractionated doses of radiation to the lymphoid tissues (total lymphoid irradiation), similar to that used in the treatment of Hodgkin's disease, is under investigation. Profound immunosuppression is produced, and low doses of azathioprine and prednisone can maintain the effect. Local irradiation of the graft may also provide some immunosuppressive effects by damaging invading lymphocytes as well as producing nonspecific anti-inflammatory effects.

Both total body irradiation and total lymphoid irradiation have been used to eliminate the immune reactivity of patients in preparation for bone marrow transplantation. Cytotoxic chemotherapy is often used in combination. The toxicity is predictable. The rapidly replicating skin and gastrointestinal tract are universally affected, and nausea, vomiting, diarrhea, and skin changes occur.

Complications of Immunosuppression

Infection, end-organ toxicities, and malignancy are the most frequent complications associated with the use of nonspecific immunosuppressives. At times, rejection cannot be controlled, and may occur in spite of combination therapy. Infection is still the most common complication of immunosuppression, and overall it is the most common cause of death in transplant recipients (Fig. 10-29).

Infection. A significantly increased incidence of infection is observed in transplant recipients who receive immunosuppressive agents. Infection remains the most common cause of mortality. Immunosuppression increases the risk of infection by viral, fungal, and bacterial agents because of the nonspecific mechanism of action. In the past, the majority of deaths occurred in transplant recipients as a result of invasive bacterial infections. Now, improved antibiotics and immunosuppressive agents have shifted the spectrum of organisms to *opportunistic* pathogens which are nor-

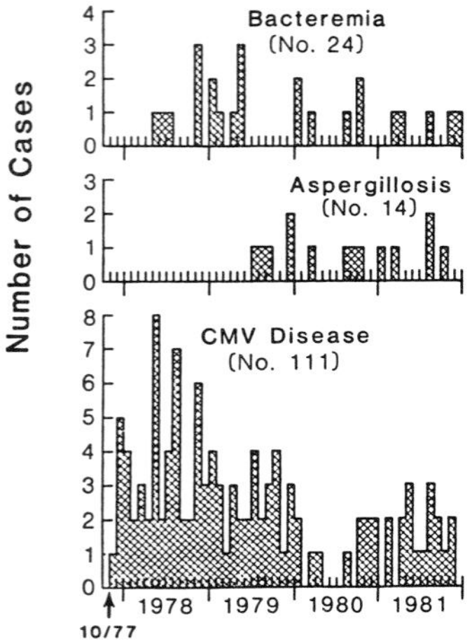

FIG. 10-29. Incidence of infections in 535 consecutive transplants performed between October 1977 and September 1981, at the University of Minnesota hospital, and followed until January 1982. The incidence varied widely, even though the rate of transplantation was the same, i.e., 10 to 15 transplants per month. The reasons for this variation are not clear. (From: *Peterson PK, Ferguson R, et al: Infectious diseases in hospitalized renal transplant recipients: a prospective study of a complex and evolving problem. Medicine 61:360, 1982, with permission.*)

mally only weakly pathogenic, if at all. Prophylactic antibiotics now eradicate the more aggressive bacteria, but infection by fungal, protozoal, and viral organisms remains a major source of morbidity and mortality in transplant recipients. *Candida albicans* is the most common cause of fungal infection in transplant patients, with *Aspergillus* species second in frequency. *Aspergillus* typically produces upper lobe pulmonary cavities. *Pneumocystis carinii*, a protozoan, is also a frequent cause of pulmonary infection, but is seen less frequently now that Bactrim prophylaxis is administered to transplant recipients. This organism characteristically produces an alveolar infiltrate with disproportionate dyspnea and cyanosis. Viral infections are also very common in transplant recipients, especially the herpes group of DNA viruses. Cytomegalovirus (CMV) is a frequently encountered offender.

Standard patient isolation precautions are of little use against these organisms, and prophylactic antibiotics are not available for most of them. Prevention is dependent upon avoiding excessive dosages of immunosuppressive agents in a futile attempt to prolong the function of a rejected graft. Some protection against *P. carinii, Nocardia*, the pneumococci, *Listeria, Legionella*, and other susceptible organisms may be provided by the prophylactic trimethoprim and sulfamethoxazole. The pneumococcal vaccine may ultimately be useful.

Viral Infections. Viral infections seem to be almost ubiquitous among kidney transplant recipients. The herpes group of DNA viruses are the most common etiologic agents. Infection or antibody response to cytomegalovirus (CMV) is found in 50 to 90 percent of patients after renal transplantation (see Fig. 10-29). Herpes simplex infection occurs in about 25 percent and zoster in 10 percent of graft recipients; both can be prevented or treated with the antiviral agent acyclovir. Epstein-Barr virus (EBV) commonly infects transplant patients, but most infections are mild. EBV is associated with posttransplant malignancy in rare patients, however. The prophylactic use of the antiviral agents acyclovir and ganciclovir has resulted in a significant reduction in viral infections.

Antigenic evidence for hepatitis B virus infection can be detected in many transplant patients and non-A, non-B hepatitis is probably a cause of liver failure in some long-term survivors. Immunosuppressed patients have both typical and atypical patterns of infection. Hepatitis is particularly illustrative. Transplantation and hemodialysis patients may have no symptoms of acute hepatitis, but antibody responses and viral elimination are unusual. For this reason, persistent active hepatitis is a common finding in long-term survivors and a common underlying cause of death years after the transplant.

Cytomegalovirus (CMV) is the most important infectious illness that afflicts immunosuppressed transplant patients. CMV infection can produce a spectrum of illness typically characterized by fever, neutropenia, arthralgias, malaise, myocarditis, pancreatitis, or gastrointestinal ulceration. The most severe illnesses are acquired as primary infections from latent virus residing in the grafted tissue. Less often, blood transfusions are the vector. Some cases of apparently new infection represent reactivation of latent intracellular viruses. Transplant recipients who do not have antibodies to CMV and who receive grafts from donors who do are at the highest risk. The use of antilymphocyte antibody preparations for immunosuppression increases the risk. Recipients of cyclosporine appear to be at lower risk.

The typical CMV infection is a mild febrile illness, followed by an antibody response and regression of viral symptoms. A rejection episode sometimes accompanies the viral infection and raises the controversy of whether the virus triggers the rejection episode. These patients usually recover but may continue to excrete CMV in urine or saliva despite the presence of antibodies to CMV. In certain patients, however, there is no effective immune response, and the infection can be lethal. The virus itself induces a profound state of immunosuppression, rendering these patients exquisitely susceptible to bacterial or fungal opportunists. Many serious infections are superinfections in patients already suffering CMV infections.

Prevention of Infection. The incidence of severe, near-fatal infections has been reduced through a number of precautions. (1) The most important precaution is to eliminate all sources of infection before transplantation, especially those in the urinary tract and dialysis access site. Other sources of infection should be sought by routine preoperative cultures and careful examination. If any source is found, it should be eliminated by the appropriate use of surgical drainage or antibiotic therapy. (2) When technical problems are avoided, wound sepsis is uncommon. Urinary, biliary, or pancreatic anastomotic breakdown especially predisposes to wound infection. (3) Organs from related and well-matched cadavers elicit less frequent and less vigorous rejection reactions. If repeated rejection can be avoided, the doses of immunosuppressive drugs can be minimized and the rate and severity of infection will diminish. (4) Many patients who die of infection develop leukopenia (especially neutropenia) at some time. Some bouts of leukopenia can be attributed to cytomegalovirus infections. Leukopenia can be prevented by careful reduction in azathioprine doses when the leukocyte count or platelet count falls. The use of other bone marrow depressants (e.g., chloramphenicol) should be avoided in patients already on azathioprine therapy. Cyclosporine A is not myelosuppressive and has reduced the incidence of neutropenia. (5) Protective isolation protocols were formerly used to minimize infections in the initial postoperative care. Most transplant units have discontinued their use because they restrict access to the patients, impose psychologic stress, and are probably ineffective against viral, fungal, or endogenous bacteria.

Malignancy. Cancer has been an unexpectedly frequent companion of clinical transplantation. The incidence of cancer is not high enough, however, to contraindicate the transplant procedure. Tumors in transplant recipients have come from two general sources. A rare cause is the inadvertent transplantation of a cancer from a cadaver donor in whom the cancer was unsuspected. These tumors can sometimes be treated simply by halting immunosuppression therapy and allowing rejection of the tumor tissue, as well as the transplant, to occur.

The more common cancers are the primary tumors that appear in the immunosuppressed recipient. Only certain tumors grow more readily in immunodepressed patients. Seventy-five percent of the spontaneous cancers are either epithelial or lymphoid in origin. Carcinoma in situ of the cervix, carcinoma of the lip, and squamous or basal cell carcinomas of the skin account for about half of this group, while B-cell lymphomas make up the remainder. It has been estimated that the risks to the transplant recipient of developing cervical cancer, skin cancer, or lymphoma are increased by 4, 40, and 350 times, respectively. The lymphomas are unusual both in their frequency and in their behavior. Almost 50 percent of the immunosuppressed patients with lymphomas have brain involvement, which occurs in only 1 percent of nontransplanted related cases of lymphoma. These lymphomas, although initially responsive to radiation therapy, are usually fatal. They have been linked to infection of transplant recipients with Epstein-Barr virus (EBV) and have been termed lymphoproliferative disease (LPD).

Recent evidence suggests that not all lymphomas are true neoplasms. Immunologic analysis has indicated that these tumors secrete several different types of immunoglobulins, i.e., they do not have the monoclonal characteristics of cancer. Most evidence suggests that some may represent uncontrolled B-cell proliferative responses to EBV in seronegative patients. At this stage, antiviral chemotherapy with acyclovir appears promising. Subsequently true lymphoid neoplasms seem to evolve from chromosomal abnormalities; such true monoclonal malignancies have not responded well to conventional cancer chemotherapy.

We do not know why transplant patients have an increased risk for these cancers. It has been postulated that the surveillance and elimination of tumor cells, as they arise, by lymphocytes is an important natural defense of human beings against cancer. Certainly this function might be abnormal in immunodepressed patients. Another possibility is the use of mutagens like azathioprine as immunosuppressive drugs. There is also growing evidence that herpes viruses, to which the immunosuppressed patient is manifestly susceptible, can induce these neoplasms. EBV is almost certainly the cause of the polyclonal B-cell lymphoproliferative disorder that evolves into a monoclonal lymphoma. All these lesions contain the EBV genome as part of the cellular DNA.

Less certain is the possibility that cancers of the epithelium may be a consequence of herpes virus transformation. This group of viruses is carcinogenic in animals and infects epithelial cells of lip, skin, and genital tissue. Circumstantial evidence exists for a role in human cervical cancer. Herpes viruses are usually dormant, but the stress of transplantation or the action of antimetabolite may activate them. The viruses might then either proliferate and cause a clinical viral illness or produce cellular transformation into cancer cells. Similarly, the papovaviruses are probably the cause of skin cancer in immunosuppressed patients.

Cushing's Disease. Most transplant patients who receive steroid therapy develop Cushing's syndrome. The appearance of the face is altered by rounding, puffiness, and plethora; fat tends to be redistributed from the extremities to the trunk and face. There is also an increased growth of fine hair over the thighs and trunk and sometimes over the face. Acne may appear or increase, and insomnia and increased appetite are noted. The underlying metabolic changes can be even more serious: The continuing breakdown of protein and diversion of amino acids to glucose increase the need for insulin and result in weight gain, fat deposition, muscle wasting, thinning of the skin with striae, and sometimes the development of steroid diabetes, cataracts, and osteoporosis. In some patients a myopathy develops, the nature of which is unknown. The cushingoid changes may represent such a problem that transplant nephrectomy will be necessary on that basis alone.

Gastrointestinal Bleeding. Gastrointestinal bleeding due to reactivation of a preexisting ulcer or diffuse ulceration of the gastrointestinal tract can be a fatal complication. The relative pathogenetic contribution of progressive uremia and steroid administration is unknown, but when bleeding appears, it can be difficult to control by nonoperative means. Occasionally the use of cimetidine or the intramesenteric arterial infusion of vasopressin is effective.

During steroid therapy of moderate dosage, episodes of gastrointestinal bleeding can be almost totally prevented by the use of antacids between meals. In patients with rejection who require high steroid dosage, antacid therapy must be intensified with each increase in steroid administration. Pretransplant antiulcer operations have been used in patients with peptic disease.

Other Intestinal Complications. A number of colonic complications, including diverticulitis, bleeding, and ulceration, are associated with immunosuppressive treatment. A syndrome of acute cecal ulceration with gastrointestinal bleeding is due to cytomegalovirus. Cytomegalovirus underlies sporadic ulcer disease in other enteric locations as well.

Cataracts. Cataracts are common in patients who require steroids. The cataracts, which develop slowly, appear to be independent of the absolute prednisone dosage.

Thrombosis and Thromboembolic Phenomena. Thrombophlebitis may occur in the renal transplant recipient, particularly on the side of the graft where the venous anastomosis may become partially or completely thrombosed. The diagnosis is difficult because swelling of the leg on the side of the transplant site is an occasional sign of rejection, associated with increases in weight, pulmonary infiltrates, and slight increases in serum creatinine level. When the differential diagnosis is difficult, a femoral venogram is indicated. The diagnosis of pulmonary embolism may also be difficult because clinical thrombophlebitis seldom precedes the embolus.

Hypertension. Many of the patients who come to renal transplantation are already hypertensive. Hypertension can usually be controlled with dialysis or, in rare refractory cases, with nephrectomy. Hypertension in most patients will develop soon after transplantation, but posttransplant hypertension can be easily controlled with dietary salt restriction and drugs. The hypertension seems to be due not only to prednisone but also to failure to regulate the normal salt and water balance in the early posttransplant period and secretion of renin by the kidney. Hypertension may be aggravated by rejection. It should be remembered, however, that significant hypertension may be due to renal arterial stenosis, and arteriography may be necessary for the differentiation. Hypertension is also a well-characterized side effect of cyclosporine.

Disorders of Calcium Metabolism. Patients frequently come to renal transplantation with renal osteodystrophy. Alterations in vitamin D metabolism and secondary hyperparathyroidism are prominent factors in the pathogenesis of skeletal disease. Long-standing acidosis may likewise be contributory. The resulting osteoporosis, osteomalacia, and osteitis fibrosa cystica in the child can lead to growth restriction, epiphysiolysis, skeletal deformities, and pathologic fractures. The bone disease in some cases can be arrested with pharmacologic doses of vitamin D or aluminum hydroxide.

Hemodialysis can correct the uremic state, but the bone disease may actually progress if the stimulus to parathyroid hormone secretion is not effectively eliminated. Great attention should be directed toward keeping the dialysate calcium concentration at a level (6 to 7 mg/dL) that does not promote calcium loss from the blood. Parathyroidectomy is sometimes required to help arrest progressive bone disease but is not indicated for hypercalcemia alone after transplant. Parathyroidectomy seems primarily indicated for patients on chronic hemodialysis in whom transplantation is not planned.

Musculoskeletal Complications. A disturbing complication from the use of chronic nonspecific immunosuppressive agents is avascular necrosis of the femoral heads and other bones. Its occurrence is most closely correlated with the dosage of steroid used. Transient rheumatoid symptoms precede changes visible by radiography by several months. The bone changes apparently occur secondarily to steroid osteopenia or osteonecrosis with resulting microfractures. Alterations in lipid metabolism caused by fluctuating high levels of steroids likewise appear to be important in the pathogenesis. The treatment is for the most part symptomatic. It is doubtful that bone lesions can revascularize sufficiently to restore normal architecture in the presence of maintenance steroids. Should symptoms increase, replacement arthroplasty is usually successful.

Migratory arthralgia, myalgia, and tendinitis are common, but persistent joint pain and swelling are most often signs of intraarticular infection. Occasionally, an unexplained septic arthritis crops up in these patients; mycobacterial infections are most commonly reported.

Pancreatitis. Pancreatitis may appear suddenly and unexpectedly in transplant allograft recipients, and recurrent bouts may prove to be fatal. It has been attributed variously to corticosteroid therapy, azathioprine, cytomegalovirus, or hepatitis virus. Steroids are known to thicken pancreatic secretions.

Growth. Since chronic renal failure itself is inhibitory to development, uremic children are usually far behind their peers in size. After successful transplantation their growth response is highly variable and may depend on age, previous growth rate, renal function, and immunosuppressive drug regimen. Many children return to a normal growth rate; unfortunately the growth that was lost during their original illness is not made up, so these children will always be smaller than their peers.

Pregnancy. Many normal children have been born to renal transplant women despite their use of mutagenic immunosuppressive drugs. The pregnancies of renal transplant recipients are frequently complicated, however, by toxemia and bacterial and viral infections, particularly of the urinary tract. Both toxemia and infection may contribute to a higher incidence of premature labor and small neonates. Another important problem that must be faced is the decreased life expectancy of the transplant recipient. Parenthood is a long-term obligation, and counseling of these patients should include a discussion of these considerations.

CLINICAL TISSUE TRANSPLANTATION

Exponential progress in clinical transplantation has occurred as a result of the availability of new immunosuppressive agents to prevent graft rejection. Combination drug therapy targeting different components of the immune response is now possible as the immunobiology of graft rejection has become better understood. Numerous tissues, solid organs, and even cellular free grafts are now transplantable with ease. There is currently a critical shortage of organs available for transplantation as a result of this success.

Allotransplants, or transplants from one individual into another genetically different one, have been carried out for an ever-expanding variety of tissues and organs, including cornea, teeth, thyroid, parathyroid, adrenal, ovary, testes, pituitary, spleen, lymph node, bone marrow, skin, bone, cartilage, fascia, tendons, nerves, arteries, valves, veins, hemopoietic tissue, pancreas, duodenum, intestine, kidney, liver, lung, and heart. Clinical allotransplants may be of several types: (1) temporary free grafts, such as skin allografts and blood transfusions; (2) partially inert struts that provide a framework for the ingrowth of host tissue, such as bone, cartilage, nerve, tendon, and fascial grafts; (3) permanent, partially privileged, structurally free grafts, such as cornea, blood vessels, and heart valves; (4) functional free grafts such as parathyroid, ovary, and testes; (5) whole organ grafts, such as pancreas, kidney, small intestine, liver, lung, and heart; (6) free cellular grafts (e.g., purified insulin-producing pancreatic islets, hepatocytes, myocytes); and (7) bone marrow that acts as a functional replacement of the entire hemopoietic and lymphopoietic systems. Bone marrow is unique in that graft take is associated with the induction of tolerance to the graft: no further immunosuppression is required. For all other living grafts, immunosuppressive agents are required to prevent graft rejection. Immunosuppression is justified only for grafts essential for life. Therefore, tooth bud, thyroid, and parathyroid grafts, which would require immunosuppression for any success, are trivial grafts and are easily replaced by prostheses or medication.

Autotransplants involve the transplantation of tissues from one individual back to that same individual. Clinical autotransplants have been carried out with hair, skin, teeth, kidney, legs, arms, veins, arteries, pericardium, valves, bone, cartilage, fascia, fat, tendons, nerves, stomach, bowel, parathyroid, thyroid, ovary, testes, adrenal, and bone marrow.

Xenografts, which are grafts between different species, have been performed in the past for skin, heart valves, heart, kidney, testes, bone, and cartilage. A renewed interest in xenotransplantation has emerged with the current shortage of organs available for transplantation, with the appeal that an unlimited supply of organs from a selected donor species (e.g., pig) could be harvested.

Skin

Autotransplants of hair-bearing skin are used to reconstrcut eyebrows or to replace the scalp after traumatic avulsion. Autotransplants of individual hair roots are sometimes used as a treatment for baldness. Skin autotransplants have been used to reconstruct the esophagus, urinary tract, vagina, and hernial weaknesses as well as the usual surface defects. The main use of skin autografts is to cover and replace areas destroyed by trauma, burn, or operation.

Skin allotransplants are also used quite extensively in burned patients when autochthonous skin is not available. They function as a biologic dressing and if left on long enough will be rejected. One cannot justify the use of immunosuppressive agents to achieve prolonged graft survival in this group of patients. In addition, skin is one of *the most* antigenic (immunogenic) of all tissues and is usually rejected aggressively in spite of immunosuppression. The theory behind this procedure, though, is that the skin allograft provides a better cover than any other material, and during the period of time when it is taking, it prevents the continued spread of sepsis.

Vascular Grafts

Autografts

Vein autografts have been used for over 50 years to replace segments of damaged arteries. They are still the best bypass grafts for occluded vessels in the lower extremities. After a period of time in the arterial circuit the vein wall thickens, and the vein becomes somewhat arterialized. Although there are occasional instances in which vein grafts weaken and rupture, by and large they make very satisfactory arterial substitutes. The two most common usages at the present time are in femoropopliteal artery–saphenous vein bypass grafts and in coronary artery bypass grafts. Pieces of autologous vein are also used as patch grafts. It is possible, too, to carry out successful autologous vein grafts to bridge defects in veins, although veins are less likely to stay open than arteries. Because they are an identical match with the recipient, rejection does not occur.

Autografted arteries are also sometimes used as vascular replacements; most often the hypogastric artery is utilized. Pieces of pericardium are sometimes used to patch defects or divert flow in the repair of intracardiac defects.

Allografts

Before the development of prosthetic graft materials, arterial allografts and xenografts were attempted, but this approach was limited for three reasons: (1) aneurysms sometimes occurred, with rupture and a fatal outcome; (2) plastic prostheses have proved so suitable for the larger blood vessels; (3) for smaller blood vessels the use of the autologous saphenous vein has proved to be better than either prostheses or allografts. Arterial allografts, even if viable, do not survive but in part are replaced by host tissue and in part persist as semi-inert material. Interestingly, neither prosthetic materials nor allografts become endothelialized. When organs are transplanted, the artery supplying the organ becomes an arterial allograft. It has been shown that the epithelium of smaller blood vessels is antigenic, and some degree of allograft rejection occurs.

Nerve

Nerve autotransplants are used to bridge defects in important motor nerves or sometimes to transfer the function of one nerve into the distal end of another, to repair a severed facial, digital, or recurrent laryngeal nerve, for instance. The autografts undergo Wallerian degeneration with proliferation of Schwann cells and are penetrated by regenerating nerve fibers after a few weeks. When the nerve graft is thick, the center of the graft may develop a zone of avascular necrosis through which regeneration fails to occur. This does not happen with thin grafts. As a consequence, some investigators have advocated the use of cable grafts consisting of several strands of smaller nerves to bridge defects in nerves of larger caliber. Experimental work is being done to evaluate the function of vascularized nerve grafts transferred with microsurgical techniques. Motor recovery can occur as well as sensory recovery.

When allografts are used, the rate and intensity of nerve fiber penetration are less, and the outcome is far inferior to that obtained with autografts. In general they should probably be used only when autografts cannot be obtained. Xenografts have been tried but appear to be of no value to human beings. It is likely that the inflammatory rejection response interferes with the passage of autologous nerve endings down the transplanted nerve sheath.

Cornea

Perhaps the most common clinical allotransplant is that of the cornea. The eye should be harvested from cadavers within 6 h after death. Eyes removed more than 36 h after death are unsuitable for corneal transplantation. The whole eye is generally preserved in a sterile container at a temperature of 3° to 5°C, and the graft is cut from the eye at the time of the transplant procedure. The eye is suspended from a suture passed through the severed optic nerve to keep it from coming in contact with the sides of the vessel. Eye banks store eyes in nutrient media at 4° or 34°C as long as 1 month.

Two types of corneal transplants are utilized: the full-thickness graft and the lamellar, or partial-thickness, graft. The full-thickness graft gives the best results, but complications such as secondary glaucoma, anterior synechiae, and a partial lifting off of the graft, causing astigmatism or opacification, can occur infrequently. These complications are avoided in lamellar keratoplasty, which is the operation of choice when the corneal opacity does not involve the full thickness of the cornea. In order to achieve a successful graft there must be good apposition between the graft and the host, the graft must be in contact with healthy cornea at some point in the circumference if it is to remain transparent, and blood vessels must not invade the graft to any appreciable extent.

The best patients for grafting are those with central corneal scars and healthy surrounding cornea with no vascularization, keratoconus (especially if the apex of the cone is beginning to break down), or corneal dystrophy. Indolent corneal abscesses, perforating ulcers of the cornea, and descemetocele have less positive outcomes. The results are also somewhat less good in acne rosacea and herpetic keratitis because of the danger of recurrence of the disease.

Corneal grafts are apparently so successful because they are in a privileged location in which they remain effectively isolated from the host's immune system as long as the graft itself and the cornea directly around it remain avascular. Unlike most other allografts, systemic immunosuppression is usually not required. Many corneal grafts remain clear indefinitely, although occasionally a graft that has remained clear for several weeks becomes opaque, suggesting rejection. A fibrous barrier that is almost impervious to blood vessels forms at the junction between the host and the graft.

Bone

Bone implants are used for the following indications: (1) to hasten the healing of defects and cavities, e.g., the use of cancellous bone chips in the residual defect after curettage of a unicameral bone cyst; (2) to supplement bony union in cases of delayed healing or pseudarthrosis arising after fracture, e.g., sliding or barrel stave grafts for nonunion of tibial shaft fractures, or to supplement the healing of certain fresh acquired or surgical fractures where skeletal continuity is problematic, e.g., cancellous autogenous implants for fractures of both bones of the forearm in an adult; (3) to reconstruct contour or major skeletal defects arising as a result of surgery trauma, disease, or congenital malformation, e.g., replacement of calvarial defects after surgery for trauma by compact bone implants.

Bone grafts are used to provide one or more of the following: (1) a source of viable osteoblasts (bone production); (2) a source of replacement for lost skeletal architecture (bone conduction); or (3) new bone formation (bone induction). Autografts of cancellous bone may provide all three: a source of living bone cells when harvested in thin strips where diffusion will provide cell nourishment, conduction of new bone formation along the cancellous surfaces, and bone induction from the matrix component diffusion that induces the differentiation of mesenchymal cells to form new bone. Autografts of cortical bone, such as fibular struts, may provide some small amount of living cells but primarily serve to reconstruct skeletal defects without the problems of antigenicity encountered in allografts. Allografts are generally reserved for large defects that cannot be filled or bridged by autografts without major disability at the donor site. Allografts are not viable and serve only only as a strut for conduction and induction of a new bone. Combinations of autogenous cancellous grafts with cortical autografts or allografts are frequently used to hasten incorporation of these grafts to the recipient sites.

A variety of grafting techniques have been devised to meet the differing clinical requirements. The most frequent types of bone grafts are autogenous grafts with or without internal fixation. These may be applied as barrel stave grafts, sliding grafts, or cancellous chips. In addition, there are vascularized pedicle grafts of two types: those with a bony base, and muscle pedicle grafts. Microvascular anastomosis to provide free viable bone grafts or composite bone and soft tissue grafts has been useful in major defects of the limbs from trauma or neoplasia. Similarly, in some locations, vascularized grafts may be mobilized and rotated on their vascular pedicle to provide a viable graft without the requirement of anastomosis.

Autografts are preferred for clinical use, since the cellular elements of bone allografts usually elicit a rejection response. Bone allografts do elicit new bone formation (osteoinduction) and serve as struts for the ingrowth of autologous bone (osteoconduction). When properly prepared, the immune response to the allograft can be substantially reduced. As such, allografts are of great clinical use.

For the most part stored or processed bone allografts are used in clinical situations. Preservation methods include (1) refrigeration, (2) freezing, (3) freeze-drying, (4) decalcification, or (5) any one of the above plus irradiation for sterilization. Such nonviable grafts mainly serve as architectural supports to stimulate and conduct new autologous bone formation.

Cartilage

It has been long known that cartilage can be successfully transferred between individuals of different genetic backgrounds without the need for immunosuppressive therapy. This immunologic privilege is attributable in adult articular cartilage to the absence of a blood supply. Under normal circumstances the fluid-nutritional needs are met via the synovial fluid. Thus, the absence of direct vascular contact and the presence of a dense proteoglycan-collagen matrix will insulate the chondrocytes from the host immune response.

Free autografts of cartilage have been used most extensively in plastic reconstructive surgery (1) to rebuild the contours of the nose after congenital or posttraumatic deformity, (2) to reconstruct the pinna, and (3) to fill out defects in the facial bones and the skull.

The fresh cartilage autograft comes closest to fulfilling the ideal: it should maintain its structure, have the potential for growth and repair, provoke no untoward reaction, and form a firm union with host tissues, persisting without loss of viability or absorption. Recent experimental and clinical application of rib perichondrial grafts as a source of new cartilage growth remains promising as an autograft technique for small joints.

The fresh cartilage allograft, however, has been reported to be a reasonable substitute for the autograft in particular circumstances because of its greater ease of procurement. The major drawback of such grafts is that despite the immunologic privilege of cartilage, the bulk of experimental and clinical evidence suggests that the tendency for late deterioration and absorption is somewhat greater than that of autografts. Furthermore, the potential for infection or transmission of virus-induced disease is similar to other living tissue transplants that are not proved sterile by culture or donor serology.

The preserved cartilaginous allograft has been used as a substitute for the fresh implant primarily because of the convenience that storage of such implants in cartilage banks provides. Refrigerated and chemically preserved frozen sections of cartilage have all been used with variable success.

Composite Grafts of Bone and Cartilage

Composite grafts involve the surgical transfer of entire functional units rather than the implantation of bits and pieces of cartilage or bone.

Epiphyseal Growth Plates. The object of the transplantation of epiphyseal growth plates is to restore longitudinal growth in hypoplastic limbs, whether congenital or acquired. This type of procedure has been used in efforts to improve the function of children with congenital deficiency of the radius. In these cases, autotransplantation of the proximal fibula has been used as a substitute for the radial deficiency. Although, in some cases, enlargement of the transplant could be demonstrated, this was always inferior to the natural growth potential and has not been sufficient to justify incorporation of this procedure into the surgical armamentarium. Microvascular transfer of epiphyseal growth plates shows continued growth and hypertrophy. This technique is now under clinical trial for restoring growth in damaged limbs.

Osteochondral Grafts. The diseases that destroy the articular cartilage are common. The osteochondral or osteoarticular graft might be a useful substitute. Transplants of articular cartilage, in conjunction with a very thin shell of subchondral supporting bone, are still in the experimental stage. Both allogenic and autogenous composites are now being applied in clinical trials in selected centers.

Transplant of Hemijoints or Whole Joints. The experimental transplantation of joints was initiated by Judet in 1908. Autografts tend to heal their osteosynthesis sites, revascularize the bony component, and in general maintain the articular surfaces in a fair state of preservation. On the other hand, both fresh and preserved allogenic transplants give unpredictable results, sometimes healing well with good function, and other times showing progressive deterioration. The latter changes in the allogenic groups are associated with delayed revascularization of the bony component, subchondral fracture and collapse, and synovial invasion of the joint surfaces. Immunosuppressive agents have not been shown to prevent this phenomenon in animal models, suggesting that rejection is the underlying mechanism. Because other options are available, the clinical use of immunosuppressive agents cannot be justified to prolong graft survival; and application of these procedures, therefore, awaits improved approaches to achieve rejection-free graft survival.

Artificial hemijoints or whole joints have superseded transplantation, at least for the present, but are more commonly used as composite replacements in major segmental defects. These composites generally use an allogenic bone segment with an artificial joint implant to allow soft tissue reattachment around the joint for better function; host tendons and ligaments will generally reattach to the allograft and do not grow into a metal implant.

Extremity Replantation

Replantation of severed extremities (autografts) has been carried out with increasing frequency in recent years. These procedures have usually involved the upper extremities, because the chances for good functional recovery are far greater in the arm than in the leg. Excellent prostheses exist for the lower extremity, but they are much less satisfactory for the upper. The major advantage of replantation is the development of useful sensation in the replanted extremity. Advances in microsurgery have made replantation of digits routine for the experienced microsurgeon.

The technique of limb replantation initially requires a general evaluation of the patient to assess other associated injuries. This should include radiography of the proximal stump as well as the amputated extremity itself, and particularly of the spine to be certain that the spinal roots to the extremity have not been avulsed. After securing hemostasis with pressure and being certain that no serious injury has been overlooked, the replantation can begin. During this initial phase the severed limb should be placed in a plastic container and packed in ice. The extremity should not be frozen, however, and for that reason, dry ice should be avoided. The limb may be replanted even though several hours have elapsed between its severance and the start of replantation. The exact critical period of ischemia has not definitely been established, but it appears that at least 12 h for a limb and up to 36 h for a finger can elapse with successful results after replantation. The more distal the amputation, the less ischemia-sensitive muscle tissue there is in the extremity, so prolonged cold ischemia is tolerated.

Before replantation a thorough debridement of grossly devitalized tissue is carried out. The bone is fixed first so that the limb will be stabilized before beginning the repairs of the vessels and nerve supply. Bones may require slight shortening to freshen up the ends and to gain additional length for relaxation of the arteries and nerves, and closure of soft tissue. Intramedullary fixation is used whenever possible to stabilize the bony fragments and therefore the vascular anastomoses. After proper fixation of the bones, and repair of the tendons, the blood vessels are joined. In a distal amputation, a microsurgical team is required. The precise sequence of repair varies from surgeon to surgeon, but often the largest vein is joined first, so that there will be outflow available at the moment when the blood is ready to flow through the artery. It is important to join normal vessels beyond the zone of injury using interposition vein grafts as necessary. If a nerve gap exists, nerve repair is delayed until healing is complete and a nerve graft can be done. If the nerve has been cleanly severed, immediate primary repair is carried out. A better result is obtained in distal nerve transections than in proximal ones, and in young people as compared with older ones. Distal sensory nerves give the most favorable results. Motor recovery in the median nerve is much more successful than in the ulnar nerve.

After completing the arterial and venous anastomoses and after either joining the ends of the nerves or deciding to perform a nerve graft as a secondary procedure, attention is turned to the soft tissues. With the blood supply restored, viability of tissues is easier to ascertain, and debridement can be completed. The shortening of the bone makes it possible to join several muscles together with a view to covering the blood vessels with living tissues. If soft tissue loss is minimal, the coverage can be achieved with the skin of the extremity, and other defects can be covered with split-thickness skin grafts. If the soft tissue defect is great and no covering is available, the defect must be covered by a pedicle flap. The newer microsurgical techniques permit the use of free tissue transfer in the form of revascularized myocutaneous flaps. This is usually done as a secondary procedure.

In the postoperative period the patient's limb must be kept in an elevated position to minimize edema. It is important to do a fasciotomy, including carpal tunnel release, at the end of the replantation to avoid compartment swelling from ischemic damage to the arm musculature. Heparin and dextran are not generally used postoperatively. Some degree of hypotension may occur as a consequence of leakage of plasma into the replanted extremity and acute blood loss. This is particularly true of proximal extremity injuries. Therefore, the surgeon must closely monitor fluid status postoperatively to prevent hypovolemia and/or hypotension.

After the blood supply is reestablished in a major limb amputation, there is a period of acute acidosis as a consequence of absorption of metabolic products from the ischemic extremity when venous return begins. This acidosis is aggressively treated with the administration of bicarbonate. Both bicarbonate and mannitol are administered to protect against myoglobin-associated renal damage; prophylactic antibiotics are also administered. If early severe sepsis supervenes, the extremity may have to be amputated. Low-grade late infection, usually consisting of osteomyelitis, is treated by drainage and irrigation. The fixation materials are left in place until the bone heals, even in the face of sepsis, because fixation must be achieved if possible.

Muscle and Musculocutaneous Grafts

Occasionally, following a severe trauma or extirpative surgery, vital structures such as brain, bone periosteum, tendon, nerve, and major vascular structures become exposed in a wound. Such wounds require full-thickness flap coverage to preserve the viability of these important structures and promote functional recovery. When no local or regional flaps are available for transfer, autogenous muscle or musculocutaneous flaps must be grafted using microsurgical techniques. The most commonly used muscles and musculocutaneous flaps are the rectus abdominis, perfused on the inferior epigastric arterial pedicle, and the latissimus dorsi, perfused by the thoracodorsal artery and vein. Microsurgical transfer of these muscles results in minimal donor site functional morbidity and provides a large volume of tissue for reconstruction of the wound.

Following harvest, the muscles are revascularized using appropriate recipient vessels in the region of wound. Care must be taken to perform the microsurgical anastomosis outside the zone of injury so that normal vessels are used to revascularize the flap. These free flap transfers are commonly done by organized microsurgical teams where technical skills are maintained by a high volume of replantation and reconstructive surgery.

Other free flaps are occasionally used for specialized situations. The skin and soft tissue of dorsum of the foot perfused by the dorsalis pedis artery, and thin skin of the volar forearm perfused by the radial artery, are occasionally used for reconstructions in the head, neck, and face where their thinness and malleability are an asset. The great toe or the second toe perfused on the dorsalis pedis axis can be transferred to reconstruct the thumb or hand where no digits are available for opposition. These transfers are extremely complex, and require reconnection of tendons, nerves, and bone, as well as successful microvascular anastomosis.

Microsurgical techniques have significantly increased the reconstructive surgeon's armamentarium. Using microsurgery, a wide variety of autogenous transplants are possible and can provide functioning tissue where it is needed. As methods to prolong graft survival improve, similar tissue transfer of allografts and even xenografts may become possible for reconstructive purposes.

Bone Marrow Transplantation

The pluripotent bone marrow stem cell is now known to provide the host with red blood cells, platelets, neutrophils, glial cells of the brain, plus all components of the immune system: T cells, B cells, natural killer (NK) cells, macrophages and other antigen-presenting cells, and monocytes. A privileged time exists early in development (up to 16 weeks in the human fetus) in which transplanted bone marrow will engraft readily. Following this time point, the host stem cells must be destroyed by irradiation, drugs, or chemicals, to "make space" for the newly transplanted bone marrow stem cells. Bone marrow transplantation has become a clinically preferred approach to treat numerous hematologic malignancies (e.g., leukemia), aplastic anemia, solid tumors with widespread metastatic disease, severe combined immunodeficiency (SCID) states, and a number of genetic and metabolic defects. Both autografts and allografts can be utilized, and the type of graft performed is dependent on the disease state. The majority of bone marrow transplants performed are for treatment of cancer, since larger doses of chemotherapy can be utilized and if the marrow is damaged the transplant can replace the damaged stem cells. In addition, replacement of an existing hematologic malignancy (e.g., leukemia) can be achieved by destruction of the cells of the recipient and transplantation of donor (or modified host) bone marrow.

Bone marrow autotransplants and transplants between identical twins have enjoyed the greatest success. They have been utilized for treatment of irradiation exposure, aplastic anemia, and leukemia. Because the bone marrow cells of the donor are an identical match with the recipient, graft take is usually readily achieved and graft-versus-host reactivity (see below) does not occur. Autologous bone marrow (self → self) transplantation may allow higher doses of chemotherapy to be utilized to treat malignancy without the limitation of untreatable bone marrow destruction, since many of the anticancer drugs have as a side effect suppression of the rapidly dividing bone marrow cells.

Allogenic bone marrow transplantation is successfully utilized for a number of disease states. The host must be prepared or conditioned to accept the donor bone marrow cells by the use of pharmacologic agents or irradiation to remove recipient stem cells. This is usually done for treatment of hematologic cancers in which the desired result is complete replacement of the recipient's bone marrow compartment (and therefore the cancer) with that of the donor. Unlike any other allograft, once bone marrow cells are accepted by the recipient, no further immunosuppression is required to permit permanent graft survival. A chimeric state results in which tissues from two genetically different sources (the donor and recipient) coexist. In fact, bone marrow grafts possess the unique ability to confer tolerance in the form of permanent graft acceptance for subsequent tissue and organ grafts. The recipient is tolerant to the donor and sees the donor as part of self. However, if mature donor T cells accompany the bone marrow graft, they can attack the host, which they see as foreign, resulting in graft-vs.-host (GVH) reactivity. The target tissues of these donor lymphocytes are those of epithelial origin and include the skin, liver, and gastrointestinal tract, resulting in signs including generalized skin rash, liver failure, diarrhea, and wasting. The greater the genetic difference between donor and recipient, the stronger the GVH reaction.

In clinical trials, depletion of the GVH-causing T lymphocytes from the donor bone marrow significantly reduced the severity and incidence of GVH disease. However, removal of those T cells from the bone marrow transplant also resulted in a significant rate of failure of graft take and in death, demonstrating for the first time that T cells must be present to help the pluripotent bone marrow stem cells to engraft. GVH, therefore, remains a major challenge in allogenic bone marrow transplantation, since most centers no longer consider depletion of T cells from the bone marrow transplant to be acceptable in view of the increased risk in failure of graft take. The use of immunosuppressive drugs such as FK506 and cyclosporine A plus steroids lessens, but does not eliminate, GVH in bone marrow transplant recipients. Studies are in progress to identify which T cells help the stem cell to engraft, allowing only the GVH-causing T cells to be removed prior to bone marrow transplantation.

Although it was once believed that GVH could not occur in the absence of donor bone marrow, it has become apparent that this is not true. Three factors are essential for the existence of GVH: (1) recognizable antigenic difference between the donor and the host; (2) immunocompetent donor T cells; and (3) a relative immunocompromise of the recipient. Recently, GVH has been identified in transplant patients who have received solid organ grafts (especially liver) and after blood transfusions in patients undergoing major operations (especially cardiac surgery). The same target tissues are affected, and bone marrow aplasia also occurs, since the stem cell is still of host origin and, therefore, a target of attack. The diagnosis is dependent on astute clinical observation (skin rash, hepatic dysfunction, intestinal symptoms, and myelosuppression) and a high index of suspicion, and can be established with a skin biopsy. Treatment is by immunosuppression, usually FK506 or cyclosporine, plus steroids. If the diagnosis is missed, the condition is almost uniformly fatal.

The use of bone marrow to induce tolerance to subsequent solid organ grafts, such as liver, heart, and kidney, has been considered as a potential approach to achieve long-term rejection-free graft survival without chronic nonspecific immunosuppression. Significant success has been achieved in a number of species, and studies are in progress to attempt this approach clinically.

Endocrine Grafts (Other Than the Pancreas)

The placement of endocrine fragments as autografts into intramuscular pockets has been successful in several clinical situations. The indications for parathyroid autotransplantation are listed in Table 10-5. When it appears possible that a patient may have insufficient parathyroid tissue following removal of the thyroid gland, or of all four parathyroid glands for chief cell hyperplasia, the glands should be diced and implanted into intramuscular pockets. The volar forearm muscle is a useful site for autotransplantation because the parathyroids are readily available for subsequent excision if hyperparathyroidism recurs. Their function can be easily assessed by hormone assay of antecubital vein blood.

Similar indications for transplantation of other endocrine organs have been suggested. None of these indications has been well defined, however, because hormonal replacement (parathyroids excepted) is simpler. Endocrine allografts would provide a more physiologic approach to treat various disease states of endocrine dysfunction. However, one cannot justify the immunosuppressive agents required to prevent rejection of endocrine allografts since replacement therapy for endocrine deficiency (except for insulin deficiency) is generally adequate. In the case of parathyroid allotransplants, there has been an insistent and recurrently hopeful effort. Parathyroid deficiency is not treated with specific hormone replacement, but rather with calcium and vitamin D, which give inadequate results. An occasionally successful parathyroid allotransplant in a patient with a functioning renal allograft already receiving immunosuppressive drugs has been reported.

ORGAN TRANSPLANTATION

Pancreas

The discovery of insulin in 1921 was hailed as the cure of diabetes; it prevented death from diabetic coma, controlled the overt symptoms of diabetes, and provided an increased life expectancy. As diabetic patients lived longer, however, previously unseen complications developed and the disease has become better understood. It has become apparent that Type I diabetes is a true autoimmune state, in which the patient loses tolerance to self, resulting in an attack on the target tissues. In essence, the patient attempts to reject himself or herself. Diabetes was responsible for at least 30,000 deaths in 1974, and it is the leading cause of new cases of blindness in adults. Diabetics are seventeen times more liable to kidney disease, five times more liable to gangrene of the extremities, and twice as likely to develop heart diseases. Diabetes is now the number one cause of renal failure requiring dialysis or renal transplantation in the United States. Obviously, new approaches to treatment are required. Pancreas and islet transplantation offer the possibility that the development and progression of diabetic lesions will be prevented by precise regulation of carbohydrate metabolism, control not yet achieved by injected insulin.

Table 10-5
Indications for Parathyroid Transplantation

1. Autotransplantation
   a. Severe secondary hyperparathyroidism
   b. Primary generalized parathyroid hyperplasia
   c. Inadvertent removal of parathyroid tissue
2. Allotransplantation
   a. Congenital absence of parathyroid glands—DiGeorge's syndrome
   b. Iatrogenic aparathyroidism that is not controllable with a medical regimen

It is well documented that tight control of glucose homeostasis reduces the complications associated with diabetes. However, it is still debated whether the complications are due only to absence of insulin or are secondary to other subcellular abnormalities such as autoimmunity. Whether normalization of carbohydrate metabolism in these patients will prevent the development of systemic lesions is being answered now with earlier pancreas and islet transplantation. Until recently, transplantation of the pancreas was performed clinically only in patients with extensive (and irreversible) complications from the disease such as renal failure.

Several observations support the hypothesis that angiopathic lesions are, in part, associated with diabetes and are secondary to abnormal metabolism:

1. Nephropathy and retinopathy occur in patients who develop diabetes as a result of other disease states (e.g., hemochromatosis) or after total pancreatectomy.
2. Numerous longitudinal clinical studies have shown a relationship between duration of the disease, control of plasma glucose, and development of lesions.
3. Nephropathy and retinopathy occur in animals with induced diabetes.
4. Studies in animals have demonstrated that reduction of hyperglycemia by insulin therapy or by transplantation of whole pancreas or islets prevents or minimizes formation of diabetic lesions in the eye, kidney, and nerve. In some patients with Type I diabetes, however, the retinopathy does not cease after transplantation of the pancreas.
5. Kidneys transplanted from normal to diabetic rats develop histologic lesions characteristic of diabetes, whereas kidneys transplanted from diabetic to normal rats showed disappearance or lack of progression of these lesions.

These observations suggest that it may be possible to prevent the systemic complications of diabetes by insulin released from transplanted pancreatic islets, a goal not achieved by tight glucose control using insulin. Alternative methods to provide precise glucose homeostasis, such as an implantable glucose sensor coupled to an insulin pump, are also possible approaches. To date, these types of approaches to achieve tight glucose control have been limited by hypoglycemia due to imperfect regulation.

It is not necessary to transplant the pancreas in order to cure diabetes; transplantation of the pancreatic islets will suffice. Because the islet tissue composes less than 2 percent of the total pancreatic mass, transplantation of the insulin-producing islet tissues is the most focused approach to treat diabetes. In addition, the vascular and ductal anastomoses required with transplantation of the whole organ are eliminated. Although it had been predicted that cellular grafts would be less antigenic than the whole organ, this has not proven true for islet grafts.

The current technique for isolation of islets from the pancreas involves mechanical disruption, enzymatic digestion, and density gradient separation (Figs. 10-30 and 10-31). Isolated adult islets infused into the portal vein will produce long-lasting control of diabetes in rats. This technique has also been successfully applied

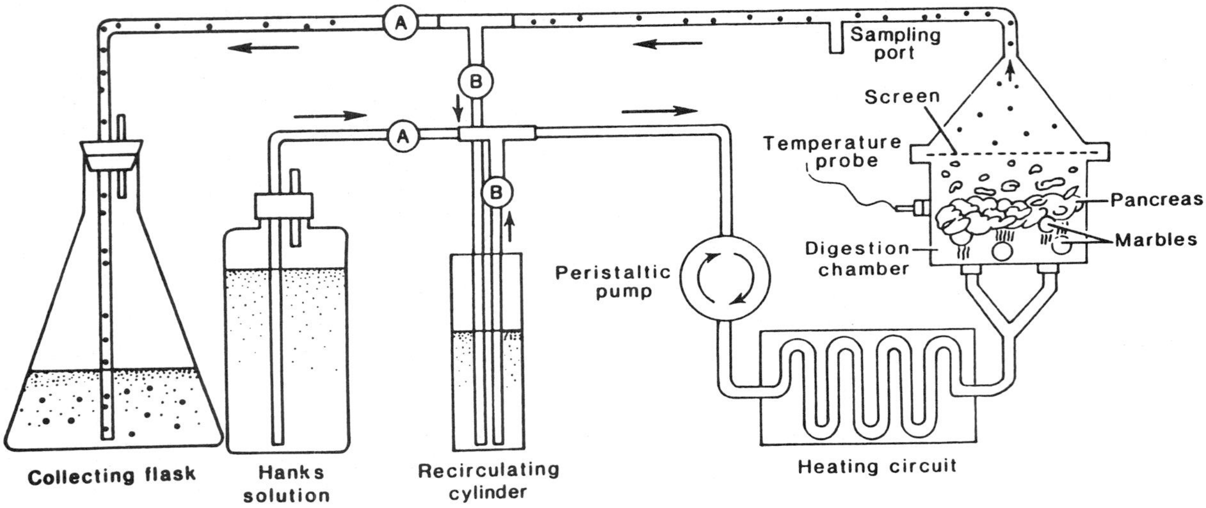

FIG. 10-30. The automated approach for isolation of islets from the pancreas involves mechanical disruption, enzymatic digestion, and density gradient separation. (Adapted from: *Ricordi C: The automated method for islet isolation, in Ricordi C [ed]: Pancreatic Islet Cell Transplantation 1892–1992: One Century of Transplantation for Diabetics. Austin, TX, RG Landes Company, 1992, p 107, with permission.*)

to the autotransplantation of islets in people who require total pancreatectomy for chronic pancreatitis. Islet allografts in nondiabetic patients remain functional and maintain glucose homeostasis if immunosuppressive agents are administered. The first successful islet allograft was performed in a fifteen-year-old female at the University of Pittsburgh for treatment of a malignancy that required en bloc resection of the liver and pancreas. It is now two years since this patient's "cluster transplant" of liver, pancreatic

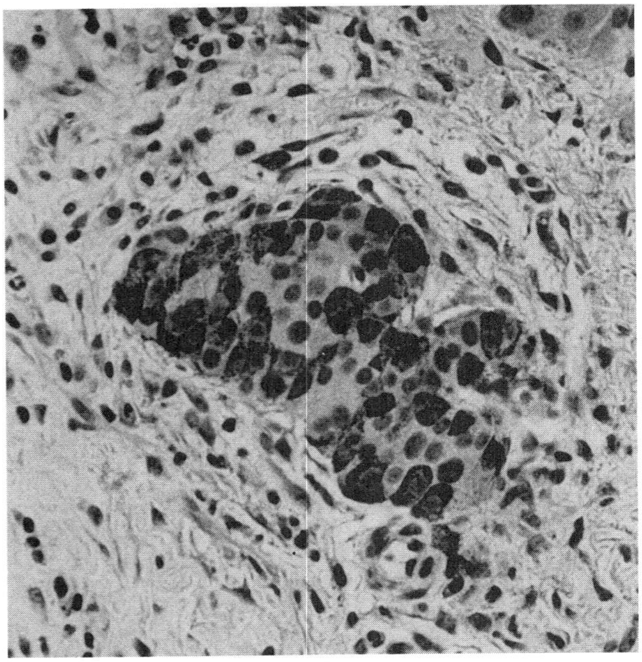

FIG. 10-31. Hepatic biopsy in recipient demonstrates viable islets in situ. (From: *Ricordi C, Tzakis A, Alejandro R, et al: Detection of pancreatic islet following islet allotransplantation in man. Transplantation 52:1080, 1991, with permission.*)

islets, and duodenum, and she remains insulin-independent. The survival of islet allografts in diabetic patients has not achieved the same success. It is currently postulated that the systemic autoimmune state associated with this disease exerts an influence on the transplanted islets and contributes to graft rejection.

Over 100 clinical islet allografts have been performed. It has now been demonstrated that transplantation of the insulin-producing islet tissue is sufficient to achieve glucose homeostasis. Clinical islet allotransplantation has been limited by the apparent increased susceptibility of islets to allograft rejection. Long-term graft survival has been difficult to achieve even when immunosuppression, which will prolong skin, kidney, or heart allografts, is used. This is especially true in diabetic recipients, in whom graft rejection appears to be accelerated. The mechanism for this action is not understood, but may be due to the autoimmunity that produces the initial disease state.

The experimental evidence that islet tissue grafts can prevent, halt, or even improve the vascular and neurologic lesions of diabetes provides a tremendous impetus to continue research, despite these limitations. The goal would be to transplant islets before the complications of diabetes (e.g., renal failure) develop or, better yet, identify methods to prevent the onset of insulin dependence.

Either whole organ or distal segmental pancreatic transplants will ameliorate experimental diabetes. In addition to the expected problems associated with the control of immunologic rejection and the need for immunosuppressive drugs, there are special technical concerns. Of these, the major problem is difficulty in establishing drainage of the pancreatic duct. Theoretically, ligation of the pancreatic duct should result in atrophy of exocrine tissue without affecting endocrine tissue, but in practice, a severe inflammatory reaction occurs and leads to a constricting fibrosis that damages even the islets. Three surgical approaches are used for pancreatic graft duct management: (1) bladder drainage; (2) ductal injection with a synthetic polymer; and (3) enteric drainage. Anastomosis of the duct with the bladder is the favored approach, with over 75 percent of all pancreatic grafts in the United States performed in this way.

As of October 1990, more than 3800 clinical pancreatic transplants had been performed. Usually cadaver organs are used, and most recipients have diabetic end-stage renal disease; both kidney and pancreas are transplanted in a single operation. Increasingly, however, as success grows, pancreatic transplantation is being carried out in patients before advanced renal disease occurs. In fact, one-fourth of all pancreatic transplants performed between 1986 and 1990 did not receive a simultaneous kidney.

Successful whole-organ or segmental pancreatic transplants produce circulating insulin and normal plasma glucose levels. When the venous drainage of the pancreatic graft is hooked up to the systemic circulation, the circulating insulin levels are higher than when the venous anastomosis is made to the portal system, although the plasma glucose levels are similar. Rejection episodes are as difficult to reverse as they are to detect. By the time glucose levels become abnormal, rejection is usually too far advanced to be reversed. Serum enzyme levels do not become elevated, and therefore do not predict graft rejection episodes. When the pancreatic duct is anastomosed to the bladder, however, the urine amylase level can be monitored. The amylase level falls early in the rejection response. Thus, the most successful technical solution also permits better immunologic monitoring of the rejection response.

Experience in human beings has shown that functioning vascularized pancreatic allograft will correct the metabolic deficiency in diabetes. The techniques (Figs. 10-32 and 10-33) are now safer and more successful. Graft survival has been steadily improving; for patients who received grafts between 1988 and 1990, slightly greater than 60 percent of grafts were functional at 36 months, in contrast with only 18 percent in 1978–1982 (Fig. 10-34). Most current clinical research continues to focus on methods of controlling pancreatic exocrine secretion without inducing pancreatitis in the transplant. Rejection, thrombosis, and fibrosis still remain challenges to widespread clinical application in the early stages of diabetes.

Transplantation of only the essential cells rather than an entire solid organ graft into a recipient is the most focused approach for treatment of a number of disorders. The field of cellular transplantation is a newly emerging specialty. Historically, bone marrow is probably the prototypic clinically successful cellular allograft. Following that, transplantation of pancreatic islets has now become an accepted clinical approach for treatment of diabetes, and clinical trials are in progress. Hepatocytes, myoblasts, and neuroendocrine cellular grafts are on the horizon.

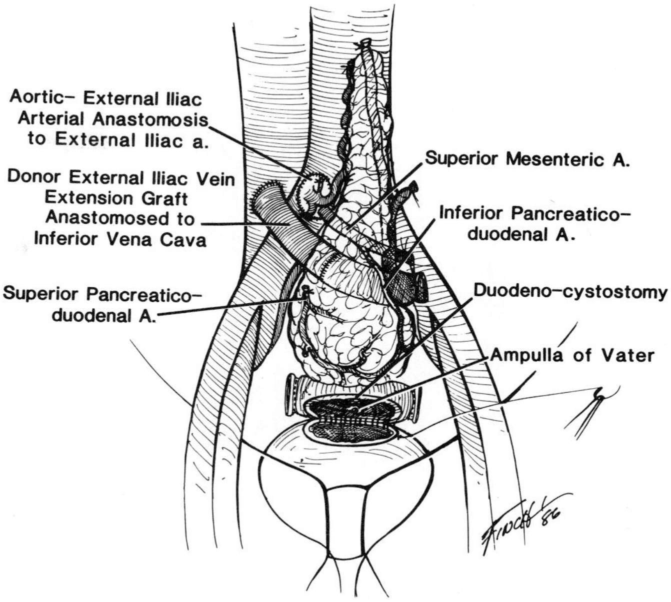

FIG. 10-33. Preferred method of pancreatic-duodenal transplantation. The whole pancreas is used. The celiac axis and superior mesenteric arteries are anastomosed to the iliac artery. The portal vein provides venous drainage. The duodenum is anastomosed to the bladder. (From: *Sutherland DER, Najarian JS, in Simmons RL, Finch M, et al [eds]: Manual of Vascular Access, Organ Donation, and Transplantation. New York, Springer-Verlag, 1984, with permission.*)

Gastrointestinal Tract

The transplantation of multiple abdominal viscera, including liver, duodenum, and pancreas or liver-stomach-duodenum-pancreas, or liver-intestine en bloc, is being performed clinically with increasing success. "Cluster" transplants have been used after removal of the recipient liver, pancreas, stomach, spleen, duodenum, and proximal jejunum (Fig. 10-35). The majority of these operations

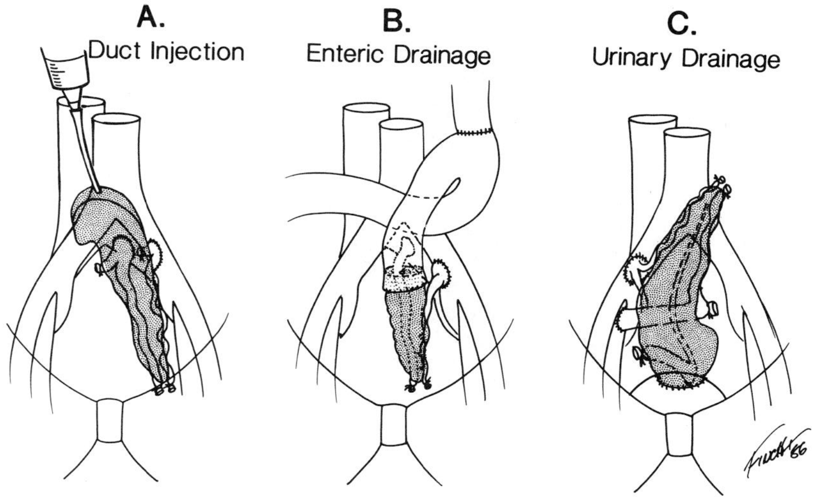

FIG. 10-32. Technique of pancreatic transplantation. The body and tail can be transplanted with anastomoses of splenic vessels of donor pancreas to iliac vessels of recipient. The duct can be injected with a polymer to occlude it, or the duct can be anastomosed to a loop of bowel or the bladder. These techniques are still in use in some centers. (Adapted from: *Sutherland DER, Kendall D, et al: Surg Clin North Am 66:557, 1986, with permission.*)

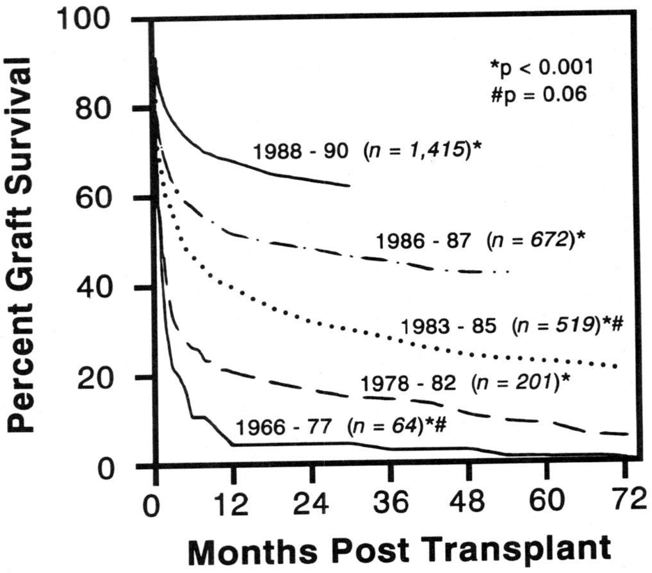

FIG. 10-34. Functional survival of pancreas allografts by year of procedure. Note steady improvement in overall graft survival, with in excess of 60% of grafts between 1988 and 1990 functioning at 36 months.

have been performed for treatment of extensive but localized intra-abdominal malignancy involving the liver or pancreas.

Various segments of intestine can be autotransplanted by removal from the body and reimplantation. Stomach, small bowel, and colon can be used to replace esophagus, with reimplantation of the vascular supply. Allotransplantation of the small bowel is now performed clinically. A number of successes have been reported. The largest series is from the University of Pittsburgh. Under FK506 treatment, the University of Pittsburgh has performed 15 small intestine transplants. Although GVH disease was anticipated due to the high lymphoid burden of the small intestine, this has not proven to be a limitation.

The most common patients are pediatric recipients who have lost their small intestine secondary to malrotation with midgut volvulus or necrotizing enterocolitis (NEC). Hyperalimentation for nutritional support is a temporizing measure, but chronic use of this method of nutritional support is associated with cirrhosis and liver failure. In addition, vascular access often becomes a limitation in patients on chronic hyperalimentation, since an indwelling foreign body predisposes to thrombosis. In most of the early recipients, combined liver plus small bowel transplantation has been required due to end-stage cirrhosis associated with chronic hyperalimentation (Fig. 10-36). Recently, small bowel transplantation has been performed before the development of hepatic failure.

Liver

Liver transplantation has become a highly successful solution to a variety of congenital and acquired hepatic disorders in thousands of patients. A liver transplant is usually positioned in the normal anatomic location (orthotopic transplantation) following a total hepatectomy of the recipient. Alternatively, the donor organ can be placed in an ectopic site (heterotopic transplantation), generally with retention of the host's liver (auxiliary transplantation). Orthotopic grafts are universally preferred by clinicians.

Indications. In theory, liver transplantation is appropriate for any disease that results in liver failure (Table 10-6). In a recent analysis of 2395 liver transplants performed at the University of Pittsburgh between 1981 and 1989, the most frequent underlying disease that resulted in liver failure was chronic active hepatitis (27 percent of total grafts), followed by cholestatic liver disease, including primary biliary cirrhosis and sclerosing cholangitis (21 percent), followed by biliary atresia (16.7 percent) and alcoholic cirrhosis (8.5 percent). In children the most common indication for transplantation is extrahepatic biliary atresia. Virtually all these patients previously have had one or more Kasai procedures.

Transplantation is contraindicated in any patient with (1) irreversible infection, (2) widespread malignancy, (3) concurrent disease (e.g., myocardial failure, old age) that would seriously impair survival, or (4) a high risk for recurrent disease in the transplant

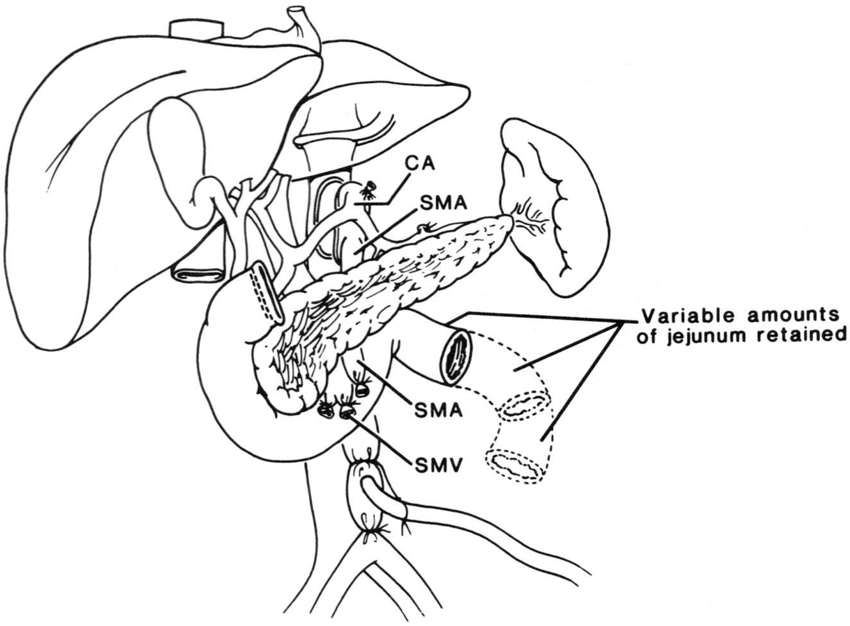

FIG. 10-35. Cluster allograft used to replace resected viscera after exenteration of the upper part of the abdomen for localized malignancy. Resection usually includes the recipient liver, pancreas, stomach, spleen, duodenum, proximal jejunum, and a portion of the colon. CA = celiac axis; SMA = superior mesenteric artery; SMV = superior mesenteric vein. (From: *Starzl TE, Todo S, Tzakis A, et al: The many faces of multivisceral transplantation. Surg Gynecol Obstet 172:339, 1991, with permission.*)

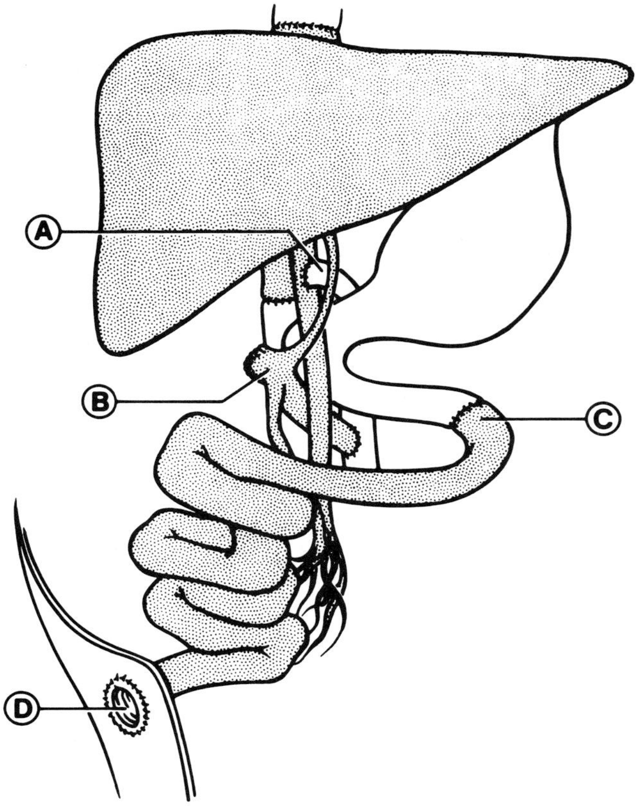

FIG. 10-36. Diagram of reconstructed small bowel/liver graft *(stippled)*. A = anastomosis with end of recipient's portal vein to side of donor portal vein; B = aortic conduit with origins of celiac artery and superior mesenteric artery; C = anastomosis of donor jejunum to the recipient's duodenum; D = ileostomy. (From: *Grant D, Wall W, Mimeault R, et al: Successful small bowel/liver transplantation. Lancet 335:182, 1990, with permission.*)

organ. Because active hepatitis also usually recurs, the presence of HBsAg or HBeAg antigenemia is a relative contraindication. The risk of recurrent alcoholism also makes alcoholic cirrhosis a relative contraindication unless the patient has abstained from alcohol for at least 2 years. In patients with sclerosing cholangitis, active ulcerative colitis also rules out liver transplantation. Patients with portal vein thrombosis cannot be successfully revascularized with orthotopic grafts.

In pediatric patients, size discrepancy has been a major limitation to hepatic transplantation and has limited the number of donor organs available. *Reduced-size liver transplants* have provided a solution to this problem, expanding the potential donor pool for pediatric recipients. The greatest success has been achieved when transplantation of the right, left, or left lateral lobe of the donor liver is carried out.

Before the technique for reduced-size liver transplantation was developed, approximately 50 percent of small children awaiting a liver transplant died before a donor of suitable size became available. Living related donor liver transplantation in children has also been performed at some centers because of the critical shortage of donor organs of appropriate size. In this approach, a portion of the donor liver is carefully removed and transplanted into the recipient. The transplant community is divided on whether subjecting the donor to the potential morbidity and mortality associated with a

Table 10-6
Common Indications for Hepatic Transplantation

Adult	*Children*
Chronic active hepatitis	Biliary atresia
Alcoholic cirrhosis	Chronic active hepatitis
Primary biliary cirrhosis	Hepatoma
Secondary biliary cirrhosis	Neonatal hepatitis
Secondary cholangitis	General hepatic fibrosis
α-1-Antitrypsin deficiency	Secondary biliary cirrhosis
Hemachromatosis	Inborn errors of metabolism
Budd-Chiari syndrome	
Acute hepatitis B	

SOURCE: Modified from Ascher NL, Simmons RL, Najarian JS: Host hepatectomy and liver transplantation, in Simmons RL, Finch ME, Ascher NL, Najarian JS (eds): *Manual of Vascular Access, Organ Donation, and Transplantation.* New York, Springer-Verlag, 1984, pp 255–284.

partial hepatic resection is justified. One hopes that in the future living related liver donation will be replaced by xenotransplantation (cross-species) or by expanding the donor pool in other ways.

Preoperative Evaluation of the Recipient. Intensive preoperative evaluation is designed to (1) characterize those physiologic defects in hepatic, pulmonary, renal, or cardiac function that will influence the patient's chance of survival, (2) determine whether the transplant is technically feasible for that particular patient, and (3) search out sites of occult infection and malignancy (Table 10-7).

During the complete history and physical examination, special attention is given to specific extrahepatic organ systems. For example, fluid overload and congestive heart failure are frequently present and must be treated with fluid restriction, diuretics, and Lanoxin. In adults, roentgenograms of the chest and electrocardiograms are obtained, and a stress exercise test is done if recommended after a formal cardiology consultation.

Attention to respiratory reserve is important. Because all patients are respirator-dependent in the early posttransplant period, knowledge of their prior pulmonary function will help during the process of weaning from the respirator. Therefore, pulmonary function tests are obtained on all adult patients but only arterial blood gases and chest roentgenograms are necessary for pediatric patients. Postoperative ascites or a marginally oversized donor liver can further compromise respiratory function.

A variety of preoperative tests are obtained to assess hepatocellular function (Table 10-7). Hepatitis screening results will determine the need for hyperimmune globulin to prevent recurrent hepatitis, and unsuspected tumors are sought using α-fetoprotein, hepatic ultrasound, and computed tomography (CT). A coagulation profile is obtained to document functional capacity of the liver and predict the need for correction. An uncorrectable prothrombin time abnormality is a poor prognostic sign. A radionuclide hepatic excretion scan will reveal unsuspected biliary calculi that must be removed from the common bile duct at the time of recipient hepatectomy. An upper gastrointestinal series and upper gastrointestinal endoscopy will reveal the presence of gastric or esophageal varices. Sclerotherapy is used to treat bleeding esophageal varices while the patient is awaiting transplantation. Transjugular intrahepatic portosystemic shunts (TIPS) can be placed percutaneously in patients with severe portal hypertension from cirrhosis. This approach results in decreased bleeding perioperatively and has been utilized in patients with variceal bleeding in place of emergency

Table 10-7
Work-up of Potential Recipients for Liver Transplantation

1. General
   a. History and physical examination
   b. Chest roentgenogram
   c. Electrocardiogram (ECG)
   d. Serum electrolytes
   e. Fasting blood sugar
2. Hematology
   a. Hemoglobin, leukocyte count, and differential count
   b. Platelet count, bleeding-clotting time, prothrombin time, partial thromboplastin time, thrombin time (factor analysis)
3. Hepatic
   a. Bilirubin, alkaline phosphatase, serum glutamic pyruvic transaminase (SGPT), aspartate aminotransferase (AST)
   b. Protein electrophoresis
   c. Serum amino acid analysis
   d. α-Fetoprotein
   e. Ultrasound
   f. Ascitic cytology and culture
4. Nutritional evaluation
   a. Transferrin, prealbumin, serum amino acid analysis
5. Renal
   a. Urinalysis
   b. Blood urea nitrogen (BUN), serum creatinine
   c. 24-h creatinine clearance
6. Calcium metabolism (primary biliary cirrhosis)
   a. (Bone roentgenograms: hands, skull, clavical, lamina dura)
   b. (Ca, PO_4, Mg, alkaline phosphatase)
   c. (Parathormone)
7. Gastrointestinal
   a. Upper GI series
   b. Upper GI endoscopy
   c. (Variceal sclerotherapy)
8. Immunologic studies
   a. Blood type (ABO)
   b. Tissue typing including serial cytotoxic antibody determinations
9. Pulmonary function studies
   a. Chest roentgenogram
   b. Blood gases
   c. Pulmonary function tests
10. Infectious work-up
    a. Chest roentgenogram
    b. Blood, urine, throat, feces, ascites cultures
    c. Hepatitis screen
    d. Dental consult
11. Financial-social rehabilitation

The tests enclosed within parentheses are not administered routinely during the potential recipient work-up, but only when the circumstances indicate.

SOURCE: Modified from Ascher NL, Simmons RL, Najarian JS: Host hepatectomy and liver transplantation, in Simmons RL, Finch ME, Ascher NL, Najarian JS (eds): *Manual of Vascular Access, Organ Donation, and Transplantation*. New York, Springer-Verlag, 1984, pp 255–284.

portacaval shunting procedures. Oral nystatin antifungal prophylaxis must be used to prevent invasive candidiasis at the sclerotherapy site.

Patency of the portal vein system must be determined before transplantation because occlusion of the portal vein contraindicates liver transplant. CT scans used to detect silent malignancy may also show portal vein patency. If either CT scan or ultrasonography fails to visualize the portal vein, celiac angiography, with special attention to the venous phase, may be required.

The value of immunologic testing has not been determined, but most centers prefer that liver donors and recipients are ABO compatible. Unlike the kidney, however, in which ABO mismatching results in immediate hyperacute rejection, liver transplantation across ABO disparities is tolerated. HLA matching is not required for hepatic transplants. In fact, there are data to suggest that HLA matching results in an inferior survival for hepatic grafts.

While the patient is awaiting transplant a program of pretransplant management is set up to optimize the patient's general condition and to improve the suboptimal function of the multiple organ systems. Nutritional and respiratory functions receive special attention. All patients, especially those with pulmonary insufficiency, are begun on an intensive program of pulmonary toilet and exercise. For example, smokers must stop smoking, and postural drainage and short courses of broad-spectrum antibiotics may be necessary to treat bacterial infection.

The patient's preoperative nutritional status may be enhanced by cautiously increasing dietary protein while monitoring the serum ammonia and serial amino acid profiles.

Immediate Pretransplant Management. A rigidly defined protocol must be set up for the recipient as soon as a potential cadaver donor is located. Most of the procedures simply reassess the patient's condition, while others are designed to prevent infection, replace blood loss, correct coagulation defects, and institute immunosuppression. Prophylactic antibiotics are begun to reduce colonization of the gastrointestinal tract, to minimize wound infection, or to provide protection against infection.

Immediate preoperative exchange transfusion is indicated in all patients with impaired coagulation parameters, even though an effective exchange often results from the replacement of lost blood during the early stages of the operation. To effect rapid replacement of blood loss or perform exchange transfusion, central venous cannulation must be carried out. Systemic arterial and pulmonary artery pressure measurements should be monitored during the administration of fresh frozen plasma and load-reducing agents. This requires both arterial and pulmonary artery cannulation (Swan–Ganz catheter).

Technique. Liver transplantation is a relatively straightforward procedure, although excessive bleeding, brought on by the extensive collateral venous system caused by the patient's portal hypertension, makes the native hepatectomy the most difficult part of the transplant process. Complications can occur if there is a septic focus, or if residual scars exist from prior operations (portosystemic shunts; attempts at biliary decompression). If technical difficulties prohibit the completion of the liver transplant, the patient will die.

The following eight precautions should be followed: (1) Do not remove the spleen (bleeding is excessive, removal obviates an important portosystemic collateral pathway, and splenic vein flow may be essential to maintain a patent portal vein); (2) minimize retroperitoneal dissection; (3) do not interfere with collateral vessels; (4) avoid thoracic incisions; (5) preserve the blood supply to the distal common duct by minimizing dissection in this region; (6) preserve as much length of suprahepatic vena cava, portal vein, hepatic artery, and infrahepatic vena cava as possible; (7) avoid clamp injury to the renal vessels; and (8) match the weights of donor and recipient ± 20 percent. In children the donor can be smaller by as much as 20 percent but only minimally larger.

The most common incision for an orthotopic liver graft is a transverse abdominal incision. The diseased liver is dissected free, and clamps are applied to the suprahepatic and intrahepatic vena cava, the portal vein, and the hepatic artery. The liver can then be removed and replaced by the cadaver liver. Many surgeons perform a portal vein–to–superior vena cava temporary shunt so that the splanchnic venous bed does not become excessively congested during clamping of the portal vein. A concurrent temporary inferior vena cava–to–superior vena cava shunt minimizes renal venous congestion and permits the return of blood to the heart during the anhepatic phase.

The allograft anastomoses are shown in Fig. 10-37. The suprahepatic caval anastomosis is the most difficult to perform. The second anastomosis is usually the portal vein to minimize venous congestion of the intestine. After the portal vein anastomosis is completed, the inferior hepatic caval clamps should be briefly removed, leaving the suprahepatic vena cava clamped. The portal vein inflow should be opened to allow the liver to be perfused with warm blood. This sequence is useful to remove the cold perfusate from the liver and prevent systemic hypothermia and heparinization. As soon as the perfusate is washed from the liver and it becomes firm and pink, the intrahepatic vena cava is clamped, and the suprahepatic vena cava clamp is removed. The remaining vascular anastomoses (hepatic artery, inferior vena cava) can then be accomplished.

Following the vascular anastomoses, biliary drainage must be obtained. A direct bile duct–to–bile duct anastomosis is preferred in adults. A choledochojejunostomy is preferred in children.

As many as 30 to 40 percent of patients have double hepatic arteries, and one of them may arise from the superior mesenteric artery. Care must be taken during the donor operation to preserve this arterial supply to the transplanted liver.

Postoperative Management. The early posttransplant management of liver recipients is so complex that protocols have been designed to guarantee that crucial details are not omitted. If renal function is satisfactory, cyclosporine and prednisone are preferred for immunosuppression. If renal function is poor, cyclosporine is omitted and antilymphoblast serum and azathioprine are used until the acute recovery period has stabilized. Recently, the use of FK506 has been applied to prevent hepatic graft rejection. In combination with steroids, it was at least as effective as cyclosporine (Fig. 10-38). One added advantage is that FK506 is often steroid-sparing, allowing one to discontinue chronic steroid use after the early period following transplantation. This is of particular benefit in children, since growth is promoted.

Some degree of acute tubular necrosis is common in the immediate postoperative period, probably because of poor perfusion due to blood loss and the clamping of the inferior vena cava, with renal venous hypertension. If renal function is already compromised, the nephrotoxic effect of cyclosporine can be minimized by delaying its use until 12 h after transplantation. Constant monitoring of renal function and cyclosporine levels will ensure the precise adjustment of the dosage.

Respiratory support is usually required for at least 24 to 48 h after extubation. Most patients can then be transferred to a regular nursing ward. Nasogastric suction is maintained until bowel function returns, and intravenous hyperalimentation is used until they can eat. Levels of BUN, creatinine, electrolytes, calcium, phosphate, white blood cell count, and hemoglobin are determined daily. Chest roentgenograms are taken daily for 5 days, and whenever the patient becomes febrile, to seek evidence for atelectasis, pneumonia, diaphragmatic paralysis, and pleural effusion. Culture samples are taken as indicated.

Monitoring liver transplant function with frequent chemical determination of coagulation parameters (especially prothrombin time, factor V levels, the serum bilirubin, transaminase, and alkaline phosphatase levels) is mandatory. Changes in these levels can signal rejection, ischemia, viral infection, cholangitis, or mechanical obstruction.

A radionuclide excretory cholangiogram is performed on postoperative day 3 and at weekly intervals; excretion of the radioisotope by the liver into the small bowel by 45 min is considered normal. A delay can reflect hepatocellular damage during death of the donor, complications of the donor operation, prolonged cold storage, vascular compromise, or rejection. Also, delayed excretion into the biliary tree can reflect rejection, hepatocellular dam-

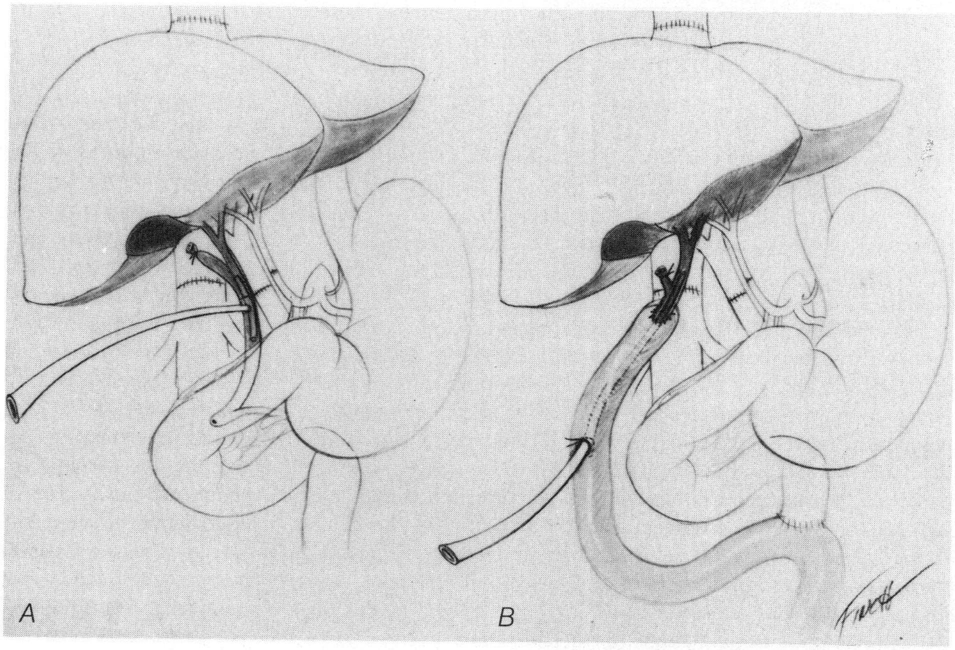

FIG. 10-37. Completed orthotopic liver transplant in *(A)* adults and *(B)* children. The two preferred methods of biliary reconstruction are illustrated. (From: *Ascher NL, Najarian JS, et al, in Simmons RL, Finch M, et al [eds]: Manual of Vascular Access, Organ Donation, and Transplantation. New York, Springer-Verlag, 1984, with permission.*)

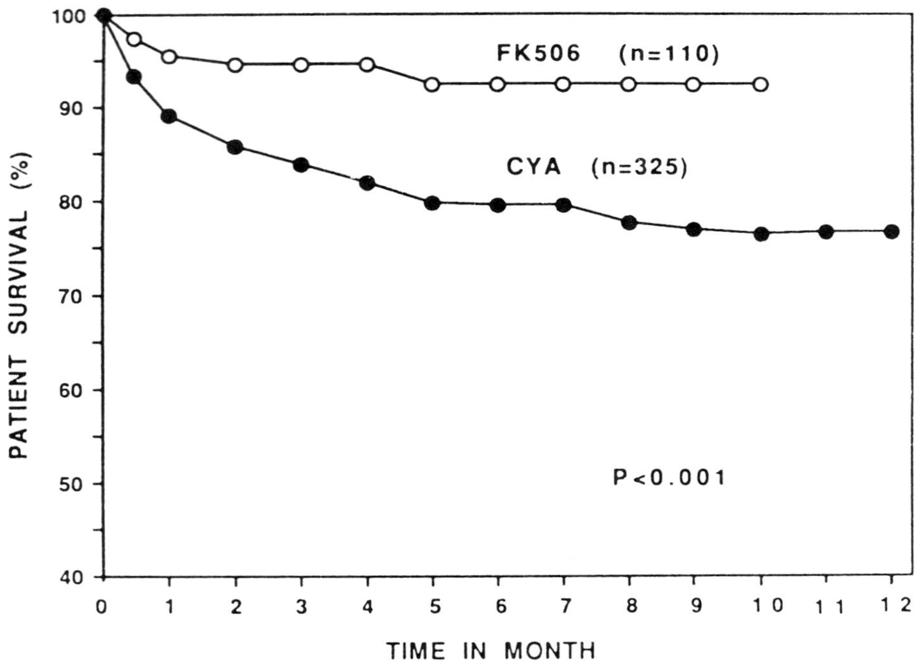

FIG. 10-38. Patient survival curves in 110 consecutive adult liver recipients treated with FK506, and 325 historical controls under conventional immunosuppression (CYA = cyclosporine). (From: *Todo S, Fung JJ, et al: One hundred ten consecutive primary orthotopic liver transplants under FK506 in adults. Transplant Proc 23:1398, 1991, with permission.*)

age from ischemia, or viral infection. Delayed passage into the small bowel can indicate mechanical obstruction or breakdown. A T-tube cholangiogram (performed with gravity) will diagnose breakdown at the site of biliary drainage, or if a T tube has not been used (e.g., with a cholecystojejunostomy), transhepatic cholangiography may be necessary to evaluate the biliary system.

During rejection, lymphocytes infiltrate portal tracts and central veins, with varying degrees of bile duct epithelial damage; therefore, a percutaneous liver transplant biopsy and culture is the only way to differentiate among rejection, ischemia, viral infection, and cholangitis. Rejection is treated initially with intravenous steroids, OKT3, or antilymphoblast globulin. The presence of polymorphonuclear leukocytes within the portal tracts indicates cholangitis. The patient is treated with antibiotics and a search is made for a mechanical obstruction as an underlying cause. Cytomegalovirus (CMV) hepatitis is treated with ganciclovir. Recent protocols which have used this drug prophylactically have demonstrated a lower incidence of life-threatening viral infections.

Postoperative Complications. The most serious complication is *primary nonfunction,* in which the liver fails to function sufficiently well to support life. This may be a result of ischemia, technical factors, or accelerated rejection. Primary nonfunction is first suspected when factor V levels in the plasma fail to return to normal.

Intraoperative bleeding results from many causes; extensive portosystemic shunts are almost always present and global coagulation defects always exist. Even when hemostasis appears adequate during operation, bleeding is a special hazard in the immediate postoperative period. Coagulation parameters, including platelet levels and serum calcium levels, must be measured during closure of the abdomen so that they can be corrected. Blood loss may continue into the postoperative period, although immediate normal transplant function will minimize these complications. A normal prothrombin time and factor V level is an early sign that normal function has returned.

Thrombotic occlusion of either the hepatic artery or portal vein will cause sudden deterioration of hepatic function. The bilirubin and transaminase values rise rapidly; coagulopathy, hyperkalemia, and hypoglycemia appear, and the liver fails to extract radionuclides during liver scan. In many centers, these catastrophes are indications for retransplantation.

Vena caval stenosis (most often the suprahepatic anastomosis) leads to edema in the lower trunk and renal insufficiency. An angiogram of the vena cava will confirm the diagnosis. Operative repair must be undertaken. Milder degrees of stenosis of the suprahepatic vena cava anastomosis in children declare themselves by nonspecific alterations in hepatic function: persistent ascites, elevated bilirubin, and hepatic enzymes. Balloon angioplasty can be used for vena cava stenosis in the late postoperative period.

Respiratory complications are common. Liver transplant recipients have ascites, pleural effusion, paralyzed diaphragms, and a new edematous liver. The operative pain and spasms of the abdominal wall add to the high risk of pulmonary complications. The atelectasis can easily become complicated by pneumonia. Prophylaxis includes both training the prospective recipients to use their accessory respiratory muscles, and vigorous pulmonary toilet in the postoperative period. Function usually returns to a paralyzed diaphragm within 3 to 4 weeks. The ascites can be drained via peritoneal dialysis catheters if care is taken to maintain asepsis. Provided that liver function is good and infection does not supervene, almost all patients can be weaned from their sometimes lengthy respirator dependence.

Renal malfunction is common both before and after transplantation, but the posttransplant problems can be minimized by attention to a number of details: (1) maintain renal perfusion in the preoperative period by maintenance of blood volume; (2) do not compromise the renal veins or the right renal artery as it courses behind the vena cava; (3) use a portosystemic shunt during the operation to reduce renal vein pressure during the anhepatic phase; (4) intravenous cyclosporine should be infused slowly in low doses during the initial periods of recovery so that peak blood cyclosporine levels remain below nephrotoxic levels; (5) stop the use of cyclosporine therapy with the first sign of renal compromise, and temporarily use conventional immunotherapy (ALG, azathioprine); (6) avoid nephrotoxic agents (aminoglycosides, amphotericin B); and (7) remove ascites to reduce intraabdominal pressure.

Although infectious complications are no longer the most common causes of death after liver transplantation, they continue to be a major problem. The nonspecific immunosuppressive agents that are required to prevent rejection of the graft also impair host immune responses to pathogens. The incidence of bacterial sepsis has diminished with the judicious use of cyclosporine, antibiotic prophylaxis, and newer methods of biliary drainage. Cholangitis and biliary anastomotic breakdown are now rare. Even so, perioperative antibiotics should be used in repeated doses during operation because the blood loss is great and the operation is long. Postoperative antibiotics should be based on intraoperative culture results of contaminated material.

Prophylactic administration of oral trimethoprim sulfamethoxazole will reduce the postoperative incidence of *Pneumocystis carinii* and *Nocardia* infections, as it does in renal transplant patients. With successful control of bacterial and protozoal infections using prophylactic antibiotic therapy, fungal and viral infections have become the most frequent infections in transplant recipients. The postoperative use of high-dose oral, esophageal, and gastric nystatin and the antiviral agents acyclovir and ganciclovir has resulted in a reduction in the incidence of these infections. Prompt institution of systemic amphotericin B for candidiasis without fungemia will minimize the adverse consequences.

Central venous pressure lines should be removed as soon as possible to decrease the chance of their colonization.

Viral infections are a major problem. The most serious is cytomegalovirus (CMV). CMV can be treated with acyclovir or ganciclovir, which are antiviral drugs. Both of these agents are being studied as prophylactic agents in clinical trials.

Cholangitis in the absence of discernible biliary obstruction is more common than previously described. Only by biopsy of the transplant can it be diagnosed. Culture of the specimen permits rational antimicrobial therapy.

Subclinical and reversible rejection episodes are commonly detected if liver biopsies are carried out at weekly intervals. Rejection may occur at any time in the postoperative period, including the first 24 h, but most cases occur at least several weeks after transplantation.

Results. Although the first liver transplant in a human being was performed in 1963, the procedure was not successful until 1967. From then until 1978 the results were generally poor, with 1-year survival figures ranging from 25 to 30 percent. The addition of cyclosporine to prednisone, or to prednisone plus azathioprine, resulted in a dramatic improvement in outcome, with a 1-year graft survival rate of approximately 80 percent. Liver transplantation is now considered a therapeutic option for an ever-expanding number of diseases that result in end-stage hepatic failure. In a series reported by Starzl's group at the University of Pittsburgh, analyzing the "Cyclosporine Decade" (1981–1988), overall survival for 1819 patients approximated 80 percent at 1 year and was in excess of 65 percent at 5 years. In preliminary studies, the use of FK506 appeared to be at least as promising (Fig. 10-38). Many other new drugs are on the horizon.

Cardiac Transplantation

Historical Development. When the first human heart transplant was performed, by Christiaan Barnard in 1967, a flurry of imitation was triggered throughout the world. Disappointing early results led to a backlash of public disparagement, and early eclipse into disfavor by 1970. More cardiac transplants were performed in 1968 (102) than were performed in any subsequent year until 1981.

Discouragement with early clinical results tended to overshadow the substantial experimental foundations of the procedure. Heterotopic transplants, in which the heart is placed in parallel in the circulation, were done as early as 1905 by Carrel and Guthrie. Orthotopic transplants, in which the donor heart replaces the recipient heart, were first done successfully in dogs by Lower and Shumway in 1959. By 1967 the operative technique was well refined, and the procedure was quite reproducible in animals. Operative technique has changed remarkably little in 25 years. After 1970 Shumway had the foresight to persevere clinically, and by 1982 Shumway's series at Stanford enjoyed 50 percent survival at 5 years.

With the clinical introduction of cyclosporine in 1982, cardiac transplantation entered a phase of exponential growth. More transplants were done in 1985 (984) than were done from 1967 to 1984. At the beginning of the 1980s, fewer than 10 centers in the world were performing cardiac transplants, a number that has grown to 145 in the United States alone.

Indications. Most patients requiring cardiac transplantation fall under a diagnosis of congestive cardiomyopathy, which is a broad category of diverse pathogenesis. The "idiopathic" cardiomyopathies are a heterogeneous group of conditions sharing common end-stage pathology characterized by dilated cardiac chambers, myocardial degeneration, and fibrosis. Viral cardiomyopathy is thought to account for the majority of "idiopathic" cases. Specific diagnoses such as familial cardiomyopathy, alcoholic cardiomyopathy, or postpartum cardiomyopathy account for a small fraction of the group, since most are ultimately idiopathic. Idiopathic cardiomyopathy primarily attacks young and otherwise healthy patients.

Ischemic cardiomyopathy is an end-stage manifestation of coronary athersclerosis. Compared to patients with idiopathic cardiomyopathy, patients with ischemic cardiomyopathy are generally older, and have a higher frequency of associated problems such as diabetes and peripheral vascular disease. Ninety percent of patients undergoing cardiac transplant have either idiopathic (49 percent) or ischemic (41 percent) cardiomyopathy. Ten percent have end-stage ventricular failure associated with valvular disease or unreconstructable congenital heart disease. In children, the proportions are different, with idiopathic cardiomyopathy (49 percent) and congenital heart disease (44 percent) accounting for 93 percent of the total.

The age range for all patients transplanted from 1967 through early 1992 is newborn to seventy-two years, with a mean age of forty-four years. The broad distribution of age over the middle decades reflects overlap between the differing age distributions of idiopathic and ischemic cardiomyopathy. If eligibility for transplant was not influenced by age, the distribution of diagnoses would shift toward that of coronary atherosclerosis, with all its associated problems, and the mean age would increase accordingly. Eighty-one percent of patients transplanted have been men. It is not clear whether this is due to differences in the expression of cardiomyopathies by gender or to differences in selection criteria favoring men.

Recipient Selection. Recipients are selected from among patients with end-stage ventricular failure, clinically NYHA Class III-IV, who are u likely to survive more than one year, and for whom there is no alternative therapy. Selection criteria (Table 10-8) continue to be strict because of the belief that heart donors are a scarce resource that must be distributed preferentially to those with the greatest chance of benefit. The proper psychosocial profile includes evidence of ability to comply with an elaborate regimen of postoperative care. Initially patients older than fifty-five years were excluded, but at present carefully selected older patients are being successfully transplanted when the other essential criteria are met.

Contraindications include systemic diseases likely to compromise long-term survival, such as malignancy, severe peripheral vascular disease or autoimmune vasculitis, and renal or hepatic dysfunction not likely to respond to an improvement in cardiac output. Diabetes and peptic ulcer disease have been considered relative contraindications.

The level of pulmonary vascular resistance in a potential recipient is given particular attention. In all patients with left ventricular failure, regardless of cause, pulmonary vascular resistance (PVR) and pulmonary artery pressure (PAP) increase as left atrial pressure rises. PVR can become extremely elevated and irreversible. A normal donor heart, accustomed to low pulmonary artery pressure and resistance, will fail immediately if placed in a recipient with sufficiently elevated PVR. Therefore right heart catheterization provides essential information regarding operative risk. PVR index equals mean PAP minus wedge pressure divided by cardiac index, and is assigned dimensionless units called Wood's units (WU). The normal range is 0 to 3 WU. Cardiac output is frequently used for the denominator, but some accuracy in prediction is lost when the patient's body surface area is significantly greater or less than 1.0 m^2. At the time of catheterization, patients with elevated PAP and PVR receive a trial infusion of nitroprusside or prostaglandin E_1, and the effect on PVR as the infusion rate is increased up to the point at which systemic pressure falls below an acceptable level is observed. If the PVR can be reduced to less than 5 WU, the patient is considered an acceptable risk. Another index frequently applied is the transpulmonary gradient (TPG), which is defined as the difference between pulmonary artery mean pressure and mean wedge pressure. TPG $>$ 15 mmHg is thought to be associated with exceptionally high risk.

Patients accepted for transplant are placed on a national donor waiting list managed by the United Network for Organ Sharing (UNOS). Patients are stratified according to urgency, blood type, waiting time, and size. To receive priority for critical illness as a UNOS Status I recipient, a patient must require intravenous pressors or inotropic agents, an intraaortic balloon pump, a respirator, or a ventricular assist device, and must be in an intensive care unit. Candidates under six months of age are Status I. All other patients are UNOS Status II. A donor is offered first to the blood group compatible Status I patients of appropriate size with the longest waiting time and closest proximity to the donor. At present Status II patients are infrequently transplanted because of the length of the waiting list for Status I patients, a direct consequence of the proliferation of transplant centers. As the list becomes crowded with critically ill Status I patients, ventricular assist devices play an increasing role in providing a ''bridge'' to transplant.

Table 10-8
Selection of Recipients for Cardiac Transplantation

Indications:	End-stage ventricular failure
	NYHA Class III–IV existence
	Poor 6- to 12-month prognosis for survival
	Medically compliant psychosocial profile
	No alternative treatment
Contraindications:	Systemic disease (vascular, autoimmune)
	Irreversible renal/hepatic insufficiency
	Neoplasia
	High, fixed pulmonary vascular resistance
	Active infection
Relative contraindications:	Age $>$ 60 years
	Diabetes mellitus
	Active peptic ulcer disease

Donor Evaluation. Estimates based on current recipient acceptance criteria suggest that about 14,000 people per year in the United States could benefit from cardiac transplantation. Estimates of the number of potential heart donors suggest that a maximum of 2,000 are available each year. Under such conditions the cornerstone of any cardiac transplant program is an effective system for identifying and managing potential donors.

Table 10-9 summarizes the process of donor evaluation. It must be emphasized that such listings are guidelines and not requirements, and a balance must be reached between the desire to use only ideal donors, and the need to minimize the mortality on the recipient waiting list.

Ischemic time (time elapsed from interruption of coronary circulation in the donor to restoration of coronary circulation in the recipient) is ideally less than 4 hours. Travel time between the donor and recipient hospitals is usually the main determinant of

Table 10-9
Elements of Heart Donor Evaluation

Age (flexible upper limit)
Gender
Size (height/weight)
ABO blood group
Travel time (major variable in ischemic time)
Cause of brain death
- Blunt trauma: rule out myocardial contusion
- Penetrating trauma and primary neurologic: look carefully at medical history
- Carbon monoxide: beware

Medical history
- Heart disease
- Hypertension
- Drug abuse
- Smoking
- Alcoholism

Hemodynamic history since admission
- Cardiac arrest, prolonged hypotension
- Cardioactive and vasoactive drug requirements
- Central venous pressure

Cardiac
- ECG: ST-T waves can be misleading in brain death
- Echocardiogram: contractility, regional wall motion
- Evaluation by cardiologist

Pulmonary
- Gas exchange
- Chest x-ray: contusion, infiltrates, pneumothorax, edema

Serology
- Hepatitis B and C
- HIV
- Cytomegalovirus

ischemic time, so expedient transportation is arranged accordingly. Age criteria are set to minimize the risk of using a heart with silent coronary atherosclerosis. Size matching is designed to avoid extreme discrepancies in the atrial and great vessel anastomoses, and to avoid any predictable mismatch in hemodynamics.

Major blood group compatibility is essential. The importance of a prospective lymphocyte cross match remains controversial in the transplantation of solid organs other than the kidney. As a practical matter, time constraints usually prohibit prospective cross matching.

Victims of blunt trauma must be assessed carefully for myocardial contusion, which can be present with few objective findings. Victims of penetrating trauma frequently have a social profile that makes attention to certain features of medical history such as I.V. drug abuse important. Patients with primary neurologic brain death (e.g., subarachnoid hemorrhage) require close scrutiny for evidence of major hypertension and its cardiac sequelae.

Features of the hemodynamic course that might be alarming in isolation, such as cardiac arrest or a high-dose dopamine infusion, need to be considered in context. A common scenario is a patient on high-dose dopamine with diabetes insipidus and a low CVP, who can be taken off dopamine after volume replacement.

The ECG should be normal, but striking ST-T changes can be associated with cerebrovascular accidents, hypothermia, and electrolyte abnormalities. Echocardiography is extremely important to assess contractility and search for focal wall motion abnormalities.

A fairly broad spectrum of pulmonary pathologic conditions can be tolerated as long as oxygenation is adequate and sepsis is avoided. Extensive traumatic injury should raise the index of suspicion for myocardial contusion but is not an independent exclusion.

Positive serology for HIV or for hepatitis B antigen excludes a potential donor. The risk associated with hepatitis B or C antibody is controversial. Knowledge of the potential recipient's cytomegalovirus (CMV) titer is required to interpret a positive CMV titer in the donor. Acute CMV infection is transmissable with the heart and can produce serious disease in a seronegative recipient. Both acute infection and reactivation can occur in a CMV-positive recipient given a CMV-positive heart, but CMV disease in such a recipient is usually less serious. In many centers prophylactic treatment for CMV disease, combining ganciclovir with passive immunization (gamma-globulin), is begun at the time of transplant when the donor is CMV positive.

Donor Operation. The procedure is timed in coordination with teams removing liver and kidneys, and with the team preparing for implantation in the recipient. The heart is exposed through a median sternotomy, and a final assessment made by visual inspection. Heparin is given. Removal begins with ligation of the superior vena cava and division of the inferior vena cava and pulmonary veins (Fig. 10-39). This is done as the first step in order to decompress the heart and avoid any ventricular distention with the aorta occluded. An aortic cross clamp is applied just proximal to the innominate artery. Preservation is begun by infusing hyperkalemic cardioplegia solution at 40°C into the aortic root to produce a prompt arrest in diastole. The cooling provided by coronary perfusion is augmented by immersion in saline solution at 4°C. The heart is observed closely for distention, which can be relieved if necessary by passing a finger across the mitral valve from the opening in the pulmonary veins. Finally the aorta and pulmonary artery are divided distally (Fig. 10-40); the heart is removed from the pericardium and wrapped in ice for transport.

Recipient Operation. Through a median sternotomy the recipient is placed on cardiopulmonary bypass under moderate systemic hypothermia using bicaval cannulation with caval snares. To minimize ischemic time, close communication is maintained with the donor team so that implantation can proceed as soon as the donor heart arrives in the recipient operating room. The recipient aorta is cross-clamped just proximal to the innominate artery, and the heart is removed by dividing the great vessels at their commissures and separating the atria from the ventricles at the

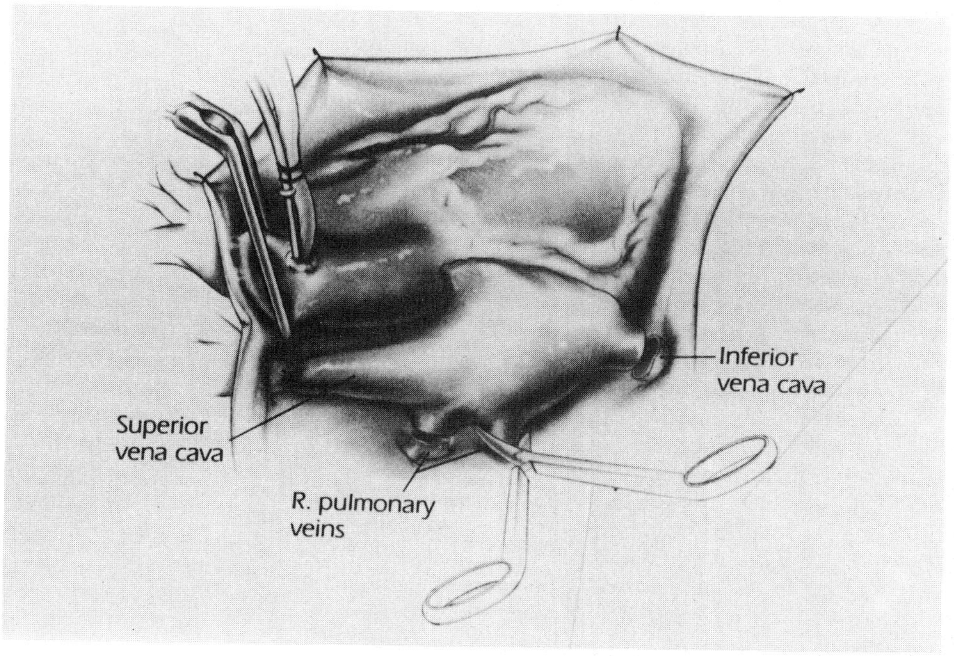

FIG. 10-39. Donor cardiectomy. The aortic cross clamp has been applied, and cardioplegia is being infused through a cannula in the aortic root. The superior vena cava has been ligated. The inferior vena cava and right superior pulmonary vein have been divided, and the scissors are about to divide the right inferior pulmonary vein. For the next few minutes attention is directed toward achieving a rapid arrest without ventricular distention, and beginning topical hypothermia with iced saline irrigation.

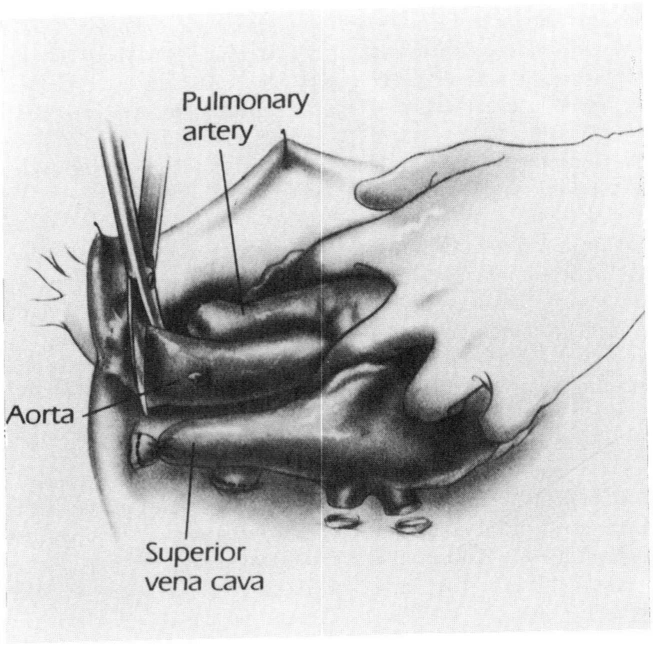

FIG. 10-40. Donor cardiectomy. The scissors are about to divide the aorta. The pulmonary artery and superior vena cava will be divided next and the donor heart removed for transport. The pulmonary artery is usually divided at or beyond the bifurcation to preserve all possible length. It is convenient to divide the right pulmonary artery just to the right of the superior vena cava *(dotted line)* and divide the left pulmonary artery at the pericardial reflection. (From: *Doty DB: Cardiac surgery: A looseleaf workbook and update service. "TRANSPL" section in Update 3. Chicago, Year Book Medical Publishers, 1986, with permission.*)

atrioventricular groove. Both atrial appendages are excised. The posterior aspects of both atria are left intact and connected by the interatrial septum. The donor heart is removed from cold storage, trimmed appropriately, and carefully inspected, looking particularly for a patent foramen ovale. If a patent foramen is left open, a significant right-to-left shunt can occur in patients with residual pulmonary hypertension. Implantation proceeds with anastomosis of the left atria, followed by the right atria, pulmonary arteries, and aortas (Fig. 10-41). Size discrepancies are easily accommodated in the atrial suture lines. Significant aortic size discrepancy is quite common, especially when there is a large age difference between donor and recipient. Remarkably large mismatches can be accommodated with a careful anastomosis, in part because of the elasticity of youthful aortic tissue. The cross clamp is removed, and a spontaneous rhythm is restored. The sinus node of the donor heart becomes the dominant pacemaker. The recipient's intrinsic rhythm frequently persists, producing regular nonconducted contractions of the native atrial tissue and a second independent P wave on the posttransplant ECG.

Early postoperative care is identical in most respects with that given any patient following open heart surgery. The denervated heart often requires a period of chronotropic support, which is usually provided by isoproterenol infusion or epicardial pacing to maintain a heart rate of 90 to 110. Most patients demonstrate a degree of right ventricular decompensation as the donor right ventricle adapts to the residual elevated PVR in the recipient. Clinical manifestations include a rising central venous pressure, a right ventricular gallop, and edema. Echocardiography done during this period typically shows decreased right ventricular contractility with chamber dilation, and may show tricuspid insufficiency. In correctly selected patients these findings will return to normal as the PVR gradually falls, but inotropic and vasodilator support may be required for many days. Occasionally a period of circulatory support with a right ventricular assist device (RVAD) will be required. An RVAD removes blood from the right atrium and pumps it into the pulmonary artery.

Immunosuppression. Maintenance immunosuppression (Table 10-10) usually uses three immunosuppressive agents ("triple therapy"). The most common combination consists of daily oral cyclosporine, azathioprine, and prednisone. Cyclosporine dosage is adjusted to maintain an appropriate serum level. Side effects of cyclosporine are significant, and include nephrotoxicity, hypertension, hirsutism, and gingival hypertrophy. Complex interactions with other medications are frequently seen, notably diphenylhydantoin (Dilantin), ketoconazole, and trimethoprim/sulfamethoxazole (Bactrim). Azathioprine is adjusted to maintain a white blood cell count of 3000 to 5000 while avoiding oversuppression of other marrow precursors. Beginning 3 to 6 months posttransplant the prednisone dose is tapered slowly to a level about one-third of the initial dose. Most features of a cushingoid habitus slowly disappear as the prednisone dose is tapered. Chronic complications of steroid administration (arthropathy, myopathy, glucose intolerance) become increasingly prevalent in long-term survivors.

Immunosuppression continues to evolve as new agents emerge offering the hope of increased or equivalent efficacy with a reduction in side effects. FK506, RS61443, and rapamycin are undergoing evaluation as substitutes for cyclosporine. Avoidance of steroids has been pursued aggressively with some success in certain centers using cyclosporine-based immunosuppression, and the newer agents may improve the success of steroid-free regimens. Cytolytic agents are potent antithymocyte and antilymphocyte globulins (OKT3, ATG, ALG) which are the mainstay of "rescue" therapy for rejection. Cytolytic agents are also used as "induction" therapy in patients at high risk for early perioperative cyclosporine nephrotoxicity, typically patients who are critically ill with serious prerenal insufficiency. The cytolytic agent is given intravenously each day in place of cyclosporine until renal function improves, and may be continued for as long as 2 weeks. Wider use of these very potent agents is limited by a predictable increase in the incidence of viral infections, particularly CMV.

Rejection. Rejection is monitored by right ventricular endomyocardial biopsy, done at least weekly in the first month, then less frequently on a tapering schedule. At the time of each biopsy a

Table 10-10
Immunosuppression

Maintenance "triple therapy":
Cyclosporine: Oral dose adjusted to maintain serum level 100–250 ng/mL
Prednisone: 0.2 mg/kg, P.O., daily, tapered after 3–6 months to ~0.1 mg/kg
Azathioprine: 1–2 mg/kg, P.O., daily
Evolving modifications:
"Induction" with cytolytic agents (OKT3, ATG, ALG)
FK506, rapamycin, RS61433 in place of cyclosporine
Steroid-free regimens

right heart catheterization is performed. Most rejection episodes have normal hemodynamics, but a low cardiac output, low mixed venous oxygen saturation, and elevated right atrial or wedge pressures raise suspicion of rejection. The biopsy is performed through the same venipuncture with a flexible biopsy forceps passed into the right ventricle. Adequate sampling is important, since the false-negative rate only drops below 5 percent when three or more pieces of muscle can be examined on the slide. The biopsy material can be fixed, stained, and examined microscopically within 24 hours.

Biopsies are graded according to a standard nomenclature (Table 10-11). Histologic evidence of myocyte necrosis (grade 2 or greater) is considered diagnostic of significant rejection. Grade 1 inflammatory cell infiltrates are considered abnormal, but are usually not treated as rejection in the absence of myocyte necrosis. All suspected rejection episodes are considered in clinical context, especially if the histologic diagnosis is ambiguous. Subjective signs are frequently subtle but may include malaise, fatigue, and frank dyspnea or orthopnea. Physical findings are usually absent, but can include tachycardia, a ventricular gallop, rales, and edema. Diminution in ECG voltage correlated with rejection in patients maintained on azathioprine and steroids, but is without value in patients on cyclosporine. Echocardiography can add suggestive findings but is not independently diagnostic. Occasionally all the evidence will suggest rejection in the presence of a repeatedly negative biopsy. In such cases, once bacterial sepsis, viral infection, constrictive pericarditis, and tamponade are excluded, a left heart catheterization is likely to show diffuse graft coronary disease.

About 95 percent of rejection episodes are treated initially with steroid (Table 10-12), either as a 3-day oral boost in prednisone followed by a 7- to 10-day taper, or as intravenous methylprednisolone (1 g/day for 3 days). The oral boost offers the advantage of outpatient treatment, and may reduce the incidence of infectious complications by reducing the total steroid dose. Rejection episodes unresponsive to one or more steroid boosts, and those associated with hemodynamic instability, receive "rescue therapy" with cytolytic agents. "Vascular" rejection, which is directed toward coronary vasculature and thought to be mediated by humoral (antibody) rather than cellular (lymphocytotoxic) immunity, may be treated with plasmapheresis, photophoresis, and methotrexate or cyclophosphamide, in addition to the first- and second-line treatments described above. Treatment with oral or intravenous steroid is effective in 90 percent of all rejection episodes, and half the remainder are salvaged with rescue therapy. Patients who present initially with hemodynamic instability are at high risk, and should receive aggressive initial treatment with intravenous steroid and a cytolytic agent.

Results. A total of 19,455 heart transplants performed from 1967 through 1991 have been recorded in the Registry of the International Society for Heart and Lung Transplantation. Figure 10-42 shows that 1-year actuarial survival for transplants performed during the most recent 5-year period is 80 percent, increased from 73 percent during the previous 5-year period. Similarly, 5-year survival has improved from 58 percent to 70 percent. In other words, survival at 5 years is essentially the same today as it was at 1 year when the decade began. Results measured by assessing functional status 2 years after transplant show that 85 percent of patients are New York Heart Association (NYHA) Class I and 13 percent are NYHA Class II.

Five years ago results in children were discouraging, with 1-year actuarial survival of 49 percent. Results have improved dramatically. One-year survival currently exceeds 80 percent for all recipients under age eighteen years, and has increased to 70 percent for patients under one year of age.

Thirty-day mortality has stabilized at 9 to 10 percent. Thirty-day mortality was attributed to rejection or infection in about 40 percent of patients, and to "cardiac" and other causes in the majority (60 percent). The most common cardiac causes of early mortality are poor donor selection, poor donor preservation, and prohibitive pulmonary hypertension in the recipient. A small number of patients suffering early donor dysfunction can be salvaged with ventricular assist devices (VADs). VADs are most likely to succeed in temporary support of the right ventricle (RVAD) during a period of adaptation to high PVR, and are least likely to succeed when used as a bridge to retransplant for unsalvageable donor failure. Cyclosporine and cytolytic agents have significantly reduced the frequency of early death due to rejection but have had no significant impact on deaths due to other causes.

For all patients, risk falls dramatically during the first year. Three-quarters of the first-year mortality occurs during the first quarter of the year. Infection, which should be viewed as a complication of immunosuppression, accounts for the highest mortality in the first year. Infectious complications in cardiac transplant recipients are most often pulmonary. Opportunistic pathogens predominate, and include *Pneumocystis carinii,* cytomegalovirus (CMV), *Legionella,* and fungi. Antibacterial and antifungal agents will control most infections if the level of immunosuppression can be tightly controlled. Use of cytolytic agents clearly increases the frequency of viral infections, of which CMV is the most pernicious.

After the first year cellular (antimyocyte) rejection and graft coronary disease become steadily increasing causes of mortality.

Table 10-11
Standardized Cardiac Biopsy Grading

Grade	*Nomenclature*	*Description*
0	No rejection	No infiltrates
1A	Mild acute, focal	Focal lymphocytic infiltrates
1B	Mild acute, diffuse	More diffuse infiltrates
2	Moderate acute, focal	Focal infiltrate, myocyte necrosis
3A	Moderate, multifocal	Multiple infiltrates, myocyte necrosis
3B	Diffuse, > moderate	Diffuse, almost severe
4	Severe acute	Diffuse aggressive necrosis, hemorrhage

Table 10-12
Treatment of Cardiac Rejection

Asymptomatic acute rejection:	Prednisone oral boost, taper over 7–10 days
Symptomatic acute rejection:	Solumedrol 1 g, I.V., daily for 3 days
Refractory rejection:	Cytolytic agent Methotrexate Photophoresis Total lymphoid irradiation

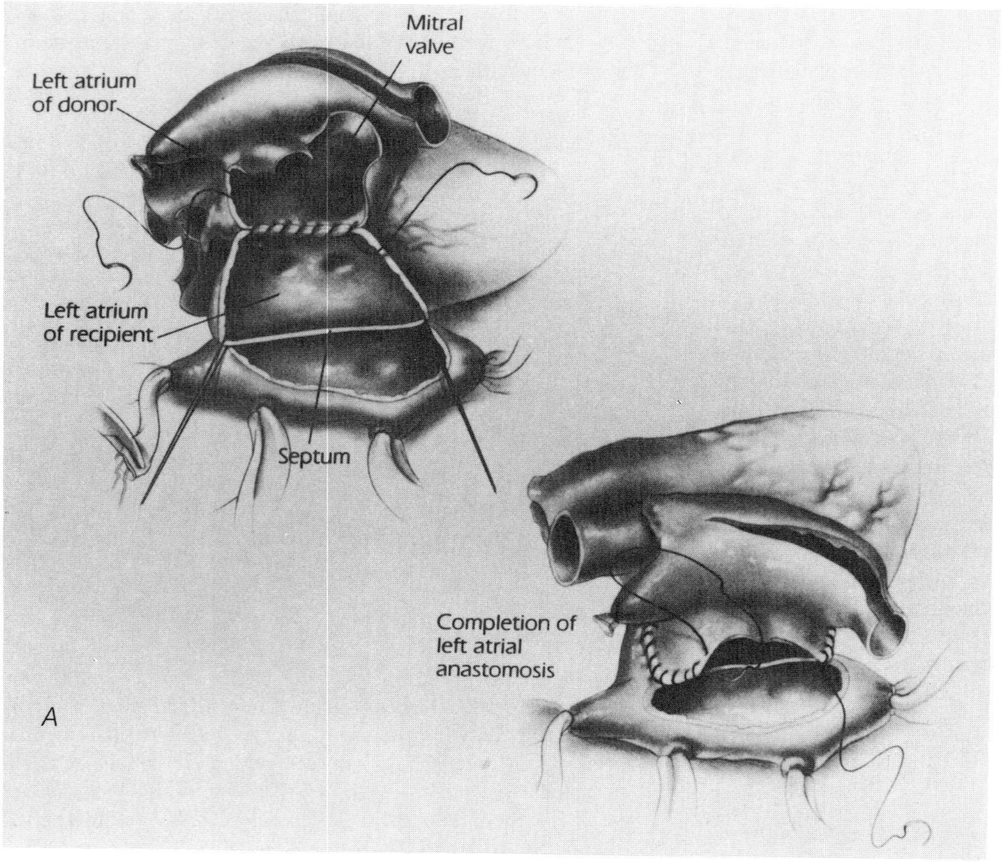

FIG. 10-41. *A.* Implantation of the donor heart. The left atrial anastomosis is begun adjacent to the left atrial appendage of the donor and the confluence of the left pulmonary veins in the recipient *(upper figure)*. It is completed by joining the right edge of the donor left atrium to the interatrial septum *(lower figure)*. Note the opening in the right atrium, which is directed from the inferior vena caval orifice toward the middle of the right atrial appendage. *B.* Implantation of the donor heart. The right atrial anastomosis is begun by rolling the posterior edge of the right atriotomy over to the interatrial septum, where the suture line overlaps the septal segment of the left atrial suture line just completed *(upper figure)*. The closure diverges from the left atrium at the inferior and superior ends of the septum and continues anteriorly *(lower figure)*. *C.* Implantation of the donor heart. The pulmonary artery *(upper figure)* and aorta *(lower figure)* are trimmed and joined with a continuous suture, beginning posteriorly. Discrepancies in circumference are taken up with careful suture spacing. (From: *Doty DB: Cardiac surgery: A looseleaf workbook and update service. "TRANSPL" section in Update 3. Chicago, Year Book Medical Publishers, 1986, with permission.*)

Graft coronary disease is a diffuse obliterative endarteritis which is presumed to be immunologically mediated and is best viewed as a vascular, rather than cellular, manifestation of chronic rejection. Graft coronary disease is rarely treatable with coronary bypass or angioplasty, and will occur in at least 30 percent of long-term survivors. To date, retransplant is the only recognized treatment for this condition, without which mortality approaches 100 percent. Most patients die before a second donor becomes available, and survival following retransplant is not as good as that expected after a first transplant. One-year actuarial survival recorded in the Registry for 448 patients undergoing cardiac retransplantation is 49 percent. These results have caused many to question whether retransplant is a justifiable use of a scarce donor organ which could be used in a primary recipient with better prospects for survival.

Many chronic complications are consequences of immunosuppression. Slowly progressive renal insufficiency and hypertension are still common in patients on long-term cyclosporine. Steroids produce osteoporosis and aseptic necrosis of joints, glucose intolerance, weight gain and fluid retention, and exacerbate hypertension. Malignant growths occur in 2 to 5 percent of patients, and have a spectrum of pathology characteristic of immunosuppressed patients. Lymphoma (especially non-Hodgkin's lymphoma), Kaposi's sarcoma, and other relatively unusual neoplasms predominate. An increase in malignant growths related to the use of cytolytic agents has been suspected, but no association has been established.

Problems related to regulatory physiology in a denervated heart, which were the subject of much speculation and experimental modeling in the early years, do not appear to be major. The adaptive mechanisms are incompletely understood, but at least partially involve increased levels of circulating catecholamines combined with receptor up-regulation. By whatever mechanism, autoregulation of cardiac output is remarkably well preserved after cardiac transplantation. Contrary to all expectations, reinnervation

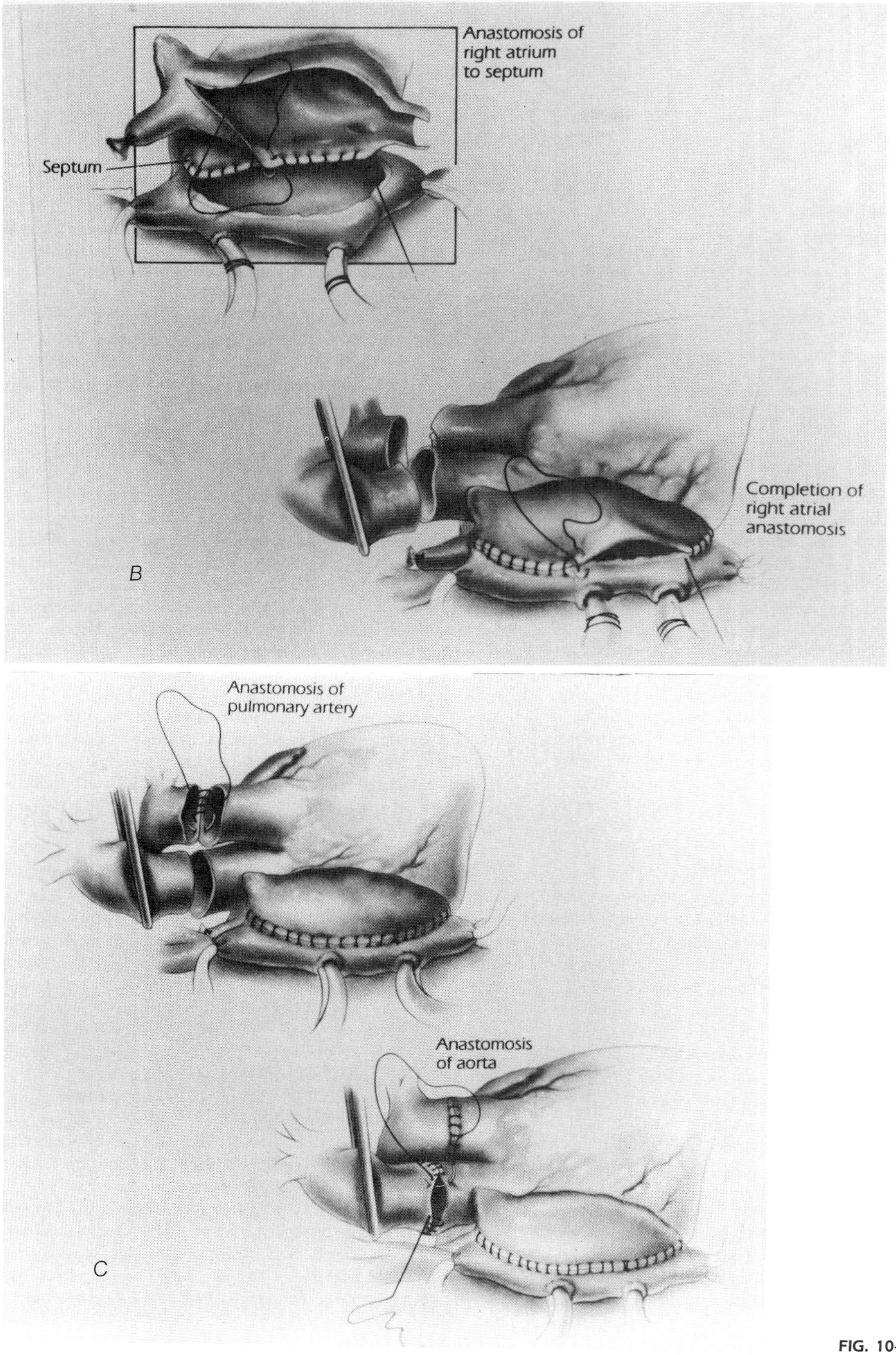
Anastomosis of
right atrium
to septum
Septum
Completion of
right atrial
anastomosis
B
Anastomosis of
pulmonary artery
Anastomosis
of aorta
C

FIG. 10-41. (cont.)

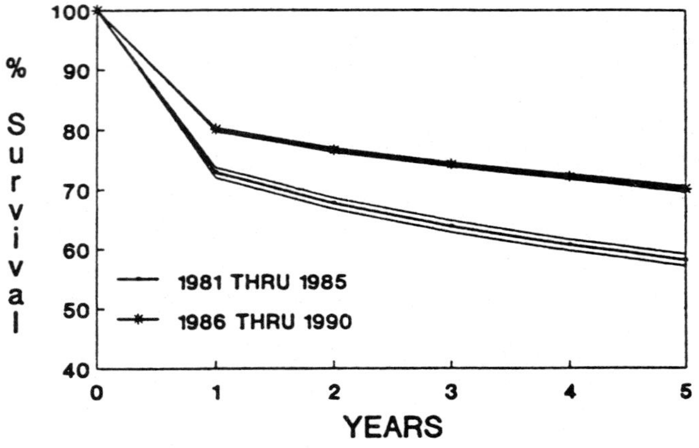

FIG. 10-42. Kaplan-Meier actuarial survival curves for heart transplants contained in the Registry of the International Society for Heart and Lung Transplant, performed during two time periods. (From: *Kaye MP: 1992, with permission.*)

of the heart has been seen in isolated cases many years following transplant, endowing the affected patients with the ability to develop angina as a symptom of graft coronary disease.

Cardiac transplantation is a well-established therapy for end-stage heart failure, but broader application continued to be limited by donor shortage, and long-term results are still limited by chronic rejection. Xenograft transplantation is the subject of an accelerating research effort in many centers which may offer hope for an improvement in donor supply, but all efforts in this area to date suffer from a need for intolerable levels of immunosuppression. The best long-term hope lies in development of artificial heart technology, which avoids rejection altogether. Remarkable technical advances have already occurred through experience gained using ventricular assist devices as bridges to transplantation. Complete mechanical replacement may become a reality within the next decade.

Lung and Heart-Lung Transplantation

Historical Development. The first human lung transplant was a single-lung transplant performed by Hardy in 1963, which resulted in early death. This attempt was followed by 46 single-lung transplants performed over the next 20 years, with $>$ 80 percent mortality at 18 days, median survival of 10 days, and 0 percent 1-year survival. Nearly all deaths were associated with dehiscence of the bronchial anastomosis.

One reaction to these events was to explore, in the laboratory, transplantation of the heart and lungs as a block, reasoning that a single tracheal anastomosis, nourished in part by coronary-bronchial collaterals, would prove more successful than a bronchial anastomosis. Reitz at Stanford developed a successful primate model of heart-lung transplant, then reported the first three patients in 1982.

Early experience confirmed that there was minimal difficulty with tracheal healing, and an outstanding functional result was achieved in patients surviving the early perioperative period. Perioperative mortality proved to be a striking 20 to 25 percent, however, and difficulty in the management of early postoperative infection and rejection contributed to a disappointing 1-year survival of 54 percent through 1988.

Another reaction to the early experience with single-lung transplant was to explore ways to improve bronchial healing. Cooper in Toronto concluded from a dog model that poor blood supply and perioperative steroids were responsible for the high incidence of bronchial dehiscence. Cooper developed a doctrine of cyclosporine-based immunosuppression, steroid abstinence during the early postoperative period, and omental wrapping of the anastomosis. With this approach Cooper's team in Toronto performed the first two successful single-lung transplants in 1983 and 1984. Single-lung transplant was less technically demanding than heart-lung transplant, offered the opportunity to benefit three recipients with each heart-lung block, and provided the hope of treatment for conditions such as pulmonary fibrosis and emphysema for which heart-lung transplant was illogical when the heart was reasonably normal. Early results with single-lung transplant fell somewhat short of the promise, with 45 percent 1-year survival in Cooper's first 20 patients with pulmonary fibrosis, and 67 percent 1-year survival for all single-lung transplants recorded in the International Registry through 1990.

Neither single-lung nor heart-lung transplant provides a perfect solution for patients requiring two lungs who have a salvageable heart. Patients with cystic fibrosis provide the best example. Transplanting only one lung in such a patient condemns the new lung to infection from the bronchiectatic, chronically infected contralateral lung. Heart-lung transplant for cystic fibrosis requires replacement of a reasonably normal heart in most cases, and the extreme scarcity of heart-lung blocks militates against this approach for any condition as common as cystic fibrosis. Patterson, working as a member of Cooper's group in Toronto, developed an experimental model of en bloc double-lung transplant, and reported the first patient in 1988. The en bloc approach proved to have exceptionally high mortality and a surprisingly high incidence of tracheal dehiscence, and was largely abandoned by 1990. At about that time groups in the United States, Canada, and France reported success with bilateral single-lung transplant performed through a bilateral anterior thoractotomy. This has become the standard approach when both lungs must be transplanted without the heart.

Recipient Selection. Lung transplant recipients have end-stage pulmonary disease which severely restricts normal activity, and have poor prospects for survival beyond 1 to 2 years. Psychosocial and general medical criteria are the same as those for cardiac transplant. Most pulmonary diseases have an end stage characterized by respiratory insufficiency, with variable degrees of secondary cor pulmonale. Obstructive/fibrotic lung diseases such as emphysema, cystic fibrosis, and idiopathic pulmonary fibrosis are the most common examples. In contrast, pulmonary vascular diseases such as primary pulmonary hypertension or Eisenmenger's syndrome are characterized by right ventricular failure with near normal bronchoalveolar function.

The first step in selection is to stratify patients by procedure (Table 10-13). Patients with unreconstructible intracardiac anatomy and end-stage Eisenmenger's syndrome must have a heart-lung transplant, and recipient selection should reflect the magnitude of the procedure by favoring young ($<$45) patients with substantial physical reserve and excellent rehabilitation potential. Patients requiring heart-lung transplant should also be placed on a waiting list early rather than late in their course because waiting time for the rare heart-lung blocks is the longest of any solid organ.

Table 10-13
Stratification of Procedures by Diagnosis

Procedure	*Diagnoses*	*Limits*
Single-lung	Emphysema	Age < 65
	Pulmonary fibrosis	RV/LV function
	Other nonseptic obstructive	Coronary disease
	Pulmonary hypertension	V/Q mismatch
Double-lung	Cystic fibrosis	Age < 60
	Bronchiectasis	RV/LV function
	Pulmonary hypertension	Coronary disease
	Correctable congenital	
	Emphysema	
Heart-lung	Uncorrectable congenital	Age < 45
	Other, RV/LV unsalvageable	Vascular adhesions
		Systemic-pulmonary collaterals

Recipients of double-lung transplant also face a major procedure, but a higher age limit is generally observed (<60). Patients with septic lung disease, most typically those with bronchiectasis from cystic fibrosis, require transplant of both lungs to prevent infection of the transplanted lung by the native lung. Patients with cystic fibrosis also require attention to the antibiotic sensitivity of their infecting flora, which are typically very resistant strains of *Pseudomonas*. Certain patients with very advanced emphysema may require transplant of both lungs to avoid serious ventilation/perfusion mismatches and mediastinal shifting, although current experience shows that most patients with emphysema do well with a single-lung transplant. There is a belief in several centers that patients with primary or secondary pulmonary hypertension should have both lungs transplanted to avoid acute and chronic problems associated with perfusion shifts to the transplanted lung. Although Cooper has recently reported excellent early results in a small series of patients with pulmonary hypertension treated with single-lung transplant, it is not yet clear that these results can be extrapolated to less carefully selected patients representing the spectrum of disease more broadly.

Recipients selected for single-lung transplant usually have emphysema or another respiratory disease not complicated by prominent septic features or serious pulmonary hypertension. Single-lung transplant offers the advantage of relative technical simplicity in comparison with double-lung or heart-lung transplant, and appropriate selection can include older patients (<65). Candidates for single- or double-lung transplant must receive a thorough evaluation for cardiac disease. Young patients at low risk for coronary disease require right heart catheterization for assessment of pulmonary artery pressures and intracardiac shunts. Older patients require left heart catheterization and coronary angiography. In candidates with emphysema, most of whom are older than forty-five years, the characteristic history of smoking habits and associated medical problems guarantees a high incidence of coronary disease. Patients with significant coronary disease are generally not accepted for transplant. Assessment of ventricular function is always important, especially when hoping to avoid heart-lung transplant in young patients with pulmonary vascular disease. Patients with normal intracardiac anatomy and those with correctable defects must have recoverable right and left ventricular function to allow consideration of single- or double-lung transplant.

Donor Operation. A lung donor must have normal gas exchange, a clear chest x-ray, and clean tracheobronchial secretions (Table 10-14). Lungs tend to deteriorate more quickly than other solid organs in patients with brain death. Contributing factors include the insults of mechanical ventilation, volume resuscitation, neurogenic pulmonary edema, and airway colonization with nosocomial organisms. Lungs are more easily contused in blunt thoracic trauma than the heart. Approximately 30 percent of suitable heart donors are also suitable lung donors. Size matching seeks to avoid compressive atelectasis in a lung too large for the thorax, to avoid large effusions and residual pneumothorax if the lung is too small, and to avoid gross discrepancies in bronchial circumference. Many centers rely on measurements of the chest x-ray to estimate lung volume. Predicted vital capacity, derived from a nomogram based on height, age, and gender, can be used equally well. If predicted vital capacity is used, distortions in recipient anatomy must be kept in mind. Recipients with emphysema, cystic fibrosis, or other conditions associated with hyperinflated lungs should have a donor with a predicted vital capacity about one liter greater than that of the recipient. Size matching is most important in double-lung or heart-lung transplant because mediastinal shift cannot be relied upon to compensate.

Methods for lung preservation that would allow distant procurement were late to develop. Cooling the entire donor to about 15°C on cardiopulmonary bypass has been practiced effectively in certain centers, but is logistically complex. In recent years cooling with pulmonary artery perfusion ("cold flush") has become the dominant method used for lung preservation. Success was first obtained using modified EuroCollins solution, which is a high-potassium "intracellular" fluid. Refinement of the flush technique and the constituents of the flush solution continues to be an active area of research. With current methods, using EuroCollins solution, preservation is reliable for 4 to 6 hours, and has been effective for as long as 8 hours of ischemic time.

The lungs are usually removed with the heart through a median sternotomy. Simultaneous with heart preservation the lungs are flushed through an infusion catheter in the main pulmonary artery with 60 mL/kg of EuroCollins solution at 4°C over a period of 4 to 6 minutes, maintaining pulmonary artery pressure below

Table 10-14
Evaluation of Lung Donor

- Pulmonary
  - Chest x-ray: infiltrates, pneumothorax, edema
  - Gas exchange: $P_{O_2} > 100$ on 40% F_{IO_2}, > 300 on 100% F_{IO_2}
  - Secretions: quantity, character, Gram stain
  - Bronchoscopy (when possible)
  - Size (predicted vital capacity, chest x-ray measurements)
- Serology
  - Hepatitis B and C
  - HIV
  - CMV
- Hemodynamics
  - CVP, volume status
- Travel time (major variable in ischemic time)
- Age (< 50, flexible upper limit)
- ABO blood group
- Medical history
  - Smoking
  - Pulmonary disease
  - IV drug abuse
  - Alcoholism

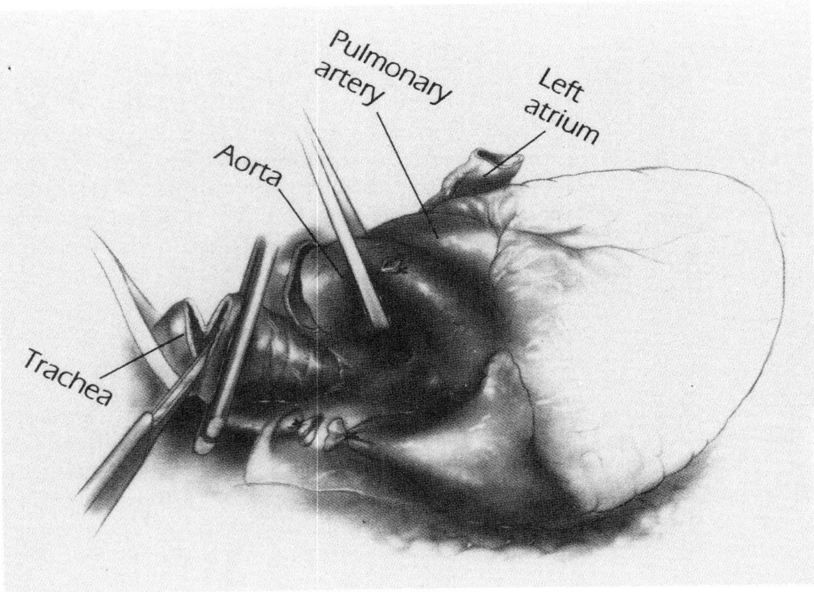

FIG. 10-43. The donor operation for removal of the heart and both lungs: Following cold cardioplegic arrest of the heart and cold perfusion of the lungs through the pulmonary artery, the aorta and both cavae are divided, and the trachea is divided several rings proximal to the carina, stapling the distal end to maintain lung inflation. Note that the tip of the left atrial appendage has been amputated to vent the left atrium, which is done to prevent distention by the large volume of cold solution flushed through the lungs. (From: *Doty DB: Cardiac surgery: A looseleaf workbook and update service. "TRANSPL" section. Chicago, Year Book Medical Publishers, 1988, with permission.*)

25 mmHg. Ventilation is continued throughout the flush. The effluent is vented through a stab wound in the left atrial appendage to prevent cardiac distention. Just before flushing, in order to facilitate rapid and uniform perfusion, a large bolus of a vasodilator (usually prostaglandin E1) is administered directly into the pulmonary artery to counteract the vasospasm induced by cold fluid and high potassium. The aorta and both cavae are divided. The trachea is divided several rings above the carina, with the distal end stapled to keep both lungs inflated (Fig. 10-43), and the lungs are separated from their remaining minor attachments by sharply developing the plane anterior to the esophagus (Fig. 10-44), taking care to avoid injury to the membranous portion of each bronchus. The organs are packed in cold solution for transport. For use in a heart-lung recipient the organ block is transported and implanted without further separation (Fig. 10-45). The heart can be separated from the lungs in the donor before lung removal or on a back table after removal. When separating the heart from the lungs, division of the left atrium must be done accurately to preserve a cuff of atrial tissue joining the confluence of the pulmonary veins on each lung while avoiding injury to structures of the atrioventricular groove in the donor heart (Fig. 10-46). When each lung is to be used separately, the left main bronchus is divided so that the tracheal carina remains attached to the much shorter right main bronchus (Fig. 10-47). When the donor bronchus is opened in the recipient operating room, airway secretions should be cultured to guide early postoperative antibiotic therapy.

Recipient Procedures. ***Single-Lung.*** In some patients the choice of side is predetermined, as in patients with one undersized hemithorax. In most patients either lung can be transplanted, but one or the other might be preferable. Patients requiring cardiopulmonary bypass are more easily cannulated through the right chest. Mediastinal shifts in emphysema may be less prevalent if a right lung is transplanted, or the underlying disease may be asymmetric in a manner favoring one lung or the other.

Split-lung ventilation is essential, and can be achieved with a double-lumen endotracheal tube or with a bronchial blocker inflated in the bronchus on the side to be transplanted. Maintenance of acceptable gas exchange in a patient with end-stage pulmonary disease ventilated on one lung in thoracotomy position is a major challenge for the anesthesiologist which should not be underestimated.

Recipient pneumonectomy is performed through a posterolateral thoracotomy. A judgment must be made about the need for cardiopulmonary bypass, preferably before division of the vessels. Bypass is clearly indicated in patients with significant pulmonary

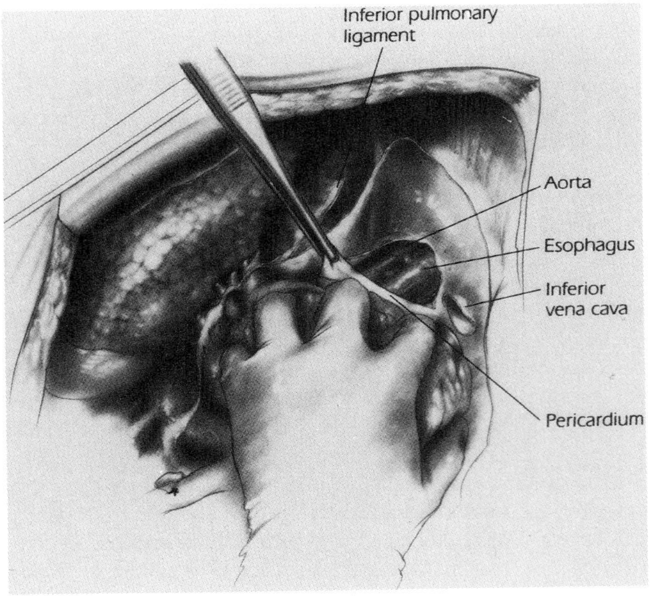

FIG. 10-44. The donor operation for removal of the heart and both lungs: The heart-lung block is freed posteriorly by sharply developing the plane anterior to the esophagus with the organs reflected cephalad. A large piece of posterior pericardium remains attached to the organ block. (From: *Doty DB: Cardiac surgery: A looseleaf workbook and update service. "TRANSPL" section. Chicago, Year Book Medical Publishers, 1988, with permission.*)

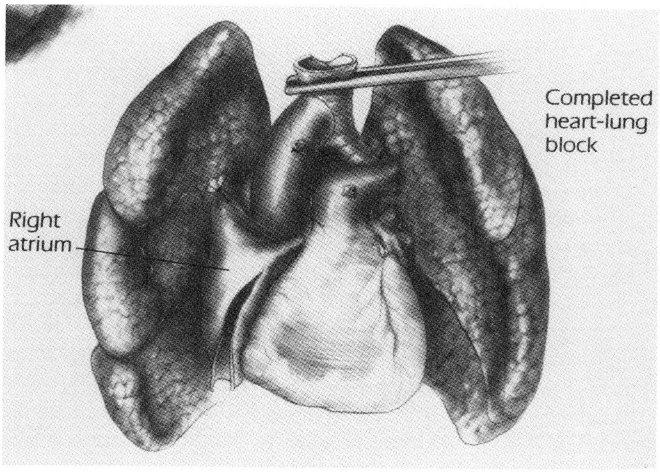

FIG. 10-45. The explanted heart-lung block: If destined for a heart-lung recipient, nothing further is done. If the organs are to be used for a heart recipient and one or two lung recipients, the heart is separated from the lungs by dividing the left atrium and the pulmonary artery, which can be done before or after removal of the organ block from the donor. (From: *Doty DB: Cardiac surgery: A looseleaf workbook and update service. "TRANSPL" section. Chicago, Year Book Medical Publishers, 1988, with permission.*)

hypertension (systolic pressures at least half systemic). In borderline situations the pulmonary artery is clamped and hemodynamics observed for at least 5 minutes. Bypass is mandated by a dramatic rise in pulmonary pressures associated with fall in cardiac output, or by transesophageal echocardiographic evidence of increased right ventricular dysfunction. Occasionally bypass will be required simply because of intolerably poor gas exchange. Cannulation for

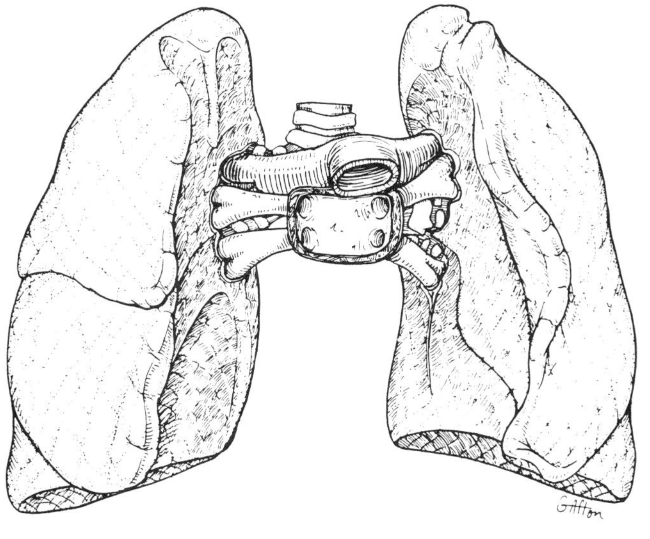

FIG. 10-46. A donor double-lung block after the heart has been removed. The left atrium was opened between the pulmonary veins and the atrioventricular groove, preserving a cuff of left atrial tissue joining the pulmonary veins on each side. To implant the lungs separately, the remaining piece of common left atrium is divided posteriorly, each pulmonary artery is divided, and the left main bronchus is divided. (From: *Bonser RS, Fragomeni LS, et al: Technique of clinical double-lung transplant. J Heart Transplant 7:299, 1988, with permission.*)

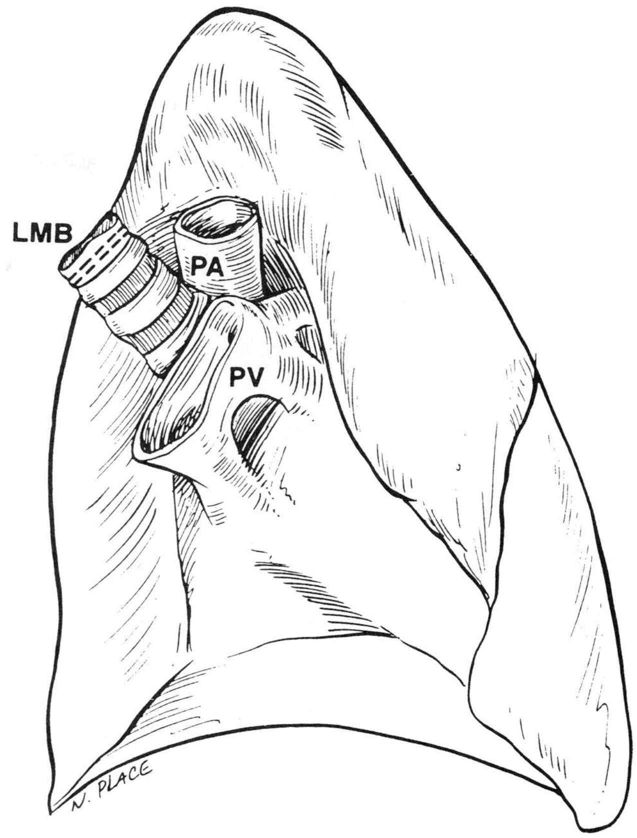

FIG. 10-47. A donor left lung. When each lung is separated from the double-lung block the left main bronchus (LMB) is divided because of its greater length; the corresponding right lung would still have the tracheal carina attached. At implantation either bronchus is divided again so that the anastomosis is placed just above the upper lobe orifice. The pulmonary artery (PA) and pulmonary veins (PV) are ready for anastomosis. (From: *Calhoon JH, Grover FL, et al: Single lung transplantation: Alternative indications. J Thorac Cardiovasc Surg 101:821, 1991, with permission.*)

bypass can be ipsilateral femoral-femoral, femoral and right atrial, or aortic and right atrial.

To preserve length the pulmonary artery and veins are divided in the hilum, and the bronchus is divided just proximal to the upper lobe origin. A clamp is placed across the left atrium encompassing the origins of the pulmonary veins (Fig. 10-48), which are opened and connected to form a circular cuff for anastomosis to the donor left atrial cuff. Either the left atrial or bronchial anastomosis can be performed first. To minimize the length of potentially ischemic donor bronchus, the donor bronchus is divided one or two cartilaginous rings proximal to the upper lobe orifice. Details of bronchial anastomotic technique are widely debated because of the importance of bronchial healing and the history of high mortality associated with dehiscence. Currently a "telescoping" technique is popular (Fig. 10-49), which relies on intussusception of the donor bronchus into the recipient to reinforce the anastomosis. Wrapping the bronchial anastomosis with omentum to improve early vascularity is common but optional. The pulmonary artery anastomosis is done last (Figure 10-50). To minimize the risk of air embolus from the left atrium, before restoring forward circulation the left

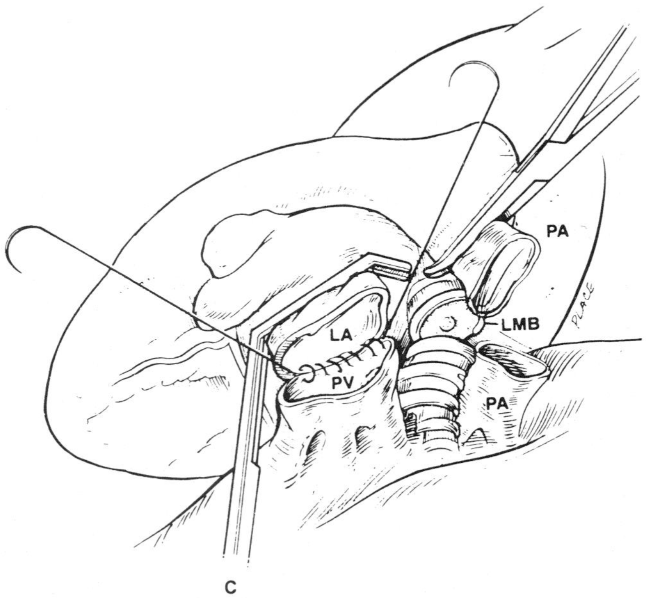

FIG. 10-48. Single-lung transplant, illustrated on the left side. A clamp across the left atrium (LA) of the recipient encompasses the origins of the recipient pulmonary veins. The recipient atrial cuff is sewn to the donor atrial cuff connecting the donor pulmonary veins (PV). The recipient pulmonary artery (PA) is clamped, and the left main bronchus (LMB) has been divided. (From: *Calhoon JH, Grover FL, et al: Single lung transplantation: Alternative indications. J Thorac Cardiovasc Surg 101:821, 1991, with permission.*)

atrial clamp is released to allow retrograde filling of the vasculature, which displaces air through the open pulmonary artery.

Double-Lung. In 1992 most double-lung transplants are performed as bilateral single-lung transplants, for which the technical description of single-lung transplant applies to each side in sequence. With the patient supine, the operation is usually done through a bilateral anterior thoracotomy placed in the fourth or fifth interspace, dividing the sternum at that level (Fig. 10-51). Management of the airway must provide alternating single-lung ventilation, either with a double-lumen tube or with bilateral bronchial blocking balloons. When the procedure is done without cardiopulmonary bypass, the first lung is transplanted with the patient supported on the contralateral native lung, which is then transplanted with the patient supported on the new lung. Bypass is frequently required. Patients having repair of an intracardiac defect, such as an atrial septal defect or ventricular septal defect, require bicaval cannulation with caval snares and a period of cardioplegic cardiac arrest. Patients with advanced septic disease, cystic fibrosis in particular, require aggressive endotracheal suctioning of purulent secretions to maintain an airway, and the technique used for each pneumonectomy must minimize opportunities for contamination of the mediastinum and pleural spaces with highly resistant bacteria.

Double-lung transplant can be performed with the lungs implanted en bloc (Fig. 10-52), but initial experience has been discouraging. Cardiopulmonary bypass is required. The heart is retracted cephalad and to the right to expose the left atrium for anastomosis with the common left atrium of the donor block (Fig.

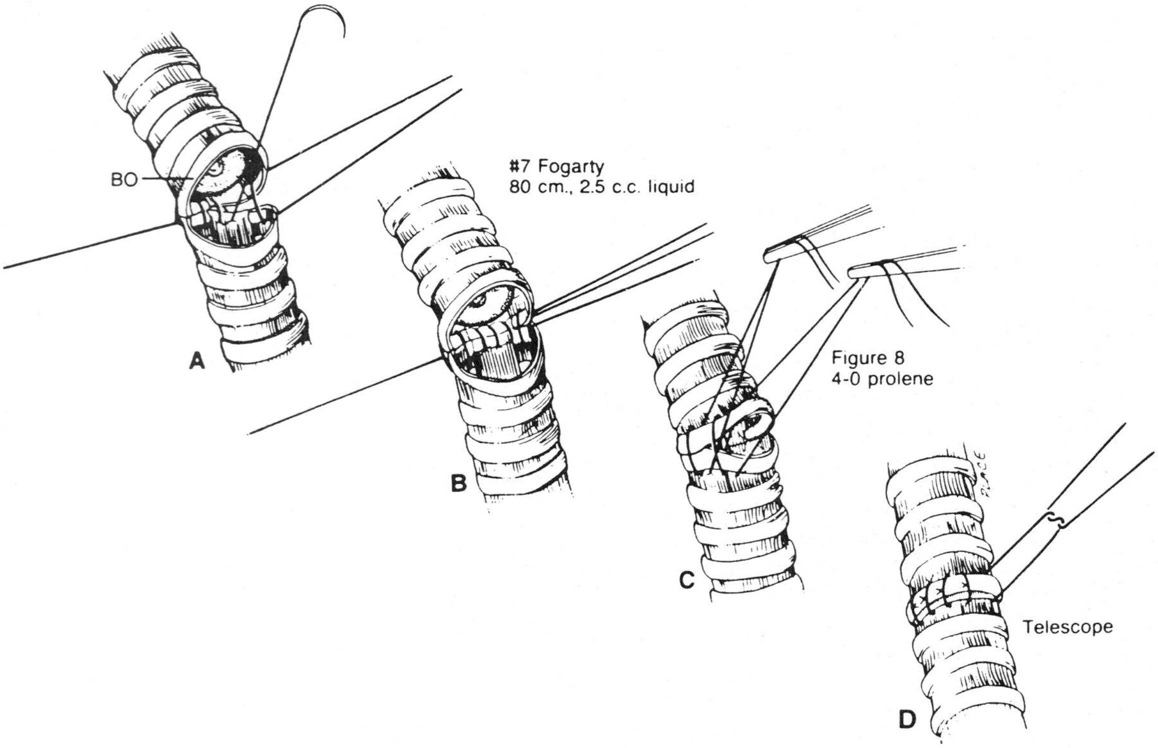

FIG. 10-49. The "telescoping" technique for bronchial anastomosis. *A.* Traction sutures are placed at each end of the membranous portion of the bronchus and a running suture begun posteriorly. *B.* The suture line in the membranous bronchus has been completed. *C.* The anterior anastomosis is completed by placing figure-of-eight sutures around the cartilages. *D.* As the anterior sutures are tied, the donor bronchus "telescopes" to a depth of one cartilage. (From: *Calhoon JH, Grover FL, et al: Single lung transplantation: Alternative indications. J Thorac Cardiovasc Surg 101:822, 1991, with permission.*)

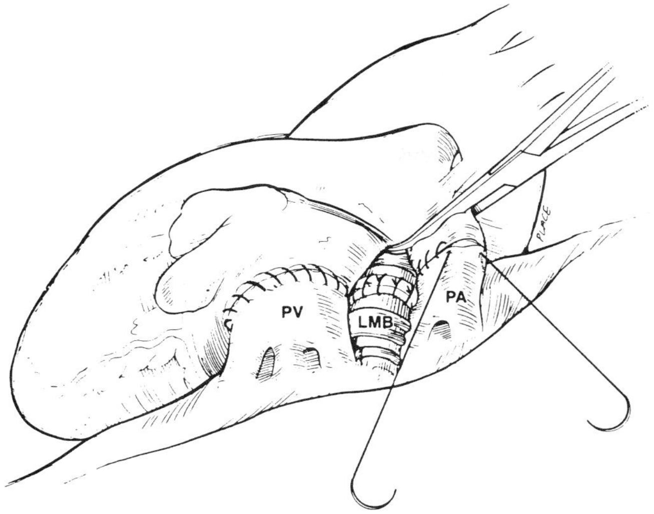

FIG. 10-50. Completion of a left single-lung transplant. After completing anastomoses between pulmonary veins (PV) and left main bronchi (LMB), the pulmonary artery (PA) anastomosis is completed. The left atrial clamp has been removed to allow retrograde filling of the lung vasculature, which will expel air through the open portion of the PA anastomosis. (From: *Calhoon JH, Grover FL, et al: Single lung transplantation: Alternative indications. J Thorac Cardiovasc Surg 101:822, 1991, with permission.*)

10-53), followed by a tracheal anastomosis placed just above the carina. Anastomosis between the main pulmonary arteries completes the procedure.

Heart-Lung. The operation is usually performed through a median sternotomy, but can be performed through a bilateral ante-

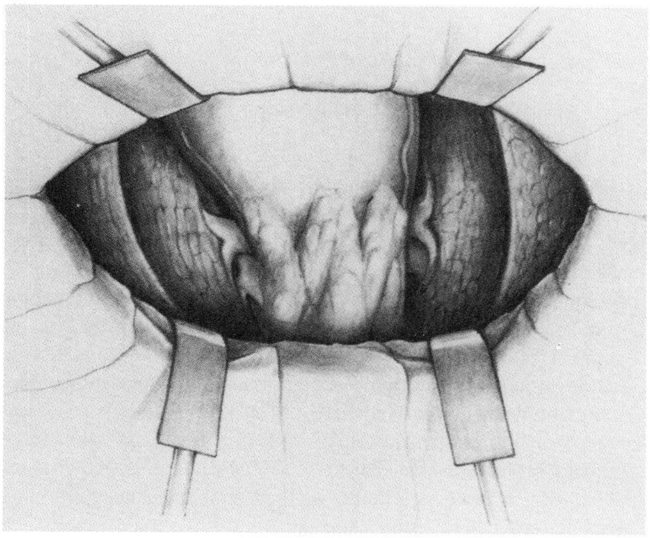

FIG. 10-51. A bilateral anterior thoracotomy provides exposure of the heart, visible in the center, and both lungs. Interspace incisions are connected across the sternum, dividing both internal mammary arteries. The fifth interspace is most frequently used, although the fourth or sixth can be advantageous in some circumstances. This approach was routinely used for open heart surgery before median sternotomy became popular, and has also been called the "clamshell," the "crossbow," and "sternal bithoracotomy." (From: *Bisson A, Bonnette P, A new technique for double lung transplantation: Bilateral single lung transplantation. J Thorac Cardiovasc Surg 103:42, 1992, with permission.*)

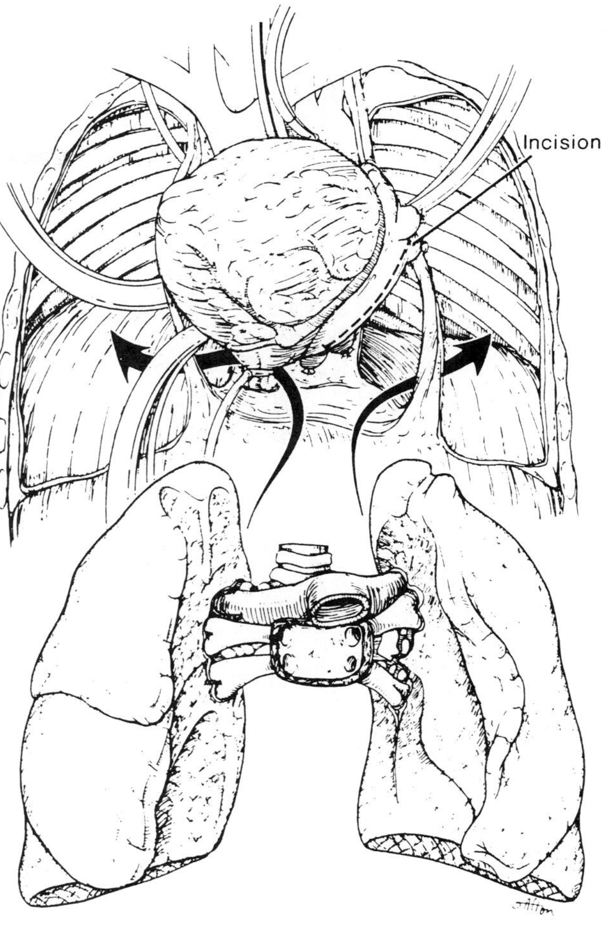

FIG. 10-52. En bloc double-lung transplant. The recipient is on cardiopulmonary bypass, which permits retraction of the heart to expose the left atrium. The incision to be made in the recipient left atrium is shown. Each lung is passed under the phrenic nerve. (From: *Bonser RS, Fragomeni, et al: Technique of clinical double-lung transplant. J Heart Transplant 7:300, 1988, with permission.*)

rior thoracotomy when there are unusual demands for posterior exposure. The patient is placed on cardiopulmonary bypass with bicaval venous cannulation. The heart is excised by dividing the great vessels at their commissures and resecting the ventricles at the level of the atrioventricular grooves (Fig. 10-54). Removing the heart improves exposure for the difficult posterior hilar and mediastinal dissection that follows. Both phrenic nerves are carefully isolated on pedicles of pericardium extending from the diaphragm to each pulmonary artery. The two lungs are excised along with the left atrium and the main pulmonary artery, leaving a small button of pulmonary artery to protect the recurrent laryngeal nerve where it passes under the ligamentum arteriosum. The right atrium and both cavae are mobilized to provide room for the right lung to pass underneath. The bronchi are followed back into the middle of the mediastinum posterior to the aorta, through dense layers of highly vascular lymphatic tissue, to expose the trachea for division just proximal to the carina (Fig. 10-55). Implantation begins by passing the left lung under the left phrenic pedicle, and by passing the right lung under the right phrenic pedicle and right atrium, followed by tracheal, right atrial, and aortic anastomoses (Fig. 10-56).

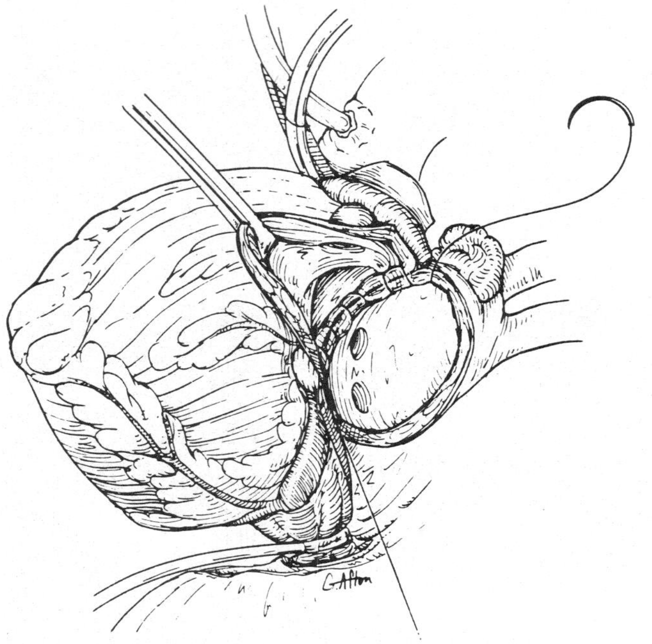

FIG. 10-53. En bloc double-lung transplant. The cephalad portion of the left atrial anastomosis is completed first. Following the left atrial anastomosis the tracheal and pulmonary artery anastomoses are carried out. (From: *Bonser RS, Fragomeni LS, et al: Technique of clinical double-lung transplant. J Heart Transplant 7:300, 1988, with permission.*)

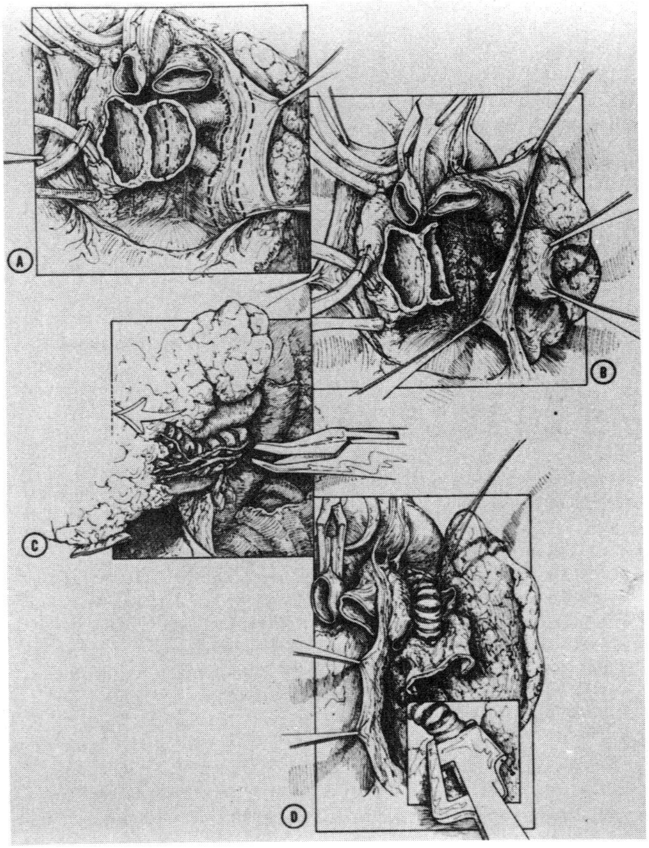

FIG. 10-54. *A.* The recipient atria after removal of the heart. Incisions are made so as to preserve the phrenic nerve in a "ribbon" of pericardium. The left and right pulmonary veins are separated by a longitudinal incision in the posterior left atrial wall and thus into the oblique sinus. *B.* The left pulmonary veins are withdrawn beneath the phrenic nerve. The vagus nerve is immediately posterior. *C.* The left lung is progressively mobilized, and the bronchial arteries are secured. *D.* The left pulmonary artery is divided and the bronchus is stapled and cut. (Copyright B. Hyams.) (From: *Jamieson SW, Stinson EB, et al: 1984, with permission.*)

The technical keys to operation are hemostasis of the middle mediastinum and protection of both phrenic nerves, both vagus nerves, and the recurrent nerve. Hemostasis can be very difficult to achieve, especially in patients with large bronchial collateral vessels. Postoperative bleeding has been a major problem, one that can begin a vicious cycle of massive transfusion and deteriorating pulmonary function. Intraoperative administration of aprotinin, a serine protease inhibitor which reduces postoperative bleeding, has become an important adjunct to heart-lung transplant. Paralyzed diaphragms and gastric dilatation can seriously interfere with ventilation.

Postoperative Management. All patients, regardless of procedure, should be extubated as soon as possible to minimize barotrauma to the lung(s) and to the tracheal/bronchial anastomoses. Before and after extubation tracheobronchial secretions can be profuse, and are aggressively managed with bronchoscopy and chest physiotherapy. During the first 2 weeks, before lymphatic drainage is reestablished and ischemic injury has healed, the lungs are kept as dry as possible with vigorous diuresis. Broad antibiotic coverage is maintained until intraoperative cultures from the donor allow discontinuation or guide modification. Gas exchange and serial chest x-rays are followed closely for evidence of change suggesting infection, rejection, or lung injury due to ischemia/reperfusion.

A problem unique to lung, in comparison to other solid organ, transplants is that infection of the transplanted organ is more common and more serious, and must always be considered when changes in the chest x-ray or in gas exchange suggest rejection. Infection was the cause of death in 34 percent of heart-lung recipients and 55 percent of single-lung recipients recorded in the Registry of the International Society for Heart and Lung Transplantation. The most difficult distinction to make is between rejection and viral pneumonia, which can be clinically indistinguishable, yet the distinction is crucial because viral pneumonia is likely to become rapidly progressive if treated as rejection with augmented immunosuppression. Bronchoscopy to obtain deep specimens for culture is essential when infection must be ruled out, and should include bronchoalveolar lavage and transbronchial biopsy. Not infrequently, the crucial diagnosis of CMV lung disease relies entirely upon the demonstration of inclusion bodies in lung tissue obtained by transbronchial biopsy. CMV disease is treated with ganciclovir, immune globulin, and reduced immunosuppression when the clinical situation allows. Fungal infections, usually *Aspergillus,* have a poor prognosis, and are treated with amphotericin.

Most centers use triple-drug immunosuppression as maintenance therapy (see Table 10-10). There is a prevalent belief that lung rejection is more frequent, more aggressive, and more difficult to reverse than cardiac rejection, and maintenance immunosuppression in lung recipients tends to be correspondingly aggressive. Many centers use cytolytic induction therapy, although

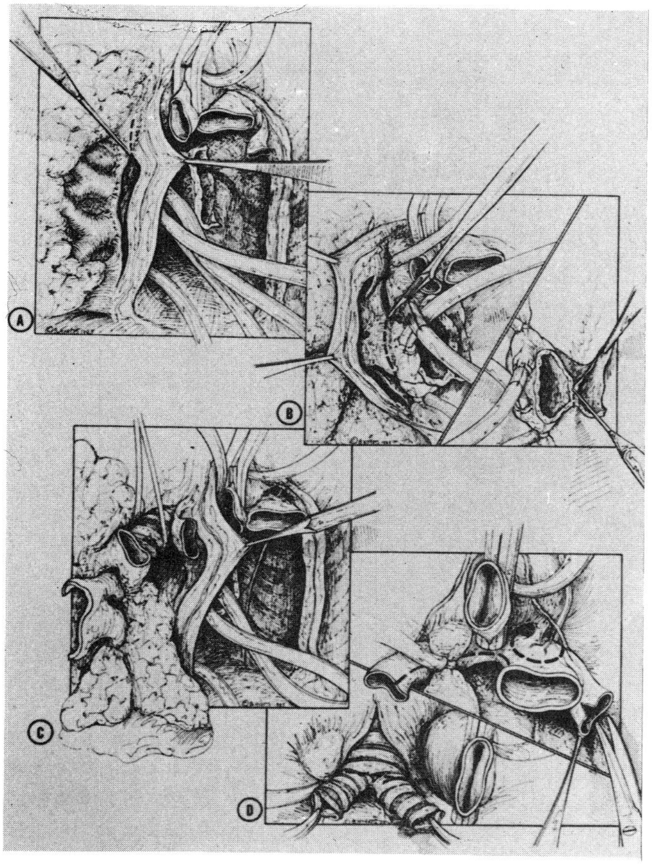

FIG. 10-55. *A.* The right phrenic nerve is separated from the hilum. *B.* The right pulmonary veins are separated from the right atrium. *C.* The right pulmonary ligament is divided, the lung is mobilized, and the pulmonary artery and bronchus are cut. *D.* The remnants of the pulmonary artery are removed, leaving the area around the ductus ligament and recurrent nerve. The trachea and bronchial remnants are exposed to the right of the aorta. The trachea is cut just above the carina. (Copyright B. Hyams.) (From: *Jamieson SW, Stinson EB, et al: 1984, with permission.*)

others feel strongly that the price paid in the incidence of fatal viral infections is too high. Although a cornerstone of the doctrine developed by Cooper to inaugurate the modern era of single-lung transplant held that steroid abstinence for the first 2 weeks was important to bronchial healing, recent trends generally favor use of steroids throughout the postoperative period. As with heart transplantation, complete steroid abstinence may become a possibility with combinations of newer immunosuppressive agents, but is not uniformly achievable with cyclosporine-based immunosuppression.

Histologic examination of transbronchial biopsy tissue specimens is the standard method for diagnosis of lung rejection. Surveillance biopsies are performed on a tapering schedule. Decrements in pulmonary function tests, particularly FEV_1, may signal rejection and call for biopsy. Rejection is graded according to standard nomenclature (Table 10-15). Taking into account the entire clinical context, rejection of Grade 2 or greater is first treated with an oral or intravenous steroid boost, and refractory rejection is treated with a cytolytic agent.

Single-lung transplant has certain unique problems related to the presence of the native lung. In patients with emphysema, the high compliance of the native lung favors overexpansion on positive-pressure ventilation, which can produce serious mediastinal shifts capable of compromising venous return and gas exchange. When early extubation is impractical, this can be corrected by maintaining the patient on split-lung ventilation with two ventilators through a double-lumen endotracheal tube, keeping tidal volume to the native lung as low as the machine will allow.

In single-lung recipients with pulmonary hypertension, 80 to 95 percent of perfusion shifts immediately to the transplanted lung, which may exacerbate early reperfusion injury and contribute to a syndrome of profound pulmonary edema. For similar reasons, any process that interferes with effective ventilation of the transplanted lung, such as pneumonia or rejection, further exacerbates a dramatic ventilation/perfusion mismatch if ventilation begins to shift back toward the native lung. This is most common in patients with primary pulmonary vascular disease who have relatively normal bronchoalveolar mechanics. Cardiorespiratory support with ECMO (extracorporeal membrane oxygenation) has occasionally salvaged patients with extreme ventilation/perfusion mismatches in the early postoperative period.

Heart-lung recipients require inotropic and chronotropic support of the denervated heart in the early postoperative period and carry the risk of cardiac rejection in addition to lung rejection. Cardiac and pulmonary rejection can occur independently. For reasons that are not entirely clear, cardiac rejection in heart-lung recipients is significantly ($p < 0.01$) less frequent than in heart recipients. Surveillance endomyocardial biopsies are performed on a tapering schedule and become unnecessary after one year.

Results. A total of 1212 heart-lung transplants performed over a 10-year period through 1991 have been recorded in the Registry of the International Society for Heart and Lung Transplantion. Numbers of heart-lung transplants have been decreasing in recent years, as many patients previously treated with heart-lung transplant have been shifted successfully to single-lung or double-lung transplant (Fig. 10-57). The mean age for those requiring double-lung transplants is 31 years versus 45 years for those requiring single-lung transplants; this is reflected by the nature of these diseases.

One-year actuarial survival for all heart-lung transplants contained in the Registry is a disappointing 64 percent (Fig. 10-58). Reports from active centers concentrating on recent experience are more encouraging; at Stanford 1-year actuarial survival is 73 percent for patients treated since 1986. Thirty-day mortality for heart-lung transplant continues to be about 20 percent, reflecting the technical challenge of the operation, while 30-day mortality has steadily decreased since 1988 for double-lung (from 44 to 14 percent) and single-lung (from 23 to 13 percent).

Appropriately selected patients who avoid early problems achieve an excellent functional result, with normal exercise function and with pulmonary function tests that often exceed 80 percent of predicted values. Obliterative bronchiolitis, which is thought to be a manifestation of chronic rejection directed against airways, limits long-term function and survival in up to 30 percent of patients.

The most recent compilation of results for single- and double-lung transplants are contained in the St. Louis International Lung Transplant Registry, with 1536 lung transplants reported through August 1992 from 81 centers around the world. Two-thirds of the procedures have been single-lung, with a slight predominance of single left lung (532 left, 472 right). One-third of the procedures

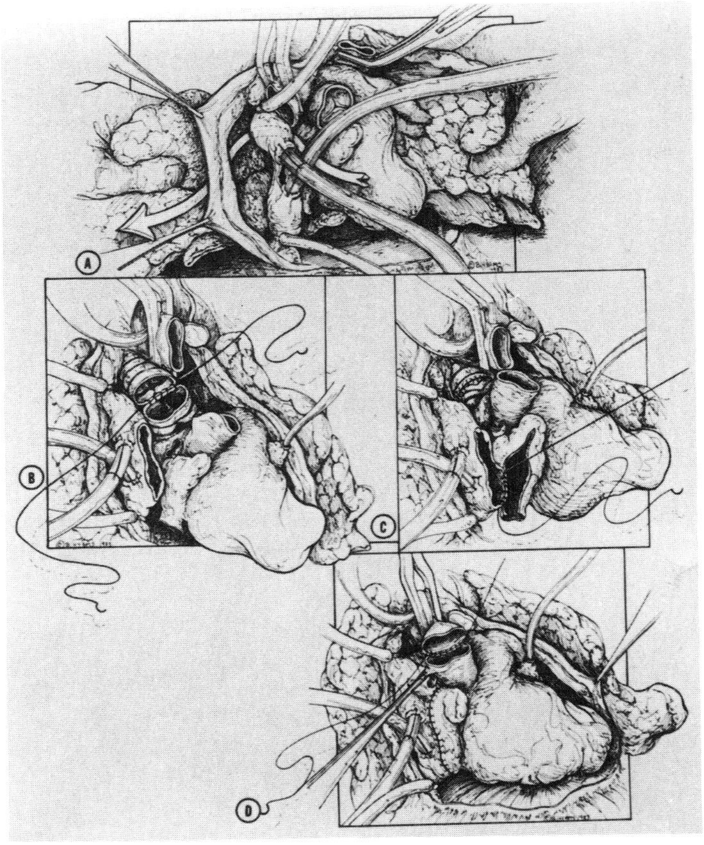

FIG. 10-56. Reimplantation: *A.* The right lung passes beneath the right atrial remnant and the phrenic nerve. *B.* The tracheal anastomosis is performed first, commencing with the posterior wall. *C.* The right atrial anastomosis. *D.* The aortic anastomosis. (Copyright B. Hyams.) (From: *Jamieson SW, Stinson EB, et al: 1984, with permission.*)

Table 10-15
Standardized Lung Biopsy Grading

Class	*Grade*	*Nomenclature*	*Description*
A. Acute rejection	**0**	No rejection	No significant abnormality
	1a,b,c,d*	Minimal acute rejection	Scattered perivascular infiltrates
	2a,b,c,d	Mild acute rejection	Frequent perivascular infiltrates
	3a,b,c,d	Moderate acute rejection	Dense infiltrates, extension into alveoli
	4a,b,c,d	Severe acute rejection	Pneumocyte necrosis, alveolar hemorrhage
B. Acute airway damage	1	Lymphocytic bronchitis	Lymphocytic infiltrates, mucosal/submucosal
	2	Lymphocytic bronchiolitis	Same, involving terminal bronchioles
C. Chronic airway rejection	1	Bronchiolitis obliterans (subtotal) (a = active, b = inactive)	Partial fibrous obliteration of airways
	2	Bronchiolitis obliterans (total)	Total fibrous obliteration of airways
D. Chronic vascular rejection			Fibrointimal thickening of arteries, veins
E. Vasculitis			Inflammatory infiltrates in vessel walls

*For each grade of acute rejection, modifiers a–d are applied:
a = With evidence of bronchiolar inflammation
b = Without evidence of bronchiolar inflammation
c = With large airway inflammation
d = No bronchioles are present in the biopsy

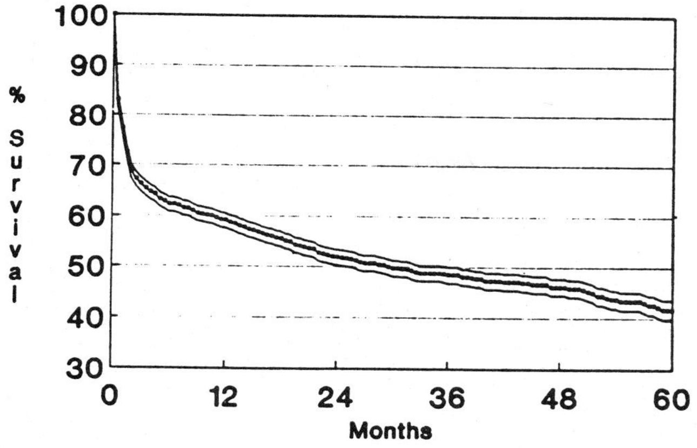

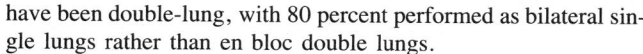

FIG. 10-57. A bar graph showing the number of heart-lung (H-L), double-lung (D-L), and single-lung (S-L) transplants done from 1986 through 1991. (From: *Kaye MP: 1992, with permission.*)

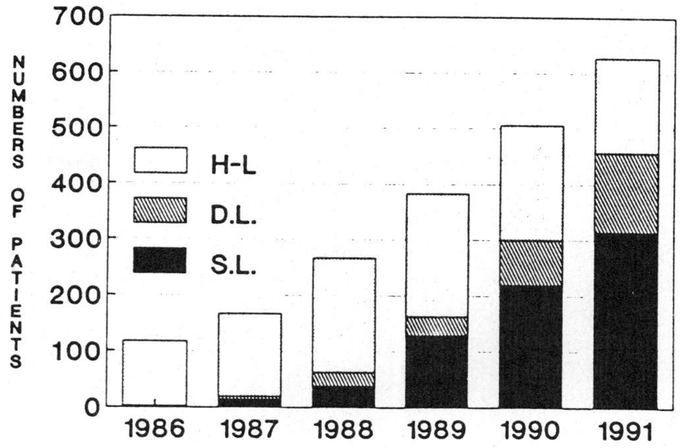

FIG. 10-58. Kaplan-Meier actuarial survival curve for all heart-lung transplants recorded in the Registry of the International Society for Heart and Lung Transplantation. (From: *Kaye MP: 1992, with permission.*)

have been double-lung, with 80 percent performed as bilateral single lungs rather than en bloc double lungs.

The period of exponential growth in lung transplantation may be ending. One-third of the entire experience recorded in the Registry occurred in 1991 (543 transplants), and 1992 appears unlikely to exceed that figure (336 transplants through August 1992). Slacking growth in total numbers reflects in part a shift toward double-lung transplant, which spreads the same number of donors across fewer recipients.

The predominant indication for single-lung transplant is emphysema (42 percent), many of whom (12 percent) have alpha$_1$-antitrypsin deficiency. Single-lung transplants for pulmonary fibrosis have continued to decrease in frequency (from 26 to 14 percent over 3 years) because results have not been as good as those obtained in patients with obstructive lung disease. The predominant indications for double-lung transplant are cystic fibrosis and similar conditions producing end-stage septic lung disease (45 percent). Emphysema (31 percent) and pulmonary hypertension (14 percent) are other common indications for double-lung transplant.

One-year actuarial survival for all lung transplants contained in the St. Louis Registry is 68 percent (Fig. 10-59). Results are virtually identical for single lungs and double lungs performed as bilateral single lungs (69 percent and 68 percent, respectively), with a poorer outcome for en bloc double lungs (57 percent). Although few statistically significant trends relating outcome to diagnosis have emerged, results of lung transplant for patients with emphysema have been consistently at the high end (74 to 81 percent

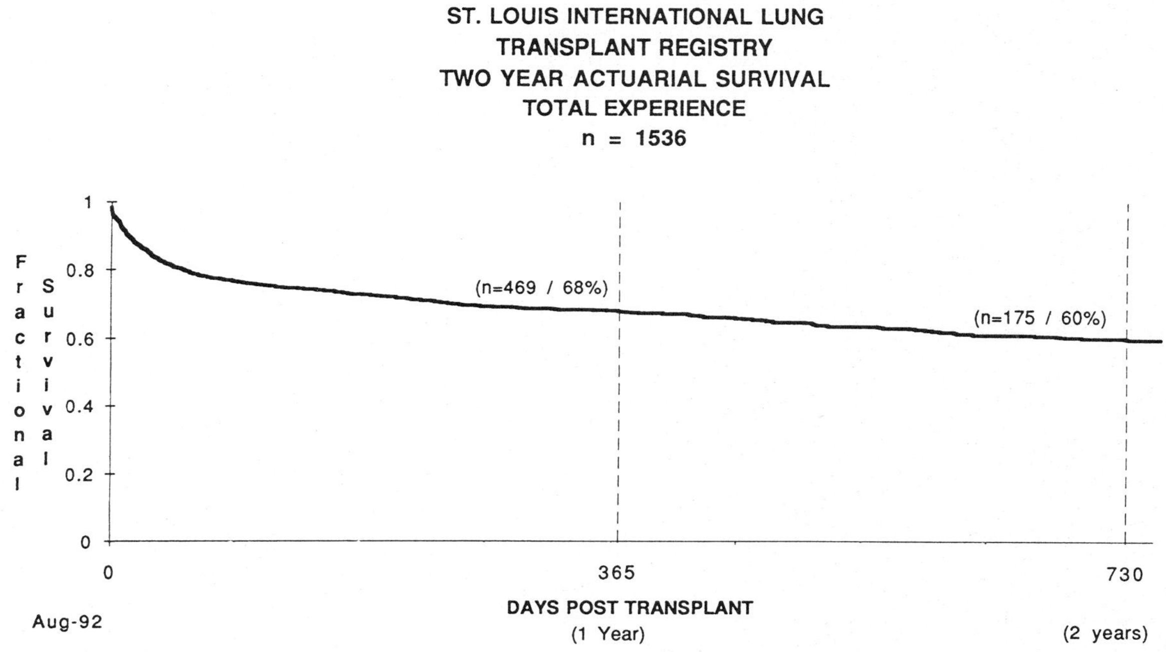

FIG. 10-59. Kaplan-Meier actuarial survival curve for all single- and double-lung transplants (n = 1536) recorded in the August 1992 report of the St. Louis International Lung Transplant Registry. (From: *Cooper JD (ed): 1992, with permission.*)

1-year survival). Although 1-year survival in 202 patients transplanted for cystic fibrosis in the St. Louis Registry is only 65 percent, results have been outstanding in certain centers reporting recent experience (> 90 percent at Columbia-Presbyterian and the University of North Carolina).

Functional results following lung transplant were thoroughly evaluated in 50 single- and 40 double-lung transplants done in Toronto. Although pulmonary function tests rarely return to 100 percent of predicted values, substantial improvement occurs in virtually all parameters. Not surprisingly, double-lung recipients demonstrate significantly greater functional improvement than single-lung recipients. Trends seen for improvement in exercise capacity (Fig. 10-60) are representative of trends equally well seen in pulmonary function tests (Fig. 10-61) and arterial blood gases.

Obliterative bronchiolitis is proving to be as prevalent in single- and double-lung transplants as in heart-lung transplants, and can be expected to limit long-term survival and functional results in up to 30 percent of recipients. It has been suggested that mortality from obliterative bronchiolitis would be lower in single-lung recipients because they could rely on the native lung. In fact, single-lung recipients with primary or secondary pulmonary hypertension tolerate bronchiolitis very poorly, because any interference with ventilation to the transplanted lung dramatically exacerbates a major underlying ventilation-perfusion mismatch.

Lung transplantation in children is performed for a different spectrum of indications. Eisenmenger's syndrome and other congenital heart disease, cystic fibrosis, and primary pulmonary hypertension predominate. As a consequence, single-lung transplant is the least frequent procedure performed in children. Combining both Registries, 212 lung transplants have been performed in children, of which 141 were heart-lungs, 50 were double lungs, and 21 were single lungs. Although 1-year survival in the Registries is ~65 percent, results have been better in centers reporting concentrated recent experience. At Stanford, 1-year survival was 82 percent for children aged one to fourteen years, and 74 percent for children under one year; and at Columbia-Presbyterian, for children ages one to sixteen years 1-year survival is currently 86 percent.

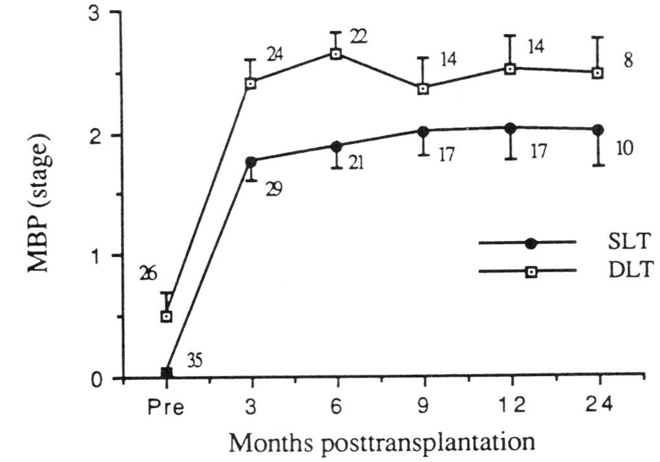

FIG. 10-60. Performance of single- (SLT) and double-lung transplant (DLT) recipients in a Modified Bruce protocol (MBP) assessment of exercise capacity. (From: *de Hoyos AL, Patterson GA, et al: Pulmonary Transplantation: Early and late results. J Thorac Cardiovasc Surg 103:302, 1992, with permission.*)

Retransplantation for acute or chronic graft failure has been associated with very low salvage. One-year survival among 63 retransplants recorded in the St. Louis Registry is only 39 percent. In view of these findings an ethical argument is often made against use of a donor lung for a retransplant when it could be used for another patient with greater probability of benefit.

Future Directions. In lung transplantation, matching the procedure to the diagnosis remains imperfect. Donor shortage is a powerful argument favoring priority for single-lung transplant for any suitable diagnosis; three recipients can benefit from a heart-lung block if each lung is transplanted singly. There seems to be

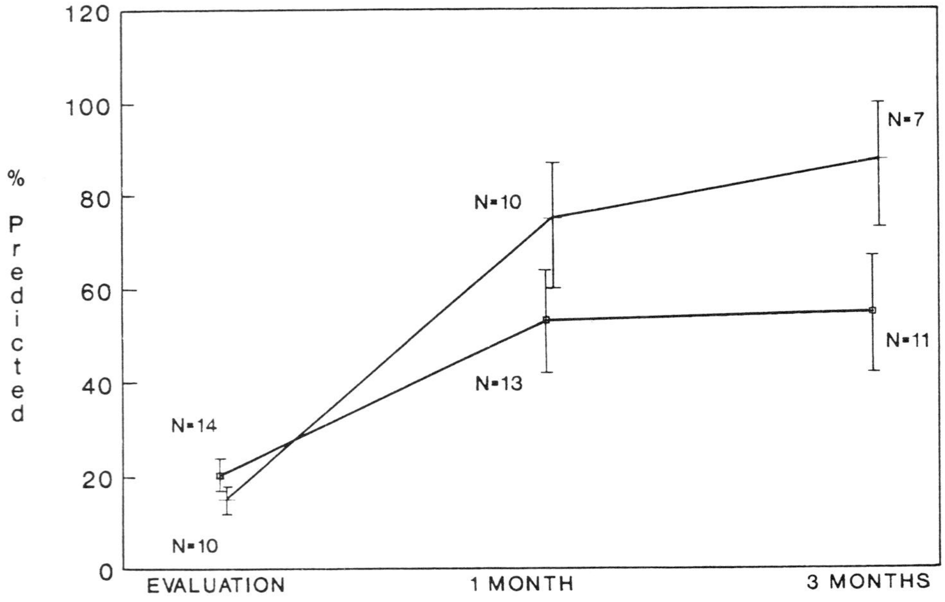

FIG. 10-61. Percent of predicted FEV_1 in patients with obstructive lung disease who underwent single (bottom curve, N = 14) or double (top curve, N = 10) lung transplant. Bars are 95 percent confidence limits. (From: *Haydock DA, Trulock EP, et al, with permission.*)

little question that most patients with emphysema do very well with single-lung transplant. Double-lung transplant clearly produces greater functional improvement, with a 30-day mortality comparable with single-lung; and double-lung transplant avoids the ventilation-perfusion mismatches seen with single-lung. Especially in the treatment of primary and secondary pulmonary hypertension, the balance may tip toward double-lung. Heart-lung will continue to be reserved for patients with unsalvageable cardiac pathology. Much remains to be learned about how to define the boundary between salvageable and unsalvageable right ventricular function.

Kidney

Renal transplantation is one of the earliest success stories for solid organ transplantation. The technical knowledge necessary to perform kidney transplants has been available since the turn of the century, when Carrel and Guthrie developed the techniques of vascular suture. Renal transplantation is now the treatment of choice for many patients with renal failure, although hemodialysis and peritoneal dialysis serve as an adequate substitute for most patients.

Indications and Contraindications. In general, irreversible renal failure is the only indication necessary for the patient with a normal urinary outflow tract and without active infection, severe malnutrition, disseminated malignancy, or life-limiting systemic disease. Lower tract abnormalities can usually be corrected. The only absolute contraindications are active infection or malignant disease that cannot be brought under control. A partial list of diseases for which transplantation has been carried out is included in Table 10-16. Diabetes is now the most common cause of renal failure in the United States: approximately one-third of all renal transplants are performed for treatment of renal failure in Type 1 diabetes.

Transplantation, when successful, offers a greater degree of rehabilitation to the uremic patient than does either hemodialysis or peritoneal dialysis. The risks are also slightly greater because immunosuppression is required for the duration of graft function. Renal transplantation has been demonstrated to be superior to chronic dialysis with respect to quality of life, medical costs, and overall health of the patient. In children, growth is better after transplantation. Diabetics seem to have fewer problems after transplantation than during dialysis. Most patients who have had a transplant—even one that has failed—prefer life with a kidney transplantation to life on dialysis.

A few renal diseases will recur in transplants but such diseases are only relative contraindications; focal glomerulosclerosis, hemolytic uremia syndrome, membranoproliferative glomerulonephritis of the dense-deposit type, and diabetes are among them. A number of metabolic diseases (gout, oxalosis, cystinosis, hyperoxaluria, nephrocalcinosis, and amyloidosis) have very little in common except for the accumulation within the kidney of abnormal deposits associated with renal failure. Transplants in most of these diseases can be successful, although recurrence after oxalosis is common.

The psychologic disturbances exhibited by some patients with chronic renal failure are not contraindications to selection. It is extremely difficult to judge the psychologic and social stability of a patient with chronic illness. Similarly, one cannot exclude, out of hand, patients with coronary disease or cerebrovascular accidents. Patients with severe liver disease, however, are more susceptible to cyclosporine or azathioprine toxicity and sepsis. Liver disease, therefore, remains a relative contraindication.

Table 10-16
Indications for Renal Transplantation

Irreversible chronic renal failure	Irreversible acute failure
Chronic pyelonephritis	Cortical necrosis
Chronic glomerulonephritis	Hemolytic-uremic syndrome
Diabetic nephropathy	Acute and subacute glomerulonephritis
Goodpasture's disease	Anaphylactoid purpura (Henoch-Schönlein)
Hypocomplementemic nephritis	Acute tubular necrosis
Steroid-resistant nephrotic syndrome	Trauma requiring nephrectomy
Hypertensive nephrosclerosis	Renal vascular diseases
Obstructive uropathy	Renal artery occlusion
Acquired	Renal vein thrombosis
Congenital	Tumors requiring nephrectomy
Congenital disorders	Renal carcinoma
Aplasia	Wilms' tumor
Hypoplasia	Tuberous sclerosis
Horseshoe kidney	Other
Hereditary nephropathies	Multiple myeloma
Alport's syndrome	Macroglobulinemia
Polycystic kidney disease	Wegner's disease
Medullary cystic disease	Scleroderma
Metabolic disorders	Lupus erythematosus
Hyperoxaluria	Polyarteritis (periarteritis nodosa)
Nephrocalcinosis	
Gout	
Oxalosis	
Amyloidosis	
Cystinosis	

SOURCE: Modified from Simmons RL, Ascher NL, Najarian JS: Host hepatectomy and liver transplantation, in Simmons RL, Finch ME, Ascher NL, Najarian JS (eds): *Manual of Vascular Access, Organ Donation, and Transplantation*. New York, Springer-Verlag, 1984, pp 255–284.

Most important than the actual selection technique of the potential recipient is the choice of time for the institution of treatment by dialysis or transplantation. Treatment by either technique should always be instituted before the development of uremic complications. Once hypertension, pericarditis, cardiac failure, severe anemia, and neuropathy appear, management is markedly complicated and rehabilitation compromised. Ideally, the conservative management of progressive renal functional deterioration should be carried out in conjunction with nephrologists associated with both dialysis and transplant centers. In this way, the complication of severe uremia can be rapidly prevented by treatment without the delays inherent in the referral process.

The traditional indication for the institution of dialysis has been a serum creatinine level greater than 15 mg/dL or a creatinine clearance less than 3 mL/min despite meticulous conservative care. It is obvious that there are exceptions to this rule. Some patients, particularly patients with polycystic kidney disease, with serum creatinine levels greater than 15 mg/dL can be maintained well for months on dietary management. In other patients, especially diabetic patients, severe complications of uremia will develop long before the serum creatinine reaches that level. The most pernicious of these complications is peripheral neuropathy. If there are signs of motor involvement, the patient should have dialysis and transplantation without delay, since very rapid progression of the disease can make it impossible ever to rehabilitate such a patient. Another indication for early dialysis-transplantation is uncontrollable hypertension, or hypertension that can be controlled only at the expense of severe orthostatic hypotension and other side effects. Severe anemia with anemic symptoms (dyspnea at the mildest exertion), severe bone disease (especially in children), and the failure of the patient to maintain a diet or carry on social and family obligations all should lead to early dialysis and transplantation. There is little to be gained by a delay of 3 to 6 months, and lives may be lost in futile attempts at conservative management. The administration of *erythropoietin,* a red-blood-cell colony-stimulating factor, has virtually eliminated the requirement for blood transfusions in patients with renal failure. The absence of production of erythropoietin by the kidney in renal failure resulted in transfusion-dependent severe anemia in the past, before the availability of exogenous sources of erythropoietin.

Since some of the complications of uremia may appear suddenly during conservative management, it is extremely important that the patient be fully evaluated as early in the course of progressive uremia as possible. In addition to the medical evaluation, this preparation should include interviews with the hospital, the rehabilitation clinic, and social service in order to ameliorate the financial and social difficulties that may accompany dialysis and transplantation. Rehabilitation of the patient can be actively pursued even before the institution of definitive treatment.

Although most patients with end-stage renal disease will undergo a period of dialysis before transplant, many patients who are carefully followed for progressive uremia can be transplanted without dialysis. In this way, the number of vascular or peritoneal access procedures necessary for dialysis can be reduced, and care can be rendered more economically. This approach is favored increasingly by many.

Preparation for Transplantation. The pretransplantation studies are listed in Table 10-17. Most of these studies are used by many transplant groups and for patients on dialysis. A few deserve elaboration.

Table 10-17
Work-up of Potential Recipients of Renal Transplantation

1. General
   a. History and physical examination
   b. Chest x-ray
   c. ECG
   d. Electrophoresis
   e. Fasting blood sugar
2. Hematologic
   a. Hemoglobin
   b. Leukocyte count and differential count
   c. Platelet count
   d. Bleeding-clotting time
   e. Prothrombin time, partial thromboplastin time, thrombin time
3. Renal
   a. Flat plate of abdomen (kidney size) (tomography)
   b. Creatinine clearance
   c. 24-h protein excretion
   d. (Electrophoresis/urine, protein excretion selectivity)
   e. Electrolyte status in blood
   f. (Electrolyte status in urine)
   g. Urinalysis ×3
   h. Urine culture ×3
   i. (Renal biopsy)
4. Signs of hyperparathyroidism
   a. Bone x-ray (hands, skull, clavicle, lamina dura)
   b. Ca, PO_4, Mg, alkaline phosphatase
5. Hypertensive work-up
   a. Chest x-ray (heart size)
   b. ECG
   c. Ophthalmic examination
   d. Serial blood pressure
6. Urologic evaluation
   a. Voiding cystogram
   b. (Retrograde pyelography)
   c. (Cystometrography)
   d. (Bladder biopsy)
   e. (Bladder stimulation)
7. Upper gastrointestinal x-ray, cholecystogram (colon x-ray in older patients)
8. Pap smear
9. Dental consultation and correction of any infectious problem
10. Typing
    a. ABO
    b. Blood pedigree
    c. Tissue typing including serial cytotoxic antibody determinations
11. (Pulmonary function studies)
12. Infectious work-up
    a. Chest x-ray
    b. Urine culture
    c. Blood culture
    d. (Sinus-teeth x-ray; ear, nose, and throat consultation)
13. Financial-social rehabilitation
    a. (Psychologic-psychiatric)

NOTE: The tests listed within parentheses are not administered routinely during the potential recipient work-up, but only when the circumstances so indicate.

The urinary tract should be evaluated for patency of its outflow and absence of ureterovesical reflux. In general, a voiding cystogram suffices. That test makes it possible to determine that the urethra is unobstructed, that the bladder empties, that there are no abnormalities of the bladder wall, and that there is no ureteral reflux. It is almost impossible to evaluate bladder emptying in the presence of ureterovesical reflux. Contraction of the bladder wall leads to reflux of the urine into the ureters, which then empty back into the bladder when the bladder wall is relaxed. It may be necessary to remove both ureters at the ureterovesical junction before evaluation of the bladder for competence.

The gastrointestinal tract should be evaluated for the possibility of a preexisting peptic ulceration and to rule out a gastrointestinal malignancy. Pretransplant treatment regimens have almost completely eliminated upper gastrointestinal tract bleeding as a complication of steroid administration after transplant.

Because so many patients with uremia also have hearing deficits, periodic audiograms should be carried out.

Tissue Typing and Cross Matching. The principles of transplantation immunogenetics have been presented in detail above. Before transplantation, tissue typing to match donor and recipient should be carried out—both for the selection for the most appropriate donor and for the determination of the prognostic implications of tissue matching. It is possible at present to type most patients completely at the HLA-A, -B, and -D/DR loci (see Table 10-1). Monoclonal antibodies to various antigenic portions of HLA antigens are highly specific, allowing more precise HLA typing. In addition, techniques of molecular biology and peptide sequencing have been applied to HLA typing. This is extremely valuable in family donor selection because HLA identity between siblings occurs 25 percent of the time. Transplants between such perfectly matched siblings have long-term success rates of 95 percent. It is now established that cadaver donor 6-antigen-match grafts have a significantly higher survival rate than grafts that are randomly matched. Therefore, in spite of new immunosuppressive agents such as cyclosporine and FK506, the value of HLA matching remains of importance. However, because of the shortage of donor kidneys, many centers do not routinely utilize HLA matching for distribution of cadaver donor kidneys.

In addition to HLA matching, it is important to determine whether a putative recipient has antibodies against antigens on donor tissue. Patients who have been presensitized by blood transfusion, pregnancy, or previous transplantation can then be identified by serum reactivity against a panel of normal leukocytes bearing known HLA specificities.

Because many patients have preformed antibodies against a potential renal allograft donor, cross matching of the patient's serum to detect antibodies against donor leukocytes must be carried out immediately before the transplant. If these preformed antibody barriers are crossed, immediate (hyperacute) or accelerated rejection frequently ensues. Varying cross-matching techniques have varying degrees of sensitivity, and the most sensitive method should be utilized. Organ preservation techniques currently permit prolonged storage of kidneys (up to 48 and frequently 72 h) so that cross-matching techniques that take several hours can always precede transplantation.

Most transplant units draw serum samples monthly on all patients awaiting transplantation in order to detect the formation of antidonor antibodies. Several of these sera for final cross matching should always be used, since antibodies appear and disappear without apparent reason in recipients. Nevertheless, if a patient has previously made antibodies against the putative donor, it is likely that an accelerated rejection will occur and that that donor should not be utilized.

Transfusion. For many years blood transfusions to prospective transplant recipients were avoided as much as possible. Physicians recognized that sensitization to the histocompatibility antigens of the blood donor would occur and that cross matching of the donor kidney to the transfused recipient would be more difficult. Paradoxically, most data now agree that transplants to transfused patients are much more successful than transplants to the untransfused. In the cyclosporine era, first cadaver graft recipients had a 4 to 5 percent increase in graft survival associated with random blood transfusion, compared with untransfused recipients ($p <$ 0.001). The reason for this effect is not clear, but much data support the idea that a degree of specific immunologic nonreactivity may be induced to the transfused histocompatibility antigens. Whatever the reason, most transplant centers permit transfusions as needed for the uremic patient awaiting transplantation. Some centers perform deliberate transfusions either from the prospective related donor or from random donors. In practice, an immunosuppressive drug (azathioprine or cyclosporine) is often administered during pretransplant transfusions to minimize sensitization and maximize the effect.

Dialysis. Dialysis is not an essential preparation for all transplant patients, but most patients do require a period of dialysis because of preexistent uremia. Dialysis removes toxic products of small molecular size from the blood and reinstitutes acid-base balance and electrolyte homeostasis. Although such treatment will not relieve all the complications of uremia, it will prevent death in most cases. In hemodialysis, blood is passed through a tubing composed of a semipermeable membrane, so that dialyzable substances within the blood pass into the dialysis bath and dialyzable materials within the bath pass into the blood. Peritoneal dialysis uses the peritoneum as the semipermeable membrane, and the peritoneal cavity as the container of the dialysis bath.

Vascular Access for Hemodialysis. The Quinton-Scribner cannula was the instrument first widely used for access to blood in dialysis. This technique used cannulation of an artery and a vein with an external arteriovenous shunt. The persistence of the cannulas within the vessels and the subsequent passage through the skin had predictable consequences—the cannulas clotted. The cutaneous fistulas became infected, and the shunt was in danger of bleeding. Similar problems occur when long-term subclavian vein cannulation is used for vascular access, but such external systems using intravascular cannulation are still very useful for short-term hemodialysis.

For prolonged vascular access without prosthetic implants the best technique uses a subcutaneous arteriovenous fistula, usually constructed between the radial artery and the cephalic vein at the wrist (Fig. 10-62). The superficial veins become dilated, and blood can be obtained for passage through the dialyzer by the use of two large-bore needles inserted into the dilated venous system.

Many modifications of these fistulas have been devised that utilize vascular or prosthetic grafts to bridge gaps between artery and vein, but all provide a dilated subcutaneous vessel for repeated puncture with large-bore needles.

Peritoneal dialysis is a useful but less efficient alternative. The dialysis fluid is alternately infused into the peritoneal cavity and drained off. This technique requires the permanent implantation of a catheter through the abdominal wall. The catheter is capped when not in use. Peritoneal dialysis is most useful for children, and its principal disadvantage is a high incidence of bacterial peritonitis. Although even repeated peritoneal infections are rarely fatal, they render the dialysis treatment increasingly inefficient.

Dialysis as a definitive treatment for end-stage renal failure is a lifesaving, effective treatment for both short- and long-term therapy. The principal disadvantages are the energy-consuming nature of the treatment that requires a continuous commitment of the patient and physician to details for daily care. For this reason, transplantation, if successful, is preferable.

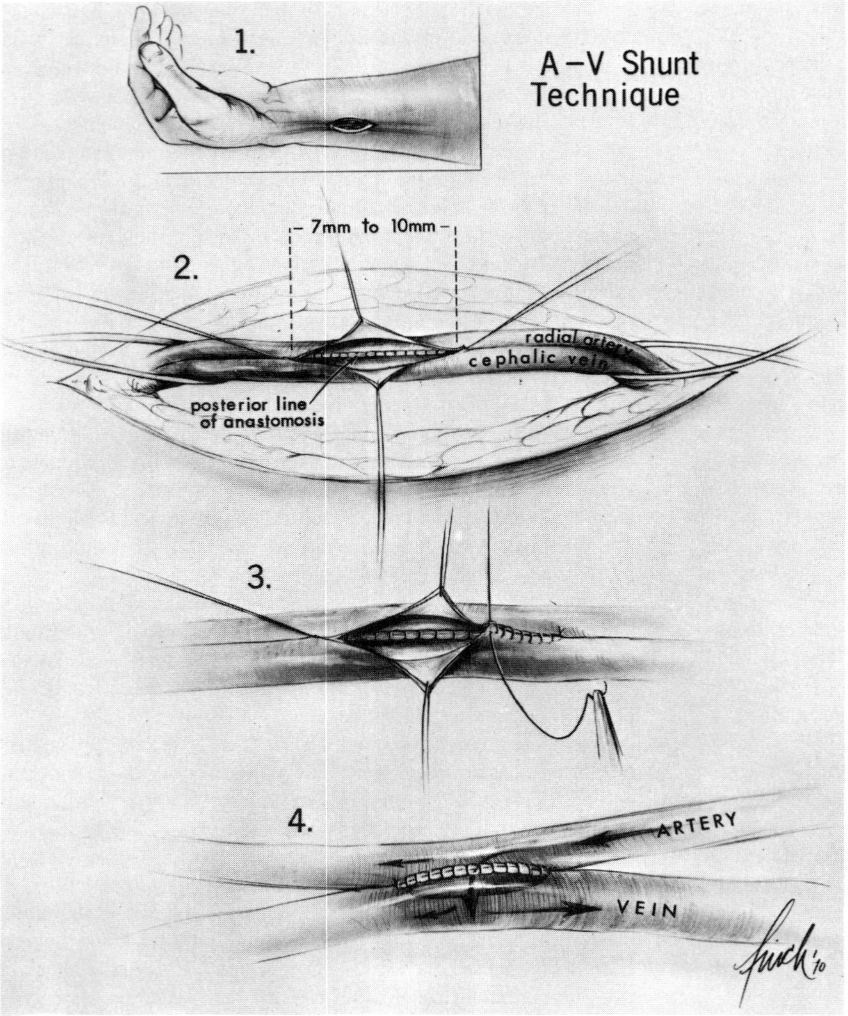

FIG. 10-62. Technique for constructing an arteriovenous anastomosis between radial artery and cephalic vein at the wrist. (From: *Kjellstrand CM, Simmons RL, et al: Kidney: I. Recipient selection, medical management, and dialysis, in Najarian JS, Simmons RL [eds]: Transplantation. Philadelphia, Lea & Febiger, 1972, p 148, with permission.*)

Selection and Evaluation of Living Donor. The principles of histocompatibility typing and matching have been described above. From the recipient's point of view it is generally preferable that the donor be a biologic relative. Even mismatched sibling and parent kidneys have survived with better function and for more prolonged periods than closely matched cadaver kidneys. Before the advent of histocompatibility typing, it was shown that kidneys from sibling donors functioned better than kidneys from parental donors. Because the genes governing the expression of histocompatibility antigens are situated at one (complex) locus, there will always be one major allelic difference between the parent and the offspring, whereas one-fourth of siblings will be identical, one-half will have a one-haplotype difference, and one-fourth will have both haplotypes different. Tissue typing can usually identify that sibling (if any) who shares all the serologically detectable antigens at the major histocompatibility complex (MHC). Such sibling grafts have a better than 95 percent chance for long-term success.

A living related donor offers other advantages to the recipient: the delay between renal failure and rehabilitation is shorter, post-transplant renal function is usually immediate, and there are fewer rejection episodes, so that smaller doses of immunosuppressive drugs are required.

The major blood group antigens (ABO) are strong transplantation antigens. Although a number of successful allotransplants have been carried out across isoantibody barriers, it is generally unwise to perform transplants into patients with known preformed isohemagglutinins against the donor blood type. The same rules apply to clinical transplantation that apply to transfusion, i.e., AB is the universal recipient and O the universal donor. When such blood type barriers are crossed, the most violent type of hyperacute rejection reaction may occur. There is some evidence to suggest that Lewis blood group factors (but not Rh, Duffy, Kell) act as histocompatibility antigens.

The living related donor should be in perfect health to minimize any risks inherent in an operation of this magnitude. Rare deaths following renal donation from a healthy person have been reported, and the utmost caution must be exerted not to harm or diminish the renal reserve of a healthy volunteer. Table 10-18 lists the examinations routinely carried out on volunteer related donors.

Ethical Problems. Selection of a related donor is made on the basis of histocompatibility testing when possible; often, however,

Table 10-18
Protocol for Living Related Donor Work-up

1. History and physical examination.
2. Hematology: hematocrit, leukocyte count, differential count, platelet count
3. Coagulation: prothrombin time, partial thromboplastin time, thrombin time
4. Chemistry: serum Na^+, K^+, Cl^-, CO^{2-}, SGOT, bilirubin, uric acid, Ca^{2+}, P, BUN, creatinine, fasting blood sugar, glucose tolerance test
5. Urine: urinalysis, 24-h urine for creatinine clearance
6. Microbiology: clean-catch urine culture ×2
7. Immunology: blood type (major and minor), tissue typing, leukocyte cross match for recipient antidonor and leukocyte antibodies; VDRL; screen for hepatitis
8. X-ray: chest x-ray, intravenous pyelogram (IVP), renal arteriograms
9. Isotope: bilateral renogram
10. Electrocardiogram

there is only one volunteer. The ethical and social problems of donor selection have been extensively discussed elsewhere, but brief consideration is pertinent here.

In practice, the recipient should be informed of the risks and benefits of receiving a kidney from a related donor. The recipient knows best which relatives can be approached and which cannot. When a volunteer appears he or she is blood-typed and tissue-typed. If the volunteer is acceptable on these grounds, the risk of donor nephrectomy is explained to him or her. The risk to life in an otherwise perfectly healthy patient has been estimated to be 0.05 percent. The long-term risk has been estimated by actuarial statistics to be similar to that incurred by driving a car 16 miles every working day. Much evidence suggests that no long-term harm results from life with a single kidney. Although risks are small, the pain, anxiety, and loss of work time are real.

It is difficult to conceive of a living related donor who is not subject to some family pressure to donate. That such pressures exist, however, is evidence that people have feelings of family and role obligations within the society. When a person freely volunteers to donate, both the benefits to the recipient and the risks to the donor are explained. No pressure is exerted to persuade or dissuade potential donors. They are not subjected to extensive psychologic interviews or testing. Careful studies of actual donors indicate a remarkably favorable psychologic response in most donors, but some ambivalence and conflict within the family occur in a minority. On occasion, when the potential donor expresses anxiety concerning the donation, it is necessary to fabricate a medical excuse not to donate that can be used by the otherwise medically and immunologically compatible donor.

Sometimes it is necessary or advisable to use donors under the age of eighteen. This has frequently been necessary for identical-twin transplants. The use of such donors, however, should be restricted to those circumstances in which other donors are not available. A court of law will find it difficult to decide whether an adolescent should donate to parents or siblings when family pressure may exist. Teen-aged donors have been used when they have insisted on donation and the court has agreed to it.

Unrelated persons are not generally encouraged to donate, since the results are no better than those achieved with cadaver donors.

Selection of Cadaver Donor. The ideal cadaver kidney donor (1) is young, (2) has remained normotensive until a short time before death, (3) is free of transmissible infection and malignant disease, and (4) has died in the hospital after observation for a number of hours, during which time blood group and tissue type have been determined and urinary function has been assessed. Under these ideal conditions the donor kidneys can be removed within minutes to minimize the warm ischemia time. It is often necessary, however, to compromise with these ideal principles. The age of the donor is not of crucial importance but kidneys from young children have decreased survival. A donated kidney can recover from long periods of shock and anuria that occur while it is still in the donor. But no more than 1 h of warm ischemia time should elapse during donation.

Criteria of Brain Death. The procurement of cadaver organs for transplantation has raised some serious moral, ethical, legal, and psychologic problems. The first problem is to establish when death occurs. Since the decision is a clinical one, made by the physician in the interest of the patient (potential donor), it should be based primarily on clinical criteria of irreversible brainstem damage—fixed, dilated pupils; absent reflexes; unresponsiveness to external stimuli; and the inability to maintain vital functions such as respiration, heartbeat, and blood pressure without artificial means. The decision should be made by physicians who are not associated with the potential recipient in any way, either as the referring physician or as a member of the transplant team. The exact criteria vary among institutions. Table 10-19 lists the guidelines for the determination of death reported to the President's Commission for the Study of Ethical Problems in Medicine and

Table 10-19
Criteria for Determination of Death

An individual with the findings in either section A (cardiopulmonary) or B (neurologic) is dead.

A. Cardiopulmonary
An individual with irreversible cessation of circulatory and respiratory functions is dead.
1. Cessation is recognized by an appropriate clinical examination . . . absence of responsiveness, heartbeat, respiratory effort.
2. Irreversibility is recognized by persistent cessation of functions during an appropriate period of observation and/or trial of therapy.

B. Neurologic
An individual with irreversible cessation of all functions of the entire brain, including the brainstem, is dead.
1. Cessation is recognized when evaluation discloses findings of *a and b*:
   a. Cerebral functions are absent.
   b. Brainstem functions are absent.
2. Irreversibility is recognized when evaluation discloses findings of *a and b and c*:
   a. The cause of coma is established and is sufficient to account for the loss of brain functions.
   b. The possibility of recovery of any brain functions is excluded.
   c. The cessation of all brain function persists for an appropriate period of observation and/or trial of therapy.

SOURCE: Report of the medical consultants on the diagnosis of death to the President's Commission for the Study of Ethical Problems in Medicine and Biomedical and Behavioral Research, Guidelines for the determination of death. *JAMA* 246:2184, 1981.

Biomedical and Behavioral Research by a panel of medical consultants.

In the past, a falling blood pressure has been used as a criterion of brain death, but this sign is frequently the result of dehydration due to diabetes insipidus. This is aggravated by loss of vasomotor tone, which produces hypotension. Almost all patients with brain death can be maintained for prolonged periods with normal vital signs using plasma and vasopressors; cardiac stimulants are rarely required. Urinary output can likewise be maintained with hydration and diuretics. Even the head injury patient who has been anuric and in shock for many hours can be restored to hemodynamic stability by restoration of a normal blood volume.

The principles of organ preservation are described in a subsequent section. The advances in organ preservation have alleviated the urgency of cadaver transplantation. It is possible to harvest kidneys at the moment of death and preserve them in iced solutions for more than 48 h until the transplant recipients are ready. Kidneys can now be routinely preserved by hypothermic perfusion for more than 48 h (see subsequent section). The use of machines for this purpose has increased the availability of cadaver kidneys because the kidneys can be transported for long distances. The development of preservation also allows for more careful typing, matching, shipping, and sharing of organs between various centers.

Organ Harvest. ***Related Living Donor.*** The actual technique of the donor operation is not as crucial as those factors that maintain urinary output in the donated kidney and in the remaining donor kidney. An active diuresis in the donor at the moment of renal artery occlusion favors prompt function in the recipient. For these reasons, the urine output is monitored throughout the donor operation and should not fall below 1 mL/min/kidney. The patient is hydrated several hours before operation, and both colloid (5 mL/kg/h) and crystalloid (5 mL/kg/h) solutions are administered during the operation, with constant attention to the central venous pressure and the urine output. Mannitol and furosemide are given shortly before the kidney is removed. In addition, systemic heparinization is carried out a few minutes before the renal artery is occluded. The heparin is then counteracted with protamine.

The donor operation is carried out through a flank incision and a retroperitoneal approach. The peritoneum is retracted, the ureter identified, and a length of ureter is dissected free. The ureter is then transected (preserving its blood supply from the renal pelvis) so that the urinary output of the donor kidney can be observed throughout the operation. The remainder of the ureter is dissected free up to the renal vein. A large lumbar vein, the ovarian or testicular vein, and the adrenal branch of the renal vein are doubly ligated on the left side. There are no major branches of the renal vein on the right side. Dissection on the renal vein is carried down to the vena cava. The artery is not dissected free until the dissection of the renal vein is complete. The kidney is not removed until urinary output from the donor kidney itself is excellent. At that time the renal artery and vein are sequentially clamped and divided.

Minor complications of nephrectomy in healthy related donors are common, but serious complications are quite rare. The function of the remaining kidney increases to about 70 percent of the preoperative value. Prolonged follow-ups indicate that the health and life expectancy of the donor are not adversely affected by donation.

Cadaver Donor. The technique of kidney harvest from a cadaver donor depends to a large degree on the status of the donor's circulation. If the cadaver is brain-dead but with intact circulation and urine output, nephrectomy can be performed at leisure via the transperitoneal route.

If the donor has a sudden irreversible circulatory collapse, the kidneys must be removed more rapidly to minimize ischemia time. Heparin is administered, and both kidneys are removed together by clamping the aorta and vena cava above the origin of the renal arteries and veins and pulling the kidneys up together, before transection of the aorta and vena cava below the origin of the renal vessels and the ureters in the pelvis. Prompt cooling of the organs is required, and both kidneys can be perfused with iced crystalloid solution before storing them in the cold or perfusing them on preservation machines.

Technique. ***Preparation.*** It is probably not necessary to remove the kidneys from most patients. Removal of the patient's diseased kidneys may be considered to control hypertension, to eliminate a source of infection, or to eliminate the nephrotic syndrome. Recurrence of the glomerulonephritis in the transplanted kidney is not known to be aggravated by the presence of the diseased kidneys. Asymptomatic polycystic kidneys rarely present a problem.

When indicated, the nephrectomy is performed at most transplantation centers sometime before transplantation in order to minimize the surgical stress at transplantation when immunosuppressant drugs are utilized and optimal transplant function desired, or to completely eliminate urinary tract infection before immunosuppression is begun.

When two-stage transplantation is carried out (i.e., nephrectomy preceding the transplantation by a week or 10 days), the postnephrectomy management is simple. Hyperkalemia is a recurrent postnephrectomy problem, but it can usually be prevented if a 20 percent glucose solution is administered prophylactically (with insulin if the patient has diabetes). Rectal ion-exchange resins may be required to control hyperkalemia. Dialysis can usually be postponed 2 or 3 days with these techniques. Delay in reinstituting dialysis is preferred if heparinization is required. Peritoneal dialysis can be resumed immediately to avoid clotting of the catheter.

During preparation for transplantation, sepsis from any source must be scrupulously removed. Frequent sources of sepsis are (1) the hemodialysis cannulas, if present, (2) the bladder in patients with preexisting urinary tract infections, (3) the skin of patients with uremic dermatitis, and (4) dental caries. The bladder of the totally anuric patient frequently becomes infected and should be irrigated with appropriate antimicrobial agents several times weekly prior to grafting.

Dialysis should be frequent and intense in the immediate pretransplantation period. Recipients of cadaver kidneys will have little preparation time prior to transplantation. Many patients will be maintained on systemic anticoagulants because of clotting problems in hemodialysis shunts; the anticoagulants must be discontinued, and vitamin K must be administered.

Transplantation. The operative technique of renal transplantation has become standardized. A retroperitoneal approach is used to the iliac vessels, and the renal artery and vein are anastomosed to the iliac vessels as shown in Figs. 10-63 and 10-64.

There must be no deficit in blood volume following the vascular anastomoses. Hypovolemia interferes with the rapid resump-

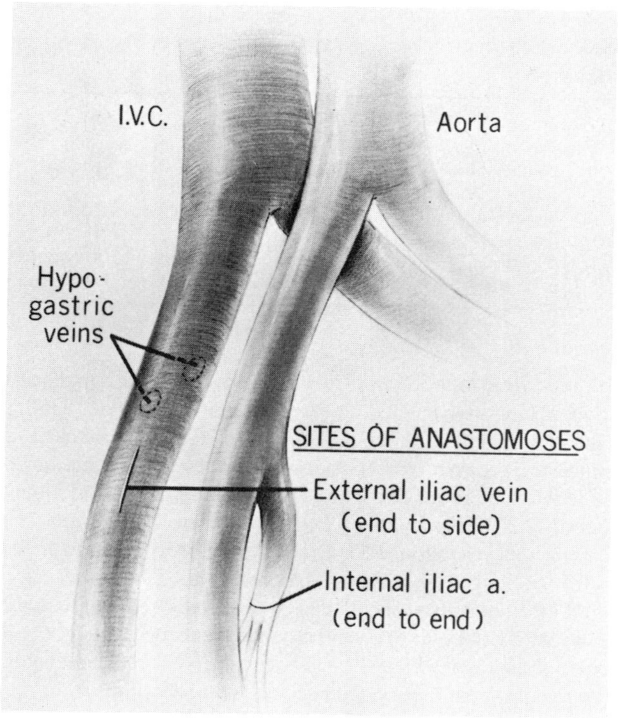

FIG. 10-63. Sites of anastomoses of renal vein to the side of the iliac vein. (From: *Simmons RL, Kjellstrand CM, Najarian JS: Kidney: II. Technique, complications, and results, in Najarian JS, Simmons RL [eds]: Transplantation. Philadelphia, Lea & Febiger, 1972, p 445, with permission.*)

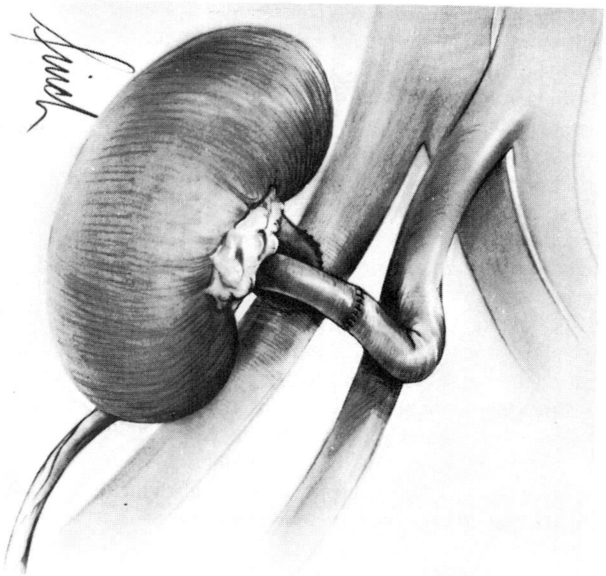

FIG. 10-64. Completed anastomosis of hypogastric artery to renal artery, and of renal vein to common iliac vein. (From: *Simmons RL, Kjellstrand CM, Najarian JS: Kidney: II. Technique, complications, and results, in Najarian JS, Simmons RL [eds]: Transplantation. Philadelphia, Lea & Febiger, 1972, p 445, with permission.*)

tion of renal function. Urine usually appears within a few minutes of completion of the vascular anastomoses in related living donor kidneys; mannitol and furosemide may be helpful in hastening the appearance of urine, a useful sign that there are no serious technical deficiencies.

Three methods are generally available for establishing urinary tract continuity. The preferred method involves ureteroneocystostomy. Pyeloureterostomy and ureteroureterostomy have also been used. Systemic or topical perioperative antibodies will help prevent wound infections.

Anesthesia in the Anephric Patient. Certain precautions are necessary during any operation on an anephric patient. In particular, certain anesthetics are excreted almost exclusively by the kidney and should not be used. These include the muscle relaxant gallamine triethiodide. Both curare and succinylcholine are metabolized by the liver, but both may also be accompanied by prolonged paralysis in the postoperative period. In the case of succinylcholine, a number of investigators have found that serum cholinesterase is broken down during hemodialysis. In such patients, succinylcholine would be expected to have prolonged action. Conduction anesthesia has been used, but most anesthesiologists prefer general anesthesia.

In the administration of anesthetics and fluids, it should always be assumed that the kidney will not function immediately after transplantation, even if dialysis is rarely required after transplantation. Similar thinking should be used with regard to hyperkalemia in the uremic patient. Other concerns of the anesthesiologist are the lowering of hypertension after induction of anesthesia and the low hematocrit in patients with chronic uremia. The hematocrit should be raised to 30 before transplantation, and hypovolemia due to excessive ultrafiltration during hemodialysis should be avoided.

Posttransplantation Care. The management of kidney allograft patients in the early posttransplant period does not differ radically from the management of other postoperative patients. Vital signs are monitored frequently for the first day, and the central venous pressure is utilized as a guide to blood volume. A Foley catheter is left in the bladder, which is not irrigated unless clots are thought to be occluding the catheter. The urine output is measured at least every hour. The volume of urine should be replaced with intravenous fluids. A convenient replacement solution consists of one-half normal saline solution with 5% dextrose and water and 10 meq of sodium bicarbonate per liter. Potassium need not be added to the intravenous fluids except in small children, whose urinary electrolytes should be replaced milliequivalent for milliequivalent. Diabetic patients should receive continuous insulin infusion intravenously to maintain blood sugars in the slightly hyperglycemic range (150 to 200 mg/dL).

The urinary output in the early postoperative period may be enormous, partly because of tubular dysfunction but primarily because of the overhydrated state of even the best-dialyzed patient. A creatinine clearance obtained on the evening of transplantation will be helpful in assessing renal function.

The Foley catheter can be removed almost any time after the first day. The tip of the catheter should be cultured at that time. Moderate hypertension is frequently seen in the early posttransplant period, and a low-sodium diet and low doses of antihypertensive medication (α-methyldopa, hydrochlorothiazide, or hydralazine) are useful to counteract this tendency. Antacids are useful in preventing the appearance of gastrointestinal ulceration of patients on immunosuppressive drugs. The patient is allowed out of bed and oral fluids are begun on the first postoperative day.

The 2-h creatinine clearance determination can be useful in interpreting early oliguria, but the test is not routine. The hematocrit should be followed at 4-h intervals, since rebleeding is a rare but severe complication that can produce oliguria and the onset of acute tubular necrosis (ATN).

A base-line sonogram and ^{131}I Hippuran renogram are usually performed soon after transplantation. Intravenous pyelography (IVP) is rarely necessary. Determinations of blood urea nitrogen (BUN), serum creatinine, and creatinine clearance suffice to estimate daily renal functions. Serum electrolyte determinations can usually be discontinued after good renal function is established. Periodic leukocyte and platelet counts are necessary to assay the state of the bone marrow during immunosuppression. Rarely, hyperglycemia and hypercalcemia are complications, and therefore blood sugar and calcium levels should be determined from time to time. The diabetic patient will require frequent blood sugar determinations and adjustments of insulin dosage.

Prophylactic Immunosuppression. Standard immunosuppressive management at most clinical transplant centers now consists of cyclosporine, azathioprine, and prednisone. At the University of Pittsburgh, a prospective trial using FK506 is under way (Table 10-20). Because of cyclosporine's nephrotoxic properties, ALG or azathioprine or both are sometimes used until renal function approaches more normal levels. When stable renal function is present, ALG is stopped and cyclosporine started. Most centers are currently individualizing the concurrent use of all four of these drugs. Combined or multimodal drug therapy allows one to maximize immunosuppression but minimize the side effects associated with the use of high concentrations of individual agents. A higher dose of prednisone or methylprednisone is used for rejection episodes. Most centers reserve the use of monoclonal antilymphocyte antibodies such as OKT3 to treat steroid-resistant rejection episodes (Table 10-21).

Table 10-20
Current Induction and Maintenance Immunosuppression for Renal Transplantation at the University of Pittsburgh

A. FK506
   1. Start at 0.15 mg/kg/day on day 0 orally as a one-time preoperative dose
   2. Postoperatively, 0.1 mg/kg/day continuous infusion I.V. over 24 h; when taking P.O., 0.15 mg/kg/b.i.d.

B. Azathioprine (evening dose after checking leukocyte count)
   1. Preoperative dose is 3 mg/kg/day
   2. Then: 3 mg/kg/day and maintain at 2–3 mg/kg as dictated by WBC count
   3. Adjust at all times with respect to WBC, platelet count, and renal function
   4. Caution: Reduce dosage to 1.5 mg/kg for severe renal functional impairment

C. Corticosteroids
   1. Solu-Medrol 1 g I.V. in OR
   2. Then slow tapering dose of I.V. Solu-Medrol 50 mg I.V. q 6 h × 4 doses; then 40 mg I.V. q 6 h × 4 doses; then 40 mg I.V. q 6 h × 4 doses; then 20 mg q 12 h × 2 doses; then 20 mg/day P.O. until 1 month postoperatively; then gradually taper to final level of 0.5 mg/kg/day or total discontinuation

Table 10-21
Standard Antirejection Therapy at the University of Pittsburgh

A. Document by biopsy

B. Therapy
   1. Prednisone: 1 g bolus, then follow by a "recycle" and end at 30 mg/day. Begin slow tapering after 30 days.
   2. In steroid-resistant rejection, 10 days of OKT3 I.V. (5 mg/day).
   3. If patients are on double therapy (no azathioprine), azathioprine is added in doses similar to those in section B of Table 10-20.

Complications. ***Renal Failure.*** The most serious complication of renal transplantation is the failure of the graft to initiate or maintain function. Although the causes of failure can easily be defined, the differential diagnosis may, at the time, be impossible. The functional failure of the kidney is best examined in relation to the time after transplantation. The kidney may (1) never function, (2) have delayed onset of functions, (3) fail to function after a brief or prolonged time, or (4) gradually lose its function over a period of months or years. In each phase, four general diagnoses should be considered: (1) ischemic damage to the kidney; (2) rejection of the kidney by reactions directed against histocompatibility antigens on the kidney; (3) technical complications; and (4) the development of renal disease, either a new disease or recurrence of the original.

The simplest and best assays for decreased renal function are the frequent determination of BUN and serum creatinine and the determination of creatinine clearance. Sonograms and renograms are also useful. The differential diagnosis of renal malfunction, however, may require percutaneous pyelography, arteriography, and renal biopsy.

Early Anuria and Oliguria. Early anuria or oliguria is a major diagnostic problem. The possibilities include (1) hypovolemia, (2) thrombosis of the renal artery or renal vein, (3) hyperacute rejection of the kidney, (4) ischemic renal damage (ATN), (5) compression of the kidney (by hematoma, seroma, or lymph), and (6) obstruction of the urinary flow.

The investigation of early posttransplant anuria should be rapidly performed in a strict sequence. The Foley catheter should first be irrigated and/or changed to remove any question of catheter obstruction. Unfortunately, whatever the cause of anuria, a clot can be obtained by bladder irrigation on the first posttransplant day. The clot may not be the primary cause of anuria, however, because blood will clot within the bladder if the urine is not copious enough to wash it out before coagulation. Therefore, even if a clot is present within the urinary catheter, the urine output should be monitored for the first 10 to 15 min after emptying the bladder to determine urine output adequacy.

If the obstructed catheter has not caused the oliguria, one must rule out hemorrhage and hypovolemia combined with compression or displacement of the kidney by the hematoma. If hypotension and tachycardia are present and the central venous pressure is low, hypovolemia is very likely. A radiograph of the abdomen will reveal displacement of the intraperitoneal contents by a massive hematoma. Echography and repeated hematocrit determinations will confirm the diagnosis. The normal degree of ischemic damage to the transplanted kidney plus hypovolemia and compression of the kidney and vessels by a hematoma all conspire to impair renal function. If anuria or severe oliguria is present, restoration of the blood volume will seldom suffice to restore renal function, even if furosemide or other diuretics are used. Many patients will require reexploration to control the bleeding point. After exploration, if the period of hypovolemia and renal compression has been relatively brief and diuretics have been used during ischemia, prompt restoration of renal function usually occurs.

The diagnosis of bleeding is frequently apparent and obviates the need for the next step in the investigation sequence—an ^{131}I Hippuran renogram (Fig. 10-65). The renogram permits assessment of the blood flow to the kidney and the ability of the kidney to concentrate and excrete the Hippuran. The results are never diagnostic. If the vascular phase and concentration are near normal, however, the renal arterial and venous anastomoses are patent. If the Hippuran uptake by the kidney is severely depressed, a renal arteriogram should be done. Arteriography will assess the renal arterial anastomosis, and if it reveals the presence of intravascular thrombosis of the kidney, the diagnosis of hyperacute rejection will be suggested.

Technical Complications. Thrombosis of the renal arterial anastomosis is rare. Partial obstruction due to torsion or kinking of the vessels is more common and should be promptly repaired. When the renogram demonstrated poor concentration of the ^{131}I Hippuran, an arteriogram should be performed to detect correctable technical complications (Fig. 10-66). Thrombosis of the renal vein occurs even more rarely than thrombosis of the renal artery. When it does occur, thrombosis of the artery ensues because the collateral venous circulation of the kidney has been interrupted by the transplant procedure. Partial thrombosis of the renal and iliac veins has occurred. Usually, this is accompanied by swelling of the ipsilateral lower extremity, fever, and evidence of pulmonary embolism.

Formerly, one of the most common, and most frequently fatal, complications following renal transplantation was urinary extravasation due to distal ureteral necrosis. Rejection was seldom at fault. The problem can generally be avoided by (1) using the ureter as short as possible; (2) avoiding tension at the ureteroneocystostomy site; (3) avoiding hematomas within the wound, which put tension on the ureter and also interfere with the developing collateral blood supply to the distal ureter; (4) avoiding transperitoneal "clotheslining" of the ureter by always placing the ureter in the retroperitoneal position where tension will be minimal and the collateral blood supply can develop.

Urinary extravasation is a serious complication that can lead to infection. It demands urgent reexploration with reimplantation of the ureter into the bladder, nephrostomy, or performance of a pyeloureterostomy to the host ureter. On occasion, the pelvis of the transplanted kidney may be involved, and nephrectomy may be required. Delay in definitive repair will frequently lead to infection, loss of the kidney, and death.

Technical errors can become manifest long after the immediate posttransplant period. Arterial stenosis, venous thrombosis, and late ureteral leaks and strictures are frequently confused with rejection (see below). Before any antirejection treatment, technical problems should be ruled out by echography, arteriography, renography, or percutaneous nephrostograms.

Hyperacute Rejection. Hyperacute rejection of the kidney is almost always mediated by humoral antibody, with the subsequent participation of the complement, coagulation, and kinin cascade systems. Platelets, PMNs, and vasospasm may also play a role. Classic hyperacute rejection is now rare because laboratory techniques can demonstrate preformed cytotoxic antibody directed against donor histocompatibility antigens as a positive cross match. A rare patient will have a hyperacute rejection in the ab-

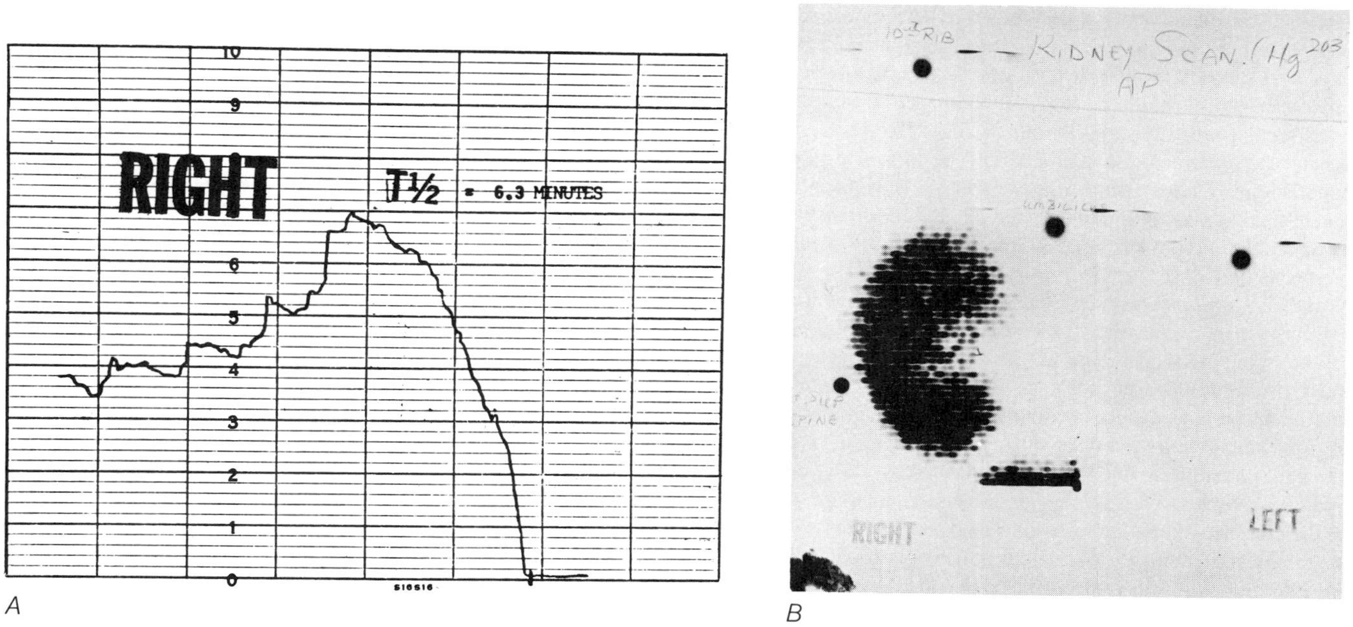

FIG. 10-65. Function of a homotransplanted kidney. *A.* A radiograph showing a half-life of 6.3 min and a completely normal-appearing curve. *B.* A scan of the same transplant showing excellent uptake in the kidney and the appearance of the radioactive material in the bladder. This transplant continued to have excellent function 5½ years later. (From: *Hume DM: Advances in Surgery, Vol II. Chicago, Year Book Medical Publishers, 1966, with permission.*)

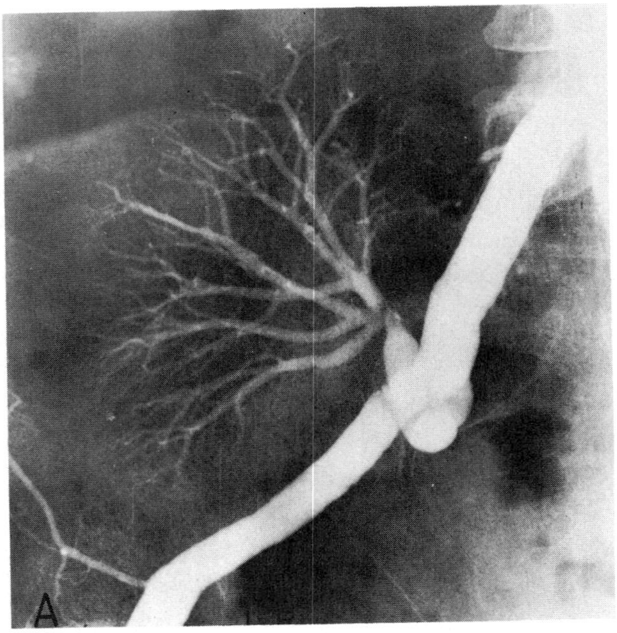

FIG. 10-66. Correctable arterial complications in the early posttransplant period. Oliguria was present in both patients. ^{131}I Hippuran revealed poor vascular phase. The arteriograms revealed torsion distal to the renal arterial anastomosis, which was corrected by a reanastomosis. (From: *Simmons RL, Kjellstrand CM, Najarian JS: Kidney: II. Technique, complications, and results, in Najarian JS, Simmons RL [eds]: Transplantation. Philadelphia, Lea & Febiger, 1972, with permission.*)

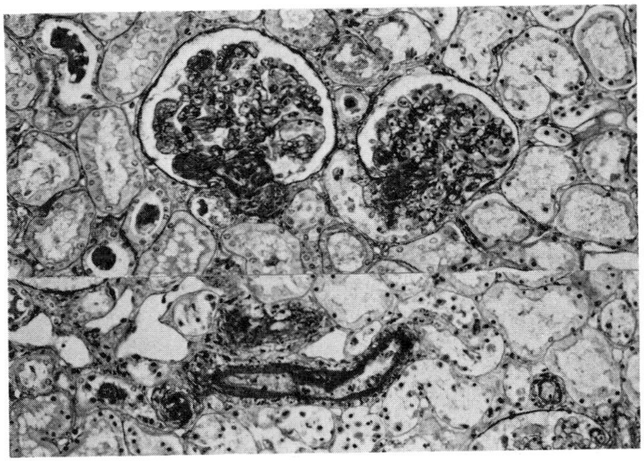

FIG. 10-67. Hyperacute renal rejection 20 h posttransplantation in a twenty-five-year-old male. Hyperacute rejection is characterized initially by fibrin and platelet thrombosis and fibrinoid necrosis of glomerular tufts, renal arterioles, and small arteries. A massive polymorphonuclear leukocyte reaction, interstitial hemorrhage, and tubular necrosis occur with subsequent cortical infarction 24 to 36 h posttransplantation. (×160.) (From: *Richard K. Sibley, personal communication.*)

sence of demonstrable cytotoxic antibody. Indeed, detectable cytotoxic antibody will appear and disappear at intervals in patients awaiting transplantation. In the classic hyperacute rejection, the kidney will fail to regain its normal turgor and healthy pink color after anastomoses are established. Biopsy and histologic study at this time may reveal leukocytes in the glomerular capillaries, and intravascular renal thrombosis follows (Fig. 10-67). Definite evidence of a hyperacute rejection should be treated by immediate nephrectomy. A less acute rejection may occur, however, and renal function may not fail until a day or two after transplantation. Such rapid rejection has been differentiated by the term *accelerated rejection*.

Acute Tubular Necrosis. The diagnosis of ischemic renal injury is one of exclusion. If all other causes of renal functional failure in the early posttransplant period have been ruled out, one must assume that the diagnosis is ATN. "Acute tubular necrosis" in clinical parlance refers to kidneys whose function is impaired from ischemia or a variety of other causes. If kidneys from this clinical spectrum are biopsied, they most frequently show only hydropic changes. The more severe the insult, the more likely will be the presence of tubular necrosis. The correlation between tubule pathology and function, however, is not always good and suggests the interplay with other mechanisms, including prolonged vasoconstriction and vascular endothelial cell swelling. Most kidneys will recover, but sometimes disruption is so severe that cellular repair is not possible.

ATN occurs most commonly in cadaver recipients when the donor had undergone long periods of stress and hypotensive insult to the kidney to be transplanted. Another cause of recipient ATN is a long period of warm ischemia preceding transplantation. Kidneys with warm ischemic intervals greater than 1 h should not be utilized for transplantation, because function will seldom return to normal. Cold ischemia is much better tolerated, and preservation up to 48 h is now very satisfactory.

Almost all transplanted kidneys have undergone some degree of damage secondary to trauma and ischemia. A second trauma (hypovolemia, hypoxemia, renal compression, bacteremia, allergic reactions to ALG) that normally might not result in ATN in normal kidneys may cause oliguria in transplanted kidneys. One must not diagnose rejection and institute massive steroid therapy in the early posttransplant period without ruling out the possibility that an additional insult to an already damaged kidney has occurred and that the diagnosis is not acute rejection but ATN. Renal biopsy may be necessary to make this differentiation.

The management of the patient with ATN is simple. Urinary flow will resume in almost all cases within 2 or 3 weeks, but anuria for as long as 6 weeks with total recovery has been observed. ^{131}I Hippuran renograms are useful in following improvement before resumption of urinary flow. Dialysis is maintained intermittently during the period of oliguria. A number of studies have shown that the long-term function of renal transplants is independent of the presence or absence of oliguria in the early posttransplant period.

Rejection. Technical errors may not become evident for several weeks postgrafting, and any trauma can aggravate the degree of ATN in a previously damaged kidney. Nevertheless most renal failure appearing after the first posttransplant week can be attributed to rejection.

With better immunosuppression, the acute rejection episodes that formerly appeared in the first month following transplantation are seen less and less frequently. The majority of patients, however, will sustain at least one acute rejection episode during the first 3 to 4 months following transplantation. Clinical rejection is rarely an all-or-nothing reaction, and the first episode seldom progresses to complete renal destruction. The functional changes induced by rejection appear to be in large part reversible; therefore, the recognition and treatment of the rejection episode before the development of severe renal damage are of extreme importance. Usually the rejection reaction responds to increased prednisone doses and local irradiation. Even with prompt treatment the creatinine clearance may be permanently impaired, however slightly, following each clinical rejection episode.

The clinical picture of a rejection reaction may be distressingly similar to several other problems: ureter leak or obstruction, hemorrhage with consequent ATN, infection, or stenosis or twist in the renal artery or vein. Classic renal rejection is characterized by oliguria, enlargement and tenderness of the graft, malaise, fever, leukocytosis, hypertension, weight gain, and peripheral edema. Laboratory studies have shown lymphocyturia, red cell casts, proteinuria, immunoglobulin fragments, fibrin fragments in the urine, complementuria, lysozymuria, decreased urine sodium excretion, renal tubular acidosis, and increased lactic dehydrogenase in the urine. The level of the blood urea nitrogen increases, as does serum creatinine. Creatinine clearance is obviously decreased; renograms will show slow uptake of the Hippuran and slow urinary excretion. Echography can show edema of the renal papillae (Fig. 10-68).

The most important parameter to follow is the serum creatinine level. Unlike the BUN, which is sensitive to a number of changes (steroid administration, fever, and high-protein diet), serum creatinine levels are relatively stable for each patient. The creatinine clearance is more sensitive, but it depends on a carefully timed collection of urine.

The most reliable clinical signs of renal functional deterioration are a slight decrease in urinary output, slow weight gain, small increases in diastolic blood pressure, and edema of the lower extremity on the side of the graft. A peripheral leukocyte count and a serum creatinine level should be determined to confirm renal functional deterioration. A renogram and echogram should be promptly performed and compared with those obtained at the peak of renal function (usually before discharge from the hospital) to rule out urinary extravasation, urinary obstruction, or ureteral stenosis. Arteriography is seldom necessary but may reveal (1) characteristic changes of decreased concentration of dye flowing into the kidney, (2) decreased nephrogram effect, (3) an irregularity of the cortical vasculature and intralobar vasculature characteristic of rejection, and (4) normal renal artery and anastomosis, eliminating the possibility of a technical problem.

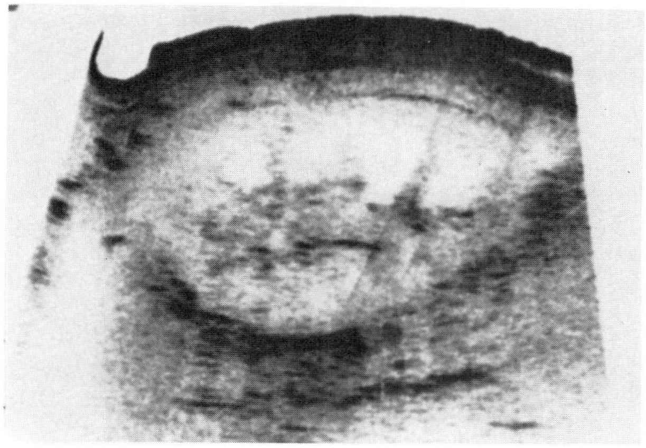

FIG. 10-68. Longitudinal sonogram of a renal transplant during episode of acute rejection (characterized clinically by anuria, fever, weight increase, and elevated creatinine levels to 0.079 mg/mL). Note enlarged pyramids of decreased echogenicity anteriorly. Interpyramidal cortex (septa of Bertin) shown as echogenic bands between pyramids. The kidney appears enlarged and more globular in shape compared with a baseline study 4 weeks earlier. Biopsy confirmed severe acute rejection requiring transplant nephrectomy 3 days after the sonogram. (From: *Frick MP, Feinberg SB, et al: Ultrasound in acute renal transplant rejection. Radiology 138:659, 1981, with permission.*)

Renal biopsy should be a definitive diagnostic tool. Both open biopsy and needle biopsy techniques have been described, and the histologic changes of rejection are characteristic. A normal kidney biopsy is diagnostic, but a biopsy that reveals renal damage may merely reflect acute rejection, a chronic ongoing process, exacerbation of the preexisting renal disease, or damage due to infection or radiation. With experience, however, needle biopsy of transplanted kidneys is a safe procedure and usually provides the diagnosis. Aspiration of the kidney to obtain cells for cytologic analysis can also be used to diagnose rejection.

Most institutions have developed a standard rejection regimen for allografted kidneys (Table 10-22). This standard regimen can be repeated as many as three times within a 2-month period in patients for whom rejection appears to be unremitting. If it is repeated more often than that, infection due to profound immunosuppression may occur. The decision to stop immunosuppression and sacrifice the transplant frequently depends on subtle factors and is difficult to make, particularly in patients who have deterioration of renal function over a period of months and years.

Renal Failure Due to Recurrent Disease. Certain diseases are known to recur in the transplanted kidney. These are listed in Table 10-23. Transplantation is not necessarily contraindicated in these diseases, since the recurrence is unpredictable and the transplant may provide long-term palliation that is superior in the individual case to dialysis. The best example is diabetes, in which the histologic features of diabetes often recur with only gradual deterioration of function.

Results. The outcome in renal transplant recipients is excellent (Figure 10-69).

Transplantation in Children. Renal failure in children is a common cause of death. Until recently, young children were not considered ideal candidates for renal transplantation. The small caliber of vessels and active social behavior of children make their management on hemodialysis extremely difficult. Long-term immunosuppressive therapy is also thought to interfere with normal growth, with resultant social problems. Long-term hemodial-

Table 10-22
Standard Antirejection Therapy at the University of Minnesota

1. Therapy
   a. Prednisone: 2 mg/kg × 3 days; then 1.5 mg/kg × 3 days; then 1.0 mg/kg × 3 days; thereafter reduce prednisone slowly to a maintenance dose.
   b. Azathioprine: Regulate dose to prevent leukopenia; do not increase.
   c. Irradiate kidney transplant: 150 rad every other day for three doses.
2. Adjuncts
   a. Reinstitute antacid therapy.
   b. Reinstitute oral nystatin (100,000 units twice daily) to prevent mucosal candidiasis.
   c. Reduce protein and fluid intake if renal function is significantly impaired.

Table 10-23
Risk of Recurrence of Primary Renal Disease Following Transplantation

High risk	
	Focal sclerosis (proliferative type)
	IgA disease
	Membranoproliferative glomerulonephritis (dense-deposit disease type)
	Hemolytic-uremic syndrome
	Diabetes mellitus
	Oxalosis
Moderate risk	
	Antiglomerular basement membrane disease
	Scleroderma
Low risk	
	Membranous glomerulonephritis
	Amyloidosis
	Rapidly progressive crescentic AP nephritis
	Lupus
	Wegener's
No risk	
	Congenital nephrosis
	Fabry's disease
	Cystinosis
	Myeloma kidney
	Polycystic kidney
	Pyelonephritis
	Glomerulonephritis
	Congenital renal disease (aplasia/dysplasia; valves)

ysis is seldom satisfactory, and a parent is almost always willing to donate a kidney. The growth of children following transplantation has been the subject of several studies. Most children with allografts grow slightly more slowly than normal; end growth is significantly superior when compared with dialysis. Multimodal immunosuppressive therapy has allowed improved growth in pediatric renal transplant recipients. Aggressive attempts are made to reduce the steroid dosage, since these agents are believed to have the greatest growth-retarding effect.

Multiple Transplants. A number of studies have shown that second and third transplants are less successful than the first. This is especially true if the graft was rejected early following placement. The rejection of one transplant may sensitize the patient to a number of weaker histocompatibility antigens that cannot be easily detected by sensitive cross-match techniques. In addition, such patients may have less compromised immune systems that permitted the rejection of the first transplant. By contrast, patients who have maintained a successful first transplant for several years will, after losing the first transplant, accept the second transplant more readily.

XENOGRAFTS

Xenografts between related species are probably not rejected by the same immune mechanism as are allografts. In allografts, most rejection responses are mediated by T lymphocytes. In contrast, rejection of xenografts is influenced by both B cells and T cells. In some species combinations, preformed cytotoxic antibodies exist which cause immediate graft destruction through activation of complement and clotting cascades. These species combinations are termed *discordant*. For those species combinations in which preformed antibody is not present, the term *concordant* is applied.

Renal xenografts using both chimpanzee and baboon donors were performed in a number of human beings in the 1950s, but this procedure was abandoned when dialysis became available. In general, the greater the genetic disparity, the stronger the rejection response. Therefore, the conventional immunosuppressive agents which control graft rejection in allografts do not prevent rejection of xenografts. Surprisingly, there were a few relatively long-term survivors with chimpanzee renal transplants, which were considerably better tolerated than baboon transplants. A renewed interest in xenotransplantation has occurred with the current shortage of organs available for transplantation. As success in solid organ transplantation occurred, the potential application of transplantation broadened, as well. As a result there is currently a critical shortage of solid organs available for transplantation. Xenotransplantation may overcome this limitation, if methods to prevent rejection of grafts from other species can be identified. Research efforts are being increasingly applied to understanding the immunobiology of xenograft rejection in an attempt to allow this goal to become a clinical reality.

ORGAN PRESERVATION

The preservation of viable whole organs is one of the essential components of any transplantation program. Only cadaver donors can be used for some organs (heart and liver), and even when the organ is expendable (as in one of a pair of kidneys), the use of cadaver donors avoids the risks inherent in removal of the organ from living persons. If tissue typing and matching ever achieve their true potential, it may be necessary to store the organ until these matching procedures can be carried out. Even more time-consuming procedures, such as tolerance induction, may ultimately become available to pretreat the recipient and make him or her unresponsive to specific histocompatibility antigens. Table 10-24 lists some of those procedures that might be useful to carry out during organ preservation.

Methods of Viable Organ Preservation

The main problem associated with preservation of organs in a viable state seems to be hypoxia. When the organ is removed from its

Table 10-24
Procedures During Organ Storage

A. Evaluation of the organ
  1. Typing and matching
    a. ABO typing
    b. Lymphocyte typing
    c. Organ cell typing
    d. Mixed lymphocyte culture with the recipient
  2. Diagnosis of disease in the donor or donor tissue
    a. Malignant tumors
    b. Infections
    c. Degenerative conditions
  3. Determination of functional state
  4. Restoration of normal function

B. Preparation of the recipient
  1. Induction of tolerance
  2. Immunosuppression
  3. Surgical procedures

C. Logistical procedures
  1. Stockpile various sizes and types
  2. Transport to a distant recipient

D. Modification of the immunogenicity of the organ

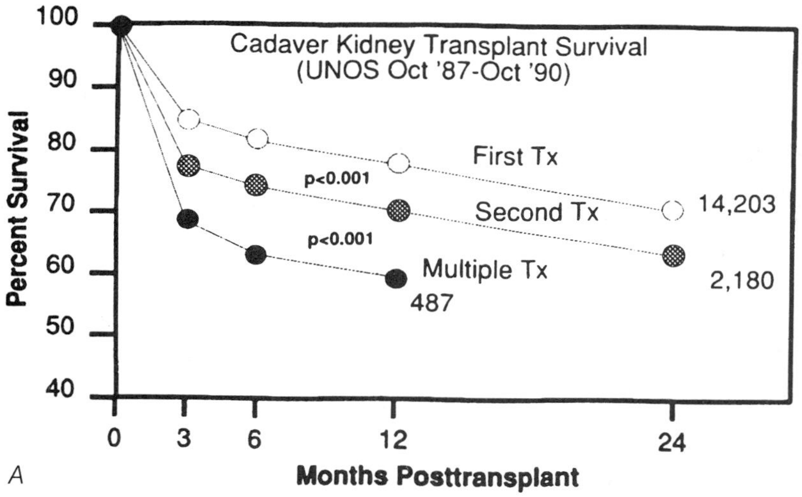

A

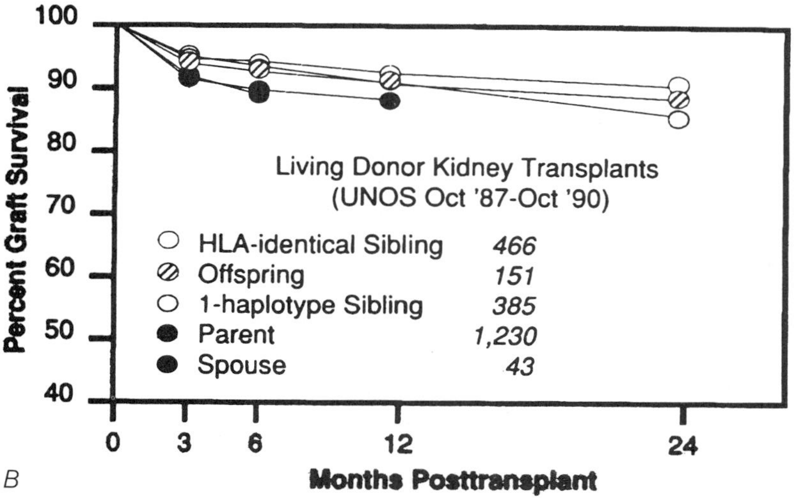

B

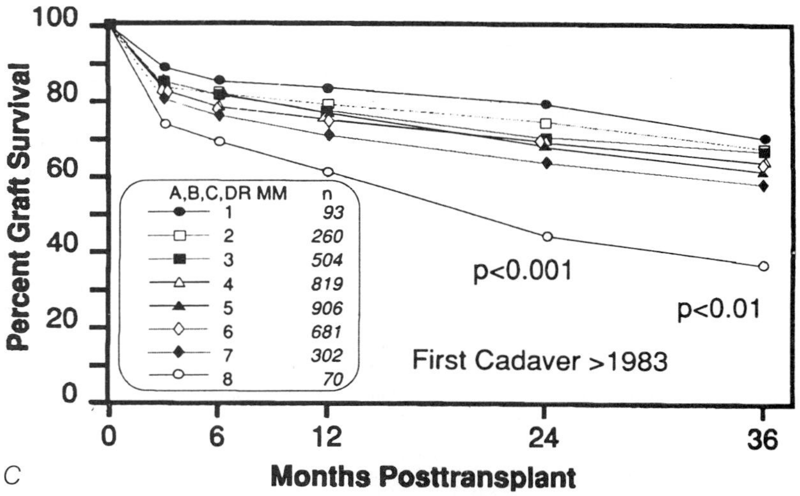

C

FIG. 10-69. *A.* UNOS cadaver kidney transplant survival for 1987–1990, comparing first grafts with second and third grafts. *B.* Graft survival among recipients of living donor transplants. *C.* Effect of HLA-A, -B, -C, and -DR mismatching on first cadaver graft survival. The number refers to number of mismatches (MM), while n = number of patients. (Adapted from: *Terasaki PI: Clinical Transplants 1990. Los Angeles, UCLA Tissue Typing Laboratory, 1991, pp 2, 8, 590, with permission.*)

physiologic state, it is deprived of its normal oxygenation. The two major approaches to organ preservation have been what might be called metabolic inhibition and metabolic maintenance.

Metabolic inhibition seeks to prevent the normal catabolic processes from causing severe or irreversible damage to the tissues during the period of preservation. It is currently best achieved by hypothermia, which protects the organ by slowing metabolic activity and decreasing oxygen need. Two techniques of cooling are currently available: (1) simple cooling of a kidney by immersing it in, or flushing it with, a cold solution, which allows many hours of preservation and is almost always used for short periods of time, before transplantation of any organ; and (2) perfusion cooling, which allows longer periods of preservation.

Metabolic maintenance, the second approach to organ preservation, attempts to sustain a level of metabolic activity as close to physiologic normalcy as is feasible. Usually it implies perfusion of the organ in vitro with a carefully controlled fluid medium, although tissue oxygenation may be attempted. In practice metabolic maintenance is always best combined with perfusion cooling. The best system, at present, utilizes a pulsatile pump and pooled homologous plasma passed through a membrane oxygenator. Excellent transplantation results are obtained after perfusion as long as 72 h. These moderately long preservation periods provide adequate time for accurate matching of donors and recipients.

Not all organs can be perfused equally well by the same approach. Certain precautions are necessary. It is necessary *to maintain optimal organ function* up to and beyond the moment of clinical death. For kidneys, adequate hydration and maintenance of systemic blood pressure are recommended. Manipulation of the organ also contributes to vasospasm, and so surgical dissection should be as rapid and efficient as possible. The *period of time* between the cessation of blood flow through the organ and the establishment of the organ in its new environment (warm ischemia time) is critical in preservation studies. *Temperature* is also important. Successful perfusion systems have incorporated hypothermia to reduce the need for oxygen and metabolic nutrients. *Oxygenation* is also critical. Oxygen dissolved in aqueous solution more readily at lower temperatures; a membrane oxygenator is incorporated into the system.

The *flow rate* necessary at 37°C can be substantially reduced when metabolic activity is lessened by hypothermia; flow rates of one-fifth to one-third of normal have been satisfactory. The *viscosity of the perfusion fluid* may have some influence on perfusion pressure and flow rate. The perfusion pressure is significant. If the flow rate is adequate to provide the nutrients and waste removal, then the absolute level of pressure is not critical, but excessive perfusion pressure invariably causes transudation of the perfusate, tissue edema, and ultimately obstruction to the flow. Another factor is *pulsation*. Perfusion results in less damage when the flow is pulsatile, particularly at normothermic temperatures. The necessity for pulsatile flow during hypothermic perfusion is less well documented. It is probably not necessary to maintain any *venous pressure gradient*. The *perfusate composition* has apparent significance. Whole plasma probably is the most physiologic perfusate and contains most of the nutrient ingredients, including fatty acids, that might be required for the metabolic activity of organs. Many other formulations have been successful, including dextran, albumin, other plasma expanders, tissue culture media, and balanced salt solutions. *Osmolarity* is important. Crystalloids are poor perfusates and lead to edema. The perfusate must be maintained at "normal" pH range of 7.35 to 7.45. CO_2 buffering may be necessary, with the addition of 2.5 to 5 percent of this gas to the oxygenator. Extremes of alkalosis and acidosis can be prevented with the addition of HCl or $NaHCO_3$ as necessary. A number of *additives* to the perfusate have been tried. These include membrane stabilizers, vasodilators, and anticoagulants. The recent development of UW (University of Wisconsin) solution has improved the outcome of cadaver organs, including liver and kidney, and prolonged the acceptable time for ischemia.

There is evidence that an adequate flow rate during perfusion is a good prognostic sign of the viability and transplantability of the organ. The most significant indication of inadequate flow rate is the swelling caused by fluid retention. This edema is usually the result of anoxia, with subsequent lysosomal and cellular damage. Poor perfusion itself can produce anoxia, so that a vicious cycle of edema-anoxia-edema can be started. Other possible causes of interstitial edema are perfusate osmolarity and excessive perfusion pressure. Even hypothermia alone may cause cellular swelling.

Another important factor in the obstruction of flow is simple blockage of the microvasculature. The many causes of this blockage have been described in detail and include bubbles in the perfusion system, fibrin, red cell agglutination, the adherence of platelets and leukocytes to endothelial cells, cell breakdown due to mechanically imperfect pumps, crystal formation, and even agglutination of bacteria. Some of this blockage can be prevented with adequate filtration, but even blood-derived perfusion media like whole plasma have been shown to contain aggregates that appear during hypothermic perfusion. This aggregated material has been identified as lipoprotein. Fortunately, these substances can be removed from plasma quite easily by freezing, which causes flocculation of the lipoprotein, and by subsequent filtration and/or ultracentrifugation to remove the aggregates.

When plasma or plasma products are used as perfusates, immunologic damage is possible. This may be due to antibodies directed against organ antigens or to the precipitation of circulating antigen-antibody complexes within the organ. Although complement cannot be activated at hypothermic temperatures, bound antibody will activate complement within the recipient's body soon after transplantation. Although this has led to few recognized complications after renal transplantation, elimination of immunoglobulins from perfusates would be preferable.

One of the major problems in organ presentation research is the lack of methods to assay the functional state of organs in vitro and the consequent inability to measure the effectiveness of innovations in organ preservation techniques. Ultimately, of course, each preservation method must be tested by reimplantation of the organ. This is an all-or-none test that requires a large number of transplants in order to get statistically valid data. What is needed is an in vitro assay technique that can predict the transplantability of an organ and provide quantitative assessment of viability as the organ is subjected to the various preservation protocols. For practical purposes, such an assay should be utilized both before preservation (to determine whether postmortem changes have rendered the organ unfit for preservation) and immediately before transplantation (to determine whether the preservation efforts have been effective).

Storage of Nonviable Tissues by Freeze-Drying

Tissue grafts have been used in human reconstructive surgery for several decades. A majority of these grafts are from connective tissue and do not require that the graft be viable to function adequately. A major constituent of most of these tissues is collagen, which seems to maintain its integrity (or at least its strength) even after long-term storage by freezing or freeze-drying. Many thousands of patients each year receive bone, fascia, dura, tendon, heart valve, or skin grafts in treatment of traumatic or surgical defects. The architecture of these grafts is used as a framework for reconstruction as the host slowly replaces the tissue.

These tissues are probably best preserved by freeze-drying, which consists of rapid freezing of the tissue and the application of vacuum for removal of the water from the frozen state to the vapor state without permitting it to become liquid. Such a process usually results in maintenance of morphologic structure and therefore maintains the strength and structural integrity of the tissue. The rapidity of the initial freeze is important, as slow freezing can result in the formation of large ice crystals that can disrupt the tissue. This is apparently not a severe problem in tissues that consist largely of collagen. Other tissues, such as vascular grafts, that contain elastic fibers can show a disruption of these fibers due to crystal formation. In this instance, the most rapid freeze possible is indicated to minimize crystal size. The graft is then dehydrated to a residual moisture of 5 percent. At this level it has been noted that tissues can subsequently be stored under vacuum at room temperature for years without further degradation or activation of metabolic processes. On reconstitution, it has been found preferable to inject water or saline solutions into a vacuum bottle containing tissue, so that the fluid can enter the tissue before it is exposed to air. Prior exposure to air apparently allows air molecules to enter the tissue and delays or prevents subsequent penetration of the water molecules necessary to rehydrate the tissue.

The usefulness of freeze-dried allografts is at least partly due to reduced antigenicity remaining in such grafts. The results of using freeze-dried allogenic bone and autografting bone are not remarkably different. The dura has also been preserved by freeze-drying and functions extremely well when used to cover large cranial defects. Flexor tendon grafts of the hand have been freeze-dried and used successfully, particularly when removed with their tendon sheaths intact. Many other freeze-dried tissues have been used with greater or lesser success. Cornea of nonpenetrating lamellar transplants, fascia, cartilage, heart valve, and nerve have all been tried.

Similarly, freeze-dried grafts have served as temporary biologic dressings to cover large burn wounds. In these instances the nonviable, freeze-dried graft "takes" and is even revascularized. It remains in place for several weeks or months, before it is finally sloughed. These grafts can be applied repeatedly without sensitization or acceleration of sloughing. Skin grafts have proved to be the best biologic dressing to prevent infection and to promote maximum granulation tissue formation in open skin wounds.

Techniques to cryopreserve viable cells are successful for single cells (bone marrow, islets) but have not been successfully extended to solid organs.

The usefulness of these techniques for the preservation of transplantable tissue led to the organization of the American Association of Tissue Banks. The purpose of this organization is to encourage research into and to standardize successful methods for the harvest, storage, and distribution of tissues and organs to needy patients.

Bibliography

General

Bach FH, Sachs DH: Transplantation immunology. *N Engl J Med* 317:489, 1987.

Clark SC, Kamen R: The human hematopoietic colony-stimulating factors. *Science* 236:1229, 1987.

Evans RS: Cost-effective analysis of transplantation. *Surg Clin North Am* 66:603, 1986.

First MR: The organ donation problem. *Lit Scan: Transplant* 7:1, 1991.

Golub ES, Green DR: *Immunology: A Synthesis*. Sunderland, Sinauer Associates, 1991.

Johnson RB: Immunology: Monocytes and macrophages. *N Engl J Med* 318:747, 1988.

Morris PJ (ed): *Kidney Transplantation: Principles and Practice*. New York, Grune & Stratton, 1984.

Park WE, Barber R, et al: Ethical issues in transplantation. *Surg Clin North Am* 66:663, 1986.

Penn I: Cancers following cyclosporine therapy. *Transplantation* 43:32, 1986.

Pirenne J, Nakhleh RE, Dunn DL: Graft-versus-host disease after multiorgan transplantation. *J Surg Res* 50:622, 1991.

Rapaport FT, Dausset J (eds): *Human Transplantation*. New York, Grune & Stratton, 1968.

Report of the Task Force on Organ Transplantation Issues and Recommendations: US Department of Health and Human Services, 1986.

Roberts AJ, Parnven GS (eds): Organ transplantation. *Surg Clin North Am* 55:1, 1986.

Simmons RL, Finch NL, et al (eds): *Manual of Vascular Access, Organ Donation and Transplantation*. New York, Springer-Verlag, 1984.

Terasak PI (ed): *Clinical Kidney Transplants 1985*. Los Angeles, UCLA Tissue Typing Laboratory, 1985.

Tilney NL, Lazarus JM: *Surgical Care of the Patient with Renal Failure*. Philadelphia, Saunders, 1982.

Transplantation Immunology

Accolla RS, Auffray C, et al: The molecular biology of MHC genes. *Immunol Today* 12:97, 1991.

Ales-Martinez JE, Cuende E, et al: Signalling in B cells. *Immunol Today* 12:201, 1991.

Calne RY (ed): *Transplantation Immunology: Clinical and Experimental*. Oxford, Oxford Medical, 1984.

Carding SR, Hayday AC, et al: Cytokines in T-cell development. *Immunol Today* 12:239, 1991.

deVries RRP, Van Rood JJ: Immunology of HLA class I and class II molecules. *Prog Allergy* 36:1, 1985.

Finkel TH, Kubo RT, et al: T-cell development and transmembrane signaling: changing biological responses through an unchanging receptor. *Immunol Today* 12:79, 1991.

Goldstein G: An overview of Orthoclone OKT3. *Transplant Proc* 17:927, 1986.

Habeshaw JA, Dalgleish AG, et al: AIDS pathogenesis: HIV envelope and its interaction with cell proteins. *Immunol Today* 11:418, 1990.

Hayry P: Intragraft events in allograft destruction. *Transplantation* 38:1, 1984.

Hayry P, von Willebrand E: Transplant aspiration cytology. *Transplantation* 38:7, 1984.

Ildstad ST, Simmons RL: Biology of organ transplantation and immunosuppression, in Starzl TE, Shapiro R, Simmons RL: *Atlas of Organ Transplantation*. New York, Gower Medical Publishing, 1992.

Kahan BD: *Cyclosporine, Diagnosis and Management of Associated Renal Injury*. Orlando, FL, Grune & Stratton, 1985.

Kirkmon RL, Berrett LV, et al: Administration of anti-interleukin 2 receptor monoclonal antibody prolongs cardiac allograft survival in mice. *J Exp Med* 162:358, 1985.

Lafaille JJ, Haas W, et al: Positive selection of $\gamma\delta$T cells. *Immunol Today* 11:75, 1990.

Lechler RI, Lombardi G, et al: The molecular basis of alloreactivity. *Immunol Today* 11:83, 1990.

Ljunggren HG, Karre K: In search of the "missing self": MHC molecules and NK cell recognition. *Immunol Today* 11:237, 1990.

Marrack P, Kappler J: The T cell and its receptor. *Sci Am* 254:36, 1986.

Mason DW, Morris PJ: Effector mechanisms in allograft rejection. *Annu Rev Immunol* 4:119, 1986.

Morris RE: Rapamycin: FK506's fraternal twin or distant cousin? *Immunol Today* 12:137, 1991.

Mosmann TR, Moore KW: The role of IL-10 in crossregulation of TH1 and TH2 responses. *Immunol Today* 11:A49, 1991.

Natvig JB: Immunology in a changing world and immunology changing the world. *Immunol Today* 11:72, 1990.

Parham P: Making just the right match. *Nature* 350:111, 1991.
Reth M, Hombach J, et al: The B-cell antigen receptor complex. *Immunol Today* 12:196, 1991.
Sablinski T, Hancock WW, et al: CD4 monoclonal antibodies in organ transplantation—a review of progress. *Transplantation* 52:579, 1991.
Sachs DH: Specific transplantation tolerance. *N Engl J Med* 325:1240, 1991.
Shevach EM: The effects of cyclosporine on the immune system. *Annu Rev Immunol* 3:397, 1985.
Strom TB: Immunosuppressive agents in renal transplantation. *Kidney Int* 26:353, 1984.
Thomson A: FK-506 enters the clinic. *Immunol Today* 11:35, 1990.
Tilney NL, Whitley WD, et al: Chronic rejection—an undefined conundrum. *Transplantation* 52:389, 1991.
Tzakis AG, Fung JJ, et al: Use of FK 506 in pediatric patients. *Transplant Proc* 23:924, 1991.
Van Buren CT: Cyclosporine: progress, problems and perspectives. *Surg Clin North Am* 66:435, 1986.
Weaver CT, Unanue ER: The costimulatory function of antigen-presenting cells. *Immunol Today* 11:49, 1990.
Westermann J, Pabst R: Lymphocyte subsets in the blood: a diagnostic window on the lymphoid system? *Immunol Today* 11:406, 1990.

Liver Transplantation

Ascher NL, Simmons RL, et al: Host hepatectomy and liver transplantation, in Simmons RL, Finch ME, et al (eds): *Manual of Vascular Access, Organ Donation, and Transplantation*. New York, Springer-Verlag, 1984, p 255.
Broelsch CE, Edmond JC, et al: Application of reduced-size liver transplants as split grafts, auxiliary orthotopic grafts, and living related segmental transplants. *Ann Surg* 212:368, 1990.
Burdick JF, Vogelsang GB, et al: Graft-vs-host disease after liver transplantation. *Hepatology* 11:144, 1990.
Busuttil RW: Living-related liver donation: CON. *Transplant Proc* 23:43, 1991.
Busuttil RW, Seu P, Millis JM: Liver transplantation in children. *Ann Surg* 213:48, 1991.
Castaldo P, Stratta RJ, et al: Clinical spectrum of fungal infections after orthotopic liver transplantation. *Arch Surg* 126:149, 1991.
Cosmini AB, Cho SI, et al: A randomized clinical trial comparing OKT3 and steroids for treatment of hepatic allograft rejection. *Transplantation* 43:91, 1987.
Demetriou AA, Chowdrury NR, et al: New method of hepatocyte transplantation and extracorporeal liver support. *Ann Surg* 204:259, 1986.
Fath JJ, Ascher NL, et al: Metabolism during hepatic transplantations. Indicators of allograft function. *Surgery* 96:64, 1984.
Foster JH: History of liver surgery. *Arch Surg* 126:381, 1991.
Fung JJ, Todo S, et al: Conversion of liver allograft recipients from cyclosporine to FK 506-based immunosuppression: benefits and pitfalls. *Transplant Proc* 23:14, 1991.
Gordon RD, Shaw BW, et al: Indications for liver transplantation in the cyclosporine era. *Surg Clin North Am* 66:541, 1986.
Gordon RD, Todo S, et al: Liver transplantation under cyclosporine: a decade of experience. *Transplant Proc* 23:1393, 1991.
Gugenheim J, Samuel D, et al: Liver transplantation across ABO blood group barriers. *Lancet* 336:519, 1990.
Hood JM, Koep LJ, et al: Liver transplantation for advanced liver disease with alpha-1-antitrypsin deficiency. *N Engl J Med* 302:272, 1980.
Indications for liver transplantation. *Transplant Immunol Ltr* 7(3):2, 1991.
Kam I, Lynch S, et al: Low flow venous bypasses in small dogs and pediatric patients undergoing replacement of the liver. *Surg Gynecol Obstet* 163:33, 1986.
Kirschner BS, Baker AL, Thorp FK: Growth in adulthood after liver transplantation for glycogen storage disease type I. *Gastroenterology* 101:238, 1991.
Koneru B, Flye MW, et al: Liver transplantation for hepatoblastoma, the American experience. *Ann Surg* 213:118, 1991.
Kretchtle SJ, Kolbeck PC, et al: Hepatic transplantation into sensitized recipients: demonstration of hyperacute rejection. *Transplantation* 43:8, 1987.
Lerut J, Gordon RD, et al: Biliary tract complication following human orthotopic liver transplantation. *Transplantation* 43:47, 1987.
McMaster P: What's new in hepatobiliary surgery. *J R Coll Surg Edinb* 36:1, 1990.
Penn I: The changing pattern of posttransplant malignancies. *Transplant Proc* 23:1101, 1991.
Perkins JD, Wiesner RH, et al: Immunohistologic labelling as an indication of liver allograft rejection. *Transplantation* 43:100, 1987.
Single lung, double lung, and heart-lung transplantation. *Transplant Immunol Ltr* 7(4):2, 1991.
So SKS, Platt JL, et al: Increased expression of class I MHC antigens on hepatocytes in rejecting human liver allografts. *Transplantation* 43:79, 1987.
Todo S, Fung JJ, et al: One hundred ten consecutive primary orthotopic liver transplants under FK 506 in adults. *Transplant Proc* 23:1397, 1991.
Wall WJ, Grant DR, et al: Liver transplantation without veno veno bypass. *Transplantation* 43:56, 1987.
Whitington PF, Balistreri WF: Liver transplantation in pediatrics: indications, contraindications, and pretransplant management, *J Pediatr* 118:169, 1991.

Pancreas Transplantation

Corry RJ, Nghiem DD, et al: Surgical treatment of diabetic nephropathy with simultaneous pancreatic, duodenal and renal transplantation. *Surg Gynecol Obstet* 162:547, 1986.
Hullett DA, Faleny JL, et al: Human fetal pancreas—a potential source for transplantation. *Transplantation* 43:18, 1987.
Nghiem DD, Gonwa TA, et al: Metabolic effects of urinary diversion of exocrine secretion in pancreatic transplantation. *Transplantation* 43:70, 1987.
Prieto M, Sutherland DER, et al: Experimental and clinical experiences with urine amylase monitoring for early diagnosis of rejection in pancreas transplantation. *Transplantation* 43:73, 1987.
Sutherland DER: Current status of pancreas transplantation. *J Clin Endocrinol Metab* 73:461, 1991.
Sutherland DER, Gillingham K, Moudry-Munns K: Results of pancreas transplantation in the United States for 1987–90, from the United Network for Organ Sharing (UNOS) registry with comparison to 1984–87 results. *Clin Transplant* 5:330, 1991.
Sutherland DER, Moudry-Munns KC, Dunn DL: Pancreas transplantation as endocrine replacement therapy in type I diabetes mellitus, in Samols E: *The Endocrine Pancreas*. New York, Raven Press, 1991, chap 24.

Bone Marrow Transplantation

Advisory Committee of the Bone Marrow Transplant Registry: Bone marrow transplantation from donors with aplastic anemia: A report from the ACS/NTH Bone Marrow Transplant Registry. *JAMA* 236:1131, 1976.
Beatty PG, et al: Marrow transplantation from related donors other than HLA identical siblings. *N Engl J Med* 313:765, 1985.
Bolman RM, Molina JE, et al: Heart transplantation, in Simmons RL, Finch ME, et al (eds): *Manual of Vascular Access, Organ Donation and Transplantation*. New York, Springer-Verlag, 1984, p 209.
Down JD, Mauch PM: The effect of combining cyclophosphamide with total-body irradiation on donor bone marrow engraftment. *Transplantation* 51:1309, 1991.
Frazier OH, Cooley DA: Cardiac transplantation. *Surg Clin North Am* 66:477, 1986.

Martin PJ, Schoch G, et al: A retrospective analysis of therapy for acute graft-versus-host disease: secondary treatment. *Blood* 77:1821, 1991.

Murawska MB, Duijvestijn AM, et al: Differential kinetics of various subsets of thymic bone marrow–derived stromal cells in rat chimeras. *Scand J Immunol* 33:473, 1991.

Wingard JR, Curbow B, Baker F: Health, functional status, and employment of adult survivors of bone marrow transplantation. *Ann Int Med* 114:113, 1991.

Yazdi B, Patel MP, et al: Vascularized bone marrow transplantation (VBMT): induction of stable mixed T-cell chimerism and transplantation tolerance in unmodified recipients. *Transplant Proc* 23:739, 1991.

Cardiac Transplantation

Armitage JM, Kormos RL, et al: Posttransplant lymphoproliferative disease in thoracic organ transplant patients: ten years of cyclosporine-based immunosuppression. *J Heart-Lung Transplant* 10:877, 1991.

Armitage JM, Kormos RL, et al: Clinical trial of FK 506 immunosuppression in adult cardiac transplantation. *Ann Thorac Surg* 54:205, 1992.

Backer CL, Zales VR, et al: Intermediate term results in infant orthotopic cardiac transplantation from two centers. *J Thorac Cardiovasc Surg* 101:826, 1991.

Barnard CN: A human cardiac transplant. *S Afr Med J* 41:1271, 1967.

Billingham ME, Cary NRB, et al: A working formulation for the standardization of nomenclature in the diagnosis of heart and lung rejection: heart rejection study group. *J Heart Transplant* 9:587, 1990.

Carrel A, Guthrie CC: The transplantation of veins and organs. *Am Med* 10:1101, 1905.

Costanzo-Nordin MR: Cardiac allograft vasculopathy: relationship with acute cellular rejection and histocompatibility. *J Heart-Lung Transplant* 11:S90, 1992.

Costanzo-Nordin MR, O'Sullivan EJ, et al: Prospective randomized trial of OKT3 versus horse antithymocyte globulin-based immunosuppressive prophylaxis in heart transplantation. *J Heart Transplant* 9:306, 1990.

Costard-Jackle A, Hill J, et al: The influence of preoperative patient characteristics on early and late survival following cardiac transplantation. *Circulation* 84:329, 1991.

Ensley RD, Hunt S, et al: Predictors of survival after repeat heart transplantation. The Registry of the International Society for Heart and Lung Transplantation, and Contributing Investigators. *J Heart-Lung Transplant* 11:S142, 1992.

Havel M, Owen AN, et al: Decreasing use of donated blood and reduction of bleeding after orthotopic heart transplantation by use of aprotinin. *J Heart-Lung Transplant* 11:348, 1992.

Kaye MP: The Registry of the International Society for Heart-Lung Transplantation: Ninth Official Report. *J Heart-Lung Transplant* 11:599, 1992.

Keogh A, Macdonald P, et al: Five-year follow-up of a randomized double-lung versus triple drug therapy immunosuppressive trial after heart transplantation. *J Heart-Lung Transplant* 11:550, 1992.

Keogh A, Macdonald P, et al: Initial steroid-free versus steroid-based maintenance therapy and steroid withdrawal after heart transplantation: two views of the steroid question. *J Heart-Lung Transplant* 11:421, 1992.

Lower RR, Shumway NE: Studies on orthotopic transplantation of the canine heart. *Surg Forum* 11:18, 1960.

Merigan TC, Renlund DG, et al: A controlled trial of ganciclovir to prevent cytomegalovirus disease after heart transplantation. *N Engl J Med* 326:1182, 1992.

Miller LW (ed): Cardiac allograft vascular disease: a basic science and clinical review, in Proceedings of an International Conference on Cardiac Allograft Vascular Disease, St Louis, Missouri, October 25–26, 1991. *J Heart-Lung Transplant* 11:S1, 1992.

Oaks TE, Pae WE Jr, et al: Combined Registry for the clinical use of mechanical ventricular assist pumps and the total artificial heart in conjunction with heart transplantation: Fifth Official Report 1990. *J Heart-Lung Transplant* 10:621, 1991.

Paris W, Woodbury A, et al: Social rehabilitation and return to work after cardiac transplantation—a multicenter survey. *Transplantation* 53:433, 1992.

Starnes VA, Oyer PE, et al: Heart, heart-lung, and lung transplantation in the first year of life. *Ann Thorac Surg* 53:306, 1992.

Teo KK, Yusuf S, et al: Preserved left ventricular function during supine exercise in patients after orthotopic cardiac transplantation. *Eur Heart J* 13:321, 1992.

Lung and Heart-Lung Transplantation

Auteri JS, Jeevanandum V, et al: Normal bronchial healing without bronchial wrapping in canine lung transplantation. *Ann Thorac Surg* 53:80, 1992.

Calhoon JH, Nichols L, et al: Single lung transplantation: factors in postoperative cytomegalovirus infection. *J Thorac Cardiovasc Surg* 103:21, 1992.

Carere R, Patterson GA, et al: Right and left ventricular performance after single and double lung transplantation. *J Thorac Cardiovasc Surg* 102:115, 1992.

Cooper JD (ed): St Louis International Lung Transplant Registry Report, August, 1992.

Dubois P, Choiniere L, et al: Bronchial omentopexy in canine lung allotransplantation. *Ann Thorac Surg* 38:211, 1984.

Goldberg M, Lima O, et al: A comparison between cyclosporine A and methylprednisolone plus azathioprine on bronchial healing following canine lung autotransplantation. *J Thorac Cardiovasc Surg* 85:821, 1983.

Hutter JA, Stewart S, et al: Histologic changes in heart-lung transplant recipients during rejection episodes and at routine biopsy. *J Heart Transplant* 7:440, 1988.

Jamieson SW, Stinson EB, et al: Operative technique for heart-lung transplantation. *J Thorac Cardiovasc Surg* 87:930, 1984.

Kaiser LR, Cooper JD, et al: The evolution of single lung transplantation for emphysema. *J Thorac Cardiovasc Surg* 102:333, 1991.

LoCicero J, Robinson PG, et al: Chronic rejection in single-lung transplantation manifested by obliterative bronchiolitis. *J Thorac Cardiovasc Surg* 99:1059, 1990.

Low DE, Trulock EP, et al: Morbidity, mortality, and early results of single versus bilateral lung transplantation for emphysema. *J Thorac Cardiovasc Surg* 103:1119, 1992.

McCarthy PM, Starnes VA, et al: Improved survival after heart-lung transplantation. *J Thorac Cardiovasc Surg* 99:54, 1990.

McGregor CGA, Dark JH, et al: Early results of single lung transplantation in patients with end-stage pulmonary fibrosis. *J Thorac Cardiovasc Surg* 98:350, 1989.

Novick RJ, Menkis AH, et al: New trends in lung preservation: a collective review. *J Heart-Lung Transplant* 11:377, 1992.

Pasque MK, Kaiser LR, et al: Single lung transplantation for pulmonary hypertension: technical aspects and immediate hemodynamic results. *J Thorac Cardiovasc Surg* 103:475, 1992.

Ramirez JC, Patterson GA, et al: Bilateral lung transplantation for cystic fibrosis. *J Thorac Cardiovasc Surg* 103:287, 1992.

Reitz BA, Burton NA, et al: Heart and lung transplantation: autotransplantation and allotransplantation in primates with extended survival. *J Thorac Cardiovasc Surg* 80:360, 1980.

Retiz BA, Wallwork JL, et al: Heart-lung transplantation: successful therapy for patients with pulmonary vascular disease. *N Engl J Med* 306:556, 1982.

Shennib H, Noirclerc M, et al: Double-lung transplantation for cystic fibrosis. *Ann Thorac Surg* 54:17, 1992.

Starnes VA, Lewiston N, et al: Cystic fibrosis: target population for lung transplantation in North America in the 1990's. *J Thorac Cardiovasc Surg* 103:1008, 1992.

Starnes VA, Theodore J, et al: Evaluation of heart-lung transplant recipients with prospective, serial transbronchial biopsies and pulmonary function studies. *J Thorac Cardiovasc Surg* 98:683, 1989.

Starnes VA, Oyer PE, et al: Heart, heart-lung and lung transplantation in the first year of life. *Ann Thorac Surg* 53:306, 1992.

Trulock EP, Cooper JD, et al: The Washington University–Barnes Hospital experience with lung transplantation. *JAMA* 266:1943, 1991.

Yousem SA, Berry GJ, et al: A working formulation for the standardization of nomenclature in the diagnosis of heart and lung rejection: lung rejection study group. *J Heart Transplant* 9:593, 1990.

Kidney Transplantation

Burlingham WJ, Grailer A, et al: Improved renal allograft survival following donor specific transfusions. II. *In vitro* correlates of early DST type rejection episodes. *Transplantation* 43:41, 1987.

Calne RY, Wood AJ: Cyclosporine in cadaveric renal transplantation: 3 year followup of a European multicenter trial, *Lancet* 2:549, 1985.

Canadian Multicentre Transplant Study Group: A randomized trial of cyclosporine in cadaveric renal transplantation. *N Engl J Med* 314:1219, 1986.

Casteneda-Zuniga WR (ed): *Radiographic Diagnosis of Renal Transplant Complications*. Minneapolis, University of Minnesota, 1986.

Chandler ST, Buckels J, et al: Indium labelled platelet uptake in rejecting renal transplants. *Surg Gynecol Obstet* 157:242, 1983.

Cho SI, Zalneraetes BP, et al: The influence of acute tubular necrosis on kidney transplant survival. *Transplant Proc* 17:16, 1985.

Fryd DS, Sutherland DER, et al: Results of a prospective randomized study on the effect of splenectomy versus no splenectomy in renal transplant patients. *Transplant Proc* 13:48, 1981.

Keown PA, Stiller CB: Kidney transplantation. *Surg Clin North Am* 66:517, 1986.

Land W, Schneeberger H, et al: Long-term results in cadaveric renal transplantation under cyclosporine therapy. *Transplant Proc* 23:1244, 1991.

Malkowicz SB, Perloff LJ: Urologic consideration in renal transplantation. *Surg Gynecol Obstet* 160:579, 1985.

Mauer SM, Barbosa J, et al: Development of diabetic vascular lesions in normal kidneys transplanted into patients with diabetes mellitus. *N Engl J Med* 295:916, 1976.

Mendez-Picon G, Posner MS, et al: The effect of delayed function on long term survival of renal allografts. *Surg Gynecol Obstet* 161:351, 1986.

Monoco AP: Clinical kidney transplantation. *Transplant Proc* 17:5, 1985.

Najarian JS, Fryd DS, et al: A single institution, randomized, prospective trial of cyclosporine, versus azathioprine–antilymphocyte globulin for immunosuppression in renal allograft recipients. *Ann Surg* 201:142, 1985.

Najarian JS, So SKS, et al: The outcome of 304 primary renal transplants in children (1968–1985). *Ann Surg* 204:246, 1986.

Najarian JS, Sutherland DER: The impact of transplantation on the understanding and treatment of diabetes and the pancreas. *Transplant Proc* 12:634, 1980.

Novick AC (ed): Renal transplantation. *Urol Clin North Am* 10:203, 1983.

Opelz G: Correlation of HLA matching with kidney graft survival in patients with or without cyclosporine treatment. *Transplantation* 40:240, 1985.

Opelz G: Current relevance of the transfusion effect in renal transplantation. *Transplant Proc* 17:1015, 1985.

Opelz G, Mytilineos J, et al: Survival of DNA HLA-DR typed and matched cadaver kidney transplants, *Lancet* 338:461, 1991.

Ortho Multicenter Study Group: A randomized clinical trial of OKT3 monoclonal antibody for acute rejection of cadaveric renal transplants. *N Engl J Med* 313:37, 1985.

Report of the medical consultants on the diagnosis of death: Guidelines for determination of death. *JAMA* 246:2184, 1981.

Simmons RG, Anderson CR: Related donors and recipients: Five to nine years post-transplant. *Transplant Proc* 14:9, 1982.

Simmons RL, Najarian JS: Kidney transplantation, in Simmons RL, Finch ME, et al (eds): *Manual of Vascular Access, Organ Donation, and Transplantation*. New York, Springer-Verlag, 1984, p 292.

Simmons RL, Sutherland DER: Transplant nephrectomy, in Simmons RL, Finch ME, et al (eds): *Manual of Vascular Access, Organ Donation, and Transplantation*. New York, Springer-Verlag, 1984, p 329.

So SKS, Simmons RL, et al: Improved results of multiple transplantation in children. *Surgery* 98:729, 1985.

Sommer BG, Henry M, et al: Sequential antilymphoblast globulin and cyclosporine for renal transplantation. *Transplantation* 43:85, 1987.

Starzl TE, Hakala TR: Variable convalescence and therapy after cadaveric renal transplantation under cyclosporin A and steroids. *Surg Gynecol Obstet* 154:819, 1982.

Stiller CR, Keown PA: Immunologic monitoring: current perspectives and clinical implications. *Transplant Proc* 13:1699, 1981.

Sutherland DER: International human pancreas and islet transplant registry. *Transplant Proc* 12:229, 1980.

Sutherland DER, Fryd DS, et al: The high-risk recipient in renal transplantation. *Transplant Proc* 14:19, 1982.

Tzakis AG, Fung JJ, et al: Use of FK 506 in pediatric patients. *Transplant Proc* 23:924, 1991.

Wing AJ, Broyer M, et al: Renal transplantation in Europe—some comparisons between national programs. *Transplant Proc* 14:5, 1982.

Transplantation of Other Organs and Cellular Grafts

Alejandro R, Tzakis A, et al: Combined liver-islet allotransplantation in man under FK 506. *Transplant Proc* 23:789, 1991.

Baird RN, Abbott WM: Vein grafts: an historical perspective. *Am J Surg* 134:293, 1977.

Cohen Z, Wassef R, et al: Transplantation of the small intestine. *Surg Clin North Am* 66:583, 1986.

Friedlander GE, Mankin HJ, et al (eds): *Osteochondral Allografts*. Boston, Little, Brown, 1983.

Hardy MA, Chabot J: Transplantation of the small intestine—its time has come. *Lit Scan: Transplant* 6:1, 1990.

Pritchford TJ, Kirkman RL: Small bowel transplantation. *World J Surg* 9:860, 1985.

Quilici PJ, Vieta JO, et al: The use of dura mater allografts in the surgical repair of the abdominal wall. *Surg Gynecol Obstet* 161:47, 1985.

Ricordi C, Tzakis A, et al: Human islet isolation and allotransplantation in 22 consecutive cases. *Transplantation* 53:407, 1992.

Then P, Sandbichler P, et al: Hepatocyte transplantation into the lung for treatment of acute hepatic failure in the rat. *Transplant Proc* 23:892, 1991.

Tzakis AG, Ricordi C, et al: Pancreatic islet transplantation after upper abdominal exenetration and liver replacement. *Lancet* 336:402, 1990.

Vrist MR: Practical application of basic research on bone graft physiology. Instructional course lectures. *Am Acad Orthoped Surg* 25:1, 1976.

CHAPTER 11

Surgical Complications

Darryl T. Hiyama and Michael J. Zinner

GENERAL CONSIDERATIONS

Optimal care of the surgical patient requires a thorough knowledge of the potential complications that might arise during the perioperative and postoperative periods. These problems may be the result of the primary disease process, concomitant medical illness, or errors in operative technique or medical therapy. On rare occasions, complications may arise from an apparently unrelated etiology, for example, the postoperative development of acute appendicitis or acute cholecystitis.

Of paramount importance is the surgeon's ability to recognize and manage the problems as they develop. For the majority of patients, the period after surgery is characterized by a predictable and orderly pattern of recovery. Any deviation from the anticipated course, however subtle, should alert the surgeon to the possible development of a complication.

Some complications are preventable. Thorough preoperative evaluation, patient preparation, meticulous operative technique, and close postoperative observation serve well to avoid potentially serious or fatal problems. Other complications may not be preventable because of the need for urgent operation which may preclude thorough preparation before operation. In these instances, assessment of the individual patient's risks for developing specific problems and the anticipation of these problems will lead to more effective prevention or earlier diagnosis.

FEVER

Fever, or pyrexia, is a common occurrence in surgical patients in the postoperative period and may arise from either infectious or noninfectious causes. Fever may represent a potentially fatal problem, such as an intraabdominal sepsis or infected aortic graft, or a more benign process, such as atelectasis or drug fever.

In healthy individuals, a core temperature of 37°C (98.6°F) is considered to be normal with an expected diurnal variation of approximately 0.8°C (1.4°F). There is, however, no uniform clinical definition of a significant fever. In a number of clinical studies, definitions of fever have included temperatures greater than 38°C, greater than 38.3°C, more than 38.5°C, and greater than 38.5°C on two or more postoperative days. Though no consensus exists, temperatures exceeding 38°C or persisting for more than two postoperative days are generally considered to be clinically significant. The incidence of postoperative fever is remarkably high. Ledger and Child reported that of 12,026 women undergoing hysterectomy, 33 percent were found to have a postoperative temperature elevation greater than 38.3°C. Garibaldi and associates prospectively studied 871 patients undergoing general surgical, thoracic, orthopaedic, and head and neck procedures, reporting that 22 percent of patients experienced temperatures exceeding 38°C on two consecutive postoperative days. In two other retrospective studies the incidence of postoperative fever was 29 percent and 40 percent. Though fever is common, infection is found as the cause in fewer than one-half of febrile patients. Swartz and Tanaree reported that of 200 hysterectomy patients, 57 developed postoperative fever, of which only 21 were subsequently found to have a documented infection. Freischlag and Busuttil, in a retrospective study of adult general surgical patients, found that only 27 percent of febrile patients have an infection as the source of the fever. However, Garibaldi and associates have reported that in 58 percent of febrile patients, an infection was identified. Galicier and Richet, in a similar prospective study, noted that 62 percent of fevers were associated with infection.

The onset of postoperative fever bears clinical diagnostic and management significance. Garibaldi and associates noted that in 81 cases of fever, no apparent cause could be identified and that 72 percent of these cases occurred within the first two postoperative days.

Numerous conditions, both infectious and noninfectious, can cause postoperative fever (Table 11-1). Determining the cause of the febrile reaction requires a thorough evaluation of the patient. A detailed history focusing on preexisting infections, perioperative blood transfusions, drug therapy, catheter use, and the details of the operative procedure should be obtained. The physical examination should specifically assess those sites most commonly involved in infectious processes such as the surgical wound, lungs, abdomen, catheter sites, and head and neck. In addition, the legs should be examined for indications of deep venous thrombophlebitis, and the skin for signs of allergic drug reactions. Rote use of multiple laboratory studies, including blood, urine, and sputum cultures, should be condemned. In the majority of patients, a diagnosis can be made based on clinical findings and subsequently confirmed by the directed use of appropriate laboratory and radiologic studies.

The time of onset of fever in relation to the operation has significant diagnostic implications. Four phases are recognized: (1) the immediate perioperative period, (2) the first 24 h after operation, (3) 24 to 72 h after operation, and (4) greater than 72 h after operation.

Table 11-1
Causes of Postoperative Fever

Infectious	*Noninfectious*
Abscess	Acute gout
Acute cholecystitis	Adrenal insufficiency
Acute sinusitis	Atelectasis
Bacteremia	Dehydration
Candidiasis	Drug fever
Endocarditis	Head trauma
Hepatitis	Malignancy
Herpes virus infections	Myocardial infarction
Infectious diarrhea	Pancreatitis
Osteomyelitis	Pheochromocytoma
Parotitis	Pulmonary embolus
Peritonitis	Thrombophlebitis
Pharyngitis	Thyrotoxicosis
Pneumonia	Transfusion reaction
Postperfusion syndrome	
Prosthetic device infection	
Suppurative thrombophlebitis	
Transfusion-related infection	
Urinary tract infection	
Wound infection	

SOURCE: Howard RJ, 1988, with permission.

Perioperative Fever. The occurrence of fever in this period may be the result of preexisting infection, intraoperative manipulation of purulent material, blood transfusion reaction, drug reactions, or malignant hyperthermia. In many instances, preexisting infection is the primary disease process for which the operation is undertaken (e.g., perforated appendicitis, colonic diverticular abscess), and the diagnosis is confirmed at the time of operation. Sudden temperature elevations may occur after the intraoperative release of infected material during abdominal surgery with contamination of the peritoneal cavity. Febrile transfusion reactions are common and may be the result of allergic reactions, major hemolytic transfusion reactions, or the infusion of contaminated blood. The occurrence of fever during blood transfusion, as well as the presence of associated signs such as excessive bleeding, hemoglobinuria, or hemodynamic instability, should lead one to the diagnosis. Under these circumstances, the transfusion should be immediately terminated and samples of the patient's blood and urine obtained to be examined for evidence of hemolysis. The remaining blood product should also be returned for bacterial culture and analysis as well as confirmation of patient-donor compatibility. Hypotension is treated with intravenous saline infusions, and an attempt should be made to prevent acute tubular necrosis with the administration of sodium bicarbonate to alkalinize the urine and of mannitol to promote diuresis. If no hemolysis or hemodynamic instability is present, a less severe nonhemolytic or allergic reaction might have occurred. In this situation, antipyretic agents can be used to control the fever, and the transfusion can be continued cautiously. Malignant hyperthermia is an uncommon but lethal cause of perioperative fever. Elicited by inhalational anesthetic agents and succinylcholine, malignant hyperthermia results in a dramatic and profound temperature elevation (up to 42°C) associated with the presence of dark blood in the operative field, metabolic acidosis, hyperkalemia, and circulatory collapse. If malignant hyperthermia is suspected intraoperatively, both the operation and anesthesia should be terminated as soon as possible, and the patient should be hyperventilated with 100% oxygen. Continuous intravenous dantrolene in a dose of 2 to 3 mg/kg is administered until symptoms subside. Hyperkalemia and acidosis should be treated and mannitol given to promote diuresis. Many of the common signs of both transfusion reactions and malignant hyperthermia may be absent in the anesthetized patient, and fever may be the sole indication of the complication.

Fever Within 24 Hours. Atelectasis is the most common cause of fever within the first 24 h following surgery, in the absence of preexisting infection. Though uncommon, necrotizing streptococcal and clostridial wound infections can also occur at this early juncture. Close examination of the surgical wound is mandatory if early fever occurs. If these infections are present, the wound appears violaceous with woody edema and spreading erythema.

Fever at 24 to 48 Hours. Febrile reactions occurring between 24 and 72 h after surgery are usually attributable to respiratory complications or catheter-related problems. Noninfectious causes such as persistent atelectasis and thrombophlebitis are commonplace. Infectious complications such as bacterial pneumonia, aspiration pneumonia, and septic thrombophlebitis can also occur.

Fever After 72 Hours. There is evidence to indicate that the occurrence of fever after the third postoperative day or fever that persists for more than 2 days is suggestive of an infectious source. Fever due to urinary tract infections often is evident at 3 to 5 days after operation and is more likely to occur in patients after bladder catheterization, instrumentation of the urinary tract, or preexisting mild urinary tract obstruction such as benign prostatic hypertrophy. Wound infections usually become clinically evident at anywhere from 7 to 10 days after operation. Typically, an intra-abdominal abscess or anastomotic leak results in fever during the fourth and seventh days following abdominal surgery. Occasionally, deep venous thrombosis will manifest as a fever during the fifth and seventh days after surgery.

The absence of obvious sources of fever in these common locations necessitates the consideration of uncommon causes of postoperative fever. Unrelated bacterial infections such as acute sinusitis, acute cholecystitis, acute parotitis, endocarditis, or pseudomembranous colitis may be present. Osteomyelitis may develop following orthopaedic procedures or extremity trauma. Hepatitis B, hepatitis C (non-A, non-B), and cytomegalovirus (CMV) may develop after blood product transfusion. Candidiasis may develop in immunocompromised patients or those on prolonged broad-spectrum antibiotic therapy. Viral infections caused by opportunistic pathogens such as herpes simplex, varicella-zoster, Epstein-Barr, and CMV also occur in immunocompromised patients, especially after transplantation. In general, the usual guideline for the time of occurrence of a fever and the underlying cause is not helpful in the immunosuppressed patient.

Rarely, noninfectious etiologies can cause postoperative fever. Despite the numerous possible causes of noninfectious fever (Table 11-1), most of these are uncommon. The clinical diagnosis is often made by the exclusion of all potential infectious causes for fever, before giving final consideration to noninfectious etiologies.

Endocrine disorders may give rise to perioperative fever. Thyroid storm, a severe form of thyrotoxicosis, can be precipitated by stress of operation or anesthesia and manifests with fever. Patients with thyrotoxicosis who are inadequately prepared for operation or patients with unrecognized hyperthyroidism are at risk. Though an uncommon tumor, pheochromocytoma can also be revealed by the stress of operation, and the patient will present with fever in addition to labile hypertension.

WOUND COMPLICATIONS

Hematomas

The formation of a hematoma can occur in any surgical wound. Hematomas impair wound healing by providing a medium for bacterial infection, as well as a mechanical barrier to the apposition of tissue edges. In addition, significant fibrosis can occur with resolution of the hematoma, leading to altered scar formation and a poor cosmetic outcome. In the neck, large hematomas may cause tracheal compression and airway compromise following thyroid or carotid artery surgery. Hematomas forming under split-thickness skin grafts prevent vascularization and adherence, with subsequent graft failure. Similarly, hematomas forming under soft tissue flaps may impair the blood supply, leading to flap necrosis.

The risk for hematoma formation appears to be increased in the presence of extensive subcutaneous dissection and poor tissue approximation. The use of local anesthetic with epinephrine also appears to increase this risk, probably due to delayed hemorrhage from vessels undergoing transient epinephrine-induced vasoconstriction. Similarly, marked coughing and retching while awakening from anesthesia can cause renewed hemorrhage from poorly controlled vessels. Underlying disorders of coagulation (see Chap. 3), both acquired and hereditary, increase the likelihood of this complication. In addition, the preoperative use of aspirin or anticoagulants such as heparin or warfarin may cause hematomas. An increased number of hematomas following plastic surgery procedures in patients experiencing postoperative hypertension has been reported. Patients undergoing operative procedures such as inguinal herniorrhaphy, umbilical herniorrhaphy, breast operations, and leg amputations appear to be prone to hematoma formation.

Wound hematomas present with pain, pressure, and swelling within the wound, often soon after the patient awakens from anesthesia. Wound drainage may be present, appearing as a sanguineous or serous discharge.

In general, significant wound hematomas recognized within 24 to 48 h after operation should be evacuated under sterile conditions by removing a few of the skin sutures. If hemostatis is achieved, the wound is closed primarily. This action should reduce the risk of subsequent infection and promote more rapid wound healing. Smaller, sterile hematomas or those recognized late in the postoperative course can be managed expectantly. The more serious situations cited above (i.e., carotid, thyroid, facial plastic, or flap operations) are exceptional, and urgent evacuation of the hematoma may be necessary to avoid airway compromise or jeopardizing the surgical graft.

Seromas

Lymph collections, or seromas, usually present as painless swelling within the wound or below flaps. These often develop in wounds involving dissection in lymph node–bearing areas (i.e., axillae, neck, or groin) or in areas where significant dead space remains, such as after abdominal-perineal resection or total mastectomy. These collections prevent adequate tissue approximation or may become secondarily infected.

The primary cause lies in the failure to identify and control lymphatic vessels during dissection. Though lymph is a protein-rich fluid, electrocauterization is ineffective because coagulation proteins are not present in sufficient quantities. Instead, ligation or the use of stainless-steel clips is preferred. In addition, lymph accumulation can be prevented by the use of closed-suction drainage. The risk for infection remains low, as long as the drains remain in place no longer than 5 days.

Wound seromas may be treated by needle aspiration under sterile technique, if no erythema or fever is present, and repeat aspirations might be required to resolve the problem. Collections refractory to repeated attempts of needle aspiration may require the placement of drainage catheters, although this situation is uncommon. The presence of erythema or fever is suggestive of an infected seroma or a primary wound infection, and in this setting, open drainage may be preferable.

Wound Infections

Though infection cannot occur without bacterial contamination, the simple presence of bacteria within the wound does not inevitably result in an infection. Multiple factors determine the potential and the incidence of infection (Table 11-2). Many of these factors can be influenced by the surgeon and are determined within the first few hours of wounding.

Bacteria may originate from several sources such as the patient, the operating room personnel, the operating room environment, and the equipment. The probability of wound infection and the most likely primary source for the infecting bacteria differs depending on the operation performed (Table 11-3). In operations classified as clean, the rate of infection is low, on the order of 1 to 2 percent. In this situation, infecting organisms originate from the skin or from exogenous sources (operating room environment or personnel). If remote infection is present, this may also provide a source of infecting organisms. For example, in patients with urinary tract infections, wound infections usually involve the same organism. Hence, elective operations should be postponed until any existing remote infection is eradicated. In clean-contaminated and contaminated cases, the incidence of infection ranges from 7 to 18 percent. The source is usually the gastrointestinal, biliary, genitourinary, or respiratory tract, whichever is entered during the operation. In these cases, the number of bacteria contaminating the wound is significantly greater than is usually seen in clean operations. In infected cases, the likelihood of a wound infection exceeds 50 percent. The degree of contamination may be on the order of 10^{10} bacteria/mL. In these wounds, delayed primary closure is the best alternative to avoid an almost certain wound infection.

Table 11-2
Influencing Factors in Wound Infection

Source of bacteria
Type of bacteria
Bacterial virulence
Bacterial antibiotic resistance
Size of bacterial inoculum
Skin preparation
Duration of operation
Extent of tissue damage
Presence of hematoma or seroma
Presence of foreign body
Inappropriate use of electrocautery
Patient age
Hypoxemia
Presence of chronic illness (e.g., renal failure, liver failure, chronic obstructive pulmonary disease, malignancy, diabetes mellitus)
Hypotension or shock
Malnutrition
Use of immunosuppressive drugs
Corticosteroids
Chemotherapeutic agents

Table 11-3
Classification of Operative Wounds

Class	*Wound Description*	*Examples*
I	Clean	Nontraumatic, uninfected operative wounds in which the respiratory, alimentary, or genitourinary tract is not entered. Usually closed without drains.
II	Clean-contaminated	Operative wounds in which the respiratory, alimentary, or genitourinary tract is entered with only minimal contamination.
III	Contaminated	Fresh traumatic wounds; wounds with a major break in sterile technique; wounds encountering nonpurulent inflammation; wounds made in or near contaminated skin.
IV	Infected	Wounds in which purulent infection is encountered.

SOURCE: Report of an Ad Hoc Committee of the Committee on Trauma, Division of Medical Sciences, National Academy of Sciences–National Research Council, 1964, with permission.

There are several preoperative techniques available to reduce or eliminate bacteria from the operative field. The patient's own bacterial flora is the most likely source of contaminating bacteria; antimicrobial showers or baths and preoperative skin decontamination are methods of reducing skin flora. Body hair, which harbors significant numbers of staphylococci, should be clipped and not shaved to avoid skin trauma and the secondary bacterial growth that occurs in the traumatized areas. The quantity of bowel bacteria can be dramatically reduced by ablutionary preparations that mechanically cleanse the bowel, as well as orally administered nonabsorbable antibiotics to decrease the number of bacteria.

The use of prophylactic systemic antibiotics has been proved to reduce wound infection rates in clean and clean-contaminated cases. It is essential that the antibiotic chosen has demonstrated activity against the likely contaminating organisms and that the preoperative dose is administered such that adequate tissue concentrations are achieved by the time of wounding (see Chap. 5).

Once wounding has occurred, the surgeon has control over several factors concerning the wound itself to reduce the susceptibility for infection. The duration of the operation influences the wound infection rate. Operations exceeding 2 h are associated with a higher infection rate and may be related to the desiccation or maceration of the wound edges, as well as to the increase in the number of bacteria that accumulate within the wound. Fewer bacteria are required to produce an infection in the presence of necrotic tissue, foreign bodies, hematomas, seromas, and poor tissue perfusion. Tissue damage can be reduced by adherence to the Halstedian principles of sharp anatomic dissection, hemostasis, gentle handling of tissues, and the use of fine sutures. Large sutures and mass ligatures should not be used. Hematomas and seromas must be avoided and necrotic tissue, if present, removed. The use of electrocautery must be judicious, providing pinpoint coagulation to avoid thermal tissue destruction and charring.

Local perfusion of the wound has significant implications for the probability of infection. Hunt and others have demonstrated the importance of maintaining adequate oxygen delivery and arterial oxygen tension in preventing wound infection. Local perfusion and oxygen delivery may be compromised by placement of an incision in an ischemic area (as in an ischemic limb) or by the development of shock.

Certain host factors are associated with an increased risk for wound infection. Advanced age, use of chemotherapeutic and immunosuppressive agents, and associated medical conditions such as diabetes mellitus, renal insufficiency, or hepatic insufficiency have been identified as potential risk factors.

Clinical Manifestations. The diagnosis of a wound infection is based on clinical findings. Presentation is usually between the seventh and tenth postoperative days, though it may occur as early as 24 h after surgery or as late as 2 weeks. Increasing local pain at a time when pain should be decreasing is a common complaint. Local signs include erythema, swelling, and drainage from the incision as well as tenderness. The presence of accompanying fever and leukocytosis varies. Wound infection occurring below muscle or fascial layers or below thick, uninfected subcutaneous tissue (in obese patients) may have a delayed presentation or lack many of the local signs noted above.

Management. The treatment of a wound infection requires opening the wound to effect drainage of purulent material and to evaluate the affected tissues. If the process is determined to be superficial, without surrounding cellulitis and systemic signs, then antibiotic therapy is not indicated. If the local reaction is severe or systemic signs are present, antibiotic therapy is advisable. Empiric antibiotic selection is determined by the likely contaminating organism. Suitable specimens for bacterial culture should always be obtained when the wound is opened and the antibiotic therapy later modified once the organism is identified (see Chap. 5).

Wounds not involving the perineum and not associated with entrance into the gastrointestinal or biliary tract are most often infected by *Staphylococcus aureus* or streptococci. By contrast, wounds involving the perineum, or associated with the gastrointestinal or biliary tract, often are infected with gram-negative bacilli and anaerobic bacteria. Under these circumstances, polymicrobial infections are common. Infrequently, a superficial wound infection may progress to necrotizing fasciitis. This potentially fatal complication almost invariably involves a polymicrobial infection and is characterized by extensive destruction of the underlying fascia. An aggressive, radical surgical debridement of the affected tissue is mandatory to control the process.

Wound Dehiscence

In any surgical incision, the long-term strength of the wound arises from the approximation and proper healing of the fascial components. Wound dehiscence is defined as the separation of approximated fascia. Though fascial dehiscence may occur in any type of incision, the term *wound dehiscence* is classically associated with laparotomy incisions, where the development of this complication has its most severe consequences. Dehiscence of thoracic incisions is rare and usually follows median sternotomy. In this situation, inadequate fusion of the bony cortex of the sternum is the primary defect.

Wound healing involves the proper interaction of many processes including inflammation, epithelialization, contraction, and collagen metabolism. Numerous biochemical and cellular events mediate these processes; consequently, factors that have an injurious effect on these biologic events will impair wound healing. Several factors are well recognized to influence the ability to heal including age, obesity, nutritional status, anemia, diabetes mellitus, renal or hepatic insufficiency, infection, hypoxia, use of corticosteroids or cytotoxic chemotherapeutic agents, and radiation therapy.

Protein-calorie malnutrition has long been associated with poor wound healing. These effects of malnutrition are probably related to the lack of an energy source, specifically glucose for inflammatory, immune, and fibroblast cell functions such as phagocytosis, cell proliferation, and collagen modeling and a lack of protein essential for tissue repair and synthesis.

Haydock and Hill recently reported that patients classified with mild, moderate, or severe protein-calorie malnutrition had a suboptimal wound response, as measured by the hydroxyproline content of the wound, compared to well-nourished patients. In addition, this effect could be reversed with parenteral nutrition. Another clinical study has shown that a decline in food intake for less than 1 week, before nutritional indicators are affected, resulted in a decreased rate of synthesis of hydroxyproline in wounds. This would suggest that recent preoperative food intake has a greater influence than the absolute degree of malnutrition. A recent prospective trial, conducted by the Veterans Affairs Total Parenteral Nutrition Cooperative Study Group, studied 395 malnourished patients requiring laparotomy or noncardiac thoracotomy. They concluded that the use of perioperative total parenteral nutrition (TPN) (7 to 15 days before and 3 days after surgery) in severely malnourished patients resulted in fewer noninfectious postoperative complications compared to similar patients who did not receive TPN. By contrast, patients with borderline or mild malnutrition had no demonstrable benefit from TPN and an increased rate of infectious complications.

Patients with advanced malnutrition may also have significant deficiencies in minerals and vitamins. Vitamin C is essential for collagen synthesis, fibroblast formation, bacterial killing, and the production of neutrophil superoxide. Though clinical scurvy is rarely seen today, it has been shown that wound dehiscence is eight times more prevalent in patients with depleted levels of vitamin C. Zinc appears to play an important role in cell mitosis and proliferation in epithelial cells and fibroblasts and is thought to play a role in the stabilization of inflammatory cell membranes. Zinc deficiency may result from stress, sepsis, diarrhea, or enterocutaneous fistulas. Serum zinc levels of less than 100 $\mu g/dL$ are associated with poor healing. It appears that zinc replacement can reverse these effects, although excess zinc replacement does not hasten the healing process and might be detrimental.

Uremia secondary to acute or chronic renal failure is associated with poor wound healing. It is unclear whether this effect is due to a direct toxic effect of urea or to malnutrition which is common in patients with renal failure. Effective dialysis and adequate nutritional supplementation can ameliorate the adverse effects on wound healing. Jaundice has long been associated with impaired wound healing. It is unclear, however, whether this is due to a direct toxic effect of bilirubin on wound healing or if the effect is due to the synthetic dysfunction, anemia, malnutrition, immunocompromise, and intravascular volume depletion that accompanies hepatic failure. Prospective trials conducted to date have shown that preoperative biliary drainage in jaundiced patients does not have any beneficial effect on postoperative wound complications.

Wound healing is essentially normal in well-controlled diabetes mellitus but poor in patients with hyperglycemia. Hyperglycemia causes impairment of essentially all aspects of leukocyte function and, thus, the inflammatory response. In addition, there appears to be a general suppression of humoral and cellular immunity. Diabetic microangiopathy, which may impair the blood supply to the healing wound, may also adversely affect wound healing.

Corticosteroids are known to interfere with wound healing at virtually every level including inflammation, wound macrophage function, capillary proliferation, and fibroplasia. These effects are seen with both topical and systemic steroid use. The use of vitamin A appears to counteract some of the deleterious effects of corticosteroids. Topical doses of 200,000 I.U. have been shown to be locally effective but should be administered at the time of or within 3 or 4 days of wounding to be effective. Prolonged use of vitamin A bears the potential complication of hypervitaminosis A.

In one animal study, azathioprine appeared to have effects similar to corticosteroids on primary wound healing. In another study, cyclosporine appeared to have no effect on skin or fascial healing. Chemotherapeutic agents have significant potential to interfere with wound healing by inducing neutropenia (increased risk of infection), suppressing inflammatory cell function, inhibiting fibroplasia, and reducing collagen deposition. While most animal studies have demonstrated that chemotherapeutic agents delay wound healing, human studies have shown few clinical effects. Nitrogen mustard in doses up to 0.4 mg/kg used in the immediate postoperative period did not result in a significant increase of wound complications. The use of 5-fluorouracil in patients with breast cancer, given during the first postoperative week resulted in an increased frequency of wound infection and a small, but statistically significant, increase in wound dehiscence. The use of 5-fluorouracil in patients with colon cancer administered during and immediately after operation did not have a deleterious effect on wound healing. The use of thio-tepa in patients with breast or colon cancer in the first 3 days of operation or the use of cyclophosphamide in patients with breast cancer did not appear to interfere with wound healing. Doxorubicin had no serious effect on wound healing if used more than 7 days before or after operation in patients with soft tissue sarcomas. These results suggest that the use of some chemotherapeutic agents during the early postoperative period may not adversely affect wound healing or that the effects may be dose-dependent.

Early exposure of the wound to radiation therapy has direct effects on cellular proliferation and collagen synthesis, although these effects are minimized if exposure is delayed until the fourth to sixth postoperative days. The late effects of radiation therapy are endarteritis obliterans and fibrosis resulting in local hypoperfusion and wound hypoxia.

Several technical factors definitely influence wound healing. Wound closure should be performed with suture material of adequate tensile strength and durability to maintain wound approximation until healing is completed. In general, monofilament suture is used in any case where contamination is possible. Multifilament suture, in theory, can entrap microorganisms within the interstices and lead to infection. Suture placement should be made such that the suture will not cut through the fascia and will not strangulate the approximated tissues when tied. It is recommended that sutures be placed 1 cm from the wound edge and no further than 1 cm apart. Sutures should be tied to achieve approximation without excessive tension. Tissues should be handled delicately to minimize damage and maintain adequate local perfusion.

Clinical Manifestations. Abdominal wound dehiscence may occur in two forms. In one presentation, usually on the fifth to tenth postoperative days, serosanguineous fluid is found leaking from the wound. If the skin sutures have been removed or any remaining sutures break or cut through the skin, the small bowel and omentum can be released from the abdominal cavity, resulting in evisceration. Though evisceration may complicate only 0.5 percent of laparotomy incisions, this complication is associated with a mortality of 15 to 20 percent.

A less dramatic presentation of fascial dehiscence often occurs in grossly infected wounds. Sutures cut through weakened, friable fascia result in areas of separation. If these areas are small, evisceration may not occur because of the size of the defect and the adherence of the underlying viscera. If evisceration is deemed to be unlikely, conservative management of the wound is acceptable, though the development of an incisional hernia is inevitable. If the situation is unclear, operative exploration of the wound under general anesthesia is warranted.

URINARY AND RENAL COMPLICATIONS

Urinary Retention

Urinary retention frequently occurs in patients who undergo inguinal herniorrhaphy and anorectal surgery, though it may occur after any surgical procedure in which general or spinal anesthesia is used. A 4 percent incidence of urinary retention in one large series of 5220 patients who had undergone general surgical procedures was reported, although the incidence may range as high as 52 percent after anorectal surgery. Significant catecholamine release is associated with general and spinal anesthesia, as well as with stress and pain. It is believed that retention occurs as a result of catecholamine stimulation of alpha-adrenergic receptors in the smooth muscle of the bladder neck and urethra, which, in turn, increases bladder outlet tone and urethral resistance.

Urinary retention is more likely to occur in older men, especially those with a previous history of symptomatic prostatic obstruction or urethral trauma. Excessive intravenous fluid administration (in excess of 1000 mL) is also associated with an increased incidence of retention. The incidence of urinary retention is also increased with spinal or epidural anesthesia, with some additional evidence to suggest that this risk is further increased with long-acting anesthetic agents.

There is increasing evidence to suggest that the incidence of urinary retention can be minimized using alpha-receptor blocking agents. Goldman and coworkers reported the absence of urinary retention in 58 older male patients following inguinal herniorrhaphy treated with phenoxybenzamine. In comparison, 26 percent of the 44 control patients developed retention. A similar study using bethanechol after anorectal surgery showed no benefit. Petersen and associates in a randomized, prospective trial of 60 male patients undergoing hip and knee prosthesis operations found that the preoperative and postoperative use of prazosin hydrochloride resulted in a significant decrease in the incidence of postoperative urinary retention, 21 percent in the treated group compared to 59 percent in the control group.

Other studies have shown that intravenous fluid restriction to less than 250 mL and the use of local anesthesia reduces the incidence of urinary retention following inguinal herniorrhaphy. Currently, there is insufficient evidence to promote the use of alpha-receptor blocking agents to prevent urinary retention. Instead, local anesthesia and a minimum volume of intravenous fluids should be utilized when possible. The clinical diagnosis of urinary retention is not difficult, as the patient will experience urgency, lower abdominal discomfort or cramping, and be unable to void. The treatment is continual urinary bladder catheterization and drainage until the patient is ambulatory, usually a period of 2 to 7 days.

Acute Renal Failure

Despite improvements in the care of patients with acute renal failure (ARF), the mortality rate associated with the development of this complication in surgical patients continues to range from 50 to 90 percent. This high mortality is attributed to the underlying causes of ARF and the high incidence of sepsis and multisystem organ failure found in these patients. Acute renal failure is defined as the abrupt decline in renal function that results in the accumulation of nitrogenous wastes, evidenced by elevation of the serum blood urea nitrogen (BUN) and creatinine. Renal failure is described as oliguric (urine output < 400 mL/24 h) or nonoliguric (urine output normal or markedly increased). Nonoliguric renal failure is associated with a lower mortality rate.

Acute renal failure is classified according to the primary cause: prerenal, intrinsic, or postrenal. Prerenal causes are those that affect cardiac output and renal perfusion. Volume depletion is the most common cause of prerenal azotemia in surgical patients and can result from dehydration, hemorrhage, or third-space sequestration of fluids as seen in burns and acute pancreatitis. Hypotension and shock, whether due to sepsis, myocardial dysfunction, or hypovolemia, is also a common cause of ARF. Less common are abnormalities of the renal vasculature such as renal artery emboli or renal vein thrombosis. The optimization of renal perfusion by volume repletion and maintenance of cardiac output are the primary goals in preventing and managing prerenal causes of ARF.

Obstructive uropathy is the postrenal cause of ARF. Obstruction of the ureter may develop due to stone, tumor, clot, or trauma. Iatrogenic ureteral injury is a serious consideration following retroperitoneal or pelvic surgery if postoperative anuria occurs. Benign prostatic hypertrophy, stricture, stone, or trauma can cause urethral obstruction. A common and easily correctable cause of urethral obstruction is an occluded or improperly placed Foley catheter. Therapy for postrenal causes of ARF is relief of the obstruction which often results in normalization of renal function.

The common intrinsic renal causes of ARF noted in surgical patients are acute tubular necrosis (ATN), pigment nephropathy, and drug nephrotoxicity. ATN results from prolonged ischemia of the renal parenchyma. In response to diminished renal perfusion, glomerular blood flow and filtration is maintained by afferent arteriolar dilatation and efferent arteriolar vasoconstriction. Continuing hypotension activates the renin-angiotensin system increasing circulating catecholamines and angiotensin, which cause afferent arteriolar vasoconstriction. The eventual result is hypoperfusion of the renal cortex and tubular ischemia. Unless renal perfusion is reestablished, tubular necrosis occurs. Further, tubular ischemia potentiates the injurious effects of other agents such as myoglobin, radiocontrast material, and nephrotoxic antibiotics.

Although neither myoglobin nor hemoglobin is a direct cellular toxin, these molecules dissociate into hematin, which is toxic to renal cells in acid urine (pH < 5.6). In addition, intratubular precipitation of these pigments may contribute to tubular injury. Myoglobin release into the circulation may occur after any condition that results in significant damage to a large quantity of muscle. Rhabdomyolysis may follow severe burns, massive crush injuries, seizures, alcohol or drug intoxication, and extended coma. Indicative laboratory abnormalities consistent with significant muscle injury include hyperkalemia, an elevated serum creatinine and serum creatinine phosphokinase, and urine analysis indicating the presence of heme pigment without red blood cells in the sediment. Hemoglobinuria results from conditions in which intravascular hemolysis occurs such as major transfusion reactions, massive blood transfusion, sepsis, and cardiopulmonary bypass.

Numerous drugs have nephrotoxic potential (Table 11-4) on various sites within the nephron. Normal reabsorption and secretion exposes the kidney to higher concentrations of drugs and other agents. This is worsened by hypovolemia where water reabsorption within the tubule further increases these concentrations. In contrast to ATN and pigment nephropathy, drug-induced ARF is often nonoliguric despite significant tubular damage. The incidence of ARF after the administration of radiographic contrast agents is from 1 to 10 percent. These agents appear to induce injury by causing hypovolemia through osmotic diuresis, as well as by a direct nephrotoxic effect. Preexisting renal insufficiency, advanced age, larger contrast load, diabetes mellitus, and congestive heart failure are recognized risk factors. There is general agreement that patients at risk to develop contrast-induced ARF should be adequately hydrated before the administration of the contrast.

The potential nephrotoxicity of aminoglycoside antibiotics is well known. Even under ideal circumstances and closely controlled serum levels, the incidence of nephrotoxicity with these drugs is approximately 10 percent. Toxicity is influenced by the daily dose and the duration of therapy and is increased by extracellular volume contraction, metabolic acidosis, and sustained high serum levels. Amphotericin B is another agent well recognized for its potential for tubular injury. Beta-lactam agents, i.e., penicillins and cephalosporins, can cause interstitial nephritis. Nonsteroidal anti-inflammatory agents are capable of blunting prostaglandin-dependent vasodilation, particularly in patients with preexisting

Table 11-4
Nephrotoxic Drugs

Glomerulus	Proximal tubule
Heroin	Aminoglycosides
Hydralazine	Amphotericin B
Penicillamine	Cephaloridine
Probenecid	Polymyxin B
Procainamide	Distal tubule
Renal arterioles	Amphotericin B
Allopurinol	Lithium
Penicillin G	Vitamin D
Propylthiouracil	Interstitial
Sulfonamides	Acetaminophen
Thiazides	Aspirin
	Methicillin
	Penicillin G
	Phenacetin

SOURCE: Adapted from Mault JR, Bartlett RH: Acute renal failure, in Greenfield LJ (ed.): *Complications in Surgery and Trauma,* 2d ed, Philadelphia, JB Lippincott, 1990, chap 12, with permission.

renal hypoperfusion. Elderly patients, and those with cirrhosis, previous renal insufficiency, and congestive heart failure are at increased risk. The appropriate treatment of drug-induced nephropathy is a reduction in dosage or, preferably, discontinuation of the drug.

A predisposition to the development of postoperative renal failure is recognized in specific surgical settings. Trauma and burn injury patients are exposed to numerous potential causes of ARF including hypovolemic shock, massive crush injury, blood transfusion, anesthetic agents, and sepsis. The risk of ARF after aortic vascular surgery appears directly related to the position and duration of aortic clamp occlusion during the operation. The incidence of ARF after thoracic aortic aneurysm resection may be as high as 50 percent and may be greater if occlusion time exceeds 30 min. In comparison, ARF after abdominal aortic aneurysm resection is 7 percent. Infrarenal occlusion in excess of 100 min is associated with 30 percent incidence of ATN. In addition to renal hypoperfusion, further damage may be caused by atheromatous emboli dislodged from the aorta and "washout" acidosis after reperfusion of the lower body. Postrenal ARF may also result from bilateral ureteral injury after aortic or iliac artery bypass surgery.

Heart operations requiring cardiopulmonary bypass may be complicated by ARF in 1 to 2 percent of cases. Preoperative chronic renal hypoperfusion due to low cardiac output significantly increases the likelihood of postoperative ARF after cardiopulmonary bypass. ARF occurs in 34 percent of cadaveric renal transplants and 9 percent of living-related donor transplants. ATN is the most common cause and may be due to hypotension occurring in the donor before procurement, extended "warm ischemia" time, inadequate organ preservation during transport, or a technical complication of the vascular or ureteral anastomoses causing graft ischemia or postobstructive uropathy.

Prevention. Prevention is the best management for ARF. Identification of patients at risk is an initial step in the prevention of the complication. Patients with preexisting renal insufficiency, cardiac failure, liver failure, advanced age, and sepsis should be considered at substantial risk. Hypovolemia, hypoxia, and hypotension should be avoided and corrected expeditiously if they occur. In some instances, use of central venous pressure monitoring or pulmonary artery catheters is necessary for accurate assessments of the intravascular volume status. The use of nephrotoxic agents such as radiographic contrast and aminoglycoside antibiotics must be judicious. In selected circumstances, the prophylactic use of diuretics may be of benefit. Induced diuresis may afford protection by clearance of the tubule and prevention of back-leakage of filtrate. Mannitol increases cortical renal blood flow, produces an osmotic diuresis, and has been proved beneficial in protecting against ARF when used before the onset of renal ischemia in cardiac bypass and aortic resection procedures.

Clinical Manifestations. Acute renal failure typically presents as oliguria (less than 0.5 mL/kg/h in an adult) in the postoperative period. Anuria is less common and indicative of an obstructive uropathy. Laboratory studies usually reveal elevated BUN levels and milder elevations of the serum creatinine.

Management. The goals are to establish the cause and initiate immediate corrective measures to minimize renal injury while simultaneously preventing complications. A physical examination is the initial and essential step to assess the patient's circulatory status and to identify the presence of urinary tract obstruction. Spurious causes of postoperative oliguria such as a plugged urinary catheter should be eliminated. Signs of hypovolemia and hypervolemia should be sought. Bladder catheterization is performed. In the event urethral obstruction is the cause, this action will be therapeutic. The catheter is subsequently used to monitor eventual therapy.

Decreased renal perfusion is the most common cause of postoperative oliguria and mild azotemia. An intravenous fluid bolus of normal saline is administered. A volume of 10 to 20 mL/kg may be used in otherwise healthy individuals; a smaller dose may be required for elderly patients or for those with cardiac insufficiency. Restoration of urine flow is indicative of prerenal azotemia due to hypovolemia. Hydration should be continued while evaluating potential sites of fluid loss, for example, hemorrhage or "third-space" losses. When oliguria or anuria persist despite the fluid bolus and bladder catheterization, or when complicating medical conditions exist such as cardiac, renal, or hepatic insufficiency, further evaluation is indicated. Central venous pressure measurement or determination of pulmonary capillary wedge pressure (PCWP) should be performed to assess intravascular volume. Placement of a pulmonary artery catheter to monitor cardiac performance may be beneficial. Both intravascular volume and cardiac output should be optimized.

An indication of both renal function and the cause of renal failure can be obtained with measurements of urine and serum electrolytes and urine analysis. The fractional excretion of sodium (FE_{Na}) is calculated using the levels of sodium and creatinine in the urine and plasma. A prerenal cause is indicated by urine specific gravity of less than 1.020, urine sodium less than 20 meq/L, and a FE_{Na} of less than 1. Intrinsic renal failure is suggested by the presence of tubular cells, as well as red blood cell (RBC) and white blood cell (WBC) casts in the urine. Urine sodium is greater than 40 meq/L, and the FE_{Na} is greater than 3. These studies have limited usefulness in the elderly, patients with previous renal insufficiency, and those receiving diuretics within the previous 24 h.

The presence of postobstructive uropathy may be confirmed by abdominal ultrasonography with findings of hydronephrosis and ureteral dilatation.

Once prerenal and postrenal causes have been eliminated, it is likely that intrinsic renal disease has occurred. Treatment at this point is directed toward maintenance of renal perfusion, promotion of diuresis if possible, and general support. Intravenous fluids should be minimized to replace only actual losses once intravascular volume and cardiac output is optimized. If hypervolemia develops in conjunction with oliguria, ultrafiltration is mandatory to avoid congestive heart failure and pulmonary edema.

The use of loop diuretics such as furosemide, bumetanide, and ethacrynic acid is advocated for promoting diuresis in ARF. Clinical studies have demonstrated that the use of furosemide increases both glomerular filtration and urine output. Brown, however, reported a prospective study of 58 surgical patients with acute oliguric renal failure in whom oliguria was prevented or reversed in one group using furosemide. Despite achieving satisfactory diuresis, no differences in the need for dialysis, the duration of the renal failure, or mortality were noted between the oliguric and nonoliguric groups indicating that the use of diuretics in oliguric renal failure does not influence outcome.

Hyperkalemia is an immediate possible complication. Exogenous potassium supplements and blood products should be avoided and frequent determinations of serum potassium performed. Metabolic acidosis is treated with sodium bicarbonate.

Patients with marked uremia (BUN > 100 mg/dL) should undergo hemodialysis until renal function and diuresis improves. Attention to provision of adequate nutrition is essential because these patients are hypermetabolic and catabolic even while receiving dialysis.

RESPIRATORY COMPLICATIONS

Respiratory complications are the primary cause of death in 25 percent of surgical patients and a significant contributory factor in another 25 percent of patients. These complications include atelectasis, pneumonia, pulmonary edema, respiratory failure, and the adult respiratory distress syndrome (ARDS).

Atelectasis

Atelectasis, or the collapse of pulmonary alveoli, is the most common complication after surgical procedures. Strandberg and coworkers reported that 100 percent of patients developed atelectasis within 5 to 10 min after anesthesia. Atelectasis continued to be present in 90 percent of patients 1 h later and in 50 percent of patients at 24 h. Under normal circumstances, alveolar collapse is minimized by the clearance of secretions to prevent airway obstruction, periodic deep inspirations to promote inflation, and the presence of pulmonary surfactant that reduces surface tension in the alveoli and prevents collapse as lung volume is decreased. Deep inspiration promotes the release of pulmonary surfactant. A prospective multicenter European study using ambroxol, an experimental drug that promotes surfactant synthesis, demonstrated a significant reduction of postoperative pulmonary complications in patients with chronic obstructive pulmonary disease (COPD) after upper abdominal surgery. The incidence of atelectasis in the control group was 24 percent versus 11 percent in the group receiving prophylactic ambroxol.

Numerous perioperative events contribute to the development of atelectasis. Anesthetic agents cause decreased mucociliary clearance and drying of secretions which may result in small airways obstruction. Pain arising from surgical incisions and drain sites restricts the patient's mobility and limits respiratory excursion, thus preventing deep inspiration. Narcotic analgesic agents decrease respiratory drive and suppress the cough reflex. Nasogastric tubes also impair coughing and the clearance of secretions. Atelectasis may also develop due to direct lung injury from trauma, or surgical manipulation, as well as compression of the lung by the accumulation of pleural fluid or air.

Atelectasis precedes pneumonia, possibly due to bacterial infection of nonventilated lung regions. Large areas of atelectasis may have more acute and dramatic physiologic effects by causing ventilation and perfusion mismatching and promoting right-to-left intrapulmonary shunting as collapsed alveoli remain perfused.

Clinical Manifestations. Atelectasis usually becomes manifest within the first 24 h after operation. In intubated patients on mechanical ventilation, atelectasis may occur at any time. Fever is almost always present and in the absence of pneumonia it resolves following reinflation. The presence and severity of tachypnea, dyspnea, and tachycardia varies with the extent of alveolar collapse. Examination may reveal diminished breath sounds, percussive dullness, and elevation of the diaphragm over the affected areas. With massive lobar involvement, the heart, mediastinum, and trachea may be shifted toward the affected side. Hypoxemia, if present, reflects the severity of the ventilation-perfusion mismatch and intrapulmonary shunting and may be accompanied by normal or mildly elevated Pa_{CO_2}. Common findings on chest radiographs are platelike linear densities in the lung bases and elevation of the ipsilateral diaphragm. Triangular densities or lobar opacification represent extensive collapse.

Management. Ideally management should begin with prevention. Patients at particular risk are those with advanced age, obesity, a current smoking habit, and preexisting chronic pulmonary disease. The incidence of atelectasis is increased after upper abdominal and thoracic operations and the use of general anesthesia. Before an elective operation, instruction in deep breathing and treatment with incentive spirometry should be given. Smoking should be discontinued for at least 3 weeks before surgery to be beneficial. Active respiratory infections such as bronchitis or pneumonia should be completely treated before operation since the effects of anesthetic agents will worsen the condition by the impairment of mucociliary clearance. Bronchodilator therapy, including theophylline and inhalational drugs such as metaproterenol, should be used to control bronchospasm before, during, and after operation.

In abdominal operations, the use of transverse or lower abdominal incisions has been associated with fewer pulmonary complications compared to longitudinal and midline incisions. Intraoperative instillation of local anesthetic to the incision site, as well as the use of continuous epidural anesthesia in the postoperative period, will lessen pain and allow increased respiratory efforts; however, prospective studies have not demonstrated a reduction in the incidence of postoperative respiratory complications. If prolonged nasogastric intubation is anticipated, placement of a tube gastrostomy should be considered.

In the postoperative period, adequate analgesia is vital to allow deep breathing and ambulation. Incentive spirometry, which uses a device to indicate volume inhaled and provides the patient with visual cues, is useful in the early postoperative period and has been shown to decrease pulmonary complications following laparotomy from 30 to 10 percent. In patients with excessive sputum production, coughing is necessary to mobilize secretions. Patients unable or unwilling to cough may require tracheal suctioning to remove secretions. While this procedure both eliminates some secretions and stimulates the cough reflex, it is traumatic and may cause bronchospasm and hypoxia. In the event the above measures are unsuccessful or if extensive lobar collapse has occurred, flexible bronchoscopic aspiration of inspissated mucus is indicated. In addition, secretions may be rendered less adherent by maintaining hydration and administering humidified air or oxygen and nebulized mucolytic agents such as acetylcysteine.

Once atelectasis has developed, coughing, deep breathing and incentive spirometry should be continued with greater intensity. Significant hypoxemia ($Pa_{O_2} < 60$ mmHg) should be corrected with oxygen therapy. The maneuvers discussed above for the clearance of secretions may be necessary. Drainage of pleural fluid or air via tube thoracostomy may be necessary to relieve compressive atelectasis.

Pneumonia

Pneumonia is the third most common nosocomial infection on surgical services following urinary tract and wound infections but is associated with a significantly higher mortality. The risk factors and predisposing conditions for both atelectasis and pneumonia in surgical patients are similar. Critically ill patients are at greatest risk, with nosocomial pneumonia occurring in up to 22 percent of intensive care unit (ICU) patients. The duration of endotracheal intubation is also influential. The incidence of pneumonia in patients intubated for up to 3 days was 8 percent, compared to 21 percent in patients intubated for 7 days, and 45 percent if the duration of intubation exceeded 14 days.

The causative organisms in nosocomial pneumonias are predominantly gram-negative aerobic bacteria including *Pseudomonas aeruginosa, Proteus mirabilis, Serratia marcescens, Escherichia coli, Klebsiella pneumoniae,* and *Enterobacter* sp. *Staphylococcus aureus* and *Streptococcus pneumoniae* are the infecting organism in about 14 percent of cases. Anaerobic organisms are found in about 2 percent of cases and are more likely to be the causative organism in aspiration pneumonia. Fungal pneumonia is uncommon.

Clinical Manifestations. Fever, productive cough, dyspnea, pleuritic chest pain, and purulent or blood-stained sputum are classic symptoms. Physical findings may be similar to those found in atelectasis and, in some cases, differentiating between the two processes may be difficult. Lung infiltrates are evident on chest films.

Management. Differentiation from other processes such as atelectasis, pulmonary embolism, congestive heart failure, or pulmonary contusion or infarction may be necessary. Supplemental oxygen may be needed for hypoxemia, while severe respiratory compromise may require intubation and mechanical ventilatory support. Sputum samples should be obtained (preferably before institution of antibiotic therapy) whether by expectoration, transtracheal needle aspiration, or endotracheal tube suctioning. From the sample, a gram-stained smear is obtained; the presence of numerous neutrophils, few squamous cells, and a dominant organism (gram-positive cocci or gram-negative rods) is suggestive of active infection. Cultures from sputum specimens should also be obtained, although these accurately identify the causative organism in only 50 percent of cases.

Empiric antibiotic therapy is begun, often consisting of an aminoglycoside and an antipseudomonal penicillin. The antibiotic selection can be modified based upon the gram-stain smear results, and once the culture results are available, specific antimicrobial therapy should be instituted.

Aspiration Pneumonitis

First described by Mendelson in 1946, the syndrome associated with the aspiration of gastric contents is a devastating and highly lethal complication. The initial pulmonary injury is airway obstruction by large and small particulate matter resulting in obstructive atelectasis and hypoxemia. The major determinant of injury is the pH of the aspirate; a pH of < 3.0 is associated with severe chemical burns of the airways.

The patients at greatest risk for aspiration are those who cannot voluntarily effect glottic closure because of depressed consciousness secondary to neurologic impairment, drugs, or anesthesia. Increased gastric volume caused by a recent meal (within 6 h of operation), gastric atony, gastric outlet obstruction, bowel obstruction, or poorly tolerated tube feedings increases the likelihood of aspiration. Conditions that increase the likelihood of regurgitation such as gastroesophageal reflux, hiatal hernia, or the presence of a large bore nasogastric tube may also predispose patients to aspiration.

Clinical Manifestations. Gastric aspiration is most likely to occur at the time of anesthetic induction and after extubation but may occur at any time. Immediately after aspiration, dyspnea, tachypnea, chest wall retraction, and noisy respirations may be evident. Coughing productive of particulate matter may be present in conscious patients, while in unconscious patients symptoms of major airway obstruction may develop. Gastric aspirate may be present in the oropharynx. In some instances, the aspiration episode may be asymptomatic.

Within several hours after the episode, the chemical burn injury results in continued dyspnea, expiratory wheezing, rhonchi, cyanosis, and tachycardia. Bronchorrhea and bronchoconstriction will develop. Chest films will demonstrate a progressing local infiltrate. Progression of the inflammatory process and pulmonary damage over the next few days results in acute respiratory failure marked by worsening atelectasis, pulmonary edema, hypovolemia, hypoxemia, and hypercapnia. Extension of the pulmonary infiltrate and consolidation will become evident on chest film. In 50 percent of patients following gastric aspiration, bacterial pneumonia will ensue.

Prevention. Before elective operations, oral intake should be prohibited for at least 6 h before surgery. In more urgent situations, nasogastric decompression may be of some benefit. The use of metoclopramide, a gastric motility agent, is thought to be beneficial in increasing lower esophageal sphincter tone and enhancing gastric emptying but is contraindicated if intestinal obstruction is present. Gastric acid neutralization using nonparticulate antacids like sodium citrate and H_2-receptor antagonists may be beneficial in reducing the severity of acid aspiration damage. Mechanical maneuvers at the time of anesthetic induction include application of cricoid pressure followed by rapid endotracheal intubation (Sellick's maneuver) and induction in the head-up or reverse Trendelenburg position.

Management. Treatment of the early phase of aspiration focuses on the immediate removal of mechanical debris and fluid from the upper airway. Endotracheal intubation to effect airway protection is advisable, with nasogastric decompression used to prevent a subsequent episode. If distal airway obstruction is evident on chest film, flexible bronchoscopic aspiration of obstructive debris is indicated. Bronchodilators may be useful in relieving bronchospasm. Steroids are not indicated. Initially, pulmonary support may be minimal to reverse hypoxia and correct hypoventilation; however, if acute respiratory failure develops, positive-pressure ventilation is required. A pulmonary artery catheter is often advisable to monitor and thereby avoid hypervolemia and consequent exacerbation of pulmonary edema.

Pulmonary Edema

Cardiogenic or high-pressure pulmonary edema occurs when circulatory overload or left heart failure causes pulmonary capillary hydrostatic pressure to exceed plasma oncotic pressure and favors transudation of fluid into the alveoli. In surgical patients, circulatory overload results from massive infusions of crystalloid fluids such as those used in the resuscitation of burn patients or trauma victims. Fluid overload can also result from the absorption of fluids used to irrigate the peritoneum or urinary bladder. In patients with preexisting left ventricular dysfunction, hepatic failure, or renal failure, the volume of fluid that results in pulmonary edema may be significantly smaller. The development of left heart failure may also lead to pulmonary edema, an occurrence most likely in elderly patients and those with a previous history of cardiac disease. Pulmonary edema may be an early manifestation of a perioperative myocardial infarction.

Low pressure or noncardiogenic pulmonary edema, results from damage to the alveolar membrane which allows exudation of fluid into the alveoli. The typical example of this condition is the pulmonary injury seen in ARDS (see Chap. 4). Noncardiogenic pulmonary edema may be a manifestation of several conditions including sepsis, fat embolism, massive blood transfusion, burn inhalation injury, gastric aspiration, severe central nervous system (CNS) injury, transfusion or drug reaction, and severe acute pancreatitis.

Clinical Manifestations. The formation of interstitial edema decreases lung compliance and increases the work of breathing causing dyspnea, tachypnea, and mild hypoxemia. Bronchial narrowing due to edema results in expiratory wheezing (cardiac asthma). If the process progresses, alveolar flooding occurs, exacerbating pulmonary dysfunction and worsening the hypoxemia. Diffuse rales become evident. If hypervolemia or heart failure is present, other signs such as distended neck veins or peripheral edema may be present. Hypertension, tachycardia, and diaphoresis often accompany pulmonary edema.

Interstitial edema may be evident on early chest radiograph as septal lines, peribronchial and perivascular cuffs, and accentuation of the interlobar fissure. ''Cephalization'' of the pulmonary vasculature and hilar opacification are characteristic findings. Progression to alveolar flooding results in diffuse bilateral ''fluffy'' infiltrates. The correlation of the radiographic findings with the physiologic status of the patient is poor.

Management. Pulmonary edema requires urgent attention. Cardiogenic pulmonary edema resolves rapidly after correction of volume overload. Young patients with normal cardiac function and obvious hypervolemia can be safely treated with fluid restriction alone or in combination with diuretic therapy. In most surgical patients pulmonary artery catheterization is necessary to distinguish between cardiogenic and low-pressure pulmonary edema. Characteristically, the PCWP, a reflection of the left ventricular end-diastolic pressure (LVEDP), is greater than 20 to 25 mmHg; cardiac output is low; and the systemic vascular resistance is elevated in cardiogenic pulmonary edema. A normal PCWP of 10 to 15 mmHg and normal or elevated cardiac output is suggestive of low-pressure pulmonary edema or ARDS.

Immediate measures include sitting the patient upright to improve lung compliance, decreasing the work of breathing, and decreasing cardiac preload. Hypoxemia is treated with the administration of 100 percent oxygen, and if this is unsuccessful, positive-pressure ventilatory support should be instituted. Hypervolemia should be corrected using fluid restriction and diuretics, using PCWP measurements to guide therapy. Low-dose dopamine, 2 to 5 μg/kg/min, increases renal blood flow and promotes diuresis; in situations where diuresis is inadequate, hemofiltration is highly effective in rapidly reducing intravascular volume. Inotropic agents such as dopamine or dobutamine can improve low cardiac output. Afterload reduction using sodium nitroprusside should be used in patients with elevated systemic vascular resistance.

Fat Embolism Syndrome

Fat embolism is an extremely common pathologic finding following trauma. In an autopsy series of 300 accident victims, the incidence rate ranged from 80 to 100 percent, with the higher incidence occurring in patients who survived for 12 h or more after injury. In view of the high volume of fat in long bones, it is not surprising that fat embolism is common after bony trauma. In other studies, the incidence of fat embolism ranged from 26 percent in patients with a single fracture to 44 percent in patients with multiple fractures.

The clinical fat embolism syndrome of pulmonary dysfunction, coagulopathy, and neurologic disturbances associated with increased circulating fat globules appears to be uncommon. Chan and associates, in a prospective series of 80 patients with tibial and femoral fractures, reported an incidence of 8.75 percent. Studying a larger series of 172 patients, ten Duis and associates identified the fat embolism syndrome in only 3.5 percent of patients. The fat embolism syndrome most commonly follows orthopaedic injuries, but it has also been reported to occur after prosthetic joint replacement, closed chest cardiac massage, blast concussion, liver trauma, burns, extracorporeal circulation, rapid high-altitude decompression, bone marrow transplantation, and liposuction. The syndrome has also been reported following acute hemorrhagic pancreatitis and carbon tetrachloride poisoning.

Pathophysiology. The origin of the circulating fat globules found in this syndrome remains controversial. The most plausible theory proposes a mechanical process involving the liberation of fat globules from a site of injury that subsequently gain access to the circulation. Such a scenario is particularly applicable to long bone fractures where fat is released from the damaged marrow and becomes intravasated via torn venules within the marrow substance. Movement at the fracture site and compression by the hematoma would generate increases in local tissue pressure that would facilitate the process. It has also been suggested that the fat globules found within the circulation form from the coalescence of plasma chylomicrons. Such a theory would account for episodes of fat embolism syndrome that occur in the absence of trauma or surgery. An analysis of the fat emboli recovered from the lungs of affected patients demonstrates a lipid profile similar to that of bone marrow. The formation of fat emboli from circulating lipids cannot be completely excluded at this time.

The pathogenesis of the fat embolism syndrome is thought to occur via numerous mechanisms. Because of the size of the fat globules, microvascular occlusion of arterioles and venules occurs. In severe instances, larger emboli may cause mechanical obstruction of the pulmonary vessels, pulmonary hypertension, and result in acute right heart failure. It is unlikely that vascular occlusion and hypoperfusion are the sole causes of many of the severe neurologic and pulmonary disturbances that are observed. Peltier has suggested that emboli, lodged in the pulmonary vasculature, become coated with platelets that subsequently release a variety of mediators such as bradykinin and serotonin. These mediators may induce localized vasospasm and bronchospasm resulting in capillary congestion, edema, and ventilation-perfusion mismatch. The local release of platelet-derived mediators can also cause an increase in tissue lipase that may act on fat globules, releasing glycerol and free fatty acids. Peltier and others have demonstrated the toxic potential of free fatty acids on lung tissue.

Dissolution of the pulmonary capillary basement membrane by free fatty acids has been well demonstrated in animal models and may well explain the local hemorrhagic changes found in the brain, lung, and skin of patients with fat embolism syndrome.

The presence of neurologic symptoms or petechial skin changes implies fat emboli to the arterial circulation which occur by passage through the pulmonary "filter" either via the alveolar capillaries or through precapillary shunts opened by increases in pulmonary artery pressure. Some authors have suggested that in contrast to the pathogenesis of the pulmonary changes, the changes noted in the brain and skin are primarily due to microvascular occlusion. The histologic features of the cerebral lesions consist of petechial hemorrhages of the cortical white matter, brainstem, and spinal cord, findings not dissimilar from the hemorrhagic lesions found in the lung. While the focal neurologic deficits can be explained by localized vascular occlusion, in some cases, the severity of the changes in consciousness do not correlate with the amount of fat emboli found at autopsy. An elevation in free fatty acids in the cerebral circulation has been proposed as a cause of the encephalopathy.

Clinical Manifestations. Respiratory insufficiency occurs in 75 percent of patients and may develop within several hours to 2 to 3 days after injury. Hypoxemia is a sensitive finding and may precede the development of dyspnea and tachypnea by several hours. Chest radiographic findings are usually absent in the early phases but will progress to bilateral fluffy alveolar infiltrates as respiratory failure develops. Ten percent of patients with fat embolism syndrome will develop respiratory failure similar to ARDS. The pulmonary findings in fat embolism syndrome are nonspecific and are not differentiated from other conditions such as pulmonary contusion, pneumonia, or ARDS due to sepsis or shock.

Neurologic involvement occurs in up to 86 percent of patients and does not develop in the absence of pulmonary abnormalities. Neurologic findings may precede respiratory symptoms by 6 to 12 h. Encephalopathy, presenting with acute confusion, is the most common finding and must be separated from traumatic conditions such as epidural hematoma or cerebral contusion and metabolic conditions such as hypoglycemia, narcotic overdose, or delirium tremens. In the encephalopathy of the fat embolism syndrome, hypoxemia will exacerbate the confusion, but the condition will not improve with oxygen administration. Focal neurologic findings will occur in a smaller group of patients and include hemiplegia, aphasia, apraxia, and visual field defects.

The classic finding of a petechial rash, which occurs in 60 percent of patients, results from embolization of fat globules into the dermal capillary network. The rash usually appears within the first 36 to 48 h and is prominent on the upper body, particularly on the neck, axillae, and skin folds. It may also be noted in the oral mucous membranes and conjunctivae. The rash itself is self-limiting and usually resolves within 7 days.

Fever and tachycardia are common but nonspecific findings. Fundoscopic examination may reveal emboli within the retinal vessels, as well as macular edema and retinal hemorrhages. Renal involvement may be manifested by lipuria, proteinuria, or, less commonly, oliguria or hematuria. Jaundice is a rare occurrence.

Diagnostic Studies. There are no specific diagnostic tests for fat embolism. Precipitous drops in the hematocrit frequently occur coincident with the onset of symptoms and may be due to pulmonary hemorrhage or to increased red blood cell aggregation and destruction. Thrombocytopenia, though less common, also occurs. Hypocalcemia may be present because of the binding of ionized calcium by free fatty acids. Hypoalbuminemia may also occur because of increased capillary permeability. Arterial blood gases will demonstrate some degree of hypoxemia.

A cryostat test for the detection of fat globules in clotted blood has been developed. Clotted blood is rapidly frozen and sections examined for the presence of fat globules. In one series, a positive test was found in 52 percent of patients. The result correlated well with clinical findings in patients with two or three major clinical signs of fat embolism syndrome. Though previously suggested to be diagnostic for fat embolism, the incidence of lipuria was found to be very low in a series of patients with clinical evidence of fat embolism syndrome. Fat in the sputum is a common finding in patients following trauma and is not specific. In patients with a rash, frozen section biopsy of the skin lesion to determine the presence of fat may be helpful.

Elevation of serum lipase levels occurs in up to 50 percent of cases of fat embolism syndrome. The rise may be detected within 2 h of injury and returns to normal within 24 h. Though high elevations were thought to bear a favorable prognosis, one series reported that of 11 patients with the highest elevations of serum lipase, seven expired and fat embolism was demonstrated at autopsy in five cases.

Treatment. Much of the treatment of fat embolism syndrome is supportive. Early immobilization and fixation of fracture sites decreases the incidence of the syndrome. Adequate fluid resuscitation is important since the presence of shock increases the susceptibility to the development of the syndrome. Respiratory support is applied as needed to maintain $Pa_{O_2} > 80$ mmHg, and O_2 saturation > 90 percent. Encephalopathy is managed by minimal sedation, periodic neurologic examinations, and maintaining adequate oxygenation and avoiding hypercapnia. There is no information about the role of intracranial hypertension in the cerebral manifestations of this syndrome or any evidence to support the use of hyperventilation or osmotic diuretics.

Clinical studies have suggested that the prophylactic administration of steroids minimizes the fall in arterial oxygen tension, but the number of patients in these studies with fat embolism syndrome is small and the efficacy of steroids in preventing the development of this syndrome is not clearly demonstrated. Heparin has potential benefits by increasing lipase activity and promoting clearance of circulating fat globules. While lipolytic activity can be achieved with doses of 2500 units every 6 h, clinical data are conflicting and the use of heparin is debatable. Low-molecular-weight dextran (40,000 MW) can reduce red cell aggregation, decrease blood viscosity, and reduce platelet adhesion. The available clinical data concerning the benefit of dextran in patients with fat embolism syndrome is conflicting, and its use, at present, is not supported. Despite the ability of ethyl alcohol to reduce lipase activity and decrease the production of free fatty acids, and encouraging results obtained in early animal studies, the findings in clinical studies have been equivocal, and the use of intravenous alcohol in this syndrome is not supported.

Acute Respiratory Failure

Acute respiratory failure is a condition caused by a number of pulmonary and nonpulmonary diseases. It is a life-threatening condition with high lethality and it is estimated that 20 to 50 percent of affected patients will die. The defining characteristic is an acute deterioration of respiratory gas exchange that results in hypoxia (inadequate oxygen delivery to meet tissue demands) and hypercapnia (excess blood carbon dioxide). The potential causes of acute respiratory failure are protean (Table 11-5).

ARDS is not the equivalent of acute respiratory failure, though it is a major cause of the condition. Older, less specific terms such as shock lung, Da Nang lung, or posttraumatic lung syndrome should be abandoned because these terms describe etiologies of the syndrome, not distinct clinical entities. ARDS may represent a final common course for a number of seemingly unrelated diseases associated with respiratory failure such as acute pancreatitis, sepsis, or massive blood transfusion.

Pathophysiology. The hallmark defects of hypoxia and hypercapnia are the result of the singular or combined effects of a number of pathophysiologic mechanisms: alveolar hypoventilation, ventilation-perfusion ($\dot{V}/\dot{Q}$) mismatch, increased pulmonary shunt, impaired membrane diffusion, pulmonary hypertension, and decreased oxygen delivery.

Hypercapnia results from alveolar hypoventilation or $\dot{V}/\dot{Q}$ mismatch. Alveolar hypoventilation may be caused by the impairment of central ventilatory drive, respiratory muscle function, or airflow obstruction. Numerous drugs such as narcotics, sedative-hypnotics, or inhalational anesthetic agents blunt the normal CNS responses to hypercapnia and can diminish respiratory drive. Occasionally, injury to the ventilatory drive center may result from direct injury or from increased intracranial pressure following head trauma. In patients with COPD, hypoxemia-driven ventilatory drive may be abolished by the correction of hypoxemia with supplemental oxygen, resulting in hypoventilation. Neuromuscular control of the respiratory muscles, the chest wall, and diaphragm may be partially or totally inhibited by skeletal muscle relaxants (e.g., pancuronium, vecuronium), antibiotics such as neomycin, spinal or epidural anesthesia, or neuromuscular disorders like myasthenia gravis. Diaphragmatic movement may be restricted by abdominal distention due to ileus, intestinal obstruction, or ascites. Alternatively, diseases causing decreased pulmonary compliance such as pulmonary edema, ARDS, or interstitial fibrosis can significantly increase the work of breathing despite normal respiratory muscle function with respiratory failure resulting from eventual fatigue. Upper airways obstruction due to gastric aspiration, foreign bodies, laryngeal trauma, or simple posterior tongue displacement prevents ventilation by impeding airflow. Less commonly, hypercapnia can result from increased dead-space ventilation with subsequent aggravation of $\dot{V}/\dot{Q}$ imbalance, a phenomenon seen in patients with COPD with extensive pulmonary capillary damage.

Hypoxemia, defined as a Pa_{O_2} less than 60 mmHg, results from inadequate intrapulmonary gas exchange and is attributable to increased $\dot{V}/\dot{Q}$ mismatch, increased pulmonary shunt, alveolar hypoventilation, and diffusion abnormalities. Ventilation and perfusion imbalance is the most common cause of hypoxemia. Diseases that increase the $\dot{V}/\dot{Q}$ ratio (reduced perfusion of ventilated areas) in essence increase physiologic dead space and cause wasted ventilation. Acute reductions in pulmonary capillary perfusion due to emboli or thrombi occur in diseases such as pulmonary embolism. Alternatively, conditions such as atelectasis, and pulmonary edema, which decrease the $\dot{V}/\dot{Q}$ ratio (reduced ventilation in perfused areas), diminish the amount of alveolar oxygen available for exchange causing hypoxemia and decreased oxygen saturation. The extreme of the latter situation is the increased intrapulmonary shunt in which hypoxemia results from admixture of nonoxygenated shunt blood with oxygenated blood from ventilated segments. Conditions that promote alveolar collapse increase the shunt. The shunt fraction can be calculated with known information of the hemoglobin, Pa_{O_2}, Sa_{O_2}, and mixed venous oxygen tension ($P\bar{v}_{O_2}$) and saturation ($S\bar{v}_{O_2}$) obtained while the patient is breathing 100% oxygen. The normal shunt fraction is 5 percent of the cardiac output, but in respiratory failure it exceeds 25 to 30 percent. Impaired diffusion of gases across the alveolar-capillary membrane may result from changes within the membrane or alterations in the diffusion surface area. Processes that alter either the pulmonary capillary or alveolar surface area have already been mentioned. Conditions that cause interstitial edema, inflammation, or fibrosis of the membrane will alter the diffusion characteristics and impair gas exchange.

The adequacy of oxygen exchange is reflected by the Pa_{O_2}; however, the efficiency of this process is better measured by the alveolar-arterial oxygen gradient (AaD_{O_2}) and the final product, arterial oxygen saturation (Sa_{O_2}). The AaD_{O_2} can be calculated with knowledge of the Pa_{CO_2} and Pa_{O_2} obtained while the patient is breathing 100% oxygen with normal values ranging from 25 to 65 mmHg. Hypoxemia with a widened gradient is suggestive of abnormalities with $\dot{V}/\dot{Q}$ mismatch, shunting, or diffusion, while a normal gradient is suggestive of hypoventilation.

Conditions affecting pulmonary blood flow and overall cardiac output also affect oxygen exchange and oxygen delivery. Increased pulmonary vascular resistance may arise from obstruction (e.g., thromboemboli, fat emboli), external compression by interstitial disease (e.g., edema, fibrosis, ARDS), the local release of vasoactive mediators (e.g., leukotrienes, thromboxane, serotonin), local hypoxia-induced vasoconstriction, or increased left atrial pressure (e.g., congestive heart failure, volume overload). This results in decreased pulmonary capillary perfusion and decreased oxygen saturation. Decreases in cardiac output due to hypovolemia, heart failure, or dysrhythmia decrease oxygen delivery and promote hypoxia.

Clinical Manifestations. Early signs are often subtle, with tachypnea and shallow respirations. Tachycardia, hypertension, and air hunger develop as hypoxemia worsens. Confusion, agitation, or obtundation may result from either hypoxia or hypercapnia. Arterial blood gases (ABGs) should be obtained immediately in patients with respiratory distress to define the degree of hypoxemia. Hypocapnia is common in the early stages due to hyperventilation but progresses to hypercapnia and respiratory acidosis as the failure worsens. Chest radiographs may be useful in identifying primary etiologies for failure, like pneumonia or ARDS.

Management. The primary goals of management are to temporarily support respiratory function while correcting the un-

Table 11-5
Causes of Acute Respiratory Failure

Postoperative atelectasis
Pneumonia
Acid aspiration
Pulmonary edema
Pulmonary embolism
Fat embolism syndrome
Smoke inhalation
Adult respiratory distress syndrome

derlying and primary problem. Support involves four features: (1) airway management, (2) ventilatory support, (3) oxygenation, and (4) cardiac support. Endotracheal intubation is indicated in patients who are unable to maintain the patency of, or protect, their airways such as those who are obtunded or comatose or in patients who have been determined to require mechanical ventilation. A minority of patients who are alert with mild hypoxemia responsive to supplemental oxygen may not require immediate intubation but must be closely monitored for potential deterioration of their clinical status. Orotracheal intubation is advantageous when urgent or emergent airway control is required, though patient tolerance of the nasotracheal route is better if intubation for longer than 1 week is required. Tracheostomy is reserved for intubation extending beyond 2 weeks to reduce the incidence of tracheal stenosis and occasionally in patients with severe facial injuries and laryngeal trauma.

The criteria for the need for ventilatory support includes the presence of apnea, a respiratory rate exceeding 30 breaths/min, Pa_{O_2} less than 70 mmHg, Pa_{CO_2} greater than 55 mmHg (except in COPD) in addition to a number of ventilatory and oxygenation parameters (Table 11-6). After intubation, patients with normal brainstem function should be placed on assist-control ventilation with a base respiratory rate of 10/min and a tidal volume of 10 to 15 mL/kg of body weight. The adequacy of ventilation is monitored using the Pa_{CO_2}, with a preferred value range of 40 to 45 mmHg and maintenance of the pH between 7.35 and 7.45. Rarely should the respiratory rate need to exceed 20/min.

The goal of oxygenation therapy is to optimize oxygen exchange while avoiding oxygen toxicity and the deleterious effects of positive end-expiratory pressure (PEEP). Increases in the fraction of inspired oxygen (FI_{O_2}) may improve hypoxemia related to $\dot{V}/\dot{Q}$ mismatch, hypoventilation, or diffusion abnormalities but will not correct poor gas exchange due to shunting. The use of 100% oxygen promotes absorption atelectasis and, if continued for greater than 48 h, is associated with oxygen toxicity. The use of PEEP increases functional residual capacity (FRC) and both promotes alveolar reexpansion and prevents alveolar collapse. This improvement in alveolar ventilation optimizes $\dot{V}/\dot{Q}$ matching, decreases shunting, and increases the diffusion surface area. Initial ventilator settings should provide an FI_{O_2} of 100 percent and PEEP of 5 cmH_2O. Adjustments are guided by measurements of the Pa_{O_2} and Sa_{O_2}, maintaining oxygen tension greater than 60 mmHg and saturation greater than 90 percent, preferably with an FI_{O_2} of 50 percent or less. PEEP adjustments should be made in increments of 2 to 3 cmH_2O. The adverse consequences of PEEP are pulmonary barotrauma and depression of cardiac output. The risk of barotrauma is greatly increased when peak inflation pressures exceed 60 cmH_2O. Tension pneumothorax is a potential hazard. Depression of cardiac output rarely occurs until PEEP exceeds 10 cmH_2O. When PEEP must be increased past this level, a pulmonary artery catheter should be inserted to measure cardiac output and sample mixed venous blood. The additional information is used to determine mixed venous saturation, intrapulmonary shunt, and oxygen delivery and consumption. PEEP should be subsequently increased to improve arterial oxygen saturation, reduce the shunt fraction to less than 15 percent, and optimize oxygen delivery. Oxygen-carrying capacity should be optimized by correcting anemia. Depression of cardiac output may require fluid administration to increase stroke volume and inotropic agents such as dopamine to improve myocardial performance.

The achievement of adequate oxygenation and correction of the primary disease process should result in an improvement in the clinical condition, at which time weaning can be begun. PEEP should be reduced by 3 to 5 cmH_2O every 12 h utilizing the above monitoring parameters until a level of 5 cmH_2O is reached. Arterial saturation should be greater than 95 percent, and Pa_{O_2} greater than 60 mmHg at an FI_{O_2} of between 0.3 and 0.4. Mechanical ventilatory support is weaned by converting the patient to intermittent mandatory ventilation (IMV) and decreasing the ventilator rate to 2/min assuming a normal Pa_{CO_2} is maintained. Indications of adequate ventilatory function include a spontaneous respiratory rate of less than 25/min, a spontaneous tidal volume of greater than 5 mL/kg, a vital capacity of greater than 10 mL/kg, a minute ventilation of less than 120 mL/kg/min, and an inspiratory force greater than −20 cmH_2O. If these conditions are met, a 30-min trial of spontaneous breathing via the endotracheal tube with humidified oxygen is conducted. In general, a patient with a respiratory rate of less than 25/min and a pulse rate of less than 120/min with a Pa_{O_2} greater than 60 mmHg and a Pa_{CO_2} less than 45 mmHg will be able to sustain adequate ventilation and oxygenation without tiring.

Table 11-6
Criteria for Diagnosis of Acute Respiratory Failure

Parameter	*Normal Range*	*Respiratory Failure*
Respiratory rate	12–20	> 35
Vital capacity (mL/kg)*	65–75	< 15
FEV_1 (mL/kg body wt.)*	50–60	≤ 10
Inspiratory force (cmH_2O)	−(75–100)	≥ −25
Compliance (mL/cmH_2O)	100	< 20
Pa_{O_2} (mmHg) (room air)	80–95	< 70
AaD_{O_2} (mmHg) (FI_{O_2} = 1.0)	25–65	> 450
Q_S/Q_T (%)	5–8	> 20
Pa_{CO_2} (mmHg)	35–45	> 55†
V_D/V_T	0.2–0.3	> 0.60

*Ideal body weight should be used.

†Chronic lung disease constitutes the exception. FEV_1—forced expiratory volume in 1 s; Pa_{O_2}—partial pressure of oxyygen in arterial blood; AaD_{O_2}—alveolar-arterial oxygen gradient; FI_{O_2}—fraction of inspired oxygen; Q_S/Q_T—shunt fraction; Pa_{CO_2}—partial pressure of carbon dioxide in arterial blood; V_D/V_T—ratio of dead space to tidal volume.

SOURCE: Bartlett R: Pulmonary dysfunction, in Wilmore DW, Brennan MF, Harken AH, Holcroft JW, Meakins JL, (eds): *Care of the Surgical Patient*. New York, Scientific American, 1990, with permission.

CARDIAC COMPLICATIONS

Based on 1988 statistics, the number of surgical patients undergoing noncardiac surgical procedures is estimated at 7 to 8 million annually; of these, 4 million will have coronary artery disease (CAD) or two or more major risk factors for CAD. In addition, the largest number of operations are now performed in the over-65 age group. The implication of these facts is an increasing number of patients who may be at risk for perioperative cardiac complications when subjected to the stress associated with anesthesia and operation. Increasingly, the surgeon will be faced with the task of assessing a patient's cardiac risk as well as managing the cardiac-related complications that can arise in the perioperative period.

Arrhythmias

Incidence. Cardiac arrhythmias are common in the general population and may occur at any time during the perioperative or postoperative periods. Two studies using continuous recording techniques in a total of 254 patients undergoing noncardiac operations reported an overall incidence of intraoperative cardiac arrhythmias of 73 percent. Kuner and associates reported an incidence of 62 percent and noted that the incidence was higher during general anesthesia, in intubated patients, and for neurosurgical and thoracic procedures. Significantly, 21 percent of the arrhythmias in this study were ventricular in origin. Bertrand and associates reported an incidence of 84 percent, with the majority of arrhythmias occurring during the intubation and extubation phases of anesthesia. In this latter study, 43 percent of arrhythmias were ventricular, with the incidence being greater in patients with heart disease.

The incidence of postoperative cardiac arrhythmias following noncardiac surgery is low. In one large study of 3000 noncardiac cases, only 2.4 percent had abnormal postoperative electrocardiograms (ECGs) and the majority of the abnormalities were asymptomatic conduction disturbances. Buckley and Jackson in a study of 100 patients following operation reported 32 percent with sinus tachycardia, 7 percent with premature ventricular contractions, 3 percent with sinus arrhythmia, 2 percent with sinus bradycardia, and 1 percent with ventricular trigeminy.

The incidence of postoperative arrhythmias after cardiac operations occurs in up to 48 percent of cases and in 20 to 30 percent of patients after thoracic procedures. The extent of the surgical procedure influences the incidence. Following pneumonectomy, arrhythmias will occur in 10 to 29 percent of cases. Krowka and associates in a study of 236 patients undergoing pneumonectomy (without digitalis prophylaxis) reported an incidence of supraventricular arrhythmias of 22 percent. In patients with persistent or recurrent dysrhythmias, 31 percent died versus 7 percent of patients without dysrhythmias. Shields and Ujiki reported that the prophylactic use of digitalis reduced the incidence of dysrhythmias after pneumonectomy but did not comment on whether this result influenced the postoperative mortality rate. The incidence of dysrhythmias after lesser pulmonary resection procedures is significantly less approximating 5 percent.

The types of arrhythmias following thoracic operations are usually supraventricular tachyarrhythmias such as supraventricular tachycardia, atrial flutter, or fibrillation. Thirty percent of these arrhythmias will occur on the first postoperative day, and 60 percent within 72 h of operation.

Etiology. Underlying cardiac disease including CAD, cardiomyopathy, valvular lesions, and organic conduction defects all predispose patients to both atrial and ventricular arrhythmias. Ischemic heart disease, in particular, increases ventricular irritability and may increase the arrhythmogenic effects of hypoxemia, hypercarbia, hypertension, and hypokalemia. Electrolyte abnormalities may cause arrhythmias. Hypokalemia may cause paroxysmal atrial contractions (PACs), paroxysmal ventricular contractions (PVCs), or ventricular fibrillation. Hyperkalemia may result in alterations in cardiac conduction and asystole. Hypocalcemia may cause increased Q-T intervals and, occasionally, ventricular arrhythmias, while hypercalcemia may cause bradycardia and heart block. Hypomagnesemia can cause resistant ventricular arrhythmias.

Various cardiac medications may cause cardiac arrhythmias. Previous treatment with digitalis predisposes surgical patients to serious dysrhythmias, and digitalis toxicity may cause PVCs, ventricular tachycardia or fibrillation, bradycardia, PACs, atrioventricular (AV) block, and supraventricular tachycardia. Common antihypertension medications such as propranolol, reserpine, methyldopa, and clonidine may cause sinus bradycardia or AV block. Anesthetic drugs and agents may produce or predispose to arrhythmias. Halothane and cyclopropane (rarely used today) both sensitize the myocardium to the arryhthmogenic effects of catecholamine stimulation.

Perioperative events such as hypoxemia, hypercarbia, light anesthesia with stimulation, anxiety and postoperative pain all result in significant catecholamine release. Parasympathomimetic drugs such as the muscle-relaxant antagonists neostigmine and pyridostigmine as well as the relaxant succinylcholine may cause profound bradycardia unless administered with an anticholinergic agent such as atropine. As noted earlier, metabolic disturbances may give rise to arrythmias. Hypoxemia can cause bradycardia, especially in pediatric patients, as well as atrial and ventricular dysrhythymias. Hypercapnia may cause suppression of sinoatrial node function and intrinsic pacemaker activity leading to atrial or ventricular arrythmias arising from ectopic pacemakers or re-entry mechanisms.

Organ manipulation during operation can cause intraoperative arrhythmias. Reflex vagal bradycardia may result from manipulation of the carotid sinus or traction on the upper gastrointestinal tract organs such as the stomach or intestinal mesentery. Manipulation of the lung or heart during thoracic or cardiac procedures may give rise to both atrial and ventricular dysrhythmias. Endocrine abnormalities can cause cardiac arrhythmias. A number of atrial arrhythmias, most commonly atrial fibrillation, may result from thyrotoxicosis. Pheochromocytoma causes elevated plasma catecholamine which may also result in arrhythmias.

Management of Preexisting Arrhythmias. Preoperatively, the existence of an arrhythmia should prompt a thorough evaluation including ECG, rhythm strip, and 24-h continuous ambulatory monitoring. Arrhythmias must be well controlled before operation. Cooperman and associates reported that 33 percent of patients with preoperative arrhythmias undergoing peripheral vascular operations developed cardiac complications compared to 9 percent of patients with normal sinus rhythm before operation. Digoxin should be used to control the ventricular rate in patients with atrial flutter or fibrillation. Though there is no consensus, supraventricular tachycardia should probably be treated with digoxin as well. Multifocal PVCs or nonsustained ventricular tachycardia, especially in elderly patients and those with preexisting coronary artery disease or congestive heart failure, should be treated aggressively. This includes correction of reversible causes such as hypoxia, electrolyte disturbances, and drug toxicity in addition to the use of intravenous lidocaine. Preoperative conduction defects may require preoperative cardiac pacing. Permanent pacing is indicated for third-degree AV block, second-degree Mobitz II block, and sick sinus syndrome. Temporary percutaneous pacing is indicated in the situation of new-onset bifascicular block with ischemia, in patients with left fascicular block who require placement of a Swan-Ganz catheter, or when bacteremia or sepsis precludes the placement of a permanent pacemaker. Before thoracic surgical operations, some surgeons use prophylactic digitalization in view of the high incidence of atrial arrhythmias following these procedures.

Management of New-Onset Arrhythmias. The management of new-onset arrhythmias essentially consists of determining (1) the hemodynamic stability of the patient, (2) the ventricular rate (rapid or slow), (3) the site of origin (atrial or ventricular) of the arrhythmia, (4) the need for electrocardioversion, and (5) identifying and correcting the underlying cause of the arrhythmia. In hypotensive patients with an acute tachyarrhythmia, cardioversion should be performed. The initial impulse should be at 100 joules (J), and if the arrhythmia is not eliminated, cardioversion should be repeated with the voltage rapidly increased to 360 J.

In stable patients, the ventricular rate should be determined. Bradycardia (heart rate < 60 beats/min) is treated only if symptomatic with chest pain, dyspnea, altered mental status, evidence of myocardial ischemia, or ventricular extrasystoles. Atropine 0.5 mg is administered intravenously (IV) and may be repeated every 5 min if the bradycardia persists (maximum dose 0.04 mg/kg). In the setting of a refractory symptomatic bradycardia, or Mobitz type II or III AV block, a temporary transvenous or transcutaneous pacemaker should be inserted to maintain the heart rate.

For patients with hemodynamic stability and tachyarrhythmias (heart rate > 100 beats/min) a 12-lead ECG with rhythm strip should be obtained. The ECG is examined for the presence and morphology of the P waves, the width of the QRS complexes, and the ratio of AV conduction. The presence of P waves indicates atrial activity, and variable morphology is indicative of ectopic atrial tachycardia, multifocal atrial tachycardia, or supraventricular tachycardia. The absence of P waves is suggestive of atrial fibrillation. Normal or narrow QRS complexes (< 0.08 s) indicate normal ventricular activation and indicates that the origin of arrhythmia is atrial or supraventricular. By contrast, wide QRS complexes indicate a ventricular origin of the arrhythmia or, less commonly, a supraventricular rhythm with aberrant conduction. Wide QRS complexes are also found in AV conduction block rhythms.

Sinus Tachycardia. By definition, this is not a true arrhythmia. Sinus tachycardia is caused by increased sympathetic stimulation and is associated with a variety of conditions including pain, hypovolemia, hypoxia, hypercapnia, sepsis, congestive heart failure, and hyperthyroidism. Treatment is directed at the identification and correction of the underlying cause.

Paroxysmal Supraventricular Tachycardia. This is a reentry arrhythmia characterized by abrupt onset with a ventricular rate between 150 and 250 beats/min. It may be caused by hypoxia, myocardial ischemia or infarction, congestive heart failure, or thyrotoxicosis. Synchronized direct current (DC) countershock is indicated if the patient is hemodynamically unstable. This arrhythmia sometimes responds to vagal stimulation by carotid sinus massage or Valsalva maneuver. Adenosine 6 mg intravenously is the drug of choice and may be repeated with 12 mg after 1 to 2 min if needed. Verapamil may be used if the arrhythmia persists. The recommended dose is 2 to 5 mg intravenous, initially. A second dose of 5 to 10 mg may be given in 15 to 30 min if needed, unless hypotension has occurred. It should be used with caution in elderly patients or those with poor left ventricular function and is contraindicated in hypotensive patients or those with high-grade AV block.

Nonparoxysmal Supraventricular Tachycardias. These include atrial fibrillation, atrial flutter, and atrial tachycardias. Multifocal or ectopic atrial tachycardia is usually due to digitalis toxicity or sick sinus syndrome. Treatment consists of discontinuing digitalis, obtaining serum potassium level, and supplementing potassium if necessary. Procainamide or quinidine may be required.

Atrial Fibrillation. It may be associated with numerous conditions including valvular heart disease, hypertension, CAD, myocardial ischemia, pulmonary embolism, thyrotoxicosis, and pulmonary resection. DC cardioversion is indicated for hemodynamic instability. Initial treatment is directed toward control of the ventricular rate; verapamil is the drug of choice. Digitalis is used to maintain control once the heart rate is reduced. In patients previously on digitalis therapy, quinidine or procainamide is effective in converting fibrillation to sinus rhythm.

Atrial Flutter. It is characterized by a rapid but regular atrial rate, while the ventricular response varies according to the degree of AV conduction. It is usually associated with mitral or tricuspid valvular heart disease and acute or chronic cor pulmonale and rarely is due to digitalis toxicity. The treatment of choice, if rapid ventricular response is present, is synchronized DC countershock; otherwise the treatment is similar to that of atrial fibrillation.

Ventricular Tachycardia. This is rarely seen in patients with normal hearts and is most often seen in the setting of CAD, cardiomyopathy, mitral valve prolapse, hypoxemia, or digitalis toxicity. The rate is variable between 100 to 220 beats/min. The rhythm may be regular or irregular with wide, bizarre QRS complexes. In patients with no palpable pulse, a precordial thump and immediate defibrillation (200 J) should be performed followed by initiation of cardiopulmonary resuscitation (CPR) and treatment analogous to that used for ventricular fibrillation. If a pulse is present, lidocaine in a dose of 1 mg/kg is given, followed by a second bolus dose of 0.5 mg/kg and a continuous infusion of 2 to 4 mg/min. If the tachycardia is refractory to lidocaine, bretylium in a dose of 5 to 10 mg/kg may be given and repeated every 15 min to a total of 30 mg/kg.

Ventricular Fibrillation. It is associated with myocardial ischemia, hypokalemia, hypoxemia, or digitalis toxicity. Ventricular fibrillation is characterized by chaotic rhythm without P waves or QRS complexes and absent cardiac output. Treatment begins with initiation of CPR and DC countershock to achieve defibrillation (repeat up to 3 times as needed). Epinephrine is given intravenously followed by countershock at maximum output. Bretylium or lidocaine is given as described above, followed by repeat countershock. Epinephrine is repeated every 3 to 5 min followed by defibrillation. Sodium bicarbonate is used in prolonged resuscitations and guided by arterial blood gas analysis.

Myocardial Infarction

Myocardial infarction (MI) associated with operation is a feared complication because of the attendant high mortality rate. Perioperative MI is now the leading cause of postoperative death in the elderly after noncardiac surgery. In two large retrospective reviews of patients undergoing general anesthesia for noncardiac operations the mortality rate associated with perioperative MI ranges from 54 to 69 percent, with 80 percent of the deaths occurring within 48 h of operation. By contrast, the in-hospital mortality rate for acute MI without shock and not associated with operation is estimated to be 12 percent.

The incidence of MI following noncardiac surgery in the general population is 0.1 to 0.7 percent. In patients with CAD the reported perioperative infarction rate is 1.1 percent, and in patients over 40 years, with or without CAD, the infarction rate is 1.8 percent. The risk for perioperative MI is increased in patients who have experienced a previous MI. For patients with a prior MI, reinfarction rates range from 5 to 8 percent. Tarhan and associates and Steen and associates reported that patients who were operated on within 3 months of previous infarction had a reinfarction rate of 27 percent; those operated on between 3 and 6 months had a reinfarction rate of 11 percent. After 6 months, the reinfarction rate stabilized at 5 percent. Rao and associates have reported a significantly lower reinfarction rate of 5.7 percent when the previous infarction occurred within 3 months of operation, and 3.5 percent in those having surgery between 3 and 6 months after an MI. Wells and Kaplan reported no recurrent infarctions in 48 patients who underwent surgical procedures within 3 months of an infarction.

Several other factors are associated with an increased risk of perioperative myocardial infarction and cardiac death. Goldman and associates used a multifactorial analysis and identifed several independent risk predictors for cardiac complications or cardiac-related deaths (Table 11-7) including recent MI within 6 months; physical signs of heart failure; significant preexisting cardiac arrhythmia; age greater than 70 years; intrathoracic, intraperitoneal or aortic operation; aortic stenosis; and poor general medical condition. Based on an index score, patients were categorized into four classes. For patients with scores greater than 25 (class IV), the rate of life-threatening nonfatal cardiac complications was 22 percent, and the mortality due to cardiac causes was 56 percent. Pasternack and associates have reported findings that a preoperative ejection fraction less than 0.35 (determined by radionuclide imaging or ventriculography) was associated with a 75 to 85 percent incidence of perioperative MI compared to a 20 percent incidence in patients with an ejection fraction greater than 0.35. Preexisting controlled hypertension does not appear to increase the risk of perioperative MI. Steen and associates, however, reported a significantly higher reinfarction rate in patients with intraoperative or postoperative hypertension compared to nonhypertensive patients. This finding may reflect the increased myocardial oxygen demand and decreased coronary blood flow that can accompany acute hypertensive episodes. Antihypertension medications such as beta-blocking agents, nitrates, or calcium-channel blockers should be continued up to and including the morning of surgery. The withdrawal of drugs such as propranolol and clonidine can result in rebound tachycardia and hypertension that causes an abrupt and potentially dangerous increase in myocardial oxygen demand. Intraoperative hypotension has significant and predictable effects on coronary blood flow in the presence of preexisting CAD. Several studies have demonstrated a strong association between intraoperative hypotension and the incidence of perioperative MI. Operations or anesthesia extending beyond 3 h, as well as emergency procedures, are also associated with a higher likelihood of perioperative MI. Previous coronary artery bypass grafting (CABG) appears to confer protection against postoperative MI. The results of several studies show the incidence of postoperative MI in patients with CABG undergoing noncardiac surgery to be 0.0 to 1.2 percent compared to 1.1 to 6 percent in patients without prior CABG.

Clinical Manifestations. The majority of MIs occur within the first 3 days after operation, with the remainder occurring between the fourth and sixth postoperative days. The peak occurrences are during the intraoperative period and on the third postoperative day. Often the presentation may be atypical; 60 percent of postoperative MIs are silent compared to 10 to 15 percent of nonsurgical infarctions. Typical chest pain may be blunted or eliminated by narcotics or sedatives or masked by competing sensory stimuli such as incisional pain. Other findings may be present such as dyspnea, cyanosis, altered mental status, tachycardia, arrhythmias, hypotension, or shock.

The ECG may be diagnostic if the characteristic interval changes consistent with MI have appeared. ST-segment elevation is most suggestive of MI, though other causes such as pericarditis and early repolarization may be present. ST segment depression and T-wave inversion is suggestive of non-Q wave infarction. The presence of Q waves, T-wave inversion, and baseline ST-segment changes are indicative of completed infarction. In view of the silent nature of perioperative MI, daily serial ECGs should be obtained during the first postoperative week in patients with a history of previous MI, known CAD, or peripheral vascular disease. Several recent studies have documented the occurrence of silent myocardial ischemia using continuous ECG monitoring in patients with or at risk for CAD. Mangano and associates reported that these ischemic episodes were silent and most frequent and severe

Table 11-7
Computation of Multifactorial Index Score to Estimate Cardiac Risk in Noncardiac Surgery

	Points
S_3 gallop or jugular venous distention on preoperative physical examination	11
Transmural or subendocardial myocardial infarction in the previous 6 months	10
Premature ventricular beats, more than 5/min documented at any time	7
Rhythm other than sinus or presence of premature atrial contractions on last preoperative electrocardiogram	7
Age over 70 years	5
Emergency operation	4
Intrathoracic, intraperitoneal, or aortic site of surgery	3
Evidence for important valvular aortic stenosis*	3
Poor general medical condition†	3

Risk of cardiac complications based on index score: class I (0–5 points): 1%; class II (6–12 points): 5%; class III (13–25 points): 11%; class IV (> 25 points): 22%.

*Findings of a cardiologist's examination, noninvasive testing, or cardiac catheterization.

†As evidenced by electrolyte abnormalities (potassium < 3.0 meq/L; HCO_3 < 20 meq/L), renal insufficiency (blood urea nitrogen > 50 mg/dL; creatinine > 3.0 mg/dL), abnormal blood gases (P_{O_2} < 60 mmHg; P_{CO_2} > 50 mmHg), abnormal liver status (elevated aspartate transaminase or signs at physical examination of chronic liver disease), or any condition that has caused the patient to be chronically bedridden.

SOURCE: Adapted from Goldman G, et al., 1988, with permission.

during the postoperative period and most common during the first three postoperative days. Ouyang and associates found that 53 percent of patients with silent postoperative ischemia subsequently suffered a clinical ischemic event. While no definite causal relation between these silent ischemic episodes and postoperative MI has yet been demonstrated, these results suggest that postoperative observation with continuous ECG monitoring (leads V_1, V_5, II, aVF) may be expedient in patients at high risk for postoperative MI.

Creatinine kinase (CPK) isoenzymes are a more reliable diagnostic tool and should be obtained in serial fashion for 3 days if MI is suspected. Soft tissue trauma due to surgery can also raise serum CPK levels though the MB fraction should not exceed 5 percent.

In the diagnosis of MI, regional wall motion abnormalities may be demonstrated by echocardiography. In addition, the technique may be useful in evaluating pericardial, valvular, or aortic root disease.

Management. Once the diagnosis is confirmed, treatment is largely supportive. Satisfactory relief of pain and anxiety is important and can be accomplished using morphine and sedation. Maintenance of optimal oxygenation is crucial, and effective pulmonary toilet to clear bronchial secretions is combined with supplemental oxygen to maintain the arterial oxygen saturation at greater than 95 percent. All patients should be initially treated in an intensive care or monitored bed unit. If evidence of hemodynamic instability or respiratory distress is present, intraarterial catheter monitoring should be utilized. Frequent determinations of fluid status and cardiac output to guide diuretic and vasopressor therapy may require pulmonary artery catheter monitoring.

Hypertension

Systemic hypertension, defined as a blood pressure greater than 140/90 mmHg, is estimated to affect 40 percent of the U.S. population and is one of the most common medical problems encountered in surgical patients. Chronic hypertension causes arteriolar medial hypertrophy and accelerates atherosclerosis. The resulting increased peripheral resistance leads to an elevated left ventricular stroke work, cardiac hypertrophy, and altered renal blood flow. The development of end-organ injury, CAD, hypertensive heart disease, renal insufficiency, and cerebrovascular disease increase the risk for perioperative morbidity and mortality. In addition, the vascular smooth muscle hypertrophy and wall thickening result in exaggerated increases in vascular resistance for given changes in muscle tone caused by sympathetic stimulation due to pain, anesthesia, or hypotension. This may be the mechanism of the extreme lability of perioperative blood pressure noted in hypertensive patients leading to episodes of hypotension. In elderly patients with chronic hypertension, cerebral autoregulation of blood flow is impaired with an increase in the lower systolic pressure limit at which perfusion is maintained, thus increasing the risk of cerebral ischemia with reductions in blood pressure.

Preoperative Hypertension. Whether preoperative hypertension is predictive of perioperative cardiac morbidity and mortality is debatable. Though mild diastolic hypertension [diastolic blood pressure (DBP) $<$ 110 mmHg] is not an independent preoperative risk factor, diastolic pressures in excess of 110 mmHg are associated with an increased incidence of significant intraoperative hypotension and myocardial ischemia but not MI or sudden cardiac death. Preoperative hypertension that is untreated, poorly controlled, or labile increases the risk of perioperative blood pressure lability, arrhythmias, myocardial ischemia, transient neurologic events, and possibly postoperative renal failure. The predictive role of preoperative systolic hypertension is less clear.

Elective operation should be delayed if there is diastolic hypertension in excess of 110 mmHg, new-onset hypertension, sudden increases in hypertension in previously well controlled patients, or recent deterioration in end-organ status (e.g., eye, heart, kidney). Secondary causes of hypertension such as pheochromocytoma, Cushing's syndrome, renovascular disease, and primary hyperaldosteronism must be considered. In women of child-bearing age, hypertension may arise from toxemia of an unsuspected pregnancy. Coarctation of the aorta is also a possible cause in patients who are less than 25 years old.

For patients with severe essential hypertension, elective operation should be postponed until adequate blood pressure control has been achieved, since the incidence of complicating events such as accelerated hypertension, congestive heart failure, cerebral vascular accidents, renal failure, retinopathy, dissecting aortic aneurysm, and sudden death can be significantly reduced.

In patients with mild to moderate hypertension and any of the following findings, elective operation should be delayed until these risk factors can be evaluated and corrected: (1) new onset or worsening angina pectoris; (2) congestive heart failure; (3) ECG evidence of myocardial ischemia or infarction, dysrhythmias, or left ventricular hypertrophy; (4) renal insufficiency; (5) neurologic deficit; (6) new appearance or enlargement of abdominal aortic aneurysm; or (7) new onset of high-grade hypertensive retinopathy. Similarly, the presence of malignant hypertension (DBP $>$ 120 mmHg and new-onset, progressive end-organ damage) requires emergent medical therapy before any operation with the exception of life-saving emergency surgery.

For patients with well-controlled hypertension, DBP less than 100 mmHg, and no evidence of significant end-organ damage, elective operation need not be delayed.

Those patients on preoperative antihypertensive therapy should continue to receive their medication up to the time of operation to reduce the likelihood of both hypertensive and hypotensive episodes during the intraoperative and postoperative periods. Prys-Roberts and associates studying patients with chronic hypertension reported that patients receiving adequate therapy maintained a constant systemic vascular resistance (SVR) and experienced moderate intraoperative reductions in blood pressure. By contrast, patients with inadequate blood pressure control had significantly decreased SVR during anesthesia. This effect, in combination with anesthetic-induced reductions in cardiac output caused extreme reductions in arterial blood pressure and may have contributed to ECG-documented episodes of intraoperative myocardial ischemia.

The abrupt withdrawal of some antihypertensive medications may result in serious "rebound" effects. In patients receiving beta-blocking agents for the treatment of angina and hypertension, unstable angina, ventricular tachycardia, MI, and sudden death have been reported following abrupt discontinuation of the agent. In patients receiving beta-blocking agents for hypertension, acute withdrawal may result in symptoms of anxiety, tremor, diaphoresis, malaise, and tachycardia. Five to 20 percent of patients receiving clonidine will develop similar symptoms within 12 to 48 h of cessation of the drug. A smaller percentage of patients will experience severe rebound hypertension, tachycardia, and premature ventricular contractions within 24 h of stopping therapy. If possible, clonidine therapy should be continued during the perioperative period. If the oral route is not available in the postoperative period due to ileus or nasogastric suction, clonidine may be administered via a transdermal patch or an alternate agent such as methyldopa or a beta-blocking agent should be substituted.

Postoperative Hypertension. In the previously normotensive patient without atherosclerotic vascular disease, moderate hypertension does not impose great risk. In the setting of preexisting CAD or myocardial dysfunction, systolic hypertension increases cardiac afterload and myocardial work. The increase in myocardial oxygen demand may result in ischemia or infarction when coronary perfusion is diminished by atherosclerosis. In patients with chronic hypertension, sustained increases in afterload cause compensatory ventricular hypertrophy and increased wall tension which reduces coronary reserve. In this setting of diminished cardiac reserve, acute increases in blood pressure are compensated for by increasing left ventricular end-diastolic volume and pressure which further reduces coronary perfusion.

The impairment of cerebral autoregulation in elderly patients renders them susceptible to both hypotensive- and hypertensive-induced cerebral injury. Acute elevations in blood pressure can induce severe intracerebral vasoconstriction and ischemia.

The incidence of postoperative hypertension ranges between 3 and 25 percent. Twenty-five percent of patients with previous hypertension will develop postoperative hypertension, regardless of the adequacy of preoperative blood pressure control. Both the significance and incidence of postoperative hypertension is higher in patients with peripheral vascular disease. Postoperative hypertension is reported to develop in 20 percent of patients after carotid endarterectomy and 57 percent after abdominal aortic aneurysm resection. After vascular surgery, systolic blood pressures greater than 200 mmHg are associated with an increased incidence of postoperative hemorrhagic cerebral infarction, bleeding at vascular anastomoses, myocardial ischemia or infarction, and acute renal failure. Following carotid endarterectomy, the incidence of neurologic deficits was higher when postoperative hypertension developed than when hypotension occurred. Cardiac operations in which cardiopulmonary bypass is used are commonly followed by hypertensive episodes. Acute blood pressure elevation in this circumstance may jeopardize the integrity of vascular anastomoses and sites repaired by suture closure. An increased incidence of wound hematomas has been reported in patients with poorly controlled hypertension undergoing plastic surgery operations.

Hypertension may develop during the intraoperative period, most commonly during the times of anesthetic induction and emergence. Hypertension should prompt an immediate assessment of the level of anesthesia, the adequacy of ventilation and oxygenation, fluid status, as well as of any manipulations that may be occurring in the operative field (e.g., aortic cross-clamping, carotid endarterectomy). The correction of reversible factors should be effective, though the use of sodium nitroprusside or nitroglycerin may be necessary in some instances.

Eighty percent of postoperative hypertensive episodes are seen in the immediate postoperative period within 30 min of operation and resolve within 3 h. Contributory factors during this period include emergence from anesthesia, tracheal stimulation by an endotracheal tube, inadequate analgesia, hypothermia, hypercapnia, hypoxemia, fluid overload, or acute urinary bladder distension. Efforts should be made to warm the patient, confirm the adequacy of ventilation and oxygenation, provide adequate analgesia, and assess for fluid overload. Fluid restriction or, if the overload is severe, diuretic therapy may be required. If urgent blood pressure control is required, intravenous sodium nitroprusside or labetalol are preferred for a rapid and controlled effect. Intravenous nitroglycerin, sublingual nitroglycerin, or nifedipine are also effective, particularly in patients with angina pectoris or heart failure. In less urgent situations, methyldopa or hydralazine may be useful.

Hypertension occurring later in the postoperative course is usually related to hypervolemia secondary to fluid mobilization into the intravascular space, inadequate analgesia, or failure to resume previous antihypertensive medications. If fluid overload is mild, fluid restriction may be sufficient. Occasionally, diuretic therapy may be necessary. Sufficient doses of analgesics should be provided. Preoperative medications should be resumed as soon as is feasible.

HYPERCOAGULABLE STATES

Thrombotic disorders, particularly in the surgical patient can cause significant morbidity and mortality from complications arising from either arterial or venous thrombosis. The patients at risk are identified either by a previous history of thrombotic events, particularly in younger patients, or the development of thrombotic complications in the perioperative period. Recurrent episodes of thrombosis or episodes occurring despite adequate anticoagulation therapy should prompt consideration of an underlying problem. Iliofemoral deep venous thrombosis is the most common manifestation, though inherited thrombotic disorders may affect unusual sites such as the mesenteric or cerebral venous systems.

Acquired Hypercoagulable States

Acquired hypercoagulable states are far more common and represent a number of clinical disorders in which the risk of thrombotic complications is increased over the general population. These disorders include the postoperative state, immobilization, advanced age, obesity, malignancy, atherosclerosis, oral contraceptive or estrogen therapy, the postpartum state, myeloproliferative disorders, hyperviscosity, thrombotic thrombocytopenic purpura, paroxysmal nocturnal hemoglobinuria, nephrotic syndrome, prosthetic cardiac valves, anticardiolipin syndrome (lupus anticoagulant), and heparin-induced thrombocytopenia.

Inherited or congenital thrombotic disorders are less common. In one study of 141 patients with a positive family history of thrombosis problems or a personal history of spontaneous venous thrombosis, 15 percent of patients were found to have deficiencies of identifiable natural anticoagulant proteins: protein S, 5 percent; protein C, 4 percent; antithrombin III, 3 percent; plasminogen, 2 percent; and fibrinogen, 1 percent.

Anticardiolipin Syndrome. Lupus anticoagulants are antibodies that interfere with the in vitro partial thromboplastin time by prolonging phospholipid-dependent clotting factors. Lupus anticoagulants may also interfere with heparin monitoring during cardiac surgery. These antibodies may occur in patients with other autoimmune diseases besides systemic lupus erythematosus, following drug exposure, malignancy, various infectious agents, and occasionally in patients without underlying disease. The presence of the antibodies is associated with an increased risk of both arterial and venous thrombosis, and one-third of patients will have a history of thrombotic events. Several specific assays are available to detect the presence of lupus anticoagulants.

The management of acute venous thromboembolism with heparin therapy in these patients is complicated by the distortion of the activated partial thromboplastin time (APTT). Ideally, plasma heparin measurements should be monitored, with a range of 0.2 to 0.5 U heparin/mL, corresponding to an APTT of 1.5 to 2.5 times greater than control values. The long-term management of these patients is confused by the clinical heterogeneity of the syndrome. Asymptomatic individuals with lupus anticoagulants and no prior history of thrombosis do not require anticoagulant therapy; however, patients undergoing major surgical procedures should receive prophylactic anticoagulation.

Heparin-Induced Thrombocytopenia. The incidence of this syndrome is estimated to be 3 to 6 percent. The syndrome is characterized by heparin-associated thrombocytopenia and in a subgroup of patients both arterial and, less commonly, venous thrombosis. The underlying mechanism is thought to be autoantibody formation directed toward heparin and platelet surface antigens that results in both platelet activation and consumption. The effect of heparin is not dose-dependent, and the syndrome can be precipitated by quantities as small as 10 units. Evidence suggests that porcine heparin may be less likely to induce thrombocytopenia.

The clinical syndrome may vary. A less severe variant is described with mild transient thrombocytopenia occurring 2 to 4 days after heparin exposure. The second variant is marked by severe thrombocytopenia 6 to 12 days after heparin exposure and thrombosis. The reported sites of arterial thrombosis include femoral artery, aortic and lower extremity vascular bypass grafts, coronary artery, and cerebral artery. Thrombosis of the iliofemoral vein, renal vein, and inferior vena cava have been reported, in addition to the related complications of phlegmasia cerulea dolens and pulmonary embolism.

The diagnosis is based on clinical suspicion and the exclusion of other causes of thrombocytopenia. Platelet aggregation studies using the patient's plasma in combination with donor platelets and pharmaceutical heparin may be helpful if the response is greater than 30 percent above control levels.

Laster and associates reported that prompt recognition of the syndrome and discontinuation of heparin can decrease the complication and mortality rates from 61 and 23 percent, respectively, to 23 and 12 percent. Earlier studies indicated a limb amputation rate of 29 percent. Arterial thrombosis may be effectively managed by surgical thrombectomy in combination with the use of alternate antithrombotic agents such as dextran and warfarin. Major venous thromboembolism has been effectively treated with placement of a Greenfield caval filter and initiation of warfarin therapy when platelet levels exceeded $50{,}000/mm^3$.

Inherited Thrombotic Disorders

In general, the presence of an inherited thrombotic disorder should be considered in patients with the following clinical features: thrombosis occurring at an early age, spontaneous venous thrombosis, a family history of thrombotic problems, thrombosis involving unusual sites such as mesenteric or cerebral veins, and recurrent thrombosis without apparent precipitating factors. Arterial thrombosis is notably absent in these disorders.

Management of thromboembolism in these patients is similar to the treatment of patients without these disorders. Heparinization should be continued until full oral anticoagulation with warfarin is achieved. Prophylactic anticoagulation is indicated before surgical procedures.

Protein C Deficiency. Protein C deficiency is an autosomal dominant gene disorder that results in a deficiency of the protein that inactivates factors V and VIIIa. It occurs in 4 to 5 percent of patients younger than 45 years with unexplained venous thrombosis. Protein C is vitamin K–dependent and levels are affected by warfarin. Thrombosis occurs with levels less than 70 percent of normal activity.

Protein S Deficiency. The clinical presentation and incidence of this disorder are similar to protein C deficiency. This disorder exists in both heterozygous and homozygous forms. Acquired protein S deficiency may occur during pregnancy, with oral contraceptives, in DIC, and in acute thromboembolic disease. Protein S assays are also affected by oral anticoagulants. Thrombotic problems occur with levels below 60 percent of normal.

Antithrombin III Deficiency. This is an autosomal dominant inherited trait characterized by a deficiency of the factor that inactivates factor Xa and thrombin. Less than one-half of patients with the disorder will have spontaneous initial thrombotic episodes. Sixty percent of patients develop recurrent thrombosis, and 40 percent develop symptoms of pulmonary embolism. Diagnosis may be difficult because of a number of conditions that can also reduce antithrombin III concentrations such as cirrhosis, nephrotic syndrome, DIC, estrogen therapy, oral contraceptives, as well as heparin and L-asparaginase. Management of thromboembolic episodes with heparin is usually successful. Instances of significant heparin resistance or recurrent thrombosis despite heparin therapy may require antithrombin III replacement. The use of the fresh frozen plasma is also indicated for patients undergoing operation. Plasma levels should be monitored and maintained above 80 percent. Warfarin should be continued indefinitely in patients with recurrent venous thrombosis.

SUPPURATIVE PAROTITIS

Acute suppurative parotitis is now an uncommon complication, although it may still occur in the elderly or debilitated patient. Under normal circumstances, bacterial infection of the parotid gland is prevented by the bacteriostatic nature of the secretions as well as the normal flow of saliva through Stensen's duct. Situations in which these natural defenses are eliminated appear to lead to the development of an ascending bacterial infection. Dry mouth secondary to decreased oral intake, operation, general anesthesia, and the use of atropinergic drugs as well as poor oral hygiene are associated with suppurative parotitis.

Clinical Manifestations. Typically, the disease develops in elderly or chronically ill patients approximately 2 weeks after operation. The onset is abrupt with unilateral pain and swelling over the affected gland. High fever and chills are often present. On physical examination, the gland is firm and tender and the overlying skin may be edematous and erythematous. Frank pus may be manually expressed from the orifice of Stensen's duct, and the specimen should be Gram-stained to identify the causative organism.

Treatment. The infecting organism is usually *Staph. aureus.* A penicillinase-resistant penicillin should be administered parenterally. In addition, attention should be paid to improving the patient's overall hydration and oral hygiene. Some authors advocate the use of gland massage and sialogogue to stimulate secretion and promote saliva flow. In rare instances, medical management may be ineffective, necessitating surgical drainage.

COMPLICATIONS OF GASTROINTESTINAL SURGERY

Anastomotic Leak

The integrity of gastrointestinal anastomoses is dependent on several critical factors, all of which are influenced by surgical technique. The initial and early integrity of the anastomosis is derived from the mechanical approximation of the edges by suture material or metallic staples to form a complete and watertight seal. Apposition of the mucosal layers of the joined organs is essential in creating this seal. The serosal layer of the organ wall, when present, possesses a high tensile strength available to support suturing. In addition, under normal circumstances, fibrin deposition occurs at the anastomotic site in response to local inflammation. Tension across the anastomosis or increased intraluminal pressure due to construction of the anastomosis proximal to a point of obstruction exerts mechanical forces that will disrupt the anastomosis. Sutures improperly placed may tear through tissues or fail to approximate the intestinal edges when tied too loosely or cause ischemic necrosis if tied too tightly.

Ensuring the availability of an adequate blood supply to support normal inflammation and healing is the most critical factor in constructing gastrointestinal anastomoses. In addition, avoiding creation of anastomoses in the presence of infection such as gross purulence, fecal contamination, or diffuse peritonitis circumvents the potential for disruption of the site by secondary infection of the inflammatory process occurring at the anastomosis.

The likelihood of anastomotic disruption as well as the physiologic effects and clinical manifestation of the event are, in part, a function of the site within the gastrointestinal tract in which the anastomosis is performed.

Esophageal Anastomoses. The risk of anastomotic disruption is thought to be higher in esophageal anastomosis. This observation has been attributed to the lack of a serosal layer in the esophagus and to the segmental nature of the blood supply of the esophagus. Esophageal anastomoses are usually performed by approximation of the esophagus to stomach, colon, or small bowel. Anastomotic leaks occurring within the thoracic cavity or mediastinum result in very high morbidity and mortality and are leading causes of death in patients following esophagectomy. This has led many authors to advocate placement of the anastomoses in the cervical esophagus where leakage, if it occurs, is better tolerated.

Disruption of an intrathoracic esophageal anastomosis often occurs within the first 10 days after surgery. The presentation is dramatic with fever, chest pain, tachycardia, tachypnea, often with evidence of impending shock. Chest roentgenogram may reveal the presence of a pneumothorax or a pleural effusion. In less dramatic situations, presence of a leak may be confirmed with contrast esophagography using a water-soluble contrast agent. Treatment consists of immediate reoperation with irrigation of the chest and mediastinum and establishment of chest tube drainage.

Gastric Anastomoses. Following gastric operations the incidence of anastomotic leak is less than 2 percent. The clinical presentation of anastomotic disruption following gastric surgery is commonly subtle and manifested by the presence of abdominal pain, prolonged ileus, fever, leukocytosis, gastrointestinal bleeding, gastric outlet obstruction, oliguria, hyperamylasemia, hyperbilirubinemia, and respiratory insufficiency. Occasionally, the presentation may be dramatic with peritonitis and shock.

Plain abdominal radiographs may be useful in demonstrating pneumoperitoneum or air-fluid levels suggestive of an intraabdominal abscess. Water-soluble contrast radiography will usually demonstrate the site of the leak. If an intraabdominal drain is in place and producing fluid, sinography may also be used to demonstrate the actual leak.

When drainage from the leak is very small and contained by omentum or adjacent structures, or if the drainage is effectively controlled by drains placed at the time of surgery in patients without sepsis, nonoperative management is acceptable. Nasogastric decompression, parenteral broad-spectrum antibiotics, and parenteral nutrition is provided. In the absence of carcinoma or obstruction distal to the site of the leak, gastrocutaneous fistulas created by the drain should resolve. If sepsis is present, or no prior drainage has been established, immediate reexploration is indicated once a leak has been confirmed. Small anastomotic disruptions may be primarily repaired; larger defects may require complete revision of the anastomosis.

Small-Intestinal Anastomoses. Anastomotic leaks from small-intestinal anastomoses are uncommon due to the rich blood supply, low bacterial content, and rapid epithelialization of the small bowel. Disruption, when it does occur, may be followed by local abscess formation or peritonitis. Enterocutaneous fistula formation may occur as the process extends from the anastomosis to the abdominal incision or drain sites. Reoperation to control the fistula is indicated if peritonitis or sepsis is present. Single well-localized abscesses may be amenable to percutaneous computed tomography–guided drainage, with acceptance of the inevitable resulting enterocutaneous fistula.

Colorectal Anastomoses. Colonic anastomoses are more prone to disruption and leakage than are those of the stomach and small intestine. This fact has been attributed to the large quantity of pathogenic bacteria within the colonic flora, the propensity of the colon to distention, and slow recovery from ileus and a single thin layer of circular muscle to support sutures. The more distal the anastomosis in the colon, the greater the risk of leakage. While leakage following ileotransverse colostomy rarely occurs, subclinical leakage can be demonstrated radiographically in 20 percent, and clinical leakage is present in 5 percent of patients with rectal anastomoses.

Colonic anastomotic leaks usually present between 7 and 14 days after operation with features of an intraabdominal or pelvic abscess. Disruption of a rectal anastomosis may occur as early as the first postoperative week. Suspicion of a colonic anastomotic leak requires reexploration with drainage of the abscess, dismantling the anastomosis, and exteriorization of the bowel ends. Rectal anastomotic leak may be confirmed by direct examination of the anastomosis using rigid sigmoidoscopy or gentle water-soluble contrast enema. Treatment consists of diversion of the fecal stream by proximal loop colostomy to prevent further soilage and the establishment of pelvic drainage.

The risk of colon and rectal anastomosis complications can be reduced by optimal preoperative preparation with mechanical cleansing of the colon and the reduction of bacterial flora using nonabsorbable antibiotics (neomycin and erythromycin). In the lower rectum where exposure is limited, the local blood supply is tenuous, and performing a hand-sewn anastomosis is difficult, use of the endorectal circular stapling device may be preferable to obtain a well-constructed anastomosis.

Ileus and Small-Bowel Obstruction

Ileus is defined as a functional, nonmechanical obstruction of the bowel. It is thought to arise from splanchnic nerve stimulation leading to neural inhibition of coordinated intrinsic bowel wall motor activity and the elimination of effective peristalsis. Ileus itself is expected after any type of abdominal operation in which the peritoneal cavity is entered and may be due to pain stimulation of the peritoneum, manipulation of the abdominal contents, or mediation via some other mechanism. The duration of ileus varies in different segments of the gastrointestinal tract. In the stomach, normal peristalsis should return within 24 to 48 h, in the small intestine within 24 h, and in the colon within 3 to 5 days. Although the presence of bowel sounds may signal return of small intestinal peristalsis, only the passage of flatus clearly indicates the resolution of colonic ileus.

The presence of ileus for greater than 5 days after operation suggests a prolonged condition and should prompt a search for alternate causes. Prolonged ileus is associated with any form of intraabdominal inflammation such as peritonitis, abscess, or hemoperitoneum. Mesenteric and retroperitoneal hematomas may also cause prolonged ileus. Ileus has also been associated with thoracic trauma, distant sepsis, occlusive mesenteric vascular disease, as well as numerous drugs. Electrolyte imbalances, specifically hypokalemia, hyponatremia, hypocalcemia, and hypomagnesemia are also known to delay the return of peristalsis. The failure of normal peristalsis to return after the fifth postoperative day should prompt the surgeon to consider treatment of potentially reversible causes such as treatment of the source of peritonitis, drainage of intraabdominal abscesses, correction of electrolyte imbalances, and elimination of offending drugs.

In some instances, distinguishing between prolonged ileus and early postoperative bowel obstruction on physical examination alone may be difficult. Some authors suggest water-soluble contrast studies, administered via the nasogastric tube to demonstrate the presence of a frank mechanical bowel obstruction. The failure of contrast to pass a fixed point is suggestive of a complete small-bowel obstruction. In the early postoperative period and in the absence of signs of ischemic bowel, the use of long nasointestinal tubes (the Baker, Leonard, Miller-Abbott, or Dennis tube) may be warranted to effect intestinal decompression and relieve edema. The presence of fever, leukocytosis, or abdominal tenderness are signs suggestive of bowel compromise, and their presence is an indication for laparotomy.

Fistulas

General Principles of Management. The majority of external gastrointestinal fistulas that develop in the postoperative period are the result of technical complications, primarily errors in construction of bowel anastomoses and inadvertent and unrecognized direct injury to the bowel that results in a full-thickness defect. The technical errors leading to breakdown of anastomoses have been discussed above. Less common but recognized causes of fistula formation include deserosalization of bowel, poor placement of drains with subsequent erosion into bowel, and the entrapment of intestine within the fascial closure.

The likelihood of spontaneous closure and the mortality associated with gastrointestinal fistulas is dependent on several factors: (1) location in the gastrointestinal tract and fistula output, (2) intestinal continuity, (3) the number of external openings, (4) the involvement of other organs, (5) the length of the fistula, and (6) the presence of local factors preventing healing. In general, the more proximal in the gastrointestinal tract the origin of the fistula, the greater the output and the less likely spontaneous closure will occur. High-output proximal fistulas from the stomach, duodenum, and proximal jejunum result in large fluid and electrolyte losses. In addition, nutritional deficits are more common due to high protein losses in the secretions, as well as to malabsorption as a result of the loss of bile salts and pancreatic enzymes. Distal fistulas, by contrast, are usually the low-output type with adequate reabsorption occurring in the intact proximal bowel.

Lateral fistulas, with intestinal continuity both proximal and distal, are likely to undergo spontaneous closure. By contrast, end fistulas may result mechanically from complete disruption of the bowel or functionally from the presence of obstruction distal to the fistula. The complete diversion of intestinal contents through the fistula makes spontaneous closure very unlikely.

In general, fistulas with multiple cutaneous openings are thought to be less likely to close spontaneously. In addition, if inadequately cared for, this situation may lead to large abdominal wall defects and, in some studies, is associated with a higher mortality rate. Fistulas arising from multiple organs (e.g., stomach, colon, pancreas) appear to have a lower spontaneous closure rate than single-organ fistulas. Fistulas longer than 2 cm are more likely to undergo spontaneous closure. This has been attributed to the higher resistance to flow generated by a longer tract as well as a decreased likelihood of epithelialization occurring. In addition, fistulas associated with bowel wall defects greater than 1 cm at the tract origin are unlikely to close spontaneously. If healing does occur, bowel stricture often ensues.

The presence of a foreign body, carcinoma, epithelialization of the tract, or irradiation of the affected bowel are local factors that inhibit healing and make fistula closure unlikely.

The principles of gastrointestinal fistula management are (1) fluid and electrolyte correction, (2) control of sepsis, (3) control of fistula drainage and skin protection, (4) bowel rest, and (5) definition of fistula anatomy. Volume deficits, as noted earlier, may be substantial with upper gastrointestinal tract fistulas. Fluid and electrolyte therapy should be guided by quantitation of fistula losses as well as by measurement of both serum and fistula electrolyte levels. Sepsis is the most common cause of death in patients with gastrointestinal fistulas and must be controlled by identifying, localizing, and draining intraabdominal abscesses when they occur. Localized abscess formation is more common with colonic fistulas; however, sepsis associated with proximal fistulas tends to be more virulent because of the corrosive nature of upper gastrointestinal tract secretions leading to widespread contamination and peritonitis. Fistula drainage is controlled by intubation of the tract with a soft rubber catheter, thus allowing quantitation of the drainage and affording protection of the skin. Once the fistula is well established and the patient stabilized, contrast fistulography is performed to determine the site of origin, fistula length, the presence of an associated abscess or cavity, and the condition of the affected bowel. In some instances, other contrast studies, such as upper gastrointestinal series or barium enema, may be of benefit. Bowel rest is accomplished by not allowing patients oral intake and providing parenteral or enteral nutrition as indicated. Gastric secretion can be significantly reduced with H_2-receptor antagonists such as cimetidine.

In general, early surgery is indicated for abscesses not amenable to percutaneous drainage techniques to control sepsis. Otherwise, 6 to 8 weeks of conservative management is recommended before operation is undertaken. The operative mortality and fistula recurrence rates are highest for operations performed between the first and sixth weeks following fistula formation.

Gastric Fistulas. Isolated gastrocutaneous fistulas are uncommon, with an incidence of 2 to 20 percent. They may arise as complications of gastrectomy most likely originating from the gastroduodenal or gastrojejunal anastomosis. In these instances, suture line failure may be due to ischemia of the gastric remnant, the presence of tumor, pancreatitis, or stomal obstruction. In one series, almost one-half of fistulas arose following splenectomy and were attributed to unrecognized iatrogenic injury of the gastric wall. In most instances, fistulas arise from the greater curvature of the stomach and can be identified by upper gastrointestinal contrast studies or fistulography. The most common complications of gastrocutaneous fistulas are fluid and electrolyte abnormalities, subphrenic abscess, malnutrition, wound infection, and sepsis. The reported mortality ranges from 15 to 22 percent, and most deaths are due to sepsis.

Treatment requires intensive fluid and electrolyte management since losses can be substantial. Nutritional support in the form of TPN or, preferably, nasoenteric feedings distal to the fistula origin is ideal. Because of the corrosive nature of gastric secretions, meticulous skin protection is essential. Conservative management results in spontaneous closure in approximately 70 percent of cases, usually within 6 weeks. In the presence of obstruction to gastric emptying, closure is unlikely and operation is indicated to resect the fistula and relieve the obstruction. Fistulas arising from gastrojejunal anastomotic disruption usually require revision or creation of a new gastrojejunostomy.

Duodenal Fistulas. Duodenal fistulas usually arise from duodenal stump leakage following subtotal gastrectomy with gastrojejunostomy for peptic ulcer disease. Suture line disruption of the duodenal closure is most often due to devascularization of the duodenum by extensive dissection. Obstruction of the afferent limb may also lead to leakage and fistula formation. Nonoperative treatment is similar to that of gastric fistulas with emphasis on fluid and electrolyte replacement and skin protection. Fluid losses from duodenal fistulas can exceed 2 L/day. Spontaneous closure has been found to occur in 37 to 100 percent of fistulas. If sepsis is present or spontaneous closure has not occurred by 6 weeks, operative repair may be warranted. Direct suture closure is usually unsuccessful in this instance, and better results have been reported using serosal patching or Roux-en-Y anastomosis to the defect.

Enterocutaneous Fistulas. The majority of enterocutaneous fistulas are the result of operative complications, either anastomotic breakdown or unrecognized injury to the bowel as described above. In 25 percent of cases, however, spontaneous fistula formation may occur due to inflammatory bowel disease, irradiation, neoplasms, and vascular disease. The typical presentation involves cellulitis and purulence in the surgical wound about 5 to 7 days after operation, with drainage of intestinal contents occurring in the next 2 to 3 days. Alternatively, bowel leakage will result in an abscess and peritonitis without establishment of a complete fistulous tract to the skin.

While the use of TPN is well accepted in the management of enterocutaneous fistulas, the benefit of its use is debated. In two separate studies the outcomes of patients whose management included the use of TPN were compared to the outcomes of historical controls treated before the availability of TPN. In both studies, no significant differences in mortality were found, though a higher spontaneous closure rate was found in the TPN group in one study. Three other studies of similar design disagree, finding a decrease in mortality and an increase in spontaneous closure when using TPN. Despite this dispute, nutritional support renders these patients better able to tolerate sepsis and operation if these occur. From the available data, the use of somatostatin in the treatment of enterocutaneous fistulas is unclear. A retrospective study of 37 patients treated with both TPN and somatostatin indicated a substantial reduction in fistula output, a spontaneous closure rate of 82 percent, and an average time to closure of 5.4 days after starting therapy. A second study comparing somatostatin and TPN therapy with historical controls treated with TPN alone reported that spontaneous closure occurred after an average of 6 days versus 27 days in the control group. These findings suggest that the use of somatostatin in addition to TPN may allow spontaneous closure to occur earlier, though the rate of spontaneous closure is not increased.

The indications and timing of operation for fistula closure are discussed above. The operation of choice is resection of the fistula-bearing segment and primary end-to-end anastomosis. The spontaneous closure rate of enterocutaneous fistulas ranges between 50 and 80 percent with a mortality rate of 28 percent. The success rate of surgical closure may approach 90 percent.

Colocutaneous Fistulas. These are generally the result of colonic anastomotic leaks or unrecognized trauma to the colon during operation. Creation of an anastomosis in the presence of infection or fecal contamination such as for acute diverticulitis or traumatic colon injuries increases the likelihood of fistula formation. In contrast to enterocutaneous fistulas, fluid and electrolyte abnormalities and skin digestion are rare. However, infectious complications are prominent with abscess formation and wound infections.

Nutritional status can be maintained by using low-residue elemental enteral diets. Localized infection should be controlled with percutaneous drainage of intraabdominal abscesses and local care of wound infections. Antibiotics are used as indicated. Spontaneous closure is very likely with colocutaneous fistulas approaching 75 percent. The presence of sepsis involving the fistula, distal obstruction, anastomotic dehiscence, Crohn's disease, or carcinoma were factors associated with persistence of the fistula. Earlier operative intervention is indicated if peritonitis or septicemia is present. The lack of spontaneous closure by 6 weeks is also an indication for surgical repair. Definitive operation involves resection of the fistula and affected colonic segment with primary anastomosis and temporary diversion of the fecal stream by colostomy. The success rate of surgical repair of colocutaneous fistulas is about 70 to 80 percent.

Pancreatic Fistulas. Pancreatico-cutaneous fistulas may develop after any operation performed in the presence of injury to the pancreas or where pancreatic resection has been performed. The incidence of fistula formation varies according to the underlying pathologic condition of the pancreas and is as high as 31 percent following the drainage of pancreatic abscesses. Pancreatic resection and internal drainage of pseudocysts are associated with a 5 to

10 percent incidence of external fistula formation. The potential complications of pancreatic fistulas include infection, abscess formation, erosion in major vessels, fluid and electrolyte imbalances, and malnutrition due to malabsorption. External pancreatic fistulas present as clear fluid originating from the surgical wound or an appropriately placed drain, and the diagnosis is confirmed by determination of the high amylase content of the drainage. High-output fistulas produce greater than 200 mL/day.

Conservative management consisting of replacement of fluid and electrolyte losses, maintenance of nutrition with TPN, and adequate local skin care at the drainage site should result in spontaneous closure of up to 80 percent of fistulas. The average time required for closure is 3 to 4 weeks. Several groups have attempted with limited success to hasten fistula closure by decreasing pancreatic secretion using various agents such as atropine, acetazolamide, epinephrine, glucagon, and terbutaline. Somatostatin has been shown to shorten the time required for fistula closure in one prospective study. Spontaneous fistula closure is unlikely in the presence of contamination with bile or enteric contents, the presence of infection or foreign bodies, and extremely remote if proximal obstruction of the pancreatic duct exists. Communication between the fistula and pancreatic duct may be evident on fistulography; however, endoscopic retrograde pancreatography (ERCP) is usually necessary to determine the patency of the ductal system. High-output fistulas persisting for longer than 4 to 6 weeks and those associated with ductal obstruction or persistent infection should be considered for operative closure.

Postgastrectomy Syndromes

Dumping Syndrome. Almost all postgastrectomy patients experience minor symptoms of dumping syndrome at some time or another after operation. However, only 5 percent of patients have symptoms severe enough to seek medical attention. There are two phases of the syndrome, early and late. While the etiology of the dumping syndrome is not well understood, the anatomic requirement appears to be bypass or removal of the pylorus. It is thought that under these circumstances, the normal function of the stomach in diluting and regulating the transfer of chyme into the small intestine is circumvented. Following partial gastrectomy, hyperosmolar chyme may be suddenly emptied into the jejunum resulting in a large influx of extracellular fluid into the bowel lumen. The subsequent bowel distention is thought to provoke an autonomic response and vasomotor symptoms. The manifestations of early dumping syndrome appear to reflect these physiologic events. Faintness, nausea and vomiting, diaphoresis, pallor, palpitations, and abdominal colic and diarrhea occur within 15 to 20 min of a meal. High-carbohydrate meals such as ice cream are especially provocative. By contrast, late dumping with similar neurologic symptoms but without diarrhea occurs 2 to 4 h after eating and is related to a delayed reactive hypoglycemia phenomenon.

Early dumping syndrome responds in most instances to dietary manipulations such as eating small, dry meals; separating solids from liquids during meals; and lying down when symptoms occur. Recent studies have addressed the observation that numerous gastrointestinal peptides such as vasoactive intestinal peptide, pancreatic polypeptide, insulin, glucagon, neurotensin, and enteroglucagon, as well as serotonin and bradykinin, are elevated in the early dumping syndrome. The long-acting somatostatin analogue antagonizes the effects of these hormones as well as alters the motility pattern of the small intestine. The clinical experience with this drug has been favorable with patients achieving significant relief of early dumping symptoms. For patients with severe, persistent symptoms remedial operations have been performed with moderate success. The most effective has been interposition of a 10-cm segment of reversed jejunum between the stomach and duodenum or jejunum, which has been reported to be successful in 85 percent of patients in which it was performed.

Late dumping syndrome is rare, occurring in less than 2 percent of patients after gastric procedures. Management is nonoperative with emphasis on the reduction of carbohydrates in meals and the addition of pectin which may prevent symptoms of hypoglycemia.

Afferent Loop Syndrome. This complication is a mechanical problem peculiar to the gastroenterostomy reconstruction after gastrectomy. Optimal function of this arrangement requires free flow of material from the duodenum (afferent loop) to the intestine draining the gastric pouch (efferent limb). Obstruction of the afferent loop may result from adhesions, kinking, intussusception, volvulus of the afferent loop, stomal ulcer, or obstruction of the efferent limb. When this occurs, bile, pancreatic juice, and duodenal secretions accumulating in the afferent loop are regurgitated into the stomach.

The clinical history is distinctive and often diagnostic. Patients experience severe epigastric pain 1 to 2 h after eating which is relieved by projectile vomiting of copious amounts of bile-stained fluid without food. In addition, they may have elevations of serum amylase and alkaline phosphatase which may reflect the degree of relative obstruction. The diagnosis can be confirmed by barium contrast radiography which may reveal a distended afferent loop or, preferably, by upper endoscopy. Endoscopy is especially useful in identifying the causative anatomic defect at the gastrojejunal anastomosis.

Preferable treatment of the afferent loop syndrome is conversion of the gastrojejunostomy either to a gastroduodenostomy (Billroth I) or to a long-limbed (60 cm) Roux-en-Y gastrojejunostomy. If stomal ulceration is present, the causes of recurrent peptic ulceration following gastrectomy should be evaluated.

Alkaline Reflux Gastritis. This complication is a poorly defined condition that affects a small number of patients following gastrectomy. Patients complain of severe, continual burning epigastric pain, usually aggravated by meals and unrelieved by vomiting. The emesis is bile-stained, undigested food. The diagnosis is aided by endoscopy which reveals a typical "beefy red," inflamed gastric mucosa with superficial erosions. Mucosal biopsy may show histologic evidence of acute or chronic inflammatory cell infiltrates, a decrease in parietal cells, an increase in mucus-secreting cells, and intestinalization of the gastric glands. There is usually no evidence of gastric outlet obstruction. Nonoperative treatment with bile salt–absorbing resins such as cholestyramine, H_2-receptor blockers, aluminum-containing antacids, or metoclopramide have not been proved effective in prospective trials. The goal of operative treatment is to divert bile from the stomach, and the preferred procedure is a 50- to 60-cm limb Roux-en-Y gastrojejunostomy.

Postvagotomy Diarrhea. Truncal vagotomy is associated with an increased incidence of diarrhea after operation. Though 70 percent of patients are noted to have an increase in bowel movements after vagotomy, the incidence of significant postoperative diarrhea is lower, ranging from 5 to 20 percent. The etiology of this problem is not well defined. Numerous factors have been proposed including gastric stasis, impaired biliary and pancreatic secretory function, small intestine dysmotility, bacterial colonization of the small intestine, and the diarrheogenic effects of bile salts and acids in the colon.

Characteristically, the diarrhea is variable in its occurrence and unassociated with food intake. Though it can be mild, postvagotomy diarrhea is often unpredictable and explosive. The symptoms may be debilitating enough to cause weight loss and malnutrition as well as severe social complications. The incidence of diarrhea seems to diminish significantly with time.

Treatment of the diarrhea should be symptomatic and is usually effective. Cholestyramine to bind bile salts and the use of neomycin or tetracycline to reduce bacterial colonization may be beneficial. For the very small number of patients who do not respond to conservative measures, moderate success has been achieved in controlling diarrhea using an operation in which a 10-cm reversed jejunal segment is placed 100 cm distal to the ligament of Treitz. It is thought that this results in increasing small-bowel transit time and improves mixture of pancreatic and biliary secretions with intestinal chyme and reduces bile salt delivery to the colon.

Stoma Complications

Complications involving intestinal stomas may result in considerable morbidity. Though some problems are functional and not preventable, a number of stomal complications are related to technical error. Other complications may arise from the recurrence of disease within the stoma, such as an ileostomy with Crohn's disease or colon cancer within a colostomy. The following discussion focuses on common complications that affect the two most common intestinal stomas encountered in general surgery, the ileostomy and colostomy.

Improper Placement. The most common technical error is poor placement of the stoma. Ideally, stomas should be positioned within the rectus sheath away from the costal margins, umbilicus, symphysis pubis, iliac crests, and any skin folds, scars, or grooves. The site should be visible to the patient and surrounded by 5 cm of flat, unencumbered skin. Pouch appliances should fit well whether the patient sits, stands, or lies down. Application of stomal appliances may be difficult with poorly positioned stomas with a tendency for leakage. Such leaks may lead to skin destruction, and the fear of such occurrences may prevent patients from pursuing active lives.

Stomal Necrosis and Retraction. Inadequate vascularization of the stoma can lead to ischemia or necrosis in the immediate postoperative period. The development of duskiness or frank necrosis of the stoma should prompt an evaluation to determine the extent of involvement. A good light and a lubricated glass or plastic test tube inserted into the stoma will allow one to determine the level of viability. If the necrosis is superficial to the fascia, no immediate action is required and the necrotic tissue will slough or require debridement. Stricture formation is the common result of this situation. If the necrosis extends below the fascia, immediate laparotomy and reconstruction of the stoma is indicated to prevent the development of peritonitis.

Inadequate mobilization of the mesentery or poor fixation of the stoma to the skin or fascia may result in retraction of the stoma usually during the early postoperative period. Retraction below the level of the fascia requires immediate laparotomy to prevent further fecal contamination of the peritoneal cavity. Retraction above the fascia does not require intervention. This will usually result in poor fitting of the appliance and leakage due to loss of the spigot configuration.

Skin Destruction. Soiling of the peristomal skin with stomal effluent may lead to maceration and skin destruction. While this is more common in ileostomies where the effluent is liquid and contains proteolytic pancreatic enzymes, identical problems can occur with colostomies proximal to the splenic flexure or colostomy diarrhea. The common and usual mechanism is a poor appliance seal. Skin destruction may also result from peristomal folliculitis, contact dermatitis due to the use of benzoin, or allergic dermatitis. High ileostomy output due to short bowel syndrome, recurrent Crohn's disease, partial small-bowel obstruction, stomal stenosis, gastroenteritis, or intraabdominal sepsis may also contribute to skin destruction.

Excoriation should be managed by applying a proper-fitting appliance to prevent further skin injury. Consultation with an enterostomal therapist is advisable, especially in severe cases. If improper stoma construction is the cause, and intensive enterostomal therapy is unsuccessful, operative reconstruction of the stoma is indicated. Attention should also be directed toward control of high ileostomy output with the use of antidiarrheal agents, dietary manipulation, and fluid and electrolyte replacement. By contrast, colostomy diarrhea is often the result of fecal impaction, which should be ruled out by examination of the stoma. In this situation, antidiarrheal agents are not indicated.

Stomal Stricture. Although stomal stricture is a late complication, it is caused by the development of serositis in the immediate postoperative period. Adoption of the technique of primary maturation, involving the approximation of the intestinal mucosa to the skin at the time of stoma construction, has drastically reduced the development of serositis. Today the most common cause of stomal stricture is necrosis or retraction, resulting in mucocutaneous separation, exposure of the serosa, and subsequent serositis.

Stomal strictures should be treated by excision of the skin and scar, with resuturing of the intestinal mucosa to the skin to form an adequate stomal orifice. Dilation of stomal strictures is usually ineffective.

Stomal Prolapse. Prolapse of a colostomy usually results from its construction at a time when the bowel is markedly dilated or edematous. Consequently, the abdominal wall opening that is created is excessive once the colon returns to normal size. Elimination of the colostomy is the best treatment. In the case of temporary loop colostomies, a definitive procedure to restore intestinal continuity can be performed. If the stoma must be permanent, conversion of the loop colostomy to an end colostomy with a mucous fistula located in a new site may be helpful. The development of prolapse in an end colostomy should be treated by resection of the redundant section, tightening of the aperture, and reconstruction of the stoma.

Prolapse of an ileostomy usually occurs due to parastomal hernia formation or placement of the stoma outside the rectus muscle. Treatment involves repair of the parastomal hernia or resection of the prolapsing segment with reconstruction of the ileostomy.

Parastomal Hernia. Formation of a parastomal hernia is the most common problem requiring surgical correction following colostomy construction. The etiology of this complication is unclear, though it is thought to result from an excessive abdominal wall opening or placement of the stoma lateral to the rectus muscle. The indications for correction are symptoms of intestinal obstruction, parastomal pain, or difficulty in maintaining the stoma or fitting of the appliance. Relocation of the stoma and closure of the hernia defect is the most effective measure and, in some cases, may be accomplished through the hernia defect. Recurrent herniation may require local reconstruction to reduce the orifice size using native tissue or synthetic mesh.

METABOLIC COMPLICATIONS

Diabetes Mellitus

In the United States approximately 5 percent of the population between the ages of 20 and 74 years are affected with diabetes mellitus. Fifteen percent of elderly patients aged 65 to 74 years of age are affected. It has been estimated that approximately one-half of the diabetic individuals in the United States will require one operation in their lifetime. These data would suggest that patients with diabetes constitute a significant portion of surgical practice. Infection, operation, anesthesia, and a number of other acute illnesses can precipitate acute hyperglycemic crises such as diabetic ketoacidosis and hyperosmolar coma in diabetic patients. In addition, there is evidence to suggest that hyperglycemia impairs granulocyte functions such as chemotaxis, phagocytosis, and intracellular bactericidal killing and may be a partial explanation to the susceptibility of diabetics to infections.

Common infections in diabetic patients include esophageal candidiasis, urinary tract infections (pyelonephritis, perinephric abscess), pneumonia, and unusual infections such as necrotizing fasciitis and mucormycosis. The long-term complications of diabetes also significantly increases operative risks. Atherosclerosis and CAD are more prevalent in diabetic compared to nondiabetic patients. Diabetic nephropathy predisposes patients to renal injury from events such as hypotension and agents such as radiographic contrast that may precipitate acute renal failure. One-third of diabetic patients may have autonomic neuropathy that can lead to gastroparesis, neurogenic bladder, esophageal dysmotility, and intractable diarrhea and steatorrhea. The risk of perioperative complications in patients with diabetes is substantial.

Pathophysiology. Diabetes mellitus is a disorder of carbohydrate metabolism, resulting from the deficiency of insulin or a resistance to the actions of insulin. Insulin, produced by the beta islet cells of the pancreas, is released in response to blood glucose levels. The primary effects of insulin promote glucose utilization and fat and muscle protein synthesis. In diabetes, hyperglycemia results from impaired glucose utilization, and ketone bodies are generated from fatty acid degradation as an alternate energy source. The hyperglycemia as well as the accumulation of ketone bodies are excreted in the urine and promote an osmotic diuresis. Unchecked, this process results in acidemia, hyperosmolarity, and dehydration. Catecholamines and glucocorticoid released by stress antagonize the effects of insulin and promote hepatic glycogenolysis and gluconeogenesis and exacerbate the pathologic process. Such a stress response can be elicited by acute illness, anesthesia, trauma, or surgery and can precipitate metabolic decompensation in diabetic patients.

Classification. The type of diabetes mellitus has implications in the management of the condition and the risks for metabolic complications. Overt diabetes mellitus is divided into two categories, insulin-dependent (type I or IDDM) and non-insulin-dependent (type II or NIDDM). Insulin-dependent diabetes represents about 20 percent of all types and has its onset in childhood or early adulthood. Total or near-total insulin deficiency necessitates a complete dependence on exogenous insulin, and there is a marked tendency to the development of both ketoacidosis and hypoglycemic episodes.

Non-insulin-dependent diabetes frequently has an insidious onset, often affecting patients after age 45. Insulin levels are normal or elevated in these patients, and the majority (80 percent) are not dependent on exogenous insulin. Obesity is common, and weight reduction and maintenance reduces hyperglycemia and glucose tolerance. Ketoacidosis is rare but may be precipitated by conditions of stress.

The diagnosis of secondary diabetes is made in patients with abnormal glucose tolerance (values between normal and diabetic levels) and fasting blood glucose levels that are elevated but lower than overt diabetic values. Secondary diabetes may result from a number of conditions including pancreatic disease, endocrine disorders, drugs, and, rarely, hereditary syndromes.

Perioperative Management. The goals of the perioperative management of the surgical patient with diabetes are to control hyperglycemia while avoiding ketoacidosis and hypoglycemia. The protocol selected for the individual patient is determined by the type of diabetes, the effectiveness of blood sugar control, and the magnitude of the planned operation. Numerous protocols for the perioperative management of diabetic patients exist. The initial assessment should include a thorough clinical and laboratory evaluation of the patient with an intent to optimize cardiac, pulmonary, and renal function before surgery. Specific attention should be paid to the recent degree of control of diabetes, the type of therapy used (diet, medication, dosage, and timing), and the presence of symptoms of uncontrolled diabetes and other medications (e.g., diuretics, calcium channel blockers, beta-blocking agents) that may affect carbohydrate metabolism.

In general, it is preferable to schedule operations for diabetic patients early in the day to minimize the effects of fasting. Patients undergoing elective, minor operations in whom diabetes is well controlled and no meals will be missed may be allowed to follow their usual dietary and insulin regimen. If a meal is to be missed, patients with diabetes controlled by oral hypoglycemic agents should withhold the drug on the day of operation until after the operation is completed and the usual diet resumed. Those patients using the longer-acting chlorpropamide agents should discontinue the drug 24 h before surgery. Patients requiring insulin should receive one-half their usual morning dose of insulin (intermediate-acting and regular) the morning of operation and a continuous 5% dextrose infusion to provide 10 g of glucose/h. Blood glucose monitoring should be performed postoperatively. Following operation, subcutaneous doses of regular insulin every 6 h, in addition to a sliding scale regimen, may be required until resumption of the usual dietary intake allows a return to the previous insulin regimen.

For major elective procedures, if diabetes is controlled with oral hypoglycemic agents, the drug should be discontinued as described above. Insulin-dependent patients who are well controlled should receive one-half of their usual morning regular insulin dose, withholding the longer-acting agent. For both types of patients, on the morning of operation a 5% dextrose infusion at 10 g/h is begun. Blood glucose is determined every 2 to 3 h both before and during the operation with intravenous regular insulin administered to maintain glucose levels between 150 to 200 mg/dL. Alternatively, the use of continuous insulin infusions can reduce wide fluctuations in blood glucose levels and decrease the risk of hypoglycemia and may be a preferable technique in patients with "brittle" diabetes. Regular insulin may be added to the dextrose infusion so that 1 to 2 units/h is given. Insulin infusions should be discontinued if the blood glucose falls below 150 mg/dL to avoid hypoglycemia. Postoperatively, glucose control can be managed using scheduled insulin doses and sliding scales or a continuous insulin infusion until oral intake is resumed. Once a diet is begun, insulin infusions should be discontinued and a conversion made to a maintenance insulin regimen.

In patients with poorly controlled diabetes evidenced by blood glucose levels greater than 200 mg/dL, operation should be delayed until adequate control is achieved. Under elective circumstances, this can be accomplished by close medical supervision, dietary management, and insulin dosage adjustments. Dietary management includes an accurate individualized determination of caloric requirements with provision of 50 to 55 percent of calories as carbohydrates, 30 to 35 percent as fat, and 20 percent as high-quality protein. A combination of regular- and intermediate-acting insulin is administered each morning. Blood glucose is determined in the morning with fasting and in the late afternoon. Once blood sugars are controlled, the perioperative regimen for insulin-dependent diabetics described above can be followed. In the emergency setting, severe hyperglycemia requires treatment with continuous insulin infusions before operation (Table 11-8).

Diabetic Ketoacidosis. Diabetic ketoacidosis (DKA) is a medical emergency characterized by hyperglycemia, dehydration, and acidosis and is more prone to affect patients with insulin-dependent diabetes. Mortality results from acidosis, shock, or iatrogenic cerebral edema if serum osmolarity is reduced too rapidly. Any major stress such as infection, MI, or operation or noncompliance with insulin dosing can precipitate the condition in a diabetic individual.

The common symptoms are polydipsia, polyuria, anorexia, nausea and vomiting, weakness, and malaise. Abdominal pain is present in 50 percent of patients and may mimic an acute abdomen. Tachycardia, orthostatic hypotension, altered mental status, or frank shock may be evident depending on the degree of dehydration. If the acidosis is severe, a "fruity" acetone breath and Kussmaul's type respirations may be present.

Laboratory findings generally reveal hyperglycemia (blood sugar > 350 mg/dL), ketonemia (ketone > 5 mmol/L), acidemia, moderate hyperosmolarity, and glycosuria and ketonuria. Serum sodium and potassium levels may be normal, elevated, or decreased. Despite this, total body potassium is often severely depleted. Leukocytosis (WBC > 20,000/mm^3) and left shift are common.

Ketoacidosis must be treated before operation with the following goals: correct fluid and electrolyte deficits, correct hyperglycemia and acidosis, and treat primary underlying cause of DKA. In the emergent setting, correction of blood pH to greater than 7.3 and serum bicarbonate to a level greater than 20 meq/L may be adequate and achieved within 8 h. Under less urgent circumstances, fluid and electrolyte abnormalities should be stabilized for 48 h before operation. All patients should be initially admitted to an intensive care unit. Obtunded or comatose patients should be endotracheally intubated for airway management.

Serious consideration to the use of central venous pressure or pulmonary artery catheters for monitoring fluid therapy should be given in elderly patients and those with cardiac or pulmonary disease. Fluid therapy is begun immediately using normal saline and later changed to one-half normal saline when the serum sodium exceeds 150 meq/L. Continuous intravenous insulin is used to correct hyperglycemia and ketosis, guided by hourly blood glucose determinations. The reduction in glucose levels should not exceed 100 mg/dL/h to avoid inducing cerebral edema. Once the glucose level is less than 250 mg/dL, the insulin infusion can be reduced and the intravenous fluids changed to 5% dextrose. Serum potassium should be monitored hourly and replacement begun when hypokalemia develops. Sodium bicarbonate should not be used to correct acidosis unless the initial blood pH is less than 7.1.

Table 11-8
Continuous Insulin Infusion Guidelines

1. Place 1 mL of U100 regular insulin in 100 mL of normal saline for a concentration of 1 U/mL
2. Preflush intravenous tubing to allow adherence of insulin to plastic
3. IVAC or IMED pump (or even pediatric)
4. Give 0.2 unit/kg as IV bolus and give 0.1 unit/kg/h as continuous drip
5. Expect initial drop in blood glucose from rehydration and then approximately 10% drop from original blood glucose level each hour (e.g., 50–70 mg/dL/h)
6. Monitor blood glucose at 1 h and then every 2–4 h. Plasma electrolytes should be checked every 2–6 h until stable
7. Double rate of infusion or shift to alternative protocol if blood glucose does not fall in 2 h
8. Stop insulin infusion when blood glucose reaches 250 ± mg/dL and change intravenous solution to contain 5% dextrose
9. Because of short half-life of intravenous insulin, insulin (regular or regular plus lente or NPH) must be given 20–30 min before discontinuing insulin infusion. Dosage adjusted according to duration of diabetes, degree of ketoacidosis, age of patient, body size, known sensitivity to insulin, amount of insulin given so far in treatment, or other factors affecting amount of insulin needed (pregnancy, renal failure, ongoing infection, etc.)

Hyperosmolar Nonketotic Coma. Hyperosmolar, nonketotic coma (HNKC) is characterized by extreme hyperglycemia, severe dehydration, and marked hyperosmolarity without ketoacidosis. This condition is usually seen in elderly patients with non-insulin-dependent diabetes precipitated by infection or stress. It may also be seen in nondiabetic obese patients and may be induced in both diabetic and nondiabetic patients by drugs such as diazoxide and phenytoin. It is also a recognized complication of TPN using hypertonic glucose solutions. The clinical presentation may be marked by the presence of obtundation, coma, seizures, or even transient hemiplegia. Blood glucose is often in excess of 1000 mg/dL and serum osmolality greater than 375 mOsm/kg. Fluid and insulin therapy is similar to that of DKA, though the fluid deficits in HNKC are usually much greater (> 10 L). Because of the massive fluid deficit and the advanced age of the affected patients, it is recommended that one-third of the fluid deficit be replaced in the first 8 h of therapy, another third during the next 16 h, and the remainder during the following 24 h.

Hypoglycemia. The most common causes of hypoglycemia are insulin overdose and prolonged effects of oral hypoglycemic agents. Hypoglycemia may also be a manifestation of severe pancreatic insufficiency, acute fulminant hepatic failure, acute adrenal insufficiency, and insulinoma. Symptoms are usually evident at blood glucose levels less than 50 mg/dL, and clinical findings may include mild confusion, somnolence, obtundation, coma, seizures, diaphoresis, hypotension, arrhythmias, and cardiac arrest. A definitive diagnosis is made rapidly by using fingerstick capillary glucose measurements. Mild symptoms may be treated with a 10% dextrose infusion, while more severe symptoms such as coma should be treated with an intravenous bolus of 50 mL of 50% dextrose. Identification and correction of the underlying cause should be performed if possible.

Thyroid Storm and Myxedema Coma

Both hyperthyroidism and hypothyroidism can predispose patients to the development of potentially severe metabolic derangements precipitated by stress events such as infection, surgery, or trauma.

Thyroid Storm. Thyroid storm or thyrotoxic crisis is a relatively uncommon event representing an acute exacerbation of hyperthyroidism. It occurs in patients with existing thyrotoxicosis and may be precipitated by a number of agents and events. These include surgery, trauma, infection, congestive heart failure, bowel infarction, pulmonary embolism, ketoacidosis, hypoglycemia, cerebrovascular accidents, parturition, and iodinated contrast agents. Potential iatrogenic causes of thyroid storm also include the sudden withdrawal of antithyroid medication and the abrupt administration of iodides without antithyroid drugs. The patient with undiagnosed hyperthyroidism undergoing operation is at greatest risk, but the condition may occur in patients with known hyperthyroidism despite adequate preoperative preparation (see Chap. 36).

High fever, tachycardia, and mental status changes are the most prominent symptoms. Mental status changes are a distinguishing diagnostic feature and include intense irritability, confusion, delirium, or coma. Hyperthermia may be as high as 42.2°C. Tachycardia may deteriorate into tachyrhythmia and high-output cardiac failure. Hypotension is a preterminal event, and irreversible cardiovascular collapse is the most common cause of death. Gastrointestinal hypermotility can cause nausea, vomiting, diarrhea, and abdominal pain in some patients.

Immediate supportive therapy using oxygen, fluid hydration with glucose-containing fluids, and fever reduction with external cooling and acetaminophen (aspirin is contraindicated) is begun. In the absence of previous cardiac insufficiency, propranolol 40 to 80 mg orally every 6 h or 1 mg/min intravenously to a maximum of 10 mg can control tachycardia and stabilize the cardiovascular system. If heart failure is present, inotropic agents and diuretics may be indicated. Propylthiouracil (PTU) 200 mg and potassium iodide 5 to 10 drops are both given orally every 8 h to decrease triiodothyronine (T_3) and thyroxine (T_4) production and release. Hydrocortisone 200 mg intravenous and 100 mg every 8 h is also given to diminish thyroid hormone release. While improvements in supportive care have decreased mortality, the death rate in thyrotoxic crises remains 10 to 20 percent.

Postoperative Myxedema Coma. This is a rare, but potentially fatal variant of hypothyroidism that bears a mortality rate of 50 percent. The condition affects patients with chronic hypothyroidism whose disease is poorly treated or unrecognized. A number of inciting factors have been identified including general anesthesia, surgery, trauma, infection, gastrointestinal bleeding, congestive heart failure, cold exposure, and drugs, particularly narcotics, phenothiazines, and sedatives. Classic findings include hypothermia with temperatures less than 32.2°C, hypoventilation, sinus bradycardia, and coma. Other neurologic signs such as psychoses, obtundation, or seizures may precede the development of coma. Hypotension is present in one-half of patients. Hypoglycemia and hyponatremia may also be present.

Diagnosis is based on clinical suspicion and confirmed by determinations of serum levels of T_4, thyroid-stimulating hormone (TSH), and serum cortisol. In most institutions, therapy cannot await laboratory confirmation of the diagnosis. Supportive care with hydration, glucose, assisted ventilation, and identification and treatment of precipitating factors is begun immediately. Hypothermia is treated by the prevention of heat loss, since the vasodilation and increased metabolism caused by active rewarming may exacerbate hypotension. The administration of an intravenous bolus of L-thyroxine 300 to 500 μg is recommended, followed by 50 to 100 μg/day. Although adrenal insufficiency is rarely associated with myxedema coma, the use of hydrocortisone 100 mg intravenously with thyroxine is recommended to prevent potential Addisonian crises.

Postoperative Adrenal Insufficiency

Conditions of stress such as those experienced during the perioperative period can precipitate potentially life-threatening adrenal crises in patients with an impaired ability to produce endogenous corticosteroids. In surgical practice this complication most commonly arises in patients receiving chronic exogenous corticosteroids when steroid therapy is withdrawn too rapidly or when there is a failure to increase steroid doses during periods of stress. Corticosteroid doses equivalent to 5 mg of prednisone daily for 2 months is sufficient to suppress the pituitary-adrenal axis. While doses of less than 10 mg of prednisone daily for less than 7 days rarely results in suppression, even brief courses of higher doses may be sufficient to induce adrenal insufficiency. While the period of adrenal recovery may vary according to the dosages and duration of steroid therapy, note that diminished adrenal responsiveness may persist for as long as 1 year after steroid therapy is discontinued.

Inadequate cortisol production may result from a number of other causes that result in destruction of the adrenal gland, or the loss of ACTH stimulation. Those of relevance to surgical patients include bilateral adrenalectomy, Addison's disease, advanced carcinoma metastases to the adrenal glands, and drug therapy. Rarely, bilateral adrenal hemorrhage may affect critically ill patients with overwhelming sepsis or those with coagulopathies or who are receiving anticoagulant therapy.

The major manifestations of acute adrenal insufficiency are fever, unexplained hypotension, and abdominal pain. Other nonspecific findings include light-headedness, weakness, nausea, vomiting, palpitations, and mental status changes. If adrenal hemorrhage has occurred, bilateral flank or back pain may be present. Though hyponatremia, hyperkalemia, and hypoglycemia compose the classic chemical abnormalities associated with adrenal failure, serum electrolytes may be normal during an abrupt episode or masked by the effects of vomiting or intravenous fluid hydration. The diagnosis of adrenal insufficiency is most likely to be missed after trauma or operation because many of the symptoms may be attributed to other causes such as sepsis or hypovolemia. A high degree of clinical suspicion is necessary to make the diagnosis and effect timely treatment. The morbidity and mortality associated with adrenal crises are due to the effects of prolonged hypotension and hypoglycemia resulting in irreversible central nervous system, cardiac, pulmonary, and renal injury.

In the situation of unexplained hypotension with the manifestations noted above, the immediate administration of hydrocortisone 200 mg intravenous may be lifesaving. If possible, blood sampling for measurements of serum cortisol, electrolytes, and glucose should be done prior to dosing; however, therapy should begin before results are available. Hydration with normal saline with dextrose should also be used. If the diagnosis is correct, hypotension should clearly improve within 1 to 2 h. Hydrocortisone 400 mg/day in divided doses should be given for the first 24 h, and the dose reduced slowly by 50 mg/day until a maintenance level is reached. The primary cause of the adrenal insufficiency should be sought.

In patients at risk, adrenal crises are prevented by a simple perioperative steroid therapy regimen. Hydrocortisone hemisuccinate or phosphate (hydrolyzable form) 100 mg intravenous bolus is given before anesthetic induction and dosing and is repeated every 6 to 8 h for the first day. In the absence of continuing stressful conditions such as sepsis, the dose should be reduced by 50 percent each day until the maintenance dose is achieved. Patients receiving high doses for prolonged periods may require slower tapering to avoid acute psychotic depression.

PSYCHIATRIC COMPLICATIONS

Delirium, dementia, depression, and functional psychoses are a number of psychiatric disorders that may complicate the postoperative course. In the few available studies, there is evidence that the prevalence of psychiatric disorders in surgical patients is remarkably high. The incidence of psychiatric illness in surgical patients before operation is estimated to be approximately 3 percent, but up to one-third of patients may be affected following operation. The incidence of each disorder in a survey of three studies is as follows: delirium in 20 percent, depression in 9 percent, dementia in 3 percent, and functional psychosis in 2 percent.

Cognitive function is defined as the process of knowing via perception, memory, imagining, and reasoning. In surgical patients, the loss or deterioration of cognitive function is most likely due to delirium but may also be caused by depression, organic mental disorders, or functional disorders. Fields and associates prospectively studied 116 medical patients and reported in-hospital mortality and morbidity rates of 17 and 39 percent, respectively, in patients identified to be cognitively ''impaired'' versus 5 percent and 18 percent in patients who were cognitively intact. The higher morbidity was attributed to respiratory complications. While the higher mortality noted in this study may be due to more severe primary illnesses in the cognitively impaired group, earlier studies have also reported mortality rates to be two to three times higher in patients with impaired cognitive function.

Delirium. Postoperative delirium is the most common psychiatric complication following surgery. Delirium is a transient organic mental disorder marked by an acute onset, global impairment of cognitive functions, and widespread disturbance of cerebral metabolism and is a signal of potentially life-threatening organic disturbance. Historically, the term delirium has been used in general reference to acute mental disorders in which consciousness is impaired and perceptual abnormalities are evident. Commonly used terms such as acute organic brain syndrome, cardiac psychosis, and ICU psychosis indicate etiology of delirium but do not necessarily describe distinctive syndromes and should be abandoned.

The onset of delirium is rapid, occasionally occurring immediately after operation but more commonly following a lucid interval of several days. The hyperactive variant of delirium is characterized by agitation, restlessness, irritability, belligerence, and, often, delusions and hallucinations. The hypoactive variant is characterized by quiet withdrawal, apathy, or somnolence. In the same patient, fluctuation between these variants during the course of delirium may occur. In addition to disturbances in the level of consciousness, patients exhibit difficulties in maintaining attention and concentration; are disoriented to time, place, or person; and have disturbance of their sleep-wake cycle. Thinking is disorganized and marked by rambling, irrelevant, or incoherent speech.

As the syndrome progresses, fluctuations in attention, perception, and intellectual functioning occur. Perceptual abnormalities commonly include illusions, hallucinations, and odd or transient physical sensations, symptoms that tend to be worse during evening hours. This phenomenon may indicate abnormal responses to environmental stimuli worsened in dim lighting and a possible explanation of the ''sundowning'' effect. Urinary incontinence, loss of motor coordination, ataxia, tremor, bilateral asterixis, and multifocal clonus may be noted. Mood disturbances may cause affective lability with crying, outbursts of panic, apathy, or depression. Such behavior may be confused with dementia or mood disorders such as depression; however, in these conditions mood changes almost always occur in clear consciousness as opposed to delirium. Electroencephalography may be helpful in diagnosis.

The etiology of delirium is multifactorial, and once the diagnosis is suspected, a complete search for contributing factors must be made (Table 11-9). Attention should be paid to drugs and drug combinations, particularly those with anticholinergic properties, cardiovascular medications, narcotics, other analgesics, and psychoactive medications such as tranquilizers and sedatives. Metabolic and physiologic disturbances such as hypoglycemia, uremia,

Table 11-9
Precipitating Organic Causes of Delirium

Drug intoxication: Anticholinergics, alcohol, analgesics, anesthesia, antiparkinsonian agents, antidepressants, antihistamines, anticonvulsants, cimetidine, digitalis, neuroleptics, sedative-hypnotics, anxiolytics
Drug withdrawal: Alcohol, sedative-hypnotics, anxiolytics
Metabolic disturbances: Electrolyte, fluid, or acid-base imbalance; hypoglycemia; hepatic or renal failure; endocrine disorders; hypothermia; paraneoplasm
Acute cerebral disorders: Edema, fat emboli, transient ischemic attack, stroke, vasculitis, epilepsy, primary or metastatic neoplasm
Infections: Pneumonia, septicemia, urinary tract infection, meningitis, bacterial endocarditis
Hemodynamic disturbance: Hypovolemia, hypotension, anemia, myocardial infarction, arrhythmia, congestive heart failure, hypertensive encephalopathy, orthostatic hypotension
Respiratory disorders: Respiratory failure, pulmonary embolus
Nutritional and vitamin deficiency
Trauma: Burns, fractures, head injury

SOURCE: Monks R, 1991, with permission.

hyperammonemia, hypoxia, acidosis, and endocrinopathies are often manifested by delirium. Sepsis, hemodynamic disturbances, and acute cerebral disorders or trauma must also be considered. Withdrawal syndromes from alcohol, benzodiazepines, and barbiturates are often indistinguishable from one another and are another possible cause of delirium.

The treatment of delirium includes the management of agitation, treatment of underlying or precipitating factors, and the correction of exacerbating conditions. For agitation associated with delirium, in general, the neuroleptic agent haloperidol is the drug of choice. Mild agitation may only require 2 to 15 mg orally twice daily. Urgent situations may require doses of 1 to 5 mg intravenously followed by doses increased by 5 to 10 mg hourly until clinical response is achieved. Less acute situations may respond to 2 to 10 mg intramuscularly each hour until agitation is controlled. Hourly doses should be held if systolic blood pressure is less than 100 mmHg. Once the patient's behavior is controlled, haloperidol should be administered via the oral route. Significant side effects of haloperidol are extrapyramidal symptoms that are relieved with parenteral benztropine.

In delirium associated with anticholinergic agents, hepatic failure, and alcohol or drug withdrawal, a neuroleptic agent is not the drug of choice and alternate management is recommended. The treatment of delirium also requires supportive care. The hospital environment should be made familiar by consistent care routines, encouraged contact with family members, and regular interaction with staff members. Visual and auditory impairments and communication deficits should be corrected if possible. Sleep deprivation must be corrected and adequate analgesia provided. The surgeon can lend further support through calm and reassuring patient education of the expected course of events, focusing on topics such as procedures, potential complications, pain and pain management, and by allowing the patient open expression of his or her fear or concerns to reduce anxiety.

The preoperative identification of patients at risk for developing delirium, in combination with early intervention, may avert the complication or reduce the severity of the episode. Certain risk factors appear to increase the risk of the development of psychiatric complications in surgical patients such as advanced age or chronic renal, hepatic, or cardiac disease. Perhaps the greatest risk arises from a prior history of psychiatric illness or behavioral disorder. In these individuals, specific preparatory measures should include (1) a review of the management of the psychiatric illness, (2) assurance of therapeutic blood levels of medications such as lithium, (3) the simplification of drug regimens with the discontinuation of unnecessary agents, (4) preempting of potential withdrawal in patients with alcohol or drug dependency using sedatives or anxiolytic agents, and (5) correct visual and auditory defects if possible to optimize sensory function. Preoperative preparation and instruction about management and coping with the stress of operation improves recovery and reduces the episodes of postoperative delirium.

Depression. Depressed feelings and thoughts are not uncommon in the postoperative patient and represent reactions to the stresses and losses that may occur in the surgical experience. Persistent and pervasive mood disturbances should raise the suspicion of the possibility of either delirium or major depression. A prior history of major depressive episodes or a strong family history may be present. In addition to a depressed mood, there is a significant change in appetite, fatigue and loss of energy, and a disturbed sleep pattern. Psychomotor agitation may be present, though retardation is more common with slowed speech, decreased spontaneity of communication and movement, and a diminished content of speech. Cognitive impairment is evidenced by feelings of worthlessness, excessive guilt, and recurrent thoughts of death or suicide.

Mild forms of depression may respond to supportive measures alone, but in the presence of cognitive impairment, tricyclic antidepressants or even electroconvulsive therapy are recommended.

Bibliography

Fever

Freischlag J, Busuttil RW: The value of postoperative fever evaluation. *Surgery* 94:358, 1983.

Galicier C, Richet H: A prospective study of postoperative fever in a general surgery department. *Infect Control* 6:487, 1985.

Garibaldi RA, Brodine S, Matsumiya S: Evidence for the non-infectious etiology of early postoperative fever. *Infect Control* 6:273, 1985.

Howard RJ: Finding the cause of postoperative fever. *Postgrad Med* 85:223, 1988.

Ledger WJ, Child MA: The hospital care of patients undergoing hysterectomy: An analysis of 12,026 patients from the Professional Activity Study. *Am J Obstet Gynecol* 117:423, 1973.

Swartz WH, Tanaree P: Suction drainage as an alternative to prophylactic antibiotics for hysterectomy. *Obstet Gynecol* 45:305, 1975.

Yeung RS, Buck JR, Filler RM: The significance of fever following operations in children. *J Pediatr Surg* 17:347, 1982.

Wound Complications

Alexander JW, Fischer JE, et al.: The influence of hair-removal methods on wound infections. *Arch Surg* 118:347, 1983.

Arbeit JM, Hilaris BS, Brennan MF: Wound complications in the multimodality treatment of extremity and superficial truncal sarcomas. *J Clin Oncol* 5:480, 1987.

Coit DG, Scalfani L: Care of the surgical wound, in Wilmore DW, Brennan ME, Harken AH (eds): *Care of the Surgical Patient.* New York, Scientific American, 1990, vol II, chap 7.

Cruse PJE, Foord R: The epidemiology of wound infection: A 10 year study of 62,939 wounds. *Surg Clin North Am* 60:27, 1980.

Davidson AIG, Clark C, Smith G: Postoperative wound infection: A computer analysis. *Br J Surg* 58:333, 1971.

Ferguson MK: The effect of antineoplastic agents on wound healing. *Surg Gynecol Obstet* 154:421, 1982.

Galandiuk S, Polk HC, Jagelman DG: Re-emphasis of priorities in surgical antibiotic prophylaxis. *Surg Gynecol Obstet* 169:219, 1989.

Garcia-Rodriguez JA, Puig-LaCalle J, Arnau C: Antibiotic prophylaxis with cefotaxime in gastroduodenal and biliary surgery. *Am J Surg* 158:428, 1989.

Haley RW, Culver DH, Morgan WM, et al.: Identifying patients at high risk of surgical wound infection: A simple multivariate index of patient susceptibility and wound contamination. *Am J Epidemiol* 121:206, 1985.

Hayden RE, Paniello RC, Yeung CST: The effect of glutathione and vitamins A, C, and E on acute skin flap survival. *Laryngoscope* 97:1176, 1987.

Haydock DA, Hill GL: Impaired wound healing in surgical patients with varying degrees of malnutrition. *JPEN* 10:550, 1986.

Hillelson RL, Glowacks J, Healey NA, et al.: Microangiographic study of hematoma formation associated flap necrosis and salvage with isoxsuprine. *Plast Reconst Surg* 66:528, 1980.

Hunt TK: Surgical wound infection: An overview. *Am J Med* 70:712, 1981.

Irvin TT, Koffman CG, Duthie HL: Layer closure of laparotomy wounds with absorbable and non-absorbable suture materials. *Br J Surg* 63:793, 1976.

Klausner JM, Lelcuk S, Inbar M: The effects of perioperative fluorouracil administration on convalescence and wound healing. *Arch Surg* 121:239, 1986.

Knight CD, Griffen FD: Abdominal wound closure with a continuous monofilament polypropylene suture. *Arch Surg* 118:1305, 1983.

Knight CD, Martin JK, Welch JS, et al.: Surgical considerations after chemotherapy and radiation therapy for inflammatory breast cancer. *Surgery* 99:385, 1986.

Knighton DR, Halliday B, Hunt TK: Oxygen as an antibiotic: A comparison of the effects of inspired oxygen concentration and antibiotic administration on in vivo bacterial clearance. *Arch Surg* 121:191, 1986.

Olson M, O'Connor M, Schwartz ML: Surgical wound infections: A 5-year prospective study of 20,193 wounds at the Minneapolis VA Medical Center. *Ann Surg* 199:253, 1984.

Ormsby MV, Hilaris BS, et al.: Wound complications of adjuvant radiation therapy in patients with soft-tissue sarcomas. *Ann Surg* 210:93, 1989.

Polk HC Jr, Lopez-Mayor JF: Postoperative wound infection: A prospective study of determinant factors and prevention. *Surgery* 66:97, 1969.

Report of an Ad Hoc Committee of the Committee on Trauma, Division of Medical Sciences, National Academy of Sciences–National Research Council: Postoperative wound infections: The influence of ultraviolet irradiation of the operating room and of various other factors. *Ann Surg* 160(suppl):1, 1964.

Richards PC, Balch CM, Aldrete JS: Abdominal wound closure: A randomized prospective study of 571 patients comparing continuous vs. interrupted suture techniques. *Ann Surg* 197:238, 1983.

Rowe-Jones DC, Peel ALG, et al.: Single dose cefotaxime plus metronidazole versus three dose cefuroxime plus metronidazole as prophylaxis against wound infection in colorectal surgery: Multicentre prospective randomised study. *Br Med J* 300:18, 1990.

Seymour DG, Vaz FG: A prospective study of elderly general surgical patients: II. Postoperative complications. *Age Ageing* 18:316, 1989.

Tadych K, Donegan WL: Postmastectomy seromas and wound drainage. *Surg Gynecol Obstet* 165:483, 1987.

Taren DL, Chvapil M, Weber CW: Increasing the breaking strength of wounds exposed to preoperative irradiation using vitamin E supplementation. *Int J Vitam Nutr Res* 57:133, 1987.

Urinary and Renal Complications

Anderson JB, Grant JBF: Postoperative retention of urine: A prospective urodynamic study. *Br Med J* 302:13, 1991.

Bowers FJ, Hartmann R, et al.: Urecholine prophylaxis for urinary retention in anorectal surgery. *Dis Colon Rectum* 30:41, 1987.

Brown CB, Ogg CS, Cameron JS: High dose furosemide in acute renal failure: A controlled clinical trial. *Clin Nephrol* 15:90, 1981.

Goldman G, Leviav A, et al.: Alpha-adrenergic blocker for posthernioplasty urinary retention: Prevention and treatment. *Arch Surg* 123:35, 1988.

Petersen MS, Collins DN, et al.: Postoperative urinary retention associated with total hip and total knee arthroplasties. *Clin Orthop* 269:102, 1991.

Petros JG, Bradley TM: Factors influencing postoperative urinary retention inpatients undergoing surgery for benign anorectal disease. *Am J Surg* 159:374, 1990.

Petros JG, Rimm EB, et al.: Factors influencing postoperative urinary retention in patients undergoing elective inguinal herniorrhaphy. *Am J Surg* 161:431, 1991.

Pritchard TJ, Bloom AD, Zollinger RM Jr: Pitfalls in ambulatory treatment of inguinal hernias in adults. *Surg Clin North Am* 71:1353, 1991.

Respiratory Complications

Becquemin JP, Piquet J, et al.: Pulmonary function after transverse or midline incision in patients with obstructive pulmonary disease. *Intensive Care Med* 11:247, 1985.

Bersten AD, Holt AW, Vedig AE: Treatment of severe cardiogenic pulmonary edema with continuous positive airway pressure delivered by face mask. *N Engl J Med* 325:1826, 1991.

Chan KM, Tham KT, et al.: Post-traumatic fat embolism: Its clinical and subclinical presentations. *J Trauma* 24:45, 1984.

Cuchieri RJ, Morran CG, et al.: Postoperative pain and pulmonary complications: Comparison of three analgesic regimens. *Br J Surg* 72:495, 1985.

Fegiz G: Prevention by ambroxol of bronchopulmonary complications after upper abdominal surgery: Double-blind Italian multicenter clinical study versus placebo. *Lung* 169:69, 1991.

Greenbaum DM, Millen JE, et al.: Continuous positive pressure without tracheal intubation in spontaneously breathing patients. *Chest* 69:615, 1976.

Kigin CM: Chest physical therapy for the postoperative or traumatic injury patient. *Phys Ther* 61:1724, 1981.

Massucci M, Louis D, et al.: Approach to the abdominal aortic: Impairment of respiratory function after supraumbilical transverse and midline laparotomy. *Ital J Surg Sci* 19:247, 1989.

O'Donohue WJ Jr: National survey of the usage of lung expansion modalities for the prevention and treatment of postoperative atelectasis following abdominal and thoracic surgery. *Chest* 87:76, 1985.

Peltier LF: Fat embolism: An appraisal of the problem. *Clin Orthop* 187:3, 1984.

Ratliff JL: Bronchoscopy in respiratory care. *Surg Clin North Am* 60:1497, 1980.

Roukema JA, Carol EJ, Prins JG: The prevention of pulmonary complications after upper abdominal surgery inpatients with noncompromised pulmonary status. *Arch Surg* 123:30, 1988.

Seidenfeld JJ, Pohl DF, et al.: Incidence, site, and outcome of infections in patients with the adult respiratory distress syndrome. *Am Rev Respir Dis* 134:12, 1986.

Strandberg A, Tokics L, et al.: Atelectasis during anaesthesia and in the postoperative period. *Acta Anaesthesiol Scand* 30:154, 1986.

ten Duis HJ, Nijsten MWN, et al.: Fat embolism in patients with an isolated fracture of the femoral shaft. *J Trauma* 28:383, 1988.

Van Besouw JP, Hinds CJ: Fat embolism syndrome. *Br J Hosp Med* 42:304, 1989.

Cardiac Complications

Asiddao CB, Donegan JH, et al.: Factors associated with perioperative complications during carotid endarterectomy. *Anesth Analg* 61:631, 1982.

Bertrand CA, Steiner NU, Jameson AG, et al.: Disturbances of cardiac rhythm during anesthesia and surgery. *JAMA* 216:1615, 1971.

Buckley JJ, Jackson JA: Postoperative cardiac arrythmias. *Anesthesiology* 22:723, 1961.

Cooperman M, Pflug B, et al.: Cardiovascular risk factors in patients with peripheral vascular disease. *Surgery* 84:505, 1978.

Emergency Cardiac Care Committee, American Heart Association: Part III. Adult advanced cardiac life support. *JAMA* 268:2199, 1992.

Foster ED, David KB, et al.: Risk of noncardiac operation in patients with defined coronary disease: The Coronary Artery Surgery Study (CASS) registry experience. *Ann Thorac Surg* 41:42, 1986.

Golden MA, Whittemore AD, et al.: Selective evaluation and management of coronary artery disease in patients undergoing repair of abdominal aortic aneurysm: A 16-year experience. *Ann Surg* 211:415, 1990.

Goldman L: Cardiac risks and complications of noncardiac surgery. *Ann Surg* 198:780, 1983.

Goldman L, Caldera DL: Risks of general anesthesia and elective operation in the hypertensive patient. *Anesthesiology* 50:285, 1979.

Goldman L, Caldera DL, et al.: Multifactorial index of cardiac risk in noncardiac surgical procedures. *N Engl J Med* 297:845, 1977.

Houston M: Pathophysiology, clinical aspects, and treatment of hypertensive crises. *Prog Cardiovasc Dis* 32:99, 1989.

Krowka MJ, Pairolero PC, et al.: Cardiac dysrhythmia following pneumonectomy: clinical correlates and prognostic significance. *Chest* 91:490, 1987.

Kuner J, Enescu V, Utsu F, et al.: Cardiac arrythmias during anesthesia. *Dis Chest* 52:580, 1967.

Mangano DT, Browner WS, et al.: Association of perioperative myocardial ischemia with cardiac morbidity and mortality in men undergoing noncardiac surgery. *N Engl J Med* 323:1781, 1990.

Mangano DT: Perioperative cardiac morbidity. *Anesthesiology* 72:153, 1990.

Mangano DT, Hollenberg M, et al.: Perioperative myocardial ischemia in patients undergoing noncardiac surgery. I. Incidence and severity during the 4 day perioperative period. *J Am Coll Cardiol* 17:843, 1991.

Mangano DT, Wong MG, et al.: Perioperative myocardial ischemia in patients undergoing noncardiac surgery. II. Incidence and severity during the 1st week after surgery. *J Am Coll Cardiol* 17:851, 1991.

Martin DE, Kammerer WS: The hypertensive surgical patient. *Surg Clin North Am* 63:1017, 1983.

Mowry FM, Reynolds EW: Cardiac rhythm disturbances complicating resectional surgery of the lung. *Ann Intern Med* 61:688, 1964.

Ouyang P, Gerstenblith G, et al.: Frequency and significance of early postoperative silent myocardial ischemia in patients having peripheral vascular surgery. *Am J Cardiol* 64:1113, 1989.

Pasternack PF, Imparato AM, Riles TS, et al.: The value of the radionuclide angiogram in the prediction of perioperative myocardial infarction in patients undergoing lower extremity revascularization procedures. *Circulation* 72(suppl II):II-13, 1985.

Prys-Roberts C, Meloche R, Foex P: Studies of anaesthesia in relation to hypertension. I. Cardiovascular responses of treated and untreated patients. *Br J Anaesth* 43:122, 1971.

Rao TK, Jacobs KH, El-Etr AA: Reinfarction following anesthesia in patients with myocardial infarction. *Anesthesiology* 59:499, 1983.

Shields TW, Ujiki GT: Digitalization for prevention of arrhythmias following pulmonary surgery. *Surg Gynecol Obstet* 126:743, 1968.

Steen PA, Tinker JH, Tarhan S: Myocardial reinfarction after anesthesia and surgery. *JAMA* 239:2566, 1978.

Tarhan S, Moffitt EA, et al.: Myocardial infarction after general anesthesia. *Anesth Analg* 56:455, 1977.

Towne JB, Bernhard VM: The relationship of postoperative hypertension to complications following carotid endarterectomy. *Surgery* 88:575, 1980.

Wells P, Kaplan JA: Optional management of patients with ischemic heart disease for noncardiac surgery by complementary anesthesiologist and cardiologist interaction. *Am Heart J* 102:1029, 1981.

Hypercoagulable States

Bauer KA: Pathobiology of the hypercoagulable state: Clinical features, laboratory evaluation, and management, in Hoffman R, Benz EJ, et al. (eds): *Hematology: Basic Principles and Practice*. New York, Churchill Livingstone, 1991, chap 116.

Kakkasseril JS, Cranley JJ, et al.: Heparin-induced thrombocytopenia: A prospective study of 142 patients. *J Vasc Surg* 2:382, 1985.

Laster J, Cikrit D, et al.: The heparin-induced thrombocytopenia syndrome: An update. *Surgery* 102:763, 1987.

Rizzoni WE, Miller K, et al.: Heparin-induced thrombocytopenia and thromboembolism in the postoperative period. *Surgery* 103:470, 1988.

Sobel M, Adelman B, Szentpetery S: Surgical management of heparin-associated thrombocytopenia. *J Vasc Surg* 8:395, 1988.

Complications of Gastrointestinal Surgery

Anselmi M, Landberg S, et al.: Assessment of the biliary tract after liver transplantation: T-tube cholangiography or IODIDA scanning. *Br J Surg* 77:1233, 1990.

Anthanassiades S, Notis P, Tountas C: Fistulas of the gastrointestinal tract: Experience with eighty-one cases. *Am J Surg* 130:26, 1975.

Ashall G: Closure of upper gastrointestinal fistulas using a Roux-en-Y technique. *J R Coll Surg Edinb* 31:151, 1986.

Di Costanzano J, Cano N, et al.: Treatment of external gastrointestinal fistulas by a combination of total parenteral nutrition and somatostatin. *JPEN* 11:465, 1987.

Fazio VW, Church JM, et al.: Colocutaneous fistulas complicating diverticulitis. *Dis Colon Rectum* 30:89, 1987.

Hill G: Operative strategy in the treatment of enterocutaneous fistulas. *World J Surg* 7:498, 1983.

Hollender L, Meyer C, et al.: Prospective fistulas of the small intestine: Therapeutic principles. *World J Surg* 7:474, 1983.

Joehl RJ, Nahrwold DL: Inhibition of human pancreatic secretion by terbutaline as a potential agent for treating patients with pancreatic fistula. *Surg Gynecol Obstet* 160:109, 1985.

Martin FM, Rossi RL, et al.: Management of pancreatic fistulas. *Arch Surg* 124:571, 1989.

McKenzie G: Extravasation of bile after operations on the biliary tract. *Aust N Z J Surg* 24:181, 1955.

Nahrwold D: Complications of biliary tract surgery and trauma, in Greenfield L (ed): *Complications in Surgery and Trauma,* 2d ed. Philadelphia, JB Lippincott, 1990, chap 35.

Nubiola P, Badia J, et al.: Enterocutaneous fistulas with long half-life somatostatin analogue SMS 201–995. *Ann Surg* 210:56, 1989.

Nubiola P, Sancho J, et al.: Blind evaluation of the effect of octreotide (SMS 201–995), a somatostatin analogue, on small bowel fistula output. *Lancet* 11:672, 1987.

Pearlstein L, Jones CE, Polk HC: Gastrocutaneous fistula: Etiology and treatment. *Ann Surg* 187:223, 1978.

Pederzoli R, Bassi C, et al.: Conservative treatment of external pancreatic fistulas with parenteral nutrition alone or in combination with continuous intravenous infusion of somatostatin, glucagon or calcitonin. *Surg Gynecol Obstet* 163:428, 1986.

Prinz RA, Pickelman J, Hoffman JP: Treatment of pancreatic cutaneous fistulas with a somatostatin analog. *Am J Surg* 155:36, 1988.

Reber HA, Roberts C, et al.: Management of gastrointestinal fistulas. *Ann Surg* 188:460, 1978.

Rombeau J, Rolandelli R: Enteral and parenteral nutrition in patients with enteric fistulas and short bowel syndrome. *Surg Clin North Am* 67:557, 1987.

Rosato F: Gallstone ileus and fistula, in Sabiston D (ed): *Textbook of Surgery,* 14th ed, Philadelphia, WB Saunders, 1991, chap 34.

Rosato FE, Berkowitz HD, Roberts B: Bile ascites. *Surg Gynecol Obstet* 130:494, 1970.

Rubelowsky J, Machiedo GW: Reoperative versus conservative management for gastrointestinal fistulas. *Surg Clin North Am* 71:147, 1991.

Saari A, Schröder T, Kivilaakso E, et al.: Treatment of pancreatic fistulas with somatostatin and total parenteral nutrition. *Scand J Gastroenterol* 24:859, 1989.

Soeters PB, Ebeid AM, Fischer JE: Review of 404 patients with gastrointestinal fistulas: Impact of parenteral nutrition. *Ann Surg* 190:189, 1979.

Spiliotis J, Vagenas K, et al.: Treatment of enterocutaneous fistulas with TPN and somatostatin, compared with patients who received TPN only. *Br J Clin Prac* 44:616, 1990.

Zajko AB, Campbell WL, et al.: Diagnostic and interventional radiology in liver transplantation. *Gastroenterol Clin North Am* 17:105, 1988.

Zinner MJ, Baker RR, Cameron JL: Pancreatic cutaneous fistulas. *Surg Gynecol Obstet* 138:710, 1974.

Metabolic Complications

Caldwell M: Diabetes mellitus, in Wilmore DW, Brennan MF, Harken AH, et al. (eds): *Care of the Surgical Patient*. New York, Scientific American, 1990.

Gavin LA, Bosker G: Reversing hypothyroid coma: Making a quick diagnosis and the right therapeutic choice. *Emerg Med Rep* 6:145, 1985.

Jordan RM: Endocrine emergencies. *Med Clin North Am* 67:1193, 1983.

Kitabchi AE, Murphy MB: Diabetic ketoacidosis and hyperosmolar hyperglycemic nonketotic coma. *Med Clin North Am* 72:1543, 1988.

Marble A, Ferguson BD: Diagnosis and classification of diabetes mellitus and the nondiabetic melliturias, in Marble A, Krall LP, Bradley RF, et al. (eds): *Joslin's Diabetes Mellitus,* 12th ed. Philadelphia, Lea & Febiger, 1985.

Mazzaferri EL: Adult hypothyroidism: II. Causes, laboratory diagnosis and treatment. *Postgrad Med* 79:75, 1986.

Nicoloff JT: Thyroid storm and myxedema coma. *Med Clin North Am* 69:1005, 1985.

Roth RN, McAuliffe MJ: Hyperthyroidism and thyroid storm. *Emerg Med Clin North Am* 7:873, 1989.

Rusnak RA: Adrenal and pituitary emergencies. *Emerg Med Clin N Am* 7:903, 1989.

Steer M, Fromen D: Recognition of adrenal insufficiency in the postoperative patient. *Am J Surg* 139:443, 1980.

Wheelock FC Jr, Gibbons GW, Marble A: Surgery in diabetes, in Marble A, Krall LP, Bradley RF, et al. (eds): *Joslin's Diabetes Mellitus,* 12th ed. Philadelphia, Lea & Febiger, 1985.

Psychiatric Complications

Fields SD, Mackenzie CR, et al.: Cognitive impairment: Can it predict the course of hospitalized patients? *J Am Geriatr Soc* 34:579, 1986.

Golinger RC: Delirium in surgical patients seen at psychiatric consultation. *Surg Gynecol Obstet* 163:104, 1986.

Gollinger RC: Psychiatric complications of surgery, in Greenfield LJ (ed): *Complications in Surgery and Trauma,* 2d ed. Philadelphia, JB Lippincott, 1990, chap 49.

Millar HR: Psychiatric morbidity in elderly surgical patients. *Br J Psychiatry* 138:17, 1981.

Monks R: Cognitive and sensory deficits, in Wilmore DW, Brennan ME, Harken AH, et al. (eds): *Care of the Surgical Patient.* New York, Scientific American, 1991, vol 2, chap 10.

Rabins PV, Folstein MF: Delirium and dementia: Diagnostic criteria and fatality rates. *Br J Psychiatry* 140:149, 1982.

Titchener JL, Zwerling I, et al.: Psychosis in surgical patients. *Surg Gynecol Obstet* 102:59, 1956.

CHAPTER 12

Physiologic Monitoring of the Surgical Patient

Albert J. Varon and Joseph M. Civetta

The primary reason for the surgeon's involvement in bedside critical care is the opportunity to understand and enhance the patient's physiologic response and to recognize and correct the pathophysiologic challenges. To do this effectively, the surgeon must understand physiologic monitoring. Without a thorough knowledge of the physics and methods of monitoring, ensuring the quality of numbers obtained, perceiving their importance, and utilizing measurements as a guide for therapy, selection of proper therapy would be difficult, without foundation, rote, or naive. Thus, there are many stimuli to obtain a fundamental knowledge of physiologic monitoring. This chapter is designed to initiate a lifelong process, one that extends the capabilities of the surgeon, improves patient outcome, and advances surgical science.

HEMODYNAMIC MONITORING

The traditional clinical evaluation, usually the initial assessment tool, is often unreliable in critically ill patients, as there may be major changes in cardiovascular function that are not accompanied by obvious clinical findings. Invasive hemodynamic monitoring at the bedside provides information about cardiorespiratory performance and guides therapy on a rational physiologic basis.

Arterial Catheterization

Indications. Arterial catheterization is indicated whenever there is a need for continuous monitoring of blood pressure and/or frequent sampling of arterial blood. States in which precise and continuous blood pressure data are necessary include shock of any etiology, acute hypertensive crisis, use of potent vasoactive or inotropic drugs, high levels of respiratory support (high intrathoracic pressure), high-risk patients undergoing extensive operations, controlled hypotensive anesthesia, and any situation in which any of the factors affecting cardiac function is rapidly changing. This is particularly true in patients with shock, because indirect measurement of blood pressure by a cuff has been proved inaccurate. Sequential analysis of blood gas tensions and pH is necessary in any acute illness involving cardiovascular or respiratory dysfunction or when hyperventilation is instituted in patients with central nervous system injuries. An indwelling arterial catheter can also provide ready access for other blood samples necessary to chart the progression of multisystemic illness.

Inserting arterial lines is a relatively safe and inexpensive procedure. There are no absolute contraindications to arterial catheterization per se, although bleeding diathesis and anticoagulant therapy may increase the risk of hemorrhagic complications. Severe occlusive arterial disease with distal ischemia, the presence of a vascular prosthesis, and local infection are contraindications to specific sites of catheterization.

Clinical Utility. With an indwelling arterial catheter and monitoring system, the systolic blood pressure (SBP), diastolic blood pressure (DBP), and mean arterial pressure (MAP) can be continuously displayed. The pulse rate can be calculated from the arterial tracing when the electrocardiogram (ECG) is not available (e.g., during electrocautery use in surgery).

Direct measurements of arterial pressure correlate rather poorly with indirect measurements. The disparities are due in part to physiologic considerations but are largely conditioned by the frequency response of the monitoring systems. Because blood pressure trends are probably more important than absolute values, the most important aspect of direct arterial pressure monitoring is that it constantly reminds the clinician to pay attention to the patient, to think about what is happening, and to reason why changes are occurring.

To obtain accurate data when measuring any pressure within the vascular system, the clinician must understand the monitoring system and methods of calibration. Minor details such as the use of long tubing and the presence of air bubbles or blood clots in the system can make the measurements unreliable.

Observation of the arterial pressure waveform obtained with an arterial catheter and monitoring system may permit a qualitative assessment of the patient's cardiovascular status. The shape of the arterial pressure tracing represents a particular stroke volume ejected at a particular state of myocardial contractility. Qualitative interpretation can be made in a hypovolemic patient with a small stroke volume that will create a smaller pressure wave. As intravascular volume is replenished, the stroke volume increases and the arterial pressure tracing will increase in size until it attains normal shape. If myocardial contractility is diminished, the rate of increase in aortic pressure will diminish, and the up slope of the arterial pressure tracing will become less vertical and assume a more tangential trajectory with the apex moved to the right.

Although quantitation of stroke volume has been attempted using computers to solve the equations necessary to relate the shape of the peripheral arterial pressure tracing to actual stroke volume ejected, critical illness introduces too many variables for this measurement to be reliable. The location of the dicrotic notch on the arterial waveform has also been advocated as an indicator of the systemic vascular resistance; however, Gerber and associates were unable to demonstrate any statistically significant correlation.

Analysis of the SBP variation during mechanical ventilation may offer important information about the nature of low-flow states. The normal decrease in SBP after a mechanical breath is more pronounced during hypovolemia but practically nonexistent during congestive heart failure.

Sites of Catheterization. Many anatomic sites have been used to access the arterial circulation for continuous monitoring. The superficial temporal, axillary, brachial, radial, ulnar, femoral, and dorsalis pedis arteries have all been used. Although the selection of anatomic site for arterial catheterization usually has an institutional bias, specific advantages and disadvantages should be considered.

The dual blood supply to the hand and the superficial location of the vessel make the radial artery the most commonly used site for arterial catheterization. Cannulation is technically easy, as is securing the catheter in place, and there is a low incidence of complications. The mean and end-diastolic radial pressures are usually accurate estimates of the corresponding aortic pressures; however, the systolic pressure at the radial artery is often much higher than that of the aorta due to overshoot caused by the resonant behavior of the radial artery. This exaggeration is accentuated in stiff, arteriosclerotic radial arteries.

Most authors recommend assessing the adequacy of collateral circulation before cannulation of the radial artery. The most commonly used test is the modified Allen test. The patient is instructed to elevate one hand, make a fist, and clench it firmly, thus squeezing the blood from the vessels of the hand. After the examiner compresses at the same time both the radial and ulnar arteries, the patient lowers and opens the hand in a relaxed fashion (carefully so as not to overextend it). The examiner then releases the pressure over the ulnar artery, and the time for return of color is noted. It is considered normal if the capillary blush of the hand is complete within 6 s. Other methods such as ultrasonic Doppler technique, plethysmography, and pulse oximetry have also been used to assess the adequacy of the collateral arterial supply.

The axillary artery has been recommended as suitable for long-term direct arterial pressure monitoring. Its use has been associated with relatively few complications and no reported permanent sequelae. The major advantages include its larger size, freedom for the patient's hand, and close proximity to the aorta so that there is better representation of the aortic pressure waveform and minimal systolic pressure overshoot. Pulsation and pressure are maintained even in the presence of shock with marked peripheral vasoconstriction. Also, because of the extensive collateral circulation that exists between the thyrocervical trunk of the subclavian artery and the subscapular artery (which is a branch of the distal axillary artery), thrombosis of the axillary artery will not lead to compromised flow in the distal arm. Major disadvantages are its rather deep location and mobility, which increase the technical difficulty for insertion, and its location within the neurovascular sheath, which may increase the possibility of neurologic compromise if hematoma occurs.

The femoral artery has also been used for continuous blood pressure monitoring. Major advantages are its superficial location and large size, allowing easier localization and cannulation when the pulses over more distal vessels are absent. The major disadvantages are the presence of atherosclerotic occlusive disease in older patients and the problems associated with maintaining a clean dressing in the presence of draining abdominal wounds and ostomies in surgical patients. Furthermore, bleeding at this site may be difficult to control or may occur in an occult manner into the abdomen or thigh. In spite of these potential disadvantages, studies have failed to demonstrate a higher complication rate in patients with femoral artery catheters.

The dorsalis pedis artery has no significant cannulation hazards if collateral flow can be demonstrated to the remainder of the foot through the posterior tibial artery. This can be done by occluding the dorsalis pedis artery and then blanching the great toe by compressing the toenail for several seconds and then releasing while observing return of color. A Doppler technique can also be used. Major disadvantages are its relatively small size (which makes it more difficult to cannulate) and overestimation of systolic pressure at this level.

The superficial temporal artery has been extensively used in infants and in some adults for continuous pressure monitoring. Because of its small size and tortuousity, however, surgical exposure is required for cannulation. Furthermore, a very small but worrisome incidence of neurologic complications due to cerebral embolization has been reported in infants.

The brachial artery is not used often because of the high complication rate associated with its use for cardiac catheterization. Although this artery has been successfully used for short-term monitoring, there is little data to support the use of prolonged brachial artery monitoring. If collateral circulation is inadequate, obstruction of the brachial artery may be catastrophic, leading to loss of the forearm and hand. Other problems include the difficulty in maintaining the site in awake active patients and the possibility of hematoma formation in anticoagulated patients. The latter may lead to median nerve compression neuropathy and Volkmann's contracture.

Complications. Common problems associated with arterial catheterization are failure to cannulate, hematoma formation, and disconnection from the monitoring system with bleeding.

The majority of reports that describe the complications following radial artery cannulation have stressed the high incidence of early radial artery occlusion and the rarity of late ischemic damage. Recannulation of the occluded artery generally occurs but may take several weeks. The incidence of radial artery thrombosis has progressively declined as a result of the understanding of the effects of different catheter size (smaller is better), material (Teflon is better), and of the use of continuous heparin flow instead of intermittent flushing. Factors associated with an increased risk of radial artery occlusion include female gender, low cardiac output states, use of vasoconstrictor drugs, severe peripheral vascular disease, small wrist circumference, insertion by surgical cut-down, multiple puncture attempts, hematoma formation, and increased duration of cannulation.

In 1979, Band and Maki studied infections related to arterial catheterization and determined that the main factors associated with an increased risk of infection were placement of the catheter for more than 4 days, insertion by surgical cut-down rather than percutaneously, and local inflammation. The rate of catheter-related infection was 18 percent and that of catheter-related septicemia was 4 percent. Seventy percent of the catheter-related infections and all septicemias occurred with catheter placements exceeding 4 days. A more recent study by Norwood and associates also supported time of arterial cannulation at a single site as an important factor and reemphasized that the risk for infection for catheter sites used less than 96 h is virtually nonexistent. In the latter study, catheter-related infection developed in 9.5 percent of radial and femoral artery sites used up to 14 days, although the risk of catheter-related septicemia was very low. The authors concluded that these sites could be used for prolonged periods if skin site colonization were controlled with strict local site care.

Other possible complications include retrograde cerebral embolization (when flushing catheters), arteriovenous fistulas, and pseudoaneurysm formation. Finally, inadvertent injection of vasoactive drugs or other agents into an artery can cause severe pain, distal ischemia, and tissue necrosis.

Central Venous Catheterization

Indications. The most common indications for central venous catheterization are to secure access for fluid therapy, drug infusions, or parenteral nutrition, and for central venous pressure (CVP) monitoring. Central venous catheters have also been used to aspirate air in case of embolism during neurosurgical procedures in the sitting position, for placement of cardiac pacemakers or inferior vena cava filters, and for hemodialysis access.

There are no absolute contraindications for CVP catheter placement although bleeding diatheses increase the risk of hemorrhagic complications. Vessel thrombosis, local infection or inflammation, and distortion by trauma or previous surgery are considered contraindications to specific sites of catheterization.

Clinical Utility. While central venous lines are placed primarily for venous access, useful information occasionally can be obtained by measuring the CVP. The CVP may be useful in a hypotensive trauma patient to differentiate a pericardial tamponade from hypovolemia. Analysis of the CVP tracing may also be helpful in the differential diagnosis of certain cardiac arrhythmias (''a'' waves are absent in atrial fibrillation) and in the diagnosis of tricuspid insufficiency (prominent ''v'' waves).

A properly placed catheter can be used to measure right atrial pressure which, in the absence of tricuspid valve disease, will reflect the right ventricular end-diastolic pressure. CVP, therefore, can give information about the relationship between intravascular volume and *right* ventricular function but cannot be used to assess either of these factors independently. CVP cannot be used to assess left ventricular function in critically ill patients, since ventricular disparity and independence of right and left atrial pressure have been confirmed repeatedly in these patients. Furthermore, CVP is only a single parameter, in contradistinction to the more complete information concerning pressures, flow, and venous gas measurements available with pulmonary artery catheters.

When monitoring CVP, the catheter should be attached to a pressure transducer for electronic measurement rather than to a water manometer. Water manometry does not permit visualization of the pressure tracing and cannot provide reliable measurements because of the frequency response limitations of a fluid-filled column that cannot respond to the full range of pressure variations.

Sites of Catheterization. There are many anatomic routes to obtain access to the central venous circulation. The most commonly chosen sites include the subclavian, internal jugular, external jugular, femoral, and brachiocephalic veins. The patient's anatomy and the operator's experience are the major factors influencing site selection.

The subclavian vein can be cannulated with a high rate of success and may be the easiest to cannulate in situations of profound volume depletion. Another advantage of this approach is the ease with which the catheter and the dressings can be secured. Disadvantages include the higher risk of pneumothorax and the inability to compress the vessel if bleeding occurs.

The internal jugular vein has been cannulated with success rates similar to that of the subclavian approach. The major advantages of internal jugular vein catheterization are the lower risk of pneumothorax and the ability to compress the insertion site if bleeding occurs. In addition, the right internal jugular provides a straight path to the superior vena cava, facilitating placement of catheters and pacemakers. The internal jugular vein, however, may be more difficult to cannulate in patients with volume depletion or shock. Fixation and dressing of catheters are also more difficult.

Cannulation of the external jugular vein has a lower incidence of complications but a higher incidence of failure. Since catheters inserted through the neck are more difficult to fix and dress than other sites, this approach is not suitable for prolonged central venous access. Although some studies have shown no higher incidence of complications from femoral cannulation than from subclavian or internal jugular sites, concerns over the risk of infection and thrombosis continue to limit general acceptance of long-term femoral cannulation in critically ill patients. Other peripheral veins, such as those in the antecubital fossa, have been used for central venous access, but the high incidence of thrombophlebitis and the fact that many catheters cannot be passed into the central venous circulation make these routes undesirable in critically ill patients.

Complications. Complications can be divided into technical or mechanical complications, usually occurring during catheter placement, and long-term complications related to the length of time that the catheter remains in place.

The list of technical and mechanical complications is truly impressive: catheter malposition, dysrhythmias, embolization (air or catheter fragments), vascular injury (hematoma, vessel laceration, false aneurysm, or arteriovenous fistula), cardiac injury (atrial or ventricular perforation, or cardiac tamponade), pleural injury (pneumothorax, hemothorax, or hydrothorax), mediastinal injury (hydromediastinum or hemomediastinum), neurologic injury (phrenic nerve, brachial plexus, or recurrent laryngeal nerve), and injury to other structures (trachea, thyroid, or thoracic duct). Pneumothorax is the most frequently reported immediate complication of subclavian vein catheterization, and arterial puncture is the most common immediate complication of internal jugular vein cannulation.

Long-term complications related to the length of time the catheter is in place are due to infection or thrombosis. Norwood and associates studied triple-lumen catheter infections in septic and nonseptic critically ill surgical patients. They found no catheter-related infections or instances of septicemia in the nonseptic patients, but the incidence of catheter-related infection in the septic group was 26.3 percent with a 9.6 percent incidence of septicemia. The catheter infection rate per 100 days, however, was only 0.9 for both septic and nonseptic patients combined, which is very similar to rates previously published for single-lumen catheters. At least three types of thrombi can develop in patients with central venous catheters: mural thrombus, catheter thrombus, and ''fibrin sleeve'' or sleeve thrombus. Any of these thrombi may spontaneously break loose or be set loose when the catheter is removed. Generally, however, symptoms or clinical consequences do not occur. Superior vena cava syndrome does occur, especially in long-term patients who have had many catheters placed.

Pulmonary Artery Catheterization

Indications. Several studies in critically ill patients have shown that the clinical assessment is inaccurate in predicting cardiac output, pulmonary artery occlusion pressure, and systemic vascular resistance, and that the information obtained from pulmonary artery catheterization prompts a change in therapy in 40 to 60 percent of the cases.

Although the pulmonary artery catheter permits a more accurate hemodynamic assessment and therapy may be modified as a result, this does not prove that knowledge of these data and alteration of the therapy improves overall patient outcome. Some studies indicate that preoperative invasive hemodynamic monitoring and cardiac function optimization in high-risk patients is associated with reduced intraoperative and postoperative cardiac complications and decreased mortality. While there are not enough carefully designed studies to definitely establish the benefit of hemodynamic monitoring to the individual patient, it is reasonable to assume that more precise bedside knowledge of fundamental cardiovascular parameters would facilitate earlier diagnosis and guide therapy. Whether morbidity can be decreased and overall survival can be improved also depends on the patient's overall response, not just improved cardiovascular function, and thus should not be considered a necessary requirement for initiating invasive monitoring.

Table 12-1
Conditions for Which Pulmonary Artery Catheterization Has Been Recommended

I. General
  A. Shock despite perceived adequate fluid therapy
  B. Oliguria that persists despite perceived adequate fluid therapy
  C. To assess the effect of intravascular volume expansion on cardiac function
  D. To delineate the cardiovascular component of multiple-organ-system dysfunction
II. Surgical
  A. Preoperative assessment and perioperative management of high-risk surgical patients
  B. Patients who need cardiac or major vascular surgery
  C. Postoperative cardiovascular complications
  D. Multisystem trauma
  E. Severe burns
III. Pulmonary
  A. To differentiate noncardiogenic (ARDS) from cardiogenic pulmonary edema
  B. To assess effects of high levels of ventilatory support on cardiovascular status
IV. Cardiac
  A. Myocardial infarction complicated by pump failure or pulmonary edema
  B. Treatment of unstable angina with intravenous nitroglycerin therapy
  C. Congestive heart failure unresponsive to simple therapy (to guide preload and vasodilator therapy)
  D. Pulmonary hypertension, for diagnosis and to monitor drug therapy

In general, a pulmonary artery catheter is indicated whenever the data obtained will improve therapeutic decision making, without unnecessary risk. Table 12-1 represents the indications most often noted in the medical literature. There are no specific contraindications to pulmonary artery catheterization, but the same cautions as those attached to central venous access apply.

Clinical Utility. The pulmonary artery catheter has provided a ''quantum leap'' in the physiologic information available for the management of critically ill patients. The information that can be obtained includes CVP; pulmonary artery diastolic (PADP), systolic (PASP), and mean (MPAP) pressures; pulmonary artery occlusion (''wedge'') pressure (PAOP); cardiac output (CO) by thermodilution; mixed venous blood gases by intermittent sampling; and continuous mixed venous oximetry. On the basis of this information, a multitude of derived parameters can also be obtained (see below).

When the pulmonary artery catheter balloon is inflated (1.5 mL), the blood flow in a distal segment of the pulmonary artery is occluded creating a conduit through which left atrial pressure (LAP) can be measured (Fig. 12-1*A*). In a tubular system, flow can only be created if there is a pressure differential at both extremes. If there is no pressure differential, flow cannot be present. Using this principle in reverse, a stagnant system in which no forward flow is present would permit an accurate measurement of a distal pressure from a proximal location (Fig. 12-1*B*). In fact,

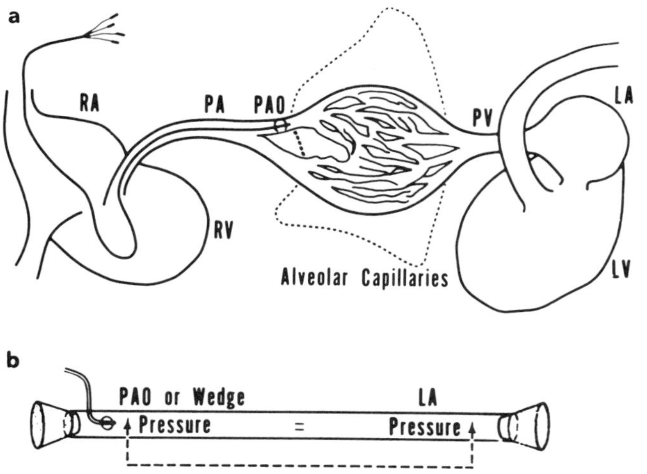

FIG. 12-1. Diagrammatic representation of a pulmonary artery catheter in the correct position *(A)*. Note that although the tip of the catheter lies in a pulmonary artery, with the balloon inflated, no flow exists in the system and that in a "closed pipe" analogy *(B)* pressure readings throughout the system would be equal.

simultaneous PAOP and LAP measurements in patients have validated this principle. The PAOP is a reliable index of the LAP even in the presence of elevated pulmonary vascular resistance. Although the PADP has also been used as an index of LAP, it is not as reliable as the PAOP particularly if there is tachycardia or increased pulmonary vascular resistance.

The PAOP represents the LAP as long as the column of blood distal to the pulmonary artery catheter tip is patent to the left atrium. This may not be so if the catheter is positioned in an area of the lung where the alveolar pressure exceeds pulmonary venous pressure (zone 2 as described by West) (Fig. 12-2) or both pulmonary artery and venous pressures (West's zone 1), causing intermittent or continous collapse of the pulmonary capillaries. The PAOP may then reflect alveolar pressure and not LAP. This is particularly important if patients have low pulmonary vascular pressures (i.e., hypovolemia) and/or are treated with high levels of positive end-expiratory pressure (PEEP). Fortunately, since the pulmonary artery catheter is flow-directed, it is most likely to pass into dependent areas of the lung where blood flow is high and both pulmonary artery and venous pressures exceed alveolar pressure (West's zone 3). In this location, the continuous column of blood between the distal lumen of the catheter and the left atrium will remain patent and the PAOP will reflect LAP. Another factor favoring appropriate catheter position is that when the patient is supine, the volume of lung located above the heart and the hydrostatic gradient favoring the formation of zones 1 and 2 are decreased. If there is any doubt, a lateral chest x-ray can be used to determine the location of the catheter tip in relation to the left atrium. If the tip of the catheter is below this chamber, zone 3 conditions will exist even if high levels of PEEP are used.

In the absence of mitral valve disease or premature mitral valve closure due to aortic regurgitation, the LAP reflects the left ventricular end-diastolic pressure (LVEDP). If there are no alterations in left ventricular compliance (the relationship between pressure and volume), LVEDP will reflect left ventricular end-diastolic volume (LVEDV). In the intact ventricle, LVEDV reflects the end-diastolic stretch of the muscle fiber, which represents the true preload (discussed later).

Raising intrathoracic pressure introduces an artifact that affects all intrathoracic vascular pressures to an extent that depends on the state of pulmonary compliance. In patients with acute respiratory insufficiency, compliance is often diminished and the "stiff" lungs do not transmit alveolar pressure as readily to the pulmonary circulation. In these patients, the PEEP artifact on the PAOP measurement should usually not exceed 1 mmHg for every 5 cmH_2O of PEEP applied. A greater discrepancy can be seen if the patient is hypovolemic or if the catheter is malpositioned as described above. Another method of evaluating the effects of PEEP on the PAOP measurement is to observe the decrement in PAOP when PEEP is briefly removed. Presumably, this decrement remains relatively constant and can be subtracted from subsequent pressure measurements. Although removal of PEEP may decrease arterial

FIG. 12-2. Model to explain the uneven distribution of blood flow in the lung based on the pressures affecting the capillaries. In zone 1, alveolar pressure (PA) exceeds pulmonary arterial (Pa) and venous (Pv) pressures so that the collapsible vessels are held closed and there is no flow. In zone 2, pulmonary arterial pressure exceeds alveolar but alveolar pressure exceeds venous. Under these conditions, there is a constriction at the downstream end of each collapsible vessel. In zone 3, pulmonary arterial and venous pressures exceed alveolar pressure and the collapsible vessels are held open. (From: *West JB, Dollery CT, Naimark A: Distribution of blood flow in isolated lung; Relation to vascular and alveolar pressures. J Appl Physiol 19:713, 1964*).

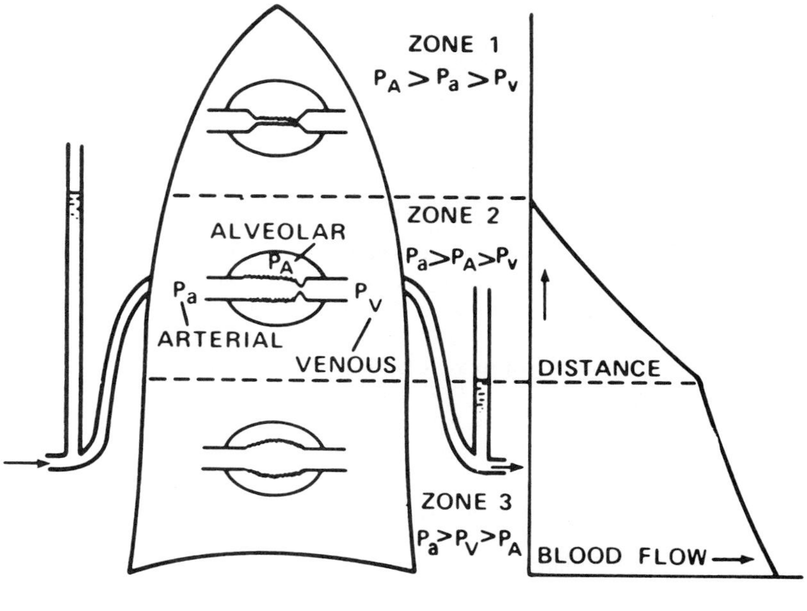

oxygen tension and increase physiologic shunt, these changes are rapidly reversible. If a physician believes that the PAOP should be measured off PEEP, this should probably be performed when PEEP is discontinued for other reasons (suctioning or changing breathing circuits), and increased concentrations of oxygen should be given before and after PEEP is stopped. Patients who are receiving very high levels of PEEP or whose condition deteriorates when PEEP is discontinued (such as immediate bradycardia) should not have PEEP removed for the exclusive purpose of measuring PAOP.

Since intravascular pressure measurements are affected by the intrathoracic pressure changes during respiration, they should be performed at end-expiration and obtained from a calibrated strip-chart recorder or oscilloscope rather than a digital display. Most digital displays are inaccurate, because the unselective nature of time-based electrical sampling and averaging includes positive and negative breathing artifacts. The digital average then contains the very respiratory variations that can be excluded by visualizing the tracing and selecting the appropriate value.

The CO is measured by the thermodilution technique, which correlates well with both the Fick and the dye dilution methods. Thermodilution represents an application of the indicator dilution principle in which a change in the heat content of the blood is induced at one point of the circulation and the resulting change in temperature is detected at a point downstream. This change is produced by a rapid injection of a known volume of fluid at a known temperature (colder than the body) into the right atrium via the proximal port of the pulmonary artery catheter. The change in temperature is registered by a thermistor located 4 cm from the catheter tip. This lowered temperature decreases the electrical resistance of the thermistor and results in a thermodilution curve.

The measurement of the cardiac output is based on a modification of the Stewart-Hamilton equation:

$$CO = \frac{V_I(T_B - T_I)K_1K_2}{\int_0^\infty \Delta\ T_B(t)\ dt}$$

where CO = cardiac output (L/min)
V_I = injectate volume (L)
T_B = blood (pulmonary artery) temperature (°C)
T_I = injectate temperature (°C)
K_1 = density factor (injectate/blood)
K_2 = computation constant (includes correction to the units of measurement)
$\int_0^\infty \Delta T_B(t)\ dt$ = change in blood temperature as a function of time (°C-s)

The variables in the formula are essentially fixed before injection, except for the denominator. The denominator of the equation is the thermodilution curve produced by the injection of the indicator. A computer integrates the area under this curve and the resulting calculation is displayed as the CO in L/min. The area under the curve is inversely proportional to the CO; that is, the larger the area under the curve, the lower the CO. In actuality, right ventricular output is being measured: In the absence of intracardiac shunting, right and left ventricular cardiac outputs are equivalent.

The injectate solution can be either 5% dextrose in water or normal saline. A volume of 10 mL of iced or room temperature injectate is recommended. The injection should be smooth, completed within 4 s, and timed with a specific phase of the respiratory cycle—i.e., injecting at peak-inspiration or end-exhalation—rather than randomly. The measurement protocol should be consistent, and three measurements should be averaged, since a single measurement is not reliable. If for any reason the fluid bolus cannot be injected through the atrial port of the catheter (e.g., obstructed lumen), it can be administered through the side port of the introducer or through the right ventricular port of a Paceport* pulmonary artery catheter.

Pitfalls in cardiac output measurement include injectate temperature different from the temperature used to determine the computer constant or that of the fluid being monitored by the reference probe, delivered volume less than the one entered in the computation constant, incorrect computer constant, rapid infusion of intravenous fluids during measurements, faulty catheter lumens, improperly positioned catheter (e.g., if the catheter is in the wedge position or if the proximal lumen is above the atrium or within the introducer sheath), and presence of intracardiac shunts or tricuspid regurgitation.

Newer approaches that allow continuous measurement of cardiac output with a pulmonary artery catheter include the use of Doppler technology and heat thermodilution. In addition, pulmonary artery catheters equipped with rapid-response thermistors and ECG electrodes have permitted the measurement of right ventricular ejection fraction at the bedside. The clinical utility of these systems in critically ill unstable patients requires further study.

Finally, the pulmonary artery catheter can also be used to obtain true mixed venous blood samples for gas analysis. The oxygen tension of mixed venous blood ($P\overline{v}_{O_2}$) and the oxygen saturation of mixed venous hemoglobin ($S\overline{v}_{O_2}$) provide valuable diagnostic information and are necessary for the calculation of various oxygen transport parameters.

Catheter Insertion. The most commonly used pulmonary artery catheter is a 7 Fr 110-cm catheter with a distal pulmonary artery lumen, a proximal lumen 30 cm from the tip, a lumen for inflation of the balloon located at the catheter tip, and a thermistor for measurement of cardiac output by the thermodilution method (Fig. 12-3). Newer catheters may contain an additional lumen for fluid administration or for passing a pacing electrode, fiberoptic bundles for continuous measurement of $S\overline{v}_{O_2}$, or a rapid-response thermistor to measure right ventricular ejection fraction.

Preparation of the electronic monitoring equipment and testing of the catheter components before insertion is essential because the displayed tracing is used to localize the position of the catheter tip during insertion. The pressure transducer must be calibrated and zeroed to the level of the left atrium. The catheter should be tested before insertion by (1) flushing the proximal and distal lumens to ensure that they are patent, (2) inflating the balloon (1.5 mL) to detect asymmetry or leaks, (3) testing the thermistor by connecting it to the cardiac output computer, and (4) shaking the catheter tip to verify that a tracing can be obtained on the oscilloscope.

Access to the central venous circulation for insertion of a pulmonary artery catheter is the same as for placement of a CVP catheter. Once an introducer sheath is in place, the pulmonary artery catheter is inserted and advanced until the tip reaches an intrathoracic vein (as evidenced by respiratory variations on the pressure tracing). The balloon is then inflated with 1.5 mL of air and the catheter advanced while the operator observes both the pressure waveform and the ECG tracing. After the right atrium is entered, the catheter is advanced through the right ventricle and into the pulmonary artery until a PAOP tracing is obtained (Fig.

*Baxter Healthcare Corp., Edwards Critical-Care Division, Santa Ana, CA.

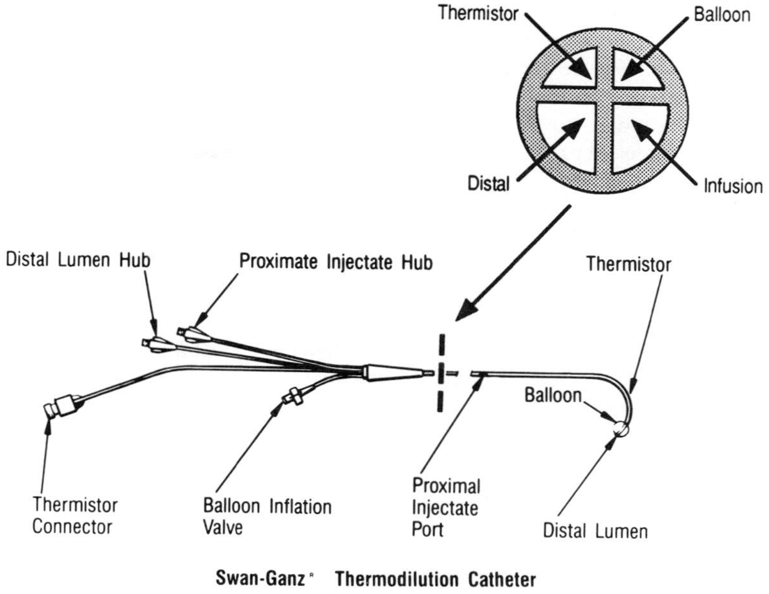

FIG. 12-3. A 7 Fr thermodilution pulmonary artery catheter. Inset cross-section, detailing lumen design. *(Courtesy of Baxter Healthcare Corporation, 1992.)*

12-4). Maneuvers often used to facilitate passage through the pulmonary valve include elevation of the head of the bed, turning the patient into the right lateral decubitus position, performance of the Valsalva maneuver, and increasing ventricular ejection in low-output states by the administration of inotropic drugs. To determine if the catheter is in the wedge position, the waveform needs to be inspected. The mean PAOP should be lower than the MPAP and lower than or equal to the PADP. In the wedged position, arterialized blood can be aspirated, or $S\bar{v}_{O_2}$ will increase to systemic arterial levels or above if an oximetric pulmonary artery catheter is used. The latter is not an absolute criterion because incomplete arterialization of the sample can occur if the tip of the pulmonary artery catheter lies wedged in a low ventilation/perfusion region.

Complications. There are risks to pulmonary artery catheterization, although they are typically infrequent and not usually life-threatening. In addition to the complications attributed to central venous cannulation, complications can occur during passage or after the catheter is in place.

The most common complication during passage of the pulmonary artery catheter is the development of dysrhythmias. They can occur in up to 50 percent of patients, but less than 1 percent of these are serious. The incidence of malignant dysrhythmias during catheterization seems to be lower when patients are in the head-up and right lateral tilt position. Transient right bundle branch block (RBBB) has been reported in 3 to 6 percent of catheterizations. Because of the rare but grave consequences of RBBB in patients with preexisting left bundle branch block, the use of standby external pacemakers and equipment for transvenous pacemaker insertion has been recommended in these patients during catheterization. Coiling, looping, or knotting in the right ventricle can occur during catheter insertion. This can be avoided if no more than 10 cm of catheter is inserted after a ventricular tracing is visual-

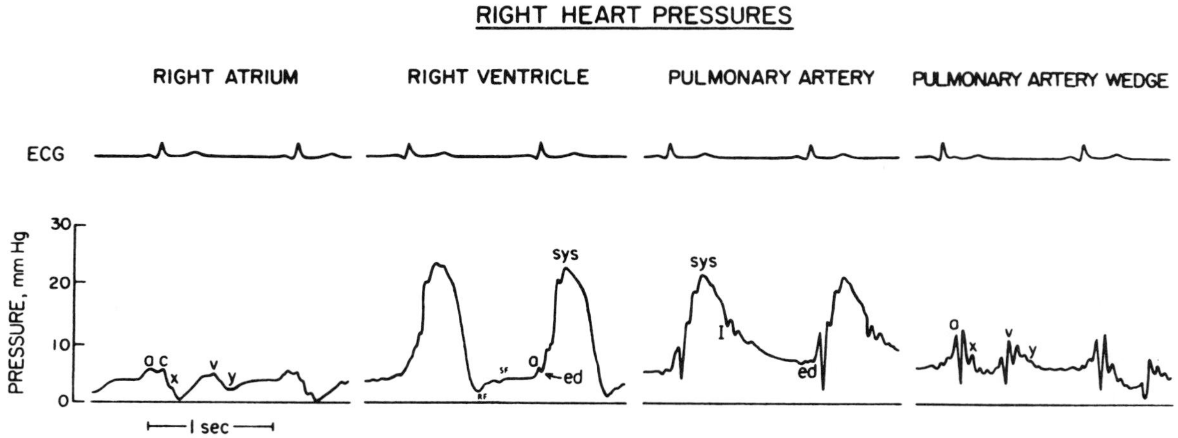

FIG. 12-4. Normal pressure waveforms from the right heart and pulmonary artery; sys = systolic, ed = end-diastolic. (From: *Grossman W, Barry WH: Cardiac catheterization. In Braunwald E (ed): Heart Disease: A Textbook of Cardiovascular Medicine, p 250. Philadelphia, WB Saunders, 1988.)*

ized and before a pulmonary artery tracing appears. Aberrant catheter location, such as pleural, pericardial, peritoneal, aortic, vertebral artery, renal vein, and inferior vena cava, have also been reported.

Complications that can occur after the catheter is in place include infections, thromboembolism, and rupture of the pulmonary artery. Infections from pulmonary artery catheters are directly related to the length and severity of illness. The risk of infectious complications has been reported between 2 and 25 percent. The higher incidence of positive cultures compared to central venous catheters has been attributed to the additional manipulation required in performing cardiac outputs, obtaining mixed venous blood samples, and repositioning the catheter. Asymptomatic thrombotic complications are frequent, but complications attributable to such thrombi are rare. Pulmonary infarction can occur due to emboli, distal migration of the pulmonary artery catheter tip, or prolonged balloon inflation occluding distal blood flow in the pulmonary artery. Pulmonary artery rupture and hemorrhage is the most serious of all the pulmonary artery catheter complications and is more likely in patients with pulmonary hypertension and in the elderly. Recurrent hemorrhage from a pulmonary artery pseudoaneurysm secondary to pulmonary artery catheter-induced perforation can also occur. Complications related to the peripheral migration of the catheter tip can be limited by continuous monitoring of the pulmonary artery tracing, avoiding prolonged balloon inflation, ensuring proximal catheter placement by review of daily x-rays, and the use of continuous heparin flush systems. Whenever the balloon is inflated, the tracing must be observed. Inflation must be stopped instantly when the waveform changes. If the catheter tip has drifted distally and is in a smaller artery, inflation with the usual 1.5 mL of air may be too much and may rupture the thin-walled pulmonary artery. Other complications that can occur after the catheter is in place include thrombocytopenia, cardiac valve injuries, catheter fracture, and balloon rupture.

In addition to the complications associated with catheter insertion and use, complications can result from delays in treatment due to time-consuming insertion problems and from inappropriate treatment based on erroneous information or erroneous data interpretation. Complications of pulmonary artery catheterization can be minimized by meticulous attention to detail and by careful evaluation of the data obtained.

Derived Hemodynamic Parameters

In addition to the information directly provided by arterial and pulmonary artery catheterization, many parameters can be calculated. The derived hemodynamic parameters (Table 12-2) aid the

Table 12-2
Measured and Derived Hemodynamic Parameters

Parameter (Abbreviation)	*Formula*	*Normal Range*	*Units*
Systolic blood pressure (SBP)	Direct measurement	100–140	mmHg
Diastolic blood pressure (DBP)	Direct measurement	60–90	mmHg
Pulmonary artery systolic pressure (PASP)	Direct measurement	15–30	mmHg
Pulmonary artery diastolic pressure (PADP)	Direct measurement	4–12	mmHg
Mean pulmonary artery pressure (MPAP)	Direct measurement	9–16	mmHg
Right ventricular systolic pressure (RVSP)	Direct measurement	15–30	mmHg
Right ventricular end-diastolic pressure (RVEDP)	Direct measurement	0–8	mmHg
Central venous pressure (CVP)	Direct measurement	0–8	mmHg
Pulmonary artery occlusion pressure (PAOP)	Direct measurement	2–12	mmHg
Cardiac output (CO)	Direct measurement	*	L/min
Mean arterial blood pressure (MAP)†	$\text{MAP} = \text{DBP} + \dfrac{\text{SBP} - \text{DBP}}{3}$	70–105	mmHg
Cardiac index (CI)	$\text{CI} = \dfrac{\text{CO}}{\text{BSA}}$	2.8–4.2	L/min/m^2
Stroke volume (SV)	$\text{SV} = \dfrac{\text{CO}}{\text{HR}}$	*	mL/beat
Stroke index (SI)	$\text{SI} = \dfrac{\text{SV}}{\text{BSA}}$	30–65	mL/beat/m^2
Left ventricular stroke work index (LVSWI)	$\text{LVSWI} = \dfrac{\text{SV} \times (\text{MAP} - \text{PAOP})}{\text{BSA}} \times 0.0136$	43–61	$\text{g} \times \text{m/m}^2$
Right ventricular stroke work index (RVSWI)	$\text{RVSWI} = \dfrac{\text{SV} \times (\text{MPAP} - \text{CVP})}{\text{BSA}} \times 0.0136$	7–12	$\text{g} \times \text{m/m}^2$
Systemic vascular resistance (SVR)	$\text{SVR} = \dfrac{\text{MAP} - \text{CVP}}{\text{CO}} \times 80$	900–1400	$\text{dyne} \times \text{s} \times \text{cm}^{-5}$
Pulmonary vascular resistance (PVR)	$\text{PVR} = \dfrac{\text{MPAP} - \text{PAOP}}{\text{CO}} \times 80$	150–250	$\text{dyne} \times \text{s} \times \text{cm}^{-5}$
Coronary perfusion pressure (CPP)	$\text{CPP} = \text{DBP} - \text{PAOP}$	60–90	mmHg

BSA = body surface area; HR = heart rate.

*Varies with size.

†Can also be measured directly.

clinician by quantitating the relationships among heart rate, filling pressures, resistance, contractility, and cardiac output.

Cardiac output is the sum of all stroke volumes ejected in a given time. It is usually represented as the product of average stroke volume and heart rate (beats per minute), where stroke volume is the amount of blood ejected by the heart with each contraction. The primary determinants of stroke volume are the ventricular preload, afterload, and contractility.

Preload is the passive load that establishes the initial muscle length of the cardiac fibers before contraction and therefore is not usually measured directly in critically ill patients. On the basis of the work by Otto Frank and others, Starling described the relationship between the resting fiber length of the myocardium and ventricular work. As resting fiber length increases, there is an increase in work performed on subsequent contraction. Beyond a certain point, however, further increases in fiber length will not increase external mechanical work, and work may decrease—a description of cardiac failure. The end-diastolic fiber length is proportional to the end-diastolic volume. If there is no change in ventricular compliance (the relationship between pressure and volume), LVEDV is proportional to LVEDP. Because in most clinical circumstances the PAOP provides a reliable measure of LVEDP, changes in PAOP are frequently used as an estimate of changes in left ventricular preload. In critically ill patients, however, changes in ventricular compliance may affect the relationship between LVEDP and LVEDV. Therefore, caution should be taken in the interpretation of the PAOP as the sole measure of left ventricular preload. In clinical practice, judgments concerning preload adequacy are often best made empirically, by observing the responses of PAOP and indices of cardiac performance to a rapid alteration of intravascular volume.

The second determinant of stroke volume is afterload. Afterload is the sum of all the loads against which the myocardial fibers must shorten during systole, including the aortic impedance, the arterial wall resistance, the peripheral vascular resistance, the mass of blood in the aorta and great arteries, the viscosity of the blood, and the end-diastolic volume of the ventricle. In the clinical setting, the most commonly used measure of ventricular afterload is the peripheral or systemic vascular resistance (SVR). Changes in SVR usually reflect either altered blood viscosity or a change in the radius of the vascular circuit. SVR, however, does not necessarily reflect left ventricular loading conditions, since the true measure of ventricular afterload must consider the interaction of factors internal and external to the myocardium. Although it is not physiologically correct to speak of afterload in terms of SVR, it is clinically useful to relate changes in SVR to changes in ventricular afterload. Since the sympathetic control of the circulation mediated by peripheral baroreceptors is designed to maintain blood pressure within relatively narrow limits, cardiac output is inversely proportional to SVR, whenever this control is functioning. In the human circulatory system, however, additional factors are so often present that this relationship should not be assumed to be a substitute for direct measurements and repeated calculations.

Contractility, the final determinant of stroke volume, may be estimated in the laboratory by the maximum velocity of contraction of the cardiac muscle fibers. At the bedside, we only have inferences based on the stroke work performed by the ventricle as filling pressure (''preload'') changes. Plotting the work done by the ventricle for each beat—the left or right ventricular stroke work index (LVSWI or RVSWI)—against an estimate of preload and comparing that point with a normal range may be a useful means of assessing overall ventricular function (Fig. 12-5). An upward shift to the left has been interpreted as an improvement in ventricular performance. A shift downward and to the right has been considered as a declining ventricular performance. The ''ventricular function curves'' are influenced by changes in ventricular afterload and compliance and therefore do not reflect true contractility. At present, the method for assessing myocardial contractility most widely considered load-independent is the end-systolic pressure-volume relationship (ESPVR). The logistical difficulty of obtaining frequent ventricular volume measurements in the intensive care unit (ICU) limits the clinical usefulness of this method. Thus, plotting PAOP and stroke work against normal curves is an appropriate use of data currently available in the ICU, but the underlying physiology is often better understood if it is considered in terms of the ventricular pressure-volume relation.

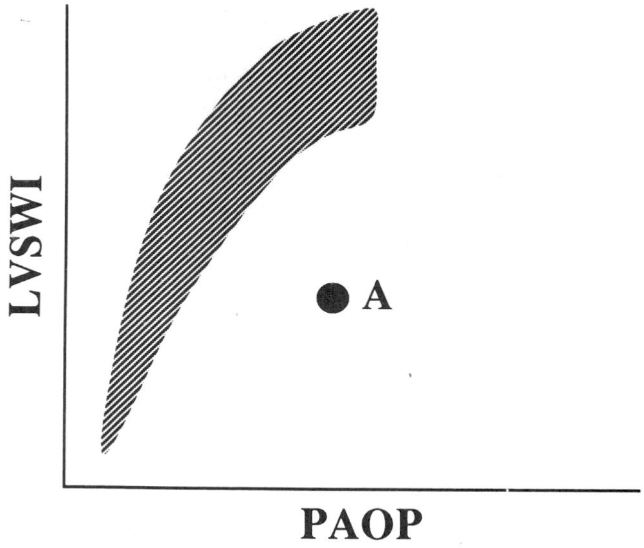

FIG. 12-5. Ventricular function curve. By comparison with the normal (shaded) area, left ventricular stroke work index (LVSWI) is seen to be depressed *(A)*. The depression could be due to a decrease in contractility, a decrease in diastolic compliance, or a significant increase in afterload secondary to increased wall tension. PAOP = pulmonary artery occlusion (wedge) pressure.

An appreciation of the determinants of stroke volume provides a rational approach in the management of patients with low perfusion states. The first and most common intervention used to increase stroke volume is to increase preload by augmentation of intravascular volume. The level of PAOP that corresponds to optimal left ventricular preload can be determined only by sequentially assessing the effects of acute hemodynamic interventions on cardiac function, and may vary over time in any particular patient. Fluid can be administered rapidly in predetermined increments while changes in PAOP and in the indices of cardiac performance are monitored. A major increase in PAOP during infusion suggests poor ventricular compliance, exhausted preload reserve, and increased risk of pulmonary edema with further volume loading. If the PAOP rises modestly, if indices of cardiac performance improve, and if PAOP returns to within several mmHg of the original value within 10 min of stopping the infusion, additional fluid can be given without high risk of exacerbating pulmonary venous congestion. After a brief observation period, this sequence can be repeated until the hemodynamic parameters are adequate or the

PAOP shows an unacceptable rise. If tissue perfusion remains inadequate after volume optimization, augmentation of stroke volume may be accomplished by increasing myocardial contractility with inotropic drugs and/or decreasing ventricular afterload with vasodilators.

RESPIRATORY MONITORING

Monitoring ventilation and gas exchange in critically ill surgical patients is of particular importance in deciding if mechanical ventilation is indicated, assessing response to therapy, optimizing ventilator management, and deciding if a weaning trial is indicated. In addition, gas monitoring permits an assessment of the adequacy of oxygen transport and calculation of derived parameters.

Ventilation Monitoring

Lung Volumes. Several lung volume measurements are useful for monitoring ventilatory function in the operating room and ICU. These include tidal volume, vital capacity, minute volume, and dead space.

Tidal volume (V_T), is defined as the volume of air moved in or out of the lungs in any single breath. If the tidal volume is depressed, the patient may have difficulty in both oxygenation and ventilation. Rapid shallow breathing, as reflected by the respiratory frequency (f) to tidal volume ratio ($f/V_T > 100$), is an accurate predictor of failure, and its absence ($f/V_T < 80$) is an accurate predictor of success, in weaning patients from mechanical ventilation. V_T can be measured at the bedside using a hand-held spirometer (Wright respirometer). Because moisture impairs its performance, the instrument is most appropriate for intermittent monitoring. Continuous V_T monitoring is facilitated by the presence of pneumotachometers in the breathing circuit of modern ventilators. In order to obtain accurate V_T measurements the spirometer must be located between the ventilator Y piece and the endotracheal tube. If the spirometer is instead positioned on the expiratory limb of the breathing circuit, the entire V_T delivered by a ventilator, not that actually received by the patient, is measured. Under conditions of decreased lung compliance or increased airway resistance, the higher peak inspiratory pressure (PIP) would result in an increase of gas volume compressed in the breathing circuit, with correspondingly less delivered to the patient. The product of PIP (cmH_2O) × 5 (mL/cmH_2O) provides an estimate of the compression volume of most circuits.

Vital capacity (VC) is defined as the maximal expiration following a maximal inspiration. It can be readily measured at the bedside in a manner similar to the one used for V_T. The VC is reduced in diseases involving the respiratory muscles or their neural pathways, in obstructive and restrictive ventilatory impairment, and in patients who fail to cooperate fully. VC is normally 65 to 75 mL/kg, and a value of 10 mL/kg or greater is commonly considered a favorable predictor of weaning outcome. This value, however, is quite dependent on patient cooperation, and its predictive power is rather poor.

Minute volume (or total ventilation) ($\dot{V}_E$) is the total volume of air leaving the lung each minute (product of V_T and f). Many ventilators display $\dot{V}_E$, or it can be measured with a Wright spirometer. An increase in the minute volume required to maintain a normal arterial blood carbon dioxide tension (Pa_{CO_2}) suggests an increased dead space relative to V_T or an abnormally high carbon dioxide (CO_2) production. A resting $\dot{V}_E$ of less than 10 L and the ability to double the resting $\dot{V}_E$ on command have been associated with successful weaning from mechanical ventilation.

The physiologic (or effective, or total) dead space (V_D) is the portion of tidal volume that does not participate in gas exchange. Physiologic dead space may be divided into two components: the volume of gas within the conducting airways (the anatomic dead space), and the volume of gas within unperfused alveoli (the alveolar dead space). The ratio of physiologic dead space to tidal volume (V_D/V_T) is calculated from the Enghoff equation (modified from the Bohr equation) as follows:

$$\frac{V_D}{V_T} = \frac{Pa_{CO_2} - P\bar{E}_{CO_2}}{Pa_{CO_2}}$$

where $P\bar{E}_{CO_2}$ is the mean partial pressure of exhaled CO_2 in the total exhaled volume of gas after thorough mixing. Normally, exhaled gas is collected in a bag over 3 min and the $P\bar{E}_{CO_2}$ is measured from the bag. The $P\bar{E}_{CO_2}$ should not be confused with PET_{CO_2}, the partial pressure of end-tidal CO_2 (discussed later). The V_D/V_T ratio provides a useful expression of the efficiency of ventilation. In healthy subjects the ratio is between 0.33 and 0.45. The V_D/V_T ratio is increased in a number of disease states associated with regions of the lung possessing high ventilation-to-perfusion ratios, such as adult respiratory distress syndrome, emphysema, pulmonary embolism, shock with low cardiac output, and the employment of positive-pressure ventilation with high V_T or excessive (more than is needed) positive end-expiratory pressure (PEEP). Patients whose V_D/V_T exceeds 0.6 are usually not weanable from ventilatory support.

By measuring $\dot{V}_E$ and calculating V_D/V_T, the alveolar (or effective) ventilation ($\dot{V}_A$) may also be calculated:

$$\dot{V}_A = \dot{V}_E - (\dot{V}_E \times V_D/V_T)$$

Pulmonary Mechanics. Various respiratory mechanical parameters can also be monitored in the operating room and ICU. These include maximal inspiratory pressure, static compliance, dynamic characteristic, and work of breathing.

Inspiratory force is measured as the maximal pressure below atmospheric that a patient can exert against an occluded airway. The measurement requires a connector to an endotracheal or tracheostomy tube and a manometer capable of registering negative pressure. A maximal inspiratory pressure (PI_{max}) value more negative than −20 to 25 cmH_2O has been used as one of the clinical parameters to confirm recovery from neuromuscular block after general anesthesia. PI_{max} values more negative than −30 cmH_2O have been used to predict successful weaning from mechanical ventilation. Recent investigations have found that PI_{max} has limited power in predicting weaning outcome, especially in patients receiving prolonged mechanical ventilation. These findings may be due in part to the fact that PI_{max} assesses only the strength of the respiratory muscle pump without taking into account the demands placed on it.

Compliance, a measure of the elastic properties of the lung and chest wall, is expressed as a change in volume divided by a change in pressure ($\Delta V/\Delta P$). In patients receiving mechanical ventilation, a rough measure of total thoracic compliance (both the lungs and chest wall) can be obtained by dividing the delivered V_T by the inflation pressure displayed on the ventilator gauge during conditions of zero gas flow. These can be achieved by using the "inspiratory hold" option on the ventilator, during which period the airway pressure falls to a plateau. If the patient is receiving PEEP, this must be first subtracted from the plateau pressure before calculating static thoracic compliance, i.e.,

$$\text{Static compliance} = \frac{\text{volume delivered}}{\text{plateau pressure} - \text{PEEP}}$$

The usual range for adult patients receiving mechanical ventilation is 60 to 100 mL/cmH_2O. Decreased values are observed with disorders of the thoracic cage or a reduction in the number of functioning lung units (resection, bronchial intubation, pneumothorax, pneumonia, atelectasis, or pulmonary edema). When the static compliance is less than 25 mL/cmH_2O, as in severe respiratory failure, difficulties in weaning are common because of the increased work of breathing (see below).

The dynamic characteristic is calculated by dividing the volume delivered by the peak (rather than the plateau) airway pressure minus PEEP. It is not correct to call this value dynamic compliance because it is actually an impedance measurement and includes compliance and resistance components. The dynamic characteristic is normally about 50 to 80 mL/cmH_2O. It may be decreased by disorders of the airways, lung parenchyma, or chest wall; if it falls to a greater extent than the static compliance, it suggests an increase in airway resistance (e.g., bronchospasm, mucus plugging, kinking of the endotracheal tube) or an excessive flow rate.

Work is calculated as force multiplied by distance, and in the pulmonary context this is translated into the product of pressure and the volume of air moved in and out of the lungs. The work of breathing in the critically ill patient who requires ventilatory support can be divided into three sections: normal physiologic work, work to overcome pathophysiologic changes in the lung, and work to overcome the imposed work of breathing created by our methods of ventilatory support. Physiologic work of breathing consists of three elements: elastic work of breathing, flow resistive work, and inertial work. Elastic work is the work necessary to overcome the elastic forces of the lung and is inversely proportional to the compliance of the lung. If compliance becomes diminished, the work of breathing increases dramatically. The second kind of physiologic work is flow resistive work or the work necessary to overcome resistance offered by the airways. This may increase the pressure change necessary to move the same tidal volume during inspiration but also adds another component of work during expiration, that necessary to expel the gas from the lungs through the narrowed airways. The third component of physiologic work is inertial work that is to overcome the tendency of gas volume to remain at rest; however, this is negligible in comparison to the elastic and flow resistive work. When a patient develops respiratory failure, in addition to the normal physiologic work, the patient must overcome the increased work of breathing associated with the disease. This is clinically manifest as a change from a relatively large tidal volume at a slow rate to a small tidal volume at a rapid rate. Finally, the patient must do additional work to breath spontaneously against a breathing apparatus that consists of the ventilator itself, demand valve, tubing, exhalation valves, and, most importantly, the endotracheal tube. In patients requiring prolonged mechanical ventilation, work of breathing may be a better indicator of successful weaning than conventional criteria. Until recently, measuring the work of breathing has been largely restricted to research studies. Although the new microprocessor ventilators allow some components of work to be measured, their accuracy has not yet been validated. A new monitoring device (CP-100 Pulmonary Monitor*) that incorporates an airway flow transducer and an esophageal balloon catheter permits bedside measurement of the work of breathing and many other respiratory parameters. Although this instrument appears to be promising, its clinical utility requires further study.

Gas Monitoring

Blood Gas Analysis. Blood gas measurements provide information about the efficiency of gas exchange, the adequacy of alveolar ventilation, and the acid-base status. Blood gas values are usually reported in terms of directly measured partial pressures (P_{O_2} or P_{CO_2}) and calculated hemoglobin oxygen saturations (S_{O_2}). Calculated S_{O_2} values are derived from the measured partial pressure and a nomogram of the oxyhemoglobin dissociation curve usually corrected for blood temperature, pH, and perhaps other factors. Because these assumptions may not be accurate in critically ill patients, actual measurements of S_{O_2} by co-oximetry are preferred. S_{O_2} can also be measured continuously by using pulse oximeters or pulmonary artery catheters that incorporate oximetric fibers (see below).

Arterial blood gas tensions are determined by the composition of the alveolar gas and the efficiency of gas transfer between the alveoli and pulmonary capillary blood. Alveolar gas tensions depend on the mixture of inspired gas, ventilation, and blood flow in the lungs, the matching of ventilation and perfusion, and the composition of mixed venous blood gases. Pathophysiologic causes of arterial hypoxemia include ventilation-perfusion inequality or venous admixture from regional alveolar hypoventilation, true intrapulmonary or intracardiac shunt, and decreased mixed venous oxygen content. Although diffusion abnormalities may lead to hypoxemia if pulmonary end-capillary blood fails to equilibrate fully with alveolar gas, such conditions are uncommon. A decreased cardiac output in the presence of a constant oxygen consumption, or an increased oxygen consumption in the presence of a constant cardiac output, or a decreased cardiac output and an increased oxygen consumption must all result in a lower mixed venous oxygen content and, therefore, can also produce arterial hypoxemia. Failure to recognize this nonpulmonary cause of hypoxemia may cause a clinician to falsely attribute a falling arterial blood oxygen tension (Pa_{O_2}) to deteriorating pulmonary function. Thus, pulmonary and cardiac function must be assessed to evaluate any given set of arterial blood gases accurately. A decreasing Pa_{O_2} without a change in Pa_{CO_2} suggests that blood oxygenation is deteriorating despite constant alveolar ventilation. In the acutely ill patient, this finding is usually attributable to ventilation-perfusion imbalance or intrapulmonary shunting. An important feature of shunting is that as it increases, supplemental oxygen has progressively less effect on Pa_{O_2} because shunted blood bypasses ventilated alveoli. Intrapulmonary shunting does not usually result in elevation of the Pa_{CO_2} because the central chemoreceptors sense any rise in Pa_{CO_2} and respond by increasing ventilation.

The relation of P_{O_2} to S_{O_2} is described by the oxyhemoglobin dissociation curve (Fig. 12-6). The flat upper portion of the dissociation curve means that even if the P_{O_2} in alveolar gas falls somewhat, loading of oxygen will be little affected. The steep lower part of the curve means that the peripheral tissues can withdraw large amounts of oxygen for only a small drop in capillary P_{O_2}. The curve shifts as the affinity of hemoglobin for oxygen changes.

*Bicore Monitoring Systems, Irvine, CA.

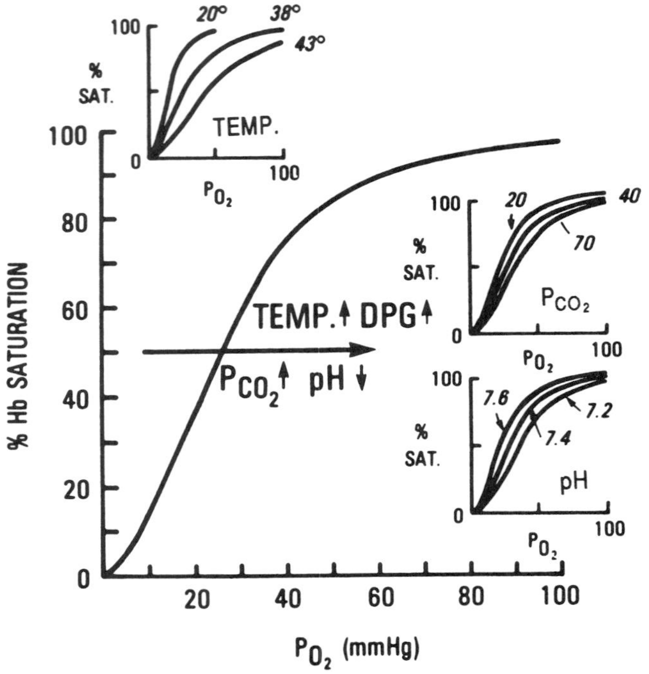

FIG. 12-6. Rightward shift of the oxyhemoglobin dissociation curve by increase of temperature, P_{CO_2}, hydrogen ion concentration, and 2,3-diphosphoglycerate (DPG). (From: *West JB: Pulmonary Physiology, 4th ed. Baltimore, Williams & Wilkins, 1990, with permission.)*

A shift to the right (decreased affinity for oxygen) helps release oxygen into the tissue. A shift to the left (increased affinity for oxygen) causes less oxygen to be available to tissue. The curve can be shifted to the right by *increased* erythrocyte 2,3-diphosphoglycerate concentration, temperature, P_{CO_2}, and concentration of hydrogen ion (decreased pH). Opposite changes shift it to the left. Other conditions such as carboxyhemoglobinemia and methemoglobinemia can also shift the oxyhemoglobin dissociation curve to the left and therefore interfere with peripheral oxygen unloading. The position of the oxyhemoglobin dissociation curve is defined by the P_{50}, that is the P_{O_2} at which hemoglobin is 50 percent saturated. Normal hemoglobin has a P_{50} of 26.5 mmHg. When it is greater than this value, the curve is shifted to the right; when it is lower, the curve is shifted to the left. In spite of a considerable amount of information, there is little evidence that shifts of the oxyhemoglobin dissociation curve are clinically significant in the majority of patients. Individuals with limited circulatory reserve, however, who cannot augment oxygen delivery by the usual compensatory mechanisms of increased cardiac output and organ blood flow, may develop local tissue hypoxia when an increased hemoglobin-oxygen affinity state (i.e., alkalemia) exists.

The Pa_{CO_2} directly reflects the adequacy with which alveolar ventilation meets metabolic demands for CO_2 excretion. The relationship between Pa_{CO_2}, CO_2 production ($\dot{V}_{CO_2}$), and alveolar ventilation ($\dot{V}_A$) in normal lungs is given by the equation:

$$Pa_{CO_2} = \frac{\dot{V}_{CO_2}}{\dot{V}_A} \times K$$

were K is a constant. In diseased lungs the denominator $\dot{V}_A$ in this equation is less than the ventilation going to the alveoli because of alveolar dead space, that is, unperfused alveoli or those with high ventilation-perfusion ratios. For this reason the denominator is sometimes referred to as the *effective alveolar ventilation*.

An increased Pa_{CO_2} (hypercapnia) reflects the failure of the ventilatory system to eliminate the CO_2 produced during metabolism. This "ventilatory failure" is traditionally described as respiratory acidosis. Hypercapnia can also occur because of hypoventilation (i.e., CNS depression), increased CO_2 production (e.g., hyperthermia, hyperthyroidism), or increased physiologic dead space resulting in inadequate alveolar ventilation. The mechanisms of hypocapnia are the reverse of those that produce hypercapnia, the most common being hyperventilation (respiratory alkalosis).

The oxygen tension of mixed venous blood ($P\bar{v}_{O_2}$) and the oxygen saturation of mixed venous hemoglobin ($S\bar{v}_{O_2}$) provide valuable diagnostic information and are necessary for the calculation of various parameters, such as arteriovenous oxygen content difference, intrapulmonary shunt, and oxygen consumption. Mixed venous blood is the mixture of all blood that has traversed the capillary beds capable of extracting oxygen. This venous effluent is thoroughly mixed, so its oxygen content is a flow-weighted representation of all the end-capillary contents of the body and as such will reflect the *total body balance* between oxygen delivery and oxygen consumption of *perfused* tissues. The mixed venous oxygen content (and therefore $S\bar{v}_{O_2}$) is determined by the variables in the Fick equation (see section on Continuous Mixed Venous Oximetry). The $P\bar{v}_{O_2}$ is determined by the same factors and the position of the oxyhemoglobin dissociation curve.

In critically ill patients, sampling of mixed venous blood can be accurately performed only in the pulmonary artery. Sampling technique is important; blood should be withdrawn from the most proximal pulmonary artery location possible and at a very slow rate. A fast rate of blood withdrawal or a malpositioned catheter (distal migration or wedging) may cause a falsely elevated $P\bar{v}_{O_2}$ and $S\bar{v}_{O_2}$. This is due to "contamination" of the mixed venous blood with arterialized pulmonary capillary blood and should be suspected if the CO_2 tension of mixed venous blood ($P\bar{v}_{CO_2}$) is equal to or lower than a simultaneously determined Pa_{CO_2}.

Proper sample handling before arterial or venous blood gas analysis is a prerequisite to accurate blood gas measurement. The two principal requirements are that the sample be obtained under strict anaerobic conditions and immediately placed on ice until analyzed. Because room air has a P_{O_2} of about 150 mmHg and a P_{CO_2} of essentially zero, equilibration of a blood sample with air bubbles may significantly alter the results. Placement of the sample on ice is necessary to reduce the metabolic rate of the red blood cells and prevent continued oxygen consumption and CO_2 production if analysis is to be delayed beyond 15 to 20 min. The addition of excessive heparin will also alter the results, and therefore after aspiration, the heparin should be expelled, leaving only the heparin wetting the barrel.

Because blood gas values can change rapidly in critically ill patients, intermittent sampling for blood gas analysis might miss significant changes. Miniaturized intravascular gas sensors based upon the principles of optical fluorescence have permitted continuous measurement of pH, P_{O_2}, and P_{CO_2}. Although this method seems to be promising, further improvements in accuracy are still needed, particularly for P_{CO_2}.

Parameters Derived From Blood Gas Analysis. Just as the derived hemodynamic parameters can be used to evaluate the choice and effects of hemodynamic interventions, parameters

Table 12-3
Parameters Derived from Blood Gas Analysis

Parameter (Abbreviation)	*Formula*	*Normal Range*	*Units*
Arterial blood O_2 tension (Pa_{O_2})	Direct measurement	70–100	mmHg
Arterial hemoglobin O_2 saturation (Sa_{O_2})	Direct measurement	> 0.92	(fraction)
Mixed venous blood O_2 tension ($P\bar{v}_{O_2}$)	Direct measurement	35–45	mmHg
Mixed venous hemoglobin O_2 saturation ($S\bar{v}_{O_2}$)	Direct measurement	0.65–0.80	(fraction)
Arterial blood O_2 content (Ca_{O_2})	$Ca_{O_2} = (Hb \times Sa_{O_2} \times 1.39) + (0.0031 \times Pa_{O_2})$	16–22	mL O_2/dL blood
Mixed venous blood O_2 content ($C\bar{v}_{O_2}$)	$C\bar{v}_{O_2} = (Hb \times S\bar{v}_{O_2} \times 1.39) + (0.0031 \times P\bar{v}_{O_2})$	12–17	mL O_2/dL blood
Arterial-venous O_2 content difference ($C(a - \bar{v})_{O_2}$)	$C(a - \bar{v})_{O_2} = Ca_{O_2} - C\bar{v}_{O_2}$	3.5–5.5	mL O_2/dL blood
O_2 delivery ($\dot{D}_{O_2}$)	$\dot{D}_{O_2} = Ca_{O_2} \times CO \times 10$	700–1400	mL/min
O_2 consumption ($\dot{V}_{O_2}$) (Fick)	$\dot{V}_{O_2} = C(a - \bar{v})_{O_2} \times CO \times 10$	180–280	mL/min
O_2 utilization coefficient (O_2UC)	$O_2UC = \dfrac{\dot{V}_{O_2}}{\dot{D}_{O_2}} = \dfrac{C(a - \bar{v})_{O_2} \times CO}{Ca_{O_2} \times CO} = \dfrac{C(a - \bar{v})_{O_2}}{Ca_{O_2}}$	0.23–0.32	(fraction)
Physiologic shunt (venous admixture) (Q_{sp}/Q_t)	$\dfrac{\dot{Q}_{sp}}{\dot{Q}_t} = \dfrac{Cc'_{O_2} - Ca_{O_2}}{Cc'_{O_2} - C\bar{v}_{O_2}}$	0.03–0.05	(fraction)
Pulmonary end-capillary O_2 content (Cc'_{O_2})	$Cc'_{O_2} = (Hb \times 1.39)^* + (0.0031 \times PA_{O_2})$	†	mL O_2/dL blood
Alveolar O_2 tension (PA_{O_2})	$PA_{O_2} = FI_{O_2}(PB - P_{H_2O}) - \dfrac{Pa_{CO_2}}{RQ}$	†	mmHg

Hb = hemoglobin concentration; CO = cardiac output; FI_{O_2} = inspired O_2 fraction; PB = barometric pressure; P_{H_2O} = partial pressure of water vapor (47 mmHg at 37°C); Pa_{CO_2} = arterial blood CO_2 tension; RQ = respiratory quotient (CO_2 production/O_2 consumption).

*Assumes 100% Hb saturation.

†Varies with FI_{O_2}.

derived from blood gas analysis (Table 12-3) yield information about the adequacy of cardiopulmonary function in meeting the tissue demands for oxygen.

The oxygen content of the blood is equal to the amount of oxygen bound to hemoglobin plus the amount dissolved in plasma. The amount of bound oxygen is directly related to the concentration of hemoglobin and to how saturated this hemoglobin is with oxygen (i.e., Sa_{O_2} or $S\bar{v}_{O_2}$). The amount of oxygen dissolved in plasma depends upon the oxygen tension (i.e., Pa_{O_2} or $P\bar{v}_{O_2}$). Oxygen delivery ($\dot{D}_{O_2}$) is the volume of oxygen delivered from the heart each minute and is calculated as the product of cardiac output and arterial oxygen content (Ca_{O_2}). Oxygen consumption ($\dot{V}_{O_2}$) is the amount of oxygen that diffuses from the capillaries into all tissues and can be calculated according to the Fick principle as the product of cardiac output and arteriovenous oxygen content difference ($C(a - \bar{v})_{O_2}$). If this equation is rearranged, the arteriovenous oxygen content difference relates oxygen consumption and cardiac output ($\dot{V}_{O_2}$/CO). An increase in the arteriovenous oxygen content difference indicates that either consumption is too high or flow is too low. Finally, the oxygen utilization coefficient or extraction ratio (O_2UC), relates oxygen consumption and oxygen delivery ($\dot{V}_{O_2}/\dot{D}_{O_2}$). This parameter has been used in many ICUs to evaluate the adequacy of oxygen transport.

The adequacy of oxygen transport must also be assessed in relation to oxygen demand, which is the amount of oxygen *required* by the body tissues to use aerobic metabolism. Although oxygen demand cannot be clinically measured, the relative balance between consumption and demand is best indicated by the presence of excess lactate in the blood. Lactic acidosis means that demand exceeds consumption and anaerobic metabolism is present.

Although precise numerical end points cannot be defined, the parameters already listed provide a framework for testing a clinical hypothesis: If oxygen delivery or consumption is low, if utilization is high, or if lactic acidosis is present, arterial oxygen content might be augmented by increasing hemoglobin concentration or oxygen saturation, or cardiac output might be increased by manipulation of preload, afterload, or contractility. A response might be considered beneficial if oxygen consumption increases, if utilization returns to the normal range, or if lactic acidosis resolves.

Physiologic right-to-left shunt or venous admixture ($\dot{Q}_{sp}/\dot{Q}_t$) estimates the fraction of total blood flow reaching the left side of the circulation without participating in gas exchange. Shunt may occur (uncommonly) in adults via intracardiac shunts. More commonly, the reason for increased venous admixture in critically ill patients is due to alterations in the balance of pulmonary ventilation and perfusion (lung areas that are perfused but not ventilated). Before calculating venous admixture, it is necessary to calculate arterial, mixed venous, and pulmonary end-capillary oxygen contents. The latter can be calculated by using the *alveolar* oxygen tension (PA_{O_2}) to estimate pulmonary end-capillary oxygen tension, and using the oxyhemoglobin dissociation curve to estimate pulmonary end-capillary hemoglobin saturation (assume 100% if $PA_{O_2} > 150$ mmHg) (Table 12-3).

Other indices, such as the alveolar-arterial oxygen partial pressure difference ($PA_{O_2} - Pa_{O_2}$) and the arterial-to-alveolar oxygen tension ratio (Pa_{O_2}/PA_{O_2}), have been suggested for evaluating the efficiency of gas exchange. These oxygen tension-based indices, however, are inaccurate in predicting efficiency of gas exchange. The relationship between physiologic shunt and the oxygen tension-based indices is nonlinear and substantially influenced by changes in inspired oxygen concentration and arteriovenous oxygen content difference.

The collection of the measured and derived cardiopulmonary parameters has been called the cardiopulmonary profile. Normal values can be seen in Tables 12-2 and 12-3. The measured and derived data can be used to formulate a plan of interventions designed to improve oxygen delivery relative to myocardial and systemic needs. This analysis is a dynamic process that evolves as new data are obtained and response to therapy is incorporated. The process of generating a cardiopulmonary profile has been greatly simplified by the use of programmable calculators and microcomputers.

Capnography. Capnography is the graphic display of CO_2 concentration as a waveform. It should not be confused with capnometry, which refers to only the numerical presentation of the concentration without a waveform. Capnography includes capnometry when the capnographic display is calibrated.

Currently available systems for CO_2 analysis include infrared spectroscopy, mass spectrometry, and Raman scattering. In addition, a disposable, noninvasive and inexpensive colorimetric device (EASY CAP*) is available. This device permits a semiquantitative measurement of the end-tidal CO_2 concentration when it is attached between an endotracheal tube and a resuscitation bag.

In the majority of stand-alone capnographs, the CO_2 concentration is measured by infrared spectroscopy. A beam of infrared light is passed through the sampled gas. CO_2 molecules in the light path absorb some of the infrared energy. The capnograph compares the amount of infrared light absorbed by the patient gas in the sample cell to the amount absorbed either by gas in a reference cell or by the sample cell during a time of known zero-gas concentration. The capnograph then displays the instantaneous CO_2 concentration.

Gas for analysis of CO_2 may be aspirated from the airway (sidestream capnography) or may be analyzed as it flows through a sensor placed in the airway (mainstream capnography). Sidestream analyzers offer advantages in that gas is sampled close to the patient's mouth with the use of an inexpensive, lightweight connector and they can be used in nonintubated patients. The major disadvantage of these systems is that analysis is delayed because gas is routed through a capillary tube to the capnograph.

Mainstream analyzers generate a capnogram practically instantaneously because the gas is analyzed as it passes through a sampling cuvette. The major disadvantage of these systems is the weight of the sensor and sampling cuvette. Because the sensor itself is a sophisticated instrument, it needs to be treated carefully: It is fragile and replacements are expensive. The volume of the cuvette adds dead space to the system.

Normally there is a fairly predictable relationship between the peak exhaled or end-tidal CO_2 (PET_{CO_2}) and the Pa_{CO_2}. In healthy subjects with normal lungs the Pa_{CO_2} is 4 to 6 mmHg higher than the PET_{CO_2}. Patients with chronic obstructive lung disease and other derangements associated with increased dead space (see section on Lung Volumes) have an increased arterial to end-tidal CO_2 gradient ($P(a - ET)_{CO_2}$). This difference occurs because the exhaled gas from the alveolar dead space, which contains little or no CO_2, dilutes the CO_2-containing gas from the normally ventilated and perfused alveoli.

Measurement of PET_{CO_2} and $P(a - ET)_{CO_2}$ provides insight into several normal and pathologic processes. PET_{CO_2} measurement is at present perhaps one of the most reliable means of determining proper endotracheal tube placement. Esophageal intubation may produce one or a few breaths containing CO_2 during expiration, but because there is no CO_2 in the stomach cavity, PET_{CO_2} rapidly decreases to zero.

PET_{CO_2} has been found to correlate with cardiac output and coronary perfusion pressure during cardiopulmonary resuscitation (CPR) and with successful resuscitation from and survival after cardiac arrest. Because circulatory arrest creates total dead space, if ventilation is continued, PET_{CO_2} disappears. An increase in PET_{CO_2} provides an immediate bedside validation of the efficacy of CPR and, if the increase is abrupt, it provides the earliest evidence of successful resuscitation. The use of PET_{CO_2} to monitor resuscitation is predicated on maintaining a constant minute ventilation so that changes in PET_{CO_2} result from changes in lung perfusion (and therefore cardiac output) and not ventilation.

PET_{CO_2} monitoring is extremely useful as a diagnostic tool in several situations unique to the operating room. These include the detection of air emboli during neurosurgical procedures requiring the sitting position, the detection of increased CO_2 production in malignant hyperthermia, and the detection of disconnection or malfunction of the anesthesia breathing circuit.

In the ICU environment PET_{CO_2} monitoring can also be used as a ventilator disconnect alarm as well as a system to determine ventilator malfunction. Measurement of PET_{CO_2} has been proposed as a substitute for arterial blood gas sampling during mechanical ventilation adjustment and weaning in critically ill patients. PET_{CO_2} trends in these patients are often misleading because the $P(a - ET)_{CO_2}$ varies greatly in a single individual as ventilation changes.

The $P(a - ET)_{CO_2}$ is primarily a reflection of dead-space ventilation, and its size can serve as a gauge of physiologic aberration. Factors related to the instrumentation and the technique used, however, may also contribute to the $P(a - ET)_{CO_2}$. For example, aspiration of room air through a loose connection or break in the circuit or sampling tube, a leak around the cuff, or aspiration of fresh gases will dilute the exhaled CO_2 and result in an increased $P(a - ET)_{CO_2}$ and an altered waveform. Finally, analysis of the CO_2 waveform can provide valuable information. A detailed review of waveform analysis is outside the scope of this chapter but can be found elsewhere (Gravenstein and associates).

Pulse Oximetry. Pulse oximetry provides a reliable, real-time estimation of arterial hemoglobin oxygen saturation. This noninvasive monitoring technique has gained clinical acceptance in the operating room, recovery room, and ICU.

Pulse oximeters estimate arterial hemoglobin saturation by measuring the absorbance of light transmitted through well-perfused tissue, such as the finger or ear. The light absorbance is measured at two wavelengths: 660 nm (red) and 940 nm (infrared) to distinguish between two species of hemoglobin—oxyhemoglobin and deoxyhemoglobin. Oxyhemoglobin absorbs less red light than deoxyhemoglobin, accounting for its red color; at infrared wavelengths the opposite is true (Fig. 12-7). Light absorbances at both wavelengths have two components: the pulsatile (or AC) component, which is attributed to the pulsating arterial blood, and the baseline (or DC) component, which represents the absorbances of the tissue bed, including venous blood, capillary blood, and nonpulsatile arterial blood (Fig. 12-8). The pulse oximeter first determines the AC components of absorbance at each wavelength and divides this by the corresponding DC component to obtain a pulse-added absorbance that is independent of the incident light intensity. It then calculates the ratio *(R)* of these pulse-added absorbances:

$$R = \frac{AC_{660}/DC_{660}}{AC_{940}/DC_{940}}$$

The ratio of the pulse-added absorbances at the two wavelengths is used to generate the oximeter's estimate of arterial saturation

*Nellcor Incorporated, Hayward, CA.

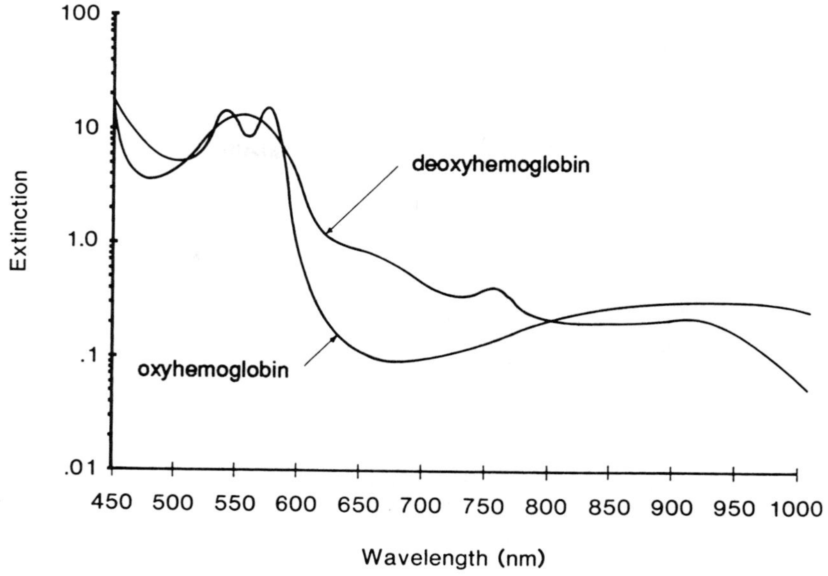

FIG. 12-7. Light absorption (extinction) as a function of wavelength for oxyhemoglobin and deoxyhemoglobin. (From: *Pologe JA: Pulse oximetry: Technical aspects of machine design. Int Anesthesiol Clin 25:137, 1987, with permission.*)

(Sp_{O_2}). The relationship between this ratio and Sp_{O_2} is empirical. The algorithm was created by measuring pulse-added absorbances in healthy, awake volunteers breathing hypoxic gas mixtures. These absorbances were then correlated with actual Sa_{O_2} as determined by a laboratory co-oximeter.

In practice, pulse oximeters use two light-emitting diodes (LEDs) and one photodiode as transmitting and sensing transducers, usually placed on opposite sides of a digit. The microprocessor of the pulse oximeter is programmed to distinguish arterial pulse waveforms, minimize the effects of ambient light, patient motion, and electrocautery, and vary the intensity of transmitted light required to obtain the waveforms.

In most studies of pulse oximetry accuracy, data have been collected only when the pulse oximeter heart rate equaled the ECG heart rate. It has been assumed that this is a necessary condition for accuracy because it implies that the pulse oximeter is detecting pulses produced by heartbeats.

Most manufacturers claim that their pulse oximeters are accurate within ± 2 percent (SD) from 70 to 100% saturation. Although pulse oximetry may provide erroneous measurements when Sa_{O_2} is less than 70 percent, these values occur quite rarely (or *should* occur quite rarely) in patients, because Pa_{O_2} would be less than 40 mmHg. Sa_{O_2} values in the range of perhaps 70 to 95 will reflect changes in Pa_{O_2}; it is in this range that pulse oximetry finds great value in monitoring cardiorespiratory disease and directing therapy. High levels of saturation give no information about Pa_{O_2}. Because of the sigmoid shape of the oxyhemoglobin dissociation curve (Fig. 12-6), Sa_{O_2} may not decrease despite a significant deterioration in pulmonary gas exchange, i.e., if Pa_{O_2} fell from 200 to 100 mmHg. Since delivery of oxygen to the tissues is proportional to Sa_{O_2}, however, pulse oximeters will detect changes before tissue oxygenation is impaired.

Various physiologic and environmental factors interfere with the accuracy of pulse oximetry. These include decreased amplitude of peripheral pulses (hypovolemia, hypotension, hypothermia, vasoconstrictor infusions), motion artifact, electrosurgical interference, backscatter from ambient light, and dyshemoglobinemias.

The pulse oximeter can only distinguish oxyhemoglobin and deoxyhemoglobin. If other hemoglobin species are present, an error is introduced. Laboratory co-oximeters, on the other hand, generally use more than two wavelengths and often can quantify other hemoglobin species directly. When dyshemoglobins such as carboxyhemoglobin and methemoglobin can be measured, it becomes meaningful to distinguish between functional saturation [100 × oxyhemoglobin/(oxyhemoglobin + deoxyhemoglobin)]

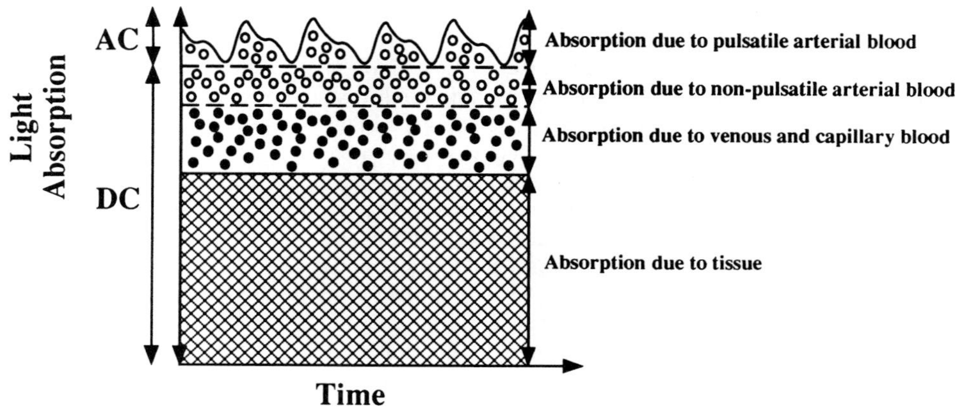

FIG. 12-8. Diagram illustrating the light absorption through living tissue. Note that the AC signal is due to the pulsatile component of the arterial blood, while the DC signal is comprised of all the nonpulsatile absorbers in the tissue. (Adapted from: *Ohmeda Pulse Oximeter Model 3700 Service Manual. Boulder, Colo., Ohmeda, 1986.*)

and fractional saturation [100 × oxyhemoglobin/(oxyhemoglobin + deoxyhemoglobin + carboxyhemoglobin + methemoglobin)]. Barker and colleagues have shown that in the presence of elevated carboxyhemoglobin or methemoglobin levels, Sp_{O_2} *overestimates* fractional saturation at all saturation values. Carboxyhemoglobinemia may occur in heavy smokers or in patients who suffer carbon monoxide inhalation. Methemoglobinemia may be induced by a large number of drugs, including local anesthetics (prilocaine, benzocaine), nitroglycerin, phenacetin, phenytoin, Pyridium, and sulfonamides.

Intravenously administered dyes, particularly methylene blue and indocyanine green, can temporarily induce artifactually low saturation readings. Deeply pigmented skin and opaque nail polish coatings may significantly decrease light transmission, rendering oximeters inoperative. The presence of fetal hemoglobin, hyperbilirubinemia, or moderate anemia (with hematocrits as low as 15 percent) do not affect the accuracy of pulse oximeters. Despite its limitations, pulse oximetry is generally acknowledged as one of the most significant advances in clinical monitoring.

Continuous Mixed Venous Oximetry. Measurement of the oxygen saturation of mixed venous hemoglobin ($S\bar{v}_{O_2}$) is helpful in the assessment of the oxygen supply-demand relationship in critically ill patients. The use of improved fiberoptic oximetry systems in conventional pulmonary artery catheters has now permitted continuous monitoring of $S\bar{v}_{O_2}$ and made bedside monitoring of this relationship practical.

$S\bar{v}_{O_2}$ can be derived from the Fick equation (Table 12-3) that relates oxygen consumption, cardiac output, and arteriovenous oxygen content difference. If the small quantity of physically dissolved oxygen in the blood is considered negligible, solving the Fick equation for $S\bar{v}_{O_2}$ yields

$$S\bar{v}_{O_2} = Sa_{O_2} - \frac{\dot{V}_{O_2}}{CO \times Hb \times 1.39 \times 10}$$

Therefore, the determinants of $S\bar{v}_{O_2}$ include the principal components of oxygen delivery [CO, hemoglobin (Hb), and Sa_{O_2}] and oxygen consumption. There is a poor correlation between $S\bar{v}_{O_2}$ and any single component of the equation ($\dot{V}_{O_2}$, CO, Sa_{O_2}, Hb)—as would be expected, because there are four separate determinants. There is, however, a good correlation between $S\bar{v}_{O_2}$ and all of these components acting at once.

With the above formula in mind, it is easy to understand that the $S\bar{v}_{O_2}$ will decrease when there is an imbalance between oxygen consumption and delivery caused by an increase in $\dot{V}_{O_2}$ or a decrease in CO, Hb, or Sa_{O_2}. $S\bar{v}_{O_2}$ will increase when the imbalance is due to changes in the opposite direction.

The normal range for $S\bar{v}_{O_2}$ in healthy subjects is 0.65 to 0.80 with an average value of 0.75 corresponding to a $P\bar{v}_{O_2}$ of 40 mmHg at a normal pH of 7.4. A rapid or prolonged fall from the normal range is indicative of a significant deterioration in the patient's clinical condition. Values below the normal range may be associated with increased oxygen consumption due to fever, shivering, seizures, exercise, and agitation, or associated with decreased oxygen delivery due to low cardiac output, anemia, or arterial hemoglobin desaturation. Values of about 0.53 correspond to a $P\bar{v}_{O_2}$ of about 28 mmHg; values at or below this level have been often associated with anaerobic metabolism, lactic acidosis, and death. Astiz and colleagues, however, were unable to identify the critical level of $S\bar{v}_{O_2}$ associated with lactic acidosis in patients with sepsis or acute myocardial infarction.

Values above the normal range indicate an increase in oxygen delivery relative to consumption and are associated with the hyperdynamic phase of sepsis, cirrhosis, peripheral left-to-right shunting, general anesthesia (when $\dot{V}_{O_2}$ is low), cellular poisoning such as cyanide toxicity (rare), marked arterial hyperoxia, or a technical malfunction of the system (e.g., wedged catheter). Normal or high $S\bar{v}_{O_2}$ values do not *ensure* that the oxygen supply-demand balance is satisfactory because accurate interpretation assumes intact and consistent vasoregulation, which is not the case in some disease states (e.g., sepsis).

Pulmonary artery catheter oximetry differs from pulse oximetry in several ways. First, the pulmonary artery catheter measures *reflected* rather than *transmitted* light. Second, being immersed in blood the pulmonary artery catheter has no need for the pulse-added signal analysis used by the pulse oximeter. Finally, one of these catheters, the Opticath* uses three wavelengths (670, 700, and 800 nm) rather than the two wavelengths (660 and 940 nm) employed by most pulse oximeters.

The Oximetrix 3 System used by the Opticath has three light-emitting diodes contained in an optical module that provide the light sources for the three selected wavelengths. Light from each of these diodes is sequentially transmitted through a single optical fiber to illuminate the blood flowing past the catheter tip. This illuminating light is absorbed, refracted, and reflected depending on the color and, therefore, oxyhemoglobin concentration of the blood. The reflected light is collected by a second fiber and returned through the catheter to a photodetector in the optical module (Fig. 12-9). Using the relative intensities of the signals representing the light levels at the various wavelengths, a computer calculates the oxygen saturation and the average for the preceding 5 s is displayed.

The saturation measured by catheter oximetry correlates well with values obtained from a laboratory co-oximeter particularly when a three-wavelength catheter is used. Accuracy of this system is maintained at hematocrits as low as 15 percent. The most common sources of error when measuring $S\bar{v}_{O_2}$ are incorrect calibration and catheter malposition. Methemoglobinemia or intravenous administration of methylene blue can also affect the measurements.

Continuous $S\bar{v}_{O_2}$ monitoring serves three major functions. First, it serves as an indicator of the adequacy of the oxygen supply-demand balance of perfused tissues. In clinically stable patients, a normal and stable $S\bar{v}_{O_2}$ may be considered an additional assurance of cardiopulmonary stability. Further assessment of cardiac output and arterial and mixed venous blood gas analyses are not necessary. Second, continuously measured $S\bar{v}_{O_2}$ may function as an early warning signal of untoward events. In this situation, although an alert has been given, the cause of the change in $S\bar{v}_{O_2}$ is not necessarily clear since the change in $S\bar{v}_{O_2}$ is sensitive but not specific. It may be necessary to measure cardiac output, Sa_{O_2}, and Hb in this setting to identify the etiology of the $S\bar{v}_{O_2}$ change. Third, continuously monitored $S\bar{v}_{O_2}$ may improve the efficiency of the delivery of critical care by providing immediate feedback as to the effectiveness of therapeutic interventions aimed at improving oxygen transport balance.

Finally, an important application of continuous venous oximetry must be one of cost containment in the ICU. The potential of cost savings lies in the decreased use of other modes for assessing oxygen transport balance, e.g., cardiac output measure-

*Abbott Critical Care Systems, Mountain View, CA.

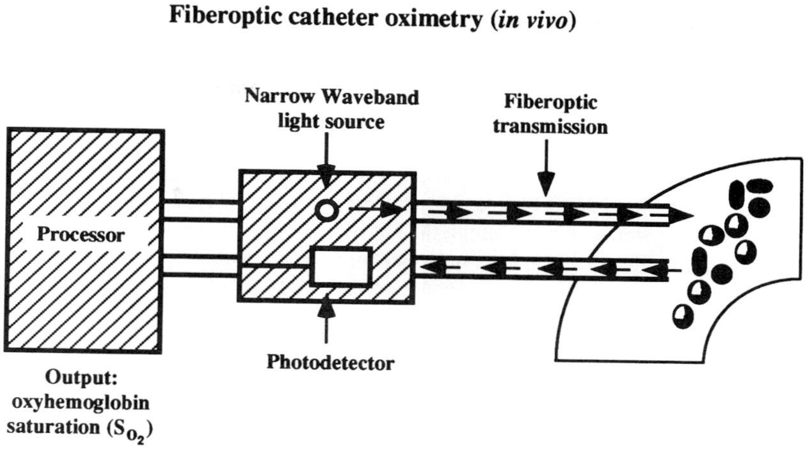

FIG. 12-9. Principle of reflection spectrophotometry used by the continuous in vivo oximeter. *(Reprinted with permission from Abbott Laboratories.)*

ments and venous blood gas analysis. The savings in some institutions are greater than the price of the catheter, and its use has been judged cost-effective.

Dual Oximetry. Pulse oximetry and continuous mixed venous oximetry can be used together (dual oximetry) to provide bedside estimates of arteriovenous oxygen content difference, oxygen utilization coefficient, and physiologic shunt.

As previously indicated, the arteriovenous oxygen content difference ($C(a - \bar{v})_{O_2}$) (Table 12-3) relates oxygen consumption with cardiac output ($\dot{V}_{O_2}/CO$). Therefore, it should be a useful bedside calculation. An initial appraisal of the total formula is somewhat intimidating: $C(a - \bar{v})_{O_2} = [(Hb \times 1.39 \times Sa_{O_2}) + (Pa_{O_2} \times 0.0031)] - [(Hb \times 1.39 \times S\bar{v}_{O_2}) + (P\bar{v}_{O_2} \times 0.0031)]$. However, the contribution of dissolved oxygen ($P_{O_2} \times 0.0031$) can be ignored in the clinically relevant ranges. The $C(a - \bar{v})_{O_2}$ can then be easily estimated at the bedside by subtracting the displayed values of pulse oximetry and continuous mixed venous oximetry and multiplying this value by the hemoglobin concentration and the constant 1.39:

$$C(a - \bar{v})_{O_2} \approx (Sa_{O_2} - S\bar{v}_{O_2}) \times Hb \times 1.39$$

The oxygen utilization coefficient (O_2UC) (Table 12-3), which relates oxygen consumption ($\dot{V}_{O_2}$) and oxygen delivery ($\dot{D}_{O_2}$), is probably the most accurate index available for routine assessment of tissue oxygen balance. This ratio can be estimated with dual oximetry by ignoring the contribution of dissolved oxygen and by eliminating CO and the factor Hb × 1.39 from the calculation (because they are present in both the numerator and denominator):

$$O_2UC = \frac{\dot{V}_{O_2}}{\dot{D}_{O_2}} = \frac{C(a - \bar{v})_{O_2} \times CO}{Ca_{O_2} \times CO} \approx \frac{Sa_{O_2} - S\bar{v}_{O_2}}{Sa_{O_2}}$$

From the above formula it is easy to understand that when the arterial blood is fully saturated with oxygen ($Sa_{O_2} = 1$), changes in oxygen utilization will be reflected by opposite changes in $S\bar{v}_{O_2}$ ($O_2UC \approx 1 - S\bar{v}_{O_2}$). Although continuous mixed venous oximetry alone can be used to estimate the oxygen utilization coefficient, the addition of pulse oximetry will increase accuracy of the estimation, particularly in patients with low and variable arterial saturation.

Calculation of physiologic shunt ($\dot{Q}_{sp}/\dot{Q}_t$) (Table 12-3) currently is one of the best methods available to accurately assess pulmonary gas exchange in critically ill patients. Assuming that hemoglobin saturations accurately reflect alterations in blood oxygen content and that pulmonary end-capillary blood is fully saturated with oxygen (i.e., $Sc'_{O_2} = 1$), an estimate of $\dot{Q}_{sp}/\dot{Q}_t$, the ventilation-perfusion index (VQI), can be obtained:

$$\frac{\dot{Q}_{sp}}{\dot{Q}_t} \approx \frac{1 - Sa_{O_2}}{1 - S\bar{v}_{O_2}} = VQI$$

The accuracy of this index is maintained as long as arterial saturation has a value other than 100 percent. Because the dissolved oxygen is not considered, the VQI fails to reflect the severity of respiratory failure at high inspired oxygen concentrations (FI_{O_2}). To minimize this effect, Räsänen and colleagues have suggested a more elaborate formula. This makes the calculation more difficult and not easily done at the bedside. In fact, the original formula for physiologic shunt might as well be used, because this can be computer-calculated as easily as the modified VQI and avoids the assumptions and inability to quantify severity. A possible compromise, then, to indicate the severity of respiratory failure, is to append the FI_{O_2} to the VQI.

Finally, newer monitoring devices (e.g., Explorer*) incorporate dual oximetry and can display on-line the arteriovenous oxygen saturation difference ($Sa - \bar{v}_{O_2}$), the modified VQI, and an estimate of the oxygen utilization coefficient.

RENAL MONITORING

The primary reason for monitoring renal function is that the kidney serves as an excellent monitor of the adequacy of perfusion. The second major indication for monitoring kidney function is to prevent acute parenchymal failure. Finally, renal function monitoring is helpful in predicting drug clearance and proper dose management.

Urine output is frequently monitored but may be misleading. Although very low urine outputs, less than 0.5 mL/kg/h, are consistently associated with low glomerular filtration rate (GFR) values, levels greater than this can also be associated with low GFR values. Diuresis created by an osmotic load (radiographic contrast or glucose), administration of diuretics, or nonoliguric renal failure may give the clinician a false sense of security while the patient has deteriorating renal function. Other methods of monitoring

*Baxter Healthcare Corp., Edwards Critical-Care Division, Santa Ana, CA.

renal function are necessary. These include tests of glomerular function and tests of tubular function.

Glomerular Function Tests

Blood urea nitrogen (BUN) has often been used to estimate renal function. BUN is affected by glomerular filtration rate and urea production. Production may be increased if large amounts of nitrogen are administered during parenteral nutritional support, as a result of gastrointestinal bleeding, or in catabolic states induced by trauma, sepsis, or steroids. Urea production may be lowered during starvation and in advanced liver disease. Because these factors are often interrelated in an unpredictable manner in critically ill patients, BUN is not a reliable monitor of renal function.

The value of plasma creatinine as a measure of renal function far exceeds the value of the BUN. The serum creatinine level is directly proportional to the level of creatinine production and inversely related to the glomerular filtration rate. In contrast to BUN concentration, plasma creatinine levels are not influenced by protein metabolism or the rate of fluid flow through the renal tubules. When creatinine production is constant, the serum creatinine level reflects glomerular filtration rate. The plasma creatinine level will double with a 50 percent reduction in glomerular filtration rate, assuming that creatinine production remains constant. Acute reductions in the glomerular filtration rate are not immediately reflected, however, because it takes 24 to 72 h for equilibration to occur.

Creatinine production is directly proportional to the muscle mass and its metabolism. In rhabdomyolysis, creatinine formation exceeds its filtration rate, such that measured serum creatinine levels increase. In conditions where the skeletal muscle mass is reduced (e.g., advanced age, immobilization), the endogenous creatinine pool is diminished and thus the serum creatinine concentration does not rise appropriately with impairment of renal function. Only with measurement of creatinine clearance can the severity of such renal function loss be determined.

Creatinine clearance is the most reliable method for clinically assessing glomerular filtration rate. Although measurements are usually performed over 24 h, 2-h creatinine clearance determinations are reasonably accurate and easier to perform. When urine output is measured in clearance studies, special efforts should be made to ensure complete bladder emptying at the beginning and end of collection periods. Creatinine clearance (C_{cr}) is calculated from the formula:

$$C_{cr} = \frac{U_{cr} \times V}{P_{cr}} \times \frac{1.73}{BSA}$$

where U_{cr} = urinary creatinine concentration, mg/dL
V = urinary volume flow, mL/min
P_{cr} = plasma creatinine concentration, mg/dL
BSA = body surface area, m^2

Clearance results are expressed as milliliters per minute per 1.73 m^2.

Tubular Function Tests

Tests that measure the concentrating ability of the renal tubules are primarily used in the differential diagnosis of oliguria to differentiate a prerenal cause unresponsive to judicious fluid therapy from intrinsic renal failure due to tubular dysfunction. Table 12-4 summarizes the differential diagnosis based on tubular function studies. The utility of each depends on the ability of the renal tubular cells to physiologically respond to a decreased extracellular fluid volume. Thus, with prerenal azotemia, the tubules can appropriately reabsorb sodium and water. In intrinsic renal failure, tubular function is markedly compromised and the ability to reabsorb sodium and water is impaired. Multifactorial renal dysfunction is most common; rarely is an isolated etiology discovered.

Table 12-4
Laboratory Findings in Prerenal Azotemia and Acute Tubular Necrosis

Test	*Prerenal Azotemia*	*Acute Tubular Necrosis*
BUN/creatinine ratio	$> 20/1$	$< 15/1$
Urine/plasma osmolar ratio	> 1.8	< 1.1
Urine/plasma creatinine ratio	> 40	< 20
Urine osmolality (mOsm/kg)	> 500	< 350
Urinary sodium concentration (meq/L)	< 20	> 40
Fractional excretion of sodium (%)	< 1	> 2

Tubular function tests are useful in oliguric patients (urine output less than 500 mL/day), because nonoliguric individuals typically have less severe tubular damage and their laboratory findings are likely to show more overlap with the values of patients with prerenal azotemia.

The fractional excretion of sodium (FE_{Na}) appears to be the most reliable of the laboratory tests for distinguishing prerenal azotemia from acute tubular necrosis. This test requires only simultaneously collected "spot" urine and blood samples. FE_{Na} can be calculated as follows:

$$FE_{Na}(\%) = \frac{U_{Na}/P_{Na}}{U_{cr}/P_{cr}} \times 100\%$$

where U_{Na} = urinary sodium concentration (meq/L), and P_{Na} = plasma sodium concentration (meq/L).

The FE_{Na} value is normally less than 1 to 2 percent. In an oliguric patient, a value of less than 1 percent is usually due to a prerenal cause. A value greater than 2 to 3 percent in this setting suggests compromised tubular function. When the value ranges between 1 and 3 percent, the test is not discriminating.

Although the FE_{Na} is very useful, it is now apparent that a number of causes of acute renal failure other than prerenal disease can, on occasion, be associated with a FE_{Na} value less than 1 percent. These include nonoliguric acute tubular necrosis, acute tubular necrosis superimposed on chronic prerenal disease (e.g., advanced cardiac or liver disease), administration of radiocontrast media or release of heme pigments (hemoglobin or myoglobin), and renal allograft rejection.

Thus, the FE_{Na} test must be interpreted in light of the specific clinical setting and other laboratory data to be useful in patient management. Correct interpretation of FE_{Na} or any of the other urinary indices is not possible if the patient had received diuretics in the 6 to 12 h preceding the test.

NEUROLOGIC MONITORING

Monitoring the function of the central nervous system may permit early recognition of cerebral dysfunction and facilitate prompt intervention in situations in which aggressive early treatment favor-

Table 12-5
Glasgow "Coma" or Responsiveness Scale

Sign	*Evaluation*	*Score*
Eye opening (E)	Spontaneous	4
	To speech	3
	To pain	2
	Nil	1
Best motor response (M)	Obeys	6
	Localizes	5
	Withdraws	4
	Abnormal flexion	3
	Extends	2
	Nil	1
Verbal response (V)	Oriented	5
	Confused conversation	4
	Inappropriate words	3
	Incomprehensible sounds	2
	Nil	1
EMV score or responsiveness sum 3–15		

SOURCE: From Jennett, Teasdale, 1977, with permission.

ably influences outcome. In the perioperative setting several methods have been used to evaluate brain function and the effects of therapy. These include the Glasgow coma score, intracranial pressure monitoring, and electrophysiologic monitoring.

Glasgow Coma Score (Scale)

The Glasgow coma score (GCS), which was initially developed to help predict outcome after closed-head injury, is now also commonly used as an objective means to measure the level of consciousness. This scoring system is extremely simple (Table 12-5), recording best possible responses to auditory or noxious stimuli as evidenced by eye opening, verbalization, and motor response. The total score ranges from 3 to 15. Head-injured patients with a GCS of 7 or less require immediate tracheal intubation and possibly hyperventilation. A GCS of 3 is assigned to ventilator-dependent patients with no response to verbal or painful stimulation.

Because of the widespread use of tracheal intubation, pharmacologically induced neuromuscular paralysis, and mechanical ventilator-induced hyperventilation, the GCS can only be accurately ascertained before and after but not during such therapy. In any event, it is artifactually low since patients' verbal responses cannot be determined while they are intubated.

Intracranial Pressure Monitoring

Physical findings are often unreliable to ascertain the presence of increased intracranial pressure (ICP). Thus, the only direct assessment of ICP is obtained by measurement.

Measuring ICP permits calculation of cerebral perfusion pressure (CPP), which is defined as the difference between the MAP and ICP. Thus, isolated increases in ICP or decreases in MAP will result in a reduction in CPP. The CPP may be insufficient if ICP increases to more than 20 mmHg. Values above 40 mmHg represent very dangerous and life-threatening levels of intracranial hypertension.

The most common indication for ICP monitoring is head injury. In this condition, ICP monitoring is recommended when the coma score following resuscitation is 7 or below. According to Narayan and colleagues an exception may be made in patients with a normal brain CT scan at admission unless two of the following features are present: systolic blood pressure under 90 mmHg, motor posturing, and age over 40 years. In those patients not monitored initially, monitoring may be initiated later in their course should they deteriorate neurologically or if they demonstrate delayed hematomas on follow-up CT scans.

Other conditions for which ICP monitoring has been recommended include subarachnoid hemorrhage, hydrocephalus, postcraniotomy, and Reye's syndrome. Although some investigators have also advocated this form of monitoring in patients with massive strokes, encephalitis, and post–cardiac arrest states, little evidence has been generated to suggest a beneficial impact.

Several methods of ICP measurement are available (Fig. 12-10). A ventricular catheter connected to a standard strain gauge transducer offers excellent waveform characteristics and permits withdrawal of cerebrospinal fluid (CSF). This catheter, however, may be difficult to insert when cerebral edema or hematoma causes shifting or collapse of the lateral ventricle system. A subarachnoid bolt is easily inserted under any circumstances, although at times may give erroneous readings, depending on its placement relative to the site of injury. Compared to ventricular catheters, the waveforms obtained are not as good and CSF drainage is usually not possible. Epidural bolts have a lower risk of complications but are less accurate than ventricular catheters or subarachnoid bolts

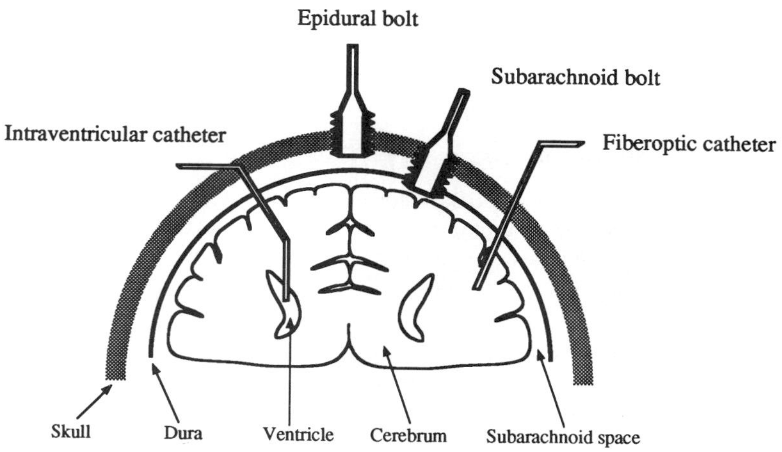

FIG. 12-10. Diagram illustrating intraventricular catheters, epidural bolts, subarachnoid bolts, and fiberoptic catheters for ICP measurement. (From: *Doyle DJ, Mark PWS: 1992, with permission.*)

and do not permit withdrawal of CSF. Fiber-optic transducer-tipped catheters can be placed into intraventricular, subarachnoid, or intraparenchymal sites. These devices appear to offer advantages over conventional ICP monitors, especially in their ability to measure brain parenchymal pressures.

The major risk of ICP monitoring is that of infection. If monitoring is conducted for less than 3 days, the infection rate is virtually zero; beyond 5 days the incidence of infection increases significantly.

Electrophysiologic Monitoring

The electroencephalogram (EEG) reflects spontaneous and ongoing electrical activity recorded on the surface of the scalp. Intraoperative EEG recording has been primarily used for monitoring the adequacy of cerebral perfusion during carotid endarterectomy. Other procedures in which EEG recording has been used include cerebrovascular surgery, open heart surgery, epilepsy surgery, and induced hypotension for a variety of surgical procedures. In the ICU, standard EEG recording is not routinely used because of insufficient technical personnel, the volume of data generated in a short period, the difficulty of on-line EEG interpretation, numerous electrically induced artifacts, and drug-induced suppression of electrical activity. To simplify EEG recording and to make it more useful for clinical application in the operating room and ICU, some monitors process the raw data automatically. The compressed spectral array (CSA) and density spectral array (DSA) are two methods of visually displaying such processed EEG information.

Sensory-evoked potentials (SEP) are minute electrophysiologic responses elicited by a stimulus and extracted from an ongoing EEG by signal averaging. They reflect the functional integrity of specific sensory pathways and serve to some extent as more general indicators of function in adjacent structures. Somatosensory evoked potentials (SSEP) reflect the integrity of the dorsal spinal columns and the sensory cortex and may be useful for monitoring during resection of spinal cord tumors, spine instrumentation, carotid endarterectomy, and aortic surgery. Brainstem auditory-evoked potentials (BAEP) reflect the integrity of the eighth cranial nerve and the auditory pathways above the pons and are used for monitoring during surgery of the posterior fossa. Visual-evoked potentials (VEP) may be used to monitor the optic nerve and upper brainstem during resections of large pituitary tumors. Several studies have promoted the prognostic value of SEP in the ICU, primarily in head trauma patients. Continuous monitoring in the ICU is still rare.

METABOLIC MONITORING

General Considerations

The necessity to substitute artificial feedings during recovery from surgery and trauma turns the simple everyday function of ingestion of food into a complicated area involving mathematics, suppositions, high technology, and the potential for creating harmful side effects.

Assessment of Caloric Expenditure. Energy requirements are dependent on a number of factors including the body surface area, age, and sex. Basal energy expenditure (BEE) can be predicted with reasonable accuracy (± 5 percent) by the Harris-Benedict equation:

$$\text{Men: } 66.47 + (13.75 \times W) + (5.00 \times H) - (6.76 \times A) = \text{BEE} \quad \text{kcal/day}$$

$$\text{Women: } 655.10 + (9.56 \times W) + (1.85 \times H) - (4.68 \times A) = \text{BEE} \quad \text{kcal/day}$$

where W = body weight, kg
H = height, cm
A = age, years

Elwyn and colleagues state that resting energy expenditure (REE) can be approximated from the BEE by increasing it by 10 percent, adding the calories necessary to compensate for the specific dynamic action of food.

The stress of illness, the change in hormonal milieu relating to the stress state, alterations in substrate utilization, and fever all can be predicted to increase REE. While early studies emphasized increases of 25 percent for multiple-trauma patients and 50 percent for burn patients, even an increase of 60 percent above BEE would only result in a need for 40 kcal/kg/day or less than 3000 kcal in a 70-kg patient. Excessive caloric administration is potentially detrimental. Carbohydrates given in excess of requirements are turned into fat resulting in an increase in CO_2 production. The liver may develop fatty infiltration resulting in hepatic dysfunction.

In addition, many patients may have protein malnutrition despite being overweight due to obesity or overhydration. In a study of critically ill patients, Makk and colleagues found that 58 percent were overweight. Forty-two percent had a kwashiorkor-like pattern of malnutrition and 11 percent had a marasmus-like pattern. Protein malnutrition necessitates administration of higher levels of protein to avoid or reverse end-organ dysfunction and impaired acute-phase protein synthesis which sets the stage for nosocomial infections and the multiple-organ-system failure syndrome.

Assessment of Oxygen Consumption. If caloric expenditures can be considered the fuel, then another aspect of metabolic monitoring is the flame. Oxidative metabolism or oxygen consumption reflects metabolic activity. Cuthbertson described the ebb-and-flow phase of the metabolic response to injury. In his terms, the ebb phase, lasting 24 to 48 h, is a period of "diminished circulatory vitality"—decreased cardiac output, diminishing oxygen delivery, and resulting decreased oxygen consumption. The recognition of the association between diminished oxygen delivery in the ebb phase with the late occurrence of sepsis and multiple-organ-system failure has focused attention on improving oxygen delivery in an attempt to forestall this seemingly inevitable progression. Thus, monitoring and maximizing oxygen delivery as described previously has been given additional significance in terms of minimizing long-term detrimental metabolic effects secondary to stress and injury.

Measurements and Uses

Oxygen delivery or cardiac output times arterial oxygen content and oxygen consumption (normally about 150 mL/min/m^2) assess oxidative metabolism. CO_2 production is a measure of a by-product of oxidative metabolism. The ratio of CO_2 production to oxygen consumption is termed the respiratory quotient (RQ). During normal oral dietary intake, carbohydrates, protein, and fat are ingested, giving an average RQ of approximately 0.8. During prolonged starvation, the body adapts to fat metabolism and the RQ may fall to as low as 0.6 to 0.7. On the other hand, during excessive carbohydrate administration, the transformation into fat releases additional CO_2 and the RQ rises above 1.0. Thus, monitoring oxygen consumption, CO_2 production, and calculating the RQ provides inferences into the adequacy of total calories as well as the mixture of substrates.

Technology

In the past few years, clinicians, recognizing the number of variables affecting REE and total energy expenditure (TEE), have attempted direct measurements in order to meet an individual patient's needs at a particular time in the course of the illness. It is clear that estimates of REE from the Harris-Benedict equation, even modified by estimates to adjust for increased metabolic activity as suggested by Elwyn and Grant, still lead to inaccurate assessment of TEE. Direct calorimetry measures body heat production and is correlated with energy use. The subject, however, must be placed in a closed chamber for measurement of heat production, and clearly this is not applicable to patient care. Indirect calorimetry permits derivation of caloric requirements from the measurements of oxygen consumption and CO_2 production. Methods used include Douglas bag collection of expired gases, use of the Fick equation, and computerized open circuit measurements.

Douglas Bag Collection. Samples of inspiratory and mixed expiratory gases are analyzed for oxygen and CO_2 concentrations. This technique is unfortunately prone to many errors. Gas leakage, incomplete emptying, inaccurate measurement of total expired gases, and incomplete mixing or leakage through incompletely sealed connections are but a few of the problems encountered. Finally, it is a tedious method that does not lend itself to frequent or routine clinical use.

The Reverse Fick Method. The classic Fick equation (Table 12-3) relates oxygen consumption to the product of cardiac output and arterial venous oxygen content difference. Repeated cardiac output determinations have an accuracy in the range of ±5 percent but are not as important as variability in the patient's physiology in which changes may exceed ±10 percent in a short time. Pulse oximetry and mixed venous oximetry show that minute-to-minute variations in these values also occur. Smithies has shown that these factors result in a 10 percent variation between measurements and lower total values compared to validated spirometric techniques. This latter difference reflects the oxygen consumption of the lung, which is included in the spirometric method but not in the reverse Fick technique.

Computerized Open Circuit Indirect Calorimetry. Several commercial indirect calorimeters have been evaluated by Makita and associates. The Datex Deltatrac Metabolic Monitor,* the Engstrom Metabolic Computer,† and the SensorMedics MMC Horizon‡ use slightly different techniques and formulas. Mean relative errors of measurement for all three monitors, however, were in the range of 1.4 to 6 percent for oxygen consumption, CO_2 production, and RQ.

*Datex Instrumentarium, Helsinki, Finland.

†Gambro Engström A.B., Broma, Sweden.

‡SensorMedics, Anaheim, CA.

In routine clinical use, however, there are many potential errors. Instruments lose calibration easily. High inspired oxygen concentrations ($F_{I_{O_2}} > 0.6$) render measurements inaccurate. Fluctuations in hospital gas line presure cause 1 to 2 percent fluctuations in inspired $F_{I_{O_2}}$, sufficient to impair the accuracy of overall oxygen consumption. Leaks at joints and connections occur frequently and must be eliminated before and during studies. Measurements of CO_2 production depend upon a steady-state relationship between CO_2 production at the cellular level, transport to lungs, and CO_2 elimination via the lungs and measured in exhaled gases. Therefore, changes in the metabolic rate, changes in cardiac output, and changes in ventilation all affect the inherent supposition that CO_2 production and CO_2 elimination measured by the metabolic monitor are equal. Minute-to-minute variations may be minimized by ensuring that measurements encompass at least 15 min twice daily.

Usefulness of Metabolic Monitoring

First, these measurements can be used to judge the end result of the interactions of all the unknowns (including degrees of illness, activity, and metabolism) in producing the current levels of oxygen consumption and CO_2 production.

Second, either too little or incorrect proportions of nutritional support are undesirable. If we remember that approximately 32 to 35 kcal/day should suffice in most clinical circumstances and that there is no outcome data suggesting that ±10 or even 20 percent has a demonstrable adverse effect on any known variable, we should ensure that we stay within this range of measured values.

Third, we could identify patients with significant hypometabolism or hypermetabolic states because clinical estimates are often incorrect. Adjusting nutritional support in these circumstances seems to be common sense although it has not been proved that these adjustments make any real difference.

Fourth, given the wide variations in caloric requirements and in substrate utilization, metabolic monitoring, allowing more appropriate partitioning of the substrates, seems more desirable than administering quantities by rote or formula.

Fifth, measurements of RQ may be useful in patients who have respiratory failure and CO_2 retention while receiving high carbohydrate loads. Identification of a high RQ due to excessive carbohydrate administration is one correctable factor.

Because commercially available indirect calorimeters now can measure oxygen consumption, CO_2 production, and calculate other parameters of metabolic cellular activity, the demonstrated accuracy in measurement can be used to support more precise prescription of nutritional therapy. Questioning whether this degree of obtainable precision alters outcome is relevant; at the same time, inaccurate prescriptions based on invalid estimates would not seem to be a viable objective. The costs of this approach are not inconsiderable, and while they may be offset by savings in wasted nutritional support, more data reflecting improvement in outcome are necessary before mandatory or daily usage even in critically ill patients can be supported.

TEMPERATURE MONITORING

Temperature, along with heart rate, blood pressure, and respiratory rate, remains one of the traditional four cardinal vital signs. Temperature is usually taken rectally in ill patients or orally when significant elevations are not expected.

Temperatures of the periphery of the body measured at the mouth, skin, or axilla are often unreliable and may be influenced by factors such as mouth breathing, temperature of recently ingested food, and/or environmental temperature. Therefore, it is recommended that deeper core temperatures be taken in the critically ill.

Core temperatures, which are relatively resistant to external influences, more accurately reflect the mean temperature of the body's vital organs. Core temperature has been measured by either placing a thermistor wire directly against the tympanic membrane, placing a thermistor probe into the esophagus, or by a special thermistor probe deep in the rectum. Esophageal and tympanic membrane wires are uncomfortable and invasive and are used exclusively in patients under general anesthesia. Rectal probes are commonly used in the operating room and ICU but may be extruded from the rectum and have a recognized risk of bowel wall perforation.

Three devices are now commercially available to measure bedside core temperature in ICU patients: pulmonary artery thermistor catheters, urinary bladder thermistor catheters, and auditory canal probes. Measurement of pulmonary artery blood temperature by the pulmonary artery thermistor catheter is increasingly being used as a reliable indicator of core temperature. The need for a catheter is an obvious disadvantage of this approach. Urinary bladder catheters have the advantage of giving both exact measurements of urine output and continuous urine temperature. Auditory canal infrared probes noninvasively measure tympanic membrane temperatures; however, further study of their accuracy in the ICU setting is needed.

Bibliography

Hemodynamic Monitoring

Band JD, Maki DG: Infections caused by arterial catheters used for hemodynamic monitoring. *Am J Med* 67:735, 1979.

Banner T, Banner MJ: Cardiac output measurement technology, in Civetta JM, Taylor RW, Kirby RR (eds): *Critical Care*. Philadelphia, Lippincott, 1988, chap 35.

Bedford RF, Wollman H: Complications of percutaneous radial artery cannulation: An objective prospective study in man. *Anesthesiology* 38:228, 1973.

Bedford RF: Invasive blood pressure monitoring, in Blitt CD (ed): *Monitoring in Anesthesia and Critical Care Medicine,* 2d ed. New York, Churchill Livingstone, 1990, chap 7.

Berglund E: Balance of left and right ventricular output: Relation between left and right atrial pressures. *Am J Physiol* 178:381, 1954.

Berlauk JF, Abrams JH, et al: Preoperative optimization of cardiovascular hemodynamics improves outcome in peripheral vascular surgery. *Ann Surg* 214:289, 1991.

Brown M, Gordon LH, et al: Intravascular monitoring via the axillary artery. *Anaesth Intensive Care* 13:38, 1985.

Bruner JMR: *Handbook of Blood Pressure Monitoring*. Massachusetts, PSG Publishing, 1978.

Bull MJ, Schreiner RL, et al: Neurologic complications following temporal artery catheterization. *J Pediatr* 96:1071, 1980.

Calvin JE, Driedger AA, Sibbald WJ: Does the pulmonary capillary wedge pressure predict left ventricular preload in critically ill patients? *Crit Care Med* 9:437, 1981.

Cederholm I, Sørensen J, Carlsson C: Thrombosis following percutaneous radial artery cannulation. *Acta Anaesth Scand* 30:227, 1986.

Civetta JM, Gabel JC, Laver MB: Disparate ventricular function in surgical patients. *Surg Forum* 22:136, 1971.

Civetta JM: Pulmonary artery catheter insertion, in Sprung CL (ed): *The Pulmonary Artery Catheter: Methodology and Clinical Applications*. Rockville, Aspen Publishers, 1983, chap 2.

Civetta JM: Invasive catheterization, in Shoemaker WC, Thompson WL (eds): *Critical Care: State of the Art*. Anaheim, CA, Society of Critical Care Medicine, 1980, chap 1.

Cohn JN: Blood pressure measurement in shock. *JAMA* 199:972, 1967.

Connors AF, McCaffree DR, Gray BA: Evaluation of right heart catheterization in the critically ill patient without acute myocardial infarction. *N Engl J Med* 308:263, 1983.

De Campo T, Civetta JM: The effect of short-term discontinuation of high level PEEP in patients with acute respiratory failure. *Crit Care Med* 7:47, 1979.

Dhainaut JF, Brunet F, et al: Bedside evaluation of right ventricular performance using a rapid computerized thermodilution method. *Crit Care Med* 15:148, 1987.

Eisenberg PR, Jaffe AS, Schuster DP: Clinical evaluation compared to pulmonary artery catheterization in the hemodynamic assessment of critically ill patients. *Crit Care Med* 12:549, 1984.

Ejrup B, Fischer B, Wright IS: Clinical evaluation of blood flow to the hand: The false-positive Allen test. *Circulation* 33:778, 1966.

Eyer S, Brummitt C, et al: Catheter-related sepsis: Prospective randomized study of three methods of long-term catheter maintenance. *Crit Care Med* 18:1073, 1990.

Forrester JS, Diamond G, et al: Filling pressures in the right and left sides of the heart in acute myocardial infarction. *N Engl J Med* 285:190, 1971.

Forrester JS, Diamond GA, Swan HJC: Correlative classification of clinical and hemodynamic function after acute myocardial infarction. *Am J Cardiol* 39:137, 1977.

Gardner RM: Direct blood pressure measurements: Dynamic response requirements. *Anesthesiology* 54:227, 1981.

Gardner RM: System concepts for invasive pressure monitoring, in Civetta JM, Taylor RW, Kirby RR (eds): *Critical Care*. Philadelphia, Lippincott, 1988, chap 28.

Gerber MJ, Hines RL, Barash PG: Arterial waveforms and systemic vascular resistance: Is there a correlation? *Anesthesiology* 66:823, 1987.

Goldenheim PD, Kazemi H: Cardiopulmonary monitoring of critically ill patients. *N Engl J Med* 311:776, 1984.

Hunn D, Gobel FL, et al: Thermodilution cardiac output values obtained by using a centrally placed introducer sheath and right atrial port of a pulmonary artery catheter. *Crit Care Med* 18:438, 1990.

Johnstone RE, Greenhow DE: Catheterization of the dorsalis pedis artery. *Anesthesiology* 39:654, 1973.

Keusch DJ, Winters S, Thys DM: The patient's position influences the incidence of dysrhythmias during pulmonary artery catheterization. *Anesthesiology* 70:582, 1989.

Kirton OC, Varon AJ, et al: Flow-directed, pulmonary artery catheter-induced pseudoaneurysm: Urgent diagnosis and endovascular obliteration. *Crit Care Med* 20:1178, 1992.

Lang RM, Borow KM, et al: Systemic vascular resistance: An unreliable index of left ventricular afterload. *Circulation* 74:1114, 1986.

Lappas D, Lell WA, et al: Indirect measurement of left-atrial pressure in surgical patients: Pulmonary-capillary wedge pressure and pulmonary-artery diastolic pressures compared with left-atrial pressure. *Anesthesiology* 38:394, 1973.

Norwood S, Ruby A, et al: Catheter-related infections and associated septicemia. *Chest* 99:968, 1991.

Norwood SH, Cormier B, et al: Prospective study of catheter-related infection during prolonged arterial catheterization. *Crit Care Med* 16:836, 1988.

Norwood SH, Jenkins G: An evaluation of triple-lumen catheter infections using a guidewire technique. *J Trauma* 30:706, 1990.

O'Quin R, Marini J: Pulmonary artery occlusion pressure: Clinical physiology, measurement, and interpretation. *Am Rev Respir Dis* 128:319, 1983.

Pearl RG, Rosenthal MH, et al: Effect of injectate volume and temperature on thermodilution cardiac output determination. *Anesthesiology* 64:798, 1986.

Perel A, Pizov R, Cotev S: Systolic blood pressure variation is a sensitive indicator of hypovolemia in ventilated dogs subjected to graded hemorrhage. *Anesthesiology* 67:498, 1987.

Pesola GR, Carlon GC: Thermodilution cardiac output: Proximal lumen versus right ventricular port. *Crit Care Med* 19:563, 1991.

Pillow K, Herrick IA: Pulse oximetry compared with Doppler ultrasound for assessment of collateral blood flow to the hand. *Anaesthesia* 46:388, 1991.

Pinsky M, Vincent J-L, De Smet J-M: Estimating left ventricular filling pressure during positive end-expiratory pressure in humans. *Am Rev Respir Dis* 143:25, 1991.

Pizov R, Ya'ari Y, Perel A: The arterial pressure waveform during acute ventricular failure and synchronized external chest compression. *Anesth Analg* 68:150, 1989.

Raper R, Sibbald WJ: Misled by the wedge? The Swan-Ganz catheter and left ventricular preload. *Chest* 89:427, 1986.

Russell JA, Joel M, et al: Prospective evaluation of radial and femoral artery catheterization sites in critically ill adults. *Crit Care Med* 11:936, 1983.

Schlant RC, Sonnenblick EH: Normal physiology of the cardiovascular system, in Hurst JW (ed): *The Heart,* 7th ed. New York, McGraw-Hill, 1990, chap 3.

Schmitt EA, Brantigan CO: Common artifacts of pulmonary artery and pulmonary artery wedge pressures: Recognition and interpretation. *J Clin Monit* 2:44, 1986.

Schwid HA, Taylor LA, Smith NT: Computer model analysis of the radial artery pressure waveform. *J Clin Monit* 3:220, 1987.

Segal J, Pearl RG, et al: Instantaneous and continuous cardiac output obtained with a Doppler pulmonary artery catheter. *J Am Coll Cardiol* 13:1382, 1989.

Shah KB, Rao TLK, et al: A review of pulmonary artery catheterization in 6,245 patients. *Anesthesiology* 61:271, 1984.

Sharkey SW: Beyond the wedge: Clinical physiology and the Swan-Ganz catheter. *Am J Med* 83:111, 1987.

Shoemaker WC, Appel PL, et al: Prospective trial of supranormal values of survivors as therapeutic goals in high risk surgical patients. *Chest* 94:1176, 1988.

Sprung CL, Elser B, et al: Risk of right bundle-branch block and complete heart block during pulmonary artery catheterization. *Crit Care Med* 17:1, 1989.

Sprung CL, Jacobs, LJ: Indications for pulmonary artery catheterization, in Sprung CL (ed): *The Pulmonary Artery Catheter: Methodology and Clinical Applications*. Rockville, Aspen Publishers, 1983, chap 1.

Sprung CL, Rackow EC, Civetta JM: Direct measurements and derived calculations using the pulmonary artery catheter, in Sprung CL (ed): *The Pulmonary Artery Catheter: Methodology and Clinical Applications*. Rockville, Aspen Publishers, 1983, chap 4.

Steingrub JS, Celoria G, et al: Therapeutic impact of pulmonary artery catheterization in a medical/surgical ICU. *Chest* 99:1451, 1991.

Stevens JH, Raffin TA, et al: Thermodilution cardiac output measurement: Effects of the respiratory cycle on its reproducibility. *JAMA* 253:2240, 1985.

Swan HJC: Monitoring the seriously ill patient with heart disease (including use of Swan-Ganz catheter), in Hurst JW (ed): *The Heart,* 7th ed. New York, McGraw-Hill, 1990, chap 120.

Tooker J, Huseby J, Butler J: The effect of Swan-Ganz catheter height on the wedge pressure-left atrial pressure relationship in edema during positive-pressure ventilation. *Am Rev Respir Dis* 117:721, 1978.

Tuman KJ, Carroll GC, Ivankovich AD: Pitfalls in interpretation of pulmonary artery catheter data. *J Cardiothor Anesth* 3:625, 1989.

Venus B, Mallory D: *Problems in Critical Care: Vascular Cannulation*. Philadelphia, Lippincott, 1988.

Verweij J, Kester A, et al: Comparison of three methods for measuring central venous pressure. *Crit Care Med* 14:288, 1986.

West JB, Dollery CT, Naimark A: Distribution of blood flow in isolated lung; Relation to vascular and alveolar pressures. *J Appl Physiol* 19:713, 1964.

Wilkins RG: Radial artery cannulation and ischemic damage: A review. *Anaesthesia* 40:896, 1985.

Yelderman M: Continuous measurement of cardiac output with the use of stochastic system identification techniques. *J Clin Monit* 6:322, 1990.

Respiratory Monitoring

Alexander CM, Teller LE, Gross JB: Principles of pulse oximetry: Theoretical and practical considerations. *Anesth Analg* 68:368, 1989.

Astiz ME, Rackow EC, Kaufman B: Relationship of oxygen delivery and mixed venous oxygenation to lactic acidosis in patients with sepsis and acute myocardial infarction. *Crit Care Med* 16:655, 1988.

Barker SJ, Hyatt J: Continuous measurement of intraarterial pHa, Pa_{CO_2}, and Pa_{O_2} in the operating room. *Anesth Analg* 73:43, 1991.

Barker SJ, Tremper KK, Hyatt J: Effects of methemoglobinemia on pulse oximetry and mixed venous oximetry. *Anesthesiology* 70:112, 1989.

Barker SJ, Tremper KK: The effect of carbon monoxide inhalation on pulse oximetry and transcutaneous P_{O_2}. *Anesthesiology* 66:677, 1987.

Birmingham PK, Cheney FW, Ward RJ: Esophageal intubation: A review of detection techniques. *Anesth Analg* 65:886, 1986.

Bone RC, Gravenstein N, Kirby RR: Monitoring respiratory and hemodynamic function in the patient with respiratory failure, in Kirby RR, Banner MI, Downs JB (eds): *Clinical Applications of Ventilatory Support*. New York, Churchill Livingstone, 1990, chap 11.

Callaham M, Barton C, Matthay M: Effect of epinephrine on the ability of end-tidal carbon dioxide readings to predict initial resuscitation from cardiac arrest. *Crit Care Med* 20:337, 1992.

Callaham M, Barton C: Prediction of outcome of cardiopulmonary resuscitation from end-tidal carbon dioxide concentration. *Crit Care Med* 18:358, 1990.

Cane RD, Shapiro BA, et al: Unreliability of oxygen tension-based indices in reflecting intrapulmonary shunting in critically ill patients. *Crit Care Med* 16:1243, 1988.

Civetta JM: Simultaneous arterial and venous oximetry, in Civetta JM, Taylor RW, Kirby RR (eds): *Critical Care Updates*. Philadelphia, Lippincott, 1990, vol 1.

Divertie MB, McMichan JC: Continuous monitoring of mixed venous oxygen saturation. *Chest* 85:423, 1984.

Edwards JD, Wilkins RG, Mayall RM: Importance of sampling site for measurement of mixed venous oxygen saturation. *Crit Care Med* 15:405, 1987.

Fiastro JF, Habib MP, et al: Comparison of standard weaning parameters and mechanical work of breathing in mechanically ventilated patients. *Chest* 94:232, 1988.

Flick GR, Berger MB: Pulmonary function testing in the critical care unit, in Civetta JM, Taylor RW, Kirby RR (eds): *Critical Care*. Philadelphia, Lippincott, 1988, chap 33.

Geha DG: Blood gas monitoring, in Blitt CD (ed): *Monitoring in Anesthesia and Critical Care Medicine,* 2d ed. New York, Churchill Livingstone, 1990, chap 15.

Gettinger A, DeTraglia MC, Glass DD: In vivo comparison of two mixed venous saturation catheters. *Anesthesiology* 66:373, 1987.

Gravenstein JS, Paulus DA, Hayes TJ: *Capnography in Clinical Practice*. Boston, Butterworths, 1989.

Hecker BR, Brown DL, Wilson D: A comparison of two pulmonary artery mixed venous oxygen saturation catheters during changing conditions in cardiac surgery. *J Cardiothor Anesth* 3:269, 1989.

Hoffman RA, Krieger BP, et al: End-tidal carbon dioxide in critically ill patients during changes in mechanical ventilation. *Am Rev Respir Dis* 140:1265, 1989.

Kasnitz P, Druger GL, et al: Mixed venous oxygen tension and hyperlactatemia. *JAMA* 236:570, 1976.

Kelleher JF: Pulse oximetry. *J Clin Monit* 5:37, 1989.

Lee S, Tremper KK, Barker SJ: Effects of anemia on pulse oximetry and continuous mixed venous hemoglobin saturation monitoring in dogs. *Anesthesiology* 75:118, 1991.

Nelson LD: Application of venous saturation monitoring, in Civetta JM, Taylor RW, Kirby RR (eds): *Critical Care*. Philadelphia, Lippincott, 1988, chap 31.

Nelson LD: Mixed venous oximetry, in Snyder JV, Pinsky MR (eds): *Oxygen Transport in the Critically Ill*. Chicago, Yearbook Medical Publishers, 1987, chap 16.

Orlando R: Continuous mixed venous oximetry in critically ill surgical patients: ''High-Tech' cost-effectiveness. *Arch Surg* 121:470, 1986.

Räsänen J, Downs JB, DeHaven B: Titration of continuous positive airway pressure by real-time dual oximetry. *Crit Chest* 92:853, 1987.

Räsänen J, Downs JB, et al: Estimation of oxygen utilization by dual oximetry. *Ann Surg* 206:621, 1987.

Räsänen J, Downs JB, et al: Oxygen tension and oxyhemoglobin saturations in the assessment of pulmonary gas exchange. *Crit Care Med* 15:1058, 1987.

Räsänen J, Downs JB, Malec DJ, et al: Real-time continuous estimation of gas exchange by dual oximetry. *Intensive Care Med* 14:118, 1988.

Rouby J-J, Poète P, et al: Three mixed venous saturation catheters in patients with circulatory shock and respiratory failure. *Chest* 98:954, 1990.

Russell GB, Graybeal JM: Stability of arterial to end-tidal carbon dioxide gradients during postoperative cardiorespiratory support. *Can J Anaesth* 37:560, 1990.

Sahn SA, Lakshminarayan S: Bedside criteria for discontinuation of mechanical support. *Chest* 63:1002, 1973.

Sanders AB, Atlas M, et al: Expired pCO_2 as an index of coronary perfusion pressure. *Am J Emerg Med* 3:147, 1985.

Sanders AB, Kern KB, et al: End-tidal carbon dioxide monitoring during cardiopulmonary resuscitation: A prognostic indicator for survival. *JAMA* 262:1347, 1989.

Scheller MS, Unger RJ, Kelner MJ: Effects of intravenously administered dyes on pulse oximetry readings. *Anesthesiology* 65:550, 1986.

Schweiss JF: Mixed venous hemoglobin saturation: Theory and application. *Int Anesthesiol Clin* 25:113, 1987.

Shapiro HM, Smith G, et al: Errors in sampling pulmonary arterial blood with a Swan-Ganz catheter. *Anesthesiology* 40:291, 1974.

Shapiro M, Wilson RK, et al: Work of breathing through different sized endotracheal tubes. *Crit Care Med* 14:1028, 1986.

Tahvanainen J, Salmenpera M, Nikki P: Extubation criteria after weaning from intermittent mandatory ventilation and continuous positive airway pressure. *Crit Care Med* 11:702, 1983.

Tobin MJ: Respiratory monitoring. *JAMA* 264:244, 1990.

Tremper KK, Barker SJ: Pulse oximetry. *Anesthesiology* 70:98, 1989.

Varon AJ, Anderson HB, Civetta JM: Desaturation noted by pulmonary artery catheter oximeter after methylene blue injection. *Anesthesiology* 71:791, 1989.

Varon AJ, Morrina J, Civetta JM: Clinical utility of a colorimetric end-tidal CO_2 detector in cardiopulmonary resuscitation and emergency intubation. *J Clin Monit* 7:289, 1991.

Veyckemans F, Baele P, et al: Hyperbilirubinemia does not interfere with hemoglobin saturation measured by pulse oximetry. *Anesthesiology* 70:118, 1989.

Weil MH, Bisera J, et al: Cardiac output and end-tidal carbon dioxide. *Crit Care Med* 13:907, 1985.

West JB: *Pulmonary Physiology*, 4th ed. Baltimore, Williams & Wilkins, 1990.

Wingarten M: Respiratory monitoring of carbon dioxide and oxygen: A ten-year perspective. *J Clin Monit* 6:217, 1990.

Woodson RD: Physiological significance of oxygen dissociation curve shifts. *Crit Care Med* 7:368, 1979.

Yang KL, Tobin MJ: A prospective study of indexes predicting the outcome of trials of weaning from mechanical ventilation. *N Engl J Med* 324:1445, 1991.

Renal Monitoring

Espinel CH: The FE_{Na} test: Use in the differential diagnosis of acute renal failure. *JAMA* 236:579, 1976.

Tonnesen AS: Monitoring the kidney and urine, in Blitt CD (ed): *Monitoring in Anesthesia and Critical Care Medicine*, 2d ed. New York, Churchill Livingstone, 1990, chap 22.

Zarich S, Fang LST, Diamond JR: Fractional excretion of sodium: Exceptions to its diagnostic value. *Arch Intern Med* 145:108, 1985.

Neurologic Monitoring

Doyle DJ, Mark PWS: Analysis of intracranial pressure. *J Clin Monit* 8:81, 1992.

Jennett B, Teasdale G: Aspects of coma after severe head injury. *Lancet* 1:878, 1977.

Judson JA, Cant BR, Shaw NA: Early prediction of outcome from cerebral trauma by somatosensory evoked potentials. *Crit Care Med* 18:363, 1990.

Kirby R: Monitoring of neurologic function, in Civetta JM, Taylor RW, Kirby RR (eds): *Critical Care*. Philadelphia, Lippincott, 1988, chap 34.

Lam AM, Manninen PH, et al: Monitoring electrophysiologic function during carotid endarterectomy. A comparison of somatosensory evoked potentials and conventional electroencephalogram. *Anesthesiology* 75:15, 1991.

Miller SM: Management of central nervous injuries, in Capan L, Miller SM, Turndorf H (eds): *Trauma Anesthesia and Intensive Care*. Philadelphia, Lippincott, 1991, chap 10.

Narayan RK, Kishore DRS, et al: Intracranial pressure: To monitor or not to monitor? *J Neurosurg* 56:650, 1982.

Metabolic Monitoring

Askanazi J, Rosenbaum SH, et al: Respiratory changes induced by the large glucose loads of total parenteral nutrition. *JAMA* 243:1444, 1980.

Cuthbertson DP: Post-shock metabolic response. *Lancet* 1:433, 1942.

Dietrich KE, Romero MD, Conrad SA: The technique of measuring energy expenditure at the bedside. *J Crit Illness* 4:65, 1989.

Elwyn DH, Kinney JM, Askanazi J: Energy expenditure in surgical patients. *Surg Clin North Am* 61:545, 1981.

Grant JP: *Handbook of Total Parenteral Nutrition*. Philadelphia, WB Saunders, 1975.

Harris JA, Benedict FG: A biometric study of basal metabolism in man. Carnegie Institute of Washington, Publication no. 279, 1919.

Kemper M, Weissman C, Hyman AI: Caloric requirements and supply in critically ill surgical patients. *Crit Care Med* 20:344, 1992.

Kinney JM: Surgical hyper-metabolism and nitrogen metabolism, in Wilkinson AW, Cuthbertson D (eds): *Metabolism and the Response to Injury*. Turnbridge Wells, Pitman Medical, 1976.

Makita K, Nunn JF, Royston B: Evaluation of metabolic measuring instruments for use in critically ill patients. *Crit Care Med* 18:638, 1990.

Makk LJK, McClave SA, et al: Clinical application of the metabolic cart to the delivery of total parenteral nutrition. *Crit Care Med* 18:1320, 1990.

Smithies MN, Royston B, et al: Comparison of oxygen consumption measurements: Indirect calorimetry versus the reversed Fick method. *Crit Care Med* 19:1401, 1991.

Temperature Monitoring

Nierman DM: Core temperature measurement in the intensive care unit. *Crit Care Med* 19:818, 1991.

PART II
SPECIFIC CONSIDERATIONS

CHAPTER 13

Skin and Subcutaneous Tissue

David M. Young and Stephen J. Mathes

INTRODUCTION

The skin is the largest and one of the most complex organs of the body. Its uniform appearance belies its great variation from region to region of the body and the complex organization and interaction of the many different cells and matrices of the skin. Although the skin functions simply as a protective barrier and interface with our environment, its structure and physiology are very complex.

The skin is an extremely good interface with our environment. It is protective against most of the noxious agents, such as chemicals (by the impermeability of the epidermis), solar radiation (by means of pigmentation), infectious agents (through efficient immunosurveillance), and physically deforming forces (by the durability of the dermis). The skin is the major organ responsible for thermoregulation, having an efficient ability to conserve or disperse heat. To direct all these functions, the skin has a highly specialized nervous structure.

These various functions are better served by different components of skin, so teleologically there developed regional variation. The palms and soles are particularly thick to bear weight. The fingertips have the highest density of sensory innervation and allow for intricate tasks. Even the lines of the skin, first described by Langer, are oriented perpendicular to the long axis of muscles to allow the greatest degree of stretching and contraction without deformity.

The relative ease of observing and obtaining skin specimens for examination and experiments has made skin one of the best-studied tissues of the human body. Thus not only is skin central to the field of dermatology, but its study launched the fields of immunology, transplantation, and wound healing. Although this chapter emphasizes surgically treated diseases of the skin, it is important for students of surgery to be familiar with the basic physiology and structure of skin since many of the future advances in medicine will predictably come from these studies.

ANATOMY AND PHYSIOLOGY

The skin has been traditionally divided into three layers: the epidermis, the basement membrane, and the dermis (Fig. 13-1). The epidermis is composed mainly of cells, with very little extracellular matrix. Each cell type serves a specific barrier function. Keratinocytes provide a mechanical barrier, melanocytes a radiation barrier, and Langerhans cells an immunologic barrier. The dermis contains mostly extracellular matrix, providing support for nerves, vasculature, and adnexal structures. The dermis allows skin to resist deforming forces and return to its resting state, thus providing durability. The basement membrane is a specialized structure that anchors the epidermis to the dermis.

The main cell type in the epidermis is the keratinocyte. The deep, mitotically active, basal cells are a single cell layer of the least-differentiated keratinocytes. Some multiplying cells leave the basal layer and begin to travel upward. In the spinous layer they lose the ability to undergo mitosis. These differentiated cells start to accumulate keratohyalin granules in the granular layer. Finally, in the horny layer, the keratinocytes senesce, the once numerous intercellular connections disappear, and the dead cells are shed. Using radioactive and fluorescence labelling, experiments estimate the keratinocyte transit time to be from 40 to 56 days. The control of keratinocyte multiplication and subsequent maturation is an area of active study, and may clarify the complex mechanism of cellular differentiation.

Melanocytes migrate to the epidermis from precursor cells in the neural crest. They lie scattered beneath basal cells and have dendritic processes that reach out to surrounding keratinocytes. They number approximately one for every 35 keratinocytes. The melanocytes produce a pigment, melanin, from tyrosine and cysteine. The pigment is packaged in melanosomes and transported to the tips of the dendritic processes. The tips are sheared off (apocopation) and then phagocytized by the keratinocyte, thus transferring the pigment to the keratinocyte. Once in the keratinocyte they aggregate on the superficial side of the nucleus in an umbrella shape. The density of melanocytes is constant between individuals of different skin color. The rate of melanin production, transfer to keratinocytes, and melanosome degradation determine the degree of skin pigmentation. These activities are influenced by genetically activated factors as well as ultraviolet radiation and hormones such as estrogen, adrenocorticotropic hormone, and melanocyte-stimulating hormone.

The Langerhans cells migrate from the bone marrow and function as the skin's macrophages. The Langerhans cells constitutively express class II major histocompatability antigens and have antigen-presenting capabilities. These cells play a crucial role in immunosurveillance against viral infections and neoplasms of the skin, and may initiate skin allograft rejection.

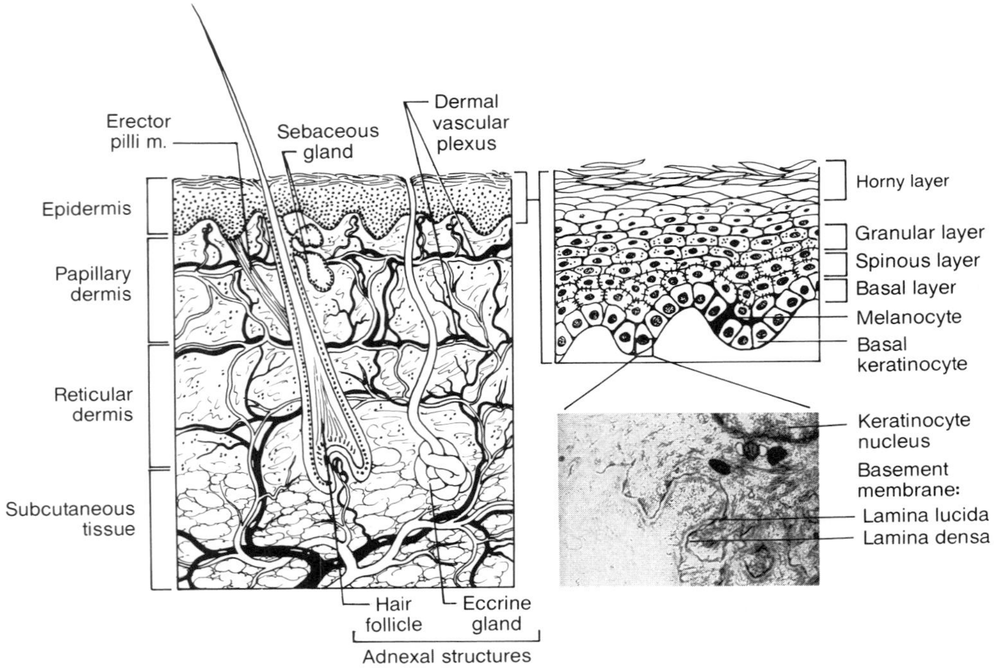

FIG. 13-1. The histologic section of skin, on the left side, demonstrates a complex organization of cells, connective tissue, blood vessels, and adnexal structures. The drawing in the upper right depicts the orderly maturation of keratinocytes in the epidermis. The lower right electron micrograph shows details of the basement membrane, which is the interface between the epidermis and the dermis.

The dermis consists mostly of several structural proteins. Collagen constitutes 70 percent of the dry weight of dermis and is responsible for its remarkable tensile strength. Tropocollagen consists of three polypeptide chains (formed mainly of hydroxyproline, hydroxylysine, and glysine) wrapped in a helix. These long molecules are then cross-linked to one another to form collagen fibers. Of the seven structurally distinct collagens, the skin contains mostly type I. Early fetal dermis contains mostly type III (reticulin fibers) collagen, but this remains only in the basement membrane zone and the perivascular regions in postfetal skin. Elastic fibers are highly branching proteins that are capable of being reversibly stretched to twice their resting length. This allows skin to return to its original form after stretching. Ground substance is an amorphous material that fills the remaining spaces. It consists of various polysaccharide-polypeptide (glycosaminoglycans) complexes. The nonsulfated form is mostly hyaluronic acid and the sulfated forms are heparin sulfate, dermatan sulfate, and chondroitin-6-sulfate. Glycosaminoglycans, which can hold up to 1000 times their own volume in water, constitute most of the volume of dermis.

Fibroblasts are scattered throughout the dermis and are responsible for production and maintenance of the protein matrix. Recently proteins that control the proliferation and migration of fibroblasts have been isolated. The study of fibroblast activity by these growth factor interactions is crucial to our understanding of wound healing and organogenesis.

The basement membrane zone of the dermal epidermal junction is a highly organized structure of proteins that anchors the epidermis to the dermis. Mechanical disruption or a genetic defect in the synthesis of this structure (epidermolysis bullosa) results in separation of the epidermis from the dermis.

In the dermis are situated the remaining structures of the skin. There is an intricate network of blood vessels that regulates body temperature. Two horizontal plexuses, one at the dermal subcutaneous junction and one in the papillary dermis, are interconnected by vertical vascular channels. Glomus bodies are tortuous arteriovenous shunts that allow a tremendous increase in blood flow to the skin when open. This large amount of blood flow in excess of its nutritional needs allows skin to dissipate a vast amount of body heat when needed.

Thermoregulation is carried out by autonomic fibers that synapse to sweat glands, the hair erector muscles, and control points in the vasculature. Sensory innervation follows a dermatomal distribution from segments of the spinal cord. These fibers connect to corpuscular receptors (pacinian, Meissner's, and Ruffini's) that respond to pressure, vibration, and touch, to "unspecialized" free nerve endings associated with Merkel cells of the basal epidermis, or to hair follicles. These nerves are stimulated by temperature, touch, pain, and itch.

The adnexal structures of the skin consist of three main structures. The eccrine glands produce sweat and are located all over the body but are concentrated on the palms, soles, axillae, and forehead. The hair follicles consist of a mitotically active germinal center that produces a cylinder of tightly packed cornified epithelial cells. Control of the growth cycle of the hair is little understood. The sebaceous glands produce an oily substance that coats the skin. Together these two structures form a pilosebaceous unit. The apocrine glands are found primarily in the axillae and the anogenital region. In lower mammals these glands produce scent hormones (pheromones).

TRAUMA

Penetrating Injuries

Disruption of the continuity of the skin allows the entry of organisms that can lead to wound infection. Sharp lacerations, bullet wounds, "road rash," and degloving injuries should be treated by gentle cleansing, debridement of all foreign debris and necrotic tissue, and application of a proper dressing. Dirty or infected wounds should be left open to heal by secondary intention or delayed primary closure. Clean lacerations may be closed primarily. Road rashes are treated as second-degree burns and degloving injuries as third-degree burns. The degloved skin can be placed back on the wound like a skin graft and assessed for survival. If the skin becomes necrotic, it is removed and the wound covered with split-thickness skin grafts.

Pressure Ulcers (Decubitus Ulcers)

Pressure ulcers, as the name implies, are caused by excessive, unrelieved pressure. In animal studies, 60-mm Hg pressure applied to the skin for 1 hour produced histologically identifiable injuries such as venous thrombosis, muscle degeneration, and tissue necrosis. The average human being lying in bed or sitting in a chair exerts 60 to 70 mm Hg pressure on such body areas as the sacrum, occiput, heels, and ischia. Healthy individuals, however, constantly shift their body weight intermittently, even while asleep. Sitting in one position causes pain in areas of increased pressure, thus stimulating movement. Patients unable to sense pain or shift their body weight, such as paraplegics or bedridden individuals, develop prolonged elevated tissue pressures and, eventually, necrosis. Muscle tissue is more sensitive to ischemia than the overlying skin. That is why the necrotic area is always wider and deeper than it appears on first inspection (Fig. 13-2).

Treatment of pressure sores requires nutritional support of the patient to promote healing and relief of pressure with special cushions and beds. The necrotic tissue should be removed, often along with the underlying bony prominence. Small ulcers may close by secondary intention but larger lesions require soft tissue and skin coverage. To prevent future breakdown of the area, stable coverage should be obtained with local myocutaneous or fasciocutaneous flaps. Prevention of ulcers is best achieved by close attention to susceptible areas, frequent repositioning of paralyzed patients, and use of special cushions.

Keloids and Hypertrophic Scars

All wounds heal by scar formation. Hypertrophic scars are raised, red, and nodular, but remain within the limits of the original incision or trauma. Keloids are much bulkier; the nodularity and firmness extend beyond the wound (Fig. 13-3). Although there are distinct histologic and biochemical differences between keloids and hypertrophic scars, the distinction is largely clinical. Children and dark-skinned individuals are more likely to develop hypertrophic scars. Wounds across joints and on the sternum are particularly susceptible.

Medical treatment includes intradermal injections of glucocorticoids (Kenalog) to reduce the itching and flatten the scar. Mechanical pressure (as with pressure garments) can also soften and flatten raised scars. Scar excision or revision is reserved for hypertrophic scars. Keloids are prone to recur after excision and are best treated medically. If surgery is done on a keloid, steroid injections should be started early.

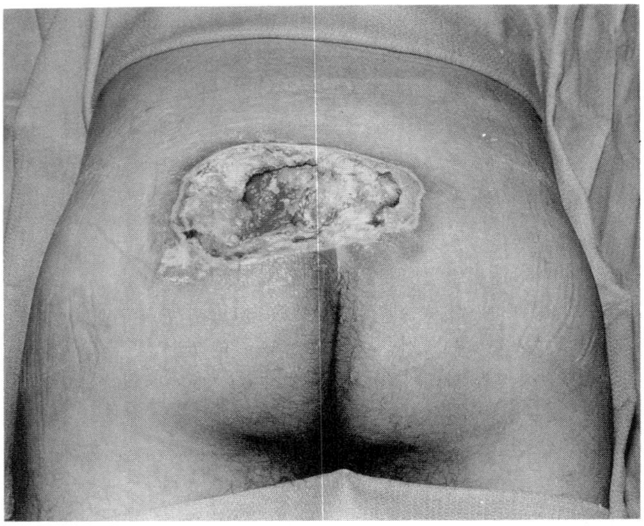

A

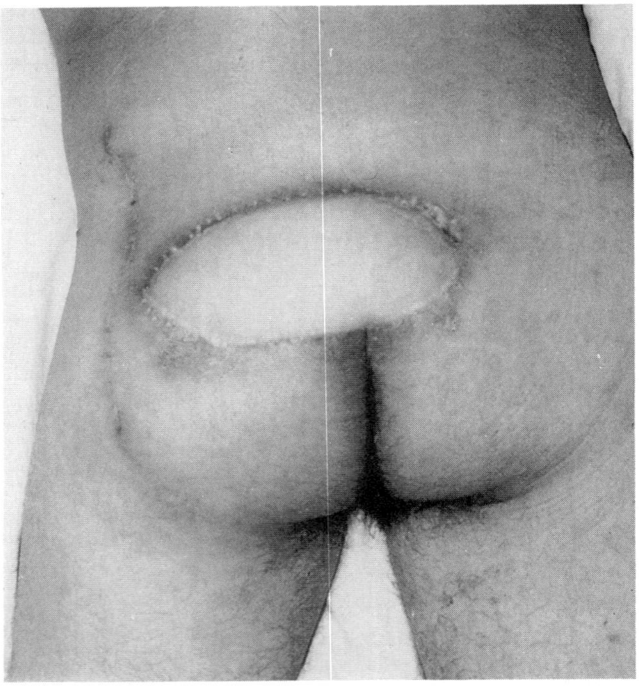

B

FIG. 13-2. Sacral decubitus ulcer is *(A)* debrided and *(B)* covered with a flap.

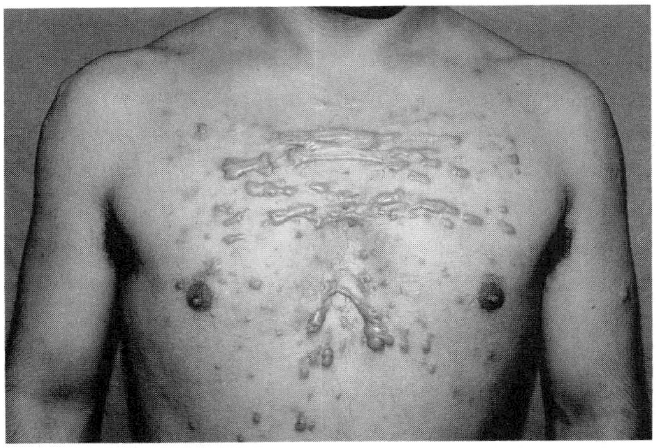

A

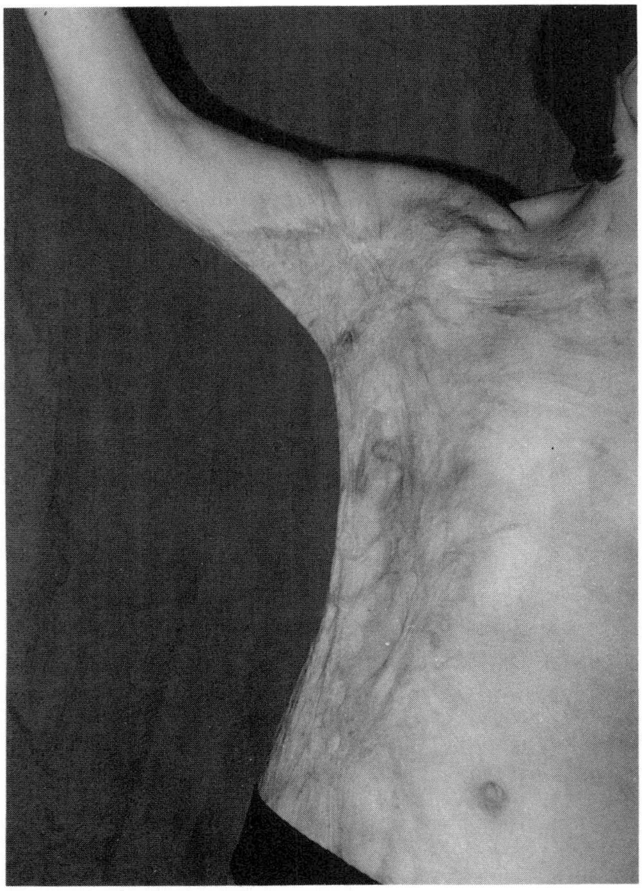

B

FIG. 13-3. *A.* Keloids of the chest. *B.* Hypertrophic scars from a burn wound.

INFECTIONS

Bacterial

Folliculitis, Furuncles, and Carbuncles

Folliculitis is infection and inflammation of a hair follicle. The causative organism is usually *Staphyloccocus* and occasionally a gram-negative organism. A furuncle (boil) begins as folliculitis but progresses to form a nodule that eventually becomes fluctuant. The abscess eventually ruptures and usually resolves. Deep-seated infections that result in multiple draining cutaneous sinuses are called carbuncles.

Folliculitis usually resolves with time and adequate hygiene. Warm soaks to a furuncle may hasten liquefaction, speed drainage, and encourage healing. Occasionally antibiotics are used to manage surrounding cellulitis. Carbuncles are more difficult to treat and require incision and drainage or wide excision of the infected tissue and sinuses.

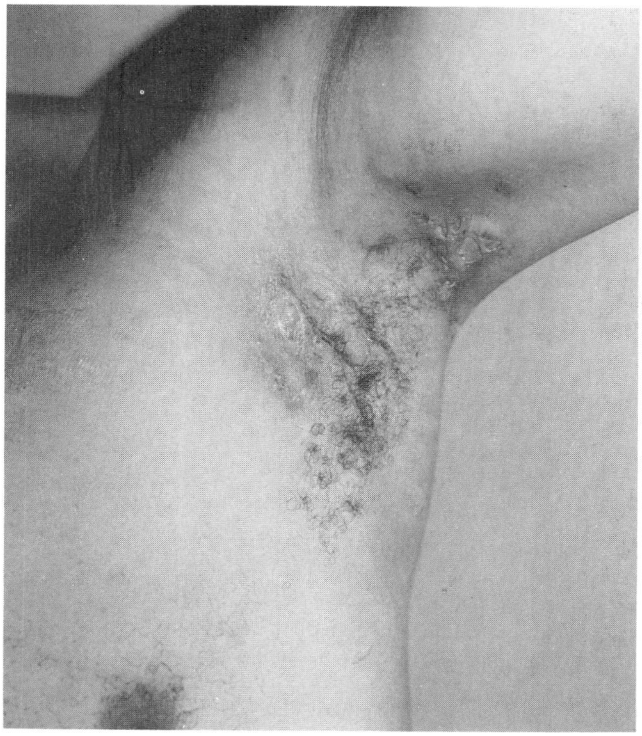

FIG. 13-4. Active hidradentis suppurativa of the axilla.

Hidradentitis Suppurativa

Bacterial infection of a plugged apocrine gland occurs most commonly in the axillae and inguinal and perianal regions. An abscess forms with subsequent drainage and sinus formation. Repeated infections create a wide area of inflamed and scarred tissue that is foul-smelling and painful (Fig. 13-4). Treatment of acute infections includes application of warm compresses, antibiotics, and open drainage. Proper hygiene and discontinuation of deodorants may prevent recurrence. Chronic hidradentitis requires excision of the entire area of infection and closure with skin grafts.

Pilonidal Disease

Infected pilonidal cysts of the sacrococcygeal region occur primarily in young adults and are four times more common in males. The pathogenesis of the disease is much debated but sweaty activity and buttock friction such as occurred in jeep drivers in World War II (Jeep driver's disease) is associated with a high incidence of pilonidal disease. The infection probably begins in a pilosebaceous unit in the natal cleft. Recurrent trauma causes obstruction of a hair follicle and leads to infection. The localized folliculitis spreads into the surrounding soft tissue and produces an abscess. This eventually drains to the surface and produces a sinus that is usually located lateral to the midline. The sinus is lined with granulation tissue but over time can epithelialize. Constant movement and friction of the buttocks causes hair and loose debris to enter the tract and incite a foreign body reaction.

Acute pilonidal abscesses should be drained. Without further therapy, many will recur. There are many different ways of treating the chronic sinus tract, including tract curettage, local excision and closure, wide excision and marsupialization, and wide excision and flap closure. Another method currently gaining favor is fistulotomy and marsupialization. Each method has its drawbacks. Primary closure has the advantage of least disrupting the patient's life-style and allows early return to normal activities, but the recurrence rate after this treatment is high. With wide excision there is a lower recurrence rate but a longer hospitalization and time to heal is required. This is more expensive in terms of medical costs and in lost income to the patient. No good controlled studies comparing the various treatments have been published, but the literature is filled with reports of individual surgeons' experiences.

Toxic Epidermal Necrolysis and Staphylococcal Scalded Skin Syndrome

These two diseases cause a similar clinical picture that includes erythema of the skin, bullae formation, and, eventually, wide areas of skin loss. Staphylococcal scalded skin syndrome (SSSS) is caused by an exotoxin produced during a staphylococcal infection of the nasopharynx or middle ear in the pediatric population. Toxic epidermal necrolysis (TEN) is thought to be an immunologic reaction to certain drugs, such as sulfonamides, phenytoin, barbiturates, and tetracycline. Diagnosis can be made with a skin biopsy since SSSS produces a cleavage plane in the granular layer of the epidermis, while TEN occurs at the dermoepidermal junction. The injury is similar to a second-degree burn and in severe cases can be life-threatening. Treatment involves fluid and electrolyte replacement and wound care as in a burn injury.

Actinomycosis

Actinomycosis is a localized inflammatory mass of the jaw that spreads by multiple fistulas and abscesses into the neck and face. The underlying bone can also become infected, as well the apex of the lung. The causative agent is *Actinomyces,* an organism of the Actinomycetes family. Other actinomycetes, including *Nocardia, Actinomadura,* and *Streptomyces,* cause mycetomas, which are deep cutaneous infections that present as nodules and spread to form draining tracts to the skin and surrounding soft tissue. Chronic disease causes fibrosis and contractures. The most common site for infection is the foot (Madura foot).

The gram-negative bacteria that cause these infections were once believed to be fungi because they grow slowly as branched filaments and chains. Diagnosis is dependent on the presence of characteristic sulfur granules on microscopic examination. Special stains should be done to exclude fungal infection. Penicillin and sulfonamides are effective against these infections. Abscesses and areas of chronic scarring may require surgical therapy.

Lymphogranuloma Venereum

Chlamydia trachomatis is a sexually transmitted, intracellular, gram-negative bacterium. After infection and a 2-week incubation period, an inconspicuous ulcer appears on the penis or labia, although over half the time this lesion is not noticed or does not appear. A few weeks later, inguinal lymphadenopathy erupts. The nodes become very large and painful (buboes) and are occasionally confused with an incarcerated inguinal hernia. Adenopathy can occur above and below the inguinal ligament, forming a characteristic groove. The matted nodes may suppurate, and occasionally rupture. Surgical drainage of unruptured abscesses is not recommended since a chronic draining sinus often develops. Active infection is treated with oral tetracyline or its derivatives. Inflammation from infection can lead to lymphatic obstruction and chronic lower extremity edema. Rectal strictures can also occur.

Viral

Warts are epidermal growths associated with human papilloma virus infection. Histologically, they are characterized by hyperkeratosis (hypertrophy of the horny layer), acanthosis (hypertrophy of the spinous layer), and papillomatosis. Koilocytes, large keratinocytes with eccentric nuclei, are present. Different morphologic types have a propensity to occur on different parts of the body. The common wart (verruca vulgaris) is found on the fingers and toes, and has a rough, gray-brown surface. Plantar warts (verruca plantaris) occur on the soles and palms, and may appear like a callus. Flat warts (verruca plana) are flat but slightly raised. They appear on the face, legs, and hands. Genital warts (condylomata acuminatum) grow on the moist areas around the vulva, anus, and scrotum. The lesions are softer than other types of warts and are transmitted by sexual contact.

Warts can be removed by a number of chemicals, including formalin, podophyllum, and phenol-nitric acid. Curettage with electrodesiccation can also be used for scattered lesions. Treatment of extensive skin involvement, especially around the genital area, requires surgical excision under general anesthesia. Unfortunately, because of the infectious etiology, recurrences are common and repeated excisions are necessary to eliminate lesions. Some warts (especially human papilloma virus types 5, 8, and 10) are associated with squamous cell cancers, therefore lesions that grow rapidly or ulcerate should be biopsied.

BENIGN TUMORS

Cysts (Epidermal, Dermoid, Trichilemmal)

Epidermal cysts are the most common type of cutaneous cyst. They occur throughout the body as a single firm nodule. On the scrotum they are often multiple and can calcify. Trichilemmal (pilar) cysts, the next most common, occur more often in females and usually on the scalp. When ruptured these cysts have a characteristic strong odor. Dermoid cysts are present at birth and may result from epithelium trapped during midline closure in fetal development. Dermoids are most often found in the midline of the face (e.g., on the nose or forehead). They are also common on the eyebrow (Fig. 13-5).

On gross examination, it is difficult to distinguish one type of cyst from another. They are all subcutaneous, thin-walled nodules containing a white, creamy center. Histologic examination is needed to differentiate them. The walls of all the cysts consist of a layer of epidermis oriented with the basal layer superficial and the more mature layers deep (i.e., with the epidermis growing into the center of the cyst). The desquamated cells (keratin) collect in the center and form the creamy substance of the cyst. Epidermal cysts have a completely mature epidermis containing a granular layer. Trichilemmal cyst walls do not contain a granular layer but do have a distinctive outer layer resembling the outer root sheath of the hair follicle (tricholemmoma). Dermoids have a squamous epithelium, eccrine glands, pilosebaceous units, and, occasionally, bone, teeth, or nerves. Surgeons often refer to cutaneous cysts as *sebaceous cysts* because they appear to contain sebum. In reality this is a misnomer since the substance is actually keratin.

Cysts are usually asymptomatic and ignored until they rupture and cause local inflammation. The area becomes infected and an abscess forms. Incision and drainage is recommended for an acutely infected cyst. After resolution of the abscess the cyst wall must be excised or the cyst will recur. Similarly, when excising an unruptured cyst, care must be taken to remove all of the wall in order to prevent recurrence.

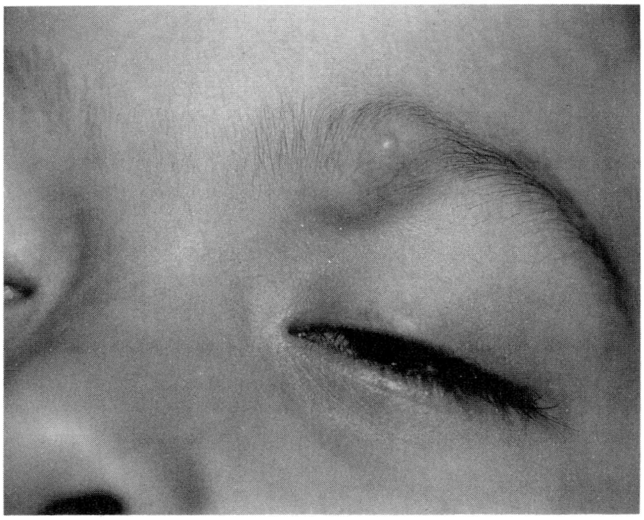

FIG. 13-5. Dermoid cysts are commonly found on the eyebrow.

Keratoses (Seborrheic, Solar)

Seborrheic keratoses commonly occur on the chest, back, and abdomen of older individuals. The lesions are light brown or yellow and have a velvety, greasy texture. They are rarely mistaken for other lesions, so biopsy and treatment are seldom needed. Sudden eruptions of multiple lesions in elderly patients may be associated with internal malignancies.

Solar keratoses (actinic) are also found in the older age group. They arise in sun-exposed areas of the body, such as the back of the hand, face, and forearms. Histologically, they contain atypical-appearing keratinocytes and evidence of solar damage in the dermis. These are thought to be premalignant lesions and squamous cell carcinoma may develop over time. Treatment is by local removal or application of topical 5-fluorouracil. Malignancies that do develop rarely metastasize.

Nevi (Acquired, Congenital)

Acquired melanocytic nevi are classified as junctional, compound, or dermal depending on the location of the nevus cells. This classification does not represent different types of nevi but rather different stages in the maturation of nevi. Initially nevus cells accumulate in the epidermis (junctional), migrate partially into the dermis (compound), and finally rest completely in the dermis (dermal). Eventually most lesions undergo involution.

Congenital nevi are much more rare, occurring in only 1 percent of neonates. These lesions are larger and may contain hair. Histologically they appear similar to acquired nevi. Congenital giant lesions (giant hairy nevi) most often occur in a bathing trunk distribution, or on the chest and back (Fig. 13-6). These lesions are a major cosmetic problem. In addition, according to some series, they develop malignant melanoma 5 to 30 percent of the time. Excision of the nevus is the treatment of choice, but often the lesion is so large that closure of the wound with autologous skin grafts is not possible due to lack of adequate donor sites. Serial excisions over several years with either primary closure or skin grafting is the present mode of therapy. Tissue expansion of nor-

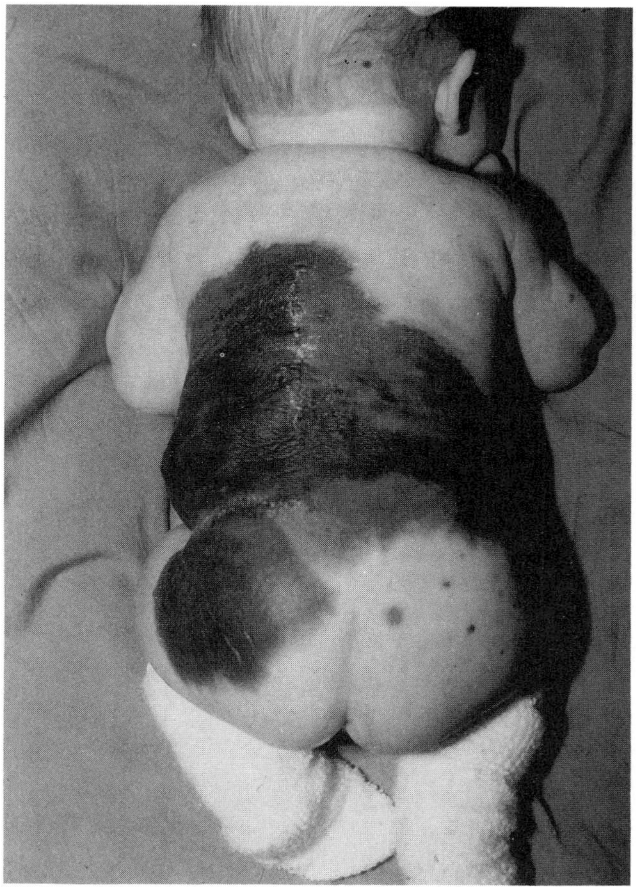

FIG. 13-6. *Giant hairy nevus in an infant.*

mal surrounding skin is now also used to accelerate the rate of nevus excision and avoid the use of skin grafts.

Vascular

Hemangiomas (Capillary, Cavernous)

Hemangiomas are benign vascular lesions that are present at birth or arise soon after. Capillary (strawberry) hemangiomas are soft, compressible papular lesions with sharp borders located mostly on the shoulders, face, and scalp. Cavernous hemangiomas are bright red or purple and have a spongy consistency. Histologically, capillary hemangiomas are composed of endothelial cells seen primarily in fetal veins. Cavernous lesions contain large, blood-filled spaces lined by normal-appearing endothelial cells.

Capillary hemangiomas can enlarge during the first year of life, and over 90 percent will involute by fibrosis over time. Allowing lesions to regress spontaneously usually gives optimal cosmetic results (Fig. 13-7). Acute treatment is limited to lesions that interfere with bodily functions, such as vision, feeding, and urination, or lead to systemic problems, such as thrombocytopenia and high-output cardiac failure. The growth of these rapidly enlarging lesions can be stopped with a short (2-week) course of prednisone, while longer periods of treatment will cause the lesions to shrink. Hemangiomas that remain after early adolescence will probably not involute further. Surgical excision or compression garment therapy are recommended.

Vascular Malformations (Port Wine Stains, Arteriovenous Malformations, Glomus Tumors)

Vascular malformations are a result of structural abnormalities formed during fetal development. Unlike hemangiomas, vascular malformations do not undergo rapid growth and involution but rather grow in proportion to the body. Histologically they contain enlarged vascular spaces lined by nonproliferating endothelium rather than the mitotically active endothelial cells of a hemangioma.

Port wine stains (nevi flammeus) are flat, dull red capillary malformations located on the trunk, extremities, and, most commonly, along a trigemminal distribution on the face. Histologically, they are ectatic capillaries lined by mature endothelium. These lesions may be part of the Sturge-Weber syndrome (leptomeningeal angiomatosis, epilepsy, and glaucoma). Unsightly lesions can be covered with cosmetics or surgically excised.

Arteriovenous malformations are high-flow lesions located on the head and neck. They appear as a mass under the skin with locally elevated temperature, a dermal stain, and a thrill and bruit. Overlying ischemic ulcers and adjacent bone destruction may occur. Large malformations can cause cardiac enlargement and congestive heart failure.

Complications of arteriovenous malformations, such as pain, hemorrhage, ulceration, cardiac effects, and cosmetic deformity, should be treated by elimination of the lesion. Therapy consists of either angiography with selective embolization or complete surgical resection. Embolization is particularly useful for lesions not accessible to surgery or when resection would cause too much mutilation. Embolization can also be used preoperatively to reduce blood loss during surgery.

Glomus tumors are blue-gray nodules that are extremely tender. They can occur anywhere on the body but the most common location is subungual. The tumor arises from a glomus body and histologically resembles the arterial portion of the glomus. Excision of the tumor will relieve the pain.

Soft Tissue (Achrochordons, Dermatofibromas, Lipomas)

Acrochordons (skin tags) are fleshy, pedunculated masses located on the axillae, trunk, and eyelids. They are composed of hyperplastic epidermis over a fibrous connective tissue stalk. These lesions are usually small and are always benign.

Dermatofibromas are usually solitary nodules measuring approximately 1 to 2 cm in diameter. They are found primarily on the legs and sides of the trunk. The lesions are composed of whorls of connective tissue containing fibroblasts. The mass is not encapsulated and vascularization is variable. Dermatofibromas can be diagnosed by clinical examination. When lesions enlarge to 2 to 3 cm, excisional biopsy is recommended to assess for a malignancy.

Lipomas are the most common subcutaneous neoplasm. They are found mostly on the trunk but may appear anywhere. They may sometimes grow to a large size. Microscopic examination reveals a lobulated tumor containing normal fat cells. Excision is performed both for diagnosis and to restore normal skin contour.

Neural (Neurofibromas, Neurilemmomas, Granular Cell Tumors)

Benign cutaneous neural tumors arise primarily from the nerve sheath. Neurofibromas can be sporadic and solitary, but are more

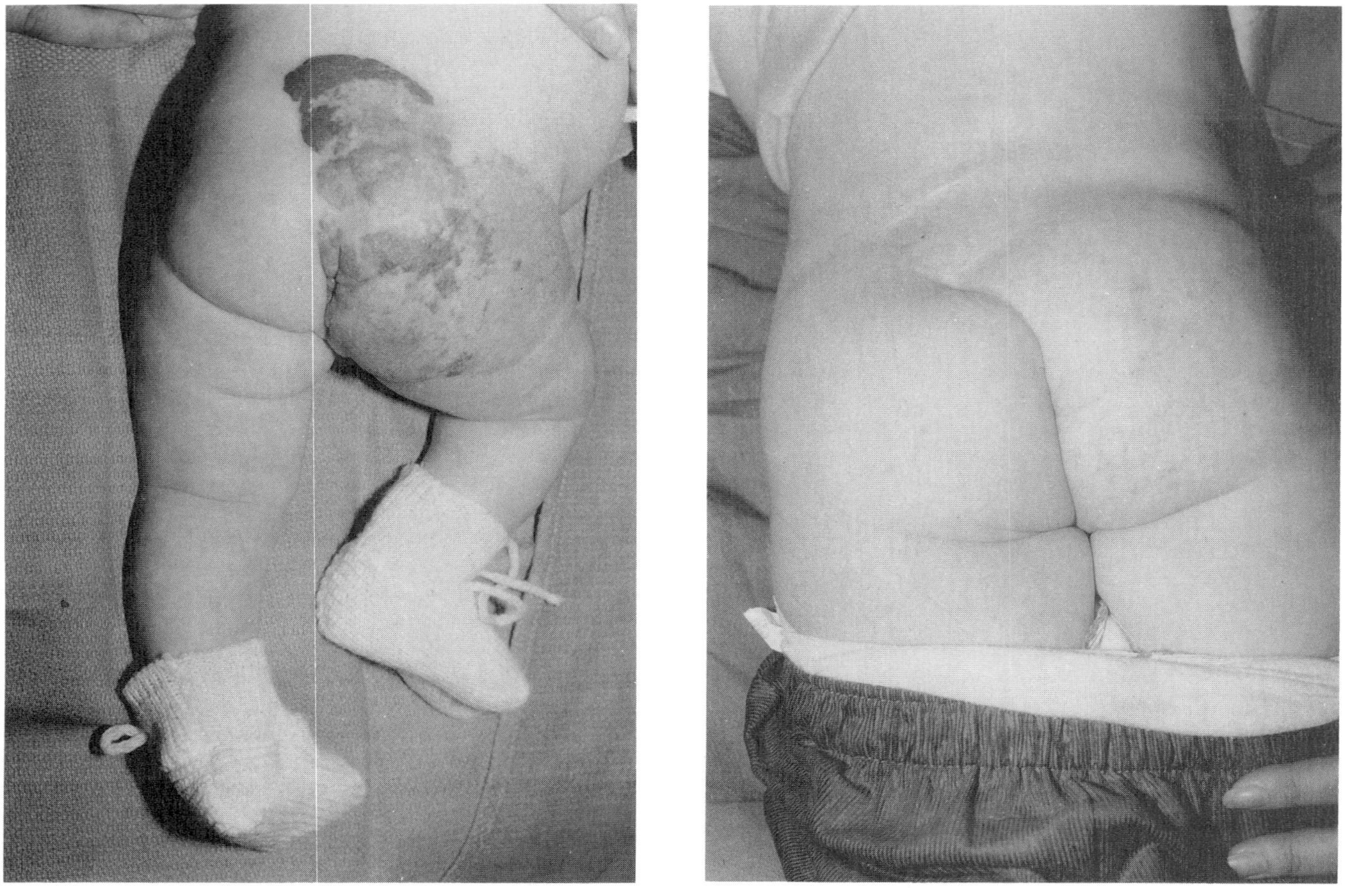

A B

FIG. 13-7. *A.* *Large hemangioma.* *B.* *Regression without therapy.*

commonly noted as multiple and associated with café-au-lait spots and an autosomal dominant inheritance (von Recklinghausen's disease). The lesions are firm, discrete nodules attached to a nerve. Histologically there is proliferation of perineurial and endoneurial fibroblasts and Schwann cells embedded in collagen. Neurilemmomas are solitary tumors found along peripheral nerves of the head and extremities. They are discrete nodules that may be locally painful or radiate along the distribution of the nerve. Microscopically, the tumor contains Schwann cells with nuclei packed in palisading rows.

Granular cell tumors are usually solitary lesions of the skin or, more commonly, the tongue. They consist of granular cells derived from Schwann cells that often infiltrate the surrounding striated muscle.

MALIGNANT TUMORS

The most common cancers of the skin arise from the cells of the epidermis, and consist of basal cell carcinoma, squamous cell carcinoma, and melanoma in order of frequency. Malignancies arising from cells of the dermis or adnexal structures are much less common.

Environmental influences and concomitant diseases are associated with an increased incidence of epidermal malignancies. These factors have been extensively studied and form some of our best understanding about the causes of cancer.

Epidemiology

Increased exposure to ultraviolet radiation is associated with an increased development of all three of the common skin malignancies. Epidemiologic studies have shown that people with outdoor occupations have skin malignancies more often than people who work indoors. Squamous cell cancer is much more common on the lower lip than the upper. People with fair complexions are more prone to skin cancer. These same people are also more likely to develop malignancies living in areas of the world that receive more sunlight, such as New Zealand compared to Great Britain. Albino individuals of dark-skinned races are prone to develop cutaneous neoplasms that are usually rare in the nonalbino members, suggesting that melanin plays a large role in protection from carcinogenesis.

Other factors associated with skin malignancies have also been identified. Chemical carcinogens have long been identified. In the 18th century, Sir Percival Pott noted the association of soot and scrotal cancer in chimney sweeps. Tar, arsenic, and nitrogen mustard are known carcinogens. Human papilloma virus has been found in certain squamous cell cancers and may be linked with oncogenesis. Radiation therapy in the past for skin lesions such as acne vulgaris that resulted in radiation dermatitis is associated with an increased incidence of both basal and squamous cell cancers in the treated areas. Any area of skin subjected to chronic irritation, such as burn scars (Marjolin's ulcers), repeated sloughing of skin from bullous diseases, and decubitus ulcers all have an increased chance of developing squamous cell cancer. One variant of this type of lesion is Karro cancer, which develops on skin that has suffered repeated burns (so named from the Japanese custom of wearing a box of ashes on the abdomen to keep warm).

Systemic immunologic dysfunction is related to an increase in cutaneous malignancies. Immunosuppressed patients receiving chemotherapy for other malignancies or organ transplant recipients have an increased incidence of basal cell and squamous cell cancers, and malignant melanoma. The acquired immunodeficiency syndrome (AIDS) is associated with a propensity to develop skin neoplasms, especially Kaposi's sarcoma (see below).

Basal Cell Carcinoma

Basal cell carcinomas contain cells that resemble the basal cells of the epidermis. It is the most common skin cancer and is subdivided into several types by gross and histologic morphology. The nodulocystic or noduloulcerative type accounts for 70 percent of basal cell carcinomas. It is a waxy, cream-colored lesion with rolled, pearly borders (Fig. 13-8). It often contains a central ulcer. When large these lesions are called "rodent ulcers." Pigmented basal cell carcinomas are tan to black and should be distinguished by biopsy from melanoma. Superficial basal cell cancers occur more commonly on the trunk and form a red, scaling lesion sometimes difficult to distinguish grossly from Bowen's disease. A rare form of basal cell carcinoma is the basosquamous type, which contains elements of both basal cell and squamous cell cancer. These lesions can metastasize more like a squamous cell carcinoma and therefore should be treated aggressively. Other types include morpheaform, adenoid, and infiltrative carcinomas.

Basal cell carcinomas are usually slow growing, and patients often neglect these lesions for years. Metastasis and death from this disease is extremely rare, but these lesions can cause extensive local destruction. The majority of small (less than 2 mm), nodular lesions may be treated by dermatologists with curettage and electrodesiccation or laser vaporization. A major drawback to these procedures is that no pathologic specimen may be obtained to confirm the clinical diagnosis. Larger tumors, lesions that invade bone or surrounding structures, and more aggressive histologic types (morpheaform, infiltrative, and basosquamous) are best treated by surgical excision with a 2- to 4-mm margin of normal tissue. Histologic confirmation that the margins of resection do not contain tumor is required. Since nodular lesions are less likely to recur, the smaller margin may be used, while the other types need a wider margin of resection. Alternative methods of treatment, such as radiation therapy and Mohs' surgery, are discussed later.

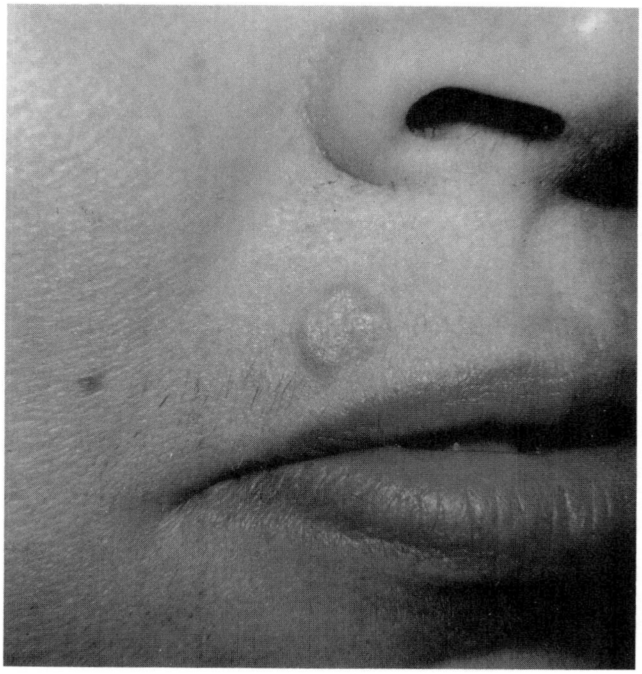

FIG. 13-8. Basal cell carcinoma with rolled, pearly borders.

Squamous Cell Carcinoma

Squamous cell carcinomas arise from keratinocytes of the epidermis. It is less common than basal cell carcinoma but is more devastating because it can invade surrounding tissue and metastasize more readily. In situ lesions have the eponym of Bowen's disease and in situ squamous cell carcinomas of the penis are referred to as erythroplasia of Queyrat. Contrary to previous reports, Bowen's disease is not a marker for other systemic malignancies.

Tumor thickness correlates well with its biologic behavior. Lesions that recur locally are greater than 4 mm thick and lesions that metastasize are 10 mm or greater. The location of the lesion is also important. Tumors arising in burn scars (Marjolin's ulcer), areas of chronic osteomyelitis, and areas of previous injury metastasize early. Lesions on the external ear frequently recur and involve regional lymph node basins early. Squamous cell cancers in areas with solar damage behave less aggressively and usually require only local excision.

Although small lesions can be treated with curettage and electrodesiccation, most surgeons recommend excision of the tumor. Lesions should be excised with a 1-cm margin, if possible, and histologic confirmation that the margins are not involved by tumor is mandatory. Tumor invading bone should be excised if recurrence is to be avoided. Regional lymph node excision is indicated for clinically palpable nodes (therapeutic lymph node dissection). Lesions arising in chronic wounds behave aggressively and are more likely to spread to regional lymph nodes. For these lesions lymphadenectomy before the development of palpable nodes is indicated (prophylactic lymph node dissection). Metastatic disease is a poor prognostic sign, with only 13 percent of patients alive after 10 years.

Alternative Therapy. Alternatives to surgical therapy for both squamous and basal cell cancers consist of radiation therapy or topical 5-fluorouracil for patients unable or unwilling to undergo surgery. Radiation therapy for small and superficial lesions obtains cure rates comparable to surgical excision. Radiation damage to surrounding normal skin with inflammation and scarring can be a problem. Also the development of cutaneous malignancies in irradiated skin is a serious long-term risk with this method.

For lesions on the face near the nose or eye, resection of a wide rim of normal tissue to remove all the tumor can cause significant functional and cosmetic problems. These lesions can be removed by Mohs' micrographic surgery. Mohs' technique, developed in 1932, is a method to serially excise a tumor by taking small increments of tissue until the entire tumor is removed. Each piece of tissue removed is frozen and immediately examined microscopically to determine whether tumorous tissue has been resected. The advantage of this method over that of standard histologic examination after wide surgical resection is that this technique evaluates the entire margin of resection. The major benefit is the ability to remove a tumor with the least sacrifice of uninvolved tissue. This technique is effective for treating carcinomas around the eyelids and nose, where tissue loss is most conspicuous. The procedure is extremely lengthy (up to several days) since complete excision may require multiple attempts; this remains its major drawback. Cure rates are comparable to those of wide excision.

Malignant Melanoma

What was a relatively rare disease 50 years ago has now become alarmingly more common. The rise in the rate of melanoma is the highest of any cancer in the United States. In 1935, the incidence of the disease was 1 in 1500 people. By 1987, 1 in 135 individuals developed melanoma. In 1987, approximately 26,000 new cases of melanoma developed in the United States. The case fatality rate has fallen over the years, probably due to earlier detection and treatment of these lesions.

Since melanoma is becoming so common, it is important for all physicians to be familiar with this disease. Surgery is still the mainstay of therapy for melanoma, so it is imperative that surgeons be aware of the latest methods of diagnosis, staging, and therapy.

Pathogenesis

Melanoma arises from transformed melanocytes and therefore can arise anywhere that melanocytes have migrated during embryogenesis. The eye, central nervous system, gastrointestinal tract, and even the gallbladder have been reported as primary sites of the disease. Over 90 percent are found on the skin, however, 4 percent of melanomas are discovered as metastases without an identifiable primary site. Many melanomas, especially in the early phases of growth, contain areas of tumor regression on histologic examination. Regression represents a host immune response to the tumor. Metastatic melanomas with unknown primaries probably arise from completely regressed lesions that are difficult to locate.

Nevi are benign melanocytic neoplasms found on the skin of most people. Dysplastic nevi are much rarer and contain a histologically identifiable focus of atypical melanocytes. This type of nevus may represent an intermediate between a benign nevus and a true malignant melanoma. It is well documented that patients with melanoma have significantly more nevi and dysplastic nevi than matched controls. The relative risk of developing melanoma increases with the number of dysplastic nevi a patient develops. This is a similar concept to the relationship of the number of colonic polyps and the development of colon cancer.

Once the melanocyte has transformed into the malignant phenotype, the growth of the lesion is radial in the plane of the epidermis. Even though microinvasion of the dermis can be observed during this radial growth phase, metastases do not occur. Only when the melanoma cells form nests in the dermis are metastasis observed. The transformed cells in the vertical growth phase are morphologically different and express different cell-surface antigens than those in the radial phase or cells of the dysplastic nevus. In addition, these cells behave differently in cell culture. They can grow in a less enriched media and have a longer life span.

Types

There are four common distinct types of melanoma. These are superficial spreading, nodular, lentigo malignant, and acral-lentiginous in order of decreasing frequency. Each has distinctly different characteristics and behaviors.

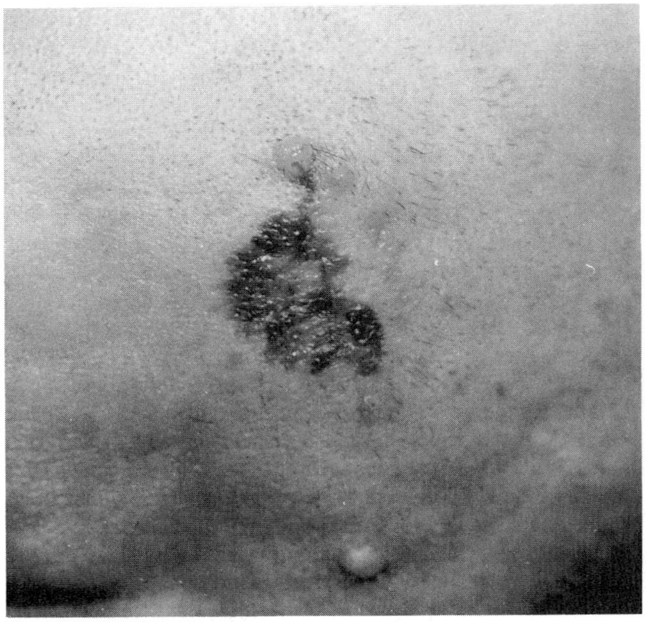

FIG. 13-9. This is the typical appearance of a superficial spreading melanoma. Note the area of regression in the center of the lesion.

The most common type (70 percent of melanomas) is superficial spreading. These lesions occur anywhere on the skin except the hands and feet. They are flat, commonly contain areas of regression, and measure 1 to 2 cm in diameter at the time of diagnosis (Fig. 13-9). There is a relatively long radial growth phase before vertical growth begins.

The nodular type accounts for 15 to 20 percent of melanomas. These lesions are darker and raised. The histologic criterion for a nodular melanoma is the lack of radial growth peripheral to the area of vertical growth; therefore all nodular melanomas are in the vertical growth phase at the time of diagnosis. Although it is an aggressive lesion the prognosis for a patient with a nodular-type lesion is no different from that of a patient with a superficial spreading lesion when the lesions are compared by depth of invasion.

The lentigo malignant type (5 to 10 percent) occurs mostly on the back of the hands, neck, and face of elderly individuals. These lesions are always surrounded by dermis with heavy solar degeneration. These lesions tend to become quite large before a diagnosis is made but also have the best prognosis since invasive growth occurs late.

The rarer acral-lentiginous type is distinctly different. It occurs on the palms, soles, and subungual regions. Although melanoma among dark-skinned people is relatively rare, the acral-lentiginous type accounts for a higher percentage in dark-skinned people than in people with less pigmented skin. The subungual lesions appear as blue-black discolorations of the posterior nailfold and are most common on the great toe or thumb.

Prognostic Factors

The original staging system classified melanoma into local (stage I), regional lymph node (stage II), and metastatic (stage III) disease. This staging system had the disadvantage of lumping most patients into stage I disease, therefore limiting its usefulness in prognostic studies. The most current staging system, from the

Table 13-1
TNM Classification of Melanoma of the Skin

Primary Tumor (T)	
TX	No evidence of primary tumor (unknown primary or primary tumor removed and histologically not examined.
T0	Atypical melanocytic hyperplasia (Clark level I), not a malignant lesion.
T1	Invasion of papillary dermis (level II) or 0.75 mm in thickness or less.
T2	Invasion of the papillary-reticular-dermal interface (level III) or 0.76 to 1.5 mm in thickness.
T3	Invasion of the reticular dermis (level IV) or 1.51 to 4.0 mm in thickness.
T4	Invasion of subcutaneous tissue (level V) or 4.1 mm or more in thickness or satellite(s) within 2 cm of any primary melanoma.

Nodal Involvement (N)

NX	Minimum requirements to assess the regional nodes cannot be met.
N0	No regional lymph node involvement.
N1	Involvement of only one regional lymph node station; node(s) movable and not over 5 cm in diameter or negative regional lymph nodes and the presence of less than five in-transit metastases beyond 2 cm from primary site.
N2	Any one of the following: (1) involvement of more than one regional node station; (2) regional node(s) over 5 cm in diameter or fixed; (3) five or more in-transit metastases or any in-transit metastasis beyond 2 cm from primary site with regional lymph node involvement.

Distant Metastasis (M)	
MX	Minimum requirements to assess the presence of distant metastasis cannot be met.
M0	No known distant metastasis.
M1	Involvement of skin or subcutaneous tissue beyond the site of primary lymph node drainage.
M2	Visceral metastasis (spread to any distant site other than skin or subcutaneous tissues).

Stage Grouping

Stage IA	T1, N0, M0
Stage IB	T2, N0, M0
Stage IIA	T3, N0, M0
Stage IIB	T4, N0, M0
Stage III	Any T, N1, M0
Stage IV	Any T, N2, M0
	Any T, Any N, M1, M2

American Joint Committee on Cancer (AJCC), contains the best method of interpreting clinical information in regard to prognosis of this disease (Table 13-1).

The T classification of the lesion comes from the original observation by Clark that prognosis is directly related to the level of invasion of the skin by the melanoma. Whereas Clark used the histologic level (I, superficial to basement membrane (in-situ); II, papillary dermis; III, papillary/reticular dermal junction; IV, reticular dermis; and V, subcutaneous fat), Breslow modified the concept to a more reproducible measure of invasion by use of an ocular micrometer. The lesions were measured from the granular layer of the epidermis or the base of the ulcer to the greatest depth of the tumor (I, 0.75 mm or less; II, 0.76 to 1.5 mm; III, 1.51 to 3.0 mm; IV, greater than 3.0 mm). These levels of invasion have been subsequently modified and incorporated in the AJCC staging system (Fig. 13-10).

Evidence of tumor in regional lymph nodes is a poor prognostic sign. This is accounted for in the staging system by advancing any T classification from stage I or II to stage III. The 10-year survival rate drops precipitously with the presence of lymph node metastasis. The number of positive lymph nodes is also correlated with survival.

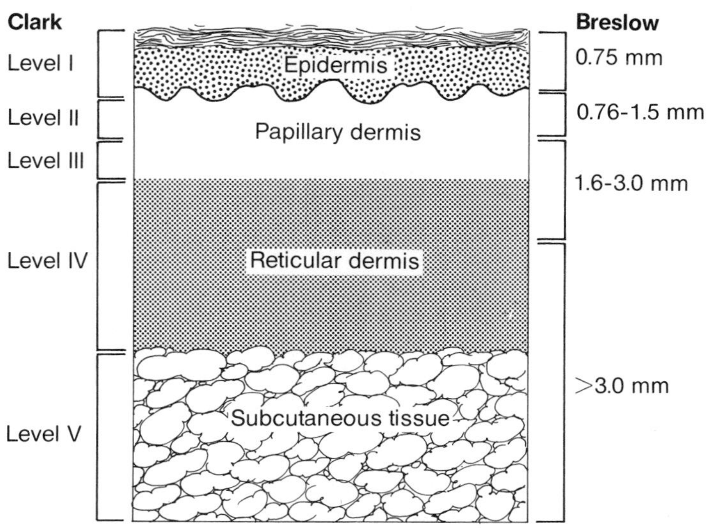

FIG. 13-10. The primary melanoma is classified according to its depth of invasion in the skin. The criteria for Clark's and Breslow's levels are illustrated. The present T classification adopted by the AJCC is a modification of these classifications.

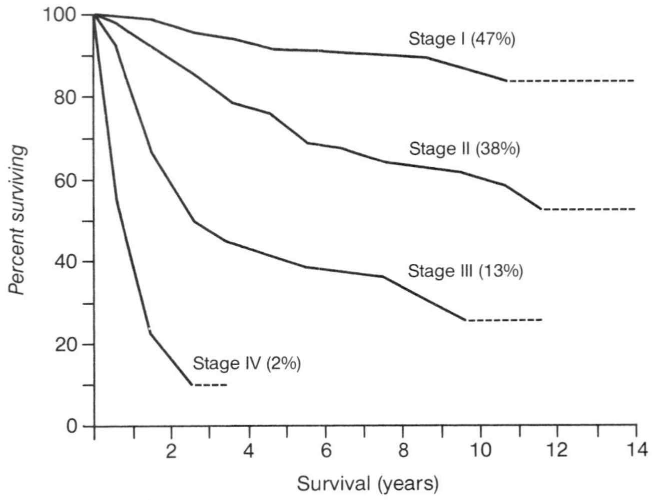

FIG. 13-11. The graph summarizes the data for 10-year survival of patients with melanoma grouped according to stage. (*From Balch CM, et al., 1992, with permission.*)

Finally, the presence of distant metastasis is a grave prognostic sign (stage IV). The median survival ranges from 2 to 7 months depending on the number and site of metastases, but survival up to a few years has been reported (Fig. 13-11).

Other independent prognostic factors have been identified:

1. Anatomic location. Independent of histologic type and depth of invasion, people with lesions of the extremities do better than people with melanomas of the trunk or face (i.e., 82 percent 10-year survival for localized disease of the extremity compared to 68 percent survival with a lesion of the face).
2. Ulceration. Presence of ulceration in a lesion carries a worse prognosis. For unknown reasons these melanomas act more aggressively than nonulcerated ones. The 10-year survival for patients with local disease (stage I) and an ulcerated melanoma was 50 percent compared to 78 percent for the same stage lesion without ulceration.
3. Inflammatory infiltrate. A large inflammatory infiltrate seen on histologic examination of a lesion is a good prognostic sign. However, the presence of regression in a lesion is not.
4. Sex. Women have melanomas in more favorable anatomic sites and these lesions are less likely to contain ulceration. Despite correction for these factors, females have a higher survival rate than men (80 percent 10-year survival in women versus 61 percent in men with stage I disease).
5. Histologic type. As noted before, nodular melanomas have the same prognosis as superficial spreading types when lesions are matched for depth of invasion. Lentigo malignant types, however, have a better prognosis even after correcting for thickness.

Treatment

The treatment of melanoma is primarily surgical. The indication for procedures such as lymph node dissection, parotidectomy, and resection of distant metastases have changed somewhat over time, but the only hope for cure and the best treatment for regional control and palliation remains surgery. Radiation therapy, regional and systemic chemotherapy, and immunotherapy are effective in limited circumstances, but none is considered to be a first option.

All suspicious lesions should undergo excisional biopsy with closure of the skin. A wide skin margin need not be taken at this point. If the lesion is large, then incisional biopsy of a representative part is recommended. Once a diagnosis of melanoma is made, the biopsy scar and any remains of the lesion need to be removed. For in situ lesions a 0.5 to 1-cm margin of normal skin is adequate for cure. A T1 melanoma (smaller than .76 mm) requires a 1 to 2-cm margin to prevent local recurrence. For thicker lesions a 3-cm margin is recommended since a wider margin does not affect local recurrence rates. The depth of excision has been traditionally designated as the deep fascia, more because it is an easily identified landmark rather than for any therapeutic benefit. The defect is closed with a skin graft or flap.

The indication for regional lymph node dissection is less straightforward. All clinically positive lymph nodes should be removed by regional nodal dissection for cure or at least palliation of the disease. For patients without lymphadenopathy and T1 lesions, the cure rate is excellent with wide excision of the primary lesion and prophylactic nodal dissection is not warranted. Patients with T4 (greater than 4 mm) lesions will die of metastatic disease and prophylactic nodal removal does not influence survival. Some surgeons would remove the lymph nodes before they are palpable (prophylactic lymphadenectomy) since approximately 40 percent of these patients develop clinically evident nodal metastases during the course of their disease if the lymph nodes are left intact at the time of the initial resection. When groin lymph nodes are removed for clinically palpable nodes (therapeutic lymphadenectomy) the deep (iliac) nodes must be removed along with the superficial (inguinal) nodes or disease will recur in that region. For axillary dissections the nodes medial to the pectoralis minor muscle must also be taken. Disruption of the lymphatic outflow does cause significant problems with chronic edema, especially of the lower extremity; therefore prophylactic node dissection is not routinely performed.

In patients with intermediate-thickness tumors (T2 and T3, 0.76 to 4.0 mm) and no clinical evidence of nodal or metastatic disease (stages IB and IIA), the benefit of prophylactic dissection is controversial. To date, two prospective randomized studies assessed patients undergoing prophylactic versus delayed lymph node dissection. For intermediate-thickness melanomas no survival difference was noted between these groups. There are hopes that ongoing trials will identify a subgroup of patients with intermediate-thickness melanomas that would benefit from elective nodal removal. These factors may include ulceration of the lesion, anatomic location, sex of the patient, and histologic type. Some surgeons still advocate lymph node removal at the time of wide local excision of the primary lesion since 20 to 25 percent of these patients with clinically negative nodes will have microscopically identifiable metastasis in the resected specimen. Lymph node dissection at the time of the first operation would save these patients a second procedure. When a cervical lymph node dissection is performed for lesions of the face a superficial parotidectomy should also be done at the same time since the preparotid nodes will contain tumor before the cervical nodes. Lesions on the trunk may drain to either the axilla or groin. Lymphoscintigraphy may be used to determine if a lesion drains to either lymph node basin or both.

Even when patients develop distant metastasis surgical therapy may be indicated. Solitary lesions in the brain, gut, or skin that are symptomatic should be excised when possible. Although cure is extremely rare, palliation can be good and asymptomatic survival prolonged. A decision to operate on metastatic lesions must be made after careful deliberation with each individual patient.

Other forms of therapy are available and are undergoing clinical trials. To date adjuvant therapy has not been shown to influence survival. All modalities of treatment other than surgery are reserved for patients with confirmed metastatic or recurrent disease. Although initially thought to be ineffective in the treatment of melanoma, radiation therapy has been shown to be useful. High dose per fraction radiation produces a better response rate than low-dose, large-fraction therapy. Radiation therapy is the treatment of choice for patients with symptomatic multiple brain metastases. The chemotherapy agent dacarbazine is the most effective agent against melanoma. It is used as a single agent since multidrug therapy has not been shown to be any more effective. Nitrosoureas and Taxol (a drug made from the Pacific yew tree) have also been shown to have activity. Unfortunately, response rates range from 10 to 20 percent in most series.

The most promising area of melanoma treatment is the use of immunologic manipulation. With the knowledge that tumor regression seen in primary lesions represented an immunologic response of the patient against the malignancy, attempts to increase or supplement that response have been attempted. Administration of interleukin-2 with lymphokine-activated killer cells has had an encouraging response rate. Vaccines have been developed with the hope of stimulating the body's own immune system against the tumor. Melanoma cells contain a number of distinctly different cell-surface antigens. Monoclonal antibodies have been raised against these antigens. These antibodies have been used alone or linked to a radioisotope or cytotoxic agent in an effort to selectively kill tumor cells. All treatments are currently investigational.

Hyperthermic regional perfusion of the limb with a chemotherapeutic agent is considered for patients with local recurrence or in-transit lesions (local disease in lymphatics) on an extremity not amenable to excision. While difficult to perform and associated with complications, it does produce a high response rate (greater than 50 percent response). The 10-year survival rate using isolated limb perfusion is estimated to be 15 percent better than that for surgical treatment alone.

Pathologic Conditions Associated with Skin Malignancies

There are several well-recognized diseases associated with an increased incidence of skin malignancies. Some are associated with a specific neoplasm, while others appear to have a less specific effect of leaving the patient susceptible to a variety of neoplasms.

Diseases linked with basal cell carcinoma include the basal cell nevus syndrome and nevus sebaceus of Jadassohn. Basal cell nevus syndrome is an autosomal dominant disorder characterized by the growth of hundreds of basal cell carcinomas during young adulthood. Palmar and plantar pits are a common physical finding and represent foci of neoplasms. Treatment is limited to excision of only aggressive and symptomatic lesions. Nevus sebaceus of Jadassohn is a lesion containing several cutaneous tissue elements and develops during childhood. These lesions are associated with a variety of neoplasms of the epidermis, but most commonly basal cell carcinoma.

Diseases associated with squamous cell carcinoma may have a causative role (see section on pathogenesis). Skin diseases that cause chronic wounds, such as epidermolysis bullosus and lupus erythematosus, are associated with a high incidence of squamous cell carcinoma. Epidermodysplasia verruciformis is a rare autosomal recessive disease associated with infection with human papilloma virus. Large verrucous lesions develop early in life and often progress to invasive squamous cell carcinoma in middle age.

Xeroderma pigmentosum is an autosomal recessive disease associated with a defect in cellular repair of DNA damage. The inability of the skin to correct DNA damage from ultraviolet radiation leaves these patients prone to cutaneous malignancies. Squamous cell carcinomas are most frequent, but basal cell carcinomas, melanomas, and even acute leukemias are seen.

Dysplastic nevi may represent a precursor to melanoma. Familial dysplastic nevus syndrome is an autosomal dominant disorder. Patients develop multiple dysplastic nevi and longitudinal studies have demonstrated an almost 100 percent incidence of melanoma. Familial dysplastic nevus syndrome is similar to familial polyposis coli and the association with colon cancer. While the development of colon cancer can be arrested with total proctocolectomy, a similar solution is not possible with familial dysplastic nevi. Close surveillance and frequent biopsy of all suspicious lesions constitutes the best therapy.

Other Malignancies

Merkel Cell Carcinoma (Primary Neuroendocrine Carcinoma of the Skin)

Originally thought to be a variant of squamous cell carcinoma, it has only recently been demonstrated by immunohistochemical markers that Merkel cell carcinomas are of neuroepithelial differentiation. These tumors are associated with a synchronous or metasynchronous squamous cell carcinoma 25 percent of the time. Because these tumors are very aggressive, prophylactic regional lymph node dissection and adjuvant radiation therapy are recommended.

Extramammary Paget's Disease

This tumor is histologically similar to the mammary type. It is a cutaneous lesion that appears as a pruritic, red patch that does not resolve. Biopsy demonstrates classic Paget cells. Paget's disease is thought to be a cutaneous extension of an underlying adenocarcinoma, although an associated tumor cannot always be demonstrated.

Adnexal Carcinomas

These consist of apocrine, eccrine, and sebaceous carcinomas. These are all rare tumors. They are locally destructive and can cause death by distant metastasis.

Angiosarcomas

Angiosarcomas may arise spontaneously, mostly on the scalp, face, and neck. They usually appear as a bruise that spontaneously bleeds or enlarges without trauma. Tumors may also arise in areas of prior radiation therapy or in the setting of chronic lymphedema of the arm, such as after mastectomy (Stewart-Treves syndrome). The angiosarcomas that arise in these areas of chronic change occur decades later. The tumors consist of anaplastic endothelial cells surrounding vascular channels. While total excision of early lesions can provide occasional cure, the prognosis is usually poor. Five-year survival rates are under 20 percent. Chemotherapy and radiation therapy are used for palliation.

Kaposi's Sarcoma

Kaposi's sarcoma (KS) appears as rubbery, bluish nodules that occur primarily on the extremities but may appear any place on the skin and viscera. These lesions are usually multifocal rather than metastatic. Histologically, the lesions are composed of capillaries lined by atypical endothelial cells. Early lesions may resemble hemangiomas, while older lesions contain more spindle cells and resemble sarcomas.

Classic KS is seen in people of Eastern Europe or sub-Sahara Africa. The lesions are locally aggressive but undergo periods of remission. Visceral spread of the lesions is rare, but a subtype of the African variety has a predilection of spreading to lymph nodes. A different variety of KS has been described for people with AIDS and patients with immunosuppression from chemotherapy. For unclear reasons, AIDS-related KS occurs primarily in male homosexuals and not in intravenous drug abusers or hemophiliacs. In this form of the disease, the lesions spread rapidly to the nodes, and the gastrointestinal tract is often involved.

Treatment for all types of KS consists of radiation to the lesions. Chemotherapy has been reported to be of some benefit. Surgical excision is reserved for lesions that cause obstruction of vital functions. Death from KS is rare.

Dermatofibromasarcoma Protuberans

Dermatofibromasarcoma protuberans consists of large nodular lesions located mainly on the trunk. They often ulcerate and become infected. With enlargement the lesions become painful. Histologically, the lesions contain atypical spindle cells, probably of fibroblast origin, located around a core of collagen tissue. Sometimes they are mistaken for an infected keloid. Metastases are rare and surgical excision can be curative. Excision must be complete because local recurrences are common.

Fibrosarcoma

Fibrosarcomas are hard, irregular masses found in the subcutaneous fat. The fibroblasts appear very anaplastic and their growth disorganized. If not excised completely metastases usually develop. Five-year survival is about 60 percent with excision.

Liposarcoma

Liposarcomas arise in the deep muscle planes and, rarely, from the subcutaneous tissue. They occur most commonly on the thigh. An enlarging lipoma should be excised and inspected to distinguish it from a liposarcoma. Wide excision is the treatment of choice, with radiation therapy reserved for metastatic disease.

FUTURE DEVELOPMENTS IN SKIN SURGERY

The major challenge facing surgical therapy for diseases of the skin is the lack of replacement for diseased or damaged tissue. The discovery of autologous skin grafts for treatment of skin defects was a tremendous advancement. However, technical limitations, such as graft contraction and donor site problems, and biologic limitations, such as the limited amount of autologous skin available, make autografts less than a universal solution. The future of surgical therapy for diseases of the skin lies in the development of skin replacement. Present research is directed at tissue expansion, cell culture expansion, and neogenesis of skin.

Techniques for tissue expansion have been reported since 1982. During skin expansion with these subcutaneous balloon implants (Fig. 13-12), new epidermis and some collagen is produced. Much of this new tissue, however, is rearrangement of the old tissue. Expansion of skin produces a limited amount of tissue for use.

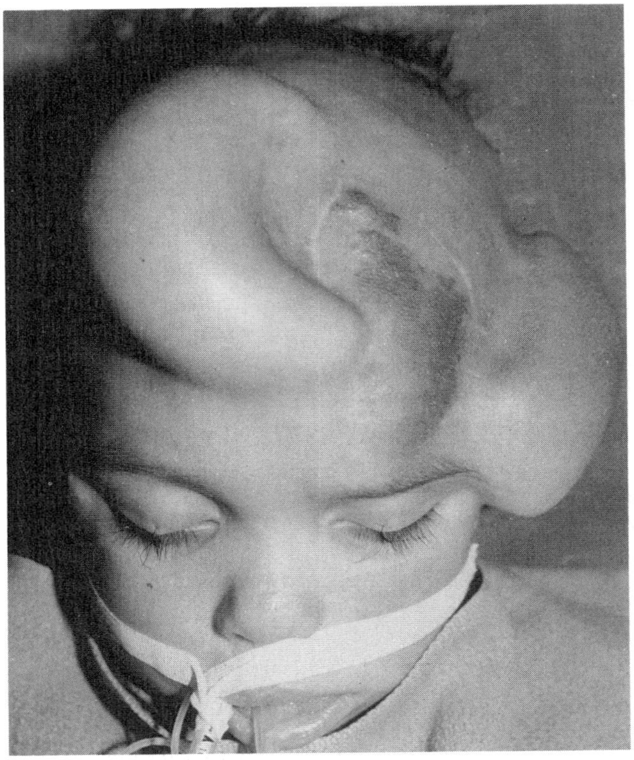

A

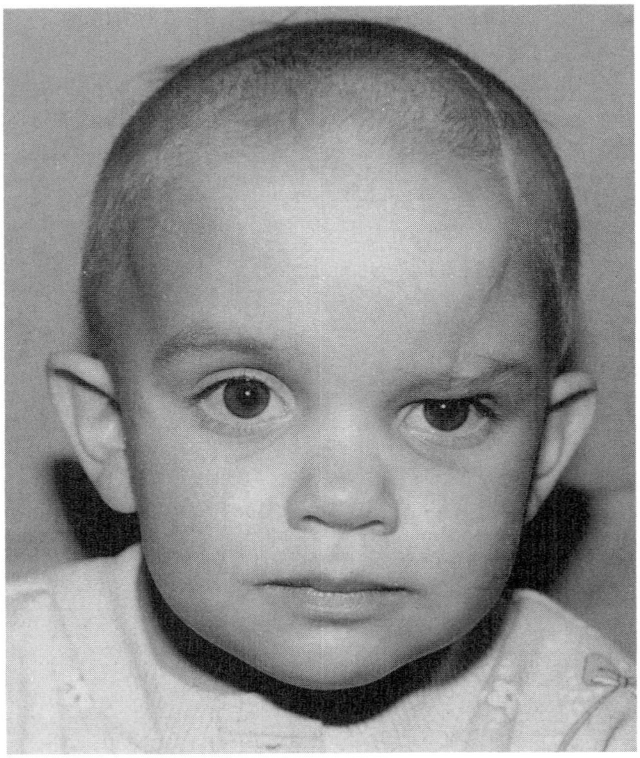

B

FIG. 13-12. *A.* Tissue expanders are used in the scalp of an infant for excision of a neurofibroma. *B.* After excision and closure of scalp defect.

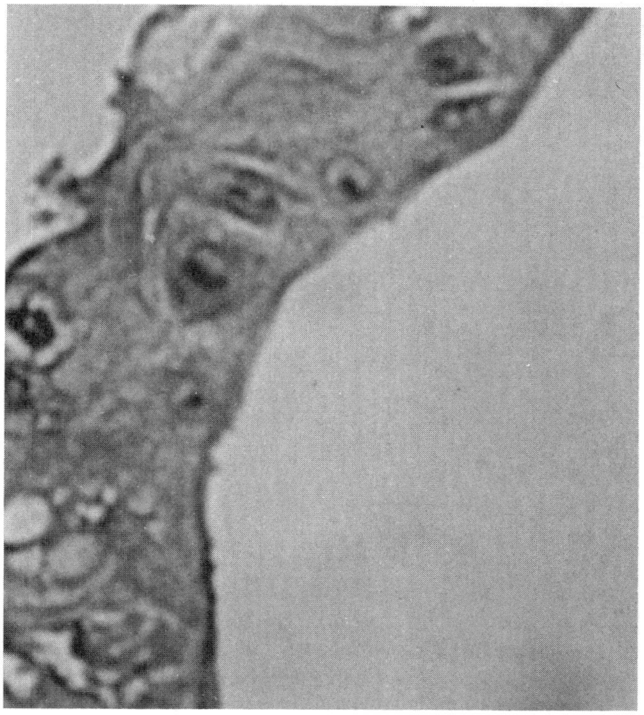

FIG. 13-13. Photomicrograph of mature cultured epithelium.

The expansion of epidermis by the growth and maturation of keratinocytes in culture can be performed. The use of a postage stamp-size biopsy to produce enough autologous epithelium to cover a greater than 90 percent total body surface area burn has been reported (Fig. 13-13). Although this was a major advancement, the shortcomings of this skin coverage are evident. Skin (comprising dermis, vasculature, adnexal structures, and pigmentation) is much more complex than epidermis. Replacement of these other structures is presently under investigation. Dermal replacements from man-made materials or cadaveric sources are being tested. Melanocytes can be cocultured with keratinocytes and may provide a way to control pigmentation. With more sophisticated methods of tissue culture a more complex skin replacement will become available.

The ultimate replacement for damaged skin will come from complete neoorganogenesis of tissue. This will come about as investigators learn more about the protein factors that control wound healing and tissue growth. Characterization of these growth factors on a structural and functional level is just beginning, but the information obtained to date has been enormous. Factors have been isolated that cause specific mesenchymal cells to proliferate (fibroblast growth factor), migrate (epidermal growth factor), and organize into structures such as capillaries (transforming growth factor-beta) or even rudimentary organoid tissue. This may eventually allow us to really generate new tissue in situ for skin replacement.

Bibliography

Introduction

Ballantyne D, Converse J: *Experimental Skin Grafts and Transplantation Immunity*. New York, Springer-Verlag, 1979.

Medawar P: The behavior and fate of skin autografts and skin homografts in rabbits. *J Anat* 78:176, 1944.

Anatomy and Physiology

Baker H, Kligman AM: Technique for estimating turnover time of human stratum corneum. *Arch Dermatol* 95:408, 1967.

Braverman IM, Yen A: Ultrastructure of the human dermal microcirculation II. The capillary loops of the dermal papillae. *J Invest Dermatol* 68:44, 1977.

Flaxman BA, Sosio AC, Van Scott EJ: Changes in melanosome distribution in caucasoid skin following topical application of N-mustard. *J Invest Dermatol* 60:321, 1973.

Frost P, Weinstein GD, Van Scott EJ: The ichthyosiform dermatosis. II. Autoradiographic studies of dermal proliferation. *J Invest Dermatol* 47:561, 1966.

Johnson, WC, Helwig EB: Histochemistry of the acid mucopolysaccharides of the skin in normal and in certain pathologic conditions. *Am J Clin Pathol* 40:123, 1961.

Meigel WN, Gay S, Weber L: Dermal architecture and collagen type distribution. *Arch Dermatol Res* 259:1, 1977.

Pessa M, Bland K, Copeland E: Growth factors and determinants of wound repair. *J Surg Res* 42:207, 1987.

Shimada S, Katz SI: The skin as an immunologic organ. *Arch Pathol Lab Med* 112:231, 1988.

Stingl G, Tamaki K, Katz S: Origin and function of epidermal Langerhans cells. *Immunol Rev* 53:149, 1980.

Tamaki K, Stingl G, Katz SI: The origin of the Langerhans cells. *J Invest Dermatol* 74:309, 1980.

Trauma

Anthony J, Huntsman T, Mathes S: Changing trends in the management of pelvic pressure ulcers: A 12 year review. *Decubitus* 5:44, 1992.

Colen SR: Pressure sores, in McCarthy JG (ed): *Plastic Surgery*. Philadelphia, WB Saunders, 1990, p. 3797.

Infection

Allen-Mersh TG: Pilonidal sinus: Finding the right track for treatment. *Br J Surg* 77:123, 1990.

Benign Tumors

Burgdorf WHC: Tumors of sebaceous gland differentiation, in Farmer ER, Hood AF (eds): *Pathology of the Skin*. Norwalk, CT, Appleton & Lange, 1990, p. 615.

Leikensohn J, Epstein L, Vasconez L: Superselective embolization and surgery of noninvoluting hemangiomas and av malformations. *Plast Reconstr Surg* 68:143, 1981.

Lister W: The natural history of strawberry naevi. *Lancet* 1:1429, 1938.

Malignant Tumors

Balch CM, Soong SJ, et al: A comparison of prognostic factors and surgical results in 1,786 patients with localized (stage I) melanoma treated in Alabama, USA, and New South Wales, Australia. *Ann Surg* 1196:677, 1982.

Balch CM, Houghton AN, et al: *Cutaneous Melanoma*. 2nd ed. Philadelphia, JB Lippincott, 1992.

Bostwick J, Pandergrast WJ, Vasconez LO: Marjolin's ulcer: An immunologically privileged tumor? *Plast Reconstr Surg* 57:66, 1976.

Breslow A: Thickness, cross-sectional areas and depth of invasion in the prognosis of cutaneous melanomas. *Ann Surg* 172:902, 1970.

Byers R, Kesler K, et al: Squamous carcinoma of the external ear. *Am J Surg* 146:447, 1983.

Carter DM, O'Keefe EJ: Hereditary cutaneous disorders, in Moscchella SSL, Hurley HJ (eds): *Dermatology*. Philadelphia, WB Saunders, 1985.

Chanda JJ: Extramammary Paget's disease: Prognosis and relationship to internal malignancy. *J Am Acad Dermatol* 13:1009, 1985.

Clark WH, Elder DE, DuPont G: Dysplastic nevi and malignant melanoma, in Farmer ER, Hood AF (eds): *Pathology of the Skin*. East Norwalk, CT, Appleton & Lange, 1990, p. 684.

Clark WH, Elder DE, Dupont G: A model predicting survival in stage I melanoma based upon tumor progression. *J Natl Cancer Inst* 81:1893, 1989.

Coburn RJ: Malignant ulcers following trauma, in *Cancer of the Skin,* vol. 2. WB Saunders, Philadelphia, 1976, p. 939.

Dutcher JP, Creekmore S, et al: Phase II study of high dose interleukin-2 and lymphokine activated killer cells in patients with melanoma. *Proc Am Soc Clin Oncol* 6:970, 1987.

Fleming MD, Hunt JL, et al: Marjolin's ulcer: A review and reevaluation of a difficult problem. *J Burn Care Rehabil* 11:460, 1990.

Friedman HI, Cooper PH, Wanebo HJ: Prognostic and therapeutic use of microstaging of cutaneous squamous cell carcinomas of the trunk and extremities. *Cancer* 56:109, 1985.

Greene MH, Clark WH, et al: High risk malignant melanoma in melanoma-prone families with dysplastic nevi. *Ann Intern Med* 102:458, 1985.

Hall AF: Relationship of sunlight, complexion and heredity to skin carcinogenesis. *Arch Dermatol* 61:589, 1950.

Harris MN, Gumport SL, Maiwandi H: Axillary lymph node dissection for melanoma. *Surg Gynecol Obstet* 135:936, 1972.

Hurwitz RM, Egan WT, et al: Bowenoid papulosis and squamous cell carcinoma of the genitalia: Suspected sexual transmission. *Cutis* 39:193, 1987.

Krementz ET, Ryan RF, et al: Hyperthermic regional perfusion for melanoma of the limbs, in Balch CM, Houghton AN (eds): *Cutaneous Melanoma,* 2nd ed, chap. 35. Philadelphia, JB Lippincott, 1992.

Lee CA, Fritz KA, Golitz L: Second cutaneous malignancies in patients with mycosis fungoides treated with nitrogen mustard. *J Am Acad Dermatol* 7:590, 1982.

Luanda J, Nenscke CI, Mohammed N: The Tanzanian human albino skin: Natural history. *Cancer* 55:1823, 1985.

Mohs FE: *Chemosurgery, Microscopically Controlled Surgery for Skin Cancer*. Springfield, IL, Charles C. Thomas, 1978.

Orth G: Epidermodysplasia verruciformis: A model for understanding the oncogenicity of human papillomaviruses. *Papillomaviruses. CIBA Found Symp* 120:157, 1986.

Overgaard J, Overgaard M, et al: Some factors of importance in the radiation treatment of malignant melanoma. *Radiother Oncol* 5:183, 1986.

Rigel DS, Kopf AN, Friedman RJ: The rate of malignant melanoma in the US: Are we making an impact? *J Am Acad Dermatol* 17:1050, 1987.

Rhodes AR, Seki Y, et al: Melanosomal alterations in dysplastic melanocytic nevi: A quantitative, ultrastructural investigation. *Cancer* 61:358, 1988.

Schwartz RA, Birnkrant AP, et al: Squamous cell carcinoma in dominant type epidermolysis bullosa dystrophica. *Cancer* 47:615, 1981.

Sim FH, Taylor WF, et al: Lymphadenectomy in the management of stage I malignant melanoma: A prospective randomized study. *Mayo Clin Proc* 61:697, 1986.

Veronesi U, Adams J, et al: Delayed regional lymph node dissection in stage I melanoma of the skin of the lower extremities. *Cancer* 49:2420, 1982.

Wick MR: Malignant tumors of the epidermis, in Farmer ER, Hood AF (eds): *Pathology of the Skin*. Norwalk, CT, Appleton & Lange, 1990, p. 568.

Zeitels J, LaRossa D, et al: A comparison of local recurrence and resection margins for stage I primary cutaneous malignant melanoma. *Plast Reconstr Surg* 81:688, 1988.

Future Developments in Skin Surgery

Austad E, Thomas S, Pasyk K: Tissue expansion: Dividend or loan. *Plast Reconstr Surg* 78:63, 1986.

Cuono C, Langdon R, et al: Composite autologous-allogeneic skin replacement: Development and clinical application. *Plast Reconstr Surg* 80:626, 1987.

Cuono C, Halaban R, et al: Mixed keratinocyte-melanocyte cultures: an approach to immediate and secondary repigmentation after burn injury. *Proc Am Burn Assoc* 20:13, 1988.

Galico G, O'Connor N, et al: Permanent coverage of large burn wounds with autologous cultured human epithelium. *N Engl J Med* 311:448, 1984.

Heimbach D, Lutterman A, et al: Artificial dermis for major burns: A multicenter randomized clinical trial. *Ann Surg* 308:313, 1988.

Radovan C: Breast reconstruction after mastectomy using the temporary expander. *Plast Reconstr Surg* 74:482, 1982.

Reinwald J. Green H: Serial cultivation strains of human epidermal keratinocytes. The formation of keratinizing colonies from a single cell. *Cell* 6:331, 1975.

Rifkin D, Moscatelli D: Recent developments in the cell biology of basic fibroblast growth factor. *J Cell Biol* 109:1, 1989.

Sporn MD, Roberts AB: The transforming growth-factor-betas, in Sporn MB, Roberts AB (eds): *Handbook of Experimental Pharmacology,* vol. 95, part I, chap. 8, *Peptide Growth Factors and Their Receptors I*. New York, Springer-Verlag, 1990, p. 419.

Thompson J, Haudenschild C, et al: Heparin-binding growth factor 1 induces the formation of organoid neovascular structures in vivo. *Proc Natl Acad Sci* 86:7928, 1989.

CHAPTER 14

Breast

Kirby I. Bland and Edward M. Copeland III

INTRODUCTION

The breast or mammary gland is a distinguishing feature of the class Mammalia. From puberty to death, the breast is subjected to constant physical and physiologic alterations that relate to menses, pregnancy, gestation, and menopause. The impact of breast disease in Western societies assumes greater importance as cancer of this organ continues to increase exponentially. Currently one of every two women will consult her physician for breast disease, approximately one of every four women will undergo breast biopsy, and one of every nine American women will develop some variant of breast carcinoma.

EMBRYOLOGY

The breast is a highly modified sudoriferous gland that develops as ingrowths from ectoderm form the alveoli and ducts. Supporting vascularized connective tissue takes derivation solely from mesenchyme. At approximately the fifth or sixth week of fetal development, two ventral bands of thickened ectoderm (mammary ridges, "milk lines") are evident in the embryo. In the majority of the class Mammalia, paired glands develop along these ridges and extend from the base of the forelimb (future axilla) to the region of the hind limb (inguinal area). These ridges are not prominent in the human embryo and disappear shortly thereafter, except for a small portion that may persist in the pectoral region. Accessory mammary glands (polymastia) or accessory nipples (polythelia) may occur along the original mammary ridge or "milk line" (Fig. 14-1) if the normal regression fails.

Each mammary gland develops as an ingrowth of ectoderm and initiates a primary bud of tissue in underlying mesenchyme. Each *primary* bud initiates the development of 15 to 20 *secondary* buds or outgrowths. In the fetus, epithelial cords develop from the secondary buds and extend into the surrounding connective tissues of the chest wall. Lumina develop in the outgrowths to form lactiferous ducts with prominent branches. By birth, lactiferous ducts open into shallow epithelial depressions referred to as the *mammary pit*. In infancy, the pit becomes elevated and transformed into the nipple as a consequence of proliferation of mesenchyme.

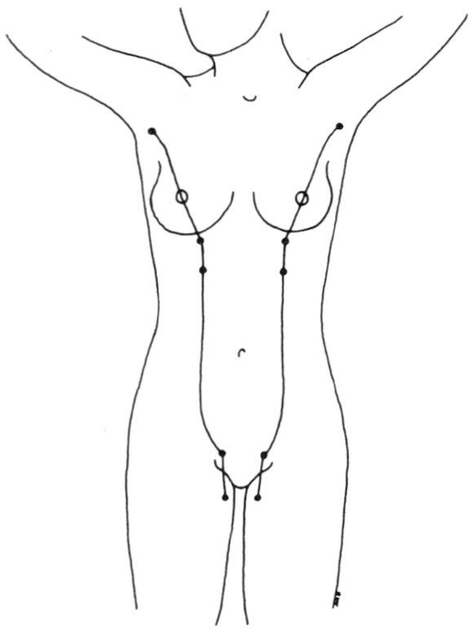

FIG. 14-1. Mammary milk line. (From: *Bland KI, Romrell LJ: 1991, Chap 4, p 70, with permission.*)

If there is failure of the pit to elevate above skin level, a congenital malformation, recognized in 2 to 4 percent of patients as inverted nipples, is evident.

In either newborn females or males, transient enlargement of the breast bud may be evident and produces a secretion referred to as "witch's milk." These transitory changes occur in response to maternal hormones that cross the fetal-maternal circulation of the placenta.

At birth, the breasts appear essentially identical in both sexes and demonstrate only the presence of major lactiferous ducts. In the female, the gland remains undeveloped until puberty. Thereafter, the organ enlarges rapidly in response to estrogen and progesterone secretion by the ovaries. Hormonal stimulation initiates proliferation of glandular tissue as well as fat and connective tissue elements associated with breast support. Glandular tissues remain incompletely developed until pregnancy occurs. With parturition, the intralobular ducts undergo rapid development and form buds that become alveoli.

Unilateral absence of the breast (*amastia*) is more common than bilateral amastia; both conditions occur more commonly in females. This rare congenital anomaly occurs as a result of an arrested mammary ridge at about the sixth week of fetal development. Typically, other abnormalities are not associated with bilateral absence of nipple and breast tissue. By contrast, Alfred Poland described the absence of musculature (pectoralis major and minor) of the shoulder girdle and malformations of the ipsilateral upper limb with unilateral amastia. Hypoplasia or complete absence of the ipsilateral breast or nipple, costal cartilage and rib defects, hypoplasia of subcutaneous tissues of the chest wall, and brachysyndactyly is referred to as *Poland's syndrome*.

Iatrogenic factors may also induce breast hypoplasia. The failure of complete development of the vestigial male or female breast (developmental hypomastia) may be initiated by therapeutic manipulation and/or injury to the mammary anlage in infancy or in the prepubertal state. Recognized iatrogenic mechanisms that initiate hypoplasia of the organ include trauma, abscess, incisions, infectious lesions, and radiation therapy.

The newly coined terminology for medial confluence of the breast is *symmastia*. This rare anomaly is recognized as webbing across the midline in breasts that are usually symmetrical. The presternal blending (confluence) of tissue that is associated with *macromastia* is more common.

Accessory or *supernumerary nipples,* polythelia, is a relatively common, minor congenital anomaly that occurs in both sexes with an estimated frequency of 1:100 to 1:500 persons. *Polythelia* may be associated with abnormalities of the urinary tract (renal agenesis and carcinoma), cardiovascular system (conduction disturbance, hypertension, congenital heart anomalies) and other conditions (pyloric stenosis, epilepsy, ear abnormalities, and arthrogryposis).

Supernumerary nipples or breasts may occur in any size or configuration along the mammary milk line; the most common site is a line that extends from the nipple to the symphysis pubis. *Turner syndrome* (ovarian agenesis and dysgenesis) and *Fleischer syndrome* (lateral displacement of nipples to the midclavicular line with bilateral renal hypoplasia) may have polymastia as a component. *Accessory* or *ectopic axillary breast tissue* is relatively uncommon but, when present, is usually bilateral.

ANATOMY AND DEVELOPMENT

Located within the superficial fascia of the anterior thoracic wall, the breast is composed of 15 to 20 lobes of glandular tissue of the tubuloalveolar type. Fibrous connective tissues connect the lobes; adipose tissue is abundantly interposed between the lobules. Subcutaneous connective tissues surround the gland and extend as septa between lobes and lobules, providing structural support for glandular elements. The deep layer of superficial fascia lies on the posterior surface of the breast adjacent to and at some points fusing with the deep (pectoral) fascia of chest wall. The *retromammary bursa* may be identified surgically on the posterior aspect of the breast between the deep layer of superficial fascia and deep investing fascia of the pectoralis major and contiguous muscles of the thoracic wall (Fig. 14-2). Fibrous bands of connective tissue interdigitate between parenchymal tissue to extend from the deep layer of the superficial fascia (hypodermis) and attach to the dermis of the skin. Described by Sir Astley Cooper, these ligaments insert perpendicular to the delicate superficial fascial layers of the dermis and permit mobility of the breast while providing structural support.

The mature breast of the female extends inferiorly from the level of the second or third rib to the inframammary fold at approximately the sixth or seventh rib. Transversely, it extends from the lateral border of the sternum to the anterior or midaxillary line. The deep or posterior surface rests on portions of deep investing fascia of the pectoralis major, serratus anterior, and external oblique abdominal muscles and the upper extent of the rectus sheath. The axillary tail (of Spence) extends superolaterally into the anterior axillary fold. The upper half of the breast, and particularly the upper outer quadrant, contains a greater volume of glandular tissue than do other sectors.

At *maturity,* glandular components of the breast take a protuberant conical form. The base of the cone is roughly circular, measuring 10 to 12 cm in diameter and 5 to 7 cm in thickness. Tremendous variations in size, contour, and density of the breast are evident at maturity. The nulliparous breast has a typical hemispheric configuration with distinct flattening above the nipple. By contrast, with *multiparity* and the hormonal stimulation that accompanies *pregnancy* and *lactation,* the organ assumes a larger and more pendulous form and increases in volume and density.

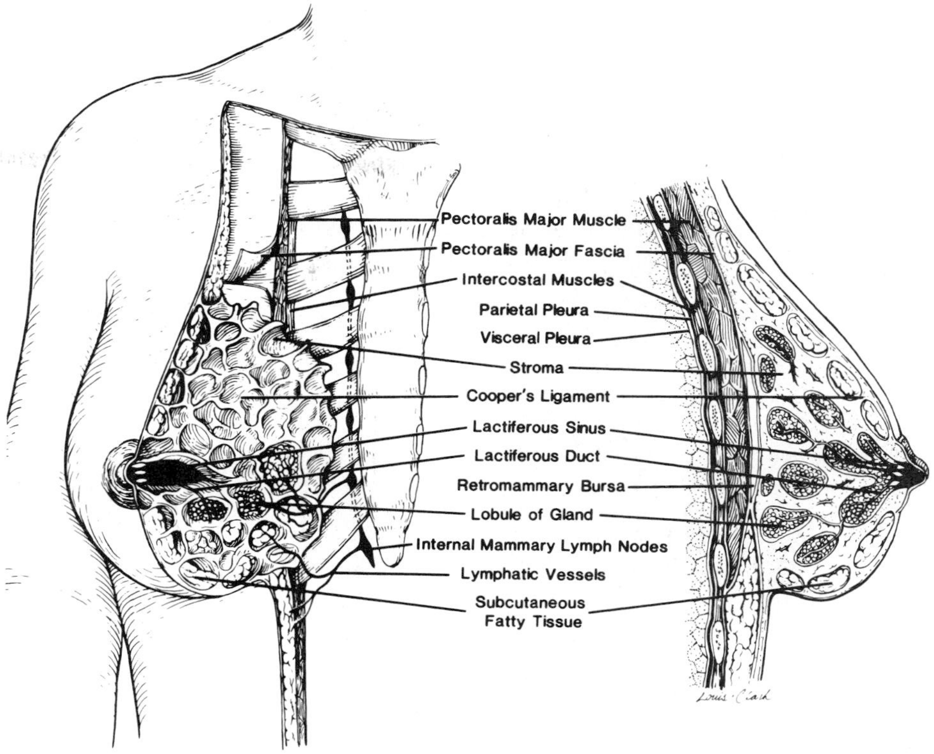

FIG. 14-2. *A tangential view of the breast on the chest wall and a cross-sectional (sagittal) view of the breast and associated chest wall. (From: Romrell LJ, Bland KI: 1991, Chap 2, p 18, with permission.)*

With *senescence,* the aging breast assumes a flattened, flaccid, and more pendulous configuration with decreased volume.

Nipple and Areola. The epidermis of the nipple and areola is highly pigmented and variably corrugated. The complex is covered by keratinized stratified squamous epithelium. During puberty, the skin becomes increasingly pigmented and the nipple assumes an elevated, prominent configuration. During pregnancy, the areola enlarges and pigmentation is enhanced. Smooth muscle bundle fibers arranged radially and circumferentially in the dense connective tissue and longitudinally along the lactiferous ducts extend upward into the nipple. These muscle fibers are responsible for erection of the nipple, which occurs with various sensory and thermal stimuli.

The areola contains sebaceous glands, sweat glands, and accessory areolar glands. These accessory glands produce small elevations on the surface of the areola (Montgomery tubercles). The tip of the nipple contains numerous sensory nerve cell endings and Meissner's corpuscles in the dermal papillae; the areola contains few of these structures. The rich sensory innervation of the breast, particularly the nipple and areola, is of great functional importance because the sucking infant initiates a chain of neurohumoral events that result in ''milk letdown.''

Inactive Mammary Tissue. The tubuloalveolar glands derived from modified sweat glands of the epidermis lie in the subcutaneous tissues. Each of the 15 to 20 irregular *lobes* of branched tubuloalveolar glands in the adult terminates in a *lactiferous duct* (2 to 4 mm in diameter), which opens into a constricted orifice (0.4 to 0.7 mm diameter) with entry into the ampulla of the nipple (see Fig. 14-2). Immediately under the areola, each duct has a dilated portion, the *lactiferous sinus.* Lined with stratified squamous epithelium, these ducts show a gradual transition to two layers of cuboidal cells which then become a single layer of columnar or cuboidal cells in the remaining duct system. Myoepithelial cells of ectodermal origin reside between surface epithelial cells in the basal lamina. In the secretory portion of the gland and in the larger ducts, these cells contain myofibrils and are microscopically similar to smooth muscle cells.

In the inactive gland, the glandular component is sparse and consists chiefly of duct elements (Fig. 14-3). During menstruation, the breast undergoes cyclical changes. In early phases of the

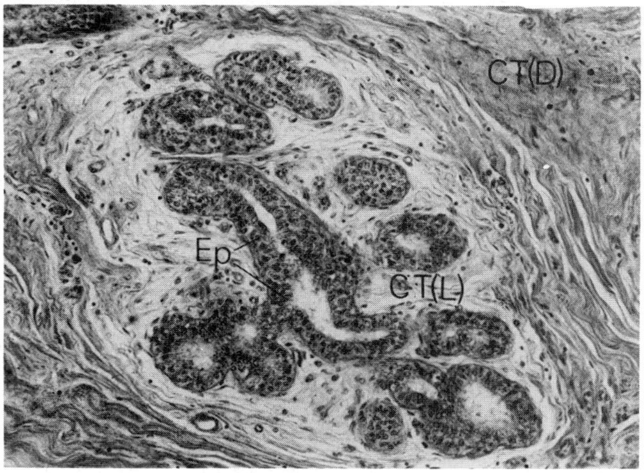

FIG. 14-3. *Inactive or resting human mammary gland. The epithelial (Ep) or glandular elements are embedded in loose connective tissue, CT(L). Within the lobule the epithelial cells are primarily duct elements. Dense connective tissue, CT(D), surrounds the lobule. (×160.) (From: Romrell LJ, Bland KI: 1991, Chap 2, p 20, with permission.)*

cycle, ductules appear as cords with sparse or absent lumina. With estrogen stimulation at or about the time of ovulation, secretory cells increase in height, lumina appear, and a small volume of secretions accumulates. Thereafter, fluid and lipids accumulate in connective tissue. In the absence of prolonged hormonal stimulation, the glandular components regress to a more inactive state throughout the remainder of the menstrual cycle.

Active Mammary Gland; Pregnancy and Lactation. With pregnancy and preparation for lactation, glands undergo marked proliferative and developmental maturation. As the breast enlarges in response to hormonal stimulation, lymphocytes, plasma cells, and eosinophils infiltrate and accumulate within fibrous components of connective tissue.

Development of glandular tissue is asymmetric; variation in degree of development may occur within a single lobule. With cellular division following mitotic phases, ductules branch and alveoli begin to develop. In the third trimester of pregnancy, alveolar development becomes more prominent (Fig. 14-4). With termination of pregnancy, proliferation declines and subsequent enlargement of the breasts occurs via hypertrophy of alveolar cells and accumulation of secretory products in lumina of the ductules.

Secretory cells contain abundant endoplasmic reticulum, moderate numbers of large mitochondria, Golgi complexes, and a number of dense lysosomes. Two distinct products produced by the cells are released by different mechanisms: (1) the protein component of milk synthesized in the granular endoplasmic reticulum; and (2) the lipid, or fatty, component of milk that forms as free lipid droplets in the cytoplasm. These components of milk are formed by merocrine secretion (protein) and apocrine secretion (lipid).

Milk released in the first few days following parturition is termed *colostrum*. Colostrum has a low lipid content but harbors considerable quantities of antibodies that are passively transferred from the mother to the fetus via the placenta. Lymphocytes and plasma cells infiltrate the stroma of the breast during proliferation

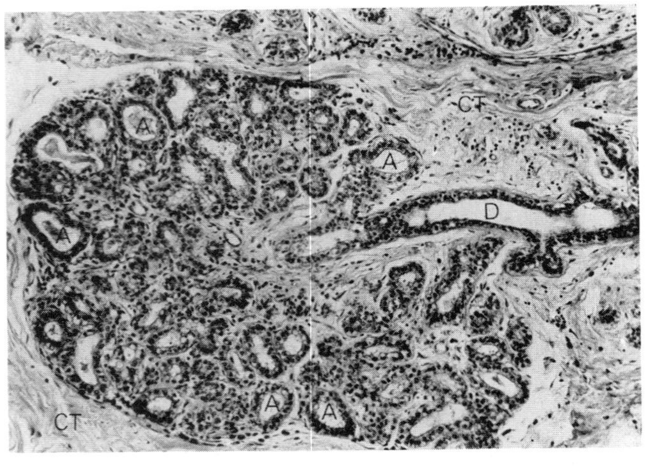

FIG. 14-4. Proliferative or active (pregnant) human mammary gland. The alveolar elements of the gland become conspicuous during the early proliferative period (compare with Fig. 14-3). Within the lobule of the breast, distinct alveoli (A) are present. The alveoli are continuous with a duct (D). The alveoli are surrounded by highly cellular connective tissue (CT). The individual lobules are separated by dense connective tissue septa. (× 160.) (From: *Romrell LJ, Bland KI: 1991, Chap 2, p 20, with permission.*)

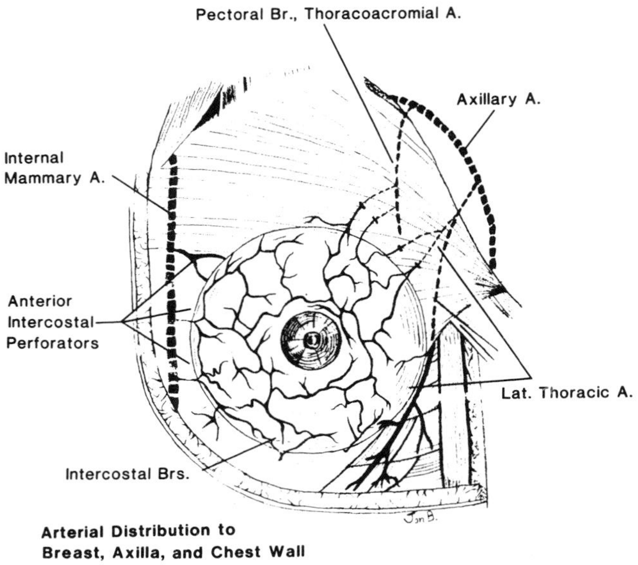

FIG. 14-5. Arterial distribution of blood to the breast, axilla, and chest wall. (From: *Romrell LJ, Bland KI: 1991, Chap 2, p 26, with permission.*)

and development and are believed to be the source of the components of colostrum. With reduction of these cellular structures, the production of colostrum is terminated and lipid-laden milk is released.

Blood Supply. The gland receives its principal blood supply from: (1) perforating branches of the internal mammary artery; (2) lateral branches of the posterior intercostal arteries; and (3) various branches from the axillary artery including the highest thoracic, lateral thoracic, and pectoral branches of the thoracoacromial artery (Fig. 14-5). The second, third, and fourth anterior perforating arteries give branches that arborize in the breast as medial mammary arteries. The lateral thoracic vessel gives branches to the serratus anterior, pectoralis major and minor, and subscapularis muscles. It also gives rise to lateral mammary branches that invest lateral portions of the pectoralis major.

Veins of the breast follow the course of the arteries; primary venous drainage is toward the axilla. Three principal groups of veins for drainage of the thoracic wall and breast include: (1) perforating branches of the internal thoracic vein; (2) tributaries of the axillary vein; and (3) perforating branches of the posterior intercostal veins. Lymphatics usually parallel the course of blood vessels.

The vertebral venous tributaries (*Batson's plexus*) may provide a secondary route for metastases of breast cancer. This plexus invests the vertebrae and extends from the base of the skull to the sacrum. Venous channels exist between this plexus and veins associated with thoracic, abdominal, and pelvic organs. These potential pathways explain metastases to the vertebrae, skull, pelvic bones, and the central nervous system in the absence of pulmonary metastases.

Innervation of the Breast. Lateral and anterior cutaneous branches of the second through sixth intercostal nerves provide sensory innervation. Nerves of the breast are principally derived from the fourth, fifth, and sixth intercostal nerves. A limited area of skin over the upper portion of the breast is supplied by nerves

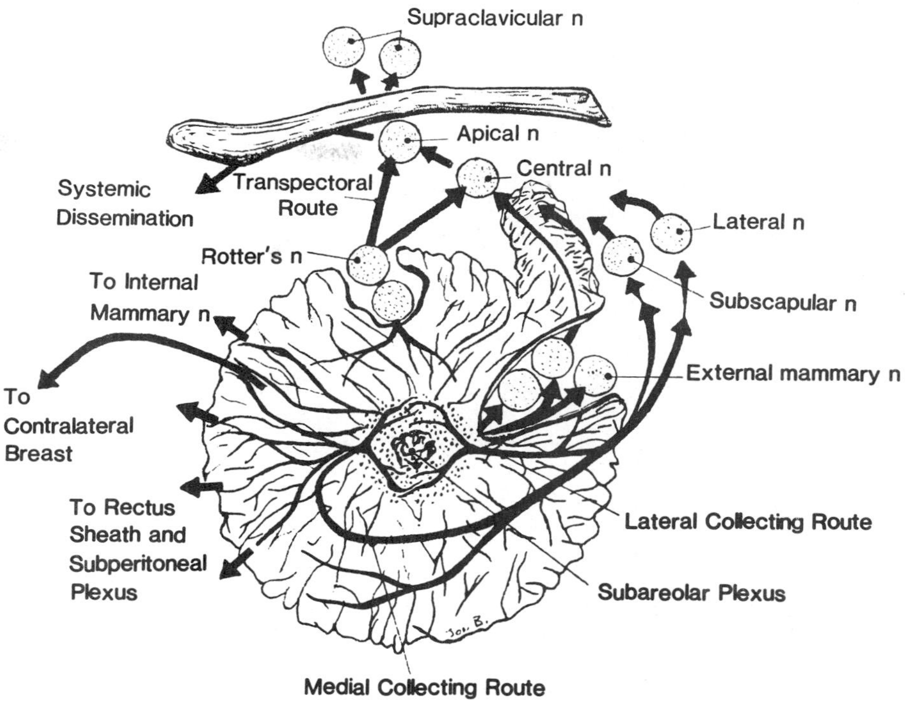

FIG. 14-6. Schematic drawing of the breast identifying the position of lymph nodes relative to the breast and illustrating routes of lymphatic drainage. The arrows indicate the routes of lymphatic drainage (see text). (From: *Romrell LJ, Bland KI: 1991, Chap 2, p 28, with permission.*)

that arise from the cervical plexus, specifically the anterior or medial branches of the *supraclavicular nerve*.

Lateral branches of the *intercostal nerves* exit the intercostal spaces through slips of the serratus anterior muscle. These nerves supply the anterolateral thoracic wall; the third through sixth branches, also known as *lateral mammary branches*, supply the breast. The *intercostal brachial nerve* represents the lateral branch of the second intercostal nerve and is commonly visualized during surgical dissection of the axilla. Resection of the intercostal brachial initiates loss of sensation from the upper medial aspect of the arm and axilla.

Lymphatic Drainage. The boundaries of lymphatic drainage of the axilla are not well demarcated. There is also considerable variation in positions of regional nodes. Anatomists usually define five groups of axillary nodes while surgeons identify six primary groups (Fig. 14-6). These groups include (1) the *axillary vein group*, or *lateral group*, which consists of 4 to 6 nodes medial or posterior to the vein (Figs. 14-6, 14-7); these receive most of the lymph drainage from the upper extremity. (2) The *external mammary group* (anterior or pectoral group) harbors 5 or 6 nodes along the lower border of the pectoralis minor contiguous with the lateral thoracic vessels. This group receives the majority of lym-

FIG. 14-7. Schematic drawing illustrating the major lymph node groups associated with the lymphatic drainage of the breast. The Roman numerals indicate three levels or groups of lymph nodes that are defined by their location relative to the pectoralis minor. Level I includes lymph nodes located lateral to the pectoralis minor; Level II, lymph nodes located deep to the muscle; and Level III, lymph nodes located medial to the muscle. The arrows indicate the general direction of lymph flow. (From: *Romrell LJ, Bland KI: 1991, Chap 2, p 30, with permission.*)

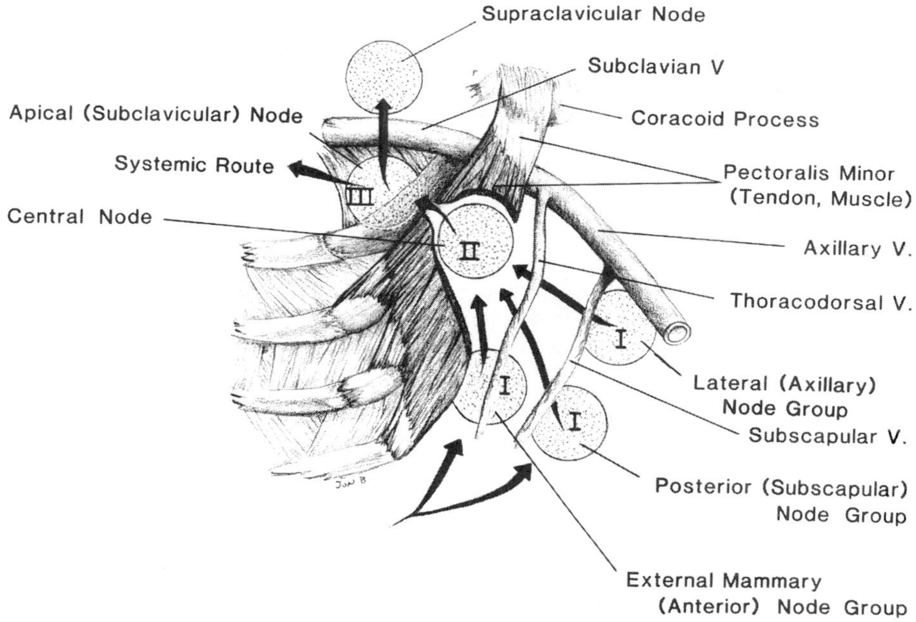

phatic drainage from the lateral breast. (3) The *scapular group* (*posterior* or *subscapular*) consists of 5 to 7 nodes from the posterior wall of the axilla at the lateral border of the scapula and is contiguous with the subscapular vessels. These nodes receive lymph principally from the lower posterior neck, posterior trunk, and posterior shoulder. (4) The *central group* consists of 3 or 4 large groups that are embedded in the fat of the axilla immediately posterior to the pectoralis minor muscle. This group receives lymph from the three preceding groups but may receive lymphatics directly from the breast. (5) The *subclavicular group* (*apical*) consists of 6 to 12 nodal groups posterior and superior to the upper border of the pectoralis minor. This group receives lymph from all groups of axillary nodes and unites with efferent vessels from the subclavicular nodes to form the *subclavian trunk*. (6) The *interpectoral* (*Rotter's*) *group* consists of 1 to 4 nodes interposed between the pectoralis major and minor muscles. Lymph from these nodes passes directly into the central and subclavicular groups.

As indicated in Fig. 14-7, relationships to the aforementioned nodal groups are assigned levels. Nodes located lateral to or below the lower border of the pectoralis minor are referred to as *Level I* and include the *external mammary, axillary vein,* and *scapular groups*. Nodes located deep to or behind the pectoralis minor are referred to as *Level II* and include the *central group*. Nodes located medial to or above the upper border of the pectoralis minor are considered *Level III* and include the *subclavicular lymph node group*.

Lymph Flow. Metastatic disease of the breast occurs predominantly by routes that are extensive and arborize in multiple directions through skin and mesenchymal lymphatics. Lymphatic flow is unidirectional except in the pathologic state and has preferential flow from the periphery toward the right side of the heart. Preferential lymphatic flow toward the axilla is observed in lesions of the upper anterolateral chest. The lymphatics of the dermis are intimately associated with deeper lymphatics of underlying fascial planes; this fact explains the multidirectional potential for drainage of superficial breast neoplasms. Two accessory directions for lymphatic flow from breast parenchyma to nodes of the apex of the axilla include the *transpectoral* and *retropectoral* routes. *Interpectoral* (*Rotter's*) *nodes,* between the pectoralis major and minor, receive lymph that terminates in the apical (Level III) group. The retropectoral pathway drains the superior and internal aspects of the breast and similarly terminates at the apex of the axilla in the apical group.

Accessory pathways provide major lymphatic drainage by way of the external mammary and central axillary node groups (Levels I and II, respectively). Internal mammary lymphatic trunks eventually terminate in subclavian node groups (see Figs. 14-6, 14-7). The presence of supraclavicular nodes (Stage IV disease) results from lymphatic permeation and subsequent obstruction of the inferior and deep cervical groups of the jugular-subclavian confluence. The supraclavicular node group represents the termination of efferent trunks from subclavian nodes of the internal mammary nodal group. Central and medial lymphatics of the breast pass medially and parallel the course of major blood vessels to perforate the pectoralis major muscle and terminate in the internal mammary nodal chain. This also represents a major pathway for metastatic spread of carcinoma into the systemic circulation.

Cross-communication from the interstices of connecting lymphatic channels for each breast provides ready access of lymphatic flow to the opposite axilla. Communicating dermal lymphatics to the contralateral breast account for occasional metastatic involvement of the opposite breast and axilla.

Lymphatic vessels that drain the breast occur in three interconnecting groups: (1) within the gland in interlobular spaces that parallel lactiferous ducts; (2) within glandular tissue and overlying skin of the central part of the gland beneath the areola (subareolar plexus); and (3) on the posterior surface of the breast, communicating with minute vessels that parallel the perimysium in deep fascia. Lymphatic vessels from deeper structures of the thoracic wall drain principally into parasternal, intercostal, or diaphragmatic nodes.

Greater than 75 percent of lymph from the breast passes to the axillary lymph nodes (Figs. 14-6, 14-7); the remainder of lymph flows into parasternal lymphatics. Although it has been suggested that parasternal nodes receive lymph principally from the medial aspects of the breast, vital-dye flow studies report that *both* the axillary and the parasternal lymphatic groups receive lymph from all quadrants of the breast.

PHYSIOLOGY

Mammary development and function are initiated by a variety of hormonal stimuli that include estrogen and progesterone, prolactin, oxytocin, thyroid hormone, cortisol, and growth hormone. Estrogen, progesterone, and prolactin have profound trophic effects that are essential to normal breast development and function. Estrogen initiates ductal development; progesterone is primarily responsible for differentiation of epithelial cells and lobular development. Progesterone also may reduce estrogen binding in mammary epithelium and limit tubular system proliferation. Prolactin is the primary hormonal stimulus for lactogenesis with late pregnancy and in the postpartum period. Prolactin increases the number of estrogen receptors and stimulates epithelial cells to act synergistically with ductular and lobuloalveolar development.

Figure 14-8 depicts secretion of neurotrophic hormones from the hypothalamus that are responsible for regulation of secretion of mammogenic hormones. Secretion of the gonadotropins—luteinizing hormone (LH) and follicle-stimulating hormone (FSH)—regulates the ovarian secretory release of estrogen and progesterone. Release of LH and FSH from basophilic cells of the anterior pituitary are further regulated by secretion of gonadotropin-releasing hormone (GnRH) from the hypothalamus. Secretion of LH, FSH, and GnRH is regulated by positive and negative feedback effects of circulating levels of estrogen and progesterone.

The secretion of these mammogenic hormones throughout the life of the normal female is responsible for alterations in the hormonal milieu and for development, function, and maintenance of lobuloalveolar tissues. In the human female *neonate,* plasma estrogen and progesterone decrease after birth. Throughout childhood these values remain low as a result of the regulatory sensitivity of the hypothalamopituitary axis to the negative feedback effects of sex steroids. With onset of *puberty* an increase in the central drive of the hypothalamus occurs, with a concurrent decrease in sensitivity to negative feedback by estrogen and progesterone. Thereafter, an increase in sensitivity to positive feedback by estrogen is evident. These physiologic events thereby initiate an increase in GnRH secretion, an increase in FSH and LH secretion, and ultimately an increase in ovarian estrogen and progesterone secretion. With development of positive feedback by estrogen, the *menses* are initiated.

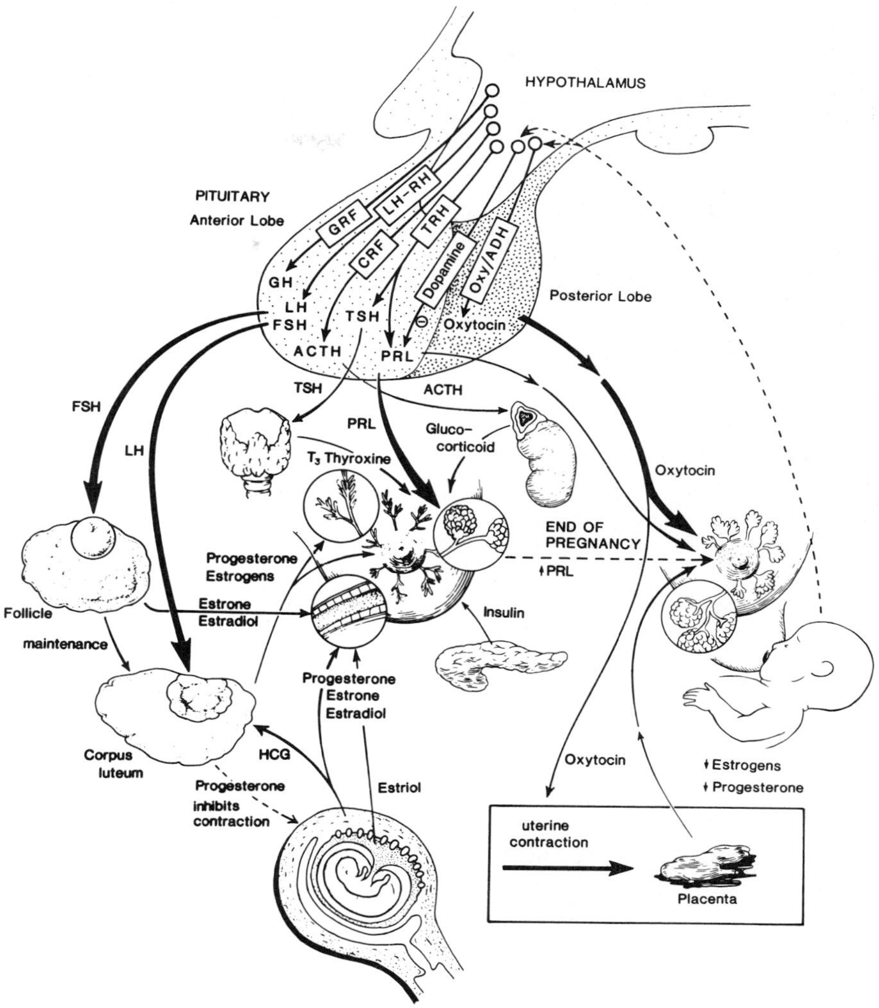

FIG. 14-8. Overview of the neuroendocrine control of breast development and function with relationship to gonadotropic hormones of the anterior pituitary and ovary. (From: *Keller-Wood M, Bland KI: 1991, Chap 3, p 37, with permission.*)

Cyclic Changes During the Menstrual Cycle (Fig. 14-9*A*). The female experiences great variations in breast volume during the menstrual cycle. Volume is greatest in the second half of the cycle, following a premenstrual increase in size, nodularity, density, and sensitivity. Progesterone may stimulate glandular growth in the luteal phase. Changes in the mitotic rate of glandular components are greater in the luteal phase than in the follicular phase. The premenstrual increase in volume occurs as a consequence of the increase in size of the lobule without any evidence of epithelial proliferation. Thereafter, engorgement of the stroma, lobules, and ducts is evident, with increase in size of ducts and acini as the lumina dilate. Parenchymal engorgement and edema subside with onset of menses.

Pregnancy (Fig. 14-9*B*). A dramatic increase in secretion and release of circulating ovarian and placental estrogens and progestins is evident with pregnancy. These hormones initiate striking alterations in form and substance of the breast. The gland enlarges, the areolar skin darkens, and the areolar glands become prominent as ducts and lobules proliferate. In the *first trimester,* lobuloalveolar formation is initiated as ducts branch to form multiple alveoli. With increase in lobular size, proliferating glandular epithelium replaces connective tissue and the components of adipose tissue. In the *second trimester,* proliferation of ductular elements increases following stimulation by estrogens and progestins secreted by the placenta. These sex steroids cause arborization of glandular structures to further develop alveoli. As this glandular system enlarges, the secretory capacity of epithelium increases, as is evident by accumulation of colloid within the alveoli.

During the *third trimester,* fat droplets accumulate in the alveolar cells and colostrum fills the alveolar and ductular spaces. Mammary blood flow increases and myoepithelial cells hypertrophy. The mammogenic action of prolactin requires the presence of cortisol, insulin, growth hormone, and epidermal growth factor. In late pregnancy, limited synthesis of milk fats and proteins is initiated. This process is stimulated by the lactogenic effects of prolactin on breast lobular tissue; other pituitary lactogenic hormones may also have trophic effects.

Postpartum Lactation (Fig. 14-9*C*). Following delivery of the placenta, progesterone and estrogen levels diminish. These quantitative decreases in the plasma estradiol and progesterone allow full expression of the lactogenic action of prolactin. Maintenance of lactation requires regular removal of milk and stimulation (''milk letdown'') of the neural reflexes to prolactin secretion. The magnitude of the suckling-induced surge of prolactin decreases

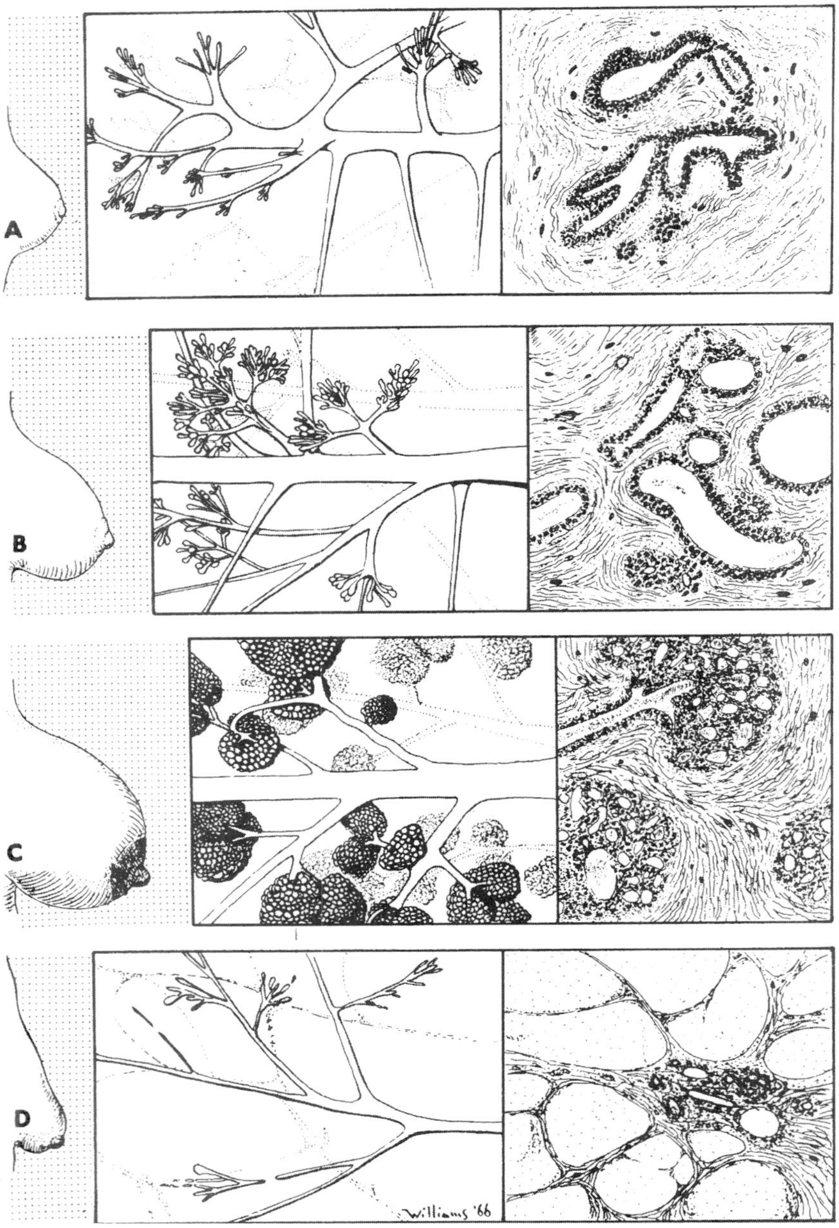

FIG. 14-9. Depiction of gross and microscopic appearance of breast at different stages of physiologic and developmental influences. Central pictures show three-dimensional projection of microscopic structure. *A.* Adolescence. *B.* Pregnancy. *C.* Lactation. *D.* Postmenopausal period.

with time, probably as a consequence of the decreased duration and frequency of nursing. Milk production and ejection in nursing women are controlled by neural reflex arcs that originate in free nerve endings of the nipple-areolar complex.

Oxytocin initiates contraction of smooth muscle components of myoepithelial cells that surround the alveoli; compression of the alveoli occurs and expulsion of milk under pressure into the lactiferous sinuses is evident. Oxytocin release can result from auditory, visual, olfactory, or other stimuli associated with nursing. Maintenance of lactation requires an intact hypothalamic-pituitary axis, adequate diet and nutrition, regular suckling release of milk, and the absence of psychologic stresses that interfere with normal control of prolactin and oxytocin release.

Following weaning of the infant, the gland returns to an inactive, nonsecretory state. Prolactin and oxytocin release subside. The secretory activity of the lactogenic epithelium decreases, and unremoved dormant milk increases pressure within the ductular and alveolar structures. The lobular structure thereafter atrophies and the secretory cells degenerate.

Postmenopausal Breast (Fig. 14-9*D*). Following menopause and the concomitant decrease in ovarian secretion of estrogen and progesterone, there is a progressive involution of ductular and glandular components. Quantitatively a decrease in number and size of glandular elements is evident; the epithelium of the lobules and ducts becomes atrophic or hypoplastic. Surrounding fibrous tissue increases in density, and the parenchyma is replaced with adipose and stromal tissue rather than supporting glandular structure. With aging there is loss of fat content and the supporting stroma, thereby initiating loss of lobular structure, density, form, and contour.

Gynecomastia

Gynecomastia implies the presence of a female-type mammary gland in the male. Most examples of gynecomastia should not be considered a disease, because enlargement of the male breast is common. *Physiologic gynecomastia* occurs mostly during three phases of life: (1) neonatal period, (2) adolescence, and (3) senescence. Common to each is an excess of estrogens in relation to circulating testosterone. Neonatal physiologic gynecomastia is due to the action of placental estrogens on neonatal breast parenchyma. In adolescence there is an excess of estradiol relative to testosterone. With aging, the plasma testosterone falls and senescent gynecomastia is caused by a relative hyperestrinism.

Pathology. The few ductal structures of the male breast enlarge, elongate, and branch with an ensheathing connective tissue. There is a combined increase in glandular and stromal elements with regular distribution of each element throughout the enlarged breast. In the pubertal male, the condition is often unilateral and typically occurs between the ages of twelve and fifteen years. By contrast, senescent gynecomastia is usually bilateral, although there may be asymmetry.

In the nonobese patient, at least 2 cm of subareolar breast tissue must be present before gynecomastia can be confirmed. Mammography and ultrasonography are used to differentiate indistinguishable or ill-defined contiguous fatty tissue from male breast lesions and soft tissue structures. Dominant nontender masses and local areas of firmness, irregularity, or asymmetry suggest the possibility of an early male breast cancer in the aging patient. Gynecomastia does not predispose the male breast to the development of cancer. By contrast, the hypoandrogenic state of primary testicular failure in Klinefelter syndrome (47,XXY) is associated with an enhanced risk for breast cancer in men.

Pathophysiology. Table 14-1 identifies the pathophysiologic mechanisms that may initiate gynecomastia. *Estrogen excess states* result from an increase in the secretion of estradiol from the testicles or nontesticular tumors. Endocrine disorders, such as hyperthyroidism or hypothyroidism, or hepatic disease (nonalcoholic and alcoholic cirrhosis) may initiate estrogen excess. Estrogen excess states may also be induced by nutritional alterations such as protein and fat starvation. "Refeeding gynecomastia" is perhaps related to the resumption of pituitary gonadotropin secretion following pituitary shutdown.

Androgen deficiency states such as aging initiate gynecomastia. Concurrent with decreased plasma testosterone is an elevation in the plasma testosterone-binding globulin resulting in a reduction of unbound testosterone. Senescent hypertrophy occurs most commonly in men between the ages of fifty and seventy years. Klinefelter syndrome of 47,XXY karyotype is manifested by gynecomastia, hypergonadotropic hypogonadism, and azoospermia. Other causes of primary testicular failure include ACTH deficiency, hereditary defects of androgen biosynthesis, and eunuchoidal males (congenital anorchia).

Secondary testicular failure as a cause of gynecomastia may result from trauma, orchitis, cryptorchidism, abdominal or genital irradiation, hydroceles, varicoceles, and spermatoceles. Renal failure, regardless of cause, may initiate gynecomastia.

Drugs with estrogenic or estrogen-related activity (digitalis, estrogens, anabolic steroids, marijuana) may be causative. Drugs that inhibit the action and/or synthesis of testosterone (cimetidine, ketoconazole, phenytoin, spironolactone, antineoplastic agents, diazepam) also may be implicated. Drugs that enhance estrogen synthesis (HCG) or drugs with idiopathic mechanisms may also induce gynecomastia (reserpine, theophylline, verapamil, tricyclic antidepressants, furosemide).

Treatment. Medical therapy of gynecomastia is rarely of value except when a specific diagnosis has been established. For disorders of androgen deficiency, testosterone administration may effect breast regression. For large, progressive gynecomastia refractory to drug discontinuance or therapy of an endocrine defect,

Table 14-1
Pathophysiologic Mechanisms of Gynecomastia

- I. Estrogen excess states
  - A. Gonadal origin
    - 1. True hermaphroditism
    - 2. Gonadal stromal (nongerminal) neoplasms of the testis
      - a. Leydig cell (interstitial)
      - b. Sertoli cell
      - c. Granulosa-theca
    - 3. Germ cell tumors
      - a. Choriocarcinoma
      - b. Seminoma, teratoma
      - c. Embryonal carcinoma
  - B. Nontesticular tumors
    - 1. Skin—nevus
    - 2. Adrenal cortical neoplasms
    - 3. Lung carcinoma
    - 4. Hepatocellular carcinoma
  - C. Endocrine disorders
  - D. Diseases of the liver—nonalcoholic and alcoholic cirrhosis
  - E. Nutrition alteration states
- II. Androgen deficiency states
  - A. Senescent causes with aging
  - B. Hypoandrogen states (hypogonadism)
    - 1. Primary testicular failure
      - a. Klinefelter syndrome (XXY)
      - b. Reifenstein syndrome (XY)
      - c. Rosewater, Gwinup, Hamwi familial gynecomastia (XY)
      - d. Kallmann syndrome
      - e. Kennedy disease with associated gynecomastia
      - f. Eunuchoidal males (congenital anorchia)
      - g. Hereditary defects of androgen biosynthesis
      - h. ACTH deficiency
    - 2. Secondary testicular failure
      - a. Trauma
      - b. Orchitis
      - c. Cryptorchidism
      - d. Irradiation
      - e. Hydrocele
      - f. Varicocele
      - g. Spermatocele
  - C. Renal failure
- III. Drug-related conditions that initiate gynecomastia
- IV. Systemic diseases with idiopathic mechanisms
  - A. Nonneoplastic diseases of the lung
  - B. Trauma (chest wall)
  - C. CNS-related causes from anxiety and stress
  - D. AIDS (acquired immune deficiency syndrome)

the most effective therapy, especially in the young adult, is transareolar mastectomy. Surgical therapy is reserved, however, for idiopathic causes of gynecomastia in which exhaustive attempts to define endocrine, metabolic, or drug-related causes fail. Attempts to reverse gynecomastia with danazol have been successful; however, side effects from the androgenic properties of the drug are significant. Tamoxifen citrate, as therapy for benign breast disorders including gynecomastia, has had encouraging initial results.

DIAGNOSIS

Presentation. A lump in the breast is a common premenopausal and postmenopausal physical finding in the female. Up to one-half of patients presenting with breast complaints have no evidence of breast pathology; 65 percent or more of all breast lumps are discovered by the patient. In patients who commonly participate in breast self-examination, greater than 85 percent of definable lesions are detected by the patient. The patient may also observe breast pain, but this symptom more commonly represents a proliferative benign breast disorder rather than carcinoma. Other presenting symptoms of breast cancer that occur less frequently include enlargement, nipple discharge, changes of the nipple, retraction or alterations of symmetry, ulceration, erythema, axillary mass, and infrequently bone or musculoskeletal discomfort. While many women recognize these symptoms, the delay in seeking medical attention persists.

Examination. The technique for examination of the breast should include inspection and palpation of the entire breast and draining lymph node sites. The clinician, standing in front of the patient, should first inspect the breast with the patient's arms by her side (Fig. 14-10*A*); with her arms straight up in the air (Fig. 14-10*C*); and with her hands on her hips with and without pectoral contraction. Symmetry, size, and shape of the breast should be documented, as well as any evidence of edema (peau d'orange), nipple inversion or change, skin retraction, or erythema. With the arms extended forward and the patient in a sitting position, a forward lean accentuates skin retraction.

Palpation. All regions of concern in the breasts that were identified by inspection should be recorded and the entire breast mass should be carefully palpated.

Examination of the patient in the supine position (Fig. 14-10*D*) is best performed with the benefit of a pillow supporting the ipsilateral hemithorax. The examiner should gently palpate the breast from the ipsilateral side, making certain to examine all quadrants of the breast from the sternum to the clavicle, laterally to the latissimus and inferiorly to the upper rectus sheath. The physician should perform the examination with the palmar aspects of the fingers; a grasping or pinching motion should be avoided. The breast may be cupped or molded in the examiner's hands to check for retraction.

A systematic search for lymphadenopathy is essential if breast cancer is suspected. Figure 14-10*B* identifies the correct position for examination of the right axilla. The shoulder girdle is stabilized by supporting the upper arm and elbow. Using gentle discrete palpation, all three levels of potential lymphatic enlargement in the axillary sites are assessed; this technique allows bimanual palpation of disease at the level of the pectoralis minor muscle. Careful palpation of subclavicular, supraclavicular, cervical, and parasternal sites is performed. A diagram of the chest and contiguous

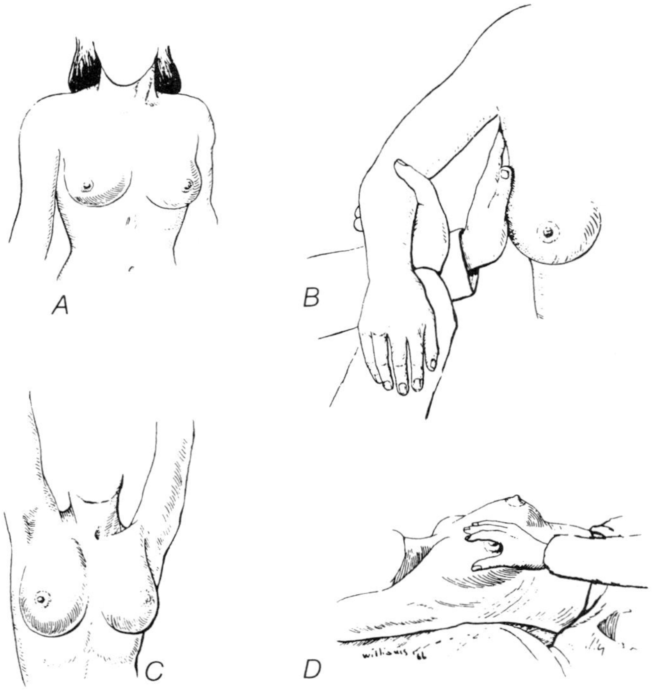

FIG. 14-10. Examination of breast. *A.* Observation with arms at side. *B.* Palpation of axilla. *C.* Observation with arms raised. *D.* Palpation with patient supine.

nodal sites is useful to record location, size, and characteristics of palpable disease (Fig. 14-11). Size, consistency, shape, mobility, and fixation of any palpable breast mass or nodal site should be documented.

Mammography. Mammography has been used in North America since the 1960s. Techniques for mammography have been modified and improved to enhance image quality. Proper utilization requires special techniques and film and a radiologist skilled in interpretation. Conventional mammography uses a low-dose film/screen technique that delivers as little as 0.1 rad per study. By comparison, each chest roentgenogram delivers one-quarter of this radiation volume. There is no proven escalation of breast cancer risk related to low-dose irradiation with screening mammography. The benefits of mammography to detect a small cancer that is often curable far outweigh any theoretical risk.

Mammography should not be considered a substitute for biopsy; rather, this technique is an adjunctive, complementary study that augments history and physical examination. The technique is useful for (1) examination of an indeterminate mass that presents as a solitary lesion suspicious of a neoplasm; (2) examination of an indeterminate mass that cannot be considered a dominant nodule, especially when multiple cysts or other vague masses are present and the indication for biopsy is uncertain; (3) follow-up examination of breast cancer treated by segmental mastectomy and irradiation; (4) follow-up examination of the contralateral breast following segmental or total mastectomy; and (5) evaluation of the large fatty breast in the symptomatic patient in whom nodules are not palpable (Fig. 14-12).

Additional value of diagnostic mammography lies in the early detection of an occult cancer before it reaches 5 mm. When abnor-

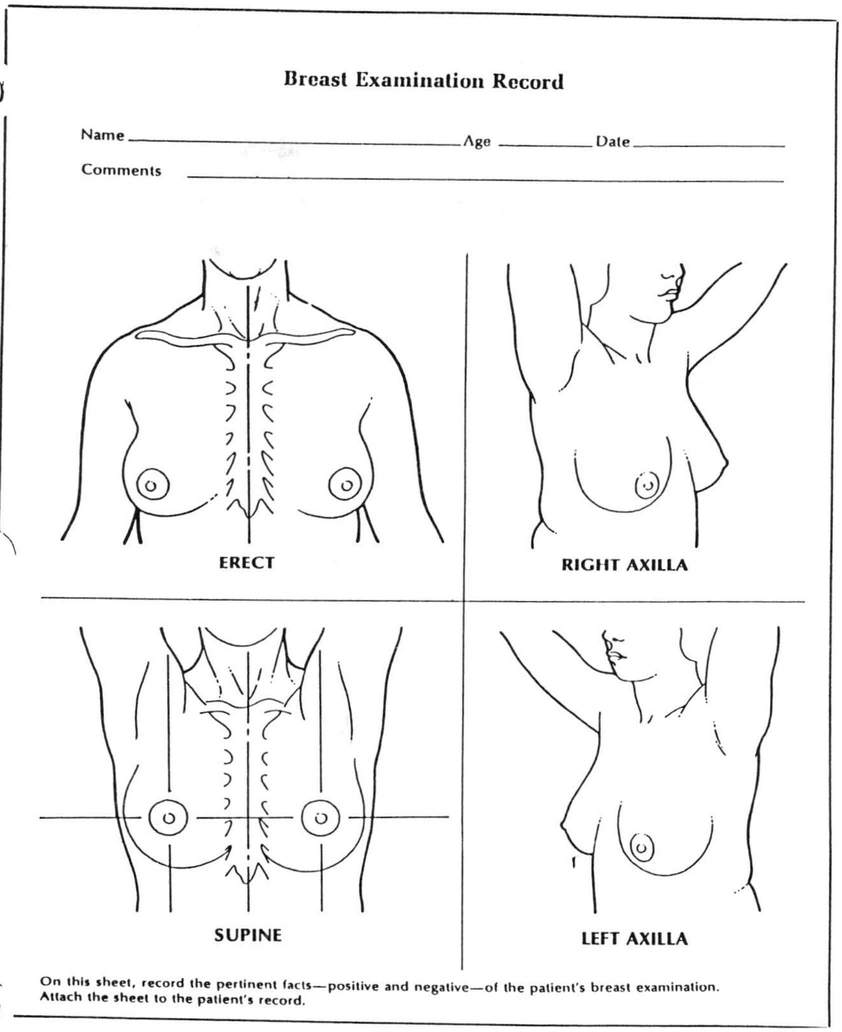

Breast Examination Record
Name ______ Age ______ Date ______
Comments ______
ERECT
RIGHT AXILLA
SUPINE
LEFT AXILLA
On this sheet, record the pertinent facts—positive and negative—of the patient's breast examination.
Attach the sheet to the patient's record.

FIG. 14-11. Breast examination record. (*With permission, Cliggott Publishing Co.*)

malities have been detected by the patient or the clinician, mammography can more precisely define the abnormality, detect multicentric disease, and identify the presence of synchronous cancers.

The presence of fine stippled calcium in the radiogram of an occult or suspicious lesion is suggestive of cancer. Calcification will occur in one-third to one-half of nonpalpable cancers, but less than one-half of these calcific foci will demonstrate the classical appearance suggestive of malignancy (Fig. 14-13). Fewer than one-half of the dominant mass lesions will have spiculated or irregular margins and approximately one-fifth of cancers will be discovered by secondary signs such as architectural distortions, duct dilatation, asymmetry, and fibronodular densities. Microcalcification, as a sign of malignancy, assumes greater importance in younger women in whom it may be the sole mammographic feature. The importance of calcification as a sign of breast cancer diminishes with age.

Careful analysis of direct and indirect signs is essential to document that the benign:malignant biopsy ratio is surgically acceptable. The positive predictive value of certain mammographic signs will dramatically increase when parenchymal distortion, poorly defined mass lesions, typical malignant-type calcifications, and stellate opacities are evident. It is estimated that a skilled radiologist can detect cancer of the breast with a false-positive rate of approximately 10 percent and a false-negative rate of 6 to 8 percent.

The clinical impetus for screening mammography came from the Health Insurance Plan (HIP) study and the Breast Cancer Detection Demonstration Project (BCDDP). The HIP study demonstrated a reduction of 33 percent in mortality in patients who were screened by mammography; these data have been verified by the BCDDP. The BCDDP confirmed that mammography conducted in an optimal environment provided a true-positive rate that exceeded 90 percent and was significantly greater in accuracy than clinical examination for detection of occult or early tumors. In both studies, 80 percent of the patients with mammographically detected carcinomas had no axillary nodal metastases. These findings contrast significantly with patients whose breast cancer was detected clinically and in whom greater than 50 percent have positive axillary nodes. Reports suggest that screening of breast cancers in women under fifty years allows earlier diagnosis and treatment of breast cancer. Disease-free, 5-year survival in this younger cohort exceeded 90 percent.

Current guidelines suggested by the American Cancer Society recommend that all women initiate breast self-examination at the

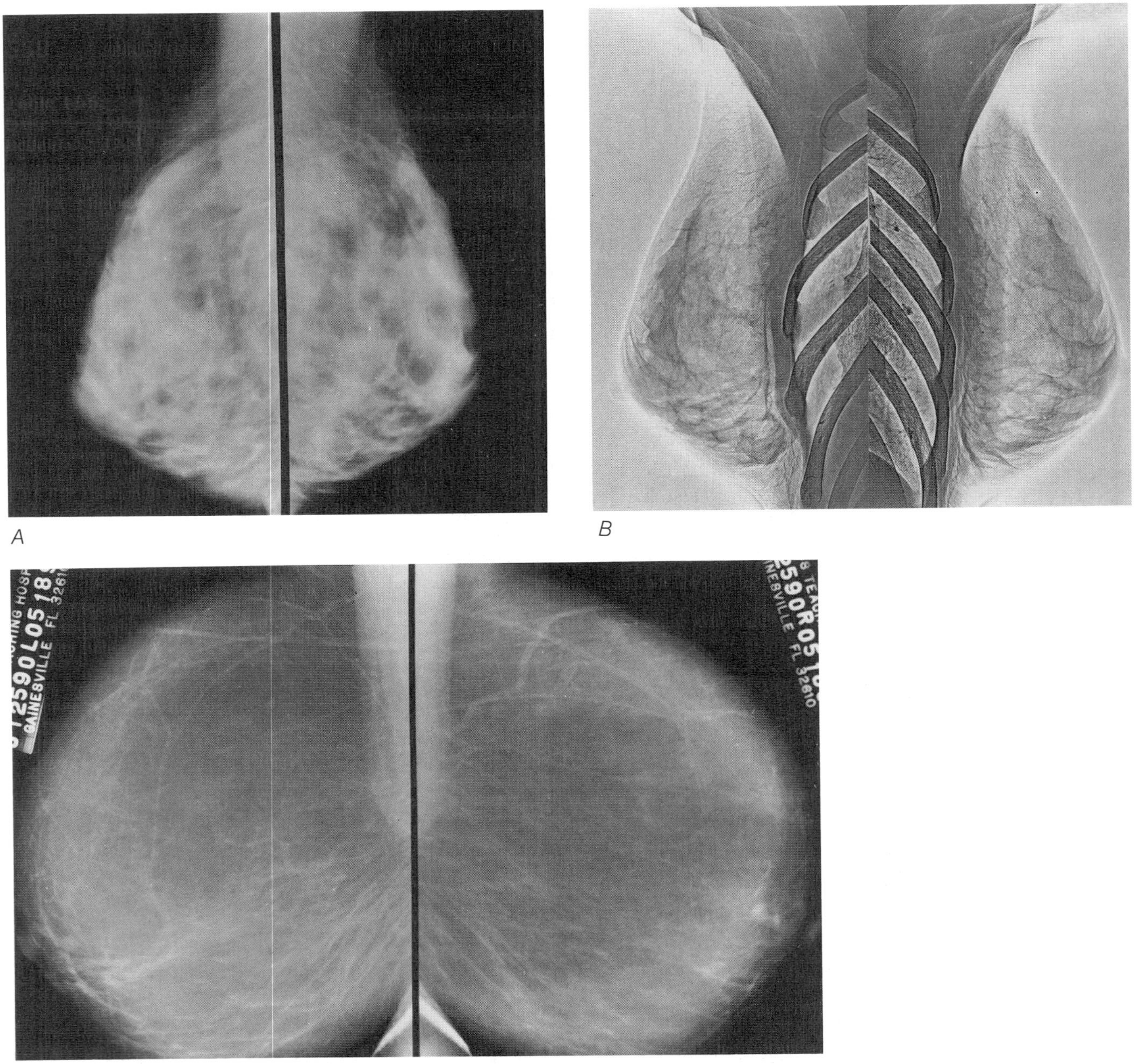

FIG. 14-12. Mammography of breast. *A.* Normal premenopausal breast with dense fibroglandular pattern evident on both film/screen mammograms. *B.* Xeromammogram of same patient (*A*). The wide recording latitude of the xeromammogram allows visualization from the nipple to the ribs. The film/screen mammogram has better contrast for visualizing masses that include the axillary tail of Spence. *C.* Normal postmenopausal breast. Oblique mediolateral views of film/screen mammogram that demonstrates sparse fibroglandular pattern with no dominant lesions. Invasive ductal carcinoma in craniocaudal (*D*) and oblique mediolateral (*E*) views. *F.* Cone-compression view of palpable mass (*D,E*) seen in upper inner quadrant of right breast. Note the spiculated margins of the mass (*arrow*) accentuated with compression. (*Courtesy of Dr. B. Steinbach.*)

age of twenty and that a ''base-line'' mammographic examination be obtained at about thirty-five years of age after consultation with a physician. The patient should consult her physician regarding the need for regular mammographic screening between the ages of forty and fifty; annual mammographic examination should be conducted thereafter.

Prospective randomized studies of routine mammographic screening confirm a 40 percent reduction for Stage II disease and more advanced cancers in the screened population; a corresponding 30 percent increase in survival was evident in patients found to have cancer. With the increasing availability of stereotactically guided biopsy for cytology and histology, the requirement for

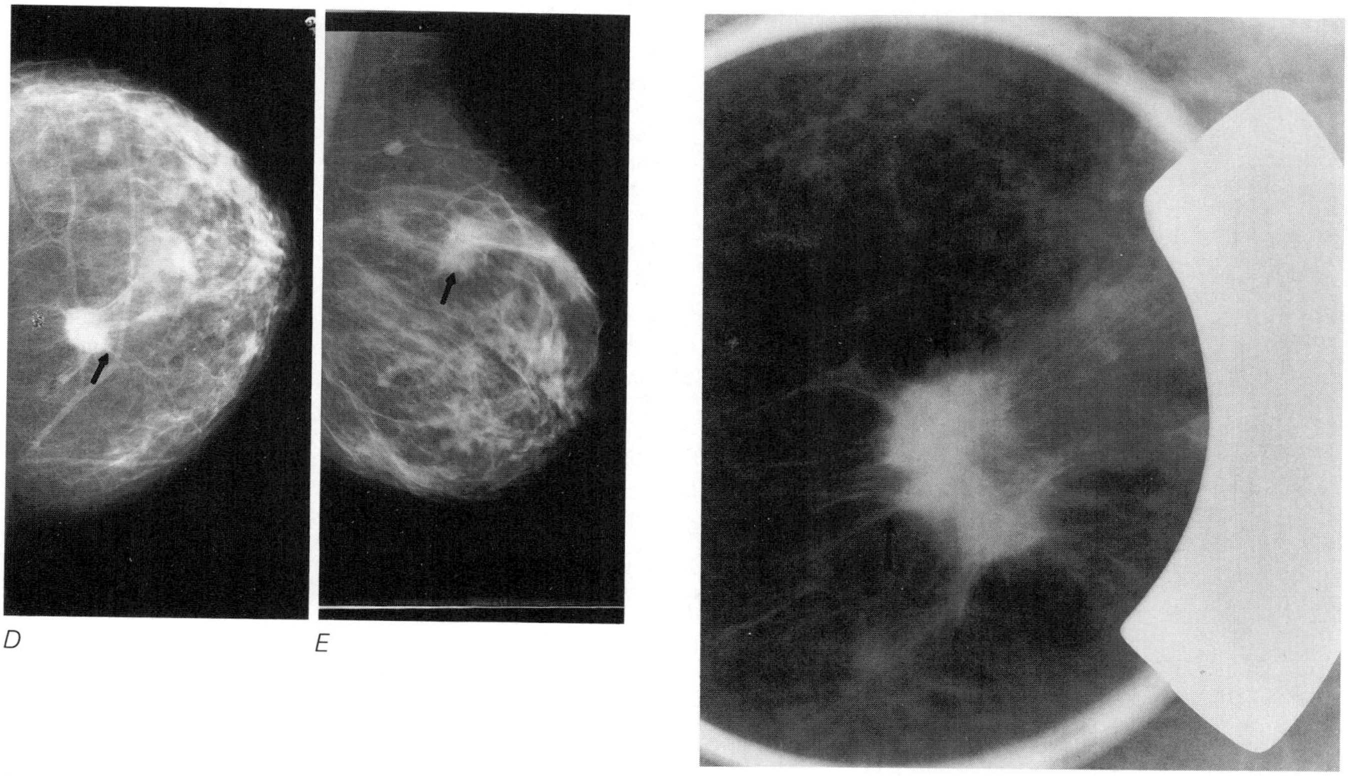

D E F

FIG. 14-12. (continued)

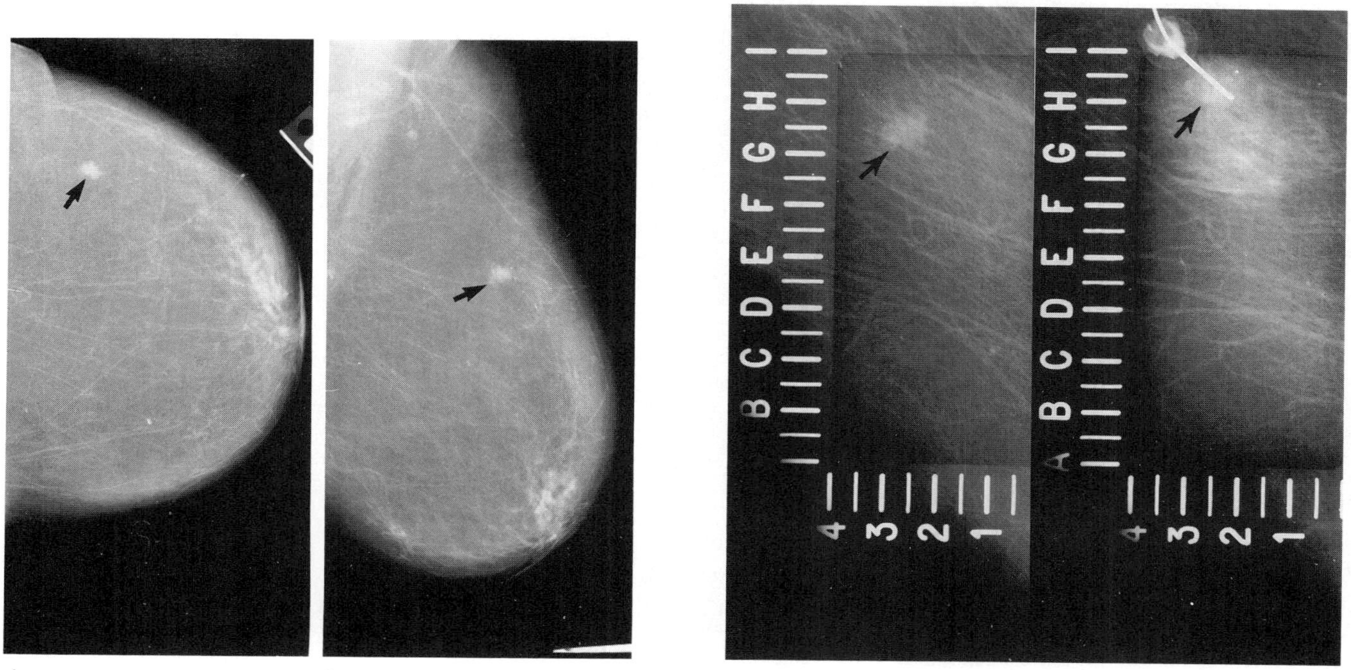

A B C D

FIG. 14-13. Early invasive ductal carcinoma of the right breast. Craniocaudal (*A*) and oblique mediolateral (*B*) views of the right breast demonstrate an 8-mm spiculated mass (*arrows*) in the upper outer quadrant. Method to determine needle localization (*C*). *D*. The numbers and letters of the plate allow biplanar dimensional positioning for placement of the localizing wire into the mass (*arrows*). (*Courtesy of Dr. B. Steinbach.*)

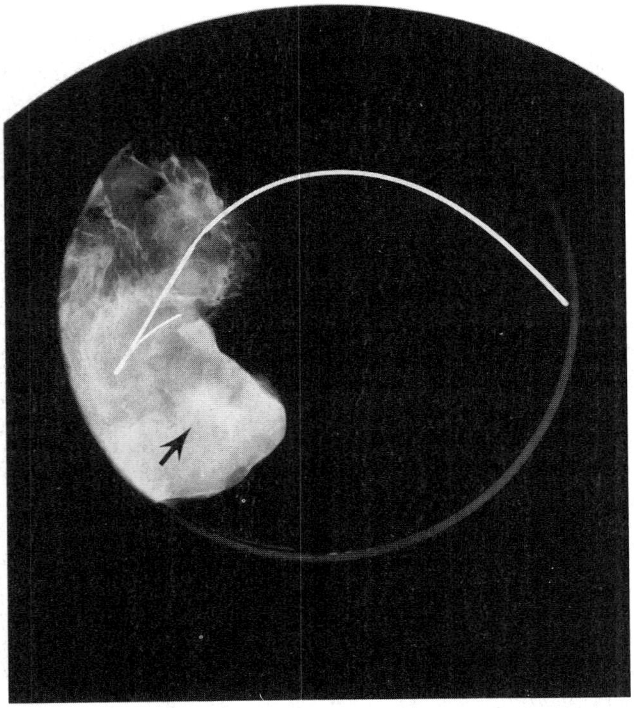

FIG. 14-14. Specimen radiograph confirms that the mass (*arrow*) is within the excised tissue depicted on the mammogram seen in Fig. 14-13. (*Courtesy of Dr. B. Steinbach.*)

open breast biopsy may be reduced. The enlarging population of patients with occult (nonpalpable) cancers detected in annual screening programs often necessitates needle-localization biopsy techniques. Postexcision confirmation of the suspicious mass and/or calcifications using specimen radiography is essential (Fig. 14-14); otherwise, histologic confirmation of benignity of the lesion cannot be assured.

Xeromammography. This technique is identical with mammography except that the image is recorded on a xerographic plate rather than a conventional transparency. The image produced is positive rather than negative (see Fig. 14-12*B*). Edge enhancement and wide recording latitude allow details of the soft tissues of the breast, chest wall, and thinner peripheral portions of the breast to be recorded with one exposure. Current opinion favors film screening techniques for routine breast radiographic examination.

Magnification Mammography. This technique enhances the sharpness of detail and increases diagnostic accuracy for breast cancer. The optimal magnification is 1.5 times life size; margins of breast masses and the degree and specificity of microcalcifications are clearly defined. This technique may significantly reduce the number of patients referred for biopsy.

Ultrasound. There is no ionizing irradiation, it is highly reproducible, and it has high patient acceptability. The importance of ultrasonography lies in the resolution of equivocal mammography, the diagnosis of cystic disease, and the demonstration of solid abnormalities with specific echogenic features. The resolution of ultrasound is inferior to high-resolution mammography, and lesions $\leq$ 1 cm in diameter, unless cystic, will not be detected. In the presence of a normal physical examination and mammogram, sonographically demonstrated abnormalities are, in the majority of cases, not significant.

Ultrasonography is also useful for guiding aspiration cysts and providing cytologic specimens. Cysts, on ultrasound, are always well circumscribed, with smooth margins, and have an echo-free center irrespective of the sensitivity setting (Fig. 14-15). Criteria distinguish benign from malignant lesions on sonography but lack specificity. Benign solid masses usually show smooth contours, round or oval shapes, with weak internal echos and well-defined anterior and posterior margins. Malignant lesions have characteristically jagged, irregular walls; malignant lesions, however, may have smooth margins with acoustic enhancement (Fig. 14-16).

Doppler Flow Studies. Blood flow in malignant breast lesions is enhanced. Doppler flow signals can be used to detect increased flow and may further distinguish benign from malignant lesions. Malignant lesions produce signals of high frequency and amplitude with continuous flow through diastole. Although Doppler flow studies may play a role in distinguishing benign from malignant lesions, this technique is not of adequate sensitivity to dictate treatment.

Thermography. Transmission of detectable heat from the breast is nonspecific, and in malignant lesions results from the hypervascularity that frequently accompanies carcinoma. Three currently available thermographic methods include telethermography, contact thermography, and computed tomography. Using special heat scanners it is possible to delineate these ''hot'' perfusion sites on film. Results were so variable and inaccurate that its use was terminated in the BCDDP. Sensitivity is $<$ 50 percent and it is not advocated as a routine screening method because it is unable to detect minimal breast cancer.

Light Scanning of the Breast. This is noninvasive and relatively inexpensive and, therefore, has attracted considerable attention as a diagnostic screening modality. This technique utilizes electromagnetic waves that impinge on a transparent medium; thereafter, the wave is scattered and absorbed. Light attenuation varies considerably depending on the biologic characteristic and hemoglobin content of the tissue studied. The most consistent and important sign of breast cancer is light absorption with a decrease in luminescence displayed in a black and white mode. In the normal breast there should be symmetrical absorption of light. Currently, sensitivity of light scanning for detection of breast cancer is limited. With lesions smaller than 1 cm in diameter, sensitivity varies from 19 to 44 percent.

Magnetic Resonance Imaging. This technique has great value in detection of vertebral body metastases and musculoskeletal pathology related to breast cancer. However, its value as a potential screening method in breast cancer is questionable. The breast is examined using conventional spin-echo T_1- and T_2-weighted sequences, preferably in the sagittal plane, but coronal and axial images can be obtained. Malignant tissue may be identified on MRI using the same morphologic criteria as mammography. Irregularly marginated spiculated masses, secondary skin changes, and enlarged glandular tissue represent signs of malignancy. MRI spectroscopy may have a role in determining the treatment rationale for patients before versus after chemotherapy.

Interventional Techniques. ***Ductography.*** Ductograms are performed by injecting radiopaque contrast media into one or more of the mammary ducts and performing subsequent mammographic imaging. The primary indication for this technique is discharge from the nipple, particularly when the fluid is serosanguineous or bloody. The duct is gently enlarged with a dilator. A small, blunt cannula is inserted under sterile conditions into the nipple ampulla, and with the patient in a supine position, 0.1 to 0.2 ml of dilute contrast media is injected until the patient experiences fullness. Craniocaudal and mediolateral mammographic views are obtained without compression. Intraductal papillomas can be demonstrated as small filling defects surrounded by contrast media (Fig. 14-17). Cysts may opacify when they communicate with ducts following injection of the contrast. Carcinomas may appear as irregular masses; invasive tumors appear as multiple intraluminal filling defects.

Localization of Nonpalpable Breast Masses. An integral part of the management of breast disease includes localization of nonpalpable (occult) breast lesions. Although surface localization and spot method identification are in use in many institutions, mammographically controlled placement of a hooked wire is more accurate and represents "state-of-the-art" technique. Under local anesthesia, the stylet is accurately placed parallel to the chest wall using acrylic plastic compression plates that contain multiple holes, each of which allows passage of a stylet needle. Following needle withdrawal, the lesion is accurately localized on mammogram and the tiny wire hook is left in position (see Fig. 14-13). Thereafter, the surgeon can adequately excise the suspicious lesion sampling minimal breast tissue. Great advances in localization and diagnosis have been made with use of stereotactic needle placement with cytologic aspiration. This technique has allowed localization of occult breast cancer successfully in more than 90 percent of patients, and the sensitivity and specificity of the cytologic aspirate for occult breast cancer exceed 95 percent.

In all cases, needle localization of suspicious occult masses and excision of the abnormal tissue must be evaluated by specimen radiography to ensure that mammographically detected abnormalities have been removed (see Fig. 14-14). Before dissection of the specimen, a radiograph of the excised tissue should be obtained using conventional mammographic equipment or, for better resolution, a dedicated specimen radiographic unit. A specimen radiograph further directs the pathologist to the precise location of the abnormality in the tissues to ensure that appropriate sampling is obtained.

INFLAMMATORY AND INFECTIOUS DISORDERS

Bacterial Infection. *Staphylococcus aureus* and other streptococci are the organisms most frequently recovered from nipple discharge in an active infection of the breast. An abscess is often related to lactation and typically occurs within the first few weeks of breast feeding. Figure 14-18 depicts the progression of an inflammatory process that may result in diffuse breast cellulitis with localized subcutaneous, subareolar, interlobular (periductal),

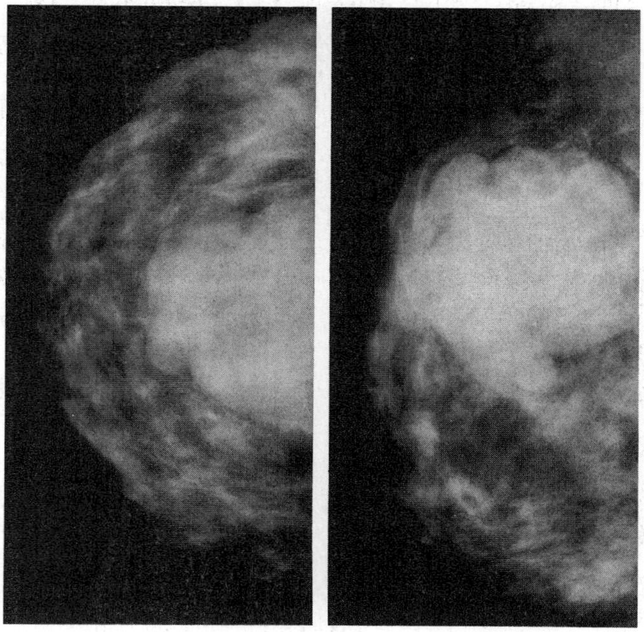

A B

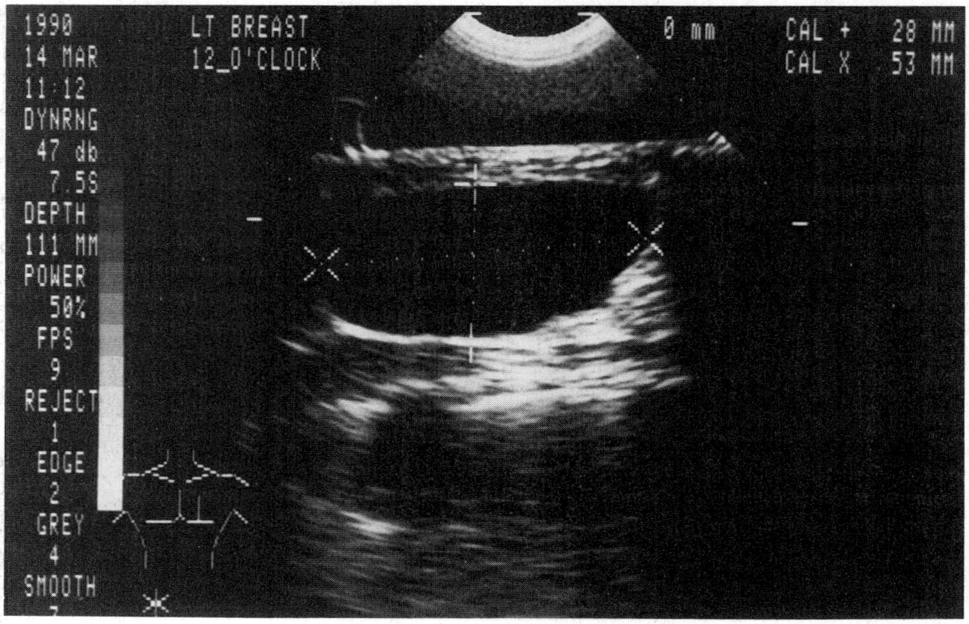

C

FIG. 14-15. Left breast cyst. Craniocaudal (*A*) and oblique mediolateral (*B*) film/screen mammograms of the left breast confirm a large lobulated mass at the 12:00 o'clock position. *C.* Ultrasound of the breast identifies the mass to be anechoic with a well-defined back wall characteristic of a cyst. (*Courtesy of Dr. B. Steinbach.*)

retromammary, or unicentric and multicentric abscesses. Streptococcal infections initiate diffuse cellulitis without localization until a more advanced stage. *S. aureus* abscesses tend to be more localized, deeply invasive, and suppurative. The multilocular abscess evident in Fig. 14-18 is typically seen in staphylococcal infections. Diffuse cellulitis of streptococcal origin with lymphatic permeation is adequately treated with local wound care, including focal heat compresses and administration of intravenous antibiotics (e.g., penicillin or cephalosporin derivatives).

All superficial or deep abscesses with overgrowth of any bacterial organism present with point tenderness, erythema, and hyperthermia. This presentation necessitates immediate and adequate operative drainage of fluctuant areas to avoid sepsis. Immediate surgical drainage is essential for the advanced breast abscess. Thorough debridement of the abscess via circumareolar or multiple nonradial incisions paralleling Langer's lines is recommended.

Breast infections may be chronic, with recurrent abscess formation. Appropriate cultures must be taken for acid-fast bacteria, fungi, and anaerobic and aerobic bacteria. Uncommon organisms might be encountered and long-term antibiotic therapy could be indicated. In extreme cases, simple mastectomy may be required to eradicate a severe chronic infection.

Puerperal (Lactational) Mastitis. Hospital-acquired puerperal infections of the breast are much less common with isolated deliveries and standardization of breast and infant hygiene. Nursing women may present with milk stasis, noninfectious inflammation, or infectious mastitis. Epidermic mastitis is initiated by highly variant strains of penicillin-resistant *S. aureus* that are transmitted via the suckling neonate. This variant of mastitis is associated with other neonatal staphylococcal infections and, in the untreated patient, may result in substantial morbidity and, occasionally, death. The patient may have pus expressed from the nipple of a very tender hyperemic breast. The infant must be rapidly weaned from breast feeding.

Nonepidemic (sporadic) puerperal mastitis refers to involvement of the interlobular connective tissue of the breast parenchyma. Such patients present with nipple fissuring and milk stasis which initiate the secondary invasive retrograde bacterial infection. Emptying of the breast has been shown to shorten duration of symptoms and improve outcome with a remarkable reduction in recurrence of the infectious mastitis. The addition of antibiotics will result in an excellent outcome for 96 percent of cases treated.

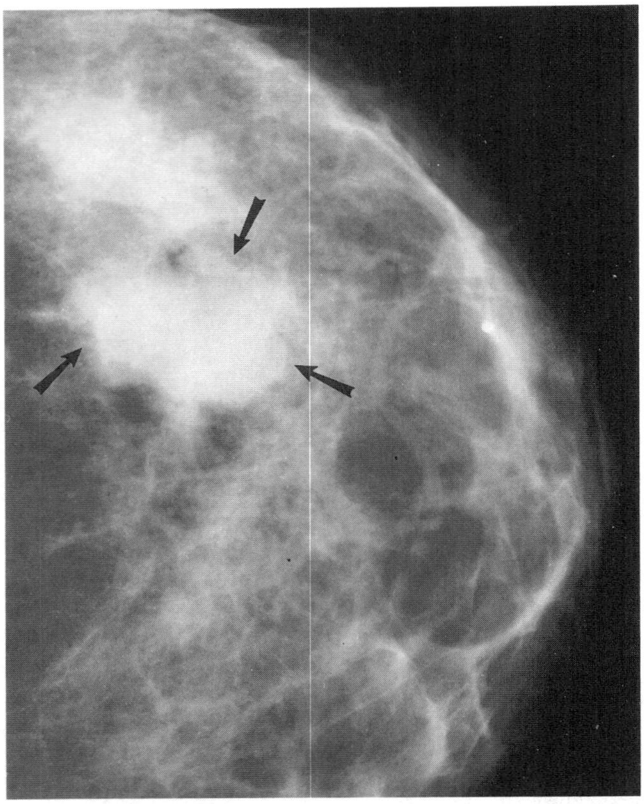

A

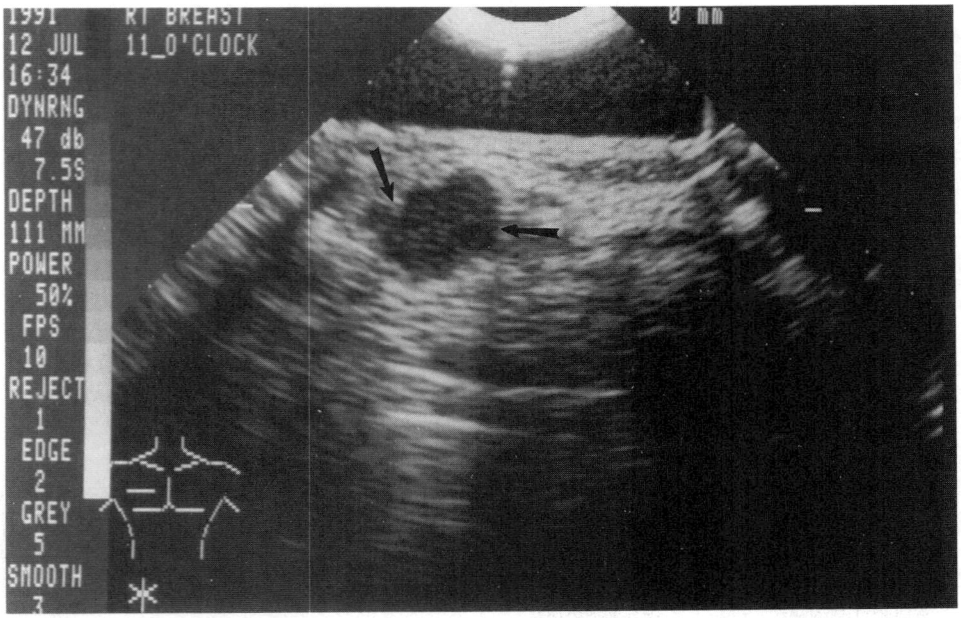

B

FIG. 14-16. Medullary carcinoma. *A.* Craniocaudal view of a palpable mass (*arrows*) in the upper outer quadrant of the right breast. *B.* Ultrasound demonstrates a solid mass with irregular borders (*arrows*) consistent with carcinoma.

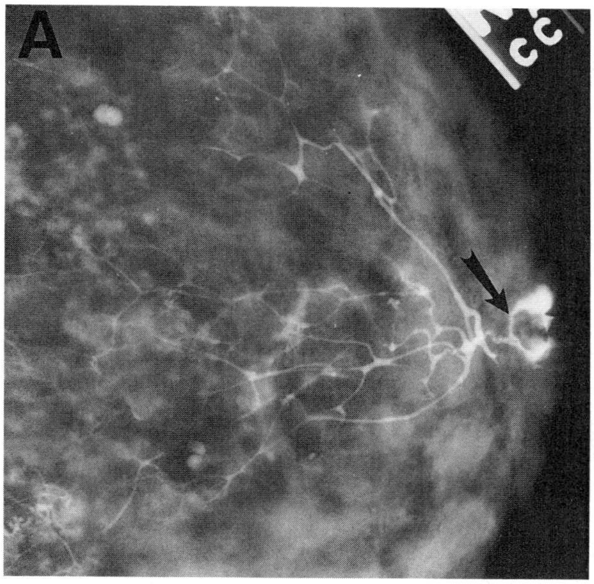

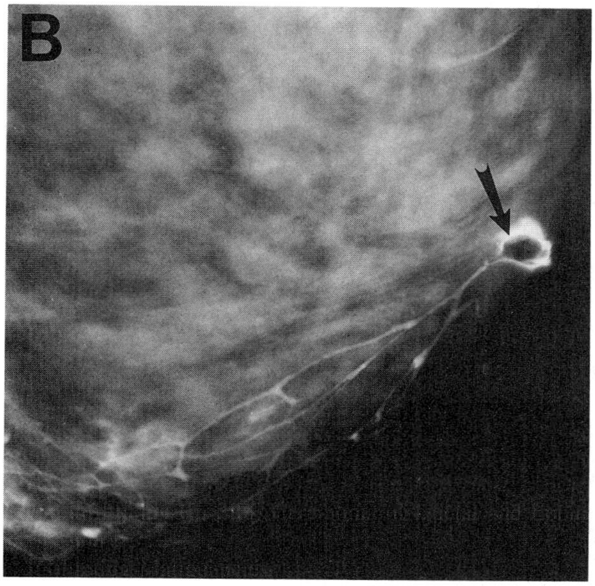

FIG. 14-17. Ductogram of right breast. Craniocaudal (*A*) and mediolateral (*B*) mammographic views demonstrate a mass (*arrows*) posterior to the nipple. The contrast injected into the draining duct outlines the mass as well as the ductal and acinar structures. (*Courtesy of Dr. B. Steinbach.*)

Discontinuance of lactation is essential to enable resolution of the inflammatory process. The use of breast suction pumps helps empty stagnant milk ducts and central abscess collections. Continuation of lactation after removal of the suckling reflex may necessitate the use of intramuscular injections of stilbestrol or testosterone/estradiol derivatives (e.g., Deladumone).

Superficial and Deep Mycoses. Fungal infestations of breast parenchyma are rare and most commonly include blastomycosis and sporotrichosis. Preoperative diagnosis is rarely established.

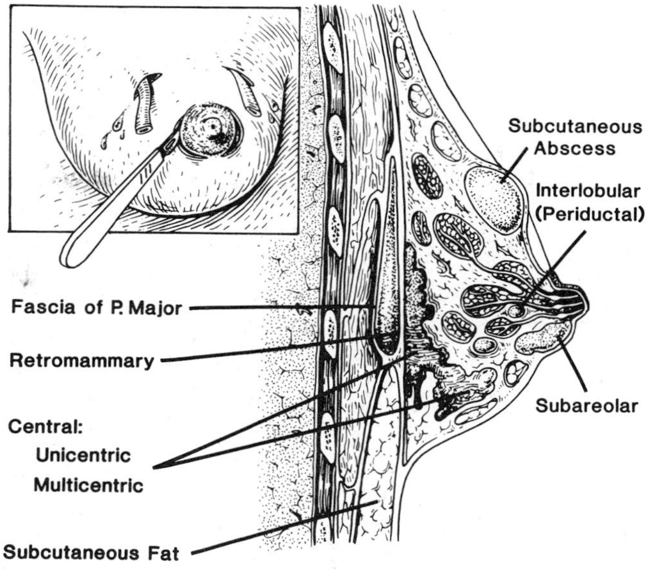

FIG. 14-18. Sagittal view of the breast with sites of potential abscess formation that include subcutaneous, subareolar, interlobular (periductal), retromammary, and central areas. Central abscesses may be focal or multicentric. Retromammary abscesses may be seen in chronic infectious or neoplastic processes (e.g., tuberculosis, carcinoma). Deep abscesses may be multilocular and may communicate with subcutaneous or subareolar sites. *Insert* depicts the necessity of thorough drainage and complete evacuation of the abscess via incisions that parallel Langer's lines.

Fungal infections are most commonly initiated by intraoral fungi inoculated into the breast parenchyma by the suckling infant. These fungal infections present as recurrent mammary abscesses juxtaposed to the nipple or areola. Pus may be expressed from the sinus tracts near the nipple and discharge may be mixed with blood.

Diagnosis of *mammary blastomycosis* is confirmed by collecting material from the abscess and demonstration of round budding organisms in a potassium hydroxide mount or a McMannus-stained smear. Staining of biopsy smears with periodic acid–Schiff reaction following digestion with diastases commonly identifies the mammary fungi of *sporotrichosis*. Serologic and sensitivity reactions may assist in the diagnosis.

Amphotericin B and stilbamidine derivatives are the most effective antifungal agents for the treatment of blastomycosis. Iodides continue to provide specific chemotherapy for the typical cutaneous variant of sporotrichosis but are ineffectual for systemic fungal disease. Amphotericin B is essential therapy for the disseminated and extracutaneous forms. Antifungal therapy, continued for months, may eliminate the necessity of surgical intervention. Drainage of the abscess, simple mastectomy, or quadrantectomy may be necessary to eradicate the fungal disorder.

Candida. *Candida albicans* affecting the breast often presents as a relatively innocuous variant of systemic mycoses. Patients demonstrate large quantities of the fungus in scrapings from the lesions or in the purulent discharge from elevated lesions that have scalloped borders with a definable margin of sodden scales. Scrapings contain an abundant quantity of filaments and budding cells. Skin tests and serologic reactions are of little value. Therapy requires removal of the predisposing factors causing maceration. Water-miscible combinations of nystatin or clotrimazole are recommended. Antibacterials and steroids should not be used.

Hidradenitis Suppurativa. Hidradenitis suppurativa of the breast areola or axilla occurs infrequently. This chronic inflammatory state originates within the large sebaceous glands (apocrine glands of Montgomery or the axilla) that are located on the epithelial surface. Patients with chronic acne have a propensity to develop hidradenitis.

When located in and about the nipple-areola complex, this chronic inflammatory state may mimic invasive carcinoma, Paget's disease of the nipple-areola, or other chronic benign inflammatory states. When confined to the nipple, the breast parenchyma is well preserved without demonstrable abscess or other lesions on mammogram. With compression of sinus tracts, scars, or pustules, purulent discharge can be expressed from sebaceous glands. The patient is frequently ill.

Therapy is directed at control of the inflammatory process by elimination of the infection in the apocrine glandular system. Excision may be accomplished under local or general anesthesia. Losses of larger areas of skin may be covered with advancement flaps from the ipsilateral breast or split-thickness skin grafts from noncontiguous sites.

Mondor's Disease. This variant of thrombophlebitis involves the superficial veins of the anterior chest wall and breast. In 1939 the classical description was provided by the French surgeon Henry Mondor. Typically this disorder occurs in an area contiguous with the breast and is detected as a thrombosed vein presenting as a tender, cordlike structure ("string phlebitis"). The cause is unknown. Surgical procedures, infectious processes, and stress-related exercise of the upper extremity, especially repetitive movements, may initiate the syndrome. Superficial veins of the anterior chest wall and abdomen that are commonly involved include the lateral thoracic vein, the thoracoepigastric vein, and, more rarely, the superficial epigastric vein.

This benign self-limited disorder is not indicative of a neoplasm. Typically the patient presents with acute pain in the lateral half of the breast or the anterior chest wall. A tender firm cord follows the distribution of one of the three major superficial veins of the chest or abdominal wall. Only rarely will bilateral presentations occur, and most patients have no evidence of thrombophlebitis in other anatomic sites.

When the clinical diagnosis is uncertain, or if a contiguous mass is present near the fibrous cord, confirmation must be established by excisional biopsy. Therapy includes liberal use of salicylates and heat compresses along the distribution of symptomatic venous involvement. Restriction of motion of the ipsilateral extremity and shoulder and brassier support are encouraged. The process usually resolves over 2 to 6 weeks. When symptoms persist or are refractory to therapy, division of the vein above and below the area of involvement or excision of smaller lesions is appropriate.

BENIGN LESIONS

Nonproliferative Lesions

Fibrocystic disease, preferably termed *fibrocystic disorder,* is an ill-defined entity. Patients present with diffuse, often bilateral breast pain. Palpation reveals multiple irregularities. When biopsied, the specimens contain "fibrocystic elements." Most lesions are not risk factors for development of cancer of the breast. The risk for cancer is increased only when there is associated dysplasia.

Patients presenting with discomfort or pain associated with multiple cystic lesions of the breast defined by palpation and/or mammography are managed conservatively. Pain is generally accentuated in the second half of their menstrual period and is diminished with the onset of menses. Analgesics usually control the pain; and in some instances, diuretics are helpful to reduce the extent of fluid accumulation.

A single dominant cyst is usually identifiable by palpation of a smooth rounded mass. The cystic nature can be substantiated by ultrasonography, but this is generally not required. The cyst should be aspirated, and if the aspirate is either clear or cloudy greenish-gray in color, it can be discarded without sending a sample for cytopathologic evaluation. If the fluid is bloody, the cyst should be excised. Recurrent cysts can be treated by recurrent aspiration, and in some patients excision is carried out if the cyst persists after multiple aspirations and is symptomatic.

Cysts

Cysts are considered foremost among all of the benign histologic changes in the breast, as are apocrine lesions that commonly accompany cysts. The size of cysts may vary from 1 mm to as great as several centimeters. Most cysts are lined by cells that harbor multiple mitochondria with secretory granules that appear pink by usual eosin staining. Cysts originate as lobular lesions in which the individual acini or terminal ductules dilate or unfold to produce solitary locules that enlarge as a cystic mass. No consistent relationship between cysts and breast cancer risk has been established. The studies of Dupont and Page demonstrate a slight elevation of risk for women with a family history of cysts and breast cancer as opposed to women with a family history of breast cancer alone. *Apocrine cytoplasmic alterations* assume minimal importance with regard to breast cancer risk. Wellings and Alpers suggested apocrine changes in breasts were associated with cancer risk. Nonetheless, this is not considered an indicator of cancer risk in a predictive manner. Neither cysts nor apocrine changes may be viewed as significant elevations for cancer risk in the absence of other established factors. *Epithelial hyperplasia,* which is related to an increased cancer risk, may coexist with cysts, and either change could be present without the other in individual biopsy specimens. It is for this reason that cysts and hyperplastic epithelial lesions should be pathologically distinguished.

Proliferative Lesions

The relationship between extensive *hyperplasia* and associated carcinoma is supported in many prospective studies. Proliferative breast disease is distinguished by epithelial hyperplasia which represents an increased number of cells ($\geq$ 2 cell layers) above the basement membrane. *Atypical ductal hyperlasic (ADH)* lesions must be differentiated from carcinoma in situ. Mild hyperplasia is characterized by three or more cells above the basement membrane in a lobular unit or duct. Such lesions commonly represent an "inflammatory" type with separation of the epithelial cells by inflammatory components. *Moderate* and *florid hyperplasia* is found in greater than 20 percent of biopsies. Moderate and florid degrees of hyperplasia are clinically important because these lesions imply a slightly increased risk (1.5 to 2 times) for subsequent invasive carcinoma.

Atypical Hyperplasia. Table 14-2 depicts the risk for development of invasive breast carcinoma based on histologic findings. Atypical hyperplasia (AH) indicates a specific pattern that

Table 14-2
Relative Risk for Invasive Breast Carcinoma Based on Histologic Examination of Breast Tissue Without Carcinoma*

No increased risk (no proliferative disease)
Apocrine change
Ductal ectasia
Mild epithelial hyperplasia of usual type
Slightly increased risk (1.5–2 times)
Hyperplasia of usual type, moderate or florid
Sclerosing adenosis,† papilloma
Moderately increased risk (4–5 times) (atypical hyperplasia or borderline lesions)
Atypical ductal hyperplasia and atypical lobular hyperplasia
High risk (8–10 times) (carcinoma in situ)
Lobular carinoma in situ and ductal carcinoma in situ (noncomedo)

*Women in each category are compared with women matched for age who have had no breast biopsy with regard to risk of invasive breast cancer in the ensuing 10 to 20 years. *Note:* These risks are not lifetime risks.

†Jensen et al. have shown sclerosing adenosis to be an independent risk factor for subsequent development of invasive breast carcinoma.

SOURCE: Modified from Hutter RVP, et al: *Arch Pathol Lab Med* 10:171, 1986, with permission.

has atypia with an increased disposition for development of subsequent breast cancer. Atypical hyperplasia represents a moderately increased risk (4 to 5 times) above that for apocrine changes, ductal ectasia, or mild epithelial hyperplasia. Atypical *ductal* hyperplasia and *lobular* hyperplasia each enhance the risk for breast cancer over the base population. These lesions have many features of carcinoma in situ (Fig. 14-19).

Localized Sclerosing Lesions. *Sclerosing adenosis* mimics invasive carcinoma. It is characterized by lobulocentric changes causing distortion and enlargement of lobular units; increased numbers of acinar structures are accompanied by fibrous changes. The lesions often contain foci of microcalcifications and, when present in an aggregate form, may be detectable mammographically (Table 14-3). Hutter et al. consider this lesion to represent a slightly increased risk (1.5 to 2 times) over that of the base population (see Table 14-2). These lesions assume a risk probability that is similar to moderate or florid hyperplastic lesions.

Radial Scar and Complex Sclerosing Lesions. These histopathologic entities are similar to sclerosing adenosis and may mimic carcinoma either histologically or clinically. The lesions are not lobulocentric but incorporate various deformed lobular units that possibly take origin from the area in which terminal ductules branch from the major duct. The lesions are characterized by central scar from which elements radiate and consist of a full array of histologic presentations that include cystic dilatation with units that demonstrate hyperplasia and lobulocentric sclerosis, similar to sclerosing adenosis. The combination of cystic and apocrine changes, as well as hyperplasia, is evident as the lesion matures. Bilaterality and multifocality may be evident. Although radial scars may represent a diverse spectrum of histologic appearances, they are not premalignant.

Ductal Ectasia. This term is reserved for conditions in which the clinical presentation includes palpable lumpiness in the region of the breast beneath the areola. Ducts are involved in a segmental fashion; nipple discharge is a common feature, with

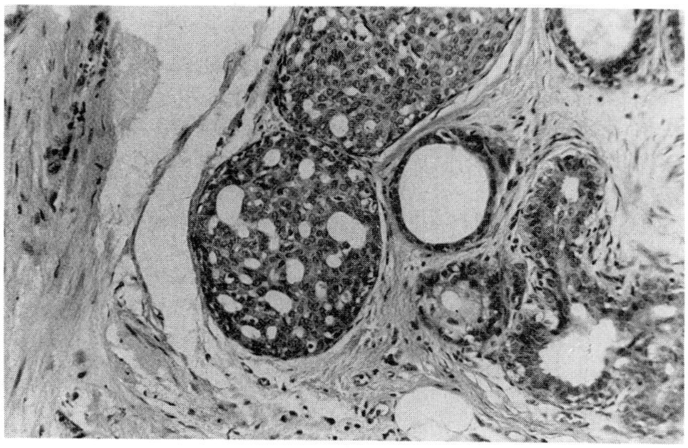

A

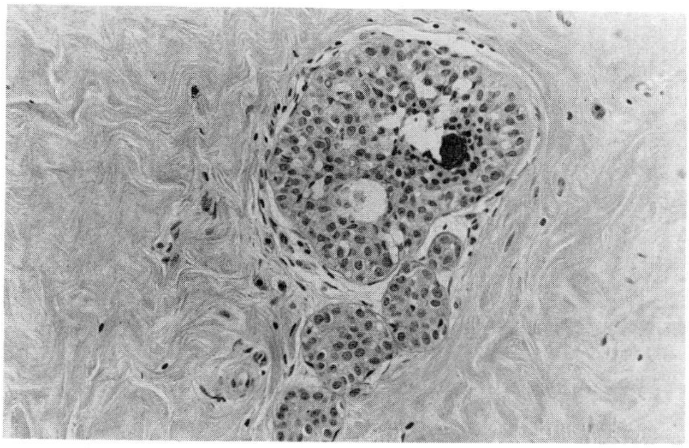

B

FIG. 14-19. *A.* Ductal epithelial hyperplasia. The irregular spaces and variable nuclei serve to differentiate this process from carcinoma in situ. *B.* Lobular hyperplasia. Lobular cells are proliferative but the presence of lumina and incomplete distention separate this process from a carcinoma in situ. Elsewhere in this biopsy, typical lobular carcinoma in situ was present. (*Courtesy of Dr. R. L. Hackett.*)

periductal scarring and inflammation an attendant finding in later stages of the process. The process is initiated with periductal inflammation and progresses to destruction and dilatation of the ductular system and, eventually, periductal fibrosis and ectasia. These lesions typically occur in perimenopausal or late premenopausal age groups; differentiation from cancer may be difficult. Plaque-like calcifications that occur within the scar wall may be visible mammographically. Localized scarring of the ectatic lesion may cause lumps that are fixed within an inflamed scar of the breast, referred to as "comedo mastitis." This refers to the grumous, pultaceous material within dilated ducts that may have many of the morphologic features of comedo carcinoma.

Fat Necrosis. This entity histologically is no different from its appearance in other organs. Although relatively uncommon, it may clinically and radiographically be confused with scirrhous or even inflammatory carcinoma. Fat necrosis may present following a history of chest wall or breast trauma. The mammographic appearance is quite characteristic and suggests benignity.

Collagenous scarring is the predominant feature in late stages of the disease; granular histiocytes surround "oil cysts" of varying

Table 14-3
Clinical Features of Benign Lesions of the Breast

Histopathologic Diagnosis	*Age*	*Palpable Mass*	*Mammographic Abnormality*
FCC + PDWA	35–50 (premenopausal)	May be present	May be present
ADH	Increases after menopause	Incidental	Rare*
ALH	Decreases after menopause	Incidental	Rare*
Sclerosing adenosis	25–50 (premenopausal)	Frequent in "aggregate adenosis"	Often with benign calcification
Fibroadenoma	20–30	More prominent in older patients	More prominent as fat increases with atrophy
CSL/RS	Not established; probably wide age range	Rare	Frequent

*Has favored relation with calcification elsewhere in the breast.
Abbreviations: ADH = atypical ductal hyperplasia
ALH = atypical lobular hyperplasia
CSL/RS = complex sclerosing lesion/radial scar
FCC = fibrocystic change
PDWA = proliferative disease without atypia

SOURCE: Page DL, Simpson JF. Chap 6, pp 113–134, in Bland KI, Copeland EM (eds): *The Breast: Comprehensive Management of Benign and Malignant Diseases*. Philadelphia, Saunders, 1991, with permission.

size. These cysts contain free lipid material that results from necrosis of lipocytes. No risk for cancer has been established.

Fibroadenoma. This generic term refers to a benign focal tumor that has mixed glandular and mesenchymal elements. Fibrous tissue composes most of the lesion; the stroma may surround rounded and easily definable ductlike epithelial structures, or epithelium may be skewed into a curvilinear arrangement (Fig. 14-20). The gross appearance is characteristic, with sharp circumscription and smooth boundaries; the cut surface is glistening white. If epithelial elements are excessive, they may appear as light brown areas.

Fibroadenomas typically stop growing when they reach 2 to 3 cm in diameter. Blacks have a greater propensity than whites to develop fibroadenomas and at a younger age. This lesion invariably has a relationship to estrogen sensitivity, and it occurs predominantly in the second and third decades of life. Pain and tenderness may be observed with pregnancy, and an inflammatory response may be accompanied by lymphadenopathy that mimics carcinoma.

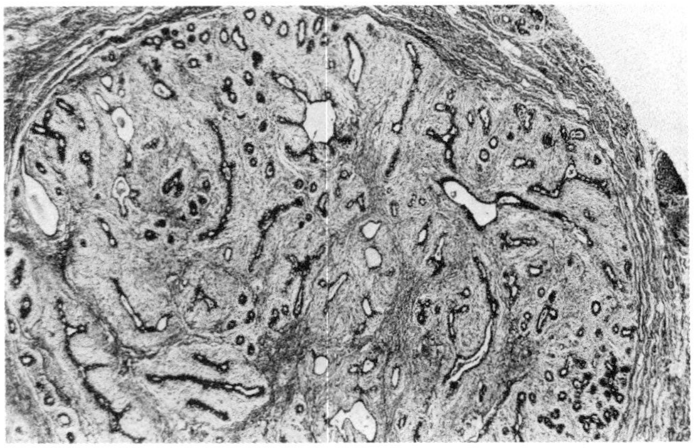

FIG. 14-20. Fibroadenoma. (×10). (*Courtesy of Dr. R. L. Hackett.*) (From: *Romrell LJ, Bland KI: 1991, Chap 2, p 18, with permission.*)

Other variants of fibroadenoma are characterized by increased cellularity of the stroma and/or epithelium. "Adolescent cellular fibroadenoma" typically occurs in adolescence and bears resemblance to *benign phyllodes tumors,* thus suggesting the term *juvenile adenofibroma*. Five to ten percent of adenofibromas occur at and about the time of menarche; they frequently have a ductal pattern of epithelial hyperplasia and stromal hypercellularity and are characterized by rapid growth.

Diagnosis of fibroadenomas can be established by fine-needle aspiration (FNA) cytologic techniques. While these tumors may evolve into phyllodes tumors, this is poorly documented. Following cytologic documentation by FNA, many clinics simply observe the characteristic 2- to 3-cm fibroadenoma. Data support this clinical approach for patients younger than twenty-five years and, perhaps, those as old as thirty-five years; however, excision is appropriate in older women to exclude carcinoma, which has an increasing incidence above age thirty-five. In most patients, excision is readily accomplished under local anesthesia. Patients with the typical clinical and histologic fibroadenoma are *not* considered at greater risk than the general population for development of subsequent carcinoma. Approximately 100 cases of carcinoma arising in the lesion have been documented. The predominant carcinoma that presents concurrently with the fibroadenoma is *lobular carcinoma in situ*.

Tubular adenoma represents a variant of fibroadenoma that possesses tubular elements arranged in a circumscribed concentric mass with minimal supporting stroma. These lesions have fine nodularity, uniform tubular structures, and the absence of lobular anatomy. The *lactating adenoma* is analogous to tubular adenomas and represents the physiologic response to pregnancy. As a consequence of estriol excess to stimulate growth, these adenomas have a more pronounced anatomic alteration of the lobule than is evident in tubular adenomas.

Phyllodes Tumors. The nomenclature, presentation, and diagnosis of phyllodes tumors historically pose many problems for clinicians. This confusion was predicated on classic terminology that placed the suffix "sarcoma" on benign and malignant examples of these lesions. Differential diagnostic problems arise with the separation of benign phyllodes tumors from closely related, but distinguishable, fibroadenomas and with recognition of the rare variant that is malignant.

No reliable histopathologic measures exist to differentiate the juvenile fibroadenoma from the benign phyllodes tumor. Typically, the latter harbors a sharp demarcation from the surrounding normal parenchyma that is considerably compressed and distorted. Connective tissue composes the bulk of the mass, which is firm with mixed areas of gelatinous, edematous, or dense areas. The cystic components owe their origin to sites of infarction, degeneration, and necrosis. These alterations give the breast surface its classic leaflike (phyllodes) appearance. The contour of the breast may assume a "teardrop" configuration with sarcomatous transformation (Fig. 14-21*A*).

Histologically, phyllodes tumor may be indistinguishable from the large fibroadenoma. The stroma of the phyllodes tumor has greater cellular activity and cellular content than the fibroadenoma (< 3 mitoses/high-power field). The epithelium is deformed into intracanalicular patterns seen in the more common fibroadenoma. Counting mitoses and evaluating margins with attention to identify infiltrating foci may predict a more aggressive behavior.

Borderline lesions are less likely to assume true malignant potential but have greater potential to recur locally than the usual phyllodes tumor. The overwhelming majority of malignant phyllodes tumors that have metastasized harbor obvious sarcomatous elements (e.g., liposarcoma, rhabdomyosarcoma) rather than fibrosarcoma.

Mammographic foci of calcification and morphologic evidence of necrosis are evident for both malignant and benign phyllodes tumors and are of little value in differentiating the entities. With comprehensive sectioning for study of the lesion to grade the mitotic rate and margins, a more predictable assessment of clinical behavior will be achieved. Local recurrence has been documented in over one-half of the cases. These recurrences are not associated with unrecognized malignant features.

Treatment options are controversial. At the very least, the small phyllodes tumor should be locally excised with an obvious margin (≥ 1 cm) of normal breast tissue. Often these lesions have been initially enucleated after clinical confusion with a fibroadenoma. When the pathologic diagnosis of a phyllodes tumor with suspicious malignant elements is made (Fig. 14-21*B*), reexcision of the biopsy scar is indicated to ensure complete local excision. With the larger phyllodes tumors, especially those with malignant elements, total (simple) mastectomy is often required for adequate treatment. Axillary dissection is generally not recommended; rarely, lymph node metastasis may occur.

Papilloma. The solitary papilloma represents a variable-sized mass that presents in epithelium of the large duct network of the subareolar breast. Peripherally, lesions may be multiple and continuous with hyperplastic alterations that occur within lobular units. These papillary lesions may harbor atypical hyperplasia and ductal carcinoma in situ that is contiguous with the papilloma.

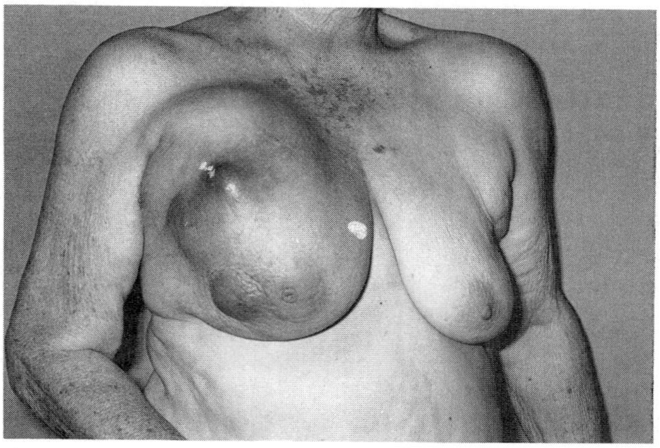

A

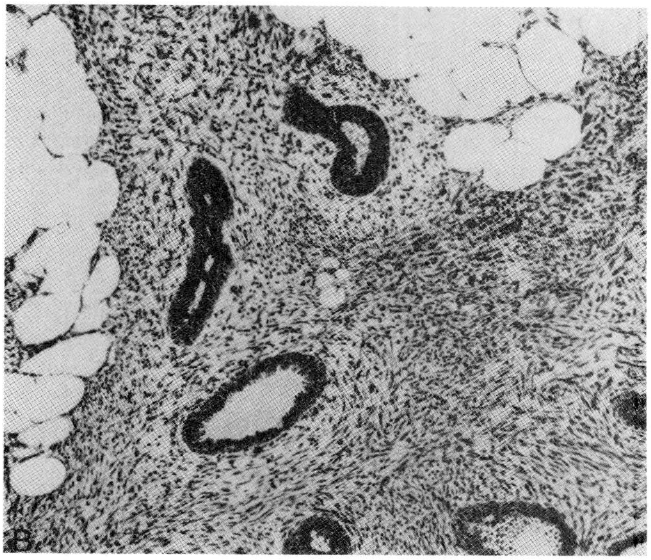

B

FIG. 14-21. *A.* Malignant cystosarcoma phyllodes. *B.* Histology of malignant cystosarcoma phyllodes. (Hematoxylin and eosin, ×100.)

The papilloma presents with a serosanguineous or bloody nipple discharge, typically unilateral. The natural history of solitary lesions suggests an increased propensity for subsequent development of carcinoma. The accompanying epithelial hyperplasia may be responsible for further elevating this risk. Multiple papillomas imply an elevated risk for cancer.

The lesions are papillary epithelial outgrowths that occupy dilated ductal spaces. The papilloma may attain several centimeters in size and may appear encysted within the duct from which it arises. Microscopically, there is branching fibrovascular tissue surmounted by epithelium. Dense sclerotic foci may be present. Focal areas of hemorrhage and necrosis are observed; sites of infarction may cause distortion and compression of epithelium that mimic the appearance of carcinoma on mammogram. When the double cell layer adjacent to the basement membrane is surmounted by excessive cellular columnar cells, the rules used for diagnosis of *atypia* and *in situ carcinoma* apply. If features of ductal carcinoma in situ are evident, the appropriate diagnosis is *noninvasive papillary carcinoma*.

Intraductal papilloma is the most common cause of bloody nipple discharge but must be distinguished surgically from adenocarcinoma, which may also present with bloody nipple discharge. The offending duct is identified by radial compression of breast tissue and observation of which lactiferous duct the discharge emerges from. Ductography may identify the involved duct. Under local or general anesthesia, a probe can be placed in the offending duct and the nipple-areola complex partially elevated via a circumareolar incision. The duct then can be identified by the contained probe and excised for pathologic confirmation of the diagnosis.

Nipple Adenoma. This lesion bears resemblance to the papilloma but presents in the nipple or tissues immediately adjacent to the ductal ampulla of the nipple. Hyperplasia and pseudoinvasion of dense stroma are basic features. *Paget's disease* of the nipple may mimic the lesion. Nipple adenomas have varying patterns of localized hyperplasia with supporting fibrous and cystic changes. Clinically the lesions are recognized when they enlarge to approximately 1 cm in size. They may demonstrate epithelial hyperplastic components and fibrosis and confusion with a malignancy is possible.

Ductal Adenoma (Nodular Adenosis). This lesion may clinically resemble the presentation of a papilloma; differentiation from carcinoma is essential. Histopathologically, adenomas are related to epithelial lesions that have unusual patterns of sclerosis and adenosis. Dense fibrous tissue within epithelial cells appears to be pseudoinvasive and may cause confusion with carcinoma.

CARCINOMA OF THE BREAST

Incidence

Carcinoma of the breast is the most common site-specific cancer in women and is the leading cause of death from cancer for females forty to forty-four years of age. Breast cancer accounts for 32 percent of all female cancers and is responsible for 19 percent of the cancer-related deaths in women. Approximately 181,000 invasive breast cancers were diagnosed in the United States in 1992; approximately 46,300 women will die because of the tumor. Cancer registries in Connecticut and upper New York State note that the age-adjusted incidence of new cases has been steadily increasing since the mid-1940s. In the 1970s the probability of a woman in the United States developing breast cancer was estimated at 1 in 13; in 1980 it was 1 in 11 and in 1992 the frequency is 1 in 9.

Until the past decade, breast cancer was the leading cause of cancer-related mortality in women. In 1985, the lung surpassed it as the leading site of cancer-related mortality in women (Fig. 14-22). Despite the steady increase in incidence, the overall breast cancer mortality has remained static. This relative decrease in mortality rate reflects the detection of an increasing percentage of early disease. Between 1960 and 1963, 5-year survival rates were 63 percent and 46 percent for white and black women, respectively; whereas, similar figures for the 1981 to 1987 interval were 78 percent and 63 percent, respectively.

Worldwide, breast carcinoma represents an epidemiologic problem. England and Wales have the highest national age-adjusted mortality for cancer of the organ (29.3 patients per 100,000 population). The United States ranks sixteenth with 22.4 cases per 100,000. For 1986 to 1988, women of the Korean Republic ranked lowest among all nations, with an incidence of 2.6

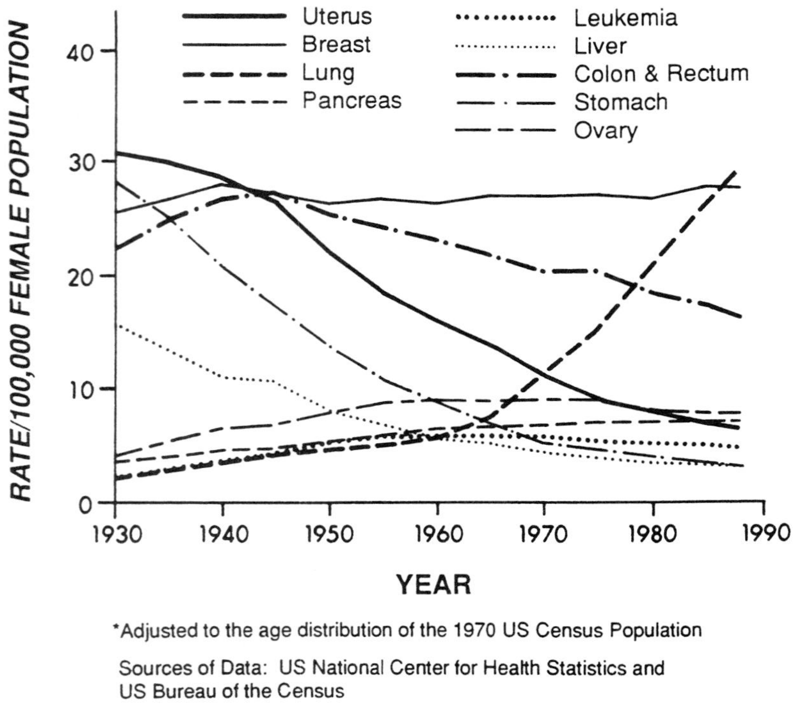

FIG. 14-22. Age-adjusted cancer death rates for selected sites in females; United States, 1930–1988. (From: *Boring CC et al: Cancer statistics. CA 42(1):28, 1992, with permission.*)

cancers per 100,000 population. Mormon, Seventh-Day Adventist, Alaskan, American Indian and Eskimo, Mexican-American, and Japanese and Filipino women living in Hawaii have a lower per capita incidence of breast cancer than other Americans; nuns and Jewish women have a higher than average incidence. There is at least a fivefold variation in the incidence of the disease reported among different countries, although this difference appears to be diminishing. Women living in less-industrialized nations tend to have lower rates of breast cancer than those living in industrialized countries, but Japan appears to be an exception.

Etiology

Genetic Factors. Henderson et al. and Lynch et al. (1991) have documented the importance of heredity and the genetic predisposition for breast cancer. Definitions suggested by Lynch et al. are as follows:

Sporadic Breast Cancer (SBC): A breast cancer patient with no family history of cancer of the breast through two generations involving siblings, offspring, parents, aunts and uncles, and both sets of grandparents.

Familial Breast Cancer (FBC): A breast cancer patient with a family history including one or more first- or second-degree relatives with breast cancer that does not fit the hereditary breast cancer definition.

Hereditary Breast Cancer (HBC): A breast cancer patient with a positive family history of breast cancer and, sometimes, related cancers (e.g., ovarian, colonic) and with high incidence and a distribution in the pedigree that is consistent with an autosomal dominant, highly penetrant, cancer susceptibility factor. Other factors supporting the HBC classification include frequent early age at premenopausal onset and an increased incidence of bilateral breast cancer and other multiple primary cancers.

Lynch and associates documented the frequency of *sporadic, familial,* and *hereditary breast cancer* variants. In an original cohort of 225 consecutive breast cancer patients, updated with 103 new patients, 68 percent of the 328 probands studied were sporadic, 23 percent were familial, and 9 percent were hereditary. The authors state that this may represent a considerable underestimation of the frequency of hereditary breast cancer. With documentation of pedigree, familial breast cancer may constitute as great as one-third of the total incidence of breast cancer cases. Approximately one-fourth of these cancers fall into the special subset of hereditary breast cancer and represent an autosomal dominant susceptibility pattern with early age of onset, with excess bilateral disease, and with other multiple primary cancers.

The risk for developing hereditary breast cancer is determined by pedigree, appears to be independent of age at first pregnancy, and is enhanced when a biopsy confirms atypical hyperplasia. Lynch considers HBC a site-specific heterogeneous entity in which other presentations may be evident. These variants include *SBLA syndrome* (*s*arcoma; *b*reast cancer and *b*rain tumors; *l*ung and *l*aryngeal carcinoma and *l*eukemia; and *a*drenal cortical carcinoma) and *Cowden's disease* (cancer-associated genodermatosis with multiple trichilemmomas, including cutaneous involvement of the face and multiple areas of the hands, feet, and forearms).

Currently biomarkers do not have the sensitivity or specificity to identify HBC individuals before cancer is expressed. Possibly, identification of oncogene expression and alleles polymorphic in DNA restriction fragment links may identify the sites on chromosomes that initiate HBC.

Dietary Influences. The committee on Diet, Nutrition and Cancer of the National Academy of Sciences concluded that a causal relationship exists between dietary mammalian fat and the incidence of breast cancer. Fried, high-fat foods can increase the risk of developing breast cancer approximately twofold. A study of five ethnic groups in Hawaii demonstrated a strong relationship between breast cancer incidence and consumption of total fat, saturated fat, animal fat, and unsaturated fat. A study conducted by the National Cancer Institute noted that dietary fat intake in breast cancer patients was contributory. Compared with controls, the highest quartile for beef or pork consumption increased the relative risk for cancer 2.7-fold over that of the lowest quartile.

Both the quality and the quantity of dietary fat intake may influence the incidence of this disease. Epidemiologic studies also suggest that Japanese and Greenland Eskimo women have a low incidence of breast cancer despite consumption of large quantities of fat. Their diets include a large volume of omega-3 fatty acids, which are unique to the marine-derived lipids. Japanese women have had a doubling of the annual breast cancer deaths over the 20-year interval 1955 to 1975. During that period, the Japanese diet became increasingly similar to that of Western societies. For second- and third-generation offspring of Japanese immigrants, the incidence approaches that of Caucasian women born in the United States.

Hormone Usage. Kalache et al. demonstrated that combined oral contraceptives have no effect on breast cancer risk when used by women in the middle of their reproductive lives (ages twenty-five to thirty-nine years). These data pertained even if oral contraceptives were taken for many years. By contrast, Lipnik et al. noted an adverse effect of these combined hormones on breast cancer risk when taken for a prolonged period of time at a very early age or when taken before the first full-term pregnancy. The World Health Organization study suggests there is neither an increase nor a decrease in the risk of breast cancer with use of the injectable contraceptive depo-medroxy-progesterone acetate (DMPA).

Vessey reviewed the epidemiologic literature and concluded that estrogen usage by perimenopausal and postmenopausal women for hormonal replacement may slightly increase the risk of breast cancer. The risk is said to be accentuated in persons with preexisting benign disease of the breast. The possibility exists that some of this excess risk is attributable to more thorough evaluation and diagnosis of breast cancer in women placed on estrogen supplement. This point of view is further supported by a favorable stage distribution in estrogen users. Very little data have been generated about the effects for cancer risk with hormonal replacement using combined estrogens and progestational agents.

Obesity. The majority of data suggest that breast cancer risk directly correlates with relative weight; obese women experience a 1.5- to 2-fold increased risk. This relative risk increase is restricted to postmenopausal individuals. The increasing incidence of breast cancer mortality in Japanese women has been paralleled by a proportionate increase in both height and weight of this population.

Breast Feeding and Menopause. Previously, breast feeding of long duration ($>$ 36 months in a lifetime) was considered a measure to reduce the risk of breast cancer. This observation is no longer considered valid. Women in whom menopause occurs after the age of fifty-five years have twice the risk of developing the disease compared with women whose menopause started before age forty-five. Artificially induced surgical menopause appears to be protective for breast cancer; protection is lifelong, and removal of endogenous estrogen dramatically reduces breast cancer risk. The earlier the surgical menopause, the lower the risk. Women having oophorectomy at age thirty-five or younger have one-third the risk for breast cancer compared with women whose natural menopause was age fifty or later.

Child Bearing and Fertility. Infertility and nulliparity confer a higher probability (30 to 70 percent) for developing breast cancer when compared with parous women. With decreasing age at the time of first pregnancy, the risk decreases proportionately. Women impregnated before eighteen years of age who have a full-term pregnancy have a breast cancer risk that approximates one-third that for women who become pregnant for the first time after thirty-five years of age. This increase in the relative risk in the latter group is related to persistent exposure to endogenous estrogens in the absence of appropriate concentrations of progesterone. Women who have their first full-term pregnancy after age thirty have an even greater risk for breast cancer than do nulliparas.

Multiple Primary Neoplasms. Harvey and Brinton concluded that women with a history of primary breast cancer have a three- to four-fold increase in risk for primary cancer in the contralateral breast. This risk for a second primary in the breast is increased in women with a positive family history of the disease. Other factors that potentially affect the risk of a second primary, including reproductive factors, body build, and prior irradiation treatment for cancer, remain undetermined. Women with a history of previous ovarian or endometrial carcinoma harbor a relative risk of about 1.3 to 1.4 for development of a primary cancer of the breast.

Irradiation. Atomic bomb survivors from Nagasaki and Hiroshima, women treated with high-dose irradiation for acute postpartum mastitis, and women who have received multiple chest fluoroscopic exams for treatment of pulmonary tuberculosis have a higher incidence of breast cancer. Risk from multiple exposures to relatively low dosages is similar to the the risk of one large dose of similar irradiation yield.

It was previously suggested that susceptibility to the carcinogenic potential of irradiation had its greatest magnitude between the ages of ten and twenty, with relative protection following exposure before age ten and after age forty. Data suggest that women exposed to ionizing irradiation from infancy to age ten have an increased risk but that this risk is within the expectant ranges for development of breast cancer. Less than 1 percent of breast cancer cases result from diagnostic radiologic procedures. Irradiation for breast cancer may increase the risk for cancer of the contralateral breast. Risk of breast cancer is reduced after irradiation treatment for cancer of the cervix and related to reduction of estrogens.

Conclusions. Table 14-4 lists the established risk factors for cancer of the breast in women and the magnitude of these factors. With the exception of age, country of birth, and history of breast cancer in both mother and sister, all of the relative risks reported to date are of modest magnitude. Inconsistent data suggest the protective effects of parity and lactation in various age groups and an increased risk associated with alcohol consumption and DES exposure with pregnancy. Physical activity has emerged as a factor worthy of study. With the exception of weight alteration and obesity, previously established risk factors have not allowed the American public to translate modification of social or environmental life-style into primary prevention.

Natural History

The natural history of breast cancer has been reported by Bloom and associates based on the records of 250 patients with *untreated* lesions cared for on cancer charity wards in Middlesex Hospital, London, between 1805 and 1933. The median survival of this population was 2.7 years after initial diagnosis (Fig. 14-23). The 5- and 10-year survival rates for these untreated patients were 18 and 3.6 percent, respectively; only 0.8 percent survive for 15 years. Autopsy data confirmed that 95 percent of these patients died of breast cancer, whereas only 5 percent died of intercurrent disease. Almost three-quarters of the patients experienced ulceration of the breast before their demise.

The mean survival in this series and for over 1000 untreated cases obtained from the world literature was 38.7 months (range 30.2 to 39.8 months). It should be noted, however, that for all reports of untreated patients, survival is calculated from onset of first symptom. The longest survivor died in the nineteenth year after the onset of symptoms. Although this suggests that the disease may not always be a rapidly lethal one, 60 percent of patients who develop metastases do so within the first 24 months after mastectomy.

Evidence from the Middlesex data and from thousands of other reports suggests that 5-year survival does not always equate with cure. Metastatic foci may become evident 20 or 30 years after treatment of the index lesion; conclusive results cannot be derived from breast cancer data until at least 5 years have elapsed following institution of a therapeutic regimen. For the breast cancer patient, metastatic cancer is the most common cause of death for years 5 through 10 following mastectomy.

The typical carcinoma of the breast (80 to 85 percent) is a scirrhous adenocarcinoma with productive fibrosis that originates in the ductules and invades the parenchyma. For the majority of lesions, there is a long preclinical (occult) period when the tumor and/or host factors can modulate metastasis. If a tumor doubled in size every 100 days, it would take more than 8 years for a solitary neoplastic cell to grow to a 1-cm detectable clinical mass (10^9) cells. Laboratory and clinical evidence suggests that growth rates are not consistent, especially within the first 30 doublings.

Metastases presumably may occur within any period of neoplastic growth following the first few doublings. Growth rates of tumors at distant sites have a wide range; this accounts for the observation that primary lesions may be diagnosed many years before the detection of metastases. Increasingly important roles of cytokines and growth factors on metastatic growth have been uncovered.

As the size of the small mass of breast cancer cells increases, numbers of these cells may be shed into cellular spaces and may be transported into the rich lymphatic network of the breast or into venous spaces. At approximately the twentieth doubling, these tiny tumor masses acquire their own blood supply as a network of neovascularization. Thereafter, these cells may be shed directly into the systemic venous blood. Fisher et al. suggest that these cells may enter the lymphatics with early crossover into the venous blood via lymphaticovenous communications. In systemic blood, tumor cells are rampantly scavenged by killer (NK) lymphocytes and macrophages. Successful implantation of metastatic foci from breast cancer rarely occurs until the index lesion exceeds 0.5 cm in

Table 14-4
Established Risk Factors for Breast Cancer in Females

Risk Factor	*High-Risk Group*	*Low-Risk Group*	*Relative Risk*
Age	Old	Young	> 4.0
Country of birth	North America Northern Europe	Asia, Africa	> 4.0
Socioeconomic status	High	Low	2.0–4.0
Marital status	Never married	Ever married	1.1–1.9
Place of residence	Urban	Rural	1.1–1.9
Place of residence	Northern US	Southern US	1.1–1.9
Race ≥ 45 years	White	Black	1.1–1.9
< 40 years	Black	White	1.1–1.9
Nulliparity	Yes	No	1.1–1.9
Age at first full-term pregnancy	≥ 30 years	< 20 years	2.0–4.0
Oophorectomy premenopausally	No	Yes	2.0–4.0
Age at menopause	Late	Early	1.1–1.9
Age of menarche	Early	Late	1.1–1.9
Weight, postmenopausal women	Heavy	Thin	1.1–1.9
History of cancer in one breast	Yes	No	2.0–4.0
History of benign proliferative lesion	Yes	No	2.0–4.0
Any first-degree relative with history of breast cancer	Yes	No	2.0–4.0
Mother and sister with history of breast cancer	Yes	No	> 4.0
History of primary cancer in endometrium or ovary	Yes	No	1.1–1.9
Mammographic parenchymal patterns	Dysplastic parenchyma	Normal parenchyma	2.0–4.0
Radiation to chest	Large doses	Minimal exposure	2.0–4.0

SOURCE: Modified from Kelsey HL, Gammon MD: *CA* 41:146, 1991, with permission.

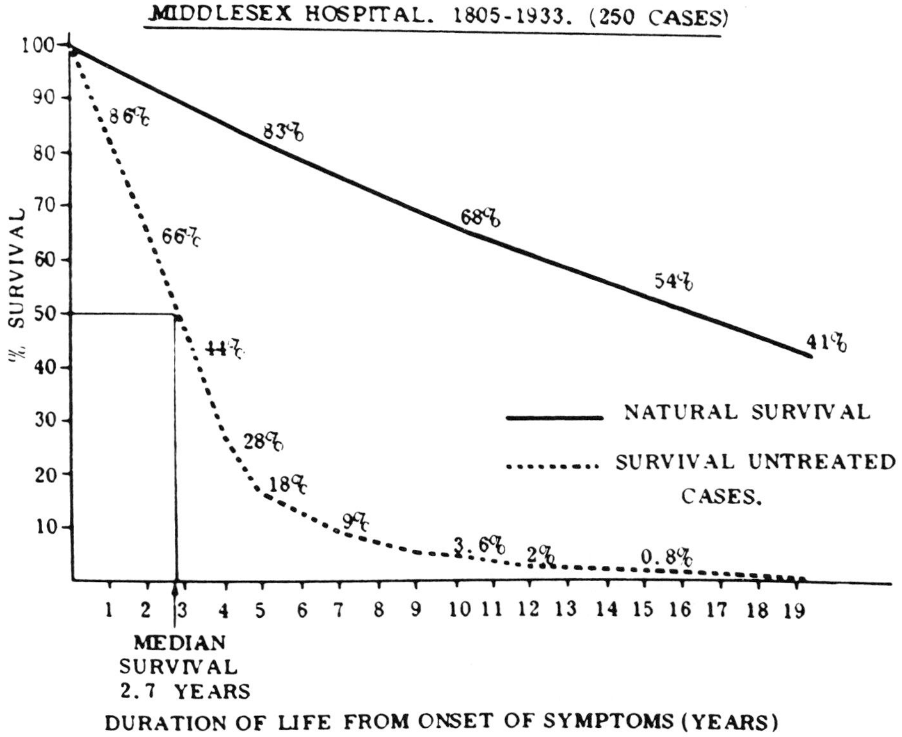

FIG. 14-23. Survival of patients with untreated cancer of breast compared with natural survival. (From: *Bloom HJG, Richardson WW, Harries EJ, with permission.*)

Table 14-5
Observed Survival for Patients with Breast Cancer Relative to Clinical and Histologic Stage

Clinical Staging (American Joint Committee)	*Crude 5-yr Survival (%)*	*Range Survival (%)*
Stage I Tumor < 2 cm in diameter Nodes, if present, not felt to contain metastases Without distant metastases	85	82–94
Stage II Tumors > 5 cm in diameter Nodes, if palpable, not fixed Without distant metastases	66	47–74
Stage III Tumor > 5 cm in diameter Tumor any size with invasion of skin attached to chest wall Nodes in supraclavicular area Without distant metastases	41	7–80
Stage IV With distant metastases	10	—

	Crude Survival (%)		*5-yr Disease-free Survival*
Histologic Staging (NSABP)	*5-yr*	*10-yr*	*(%)*
All patients	63.5	45.9	60.3
Negative axillary lymph nodes	78.1	64.9	82.3
Positive axillary lymph nodes	46.5	24.9	34.9
1–3 positive axillary lymph nodes	62.2	37.5	50.0
> 4 positive axillary lymph nodes	32.0	13.4	21.1

Abbreviation: NSABP = National Surgical Adjuvant Breast and Bowel Project

SOURCE: Reprinted with permission from Henderson IC, Canellos GP: *N Engl J Med* 302:17, 1980.

transverse diameter; this size corresponds to the twenty-seventh doubling of the tumor mass.

Table 14-5 relates observed survival for patients with breast cancer to the clinical and histologic stage. The number of lymph nodes that are involved with metastatic disease is inversely proportional to patient survival. Tumor size is another important prognostic indicator and directly correlates with probability of nodal metastases. Occult (micrometastatic) axillary lymph node metastases of 5-year survivors closely parallel those for patients whose nodes are free of disease.

With tumor enlargement and invasion of the surrounding breast parenchyma, the accompanying fibrosis and desmoplastic response entrap and shorten Cooper's ligaments to produce characteristic peau d'orange or retraction of the skin. Subdermal emboli of neoplastic cells fill the endolymphatic spaces and ultimately invade the corium. Skin invasion is preceded by localized edema; effective drainage of lymphatic fluid from the skin is disrupted. Should tumor cells in the corium continue to grow, ulceration of epithelium will occur. As new areas of skin are invaded, small satellite nodules are evident near the ulcer crater. Venous capillaries are invaded and tumor cells seed the circulation passing via lateral, axillary, or medial central intercostal veins to enter the pulmonary circulation or via vertebral veins that course up and down the spinal column (Batson's plexus).

With expansion of the tumor mass following cellular doubling, tumor cells exfoliate and transgress along lymphatic spaces toward the upper-outer quadrants or enter the rich capillary plexus to communicate with parasternal nodes of the systemic circulation. Local, regional, or distant lymphatic implantation and growth are possible. With involvement of any regional lymphatic area, the nodes are at first shoddy and soft, and then assume a firm, hard, or fixed configuration with increasing expansion of tumor growth. Eventually nodes adhere to each other and form a large conglomerate (fixed) mass. Tumor cells may break through the capsule with fixation of lymphatics to soft tissues and/or contiguous structures of the axilla or chest wall. Typically, axillary nodes are involved progressively from low (Level I) to central (Level II) to apical (Level III) regions.

Systemic dissemination is critical because more than 95 percent of patients who die of uncontrolled breast cancer have distant metastases. The most important prognostic correlate for recurrent disease and survival is the nodal status (Fig. 14-24*A*). *Node-negative patients* have a 20 to 25 percent incidence of relapse compared with node-positive patients, who have a 50 to 75 percent incidence of same. *Node-positive patients* experience recurrence preferentially in distant organs and tissues. The more common sites of disseminated disease include bone (49 to 60 percent), lung (15 to 20 percent), pleura (10 to 15 percent), soft tissues (7 to 15 per-

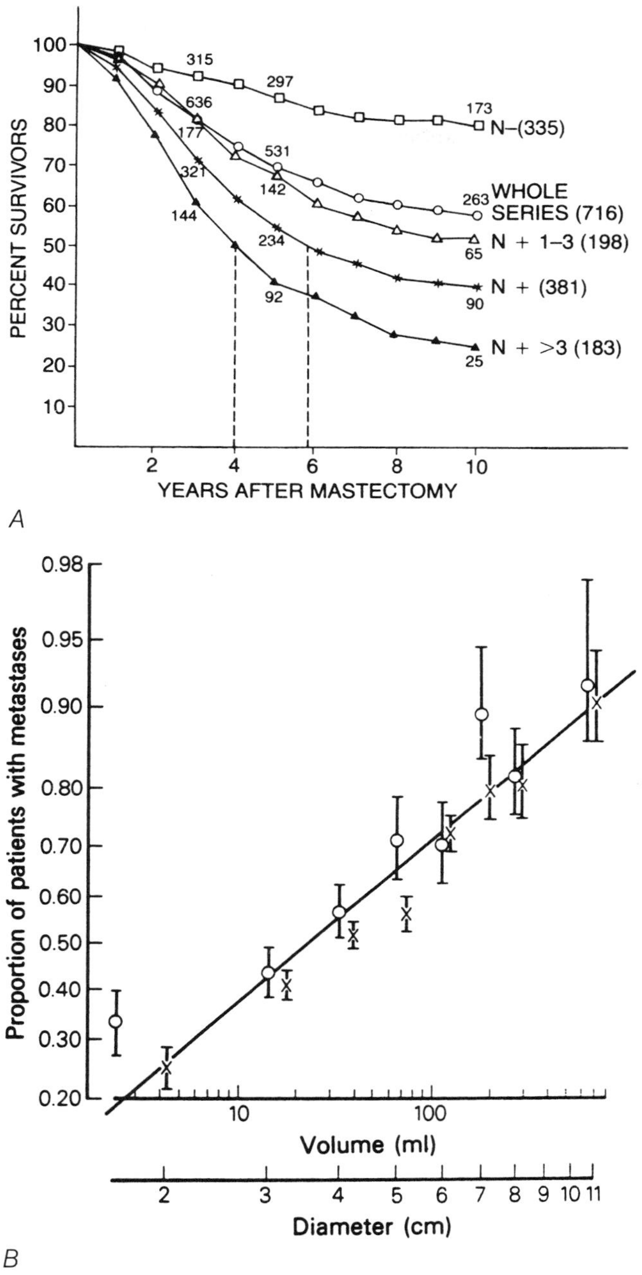

FIG. 14-24. *A.* Breast cancer treated with radical mastectomy. Overall survival according to nodal status. (From: *Valagussa P, Bonadonna G, Veronesi U, with permission.*) *B.* A linear relationship exists between tumor size (volume or diameter) and potential for metastasis. (From: *Koscielny S, Tubiana M, et al, with permission.*)

cent), and liver (5 to 15 percent). In general, 10 to 30 percent of recurrences are local, 60 to 70 percent are distant, and 10 to 30 percent are both local and distant.

Staging of Breast Cancer

The staging of breast cancer is an attempt to predict potential survival rates from objective data.

Tumor Characteristics and Lymph Node Metastases. Koscielny et al. demonstrated that metastases correlate positively with tumor size; this correlation does not occur in half the cases until the primary tumor attains a size of 3.6 cm in diameter (Fig. 14-24*B*). Nemoto et al. and Fisher et al. have shown a distinct relationship between the increase in tumor size, the probability of axillary nodal metastasis, and disease-free survival.

The single most significant predictive factor of 10- and 20-year survival is the absolute *number* of lymph nodes involved with metastatic neoplasm. Physical examination is notoriously inaccurate in determining the presence of lymphatic involvement and may have false-positive rates and false-negative rates for detection of axillary metastasis that range from 25 to 31 percent and from 27 to 33 percent, respectively. Henderson and Canellos report that patients with negative axillary lymphatics have 5-year and 10-year survival rates of 78 and 65 percent, respectively; patients with four or more positive lymphatics have survival rates of 32 and 13 percent, respectively. Fisher et al. observed that the number of positive nodes correlated with the percent of 5-year and 10-year treatment failures. The absence of positive nodes was associated with a 20 percent failure rate at 10 years; greater than four positive nodes was associated with a 71 percent treatment failure rate. Greater than 13 positive nodes increased the failure rate to 87 percent. Patients with occult micrometastasis in lymph nodes initially reported as histologically negative may have survival rates that are not significantly different from those with negative nodes.

The location of the nodes is important; apical axillary (Level III) node metastases carry an ominous prognosis that is distinctly worse than Level I involvement. Level I dissection can be predictive of axillary nodal involvement of the residual contents. Fisher et al. have determined that dissection of Levels I and II is more than adequate in most cases to predict systemic spread of disease. This report suggests that to quantitatively determine accuracy of axillary nodal involvement, sampling of more than ten nodes is necessary.

We do not recommend the sampling of internal mammary nodes in routine dissections. Positive internal mammary nodal metastasis may be expected in central and medial quadrant primaries; this frequency increases proportionately with size of the index tumor. Clinical or pathologic evidence of lymph node extension to supraclavicular sites is indicative of advanced (Stage IV) disease considered systemic. Routine scalene or supraclavicular nodal biopsies are generally not indicated.

Evolution of Staging. Three commonly used staging systems evolved: The Manchester, The Columbia Clinical Classification, and the TNM (tumor, nodes, metastasis) systems. The American Joint Committee on Cancer Staging and End Results Reporting (SEER) has since modified the TNM system for breast cancer (Table 14-6).

A number of physical and radiologic parameters must be reevaluated: (1) comprehensive history and physical examination; (2) bilateral breast imaging (e.g., film screen mammography or xeromammography; (3) clinical pathology laboratory evaluations including hemogram and hepatic function; (4) chest x-ray (PA and lateral); and (5) skeletal roentgenologic survey (indicated if symptomatic).

Select examinations include the following:

1. Abdominal computed tomography (CT) when the following are evident:
   a. Abnormal liver function
   b. Hepatosplenomegaly

Table 14-6

Definitions: TNM Classification

Primary Tumor (T)
[ ] TX Minimal requirements to assess the primary tumor cannot be met
[ ] T0 No evidence of primary tumor
[ ] Tis Paget's disease of the nipple with no demonstrable tumor
(*Note:* Paget's disease with a demonstrable tumor is classified according to the size of the tumor)
T1* Tumor 2 cm or less in greatest dimension
[ ] T1a No fixation to underlying pectoral fascia or muscle
[ ] T1b Fixation to underlying pectoral fascia or muscle
(Check below in addition to T1a or T1b)
[ ] i Tumor $\leqq$ 0.5 cm
[ ] ii Tumor $> 0.5 \leqq 1.0$ cm
[ ] iii Tumor $> 1.0 \leqq 2.0$ cm
T2* Tumor more than 2 cm but not more than 5 cm in its greatest dimension
[ ] T2a No fixation to underlying pectoral fascia or muscle
[ ] T2b Fixation to underlying pectoral fascia or muscle
T3* Tumor more than 5 cm in its greatest dimension
[ ] T3a No fixation to underlying pectoral fascia or muscle
[ ] T3b Fixation to underlying pectoral fascia or muscle
T4 Tumor of any size with direct extension to chest wall or skin
(*Note:* Chest wall includes ribs, intercostal muscles, and serratus anterior muscle but not pectoral muscle)
[ ] T4a Fixation to chest wall
[ ] T4b Edema (including peau d'orange), ulceration of the skin of the breast, or satellite skin nodules confined to the same breast
[ ] T4c Both of the above

Lymph Nodes (N)
Definitions for clinical-diagnostic stage
[ ] NX Minimal requirements to assess the regional nodes cannot be met
[ ] N0 Homolateral axillary lymph nodes not considered to contain growth
[ ] N1 Movable homolateral axillary nodes considered to contain growth
[ ] N2 Homolateral axillary nodes considered to contain growth and fixed to one another or to other structures
[ ] N3 Homolateral supraclavicular or infraclavicular nodes considered to contain growth, or edema of the arm

Lymph Nodes (N)
Definitions for surgical-evaluative and postsurgical resection-pathologic stages
[ ] NX Minimal requirements to assess the presence of distant metastasis cannot be met
[ ] N0 No evidence of homolateral axillary lymph node metastasis
[ ] N1 Metastasis to movable homolateral axillary nodes not fixed to one another or to other structure
[ ] N1a Micrometastasis $\leqq$ 0.2 cm in lymph node(s)
[ ] N1b Gross metastasis in lymph node(s)
[ ] i Metastasis more than 0.02 cm but less than 2.0 cm in one to three lymph nodes
[ ] ii Metastasis more than 0.2 cm but less than 2.0 cm in four or more lymph nodes
[ ] iii Extension of metastasis beyond the lymph node capsule (less than 2.0 cm in total dimension)
[ ] iv Metastasis in lymph node 2.0 cm or more in dimension
[ ] N2 Metastases to homolateral axillary lymph nodes that are fixed to one another or to other structures
[ ] N3 Metastasis to homolateral supraclavicular or intraclavicular lymph node(s)

Distant Metastasis (M) All time periods
[ ] MX Not assessed
[ ] M0 No (known) distant metastasis
[ ] M1 Distant metastasis present
Specify ______________________

Indicate on diagram primary tumor and regional nodes involved.
Examination by ______________________ M.D.
Date ______________________

Tumor Size __________ × __________ × __________ cm.

Predominant Lesion
Measured on [ ] Patient [ ] Mammogram
[ ] Pathologic specimen
Location [ ] OUQ [ ] Nipple/areola
(multiple when necessary) [ ] OLQ [ ] IUQ [ ] ILQ

Lymph Nodes Total number ______________________
Number with metastasis ______________________

Table 14-6 *(continued)*

Stage Grouping
[ ] Clinical-diagnostic (cTNM)
[ ] Surgical-evaluative (sTNM)
[ ] Postsurgical resection-pathologic (pTNM)

[ ] Stage Tis	in situ
Stage X	Cannot stage
[ ] Stage I	[ ] T1ai, N0, M0
	[ ] T1aii, N0, M0
	[ ] T1aiii, N0, M0
	[ ] T1bi, N0, M0
	[ ] T1bii, N0, M0
	[ ] T1biii, N0, M0
[ ] Stage II	[ ] T0, N1a or N1b; M0
	[ ] T1a or T1b; N1a or N1b; M0
	[ ] T2a or T2b; N0, M0
	[ ] T2a or T2b; N1a or N1b; M0
[ ] Stage IIIA	[ ] T0, N2, M0
	[ ] T1a or T1b; N2, M0
	[ ] T2a or T2b; N2, M0
	[ ] T3a or T3b; N0, M0
	[ ] T3a or T3b; N1, M0
	[ ] T3a or T3b; N2, M0
[ ] Stage IIIB	[ ] Any T, N3, M0
	[ ] Any T4, any N, M0
[ ] Stage IV	[ ] Any T, any N, M1

*Dimpling of the skin, nipple retraction, or any other skin changes except those in T4b may occur in T1, T2, or T3 without affecting the classification. (*Note:* Cases of inflammatory carcinoma should be reported separately.)

2. Radionuclide bone scans for any of the following lesions:
   a. Advanced local disease (T3, T4)
   b. Lymph node metastasis (N1, N2, N3)
   c. Distant metastases (M1)
   d. Osseous symptoms in the absence of *a, b,* or *c*

Bone Scans. Bone scanning remains controversial. These radionuclide tests do not precisely identify metastatic disease. Inflammation associated with degenerative joint disease, osteoarthritis, or overlying soft tissues may provide false-positive results. The presence of a positive scan is indicative of advanced stages. Application of the technique should be applied in a cost-effective manner only for patients with T1, T2 or T1,N1 lesions. Scans are indicated in the presence of positive skeletal roentgenograms, bone pain, or palpable regional or metastatic disease.

CT/MRI. Computed tomographic imaging (CT) and magnetic resonance imaging (MRI) are equivalent methods for diagnosis of visceral metastases. Extracavitary ultrasonography and radionuclide scans for detection of hepatic or pulmonary metastases may complement CT/MRT. CT and/or MRI scanning is indicated for patients who have suspected distant metastatic disease as evidenced by symptomatology, abnormal roentgenograms, abnormal liver function, bone metastases, or supraclavicular adenopathy. These modalities represent state-of-the-art techniques for detection of brain, chest, liver, abdominal, and pelvic metastases.

Future Staging Trends. New technology data allow the detection of hormonal, cytosol protein receptor and functional characteristics in the cytoplasm of breast tumor cells. Flow cytometry, which evaluates both cell surface and nuclear characteristics, has provided prognostic implications. Cytokine and growth factor analyses and the use of genetic information (e.g., on proto-oncogenes) will have increasing application in the staging process. Physical and cellular measurements of the primary tumor growth rate and percentage of malignant involvement of the breast have been developed. These refinements will potentially be included in future staging systems.

Histopathology

Noninfiltrating (In Situ) Carcinoma of Ductal and Lobular Origin

General Considerations. The literature suggests that all cases of invasive breast cancer go through a period in which normal epithelial cells undergo malignant transformation but do not "invade" beyond the investing basement cell membrane. There is reason to question whether in situ carcinoma is truly a malignancy, whether it merits substantial efforts at detection, whether treatment affects the subsequent development of invasive cancer, and what form of therapy, if any, should be applied.

Foote and Stewart published the landmark description of lobular carcinoma in situ (LCIS) in 1941, and distinguished this pathologic entity, with its unique biological behavior, from ductal carcinoma in situ (DCIS). DCIS represents the most common histologic variant of the noninvasive stage of carcinoma that takes origin from the major lactiferous ducts. In the late 1960s, Gallagher and Martin published the results of their whole organ section studies and affirmed the transition that established a stepwise evolution of invasive breast cancer from benign epithelium through the in situ and subsequent invasive stages. This recognition allowed them to coin the term *minimal breast cancer* and to stress the importance of early detection of malignancy at a stage when proper therapy would translate into a 90 percent-plus 10-year cure probability. These authors further acknowledged that minimal breast carcinoma included LCIS, DCIS, and minimally invasive cancers <0.5 cm in size.

We now recognize that all of these entities have distinct clinical and biologic implications and that each entity deserves unique

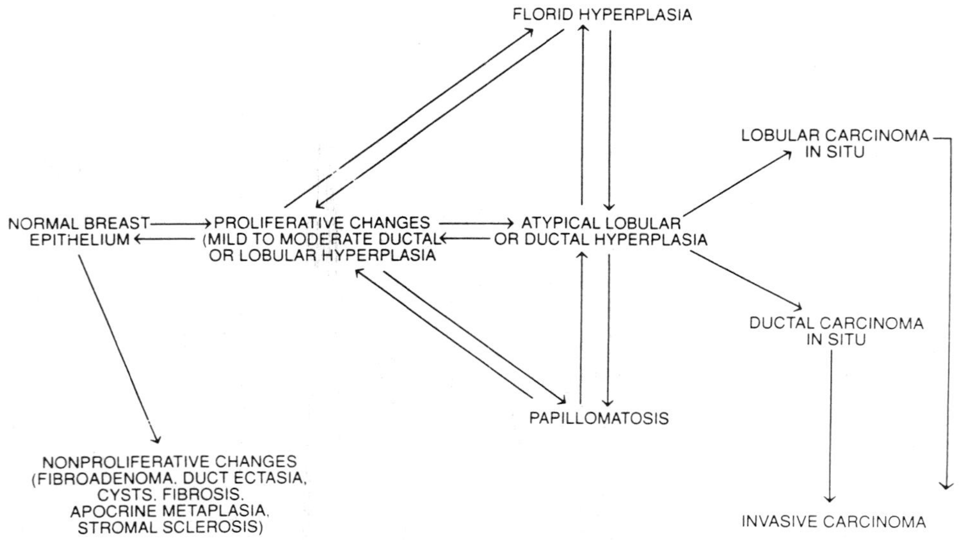

FIG. 14-25. Algorithm of histopathologic phases of proliferative changes for transformation to atypical hyperplasia and in situ cancer as a continuum to invasive carcinoma. (From: *Frykberg E, Bland KI: Adv Surg, 1992, in press.*)

therapeutic considerations. Figure 14-25 denotes the histopathologic phases of proliferative changes that transform to atypical lobular or ductal hyperplasia and the potential pathway to initiate LCIS or DCIS, respectively. Although probably irreversible to normal epithelium, all in situ carcinoma stages do not inevitably transform to invasive disease.

Epidemiology. The increasing frequency of diagnosis of LCIS and DCIS is attributable primarily to mammography. When physical examination was the most common initiator for breast biopsy, in situ lesions constituted only 1.4 percent of all biopsies and only 3 to 6 percent of all breast malignancies. LCIS was more commonly diagnosed than DCIS by ratios of 2:1 or 3:1 in these series. Of 21 clinical series reported by Frykberg and Bland, a total of 9472 mammographically detected nonpalpable breast lesions demonstrated a sevenfold increase in the incidence of in situ disease among all biopsies (9.6 percent) and a fourteenfold increase in incidence of in situ disease among all breast cancers (45 percent). Mammography has detected a predominance of DCIS over LCIS, averaging a 3:1 ratio in many series.

Lobular Carcinoma In Situ. Lobular elements of the breast from which LCIS assumes origin are not noted in males; this form of noninvasive cancer is observed only in females. The average age at diagnosis is forty-four to forty-seven years, which is 15 years *younger* than the age at which invasive breast cancer is diagnosed. Over 90 percent of women with LCIS are premenopausal; this is distinctively different from the incidence (30 percent) for women with invasive cancer. This epidemiologic observation emphasizes the importance of estrogen influence on the biologic behavior of LCIS. Ninety percent of the invasive lobular cancers have estrogen receptor activity, compared with only 55 percent in duct carcinoma.

The frequency of LCIS in the base population cannot be reliably determined because it usually presents as an incidental finding. Published series suggest a wide frequency that ranges from 0.8 to 8 percent of all breast biopsies. There is a distinct racial predilection for LCIS since it occurs twelve times more frequently in white subjects than in the black population; black women, however, have a tenfold increase in the recurrence rate following therapy. A review of 1455 nonpalpable breast malignancies in 18 recent series indicates that LCIS constitutes 2.3 percent of 6287 biopsies and 9.8 percent of all malignancies.

Ductal Carcinoma In Situ. This histologic variant of in situ carcinoma of the breast is observed predominantly in the female but constitutes approximately 5 percent of all male breast cancer. Most patients present with DCIS in early menopausal years. A DCIS occurred in almost 7 percent of 6287 breast biopsies and in nearly one-third of 1455 nonpalpable breast malignancies. The predominance of this lesion among all in situ breast cancers is related to its mammographic definition and its presentation as a clinically palpable mass in over one-half of all cases.

Pathology of In Situ Disease. The original description of in situ carcinoma by Broders stressed the absence of invasion of cells into surrounding stroma and their confinement within the natural ductal or lobular boundaries of the cell membrane. The basement membrane represents the crucial anatomic structure that defines the presence or absence of invasion. Diagnosis of an in situ lesion necessitates multiple sections to exclude invasion; frozen section is rarely relied on.

Evidence suggests that LCIS originates from the terminal duct-lobular apparatus. This explains its tendency to present as a nonpalpable mass and its diffuse distribution throughout the breast. The normal lobular anatomy undergoes a disorderly proliferation of epithelial cells to the point of filling and distending the terminal lobular lumina while the overall lobular architecture is maintained. Cells remain uniformly homogeneous, with a normal nuclear:cytoplasmic ratio and the absence of necrosis and mitoses. The cells are enlarged without loss of cohesion. Cytoplasmic mucoid globules represent a distinctive cytologic feature of LCIS that distinguishes it from DCIS. The disease process is frequently observed in breast biopsy specimens that harbor microcalcifications; however, the process is not generally associated with the calcific sites. The process typically occurs in surrounding tissues that are clinically and radiologically normal. The "neighborhood calcification" represents a unique feature of LCIS and contributes to its diagnosis.

The earliest phases of DCIS are characterized by proliferation of the inner cuboidal layer of the epithelial cells in major lactiferous ducts to form papillary ingrowths within the lumen. Cells in

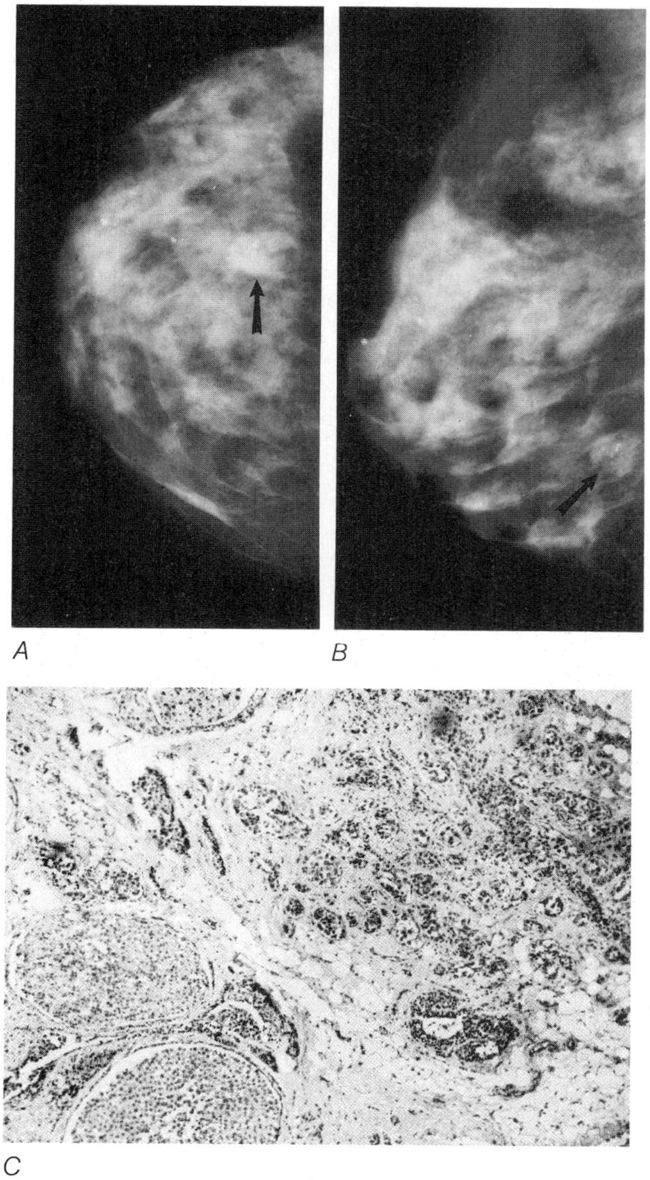

FIG. 14-26. Craniocaudal (*A*) and oblique mediolateral (*B*) mammograms of the left breast that demonstrate a poorly defined 1.2-cm mass (*arrow*) containing microcalcifications in the lower midbreast. (*C*) Histopathology of mass confirms ductal carcinoma in situ (intraductal carcinoma) with sites of stromal invasion. Field shows entire extent of this early (1.2-cm) lesion. (Hematoxylin and eosin, ×32.)

DCIS are well differentiated without evidence of significant pleomorphism, mitoses, or atypia. This may lead to difficulty in differentiating DCIS from benign hyperplasia (Fig. 14-26). With growth of the ''papillary pattern'' of DCIS, ingrowths coalesce to fill the ductal lumen until scattered rounded spaces remain interspersed among solid clumps of cells, which themselves tend to show atypia, hyperchromasia, and loss of polarity. This event was termed by Schultz-Brauns the ''crubriform'' growth pattern of DCIS. By contrast, a ''solid'' histologic pattern of DCIS is recognized when cellular growth obliterates these spaces and the ducts become distended with more anaplastic cells and mitotic figures.

With continued growth, these cells outstrip their blood supply, become necrotic, and lead to the classic example of the ''comedo'' pattern that has been confused with benign inflammatory diseases. In the comedo variant, calcium deposition generally occurs in areas of necrosis, leading to typical DCIS radiographic manifestations. This latter pattern of DCIS has a significantly higher degree of nuclear grade, multicentricity, and microinvasion, suggesting that its biologic behavior is more aggressive than the papillary or solid types. Aneuploid DNA patterns evident on flow cytometry of DCIS, particularly in the comedo forms, are correlated with poor prognosis and a strong potential for invasion. Estrogen receptor activity has been detected in this variant with the same frequency as in invasive cancer.

LCIS and DCIS may coexist and their cytologic similarities may lead to diagnostic and therapeutic confusion. Histochemical and ultrastructural studies, as well as monoclonal antibody technology, have been used to distinguish the two pathologic entities. The term *intraductal* carcinoma is commonly applied to DCIS and denotes the basic pathologic features of ductal elements and their containment within the basement membrane.

Natural History of In Situ Carcinoma. Between 10 and 37 percent of women with LCIS will develop a breast malignancy, representing a risk ratio of six- to twelvefold that of the base population. The majority of cancers that develop subsequent to LCIS occur more than 15 years following diagnosis, and over one-third occur more than 20 years later. Future malignancies are recognized in either or both breasts, regardless of which breast harbors the focus of LCIS. Invasive cancers may be discovered synchronously with LCIS in approximately 5 percent of cases.

A confounding variable is the evidence that 50 to 65 percent of future *invasive* malignancies are not lobular carcinoma but of ductal origin. This raises speculation about the validity of the transition theory. Invasive lobular carcinoma also occurs, however, in this setting at eighteen times the expected rate, and it is presumed that this entity does develop from LCIS. The distinctive pathologic and behavioral characteristics of LCIS are regarded as a ''marker'' of increased risk rather than an anatomic precursor that develops into an invasive lesion.

Since DCIS has been recognized as a distinct entity for a shorter period than LCIS, less evidence is available for the natural history of DCIS. The risk for invasive cancer from DCIS is considered to be in the range of 30 to 50 percent over 10 years. The risk of a subsequent malignancy is increased elevenfold following the diagnosis of DCIS. The future cancers are observed in the ipsilateral breast, usually in the same quadrant as the original biopsy, suggesting that DCIS represents a true precursor to its invasive counterpart. Table 14-7 depicts the salient clinical and pathologic characteristics of DCIS compared with LCIS. The report of the American College of Surgeons suggests a lower survival rate for DCIS than LCIS, suggesting the need for distinct management of the two entities.

Studies of mastectomy specimens from patients with a diagnosis of DCIS confirm that residual disease in the biopsy site existed in as many as three-quarters of patients. These data suggest that a more complete excision of the primary lesion may reduce the future risk of recurrent disease. By contrast, resection of smaller, nonpalpable specimens of DCIS for diagnosis have been observed to completely obviate risk.

Data suggest the necessity of distinguishing grossly palpable and microscopically nonpalpable variants of DCIS to more ration-

Table 14-7
Salient Characteristics of In Situ Ductal (DCIS) and Lobular (LCIS) Carcinoma of the Breast

	LCIS	*DCIS*
Age (years)	44–47	54–58
Incidence*	2%–5%c	5%–10%
Clinical signs	None	Mass, pain, nipple discharge
Mammographic signs	None	Microcalcifications
Premenopausal	2/3	1/3
Incidence synchronous invasive carcinoma	5%	2%–46%
Multicentricity	60%–90%	40%–80%
Bilaterality	50%–70%	10%–20%
Axillary metastasis	1%	1%–2%
Subsequent carcinomas:		
Incidence	25%–35%	25%–70%
Laterality	Bilateral	Ipsilateral
Interval to diagnosis	15–20 years	5–10 years
Histology	Ductal	Ductal

*Among biopsies of mammographically detected breast lesions

SOURCE: Frykberg ER, Ames FC, Bland KI: Current concepts for management of early (in situ and occult invasive) breast carcinoma, in Bland KI, Copeland EM (eds): *The Breast*. Philadelphia, Saunders, 1991, p 736, with permission.

ally plan appropriate therapy. Large palpable forms of DCIS have been observed to have occult invasive rates as great as 46 percent, higher rates of local recurrence, multicentricity, axillary nodal metastases, and evidence of poor survival when compared with nonpalpable or microscopic presentation. A more cautiously optimistic view of DCIS suggests that an occult microscopic presentation is important but, if left unresected, invasive carcinoma may develop.

Bilaterality and Multicentricity of In Situ Cancer. The frequency of synchronous bilaterality is dependent on the extent to which it is sought, suggesting that the published rates probably underestimate the true incidence. LCIS has a known statistically significant rate of bilaterality which has been reported to be as great as 90 percent. In contradistinction, DCIS is associated with only a 10 to 15 percent incidence of bilaterality with an occasional series reporting an incidence as high as 30 percent.

Cancer of the breast originates and develops from multiple foci diffusely scattered throughout the breast. This explains both the heterogeneity of histologic forms found within individual tumors and the presence of other foci of malignancy in breasts that harbor noninvasive cancer. This frequency has been known to range from 10 to 90 percent. These foci of cancer consist largely of the in situ disease identified within the index lesion and the frequency is not dependent on histology.

Multicentricity refers to occult malignancies found outside the quadrant of the primary (index) tumor, whereas *multifocality* and *residual disease* are appropriate terms for sites within the same quadrant as the index lesion. Studies that adhere to the true definition of multicentricity report that this phenomenon occurs in approximately one-third of patients with DCIS; some series note that LCIS has a much higher rate of true multicentricity that may approach 100 percent. A lower incidence of multicentricity is associated with invasive cancer compared with in situ disease. This supports the theory that breast malignancies develop from a coalescence of multiple sites of origin. The small number of valid long-term studies of treatment of DCIS, and the greater frequency of multicentricity for the lesion, suggest caution in recommending conservation therapy that has been designed and implemented for invasive disease.

Infiltrating Malignancies

General Considerations. Cancers of the mammary ducts may be classified according to histogenesis (duct, lobule, acini), histologic characteristics (adenocarcinoma, epidermoid carcinoma, sarcoma, etc.), gross characteristics (scirrhous, colloid, medullary), and invasive criteria (infiltrating, in situ). Approximately three-quarters of infiltrating carcinomas of the breast have been included in the imprecise characterization of ''infiltrating ductal'' or ''adenocarcinoma, not otherwise specified'' (NOS) category. The term ''adenocarcinoma NOS'' is preferred to ''ductal carcinoma'' because the site of origin of most breast adenocarcinomas remains indeterminate. The terminal ductal lobular unit is the most probable site for origin of the majority of breast adenocarcinomas. Based on pure morphologic features, no clinically significant differences have been observed between the less differentiated ''unspecified'' breast carcinomas and mixed variants, unless qualified by the objective assessment of nuclear and architectural degrees of differentiation, i.e., grade.

Current terminology describes histology that is based on the dominant architecture of the lesion, but many patterns may be observed in any one breast cancer. The following classification was originally proposed by Foote and Stewart:

- I. Paget's disease of the nipple
- II. Carcinoma of duct origin
  - A. Noninfiltrating (in situ, intraductal)
  - B. Infiltrating
    1. Adenocarcinoma with productive fibrosis (scirrhous, simplex)
    2. Medullary
    3. Comedo
    4. Colloid
    5. Papillary
    6. Tubular
- III. Carcinoma of mammary lobules
  - A. Noninfiltrating (in situ)
  - B. Infiltrating
- IV. Relatively rare carcinomas
- V. Sarcoma of the breast

The rarely encountered histologic patterns include melanoma, adenoid cystic carcinoma, squamous cell carcinoma, sweat gland carcinoma, and carcinoma with mesenchymal metaplasia of chondromatous or osseus types.

Approximately 40 to 50 percent of breast carcinomas are located in the upper outer quadrant, owing to the relatively larger volume of breast tissue in this sector. Almost one-quarter occur in the juxtaareolar area; the remainder are randomly distributed throughout medial and lower outer quadrants of the breast.

Paget's Disease of the Nipple. Described by Sir James Paget in 1874, this lesion presents as a chronic, eczematoid eruption of the nipple. Paget's disease constitutes approximately 2 percent of histologic types, and is almost always associated with an underlying intraductal or invasive carcinoma. It presents as an encrusted, scaly, hyperemic, and enlarged tumor that occupies the surface of the nipple-areola complex.

Symptoms include tenderness, itching, burning, and intermittent hemorrhage. Intraductal adenocarcinomas often involve the epidermis of the nipple and areola by intraepithelial dissemination.

Table 14-8
Relationship Between Morphologic Types of Invasive Breast Cancer, Lymph Node Involvement, and Patient Survival

Type	*Frequency*	*% With Nodal Involvement*	*% Survival*	
			5 Yr	*10 Yr*
Ductal with productive fibrosis	78	60	54	38
Lobular	9	60	50	32
Medullary	4	44	63	50
Comedo	5	32	73	58
Colloid	3	32	73	59
Papillary	1	17	83	56

SOURCE: Modified from McDivitt, RW, et al: Tumors of the breast, in *Atlas of Tumor Pathology*, Series 2, Fascicle 2. Washington, DC, Armed Forces Institute of Pathology, 1968, with permission.

Physical findings in the nipple-areola complex precede the identification of a palpable mass in the subareolar area. One-quarter to one-third of patients have axillary node metastasis at diagnosis. In general, this breast cancer has a better prognosis than the majority of lesions because the nipple-areola changes promote early consultation, biopsy, and diagnosis.

Microscopically, Paget's disease presents as an intraepithelial tumor composed of small groups of or single clear cells with large vesicular and prominent nuclei. The intraductal lesion is often multifocal; ducts throughout the entire breast may be dilated as a result of obstruction of central collecting ducts at the ampulla of the nipple. Pathognomonic of the entity is the presence of very large, pale, vacuolated cells (Paget's cells) in the rete pegs of the epithelium. The lesion may be confused with superficial melanoma; differentiation between pagetoid intraepithelial malignant melanoma and Paget's disease of the nipple is difficult. The diagnosis is differentiated by demonstration of S-100 protein or melanoma-specific antigen immunoreactivity in malignant melanoma. The application of immunohistochemistry, specifically demonstrating carcinoembryonic antigen (CEA) within the Paget cells, has greatly facilitated diagnosis of the lesion. Melanoma does not contain CEA.

The origin of the Paget cell remains controversial and two hypotheses are considered: (1) *epidermotrophism* of underlying tumor cells and (2) *intraepithelial carcinomatous metaplasia*. The presence of typical Paget cells and the associated findings are diagnostic of the entity even in the absence of a subareolar mass. The ductal malignancy is most commonly invasive; but Paget's disease may be associated with carcinoma in situ of ductal origin.

Infiltrating Ductal Carcinoma with Productive Fibrosis. The frequency of adenocarcinoma of the breast (ductal carcinoma) with productive fibrosis (*scirrhous, simplex, NOS*) is shown in Table 14-8. One-third of these tumors have recognizable elements of a specific histologic type, but the presence of specific tumor types in small volumes does not appear to affect prognosis. The prototypical common adenocarcinoma of the breast presents in a perimenopausal or postmenopausal woman in the sixth decade as a solitary, nontender, firm, ill-defined mass.

The tumor characteristically possesses a poorly defined border that is typically better defined by palpation than inspection. Cut surfaces suggest a central radiating stellate tumor with a chalky-white or yellow streak extending into surrounding parenchyma. The histologic picture may reveal variable cellular and nuclear grade. A broad spectrum of in situ to highly anaplastic variants are observed, suggesting significant heterogeneity (Fig. 14-26). Other lesions can possess bland homogeneity of cellular differentiation throughout the specimen. Neoplastic cells are arranged in small clusters or stacked in single rows (to produce "Indian filing") that occupy irregular cleft spaces between collagen bundles (Fig. 14-27).

With profound desmoplastic response of tumor growth, resultant fibrosis and tumor infiltration can shorten Cooper's ligaments as they course from the deep layer of clavicopectoral fascia to the superficial fascia of the corium. With hyalinization, these ligaments become entrapped within the expanding desmoplastic border of the tumor. With progressive growth, Cooper's ligaments are further shortened to initiate the classic physical finding of skin dimpling directly over the tumor and to initiate advanced local and regional presentations. This physical characteristic is exaggerated when the patient's arms are elevated above her head. This variant of skin dimpling and fixation does not represent a "grave sign" because it does not indicate direct involvement of the skin by the

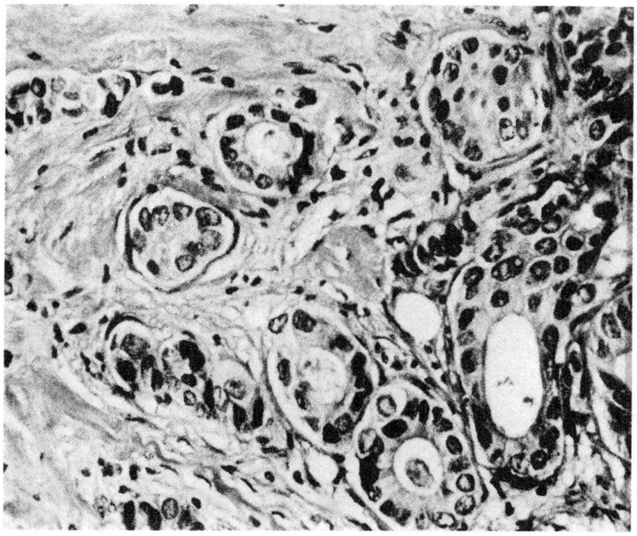

FIG. 14-27. Photomicrograph of infiltrating ductal carcinoma with productive fibrosis (scirrhous carcinoma). Ductal formation is recognized in multiple sites with stromal invasion. (×62.5.) (*Courtesy of Dr. R. L. Hackett.*)

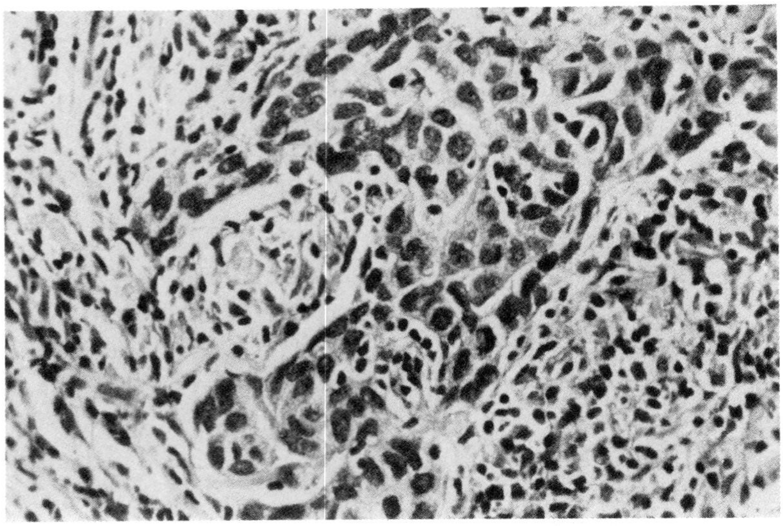

FIG. 14-28. Medullary carcinoma of breast. (×250.)

tumor. With progressive diffuse skin infiltration in the subdermal plexus and the characteristic involvement of Cooper's ligaments, there is extensive edema of the skin, referred to as peau d'orange.

Medullary Carcinoma. This cancer represents 2 to 15 percent of the histopathologic types and takes origin from large ducts. Grossly, the tumor is characterized by its soft, hemorrhagic bulky presentation. Commonly, the lesion is positioned deeply within the breast and is mobile. The skin is often stretched over a bulky, spherical mass that exceeds 3 cm in diameter. There is usually delay in its initial progression, although rapid growth may occur secondary to tumor necrosis and/or hemorrhage. Bilaterality is reported in less than one-fifth of cases; less than 10 percent of these neoplasms contain detectable estrogen or progesterone receptors.

Microscopically, medullary carcinoma is characterized by (1) a dense lymphoreticular infiltrate composed predominantly of lymphocytes and a variable number of plasma cells; (2) large pleomorphic nuclei that are poorly differentiated and accompanied by active cellular mitosis; and (3) a syncytial sheetlike growth pattern with minimal or absence of tubuloacinar differentiation (Fig. 14-28). Approximately one-half of these tumors are associated with intraductal cancer, with the intraductal component characteristically present at the periphery of the tumor mass. In rare circumstances, mesenchymal metaplasia or transformational anaplasia is noted.

Diagnosis of this lesion connotates a better 5-year survival than pure invasive ductal or lobular carcinoma. The most important prognostic determinant of medullary carcinoma is the presence or absence of axillary node metastasis. Due to the intense lymphohistiocytic response in and about the tumor, benign or hyperplastic enlargement of the nodes of the axilla may contribute to erroneous clinical staging. Metastases to axillary lymphatics are reported in more than 40 percent of patients.

Mucinous Carcinoma (Colloid Carcinoma). This adenocarcinoma of ductal origin constitutes approximately 2 percent of all breast cancers and typically presents as a bulky, mucinous (colloid) tumor that is largely confined to the elderly population. The pathologic features of mucinous carcinoma are quite distinctive: the cut surface is glistening, glaring, and gelatinous. Fibrosis is variable and, when abundant, imparts a firm consistency to the tumor. Approximately one-third of patients have axillary metastases, and 5- and 10-year survival rates are reported at 73 and 59 percent, respectively.

Characteristic microscopic features that are identifiable include large pools of mucin that surround variable groups of tumor cells. Tumor cells may not be evident in all sections. *Signet-ring cells* are not generally seen in mucin-producing breast adenocarcinomas of the breast. Approximately two-thirds of pure mucin-producing breast adenocarcinomas contain detectable ER receptors.

The lesion should be distinguished from benign *granular cell myoblastoma*. To confirm the malignant features of colloid carcinoma, multiple microscopic sections are essential. Frozen-section analyses are infrequently diagnostic; relying on this technique is inadvisable.

Tubular Carcinoma. This lesion represents a well-differentiated variant of breast carcinoma with an incidence of approximately 2 percent. Increasingly diagnosed mammographically, this tumor is reported in as many as one-fifth of women whose cancers are diagnosed by screening. Microscopically, tubular differentiation is distinctive. Under low magnification a haphazard array of small, randomly arranged tubular elements are identifiable. The small glandular (tubular) pattern and single-cell lining of neoplastic tubules provide important histologic characteristics of the tumor. Absence of myoepithelial cells and a well-defined basement membrane serve to distinguish common proliferative, microglandular, and sclerosing adenosis lesions from tubular carcinoma. Most commonly, the lesion is diagnosed in the perimenopausal or early menopausal population. These lesions are typically discovered mammographically when small (i.e., $\leq$ 1 cm maximum dimension).

Approximately 10 percent of patients with typical lesions develop axillary metastasis. Long-term survival approaches 100 percent if the carcinoma contains 90 percent or more of the tubular components. Metastases are generally confined to small numbers in low axillary nodes (Level I). Rosen and associates confirmed lower recurrences (3.5 percent) in patients treated for this disease.

Papillary Carcinoma. Papillary carcinoma accounts for less than 2 percent of all breast carcinomas and generally presents in the seventh decade. The lesion has been observed in a disproportionate number of non-Caucasian patients. Typically papillary cancer is small and rarely attains sizes greater than 2 to 3 cm in diameter. Morphologically, these cancers are well circumscribed; papillary differentiation in the form of papillae with well-defined fibrovascular stalks and multilayered epithelium may harbor moderately pleomorphic cells. McDivitt and colleagues note that this tumor had the lowest frequency of axillary nodal involvement and the best 5- and 10-year survival rates. Disease-free survival is similar to that for mucinous and tubular carcinoma. Despite the presence of axillary metastases, which may occur in up to one-third of patients, papillary carcinoma represents a more indolent, slowly progressive disease than the common adenocarcinoma.

Adenoid Cystic Carcinoma. This lesion is very rare, accounting for < 0.1 percent of all types of breast cancer. It is typically indistinguishable from the more common adenoid cystic carcinoma that occurs in salivary glands. The age distribution is similar to that for typical adenocarcinoma. These cancers present as small lesions, 1 to 3 cm in diameter, characteristically well circumscribed with well-defined margins. On close inspection the tumors contain dense mucoid material within glandular spaces that ultrastructurally mimics the lamina densa of the basement membrane. Axillary metastases are rare with adenoid cystic carcinoma. Only seven deaths from pulmonary metastases from this tumor have been confirmed.

Apocrine Carcinoma. These lesions present a ductal or acinar growth pattern with the unusual tendency to involve the lobular epithelium, and are well-differentiated with rounded vesicular nuclei and prominent nucleoli. There is a very low mitotic rate and little variance in cytomorphologic features. These lesions can contain potentially aggressive biologic behavior; low to absent levels of estrogen and progesterone receptors are frequent.

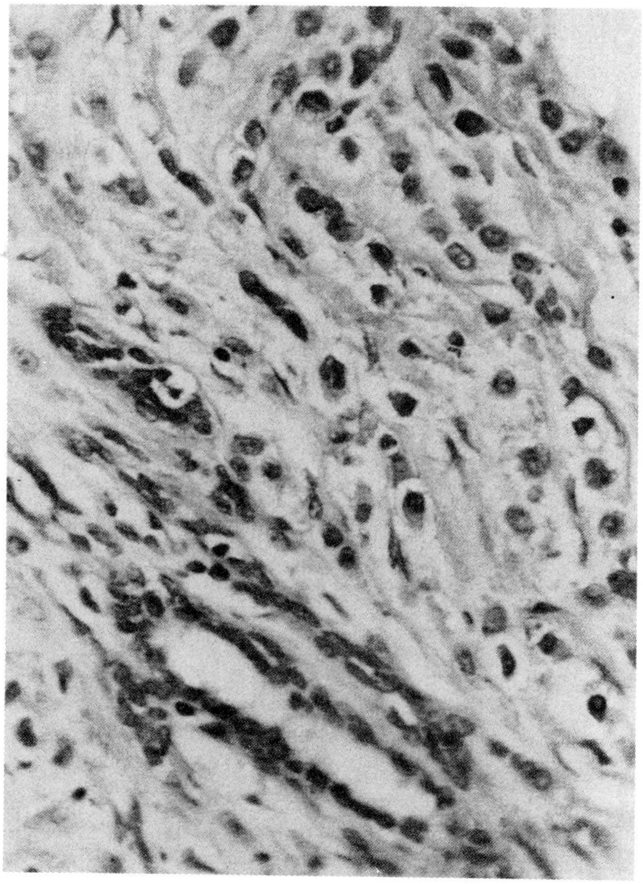

FIG. 14-29. Lobular carcinoma of the breast. (×250.) The uniform, relatively small tumor cells of lobular carcinoma are seen arranged in a single-file orientation ("Indian filing").

Carcinoma of Lobular Origin. The histopathologic features include characteristic small cells with rounded nuclei, inconspicuous nucleoli, and scant indistinct cytoplasm (Fig. 14-29). Special stains confirm the infrequent presence of intracytoplasmic mucin. Similar to colloid carcinoma, mucin may displace the nucleus, resembling *signet-ring carcinoma* of the gastrointestinal tract. These carcinomas originate in terminal ductules of the lobule and possess characteristic features that distinguish them from lesions of the larger, lactiferous ducts. The noninvasive variant is referred to as lobular carcinoma in situ (LCIS). In LCIS, lobules are packed with small hyperplastic cells of significant uniformity, arranged in rows or beads with few mitoses. Hyperchromatism, nuclear anaplasia, and other variants of invasive breast cancer are characteristic of the malignancy. The incidence of the in situ variant approximates 3 percent of breast cancers; infiltrating lobular carcinoma constitutes approximately 10 percent of breast cancers.

Grossly, the infiltrating lobular variant deserves consideration, as these lesions vary from clinically inapparent microscopic tumors to those that replace the entire breast with a poorly defined, somewhat firm mass. On occasion, this cancer may mimic inflammatory or benign lesions. Because the lesions have a high propensity for bilaterality, multicentricity, and multifocality, their presentation can present perplexing problems.

Squamous Cell (Epidermoid) Carcinoma. This infrequently observed cancer of epithelial origin arises from metaplasia within the lactiferous duct system. These cancers are typically devoid of distinctive clinical or radiographic characteristics. Similar to epidermoid carcinoma of the skin, metastases occur almost exclusively via the lymphatic route and are evident in approximately one-quarter of patients.

Sarcomas. Sarcomas of breast origin represent a heterogeneous group of lesions. These tumors include *fibromatosis* (*low-grade fibrosarcoma or desmoid tumor*), *fibrosarcoma, malignant fibrous histiocytoma, liposarcoma, leiomyosarcoma, osteogenic sarcoma,* and *chondrosarcoma*. *Stromal sarcoma* is a term that describes the diverse array of tumors of this type that are histologically identical with comparable soft tissue tumors arising in extramammary sites.

The clinical presentation is typically that of a large, painless breast mass with rapid growth. Routine mammography is not a useful diagnostic aid; false-negative rates are high.

Morphologically, the tumors are predominantly of a solid type, although small cysts in degenerative areas may be observed. The typical sarcoma lacks the "cut cabbage" or leafy laminated surface configuration of the benign cystosarcoma phyllodes. Some sarcomas are well circumscribed while others have infiltrative, ill-defined margins. Histologically these lesions assume cellular features identical with malignancies of other body parts. These spindle cell neoplasms grow as expansile, solid masses with microscopic margins that are sharp, pushing, or infiltrative. As a consequence, the lesions invade fat and tend to intervene between glandular aspects of the breast parenchyma to expand the lobules and intralobular spaces. Tumors are graded based on cellularity, degree of cellular pleomorphism and nuclear atypia, evidence of differentiation, and mitotic activity.

Angiosarcoma. In 1948, Stewart and Treves described the syndrome of lymphangiosarcoma in patients with ipsilateral lymphedema following radical mastectomy. Angiosarcoma is the preferred term. It develops in a lymphedematous extremity that locally initiates an impaired immune mechanism. The average interval between the mastectomy and onset of the angiosarcoma is 10.5 years; 60 percent of patients have a history of postoperative radiotherapy to the operative site. Irradiation is considered a cofactor in the development of angiosarcoma only in the respect that it contributes to the development of lymphedema. The overall incidence of lymphedema following radical mastectomy is 15 to 25 percent compared with 5.5 percent after modified radical mastectomy.

Poorly differentiated variants grow as solid nests and masses of either spindle-shaped or epithelioid cells, the former mimicking Kaposi's sarcoma and the latter carcinoma. Exuberant mitotic activity, necrosis, and hemorrhage are evident in high-grade tumors. Less well-differentiated tumors grow as complex papillary proliferations of malignant cells forming anastomotic vascular channels. The typical presentation is a spectrum of differentiation with small capillary-sized vessels formed by atypical endothelial cells.

Ultrastructural features of postmastectomy angiosarcoma are identical with those of other types of angiosarcoma. Factor VIII–related antigen, a protein produced by endothelial cells, has been identified in this tumor and constitutes a reliable marker. This marker is not useful for distinguishing benign and malignant vascular proliferations; however, demonstration of factor VIII in an anaplastic cutaneous neoplasm excludes the diagnosis of carcinoma and melanoma.

The prognosis for patients with angiosarcoma is dismal; median survival is 19 months. No correlation has been observed between histologic features and survival. Radical forequarter amputation of the involved extremity has been proposed to manage the ulcerative complications of the arm and axilla and to palliate the massive progressive lymphedema. Five-year survivals are extremely rare.

Lymphomas. Primary lymphomas of the breast are rare. Presentation is that of a large lesion (mean size 4 cm) in the postmenopausal patient. DeCosse et al. noted a high incidence of tumor-positive axillary nodes. An occult breast lesion may be diagnosed following detection of palpable axillary lymphadenopathy.

Mammary lymphomas are identical with other malignant lymphomas, with tumor cells that are densely infiltrative throughout the breast parenchyma. There is predominance of diffuse histiocytic lymphomas. Total mastectomy and axillary node sampling are advocated for large lymphomas of the breast. Recurrent or progressive local disease and/or regional disease is best managed by radiotherapy and multimodal systemic chemotherapy using protocols standard for non-Hodgkin's lymphoma. Prognosis is favorable, with 5- and 10-year survival rates of 74 and 51 percent, respectively.

Inflammatory Carcinoma. The presence of lymphatic or vascular invasion portends a reduction in survival rate and a shorter disease-free interval. In *inflammatory carcinoma,* characteristic clinical features of erythema, peau d'orange, and skin ridging with or without the presence of a palpable mass are evident. This relatively rare entity constitutes approximately 1.5 to 3 percent of breast cancers. No specific histologic type predominates.

Typically the skin over the lesion is warm, diffusely scaly, and indurated with ridging. It may present with the characteristics of a cellulitis. An interval of treatment with antibiotics by the physician who mistakes this for a breast abscess is common. The tumor mass may be diffuse or nondefinable. The breast is diffusely "brawny" and the nipple is often retracted when the index lesion is subareolar. Diagnosis is established by generous biopsy of skin, subcutaneous tissue, and parenchyma.

Pathologically, subdermal lymphatics and vascular channels are permeated with microscopic foci of highly undifferentiated tumor. As many as 15 percent of patients free of axillary metastases have microscopic tumor emboli in tissues that surround the primary neoplasm. Inflammatory carcinoma refers to a clinicopathologic entity with characteristic absence of polymorphonuclear leukocytes and lymphocytes near the tumor.

This disease progresses rapidly, and more than three-quarters of patients have palpable axillary metastases at the time of presentation. It is important to distinguish inflammatory carcinoma from the contiguous extension of a scirrhous carcinoma that invades subdermal lymphatic spaces and skin to produce characteristic peau d'orange and lymphangitis of locally advanced disease (Fig. 14-30). Patients with inflammatory carcinoma have distant metastatic disease evident at a much higher frequency than that for more common breast cancers. Taylor and Meltzer found bone and visceral metastases in 36 percent of their patients. The extensive report of the SEER Program by Levine et al. revealed metastatic disease at diagnosis in one-quarter of 3171 white patients with inflammatory carcinoma.

Treatment

Historical Perspectives

The Edwin Smith Surgical Papyrus (3000–2500 BC) was the first document that referred to carcinoma of the breast. The lesion was in a man, but the description encompassed most of the clinical features of breast carcinoma. The author of the papyrus concluded "there is no treatment [for cancer of the breast]." Few writings referred to tumors of the breast until the first century AD. Direct reference to treatment of breast cancer is conspicuously absent in the Corpus Hippocraticum.

Celsus recognized the value of operations for early breast cancer in his early Roman writings of the first century AD. A translation notes: "None of these can be removed but the cacoethes [early lesion], the rest are irritated by every method of cure. The more violent the operations are, the more angry they grow." In the second century AD, Galen inscribed one of the classic clinical observations:

> *We have often seen in the breast a tumor exactly resembling the animal the crab. Just as the crab has legs on both sides of his body, so in this disease the veins extending out from the unnatural growth take the shape of a crab's legs. We have often cured this disease in its early stages, but after it has reached a large size no one has cured it without operation. In all operations we attempt to excise a pathological tumor in a circle in the region where it borders on the healthy tissue.*

The Galenic system of medicine ascribed neoplasms to an excess of "black bile," and concluded that excision of a local out-

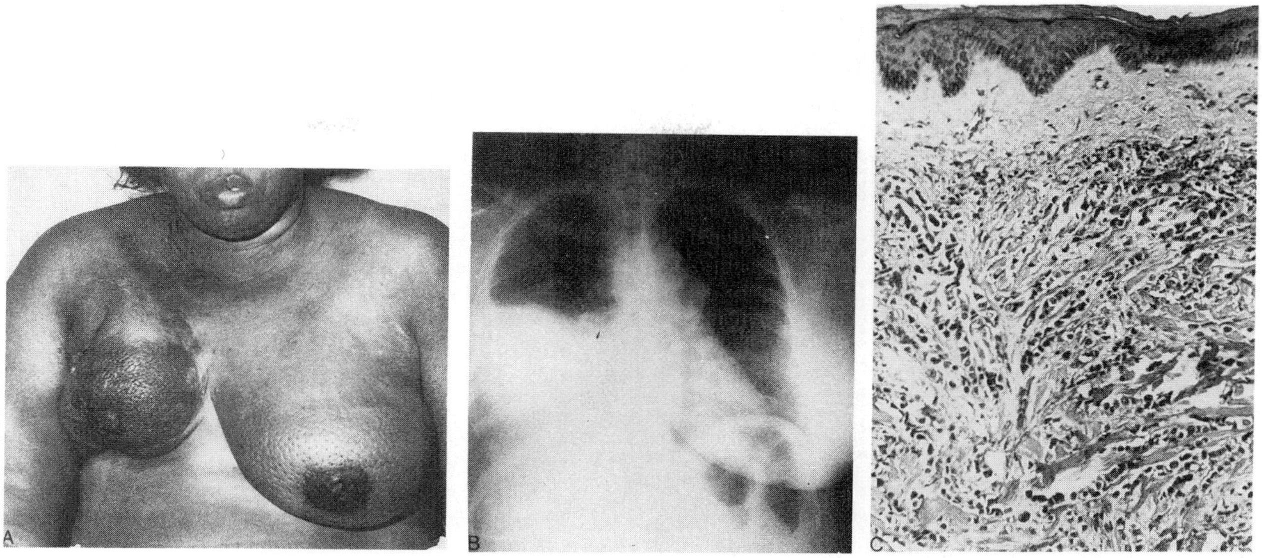

FIG. 14-30. *A.* Advanced inflammatory carcinoma. *B.* Right pleural effusion. *C.* Infiltrating adenocarcinoma within dermis (× 100) without involvement of epithelium.

break could not cure the systemic imbalance. Theories espoused by Galen dominated medicine until the Renaissance. Operative intervention was considered a misdirected, futile, ill-advised approach by the majority of established and respected physicians.

Beginning with Morgagni's systematic approaches, modalities that varied from those espoused by Galen were acceptable. More radical approaches for treatment of the breast became acceptable, including some early and primitive attempts at total mastectomy and axillary dissection. The procedure evolved slowly from simple amputation of the breast. LeDran repudiated Galen's humoral theory in the eighteenth century and stated that cancer of the breast was a local disease that spread by way of the lymphatics to regional nodes. He removed large axillary nodes in his operations on patients with cancer.

In the nineteenth century, Moore, of the Middlesex Hospital of London, emphasized wide removal of the breast and felt that the axillary contents should be removed en bloc, together with the breast, when neoplasm was evident in the axilla. In a presentation before the British Medical Association in 1877, Banks supported Moore's concepts and also advocated en bloc resection of axillary contents with the breast even when palpable nodes were not evident. Banks recognized that occult involvement of axillary nodes could be present.

In 1894, Halsted and Meyer simultaneously reported their operations for treatment of cancer of the breast. By demonstrating superior local and regional control rates following en bloc radical resection, these eminent surgeons established radical mastectomy as "state of the art" for that era. Both Halsted and Meyer advocated complete axillary dissection of all nodal levels from the latissimus dorsi laterally to the thoracic outlet medially. Both routinely resected the long thoracic nerve and the thoracodorsal neurovascular bundle en bloc with the axillary contents.

D. H. Patey of Middlesex Hospital, London, is credited with the demonstration of the worth of the "modified radical mastectomy" technique. In the 1930s, Patey was able to refute the unproved postulates on which the original radical operations were based for cases in which advanced local disease was not evident. Thereafter, Patey and colleagues developed the technique for in-continuity removal of the breast and axillary contents with preservation of the pectoralis major muscle. Removal of the pectoralis minor with retraction of the major allowed access and clearance of the axillary contents. Madden and Auchincloss advocated the modified radical approach with preservation of *both* the pectoralis major and minor muscles. This restricts the dissection of the apical (Level III) nodes, and nodal recovery is less than with the Patey modified technique.

Patient Selection. As late as the 1960s, radical mastectomy was the only procedure used for the treatment of breast cancer. Surgeons attempted to exclude from operation those patients who would almost certainly develop distant metastasis at a subsequent date. These concepts led to adoption of the generally accepted principles espoused by Haagensen, which he referred to as "criteria of inoperability." These general criteria included fixation of the local breast cancer to the chest wall, fixation of the involved lymph nodes of the axilla, and inflammatory carcinoma. This detailed list of criteria included

1. Extensive edema of the skin over the breast (Fig. 14-31)
2. Satellite nodules in the skin over the breast
3. Carcinoma of the inflammatory type (Fig. 14-30)
4. Parasternal tumor nodules
5. Proved supraclavicular metastases
6. Edema of the arm
7. Distant metastases
8. Any two or more of the following grave signs of locally advanced carcinoma:
   a. Ulceration of the skin
   b. Edema of the skin of limited extent (less than one-third of breast skin involved)
   c. Solid fixation of tumor to the chest wall
   d. Axillary lymph nodes measuring 2.5 cm or more in transverse diameter
   e. Fixation of the axillary nodes to the skin or deep structures of the axilla

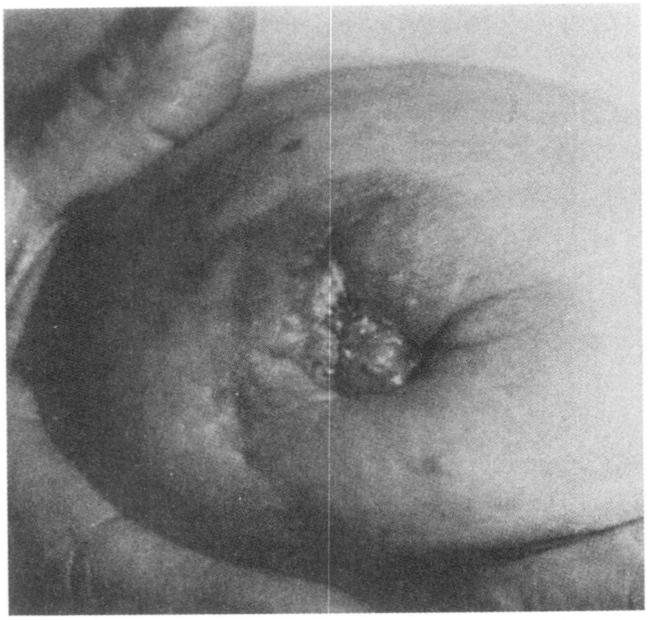

FIG. 14-31. Large cancer of breast with retraction of nipple, skin edema, and several satellite skin nodules.

At the time these criteria were developed, more than one-quarter of patients were excluded from surgical therapy. Currently, more than 10 percent of patients would be found to have such advanced tumors, and the utility of combined modality therapy would, perhaps, revert the majority to a simple extended procedure. Today, the success of adjuvant chemotherapy and irradiation has greatly altered the perspective for therapy; the majority of patients (80 percent) can, at least, expect local-regional control despite systemic metastases.

Current Therapy

Both patient and physician should have a clear perspective of the planned course of therapy. The physician should discuss with the patient that the suspicious lesion may be a cancer that necessitates a therapeutic regimen, including surgical options and the proposed multimodal therapy. The duration of therapy and the issue of irradiation also must be addressed.

Biopsy. The morbidity and the mortality related to breast biopsy is acceptably low. Local anesthesia can be used. A 1980 study on the cost-effectiveness of breast cancer management demonstrated that the most effective measure for containing economic morbidity of the illness is via targeted selection of high-risk patients for biopsy under local anesthesia. Although most (60 to 80 percent) biopsies of "suspicious" breast lesions prove to be benign, specific clinical and mammographic characteristics are associated with a high probability of malignancy.

Medical history, physical examination, and results of clinical staging will each influence the timing and method of breast biopsy. Properly done, the biopsy is of immense value to determine subsequent work-up and definitive therapy. By contrast, inconclusive data derived from inadequately sampled tissue or a skin biopsy incision placed in the inappropriate skin contour or quadrant may limit therapeutic options and alter subsequent management.

Nonpalpable Lesions. The mammographically detected nonpalpable lesion may present in the "normal" breast without physical signs of an underlying cancer. In recent decades, the wide application of screening mammography has resulted in the detection of increasing numbers of nonpalpable lesions. Specific criteria that commonly lead to the diagnosis of the nonpalpable breast mass include (1) localized soft tissue mass within the breast parenchyma; (2) architectural distortion, including contracture of trabeculae, which produces stellate alterations, and asymmetry with thickening of the lobular or periductal architecture; and (3) clustered microcalcification.

Despite the simplicity of mammographic techniques using craniocaudal and mediolateral views, intraoperative localization with adequate excision presents challenges that have led to the development of several methods including noninvasive and invasive localization. *Noninvasive techniques for localization* include visual estimation, external breast markers, stereomammograms, plotted coordinates on a breast diagram, and grid compression devices. *Invasive localization methods* have improved remarkably over the past decade with use of small radiopaque needles that may be radiographically guided into the suspicious lesion. After insertion of the localization needle, subsequent mammograms will demonstrate orientation of the needle tip to the suspect mass. This technique requires cooperation and communication between the radiologist and surgeon, and specimen radiography is necessary. Figure 14-32 demonstrates the operative technique for needle localization biopsy.

Palpable Lesions. The biopsy technique for a palpable lesion is often influenced by the physical characteristics of the tumor, size of the breast mass, location of the suspicious lesion, the type of anesthesia desired by the patient, and the therapy planned if a malignancy is confirmed. An *incisional biopsy* of a large breast mass can be performed under local anesthesia if the patient presents with bony metastasis. This technique provides histologic confirmation of the malignancy and adequate tissue for hormonal receptor analysis before initiation of radiation or chemotherapy. *Fine-needle aspiration* of a small, suspicious palpable lesion is appropriate in an outpatient setting for the patient with clinical Stage I breast cancer. Regardless of the method, it is essential that the biopsy specimen be handled expeditiously and appropriately in both clinical situations to render a valid specimen for histologic and hormone receptor analyses.

Fine-Needle Aspiration (FNA). This technique is not performed unless a palpable mass is evident. The combination of physical examination, mammography, and FNA provides a diagnostic accuracy that approaches 100 percent. A negative FNA in the presence of a palpable mass, however, does not conclusively exclude carcinoma. When the mass is clinically and mammographically suspicious, the sensitivity (true-positive) of FNA approximates 80 to 98 percent. The false-negative rate of FNA approximates 2 to 10 percent. Sensitivity and efficacy are influenced primarily by false-negative results. The specificity and predictive value of FNA approach 100 percent because false-positive results are rare.

Cutting Needle Biopsy. The standard Tru-Cut (Travenol, Deerfield, IL) needle is the most commonly used cutting needle for biopsy of breast masses. False-positive diagnostic rates are lower with tissue procured by cutting needles than with FNA specimens because more tissue is submitted for analysis. But a core biopsy without malignant tissue cannot be conclusively considered a "negative" biopsy and might represent a sampling error.

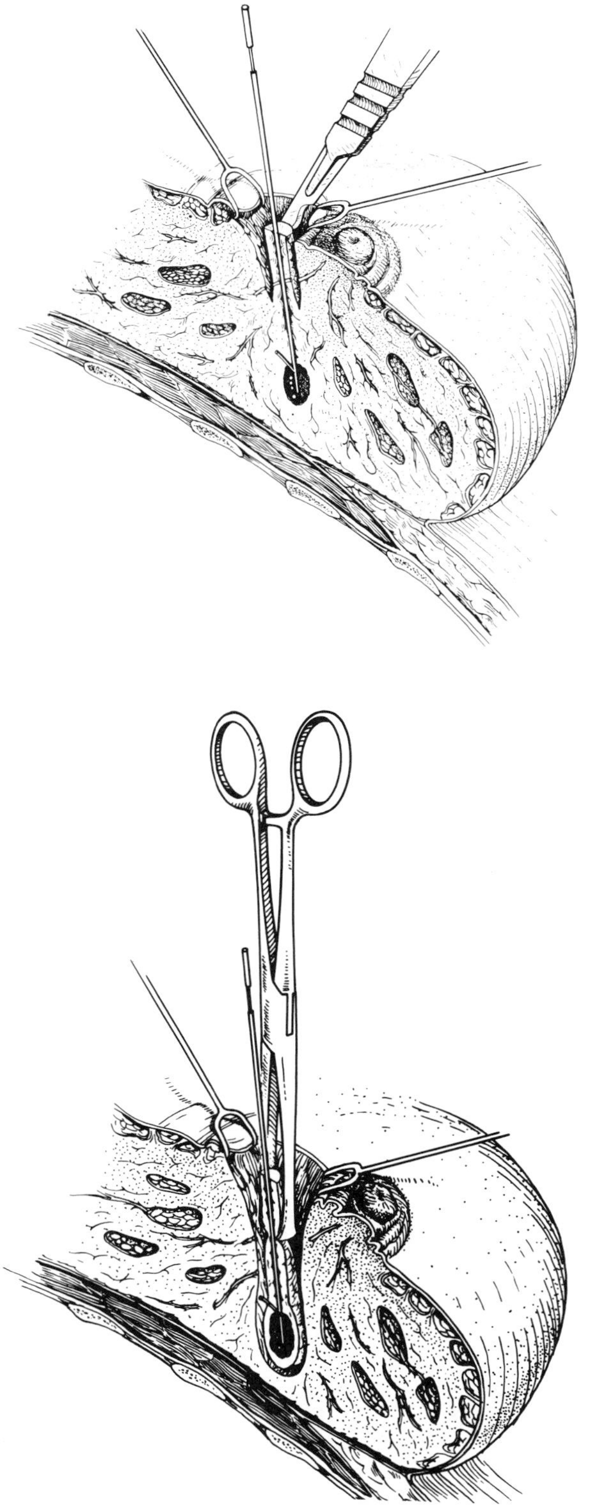

A

B

FIG. 14-32. Needle localization biopsy: the lesion is "localized" on the mammogram immediately before surgery. *A.* The needle serves as a guide to perform the biopsy, with development of tissue planes circumferential and parallel to the localization wire. *B.* Controlled dissection of the wire, with the suspicious lesion incorporated in the dissection. Specimen radiography confirms excision of the suspicious, nonpalpable mammographically identified lesion.

Incisional and Excisional Biopsies. Both techniques procure suspicious breast tissue submitted for microscopic examination. The *incisional technique* is indicated for patients with large ($\geq$ 4 cm) primary lesions for whom preoperative chemotherapy and/or radiation therapy is desirable. The incisional technique for large lesions should carefully incise tissues that are not necrotic to permit histologic and hormonal receptor analyses. Tissue procured from both incisional and excisional techniques should be obtained with the cold scalpel because electrocautery may distort histologic features of the tumor and possibly invalidate tissue levels of hormonal receptors.

Excisional biopsy implies removal of the entire lesion and generally a margin of normal breast parenchyma surrounding the suspicious lesion. The surgeon should avoid transection or disruption of the lesion for fear of tumor implantation. When the volume of tissue excised is small (< 1 cm^3) permanent histologic sections should be planned as it may be difficult pathologically to differentiate an invasive carcinoma from severe atypia or in situ disease on frozen section specimens. Both incisional and excisional biopsies can be closed in layers with absorbable sutures.

Planning Incisions. Figure 14-33 documents nonradial approaches for cosmetically acceptable scars of the breast. Radial incisions in the upper halves of the breast are ill-advised owing to scar contracture and asymmetric displacement of the nipple-areola and parenchyma. Incisions should be cosmetically designed, since approximately 70 percent of the biopsies confirm benign (proliferative and nonproliferative) disease. Lines of tension in the skin of the breast (Langer's lines) are generally concentric with the nipple (see Fig. 14-33). Incisions that parallel these lines generally result in thin, cosmetically acceptable scars. It is important to keep incisions within the boundaries of potential incisions for future mastectomy or wide-local excision that may be required for definitive treatment (Fig. 14-34). The most cosmetically acceptable scars result from circumareolar (curvilinear) incisions. Centrally located subareolar lesions are best approached in this manner.

Biopsy is best performed with a scalpel rather than electrocautery. Hormonal receptor profiles should be obtained from index tumor tissue. Use of residual tumor from the mastectomy specimen for ER/PR data may provide invalid hormone receptors, especially when warm ischemia time is prolonged in the course of the procedure.

Following scalpel removal of the lesion, electrocautery of bleeding sites or absorbable suture ligatures achieve hemostasis. Wound drainage with soft rubber Penrose drains (one-quarter inch) is optional. Although closure of the breast tissue defect is not mandatory, we recommend closure with interrupted 2-0 or 3-0 absorbable chromic, gut, or polygycolic sutures. Subcutaneous tissues can be closed with 3-0 or 4-0 absorbable sutures. A running subcuticular suture of the skin using 5-0 synthetic suture is performed, followed by Steri-Strip approximation of the defect. A light occlusive dressing is applied.

For most palpable and nonpalpable breast masses, local anesthesia and sedation incur minimal morbidity and no mortality. When general anesthesia is required for biopsy of a suspicious breast mass, a full work-up with clinical staging and plans to implement comprehensive therapy should be completed before the procedure to avoid a secondary operation. If needle localization is required, the operating room personnel must arrange, preoperatively, for *specimen radiography* to be performed as soon as the tissue is procured. In the case of a suspicious lesion, an informed consent for the previously agreed treatment should be obtained; if

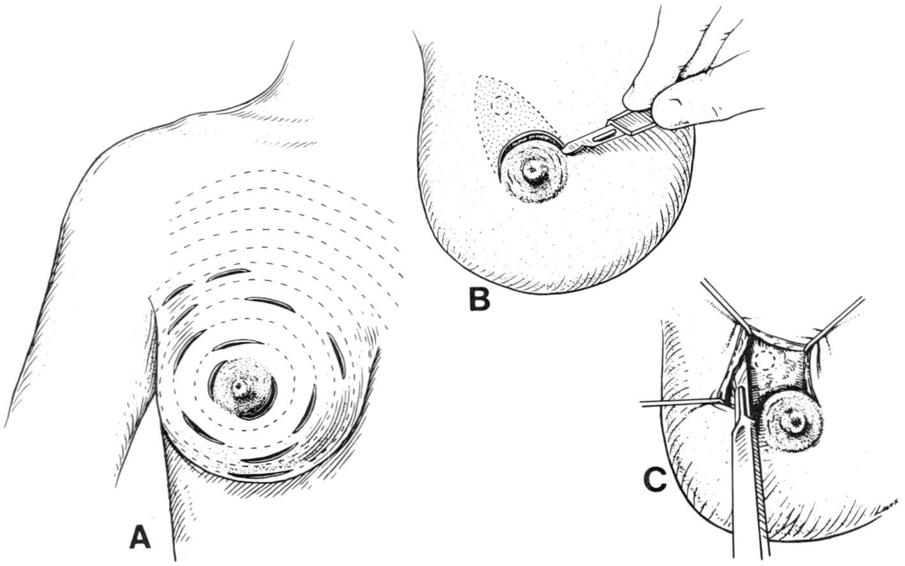

FIG. 14-33. Recommended locations for breast biopsy incisions. Thin skin flaps must be avoided to ensure cosmetically contoured and viable tissues about the areola.

frozen section confirms an invasive neoplasm, this allows the surgeon to proceed with definitive therapy. Following biopsy excision of breast tissue, three dimensions of the tumor should be carefully marked (suture or clips) and recorded; the surgeon should orient the pathologist to these findings if subsequent margins are questioned on final pathologic review.

Therapeutic Options. The past three decades have witnessed significant progress in multimodality therapy for the treatment of breast cancer and have allowed integration of these modalities to enhance survival and, in appropriate patients, to utilize conservation surgical principles. In addition, large breast cancers (> 3 cm) with matted axillary metastases are usually treated with preoperative chemotherapy to initiate a cytoreductive effect for the index tumor and the metastases. This approach allows the surgeon to complete a planned mastectomy without the use of skin grafts. Following mastectomy, irradiation to the chest wall, internal mammary and supraclavicular nodes will eradicate residual microscopic disease in the skin flap or regional nodes outside the operative field. This combination multimodal approach enhances local-

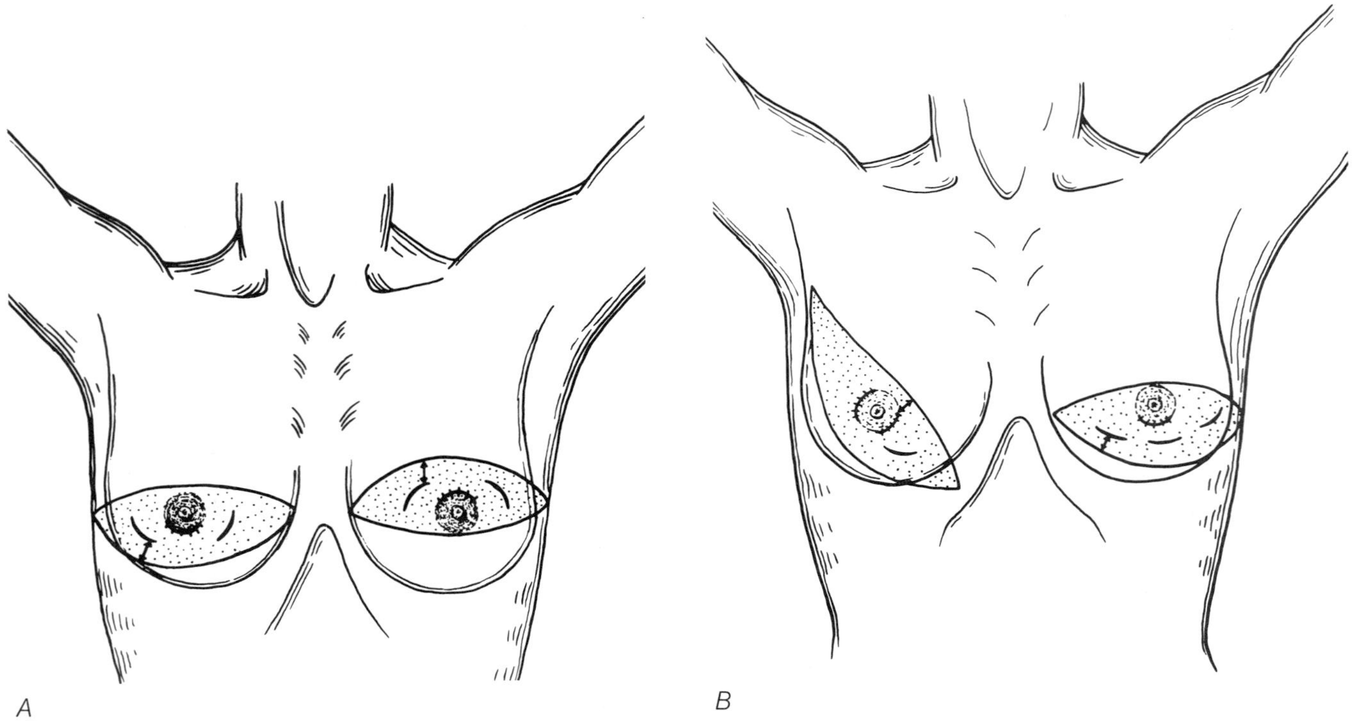

FIG. 14-34. Incisions for breast biopsy placed within the boundaries of skin flaps. Mastectomy incisions are designed at least 3 cm from the margins of the breast biopsy (*arrows*).

regional control of the advanced primary and has the additional benefit that potential systemic metastases will be treated with the preoperative chemotherapy.

The therapeutic objective of the surgeon and the radiation therapist is local-regional control; the objective of the medical oncologist is control of systemic disease. While cytotoxic agents, especially in combination, are effective for breast cancer metastases, *complete eradication* of documented metastasis is theoretically impossible due to the log-kill cytokinetics of chemotherapeutics. A small fraction of cells that enter the G_0 phase outside the cell cycle and are nonreplicating will potentially develop resistance or become refractory when exposed to these cytotoxic agents. Prospective trials in North America and Europe have allowed the clinician to predict control rates, survival rates, and prevailing toxicities. It is the integration of surgery, radiation therapy, and chemotherapy that has presently achieved the unprecedented response rates afforded patients with this disease.

Therapy of Early Breast Cancer and In Situ Disease

Adenocarcinomas of the breast in which the diameter is < 5 cm, limited to the lateral aspect of the breast, and with involvement of the pectoral fascial or skin fixation (T1a, T2a) are often treated by surgery alone, provided lymph node metastases are absent in the pathology specimen. Ductal and lobular carcinoma in situ do not represent invasive lesions and, therefore, do not have nodal metastases. These are also treatable by surgery alone, and in most clinics axillary node dissections are not performed. By contrast, when lymphatic metastases are evident pathologically and when the adenocarcinoma is medially or centrally positioned in the breast, the combination of surgery and postoperative RT is often utilized to ensure local and regional chest wall control.

LCIS. LCIS is considered a *marker* for increased risk rather than an inevitable *precursor* of invasive disease. The goal of observation is to detect subsequent invasive cancers that apparently develop in a minority of these persons. In that circumstance bilateral mastectomy will have a high probability of cure. There is no demonstrable benefit to widely excising LCIS and obtaining clear margins if nonoperative observation is chosen because the disease is assumed to diffusely involve all breast tissue as well as the contralateral breast.

A 5 percent rate of associated invasive carcinoma and a high rate of multicentricity and bilaterality represent the major arguments that support operative therapy of the disease. Routine bilateral mastectomy for LCIS appears to be an aggressive radical approach for a lesion that has a low risk potential. Routine contralateral biopsy in the absence of standard indications is not justified because the likelihood of identifying a lesion requiring therapy (i.e., invasive carcinoma or DCIS) is minimal and the clinical significance of other foci of LCIS is negligible. If operation is chosen, anything less than total mastectomy is inappropriate because the disease process is diffuse and often bilateral. In some instances bilateral mastectomy and reconstruction are applicable. The incidence of axillary node metastasis is generally less than 1 percent; routine dissection is not advised, but sampling of level I nodes in conjunction with the mastectomy adds virtually no morbidity to the procedure.

DCIS. For many decades unilateral mastectomy has been used for this lesion. Mastectomy is still considered the ''gold'' standard against which lesser procedures must be evaluated. In combined data from seven series, a total of 387 women with DCIS were treated with mastectomy; a local recurrence rate of only 3.1 percent and a mortality of 2.3 percent were demonstrated. Ipsilateral therapy is adequate because the overall incidence of occult disease (10 to 15 percent) is essentially equivalent to that for invasive carcinoma. Breast reconstruction can be performed at the time of the ipsilateral mastectomy.

The excellent results achieved with breast-sparing therapy of invasive disease have led to its use for DCIS. Rosner et al. showed that wedge resection of DCIS was equivalent to mastectomy with regard to overall survival. Follow-up intervals of up to 14 years for DCIS treated by local excision alone suggest local recurrence rates that range from 10 to 63 percent. Lagios et al. and Gump et al. note that recurrence is greatest for palpable tumors of large size (> 25 mm), when the criteria for confirmation of pathologically clear margins are less rigorously applied and the histology is the comedo type. Recurrences are most often noted within the original biopsy site, implicating inadequate marginal clearance rather than intrinsic biologic behavior of DCIS. The only randomized clinical trial comparing local excision alone versus local excision *with* radiation therapy for DCIS demonstrated a significant reduction in local recurrence (7 versus 23 percent) with the addition of irradiation. The mean follow-up (only 39 months) and the large size of the tumors in these patients suggest that firm conclusions cannot be drawn. Some of these problems are currently being addressed in the National Surgical Adjuvant Breast Project (NSABP) B-17 comparing segmental mastectomy alone with segmental mastectomy plus irradiation for DCIS. This trial, however, will not answer the crucial question of whether breast-sparing therapy for DCIS is comparable with mastectomy.

An additionally important issue with use of breast-sparing treatment for DCIS is that over one-half of all recurrences are invasive. Studies suggest that local recurrence following conservation treatment may be successfully treated with ''salvage mastectomy,'' a technique that does not carry the ominous prognosis documented following recurrence after mastectomy. Other studies suggest that local/regional recurrence in this setting may result in diminished survival. In the absence of conclusive evidence, caution is warranted as safety and efficacy of breast-sparing therapy for DCIS are less certain. Until data are available from ongoing prospective trials, it appears prudent to offer mastectomy for lesions that suggest a substantial risk of local/regional recurrence and reduced survival (palpable mass > 25 mm, comedo histology, extensive multicentricity, multifocality, high nuclear grade, negative ER/PR, aneuploid DNA pattern, high proliferative index, etc.). Breast-sparing therapy may be offered to women with DCIS when uncertainties and risks are fully discussed. Mastectomy is recommended when attempts at wide local excision reveal extensive foci of residual DCIS and when margins cannot be cleared pathologically. We continue to recommend postoperative irradiation following conservation treatment. No role currently exists for use of cytotoxic chemotherapy in this disease. Axillary nodal dissection beyond Level I is generally not recommended in view of the low yield of positive nodes (< 2 percent). Comprehensive lifelong surveillance is indicated for the contralateral breast in women previously treated for DCIS.

Stages I and II Breast Cancer. In the United States in 1972, 48 percent of patients were reported to have had a Halsted-type radical mastectomy; only 3 percent of patients underwent the

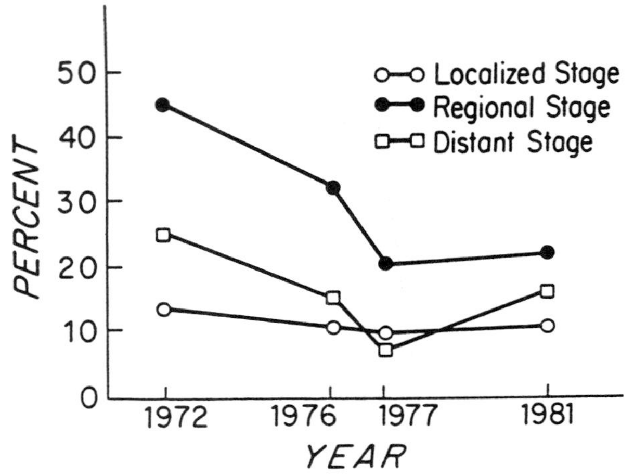

FIG. 14-35. Trends in the use of radiotherapy from 1972 to 1981 as reported in the 1982 National Survey of Carcinoma of the Breast in the United States by the American College of Surgeons. (From: *Wilson RE, Donegan WL, et al: 1984, with permission.*)

procedure in 1981. Trends in the application of radiation therapy showed a dramatic alteration in application from 1972 to 1981 (Fig. 14-35). Trends for chemotherapy are seen in Fig. 14-36. The proportion of patients at all stages reported to have received irradiation decreased from 33 percent in 1972 to 18 percent in 1981. This trend was coincident with the introduction of effective adjuvant and systemic chemotherapy. Application of multimodal chemotherapy alone has increased from 7 percent in 1972 to 22.9 percent in 1981. This exponential increase in the application of chemotherapy was limited to patients with regional and distant sites of diseases. Currently the use of adjuvant therapy for treatment of localized disease (Stages O and I) is increasing.

Evaluation of Modified Radical Mastectomy

These reports note variations in survivorship at 5 and 10 years for Stages I and II disease. In the American College of Surgeons Survey conducted in 1982, 5-year survival rates by stage, type of treatment, and type of adjuvant therapy were evaluated. Similar survival rates for patients with localized disease were observed for treatment by partial mastectomy alone and by partial mastectomy *plus* irradiation to either the breast, the axilla, or both. Five-year survival rates for patients treated by modified radical mastectomy technique were equivalent to those treated by the Halsted radical mastectomy. Wilson et al. noted that survival rates were also similar for those who received additional irradiation therapy or chemotherapy with either of the two procedures.

There has been a transition for curative surgical procedures used by American surgeons from the Halsted radical to the modified radical procedure. This transition was apparent at the time of the 1977 survey reported by Nemoto et al. and a 1981 analysis confirmed that the vast majority of patients treated had a modified rather than a radical mastectomy (77 percent versus 3 percent). This change was based on the conclusion that extirpation of the pectoralis major muscle is not essential to provide local/regional control for Stages I and II disease. Also, either the modified radical mastectomy or the Halsted procedure *alone* is an inadequate procedure for achieving local/regional control of TNM Stage III and Columbia Clinical Classification C and D tumors.

Subsequent prospective trials for modified radical mastectomy compared with the radical procedure have included the Manchester Trial, reported by Turner et al., and the University of Alabama Trial, reported by Maddox and associates. In both studies, recurrence rates for Stages I and II patients were comparable at 5 years. Disease-free survival was different at 10 years in the analysis by Maddox et al., and trends favored the more radical procedure.

Fisher, Saffer, and Fisher confirm that biologic rather than anatomic factors are responsible for metastatic dissemination. These investigators demonstrated that hematogenously carried tumor cells enter the lymph nodes; the authors concluded that hematopoietic and lymphatic systems are unified as routes of tumor cell dissemination. Because total (simple) mastectomy is designed to treat local or regional disease, some authors have proposed that the addition of the regional node dissection should *not* influence survival. These series have made comparisons of total mastectomy with and without radiation.

Five-year survival rates for clinical TNM Stage I tumors range from 51 to 78 percent; for clinical TNM Stage II cancers the range was 33.7 to 71 percent. Radical radiotherapy administered to the peripheral lymphatics in these nine series appeared to have had little overall benefit at 5 years. At 10 years the absolute survival appeared to be improved for patients who underwent radical irradiation of peripheral lymphatics. From the data it is evident that survival rates achieved with total mastectomy (± radiotherapy) are comparable with those obtained with radical mastectomy.

In the original report of the Cancer Research Campaign of the United Kingdom, Kyle and associates compared results of a "radical" therapeutic regimen (total mastectomy plus radiotherapy) with those of a conservative policy (total mastectomy alone) in a prospectively controlled study of 2268 patients. At the 5-year follow-up interval, although there was no evidence that routine postoperative radiation therapy was detrimental to wound repair, this modality conferred no additional benefit for survival or distant recurrence. The addition of radiotherapy, however, significantly reduced the incidence of local/regional recurrence. Further, a fourfold reduction in chest wall recurrence and a threefold reduction in supraclavicular recurrence was evident at 5 years in the treatment group. Similar trends were observed for recurrence in the operative site.

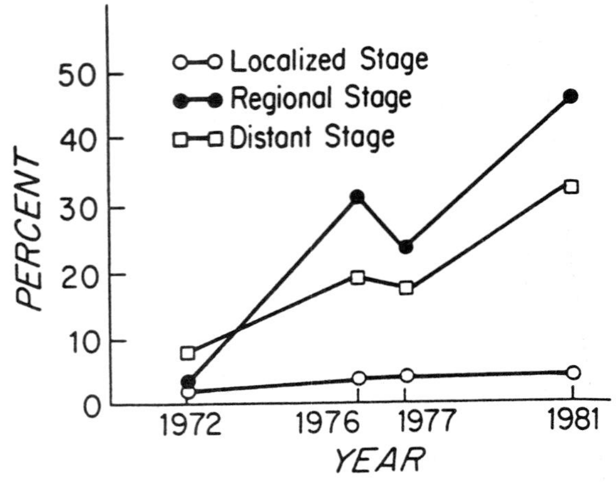

FIG. 14-36. Trends in the application of systemic chemotherapy from 1972 to 1981 as reported in the 1982 National Survey of Carcinoma of the Breast in the United States by the American College of Surgeons Survey. (From: *Wilson RE, Donegan WL, et al: 1984, with permission.*)

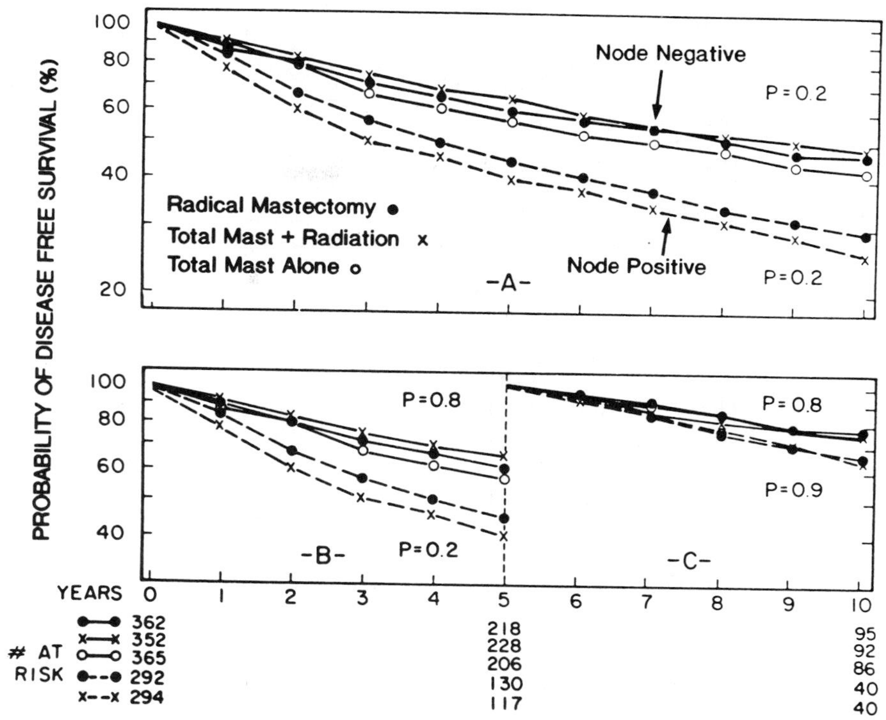

Survival Free of Disease through 10 Years (A), during the First 5 Years (B), and during the Second 5 Years for Patients Free of Disease at the End of the 5th Year (C).

FIG. 14-37. Disease-free survival for patients treated by radical mastectomy (*solid circle*), total mastectomy plus radiation (x), or total mastectomy alone (*open circle*). (From: *Fisher B, Redmond C, et al: 1985, with permission.*)

An identical trial was continued by Berstock and associates with follow-up ranging from 9 to 14 years (median 11.4). Analysis confirmed no significant difference in survival and distant recurrence between the two treatment groups. Prophylactic postoperative irradiation reduced the risk for development of local recurrence.

In the randomized trial conducted by Langlands, Prescott, and Hamilton, simple mastectomy and irradiation had overall survival equivalent to radical mastectomy. At 12 years follow-up, these authors confirmed that survival in the radical mastectomy treatment group was significantly better ($p < 0.05$), but only for those with clinical Stage I disease. There was a significant prolongation of survival after detection of recurrence in the radical mastectomy group ($p < 0.05$); this was greatest when local recurrence and distant metastases coincided ($p < 0.01$).

The National Surgical Adjuvant Breast Project B-04 trial conducted by Fisher and collaborators compared local and regional treatments of breast cancer. Life table estimates were obtained for 1665 women enrolled for a mean 120 months. This NSABP trial randomized patients with *clinically negative* axillae into three arms: (1) Halsted radical mastectomy (RM); (2) total mastectomy plus local/regional irradiation (TM + RT); or (3) total mastectomy alone (TM). Removal of axillary regional nodes was to be completed only when nodes became clinically positive. *Clinically node-positive* patients were treated with RM or TM + RT. Adjunctive chemotherapy was not given to patients in any of the three randomization arms.

For patients treated by total mastectomy and regional irradiation versus those treated by total mastectomy alone, no differences were observed between treatment groups for patients with clinically positive nodes or clinically negative nodes with respect to disease-free, distant disease-free, or overall survival at 10 years follow-up. Ten-year survival was approximately 57 percent for node-negative patients and 38 percent for node-positive. These investigators conclude that *variations of local and regional therapy were not important in determining survival of patients with breast cancer*. Further, results obtained at 5 years accurately predicted outcome at 10 years. Despite similarity in survival, chest wall recurrence was significantly greater at 10-year follow-up for Stage I patients treated with mastectomy alone (5.2 percent) versus patients treated with total mastectomy and radical irradiation (0.9 percent).

Figure 14-37 confirms that there was no significant difference ($p = 0.2$) in disease-free survival during the entire period of follow-up among groups of patients with *clinically negative nodes* treated by RM, TM + RT, or TM (panel A of Fig. 14-37). When disease-free survival was evaluated in the first and second 5-year periods of follow-up, Fisher and colleagues observed no differences among groups within the first 5 years following surgery (panel B). Panel C of Fig. 14-37 confirms no statistical differences in the probability of failure among the three groups during the *second* 5 years of follow-up ($p = 0.8$). For each group, approximately 75 percent of patients who were free of disease at the end of 5 years remained so at the end of the tenth year. Patients undergoing TM + RT also had a lower incidence of local and regional recurrence than did those in the other two treatment groups.

Figure 14-37 further confirms no significant differences in disease-free survival among patients treated with RM or TM + RT for individuals who presented with *clinically positive nodes* ($p = 0.2$). These data were consistent for the first and second 5-year

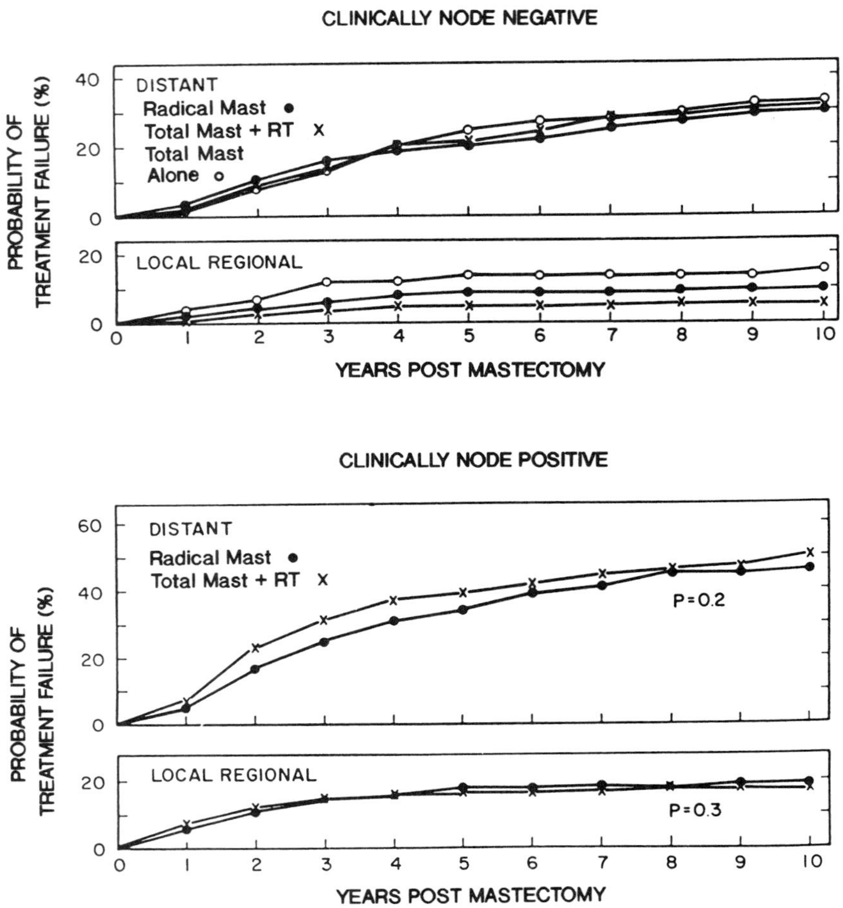

FIG. 14-38. Local or regional and distant treatment failures as the first evidence of disease in patients with clinically negative and positive nodes who were treated by radical mastectomy (*solid circle*), total mastectomy and radiation (x), or total mastectomy alone (*open circle*). (From: *Fisher B, Redmond C, et al: 1985, with permission.*)

intervals of follow-up. In this NSABP study, little difference between the two groups was observed with respect to occurrence of distant, local, or regional disease (Fig. 14-38).

Finally, Figure 14-39 relates the probability of survival for node-negative and node-positive patients. For node-negative patients among the three treatment groups, no significant differences were evident for distant disease-free or overall survival. These data also were confirmed for the two treatment groups with positive nodes. Approximately 75 percent of patients with negative nodes who were alive in the first 5 years of follow-up remained alive at 10 years. Approximately 65 percent of patients with positive nodes who lived 5 years survived an additional interval.

Figure 14-40 further confirms the relationship of treatment to survival according to tumor *location* in the NSABP B-04 study. For patients with clinically negative nodes in medial-central or laterally located tumors, no statistical differences ($p = 0.6$) were observed in outcome among the three treatment groups. For patients with clinically positive nodes, treatment was not observed to affect survival in those with lateral ($p = 0.8$) or medial-central tumors ($p = 0.3$). Thus, location of breast tumor does not influence prognosis, and irradiation of the internal mammary chain in patients with inner quadrant lesions does not improve survival. This study further reiterated the important principle that variations of local and regional treatment parameters have less importance in determining survival of the patient with breast cancer than originally presumed.

Mastectomy

Both the Halsted radical mastectomy and the Patey modified radical mastectomy necessitate en bloc resection of the breast, the axillary lymphatics, and overlying skin near the tumor with a 3-cm to 5-cm margin that ensures histologic clearance of the tumor. The Patey mastectomy acknowledges the importance of the complete axillary dissection and the anatomic necessity for preservation of the medial and lateral pectoral (anterior thoracic) nerves which may provide dual innervation to the pectoralis major. The Halsted mastectomy necessitates resection of the pectoralis major by virtue of size of the lesions (T2, T3, T4) that present with gross infiltration (fixation) of the skin or pectoralis major and for peripheral (high-lying) lesions near the clavicle in patients who are otherwise not candidates for irradiation. Major considerations for operations less extensive than the classic Halsted mastectomy are based on tissue preservation to enhance the cosmetic result. The modified radical mastectomy, with removal of the pectoralis minor muscle (Patey dissection), allows access to Level III nodes. The Patey modified technique is intended for lesions that cannot be removed with clear margins by segmental mastectomy and for lesions of large size (> T2, > 5 cm) in which cosmetic reconstruction and regional control cannot be accomplished. The modified radical technique is not intended for large tumors with evidence of skin or pectoral muscle fixation for which resection of the muscle is necessary to achieve adequate margins.

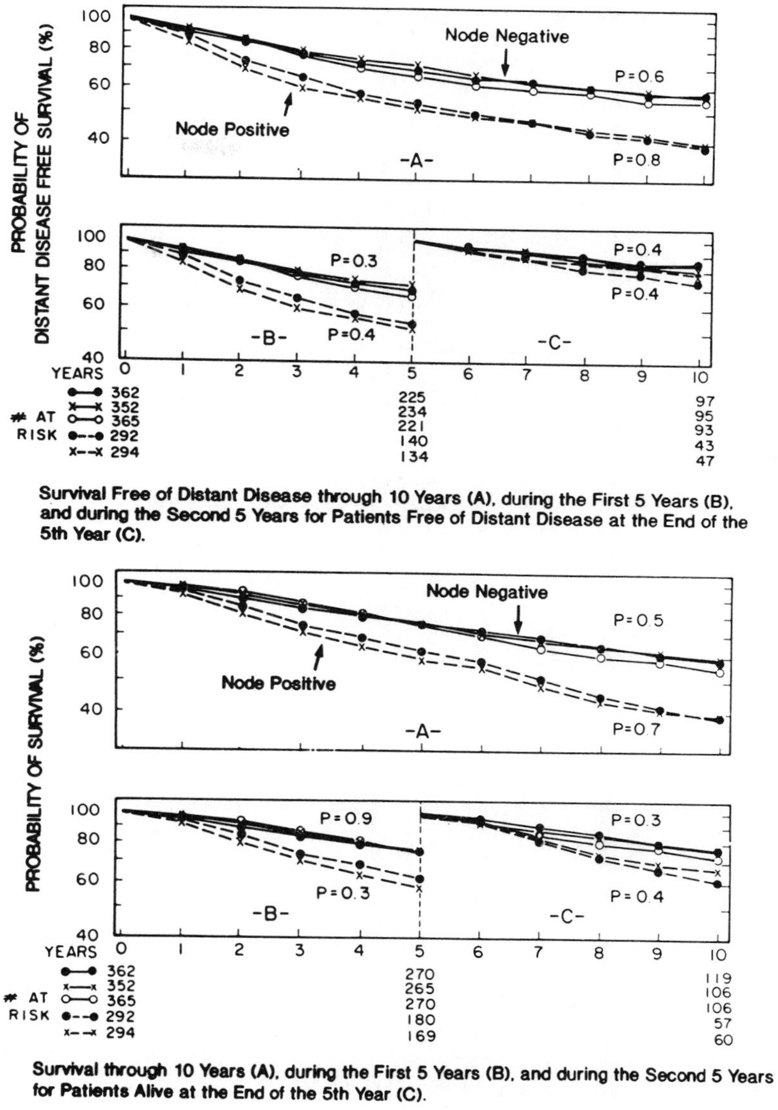

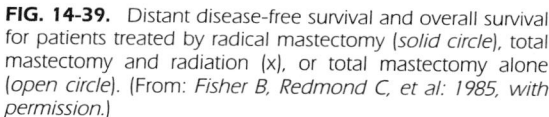

FIG. 14-39. Distant disease-free survival and overall survival for patients treated by radical mastectomy (*solid circle*), total mastectomy and radiation (x), or total mastectomy alone (*open circle*). (From: *Fisher B, Redmond C, et al: 1985, with permission.*)

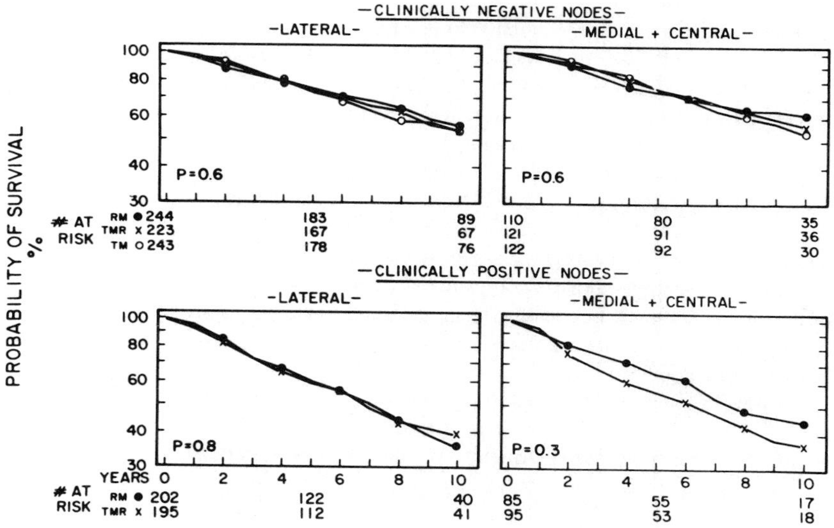

FIG. 14-40. Relation of treatment to survival according to tumor location. Patients were treated by radical mastectomy (*solid circle*), total mastectomy and radiation (x), or total mastectomy alone (*open circle*). (From: *Fisher B, Redmond C, et al: 1985, with permission.*)

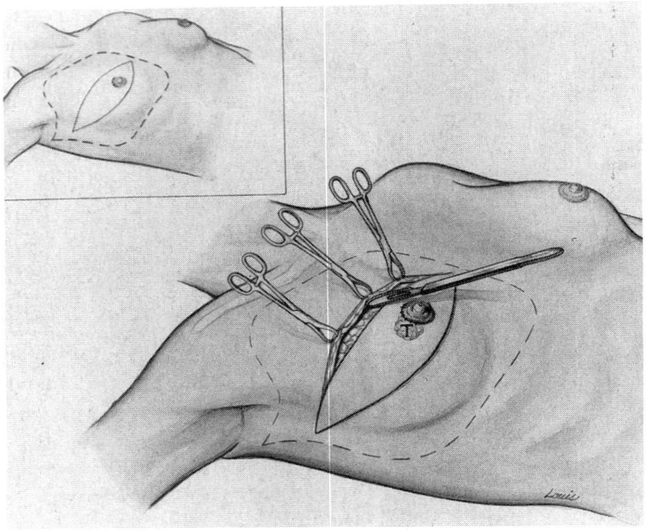

FIG. 14-41. *Inset:* Limits of the modified radical mastectomy. Flaps should be 7 to 8 mm in thickness, inclusive of the skin and tela subcutanea. (From: *Bland KI, Copeland EM III (eds): The Breast: Comprehensive Management of Benign and Malignant Diseases. Philadelphia, Saunders, 1991, Chap 29, p 616, with permission.*)

Both the Madden and Auchincloss mastectomies advocate preservation of *both* pectoralis major and minor muscles, thus allowing adequate access to Level II lymphatics with incomplete dissection (or preservation) of apical (Level III) nodes. These approaches (Figs. 14-41, 14-42, 14-43, 14-44) both require total mastectomy with at least partial axillary lymph node dissection. With limitation for dissection of the apical (subclavicular) nodal group, the Auchincloss and Madden procedures allow higher probability for preservation of the medial (anterior thoracic) pectoral nerve, which courses in the lateral neurovascular bundle of the axilla and commonly penetrates the pectoralis minor to supply the lateral border of the pectoralis major.

Regardless of the skin incisions chosen, the limits of the modified radical mastectomy are delineated *laterally* by the anterior margin of the latissimus dorsi muscle, medially by the midline of the sternum, *superiorly* by the subclavius muscle, and *inferiorly* by the caudal extension of the breast some 2 to 3 cm inferior to the inframammary fold (see Fig. 14-41, *inset*). The operator should be cognizant of the thoracodorsal nerve, whose origin is medial to the thoracodorsal artery and vein en route to innervation of the latissimus. With medial dissection, the operator encounters the chest wall deep in the medial axillary space and is able to identify the long thoracic nerve (respiratory nerve of Bell) in the deep investing fascia of the serratus anterior. This nerve is constant in its location anterior to the subscapularis muscle and is closely applied to this fascial compartment. Every effort should be made to preserve the long thoracic nerve; otherwise, permanent disability with a "winged" scapula and shoulder apraxia will follow denervation of the serratus anterior.

Following completion of the extirpation of breast tissue from the chest wall, the entire mastectomy specimen and axillary contents are submitted en bloc for pathologic analysis. Estrogen (ER) and progesterone receptor (PR) activity should be obtained on all pathologic breast cancer specimens to aid therapeutic planning of endocrine replacement treatment should metastatic disease occur. These receptors will guide future management for neoadjuvant therapy as well. Despite the importance of ER and PR activity to guide future therapies, processing of neoplastic tissue for pathologic examination, in all cases, must take precedence over determination of steroid receptor activity. Procurement of tissues for pathologic diagnosis and determination of qualitative and quantitative steroid receptor activity is best accomplished with the cold scalpel. This technique avoids the possibility of heat-induction artifact, tissue necrosis, cellular death, and temperature-dependent inactivation in steroid receptor activity and in procured tissues.

The responsibilities of the surgeon and the radiation therapist are to provide the patient with the greatest probability for control of chest wall disease and to ensure minimal morbidity and mortality related to the therapy. After complete dissection of the axilla for Levels I, II, and III nodes, axillary irradiation should *not* be used, as the incidence of lymphedema to the ipsilateral extremity is enhanced some six to eight fold with these combination modalities. Major lymphatics are removed surgically and residual lymphatic collaterals may be destroyed by irradiation. In addition, the axilla dissected for operable disease should not require irradiation following modified radical or radical mastectomy unless extracapsular involvement of the lymphatics or tumor implantation in soft tissues of the axilla is evident.

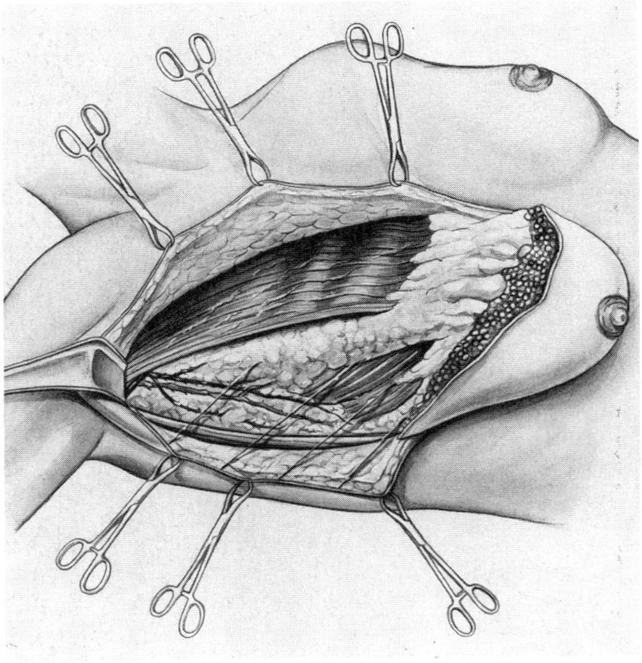

FIG. 14-42. The completed superior and inferior flap with breast parenchyma intact with the axillary tail of Spence and the axillary contents. The pectoralis major is completely cleared of its fascia en bloc with the breast parenchyma. The latissimus dorsi muscle has been dissected on its anterior surface to delineate the lateral boundary of dissection. Illustrated in this view is the cutaneous innervation of the skin of the lateral chest, axilla, and medial arm by intercostobrachial sensory nerves. (From: *Bland KI, Copeland EM III (eds): The Breast: Comprehensive Management of Benign and Malignant Diseases. Philadelphia, Saunders, 1991, Chap 29, p 618, with permission.*)

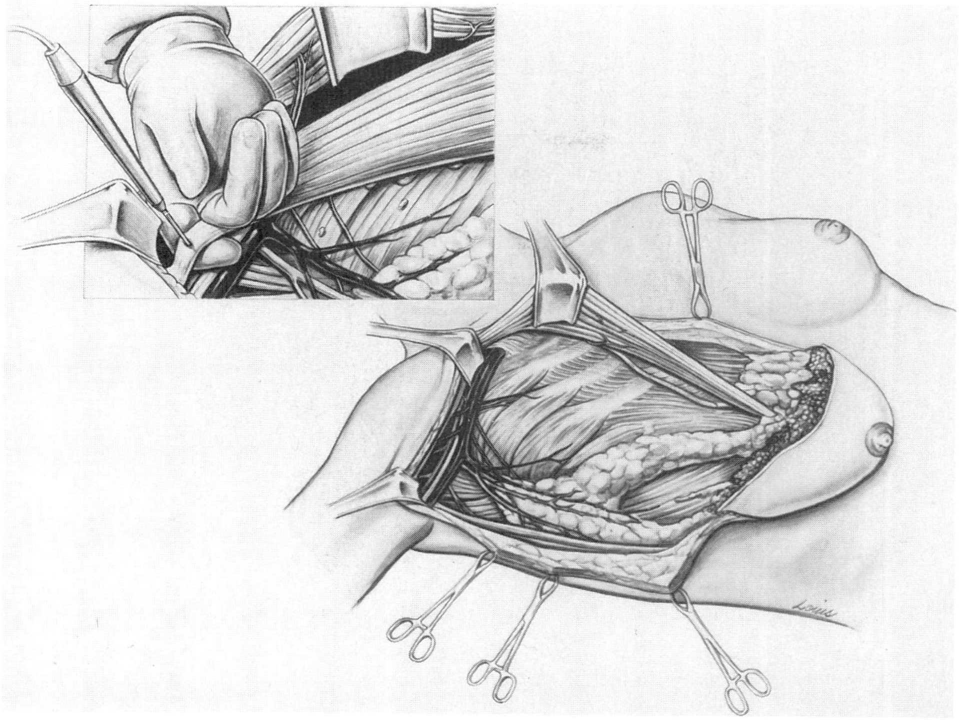

FIG. 14-43. *Inset:* Digital protection of the brachial plexus for division of the insertion of the pectoralis minor muscle on the coracoid process. Dissection commences lateral to medial, with complete visualization of the anterior and ventral aspects of the axillary vein. Dissection craniad to the axillary vein is inadvisable, for fear of damage to the brachial plexus and the infrequent observation of gross nodal tissue cephalic to the vein. Caudal to the vein, loose areolar tissue at the junction of the vein with the anterior margin of latissimus is swept inferomedially inclusive of the lateral (axillary) nodal group (Level I). Care is taken to preserve the neurovascular thoracodorsal artery, vein, and nerve in the deep axillary space. Lateral axillary nodal groups are retracted inferomedially and anterior to this bundle for dissection en bloc with the subscapular (Level I) nodal group. Preferentially, dissection commences superomedially before completion of dissection of the external mammary (Level I) nodal group. Superomedial dissection over the axillary vein allows extirpation of the central nodal group (Level II) and apical (subclavicular) Level III group. The superomedialmost extent of the dissection is the clavipectoral fascia (Halsted's ligament). This level of dissection with the Patey technique allows the surgeon to mark, with metallic clip or suture, the superiormost extent of dissection. All loose areolar tissue just inferior to the apical nodal group is swept off the chest wall, leaving the fascia of the serratus anterior intact. With dissection parallel to the long thoracic nerve (respiratory nerve of Bell), the deep investing serratus fascia is incised, and the nerve is preserved. (From: *Bland KI, Copeland EM III (eds): The Breast: Comprehensive Management of Benign and Malignant Diseases. Philadelphia, Saunders, 1991, Chap 29, p 619, with permission.*)

Conservation Surgery

Conservation surgery of the breast implies the resection of minimal volumes of diseased breast tissue to achieve control rates equivalent to that accomplished by mastectomy. It has the goal of preservation of cosmesis and function. These procedures are variously termed *segmental resection, lumpectomy,* or *tylectomy*.

The breast may be preserved when adequate removal of all primary breast cancer can be accomplished without incision into cancerous tissue in appropriately selected patients. In all circumstances, frozen-section evaluation and permanent-section analyses of resected margins should be performed to ensure that all breast cancer has been removed en bloc with the specimen. Margins that harbor residual breast cancer warrant further excision. If clearance of tumor margins is not possible, or if multicentric disease is evident, total mastectomy is appropriate.

After reconstruction of the peripheral breast tissues in the operative site, sampling of ipsilateral axillary lymphatics is completed. To determine the necessity for adjuvant chemotherapy, the status of the axillary lymphatics must be determined. Adequate sampling is accomplished via a curvilinear incision between the lateral border of the pectoralis major and latissimus dorsi muscles 4 to 6 cm below the apex of the axilla. Lateral axillary contents that would be removed with an extended simple mastectomy (Level I) are taken with approximately 10 to 15 lymph nodes in the sampling. This volume of lymph nodes assures adequate sampling that is indicative of the regional nodal status. Some clinics demand complete axillary dissection of Level I through Level III. Subsequent irradiation to the axilla should be avoided to obviate lymphedema of the ipsilateral extremity.

Indications for lumpectomy, axillary sampling, and comprehensive irradiation to the ipsilateral breast include (1) a small

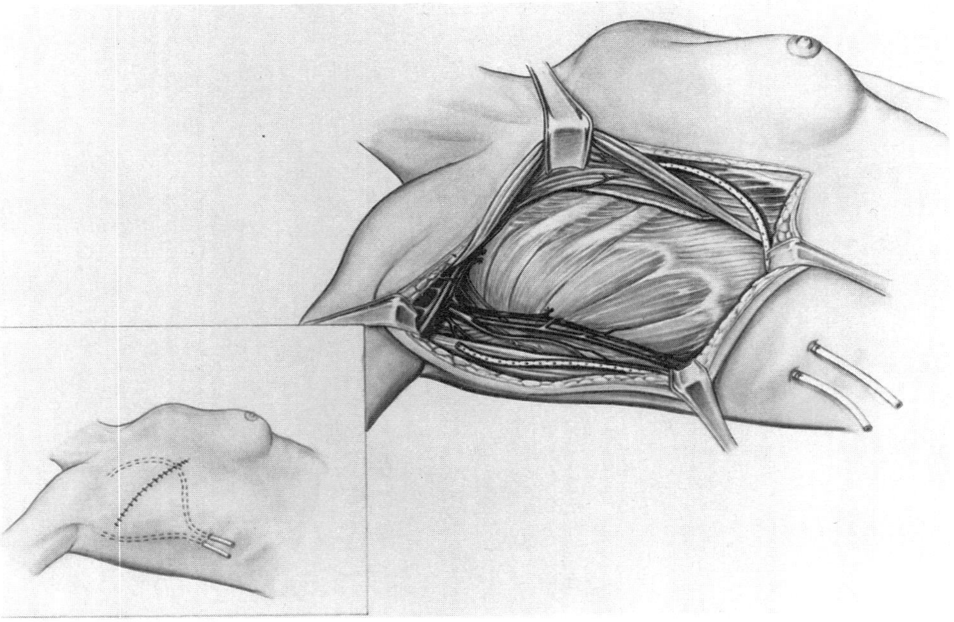

FIG. 14-44. The completed Patey axillary dissection variant of the modified radical technique. The dissection is inclusive of the pectoralis minor muscle from origin to insertion on ribs 2 to 5. Both medial and lateral pectoral nerves are preserved to ensure innervation of the lateral and medial heads, respectively, of the pectoralis major. With completion of the procedure, remaining portions of this muscle are swept en bloc with the axillary contents to be inclusive of Rotter's interpectoral and the retropectoral groups. *Inset:* Following copious irrigation, closed-suction Silastic catheters (18 to 20 French) are positioned via stab incisions placed in the inferior flap at the anterior axillary line. The lateral catheter is placed approximately 2 cm inferior to the axillary vein. The superior, longer catheter, placed via the medial stab wound, is positioned in the superomedial aspect of the defect anterior to the pectoralis major muscle beneath the skin flap. The wound is closed in two layers with 2-0 absorbable synthetic sutures placed in subcutaneous planes. The skin is optionally closed with subcuticular 4-0 synthetic absorbable sutures or stainless steel staples. (From: *Bland KI, Copeland EM III (eds): The Breast: Comprehensive Management of Benign and Malignant Diseases. Philadelphia, Saunders, 1991, Chap 29, p 621, with permission.)*

breast cancer ($<$ 4 cm in transverse diameter); (2) clinically negative axillary lymphatics; (3) breast volume of adequate size to allow a uniform dosage of irradiation; and (4) a radiation therapist experienced with the technique. Excessive irradiation doses or nonhomogeneous distribution of the radiotherapeutic field may initiate painful, edematous, ulcerative and/or fibrotic residual breast tissue. As experience with this treatment modality has increased, the indications have been extended successfully to larger-breasted women and to women with small, but clinically positive, axillary lymph nodes.

It is the surgeon's responsibility to ensure complete removal of the cancer within the breast. If viable cancer cells remain within the breast parenchyma at the periphery of the resection, they will be incorporated into the desmoplastic response of scarring and become poorly oxygenated. Marginally or poorly oxygenated anoxic cells entrapped within scar tissue may not be eradicated by irradiation; recurrence of breast cancer in the scar would be anticipated. Data confirm that clearance of the surgical margins of the index lesion is required to reduce local recurrence and to enhance cure and control rates. It is the practice of most North American and European clinics to reexcise scar in such patients and complete the axillary sampling procedure. If reexcision with histologically negative margins is not obtainable, these patients are best treated by total mastectomy. Approximately one-half of patients who have had scars reexcised were determined to have viable cancer cells present in the wound margins after what was originally deemed an adequate segmental mastectomy. For patients in whom reexcision of the scar has not been advocated, external beam irradiation boosted by implantation of iridium (^{192}Ir) needles in the area of the scar has been used.

Conservation surgery for patients who meet the above criteria results in long-term disease control and survival data that are equivalent to those achieved in patients treated by modified radical mastectomy. The important contributions of Fisher et al. for protocol B-06 of the NSABP are detailed in Table 14-9. The long-term effects of irradiating the breast are not yet known, and patients wishing conservation surgery should be apprised of the uncertainty of the prolonged effects of radiobiologic injury. Properly done, lumpectomy, axillary sampling, and comprehensive irradiation to the remaining breast can give a very satisfactory functional and cosmetic result. Breast cancer cannot be considered cured, however, by lumpectomy alone. Several studies have shown the disease to be potentially multicentric within the ipsilateral breast, requiring irradiation for sterilization of residual foci of invasive microscopic disease.

If lymphatics removed at the time of axillary sampling confirm histologic metastases, *adjuvant chemotherapy* should be considered in the postoperative period. For approximately 20 to 30 percent of patients, clinically negative axillary lymph nodes will be proved pathologically positive. In many clinics, the concomitant

Table 14-9
NSABP Protocol B-06. Comparison of Total Mastectomy, Lumpectomy, and Lumpectomy Plus Radiation Therapy According to Nodal Status Life Table Estimates 8 Years After Surgery

Treatment Group	*Disease-free Survival (%)*	*Distant Disease-free Survival (%)*	*Survival (%)*
NETATIVE-NODE PTS.			
Total mastectomy (N = 366)	65.5 ± 3.3*	73.8 ± 3.2	78.7 ± 3.2
Lumpectomy (N = 392)	60.7 ± 2.8	69.6 ± 2.6	76.6 ± 2.8
Lumpectomy and irradiation (N = 399)	65.6 ± 3.3	70.7 ± 3.2	82.9 ± 2.3
POSITIVE-NODE PTS.[†]			
Total mastectomy (N = 224)	45.5 ± 4.0	50.7 ± 4.2	59.9 ± 4.1
Lumpectomy (N = 244)	41.6 ± 4.1	49.1 ± 4.6	60.3 ± 4.5
Lumpectomy and irradiation (N = 230)	46.6 ± 4.1	53.1 ± 3.9	68.3 ± 3.9

*Mean ± S.E.

[†]Values are adjusted for the number of positive nodes (1 to 3, 4 to 9, or ≥).

SOURCE: Modified from Fisher B, Redmond C, et al: *N Engl J Med* 320(13):822, 1989, with permission.

administration of adjuvant therapy (CMF—cyclophosphamide, methotrexate, and 5-fluorouracil) with comprehensive irradiation is being used with minimal toxic systemic effects.

QU.A.RT. Procedure (Quadrantectomy, Axillary Dissection, and Radiation Therapy). Quadrantectomy implies that a quadrant of the breast that harbors carcinoma is resected. Resection of an entire quadrant in a small- or medium-sized breast can produce an unacceptable cosmetic result. This procedure has yielded excellent local control and survival results when followed by radiation therapy and axillary dissection. The technique aims to remove an entire quadrant of the breast, including the skin and superficial pectoralis fascia. The objective is radical removal of the primary tumor and potential foci of infiltration via en bloc excision of one-fourth of the entire breast. Veronesi notes that it is difficult to do an appropriate operation for tumors whose diameter exceeds 2 to 3 cm unless the breast is large. The segmental mastectomy, however, has been applied in moderate-size breasts for lesions as great as 4 cm, so long as 1-cm margins are obtained. The QU.A.RT. procedure provides a more radical resection (≥ 2 cm from the biopsy incision) of the tumor.

Veronesi suggests that the axillary dissection be performed in continuity; excision of a previously made biopsy incision allows adequate exposure of the axilla. The en bloc operation is generally performed when the primary tumor is situated in the upper outer quadrants close to the axilla. For index lesions in other quadrants, quadrantectomy is performed separately from the axillary dissection, which incorporates Levels I through III nodes (Figs. 14-45 and 14-46). Comprehensive irradiation of the intact breast is an important component of therapy. A dose of 50 Gy is delivered through two opposing tangential fields with high-energy photons (cobalt unit or a 6 MeV linear accelerator), and another dose of 10 Gy is given with orthovoltage radiotherapy as a booster to the skin surrounding the scar.

Figure 14-47 depicts equivalent disease-free survival curves for the QU.A.RT. procedure and the classic Halsted radical mastectomy. These data apply to node-negative and node-positive disease confirmed at axillary dissection (Fig. 14-48).

Future Developments. Prospective trials conducted by Veronesi for the QU.A.RT. procedure and Fisher et al. of the NSABP for segmental mastectomy indicate that conservation surgery results in equivalent disease-free and overall survival compared with more radical procedures. Veronesi makes two important conclusions about the value of these procedures: (1) with specific reference to QU.A.RT., the operation appears to be safe and allows preservation of the majority of breast substance and form and (2) the patient treated with *inadequate* local-regional

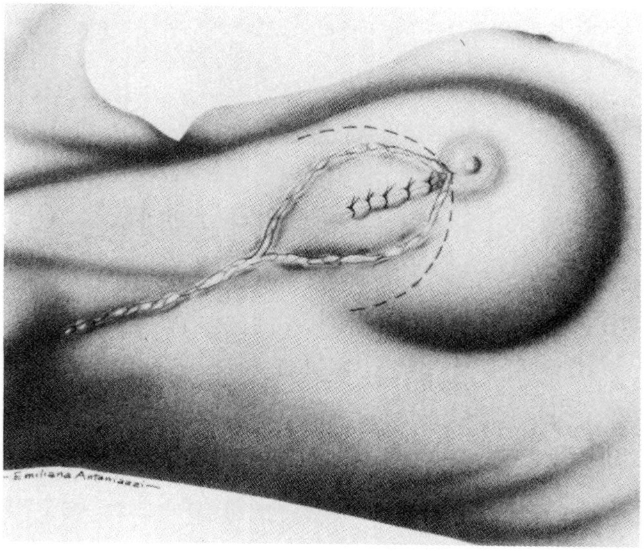

FIG. 14-45. Quadrantectomy and in-continuity axillary dissection lines of skin incision. (From: *Veronesi U: 1991, Chap 29, p 632, with permission.*)

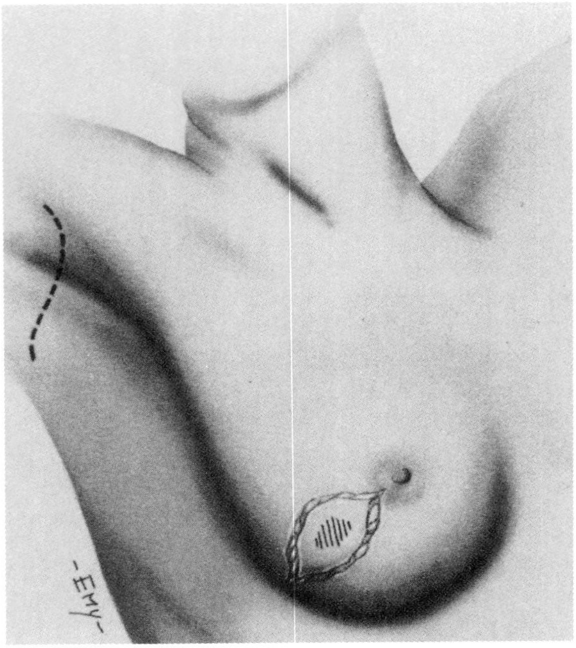

FIG. 14-46. Quadrantectomy and axillary dissection with separate incision. (From: *Veronesi U: 1991, Chap 29, p 633, with permission.*)

surgery or *inadequate* radiotherapy may be exposed to an excess of local-regional recurrences which may, thus, convert to a diminished overall and disease-free survival.

International trends favor a reduction in radical procedures, with increasing selection of breast conservation. An increasing realization has emerged that lumpectomy *without* radiation may be suitable for an undefined proportion of patients with early breast cancer. At 8 years, the B-06 protocol of the NSABP demonstrated no statistically significant reduction in survival (distant disease-free or overall) for patients who had local excision *alone* compared with those who underwent local excision with radiation therapy for cancers $\leq$ 4 cm in transverse diameter. The trend for management of this disease over the past decade has been toward selective breast-sparing procedures with restriction of radiation therapy (i.e., elimination of irradiation to axillary, supraclavicular, and internal mammary node sites), and more liberal application of systemic adjuvant therapy.

We can expect the subset of patients treated by local excision *without* irradiation to increase. These patients will be the product of early detection, definition of risk for local recurrence, pathologic analysis, and the emerging application of the adjuvant antiestrogen tamoxifen. Expanded therapeutic regimens will invoke the application of sophisticated genetic, biochemical, and pathologic prognostic indicators to verify and predict recurrence following conservative management parameters.

Limitations. Kurtz et al. and Recht et al. identified patients at risk for failure after breast-preserving techniques. There is every expectation that recurrence after conservation surgery might be reduced to approximately 3 percent for the majority of patients who do not have an *extensive intraductal component* (*EIC*) and who are older than thirty-five years (Fig. 14-49). Certain morphologic and histochemical features allow the selection of patients in whom breast conservation can be performed with increasing confidence: (1) mammographically detected lesions; (2) decreasing size of the primary invasive cancer; and (3) low S-phase component of DNA flow cytometry.

Despite the importance of breast preservation to enhance cosmesis and allow control and survival rates equivalent to radical procedures, certain women will desire total mastectomy for a variety of economic and psychosocial reasons. Patients less concerned about the cosmetic or functional importance of the breast may desire total mastectomy as the most expeditious and desirable therapeutic option, especially with the economic morbidity and inconvenience of irradiation therapy. Women who have EIC within and surrounding the index lesion should undergo total mastectomy because of the very high local failure rates in the remaining irradiated breast. This high local recurrence rate for EIC was observed despite extensive lumpectomy and evidence of pathologically negative margins with frozen section control of the inked specimen.

For large lesions that occupy the central, subareolar portion of the breast, margins sufficient to achieve local control require sacri-

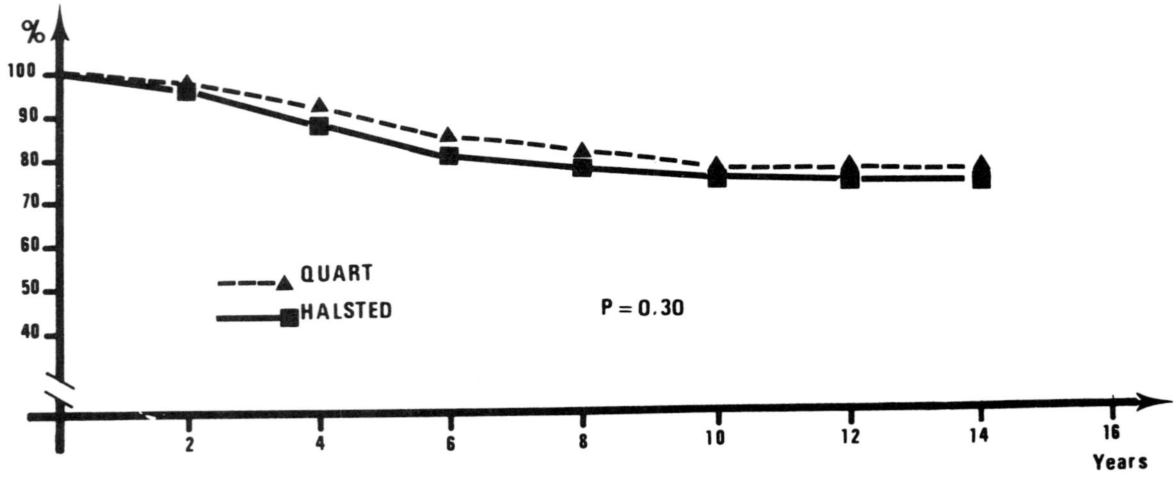

FIG. 14-47. Disease-free survival curves according to type of treatment (Milan Trial I). (From: *Veronesi U: 1991, Chap 38, p 806, with permission.*)

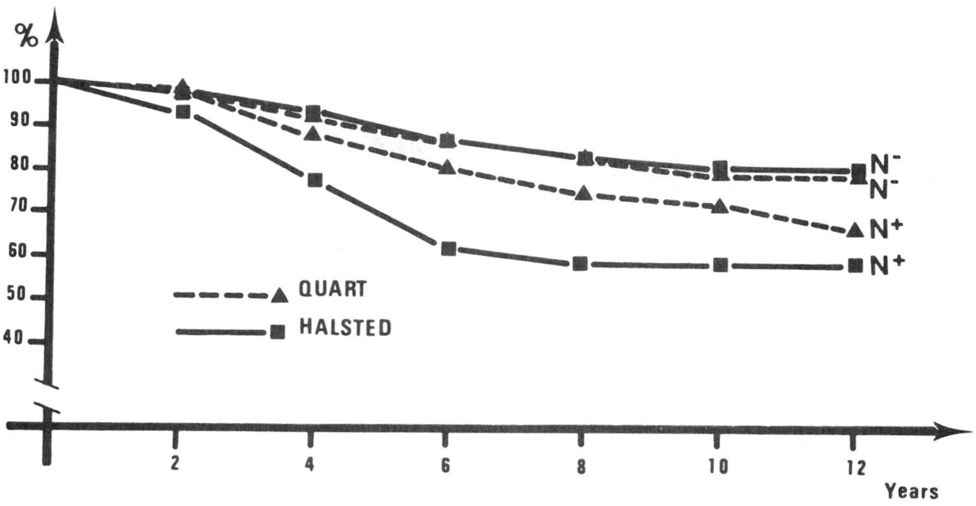

FIG. 14-48. Disease-free survival curves of patients treated with Halsted mastectomy and with quadrantectomy, axillary dissection, and radiotherapy (QU.A.RT.), according to absence (N−) or presence (N+) of axillary node metastases (Milan Trial I). (From: *Veronesi U: 1991, Chap 38, p 807, with permission.*)

fice of large volumes of breast tissue, which may yield an unsatisfactory cosmetic deformity. These patients are best treated by total mastectomy and autogenous tissue reconstruction. Patients with two or more primary lesions in the same breast have a higher probability of local recurrence after local excision and irradiation. Patients with synchronous, multiple primaries have a higher likelihood of EIC. Very young age (under thirty-five years) patients also have increased breast recurrence in the presence of the EIC component following local excision and radiotherapy (see Fig. 14-49).

Advanced Local Disease (Stage IIIA, IIIB, and Inflammatory Carcinoma). *Inflammatory breast carcinoma* (see Fig. 14-30) represents an ominous clinicopathologic variant with limited 5-year survival rates of 3 to 5 percent. Combination chemotherapeutic regimens (e.g., CAF—cyclophosphamide [Cytoxan], doxorubicin [Adriamycin], and 5-fluorouracil) have effected dramatic regressions of the breast lesion in approximately 60 to 75 percent of these patients. The index lesion and the associated breast changes related to subdermal lymphatic infiltration, as well as any

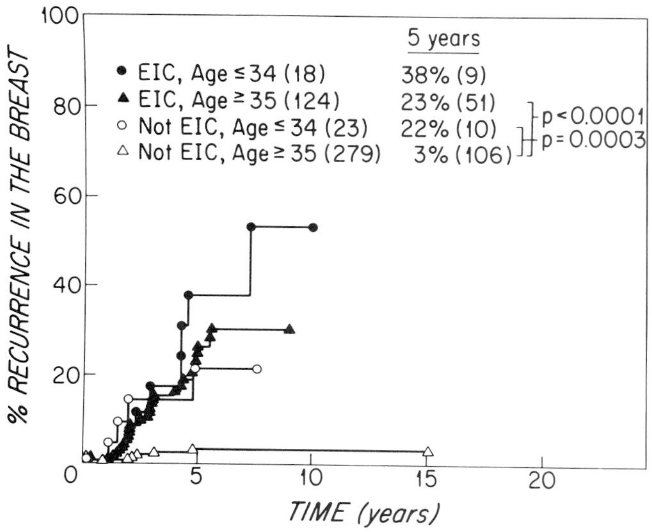

FIG. 14-49. Breast cancer recurrence as a function of age at diagnosis and presence of an extensive intraductal component (EIC). (From: *Recht A, Connolly JC, et al: 1988, with permission.*)

axillary metastases, may disappear. With induction responses following two to six drug cycles of CAF, an extended simple mastectomy (inclusive of Level I nodes) is performed to remove residual malignant disease from the chest wall. Thereafter, peripheral lymphatics, skin flaps, and the central-apical axilla (Levels II and III) are treated with comprehensive radiation therapy. This multimodal approach may result in a 5-year survival with inflammatory breast cancer that approximates 30 percent.

Polychemotherapy has been valuable in the therapy of Stage III disease. In patients with large matted axillary metastases and "grave signs" (edema, ulceration, peau d'orange, and skin or pectoralis major muscle fixation), extended simple mastectomy might not be technically possible. Preoperative chemotherapy allows a regression in size of the index lesion and of axillary metastasis. Sites of tumor infiltration and fixation to skin with ulceration also may undergo regression. Subsequently, an extended simple mastectomy might be feasible. Comprehensive irradiation to the chest wall defect and peripheral lymphatics is important to enhance local and regional control. These multimodal approaches may reduce chest wall recurrence to 4 to 10 percent; 5- and 10-year survival rates are reported as 45 and 28 percent, respectively.

Breast Reconstruction

The use of immediate chest wall reconstruction at the time of mastectomy for invasive carcinoma has increased. In most instances, when radiation therapy or chemotherapy is planned, breast reconstruction can be delayed until these treatments have been completed. Increasingly, chest wall irradiation is being used in persons with implants, although planning and implementation of radiation physics are less precise. Optimally, reconstruction should be deferred until radiation is completed because capsular scarring around the breast prosthesis may be stimulated by irradiation and various types of chemotherapy, particularly with doxorubicin. In 1992, the Food and Drug Administration allowed the placement of gel prostheses for reconstruction purposes only in the patient with neoplastic disease. The increasing use of autogenous tissue transfers for reconstruction does not appear deleterious to the radiation therapy.

Immediate breast reconstruction can also be considered in persons having total mastectomies for ductal carcinoma in situ or lobular carcinoma in situ, as well as individuals who, because of high risk, undergo prophylactic mastectomy. The use of autogenous tissues for reconstruction is highly desirable in these clinical settings.

The mastectomy is ideally performed via a transverse or oblique incision (see Fig. 14-34). If the oblique incision is used, off-shoulder gowns may be worn without the medial portion of the scar visible. Laterally, however, the oblique scar should not extend into the apex of the axilla, as scarring may limit mobility of the arm and shoulder.

The major criticism of breast reconstruction has been the potential for delay in diagnosis of recurrent chest wall disease. For Stage I breast cancer, chest wall recurrence as the first sign of failure is unusual. When proper local therapy of breast cancer has been completed, local chest wall recurrence of Stage I and early Stage II disease will approximate 0 to 2 percent. As the breast prosthesis is placed in the subpectoral position, superficial recurrence of the skin and subdermal connective tissues is usually palpable and is not obscured clinically or radiographically by the prosthetic implant.

Adjuvant Therapy

No solid tumor has been as extensively studied to determine the effects of systemic therapy as has carcinoma of the breast. Clinical trials indicate that *adjuvant cytotoxic therapy* and, possibly, *hormonal therapy,* when used in patients with axillary metastasis but without established distant metastasis, prolong the disease-free interval and, perhaps, enhance survival rates. For patients with established distant metastasis (Stage IV), therapy with several drugs that are less effective as single agents has resulted in greater than 50 percent response rates when used in combination (polychemotherapy). The most prevalent and studied polychemotherapy combinations include (1) cyclophosphamide (Cytoxan), methotrexate, and 5-fluorouracil (CMF) and (2) cyclophosphamide, doxorubicin (Adriamycin), and 5-fluorouracil (CAF). Prednisone and vincristine have sometimes been added to these regimens to potentially enhance response rates. Liberal use of these agents, however, is not justified because of their profound neurotoxicity.

Response rates for cytotoxic combinations vary from 20 to 70 percent. Complete response rates (patients in whom all evidence of disease resolves) are rare and consistently are lower than 20 percent. Complete responses with combination cytotoxic therapy are rare because heterogeneity of the breast cancer cell population often denies response by cells that are in a resting (G_0) phase of the cell cycle. With reentry into the cell cycle, neoplastic cell growth and mitosis are evident. Heterogeneous cell populations have variable response rates to the administered agents. This heterogeneity of cell population may explain why multiple drug combinations, with different sites of cytotoxic action within the cell, have a better overall response rate than is associated with single-agent therapy.

The toxicity noted with cytotoxic agents for breast cancer is similar to that observed with chemotherapy of other malignancies, and includes nausea, vomiting, myelosuppression, alopecia, thrombocytopenia, and exercise intolerance. These toxic events may be reversible with discontinuance of the cytotoxic agents. Doxorubicin initiates a profound and predictable cardiomyopathy with cumulative, dose-limiting side effects. Only 550 mg/m^2 may be given to a patient because cardiomyopathy, if it occurs, is irreversible.

Hormonal Receptors. Within the cytosol of breast cancer cells are specific proteins that bind and transfer steroid moities into the cell nucleus to exert specific hormonal effects. The most widely studied and available receptor proteins are the estrogen (ER) and progesterone (PR) receptor proteins. To obtain a quantitative hormonal assay of either hormone receptor, one gram of fresh tissue obtained from the tumor is essential; the receptors are thermal and ischemia labile. Use of the electrocautery current near the fresh tumor at the time of excision should be avoided, as ER and PR activity will be measurably invalidated. It is advisable to use the cold scalpel for obtaining tissue useful for valid analyses.

Specimens must be rapidly frozen (−70°C) tissue for ER and PR assay because decay in activity is evident within 20 to 30 minutes after extirpation of the neoplasm. Tissue cytosol is obtained by homogenation and centrifugation of the prepared specimen, which is then incubated with ^{3}H-tritium-labeled estradiol-17β. Labeled unbound hormone is removed from the incubation mixture and the bound estrogen sediment is measured by multipoint titration with Scatchard plot analysis. Binding capacity is expressed in femtomoles of ^{3}H-estradiol bound tissue per milligram cytosol protein.

Values $\geq$ 10 fmol/milligram cytosol protein are considered *receptor-positive;* values $<$ 3 to 4 fmol/mg are *receptor-negative.* Intermediate values are considered *borderline.* In all cases the laboratory analysis values should be reviewed to ensure appropriate interpretation.

The degree of positivity is proportional to the differentiation and histologic subtype of the lesion. Ninety percent or more of well-differentiated ductal and lobular carcinomas are ER-positive. Sequential studies of ER activity in the same patient usually reveal no significant difference between lesions of the primary and metastatic sites. There also appears to be no evolution or change of activity in metastatic sites from that of the index lesion.

Clinical response to various forms of endocrine manipulation is evident in patients who have ER activity. Less than 10 percent of ER-negative patients are responders; greater than 60 percent of ER-positive patients respond to exogenous estrogens or endocrine ablative measures.

In the past, oophorectomy, adrenalectomy, and/or hypophysectomy were the primary *endocrine ablative procedures* commonly used to treat metastatic foci. *Oophorectomy* was primarily used for premenopausal patients who presented with skin and/or bony metastasis with a prolonged disease-free interval that exceeded 18 months between treatment of the primary and the discovery of metastases. Visceral metastasis (e.g., lung, liver) were infrequently observed to respond to any form of hormonal manipulation. Pharmacologic doses of exogenous estrogens were provided for postmenopausal women who were observed to have an 18-month disease-free interval and metastasis primarily to bone or skin. Response rates for each of these subgroups approximated 30 percent. *Adrenalectomy* and *hypophysectomy* were effective in individuals who had previously responded to either oophorectomy or exogenous estrogen therapy. The response rates of these additional ablative techniques were also seen in one-third of the treated population.

Receptor activity is the most commonly utilized measure for determining the applicability and selection of additive hormonal or ablative endocrine procedures. Correlations exist between tumor differentiation characteristics and reactivity of ER. In one review, only 8 percent of patients with ER-positive tumors were observed to have relapse. Ninety-one percent of patients with ER-positive tumors were free of disease at 24 months, compared with only 62 percent of ER-negative patients.

Other prognostic variables potentially account for differences in recurrence rates according to ER activity. Younger patients were observed to have trends toward positive nodes and greater need for adjuvant chemotherapy and more commonly had ER-negative tumors.

PR activity in the cytosol is also a measure of hormonal responsiveness of the index tumor or metastatic foci of disease. This receptor is measured concomitantly with ER from the primary tumor. Premenopausal patients have a lower incidence of ER-positive activity (30 percent) compared with postmenopausal patients (60 percent). These data suggest that premenopausal patients have a reduced responsiveness to hormonal manipulation. However, response rates of premenopausal and postmenopausal patients are similar, and PR activity may be more indicative of an opportunity for hormonal manipulation in the premenopausal patient. Commonly, the premenopausal patient may have a tumor that is strongly PR-positive, yet may be ER-negative. This profile may indicate a high clinical correlation for response of the malignancy to hormonal manipulative therapy.

Premenopausal patients with nondetectable ER have a threefold increase in PR as compared with postmenopausal groups. Since high endogenous estrogens in premenopausal patients may mask ER in tumor biopsies, it appears advantageous to perform PR determinations to identify an additional 15 percent of women with metastatic breast cancer who may benefit from endocrine therapy (Table 14-10). McGuire observed a correlation for level of ER (fmol/mg cytosol protein) in breast neoplasms with the response rate to endocrine therapy. He observed that synthesis of PR is strictly estrogen-dependent and represents the end product of estradiol-stimulated pathways in breast cancer tissues. An 80 percent objective response was observed in patients whose ER was ≥ 100 fmol/mg cytosol protein. A response rate of 46 percent was observed in women with lesser values. This objective response rate to endocrine therapy as a function of content of ER has been confirmed by others. Studies also correlate a trend toward higher quantitative values of ER and PR in tumors that are histologically well differentiated. These correlations have been confirmed as high mean ER and PR values in tissues harboring low-grade (grade 1) neoplasms when both receptors are positive.

Antiestrogen Therapy

The antifertility drug tamoxifen was originally observed to have antiestrogen activity and initiate regression of breast cancer. Approximately one-third of patients initially treated with the drug showed objective regression of metastatic disease. Antitumor activity correlated closely with the reactivity of ER and/or PR. Antiestrogens block the uptake of estrogen by the target tissue following cytosol binding to the ER. Diminished responsiveness at one dose level may be reversed by escalation of the dose.

The most striking advantage of tamoxifen over chemotherapy is the absence of toxicity and profound side effects. There may be, however, a ''flare'' of bone pain with induction of hypercalcemia when therapy is initiated; this effect is usually short-lived. Therapeutic estrogens also produce bony pain; nausea, vomiting, and fluid retention are also induced.

Adrenalectomy

The initial application of adrenalectomy was in postmenopausal females after ablation of all other sources of estrogen, particularly in individuals who initially responded to exogenous estrogens. Following menopause, the adrenals represent the major site for production of endogenous estrogens. Aminoglutethimide blocks enzymatic conversion of cholesterol to γ-5-pregnenolone and inhibits the conversion of androstenedione to estrogen in peripheral tissues. Following treatment with this agent, adrenal suppression is evident, with a reduction of cortisol secretion and feedback increase in ACTH that may override the aminoglutethimide blockade. Thereafter, glucocorticoid therapy is required for suppression of ACTH secretion by the adrenal cortex. This therapy amounts to a ''medical adrenalectomy'' and has been compared prospectively with surgical adrenalectomy and hypophysectomy.

Table 14-10
Proposed Therapeutic Options and Frequency of Steroid Receptors for Premenopausal and Postmenopausal Patients with Breast Cancer

	Premenopausal		*Postmenopausal*	
Receptor Status	*No. (%)*	*Proposed Therapy*	*No. (%)*	*Proposed Therapy*
ER +/PR +	222 (45)	O,A,H,T T + CT Horm	520 (63)	T,A,H,CT Horm
ER +/PR −	58 (12)	O,A,H T → T + CT Horm	128 (15)	T,A,H T + CT Horm
ER −/PR −	136 (28)	CT	137 (17)	CT
ER −/PR +	72 (15)	O,A,H,T ?T + CT ?Horm	41 (5)	CT,T + CT Horm

O, oophorectomy; T, tamoxifen; A, adrenalectomy; H, hypophysectomy; ER, estrogen receptor; PR, progesterone receptor; Horm, hormonal (estrogen, progesterone, androgen); CT, cytotoxic chemotherapy; +, ≥10 fmol/mg cytosol protein; −, <10 fmol/mg cytosol protein.

SOURCE: Adapted from Bland KI, et al: *Surg Forum* 32:410, 1981, with permission.

Medical therapy is equivalent to surgical ablation and represents an alternative. Neither permanent adrenal insufficiency nor acute crises were observed. Side effects included ataxia, dizziness, and lethargy; these effects were dose-dependent and transient.

Applications

Fisher and associates, and Bonnadonna et al. suggested that disease-free and overall survival may be enhanced when additive therapy is initiated before clinically detectable distant disease. The goal of therapy is eradication of well-established but, as yet, unidentified micrometastases. Original recommendations were for adjuvant chemotherapy using multiple combinations in premenopausal women with ≥ 3 positive axillary lymph nodes. Data suggest that this approach may also be applicable for women with 1 to 3 positive nodes regardless of the menopausal status. The recent addition of the antiestrogen tamoxifen to the chemotherapeutic regimen for ER-positive patients appears to provide even greater protection against the development of distant disease.

An enhancement in survival of at least 5 to 20 percent over that anticipated for untreated patients with either Stage II or III disease is being realized in most clinical trials.

Node-Negative Breast Cancer. Data from the NIH Consensus Conference in 1991 note that (1) the majority of patients with node-negative cancers are cured by breast conservation treatment or total mastectomy and axillary dissection; and (2) the prevailing evidence suggests that rate of local and distant recurrence is decreased by *both* adjuvant combination cytotoxic chemotherapy and adjuvant tamoxifen. Ten randomized trials confirm that adjuvant systemic therapy reduces the observed rate of recurrence by approximately one-third.

At present, prospective randomized trials are too immature and often lack sufficient numbers to estimate with acceptable precision the correlation between menopausal status or steroid reactivity and the effects of adjuvant therapy in these node-negative patients. Few patients with ER-negative tumors have been included in tamoxifen studies. Reduced mortality, however, is seen in nearly all trials, although this has not reached statistical significance in most trials. The rate of death in patients with node-negative disease is low; thus, a clinically important reduction in mortality will obviously require prolonged follow-up with large numbers of patients to achieve statistical significance.

The major benefits of chemotherapy are seen when the antimetabolites (5-fluorouracil and methotrexate) are administered intravenously, rather than given orally. Trials with tamoxifen suggest the use of this drug for more than 2 years (usually 5 years) results in greater reduction in the risk of recurrence.

In all prospective-study patients who are node-negative, the antiestrogen tamoxifen reduces the clinical incidence of contralateral primary breast cancer. Overall benefits from tamoxifen in postmenopausal patients clearly outweigh the described toxic side effects encountered. For premenopausal patients, the administration of tamoxifen may initiate endocrine abnormalities that have not been defined by long-term analysis (e.g., endometrial carcinoma, effect on the developing fetus). Data are nonexistent with regard to the effects of combination cytotoxic agents with tamoxifen for treatment of node-negative breast cancer patients.

The NIH Consensus Conference recommended that patients who are not candidates for prospective trials or who are noncompliant for participation in these trials should be made aware of the benefits and risks of adjuvant systemic therapy. Adjuvant therapy should consist of either combination chemotherapy in these patients or tamoxifen (20 mg/day for at least two years). Comprehensive prospective studies have not directly compared tamoxifen and chemotherapy (± tamoxifen) in the node-negative subset.

Prognostic Factors. The majority of node-negative patients should be cured following local-regional therapy. Factors considered of importance to the risk for recurrence include tumor size, ER and PR receptor status, tumor grade, histologic type, proliferative rate (thymidine labeling indices, S-phase fraction), as well as other incompletely defined risk parameters (protease, cathepsin, HER-2/neu, EGF receptors, stress-response proteins). Despite the proliferation of definable risk factors and biologic markers, tumor size and the axillary nodal status maintain primacy as the most important of these risk variables (Table 14-11).

The incorporation of such prognostic parameters into summation equations that mathematically and logarithmically estimate risk proportion in numerical form are gaining attention and may have theoretical and clinical investigational value. With the exception of clinical trials, it is not reasonable to treat patients with tumors ≤ 1 cm in diameter because the chance of recurrence in 10 years is < 10 percent. With increasing tumor diameter ± positive nodes, other prognostic variables must be considered in deciding whether to use adjuvant therapy.

Systemic Therapy Trials for Early Breast Cancer. Surgery for early breast cancer allows all clinically apparent (macroscopic) disease to be removed. Various forms of systemic "adjuvant" therapy should be considered postoperatively, namely antiestrogen therapy (tamoxifen) and those that involve a cytotoxic agent or a combination of the two drugs. Analysis of collected data for 15,000 cases confirmed highly significant reductions in annual rates both for recurrence and for death with tamoxifen-treated patients, with ovarian ablation below age fifty, and with polychemotherapy-treated patients, but no enhancement in survival or reduction in recurrence for patients treated by immunotherapy.

Tamoxifen was also shown to have the added benefit of reduction in risk for development of contralateral breast cancer by 39 percent. The salient benefits of reduction in *recurrence* by both polychemotherapy and tamoxifen were seen chiefly during years 0 to 4 postoperatively; the reduction of *mortality* was highly significant both during and after years 0 to 4 with these relatively brief treatments. The Cancer Trial Collaborative Group provided little information beyond year 10, except for ovarian ablation, which produced significant mortality reductions both during and after years 0 to 9 postoperatively. These collaborators verified that long-term (12 months) polychemotherapy was no better than shorter (6 months) regimens. Polychemotherapy provided reduction of recurrences and overall survival that was superior to single-agent chemotherapy. There was no significant difference between various forms of polychemotherapy or different tamoxifen doses, but long-term tamoxifen (e.g., two years, or even five years) was significantly more effective than short-term regimens.

Tamoxifen was effective in older patients (over seventy years); chemotherapy has not been properly evaluated in this geriatric group. Between ages fifty and sixty-nine, direct comparisons confirm that chemotherapy *plus* tamoxifen is superior to chemotherapy alone or tamoxifen alone, for both recurrence and survival. In younger women (under fifty years), chemotherapy and ovarian ablation have comparable effects. Trends suggest that the combination of chemotherapy and ovarian ablation might be superior to either alone.

Table 14-11
Prognostic Variables for Breast Cancer That Determine Recurrence and Overall Survival

Prognostic Factors	*Status*	*Effect on Recurrence (R) and Survival (S)*
Tumor size	≤ 1 cm	R = <10%, 10 years
	1.1–2 cm	R = 10–30%, 10 years
	> 5 cm	S = 41%, 5 years
Nodal status* (metastases)	0	S = 65%, 10 years
	1–3	S = 38%, 10 years
	> 4	S = 13%, 10 years
Estrogen-progesterone receptor	Positive versus negative	R = 8–10%
Histologic type	Variable:	
	Scirrhous	R = High
	Tubular, Colloid	R = Low
	Papillary	R = Low
Proliferative rate (DNA flow cytometry)	Ploidy:	Indeterminate
	Low S-phase	Favorable
	Aneuploid	Unfavorable
Growth factors and chromosomal/oncogene abnormality		
A. Chromosomal defect	Deletion/alteration	
	1,3,6,7,9	Unfavorable
	Loss of length of allele on chromosome 11	Highly unfavorable
B. Proto-oncogenes (when expressed)	*c-myc*	Unknown
	c-erb-B (EGF)	Unfavorable
	c-erb-B_2 (*neu*/HER2)	Unfavorable
	c-H-*ras*	Highly unfavorable
C. Growth factors present	EGF	Unfavorable
	TGF-α	Unfavorable
	TGF-β	Highly favorable
	IGF-I	Unfavorable
	PDGF	Unfavorable
	FGF	Unknown

*NSABP data

EGF = epidermal growth factor; TGF = transforming growth factor; IGF = insulinlike growth factor; PDGF = platelet-derived growth factor; FGF = fibroblast growth factor

A 30 to 40 percent proportional reduction in risk was achieved with combination chemoendocrine therapy for middle-aged patients. This risk reduction was evident for node-positive and for node-negative patients. The improvement in absolute 10-year survival was twice as great for the node-positive patients as for the node-negative groups (see Table 14-11).

Metastatic Disease. Polychemotherapy was designed for therapy of metastasis to bone, liver, soft tissue, lung, and occasionally brain. The combinations of cytotoxic agents most commonly used were 5-fluorouracil, Cytoxan, methotrexate, vincristine, and Adriamycin. Randomized trials comparing cytotoxic agents indicated an increase in response rates from approximately 25 percent with single agents to between 50 percent and 60 percent with combination therapy. Further, median survival for combination therapy in those individuals who do not respond is longer than that obtained with single agents. While relationships between responsiveness to chemotherapy and the ER-PR status have been controversial, more recent studies confirm that hormonal receptor data properly guide anticipated response rates. The heterogeneity of the cellular population within the breast cancer primary and metastatic sites probably dictates therapeutic response cytokinetics and cell kill relative to the cell cycle. No reproducible parameters to evaluate heterogeneity of the cell population are as yet available. The majority of trials identify significant prolongation of chemotherapy-induced responses for patients who previously were responders to hormone therapy and who have ER-positive tumors.

Age, menstrual status, family history, number of positive nodes, tumor size, and type of surgery have been poor predictors for objective response to chemotherapy. A prolonged disease-free interval usually does not indicate a response advantage. The median duration of response to combination chemotherapy ranges between 12 to 18 months. Once failure has occurred, the use of an additional combination of agents may initiate a remission (partial or complete). Stage IV patients who ultimately achieve complete remissions have a median survival of 32 months.

Patients who experience relapses from combination therapy remain eligible for hormonal manipulation, particularly if their tumors are hormone-receptor positive and they have not previously been treated by hormonal manipulation. Patients who have rapidly progressive disease and a short disease-free interval should be treated initially with combination cytotoxic agents before therapy with hormonal manipulation. As tamoxifen has shown therapeutic advantage when combined with chemotherapy in the age group fifty to sixty-nine, this antiestrogen will possibly prolong survival in advanced disease as well.

A relationship exists between *response* to chemotherapy and *dose* of the cytotoxic agent used, but there is dose-limiting toxicity. For the majority of chemotherapeutic agents this toxicity factor is myelosuppression. Recent trials using transplantation of normal autologous bone marrow cells have allowed dose-intensive chemotherapy regimens to overcome this limitation.

In the setting of advanced local disease (Stage III), the cytotoxic dose may be escalated as great as tenfold, depending upon the toxicities encountered. Anteman and Gale reviewed 27 trials of high-dose therapy in which 172 patients received single- or multiple-agent therapy, radiation, or both. Many had been treated extensively with multiple agents before receiving high-dose intensive therapy after marrow transplantation. The multiple alkylating agents offer the best response rate (76 percent). Although response rates are high, duration of response may be short and is often less than 6 months.

In a trial with high-dose cyclophosphamide, cisplatin, and carmustine (melphalan) and bone marrow support as initial therapy, a *complete response* was evident in 55 percent with an *overall response* rate of 73 percent. The median duration of response for patients receiving complete remission was 9 months. These studies suggest that a large cell kill can be obtained with single intensive therapy using autologous marrow rescue. This therapy, however, appears to be inadequate to eliminate adequate cell populations in order to provide durable remission responses. The use of hematopoietic growth factors (GM-CSF—granulocyte-macrophage–colony-stimulating factor) may allow applications of multiple-dose intensive regimens to obtain an enhanced cell kill with autologous marrow rescue. The future of successful therapeutic interventions for Stage IV disease is dependent upon innovative approaches that provide high cell kill with reduced myelosuppression and systemic toxicities.

Carcinoma of the Male Breast

Less than 1 percent of all breast cancer occurs in men. The incidence appears to be highest among North Americans and the British, in whom it constitutes 0.4 to 1.5 percent of all male cancers. Gynecomastia precedes approximately one-fifth of these malignancies. Male breast cancer has been associated with Klinefelter syndrome (XXY), estrogen therapy, high endogenous estrogen levels related to testicular feminizing syndromes, irradiation, and trauma.

This tumor is rarely seen in young males; the incidence peaks between sixty and sixty-nine years of age. Hormonal dependence of the neoplasm is typical and the tumor is commonly estrogen-receptor positive. An increased incidence occurs in Jewish and black males. Clinical presentations of the disease are similar to those for women except that the diagnosis is delayed owing to infrequent recognition in the male patient.

Clinical characteristics include breast mass, nipple retraction, discharge, skin fixation, ulceration, and pain. Stage for stage, men with this neoplasm appear to have the same survival rate as women, but the overall prognosis is poor because of the advanced stage of disease (Stages III, IV) at the time of diagnosis. Overall survival rates for node-negative patients correspond favorably with those for women; survival in node-positive males is poor, suggesting the necessity of adjuvant therapy in this group.

The preferred treatment is modified radical mastectomy and use of postoperative irradiation for ulcerative and/or high-grade anaplastic tumors to reduce local recurrence. Orchiectomy and administration of estrogenic steroids may induce remissions of metastatic disease. Hormonal manipulation, by either medication or ablation, often provides objective responses in the management of metastatic disease. Cytotoxic chemotherapeutic agents have been used infrequently in the therapy of male cancer. Early trials suggest response rates similar to those for female breast cancer patients.

Breast Cancer During Pregnancy and Lactation

From the time of Billroth until Halsted's pioneering work, carcinoma of the breast diagnosed during pregnancy was considered incurable. White and White reported an incidence of approximately 2.8 percent for cases occurring during pregnancy. Recent reviews suggest an incidence of 3 cancers per 10,000 pregnancies, or a range from 0.4 to 3.8 percent of reported breast cancers. The average age of a pregnant patient with concomitant breast cancer is thirty-four years.

In the past, the association of cancer with pregnancy was considered ominous. The profound estrogen and progesterone stimulation of breast cancer cells from the placenta and corpus luteum reportedly increases the risk of distant disease with provision of an excellent hormonal milieu to support cellular growth of the neoplasm. More recent data indicate that, stage for stage, carcinoma of the breast in pregnancy is associated with a prognosis similar to that of the nonpregnant female. There are, however, proportionally more patients with Stages II and III breast cancers diagnosed in pregnancy than in the general population. Whether this late stage at diagnosis is secondary to the hormonal stimulation of pregnancy or to delay because of the coincident physiologic changes expected with pregnancy has not been determined.

Diagnosis. A careful breast exam should be performed at the initial obstetric visit and, at least, in each trimester of the pregnancy. Diagnostic work-up in pregnancy and lactation is similar to that in the nonpregnant patient, although breast mammography tends to be less reliable due to the extensive parenchymal changes associated with gestation. Radiation exposure of the fetus should be negligible with modern techniques for proper shielding of the abdomen. Regardless of the mammographic findings, any dominant mass should be evaluated promptly in the pregnant or lactating patient. Evaluation may begin with fine-needle aspiration to distinguish cysts from solid lesions. Any solid, discrete mass requires biopsy, which can usually be completed under local anesthesia. Risk of spontaneous abortion during mastectomy is approximately 1 percent and correlates with stage of gestation.

Treatment. Therapy is identical with that for the nonpregnant individual. Patients who have advanced cancer require appropriate chemotherapy and irradiation. Modified radical mastectomy is optimal therapy for Stage I or Stage II patients. When segmental mastectomy is selected, it must be followed by whole breast irradiation, after delivery if the diagnosis is established late in the third trimester. In patients with positive axillary lymph nodes, chemotherapy should be delayed until the second trimester of pregnancy to diminish fetal toxicity and spontaneous abortion.

Termination of pregnancy has no role in the management of Stage I or Stage II disease. No evidence exists to substantiate that oophorectomy influences the course of breast cancer during pregnancy and lactation. With mastectomy, normal pregnancy is allowed to continue, with minimal risk to the mother or the fetus. Modern series do not provide evidence that abortion benefits control or survival rates for patients with the disease. For Stage I and Stage II disease some patients with early disease will elect breast conservation. Segmental mastectomy should be strongly discouraged except in the third trimester, when irradiation could be reasonably delayed (4 to 6 weeks) until delivery.

Risks associated with chemotherapy during pregnancy have not been established. Schapira and Chudley found the incidence for teratogenicity of chemotherapeutics given to humans in the first trimester to be 12.7 percent, whereas Sweet and Kinzie noted an 11.5 percent incidence. There was no evidence of teratogenicity from administration of chemotherapeutic agents in the second and third trimesters. Little data exist with regard to combination regimens, as most of the reports considered single-agent usage. Long-term consequences of fetal exposure to chemotherapeutic agents are unavailable.

In general, the use of cytotoxic agents during the first trimester should be discouraged; usage during the second and third trimesters probably induces very few fetal abnormalities. For patients with positive lymph nodes at mastectomy, chemotherapy may be delayed until the second trimester. In the third trimester, after determination of fetal age and maturity, consideration should be given to early cesarean section to minimize delay in initiating cytotoxic therapy for Stages II and III disease.

Lactation should be suppressed promptly in the postpartum state, even if the biopsy identifies a benign lesion, as milk from transected lactiferous ducts will drain via the biopsy site. If the infant is breast feeding, rapid weaning is desirable.

During postoperative irradiation or chemotherapy to control an aggressive primary lesion (Stage III, inflammatory cancer), the patient who becomes pregnant should consider therapeutic abortion. In the first trimester, both irradiation and chemotherapy are potentially teratogenic, particularly in the first 9 weeks of gestation. Irradiation in doses greater than 500 millirads, by itself, administered in early fetal development may be teratogenic.

Recurrence During Pregnancy. Data do not convincingly establish that survival is diminished nor that recurrence is enhanced for women who subsequently become pregnant following treatment of a breast cancer. In contradistinction, studies suggest an improved survival among breast cancer patients who later become pregnant. These data document no detrimental effect of subsequent pregnancy even among patients with positive nodes or of pregnancies that occur less than 2 years following mastectomy. Abortion does not appear to provide an improvement in the survival rate.

While no therapeutic grounds exist for recommending avoidance or termination of pregnancy among patients without documented recurrence, theoretically the disease-free interval may be shortened particularly in ER-positive patients in whom the enhanced estrogen milieu will support growth of tumor cells. Thus, child bearing or estrogen-containing compounds must be considered cautiously before either is recommended to the patient at high risk for recurrent disease (e.g., Stages II and III, inflammatory cancer). For patients at enhanced risk for recurrent disease, and in whom estrogen antagonists may be useful as an antineoplastic agent, the use of oral contraceptives and estrogen-containing compounds should be avoided.

References

Embryology

Bland KI, Romrell LJ: Congenital and acquired disturbances of breast development and growth, in Bland KI, Copeland EM III. *The Breast: Comprehensive Management of Benign and Malignant Diseases*. Philadelphia, Saunders, 1991, Chap 4.

Anatomy and Development

Romrell LJ, Bland KI: Anatomy of the breast axilla, chest wall and related metastatic sites, in Bland KI, Copeland EM III. *The Breast: Comprehensive Management of Benign and Malignant Diseases*. Philadelphia, Saunders, 1991, Chap 2.

Physiology

Keller-Wood M, Bland KI: Breast physiology in normal, lactating, and diseased states, in Bland KI, Copeland EM III. *The Breast: Comprehensive Management of Benign and Malignant Diseases*. Philadelphia, Saunders, 1991, Chap 3.

Gynecomastia

Bland KI, Page DL: Gynecomastia, in Bland KI, Copeland EM III. *The Breast: Comprehensive Management of Benign and Malignant Diseases*. Philadelphia, Saunders, 1991, Chap 7.

Haagensen CD: *Diseases of the Breast*. Philadelphia, Saunders, 1986, pp 502, 505, 574.

Nuttall FQ: Gynecomastia as a physical finding in normal men. *J Clin Endocrinol Metab* 48(2):338, 1979.

Mammography

Bartrum RJ, Crowe HC: Transillumination light scanning to diagnose breast cancer: a feasibility study. *AJR* 142:409, 1984.

Bland KI, Buchanan JB, et al: Analysis of breast cancer screening in women younger than fifty years of age. *JAMA* 245:1037, 1981.

Ciatto S, Cataliotti L, Distante V: Non-palpable lesions detected with mammography: review of 512 consecutive cases. *Radiology* 165:99, 1987.

Sickles EA: Breast cancer detection with transillumination in mammography. *AJR* 142:841, 1984.

Nonproliferative Lesions

Dupont WD, Page DL: Risk factors for breast cancer in women with proliferative breast disease. *N Engl J Med* 312:146, 1985.

Wellings SR, Alpers CE: Apocrine cystic metaplasia: subgross pathology and prevalence in cancer-associated versus random autopsy breasts. *Hum Pathol* 18:381, 1987.

Benign Proliferative Lesions

Carter CL, Corle DK, Micozzi MS: A prospective study of the development of breast cancer in 16,692 women with benign breast disease. *Am J Epidemiol* 128:467, 1988.

Dupont WD, Rogers LW, et al: The epidemiologic study of anatomic markers for increased risk of mammary cancer. *Pathol Res Pract* 166:471, 1980.

Eusebi V, Foschini MA, et al: Long-term follow-up of in situ carcinoma of the breast with special emphasis on clinging carcinoma. *Semin Diagn Pathol* 6:165, 1989.

Kodlin D, Winger EE, et al: Chronic mastopathy and breast cancer. A follow-up study. *Cancer* 39:2603, 1977.

Moskowitz M, Gartside P, et al: Proliferative disorders of the breast as risk factors for breast cancer in a self-selected screened population: pathologic markers. *Radiology* 134:289, 1980.

Wellings SR, Jensen HM, Marcum RG: An atlas of subgross pathology of the human breast with special reference to possible precancerous lesions. *J Natl Cancer Inst* 55:231, 1975.

Localized Sclerosing Lesions

Hutter RVP, et al: Consensus meeting. Is "fibrocystic disease" of the breast precancerous? *Arch Pathol Lab Med* 110:171, 1986.

Radial Scar and Complex Sclerosing Lesions

Anderson TJ, Battersy S: Radial scars of benign and malignant breasts: comparative features and significance. *J Pathol* 147:23, 1985.

Fat Necrosis

Page DL, Simpson JF: Benign, high-risk, and premalignant lesions of the mamma, in Bland KI, Copeland EM III. *The Breast: Comprehensive Management of Benign and Malignant Diseases*. Philadelphia, Saunders, 1991, Chap 6.

Fibroadenoma and Phyllodes Tumors

Cant PJ, Madden MV, et al: Case for conservative management of selected fibroadenomas of the breast. *Br J Surg* 74:857, 1987.

Fechner RE: Fibroadenoma and related lesions, in Page DL, Anderson TJ: *Diagnostic Histopathology of the Breast*. Edinburgh, Churchill Livingstone, 1987, pp 72–88.

Fondo EY, Rosen PP, et al: The problem of carcinoma developing in a fibroadenoma. Recent experience at Memorial Hospital. *Cancer* 43:563, 1979.

Hajdu SI, Espinosa MH, Robbins GF: Recurrent cystosarcoma phyllodes: a clinicopathologic study of 32 cases. *Cancer* 38:1402, 1976.

Lindquist KD, van Heerden JA, et al: Recurrent and metastatic cystosarcoma phyllodes. *Am J Surg* 144:341, 1982.

Oberman HA: Breast lesions in the adolescent female. *Ann Pathol* 14:175, 1979.

Pick PW, Iossifedes IA: Occurrence of breast carcinoma within a fibroadenoma. A review. *Arch Pathol Lab Med* 108:590, 1984.

West TL, Weiland JH, Clagett OT: Cystosarcoma phyllodes. *Ann Surg* 173:520, 1971.

Papilloma

Carter D: Intraductal papillary tumors of the breast: a study of 78 cases. *Cancer* 39:1689, 1977.

Haagensen CD: *Diseases of the Breast,* 3rd ed. Philadelphia, Saunders, 1986, pp 136–191.

Ductal Adenoma (Nodular Adenosis)

Azzopardi JG, Salm R: Ductal adenoma of the breast: a lesion which can mimic carcinoma. *J Pathol* 144:11, 1984.

Carcinoma of the Breast

Boring CC, Squires TS, Tong T: Cancer statistics, 1992. *CA* 42(1):19, 1992.

Henderson BE, Pike MC, Ross RK: Epidemiology and risk factors, in Bonadonna G (ed): *Breast Cancer: Diagnosis and Management*. Chichester, MA, John Wiley & Sons, 1984, pp 15–33.

Hirayama T: Epidemiology of breast cancer with special reference to the role of diet. *Prev Med* 7:173, 1978.

Kolonel LN, Hankin JH, et al: Nutrient intakes in relation to cancer incidence in Hawaii. *Br J Cancer* 44:332, 1981.

Lubin JH, Burns PE, et al: Dietary factors and breast cancer risk. *Int J Cancer* 28:685, 1981.

Lynch HT, Albano WA, et al: Genetics, biomarkers, and breast cancer: a review. *Cancer Genet Cytogenet* 13:43, 1984.

Lynch HT, Lynch JF: Breast cancer genetics in an oncology clinic: 328 consecutive patients. *Cancer Genet Cytogenet* 22:369, 1986.

Lynch HT, Marcus JN, et al: Familial breast cancer, family cancer syndromes, and predisposition to breast neoplasia, in Bland KI, Copeland EM III. *The Breast: Comprehensive Management of Benign and Malignant Diseases*. Philadelphia, Saunders, 1991, Chap 13.

National Academy of Sciences, Committee on Diet, Nutrition and Cancer: Dietary factors in cancer. Washington, DC, National Academy Press, 1982, p 496.

Phillips RL: Role of life-style and dietary habits in risk of cancer among Seventh Day Adventists. *Cancer Res* 35:3513, 1975.

Willett WC, Stampfer MJ, Colditz GA: Dietary fat and the risk of breast cancer. *N Engl J Med* 316:22, 1987.

Hormone Usage

Brinton LA, Hoover R, Fraumeni JF: Epidemiology of minimal breast cancer. *JAMA* 249(4):483, 1983.

Hunt K, Vessey M, et al: Long-term surveillance of mortality and cancer incidence in women receiving hormone replacement therapy. *Br J Obstet Gynaecol* 94:620, 1987.

Kalache A, McPherson K, et al: Oral contraceptives and breast cancer. *Br J Hosp Med* 30:278, 1983.

Lipnick R, Speizer FE, et al: Case control study of risk indicators among women with premenopausal and early postmenopausal breast cancer. *Cancer* 53:1020, 1984.

McPherson K, Neil A, et al: Oral contraceptives and breast cancer. *Lancet* 2:1414, 1983.

Vessey MP: Exogenous hormones in the aetiology of cancer in women. *J R Soc Med* 77:542, 1984.

Obesity

Willett WC, Brown ML, Bain C: Relative weight and risk of breast cancer among premenopausal women. *Am J Epidemiol* 122(5):731, 1985.

Multiple Primary Neoplasms

Curtis RE, Hoover RN, et al: Second cancer following cancer of the female genital system in Connecticut, 1935–82. *NCI Monogr* 68:113, 1985.

Harvey EB, Brinton LA: Second cancer following cancer of the breast in Connecticut, 1935–82. *NCI Monogr* 68:99, 1985.

Irradiation

Boice JD Jr, Blettner M, et al: Radiation dose and breast cancer risk in patients treated for cancer of the cervix. *Int J Cancer* 44:7, 1989.

Boice JD Jr, Land CE, et al: Risk of breast cancer following low-dose radiation exposure. *Radiology* 131:589, 1979.

Evans JS, Wennberg JE, McNeil BJ: The influence of diagnostic radiography on the incidence of breast cancer and leukemia. *N Engl J Med* 315:810, 1986.

Harvey EB, Brinton LA: Second cancer following cancer of the breast in Connecticut, 1935–82. *NCI Monogr* 68:99, 1985.

Hildreth NG, Shore RE, Dvoretsky PM: The risk of breast cancer after irradiation of the thymus in infancy. *N Engl J Med* 321:1281, 1989.

Hildreth NG, Shore RE, et al: Risk of extrathyroid tumors following radiation treatment in infancy for thymic enlargement. *Radiat Res* 102:378, 1985.

Hoffman DA, Lonstein JE, et al: Breast cancer in women with scoliosis exposed to multiple diagnostic x-rays. *J Natl Cancer Inst* 81:1307, 1989.

Horn PL, Thompson WD: Risk of contralateral breast cancer: associations with histologic, clinical and therapeutic factors. *Cancer* 62:412, 1988.

Hrubec Z, Boice JD Jr: Breast cancer after multiple chest fluoroscopies: second follow-up of Massachusetts women with tuberculosis. *Cancer Res* 49:229, 1989.

Kelsey JL, Gammon MD: The epidemiology of breast cancer. Reprinted from *CA* 41:146, 1991.

Land CE, Boice JD Jr, et al: Breast cancer risk from low-dose exposures to ionizing radiation: results of parallel analysis of three exposed populations of women. *J Natl Cancer Inst* 65:353, 1980.

Modan B, Chetrit A, et al: Increased risk of breast cancer after low-dose irradiation. *Lancet* 1:629, 1989.

Tokunaga M, Land CE, et al: Breast cancer in Japanese A-bomb survivors (letter). *Lancet* 2:924, 1982.

Natural History

Bloom HJG, Richardson WW, Harries EJ: Natural history of untreated breast cancer (1805–1933): comparison of untreated and treated cases according to histological grade of malignancy. *Br Med J* 5299:213, 1962.

Hietanen P: Relapse pattern and follow-up of breast cancer. *Ann Clin Res* 18:134, 1986.

Lee YTN: Breast carcinoma: pattern of recurrence and metastasis after mastectomy. *Am J Clin Oncol* 7:443, 1984.

Valagussa P, Bonadonna G, Veronesi U: Patterns of relapse and survival following radical mastectomy. Analysis of 716 consecutive patients. *Cancer* 41:1170, 1978.

Wilkinson EJ, Hause LL, et al: Occult axillary lymph node metastases in invasive breast carcinoma: characteristics of the primary tumor and significance of the metastases, in Sommers SC, Rosen PP (eds): *Pathology Annual II*. New York, Appleton-Century-Crofts, 1982, p 67.

Staging of Breast Cancer

Boova RS, Roseann B, Rosato F: Patterns of axillary nodal involvement in breast cancer. Predictability of level one dissection. *Ann Surg* 196:642, 1982.

Fisher B, Slack NH: Number of lymph nodes examined and prognosis of breast carcinoma. *Surg Gynecol Obstet* 131:79, 1970.

Fisher B, Wolmark N, et al: The accuracy of clinical nodal staging and of limited axillary dissection as a determinant of histologic nodal status in carcinoma of the breast. *Surg Gynecol Obstet* 152:765, 1981.

Fisher ER: Prognostic and therapeutic significance of pathological features of breast cancer. *NCI Monogr* 1:29, 1986.

Henderson IC, Canellos GP: Cancer of the breast. The past decade. *N Engl J Med* 302(1):17, 1980.

Koscielny S, Tubiana M, et al: Breast cancer: relationship between the size of the primary tumor and the probability of metastatic dissemination. *Br J Cancer* 49:709, 1984.

Mambo NC, Gallagher HS: Carcinoma of the breast. The prognostic significance of extranodal extension of axillary disease. *Cancer* 39:2280, 1977.

Nemoto T, Vana J, et al: Management and survival of female breast cancer: results of a national survey by the American College of Surgeons. *Cancer* 45:2917, 1980.

CT/MRI

Feig SA: The role of new imaging modalities in staging and follow-up of breast cancer. *Semin Oncol* 13:402, 1986.

Harris JR, Hellman S, et al: Cancer of the breast, in DeVita VT Jr, Helman S, Rosenberg SA (eds): *Cancer: Principles and Practice of Oncology*, 2nd ed. Philadelphia, Lippincott, 1985.

Histopathology of Noninfiltrating (In Situ) Carcinoma

Broders AC: Carcinoma in situ contrasted with benign penetrating epithelium. *JAMA* 99:1670, 1932.

DeOme K: Formal discussion of multiple factors in mouse mammary tumorigenesis. *Cancer Res* 25:1348, 1965.

Foote FW Jr, Stewart FW: Lobular carcinoma in situ: a rare form of mammary carcinoma. *Am J Pathol* 17:491, 1941.

Gallagher HS, Martin JE: The study of mammary carcinoma by mammography and whole organ sectioning. *Cancer* 23:855, 1969.

Gallagher HS, Martin JE: An orientation to the concept of minimal breast cancer. *Cancer* 28:1505, 1971.

Gillis DA, Dockerty MB, Clagett OT: Preinvasive intraductal carcinoma of the breast. *Surg Gynecol Obstet* 110:555, 1960.

Ketcham AS, Moffat FL: Vexed surgeons, perplexed patients, and breast cancers which may not be cancer. *Cancer* 65:387, 1990.

Rosen PP: Lobular carcinoma in situ and intraductal carcinoma of the breast. *Monogr Pathol* 25:59, 1984.

von Rueden DG, Wilson RE: Intraductal carcinoma of the breast. *Surg Gynecol Obstet* 158:105, 1984.

Epidemiology

Anderson JA, Schiodt T: On the concept of carcinoma in situ of the breast. *Pathol Res Pract* 166:407, 1980.

Blichert-Toft M, Graversen HP, et al: In situ breast carcinomas: a population-based study on frequency, growth pattern, and clinical aspects. *World J Surg* 12:845, 1988.

Carter D, Smith RRL: Carcinoma in situ of the breast. *Cancer* 40:1189, 1977.

Farrow JH: Current concepts in the detection and treatment of the earliest of early breast cancers. *Cancer* 25:468, 1970.

Rosner D, Bedwani RN, et al: Noninvasive breast carcinoma: results of a national survey by the American College of Surgeons. *Ann Surg* 192:139, 1980.

Smart CR, Myers MH, Gloeckler LA: Implications from SEER data on breast cancer management. *Cancer* 41:787, 1978.

Swain SM, Lippman ME: Intraepithelial carcinoma of the breast, in Lippman ME, Lichter AS, Danforth DN (eds): *Diagnosis and Management of Breast Cancer*. Philadelphia, Saunders, 1988, pp 296–325.

Lobular carcinoma in situ

Bland KI, Frykberg ER: In situ carcinoma of the breast: ductal and lobular cell origin, in Cameron JL (ed): *Current Surgical Therapy*, 4th ed. St Louis, MO, Mosby Yearbook, 1992, pp 612–621.

Giodano JM, Klopp CT: Lobular carcinoma in situ: incidence and treatment. *Cancer* 31:105, 1973.

Rosen PP: Lobular carcinoma in situ and intraductal carcinoma of the breast. *Monogr Pathol* 25:59, 1984.

Rosen PP, Senie RT, et al: Epidemiology of breast carcinoma: age, menstrual status, and exogenous hormone usage in patients with lobular carcinoma in situ. *Surgery* 85:219, 1987.

Schwartz GF, Feig SA, et al: Staging and treatment of clinically occult breast cancer. *Cancer* 53:1379, 1984.

Wheeler JE, Enterline HT, et al: Lobular carcinoma in situ of the breast: long-term follow-up. *Cancer* 34:554, 1974.

Ductal carcinoma in situ

Heller KS, Rosen PP, et al: Male breast cancer: a clinicopathologic study of 97 cases. *Ann Surg* 188:60, 1978.

Schuh ME, Nemoto T, et al: Intraductal carcinoma: analysis of presentation, pathologic findings, and outcome of disease. *Arch Surg* 121:1303, 1986.

Westbrook KC, Gallagher HS: Intraductal carcinoma of the breast: a comparative study. *Am J Surg* 130:667, 1975.

Pathology of in situ disease

Andersen JA, Fechner RE, et al: Lobular carcinoma in situ (lobular neoplasia) of the breast (a symposium): *Pathol Annu* 15:193, 1980.

Andersen JA, Schiodt T: On the concept of carcinoma in situ of the breast. *Pathol Res Pract* 166:407, 1980.

Carpenter R, Gibbs N, et al: Importance of cellular DNA content in premalignant breast disease and pre-invasive carcinoma of the female breast. *Br J Surg* 74:905, 1987.

Cooke TG: Ductal carcinoma in situ: a new clinical problem. *Br J Surg* 76:660, 1989.

Jones EL, Codling BW, Oates GD: Necrotic intraduct breast carcinomas simulating inflammatory lesions. *J Pathol* 110:101, 1973.

Rosen PP: Lobular carcinoma in situ and intraductal carcinoma of the breast. *Monogr Pathol* 25:59, 1984.

Natural history of in situ carcinoma

Bland KI, Frykberg ER. In situ carcinoma of the breast: ductal and lobular cell origin, in Cameron JL (ed): *Current Surgical Therapy*, 4th ed. St Louis, MO, Mosby Year Book, 1992, pp 612–621.

Brown PW, Silverman J, et al: Intraductal "noninfiltrating" carcinoma of the breast. *Arch Surg* 111:1063, 1976.

Carter D, Smith RRL: Carcinoma in situ of the breast. *Cancer* 40:1189, 1977.

Fisher ER, Sass R, et al: Pathologic findings from the National Surgical Adjuvant Breast Project (Protocol 6). I. Intraductal carcinoma (DCIS). *Cancer* 57:197, 1986.

Frykberg ER, Bland KI: Evolution of surgical principles for the management of breast cancer, in Bland KI, Copeland EM (eds): *The Breast: Comprehensive Management of Benign and Malignant Diseases*. Philadelphia, Saunders, 1991, Chap 29, pp 539–569.

Gillis DA, Dockerty MB, Clagett OT: Preinvasive intraductal carcinoma of the breast. *Surg Gynecol Obstet* 110:555, 1960.

Gump FE: In situ cancers, in Harris JR, Hellman S, Henderson IC, et al (eds): *Breast Diseases*. Philadelphia, Lippincott, 1987, pp 359–368.

Gump FE, Jicha DL, Ozello L: Ductal carcinoma in situ (DCIS): a revised concept. *Surgery* 102:790, 1987.
Haagensen CD: *Diseases of the Breast,* 3rd ed. Philadelphia, Saunders, 1986.
Haagensen CD, Lane N, Lattes R: Neoplastic proliferation of the epithelium of the mammary lobules: adenosis, lobular neoplasia, and small cell carcinoma. *Surg Clin North Am* 52:497, 1972.
Hutter RVP: The management of patients with lobular carcinoma in situ of the breast. *Cancer* 53:798, 1984.
Ketcham AS, Moffat FL: Vexed surgeons, perplexed patients, and breast cancers which may not be cancer. *Cancer* 65:387, 1990.
Lagios MD, Westdahl RP, et al: Duct carcinoma in situ: relationship of extent of noninvasive disease to the frequency of occult invasion, multicentricity, lymph node metastases and short-term treatment failures. *Cancer* 49:751, 1982.
Pagana TJ, Lubbe WJ, et al: A comparison of palpable and nonpalpable breast cancers. *Arch Surg* 124:26, 1989.
Page DL, Dupont WD, et al: Intraductal carcinoma of the breast. *Cancer* 49:751, 1982.
Powers RW, O'Brien PH, Kreutner A: Lobular carcinoma in situ. *J Surg Oncol* 13:269, 1980.
Rosen PP, Senie R, et al: Noninvasive breast carcinoma: frequency of unsuspected invasion and implications for treatment. *Ann Surg* 189:377, 1979.
Rosner D, Bedwani RN, et al: Noninvasive breast carcinoma: results of a national survey by the American College of Surgeons. *Ann Surg* 192:139, 1980.
Rosner D, Bedwani RN, Vana J, et al: Noninvasive breast carcinoma: results of a national survey by the American College of Surgeons. *Ann Surg* 192:139, 1980.
Wheeler JE, Enterline HT: Lobular carcinoma of the breast in situ and infiltrating. *Pathol Annu* 11:161, 1976.
Wobbes T, Tinnemans JGM, van der Sluis RF: Residual tumor after biopsy for non-palpable ductal carcinoma in situ of the breast. *Br J Surg* 76:185, 1989.

Bilaterality and multicentricity of in situ cancer
Brown PW, Silverman J, et al: Intraductal ''noninfiltrating'' carcinoma of the breast. *Arch Surg* 111:1063, 1976.
Farrow JH: Current concepts in the detection and treatment of the earliest of early breast cancers. *Cancer* 25:468, 1970.
Fracchia AA, Robinson D, et al: Survival in bilateral breast cancer. *Cancer* 55:1414, 1985.
Frazier TG, Copeland EM, et al: Prognosis and treatment in minimal breast cancer. *Am J Surg* 133:697, 1977.
Gallager HS, Martin JE: The study of mammary carcinoma by mammography and whole organ sectioning. *Cancer* 23:855, 1969.
Gump FE, Shikora S, et al: The extent and distribution of cancer in breasts with palpable primary tumors. *Ann Surg* 204:384, 1986.
Holland R, Veling SHJ, et al: Histologic multifocality of Tis, T1-2 breast carcinoma. *Cancer* 56:979, 1985.
Ringberg A, Palmer B, Linell F: The contralateral breast at reconstructive surgery after breast cancer operation—a histological study. *Breast Cancer Res Treat* 2:151, 1982.
Rosen PP: Lobular carcinoma in situ contrasted with benign penetrating epithelium. *JAMA* 99:1670, 1932.
Rosen PP: Lobular carcinoma in situ and intraductal carcinoma of the breast. *Monogr Pathol* 25:59, 1984.
Schwartz GF, Patchefsky AS, et al: Clinically occult breast cancer: multicentricity and implications for treatment. *Ann Surg* 191:8, 1980.
Sunshine JA, Moseley HS, et al: Breast carcinoma in situ: a retrospective review of 112 cases with a minimum 10 year followup. *Am J Surg* 150:44, 1985.
Tulusan AH, Egger H, et al: A contribution to the natural history of breast cancer: lobular carcinoma in situ and its relation to breast cancer. *Arch Gynecol* 231:219, 1982.
Urban JA: Bilaterality of cancer of the breast. *Cancer* 20:1867, 1967.
Webber BL, Heise H, et al: Risk of subsequent contralateral breast carcinoma in a population of patients with in situ breast carcinoma. *Cancer* 47:2928, 1981.
Westbrook KC, Gallager HS: Intraductal carcinoma of the breast: a comparative study. *Am J Surg* 130:667, 1975.

Therapy of in situ cancer
Hutter RVP: The management of patients with lobular carcinoma in situ of the breast. *Cancer* 53:798, 1984.
Rosen PP, Senie R, et al: Noninvasive breast carcinoma: frequency of unsuspected invasion and implications for treatment. *Ann Surg* 189:377, 1979.

DCIS
Ashikari R, Hajdu SI: Intraductal carcinoma of the breast (1960–1969). *Cancer* 28:1182, 1971.
Bland KI, Frykberg ER: In situ carcinoma of the breast: ductal and lobular cell origin, in Cameron JL (ed): *Current Surgical Therapy,* 4th ed. St Louis, MO, Mosby Year Book, 1992, pp 612–621.
Bradley SJ, Weaver DW, Bouwman DL: Alternatives in the surgical management of in situ breast cancer: a meta-analysis of outcome. *Am Surg* 56:428, 1990.
Brown PW, Silverman J, et al: Intraductal ''noninfiltrating'' carcinoma of the breast. *Arch Surg* 111:1063, 1976.
Carter D, Smith RRL: Carcinoma in situ of the breast. *Cancer* 40:1189, 1977.
Cooke TG: Ductal carcinoma in situ: a new clinical problem. *Br J Surg* 76:660, 1989.
Fentiman IS, Fagg N, et al: In situ ductal carcinoma of the breast: implications of disease pattern and treatment. *Eur J Surg Oncol* 12:261, 1986.
Fisher ER, Sass R, et al: Pathologic findings from the National Surgical Adjuvant Breast Project (Protocol 6). I. Intraductal carcinoma (DCIS). *Cancer* 57:197, 1986.
Frykberg ER, Ames FC, Bland KI: Current concepts for management of early (in situ and occult invasive) breast carcinoma, in Bland KI, Copeland EM (eds): *The Breast: Comprehensive Management of Benign and Malignant Diseases*. Philadelphia, Saunders, 1991, Chap 35, pp 731–751.
Gilliland MD, Barton RM, Copeland EM: The implications of local recurrence of breast cancer as the first site of therapeutic failure. *Ann Surg* 197:284, 1983.
Gump FE: In situ cancers, in Harris JR, Hellman S, Henderson IC, et al (eds): *Breast Diseases*. Philadelphia, Lippincott, 1987, pp 359–368.
Gump FE, Jicha DL, Ozello L: Ductal carcinoma in situ (DCIS): a revised concept. *Surgery* 102:790, 1987.
Harris JR: Clinical management of ductal carcinoma in situ, in Harris JR, Hellman S, Henderson IC, et al (eds): *Breast Diseases*. Philadelphia, Lippincott, 1991, pp 233–239.
Kurtz JM, Amalric R, et al: Local recurrence after breast-conserving surgery and radiotherapy: frequency, time course, and prognosis. *Cancer* 63:1912, 1989.
Lagios MD, Margolin FR, et al: Mammographically detected duct carcinoma in situ: frequency of local recurrence following tylectomy and prognostic effect of nuclear grade on local recurrence. *Cancer* 63:618, 1989.
Lagios MD, Westdahl PR, et al: Duct carcinoma in situ: relationship of extent of noninvasive disease to the frequency of occult invasion, multicentricity, lymph node metastases and short-term treatment failures. *Cancer* 50:1309, 1982.
Rosen PP, Braun DW, Kinne DE: The clinical significance of pre-invasive breast carcinoma. *Cancer* 46:919, 1980.
Rosner D, Bedwani RN, et al: Noninvasive breast carcinoma: results of a national survey by the American College of Surgeons. *Ann Surg* 192:139, 1980.
Schnitt SJ, Silen W, et al: Ductal carcinoma in situ (intraductal carcinoma) of the breast. *N Engl J Med* 318:898, 1988.

Silverstein MJ, Gierson ED, et al: Axillary lymphadenectomy for intraductal carcinoma of the breast. *Surg Gynecol Obstet* 172:211, 1991.

Stotter AT, Atkinson EN, et al: Survival following locoregional recurrence after breast conservation therapy for cancer. *Ann Surg* 212:166, 1990.

Stotter AT, McNeese MD, et al: Predicting the rate and extent of locoregional failure after breast conservation therapy for early breast cancer. *Cancer* 64:2217, 1989.

Sunshine JA, Moseley HS, et al: Breast carcinoma in situ: a retrospective review of 112 cases with a minimum 10 year followup. *Am J Surg* 150:44, 1985.

Swain SM, Lippman ME: Intraepithelial carcinoma of the breast, in Lippman ME, Lichter AS, Danforth DN (eds): *Diagnosis and Management of Breast Cancer*. Philadelphia, Saunders, 1988, pp 296–325.

Von Rueden DG, Wilson RE: Intraductal carcinoma of the breast. *Surg Gynecol Obstet* 158:105, 1984.

Histopathology of Infiltrating Malignancies

Wellings SR, Jensen HM: On the origin and progression of ductal carcinoma in the human breast. *J Natl Cancer Inst* 50:1111, 1973.

Mucinous carcinoma (colloid carcinoma)

McDivitt RW, Stewart FW, Berg JW: Tumors of the breast, in *Atlas of Tumor Pathology*. Series 2, Fascicle 2. Washington, DC, Armed Forces Institute of Pathology, 1968.

Robinson RR: Gelatinous cancer of the breast. *Trans Pathol Soc Lond* 4:275, 1852.

Tubular carcinoma

Rosen PP: The pathology of breast carcinoma, in Harris J, Hellman S (eds): *Breast Diseases*. Philadelphia, Lippincott, 1987, pp 147–209.

Papillary carcinoma

Devitt JE, Barr JR: The clinical recognition of cystic carcinoma of the breast. *Surg Gynecol Obstet* 159:130, 1984.

Fisher ER, Palekar AS, et al: Pathologic findings from the National Surgical Adjuvant Breast Project (Protocol No. 4). VI. Invasive papillary cancer. *Am J Clin Pathol* 73:313–322, 1980.

McDivitt RW, Stewart FW, Berg JW: Tumors of the breast, in *Atlas of Tumor Pathology*. Series 2, Fascicle 2. Washington, DC, Armed Forces Institute of Pathology, 1968.

Adenoid cystic carcinoma

Jundt G, Schultz A, et al: Small cell neuroendocrine (oat cell) carcinoma of the male breast. *Virchows Arch [Pathol Anat]* 404:213, 1984.

Sarcomas

Berg JW, DeCosse JJ, et al: Stromal sarcomas of the breast: a unified approach to connective tissue sarcomas other than cystosarcoma phyllodes. *Cancer* 13:418, 1962.

Golematis BC, Delikaris PG, et al: Lymphedema of the upper limb after surgery for breast cancer. *Am J Surg* 129:286, 1975.

Miettinen M, Lehto V-P, Virtanen I: Post-mastectomy angiosarcoma (Stewart-Treves syndrome). Light microscopic, immunohistological and ultrastructural characteristics of two cases. *Am J Surg Pathol* 7:329, 1983.

Sordillo PP, Chapman R, et al: Lymphangiosarcoma. *Cancer* 48:1674, 1981.

Woodward AH, Ivins JC, Soule EA: Lymphangiosarcoma arising in chronically lymphedematous extremities. *Cancer* 30:562, 1972.

Lymphomas

Brustein S, Kimmel M, et al: Malignant lymphoma of the breast. A study of 53 patients. *Ann Surg* 205:144, 1987.

DeCosse J, Berg J, et al: Primary lymphosarcoma of the breast. A review of 14 cases. *Cancer* 15:1264, 1962.

Inflammatory carcinoma

Bozzetti F, Saccozzi R, et al: Inflammatory cancer of the breast: analysis of 114 cases. *J Surg Oncol* 18:355, 1981.

DeLarue JC, Levin F, et al: Estrogen and progesterone cytosolic receptors in clinically inflammatory tumors of the human breast. *Br J Cancer* 44:911, 1981.

Haagensen CD: *Diseases of the Breast,* 2nd ed. Philadelphia, Saunders, 1971, pp 576–584.

Levine PH, Steinhorn SC, et al: Inflammatory breast cancer: the experience of the Surveillance, Epidemiology, and End Results (SEER) Program. *J Natl Cancer Inst* 74:291, 1985.

Rosen PP: Tumor emboli in intramammary lymphatics in breast carcinoma: pathologic criteria for diagnosis and clinical significance. *Pathol Annu* 18(Pt 2):215, 1983.

Rosen PP, Saigo PE, et al: Predictors of recurrence in Stage I (TINOMO) breast carcinoma. *Ann Surg* 193:15, 1981.

Taylor GW, Meltzer A: Inflammatory carcinoma of the breast. *Ann Surg* 33:33, 1938.

Treatment

Baker RR, Montague ACW, Childs JN: A comparison of modified radical mastectomy to radical mastectomy in the treatment of operable breast cancer. *Am Surg* 189(5):553, 1979.

Gray JH: The relation of lymphatic vessels to the spread of cancer. *Br J Surg* 26:462, 1939.

Haagensen CD: Anatomy of the mammary gland, in Haagensen CD (ed): *Diseases of the Breast,* 2nd ed. Philadelphia, Saunders, 1971, pp 1–28.

Halsted WS: Results of operation for cure of cancer of breast performed at Johns Hopkins Hospital from June 1889 to January 1894. *Ann Surg* 20:497, 1894.

Madden JL: Modified radical mastectomy. *Surg Gynecol Obstet* 121(6):1221, 1965.

Mahler F: Ueber die in der Heidelberger Klinik 1887–1897 behandelten Falle von Carcinoma Mammae. *Beitr Klin Chir* 26:681, 1900.

Meyer W: An improved method of the radical operation for carcinoma of the breast. *Med Rec NY* 46:746, 1894.

Patey DH: A review of 146 cases of carcinoma of the breast operated upon between 1930–1946. *Br J Cancer* 21:260, 1967.

Patey DH, Dyson WH: Prognosis of carcinoma of the breast in relation to type of operation performed. *Br J Cancer* 2:7, 1948.

Nonpalpable lesions

Egan RL: Breast biopsy priority: cancer versus benign preoperative masses. *Cancer* 35(3):612, 1975.

Egeli RA, Urban JA: Mammography in symptomatic women 50 years of age and under, and those over 50. *Cancer* 43:878, 1979.

Gallager HS: Breast specimen radiography: obligatory, adjuvant and investigative. *Am J Clin Pathol* 64:749, 1975.

Palpable lesions—fine-needle aspiration (FNA)

Hermansen C, Poulsen HS, et al: Palpable breast tumours: ''triple diagnosis'' and operative strategy. *Acta Chir Scand* 150:625, 1984.

Silverman JF, Lannin DR, et al: Fine needle aspiration cytology of subareolar abscess of the breast. Spectrum of cytomorphologic findings and potential diagnostic pitfalls. *Acta Cytol* 30(4):413, 1986.

Silverman JF, Lannin DR, et al: The triage role of fine needle aspiration biopsy of palpable breast masses. *Acta Cytol* 31:731, 1987.

Wilkinson EJ, Schuettke CM, et al: Fine needle aspiration of breast masses: analysis of 276 aspirates. *Acta Cytol* 33:613, 1989.

Wollenberg NJ, Caya JG, Clowry SJ: Fine needle aspiration cytology of the breast. A review of 321 cases with statistical evaluation. *Acta Cytol* 29(3):425, 1985.

Zajicek J: Aspiration biopsy cytology. Part I: Cytology of supradiaphragmatic organs. *Monogr Clin Cytol* 4:1, 1974.

Therapy of early breast cancer and in situ disease

Berstock DA, Houghton B, et al: The role of radiotherapy following total mastectomy for patients with early breast cancer. *World J Surg* 9:667, 1985.

Fisher B, Redmond C, et al: Ten-year results of a randomized clinical trial comparing radical mastectomy and total mastectomy with or without radiation. *N Engl J Med* 312(11):674, 1985.

Fisher B, Saffer EA, Fisher ER: Studies concerning the regional lymph node in cancer. VII. Thymidine uptake by cells from nodes of breast cancer patients relative to axillary location and histopathologic discriminants. *Cancer* 33:271, 1974.

Forrest APM, Roberts MM, et al: The Cardiff–St. Mary's trial. *Br J Surg* 61:766, 1974.

Forrest APM, Stewart HJ, et al: Simple mastectomy and axillary node sampling (pectoral node biopsy) in the management of primary breast cancer. *Ann Surg* 196(3):371, 1982.

Grace E: Simple mastectomy in cancer of the breast. *Am J Surg* 35:512, 1937.

Halsted WS: The results of operations for the cure of cancer of the breast performed at the Johns Hopkins Hospital from June 1889 to January 1894. *Arch Surg* 20:497, 1894.

Hermann RE, Esselstyn CB Jr, et al: Results of conservative operations for breast cancer. *Arch Surg* 120:746, 1985.

Kyle J, et al: Management of early cancer of the breast: report on an international multicentre trial supported by the Cancer Research Campaign. *Br Med J* 1:1035, 1976.

Langlands AO, Prescott RJ, Hamilton T: A clinical trial in the management of operable cancer of the breast. *Br J Surg* 67:170, 1980.

Maddox WA, Carpenter JT Jr, et al: A randomized prospective trial of radical (Halsted) mastectomy versus modified radical mastectomy in 311 breast cancer patients. *Ann Surg* 198(2):207, 1983.

Maddox WA, Carpenter JT Jr, et al: Does radical mastectomy still have a place in the treatment of primary operable breast cancer? *Arch Surg* 122:1317, 1987.

McWhirter R: The value of simple mastectomy and radiotherapy in the treatment of cancer of the breast. *Br J Radiol* 21:599, 1948.

Meyer W: An improved method for the radical operation for carcinoma of the breast. *Med Rec NY* 46:746, 1894.

Murphy JB: Carcinoma of breast. *Surg Clin JB Murphy* I(6):779, 1912.

Nemoto T, Vana J, et al: Management and survival of female breast cancer; results of a national survey by the American College of Surgeons. *Cancer* 45:2917, 1980.

Nemoto T, Vana J, et al: Observations on short-term and long-term surveys of breast cancer by the American College of Surgeons. In Murphy GP (ed): *International Advances in Surgical Oncology,* Vol IV. New York, Alan R Liss, 1981, pp 209–239.

Turner L, Swindell R, et al: Radical vs modified radical mastectomy for breast cancer. *Ann R Coll Surg Engl* 63:239, 1981.

Williams IG, Murley RS, Curwen MP: Carcinoma of the female breast: conservative and radical surgery. *Br Med J* 2:787, 1953.

Wilson RE, Donegan WL, et al: The 1982 National Survey of Carcinoma of the Breast in the United States by the American College of Surgeons. *Surg Gynecol Obstet* 159:309, 1984.

QU.A.RT.

Greening WP, Montgomery CV, et al: Quadrantic excision and axillary node dissection without radiation therapy: the long-term results of a selective policy in the treatment of Stage I breast cancer. *Eur J Surg Oncol* 14:221, 1988.

Lagios MD, Richards VE, et al: Segmental mastectomy without radiotherapy. Short-term follow-up. *Cancer* 52:2173, 1983.

Veronesi U: Quadrantectomy, in Bland KI, Copeland EM III (eds): *The Breast: Comprehensive Management of Benign and Malignant Diseases*. Philadelphia, Saunders, 1991, Chap 29, pp 631–634.

Limitations for conservation procedures

Doets CJ: *De heelkunde van Petrus Camper 1722–1789*. Thesis. Leiden, 1948, p 25.

Donegan WL: Introduction to the history of breast cancer, in Donegan WL, Spratt JS (eds): *Cancer of the Breast,* 3rd ed. Philadelphia, Saunders, 1988, pp 1–15.

Fisher B: Lumpectomy (segmental mastectomy) and axillary dissection, in Bland KI, Copeland EM III (eds): *The Breast: Comprehensive Management of Benign and Malignant Diseases*. Philadelphia, Saunders, 1991, Chap 29, pp 634–652.

Fisher B, Fisher ER: Transmigration of lymph nodes by tumor cells. *Science* 152:1397, 1966.

Fisher B, Redmond C, et al: Eight year results of the NSABP randomized clinical trial comparing total mastectomy and lumpectomy with or without radiation in the treatment of breast cancer. *N Engl J Med* 320(13):822, 1989.

Kurtz JM, Amalric R, et al: Local recurrence after breast-conserving surgery and radiotherapy. Frequency, time course, and prognosis. *Cancer* 63:1912, 1989.

Recht A, Connolly JC, et al: The effect of young age on tumor recurrence in the treated breast after conservative surgery and radiotherapy. *Int J Radiat Oncol Biol Phys* 14:3, 1988.

Breast reconstruction

Gilliland MD, Barton RM, Copeland EM III: The implications of local recurrence of breast cancer as the first site of therapeutic failure. *Ann Surg* 197:284, 1983.

Hormonal receptors

Allegra JC: The use of steroid hormone receptors in breast cancer, in Margolese R (ed): *Contemporary Issues in Clinical Oncology: Breast Cancer*. New York, Churchill Livingstone, 1983.

Bonadonna G, Brusamolino E, et al: Combination chemotherapy as an adjuvant treatment in operable breast cancer. *N Engl J Med* 294:405, 1976.

Clark GM, McGuire L: New biologic prognostic factors in breast cancer. *Oncology* 3(5):49, 1989.

Ellis LM, Bland KI: Techniques for obtaining the diagnosis of malignant breast lesions. *Surg Clin North Am* 70:815, 1990.

Fisher B, Carbone P, et al: L-Phenylalanine mustard (L-PAM) in the management of primary breast cancer. *N Engl J Med* 292:117, 1975.

Horwitz KB, McGuire WL: Estrogen and progesterone: their relationship in hormone-dependent breast cancer, in McGuire WL, Raynaud P, Baulieu EE (eds): *Progesterone Receptors in Normal and Neoplastic Tissues*. New York, Raven Press, 1977.

Lippman ME, et al: The relation between estrogen receptors and response rate to cytotoxic chemotherapy in metastatic breast cancer. *N Engl J Med* 298:381, 1978.

Martin PM, Rolland PH, et al: Multiple steroid receptors in human breast cancer. III. Relationships between steroid receptors and the state of differentiation and the activity of carcinomas throughout the pathologic features. *Cancer Chemother Pharmacol* 2:115, 1979.

McCarty KS Jr, et al: Correlation of estrogen and progesterone receptors with histologic differentiation in mammary carcinoma. *Cancer* 46:2851, 1980.

McGuire WL: Steroid receptors in human breast cancer. *Cancer Res* 38:4289, 1980.

NIH Consensus Conference: Treatment of Early-Stage Breast Cancer. *JAMA* 265(3):391, 1991.

Savlov ED, Witliff JL, Hilf R: Further studies of biochemical predictive tests in breast cancer. *Cancer* 39:539, 1977.

Silva JS, et al: Biochemical correlates of morphologic differentiation in human breast cancer. *Surgery* 92:443, 1982.

Metastatic disease

Anteman K, Gale RP: Advanced breast cancer: high-dose chemotherapy and bone marrow antotransplants. *Ann Int Med* 108:570, 1988.

Peters WP, Shpall EJ, et al: High-dose combination alkylating agents with bone marrow support as initial treatment for metastatic breast cancer. *J Clin Oncol* 6(9):1368, 1988.

Breast cancer during pregnancy and lactation

Donegan WL: Mammary carcinoma and pregnancy, in Dunphy JE (ed): *Major Problems in Clinical Surgery*. Philadelphia, Saunders, 1967, pp 170–178.

Donegan WL: Mammary carcinoma in pregnancy, in Hall EJ (ed): *Radiobiology for the Radiologist*. New York, Harper & Row, 1978, pp 397–410.

Schapira DV, Chudley AE: Successful pregnancy following continuous treatment with combination chemotherapy before conception and throughout pregnancy. *Cancer* 54:800, 1984.

Sweet DL, Kinzie J: Consequences of radiotherapy and antineoplastic therapy for the fetus. *J Reprod Med* 17:241, 1976.

White TT, White WC: Breast cancer and pregnancy, a report of 49 cases followed 5 years. *Ann Surg* 144:384, 1956.

Recurrence during pregnancy

Harvey EB, Borce JD, et al: Prenatal x-ray exposure and childhood cancer in twins. *N Engl J Med* 315:541, 1985.

Jablon S, Kato H: Childhood cancer in relation to pre-natal exposure to atomic bomb radiation. *Lancet* 2:1000, 1970.

CHAPTER 15

Tumors of the Head and Neck

John J. Coleman III and Mark R. Sultan

CONGENITAL LESIONS

Thyroglossal Duct Cysts

The thyroid gland originates from the pharyngeal floor at the foramen cecum during the fourth week of gestation. It enlarges, becomes bilobed, and descends ventrally in the midline of the neck in close approximation to the developing hyoid bone. During this descent the patent diverticulum is called the thyroglossal duct. The duct normally resorbs by the tenth week of gestation. When all or a portion of this duct persists, thyroglossal duct cysts or sinuses are formed.

Classically these cysts present as midline masses in childhood, although they have been reported to be as much as 2 cm from the midline and may present for the first time in adults. Eighty percent occur at or just below the hyoid bone. A maneuver to differentiate them from Delphian lymph nodes or other central masses is to have the patient protrude the tongue. The level of the cyst is elevated by protrusion, demonstrating its embryologic origin from the base of the tongue. Unlike branchial cleft remnants, thyroglossal duct cysts generally do not have external sinuses. A significant percentage, however, do become infected, usually during the course of an upper respiratory tract infection. Approximately 5 percent of the cysts contain functional thyroid tissue, and rare cases of thyroglossal duct carcinoma have been reported.

The differential diagnosis for midline neck masses about the hyoid bone includes lingual thyroid tissue. Rarely this may be the patient's only active thyroid gland. Therefore, the presence of thyroid tissue in its normal anatomic location must be confirmed either clinically or by radioactive scan before any midline neck mass is excised, and careful postoperative observation for hypothyroidism is imperative.

Sistrunk is credited with the development of a technique for excising thyroglossal duct cysts and sinuses which minimizes the risk of recurrence. He describes resection of the cyst with the central portion of the hyoid bone, following the sinus superiorly to its putative site of origin, the foramen cecum, and excising it in its entirety.

Branchial Cleft Anomalies

Branchial cleft cysts, sinuses, and cartilaginous remnants result from the incomplete fusion of the branchial clefts. The branchial clefts, appearing in week 4 of embryonic life and normally involuting fully by week 7, contribute to the formation of various head and neck structures in the developing embryo. When a portion of a cleft persists, epithelium-lined cysts or sinuses, with or without cutaneous openings and cartilaginous rests, may manifest. These anomalies usually present in the first decade of life but may go undetected until adulthood. The majority of branchial cleft cysts and sinuses are lined by squamous epithelium, although ciliated columnar epithelium has been reported as well. Branchial cleft carcinoma occurs rarely when there is a history of a branchial cleft cyst, the subsequent development of epidermoid cancer at that site, and no other primary lesion. Branchial cleft cysts also contain lymphoid tissue and may enlarge in response to upper respiratory infections.

The most common types of branchial cleft anomalies are those of the second cleft. These are present at the middle and lower thirds of the sternocleidomastoid muscle. Cartilaginous rests from the first branchial cleft typically are subcutaneous, usually appear medial to the tragus, and may be managed by simple excision. Cysts and sinuses often extend more deeply into the neck. The fistulous tract courses superiorly along the carotid sheath and then medially over the hypoglossal nerve between the internal and external carotid arteries to end at the pharynx adjacent to the tonsillar fossa. A stair-step incision is sometimes needed to follow this circuitous route. First branchial cleft cysts and sinuses are located above the level of the hyoid just below the body of the mandible and extend superolaterally through the parotid gland to end within the membranous external auditory canal. Excision of these cysts and sinuses is recommended to avoid the complications associated with recurrent infection. Dissection must be meticulous to avoid injury to the facial, hypoglossal, vagus, and lingual nerves and to the carotid vessels. Anomalies of the third branchial cleft are rare. Like second cleft anomalies they arise anterior to the middle and lower thirds of the sternocleidomastoid muscle. However, they course behind the carotid artery to end at the pyriform sinus.

Hemangiomas and Vascular Malformations

Congenital vascular lesions must be clearly classified as hemangiomas or vascular malformations in order to assess their prognosis and establish appropriate management plans. Recently the distinctions between the two have been clarified on the basis of cellular and clinical characteristics. Hemangiomas have an increased mitotic activity and as such may be considered true neoplasms. They are typically absent at birth or may be present as a faint vascular blush. During the first several months of life they may undergo a rapid proliferative phase during which they sometimes grow to large size. Although the majority of hemangiomas undergo spontaneous involution by the age of seven, complications such as ulceration and bleeding, obstruction of the eye with subsequent amblyopia, nasal airway obstruction, and rarely thrombocytopenia (Kasabach-Merritt syndrome) may mandate early surgical resection. Systemic dexamethasone therapy for a short course has been found to arrest the growth of large lesions during their proliferative phase. The use of intralesional steroid injections or sclerosing agents may be successful in achieving temporary control of smaller hemangiomas in strategic locations such as the lip or eyelid. Photodynamic laser therapy may be helpful in preventing the onset of the proliferative phase of hemangiomas.

Vascular malformations, unlike hemangiomas, have a normal rate of endothelial cell turnover. They result from congenital errors in vascular morphogenesis and are classified by their vessel of involvement—namely capillary, venous, arterial, lymphatic, or combined. High-flow lesions result from gross abnormalities connecting the arterial and venous systems and may cause catastrophic problems of massive hemorrhage, high-output congestive heart failure, and hemolytic anemia. Chronic increased blood flow may be associated with skeletal abnormalities such as bone hypertrophy and distortion. Capillary, venous, and arterial malformations may occur anywhere in the head and neck. Lymphatic malformations (cystic hygromas) classically occur in the neck or floor of mouth. Malformations are always present at birth although they may not be clinically evident until the ectatic vessels suddenly dilate under hormonal or other physiologic influences. They normally grow proportionately to the child and do not regress spontaneously, unlike hemangiomas. Therefore, the management of malformations is often surgical. Indications for early surgical resection include recurrent infections, obstructive symptoms (e.g., respiratory distress), hemorrhage, and significant aesthetic deformities.

Because vascular malformations of the head and neck are often highly infiltrative, a complete preoperative evaluation of the extent of the lesion and its vascularity must be obtained. Angiography is usually necessary, sometime for diagnosis but usually to determine the contributory vessels. When technically possible, complete extirpation of the malformation should be performed while preserving normal anatomic structures. Preoperative embolization by arteriographic technique may decrease blood flow temporarily, making surgical resection safe and more practical.

Vascular birthmarks, in the past descriptively named "strawberry" or "capillary" hemangioma, "port-wine stains," "cavernous hemangiomas," and "cystic hygromas," are now classified by their major vessel of involvement, namely "capillary," "venous," or "lymphatic malformation," respectively. Since the prognosis and management of vascular birthmarks are directly dependent on their correct classification as hemangiomas or malformations, the importance of accurate description is obvious.

In deep-seated subcutaneous vascular malformations such as those sometimes occurring in the cheek or pharynx, physical examination may be inadequate for accurate delineation. Further evaluation is often necessary and may include CT or MRI, angiography, or technetium-labeled red blood cell scintigraphy. Definitive diagnosis in any patient with a vascular mass may require open biopsy to rule out a malignancy, which may occasionally have similar radiographic characteristics.

BENIGN LESIONS

Lip

The lower lip may be subject to chronic irritants such as pipe smoking or lip biting and, more important, to the damaging effects of chronic actinic exposure. In affected individuals the epidermis of the vermilion becomes atrophic and the dermis reveals elastosis. The basal layer of the epidermis then develops dysplasia creating thickening of the superficial mucosal layer, the stratum corneum. This thickening or hyperkeratosis is clinically visible and palpable. With progression the dysplasia extends upward into the epithelium, producing parakeratosis, the accumulation of nucleated cells, near the epithelial surface. This is manifested clinically by scaling of the lip. A proliferation and abnormal orientation of epithelial cells, dyskeratosis, may then follow, ultimately leading to carcinoma in situ. With penetration of the basement membrane, an invasive squamous cell carcinoma develops. When *dyskeratosis* or *carcinoma in situ* is present over a large extent of the surface of the lower lip, excision of the entire vermilion (''lip shave'') should be considered. The lip is then resurfaced by advancing the buccal mucosa to the mucocutaneous junction.

Oral Cavity

A variety of benign lesions arise in the oral cavity. They may be grouped by location into those affecting the buccal mucosa, gingiva, or tongue or by their causation, such as inflammatory or ulcerative. For many, their significance lies in their possible premalignant potential or in their mimicking of true malignancies.

The oral lining contains countless mucous glands, the minor salivary glands. A submucosal accumulation of mucus results in a mucous retention cyst. Since the majority of these cysts have no epithelial lining, it is now believed that they are most often caused by rupture of the duct system, with extravasation of mucus, and not by ductal obstruction, as was previously thought. The most common location for a mucous cyst or mucocele is the labial mucosa of the lower lip (Fig. 15-1). These lesions are typically less than 1 cm in diameter, smooth, rounded, and have a bluish hue. The treatment of choice is excision. Marsupialization alone is reserved for extensive lesions. A *ranula* is a type of mucous retention cyst that arises from major salivary glands, most commonly the sublingual. This too is managed by excision, but due to its occasional large size and location in the floor of the mouth, it may require a meticulous dissection to avoid nerve injury and postoperative hemorrhage. It is frequently necessary to resect the affected sublingual gland in-continuity to prevent recurrence.

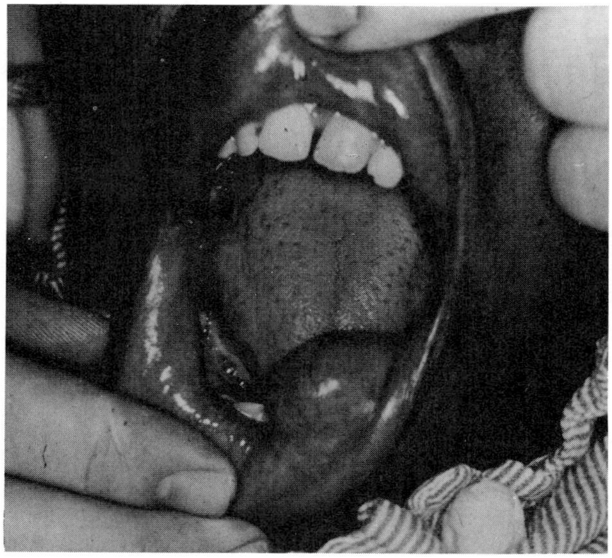

FIG. 15-1. Mucous cyst of the lip, the most common location for the lesion. The mucocele has resulted from rupture of a minor salivary gland duct with spillage of mucus into the surrounding tissue.

An *epulis* is a granulomatous lesion of the gingiva, and as elsewhere in the body, it represents an exaggerated inflammatory response to minor injury. Two subtypes exist: namely, congenital epulis, which is typically found in the anterior maxilla of newborns, and epulis gravidarum, which occurs in approximately 1 percent of pregnant women and normally resolves spontaneously when the pregnancy is concluded. Only symptomatic epulides need be excised.

Peripheral giant cell reparative granulomas also occur most commonly on the gingiva. The ''giant'' cell of origin resembles an osteoclast. These granulomas are polypoid, submucosal, and fibrous. They can create ulceration and hemorrhage of the overlying musosa. Radiographs may reveal erosion of the underlying bone. Excision must be complete to prevent recurrence. The term ''peripheral'' refers to the soft tissue origin of these tumors as opposed to the *central giant cell reparative granulomas,* which, although similar histologically, arise within bone. The peripheral giant cell reparative granulomas are four times more common than central type. The latter are expansile endosteal lesions which typically present within the mandible of young adults. They have also been reported in the paranasal sinuses, orbit, cranial vault, and temporal bone. They must be distinguished from true giant cell tumors of bone (which have malignant potential), brown tumors of hyperparathyrodism, traumatic bone cysts, and fibrous dysplasia. Thorough curettage is generally curative.

The tongue and the larynx are common locations for the development of *papillomas*. They are caused by the human papilloma virus which induces squamous epithelial proliferation into soft, irregular, pedunculated lesions. Eradication may be accomplished by excision or cauterization. Other common benign masses of the tongue include fibromas, neurofibromas, and lingual thyroid nodules. The last may lie dormant through childhood and yet rapidly enlarge during puberty.

In 1926, Abrikossoff described rare benign tumors involving the tongue which he named *granular cell myoblastoma* because of their presumed embryonal muscle cell of origin. They are now believed to derive from Schwann cells and have been found to arise throughout the aerodigestive tract, particularly in the larynx. In the tongue they typically occur as firm, submucosal swellings in the middle one-third and may therefore mimic squamous cell carcinoma. Wedge excision is curative.

The oral lining is subject to a number of ulcerative conditions. The *idiopathic aphthous ulcer* is the most common type. The cycle of painful ulceration and spontaneous healing may occur several times a year and persist for many years. Other similar ulcers have identifiable etiologic factors, including viral infection with herpes simplex, nutritional deficiencies including vitamin B, folate or iron, and emotional stress. These ulcers often respond to topical steroids. Multiple painful oral ulcerations may be a manifestation of *pemphigus vulgaris*. This may be accompanied by severe, generalized toxicity. The disease typically occurs in the fifth to seventh decade of life in patients of Mediterranean descent. The ulcers begin as intraepithelial bullae which subsequently rupture and ulcerate. The overlying epithelium may be rubbed off easily (Nikolsky's sign). In *erythema multiforme,* persistent or recurrent painful oral ulcerations arise within a background of diffuse oral erythema. Biopsy reveals a perivascular lymphocytic cellular infiltrate. Separate skin involvement may or may not be present. A variety of causes have been proposed. Management with systemic steroids and antimetabolites is often necessary.

Discrete, painful ulcers are also present in *necrotizing sialometaplasia*. This is a benign inflammatory disease of minor salivary glands which usually occurs on the hard palate. It is believed that local trauma leads to progressive local ischemia and ulceration. The histologic differentiation from squamous cell cancer or mucoepidermoid carcinoma can be extremely difficult by incisional biopsy. Therefore, although these ulcers will ordinarily heal spontaneously in 6 to 10 weeks without specific treatment, in cases where the correct diagnosis remains unclear after incisional biopsy, complete excision of the ulcer is prudent.

The description and significance of leukoplakia and erythroplasia will be reviewed later in this chapter. Other white plaque-like lesions of the oral cavity include *white sponge nevus, lichen planus,* and *oral hairy leukoplakia*. Histologically, all reveal parakeratosis. White sponge nevus is a rare familial ectodermal disease which diffusely involves the oral cavity in a benign, self-limited manner. Lichen planus is a degenerative mucocutaneous disease with a probable autoimmune basis. Oral lesions may appear with or without cutaneous manifestations and may at times become erosive. Oral squamous cell carcinoma has been found in association with lichen planus with an incidence varying between 0.09 and 10 percent in different series. Therefore, as in oral leukoplakia, systemic and topical retinoids are being evaluated in the treatment of oral lichen planus to reverse the condition itself and, more important, to suppress the presumed heightened potential of the oral mucosa toward degeneration into invasive carcinomas in these conditions. Oral hairy leukoplakia is a form of parakeratosis recently described in patients with AIDS or other forms of immunosuppression such as renal transplants and leukemia. Thick shaggy plaques typically appear on the lateral surface of the tongue and become symptomatic when superinfected with *Candida*. Management includes antifungal medication, antiviral agents, or surgical excision.

Nose

Polyps arise commonly within the nasal cavity and paranasal sinuses. They occur with equal frequency in males and females and in all age groups after adolescence. Ten percent of children with cystic fibrosis may also develop nasal polyps. The polyps are often multiple, involving both sides of the nasal cavity and the paranasal sinuses. They may present with nasal obstruction, mucoid nasal discharge, or anosmia. Those that arise in the region of the turbinates and ethmoids are mainly allergic in origin, while those of the posterior nasal cavity are most often infectious. Medical management should include an evaluation for allergies. Aspirin should be stopped or avoided, since an association exists between aspirin use and the formation of nasal polyps. If the allergic evaluation is negative, an empiric trial of antimicrobials is begun. Steroid nasal sprays may also be helpful. When medical management fails, surgical intervention may be necessary. Simple polypectomy carries a high rate of recurrence, and more extensive endoscopic or open excision may be necessary.

Papillomatous growths may occur on the nasal skin or within the nasal cavity. The *squamous papilloma* is an exophytic verrucous lesion caused by the papilloma virus and is present on the skin of the nasal sills, columella, or alae. It is managed as are other cutaneous warts. The *inverted papilloma* (also called schneiderian papilloma, squamous papilloma, or papillomatosis) is a polypoid mass occurring on the lateral nasal wall, typically in middle-aged men. The name is derived from its histologic appearance of an "inverted" proliferative growth pattern. The significance of this lesion lies in its presentation with symptoms of nasal obstruction, its recurrence rate of 50 percent with polypectomy alone, and its association with concurrent and subsequent invasive squamous cell carcinoma in 8 and 4 percent of patients, respectively. More extensive resection and close follow-up are therefore indicated and can lower the recurrence rate to 6 percent.

Juvenile nasopharyngeal angiofibromas are benign but highly expansible and destructive fibrovascular neoplasms which typically arise in adolescent males, between ten and twenty years of age. Originating in the superior nasal cavity they can erode widely into the paranasal sinuses, orbit, pterygomaxillary fossa, and middle cranial fossa. Early symptoms include nasal obstruction and epistaxis, while more advanced lesions can produce anosmia, proptosis, or cranial nerve dysfunction. Management commonly requires preliminary angiographic embolization followed by surgical extirpation. Approximately 10 percent require a combined intracranial/extracranial approach. Radiation therapy is generally reserved for residual or recurrent disease, although its successful use as a primary modality has also been reported.

Paranasal Sinuses

Although the terms are often used interchangeably, mucous retention cysts and mucoceles of the paranasal sinuses are different entities with distinct pathogeneses, natural histories, and connotations. *Mucous retention cysts* arise as a result of blockage of secretion from *microscopic* secretory ducts of mucous glands within the lining of the paranasal sinus cavity, possibly as a sequela of sinusitis. The fluid mass that results remains separate from the bony wall of the sinus and so continues to be surrounded by air within the sinus, except at its base. Rarely, they can enlarge to occupy the entire sinus, at which point it would be difficult to distinguish them from the more virulent mucoceles. Radiographically they appear as discrete masses which are profiled by sinus air. The most common location for mucous retention cysts of the paranasal sinuses is within the maxillary sinus, where they usually present as an asymptomatic incidental finding on x-ray. Ten percent of routine sinus radiographs reveal evidence of these cysts in the maxillary sinus. They are considered the most common benign lesions of the maxilla. Treatment is rarely necessary.

As opposed to the indolent mucous cyst, *mucoceles* of the paranasal sinuses, although benign, can be expansile, highly destructive lesions. These result from *macroscopic* blockage of a sinus ostium by epithelial or osseous neoplasms, inflammatory processes, or as a result of trauma (e.g., facial bone fractures). Mucinous secretions then accumulate within the entire sinus. With persistent secretion a pressure effect on the entire sinus wall is produced, displacing both the epithelial lining and bony wall. This can ultimately result in thinning and destruction of the wall such that the mucocele can "invade" adjacent vital structures. CT scans or MRI scans are needed to delineate the complete extent of the process, but clinical distinction from a carcinoma can be difficult. Mucoceles most commonly arise within the frontal sinuses followed in order by the ethmoidal, maxillary, and sphenoidal sinuses. In the frontal sinus location they most often present with frontal headaches. Sixty percent of frontal sinus mucoceles erode through the floor of the sinus (the orbital roof) causing proptosis and frontal swelling. Left untreated, diplopia and even blindness can result. Symptoms resulting from mucoceles of the remaining sinuses depend on their direction of spread. Fortunately, intracranial extension is rare. Mucoceles that become infected are called pyoceles and present with the additional signs and symptoms of sinusitis. The most definitive treatment of a mucocele includes the evacuation of the contents of the sinus through an open approach. The entire mucosal lining on the sinus must then be removed and the sinus duct occluded with muscle or bone. The need to then obliterate the remaining sinus itself and, if so, with what material (e.g., muscle, fat, or cancellous bone) remains controversial.

Larynx

The most common benign neoplasm of the larynx is the *pappiloma,* accounting for more than 90 percent of such tumors. Papillomas usually arise on the true vocal cords and usually present with hoarseness. They may be found at any site within the larynx as well as on the hypopharyngeal or pharyngeal walls. They are likely caused by the human papilloma virus and present as predunculated exophytic masses. Laryngeal papillomas may be grouped into juvenile or adult types depending on the age of onset. In the juvenile group there is a 2:1 female predominance, whereas the opposite is true in the adult group. The typical course of each type is also distinctly different. In adults the masses are most often solitary and rarely recur after excision. In the juvenile group the lesions tend to be multiple and may recur and spread rapidly after excision. The reason for these differences is not known. Laryngeal papillomas are most often treated today with laser obliteration.

Other less common benign tumors of the larynx include oncocytic tumors and granular cell myoblastomas. The former present as a smooth submucosal mass and the latter as a sessile mucosal mass. The most common location for each is the true vocal cords, and so they too typically present with hoarseness. Chondromas of the larynx are rare benign cartilaginous neoplasms most commonly occurring on the cricoid cartilage. They can cause hoarseness, respiratory obstruction, or dysphasia. All of these benign neoplasms are managed by conservative excision.

A *laryngocele* is a herniation of the laryngeal ventricle. Three forms exist, categorized by their site of presentation. An internal laryngocele remains confined to the larynx and presents as an enlargement of the false cord. An external laryngocele protrudes through the thyrohyoid membrane causing swelling in the anterior neck. Combinations of these two types, called mixed laryngoceles, exist as well. The pathogenesis is believed to be associated with chronic increases in intralaryngeal pressure. Corroborative evidence for this theory includes the fact that singers and musicians have a propensity for their development. Symptoms depend on the site of presentation, with the internal variety often causing hoarseness and the external most commonly remaining asymptomatic. Treatment includes ligation of the stalk of the laryngocele and repair of the ventricular weakness.

Odontogenic and Bone Tumors

Odontogenic Tumors

A variety of cysts and tumors of the mandible and maxilla may arise from the progenitor cells of tooth development. The majority of these odontogenic lesions are benign and may be treated conservatively. Ameloblastomas (adamantinomas) arise from dental lamina and are often associated with impacted teeth in young patients. Their usual presentation is that of a painless mass of the jaw with a multilocular radiolucent appearance on x-ray. They occur four times more frequently in the mandible than in the maxilla. Although slow-growing, they may grow to large size and erode adjacent bone (Fig. 15-2). Treatment consists of resection of the entire lesion with a margin of bone to prevent local recurrence. Myxomas and Pindborg tumors (calcifying epithelial odontogenic tumors) are similar in their presentation and management in that they too require an en bloc resection for cure.

A second group of odontogenic tumors, including calcifying odontogenic cysts (Gorlin's cysts), ameloblastic fibromas, cementomas, and keratocysts, are generally less aggressive than those discussed above and are treated effectively by enucleation and excision of the entire lining of the lesion.

Nonodontogenic Tumors

This group of tumors arise from bone that is not involved in tooth development. Torus is a benign, slow-growing projection from the surface of bone. The torus palatinus occurs in the midline of the hard palate, and the torus mandibularis usually develops on the lingual surface of the mandible opposite the premolars, often bilaterally. They are both common lesions. In the United States 20 percent of the population have a torus palatinus and 8 percent a torus mandibularis. Evidence exists that they are genetically inherited by autosomal dominant genes with incomplete penetrance. Tori often begin around puberty and are slow-growing. They can induce ulceration of the overlying mucosa, thereby mimicking a mucosal neoplasm. No therapy is needed unless they interfere with speech, mastication, or the use of dentures, at which time simple excision is performed.

Exostoses are similar to tori and also commonly occur in the jaws. There are localized overgrowths of bone which may be nodular, pedunculated, or flat and are often multiple. They most often present in the maxilla at the canine fossa as a hard, discrete, submucosal mass. Only symptomatic masses require excision.

Osteomas are slow-growing tumors of mature bone that arise within (intraosseous) or at the periphery of the involved bone. The peripheral lesions are often attached to the cortical bone by a dense pedicle. Involvement of the bones outside of the face and skull is rare. They most commonly arise on the mandible on the lingual aspect of the ramus or on the lower border of the angle of the

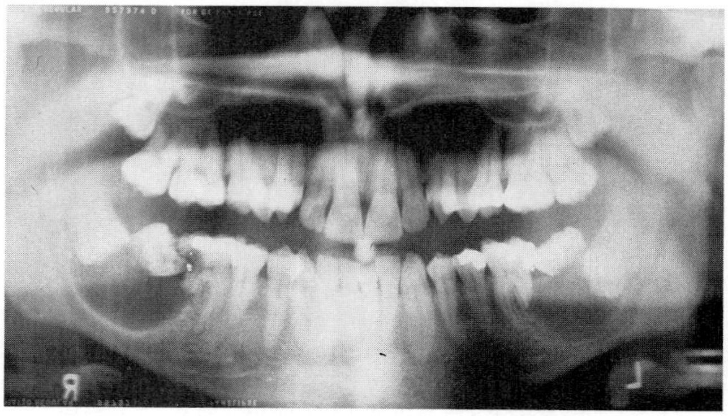

FIG. 15-2. Bilateral dentigerous (odontogenic) cysts of the mandibular alveolus showing resorption of tooth roots.

mandible. Osteomas may also occur in the paranasal sinuses, where they may achieve a large size. Excision is advised when continued growth encroaches upon vital structures or becomes cosmetically unacceptable. Multiple osteomas are one of the manifestations of Gardner's syndrome, the others being multiple inclusion cysts of the skin, supernumerary teeth, and familial polyposis.

Fibrous dysplasia is a benign bone disorder of unknown cause in which cortical bone is replaced by immature fibrous tissue. The fibrous tissue often proliferates and extends beyond normal boundaries, distorting and compressing vital structures. Seventy percent of patients have involvement of a single bone (monostotic) and 30 percent have the polyostotic form. In the head and neck, the mandible or maxilla is most often involved. Albright's syndrome includes polyostotic fibrous dysplasia, precocious puberty, café au lait spots, and several endocrine abnormalities. The management of the patient with fibrous dysplasia is dictated by the aggressiveness of the disease and ranges from observation only to extensive local resection and reconstruction. Malignant degeneration occurs in 1 percent of cases and may be related to prior radiation therapy. Malignant degeneration should be suspected in any lesion that undergoes rapid growth or significant pain.

CARCINOMAS

General Considerations

Malignant neoplasms that arise in the head and neck area or upper aerodigestive tract share the general behavior of most solid tumors: local growth, locoregional spread, and distant metastasis. Their effect, however, on the human organism both before therapy and as a consequence of therapy depends much more than most other neoplasms' on local disruption of function. The two main vegetative functions of the human—alimentation and respiration—are effected by the intricate synergy of the bone, nerve, muscle, and the mucosa-lined cavities that make up the head and neck. Invasive carcinoma disrupts this fine balance, resulting not only in the proliferation of abnormal cells but also in the derangement of feeding, breathing, and speaking, which may present as malnutrition, upper airway obstruction, and recurrent aspiration pneumonia. Thus unlike adenocarcinoma of the breast, colon, stomach, malignant melanoma, squamous cell carcinoma of the lung, and most other solid tumors where the fatal event is virtually always disseminated malignancy, as many as 60 percent of patients dying with head and neck malignancy expire without clinical evidence of metastasis beyond the local/regional disease. Central nervous system invasion, rupture of the great vessels, airway obstruction, and invasive local infection are common causes of death in these patients (Fig. 15-3). Because of the predominant local and locoregional natural history of this disease, significant attention must be paid to local diagnosis and therapy.

Most malignant tumors that develop in the anatomic area above the clavicles are squamous cell carcinomas (epidermoid carcinomas) originating from the respiratory and stratified squamous epithelium of the upper aerodigestive tract. Although there are some differences in the natural history of tumors arising at the various sites of the upper aerodigestive tract, probably dependent on characteristics of blood supply, lymphatic drainage, or histologic variation specific to that area, most squamous cell carcinomas of the head and neck behave similarly. Their unique clinical expression then depends on the interruption of normal activity inherent in their epicenter and those areas to which they spread (Fig. 15-4). So nasopharyngeal carcinoma may present with nasal stuffiness and progress to cranial nerve dysfunction and central nervous system invasion as well as neck metastasis; and carcinoma of the floor of

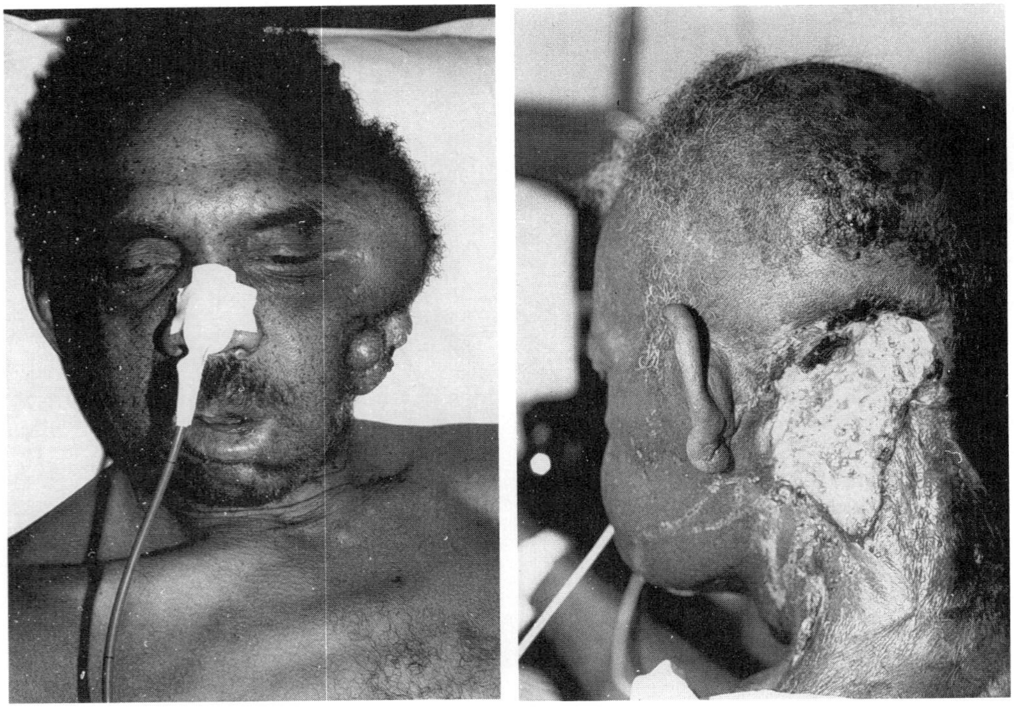

A B

FIG. 15-3. *A.* Local recurrence of squamous cell carcinoma of oral cavity, involving retromolar trigone with infiltration of pterygoid muscles, infratemporal fossa, trigeminal nerve, and cutaneous satellitosis. No evidence of distant metastasis. *B.* Uncontrolled regional recurrence in the neck from squamous cell carcinoma of tonsil treated with neck dissection and radiation showing ulceration and invasion of mastoid and occipital bones.

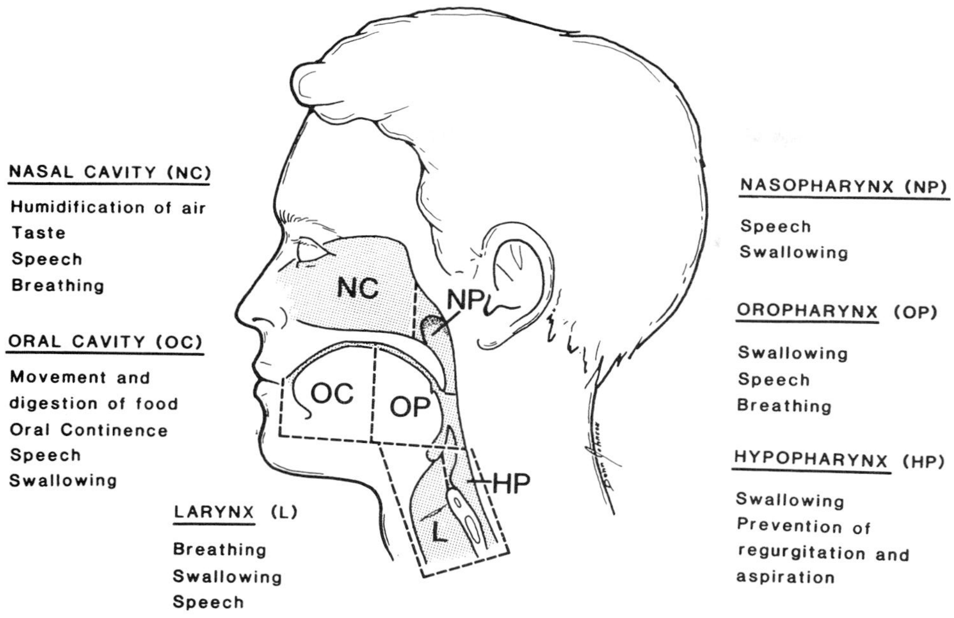

FIG. 15-4. Functional role of the anatomic divisions of the upper aerodigestive tract (From: *Coleman JJ III, Searles JM: Anatomical reconstruction after resection (surgical removal) of cancer. New Developments in Medicine 4(2):37, 1989, Figure 1, with permission.*)

the mouth may present with pain, tethering of the tongue, and dysphagia, resulting in malnutrition and possible aspiration.

Moreover, the therapeutic approach to the malignancy may interfere with normal function. Laryngectomy and glossectomy obviously impair speech and swallowing to a great degree. Radiotherapy, used alone or in combination with surgery, may result in deficiencies of olfaction, salivation, and infection control in the upper aerodigestive tract. Survival of the patient with head and neck cancer then requires consideration of both tumor growth and residual local function in formulation of the therapeutic plan. The appropriate selection of radiotherapy, extirpative surgery, chemotherapy, and reconstructive surgery is crucial to the patient in the physician's attempt to prolong life and restore reasonable function and appearance. A multidisciplinary approach to this group of tumors is essential.

Both in children and in adults neoplasms other than squamous cell carcinoma, benign and malignant, and other clinically important masses arise in the head and neck area (Fig. 15-5). Although some of these are more likely to progress to early metastatic disease, most have significant local effect in both their clinical expression and therapy. In adults, salivary neoplasms are the next most important group of lesions in the head and neck.

Epidemiology

Squamous cell carcinoma of the head and neck is not a major public health problem in the United States of America. Combined upper aerodigestive tract sites account for approximately 23 new cases per 100,000 males and 8 per 100,000 females, or roughly 6 percent of new cancers in males and 2 percent in females. There are between 30,000 and 40,000 new cancers of the head and neck and 10,000 to 15,000 deaths per year. Approximately one-third of patients who develop a squamous cell carcinoma of the upper aerodigestive tract will die from it. Incidence and mortality rates in the United States have remained relatively stable over the past 40 years in white males but have increased dramatically for most sites in nonwhite males and in females of both groups (Fig. 15-6). Like many solid tumors, the incidence of disease increases with age in both sexes, being very rare below age thirty except in immunocompromised patients. In the United States there seems to be a clear-cut relationship between squamous carcinoma of the upper aerodigestive tract and the chronic use of tobacco and alcohol together. Although the use of either tobacco or alcohol alone increases the likelihood of squamous cell carcinoma of the upper aerodigestive tract, the cumulative abuse greatly increases the risk (Fig. 15-7). Previously noted increases in the incidence of squamous cell carcinoma in females were probably due to the more widespread acceptance of cigarette smoking among women over the past 30 years. In the Western world the combination of tobacco and alcohol of various forms seems to be the predominant cause of this disease; and though there is some slight variation, the mortality rate is similar from country to country. Cigarette, cigar and pipe smoking, chewing tobacco, and snuff have all been implicated, as have distilled beverages, beer, wine, and even mouthwash, which in many forms has a high content of alcohol. The previously demonstrated relationship of asbestos and tobacco in the carcinogenesis of lung cancer is probably operant in squamous cell carcinoma of the upper aerodigestive tract as well.

Squamous cell carcinoma of the head and neck is endemic in other parts of the world, with incidences reaching as high as 50 percent of new cancers in Bombay, India, where chewing of *pan*, a combination of local tobacco, betel nut, and lime ($CaOH_2$), causes buccal carcinoma. Throughout southeast Asia the use of betel nut and tobacco combinations similarly results in a high frequency of oral cancers. In cultures such as those of south Asia and southeast Asia, where alcohol is not commonly used, the prevalence of vitamin deficiency and local submucosal fibrosis of the oral mucosa may play an important adjuvant role. Reverse smoking (smoking of cigarettes and cigars with the lighted end inside the mouth) similarly contributes to the high incidence of palate and oral cancers seen in India and some parts of Central and South America. In South Africa unusually high rates of nasal and paranasal cancers have been discovered, where nickel contaminates the tobacco inhaled as snuff, and where it and other substances are

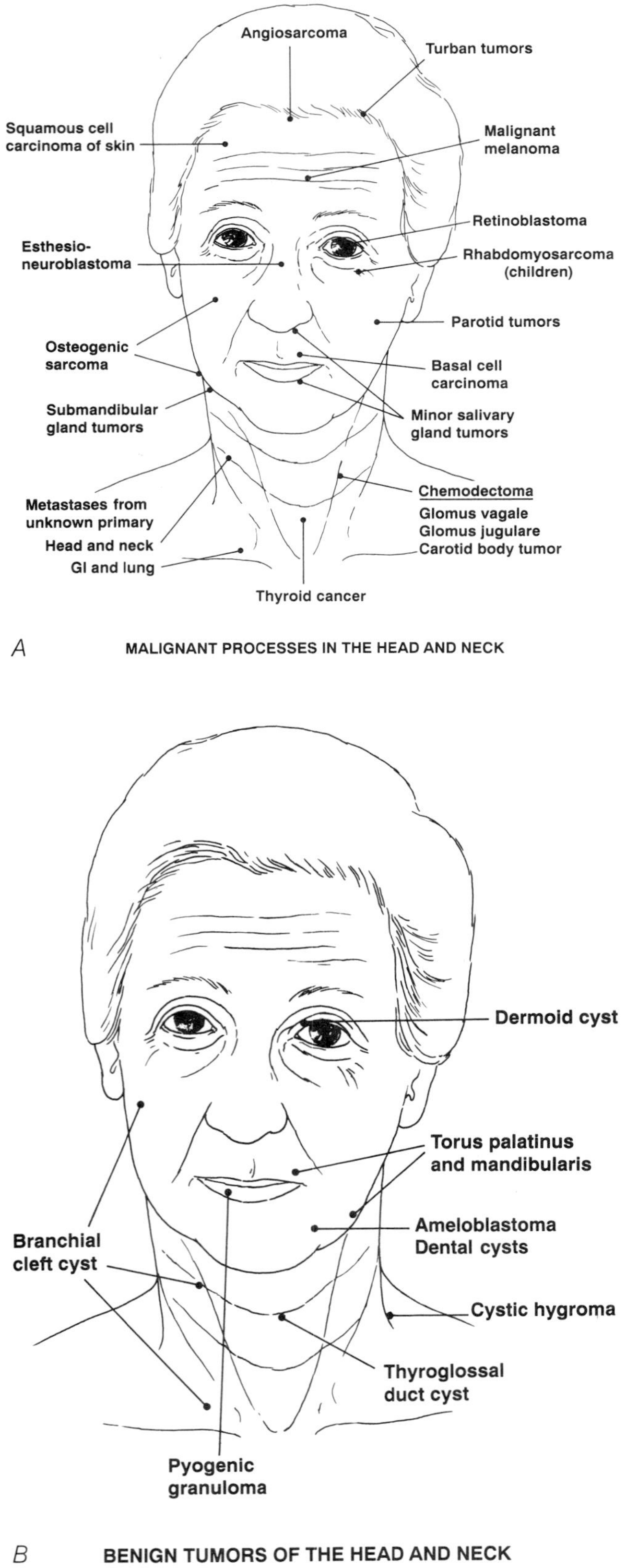

FIG. 15-5. Although squamous cell carcinoma makes up 95 percent of malignancies in the head and neck, other malignant (*A*) and benign (*B*) masses may be seen in the adult population.

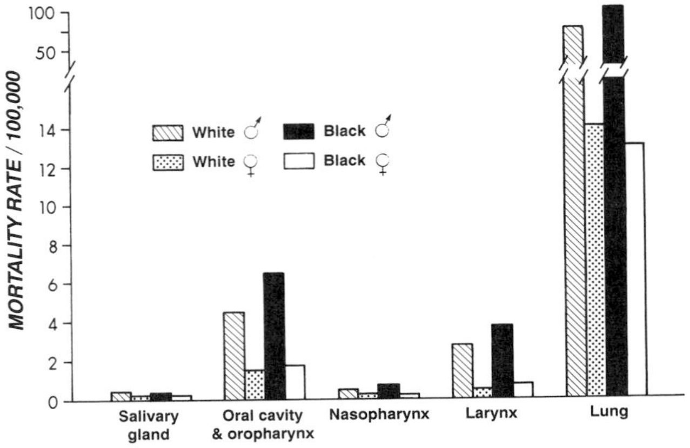

FIG. 15-6. Mortality rates/100,000 persons, 1970–1979, by site of primary disease, race, and sex with percent change from 1950 to 1959 (Derived from: *Blitzer PH: 1988, with permission.*)

industrial contaminants as among nickel workers, furniture workers and shoe workers.

In southern China and the Pacific rim countries, carcinoma of the nasopharynx is extremely common in both men and women, up to 20 times more common than in the United States. The etiologic factors are unclear, although inhaled fumes, cooking smoke, chemical pollutants, or others have been proposed, as has the ingestion of salted fish. The role of the Epstein-Barr virus in the causation and natural history of nasopharyngeal carcinoma is unclear. Infection with EBV is prevalent in this group, and there seems to be a close relationship between elevated serum EBV titers and risk. Despite the differences in proposed causative agents throughout the world, it appears clear that an important factor in the origin of squamous cell carcinoma is a chemical carcinogen and that a linear dose-time risk ratio is likely. Prevention should be possible.

Carcinogenesis

The simplest explanation of the causation of squamous cell carcinoma falls within the accepted principles of chemical carcinogenesis, more specifically cocarcinogenesis, where an *initiating* agent (perhaps some contaminant or metabolite of tobacco) induces an irreversible change in the DNA of the affected cell. A *promoting*

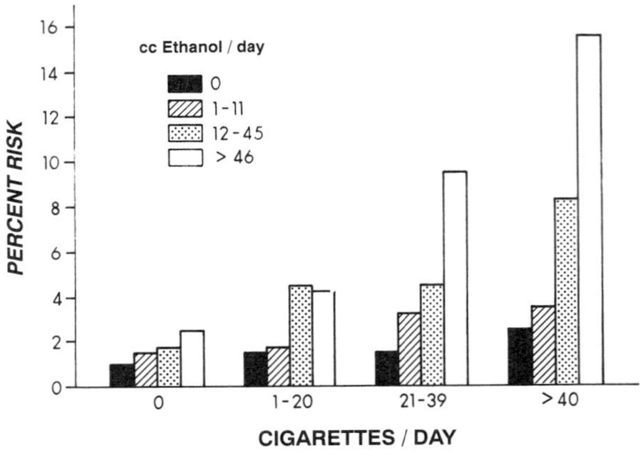

FIG. 15-7. Relative risk of developing squamous cell carcinoma as a function of daily cigarette and alcohol consumption.

agent (perhaps alcohol, vitamin deficiency, local inflammation secondary to trauma, poor hygiene, or submucosal fibrosis) allows that irreversible change to manifest itself as a histologically and clinically identifiable malignancy. Initiation involves alteration of the DNA by either addition through covalent bonding, replacement, deletion, or other mechanism. Promotion theoretically involves facilitation of expression of the abnormal DNA via activation of cell surface and cytoplasmic protein receptors or other reactions with the epithelial cell. This theory is consistent with many of the epidemiologic and clinical characteristics of squamous cell carcinoma of the upper aerodigestive tract. The necessity for chronic use implies that initiation alone is not sufficient for malignancy. In addition to the sites in the nasopharynx and larynx where inhaled and exhaled tobacco smoke contact, high-dose exposure is possible to the mouth, tongue, and buccal mucosa as metabolites of tobacco are secreted into saliva and sit pooled in the lingual and buccal sulci. The chronic inflammation attendant on frequent alcohol use may stimulate local proliferation of epithelial cells and react with reproducing cells to allow expression of the previously altered DNA.

The role of viral carcinogenesis via initiation or promotion is unclear but certainly suspicious. Patients with papillomatosis caused by human papilloma virus of the nasal cavity and larynx have been observed to be at higher risk for development of invasive squamous cell carcinoma. Recent studies of DNA from squamous cell carcinoma of the nasal cavity and paranasal sinuses using the polymerase chain reaction have identified human papilloma virus (HPV) types 16 and 18, whereas they were not identified in tumors of other histologic type (adenocarcinoma, adenoid cystic, etc). HPV 16 genomes have also been found in squamous cell carcinoma of the larynx, buccal mucosa, tongue, and cervical lymph node metastases. Elevated antibody to Epstein-Barr virus is associated with the presence of nasopharyngeal carcinoma but is not specific enough to be of clinical use, since viral infection is common. That the virus plays either an initiating or a promoting role in carcinogenesis is suggested by the presence of the EB viral genome in cervical metastases as well as the primary tumor arising in the nasopharynx but its absence in lymph nodes of EB antibody seropositive patients that did not contain tumor and its absence in metastatic tumors of other histology.

Although malignancy of the head and neck is not commonly associated with familial syndromes, benign tumors such as exostoses, sebaceous cysts, and sebaceous adenomas may be seen in the genetic alteration that causes Gardner's and Muir-Torres' syndrome. Of the identified oncogenes, several have been discovered in squamous cell carcinoma. The *int-2* oncogene related to fibroblast growth factor and the *C-myc* gene which codes for a DNA binding protein concerned with regulation of cell growth have been demonstrated in 11 of 21 and 2 of 21 squamous cell carcinoma tumors studied. Improved methods of DNA characterization will certainly clarify the role of viral transformation, heredity, and increased susceptibility in the pathogenesis of squamous cell carcinoma.

The protean manifestations of AIDS include a number of abnormalities in the head and neck. Proliferative lymphocyte deposits in the nasopharynx have been noted to cause eustachian tube dysfunction and may be precursors of the commonly seen extranodal lymphomas. Squamous cell carcinomas of the upper aerodigestive tract appear to be disproportionately common and unusually aggressive in patients with AIDS, as in other immunodeficient states such as chronic lymphocytic leukemia. Oral and pharyngeal presentations of Kaposi's sarcoma are common in HIV-positive patients and may require surgical or radiotherapeutic intervention occasionally (Fig. 15-8). Cystic degeneration of lymph nodes in the parotid and submandibular glands is also seen, and in one series was the presenting symptom of newly diagnosed HIV infection.

Natural History

Malignancy in the head and neck follows a relatively predictable course along the continuum of histologic changes from early evidence of hyperplasia with atypia to poorly differentiated invasive malignancy. The sequential presentation of these abnormalities fits well with a theory of chronic exposure to one or several chemical carcinogens. The normal oral and oropharyngeal cavities are lined with stratified squamous epithelium similar to the skin but without the characteristic keratinization. Another difference between the skin and oral mucosa is the lack of distinct rete ridges in the mouth in normal states. Immediately subjacent is the basement membrane, beneath which lies the submucosa, containing lymphoid aggregates and lymphatic channels, blood vessels, and mucous and serous glands. In most areas of the oral cavity and oropharynx, mucosa and submucosa cover muscle. Within the epithelial layer are terminations of the nerves mediating the special senses of olfaction and taste as well as other nerve fibers. The larynx, nasal cavity, and paranasal sinuses are lined by pseudostratified columnar ciliated epithelium, which overlies a similar arrangement of minor salivary glands, nerves, and blood vessels.

Viral infection, chronic irritation by ill-fitting dentures, trauma, or infection from poor dental hygiene may elicit a response from the epithelium known as hyperplasia or papillomatosis, in which cells with normal DNA configuration and organelle structure proliferate, resulting in more prominent intraluminal projection as well as extension of the mucosa deeper into the submucosa. Despite these changes there are none of the cellular manifestations of malignancy (mitoses, pyknotic nuclei, prominent nucleoli, etc.), and the basement membrane beneath to the mucosa remains intact.

Most of the clinical changes that reflect these histologic alterations, including hyperplasia, hyperkeratosis, and pseudoepitheliomatous hyperplasia (the aggressive end of this spectrum which

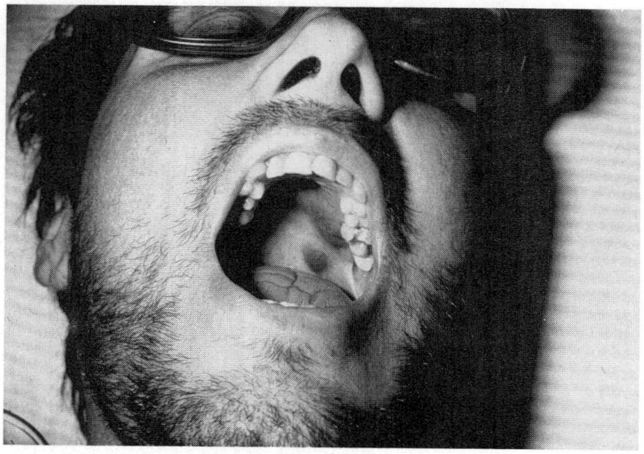

FIG. 15-8. Purplish nodules on the hard and soft palate of Kaposi's sarcoma in patient with ARC (AIDS-related complex).

may be confused clinically with malignancy), have been grouped under the term *leukoplakia* (white patch). Histologic analysis shows hyperkeratosis and parakeratosis or orthokeratosis (appearance of nuclei in the most superficial layers of the mucosa with or without inflammatory cell infiltrate and acanthosis). Early dictates required removal of all leukoplakia, since it was felt to be a precursor of invasive malignancy. More recent thinking, however, suggests that this change is not in itself premalignant but simply evidence of chronic irritation.

Cellular manifestations of malignancy result in the diagnosis of epithelial dysplasia. Lack of a normal cellular progression to maturation characterizes dysplastic epithelium. Nuclei are larger, are hyperchromatic, and show mitotic activity. Cells may be pleomorphic with basophilic cytoplasm. Cell layers become disorganized, with loss of the gradual ascent to the epithelial surface and the presence of immature cells at the basement membrane as well as the epithelial surface. The extent of the individual cellular changes and loss of normal polarity determines whether the entity is termed dysplasia, severe dysplasia, or carcinoma in situ. All of these changes, however, overlie an intact basement membrane. The change from hyperplasia to dysplasia is thought to be irreversible and the initial step in ultimate carcinogenesis. The clinical manifestation of these histologic changes has been termed *erythroplasia* or *erythroplakia* or red patch. These lesions appear reddish, frequently exudative, and may have associated leukoplakia. Biopsy or excision is mandatory since they are premalignant and may also indicate the presence of another adjacent malignancy.

The cellular changes of carcinoma in situ with loss of the integrity of the basement membrane become invasive squamous cell carcinoma. Deranged cellular function results in intracellular keratinization or keratin pearl formation (Fig. 15-9). Growth into the oral cavity may manifest grossly as an exophytic carcinoma, whereas invasion into the adjacent muscle or bone produces ulcerative lesions.

In addition to the continuum of changes from hyperkeratosis to invasive carcinoma, patients with squamous cell carcinoma frequently demonstrate another phenomenon consistent with the theory of chemical carcinogenesis. Field *cancerization* or the *condemned mucosa* phenomenon is the finding of epithelial abnormalities throughout the entire upper aerodigestive tract in a patient with squamous cell carcinoma at one site (Fig. 15-10). Erythroplakia in the oral cavity increases the risk of invasive carcinoma in the pharynx, larynx, esophagus, and lung. The presence of synchronous malignancies in the upper aerodigestive tract has been reported to range from 4.4 to 10 percent or higher, with lung, esophagus, and other head and neck sites being most common.

Other anatomic abnormalities and functional disorders are also more frequent in patients with upper aerodigestive tract malignancy. Barrett's esophagus and esophagitis have been reported to occur in 33 percent of patients undergoing laryngoesophagectomy for advanced laryngeal carcinoma. An overall incidence of esophageal disease of 54 percent was found, with synchronous esophageal cancer in 25 percent of these patients. Metachronous or subsequent malignancies also appear at a higher frequency than in the

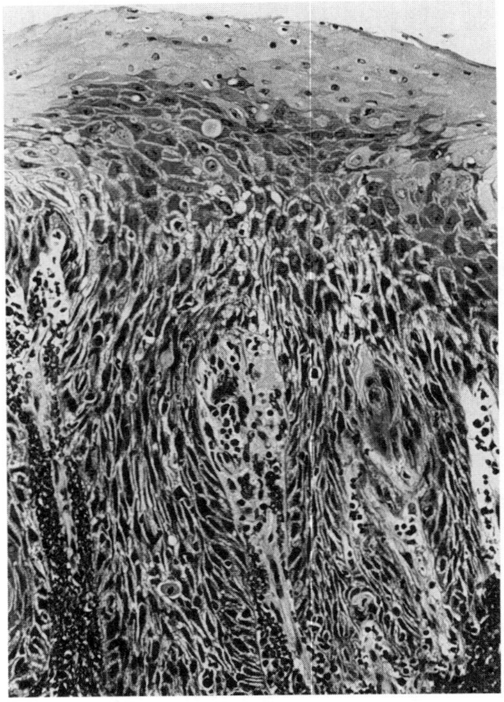

A

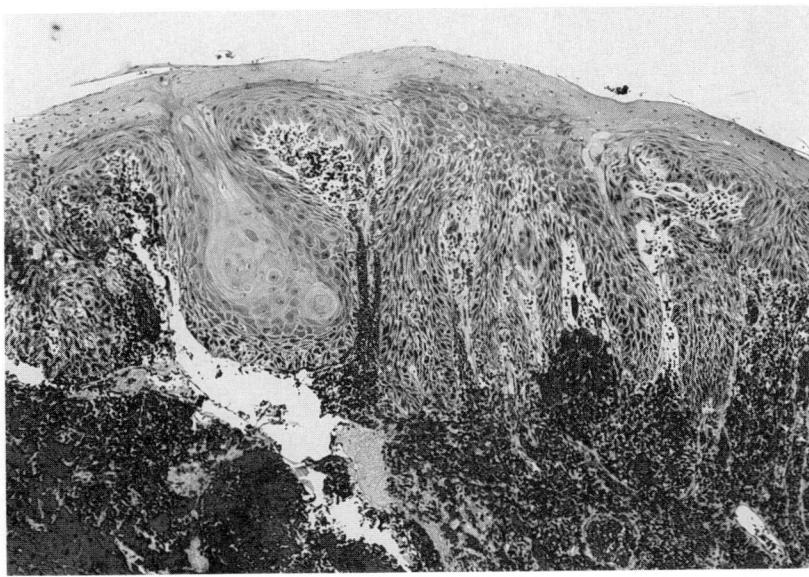

B

FIG. 15-9. *A.* Squamous cell carcinoma in situ with adjacent epithelial dysplasia. Hyperkeratosis at surface with keratin pearl but no evidence of penetration of basement membrane. Dense mononuclear inflammatory response. (Hematoxylin and eosin.) *B.* Squamous cell carcinoma in situ of tongue showing cellular changes of malignancy, parakeratosis, cellular pleomorphism, loss of cellular polarity, severe dysplasia in rete ridges, keratin at lower levels than normal. (Hematoxylin and eosin.) (*Courtesy of C. Whitaker Sewell.*)

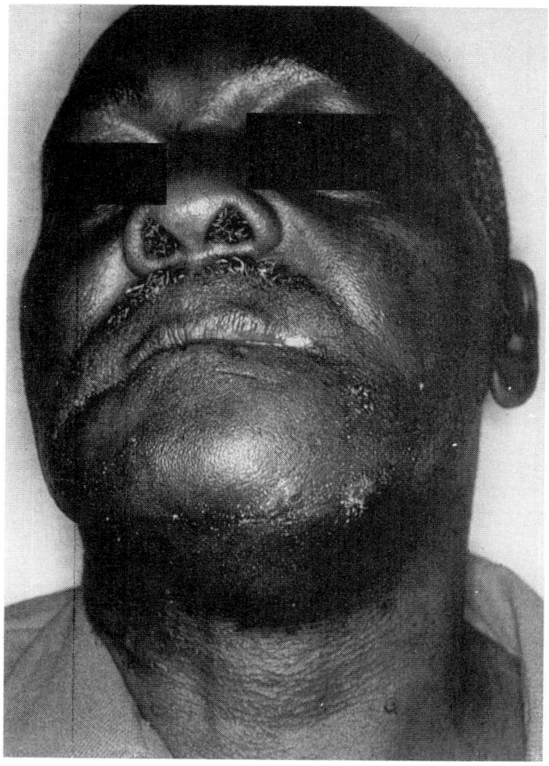

A

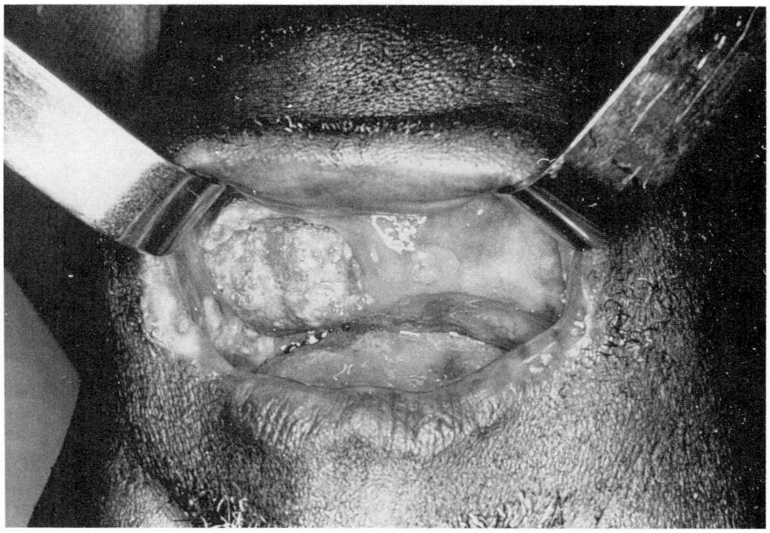

B

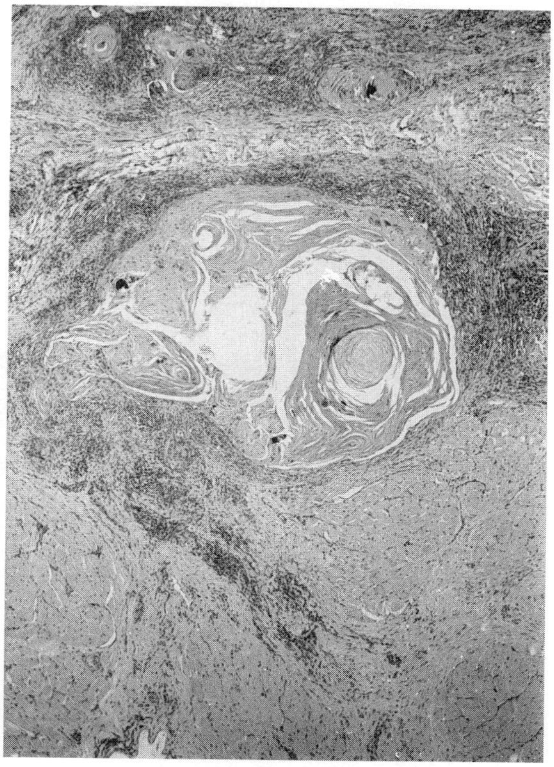

C

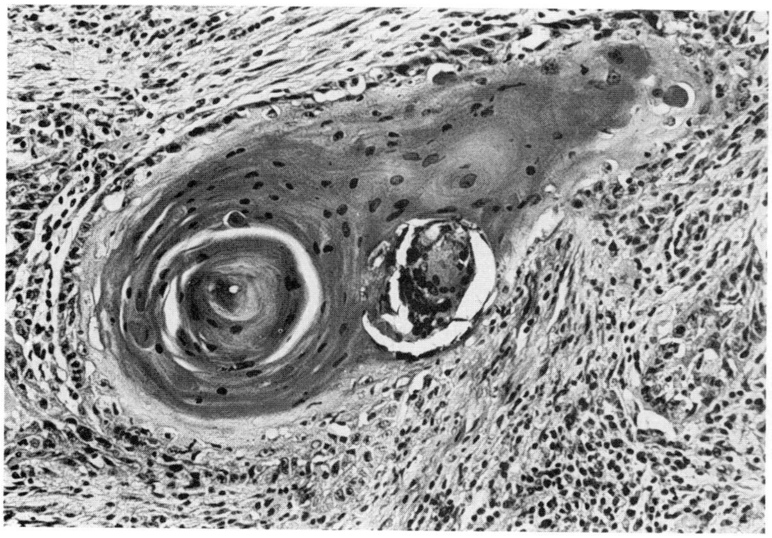

D

FIG. 15-10. *A.* Fifty-six-year-old male with 40-year history of constant use of chewing tobacco and moderate to heavy alcohol intake. Submandibular fullness and excoriated area in skin represent local growth of invasive squamous cell carcinoma of the mandibular alveolus (gum). T4,N0,M0 therapy required radical excision of jaw, floor of mouth, skin of the submental and submandibular areas and reconstruction with pectoralis major musculocutaneous flap. *B.* Invasive squamous cell carcinoma of alveolus. *C* and *D.* Photomicrographs of lesion showing tumor invading subjacent muscle and nerve. Enlargement shows cellular and nuclear pleomorphism, microvascular invasion, and keratin pearl formation. *E.* This patient demonstrates the phenomenon of field cancerization. On his right buccal mucosa he had an exophytic lesion, a verrucous carcinoma. *F.* Photomicrograph of verrucous carcinoma showing sharp demarcation of border of normal epithelium and tumor (*left*), the pushing border. Despite marked epithelial proliferation and abnormality there is no invasion into the submucosa. *G.* Further manifestation of field cancerization with leukoplakia and erythroplakia on the dorsal surface of the tongue. *H* and *I.* Cellular features of leukoplakia include thickening of the epithelial layer, hyperkeratosis, loss of normal progression from the basal layers to the surface, with nuclei present in most superficial layers, and submucosal inflammatory infiltrate. The basement membrane, however, remains intact and there is no evidence of malignancy in the submucosal layers.

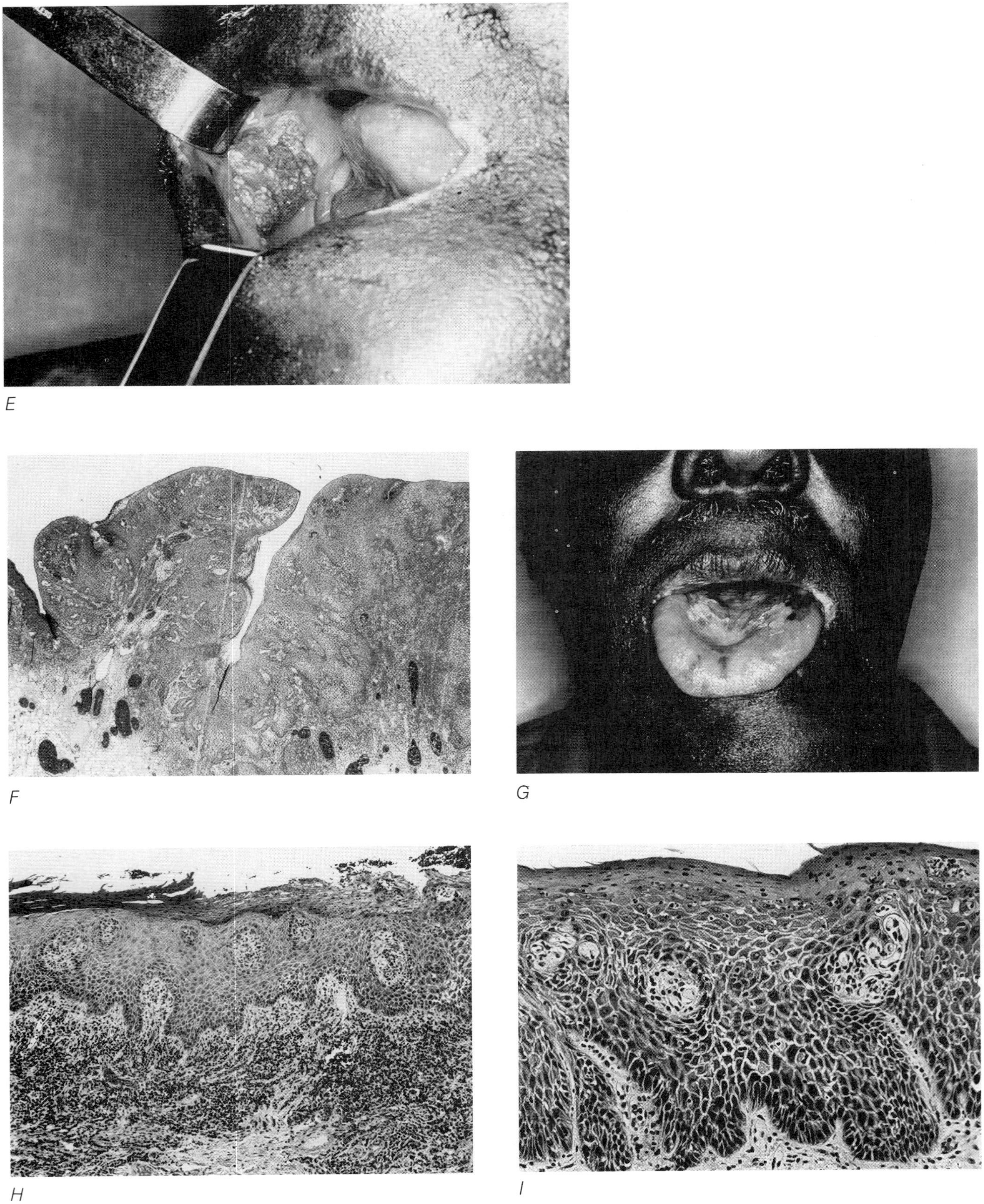

E F G H I

FIG. 15-10. Continued.

general public in patients with squamous cell carcinoma of the upper aerodigestive tract. Lung, esophagus, and other head and neck sites are more common, with a risk of up to 27 percent. Cessation of smoking and alcohol intake may or may not be protective.

The phenomenon of field cancerization and the high frequency of synchronous and metachronous malignancies in patients with squamous cell carcinoma of the head and neck fit nicely the current theories of oncogenesis. Within the condemned mucosa there may be multiple subpopulations of neoplastic cells, each the clonal expression of a common initial abnormality. Different environmental conditions, subsequent mutations caused by the chronic insult of chemical carcinogens, amplification of genetic abnormalities at one site more than another may explain the simultaneous appearance of erythroplasia, well-differentiated local carcinoma, and poorly differentiated lymph node metastasis as the disease progresses both clinically and histologically. The application of the theory of *tumor heterogeneity* to the entire mucosal surface explains many of the characteristics of individual tumors such as resistance to chemotherapy and radiotherapy as well as the patient's systemic response to disease.

Although theories of malignancy that espouse a stepwise progression from local to locoregional to metastatic disease have been shown to be inaccurate for breast and gastrointestinal solid tumors, squamous cell carcinoma of the head and neck does seem to spend a considerable portion of its natural history in the local or locoregional stages. After passage through the basement membrane, malignancy invades the surrounding mesenchymal tissue, be it muscle, cartilage, or bone. Proteases and collagenolytic and osteoclastic enzymes facilitate the destruction of the adjacent tissues. Invasion of subjacent nerves opens the perineural spaces, and tumor emboli may pass in the perineural lymphatics. The usual spread of tumor is from the primary site via the subjacent lymphatics (Fig. 15-11) to the neck or by continued local invasion through nerve and bone to the base of the skull. The virulence of the primary tumor and its likelihood of metastasis or ability to cause the demise of the host have been estimated by a number of methods. Size of the primary tumor is the main parameter determining its clinical stage in the TNM staging system adopted by the American Joint Committee on Cancer and other worldwide organizations (Fig. 15-12). Although a crude method, it is fairly reliable in suggesting the prognosis of the patient and the appropriate form of therapy.

Histologic characteristics such as degree of differentiation (primarily a function of nuclear morphology) pattern of invasion (blunt pushing borders vs. noncohesive jagged borders), microvascular invasion, perineural invasion, and tumor thickness have been used to predict the likelihood of lymph node metastasis and overall prognosis. Advances in biochemical and molecular investigation have allowed more careful consideration of the primary tumors. Flow cytometric analysis of tumor suspensions shows that aneuploidy is common in primary tumors (68 percent) and in cer-

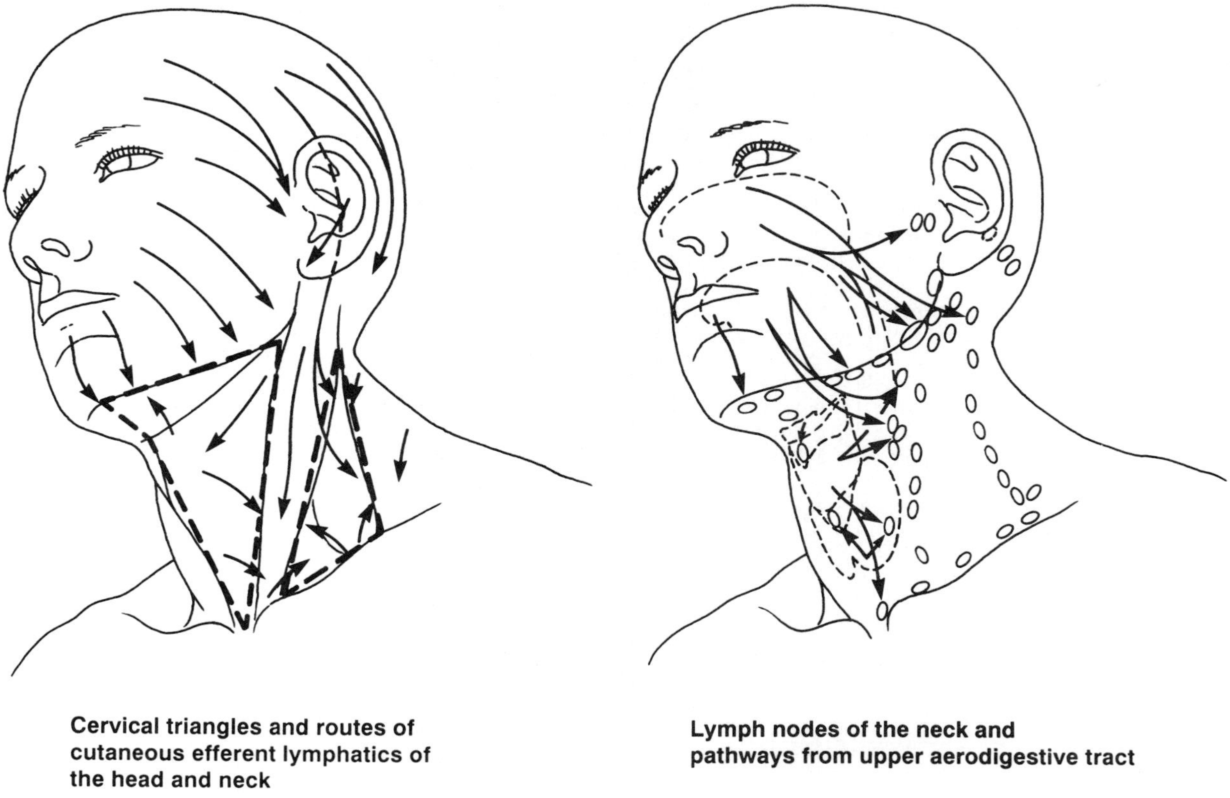

Cervical triangles and routes of cutaneous efferent lymphatics of the head and neck
Lymph nodes of the neck and pathways from upper aerodigestive tract

FIG. 15-11. Lymphatic drainage pathways from external and internal structures in the head and neck region. The jugulodigastric lymph nodes are the way station for a considerable part of this area. The locations of the lymph nodes correspond in great degree to the anatomic triangles of the neck. (Adapted from: *Haagensen CD, Feind C, et al: The Lymphatics in Cancer. Philadelphia, WB Saunders, 1972, Fig 5-10, p. 88, with permission.*)

Data Form for Cancer Staging

Patient identification
Name ____________________
Address ____________________
Hospital or clinic number ____________________
Age ______ Sex ______ Race ____________________

Institutional identification
Hospital or clinic ____________________
Address ____________________

Oncology Record

Anatomic site of cancer ____________________

Histologic type† ______________ Grade (G) ______________

Chronology of classification* [ ] Clinical-diagnostic (cTNM) [ ] Surgical-evaluative (sTNM) [ ] Postsurgical resection–pathologic (pTNM) [ ] Retreatment (rTNM) [ ] Autopsy (aTNM)

Date of classification ____________________

Definitions for all Time Periods

Primary Tumor (T)

[ ] TX Minimum requirements to assess the primary tumor cannot be met.
[ ] T0 No evidence of primary tumor
[ ] Tis Carcinoma *in situ*
[ ] T1 Greatest diameter of primary tumor 2 cm or less
[ ] T2 Greatest diameter of primary tumor more than 2 cm but not more than 4 cm
[ ] T3 Greatest diameter of primary tumor more than 4 cm
[ ] T4 Massive tumor more than 4 cm in diameter with deep invasion to involve antrum, pterygoid muscles, base of tongue, skin of neck

Lymph Nodes (N)

Same definitions to be used if postsurgical treatment–pathologic staging is used:

[ ] NX Minimum requirements to assess the regional nodes cannot be met.
[ ] N0 No clinically positive node
[ ] N1 Single clinically positive homolateral node 3 cm or less in diameter
[ ] N2 Single clinically positive homolateral node more than 3 but not more than 6 cm in diameter or multiple clinically positive homolateral nodes, none more than 6 cm in diameter
  [ ] N2a Single clinically positive homolateral node more than 3 cm but not more than 6 cm in diameter
  [ ] N2b Multiple clinically positive homolateral nodes, none more than 6 cm in diameter
[ ] N3 Massive homolateral node(s), bilateral nodes, or contralateral node(s).
  [ ] N3a Clinically positive homolateral node(s), one more than 6 cm in diameter
  [ ] N3b Bilateral clinically positive nodes (in this situation, each side of the neck should be staged separately; (*i.e.*, N3b: right, N2a; left, N1)
  [ ] N3c Contralateral clinically positive node(s) only

Distant Metastasis (M)

[ ] MX Minimum requirements to assess the presence of distant metastasis
[ ] M0 No (known) distant metastasis
[ ] M1 Distant metastasis present
Specify ____________________

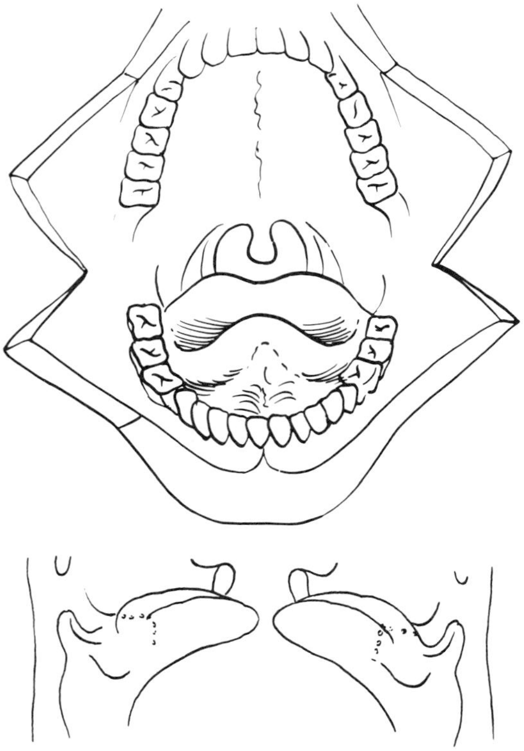

Tumor size: ________ cm

Location of Tumor

[ ] Lips: Upper
Lower
[ ] Buccal mucosa
[ ] Floor of mouth
[ ] Oral tongue
[ ] Hard palate
[ ] Gingivae: Upper
Lower
Retromolar trigone

Examination by ____________________ M.D.
Date ____________________

*Use separate form each time a case is staged.
†See reverse side for additional information.

American Joint Committee on Cancer Manual for Staging of Cancer

A

FIG. 15-12. American Joint Committee on Cancer staging system for carcinoma of the oral cavity shows anatomic sites, extent of disease, and disease in the neck in both diagrammatic and verbal form.

Characteristics of Tumor

[ ] Exophytic
[ ] Superficial
[ ] Moderately infiltrating
[ ] Deeply infiltrating
[ ] Ulcerated
[ ] Extends to or overlies bone
[ ] Gross erosion of bone
[ ] Radiographic destruction of bone

Involvement of Neighboring Regions

[ ] Tonsillar pillar or soft palate
[ ] Nasal cavity or antrum
[ ] Nasopharynx
[ ] Pterygoid muscles
[ ] Soft tissues or skin of neck

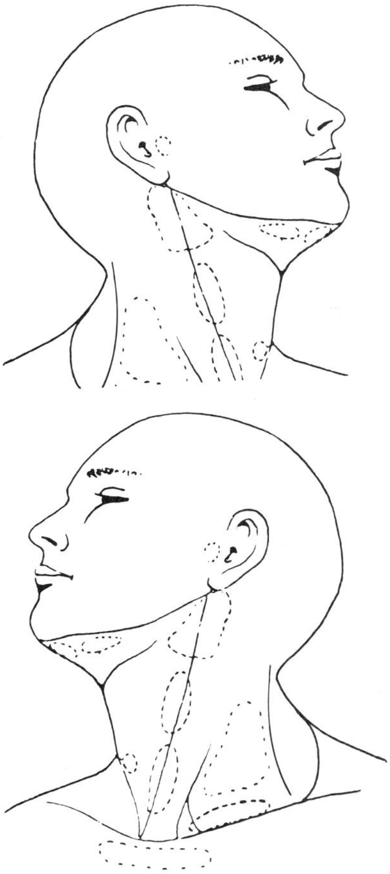

Indicate on diagram primary tumor and regional nodes involved.

Stage Grouping

[ ]	Stage I	T1, N0, M0
[ ]	Stage II	T2, N0, M0
[ ]	Stage III	T3, N0, M0
		T1, T2, T3; N1, M0
[ ]	Stage IV	T4, N0, N1; M0
		Any T, N2, N3; M0
		Any T, any N, M1

B

FIG. 15-12. Continued.

Staging Procedures

A variety of procedures and special studies may be employed in the process of staging a given tumor. Both the clinical usefulness and cost efficiency must be considered. The following suggestions are made for staging a cancer of the oral cavity.

Essential for staging

1. Complete physical examination of the head and neck including indirect laryngoscopy and nasopharyngoscopy
2. Biopsy of primary tumor
3. Chest roentgenogram
4. Panorex films or other x-ray films for tumors overlying the jaws
5. Roentgenograms of paranasal sinuses for tumors overlying the palate

May be useful for staging or patient management

1. Multichemistry screen
2. Staining of surface mucosa with toluidine blue
3. Performance status (Karnofsky or ECOG scale)

May be useful for future staging systems or research studies

1. Panendoscopy (direct laryngoscopy, bronchoscopy, esophagoscopy)
2. Studies of immune competence

Histologic Type of Cancer

Predominant cancer is squamous cell carcinoma.

Histologic Grade

[ ]	G1	Well differentiated
[ ]	G2	Moderately well differentiated
[ ]	G3–G4	Poorly to very poorly differentiated

Postsurgical Resection–Pathologic Residual Tumor (R)

This does not enter into staging but may be a factor in deciding further treatment.

[ ]	R0	No residual tumor
[ ]	R1	Microscopic residual tumor
[ ]	R2	Macroscopic residual tumor
		Specify ____________

Performance Status of Host (H)

Several systems for recording a patient's activity and symptoms are in use and are more or less equivalent, as follows:

AJCC	*Performance*	*ECOG Scale*	*Karnofsky Scale (%)*
[ ] H0	Normal activity	0	90–100
[ ] H1	Symptomatic but ambulatory; cares for self	1	70–80
[ ] H2	Ambulatory more than 50% of time; occasionally needs assistance	2	50–60
[ ] H3	Ambulatory 50% or less of time; nursing care needed	3	30–40
[ ] H4	Bedridden; may need hospitalization	4	10–20

vical metastases (82 percent). Aneuploid tumors are more likely to metastasize than are diploid tumors. Correlation has also been found between thymidine labeling index and T stage of squamous cell carcinomas, with T3 lesions having significantly more activity than T1. Further subcellular analysis of squamous cell carcinoma has attempted to correlate abnormalities and thus predict behavior.

Expression of both histocompatibility antigens HLA-1 and HLA-2 on squamous cell carcinoma demonstrated marked tumor heterogeneity, particularly in poorly differentiated tumors. The relationship of growth factors to primary tumor development and progression is unclear at present, but as in other tumors, such as breast and brain, growth factor receptors have been identified on squamous cell carcinoma of the head and neck. Higher absolute levels of epithelial growth factor receptor and demonstration of amplification of the gene for epithelial growth factor receptor in squamous cell carcinoma of the upper aerodigestive tract may indicate that epithelial growth factor plays an important role in local tumor behavior. The histologic, biochemical, and genetic characteristics of head and neck tumors have also been used in an attempt to predict response to radiotherapy and chemotherapy.

As with most solid tumors, the most cogent prognosticator of head and neck cancer is the presence or absence of lymph node metastases. In the unoperated patient, passage of tumor emboli through the lymphatics follows an orderly pattern, with the anatomic triangles of the neck reflecting the site of primary disease. In the patient who has undergone previous surgical therapy or radiotherapy or who has extensive tumor which may block normal lymphatic flow, metastasis from a primary tumor may not follow the usual pathways, and a neck mass may not predict accurately the site of recurrence or new primary disease (see Fig. 15-3*B*). Clinical and ultimately pathologic staging of the neck according to the AJCC system depends on number of lymph nodes, size of lymph nodes, fixation to the skin or subjacent neck muscles, and laterality with respect to the primary tumor (ipsilateral, contralateral, and bilateral). Although there are certainly many determinants of primary tumor behavior, size and differentiation are useful predictors of risk of metastases. Increasing T stage is generally reflected by increasing N stage. Distant metastasis, however, is more closely related to N stage than to T stage. In a study of 160 patients with extensive disease in the neck, N3a, only 63 completed combined therapy with surgery and radiation and, of these, only 13 showed no evidence of disease at 2 years. Disseminated disease was the most common cause of death, followed by failure at the primary site and in the neck.

Lymph node metastases appear to behave in some ways similarly to primary disease in that micrometastases are not as poor a prognostic indicator as clinically palpable metastatic disease. Spread of the tumor outside the capsule of the lymph node may occur in clinically negative and positive lymph nodes and is a poor prognostic sign, indicating a more aggressive tumor. In a study of Stage III carcinoma of the oral cavity, the 2-year survival of patients with no lymph node metastases was 87 percent; with intracapsular lymph node metastases 75 percent; and with cervical metastases with extracapsular spread was only 39 percent. The incidence of extracapsular spread (ECS) of cervical disease increases with the size of the lymph node. Proportionate to increase in ECS is the likelihood of recurrent disease and thus death.

Uncontrolled growth of squamous cell carcinoma in the neck results in carotid artery hemorrhage, invasion of the sympathetic ganglia resulting in Horner's syndrome, erosion of the cervical vertebrae, invasion of cranial nerves IX, X, XI, and XII at the base of the skull (jugular foramen syndrome), airway obstruction, and brachial plexus palsy. The site of the primary tumor dictates not only the site of cervical metastasis but the frequency as well. Although the size of the primary lesion at presentation is important, it seems that independent of size, tonsil and base of tongue squamous carcinomas have high rates of metastasis to the neck, and buccal mucosa and palate lesions have low rates.

Distant metastases from squamous cell carcinoma may be present in from 31 percent of patients with no evidence of cervical metastases to 59 percent of those with extensive neck disease. Despite this relatively high incidence they are not uniformly the cause of death. Although any site is possible, lung, bone, skin, and liver are the most common metastases. Systemic effects of both local and systemic disseminated tumors include hypercalcemia from bone metastasis and elaboration of parathormonelike peptides as well as SIADH from vasopressinlike substances. There is some evidence that the widespread use of chemotherapy has changed the natural history of metastatic squamous cell carcinoma, increasing the frequency of patients dying with disseminated disease.

Diagnosis and Evaluation

History and physical examination are the most important considerations in the diagnosis of carcinoma of the upper aerodigestive tract. The history of chronic tobacco and alcohol abuse places the patient into a high-risk category. Males over forty with such history make up 70 to 80 percent of most series of patients with head and neck cancer. The previous occurrence of lung cancer, esophageal cancer, or other head and neck malignancy, as well as diseases causing immunodeficiency such as renal failure with its therapy by transplantation, malnutrition, and AIDS, is also significant.

Symptoms referable to the tumor itself are usually mild and not commensurate with the size of the tumor, probably because of the patient's generally stoic personality characterized by denial. Late-stage presentation is common in these patients. Barkley noted that 36 percent of patients presenting with oropharyngeal lesions had local disease alone and that the remaining 64 percent already had cervical or disseminated metastases. Pain at the site of the tumor is not a frequent complaint. Because otitis media and externa are relatively rare problems in adults, pain in the ear in a patient over forty may be a manifestation of tumor in the oral cavity, oropharynx, or larynx via referred pain pathways including the lingual to auriculotemporal nerves, glossopharyngeal to tympanic nerve, or vagus to auricular nerve. Prograde neural symptoms such as formication (the feeling of ants crawling along the lip or cheek) may represent mental or infraorbital nerve invasion by buccal, labial, or alveolar carcinoma. Family members or the patient may note change of speech due to tethering of the tongue (Fig. 15-13). Constant or variable hoarseness is the sign of vocal cord impairment by local growth of laryngeal or hypopharyngeal cancer or by paralysis in the neck of the recurrent laryngeal nerve. The sensation of scratchiness or tickling in the throat, gagging on food, or nocturnal choking secondary to aspiration may all represent interference with the synergistic mechanisms of swallowing and breathing. Airway compromise is usually a late symptom but occasionally may be the first presentation in an emergency setting. The typical American patient, then, is male, over forty, with a long history of tobacco and alcohol abuse, frequently with underlying psychologic or behavioral disorder such as depression or antisocial personality with withdrawal.

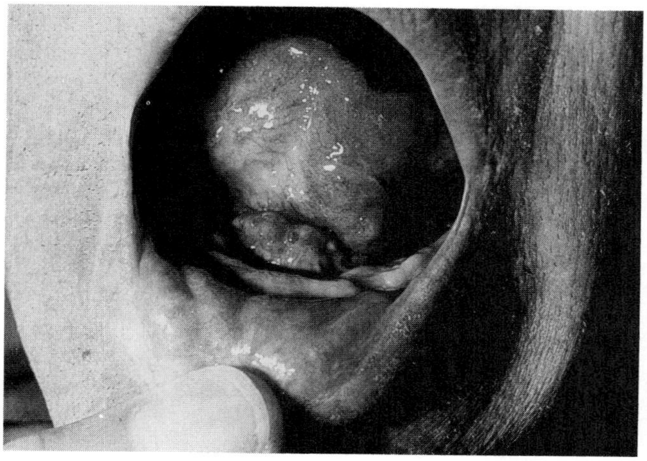

FIG. 15-13. T2,N0 squamous cell carcinoma of floor of mouth demonstrating the tendency for the lingual sulcus to be filled, pushing the tongue cephalad but inhibiting its protrusion.

Visualization of the entire upper aerodigestive tract is the sine qua non of diagnosis. A systematic approach that includes inspection of the facial and cervical surface anatomy and contour, intraoral examination, and indirect (mirror) laryngoscopy with nasopharyngoscopy is essential for diagnosis and staging (Fig. 15-14). In addition to size, shape, and projection into the cavity (exophytic or degree of ulceration), it is important to note mobility of the tongue, its position with relation to the midline (hypoglossal nerve function), fixation of the tongue to the adjacent mandible, or direct invasion of the mandible. Mirror examination of the oropharynx and hypopharynx and larynx should note the patency of the vallecula, the distensibility of the pyriform sinuses, and the normal adduction to the midline of the vocal cords. Interference with vocal cord function may result as hypopharyngeal lesions invade the medial wall of the pyriform sinus or by paralysis of the recurrent laryngeal nerve. By retracting the soft palate forward with a transnasal catheter, visualization of the nasopharynx is possible with the mirror. The vault of the nasopharynx, the choanae, and the eustachian tube should be examined. The condition of the teeth and gums should also be evaluated and the presence of torus palatinus or torus mandibularis. Limited motion of the mandible may come from direct tumor invasion or more frequently from invasion of tumor through the retromolar trigone area or tonsillar fossa to the pterygoid muscles. Infiltration or occasionally inflammation of the internal and external pterygoids limit jaw motion and cause the uncomfortable symptom of trismus, an ominous clinical sign. Compilation of the appropriate information about the primary tumor allows clinical staging. The distinct anatomic site, size, pattern of growth and invasion of adjacent structures are all necessary to assign the appropriate T stage.

Examination of the neck will reveal the presence or absence of metastatic lymph nodes. The site of the primary tumor should predict the most likely site of disease (see Fig. 15-11). Enlargement or inflammation of the submandibular gland may interfere with evaluation of the neck. Careful palpation, preferably performed with the patient sitting and the examiner standing behind him or

FIG. 15-14. Indirect laryngoscopy (*A*) and nasopharyngoscopy (*B*) using mirror. Good visualization of larynx, pharynx, and nasopharynx is usually possible without anesthesia, and assessment of function is possible during inspiration and expiration.

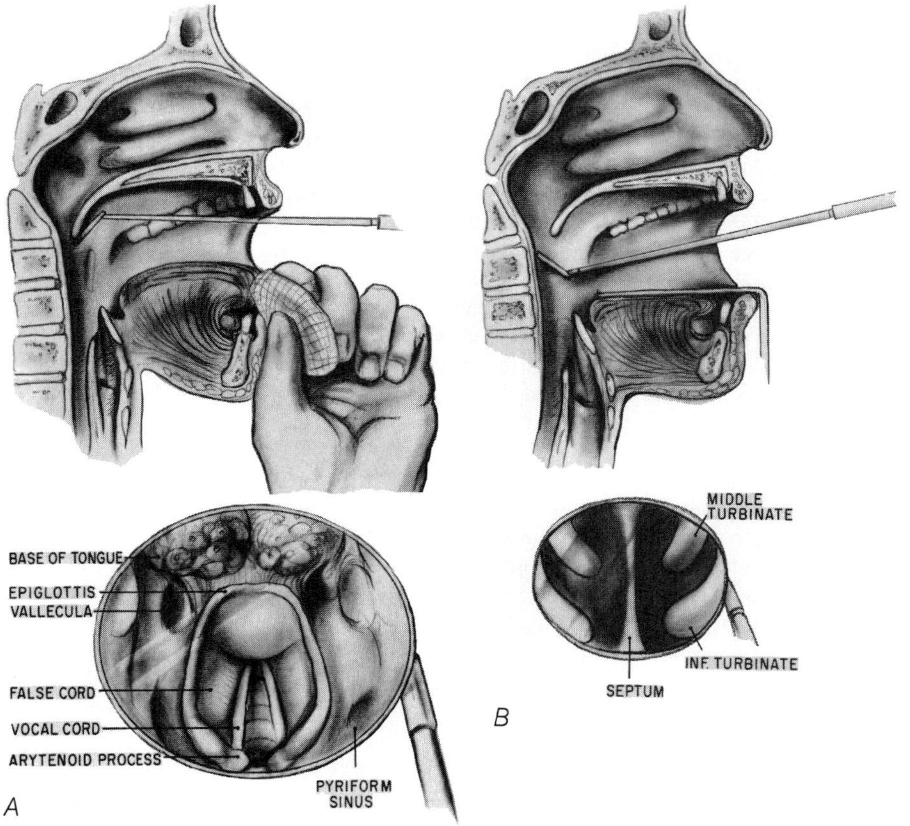

her, will allow systematic and sequential evaluation of the submental, submandibular, jugulodigastric, midjugular, jugulo-omohyoid, posterior triangle, and supraclavicular lymph node stations. The number of lymph nodes, size, and fixation to the skin or subjacent muscle will allow the examiner to assign an N stage to the patient. Tumors with no evident primary site manifest as lymph node metastases in 3 to 4 percent of malignancies. Cervical metastases of squamous cell carcinoma make up two-thirds of these cases. Furthermore, the initial manifestation of the subsequently discovered disease is a neck mass in 25 percent of the patients with carcinoma of the oral cavity, oropharynx, and thyroid, and 50 percent of patients with carcinoma of the nasopharynx. Because of variable extension into the neck, parotid gland masses may present as a cervical lymph node. The characterization of masses in the neck can be guided to a great degree by age. In children congenital and inflammatory masses predominate, in young adults inflammation or proliferative disorders of the lymphatic system, and in adults metastatic disease form the upper aerodigestive tract and skin.

Careful physical examination, including neurologic examination of the remainder of the head and neck area, may reveal evidence of more extensive disease such as cavernous sinus invasion, as documented by extraocular movement disorders, or Horner's syndrome from invasion of the cervical sympathetics.

Distant metastases are evaluated by history, physical examination, laboratory procedures, and radiology. Pleuritic pain or shortness of breath may indicate lung involvement, and distinct pain at a specific site spread to distant bone.

Before treatment planning, definitive histologic confirmation of disease is necessary. If a primary site is visible, a wedge biopsy should be taken at the edge of the tumor to include some adjacent normal tissue, fixed in formalin, and examined histologically. Touch preps and other cytologic methods are occasionally helpful but suffer from lack of specificity and also sensitivity. Although the extent of the tumor can usually be assessed by direct visualization, the use of vital dyes such as toluidine blue may help to delineate the extent of the disease, staining only the malignant and dysplastic epithelium and washing off the surrounding inflamed tissue. Hematoporphyrin dyes share this characteristic of differential uptake by tumor and normal cells and have occasionally been of use in demarcating index tumors and identifying and sometimes treating multicentric disease. Because of the significant incidence of synchronous primaries, evaluation of the rest of the upper aerodigestive tract may be useful. The value of triple endoscopy—bronchoscopy, esophagoscopy, and direct laryngoscopy—has been debated but is advisable for the ideal work-up of an advanced head and neck cancer in a patient with a long history of tobacco and alcohol use.

Since treatment planning depends to a great degree on the clinical stage of disease, and since therapies vary greatly in morbidity to the patient, precise and accurate staging is essential. Extent of resection and volume of radiotherapy depend on a reliable assessment of the degree of invasion of the primary tumor. The use of adjuvant chemotherapy or radiotherapy or the inclusion of neck dissection in the surgical plan is usually determined after careful analysis of the neck. Various radiologic studies may help define the extent of the disease.

Radiologic evaluation of intraoral disease usually involves assessment of the mandible. If tumor abuts the mandible in the lingual or buccal sulcus and is not easily mobile, it may penetrate the cortex. In edentulous patients, tumor descends through the cortical defects left by the previous teeth along the occlusal ridge. Once the medullary canal has been invaded, spread may occur locally or by way of the inferior alveolar nerve. In dentulous patients, direct invasion of the lingual plate occurs, and spread usually does not extend within the bone beyond the extent of the soft tissue tumor. Dental films taken directly at the site of tumor contact show cortical invasion or widening of the periodontal membrane. Panoramic films and mandibular series show the extent of disease within the mandible by cortical disruption and widening of the inferior alveolar canal or mental foramen. Simple plain film radiographic analysis of the mandible may, however, be inaccurate, with one series of 111 patients revealing a false-negative rate of 44 percent and a false-positive rate of 9 percent. Technetium 99m radionuclide bone scans have been advocated for diagnosis of mandibular invasion. Although their sensitivity is greater in general than in plain films, their specificity is not great, with false-positive rates of 53 percent and false-negative rates of 12 percent. In large tumors bone scans are even more likely to be false positive because of surrounding inflammation. Computed tomography is a highly sensitive method of diagnosing cortical invasion, but the presence of metal tooth fillings interferes with its accuracy (Fig. 15-15). Magnetic resonance imaging (MRI) is probably the most accurate and useful method of evaluating the mandible in suspicious but not definitive cases, since it can accumulate and reformat data in any plane without repositioning the patient, there is superior separation of cortical and marrow images, and there is no interference produced by dental fillings.

Analysis of the extent of intraoral and paranasal sinus tumors in difficult-to-examine areas such as the parapharyngeal space, larynx, and nasopharynx is assisted by both computed tomography and MRI. Correlation between extent of disease determined at operation and preoperative CT scanning was found in 78 percent of 26 patients evaluated by high-resolution computed tomography, improving to 94 percent when MRI with contrast enhancement by gadolinium DTPA was used. Particular advantage is obtained in evaluation of muscle and bone invasion but mucosal detail is difficult to assess with both CT and MRI (Fig. 15-16).

Since survival seems to depend on eradication of regional as well as local disease, evaluation of the neck for the risk of metastatic disease is crucial to the overall treatment plan. Surgery or radiotherapy may be used to remove regional disease in the lymph nodes if there is disease that is clinically apparent (palpable N+) or if there is high risk of disease in a clinically negative neck (N0). As has been previously discussed, size of the primary tumor (T stage), histologic parameters, and site may all suggest the increased likelihood of subclinical disease in the neck. Unfortunately, physical examination of the neck may be faulty, with false-negative rates ranging from 16 to 60 percent. Although of some importance, the rates of false positivity are generally lower and usually not as clinically relevant. Lymphangiography has been unrewarding in the evaluation of the neck. Computed tomography has recently been evaluated and found in most studies to be slightly more sensitive than physical examination: 82 percent sensitivity vs. 75 percent, 93 percent vs. 70 percent and 90 percent vs. 82 percent. Implicit in this advantage is the ability of computed tomography to upstage disease from N0 to N+ and suggest the necessity for neck dissection. Gadolinium-enhanced MRI scanning appears even more sensitive—92 percent sensitivity vs. 82 percent for CT scanning and 75 percent for physical examination—and is also useful in upstaging disease. Although these technologies are not necessary in every case of clinical staging, they are of

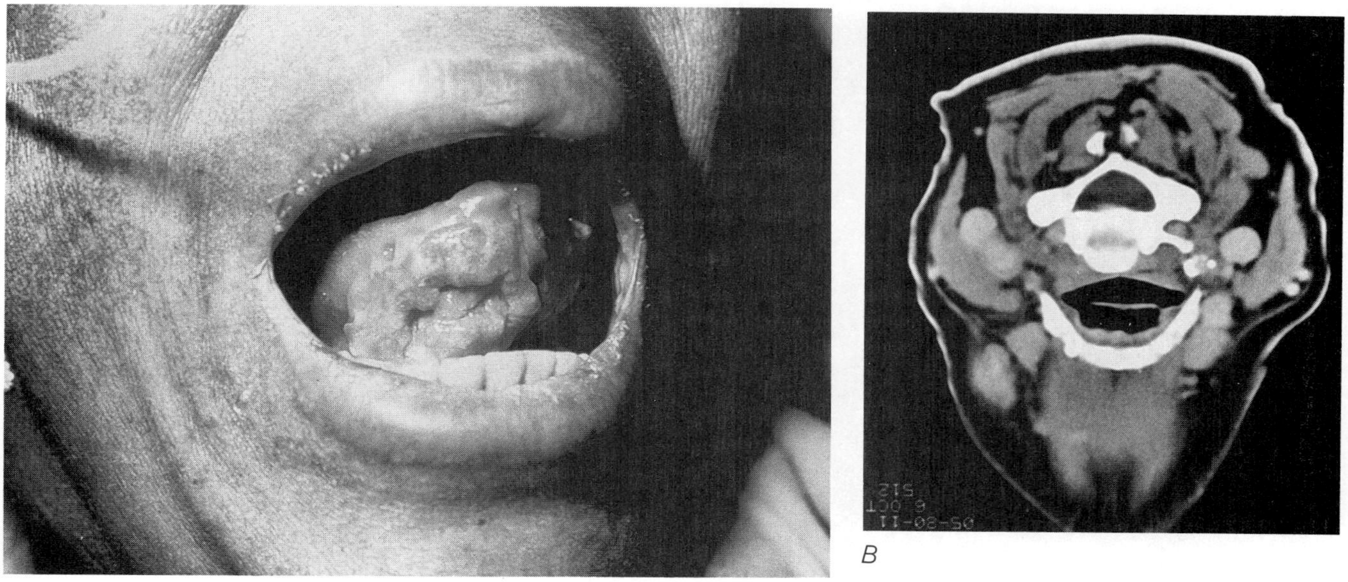

A B

FIG. 15-15. *A.* Invasive squamous cell carcinoma of ventral surface of tongue with submandibular adenopathy T2,N1,M0. Note central ulceration and irregular infiltrative borders. *B.* CT scan of neck with contrast demonstrating enlarged submandibular lymph node.

significant value in decision making where physical examination of the neck is difficult because of obesity, anatomic variation, or previous therapy, either surgery or radiotherapy. Micrometastases of less than 3 mm are still, however, undetectable by any available technology.

Therapy

Decision making concerning therapy is based almost completely on the clinical stage (TNM) of the tumor at the time of presentation. Although histologic characteristics may to a slight degree influence the treatment, the size of the local tumor and extent of invasion of adjacent structures (T stage); the presence or absence, number, and laterality of cervical metastases (N stage); and the presence or absence of distant metastatic disease (M stage) dictate therapy. Definitive or curative treatment methods are all oriented toward total extirpation of local and locoregional disease, with the expected subsequent decrease in disseminated disease. Palliative procedures, which may produce relief of pain, relief of airway obstruction, or improvement in local function and hygiene, similarly require complete macroscopic tumor removal at the primary site and in the neck and may occasionally be justifiable in the presence of distant metastases. Subtotal resection of local or locoregional disease is unlikely to be of benefit in any situation.

Definitive therapy may consist of surgery alone, radiotherapy alone, surgery with radiotherapy as a preoperative or postoperative adjuvant, or chemotherapy delivered either systemically by intravenous route or locally by intraarterial infusion before either or both modalities as neoadjuvant therapy. For small tumors (less than 2 cm, T1) in most cases surgery or radiotherapy, well planned and appropriately executed, will have equivalent local control and survival rates (Fig. 15-17). Choice, then, of the method depends on patient compliance, volition, associated disease, expense, interference with normal function, and available facilities. As the size of the tumor increases, T2 or greater, the likelihood of local control and ultimate cure with radiotherapy alone decreases, so surgery or surgery with adjuvant radiotherapy becomes preferable (Fig. 15-18). In the larynx, where staging is more a function of invasion of adjacent structures than size, and where function is completely dependent on preservation of structure, radiotherapy is usually the first choice for T1 and T2 lesions and is occasionally used as definitive therapy for T3 lesions as well. Advanced disease has a poor prognosis even with combined treatments of surgery and radiotherapy.

Unfortunately postoperative adjuvant chemotherapy has been unsuccessful in prolonging life in controlled randomized trials. Despite high response rates to preoperative administration of *cis*-platinum and 5-FU there has not been a survival advantage as has been demonstrated with chemotherapy for breast disease. One possible role, however, for chemotherapy is as a predictor of successful therapy and thus an indicator of which patient may be treated with radiotherapy instead of surgery with better preservation of function. In several prospective studies patients with T3 or T4 laryngeal tumors have been treated with *cis*-platinum, 100 mg/m^2, and 5 FU, 100 mg/m^2/day $\times$ 4 for three courses. Patients with complete response (disappearance of all tumor) were then treated by either radiotherapy alone or the more conventional approach of surgery (laryngectomy) with postoperative adjuvant radiotherapy. Patients with less than complete responses were treated with surgery plus radiotherapy. Early results show no difference in survival between patients who respond completely to chemotherapy whether they had been treated with surgery, radiation therapy, or not. Patients with incomplete response to chemotherapy had much poorer survival than either group of complete responders. These preliminary findings may indicate that the natural history of tumors that respond completely was more benign and that they can be treated less aggressively, preserving function. Nonresponders probably demonstrate greater tumor heterogeneity or clonal resistance to therapy and are thus unlikely to be con-

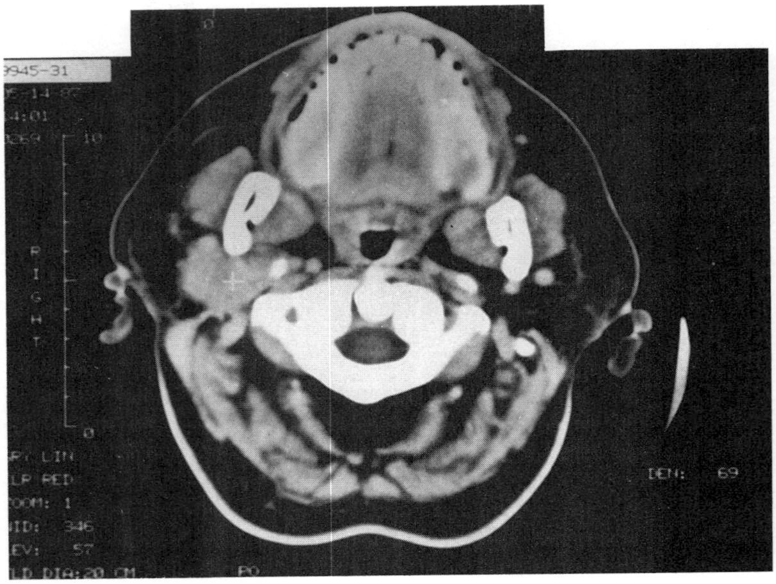

A

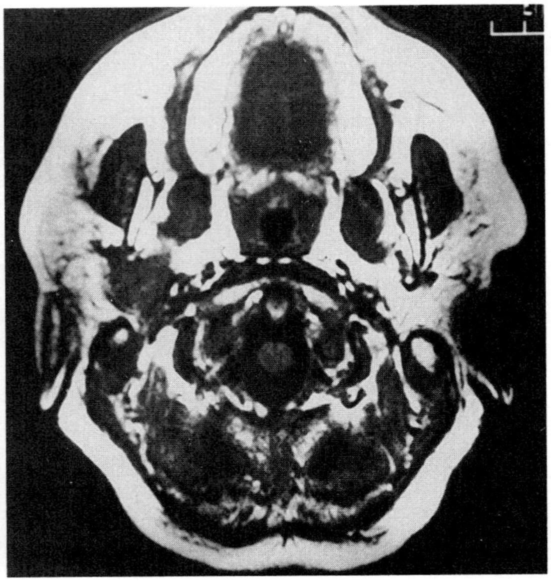

B

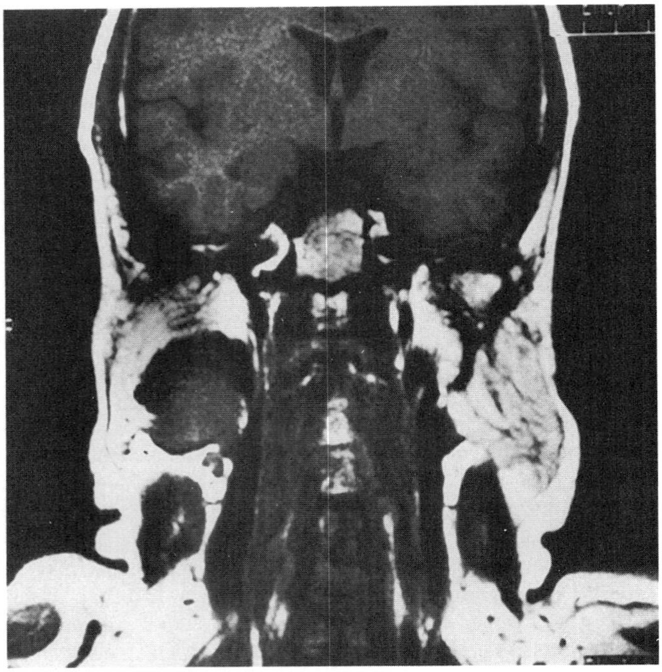

C

FIG. 15-16. *A.* CT scan of head and neck in patient with adenoid cystic carcinoma of the right parotid gland arising in the deep lobe extending into the pterygopalatine space. *B.* Axial magnetic resonance imaging shows similar detail. *C.* Coronal scans with MRI show more clearly relationship to great vessels of neck.

trolled by any therapy. Long-term results, however, are not presently available and the role of chemotherapy in head and neck cancer treatment thus remains unclear.

The basic principle of solid tumor therapy is en bloc treatment, either resection or radiotherapy of the primary tumor and the regional disease in the neck. The decision whether to treat the neck or not depends on the presence of clinically discernible metastatic disease or the risk of micrometastases to the neck. As primary tumor size increases, risk of neck disease increases at a greater rate with some primary sites than others (Fig. 15-19). When palpable lymph nodes are present in the neck, confirmation of metastatic disease may be obtained with fine-needle aspiration and cytologic examination, or the decision to proceed with therapy may be made on purely clinical grounds. Palpable or radiologically positive lymph node metastases require surgical therapy in the form of some type of neck dissection, usually performed in continuity with the resection of the primary tumor. Subclinical disease or micrometastases may be treated by a modification of neck dissection or radiotherapy, depending on the modality chosen for treatment of the primary site.

The lymph nodes draining the head and neck area are contained in a fascial envelope, between the superficial and deep layers of

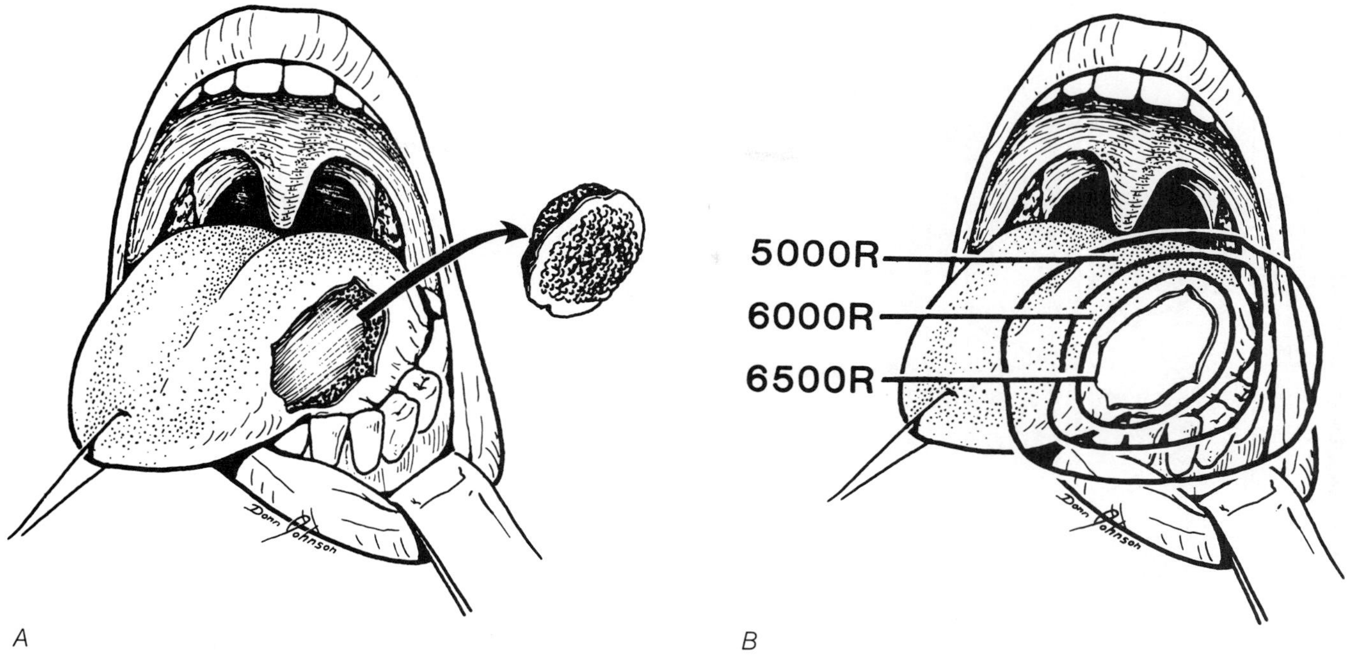

FIG. 15-17. *A.* The therapeutic principle of surgical oncology is resection of the primary tumor with a margin (1 to 2 cm) of normal tissue, with or without removal of the draining lymph nodes. (From: *Coleman JJ III, Searles JM: New Developments in Medicine. 1989, with permission.*) *B.* Therapeutic radiology is based on delivery of a tumoricidal dose for squamous cell carcinoma, 5500 to 6500 R to the entire tumor with slightly lower doses to the surrounding tissues. (From: *Coleman JJ III, Searles JM: New Developments in Medicine. 1989, with permission.*)

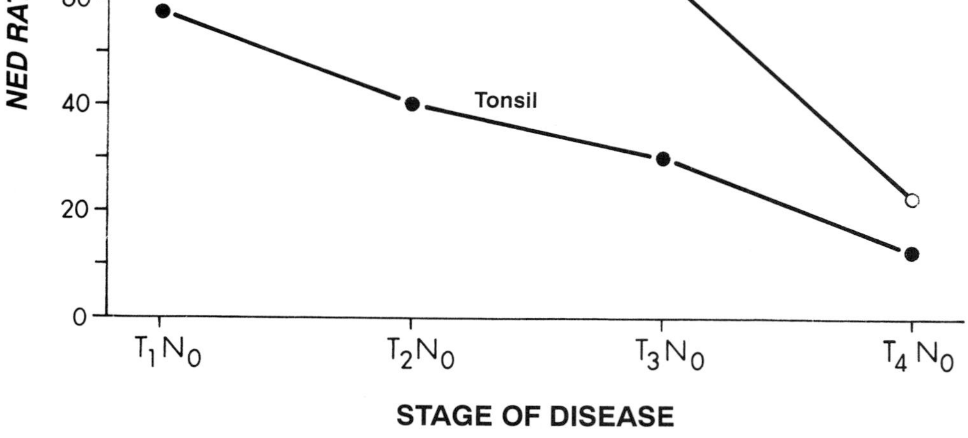

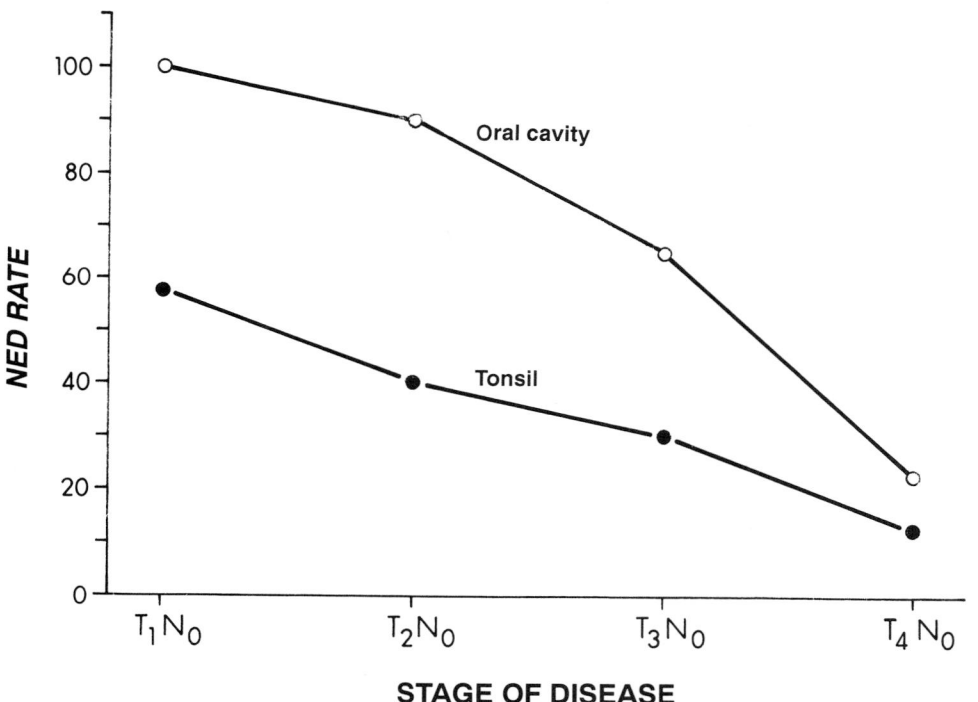

FIG. 15-18. Survival rates with no evidence of disease (NED) by T stage for patients with carcinoma of the oral cavity (3-year rates) and tonsil (2-year rates) treated by radiotherapy alone (Adapted from: *Perez CA, in Brady LW, Principles and Practice of Radiation Oncology, Philadelphia, Lippincott, 1987, pp 529–568, with permission.*)

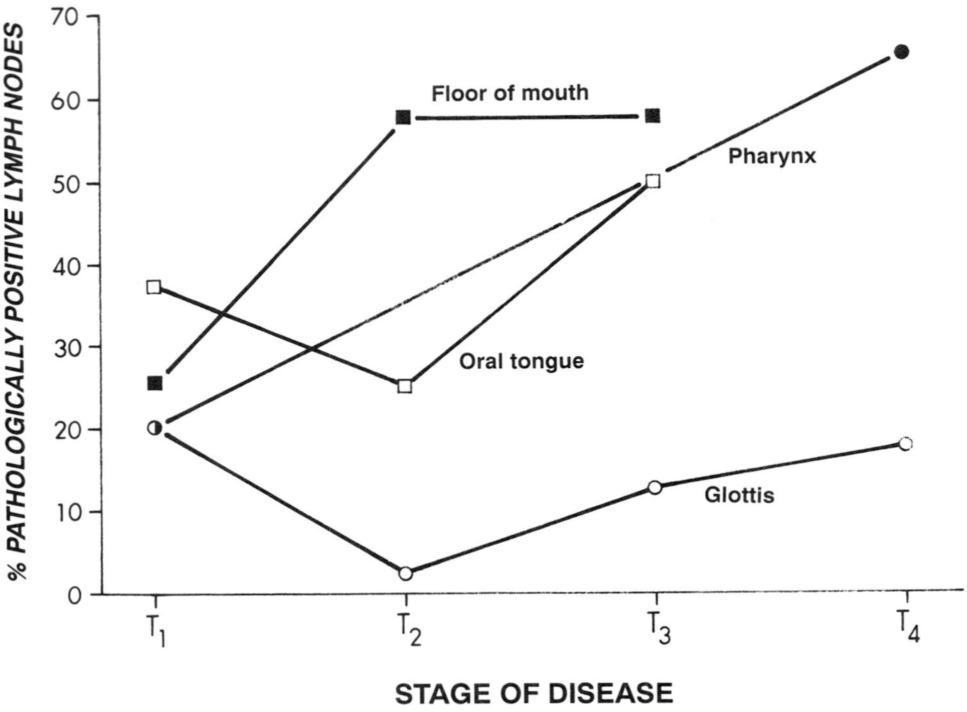

FIG. 15-19. Incidence of pathologically positive lymph nodes in clinically negative necks (N0) by stage of primary disease and site. In general as the primary tumor increases in size, the likelihood of micrometastases increases, as does the presence of palpable metastatic disease.

the investing fascia of the neck. Within the layers of the investing fascia lie the sternocleidomastoid muscle and the accessory nerve. The cervical lymph nodes lie between the investing fascia and the deep cervical fascia (Fig. 15-20) or prevertebral fascia and can be removed in toto with the jugular vein, sternocleidomastoid, and accessory nerve, as in the classical radical neck dissection described by Crile in 1906 (Fig. 15-21). The lymphatic connections between the tumor and the cervical metastases should remain intact with en bloc resection, and all the lymph-node-bearing tissue of the exposed side of the neck, including the anterior and posterior triangle, is removed.

The major morbidity of neck dissection is secondary to paralysis of the trapezius muscle by resection of the accessory nerve. Because of this, Bocca, in 1967 suggested preservation of the accessory nerve. Other surgeons have demonstrated techniques where the jugular vein and the sternocleidomastoid can also be left intact. These methods are particularly useful in prophylactic (elective) neck dissections where there is no clinical evidence of meta-

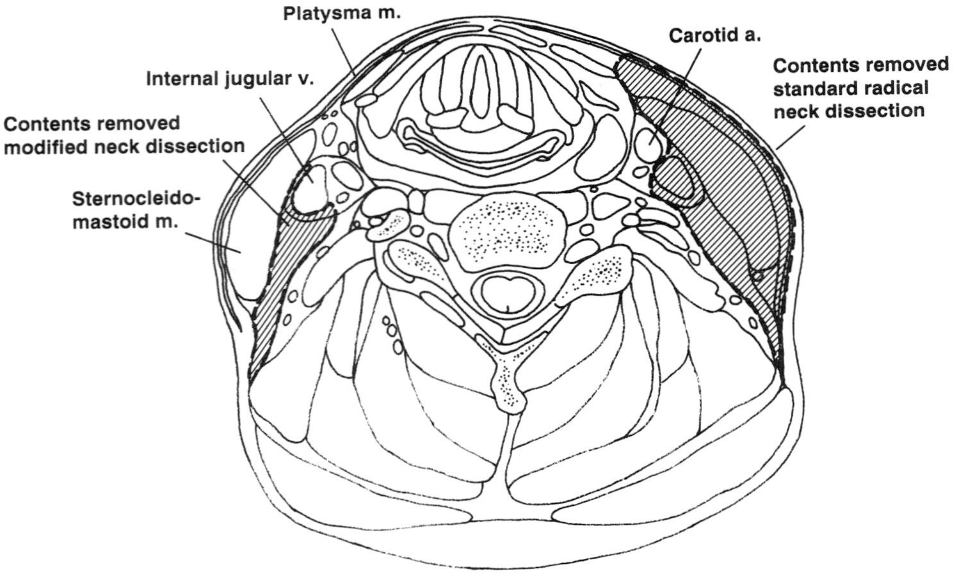

FIG. 15-20. Cross section of the neck highlighting the fascial envelope. Structures within the investing fascia and the internal jugular vein are removed during standard radical neck dissection. (Adapted from: *Cummings CW [ed]: Otolaryngology Head and Neck Surgery. St Louis, CV Mosby, 1986, with permission.*)

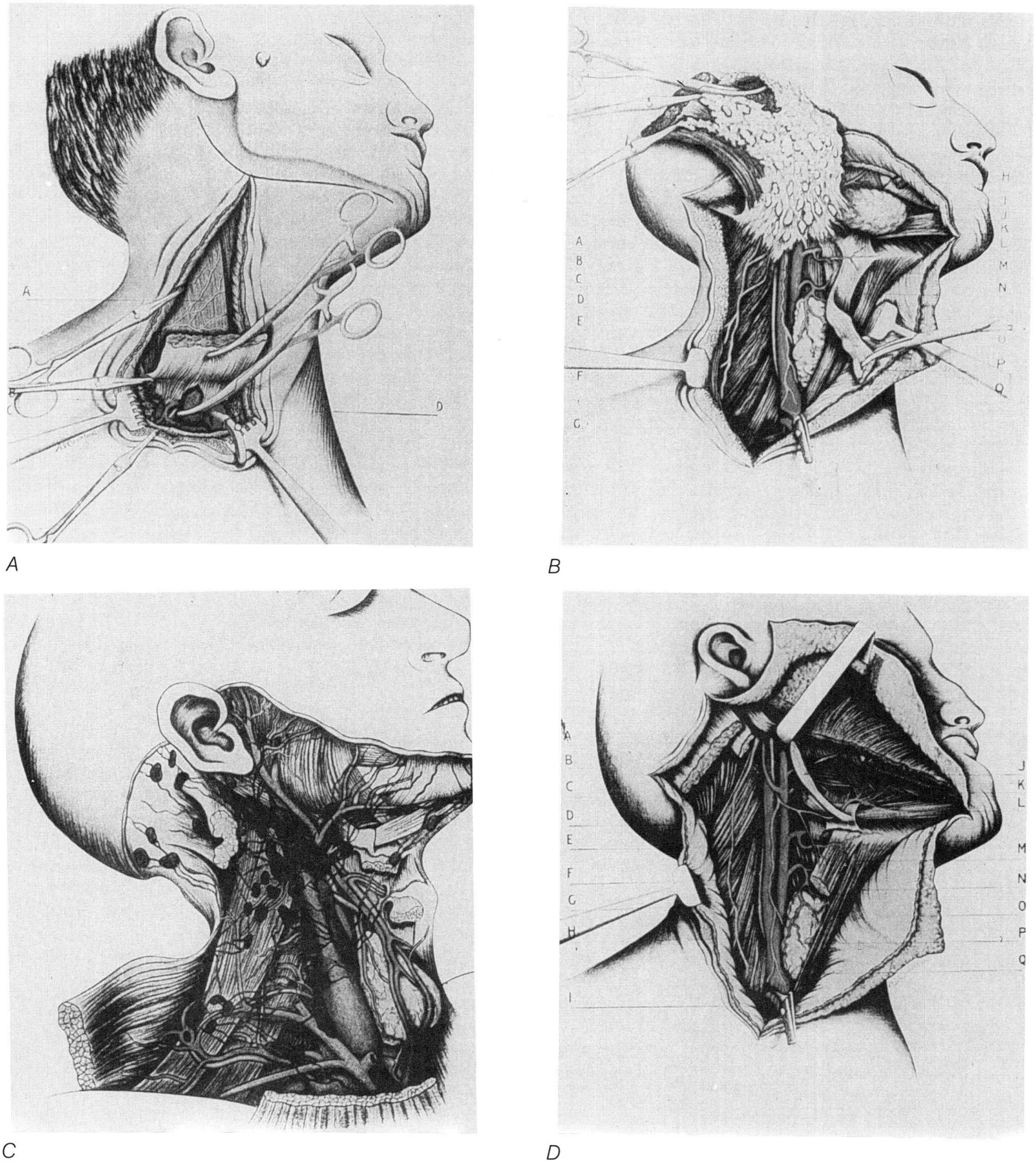

FIG. 15-21. *A.* Standard radical neck dissection as described by Crile in 1906 is performed in a very similar way today. Access to the neck may be through a number of skin incisions, and dissection is carried out below the level of the platysma from the medial border of the trapezius to the strap muscles. *B.* The sternocleidomastoid muscle is divided to gain access to the lymph nodes of the neck which are situated within the investing fascia. *C.* The lymph nodes are clustered along the internal jugular vein, along or within the submandibular triangle and along the accessory nerve. *D.* En bloc resection of the lymph nodes is achieved by transecting the sternocleidomastoid muscle, the jugular vein, and the fatty tissue of the posterior triangle and the submandibular triangle. The branches of the external carotid artery and the accessory nerve which passes through the jugulodigastric area are resected. Unless invaded by tumor, the hypoglossal and vagus nerves and the carotid artery are preserved.

static disease to the neck. Although there is some debate about the quality of function after modified neck dissection, it seems likely that long-term function is improved when the spinal accessory nerve is preserved, and the likelihood of survival is not significantly impaired by the lesser procedure.

Since the site of potential neck metastasis can be fairly accurately predicted by the location of the primary squamous cell carcinoma, and since the lymph-node-containing areas of the neck have been described as discrete anatomic areas demarcated by muscles, fascial condensations, and the triangles of the neck, there has been suggestion that in addition to leaving the accessory nerve and sternocleidomastoid muscle intact, only those lymph nodes at risk should be resected. The concept of *selective neck dissection,* customized to the site of primary disease, has gained recent support. Thus for carcinoma of the lip, anterior tongue, floor of the mouth, and buccal mucosa *supraomohyoid neck dissection* might be used, removing the submental, submandibular, upper and mid jugular lymph nodes (Levels I, II, and III). If a nasopharyngeal lesion or posterior scalp melanoma was the primary site, the suboccipital, retroauricular and upper mid jugular, and posterior triangle lymph nodes (Levels II, III, IV, and V) would be removed via a *posterolateral neck dissection.* In primary sites of the pharynx or larynx, a *lateral neck dissection* including upper, middle, and lower jugular nodes (Levels II, III and IV) might be appropriate. In thyroid disease, removal of the paratracheal, perithyroidal, and precricoid nodes, the *anterior compartment neck dissection,* may be appropriate (Fig. 15-22). Although it seems obvious that control of disease in the neck by its surgical removal with some form of neck dissection should improve survival, there is no well-designed prospective study to prove the equivalency or superiority of neck dissection or radiotherapy for the clinically negative (N0) neck or to suggest which operation of the several described should be utilized.

Approximately 70 percent of patients in the United States who present with squamous cell carcinoma of the upper aerodigestive tract have advanced disease, Stage III or IV. Even with aggressive therapy late-stage disease has a high recurrence rate. Recurrent disease may manifest at the primary site in the previously treated neck and in the contralateral neck. Just as with primary disease, the therapy of recurrence is based on wide local resection and clearance of the involved or at-risk regional lymph nodes. The extent of resection depends on involvement by tumor and the proximity to the great vessels and the central nervous system. If tissue tolerance to ionizing radiation allows, postoperative adjuvant radiotherapy may be useful, even as a second course. For unresectable recurrent disease, combinations of chemotherapy and radiation therapy or chemotherapy alone may provide some palliation in reducing bulk, alleviating pain and airway compression, but long-term survival does not appear to be improved.

The therapy of distant metastases of squamous cell carcinoma of the upper aerodigestive tract has been very unsuccessful. The lung is a common site of metastasis for head and neck cancer, but it must be realized that a solitary lesion in the lung of a patient with a previous squamous cell carcinoma of the head and neck is more likely to be a primary lung cancer than a metastatic deposit. The patient should be aggressively evaluated and treated for that primary cancer. Resection of metastatic disease to the lung, however, has not proven salutary in most cases. Second primary tumors or

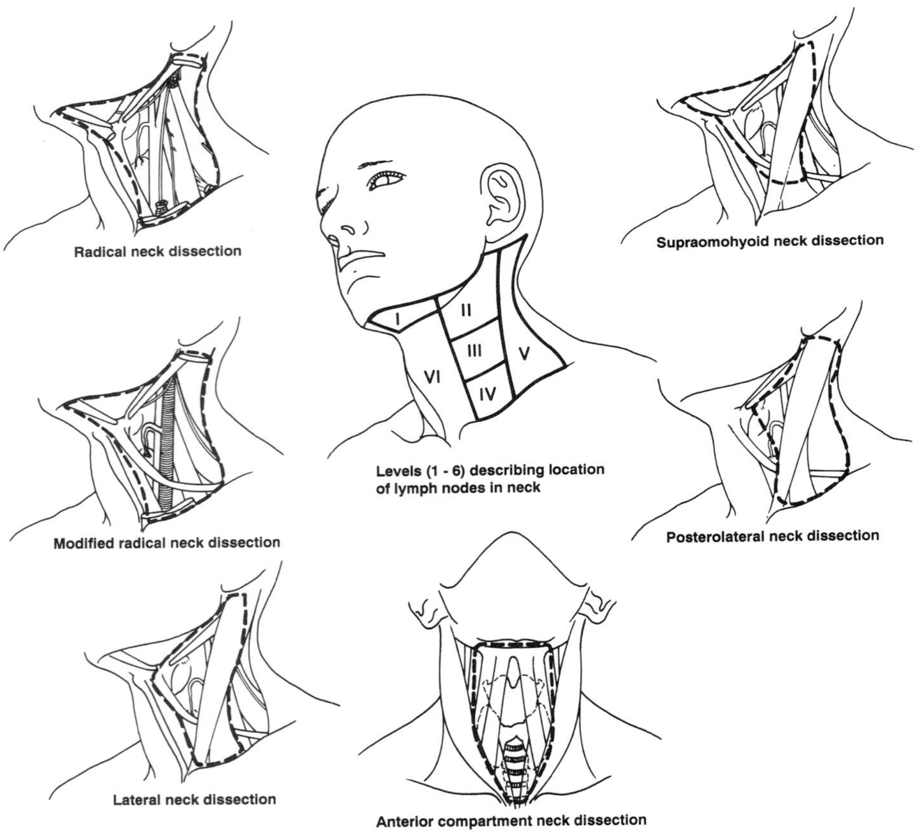

FIG. 15-22. System of pathologic classifications of lymph node anatomy. Specimens from neck dissections are usually described as involved or not involved according to these levels. This system has been used to justify the concept of selective neck dissections for certain primary tumor sites in an attempt to decrease morbidity. (From: *Robbins KT, Medina JE, et al: 1991, with permission.*)

metachronous tumors are a significant problem in head and neck cancer. Prevention of recurrent disease and of new primary disease and reversion of possible premalignant entities may be possible with chemoprevention. Isotretinoin, a vitamin A analogue, has been shown to decrease the incidence of second primary tumors in select groups of head and neck cancer patients.

Immunotherapy

Because of prolonged alcohol abuse and coincident malnutrition, many patients with squamous cell carcinoma of the head and neck present with various manifestations of immunodeficiency. There is evidence that anergy and deficient cellular immunity result in poorer survival rates for squamous cell carcinoma of the head and neck as well as for other malignancies.

Cell-mediated immunity has been demonstrated to be depressed in head and neck cancer patients. The cause of this depression is, however, uncertain, and surgery, radiotherapy, the malignancy itself, and suppression of natural killer cell function by circulating immune complexes have all been implicated. Natural killer cells have been shown to function as a recognition and defense mechanism against metastatic disease from primary squamous cell carcinoma. The effects of humoral or B-cell-mediated immunity on the progression of head and neck carcinoma are not as clear. Unlike some malignant cells, the squamous cell carcinoma tumor cultures have not been particularly immunogenic, and cell-specific immune manipulation has been impossible to date.

Nonspecific cellular immunostimulation with various agents such as levamisole, thymosin, and interferon has, however, shown some promise as both an adjuvant and palliative method. Natural killer cells from patients with head and neck cancer treated in vitro with interleukin-2 show increased activity after therapy suggesting that IL-2 negates some of the suppressive agents in the serum. The use of IL-2 has been extended to the clinical arena, with infusion of this agent with intramuscular interferon alpha reversing in vivo natural killer cell depressed activity. Perilesional injection of IL-2 in recurrent inoperable head and neck carcinoma resulted in temporary but dramatic response in 65 percent of 20 patients treated. Systemic recombinant interferon alpha given intramuscularly resulted in 1 complete response, 1 partial response and 2 stabilizations of disease in 14 patients treated with a second cycle, with salutary effect being attributed to a rise in natural killer cell activity.

Although the benefit is as yet uncertain, it appears likely that more specific characterization of the antigenic identity of squamous cell carcinoma and more precise manipulation of effector cells through natural or synthetic lymphokines will ultimately help in the adjuvant therapy of head and neck cancer.

Reconstruction

In the treatment of head and neck cancer, as in any other disease, there is a hierarchy of priorities. *Survival* is obviously of first concern and to a great degree depends on adequate surgical or radiotherapeutic ablation and possibly adjuvant chemotherapy or immunotherapy. *Freedom from pain* is fortunately accomplished in most cases of successful ablative therapy. Preservation or restoration of *function* as well as *appearance* is the next consideration and relies to a great degree on the ability of the surgeon to repair the created defect with local, regional, or distant tissues. Finally, but perhaps most practically important to the patient, is the *efficiency* of the treatment regimen. Efficiency is the characteristic that dictates the therapy be delivered in a time period commensurate with the natural history of the disease.

Advanced squamous cell carcinoma has a high recurrence rate. Eighty-nine percent of patients whose local or regional disease recurs manifest this within 2 years of therapy. Thus restoration of function and appearance in this group of patients with high failure rate and short disease-free intervals should be performed as quickly as possible. A multiple-stage method of reconstruction carried out over several months may prolong recovery. The most efficient methods are single-stage reconstructions performed at the time of the ablative surgery.

In the past there was considerable reluctance to perform immediate reconstruction after resection of malignancy. Fear of cloaking persistent or recurrent disease, coupled with realistic assessment of the poor results from multiple procedures, led to recommendations that the patient be observed for 1 to 5 years after surgery. The functional disability inherent in major oral or oropharyngeal resection usually mandated permanent gastrostomy for feeding and tracheostomy for safe maintenance of the airway. The attendant loss of taste, speech, swallowing, and other corollary functions made the postoperative state of the patient with head and neck cancer miserable.

Improved methods of reconstruction, better pathologic analysis at surgery, and a more comprehensive understanding of the natural history of the disease have made single-stage reconstruction at the time of the initial surgical resection the present standard of care in most instances. Resection of the primary disease and regional metastatic disease, confirmation of disease clearance by frozen section of the margin of resection, and immediate reconstruction are usually possible for squamous cell carcinoma of the upper aerodigestive tract. In malignancies where frozen-section analysis may be inaccurate when bone is involved or in recurrent disease with previous radiotherapy, or when there is uncertainty about other aspects of the resection, secondary reconstruction may be more appropriate.

The upper aerodigestive tract is a complex mixture of cutaneous cover, epithelial lining, bone and cartilaginous framework all joined in complex arrangement by muscle and driven in intricate synergy to facilitate the main vegetative functions of the organism, alimentation and respiration. This complex mobile structure and the heavy colonization of the mucosal surfaces by bacteria, as well as the deleterious effects of adjuvant radiotherapy (acute inflammation in the early stages and fibrosis and vasculitis in later stages), make reconstruction extremely difficult.

The basic needs presented by surgical resection are restoration of continuity of the alimentary tube with epithelial lining, provision of reliable external coverage for protection of the great vessels and bony structures, and separation of the central nervous system and upper aerodigestive tract. Restoration of oral continence, facilitation of the coordinated motions of the tongue and larynx, and maintenance of an open passage for swallowing while separating the oral, oropharyngeal, and nasal cavities are refinements on the basic demand that are necessary for a reasonable quality of life. Accurate *analysis of the wound* created by the surgical resection is the first element required for successful reconstruction. Size, exposure of the central nervous system, mobility of the removed parts, presence of bacterial colonization or invasive infection, type of tissue removed (mucosa, bone, cartilage), history of previous surgery or radiotherapy, likelihood of subsequent surgery or radiotherapy, exposure of the carotid or jugular vessels, and effect of external appearance will all be important wound characteristics that will modify the choice of reconstructive techniques. Whether to attempt to satisfy only the basic reconstructive needs or to restore as many missing elements as possible is a difficult decision involving patient desire and compliance, surgical skill, consideration of disease stage, and many other complex factors.

The past 15 years have brought enormous advances in reconstructive techniques which have impacted mainly on *efficiency* of therapy, to restore the patient to reasonable function and appearance rapidly. Indirectly, however, improved reconstructive techniques have an impact on survival since more aggressive resections, salvage of radical radiotherapy, and decrease in postoperative complications with attendant infection and malnutrition are accomplished with relative safety. The fundamental improvement has been the ability to transfer large volumes of well-vascularized tissue to the area.

Although flap reconstruction of the external surface of the nose was taught by the early Hindu surgeon Susruta, and the Renaissance saw a number of reconstructive attempts at nasal and other external defects (by distant flaps attached to the defect and divided after parasitizing their blood supply from local tissues), major reconstructions have been a relatively recent phenomenon. Throughout the development of surgical technique that followed the introduction of general anesthesia in 1846, the principle of random flaps of skin being attached and divided remained the mainstay of the reconstructive effort. Large segments of tissue from the thorax and back were moved in multiple stages to the oral cavity, face, and pharynx.

In 1965 Bakamjian described the deltopectoral flap, which possessed an *axial* or direct arterial blood supply from the perforating vessels of the internal mammary artery and vein to the skin of the chest and shoulder. This provided a relatively reliable large segment of tissue that was particularly useful in the reconstruction of the pharynx. The forehead flap, another axial pattern flap, based on the superficial temporal vessels, was described in 1963 and, despite its disfigurement of the donor site, became a useful method of reconstruction of the oral cavity. With the realization in the 1970s that the blood supply to the skin came not only from the randomly oriented subdermal plexus vessels and axial cutaneous vessels but also from perforating vessels from the subjacent muscles, the *musculocutaneous concept* transformed reconstruction, particularly that of head and neck defects. Large flat muscles of the thorax could be rotated on their long vascular pedicles to supply a large volume of well-vascularized tissue in a single operation on the oral cavity, pharynx, or soft tissues of the face. Moreover, if recurrence of disease mandated a subsequent resection, another thoracic musculocutaneous flap was available to repair the defect. The pectoralis major, latissimus dorsi, trapezius, sternocleidomastoid, and platysma muscles are all useful, either alone or with their overlying skin. Now much larger and more complex wounds could be addressed at a single operation, returning the patient to reasonable function and appearance promptly.

Some of the problems with the thoracic musculocutaneous flaps are the effect of gravity on bulky flaps, additive morbidity to the shoulder girdle when neck dissection is performed, and variable blood supply to the skin, particularly in the pectoralis major musculocutaneous flap, depending on where the skin portion of the flap is located. Furthermore, there is no reliable method of transporting vascularized bone on a regional musculocutaneous flap.

Despite these disadvantages, the musculocutaneous concept has made immediate reconstruction of the head and neck resection the accepted procedure in most cases.

An offshoot of the success of reconstructive efforts with musculocutaneous flaps has been the increased interest in vascular anatomy (Fig. 15-23). Subsequent research and improvements in microscope and instrument technology have resulted in the ability to transfer tissue of many different types from various sites of the body by separating arterial supply and venous drainage of the tissue and reattachment to blood vessels in the head and neck. Bone, muscle, skin, fascia, and combinations of these are available for various sites, as are intraabdominal viscera. Microvascular reconstruction or free tissue transfer has made it possible for the surgeon to close virtually any defect in the head and neck, no matter how large or complex. Even more important, however, the large number of methods available allows the reconstructive surgeon to choose the method or methods most suitable to a specific site and analyze the results (Table 15-1). Just as each wound has its own characteristics, so does each flap. Vascular pedicle length, bulk,

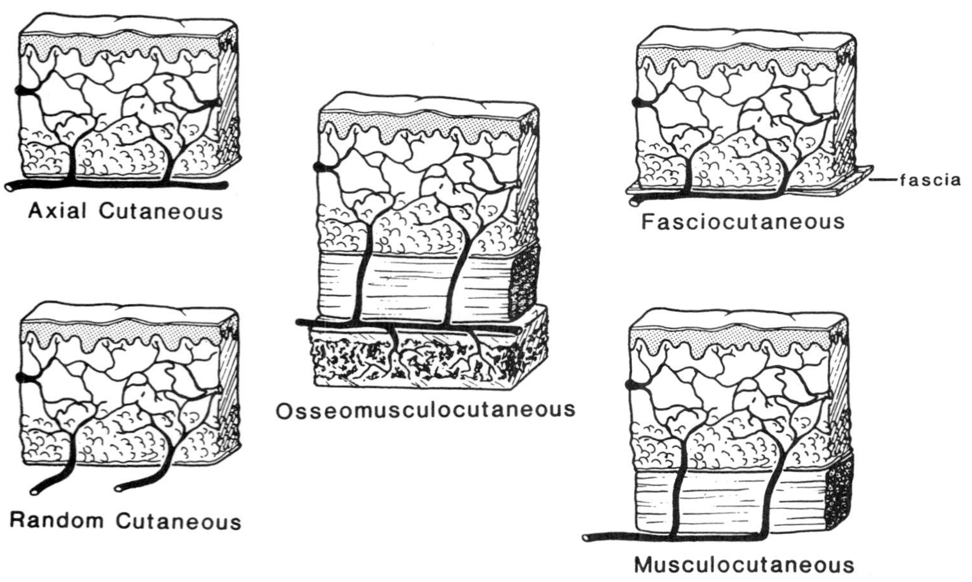

FIG. 15-23. Classification of flaps used for reconstructive purposes based on their vascular anatomy. The musculocutaneous concept states that skin is supplied not only by the direct skin vessels but also by perforating vessels from the subjacent muscle which come from the main vessels supplying the muscle.

Table 15-1
Available Methods of Reconstruction of Various Head and Neck Defects

Epithelial lining	*Soft tissue coverage*	*Bone*
Deltopectoral flap	Pectoralis major*†	Fibula*
Platysma	Deltopectoral	Scapula*
Pectoralis major*†	Trapezius†	Lateral arm*
Trapezius*†	Latissimus dorsi*†	Radial forearm*
Latissimus dorsi*†	Radial forearm*	Groin flap (DCIA)*
Radial forearm*	Rectus abdominis*	Dorsalis pedis (metatarsal)*
Lateral arm*	Omentum*	Serratus*
Medial arm*	Lateral arm*	
Lateral thigh*	Scapula*	
Jejunum*	Serratus*	
Gastroepiploic*		
Scapula*		

*Possible free flaps

†Thoracic musculocutaneous flaps

type of epithelium, presence and durability of bone, and thickness of soft tissue all can be evaluated to select the most appropriate replacement for the individual problem (Fig. 15-24).

Complications

The therapy of squamous cell carcinoma of the head and neck usually requires two potent modalities—surgery and radiotherapy—directed at an area that is heavily contaminated with saprophytic and pathogenic organisms in a patient who is frequently malnourished and immunodeficient, and may be noncompliant. Since many patients present with advanced disease, the failure rate even for combined therapy is high due to disseminated disease as well as local or locoregional failure. It is, therefore, imperative to deliver the therapy in a form that is efficient and results in a rapid return of the patients to function, reasonable appearance, and whatever social situation they may be able to recover. Recognition of the inevitable sequelae of therapy *(complications)* and rapid resolution or preferably prevention are thus of great importance.

Complications specific to head and neck cancer therapy can be categorized as *anatomic,* injury to nerves or blood vessels within the field of surgery; *physiologic,* the results of interference with blood or lymphatic supply to the area secondary to surgery or radiotherapy; *technical,* surgical rearrangements that result in secondary problems; and *functional* derangements of normal behavior secondary to therapy. All of these can then be grouped into catastrophic or noncatastrophic complications, which will to a great degree dictate the surgeon's approach to them, both preventive and therapeutic.

The most appropriate approach to complications is prevention. Restoration of positive nitrogen balance, preoperative pulmonary hygiene, control of diabetes mellitus, and weaning from alcohol and tobacco are important nonspecific measures. Preoperative antibiotics decrease the likelihood of wound infection and its sequelae. Numerous studies have shown that previously administered radiotherapy, particularly if given in definitive therapeutic doses, increases the risk of complication. Dental hygiene or rehabilitation before definitive surgery is important in patients whose mandible has been previously irradiated to prevent subsequent osteoradionecrosis. Patient education is crucial to ensure cooperation in what may be a difficult postoperative rehabilitation.

Other than injury to the thoracic duct, which may result in significant fat and protein loss through chylous fistula, most *anatomic* complications are nerve injuries, either purposeful or otherwise secondary to primary tumor resection or radical neck dissection. The accessory, marginal mandibular, mylohyoid and cervical plexus sensory branches are frequently sacrificed in neck dissection. Injuries due to traction, electrocautery, or other technical misadventure may occur to any structure but are most likely to affect hypoglossal, lingual, mandibular, vagus, phrenic, facial, recurrent laryngeal, motor branches to the cervical plexus and cervical sympathetic chain. Careful technique during surgery, adequate hemostasis to allow good visualization, and knowledge of normal and pathologic anatomy will decrease the likelihood of anatomic complications.

Previous surgery, the planned surgery, and radiotherapy all may interfere with blood supply to the head and neck area, resulting in local and systemic problems. Irradiation alone or combined with surgery may result in a 22 to 30 percent incidence of clinical hypothyroidism, particularly when surgery is on the larynx. Hypoparathyroidism, transient or permanent, may result in up to 10 percent of cases of thyroidectomy and must be considered after laryngopharyngectomy. Obstruction of one or both jugular veins, particularly when combined with lymphadenectomy, results in lymphedema of the face and may result in intracerebral edema, particularly if excessive fluid is administered during surgery. Head elevation, diuretics, and judicious fluid management will, however, usually allow collateral flow through the vertebral veins to resolve these problems.

Surgical misadventure, poor planning or execution, or the presence of infection will result in technical complications. Respiratory problems can result from pneumothorax precipitated while operating in the mediastinum or supraclavicular fossa. Hematoma may cause acute upper airway obstruction. Tracheostomy may cause subcutaneous emphysema, tracheoinnominate fistula, or subglottic stenosis. The combination of infection and local ischemia of skin or mucosa may result in wound infection, suture line breakdown, flap necrosis, osteomyelitis, and osteoradionecrosis. Exposure of a previously irradiated carotid artery will usually result in a bacterial infection and rupture and must be treated as a surgical emergency. Careful planning, meticulous attention to watertight closure of the pharynx and oral cavity, and provision of adequate independently well-vascularized tissue for reconstruction will minimize the likelihood of *technical* complications.

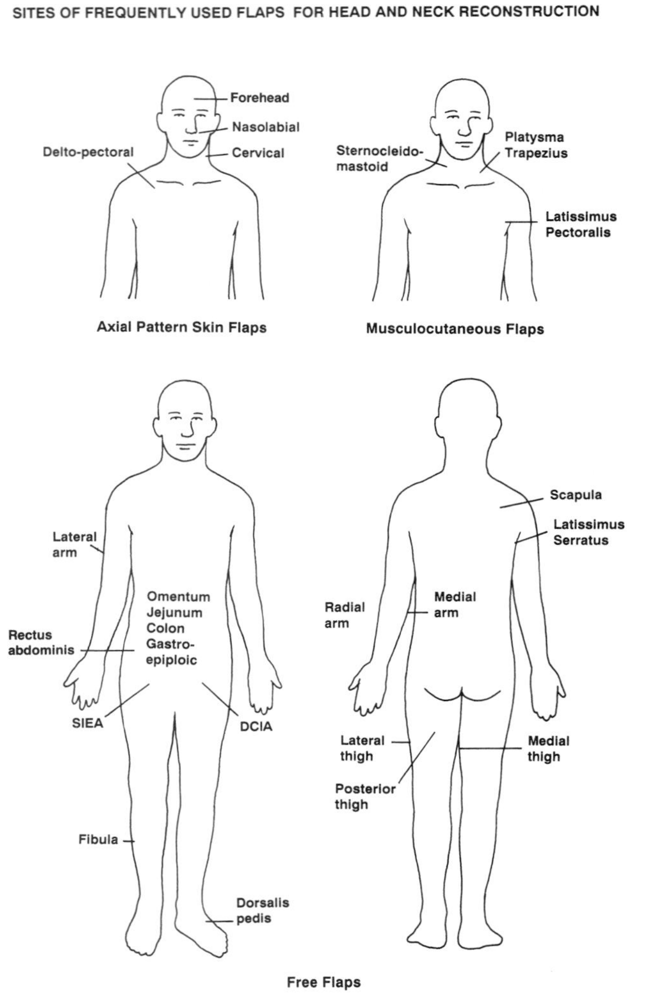

FIG. 15-24. Axial pattern flaps, thoracic and cervical musculocutaneous flaps, and free flaps frequently used for reconstruction of defects after resection of cancer of the head and neck.

Restoration of function is one of the main goals of head and neck cancer therapy. Although some dysfunction is inherent in all therapy, proper selection of reconstructive methods, attention to intrinsic function of the structures resected and those remaining, and careful and patient postoperative rehabilitation will decrease the severity of the common functional complications: chronic airway obstruction, aspiration pneumonia, dysphagia, dysphonia, and mental depression.

The potential for catastrophe is great in head and neck cancer surgery. Recognition of a complication and realization of the likelihood of rapid deterioration are important to prevent *catastrophic* complications. Tetany from hypoparathyroidism, acute airway obstruction from hematoma or a dislodged tracheostomy tube, tracheoinnominate fistula, and carotid hemorrhage can all lead to rapid death. Any complication that occurs in a patient who has been previously irradiated must be aggressively resolved. Carotid artery exposure, oropharyngocutaneous fistula, or skin flap necrosis in the irradiated neck could result in subsequent invasive infection of the great vessels and death (Fig. 15-25). Oropharyngocutaneous fistula is relatively common, ranging from 6 to 38 percent of head and neck cancer cases, and can be treated expectantly if salivary flow can be diverted and the carotid arteries protected by well-vascularized tissue. The pectoralis major musculocutaneous flap is a useful method of closing major fistulas and covering the great vessels at the same time. Pharyngocutaneous fistulas of moderate size may be treated by the sternocleidomastoid musculocutaneous flap (Fig. 15-26).

Oral Cavity

Anatomy and Physiology. The anatomic borders of the oral cavity are the mucosal surfaces of the lip externally and the anterior tonsillar pillar posteriorly. The oral cavity is usually considered as a number of distinct entities: the lips, the buccal mucosa, the gums, mandibular and maxillary including the retromolar trigone, the floor of the mouth, the mobile tongue, and the hard palate. Thus the oral cavity is the aditus of the long seromuscular-mucosal tubular conduit of food and liquid that allows the organism to obtain nourishment. As such it is modified in several ways to facilitate the initiation of alimentation. The lips are a sphincter which allow the oral cavity to be sealed after intake of food and liquid. The buccal surfaces with the buccinator muscles help collapse and expand the oral cavity to facilitate passage of food back to the pharynx. The hard palate provides a stable platform against which the mobile tongue can push and separates the oral and nasal cavities. The floor of the mouth and the gums are structural components of the reservoir and aid in the preparation functions of the oral cavity in the process of eating; the mobile tongue is the main propulsive agent in the oral cavity. Each site also has a distinct contribution to the modulation of air expelled from the lungs that results in speech.

Therapy. Carcinogenesis in the oral cavity and the natural history of subsequent disease are generally similar independent of anatomic area, although TNM staging has not been a perfect prognosticator for all sites, and histology and site play an important role in outcome. The consequences to the patient of therapy, particularly surgical therapy, are, however, very different and depend very much on the function of the area involved and the success with which it can be reconstructed.

Lip

Etiology. In the United States and Canada, carcinoma of the lip is very common, with a marked male predominance of 20:1. The lower lip is by far the most common site, being involved in approximately 95 percent of cases, and has squamous cell carcinoma as the most common histology. Basal cell carcinoma predominates in the upper lip. The habit of pipe smoking, with chronic thermal injury, was for many years felt to be the carcinogenic stimulus. Recently, however, it has become clear that the protuberant lower lip is exposed to higher doses of ultraviolet radiation, resulting in malignancy that behaves similarly to UV-induced skin cancer. Farmers and other outdoor workers in their sixth to ninth decades, of Celtic and northern European origin, who live in areas of high sunlight exposure are at highest risk. Chronic ex posure to sun results in loss of the anatomic vermilion border, the junction between the skin and mucosa of the lip, followed by leukoplakia or carcinoma in situ and by invasive malignancy (Fig. 15-27).

Pathology. Well-differentiated Stage I lesions make up the vast majority, 60 to 80 percent of most clinical series. Local recur-

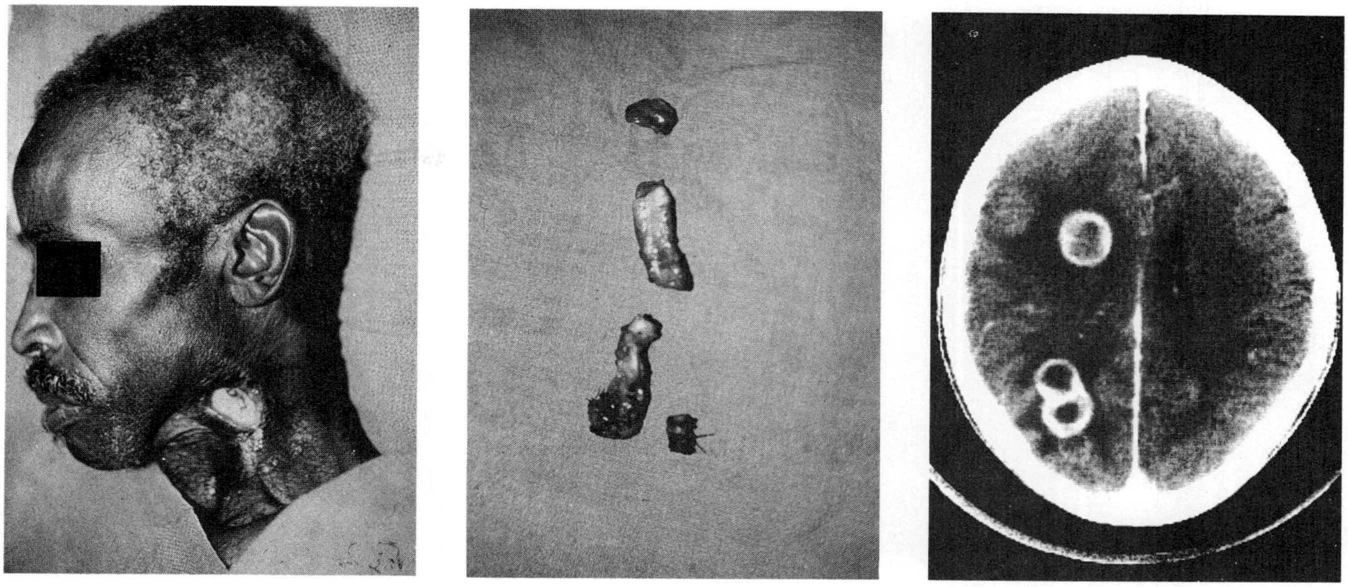

A B C

FIG. 15-25. *A.* Patient who had been previously treated for squamous cell carcinoma of the retromolar trigone with surgical resection, radical neck dissection, and postoperative adjuvant radiotherapy. One year after treatment he presented with an ulceration in the neck. Work-up revealed no evidence of recurrent malignancy. He subsequently had a bleeding episode from his common carotid artery which was treated by arteriography (suture visible in center of ulcer). *B.* Definitive therapy required resection of necrotic common external and internal carotid arteries and coverage of neck with a pectoralis major muscle flap. *C.* The neck wound was resolved, but the patient expired from multiple brain abscesses secondary to septic emboli from the infected carotid vessels. CT scan showing numerous ipsilateral abscesses (From: *Coleman JJ: Surg Clin North Am 66:149, 1986, with permission.*)

rence after either surgery or irradiation occurs in 10 to 20 percent of cases, but salvage therapy (subsequent surgery ± radiation or chemotherapy) may be successful. Nodal metastases, usually to the submental or submandibular nodes, are present in 10 to 15 percent of cases and occur in tumors of all histologic differentiation. Treatment by local excision or radiation results in cure rates of approximately 90 percent for Stage I disease and 55 to 80 percent in Stage II locoregional disease. Aggressive carcinoma of the lip seems to follow a pattern of perineural invasion, down the mental nerve to involve the mandible and pterygoid space, and ultimately extends via the trigeminal nerve to the base of the skull.

Therapy. Surgical therapy requires resection of the disease with a clear margin of normal tissue around it. If lymph nodes are involved, ipsilateral or bilateral neck dissection is indicated. Elective or prophylactic node dissection for the patient with the N0 neck is usually not recommended in epidermoid carcinoma of the lip. The functional goal in lip reconstruction is to restore oral continence and reasonable appearance. Because the lower lip is longer and more protuberant than the upper lip, primary closure of defects of approximately 25 percent of the upper lip and 35 percent of the lower lip will result in satisfactory appearance and function. The lip opposite the resection is an important donor site for larger defects. Cross lip flaps from either the upper or lower lip of the Abbé or Estlander type, as well as advancement of lateral labial and buccal elements, are useful depending on the size and site of the defect. Preservation of sensory and motor function of the remaining orbicularis oris muscle is also possible, to maintain the most efficient sphincter mechanism, using the Karapandzic principle. When the entire lower lip is resected, the damming function can be restored by a radial forearm free flap including palmaris longus tendon, which is inset to the adjacent oral musculature to serve as a dynamic sling. Since the tissue at risk is oral mucosa on the protuberant area of the lip, preneoplastic changes of leukoplakia or dysplasia should be treated by mucosal resection, vermilionectomy (lip shave), and advancement of the labial mucosa to the sun-exposed margin of the skin (mucosal advancement).

Buccal Mucosa

Anatomy and Physiology. The buccal mucosa extends from the commissures of the lips to the pterygomandibular raphe and from the maxillary (upper) to the mandibular (lower) alveoli on both sides. The subjacent structures include the buccal fat pad and buccinator muscle, and the surface of the buccal mucosa permits entry to the oral cavity of Stensen's duct from the parotid gland. This area modulates speech and oral capacitance to a great degree.

Pathology. Buccal mucosa cancer makes up about 5 percent of all oral cancers and like other sites there is a significant male predominance (3:1). There is a high incidence of advanced disease on presentation, with 18 percent Stage I, 36 percent Stage II, and 44 percent Stage III with 56 percent incidence of nodal metastasis. Large cancers of the buccal mucosa are less likely than tumors of other oral sites to have subclinical metastases to the neck. A subset of lesions arising in the buccal mucosa is *verrucous carcinoma,* which presents as an exophytic mass that has the cellular histology characteristic of malignancy but lacks the invasive as-

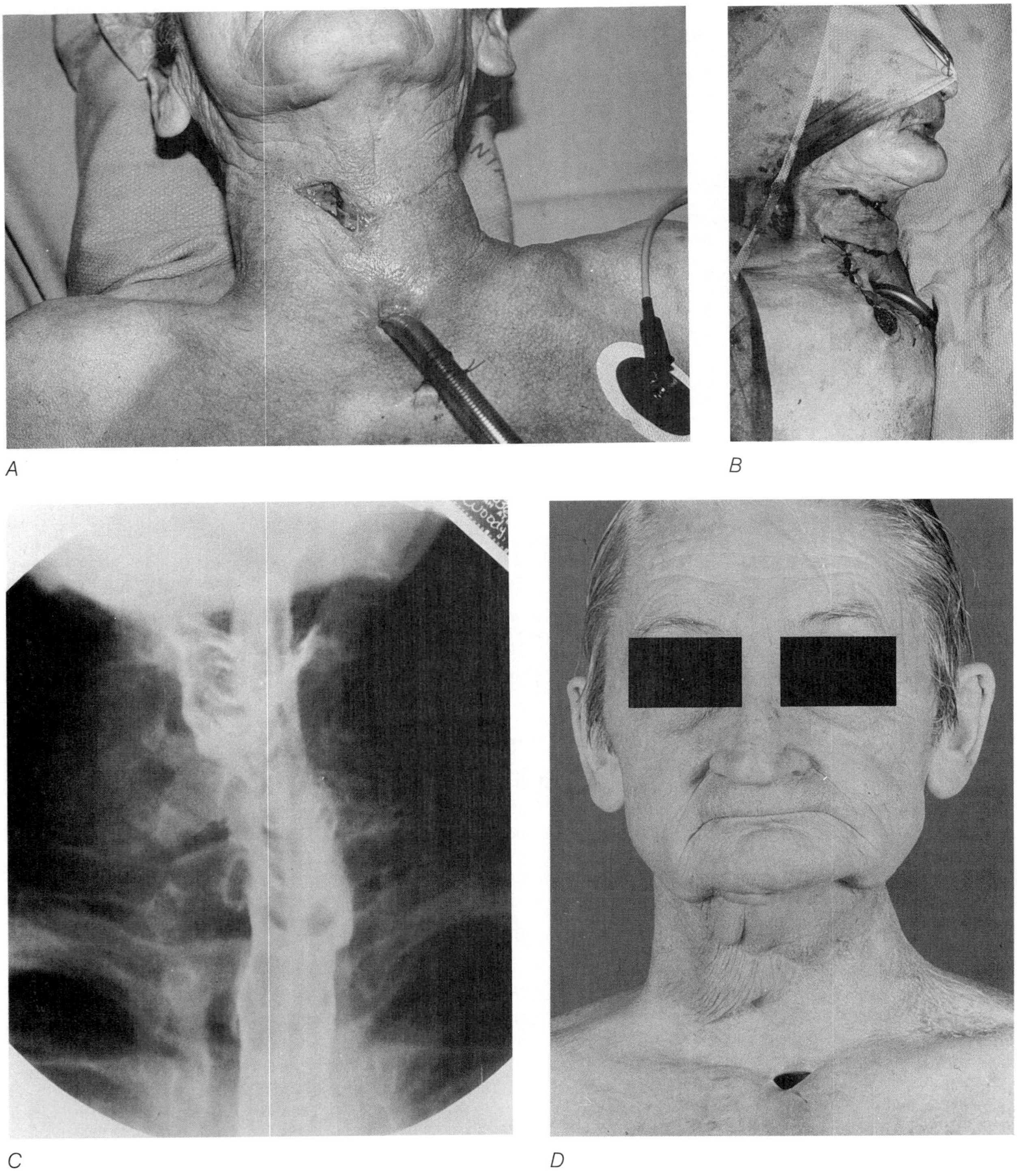

FIG. 15-26. *A.* Fistula (communication between neopharynx and skin of neck) after laryngopharyngectomy and reconstruction with jejunal free flap. *B.* Closure of fistula was performed by approximation of the mucosal defect and coverage with a sternocleidomastoid musculocutaneous flap. *C.* Barium swallow after repair shows passage of oral contents through jejunal segment without extravasation. *D.* Patient with healed neck after completing his adjuvant radiotherapy.

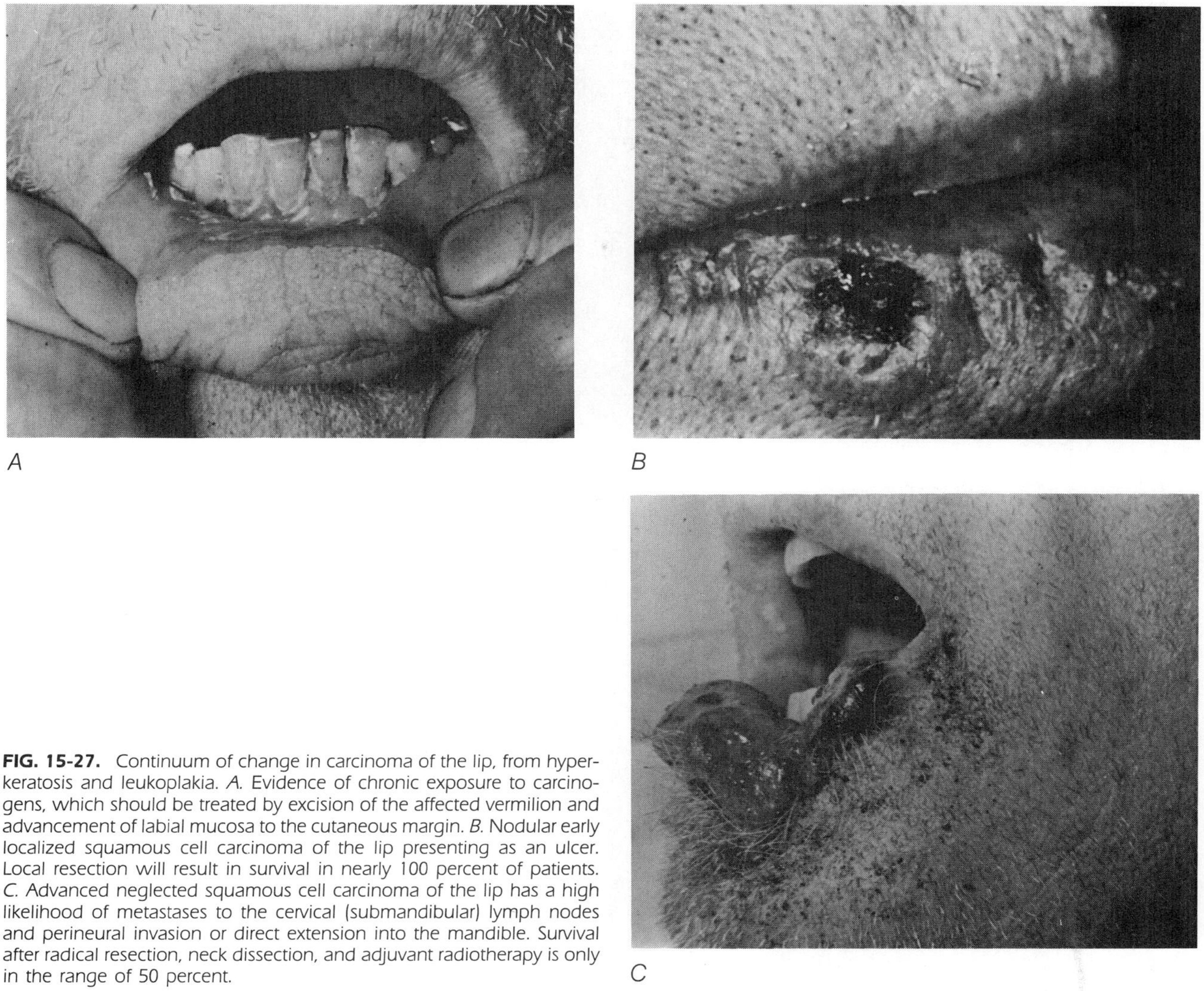

FIG. 15-27. Continuum of change in carcinoma of the lip, from hyperkeratosis and leukoplakia. *A.* Evidence of chronic exposure to carcinogens, which should be treated by excision of the affected vermilion and advancement of labial mucosa to the cutaneous margin. *B.* Nodular early localized squamous cell carcinoma of the lip presenting as an ulcer. Local resection will result in survival in nearly 100 percent of patients. *C.* Advanced neglected squamous cell carcinoma of the lip has a high likelihood of metastases to the cervical (submandibular) lymph nodes and perineural invasion or direct extension into the mandible. Survival after radical resection, neck dissection, and adjuvant radiotherapy is only in the range of 50 percent.

pects. Verrucous carcinoma is more common in females than in males and may be related to papilloma virus. The buccal mucosa is the most common site of this variant of squamous cell carcinoma, which shows warty dense keratinization, sharply circumscribed deep margins, pushing borders, and inflammatory infiltrate. There is a high incidence of multicentricity of malignancy in patients with verrucous carcinoma, with up to 40 percent having other sites of invasive carcinoma, so it probably represents a part of the spectrum of field cancerization (see Fig. 15-10*E*). There is some concern that radiation of this lesion may result in dedifferentiation or change to a more malignant histology, but this observation may be a manifestation of tumor cell heterogeneity and clonal resistance to radiotherapy rather than actual malignant degeneration. Carcinoma of the buccal mucosa, both verrucous and infiltrative, occurs commonly in chronic tobacco chewers and snuff dippers in the United States and in people who use *pan* in India and southeast Asia.

Therapy. Surgical resection with or without adjuvant radiotherapy results in survival rates of 50 to 60 percent, with 60 to 75 percent for localized disease and 25 to 45 percent for locoregional disease. The route of invasion of epidermoid carcinoma of the buccal mucosa is through the buccinator muscle and buccal fat pad dorsal toward the pterygoid musculature or lateral to the skin. In either case significant limitation of oral motion and discomfort on chewing (trismus) occurs.

Surgical resection frequently creates a full-thickness defect of mucosa, muscle, and skin with or without adjacent mandible or maxillary tuberosity. For extensive lesions, restoration of function requires replacement of internal lining as well as external skin coverage. Although the forehead flap based on the superficial temporal vessels and the deltopectoral flap from the shoulder were the standard in the 1960s and 1970s, recent methods have included the combined use of pectoralis major musculocutaneous flap for lining and deltopectoral skin flap for skin coverage or the latissimus dorsi musculocutaneous flap folded on itself to provide both internal and external surfaces (Fig. 15-28). Fasciocutaneous flaps such as the scapula and radial forearm can provide ample tissue for both defects and vascularized bone as well when transferred as a microvascular free flap. For smaller defects, intraoral flaps of mucosa and muscle such as tongue flaps, palate mucoperiosteal flaps, or advancement flaps have been useful. Split-thickness skin grafts, though successful in the short term, ultimately result in fibrosis and difficulty with chewing. For superficial lesions that extend

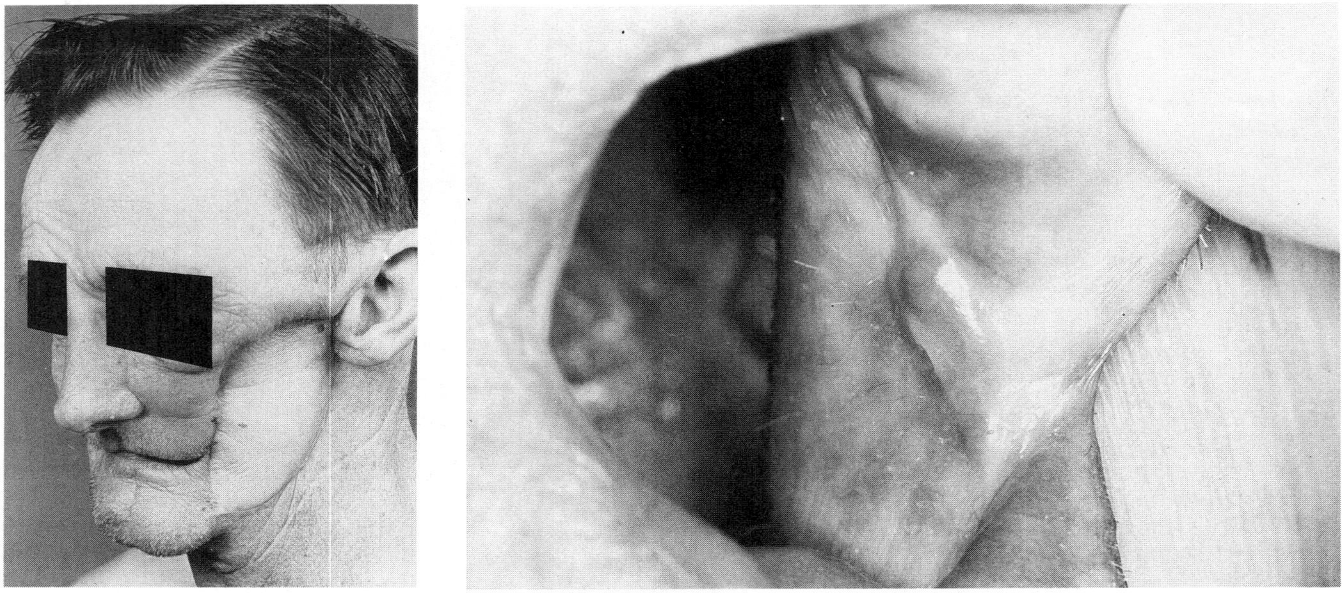

A *B*

FIG. 15-28. *A.* Patient underwent resection of recurrent cancer of the mandibular alveolus after radiotherapy which involved bone, muscle, and skin. Internal lining and external skin coverage were provided with a latissimus dorsi musculocutaneous flap brought beneath the cervical skin flap and turned on itself. *B.* Replacement of buccal mucosa with skin from the back carried on the latissimus dorsi muscle.

over the mandibular alveolus and require supple coverage, the platysma musculocutaneous flap is an excellent choice (Fig. 15-29).

Hard Palate

Pathology. The roof of the mouth, bounded by the soft palate posteriorly and the teeth anteriorly and laterally, is not a common site of intraoral squamous cell carcinoma. More common in this area are tumors, both benign and malignant, of the minor salivary glands (Fig. 15-30). Squamous cell carcinoma in the United States is usually a disease of elderly male smokers and remains superficial for prolonged periods before extending through periosteum and bone and spreading either cephalad into the nasal cavity or maxillary antrum or dorsally through the pterygopalatine fossa area. Epidermoid carcinoma of the hard palate is more common in India and Venezuela where reverse smoking (with the lighted end of the cigarette inside the mouth) is practiced.

Therapy. Treatment is surgical resection with or without adjuvant radiotherapy. Because of the underlying bone, definitive radiotherapy is rarely useful. Cervical metastases are relatively rare in disease of the hard palate, with only 10 to 25 percent of patients presenting with disease at either the prevascular facial nodes or the jugulodigastric nodes. Occult metastases are rare, so elective neck dissection is not part of the therapeutic regimen. Five-year survival rates range from 33 to 75 percent depending on stage, with an average of 55 to 60 percent for all patients.

Small to moderate-size defects of the hard palate are best treated with a dental prosthesis in both the dentate and edentulous patients; massive defects may require temporalis muscle flap or local flaps and skin grafting or free tissue transfer, since support for the prosthesis may not be available. The inflammatory process of the minor salivary glands of the hard palate, necrotizing sialometaplasia, which produces an ulcerative lesion with erythematous borders similar to squamous cell carcinoma, may be confused with malignancy. Biopsy, however, will show no evidence of malignancy, and the disease is self-limited, usually requiring no therapy.

Floor of Mouth

Anatomy and Physiology. The floor of the mouth is the horseshoe-shaped area between the mobile tongue and the lingual surface of the mandible. The papillae that allow Wharton's ducts to empty into the oral cavity lie at the anterior border of this area, and posteriorly the floor of mouth blends into the glossopalatine fold and the retromolar trigone. In this natural reservoir there may be prolonged contact of the floor of mouth mucosa with carcinogenic agents dissolved in the saliva after oral ingestion or inhalation. This area provides capacity, allowing the tongue to sit low in the mouth, thus increasing the volume of the oral cavity and preventing obstruction of the direct route between the lips and the pharynx.

Pathology. Approximately 13 to 17 percent of oral lesions arise in this area, the third most common site after the lip and mobile tongue. Because of the proximity of the mucosa to the hyoglossus and mylohyoid muscles of the submandibular triangle, and because of the rich lymphatic supply, direct extension of tumor into the neck and bilateral cervical metastases are frequent, especially in anteriorly located lesions. Medial growth at the primary site also invades the ventral surface of the tongue and lateral growth invades the mandible. Advanced-stage disease is common, with 46 to 52 percent of patients presenting with Stage III or IV disease. Subclinical disease in the neck or micrometastases in the clinically negative neck are common, with overall neck involvement increasing with primary tumor size and ranging from 15 per-

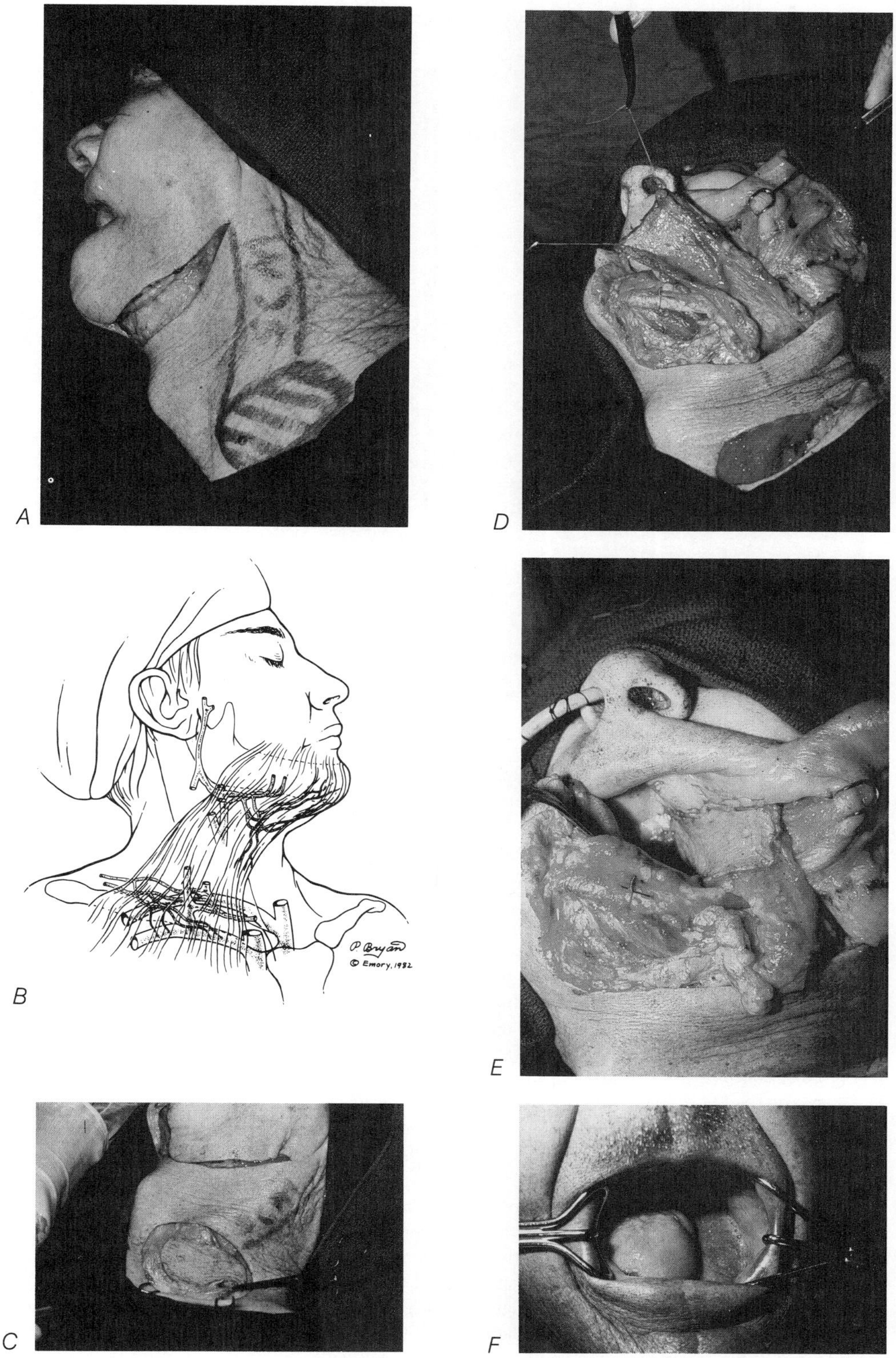

FIG. 15-29. *A.* Seventy-eight-year-old man who chronically used chewing tobacco underwent resection of T2,N0,M0 superficial carcinoma of buccal mucosa. Reconstruction was to be carried out with a superiorly based platysma musculocutaneous flap. *B.* Diagram of platysma muscle demonstrating superior blood supply from the facial artery and inferior blood supply from the transverse cervical blood supply. *C.* Island musculocutaneous flap of platysma. Hemostat is on the cutaneous branch of the transverse cervical vessels. *D.* Thin and supple musculocutaneous flap based on the submandibular branch of the facial artery are transposed beneath the cervical skin flap. *E.* Skin sutured to remaining buccal and alveolar mucosa to close defect from resection. *F.* At three months skin covering alveolus allows wearing of a denture and does not interfere with tongue motion (From: *Coleman JJ, in Jurkiewicz MJ, et al: Plastic Surgery: Principles and Practice, 1990, with permission.*)

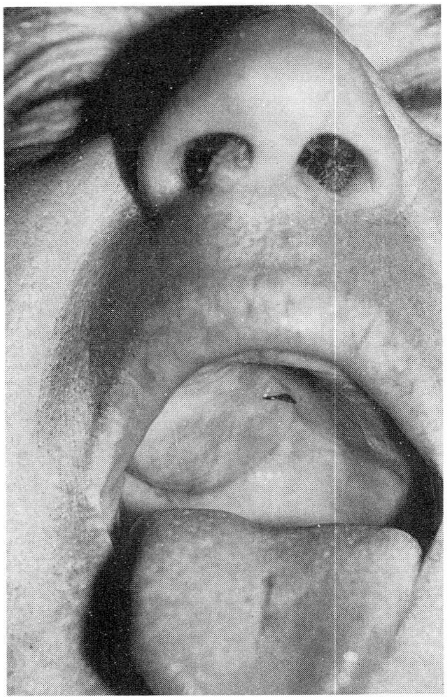

A

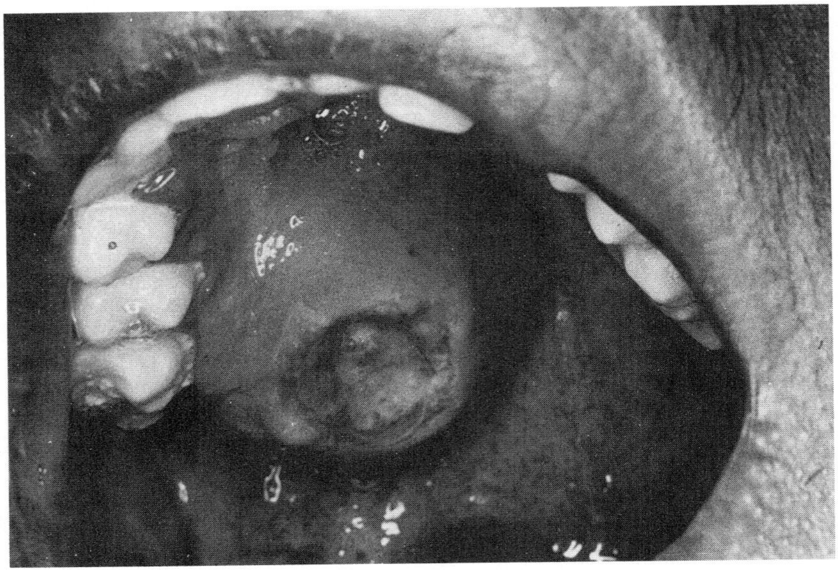

B

FIG. 15-30. *A.* Adenoid cystic carcinoma of the palate arising from a minor salivary gland with extensive submucosal extension and no ulceration. *B.* Ulcerated pleomorphic adenoma (benign mixed tumor) of the palate arising from a minor salivary gland. Despite the ulceration and size, this is a benign neoplasm.

cent for tumors less than 2 cm (T1) to 50 percent for tumors greater than 4 cm (T3).

Therapy. Because the tumor may abut or actively invade the mandible, resection with an adequate margin of normal tissue in this area frequently requires removal of the mandibular periosteum or actual resection of a segment of mandible. Uncertainty about invasion of the mandible or proximity may require removal of the medial cortex (marginal mandibulectomy) or a segment of the mandible. Because of the proximity of the mandible, therapeutic doses of radiation may result in ischemic necrosis of the bone, osteoradionecrosis. Combined therapy, surgical resection of the primary with neck dissection en bloc or pull-through resection followed by adjuvant radiotherapy, is appropriate for advanced disease. Survival rates are to a great degree dependent on stage, ranging from 68 to 91 percent for Stage I to 35 to 46 percent for Stage III. Recurrence at the primary site frequently involves the mandible or the suprahyoid complex of muscles and may require laryngectomy because of invasion of the preepiglottic space.

Reconstruction of the floor of the mouth presents a number of challenges. The watertight seal of the oral cavity, the continuity of the mandibular arch, and the mobility of the tongue all depend on this area. For superficial lesions with normal well-vascularized muscle beneath them, split-thickness skin grafts have been advocated. Although they may be successful initially in covering the area, the contracture inherent in this method may result in tethering of the mobile tongue to the subjacent muscle or to the mandibular periosteum. If the neck is not involved by tumor, a musculocutaneous island flap of platysma muscle based on the facial artery provides supple skin coverage. Bulky thoracic musculocutaneous flaps, such as pectoralis major, provide skin for lining but may be compressed by the intact mandible, resulting in ischemic necrosis, or may push the tongue back in the oral cavity, limiting movement and obstructing the pharynx and airway. The thin pliable skin of the volar forearm carried on the radial artery and its venae comitantes, as the radial forearm free flap, provides an excellent lining for this area which can drape over the mandible and allows free movement of the tongue while providing a watertight seal. Vascularized segments of bone and skin of varying size are also available as free tissue transfers from the fibula, scapula, dorsum of the foot, and other sites with high success rate if the mandible must be resected (Fig. 15-31).

Gums, Gingivae, Alveolar Ridge

Pathology. Squamous cell carcinoma arising on the gums constitutes between 10 and 17 percent of oral cavity malignancies. Eighty percent of lesions arise on the mandibular alveolus. Although the male predominance persists at this site, there seems to be a less direct relationship with tobacco and alcohol, and the causation may be related in some cases to chronic trauma from poorly fashioned dentures or jagged teeth. The thin layer of mucosa allows invasion of the underlying mandibular or maxillary bone in 35 to 50 percent of cases. Direct invasion through the periosteum is most common in patients with teeth, but spread through the empty sockets along the occlusal ridge and subsequent perineural invasion are common in edentulous patients. Cervical metastases occur in 30 to 45 percent of the cases, depending to a great degree on the size of the primary.

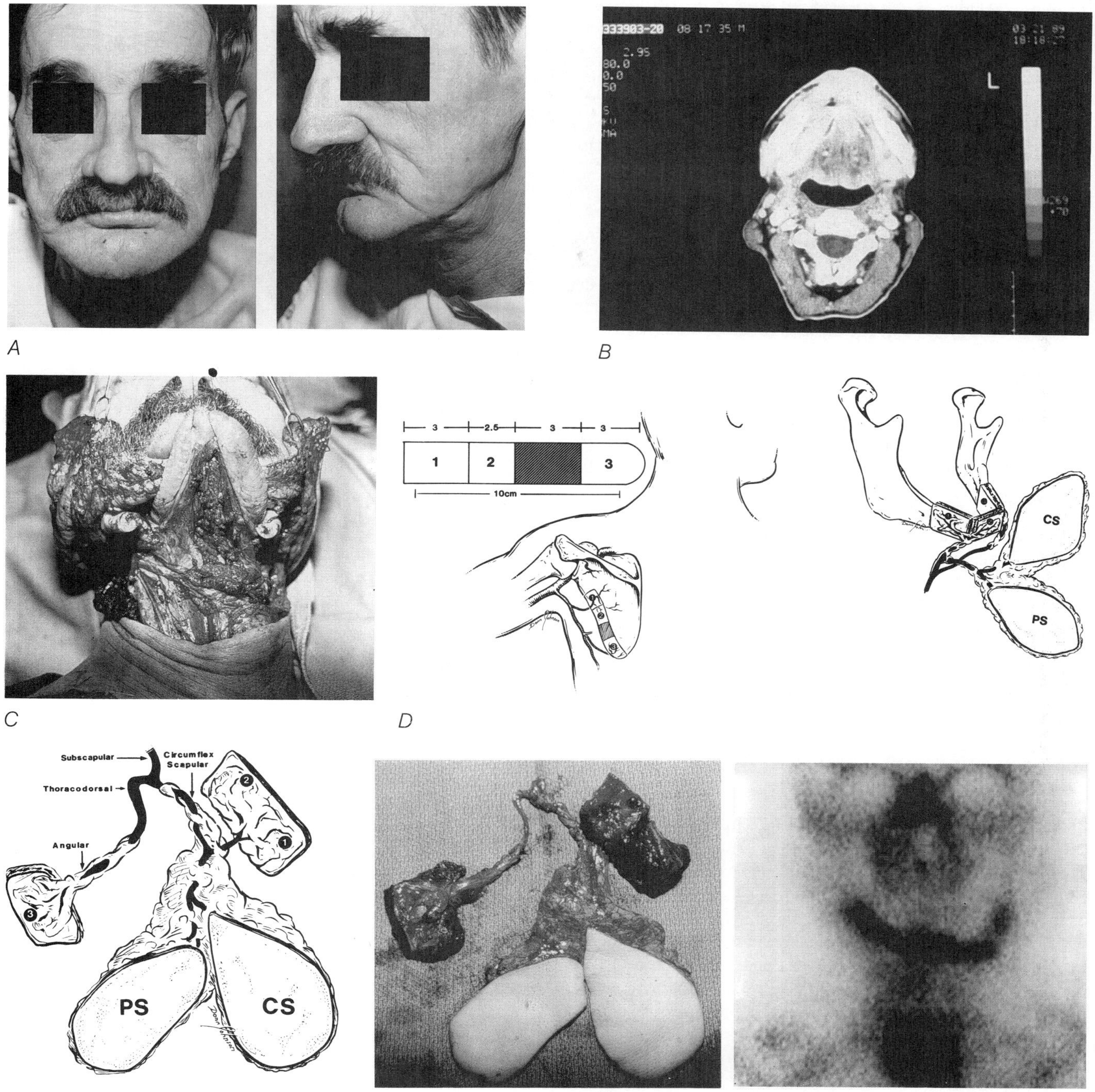

A *B* *C* *D* *E* *F*

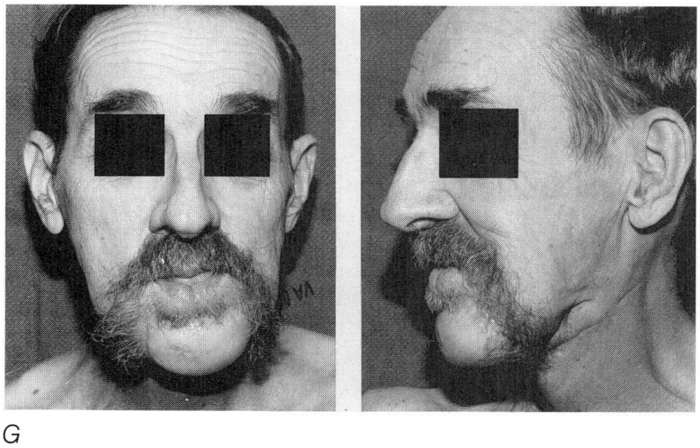

G

FIG. 15-31. *A.* Patient with recurrent squamous cell carcinoma of the floor of the mouth after previous radiotherapy for that lesion and another squamous cell carcinoma of the larynx. *B.* CT scan showing invasion of mandibular symphysis, the overlying skin, the floor of the mouth, and the ventral surface of the tongue. *C.* Surgical defect after en bloc resection of symphysis, skin of the mentum, ventral tongue, and bilateral neck dissections. Note that the suprahyoid muscles have been resected, disrupting the connection between the larynx, the tongue, and the mandibular symphysis. *D* and *E.* Reconstructive plan for the mandible and skin, for the floor of mouth mucosa and skin of mentum. The bipedicle osteocutaneous scapula flap provided two segments of bone based on the circumflex scapular and the angular branches of the subscapular artery and two segments of skin based on the circumflex scapular artery (CS) (horizontal branch) and parascapular branch (PS). The osteotomized scapula was fixed with titanium miniplates. Microvascular anastomosis was performed between the facial artery and subscapular artery and the external jugular and subscapular vein. *F.* Technetium 99m bone scan 3 days after surgery shows good perfusion of reconstructed symphysis. *G.* One month after surgery patient has comprehensible speech and is able to take his entire diet by mouth.

Therapy. Surgical resection requires removal of the subjacent bone by partial or total maxillectomy or total mandibulectomy. Maxillary defects of moderate size can be treated with dental prostheses, and mandibular defects reconstructed with various combinations of skin and bone as previously described.

Oral Tongue

Anatomy and Physiology. The tongue is a complex muscular structure covered with mucosa and receiving motor innervation from the hypoglossal nerve. The bulk of the tongue is made up of the superior and inferior longitudinal muscles joined by the vertical and transverse intrinsic muscles. Inferoposteriorly and laterally the tongue is connected to the hyoid bone by the hyoglossus muscle, and superiorly and anteriorly to the mandible by the genioglossus muscles. The styloglossus and palatoglossus muscles attach the tongue superiorly to the base of the skull. These junctions allow great mobility of the tongue wall, promoting synergy with the larynx and the pharyngeal and palatine muscles. Beneath the smooth ventral surface of the tongue, along the floor of the mouth, are the numerous openings of the sublingual ducts. On the dorsal surface are papillae, with specialized sensory organs for taste at the base. Also opening onto the tongue are the ducts of the minor salivary glands. Sensation is provided to the tongue by the lingual nerve carrying fibers of cranial nerve V, and taste by the glossopharyngeal and chorda tympani of VII. Differentiation of sweet, sour, salt, and bitter taste relies to a great degree on intact function of the tongue. As a mucosa-covered muscle, the tongue is the major propulsive force in the oral cavity. It initiates and continues movement of the food bolus to the pharynx, generating pressure of up to 120 mmHg. Numerous investigators have demonstrated that dysfunction after surgery for oral cancer depends almost exclusively on the amount of tongue resected.

Pathology. In most series of oral cancers, the oral or mobile tongue is second only to the lip as the most common primary site. Tobacco and alcohol are the most common associated factors but chronic irritation from jagged teeth or dental appliances may also be involved. Although the sixth and seventh decades are the peak periods, sporadic occurrence of squamous cell carcinoma in the tongue has been described in patients under thirty and in renal transplant and other immunosuppressed patients and may not be linked to the usual carcinogenic stimuli. In India, submucosal fibrosis seems to be a predisposing influence; and in Scandinavia, Plummer-Vinson syndrome, glossitis, iron-deficiency anemia, and achlorhydria may be related.

Malignancy of the mobile tongue occurs most frequently at the midportion of the lateral tongue and is frequently asymptomatic (Fig. 15-32). Radial spread through the tongue may extend submucosally to the base of the tongue and across the midline or laterally to the floor of the mouth. Because of the rich lymphatic supply, ipsilateral metastases are common to the submandibular and submental nodes. Clinical evidence of cervical metastasis is present in 40 to 61 percent of patients, and subclinical disease in the N0 neck is found in 25 to 31 percent. As in other sites, the presence of lymph node metastases seems to be the most important prognosticator, with survival rates of 73 to 92 percent for localized disease (T1, T2, N0) and only 31 to 45 percent with regional metastasis.

Therapy. Definitive therapy for carcinoma of the oral tongue can be attempted with either external beam radiotherapy or

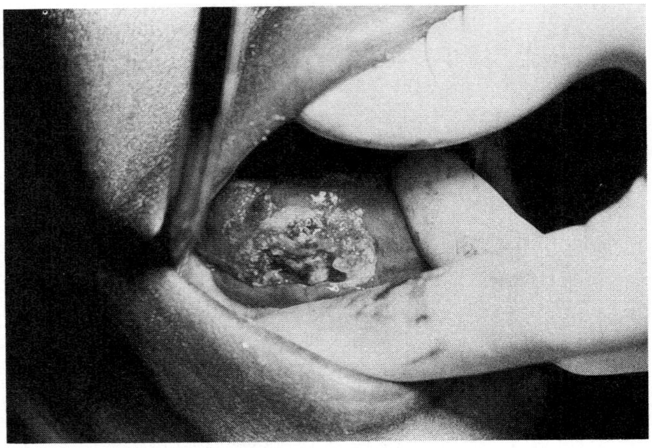

FIG. 15-32. T2,N1,M0 squamous cell carcinoma of the mobile tongue arising in the characteristic middle third of the lateral tongue.

interstitial radiotherapy. External radiation in doses to 6500 R may be useful, but implantation of afterloading devices (tubes into which iridium 192 or radium needles can be placed) can deliver doses in the range of 10,000 to 15,000 R over a small area with greater effect.

The surgical therapy of carcinoma of the tongue consists of resection of the tumor with a margin of normal tissue and en bloc removal of the regional lymph nodes. Unfortunately, evaluation of the extent of local disease is difficult in tongue cancer. Although several authors have demonstrated respectable 5-year survivals (48 to 62 percent) with partial glossectomy with or without en bloc or discontinuous neck dissection, a generally accepted uneasiness about the ability to obtain clear margins has led to the common use of adjuvant radiotherapy. Hemiglossectomy, or resection to the median raphe, has been advocated by some for lesions involving any part of the lateral tongue.

Extensive lesions of the tongue may extend posteriorly to involve the larynx. Even in those patients who do not demonstrate invasion of the larynx, widespread involvement of the tongue or resection of the base of the tongue may predispose the patient to aspiration and ultimate respiratory failure. Despite skepticism on the part of some surgeons, total glossectomy with or without laryngectomy has been shown to be a valuable procedure for both cure and palliation. A 3-year survival of 53 percent has been achieved in one series, with 80 percent of patients demonstrating intelligible speech if the larynx is preserved and 93 percent regaining the ability to maintain their nutritional status by oral alimentation.

Although attempts have been made to innervate muscle of various types transplanted to replace the tongue, there is no satisfactory way to reconstruct the tongue. Denervation of the tongue by resection of, or injury to, both hypoglossal nerves usually renders the patient incapable of swallowing or of effective speech. After surgical resection of a portion of the tongue, the reconstructive goal is to allow free mobility of the remaining tongue while providing a watertight seal to the oral cavity. If the floor of the mouth is not involved in the resection, simply skin grafting of the raw surface may suffice. Suturing the edge of the resected tongue to alveolar or buccal mucosa usually tethers the tongue, impeding its mobility. Advancing the posterior mobile tongue or setting back the excess anterior tongue may provide the optimal solution. Although the pectoralis major flap has been advocated for intraoral reconstruction, its bulk tends to push the tongue back or pull it down into the neck, interfering with its motion and the subsequent elevation of the larynx necessary for effective swallowing and speech. Furthermore, its thickness and weight effectively fix the tongue to the adjacent mandible, further interfering with its motion. The lateral arm or radial forearm free flap provides lightweight supple tissue more appropriate for restoring tongue, floor of mouth and mandibular alveolar epithelial lining.

The defect of total glossectomy consists of the tongue, floor of the mouth, and sometimes pharyngeal and laryngeal mucosa. Restoration of oral continence usually requires significant soft tissue. The pectoralis major flap serves well to replace the entire floor of the mouth, as does the jejunal free flap, which can also replace the pharynx and cervical esophagus. If the larynx is preserved in total glossectomy, the radial forearm free flap serves as an excellent diaphragm to pull the hyoid anteriorly toward the mandible and assist in swallowing.

When a portion of mandible must be resected for carcinoma of the oral tongue, the urgency of reconstruction depends on what part of the mandible has been resected. Although any mandibulectomy results in some dysfunction, partial mandibulectomy lateral to the mental foramen is usually well tolerated, the main morbidity being weakness of chewing and malocclusion of the remaining teeth. Resection of the symphysis or anterior segment of the mandible is, however, a much more devastating problem and requires immediate reconstruction. Vascularized bone from scapula, fibula, iliac crest, radius, or metatarsal is excellent for reconstruction. If appropriate soft tissue is not available, two free tissue transfers can be performed to satisfy the individual needs of the wound.

Pharynx

Anatomy and Physiology. The pharynx is the continuation of the muscular tube that constitutes the alimentary tract. It is anatomically divided into three sections, each with a slightly different function: the nasopharynx, the oropharynx, and the hypopharynx (See Fig. 15-4). An important role of the pharynx is separating the respiratory and the alimentary tracts, and its specialized structures reflect this function. The nasopharynx is unique in the pharynx in that it is a rigid cavity bounded on three sides by bone—superiorly by the base of the skull and posterior sphenoid sinus, anteriorly by the posterior rim of the ethmoid plate and the choanae, passages from the nasal cavity into the nasopharynx, and posteriorly by the pharyngeal tubercle of the occipital bone and the atlas and axis, with their prevertebral fascial and muscular coverings. The inferior surface is the nasal side of the soft palate. The lateral sides of the nasopharynx give entry to the eustachian tubes (to decompress the middle ear) and the roof is the site of a collection of lymphoid tissue, the pharyngeal tonsil.

The oropharynx is the muscular tube that serves as transit area from the propulsive oral cavity and the recipient nasal cavity to the alimentary and respiratory tracts. This mucosa-lined muscular tube contains the base of the tongue (from the circumvallate papillae back), the tonsils, the oral soft palate, the lateral pharyngeal walls, and the posterior pharyngeal wall. The dominant muscular entity that receives the propulsive energy of the tongue is the superior constrictor muscle, attached on both sides to the pterygomandibular raphe and wrapping 270 degrees to constitute the posterior and lateral walls. Contraction of this muscle closes the palatopharyngeal sphincter, or Passavant's ridge, elevating the palate. This action closes the nasopharynx and pushes the bolus of food into the hypopharynx. Up and down motion of the palate is regulated by the tensor and levator veli palatini muscles (attached to the base of the skull) and the palatopharyngeus muscle (attached to the lateral pharyngeal wall). Lack of synergy in these muscles is seen in patients with cerebrovascular accidents and hypoxia neonatorum and markedly interferes with speech and swallowing.

The anatomic boundaries of the hypopharynx are reflections of the anatomy of the larynx. The posterior pharyngeal wall runs from the tip of the epiglottis to the inferior border of the cricoid cartilage. The anterior border is the postcricoid mucosa, and the lateral surfaces the mucosal cavities on both sides of the larynx known as the pyriform sinuses. The middle pharyngeal constrictor muscle, with its attachments to the hyoid bone and prevertebral fascia, and the inferior pharyngeal constrictor, with its distal condensation of the cricopharyngeus muscle attached to the lateral surfaces of the thyroid and cricoid cartilages, serve as the pharyngeal sphincters. When they contract they close off the entrance of the cervical esophagus to air and direct it through the larynx. When they relax they allow food through the pharynx and into the cervical esophagus. The inferior constrictor and cricopharyngeus muscles serve as the upper esophageal sphincter and may become hypertonic, a condition known as cricopharyngeus spasm. Zenker's diverticulum, a lateral outpouching of the pharyngeal wall which may collect undigested food and result in chronic aspiration, is the consequence of chronic hypertension of the upper esophageal sphincter (Fig. 15-33).

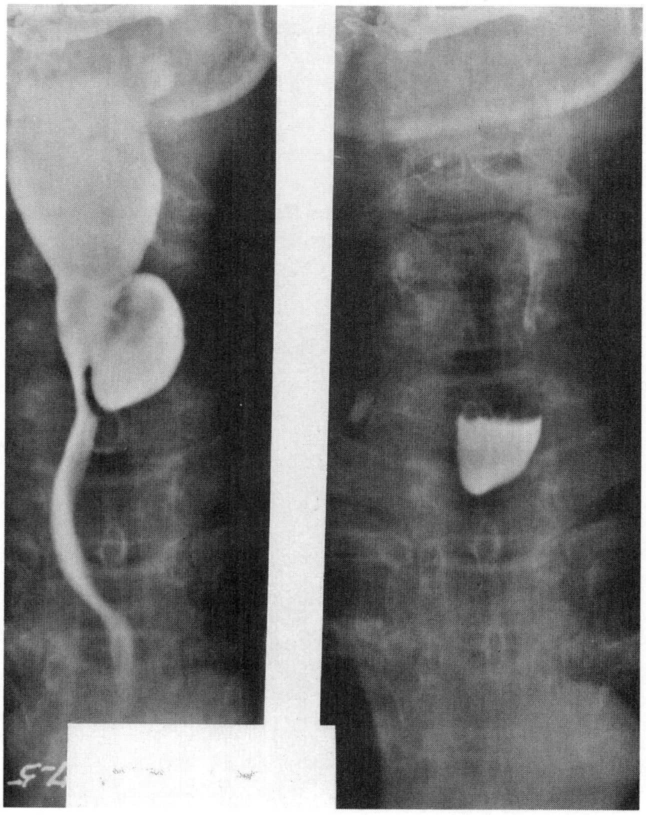

FIG. 15-33. Barium swallow showing Zenker's diverticulum and cricopharyngeus spasm distal to it. After swallowing, barium or food remains in the diverticulum and may be aspirated, resulting in pneumonitis.

Base of Tongue

Pathology. Carcinoma arising behind the circumvallate papillae in the base of the tongue frequently remains asymptomatic and undiagnosed until late-stage disease is present. Even when patients complain of pain, either local or referred, as with otalgia, difficulty in examination or reluctance of primary care physicians to perform indirect laryngoscopy and palpation of the base of the tongue results in misdiagnosis and prolonged therapy for pharyngitis, tonsillitis, and other less serious problems. The central location gives rise to cervical lymphatic metastases in up to 70 percent of patients, and there are bilateral metastases in 17 to 25 percent of cases.

Histology and gross morphology in this region predict to some degree the behavior of the lesion and the appropriate therapy. In addition to epidermoid carcinoma, minor salivary gland lesions are also seen. Exophytic lesions, with cells resembling lymphocytes and absence of keratin pearls, arise in the tissues of Waldeyer's ring, the tonsils (lingual and palatine), and base of tongue. These lymphoepitheliomas behave like nasopharyngeal carcinoma and have been characterized as undifferentiated carcinomas with lymphocytic infiltration. Such lesions are more radiosensitive, both at the primary site and as cervical metastasis, than most other infiltrative keratin-producing squamous cell carcinomas resulting in 2-year local control rates of 75 percent for T1 lesions and 67 percent for T2 lesions.

Carcinoma arising in the base of the tongue spreads anteriorly into the oral tongue, superiorly up to the tonsillar pillar, and inferiorly into the lateral pharyngeal wall and into the vallecula, preepiglottic space, and larynx. Because of the proximity and functional relationship of the base of the tongue to the larynx, interference with laryngeal elevation and closure of the epiglottis, with the attendant aspiration pneumonitis, is a hallmark of carcinoma of the base of the tongue.

Therapy. Advanced disease at the primary site or disease with cervical metastases requires surgical therapy. If the lesion is lateral enough, partial glossectomy may be adequate. Since resection of the base of the tongue usually removes the hypoglossal nerve to the tongue in that area, subtotal or posterior glossectomy is unlikely to leave functional tongue. Radical resection may require total glossectomy with or without laryngectomy (Fig. 15-34). In most patients, if the oncologic requirements of the resection do not dictate removal of the larynx, reconstruction with the larynx in situ is appropriate. Surgical therapy or surgery combined with postoperative adjuvant radiotherapy results in 5-year survivals of 50 to 60 percent for Stage III disease and 20 to 25 percent for Stage IV disease. Advanced primary disease or disease in the neck is unlikely to be successfully controlled locally with radiotherapy alone, and surgical salvage after radiotherapy has been dismal, with a high incidence of osteoradionecrosis of the mandible.

Reconstruction of defects arising from resection of the base of the tongue should attempt to close the pharynx and oral cavity with tissue that will heal to previously irradiated mucosa or withstand subsequent irradiation and still not interfere with the function of tissues left intact by the curative resection. Elevation of the larynx, the normal motion that occurs during the early pharyngeal phase of swallowing to close the epiglottis, cannot occur if the tongue is tethered to the side of the pharynx or oral cavity or if bulky tissue such as the pectoralis major flap is interposed into the area of the resection. The provision of sensate tissue into the area surrounding the larynx, to prevent aspiration, is also an important consideration. Occasionally local tissue can be mobilized for closure without tension to avoid fistula and provide sensate mucosa. More commonly, however, mucosa or skin to line the tongue, mandible, and pharyngeal wall is necessary. Buccal and palatal flaps have been described for small and moderate-size defects, but free tissue transfer of skin from radial forearm or lateral arm or lateral thigh flaps are more appropriate for the more common extensive defects.

Tonsil

Pathology. Squamous cell carcinoma of the tonsil may arise in the tonsil, the tonsillar bed, or the tonsillar pillars (Fig. 15-35). As one of the Waldeyer's ring structures, the tonsil shows a higher incidence of lymphoepithelioma than other sites. Whatever the histology, it is second only to the larynx in frequency as a site of upper aerodigestive tract primary malignancy, with 12,000 new

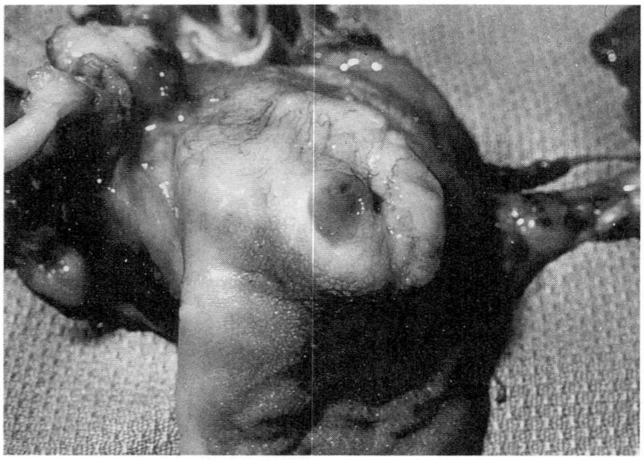

A

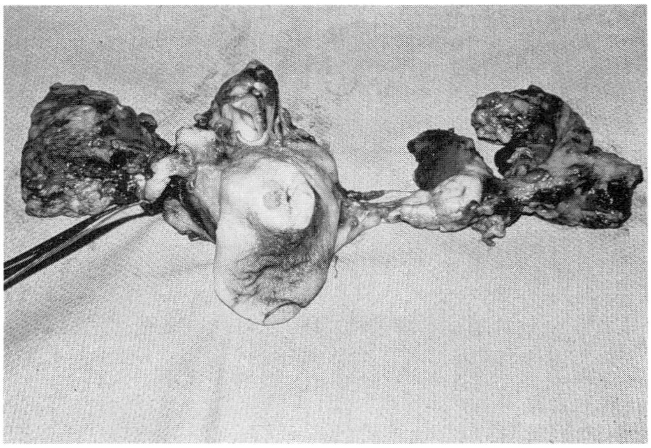

B

FIG. 15-34. *A* and *B*. Adenocarcinoma of the base of the tongue with bilateral lymph node metastases and invasion of the lingual nerve (*left part of A*) treated by total glossectomy, bilateral neck dissection, and reconstruction of the defect with a pectoralis major musculocutaneous flap.

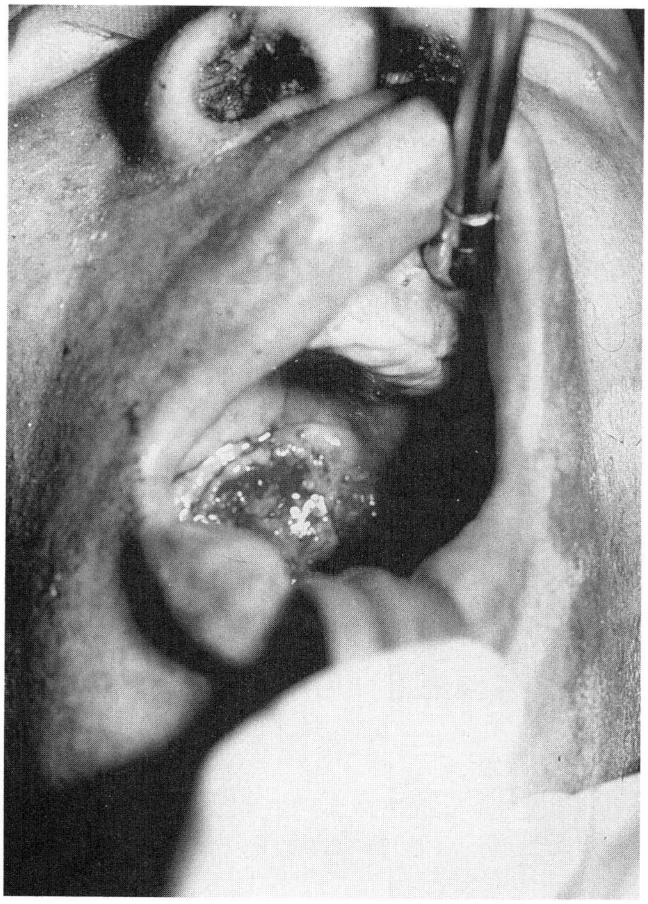

FIG. 15-35. Extensive T3,N2 squamous cell carcinoma of tonsil with extension up to the soft palate and uvula.

cases per year in the United States. Like most upper aerodigestive tract tumors tonsillar carcinoma presents with predominately late-stage disease, with 28 to 32 percent of patients presenting with Stage I or II disease, 35 to 40 percent Stage III, and 40 to 45 percent Stage IV. Cervical metastases at the time of presentation were seen in up to 67 percent of patients, and subclinical disease in the N0 neck was found in 10 percent of patients. Determination of the extent of local disease in advanced tumors is of considerable importance in decision making and execution of therapy. Growth of the tumor upward into the soft palate occurs in 60 percent of patients, downward to the base of the tongue in 56 percent, into the nasopharynx in 9 percent, and down the lateral pharyngeal wall to the epiglottis in 27 percent of cases. The site of local extension is particularly important because in treating patients with radiotherapy, geographical misses secondary to underestimation of local extent of disease were a common reason for failure.

Therapy. Carcinoma of the tonsil appears to be more radiosensitive than other primary-site squamous cell carcinomas. The usual approach to disease originating at this site is to treat for curative intent with radiotherapy ranging from 5500 to 7000 R to the primary site and bilateral cervical lymph node drainage areas (Fig. 15-36). If there is bulky neck disease or extension of the primary tumor into adjacent bone or pterygoid muscles, surgical resection, reconstruction, and postoperative adjuvant radiotherapy are safe and more effective. Risk of local recurrence is directly related to increasing size of the primary tumor and appears even more likely to occur when the predominant spread of tumor was into the base of the tongue.

The challenge of reconstruction in tonsillar disease is a function of the dimensions of local growth of the lesion and the history of previous radiation. The soft tissue defect in the lateral wall of the pharynx created by a superficial lesion can easily be resurfaced with a skin graft, deltopectoral flap, or fasciocutaneous free flap. Radial spread up to the soft palate or down into the pharynx demands that the surface of the flap contour in several planes without obstructing the pharynx, usually requiring a free tissue transfer of relatively pliable skin, such as the radial forearm, lateral arm, or lateral thigh. Invasion of the ascending ramus of the mandible can be treated by addressing the soft tissue defect alone by transposing a pectoralis major musculocutaneous flap into the lateral pharynx, using the skin for internal lining and the muscle for coverage of the carotid vessels in the neck. In the patient with teeth, soft tissue reconstruction alone will lead to malocclusion of the dental arches and other problems. Skin and bone together are available with a number of methods. Particularly suited to the lateral defect created by radical resection of the tonsil and mandible are the scapula and deep circumflex iliac artery free flaps.

Soft Palate

Anatomy and Physiology. The soft palate is the mucosa-lined fusion of the inferiorly based palatopharyngeus and palatoglossus muscles and the superiorly based levator and tensor veli palatini muscles. Extending backward from the posterior margin the palatine bone, directly opposite the superior constructor muscle and its bulge which creates Passavant's ridge, its main function is to open and close the passageway between the nasal cavity and nasopharynx and the oral cavity and oropharynx. This obturating and modulating effect has obvious importance in both speech and swallowing.

Pathology. Isolated carcinoma of the soft palate is rare, the disease usually occurring in combination with other frank malignancies or premalignant entities such as leukoplakia or erythroplakia and not showing the usual male predominance.

The oral side of the soft palate is by far the most common site for malignancy, which usually extends down the tonsillar pillars to the base of the tongue. Superior and posterolateral spread to the nasopharynx and posterior pharyngeal wall is less common. Ipsilateral cervical lymph node metastases to the jugulodigastric nodes occur in 40 to 50 percent of cases, and because tumors often pass over the midline, bilateral metastases are seen in 15 percent of cases.

Therapy. Treatment of soft palate carcinoma follows the usual principle that small primary lesions are effectively eradicated by radiotherapy in the range of 6500 R and that combined therapy, surgery with adjuvant radiotherapy, is necessary for best results in larger tumors. The importance of radiotherapy as a treatment was particularly emphasized in the past because of inability to reconstruct the soft palate and the devastating functional result. Nonrandomized studies of surgery and radiotherapy have shown 5-year survival rates of 31 to 44 percent, with the size of the primary lesion, the absence of a synchronous primary upper aerodigestive tract tumor, the absence of cervical metastases, and moderately to well differentiated histology being favorable prognostic features.

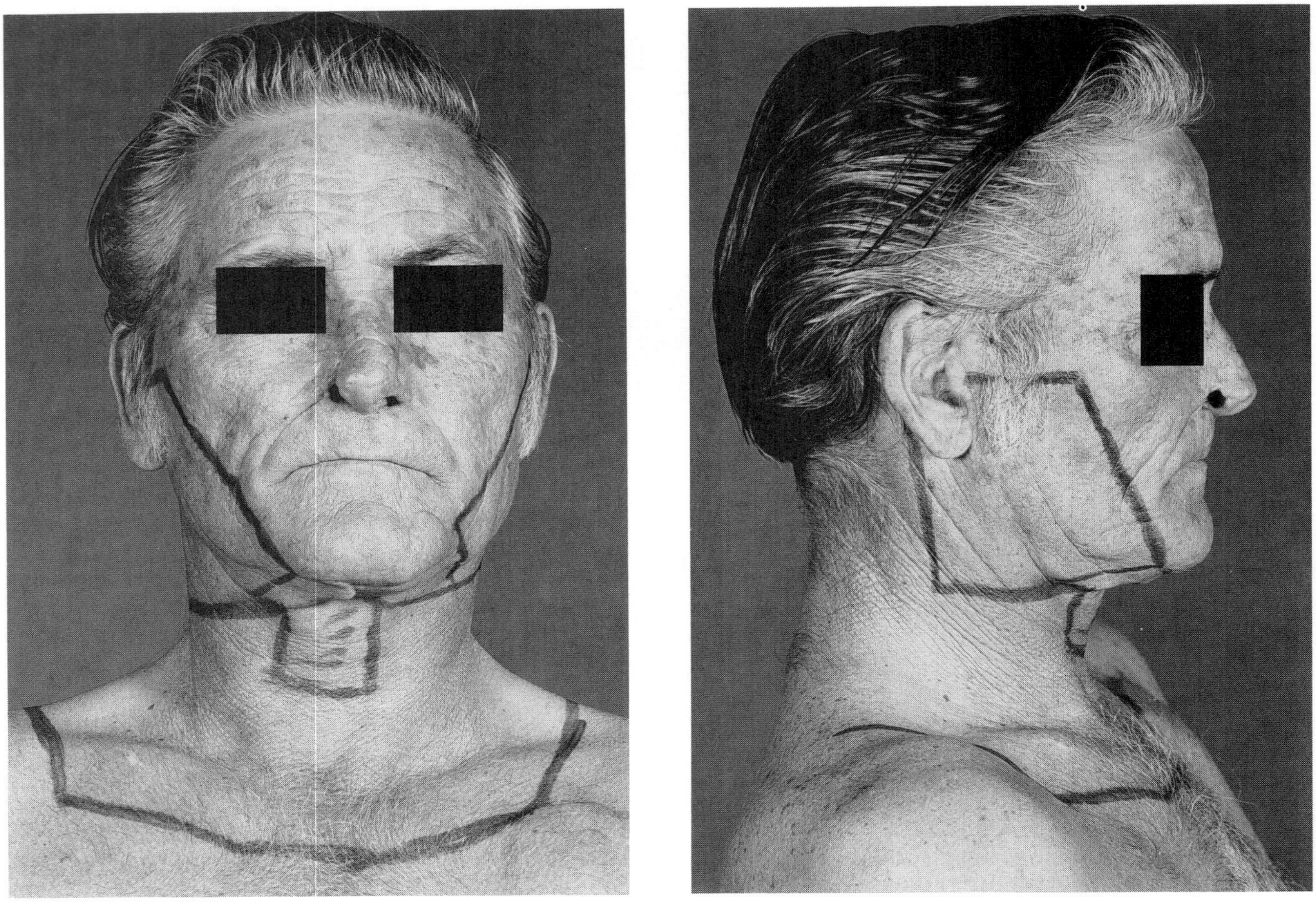

A *B*

FIG. 15-36. *A.* Anterior view of radiation portals for treatment of patient with squamous cell carcinoma of the tonsil. *B.* Primary site treated through lateral ports, and lymphatic drainage in the neck treated from mandibular borders to clavicles.

Resection or dysfunction of the soft palate results in escape of air and oral contents into the nasal cavity and ultimately out the nares. Advances in prosthetic technology have made the use of a dental prosthesis a possible solution in some cases. For those defects that do not include the lateral and posterior pharyngeal wall, a superiorly based flap of pharyngeal mucosa and muscle sutured into the margin of the palatal resection will obturate the opening between the nasopharynx and oropharynx. More extensive defects require the introduction of epithelium-lined soft tissue, the lateral arm, lateral thigh, and radial forearm free flaps being ideal when soft tissue alone is needed and the scapula free flap when both skin and bone are necessary (Fig. 15-37).

Posterior Pharyngeal Wall

Anatomy. The posterior and lateral pharyngeal walls extend from the oropharynx down into the hypopharynx, where the lateral pharyngeal walls end as the lateral walls of the pyriform sinus and the posterior wall extends to the cervical esophagus. The lymphatic drainage of the posterior pharyngeal walls is to the jugulodigastric, midjugular, and juguloomohyoid nodes but also directly to the retropharyngeal group of lymph nodes.

Pathology. Because of its location and the nonspecific symptoms of mild dysphagia and odynophagia, squamous cell carcinoma of the posterior pharynx is usually detected at a late stage, with 39 to 55 percent of patients presenting with palpable cervical metastases. Local spread of disease is cephalad toward the nasopharynx and lateral to the lateral pharyngeal walls and larynx.

Therapy. Using combinations of surgery and radiotherapy, 3- to 5-year survival rates of 25 to 32 percent overall have been reported.

The location of the posterior pharyngeal wall as the farthest border of the aerodigestive tract and its proximity to the larynx have presented some problems both of access for surgical resection and of potential for appropriate reconstruction. Accurate resection of local disease requires visual access. Midline division of the lip, mandible and tongue, the median labiomandibular glossotomy, allows visualization of the posterior pharynx. If disease is limited to the posterior wall, the surface can be relined with a split-thickness skin graft or allowed to epithelialize. Circumferential disease requires more complete pharyngeal resection and sometimes pharyngolaryngectomy. Reconstruction of the complete or partial circumferential defect may be accomplished with a free autograft

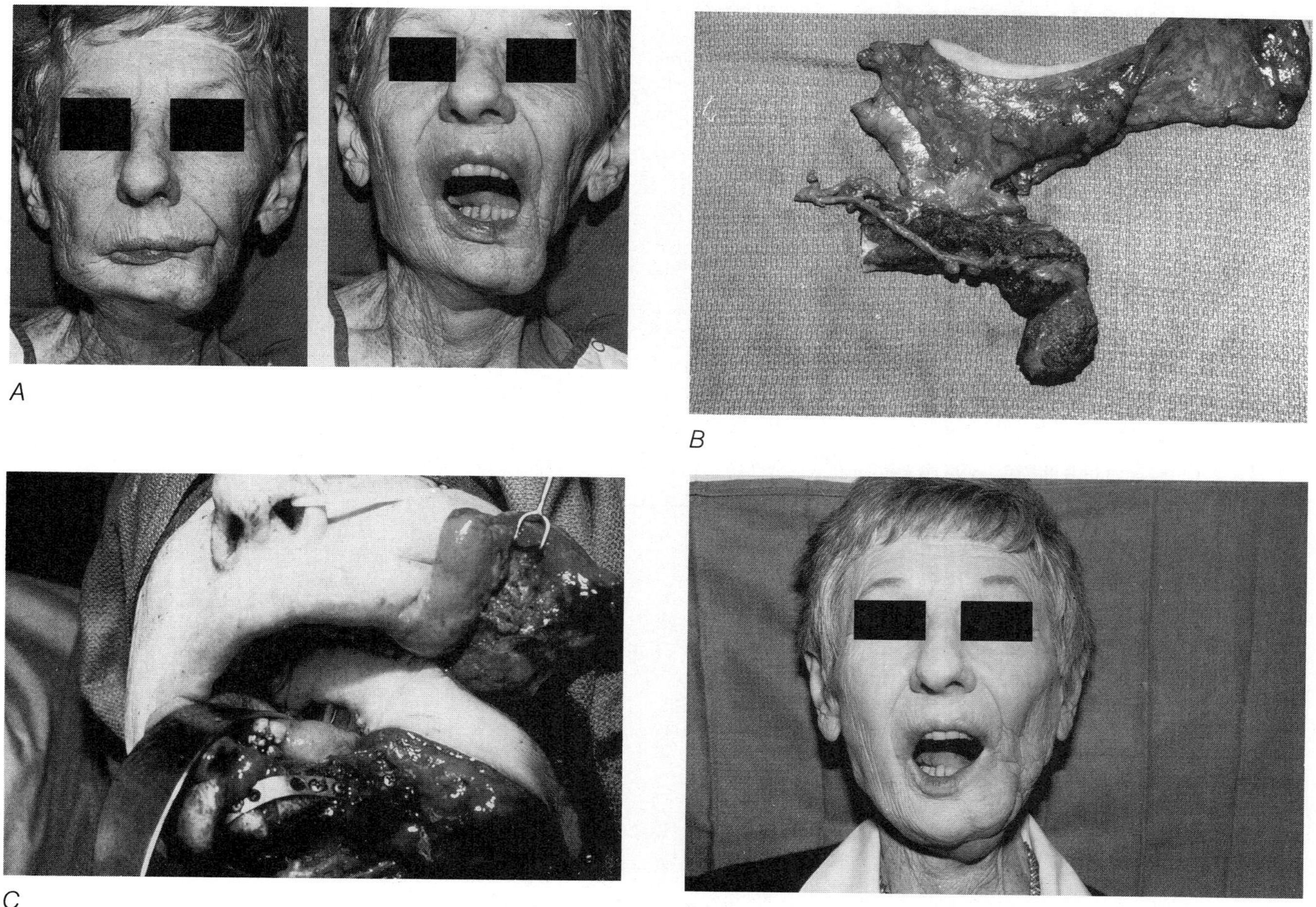

A B C D

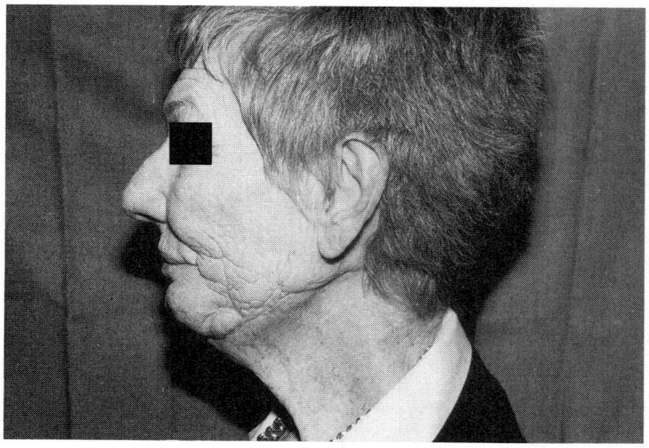

E

FIG. 15-37. *A.* Patient with marked deformity and lateral shift of jaw after hemimandibulectomy and neck dissection for squamous cell carcinoma of the tonsil originally treated by radiotherapy. This patient complained of pain in the right temporomandibular joint, inability to chew, hypernasal speech, dry mouth, and difficulty in swallowing. *B.* Reconstruction of the bony and soft tissue defects was performed with a scapula osteocutaneous free flap. Saphenous vein grafts were used to allow microvascular anastomosis to the facial artery and external jugular vein in the right neck, which had not previously been dissected. *C.* Intraoperative photograph showing fixation of scapula to mandible with titanium plates and screws. Adequate soft tissue was available for reconstruction of the palate, buccal and alveolar surfaces with skin from the back. *D* and *E.* Postoperative photographs demonstrate improved function and appearance (From: *Coleman JJ III, Wooden WA: 1990, with permission.*)

of jejunum or radial forearm free flap. If the larynx can be preserved, aspiration will be less likely if free mobility of the larynx is maintained and sensate epithelium is restored, by either sensory innervated free tissue transfer or skin grafting.

Hypopharynx

Pathology. In addition to the posterior pharynx, the hypopharynx contains the pyriform sinuses and the postcricoid area. Tumor growth in this area, the lateral and posterior mucosal border of the larynx, is intimately related to the function of the larynx, a facet recognized in the staging systems used in assessing the extent of hypopharyngeal disease (Fig. 15-38). So rather than with size, the T stage of the pyriform sinus lesion increases with extent into the medial wall or with fixation of the vocal cord caused by direct extension of disease. Another consideration in hypopharyngeal carcinoma, as in disease of the cervical esophagus, is the problem

Data Form for Cancer Staging

Patient identification
Name ______
Address ______
Hospital or clinic number ______
Age ____ Sex ____ Race ______

Institutional identification
Hospital or clinic ______
Address ______

Oncology Record

Anatomic site of cancer ______
Chronology of classification* [ ] Clinical-diagnostic (cTNM)
[ ] Surgical-evaluative (sTNM)

Histologic type† ______ Grade (G) ______
[ ] Postsurgical resection–pathologic (pTNM)
[ ] Retreatment (rTNM) [ ] Autopsy (aTNM)

Date of classification ______

Definitions: TNM Classification

Primary Tumor (T)

[ ] TX Minimum requirements to assess the primary tumor cannot be met.
[ ] T0 No evidence of primary tumor

Oropharynx

[ ] Tis Carcinoma *in situ*
[ ] T1 Tumor 2 cm or less in greatest diameter
[ ] T2 Tumor more than 2 cm but not more than 4 cm in greatest diameter
[ ] T3 Tumor more than 4 cm in greatest diameter
[ ] T4 Massive tumor more than 4 cm in diameter with invasion of bone, soft tissues of neck, or root (deep musculature) of tongue

Nasopharynx

[ ] Tis Carcinoma *in situ*
[ ] T1 Tumor confined to one side of nasopharynx or no tumor visible (positive biopsy only)
[ ] T2 Tumor involving two sites (both posterosuperior and lateral walls)
[ ] T3 Extension of tumor into nasal cavity or oropharynx
[ ] T4 Tumor invasion of skull, cranial nerve involvement, or both

Hypopharynx

[ ] Tis Carcinoma *in situ*
[ ] T1 Tumor confined to one site
[ ] T2 Extension of tumor to adjacent region or site without fixation of hemilarynx
[ ] T3 Extension of tumor to adjacent region or site with fixation of hemilarynx
[ ] T4 Massive tumor invading bone or soft tissues of neck

Nodal Involvement (N)

[ ] NX Minimum requirements to assess regional nodes cannot be met.
[ ] N0 No clinically positive node
[ ] N1 Single clinically positive homolateral node 3 cm or less in diameter
[ ] N2 Single clinically positive homolateral node more than 3 but not more than 6 cm in diameter or multiple clinically positive homolateral nodes, none more than 6 cm in diameter
  [ ] N2a Single clinically positive homolateral node more than 3 cm but not more than 6 cm in diameter
  [ ] N2b Multiple clinically positive homolateral nodes, none more than 6 cm in diameter
[ ] N3 Massive homolateral node(s), bilateral nodes, or contralateral node(s).
  [ ] N3a Clinically positive homolateral node(s), one more than 6 cm in diameter
  [ ] N3b Bilateral clinically positive nodes (in this situation, each side of the neck should be staged separately; *i.e.*, N3b: right, N2a; left, N1)
  [ ] N3c Contralateral clinically positive node(s) only

Distant Metastasis (M)

[ ] MX Minimum requirements to assess the presence of distant metastasis cannot be met.
[ ] M0 No (known) distant metastasis
[ ] M1 Distant metastasis present
Specify ______

Location of Tumor

Oropharynx

[ ] Faucial arch
[ ] Tonsillar fossa, tonsil
[ ] Base of tongue
[ ] Pharyngeal wall

Nasopharynx

[ ] Posterosuperior wall
[ ] Lateral wall

Hypopharynx

[ ] Piriform fossa
[ ] Postcricoid area
[ ] Posterior wall

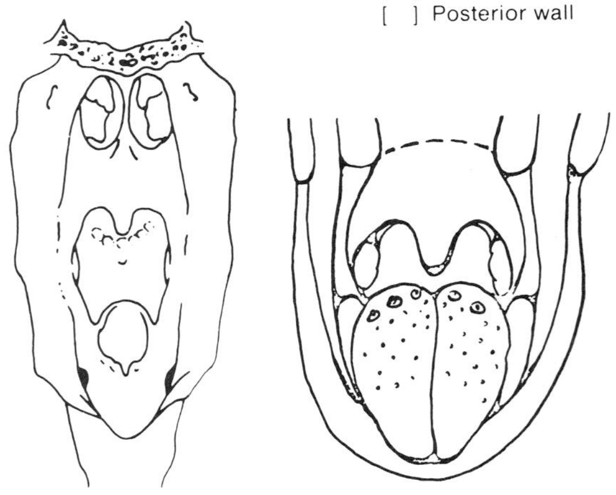

Size of primary tumor: ____ cm

Examination by ______ M.D.
Date ______

*Use a separate form each time a case is staged.
†See reverse side for additional information.

American Joint Committee on Cancer Manual for Staging of Cancer

FIG. 15-38. AJCC staging system for carcinoma of the pharynx.

of submucosal extension of tumor. Spread of disease into the cervical esophagus discovered at surgery may simply represent clinical understaging of disease but also multifocal disease or field cancerization. Local spread of disease is cephalad toward the nasopharynx or distal into the cervical esophagus, as well as medial and lateral toward the larynx. Advanced-stage local disease is common, with only 10 to 15 percent of cases confined to only one site in the hypopharynx.

The lymphatic drainage of the area is luxurious, with primary nodal stations in the midjugular, juguloomohyoid, and retropharyngeal lymph node chains. Even in small lesions there is a likelihood of lymph node metastasis, with 55 to 64 percent of patients presenting with palpable lymphadenopathy, and 41 percent of patients with clinically negative N0 necks demonstrating metastatic disease after elective neck dissection. Even in small primary lesions (T1) localized to one part of the hypopharynx, the risk of cervical micrometastases in the clinically negative neck is high (40 percent). Distant metastases at presentation and with treatment of disease appear to be more common than at other primary sites, occurring in up to 47 percent of the cases.

Therapy. Since it is unusual for hypopharyngeal lesions to present at an early stage, the treatment is usually combined, consisting of surgery followed by adjuvant radiotherapy. The extent of the operation depends on the proximity to the larynx, and the laryngopharyngectomy with bilateral modified neck dissection is the procedure that is most frequently necessary. With such an approach, survival rates of 20 to 40 percent have been achieved.

When the larynx can be saved, primary closure of the surgical defect is the most effective method. Preservation of the superior laryngeal nerves, the sensory innervation to the area, is an important consideration to allow swallowing to proceed without aspiration. When, however, the larynx is removed with the hypopharyngeal lesion, the goals of reconstructive surgery change somewhat to simple restoration of alimentary continuity with the least likelihood of fistula or other devastating problems and with the ability to restore esophageal speech. Primary closure of the pharyngeal mucosa after partial laryngopharyngectomy for pyriform sinus lesions results in a high likelihood of fistula, 43 percent, and stenosis (Fig. 15-39), 48 to 73 percent, both of which interfere with swallowing and esophageal speech.

Although use of local tissue, including the anterior wall of the larynx and the base of the tongue, and skin of the neck has been described, the extent of surgery, the history of previous radiotherapy, or the likelihood of subsequent adjuvant radiotherapy usually require the importation of distant tissue. The deltopectoral flap from the chest was the mainstay of pharyngeal reconstruction after laryngectomy but is at least a two-stage procedure with a fairly high risk of failure or persistent fistula. The pectoralis major musculocutaneous flap has been advocated for both circumferential and partial defects of the pharynx. The effect of gravity, the inhomogeneous blood supply, and the bulk of the flap result in a high rate of fistula and dysphagia, making a free autograft of bowel or skin a preferable method. When a circumferential defect is present, the problem of bulk and gravity can be circumvented somewhat by skin grafting the prevertebral fascia as the posterior wall of the neopharynx (new pharynx) and using the pectoralis major muscle and its overlying skin as a 270-degree reconstruction to complete the pharyngeal conduit.

When total esophagectomy is part of the treatment for carcinoma of the hypopharynx, transposition of the stomach or colon through the thorax can reconstitute the alimentary canal. Gastric pull-up—where the stomach, based on the right gastric and gastroepiploic vessels, is brought through the chest, and the fundus or cardia sutured to the base of the tongue or pharyngeal remnant—is a fairly reliable technique but has a mortality rate of 10 to 20 percent in most series. Right or left colon interposition is usually reserved for caustic strictures but is occasionally useful in hypopharyngeal or cervical esophageal lesions.

Reconstruction of the circumferential defect resulting from pharyngolaryngectomy by transfer of a free autograft of bowel and revascularization of microvascular anastomosis was first performed in the early 1960s. Although colon, stomach, and jejunum have all been used, the greatest experience has been with jejunal free autograft. Successful reconstruction using the jejunum has been achieved in 92 percent of patients approached with this method, allowing 83 percent of the total group to achieve total oral alimentation. Mortality with this method, used either as a tube reconstruction for circumferential defects or as a patch for partial defects, has been less than 5 percent, with few abdominal or thoracic problems. Complications in the neck, though frequent, usually resolved without further surgery, and the segment of bowel was able to withstand radiotherapy without major problems (Fig. 15-40). Although segments of jejunum may be used in the unusual situation where the larynx has been left in situ, the secretory nature of the mucosa sometimes makes aspiration a problem, and another method may be preferable. In addition to segments of bowel, fasciocutaneous free flaps, from the radial forearm, lateral arm, lateral thigh, and posterior thigh, have been used as either a tube or a patch for hypopharyngeal reconstruction.

Squamous carcinoma of the cervical esophagus presents the same reconstructive demands as that of the hypopharynx and, when localized, may be replaced with a patch of skin as either a vascularized transposition flap or a free tissue transfer. The mode of spread, however, of the local disease may involve submucosal skip areas and thus require total esophagectomy. The lymphatic drainage of the cervical esophagus is oriented more toward the mediastinum and parapharyngeal nodes than laterally into the neck and requires a different approach for lymphadenectomy.

Nasopharynx

Etiology. Carcinoma of the nasopharynx is seen intermittently in the Western world, making up about 0.25 percent of new cancers in the United States. It is, however, endemic in southeastern Asia, particularly in southern Chinese populations such as those originating from Kwantung province and constitutes 21 percent of cancers in Taiwan, 18 percent in Hong Kong, and 14 percent in Indonesia. The incidence is much lower in Asians who have immigrated to North America but still seven times higher than in the white population, suggesting genetic susceptibility to an environmental carcinogen. The sporadic and genetically linked cases of nasopharyngeal carcinoma behave in the same manner. There is a high association of the Epstein-Barr virus with this malignancy.

Pathology. The nasopharynx is a small, mucosa-lined, boxlike cavity at the base of the skull containing the pharyngeal tonsil and the openings of the eustachian tubes and the sphenoid sinus. Tumors arising in this area present local symptoms depending on their pattern of growth and spread. Lesions that are exophytic and grow out into the cavity may obstruct the eustachian orifices or the choanae, leading to hearing loss (15 percent), nasal stuffiness or

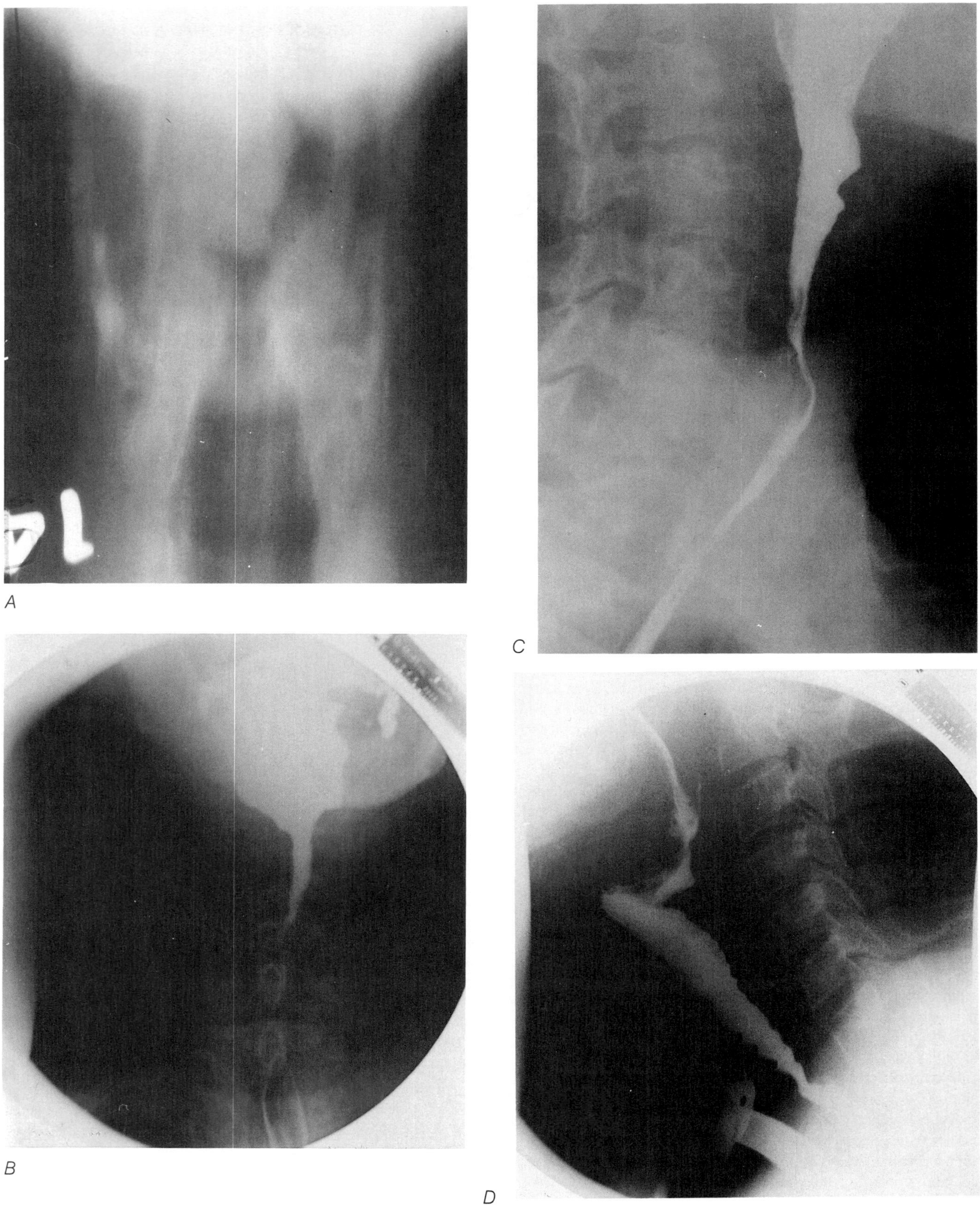

A

B

C

D

FIG. 15-39. *A.* Tomograms showing exophytic mass filling pyriform sinus, which on biopsy revealed squamous cell carcinoma. This patient was treated with laryngopharyngectomy and radical neck dissection, primary closure of the mucosa, and postoperative adjuvant radiotherapy. *B* and *C.* Eighteen months after completion of therapy the patient presented with difficulty in swallowing. Barium swallow demonstrates a significant stenosis obstructing the flow of oral contents and allowing only clear liquids to pass. Multiple biopsies of the stricture showed no evidence of malignancy. *D.* The patient was treated by resection of the stricture and replacement of that segment with a jejunal free autograft. Barium swallow shows free flow of contrast through the bowel in the area of stenosis.

obstruction (30 percent), and epistaxis (22 percent). Infiltration and bony erosion of the base of the skull into the cavernous sinus results in cranial nerve palsies in 16 to 25 percent of cases, the most commonly involved being the abducens nerve, followed by the trigeminal nerve and the oculomotor nerve, resulting in paresthesias and diplopia. The most common presenting sign of nasopharyngeal carcinomas is a mass in the neck secondary to cervical metastasis (60 percent). The site of cervical metastasis may be the jugulodigastric nodes or posterior triangle. Obviously mirror examination of the nasopharynx is an important part of any evaluation of suspicious cervical adenopathy.

Staging of nasopharyngeal carcinoma in the past has been relatively inaccurate because of difficulty with examination. Computed tomography has helped delineate invasion of both the paranasopharyngeal fascial planes and the bony skull in the absence of cranial nerve palsy. Recent staging systems have included histology, multiple symptoms, interval from onset of symptoms, location of cervical adenopathy (supraclavicular), as well as local extent of disease. Variance of histology has also been related to survival and thus is important in prognosis. Keratinizing squamous cell carcinoma has the worse 5-year survival with 21 percent, spindle cell 41 percent, round cell 51 percent, and mixed nonkeratinizing 54 percent. These histologic predictors of therapeutic response are consistent with the subset of tumors arising as variants from Waldeyer's ring, the lymphoepitheliomas.

Therapy. Despite the frequent presence of cervical lymph node metastases, nasopharyngeal carcinoma is a curable disease. Radiotherapy in doses varying from 5000 to 8400 cGY to the primary site with 5000 to 7000 to both necks results in 5-year survival rates varying from 100 percent for Stage I disease to 34 percent for Stage IV, with overall survival rates ranging from 29 to 49 percent. The total dose of radiotherapy has an effect on survival, with those patients receiving lower total doses having poorer survival. Even the presence of skull-base invasion and cranial nerve dysfunction is not a sign of incurable disease. Sixty-two percent of cranial nerve defects can be reversed by radiotherapy with an overall 31 percent survival in this subset of patients. Residual disease at the primary site may occasionally be resected by craniofacial technique, and residual neck disease may be eradicated by radical neck dissection. Distant metastatic disease in nasopharyngeal carcinoma is common, particularly in patients who have bulky cervical metastases. At present, however, adjuvant chemotherapy has not been particularly successful in improving survival.

Nasal Cavity and Paranasal Sinuses

Etiology. The nasal cavity and paranasal sinuses (maxillary, ethmoid, frontal, and sphenoid) are the aditus to the respiratory tract and function to filter impurities from the inspired air, regulate its temperature, and humidify it. As such they are exposed to the many carcinogens in the air, and yet malignancies in these sites are rare. In the Western world they constitute 0.3 percent of all malignancies, with a slightly higher incidence in men than in women. In the Orient this is a more common primary site, making up 1 percent of new cancers and 23 percent of head and neck cancers in Japan. Endemic areas are found in South Africa where inspired snuff has a high concentration of nickel. There may also be an increased risk of adenocarcinoma of the paranasal sinuses in woodworkers secondary to inspired wood dust. The disease presents most frequently in the fifth to seventh decades.

Pathology. Squamous cell carcinoma is the most common histology (60 to 80 percent), although minor salivary gland lesions, adenocarcinoma, adenoid cystic carcinoma, and mucoepidermoid carcinoma make up about 20 percent of the tumors. Other malignancies such as teratocarcinoma, lymphoma, osteogenic sarcoma, schwannoma, fibrous dysplasia, carcinosarcoma, and melanoma are occasionally encountered. Lymph node metastases are uncommon, with only 15 percent of cases presenting in the neck, since the retropharyngeal lymph nodes are the first station of drainage. There is a questionable relationship between nasal and sinonasal malignancy and the inverting papilloma of the nasal cavity.

Late-stage disease is common, since symptoms are usually rather diffuse, including nasal obstruction (35 percent), local pain (16 percent), epistaxis (12 percent), and cheek swelling (29 percent). Loosening of maxillary teeth or paresthesias also may occur. Diagnosis is made by intranasal biopsy through a speculum or by antrostomy through the lateral nasal wall or labial buccal sulcus (Caldwell-Luc procedure). The maxillary sinus is by far the most common site of origin of the disease (62 percent), followed by the nasal cavity (26 percent), ethmoid sinus (10 percent), and sphenoid sinus (2 percent).

Therapy. Treatment of paranasal sinus tumors includes a combination of radiotherapy and surgery. Radiotherapy alone provides poor palliation and unacceptably low survival rates. Preoperative radiotherapy to 6000 R combined with radical surgery has been the usual approach, resulting in 3-year survivals in the vicinity of 13 to 32 percent for all sites, 35 to 40 percent for nasal cavity, and 38 to 53 percent for maxillary sinus. Failure of therapy is most commonly manifested by local recurrence (70 percent) and only rarely disease in the neck (5 percent).

Surgical resection involves en bloc removal of the affected sinus and the surrounding involved structures. Total maxillectomy with or without orbital exenteration may be required for adequate clearance. The introduction in 1963 of the intracranial-extracranial approach to tumors, the craniofacial technique, has improved the ability to safely remove tumors of the ethmoid and other paranasal sinuses and has increased 5-year survival rates from the range of 30 percent to 58 percent.

Reconstruction of the postoperative defect that has been previously irradiated is a difficult problem. Unnatural passageways among the paranasal sinuses, oral cavity, nasal cavity, and external environment interfere with the normal flow of air, drying the mucosa and causing discomfort and bleeding as well as interfering with alimentation and speech. Small defects can be obturated with nasal or dental prostheses. Larger defects, however, require three-dimensional reconstruction with free tissue transfer (Fig. 15-41).

Larynx

Anatomy and Physiology. The larynx is a complex, mucosa-lined, bony and cartilaginous box whose function depends on motion coordinated with the adjacent tongue and pharynx. The larynx is divided into three anatomic areas—the supraglottic larynx, from the epiglottis to the ventricle, including the preepiglottic space, hyoid bone, arytenoid processes, and false vocal cords; the glottic larynx, including the true cords and the anterior commissures; and the subglottic area, surrounded by the cricoid cartilage. The different clinical behavior of supraglottic lesions comes in part from their separate embryologic origin. The supraglottis is a derivative of the pharyngobuccal anlage, and malignancy arising in this

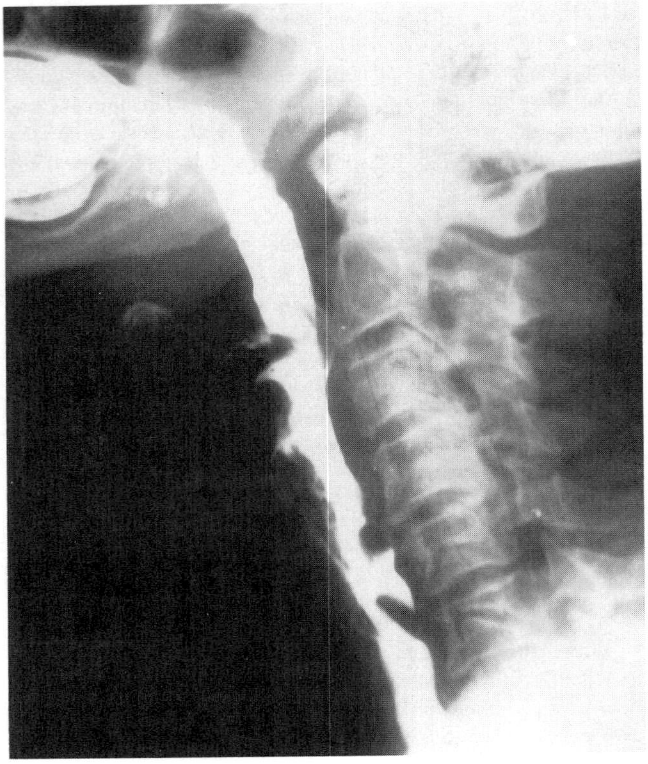

A

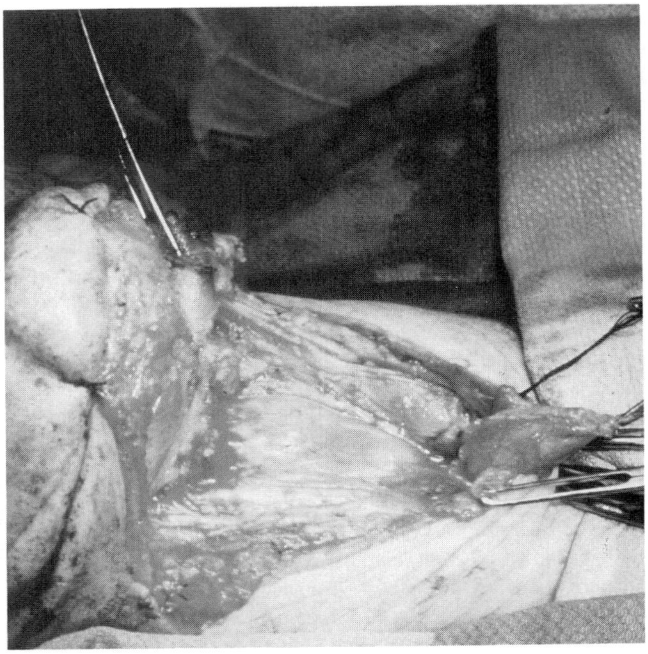

B

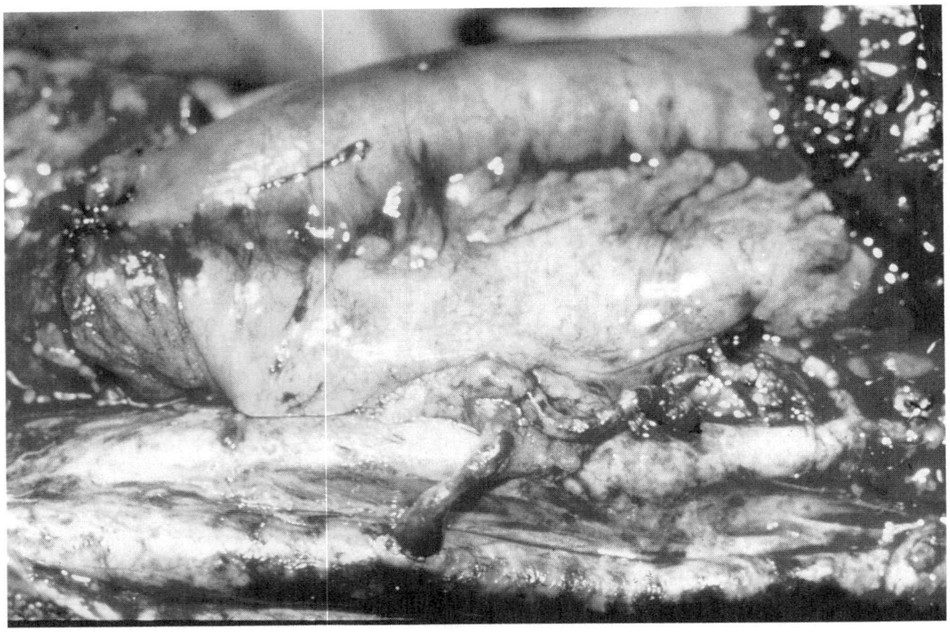

C

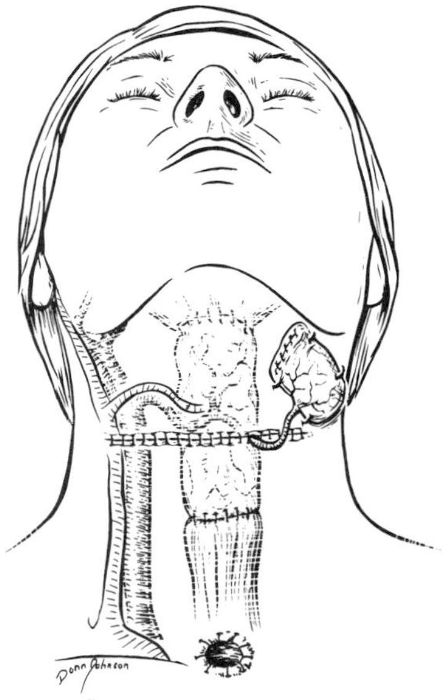

D

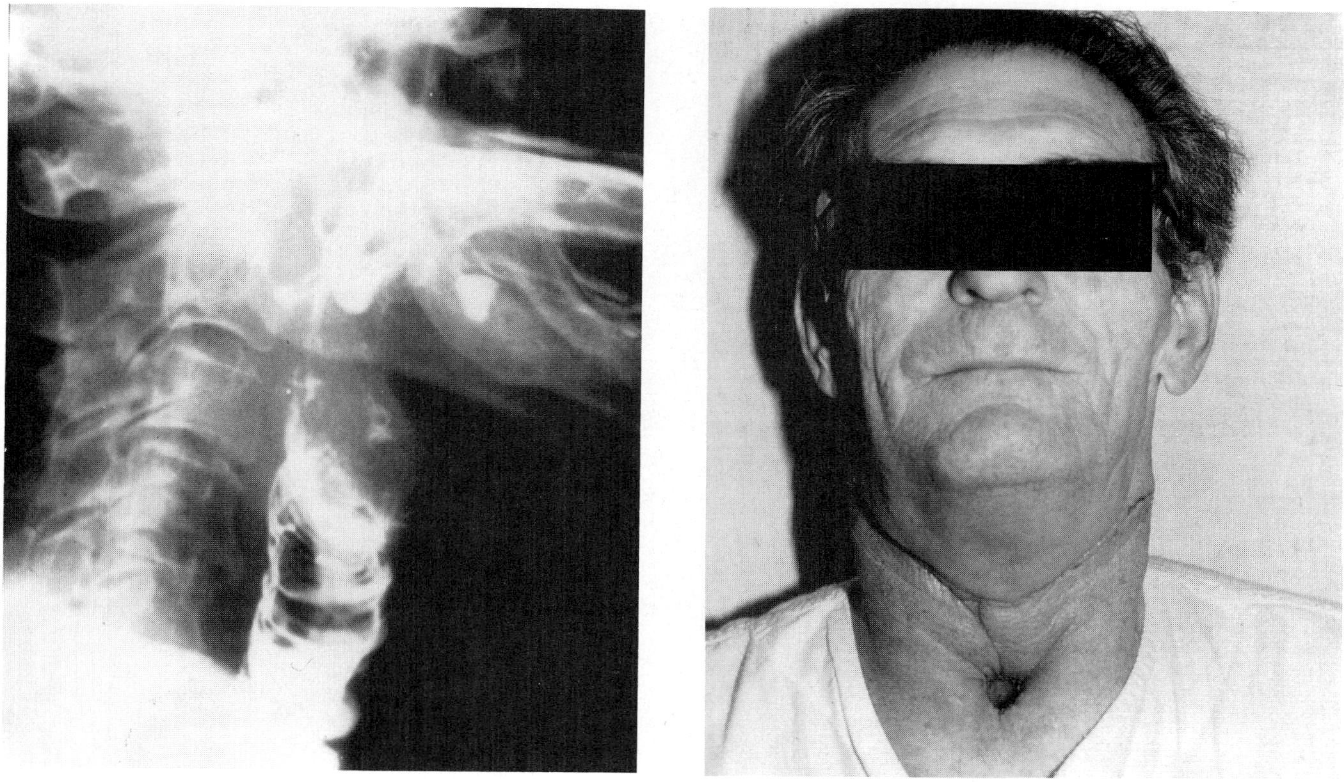

E *F*

FIG. 15-40. *A.* Recurrent squamous cell carcinoma of the cervical esophagus 9 months after definitive radiotherapy. *B.* Defect after laryngopharyngoesophagectomy extends from the base of tongue to the inlet of the thoracic esophagus. Note prevertebral fascia. *C* and *D.* Segment of jejunum with its mesenteric vessels is harvested from abdomen. Microvascular anastomosis performed between mesenteric artery and superior thyroid artery end to end and between mesenteric vein and internal jugular vein end to side. *E.* Lateral view barium swallow at 10 days shows rapid passage of barium from mouth to esophagus without extravasation. *F.* Patient at 10 days.

area behaves similarly to pharyngeal carcinoma, with early metastatic disease to the neck. The glottis arises from the tracheobronchial anlage, and malignancy is more likely to be indolent, with lower incidence of cervical metastases.

The predominant function of the larynx is the modulation of air inspired through the nose and nasopharynx and expired from the lungs. Coordination of respiration with swallowing is a complex function which prevents food from entering the respiratory tree and air from entering the digestive tract. As air enters the pharynx it is shunted to the larynx, which sits in its neutral position with the epiglottis open. Air is then drawn through the larynx by negative pressures from the thorax and prevented from entering the esophagus by the sphincter action of the middle and inferior constrictor muscles. Saliva and other oral contents are prevented from entering the larynx by sensitive reflexes mediated by the sensory component of the superior and recurrent laryngeal nerves and the intrinsic and extrinsic muscles of the larynx. In the act of swallowing the food bolus is prevented from entering the larynx by the simultaneous relaxation of the middle constrictor and the elevation of the larynx toward the relatively fixed epiglottis, which seals the aditus. This elevation is initiated as the food passes through the faucial arch by the intrinsic and extrinsic muscles of the tongue pulling through the hyoid bone. Speech is produced by air expired from the lungs through the larynx, mouth, and nose. The thickness and degree of abduction or adduction of the cords produce tone and volume, and the actions of the tongue, palate, lips, and buccal mucosa modify the expelled air into an articulated pattern, speech. Although the respiratory tract can be short-circuited and separated from the digestive tract by tracheostomy, either with or without laryngectomy, the maintenance of normal speech and swallowing depends on adequate synergy in the pharyngolarynx and oral cavity of tongue, larynx, and pharyngeal musculature and normal central nervous system afferent and efferent signals. Perhaps more than at any other body site, therapeutic decision making in laryngeal carcinoma by both patient and physician has been influenced by the desire to preserve communicative ability.

Etiology. Carcinoma of the larynx is the most common malignancy of the upper aerodigestive tract in the United States with about 10,000 new cases presenting each year. As with most other head and neck cancers the risk for development for laryngeal cancer is directly proportional to the amount of exposure to tobacco, with a lesser relationship to alcohol intake. Changing mores have decreased the male-to-female ratio for incidence of laryngeal carcinoma from 11:1 in 1960 to 4.5:1 in 1990. Furthermore, women with carcinoma of the larynx are more likely to have supraglottic

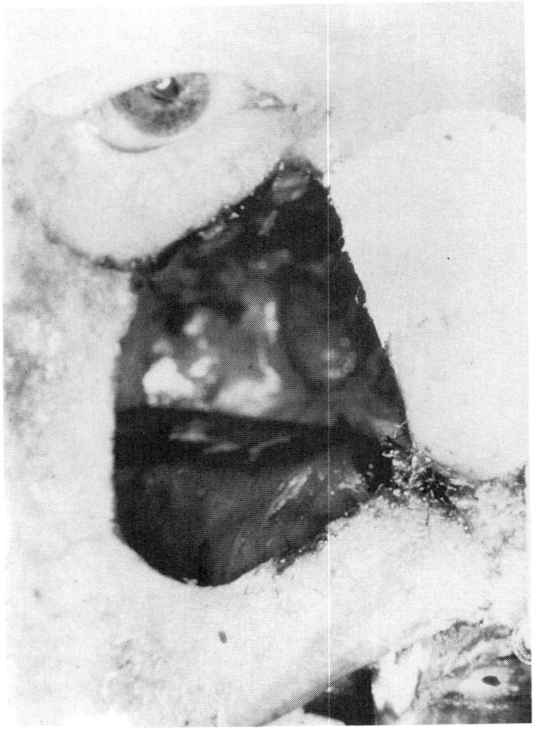

A

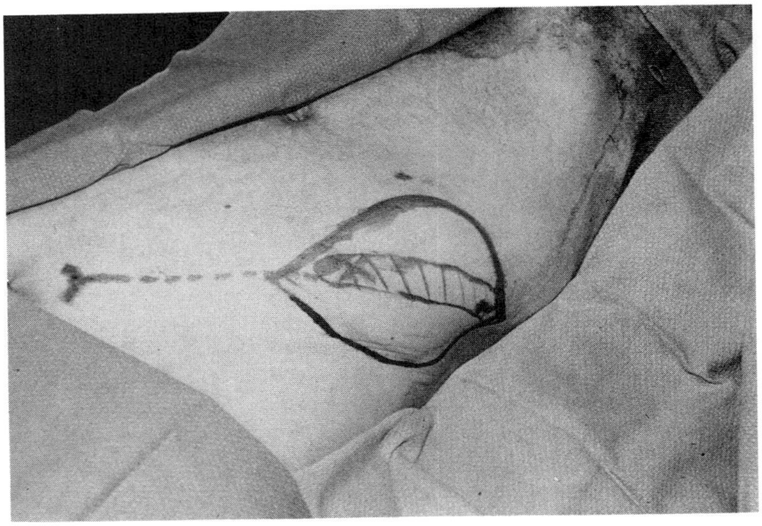

B

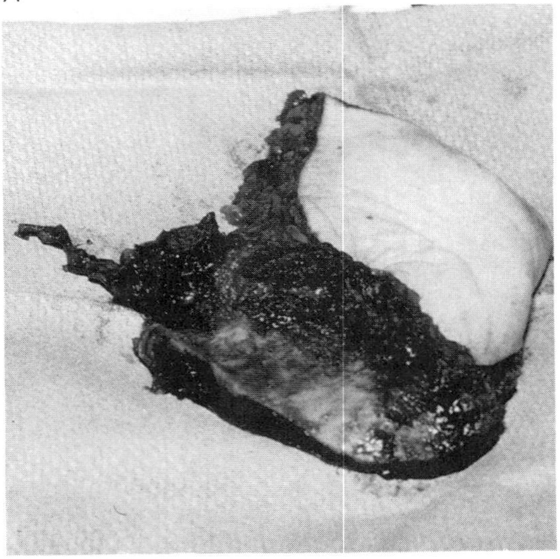

C

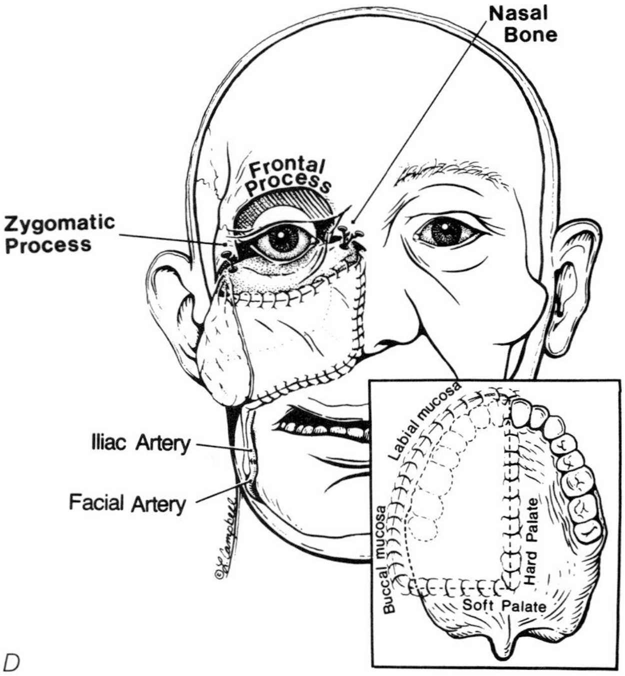

Nasal Bone
Frontal Process
Zygomatic Process
Iliac Artery
Facial Artery
Labial mucosa
Buccal mucosa
Hard Palate
Soft Palate

D

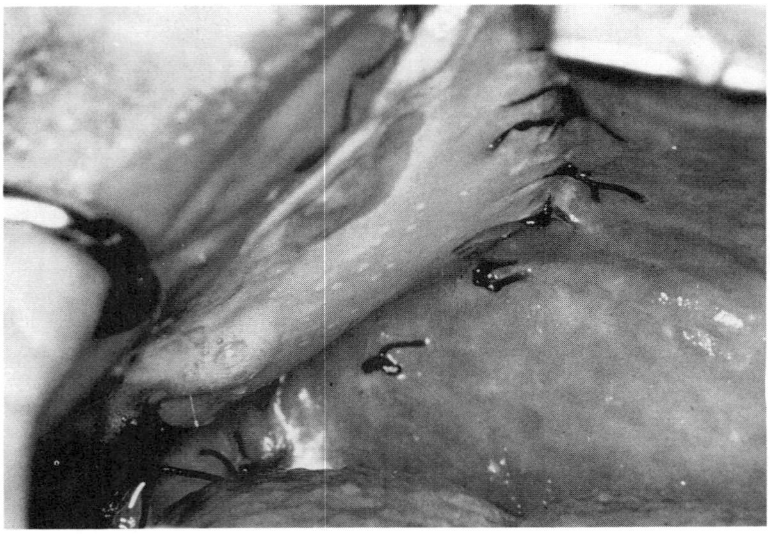

E

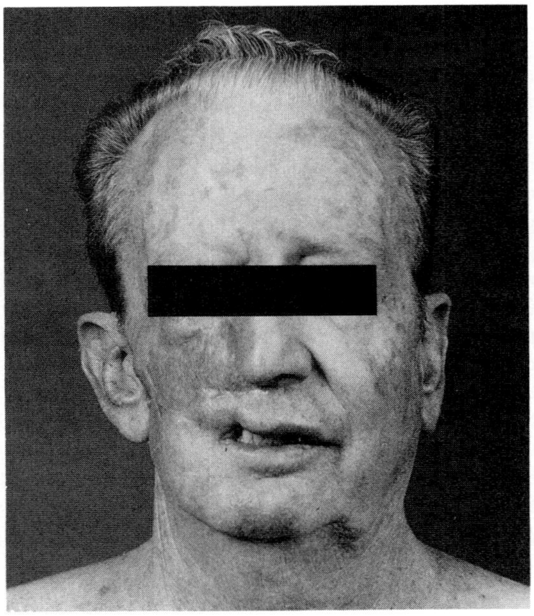

F

than glottic laryngeal cancers. Increasing age is also a risk factor, although disease in young patients has been reported and likewise is related to tobacco use. Black patients in the United States have an increased risk of developing laryngeal carcinoma at a younger age and there is a 3.5:1 male-to-female ratio. Other risk factors suggested have been metal dust, particularly nickel, asbestos, hair dyes, and wood dust, but these are likely cofactors to the insult created by tobacco smoke. The relationship of papillomas of juvenile or adult onset in the causation of the larynx is unclear.

Diagnosis. Because of the obvious symptoms of hoarseness, other voice changes, tickling in the throat, and coughing, carcinoma of the glottic larynx is more likely than many upper aerodigestive tract malignancies to present with early-stage disease. Evaluation of the patient includes indirect (mirror) laryngoscopy as well as physical examination of the neck (Fig. 15-42). The geographic site and extent of the lesion, whether confined to the larynx or spreading beyond, are of importance, but the mobility of the vocal cords is also crucial, since it represents invasion of the tumor into the deep structures of the larynx. Computed tomography and MRI are useful in documenting invasion of the thyroid cartilage in the staging process (Fig. 15-43). Definitive staging and diagnosis to clearly define extent usually require direct laryngoscopy and biopsy, which can be performed with a rigid laryngoscope, with the patient anesthetized or with a flexible fiberoptic scope with the patient awake and able to inspire and vocalize.

Pathology. The biologic behavior of malignancy in the various areas of the larynx is somewhat different and drives to great degree the choice of therapy. Supraglottic laryngeal carcinoma or extrinsic laryngeal carcinoma is more likely than glottic cancer to present with advanced-stage disease. There is an abundant lymphatic supply that extends anteriorly through the preepiglottic space as well as laterally to the midjugular and paratracheal lymph nodes. Involvement of the preepiglottic space occurs in 29 percent of clinically unremarkable supraglottic tumors. Micrometastases in the clinically negative neck are also common, with 26 to 33 percent of necks showing metastases and 25 percent bilateral metastases. Patients with inadequate primary therapy for supraglottic carcinoma are more likely to fail from recurrence in the neck and distant metastases than from local recurrence alone.

The vocal cords (glottis) or intrinsic larynx is a small area that is in constant use and thus regularly exposed to carcinogenic stimuli. When confined to the small cartilaginous box with its paucity of lymphatics, tumors usually behave indolently. When extending outside the glottis, transglottic lesions, a more aggressive pattern is noted. Unlike supraglottic cancer, early changes are noticeable and appear to have a long natural history, making them amenable to less radical therapy. Keratosis or thickening of the keratin layer of the squamous mucosa results in transformation to carcinoma in situ in 14 percent of cases and microinvasive cancer in 28 percent of cases over a period of 2 to 24 months. Keratosis with atypia progresses to carcinoma in situ in 18 percent and invasive carcinoma in 25 percent in 1 to 24 months, and carcinoma in situ progresses to invasive carcinoma in 38 percent of cases in 8 to 48 months.

FIG. 15-41. *A.* Patient presenting with surgical defect after resection of carcinoma of nasal vestibule and adjuvant postoperative radiotherapy. Surgical procedure removed hemipalate, lateral nasal wall, maxilla and maxillary sinus, malar skin, and bony orbital floor. The patient complained of inability to speak or eat, discomfort secondary to crusting of nasal mucosa, and abnormal appearance. *B.* The reconstruction was carried out with a deep circumflex iliac artery osteocutaneous free flap from the groin area. *C.* Flap dissected free, showing skin of the groin and bone from the iliac crest, both obtaining blood supply from the deep circumflex iliac artery and vein. *D.* Anastomosis of the vessels was performed to the facial artery and vein. By folding the tissue in three dimensions, the defects in the palate, lateral nasal wall, and malar skin were closed with skin, and the floor of orbit was restored with vascularized bone. *E.* Palatal reconstruction intact at 10 days. *F.* Frontal view of patient at 3 months.

Therapy. This rather indolent behavior and the low likelihood of clinically evident or micrometastatic cervical disease (1 to 7 percent in T1 and T2 lesions, 13 percent with T3 lesions) make glottic cancer more suitable for less radical therapies, with a high probability of salvage after failure of primary therapy. Because, however, of the propensity for submucosal extension, advanced-stage disease with cartilage invasion requires initial radical therapy.

Subglottic carcinomas are rare, making up only 1 to 2 percent of all laryngeal carcinomas and tend to spread by submucosal extension down the trachea and through the cricoid cartilage and cricothyroid membrane into the soft tissues of the neck. Because of their rarity, they frequently present with advanced-stage local disease, although cervical metastasis is not as common as in supraglottic disease. Radical combined therapy, surgery and radiotherapy, is necessary.

Despite the peculiarities of growth of squamous cell carcinoma of the glottic larynx, prognosis for carcinoma at all sites is related to similar variables predicting other sites. Unifactorial and multifactorial analyses have identified the presence of lymph node metastases, advanced local disease, vocal cord fixation, histologic grade, ulceration, site within the larynx, male gender, and ^{3}H-thymidine labeling index as significant factors in survival after therapy with both surgery and radiotherapy.

Because of the importance of preserving the voice and because of the low incidence of subclinical cervical metastases in glottic cancer, radiotherapy has become the accepted treatment for most early squamous cell carcinomas of the larynx. Conventional radiotherapeutic techniques that deliver doses of 6000 cGy over 30 fractions over 6 weeks result in cure rates of 80 to 90 percent for T1,N0 carcinoma of the glottis and 70 to 90 percent for T2,N0. Furthermore, salvage of radiotherapy failures with voice preservation by less-than-total laryngectomy is possible in 75 percent and overall surgical salvage in 92 percent of T1 patients and 82 percent of T2 patients. More advanced T3 lesions have also been approached with standard radiotherapy and hyperfractionation (more than one course per day) in doses of 6500 to 7680 cGy through ports that include the cervical lymphatics, resulting in local control rates of 36 to 67 percent over 2 to 4 years and surgical salvage of 67 to 83 percent. Such high-dose radiotherapy does, however, result in significant complication rates, such as persistent laryngeal edema and chondronecrosis.

Radiotherapy as treatment for supraglottic carcinoma is somewhat more controversial because of the late-stage presentation and predilection for bilateral cervical metastases. Although control rates of 74 percent for T1 and T2 supraglottic lesions have been obtained, and 40 percent for T3 and T4 with radiation and surgery held as a salvage method, the possibility of preserving the voice with supraglottic laryngectomy and treatment with preoperative or postoperative adjuvant radiotherapy has made this combined ap-

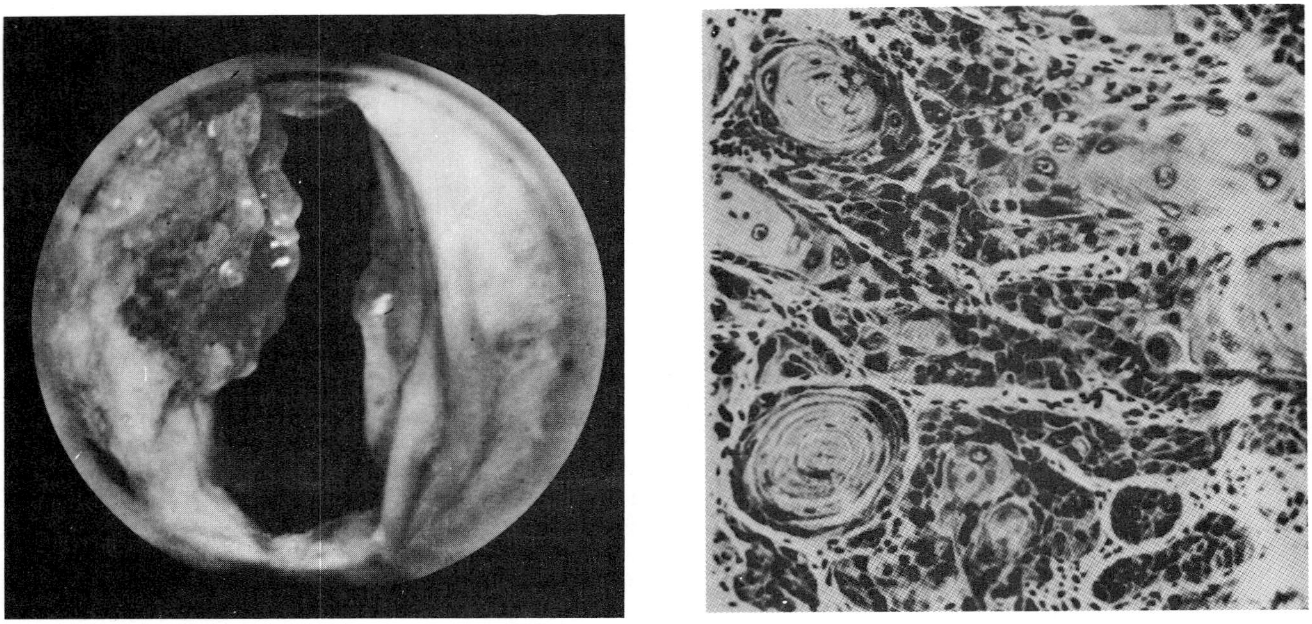

FIG. 15-42. Carcinoma involving the left side of the larynx and anterior commissure. (From: *Holinger PH, et al: Ann Otol Rhinol Laryngol 56:583, 1947, with permission*).

proach more popular for late-stage disease or disease with ominous histologic features.

The surgical approach to the larynx is varied, with the unifying principle that local and locoregional disease may be eradicated with preservation or restoration of whatever function is possible. Early lesions of the glottis, such as keratosis with atypia, carcinoma in situ, or minimally invasive carcinoma, that involve the mobile cord and do not extend to the anterior or posterior commissures may be treated with reasonable success by removal of the mucosa over the cord by vocal cord stripping. Performed transorally, by either laser diathermy or sharp dissection, this technique has minimal morbidity, leaving good voice quality. T1 lesions of more bulk but confined to one cord may be removed by cordectomy, occasionally performed transorally but usually by opening the larynx through laryngofissure. Although this interferes with voice quality, most patients will be cured, and surgical salvage by total laryngectomy is a successful backup procedure.

The conventional therapy for cancers that cross the anatomic boundaries of the supraglottis and glottis or the glottis and subglottis, and the so-called transglottic lesions, is total laryngectomy. Glottic lesions that cross the anterior or posterior commissure and are not felt to be amenable to radiotherapy similarly require total laryngectomy. Depending on the presence of palpable lymph nodes or suspicion of metastatic disease because of the site of primary disease, radical or modified radical neck dissection may be indicated. Removal of all disease is the aim of total laryngectomy, although whole-organ pathologic examinations have shown presence of microscopic disease at the margins in up to 30 percent of cases, with anterolateral (19 percent), posterolateral (11 percent), postcricoid (7 percent), and superior margins being most commonly involved. Free margin status is the most reliable predictor of local control, with 48 percent of those patients having positive margins developing local recurrence. When total laryngectomy is used as definitive therapy for advanced-stage disease, 3- to 5-year survival rates of 65 to 69 percent for T3,N0 and T3,N1 lesions and 45 to 54 percent for T4,N0 lesions have been reported.

The goal of voice preservation when surgical extirpation is a necessary part of therapy is met in two ways—by conservation surgery, removing only part of the larynx, or by reconstruction of a voice-producing mechanism after total laryngectomy.

Conservation surgery relies for its rationale on the premise that lesions confined to one part of the larynx can be removed leaving enough larynx behind to allow speech that is superior to esophageal or mechanical speech. Standard supraglottic laryngectomy or horizontal hemilaryngectomy is appropriate in patients where lesions are less than 3 cm, the vocal cords are mobile and a margin of 5 mm is possible at the anterior commissure, there is no cartilage or preepiglottic space invasion, the pyriform sinus apex and postcricoid and interarytenoid areas are clear, and tongue mobility is normal. The approach to the larynx is through the thyroid cartilage, removing the epiglottis, false cords, and ventricular mucosa en bloc with the hyoid bone. If posterior extension involves the arytenoid cartilage on one side, this may be included with specimen. Although postoperative aspiration for a limited period of time is frequently seen, good voice quality is usually obtained and the temporary tracheostomy can almost always be removed. Total laryngectomy as a salvage procedure for intractable aspiration, fistula, or recurrent disease is successful in 33 to 50 percent of cases. Five-year survival rates in the range of 70 to 85 percent for supraglottic carcinoma make it superior to radiotherapy, although no prospective randomized studies have tested this thesis.

Vertical hemilaryngectomy is the standard conservation procedure carried out for invasive carcinoma of one vocal cord or a vocal cord and the anterior commissure that does not invade the thyroid cartilage. Total resection of the cord and its subjacent muscle and adjacent cartilage is necessary. Access to the larynx is

Data Form for Cancer Staging

Patient identification
Name ____
Address ____
Hospital or clinic number ____
Age ____ Sex ____ Race ____

Institutional identification
Hospital or clinic ____
Address ____

Oncology Record

Anatomic site of cancer ____
Chronology of classification* [ ] Clinical-diagnostic (cTNM)
[ ] Surgical-evaluative (sTNM)
Date of classification ____

Histologic type† ____ Grade (G) ____
[ ] Postsurgical resection–pathologic (pTNM)
[ ] Retreatment (rTNM) [ ] Autopsy (aTNM)

Definitions: TNM Classification

Primary Tumor (T)

[ ] TX Minimum requirements to assess the primary tumor cannot be met.
[ ] T0 No evidence of primary tumor

Supraglottis

[ ] Tis Carcinoma *in situ*
[ ] T1 Tumor confined to site of origin with normal mobility
[ ] T2 Tumor involves adjacent supraglottic site(s) or glottis without fixation
[ ] T3 Tumor limited to larynx with fixation or extension to involve postcricoid area, medial wall of piriform sinus, or preepiglottic space
[ ] T4 Massive tumor extending beyond the larynx to involve oropharynx, soft tissues of neck, or destruction of thyroid cartilage

Glottis

[ ] Tis Carcinoma *in situ*
[ ] T1 Tumor confined to vocal cord(s) with normal mobility (including involvement of anterior or posterior commissures)
[ ] T2 Supraglottic or subglottic extension of tumor with normal or impaired cord mobility
[ ] T3 Tumor confined to the larynx with cord fixation
[ ] T4 Massive tumor with thyroid cartilage destruction or extension beyond the confines of the larynx, or both

Subglottis

[ ] Tis Carcinoma *in situ*
[ ] T1 Tumor confined to the subglottic region
[ ] T2 Tumor extension to vocal cords with normal or impaired cord mobility
[ ] T3 Tumor confined to larynx with cord fixation
[ ] T4 Massive tumor with cartilage destruction or extension beyond the confines of the larynx, or both

Nodal Involvement (N)

[ ] NX Minimum requirements to assess the regional nodes cannot be met.
[ ] N0 No clinically positive nodes
[ ] N1 Single clinically positive homolateral node 3 cm or less in diameter
[ ] N2 Single clinically positive homolateral node more than 3 but not more than 6 cm in diameter or multiple clinically positive homolateral nodes, none more than 6 cm in diameter
[ ] N2a Single clinically positive homolateral node more than 3 cm but not more than 6 cm in diameter
[ ] N2b Multiple clinically positive homolateral nodes, none more than 6 cm in diameter
[ ] N3 Massive homolateral node(s), bilateral nodes, or contralateral node(s)
[ ] N3a Clinically positive homolateral node(s), one more than 6 cm in diameter
[ ] N3b Bilateral clinically positive nodes (in this situation, each side of the neck should be staged separately; *i.e.*, N3b: right, N2a; left, N1)
[ ] N3c Contralateral clinically positive node(s) only

Distant Metastasis (M)

[ ] MX Minimum requirements to assess the presence of distant metastasis cannot be met.
[ ] M0 No (known) distant metastasis
[ ] M1 Distant metastasis present
Specify ____

Location of Tumor

Supraglottis

[ ] Ventricular band
[ ] Arytenoid
[ ] Suprahyoid epiglottis
[ ] Infrahyoid epiglottis
[ ] Arytenoepiglottic fold

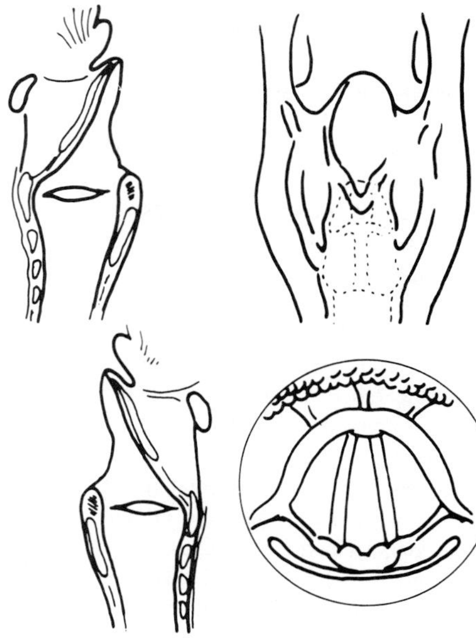

Examination by ____ M.D.
Date ____

*Use a separate form each time a case is staged.
†See reverse side for additional information.

FIG. 15-43. AJCC staging system for carcinoma of the larynx.

obtained posterior to the cord by cutting through the thyroid cartilage, leaving the external perichondrium sutured to the sternothyroid muscle. The cord with or without the ipsilateral arytenoid cartilage is resected, and if the commissure is involved, the keel of the thyroid cartilage is as well. The strap muscles and perichondrium or a cartilage graft provides a buttress against which the normal cord can appose. Five-year survival rates of 75 to 87 percent for Stages I to III treated in this fashion have been reported, again superior to radiotherapy alone. As with supraglottic laryngectomy, removal of the temporary tracheostomy and resumption of oral nutrition without aspiration is usually possible, with voice preservation. Extended hemilaryngectomy has been described for T3 lesions, where a small segment of vocalis muscle with its overlying cartilage, with sensory and motor innervation left intact, is used with the adjacent hypopharyngeal mucosa to create a phonatory shunt through which air from the lungs can be forced to provide speech. Although permanent tracheostomy is necessary, voice quality has been described as superior to esophageal speech and obtainable in a high percentage of cases.

Voice restoration after surgery that removes the entire larynx is a difficult problem. Despite widespread availability of speech therapy and extensive preoperative teaching and aggressive postoperative rehabilitation, only 24 to 45 percent of alaryngeal patients acquire esophageal speech. Inability to expel air from the stomach, cricopharyngeus spasm, and other physiologic reasons have been cited, but depression and social and emotional withdrawal play an important part as well. Mechanical devices inserted into the airway have been remarkably unsuccessful, although external vibrators do allow intelligible speech of low volume. Various attempts have been described to create a neolarynx or neoglottis, a mucosal or epithelial diaphragm which fits over the transected end of the cricoid or trachea and serves as a pathway for air inspired through the tracheostomy to exit through the oral cavity as speech. With these various methods, good speech quality may be obtained in 50 to 75 percent of cases, but there is a significant risk of aspiration, requiring takedown of the reconstruction. A simple tracheoesophageal puncture described by Singer, maintained patent by a small tube, allows pulmonary air to enter the esophagus and thus the pharynx, to be modulated by the tongue, lips and buccal mucosa. This method has allowed fluent speech restoration in 71 to 88 percent of patients with little risk of aspiration or other serious complication. This procedure may be performed either at a second stage after healing of the wound or at the time of laryngectomy, whether closed by primary approximation or reconstructed with pectoralis major, gastric pull-up, or free tissue transfer. Transplantation of the larynx has as yet been unsuccessful, but research is continuing with this method.

Extensive surgery on the larynx is associated with complications. Pharyngocutaneous fistula occurs in up to 38 percent of laryngectomies and has been associated with previous radiotherapy, malnutrition, and cell-mediated immunodeficiency. Prophylactic metronidazole has been suggested as a method to prevent fistula, but prompt recognition and closure with well-vascularized tissue will prevent prolonged drainage and rupture of the adjacent irradiated carotid vessels. Problems specific to the method of reconstruction also occur, such as regurgitation of acid and food after pharyngogastrostomy after gastric pull-up or hypersecretion of mucus after jejunal autograft. The problem of stenosis after laryngectomy, particularly in the patient who receives adjuvant radiotherapy, is similar to that after pharyngolaryngectomy. Combined with the alterations in cricopharyngeus function (upper esophageal sphincter mechanism), stenosis greatly impedes the acquisition of esophageal speech. Interposition of well-vascularized soft tissue, such as the radial forearm or lateral arm free flap, can decrease the likelihood of postlaryngectomy speech and swallowing problems (Fig. 15-44).

Nonepidermoid malignancies of the larynx are uncommon. Adenosquamous carcinoma is a poorly differentiated aggressive lesion which behaves in a manner similar to advanced squamous carcinoma. Rhabdomyosarcoma, chondrosarcoma, schwannoma, and other mesenchymal malignancies have been reported in both children and adults. Carcinoid or moderately differentiated neuroendocrine carcinoma behaves in a fashion similar to malignancy in other sites and may be treated by partial or total laryngectomy, depending on its stage. Adjuvant radiotherapy and chemotherapy do not seem to contribute to the cure of the patient. Anaplastic small cell carcinoma (oat cell) also occurs in the larynx rarely and, like its counterpart in the lung, is associated with smoking and increased age. Prognosis is also similar to lung disease, with average survival of 10 months after diagnosis. Multimodal therapy with chemotherapy as the basis is the most appropriate approach.

One of the most difficult problems associated with laryngectomy is recurrence of disease at the stoma. Occurring in approximately 5 percent of patients, it may be the result of submucosal subglottic extension or unresected pretracheal or paratracheal lymph node metastasis. Resection of disease is possible in some patients by mediastinal dissection, repositioning the stoma lower and removing the soft tissues of the superior mediastinum to the innominate vessels. Esophageal reconstruction may be performed by gastric pull-up or jejunal free autograft, and interposition of vascularized pectoralis major muscle is usually necessary to separate the great vessels from the stoma. With this aggressive surgical approach, 17 to 28 percent of patients can be salvaged.

Benign lesions of the larynx may present a diagnostic problem but are usually seen in different age groups and rarely affect mobility of the cords. Tuberculosis of the larynx, though rare, may mimic malignancy. Papillomatosis may present in children, possibly secondary to contamination of the fetus at delivery by the human papilloma virus, a DNA virus. This persistent problem may require tracheostomy, since repeated excisions by laser or otherwise may result in laryngeal or subglottic stenosis. Adult-onset papillomatosis of the larynx may come with immunosuppression of various types as recurrent disease or as an opportunistic infection. Immunotherapy with BCG has been suggested as an adjuvant for surgery. Vocal nodules or singer's nodules and polyps and sebaceous cysts may also occur in the mobile cords and may be treated by simple excision.

CONNECTIVE TISSUE NEOPLASMS

Soft Tissue Sarcomas

General Considerations. Soft tissue sarcomas arise within tissues that develop embryologically from the mesoderm, such as skeletal and smooth muscle, adipose and fibrous tissue, and endothelial cells. They are uncommon tumors overall, with less than 5,000 new cases diagnosed each year in the United States. Less than 10 percent of all sarcomas arise in the head and neck; they represent less than 1 percent of all head and neck malignancies. This low incidence, with the attendant difficulty in developing a comprehensive management plan, may partially account for the poor survival rates in adults with soft tissue sarcomas. Unlike epi-

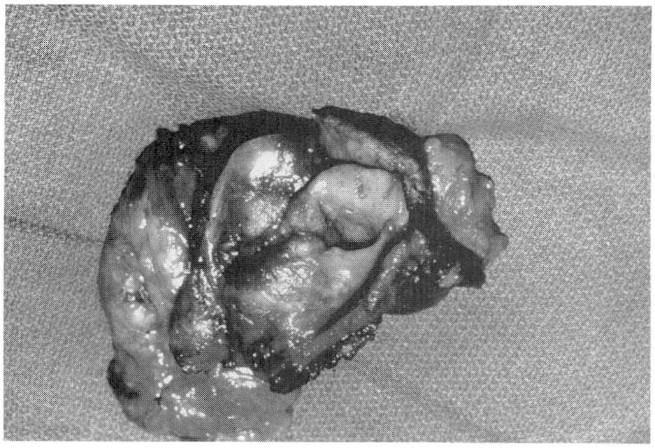

A

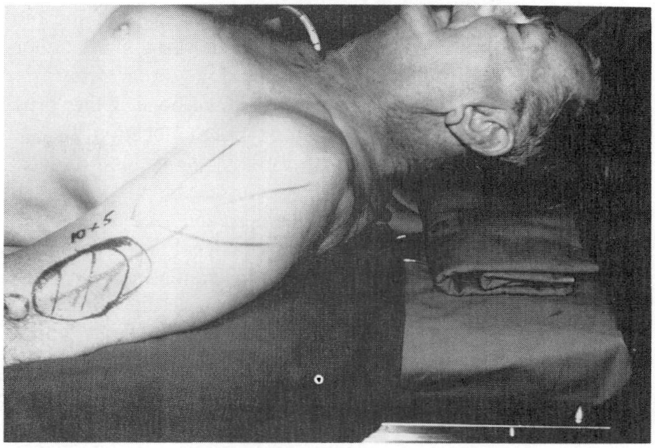

B

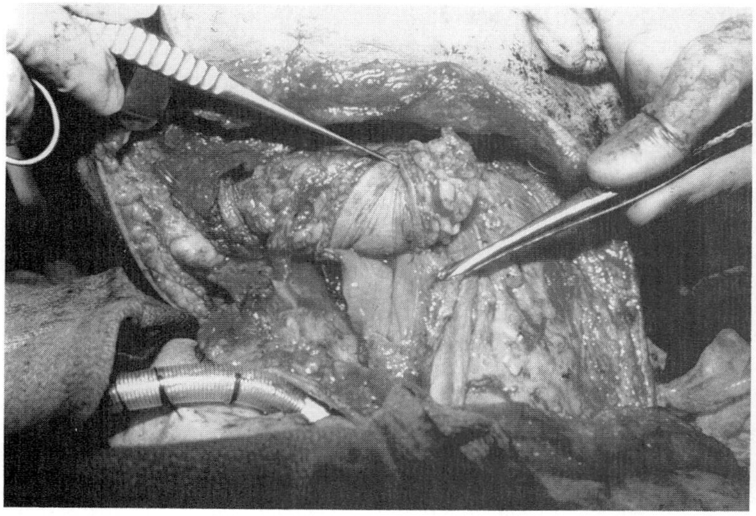

C

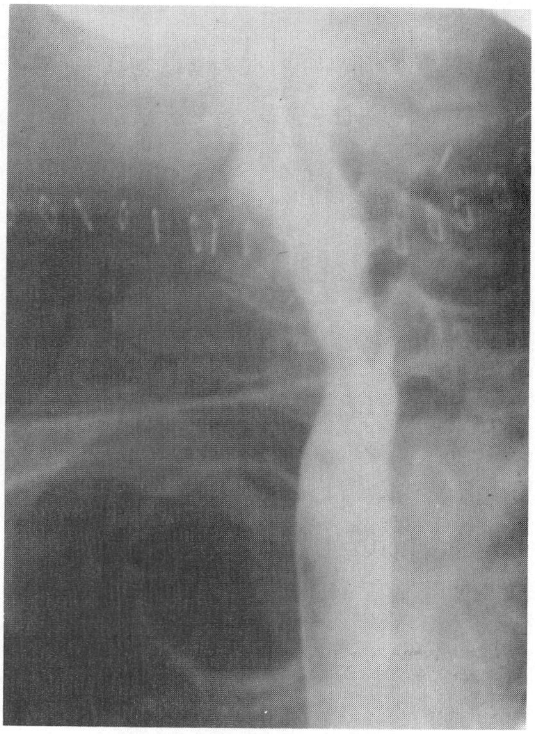

D

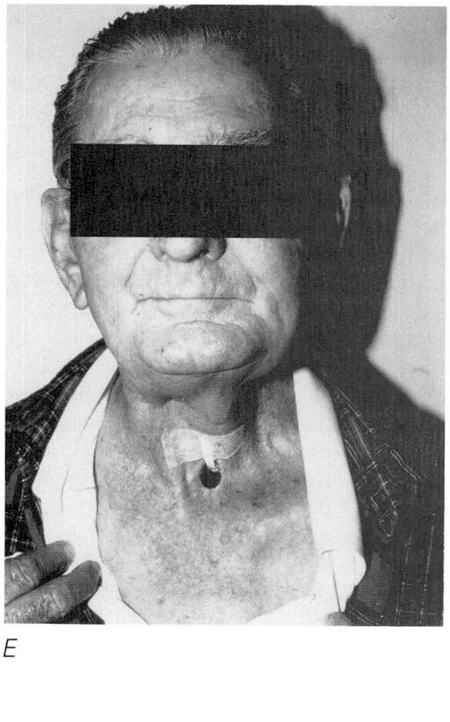

E

FIG. 15-44. *A.* Surgical specimen from laryngopharyngectomy and neck dissection on a sixty-eight-year-old male diabetic smoker showing medial wall invasion of squamous cell carcinoma of pyriform sinus, which resulted in paralysis of left vocal cord. *B.* Lateral arm fasciocutaneous free flap designed to provide epithelial lining for anterior wall of neopharynx. *C.* After vascular anastomosis, lateral arm flap provides adequate lumen of neopharynx. *D.* Barium swallow shows no evidence of stenosis. Thirteen months after postoperative adjuvant radiotherapy, a normal solid diet is tolerated. *E.* Tracheoesophageal puncture with Blom-Singer valve allows patient reasonable speech.

dermoid carcinoma, the most important determinant of the biologic behavior of sarcomas is histologic grade. Low-grade tumors tend to recur locally while high-grade lesions often metastasize early to distant sites including lung, liver, and bone. Other prognostic indicators include the histologic type, the location, the size and the degree of local invasion of primary lesions, and the presence of locoregional or distant metastatic disease.

Typically soft tissue sarcoma of the head and neck presents as a painless mass. The more advanced or more deeply invasive lesions may cause pain, obstructive symptoms, or cranial nerve deficits. Evaluation of local extent of disease in soft tissue sarcomas is similar to that of squamous cell carcinoma and includes indirect laryngoscopy, palpation endoscopy, and a CT or MRI. Depending on histology and stage of disease, a metastatic work-up should be performed. Pleomorphic sarcomas of the head and neck, like those arising in other areas, frequently demonstrate cellular changes consistent with indolent disease in one part of the tumor and characteristic of very aggressive disease in another part. A generous incisional biopsy is often necessary to confirm the diagnosis. The mainstay of treatment for the majority of these lesions in adults remains extensive local resection with clearly negative margins (tumor no less than 1 mm from the surgical margin). Regional node dissections are usually performed only if nodal disease is clinically evident. In adults, adjuvant radiation therapy and chemotherapy may be of some worth, whereas in children their therapeutic value has now been clearly established.

Fibrosarcoma. This is the most common type of soft tissue sarcoma in adults. There is a bimodal age distribution with the first peak in infants under two years old and the second in adults forty to sixty years old. Fibrosarcoma often presents as a painless mass of the face or neck. Histologically, many fibrosarcomas are low grade. The rate of metastasis to regional nodes is 5 percent, but 50 percent metastasize to lungs, liver, or bone. With aggressive local resection, 5-year survival rates approximating 45 percent have been reported.

Malignant Fibrous Histiocytoma. The reported incidence of these tumors in the head and neck has grown in recent years due to the reclassification of other high-grade sarcomas as malignant fibrous histiocytomas. Two histologic variants exist, myxoid and inflammatory, with the latter carrying a poorer prognosis. Whereas local recurrence remains the most common manifestation of treatment failure, the incidence of nodal metastasis may approach 50 percent. Therefore, in addition to aggressive local resection, prophylactic neck dissections are advocated in some centers, depending to a great degree on stage of disease. Five-year survival is approximately 50 percent.

Angiosarcoma. These rare cutaneous malignancies most often present as an ulcerated painless mass of the scalp or face in middle-aged men. They are highly aggressive tumors, with perivascular extension most often cited as the cause of local failure as well as of distant metastasis. Radiation therapy and chemotherapy have both been used as adjuvants to local resection, but 5-year disease-free survival is rare.

Rhabdomyosarcoma. This is the most common type of soft tissue sarcoma in children, and after lymphoma is the second most common malignancy of the head and neck in children. Two important histologic subtypes have been identified. The embryonal variant occurs in young children (average age four) and carries the better prognosis. Seventy-nine percent of orbital rhabdomyosarcomas are of the embryonal type. Most of these neoplasms are now treated successfully with a combination of radiation therapy and chemotherapy (vincristine, Adriamycin D, and cyclophosphamide), yielding survival rates of 77 to 90 percent. Alveolar rhabdomyosarcoma occurs in older children (average ten) and in the cervical soft tissues. While the initial response rate to radiation therapy and chemotherapy is comparable with that of embryonal rhabdomyosarcoma, the rate of local recurrences and of distant metastasis is significantly higher, decreasing survival rates to approximately 50 percent at 5 years. The Intergroup Rhabdomyosarcoma Study has established specific multimodal treatment protocols for each type and stage of disease. To date the improvements in management of rhabdomyosarcoma in children have not yet been realized in adults.

Neural Tumors

Esthesioneuroblastoma (Olfactory Neuroblastoma). This rare tumor arises from the supporting cells of the olfactory neuroepithelium at the apex of the nasal cavity. In its earlier stages it may present as a fleshy upper nasal mass causing epistaxis, unilateral nasal obstruction, or rhinorrhea. In its more advanced stages the tumor may extend throughout the cribriform plate into the anterior cranial fossa, invading the frontal lobe and leading to anosmia, rhinorrhea, headaches, or even personality changes. While this tumor may arise in all age groups, it has higher incidence in the third and fourth decades of life and a slight male predominance. When suspected on the basis of the history or CT scans showing bony erosion, the nasal mass should be biopsied in the operating room due to its highly vascular nature. Metastasis may occur in 20 percent of cases, most commonly to the cervical lymph nodes (often bilateral), lungs, and bone, but the majority of patients succumb to aggressive intracranial extension. Therefore, surgical treatment is directed to complete local control. Early lesions may be resected through a lateral rhinotomy and complete ethmoidectomy. More extensive tumors require a combined neurosurgical-craniofacial effort, with exposure and complete resection of the cribriform plate and ethmoid sinuses from both a superior and inferior approach. Adjuvant radiation therapy may improve local control and survival, while inoperable tumors are often treated with radiation therapy alone.

Paraganglionoma. Paraganglionomas or chemodectomas are neoplasms that arise from neural crest cells and histologically resemble their adrenal gland counterpart, the pheochromocytoma. They are classified by their location: carotid body, jugular (arising from the glomus jugulare), vagal body, orbital, and laryngeal. Although these extraadrenal paraganglionic cells do contain small amounts of catecholamines, it is rare for them to produce a clinically significant excess of catecholamines. The most common of the paraganglionomas, the carotid body tumor, usually presents as an asymptomatic neck mass. Chemodectomas at other sites often produce compressive symptoms resulting in hearing loss, tinnitus, or facial nerve paralysis. Only 6 percent of these tumors are malignant, and only 4 percent metastasize. Malignancy is determined by clinical behavior rather than histology. They are highly vascular and have a characteristic appearance on angiography. When technically feasible, treatment should include complete resection, which in the carotid body tumor requires subadventitial dissection.

The poor-risk patient with an asymptomatic mass may be managed more conservatively.

Osteogenic Sarcoma

Ten percent of osteogenic sarcomas occur in the head and neck. Most arise in the mandible or maxilla in the third or fourth decade of life. Risk factors include prior radiation therapy, fibrous dysplasia, and retinoblastoma. These malignancies present most frequently as a hard mass with radiographic changes of cortical destruction as well as new bone formation. These tumors are highly infiltrative not only of bone but of secondary mucosa and muscle and must be resected with a wide zone of adjacent soft tissue. Nodal metastasis is uncommon; however, distant metastasis to lung occurs in a percentage of patients if local control is not achieved. Nevertheless there has been some enthusiasm for chemotherapy administered after surgical resection. Radiation therapy is generally reserved for salvage situations. As with rhabdomyosarcoma, the use of neoadjuvant or adjuvant chemotherapy has been very effective in children with osteogenic sarcoma; the same success has not translated to adults.

AIDS-RELATED DISORDERS

HIV infection and its consequence, AIDS, produce a large number of abnormalities in the head and neck region, both neoplastic and nonneoplastic.

Symbiotic Infections. The generalized immunosuppression allows normally symbiotic or latent organisms to cause serious disease and morbidity. Oral candidiasis may be one of the earliest manifestations of AIDS. The combination of xerostomia, which may be related to the chronic fibrosis of the salivary glands or benign lymphoepithelial lesions seen in HIV-positive patients, and the disturbance of normal flora of the oral cavity results in the proliferation of yeast and other fungi to pathogenic levels. Herpes simplex virus infections, resulting in painful ulcerations of the lips, oral mucosa, and oropharynx, as well as varicella-zoster, with its painful distribution along the Vth cranial nerve, are also common in patients afflicted by AIDS, again a probable result of generalized immunosuppression. Other infectious disorders less commonly seen are human papilloma virus, cytomegalovirus, cat-scratch disease, tuberculosis, and opportunistic bacterial infection localized to the oral cavity and oropharynx.

Leukoplakia. Oral hairy leukoplakia is similar to the leukoplakia seen in chronic smokers except that it has a shaggy or more nodular appearance and is more likely to present on the lateral border of the tongue, frequently as a bilateral lesion. Cellular hyperplasia with parakeratosis is seen, and there is a high correlation, both serologically and by electron microscopy, with the Epstein-Barr virus. This lesion may be an early sign of ultimate HIV positivity, again as an expression of decreased immunosurveillance.

Lymphoproliferative Disorders. Lymphoproliferative disorders are characteristic of AIDS and frequently manifest in the head and neck area. Obstruction of the nasopharynx secondary to overgrowth in the Waldeyer's ring area has been reported. Cervical lymphadenopathy is commonly a part of the AIDS-related complex (ARC), and involvement of the intraparotid and submandibular lymph nodes, with cystic degeneration and symptomatic accumulation of fluid within them, causes enlargement of the nodes and is an early indicator of the full-blown disease. Malignant lymphomas, most commonly of the B-cell type, have also been reported and are second only to Kaposi's sarcoma in frequency, occurring in up to 10 percent of AIDS patients. The occurrence of these lymphomas is usually extranodular, with an unusual frequency of primary central nervous system disease. Lymphoma has also been reported in the neck, oral cavity, and paranasal sinuses. Although the predilection for dissemination is less than in other lymphomas, the disease course is rapid and lethal. Lymphoma occurs more commonly in intravenous drug users than in patients who have developed AIDS from other sources. Again there is a high correlation of lymphoma with elevated antigen titers for Epstein-Barr virus and electron microscopic evidence of its presence. T-cell lymphomas also occur but are less common. For disease localized to one area, radiotherapy may be an effective form of treatment. Multidrug systemic chemotherapy is also effective but places the already immunosuppressed patient at higher risk of disseminated infection.

Kaposi's Sarcoma. Kaposi's sarcoma is the most common malignancy in AIDS, arising in 15 percent of patients. There is probably a sexual mode of transmission, since it is much more common in homosexual AIDS patients than in those acquiring the disease from intravenous drug use or contaminated blood products. Unlike the classical form of Kaposi's sarcoma, which occurs in elderly males usually on the lower extremities, this form of the disease manifests in oral or perioral mucosa in 55 percent of cases. The palate is the most common site, although the tongue, pharynx, and larynx have been described. Usually multifocal within the region, it may arise in or metastasize to the cervical lymph nodes or the salivary glands. The tumor initially presents as a flat blue to purple patch and may appear to be a submucosal hematoma secondary to trauma. Later in the course of growth it becomes nodular. Biopsy reveals endothelial cell and fibroblast proliferation, with increased capillary growth, prominent spindle cells, few mitoses, and extravasation of erythrocytes. The causation of Kaposi's sarcoma is unclear, although there is some evidence linking it to cytomegalovirus infection or viral induction of local angiogenic factors.

As with all malignancies in AIDS patients, the use of conventional multidrug systemic therapy is somewhat hazardous because of chronic infection. Single-drug treatment with vinblastine or VP-16, either systemically or by intralesional injection, will result in partial regression of tumor and significant palliation in up to 30 percent of patients. Interferon alpha, either systemically or as an intralesional injection, has also been moderately effective. Local radiotherapy with an energy source, such as electrons, that has low penetration, in total doses of 800 to 1500 cGy, delivered in ten fractions, is also effective in shrinking lesions and allowing significant palliation. With all therapies, median survival of patients is 2 years, with only 10 percent 5-year survival.

Carcinoma. Squamous cell carcinoma of the upper aerodigestive tract has been reported in the mouth, tongue, larynx, and other sites. Although the true risk is at present uncertain, squamous cell carcinoma has appeared in patients of earlier age and without the usual risk factors of smoking and ethanol intake. This pattern is suggestive of a defect in immunosurveillance similar to that seen in patients having undergone organ transplantation. In AIDS patients, the median age of presentation of squamous cell carcinoma is thirty-two years, in contrast to sixty years in the noninfected patient, and the clinical course seems to be somewhat more aggressive.

SALIVARY GLANDS

Physiology. The production and excretion of the mixture of mucus, water, and electrolytes known as saliva into the entrance to the upper aerodigestive tract are the function of the salivary glands. The major salivary glands are the symmetrically paired parotid, submandibular, and sublingual glands which discharge saliva into the oral cavity via Stensen's ducts, Wharton's ducts, and the numerous small orifices in the floor of the mouth, respectively. Clustered primarily in the soft and hard palates but also found in the sinuses and other sites of the upper aerodigestive tract are the minor salivary glands, which produce mucus for lubrication. Saliva consists of varying concentrations of numerous substances. To some degree its composition reflects the osmolality and electrolyte concentration of the extracellular fluid, but its specific functions require other components as well.

The normal volume of salivary secretion in the adult male ranges from 1000 to 1500 mL per day, mainly as serous fluid from the parotid and submandibular glands (95 percent) but also composed of mucus (5 percent) from the sublingual and minor salivary glands. Active water resorption, sodium and potassium ion exchange, and bicarbonate production couple with passive diffusion of urea and uric acid to determine the inorganic content of saliva. Immunoglobulins A, G, M, albumin, lysozyme and other enzymes also are secreted. In addition to its lubricating properties, which allow food to be moved through the mouth, saliva has antibacterial and antiviral properties, which protect the soft tissue of the oral cavity as well as the teeth.

The neurogenic control of salivary secretion depends on reflex arcs which carry afferent stimuli from the specialized sense organs via cranial nerves I, V, VII, and IX to the brainstem and hypothalamus and efferent signals, both sympathetic and parasympathetic, along the branches of the external carotid nerve, the superficial petrosal nerve and the chorda tympani.

Anatomy. ***Parotid Gland.*** The parotid gland is shaped like a flattened pyramid, with its apex in the parapharyngeal space behind the mandible adjacent to the pterygoid muscles and its base extending into the preauricular area from below the angle of the mandible in the neck, sometimes as low as the midsternocleidomastoid muscle, to just below the zygomatic arch. The medial extent of the gland usually reaches over the masseter and vertical ramus of the mandible. The parotid gland is surrounded by the continuation of the investing layer of the cervical fascia, the superficial layer of which is continuous with the platysma. The parotid gland parenchyma is arbitrarily divided into the deep and superficial lobes by the facial nerve, which exits from the stylomastoid foramen and passes through the substance of the gland. Approximately 70 percent of the gland lies superficial to the plane of the nerve and 30 percent deep to it.

The lymphatic drainage of the midface, forehead, and anterior portion of the scalp empties into lymph nodes that lie superficial to the fascia of the parotid and within the gland itself before sending efferent channels to the jugulodigastric area. Sensory supply to the gland derives from branches of the trigeminal nerve and from the great auricular nerve, carrying cervical plexus axons. Stensen's duct, the parotid duct, condenses from the larger intralobular ducts and passes adjacent to the buccal branch of the facial nerve on a line between the tragus of the ear and the midline of the upper lip. It enters the oral cavity adjacent to the second maxillary molar tooth.

The facial nerve, which supplies motor innervation to the posterior belly of the digastric and the muscles of facial animation, exits the base of the skull from the stylomastoid foramen, passing deep to superficial and caudad to cephalad before branching at the *pes anserinus* into an upper and lower division. Although there is some variability in branching patterns, particularly with relationship to the buccal branch, the upper division usually includes the temporal, zygomatic, and buccal branches, and the lower division, the marginal mandibular and cervical branches.

Submandibular Gland. The submandibular salivary gland is surrounded by a condensation of the cervical fascia that lies beneath the platysma muscle, connecting to the parotid fascia and known as the *pars interglandularis,* separating the parotid and jugulodigastric areas from the submandibular triangle. The anatomic boundaries of the submandibular triangle are the anterior belly of the digastric muscle medially, the posterior belly laterally, and the mandible cephalad. The gland lies on the hyoglossus muscle and wraps both superficial and deep to the mylohyoid muscle medially. The submandibular ganglion of the lingual nerve carries efferent nerve supply via the chorda tympani. Wharton's duct conveys the secretions of the submandibular salivary gland into the oral cavity.

Sublingual Glands. The sublingual salivary glands lie immediately beneath the mucosa of the floor of the mouth, intimately related to the lingual artery, and release their mucous secretions into the oral cavity through numerous orifices along the alveololingual sulcus.

Inflammatory and Infectious Disorders. Inflammation usually presents as diffuse enlargement or firmness of the gland, unilateral or bilateral, associated with tenderness and erythema. Bacterial infection is usually the result of duct obstruction and retrograde infection with oral bacteria. Acute bacterial parotitis may be seen in the elderly postoperative patient who becomes dehydrated and is usually caused by *Staphylococcus aureus*. Although rehydration and antibiotic therapy may be successful, drainage of localized abscesses and even total parotidectomy may be required for ultimate resolution. Because of the septate nature of the parotid, simple drainage of the gland is frequently unsuccessful. Acute sialadenitis of the submandibular gland may also require gland resection.

Mumps, coxsackie, and echo viruses may also cause acute parotitis, usually panglandular but manifesting only as unilateral gland enlargement. Tuberculosis, actinomycosis, and cat-scratch disease may also present with enlargement of either the salivary glands or their adjacent lymph nodes. Systemic disorders such as sarcoidosis, Sjögren's syndrome, and cirrhosis with liver failure also result in salivary gland enlargement. Mikulicz's syndrome, enlargement of the gland with histologic changes reflecting loss of acinar epithelium and replacement with chronic inflammatory cells, is a nonspecific accompaniment of several diseases, such as leukemia, lymphoma, and tuberculosis.

Tumors. ***Pathology.*** The clinical problem most frequently presented to the surgeon is that of a discrete mass in the salivary gland, particularly the parotid gland. Of salivary gland tumors, 70 to 80 percent present in the parotid gland. Of parotid gland tumors, 70 to 80 percent are benign and, of the benign tumors, 80 percent are pleomorphic adenomas. Although lymph nodes, lipomas, cysts, or other benign entities may present as solitary masses, the benign pleomorphic adenoma is by far the most common mass.

Occurring most frequently in the fifth decade, with a slight female predominance, the benign mixed tumor or pleomorphic adenoma is the proliferation of both epithelial and myoepithelial cells of the ducts, as well as an increase in the stromal component, which histologically may appear similar to cartilage. A true epithelial benign neoplasm, it may grow to a large size without causing facial nerve symptoms (Fig. 15-45). Pleomorphic adenomas usually present as a solitary painless mass in the superficial lobe of the gland. Deep lobe growth may manifest as an intraoral pharyngeal mass as growth extends into the pharynx via the parapharyngeal space. Malignant degeneration of pleomorphic adenomas occurs in 2 to 10 percent of adenomas followed for long periods, with carcinoma ex pleomorphic adenoma manifesting most frequently as adenocarcinoma.

The second most frequent benign neoplasm of the salivary glands is the papillary cystadenoma lymphomatosum or Warthin's tumor. With a marked male predominance, it usually occurs in the tail of the parotid gland and presents a lymphocytic infiltrate as well as cystic epithelial proliferation. There is a 10 percent incidence of bilaterality and multicentricity. A subset of the group monomorphic adenomas, Warthin's tumors make up 4 to 8 percent of all parotid tumors. Other benign monomorphic adenomas include oxyphilic adenomas, oncocytomas and basal cell adenomas, sebaceous adenoma, sialadenoma papilliferum, and canalicular adenoma, all of which are rare. Pleomorphic adenoma is the most common benign tumor of the parotid, submandibular, and minor salivary glands.

Malignant tumors of the salivary glands rarely (4 percent) present as a diffuse enlargement of a gland, almost always as a discrete mass. Pain is associated with malignancy in 12 to 24 percent of cases. Other symptoms include formication (a paresthesia that is described as the feeling of ants crawling on the skin), facial nerve dysfunction (8 to 26 percent), or complete paresis of the nerve (7 to 9 percent). All of these symptoms and signs carry a poorer prognosis than asymptomatic disease (Fig. 15-46). Facial nerve palsy is almost never seen with benign disease, so the presence of peripheral nerve palsy, even without a discrete mass, must be considered a possible sign of malignancy.

Fixation to the masseter or pterygoids occurs in approximately 17 percent of cases and skin ulceration in 9 percent. The risk of clinical or subclinical metastases to the cervical lymph nodes from salivary gland cancers depends to a great degree on the histology and grade of the primary tumor. High-grade mucoepidermoid adenocarcinoma and squamous cell carcinoma have a high risk of metastatic disease (Fig. 15-47), whereas adenoid cystic acinic cell and lower grades of mucoepidermoid and squamous cell are at low risk of metastasis. Approximately 20 percent of parotid gland neoplasms are malignant. As the salivary gland becomes smaller, the

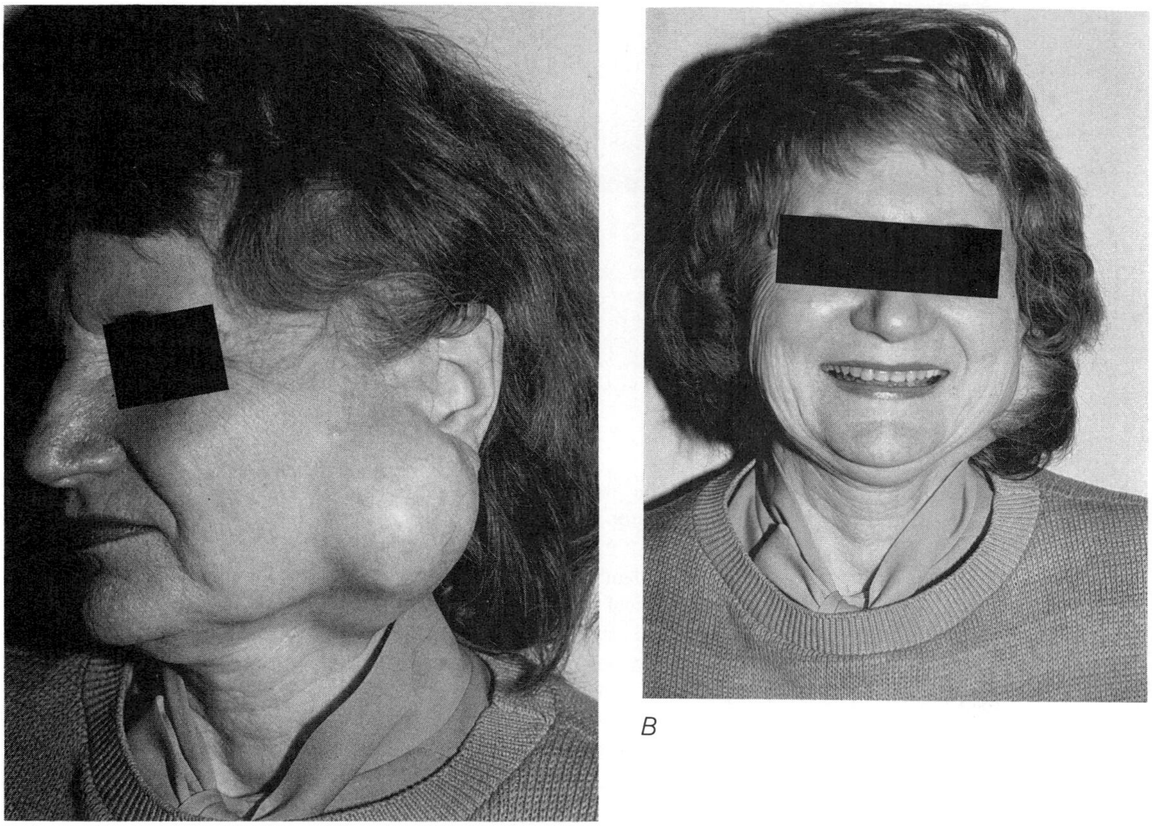

A

B

FIG. 15-45. *A* and *B*. Pleomorphic adenoma of 19 years' duration. Despite its large size it did not affect facial nerve function, and patient concealed it beneath her hair. (From: *Coleman JJ, in Jurkiewicz MJ, et al: Plastic Surgery: Principles and Practice, 1990, with permission.*)

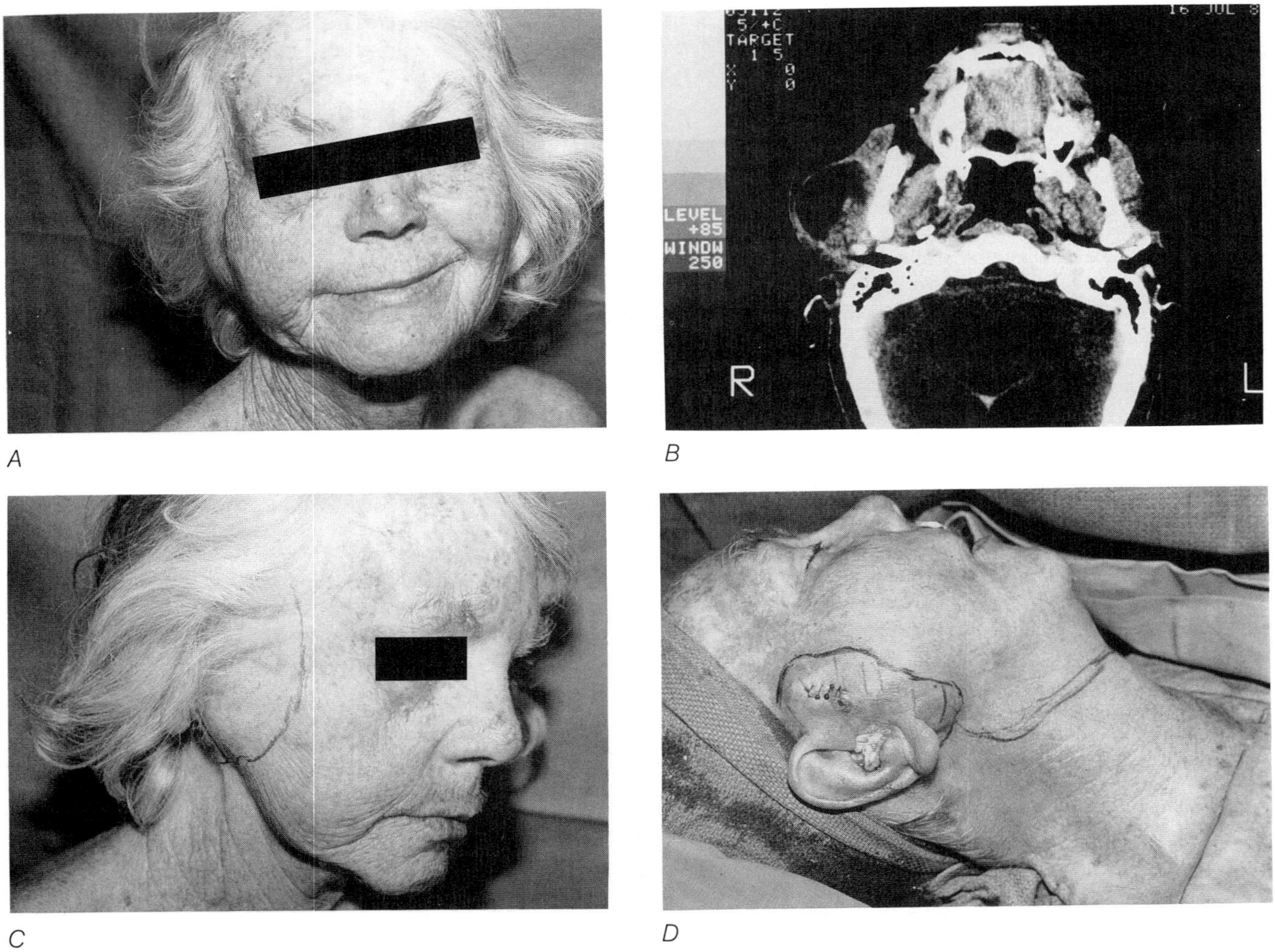

FIG. 15-46. *A.* Squamous cell carcinoma of parotid gland presenting as a diffuse mass in the cheek. (From: *Coleman JJ, in Jurkiewicz MJ, et al: Plastic Surgery: Principles and Practice, 1990, with permission.*) *B.* CT scan showing large necrotic mass fixed to masseter. *C.* Invasion of the facial nerve suggested malignant nature of mass. Note ectropion, flattened nasolabial fold. (From: *Coleman JJ, in Jurkiewicz MJ, et al: Plastic Surgery: Principles and Practice, 1990, with permission.*) *D.* Therapy was total parotidectomy with resection of the facial nerve and radical neck dissection through McFee incisions, followed by adjuvant radiotherapy.

risk of malignancy is higher, with the submandibular glands having 40 percent malignant tumors and the minor salivary glands 60 percent.

Diagnosis. The discrete mass in the salivary gland must be considered a possible malignancy. History and physical examination may provide some indication that the lesion is malignant. Complete resolution after 10 days of antibiotics in a setting consistent with inflammation may constitute an adequate therapeutic trial. Definitive histologic diagnosis is, however, ultimately necessary. Fine-needle aspiration may be helpful in planning surgery, but any uncertainty should be treated with adequate surgical excision. CT scan of the parotid is helpful in determining extension of the tumor into the deep lobe. MRI can be formatted in both axial and coronal planes, giving even better anatomic information. Contrast-enhanced studies may allow separation of the gland from metastatic lymph nodes, particularly in the submandibular area, differentiating metastases from the head and neck site to an intraglandular or epiglandular lymph node from intrinsic malignancy of the salivary gland. Sialography, or injection of contrast material into Stensen's or Wharton's ducts, is useful in demonstrating the chronic stenotic changes of a benign lymphoepithelial lesion or chronic parotitis and in showing complete occlusion from stones. Eighty percent of parotid duct stones are radiolucent. Eighty percent of submandibular gland stones are radiopaque.

Treatment. The surgical approach to a salivary gland mass is predicated on the assumption that it is malignant. The major confounding factor is the presence of the facial nerve in the parotid gland. Since the facial nerve passes through the gland, the usual surgical oncologic approach to head and neck malignancy, en bloc resection, would require excision of the nerve in all cases. This approach, however, is not appropriate in most situations. If there is no evidence of nerve involvement, the tumor should be excised by superficial lobectomy, removal of the parenchyma above the nerve with a margin of normal tissue, preserving the nerve.

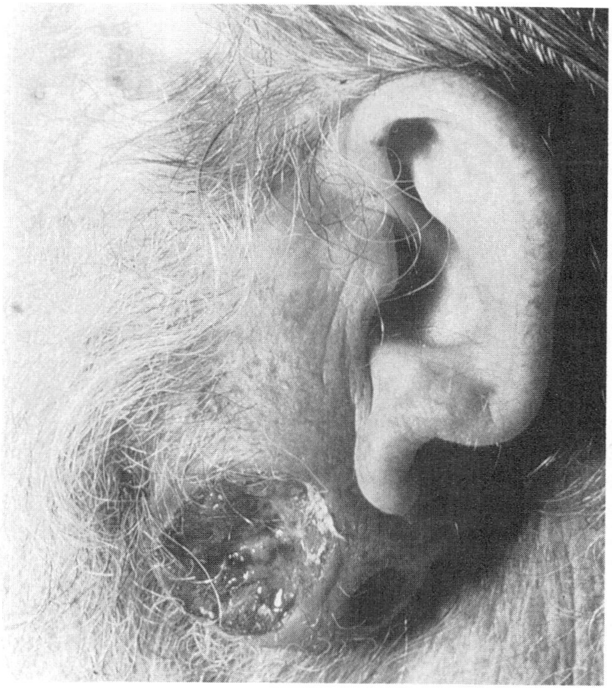

A

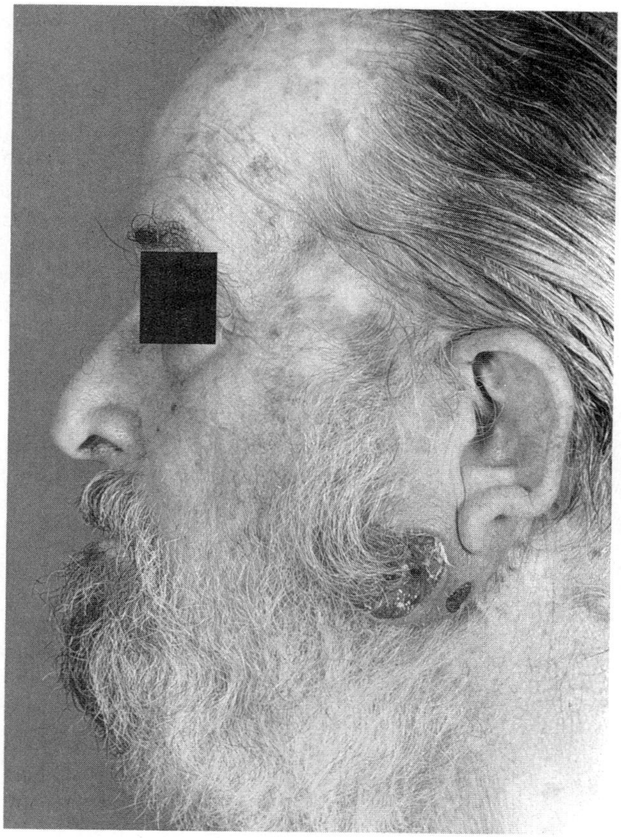

B

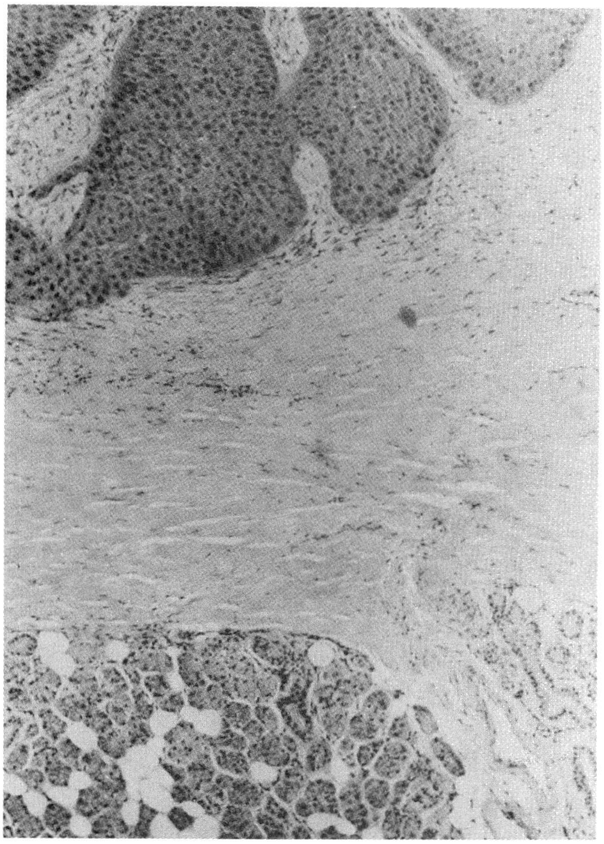

C

FIG. 15-47. *A* and *B*. Extensive squamous cell carcinoma of the parotid in a sixty-year-old male. Subsequent neck dissection revealed numerous cervical metastases. *C*. Photomicrograph shows invasive squamous cell carcinoma and parotid parenchyma.

If the tumor is malignant, total parotidectomy with preservation of the nerve is indicated, though it is a piecemeal procedure (Fig. 15-48). Involvement of a branch of the nerve or the whole nerve requires removal of that branch of the nerve. In young patients, nerve graft should be used to replace the resected nerve segment to hopefully avoid the sequelae of facial nerve palsy. In the event of invasion of the nerve by tumor, proximal extension of the malignancy to the base of the skull should be evaluated, and in some cases resection of the nerve to clear margin in the stylomastoid foramen or facial canal may improve survival. If the facial nerve is not involved by malignancy but preservation of the nerve would result in gross disruption of the tumor, the nerve should be removed and replaced with a nerve graft.

When clinical examination, with or without fine-needle aspiration, does not clearly define the problem, biopsy should be obtained by superficial lobectomy, with identification and preservation of the main trunk of the facial nerve and its branches. Benign tumors of the superficial lobe should be removed with a clear margin by superficial lobectomy. If the deep lobe is involved, total parotidectomy may be required even for benign disease, although partial parotidectomy is sometimes possible.

Treatment of the neck in patients with malignant disease of the parotid depends to a great degree on the histologic type and grade of the tumor and its risk of metastatic disease or the presence of the metastatic disease itself. N+ necks are treated by the appropriate neck dissection—radical neck dissection if there is involvement in the sternocleidomastoid or jugular vein or modified or selective neck dissection depending on the site of metastasis. Although elective or prophylactic neck dissections are not as frequently necessary as in mucosal malignancy, they are indicated in high-grade mucoepidermoid carcinoma, squamous cell carcinoma, and high-grade adenocarcinoma.

Neoadjuvant (preoperative) or adjuvant chemotherapy has not been effective in malignancy of the salivary glands-parotid, submandibular, or minor. Adjuvant postoperative radiotherapy, however, is effective. Radiation portals should include the entire site of surgery, the foramen ovale and base of the skull including mastoid and stylomastoid foramina, and the ipsilateral neck depending on the risk of metastasis.

Risk of recurrent disease and pattern of recurrence are also dependent on histology and grade. Mucoepidermoid carcinoma, squamous cell carcinoma, and high-grade adenocarcinoma have a high frequency of cervical and distant metastasis as well as local recurrence. Adenoid cystic carcinoma is characterized by an indolent course but relentless local progression and perineural invasion, with disease ultimately extending to the base of the skull and brain. Both adenoid cystic and mucoepidermoid carcinoma may demonstrate extensive pulmonary metastasis that remains asymptomatic for relatively prolonged periods, and the patient's demise may be caused by locoregional disease rather than by disseminated disease. Just as adjuvant chemotherapy has been unsuccessful, so is treatment of disseminated disease, although both Adriamycin and cis-platinum have demonstrated finite response rates without prolongation of survival. Local recurrence may be successfully treated by radical resection with or without adjuvant radiotherapy.

Treatment of submandibular gland abnormalities follows the same basic rule as for the parotid gland. If definitive diagnosis cannot be made before surgery, total excision of the gland, with

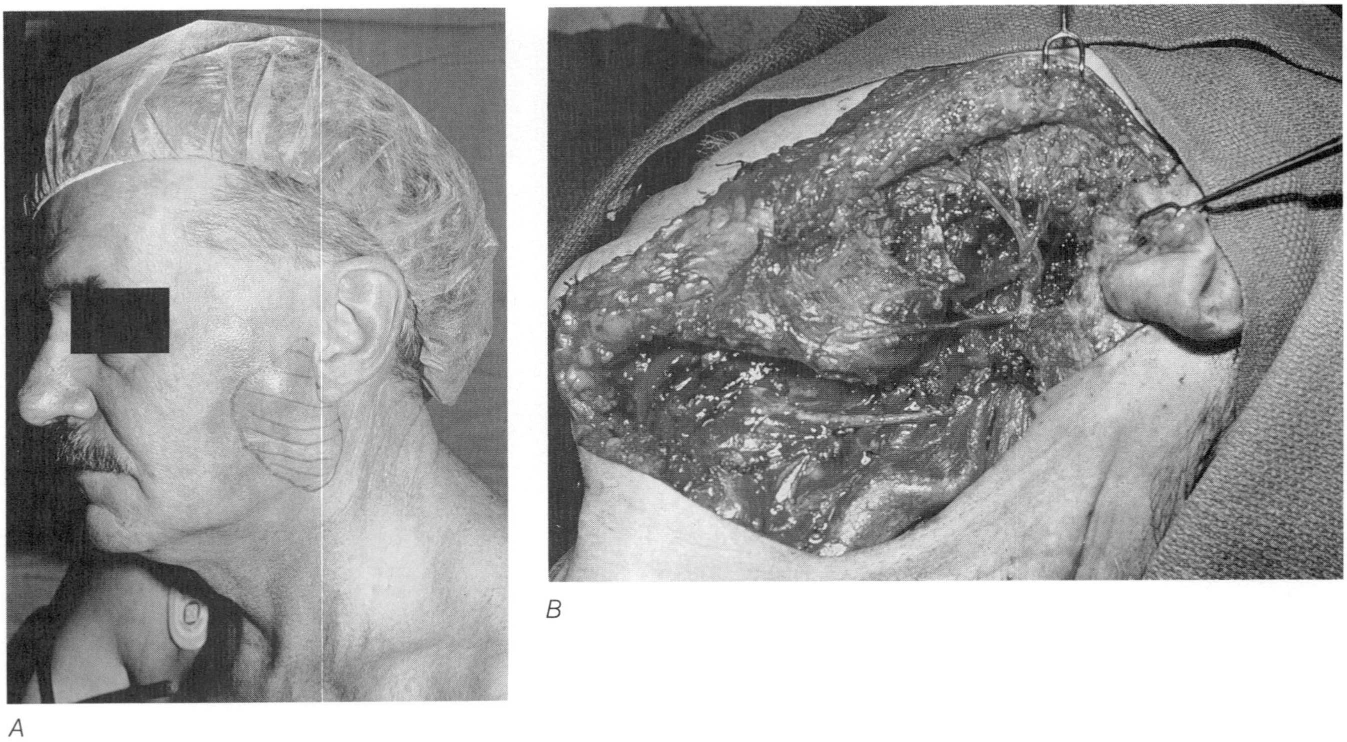

FIG. 15-48. *A.* Poorly differentiated mucoepidermoid carcinoma of the parotid gland without evidence of facial nerve palsy but with multiple cervical metastases. *B.* Therapy included total parotidectomy with preservation of the facial nerve and radical neck dissection. The main trunk and branches of the facial nerve and their proximity to the jugulodigastric area (carotid bifurcation) are apparent here.

preservation of the uninvolved marginal mandibular, hypoglossal, and lingual nerves, is indicated and is adequate therapy for benign tumors and inflammatory or autoimmune disorders. Radical resection of the nerves, platysma, skin, and underlying muscle is reserved for extensive local invasion. Adenoid cystic carcinoma is the most common malignant histology of the submandibular gland and pleomorphic adenoma the most common benign tumor. Adjuvant postoperative radiotherapy appears to be helpful in the malignant tumor.

Minor salivary gland disorders reflect the spectrum seen in the major salivary glands. Mucocele is a cystic enlargement of the intraoral glands usually seen in the lip or the floor of the mouth. Sjögren's syndrome of keratoconjunctivitis sicca is diagnosed by lip biopsy and histologic confirmation of the chronic inflammatory changes seen in the minor salivary glands. Necrotizing sialometaplasia, an ulcerative but self-limited disorder affecting the junction of the hard and soft palates, clinically mimics malignancy but eventually heals; biopsy shows no evidence of malignant change.

Tumors of the minor salivary glands, either benign or malignant, may manifest in any of the mucosa-lined areas of the upper aerodigestive tract but are most common in the hard and soft palates. Their presentation may be as a submucosal or ulcerative mass. Pleomorphic adenoma is the most common benign tumor, and mucoepidermoid and adenoid cystic carcinoma (Fig. 15-49) roughly equal in frequency as malignancies. Therapy is wide local resection, including subjacent bone if the hard palate is involved, with adjuvant radiotherapy for malignancy. Since subclinical metastases to the neck are rare, cervical lymphadenectomy is reserved for patients with histologically proven lymph node metastases. Palatal defects can usually be rehabilitated with dental prostheses, though local or distant tissue transfer may be necessary for extensive disease.

Bibliography

Ali S, Tiwari RM, Snow GB: False-positive and false-negative neck nodes. *Head Neck Surg* 8:78, 1985.

Al-Sarraf M: Head and neck cancer: Chemotherapy concepts. *Semin Oncol* 15(1):70, 1988.

Archer CR, Yeager VL: Computed tomography of laryngeal cancer with histopathological correlation. *Laryngoscope* 92:1173, 1982.

Ariyan S: Functional radical neck dissection. *Plast Reconstr Surg* 65(6)768, 1980.

Ator GA, Abemayor E, et al: Evaluation of mandibular tumor invasion with magnetic resonance imaging. *Arch Otolaryngol Head Neck Surg* 116:454, 1990.

Austin Lt, Dahlin DC, Royer RQ: Giant cell reparative granuloma and related conditions affecting the jawbones. *Oral Surg* 12:1285, 1959.

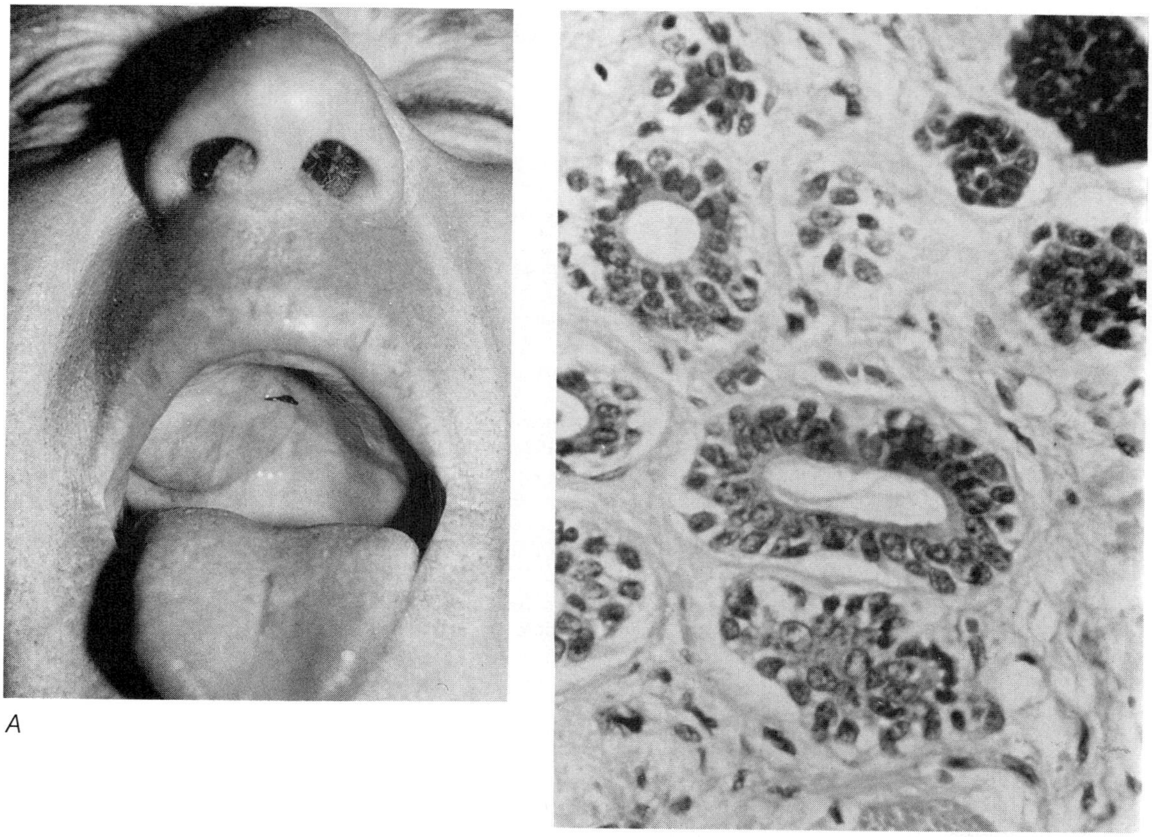

A B

FIG. 15-49. *A.* Extensive adenoid cystic carcinoma of a minor salivary gland presenting as a submucosal mass. Resection included the palate bone. A palatal prosthesis was used after surgery to allow speech and alimentation. (From: *Coleman JJ, in Jurkiewicz MJ, et al: Plastic Surgery: Principles and Practice, 1990, with permission.*) *B.* Photomicrograph of adenoid cystic carcinoma showing regular tubulelike pattern characteristic of cylindroma. (From: *Coleman JJ, in Jurkiewicz MJ, et al: Plastic Surgery: Principles and Practice, 1990, with permission.*)

Bakamjian VY: A two-stage method for pharyngoesophageal reconstruction with a primary pectoral skin flap. *Plast Reconstr Surg* 36:173, 1965.

Baker SR: Nasopharyngeal carcinoma: clinical course and results of therapy. *Head Neck Surg* 3:8, 1980.

Baker SR, Makuch RW, Wolf G: Preoperative cisplatin and bleomycin therapy in head and neck squamous carcinoma. Prognostic factors for tumor response. *Arch Otolaryngol* 107:683, 1981.

Balzi M, Ninu BM, et al: Labeling index in squamous cell carcinoma of the larynx. *Head Neck Surg* 13:344, 1991.

Barkley HT, Fletcher GT, et al: Management of cervical lymph node metastases in squamous cell carcinoma of the tonsillar fossa, base of tongue, supraglottic larynx and hypopharynx. *Am J Surg* 124:462, 1972.

Barton RT, Ucmakli A: Treatment of squamous cell carcinoma of the floor of the mouth. *Surg Gynecol Obstet* 145:21, 1977.

Bataini JP, Jaulerry C, et al: Significance and therapeutic implications of tumor regression following radiotherapy in patients treated for squamous cell carcinoma of the oropharynx and pharyngolarynx. *Head Neck Surg* 12:41, 1990.

Batsakis JG: Primary squamous cell carcinomas of major salivary glands. *Ann Otol Rhinol Laryngol* 92:97, 1983.

Beahrs OH: Surgical anatomy and technique of radical neck dissection. *Surg Clin North Am* 57:663, 1988.

Becker GD, Welch WD: Quantitative bacteriology of intra-operative wound tissue in contaminated surgery. *Head Neck Surg* 12:293, 1990.

Berman JM, Coleman BM: Nasal aspect of cystic fibrosis in children. *J Laryngol* 91:133, 1977.

Biller HF, Lucente FE: Conservation surgery of the head and neck. *Semin Oncol* 4(4):365, 1977.

Blazar BA, Fried MP, et al: Circulating immune complexes and chemotherapy response in patients with head and neck cancer. *Head Neck Surg* 11:431, 1989.

Blitzer PH: Epidemiology of head and neck cancer. *Semin Oncol* 15(1):2, 1988.

Bloom ND, Spiro RH: Carcinoma of the cheek mucosa. A retrospective analysis. *Am J Surg* 140:556, 1980.

Bocca E, Pignataro O, Oldini C: Supraglottic laryngectomy: 30 years experience. *Ann Otol Rhinol Laryngol* 92:14, 1983.

Brady LW, David LW: Treatment of head and neck cancer by radiation therapy. *Semin Oncol* 15(1):29, 1988.

Briant TDR, Fitzpatrick PJ, Berman J: Nasopharyngeal angiofibroma. A 20 year study. *Laryngoscope* 88:1247, 1978.

Brown PF, Coleman JJ: The role of radiotherapy and musculocutaneous flaps in oropharyngocutaneous fistulas. *Am J Surg* 156:256, 1988.

Bunkis J, Mulliken JB, et al: The evolution of techniques for reconstruction of full-thickness cheek defects. *Plast Reconstr Surg* 70(3):319, 1982.

Byers RM: Modified neck dissection. A study of 967 cases from 1970 to 1980. *Am J Surg* 150:414, 1985.

Byers RM, Krueger WWO, Saxton J: Use of surgery and postoperative radiation in the treatment of advanced squamous cell carcinoma of the pyriform sinus. *Am J Surg* 138:597, 1979.

Byers RM, Wolf PF, Ballantyne AJ: Rationale for elective modified neck dissection. *Head Neck Surg* 10:160, 1988.

Canalis RF, Maxwell DS, Hemanwat WC: Laryngocele—an updated review. *J Otol Laryngol* 6:191, 1977.

Candela FC, Shah J, et al: Patterns of cervical node metastases from squamous carcinomas of the larynx. *Arch Otolaryngol Head Neck Surg* 116:432, 1990.

Chatani M, Teshima T, et al: Radiation therapy for nasopharyngeal carcinoma. Retrospective review of 105 patients based on a survey of Kansai Cancer Therapist Group. *Cancer* 57:2267, 1986.

Christensen WN, Smith RR: Schneiderian papillomas: A clinicopathologic study of 67 cases. *Hum Pathol* 17:393, 1986.

Chung CK, et al: Radiotherapy in the management of primary malignancies of the hard palate. *Laryngoscope* 90:576, 1980.

Clark L, Unni KK, Dahlin DC: Osteosarcoma of the jaw. *Cancer* 51:2311, 1983.

Clayman GL, Savage HE, et al: Serologic determinants of survival in patients with squamous cell carcinoma of the head and neck. *Am J Surg* 160:434, 1990.

Close LG, Brown PM, et al: Microvascular invasion and survival in cancer of the oral cavity and oropharynx. *Arch Otolaryngol Head Neck Surg* 115:1304, 1989.

Coleman JJ: Complications in head and neck surgery. *Surg Clin North Am* 66(1):149, 1986.

Coleman JJ: Microvascular approach to function and appearance of large orbital maxillary defects. *Am J Surg* 158:337, 1989.

Coleman JJ: Reconstruction of the pharynx after resection for cancer. A comparison of methods. *Ann Surg* 209(5):554, 1989.

Coleman JJ: Salivary gland disorders, in Jurkiewicz MJ, Krizek J, et al (eds): *Plastic Surgery: Principles and Practice*. St Louis, CV Mosby, 1990, pp 379–418.

Coleman JJ, Searles JM, et al: Ten years experience with the free jejunal autograft. *Am J Surg* 154:394, 1987.

Coleman JJ, Sultan MR: The bipedicled osteocutaneous scapula flap: a new subscapular system free flap. *Plast Reconstr Surg* 87(4):682, 1991.

Coleman JJ III, Wooden WA: Mandibular reconstruction with composite microvascular tissue transfer. *Am J Surg* 160:390, 1990.

Conley J, Myers E, Cole R: Analysis of 115 patients with tumors of the submandibular gland. *Ann Otol* 81:323, 1972.

Cortesina G, De Stefani A, Galeazzi E: Interleukin-2 injected around tumor-draining lymph nodes in head and neck cancer. *Head Neck Surg* 13:125, 1991.

Crissman JD, Liu WY, et al: Prognostic value of histopathologic parameters in squamous cell carcinoma of the oropharynx. *Cancer* 54:2995, 1984.

Cusumano RJ, Persky MS: Squamous cell carcinoma of the oral cavity and oropharynx in young adults. *Head Neck Surg* 10(4):229, 1988.

Dado DV, Angelats J: Upper and lower lip reconstruction using the step technique. *Ann Plast Surg* 15:(3)208, 1985.

deLangen ZJ, Vermey A: Posterolateral neck dissection. *Head Neck Surg* 10(4):252, 1988.

DeSanto LW: Current concepts in otolaryngology. The options in early laryngeal carcinoma. *N Engl J Med* 306(15):910, 1982.

DeSanto LW, Devine KD, Weiland LM: Cysts of the larynx—classification. *Laryngoscope* 80:145, 1970.

DeSanto LW, Lillie JC, Devine KD: Cancers of the larynx: supraglottic cancer. *Surg Clin North Am* 57(3):505, 1977.

Dickson RI: Nasopharyngeal carcinoma: an evaluation of 209 patients. *Laryngoscope* 91:333, 1981.

Effron MZ, Johnson JT, et al: Advanced carcinoma of the tongue. Management by total glossectomy without laryngectomy. *Arch Otolaryngol* 107:694, 1981.

Eiband JD, Elias EG, et al: Prognostic factors in squamous cell carcinoma of the larynx. *Am J Surg* 158:314, 1989.

Emani B, Bignardi M, ET al: Reirradiation of recurrent head and neck cancers. *Laryngoscope* 97:85, 1987.

Epstein JB, Silverman S: Head and neck malignancies associated with HIV infection. *Oral Surg* 73:193, 1992.

Farhood AI, Hajdu SI, et al: Soft tissue sarcomas of the head and neck in adults. *Am J Surg* 160:365, 1990.

Feinmesser R, Miyazaki I, et al: Diagnosis of nasopharyngeal carcinoma by DNA amplification of tissue obtained by fine-needle aspiration. *N Engl J Med* 326(1):17, 1992.

Ficarra G, Gaglioti D, et al: Oral hairy leukoplakia: clinical aspects, histologic morphology and differential diagnosis. *Head Neck Surg* 13(6):514, 1991.

Franklin CD, Pindborg JJ: The calcifying epithelial odontogenic tumor: a review and analysis of 113 cases. *Oral Surg* 42:753, 1976.

Friedman M, Shelton VK, Mafee MM: Metastatic neck disease: evaluation by CT. *Arch Otolaryngol Head Neck Surg* 110:443, 1984.

Fu KK, Ray JW, et al: External and interstitial radiation therapy of carcinoma of the oral tongue. *Am J Roentgenol* 126:107, 1976.

Garrett PG, Beale FA, et al: Cancer of the tonsil: results of radical radiation therapy with surgery in reserve. *Am J Surg* 146:432, 1983.

Gillis TM, Incze J, et al: Natural history and management of kerotosis, atypia, carcinoma in situ, and microinvasive cancer of the larynx. *Am J Surg* 146:510, 1983.

Givens CD, Johns ME, Cantrell RW: Carcinoma of the tonsil. Analysis of 162 cases. *Arch Otolaryngol* 107:730, 1981.

Grandi C, Alloisio M, et al: Prognostic significance of lymphatic spread in head and neck carcinomas: therapeutic implications. *Head Neck Surg* 8:67, 1985.

Greager JA, Patel HK, et al: Soft tissue sarcomas of the adult head and neck. *Cancer* 56:820, 1985.

Harper CS, Mendenhall WM, et al: Cancer in neck nodes with unknown primary site: role of mucosal radiotherapy. *Head Neck Surg* 12:463, 1990.

Heller KS, Shah JP: Carcinoma of the lip. *Am J Surg* 138:600, 1979.

Happner GH, Miller BE: Therapeutic implications of tumor heterogeneity. *Semin Oncol* 16:91, 1989.

Hillsmer PJ, Schuller DE, et al: Improving diagnostic accuracy of cervical metastases with computed tomography and magnetic resonance imaging. *Arch Otolaryngol Head Neck Surg* 116:1297, 1990.

Hintz B, Charyulu K, et al: Randomized study of control of the primary tumor and survival using preoperative radiation, radiation alone or surgery alone in head and neck carcinomas. *J Surg Oncol* 12:75, 1979.

Hirata RM, Jaques DA, et al: Carcinoma of the oral cavity. An analysis of 478 cases. *Ann Surg* 182(2):98, 1975.

Hong WK, Lippman SM, et al: Prevention of second primary tumors with isotretinoin in squamous-cell carcinoma of the head and neck. *N Engl J Med* 323(12):795, 1990.

Hsairi M, Luce D, et al: Risk factors for simultaneous carcinoma of the neck and neck. *Head Neck Surg* 11:426, 1989.

Ildstad ST, Bigelow ME, Remensynder JP: Intra-oral cancer at the Massachusetts General Hospital. Squamous cell carcinoma of the floor of the mouth. *Ann Surg* 197(1):34, 1983.

Ildstad ST, Bigelow ME, Remensnyder JP: Squamous cell carcinoma of the alveolar ridge and palate. A 15-year survey. *Ann Surg* 199(4):445, 1984.

Irons GB, Weiland LH, Brown WL: Paragangliomas of the neck: clinical and pathologic analysis of 116 cases. *Surg Clin North Am* 57:575, 1977.

Isaacs JH, Schnitman JR: Outcome of treatment of 160 patients with squamous cell carcinomas of the neck staged N3a. *Head Neck Surg* 12:483, 1990.

Jacobs C: Adjuvant and neoadjuvant treatment of head and neck cancers. *Semin Oncol* 18(6):504, 1991.

Johansen LV, Overgaard J, Elbrond O: Pharyngo-cutaneous fistulae after laryngectomy. *Cancer* 61:673, 1988.

Kaufman S, Lore JM: TNM classification and disease description in head and neck cancer. *Am J Surg* 136:469, 1978.

Ketcham AS, Van Buren JM: Tumors of the paranasal sinuses: a therapeutic challenge. *Am J Surg* 150:406, 1985.

Kish JA, Weaver A, et al: Cisplatin and 5-fluorouracil infusion in patients with recurrent disseminated epidermoid cancer. *Cancer* 53:1819, 1984.

Kristensen S, Voore P, et al: Nasal schneiderian papillomas: a study of 83 cases. *Clin Otolaryngol* 10:125, 1985.

Lack EE, Upton MP: Histopathologic review of salivary gland tumors in childhood. *Arch Otolaryngol Head Neck Surg* 114:898, 1988.

Lam KH, Lau WF, Wei WI: Tumor clearance of resection margins in total laryngectomy. A clinicopathologic study. *Cancer* 61:2260, 1988.

Larson DL, Kroll S, et al: Long-term effects of radiotherapy in childhood and adolescence. *Am J Surg* 160:348, 1990.

Lefebvre JL, Coche-Dequeant B, Ton Van J: Cervical lymph nodes from an unknown primary tumor in 190 patients. *Am J Surg* 160:443, 1990.

Levine LS, Johns ME: Lesions of the oral mucous membranes. *Otolaryngol Clin North Am* 19:87, 1986.

Loree TR, Strong EW: Significance of positive margins in oral cavity squamous carcinoma. *Am J Surg* 160:410, 1990.

Maran AGD, Mackenzie IJ, Stanley RE: Carcinoma in situ of the larynx. *Head Neck Surg* 7(1):28, 1984.

Mark RJ, Sercarz JA, et al: Osteogenic sarcoma of the head and neck. *Arch Otolaryngol Head Neck Surg* 117:761, 1991.

Matloub HS, Larson DL, et al: Lateral arm free flap in oral cavity reconstruction: a functional evaluation. *Head Neck Surg* 11:205, 1989.

Mazer TM, Robbins T, et al: Resection of pulmonary metastases from squamous carcinoma of the head and neck. *Am J Surg* 156:238, 1988.

McCraw JP, Dibbel DG, Carraway JH: Clinical definition of independent myocutaneous vascular territories. *Plast Reconstr Surg* 60:341, 1977.

McGregor AD, MacDonald DG: Patterns of spread of squamous cell carcinoma within the mandible. *Head Neck Surg* 11:457, 1989.

McQuarrie DG: Cancer of the tongue: selecting appropriate therapy, in Ravitch MM (ed): *Current Problems in Surgery*. Chicago: Year Book Medical Publishers, 1986, pp 562–653.

Medina JE, Myers RM: Supraomohyoid neck dissection: rationale, indications, and surgical technique. *Head Neck Surg* 11:111, 1989.

Neel HB, Taylor WF: New staging system for nasopharyngeal carcinoma: long-term outcome. *Arch Otolaryngol Head Neck Surg* 115:1293, 1989.

Newburg J, Hengerer AS: Benign diseases of the nose and paranasal sinuses, in *Textbook of Otolaryngology and Head and Neck Surgery*, Chap 16. New York, Elsevier Science Publishing Company, 1989, pp 290–303.

O'Brien CJ, Carter RL, et al: Invasion of the mandible by squamous carcinomas of the oral cavity and oropharynx. *Head Neck Surg* 8:247, 1986.

Ogura JH, Marks JE, Freeman RB: Results of conservation surgery for cancers of the supraglottis and pyriform sinus. *Laryngoscope* 90:591, 1980.

Overly WL, Jakubek DJ: Multile squamous cell carcinomas and human immunodeficiency virus infection. *Ann Intern Med* 106:334, 1987.

Papac RJ: Distant metastases from head and neck cancer. *Cancer* 53:342, 1984.

Parsons JT, Million RR, Cassisi NJ: Carcinoma of the base of the tongue: results of radial irradiation with surgery reserved for irradiation failure. *Laryngoscope* 92:689, 1982.

Pera E, Moreno A, Galindo L: Prognostic factors in laryngeal carcinoma. A multifactorial study of 416 cases. *Cancer* 58:928, 1986.

Perez CA, Simpson JR, et al: Carcinoma of the tonsillar fossa: a nonrandomized comparison of irradiation alone or combined with surgery: long-term results. *Head Neck Surg* 13(4):282, 1991.

Racz T, Sacks PG, Taylor DL: Natural killer cell lysis of head and neck cancer. *Arch Otolaryngol Head Neck Surg* 115:1322, 1989.

Raney RB, Handlee SD: Management of neoplasms of the head and neck in children: II. Malignant tumors. *Head Neck Surg* 3:500, 1981.

Rentschler RE, Wilbur DW, et al: Adjuvant methotrexate escalated to toxicity for resectable stage III and IV squamous head and neck carcinomas—a prospective, randomized study. *J Clin Oncol* 5:278, 1987.

Ring AH, Sako K, et al: Nasopharyngeal carcinoma: results of treatment over a 27 year period, 1950 through 1977. *Am J Surg* 146:429, 1983.

Robb PJ, Girling A: Granular cell myoblastoma of the supraglottis. *J Laryngol Otol* 103(3):328, 1989.

Robbins KT, Davidson W, et al: Conservation surgery for T2 and T3 carcinomas of the supraglottic larynx. *Arch Otolaryngol Head Neck Surg* 114:421, 1988.

Robbins KT, Medina JE, et al: Standardizing neck dissection terminology. Official report of the Academy's committee for head and neck surgery and oncology. *Arch Otolaryngol Head Neck Surg* 117:601, 1991.

Sanger JR, Matloub HS, Yousif NJ: Sequential connection of flaps: a logical approach to customized mandibular reconstruction. *Am J Surg* 160:402, 1990.

Santini H, Byers RM, Wolf PF: Melanoma metastatic to cervical and parotid nodes from an unknown primary site. *Am J Surg* 150:510, 1985.

Schaefer SD, Johns DF: Attaining functional esophageal speech. *Arch Otolaryngol* 108:647, 1982.

Schantz SP, Savage HE, et al: Natural killer cells and metastases from pharyngeal carcinoma. *Am J Surg* 158:361, 1989.

Schramm VL, Ettron MZ: Nasal polyps in children. *Laryngoscope* 90:1488, 1980.

Schuller DE, Reiches NA, et al: Analysis of disability resulting from treatment including radical neck dissection or modified neck dissection. *Head Neck Surg* 6:551, 1983.

Shah JP: Patterns of cervical lymph node metastases from squamous carcinoma of the upper aerodigestive tract. *Am J Surg* 160:405, 1990.

Shah JP, Loree TR, Lowalski L: Conservation surgery for radiation-failure carcinoma of the glottic larynx. *Head Neck Surg* 12:326, 1990.

Shindo ML, Stanley RB, Kiyabu MT: Carcinosarcoma of the nasal cavity and paranasal sinuses. *Head Neck Surg* 12:516, 1990.

Sigurgeirsson B, Lindelof B: Lichen planus and malignancy. *Arch Dermatol* 127:1684, 1991.

Silverman S, Gorsky M, Lozada F: Oral leukoplakia and malignant transformation. A follow-up study of 257 patients. *Cancer* 53:563, 1984.

Singer MI: Tracheoesophageal speech: vocal rehabilitation after total laryngectomy. *Laryngoscope* 93:1454, 1983.

Smith DB, Arnold JE, et al: Hereditary carcinoma syndromes associated with benign head and neck tumors. *Head Neck Surg* 11:247, 1989.

Spanos WJ Jr, Shukovsky LJ, Fletcher GH: Time, dose, and tumor volume relationships in irradiation of squamous cell carcinomas of the base of the tongue. *Cancer* 37:2591, 1976.

Spaulding CA, Krochak RJ, et al: Radiotherapeutic management of cancer of the supraglottis. *Cancer* 57:1292, 1986.

Spiro RH, Kelly J, et al: Squamous carcinoma of the posterior pharyngeal wall. *Am J Surg* 160:420, 1990.

Sprio JD, Soo KC, Spiro RH: Squamous carcinoma of the nasal cavity and paranasal sinuses. *Am J Surg* 158:328, 1989.

Sprio JD, Sprio RH: Carcinoma of the tonsillar fossa. An update. *Arch Otolaryngol Head Neck Surg* 115:1186, 1989.

Spitz MR, Fueger JJ, et al: Salivary gland cancer. *Arch Otolaryngol Head Neck Surg* 116:1163, 1990.

Stern SJ, Thomsen S, et al: Photodynamic therapy with chloroaluminum-sulfonated phthalocyanine. *Arch Otolaryngol Head Neck Surg* 116:1259, 1990.

Sultan MR, Coleman JJ III: Oncologic and functional considerations of total glossectomy. *Am J Surg* 158:297, 1989.

Telander RL, Deane SA: Thyroglossal and brachial clef cysts and sinuses. *Surg Clin North Am* 57:779, 1977.

Thawley SE, May M, Ogura JM: Granular cell myoblastoma. *Laryngoscope* 84:1545, 1974.

Toroledo ME, Luna MA, Batsakis JG: Carcinomas ex pleomorphic adenoma and malignant mixed tumors: histomorphologic indexes. *Arch Otolaryngol* 110:172, 1984.

van den Brekel MWM, Castelijns JA, et al: Magnetic resonance imaging vs palpation of cervical lymph node metastasis. *Arch Otolaryngol Head Neck Surg* 117:666, 1991.

Vikram B, Strong EW, et al: Failure in the neck following multimodality treatment for advanced head and neck cancer. *Head Neck Surg* 6:724, 1984.

Wald RM, Calcaterra TC: Lower alveolar carcinoma. *Arch Otolaryngol* 109:578, 1983.

Wang RC, Geopfert H, et al: Unknown primary squamous cell carcinoma metastatic to the neck. *Arch Otolaryngol Head Neck Surg* 116:1388, 1990.

Weber RS, Gidley P, et al: Treatment selection for carcinoma of the base of the tongue. *Am J Surg* 160:415, 1990.

Weichselbaum RR, Dunphy EJ, et al: Epidermal growth factor receptor gene amplification and expression in head and neck cancer cell lines. *Head Neck Surg* 11:437, 1989.

Wenig BM, Hyams VJ, Heffner DK: Moderately differentiated neuroendocrine carcinoma of the larynx. A clinicopathologic study of 54 cases. *Cancer* 62:2658, 1988.

Wenig B, Kurtzman DM, et al: Photodynamic therapy in the treatment of squamous cell carcinoma of the head and neck. *Arch Otolaryngol Head Neck Surg* 116:1267, 1990.

Woods JE, Chong GC, Beahrs OH: Experience with 1,360 primary parotid tumors. *Am J Surg* 130:460, 1975.

Yamamoto E, Miyakawa A, Kohama G: Mode of invasion and lymph node metastasis in squamous cell carcinoma of the oral cavity. *Head Neck Surg* 6:938, 1984.

Zarbo RJ, Crissman JD: The surgical pathology of head and neck cancer. *Semin Oncol* 15(1):10, 1988.

Zelefsky MJ, Harrison LB, et al: Postoperative radiotherapy for oral cavity cancers: impact of anatomic subsite on treatment outcome. *Head Neck Surg* 12:470, 1990.

Zunt SL, Tomich CE: Oral hairy leukoplakia. *J Dermatol Surg* 16(9):812, 1990.

CHAPTER 16

Chest Wall, Pleura, Lung, and Mediastinum

Thomas C. King and Craig R. Smith

INTRODUCTION

Life depends on a delicate sequence of events that moves air to blood and blood to tissues. The cardiorespiratory system functions to assure that those events occur dependably; the margin of error is extremely small. The analysis and management of surgical concerns involving the chest and its contents, whether relating to tumors, trauma, or infection, all focus on the mechanical transport of oxygen to the vital organs and the necessary exchange of gases. Air with adequate oxygen content must pass through the upper airway, the trachea, and the bronchi to reach the alveoli properly warmed and humidified for movement across alveolar membranes. Those membranes must be in condition to allow efficient diffusion of oxygen and carbon dioxide. Blood with sufficient oxygen-carrying capacity must be circulating through the alveolar capillaries in adequate volumes and at the proper speed to allow pickup of oxygen and discharge of carbon dioxide; it must also be at the proper pH and temperature and must have the proper biochemical characteristics for optimum exchange. The vascular system must have the appropriate integrity, pressure gradients, volume, and flow dynamics to traverse the pumps and conduits from alveolar capillaries to vital organ capillaries and back. At the vital organ interface, the characteristics for release from the blood to the tissues of oxygen, and recapture of carbon dioxide must be present. Irreparable damage to vital organs may occur in minutes if any part of the system fails.

The early history of thoracic surgery was limited to the management of trauma and was closely linked to the history of weaponry. Management of chest wounds received in battle was recorded in ancient writings, including the *Iliad* (ca. 950 B.C.). Galen described a patient who recovered after partial excision of the sternum and pericardium for recurrent abscess due to an injury. Writing about chest wounds in the thirteenth century, Theodoric noted that "the stitches should be placed . . . so that the natural heat cannot escape in any way nor the air outside be able to enter."

The introduction of firearms in the fourteenth century complicated the management of chest wounds. The proper care of the open pneumothorax remained unsettled for centuries. Consistent with many of his other revolutionary insights, Napoleon's surgeon, Baron Larrey, confirmed the sporadic observations of other surgeons about the lifesaving value of closing an open wound of the thorax. His description of the cardiopulmonary effects of an open chest wound can hardly be improved upon:

> *A soldier was brought to the hospital of the Fortress of Ibrahyn Bey, immediately after a wound penetrated the thorax, between the fifth and sixth true ribs. It was about 8 cm in extent. A large quantity of frothy and vermilion blood escaped from it with a hissing noise at each inspiration. His extremities were cold, pulse scarcely perceptible, countenance discolored, and respiration short and laborious; in short, he was every moment threatened with a fatal suffocation. After having examined the wound, the divided edges of the part, I immediately approximated the two lips of the wound, and retained them by means of adhesive plaster and a suitable bandage around the body. In adopting this plan, I intended only to hide from the sight of the patient and his comrades, the distressing spectacle of a hemorrhage, which would soon prove fatal; and I, therefore, thought that the effusion of blood into the cavity of the thorax, could not increase the danger. But the wound was scarcely closed, when he breathed more freely, and felt easier. The heat of the body soon returned, and the pulse rose. In a few hours he became quite calm, and to my great surprise grew better. He was cured in a very few days, and without difficulty.*

The development of elective thoracic surgery over the past century has followed closely the history of airway management, particularly techniques for tracheal intubation and positive-pressure ventilation. By the late nineteenth century, open thoracic procedures were successfully performed on large animals along with experimentation on mechanical maintenance of ventilation. In 1904, Sauerbruch developed a negative-pressure chamber in which the operating team and the patient could be housed during operation. Under these conditions, the lung would not collapse when the chest was open. Although animal experiments produced some success, operations on patients were not rewarding. Orotracheal intubation with metal tubes for the treatment of croup and for the prevention of aspiration during oral surgical procedures provided the early experience that led to positive-pressure endotracheal anesthesia for thoracic surgery.

Over the first third of this century individual surgeons were devising and reporting imaginative techniques to control the open pneumothorax associated with chest operations. These included hand bellows and tracheostomy devices as developed and modified by Fell (1883), O'Dwyer (1896), and Matas (1900), as well as various packing techniques, preoperative pneumothorax for "conditioning," and suturing the lung to the parietal pleura. Improvements in laryngotracheal intubation techniques, in design and materials of endotracheal tubes, and in anesthesia gradually displaced these improvisations.

Though somewhat overshadowed by the dramatic developments in cardiac surgery, significant recent diagnostic, technical, and therapeutic progress has been occurring in other areas of thoracic surgery. The terrible public health consequences of tobacco addiction continue to dominate clinical practice as the long-predicted increase in cancers among smoking women has finally succeeded in making lung cancer the most common cancer killer of women as well as men. The evidence implicating side-stream smoke in health problems of nonsmokers, particularly children is now believed firmly. New imaging techniques are making important improvements in the accuracy of diagnosis and staging of intrathoracic diseases. Our evolving skills in fiberoptic endoscopy have opened new diagnostic and therapeutic opportunities in an increasing variety of intrathoracic disorders. These techniques are resulting in early detection and surgical resection of some tumors in a preclinical stage and yielding "cure" rates previously considered unobtainable. Some unanticipatedly encouraging results appear after multimodal therapy with chemotherapy and radiation therapy as pre- or postoperative adjuvant therapy for patients with lung cancer. The diagnostic and/or therapeutic role of immunohistochemical techniques, including monoclonal antibodies, remains uncertain, although research in the field continues to provide encouraging findings that predict exciting future contributions. Many centers report success with heart-lung and single- or double-lung transplantation applied to the management of patients with a variety of end-stage cardiopulmonary and pulmonary diseases. Donor shortage remains the factor limiting a wider application of this therapeutically successful approach.

ANATOMY OF THE THORAX AND PLEURA

The clinician's ability to correlate thoracic diseases with underlying anatomy is improved because many of the bony parts of the

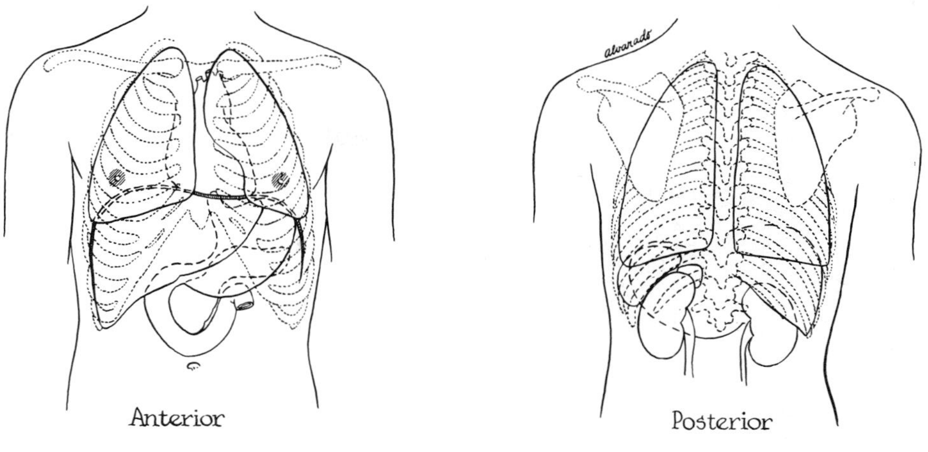

FIG. 16-1. The relationship of the thoracic cage to the upper abdominal viscera must be remembered to avoid overlooking concomitant abdominal injuries in patients with thoracic trauma.

thoracic cage are palpable and cardiac and breath sounds are transmitted through the chest wall. There are a number of anatomic factors that can be quite misleading and lead to errors of analysis and judgment. The ''squaring off'' effect of the shoulder girdle gives the chest the physical appearance of a rectangle, tempting the examiner to forget that the skeletal chest wall is conical in shape, tapering quite sharply in the upper chest. The diaphragm rises as high as the level of the nipple; the upper part of the abdomen is overlapped by six of the ten anterior ribs and the lower four posterior ribs. The lung apices rise well above the level of the clavicles anteriorly and the scapula posteriorly. These easily overlooked anatomic facts can lead to serious errors, especially in patients with penetrating trauma (Fig. 16-1). The lower ribs and costal margin overlap the liver, spleen, stomach, the upper pole of both kidneys, and the distal part of the pancreas.

The framework of the thoracic cage consists of the sternum, twelve thoracic vertebrae, ten pairs of ribs that end anteriorly in segments of cartilage, and two pairs of floating ribs. The thoracic inlet is characterized by having a rigid structural ring formed by the sternal manubrium, the short, semicircular first ribs, and the vertebral column. As a result of its articulation with the manubrium and the attachment of the costoclavicular ligament, the clavicle participates in providing protection for the underlying vascular and neural structures that traverse the thoracic inlet. The same rigidity that provides protection from trauma, however, leaves little room for pathologic swelling, enlarging masses, or postural adjustments with age.

The cartilages of the first six ribs have separate articulations with the sternum; the cartilages of the seventh through the tenth ribs fuse to form the costal margin before attaching to the lower margin of the sternum. As there is significant flexibility of the chest wall in children, serious trauma can be transmitted to the intrathoracic structures with little injury to the bony framework. Even though this flexibility decreases progressively with age, surprising damage can occasionally occur in the chest of adults without evidence of skeletal injury.

The pectoralis major and minor muscles constitute the principal muscular covering of the anterior thorax, and the lower margin of the pectoralis major forms the anterior axillary fold. Auscultation of the chest in the axilla often allows the best determination of breath sounds, because the thoracic cage is covered only by the origins of the serratus anterior muscle in that location. The long thoracic nerve passes vertically on the axillary surface of that muscle—a point to be remembered when doing a thoracentesis or tube thoracostomy. A convergence of the latissimus dorsi and teres major muscles forms the posterior axillary fold on each side. The triangle of auscultation can often be palpated near the inferior medial border of the scapula, but the latissimus, trapezius, rhomboid, and other shoulder girdle muscles form a strong muscular coat for the posterior thorax. A disadvantage of the heavy muscle coat is the difficulty in accurately identifying specific ribs by palpation of the posterior chest wall.

The sternal angle is almost always palpable, and this allows quick identification of the second rib because of its articulation with the sternum at this location. A plane that is parallel to the floor and passes through the sternal angle of an upright patient will also pass through the fourth or fifth thoracic vertebra. The tracheal bifurcation lies in this same plane, while the apex of the aortic arch is located slightly higher. There is a gradual increase in the length of ribs from the first to the seventh and a progressive lateral displacement of the rib–costal cartilage junctions. Because of the radiolucency of the cartilages, standard anteroposterior chest x-rays may fail to document injury to the thoracic cage even though a severe blunt injury to the chest has disarticulated and fractured multiple costal cartilages.

The pleura is a serous membrane of flat mesothelial cells overlying a thin layer of connective tissue in which a vascular and lymphatic network is distributed. That part covering the lungs is referred to as the visceral pleura, and it is continuous over the pulmonary hilus and the mediastinum with the parietal pleura, which covers the inside of the chest wall and the diaphragm. While it is convenient to consider the pleura as a closed sac around the pleural cavity, that model encourages a static model that misrepresents a highly dynamic structure. The pleural surfaces behave more like a flowing syncytium across which fluids actively move (from visceral pleura to parietal pleura), actively phagocytosing cells and debris and sealing air leaks and capillary leaks. It is this physiologically active membrane that contributes to the general resistance of the pleural space to infection and the lung's remarkable ability to tolerate the trauma of surgery or injury with such a low frequency of persisting air-leak problems. With normal lung expansion the pleural cavity is completely filled and only a potential space exists. As shown in Fig. 16-2, the line of pleural reflection extends slightly beyond the lung border in each direction. This is expected because of the dynamic process of respiration and the need for the pleural sac to accommodate maximum lung expansion with deep inspiration. Conversely, with acute decreases in lung volume, such as that with lobar atelectasis, there is a limit to the

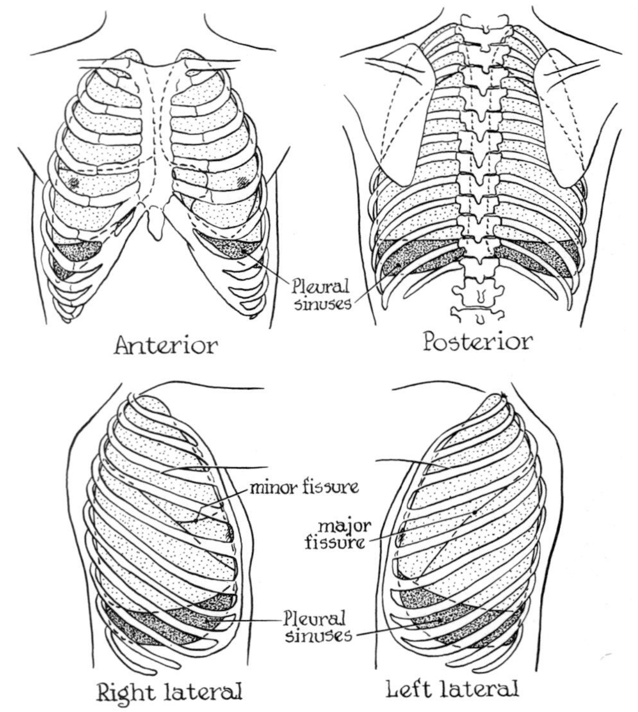

FIG. 16-2. The relation of the pulmonary lobes and pleural sinuses to the chest wall.

pleural accommodation and fluid may be drawn into the pleural cavity to replace partially the lost lung volume.

There is no communication between the pleural cavities, but the anteromedial borders of the two pleural sacs come nearly into apposition behind the sternum. The interior border of each pleural cavity is located at the ninth rib in the midaxillary line, and the borders continue posteriorly in the eleventh intercostal space. Occasionally the pleural sac extends as low as the twelfth rib. Posteriorly, the margins of the two pleural sacs lie on the anterolateral surfaces of the vertebrae, separated by the esophagus. A retroesophageal recess is occasionally formed when the pleural margins are in near apposition, and pulmonary lesions arising in the recess are easily mistaken for mediastinal tumors or cysts. At the inferior margin of the lung hilus on each side, a double layer of mediastinal pleura is formed, the inferior pulmonary ligament.

The structures that occupy the intercostal spaces have considerable significance in relation to thoracic function, disease, and diagnostic procedures. The parietal pleura, for example, is well supplied with nerve endings for pain, while the visceral pleura is insensitive. Only when pulmonary disease extends to involve the parietal pleura or chest wall is pain produced. Figure 16-3 shows the structures in an intercostal space and emphasizes the layering effect of the muscles and fascia. Three layers of intercostal muscles are present in a major part of the thoracic wall, but some anatomists consider the innermost and the internal intercostals to be a single muscle entity. With quiet respiration the ribs are elevated by synchronous contraction of the intercostal muscles. Because the ribs of each side move as a unit in respiration, a localized painful lesion may eliminate effective function of the entire side. During quiet respiration, however, movements of the diaphragm provide approximately 75 percent of pulmonary ventilation, and temporary loss of unilateral intercostal muscle function is not a threat to breathing. With labored breathing, the muscles of the upper extremity and those cervical muscles that attach to the chest wall assist in elevation and expansion of the thorax.

The endothoracic fascia is a layer of light areolar tissue subjacent to the parietal pleura. At the apex of each hemithorax it is thickened into a more substantial layer referred to as Sibson's fascia.

The vein, artery, and nerve of each interspace are located deep to the external and internal intercostal muscles and lie just behind the lower margin of the rib. For most interspaces a smaller collateral artery runs along the top border of the rib below. There is significant overlap of neural supply by adjacent nerves, and complete anesthesia in an interspace will generally not occur unless the intercostal nerve of the adjacent space above and below and the space in question are anesthetized. To minimize the risk of lacerating the intercostal artery, a thoracentesis needle or a clamp used to perforate the pleura for insertion of a catheter should be passed across the top of the lower rib of the selected interspace.

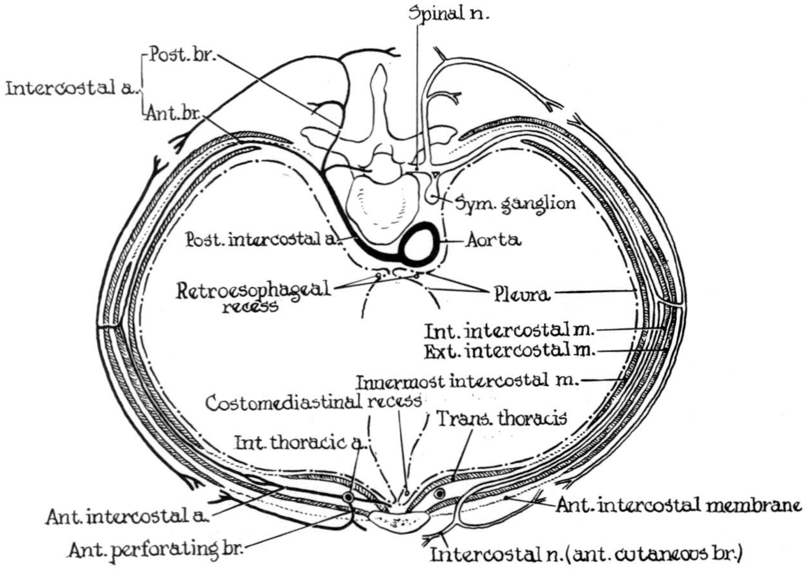

FIG. 16-3. An illustration of the structures within an intercostal space. (Modified from: *Blevins CE: Anatomy of the thorax and pleura, in Shields TW (ed): General Thoracic Surgery, 2d ed. Philadelphia, Lea & Febiger, 1983, with permission.*)

The lymphatic drainage of the chest wall extends in both anterior and posterior directions. Lymph draining from the anterior region of the first four or five intercostal spaces passes to lymph nodes along the internal thoracic arteries. These nodes may be connected by cross anastomoses before draining into a single or double trunk that joins the thoracic duct, a right lymphatic duct, or a bronchomediastinal trunk. Lymphatics that drain the posterior and lateral regions of the intercostal spaces are tributary to lymph nodes that lie near the vertebral ends of each interspace. In the lower part of the thorax these nodes join the drainage from the posterior mediastinum to contribute to the cisterna chyli. The posterior lymph nodes of the upper thorax drain into the thoracic duct or a right lymphatic duct.

A musculofibrous floor is provided for the thorax by the diaphragm. The peripheral muscular portions of the diaphragm arise from the lower six ribs and costal cartilages, from the lumbar vertebrae (right and left crus), and from the lumbocostal arches. Additional fibers arise from the xiphoid cartilages, and all the muscular elements converge into the central tendon. The central part of the tendon underlies the pericardium, while the right and left divisions extend posteriorly. Some of the lower intercostal nerves are thought to contribute to the sensory innervation of the diaphragm, but motor innervation is supplied by the phrenic nerve on each side.

Of the three major openings in the diaphragm the aortic hiatus is most posterior. The aorta, azygos vein, and thoracic duct pass through this opening. The esophageal hiatus transmits the esophagus and vagus nerves, and only the inferior vena cava goes through the foramen of that name.

Contemporary imaging techniques (including computer-analyzed tomographic and nuclear-magnetic resonance scanning) have increased the clinician's ability to identify anatomic relationships and their clinical significance. They have dramatically altered the preoperative assessment of both pulmonary and mediastinal lesions.

Figure 16-4 shows the cross-sectional anatomy at four different levels in the thorax associated with identifiable topographical landmarks. These studies provide considerable anatomic clarification of intrathoracic problems.

THORACIC INCISIONS

A basic knowledge of the incisions used to perform thoracic operations is helpful in understanding the postoperative course of patients and in managing complications. Because of the rigidity of the thoracic cage, most incisions for major procedures are relatively large and disrupt the integrity of muscles and bone, or cartilage, although contemporary anesthetic intubation techniques allowing single-lung anesthesia have made less destructive incisions feasible in most cases.

There are three principal approaches to the intrathoracic contents: (1) lateral thoracotomy, performed as either an anterolateral, midlateral (muscle-sparing), or posterolateral incision; (2) median sternotomy, performed as a vertical, sternal-splitting incision; and (3) minimally invasive video-thoracoscopy.

Other incisions are infrequently used, either because experience has shown them to be inferior, or because they are useful only in unusual circumstances. The thoracoabdominal incision combines an upper abdominal incision with an incision in a lower intercostal space (sixth, seventh, or eighth) that may be carried as far posteriorly as the posterior axillary line. The costal margin and diaphragm are divided to provide an extensive exposure of the upper part of the abdomen and the retroperitoneal and posterior thoracic structures. Prolonged pain associated with incomplete healing of the costal margin, as well as complicated wound management involving two body cavities if infection occurs, has reduced the enthusiasm for this incision. Though elective use of this disabling incision is becoming less common, it is still useful for certain operations involving retroperitoneal structures (kidney, thoracoabdominal aorta), and it may be appropriate for hepatic or thoracoabdominal trauma under emergency conditions.

A bilateral anterior thoracotomy incision with transection of the sternum was the routine operative approach to the heart and mediastinum before confidence was gained in the median sternotomy. It has now resurfaced as the preferred incision for double-lung transplantation. It is also useful in circumstances where the instruments necessary to perform median sternotomy are not available and there is urgent need to have access to both sides of the mediastinum. It also provides some cosmetic advantage in young women where bilateral submammary incisions leave much less disfiguring scars than the median sternotomy. The median sternotomy can be carried out through a submammary incision with large skin flaps, although an hypesthetic nipple is a relatively frequent complication of this approach.

The lateral muscle-sparing incision is rapidly gaining favor, but the anterolateral and posterolateral thoracotomy incisions remain the most frequently used for general thoracic operations. Each one requires division of one or more major shoulder-girdle muscles and this results in voluntary restriction of shoulder motion in the early postoperative period. All patients must be encouraged to begin active shoulder and arm motion after operation, but elderly patients are especially likely to develop a restricted range of shoulder motion if not supervised carefully. The distal parts of the transected muscles lose their nerve supply and atrophy to a significant degree postoperatively. Commonly, patients note a zone of reduced sensation in the skin on the caudal side of the incision for months after operation.

The posterolateral thoracotomy has traditionally been used for the majority of pulmonary resections (except lung biopsy), for esophageal operations, and for the approach to the posterior mediastinum and the vertebral column (Fig. 16-5). When the intent is to enter the pleural cavity in the fifth intercostal space, the most common selection, the skin incision is begun at the anterior axillary line just below the nipple level in the male, and at the corresponding position in the female. The incision extends posteriorly below the tip of the scapula and ascends midway between the vertebral border of the scapula and the spinous processes of the vertebrae. To expose the thoracic cage it is necessary to divide part of the serratus anterior, latissimus dorsi, trapezius, and rhomboid major muscles. The pleural cavity can be entered by dividing the intercostal muscles in the chosen interspace, or by resecting the posterior two-thirds of the corresponding rib. The division of the rib posteriorly before the mechanical rib spreader is put in place may avoid accidental fracture of one or more ribs or a costochondral separation by the instrument. The injury to the rib or cartilage may increase postoperative incisional pain and prolong the restricted motion of the chest cage.

Two advantages of the anterolateral thoracotomy may be important for trauma victims and for patients with unstable cardiovascular systems. The incision allows rapid entry into the chest, and the patient may be placed in the semisupine position on the operating table. This is tolerated better than the lateral decubitus position, and it gives the anesthesiologist maximum control over the patient's cardiorespiratory system. The incision may be used

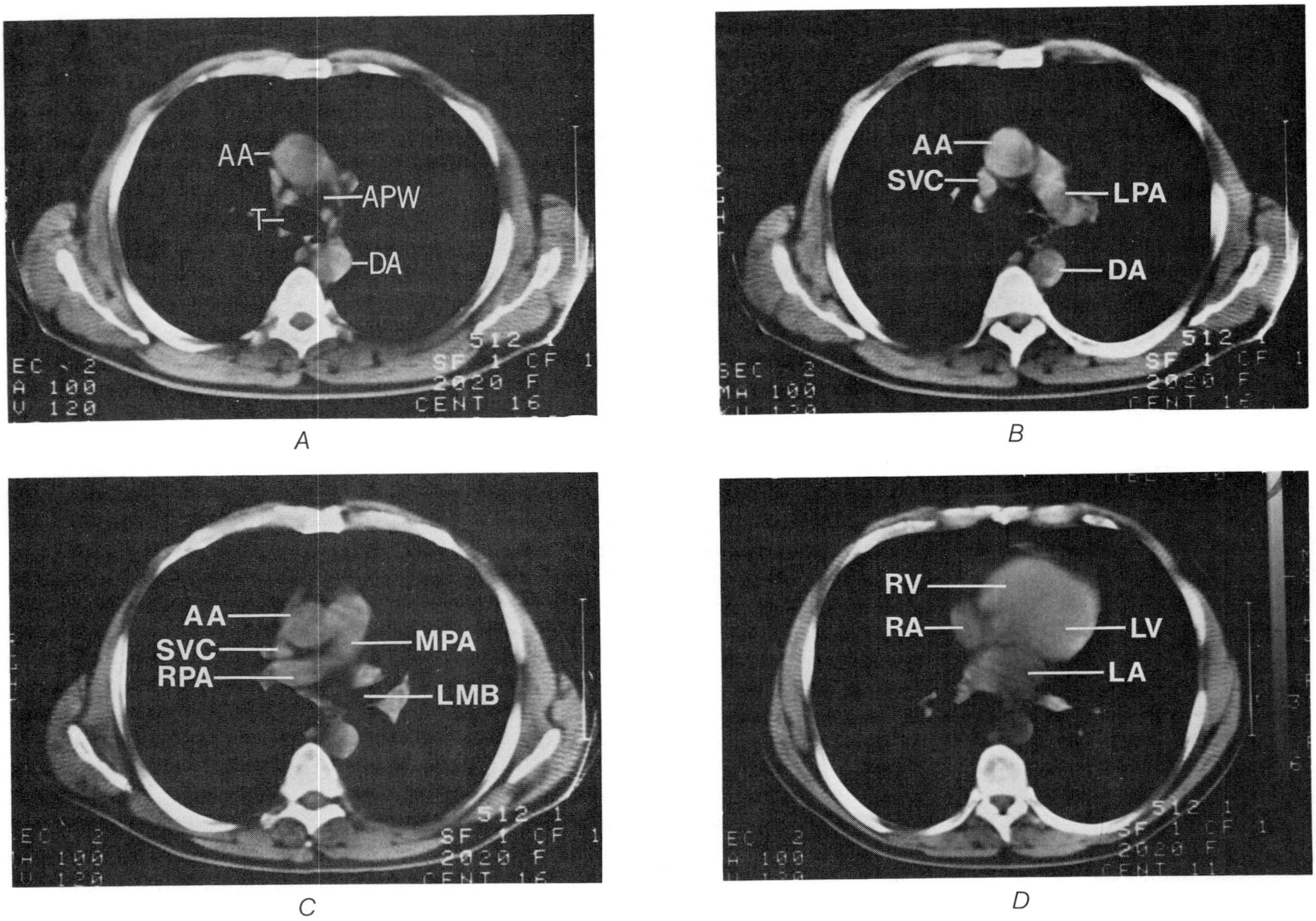

FIG. 16-4. Transverse sectional anatomy at four levels as shown by a CT scan of the thorax in a normal person. *A.* A transverse section at the level of the tracheal bifurcation outlines the aortico-pulmonary window, a frequent site of mediastinal lymph-node metastases in patients with bronchogenic carcinoma arising in the left lung. *B.* A section 1 cm inferior to *A* shows the origin of the left pulmonary artery and an air bubble in the esophagus as it lies immediately posterior to the origin of the left main-stem bronchus. *C.* The origin and course of the right pulmonary artery are shown at this level, and the left-upper-lobe bronchus is seen at its origin from the left main bronchus. *D.* At a lower level in the thorax the more complex mediastinal anatomy gives way to the cardiac chambers and pulmonary veins. AA = ascending aorta, DA = descending aorta, APW = aortico-pulmonary window, T = trachea, SVC = superior vena cava, LPA = left pulmonary artery, MPA = main pulmonary artery, RPA = right pulmonary artery, LMB = left main bronchus, RA = right atrium, RV = right ventricle, LA = left ventricle.

for mediastinal operations, for some cardiac procedures, and for wedge resections of the upper and middle lobes of the lung. The preferred approach is a submammary skin incision starting at the sternal border overlying the fourth intercostal space and extending to the midaxillary line. The pectoralis major muscle and part of the pectoralis minor are divided at the level of the fourth or fifth intercostal space, and the incision is extended into the serratus anterior. By extending the chosen intercostal muscle incision posteriorly along the top of the subjacent rib it is possible to obtain a wider opening in the chest than the length of the skin incision would suggest. Still more exposure can be obtained by transecting the sternum.

Because most advances in thoracic surgery have followed improvements in techniques of managing the airway, the recent widespread introduction of the double-lumen endotracheal tube has made it possible to utilize a less destructive midlateral thoracotomy incision. This incision has evolved from the transaxillary approach through the bed of the third rib that has been used extensively in some clinics for upper-lobe biopsies, for resection of small apical pulmonary blebs and pleural abrasion in patients with recurrent pneumothorax, for upper thoracic sympathectomy, and for biopsy of upper mediastinal lymph nodes or masses. By moving down the lateral chest wall several ribs, and with the advantage that single-lung anesthesia allows, good exposure can be obtained for most pulmonary resections and hilar dissections. The incision has the advantage that it requires cutting no major muscles, can be rapidly made and closed, and results in significantly less postoperative discomfort. An important requirement for adequate exposure in the incision is proper positioning of the patient. The patient is placed in a straight lateral position with the arm at right angles (in order to facilitate mobility of the scapula). The skin incision parallels the course of the fifth rib extending from a few centimeters

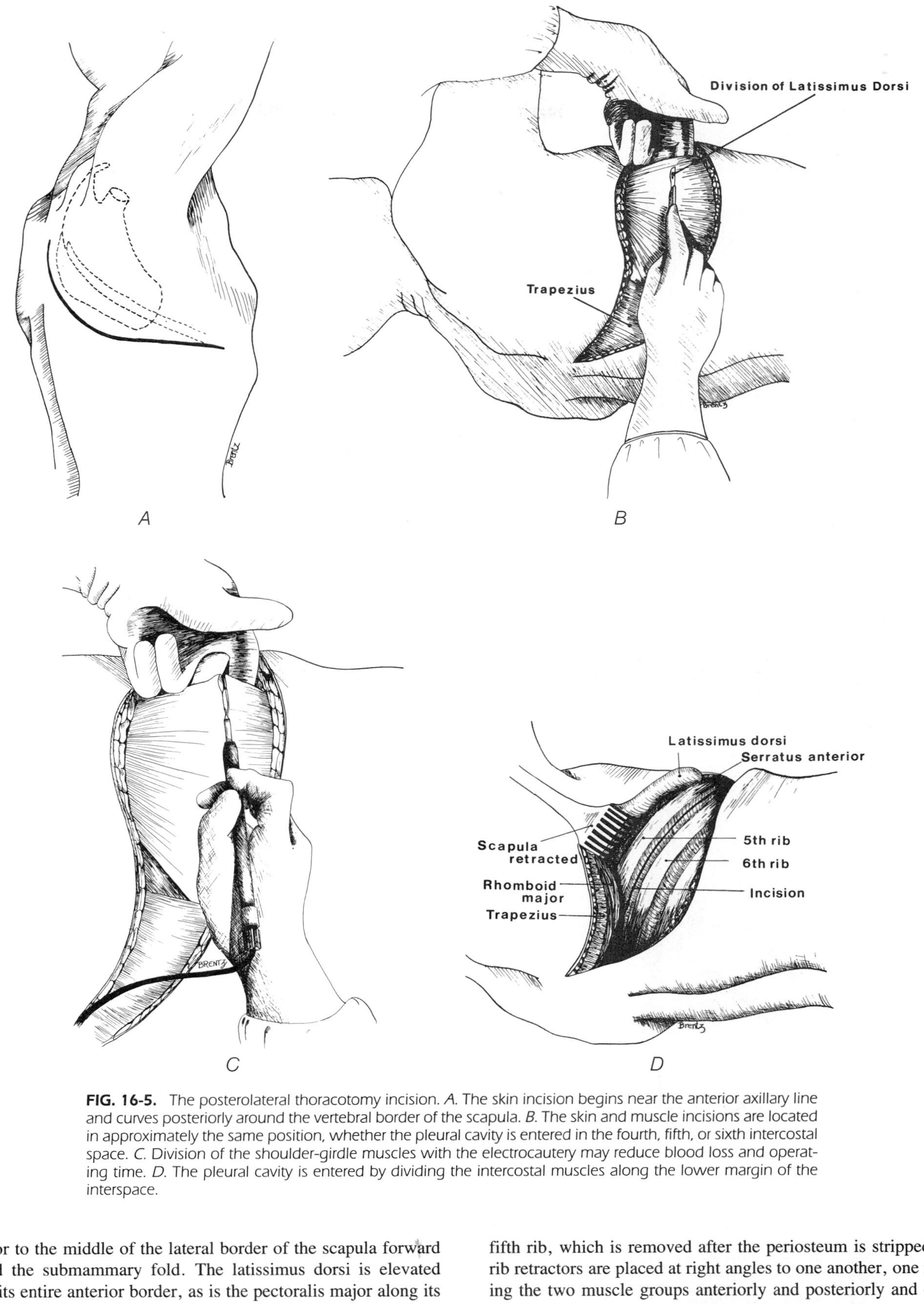

FIG. 16-5. The posterolateral thoracotomy incision. *A.* The skin incision begins near the anterior axillary line and curves posteriorly around the vertebral border of the scapula. *B.* The skin and muscle incisions are located in approximately the same position, whether the pleural cavity is entered in the fourth, fifth, or sixth intercostal space. *C.* Division of the shoulder-girdle muscles with the electrocautery may reduce blood loss and operating time. *D.* The pleural cavity is entered by dividing the intercostal muscles along the lower margin of the interspace.

anterior to the middle of the lateral border of the scapula forward toward the submammary fold. The latissimus dorsi is elevated along its entire anterior border, as is the pectoralis major along its axillary border. The serratus is separated from its insertion into the fifth rib, which is removed after the periosteum is stripped. Two rib retractors are placed at right angles to one another, one retracting the two muscle groups anteriorly and posteriorly and one retracting the ribs caudad and cephalad (Fig. 16-6).

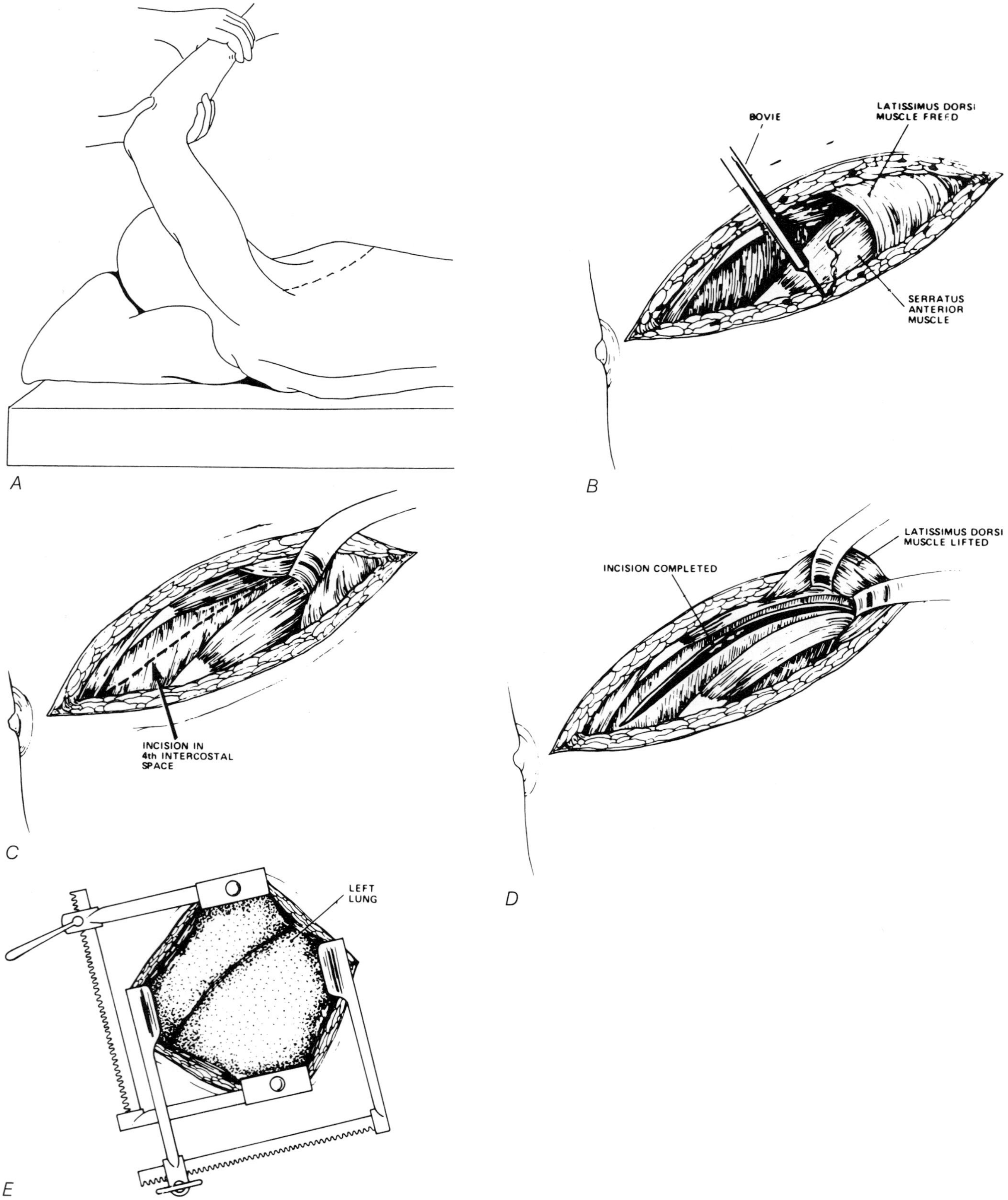

FIG. 16-6. *A.* Approach to the left pleural space via modified lateral thoracotomy. The modified lateral (axillary) thoracotomy requires minimal muscle division and yields good exposure of the pleural cavity. Entry is made through the bed of the fifth rib. The anterior end of the skin incision is in the submammary fold. One-lung anesthesia (the double-lumen endotracheal tube) is essential for adequate exposure. (From: *Mitchell R, Angell W, et al, with permission.*)

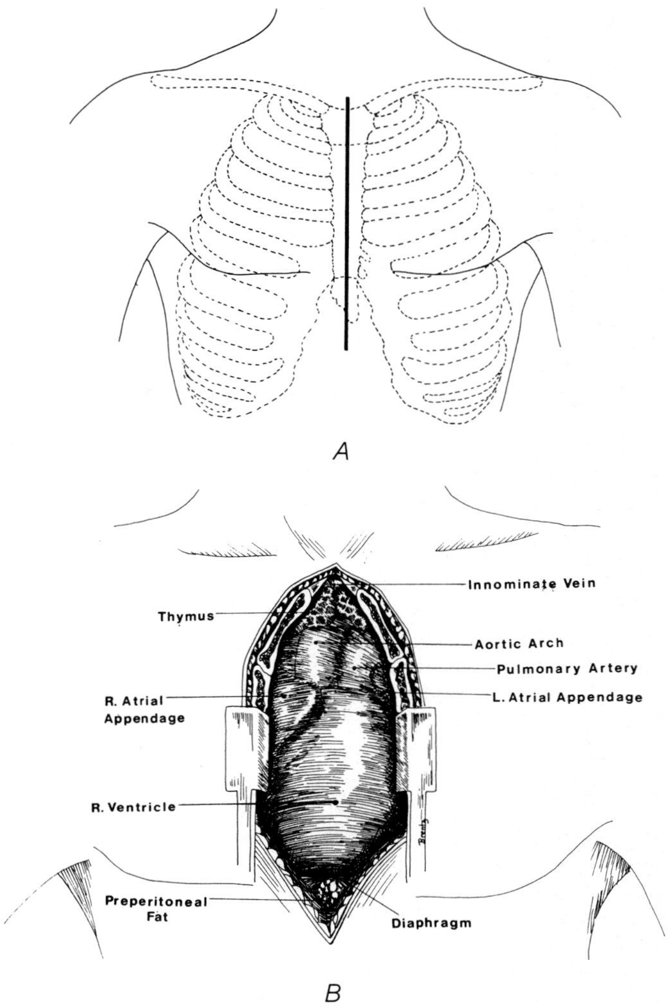

FIG. 16-7. *A.* A median sternotomy incision is outlined. *B.* Exposure of a pleural space would be made optimum by placement of mechanical retractor, rotating the patient slightly, and the use of single-lung anesthesia.

A hazard that is common to all the lateral thoracotomy incisions is the potential for injury to the brachial plexus and the axillary neurovascular structures from excessive displacement of the shoulder in positioning the patient on the operating table after anesthesia has been induced. By preventing posterior displacement of the shoulder this complication can be minimized.

The median sternotomy incision provides optimum exposure for anterior mediastinal lesions, and it is the principal incision used for cardiac operations. Either pleural cavity may be entered, or incision into the pleural cavity may be avoided if it is unnecessary. Disadvantages of the incision include an increased risk of infection if it is necessary to do a tracheostomy within a few days after operation, and the protracted course that occurs with infection because of involvement of the sternal fragments. An occasional patient who develops an acute wound infection also develops a severe mediastinitis associated with dehiscence of the sternal wound. The morbidity of this complication is high but has decreased with the evolution of effective treatment, including particularly mobilization of vascularized pedicle flaps of various trunk muscle groups.

The skin incision extends from just below the suprasternal notch to a point several centimeters below the xiphoid process (Fig. 16-7). Either an oscillating saw or a Lebsche knife and mallet may be used to split the sternum. A mechanical retractor is used to spread the incision, but the retractor blades may fracture the sternal halves with excessive pressure. Less commonly, there may be injury to the C_8–T_1 component of the brachial plexus, thought to be due to excessive spreading of the sternal halves and high placement of the retractor blades. In some instances a posterior fracture of the first rib can be demonstrated with special rib radiographs. After operation, patients who have had a sternotomy have less pain and less interference with pulmonary function than those who have had a lateral thoracotomy.

The rigid thoracoscope has been used for many years, particularly in Europe, for diagnostic visualization of the pleural space. Following upon the dramatic recent successful applications of video-endoscopic technology and techniques to surgery of the joints, gallbladder, and an increasing variety of intraperitoneal procedures, thoracic surgeons throughout Europe and North America have been searching to define the proper place for application of video-thoracoscopy to definitive resective and reparative surgery within the pleural space. Many reports have validated its use for the management of recurring pneumothorax with and without persisting air leaks as well as in performing biopsies of the lung and of pleural-based tumors. Isolated reports of major lobar resections and mediastinal nodal dissections have suggested we will be expanding our capability in this direction significantly over the next few years as surgeon-engineers direct their attention toward the development of specialized tools that may allow the surgeon to safely perform many of the current operations we do in the chest without subjecting all patients to the fear and morbidity of the formal thoracotomy.

The pleural cavity is usually drained with one or two chest tubes connected to an underwater seal system at the conclusion of the intrathoracic portion of the operation. Each chest tube should be brought through a separate stab wound in the chest wall at least two interspaces away from the incision. If the pleural cavity is not entered in operations through a median sternotomy, it is advisable to drain the retrosternal space for 24 h with an intercostal tube that is brought out through a stab wound in the epigastrium.

PATIENT EVALUATION

Since all operations on the chest result in some short-term respiratory disability, and many require removal or permanent alterations in function of intrathoracic organs, the surgeon must make a careful assessment of the patient's ability to withstand the contemplated procedure. This assessment includes most components of the patient's overall state of health.

The history and physical examination, with the consequence of thoracotomy in mind, constitute the foundation of each patient's evaluation. If the patient is in good health, young, and has normal values for the hospital admission blood tests and urinalysis, little further evaluation may be necessary. Since most candidates for thoracic operations, however, are beyond middle age, are former or active smokers, have chronic bronchitis, and have some symptoms or signs of chronic obstructive pulmonary disease (COPD), careful inquiry and examination for evidence of preexisting impairment in pulmonary or cardiac reserve is essential. The patient who can climb two flights of stairs at a steady pace without dyspnea or wheezing probably has the strength, endurance, and reserve for an uncomplicated postoperative course. Any history of exercise intolerance, dyspnea on exertion, wheezing, smoking, productive cough or physical findings of obesity, clubbing, tobacco-stained fingers, or poor oral hygiene require further evaluation and preoperative preparation. All thoracotomy patients experience some compromise in their cardiopulmonary function postoperatively, particularly if some lung tissue is resected. For those with preexisting impairment, this additional deterioration in pulmonary reserve may lead to critical operative and postoperative problems unless carefully evaluated preoperatively in order to give the surgeon reliable guidelines about how much pulmonary tissue the patient can safely lose. During an operation, one lung will be unventilated during isolation by use of the double-lumen endotracheal tube by retraction or displacement during the procedure and will contribute little, if any, to respiratory gas exchange. Further, it may be necessary to retract intermittently against the pericardium interfering with venous return to the atria or precipitating brief arrhythmias. Therefore, the functional status of the contralateral lung and the presence of preexisting cardiac disease are major determinants of the safety of the operation.

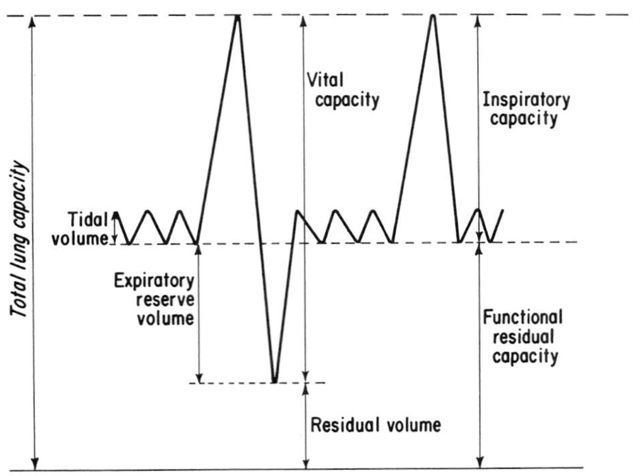

FIG. 16-8. The lung volumes and their subdivisions related to a spirograph tracing. Functional residual capacity and residual volume must be measured by other techniques.

Pulmonary Function. The major consideration in evaluating the potential thoracotomy patient is whether or not the pulmonary function is adequate to tolerate the operation, the handicaps of the postoperative period, and the long-term functional demands. There are few frustrations that match that experienced by the surgeon and patient who have successfully struggled through a difficult operation and postoperative course to discover the patient is a bed-to-chair pulmonary cripple. When the planned operation will result in a loss of functioning pulmonary tissue (lobectomy, pneumonectomy), there is a hazard that such postoperative respiratory insufficiency could result if the patient's preoperative pulmonary function is already compromised. Carefully performed spirometry forms the basis of the pulmonary-function data most used by thoracic surgeons, and the advances in technology with automated data processing allow most hospitals to have excellent pulmonary-function capability. Also, the development of electronic spirometers for office use makes it possible to perform screening tests during outpatient evaluation. If a patient has reduced pulmonary function, it is possible to begin a plan of management and determine progress before hospitalization. Figure 16-8 illustrates the subdivisions of lung volume in relation to a spirographic tracing.

Vital capacity (VC), the amount of air that can be forcefully expelled from a maximally inflated lung position, can be a useful determination if its limitations are accepted. The predicted value decreases with age, and its measurement requires understanding as well as full cooperation from the patient.

The VC is an indicator of the volume of air that a patient is able to move, but the ability to move postoperative secretions is more closely related to the velocity of forced air movement. The forced expiratory volume in 1 s (FEV_1) is a dynamic measurement of a patient's ability to move volumes of air during units of time. In practice the FEV_1 is usually reported as a percentage of the VC (FEV_1/VC) as well as an actual volume. It is important to note its value both ways. If the VC is significantly reduced, the ratio FEV_1/VC may be satisfactory while the actual volume exhaled is markedly abnormal. While VC is found to be normal or near normal in patients with moderately severe obstructive airway disease, it is reduced in individuals with restrictive pulmonary disease and those weakened by neuromuscular disease. The FEV_1 is reduced in obstructive airway disease, but the degree of reduction may vary from day to day or week to week in the same individual. The FEV_1 may be the most useful test to monitor in patients with marginal pulmonary function who are being prepared for operation by aggressive respiratory therapy programs.

Blood-Gas Determination. A measurement of the arterial blood gases and pH should be routine in the preoperative evaluation of a candidate for thoracic surgery. It would be an unusual situation in which the decision to advise operation depended solely on a single measurement of arterial oxygen or carbon dioxide tension. Even so, an occasional patient is discovered to have hypoxemia or CO_2 retention that was not suspected on the basis of clinical examination or spirometry. A measurement of the Pa_{CO_2} provides an immediate indication of the patient's alveolar ventilation; any value above 46 torr means that there is hypoventilation. There are multiple causes for this, and the specific reason should be sought in each patient. The ability of the lungs to excrete CO_2 is remarkable, and any persistent elevation of Pa_{CO_2} in a patient who might otherwise be considered a candidate for a major thoracotomy suggests serious abnormalities in distribution of ventilation and perfusion. Most operations will temporarily increase the ventilation-perfusion abnormality. A mild elevation of the Pa_{CO_2} in a patient with chronic lung disease may be treated aggressively to improve pulmonary function and allow the patient to be considered for operation. If pulmonary resection is contemplated in such an individual, the risk of postoperative respiratory failure is high and the decision to operate may depend on whether functioning pulmonary tissue would be removed.

The measurement of arterial Pa_{O_2} is valuable in the preoperative assessment of pulmonary function, but the number reported must be viewed with a consideration of the possibilities for error in its measurement. At sea level the normal Pa_{O_2} is above 85 torr. The majority of patients considered by a thoracic surgeon have a Pa_{O_2} of 80 torr or below, and values in the range of 70 to 80 torr do not suggest unusual risk in the absence of other signals of caution. If the Pa_{O_2} is below 70 torr, an attempt should be made to determine the cause and to improve the patient's respiratory exchange. The most usual cause is uneven distribution of ventilation and perfusion (V/Q mismatch), but other possibilities include right-to-left shunting as a result of the thoracic disease for which the patient is being considered (e.g., shunting through the tumor in alveolar cell carcinoma). More sophisticated pulmonary function tests may be indicated, including determination of alveolar-arterial oxygen difference, calculation of right-to-left shunt fraction, and split pulmonary function.

The major concern in assessing the reserve in prethoracotomy patients in whom parenchymal resection is contemplated is determination of the amount of lung tissue that can safely be removed. The surgeon must begin the operation knowing the maximum amount of lung tissue that can be removed without leaving a pulmonary cripple. The ''split-function'' specialized test of lung function that has been especially helpful in making this decision is radionuclide perfusion scanning for regional lung function. The data is obtained by comparing the counts over each lung during 99 mTc perfusion scanning. Perfusion scans can be performed concurrently with ventilation scanning for additional data.

The practical value of the split-function studies is that postoperative VC and FEV_1 can be predicted for the patient who may require pneumonectomy for adequate resection of a bronchial neoplasm (predicted postoperative FEV_1 = preoperative $FEV_1 \times$ percent perfusion in noninvolved lung). Even though a patient may require only a lobectomy for resection of a pulmonary neoplasm, the effects of a major thoracotomy can be likened to a ''functional pneumonectomy'' in the early postoperative period and can be expected to reduce pulmonary function by approximately 50 percent. This is particularly true if there is significant preoperative reduction in pulmonary function.

An important prospective study by Boysen and associates demonstrated the validity of the split-function concept in a group of patients with impaired ventilatory function (preoperative FEV_1 <2.0 L). If the predicted postoperative FEV_1 exceeded 800 mL, they considered the patients acceptable candidates for pulmonary resection up to and including a pneumonectomy. The perioperative mortality in their series was 15 percent, a figure considered acceptable for major pulmonary resections in extremely high-risk patients. Other investigators have corroborated their data and have shown the measured values for FEV_1 after a pneumonectomy correlated closely with the predicted values. Figure 16-9 illustrates the use of a split-function study to decide that a patient with severely decreased pulmonary function is a reasonable risk for pneumonectomy.

In recent years there has been increasing interest in exercise testing for patients who are candidates for pulmonary resection but have impaired pulmonary function. It is particularly indicated for those patients who have reasonable exercise capability despite severe obstructive airway disease. By using these tests, patients can be selected who are good risks to tolerate pneumonectomy even with significant impairment on spirometry. By combining respiratory gas analysis with ergometer testing, more sophisticated data can be obtained for correlation of oxygen consumption with work capacity.

Unilateral balloon occlusion of the pulmonary artery with right-heart catheterization is only rarely indicated in the preoperative evaluation of patients who require a major pulmonary resection. Normally, pulmonary vascular resistance decreases with exercise, and with pneumonectomy the remaining lung accepts the entire pulmonary blood flow without development of pulmonary hypertension. In a very occasional patient, occlusion of one pulmonary artery results in pulmonary hypertension to levels above 30 torr, and this has been correlated with excessive mortality after pneumonectomy. This test is done only in circumstances where there is conflicting information from other pulmonary function tests.

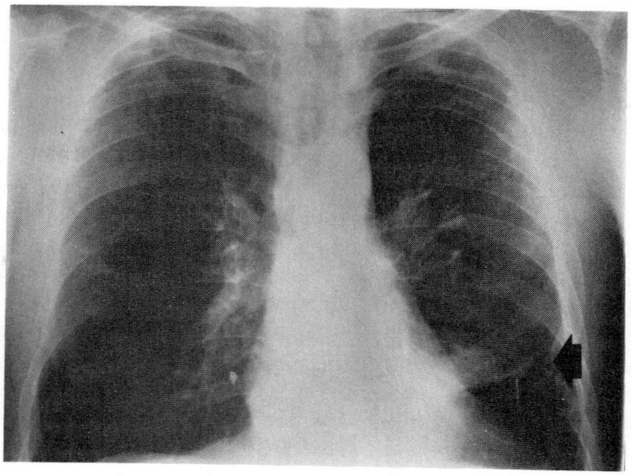

A

Patient - 58 y.o. white male

Spirometry	Measured	Predicted	% Predicted
FEV_1	1.72 liters	3.14 liters	55
FVC	2.47	4.37	57
Peak Flow	2.90 liters/s	8.63 liters/s	34
MVV	66.0 liters/min	130.0 liters/min	49

B

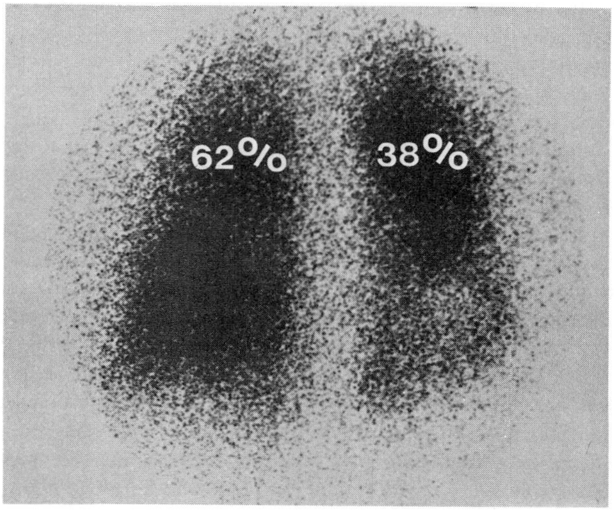

C

FIG. 16-9. An example of the use of radioisotope lung scanning for the prediction of postpneumonectomy pulmonary function. *A.* The P-A chest x-ray of a 58-year-old man with a recurrent bronchioloalveolar cell carcinoma in the left lower lobe. *B.* The results of preoperative spirometry show marked reduction in measured values for expiratory flow rates, vital capacity, and maximum voluntary ventilation. *C.* A lung perfusion scan with macroaggregated radioalbumin shows that approximately 62 percent of pulmonary blood flow is directed to the right lung. Therefore, the predicted values for postoperative vital capacity and FEV_1 after left pneumonectomy would be 1.5 and 1.0 L, respectively. These values were marginal but acceptable, and the patient underwent successful pneumonectomy. The actual measured FEV_1 2 weeks after operation was 1.02 L.

Numerous studies have shown that there is no data-analysis technique that will absolutely separate the operable patient from the inoperable. Instead, the goal of preoperative evaluation is to separate patients into low- and high-risk groups. Of the standard function tests, surgeons have come to place the greatest reliance on the expiratory flow rates (FEV_1) and maximum voluntary volume (MVV) as the critical determinants of operability for the patient with reduced function from respiratory disease, advanced age, or chronic illness. The MVV is performed by having the patient inhale as deeply and rapidly as possible for 10, 12, or 15 s. The MVV measures the status of the respiratory muscles, the compliance of the lung-thorax system, and the airway resistance. Mittman reported a 9 percent cardiopulmonary mortality rate in patients with a maximum breathing capacity (MBC—now called the maximal voluntary ventilation) greater than 50 percent of the predicted value. Those patients whose MBC was less than 50 percent had a 45 percent cardiopulmonary mortality rate after thoracotomy.

Although studies have failed to support a precise correlation between a given level of reduced pulmonary function and surgical outcome, guidelines suggested in a recent review by Zibrak and colleagues predict which patients being evaluated for resective surgery are at high risk (Table 16-1).

Zibrak and colleagues further recommended that patients should not be considered candidates for resective surgery if during balloon occlusion and exercise the mean pulmonary artery pressure exceeded 35 mmHg or the systemic Pa_{O_2} fell below 45 mmHg. The predicted postresection FEV_1 should be more than 0.8 L. The continuing improvements in facilities and technology for postoperative care have allowed surgeons to become more aggressive in recommending thoracotomy to selected patients with compromised pulmonary function. Several recent reports provide encouraging indications that of suitably selected and well-managed patients with FEV_1 less than 70 percent can expect satisfactory results after lung resection if vital capacity is preserved by limiting resection to the wide local removal of tumors rather than performing the more classic anatomic lobectomy or pneumonectomy.

The interest in providing a satisfactory evaluation of the patient before thoracic operation must not obscure the ultimate purpose of the evaluation—to provide the patient with whatever physical and mental preparation is needed. Many patients are smokers, and every effort should be made to persuade them to stop smoking before operation, preferably for 2 weeks or more. All authors agree that the character and amount of bronchial secretions have a major impact on postoperative morbidity. Aggressive attention to reducing the amount and tenacity of the secretions must be made before the operation. The etiology of pulmonary infection should be identified and treated intensively, using respiratory therapy, physical therapy, or appropriate techniques.

"Normal" pulmonary function tests are highly variable depending on age, height, weight, patient compliance, understanding, and cooperation. Table 16-2 lists the expected values for healthy young males with body surface area of 1.7 m^2.

Table 16-1
Criteria Suggesting High Risk for Resective Surgery

FVC < 50% of predicted
FEV_1 < 50% of FVC or < 2 L
MVV < 50% of predicted
Residual volume/total lung capacity > 50%

Table 16-2
Typical Values in Pulmonary Function Tests*

Lung volumes:	
Inspiratory capacity, mL	3600
Expiratory reserve volume, mL	1200
Vital capacity, mL	4800
Residual volume (RV), mL	1200
Functional residual capacity, mL	2400
Thoracic gas volume, mL	2400
Total lung capacity (TLC), mL	6000
RV/TLC ×100, %	20
Ventilation:	
Tidal volume, mL	500
Respiratory dead space, mL	150
Respirations/min	12
Minute volume, mL/min	6000
Alveolar ventilation, mL	4200
Mechanics of breathing:	
Maximal voluntary ventilation, L/min	125–170
Forced expiratory volume, % in 1 s	83
Forced expiratory volume, % in 3 s	97
Maximal expiratory flow rate (for 1 L), L/min	400
Maximal inspiration flow rate (for 1 L), L/min	300
Compliance of lungs and thoracic cage, L/cmH_2O	0.1
Compliance of lungs, L/cmH_2O	0.2
Airway resistance, cmH_2O/L/s	1.6
Alveolar ventilation/pulmonary capillary blood flow:	
Alveolar ventilation, L/min/blood flow, L/min	0.8
Physiologic shunt/cardiac output ×100, %	<7
Physiologic dead space/tidal volume ×100, %	<30
Arterial blood:	
Oxygen tension, torr	100
Carbon dioxide tension, torr	40
Oxygen tension (100% inhaled oxygen), torr	640
Alveolar-arterial P_{O_2} difference (100% inhaled oxygen), torr	33
Oxygen saturation (% saturation of hemoglobin)	97.1
pH	7.4

*The values shown are those of a resting young male, 1.7 m^2 body surface area, breathing room air at sea level, except where specified otherwise.

SOURCE: Modified from Comroe JH Jr: *The Lung*, 2d ed. Year Book Medical Publishers, Chicago, 1962, with permission.

Cardiac Evaluation. The need for preoperative cardiac evaluation is based on the expected postoperative demand for increased cardiac output, the frequency of coincidental cardiac disease, and the likelihood of cardiopulmonary complications after thoracic operations. Because cardiac symptoms are sometimes masked by the symptoms of the primary thoracic disease for which the patient is being considered, the screening evaluation must be precise. A preoperative electrocardiogram must be obtained. If the history, examination, or electrocardiogram reveals any abnormality, a consultation with a cardiologist is usually in order. The development of nuclear medicine techniques for myocardial imaging and for gated radionuclide angiocardiograms has provided noninvasive methods for evaluation of suspected myocardial ischemia and for determination of ventricular functions such as cardiac output, stroke volume, and ejection fraction. Dipyridamole thallium studies are valuable in predicting patients at high risk for postoperative cardiac events. Echocardiography is also useful for estimates of ventricular function. For patients with evidence of significant coronary artery occlusive disease it may be appropriate to proceed to coronary arteriography if the circumstances suggest that coronary revascularization may be necessary.

Mangano and colleagues in reviewing the epidemiology of postoperative cardiac events have pointed out that one in every eight of the 25 million patients in the United States who undergo noncardiac surgery have coronary artery disease and that 50,000 of these will have perioperative myocardial infarctions. Half of the 40,000 annual postoperative deaths in this country are the result of cardiac disease. Careful history and appropriate selective screening should allow the surgeon to identify those at highest risk and to protect them by collaboration with the anesthesiologist to make special efforts to avoid perioperative hyper- or hypotension and by judicious use of the data derivable from the Swan-Ganz catheter monitoring of preload pressures and cardiac output during the early recovery period.

Other Organ Systems. The preoperative evaluation should include screening tests for renal and hepatic function even in the absence of historical data that would suggest disease of those organs. Under ordinary circumstances a hospital admission biochemical profile that includes measurements of blood urea nitrogen, creatinine, serum proteins, transaminases, lactic dehydrogenase, alkaline phosphatase, and bilirubin is adequate for initial investigation. The discovery of any abnormality mandates a more detailed evaluation.

Malnutrition. Malnutrition increases the morbidity and mortality rate of any major surgical procedure, and an assessment of the preoperative nutritional state is important. In clinical practice it may be difficult to separate the effects of total calorie deficit from a deficiency of protein alone. There is a reduced blood volume and reduced tolerance for intraoperative bleeding in hypoproteinemic patients. Impaired antibody production, reduced host resistance to infection, decreased lymphocyte proliferative response, and depression of the delayed skin reactivity to antigens are associated with weight loss and hypoalbuminemia.

Particularly important in thoracic surgical patients are the adverse effects of protein depletion on pulmonary functions and ventilatory capacity. As skeletal muscle is catabolized during starvation, the muscle groups in the thorax, abdomen, shoulder, and diaphragm involved in respiration and coughing share in the unselective loss of strength that is seen in all muscles and results in an increased risk of a major thoracic operation.

POSTTHORACOTOMY CONSIDERATIONS

Pulmonary Function Changes. Significant pathophysiologic changes in pulmonary function occur after major thoracic and upper abdominal operations. Each produces similar changes in pulmonary function and has similar initial complications; with lung resections, some of these changes may be permanent. The magnitude of the changes is affected by preexisting bronchopulmonary disease, length of the operation, postoperative analgesics, and immobilization in bed. Patients without pulmonary disease develop similar changes and are subject to similar complications although the risks are much less. The pulmonary changes seen relate to (1) lung volumes, (2) ventilatory patterns, (3) respiratory gas exchange, and (4) defense mechanisms.

Lung Volume. Total lung capacity and each of its subdivisions are significantly reduced after abdominal or thoracic operations. Vital capacity is reduced by 25 to 50 percent or more, with the maximum reduction occurring during the first 4 days after operation. Similarly, functional residual capacity and expiratory reserve volume are decreased, with a gradual return toward normal beginning in the second week after operation. The reduction in lung volume is often accompanied by an increase in the closing volume to potentiate the development of atelectasis. If a pulmonary resection has been performed, the magnitude of change is even greater and is proportional to the amount of functioning lung that was removed.

Ventilatory Pattern. The sedative effect of the anesthetic agent and the postoperative analgesics, combined with the severe pain of the thoracotomy incision, produces sharp reductions in tidal volume after operation. The expected response is an increase in respiratory rate sufficient to maintain minute ventilation. Unfortunately, the parenteral narcotics ordinarily used to manage postoperative pain all depress the respiratory center, inhibiting the compensatory rate increase and leading to carbon dioxide retention and hypoxemia. An injectable nonsteroidal anti-inflammatory agent (ketorolac tromethamine) has recently been introduced that reportedly provides narcotic-equivalent pain relief without respiratory depression. These drugs are 30 to 40 times as expensive as the equivalent narcotics.

An equally important effect of the changes in ventilatory pattern is the sharp reduction or elimination of the normal periodic hyperinflations (sighs). Normal adults sigh at the rate of nine or ten times per hour under quiet conditions. With loss of periodic hyperinflations, there is closure of lung units and a reduction in compliance.

Gas Exchange. Decreases in Pa_{O_2} and mild elevations of Pa_{CO_2} are frequent as patients recover from anesthesia. However, Pa_{CO_2} generally returns to normal or below normal in the early postoperative period, while Pa_{O_2} remains depressed during the first week. The factors responsible for reduction in the Pa_{O_2} include abnormal ventilation-perfusion relationships and intrapulmonary shunting associated with atelectasis.

Pulmonary Defense Mechanisms. The lung is normally protected against inhaled particulate matter and microbes by several mechanisms. The cough reflex defends the upper airways against inhaled or aspirated material in the tracheobronchial tree. Clearance of inhaled particles and microbes from the lower airways is dependent on the mucociliary system, and the alveoli are defended by mucociliary transport, lymphatic drainage, and the alveolar macrophages. Since coughing is inhibited by several mechanisms in the postoperative period, there is significant impairment of that defense mechanism. Ciliary function is decreased, and multiple factors, including arterial hypoxemia, depress the activity of alveolar macrophages. Finally, the composition and physical properties of mucus are altered in a way that reduces the effectiveness of the mucociliary transport system.

Complications. Pulmonary complications of thoracic operations have their origins in these changes and usually begin in the operating room or soon thereafter. The principal pulmonary complications consist of obstructive atelectasis and respiratory infections, and it is possible to consider each of these problems in terms of the complex of factors that contribute to their development.

Atelectasis means closure of lung units, and it exists as microatelectasis, a diffuse sublobular form not visible on chest x-rays, and macroatelectasis, the collapse of a segment, lobe, or entire lung. The three mechanisms that are considered responsible for atelectasis are accentuations of the postoperative pathophysiologic changes described earlier: (1) retained bronchopulmonary secretions, (2) decreased sighing, and (3) decreased expiratory reserve volume.

Retention of secretions is a major cause of atelectasis in patients with chronic bronchitis. It is more subtle in patients with normal lungs though they also develop either microatelectasis or macroatelectasis. Decreased sighing and reduced tidal volume contribute to the reduced compliance in the postoperative period. Unless reversed by voluntary efforts at deep breathing, induced coughing, or attentive respiratory care techniques, these changes will contribute to the development of both forms of atelectasis. Similarly, the postoperative reductions in lung volumes are related to airway closure that is associated with the changes in ventilatory pattern. The critical relationship may be between the reduced expiratory reserve volume (ERV) and closing volume (CV). Normally, CV is above residual volume but below the end-tidal point. In the postoperative state with the expected reduction in ERV, the CV may exceed the ERV and be located above the end-tidal point. Under these circumstances, the peripheral airways are subjected to compression and closure during tidal breathing. For some patients the risk of atelectasis is greater because of preexisting abnormalities in ERV and CV. For example, elderly patients and smokers have an increased CV and patients with obstructive airway disease have an increased CV and a decreased ERV. These circumstances potentiate the opportunity for airway closure and significant atelectasis.

Postoperative bronchopulmonary infectious complications consist of tracheobronchitis and pneumonitis. While these complications occur in normal persons, their incidence is higher in patients with preexisting chronic airway disease. Decreased cough, atelectasis, reduced mucociliary clearance of inhaled particles and bacteria, pain, and analgesic drugs all contribute to these infectious complications. Interference with the mucociliary clearance mechanism leads to rapid bacterial proliferation distal to obstruction in an area of atelectasis. Of equal importance has been the demonstration that the respiratory tract becomes colonized with gram-negative bacilli, particularly in the presence of tracheal intubation, coma, hypotension, hypoxia, acidosis, and azotemia. Many of these conditions exist in the postoperative period of patients subjected to major thoracic procedures.

Pain Control. In the first few postoperative days effective management of incisional pain is of central importance in the maintenance of adequate ventilation. The pain that accompanies the thoracotomy is often severe and may be disabling. Unless well managed, it will cause hypoventilation, retention of secretions, atelectasis, hypoxia, hypoxemia, shallow and ineffective respiratory effort, and pneumonia. It is a constant challenge to find the delicate balance between giving patients enough pain medication so that they are able to cough, without giving them so much that they lose their drive to do so.

Pain is frequently managed by parenteral narcotics administered intramuscularly or intravenously, on a fixed schedule (by-the-clock) or on-demand (p.r.n.). Particularly when given p.r.n., these techniques are associated with the likelihood of swings in levels from obtundation with respiratory depression and suppression of cough to frightened and agitated patients who hurt too much to move. If parenteral narcotics are to be the primary means for postthoracotomy pain control, they should probably be given by I.V. drip in a dose carefully regulated by observation or by patient-controlled analgesia (PCA) techniques to provide adequate continuous pain relief without undue somnolence. Success with this approach requires careful preoperative education of the patient and close nursing care. Nausea, vomiting, and respiratory depression are potential side effects.

The search continues for satisfactory means to control the local incisional and pleural pain without the deleterious consequences of systemic narcotics. Either short-acting (lidocaine) or long-acting (bupivacaine) agents can be given as one-shot intercostal blocks before closing the chest or by intermittent injections through catheters left in place in the pleural space at the completion of the thoracotomy. When these methods are used, great care must be taken to avoid inadvertent intravascular or subdural injection. Severe vasomotor hypotension has occasionally been reported after this technique, and the patient should be monitored closely whenever it is used. Several investigators advocate use of intercostal nerve cryoanalgesia and have reported excellent incisional pain relief by this nerve-freezing approach (each appropriate nerve receives one 30-s exposure to the probe).

There are opiate receptors in the spinal cord with specific endorphins and enkephalin mediators. The use of continuous epidural infusion of perservative-free morphine or fentanyl administered either through a thoracic or lumbar epidural catheter has been widely reported as providing good pain control, though earlier hopes that this approach might improve postoperative pulmonary function have not been confirmed in controlled comparative studies.

Advances in anesthesia techniques, particularly improvements in the design of the various double-lumen endotracheal tubes used with or without high-frequency jet ventilation, have offered the surgeon new options for reducing postthoracotomy pain. The need for wide exposure for delicate hilar dissection was clear when the dissection was carried out around a retracted but filled, moving lung. The ability to work in the chest with a fully deflated lung encourages surgeons to seek less traumatic means for entry into the chest. Urschel has reported a large series of lobar resections in both chest cavities through a median sternotomy. The extensive experience with this incision in the open-heart surgery population has demonstrated that it is much less painful and much better tolerated physiologically. Others have worked to improve the straight lateral, or modified muscle-sparing incision to allow major resections without the necessity of dividing the muscles to the shoulder girdle. This incision is rapidly opened, rapidly closed, and leaves a chest wall with more functional integrity. The combination of these less traumatic incisions and intrapleural bupivacaine infusions as an approach to pain control is gaining favor.

THORACIC INJURIES

General Considerations

The leading cause of death, hospitalization, and short- and long-term disability for all ages from the end of the first year through the forty-fifth year of life is trauma. Twenty-five percent of all trauma deaths are due to chest injuries alone, and respiratory problems contribute significantly in 75 percent of traumatic deaths. It is not surprising that this should be so, for the respiratory system is basically a simple mechanical system of bellows, pumps, and hydraulics that requires smooth coordination of all its elements and that works on a very small margin of safety. Physical disruption of the integrity of the system, as may be expected in trauma, must be corrected rapidly or irreversible damage resulting from hypoxia in vital structures will occur. With complete loss of oxygen and with normal tissue oxygen demands (e.g., normal ambient temperature), such damage occurs after only 4 min. Lesser disruptions of delivery extend the tolerance time, but it should be apparent that accurate diagnosis of the failing or disrupted elements of the system and their prompt correction is delayed at progressive peril to the patient. Fortunately, as emphasized in the Trauma Life Support Program of the American College of Surgeons, 85 percent of patients with life-threatening thoracic injuries can be managed by simple interventions easily mastered by physicans and emergency medical service personnel.

Progressing Trauma. Trauma is a dynamic event. Injury does not stop at the moment of impact or penetration. Continued muscular effort by the patient, or movement of disrupted parts during resuscitation or transport, can quickly convert a stabilized cardiorespiratory system into an unstable one with the development of new life-threatening factors. There is always some progressive evolution of the acute injury that can create tension or fluid in spaces unable to accommodate them without dire consequences. In assessing and managing the patient with chest injury, it is especially important to recognize this propensity for continuing alterations in physiology and function.

General considerations about the management of the injured patient are discussed in Chap. 6. The preinjury cardiopulmonary functional status must be carefully considered. The rib fracture or modest pneumothorax that is well tolerated without hospitalization in a healthy young man may lead to pneumonia, empyema, or death in an older patient with chronic airway disease. The patient with preexisting cardiac disease is particularly vulnerable to the development of pulmonary edema and hypoxia that may occur with the rapid administration of intravenous fluids during resuscitation.

A rapid but perceptive overall evaluation of the patient must be carried out whether the injury is thought to be serious or not. Chest trauma is usually associated with other injuries, and the overlap of the upper part of the abdomen by the thoracic cage provides a border zone that is difficult to assess and is often the site of combination injuries. Particularly challenging are those patients who cannot describe symptoms, because of associated head injuries or profound shock. The importance of attending to the whole patient and the other progressive or subtle injuries must be emphasized, but this section will focus on those problems that result from injuries to the chest and most of its contents.

Types of Injuries. Injuries to the chest are often classified according to the type of insult that caused the damage. Depending on the setting (military or civilian, urban or rural), the predominant injury will differ. High-velocity penetrating wounds produce most of the military injuries; low-velocity gunshot wounds are replacing knife wounds as the most common in urban civilian populations; blunt injuries from motor vehicular accidents make up the majority of nonurban injuries. Penetrating wounds are becoming more frequent in suburban and rural areas as violent personal crimes increase, and blunt injuries are increasing in frequency in urban areas as the incidence of falls and jumps from buildings increases.

The mortality rate of major blunt injuries has been reduced steadily during the past quarter century, but complications and death associated with pulmonary contusion, posttraumatic pulmonary insufficiency, and trauma to the heart and great vessels are still impressive. It is especially characteristic of blunt injuries that the maximal extent of cardiopulmonary functional loss and often the complete diagnosis require several days for development.

Among the penetrating wounds that are especially treacherous are those in the lower thoracic region. The diaphragm rises to the level of the nipples in normal expiration and management of penetration in this region is dominated by concern that subdiaphragmatic viscera may have been penetrated. Some surgeons believe that a stab wound of the left lower part of the chest mandates early abdominal exploration on the basis that the knife may have injured the spleen, stomach, or colon. As the negative pressure in the chest aspirates fluid into the chest through the diaphragm wound, the abdominal findings in these cases may be missing or late in coming and peritoneal lavage is notoriously misleading. The consequence of error is costly. Because the liver is usually the abdominal structure injured by right-sided stab wounds that penetrate the diaphragm, it may be reasonable to delay exploration until the patient is more stabilized. Early abdominal exploration is indicated if there is evidence of continuing blood loss. The late consequence of holes in the diaphragm probably justifies operative repair as soon as safe in all but a few highly selected patients.

Whatever the cause, the principles of management should remain focused on the mechanical systems involved: the pump (the heart, see Chap. 18), the hydraulics (the vessels, see Chap. 19), and the bellows (the suction-blow system that draws atmospheric air into the alveoli and expels it). We will discuss the problems associated with traumatic failure of the bellows and the delivery and removal of certain gases to and from the blood, but obviously the pump must be working and the vessels must have the integrity and suitable contents to transport the gases to and from the tissues.

Conditions Requiring Urgent Correction

Airway Obstruction. Most patients with major disruption of the airway leading to obstruction will not survive initial accident; the leading cause of death at the accident site is airway obstruction. At any stage of the early resuscitation and transportation of the patient, correctable airway obstruction may occur. The oropharynx should be cleared of mechanical debris and the chin and neck positioned to facilitate opening the posterior pharynx. Until the stability of the cervical vertebrae has been ascertained, the neck should only be positioned by an anterior chin-thrust motion while applying continuous cephalad traction to the head (Fig. 16-10). If the upper airway remains at risk after clearing and positioning, access to the endotrachea for control is indicated. If cervical spine injury is suspected and midface soft tissue damage is not extensive, nasotracheal intubation is preferred, even though the small caliber of the nasotracheal tube prevents subsequent flexible bronchoscopic examination. If it can be safely done, orotracheal intubation with a size 8 mm or larger endotracheal tube is indicated.

If the equipment or expertise is not available, or if the upper airway injury precludes safe access to the cords from above, cricothyroidotomy should be performed. If high-pressure oxygen is available, catheter jet ventilation may be used (percutaneous passage of cricothyroid membrane catheter, 12 gauge or larger) while the patient is being stabilized and arrangements for tracheal intubation are being completed.

Tension Pneumothorax. When an injury to the lung parenchyma has occurred that allows air to enter the pleural space with each respiratory effort, and when the flap-valve effect of the

Aligning the airway for intubation

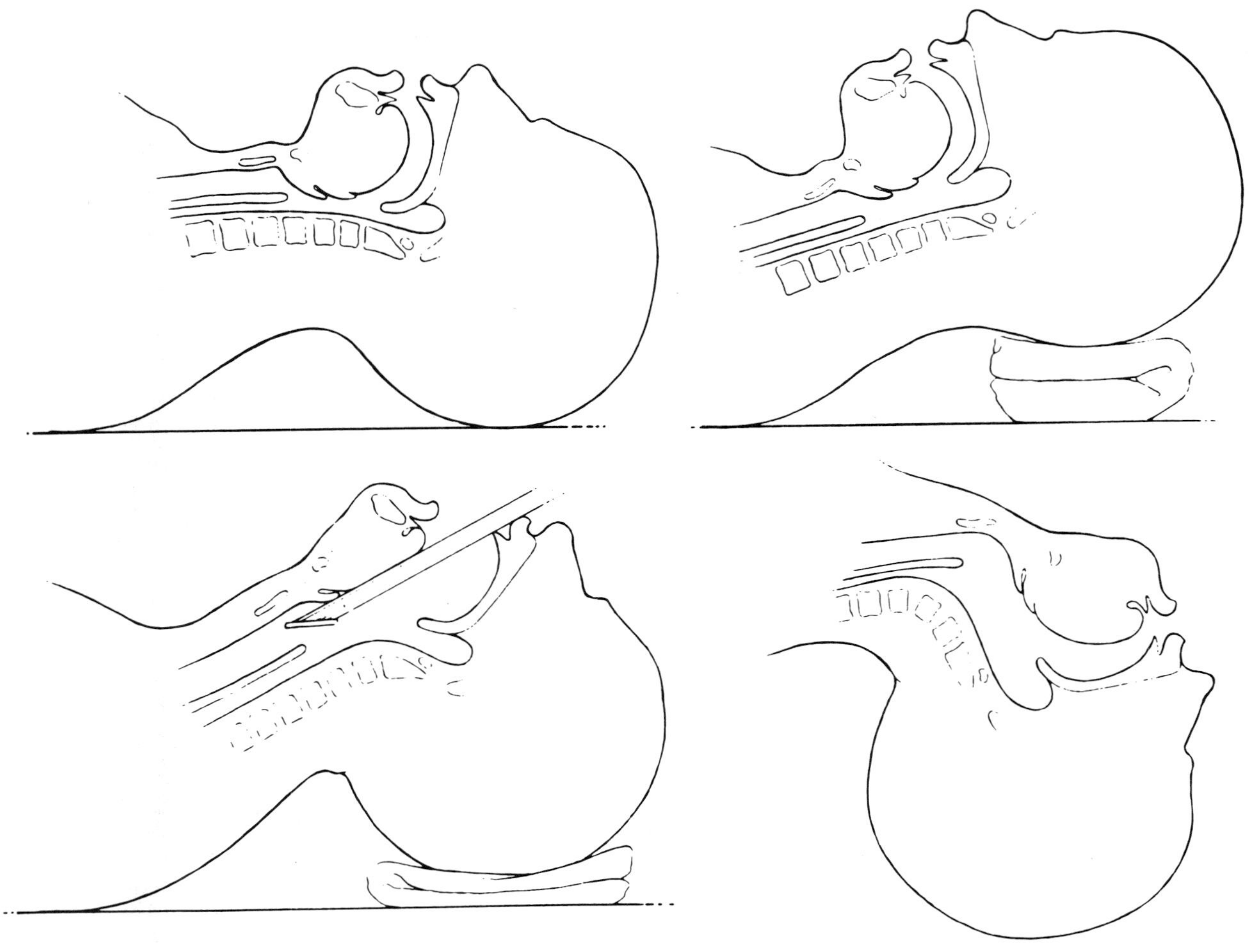

FIG. 16-10. Extension of the neck is commonly misunderstood to be the proper position for airway access. As shown, the neck should be *flexed* with the chin elevated in order to straighten the airway for visualization of cords of optimum clearing of supralaryngeal obstructions.

injury prevents that air from reentering the bronchial tree for egress through the trachea during expiration, tension develops within the pleural space until equilibration with the negative pressures the patient is able to generate is reached; at that time effective ventilation ceases and venous blood can no longer enter the chest. The mechanics of a developing tension pneumothorax may not be obvious when the patient is first seen. Pain may be the primary complaint, with no evidence of respiratory distress. But if the lung wound is behaving as a check valve, some air will escape into the pleural cavity with each inspiration or with each cough. Gradually, intrapleural pressure will build up, the lung collapses, and tension pneumothorax may develop. A shift of the mediastinum and compression of the large veins result in a decreased cardiac output that may lead to sudden death.

The diagnosis should be instantly made by the observation of a patient with dilated neck veins making respiratory effort but not respiratory motions, and unable to move air. It is immediately confirmed by the hyperresonant percussion note over the injured hemithorax and absent or distant breath sounds. The immediate release of the tension by placement of a large-bore needle followed immediately by insertion of a thoracostomy tube is lifesaving.

Open Pneumothorax. The sucking chest wound is one in which a segment of the chest wall has been destroyed such that negative intrapleural pressure sucks air directly through the chest wall defect rather than through the trachea into the alveoli. Whenever the cross-sectional area of the defect exceeds that of the trachea, the undesirable preferential air movement takes place. It occurs most commonly after shotgun blasts, explosions with flying debris, or impalement injuries. It may or may not be associated with underlying parenchymal damage.

The diagnosis can be made by noting a patient with normal or collapsed neck veins who is making respiratory motions but not moving air. Confirmation is immediate on inspection of the patient's chest and observation of the wound. The patient is stabilized by any mechanical covering over the open wound. As soon as convenient, a watertight dressing should be placed and an intercostal catheter inserted into the pleural cavity. Early debridement and closure of the wound should then be scheduled.

Massive Flail Chest. Whenever severe blunt injury results in two-point fractures of four or more ribs, a large segment of the chest wall becomes flail. On inspiratory effort, the negative pressure in the chest pulls the unstable segment of the wall inward in a paradoxical motion. The patient may be unable to develop sufficient intratracheal negative pressure to maintain adequate ventilation, and atelectasis, hypoxia, and hypercapnia occur. A patient who is conscious may splint the segment sufficiently to make it inapparent to cursory examination, but the continuing extra effort in the attempt to move air soon leads to tiring and may result in sudden respiratory decompensation. The progressing failure is aggravated by the developing pulmonary contusion that accompanies blunt trauma sufficient to break that many ribs. In the unconscious patient, the lesion may be less dangerous, because it is more readily recognized and more apt to be treated early.

In the massive flail chest, the diagnosis may be difficult unless the chest wall is visualized during the respiratory effort. If unconscious, the patient is ordinarily making vigorous respiratory motions, but moving little air; the paradoxical segment should be obvious. The patient who is awake may exhibit a very rapid shallow breathing pattern at or above 40 breaths/min. Other aspects of the management of lesser flail injuries are discussed below, but when massive flail is diagnosed, endotracheal intubation and positive-pressure controlled ventilation is mandatory.

Massive Hemothorax. When 1500 mL or more of blood is acutely removed from the pleural space as a thoracostomy tube is placed, Rene has shown that urgent thoracotomy will find a surgically correctable lesion in a high proportion of the cases. If a patient with penetrating injury or multiple rib fractures is found to have a complete hemithorax dull to percussion in association with hypotension, a chest tube should be inserted. If massive hemothorax is found, the patient should be taken directly to the operating room as blood volume resuscitation is taking place.

Conditions Requiring Urgent Thoracotomy

Continued Intrapleural Bleeding. If bleeding continues from a thoracostomy tube after initial placement at a rate exceeding 100 mL/h for 6 h or more, most surgeons would now agree that a surgically correctable lesion is present. Ordinarily it will be a bleeding intercostal vessel, since bleeding from the lower-pressure pulmonary system will almost always stop when the lung is reexpanded after the pleural space is evacuated. The rate and pattern of bleeding are more important than the amount in deciding to explore.

Massive Air Leak. This is an increasingly commonly recognized injury resulting from steering wheel compression of the trachea against the vertebral bodies following high-speed head-on collisions. Complete disruption of the trachea or a major bronchus may occur. The injury is often fatal but may be surprisingly well tolerated for a brief period. All levels of the trachea and all major bronchi have been involved; however, greater than 80 percent of these injuries are within 2.5 cm of the carina. Patients with intrathoracic tracheal or central bronchial disruption may exhibit a variety of signs and symptoms depending on whether there is free communication between the site of injury and the pleural cavity. A particularly important diagnostic finding is complete unilateral atelectasis in the face of a large air leak, or the symmetrical downward displacement of the bilateral hila. Distal injuries often result in pneumothorax, which is manageable by tube thoracostomy alone since the air leak is small. Lazar and colleagues have reported a case in which a complete tracheal disruption just above the carina with 6 cm of discontinuity was tolerated in a young athlete for 24 h before accurate diagnosis and repair. Extreme care must be taken in the evaluation of patients with massive air leaks, since overly aggressive diagnostic bronchoscopy or endotracheal intubation and positive-pressure ventilation before accurate location of the defect and careful operative preparation for approaching it have been made could result in rapid death. Occasionally, as in other tracheobronchial injuries discussed below, an injury may seal itself off and fail to be recognized until severe stenosis develops.

Other Indications. Several other important causes are listed here, but discussed elsewhere.

Acute or rapidly recurring pericardial tamponade
Acute heart failure secondary to valve or septal injury
Widened or widening mediastinum
Perforation of the intrathoracic esophagus

Dangerous but Less Compelling Injuries

Diaphragm Rupture. Urgent repair of massive diaphragmatic rupture is sometimes necessary if high-volume herniation of abdominal contents into the chest prevents adequate ventilation. Ordinarily, however, the acute problems associated with diaphragm rupture are related to the associated injuries to abdominal viscera resulting from the force necessary to rupture the diaphragm. Penetrating trauma to the lower chest or upper abdomen and crush injuries, most often secondary to automobile accidents, are the usual causes of traumatic rupture of the diaphragm. The left hemidiaphragm is ruptured more frequently by blunt trauma than the right, the ratio being about 9:1. The right hemidiaphragm is said to be protected by two mechanisms: the liver on the right and the heart in the center have a buffering effect that diffuses the sudden increase in intraabdominal pressure; and cadaver studies have shown an inherent weakness in the posterior lateral aspect of the left diaphragm. When rupture of the right side does occur, the liver is usually the only abdominal structure that herniates into the chest early, though gradual aspiration of the stomach into the right chest through the diaphragmatic defect can occur over time. With rupture of the left hemidiaphragm, the stomach, spleen, left transverse colon, and omentum in any combination may enter the left pleural cavity. When the diagnosis is delayed for several days or longer, there is often a progressive displacement of the abdominal viscera into the chest or progressive gaseous distention of the herniated stomach. The latter may occur despite an indwelling nasogastric tube, and it may precipitate respiratory distress (Fig. 16-11).

Patients with diaphragmatic rupture due to blunt trauma usually have associated injuries that demand first attention and prevent a detailed initial evaluation. The first chest x-ray after rupture of either hemidiaphragm may show nothing more than a blurring of the diaphragm with or without evidence of a small hemothorax. In some patients the diagnosis is made very early because the nasogastric tube is seen to lie within the confines of the left pleural cavity. Injection of air through the nasogastric tube during auscultation of the left side of the chest may add support to the diagnosis.

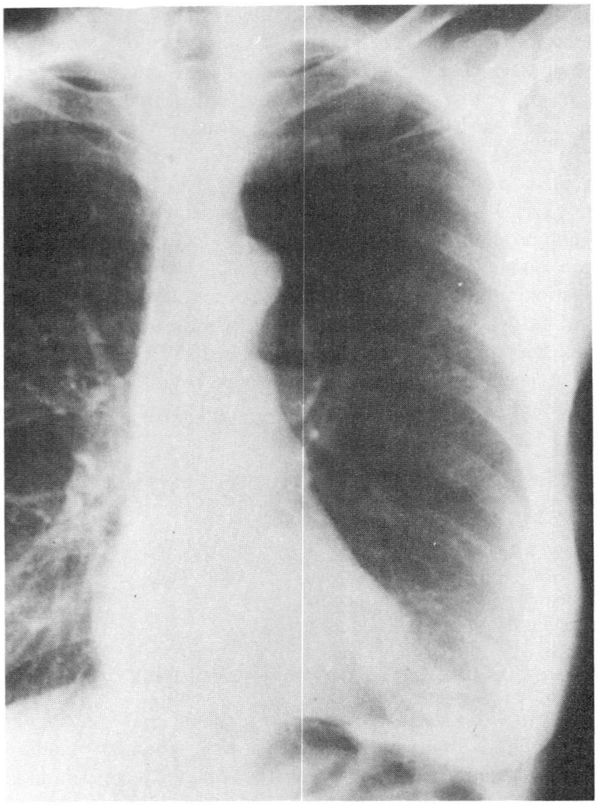

A

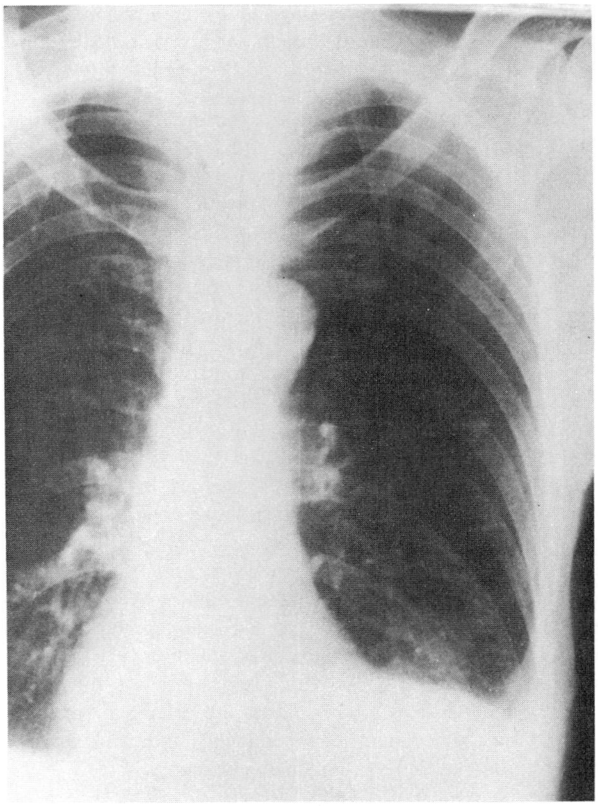

B

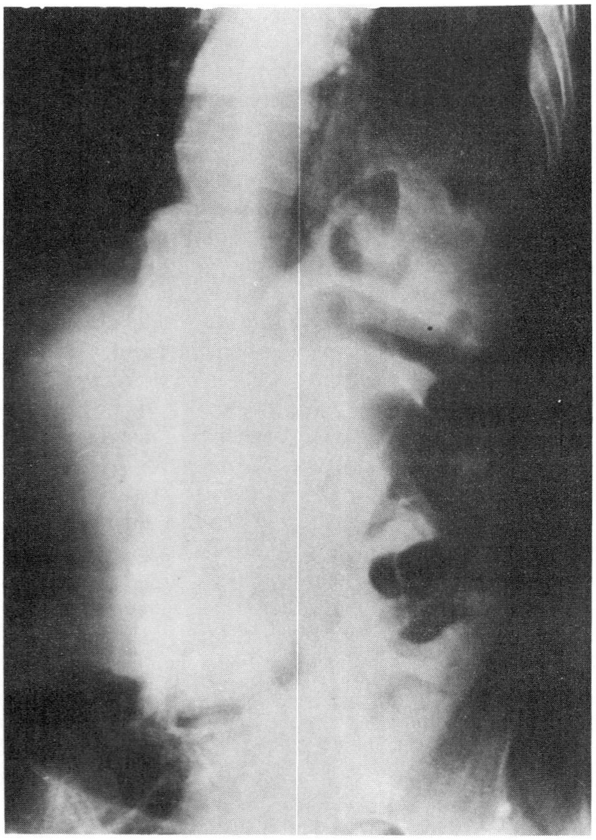

C

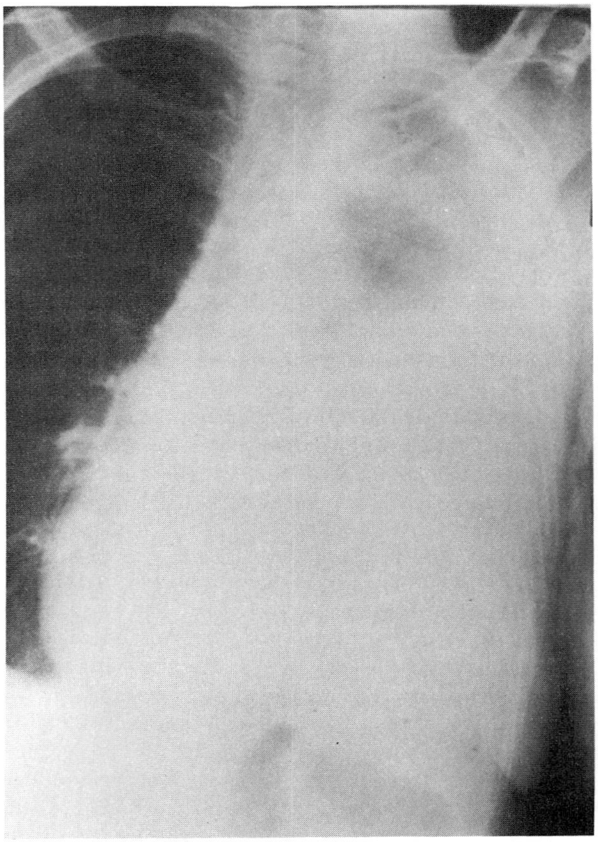

D

Penetrating diaphragmatic injuries rarely produce early symptoms except those related to other structures that may be injured. After several months or years, gastrointestinal obstruction may develop and lead to strangulation of herniated viscera. The hole in the diaphragm is small, and herniation occurs slowly. Early transabdominal operation is indicated when the diagnosis is confirmed, and associated intraabdominal injuries may be repaired at the same time. The wound in the hemidiaphragm may vary from a simple radial tear to an extensive and complex laceration. Repair can usually be accomplished by direct suture, but a prosthetic patch is occasionally required. If the diagnosis is delayed, a transthoracic approach may be preferred. It provides better exposure to (1) reduce the hernia, (2) free adhesions between the abdominal viscera and intrathoracic structures, and (3) repair the defect in the diaphragm.

Pneumothorax. Pneumothorax is usually the result of injury to the lung or the tracheobronchial tree. Esophageal perforation may be followed by a pneumomediastinum that ruptures into the pleural cavity. Whether the pneumothorax is associated with blunt injury and fractured ribs or is due to a penetrating wound, there is a variable amount of bleeding into the pleural cavity. The decision to use the term hemopneumothorax depends on the amount of blood in the pleural cavity and the likely consequences. If sufficient blood is present to require a concerted effort to assure its removal, or if its loss from the circulating volume requires transfusion replacement, it seems proper to use the double term.

Pneumothorax varies from that which is so slight that it may be missed on the initial x-ray examination to a massive, continuing air leak that displaces the mediastinum, depresses the diaphragm, and compresses the opposite lung, the tension pneumothorax discussed previously (Fig. 16-12). A pneumothorax due to a parenchymal lung injury tends to be self-limited because the developing lung collapse combines with blood clotting in the wound for a sealing effect. For some patients extensive adhesions already present between the visceral and parietal pleura may localize the pleural air and prevent a collapse of the lung (Fig. 16-13).

With any chest injury it is wisest to presume that a pneumothorax is present until proved otherwise. Because of pain and limited chest motion on the injured side, physical examination may be inadequate for diagnosis of a minimal pneumothorax. Since attention may be diverted to the management of other injuries, and because of the risks of tension developing should a general anesthetic with positive-pressure ventilation be given, prophylactic thoracostomy catheters should usually be placed whenever there is significant chest injury. The catheter is usually best placed in the lateral axillary line, just above the fifth rib, after finger exploration has induced a temporary pneumothorax or otherwise assured the pleural space to be free at the site of insertion.

Treatment of the more usual pneumothorax depends on symptoms of respiratory insufficiency, the extent of the pneumothorax, and the presence of significant hemothorax. There is a tendency to think of pneumothorax in terms of a two-dimensional concept that is conveyed by the anteroposterior chest x-ray. Instead, the hemithorax must be considered a modified cone, and when the lung surface is separated from the chest wall by 3 cm or more, the patient may have a 50 percent lung collapse (by volume) rather than the 25 or 30 percent collapse that the chest x-ray suggests. With a pneumothorax that is less than this amount, due to a nonpenetrating injury (theoretically, no contamination of the pleural space), and not accompanied by significant blood or fluid in the pleural cavity, treatment may not be required. A decision not to remove the pleural air implies that the patient has had a simple injury and that conditions for observation are ideal. Approximately 1.25 percent of the air will be absorbed each day, with full expansion expected in 3 to 6 weeks.

FIG. 16-11. *A–D.* Traumatic rupture of the diaphragm can present rapidly progressive and life-threatening complications early or late after injury. The patient whose films are pictured here developed increasing herniation of abdominal contents into the left chest over a 3-day period before findings led to urgent thoracotomy for removal of infarcted small intestine. (*Courtesy of Dr. John H.M. Austin.*)

Aspiration of the air with a needle and insertion of an intercostal catheter only if lung collapse recurs is a reasonable method of treatment advocated by some physicians even when the pneumothorax amounts to as much as 50 percent. In all cases with greater than 50 percent collapse, in those with hemopneumothorax, and in patients whose pneumothorax is the result of penetrating trauma, an intercostal catheter should be inserted and attached to a water seal with 10 to 25 cmH_2O negative pressure. In the majority of patients, lung reexpansion and cessation of the air leak will occur within a few hours or a few days. If not, a major bronchial injury may be present, and a thoracotomy may be required after appropriate diagnostic procedures.

The use of prophylactic systemic antibiotics in patients with chest trauma is a subject of current debate, but their use in cases of nonpenetrating trauma seems unjustified. The simple insertion of an intercostal catheter does not justify prescribing antibiotics.

Interstitial Emphysema. Disruption of the respiratory tract at any level will result in the passage of air into the surrounding tissues. Mediastinal emphysema occurs when air enters the areolar tissue planes from a tracheobronchial wound or from a perforation of the esophagus. Occasionally, blunt injuries to the chest may disrupt the integrity of a group of bronchioles or alveolar units without disrupting the visceral pleura. As air escapes into the pulmonary interstitium, it dissects centrally along the bronchi and pulmonary vessels to reach the mediastinum. When the mediastinal pleura remains intact, progressive loss of air into the tissue carries the dissection into the neck, where the air escapes the deep tissue planes and spreads in the subcutaneous tissue. The development of subcutaneous emphysema may cause marked distortion of the patient's appearance, but there is no reason to "treat" the condition, except to take whatever steps are appropriate to stop the air leak. The source of the leak must be found, since some potential causes (esophageal perforation or major bronchial injury) require early intervention.

Rib Fractures and Lesser Flail Injuries. The most common injury of the chest is a fracture of one or more ribs, including fracture at the costochondral junction ("separation"). Children seem less liable to rib fractures, but chest x-rays are made less frequently in those young age groups with minor trauma. Fractures occur most commonly in the middle and lower ribs with blunt trauma, but the distribution with penetrating wounds varies with the distribution of the penetrating objects.

First Rib Fractures. First rib fractures have historically been associated with high probability of associated upper rib fractures and major vessel injuries. Recent reports by many authors, however, have demonstrated isolated first rib fractures without other significant injuries in the thoracic outlet in a wide variety of pa-

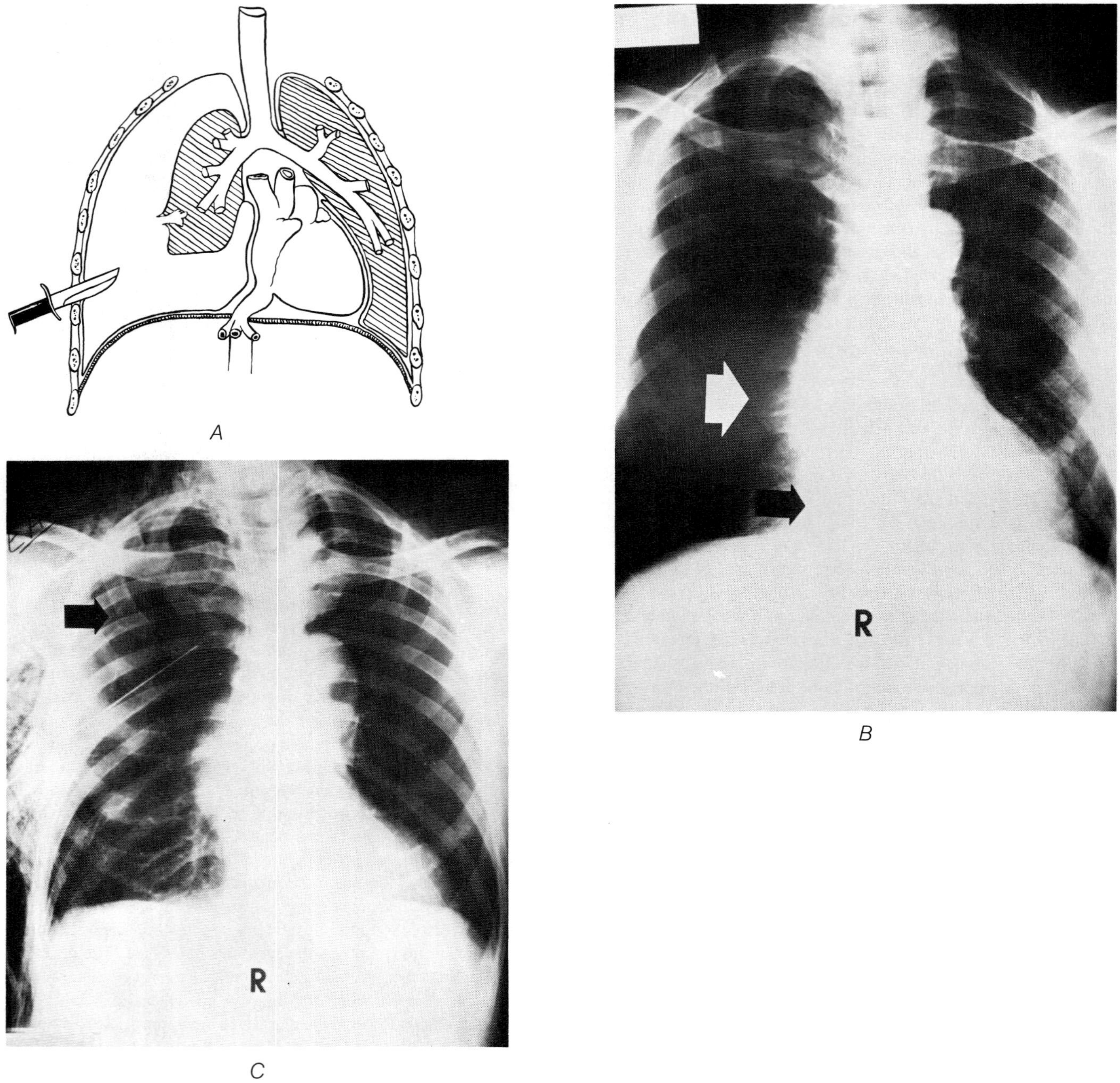

FIG. 16-12. *A.* In a tension pneumothorax there is compression of the contralateral lung and a displacement of the mediastinum that may sharply reduce venous return to the atria. *B.* If the diagnosis is strongly suspected, needle aspiration of the pleural space should be done without waiting for the chest x-ray. In this patient, the tension pneumothorax developed slowly and became symptomatic shortly after this film was taken. The lower arrow points to the displacement of the right heart border, and the lung is completely collapsed (*upper arrow*). *C.* Following needle aspiration a large intercostal tube was put in place, but a major air leak continued for several days and eventually required insertion of an additional chest catheter. The arrow points to the visceral pleura, showing incomplete expansion of the lung.

tients. Because of the relative high frequency in association with cranial and maxillofacial injuries, and in the ''surfer's'' rib (an injury occurring in surfers performing the so-called lay-back maneuver), it seems probable that isolated first rib injuries are secondary to avulsion of the first rib by its muscular attachments rather than direct trauma to the relatively protected first rib. There is inconclusive evidence that a direct relationship exists between first and second rib fractures and trauma to major vessels at the apex of the hemithorax (Fig. 16-14). Consider arteriography in stable patients with first rib fracture who have (1) absent or de-

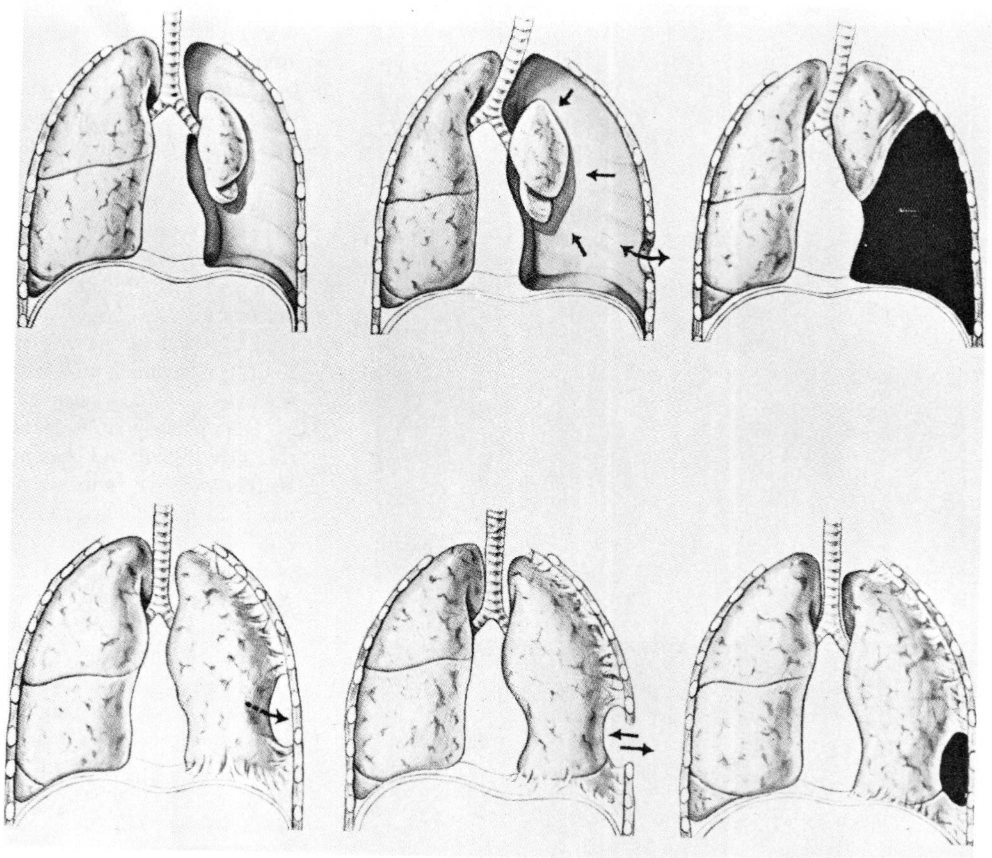

FIG. 16-13. A free pleural space will allow the development of a complete pneumothorax or a massive hemothorax. These potentially fatal complications cannot occur in patients with an obliterated pleural space. (Reproduced from: *Naciero EA: Chest Injuries. New York, Grune & Stratton, 1971, with permission.*)

creased upper extremity pulses, (2) hemorrhage, especially large extrapleural hematoma or hemothorax, and (3) brachial plexus injury. Additional criteria for angiography include displacement of fragments and multiple thoracic injuries.

Multiple Fractures. The problem of massive flail chest has been briefly discussed previously. Lesser degrees of flail occur whenever there are multiple fractures of the chest wall skeletal structure. Flail chest is appropriately diagnosed whenever there is paradoxical respiratory movement in a segment of the chest wall. This generally requires at least two segmental fractures in each of three adjacent ribs or costal cartilages or other multiple combinations of rib or sternal fractures with costochrondral or chondrosternal separations. Posterior flail segments, in the absence of disrupted intrathoracic structures, are easier to manage because of the strong muscular and scapular support, and because of patients' natural tendency to lie with their backs against the mattress.

Chest wall stabilization and reduction of respiratory dead space are major goals of treatment. Improvements in respiratory therapy, including bedside measurements of pulmonary mechanics and the widespread availability of arterial blood-gas determinations, have allowed greater individualization in the treatment of patients with flail-chest injuries. For many years endotracheal intubation or early tracheostomy has been recommended for the management of patients with flail chest, because it allows easy access for tracheobronchial suctioning, it reduces dead space, and it facilitates internal stabilization of the chest wall through mechanical ventilation. Intubation is often delayed now until evidence of a need for ventilatory support develops: a respiratory rate of 40 breaths/min, a falling Pa_{CO_2} is evidence of excessive work of breathing to maintain adequate oxygenation, or a Pa_{O_2} below 60 torr on inspired oxygen fractions of over 0.5. Other techniques for stabilizing the flail segment, such as the use of external compression dressings or the application of traction by encircling the fractured ribs with towel clips or wire, are historical oddities. For some patients with a small flail area and minimal pulmonary injury, close observation alone may allow satisfactory recovery without the use of assisted ventilation. In these patients treatment should be directed at the respiratory dysfunction rather than at stabilizing the area of paradoxical motion. A rare patient presents with localized chest wall fractures amenable to direct operative stabilization. When feasible, this approach can considerably shorten convalescence.

Several long-term follow-up studies have recently been published analyzing the late consequences of flail-chest injuries. Significant disability was reported in 50 to 64 percent of the patients with pain as the common residual complaint. In one study, 40 percent of examined patients had found it necessary to change their life style as a result of the chest injury. Much better attention to the early and continuing rehabilitation of these injured patients is undoubtedly indicated by these findings.

Other Rib Fractures. An inward displacement of the fracture fragments at the time of injury may lacerate the lung parenchyma and produce a pneumothorax with bleeding into the pleural cavity. With a single rib fracture the incidence of pneumothorax is not high, but there is an increasing likelihood of this complication as the number of fractured ribs increases. The occurrence of pneumothorax may be delayed for some hours or even days after the injury

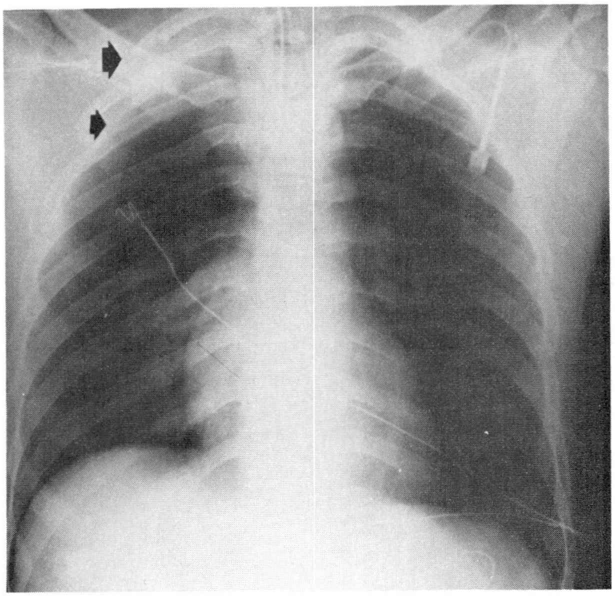

A

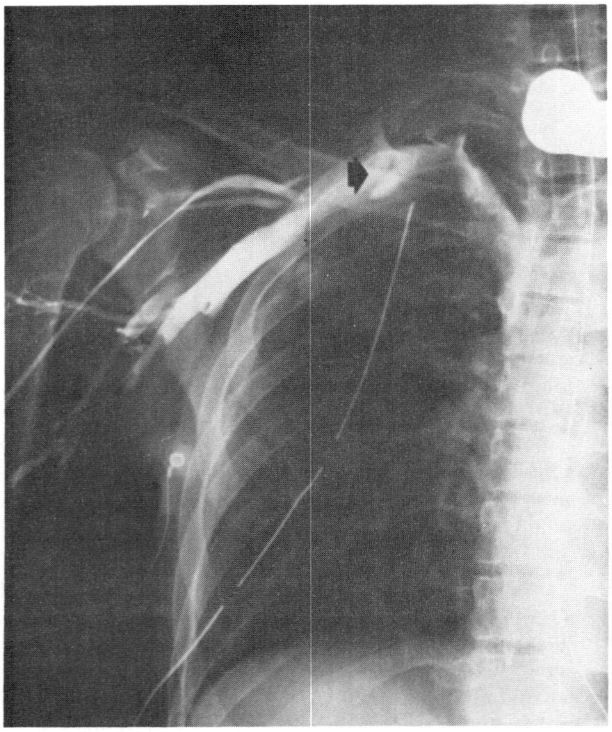

B

FIG. 16-14. *A.* The first chest x-ray of a 25-year-old man who was injured in a motorcycle accident shows a fracture of the right first rib (*upper arrow*) and a small extrapleural hematoma at the right apex (*lower arrow*). *B.* A subclavian arteriogram and venogram were done 3 days after admission because of the sudden development of a massive hemothorax (2000 mL blood) on the right side. Bleeding stopped spontaneously, and the venogram shows a tear in the subclavian vein at the rib fracture site.

has occurred. As noted previously, hemothorax of a significant degree occurring with rib fractures is usually due to laceration of an intercostal artery rather than to bleeding from the lung. Again, bleeding may be delayed in onset or it may recur after an interval of several days, and it may be life-threatening. Especially in the patient who has multiple rib fractures with segmental fractures of one or more ribs, a delayed pneumothorax or hemothorax may coincide with some shift of the rib fragments demonstrated in serial chest x-rays.

In elderly or chronically ill patients rib fractures may occur with severe coughing or hard straining. The occurrence of a spontaneous fracture should alert the physician to the possibility of a bone abnormality such as metastatic neoplasm or hyperparathyroidism. Pneumothorax and hemothorax are infrequent with rib fractures that do not result from external trauma.

The diagnosis of a rib fracture may be implied from the pleuritic type of pain and marked tenderness over the fracture area. A sharply localized contusion of the chest wall structures may mimic the findings, including shallow respirations with chest wall splinting. Green-stick fractures are those not associated with separation of the fragments, and they may not be demonstrated by the initial chest x-ray examination. Several weeks may elapse before a suspected fracture is confirmed. When the patient has two or more adjacent fractured ribs, especially if the ribs are broken in more than one place (segmental fractures), the diagnosis is made with greater certainty by examination alone. Cartilage fractures and separation from either the rib or sternum are not demonstrated by chest x-rays. In a review of emergency room practice, Thompson and coworkers emphasized how infrequently management is influenced by rib radiographs and urged higher reliance on physical findings and avoidance of efforts to obtain confirmatory radiographs, unless findings might alter treatment.

The principal goal of treatment for patients without serious injury is relief of pain. If this is accomplished, patients may resume their normal activities except those that require a vigorous work effort. Adhesive strapping of the chest or chest binders to splint the fracture area should be avoided in all but the very young. In the majority of other patients, an adequate oral analgesic or an intercostal nerve block plus oral analgesics provides reasonable pain relief with minimal risk of side effects (Fig. 16-15). Binders or strapping are particular hazards in the elderly and in patients with chronic lung disease. The nerve block may need to be repeated once daily for several days, but a single injection may suffice for individuals whose injury does not require hospitalization. A patient whose rib fractures are accompanied by minimal pneumothorax (less than 1.5 cm separation between the lung and the inner chest wall by x-ray) may be treated as an outpatient under ideal conditions of observation and follow-up.

Sternal Fractures. Any major blunt trauma to the anterior chest wall may cause a fracture of the sternum. Such fractures may occur alone or in combination with multiple rib fractures. The fractures are usually transverse and most often occur in the body of the sternum at or near the junction with the manubrium (Fig. 16-16). The injury is extremely painful and can usually be pinpointed by the conscious patient. The diagnosis should be made on physical examination and confirmed by lateral x-rays of the sternum or tomography. It is essential to rule out significant injury to underlying structures, especially the heart. In the absence of other major injury, the treatment of the fracture is aimed toward relief of pain and observation for signs of respiratory embarrassment. In patients

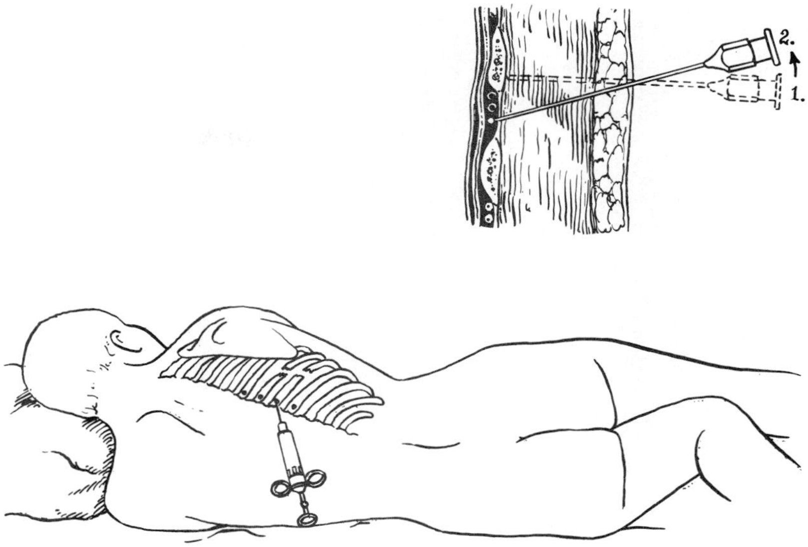

FIG. 16-15. Intercostal nerve blocks may be very effective in relieving the pain of rib fractures. The nerves above and below the fractured ribs must be blocked, in addition to those corresponding to the ribs fractured.

with compromised pulmonary function or obvious instability of the fragments, more vigorous treatment is required, e.g., positive-pressure ventilation and/or operative reduction and stabilization of the fragments. When the pain of a sternal fracture persists for a long period of time, a nonunion should be suspected. Most often, this is the result of persistent displacement of the proximal fragment. In this instance open reduction is usually required.

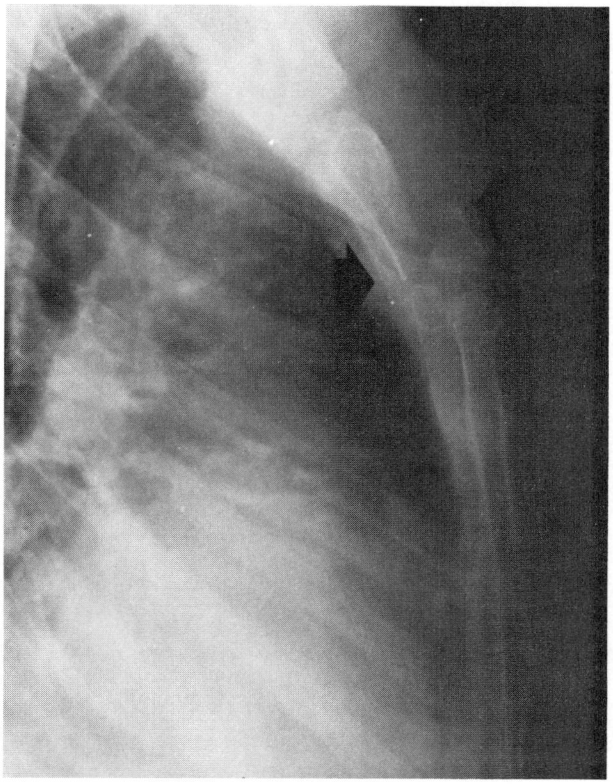

FIG. 16-16. A lateral chest x-ray demonstrates the type of sternal fracture that occurs when the driver of a car is thrown against the steering wheel.

Hemothorax. Intrathoracic bleeding occurs with any form of chest injury that disrupts the tissues. Hemothorax usually develops at the time of injury, but the bleeding may be delayed for several days. Occasionally an extrapleural hematoma will break into the pleural cavity and give the impression of delayed hemorrhage.

Bleeding from the lung as a result of rib fractures, stab wounds, or small-missile wounds will generally stop before a sufficient volume has been lost to mandate an emergency thoracotomy. From accumulated military and civilian experience it can be estimated that slightly more than 10 percent of patients with traumatic hemothorax will require thoracotomy for control of bleeding or determination of the extent of injury.

Movement of the diaphragm and thoracic structures causes partial defibrination of blood that is shed into the pleural cavity, and clotting is usually incomplete. Sufficient coagulation does occur to interfere with efficient drainage of the pleural blood through intercostal catheters, and the latter often become plugged with blood clot. Pleural enzymes begin to produce clot lysis within a few hours after bleeding stops, and the process of hemolysis with protein breakdown increases the osmotic pressure. Unless the pleural space is drained adequately, the transudation of fluid into the space can produce a significant compression of the lung and a shift of the mediastinum toward the opposite hemithorax.

The main diagnostic concerns in the management of the patient with traumatic hemothorax are how much bleeding has occurred, is it continuing, and, if stopped and clotted, when should clot be removed. Consideration of the type and extent of injury, general signs of blood loss, physical signs of fluid in the pleural cavity, and chest x-ray findings are guides to the assessment of the extent of hemothorax. Four to five hundred milliliters of blood may be hidden by the diaphragm on the upright chest x-ray, and 1 L or more may be overlooked on a supine film. A large hemothorax may even be missed on the upright chest x-ray unless the observer is aware of the phenomenon of subpulmonary trapping of the

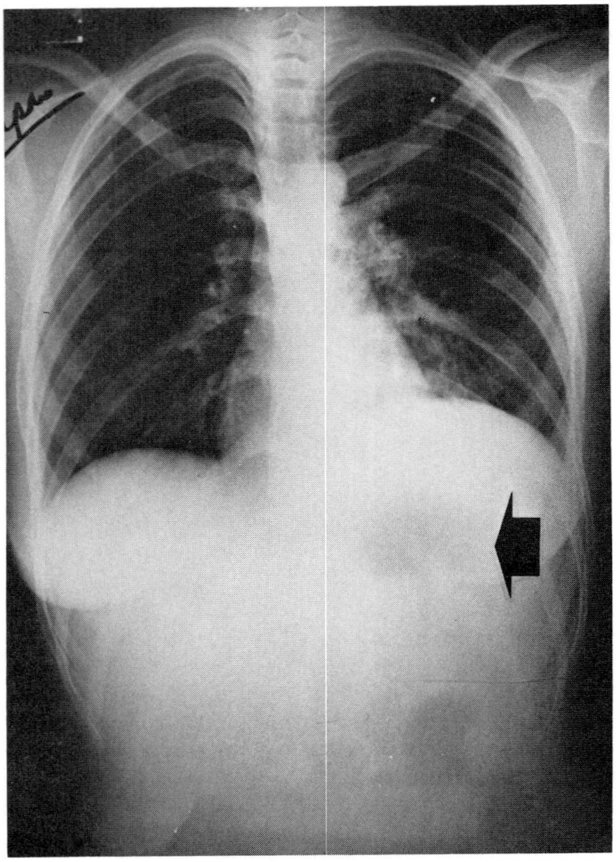

A

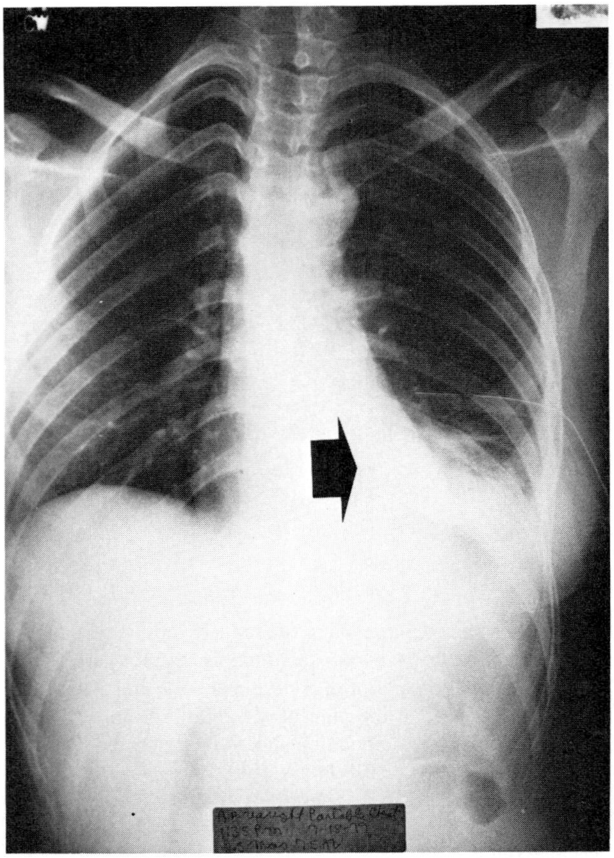

C

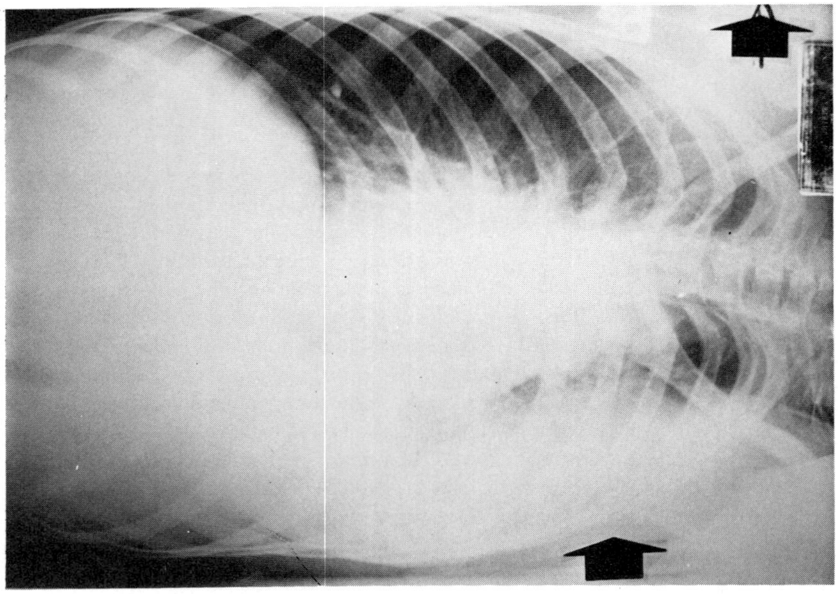

B

FIG. 16-17. Traumatic hemothorax due to a stab wound of the left chest in a 32-year-old woman. *A.* The first chest x-ray suggests an elevation of the left diaphragm, and the emergency-room physician did not suspect a hemothorax. The surgical consultant was suspicious of subpulmonary trapping of a hemothorax because of the distance between the top of the apparent diaphragm and the gastric air bubble (*arrow*). *B.* A lateral decubitis x-ray shows a large collection of blood in the left hemithorax. *C.* Insertion of an intercostal tube resulted in drainage of 600 mL of blood. However, the chest x-ray suggests the presence of residual blood and clots in the pleural cavity (*arrow*).

blood (Fig. 16-17). Lateral decubitus x-ray can confirm the diagnosis of hemothorax and guide placement of an appropriate drainage catheter.

A small hemothorax that produces little more than blunting of the costophrenic angle on the chest x-ray does not require initial treatment; follow-up x-rays at appropriate intervals will assist with the decision to drain the pleural cavity if there is a progressive accumulation. When the hemothorax exceeds an amount that fills the costophrenic sulcus, or when there is associated pneumothorax, one or more large catheters should be placed in the pleural cavity through the seventh, eighth, or ninth intercostal space in the posterior-axillary line. Underwater drainage alone may be sufficient, but low suction applied to the catheters is often helpful when combined with active efforts at stripping the tubes of blood clot. If the initial drainage of blood is followed by continued bleeding in the absence of a clotting defect, a decision to operate must be made, with a broad consideration of the possible sources of the bleeding.

With a major hemothorax the success of tube drainage is often frustrated by extensive clot that obstructs the tubes. An attitude should be adopted that a nonfunctioning chest tube represents a liability to the patient because of discomfort and the risk of carrying infection from the skin wound into the pleural clot. Especially with penetrating trauma, a hemothorax that fails to drain adequately through intercostal catheters may develop into empyema. An additional hazard is the organization of residual clot to form a fibrothorax. Coselli and colleagues in Houston have reviewed their experience with clotted hemothorax and found early thoracotomy substantially reduces hospitalization time and empyema rates.

Tracheobronchial Injury. The management of massive tracheobronchial injuries is discussed above. For small penetrating injuries of the intrathoracic trachea and major bronchi, tracheostomy and effective pleural decompression may provide satisfactory definitive treatment. Those injuries that are associated with an actual defect in the tracheobronchial wall, including partial disruption, require operative exploration and repair. Tracheostomy may be necessary to prevent high intratracheal pressures and to allow tracheal care postoperatively, but positive-pressure assisted ventilation should be avoided.

Penetrating injuries of lobar or segmental bronchi may produce a similar clinical picture to proximal tracheobronchial injuries. Bilateral pneumothorax is rare, and the principal immediate problem is to begin management of the major air leak and confirm the presence of a major bronchial injury. The bronchial air leak often stops soon after an intercostal catheter is put in place. The definitive diagnosis may be delayed if the bronchus becomes obstructed by blood clot or mucus and the air leak ceases. Under these conditions the pulmonary lobe or segment becomes atelectatic and resists conservative methods to produce reexpansion. If infection does not occur, the injured bronchus may heal with significant distortion and obstruction, or the atelectasis may persist and lead subsequently to a correct diagnosis. Operative repair of the disrupted bronchus can be achieved even years after injury. If infection occurs at the site of the bronchial injury, the patient may develop pneumonia, distal bronchiectasis, and empyema. Resection of the bronchus and the involved pulmonary lobe is then required.

Pulmonary Injury. The lungs have a remarkable ability to tolerate penetrating injuries and blunt trauma without long-term residual effects. Civilian gunshot wounds of the chest penetrate a lung more frequently than any other structure, but the majority of patients with no other significant injury can be treated without a thoracotomy. Any penetrating object produces an air leak with a variable degree of pneumothorax. The disruption of tissue along the missile track causes bleeding, which usually ceases as the damaged parenchyma becomes swollen and filled with blood clot. With small-caliber and low-velocity bullet wounds that pass through the lung periphery, the amount of tissue damage produced may be sufficiently small that late follow-up chest x-rays fail to demonstrate the area of injury. With high-velocity bullets, the tissue destruction extends more widely, and even a peripheral bullet pathway may result in irreversible damage to a lobar or lung hilus.

The immediate management of the patient with a penetrating injury is the insertion of at least one intercostal catheter for evacuation of the associated hemopneumothorax. Serial arterial blood gases and frequent evaluation of the patient's ventilatory ability allow an overall estimate of the effect of the injury on respiratory exchange. Civilian penetrating wounds rarely require ventilatory assistance. Only rarely is there a need for thoracotomy to control bleeding or to perform pulmonary resection for an irreversibly injured lung.

Pulmonary Contusion. Pulmonary contusion is the consequence of blunt trauma to the lung. The frequent causes of contusion include rapid deceleration of the chest against an automobile steering wheel, falls from a height, and blast injuries. Particularly in young persons, severe pulmonary contusion can occur by transmission of force through the chest wall with minimal fractures of the ribs or sternum. In middle-aged or elderly persons significant pulmonary contusion is usually accompanied by multiple fractures of the thoracic cage.

The contused lung is characterized by capillary disruption that results in intraalveolar and interstitial hemorrhage, edema, protein and fluid obstruction of small airways, and leukocyte infiltration. Serial chest x-rays begun right after injury show a fluffy infiltrate that progresses in extent and in density over a period of 24 to 48 h. Although the maximum lung injury is directly related to that region of the chest wall that receives the trauma, a "contrecoup" effect may be responsible for a wider distribution of the pulmonary damage. Unless the contusion involves only a small region of one lung, it may result in serious loss of respiratory function. The associated injury to the chest wall is aggravated by the loss of pulmonary compliance, increasing the work of breathing. Small areas of atelectasis become confluent, and progressive hypoxia further diminishes the patient's ability to compensate for the loss of function.

Pulmonary contusion is often part of a major chest injury that includes one or more fractures of the thoracic cage, pneumothorax, and hemothorax. If not present initially, a pneumothorax may subsequently develop from actual disruption of the contused pulmonary parenchyma. Although it is infrequent in patients who survive to reach the hospital, a major pulmonary laceration may represent the maximum extent of pulmonary contusion. In some instances the tissue disruption is the result of extensive penetration by rib fragments, but in others the causative factor is probably a severe shearing force. The clinical and x-ray findings suggest a serious chest injury but do not differentiate the patient with a major lung laceration from those with pulmonary contusion and associated hemopneumothorax. Continued or uncontrolled hemorrhage and massive air leak generally mandate an early thoracotomy. A major pulmonary resection is often necessary, and the mortality rate is high.

Treatment of pulmonary contusion must include an accurate clinical assessment of the patient's respiratory exchange and careful monitoring by serial measurements of the arterial blood gases. Steroids probably have no role in the management of pulmonary contusion.

A high percentage of patients require temporary assisted ventilation, and it may be evident at the time of admission that endotracheal or nasotracheal intubation should be performed. Without

Table 16-3
Criteria for Assisted Ventilation

Function	*Normal Values*	*Ventilate*
Pulmonary mechanics:		
Respiratory rate	12–20	>35
Vital capacity, mL/kg	65–75	<15
Maximum inspiratory force, cmH_2O (negative values)	75–100	<25–35
Gas exchange		
Pa_{O_2}, torr	76–100 (room air)	<65–70 (added oxygen)
Alveolar-arterial oxygen difference, torr (100% oxygen)	30–70	>350
Pa_{CO_2}, torr	35–45	>50
Dead space/tidal volume ratio	0.25–0.40	>0.6

question, aggressive respiratory therapy, including ventilatory support, should be initiated before cardiopulmonary decompensation requires treatment measures that add additional risks. Criteria for instituting assisted ventilation are shown in Table 16-3. For most patients the need for assisted ventilation does not extend beyond 48 to 72 h unless there is major injury to the chest wall or to other body regions.

Posttraumatic Pulmonary Insufficiency. The development of acute respiratory failure can be expected in a high percentage of patients who suffer major thoracic trauma. Preexisting pulmonary status will influence the severity of respiratory insufficiency, and the extent of actual pulmonary damage will determine whether the patient survives. An initial evaluation of respiratory exchange and ventilatory ability, confirmed by measurement of pulmonary mechanics and arterial blood gases, should be followed by serial reevaluations.

Especially in patients who have suffered multiple trauma, a respiratory-distress syndrome may develop that is out of proportion to the extent of thoracic injury. A series of terms has evolved over the years to designate several forms of respiratory insufficiency that follow trauma and may be associated with a constellation of causative factors. Such terms as "wet lung," "shock lung," "congestive atelectasis," and "adult respiratory-distress syndrome" reflect some principal features that seemed to be characteristic of the cases that came to the attention of those who coined the terms. There is certainly some overlap in the causation of the several forms of respiratory failure that follow major trauma, and it is important to determine the specific causes in individual patients. Blaisdell and Lewis have presented a thorough discussion of posttraumatic pulmonary insufficiency, choosing the term respiratory-distress syndrome of shock and trauma for those cases not due to a specific cause. They suggest that eight different explanations for respiratory failure other than the respiratory-distress syndrome occur with reasonable frequency in patients who suffer major injury. These include aspiration, simple atelectasis, lung contusion, fat embolism, pneumonia, pneumothorax, pulmonary edema, and pulmonary embolism.

On the basis of their experience with a large number of cases, Blaisdell and Lewis have concluded that the respiratory-distress syndrome (RDS) is one and the same as the fat-embolism syndrome. Originally thought to result from fat embolism from fracture of long bones, the syndrome consists of pulmonary, neurologic, and systemic manifestations. The pulmonary manifestations appear first, generally within 24 to 36 h after injury, and consist of dyspnea, tachycardia, fever, and cyanosis. Documentation that much of the fat that appears in the blood following injury represents a mobilization of free fatty acids from body neutral fat as a result of shock and increased levels of catecholamines has helped in understanding the mechanism of this condition. Because some degree of intravascular coagulation can be demonstrated in all cases, this is almost certainly a factor in development of the syndrome.

For patients who suffer major chest injury it may be impossible to define what part of their respiratory failure is a result of direct trauma and how much is a consequence of the RDS. Treatment must be based on correction of the direct results of injury and on the anticipation or early recognition of respiratory insufficiency. The radiologic changes of RDS, consisting of diffuse lung infiltrates that progress to become confluent, may be superimposed on the effects of pulmonary contusion and atelectasis. Changes observed on serial chest x-rays lag behind the changes in pulmonary function, and a patient may be in critical respiratory failure before the films suggest a progressive pulmonary lesion.

Management of the RDS requires maintenance of good cardiovascular function and prompt institution of ventilatory support. An adequate volume replacement for external fluid and blood losses is complicated by the internal fluid losses due to increased capillary permeability in the lung, in all areas of direct tissue trauma, and to a varying degree throughout the body. Monitoring central venous pressures is the minimum for guidance of fluid and diuretic therapy in these patients, but placement of a Swan–Ganz catheter to allow left atrial and pulmonary artery pressures is superior. The need for inotropic myocardial support can be detected earlier by this access to left-sided heart pressures.

Ventilatory support techniques have advanced to allow a wider selection of ventilators and methods of assisted respiration. Attention to detail can offer the patient a maximum chance of survival with a minimum risk of complications. An unanswered question is the place of steroid therapy. The experience with these agents has been variable, and their employment is generally delayed until the patient appears to be nearing an irreversible state of progressive respiratory failure. This is probably too late for a reasonable drug effect. Sladen has described an approach that probably justifies a clinical trial. He used pharmacologic doses of methylprednisolone (30 mg/kg) intravenously every 6 h for 48 h in combination with ventilatory support and reported a significant reduction in mortality rate when compared with historical controls.

CHEST WALL

Congenital Deformities

Pectus Excavatum

The most common congenital deformity of the chest wall is pectus excavatum, in which the body of the sternum is displaced posteriorly to produce a funnel-shaped depression (Fig. 16-18). The etiology is not certain, but most authors ascribe to the notion that overgrowth of the lower costal cartilages and ribs is responsible. The defect varies widely in expression. The depression is most often centered at the xiphisternal junction but may extend to the manubrium in rare cases. In lateral extent the presentation var-

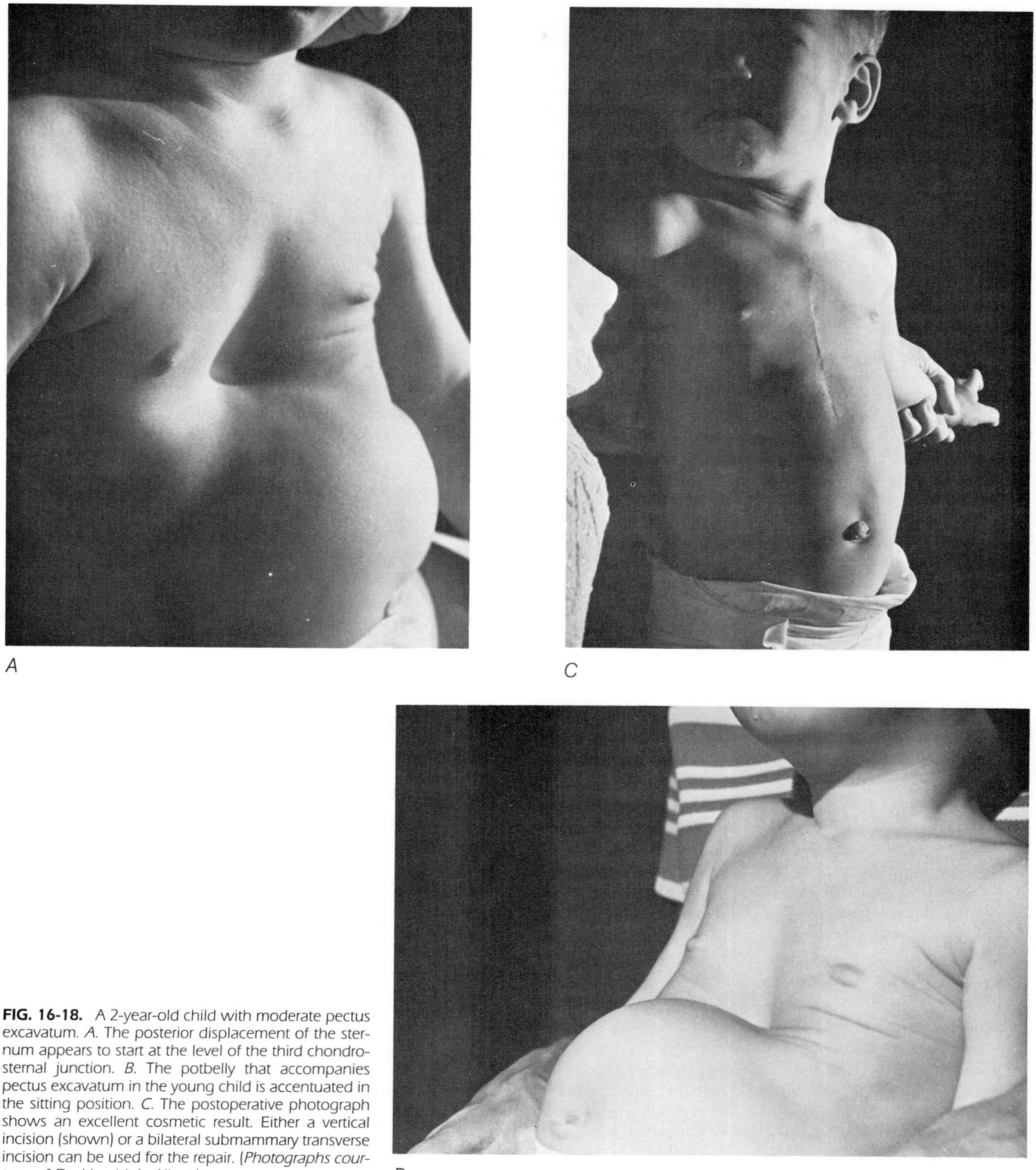

FIG. 16-18. A 2-year-old child with moderate pectus excavatum. *A.* The posterior displacement of the sternum appears to start at the level of the third chondrosternal junction. *B.* The potbelly that accompanies pectus excavatum in the young child is accentuated in the sitting position. *C.* The postoperative photograph shows an excellent cosmetic result. Either a vertical incision (shown) or a bilateral submammary transverse incision can be used for the repair. (*Photographs courtesy of Dr. Harold A. Albert.*)

ies from a narrow central cleft to a broad dish-shaped defect extending from nipple to nipple. The depth of the depression is equally variable, with the sternum reaching or even overlapping the spine in extreme forms. Asymmetry is common, and always involves greater depression of the right costal cartilages with rotation of the sternum to the right.

Pectus excavatum is present at birth and progresses at a variable and unpredictable rate through childhood. Infants and young children often have a protuberant abdomen that accentuates the deformity. Later in childhood a characteristic posture has been described, with rounded and forward-sloping shoulders, forward angulation of the head and neck, and dorsal kyphosis of the spine. Breast development in young women is frequently asymmetric, with a smaller breast on the right.

Although most cases appear in isolation, a familial tendency has been noted, and the defect is frequently seen in more than one sibling. The anomaly is about three times more frequent in males. Pectus excavatum is frequently seen in Marfan's syndrome and is one of a variety of chest wall deformities seen with increased frequency in patients with congenital heart disease.

A variety of classifications based on radiographic findings has been proposed. Haller and associates have used a "pectus index" based on the ratio of transverse to anterior-posterior diameter measured on a single standard CT scan image. In their series all patients undergoing operative correction had a pectus index > 3.25.

That pectus excavatum produces a cosmetic deformity is not a matter of debate. Thirty to seventy percent of patients are reported to be symptomatic, with a broad range of presentations including exercise intolerance, atypical chest pain, dyspnea, bronchospasm, poor feeding, and arrhythmias. In all reported series, symptoms are almost always relieved by operative correction. Systolic ejection murmurs are frequently reported, and are thought to reflect compression of the right ventricular outflow tract. Electrocardiographic abnormalities are frequent and usually resolve after repair, but are thought to reflect changes in axis due to rotation and displacement rather than any fundamental electrophysiologic disturbance.

Whether or not a physiologic defect is responsible for the characteristic symptomatology is still quite controversial. Wynn and associates and Ghory and associates have reviewed previous reports spanning 70 years and added their own observations. Ghory and associates studied 14 children with pectus excavatum and 14 normal controls and found a higher diastolic blood pressure and a decreased preejection period with exercise in older children ($>$ age 11) with pectus. No differences were seen in maximal work load, oxygen consumption, cardiac output, and stroke volume. Wynn and associates studied 12 patients with pectus excavatum. Eight were studied before and after operative correction, and four were tested twice but not corrected. No significant differences were observed in most parameters, such as maximal oxygen uptake, cardiac output, and stroke volume. The only difference that resulted in statistical significance was an 8 percent decrease in total lung capacity after operation; total lung capacity was unchanged in the nonoperated group ($p < 0.01$).

Pectus excavatum is primarily a cosmetic defect with a very broad anatomic and symptomatic spectrum. There is no conclusive evidence supporting the existence of a consistent functional defect. Operation is indicated to correct the cosmetic defect and can be expected to eliminate symptoms in the majority of patients, even though a physiologic basis for the symptomatology cannot be defined.

Operative Treatment. Most authors recommend operative correction during the preschool years (before 5 years of age) but not before 18 months. Operation at that age is thought to prevent the secondary postural, physiologic, and psychological consequences of the defect.

The technique most widely used is that described by Ravitch. All the deformed costal cartilages are excised, the xiphisternal joint is disarticulated, and intercostal muscle bundles are separated from the sternum, and transverse posterior osteotomy of the sternum is performed above the point of depression. The osteotomy can be combined with a forward fracture of the sternum and insertion of a bone wedge in the osteotomy site to provide an overcorrection of the deformity.

In certain cases the repair is reinforced with a metal strut that can be removed several months later. In recent large series, excellent short- and long-term results have been reported. Haller and associates achieved excellent long-term results in 95 percent of 664 patients followed for 1 to 40 years. Shamberger and Welch achieved satisfactory long-term results in 98 percent of 704 patients followed for 1 to 27 years.

Excellent results have also been reported with a very different operative approach. *Sternal eversion* involves transverse division of the sternum, division of the costal cartilages, 180° axial rotation of the sternum (sternal eversion), and suture reattachment. In essence, the concave deformity is made convex. The sternal plastron can be rotated on a mammary artery vascular pedicle or as a free graft. Although the series has not been recently updated, with sternal eversion Wada and associates achieved satisfactory results in 97 percent of 199 patients followed for 15 years.

Pectus Carinatum

The protrusion deformities of the sternum are much less common than pectus excavatum, accounting for less than 10 percent of patients presenting for repair. This group of "bird chest" deformities varies considerably in specific manifestations. The most common type is characterized by a deep depression of the costal cartilages along each side of the sternum, which accentuates the mild protrusion of the sternum by creating an illusion of greater anterior projection in relation to the ribs. The deformity is usually maximal below the nipple level; asymmetry is common, most often producing mild rotation of the sternum to the right.

Although symptoms reminiscent of pectus excavatum have been associated with the protrusion defects, it appears that most are asymptomatic, and the condition has seldom been studied physiologically. Operative correction is done through a curved submammary incision that allows broad exposure of the deformed cartilages and costochondral junctions (Fig. 16-19). Subperichondral and subperiosteal resection of all deformed cartilages and ribs is performed throughout the length of their deformity. The excessive length of each perichondral bed is obliterated with reefing sutures, and the sternal contour is adjusted with a transverse osteotomy if necessary. In the only reported series of any size, Shamberger and Welch achieved 98 percent satisfactory results in 152 patients followed for 1 to 12 years.

Sternal Fissures

The sternum is formed when two lateral plates of mesoderm fuse in the midline during the tenth week of embryonic development. The clavicular heads also contribute primordia to the manubrium. Failure of fusion can be complete, or it can be confined to the superior end or the inferior end of the sternum.

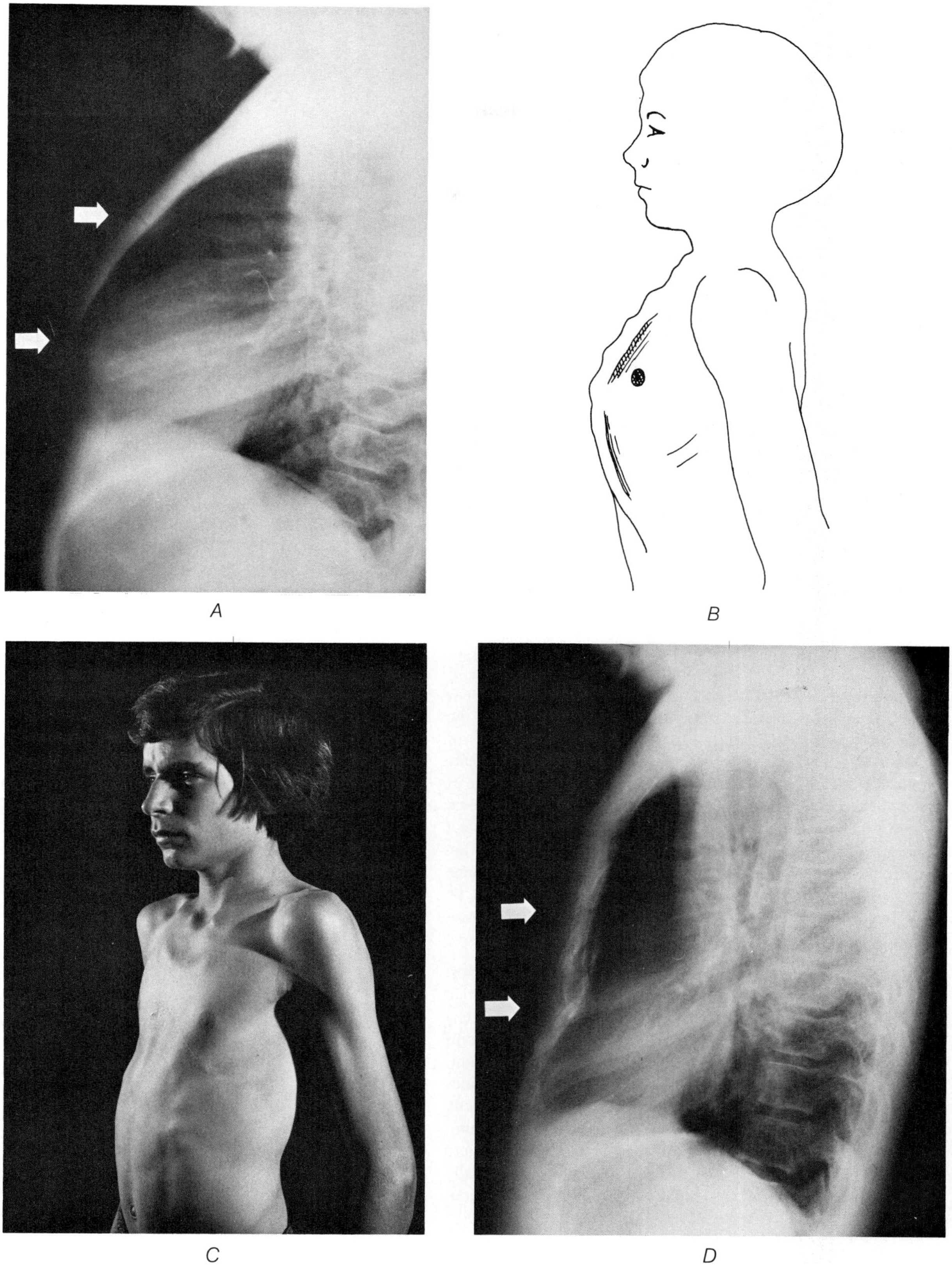

FIG. 16-19. A 14-year-old boy with pectus carinatum. *A.* The preoperative lateral chest x-ray shows remarkable anterior projection of the sternum. *B.* A line drawing demonstrates the forward projection of the sternum that is accentuated by the prominence of the knoblike costal cartilages. *C.* The postoperative photograph of the patient demonstrates a very satisfactory result. *D.* The postoperative lateral chest x-ray contrasts sharply with the preoperative film.

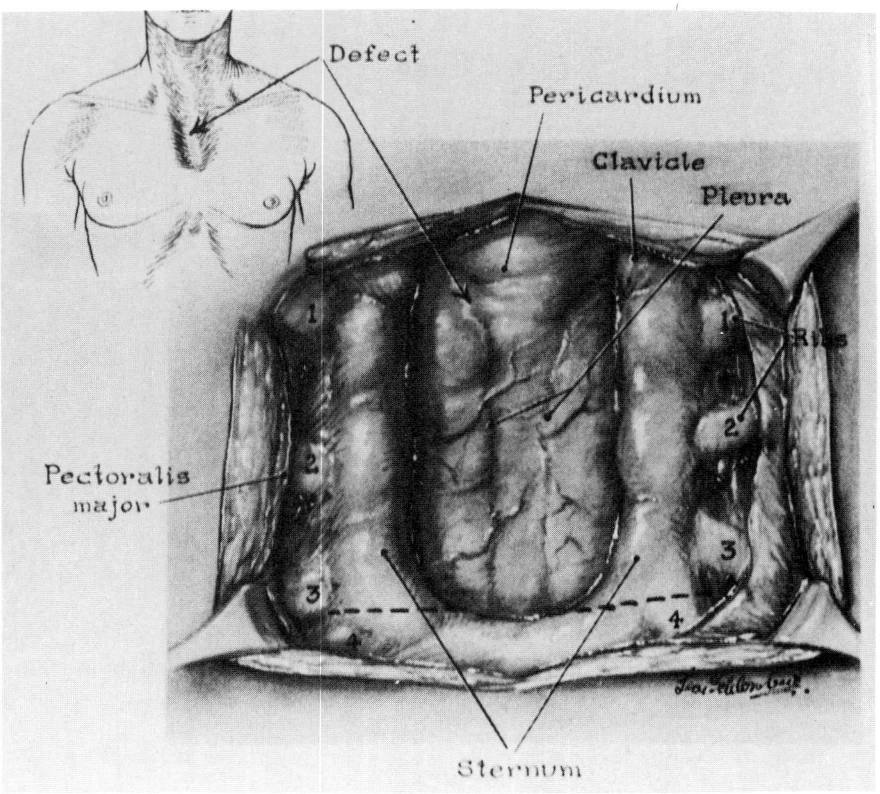

FIG. 16-20. A superior sternal cleft, presenting clinically with striking pulsation at the base of the neck, where the pericardium bulges out through the defect. It is frequently possible to pull the two sternal halves together by transecting the inferior end of the defect (dotted lines), combined with oblique chondrotomies of the costal cartilages. In the case illustrated, an 11-year-old girl, reduction was not possible, and the defect was successfully repaired with a steel wire mesh covering. (From: *Ravitch MM, with permission.*)

Superior Sternal Cleft. In this type of defect the cleft is broad and U- or V-shaped, usually extending down to about the fourth costal cartilage (Fig. 16-20). The prominent pulsations of the heart, which is covered only by thoracic fascia and skin, create the illusion of cardiac displacement into the neck. In fact, the heart usually lies in approximately normal position, and the two separate halves of the sternum can be located at the periphery of the defect and reapproximated. Osteotomies in each half or distal transection of each half is usually necessary to bring them together. In some cases, especially those repaired after infancy, there will not be room for the heart, and coverage with prosthetic material is required.

Distal Sternal Cleft. A defect in the distal sternal is almost invariably part of a syndrome called Cantrell's pentalogy, which consists of the following five components: (1) a cleft distal sternum, (2) a ventral abdominal wall defect that may be a true omphalocele, (3) an anterior crescentic deficiency of the diaphragm, (4) communication between the parietal and peritoneal cavities through the diaphragm, and (5) congenital heart disease, usually with a ventricular septal defect and a left ventricular diverticulum.

Operative correction requires a staged approach taking into account the priorities of each defect. The omphalocele is usually repaired first. As with other forms of sternal cleft, early reconstruction offers the best chance for primary closure.

Complete Sternal Cleft. In this rarest form of sternal cleft, failure of midline fusion is complete, leaving the mediastinal contents bulging through a thin covering of skin and fascia. In the few cases described, an associated failure of midline abdominal fusion has been frequent, and communication between the peritoneum and pericardium common. Repair in infancy is highly desirable and can be quite satisfactory.

Miscellaneous Anomalies of Rib and Costal Cartilage

The simplest anomalies consist of deformed, deficient, or enlarged cartilage or rib presenting as an isolated finding in an asymptomatic patient. More complex anomalies include absence or wide divergence of one or more lower ribs and are commonly associated with hemivertebrae, fused bony paravertebral bars, and progressive scoliosis. The chest wall defect can manifest obvious paradoxic respiratory motion and even true lung herniation, but the spinal anomalies are usually more functionally significant and demand more therapeutic attention.

Poland's syndrome consists of absence or hypoplasia of the pectoralis major and minor muscles, breast hypoplasia, and partial absence of the upper costal cartilages (Fig. 16-21). Brachysyndactyly, ectrodactyly, and ectromelia are frequently described associations. It is invariably unilateral. Depending on the extent of cartilage deficiency there may be an impressive lung hernia, paradoxical respiratory motion, or simple flattening of the anterolateral chest wall. When the anomaly is on the left side, the underlying heart and lung are significantly vulnerable, since they are covered only by skin, fascia, and pleura. As the child grows, the concavity tends to become more severe on either side.

Operative reconstruction is recommended for cosmetic reasons, to eliminate paradoxical motion, and to protect intrathoracic structures. Staged procedures involving split rib grafts from the contralateral side combined with Teflon felt or Marlex mesh have been advocated in the past. A logical outgrowth of the increasing popularity of pedicled myocutaneous flaps has been their applica-

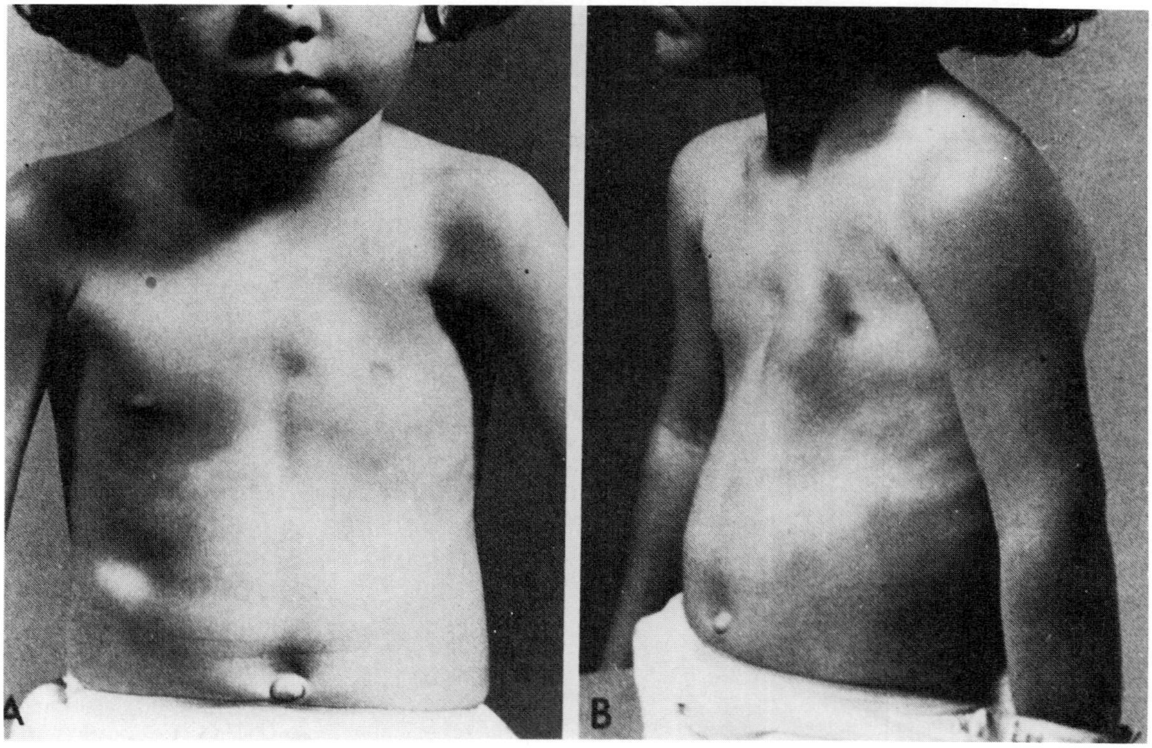

FIG. 16-21. Poland's syndrome in a child. The sternocostal portion of the pectoralis major, the pectoralis minor, and cartilages 2 to 4 are absent on the left side. The nipple, breast, and subcutaneous tissue are hypoplastic. (From: *Ravitch MM, with permission.*)

tion in the reconstruction of this anomaly. Urschel and associates described successful single-stage reconstruction in two patients using a latissimus dorsi flap and simultaneous augmentation mammoplasty.

Chest Wall Tumors

In reviewing this topic in 1949, Brian Blades observed, ". . . available statistical data concerning the exact incidence of thoracic wall tumors are incomplete and probably unimportant. Moreover accurate histological classification of the tumors is often confusing." If he were writing today, he would probably add that the accurate histologic classification is unimportant. Now as then, most reports in the literature are limited case reports, the few larger series are reported from major tertiary referral hospitals with the highly selected patient population that characterizes those institutions; the available statistical data relating to the actual frequency of the various types probably remain inaccurate. Depending on the referral characteristics of the reporting institution, the incidence of primary malignancy of chest wall tumors ranges from 13 percent (Cavanaugh) to over 50 percent (Sabanathan et al). It seems likely that the true incidence of malignancy in the general population may be nearer the lower figure. Whatever the true frequency, malignancies are common enough and clinical or laboratory findings are sufficiently uncertain that speculating about the probabilities of any given chest wall mass being benign or malignant is usually an unimportant exercise. It should be considered malignant until proved otherwise by detailed analysis by an experienced surgical pathologist.

The reported experience confirms that chest wall malignancies are often mismanaged. Inadequate biopsies are untrustworthy, fears about chest wall reconstruction difficulties may encourage inadequate local resection, and recurrence after inadequate initial resection is a common cause of failure. Most authors now agree that an adequate biopsy should be undertaken early in the evaluation of the suspicious mass. Multimodality therapy has increasingly become a standard treatment for many adult soft tissue malignancies. Contemporary diagnostic capabilities of surgical pathologists including electron microscopy, immunohistochemistry, flow cytometry, cytogenetics, and tissue culture techniques have improved diagnostic accuracy and have resulted in the addition of tumor grade classificiation, G1 (well differentiated) through G4 (undifferentiated), to the American Joint Committee Tumor–nodal involvement–metastasis (TNM) grading system. With advances in reconstruction techniques (e.g., myocutaneous flaps, improved synthetic materials), virtually any defect in the chest wall can be repaired. A logical approach at present would seem to call for an aggressive effort to ascertain an accurate diagnosis before embarking on extensive ablative therapy and to consider a multimodal approach at the outset. Accurate diagnosis requires adequate tissue; needle biopsies should be avoided and frozen sections should be performed on removed tissue before leaving the operating room, not to establish a diagnosis but to be sure suitable tissue for eventual diagnosis has been submitted. Metastatic tumors, especially to the ribs, and direct invasion of the chest wall from primary lung and breast carcinomas easily outnumber the tumors arising from the chest wall. Therefore, while the biopsy is being processed, careful search for primary neoplasm elsewhere should be made. Neoplasms originating in the thyroid, breast, and kidney are the most common to metastasize to the ribs.

The primary tumors that occur in the chest wall are those, both benign and malignant, that occur in the soft tissue and skeletal structures that are present there.

The clinical manifestation of a chest wall neoplasm is most often either pain, a palpable mass, or an abnormality detected on a chest x-ray. Surprisingly, with either benign or malignant lesions the discomfort is relatively mild, and patients often present with tumors that have been enlarging for months or years. Many patients will attribute the tumor origin to some episode of localized trauma, or they will state that they discovered the mass while rubbing their chest after a minor injury. A differential diagnosis will include the less frequent pulmonary infections that invade the chest wall, such as actinomycosis and nocardiosis, tuberculous chondritis, costochondral separation, and Tietze's syndrome (nonspecific chondritis). A suspicion of fluctuation in the mass and a corresponding pulmonary lesion may suggest that a diagnostic aspiration should be done anticipating probable infection. A true history of trauma and the ability to reproduce a clicking sensation with local pressure may reinforce the diagnosis of a suspected costochondral separation.

Work-up of the patient with a chest wall mass should focus on a search for other areas of neoplastic involvement by radioisotope studies and other imaging studies along with careful computer-assisted tomographic scans to accurately map the local extent of the tumor invasion and to plan resection and reconstruction of the chest wall defect. It must also include evaluation of pulmonary function and assessment of the patient's ability to tolerate the physiologic deficit that might result from the procedure. Defining the clinical characteristics that might improve the diagnostic guess regarding the specific cellular origin of the tumor is probably unimportant and has little prognostic significance.

Benign Tumors

Among the more likely benign tumors are fibrous dysplasia, eosinophilic granuloma, osteochondroma, desmoid tumor, and chondroma.

Fibrous Dysplasia. The ribs are the most common site of solitary fibrous dysplasia (osteofibroma, bone cyst). Located most frequently in the posterior or lateral portion of a rib, it usually presents as a slowly enlarging nonpainful mass. Diagnostic radiographs show expansion and thinning of the bony cortex, with a central trabeculated appearance. Fibrous dysplasia in ribs as well as other bones forms part of Albright's syndrome, a condition that includes skin pigmentation and precocious puberty in girls.

Eosinophilic Granuloma. The lesions of eosinophilic granuloma are sometimes part of a disease that includes pulmonary lesions called histiocytosis X or eosinophilic granuloma of the lung. When it occurs in a rib, the granuloma is a solitary destructive process, often associated with pain and localized tenderness. Radiographs reveal a punched-out osteolytic lesion, which, when subjected to excision and microscopic examination, is found to consist of a chronic granuloma. Healing may occur spontaneously, or a pathologic fracture may develop through the area of osteolysis.

Osteochondroma. These slow-growing tumors generally arise from the cortex of a rib. As with other neoplasms, the occurrence of pain may signal accelerated growth, which produces concern over the possibility of malignant change. The radiographic appearance is often that of a distorted rib cortex with an overlying mass that has a thin rim of calcification.

Chondroma. They occur at the costochondral junction, primarily in children or young people, and may be difficult to differentiate from chondritis or the sequela of traumatic costochondral separation. Chest and rib x-rays show an expansion of bone with thinned but intact cortex. Probably because of the abundance of cartilage in the chest wall, chondromas and chondrosarcomas are the most common benign and malignant tumors of the skeletal components of the thorax. Chondrosarcoma is usually a well-differentiated tumor easily misdiagnosed as a benign chondroma resulting in inadequate local resection and consequent local recurrence.

Desmoid Tumors. Whether these tumors are a form of benign fibromatosis or a low-grade fibrosarcoma, they have a high propensity to recur locally and should be resected with the same wide margins recommended for primary malignant tumors.

Malignant Tumors

Although the sarcomas arising in the adult chest wall are usually classified by the cell type of origin, prognosis is related to the histologic grade rather than cell classification. The grading system currently recommended by the American Joint Committee on Cancer no longer considers the cell of origin relevant and groups the wide variety of reported tumors under the general label of adult soft tissue sarcomas, although they may arise from any of the mesodermal tissues found in the chest wall. These tumors are potentially curable and should be approached initially by a multidisciplinary team of cancer specialists. Since the selection of treatment is dependent on accurate determination of the degree of differentiation for histologic grading, adequate biopsy and its review by an experienced pathologist is essential.

The factors that influence prognosis include age, size of tumor, histologic grade, and the stage. If the patient is over 60, the tumor is more than 5 cm, has poorly differentiated cells, or has spread to the lymph nodes or distant sites, the prognosis is poor. If the tumor has a low mitotic index, is free of hemorrhage or necrosis, and is under 5 cm in largest diameter, it is likely to be curable by surgery alone. Higher-grade tumors are associated with a higher local treatment failure rate and should be treated by pre- and/or postoperative radiation therapy or chemotherapy. Because the optimum therapy for this family of tumors is changing with increasing experience with multimodality treatment, patients should be in formal clinical protocols whenever possible.

Staging plays a central role in planning the therapeutic approach. Stages are based on the GTNM classification as defined by the American Joint Committee on Cancer.

TNM Definitions.

Primary tumor (T)
- TX: Minimum requirements to assess primary tumor cannot be met
- T0: No demonstrable tumor
- T1: Tumor 5 cm or less in diameter
- T2: Tumor more than 5 cm in diameter

Tumor grade (G)
- G1: Well differentiated
- G2: Moderately well differentiated
- G3: Poorly differentiated
- G4: Undifferentiated

Nodal involvement (N)

NX: Minimum requirements to assess regional nodes cannot be met
N0: No lymph node metastasis
N1: Regional lymph node metastasis

Distant metastasis (M)

MX: Minimum requirements to assess the presence of distant metastasis cannot be met
M0: No distant metastasis
M1: Distant metastasis present

Stage	*Classification*	*5-Year Survival*
I	G1, T1–2, N0, M0	>90%
II	G2, T1–2, N0, M0	70%
III	G3–4, T1–2, N0, M0	20–50%
IVA	Any G or T, N1, M0	<20%
IVB	Any G, T, or N, M1	<5%

In all but stage I tumors, preoperative and/or postoperative radiotherapy is being increasingly recommended. A wide variety of adjuvant chemotherapeutic protocols are currently under investigation for stage III and IV tumors.

These tumors can occasionally grow at extremely rapid rates. The case depicted in Figs. 16-22 and 16-23 was believed to be a walnut-sized breast mass 4 months before the CT scan was taken. Resection required complete removal of ribs 4 through 11 along with the lateral portion of the diaphragm and a generous wedge of lung.

Chest Wall Reconstruction

Because of the high rate of malignancy in chest wall neoplasms, there is need for an aggressive attitude toward management of any mass that likely represents a primary tumor. When malignancy is suspected, preliminary plans must be made for chest wall reconstruction that will allow resection of a generous margin of normal tissue around the neoplasm. The resection should include at least one normal adjacent rib above and below the tumor with all intervening intercostal muscles and pleura. In addition, it is often necessary to include an en bloc resection of overlying chest wall muscles such as the pectoralis minor or major, the serratus anterior, or the latissimus dorsi. When the periphery of the lung is involved with the neoplasm, it is appropriate to resect the adjacent part of the pulmonary lobe in continuity (Fig. 16-23*C*). Involvement of the sternum by a malignant tumor requires a total resection of the sternum with the adjacent cartilages. Techniques for postoperative respiratory support are sufficiently good that resection should not be compromised because of a concern about the patient's ability to ventilate adequately in the early postoperative period.

Reconstruction of a large defect in the chest wall requires the use of some type of material to prevent lung herniation and to provide stability for the chest wall (Fig. 16-23*D*). Mild degrees of paradoxical motion are often well tolerated if the area of instability is relatively small. Pairolero and Arnold have reported an extensive experience at the Mayo Clinic of over 200 chest wall reconstructions after removal of significant portions of the bony thorax. They emphasize that both adequate resection and dependable reconstruction are essential ingredients to a successful operation and express the strong belief that a thoracic surgeon–plastic surgeon team is an important collaboration if these complicated problems are to be undertaken. While a wide variety of materials has been used to reestablish chest wall stability including rib autografts, steel struts, acrylic plates, and various synthetic meshes, current preference is a 2-mm-thick polytetrafluoroethylene (Gore–Tex) soft tissue patch with rotation or myocutaneous flaps for coverage.

DISEASES OF THE PLEURA AND PLEURAL SPACE

The inner surface of each hemithorax has a mesothelial lining, the parietal pleura, which is invaginated at each pulmonary hilum to form the visceral pleura. The two surfaces are normally in apposition, lubricated by a thin layer of serous fluid secreted by the mesothelium, so that the steady motion of normal respiration is accomplished without friction. Therefore, the pleural ''space'' is normally only a potential space lying between the visceral pleura investing the lung and the parietal pleura of the chest wall. The elastic recoil of the lung and the rapid continuous absorption of fluid from the pleural space create a balance of opposing forces that favor apposition of the visceral pleura to the parietal pleura. The introduction of fluid or air breaks this dynamic coupling and converts the potential space to a real space. Normal respiratory mechanics are impaired in proportion to the size of the space created and the pressure within it. Many of the processes affecting the pleural space are essentially mechanical, such as spontaneous pneumothorax or congestive heart failure, and are not associated with any pathologic alteration in either pleural surface. However, virtually any chronic form of pleural space disturbance is associated with pathologic changes that produce thickening and adherence of the visceral and parietal surfaces. The end results vary from a few filmy adhesions of no consequence to a dense fibrous and calcific obliteration of the pleural space with a permanent restrictive defect in pulmonary function.

Pleural Effusion

A pleural effusion is an accumulation of fluid in the pleural space. It is not a disease entity but signals the effect of pleural or systemic disease on the normal daily passage of fluid through the pleural space. Normally, the balance of hydrostatic and colloid osmotic forces favors movement of fluid from systemic capillaries in the parietal pleura to pulmonary capillaries. It is estimated that between 5 and 10 L of protein-free fluid traverses the pleural space in 24 h. Simultaneously, lymphatics drain smaller volumes of fluid containing protein, which would otherwise remain in the pleural space as a source of colloid osmotic pressure favoring retention of fluid. Alterations in systemic hydrostatic or colloid osmotic pressure that disturb the balance of forces across normal pleural surfaces produce an effusion consisting of a protein-poor ultrafiltrate of plasma classified as a transudate. Changes in capillary permeability caused by inflammation or infiltration of the pleura produce a protein-rich effusion classified as an exudate. Common causes of transudates and exudates are listed in Tables 16-4 and 16-5. The distinction between transudate and exudate has diagnostic relevance, as noted in one series in which effusions were malignant in 42 percent of patients with an exudate and were caused by congestive heart failure in 83 percent of patients with a transudate.

Characteristics of fluid obtained by diagnostic thoracentesis that can help to make the distinction between transudative and exudative effusions are summarized in Table 16-6. Few findings are independently diagnostic, with the exception of positive cultures (empyema) and positive cytology (malignancy). Certain gross findings can be nearly diagnostic, such as the milky white

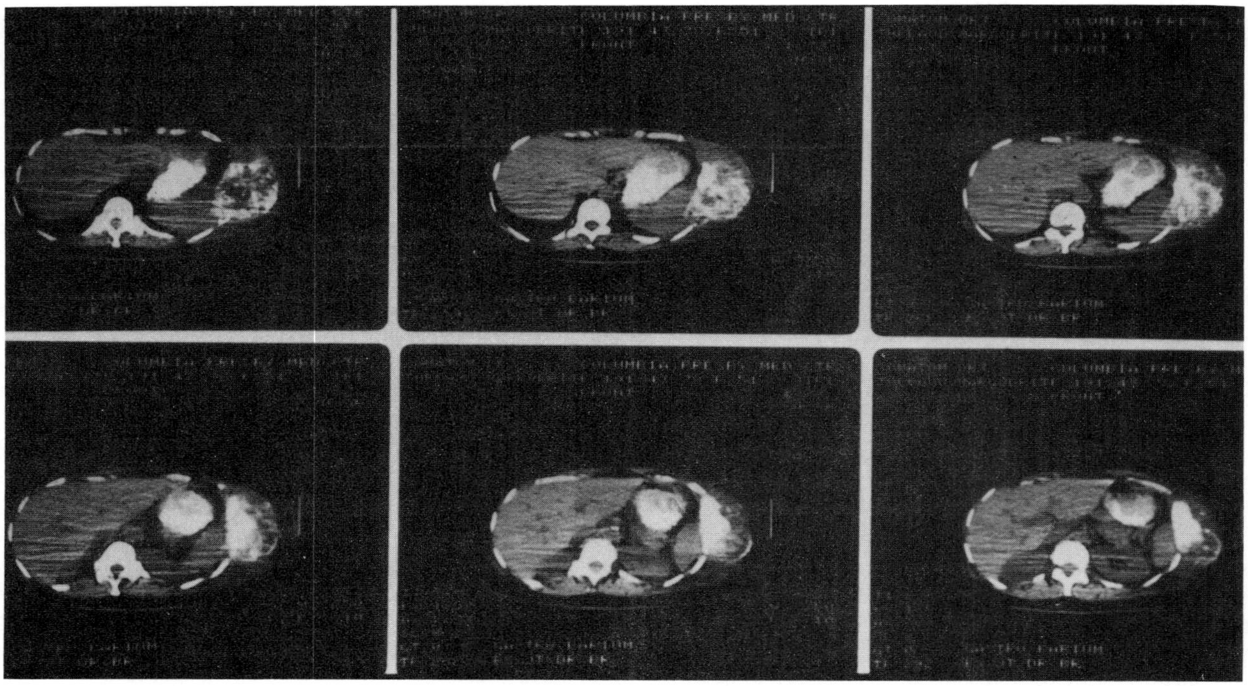

A

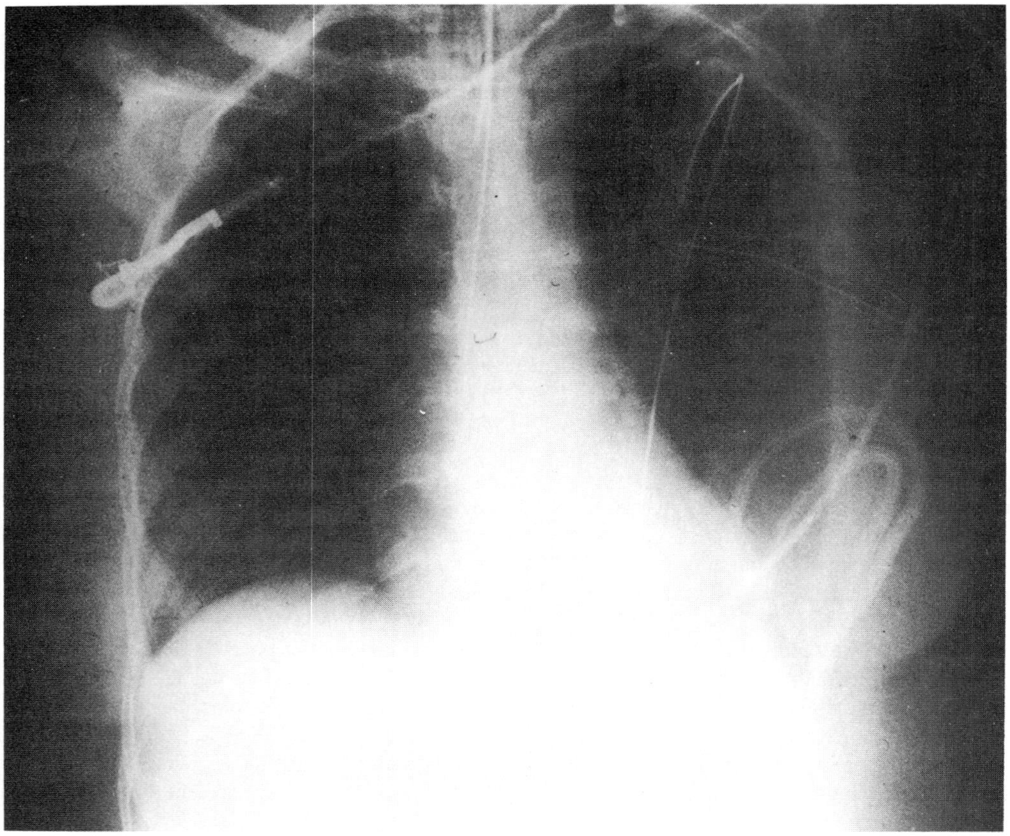

B

FIG. 16-22. Preoperative CT and first postoperative chest x-ray of explosively enlarging chest wall tumor (osteogenic sarcoma) in the left chest of a forty-year-old woman. Only 4 months earlier a small nodule thought to be a breast tumor was felt.

Table 16-4
Causes of Transudative Effusion

Congestive heart failure
Nephrotic syndrome
Cirrhosis
Hypoproteinemia
Myxedema
Peritoneal dialysis

Table 16-5
Causes of Exudative Pleural Effusion

Malignancy (primary and metastatic)
Infection
Infarction
Sympathetic (pancreatitis, subphrenic abscess, etc.)
Traumatic
Collagen vascular diseases (rheumatoid arthritis, lupus)

Table 16-6
Some Distinguishing Characteristics of Transudate and Exudate

	Transudate	*Exudate*
Color	Clear, serous	Cloudy, tan
WBC count	$<1000/mm^3$	$>10{,}000/mm^3$
RBC count	$<10{,}000/mm^3$	$>10{,}000/mm^3$—blood tinged $>100{,}000/mm^3$—grossly bloody
Glucose	Normal	Low in certain conditions
Protein	<3.0 g/dL	>3.0 g/dL
Protein ratio*	<0.5	>0.5‡
Specific gravity	<1.016	>1.016
LDH	Normal	>67% of upper limit of normal‡
LDH ratio†	<0.6	>0.6‡
pH	Same as arterial	<7.20 suggests empyema
Culture	Negative	May be positive (empyema)
Cytology	Negative	May be positive (malignant)

*Pleural fluid protein divided by serum protein.
†Pleural fluid LDH divided by serum LDH.
‡From Light RW, MacGregor MI, et al.

fluid of chylothorax or the foul purulence of an empyema. Other findings can narrow the possibilities considerably. For example, grossly bloody fluid (red cell count > 100,000 per mm^3) is almost always caused by trauma, pulmonary infarction, or malignancy. Markedly elevated amylase can be found in sympathetic effusions associated with pancreatitis, pancreatic pseudocyst, and esophageal perforation. Pleural fluid pH < 7.20 (with an arterial pH > 7.35) strongly suggests bacterial infection and may appear before culture and Gram's stain are positive in some cases. Low pH has also been reported in some malignant effusions, and in effusions associated with connective tissue disease.

There can be considerable overlap in the findings ostensibly separating exudate from transudate, and any chronic effusion tends to develop "exudative" characteristics. Too much can be made of laboratory distinctions, and it is rare for pleural effusion to be the sole manifestation of disease such that diagnosis hinges exclusively on pleural fluid analysis. The etiology of most effusions is best recognized by simply looking carefully at the rest of the patient.

A concave meniscus in the costophrenic angle on an upright chest x-ray suggests the presence of at least 250 mL of pleural fluid. A lateral decubitus view can detect a smaller volume, and confirms that the fluid is free in the pleural space if it is shown to layer out along a dependent surface. In some cases an effusion is completely contained between the base of the lung and the diaphragm (a subpulmonic effusion) and can be difficult to distinguish from an elevated hemidiaphragm or a subdiaphragmatic process. When this occurs on the left side, the position of the stomach bubble can provide a useful clue. On a supine film a small to moderate effusion will be completely inapparent, and a large effusion only produces a uniform hazy appearance of the affected hemithorax that can be difficult to detect unless the process is unilateral. A very large effusion can produce complete opacification of one hemithorax that does not change in appearance with changes in position (Fig. 16-24). Adhesions can compartmentalize an effusion into loculations that assume a wide variety of radiographic configurations, frequently requiring multiple views or CT scanning for definition. Presence of an air-fluid level has specific connotations, since the air can only come from the tracheobronchial tree, from the esophagus, or directly through the chest wall.

Thoracentesis is the mainstay of diagnosis. Needle biopsy of the pleura can provide diagnostic tissue but has a high frequency of false-negative results because of sampling difficulties in diseases that do not involve the pleura uniformly. Thoracoscopy can increase the specificity of pleural biopsies in selected cases.

Pleural effusions can produce dyspnea but can also be surprisingly asymptomatic at rest. Therapeutic drainage is rarely indicated for transudative effusions since the fluid will rapidly reaccumulate until the underlying condition is improved. Most exudative effusions warrant a more aggressive approach. The treatment of hemothorax is considered elsewhere, and empyema, malignant effusion, and chylothorax are considered separately below. A variety of nonmalignant, uninfected exudative effusions are frequently treated as if they were transudative; examples include collagen vascular disease, pulmonary infarction, and sympathetic effusion secondary to abdominal pathology.

Malignant Pleural Effusion

More than half of all patients with malignancy will have a pleural effusion at some time in their course. The effusion is frequently massive and symptomatic. The pathophysiology is thought to be interference with venous and lymphatic drainage by direct tumor invasion. Although pleural biopsy is most often normal, the fluid contains malignant cells in at least 80 percent of the patients. Lung carcinoma is the most common primary, with breast and gastrointestinal malignancies close behind. The fluid is exudative in character, and often bloody. Grossly bloody fluid (red cell count > 100,000/mL) has a 90 percent probability of being malignant, once trauma and pulmonary infarction are excluded. The presence of a malignant effusion is a poor prognostic sign, with mean survival after diagnosis of 3 to 11 months in most series.

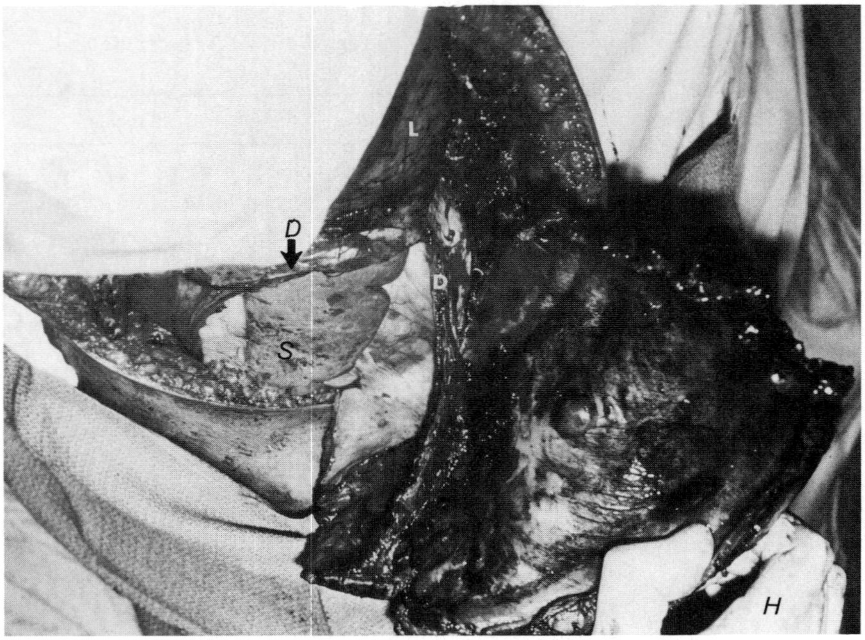

A

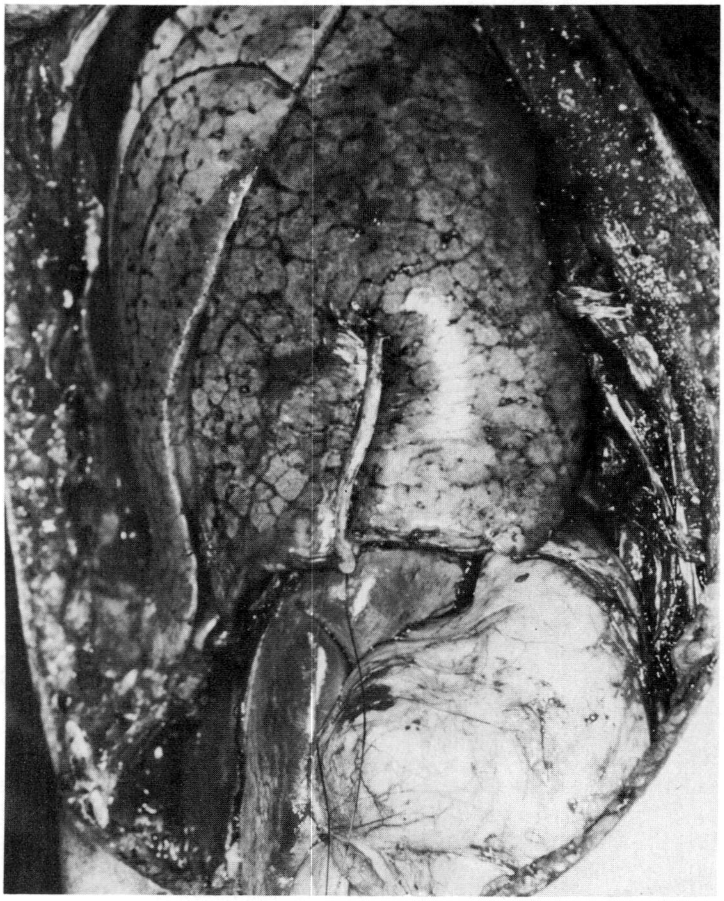

B

FIG. 16-23. Photographs taken in the operating room from the case noted in Fig. 16-22. *A.* The tumor is being resected with two grossly normal ribs above and below the lesion. This required removal of most or all of ribs 3 through 10. H indicates the surgeon's hand retracting the lesion; D marks the cut edge of the diaphragm on both specimen and patient side; S indicates the spleen; L is the lung. *B.* A wedge of lung was removed where pleural adhesions attached to the tumor. The large defect included the lateral third of the diaphragm. This operative view reveals the spleen and abdominal viscera and huge chest wall defect that existed after resection. *C.* The resected specimen. *D.* The prosthesis has been sewed in place. The line of reattachment of the diaphragm is seen in the lower third of the prosthesis. A myocutaneous flap from the left rectus muscle was used to close the skin defect.

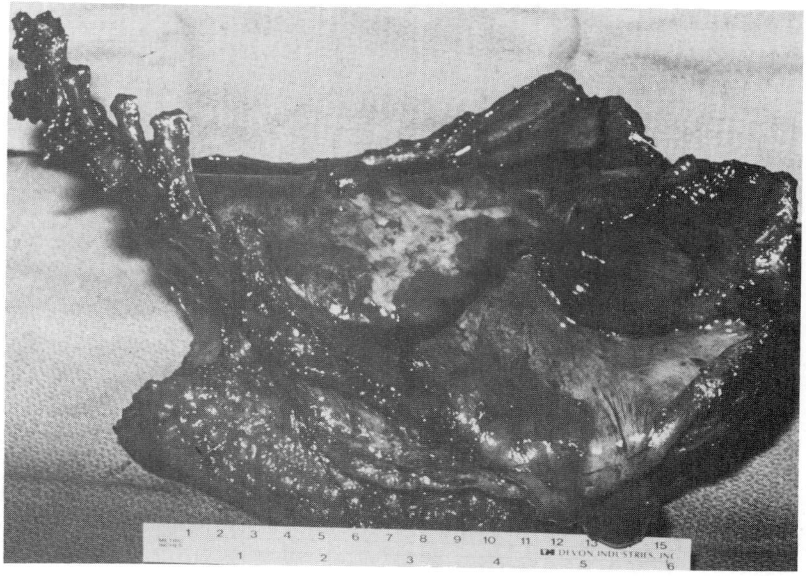

C

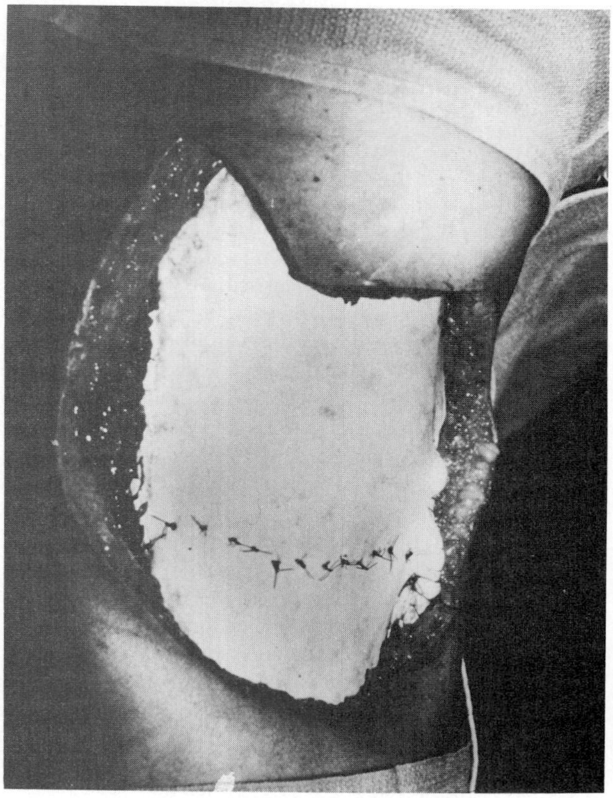

D

FIG. 16-23. *(continued)*

Treatment. Treatment is palliative. Repeated thoracentesis has a high failure rate. Chest wall radiation, thoracotomy with decortication and pleurectomy, and even pleuropneumonectomy have been described but carry unacceptable mortality and morbidity to be considered standard treatment. At present the standard therapy is tube thoracostomy and pleurodesis.

Pleurodesis creates an inflammatory fusion between visceral and parietal pleura that eliminates the potential pleural space. An essential first step is complete evacuation of the fluid and reexpansion of the lung accomplished by inserting a chest tube connected to a water seal drainage system (Fig. 16-25). If loculations or inaccurate tube placement prevent complete fluid removal and

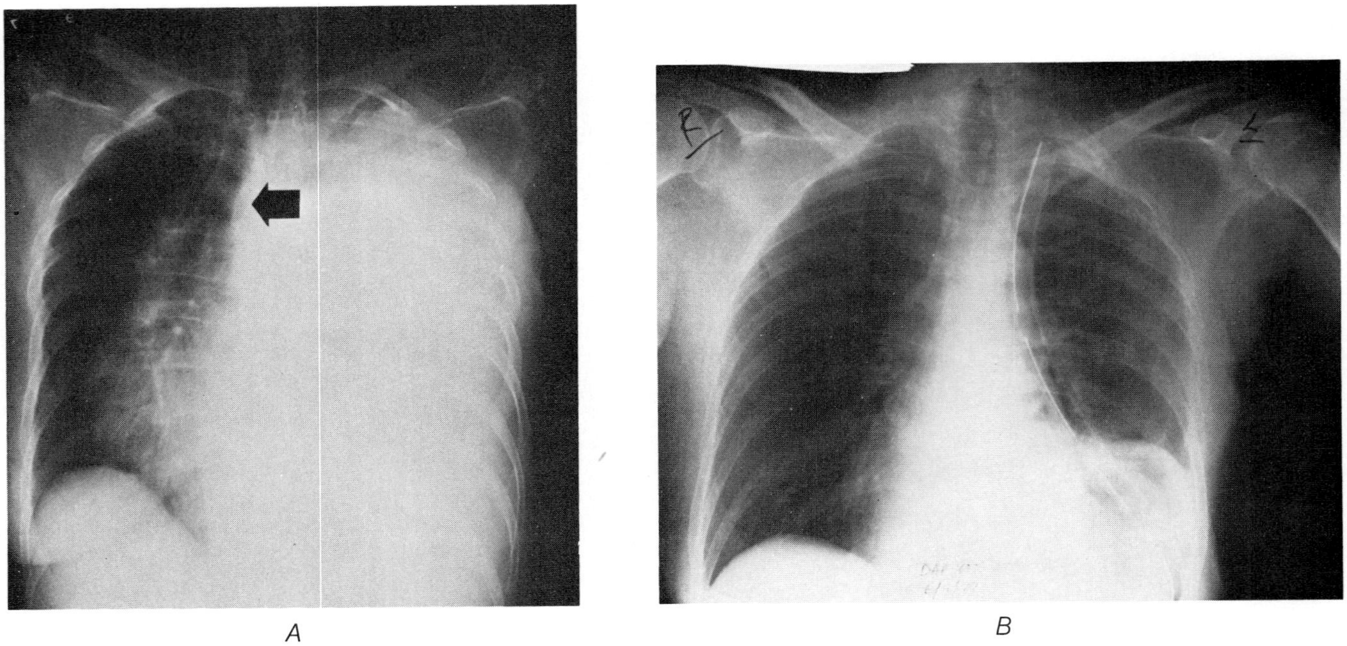

FIG. 16-24. A massive pleural effusion due to metastases from breast carcinoma. *A.* The arrow shows the tracheal displacement to the opposite side. *B.* The malignant effusion has been completely evacuated with a thoracostomy tube, and the mediastinum has shifted back to the midline. The left hemidiaphragm is elevated because of phrenic nerve invasion by pleural metastases.

lung expansion, pleural symphysis will not occur uniformly and pleurodesis is much less likely to succeed; this is probably more important than the choice of the chemical agent used in the next step. Innumerable agents have been used to induce the inflammation, including talc, nitrogen mustard, Adriamycin, quinacrine, and tetracycline. Recently a preparation of heat-killed, freeze-dried *Corynebacterium parvum* has been tried, reportedly with great success. Tetracycline is the agent most commonly used in the United States. The agent selected is usually administered through the chest tube, which is removed shortly thereafter. Although each agent has its staunch advocates, reported results suggest that the effusion will not recur in 60 to 90 percent of patients, regardless of which agent is used.

Use of an indwelling shunt connecting the pleural cavity to the peritoneum through a one-way valve has received attention recently. The system is analogous to a LaVeen or Denver shunt, except that the normal pressure gradient between the abdomen and chest is overcome with a subcutaneous squeeze bulb pump. The method has the theoretical disadvantage of continuously circulating malignant cells but does appear capable of producing satisfactory palliation in refractory cases.

Empyema

Empyema is a suppurative infection confined to a natural anatomical space by normal epithelial boundaries; in the thoracic cavity this is the potential space existing between visceral and parietal pleura. Empyema was carefully studied 2400 years ago by Hippocrates, who first described open drainage with rib resection. In the early 1900s empyema complicated pneumonia in 5 to 10 percent of cases, and Sir William Osler required open drainage and rib resection in 1919 for a postpneumonic empyema.

In the postantibiotic era, empyema has become a less frequent complication of pneumonia, now occurring in about 1 percent of cases, and the bacteriologic spectrum has shifted from *Pneumococcus* and *Streptococcus* to *Staphylococcus, Streptococcus,* and gram-negative organisms. Although pneumonia is the most frequent association with empyema, it can also occur following trauma, pulmonary infarction, or pulmonary resection, and can be caused by spread from an intraabdominal source.

Infection of the pleural space initially produces a large, exudative effusion with a high concentration of leukocytes. In hours to days fibrinous adhesions succeed in limiting involvement to one or more loculated compartments. The ability of the lung to expand and obliterate potential space becomes very important in confining the infection, and prevents formation of a fibrous "peel" over the visceral pleura that can permanently restrain the lung in a partially collapsed configuration ("trapped lung"). The pleura actually has remarkable ability to resolve infection when assisted by an expanded lung. A persistent air leak (bronchopleural fistula) potentiates infection both by providing a route for constant inoculation of the pleural space, and by promoting lung collapse. The difficulty of obliterating space following pulmonary resection, particularly pneumonectomy, accounts in part for the seriousness of postresection empyema.

Clinical Manifestations. Empyema should be suspected in a patient with a febrile illness and pleural effusion on chest x-ray. Thoracentesis with Gram's stain and culture of the fluid obtained confirms the diagnosis and guides selection of antibiotics. The gross appearance of the fluid is usually unambiguous, although some seropurulent parapneumonic effusions are sterile. Pleural fluid with pH < 7.20 and glucose < 40 mg/dL strongly suggests

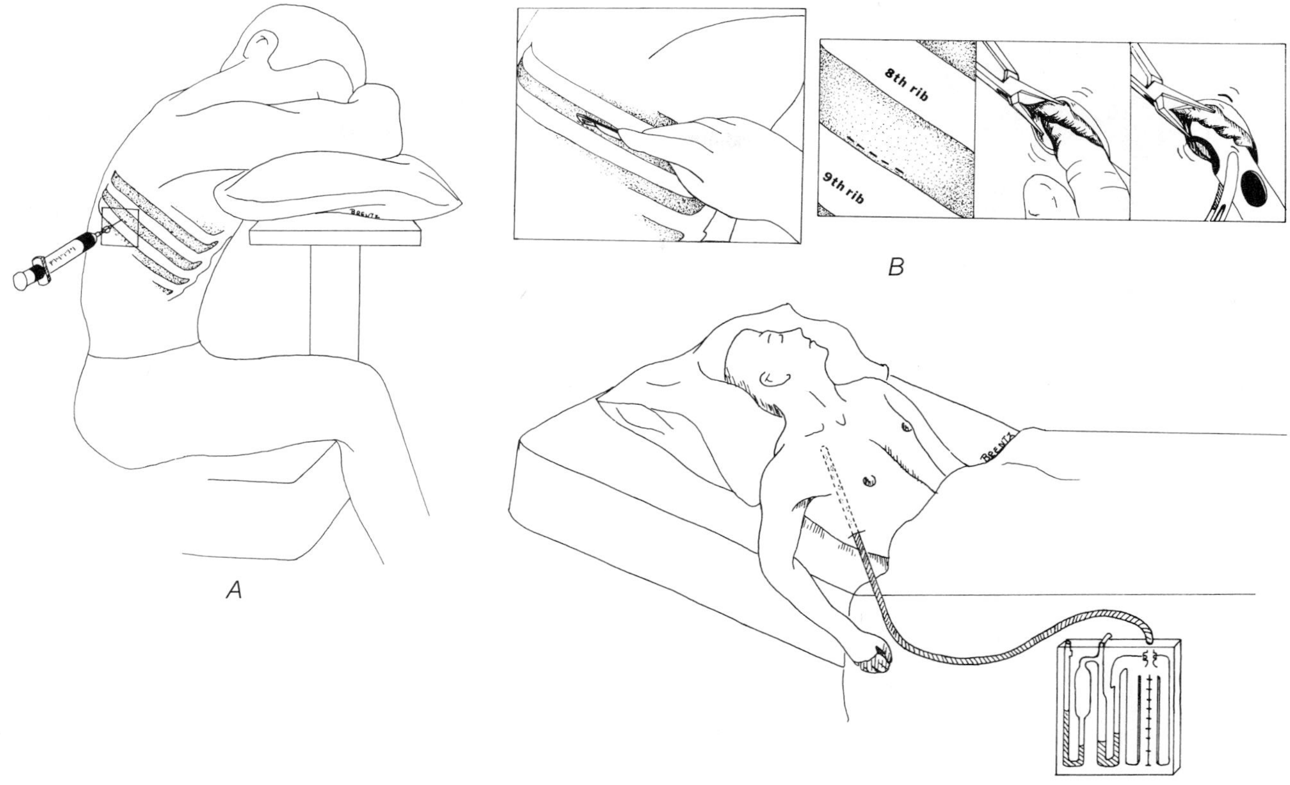

FIG. 16-25. Techniques for aspiration and drainage of a pleural effusion. *A.* Needle aspiration: Based on careful appraisal of the x-ray findings, the best interspace is selected, and fluid is aspirated with a needle and syringe. Large volumes of fluid can be removed with a little patience and a large-bore needle. *B.* Chest tube insertion: After careful skin preparation and draping, and administration of local anesthesia, a short skin incision is made over the correct interspace. The incision is deepened into the intercostal muscles, and the pleura is penetrated, usually with a clamp. When any doubt exists about the status of the pleural space at the site of puncture, the wound is enlarged bluntly to admit a finger, which can be swept around the immediately adjacent pleural space to assess the situation and break down any adhesions. The tube is inserted, with the tip directed toward the optimum position suggested by the chest x-rays. In general, a high anterior tube is best for air (pneumothorax) and a low posterior tube is best for fluid. A 28 to 32F tube is adequate for most situations. A 36F tube is preferred for hemothorax or for a viscous empyema. Many surgeons prefer a very small tube (16 to 20F) for drainage of simple pneumothorax. *C.* The tube is connected to a water seal drainage system. Suction is added if necessary to expand the lung and will usually be required in a patient with a substantial air leak (bronchopleural fistula).

empyema requiring drainage. Loculations and/or air-fluid levels on chest x-ray suggest empyema, but CT examination is usually required to distinguish simple empyema from an intraparenchymal process such as lung abscess, an infected congenital cyst, or an infected bulla (pyocyst).

Treatment. Successful treatment depends upon early recognition of the problem, selection of appropriate antibacterial therapy based on identification of the organism, and complete obliteration of the emypema space (Table 16-7). Thoracentesis alone, even in the preantibiotic era, provides adequate treatment in only about 10 percent of empyemas because the space is rarely obliterated. The first step should be insertion of a chest tube connected to a closed drainage system, applying suction as necessary to fully evacuate the space and promote lung expansion. Image guidance during tube or catheter insertion, with CT or ultrasound, can be important when the empyema space is small or has complex loculations. Lung expansion is especially important in empyema associated with bronchopleural fistula. Lysis of loculations with streptokinase, and thoracoscopic evacuation of the cavity have been reported to improve the success of treatment with simple closed-tube drainage.

Table 16-7
Treatment Options for Empyema

1. Antibiotic alone
2. Thoracentesis
3. Closed-tube thoracostomy (drainage to water seal, +/− suction)
4. Closed-tube/catheter drainage with antibiotic irrigation
5. Closed-tube thoracostomy converted to open drainage (no water seal, tubes cut off at the skin and slowly extruded)
6. Formal open drainage with rib resection
7. Thoracotomy and decortication
8. Thoracotomy, decortication, pulmonary resection, thoracoplasty, intrathoracic rotation of pedicled muscle flaps

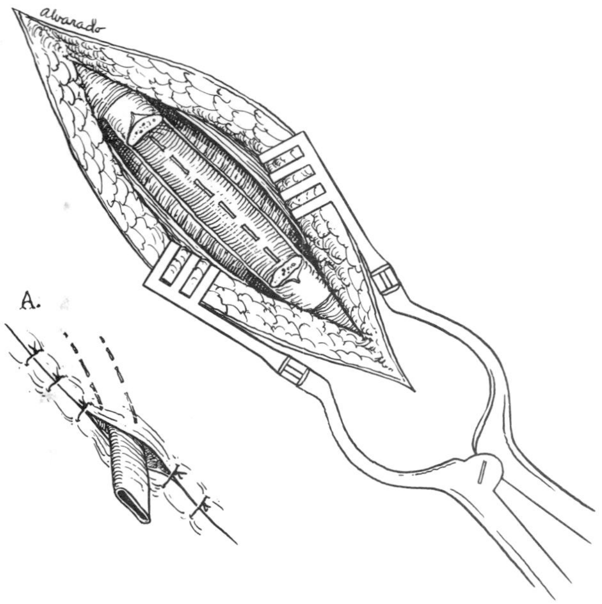

FIG. 16-26. Open drainage through the bed of a resected rib. For an empyema dependent drainage is important and the site is selected accordingly. A tube can be left in place as shown to prevent closure of the skin opening, or the skin edges can be sewed to the parietal pleura to create an epithelialized tract (a modification of an Eloesser flap). Progress can be gauged by periodically measuring the volume of the cavity, which can be done simply by measuring the volume of saline required to overflow it.

Failure of simple drainage is marked by persistent purulent drainage and persistence of an empyema space overlying incompletely expanded lung. The simplest option is to convert to open-tube drainage by cutting the existing tubes off near the skin, allowing chronic drainage into dressings. When this approach is successful, the cavity will gradually shrink and obliterate over weeks to months, slowly extruding the tubes, which are progressively shortened.

It is important that open drainage not be attempted before a secure pleural symphysis has occurred at the margins of the cavity, a process that requires at least 10 to 14 days. If this rule is violated, the resulting pneumothorax can cause a rapid spread of the infection throughout the pleural space. A simple test is to disconnect the tubes from the water seal and obtain a chest x-ray. If the space is ready for conversion to open drainage, the x-ray will be unchanged. Open drainage is most effective when the tubes are in a very dependent position, because suction cannot be used to augment gravity drainage. Conversion to open drainage is also less attractive in the presence of an air leak, because the bronchopleural fistula is converted to a more chronic bronchopleurocutaneous fistula. A combination of closed-tube and open-tube drainage is successful in at least 60 percent of patients.

Formal open drainage with rib resection (Fig. 16-26) was done more frequently in the preantibiotic era but is still useful today in the treatment of chronic, mature empyemas with a thick fibrous capsule (Fig. 16-27). Drainage is assured by marsupialization of the empyema cavity. The same cautions important in conversion of closed-tube to open-tube drainage still apply—the cavity must be mature, the drainage site should be dependent, and production of a bronchopleurocutaneous fistula is best avoided. The larger wound allows easier access to the cavity, and drainage can be augmented with irrigation.

If drainage fails to expand the lung, a permanent restrictive defect in ventilation on the affected side is likely to result as the inflammatory membrane heals and contracts over the surface of the lung. Failure of expansion is frequent with a bronchopleural fistula. Four to seven days of high-suction drainage is generally considered an adequate trial, after which thoracotomy and decortication should be performed (Fig. 16-28). The empyema space is completely evacuated under direct vision, and drainage tubes are accurately placed in the most dependent position. The inflamma-

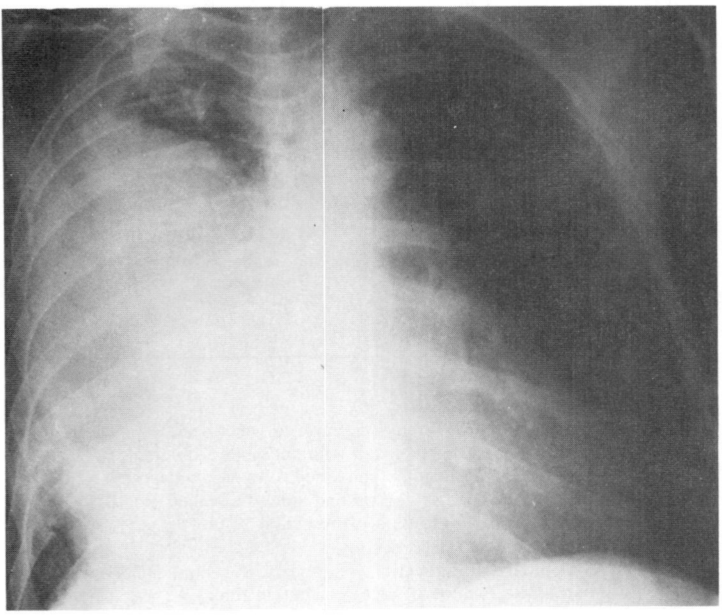

A

FIG. 16-27. *A.* This 54-year-old homeless man presented to the emergency room with a massive consolidation of the right lung. *B.* On antibiotics the radiographic picture slowly evolved into a large cavity with an air-fluid level. *C.* Uncertainty about whether the cavity might be a large lung abscess or infected bulla was largely relieved by the CT scan, which shows a plate of consolidated lung compressed medially by a large empyema cavity. Note the degree of pleural thickening, which contributed to the difficulty encountered obtaining adequate drainage with thoracostomy tubes. Formal open drainage with rib resection was ultimately performed, with gradual resolution of the cavity over several months. At operation the fibrous wall of the cavity was 2 to 3 cm in thickness, precluding any thought of decortication.

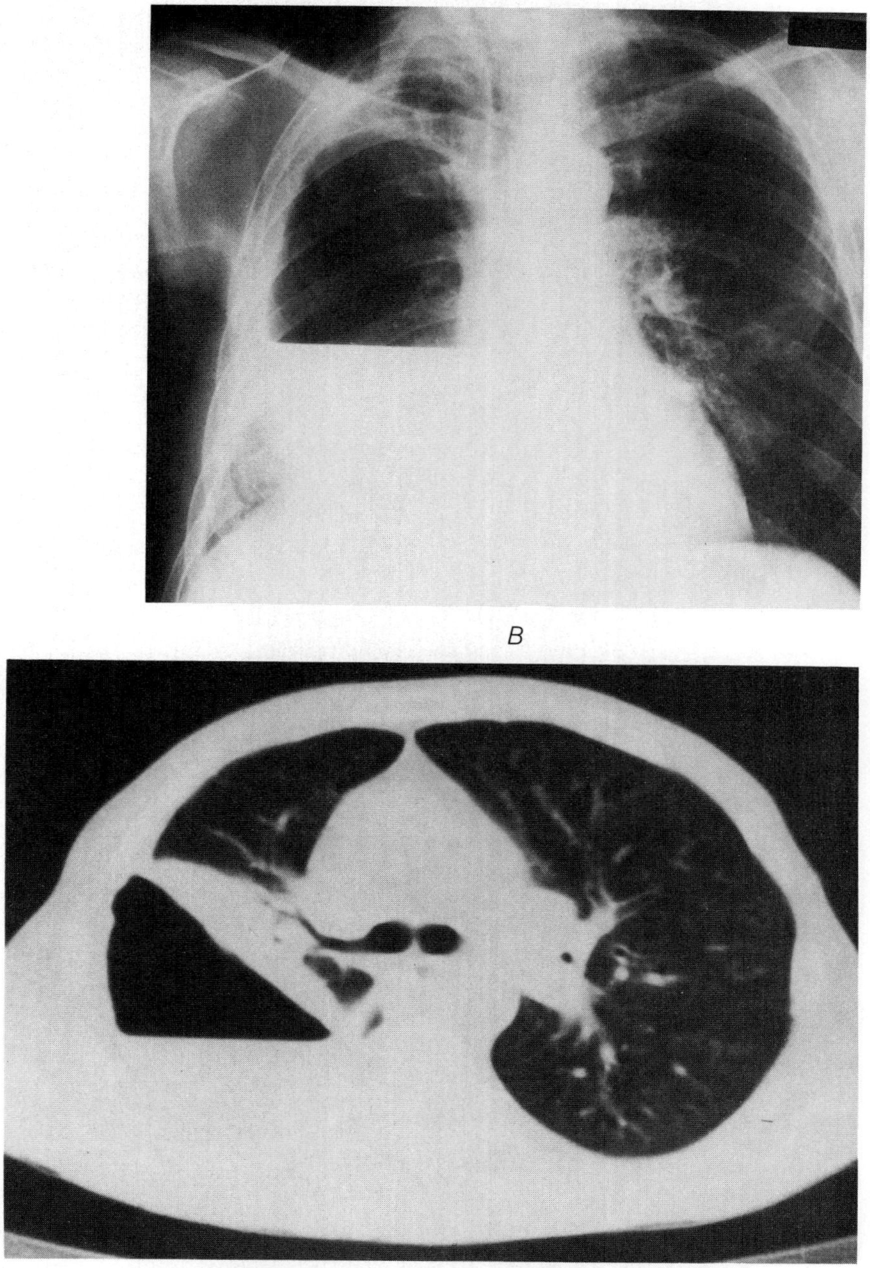

B

C

FIG. 16-27. *(continued)*

tory "peel" is tightly adherent to the visceral pleura and should be entirely removed, a tedious process that must be done carefully to prevent development of new air leaks from tears in the lung. When an intraparenchymal abscess coexists with a large air leak, pulmonary resection is necessary. Thoracoplasty and intrathoracic rotation of muscle flaps can be added to help obliterate the remaining space.

Decortication has been successful in 80 to 100 percent of cases in reported series, and often shortens hospitalization. It has the disadvantage of requiring general anesthesia and a thoracotomy in patients who frequently have limited ventilatory reserve and are suffering the systemic consequences of chronic infection. Even so, in the long run, thoracotomy is often better tolerated than a chronic, drainage infection.

Pleural Plaques and Calcification

Pleural plaques are idiopathic thickenings of parietal pleura, usually smooth and white, and frequently calcified. Most are small (1 to 5 mm) and irregular densities that are frequently bilateral and symmetric and do not occur at the apex or on the visceral pleura. They have no documented relationship to mesothelioma or other neoplasms. Localized inflammatory or traumatic events can heal with production of calcified plaquelike lesions, but they are usually larger and unilateral.

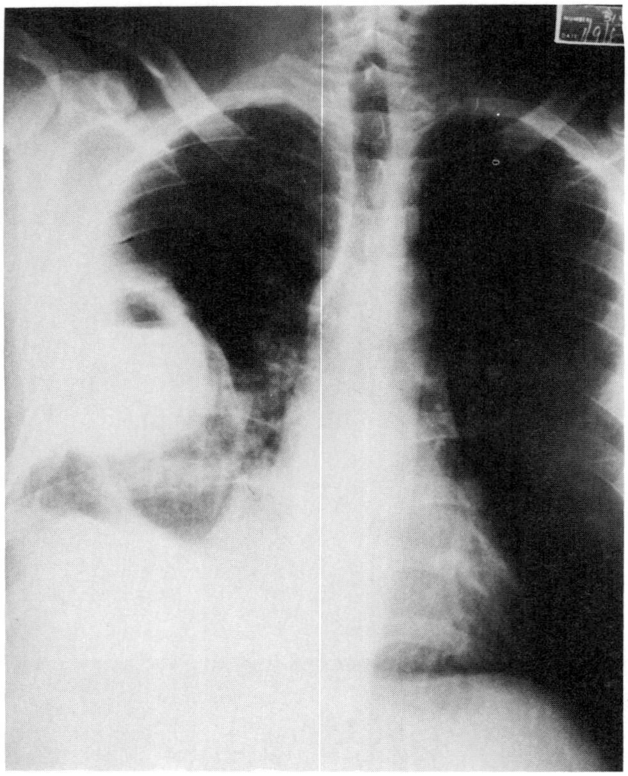

A

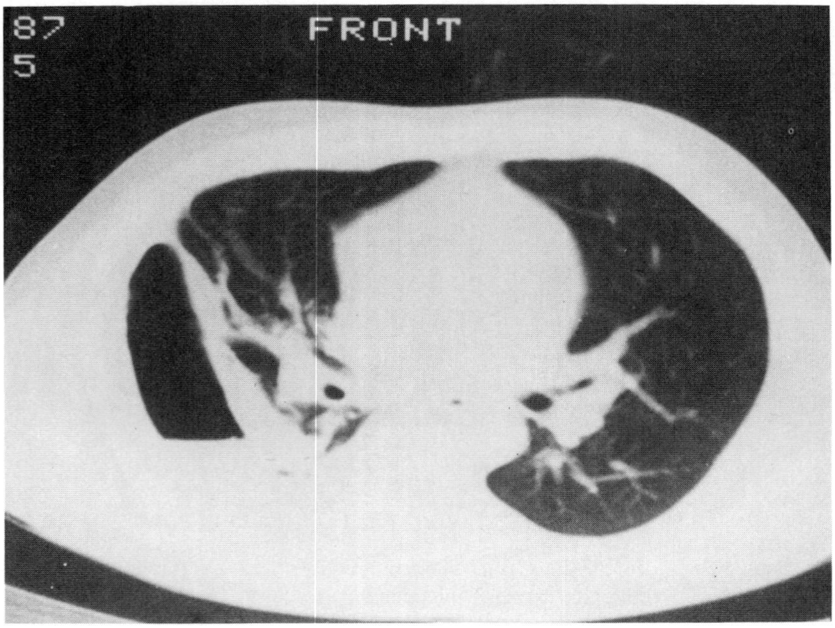

B

FIG. 16-28. *A.* This 37-year-old intravenous drug abuser presented with pneumonia that evolved into a cavitary process in the right lung, thought to be a lung abscess. *B.* The CT scan showed consolidated right lung compressed medially by a large, thick-walled empyema cavity with an air-fluid level. A decortication was performed through a right posterolateral thoracotomy with excellent results.

Chronic pleuritis can result in diffuse, remarkably uniform thickening and calcification of parietal pleura. The original pleuritis may result from an unresolved hemothorax, from tuberculous or nontuberculous empyema, and from viral or bacterial pleuritis or pleuropneumonitis. When the wall of a chronic but active empyema becomes calcified, resolution by drainage alone will never occur, and resection, decortication, pleurectomy, and thoracoplasty are likely to be required.

Chylothorax

Leakage of lymphatic fluid (chyle) from the thoracic duct produces a characteristic milky effusion called a chylothorax. The

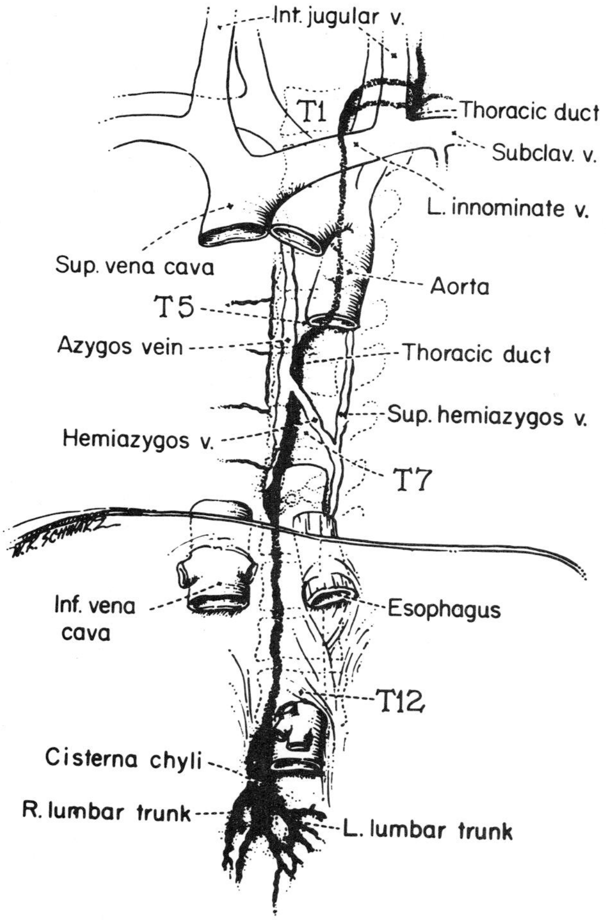

FIG. 16-29. The most common anatomy of the thoracic duct is shown. Anomalous patterns are frequently encountered. After passing through the diaphragm at the aortic hiatus, the duct lies between the aorta and the azygous vein on the anterior surface of the vertebral column, behind the esophagus. Ligation of the duct is most easily performed just above the diaphragm on the right. Although it can be ligated from the left side, the aorta must be mobilized for exposure. At about T_5 the duct crosses to the left side and ascends in the posterior mediastinum, where it is vulnerable to injury during any procedure involving dissection behind the distal transverse aorta. (From: *Bessone LN, Ferguson TB, et al: Chylothorax. Ann Thorac Surg 12:527, 1971, with permission.*)

most common cause is surgical trauma to the thoracic duct, most frequently seen following procedures that involve dissection in the vicinity of the proximal descending thoracic aorta and left subclavian artery (Fig. 16-29), such as ligation of patent ductus or Blalock-Taussig shunt. Traumatic chylothorax is almost always unilateral, usually on the left side. Nontraumatic chylothorax is less common, accounting for about one-third of cases in most series. Because venous hypertension in the brachiocephalic system is the most common cause of nontraumatic chylothorax, the process is usually bilateral. Underlying causes include superior vena cava thrombosis complicating central intravenous line placement, and chronic elevation of central venous pressure following the Fontan procedure. The least common variety of nontraumatic chylothorax is that associated with malignancy, which is frequently accompanied by chylous ascites and is thought to be caused by neoplastic obstruction or erosion of lymphatic channels.

Table 16-8
Normal Composition and Characteristics of Chyle

General:	
Opaque, milky, odorless	
Opacity clears with alkali/ether extraction	
Sterile	
pH 7.4–7.8	
Specific gravity 1.012–1.025	
Total protein 2.20–5.98 g/dL	
Glucose 48–200 mg/dL	
Cell counts:	
Lymphocytes 400–6800/mm³ (average 70% of total WBC count)	
Erythrocytes 50–600/mm³	
Fats:	
Fat globules stain with Sudan III	
Total fat 0.4–6.0 g/dL	
Triglycerides: Higher than serum value; Average 10-fold higher than upper limit of normal	
Cholesterol: Same or lower than serum value	
Triglyceride/cholesterol ratio: >1	
Electrolytes:	
Sodium	104–108 meq/L
Potassium	3.8–5.0 meq/L
Chlorine	85–130 meq/L
Calcium	3.4–6.0 meq/L
Total protein 2.20–5.98 g/dL	
Glucose 48–200 mg/dL	

Aspiration of milky-white, odorless fluid from the pleural space is virtually diagnostic. Pseudochyle, which has a similar appearance, is a rare source of confusion seen in certain malignancies, infections, and connective tissue diseases. In comparison with chyle, pseudochyle has a lower fat content and lymphocyte count, and its opalescent appearance is caused by the presence of lecithin-globulin complexes. If the patient is not eating, or if a coexisting problem could significantly dilute the chylous drainage, the gross appearance of the fluid may not be distinguishable from many other effusions. Table 16-8 summarizes characteristics of chyle that can be diagnostically helpful when gross appearance is ambiguous. The lymphocyte count and triglyceride level are most useful. Lymphangiography will occasionally define the site of leak with precision and is most useful in cases of nontraumatic chylothorax. It is rarely indicated in the traumatic variety.

Normal chyle flow ranges between 1.5 and 2.5 L/day but can vary much more widely depending on diet and on the fat content of the diet. During starvation or intravenous feeding flow falls to about 250 mL/day of clear fluid. Chylothorax is frequently massive (Fig. 16-30) and symptomatic, and significant volume losses can occur through thoracentesis or chest tube drainage. In one recent series, the average amount of fluid lost per day was 756 mL, ranging up to 1720 mL in one 9-year-old patient. Dehydration, nutritional losses, and a steady decline in circulating lymphocytes can produce significant disability and an increased susceptibility to infection.

Treatment. Until Lampson described successful treatment of chylothorax by ligation of the thoracic duct in 1948, mortality for the condition averaged 50 percent. Since that time, better understanding of fluid and electrolyte management, and the development of total parenteral nutrition have introduced additional options. Spontaneous resolution can occur, so a trial of nonoperative treatment is usually justified. Conservative treatment has two goals: one is to decrease chyle production; the other is to keep the

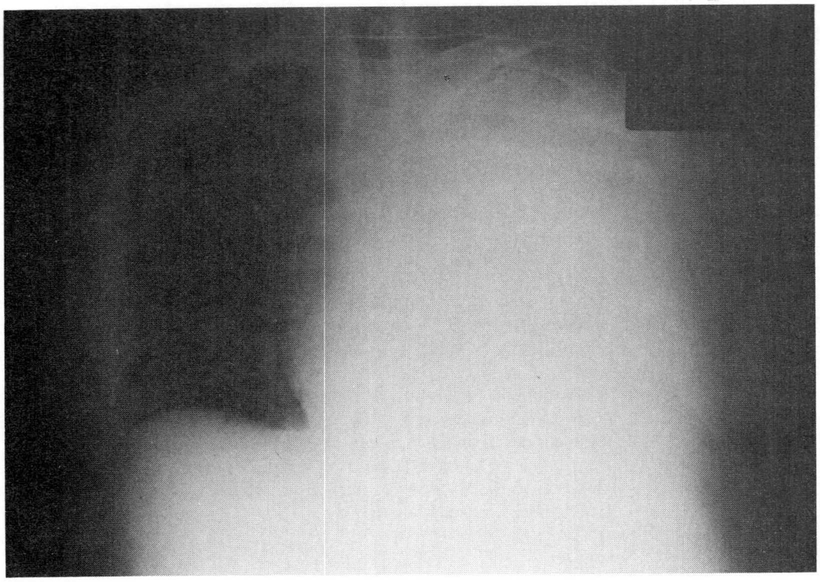

FIG. 16-30. Massive chylothorax in a patient with lymphoma. The mediastinum appears shifted to the right.

lung expanded against the mediastinum. Maximal reduction in chyle production is achieved by eliminating oral intake, while the patient is supported by total parenteral nutrition. A possible compromise is replacement of dietary fat with medium-chain triglycerides, which are not absorbed by lymphatics. Fluid can be removed intermittently by thoracentesis, but continuous evacuation with a chest tube is much more effective. It is generally accepted that a 2-week trial of drainage and diet manipulation is justified. Experience in renal transplantation has shown that thoracic duct drainage produces measurable immunosuppression after 2 weeks. An occasional patient will have such massive drainage that persistence for more than a few days is unacceptably debilitating. A commonly accepted criterion is that drainage exceeding 500 mL/day in an adult or more than 100 mL/day/year of age in a child is an indication for abandonment of conservative therapy.

When conservative treatment fails, the operative approach is dictated by the etiology and the location of the leak. In the most common situation, involving iatrogenic injury near the aortic arch, the left thorax is explored, the site identified, and the injury controlled with suture, clips, or fibrin glue. If the site of injury cannot be clearly identified, the thoracic duct can be ligated at the diaphragm where it enters the thorax, and a pleural abrasion performed. An alternative gaining in popularity is insertion of a pleuroperitoneal shunt.

Ligation of the duct is most easily done through a right thoracotomy, but it can be accomplished through a left thoracotomy when necessary. If the problem is bilateral, the right side is approached first, since ligation will usually resolve the problem on both sides. Direct operative approaches through thoracotomy are successful in approximately 80 percent of cases. Treatment failures are most common in nontraumatic chylothorax. Based on early experience with thoracoscopy, thoracotomy may become a last resort for exploration.

The use of a pleuroperitoneal shunt has been added recently to the list of effective treatment options for chylothorax. Fluid is pumped from the pleural cavity to the peritoneal cavity with a small subcutaneous squeeze bulb on a one-way valve. Excellent results were obtained with Denver pleuroperitoneal shunts in 12 of 16 patients (75 percent recently reported by Murphy and associates), and it was possible to remove the shunt in 10 of the 12 patients with good outcomes.

Tumors

Mesothelioma

Mesothelioma is a neoplasm originating in the mesothelial lining of serosal cavities. Tumor presents in the pleura in 80 percent and in the peritoneum in 20 percent of cases. Although mesothelioma is a rare tumor (2.2 cases/million per year), an increased incidence has been anticipated since an association with asbestos exposure was recognized in the 1970s. In several large series, a history of asbestos exposure has been documented in 10 to 77 percent of patients. The disease has been most widely recognized in geographical areas having local industries associated with high risk of exposure, such as shipbuilding or manufacturing processes using asbestos. Exposure to asbestos particles carried on the clothing of workers at risk has been implicated as a cause of increased incidence of mesothelioma in family members. The epidemiology is complicated by the fact that asbestos is nearly ubiquitous in any urban environment, and the characteristic refractile particles can be identified in many people without disease. Some evidence has suggested that smoking is an important etiologic cofactor, and the latency period from exposure to clinical disease is very long.

Mesothelioma exists in a benign and malignant form. The benign form accounts for only 10 to 15 percent of the total, presents as an intrathoracic mass on chest x-ray, and is usually asymptomatic. Pleural effusion is rare. Pathologically the tumor arises from visceral or parietal pleura as an encapsulated mass that is pedunculated (Fig. 16-31). Resection is the treatment of choice, if only because thoracotomy has almost always been required for accurate diagnosis.

In contrast, malignant mesothelioma is a locally aggressive neoplasm usually appearing after age forty, with a male predominance of more than 2:1. The tumor usually appears to be multicentric, with multiple pleural-based nodules coalescing to form sheets of desmoplastic mass separated by loculated, cystic spaces.

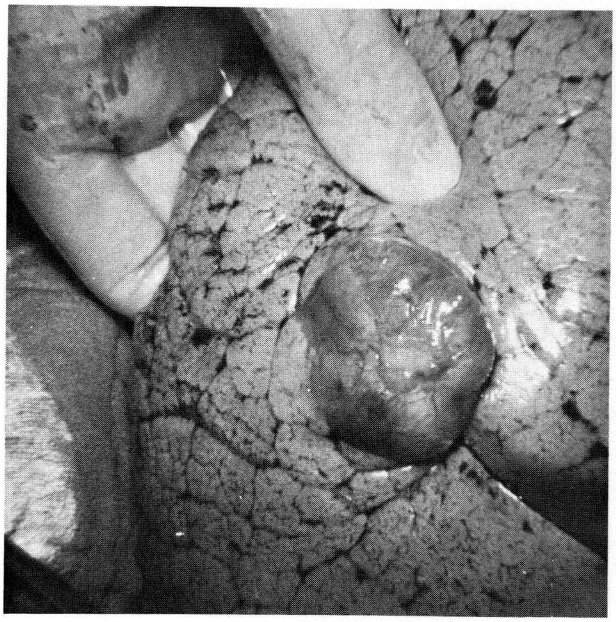

FIG. 16-31. A localized benign mesothelioma arising from the juncture of the right upper and lower lobes. The tumor was removed by wedge resection with a margin of normal lung.

Table 16-9
Clinical Staging of Malignant Mesothelioma

Stage I:	Tumor confined to ipsilateral pleura or lung
Stage II:	Tumor involving chest wall, mediastinum, pericardium, or contralateral pleura
Stage III:	Tumor on both sides of the diaphragm, or in lymph nodes outside the thorax
Stage IV:	Hematogenous metastases outside the thorax

There are two cell types: fibrosarcomatous and epithelial. The fibrosarcomatous variety is less common and has a better prognosis.

Although hematogenous and lymphatic spread occur in at least one-third of cases, the predominant feature is aggressive tissue invasion. Involvement of lung, chest wall, diaphragm, and mediastinal structures is common. In one series of 69 patients only 3 of 14 patients autopsied had disease limited to the thorax, and 9 patients developed tumor in a needle biopsy tract. Local spread can produce a Horner's syndrome and spinal cord compression. Most patients die of the primary tumor rather than metastases. For unexplained reasons, thrombocytosis is frequently seen and may account for a high incidence of thromboembolic complications. In one series the platelet count was more than $400{,}000/mm^3$ in 90 percent of patients and greater than $1{,}000{,}000/mm^3$ in 14 percent.

Clinical Manifestations. Chest pain, dyspnea, or both are present in virtually all patients with malignant mesothelioma. Pleural effusion is present at some time in 85 to 95 percent of cases, although as the disease progresses the pleural space tends to become obliterated with solid tumor. Radiographic findings other than effusion cover a wide spectrum including pleural thickening, lung nodules, chest wall masses, and mediastinal masses (Fig. 16-32). CT scan of the chest can add important anatomic detail regarding mediastinal involvement or contralateral pleural involvement, and one should always be obtained unless no treatment is planned (Fig. 16-33).

A tissue diagnosis is difficult to obtain without thoracotomy. In a series of 123 patients reported by Brenner and associates thoracentesis in 60 patients revealed malignant cells in only 22, and a definitive diagnosis of mesothelioma could only be made in 7. Needle biopsy and thoracoscopy have similar yield, and bronchoscopy almost never provides diagnostic tissue. Unless a representative specimen of adequate size is obtained, the epithelial cell type in particular can be easily confused with adenocarcinoma. A recently developed monoclonal antibody (ME1) that recognizes malignant mesothelial cells appears capable of greatly increasing the accuracy of histologic diagnosis.

Treatment. For benign mesothelioma, resection is the treatment of choice and is generally curative. For diffuse malignant mesothelioma, treatment is controversial. Since thoracotomy is likely to be required for accurate diagnosis, careful preoperative clinical staging (Table 16-9) should be done to help estimate prognosis. Stages II to IV have a dismal prognosis regardless of treatment, with median survival measured in months. In such cases radiotherapy and chemotherapy are usually given, but protocols with significant benefit have not been established. Even in Stage I disease, a 1986 retrospective analysis of 328 Canadian patients demonstrated median survival of only 17 months regardless of treatment.

Radical surgery in Stage I disease is favored by some authors, who feel that meaningful palliation and an occasional long-term survival can be achieved with acceptable mortality and morbidity. At the most radical extreme, DaValle and associates reported their experience with 33 patients treated with extrapleural pneumonectomy, including resection of pericardium and diaphragm; 8 patients (24 percent) survived more than 24 months, and 5 survived more than 36 months. Operative mortality was 9 percent, and serious complications occurred in 24 percent. This contrasts with experience reported from a multi-institutional trial in which 20 patients treated with extrapleural pneumonectomy had 15 percent perioperative mortality and were improved in comparison to nonoperative management only with respect to recurrence-free survival. Twenty-four-month survival was 33 percent, not significantly different from that obtained with nonoperative or limited palliative treatment. A less radical approach is favored at Memorial Sloan-Kettering Cancer Center in New York, where pleuropneumonectomy has been abandoned in favor of radical pleurectomy, preserving the lung but resecting diaphragm and pericardium when necessary. They emphasize the importance of combined treatment with systemic chemotherapy and radiation, administered as a combination of intraoperative implantation of radioactive material and postoperative external beam. In 94 patients there was no operative mortality, 40 percent survived more than 2 years, and median survival was 21 months. All authors agree that long-term survival in malignant mesothelioma remains a rare occurrence.

Metastatic Pleural Tumors

Over 90 percent of pleural tumors are metastatic. Lung and breast carcinoma are the most common primaries. In more than half of all cases, gross tumor is not visible but produces a malignant pleural effusion, which is discussed elsewhere. When multi-

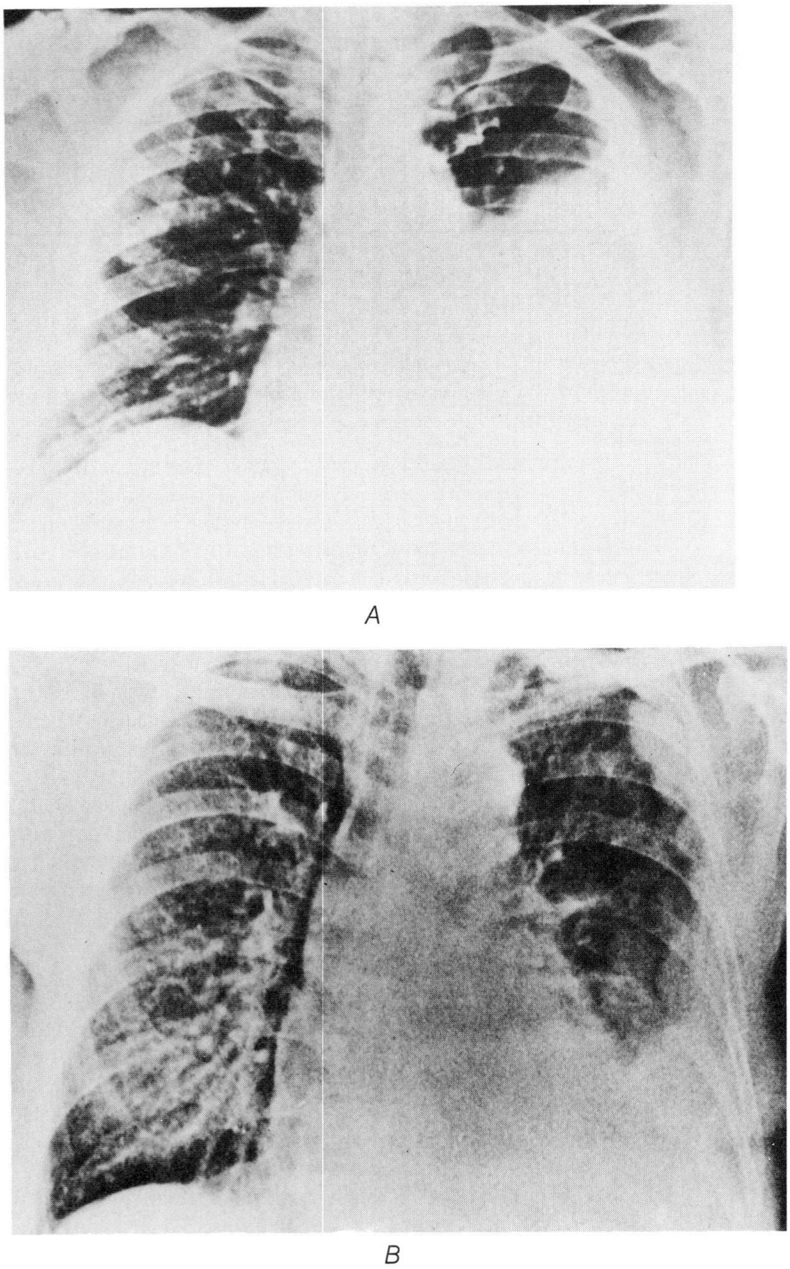

FIG. 16-32. Three common radiographic presentations of malignant mesothelioma. *A.* Large pleural effusion without a discrete mass. *B.* Multiple pleural-based masses without an effusion. While the appearance of the left lower lung field is consistent with effusion or mass, the two can be distinguished on the basis of lateral decubitus views and CT scan. *C.* Large pleural-based mass with pleural effusion and thickening. (From: *Martini N, McCormack PM, et al: Ann Thorac Surg 43:113, 1987, Fig 3A–C, p 116, with permission.*)

ple nodules or diffuse obliterative spread occur, differentiation from mesothelioma is impossible without biopsy.

Spontaneous Pneumothorax

Nontraumatic pneumothorax most commonly results from rupture of a pulmonary bleb or bulla. Negative intrathoracic pressure throughout the respiratory cycle favors movement of air into the pleural space, with egress prevented by the ball-valve effect of collapsing tissue during expiration. The pneumothorax will continue to progress until the leak seals with fibrin, at a rate directly related to the size of the bleb. Large leaks can produce life-threatening tension pneumothorax. Spontaneous resolution can occur once the leak stops, but the gas in the space is mostly nitrogen and is very slowly reabsorbed by the pleural surfaces.

Up to 80 percent of patients with spontaneous pneumothorax are young adults, usually male, without clinically significant pulmonary disease. A tall, asthenic habitus is common. In 85 percent of cases blebs or bullae of varying sizes are found in the lung apices (Fig. 16-34), and it is not known whether their origin is congenital or acquired. After the first episode, the chance of ipsilateral recurrence is 50 percent, and the risk rises with each recurrence to 62 percent after a second episode and 80 percent after a third episode. The risk of a contralateral pneumothorax after the first episode is about 10 percent.

In patients over age forty, significant pulmonary disease is usually present, most frequently emphysema in a tobacco addict. Catamenial pneumothorax is a rare condition in which pneumothorax occurs predictably within a few days of menses, usually in women

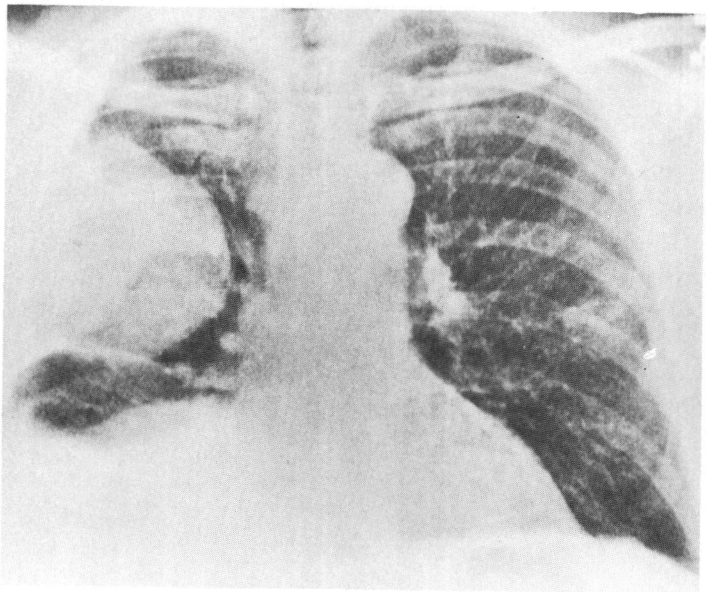

FIG. 16-32. *(continued)*

C

over thirty, and almost always on the right side. The mechanism is not known. The two most frequently cited possibilities are pleural endometriosis and small perforations of the diaphragm.

Clinical Manifestations. Chest pain is the most common presenting symptom, followed by dyspnea. If the lung is more than about 25 percent collapsed, a decrease in breath sounds will be evident to auscultation, and the affected side will be hyperresonant to percussion. Young patients without underlying lung disease can be asymptomatic at rest with nearly complete collapse of one lung, and arterial blood gases will be nearly normal. A more dramatic presentation, including tachypnea, cyanosis, and hypoxia, is seen in patients with underlying lung disease and limited ventilatory reserve. An occasional patient with extensive lung disease and a pleural space obliterated with adhesions will present with massive subcutaneous emphysema and pneumomediastinum, because air escaping from the ruptured bleb follows the path of least resistance retrograde through the peribronchial soft tissue.

The characteristic radiographic finding is absence of lung markings and a faint visible line defining the edge of the lung. When the lung collapses almost completely, it is visible as an irregular density attached to the hilus (Fig. 16-35). Presence of a small amount of fluid with an air-fluid level is common. The fluid is usually serosanguinous and insignificant. On occasion bleeding from a torn pleural adhesion will produce a large and increasing hemothorax that can require urgent exploration. The lung fields must be closely examined for evidence of gross abnormalities, such as apical blebs or bullae. Although blebs and bullae are frequently obvious at thoracotomy, only about 15 percent are visible radiographically.

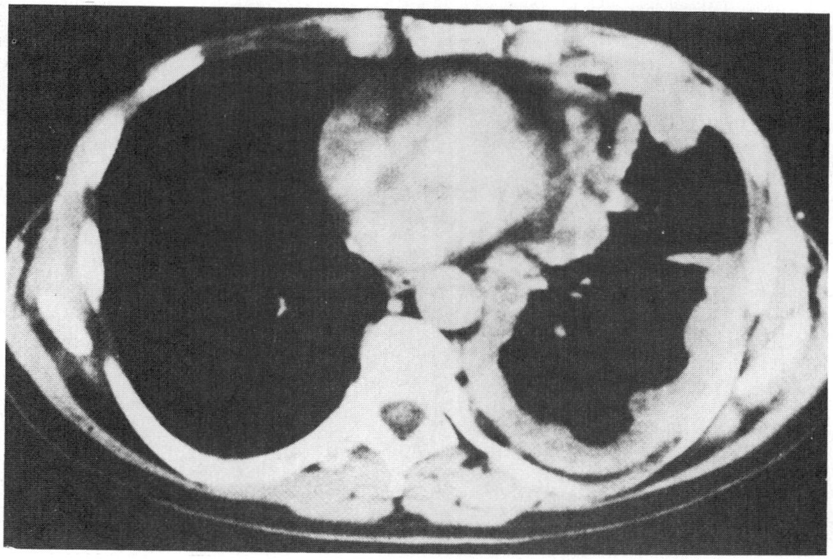

FIG. 16-33. CT scan of a diffuse pleural mesothelioma encasing the lung and extending into the major fissure, but without evidence of mediastinal involvement. (From: *Martini N, McCormack PM, et al: Ann Thorac Surg 43:113, 1987, Fig 3A–C, p 116, with permission.*)

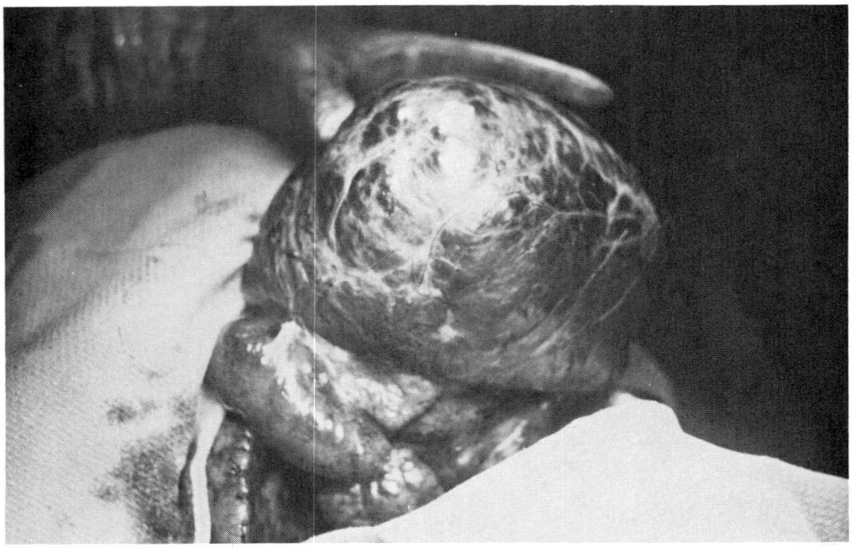

FIG. 16-34. An operative photograph showing a giant bulla arising from the upper lobe of an 18-year-old man with no symptoms of obstructive airway disease.

An asymptomatic or mildly symptomatic pneumothorax with less than 30 percent collapse that is shown not to increase in size over 6 to 8 h can safely be observed. Simple needle aspiration of the air space can nearly eliminate the space in a stable pneumothorax and will greatly reduce the amount of time required for spontaneous resolution. In a report by Delius and associates, aspiration through an 8F Teflon catheter was successful in 69 percent of 114 patients and in 87 percent of patients with simple pneumothorax. The average cost was comparatively low. Needle aspiration of a tension pneumothorax can be a lifesaving temporizing manuever.

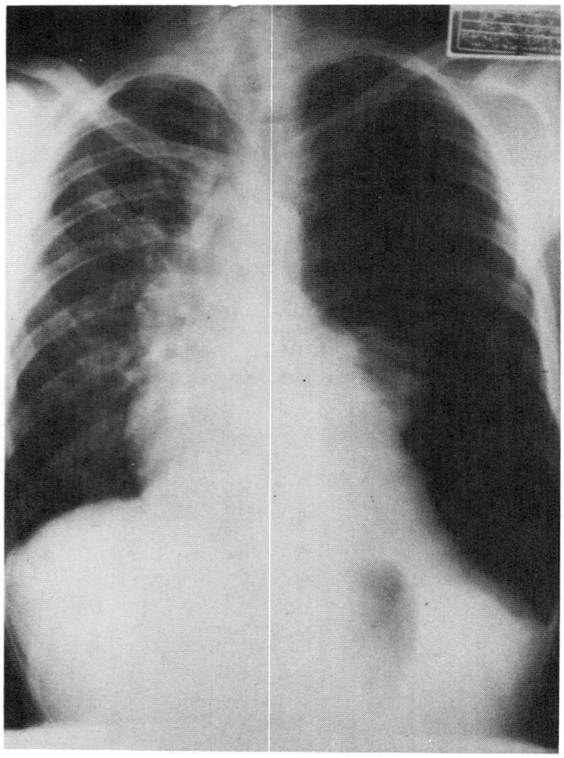

FIG. 16-35. Spontaneous pneumothorax in a young male. The lung is visible as a density collapsed against the mediastinum. The mediastinum is shifted to the right, the diaphragm is pushed down, and the intercostal spaces are wider on the left than on the right—findings that suggest an element of tension pneumothorax. In fact, the patient was hemodynamically stable and only mildly symptomatic.

Thoracostomy tube drainage is the most common treatment. The tube is inserted either anteriorly (second interspace, midclavicular line) or laterally in a lower interspace (mid to anterior axillary line), with the tip directed toward the apex. The tube is connected to water seal, to which suction can be added to increase the gradient favoring removal of air from the pleural space. Water seal alone will suffice in many cases. As the lung reexpands, the patient will feel pain as the visceral and parietal surfaces reoppose. The pain gradually subsides but is usually much more acute and severe when suction is applied initially. Rapid reexpansion occasionally leads to reexpansion pulmonary edema involving the ipsilateral lung, which was seen in 21 of 146 cases (14 percent) reported by Matsuura and associates. Those at greatest risk were patients 20 to 39 years of age with large pneumothoraces. Although the cause is not understood, the entity needs to be kept in mind because mortality has been as high as 20 percent. Some authors favor attaching the tube to a one-way flutter valve (Heimlich valve) that permits outpatient treatment of a pneumothorax in a reliable patient with a small leak.

Serial check x-rays are followed to assess reexpansion, and the size of the air leak is monitored by observing the rate of bubbling in the water seal chamber. Air will cross the water seal only with cough or valsalva in a pneumothorax caused by a leak that has already sealed, and the bubbling will usually cease altogether within 24 h. At the opposite extreme, continuous bubbling occurring through both phases of respiration reflects a large active leak that may take days to seal, if it will seal at all. With large air leaks a single tube may be inadequate. If two tubes connected to suction still fail to expand the lung, thoracotomy is required. Even a large leak can seal if the lung can be fully expanded, which promotes adhesion formation between parietal pleura and the site of the leak in the visceral pleura. Intrapleural instillation of tetracycline appears effective in reducing the recurrence rate. In a recent multicenter controlled trial reported by Light and associates, the recurrence rate after tetracycline was 25 percent as opposed to 41 percent in the control group.

Operation is indicated for a massive air leak with failure of lung reexpansion or for a smaller leak that has persisted for more than a week. Because of the frequency of recurrence after one episode, operation is recommended after any second episode and in any patient with a previous contralateral pneumothorax. Operation might be recommended after a first episode to anyone with large apical bullae visible on chest x-ray, to persons likely to be exposed to dangerous changes in atmospheric pressure (airline pilots, scuba divers), or to persons living in remote areas. Complications such as empyema or hemothorax occasionally develop and mandate operation. In general, conservative treatment is continued as long as possible in older patients with underlying lung disease because of their limited ventilatory reserve.

At thoracotomy or thoracoscopy the site of the leak can be identified and resected, oversewn, closed with staples, or ablated with laser energy. Pleural abrasion should also be performed to promote formation of adhesions between visceral and parietal pleura, an especially important manuever if no leak site can be identified. Pleurectomy, accomplished by stripping all the parietal pleura off the underlying ribs and intercostal muscles, is undeniably effective but has substantially greater morbidity and is reserved for extreme cases. Either method is 90 to 95 percent effective.

LUNG

Development and Anatomy

In the 4-mm (3-week) embryo, an outpouching from the primitive foregut appears caudad to the paired pharyngeal pouches and bifurcates into the right and left primitive bronchial buds. Over the next two weeks, further branching occurs with 10 segmental tubes on the right and 8 on the left, providing an early indication of the lobar development that will continue in each lung. Progressive branching of epithelial tubes results in a rich arborization of bronchioles, and alveolar ducts and sacs. It is estimated that 300 million alveolar sacs eventually develop. As the structural maturation is taking place, histologic differentiation progresses from the cuboidal epithelium that lines the terminal buds during the first four fetal months to the flattened epithelium present at birth. It is likely that the basic architecture of the lungs is completely developed at birth. As the lungs grow, they bulge into the lateral pleural cavities, leaving a dorsal mesentery to encase the developing mediastinal structures. The most caudal pair of aortic arches (the sixth) gives rise to the pulmonary arteries, with the remnant of the left sixth arch persisting as the ductus arteriosus. Vascular sprouts from the unilocular atrium fuse with the developing capillary vasculature in the lung mesenchyma to become the pulmonary veins.

Although the number of respiratory units may not increase after birth, it does seem apparent that the newborn's lung is structurally immature. In place of alveoli, the lungs are made up of primitive air sacs that differentiate into alveolar ducts and sacs. Alveoli develop by outpouching and compartmentalization, and maturation continues throughout the first eight years of life. The fully developed alveoli give a surface area of 70 to 80 m^2 at three-fourths maximal inflation of the adult lung.

Segmental Anatomy. The segmental anatomy of the lungs and bronchial tree is illustrated in Fig. 16-36. Although there is continuity of the pulmonary parenchyma between adjacent seg-

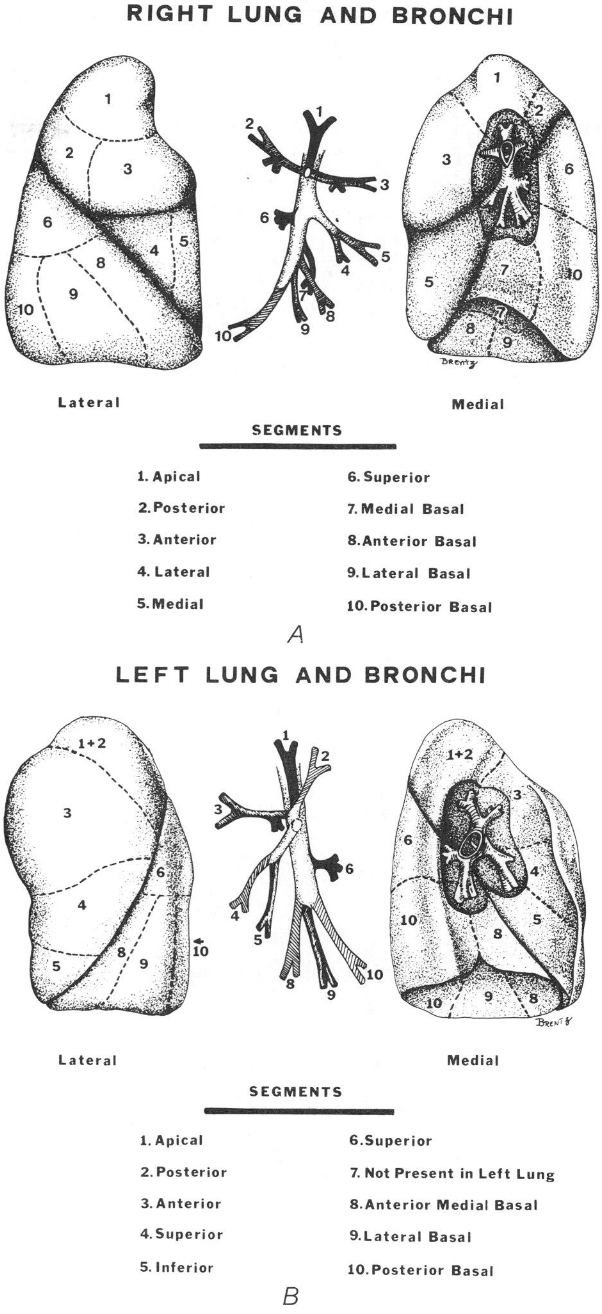

FIG. 16-36. *A* and *B*. The segmental anatomy of the lungs. An appreciation of these anatomic divisions often makes it possible to preserve pulmonary tissue by performing segmental resections for localized disease.

ments of each lobe, the separation of the bronchial and vascular stalks allows subsegmental and segmental resections whenever the clinical situation requires or allows preserving lung tissue. This may be particularly important in patients with impaired pulmonary function or in those with disease processes that are apt to be or to become multifocal, requiring multiple resective procedures. Less-than-lobar resections are desirable when dealing with localized inflammatory diseases such as tuberculosis and bronchiectasis that characteristically involve segmental units of the upper and lower lobes, respectively, but often do so in a way that leaves one or more segments of the same lobe unaffected. Both these diseases, as well as metastatic pulmonary neoplasms, may involve more than one pulmonary lobe, either synchronously or metachronously. Many surgeons doubt the necessity of extending the resection even of primary lung neoplasms beyond the field necessary for adequate margins around the tumor. The advantages of a segmental concept of surgical treatment are important in all these circumstances.

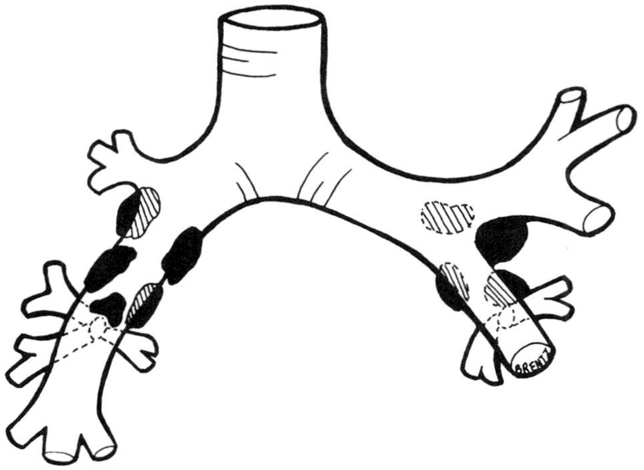

FIG. 16-38. The lymphatic sump of Borrie represents those lymph nodes on each side that receive lymphatic drainage from all lobes of the corresponding lung.

Lymphatic Drainage. Abundant lymphatic vessels are located beneath the visceral pleura of each lung, in the interlobular septums, in the submucosa of the bronchi, and in the perivascular and peribronchial connective tissue. The lymph nodes that drain the lungs are divided into two large groups, the pulmonary lymph nodes and the mediastinal nodes, referred to as N1 and N2 nodes, respectively, in the TNM system of staging of lung cancer (Fig. 16-37). In turn, the pulmonary (N1) lymph nodes consist of (1) intrapulmonary, or segmental, nodes that lie at points of division of segmental bronchi or in the bifurcations of the pulmonary artery, (2) lobar nodes that lie along the upper-, middle-, and lower-lobe bronchi, (3) interlobar nodes, situated in the angles formed by the bifurcation of the main bronchi into lobar bronchi, and (4) hilar nodes located along the main bronchi.

The interlobar lymph nodes lie in the depths of the interlobar fissure on each side and have special surgical significance because they constitute a lymphatic sump for each lung, referred to as the lymphatic sump of Borrie (Fig. 16-38). This designation results from the fact that all the pulmonary lobes of the corresponding lung drain into that group of nodes. On the right side the nodes of the lymphatic sump lie around the bronchus intermedius, bounded above by the right-upper-lobe bronchus, and below by the middle lobe and superior-segmental bronchi. The lymphatic sump on the left side is confined to the interlobar fissure, with the lymph nodes disposed in the angle between the lingular and lower-lobe bronchi, and in apposition to the pulmonary artery branches.

The mediastinal (N2) lymph nodes consist of four principal groups: (1) anterior mediastinal, (2) posterior mediastinal, (3) tracheobronchial, and (4) paratracheal. The anterior mediastinal nodes are located in association with the upper surface of the pericardium, the phrenic nerves, the ligamentum arteriosum, and the left innominate vein. Within the inferior pulmonary ligament on each side are found the paraesophageal lymph nodes that constitute a major part of the posterior mediastinal group. Additional paraesophageal nodes may be located more superiorly between the esophagus and trachea in the region of the arch of the azygos vein.

The tracheobronchial lymph nodes are made up of three subgroups that are located about the bifurcation of the trachea. Included are the subcarinal nodes, the lymph nodes lying in the obtuse angle between the trachea and each main-stem bronchus, and a few nodes that lie anterior to the lower end of the trachea. The paratracheal lymph nodes are located in proximity to the trachea in the superior mediastinum. Those on the right side form a chain with the tracheobronchial nodes inferiorly and with some of the deep cervical nodes above. A few of the latter are referred to as the scalene lymph nodes because they lie on the anterior scalene muscle. Lymphatic drainage of the right lung is ipsilateral except for an occasional incidence in which drainage to the superior mediastinum is bilateral. Drainage from the left lung to the superior mediastinum is as frequently ipsilateral as it is to the opposite side.

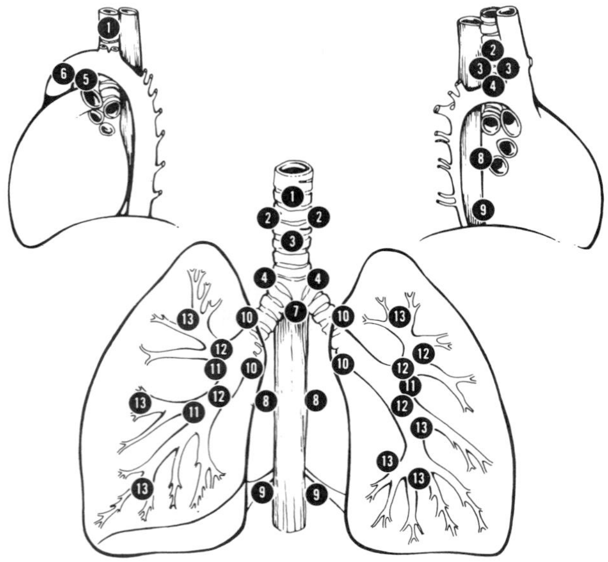

N2 Nodes

- Superior Mediastinal Nodes
  1. Highest Mediastinal
  2. Upper Paratracheal
  3. Pre- and Retrotracheal
  4. Lower Paratracheal (including Azygos Nodes)
- Aortic Nodes
  5. Subaortic (aortic window)
  6. Para-aortic (ascending aorta or phrenic)
- Inferior Mediastinal Nodes
  7. Subcarinal
  8. Paraesophageal (below carina)
  9. Pulmonary Ligament

N1 Nodes

10. Hilar
11. Interlobar
12. Lobar
13. Segmental

FIG. 16-37. The American Joint Committee classification of regional lymph nodes. (From: *Staging of Lung Cancer, American Joint Committee for Cancer Staging and End-Results Reporting, Task Force on Lung Cancer, Chicago, 1979, with permission.*)

Diagnostic Evaluation

Two factors make diagnostic evaluation of disorders of the lung more logical than is often the case in other anatomic regions. There is direct communication between the oropharynx and the respiratory system, and the contrasting densities of the contents of the thorax provide exceptional opportunities for a variety of imaging techniques. The first factor allows collection of secretions, abnormal drainage or purulent material, and desquamated cells that may provide a definitive diagnosis. It also allows an orderly sequence of progressively more invasive diagnostic endoscopic procedures for visualization, culture, or biopsy. The ''window'' into the thoracic cavity provided by fluoroscopy, conventional radiography, CT, and MRI allows remarkably clear anatomical definition, opportunities for serial observations, and precise guidance of biopsy needles and forceps.

Airway Investigation. In most acquired pulmonary diseases sputum collection and examination are indicated as an initial diagnostic procedure. The specific etiologic agent of infections is sought by examination of smears and by culture techniques. The flora of the upper part of the respiratory tract stops abruptly at the level of the larynx, and the tracheobronchial tree is normally sterile. Not frequently, either the patient's sputum is scant, or because it is mixed with saliva and an oral bacterial flora, its diagnostic usefulness is reduced. To bypass these problems, percutaneous transtracheal aspiration may be performed through the cricothyroid membrane. A 16- or 14-gauge intracatheter needle is used for the procedure after preparation of the skin with soap or iodine solution and local infiltration anesthesia with lidocaine. Coughing may be induced by injecting 5 to 10 mL sterile saline solution without preservative into the trachea. Aspiration of the diluted secretions into a 10- or 20-mL syringe should be followed by immediate delivery of the material to the laboratory.

Bronchoscopy. Whenever malignancy is a diagnostic consideration, or when the preceding studies have failed to yield adequate information, direct visual examination of the tracheobronchial tree is indicated. Information can be gained from this procedure that is available from no other source: cell type of bronchial neoplasms by direct biopsy, mobility of surrounding structures, extent of endobronchial involvement in neoplasms and inflammatory disease, and on occasion, source of bleeding. In addition, the therapeutic aspects of bronchoscopy should not be overlooked. The removal of thick, inspissated secretions from the postoperative patient can be lifesaving. The benefit of foreign body extraction by endoscopic means is obvious.

While the vast majority of endotracheal endoscopic examinations are now made with the flexible bronchoscope, there are still some important uses for the rigid scope, particularly for the removal of certain foreign bodies and the performance of endobronchial resections. The rigid scope provides a large, controlled airway with superb suction capabilities, and room for limited use of snares, scissors, lasers, and forceps. In small children, the restricted caliber of the airway may require use of the rigid scope.

The introduction of the flexible bronchoscope in 1967 by Ikeda has greatly extended indications for this procedure. Optically enhanced visualization of tracheobronchial tree to the subsegmental level is now possible and with the addition of fluoroscopic guidance, brush biopsy of many peripheral lesions has become practical.

Both rigid and flexible bronchoscopy may be performed using either topical or general anesthesia, on conscious or unconscious patients, and with patients breathing either spontaneously or with ventilator support. With the rigid scope, a ventilating scope is used that has a side arm for attachment of the ventilator connectors. A size 8 or larger endotracheal tube will allow passage of the flexible scope through a special attachment. Topical anesthesia is the preferred method under most circumstances. The flexible scope can play a major therapeutic role in intubated patients in an intensive care setting where specific suctioning of the segmental bronchi can prevent obstructive atelectasis and provide specific culture information by gathering secretions from localized infected areas. The sputum coughed up immediately after bronchoscopy is especially valuable for cytologic examinations. Chest physical therapy, ultrasonic nebulizers, and bronchodilators are additional techniques to facilitate the collection of sputum.

Imaging. The juxtaposition in the chest of tissues of widely differing densities makes radiography especially useful in the diagnosis of diseases involving the thorax and its contents. The standard posteroanterior (PA) chest film along with a companion lateral view, each taken at 6-m tube-to-film distance, remains the most frequently used study. When correlated with symptoms, physical findings, and previous radiographs, it provides most of the information needed for the diagnosis and management of a high proportion of disorders of the lung and its major support systems. With the addition of CT and MRI, the ability to accurately map and characterize abnormalities in the lung parenchyma, pleura, and hilar and mediastinal nodal areas is excellent, and the wide application of these techniques has simplified significantly the work-up and preoperative staging of patients with intrathoracic neoplasm. Templeton and associates have reviewed the role of these techniques in the staging of lung cancer and has suggested some useful simplifying generalizations. Clinicians now rely heavily on CT scans to assess intrathoracic pathology, particularly in evaluating the patient with lung cancer, though agreement is still lacking regarding the proper size criteria and axis length in nodal assessment. For most workers, lesions larger than 1.5 cm are presumed to be positive until biopsy proves otherwise. No other imaging test is as comprehensive in evaluating the patient with lung cancer. MRI is useful mainly in resolving specific questions relating to invasion of the chest wall, vascular structures, brachial plexus, adrenal masses, and the hilum and mediastinum in patients who cannot receive intravenous contrast during CT studies. The overall accuracy of CT and MRI is disappointing in distinguishing operability in patients with Stage IIIA or IIIB disease. MRI can often detect encasement or invasion of hilar or mediastinal vessels (see Fig. 16-84C). CT diagnostic accuracy is not apt to increase significantly; there is substantial potential for improved diagnostic accuracy with MRI as continued research and interpretive experience moves this technology forward. The Radiologic Diagnostic Oncology Group has recently reported recommendations concluding that there is little difference between the two techniques in their present generations of development with the exception of the resolution of hilar vessels by MRI.

The increased time it takes to perform MRI sequences gives CT a decided advantage in most clinical settings, particularly when, as is usually the case, it is desirable to evaluate the upper abdominal organs to which lung tumors commonly metastasize.

The indications for other more invasive radiographic procedures have been sharply reduced by these new techniques. Bronchography is now rarely useful in the assessment of bronchiectatic dilations but may aid in demonstrating occult esophageal fistulae.

Pulmonary angiography has been disappointing as a general diagnostic technique, but it can be important in defining congenital abnormalities. Bronchial arteriography can be a useful technique in the diagnosis and treatment of chronic or massive hemoptysis. Intractable hemoptysis associated with chronic pulmonary inflammatory diseases such as bronchiectasis, cystic fibrosis, or tuberculosis may be due to an eroded bronchial artery. In carefully selected cases, selective bronchial arteriography may identify the site of bleeding and allow embolic occulsion of the bleeding vessel through the arteriographic catheter.

Nuclear medicine has played an increasingly important role in clinical diagnosis and in the evaluation of the patient with neoplastic disease. Lung ventilation and perfusion scanning has been important in the diagnosis of pulmonary embolism and for evaluation of split-pulmonary function. While a few groups advocate a program of routine multiorgan scanning to evaluate potential lung cancer patients, most studies have concluded that only in the presence of symptoms focusing on a specific organ should radionuclide scans be done.

Biopsies. There are many indications for biopsy of intrathoracic tissues for the diagnosis of nonneoplastic diseases. There are also several research protocols involving pretreatment of patients with certain stages of lung cancers. In each of those situations, efforts to obtain diagnostic tissue and to sample certain lymph-node beds seem clearly indicated. It is logical to outline a sequence of biopsy efforts based on the invasiveness and risk of the studies. Controversy exists concerning the appropriateness of preoperative invasive procedures if they will not alter the immediate operative plan. Metastatic disease in the mediastinum sharply worsens the prognosis for lung cancer patients. There is little consensus among thoracic surgeons, however, about the impact this observation should have on the initial clinical management of the individual patient. Five-year survival of up to 28 percent has been reported from some centers in patients with positive mediastinal (N2) nodes; surgeons in these institutions recommend that the presence of nodes in that area does not preclude resection. These surgeons emphasize that the most economic, expeditious, and accurate staging can be done at the time of thoracotomy for resection. They suggest that, once the probability of extra thoracic metastases has been assessed and the appropriate search made, it is best to proceed with exploration for resection and staging. While this controversy has not been resolved, it seems likely that as multimodal therapy becomes a more usual approach to neoplastic disease, careful staging and preoperative planning will justify efforts to establish the extent of the disease at the onset of therapy, before thoracotomy.

Needle Biopsies. Both transbronchial and percutaneous needle biopsy techniques have become increasingly productive diagnostic tools. Our surgical pathology colleagues have become extremely skillful in obtaining information from isolated cell clusters. Instrumental advances have created a variety of flexible and highly versatile needles. Radiologists can assist us with accurate mapping of the mediastinal and parabronchial nodes, and with fluoroscopic guidance to high-yield areas. With careful technique, tissue samples can be obtained sufficient to allow diagnosis of diffuse pulmonary diseases such as sarcoidosis, pulmonary alveolar proteinosis, and *Pneumocystis carinii* pneumonia. The morbidity rate of transbronchial lung biopsy has been low, with pneumothorax as the principal complication. Though the incidence of pneumothorax has varied from 5 to 20 percent, few patients require active treatment.

Whether the patient has a diffuse lung disease or a tumor, percutaneous transthoracic needle biopsy (TTNB) can provide a rapid diagnosis that expedites overall evaluation and avoids the need for diagnostic thoracotomy in those individuals for whom operation is not indicated; several investigators in this country have reported diagnostic accuracy of 80 to 90 percent in accessible parenchymal lesions. For the candidate for operative treatment, some recommend proceeding with the thoracotomy without biopsy, since negative results cannot be relied on. On the other hand, if the needle biopsy confirms a suspected primary malignancy, the established diagnosis allows planning the operative procedure and fully informing the patient of the plans; the psychologic climate provided by certainty in diagnosis may be very important for some patients.

Figures 16-39 and 16-40 show the close correlation between cytologic material obtained with needle biopsy and the histology of the resected specimens. TTNB is performed under local anesthesia, usually with fluoroscopic control. Aspirated material must be immediately smeared or cultured, but pathology departments vary in their preference for the handling of tissue removed with cutting needles. The complications include hemoptysis, pneumothorax, and rarely hemothorax. Although an incidence of pneumothorax as high as 30 percent has been reported, only an occasional patient requires tube thoracostomy for treatment. The theoretic possibility of implanting the needle track through the chest wall with malignant cells has not been confirmed even with extensive experience in a number of major cancer centers.

Contraindications to needle biopsy include (1) coagulopathies, (2) pulmonary hypertension, (3) severe bullous lung disease, (4) a patient receiving continuous positive-pressure breathing, and (5) a suspected vascular lesion.

Mediastinoscopy. Following its introduction by Carlens in 1959 and until the recent increasing dependence on CT scanning of the mediastinum, mediastinoscopy gained increasing use as a technique for exploring the routes of mediastinal spread of pulmonary neoplasms. Controversy persists among thoracic surgeons over the significance of positive mediastinal nodes. For those who would alter management with confirmation of tumor involvement in the mediastinum, and when the imaging studies identify enlarged (>1.5 cm) nodes in the paratracheal (particularly on the right side) and the anterior subcarinal areas, these nodes can be satisfactorily explored and biopsied by passing a mediastinoscope or laryngoscope along the pretracheal plane for direct visualization and sampling of the suspicious nodes. The procedure is usually performed under general endotracheal anesthesia with a small transverse incision in the suprasternal notch. Digital exploration is carried inferiorly in the plane between the anterior surface of the trachea and the posterior surface of the innominate artery and the aorta. The paratracheal, tracheobronchial, and subcarinal lymph nodes are accessible to visualization and biopsy through the mediastinoscope; tumor masses such as thymomas or thyroid lesions may be biopsied directly. The technique provides a positive diagnosis in almost all patients with lymphoma who have radiographic evidence of enlarged mediastinal lymph nodes, and the yield is similarly very high for patients with infectious disease. Mediastinoscopy is considered the procedure of choice for diagnosis of sarcoidosis in most institutions, and it has largely replaced scalene lymph-node and fat-pad biopsy for both benign and malignant lesions (Fig. 16-41). Unfortunately, metastases to lymph nodes between the trachea and esophagus and to posterior mediastinal lymph nodes cannot be determined by mediastinoscopy. Similarly, suspected lesions on the left side are difficult to evaluate by this technique because of the location of the aortic arch.

Parasternal Mediastinotomy. Additional methods for exploring the mediastinum have been developed, and the procedure referred to as anterior mediastinotomy has been used most frequently. Through either a transverse or vertical parasternal incision the second costal cartilage is removed on the side of the lesion. An effort is made to avoid opening the pleural cavity as the mediastinal pleura is freed from the undersurface of the sternum and dissected away from the mediastinum. By additional removal of the third costal cartilage a wider exploration can be performed; the reason is to sample mediastinal lymph nodes and determine the extent of mediastinal spread of a centrally located bronchial neoplasm. If it is pertinent to the confirmation of the diagnosis, the mediastinal pleura can be opened to allow direct lung or pleural biopsy. Several authors have recommended the combination of the parasternal approach to the mediastinum with the mediastinoscopic examination for improved exposure, control, and flexibility in evaluating suspicious mediastinal findings. The left mediastinotomy is particularly useful for the evaluation of nodes in the left aortic window and hilus.

Thoracoscopy. In 1910, H.C. Jacobaeus adapted the cystoscope to investigate ''pleurisy,'' to biopsy pleural masses, and to lyse adhesions to facilitate the therapeutic induced pneumothorax then being used as collapse therapy for tuberculosis. Surgeons are adapting the laparoscope, which has had such a dramatic impact on intraperitoneal surgery, to intrathoracic concerns. The thoracoscope has been found useful in diagnosing those chronic or recurrent pleural effusions that remain enigmas after pleurocenteses and needle pleural biopsies, in visualizing and obtaining tissue samples from pleural masses, in staging tumors, in removing foreign bodies, in assisting in therapeutic pleurodesis for malignant effusions or resistant pneumothorax, and in evacuation of posttraumatic clotted hemothorax when indicated. Wakabayashi along with several others has been dramatically expanding the scope of the video-assisted thoracoscopic approach to intrathoracic lesions. It is a rapidly developing area of surgical endeavor. There are some ambitious projections that major resective surgery might be feasible by this approach, and several thoracoscopic lobectomies have

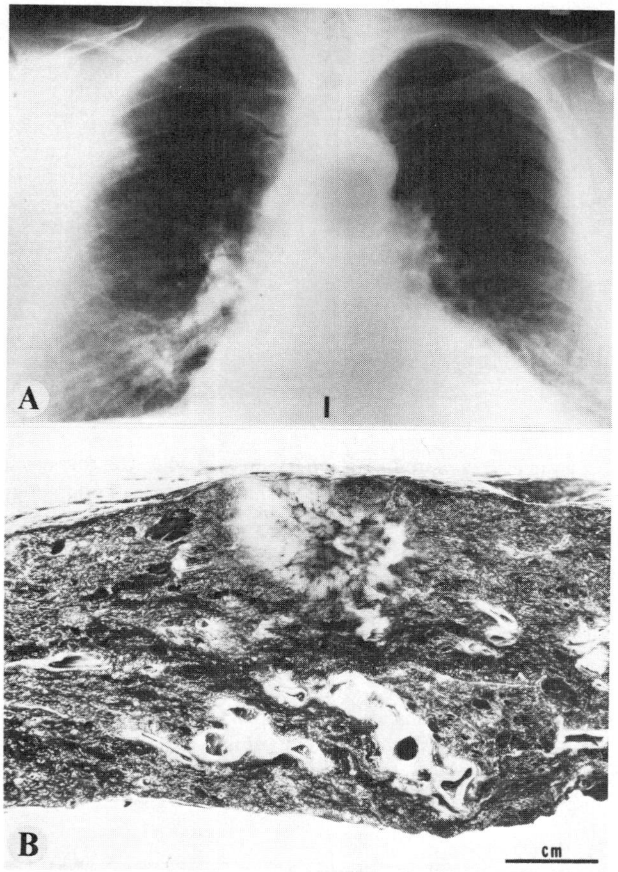

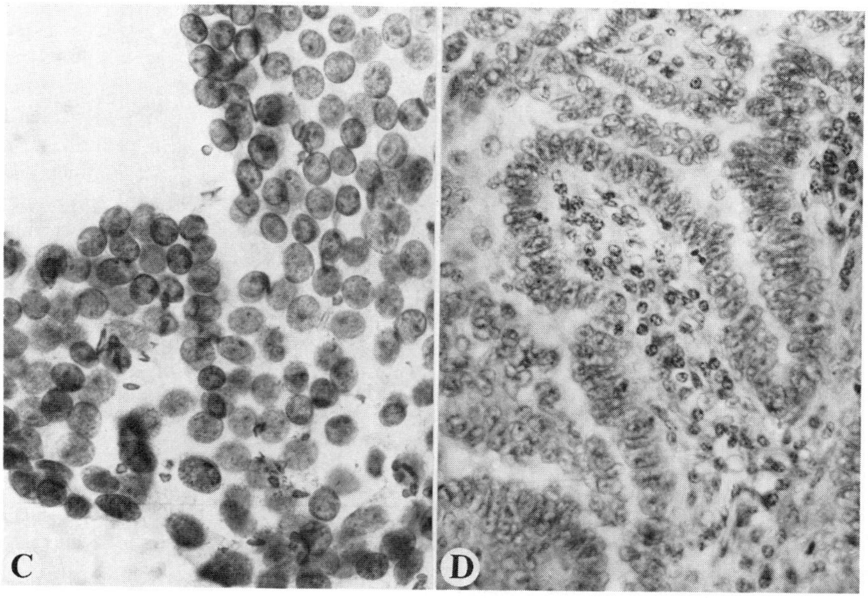

FIG. 16-39. A 63-year-old male with an adenocarcinoma of the right upper lobe of the lung. *A.* The P-A chest x-ray shows a peripheral mass near the lateral chest wall in the right upper lobe. *B.* The right-upper-lobe specimen shows a 2-cm subpleural mass arising from within an anthracotic scar. *C.* Chiba fine-needle aspiration cytology from percutaneous needle biopsy: adenocarcinoma showing a papillary projection extending from a sheet of overlapping large cells with bland vesicular nuclei, prominent nuclear rim, and conspicuous nucleoli (×471). *D.* Tissue section histology: papillary adenocarcinoma, showing a papillary fibrovascular core lined by an irregular border of malignant epithelial cells (×471).

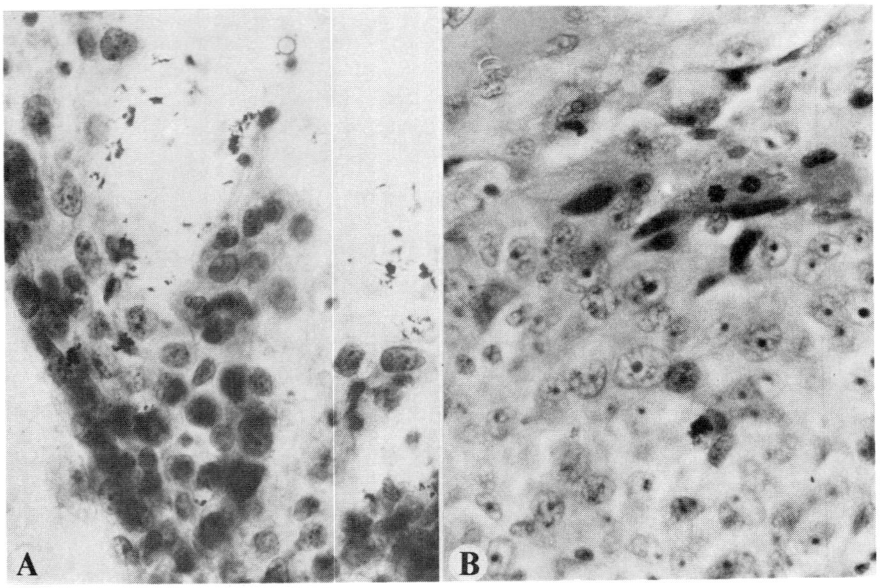

FIG. 16-40. Percutaneous needle biopsy and histology of the resected specimen from a 55-year-old male with a right-lower-lobe mass. *A*. The Chiba fine-needle aspiration cytology shows a mosaic sheet of large pleomorphic cells with irregular, hyperchromatic granular nuclei and macronucleoli, interpreted as squamous carcinoma (×471). *B*. Resection specimen tissue histology: squamous carcinoma showing large pleomorphic cells with macronucleoli and a contrasting smaller population of cells with angular hyperchromatic nuclei and cytoplasmic keratinization (×471).

been done. It is more likely, however, that when the role has been fully clarified, its use will likely include resection of nonmalignant nodules, diagnostic node and lung biopsies, definitive treatment of difficult persisting air-leak problems in the postresection, post-trauma, and resistant spontaneous pneumothorax patient. The carbon dioxide laser shows promise as a tool that might seal air and blood leaks from the lung surface.

The thoracoscopic procedure is usually performed after the patient has been intubated with a double-lumen tube and is under general anesthesia and after the lung on the ipsilateral side is selectively deflated. In the series reported by various authors, complications have been exceedingly rare, usually minor and non-life-threatening.

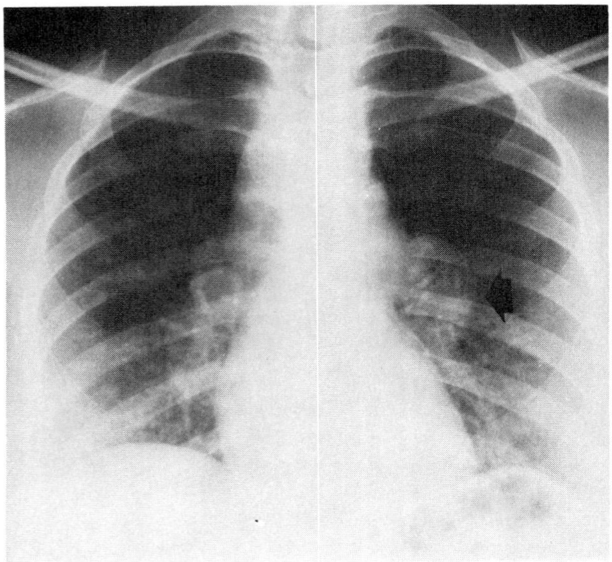

FIG. 16-41. This chest x-ray of a 24-year-old woman shows bilateral hilar masses that could be lymphoma or sarcoidosis. Mediastinoscopy was performed to obtain tissue that confirmed the diagnosis of sarcoidosis.

Open Lung Biopsy. The chief indications for open lung biopsy are failure of less invasive closed or semi-closed methods for diagnosis. The video-assisted thoracoscope should sharply decrease the indication for open thoracotomy for biopsy or resection of nodules, particularly in patients physiologically poorly suited for a formal thoracotomy.

Congenital Lung Lesions

Developmental Anatomy. The respiratory system begins to differentiate in the third week of gestation as an outpouching in the floor of the primitive foregut. As the outpouching lengthens it bifurcates into two distinct buds, which promptly elongate and begin to form the secondary buds that will become the lobar and segmental bronchi. Rapid dichotomous branching of the terminal bud proceeds such that the lobes of each lung are well defined by 12 weeks, and by 16 weeks development of the bronchial system is complete.

Alveolar development proceeds more slowly. The alveolar or terminal sac stage of development only begins in about the seventh month of gestation, when primitive air sacs surrounded by capillary loops can be identified. Most alveolar development occurs after birth. At birth, the lung contains approximately 20 million large, thick-walled terminal air sacs, which proliferate rapidly until 300 million alveoli have been formed, with most of the increase occurring during the first 4 years of life, and with no further proliferation after about 10 years of age.

The pulmonary arterial circulation begins in a rich capillary network surrounding the developing lung buds, which is joined by the primitive pulmonary arteries budding off the sides of the aortic sac at about 5 weeks of gestation. The left sixth aortic arch extends to join the developing pulmonary artery, and persists as the ductus arteriosus. Each pulmonary artery develops in close relationship to the bronchi, and follows the course of the branching airways, although it gives off many more branches than the airway it accompanies. Normally, the only persistent connections with the aorta are the ductus arteriosus and the bronchial arteries.

Anatomic Variants. The most common variation of segmentation is the azygous lobe, which is present in about 0.5 percent of routine chest x-rays. In this anomaly the azygous vein lies in the substance of the right upper lobe, on a pleural mesentery that separates the azygous lobe from the remainder of the lung. It appears on chest x-ray as an ''inverted comma'' in the medial apex of the right upper lobe. On rare occasions an azygous lobe can be the site of an infection or neoplasm that does not involve the remainder of the right upper lobe.

Situs inversus is a rare entity in which the thoracic viscera alone (situs inversus thoracis) or the thoracic and abdominal viscera (situs inversus totalis) undergo complete mirror-image reversal in position during development. The anomaly may exist in isolation or may be associated with other conditions. One example of the latter is Kartagener's syndrome, a familial association of situs inversus with sinusitis and bronchiectasis. Abnormal ciliary function is thought to explain the syndrome.

Aberrant origin of a normal major bronchus is infrequent but can have major significance when pulmonary resection is required for another reason. The most common example is origin of the right upper lobe bronchus or the apical segmental bronchus from the lateral wall of the trachea just above the carina.

Developmental Anomalies

Agenesis. Many tracheobronchial anomalies reflect an arrest in embryonic development. The most complete example is bilateral pulmonary agenesis, which is obviously incompatible with life and is often seen in anencephalic monsters. Unilateral pulmonary agenesis has a low survival rate when associated with other congenital anomalies, which are present in about 50 percent of cases. When seen as an isolated lesion, it is compatible with relatively normal life. Seventy percent of cases occur on the left side. The single lung fills both hemithoraces, and the condition is often detected in otherwise normal individuals by findings suggesting mediastinal shift or asymmetric thoracic development. Pulmonary arteriography demonstrating single pulmonary artery confirms the diagnosis in such patients and may protect them against therapeutic misadventures. Lobar agenesis is rarely reported and is most often discovered during evaluation for other conditions.

Hypoplasia. Hypoplasia of the lung is most often seen in association with anomalies that compete with the lungs for space, such as diaphragmatic hernia. It has been postulated that the defect arises from arrested alveolar development occurring during the last 2 months of gestation. The scimitar syndrome is a condition difficult to classify, which has as one of its features hypoplasia of the right lung. The syndrome takes its name from the radiographic finding of a scimitar-like shadow running parallel to the right heart border that represents an anomalous pulmonary vein entering the inferior vena cava. The hypoplastic right lung also has an aberrant pulmonary arterial origin from the aorta.

Tracheoesophageal Fistulae. See Chap. 37.

Diverticula. These are usually asymptomatic, small, and in free communication with the airway, usually the distal trachea.

Cystic Adenomatoid Malformation. Cystic adenomatoid malformation is one cause of respiratory distress in the newborn period that can require emergent operation. Other congenital anomalies, prematurity, and stillbirth are common associations. Surviving neonates present with acute respiratory distress in the first few hours of life. The chest x-ray shows a multicystic ''swiss cheese'' configuration with overexpansion of the involved region and mediastinal shift toward the normal lung. The pattern on chest x-ray can be confused with dilated loops of intestine suggesting diaphragmatic hernia. This lesion is diagnosed with increasing frequency in prenatal ultasound examinations, and prenatal transthoracic cyst aspiration has been attempted in the hope of allowing growth of normal lung elements. Any lobe of either lung can be involved, although the process has a predilection for the lower lobes. About half the reported cases have escaped crisis in the newborn period to present later in infancy or during childhood with a more indolent course of chronic recurrent pulmonary infection, and can be difficult to distinguish clinically from sequestration, infected congenital cysts, and bronchiectasis.

Thoracotomy reveals a dense, meaty mass studded with cysts that may appear to be partially aerated but have no ventilatory function. Anomalous vessels are very rare. Histopathology reveals multiple components of respiratory tissue including a maze of irregular tubules resembling fetal bronchioles lined with disorganized respiratory epithelium that can resemble an adenoma. Lobectomy is the treatment of choice, although pneumonectomy has been necessary in some cases. The prognosis is excellent with a successful early operation.

Pulmonary Sequestration. A portion of lung may be isolated during development from the remainder of the lung and receive its blood supply from an aberrant branch of the aorta instead of the pulmonary artery. Intralobar sequestrations rest within a lobe and do not have their own visceral pleural envelope, but usually have a communication with the tracheobronchial tree producing a cystic appearance. They occur invariably in the posterobasal portion of the lower lobes, most frequently on the left side. The sequestered lung is supplied by an anomalous branch of the aorta that is usually tortuous and disproportionately large, arising from the thoracic aorta in 70 percent of cases and from the abdominal aorta or its branches in the remainder. The vessel reaches the sequestered lung by passing through the inferior pulmonary ligament. Venous drainage is through the pulmonary veins. The radiographic appearance is that of a dense mass usually containing cysts with air-fluid levels, not distinguishable from cystic adenomatoid malformation or other congenital cystic abnormalities without an arteriogram (Fig. 16-42). Intralobar sequestration often remains asymptomatic until childhood or young adulthood, when it presents as pulmonary infection.

Extralobar sequestration is a much less common entity in which the sequestered lung is enclosed by a separate pleural envelope sitting in the inferoposterior mediastinum adjacent to lung and esophagus, usually on the left side (Fig. 16-43). Association with other congenital anomalies, especially diaphragmatic hernia, occurs in over 50 percent of patients. Although tracheobronchial communication is said not to occur, an esophageal communication is occasionally seen. Extralobar sequestration is more likely to be detected early in childhood, appearing as an unexplained dense triangular mass in the posterior lower lung field (Fig. 16-44). Venous drainage is to the azygous or portal venous system.

If either type of sequestration is suspected, an arteriogram should be done to confirm the diagnosis and define the aberrant systemic blood supply. A barium esophagram should be done to exclude the possibility of a communication with the esophagus. CT scanning can help to define lobar and mediastinal relationships. The treatment of choice is lobectomy for the intralobar types, and resection for the extralobar types.

An accessory lobe is distinguished from sequestration by the fact that it communicates with the trachea or a major bronchial

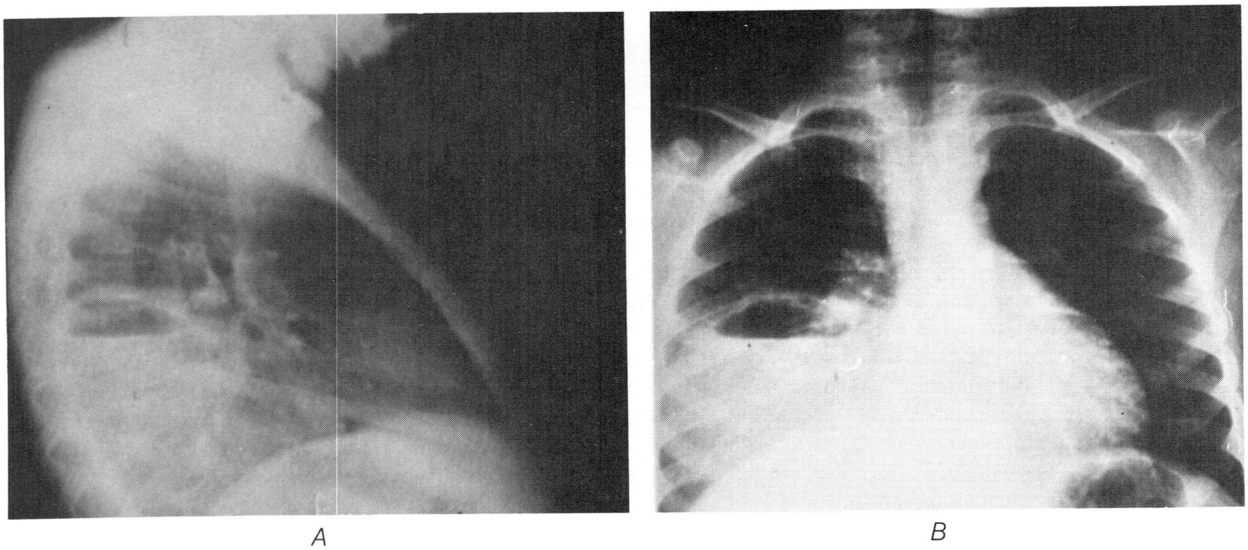

FIG. 16-42. An example of intrapulmonary sequestration. Consolidation and an air-fluid level are evident posteriorly in the right lower lobe. Lobectomy revealed an infected sequestration.

branch, most commonly on the left side. The accessory lobe can be supplied by either the pulmonary or systemic circulation.

Congenital Cysts. These are a diverse group of abnormalities that can be single or multiple, and vary greatly in size. They are usually confined to a segment or lobe and almost invariably present with infection (Fig. 16-45). Etiology is poorly understood and may be equally diverse. Unilateral absence of a pulmonary artery branch may produce hypoplastic development of the lung, leading to cystic transformation. The lesions may begin as intrapulmonary bronchogenic cysts, which are thought to represent remnants of developing bronchial buds pinched off in the lung periphery. A region of cystic lung can develop distal to congenital or acquired bronchial obstruction. The cysts are typically lined with respiratory epithelium and are filled with a viscid opaque fluid until they develop communication with the airway, after which they become partially air-filled and infected. The presence of respiratory epithelium is thought to indicate true congenital origin, but once chronic infection destroys the epithelium it becomes impossible to separate a congenital cyst from a chronic pulmonary abscess or bronchiectasis, grossly or histopathologically. Resection is indicated for large or chronically infected cysts. Preoperative evaluation includes bronchoscopy and arteriography, to exclude sequestration.

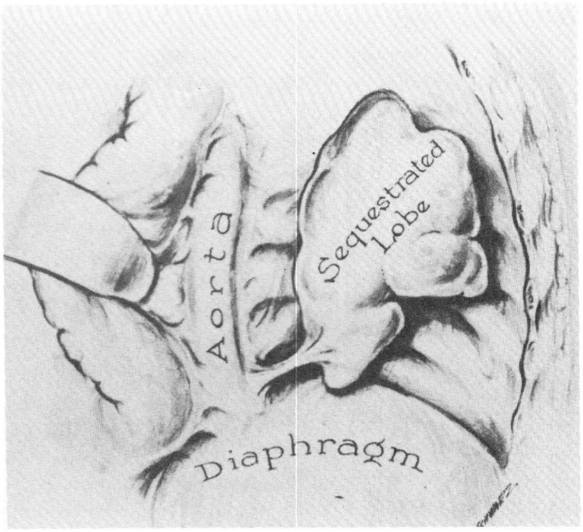

FIG. 16-43. Artist's conception of an extralobar sequestration as seen at operation through a left posterolateral thoracotomy. Anterior is to the left. Note the anomalous systemic artery arising directly from the aorta, a feature common to both extralobar and intralobar sequestrations. (From: *Ferguson TB, in Gibbon's Surgery of the Chest, 4th ed, Fig 22-28, p 685, with permission.*)

Arteriovenous Malformation. Pulmonary arteriovenous malformation is a fistula between pulmonary arteries and pulmonary veins. One or more thin-walled saccular channels with an endothelial lining are present, without reaction in the surrounding lung tissue. The lesions are somewhat more frequent in the lower lobes. Multiple small (<1 cm) lesions associated with capillary abnormalities elsewhere, a feature of hereditary hemorrhagic telangiectasia (Osler–Weber–Rendu syndrome), account for half of all reported cases. In the other half the lesions are singular or few in number, and larger (1 to 5 cm) in size. Although the vascular pattern is variable, one afferent pulmonary arterial branch with two or more efferent venous branches is the most common arrangement (Fig. 16-46). The lesions are frequently very superficial and vulnerable to erosion and can present with spontaneous hemothorax.

Diagnosis is easiest in the 20 percent of patients presenting with cyanosis, polycythemia, and clubbing. Cyanosis is said to develop when the shunt fraction exceeds 25 percent of the total blood flow and is usually not seen until adolescence or early adulthood. There is an interesting difference between the right-to-left shunt seen in congenital heart disease and that seen with a pulmonary arteriovenous malformation. In the latter condition, vascular resistance in both the pulmonary capillary bed and the fistula are negligible, so the total volume returned to the left atrium is not increased, it is simply desaturated in proportion to the amount of

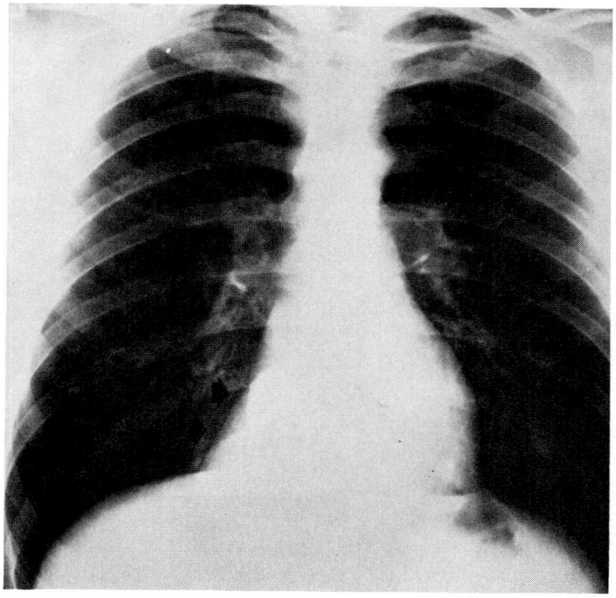

A

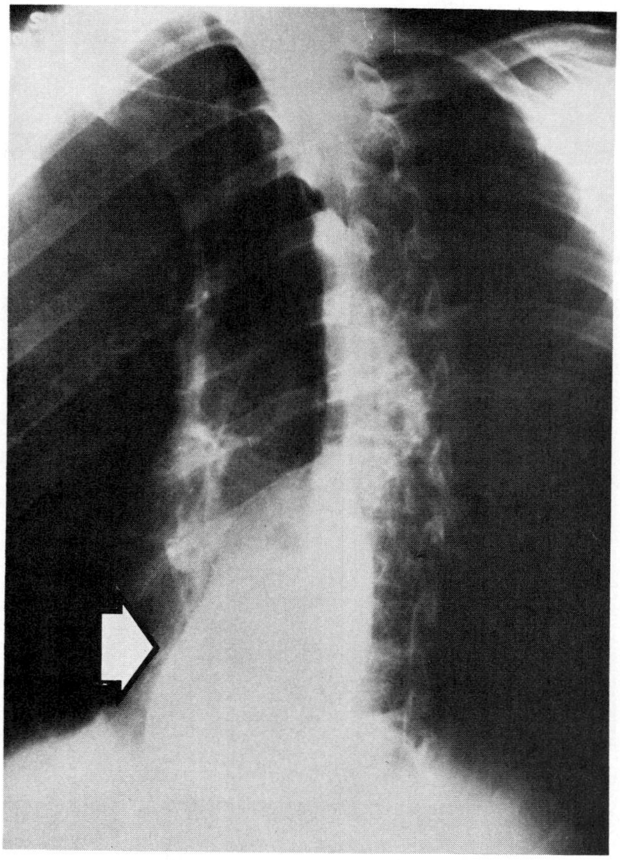

B

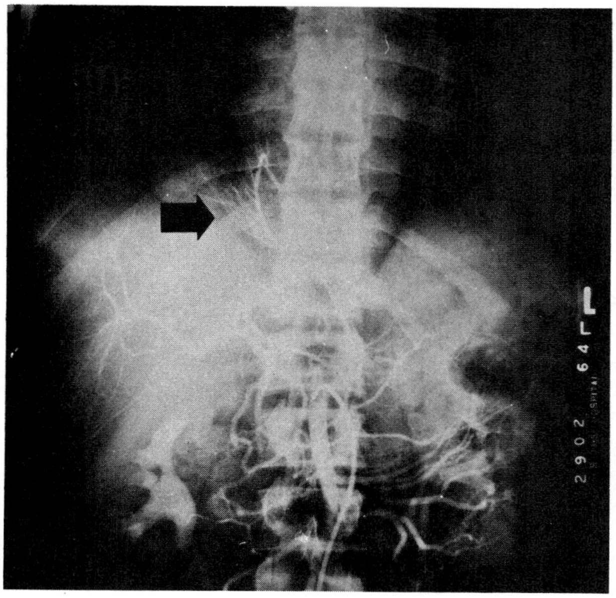

C

FIG. 16-44. An extrapulmonary sequestration discovered on a routine chest x-ray in a 20-year-old male. *A.* The posteroanterior chest x-ray shows a triangular density adjacent to the right heart border and based on the diaphragm. *B.* An oblique view shows the density to be a large mass with sharp borders. *C.* An aortogram shows several arteries passing retrograde from the infradiaphragmatic aorta to supply the sequestration.

flow going through the fistula. Therefore, in contrast to the patient with an intracardiac shunt, the patient with the fistula has normal cardiac output, pulse, blood pressure, venous pressure, electrocardiogram, and heart size. No murmur is audible over the heart, but in over half the cyanotic patients a continuous murmur can be heard peripherally over the fistula. Patients with either condition have arterial desaturation and polycythemia.

Diagnosis is more difficult in the asymptomatic, acyanotic patient. Small, single malformations can be indistinguishable from all other solitary pulmonary nodules. Larger lesions may have a more characteristic lobulated appearance, and the afferent and efferent vessels can often be demonstrated on plane tomography or CT scan. Pulmonary angiography confirms the diagnosis (Fig. 16-47). Both lungs should be examined carefully for multiple lesions.

Significant complications occur in at least 25 percent of all patients, and in a higher percentage of patients with hereditary telangiectasis and multiple fistulas. Complications can be local effects such as hemothorax, but consequences of polycythemia, such as cerebral thrombosis, are more common. Resection is indicated in all patients with solitary nodules, and in selected patients with multiple nodules when adequate lung tissue can be preserved. Cyanotic patients with widespread multiple small fistulas are inoperable, although improvement with embolization has been reported in a few cases.

Lobar Emphysema. Lobar emphysema presents with massive distention of a lobe or segment that shifts the mediastinum and compresses the contralateral lung. It is the most common of the

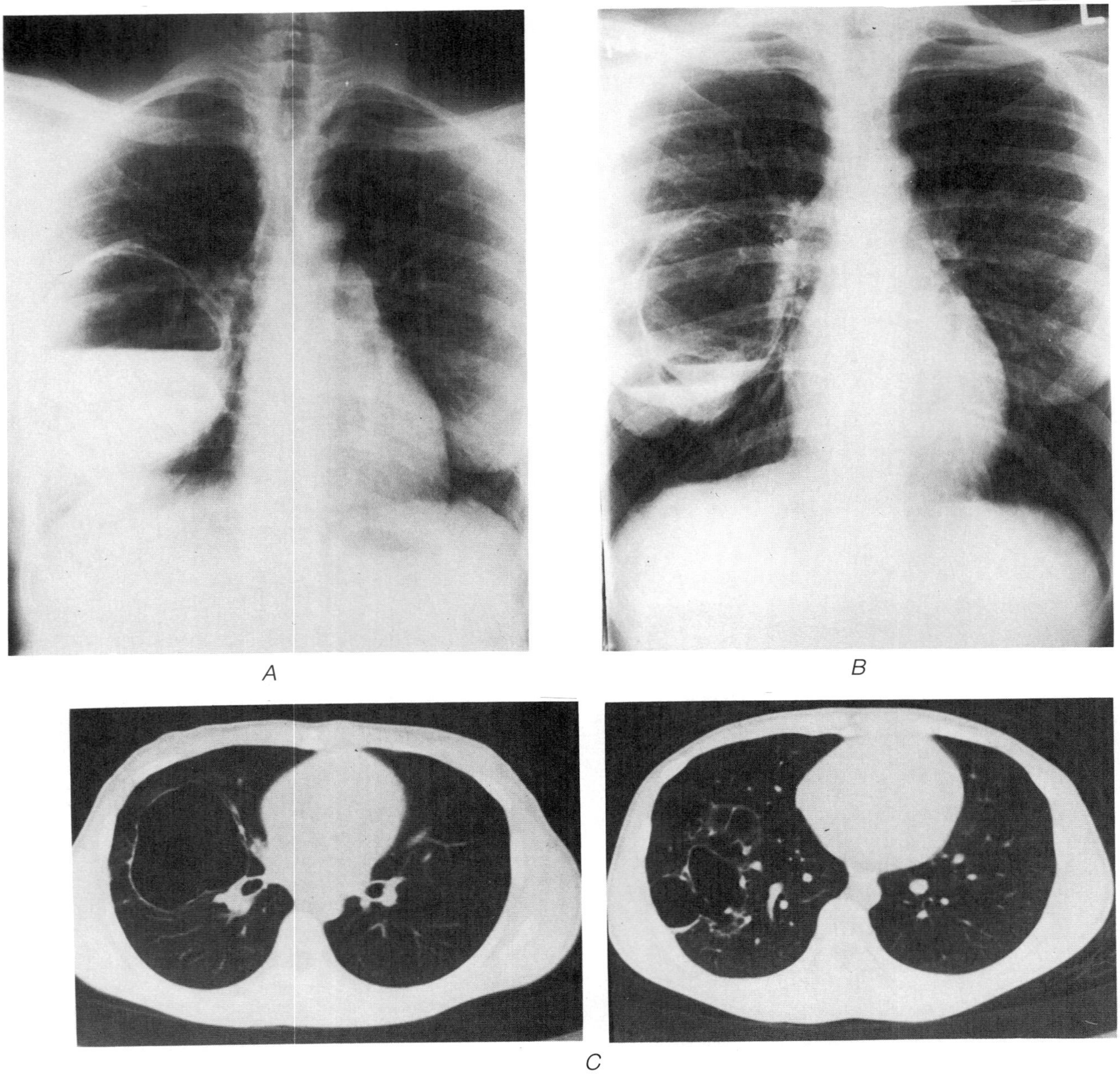

FIG. 16-45. *A.* This young woman had a long history of recurrent respiratory infections with foul, copious sputum production. *B.* The large cavity in the right lung would partially empty after each period of aggressive medical management, revealing a more complex array of cystic spaces with air-fluid levels. *C.* A similar appearance is evident on CT scan. After several years the patient was persuaded to undergo surgery. A preoperative arteriogram did not demonstrate anomalous vessels, suggesting sequestration. At operation, only the right upper lobe could be salvaged.

four structural lesions usually considered in the differential diagnosis of respiratory distress in the newborn. The other three are sequestration, cystic adenomatoid malformation, and bronchogenic cyst. Etiology has been a matter of continuing debate, and the clinical syndrome may represent the final common pathway of several distinct processes. Dysplasia of bronchial cartilage has been most frequently recognized, occurring in about 25 percent of cases. Acute bronchiolitis, extrinsic compression by lymph nodes or anomalous vessels, bronchial atresia, and several other possible causes of bronchial obstruction have been cited. No specific cause can be identified in more than 50 percent of cases. Associated malformations, mostly cardiovascular, are present in about 40 percent of patients, a fact that some authors interpret as support for a congenital etiology.

Respiratory distress typically appears from 4 days to 6 months postpartum. Half of all reported cases have occurred within the first 4 weeks of life. Physical findings of hyperresonance and decreased breath sounds mimic pneumothorax, which is a dangerous

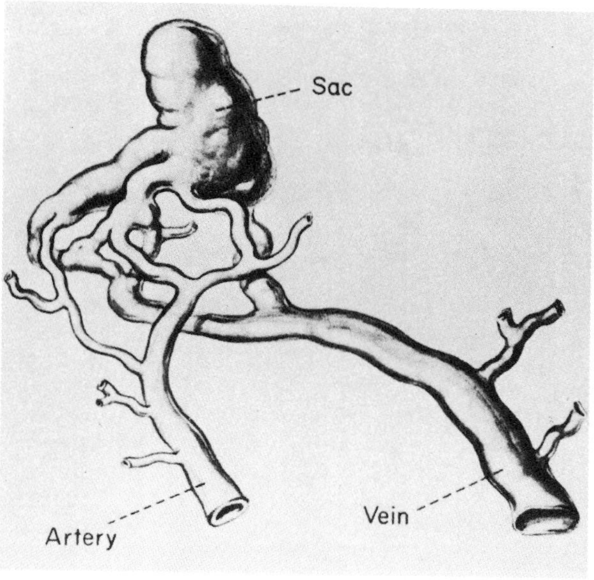

FIG. 16-46. Anatomy of a typical arteriovenous fistula in the lung. (From: *Ferguson TB, in Gibbon's Surgery of the Chest, 4th ed, Fig 22-42, p 694, with permission.*)

misapprehension if it leads to impulsive chest tube insertion. The chest x-ray can also mimic pneumothorax because the distended lung is very hyperlucent. Another common misinterpretation occurs when the compressed normal lung is thought to be atelectatic and the distended lung compensatory. An important radiographic clue is that the diaphragm is usually depressed on both sides with lobar emphysema but is normal or elevated on the side of primary atelectasis (Fig. 16-48).

In an infant with florid, progressive respiratory distress and a characteristic chest x-ray, emergency thoracotomy and lobectomy is indicated without further study. In such circumstances the mortality without operation approaches 50 percent. Involvement of an upper lobe or the right middle lobe is the most frequent finding. Lower lobe involvement is rare. Resection is ordinarily straightforward anatomically and completely curative. When the clinical presentation is less fulminant, the decision is more difficult. There is no question that varying degrees of lobar emphysema can be produced by aspiration of mucus or amniotic fluid, or by acute bronchiolitis. In such cases the emphysema almost always resolves in a few days with appropriate medical therapy.

Emphysematous Blebs and Bullae

Emphysema is characterized by enlarged air spaces produced by a complex process of elastic tissue destruction, alveolar wall breakdown, and coalescence of damaged alveoli, resulting in impaired alveolar ventilation and gas exchange. The disease represents one characteristic expression of advanced chronic obstructive pulmonary disease, overlapping considerably with the secretory, fibrotic bronchiolar obstructive pattern of chronic bronchitis, and with the reactive, atopic pattern of asthma. Pathogenetic differences promoting a predominant pattern of alveolar breakdown are difficult to isolate, and the response to a common mechanism of injury such as cigarette smoking is not predictable. An exception is the emphysematous pattern produced by the loss of normal restraints on tissue destruction seen in alpha$_1$-antitrypsin deficiency.

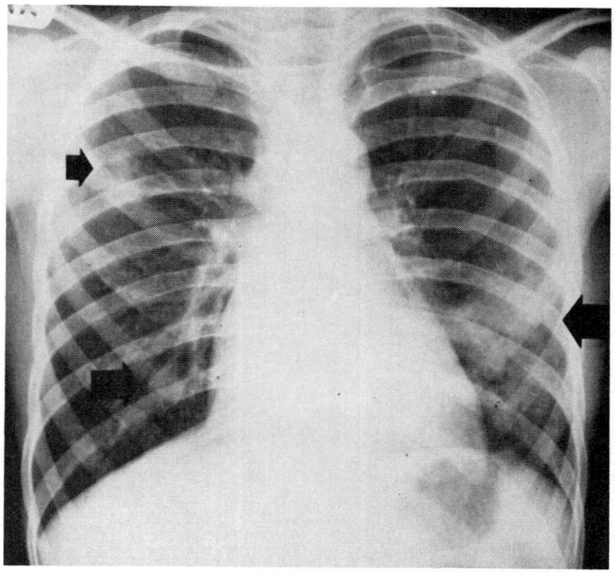

A

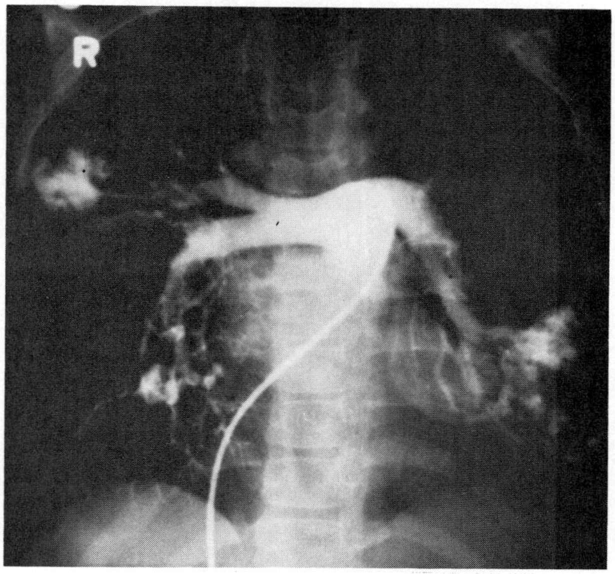

B

FIG. 16-47. *A.* Three lesions (*arrows*) thought to be compatible with pulmonary arteriovenous aneurysms are visible on the chest x-ray in this 8-year-old boy. *B.* A pulmonary arteriogram confirms the diagnosis. The lesions were subsequently removed through staged bilateral thoracotomies.

The surgeon has the luxury of ignoring the confusion of pathogenesis in this complex disorder to concentrate on the parts of the spectrum that have surgical significance. Emphysema is usually not truly diffuse, and involved areas may be quite localized into collections of small cysts (blebs) or very large ones (bullae). Blebs are usually subpleural, do not extend deeply into more central parenchyma, and consequently may have little effect on gas exchange or overall pulmonary function, even when multiple discrete collections of considerable size are present. Their chief significance relates to their potential for rupture with production of pneumothorax. The localized collection of blebs frequently en-

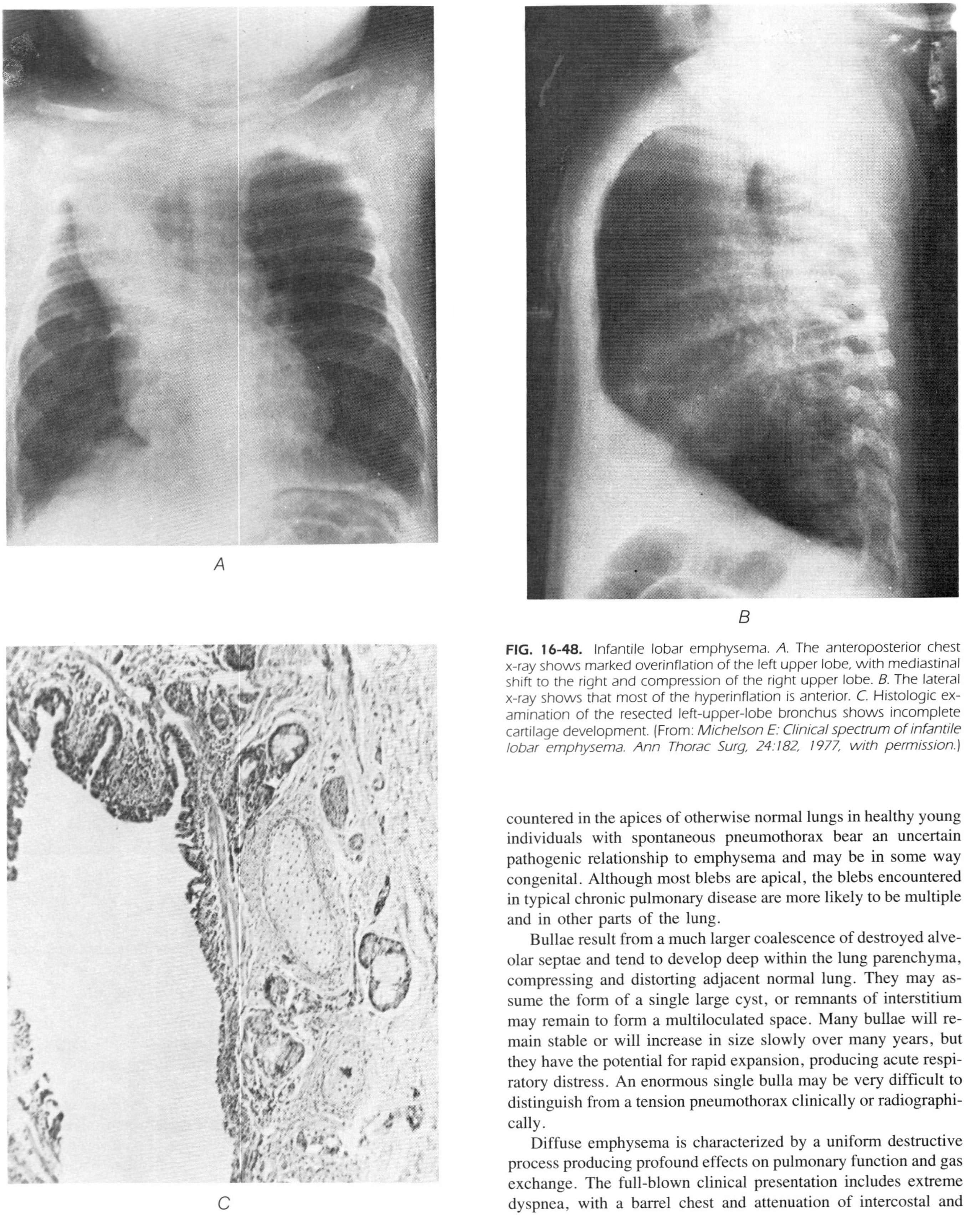

FIG. 16-48. Infantile lobar emphysema. *A.* The anteroposterior chest x-ray shows marked overinflation of the left upper lobe, with mediastinal shift to the right and compression of the right upper lobe. *B.* The lateral x-ray shows that most of the hyperinflation is anterior. *C.* Histologic examination of the resected left-upper-lobe bronchus shows incomplete cartilage development. (From: *Michelson E: Clinical spectrum of infantile lobar emphysema. Ann Thorac Surg, 24:182, 1977, with permission.*)

countered in the apices of otherwise normal lungs in healthy young individuals with spontaneous pneumothorax bear an uncertain pathogenic relationship to emphysema and may be in some way congenital. Although most blebs are apical, the blebs encountered in typical chronic pulmonary disease are more likely to be multiple and in other parts of the lung.

Bullae result from a much larger coalescence of destroyed alveolar septae and tend to develop deep within the lung parenchyma, compressing and distorting adjacent normal lung. They may assume the form of a single large cyst, or remnants of interstitium may remain to form a multiloculated space. Many bullae will remain stable or will increase in size slowly over many years, but they have the potential for rapid expansion, producing acute respiratory distress. An enormous single bulla may be very difficult to distinguish from a tension pneumothorax clinically or radiographically.

Diffuse emphysema is characterized by a uniform destructive process producing profound effects on pulmonary function and gas exchange. The full-blown clinical presentation includes extreme dyspnea, with a barrel chest and attenuation of intercostal and diaphragmatic musculature. Lungs with diffuse emphysema frequently contain areas of bleb or bullous disease as well.

Surgical Considerations. The surgeon confronts emphysema in two principal situations: in operations performed on patients with emphysema, and in operations performed for emphysema. In the former category, patients with emphysema undergoing procedures with general anesthesia have an increased operative risk due to their abnormal gas exchange and are at higher risk for barotrauma during mechanical ventilation. Postoperative pulmonary toilet can be a major challenge in a patient with greatly reduced expiratory forces whose ability to cough is further compromised by postoperative pain. Every surgeon has seen patients with marginally compensated emphysema become ventilator-dependent, with a tracheostomy and bilateral chest tubes, following routine abdominal surgery. Elective operation in such patients requires cautious assessment of risks and careful attention to preoperative pulmonary physiotherapy.

Thoracic operations designed to correct specific manifestations of emphysema carry similar risks but also offer the expectation of improvement. The history of operations for emphysema illustrates the danger of allowing surgical intuition to precede an understanding of pathophysiology. Some of the earliest procedures were designed to "make room" for the hyperinflated lung by further enlarging the barrel chest with sternotomy or chondrectomy. Upon observation that such procedures were ineffective at best, attempts were made to decrease lung volume by phrenic nerve destruction or thoracoplasty, with counterproductive results that would be considered predictable today.

Selection for operation is directed toward identifying patients in whom resection of localized bullous disease is likely to improve pulmonary function. Ventilation-perfusion scans and pulmonary angiography can help define areas of normal lung adjacent to large bullae that are compressed and nonventilated but normally perfused (Fig. 16-49). The most favorable patients are young (under 55 years of age), with unilateral disease and marked asymmetry of function, recently progressive symptoms, well-defined bullae, and evidence of crowded vessels in adjacent parenchyma. Large bullae displacing more than half the hemithorax are more likely to produce symptomatic improvement after resection than smaller bullae. Patients under age 60 with end-stage diffuse disease are candidates for lung transplantation when other therapeutic options have been exhausted.

In all patients every effort is made preoperatively to maximize pulmonary function and eliminate chronic bronchial infection. The disease is usually approached through a posterolateral thoracotomy, although some authors have favored median sternotomy for anterior and superior bullae, claiming that postoperative morbidity is reduced. The resection is carefully tailored to preserve all adjacent vascularized parenchyma. Mechanical stapling devices are extremely helpful. Planes of division through emphysematous lung are friable and prone to air leak. Elimination of any residual pleural space by careful placement of chest tubes and judicious use of pleural tents or thoracoplasty can be essential to success.

Pulmonary Infections

As recently as the early 1960s, thousands of patients each year in the United States required pulmonary resection for lung abscess, bronchiectasis, and chronic granulomatous disease. Since that time effective antibiotics, aggressive methods for accurate early diagnosis, an increased standard of living, and public health programs are among the factors that have diminished the surgeon's role dramatically. Fifteen or twenty years ago it seemed reasonable to hope that suppurative pulmonary infections would remain a common surgical problem only in areas of the world with limited medical technology and limited access to antibiotics. Ironically such problems are becoming increasingly frequent at the high-technology frontiers—patients immunosuppressed following transplant or as part of cancer chemotherapy, and patients with AIDS all too commonly develop serious pulmonary infections.

The pathologic spectrum of pulmonary infections is very broad, ranging from the indolent bronchiolar and peribronchial suppuration of bronchiectasis, to the contained parenchymal necrosis of lung abscess, to the pleural space infection of empyema. The clinical expression of pulmonary infection is determined by the route of inoculation, the competence of host defenses, and the specific organism(s) involved, which can include aerobic and anaerobic bacteria, viruses, and fungi, often in synergistic combinations. This broad spectrum of pathology has an equally broad spectrum of treatment in which surgical management remains important.

Lung Abscess

Spectrum of Disease. Lung abscess may be defined as a focus of infection with parenchymal necrosis, usually with cavitation. Distinction between a lung abscess and a consolidated pneumonia is made as areas of cavitation appear on the chest x-ray, and as the peripheral margins of the infection develop sharper definition. Lung abscess and empyema can coexist as confluent or separate processes. Causes of lung abscess are outlined in Table 16-10.

Lung abscess is most commonly a complication of necrotizing pneumonia. Aspiration of gastric contents or saliva produces an infectious focus with enzymatic tissue degradation, mixed aerobic and anaerobic bacterial contamination, and frequently particulate

Table 16-10
Causes of Lung Abscess

I. Primary necrotizing pneumonia
  A. Aerobic infection
    1. *Staphylococcus aureus*
    2. *Klebsiella, Pseudomonas,* other gram negatives
    3. *Mycobacteria (M. tuberculosis* and atypical *Myobacteria)*
  B. Anaerobic infection
    1. *Bacteroides (B. fragilis, B. melaninogenicus)*
    2. *Fusobacterium* species
    3. *Actinomyces*
  C. Parasitic infection
    1. *Entamoeba histolytica*
    2. *Echinococcus (E. granulosus, E. multilocularis)*
II. Aspiration pneumonia
III. Bronchial obstruction
  A. Neoplasm
  B. Foreign body
IV. Complication of systemic sepsis
  A. Septic pulmonary emboli
  B. Seeding of pulmonary infarct
V. Complication of pulmonary trauma
  A. Infection of hematoma or contusion
  B. Contaminated foreign body or penetrating injury
VI. Direct extension from extraparenchymal infection
  A. Pleural empyema
  B. Mediastinal, hepatic, subphrenic abscess

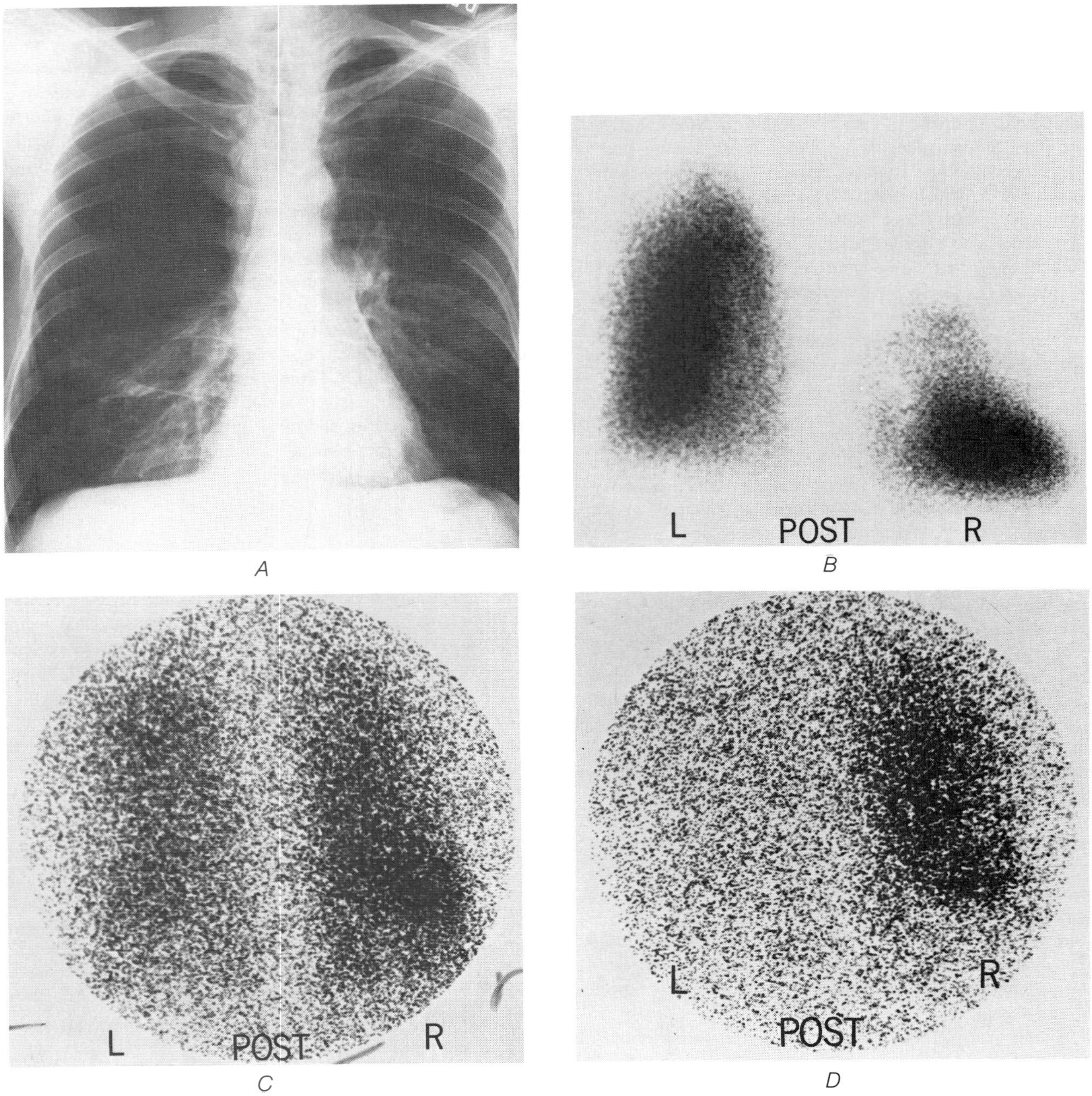

FIG. 16-49. A 49-year-old man with obstructive airway disease (FEV$_1$ = 50% of predicted) and dyspnea with minimal exertion. *A.* The chest x-ray shows marked radiolucency in the upper half of the right hemithorax, due to giant bullae compressing the remaining normal parenchyma into the lower part of the hemithorax. *B.* A lung perfusion scan with ^{99m}Tc macroaggregated albumin shows loss of perfusion in the right upper and middle lobe regions. *C.* The ventilation scan with ^{33}Xe shows early delay in washout of the radioisotope from the right lung after equilibration. *D.* After 3 min of the washout phase of the ventilation scan, there is marked trapping of the radioisotope in the giant bullae of the right lung. The patient underwent successful resection of the bullae with considerable subjective improvement in symptoms.

matter that combine to promote abscess formation. Aspiration remains the most common single cause of lung abscess, and has a well-recognized association with altered states of consciousness (Fig. 16-50). Alcoholic stupor is most frequently cited, but drug overdosage, head trauma, cardiopulmonary resuscitation, and general anesthesia can also set the stage for aspiration leading to lung abscess. Because most episodes of aspiration occur with the person supine, the abscess is characteristically located in the lung segments that are dependent in the supine position—the posterior segments of the upper lobes, and the superior segments of both

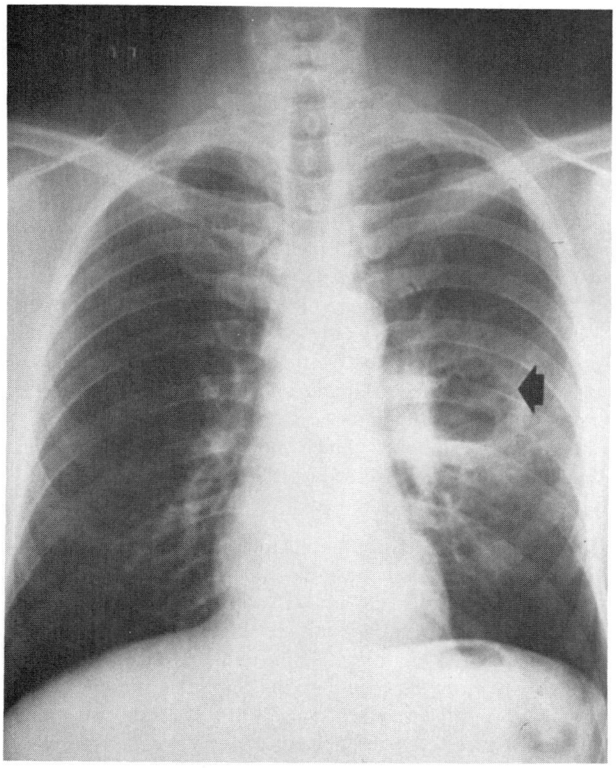

A

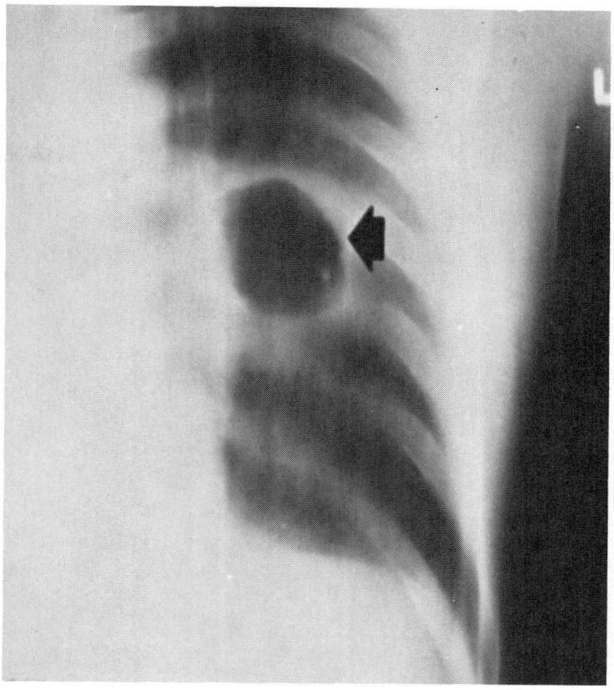

B

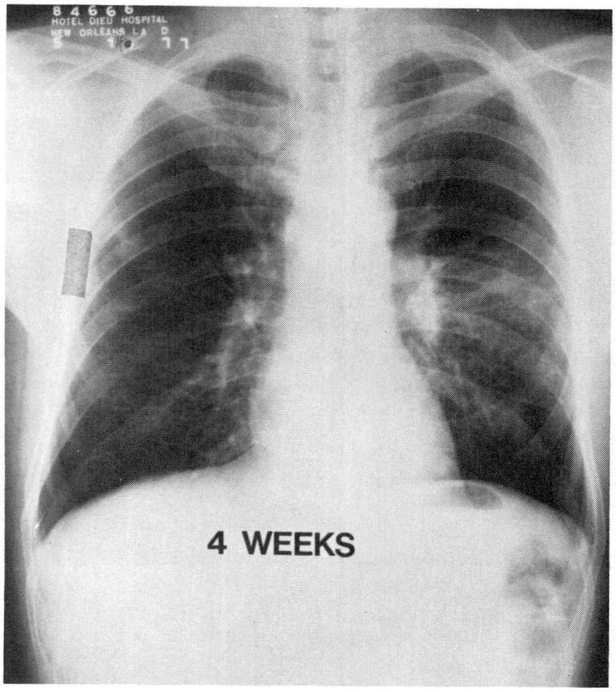

C

FIG. 16-50. Lung abscess due to vomiting and aspiration after an alcoholic binge. *A.* The chest x-ray shows an abscess cavity in the superior segment of the left upper lobe. *B.* A tomogram confirms the thin wall of the abscess, reducing the probability that the lesion could be a cavitated carcinoma. *C.* After 4 weeks of antibiotic therapy and postural drainage the abscess cavity appears to be healing.

lower lobes. Bacteriologically the infection is usually mixed, with anaerobic mouth organisms such as *Bacteroides* species frequently predominating.

The tissue necrosis that is the hallmark of "necrotizing" pneumonia is a function of the specific organism involved and is most prominent with *Klebsiella, Pseudomonas,* and other gram-negative organisms. Tissue necrosis is rare with Group B streptococcal pneumonia (*Pneumococcus*), whereas necrosis and abscess formation are frequent with *Staphylococcus aureus* and Group A streptococci. Staphylococcal lung abscess is most common in the first year of life and has characteristic pathology, most frequently with pyopneumothorax and pneumatoceles. The latter are large cystic spaces, typically not containing true pus, that are thought to result from air trapping distal to bronchiolar obstruction. Staphylococcal lung abscess in infancy is also characterized clinically by a remarkable tendency to resolve completely with antibiotics alone, even when temporary drainage of the pleural space has been required.

Establishment of a gram-negative pneumonia begins with major alteration in the bacteriologic composition of upper respiratory flora. The mechanisms that reduce gram negatives to transient visitors in normal individuals are seriously impaired in many hospitalized patients. For example, experiments in mice suggest that an *Escherichia coli* peritonitis interferes with recruitment of polymorphonuclear leukocytes in the lung, increasing susceptibility to gram-negative (*Pseudomonas*) but not to gram-positive infections. Over half the pneumonias seen in seriously ill hospitalized patients are gram-negative, and a significant proportion of such patients manifest a necrotizing infection leading to lung-abscess formation.

Systemic sepsis can produce multiple bilateral foci of parenchymal infection that are radiographically quite discrete and are most frequently caused by *Staphylococcus* and other gram-positive

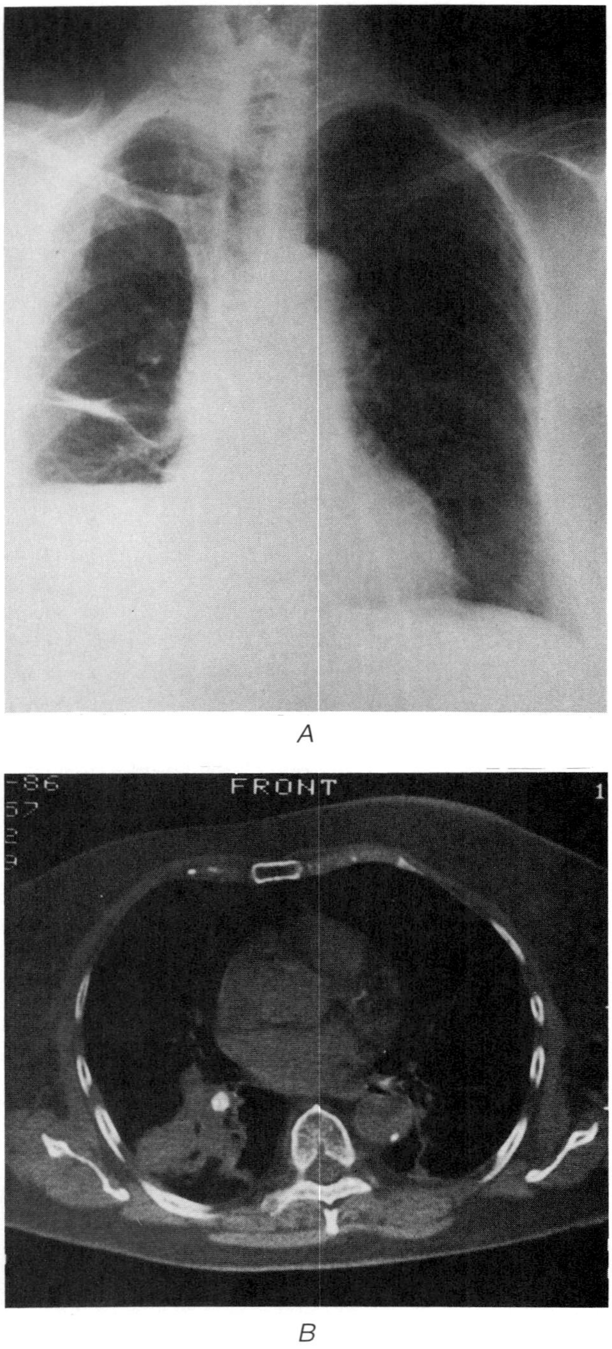

FIG. 16-51. *A.* This 72-year-old woman presented with a clinical picture of slowly progressing pneumonia, and chest x-ray revealed right lower lobe consolidation with a pleural effusion. *B.* CT scan demonstrated a large area of consolidation and early abscess formation in the right lower lobe, and a small bone-density mass lying medially within. An obstructing chicken bone was identified by bronchoscopy but could not be removed. A successful right lower lobectomy was performed.

organisms. One or more of the foci can become an abscess, although most resolve without a trace. Unlike staphylococcal pneumonia of tracheobronchial origin, hematogenous infection does not tend to form pneumatoceles and can be seen in septic patients of any age. Lung abscess developing in a pulmonary infarction following pulmonary embolus is most frequently a special case of hematogenous infection seeding an area of devitalized or injured tissue.

A cavitary necrotizing infection can also form distal to an obstructive lung carcinoma or intrabronchial foreign body (Fig. 16-51), a reminder that bronchoscopy is an important diagnostic manuever. Not infrequently a carcinoma becomes visible as the distal infection responds to antibiotic treatment.

In certain parts of the world parasitic infection is a common cause of lung abscess. *Entamoeba histolytica* can produce lung abscess by hematogenous spread or by direct extension from the liver, in which case it is almost always associated with empyema. Metronidazole is usually effective treatment, and operative intervention is rarely required. Hydatid infection (*Echinococcus* species) is associated with lung abscess in some cases (Fig. 16-52). Intraabdominal pathology is much more prominent. Treatment with oral mebendazole or albendazole has been moderately successful, but resection has frequently been required.

Clinical Manifestations. Regardless of etiology, the clinical presentation is relatively uniform. The patient appears chronically ill, is likely to be febrile, and will often describe recent onset of copious foul sputum production, reflecting decompression of the abscess into the airway. Whether the initial infection originated from the airway or the bloodstream, the necrotizing process tends to find its way into the tracheobronchial tree, a development heralded radiographically by the appearance of cavitation on chest x-ray. Because of the necrotizing, erosive nature of the communication with the airways, hemoptysis can occur and can be massive. In contrast to pneumonia, dyspnea is not a prominent symptom. Auscultatory findings, if any, are more likely to be attributable to coexistence of a pleural effusion or empyema than to the presence of lung abscess. In the acute phase of abscess development, constitutional symptoms will overlap with those of acute pneumonia. As the process becomes more chronic, symptoms frequently ameliorate as the abscess becomes walled off.

In a febrile patient with copious production of foul sputum, the differential diagnosis can be reduced to three entities: lung abscess, bronchiectasis, and cavitating carcinoma. Chronic copious sputum production is most characteristic of bronchiectasis; the other two entities tend to have acute or episodic sputum production. A dramatic febrile illness is most consistent with lung abscess, reflecting its origins in a necrotizing pneumonia, although bronchiectasis and carcinoma can have febrile episodes associated with exacerbations of the inflammatory process surrounding the primary pathology. A chest x-ray showing a well-delineated cavity is against bronchiectasis alone, but the chest x-ray is usually of little help in distinguishing carcinoma from lung abscess, for which bronchoscopy and biopsy are essential. Bronchiectasis is confirmed by bronchography.

Treatment. The options for treatment of lung abscess are outlined in Table 16-11. Primary treatment consists of antibiotics and drainage. Antibiotics are administered intravenously in high doses based on the sensitivities of the infecting organism. In the most fortunate cases, spontaneous drainage by expectoration is adequate. More commonly, drainage must be achieved by other means, the least invasive of which is bronchoscopic aspiration. Proponents of nonoperative treatment favor at least 8 weeks of antibiotics and "internal" (cough and bronchoscopy) drainage before proceeding to external drainage or resection. Such methods are successful in more than 75 percent of all patients with lung

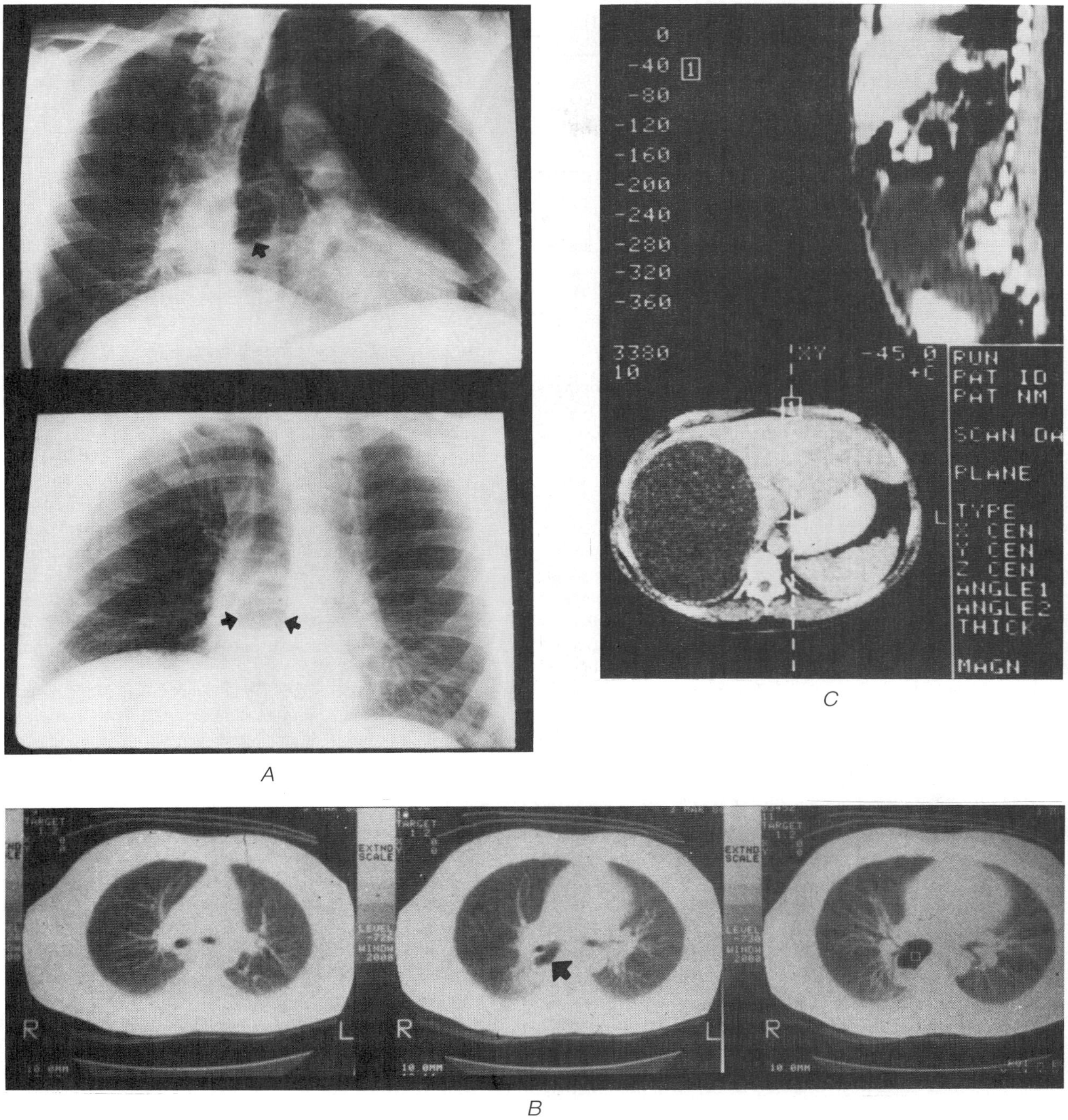

FIG. 16-52. *A.* This 48-year-old Yugoslavian immigrant was completely asymptomatic until he presented with a transient episode of copious, foul productive cough. A mediastinal cavity is visible in the oblique views shown (*see arrows*). *B.* A CT scan of the chest shows the cavity lying just below the right main-stem bronchus and that the mediastinal cavity does not communicate with the abdomen. *C.* A CT scan of the abdomen shows further evidence of widespread infection with *Echinococcus granulosus.* The sagittal view shows a large pelvic mass, and the transverse section shows a huge mass in the right lobe of the liver, containing several daughter cysts.

abscess (see Fig. 16-50), although convalescence can be prolonged. In one representative nonoperative series the average duration of therapy was 4 months. Numerous surgical series have demonstrated that convalescence can be shortened dramatically in properly selected patients.

When antibiotics and internal drainage are ineffective, there are three options for operative treatment: (1) tube pneumonostomy, (2) pneumonotomy, and (3) pulmonary resection. Tube pneumonostomy and pneumonotomy depend on the development of a secure pleural symphysis between the parietal pleura and the visceral

Table 16-11
Options for Treatment of Lung Abscess

1. Antibiotics and internal drainage (cough, bronchoscopy)
2. External drainage
   a. Pneumonostomy
   b. Pneumonotomy
3. Pulmonary resection

pleural surface closest to the abscess cavity. Both techniques establish external drainage through the area of symphysis to avoid spilling a contained infection into the free pleural space. Therefore, it is critical to localize the abscess in relationship to the chest wall. CT or MRI scans should be obtained if possible. Markers can be placed on the skin overlying the site for drainage.

Tube pneumonostomy is usually adequate and is enjoying a resurgence of popularity, as recent reports indicate (Fig. 16-53). The technique involves insertion of a percutaneous drainage tube that is usually connected to a water seal with or without suction. Tube drainage is theoretically limited by the viscosity and particulate content of the pus and by the presence of a foreign body. As reports from vanSonnenberg and associates and Yang and associates illustrate, CT and ultrasound guidance can be used to localize the abscess and accomplish effective tube drainage in a single stage. With any form of external drainage the possibility of erosive injury to large-caliber bronchioles and vascular structures that lay close to the soft inner surface of the abscess cavity imposes a risk of bronchopleurocutaneous fistula or hemorrhage. Fortunately, most abscesses are more peripheral than central, which reduces this risk somewhat, and peripheral location helps promote the kind of aggressive pleural symphysis that favors external drainage when necessary.

Pneumonotomy avoids the risk associated with an indwelling foreign body and is favored for the most organized cavities containing large volumes of especially viscid pus mixed with large amounts of necrotic debris. Drainage is achieved through a generous incision with rib resection. If inspection of the parietal pleura suggests that adequate symphysis has not taken place, the wound is packed open without opening the pleura. After several days, this usually results in an exuberant pleural reaction and symphysis allowing safe access to the abscess cavity.

The most definitive operative treatment for lung abscess is pulmonary resection. Standard indications for resection are chronicity with symptoms, serious hemorrhage, and suspicion of associated carcinoma. Lobectomy is ordinarily preferred to simplify dissection and preserve protective tissue planes. Resection has the advantage of removing the entire infection promptly and is less hazardous than external drainage when the abscess is very large or centrally located. On the other hand, resection does not eliminate the risk of pleural space contamination. It can be technically difficult to remove a thin-walled abscess presenting close to the visceral pleura without spillage, and empyema following lobectomy is far more serious than primary empyema. Anesthetic technique and patient positioning are critical to prevent spillage of pus through the tracheobronchial tree across to the dependent lung. In the past, the patient was often positioned prone or supine. Currently use of a double-lumen endotracheal tube, which can effectively isolate the two sides, generally allows use of the lateral decubitus position. Safety can be further augmented by frequent intraoperative bronchoscopy performed from the head of the table through the endotracheal tube, providing accurate irrigation and aspiration of the airways.

Life-threatening hemorrhage requires prompt resection once the bleeding site is unequivocally localized by bronchoscopy. Unfortunately, this complication most frequently arises in patients least able to tolerate thoracotomy, who are often bleeding because of coagulopathy secondary to sepsis and multiple organ failure. Acceptable temporizing measures designed primarily to protect the uninvolved lung include insertion of a double-lumen endotracheal tube, placement of a bronchial blocker on the affected side, and aggressive toilet of the unaffected side with rigid or flexible bronchoscopy. Bronchial artery embolization is worth consideration but is limited by the rich collateral circulation of the lung.

The Immunocompromised Host

Cancer chemotherapy and organ transplantation are creating a steadily increasing population of immunologically compromised individuals who would not have been alive 20 years ago. Patients nursed through major trauma or complications of surgery exhibit a characteristic spectrum of immunologic compromise. In only a decade, AIDS has become epidemic. All categories of immunocompromised patients share a predilection for pulmonary infections caused by familiar agents and by pathogens rarely seen in healthy individuals. Perhaps reflecting the fact that the lung is the only organ capable of presenting pathogens to a delicate nonsquamous epithelium many times each minute, pulmonary infections are the most common infections seen in immunocompromised patients.

Currently AIDS is the most relevant model of pulmonary infection in the immunocompromised host. AIDS was first described in 1981 in a group of homosexual men with *Pneumocystis carinii* pneumonia and mucosal candidiasis. The causative agent, a retrovirus named the human immunodeficiency virus (HIV), was identified in 1983. Seventeen thousand cases had been reported in the United States by 1986, a figure that has ballooned to nearly 300,000, with deaths approaching 200,000. Although improved medical treatment has lengthened the average survival time after diagnosis to longer than 1 year, mortality remains virtually 100 percent. The disease has clearly escaped the confines of the originally recognized risk groups (homosexual males and intravenous drug abusers) to become a venereal scourge threatening the general population.

Numerous examples of transmission through blood transfusion during the 1980s accelerated development of techniques for blood conservation, although blood donors screened using currently available serological testing for presence of HIV infection pose a very small risk (about 1 in 100,000 per unit of blood).

Opportunistic infection and Kaposi's sarcoma are hallmarks of active disease. *Pneumocystis carinii,* the most common pathogen, is present in 50 to 60 percent of all patients. *Pneumocystis carinii* is a protozoan originally thought to be a trypanosome, and not recognized in human beings until 1938. Characteristic interstitial pneumonitis thought to be caused by *Pneumocystis* was recognized in epidemics among undernourished infants and among the very elderly. In the United States *Pneumocystis* emerged as an infection confined to iatrogenically immunosuppressed patients on chemotherapy, until its dominant role as a pulmonary pathogen in AIDS was recognized in 1981. The characteristic clinical presentation consists of diffuse interstitial infiltrates on chest x-ray, dyspnea, and an increased A-aO2 gradient.

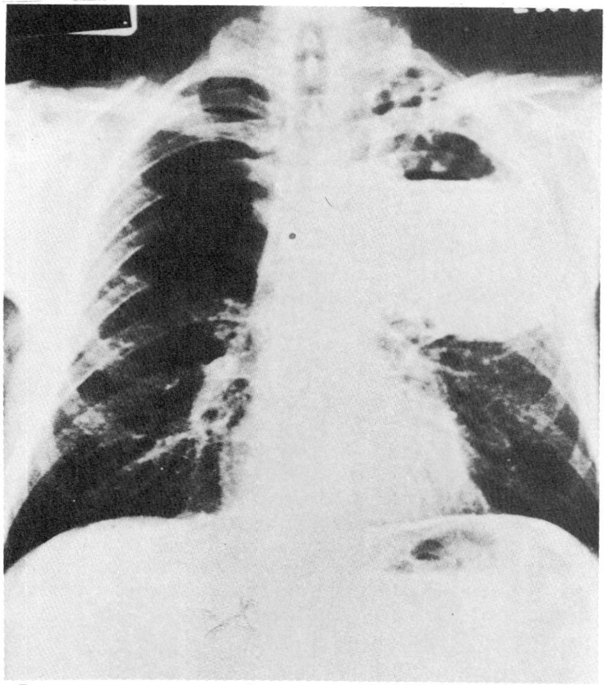

A

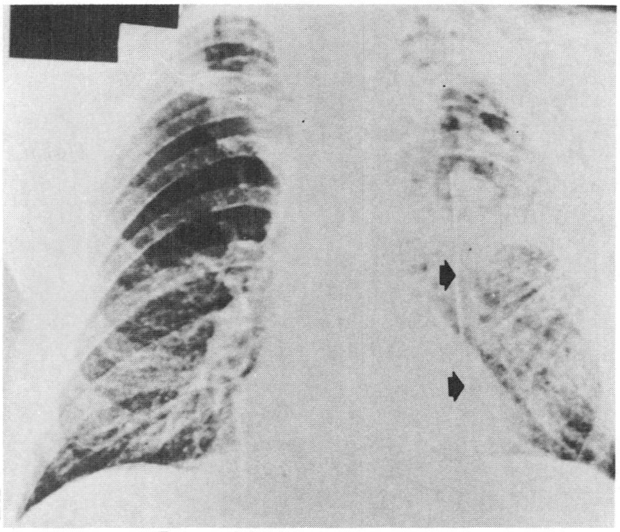

B

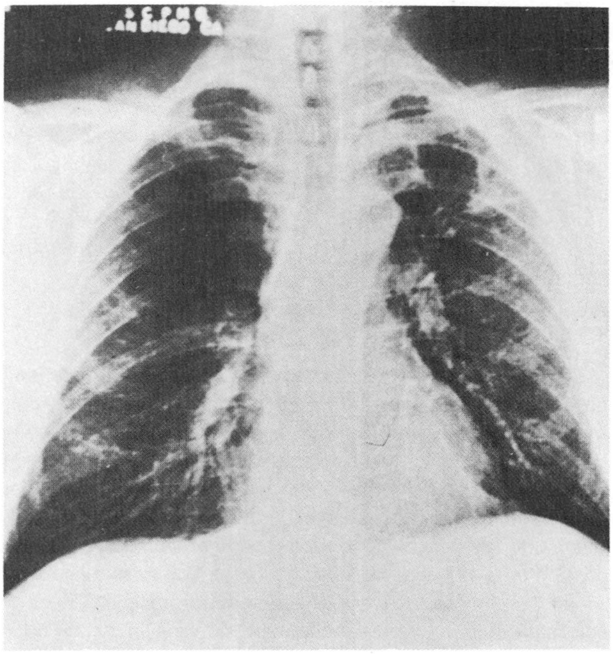

C

FIG. 16-53. *A.* Chest x-ray shows a large abscess cavity in the left upper lobe. The abscess appeared very anterior and adherent to the parietal pleura in lateral views (not shown), making it ideal for percutaneous drainage. *B.* At the bedside, a chest tube (*see arrows*) was inserted in the abscess cavity, and drained 900 mL of thick pus in the first 48 h. After 1 week the tube was amputated, leaving a short segment in the cavity as a straight drain. The patient was discharged on oral antibiotics, and the tube was removed 4 weeks later. *C.* A chest x-ray done 3 months after discharge showed mild residual scarring and a vague outline of the cavity in the left upper lobe. (From: *Mengoli L: J Thorac Cardiovasc Surg 90:189, 1985, Figs 8, 9, 10, with permission.*)

Trimethoprim-Sulfasoxisole (TMP-SFX) is effective treatment in most cases. Pentamidine is equally effective but is usually reserved for resistant cases or patients allergic to TMP-SFX. Medical treatment, and medical prophylaxis with TMP-SFX or aerosolized pentamidine, is quite effective in transplant recipients, in part because the level of immune suppression can be modulated. Medical treatment is considerably less successful in AIDS patients, with mortality approaching 50 percent.

Role of Operations. The surgeon's role in the treatment of immunocompromised patients with pulmonary infection can be both diagnostic and therapeutic. Transbronchial biopsy combined with bronchoalveolar lavage can establish a specific infectious diagnosis, which has markedly reduced the need for open lung biopsy. In a report by Bonfils-Roberts and associates the need for open biopsy in AIDS patients dropped from 28 percent during 1983 to 0.7 percent in 1987, and a successful change in therapy based on the results of open biopsy was possible in only 1 of 66 patients biopsied (1.5 percent). Open lung biopsy and thoracoscopic biopsy should be reserved for confusing mixed infections with inadequate response to empirical treatment.

In patients with AIDS, the most frequent therapeutic procedure is insertion of a chest tube for control of an air leak from infected lung. Frequently several tubes are required (Fig. 16-54), and on occasion thoracotomy or thoracoscopy for direct control of the leak and pleural abrasion or pleurectomy will be justified (Fig. 16-55). Gerein and associates illustrate that satisfactory palliation can be achieved with operation, but the overall prognosis remains very poor and is dictated by the activity of the underlying lung disease rather than by the surgical treatment.

Operative therapy in immunocompromised patients without AIDS can be applied with greater optimism. The spectrum of infections includes *Pneumocystis* and the other organisms seen in AIDS but also includes a greater number of infections with more common pyogenic bacteria and *Aspergillus*. The role of open biopsy is controversial, with opinion dividing between those favoring initial reliance on empiric therapy and those whose open biopsy results alter therapy in up to 65 percent of cases. Empyemas

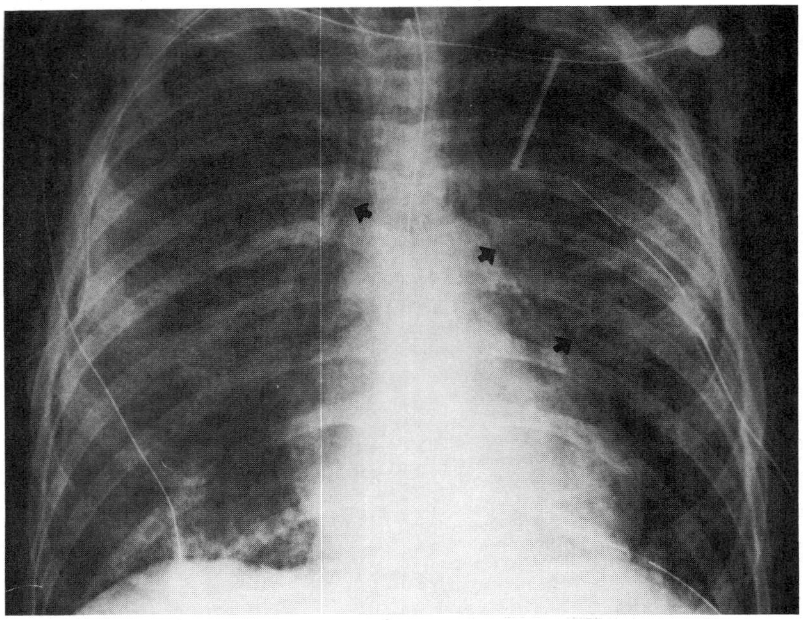

FIG. 16-54. This 31-year-old male homosexual with AIDS developed *Pneumocystis* pneumonia. The typical bilateral hazy, diffuse infiltrates are clearly evident. In spite of having one chest tube on the right side and two on the left side, the patient has large amounts of subcutaneous and mediastinal air (see arrows), as well as a persistent pneumothorax at the left apex. The patient expired with *Pseudomonas* and *Staphylococcus aureus* superinfection and a total of six chest tubes in place.

and intraparenchymal infections should be approached aggressively using indications for operation that are the same as those applied to normal hosts with similar infections. Although mortality and morbidity has generally been higher in immunosuppressed patients, it has been possible to perform major pulmonary resection, thoracoplasty, and decortication with excellent long-term results (Fig. 16-56).

Bronchiectasis

Bronchiectasis is characterized by bronchial dilatation, a chronic course, and variable involvement of surrounding parenchyma. Second- to fourth-order segmental bronchi in the basal segments of the lower lobes, the right middle lobe, and the lingula are most frequently involved. Isolated upper-lobe involvement is very rare and is usually associated with tuberculosis or bronchial obstruction. Approximately one-third of bronchiectasis is unilobar, one-third is unilateral bilobar, and one-third is bilateral. Although the bronchial mucosa usually remains intact and lined with pseudostratified columnar epithelium, the bronchi are filled with mucus, pus, and an occasional broncholith. The changes vary in degree from mild tubular dilation to cystic or saccular changes with almost unrecognizable gross architecture (Fig. 16-57). Collateral air circulation is only partially effective in maintaining expansion of alveoli distal to chronically obstructed segments, and a resected lobe will usually be shrunken and fibrotic. Hypertrophy of bronchial arteries occurs as part of the inflammatory process, producing a locally extensive precapillary left to right shunt into the pulmonary venous system, and laying the substrate for erosive hemorrhage and hemoptysis.

In most cases the disease has to be considered idiopathic. It is occasionally associated with chronic bronchial obstruction by tumor, foreign body, or bronchostenosis. Immune deficiency states have been implicated in certain instances. Kartagener's syndrome (situs inversus, pansinusitis, bronchiectasis) is a rare congenital disorder possibly related to a defect in ciliary function. In many patients afflicted during childhood a history of recurrent bronchitis and bronchopneumonia, presumed to be viral, is present. Bronchiectasis is the most common cause of death in cystic fibrosis.

Clinical Manifestations. The clinical picture is dominated by cough and production of mucopurulent sputum, varying in volume from scant to as much as 500 to 1000 mL/day. Fever is usually low-grade with acute exacerbations. The systemic effects of chronic infectious illness can dominate the picture to produce a broad spectrum of constitutional symptoms, weight loss, and retarded development. The disease can occur at any age and is seen equally in both sexes. In the United States an unusually high incidence has been identified in Alaskan Native children, many of whom have required aggressive surgical treatment (Fig. 16-58). Dyspnea is not common except in diffuse disease or in late disease with cor pulmonale. Hemoptysis occurs in about 50 percent of patients, usually late in the disease, and is only major in about 10 percent. Serious hemoptysis is more frequent in association with lung abscess than with bronchiectasis.

Physical findings are dominated by stigmata of chronic disease and can include digital clubbing and pulmonary osteoarthropathy, even though cyanosis is rare. Auscultatory findings are primarily related to presence or absence of associated pneumonitis and to the effectiveness of pulmonary toilet. A history of chronic profuse sputum production will strongly suggest the diagnosis, and in children associations such as cystic fibrosis, immune deficiency, and $alpha_1$ antitrypsin deficiency should be ruled out. Chest x-rays tend to be nonspecific but may show linear streaking and volume loss in the affected areas. Bronchiectasis is one possible explanation for the ''middle-lobe syndrome,'' which is isolated middle-lobe atelectasis (Fig. 16-59). Bronchoscopy should be done to exclude the rare case of correctable bronchial obstruction or carcinoma, to obtain accurate cultures, and to aspirate the tracheobronchial tree. Careful bronchoscopic pulmonary toilet can achieve surprisingly durable symptomatic benefit. Complete bronchography remains the definitive test and is essential to define the anatomy if resection is contemplated. CT scanning has been exten-

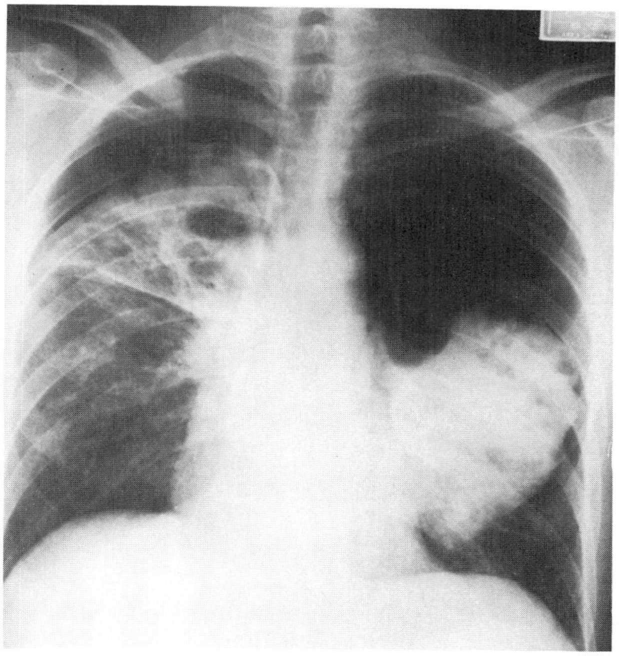

A

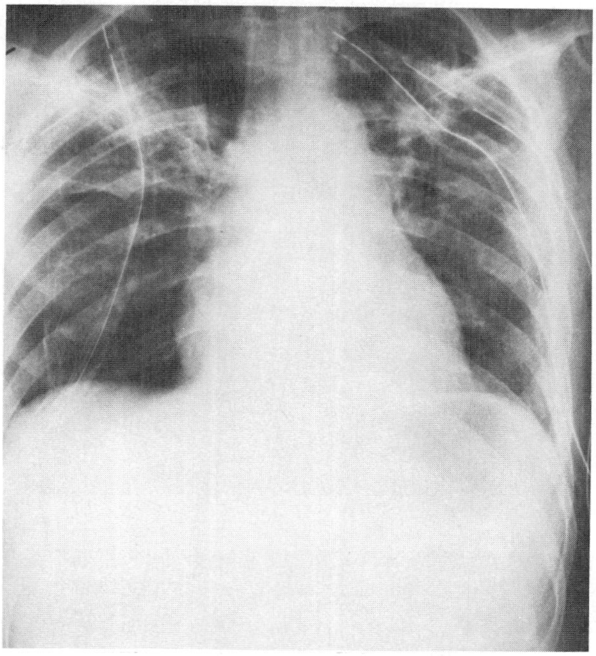

B

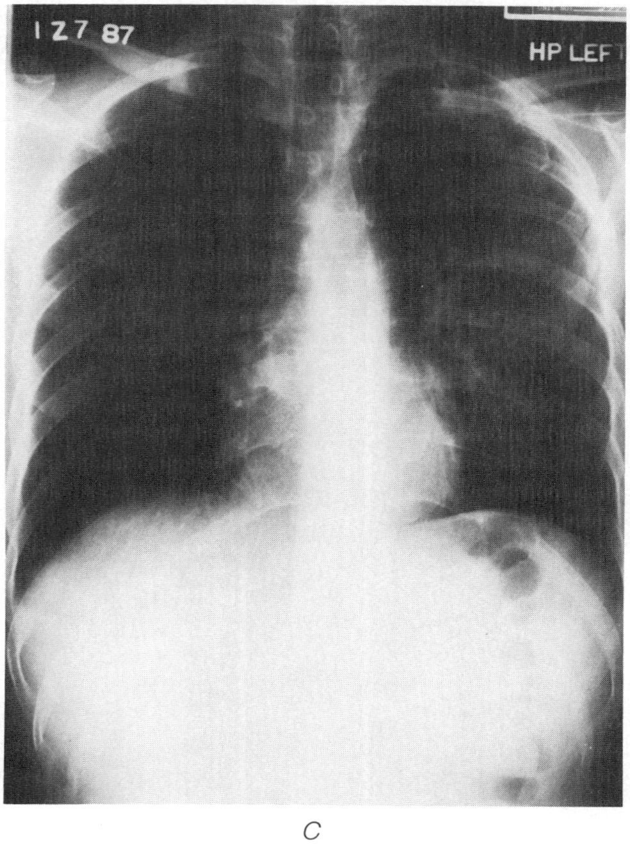

C

FIG. 16-55. *A.* This 24-year-old male intravenous drug abuser with AIDS developed *Pneumocystis* pneumonia and bilateral pneumothoraces. *B.* With two chest tubes on each side, the right side eventually resolved. A large air leak persisted on the left. Because the infection was resolving remarkably well on medical treatment, operation was elected. Through a left thoracotomy a large collection of leaking apical blebs were stapled, and pleural abrasion was performed. *C.* This chest x-ray obtained after discharge from the hospital shows an unusually successful early result in the treatment of AIDS.

sively evaluated as an alternative to bronchography. A report by Munro and associates compared thin-section (3 mm) scanning to bronchography and found equivalent accuracy for the two techniques. Nonetheless, thin-section CT can entail a large radiation dose and does not provide the kind of "road map" most useful in planning resection. Even bilateral bronchography is usually well tolerated but can produce a febrile response due to chemical and bacterial pneumonitis. It should not be done within about 3 months of an acute episode of pneumonia to reduce this risk, and to avoid overinterpretation of changes that may be reversible.

Treatment. The majority of patients with bronchiectasis do not require operative treatment. Postural drainage and chest physical therapy (see Fig. 16-60) minimize retention of purulent sputum, and antibiotic treatment of all episodes of pneumonitis should be pursued indefinitely. When debilitating effects of chronic infection become prominent, the anatomy should be carefully defined with bronchography, and resection planned. When extensive saccular disease is confined to one lobe or segment in a sufficiently symptomatic patient, resection is a clear choice. In children, interference with growth should suggest resection. Frequent hemoptysis associated with localized disease deserves operation. Patients with diffuse bilateral disease, of which cystic fibrosis is the best example, should be considered for lung transplantation as they approach end-stage disease.

All patients should receive a maximal preoperative effort to reduce sputum volume and infection. Care must be taken during anesthesia to prevent spillage of infected secretions into uninvolved segments. A double-lumen endotracheal tube can be used to protect the contralateral lung, and intraoperative flexible fiberoptic bronchoscopy can be used to aspirate uninvolved segments in

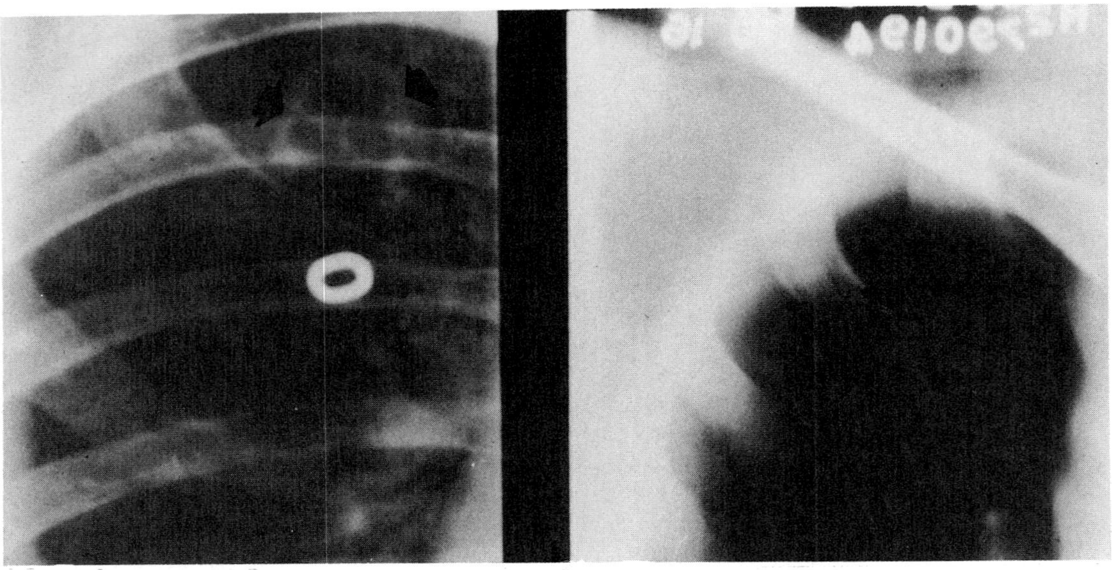

A

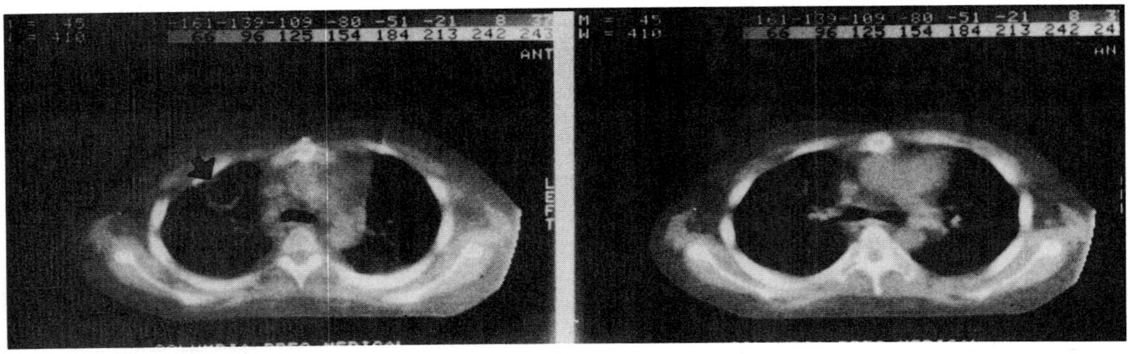

B

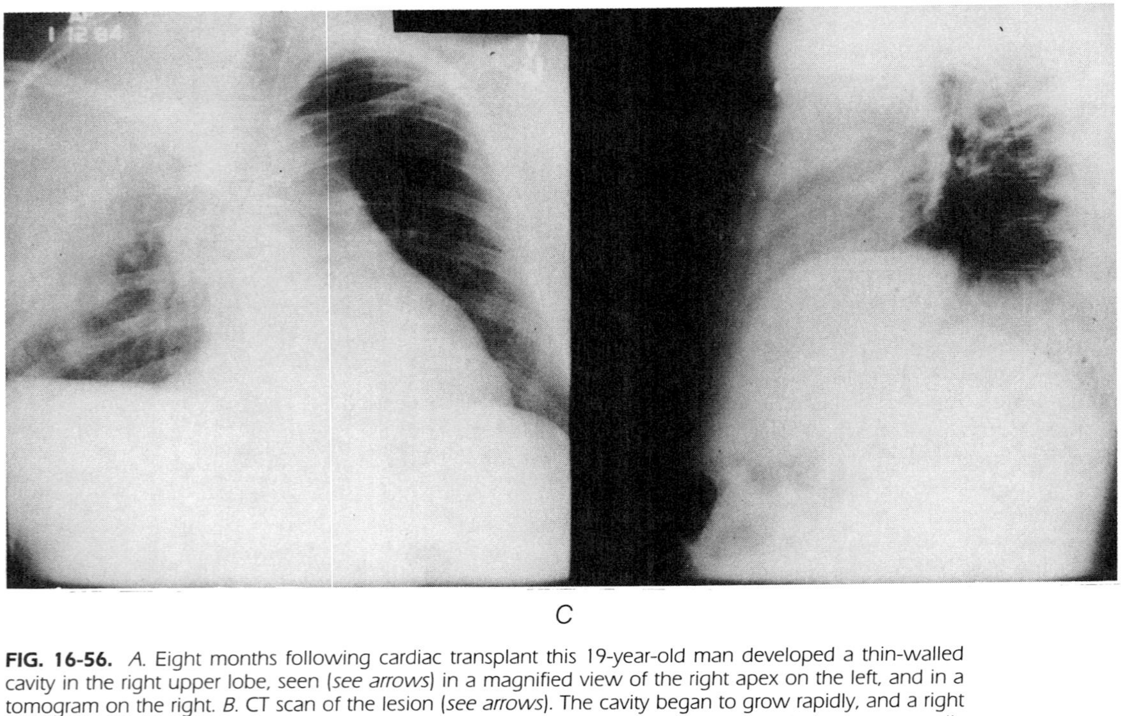

C

FIG. 16-56. *A.* Eight months following cardiac transplant this 19-year-old man developed a thin-walled cavity in the right upper lobe, seen (*see arrows*) in a magnified view of the right apex on the left, and in a tomogram on the right. *B.* CT scan of the lesion (*see arrows*). The cavity began to grow rapidly, and a right upper lobectomy was performed. The lesion proved to be an aspergilloma. *C.* A thoracoplasty was eventually required for control of a persistent air leak and pneumothorax. A late postoperative chest x-ray is shown. The infection never recurred and the patient was able to resume near-normal activity.

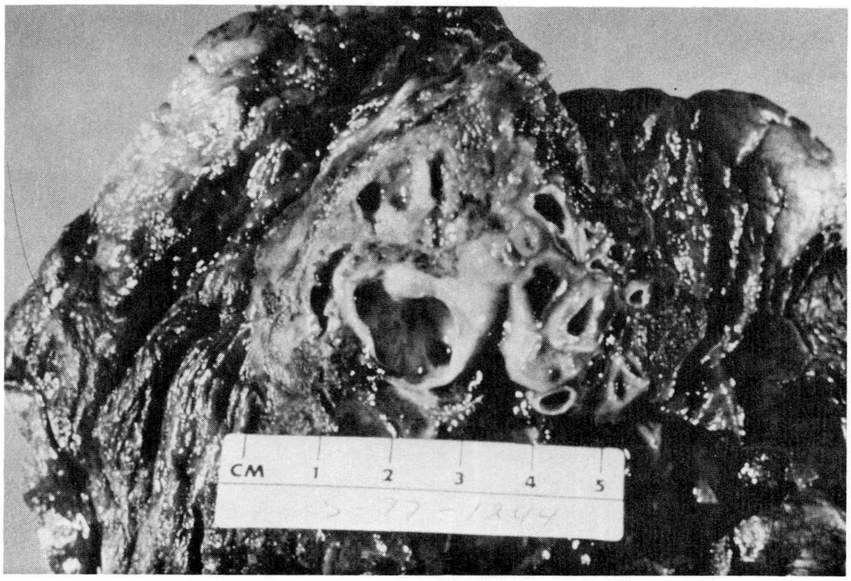

FIG. 16-57. The cut section of this right lower lobe shows one of several cystic bronchiectatic cavities with surrounding localized pneumonia.

the ipsilateral lung. As with operation for lung abscess, the risk of postoperative empyema is higher than for clean surgery, and considerable effort must be expended in postoperative pulmonary toilet to assure that residual infected secretions are not allowed to pool in the bronchial stump. The operative strategy is to remove as little normal lung as possible without entering the central focus of infection. This usually requires segmentectomy or lobectomy. Disease so localized as to be treatable with wedge resection probably should not come to operation. Pneumonectomy is almost never indicated for bronchiectasis.

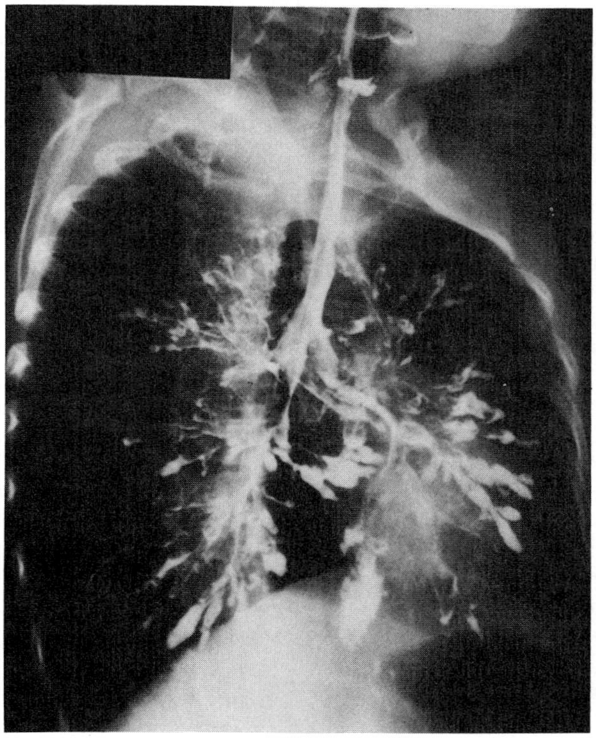

FIG. 16-58. Bronchogram obtained in an eight-year-old Alaskan native, demonstrating widespread saccular and cystic bronchiectasis. This otherwise normal child had a history of repeated respiratory infections, presumed to be viral, during infancy and early childhood. *(Courtesy of JP Wilson.)*

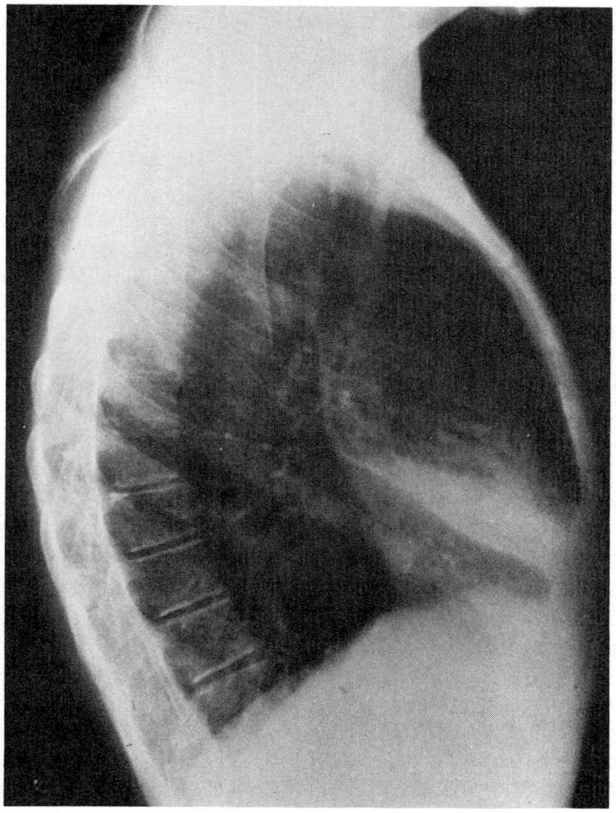

FIG. 16-59. This lateral chest x-ray shows a wedge-shaped density overlying the cardiac shadow and corresponding to a collapsed middle lobe. Resection of the fibrotic lobe showed marked bronchiectasis of the segmental bronchi (middle-lobe syndrome).

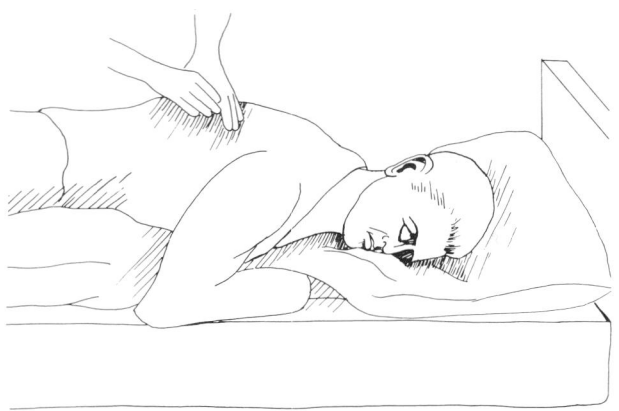

FIG. 16-60. Postural drainage combined with chest physical therapy is important in the medical management of bronchiectasis and in the preoperative care of patients who require pulmonary resection.

As with many clinical situations in which choice of therapy is based largely on quality of life decisions, there are no prospective controlled series to compare relative benefits of medical versus surgical treatment. In a Turkish series of 487 patients treated over a 12-year period, including 190 treated with pneumonectomy, mortality was 3.5 percent and 71 percent were asymptomatic (follow-up 4 months to 10 years). Surprisingly good quality of life has been described by Laros and associates from the Netherlands in 30 patients treated with unusually extensive bilateral resections (11 to 13 segments) and followed for 30 years. As a comparison, other authors have estimated that 70 percent of patients treated medically will develop persistent or progressive symptoms.

Tuberculosis

Sanskrit written in 6000 B.C. refers to tuberculosis as the "King of Diseases." Tuberculosis, then called "phthisis," was well known to Hippocrates. A generation beginning to face an uncertain battle with the AIDS complex would do well to recall that pulmonary tuberculosis was epidemic in Europe during the eighteenth and nineteenth centuries and took an extraordinary toll on young adults in the prime of life. In the United States in the 1940s pulmonary resection for tuberculosis carried a mortality rate of about 25 percent, and effective chemotherapy did not exist until streptomycin was discovered in 1944. Tuberculosis remained epidemic in part of the United States (Alaska) as recently as the early 1960s. Over the next 20 years the treatment of tuberculosis was largely reduced to a straightforward recipe of medical therapy. Tragically, the past decade has seen a recrudescence of tuberculosis as a significant public health concern. Noncompliance with drug therapy among those populations at particular risk, prisoners and drug addicts, has given rise to a more virulent multiple drug resistant (MDR) organism. The expanded population of immunocompromised patients, whether from AIDS or post-transplantation drug therapy, has increased the pool of the highly susceptible. Many authorities are anticipating a return to the need for relatively long term isolation of the MDR infected patient with active disease, and a resurrection of the challenging if nearly forgotten surgical techniques characteristic of the pre-drug treatment era.

Pathophysiology and Clinical Manifestations. In broad outline a pulmonary infection with *Mycobacterium tuberculosis* behaves like a lung abscess, with notable differences based primarily on the peculiar growth characteristics of the organism and the nature of the host response. The disease usually becomes clinically apparent when a previously acquired and quiescent infection is reactivated, usually in the apical or posterior segments of an upper lobe or in the superior segment of a lower lobe. In an immunocompetent host the characteristic cycle of caseous necrosis and scar formation will eventually produce what amounts to a tuberculous lung abscess. Just as with pyogenic lung abscess, the smouldering central focus of infection tends to find communication with the tracheobronchial tree, providing a route for drainage and expectoration of purulent sputum loaded with tubercle bacilli, and allowing ingress of air to produce cavitation. The ultimate extent of infection is determined by the size of the inoculum, the immune competence of the host, and the success of antituberculous drugs. Rapid progression can produce a tuberculous empyema surrounding a destroyed lung. If growth of the bacillus is controlled, the cavity may collapse and obliterate or may remain open indefinitely. Such cavities ("open negative") are no longer sites of tuberculous infection but remain potential sites for secondary infection, the classic example of which is an *Aspergillus* "fungus ball" (mycetoma).

As with lung abscess and bronchiectasis, the intense inflammatory process in the periphery of a cavity tends to promote hypertrophy of bronchial arterial and pulmonary arterial branches. These may be eroded by the necrotizing process in the center of the cavity to produce hemoptysis, which can be life-threatening. The vessel responsible is most frequently a dilated pulmonary arterial branch, referred to as a Rasmussen aneurysm. The management of massive tracheobronchial hemorrhage has been discussed in connection with lung abscess. Because a tuberculous cavity is likely to be more chronic, when major hemoptysis occurs the vessel involved is likely to be larger than that seen in a pyogenic lung abscess, and emergency pulmonary resection is often necessary.

On occasion the most intense inflammatory process is confined to regional lymph nodes, which can enlarge enough to produce bronchial stenosis and distal atelectasis—one cause of the middle-lobe syndrome. If this occurs distal to an evolving cavity, rapid expansion can occur due to air trapping, to produce a "tension cavity." The responsible nodes are choked with caseating granulomata. Discrete bronchial stenosis can also be seen without evidence of extrinsic compression, in which case it is usually ascribed to an intense tuberculous bronchitis occurring in a segment draining an active parenchymal infection.

In a typical case of pulmonary tuberculosis the diagnosis is easily made on the basis of characteristic cavitary changes in an upper lobe on chest x-ray, occurring in a patient with a positive PPD whose sputum has grown *Mycobacterium tuberculosis*. A suggestive x-ray without positive cultures does not confirm the diagnosis, and a negative PPD does not rule out active tuberculosis. Definitive diagnosis rests on growth of the organism in culture (Fig. 16-61). A positive acid-fast stain provides a highly suggestive provisional diagnosis but cannot discriminate completely between *Nocardia* and *M. tuberculosis*.

Culture also allows identification of "atypical" *Mycobacteria*, which deserve special mention. Clinically and pathologically, infection with an atypical *Mycobacterium* can be indistinguishable from infection with *M. tuberculosis*. Resistance to multiple antituberculous drugs is common among the atypical *Mycobacteria*, and chances for a nonoperative cure depend on accurate assessment of appropriate medical therapy. Culture becomes important for identification of a specific species, and for characterization of its drug

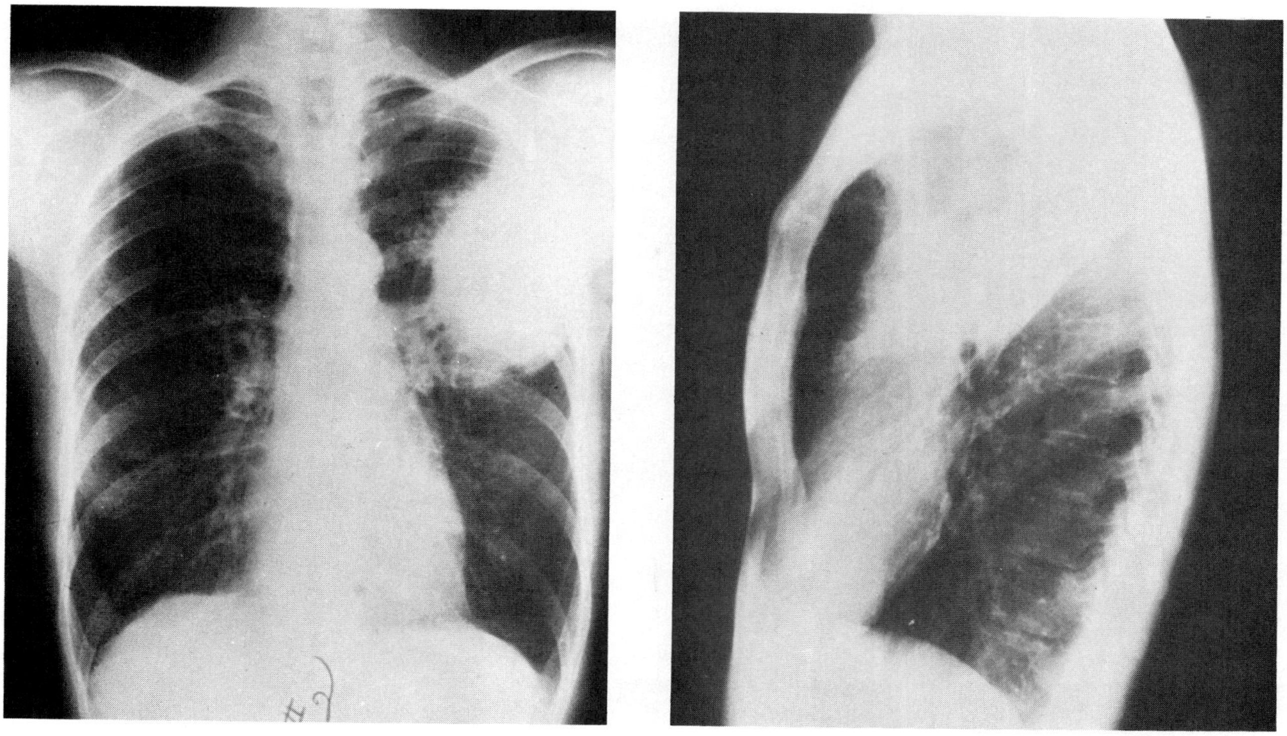

A B

FIG. 16-61. Pulmonary tuberculosis, active. *A* and *B*. A large mass in the left upper lobe that was associated with marked atypia of cells obtained by bronchoscopy, and negative sputum smears for acid-fast bacilli. The resected lobe showed active tuberculosis without cavitation.

sensitivities. Even with successful medical treatment the use of three or four drugs for 2 to 4 years can be anticipated. Because of drug resistance, a higher proportion of atypical than of typical mycobacterial pulmonary infections will require operation. *Mycobacterium kansasii* and *M. intracellulare-avium* are the species most often associated with pulmonary disease (Table 16-12).

Treatment. Operative treatment of tuberculosis is ordinarily an elective procedure performed after a period of treatment with antituberculous drugs. Emergency operation is only required for life-threatening hemorrhage or massive air leak with tension pneumothorax. The procedure of choice is almost always lobectomy or segmentectomy. The technical precautions necessary to minimize the risk of tracheobronchial or pleural spread of infection are the same as those discussed with regard to resection for lung abscess. Noncontroversial indications for resection include (1) extensive pulmonary destruction with bronchopleural fistula and empyema, (2) persistently active disease with drug-resistant organisms, (3) inability to rule out coexisting bronchogenic carcinoma, (4) pulmonary hemorrhage, and (5) posttuberculous bronchostenosis with recurrent nontuberculous infection. There has always been some controversy regarding resection of an ''open negative'' cavity. In these patients with negative sputum, the goal of treatment is to ensure that the cavity itself is made truly negative. There is considerable evidence that well-managed long-term medical therapy can produce results at least as good as those following resection. Partial adherence to a drug regimen can encourage emergence of resistant strains, so that noncompliant patients are poor candidates for medical treatment of large residual cavities and should have a resection. This discussion applies equally to typical and atypical Mycobacterial infections.

An occasional patient will have persistent active infection but such limited ventilatory reserve that resection would not be tolerated. Under these circumstances thoracoplasty remains a valid alternative. Thoracoplasty is designed to collapse the affected lung, which can be remarkably effective. Collapse is achieved without

Table 16-12
Classification of Atypical Mycobacteria

Group	*Example*	*Principal Lesion*
I. Photochromogens	*Mycobacterium kansasii*	Pulmonary disease
II. Scotochromogens	*Mycobacterium scrofulaceum*	Cervical lymphadenitis
III. Nonchromogenic	*Mycobacterium intracellulare* (Battey bacillus)	Pulmonary disease
IV. Rapid growers	*Mycobacterium marinum*	Swimming pool skin granuloma

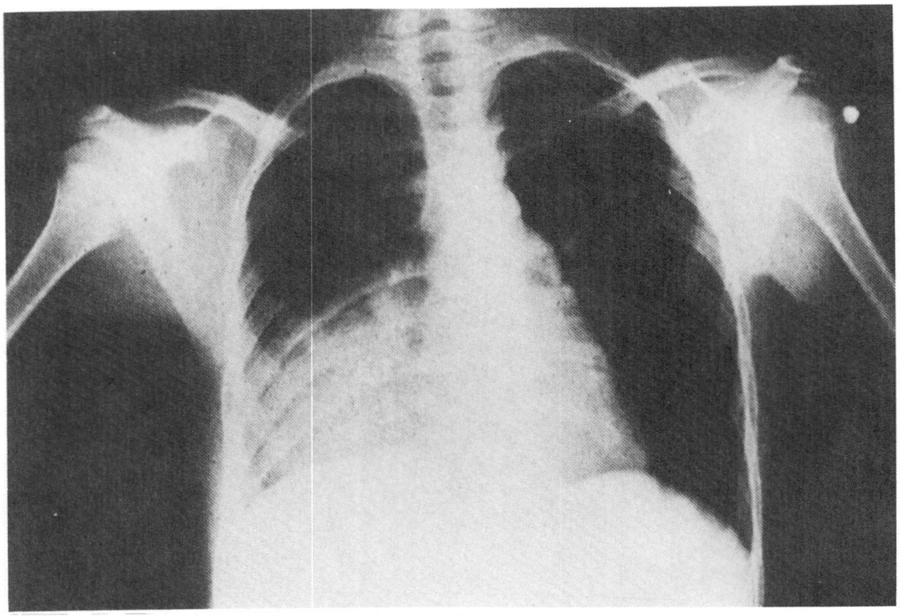

A

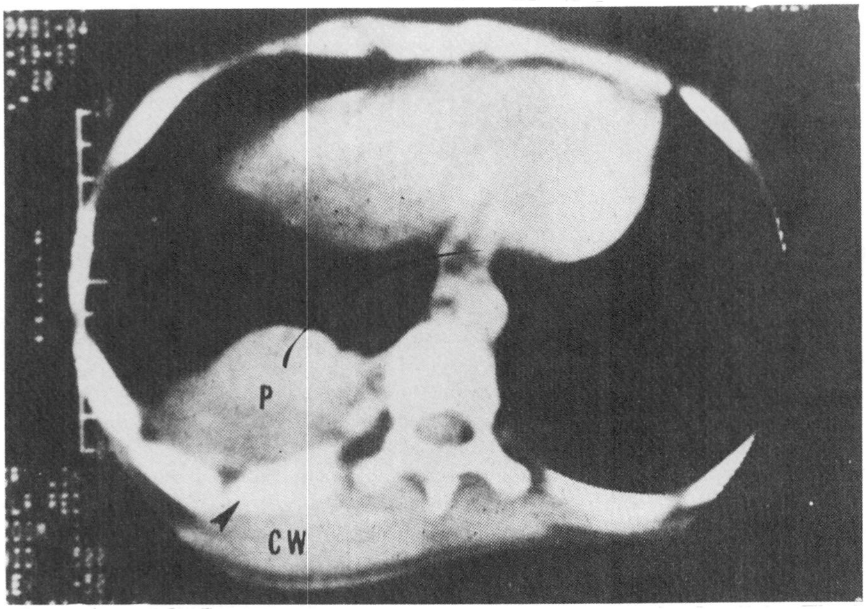

B

FIG. 16-62. A 14-old boy presented to his local hospital complaining of a "lump" on his back that had been growing for about 1 month. He recalled an episode of right lung pneumonia 10 months previously. *A.* Chest x-ray on admission showed a density in the right lower lung field and mild levoscoliosis. *B.* A CT scan of the lower thoracic region revealed a mass involving the pleura (P) and the chest wall (CW) with thickening of the eighth rib (*arrow*). CT sections of the first lumbar vertebra showed lucent bony lesions (not shown). *C.* Biopsy of the mass revealed the characteristic clumped colonies of *Actinomyces.* The patient was treated with 6 weeks of intravenous and 12 months of oral penicillin. The chest x-ray was normal in 3 months. (From: *Golden N, Cohen H, et al: Clin Pediatr 24:646, 1985, Figs 2, 3, 5, with permission.*)

entering the pleural space by performing an extrapleural resection of the first five ribs, followed in 10 to 14 days by resection of the sixth and seventh ribs. Although this procedure has its origins in the treatment of tuberculosis, the principle of chest wall collapse is occasionally used to obliterate pleural space following pulmonary resection as well.

Fungal Infections

By about 1900 all the major fungal pathogens had been isolated and named, but recognition of their role in disease underwent a very characteristic evolution. They were initially thought to be rare and fatal infections, but as diagnostic acumen increased, it became clear that mild asymptomatic infection was far more common. Now the pendulum is beginning to swing back somewhat, as fungal infections find their way into our enlarging reservoir of iatrogenically immunocompromised patients. Features common to all fungal infections include protean manifestations in compromised hosts, sensitivity to amphotericin B, and mimicry of carcinoma and tuberculosis. Amphotericin B is a very important drug that has rendered most fungal infections medically treatable, but it is also a highly toxic drug that cannot be administered as casually as antituberculous drugs are given.

Actinomycosis. For many years the actinomycetes were misclassified as fungi because they form branching hyphae and spores. Only in the past 20 years has it been recognized that the

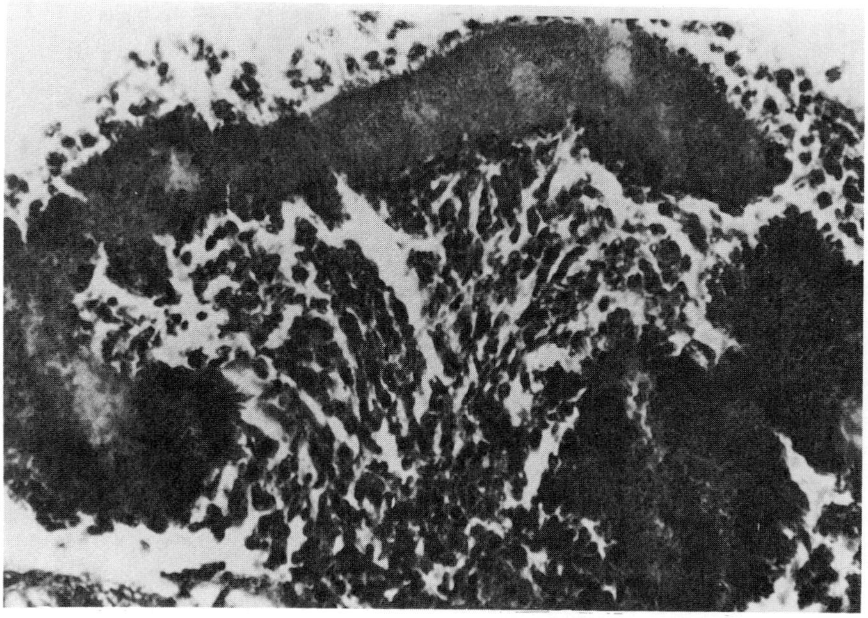

FIG. 16-62. (continued) C

actinomycetes are bacteria. This taxonomic distinction has therapeutic relevance, because the pathogens in this group are sensitive to penicillin and sulfonamides but not to amphotericin B.

Actinomycosis is caused by *Actinomyces israelii,* an anaerobic filamentous bacillus that is not found in nature but is a normal commensal inhabitant of the oral cavity and tonsillar crypts. It is not known what causes this organism to become an invasive pathogen, but in about three-fourths of cases some kind of predisposing factor can be identified, such as immunosuppression or breakdown of local tissue barriers (i.e., tooth extraction). About 60 percent of cases are cervicofacial, and only 15 percent are thoracic. Thoracic infection is presumed to result from aspiration of infected secretions. Classically the disease is characterized by suppuration, abscess and sinus tract formation, and relentless invasion with complete disregard for tissue planes. Multiple sinus tracts are observed today in only one-third of cases, and the lesion is more commonly seen as a parenchymal process mimicking bronchogenic carcinoma. Nonetheless, when involvement of ribs or extension into mediastinal structures is seen, actinomycosis must be high on the list of possible causes (Fig. 16-62).

Expectorated sputum, material from a sinus tract, and biopsy material can demonstrate sulfur granules, which are yellow-brown clusters of microcolonies. This finding is highly suggestive, but since *Nocardia,* certain fungi, and *Staphylococcus aureus* are also capable of producing clumps of material resembling sulfur granules, diagnostic confirmation rests on identification of the bacillus within the granules, for which special stains are required. Cultures are positive in only about one-fourth of cases.

The organism is sensitive to penicillin, although large doses are required to penetrate the dense colonies, and medical treatment is most often quite successful. Therefore, the surgical strategy is to make an accurate diagnosis at an early stage of disease. Because the disease can have gross resemblance to fungal infections and to carcinoma, and because tissue stains are essential to the diagnosis, operation is frequently required to obtain adequate biopsy material. Successful diagnosis is followed by high-dose intravenous penicillin and a long subsequent course of oral administration. Resection should rarely be necessary except in unusually advanced presentations with an inadequate response to penicillin.

Nocardiosis. Nocardiosis is caused by *Nocardia asteroides,* an aerobic acid-fast filamentous bacillus widely distributed in nature as a saprophyte in soil and domestic animals. It is a rare pathogen except in an immunocompromised host and is most often thoracic, beginning as a pneumonic process difficult to distinguish grossly from tuberculosis, fungal infections, and carcinoma. It can also closely mimic actinomycosis, with chest wall involvement, sinus tract formation, and production of sulfur granules. The acute infection is often much more aggressive than actinomycosis, with extensive pulmonic necrosis and abscess formation, and metastatic dissemination to the central nervous system and elsewhere.

Nocardia is relatively easy to culture and to identify with standard stains, so the diagnosis can frequently be made by brush or needle biopsy, and even from expectorated sputum. The organism is sensitive to sulfonamides, which usually provide successful therapy. Other drugs can be added in poorly responsive cases (trimethoprim-sulfamethoxasole, minocycline) with good results, and surgery remains purely adjunctive in the majority of cases. Pulmonary resection, drainage of empyema, and similar procedures can be performed safely when necessary.

Histoplasmosis. Histoplasmosis is the most common systemic fungal infection in the United States. *Histoplasma capsulatum* is a dimorphic fungus common in the great river valleys of the midwest, where it lives in mycelial form in soil, decaying organic material, and guano. It assumes yeast form in the cytoplasm of pulmonary alveoli after inhalation. It is extremely common in endemic areas as an asymptomatic infection; the severity of disease is determined by the size of the inoculum and the immune competence of the host. Release of a large inoculum can produce outbreaks of acute pneumonic illness in normal hosts, and usually occurs following an environmental disruption such as excavation or demolition. Such infections ordinarily resolve without specific treatment, but not before widespread lymphatic and hematogenous

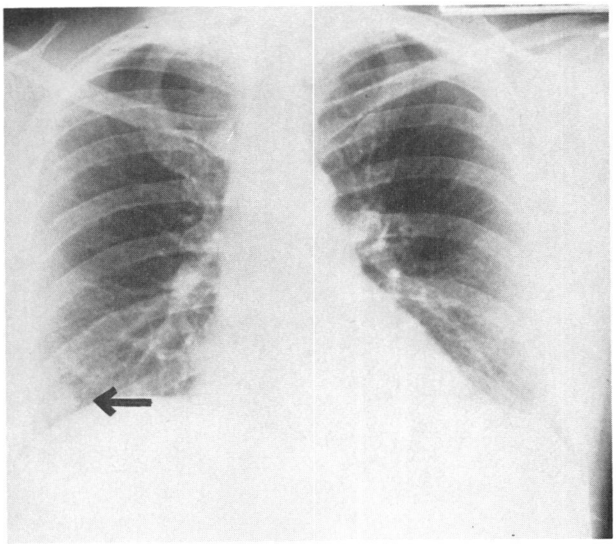

A

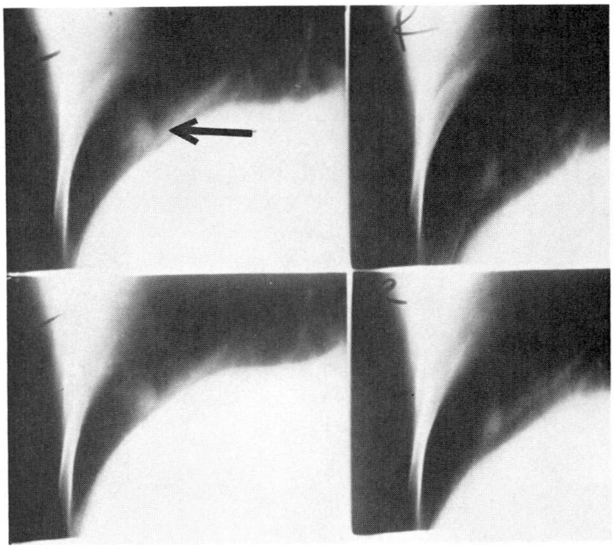

B

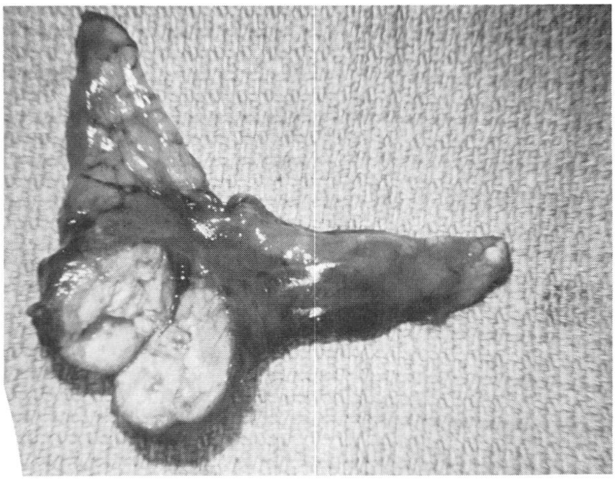

C

FIG. 16-63. Histoplasmosis. *A.* The chest x-ray shows a faint round lesion in the right lower lung field (*arrow*). *B.* Conventional tomography demonstrates the lesion clearly and shows that it has sharp borders. *C.* The lesion was removed by wedge resection; the cut surface shows a histoplasmoma.

dissemination has occurred, apparent later as scattered calcific nodules in lungs, mediastinum, spleen, and liver. In symptomatic patients the disease can take many forms and is often distinguishable from tuberculosis only by culture. Skin testing reagents are available but are not as reliable as PPD. Serologic diagnosis is also available but is no more reliable and can be misleading if obtained following skin testing. As with tuberculosis, definitive diagnosis requires growth of the organism from pathologic specimens.

Amphotericin B is effective treatment in the majority of cases and is always the treatment of choice in a serious illness once the diagnosis is made. Most infections are asymptomatic or moderately symptomatic and self-limited, and chemotherapy is not recommended for skin test conversion as it is in tuberculosis. Operation is applied much as it is in tuberculosis. Cavitary disease is quite common, and in a recent large series from an endemic area (Tennessee) this was the most frequent indication for resection. Large, thick-walled cavities that have failed to improve after a course of amphotericin B are likely to progress and can be resected with low morbidity and mortality. Another frequent indication for operative intervention is inability to establish a definitive diagnosis, especially when the lesion presents as a solitary pulmonary nodule grossly consistent with carcinoma (Fig. 16-63). As in tuberculosis, hemoptysis can require operation, and bronchostenosis produced by extrinsic nodal compression can require resection. The lymphogenous phase of *Histoplasma* dissemination leads to remarkable nodal enlargement in some patients, producing symptoms related to compression of mediastinal structures, and a radiographic appearance resembling mediastinal malignancies. Mediastinal involvement can also produce a sclerosing mediastinitis with obstruction of the superior vena cava, pulmonary arteries or veins, esophagus, or tracheobronchial tree. The pathophysiology of this desmoplastic response to infection is not completely understood but appears to be an idiosyncratic reaction.

Coccidiomycosis. Coccidiomycosis is the second most common fungal infection encountered in the United States. *Coccidioides immitis* is a dimorphic fungus found in mycelial form as a saprophyte in the arid soil of the American Southwest. Arthrospores released by the hyphae are inhaled and initiate the parasitic phase by becoming spherules that release infective endospores. In the normal host most infections are asymptomatic, but some will manifest ''valley fever,'' essentially a mild pneumonic form of the illness. The organism is not difficult to recover from sputum or pathologic specimens. The skin test and serologic titers are almost always positive in active disease but are more ambiguous in the more chronic and indolent forms of infection. Except for a propensity to form thin-walled cavities, the spectrum of gross and microscopic pathology is similar to that seen in histoplasmosis, tuberculosis, and other fungal infections.

For patients with symptomatic illness requiring treatment, amphotericin B is the primary therapy. As with histoplasmosis, the lungs provide an effective barrier against serious systemic illness in most patients, and specific treatment is frequently not required. Aggressive necrotizing pulmonary infection and disseminated disease are usually seen in immunocompromised hosts, and require early and aggressive medical treatment.

Indications for operation are virtually identical to those applied to histoplasmosis. Resection of cavitary disease and resection for definitive diagnosis of a solitary pulmonary nodule are most frequently performed. Specific indications in cavitary disease include progressive enlargement, hemoptysis, rupture, and secondary infection.

Blastomycosis. Blastomycosis is caused by *Blastomyces dermatitidis,* a round, single budding yeast endemic in the southeastern United States and other scattered areas. Although there is a common cutaneous form, the disease is always acquired through aspiration of spores into the lungs, where it can assume a variety of appearances—pneumonic infiltrates, cavitation, solitary granulomatous nodules, and disseminated disease. The cutaneous form is characterized by crusty, ulcerative lesions from the margins of which the organism can readily be cultured. Cutaneous and pulmonary infection can occur together, and the cutaneous form has a better prognosis. Diagnosis rests on identification of the organism, which can be done with a sputum Papanicolaou stain.

Although it can mimic tuberculosis and other fungal infections, in endemic areas it most frequently mimics bronchogenic carcinoma, and resection will frequently be required if a definitive diagnosis cannot be established (Fig. 16-64). Aggressive infection is treated with amphotericin B. Cutaneous infection and mild pulmonary infection also respond well to 2-hydroxystilbamadine. As with other fungal infections, treatment with amphotericin B can often be avoided in mild presentations of illness, especially in normal hosts during outbreaks in endemic areas.

Aspergillosis. *Aspergillus* is a filamentous fungus with septate hyphae that is ubiquitous in nature. Inhalation of spores from *A. fumigatus, A. niger,* and other species initiates infection in susceptible individuals. Aspergillosis presents in three forms: allergic bronchopulmonary, saprophytic, and invasive. The first is characterized by asthmatic symptoms resulting from host response to fungus in the airways and is of no surgical importance. The invasive form is usually seen in the immunocompromised host, can involve any organ system, and is almost always fatal. Surgical attention focuses on the saprophytic form, produced by colonization of a preexisting pulmonary cavity (an aspergilloma, mycetoma, or "fungus ball"). On chest x-ray the aspergilloma appears as a solid, rounded mass within a cavity, surrounded by a crescent of air between the fungus and the cavity wall (Fig. 16-65). *Aspergillus precipitins* are almost always detectable in patients with aspergilloma. Skin testing is available but is positive in only 30 to 75 percent of cases. The value of sputum cultures has been debated, but recent evidence suggests that two or more positive cultures carry excellent specificity and sensitivity.

For disseminated disease amphotericin B is the mainstay of therapy. Penetration of the drug into a cavity containing an aspergilloma is very poor, so resection is considered the treatment of choice for a significant aspergilloma. Operative treatment most frequently requires lobectomy, segmentectomy, or pneumonectomy. Cavernostomy (open drainage through the chest wall) is occasionally performed in patients with poor ventilatory reserve and can be augmented by intracavitary instillation of antifungal agents. Operation is most often justified as prevention for hemoptysis, which occurs in 50 to 83 percent of cases and can be life-threatening in a fraction of that total. Even so, operation remains somewhat controversial because it is associated with considerable

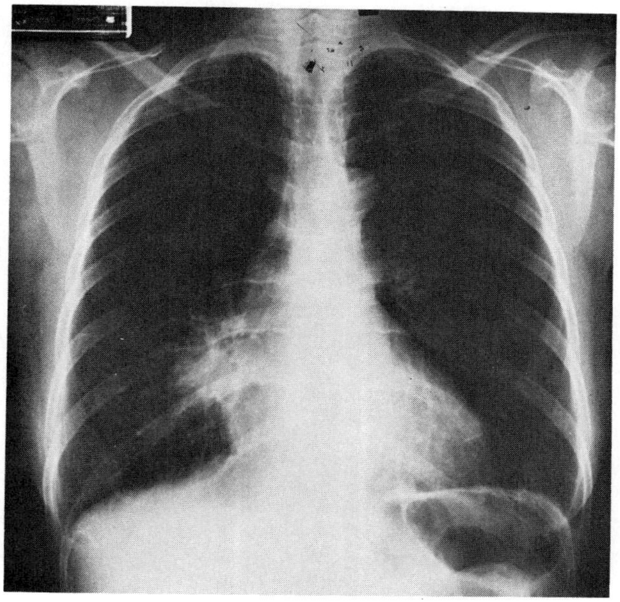

A

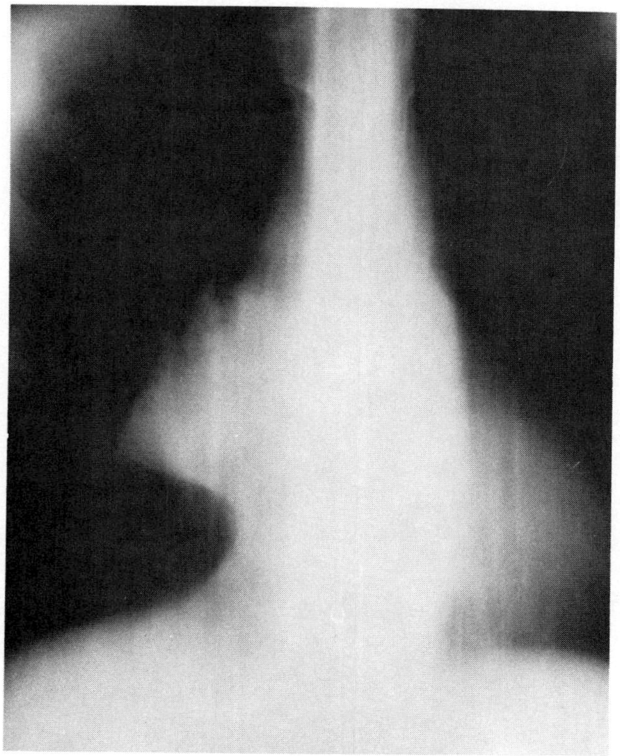

B

FIG. 16-64. North American blastomycosis. *A.* Chest x-ray shows a mass in the right lung field adjacent to the heart border. *B.* Conventional tomography defines the mass more clearly, but neoplasm cannot be excluded. A pulmonary resection revealed active blastomycosis in the right middle lobe.

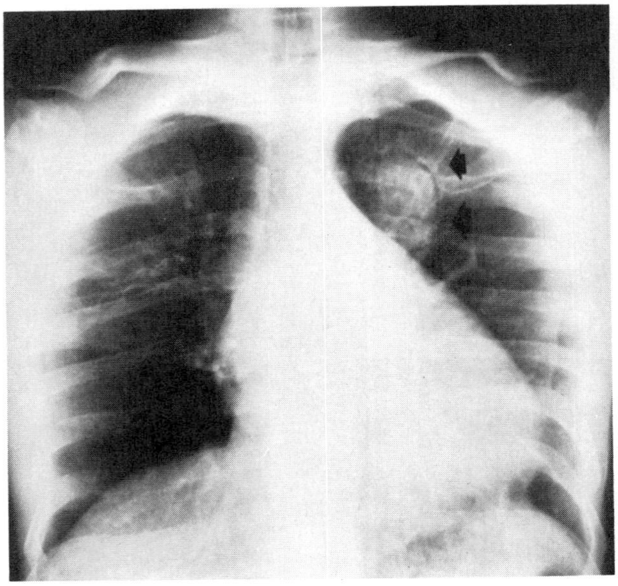

A

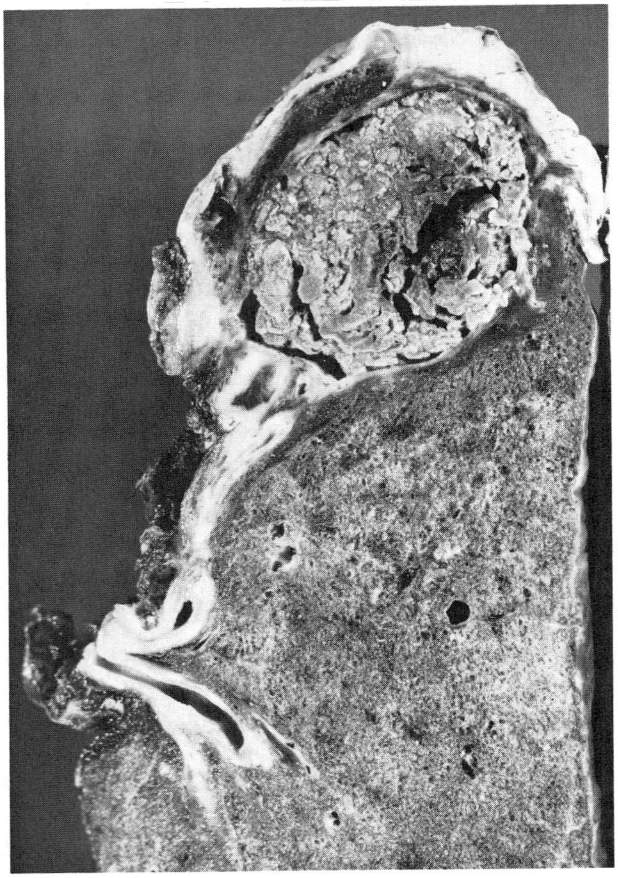

B

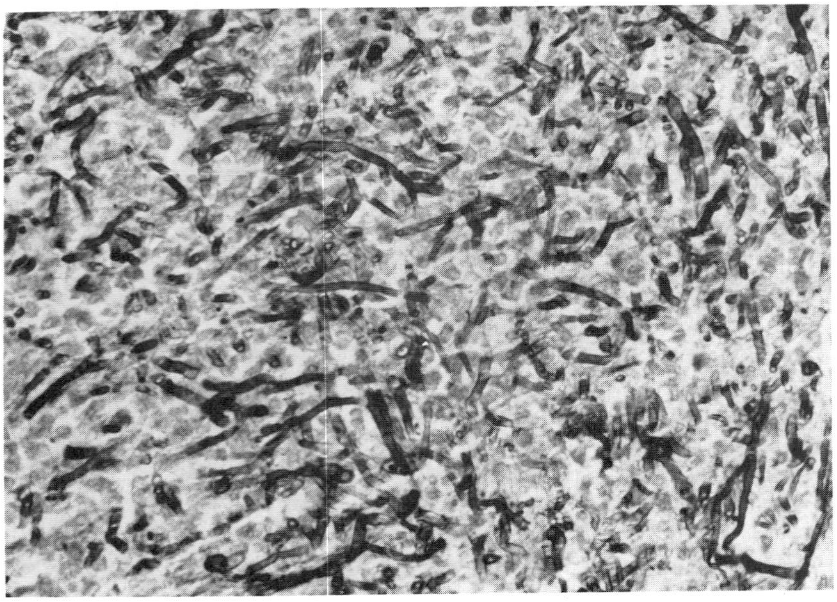

C

FIG. 16-65. A *Aspergillus fumigatus* "fungus ball." *A.* In a patient presenting with recurrent hemoptysis, a lordotic chest x-ray shows a solid mass within a cavity surrounded by a rim of air between the mass and the cavity wall (*arrows*), a finding highly suggestive of an aspergilloma. *B.* After resection of the left upper lobe, cut section reveals the fungus ball filling an old fibrotic cavity. *C.* The histopathology with special stains for fungus demonstrates mycelia infiltrating the tissue in the wall of the cavity.

mortality and morbidity. This is related to the poor health of most susceptible hosts and the technical difficulty of resection through dense inflammatory tissue. In a recent series from the Mayo Clinic, for example, either underlying lung disease or immunologic risk factors were present in 92 percent of patients, and complications occurred in 78 percent of patients with complex aspergillomas. In this series and others, operative mortality has been 5 to 10 percent, and complications in "simple" aspergilloma resection have ranged from 25 to 34 percent. Nonetheless, in the Mayo Clinic series the late results were excellent in about 75 percent of cases. In conclusion it is probably prudent to observe small asymptomatic aspergillomas, but in most cases resection should be performed, accepting increased risk in favor of potential benefits.

Cryptococcosis. Cryptococcosis is caused by *Cryptococcus neoformans,* a round, budding yeast found in soil and pigeon droppings. Infection occurs through inhalation of the organism and in most individuals produces a comparatively benign bronchopulmonary illness. The chief radiologic finding is a granulomatous complex with hilar node involvement, indistinguishable from the Ghon complex of tuberculosis. It is rarely of surgical significance except in the compromised host, when the entire spectrum of fungal pulmonary pathology seen in more inherently virulent infections can be seen on occasion (Fig. 16-66). The best-known disseminated manifestation is meningitis. Infection can be controlled in many cases with amphotericin B and 5-fluorocytosine, even with meningeal involvement.

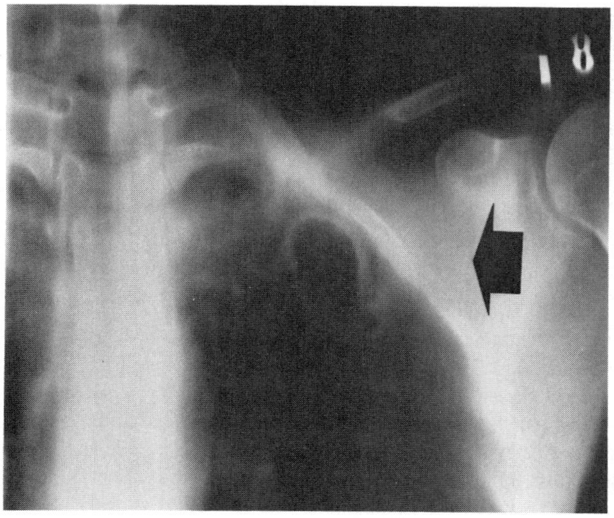

A

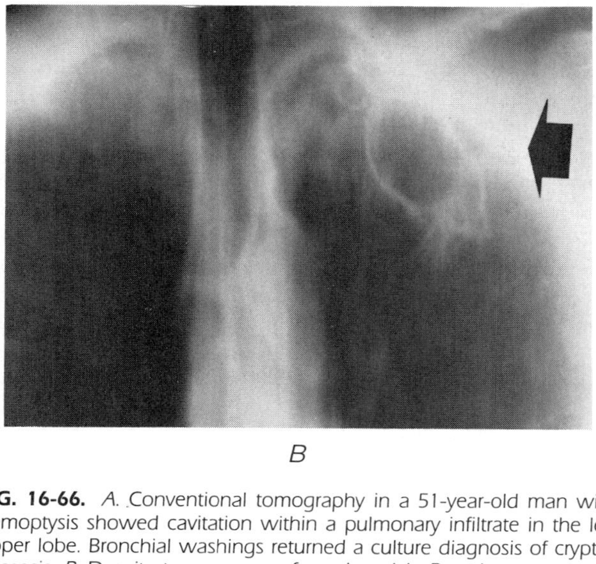

B

FIG. 16-66. *A.* Conventional tomography in a 51-year-old man with hemoptysis showed cavitation within a pulmonary infiltrate in the left upper lobe. Bronchial washings returned a culture diagnosis of cryptococcosis. *B.* Despite two courses of amphotericin B and one course of ketoconazole, tomograms repeated 2 years later demonstrated progressive cavitation. A left upper lobectomy was performed for recurrent hemoptysis and failure of drug therapy.

Innumerable other fungi can be associated with pulmonary disease in human beings, but as the list diverges further and further from the recognized pathogens, it becomes increasingly confined to immunocompromised hosts. *Candida,* mucormycosis, sporotrichosis, monospirosis, *Torulopsis,* even *Penicillium*—all have been described. Surgical treatment is rarely indicated and seldom definitive.

Tumors

Primary Carcinoma of the Lung

Tobacco addiction (cigarette smoking) is the predominant factor in the etiology of lung cancer. It must puzzle any logical person to observe the paradoxes in the way our society deals with its addiction problems. On the one hand are several substances that, though distressing in individual cases, pose a modest public health problem but are aggressively discouraged with heavy criminal sanctions against production, distribution, or use. On the other hand, we have long subsidized by tax dollars the production and distribution of an addicting drug that is by far this nation's most serious public health problem.

Each year in the United States there are 450,000 excess and preventable deaths at immense direct cost for nonsmokers in extra taxes and health insurance premiums. Demographic data consistently reveal that tobacco addicts are 9 to 10 times more likely to die before age seventy than are nonsmokers. Furthermore, there is no longer any reasonable doubt that those who live or work with tobacco addicts are forced to share a substantial health risk. Physicians must speak clearly on the importance of educating patients and public regarding the consequences of tobacco addiction and on the importance of establishing a smoke-free environment in public and work places for the nonsmoking 70 percent of the population who must not be subjected to this unnecessary health hazard.

Even with the best available air-moving and ventilating equipment, Environmental Protection Agency engineers demonstrated that it was not possible to reduce carcinogenic air contamination to an acceptable level for a nonsmoker sharing work space with a tobacco addict. Physical isolation of the addict while engaging in the habit is essential.

Tobacco addiction causes four times as many excess deaths each year as all other drug and alcohol abuse deaths combined; ten times more than all automobile fatalities per year; twelve times as many as are caused by the acquired immunodeficiency syndrome; and more than all American military fatalities in this century put together.

From a trivial health problem at the beginning of this century, and a minor one by 1930 (a death rate of 5 per 100,000), lung cancer has now become the main cancer killer in both men and women. Reflecting the changing smoking habits in women that have occurred since the early 1950s, and the long exposure required for the development of this malignancy, the rate in women is rising at an alarming pace (Fig. 16-67). The histologic changes in the bronchial mucosa occur gradually over many years, an observation that provides important and reasuring information for the addict; those who stop smoking will sharply reduce their risk. It also provides a strong incentive for the disease-prevention oriented physician to campaign to educate patients, their families, and society to the urgency of creating a smoke-free environment.

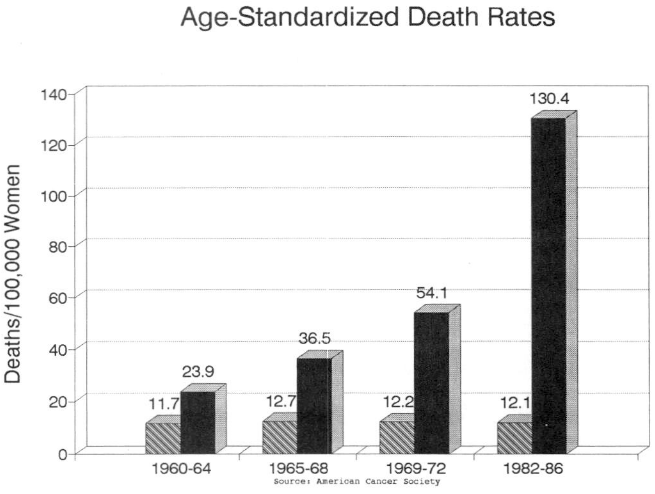

FIG. 16-67. Rising rate for female lung cancer, 1960–1986. (From: *American Cancer Society, with permission.*)

The labels currently used to represent the predominate cellular components of lung carcinoma are as follows:

Squamous cell (epidermoid) carcinoma
- Spindle cell variant

Adenocarcinoma
- Acinar
- Papillary
- Bronchioloalveolar
- Solid tumor with mucin

Large-cell carcinoma
- Giant cell
- Clear cell

Adenosquamous carcinoma

Since some cases of small-cell lung cancer might respond to chemotherapy, and because they can be confused on microscopic examination with some non-small-cell carcinomas, it is essential that the pathologic material be reviewed by a pathologist experienced in lung cancer diagnosis. There are some general characteristic differences in the clinical behavior of those tumors with a recognizable predominance in cell type.

Nonsquamous cancers are more likely to recur after surgical resection of early Stage I tumors. Bronchioalveolar carcinoma has a distinct presentation and biologic behavior. Most patients present with disease confined to the lung without nodal metastases. Prognosis is determined primarily by local factors such as size (T1 versus T2), histologic subtypes (nonmucinous versus mucinous), and tumor collagen content (collagen versus none). Resection of the solitary or localized tumor has resulted in a 5-year survival rate of 50 to 75 percent. This contrasts markedly with the diffuse form of bronchioalveolar cell carcinoma, in which there is rapid dissemination of the neoplasm in one or both lungs, with no possible consideration of operative treatment.

A few patients (about 10 percent) present with multiple unilateral lesions; about one-third of such patients may undergo resection with curative intent if the nodes are negative. Up to one-third of the patients with this relatively rare form of lung cancer may have no significant smoking history.

Small-Cell Lung Cancer (SCLS). Untreated small-cell (oat cell) carcinoma of the lung has the most rapidly adverse clinical course of any type of pulmonary tumor, with median survival from diagnosis of only 2 to 4 months. It has a high likelihood of being widely disseminated by the time of diagnosis. The SCLS is most often central in location because of origin from a proximal bronchus. It aggressively invades local structures and is disseminated by early vascular invasion. Even though it grows and spreads rapidly, it has become apparent that certain histologic subtypes of small-cell undifferentiated carcinoma have a better prognosis after curative resection (Fig. 16-68).

Non-Small-Cell Lung Cancers (NSCLC). There is frequently a high degree of overlap in the histopathology of most of the various primary lung cancers. Particularly as they become less differentiated, many mixed elements may appear that are suggestive of any of the NSCLCs. Except in the most typical situation, the classifications should not be overinterpreted. The therapeutic decisions are largely made on the basis of nodal metastases and other aspects of the clinical behavior of the tumor rather than the specific label assigned.

In view of the long exposure to carcinogens in smoke that is required and the progressive mucosal abnormalities that occur, it is likely these cancers are very slow-growing and are present for several years before symptoms occur. It has been estimated that a tumor nodule must go through approximately 30 doublings to become 1 cm in diameter, a size that is large enough to be seen on the routine chest x-ray. This could mean pulmonary tumors may have been present for as long as 8 years before discovery.

Staging. To share information and to standardize evaluation of protocols, the recommendations of the American Joint Committee on Cancer (AJCC) and the International Union Against Cancer (IUCC) have had their systems reconciled with Mountain's staging and the American Joint Committee Task Force on Lung Staging Revision. Recommended variations from the previous AJCC scheme include several modifications of the TNM descriptors. A T4 category denoting local mediastinal, visceral, great vessel, or bony invasion, or the presence of cytologically malignant pleural effusion has been added and N3 has been redefined to include contralateral mediastinal, contralateral hilar, or scalene-supraclavicular nodal involvement. Stage III has been subclassified as a and b (b meaning T4 or N3 disease). Stage IV has been added to include all M1 tumors.

Since this classification deviates from the more usually reported earlier AJCC classification, it is worth emphasizing the modifications from that version. Stage I no longer includes any patients with any nodal metastases. Stage III has been divided into one group with large locally invasive tumors but with nodes confined to the ipsilateral chest (IIIa) and a second group including contralateral nodal involvement or invasion of mediastinal viscera (IIIb). All tumors metastasizing beyond the thoracic and low cervical lymph nodes are now designated as Stage IV. Using the grading system, patients with NSCLC can be divided clinically into logical treatment groups, whatever the cell type. According to the NCI's current prognosis and treatment recommendations, Stages 0, I, and II tumors are usually surgically respectable. The prognosis in this group is 30 to 80 percent 5-year survival, with the range depending on a variety of tumor and host factors. If the patients in these groups have medical conditions that preclude an attempt at curative surgery, radiation therapy can be expected to result in a 20

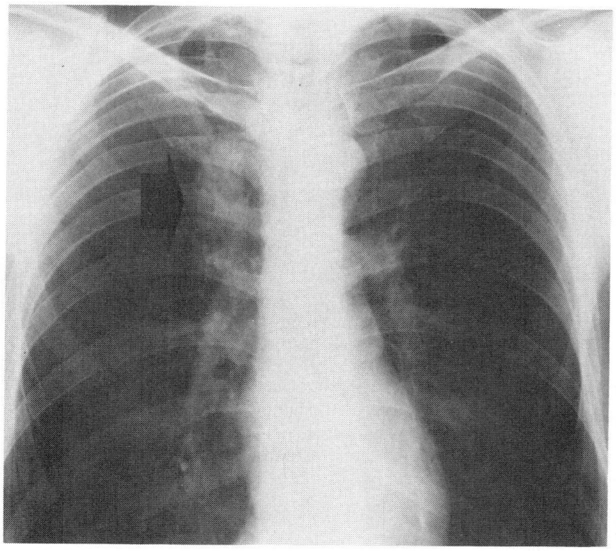

A

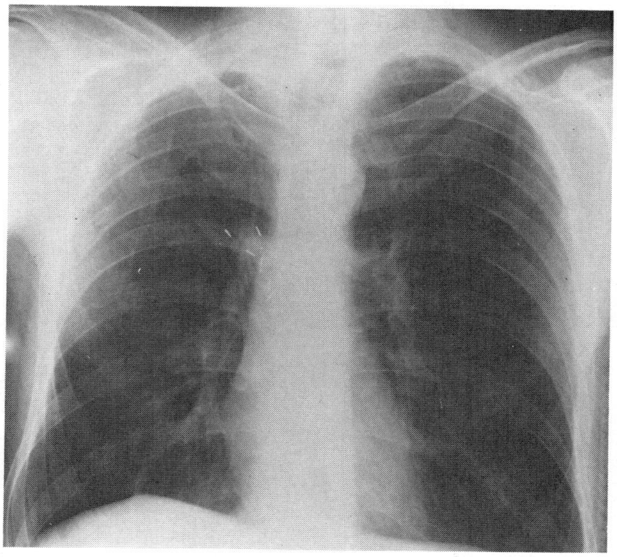

C

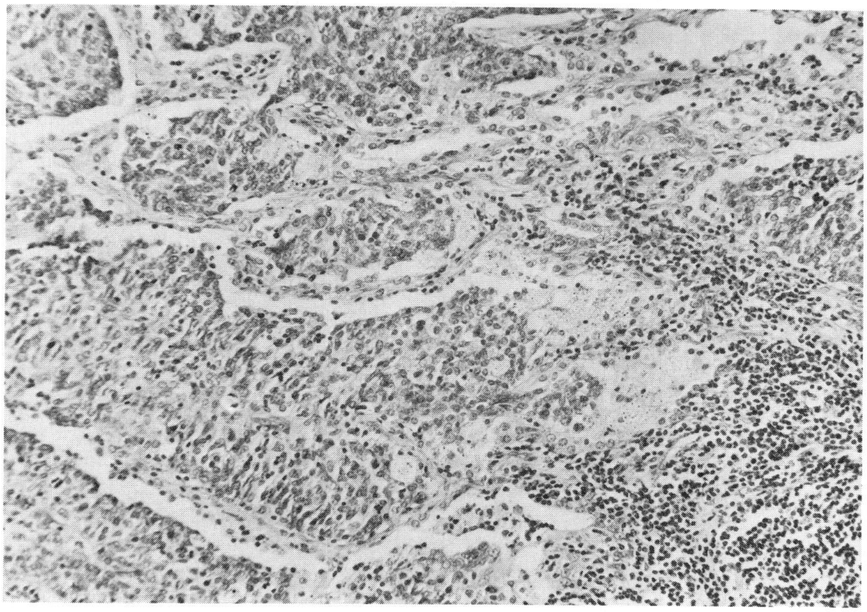

B

FIG. 16-68. Undifferentiated small-cell carcinoma, intermediate-cell type, in a 55-year-old man. *A.* The preoperative chest x-ray shows a mass above the right hilus. Mediastinoscopy failed to show evidence of mediastinal lymph-node involvement, and the patient underwent right upper lobectomy. *B.* Histological examination of the resected lobe showed an undifferentiated small-cell carcinoma, intermediate-cell type, invading the lung parenchyma. Note the size of tumor cells in comparison with the mature lymphocytes in the lower right corner (×188). *C.* A follow-up chest x-ray 4 years after operation shows no evidence of tumor recurrence, and the patient is well.

percent survival at 5 years. A second group of patients with locally advanced cancers (T3) or certain patterns of regional extension (N2) may respond favorably to extended local resection (the T3 lesions) combined with radiation and/or chemotherapy, or curative radiation doses directed at the involved nodal areas. Though the overall 5-year survival for this group is 10 percent or less and the median survival is less than a year several centers have achieved better results in selected subsets of this group. In Stage IV patients (those with distant metastases at the time of diagnosis), radiation for palliation of symptoms from the primary tumor may be useful. Though progress is being made in the oncology field, at present chemotherapy has not produced much survival benefit. Patients with lung cancer who have extrathoracic disease rarely survive for any significant period. The median survival is less than 6 months.

Clinical Manifestations. Bronchogenic carcinoma is seen predominantly in men of 45 to 65 years of age, with a peak incidence at 55 to 60 years. It is not rare in men less than 45 years old, and the diagnosis is being made with increasing frequency in women who are in their fifth decade. In a few cases, the disease is discovered incidentally in asymptomatic patients. Such discovery is by means of chest x-ray for the greatest number of patients, but sputum cytology occasionally leads to the eventual identification of an otherwise occult tumor.

Because intermittent or chronic cough is so common among tobacco addicts, it may be difficult to establish an onset of symptoms. Nevertheless, about three-fourths of patients with bronchogenic carcinoma must be said to have coughing as a principal symptom. Hemoptysis in the form of blood streaking of sputum

The Revised (1986) AJCC Staging System

	Primary Tumor (T)
TX	Tumor proved by the presence of malignant cells in bronchopulmonary secretions but not visualized roentgenographically or bronchoscopically, or any tumor that cannot be assessed as in a retreatment staging
T0	No evidence of primary tumor
T_{is}	Carcinoma in situ
T1	A tumor that is 3.0 cm or less in greatest dimension, surrounded by lung or visceral pleura, and without evidence of invasion proximal to a lobar bronchus at bronchoscopy
T2	A tumor more than 3.0 cm in greatest dimension, or a tumor of any size that either invades the visceral pleura or has associated atelectasis or obstructive pneumonitis extending to the hilar region. At bronchoscopy, the proximal extent of demonstrable tumor must be within a lobar bronchus or at least 2.0 cm distal to the carina. Any associated atelectasis or obstructive pneumonitis must involve less than an entire lung.
T3	A tumor of any size with direct extension into the chest wall (including superior sulcus tumors), diaphragm, or the mediastinal pleura or pericardium without involving the heart, great vessels, trachea, esophagus or vertebral body, or a tumor in the main bronchus within 2.0 cm of the carina without involving the carina
T4	A tumor of any size with invasion of the mediastinum or involving heart, great vessels, trachea, esophagus, vertebral body, or carina, or presence of malignant pleural effusion
	Nodal Involvement (N)
NX	Minimum requirements to access the regional nodes cannot be met
N0	No demonstrable metastasis to regional lymph nodes
N1	Metastasis to lymph nodes in the peribronchial or the ipsilateral hilar region, or both, including direct extension
N2	Metastasis to ipsilateral mediastinal lymph nodes and subcarinal lymph nodes
N3	Metastasis to contralateral mediastinal lymph nodes, contralateral hilar lymph nodes, ipsilateral or contralateral scalene, or supraclavicular lymph nodes
	Distant Metastasis (M)
MX	Minimum requirements to assess the presence of distant metastasis cannot be met
M0	No (known) distant metastasis
M1	Distant metastasis present

Stage Grouping

Occult stage	TX	N0	M0
Stage 0	T_{is}	N0	M0 (in situ)
Stage I	T1	N0	M0
	T2	N0	M0
Stage II	T1	N1	M0
	T2	N1	M0
Stage IIIa	T3	N0	M0
	T3	N1	M0
	T1–3	N2	M0
Stage IIIb	Any T	N3	M0
	T4	Any N	M0
Stage IV	Any T	Any N	M1

Summary of Staging Definitions

Occult stage	Microscopically identified cancer cells in lung secretions on multiple occasions (or multiple daily collections); no discernible primary cancer in the lung
Stage 0	Carcinoma in situ
Stage I	Tumor surrounded by lung or visceral pleura arising more than 2 cm distal to the carina (T1–2, N0)
Stage II	Tumor not extending to adjacent organs, pleura, or chest wall, with hilar lymph-node involvement (T1–2, N1)
Stage IIIa	Tumor invading chest wall, pleura, or pericardium or within 2 cm but not involving carina; nodes in hilum or ipsilateral mediastinum (T3, N0–1; T1, N2)
Stage IIIb	Direct extension to adjacent organs (pleura, heart, chest wall, diaphragm, or mediastinum); or associated with contralateral mediastinal or supraclavicular lymph-node involvement (T4 or N3)
Stage IV	Any tumor with distant metastases (M1)

occurs in about half of all patients, but massive hemoptysis or spitting of blood clots is unusual. Chest pain of dull, nonspecific type is described by some patients whose tumor is subsequently found to be free of chest wall involvement. When there is invasion of the parietal pleura or chest wall, the patient may have mild to severe pain that is either localized or radicular in form. Fever and purulent sputum may mark an increase of symptoms in the patient whose tumor is producing major bronchial obstruction, and wheezing or stridor may also be present.

Involvement of the left recurrent laryngeal nerve (rarely the right nerve), either by direct tumor invasion or by extension from a metastatic lymph node, may result in hoarseness that is often minimized by the patient. Direct tumor extension into the superior vena cava or its compression by the expanding neoplasm produces early symptoms of edema of the eyes and prominence or distension of the superficial veins over the upper part of the body. Dyspnea occurring as a symptom of bronchogenic carcinoma is usually associated with a large pleural effusion, paralysis of a hemidiaphragm due to phrenic nerve invasion, or major bronchial obstruction.

A loss of appetite accompanied by weight loss of more than a few pounds is a particularly ominous sign in the patient with a bronchial neoplasm; such patients usually have either an unresectable tumor or systemic metastases. An aggressive search should be made for evidence of spread by isotope scanning and CT. Because the metastatic spectrum of these tumors is so wide, almost any imaginable symptom can be produced. A rare patient may develop pulmonary hypertrophic osteoarthropathy with clubbing of the digits (Fig. 16-69). Evidence of metastases may be absent, and the process may be dramatically reversed when the tumor is resected.

A small percentage of patients with bronchogenic carcinoma present with extrapulmonary nonmetastatic manifestations that are considered due to elaboration of hormonelike substances by the neoplastic cells. The occurrence of these signs and symptoms does not imply systemic spread of the bronchogenic tumor, and resection of the lesion is generally associated with a regression of the symptoms. Ultrastructural studies have demonstrated the presence of neurosecretory-type granules in the cells of many anaplastic tumors, and the more striking clinical symptoms are associated with oat cell carcinomas. An example is a Cushing-like syndrome that differs from the classic Cushing's syndrome by an older age incidence, a greater frequency in males, and a more rapid clinical course. The ectopic adrenocorticotropic hormone that has been demonstrated in the oat cell tumors appears indistinguishable from the normal hormone. An inappropriate antidiuresis associated with the anaplastic small-cell carcinoma occasionally results in the symptoms of water intoxication with hyponatremia and increasing cerebral symptoms. The carinoid syndrome has been reported in a few patients with oat cell carcinoma, and either 5-hydroxytryptamine or 5-hydroxytryptophan may be secreted.

Hypercalcemia caused by a parathormone-like polypeptide has most often been associated with squamous bronchogenic carcinoma. Tender gynecomastia and ectopic gonadotropin secretion have been identified with large-cell anaplastic carcinoma. Satisfactory resection of the squamous neoplasm reverses the hypercalcemia, but it may return if the tumor recurs. A group of carcinomatous neuromyopathies is included in the nonmetastatic manifestations of lung cancer, and their incidence is thought to be as high as 15 percent. The symptoms may be subtle or somewhat overshadowed by the pulmonary complaints. The patient with bronchogenic carcinoma who mentions weakness along with cough and chest pain is usually not questioned in detail about the characteristics of the weakness. This is the principal symptom, however, of a myasthenia-like syndrome that is probably due to a defect in neuromuscular conduction. Peripheral and central neuropathies also occur, and their differentiation from the symptoms of metastatic lesions can be important. With the former, pulmonary resection may be possible and may result in disappearance of the symptoms.

Diagnosis and Work-up. Approximately 50 percent of patients with bronchogenic cancer are beyond consideration for operative treatment when the opportunity for definitive diagnosis is first presented. For this reason diagnostic evaluation must include an effort to determine whether localized or metastatic spread has occurred. The key to this effort is a meticulous history. If carefully sought, symptoms can almost always be found that will direct attention to involved organ systems. A thorough examination for suggestive lymph nodes must also be made. Though the yield is low in the absence of symptoms, any or all of the scanning techniques should be used to search for metastatic spread in the presence of suggestive symptoms, or if the patient's general condi-

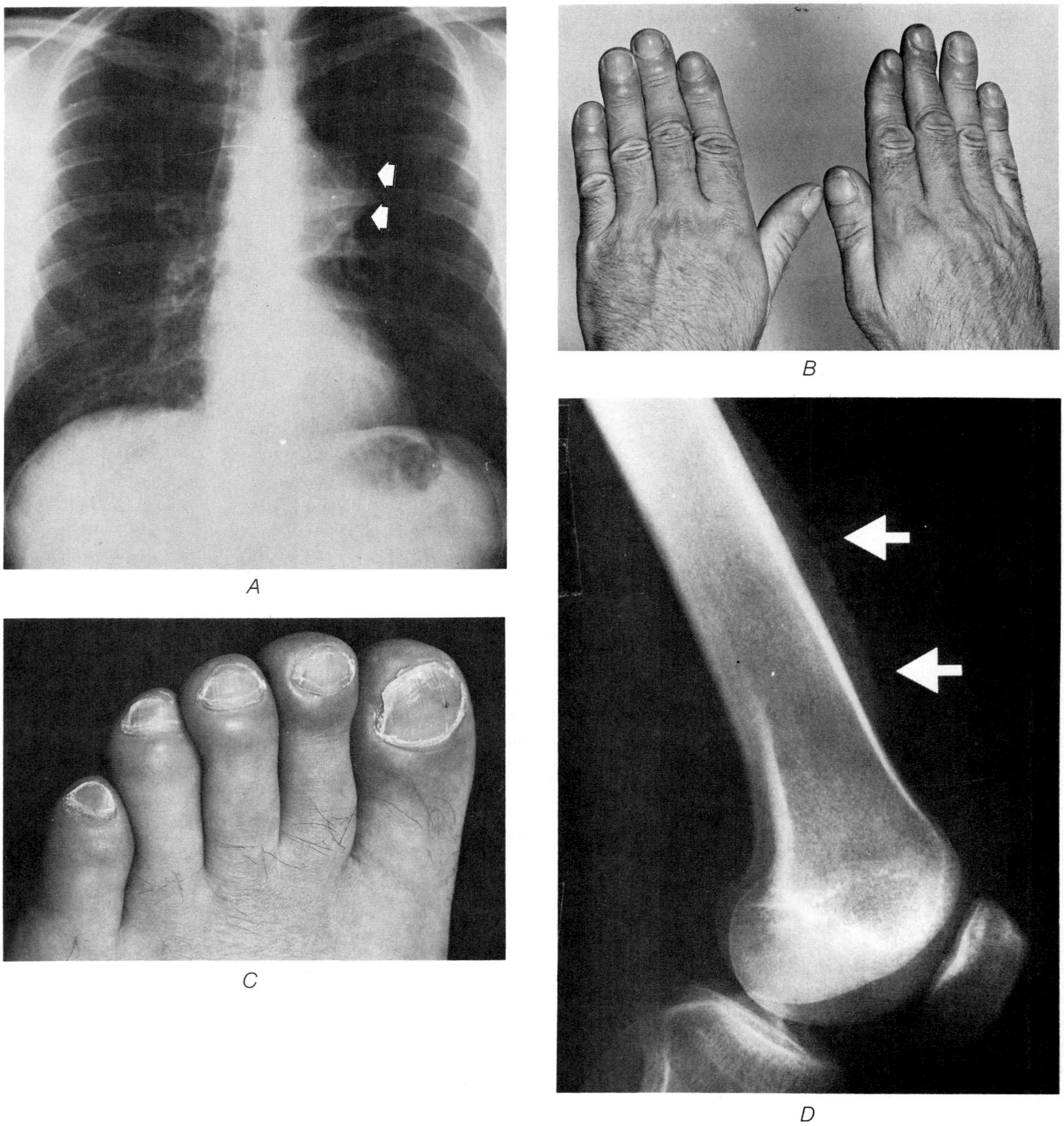

FIG. 16-69. Pulmonary hypertrophic osteoarthropathy associated with oat cell carcinoma. *A.* The chest x-ray in a 39-year-old man shows a left hilar mass that proved to be oat cell carcinoma on bronchial biopsy. *B.* Painful clubbing of the fingers and toes developed during an interval of approximately 3 months. *C.* A close-up of the patient's foot demonstrates clubbing of the toes. *D.* The arrow points to the new bone formation on the femur.

tion suggests systemic spread. With any question of metastasis, an attempt at biopsy should be considered before treatment for the primary neoplasm is planned.

Whenever the differential diagnosis includes lung cancer, aggressive efforts to obtain cytologic or biopsy tissue diagnosis are indicated. Almost any type of pulmonary infiltrate, nodule, mass, or atelectasis should be considered cancer until it can be proved otherwise. This is particularly true if the patient is, has been, or lives with a tobacco addict. As previously discussed, there is an orderly and progressively invasive series of investigative studies that can be undertaken to obtain diagnostic tissue. The degree to which a search should be made for extra thoracic disease is a matter of controversy among those who care for lung cancer patients. Radioactive scans of liver, brain, and bones are recommended by many, but evidence is lacking that such searches are fruitful in the absence of symptoms. The demonstrated value of the CT in visualizing the mediastinum has greatly reduced the indication for staging mediastinoscopy. Most surgeons now reserve exploration of the mediastinum for those patients with nodes identified on CT as being larger than 1 cm (Fig. 16-70).

Along with CT mapping, bronchoscopy is the fundamental diagnostic technique for patients with suspected carcinoma, and the development of the flexible fiberscope has increased the positive diagnosis yield to better than 70 percent in most centers. These results include bronchial brushing and cytologic studies of bronchial washings that may be obtained at the same time. The endoscopist must determine the proximal extent of a visualized neoplasm because the patient's operability may be governed by the closeness of the tumor to the tracheal carina.

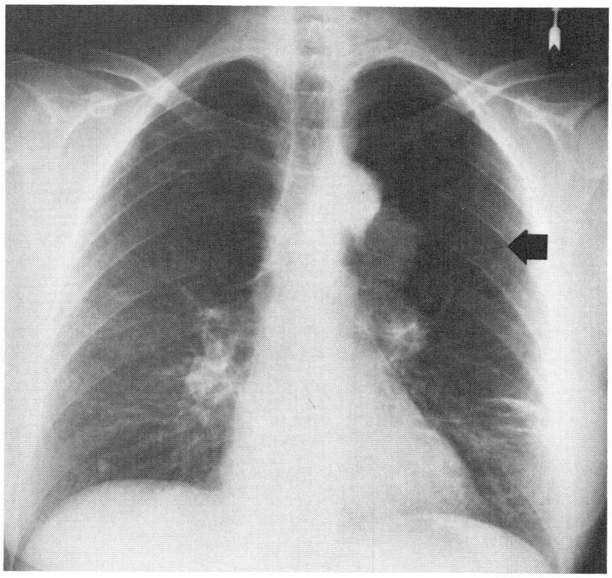

A

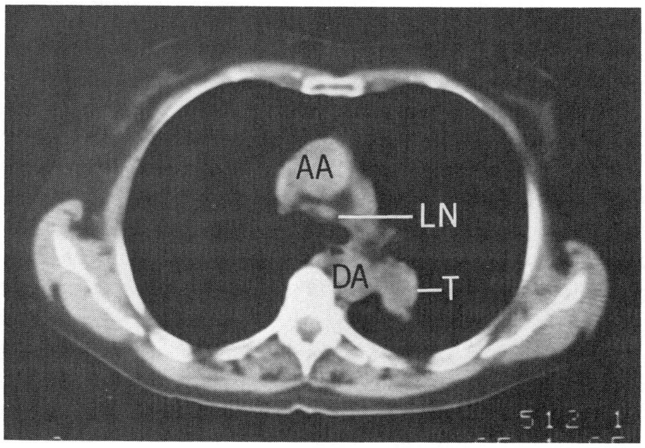

B

FIG. 16-70. The use of computed tomography for preoperative staging of bronchogenic carcinoma. *A.* The P-A chest x-ray in a 62-year-old woman shows a mass between the aortic knob and the left hilus. On the lateral chest x-ray the mass was seen to be located in the posterior segment of the left upper lobe. *B.* A CT scan at the level of the tracheal carina shows the tumor in juxtaposition to the descending aorta. The lymph nodes just in front of the carina and posterior to the ascending aorta were interpreted to be at the upper limit of normal size. At operation all lymph nodes were negative for metastases, confirming the CT impression. AA = ascending aorta, LN = lymph nodes, T = tumor, DA = descending aorta.

A primary goal of the patient's work-up is to confirm the suspected diagnosis of carcinoma by means other than exploratory thoracotomy. Diagnostic procedures should be carried out as techniques for establishing the patient's suitability for operation are completed. Despite a proper application of all reasonable diagnostic procedures, 10 to 20 percent of patients usually undergo thoracotomy without a proved diagnosis before operation. The role to be played by video-assisted thoracoscopy in prethoracotomy evaluation is currently being clarified.

An infrequent but clinically frustrating dilemma occurs when a patient is found to have recurring positive sputum cytology without a visible lesion on the chest x-rays. Other sources of the malignant cells, such as the nasopharynx or piriform sinuses, have to be eliminated, and careful flexible bronchoscopic examination may need to be performed at intervals of 4 to 8 weeks. Selective bronchial brushing or selective washing may localize the lesion, but exfoliated cells can become displaced into a bronchus other than the one of origin. This suggests caution in planning a major resection on the basis of these techniques alone. As new generations of CT scanners are developed, it may become possible to localize a so-called occult carcinoma by noninvasive techniques. The use of photoelectric endoscopic markers has shown some promise in detecting early, occult cancers. Unfortunately, the false-positive rate is high because the agent used currently (a hematoporphyrin derivative—HpD) is concentrated in areas of atypical squamous metaplasia as well as in cancer tissue.

There is now less resistance to needle biopsy than there used to be because of the decreasing fear of implanting tumor cells in the needle tract. In some institutions, needle biopsy is among the first procedures performed in the diagnostic work-up of the patient with a suspicious pulmonary lesion. Pneumothorax is the most frequent problem following needle biopsy, but less than half of the patients with this complication require treatment.

A pleural effusion in the presence of a suspected or confirmed pulmonary cancer is generally an indication of extensive tumor that is producing pleural or mediastinal invasion. An effusion can occur as a consequence of bronchial obstruction with atelectasis or infection. The fluid should be examined for the presence of blood and malignant cells with a simultaneous pleural needle biopsy if feasible. A demonstration of malignant cells in the effusion occurs in approximately half the patients with visceral or parietal pleural invasion by the neoplasm.

Treatment and Prognosis. An orderly approach to consideration of treatment of lung cancer involves deciding what is best for the given tumor according to its stage and cell type, and deciding what is best for the given patient according to the physical capabilities to withstand what might be optimal tumor treatment. In general, results of standard treatment are discouraging except in the most localized cancers. At this time, surgery is the only therapeutic option with cure potential; though radiotherapy may provide occasional long disease-free survival, its role is currently mostly adjunctive or palliative. While it is likely future treatment will combine surgery, radiotherapy, chemotherapy, and immunotherapy, there are currently no specific chemotherapy programs that can be recommended nor is there any established reproducible benefit from immunotherapeutic regimens.

The Tumor. The material in this section draws upon the recommendations made by the National Cancer Institute (NCI) and the National Library of Medicine (NLM) as reported in their computer-based information resource, PDQ. This excellent source of up-to-date information reports *current research protocols* and consensus recommendations for therapy and outlook and includes current bibliographic citations.

Non-Small-Cell Lung Cancer (NSCLC). Occult NSCLC (TONOMO). Aggressive diagnostic efforts are required to define the site and nature of the primary tumor since these tumors are generally curable with surgery. Localized endoscopic cytologic or photoactive marker methods may be useful. Repeated chest imaging studies, at monthly intervals if necessary, should be considered. Once properly staged, appropriate therapy is as outlined below.

Stage 0 (NSCLS). Carcinoma in situ. These tumors are noninvasive and do not metastasize; they should be curable by surgical resection. Second primary cancers are common. Endoscopic phototherapy with a hematoporphyrin derivative may be an alternative to surgical resection in selected patients. The least extensive resection possible should be done, conserving the maximum amount of lung tissue since these patients are at high risk for second lung cancers.

Stage I (NSCLC). Surgical resection should be carried out on all patients with Stage I NSCLC who can medically tolerate the procedure. Preoperative assessment of the patient's medical condition, particularly the pulmonary reserve, must be considered in assessing the benefits of surgery. Early postoperative mortality rates of 5 to 8 percent following pneumonectomy or 3 to 5 percent following lobectomy are generally reported, though risk is clearly age-related. Patients with impaired pulmonary function may be candidates for removal of the primary tumor by segmental or wedge resections. There is increasing interest in wide local excision by less than lobectomy in appropriate good-risk patients with Stage I lung cancers. Patients with insufficient pulmonary reserve for surgical approach may be considered for radiation therapy with curative intent. Patients over the age of 70 with Stage I lesions who are medically inoperable or who refuse surgery and undergo radiation with curative intent can expect survival at 5 years comparable to that for persons of similar age operated on for cure. Because of the high rates of brain metastases in adenocarcinoma and large-cell carcinoma, some have advocated prophylactic cranial irradiation to patients with these types of cancer. Most of the recent reports analyzing this approach have concluded that the benefits do not justify the neurologic sequelae reported. Prophylactic cranial irradiation is not usually recommended in patients with NSCLC without symptoms.

Several more recent reports of fewer survivors in general confirm their observations. A recent clinical trial demonstrated that nonspecific stimulation of the immune system (levamisole) has no effect as adjuvant therapy to radiation in patients with medically inoperable disease. Active investigation continues in immunotherapy protocols, although results remain unimpressive.

Mountain and associates have reported survival of 1533 patients surgically treated for Stage I non-small-cell bronchogenic carcinoma, and projected a 5-year survival of 50 percent overall. Figure 16-71, taken from their report, compares the survival according to stage and shows the effect of pulmonary lymph-node metastases. These authors made several other comparisons by

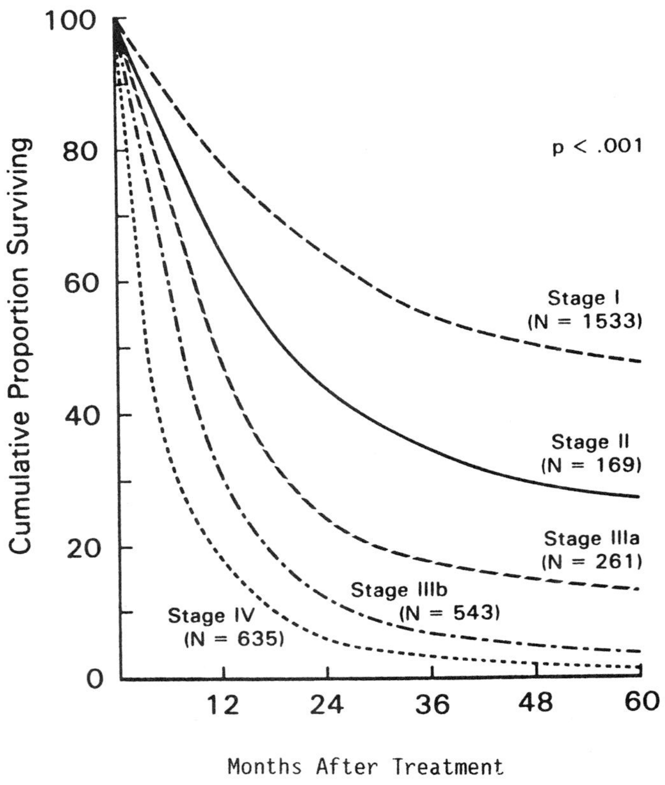

FIG. 16-71. Survival experience according to stage. (*Reproduced from: Mountain CF: A new international staging system for lung cancer. Chest 89:232S, 1986, with permission.*)

analysis of this extensive experience. They found the survival of women to be better than that of men in this series, and survival was better for patients less than 70 years of age than for those who were beyond 70 years. There were no overall significant differences in survival based on cell type.

Stage II NSCLC. Surgery is also the treatment of choice for Stage II tumors, and 30 percent of resected patients should expect 5-year survival. As with Stage I patients, those who are medically unacceptable for operation but who have sufficient pulmonary reserve to tolerate high-dose irradiation (5500 to 6000 cGy) can anticipate up to 20 percent 3-year survival. Careful target volume definition and avoidance of critical normal structures is important for optimal results.

Approximately 70 percent of surgically treated patients develop regional or distant metastatic disease. Therefore, most patients should be considered for adjuvant therapy, preferably through entry into an investigative clinical trial. As in several other controlled trials, Cox has shown a reduction in local recurrences after postoperative irradiation to N1 patients, but failed to demonstrate a survival benefit in squamous cell tumors although local recurrences were reduced.

Several trials in surgically resected patients who received adjuvant combination chemotherapy (cisplatin, doxorubicin, and cyclophosphamide) have reported a slight increase in disease-free survival and a trend toward improved survival. Further carefully conducted clinical trials are needed evaluating adjuvant chemotherapy after surgical resection before recommending such therapy routinely.

Stage IIIa NSCLC. The presence of lymph-node metastases has a profound effect on survival in bronchogenic carcinoma. In most patients with N2 (ipsilateral mediastinal node) involvement, definitive surgery is not indicated. When N2 disease is documented by prethoracotomy biopsy, the 5-year survival rate after definitive surgery is only about 2 percent. Surprisingly, patients with small primary squamous tumors (T1, T2), whose mediastinal lymph node involvement (N2) is discovered at thoracotomy, may benefit from resection of the primary and all gross nodal tumors with 5-year survival rates of 15 to 30 percent. In this situation, postoperative radiation therapy reduces local recurrences. A new approach to the treatment of patients with T1 to T3 and N2 tumors has recently been reported. In this study, preoperative chemotherapy (cisplatin and vindesine with or without mitomycin C) was administered for 2 to 3 cycles. Resection was subsequently accomplished in 50 percent of the patients with a 54 percent 3-year survival rate. These results are encouraging, and preoperative chemotherapy in patients with T1, T2 and N2 disease should be further evaluated.

Depending on the clinical situation, some combination of radiation therapy and surgery is the mainstay in treating patients with locally or regionally advanced tumors. Surgery remains an important modality; the only chance for "cure" may be in those who have resectional surgery. Several groups have reported 5-year survival of approximately 50 percent in T3, N0, M0 patients with chest wall invasion and wide resection. A special subset of these locally invasive tumors, the superior sulcus tumor (Pancoast tumor), has long been known to have a potential for satisfactory response to combined radiation and resection. In many reports of long-term survivors from large series, a few of the patients would appear to have had Stage III tumors. Though few patients achieve complete response to radiation, most have significant palliation and 5 to 10 percent will experience long-term survival benefit.

Stage IIIb NSCLC. In the special clinical setting of superior vena cava syndrome, prompt radiation therapy is indicated regardless of stage. The response to chemotherapy is too infrequent to rely on for routine management of this syndrome. Symptoms relating to specific local mechanical compression by growing tumor mass (tracheal, esophageal, bronchial, or superior vena caval obstruction, vocal cord paralysis, or hemoptysis) might respond to palliative radiation therapy. Appropriately timed radiation can maintain an acceptable life-style for a brief period in otherwise functional patients.

Stage IV (NSCLC). None of the currently reported therapeutic programs appears to offer any significant survival benefit for patients with distant metastases (M1). The only justification for administering toxic chemotherapeutic agents to lung cancer patients with distant metastases at this time is in those patients with good performance status who are able to be included in an investigational protocol. Only a small percentage of these patients can be expected to survive 5 years, though several selected subgroups may do reasonably well if aggressively treated, and an occasional long-term survivor is reported against all odds. Pending new evidence to support its use, chemotherapy should be given only to patients in a clinical trial setting who desire such treatment after being fully informed of its experimental status, anticipated risks, and limited benefits.

In some cases, endobronchial laser and/or brachytherapy has been used to alleviate proximal obstructing lesions. Such therapeutic intervention may prolong acceptable life-style in otherwise functional patients.

Solitary pulmonary metastases from a resected bronchogenic carcinoma are unusual, but second primary malignancies are relatively common in patients with primary lung cancers. Recent studies confirm that newly appearing lesions are most likely second primaries, and patients might achieve long-term survival after resection; if the first primary is controlled, the second primary should be resected.

Small-Cell Lung Cancer (SCLC). Patients with small-cell lung cancer should receive combination chemotherapy regardless of tumor dissemination. Current chemotherapy regimens prolong survival with a four- to five-fold increase in median survival and an overall survival at 10 years of about 5 percent. Most survivors are patients who have tumor confined to one hemithorax. If the tumor extends beyond the pleural space of origin, median survival falls to 6 to 12 months and long-term disease-free survival is anecdotal. Despite the dramatic improvements made over the past 10 to 15 years in diagnosis and therapy, the prognosis for more than short-term survival in patients with small-cell lung cancer is extremely poor regardless of stage. There are several encouraging multimodal therapy investigative protocols under way that are providing some encouraging improvements in short-term outlook. It is a rare patient with disease sufficiently localized to allow resection for cure by standard surgical criteria; these patients may have a reasonable prognosis if medically suitable for a radical surgical approach combined with chemotherapy and radiation. The Toronto Lung Oncology group projects 50 percent 5-year survival for Stage I disease, 25 percent for Stage II, and 19 percent for Stage III after combined treatment.

The Patient. Careful preoperative assessment of the patient's overall medical condition and especially the patient's pulmonary reserve are critical issues in considering the benefits of surgery. Unfortunately, by the time the diagnosis is made the opportunity for curative surgery has passed in about half of all patients with bronchogenic carcinoma. These patients have centrally located neoplasms with evidence of mediastinal extension, symptoms of distant metastases, or compromised cardiopulmonary function that precludes a major pulmonary resection.

Factors such as the patient's age, impaired pulmonary function, and tumor extension outside the lung vary in their influence on the decision of individual surgeons to attempt pulmonary resection. Though there is increasing risk of morbidity and mortality for those who undergo major pulmonary resection after 60 years of age, it has been demonstrated that patients of 70 years and beyond tolerate lobectomy with an acceptable mortality rate (Table 16-13). Similarly, impaired pulmonary function does increase the risk of operation, but Peters and associates have demonstrated an acceptable mortality and complication rate by careful analysis of the pulmonary-function data to allow the selection of patients who can be brought through the surgical experience. Invasion of either the phrenic or recurrent laryngeal nerve is considered a contraindication to thoracotomy by most surgeons, but this is not totally accepted. In particular, phrenic nerve involvement is usually along its course over the pericardium, and some surgeons advocate an en bloc resection of the involved area along with the pulmonary resection.

Surgical Considerations. Several technical advances have made it possible to extend the indications for surgical resection to a higher-risk group of patients. Less physiologically damaging incisions (the median sternotomy and the straight lateral-modified transaxillary), better anesthetic tools (double-lumen tubes, jet ven-

Table 16-13
Mortality and Age-risk Factors in Resections for Lung Cancer

LCSG mortality rates for pneumonectomy, lobectomy, and lesser resections

	No. of Resections	Deaths No.	Deaths Percent, %	
Pneumonectomy	569	44	6.2	
				$p < 0.001$*
Lobectomy	1058	35	2.9	
				$p =$ NS*
Lesser resection (segmentectomy or wedge excision)	143	2	1.4	

*Chi square, NS = not significant.

Age-risk factors obtained from LCSG data

Age, years	Mortality Rate, %	
< 60	1.3	
		$p < 0.001$*
60–69	4.1	
		$p = 0.014$*
> 70	7.1	

*Chi square.

SOURCE: From Ginsberg, Hill, et al, with permission.

tilation), and the increasing use of parenchyma-saving resections (sleeve resections, wedge resections, and segmental resections) have made it possible to offer potentially curative operations to patients previously considered inoperable.

Within recent years, some chest surgeons have followed the trends established in some other areas of surgical oncology by reconsidering the question of extent of resection. Historically, the total pneumonectomy has been considered the optimal operation for lung cancer (Fig. 16-72), but the increased mortality and morbidity of that operation lead to the wide acceptance of the lobectomy as an acceptable compromise. As the evidence accumulated that the prognosis did not seem to be compromised by the lesser resection, the lobectomy became the operation of choice whenever it was possible to adequately remove the primary without pneumonectomy. As experience has grown with sleeve and segmental resections, largely stimulated by the work of Jensik, a similar evolution in thinking seems to be taking place. A dozen reports have appeared in the past several years indicating comparable survival figures in selected bad-risk patients undergoing lung-salvaging procedures because they could not safely undergo more extensive resections. As anticipated, the short-term survival was improved; less expected was the equivalent or improved long-term control of tumor. Particularly noteworthy has been the comparable incidence of local recurrence among these patients and those with more traditional resections.

Adjuvant Therapy. Multiple-agent therapy has shown considerable success in the control of small-cell carcinoma, particularly when combined with radiation therapy to the primary disease in the thorax and prophylactic radiation therapy to the brain. The current treatment protocols for small-cell carcinoma generally include cyclophosphamide, doxorubicin, and vincristine. VP-16 has become an important chemotherapeutic agent and is being evaluated in combination protocols with doxorubicin and vincristine.

Chemotherapy for non-small-cell bronchogenic carcinoma has appeared to be more effective for adenocarcinoma and large-cell carcinoma than for squamous tumors. Five-year survival rates of up to 20 percent have been reported in adenocarcinoma using combinations of radiation therapy and chemotherapy with cyclophosphamide, Adriamycin, methotrexate, and procarbazine. More recently, cisplatinum is being substituted for procarbazine in the four-drug regimens. Most studies have confirmed that if the patients with unresectable lung cancer have a good performance status, they are likely to benefit from carefully administered chemotherapy.

Immunodeficiency. Recent studies have emphasized the important but not clearly defined role of immunodeficiency in the prognosis of patients with many forms of cancer. An impaired reaction to delayed cutaneous hypersensitivity testing with 2,4-dinitrochlorobenzene has been demonstrated in many lung cancer patients, and those who are unable to become sensitized to this antigen often have unresectable neoplasms. Impaired lymphocyte transformation with in vitro stimulation by several antigens and mitogens has also demonstrated a marked decrease in immunocompetence in patients with pulmonary carcinoma. One of the mechanisms of immunodeficiency is thought to be the presence of circulating immunosuppressive factors in the serum of the lung cancer patient. Whether such factors might be produced by the neoplasm is only speculative.

Hyman and associates made some provocative inferences about the protective effect of blood transfusions on the host acceptance of renal transplants which led them to evaluate the effect of transfusions on survival of lung cancer. In their small series, intraoperative blood transfusion seemed to worsen prognosis, as predicted. If verified, this observation could have important implications for host defense relationship to early dissemination of tumor cells.

Solitary Pulmonary Nodules

Among those patients with lung cancer, the best survival can be expected from that group of patients where the cancer is first found as an asymptomatic solitary peripheral pulmonary nodule on the chest x-ray. Because of this relatively favorable outlook if the nodule is a cancer, and because of the variety of nonmalignant lesions that also present in this fashion, there is considerable inter-

FIG. 16-72. Resection of lung. *A.* Opening into pleural cavity: (1) periosteum incised over the rib; (2) subperiosteal resection being performed; (3) pleura opened through bed of resected rib. *B.* Freeing of pulmonary artery from adjacent structures. *C.* Ligation and division of pulmonary artery: (1) artery doubly ligated with an adequate distance between the two ligatures; (2) artery transected between two ligatures. *D.* Peripheral dissection of pulmonary artery to increase safety factor: (1) branches of pulmonary artery and main pulmonary artery identified; (2) branches individually double-ligated and transected. *E.* Division of pulmonary vein. Double ligatures are on inferior pulmonary vein which is to be transected. *F.* Transection of bronchus. This is performed after ligation of pulmonary arteries and veins. Diagram indicates bronchial transection during a left pneumonectomy. (1) Clamp is applied to bronchus distad, and as the bronchus is transected, the proximal end is closed with interrupted sutures in order to avoid a widely open bronchus with its associated ventilatory disturbance; alternately, the bronchus may be closed with an automatic stapler. (2) Progression of bronchial transection. *G.* Pleural flap placed over sutured bronchial stump.

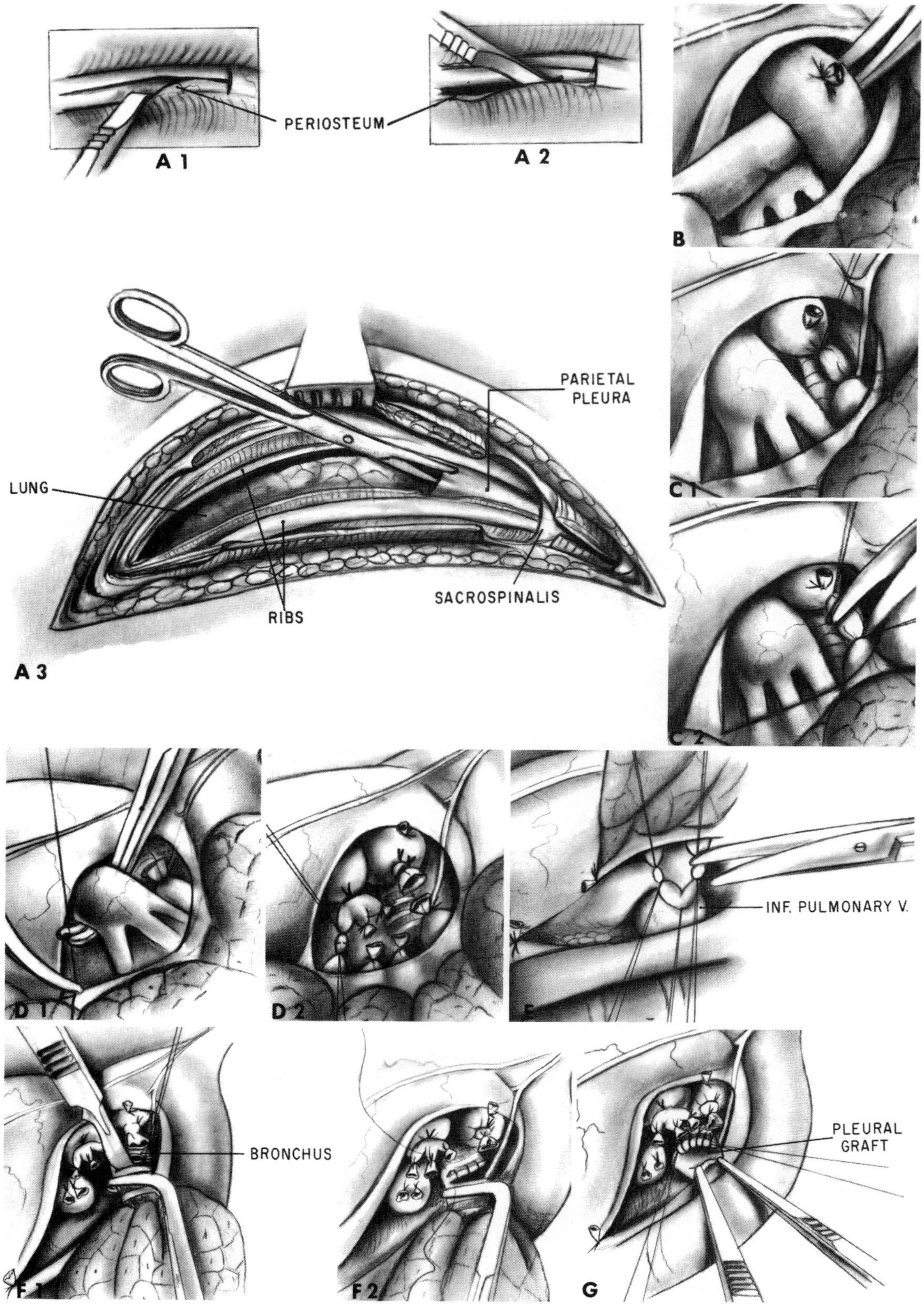
PERIOSTEUM
A 1
A 2
B
PARIETAL PLEURA
LUNG
RIBS
SACROSPINALIS
A 3
C 1
C 2
D 1
D 2
INF. PULMONARY V.
E
BRONCHUS
F 1
F 2
PLEURAL GRAFT
G

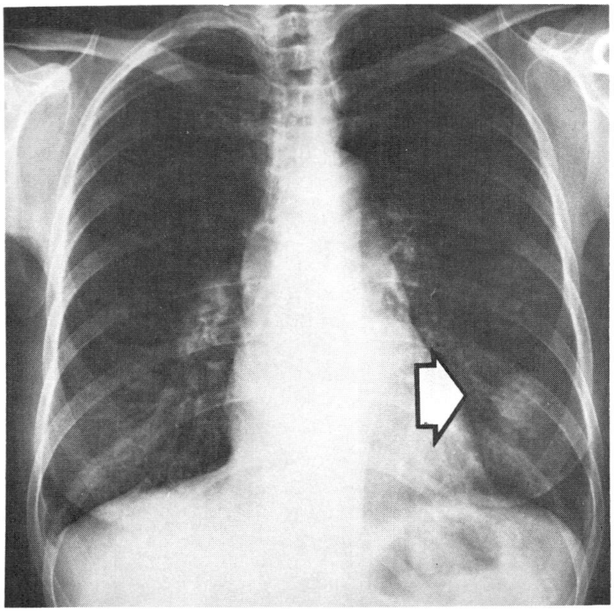

A

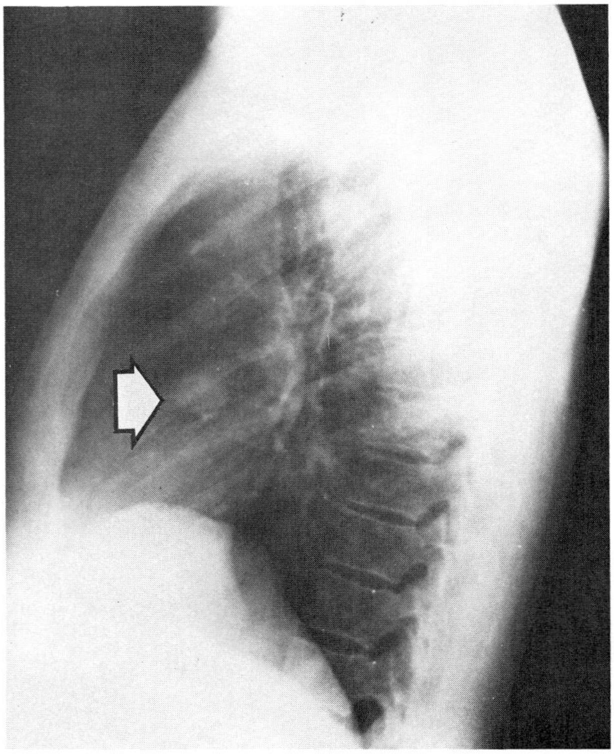

B

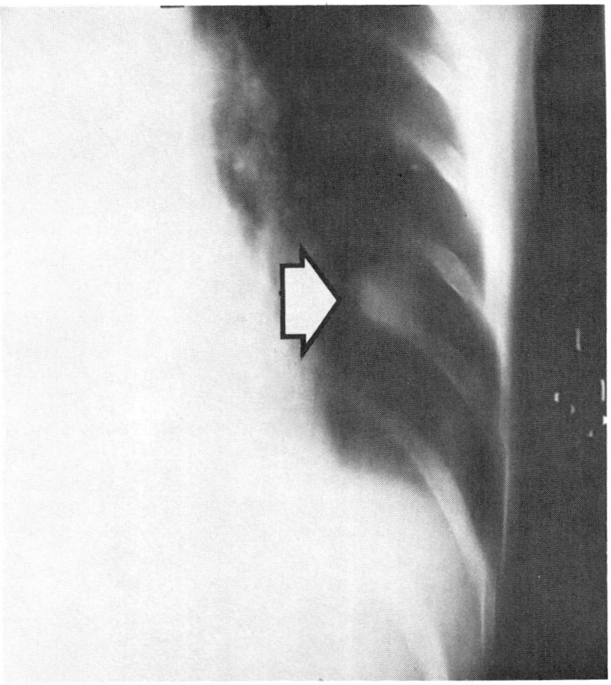

C

FIG. 16-73. A solitary pulmonary nodule. *A* and *B*. The posteroanterior and lateral chest x-rays show a round density in the lingula that had not been present on the patient's previous x-rays. *C*. The lesion is homogeneous, with smooth borders, on tomograms. A wedge resection showed the lesion to be a resolving pulmonary infarct.

est in the differential diagnosis of these "coin lesions." For convenience in discussion the solitary pulmonary nodule (SPN) has been defined by general agreement to be an abnormal density up to 4 cm in diameter, rounded or ovoid in appearance (Figs. 16-73 and 16-76), surrounded by a zone of lung tissue by x-ray, and free of cavitation or associated lung infiltrates. Eccentric flecks of calcium may be present, but lesions that are largely calcified or that have concentric calcium rings are not considered.

Whereas earlier reports suggested a malignancy rate of about 40 percent in the SPNs, in more recent analyses approximately 80 percent of all coin lesions were malignant in patients over 50 years. Only when the nodule is known to have been present for a long period with absence of growth and with a pattern of calcification characteristic of the several benign lesions that can occur should histologic diagnosis of these nodules be delayed.

Proof that the lesion has not recently developed requires inspection of old chest x-rays because faint, small lesions are frequently overlooked in screening films, and a negative official report has often been in error. Even when previous x-rays document radiologic stability of a solitary nodule for up to 2 years, malignancy must be suspected.

The differential diagnosis of an SPN includes many entities, among which are pulmonary hamartoma, granuloma, pulmonary arteriovenous fistula, pulmonary infarct, and several benign and malignant tumors. Since surgery is rarely indicated for the nonmalignant lesions under consideration, many clinics have recommended extensive diagnostic efforts to ascertain the correct diagnosis before thoracotomy. Unfortunately, there is a significant false-negative rate in virtually all the studies short of excisional biopsy. With improving imaging techniques, the odds of a correct preoperative diagnosis are improving, but with the consequences of error so high and with the reasonably good results following surgical resection, many surgeons feel it is unwise to gamble on a determination of benignancy unless the lesion is in a young (under 35), nonsmoking patient with a known history of radiographic stability.

Where calcification is present, CT is especially useful in improving the preoperative guess or in selecting the rare patient who can be safely observed. CT scans have the capacity to measure absorption coefficients and therefore indicate tissue density. Siegelman and associates used CT with thin sections to assess tissue density in 91 apparently noncalcified pulmonary nodules in 88 patients. They established a separation between benign and malignant lesions on the basis of high attenuation values in the benign SPN. The high values were presumably due to diffusely distributed calcium deposits within the lesions but not visible on standard radiographs. In the absence of calcium, however, benign SPN may have attenuation values in the same range as malignant lesions. Similarly, in a small proportion of cases, malignant lesions may have sufficient calcium to result in the high values characteristic of benign nodules.

For many years there has been a difference of opinion regarding the management of patients with solitary nodules with some groups advocating early thoracotomy with resection of the lesion for all patients above 35 years of age and others urging a more conservative approach with greater emphasis on diagnostic studies and observation. Though the resection policy did result in a 50 percent frequency of removal of benign lesions, excellent cure rates were expected if primary malignancies were found. With the sharply falling frequency of tuberculous granulomata and the continuing rise in lung cancer rates, current odds favor early resection unless there is strong evidence of a benign process. Sputum cytology, bronchoscopic washings and brushings, and percutaneous needle biopsies each provide clear-cut positive information if malignant cells are found but cannot exclude malignant disease.

If previous films are available for comparison, or if a course of observation is elected for other reasons, calculation of the time necessary for doubling of the tumor volume is a useful indicator of the nature of the lesion. Serial radiographs provide the data for calculation of growth rate, and it is generally possible to detect that a lesion is growing within a few weeks. The doubling time of malignant nodules is usually between 37 and 465 days. If the lesion is growing more slowly or more rapidly than this, the evidence is in favor of benignancy. Advocates of a conservative approach insist that present knowledge supports the concept that a pulmonary nodule can be watched safely for a period of time to determine whether it is growing.

A logical approach to the SPN would include early thoracotomy for lesions in known risk populations: age over 50, smoking history, absence of certain knowledge of a similar lesion on chest film more than 2 years old. A careful review should be made of systems for suggestion of symptoms that might justify a search for a primary elsewhere, but extensive (and expensive) screening in asymptomatic patients is probably not warranted. If the patient is under 35 and a nonsmoker, and the chance of malignancy is small, needle biopsy and bronchial brush biopsy are appropriate, with watchful waiting and close observation for growth or change. It is likely the next few years will see an enlarging role for video-assisted thoracoscopy to aid in diagnosis and resective therapy of these lesions.

Other Lung Tumors

Bronchopulmonary Neuroendocrine Tumors. Both Warren and associates and Benfield's group have recently presented analyses utilizing contemporary electron microscopic and immunohistochemical techniques to demonstrate the continuum that exists from carcinoids to small-cell undifferentiated lung cancers (SCLC). It now seems clear that this group of tumors are all neuroendocrine neoplasms arising from Kulchitsky cells. At the benign end of the spectrum, the bronchopulmonary carcinoid histologically resembles the carcinoid tumors of the small intestine. Along with cylindroma and mucoepidermoid tumors, the bronchial carcinoid was formerly referred to as a bronchial adenoma. This designation was awkward because the term adenoma implied a fundamental quality of benignancy that was not in keeping with the high incidence of malignant behavior shown by cylindroma and mucoepidermoid tumors. Further, a small proportion of bronchial carcinoids will metastasize to regional lymph nodes, with the result that reference was occasionally made to "metastasizing bronchial adenomas."

Over 80 percent of carcinoids arise in proximal bronchi, but peripheral origin beyond cartilage-containing bronchi does occur. The tumors grow slowly and protrude into the bronchial lumen making signs and symptoms of bronchial obstruction the principal clinical presentation. Unusual vascularity may cause hemoptysis as a presenting complaint (Fig. 16-74). The vascularity gives the tumor a deep pink or red color when visualized through a bronchoscope.

The extent of bronchial-wall involvement is variable, but there is usually invasion of the underlying cartilages. Rarely, direct extension through the bronchial wall can result in invasion of mediastinal structures. Regional lymph-node deposits are found in approximately 10 percent of patients, liver metastases more rarely. In keeping with the neuroendocrine origin of these tumors, a few patients with bronchial carcinoid have Cushing-like syndromes that seem attributable to the tumor.

Although the average age of patients with a carcinoid tumor is approximately 40 years, the neoplasm does occur in children. Commonly, the clinical presentation is a result of bronchial obstruction with infestation and pulmonary atelectasis. Sputum cytology is negative, but more than 80 percent of the lesions can be visualized by bronchoscopy. The carcinoid syndrome is seen rarely and can occur without extrathoracic metastases. It is wise to measure urinary 5-HIAA excretion and blood serotonin level, but these can be clearly elevated without corresponding symptoms.

The treatment for bronchial carcinoid tumor is surgical resection. Neither the primary neoplasm nor lymph-node metastases, when they occur, are sensitive to radiation therapy. Though lobectomy is an acceptable operation, most surgeons, in view of the low potential for malignancy of the carcinoid neoplasm, now recommend more conservative procedures such as sleeve resection or local bronchial excision with bronchoplasty whenever feasible (Fig. 16-75). The expected long-term survival rate is over 90 percent.

Tumors of Bronchial Gland Origin. Cylindroma, or adenocystic carcinoma, and mucoepidermoid tumors are the commonest neoplasms arising from the bronchial glands. Their location is predominantly central, and they are said to take origin only from bronchi containing cartilage. Both neoplasms may show a spectrum of behavior from benign to malignant, with regional and distant metastases. The treatment is surgical resection, including en bloc removal of regional lymph nodes when possible. Though the long-term cure rate is considerably higher than that of primary carcinoma of the lung, it does not equal the results in bronchial carcinoid.

Other rare tumors of bronchial gland origin are occasionally reported; the majority seem to be forms of adenocarcinoma.

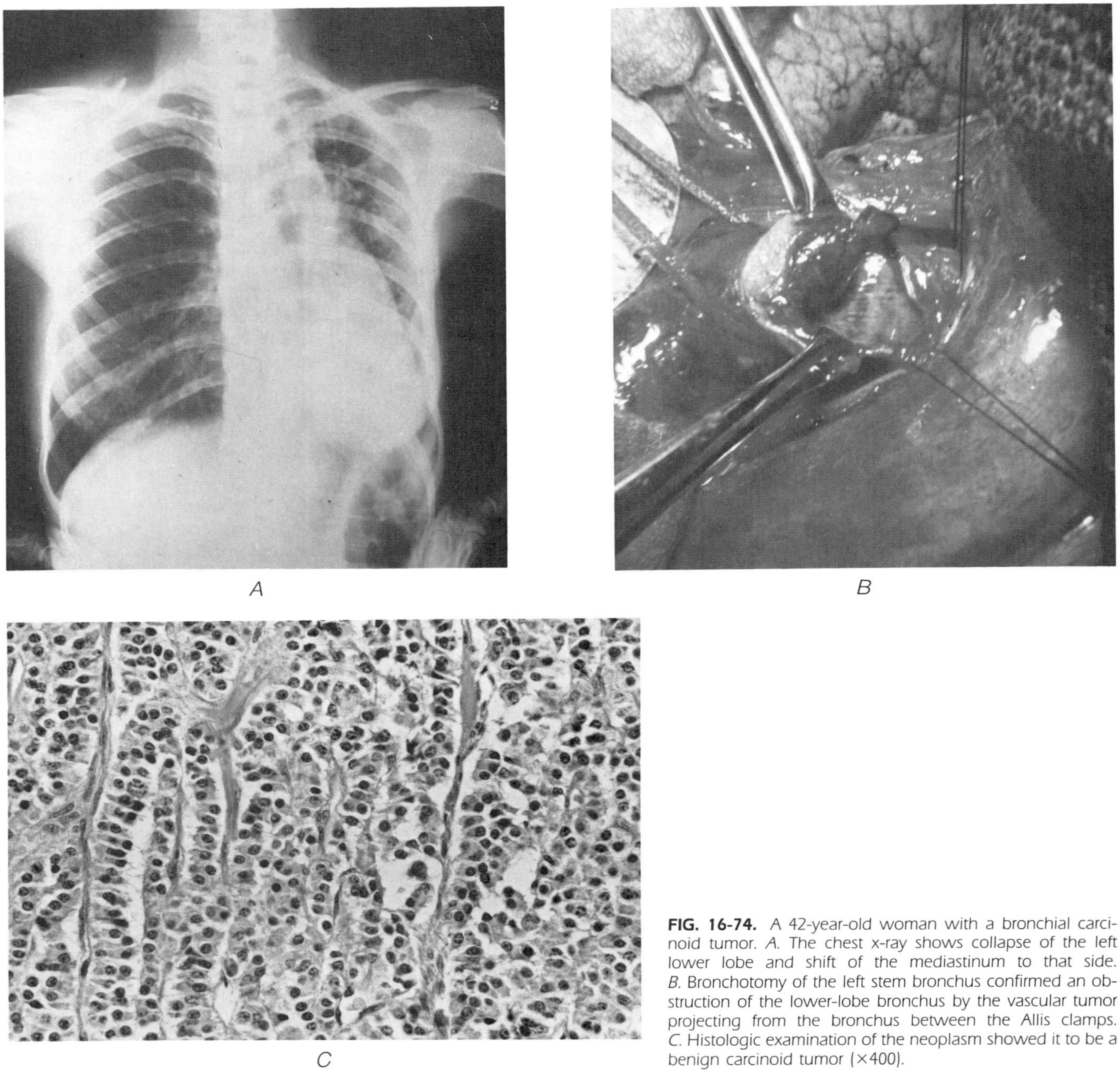

FIG. 16-74. A 42-year-old woman with a bronchial carcinoid tumor. *A.* The chest x-ray shows collapse of the left lower lobe and shift of the mediastinum to that side. *B.* Bronchotomy of the left stem bronchus confirmed an obstruction of the lower-lobe bronchus by the vascular tumor projecting from the bronchus between the Allis clamps. *C.* Histologic examination of the neoplasm showed it to be a benign carcinoid tumor (×400).

Carcinosarcoma. Making up less than 1 percent of lung cancers, the carcinosarcoma consists of both epithelial and mesenchymal types of tissue, and electron microscopy has confirmed that the sarcomatous elements are not simply transformed components of epithelial origin. The term blastoma has recently been used for some tumors that show histologic evidence of association with embryonal tissue.

Carcinosarcomas may be located in the lung periphery or in proximal bronchi, and they have been reported in a wide age range, including children. They most commonly are found in patients with tobacco addiction, in the sixth decade. Afflicted patients rarely survive into their second year after diagnosis.

Sarcoma. A variety of mesodermal sarcomas and tumors of reticuloendothelial origin may occur in the lungs. As a group these tumors represent approximately 1 percent of all primary neoplasms removed at operation. The age range of presentation is considerably wider than that for bronchogenic carcinoma, and the tumors may arise anywhere in the lung or bronchial tree. Difficulty with true histologic identification of the neoplasms is not rare, and they may be mistaken for highly undifferentiated carcinomas or metastatic neoplasms.

In general, the symptoms may be the same as those expected with primary carcinomas, but there is no distinct association with cigarette smoking. When the tumors develop as intrabronchial pol-

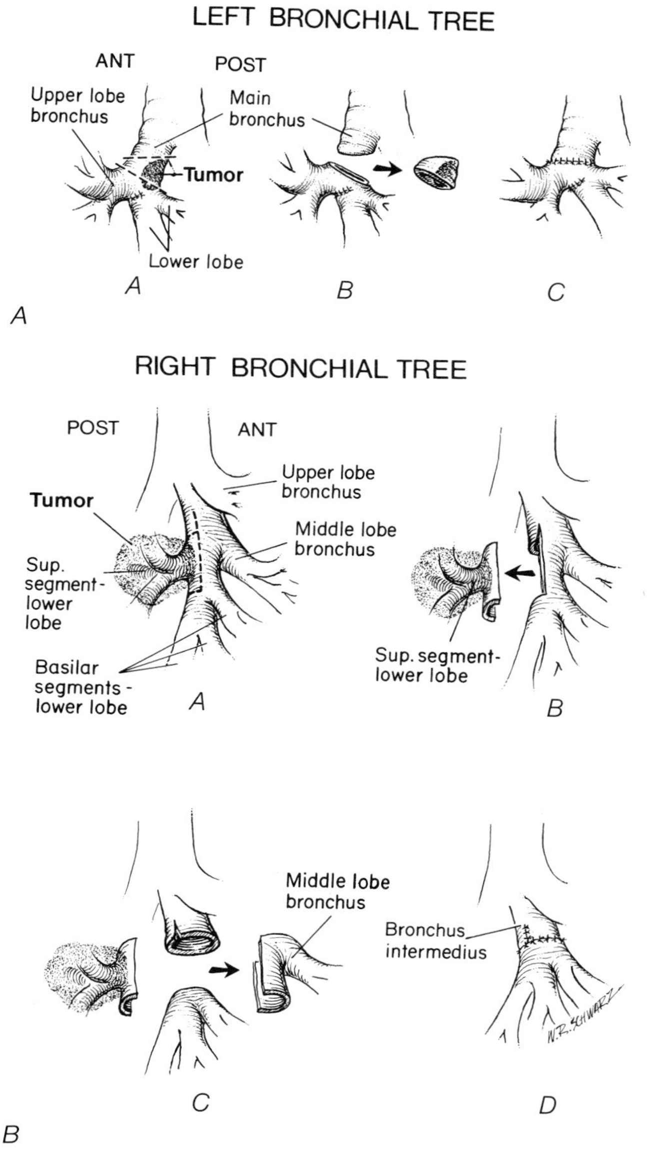

FIG. 16-75. Operative procedures to conserve pulmonary tissue in patients with bronchial carcinoid. *A.* Sleeve resection of tumor from left main bronchus. *B.* Superior segmentectomy and middle lobectomy with bronchial anastomosis. (From: *Jensik RJ, Faber LP, et al: Bronchoplastic and conservative resectional procedures for bronchial adenoma. J Thorac Cardiovasc Surg 68:556, 1974, with permission.*)

ypoid neoplasms, the symptoms of bronchial obstruction lead to earlier diagnosis and, therefore, a relatively higher cure rate after resection. Leiomyosarcomas, for example, had a 5-year cure rate of approximately 40 percent in McNamara's report.

Lymphosarcoma and reticulum cell sarcoma may rarely develop in the lung without evidence of tumor elsewhere. Routine chest x-rays discover an asymptomatic pulmonary lesion in a number of patients; other lesions become symptomatic because of pressure of the growing tumor or lymph nodes on adjacent structures. There is no characteristic radiographic appearance, and the diagnosis is rarely suspected from sputum cytology or bronchoscopy. Percutaneous needle biopsy may give the diagnosis with either neoplasm.

A sufficient number of lymphosarcomas are localized to make the prognosis good after pulmonary resection. A 5-year survival exceeding 50 percent may be anticipated, but the results with reticulum cell sarcoma are not as good because the neoplasm is less often resectable.

Hodgkin's disease frequently involves the lung, and a rare patient is seen in whom a solitary pulmonary lesion is unassociated with other evidence of tumor. If resection has been performed, the patient should have complete staging of the disease so that decisions regarding additional therapy can be made.

Fibrosarcoma, rhabdomyosarcoma, neurofibrosarcoma, and other tumors of mesodermal origin may occur rarely in the lung but without specific clinical presentation. The treatment is surgical resection, and the prognosis depends on the stage at which the neoplasm was discovered.

Benign Tumors. Primary or metastatic cancers make up 99 percent of all pulmonary tumors, and benign tumors are a relatively small fraction of the other 1 percent. Among that group of rare tumors, the hamartoma (chondroadenoma) is the commonest. Though occasionally seen in children, they usually appear in men in their fifth to sixth decades, produce no symptoms, and are found in the periphery of dependent portions of the lungs (Fig. 16-76). The characteristic marblelike feel of these cartilaginous tumors makes it is usually possible to simply enucleate them; wedge resection may be preferred if the physical findings leave the surgeon uncertain about the diagnosis. Epithelial elements are generally present, and there may be fat, muscular, or fibrous tissue interspersed.

Since benign tumors can theoretically occur wherever the cells from which they might arise are present, a wide variety of other exceedingly rare tumors are occasionally reported. They can be

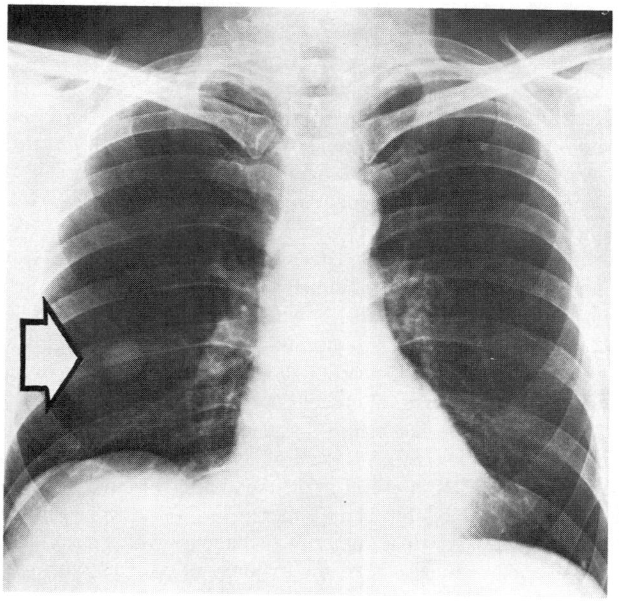

FIG. 16-76. This posteroanterior chest x-ray shows a smooth round density in the midlung field that proved to be a hamartoma when removed by wedge resection.

epithelial (tumorlet and papilloma), mesenchymal (fibroma, leiomyoma, lipoma, hemangioma, lymphangioma, neuroma, and rhabdomyoma), or lymphoid (plasmacytoma, lymphocytoma, plasma cell granuloma). Neurofibromas may occur, particularly in patients with neurofibromatosis. The significance of these tumors is almost exclusively related to the differential diagnosis from malignancies. When these neoplasms develop in a major bronchus, they may obstruct and present with the effects of chronic infection.

Metastatic Tumors

Metastases to the lung are common during the clinical course of many uncontrolled primary neoplasms of extrathoracic origin. Cells are shed into the vascular system and are trapped in the first capillary bed encountered; for primary sites not in contact with the venous portal system, this is the lung. Surgical manipulation of primary tumors might contribute to the shedding of cells, but metastases can appear at any time, even long after the primary seems controlled. Five-year survival rates following resection of one or more pulmonary metastases can result in 25 to 45 percent 5-year survival rate for patients with several types of carcinoma or sarcoma.

Since the treatment of solitary pulmonary metastases in patients with controlled primaries has been aggressive surgery, randomized, prospective clinical trials comparing surgical resection with medical management have not been done and today would probably be considered unethical. Because of the relatively good results of resection, and the absence of evidence that other therapeutic modalities are curative, surgical removal of isolate pulmonary metastases remains the accepted treatment for many tumors.

Evidence is ambiguous about tumor characteristics that correlate with 5-year survival. While it seems logical that long tumor doubling times (greater than 40 days) should portend a better outcome, shorter doubling times do not contraindicate surgery if other criteria are met. Equivalent survival rates are found when unilateral and bilateral disease are compared. Contrary to expectations, the disease-free interval (time between initial treatment of the primary and appearance of the metastasis) lacks verifiable predictive value. Only the cell type of the original tumor and its biologic behavior has been firmly linked to prognosis. Table 16-14 summarizes Mountain's results with individual tumor types. Nonseminomatous testicular carcinomas and osteogenic sarcomas have particularly encouraging outlooks with long-term survival near 50 percent. Patients with malignant melanomas do poorly; only one in eight can be expected to survive 5 years.

The problem to be considered when a patient presents with a solitary pulmonary nodule, either synchronous or metachronous from an extrathoracic tumor, is whether it is a metastasis, a primary pulmonary tumor, or a non-neoplastic lesion. When lesions are picked up on a routine chest radiograph following patients with resected colon cancers, almost 90 percent will be malignant. CT scans, which can locate lesions 2 mm in size, have a lower specification for tumor—only 45 percent of lesions picked up on CT will be neoplastic. MRI is useful in differentiating vascular structures from solid structures but is not superior to CT for evaluating pulmonary metastases. The majority of patients with breast cancer have a primary lung cancer; the majority of patients with melanoma have metastases; patients with colon or other gastrointestinal cancers have an equal frequency of each.

The work-up of a pulmonary metastasis should primarily consist of an aggressive search for other metastases from the original tumor. Besides the standard radiographic and radioisotopic surveys for metastatic disease, other special procedures are indicated depending on the known biologic behavior of the primary neoplasm. It is not mandatory to establish the diagnosis of a presumed metastasis before thoracotomy. In the absence of strong evidence that the lesion is non-neoplastic, that there are extra-thoracic metastases, that the primary is uncontrolled, or that the patient is unable to medically tolerate a limited resection, an aggressive surgical approach is the mainstay of treatment.

Table 16-14
Survival by Cell Type Following Resection for Metastases to the Lung

Cell Type	No. of Patients		Cumulative Percent Surviving 5 Years	
Carcinoma (N = 242)				
Squamous cell carcinoma	75		31.7	
Adenocarcinoma	79		40.4	
All other carcinoma	88		43.5	
Embryoma		9		33.3
Transitional cell		14		41.3
Teratoma		9		63.5
Sarcoma (N = 141)				
Osteogenic sarcoma	56		50.7	
Fibrosarcoma	16		37.5	
All other sarcoma	69		26.9	
Ewing's tumor		7		21.4
Rhabdomyosarcoma		6		16.7
Neurofibrosarcoma		5		60.0
Fibrohistiocytoma		8		37.5

SOURCE: From Mountain, McMurtrey, Hermes, with permission.

Metastases can usually be adequately removed by a wedge or segmental resection. Lobectomies or pneumonectomies are rarely justified. A more extensive resection is considered only if the lesion is near the hilus and cannot be safely removed by wedge or sleeve resection. It is important to conserve as much lung tissue as possible because a certain percent of these patients will undergo multiple resections.

Some authors advocate median sternotomy as the preferred approach for pulmonary metastatic disease. Median sternotomy allows for palpation of both lungs and provides adequate exposure for most resections. Patients with median sternotomy have less postoperative pain, a shorter convalescence, and can start or resume chemotherapy faster.

With the increased effectiveness of chemotherapy in selected tumors, the role of surgery for pulmonary metastases is changing. With nonseminomatous testicular cancer, chemotherapy has been so successful that surgical resection of metastases is used primarily to establish the diagnosis, to resect metastases proved unresponsive to chemotherapy, and to reclassify lesions that do not disappear totally following chemotherapy. The role of the video-assisted thoracoscope may prove particularly valuable in the diagnosis and removal of metastatic lesions.

In the treatment of metastatic carcinoma of the colon, Kemeny and associates have reported encouraging results with chemotherapy. Thirty-four patients with colonic cancer metastasized to the lung showed a complete or partial response to treatment with methyl-CCNU, 5-FU, and streptozotocin. If further data confirm this trend, the role of surgery for metastatic colon carcinoma to the lungs may change.

Though resection remains the standard treatment in suitable patients with limited pulmonary metastatic disease and in patients with a variety of controlled primary malignant tumors, thoracotomy and resection may assume new roles as chemotherapeutic advances occur.

TRACHEA

Anatomy. The trachea is a centrally located unpaired organ that shares with the heart singular importance in the physiologic matters of moment-to-moment survival. It follows an oblique course from a vulnerable superficial position in the neck deep into the cloistered recesses of the middle mediastinum. The adult trachea has an average length of 11 cm (range 10 to 13 cm) segmented by 18 to 22 cartilaginous rings, and has elliptical internal dimensions averaging 2.3 cm in lateral diameter and 1.8 in anteroposterior diameter. The cricoid cartilage of the larynx, which merges with the first tracheal ring, is the only complete cartilaginous ring. The membranous trachea is a flexible sheet of tissue forming the posterior wall of the trachea between the ends of the rings, and lies against the esophagus. The rigid rings of the anterior two-thirds of the trachea combined with the flexible posterior third impart great flexibility without collapse over a broad range of flexion, extension, and torsion, and maintains patency of the lumen through the extremes of coughing and forced respiration. The loss of cartilaginous support in tracheomalacia allows dynamic collapse and airway obstruction.

The important anterior relationships of the trachea are the thyroid isthmus, lying across the second to third rings, the innominate artery crossing obliquely several more rings distally, and the aortic arch crossing just above the carina. Laterally, the recurrent nerves lie close to the trachea in the tracheoesophageal groove, with the left recurrent following a longer course, joining the trachea just above the carina after passing around the ligamentum arteriosum. Since the blood supply enters laterally, dissection along the trachea is safest when confined to anterior and posterior planes. The major arterial inflow for the cervical trachea comes from the inferior thyroid artery. Lower portions of the trachea are supplied by branches of the bronchial arteries. Small branches from other mediastinal arteries can assume importance following tracheal division, as, for example, the coronary arterial branches that have been shown to provide blood supply to the tracheal anastomosis following heart-lung transplant.

Congenital Lesions

The most common congenital lesion involving the trachea is a tracheoesophageal fistula, the management of which is discussed in detail elsewhere. Congenital tracheal stenosis presents in several variants, all of which are uncommon. Simple weblike diaphragms can be seen, usually at the subcricoid level. Segments of functional stenosis due to tracheomalacia can be seen at sites of compression by a vascular ring or an anomalous pulmonary artery (pulmonary artery sling). Another variant is characterized by absence of the membranous trachea with fusion of the cartilaginous rings posteriorly over a variable distance, presenting in three principal forms: (1) segmental stenosis; (2) funnel stenosis, in which the distal trachea tapers to a tight stenosis just above the carina; and (3) diffuse hypoplasia of the entire trachea.

Diagnosis. Congenital stenosis should be suspected in any infant with noisy breathing, wheezing, and retractions occurring shortly after birth. The necessary diagnostic evaluation is exhaustive, reflecting the broad differential diagnosis and the association with other anomalies. Radiographic studies include chest films with magnification focused on the trachea, in inspiration and expiration, barium swallow, xeroradiography, CT scan of the neck and mediastinum, and angiography. Inspiratory and expiratory flow-volume curves, echocardiography, bronchoscopy, and bronchography are also frequently helpful. Great care is taken during bronchoscopy to prevent mucosal irritation and edema from converting partial to total obstruction.

Treatment. Therapy is individualized to suit the anatomy and the age of the child. Operative treatment is indicated if repeated dilatations or tracheostomy fail to allow growth, and every attempt is made to postpone reconstruction during infancy. When possible, the stenotic segment is resected and the trachea reconstructed with an end-to-end anastomosis. Diffuse involvement presents a greater technical challenge in which successful results have been rare, although Kimura and associates have shown that satisfactory reconstructions can be performed using splints constructed from rib or costal cartilage to patch the length of the stenotic segment (Figure 16-77) reinforced with an omental pedicle flap. Perioperative airway management and the maintenance of lumenal patency during healing and remodeling pose major challenges. Relief of tracheal stenosis related to vascular anomalies requires more than simple correction of the vascular anomaly in about half of the cases. Simple congenital webs can occasionally be removed bronchoscopically.

Trauma

Blunt and penetrating trauma produce a spectrum of tracheal injury ranging from simple laceration or contusion to complete transection. Hemoptysis, stridor, wheezing, or the presence of subcutaneous air following trauma require that the possibility of tracheal injury be evaluated by bronchoscopy or exploration. Occasionally a primary reconstruction will be indicated, but the more conservative approach of inserting a tracheostomy tube at the site of injury is often more rational.

Currently the most common tracheal injury requiring treatment is that occurring as a complication of tracheal intubation for mechanical ventilation (Fig. 16-78). Modern endotracheal tubes and tracheostomy tubes with soft, low-pressure cuffs have reduced but not eliminated the problem. Ischemic necrosis at the site of the tube cuff or the tube tip can produce a segment of ischemic stricture, a segment of tracheomalacia with functional obstruction during expiration, or erosion and fistula formation with the esophagus or the innominate artery. At the site of a tracheal stoma, exuberant granulations can form a bulky obstruction, or cicatricial healing may form an anterolateral stricture.

Areas of stricture should be carefully defined with radiographic studies that include magnified air contrast examination of the trachea, xeroradiography, and CT scan of the cervical region and upper mediastinum. Particular attention is paid to definition of laryngeal function, which can be done by fluoroscopy. Bronchoscopy is essential but is often deferred to the time of operation to avoid precipitation of tracheal obstruction in an uncontrolled setting.

Treatment. The operative approach for reconstruction of tracheal strictures is similar to that described below for the resec-

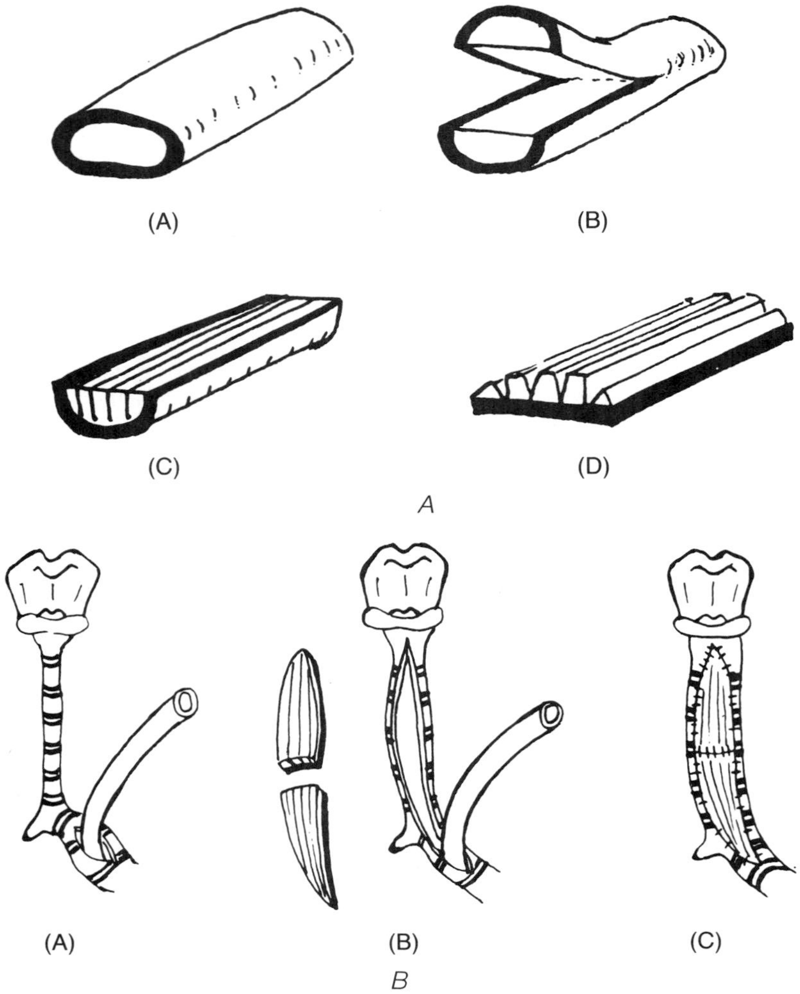

FIG. 16-77. One technique for reconstruction of congenital tracheal stenosis using autologous costal cartilage. *A.* The costal cartilage (A) is longitudinally split (B). Parallel longitudinal slits are made (C) to render the graft flexible (D). *B.* The stenotic trachea (A) is longitudinally opened (B), and the anterior wall reconstructed with the grafts (C). The long-term results with this method are not yet known. (From: *Kimura K, Mukohara N, et al: J Pediatr Surg 17:869, 1982, Figs 3 and 4, with permission.*)

tion of tracheal neoplasms (Fig. 16-79). The endoscopic laser can be useful for removal of granulation tissue but has no place in the treatment of stricture. Tracheoesophageal and tracheoinnominate fistulas are repaired by separating the two structures, closing the defects, and interposing muscle. For tracheoinnominate fistulas it is usually not necessary to reconstruct the innominate artery; rather the involved segment is resected and the two ends ligated.

Neoplasms

Primary tracheal neoplasms are uncommon and are outnumbered by tumors that involve the trachea by direct extension from a bronchial, laryngeal, esophageal, or thyroid primary. More than 80 percent of primary tracheal neoplasms are malignant, with squamous cell carcinoma and adenoid cystic carcinoma accounting for the vast majority of histological types. Adenoid cystic carcinoma is radiosensitive and usually slow-growing, even when metastatic, so resection combined with radiotherapy offers excellent long-term results. Squamous papillomas and fibromas are the most common benign tumors. A variety of rare benign and malignant neoplasms have been identified in the trachea, including carcinoid, chondroma, adenocarcinoma, mucoepidermoid carcinoma, and many others.

Diagnosis. Symptomatic patients with tracheal tumors present with some combination of dyspnea, cough, wheezing, inspiratory stridor, hemoptysis, and recurrent respiratory infections. Chest x-rays can have the detrimental effect of delaying further evaluation because the lung fields are clear, but an alert physician will obtain magnification laminagrams of the trachea and a CT scan of the cervical region and upper mediastinum. Standard pulmonary function testing may be normal, but flow-volume loops can detect airway obstruction. Bronchoscopy is an essential part of the evaluation but is best approached cautiously after maximum information has been obtained from noninvasive methods, because of the potential for precipitation of acute airway obstruction. When approached carefully, most tumors can be biopsied endoscopically and a tissue diagnosis confirmed before proceeding with further treatment.

Treatment. Resection, tracheostomy, and endoscopic ablation are the invasive options for treatment of tracheal neoplasms. Tracheostomy is pure palliation in patients with inoperable disease. Endoscopic ablation has been gaining favor in recent years because of advances in laser technology.

Laser Endoscopy. Developed in 1960, lasers produce coherent, low-divergence, high-intensity light capable of destroying tis-

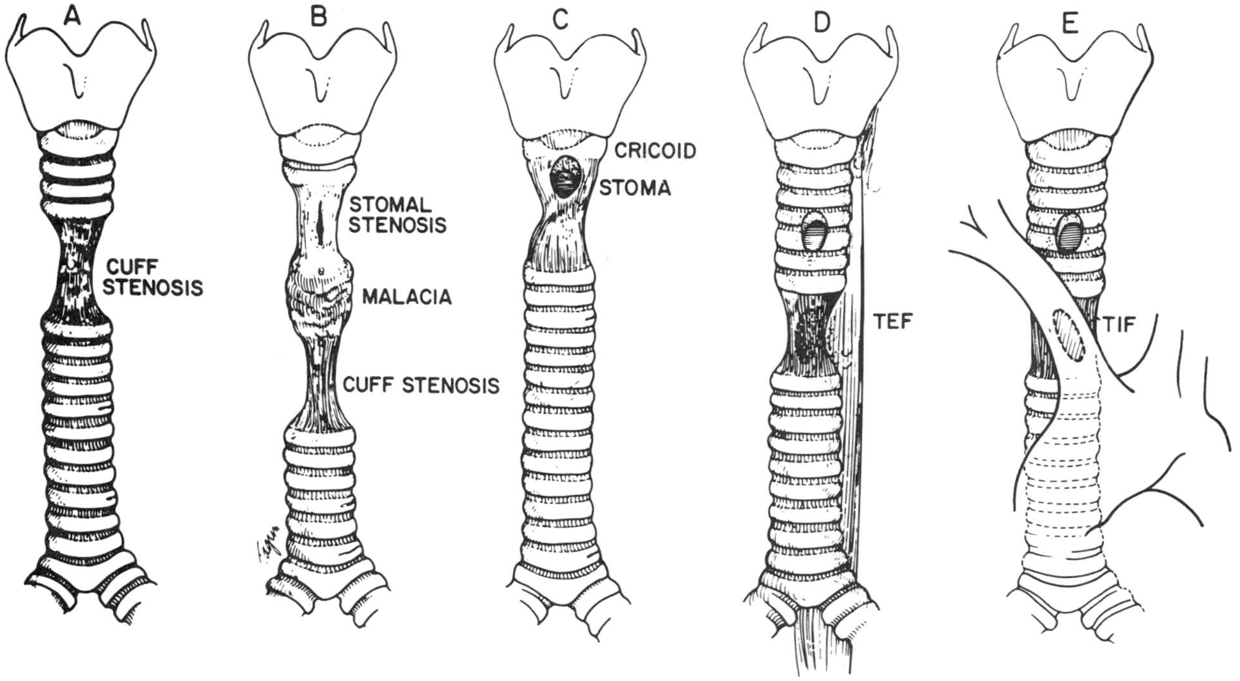

FIG. 16-78. Diagram of principal postintubation lesions. *A.* Lesion at cuff site in a patient who has been treated with an endotracheal tube alone. The lesion is high in the trachea and circumferential. *B.* Lesions that occur with tracheostomy tubes. At the stomal level, anterolateral stenosis is seen. At the cuff level, lower than with an endotracheal tube, circumferential cuff stenosis occurs. The segment between is often inflamed and malacic. *C.* Damage to the subglottic larynx. A high tracheostomy or one that erodes back by virtue of the patient's anatomy may damage the inferior cricoid and produce a low subglottic stenosis as well as an upper tracheal injury. *D.* Tracheoesophageal fistula (TEF). The level of fistulization is usually where the cuff has eroded posteriorly. Occasionally, angulation of the tip of the tube may produce erosion of the tip. There is also usually circumferential damage at this level by the cuff. *E.* Tracheoinnominate fistula (TIF). A high-pressure cuff frequently rests on the trachea directly behind the innominate artery. Erosion may occur, although rarely. The more common innominate artery injury is from a low tracheostomy where the inner portion of the curve of the tube rests in proximity to the artery and causes direct erosion. (From: *Grillo H: J Thorac Cardiovasc Surg 78:860, 1979, Fig 2, with permission.*)

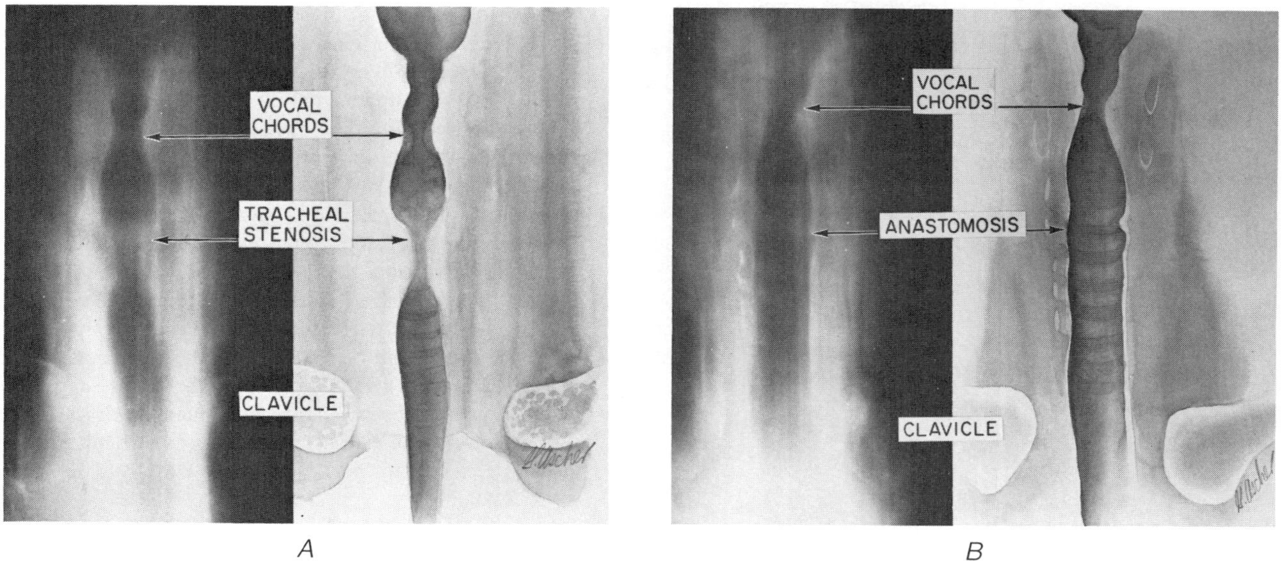

FIG. 16-79. Resection and the anastomosis of the trachea for tracheostomy stomal stenosis. *A.* A tomogram of the cervical trachea demonstrates the area of stenosis. *B.* A postoperative tomogram shows restoration of a normal tracheal lumen after resection and end-to-end anastomosis.

sue. As early as 1964, lasers were used experimentally to kill tumor cells. The CO_2 laser was the first of the five major types of laser to be used extensively for resection of neoplasms. The CO_2 laser is very effective for tissue cutting and vaporization, but use in the trachea requires a rigid bronchoscope because the beam cannot be passed through fiberoptic systems. The neodymium-yttrium aluminum garnet (Nd-YAG) laser is currently favored because it is almost as effective as the CO_2 laser and can be used through fiberoptic systems. In several large series excellent results have been obtained in up to 92 percent of patients treated for unresectable obstructing tumors of the trachea (Fig. 16-80). Laser resection, however, is not always better than more traditional methods of palliative endoscopic resection using forceps and cautery. Use of laser ablation as the sole treatment for benign tracheal neoplasms is also controversial.

Another interesting application of laser technology as a preoperative means of increasing resectability has been reported by Kato

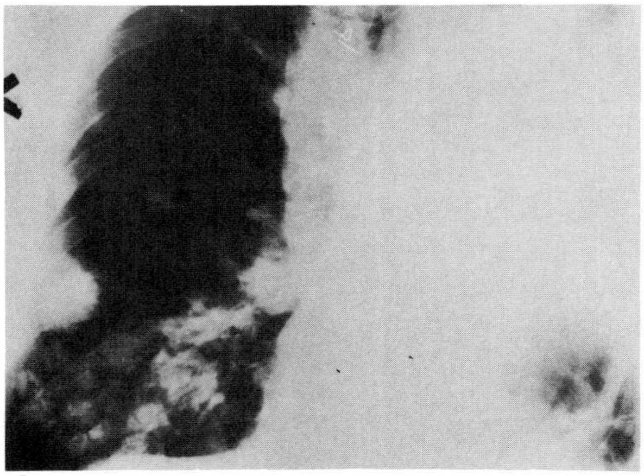

A

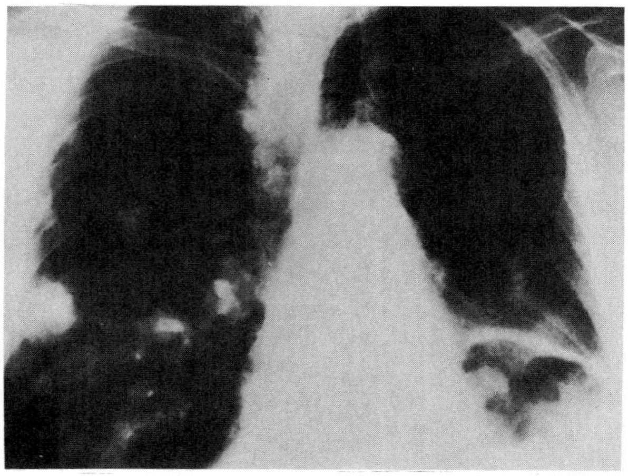

B

FIG. 16-80. *A.* Chest x-ray of a patient with metastatic renal cell carcinoma obstructing the left main-stem bronchus. Note the complete atelectatic opacification of the left lung, and the parenchymal metastases in the right lung. *B.* After Nd-YAG laser ablation of the bronchial lesion, the left lung is reexpanded. (From: *Unger M, Atkinson GW: Nd:YAG applications in pulmonary and endotracheal lesions, in Joffe SN, Muckerheide MC, Goldman L (eds): Neodymium-YAG Laser in Medicine and Surgery, chap 9, p 78, Elsevier, 1984, with permission.*)

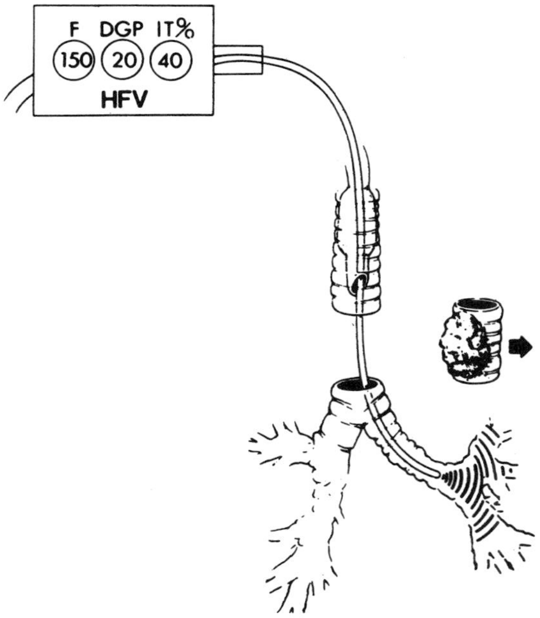

FIG. 16-81. Catheter for high-frequency positive-pressure ventilation ("jet" ventilation) shown passing through the endotracheal tube, across the tracheal lesion, and into the distal left main-stem bronchus. Ventilation is satisfactory with the trachea open, and the field is relatively unobstructed. In the illustration, the high-frequency ventilator (HFV) is set for a frequency of 150 breaths/min. (From: *El-Baz N, Jensik R, et al: Ann Thorac Surg 34:564, Fig 4, with permission.*)

and associates. Hematoporphyrin derivatives, which are tumoricidal when stimulated by light and are reported to be preferentially retained by malignant tissues, were injected into 15 patients with lung cancer involving the proximal tracheobronchial tree. After 48 to 72 h photodynamic therapy was performed by directing an argon laser beam on the tumors. The authors assert that four out of five originally inoperable cases became operable and that seven out of ten patients originally thought to require pneumonectomy were treated with lesser resections.

The ease of ventilation during tracheal reconstruction has been greatly facilitated by the development of high-frequency "jet" ventilation, which is delivered to the distal airway through a small catheter passed through the endotracheal tube (Fig. 16-81). A small tidal volume is delivered at high frequency (60 to 150 breaths/min), maintaining lung expansion, alveolar ventilation, and oxygenation in the normal range. The catheter is small enough to pass through most stenoses and interferes little with exposure.

The choice of incision for tracheal reconstruction depends on the level of involvement, and somewhat on the age of the patient. In a young patient hyperextension of the neck brings more than half the trachea above the suprasternal notch, accessible through a cervical incision. In older patients, it can be difficult to bring more than the first few tracheal rings above the notch. In general, lesions involving the upper half of the trachea are approached through a cervical collar incision, augmented as necessary with a midline upper sternal extension. Lesions involving the lower half can be approached through a right posterolateral thoracotomy (Grillo), entering the hemithorax at or above the fifth rib, or through a median sternotomy (Pearson). All cases are preceded by bronchoscopy in the operating room, at which time particularly tight stenoses (lumenal diameter < 5 mm) should be dilated to temporarily facilitate anesthesia.

Surprising lengths of trachea can be resected and reconstructed with end-to-end anastomosis. Minimizing tension on the anastomosis is critical and is accomplished by holding the neck in hyperflexion for at least 7 days postoperatively and by performing a laryngeal release procedure. Care is taken to avoid disturbance of the lateral blood supply, and only 1.5 cm of trachea should be circumferentially dissected on either side of the anastomosis. In most cases, 4.5 to 5 cm of trachea (at least eight rings) should be resectable. A wide variety of complex reconstructions involving the larynx, carina, and both main-stem bronchi have been described in detail by Grillo and others. The use of prosthetic materials for tracheal reconstruction remains anecdotal and experimental. Methods that appeared promising in series reported more than 10 years ago by Neville and by Moghissi have failed to achieve widespread application.

MEDIASTINUM

The mediastinum is the central cavity of the thorax, bounded on either side by the pleural cavities, bounded inferiorly by the diaphragm, and merging superiorly with the thoracic inlet. No compartment of the body carries more physiologic traffic. Many liters of blood pass through the mediastinum each minute, as liters of air, all ingested material and saliva, most autonomic nervous activity, and all the body's lymphatic fluid pass through the same confined space. Much of the embryologic development of the circulatory, respiratory, and digestive systems takes place within the mediastinum. Congenital, traumatic, inflammatory, and neoplastic processes all find frequent expression in this complex compartment, and produce a broad spectrum of pathology in which anatomic relationships assume paramount importance.

The mediastinum is conveniently divisible along rough anatomic boundaries into subcompartments that contain characteristic lesions. The most traditional classification recognizing four spaces has largely given way to a system recognizing three spaces, which divides the highly overlapping contents of the superior compartment between the more surgically relevant anterior and posterior compartments (Fig. 16-82). In this system the anterior mediastinum lies anterior to the heart and extends cephalad into the anterior half of the thoracic inlet, where it meets the posterior mediastinum. The posterior mediastinum lies behind the heart, extending cephalad into the thoracic inlet where the anterior borders of the upper thoracic vertebrae form its boundary with the anterior mediastinum. The middle mediastinum is the wedge in between, with its base lying on the diaphragm and its apex at the top of the aortic arch.

The anterior mediastinum contains the thymus, along with a variable amount of adipose, areolar, and lymphatic tissue. The middle mediastinum contains the heart and pericardium, aorta, trachea and main-stem bronchi, and associated lymph nodes. The posterior mediastinum contains the descending aorta, the esophagus, autonomic nerve trunks, and the thoracic duct.

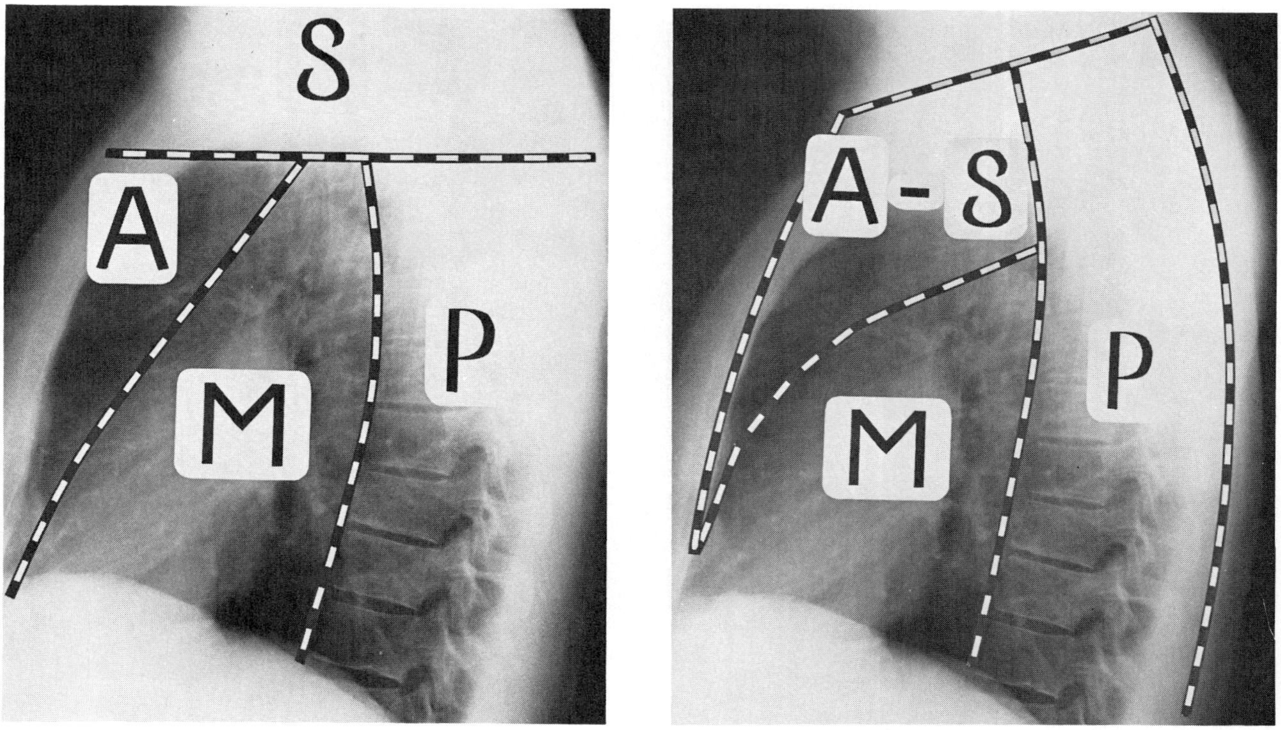

A B

FIG. 16-82. The anatomic divisions of the mediastinum. *A.* The traditional classification divides the mediastinum into superior (S), anterior (A), middle (M), and posterior (P) compartments. *B.* A more clinically relevant classification divides the superior compartment between the anterior and posterior compartments. (From: *Burkell CC, Cross JM, et al: Mass lesions of the mediastinum, in Ravitch MM (ed): Current Problems in Surgery. Year Book Medical Publishers, Chicago, 1969, with permission.*)

The great majority of mediastinal lesions appear as mass lesions radiographically, and most are neoplasms or cysts. A small number of mediastinal mass lesions are inflammatory or infectious. Vascular lesions, such as aneurysms, are considered elsewhere.

Tumors and Cysts

Mediastinal tumors and cysts in adults are distributed by type with similar frequencies in most large series. Among 400 patients with mediastinal masses reported on by Davis and associates 25 percent had primary cystic lesions; thymic neoplasms were the most common primary tumors (17 percent), followed closely by lymphoma (16 percent), neurogenic tumors (14 percent), and germ cell tumors (11 percent). Malignant neoplasms have increased to 42 percent of the total over the 56 years encompassed by the series. Among the 62 percent of asymptomatic patients the fraction of benign neoplasms has decreased from 93 percent before 1967 to 76 percent. This trend toward more frequent detection of occult malignancies probably reflects improved sensitivity of diagnostic techniques. In childhood series the distribution of neoplasms is skewed toward malignancy, with nearly 50 percent having Hodgkin's or non-Hodgkin's lymphoma, while neurogenic tumors are a distant second. Lymphoma is the most common malignant neoplasm in all age groups.

Manifestations and Diagnosis. Mediastinal masses produce a wide variety of signs and symptoms, and one-half to one-third of patients are asymptomatic. The most common symptoms are nonspecific (chest pain, cough, dyspnea), and most can be ascribed to compression of adjacent structures, trachea and esophagus in particular. Superior vena caval obstruction, recurrent nerve palsy, and Horner's syndrome are less common examples, but their presence focuses diagnostic attention on the mediastinum. Certain mediastinal tumors are associated with symptomatic endocrine syndromes, such as hypertension (pheochromocytoma), hypercalcemia (parathyroid tumor), thyrotoxicosis (intrathoracic goiter), and gynecomastia (choriocarcinoma). In such cases symptoms have nothing to do with mediastinal location but are systemic consequences of the disease. Pel-Ebstein fevers associated with Hodgkin's disease are a similar example.

The presence of symptoms correlates with malignancy. Ninety-five percent of mediastinal masses that are discovered as incidental radiographic findings are benign, whereas symptomatic lesions are about half benign and half malignant. This correlation is less meaningful in children, whose airways are more vulnerable to compression. In a large series (188 children) from the Mayo Clinic, 78 percent of patients with benign mediastinal masses under age 2 had symptoms and signs of tracheal compression. Signs and symptoms of nerve compression, such as Horner's syndrome, vocal-cord paralysis, or hemiplegia usually reflect aggressive direct invasion and carry a poor prognosis.

Diagnostic evaluation begins with chest radiography in several views. Simply localizing the mass to one of the three subcompartments of the mediastinum narrows the possibilities (Fig. 16-83) and guides selection of further studies. In most patients the next step is CT, which can sort out the uniform radiographic densities

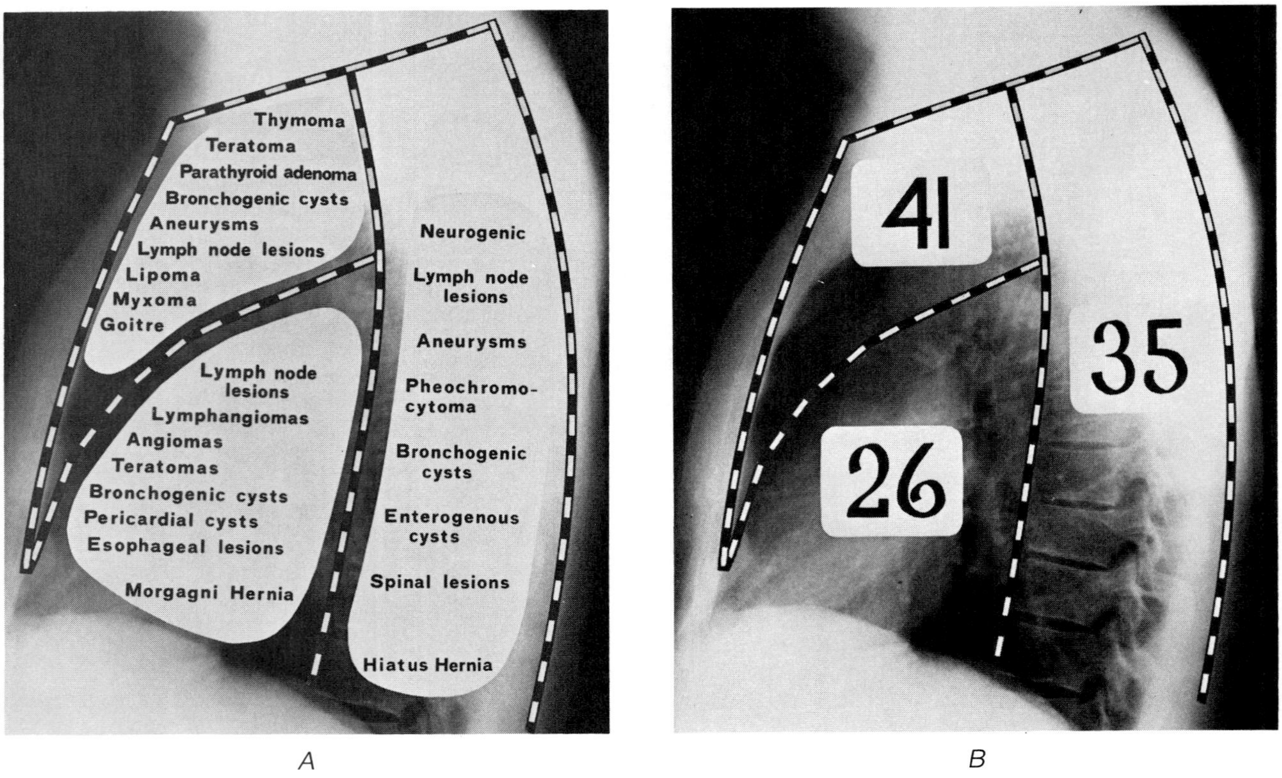

FIG. 16-83. *A.* Mediastinal lesions tend to occur within specific compartments, although some overlap is evident. *B.* The numbers shown indicate the distribution of lesions in 102 patients reported by Burkell and associates. (From: *Burkell CC, Cross JM, et al: Mass lesions of the mediastinum, in Ravitch MM (ed): Current Problems in Surgery. Year Book Medical Publishers, Chicago, 1969, with permission.*)

of the mediastinum, identifying normal vascular and soft tissue structures with great cross-sectional clarity. CT of the mediastinum is most diagnostic of benign pathology, such as a cystic mass with an attenuation coefficient close to that of water. The CT appearance of solid malignancies is less definitive, but malignant characteristics such as extension, compression, or invasion are often readily demonstrated. The diagnostic power of CT can be further enhanced by intravascular or intraesophageal injection of contrast. In one series of children with mediastinal abnormalities, CT provided additional diagnostic information in 82 percent of patients, and in 65 percent the CT findings contributed to a change in clinical management.

MRI is a noninvasive diagnostic modality thought to have great potential for imaging the mediastinum, especially for vascular lesions. Remarkable definition of vascular structures is obtainable in several views, entirely without the need for contrast injection (Fig. 16-84). Early experience has shown somewhat greater difficulty defining soft tissue masses, which tend to appear inhomogeneous or multifocal. The powerful magnetic field employed contraindicates the use of MRI in patients with pacemakers or cerebrovascular metal clips, and complicates examination of critically ill patients on monitors and elaborate life support systems. Fortunately, most metallic hardware likely to occur in the mediastinum (prosthetic valves, vascular clips, sternal wires) does not appear to pose a major hazard.

Plane tomography has been virtually replaced by CT and MRI but can still add useful information, especially in the vicinity of the pulmonary hila. A barium swallow can demonstrate invasion, compression, or displacement of the esophagus, resulting from intrinsic or extrinsic lesions. Arteriography is less frequently necessary with CT and MRI available, but contrast injection of the aorta or pulmonary artery provides information regarding blood supply and anatomic relationship to critical vascular structures that is sometimes not obtainable by any other method. For preoperative evaluation of major vascular disorders (aneurysms), which are discussed elsewhere, angiography is still the diagnostic standard. Venous angiography can provide specific information about the extent of involvement and nature of collateral channels in superior vena caval obstruction but is difficult to justify unless operation and reconstruction are anticipated. Myelography has been considered an essential part of the evaluation of posterior mediastinal tumors lying very close to the vertebral foramina, but this invasive procedure has also been replaced in many cases by CT of the spine.

Radioisotope scanning can provide very specific information when substernal goiter is suspected. Endoscopy of the esophagus or tracheobronchial tree can add observations on gross displacement or erosion by adjacent mass lesions and can occasionally provide biopsy material. Percutaneous needle biopsy, especially with direct fluoroscopic, ultrasonographic, or CT guidance, can be done safely in cases with favorable anatomy. Mediastinoscopy and mediastinotomy can also be employed for diagnosis.

Recitation of the expanding list of potentially applicable diagnostic procedures promotes the impression that operation is being avoided by assiduous diagnosis. On the contrary, there are still few mass lesions that do not come to operation. The operative mortality for resection of mediastinal lesions is very low. In the large series reported by Davis and associates from Duke, mortality has been 0.8 percent since 1930, without a single death in 236 patients over the most recent period of 26 years. Operation provides definitive diagnosis and frequently simultaneous definitive treatment, and remains an important part of most combined protocols for chemotherapy and radiation. In most cases the diagnostic armamentarium should be viewed as a means to a comprehensive preoperative evaluation.

Neurogenic Tumors

Neurogenic tumors typically arise from sympathetic ganglia or intercostal nerves and are almost always found in the posterior mediastinum lying in the paravertebral gutter. Peak incidence is in adulthood. Since only 10 to 20 percent of adult neurogenic tumors are malignant, presentation as an incidental finding in an asymptomatic young adult is quite common. A higher proportion (20 to 40 percent) of childhood tumors are malignant. Chest wall pain due to nerve compression or bony erosion is the most common symptom. Hemiparesthesia, hemiparesis, and other signs of spinal cord compression can be seen in tumors with "dumbbell" extension through the intervertebral foramina. Hormonally active tumors are most often childhood malignancies, which can produce hypertension, flushing, diarrhea, diaphoresis, anorexia, and fever.

Neurilemoma. Neurilemomas (schwannomas) account for 40 to 60 percent of all neurogenic tumors. They arise from mature Schwann cells in intercostal nerves and have a hard, yellowish, well-encapsulated gross appearance consistent with the fact that most are benign. Some form dumbbell extensions through the intervertebral foramina (Fig. 16-85).

Neurofibroma. Neurofibromas contain elements of both nerve sheath and nerve cells, and account for about 10 percent of all neurogenic tumors. They are poorly encapsulated, but radiographically resemble neurilemomas. Mediastinal neurofibromas can be one feature of generalized neurofibromatosis (von Recklinghausen's disease), in which case the risk of malignant degeneration to neurosarcoma is increased. Advanced age also increases the risk of malignancy. Malignancy is present in 25 to 30 percent of tumors of this type and carries a poor prognosis because of rapid growth and aggressive local invasion.

Neuroblastoma. Neuroblastomas are the most poorly differentiated tumors arising from the sympathetic nervous system. Only about 10 percent occur as a primary lesion in the mediastinum. More than 75 percent occur in children under 4 years of age, and many are hormonally active, producing vanillylmandelic acid in sufficient quantity to present with a systemic symptom complex often consisting of hypertension, fever, vomiting, and diarrhea. Bone, liver, and lymph-node metastases, as well as direct spinal cord invasion with neurologic deficits, are not infrequent at the time of diagnosis. Tumors presenting in such advanced stages are usually unresectable, but the tumors are generally radiosensitive, and debulking followed by radiation therapy can produce long-term survival. Tumors presenting in the mediastinum and those presenting in the first year of life have a more favorable prognosis.

Ganglioneuroma, Ganglioneuroblastoma. Ganglioneuromas arise from mature nerve cells in sympathetic ganglia and are benign tumors that usually present in a younger age group than tumors of neural sheath origin. Radiographically, ganglioneuromas have a triangular configuration, with the base toward the mediastinum, and may be completely obscured by the vertebrae in the lateral projection. They tend to be poorly encapsulated and can be difficult to resect because of adherence to adjacent structures. Ganglioneuroblastomas consist of a mixture of mature and immature cells and are rare tumors that share features of neuroblastoma. These are usually seen in patients who are under 3 years of age and are rare in adults.

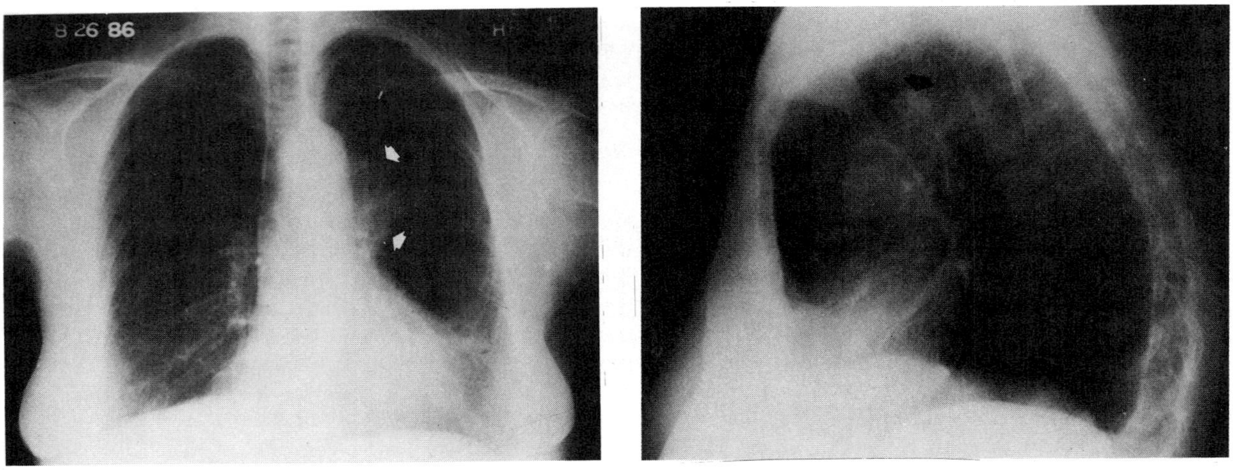

A

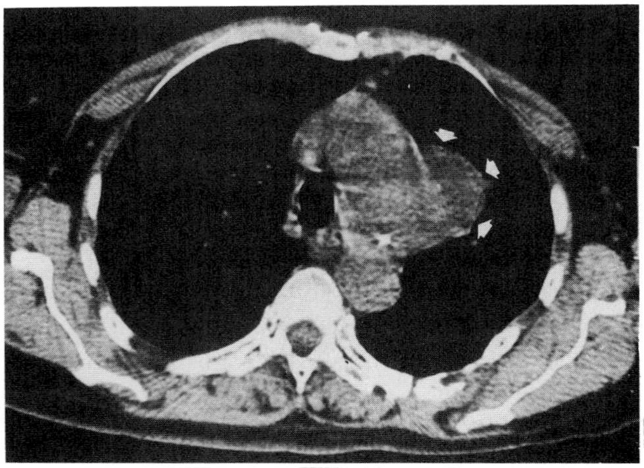

B

FIG. 16-84. *A.* This 64-year-old woman was explored through a left thoracotomy for resection of the mass seen in the middle mediastinum on this chest x-ray (*arrows*). The gross findings were confusing to the surgeon, and the patient was closed and transferred to another institution. *B.* On CT scan the mass could be seen adjacent to the aorta (*see arrows*). *C.* An MRI scan demonstrated unequivocally that the mass was an aneurysm of the aortic arch, arising proximal to the left subclavian artery. 1 = ascending aorta, 2 = aneurysm, 3 = descending aorta, 4 = left subclavian artery, P = pulmonary artery, L = left atrium. The patient died suddenly while awaiting reoperation.

Paraganglionic Tumors. Pheochromocytomas are chromaffin paraganglionic tumors that characteristically secrete catecholamines. Intrathoracic primaries are unusual, occurring in about 1 percent of all pheochromocytomas. As with all extraadrenal locations, intrathoracic tumors are more frequently ''silent'' (nonsecreting) than their adrenal counterparts but are also more often malignant—about 30 percent of extraadrenal pheochromocytomas are malignant. Chemodectomas are nonchromaffin paraganglionic tumors that rarely secrete catecholamines, and arise from chemoreceptor tissue around the aortic arch, vagus, and aorticosympathetics. They are quite rare, and 15 to 30 percent are malignant.

Treatment. Operation is indicated in virtually all posterior mediastinal neurogenic tumors. The region is best approached through a standard posterolateral thoracotomy. Benign tumors should be completely excised. Preoperative evaluation of all posterior mediastinal tumors includes careful evaluation of the intervertebral foramina and vertebral bodies, which is most easily done initially with a CT scan, using magnified views as necessary. Myelography may still be required to confirm intraspinal extension (see Fig. 16-85). When intraspinal extension exists, it is best to excise that portion first through a laminectomy, to avoid cord compression from intraspinal hemorrhage during the thoracic excision.

Malignant tumors are excised if possible. Radical operations for neuroblastoma are approached selectively, keeping clearly in mind the age of the patient, the radiosensitivity of the tumor, and the possibility of spontaneous maturation. Resection of an active (secretory) pheochromocytoma requires attention to the perioperative medical management of paroxysmal hypertension.

Thymoma

In adults thymoma is the most common anterior mediastinal mass, and ranks second in frequency among tumors and cysts of the mediastinum. Thymoma is rare in children and has equal sex distribution, with a peak age incidence between 40 and 60 years. About one-third of patients are asymptomatic at the time of diagnosis. Symptomatic patients present either with mass effects on adjacent organs or with systemic effects referable to one of the paraneoplastic syndromes associated with thymoma. Of the former, common examples include cough, chest pain, dyspnea, and superior vena caval obstruction. Of the latter, myasthenia gravis is the most common, although hypogammaglobulinemia and red cell aplasia have been described. It is most often stated that the incidence of myasthenia gravis is 10 to 50 percent in patients with thymoma. Conversely, thymoma is seen in only 8 to 15 percent of patients with myasthenia gravis. Myasthenic patients with

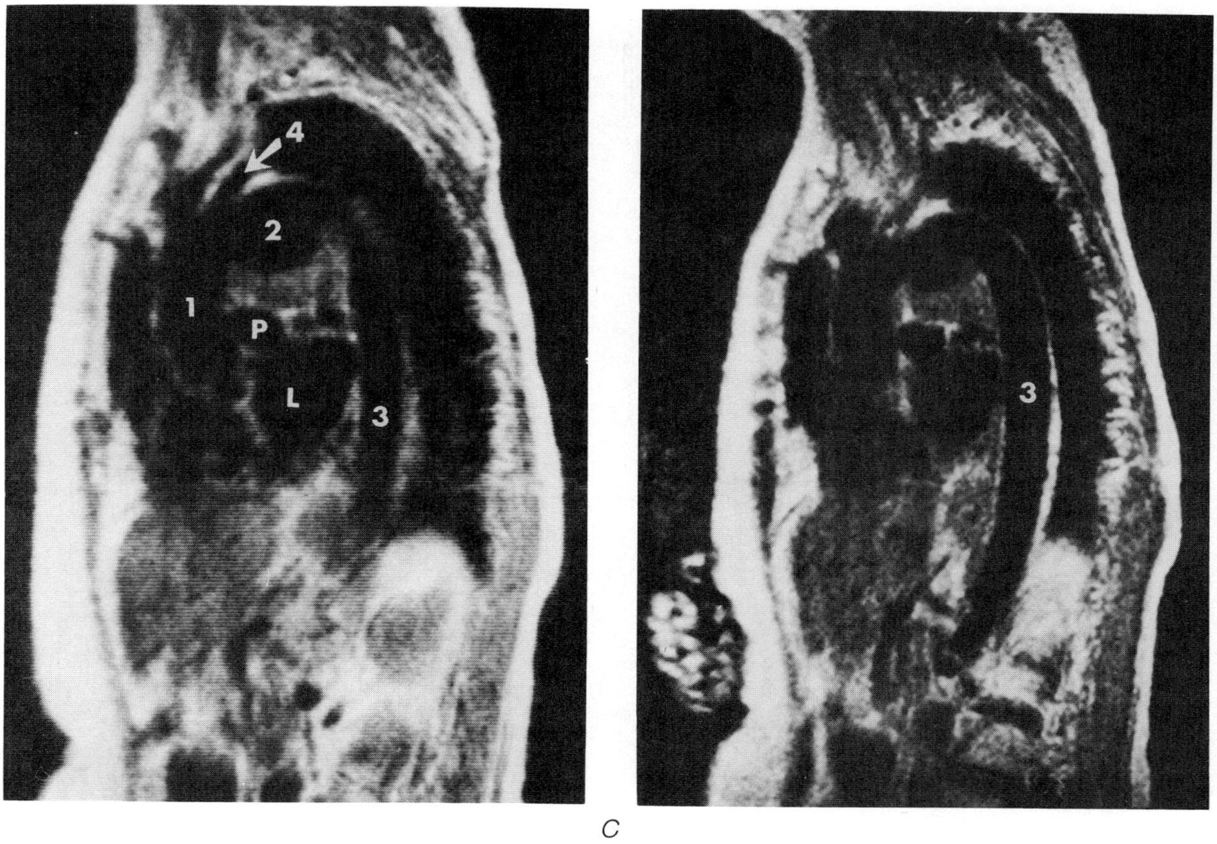

FIG. 16-84. *(continued)*

thymoma have a poorer prognosis than patients without thymoma and are less likely to benefit from thymectomy.

Thymoma does not have a characteristic radiographic appearance, and diagnosis is usually made when the mass is excised (Fig. 16-86). The most prevalent histologic classification is based on the relative proportions of lymphocytic and epithelial elements, so the tumor is described as lymphocytic, epithelial, or mixed. Histology, however, contributes nothing to the distinction between benign and malignant, which is based entirely on invasive gross characteristics. Distant metastases occur but are uncommon. CT scanning can add valuable preoperative radiographic evidence of invasive behavior. Biopsy is not usually recommended because of fear that violation of the capsule might promote invasive behavior, and because almost all such masses deserve an attempt at resection. When the findings suggest that complete resection might be difficult, it is perfectly rational to perform a biopsy followed by radiation or chemotherapy designed to shrink the tumor and simplify later resection.

In most cases resection through a median sternotomy provides the definitive diagnosis. Fifty to sixty-five percent of thymomas are benign and subject to curative resection, which should encompass the entire thymus and all adjacent mediastinal adipose tissue. Truly complete resection is best accomplished with a generous extension into the neck to follow tongues of thymic tissue that commonly extent cephalad. All adjacent nonvital structures invaded by malignant thymoma should also be resected. Postoperative irradiation is of unproved benefit but is generally recommended for patients who have had incomplete resection of a malignant thymoma (Fig. 16-87).

Lymphoma

Mediastinal involvement is present in about 50 percent of patients with Hodgkin's and non-Hodgkin's lymphoma, and lymphoma is the most common mediastinal malignancy. Lymphoma is most frequently located in the anterior mediastinum (Fig. 16-88). Hilar nodes in the middle mediastinum are less commonly involved, and posterior mediastinal location is rare. Radiation is the standard treatment for most lymphomas, and resection is indicated only for the 5 percent of patients with lymphoma whose disease is confined to the mediastinum, underscoring the importance of a thorough search for involved lymphatic tissue elsewhere.

Teratodermoid Tumors

Teratomas account for less than 10 percent of all mediastinal tumors, with almost all found in the anterior mediastinum. By definition teratomas consist of multiple tissue types not normally found at the site of the tumor. They are most often partially cystic and consist primarily of ectodermal elements that can include hair, teeth, and sebaceous glands. Teratomas are thought to arise from branchial cleft and pouch cells associated with the thymus. The mediastinum is second to the gonads as the most frequent location of teratomas in adults. The sex ratio is roughly equal, and age distribution peaks in early adulthood.

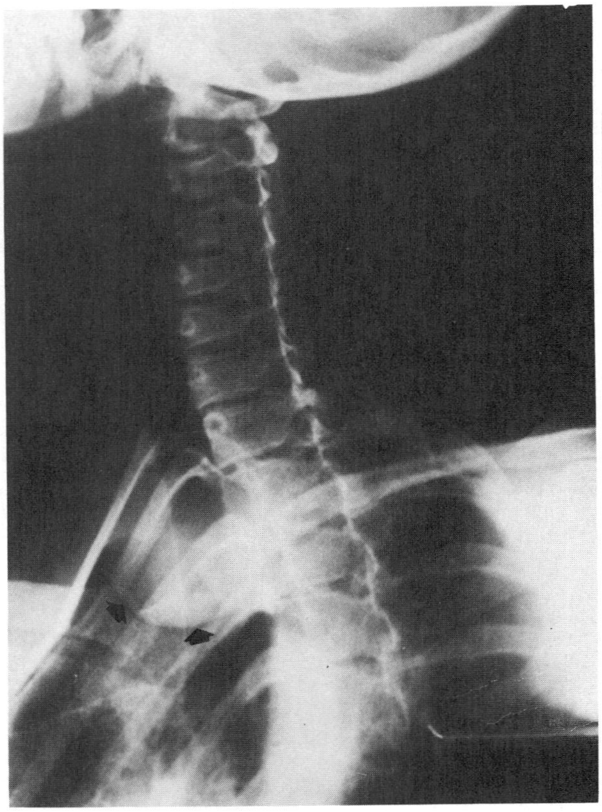

A

FIG. 16-85. This 35-year-old woman complained of neck pain following a minor accident, and had x-rays taken of her cervical spine. *A.* The cervical spine was normal, but a smooth, hemispherical mass (*see arrows*) was noted incidentally in the apex of the right hemithorax. *B.* Standard views of the chest confirmed the presence of a mass lying high in the posterior mediastinum. *C.* The CT scan showed a homogeneous solid mass lying against the spine. Extension into the intervertebral foramen could not be excluded. *D.* A CT myelogram was obtained. The spinal cord (S) is the radiolucent circle in the center of the spinal canal, surrounded by the dense opacity of myelographic contrast medium. The mass (M) can be seen to enter the T_2–T_3 neural foramen (*large arrow*), but with no impingement on the spinal canal (*small arrow*). The mass was resected uneventfully through a high right posterolateral thoracotomy. Pathologic examination proved it to be a neurilemoma. (*Courtesy of Alfred Jaretzki III.*)

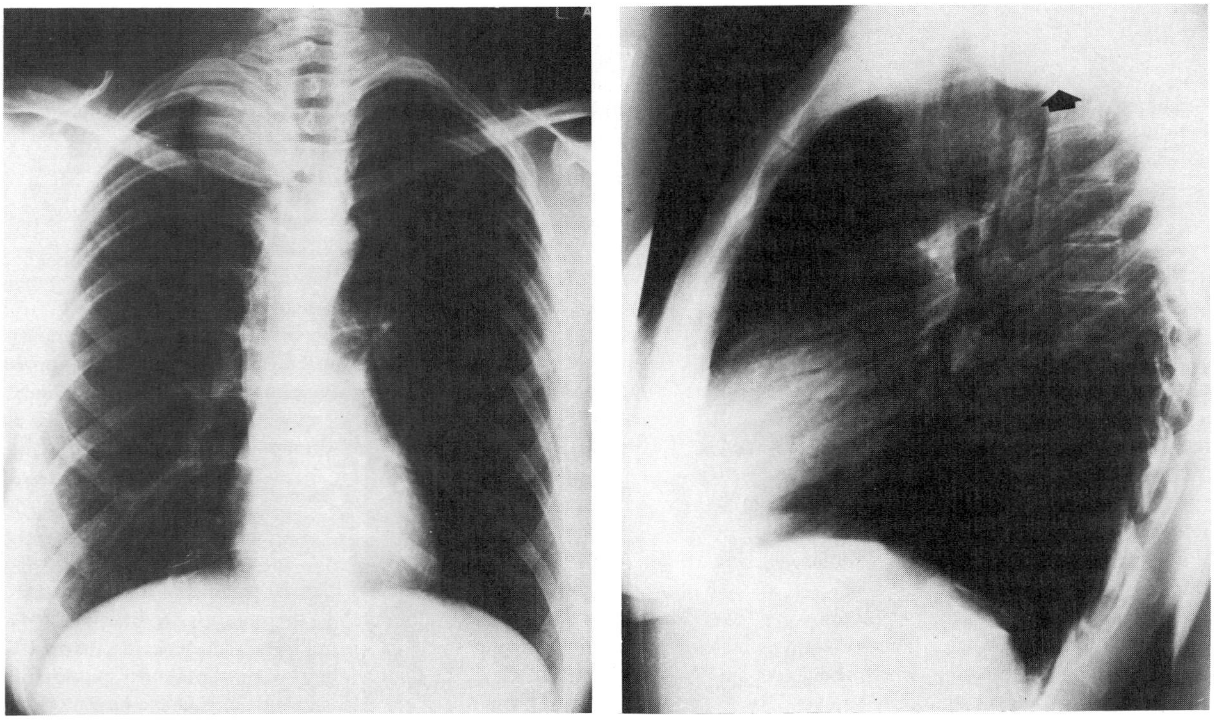

B

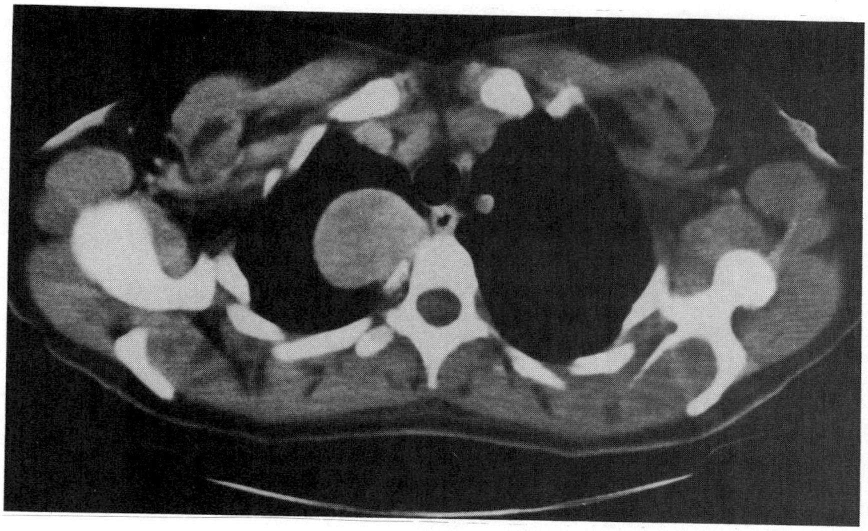

C

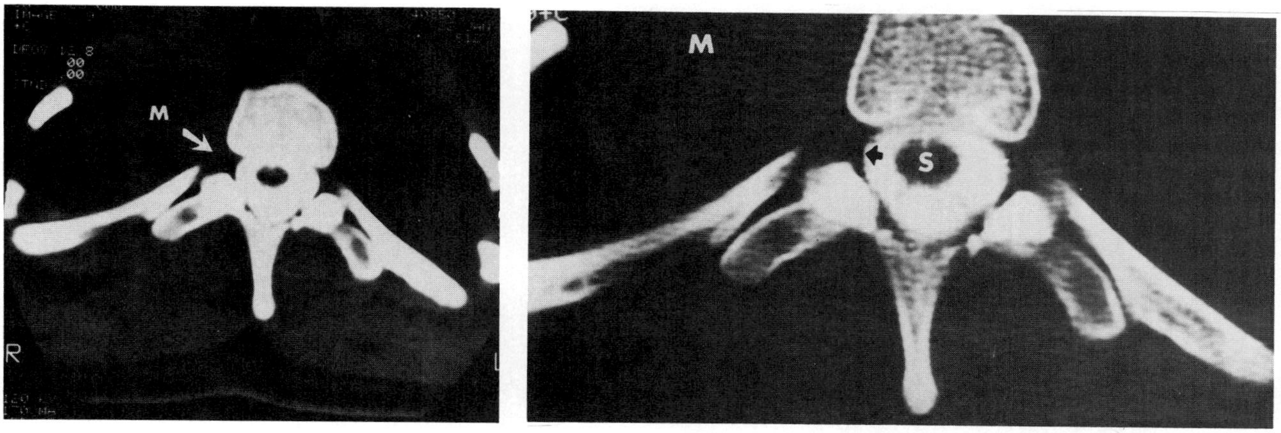

D

FIG. 16-85. *(continued)*

In modern series about two-thirds of patients are asymptomatic at presentation, and the majority of symptoms are nonspecific mass effects such as chest pain, cough, and dyspnea. The classic pathognomonic presentation with cough productive of hair and sebum has become a rarity, as most tumors are detected before eroding into the tracheobronchial tree. As with other neoplasms of the region, malignant teratocarcinomas are more likely to present with symptoms related to aggressive invasion of adjacent vital structures.

Typical radiographic appearance is that of a large, well-circumscribed anterior mediastinal mass. Twenty to forty percent of teratomas are calcified, most often appearing as a nonspecific opacity in the cyst wall, although occasionally due to the presence of teeth or bone. CT scanning is very helpful in delineating involvement of adjacent structures, and in confirming fat density in the center of the cystic mass (Fig. 16-89). Elevated serum levels of alpha-fetoprotein and carcinoembryonic antigen suggest malignancy.

Surgical excision through a median sternotomy is the best method of diagnosis and treatment. Eighty percent are benign, and resection is curative. Even with benign forms resection is made more difficult by the tendency for the tumors to be densely adherent to surrounding structures, most commonly pericardium, lung, great vessels, and thymus, and incomplete resection is occasionally necessary. For benign tumors recurrence is rare even following partial excision. The prognosis for malignant tumors is poor because of local recurrence and distant metastasis.

Germ-Cell Tumors

Primary extragonadal germ-cell tumors are rare. Although they can be seen in the pineal, sacrococcygeal, and paraaortic regions, they are most often found in the anterior mediastinum, where they comprise less than 1 percent of all mediastinal tumors. The histogenesis of germ-cell tumors outside the gonads is poorly understood, but a theory of origin from pluripotential primordial germ

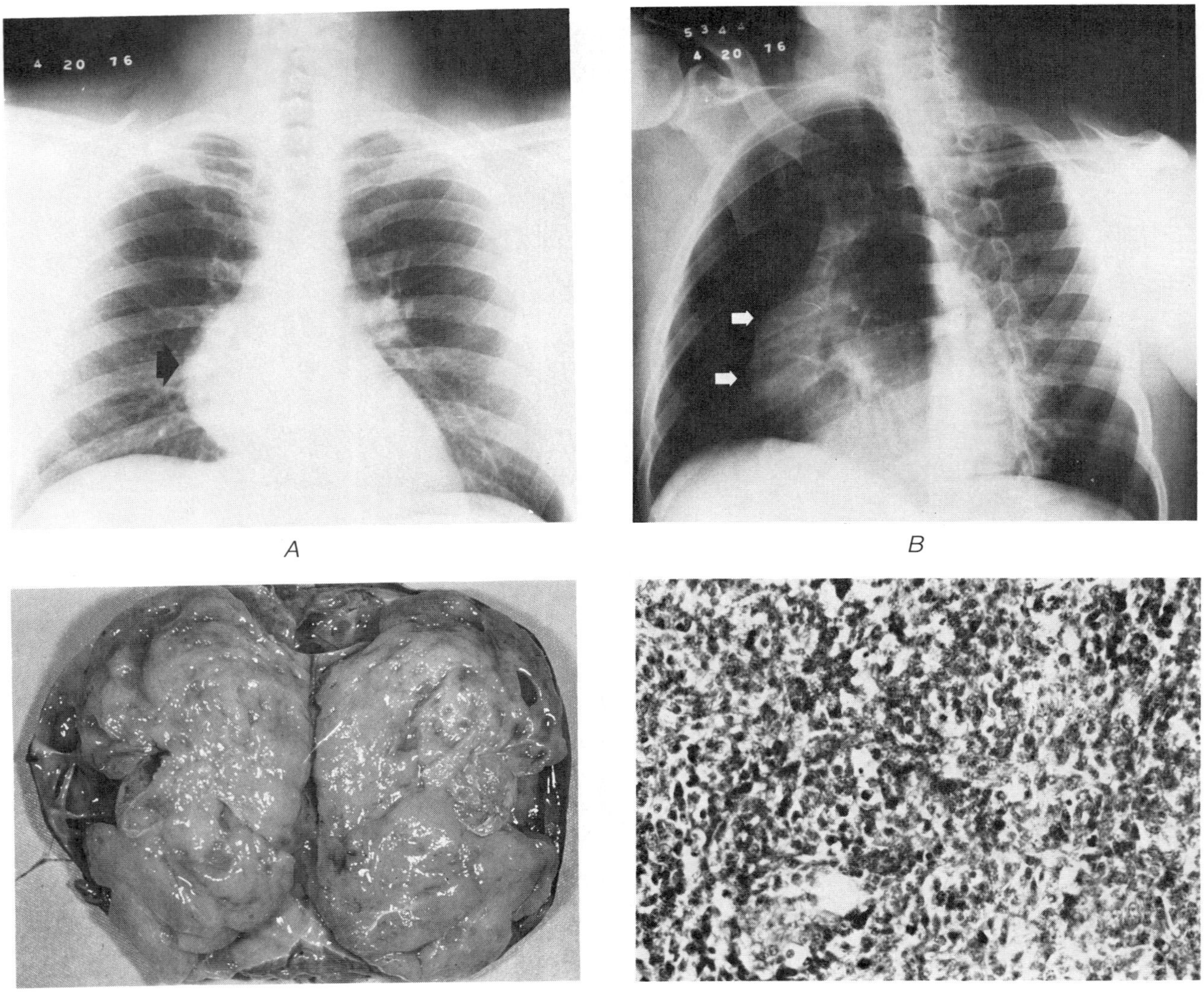

FIG. 16-86. A benign thymoma in a 30-year-old man who presented with a persistent cough. *A.* Chest x-ray shows a large smooth mass contiguous with the right heart border. *B.* An oblique view suggests that the mass is closely related to the pericardium. *C.* The tumor was removed, along with remnants of the thymus, through a high right thoracotomy. This photograph of the bisected tumor shows that it was a well-encapsulated fleshy neoplasm. *D.* Histologic examination of the tumor shows a predominance of lymphocytic elements that justifies its classification as a lymphocytic type of thymoma.

cells in the mediastinum is favored. Mediastinal teratoma should probably be viewed as the end point of benign differentiation in this germ-cell line but is usually considered separately because clinical behavior is quite different.

Five distinct cell types are recognized. Seminoma and embryonal cell carcinoma are most common, followed by choriocarcinoma, malignant teratoma, and endodermal sinus (yolk sac) carcinoma. These tumors are usually seen in young adults, with a male to female ratio of at least 4:1. Since the tumors are highly malignant, it is not surprising that 80 to 90 percent of patients are symptomatic when the diagnosis is made. The most frequent symptoms are nonspecific and result from tumor expansion encroaching on adjacent structures to produce cough, dyspnea, chest pain, or superior vena caval syndrome.

Standard posteroanterior and lateral chest roentgenograms will detect over 90 percent of such tumors. A CT scan can provide very helpful preoperative information regarding anatomic relationships and local invasion but does not substitute for exploration or biopsy. Serum tumor markers, while not specifically diagnostic, are important to obtain prior to treatment as a basis for monitoring relapse and response to treatment. All patients with choriocarcinoma have elevated serum human chorionic gonadotropin (HCG) levels, as will some patients with seminoma and embryonal cell carcinoma. Alpha fetoprotein levels can be elevated, most com-

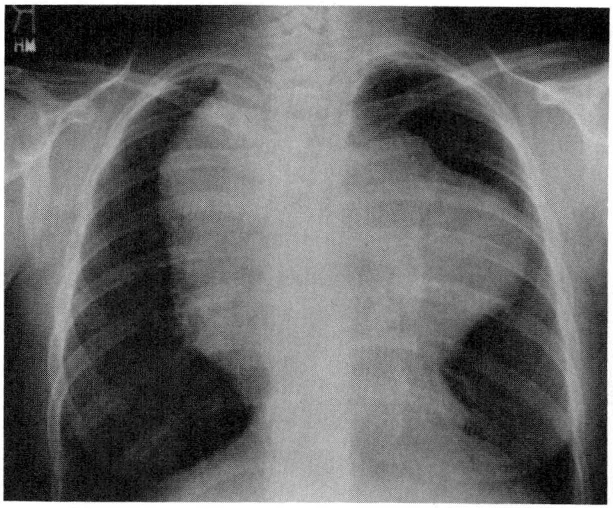

A

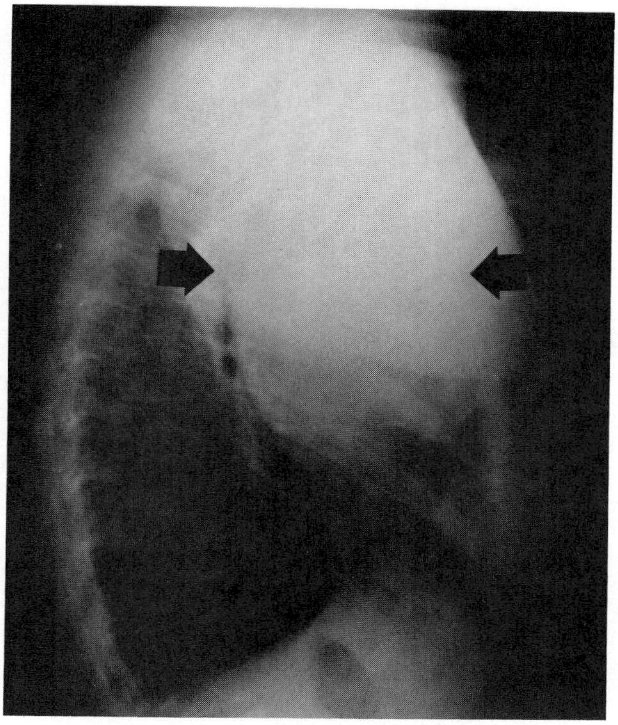

B

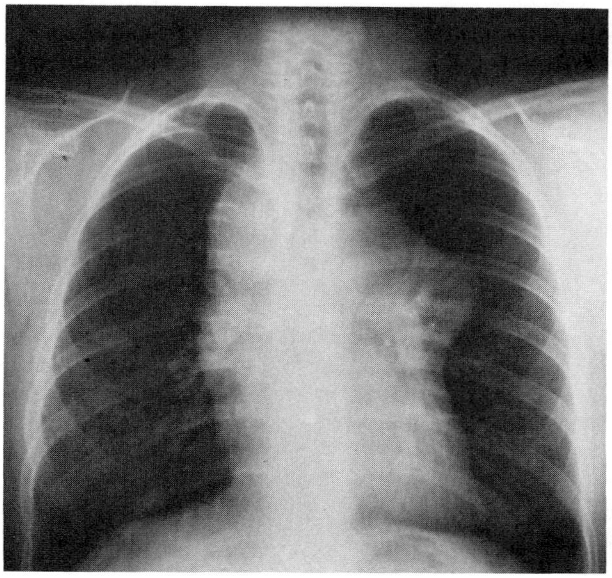

C

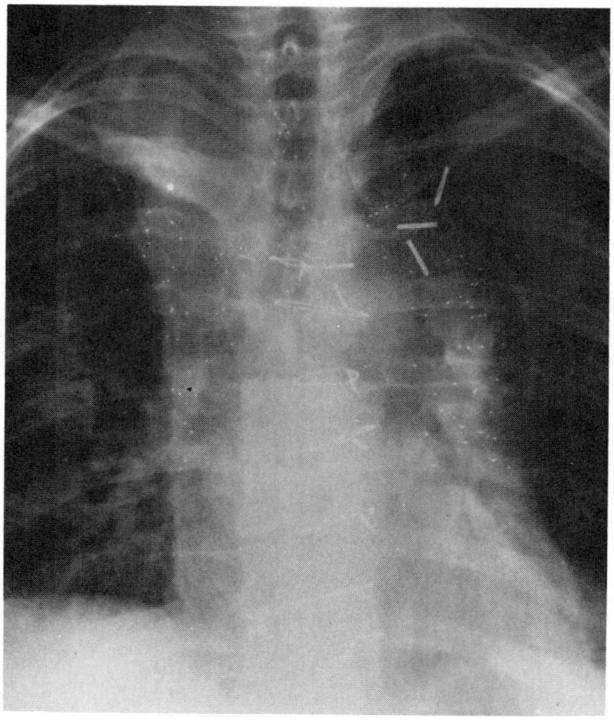

D

FIG. 16-87. A malignant thymoma in a 29-year-old woman who presented with superior vena caval obstruction and marked tracheal compression. *A.* The initial chest x-ray shows a huge mediastinal mass projecting into both hemithoraces. *B.* In lateral view the mass is seen to lie in the anterior mediastinum, compressing and posteriorly displacing the trachea. A mediastinal biopsy showed thymoma. *C.* After the patient received 2500 rad of external radiation therapy, a repeat chest x-ray shows a significant reduction in the size of the tumor. Symptoms were similarly improved. A subtotal resection was performed through a median sternotomy. The thymoma was found to invade the upper lobes of both lungs, the pericardium, and the areolar tissues of the mediastinum. Residual tumor was implanted with seeds of ^{125}I. *D.* A chest x-ray 1 month after operation shows further reduction in tumor size. The metallic markers of the isotope seeds can be seen throughout the tumor area. The patient has returned to work and is asymptomatic except for a chronic cough.

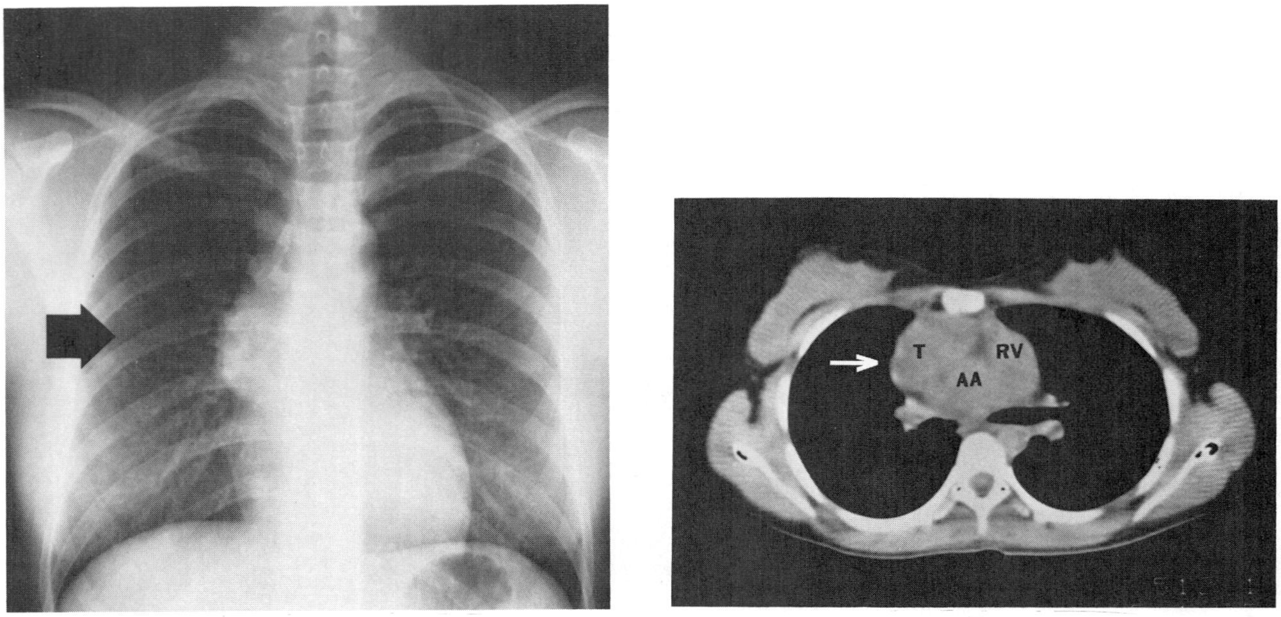

A B

FIG. 16-88. Nodular Hodgkin's disease of the mediastinum in an eighteen-year-old woman. *A.* The chest x-ray shows a right mediastinal mass overlying the superior vena cava–right atrial junction. *B.* A CT scan section at the level of the right ventricular outflow tract (RV) shows the intimate relationship of the mass (T) to the ascending aorta (AA).

monly in embryonal cell tumors, and carcinoembryonic antigen levels are occasionally elevated in all cell types.

The possibility of metastasis from a gonadal tumor must be excluded before a mediastinal germ-cell tumor is declared primary. Primary gonadal tumors rarely metastasize only to the mediastinum, and most often spread through retroperitoneal lymphatics. A gonadal primary can be excluded with reasonable accuracy if there is no evidence of retroperitoneal involvement by CT scan or lymphangiography, and if gonadal nodules are not detectable by palpation or ultrasound examination.

Most patients with mediastinal germ-cell tumors deserve exploration through a median sternotomy and an attempt at complete

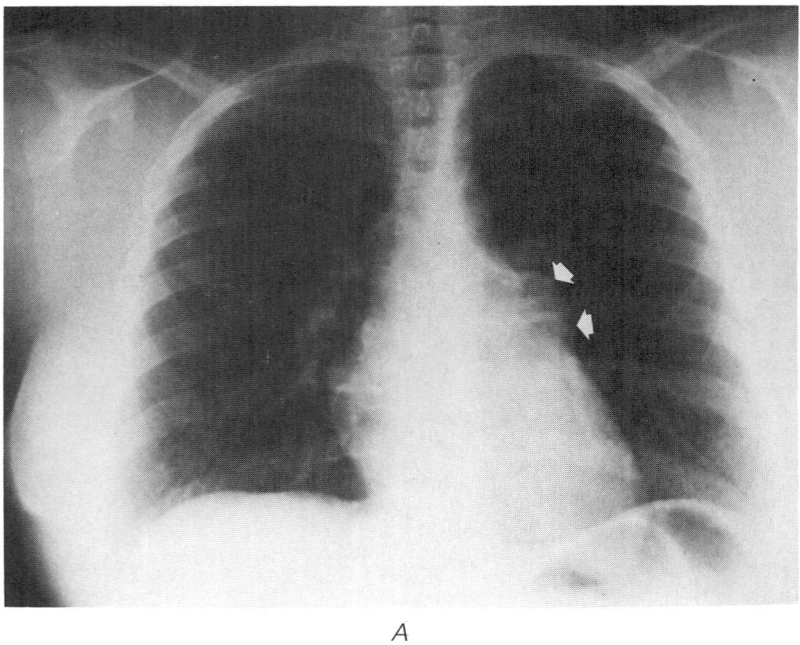

A

FIG. 16-89. *A.* Chest x-ray in an asymptomatic 19-year-old woman, demonstrating a mass along the left heart border in the vicinity of the left hilum (*see arrows*). The lateral (not shown) suggested that the mass was in the anterior mediastinum. *B.* A CT scan without contrast shows a mass with small islands of calcification lying in the anterior mediastinum against the left side of the heart. There is a faint lucency (*see arrows*) suggesting that pericardium separates the mass from the heart. *C.* A CT scan with intravascular contrast injection suggests that the mass (M) is adjacent to but separate from the pulmonary artery (P) and right ventricular outflow tract. Through a median sternotomy a benign teratoma was removed easily along with the left lobe of the thymus. (*Courtesy of Alfred Jaretzki III.*)

resection. In a recent large series from the Mayo Clinic, complete resection was achieved in 44 percent of 56 cases. The remainder frequently present with evidence of widespread local invasion or distant metastasis and are subject to partial resection or to biopsy alone. It is important to separate seminoma from the other tissue types because of its radiosensitivity and generally better prognosis. Five-year survival is about 75 percent for seminoma treated with aggressive resection, followed by irradiation for local disease left behind, and chemotherapy for distant metastases. Prognosis remains poor in the other tissue types, although various protocols of combination chemotherapy have provided increasingly successful palliation.

Mesenchymal Tumors

Tumors of mesenchymal origin constitute about 7 percent of all mediastinal tumors and cysts, with most occurring in the anterior mediastinum. Lipomas are most common and are characteristically soft masses without fixation to surrounding structures that can reach enormous size without producing symptoms. Fibromas are more dense and less common but have similar clinical behavior. The malignant forms (liposarcoma and fibrosarcoma) are seen rarely.

Tumors of lymph-vascular and blood-vascular origin are also classified as mesenchymal neoplasms. Tumors of blood-vascular

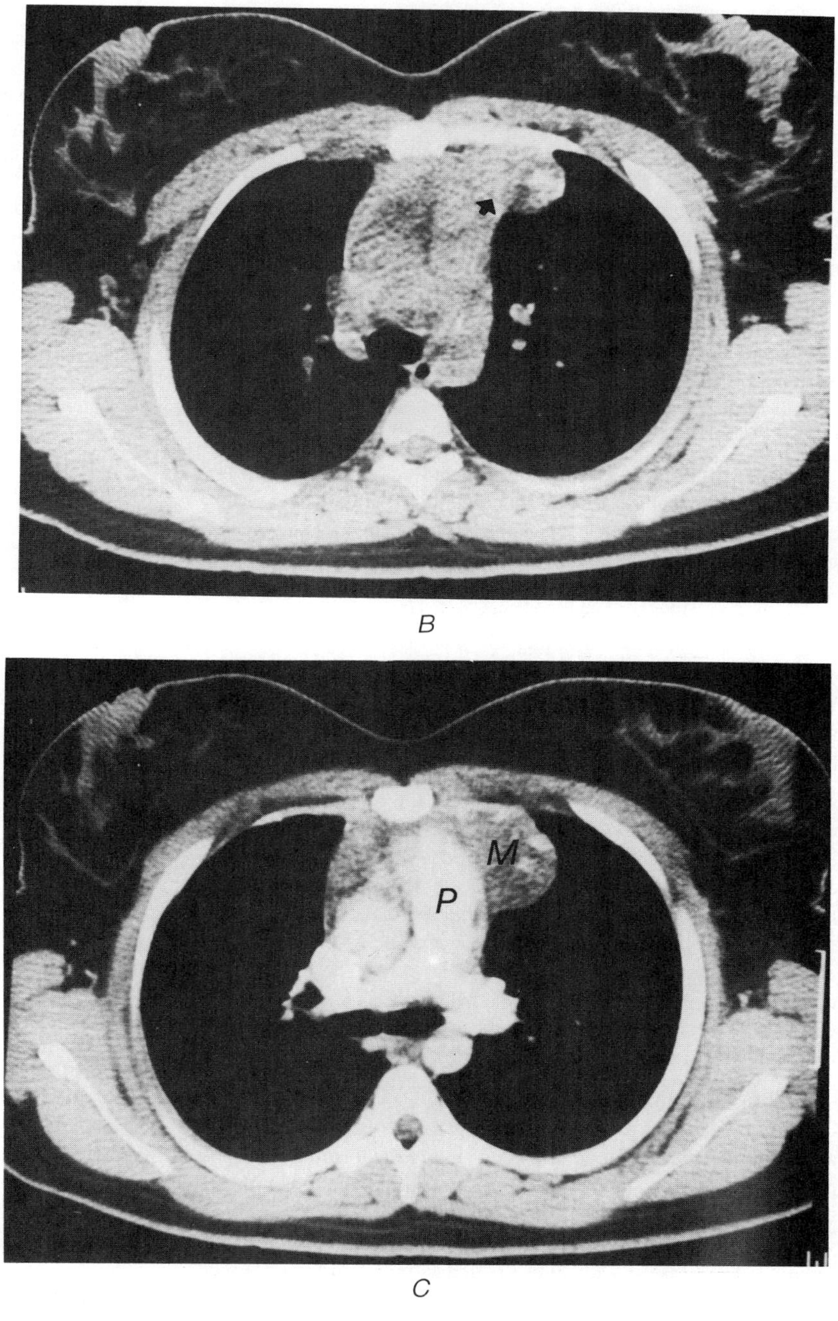

FIG. 16-89. *(continued)*

origin consist of hemangiomas (capillary, cavernous, and venous) and rare malignant hemangiopericytomas. The most common lymph-vascular tumor is a lymphangioma (cystic hygroma). Most vascular tumors present as smooth, often lobulated masses of uniform density on chest x-ray, and will appear as cystic masses on CT scan.

The complete list of mesenchymal mediastinal tumors also includes mesothelioma, hamartoma, myxoma, mesenchymoma, leiomyoma, and leiomyosarcoma, xanthogranuloma, and rhabdomyosarcoma.

Endocrine Tumors

Thyroid and parathyroid tumors appearing in the mediastinum are most properly considered within the context of their usual cervical manifestations. Less than 10 percent of parathyroid adenomas are located in the mediastinum, and most are approachable through a cervical incision. Because of their embryologic origin from the third branchial cleft they are usually in close association with the upper pole of the thymus gland. Parathyroid tumors rarely present as a mediastinal mass.

Similarly, mediastinal thyroid tissue is usually a direct substernal extension of the cervical gland. Aberrant mediastinal thyroid tissue with agenesis of the cervical gland is exceedingly rare but does provide the rationale for obtaining a radionuclide thyroid scan in any patient with an undiagnosed mass high in the anterior mediastinum.

Mediastinal Cysts

Congenital cysts constitute approximately 20 percent of all primary mediastinal mass lesions, and account for the vast majority of middle mediastinal primary lesions. On chest x-ray they appear as opaque densities that may be indistinguishable from neoplasms except on the basis of typical location. On CT scan a mass with near water density occurring in a characteristic location is virtually diagnostic and provides a strong rationale for routine use of CT scanning in mediastinal lesions. In a recent review of experience with mediastinal cysts in 34 children, Snyder and associates found that the accuracy of their preoperative diagnosis increased from 50 percent before the use of CT scanning to 100 percent thereafter.

Pericardial Cysts. These cysts are the most common type occurring in the mediastinum. They are usually detected as an incidental finding in an asymptomatic patient, and very frequently appear at the right costophrenic angle as a smooth-walled cystic mass 3 to 6 cm in diameter. They contain a clear fluid and occasionally communicate with the pericardium. Histologically they are lined with a single layer of mesothelial cells. The location and appearance of pericardial cysts are so characteristic, especially on CT scan, that close observation is becoming a defensible option, although most are still resected for diagnosis.

Bronchogenic Cysts. Bronchogenic cysts are most frequently located just posterior to the carina or main-stem bronchi, although they can be found elsewhere in the mediastinum or more peripherally in the lung (Fig. 16-90). Communication with the tracheobronchial tree can occur to produce an air-fluid level, serving to distinguish them completely from pericardial cysts but allowing for confusion with lung or mediastinal abscess in certain cases. Chest x-ray and CT scan will usually demonstrate a cystic mass in the characteristic location, although bronchogenic cysts can contain a viscid fluid difficult to distinguish from a solid mass by CT scan alone. A contrast esophagram may show compression of the esophagus by an anterior mass. Histologically they are lined with ciliated respiratory epithelium and contain varying amounts of cartilage, smooth muscle, and mucous glands. They are most frequently symptomatic in children, producing cough, dyspnea, and stridor in more than half. All bronchogenic cysts should be resected and are usually approached through a posterolateral thoracotomy. Especially when they have formed a communication with the tracheobronchial tree, the chronic infection that frequently results can make resection through dense inflammatory adhesions very difficult.

Enteric Cysts. Enteric cysts are located in the posterior mediastinum adjacent to the esophagus. They are occasionally embedded in the muscularis of the esophagus but rarely communicate with the esophageal lumen. The cysts have a smooth wall with a muscular coat and a lining recognizable as intestinal mucosa, although it may be ciliated, and they contain a clear, colorless mucoid fluid. When lined with an aberrant gastric mucosa, peptic ulceration can lead to perforation of adjacent bronchus or esophagus, producing hemoptysis or hematemesis, and erosion into adjacent lung can produce a lung abscess. A rare association with vertebral anomalies has been described in which the enteric cyst is attached to the spinal cord of meninges, and a patent tract may exist that can be demonstrated by myelography.

Approximately 60 percent of enteric cysts are recognized in patients under 1 year of age, when symptoms of tracheal and esophageal compression are prominent. Less than one-third of children with enteric cysts are asymptomatic. Complete evaluation of children with a suggestive presentation includes chest x-ray and esophagram followed by a CT scan with contrast in the esophagus. Resection is always indicated. The lesions are approached through a posterolateral thoracotomy with the choice of side determined by the level of involvement and the appearance of projection into either hemithorax.

Mediastinitis

Acute Mediastinitis

Acute mediastinitis is a fulminant infectious process with high morbidity and mortality characterized by rapid spread through the areolar planes of the mediastinum. The mediastinal pleura confines the process to the mediastinum only temporarily, with a breach occurring into one or both pleural cavities early in the course of the infection in most cases, after which the negative pressure of the pleural space helps to rapidly spread the infection throughout. The rapid spread of infection is promoted by several factors. One is the separation of tissue planes produced by air forced into soft tissues adjacent to a perforated hollow viscus, most often the esophagus, further promoted by the digestive action of salivary and gastric enzymes. Another is the pressure gradient established from the atmosphere to the negative pressure of the pleural space once the pleura is penetrated, which tends to pull the infection through the mediastinum from its source and into the pleural space. A third factor is the presence of naturally continuous fascial planes connecting the deep cervical compartments with the mediastinum, along which oropharyngeal infection can spread.

The infection is initiated most frequently by esophageal perforation, resulting from instrumentation, trauma, foreign body, su-

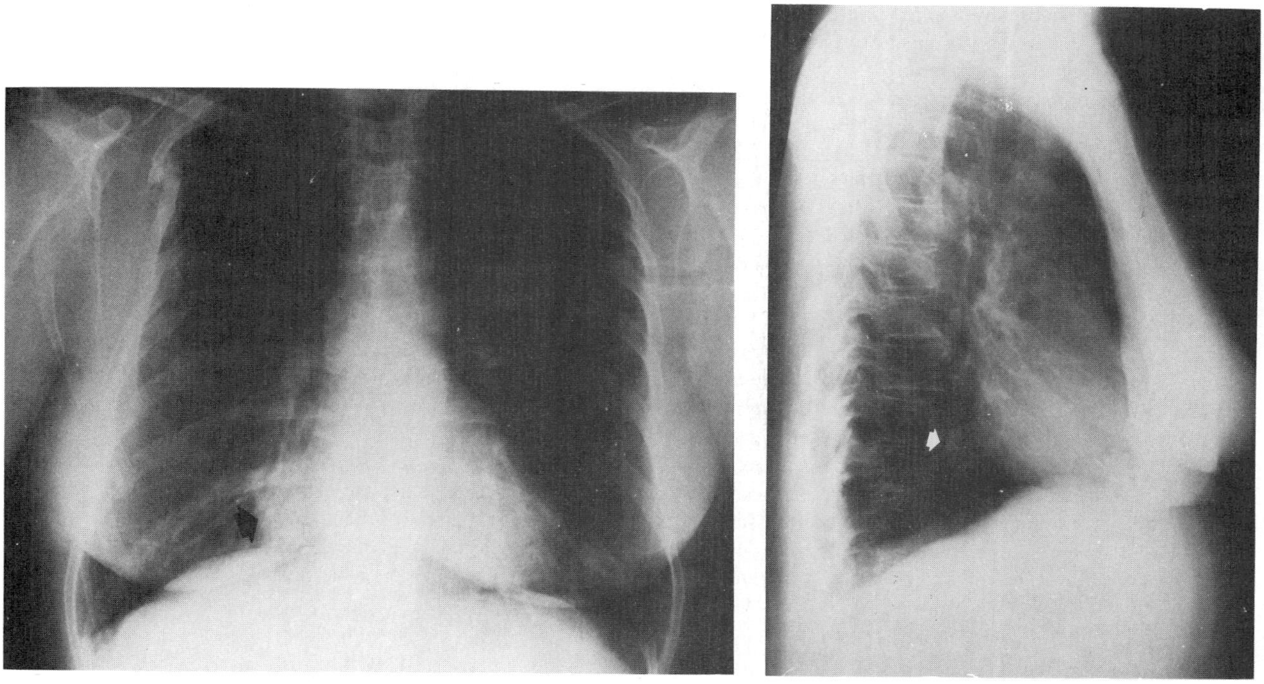

A

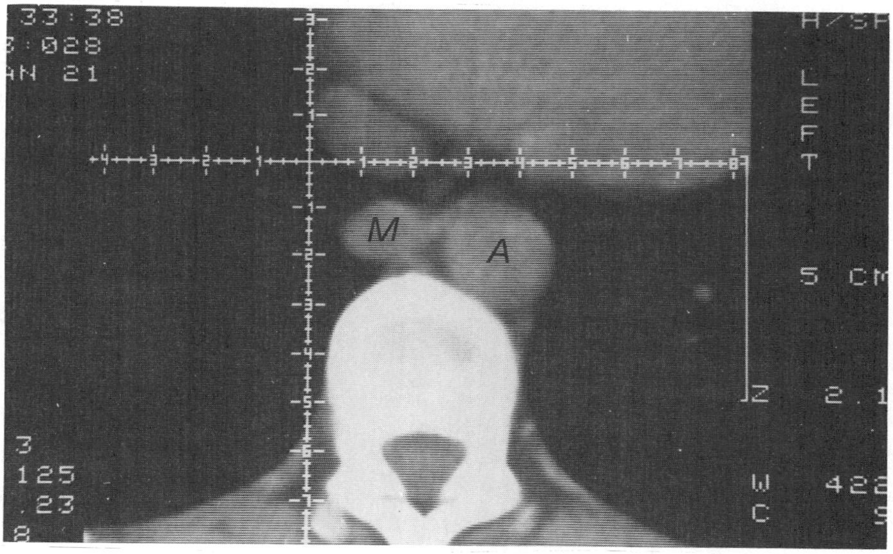

B

FIG. 16-90. This 41-year-old woman had chest x-rays obtained during a mild respiratory illness. She was otherwise asymptomatic. *A.* A smoothly circumscribed mass is visible along the right heart border near the pericardiophrenic angle and is seen in the middle mediastinum on the lateral view (*see arrows*). *B.* A magnified view from the CT scan shows a mass (M) of intermediate density lying just anterior to the spine and just to the right of the aorta (A). The mass was resected through a right posterolateral thoracotomy and was found to be a bronchogenic cyst, lined with respiratory epithelium. (*Courtesy of DM Carberry.*)

ture line leak, or spontaneous postemetic rupture (Boerhaave's syndrome). Tracheal rupture or perforation is a less common cause in which dissemination of air through the soft tissues is massive, and infection is likely to be a secondary development. Direct necrotizing spread of infection without violation of an intrathoracic viscus is seen most commonly with aggressive oropharyngeal infections involving the deep cervical space but has also been described in association with infections of ribs, sternum, and vertebrae.

Chest pain, dysphagia, respiratory distress, and cervical–upper thoracic subcutaneous crepitus are the chief hallmarks of the process during the earliest stages of infection, when it is most important to diagnose the problem and begin treatment. Evidence of fulminant systemic infection is certain to appear within 24 h, and florid sepsis with hemodynamic instability supervenes rapidly in untreated cases.

The chest x-ray may be normal very early in the process, although mediastinal and subcutaneous air becomes apparent in most cases. The mediastinal contour is usually wide, and pleural effusion with or without pneumothorax appears very frequently. A contrast esophagram, for which water-soluble contrast is usually recommended, is essential when esophageal perforation is known or suspected. Esophagoscopy is rarely indicated in acute perforation. Specific diagnostic and therapeutic approaches to esophageal perforation are dealt with elsewhere.

Infections resulting from esophageal perforation and those descending from a perioral source are usually caused by a mixture of gram-positive and gram-negative aerobic and anaerobic organisms representing the spectrum of oral flora. Initial antibiotic coverage should be broad enough to cover all possibilities until cultures are available.

Treatment must be early and aggressive. Antibiotics and fluid resuscitation are begun immediately. Chest tubes are placed for pneumothorax or effusion. The primary problem, such as esophageal perforation, is treated according to accepted principles, either separately or in combination with drainage procedures. Direct drainage of the neck is occasionally required, entering the deep cervical space through an incision parallel to the sternocleidomastoid muscle and retracting the muscle laterally to expose the carotid sheath and pretracheal and retrovisceral spaces. Unilateral and often bilateral thoracotomy is frequently necessary for direct mediastinal drainage, debridement, and accurate placement of drainage tubes. In rare instances, especially in chronic contained posterior mediastinal infection, drainage is established by approaching the mediastinum extrapleurally through the bed of the posterior end of an overlying rib.

Mediastinitis is seen in 1 to 4 percent of patients following open heart surgery and has accounted for an increasingly large proportion of all cases of mediastinitis as open heart procedures have increased in frequency. It follows a more indolent course than the entities discussed above, is rarely associated with crepitus and mediastinal air on x-ray, and has the bacteriologic spectrum of other wound infections, with *Staphylococcus aureus* and *S. epidermidis* predominating. In recent years the use of muscle flaps rotated into the sternal defect has greatly improved the treatment of this complication, which is discussed more properly in detail as a specific complication of open heart surgery.

Chronic Mediastinitis

Chronic inflammation and fibrosis in the mediastinum (sclerosing mediastinitis, fibrosing mediastinitis) are thought to result most often from granulomatous infection such as tuberculosis or histoplasmosis, although identification of an organism in individual patients is rare. It has been postulated that the process begins as

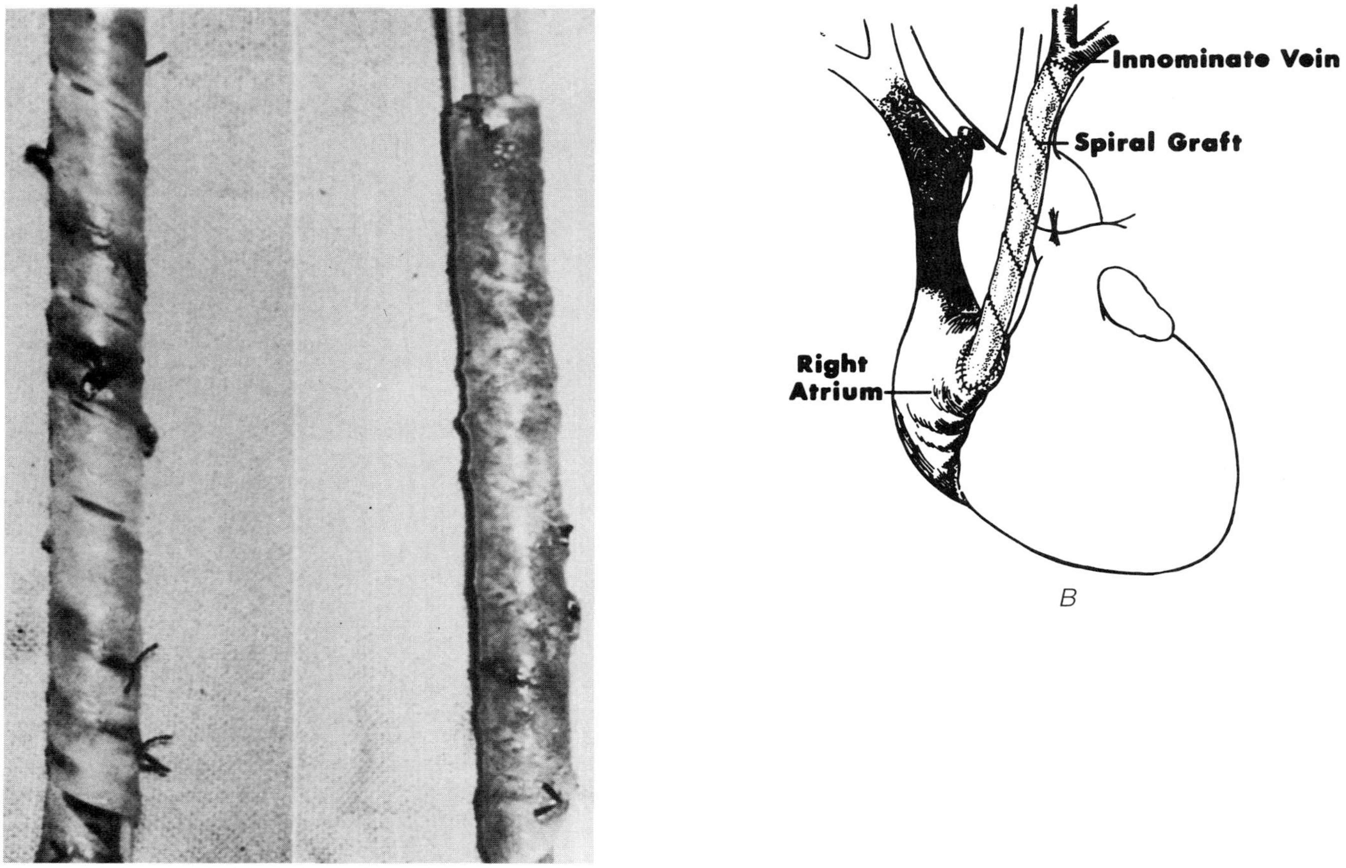

A

FIG. 16-91. Technique of spiral vein graft for bypass of superior vena caval obstruction. *A.* The spiral vein graft is constructed from a saphenous vein that has been opened from one end to the other and wrapped around a tubular stent (left). The opposing edges of vein are sewed together in a continuous spiral with fine monofilament suture (right). *B.* The spiral graft connects the innominate vein to the right atrial appendage. (From: *Doty DB, Baker WH: Bypass of the superior vena cava with spiral vein graft. Ann Thorac Surg 22:492, 1976, with permission.*)

an inflammatory reaction in the tissues surrounding involved lymph nodes. The process is likely to remain clinically silent unless it progresses to produce obstruction of the esophagus, airways, superior vena cava, or other mediastinal vascular structures. The chest x-ray may show mediastinal widening but is often normal. CT scanning combined with angiography may be necessary to define the process. Operative exploration is frequently required just to establish a diagnosis and can also be undertaken to relieve obstruction. In a series of 22 patients, medical treatment with the antifungal agent ketoconazole was surprisingly effective at controlling progression of disease when combined with operation.

Superior Vena Caval Obstruction

Superior vena caval obstruction is caused by bronchogenic carcinoma in 85 percent of cases. In the remainder the cause is another mediastinal tumor, fibrosing mediastinitis, thoracic aortic aneurysm, or caval thrombosis secondary to chronic indwelling catheters or instrumentation. At least 40 percent of bronchogenic carcinomas producing superior vena caval obstruction are small-cell tumors. Obstruction can be caused by compression or direct invasion. The clinical syndrome produced is easily recognizable, consisting of venous distention, facial edema, and plethora, often accompanied by headache and respiratory symptoms. In rare cases, associated airway compression or laryngeal edema can be life-threatening, but there is otherwise little evidence to support the commonly held notion that superior vena caval obstruction is inherently dangerous. Seizures, intracranial venous thrombosis, and other nonspecific cerebral consequences are unusual and highly associated with the presence of brain metastases. Survival in patients with obstruction due to carcinoma is usually measured in weeks to months, and it can be difficult to separate the dismal prognosis and aggressive behavior of the primary disease from the effects of superior vena caval obstruction alone. As with venous obstruction elsewhere in the body, compensatory venous collaterals develop promptly and largely ameliorate the condition, a fact that also complicates objective assessment of treatment modalities.

The vascular diagnosis can be confirmed by venography, but CT scanning with venous contrast is equally effective and provides additional information regarding surrounding structures that can be diagnostically valuable. More invasive diagnostic procedures, such as mediastinoscopy, bronchoscopy, and lymph-node biopsy, have long been considered hazardous because of elevated venous pressure. Invasive procedures can be done with a low incidence of excessive bleeding. Respiratory complications related to venous engorgement and edema of the tracheobronchial mucosa can occur but are almost always manageable in the hands of a careful anesthesiologist. The very dominant clinical tradition favoring emergency radiation therapy for the clinical syndrome prior to obtaining a tissue diagnosis deserves reappraisal.

Especially since the vast majority of cases are caused by an incurable neoplasm, palliative radiation with or without combination chemotherapy is by far the most common treatment modality. The rare cases of benign etiology have occasionally been treated with venous bypass, but without large numbers of reportable patent conduits. Bypasses from the jugular vein to the atrium or distal superior vena cava have been accomplished with femoral vein and with a spiral graft constructed from excised saphenous vein (Fig. 16-91). Saphenojugular bypass has also been described, in which the saphenous vein is routed to the neck through a subcutaneous tunnel and left attached at the saphenous bulb for outflow. All invasive treatments have in common the difficulty of predicting which patients will be unable to establish sufficient venous collaterals over time without operation.

Bibliography

Introduction

Meade RH: *A History of Thoracic Surgery*. Springfield, IL, Charles C Thomas, 1961.

Ravitch MM: *A Century of Surgery 1880–1980*. Philadelphia, Lippincott, 1981.

Anatomy of the Thorax and Pleura

Anderson JE: *Grant's Atlas of Anatomy,* 8th ed. Baltimore, Williams & Wilkins, 1983.

Shields TW (ed): *General Thoracic Surgery,* 3d ed. Philadelphia, Lea & Febiger, 1989.

Netter FH: *Atlas of Human Anatomy*. Summit, NJ, CIBA-GEIGY Corp., 1989.

Thoracic Incisions

Gibbon JH, Sabiston DC, Spencer FC: *Gibbon's Surgery of the Chest*. Philadelphia, WB Saunders, 1983.

Hazelrigg SR, Landreneau RJ, et al: The effect of muscle-sparing versus standard posterolateral thoracotomy on pulmonary function, muscle strength, and postoperative pain. *J Thorac Cardiovasc Surg* 101:394, discussion 400, 1991.

Lewis RJ, Caccavale RJ, Sisler GE: Special report: video-endoscopic thoracic surgery. *N Engl J Med* 88:473, 1991.

Martinez-Sanz R, Fleitas MG, et al: Submammary median sternotomy. *J Cardiovasc Surg* 31:578, 1990.

Pairolero PC, Arnold PG, Harris JB: Long-term results of pectoralis major muscle transposition for infected sternotomy wounds. *Ann Surg* 213:583, discussion 589, 1991.

Urschel HC Jr, Razzuk MA: Median sternotomy as a standard approach for pulmonary resection. *Ann Thorac Surg* 41:130, 1986.

Wakabayashi A: Expanded applications of diagnostic and therapeutic thoracoscopy. *J Thorac Cardiovasc Surg* 102:721, 1991.

Evaluation of the Thoracic Surgical Patient

Ali MK, Mountain CF, et al: Predicting loss of pulmonary function after pulmonary resection for bronchogenic carcinoma. *Chest* 77:337, 1980.

Boysen PG, Clark CA, Block AJ: Graded exercise testing and postthoracotomy complications. *J Cardiothorac Anesth* 4:68, 1990.

Breyer RH, Karstaedt N, et al: Computed tomography for evaluation of mediastinal lymph nodes in lung cancer: Correlation with surgical staging. *Ann Thorac Surg* 38:215, 1984.

Detsky AS, Abrams HB, et al: Predicting cardiac complications in patients undergoing non-cardiac surgery. *J Gen Intern Med* 1:211, 1986.

Goldman L: Cardiac risks and complications of noncardiac surgery. *Ann Intern Med* 98:504, 1983.

Gowda K, Zintel T, et al: Diagnostic value of maximal exercise tidal volume. *Chest* 98:1351, 1990.

Johnson JC: Surgical assessment in the elderly. *Geriatrics* 43(suppl):83, 1988.

Mangano DT: Perioperative cardiac morbidity. *Anesthesiology* 72:153, 1990.

Markos J, Mullin BP, et al: Preoperative assessment as a predictor of mortality and morbidity after lung resection. *Am Rev Respir Dis* 139:902, 1989.

Mittman C: Assessment of operative risk in thoracic surgery. *Am Rev Respir Dis* 84:197, 1961.

Olsen GN: The evolving role of exercise testing prior to lung resection. *Chest* 95:218, 1989.

Olsen GN, Weiman DS, et al: Submaximal invasive exercise testing and quantitative lung scanning in the evaluation for tolerance of lung resection. *Chest* 95:267, 1989.

Petty TL: *Pulmonary Diagnostic Techniques*. Philadelphia, Lea & Febiger, 1975.

Putnam JB Jr, Lammermeier DE, et al: Predicted pulmonary function and survival after pneumonectomy for primary lung carcinoma. *Ann Thorac Surg* 49:909, discussion 915, 1990.

Ritchie AJ, Bowe P, Gibbons JR: Prophylactic digitalization for thoracotomy: a reassessment. *Ann Thorac Surg* 50:86, 1990.

Zibrak JD, O'Donnell CR, Marton K: Indications for pulmonary function testing. *Ann Intern Med* 112:763, 1990.

Postthoracotomy Considerations

Badner NH, Sandler AN, et al: Lumbar epidural fentanyl infusions for post-thoracotomy patients: analgesic, respiratory, and pharmacokinetic effects. *J Cardiothorac Anesth* 4:543, 1990.

Brodsky JB, Chaplan SR, et al: Continuous epidural hydromorphone for postthoracotomy pain relief. *Ann Thorac Surg* 50:888, comments 862, 1990.

Chan VW, Chung F, et al: Analgesic and pulmonary effects of continuous intercostal nerve block following thoracotomy. *Can J Anaesth* 38:733, 1991.

Ferrante FM, Chan VW, et al: Interpleural analgesia after thoracotomy. *Anesth Analg* 72:105, 1991.

Grant RP, Dolman JF, et al: Patient controlled lumbar epidural fentanyl for post thoracotomy pain. *Can J Anaesth* 37:S45, 1990.

Kirsh MM, Rotman H, et al: Complications of pulmonary resection. *Ann Thorac Surg* 20:215, 1975.

Maiwand MO, Makey AR, et al: Cryoanalgesia after thoracotomy. Improvement of technique and review of 600 cases. *J Thorac Cardiovasc Surg* 92:291, 1986.

Peters RM: Pulmonary resection and gas exchange. *J Thorac Cardiovasc Surg* 88:872, 1984.

Roxburgh JC, Thompson J, Goldstraw P: Hospital mortality and long-term survival after pulmonary resection in the elderly. *Ann Thorac Surg* 51:800, 1991.

Safran D, Kuhlman G, et al: Continuous intercostal blockade with lidocaine after thoracic surgery. Clinical and pharmacokinetic study. *Anesth Analg* 70:345, 1990.

Salomaki TE, Laitinen JO, Nuutinen LS: A randomized double-blind comparison of epidural versus intravenous fentanyl infusion for analgesia after thoracotomy. *Anesthesiology* 75:790, 1991.

Thoracic Injuries

Albers JE, Rath RK, et al: Severity of intrathoracic injuries associated with first rib fractures. *Ann Thorac Surg* 33:614, 1982.

Barone JE, Pizzi WF, et al: Indications for intubation in blunt chest trauma. *J Trauma* 26:334, 1986.

Beal SL, Oreskovich MR: Long-term disability associated with flail chest injury. *Am J Surg* 150:324, 1985.

Blaisdell FW, Lewis FR Jr: *Respiratory Distress Syndrome of Shock and Trauma*. Philadelphia, WB Saunders, 1977.

Borg UR, Stoklosa JC, et al: Prospective evaluation of combined high-frequency ventilation in post-traumatic patients with adult respiratory distress syndrome refractory to optimized conventional ventilatory management. *Crit Care Med* 17:1129, 1989.

Coselli JS, Mattox KL, et al: Reevaluation of early evacuation of clotted hemothorax. *Am J Surg* 148:786, 1984.

Greene R: Lung alterations in thoracic trauma. *J Thorac Imaging* 2:1, 1987.

Johnson JA, Cogbill TH, et al: Determinants of outcome after pulmonary contusion. *J Trauma* 26:695, 1986.

Kelly JP, Webb WR, et al: Management of airway trauma. I: Tracheobronchial injuries. *Ann Thorac Surg* 40:551, 1985.

Lazar HL, Thomashow B, King TC: Complete transection of the intrathoracic trachea due to blunt trauma. *Ann Thorac Surg* 37:505, 1984.

Mandal AK, Montano J, et al: Prophylactic antibiotics and no antibiotics compared in penetrating chest trauma. *J Trauma* 25:639, 1985.

Mattox KL: Prehospital care of the patient with an injured chest. *Surg Clin North Am* 69:21, 1989.

Pate JW: Chest wall injuries. *Surg Clin North Am* 69:59, 1989.

Poulton TJ, Haldeman LW, et al: Cardiopulmonary effects of severe thoracic subcutaneous emphysema. *J Trauma* 26:396, 1986.

Regel G, Sturm JA, et al: Occlusion of bronchopleural fistula after lung injury—a new treatment by bronchoscopy. *J Trauma* 29:223, 1989.

Ross RM, Cordoba A: Delayed life-threatening hemothorax associated with rib fractures. *J Trauma,* 26:576, 1986.

Shorr RM, Rodriguez A, et al: Blunt chest trauma in the elderly. *J Trauma* 29:234, 1989.

Sladen A: Methylprednisolone. Pharmacologic doses in shock lung syndrome. *J Thorac Cardiovasc Surg* 71:800, 1976.

Thompson BM, Finger W, et al: Rib radiographs for trauma: Useful or wasteful? *Ann Emerg Med* 15:261, 1986.

Turney SZ, Rodriquez A, Cowley RA, (eds): *Management of Cardiothoracic Trauma*. Baltimore, Williams & Wilkins, 1990.

Wagner RB, Crawford WO, Schimpf PP: Classification of parenchymal injuries of the lung. *Radiology* 167:77, 1988.

Chest Wall—Congenital Deformities

Ghory MJ, James FW, Mays W: Cardiac performance in children with pectus excavatum. *J Pediatr Surg* 24:751, 1989.

Haller JA, Kramer SS, Lietman SA: Use of CT scans in selection of patients for pectus excavatum surgery: A preliminary report. *J Pediatr Surg* 22:904, 1987.

Haller JA Jr, Scherer LR, et al: Evolving management of pectus examination based on a single institutional experience of 664 patients. *Ann Surg* 9:581, 1989.

Ravitch MM: Disorders of the sternum and the thoracic wall, in Sabiston DC, Spencer FC (eds): *Gibbon's Surgery of the Chest,* 4th ed. Philadelphia, Saunders, 1983.

Shamberger RC, Welch KJ: Surgical correction of pectus carinatum. *J Pediatr Surg* 22:48, 1987.

Shamberger RC, Welch KJ: Surgical repair of pectus excavatum. *J Pediatr Surg* 23:615, 1988.

Wada J, Ikeda K, et al: Results of 271 funnel chest operations. *Ann Thorac Surg* 10:526, 1970.

Wynn SR, Driscoll DJ, et al: Exercise cardiorespiratory function in adolescents with pectus excavatum. *J Thoracic Cardiovasc Surg* 99:41, 1990.

Chest Wall—Tumors and Thoracic-Outlet Syndrome

Ala-Kulju, Ketonen P, et al: Primary tumours of the ribs. *Scand J Thorac Cardiovasc Surg* 22:97, 1988.

Arlen M, Marcove RC: Surgical treatment of soft tissue sarcomas. *Cancer Treat Res* 29:45, 1986.

Cavanaugh DG, Cabellon S Jr, Peake JB: A logical approach to chest wall neoplasms. *Ann Thorac Surg* 41:436, 1986.

Devereux DF, Wilson RE, et al: Surgical treatment of low grade soft tissue sarcomas. *Am J Surg* 143:490, 1982.

Edmonson JH, Fleming TR, et al: Randomized study of systemic chemotherapy following complete excision of nonosseous sarcomas. *J Clin Oncol* 2:1390, 1984.

Elias A, Ryan L, et al: Response to mesna, doxorubicin, ifosfamide, and dacarbazine in 108 patients with metastatic or unresectable sarcoma and no prior chemotherapy. *J Clin Oncol* 7:1208, 1989.

Hasse J: Surgery for primary, invasive and metastatic malignancy of the chest wall. *Eur J Cardiothorac Surg* 5:346, 1991.

Heise HW, Myers MH, et al: Recurrence-free survival time for surgically treated soft tissue sarcoma patients: Multivariate analysis of five prognostic factors. *Cancer* 57:172, 1986.

King RM, Pairolero PC, et al: Primary chest wall tumors: Factors affecting survival. *Ann Thorac Surg* 41:597, 1986.

Manual for Staging of Cancer: American Joint Committee on Cancer. Part II: Staging of Cancer at Specific Anatomic Sites, 3d ed. Philadelphia, JB Lippincott, 1988.

Pairolero PC, Arnold PG: Thoracic wall defects: Surgical management of 205 consecutive patients. *Mayo Clin Proc* 61:557, 1986.

Ramming KP, Holmes EC, et al: Surgical management and reconstruction of extensive chest wall malignancies. *Am J Surg* 144:146, 1982.

Sabanathan S, Salama FD, et al: Primary chest wall tumors. *Ann Thorac Surg* 39:4, 1985.

Salmon SE (ed): *Adjuvant Therapy of Cancer IV*. Philadelphia, WB Saunders, 1990.

Suit HD, Mankin HJ, et al: Preoperative, intraoperative, and postoperative radiation in the treatment of primary soft tissue sarcoma. *Cancer* 55:2659, 1985.

Tepper JE, Suit HD: Radiation therapy of soft tissue sarcomas. *Cancer* 55(suppl):2273, 1985.

Diseases of the Pleura

Agostini E: Mechanics of the pleural space. *Physiol Rev* 52:57, 1972.

Azizkhan RG, Canfield J, et al: Pleuroperitoneal shunts in the management of neonatal chylothorax. *J Pediatr Surg* 18:842, 1983.

Brenner J, Sordillo PP, et al: Malignant mesothelioma of the pleura. *Cancer* 49:2431, 1982.

Cattaneo SM, Sirak HD, et al: Recurrent spontaneous pneumothorax in the high-risk patient. *J Thorac Cardiovasc Surg* 66:467, 1973.

Chahinian AP, Pajak TF, et al: Diffuse malignant mesothelioma. *Ann Intern Med* 96:746, 1982.

DaValle MJ, Faber LP, et al: Extrapleural pneumonectomy for diffuse, malignant mesothelioma. *Ann Thorac Surg* 42:612, 1986.

de la Rocha AG: Empyema thoracis. *Surg Gynecol Obstet* 155:839, 1982.

Ferguson MK, Little AG, et al: Current concepts in the management of postoperative chylothorax. *Ann Thorac Surg* 40:542, 1985.

Lampson RS: Traumatic chylothorax. *J Thorac Surg* 17:778, 1948.

Martini N, McCormack PM, et al: Pleural mesothelioma. *Ann Thorac Surg* 43:113, 1987.

McLeod DT, Calverley PMA, et al: Further experience of corynebacterium parvum in malignant pleural effusion. *Thorax* 40:515, 1985.

Milsom JW, Kron IL, et al: Chylothorax: An assessment of current surgical management. *J Thorac Cardiovasc Surg* 89:221, 1985.

Murphy MC, Newman BM, Rodgers BM: Pleuroperitoneal shunts in the management of persistent chylothorax. *Ann Thorac Surg* 48:195, 1989.

Reshad K, Inui K, et al: Treatment of malignant pleural effusion. *Chest* 88:393, 1985.

Diseases of the Pleura—Mesothelioma

O'Hara CJ, Corson JM, et al: A monoclonal antibody that distinguishes epithelial-type malignant mesothelioma from pulmonary adenocarcinoma and extrapulmonary malignancies. *Am J Pathol* 136:421, 1990.

Rusch, VW, Piantadosi S, Holmes EC: The role of extrapleural pneumonectomy in malignant pleural mesothelioma. *J Thorac Surg* 102:1, 1991.

Diseases of the Pleura—Empyema

Arnold PG, Pairolero PC: Intrathoracic muscle flaps: An account of their use in the management of 100 consecutive patients. *Ann Surg* 211:656, 1990.

Aye RW, Froese DP, Hill LD: Use of purified streptokinase in empyema and hemothorax. *Am J Surg* 161:560, 1991.

Horrigan TP, Snow NJ: Thoracoplasty: Current application to the infected pleural space. *Ann Thorac Surg* 50:695, 1990.

Houston MC: Pleural fluid pH: Diagnostic, therapeutic, and prognostic value. *Am J Surg* 154:333, 1987.

Light RW: Management of parapneumonic effusions. *Chest* 100:892, 1991.

Ridley PD, Braimbridge MV: Thoracoscopic debridement and pleural irrigation in the management of empyema thoracis. *Ann Thorac Surg* 51:461, 1991.

Silverman SG, Mueller PR, et al: Thoracic empyema: Management with image-guided catheter drainage. *Radiology* 169:5, 1988.

Diseases of the Pleura—Spontaneous Pneumothorax

Delius RE, Farouck N, et al: Catheter aspiration for simple pneumothorax. *Arch Surg* 124:833, 1989.

Light RW, O'Hara VS, et al: Intrapleural tetracycline for the prevention of recurrent spontaneous pneumothorax. *JAMA* 264:2224, 1990.

Matsura Y, Nomimura T, et al: Clinical analysis of reexpansion pulmonary edema. *Chest* 100:1562, 1991.

Wakabayashi A, Brenner M, et al: Thoracoscopic treatment of spontaneous pneumothorax using carbon dioxide laser. *Ann Thorac Surg* 50:786, 1990.

Diseases of the Pleura—Chylothorax

Le Coultre C, Oberhansli I, et al: Postoperative chylothorax in children different between vascular and traumatic origin. *J Pediatr Surg* 25:519, 1991.

Murphy M, Newman BM, Rodgers BM: Persistent chylothorax. *Ann Thorac Surg* 48:195, 1989.

Shirai T, Amano J, Takabe K: Thoracoscopic diagnosis and treatment of chylothorax after pneumonectomy. *Ann Thorac Surg* 52:306, 1991.

Lung—Anatomy and Diagnosis

Boyden EA, Tomsett DH: Congenital absence of the medial basal bronchus in a child: With preliminary observations on postnatal growth of the lungs. *J Thorac Cardiovasc Surg* 43:517, 1962.

Garfinkel L, Auerbach O, et al: Involuntary smoking and lung cancer. A case control study. *J Natl Cancer Inst* 75:463, 1985.

Ginsberg RJ: Invasive and noninvasive techniques of staging in potentially operable lung cancer. *Semin Surg Oncol* 6:244, 1990.

Hirayama T: Nonsmoking wives of heavy smokers have a high risk of lung cancer: A study from Japan. *Br Med J* 282:183, 1981.

Martini N, Heelan R, et al: Comparative merits of conventional, computed tomographic, and magnetic resonance imaging in assessing mediastinal involvement in surgically confirmed lung cancer. *J Thorac Cardiovasc Surg* 90:639, 1985.

Mutz N, Baum M, et al: Intraoperative application of high-frequency ventilation. *Crit Care Med* 12:800, 1984.

Pollin W, Ravenholt RT: Tobacco addiction and tobacco mortality. *JAMA* 252:2849, 1984.

Replace JL, Lowrey AH: An indoor air quality standard for ambient tobacco smoke based on carcinogenic risk. *NY State J Med* 85:381, 1985.

Shields TW: The dilemma of the mediastinal node, in Kittle RE (ed): *Current Controversies in Thoracic Surgery*. Philadelphia, WB Saunders, 1986.

Templeton PA, Caskey CI, Zerhouni EA: Current uses of CT and MR imaging in the staging of lung cancer. *Radiol Clin North Am* 28:631, 1990.

Webb WR, Gamsu G, et al: Magnetic resonance imaging of the normal and abnormal pulmonary hila. *Radiology* 152:89, 1984.

Lung—Congenital Disorders, Emphysema

Bailey PV, Tracy T Jr, et al: Congenital bronchopulmonary malformations. *J Thorac Cardiovasc Surg* 99:597, 1990.

Brown SE, Wright PW, et al: Staged bilateral thoracotomies for multiple pulmonary arteriovenous malformations complicating hereditary hemorrhagic telangiectasis. *J Thorac Cardiovasc Surg* 83:285, 1982.

Dines DE, Arms RA, et al: Pulmonary arteriovenous fistulas. *Mayo Clin Proc* 49:460, 1974.

FitzGerald MX, Keelan PJ, et al: Long-term results of surgery for bullous emphysema. *J Thorac Cardiovasc Surg* 68:566, 1974.

Haddon MJ, Bowen AD: Bronchopulmonary and neuroenteric forms of foregut anomalies. *Radiol Clin North Am* 29:241, 1991.

Haller JA Jr, Golladay ES, et al: Surgical management of lung bud anomalies: Lobar emphysema, bronchogenic cyst, cystic adenomatoid malformation, and intralobar pulmonary sequestration. *Ann Thorac Surg* 28:33, 1979.

Iwa T, Watanabe Y, et al: Simultaneous bilateral operations for bullous emphysema by median sternotomy. *J Thorac Cardiovasc Surg* 81:732, 1981.

John PR, Beasley SW, Mayne V: Pulmonary sequestration and related congenital disorders. *Pediatr Radiol* 20:597, 1990.

Neilson IR, Russo P, et al: Congenital adenomatoid malformation and prognosis. *J Pediatr Surg* 26:975, 1991.

Tenholder MF, Jones PA, et al: Bullous emphysema: Progressive incremental exercise testing to evaluate candidates for bullectomy. *Chest* 77:802, 1980.

Wesley JR, Heidelberger KP, et al: Diagnosis and management of congenital cystic disease of the lung in children. *J Pediatr Surg* 21:202, 1986.

Lung—Pulmonary Infections

Alexander JC, Wolfe WG: Lung abscess and empyema of the thorax. *Surg Clin North Am* 60:835, 1980.

Amnest LS, Knatz JM, et al: Current results of treatment of bronchiectasis. *J Thorac Cardiovasc Surg* 83:546, 1982.

Confronting AIDS: *Directions for Public Health, Health Care, and Research.* Report of the Institute of Medicine, National Academy of Science, National Academic Press, Washington, 1986.

Cooper DKC, Lanza RP, et al: Infectious complication after heart transplantation. *Thorax* 38:822, 1983.

Cunningham RT, Einstein H: Coccidioidal pulmonary cavities with ruptures. *J Thorac Cardiovasc Surg* 84:172, 1982.

Daly RC, Pairolero PC, et al: Pulmonary aspergilloma. *J Thorac Cardiovasc Surg* 92:981, 1986.

Edson RS, Keys TF: Treatment of primary pulmonary blastomycosis. *Mayo Clin Proc* 56:683, 1981.

Elkadi A, Salas R, et al: Surgical treatment of atypical pulmonary tuberculosis. *J Thorac Cardiovasc Surg* 72:435, 1976.

Fuller J, Levinson MM, et al: Legionnaires' disease after heart transplantation. *Ann Thorac Surg* 39:308, 1985.

Golden N, Cohen H, et al: Thoracic actinomycosis in childhood. *Clin Pediatr* 24:646, 1985.

Kosloske AM, Ball WS, et al: Drainage of pediatric lung abscess by cough, catheter, or complete resection. *J Pediatr Surg* 21:596, 1986.

Lemmer JH, Botham MJ, et al: Modern management of adult thoracic empyema. *J Thorac Cardiovasc Surg* 90:849, 1985.

leRoux BT, Mohlala ML, et al: Suppurative diseases of the lung and pleural space. Part I: Empyema. *Curr Probl Surg* 23:1, 1986.

Mammana RB, Eskild AP, et al: Pulmonary infections in cardiac transplant patients: Modes of diagnosis, complications, and effectiveness of therapy. *Ann Thorac Surg* 36:700, 1983.

Newsom BD, Hardy JD: Pulmonary fungal infections. *J Thorac Cardiovasc Surg* 83:218, 1982.

Nonoyama A, Tanaka K, et al: Surgical treatment of pulmonary abscess in children under ten years of age. *Chest* 85:358, 1984.

Pohlson EC, McNamara JJ, et al: Lung abscess: A changing pattern of the disease. *Am J Surg* 150:97, 1985.

Prober CG, Whyte H, et al: Open lung biopsy in immunocompromised children with pulmonary infiltrates. *Am J Dis Child* 138:60, 1984.

Rao RS, Curzon PGD, et al: Cavernoscopic evacuation of aspergilloma: An alternative method of palliation for haemoptysis in high risk patients. *Thorax* 39:394, 1984.

Rubinstein A, Morecki R, et al: Pulmonary disease in children with acquired immune deficiency syndrome and AIDS-related complex. *J Pediatr* 108:498, 1986.

Shamberger RC, Weinstein HJ, et al: The surgical management of fungal pulmonary infections in children with acute myelogenous leukemia. *J Pediatr Surg* 20:840, 1985.

Solomon NW, Osborne R, et al: Surgical manifestations and results of treatment of pulmonary coccidioidomycosis. *Ann Thorac Surg* 30:433, 1980.

Sterling RP, Bradley BB, et al: Comparison of biopsy-proven *Pneumocystis carinii* pneumonia in acquired immune deficiency syndrome patients and renal allograft recipients. *Ann Thorac Surg* 38:494, 1984.

Treger TR, Visscher DW, et al: Diagnosis of pulmonary infection caused by Aspergillus: Usefulness of respiratory cultures. *J Infect Dis* 152:572, 1985.

Weiland D, Ferguson RM, et al: Aspergillosis in 25 renal transplant patients. *Ann Surg* 198:622, 1983.

White JC, Nelson S, et al: Impairment of antibacterial defense mechanisms of the lung by extrapulmonary infection. *J Infect Dis* 153:202, 1986.

Wilson JF, Decker AM: The surgical management of childhood bronchiectasis: A review of 96 consecutive pulmonary resections in children with non-tuberculous bronchiectasis. *Ann Surg* 195:354, 1982.

Lung Abscess

Rice TW, Ginsbert RJ, Todd TRJ: Tube drainage of lung abscesses. *Ann Thorac Surg* 44:356, 1987.

VanSonnenberg E, D'Agostino HB, et al: Lung abscess: CT-guided drainage. *Radiology* 178:347, 1991.

Yang PC, Luh KT, et al: Lung abscesses: US examination and US-guided transthoracic aspiration. *Radiology* 180:171, 1991.

Lung—Bronchiectasis

Dogan R, Alp M, et al: Surgical treatment of bronchiectasis: A collective review of 487 cases. *J Thorac Cardiovasc Surg* 37:183, 1989.

Laros CD, Van den Bosch JMM, et al: Resection of more than 10 lung segments. *J Thorac Cardiovasc Surg* 95:119, 1988.

Munro NC, Cooke JC, et al: Comparison of thin section computed tomography with bronchography for identifying bronchiectatic segment in patients with chronic sputum productions. *Thorax* 45:135, 1990.

Lungs—Acquired Immune Deficiency Syndrome (AIDS)

Bonfils-Roberts EA, Nickodem A, Nealon TF Jr: Retrospective analysis of the efficacy of open lung biopsy in acquired immunodeficiency syndrome. *Ann Thorac Surg* 49:115, 1990.

Gerein AN, Brumwell ML, et al: Surgical management of pneumothorax in patients with acquired immunodeficiency syndrome. *Arch Surg* 126:1272, 1991.

Lung—TB Fungal Infections

Garrett HE Jr, Roper CL: Surgical intevention in histoplasmosis. *Ann Thorac Surg* 42:711, 1986.

Horrigan TP, Snow NJ: Thoracoplasty: Current application to the infected pleural space. *Ann Thorac Surg* 50:695, 1990.

Iseman MD, Madsen L, et al: Surgical intervention in the treatment of pulmonary disease caused by drug-resistant mycobacterium tuberculosis. *Am Rev Respir Dis* 141:623, 1990.

Shapiro MJ, Albelda SM, et al: Severe hemoptysis associated with pulmonary aspergilloma. *Chest* 94:1225, 1988.

Shirakusa T, Ueda H, et al: Surgical treatment of pulmonary aspergilloma and aspergillus empyema. *Ann Thorac Surg* 48:779, 1989.

Urschel HC Jr, Razzuk MA, et al: Sclerosing mediastinitis: Improved management with histoplasmosis titer and ketoconazole. *Ann Thorac Surg* 50:215, 1990.

Lung—Tumors

Belli L, Meroni A, et al: Bronchoplastic procedures and pulmonary artery reconstruction in the treatment of bronchogenic cancer. *J Thorac Cardiovasc Surg* 90:167, 1985.
Benfield JR, Yellin A: New horizons for lung cancer. *Surg Rounds* April 1985:26–52.
Brock L: Long survival after operation for cancer of the lung. *Br J Surg* 62:1, 1975.
Cortese DA: Endobronchial management of lung cancer. *Chest* 89:234S, 1986.
Cox JD: Non-small cell lung cancer. Role of radiation therapy. *Chest* 89:284S, 1986.
Deslauriers J, Gaulin P, et al: Long-term clinical and functional results of sleeve lobectomy for primary lung cancer. *J Thorac Cardiovasc Surg* 92:871, 1986.
Errett LE, Wilson J, et al: Wedge resection as an alternative procedure for peripheral bronchogenic carcinoma in poor-risk patients. *J Thorac Cardiovasc Surg* 90:656, 1985.
Faber LP, Jensik RJ, Kittle CF: Results of sleeve lobectomy for bronchogenic carcinoma in 101 patients. *Ann Thorac Surg* 37:279, 1984.
Firmin RK, Azariades M, et al: Sleeve lobectomy (lobectomy and bronchoplasty) for bronchial carcinoma. *Ann Thorac Surg* 35:442, 1983.
Ginsberg RJ, Hill LD, et al: Modern thirty-day operative mortality for surgical resections in lung cancer. *J Thorac Cardiovasc Surg* 86:654, 1983.
Hilaris BS, Gomez J, et al: Combined surgery, intraoperative brachytherapy, and postoperative external radiation in stage III non-small cell lung cancer. *Cancer* 55:1226, 1985.
Hyman NH, Foster RS Jr, et al: Blood transfusions and survival after lung cancer resection. *Am J Surg* 149:502, 1985.
Immerman SC, Vanecko RM, et al: Site of recurrence in patients with stages I and II carcinoma of the lung resected for cure. *Ann Thorac Surg* 32:23, 1981.
Jensik RJ, Faber LP, et al: Segmental resection for bronchogenic carcinoma. *Ann Thorac Surg* 28:475, 1979.
Jensik RJ, Faber LP, et al: Survival following resection for second primary bronchogenic carcinoma. *J Thorac Cardiovasc Surg* 82:658, 1981.
Komaki R, Cox JD, et al: Characteristics of long-term survivors after treatment for inoperable carcinoma of the lung. *Am J Clin Oncol* 8(5):362, 1985.
Libshitz HI, McKenna RJ Jr, et al: Patterns of mediastinal metastases in bronchogenic carcinoma. *Chest* 90:229, 1986.
Martini N, Flehinger BJ, et al: Prospective study of 445 lung carcinomas with mediastinal lymph node metastases. *J Thorac Cardiovasc Surg* 80:390, 1980.
McCaughan BC, Martini N, et al: Chest wall invasion in carcinoma of the lung. Therapeutic and prognostic implications. *J Thorac Cardiovasc Surg* 89:836, 1985.
Mountain CF: The new international staging system for lung cancer. *Chest* 89(4 suppl):225S, 1986.
Mountain CF, McMurtrey MJ, et al: Surgery for pulmonary metastasis: A 20-year experience. *Ann Thorac Surg* 38:323, 1984.
Osterlind K, Hansen HH, et al: Mortality and morbidity in long-term surviving patients treated with chemotherapy with or without irradiation for small-cell lung cancer. *J Clin Oncol* 4(7):1044, 1986.
Paladugu RR, Benfield JR, et al: Bronchopulmonary Kulchitzky cell carcinomas. A new classification scheme for typical and atypical carcinoids. *Cancer* 55:1303, 1985.
Paulson DL, Reisch JS: Long term survival after resection for bronchogenic carcinoma. *Ann Surg* 184:324, 1976.
Paulson DL: Carcinomas in the superior pulmonary sulcus. *J Thorac Cardiovasc Surg* 70(6):1095, 1975.
Pearson FG: Lung cancer. The past twenty-five years. *Chest* 98(4 suppl):200S, 1986.
Peters RM, Clausen JL, et al: Extending resectability for carcinoma of the lung in patients with impaired pulmonary function. *Ann Thorac Surg* 26:250, 1978.
Siegelman SS, Khouri NF, et al: Solitary pulmonary nodules: CT assessment. *Radiology* 160:307, 1986.
Stair JM, Womble J, et al: Segmental pulmonary resection for cancer. *Am J Surg* 150:659, 1985.
Temeck BK, Flehinger BJ, et al: A retrospective analysis of 10-year survivors from carcinoma of the lung. *Cancer* 53:1405, 1984.
Warren WH, Gould VE, et al: Neuroendocrine neoplasms of the bronchopulmonary tract. A classification of the spectrum of carcinoid to small cell carcinoma and intervening variants. *J Thorac Cardiovasc Surg* 89:819, 1985.
Zelen M: Keynote address on biostatistics and data retrieval. *Cancer Chemother Rep* 4(2):31, 1973.
Zimmerman PV, Bint MH, et al: Ploidy as a prognostic determinant in surgically treated lung cancer. *Lancet* 2:530, 1987.

Lung—Non-Small-Cell Lung Cancer

Cellerino R, Tummarello, et al: A randomized trial of alternating chemotherapy versus best supportive care in advanced non-small-cell lung cancer. *J Clin Oncol* 9:1453, 1991.
Cox JD, Azarnia N, et al: A randomized phase I/II trial of hyperfractionated radiation therapy with total doses of 60.0 Gy to 79.2 Gy: Possible survival benefit with ≥ 69.6 Gy in favorable patients with Radiation Therapy Oncology Group stage III non-small-cell lung carcinoma: Report of Radiation Therapy Oncology Group 83-11. *J Clin Oncol* 8:1543, 1990.
Daly RC, Trastek VF, et al: Bronchoalveolar carcinoma: Factors affecting survival. *Ann Thorac Surg* 51:368, 1991.
Edell ES, Cortese DA: Bronchoscopic phototherapy with hematoporphyrin derivative for treatment of localized bronchogenic carcinoma: A 5-year experience. *Mayo Clin Proc* 62:8, 1987.
Hoffmann TH, Ransdell HT: Comparison of lobectomy and wedge resection for carcinoma of the lung. *J Thorac Cardiovasc Surg* 79:211, 1980.
Holmes EC: Adjuvant treatment in resected lung cancer. *Semin Surg Oncol* 6:263, 1990.
Grover FL, Piantadosi S: Recurrence and survival following resection of bronchioloalveolar carcinoma of the lung: The Lung Cancer Study Group experience. *Ann Surg* 209:779, 1989.
Komaki R, Mountain CF, et al: Superior sulcus tumors: Treatment and results for 85 patients without metastasis at presentation. *Int J Radiat Oncol Biol Phys* 19:31, 1990.
Martini N, Kris MG, et al: The effects of preoperative chemotherapy on the resectability of non-small cell lung carcinoma with mediastinal lymph node metastases (N2MO). *Ann Thorac Surg* 45:370, 1988.
McCaughan JS, Hawley PC, et al: Photodynamic therapy of endobronchial malignancies. *Cancer* 62:691, 1988.
Miller JI, Phillips TW: Neodymium: YAG laser and brachytherapy in the management of inoperable bronchogenic carcinoma. *Ann Thorac Surg* 50:190, 1990.
Patchell RA, Tibbs PA, et al: A randomized trial of surgery in the treatment of single metastases to the brain. *N Engl J Med* 322:494, 1990.
Rapp E, Pater JL, et al: Chemotherapy can prolong survival in patients with advanced non-small-cell lung cancer—report of a Canadian multicenter randomized trial. *J Clin Oncol* 6:633, 1988.
Rusch VW, Griffin BR, Livingston RB: The role of prophylactic cranial irradiation in regionally advanced non-small cell lung cancer. *J Thorac Cardiovasc Surg* 98:535, 1989.
Shields TW: The significance of ipsilateral mediastinal lymph node metastasis (N2 disease) in non-small cell carcinoma of the lung: A commentary. *J Thorac Cardiovasc Surg* 99:48, 1990.
Weick JK, Crowley J, et al: A randomized trial of five cisplatin-containing

treatments in patients with metastatic non-small-cell lung cancer: A Southwest Oncology Group study. *J Clin Oncol* 9:1157, 1991.

Weisenburger TH, Holmes EC, et al: Effects of postoperative mediastinal radiation on completely resected stage II and stage III epidermoid cancer of the lung. *N Engl J Med* 315:1377, 1986.

Lung—Small-Cell Cancer

Johnson BE, Grayson J, et al: Ten-year survival of patients with small-cell lung cancer treated with combination chemotherapy with or without irradiation. *J Clin Oncol* 8:396, 1990.

Prasad US, Naylor AR, et al: Long-term survival after pulmonary resection for small cell carcinoma of the lung. *Thorax* 44:784, 1989.

Rawson NS, Peto J: An overview of prognostic factors in small cell lung cancer: A report from the subcommittee for the management of lung cancer of the United Kingdom Coordinating Committee on Cancer Research. *Br J Cancer* 61:597, 1990.

Wolf M, Holle R, et al: Analysis of prognostic factors in 766 patients with small cell lung cancer (SCLC): The role of sex as a predictor for survival. *Br J Cancer* 63:986, 1991.

Zelen M: Keynote address on biostatistics and data retrieval. *Cancer Chemother Reports* 4:31, 1973.

Lung—Metastatic Tumors

Ballantine TV, Wiseman NE, Filler RM: Assessment of pulmonary wedge resection for the treatment of lung metastases. *J Pediatr Surg* 10:671, 1975.

Kemeny N, Reichman B, et al: Implementation of the group sequential methodology in a randomized trial in metastatic colorectal carcinoma. *Am J Clin Oncol* 11:66, 1988.

Kodama K, Doi O, et al: Surgical management of lung metastases. Usefulness of resection with the neodymium:yttrium-aluminum-garnet laser with median sternotomy. *J Thorac Cardiovasc Surg* 101:901, 1991.

Marincola FM, Mark JB: Selection factors resulting in improved survival after surgical resection of tumors metastatic to the lungs. *Arch Surg* 125:1387, discussion 1392, 1990.

Pastorino U, Valente M, et al: Median stenotomy and multiple lung resections for metastatic sarcomas. *Eur J Cardiothorac Surg* 4:477, 1990.

Pastorino U, Valente M, et al: Results of salvage surgery for metastatic sarcomas. *Ann Oncol* 1:269, 1990.

Pogrebniak HW, Roth JA, et al: Reoperative pulmonary resection in patients with metastatic soft tissue sarcoma [see comments]. *Ann Thorac Surg* 52:197, 1991.

Roth JA, Pass HI, et al: Comparison of median stenotomy and thoracotomy for resection of pulmonary metastases in patients with adult soft-tissue sarcomas. *Ann Thorac Surg* 42:134, 1986.

Snyder CL, Saltzman DA, et al: A new approach to the resection of pulmonary osteosarcoma metastases. Results of aggressive metastasectomy. *Clin Orthop* 270:247, 1991.

Venn GE, Sarin S, Goldstraw P: Survival following pulmonary metastasectomy. *Eur J Cardiothorac Surg* 3:105, discussion 110, 1989.

Trachea

Cavaliere S, Foccoli P, Farina PL: Nd:YAG laser bronchoscopy. *Chest* 94:15, 1988.

Ein SH, Friedberg J, et al: Tracheoplasty—a new operation for complete congenital tracheal stenosis. *J Pediatr Surg* 17:872, 1982.

El–Baz N, Jensik R, et al: One-lung high-frequency ventilation for tracheoplasty and bronchoplasty: A new technique. *Ann Thorac Surg* 34:564, 1982.

Grillo HC, Zannini P: Management of obstructive tracheal disease in children. *J Pediatr Surg* 19:414, 1984.

Grillo HC: Congenital lesions, neoplasms, and injuries of the trachea, in Sabiston DC, Spencer FC (eds): *Gibbon's Surgery of the Chest,* 5th ed. Philadelphia, WB Saunders, 1990, chap 12.

Grillo HC: Surgical treatment of postintubation tracheal injuries. *J Thorac Cardiovasc Surg* 78:860, 1979.

Kato H, Konaka C, et al: Preoperative laser photodynamic therapy in combination with operation in lung cancer. *J Thorac Cardiovasc Surg* 90:420, 1985.

Kimura K, Mukohara N, et al: Tracheoplasty for congenital stenosis of the entire trachea. *J Pediatr Surg* 17:869, 1982.

Mathiesen DJ, Grillo HC, et al: Management of acquired nonmalignant tracheoesophageal fistula. *Ann Thorac Surg* 52:759, 1991.

Moghissi K: Tracheal reconstruction with a prosthesis of marlex mesh and pericardium. *J Thorac Cardiovasc Surg* 69:499, 1975.

Nakayama DK, Harrison MR, et al: Reconstructive surgery for obstructing lesions of the intrathoracic trachea in infants and small children. *J Pediatr Surg* 17:854, 1982.

Neville WE: Prosthetic reconstruction of trachea: Technic and results in 54 patients. *Ann Chir Thorac Cardiovasc* 35:636, 1981.

Pearson FG, Todd TRJ, et al: Experience with primary neoplasms of the trachea and carina. *J Thorac Cardiovasc Surg* 88:511, 1984.

Tsugawa C, Kimura K, et al: Congenital stenosis involving a long segment of the trachea: Further experience in reconstructive surgery. *J Pediatr Surg* 23:471, 1988.

Tsugawa C, Nishijima E, et al: The use of omental flap for tracheobronchial reconstruction in infants and children. *J Pediatr Surg* 26:762, 1991.

Mediastinum

Allan A, Sethia B, et al: Investigation of superior vena caval obstruction. *Thorax* 39:878, 1984.

Aygun C, Slawson RG, et al: Primary mediastinal seminoma. *Urology* 23:109, 1984.

Baron RL, Levitt RG, et al: Computed tomography in the evaluation of mediastinal widening. *Radiology* 138:107, 1981.

Bechtold RE, Wolfman NT, et al: Superior vena caval obstruction: Detection using CT. *Radiology* 157:485, 1985.

Berry DF, Buccigrossi D: Pulmonary vascular occlusion fibrosing mediastinitis. *Chest* 89:296, 1986.

Cohen DJ, Ronnigen LD, et al: Management of patients with malignant thymoma. *J Thorac Cardiovasc Surg* 87:301, 1985.

Filler RM, Troggis DG, et al: Favorable outlook for children with mediastinal neuroblastoma. *J Pediatr Surg* 7:136, 1972.

Gladstone DJ, Pillai R, et al: Relief of superior vena caval syndrome with autologous femoral veni used as a bypass graft. *J Thorac Cardiovasc Surg* 89:750, 1985.

Ham RJ, Bulstrode C, et al: Saphenous jugular bypass for superior vena caval obstruction. *Br J Surg* 72:194, 1985.

King RM, Telander RL, et al: Primary mediastinal tumors in children. *J Pediatr Surg* 17:512, 1982.

Knapp RH, Hurt RD, et al: Malignant germ cell tumors of the mediastinum. *J Thorac Cardiovasc Surg* 89:82, 1985.

Lack EE, Weinstein HJ, et al: Mediastinal germ cell tumors in childhood. *J Thorac Cardiovasc Surg* 89:826, 1985.

Lewis BD, Hurt RD, et al: Benign teratomas of the mediastinum. *J Thorac Cardiovasc Surg* 86:727, 1983.

Livesay JJ, Mink JH, et al: The use of computed tomography to evaluate suspected mediastinal tumors. *Ann Thorac Surg* 27:305, 1979.

Monden Y, Nakahara K, et al: Myasthenia gravis with thymoma: Analysis of and postoperative prognosis for 65 patients with thymomatous myasthenia gravis. *Ann Thorac Surg* 38:46, 1984.

Parish JM, Marschke RF, et al: Etiologic considerations in superior vena cava syndrome. *Mayo Clin Proc* 56:407, 1981.

Sabiston DC, Oldham HN: The mediastinum, in Davis DR, Oldham NH, Sabiston DC, Spender FC (eds): *Gibbon's Surgery of the Chest,* 5th ed. Philadelphia, WB Saunders, 1990, chap. 17.

Schaefer S, Peshock RM, et al: Nuclear magnetic resonance imaging in Marfan's syndrome. *J Am Coll Cardiol* 9:70, 1987.

Siegel MJ, Sagel SS, et al: The value of computed tomography in the diagnosis and management of pediatric mediastinal abnormalities. *Radiology* 142:149, 1982.

Snyder ME, Luck SR, et al: Diagnostic dilemmas of mediastinal cysts. *J Pediatr Surg* 20:810, 1985.

von Schulthess GK, McMurdo K, et al: Mediastinal masses: MR imaging. *Radiology* 158:289, 1986.

Wychulis AR, Payne WS, et al: Surgical treatment of mediastinal tumors. A 40-year experience. *J Thorac Cardiovasc Surg* 62:379, 1971.

Mediastinum—Thymoma

Davis D Jr, Oldham HN Jr, Sabiston DC Jr: Primary cysts and neoplasms of the mediastinum: Recent changes in clinical presentation, methods of diagnosis, management and results. *Ann Thorac Surg* 44:229, 1987.

Jaretzki A III, Wolff M: ''Maximal'' thymectomy for myasthenia gravis. *J Thorac Cardiovasc Surg* 96:711, 1988.

Maggi G, Casadio C, et al: Thymoma: Results of 241 operated cases. *Ann Thorac Surg* 51:152, 1991.

Wilkins EW Jr, Grillo HC, et al: Role of staging in prognosis and management of thymoma. *Ann Thorac Surg* 51:888, 1991.

Mediastinum—Teratoma

Loehrer PJ, Mandelbaum I, et al: Resection of thoracic and abdominal teratoma in patients after cisplatin-based chemotherapy for germ cell tumor. *J Thorac Cardiovasc Surg* 92:676, 1986.

Mediastinum—Mesenchymal Tumors

St-Georges R, Deslauriers J, et al: Clinical spectrum of bronchogenic cysts of the mediastinum and lung in the adult. *Ann Thorac Surg* 52:6, 1991.

Mediastinum—Mediastinitis

Urschel HC, Razzuk MA, et al: Sclerosing mediastinitis: Improved management with histoplasmosis titer and ketoconazole. *Ann Thorac Surg* 50:215, 1990.

Mediastinum—Superior Vena Cava Syndrome/Obstruction

Moore WM Jr, Hollier LH, Pickett TK: Superior vena cava and central venous reconstruction. *Surgery* 110:35, 1991.

Doty DB, Doty JR, Jones KW: Bypass of superior vena cava. *J Thorac Cardiovasc Surg* 99:889, 1990.

CHAPTER 17

Congenital Heart Disease

Aubrey C. Galloway, Stephen B. Colvin, and Frank C. Spencer

INTRODUCTION

Because rheumatic fever is now rare, congenital heart disease is the most common form of heart disease seen in children. In several studies the frequency has been found to be three to four cases of congenital heart disease occurring in every 1000 live births. The frequency is about ten times greater in members of the same family than in the normal population. The risk of occurrence in younger siblings of a child with congenital heart disease is about 2 percent. In most patients the etiologic factor is unknown.

Rubella occurring in the first trimester of pregnancy is one of the few infectious diseases known to cause congenital heart disease. It produces the well-recognized syndrome of mental deficiency, deafness, cataracts, and congenital heart disease, usually a patent ductus arteriosus. Trisomy 21 is a genetic abnormality associated with a high incidence of congenital heart disease. Usually congenital heart disease occurs as an isolated malformation resulting from defective embryonic development without known cause.

The surprisingly short period of time during which cardiac development occurs in uterine life should be emphasized, for virtually all fetal heart structures are formed between the third and eighth week of pregnancy, a time interval of only 5 weeks. Atrial or ventricular septal defects result from incomplete formation of the respective septa, while transposition and other anomalies of the aorta result from abnormalities in the spiral division of the primitive bulbus cordis. Although there are six branchial aortic arches, all atrophy with the exception of the fourth left arch, which becomes the aorta, and the sixth left arch, remaining as the ductus arteriosus. Vascular ring malformations arise from different remnants of these embryonic branchial arches.

The fetal circulation has several distinctive features that may influence association with congenital heart disease. In embryonic life the lungs are collapsed, with a high vascular resistance, and pulmonary blood flow is small. Most of the blood returning through the inferior vena cava to the right atrium goes through the foramen ovale into the left atrium and thence to the left ventricle. Also, most of the blood expelled from the right ventricle into the pulmonary artery is shunted through the ductus arteriosus into the descending thoracic aorta. At birth, with expansion of the lungs, there is a fall in pulmonary vascular resistance, although the vascular resistance does not decrease to that normally found in older individuals for the first 1 to 3 years of life. There is a corresponding persistence during this time of the fetal histologic structure of the pulmonary arteries, characterized principally by an abundance of smooth muscle in the media of the arterial wall. Persistence of the fetal histologic structure of the pulmonary arterioles is associated with pulmonary hypertension.

With expansion of the lungs and increased oxygen tension, the ductus arteriosus normally closes in the first few days after birth. Oxygen constricts the ductus and prostaglandins relax it, with the mature fetus being more sensitive to the former and the immature fetus being more sensitive to the latter. The ductus remains patent in only a small percentage of individuals but is one of the most common forms of congenital heart disease. The foramen ovale is a slitlike channel that is automatically sealed when left atrial pressure becomes higher than right atrial pressure; it normally permits the flow of blood only from the right atrium to the left atrium, not in the reverse direction. Patency of the foramen ovale, usually an innocuous defect, remains throughout adult life in at least 10 to 20 percent of patients. With elevation of right atrial pressure above left atrial pressure from any cause, the foramen ovale may be stretched open and create a right-to-left shunt from the right atrium to the left atrium, resulting in cyanosis from shunting of unoxygenated blood. This characteristically occurs in patients with pulmonic valvular stenosis when right ventricular failure elevates right atrial pressure.

Although a large number of congenital heart defects have been recognized and classified, in a large pediatric cardiac clinic seven malformations will comprise the majority of abnormalities seen. Ventricular septal defect, with or without pulmonic stenosis, is by far the most common, representing 20 percent or more of all patients. The other six malformations, each occurring in 10 to 15 percent of patients, are patent ductus arteriosus, atrial septal defect, pulmonic stenosis, aortic stenosis, coarctation of the aorta, and transposition of the great vessels. The frequency of different defects varies somewhat with the age group evaluated; transposition of the great vessels is more common in the newborn but many do not survive beyond 6 months of age without an operation.

This gradual evolution of symptoms is an important consideration in evaluating children with congenital heart disease, for parents are normally apprehensive about consenting to complex diagnostic studies or operative procedures on a child who seems, to the inexperienced eye, to have little disability. Postponing therapy until a child is disabled to a point that is clinically obvious may result in irreversible changes in ventricular muscle, for severe hypertrophy of the right or left ventricle often does not regress completely following surgical correction of the basic cause, such as pulmonic or aortic stenosis. Even more serious is an increase in pulmonary vascular resistance, which is usually irreversible.

The three main physiologic disturbances resulting from congenital heart disease are (1) obstruction to emptying of the ventricles, (2) left-to-right shunts with increase in pulmonary blood flow and corresponding decrease in systemic blood flow, and (3) right-to-left shunts with cyanosis. Each of these physiologic disturbances is considered in detail in subsequent sections. With almost all forms of congenital heart disease there is an increased susceptibility to bacterial endocarditis, because the anatomic malformation creates a localized turbulent flow of blood, predisposing to local deposition of bacteria during a transient bacteremia.

Classification

Congenital heart disease may be classified by the type of anatomic abnormality present, which in turn produces a distinct physiologic disturbance. Four major groups exist: (1) left-sided obstructive lesions that restrict systemic blood flow and cardiac output, resulting in diminished peripheral perfusion and pulmonary congestion; (2) left-to-right shunts through uncomplicated septal defects or aortopulmonary connections, resulting in increased pulmonary blood flow; (3) right-to-left shunts with cyanosis, usually due to right-sided obstructive lesions with a coexisting septal defect, with mixing of blood and decreased pulmonary blood flow, but occasionally due to mixed blood exiting the aorta with coexisting increased pulmonary blood flow; and (4) complex malformations.

Pathophysiology

The physiologic consequences of congenital heart disease vary from mild to severe, depending on the anatomy. The mildest form consists of abnormal physical findings with minimal derangement of physiology. In some instances, such as with mild stenotic lesions, treatment may be unnecessary or may be delayed until late in life. In the second stage of severity, symptoms are mild to moderate. Physiologic abnormalities, such as pressure gradients across stenotic valves, shunts through septal defects, and elevated pulmonary artery pressure, can be documented by echocardiography or measured by cardiac catheterization. Eventually physiologic abnormalities worsen and corresponding anatomic changes occur, such as cardiac hypertrophy of fixed pulmonary vascular changes (the third stage of severity). The fourth stage is manifest by late-stage cardiac failure or functional disability, at times compounded by hypoxia.

Left-Sided Obstructive Lesions. The most common disorders are aortic valvular stenosis and coarctation of the aorta. These impede emptying of the left ventricular chamber, resulting in what has been termed *systolic* overloading and corresponding concentric hypertrophy of the ventricle. As the ventricular response is predominantly concentric hypertrophy, cardiac enlargement cannot be detected by clinical means, and often the chest radiograph is only slightly abnormal. The electrocardiogram and echocardiogram, however, can measure the degree of ventricular hypertrophy that has occurred. With progressive left ventricular hypertrophy angina pectoris may occur, with susceptibility to arrhythmias and even sudden death. Cardiac failure is often a late and preterminal manifestation. With severe levels of neonatal obstruction congestive heart failure is life-threatening and emergency operation is indicated.

Left-to-Right Shunts. As pressures in the left atrium and left ventricle are normally greater than those in the right atrium and right ventricle, a defect in either the atrial or ventricular septum results in a shunt of oxygenated blood from the left side of the heart to the right side. This causes pulmonary congestion from an increase in pulmonary blood flow and often a corresponding decrease in systemic blood flow. Cyanosis, of course, does not occur. With the increase in pulmonary blood flow there is a tendency to develop pulmonary hypertension, varying both with the type of defect and with the individual patient. The most common defects producing left-to-right shunts are ventricular septal defects, atrial septal defects, with or without anomalous pulmonary veins, patent ductus arteriosus, and atrioventricular canal defects.

Pulmonary Congestion. A shunt becomes physiologically significant when the pulmonary blood flow

$$Q_p = \frac{\text{Oxygen consumption}}{\text{Pulmonary venous oxygen content} - \text{Pulmonary arterial oxygen content}}$$

is one and one-half to two times as great as the systemic blood flow

$$Q_s = \frac{\text{Oxygen consumption}}{\text{Arterial oxygen content} - \text{Mixed venous oxygen content}}$$

Large shunts may produce a pulmonary blood flow three to four times greater than systemic blood flow, with a pulmonary blood flow exceeding 10 to 15 L/min/m^2 of body surface. The resulting pulmonary congestion produces a susceptibility to bacterial infection; recurrent bouts of pneumonia may occur in the first few years of life. Beyond early childhood, however, high pulmonary blood flows may produce surprisingly little disability for a period of time. With the increase in pulmonary blood flow there is a corresponding enlargement of the involved ventricle (right ventricle with atrial septal defect, left ventricle with patent ductus arteriosus, both ventricles with ventricular septal defect), resulting in so-called diastolic overloading of the ventricle, with cardiac dilatation rather than hypertrophy. The dilatation can be more easily recognized on clinical examination and on the chest radiograph than its counterpart, concentric hypertrophy. The changes in the electrocardiogram are often less prominent than those seen with concentric hypertrophy, but echocardiography can measure cardiac chamber size precisely. Cardiac failure tends to occur somewhat earlier in the course of the disease than with concentric hypertrophy, and the response to medical therapy is somewhat better than that for predominantly obstructive lesions.

Increased Pulmonary Vascular Resistance. With the increase in pulmonary blood flow, pulmonary vascular resistance may increase. The mode of development remains incompletely determined. An excellent analysis of the functional pathology of the pulmonary vascular bed was published by Edwards in 1957. Pulmonary hypertension may result from at least three factors: (1) an increase in pulmonary blood flow, (2) histologic changes in the pulmonary vascular bed with corresponding anatomic restriction of distensibility of the pulmonary vessels, and (3) pulmonary venous obstruction. The most important consideration is the pulmonary vascular resistance, not the systolic pulmonary arterial pressure per se. Pulmonary vascular resistance is calculated from the following formula:

$$\text{PVR} = \frac{\text{Mean pulmonary artery pressure} - \text{Mean left atrial pressure}}{Q_p \text{ (Pulmonary blood flow)}}$$

Normal pulmonary vascular resistance is less than 2.5 Wood units by this formula. Pulmonary hypertension resulting from an increase in pulmonary blood flow subsides as soon as the cardiac defect producing the increase in blood flow is corrected. Pulmonary hypertension caused by increased pulmonary vascular resistance caused by thickening of the media and intima is often irreversible due to fixed pulmonary vascular disease. When pulmonary vascular resistance is fixed above 10 Wood units and the shunt is balanced or right-to-left, surgical therapy is ineffective or contraindicated. Hence, in evaluating pulmonary hypertension, the significant physiologic measurement is the degree of change in the pulmonary vascular resistance, as calculated from the relation between flow and pressure, and not the absolute level of the pulmonary artery pressure per se.

Normally pulmonary arterioles are very distensible and can accommodate an increase in pulmonary blood flow up to three times normal values without any increase in pressure. Further distensibility is limited by the fibrous tissue in the adventitial sheath surrounding the arterioles. In infants and young children with pulmonary hypertension the prominent histologic change in the pulmonary arterioles is hypertrophy of the smooth muscle of the media of the arteriolar wall, which is similar to that normally found in embryonic life. Some consider these histologic changes a failure of involution of the normal fetal pattern. With more severe disease thickening of the intima occurs also. With associated fibrosis this has a serious prognosis, for such histologic changes are usually irreversible, remaining after the underlying cause has been corrected.

More significant than the increase in pulmonary blood flow, however, is the pressure under which blood is expelled into the pulmonary artery. Pulmonary hypertension is much more frequent with ventricular septal defects than with atrial septal defects that produce a similar increase in pulmonary blood flow. The incidence of pulmonary hypertension with secundum atrial septal defects in children is about 5 percent; the incidence is about 25 percent in young adults with ventricular septal defects and over 70 percent with large ventricular septal defects or atrioventricular canal defects.

There is also an individual variation in susceptibility to development of pulmonary hypertension. Some children with a large ventricular septal defect and a large increase in pulmonary blood flow will not develop any increase in pulmonary vascular resistance, while others with a smaller septal defect will develop significant pulmonary hypertension at an early age.

Defects such as truncus arteriosus, transposition, or atrioventricular canal defects may produce permanent injury in some infants before 6 months of age. Most lesions producing an increase in pulmonary vascular resistance, such as ventricular septal defect, patent ductus arteriosus, or atrioventricular canal defect should be surgically corrected in the first 3 to 12 months of life. The more serious defects, such as transposition or truncus arteriosus, may require operation in the first few weeks of life. With a simple atrial secundum defect, however, operation at such an early age is virtually never necessary, illustrating the unknown etiologic factors in producing an increase in pulmonary vascular resistance.

Restriction in Systemic Blood Flow. With large left-to-right shunts there is often a decrease in systemic blood flow, frequently associated with a retardation in normal growth and development. This is more prominently seen in children with a patent ductus arteriosus or an atrial septal defect. The appearance of frail, underweight children with atrial septal defect has been termed the *gracile* habitus. Although mental retardation is slightly more common in children with congenital heart disease, beyond this association there is no evidence that congenital heart disease retards mental development. After operation there is often a substantial increase in growth and weight.

Right-to-Left Shunts. Right-to-left shunts of venous blood directly into the systemic circulation, producing arterial hypoxemia and cyanosis, result from the combination of an intracardiac septal defect with obstruction to normal flow of blood into the pulmonary artery. The classic example is the tetralogy of Fallot, a combination of ventricular septal defect and pulmonic stenosis. Other cyanotic disorders include pulmonary stenosis-pulmonary atresia with intact ventricular septum, and tricuspid atresia, or the more complex malformations, such as transposition of the great vessels, truncus arteriosus, and double-outlet right ventricle. Most conditions have a combination of mixing of blood and decreased pulmonary blood flow, although some forms of transposition, truncus arteriosus, and double-outlet right ventricle have mixing with right-to-left shunting and cyanosis despite increased pulmonary blood flow. Right-to-left shunts produce a large number of physiologic disturbances because of the anoxia resulting from chronic hypoxemia. These are considered in detail in the following paragraphs. It should be emphasized that many disturbances result from deficient oxygen transport to tissues of the body. With right-to-left shunts there is no increase in cardiac output; the pulmonary blood flow is usually less than normal. Hence cardiac failure is rare with an uncomplicated right-to-left shunt, in contrast to its inevitable eventual occurrence with left-to-right shunts. The combination of cardiac failure and cyanosis can occur, however, with some types of transposition, with truncus arteriosus, and with double-outlet right ventricle.

Cyanosis. This is the most prominent feature of a right-to-left shunt. The degree of cyanosis depends on both the degree of anoxia and the blood hemoglobin concentration, for the visible intensity of cyanosis is determined by the number of grams of reduced hemoglobin in the circulation. It has been estimated that about 5 g of reduced hemoglobin is required to produce visible cyanosis. Normally in the capillaries about 2.25 g of reduced hemoglobin is present, so with an average hemoglobin concentration of 15 g/dL of blood, a decrease in arterial oxygen from the normal range of nearly 95 to 75 percent is needed to produce visible cyanosis. In the presence of anemia, however, a more severe degree of anoxia is required to produce visible cyanosis, while with polycythemia and hemoglobin concentrations of 20 g/dL of blood or more, severe cyanosis occurs with lesser degrees of anoxia.

Cyanosis has been conveniently grouped into "central" and "peripheral" types. *Peripheral* cyanosis results simply from a decrease in cardiac output with sluggish regional flow of blood through the capillary circulation, as a result of which more oxygen is extracted and a greater amount of reduced hemoglobin is present. This type of cyanosis occurs with conditions producing a low cardiac output, such as mitral stenosis, and varies with the condition of the patient. It is usually more prominent in certain regions of the body, such as the tips of the fingers, the lips, and the lobes of the ears.

Central cyanosis results either from a defect in oxygenation of blood in the lungs or from an intracardiac shunt. Cyanosis resulting from ventilatory insufficiency can usually be recognized from its prompt improvement when the patient breathes 100 percent oxygen, increasing the efficiency of pulmonary ventilation. In the catheterization laboratory it can be recognized from the finding that oxygen saturation of blood in the left atrium is less than 95 percent. Pulmonary insufficiency from cardiac disease occurs only with severe pulmonary congestion from cardiac failure or far-advanced pulmonary vascular disease.

An intracardiac shunt, permitting direct entry of venous blood into the systemic circulation, is the cause of central cyanosis in most patients. The intensity of the cyanosis is related to the volume of pulmonary blood flow, for ultimately cyanosis depends on the relative proportions of unoxygenated and oxygenated blood in the arterial circulation. Even though a large intracardiac shunt is present, an increase in pulmonary blood flow to produce a larger amount of oxygenated blood can substantially reduce cyanosis and improve oxygen transport. This was dramatically demonstrated by Blalock with the systemic-pulmonary artery anastomosis for tetralogy of Fallot.

The two distinctive changes that inevitably appear with chronic cyanosis are clubbing of the digits and polycythemia. The triad of cyanosis, clubbing, and polycythemia is a familiar one in children with congenital heart disease. Clubbing of the digits, or hypertrophic osteoarthropathy, is an unusual change in the appearance and structure of the digits, consisting of a rounding of the tips of the fingers and toes, as well as a thickening of the ends, associated with deposition of fibrous tissue. In addition, there may be a pronounced convexity of the fingernails. Histologically, the fingers have increased numbers of capillaries, with a large number of tiny arteriovenous aneurysms. Clubbing is usually not prominent until a cyanotic child is 1 to 2 years of age, but in some instances of severe anoxia it may evolve within several weeks. Clubbing gradually subsides following correction of the intracardiac defect.

Polycythemia is a fortunate physiologic response of the bone marrow to chronic anoxia, as an increase in red cell and hemoglobin concentration increases the ability of the blood to transport oxygen. Hematocrits of 60 to 70 percent are frequent with chronic cyanosis; values exceeding 80 percent are noted in extreme cases. There is a parallel rise in viscosity of the blood, with restriction to the flow of blood as the hematocrit rises. Once the hematocrit exceeds 75 to 80 percent, the increased viscosity constitutes a significant hazard, for transitory dehydration in an infant with a hematocrit above 80 percent may precipitate cerebral venous thrombosis and permanent neurologic injury, apparently from formation of thrombi in the viscous blood.

Limitation of Exercise Tolerance. A decrease in exercise tolerance, with dyspnea on exertion, is characteristic of cyanotic heart disease, for the circulation is unable to increase oxygen transport with exercise. The severity of the disability, or its progression, can be conveniently measured in terms of the patient's ability to walk a measured distance. Associated with exertional dyspnea is squatting, a phenomenon first emphasized by Taussig. The cyanotic child quickly learns that dyspnea on walking can be lessened by assuming a squatting position. Physiologic studies indicate that squatting produces an increase in peripheral vascular resistance, with a corresponding increase in pulmonary blood flow by diminishing the degree of right-to-left shunt. Squatting is most commonly seen in tetralogy of Fallot, less frequently in other cyanotic conditions.

Neurologic Damage. Periodic episodes of unconsciousness, termed *cyanotic spells,* are grave signs of cerebral anoxia. They often appear in the third to fourth month of life in severely cyanotic children, even in the first few weeks of life with extreme anoxia, but are rare after the fifth to sixth year of life. They characteristically occur at different times, not always associated with exertion, and evolve as episodes of crying, deepening cyanosis, and coma, lasting a few minutes to a few hours. Such episodes are extremely grave, for although recovery may ensue promptly, the spells are recurrent, and any spell may either terminate fatally or result in permanent neurologic injury. Emergency surgical treatment to improve the oxygen content of the arterial blood is strongly indicated.

Another cause of neurologic injury in cyanotic children is brain abscess, for which there is an increased susceptibility especially in children with tetralogy of Fallot. The increased susceptibility is partly related to direct access of bacteria in the venous circulation to the arterial circulation through the right-to-left shunt. This is probably not the entire explanation, however, for a similar increased frequency does not occur in other cyanotic conditions. A localized infarct with subsequent bacterial infection may explain the evolution in some patients.

Another rare cause of cerebral injury is paradoxical embolism through an intracardiac defect, in which a thrombus migrating in the venous circulation, which would normally produce a pulmonary embolus, traverses an intracardiac defect and lodges in the cerebral circulation. Hence permanent neurologic injury, most often seen as hemiplegia, is not uncommon in children with chronic severe cyanosis, constituting a strong indication for early surgical therapy when possible.

Other Changes. In older children with severe cyanosis there is a striking increase in bronchial circulation, apparently a compensatory response to the chronic decrease in pulmonary blood flow. The myriad of collateral vessels, often constituting a mass of varicosities in the mediastinum, are principally of surgical significance because of the risk of bleeding during operation. They may be associated with epistaxis in some children, but hemoptysis is rare because the pulmonary blood flow is usually less than normal, even though the bronchial circulation is greatly increased.

Eventually, with chronic polycythemia in children older than 10 to 15 years of age, multiple defects in blood coagulation occur, with abnormalities in several components of the blood-clotting mechanism. Clinically this may result in mild gastrointestinal bleeding, but the major significance is the increased susceptibility to hemorrhage following surgical procedures.

Clinical Examination

History. In obtaining the history of a patient with congenital heart disease, the presence of abnormal factors during pregnancy, especially during the first trimester, should be noted. Rubella in the first trimester has been emphasized because of the high incidence of cardiac and other defects. In some disorders, notably hypertrophic muscular aortic stenosis, there is a definite familial history of the disorder. Also, with the majority of patients with congenital heart disease there is about a 2 percent associated occurrence of congenital heart disease in other members of the same family. In most patients, however, no etiologic factors can be found.

The age at which a cardiac murmur was detected for the first time should be carefully noted. Similarly the time of appearance of cyanosis is of significance, whether at birth or subsequently during infancy. Variations in the appearance of cyanosis, as well as its location, are also important. In some patients cyanosis may be recognized at birth, then disappear for months or years, and finally appear again.

A decrease in exercise tolerance, manifested by dyspnea on exertion, is a common symptom and a convenient indication of the severity of the disorder in patients with right-to-left shunts. Squatting can be readily identified by the parents. Symptoms of lesser degrees of restriction in physical capacity, such as undue fatigability or inability to participate in exercise, should be noted, although the ability of many children with large left-to-right shunts to participate vigorously in athletics is impressive. Feeding habits and the pattern of weight are also important features.

Previous neurologic episodes such as cyanotic spells, cerebral embolism, brain abscess, or other signs of cerebral injury should be noted.

An inquiry should be made about infections such as pneumonia, bacterial endocarditis, or rheumatic fever.

Physical Examination. Abnormalities in growth and development should be particularly assessed, because these are among the most common signs of cardiac disease. Cyanosis, with clubbing or polycythemia, may be obvious or may require close scrutiny for detection. On examination of the heart, any deformity of the left costal cartilages, indicating long-standing cardiac enlargement, should be noted. A palpable thrill is particularly important, for it almost uniformly indicates significant underlying cardiac disease. Cardiac size should be estimated, although this is difficult in small children and infants and is best determined by the radiograph and echocardiogram. Systolic murmurs are commonly found but often are of little diagnostic significance. Basal systolic murmurs occur with pulmonic stenosis, aortic stenosis, patent ductus arteriosus in infants, and coarctation of the aorta. A murmur along the left sternal border is particularly prominent with ventricular septal defect. With systolic murmurs the type of murmur, location, and transmission are of particular importance. Diastolic murmurs are infrequent in infants but when present are especially significant. They may occur from aortic insufficiency with prolapse of an aortic cusp, with pulmonic insufficiency from long-standing pulmonary hypertension, or in association with a systolic murmur as the continuous murmur of a patent ductus arteriosus. The cardiac sounds, especially the second sound at the base, may be of importance in certain conditions. The pulmonic second sound is increased with pulmonary hypertension, and decreased or absent with pulmonic stenosis or atresia. Variation in splitting of the second sound may be recognized by experienced observers. A pulmonary flow murmur and a fixed split second heart sound is characteristic of atrial septal defect. Disturbances of rhythm are infrequent. The gallop rhythm with its ominous prognosis is seen in terminal forms of cardiac disease.

Examination of the lungs may detect rales from cardiac failure in large left-to-right shunts, but characteristically no abnormalities are found in the lungs with right-to-left shunts producing cyanosis. The hallmark of congestive failure in children is hepatic enlargement, occurring with surprising rapidity and regressing rapidly as failure improves. Hence estimation of the presence and extent of hepatic enlargement is of particular importance. Often hepatic enlargement precedes the detection of audible rales, in contrast to adult forms of cardiac disease. Similarly, edema is usually less prominent clinically than hepatic enlargement.

In the extremities, the presence and quality of the radial, femoral, and pedal pulses should be noted. Faint pulses are characteristic of aortic stenosis. With coarctation, radial pulses are prominent, while femoral pulses are weak or absent. Easily palpable, bounding pulses are characteristic of defects producing an abnormal exit of blood from the aorta during diastole, such as patent ductus arteriosus, aortic insufficiency, or a ruptured aneurysm of the sinus of Valsalva. These are associated with an increase in pulse pressure, usually due to a decrease in diastolic pressure. Normally the systolic blood pressure in infants is in the range of 70 to 90 mmHg, rising to about 100 mmHg in the first 5 years of life and subsequently to the normal adult level of 120 mmHg in the next few years. Diastolic pressures are usually in the range of 55 to 60 mmHg.

Examination of the digits is particularly useful with cyanosis, because clubbing is inevitable with chronic severe cyanosis. Temperature and perfusion of the extremities is extremely useful in assessing cardiac function or left-sided cardiac output in children.

Diagnostic Tests

The basic noninvasive studies are the chest radiograph, electrocardiogram, and echocardiogram. On the chest radiograph, cardiac size, contour, and vascularity of the lung fields should be noted. Unusual abnormalities include pleural effusion and notching of the ribs, seen in coarctation of the aorta. Cardiac size is best expressed as the cardiothoracic ratio, with a ratio greater than 0.5 indicating cardiac enlargement. In oblique views, enlargement of specific cardiac chambers can be estimated, though this is more precisely done with echocardiography, measuring in centimeters the exact dimensions of the atria and ventricles. Enlargement of the left atrium occurs with mitral insufficiency, ventricular septal defect, patent ductus arteriosus, or any form of left ventricular failure. Left ventricular enlargement is characteristic of aortic disease, mitral insufficiency, coarctation of the aorta, patent ductus arteriosus, and ventricular septal defect. Right atrial enlargement is especially prominent in Ebstein's malformation and also occurs in tricuspid atresia, atrial septal defect, and pulmonic stenosis. Selective enlargement of the right ventricle is frequently seen with pulmonic stenosis, pulmonary hypertension from any cause, atrial septal defect, and ventricular septal defect.

Characteristic changes in contour are seen in certain malformations. The sabot-shaped heart of tetralogy of Fallot results from hypertrophy of the right ventricle in association with a small pulmonary conus. The egg-shaped heart of transposition of the great vessels is caused by enlargement of the right ventricle and right atrium, with a narrow shadow at the base from the anterior-posterior relation between the aorta and pulmonary arteries. With total anomalous drainage of the pulmonary venous return, a figure-of-eight abnormality, composed of a large left superior vena cava in the upper mediastinum separate from the cardiac shadow, is characteristic. The size of the pulmonary vessels and the pulmonary vascularity are also important. With left-to-right shunts producing a significant increase in pulmonary flow, the vessels are enlarged with engorgement of the lung fields. The appearance may be strikingly different from conditions with a normal or decreased pulmonary blood flow, as in tetralogy of Fallot.

The electrocardiogram is the best guide to the presence of ventricular hypertrophy. Selective hypertrophy of the left ventricle, as in aortic valvular stenosis, or selective hypertrophy of the right ventricle, as in pulmonic valvular stenosis, can be identified and correlated with the degree of stenosis.

The echocardiogram has become the most valuable diagnostic test. Noninvasive two-dimensional color and Doppler echocardiography produces extremely accurate internal cardiac imaging, allowing measurement of the following: ventricular wall thickness; chamber size and configuration; shunt flow and direction; valvular location, size, and degree of regurgitant flow; and aortic or pulmonary artery size and diameter. From Doppler velocity measurement an estimate of the peak systolic gradient across a stenotic valve or coarctation is obtainable. Newer transesophageal echocardiography has increased the accuracy of this modality. Accordingly, many cases are currently treated medically or surgically based on echocardiographic studies alone. Patients with straightforward obstructive lesions, atrial septal defect, ventricular defect, or patent ductus arteriosus, or those requiring palliative emergency systemic to pulmonary shunts, are often in this category.

For more complicated procedures or for cases in which precise measurement of pulmonary vascular resistance is necessary, cardiac catheterization is still recommended. With cardiac catheterization intracardiac pressures and pressure gradients from obstructive lesions can be determined, shunts can be accurately calculated, and ventricular or vascular morphology can be clearly visualized. In the normal heart the right atrial systolic pressure is less than 5 mmHg; the right ventricular systolic pressure ranges from 15 to 30 mmHg; the left atrial pressure and the left ventricular diastolic pressure each range from 5 to 10 mmHg; and the left ventricular systolic pressure ranges from 80 to 120 mmHg. Pressure gradients, determined by continuous pressure recording as a catheter is withdrawn from one cardiac chamber to another, should normally not be present across valves. Combined right- and left-heart catheterization is usually done.

Accurate detection and quantification of any intracardiac shunt is essential. Variations from the normal pulmonary or systemic flow of 2.5 to 3.0 L/min/m^2 of body surface may occur with intracardiac shunts. A rise in oxygen saturation of 1% between cardiac chambers is usually sufficient evidence to diagnose an intracardiac left-to-right shunt. Smaller shunts may be detected with a hydrogen electrode known as hydrogen arrival time. A pulmonary blood flow (Q_p) one and one-half to two times greater than systemic blood flow (Q_s) is associated with mild physiologic disturbances and is on the borderline of indications for surgical correction. Defects producing increased pulmonary blood flows to this degree or higher are usually recommended for operation. From the combination of pulmonary blood flow and pulmonary pressure, pulmonary vascular resistance can be calculated (see section above on Pulmonary Vascular Resistance), which in the presence of pulmonary hypertension is one of the most significant physiologic measurements influencing prognosis.

The most precise physiologic evaluation of the degree of valvular stenosis is obtained by calculation of the functional cross-sectional area of the stenotic valve orifice. This is calculated by knowing the flow and pressure differential across the involved orifice using Gorlin's formula.

$$\text{Area} = \frac{\text{Flow}}{\text{Constant} \times \sqrt{\text{Pressure}_1 - \text{Pressure}_2}}$$

A valvular diameter more than 50 to 75 percent below the predicted normal for the child's body surface area is markedly abnormal. For example, a normal cross-sectional aortic valve area is 2 cm^2/m^2, while an area less than 0.5 cm^2/m^2 represents severe aortic stenosis. Similar calculations are possible for mitral valve disease, with a normal area of 2.5 to 3.0 cm^2/m^2. Significant symptoms are noted with a mitral valve diastolic gradient greater than 10 mmHg and with a mitral valve area of less than 0.8 cm^2/m^2.

Principles of Operative and Postoperative Care

Certain principles of management specifically pertain to infants undergoing cardiovascular surgery. For general principles of operative monitoring, extracorporeal circulation, cardiac massage, and defibrillation, Chap. 18 on acquired heart disease should be consulted.

Operative Management. Four important aspects of operative care are temperature control, fluid administration, prevention of air emboli, and serial blood-gas monitoring. Temperature control is essential in infants, especially in air-conditioned operating rooms, because body temperature will quickly decrease to below 32°C when the infant is anesthetized and shivering mechanisms are abolished. Constant recording of the temperature with an electric esophageal or rectal probe is mandatory, and some method of warming the infant, preferably a water mattress, should routinely be used.

Fluids must be administered with unusual precision; a 3-kg infant in cardiac failure should have no more than 20 to 40 mL of fluid in excess of measured losses during an operative procedure.

The danger of air embolism is frequently overlooked in cyanotic infants with right-to-left shunts, in whom air emboli can bypass the heart and lungs to enter the cerebral or the coronary circulation. With intravenous therapy, much care is required to prevent small air emboli, which can easily occur with the usual intravenous therapy during an operation. Only a few small bubbles, if lodged in a coronary artery, can precipitate ventricular fibrillation.

Serial measurement of the pH and the oxygen and carbon dioxide tensions of arterial and central venous blood, usually at 20- to 30-min intervals during an operation, is perhaps the most essential part of monitoring. Metabolic and respiratory acidosis are extremely frequent in seriously ill infants and may quickly become intensified with compression of the lung, ineffective cardiac contraction, or hypovolemia. A pH of central venous blood below 7.30 should be promptly corrected by appropriate ventilation, bicarbonate infusion, cessation of anesthesia, or other measures to increase cardiac output. In the authors' experiences, changes in pH almost always antedate cardiac arrest or ventricular fibrillation. This is particularly important in emergency palliative or closed procedures, because acidosis is often severe, requiring frequent treatment. With serial monitoring of blood-gas tensions during operation, desperately ill anoxic children may tolerate procedures that ordinarily would terminate in cardiac arrest or fibrillation.

The main advance responsible for the current good results obtainable with total correction of congenital heart problems is the routine use of systemic cooling during cardiopulmonary bypass, allowing low flow perfusion of the body during the operative procedure or deep hypothermia and circulatory arrest. While a full discussion of this modality is beyond the scope of this text, the technique is based on the principle that energy requirements and oxygen consumption of the body are reduced relative to decreases in body temperature. For example, at normothermia systemic flow rates during cardiopulmonary bypass must approach the normal cardiac index of 2.5 to 3.0 L/min/m^2 to supply the oxygen demands of the body. However, at 25°C total-body oxygen consumption drops by more than 50 percent and pump flow rates of 1.5 to 1.7 L/min/m^2 are adequate for tissue and organ perfusion. More strikingly, at 15°C oxygen consumption is less than 25 percent of normal. At this temperature low pump flow rates of 1.0 to 1.5 L/min/m^2 are adequate, and total cessation of flow (circulatory arrest) is safe for 45 to 60 minutes. Use of low flow or circulatory arrest allows precise intracardiac correction of complex abnormalities in small infants or neonates with a still, dry, bloodless field. This technique, first introduced experimentally by Bigelow in 1950, and adopted clinically by Dubost in 1960 and Kirklin in 1961, is one of the major advances in the modern era of cardiac surgery.

Postoperative Care. Important principles in a pediatric intensive care unit are constant observation; monitoring of the electrocardiogram; continuous measurement of central venous, left atrial, and arterial pressure; routine measurement of blood-gas tensions and urine output; and respiratory therapy (Fig. 17-1).

Constant observation of the seriously ill infant by experienced staff on a 24-h basis is mandatory. This includes observation of adequacy of ventilation with blood-gas tensions and continuous monitoring of oxygen saturation with a pulse oximeter, fluid therapy, and monitoring for arrhythmias detected on the electrocardiogram. Ventricular fibrillation can appear virtually without warning but can be corrected, usually with electric cardioversion (2 watt-sec/kg), if therapy can be started within 1 to 3 min. Hence, intensive care unit monitors with electrical alarms are essential.

Hemodynamic monitoring of the postoperative patient is best accomplished by continuous measurement of arterial pressure and by physical examination. Forward cardiac output and adequacy of

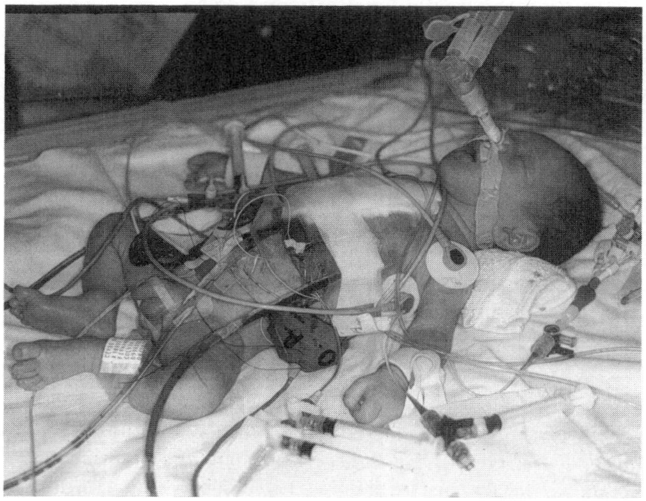

FIG. 17-1. Photograph of a 10-day-old, 1.8-kg premature child with transposition of great vessels who underwent successful arterial switch operation at New York University Medical Center. An endotracheal tube is in place and chest tubes are draining each pleural cavity and substernal space. Electrocardiograph leads sense cardiac activity and temporary pacemaker wires are in place for backup pacing. Central venous, left atrial, and arterial pressure lines are used for monitoring and blood gas determination. A catheter is in the bladder to collect urine output and a rectal probe continuously monitors core temperature, while overhead lights aid in warming.

perfusion is reflected by the temperature and color of the extremities in infants and neonates. Well-perfused children have warm feet and legs, whereas cool extremities reflect a modest reduction in cardiac output, and cold feet and legs often indicate a severe depression in cardiac output. A drop in mixed venous oxygen content indicates increased extraction due to low cardiac output, with a mixed venous oxygen pressure of less than 25 mmHg suggestive of impending circulatory collapse. Cardiac output can be measured directly in selected patients using thermodilution techniques with a pediatric Swan-Ganz catheter.

Cardiac preload and intravascular volume status should be assessed by monitoring of central venous pressure, pulmonary artery pressure, and left atrial pressure as indicated. These measurements also serve as a reflection of cardiac function. Separate monitoring of various chambers is often necessary since the left-sided cardiac function and the right-sided cardiac function may respond differently after repair of complicated congenital lesions.

Careful monitoring of fluid input and output is essential. This process balances fluid and blood administration with urine output, blood losses, and insensible losses. Maintenance fluids are usually given with D5.2NS to restrict sodium intake, although D10.2NS is sometimes used in neonates to maintain adequate serum glucose. Total fluids are restricted over the first 48 hours. Normal maintenance fluid requirements are calculated as 100 mL/kg/24h for the first 10 kg, plus 50 mL/kg/24h for the second 10 kg, plus 20 mL/kg/24h for weight above 20 kg. Children are then given 50 to 75 percent of maintenance calculations. Potassium is seldom replaced in the early postoperative phase unless serum potassium is less than 3.0 meq/L in the presence of good cardiac output and urine output. When necessary, potassium chloride is given in a dose of 0.1 meq/kg over 30 to 60 minutes, after which serum potassium is remeasured.

Urine output is a very good indicator of organ perfusion, as low cardiac output often results in an immediate drop in urine output in infants. Poorly perfused, cool extremities and a dropping urine output are sufficient indications for inotropic support in most cases. Transient renal insufficiency is not uncommon after open cardiac repair and hypothermic cardiopulmonary bypass. In recent years we have recommended early peritoneal dialysis with the first sign of renal insufficiency, as this allows control of volume status and hyperkalemia, minimizes edema, and maximizes the child's chances of early recovery.

Serial measurement of blood-gas tensions by analysis of blood samples withdrawn through arterial and central venous catheters is the best measurement of adequacy of ventilation and circulation. Arterial carbon dioxide tensions above 40 mmHg promptly develop with inefficient ventilation, and pH values below 7.30 quickly occur with either metabolic or respiratory acidosis. These changes far antedate any obvious clinical alteration in pulse or blood pressure and accordingly permit more effective therapy. Whether changes in pH and gas tensions are due to metabolic or respiratory causes can be determined by clinical evaluation and by gas analysis of peripheral arterial blood.

Proper ventilation may be a difficult postoperative problem in an infant following a thoracotomy or sternotomy. Secretions are difficult to remove and the tracheobronchial passages are so small that instrumental manipulation is difficult. The most common cause of acute bradycardia or cardiac arrest in the postoperative period is a plugged endotracheal tube, which should be promptly changed. Many advances in respiratory therapy of infants have been made in the past several years. These include mechanical respirators specifically designed for infants, the continuous positive-pressure breathing system developed by Gregory, and intermittent mandatory ventilation.

The following methods of management have been found useful, but the mode of application varies widely with individual patients. Adequate humidity, with a moist oxygen mist following operation, is essential. An endotracheal tube may be left in place for an indeterminate length of time following operation to assist ventilation and removal of secretions. Some have left endotracheal tubes in position for days or weeks, but the authors prefer a much shorter period when possible, usually less than 24 to 48 h. When an endotracheal tube is left in position, it may require changing if inspissated secretions occlude the tip of the tube.

Tracheostomy should be avoided if possible but should be done if secretions cannot be adequately removed otherwise and long-term ventilation is necessary. With a precise technique avoiding excision of any tracheal cartilage, complications are far less frequent than in the past. An extensive experience with tracheostomy and mechanical ventilation for several weeks in the treatment of neonatal tetanus has clearly demonstrated the safety of a properly performed tracheostomy in infants.

OBSTRUCTIVE LEFT-SIDED LESIONS

Coarctation of the Aorta

Historical Data. The characteristic features of coarctation were clearly outlined by Abbott in her classic analysis in 1928. In 1944 and 1945 Blalock and Park, Gross, and Crafoord and Nylin all independently contributed to the first surgical treatment of coarctation by excision and direct anastomosis. Subsequently Gross provided a strong stimulus to the study of vascular grafts by successfully using aortic homografts for patients with coarctation in whom direct anastomosis could not be done.

Incidence and Etiology. Coarctation is a common congenital malformation, occurring in 10 to 15 percent of patients with congenital heart disease. It is more common in males (3:1 ratio). Although the cause is unknown, the proximity of the coarctation to the ligamentum arteriosum supports the most plausible theory, that coarctation is an extension of the same fibrotic process that converts the patent ductus into a ligamentum arteriosum.

Pathologic Anatomy. In most patients the coarctation consists of a localized stenosis in the first 2 to 4 cm of thoracic aorta beyond the left subclavian artery. Usually there is a 1- to 3-mm lumen, though complete occlusion is present in 20 to 25 percent of patients. The ligamentum arteriosum is attached to the medial surface of the aorta near the site of coarctation. It clearly influences the coarctation, for when surgically divided, the two ends retract sharply, indicating the degree of tension previously exerted.

The stenotic area may have two or three component parts. The most frequent is a localized "shelf," consisting of an infolding of the aortic media into the lumen. This is most visible on the aortic wall opposite the ligamentum arteriosum. In the lumen, a thickened ridge of intima may be present and may increase the severity of the stenosis. In addition, a varying degree of "tubular hypoplasia" consisting of a narrowing of the aorta between the coarctation and the left subclavian artery, often extending to the left common carotid artery, is common. Coarctation of the aorta often represents a spectrum of disease, from isolated obstruction to diffuse hypoplasia of the proximal aorta and aortic arch. Arbitrary classifications, such as preductal or postductal, have not been helpful in the opinion of the authors.

Distal to the coarctation, the aorta is usually dilated. In adults a true aneurysm forms in a small percentage of patients. Large, dilated intercostal arteries entering the distal aorta, providing collateral circulation around the site of obstruction, are a striking feature. In older patients these large arteries produce "notching" of the ribs. Rarely they may become aneurysmal and rupture.

Unusual varieties of coarctation include a more proximal site of obstruction, involving the left subclavian artery, or even the left carotid and innominate artery. In some instances there is complete interruption of the aortic arch.

Patients with neonatal coarctation, previously referred to as infantile or preductal coarctation, present early in life. The condition is usually fatal unless treated, and is associated with other cardiac defects, such as ventricular septal defect, bicuspid aortic valve, and mitral valve anomalies in 75 percent of the cases. In this condition, a large patent ductus perfuses the distal aorta with blood from the pulmonary artery. The coarctation is located proximal to this. In the few patients who survive infancy without operation, cyanosis may be recognized as localized to the lower half of the body.

Pathophysiology. In 5 to 10 percent of infants, left ventricular failure may be severe, even fatal, unless operation is performed. This most frequently occurs in neonates, who present in critical condition with congestive heart failure. After the first year of life, congestive heart failure rarely occurs before the age of twenty.

The hypertension from the coarctation causes rapid degenerative changes in the proximal aorta. Children in their early teens might have obvious fibrosis and rigidity in the aortic wall, or the aorta might be extremely thin. Without treatment the average life expectancy is only 30 to 40 years. The four most common causes of death in unoperated patients are rupture of the aorta, cardiac failure, rupture of intracranial aneurysms, and bacterial endocarditis.

Clinical Manifestations. ***Symptoms.*** Congestive heart failure is usually quite severe and life-threatening with neonatal coarctation. Most older children have minimal or no symptoms despite severe hypertension. The diagnosis is often made by a routine school physical examination uncovering hypertension. Headache, epistaxis, and leg fatigue are the most frequent symptoms. Claudication in the lower extremities is uncommon.

Physical Findings. The classic combination of hypertension in the upper extremities with absent or decreased pulses in the lower extremities in a child immediately suggests coarctation. If weak femoral pulsations are present, direct measurement of the blood pressure in the upper and lower extremities may be necessary to confirm the diagnosis. Prominent pulsations from collateral circulation may be visible in the neck and over the muscles of the shoulder girdle. A systolic murmur is usually audible over the left hemithorax.

Laboratory Studies. With neonatal coarctation the diagnosis is accurately established with echocardiography, and emergency repair is usually done based on this test alone. In older patients the chest radiograph may automatically establish the diagnosis by demonstrating bilateral notching of the ribs posteriorly (Fig. 17-2). Notching is unusual before age six but is almost always present by age fourteen. The electrocardiogram characteristically shows signs of left ventricular hypertrophy, often left ventricular strain. In most patients the diagnosis can be made from the clinical findings in combination with the radiograph, electrocardiogram, and echocardiogram. Cardiac catheterization and aortography should be done routinely in older children or adults to define the location and extent of the obstruction.

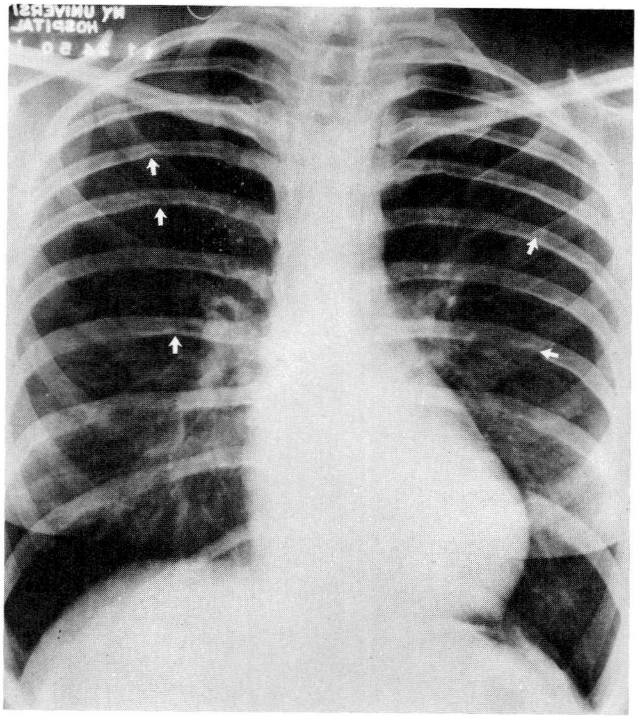

FIG. 17-2. Chest radiograph of a patient with coarctation of aorta, demonstrating classic notching of ribs from enlarged intercostal arteries. This radiographic appearance is virtually pathognomonic of coarctation of aorta, as it is rarely produced by any other condition. *(Courtesy of Dr. Raymond M. Abrams, Department of Radiology, New York University Medical Center.)*

Treatment. The ideal age for operation is between 3 and 4 years. In infants with congestive failure, operation should be performed urgently, often within the first few weeks of life, because of the high fatality rate. With severe congestive failure, other cardiac anomalies are almost always present. These may require correction during the same hospitalization. The subclavian flap technique is usually the procedure of choice in the first year of life (Fig. 17-3). Renewed interest and improved results have been achieved with resection and end-to-end anastomosis, using absorbable vascular sutures to allow for growth. The technique used depends on the particular anatomy and the length of coarctation (Fig. 17-4).

Operative Technique. A left posterolateral thoracotomy in the fourth intercostal space is used, dividing the fourth rib posteriorly in older patients. The coarctation is usually readily seen, with the typical medial indentation at the site of insertion of the ligamentum arteriosum, with large, tortuous intercostal arteries entering the distal aorta (Fig. 17-5).

Initially the mediastinal pleura is incised, after which the vagus nerve is retracted medially, noting the course of the recurrent nerve encircling the ligamentum arteriosum. The aorta proximal to

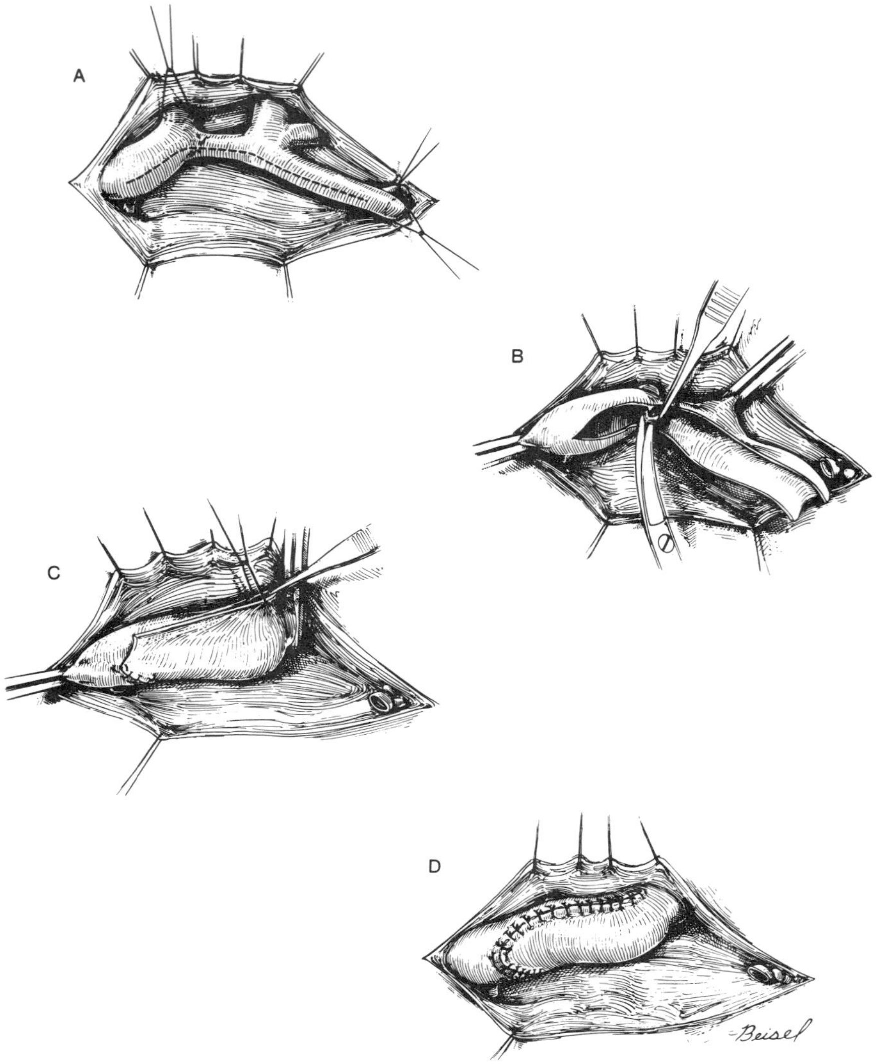

FIG. 17-3. Details of operation. (From: *Campbell DB, Waldhausen JA, et al: 1984, with permission.*)

the left subclavian artery, the left subclavian, the ligamentum arteriosum, and the distal aorta are serially mobilized. Dissection should be kept in the adventitial plane next to the aorta. This minimizes bleeding and also avoids the occasional complication of inadvertent injury to the thoracic duct.

Dissection of the distal aorta is hazardous in older patients when friable dilated intercostal arteries are present. Intercostal aneurysms, now rare, were found in 45 of 487 patients operated on by Gross and associates. Usually the aorta can be mobilized sufficiently between the intercostal arteries, individually isolating these and separately occluding them during performance of the anastomosis. The intercostal arteries can also be divided, but this is seldom necessary.

Once the vessels have been adequately mobilized, the proximal aorta, the left subclavian, and the distal aorta are all occluded with vascular clamps, after which the coarctation is excised. The objective, of course, is to obtain an anastomotic lumen as large as the proximal aorta. In children, the widest anastomosis can be obtained by excising the aorta up to the level of the left subclavian. As much as 5 cm of aorta can be excised in a child. In older children, as fibrosis decreases elasticity of the aorta, only 2.5 to 3 cm of aorta can be removed.

An end-to-end anastomosis is usually done with continuous sutures of absorbable monofilament in the posterior row of the anastomosis. Interrupted sutures can be used in small children in the anterior row to permit subsequent growth of the anastomosis. For subclavian flap repair continuous absorbable monofilament suture is used throughout the anastomosis. Following completion of the anastomosis and removal of vascular clamps, the blood pressure should be measured proximal and distal to the anastomosis to confirm that no significant gradient remains. If repair is done for neonatal coarctation in association with ventricular septal defect, pulmonary artery pressure is measured after repair of the coarctation. If the pulmonary artery pressure remains elevated either immediate pulmonary artery banding is done to restrict pulmonary blood flow, or alternately, formal repair of the ventricular septal defect is performed in 7 to 10 days.

In adults, extensive degenerative changes in the aorta from calcification and fibrosis make insertion of a prosthetic graft necessary because direct anastomosis cannot be done. A simpler ap-

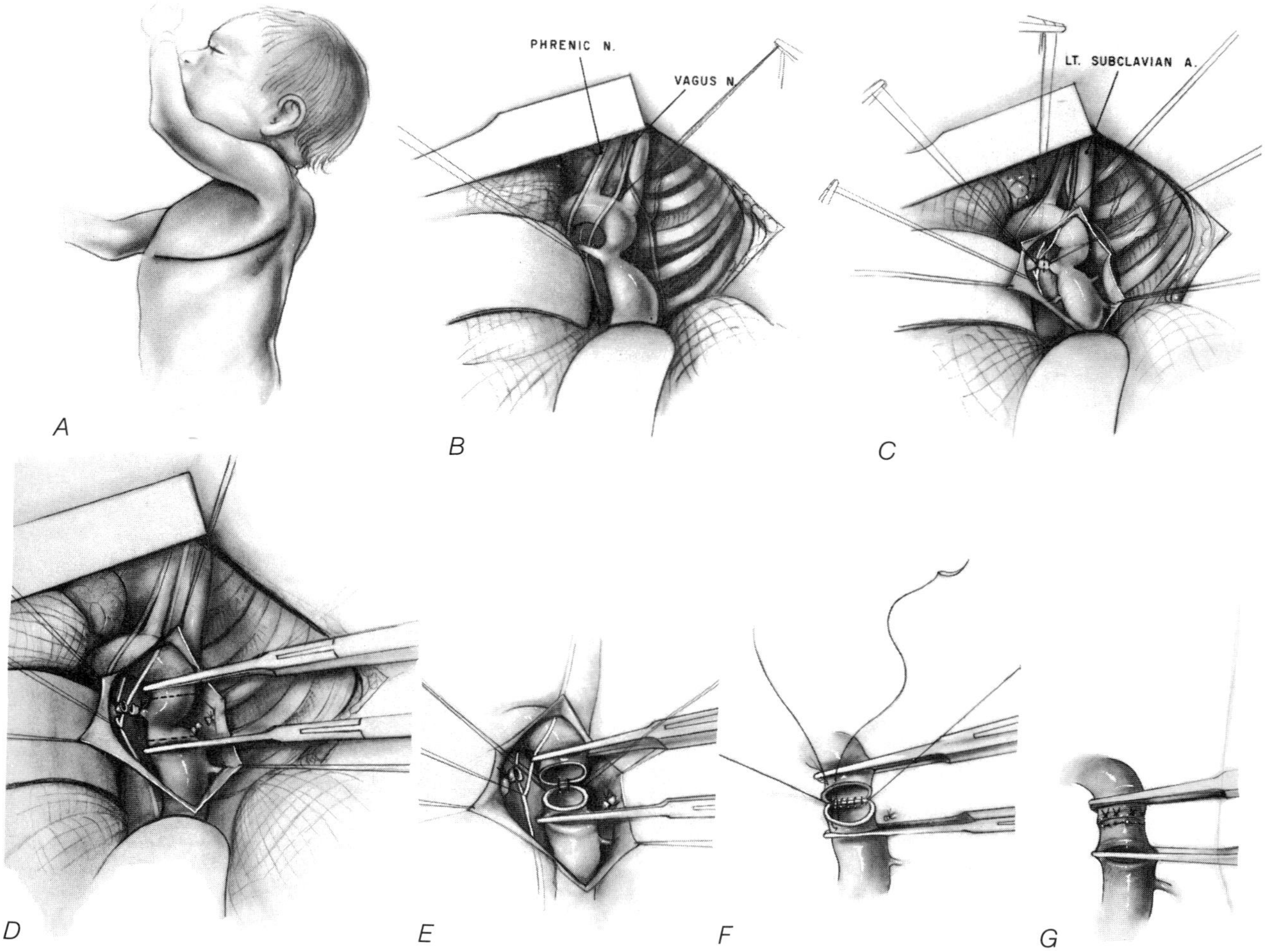

FIG. 17-4. Excision of coarctation of aorta. *A.* Chest is opened with posterolateral incision in fourth intercostal space. *B.* Once chest has been opened and lung retracted, site of coarctation is often visible where aorta is angulated inward toward mediastinum just distal to left subclavian artery. This is site where ligamentum arteriosum is inserted. *C.* After incision of mediastinal pleura overlying coarctation, vessels are isolated proximal and distal to coarctation and ligamentum arteriosum is mobilized and divided. Recurrent laryngeal nerve, often not seen during operative procedure, is displaced mediad with vagus nerve. *D.* After division of ligamentum arteriosum, vascular occlusion clamps are applied to aorta proximal and distal to site of coarctation. Often it is necessary to apply proximal clamp to aorta between left carotid and left subclavian arteries, separately occluding left subclavian artery, in order to excise widely the narrowed segment of aorta. *E.* End-to-end anastomosis is constructed with continuous or interrupted sutures of silk. *F.* After completion of posterior row of anastomosis, interrupted sutures are often used in anterior row in young children to permit growth of anastomosis. *G.* Final view of completed anastomosis.

proach in such instances is to insert a bypass graft of Dacron around the obstruction, without attempting to excise the coarctation. This relieves the obstruction without risking the hazards of excision.

Postoperative Course. Operative mortality for repair of neonatal coarctation ranges from 5 to 20 percent, depending on the severity of associated conditions. With present techniques, the risk of operation after one year of age is less than 1 percent. Antibiotics are given routinely during operation and postoperatively for 1 to 3 days. Patients usually recover rapidly and are discharged in 7 to 8 days.

The most feared operative complication is paraplegia. Current data indicate that paraplegia is due to ischemia of the spinal cord during cross-clamping in the majority of instances, and not due to ligation of intercostal arteries or other factors. In a survey of published reports by Brewer et al., paraplegia was found to occur in approximately 0.5 percent of patients. For over a decade at New York University the pressure in the distal aorta has been monitored during excision of the coarctation by inserting a small catheter or needle into the distal aorta before the aorta is clamped. Though it cannot be proved, it seems reasonable that neurologic injury probably should not occur if the distal aortic pressure remains above 50 to 60 mmHg. Distal aortic pressure following occlusion of the aorta and the left subclavian artery varies widely, from as low as 30 mmHg to levels greater than 60 mmHg.

Neurologic injury is virtually unknown if the aorta is occluded for less than 20 min or when the distal pressure remains over 50 to 60 mmHg. Hence, it seems wise to limit periods of aortic occlu-

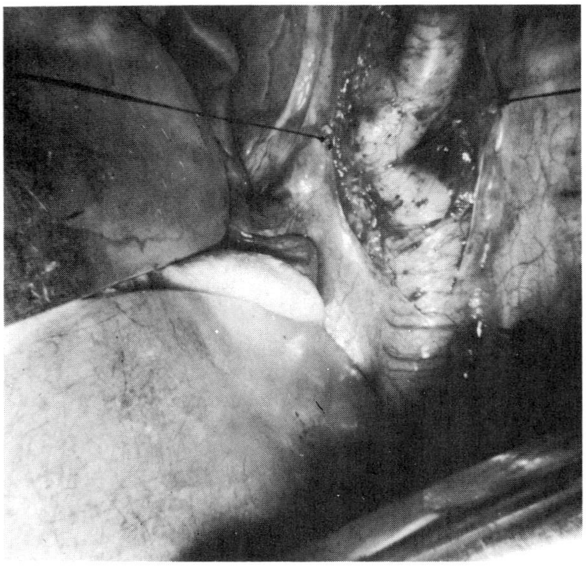

A

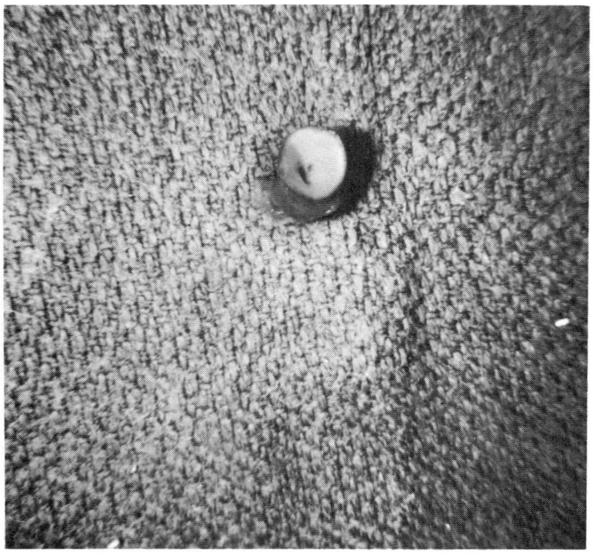

B

FIG. 17-5. *A.* Typical coarctation of aorta in child. Dilated subclavian artery is visible at top of field. At area of coarctation, aorta is angulated into mediastinum, where ligamentum arteriosum is inserted. *B.* Resected coarctation of aorta, showing narrow lumen that was present.

sion to less than 20 to 30 min if the distal pressure is less than this. This should be achievable in the majority of cases. If the planned operation takes more than 30 min and the distal pressure is low a temporary shunt can be used. The importance of pressure monitoring cannot be overemphasized.

Often there is a ''paradoxical'' hypertension in the first 48 to 72 h after operation, occurring to a greater degree in older patients with a severe coarctation. Frequently this is associated with abdominal pain. This syndrome was first described by Sealy. It seemingly is related to an increase in arterial pressure in visceral arteries, previously functioning with a lower mean pressure. Rarely, serious problems such as intestinal necrosis can occur. Prompt treatment with appropriate hypertensive medications, usually beta-adrenergic blockers and sodium nitroprusside, virtually eliminates the problem.

Some residual hypertension is common in patients operated on after five years of age and seems to increase with age. Barratt-Boyes found that 90 percent of patients were normotensive 5 years after operation, but only 50 percent at 20 years and 25 percent at 25 years. A key question is whether residual hypertension will be significantly less in patients operated on at 1 to 4 years.

Interrupted Aortic Arch

Interrupted aortic arch (IAA) is a rare defect. Neonates with this condition present with severe congestive heart failure and acidosis, with hypoperfusion of the lower half of the body. These symptoms begin 2 to 3 days after birth, when the patent ductus arteriosus begins to close. Without surgery death usually occurs within 7 to 10 days.

Pathologic Anatomy. IAA is classified by the anatomic site of aortic interruption. With Type A IAA, which occurs in 40 percent of the cases, the interruption is distal to the left subclavian artery, similar to aortic coarctation. At times it is difficult to differentiate between severe neonatal coarctation and Type A IAA, which occurs at this level, as they are physiologically similar. Type B, the most common form (55 percent), results in total arch interruption between the left carotid and left subclavian artery. Type C accounts for only 5 percent of the cases, with the interruption occurring proximally between the innominate artery and the left carotid artery. The majority of cases of IAA have associated intracardiac defects, most commonly a larger ventricular septal defect.

Pathophysiology. Children with IAA are totally dependent on ductal flow for perfusion of the lower half of the body, but the condition is often not apparent immediately after birth as long as the ductus remains patent. As systemic oxygen levels begin to rise and pulmonary vascular resistance falls the patent ductus begins to close, resulting in severe underperfusion of the lower part of the body, with acidosis and rapidly progressive renal insufficiency. Due to the high afterload and impedance to forward blood flow produced by the interrupted aorta, severe pulmonary congestion and heart failure rapidly progress. Pulmonary congestion is worsened by left-to-right shunting across the ventricular septal defect. These children are critically ill so prompt diagnosis and treatment are essential. Once the diagnosis of IAA is made an immediate infusion of prostaglandin E_1 is begun to maintain ductal patency. Acidosis should be corrected and inotropes are often necessary prior to urgent operation.

Diagnosis. Newer echocardiographic techniques are increasingly accurate in making the diagnosis of IAA. Unless the diagnosis and anatomy are completely clear by echocardiography, cardiac catheterization and angiography are recommended in order to define the anatomy and rule out associated pathology. These tests should be done emergently in order to proceed promptly with operative repair.

Operative Treatment. Type A lesions are corrected through the left chest with an incision in the fourth intercostal space. The proximal aortic arch, left subclavian artery, and distal aorta are mobilized widely. Resection and end-to-end anastomosis with absorbable suture is done, much as for neonatal coarctation. Occasionally the length between the two aortic segments is such that end-to-end anastomosis is impossible, in which case a prosthetic graft is placed from the left subclavian artery to the distal aorta. If a ventricular septal defect is present placement of a pulmonary artery band may be considered.

Children with IAA Types B and C should undergo single-stage repair via a sternotomy incision, utilizing deep hypothermia and circulatory arrest with primary end-to-end anastomosis. The associated ventricular septal defect is repaired through a right atriotomy incision, and other cardiac defects are simultaneously corrected. When severe left ventricular outflow tract obstruction is present in association with IAA, palliative treatment through the left chest is recommended, with placement of a graft from the main pulmonary artery to the descending thoracic aorta.

Results. The operative mortality for Type A IAA is less than 10 percent, while single-stage repair of Types B and C has an operative risk of 10 to 30 percent. Late survival ranges from 60 to 90 percent at 5 years, and 20 to 40 percent of the patients may require reoperation for stenosis and recurrent obstruction at the repair site.

Congenital Aortic Stenosis (Valvular/Subvalvular)

Incidence and Etiology. The condition is a common congenital abnormality, representing 8 to 10 percent of all patients with congenital heart disease. For unknown reasons, it is three to four times more frequent in males. Congenital aortic regurgitation, however, is uncommon. No causative factors are known. In the unusual variants of supravalvular or diffuse muscular stenosis associated factors suggest a genetic origin.

Pathologic Anatomy. Over four types of congenital valvular stenosis have been described; the majority are either a bicuspid valve or a tricuspid valve with fusion of commissures. A bicuspid valve is a very common anomaly, occurring in nearly 2 percent of the normal population, although such valves are not always stenotic. A common variety of bicuspid valve is failure of separation of the right and left cusps, with the undeveloped commissure being represented by a median raphe that may or may not extend to the ventricular well. Thickening of the valve cusp is common and may, when severe, contribute to the stenosis. Calcification is frequent in adults but almost never seen before 18 years of age. Mild poststenotic dilatation of the ascending aorta is common. In infants with severe valvular stenosis, more severe deformities are common, often a unicuspid valve. Other cardiac malformations commonly accompany this lesion.

Subvalvular stenosis is rare and ranges from a narrow ring of fibrous tissue to a diffuse fibromuscular tunnel with gradation between these two extremes. The discrete ringlike stenosis is present in about one-half of patients. The proximal aortic outflow tract is usually narrowed from muscular hypertrophy. Distally, the stenotic ring is adjacent to the base of the aortic cusp, often connected to the base of one cusp with a small raphe of fibrous tissue.

Two other anatomic relationships are of particular surgical importance. Beneath the noncoronary cusp the stenotic ring is attached to the ventricular septum, which can be perforated and the conduction bundle injured if appropriate landmarks are not observed. Beneath the left coronary cusp, the ring is attached to the base of the aortic leaflet of the mitral valve, which must be protected during excision.

Associated cardiac malformations are found in 15 to 20 percent of patients, more often with valvular stenosis. The most frequent ones are patent ductus, coarctation of the aorta, ventricular septal defect, and pulmonic stenosis.

Pathophysiology. The physiologic abnormality is directly related to the severity of the obstruction. Mild stenosis of little physiologic significance can occur in the presence of typical physical findings. At the other extreme, severe obstruction can cause death from congestive heart failure in infants or sudden death in older children.

Progressive stenosis leads to concentric left ventricular hypertrophy, cardiomegaly, and congestive heart failure. A gradient less than 50 mmHg usually does not produce enough disability to require operation. The more precise measurement is to calculate the functional cross-sectional area of the aortic valve from the combination of pressure gradient and cardiac output by Gorlin's formula, as noted above under Diagnostic Tests. A cross-sectional area less than 0.5 cm/m^2 of body surface should be surgically corrected. Depending on the degree of stenosis, there is a varying degree of hypertrophy of the left ventricle. Severe cardiac failure in infants is often fatal unless corrected.

Often between the ages of two and ten there are few signs of impaired ventricular function. As children grow, however, there may be a progressive decrease in cardiac reserve, with restriction of coronary and cerebral blood flow. Overt congestive failure at this age is rare. In some patients, as a consequence of fibrosis, there is an increase in the severity of the stenosis. Sudden death may occur, at times with a normal electrocardiogram. The risk of sudden death varies with different reports, and also with the signs of severity of obstruction. The mortality rate ranges from 4 to 9 percent.

In young adults with aortic stenosis calcification of the fused cusps develops with increasing frequency, approaching 100 percent in the third and fourth decades. Calcification superimposes rigidity of the leaflets onto the obstruction from the narrow orifice. Thus patients who have a history of an asymptomatic cardiac murmur during childhood may develop severe symptoms due to calcification. It is surprising how long some patients may function before calcification and rigidity precipitate cardiac failure. The authors have frequently operated on patients over 70 years of age with calcific aortic stenosis and the classic commissural abnormalities of a congenital bicuspid valve.

Trivial aortic insufficiency is present in about 50 percent of patients with subaortic stenosis. This apparently arises from thickening of the aortic cusps. Fortunately, it is rarely of any consequence. Endocarditis is a rare complication, occurring in only 1 to 3 percent of patients.

Clinical Manifestations. ***Symptoms.*** Neonates with severe aortic stenosis present in the newborn period or within the first few weeks of life with cardiomegaly, congestive heart failure, and low-output syndrome. Many older children with significant stenosis are asymptomatic, emphasizing the importance of echocardiography or catheterization to measure the severity of the abnormality. The most common symptoms are fatigue, dyspnea, angina, and syncope, found in 30 to 50 percent of patients. Usually these are found with a gradient above 50 mmHg.

Physical Examination. The four most frequent physical findings are a basal systolic murmur, a palpable thrill, a forceful left ventricular impulse, and a narrow pulse pressure. The systolic murmur is a harsh, ejection-type murmur heard best in the second right interspace, widely transmitted to the neck and arms. A palpable thrill is present in over 80 percent of patients. The left ventricular impulse is forceful and heaving. Pulse pressure is decreased in 30 to 40 percent of patients. An early diastolic murmur can be heard in 15 to 20 percent of patients; it is apparently of no physiologic significance.

Laboratory Findings. The electrocardiogram, indicating the severity of left ventricular hypertrophy, provides a moderately sensitive noninvasive guide to the severity of aortic stenosis, but has distinct limitations. The usual abnormalities are signs of left ventricular hypertrophy, and subsequent depression of the ST segment and inversion of T waves. With a gradient above 50 mmHg, a left ventricular strain pattern is common. Some patients may have severe obstruction with few electrocardiographic abnormalities.

The chest radiograph is frequently normal, because concentric hypertrophy of the left ventricle, rather than dilatation, is present. About one-half of patients will have a cardiothoracic ratio slightly greater than 50 percent. Mild dilatation of the ascending aorta is often noted. Two-dimensional echocardiography is very useful. Myocardial hypertrophy and chamber size can be accurately measured with this test. Doppler measurements define the systolic gradient with accuracy.

Diagnosis. The diagnosis can be made with reasonable certainty with the findings of the characteristic systolic murmur, palpable thrill, left ventricular impulse, and narrow pulse pressure. Confirmatory evidence can be obtained from the chest radiograph and the electrocardiogram. Echocardiography is now very accurate in establishing the diagnosis. Cardiac catheterization should be done to evaluate the severity of the obstruction in borderline cases. In infants the murmur may be loudest to the left of the sternum, requiring catheterization to establish the diagnosis. Critical aortic stenosis has been diagnosed by echocardiography in utero.

Treatment. Critical aortic stenosis in neonates usually requires emergency operative treatment. In most children, operation is performed on an elective basis after catheterization has demonstrated the severity of the obstruction or after echocardiography has demonstrated progression of disease with left ventricular hypertrophy.

Operative Technique. Occasionally neonatal aortic stenosis is treated by valvulotomy with temporary vena caval "inflow" occlusion. The more standard approach includes a median sternotomy incision, cardiopulmonary bypass, and cardioplegic myocardial protection.

Once bypass has been established, and the heart cooled and arrested, the ascending aorta is incised with a curved incision extending down into the noncoronary sinus. Calibrated Hegar dilators are useful for measuring the diameter of the stenotic orifice both before and after commissurotomy. Nomograms help estimate the length of commissural incision necessary to produce an adequate valve orifice. An attempt is made to establish an aortic valve orifice diameter that is normal for the child's body surface area. An opening larger than necessary should be made only if there is negligible risk of producing aortic insufficiency. In older children, the orifice should be enlarged so that a size 18 or 20 Hegar dilator can be inserted.

With valvular stenosis, the fused commissures are carefully incised with a small (#15) knife blade, carefully dividing the fused commissures exactly along the center of the fibrous raphe in order to leave a thick margin on each of the two cusps that are separated (Fig. 17-6). Inappropriate division of the fused commissures may result in an incision to one side of the area of fusion, increasing the likelihood of insufficiency. As far as possible, commissural incisions should be limited to where the commissures are well formed. When necessary, the incisions may be carried to the aortic wall. If not necessary, these may be terminated 1 to 3 mm from the wall.

With the classic bicuspid valve, the commissure between the right and left cusps is not well developed. Usually no incision at all is made in this area, leaving the valve as a bicuspid valve. Rarely, a short 2- to 4-mm incision may be cautiously made, but it has the hazard of producing insufficiency. *It is far better to leave some residual stenosis than to produce aortic insufficiency.* Long-term results have been disappointing if significant insufficiency was produced at operation, the patients often requiring aortic valve replacement within a few years because of cardiac failure.

In most patients the stenosis can be adequately relieved without producing significant insufficiency. The technique of commissurotomy has been emphasized in some detail because most difficulties with aortic insufficiency following aortic valvulotomy have resulted from inept valvulotomies rather than from the pathologic anatomy. Good results have also been obtained in selected cases of neonatal valvular aortic stenosis with percutaneous balloon valvuloplasty.

With subvalvular stenosis operative treatment is always necessary. The valve cusps can be carefully retracted and the fibrotic ring excised. Excellent visualization is required to prevent injury to the base of the valve cusps. The ring may consist of thin, fibrous tissue, easily removed, or it may be a thick, fibrotic structure re-

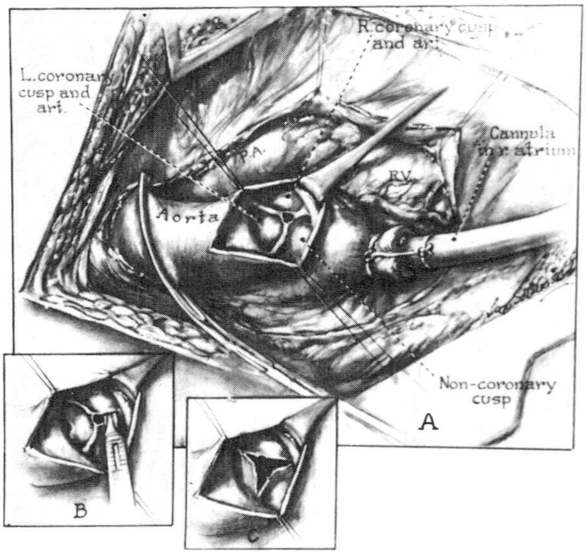

FIG. 17-6. *A.* Operative exposure of congenital aortic stenosis. Stenotic aortic valve has been exposed through longitudinal aortotomy. Fused commissures between three aortic cusps are clearly seen, with small central opening. *B* and *C.* Commissurotomy performed with knife, with center fused commissures carefully incised and incision avoided in areas where commissures are not well developed. (From: *Spencer FC, Neill CA, Bahnson HT: The treatment of congenital aortic stenosis with valvulotomy during cardiopulmonary bypass. Surgery 44:116, 1958, with permission.*)

quiring excision with a knife and rongeur (Fig. 17-7). Excellent exposure is required because the proximity of the mitral valve and the conduction bundle restricts excision of the ring out to the ventricular muscle to a narrow zone comprising less than 20 percent of the circumference of the ring. This "safe" area corresponds to the area of muscular septum beneath the commissures between the right and left coronary cusps, to the left of the right coronary ostium (Fig. 17-7). An adequate rectangular block of hypertrophied muscle must be removed similar to the operation for hypertrophic myopathy. Radical excision of the fibrotic ring beneath the left coronary cusp may perforate the aortic leaflet of the mitral valve, while radical excision beneath a noncoronary cusp may injure the ventricular septum, creating either a heart block or ventricular septal defect. With good exposure, an unhurried approach, and appropriate instruments, the area of stenosis can regularly be excised satisfactorily. Optical magnification and focal illumination with a headlight are excellent adjuncts in small children.

Subsequently the aortotomy is closed with a continuous suture, leaving a small opening for removal of air. Ventricular fibrillation is induced before removal of the clamp on the aorta, permitting the heart to fill with blood and displace air through the aortotomy before the heart is allowed to beat. Following meticulous removal of air from the heart, defibrillation can be done. Following bypass, with a systemic pressure over 100 mmHg, the pressure gradient across the aortic valve should be measured by needle puncture, preferably obtaining a gradient well under 40 mmHg.

Some rare cases of extreme left ventricular outflow tract obstruction have a combination of severe annular hypoplasia and diffuse subvalvular stenosis. These are treated with aortoventriculoplasty to enlarge both the annulus and the outflow tract. Konno

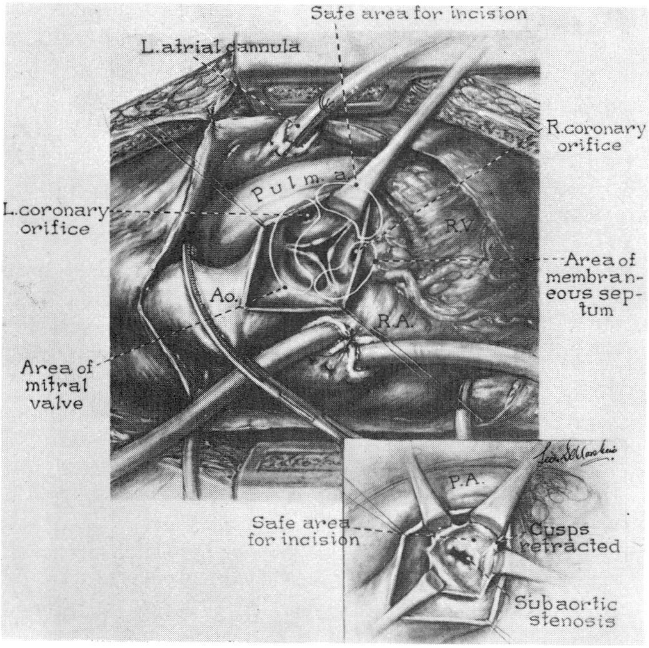

A

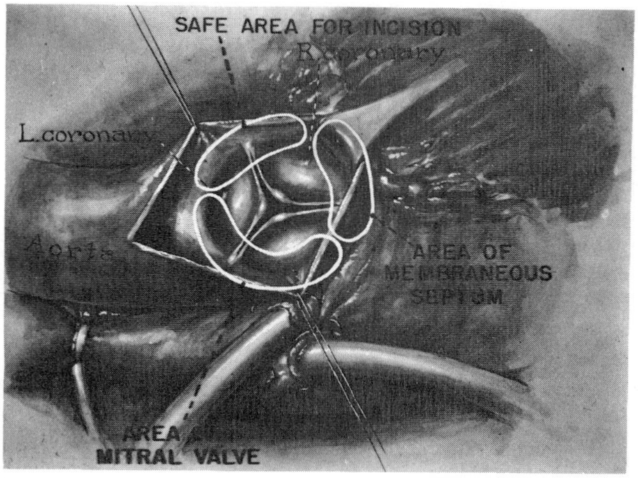

B

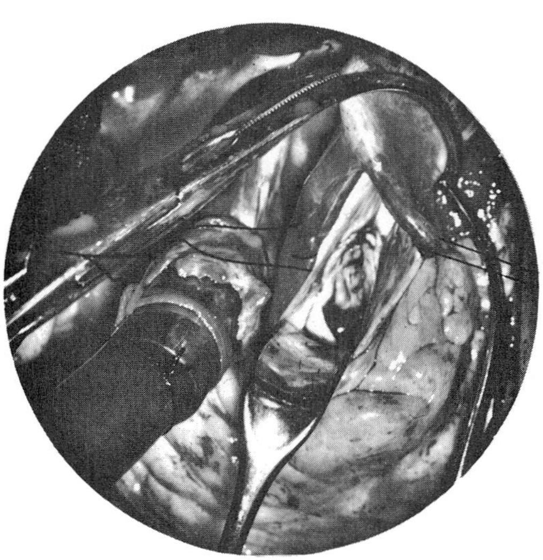

C

FIG. 17-7. *A.* Operative exposure of congenital subaortic stenosis. Valve cusps are normal. Insert shows membrane-like subaortic stenosis exposed by retraction of valve cusps. (From: *Am Surg 26:210, 1960, with permission.*) *B.* Diagram of pertinent surgical anatomy with subaortic stenosis. Beneath noncoronary cusps and part of left coronary cusp is aortic leaflet of mitral valve. Beneath part of right coronary cusp is membranous septum. Only in area beneath commissure between right and left coronary cusps is limited zone where underlying ventricular muscle can be safely excised. Failure to observe these landmarks can result in injury to mitral valve or to membranous septum with conduction bundle. *C.* Subaortic stenosis exposed at operation. Aorta has been opened with longitudinal aortotomy and retractor inserted to retract normal aortic cusps. Diaphragm-like subaortic stenosis can be clearly seen with small pinpoint central opening. (From: *Spencer FC, Neill CA, Bahnson HT: The treatment of congenital aortic stenosis with valvulotomy during cardiopulmonary bypass. Surgery 44:117, 1958, with permission.*)

(Fig. 17-8) described Dacron patch enlargement of the outflow septum and aortic annulus with associated valve replacement. More recently extended aortic root replacement and outflow enlargement has been performed with homografts.

The risks of operation are small, about 1 percent, except in the neonatal period, where operative repair of critical stenosis has an operative risk of 20 to 30 percent. Selected use of percutaneous valvuloplasty has given similar results in this group of patients. Although several reports express pessimism with operations for aortic stenosis, considering them "palliative," our experience has been most favorable. In the past 15 years there have been no deaths following elective operation in children or young adults with uncomplicated valvular or subvalvular stenosis. A satisfactory reduction in systolic gradient has been achieved in almost all patients; only a few had mild aortic insufficiency. Prosthetic valve placement or primary replacement with a homograft valve is sometimes necessary and has been required as a secondary procedure in 10 to 15 years after the initial valvulotomy. Subvalvular obstruction can recur.

In 1986, Hsieh reported long-term results in 59 patients with a mean follow-up of 18 years. Forty-six patients were alive. Sudden death occurred in seven patients, at least four of whom were known to have significant residual disease. Actuarial analysis revealed the probability of reoperation to increase from 2 percent at 5 years to 44 percent at 22 years. Dobell had reported more discouraging results; one-third of the group required a repeat operation within 10 years.

In patients with severe hypoplasia of the left ventricular outflow tract, the best results follow the Konno procedure. Ebert and associates reported results for 14 patients with no operative deaths and one late death from bacterial endocarditis, while Schaffer and associates reported long-term survival in 13 of 16 patients with aortoventriculoplasty. This procedure seems to be preferable to the once-popular insertion of an apical left ventricular-aortic conduit.

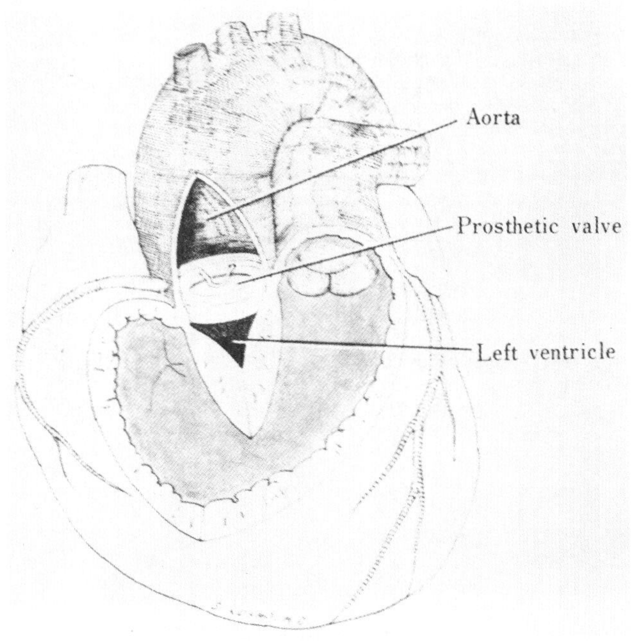

FIG. 17-8. Prosthetic valve is placed in subcoronary position as a part of an aortoventriculoplasty to enlarge the subvalvular area, annulus, and aorta. (From: *Konno S, Imai Y, et al: 1975, with permission.*)

Operative risk is generally 10 to 20 percent for both the standard Konno aortoventriculoplasty and extended aortic root replacement using homograft tissue.

Subsequently the patient should be seen at periodic intervals indefinitely because of the abnormal valve. Long-term prognosis is uncertain, although some patients are now over 20 years since operation without subsequent problems. However, the reports cited in the earlier paragraphs indicate that in some centers 20 to 30 percent of patients have required a subsequent operative procedure within 10 years. In all likelihood, eventually fibrosis and calcification of the thickened aortic cusps will lead to stenosis or insufficiency. This may also be true after homograft valve replacement.

Supravalvular Aortic Stenosis

Supravalvular aortic stenosis is the rarest form of congenital aortic stenosis. Although the first successfully treated patient was reported by McGoon and Kirklin in 1956, 10 years later Rastelli et al., reporting a personal experience with 16 patients, could only find a total of 88 cases in the medical literature, 51 of which had been treated surgically.

There is considerable variation in the type of aortic obstruction in different patients (Fig. 17-9). Peterson et al., reviewing 68 cases, found three types: hourglass, 45 cases; diffuse hypoplastic, 14 cases; and membranous, 9 cases. Associated abnormalities are frequent. In about one-third of the patients abnormalities of the aortic valve cusps are present, frequently consisting of adherence of part of one of the free margins of a cusp to the aortic wall, causing aortic regurgitation. Abnormal coronary arteries are found in over one-half of the patients. Often the right coronary artery is markedly dilated and tortuous. Focal stenotic lesions of branches of the aortic arch and peripheral branches of the pulmonary arteries have also been found.

The usual symptoms, as with other forms of aortic stenosis, are angina and syncope. Supravalvular aortic stenosis may be associated with an unusual "elfin" facies and mental retardation. Multiple peripheral pulmonary artery stenoses are also frequently noted. As physical examination provides no clues to the diagnosis except when the typical facies is present, aortography is required to establish the diagnosis. Sudden death is not uncommon in childhood, probably resulting both from the left ventricular outflow obstruction and from the coronary artery disease. It may be that most

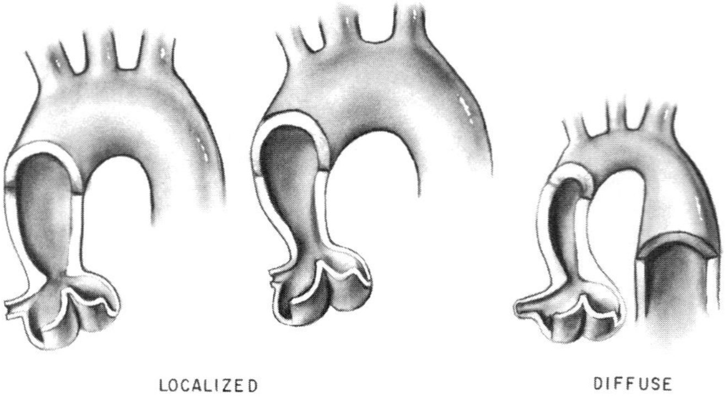

FIG. 17-9. Different types of supravalvular aortic stenosis, obstruction varying from localized constriction near aortic valve to diffuse hypoplasia of ascending aorta. (From: *Rastelli GC, McGoon DC, et al: 1966, with permission.*)

untreated patients, especially those with the characteristic facies, die before reaching adult life, because the syndrome is uncommon in adults.

Treatment. With the hourglass type, widening the stenotic area by inserting a patch of Dacron or pericardium is satisfactory. Before the patch is inserted, the intimal ridge lying above the valve cusps should be excised as completely as possible. Often a bilobed patch is placed, with extension into both the right and the noncoronary sinuses as described by Doty (Fig. 17-10). Sudden death has been described in some patients after operation, though the report by Rastelli et al. stated that a follow-up of 15 patients surviving operation found 13 with a good result. All 19 patients in the Kirklin and Barratt-Boyes series have had good short-term results.

Results have been less favorable with the diffuse hypoplastic type of obstruction. Enthusiasm has waned for a left ventricular-aortic conduit because of the high frequency of late complications. Extensive patch grafting of the ascending aorta and transverse aortic arch seems to be the most reasonable approach, though significant data are not available.

Idiopathic Hypertrophic Subaortic Stenosis

This disease is a hypertrophic myopathy of the left ventricular muscle, with secondary obstruction of the outflow tract developing from hypertrophy of the septum in about 20 percent of patients. The disease was first characterized in 1960. Diagnosis was greatly facilitated with the development of echocardiography, which has recognized asymmetric septal hypertrophy and abnormal systolic anterior motion of the mitral leaflets as characteristic findings. Recognition of patients with few or no symptoms led to confirmation of the fact that the disease is almost always genetic.

Symptoms gradually increase with age, probably as the septal hypertrophy increases. The symptoms are similar to those associated with the more common forms of aortic stenosis and include syncope, angina, and dyspnea. A systolic murmur of medium intensity near the apex, but not prominent at the base of the heart, may be the first clue to the diagnosis. With progressive disease, atrial fibrillation systemic emboli and sudden death are the most significant events. Sudden death is distressingly common, presumably from an arrhythmia. The chest radiograph and electrocardiogram are not diagnostic, but the two-dimensional echocardiogram precisely defines the abnormality and establishes the diagnosis. It can be further clarified with catheterization and angiography. On catheterization a gradient varying from 50 to 150 mmHg can be demonstrated in the proximal outflow of the left ventricle. The pressure gradient characteristically increases with the infusion of isoproterenol because of more forceful contraction of the left ventricle.

Treatment. Many patients are treated medically, reserving operation for those with symptomatic severe obstruction not improving with medical therapy. Beta blockade or calcium blockade is usually used.

Surgical myomectomy, as developed by Morrow, is clearly indicated with symptomatic patients and a gradient of 50 mm or greater. Morrow reported excellent results in a series exceeding 200 patients. Using a transaortic approach, a rectangular block of ventricular muscle is excised from the septum, extending down

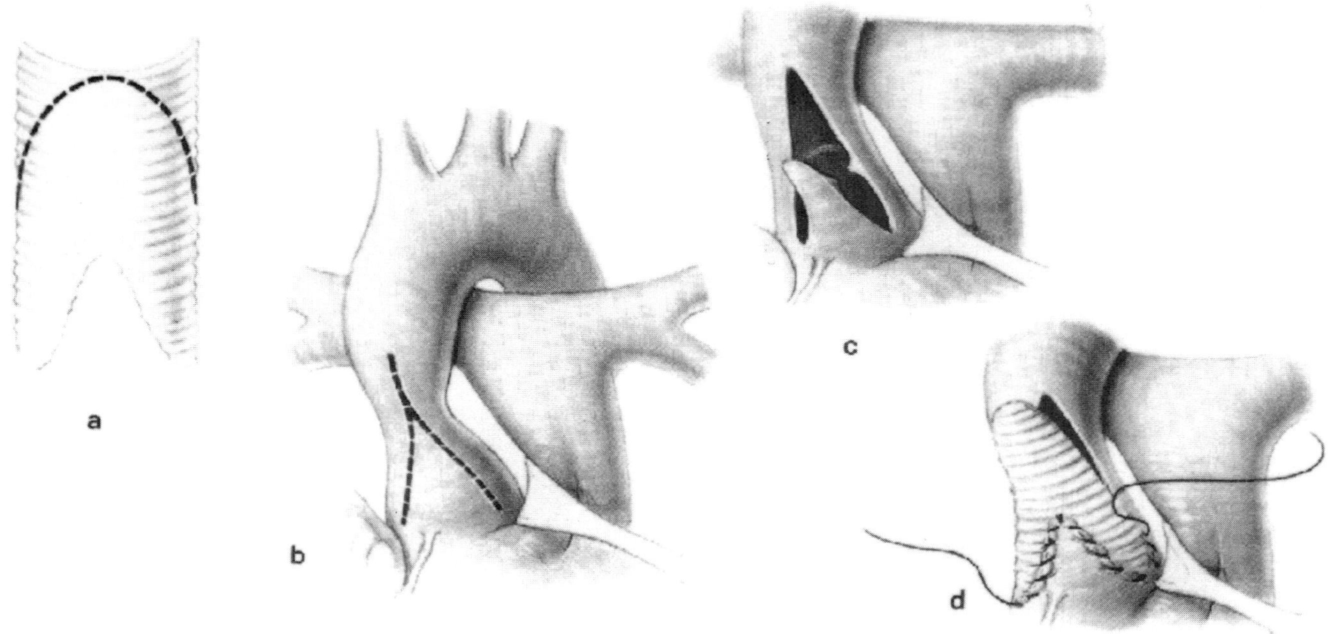

FIG. 17-10. Bilobed patch aortoplasty as described by Doty et al. for supravalvular aortic stenosis. *A.* A bilobed patch is cut. *B.* Aortic incision extends down into noncoronary sinus, with second incision extending down between left and right coronary arteries. *C.* Fibrous aortic ring is incised in two separate places. Posteriorly fibrous ring on the aortic wall is excised. *D.* Dacron, or pericardial, patch is sutured into aortotomy, placing tips down into apex of each incision, effectively enlarging aortic root. (From: *Doty et al: 1977,* and *Stark J, de Leval M (eds): Surgery for Congenital Heart Disease. Orlando, FL, Grune & Stratton, 1983, p. 449, with permission.*)

from the base of the aortic cusp into the ventricular cavity for several centimeters, staying to the left of the right coronary ostium (Fig. 17-11). Late catheterization studies following the radical myomectomy clearly document permanent relief of the outflow tract obstruction.

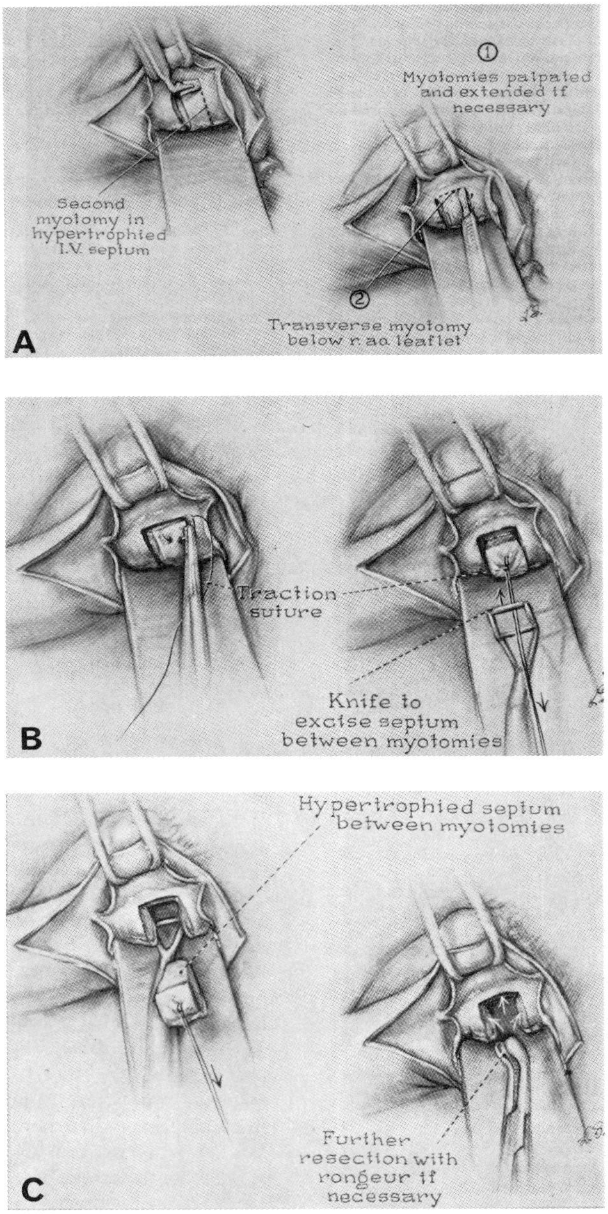

FIG. 17-11. *A.* Second myotomy is made about 1 cm to right (clockwise) of first. Incisions are then deepened if necessary by digital splitting of muscle fibers. Myotomies are usually 12 to 15 mm in depth at most prominent aspect of septum. Transverse incision is then made at base of valve leaflet connecting proximal portions of the myotomies. *B.* Bar of muscle isolated between incisions is held by traction suture as shown or by suitable clamp. Muscle is freed with rectangular knife (devised by Stinson) or with special angled rongeur. *C.* As traction is made on muscle bar, rectangular knife is pushed toward apex, freeing muscle bar from its anterior attachments to septum. Apical portion of resection is often more easily accomplished with rongeur, which may be introduced via aorta or via apical stab wound. In latter case, rongeur is positioned and directed by left index finger passed through valve ring. (From: *Morrow AG et al: Circulation 52:88, 1975, with permission.*)

Kirklin and Barratt-Boyes have reported a combined surgical experience including over 160 patients, with a low operative mortality and excellent long-term results. Symptoms are relieved. Sudden death continues to occur but much less frequently than in nonoperated patients. Operative risk is generally less than 5 percent.

Congenital Mitral Valve Disease

Congenital abnormalities of the mitral valve are rare, accounting for less than 1 percent of all cases of congenital heart disease. Rheumatic heart disease with mitral valve involvement can also occur in the childhood population but will be covered in Chapter 18, Acquired Heart Disease.

Pathology. Four types of congenital mitral stenosis were described by Ruckman and Van Praagh: (1) typical congenital mitral stenosis (49 percent) has varying degrees of annular hypoplasia with obliteration or virtual absence of the chordae and subvalvular apparatus; (2) hypoplastic congenital mitral stenosis (41 percent) results in a severely hypoplastic mitral annulus and is often associated with fatal hypoplastic left heart syndrome; (3) supramitral ring (12 percent) is a circumferential connective tissue ridge occurring above the valve in the left atrium, resulting in mitral inlet obstruction; and (4) parachute mitral valve (8 percent) occurs due to insertion of all chordae tendinea into a single, shortened papillary muscle, causing decreased valve leaflet mobility and obstruction.

Associated cardiac malformations occur in 75 percent of the cases, and include left ventricular outflow tract obstruction (40 to 60 percent), ventricular septal defect (30 percent), aortic stenosis (29 percent), aortic atresia (29 percent), and aortic coarctation (27 percent). The combination of a supramitral ring, parachute mitral valve, left ventricular outflow obstruction, and aortic coarctation is called *Shone's complex.* Abnormal left ventricular muscle with endocardial fibroelastosis occurs in nearly one-half of the cases.

Isolated mitral insufficiency may result from the annular dilation, cleft leaflets, prolapsing leaflets, and deficiency in valvular tissue.

Clinical Manifestations. Symptoms of pulmonary venous congestion often appear in infancy and include dyspnea, orthopnea, and pulmonary edema. After the appearance of symptoms approximately one-half of the patients die within 6 months if untreated. Those with less severe obstruction, better left ventricular development, and fewer associated lesions may not develop symptoms until 2 to 4 years, and rarely remain asymptomatic until 10 to 12 years of age.

The chest radiograph and electrocardiogram often demonstrate an enlarged left atrium, pulmonary congestion, and p-mitrale for stenotic lesions. With mitral insufficiency cardiomegaly and pulmonary congestion are often present. Echocardiography has evolved into an excellent diagnostic test, and recently transesophageal echocardiography has proven to be extremely accurate in identifying lesions in the mitral valve or left atrium. Cardiac catheterization is recommended before operative repair.

Treatment. Operation should be postponed as long as possible because of the strong probability of the need for repeat operation as the child grows older. When severe congestive heart failure or chronic dyspnea occurs operation is clearly indicated. Coles reported operative experiences with reparative procedures in 48 patients, with an operative mortality of only 2.9 percent since 1975. This study suggested improved late results when valve repair was possible compared with a similar group of patients undergoing mitral valve replacement. Kodoba reported a 5-year survival of only 43 percent after mitral valve replacement in the first year of life, and a 3-year freedom from reoperation of only 45 percent. The most important factors affecting survival are the severity of associated defects and the adequacy of the left ventricle. After operation late trends suggest improved results when mitral valve repair is feasible, and this is preferred over valve replacement whenever possible. The authors' experiences with over 30 cases of congenital mitral valve abnormalities in the last 10 years suggest that valve repair should be feasible in over 75 percent of the cases.

Hypoplastic Left Heart Syndrome

Hypoplastic left heart syndrome, combining the features of aortic and mitral atresia, was described by Noonan and Nadas in 1958. The syndrome produces the most extreme combination of left-sided obstruction and is incompatible with life, with most children dying within 7 to 10 days.

Pathology. Children with this syndrome have significant cardiac enlargement due to enlarged right-sided chambers. As the name implies, the left-sided structures are markedly hypoplastic. The aortic valve is totally absent with rudimentary sinuses of Valsalva giving rise to the coronary arteries. The ascending aorta and proximal aortic arch are diminutive, providing retrograde flow to the coronary arteries. The left ventricle is severely hypoplastic and the myocardial muscle fibers are in disarray, similar to the histology noted in hypertrophic cardiomyopathy. Endocardial fibroelastosis is also present. The mitral valve is either hypoplastic or totally atretic.

Mixing of blood must occur at the atrial level, as no forward blood flow occurs through the hypoplastic left heart. Blood leaves the heart through the large right ventricle and pulmonary artery, proceeding to the lungs and through the patent ductus to the systemic circulation.

Clinical Manifestations. These children present shortly after birth with respiratory distress, tachycardia, congestive heart failure, and mild cyanosis. Death occurs with physiologic closure of the ductus arteriosus. Children with this syndrome seldom survive for more than 1 week.

Physical examination demonstrates signs of congestive heart failure such as rales and hepatomegaly. Peripheral pulses are often diminished and perfusion is poor. The chest radiograph shows cardiomegaly with significant pulmonary congestion, while the electrocardiogram shows an absence of left-sided forces, with right axis deviation and right ventricular hypertrophy. The echocardiogram is usually diagnostic.

Treatment. The initial treatment is to maintain ductal patency with prostaglandin E_1. Acidosis is corrected with sodium bicarbonate. Since the outlook is extremely poor even with surgical therapy, immediate and detailed counseling with the family is done to determine a treatment plan. On many occasions no treatment is recommended in view of the abysmal results. Some centers recommend heart transplantation if this option is available. The best results have been obtained with a two-staged palliative treatment plan described by Norwood. The end goal of this staged treatment is to eventually provide pulmonary blood flow without a ventricular pump in the system. This is known to be feasible based on work by Fontan with tricuspid atresia. However, this is not possible until later in life, when the pulmonary vascular resistance drops. The initial palliative Norwood procedure involves establishing unobstructed flow from the right ventricle to the systemic circulation by anastomosis of the pulmonary artery to the aortic arch. Atrial mixing is established by resecting the atrial septum, and controlled pulmonary blood flow is established by a systemic subclavian artery-pulmonary artery shunt. The second stage of the Norwood plan is performed at 6 to 18 months of age after the pulmonary vascular resistance drops to normal. The second stage involves takedown of the systemic subclavian artery-pulmonary artery shunt and establishment of a direct atrial-pulmonary artery connection, with "Fontan-like" passive blood flow to the lungs.

Despite this innovative surgical approach the results have been less than encouraging. In most centers the operative mortality for the first stage of the Norwood procedure remains high (30–50 percent). Of those patients surviving the first palliative stage less than one-half survive to undergo the second-stage Fontan procedure. Long-term survival is probably less than 20–25 percent.

LEFT-TO-RIGHT SHUNTS (ACYANOTIC GROUP)

Atrial Septal Defects

A variety of malformations involve the atrial septum or the pulmonary veins and result in a left-to-right shunt of blood from the systemic to the pulmonary circulation. These include atrial septal defects of the secundum type, sinus venosus type with partial anomalous drainage of the pulmonary veins, and ostium primum atrial defects. Complete atrioventricular canal malformations have a combination of an ostium primum atrial septal defect with an endocardial cushion-type ventricular septal defect. These are individually discussed in the following sections. The physiologic abnormality is identical with secundum-type atrial defects and with sinus venosus defects with partial anomalous pulmonary veins, consisting simply of a left-to-right shunt. Hence, these two anomalies are discussed together. Total anomalous drainage of pulmonary veins, a more complex anomaly, is discussed later under Complex Malformations, as it usually presents with a combination of left-to-right shunt and pulmonary venous obstruction. With ostium primum defects and atrioventricular canals, mitral and tricuspid insufficiency can be present in addition.

Secundum Defects/Sinus Venosus Defects and Partial Anomalous Pulmonary Venous Return

In 1953 Lewis successfully closed a defect under direct vision, using hypothermia and inflow occlusion. In the same year, Gibbon used the pump oxygenator successfully for the first time to suture an atrial septal defect. Gross, in Boston, developed the ingenious atrial well, which was used for several years. For the next 5 to 10 years patients were usually operated on with hypothermia and circulatory arrest for 8 to 10 min, or with the atrial well. As soon as extracorporeal circulation became safe, it was routinely adopted.

Incidence and Etiology. Atrial septal defects are among the most common cardiac malformations, representing 10 to 15 percent of all cases of congenital heart disease. They are more than twice as frequent in females. Embryologically, the secundum defects result from failure of the septum secundum to develop completely.

Pathologic Anatomy. Atrial septal defects vary widely in size and location. A "high" subcaval defect near the orifice of the superior vena cava is commonly referred to as a sinus venosus type of defect and it is usually associated with anomalous entry of one or more superior pulmonary veins into the vena cava. The majority of secundum defects are located in the midportion of the atrial septum in the area of the ostium secundum (Fig. 17-12). "Low" defects are near the point of entry of the inferior vena cava. Defects vary from as small as 1 cm in diameter to virtual absence of the atrial septum with a common atrium, but most are 2 to 3 cm. A patent foramen ovale should not be considered an atrial septal defect, for it is a normal opening in 15 to 25 percent of adult hearts. Because of its slitlike construction, a normal foramen ovale allows shunting of blood only from right to left. Unusual defects include different forms of "unroofing" of the coronary sinus. Multiple defects are very rare.

A very detailed report of the pathologic anatomy of anomalous pulmonary veins was published by Blake and Manion. A total of 27 different variations were found. Anomalous veins entering the superior vena cava are usually associated with a characteristic high atrial septal defect, termed a sinus venosus defect. This is the most common form of partial anomalous pulmonary venous return and usually involves drainage of the upper and middle lobe veins, which enter the superior vena cava below the entry site of the azygos vein. Pulmonary veins entering the right atrium directly are usually found with a septal defect in a posterior location.

An unusual variant of partial anomalous pulmonary veins entering the inferior vena cava has been described as a "scimitar" syndrome, emphasizing a characteristic radiologic appearance resulting from the shadow of the anomalous vein, which is parallel to the right border of the heart. The malformation is associated with hypoplasia of the right lung and anomalous origin of the pulmonary arteries from the aorta. A left-to-right shunt is present.

A rare variant of atrial septal defect is a secundum defect combined with mitral stenosis, the Lutembacher syndrome. The mitral stenosis retards flow of blood from the left atrium to the left ventricle and produces an enormous left-to-right shunt through the septal defect, with massive dilatation of the pulmonary arteries. Some mitral valve prolapse occurs in 10 to 20 percent of patients with atrial septal defects, only a small part of whom (less than 5 percent) have significant mitral insufficiency that must be corrected at operation.

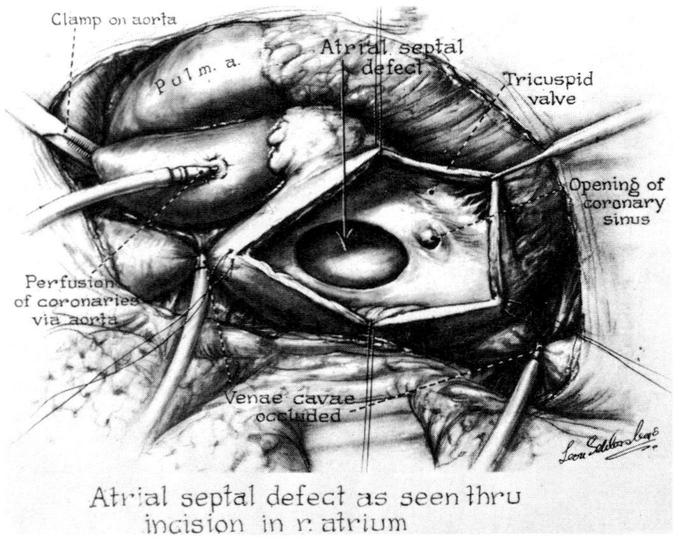

FIG. 17-12. Atrial septal defect of secundum type exposed at operation. Large oval opening in atrial septum superior to coronary sinus is the type usually found with secundum-type defects.

Pathophysiology. An atrial septal defect results in a left-to-right shunt of blood from the left atrium to the right atrium because of the pressure-volume and compliance characteristics of the left and right ventricles. The thick-walled left ventricle is less distensible than the right ventricle; with a closed atrial septum, left atrial pressure is normally 8 to 10 mmHg, while right atrial pressure is normally 4 to 5 mmHg. This difference in distensibility of the two ventricles results in a left-to-right shunt when an atrial septal defect is present. During infancy and the first few years of life the structure of the right ventricle more closely resembles that of the left ventricle, so the volume of the left-to-right shunt remains small until compliance of the right ventricle decreases 2 to more years after birth. Vascular resistance in the pulmonary bed also decreases at approximately one year of age, further increasing the degree of left-to-right shunt.

The volume of the left-to-right shunt depends primarily on the pulmonary vascular resistance and the compliance of the two ventricles. The size of the defect exerts little influence. Most significant shunts have a pulmonary blood flow two to four times greater than systemic flow. Systemic blood flow is decreased and may result in retardation of normal growth and development, the so-called gracile habitus seen in some children with a large defect. The large pulmonary blood flow increases susceptibility to pneumonia and also causes dyspnea on exertion. For unknown reasons patients are susceptible to rheumatic fever, but bacterial endocarditis is rare.

With the increased pulmonary blood flow, pulmonary vascular resistance in children is usually less than normal. Pulmonary hypertension is found in less than 5 percent of children but occurs in 10 to 15 percent of adult patients, as pulmonary vascular resistance increases as a result of years of high flow. Cardiac failure is unusual in children but becomes more frequent in adult life. Pulmonary hypertension and congestive heart failure develop much later in life than with ventricular septal defects. Arrhythmias become more common during the third to fourth decades. Without treatment it has been estimated that 75 percent of patients would die by age fifty, 90 percent by age sixty.

Some patients are initially seen in their fourth, fifth, or sixth decade with a previously undetected atrial septal defect. In these patients, arrhythmias are common, a result of long-standing hypertrophy of the right atrium. Even in patients over 60 to 70 years of age a good result may be obtained following operation if pulmonary vascular resistance is not greatly increased. Arrhythmias, however, often continue.

Clinical Manifestations. ***Symptoms.*** Symptoms are uncommon in the first few years of life because the shunt is small until the right ventricular hypertrophy of infancy has subsided. Frequently children with large shunts are physically active and asymptomatic. In a report of 275 surgically treated patients, Sellers et al. found 113 asymptomatic. The most frequent symptoms are fatigue, palpitations, and exertional dyspnea. Slow growth and development may also occur. In adults, overt signs of congestive heart failure gradually appear, often with the first pregnancy.

Physical Examination. A soft systolic murmur is usually audible in the second or third left intercostal space. In the first few years of life this murmur may be faint or considered a functional murmur. The murmur arises at the pulmonary valve from the increased flow of blood. The second pulmonic sound is characteristically widely split, and "fixed." Slight to moderate cardiac enlargement is present with large defects. Patients are often thin, with long, narrow bones and limited muscular development—the gracile habitus.

Laboratory Findings. The chest radiograph shows mild to moderate cardiac enlargement, principally due to a large right ventricle. The right atrium and pulmonary artery are also prominent, with increased vascularity in the lung fields. The electrocardiogram is usually characteristic, with a right axis deviation with a right bundle branch block. Two-dimensional echocardiography is usually diagnostic; cardiac catheterization is often not done in routine patients. If omitted, particular care must be taken at operation to explore the heart for additional anomalies, especially aberrant pulmonary veins.

Diagnosis. Certain diagnoses in infancy may not be possible on clinical examination because the systolic murmur is not distinctive. In older children the diagnosis can be made with reasonable certainty from the combination of a soft systolic murmur with fixed splitting of the pulmonic second sound. These auscultatory findings, combined with the chest radiograph and electrocardiogram, virtually establish the diagnosis. A left axis deviation on the electrocardiogram immediately suggests that an ostium primum malformation is present. The diagnosis is confirmed by echocardiography, although occasionally cardiac catheterization is required.

Treatment. ***Indications.*** Since many children are asymptomatic, operation is frequently recommended on the basis of clinical findings and the demonstration of a large shunt. Operation is usually performed if the pulmonary blood flow is more than one and one-half to two times greater than systemic flow. Most defects 1 to 2 cm in size or larger should be closed before the development of symptoms, preferably at 3 to 4 years of age. The only contraindication to operation is a severe increase in pulmonary vascular resistance, equaling or exceeding systemic vascular resistance (the Eisenmenger syndrome) or greater than 8 to 10 units/m^2 with Qp/Qs less than 1.2/1. This condition is very rare in children but is an ever-present danger after the third decade. Operation in patients with a pulmonary vascular resistance near systemic resistance is hazardous and may produce little improvement.

Operative Technique. All patients are operated on with extracorporeal circulation. A sternotomy or a right thoracotomy in the fourth intercostal space is used. Once bypass has been established, a finger is introduced into the right atrium through a stab wound to identify the pathologic anatomy, noting the atrial septal defect, the coronary sinus, the location of the pulmonary veins, the mitral and tricuspid valves, and the ventricular septum. Palpation beforehand minimizes the need for exploration of the heart once it has been opened and similarly lessens the hazards of air embolism.

The heart is then arrested with the cold blood-potassium technique. The atrium is then opened widely (Fig. 17-13). Small defects can be closed with a simple continuous suture, usually polypropylene. In fact most secundum defects in children can be closed by direct suture. Larger defects in adults or older children can be sutured, but patch closure with autogenous pericardium seems safer (Fig. 17-14).

Aspiration of blood from the left atrium is avoided to protect from air embolism. As the suture line is completed, fibrillation is induced; the aorta is unclamped to expel blood from the left atrium into the right atrium and to protect from air embolism. The lungs are ventilated to displace air from the pulmonary veins and left atrium. Gentle suction is also kept on a plastic needle vent in the ascending aorta for a short time after the heart starts to beat.

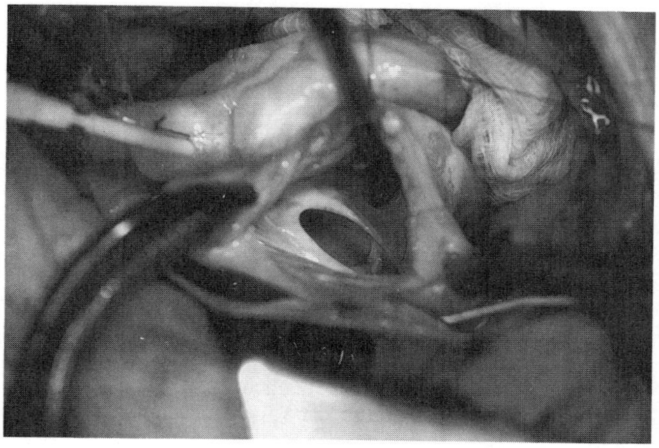

FIG. 17-13. Operative photograph of a low secundum-type atrial septal defect with the right atrium open. (From: *New York University Medical Center.*)

Subsequently, after bypass has been stopped, correction of the left-to-right shunt can be confirmed by aspirating blood from the superior vena cava and pulmonary artery and demonstrating similar oxygen concentration in the two samples. Left atrial pressure should be measured afterward in adult patients since the left heart may have decreased compliance, and serially monitored if elevated.

Anomalous veins entering the right atrium can be corrected by insertion of a pericardial patch so the defect is closed and the pulmonary veins enter the left atrium. Pulmonary veins entering the superior vena cava with a sinus venosus defect require a more complex correction to avoid obstructing either drainage of the

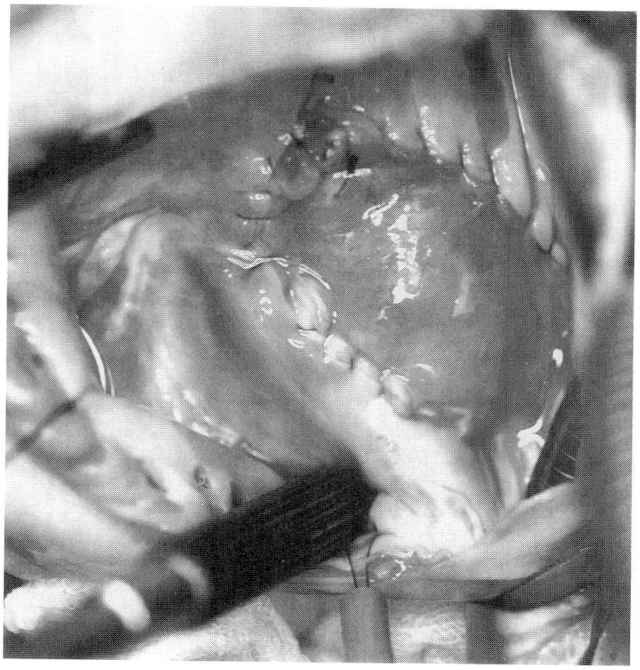

FIG. 17-14. Operative photograph of a secundum atrial septal defect closed with a pericardial patch and continuous suture. (From: *New York University Medical Center.*)

anomalous veins or the superior vena cava. This can be done satisfactorily with application of a pericardial patch. This is sutured superiorly around the point of entry of the anomalous veins and a baffle constructed that channels the blood from the pulmonary veins through the atrial septal defect into the left atrium (Fig. 17-15). This simultaneously corrects the partial anomalous venous drainage and the septal defects. The right atrium is often used to enlarge the caval-atrial junction, using an inverted "Y" to "V" advancement flap to prevent caval obstruction after repair of sinus venosus defect with partial anomalous pulmonary venous return. Anomalous veins entering the inferior vena cava, the most unusual type, are usually treated with construction of an appropriate intra-atrial pericardial baffle.

Postoperative Course. Postoperative convalescence is uncomplicated and recovery from any cardiac disability is prompt. The risk of operation with extracorporeal circulation is surprisingly small. Several groups have reported series of more than 100 patients operated upon with a mortality of under 1 to 3 percent. In the authors' experiences with more than 200 secundum defects, mortality has been near zero for over 15 years.

Ostium Primum Defects (Partial Atrioventricular Canal)

These defects are uncommon, occurring in 4 to 5 percent of patients with defects in the atrial septum. They are especially common in children with Down syndrome, occurring with a frequency of 20 to 25 percent. Except for this unusual association, no etiologic factors are known.

At least three terms have been used interchangeably: ostium primum, partial atrioventricular canal, and partial endocardial cushion defect. "Ostium primum" is an older term, commonly used before the relation to complete atrioventricular canals was recognized. The proper generic name is either endocardial cushion defect (partial or complete) or atrioventricular canal (partial or complete).

Pathologic Anatomy. The two significant defects are a defect (cleft) in the anterior leaflet of the mitral valve and a low, crescent-shaped defect in the atrial septum (Figs. 17-16 and 17-17). The sickle-like superior border of an ostium primum defect can be easily recognized on palpation at the time of operation. The cleft in the anterior leaflet of the mitral valve may be partial, extending for a short distance from the ventricular septum, or complete, separating the mitral valve anterior leaflet into halves.

Chordae tendineae are usually attached to the margins of the cleft constituting a "trileaflet valve," with little or no mitral insufficiency. In other patients significant mitral insufficiency occurs. As described by Perloff, failure of the endocardial cushions to fuse produces an abnormally low position of the atrioventricular valves with an abnormally high anterior position of the aortic valve, resulting in the characteristic "gooseneck" deformity seen on the left ventricular angiogram.

The defect in the atrioventricular septum results in inferior displacement of the conduction system, which, in turn, produces characteristic abnormalities on the electrocardiogram.

Primum defects are anatomically distinguished from the more severe atrioventricular canal malformation by the presence of distinct, separate mitral and tricuspid valve rings and an intact ventricular septum. Complete atrioventricular canals have an absence of the atrioventricular septum with free communication between the atrial and ventricular cavities.

Pathophysiology. The physiologic abnormalities are a left-to-right shunt combined with mitral insufficiency. When mitral insufficiency is minimal, physiologic abnormality is identical to that of a large atrial septal defect of the secundum type. When mitral insufficiency is moderate or severe, left ventricular failure and pulmonary hypertension appear early in life and produce a much more severe impairment of cardiac function than is seen in secundum-type septal defects. Increase in pulmonary vascular re-

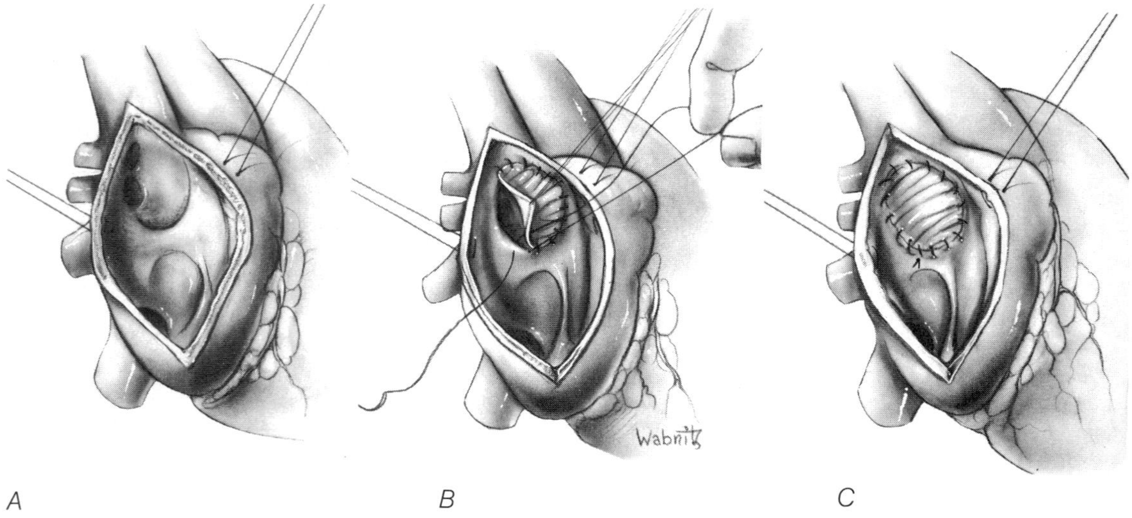

FIG. 17-15. *A.* Sinus venosus-type atrial septal defect located near junction of superior vena cava with right atrium. Defect is partly obscured by crescentic lower margin. Anomalous pulmonary veins from right upper lobe enter superior vena cava near its junction with right atrium. *B.* Prosthetic or pericardial patch can be applied to encompass both atrial septal defect and ostia of anomalous pulmonary veins, avoiding undue constriction of point of entry of superior vena cava into right atrium. *C.* Final view of patch that excludes anomalous veins and atrial septal defect from right atrium. (From: *Benson CD, et al: Pediatric Surgery. Vol. I. Chicago, Year Book Medical Publishers, 1962, p. 439, with permission.*)

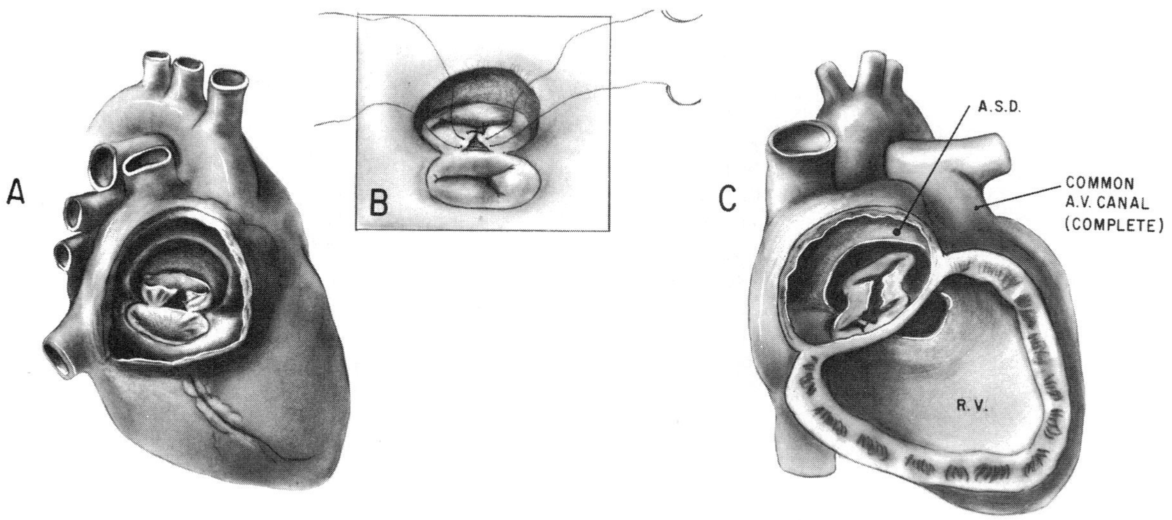

FIG. 17-16. *A.* Ostium primum-type defect. There is a cleft in anterior mitral leaflet, but ventricular septum is intact. *B.* Method of repair of cleft valve with interrupted sutures to produce competent mitral valve. Classic crescent-shaped atrial septal defect superior to valve ring is shown. *C.* Appearance of complete atrioventricular canal, showing complete division of mitral and tricuspid valves in association with atrial septal defect and ventricular septal defect. (From: *McGoon DC, et al: Am J Cardiol 6:598, 1960, with permission.*)

sistance with pulmonary hypertension may develop but is more frequent with complete atrioventricular canals.

Clinical Manifestations. ***Symptoms.*** A variety of clinical profiles occur, varying with the degree of mitral insufficiency. When mitral insufficiency is minimal, the clinical picture is similar to that of atrial septal defect of the secundum type. With significant mitral insufficiency, cardiac failure with pulmonary congestion and dyspnea may be fatal in the first year of life unless surgically corrected.

Physical Examination. Moderate cardiac enlargement is often present, with a thrill near the apex. A harsh apical systolic murmur from mitral insufficiency is usually obvious and should arouse suspicion of an ostium primum defect. An additional systolic murmur may be heard along the left sternal border. The intensity of the pulmonic second sound is often increased. With cardiac failure, signs of pulmonary congestion and hepatic enlargement are found. Growth is frequently retarded.

Laboratory Findings. The chest radiograph usually shows a moderate cardiac enlargement, involving both the right and the left ventricle. Increased pulmonary vascularity is common. The most useful diagnostic clues are found in the electrocardiogram and the vector cardiogram. The former shows abnormalities with a "left axis deviation," while the latter shows an abnormality in the frontal plane, a counterclockwise loop, that is almost pathogno-

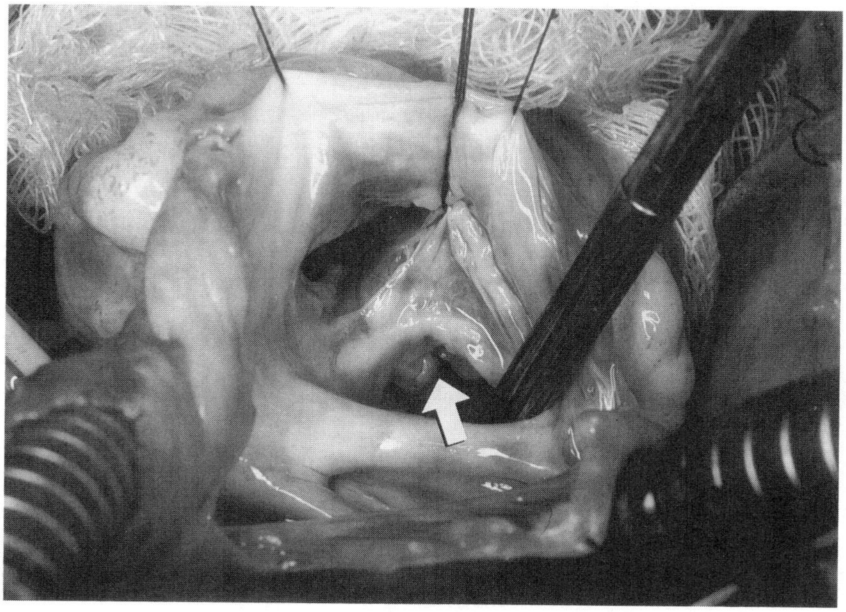

FIG. 17-17. Operative photograph of an ostium primum atrial septal defect (incomplete atrioventricular canal defect). Note upper atrial septum is retracted by suction. Lower atrial septum is absent down to annulus of mitral and tricuspid valves. More posterior structure is mitral valve, demonstrating classic cleft *(arrow)* in anterior leaflet. (From: *New York University Medical Center.*)

monic. The two-dimensional echocardiogram shows classic abnormalities. Some clinicians believe that these findings are sufficient to confirm the diagnosis and do not routinely perform cardiac catheterization.

Cardiac catheterization, however, defines the characteristic left-to-right shunt at the atrial level with the associated increase in pulmonary blood flow and pulmonary hypertension. Mitral insufficiency is best evaluated with the left ventriculogram.

Treatment. In most patients operative correction of the defect should be performed between the ages of 1 and 4 years. With pulmonary hypertension and cardiac failure, operation may be necessary in infancy. Rarely, an adult is seen in the third or fourth decade with a history of little disability from a primum defect. These patients are those in whom mitral insufficiency has been minimal, with a clinical course similar to a secundum-type defect. In most patients the combination of a left-to-right shunt with mitral insufficiency results in progressive cardiac enlargement and failure in childhood.

Operative Technique. Operation is performed with extracorporeal circulation, using a median sternotomy incision. The three principal objectives are correction of the mitral insufficiency, closure of the septal defect, and avoidance of the production of heart block from injury to the conduction bundle along the posterior margin of the septal defect.

Cardiac arrest is produced by the cold blood-potassium technique. The right atrium is widely opened, and the septal defect, cleft in the mitral valve, the tricuspid valve, and ventricular septum are carefully examined. Initially the cleft in the mitral valve is closed with interrupted sutures placed from the ventricular septum out to the free margin of the mitral orifice, the points of insertion of the chordae tendineae being carefully noted. Usually two or three sutures are necessary, but the cleft is not totally closed to the free margin in order to avoid restriction of the leaflet. After repair of the cleft mitral valve, the septal defect is repaired with a patch of pericardium inserted with continuous sutures. Along the condition bundle the sutures are inserted superficially to the left of the rim of the defect along the annulus of the mitral valve or well to the right of the coronary sinus to totally avoid conduction tissue. The latter technique is usually preferred by the authors and it results in leaving the coronary sinus as part of the left atrium. With this technique conduction problems and heart block are rare. It is usually not necessary to repair any abnormalities in the tricuspid valve.

Postoperative Course. If adequate correction of the mitral insufficiency is accomplished and production of heart block avoided, postoperative recovery is usually uneventful and similar to that for closure of other septal defects. Heart block is rare, occurring in less than 1 percent of cases with the current technique. Some mitral insufficiency remains in less than 10 percent of patients. When significant or progressive, this may require reoperation in later years. The functional results in the majority of patients, however, are excellent. At the Mayo Clinic, King and associates in 1986 reported long-term results in 199 patients, the majority of whom had maintained an excellent result following operation. The operative mortality is 3 percent since 1980. Late survival was 98 percent at 1 year and 96 percent at 20 years. Reoperation was required in less than 10 percent. Ceithaml et al. reported results in 56 children, with an operative mortality rate of 1.8 percent. Late reoperation was required in 22 percent. Late New York Heart Association (NYHA) functional status was class I or II in 89 percent.

In early experiences with surgical repair, an unusual syndrome of severe hemolytic anemia was recognized in a small percentage of patients following repair of an ostium primum defect. This striking clinical picture resulted from residual mitral insufficiency accidentally oriented so that the regurgitant jet of blood struck the Dacron prosthetic patch closing the septal defect and intermittently dislodged fibrin from the surface of the patch with each systolic jet. Although rare, such a syndrome should be recognized, for prompt reoperation and correction of the residual insufficiency is curative. This is now avoided by using pericardium as the patch material.

Complete Atrioventricular Canal

This severe malformation results from extensive failure of development of the endocardial cushions, resulting in a large atrioventricular defect involving both the atrial and ventricular septums with defects in the mitral and tricuspid valves (Fig. 17-16C) which instead of forming separately develop as an abnormal single atrioventricular valve. The great variation in valve deformities was well described by Rastelli in 1966 in an analysis of 30 postmortem specimens. Subsequently, the deformity present was often classified into one of three groups, Rastelli types A, B, and C, which are based on differing pathology of the superior leaflet. Currently this classification is less useful because a more practical approach is to visualize the common atrioventricular valve as a six-leaflet structure that provides a common inlet to the ventricles, overlying a large ventricular septal defect and contiguous with an ostium primum atrial septal defect.

Pathophysiology. The physiologic defect is a large left-to-right shunt at both the atrial and ventricular levels, resulting in pulmonary hypertension and cardiac failure in infancy. The severity of the malformation depends on the extent of atrioventricular valvular insufficiency and the size of the ventricular septal defect. In infants with severe deformities the course is a severe one, with death in the first few months of life, unless operation is performed.

A complete atrioventricular canal, rather than a partial one, may be suspected from the malignant clinical course of severe cardiac failure in infancy. These patients often have severe pulmonary hypertension early in life, and 65 percent will die before 1 year of age. Down syndrome is present in over 50 percent of the patients with complete atrioventricular canal defects. Diagnosis is established principally by the electrocardiogram and the echocardiogram. Cardiac catheterization should also be done for a complete evaluation. The catheterization shows a typical "gooseneck" deformity.

Treatment. The use of pulmonary artery banding to diminish pulmonary blood flow in patients with atrioventricular canal defects currently has little value and is not indicated except in extremely "unbalanced" atrioventricular canals that have only a single functional ventricle. Definitive operation is indicated in the first year of life, usually before 6 to 9 months of age, when repair can be done electively. With refractory congestive failure, repair must be done earlier. The corrective procedure consists of insertion of a prosthetic patch that is attached to correct the underlying ventricular septal defect, taking precautions to avoid injury to the conduction bundle (see Fig. 17-18). The abnormal mitral and tricuspid leaflets are then reconstructed and attached to the patch (see Fig. 17-18) at an appropriate level, following which the atrial septal defect is closed (Fig. 17-19). The atrial septal defect is closed either with a continuation of the single ventricular septal defect

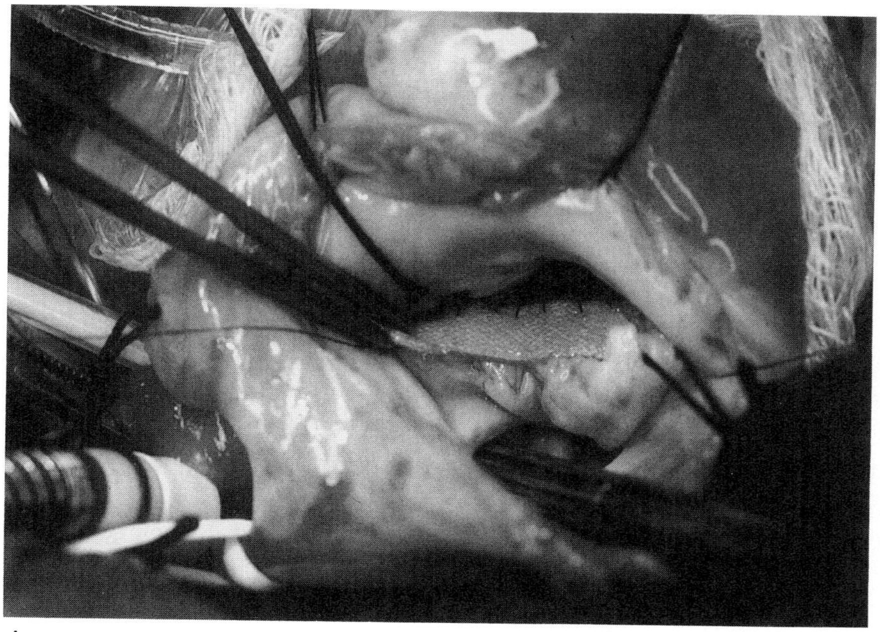

A

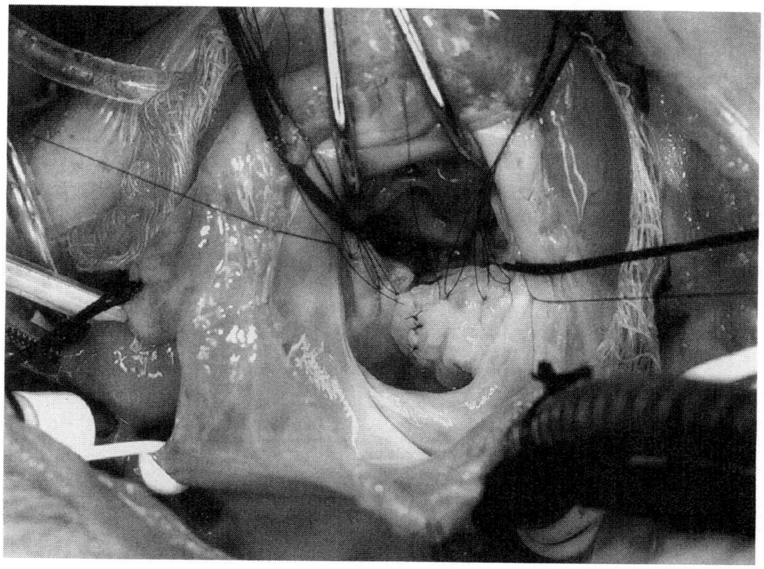

B

FIG. 17-18. Operative photograph of repair of a complete atrioventricular canal defect. *A.* Ventricular septal defect is closed with Dacron patch. *B.* New annulus between left-sided (posterior) and right-sided components of common valve has been constructed by resuspending leaflet tissue to top of Dacron patch, which was used to close ventricular septal defect. New left-sided atrioventricular valve is posterior, seen through unclosed atrial septal defect. Cleft in three-leaflet left-sided atrioventricular valve has been partially closed with interrupted sutures. (From: *New York University Medical Center.*)

prosthetic patch or with a separate pericardial closure of the atrial defect. The authors prefer the two-patch technique because this allows more precise correction of atrioventricular valvular insufficiency and is associated with less late dehiscence (see Figs. 17-18 and 17-19).

For several years operative results were poor, with a mortality exceeding 75 percent in infants. Great advances were subsequently made with the techniques of surgical correction developed by Rastelli, McGoon, and Kirklin. Operative mortality is now between 5 and 15 percent, varying with the severity of the abnormality present. The authors' experience with over 45 patients undergoing complete repair since 1981 demonstrated an operative risk of less than 5 percent despite significant preoperative pulmonary hypertension and atrioventricular valvular insufficiency. At follow-up 75 percent were functionally NYHA class I or II, and over 97 percent were free of significant late valvular insufficiency.

Ventricular Septal Defects

Historical Data. The description by Roger in 1879 of two patients with ventricular septal defect is a medical classic. It led to the designation *Roger's disease,* focusing emphasis on the asymptomatic nature of the disease when the ventricular septal defect is small. Surgical closure became possible with the development of cardiopulmonary bypass in the mid 1950s.

Incidence and Etiology. Ventricular septal defect (VSD) is a common form of congenital heart disease, constituting 20 to 30

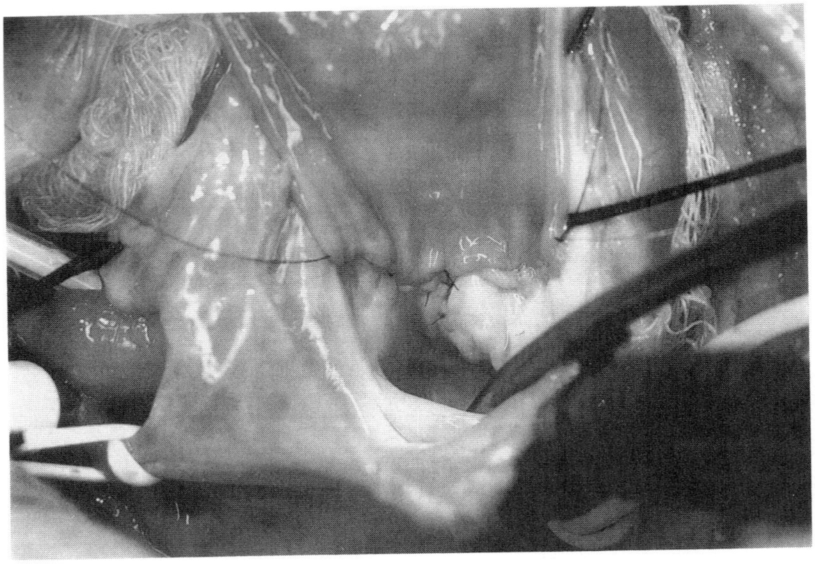

FIG. 17-19. Operative photograph of repair (continued) of complete atrioventricular canal defect. Patient seen in Fig. 17-18 now has a pericardial patch placed between the new left-sided atrioventricular valve (posterior) and new right-sided atrioventricular valve (not seen). Left atrium is seen through open atrial septal defect. Pericardial patch will be used to close remaining atrial septal defect, redirecting left atrial flow into new left-sided atrioventricular valve and completing two-patch repair. (From: *New York University Medical Center.*)

percent of congenital defects. There are no known etiologic factors.

Pathologic Anatomy. Four major anatomic types of ventricular septal defect have been recognized, depending on the location in the ventricular septum: perimembranous septal defect, infundibular outflow defect superior to the crista supraventricularis (conal or supracristal), posterior inlet inflow defects near the tricuspid (atrioventricular canal type), and muscular defect in the muscular ventricular septum (Fig. 17-20). Defects in the membranous septum are by far the most frequent requiring operation (80 percent of patients). Malignant defects are a subgroup of this conotruncal group.

Perimembranous septal defects (see Fig. 17-20, Type B) are located in the membranous septum and often extend into adjacent structures. The bundle of His, of critical importance to the surgeon, is located at the posterior superior rim of the defect, where it bifurcates into the right and left conduction bundles. The defect often extends beneath the aortic valve, which is visible through the defect. Dacron patch closure working through the right atrium is almost always possible.

Outflow (infundibular or supracristal) septal defects (see Fig. 17-20, Type A) are anterior and superior to the crista supraventricularis near the pulmonic valve. The defect is safely away from the conduction bundle. Posterior inlet (atrioventricular canal type) septal defects (see Fig. 17-20, Type C) are posterior to the papillary muscle of the conus, beneath the tricuspid valve.

Muscular ventricular septal defects are common but many close spontaneously (see Fig. 17-20, Type D). They are located inferiorly in the ventricular septum and are often multiple. The rare "Swiss cheese" type of septum consists of many serpentine communications, making surgical closure difficult, perhaps impossible. An approach through the left ventricle has been used as a last resort in some complex lesions but has the serious hazard of permanent left ventricular dysfunction. Usually muscular defects can be closed through the standard right atrial incision, working through the tricuspid valve.

Left ventricular-right atrial defects are the rarest of all, consisting of a communication between the left ventricle and the right atrium through the membranous septum superior to the annulus of the tricuspid valve. Although the defects are small, the resulting shunt is large because of the great difference in pressure between the left ventricle and right atrium. Closure can be easily done by direct suture or patch through the right atrium.

The size of septal defects varies from as small as 3 to 4 mm to greater than 3 cm. Such defects are commonly classified as "restrictive" or "nonrestrictive," depending on whether the defect is smaller than the orifice of the aortic valve. In nonrestrictive defects, right and left ventricular systolic pressures are equal, and flow is influenced by pulmonary vascular resistance. Small restrictive defects have a normal right ventricular systolic pressure with little or no hemodynamic disturbances. In larger "restrictive" defects right ventricular systolic pressure is increased but does not equal that in the left ventricle. The hemodynamic significance of nonrestrictive defects is determined by the pulmonary vascular resistance and the size of the defect.

With nonrestrictive defects and a right ventricular systolic pressure equaling that in the left ventricle, deadly histologic changes soon develop in the pulmonary arterioles, at times appearing in the first year of life. These were classically described by Heath and Edwards in 1958. The initial change is hypertrophy of the smooth muscle in the media, followed by proliferation in the intima; unfortunately, the intimal changes seem irreversible. The early evolution of these irreversible changes is the major reason for performance of operation in patients with nonrestrictive defects during the first year of life. Irreversible pulmonary vascular changes are reflected by a rise in the pulmonary vascular resistance, which is normally less than 2.5 Wood units. A pulmonary vascular resistance of 4 to 6 units is mildly elevated. With a resistance of greater than 10 units the shunt often becomes right-to-left and pulmonary vascular changes may quickly become irreversible.

Associated anomalies are common. These include patent ductus arteriosus, coarctation, atrial septal defect, mild infundibular stenosis of the right ventricle, double-outlet right ventricle, and aortic insufficiency from prolapse of an aortic valve cusp into the ventricular septal defect.

Pathophysiology. The two major consequences of a ventricular septal defect are cardiac failure and pulmonary hypertension. Normally systolic left ventricular pressure is about four times

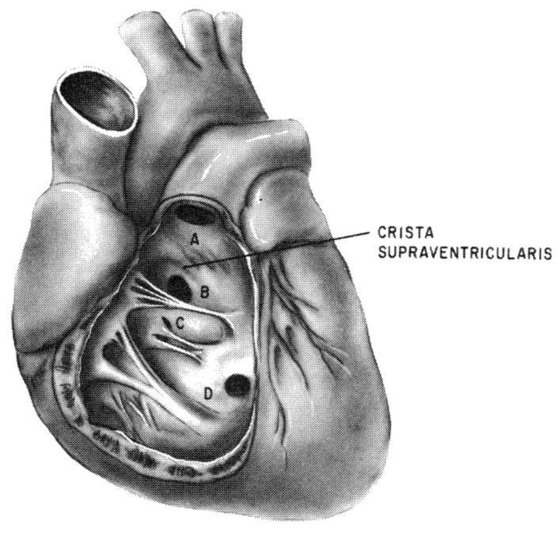

FIG. 17-20. Common types of ventricular septal defects. Most common type is Type B, a perimembranous ventricular septal defect. Type A represents an infundibular or outlet (supracrystal) defect. Type C is located posteriorly and is termed a *posterior inlet* or *atrioventricular canal-type* defect. Type D represents a muscular defect within muscular portion of ventricular septum. Muscular defects are often multiple. (From: *Kirklin JW, et al: J Thorac Surg 33:45, 1957, with permission.*)

greater than systolic right ventricular pressure. Hence, a ventricular septal defect results in a left-to-right shunt of blood from the left ventricle into the pulmonary circulation, producing an increased pulmonary blood flow. The size of the left-to-right shunt varies with both the size of the defect and the pulmonary vascular resistance.

A small increase in pulmonary blood flow is well tolerated, but a pulmonary blood flow more than twice systemic flow may produce cardiac failure. With large nonrestrictive defects, pulmonary blood flow may be four to five times greater than systemic flow, producing severe pulmonary congestion and heart failure in infancy.

After the first year of life, overt cardiac failure is uncommon, but large defects produce chronic pulmonary congestion with recurrent episodes of pneumonia and limitation of growth and development.

The other major pathologic change is an increase in pulmonary vascular resistance, produced by the changes in the media and intima of the pulmonary arterioles described in the previous paragraphs. As pulmonary vascular resistance rises, the left-to-right shunt gradually reverses with an increasing degree of right-to-left shunting, producing arterial hypoxemia. Eventually this produces a ''balanced'' shunt, and then progresses to *reversal* of the shunt with severe cyanosis. This condition exists when pulmonary vascular resistance has increased to levels greater than systemic vascular resistance. The classic term *Eisenmenger syndrome* refers to this pathologic condition. It is inoperable by present techniques except for heart-lung or isolated lung transplantation.

Small restrictive septal defects, not increasing right ventricular systolic pressure, have no known physiologic handicap except a small increase in susceptibility to bacterial endocarditis, apparently resulting from the jet of blood through the defect striking the right ventricular wall. The endocarditis usually responds to antibiotic therapy.

The life expectancy of adult patients with a ventricular septal defect depends on the degree of heart failure, the pulmonary blood flow, and the pulmonary vascular resistance. The only known hazard with small defects is endocarditis. With large defects the critical question is the pulmonary vascular resistance. Patients with a significant increase in pulmonary vascular resistance may progress to the complete Eisenmenger syndrome. The natural history of such patients has been well documented by Wood. Death usually occurs near 40 years of age, often from massive hemoptysis. At present heart-lung transplantation has been used for a few such patients with encouraging short-term results. Patients with a large defect without increased pulmonary vascular resistance usually have a pulmonary blood flow over twice normal. They gradually develop cardiac enlargement and cardiac failure, much like patients with moderate aortic insufficiency. These patients respond nicely to VSD closure.

Clinical Manifestations. Patients with small defects are usually asymptomatic even though a loud murmur and thrill are present. With large defects, dyspnea on exertion with pulmonary congestion, often with frequent episodes of pneumonia, are common. Severe cardiac failure usually occurs within the first year of life or in adults. Patients with a large increase in pulmonary vascular resistance are deceptively asymptomatic for several years until cyanosis and hemoptysis evolve as the shunt reverses and produces peripheral hypoxia.

A loud harsh pansystolic murmur is usually present along the left sternal border in the third and fourth intercostal spaces, often with a thrill. With pulmonary hypertension the pulmonic second sound is increased. Growth retardation may be significant with chronic congestive failure, accompanied by cardiac enlargement, rales, and hepatic enlargement. Basal diastolic murmurs are infrequent but can originate from two sources. A murmur of aortic insufficiency may develop from prolapse of an aortic cusp into the underlying septal defect. Alternately, a murmur from pulmonic insufficiency may appear with pulmonary hypertension.

Diagnosis. The chest radiograph with small defects is normal, while in large defects, enlargement of both ventricles occurs, especially with a rise in pulmonary vascular resistance. Enlargement of the pulmonary arteries with pulmonary congestion is often prominent. The electrocardiogram shows signs of left ventricular hypertrophy and also right ventricular hypertrophy with pulmonary hypertension. The two-dimensional echocardiogram is of particular value, for the location and size of the septal defects may be determined with reasonable accuracy. The most precise information is obtained by cardiac catheterization, documenting the volume of the shunt and the pulmonary vascular resistance, and by selective angiography.

Treatment. Small defects should simply be observed because 60 to 70 percent will close in early life. The risk of endocarditis is small. Over half of such defects close before 3 years of age, and about 90 percent by 8 years. Closure most commonly occurs with muscular defects and with small perimembranous defects, rarely with posterior inlet or outflow defects.

The treatment of large defects depends on the presence of cardiac failure or increasing pulmonary vascular resistance. Severe cardiac failure in infancy may be fatal unless operation is performed in the first few weeks or months of life. Banding of the pulmonary artery was popularly used for such critically ill infants for some years but is now used very infrequently because of the safety of definitive operation in infants. Infants with significantly increased pulmonary vascular resistance should be operated on promptly, no later than 6 to 8 months of age. Barratt-Boyes has clearly documented irreversible changes in the pulmonary vascular bed of some infants who were operated on even during the first year of life. With the safety of operation, and the ominous uncertain course of an increase in pulmonary vascular resistance, it is becoming increasingly clear that most infants with a large ventricular septal defect should be operated on during the first year of life. This is a significantly earlier age than previously recommended, based on both the safety of operation and the realization of the early development of pulmonary hypertension. When pulmonary vascular resistance is increased to near systemic levels (8 to 10 resistance units), the hazard of operation is increased and the benefit decreased. Criteria of inoperability vary significantly. In general, in about one-third of older patients successfully operated upon with a major increase in pulmonary vascular resistance, the changes continue nonetheless, producing death within a few years. A significant percentage of the other patients remain with a permanent increase but without progression, while a small group have a decrease in resistance, either for regression of the existing changes or from the growth of new arterioles. When operation is done at less than 1 year of age much more reversibility is seen.

Technique of Operation. Operation is performed through a median sternotomy with extracorporeal circulation. If a patent ductus is present, it must be closed at the beginning of operation. The ventricular septal defect may be closed through a right atrial approach or through a short transverse ventriculotomy (Fig. 17-21). For the past 8 years the authors have almost exclusively used the right atrial approach, because this minimizes ventricular dysfunction and arrhythmias (Figs. 17-21 and 17-22). A prosthetic patch is routinely used. The critical part of the operation is to avoid heart block by identifying key anatomic guides at the posterior superior margin of the defect. A useful surgical guide was described by Barratt-Boyes. With a still, dry field, the fibrous trigone located at the bottom of the noncoronary sinus can be identified on inspection through the ventricular septal defect. The conduction bundle passes through this trigone and then along the area where the membranous septum joins the muscular septum posteriorly. Placing sutures to the right of an imaginary line projected between the fibrous trigone and the papillary muscle of the conus usually avoids injury to the conduction bundle. With present techniques, the risk of heart block is very small. Outflow defects (infundibular) can be readily repaired with a prosthetic patch because there is no danger of injury to the conduction bundle. Fol-

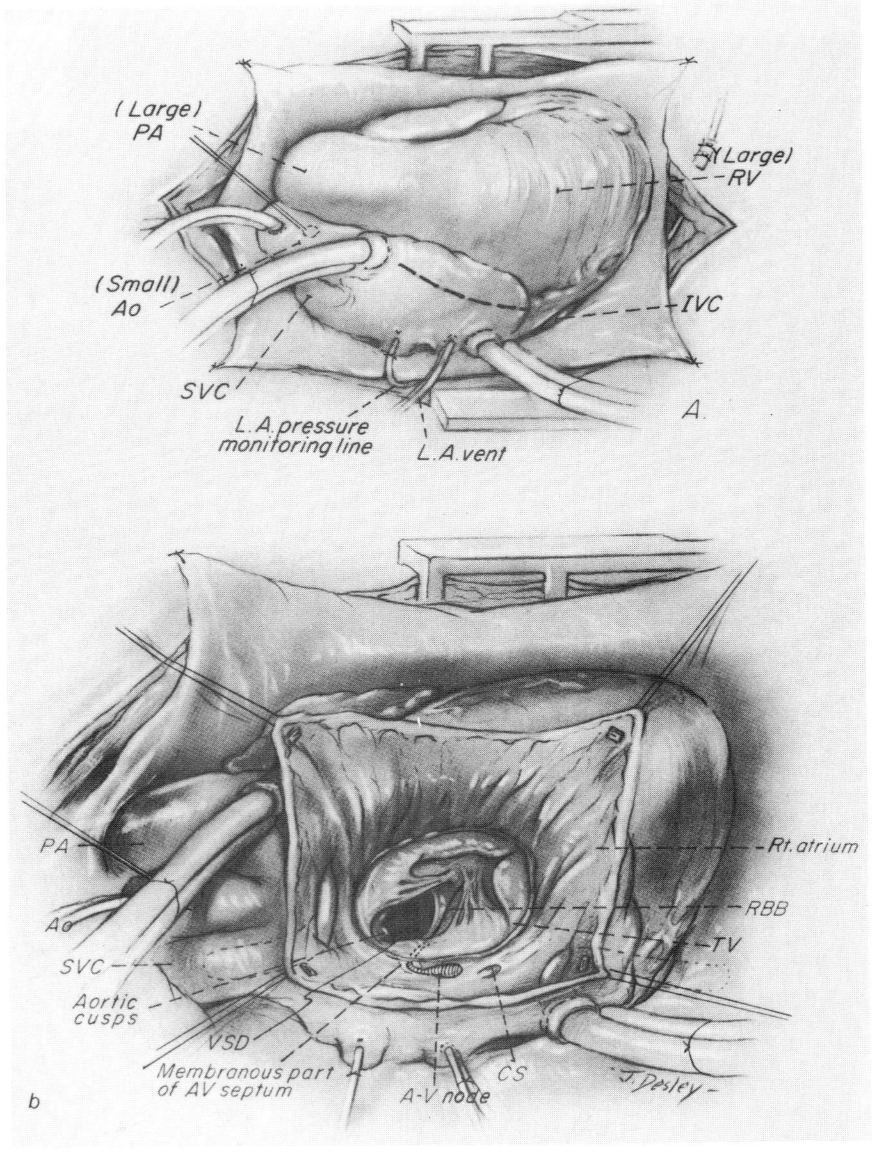

FIG. 17-21. Repair of perimembranous ventricular septal defect from right atrium. A_o, aorta; AL, anterior leaflet; AV node, atrioventricular node; CS, coronary sinus; IVC, inferior vena cava; PA, pulmonary artery; RBB, right bundle branch, SVC, superior vena cava; TV, tricuspid valve. (From: *Kirklin JW, Barratt-Boyes BG: 1986, with permission.*)

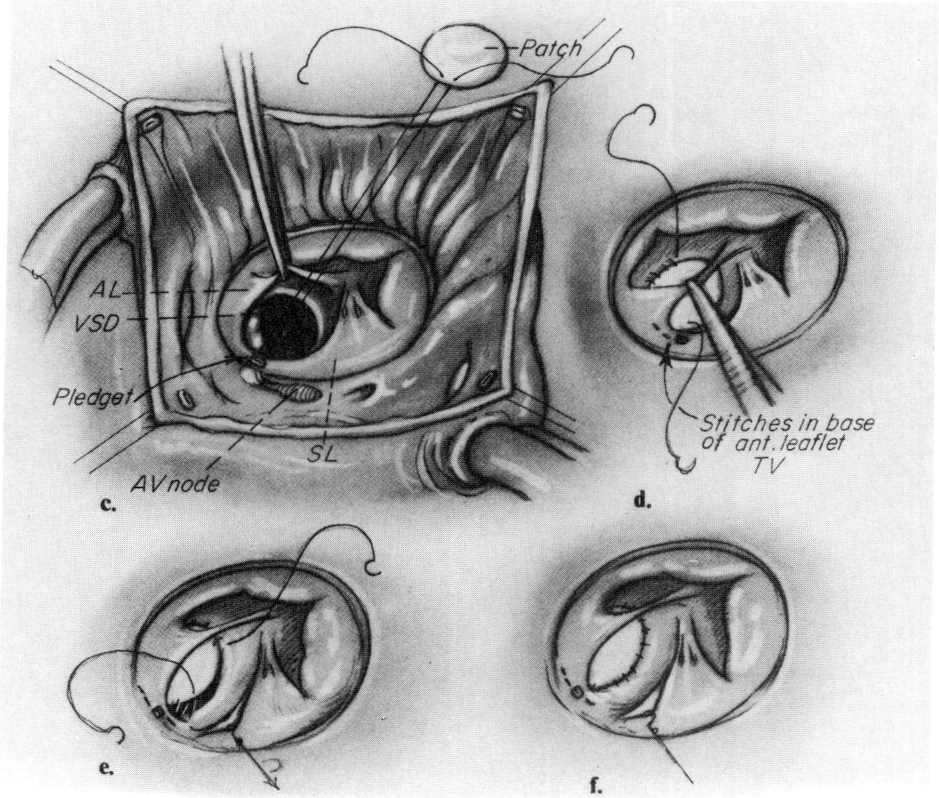

FIG. 17-21. Continued.

lowing bypass, residual shunts may be detected by measurement of oxygen content of blood samples drawn simultaneously from the right atrium and pulmonary artery.

A small percentage of patients with ventricular septal defects develop severe aortic insufficiency from prolapse of an aortic valve cusp into the underlying defect. The lesion is a progressive one as the aortic cusp herniates to a greater degree, often virtually tamponading the underlying septal defect. Surgical correction can often be done without insertion of a prosthetic aortic valve. A detailed report of the experience of Spencer and associates was published in 1973 (Fig. 17-23). Subsequent experience has remained quite satisfactory and a similar aortic valve repair technique is still used today, although the ventricular septal defect is often repaired transatrially.

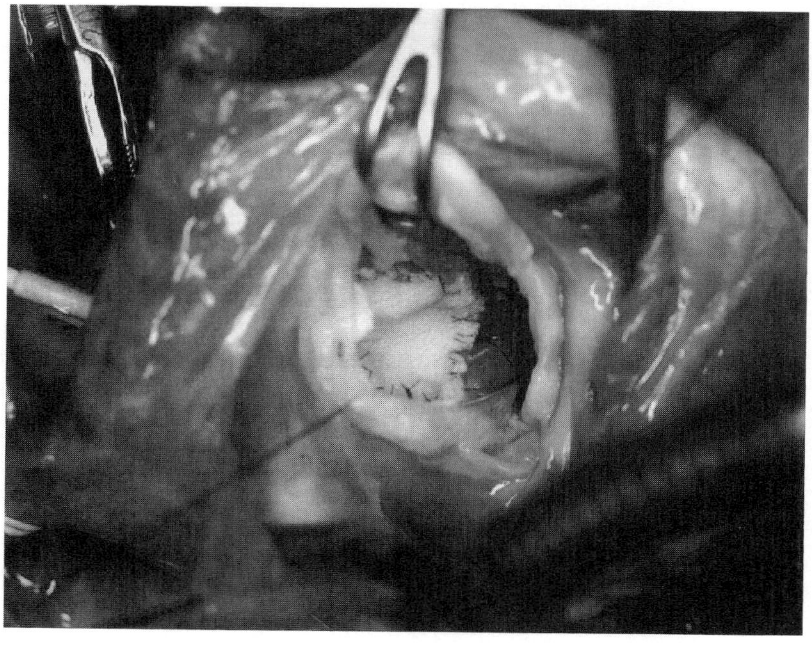

FIG. 17-22. Operative photograph of transatrial closure of perimembranous ventricular septal defect. Dacron patch is used to close defect, with proximal portion of patch sutured into base of tricuspid valve leaflet. Care is taken to avoid conduction tissue along inferior, posterior rim of adjacent ventricular septum. (From: *New York University Medical Center.*)

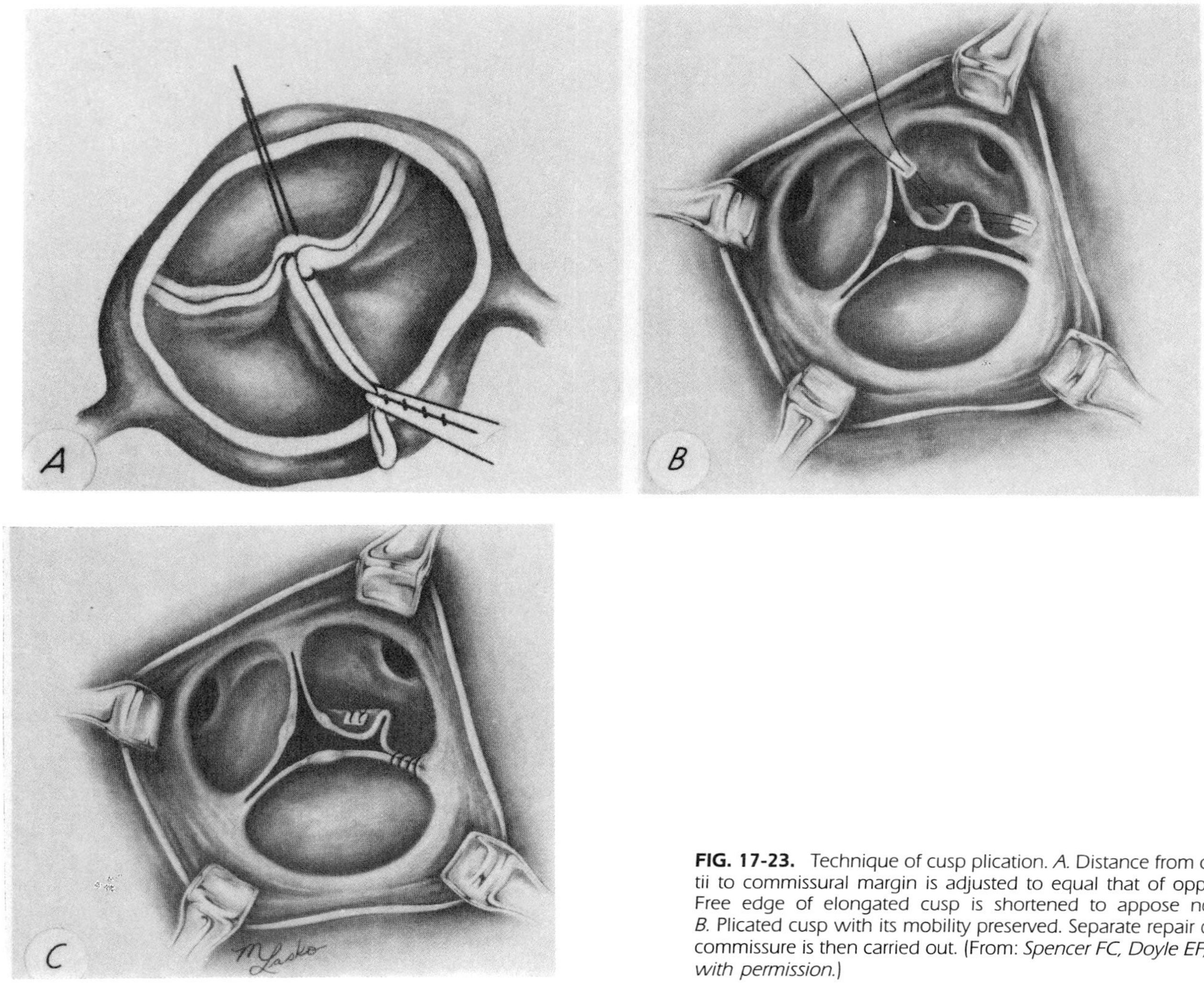

FIG. 17-23. Technique of cusp plication. *A*. Distance from corpus arantii to commissural margin is adjusted to equal that of opposing cusp. Free edge of elongated cusp is shortened to appose normal cups. *B*. Plicated cusp with its mobility preserved. Separate repair of abnormal commissure is then carried out. (From: *Spencer FC, Doyle EF, et al: 1973, with permission.*)

Defects in the muscular septum may be single or multiple. Extensive muscular defects have been described as a "Swiss cheese septum," although the true occurrence of this entity is debatable. Successful closure of muscular defects requires careful preoperative study, combined with evaluation at operation of the presence of residual defects. Apparent multiple defects often originate from only one opening in the left ventricle, providing a better surgical approach, but unfortunately left ventriculotomy may produce significant ventricular injury. Hence, different forms of approach through the right atrium or right ventricle are preferred, utilizing a left ventriculotomy reluctantly after other methods have been found unsatisfactory.

Rizzoli and associates reported in 1980 that in the past 5 years only one death occurred among 94 patients with a single large ventricular septal defect, and only one death (7 percent mortality) in 14 patients with multiple ventricular septal defects. There was only one death in 35 infants less than 1 year of age. Neither the location of the ventricular septal defect nor the surgical approach (via the right atrium or right ventricle) were significant factors. Only one heart block developed among 261 patients. Richardson et al. also described excellent results following operation upon 32 infants between 1 and 24 months of age. In 1984, Yeager reported operative experiences with 128 patients less than 1 year of age, with a hospital mortality of 7.8 percent. In 1992 we reported results from urgent or emergent repair for 54 symptomatic infants less than 1 year of age. Nine had multiple defects and 17 had associated cardiac defects. Operative risk was 6 percent and two patients required pacemakers for heart block. Late results have been excellent.

Following recovery from operation, patients without a marked increase in pulmonary vascular resistance usually have a dramatic regression of all signs of cardiac disease. Heart size and vascularity of lung fields both return to normal. Life expectancy appears to be that of a normal person. If there is a persistent increase in pulmonary vascular resistance following recovery from operation, long-term prognosis is much less favorable, but this usually only occurs in patients who are operated on later in life. Regression of the increased pulmonary vascular resistance occurs in about one-third of patients; there is no significant change in about one-third, and a gradual decrease in the remainder.

Patent Ductus Arteriosus

Historical Data. Gibson, in Edinburgh, in 1900 described the clinical features of a patent ductus arteriosus. In 1937 Strieder first attempted ligation of the ductus in a patient with bacterial endocarditis. This patient died on the fourth postoperative day, but the following year Gross successfully ligated the patent ductus of a 7-year-old girl.

Incidence and Etiology. Patent ductus arteriosus is one of the most common forms of congenital heart disease, occurring once in about every 2000 births and constituting about 10 percent of all cases of congenital heart disease. It is two to three times more frequent in females than in males.

The patent ductus arteriosus, which develops as an embryologic remnant of the sixth left aortic arch, is an important normal fetal pathway connecting the pulmonary artery at its bifurcation to the aorta just beyond the origin of the left subclavian artery. Through this channel in embryonic life blood bypasses the collapsed lungs, flowing directly from the pulmonary artery into the aorta. With the expansion of the lungs at birth, the ductus normally closes within a few days, becoming the fibrotic ligamentum arteriosum. The physiologic stimuli responsible for closure of the ductus have been studied in detail. Apparently changes in oxygen tension of the arterial blood exert a profound stimulus on the closure. An important cause of closure is probably related to the distinctive histologic structure of the wall of the ductus, which is different from that of either the pulmonary artery or the aorta. As the ductus closes, the wall of the ductus contracts, the internal elastic membrane fragments, and smooth muscle projects into the lumen as progressive fibrosis obliterates the patent channel. Naturally occurring prostaglandins oppose closure of the ductus. In term infants the ductus is more responsive to oxygen, while with premature infants the prostaglandin effect is more prominent.

If rubella occurs during the first trimester of pregnancy, a well-recognized syndrome of congenital defects can occur, including mental retardation, cataracts, and a patent ductus. For the majority of nonpremature infants, however, the cause of persistent patency is unknown.

Pathologic Anatomy. The diameter of a ductus ranges from as small as 2 to 3 mm to greater than 1 cm. Usually it is 5 to 7 mm. The length ranges from 5 to 10 mm (Fig. 17-24).

Associated anomalies occur in approximately 15 percent of cases; the most common are ventricular septal defect and coarctation of the aorta.

Pathophysiology. Depending on the diameter of the ductus, a varying amount of blood is shunted from the aorta to the pulmonary artery, constituting a left-to-right shunt. In a large ductus, the shunt may constitute 50 to 70 percent of the output from the left ventricle, with resulting decrease of blood flow to other tissues and retardation of development. With such large shunts, the pulmonary blood flow may reach levels as high as 10 to 15 L/min. The symptomatology is directly proportional to the size of the shunt.

A large patent ductus in infants may result in serious or even lethal heart failure. Without surgical treatment, 25 to 30 percent of infants may die in the first year of life. Beyond 1 year of age, heart failure is rare until adult life.

In infancy the high pulmonary vascular resistance of fetal life subsides gradually in the first 1 to 2 years after birth. During this time only a systolic murmur may be audible. In some infants the increased pulmonary blood flow from the ductus causes the pulmonary vascular resistance to remain elevated and even increase, with resulting pulmonary hypertension. Usually the pulmonary vascular resistance will decrease to normal levels following surgical division of the ductus, but in older patients only a partial regression toward normal levels may occur. With a large patent ductus (diameter larger than the aorta) pulmonary vascular resistance may increase to exceed systemic vascular resistance, as early as 5 to 6 years of age. This produces a "reversed" ductus, with blood flowing from the pulmonary artery to the descending thoracic aorta to produce cyanosis in the lower half of the body (the Eisenmenger syndrome). With early diagnosis and treatment, this condition is now rarely seen.

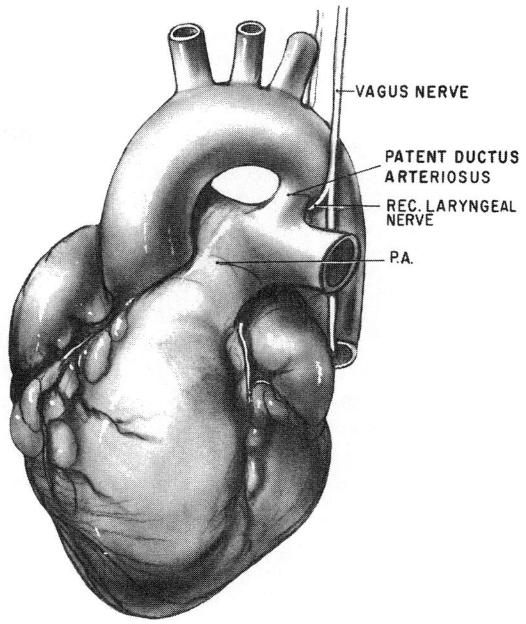

FIG. 17-24. Patent ductus arteriosus is regularly found just distal to left subclavian artery between aorta and pulmonary artery. It is encircled by recurrent laryngeal nerve, a useful surgical landmark in isolating patent ductus in mediastinal tissues. (From: *Gross RE: The Surgery of Infancy and Childhood. Philadelphia, Saunders, 1953, p. 807, with permission.*)

An unusual feature of a patent ductus is susceptibility to development of bacterial endocarditis from *Streptococcus viridans*. This is most common after the first decade; it may occur rarely in children. It has been estimated that in untreated cases such an infection would ultimately develop in 20 to 25 percent of patients. The localization of the infection apparently is related to turbulent blood flow, where blood forcefully ejected from the aorta through the ductus strikes the wall of the pulmonary artery. The vegetations of bacterial endocarditis usually begin in this location. Fortunately such infections can usually be promptly controlled with antibiotic therapy.

With the dual tendency to develop either heart failure or bacterial endocarditis, the estimated life expectancy of a 17-year-old patient with a patent ductus is approximately one-half that of a normal individual.

Clinical Manifestations. ***Symptoms.*** In infants a large patent ductus may cause serious heart failure, and children over 1 year of age are usually asymptomatic. When symptoms are present, the most common are palpitations, fatigue, and dyspnea. Approximately 30 percent of patients born with a patent ductus die before 1 year of age, often in the first few months of life if untreated. Symptoms of congestive heart failure are again seen in adult patients, usually in the third or fourth decade. In the female symptoms often appear during the first pregnancy. Over 40 percent of patients with patent ductus will die before age 45 from congestive heart failure.

Physical Examination. The hallmark of a patent ductus is the continuous murmur, one of the most distinctive signs in clinical medicine. Usually a patent ductus can be diagnosed with certainty simply on this basis. Because of the continuous quality of the murmur it is often described as a "machinery" murmur. It is a harsh, rasping sound, accentuated in systole and diminishing in diastole. It is best heard in the second left intercostal space but is normally widely transmitted over the chest and into the neck. In many patients the murmur is so loud that it is associated with a palpable thrill. Often in infants either no murmur or only a systolic murmur can be heard until the age of 1 or 2 years, after which a continuous murmur is audible. The absence of the diastolic component of the murmur during infancy is due to persistent elevation of the pulmonary vascular resistance, which limits flow of blood through the ductus during diastole.

A wide pulse pressure is usually found with a large ductus, produced by a decrease in diastolic pressure. In the extremely large ductus the diastolic pressure may approach very low levels and be associated with peripheral vascular findings similar to those of severe aortic insufficiency.

Cyanosis is never present with an uncomplicated patent ductus. The presence of cyanosis indicates either an associated cardiac anomaly, such as tetralogy of Fallot, or a marked increase in pulmonary vascular resistance from progressive sclerosis of the pulmonary arteriolar bed.

Diagnosis. With a small patent ductus the chest radiograph may be normal. With a larger ductus the pulmonary conus is prominent, the left ventricle is enlarged, and the pulmonary vascular markings are increased, all indicating a large left-to-right shunt. The electrocardiogram is often normal with a small ductus but will show left ventricular hypertrophy with a larger one. Two-dimensional Doppler echocardiography outlines the size and shunt pattern with accuracy. Cardiac catheterization can readily localize the left-to-right shunt to the pulmonary artery and differentiate the condition from a ventricular septal defect or an atrial septal defect but is seldom necessary with today's echocardiographic techniques. Catheterization is recommended primarily in adult patients to measure pulmonary vascular resistance.

There are several rare conditions that may produce a continuous murmur simulating a patent ductus arteriosus, requiring cardiac catheterization and angiography for differentiation from a patent ductus. These include an aortic-pulmonary window, a ventricular septal defect with a prolapsed cusp causing aortic insufficiency, a ruptured aneurysm of the sinus of Valsalva, and a coronary arteriovenous fistula. Most of these conditions create a physiologic left-to-right shunt and hence a continuous murmur simulating a patent ductus.

Treatment. Infants with congestive failure should be operated on promptly; otherwise, operation can be electively performed between 6 months and 2 years of age. The operative risk approaches zero, and the results are excellent. Fortunately with early operations for patent ductus advanced pulmonary vascular disease is almost unknown. Operation later in adulthood can be extremely dangerous because of pulmonary vascular changes, ventricular dysfunction, and calcification of both the ductus and the adjacent aorta. Hence, prompt operation is recommended in all cases once the diagnosis is made.

With bacterial endocarditis, intensive antibiotic therapy will effect cure in most patients; operation can then be more safely performed several weeks later. It is rarely necessary to operate in the presence of active infection.

Operative Technique. The operation is preferably done through a posterolateral thoracotomy in the fourth intercostal space, although a left anteriolateral thoracotomy in the third intercostal space has been satisfactorily used in previous years. The preferred operative technique is shown in detail in Fig. 17-25.

Patients in the third and fourth decade with pulmonary hypertension and sclerosis or calcification of the ductus constitute a difficult and dangerous technical problem because of friability of the ductus, especially at its junction with the pulmonary artery. Lacerations in this artery may quickly result in fatal hemorrhage. A temporary aortic shunt, either a left atrial-femoral artery bypass or a femoral-femoral bypass, can be employed to permit temporary occlusion of the aorta above and below the ductus, which can then be occluded with a single clamp placed near its junction with the aorta. The ductus can then be divided at its point of origin from the aorta. Usually a shunt or temporary bypass is not necessary, but should be on "standby" for repair of adult patients with patent ductus.

Ligation of a patent ductus with multiple ligatures was developed and widely used by Blalock. It is now primarily used only in premature infants. The current preferred technique involves application of a partial-occlusion vascular clamp on the aorta a few millimeters from the ductus, and placement of an angled vascular clamp on the ductus adjacent to the pulmonary artery. The ductus is divided sharply. Each side is oversewn with a continuous double layer of monofilament suture. On the aortic side the suture line is flush with the aorta to avoid late aneurysm formation in an unobliterated ductus diverticulum. Even a very short ductus can be effectively divided with this technique.

Postoperative Course. With an uncomplicated ductus, the operative risk is near zero. As early as 1953 Gross reported experience with 611 patients, with a mortality rate of less than 0.5 percent in those with neither cardiac failure nor infection. Similar figures were described by Jones in a total series of 909 patients. At New York University there has been no mortality or serious complications following division of an uncomplicated patent ductus in the past 15 years.

Convalescence following operation is usually uneventful. A functional systolic murmur may remain audible in a few patients. The electrocardiogram usually returns to normal within a few months. From data now available from over 40 years' experience, it seems certain that cardiac function becomes normal once the ductus has been surgically obliterated.

FIG. 17-25. Division of patent ductus arteriosus. *A.* Chest is opened with left posterolateral incision in fourth intercostal space. *B.* Once lung has been retracted, mediastinal pleura is incised longitudinally parallel to vagus nerve. *C.* Initial dissection is along vagus nerve to expose widely recurrent laryngeal nerve originating from vagus and passing beneath ductus. Wide exposure of recurrent laryngeal nerve is essential part of operative procedure. *D.* After dissection of recurrent laryngeal nerve, lappet of pericardium overlying ductus is freed by sharp dissection proximally to expose pulmonary artery. *E.* Subsequently ductus is encircled, and vascular occlusion clamps are applied. *F.* Ductus is gradually divided and sutured, employing two rows of sutures. *G.* Final view of divided ends of ductus with recurrent laryngeal nerve well exposed.

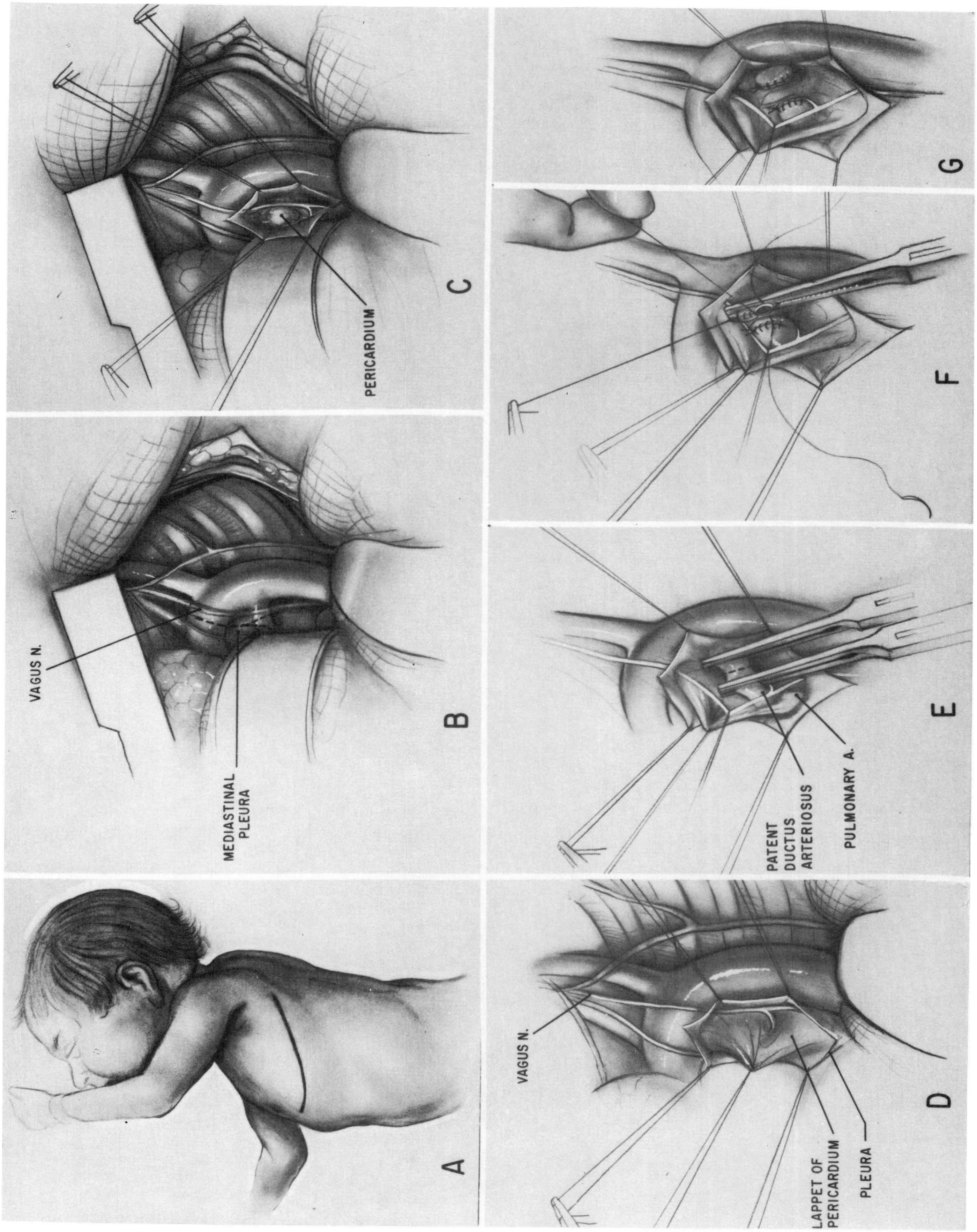
A
B
VAGUS N.
MEDIASTINAL PLEURA
C
PERICARDIUM
D
VAGUS N.
LAPPET OF PERICARDIUM
PLEURA
E
PATENT DUCTUS ARTERIOSUS
PULMONARY A.
F
G

Patent Ductus in the Premature Infant

In recent years the frequency and significance of the patent ductus in premature infants has become widely recognized. Closure can be significantly hastened by the administration of indomethacin. Indomethacin acts by blocking the synthesis of prostaglandins, which normally oppose contraction of the smooth muscle that obliterates the patent ductus. The frequency of patent ductus in premature infants varies inversely with the birth weight and gestational age, ranging from a frequency of 15 to 80 percent.

Diagnosis may be made from the widened pulse pressure detected through an umbilical arterial catheter. The echocardiogram may be helpful in confirming the diagnosis.

Most patients can be treated with medical therapy, combined with indomethacin. In the 1983 National Cooperative Study of 3559 patients, this therapy produced ductus closure in 79 percent of the group.

Surgical occlusion is usually not the initial choice, because the ductus will eventually close in most patients. With severe respiratory insufficiency and pulmonary edema, however, an operation should be done. The ductus is exposed through a short lateral incision and occluded with either double ligation using heavy silk or double metallic clip occlusion; operating time is usually less than 30 min.

Operation is surprisingly safe. Mikhail reported experiences with 306 patients, average age 11 days, without any deaths.

Aortopulmonary Window

This is a rare abnormality. At the Toronto Children's Hospital, only 23 of 15,000 patients with congenital heart disease who were seen over a period of 20 years had an aortopulmonary window. Synonyms referring to the same lesion include aortopulmonary fistula and aortic sepal defect.

The first successful case was treated by ligation by Gross in 1948, and another by division and suture by Scott and Sabiston in 1951 (Fig. 17-26). Effective safe correction became possible only with the development of extracorporeal circulation.

Pathologic Anatomy. Embryologically, the defect results from incomplete development of the spiral septum dividing the primitive truncus arteriosus into the aorta and pulmonary artery. Persistent truncus arteriosus is a more severe malformation of similar cause. The opening, or "window," between the aorta and pulmonary artery may vary in diameter from 5 to 30 mm. It is usually located proximally near the ostium of the coronary arteries. At least 30 percent of patients have a severe additional cardiac malformation.

Pathophysiology. The large left-to-right shunt is similar to that of a large patent ductus arteriosus or ventricular septal defect. The course is a malignant one because an increase in pulmonary vascular resistance quickly occurs, similar to a large ventricular septal defect or truncus arteriosus.

Clinical Manifestations. The clinical findings may be identical to those of patent ductus arteriosus, with a continuous murmur and wide pulse pressure. Often, however, only a systolic murmur is present because of the severe pulmonary hypertension. Differential diagnosis includes large patent ductus, ventricular septal defect, and truncus arteriosus.

Diagnosis. Echocardiography can usually confirm the diagnosis. CT and MRI scans also are usually diagnostic. Cardiac catheterization and aortography should be done to define precisely the relationship to adjacent structures and also confirm that the aortic and pulmonic valve rings are intact. The degree of elevation of pulmonary vascular resistance can also be determined.

Treatment. Operation should be performed as soon as the diagnosis has been established because of the rapidity of development of irreversible pulmonary vascular disease. At operation a transaortic approach has usually been employed, closing large defects with a prosthetic patch. The pulmonary artery is clamped separately. Care is taken to avoid injury to the coronary arteries or the pulmonary valve. In patients operated on in infancy or before the development of severe pulmonary vascular disease, results have been excellent. Operative risk should currently be less than 10 percent. Little information is available about those surviving with severe elevation in pulmonary vascular resistance, but with early repair long-term survival should be normal.

Doty in 1983 reported 25 patients and reviewed 50 previous reported operative repairs. He concluded that a transaortic approach was preferable with patch closure of the defect. The risk of operation was proportional to the increase in pulmonary vascular resistance.

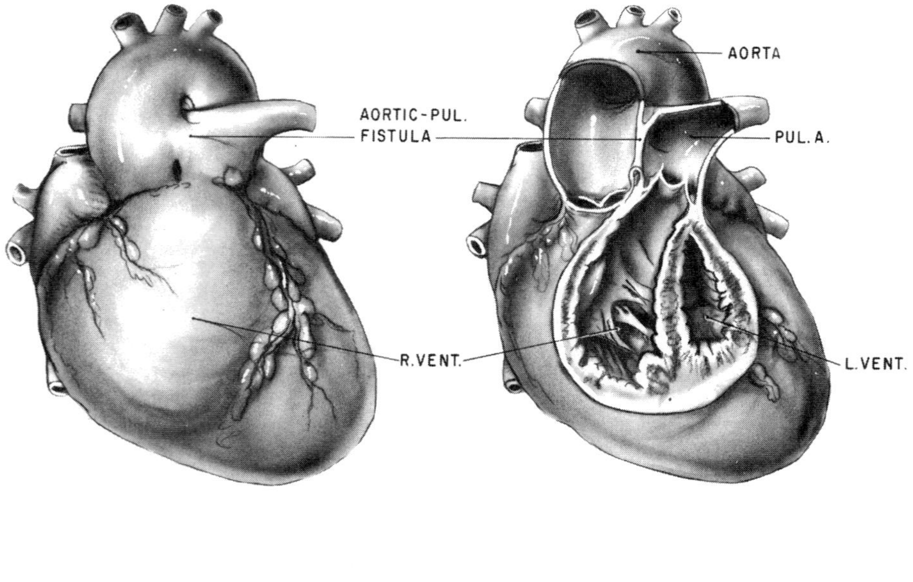

FIG. 17-26. Aorto-pulmonary window, showing large communication between aorta and pulmonary artery near base of heart. (From: *Scott HW, Sabiston DC: 1953, with permission.*)

RIGHT-TO-LEFT SHUNTS (CYANOTIC GROUP)

Any condition with a right-to-left shunt results in cyanosis. Some conditions, such as tetralogy of Fallot, pulmonary atresia, and tricuspid atresia, have decreased pulmonary blood flow and may require a palliative shunt to improve oxygenation. Other conditions, such as transposition of the great vessels, double-outlet right ventricle, and truncus arteriosus, may be cyanotic from right-to-left shunting, yet they may have increased pulmonary blood flow.

Palliative Shunts for Cyanotic Disease

The concept of improving pulmonary blood flow surgically for patients with cyanotic heart disease was introduced in 1944 when Blalock dramatically demonstrated that much benefit could be obtained by anastomosis of the subclavian artery and pulmonary artery to create an artificial systemic-to-pulmonary shunt. The operation was developed after the suggestion of Taussig, who had noted an increase in symptoms in infants with tetralogy of Fallot when a patent ductus spontaneously closed. Thereafter the procedure was termed the *Blalock-Taussig operation* (Fig. 17-27). It constituted one of the milestones in cardiac surgery, far exceeding in importance the benefit for tetralogy patients. It demonstrated for the first time that complex cardiac procedures could be performed on cyanotic infants, launching the modern era of cardiac and vascular surgery. In 1946 Potts described a direct anastomosis between the descending aorta and the left pulmonary artery, and Glenn subsequently described a cavopulmonary shunt in 1954 (Fig. 17-28). In 1962 Waterston published a technique for anastomosis between the ascending aorta and the right pulmonary artery.

The Potts and Waterston shunts are infrequently used today. Both tend to flood the lungs, while the Waterston tends to distort the pulmonary artery and the Potts is difficult to close, making subsequent operations more difficult. The Glenn shunt, which is an anastomosis between the superior vena cava and the right pulmonary artery, is used primarily for tricuspid atresia, and cannot be performed until after approximately 1 year of age since the pulmonary vascular resistance must drop before venopulmonary flow is possible. The Glenn shunt is associated with significant intrapulmonary arteriovenous fistula formation for unexplained reasons.

In recent years central palliative aortopulmonary shunts using prosthetic material have been occasionally used. Currently the most widely used systemic-pulmonary shunt is the modified Blalock-Taussig shunt popularized at Great Ormond Street Hospital (Fig. 17-29). This shunt involves placement of an interposition graft, usually of 5-mm Gore-Tex, between the subclavian artery and the pulmonary artery. With microvascular techniques and optical magnification this shunt is highly effective even in neonates with small pulmonary arteries. The classic Blalock-Taussig operation, performed on the side opposite the aortic arch to avoid kinking, is still occasionally used in older patients in whom long-term palliation is desirable. Overall palliative shunts have been highly effective in improving the well-being of cyanotic patients, but the use of palliative shunts is diminishing, as early corrective operation is increasingly becoming the treatment plan of choice for many conditions.

Tetralogy of Fallot

Historical Data. Tetralogy of Fallot was described in 1673 by Steno, but became well known in 1888 when the combination of abnormalities regularly present was emphasized by Fallot; subsequently it was known as the tetralogy. Effective therapy first became possible in 1944 with the Blalock-Taussig operation, described above under Palliative Shunts. The Blalock-Taussig operation was done over 1500 times at the Johns Hopkins Hospital. Experience with these operations led to the development of many other aspects of cardiac surgery. With the development of extracorporeal circulation, total correction of tetralogy of Fallot became possible and was first performed by Lillehei in 1954. The first repair was done using "cross circulation" with another human being serving as the pump-oxygenator. The first repair using the "heart-lung machine" pump-oxygenator was done shortly thereafter in 1955 at the Mayo Clinic.

Incidence and Etiology. Tetralogy of Fallot is the most common cyanotic malformation, constituting over 50 percent of all cases of cyanotic heart disease. Among cyanotic children who survive beyond the first 2 years of life, a tetralogy is present in 70 to 75 percent. There are no known etiologic factors.

Pathologic Anatomy. The four features of tetralogy from which the name originates are obstruction of the outflow tract of the right ventricle, a ventricular septal defect, dextroposition of the aorta, and hypertrophy of the right ventricle. It is now known that these four abnormalities are not coincidental but result from a specific developmental abnormality—anterior malalignment of the infundibular septum, the anatomic hallmark of tetralogy. In normal embryonic development the developing infundibular septum aligns inferiorly with the muscular septum. In tetralogy the infundibular septum deviates anteriorly and cephalad, creating the large ventricular septal defect at the point of nonunion. The anterocephalad rotation of the septum both narrows the right ventricular outflow tract and enlarges the aortic root in a rightward direction, hence the "overriding." The nonrestrictive ventricular septal defect results in systemic systolic pressure in the right ventricle. The concentric right ventricular hypertrophy results from outflow tract or pulmonary valve obstruction.

The right ventricular obstruction may be produced by a wide variety of abnormalities. These include valvular stenosis or hypoplasia, diffuse hypoplasia of the right ventricular outflow tract, a localized infundibular stenosis, and pulmonary atresia. A discrete infundibular stenosis is present in about 15 percent, and pulmonary atresia in about 20 percent. Pure valvular stenosis is unusual. In most patients a combination of infundibular and valvular stenosis is present (Fig. 17-30).

The ventricular septal defect is large, 2 to 3 cm in diameter, is almost always located proximal to the crista supraventricularis in the membranous septum, and is classified as a perimembranous defect. The aortic cusps are readily visible through the defect, varying with the degree of dextroposition.

There is striking enlargement of the bronchial arteries, aortopulmonary collateral arteries, and other routes of collateral circulation to the lungs, creating extensive varicosities throughout the mediastinum and chest wall.

Anomalous coronary arteries are found in 5 percent of patients, especially in the outflow tract of the right ventricle, where they are of particular surgical significance. A right aortic arch, for unknown reasons, occurs in about 25 percent of patients. Atrial septal defect is found in 10 to 15 percent of patients. Such patients have what has been termed a *pentology of Fallot,* though the name has negligible physiologic significance. It is curious that although a patent ductus arteriosus may be essential to life, it gradually

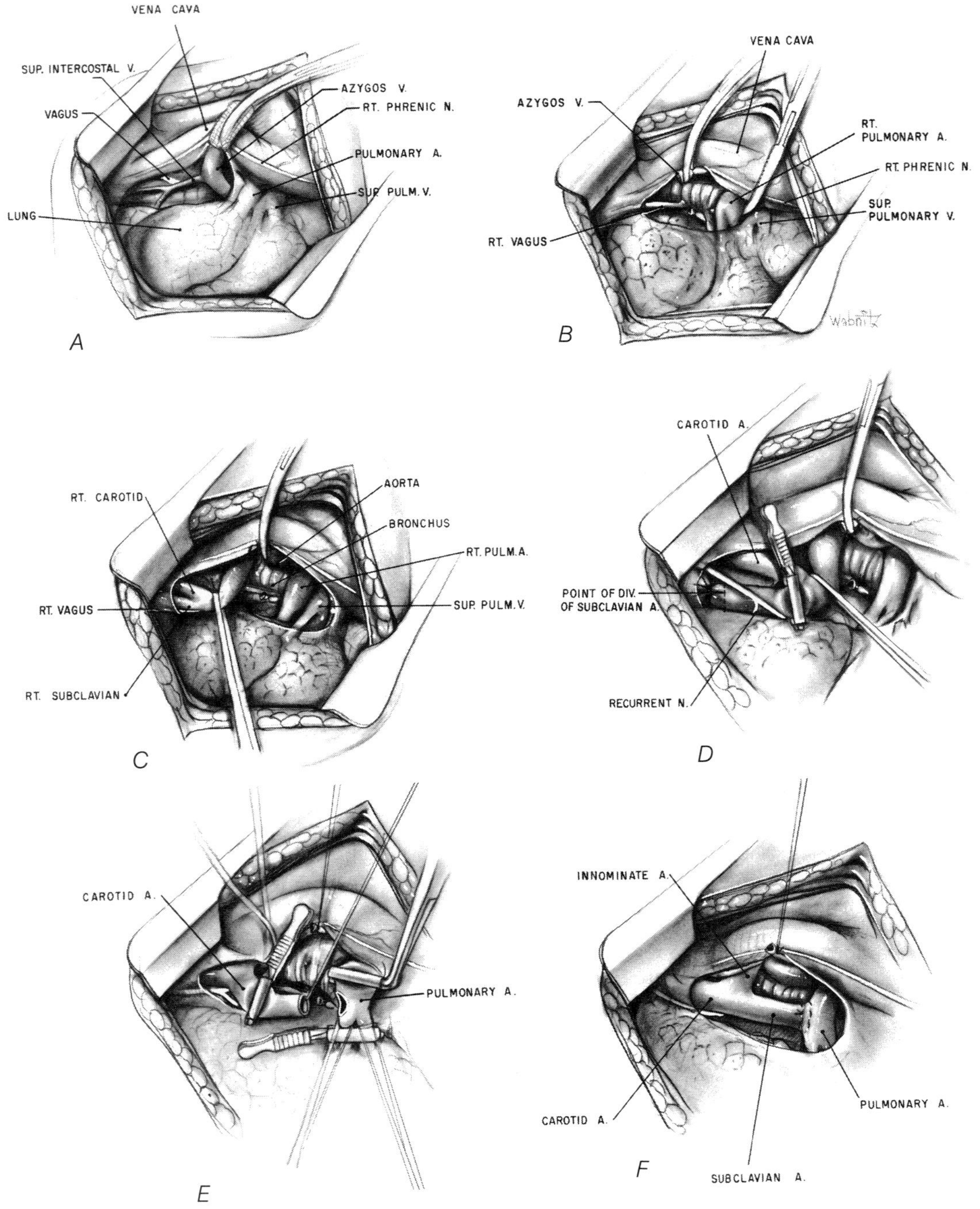

FIG. 17-27. Blalock-Taussig procedure. *A.* Dissection is begun by isolation and division of azygos vein, followed by incision of mediastinal pleura in front of pulmonary artery. *B.* Pulmonary artery is isolated in hilus, dissecting artery distally to beyond point of origin of upper lobe branch. Medially, artery is freed well into mediastinum in order to permit displacement of artery superiorly during construction of anastomosis. Traction on stump of divided azygos vein retracts superior vena cava to expose pulmonary artery in mediastinum. *C.* Subclavian artery is mobilized at apex of thorax, mobilizing carotid artery and subclavian artery down into mediastinum. Wide mobilization of carotid artery greatly facilitates subsequent performance of anastomosis. Vagus and recurrent nerves are protected during this dissection. *D.* After mobilization of carotid and subclavian arteries, tributaries of subclavian arteries are ligated, vertebral artery being ligated separately to avoid retrograde flow of blood from vertebral artery distad into arm, producing subclavian "steal" abnormality. *E.* After division of subclavian artery, longitudinal arteriotomy is made in pulmonary artery. Adventitia is carefully cleared from subclavian artery before performance of anastomosis. *F.* Appearance of completed anastomosis. With wide mobilization of carotid artery superiorly and pulmonary artery inferiorly, satisfactory anastomosis can be accomplished with subclavian artery as short as 1 to 1.5 cm in length.

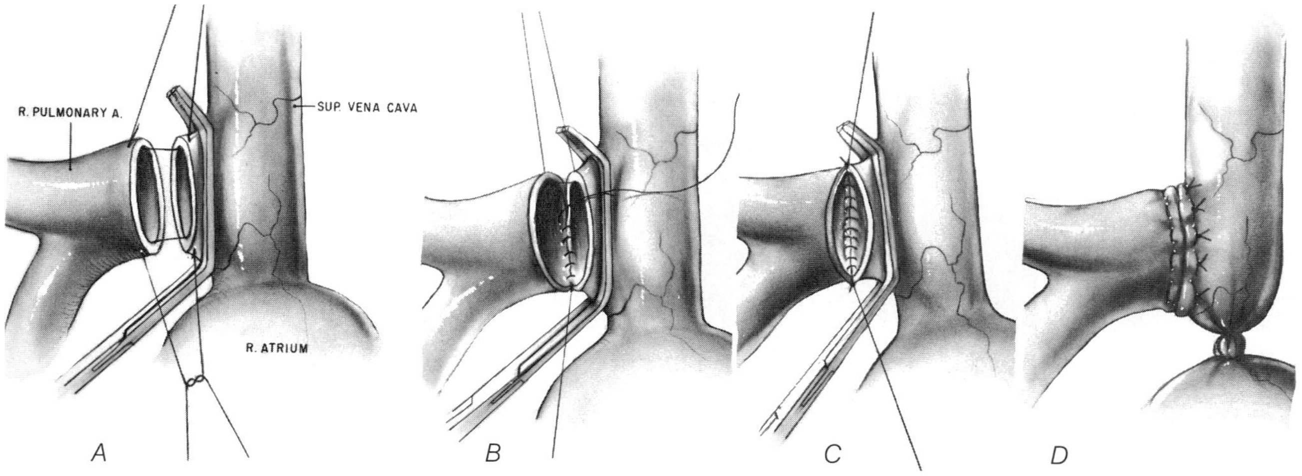

FIG. 17-28. Anastomosis between superior vena cava and right pulmonary artery (Glenn procedure). *A.* Tangential clamp has been applied to superior vena cava to include origin of azygos vein. Right pulmonary artery has been divided, and end-to-end anastomosis will be constructed. *B.* Posterior row of anastomosis is constructed. *C.* Completed posterior row of anastomosis. *D.* Anterior row of anastomosis is constructed. After removal of occluding clamps, superior vena cava is doubly ligated at point of juncture with right atrium. (From: *Glenn WWL: 1958, with permission.*)

closes in most patients during the first few months of life, often with a disastrous increase in the severity of anoxia.

The pulmonary valve leaflets are often thickened, with fused commissures; in addition one or more leaflets may be tethered to the arterial wall with resulting limitation of motion.

Pathophysiology. Physiologically, a tetralogy of Fallot is a combination of a large ventricular septal defect and an obstruction in the right ventricular outflow tract of sufficient severity to elevate right ventricular systolic pressure to equal left ventricular systolic pressure. Venous blood entering the right ventricle is then

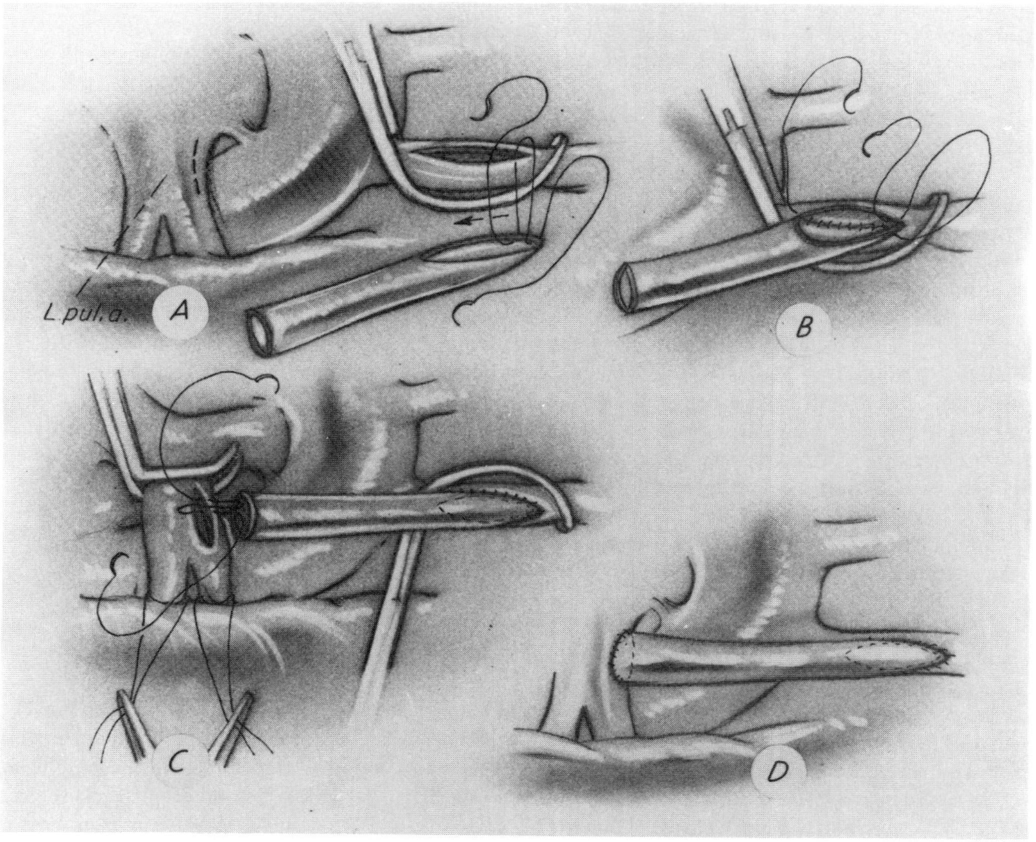

FIG. 17-29. Modified Blalock-Taussig operation with a Gore-Tex interposition shunt. *A.* The Gore-Tex graft has been trimmed for insertion. End-to-side anastomosis is made between the Gore-Tex and the left subclavian artery. The first portion of the suture line is being made by sewing from within as shown. *B.* With the other end of the double-armed suture, the second portion of the suture is begun. *C.* The distal anastomosis is made in a similar fashion. The direction of suturing at both anastomoses minimizes the possibility of tearing the delicate subclavian or pulmonary artery. *D.* Completed anastomosis. (From: *Kirklin JW, Barratt-Boyes BG (eds): 1986, with permission.*)

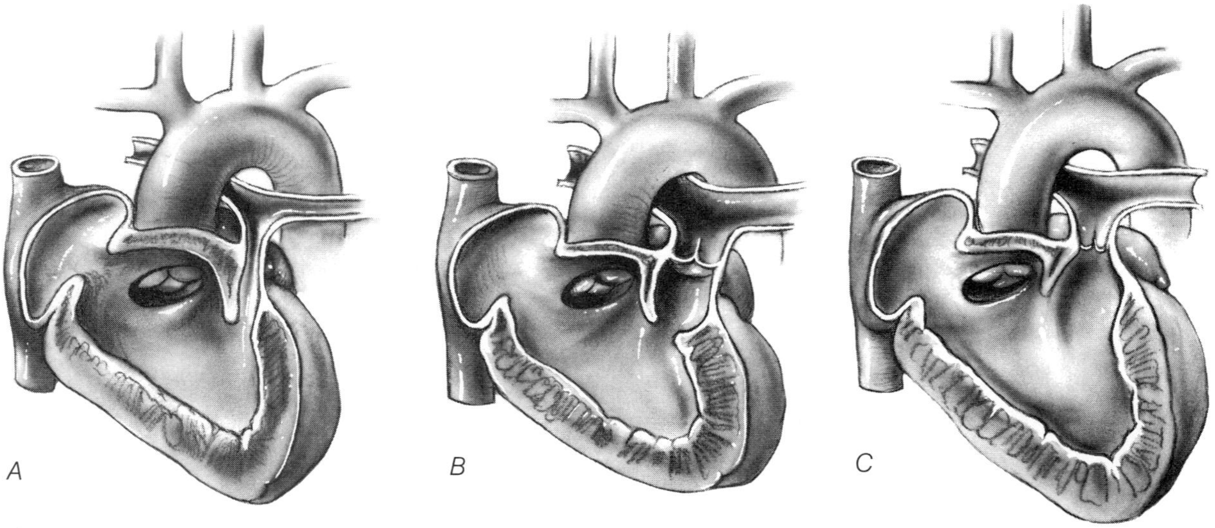

FIG. 17-30. Different types of right ventricular obstruction in tetralogy of Fallot. *A.* Combined obstruction from hypoplasia of pulmonic annulus in association with diffuse stenosis of outflow tract of right ventricle. This type of diffuse stenosis is commonly found and often requires insertion of prosthetic patch to widen annulus. *B.* Localized stenosis of infundibulum of right ventricle, with "infundibular chamber" distal to this which is proximal to normal pulmonic valve. *C.* Pulmonic stenosis of valvular type in association with normal right ventricular outflow tract. (From: *Benson CD, et al: Pediatric Surgery. Vol. I. Chicago, Year Book Medical Publishers, 1962, p. 463, with permission.*)

shunted directly into the left ventricle and aorta to produce cyanosis. The degree of right-to-left shunting is dependent on the severity of outflow tract obstruction. In addition to cyanosis, the malformation decreases pulmonary blood flow and hence limits the capacity of the lungs to absorb oxygen. The inability to increase pulmonary blood flow constitutes the basis for the severe intolerance to exercise. The large ventricular septal defect has a separate influence, in that right ventricular pressure almost never exceeds left ventricular pressure, in contrast to isolated pulmonic valvular stenosis. For this reason, cardiac enlargement and failure are rare.

The severity of the anoxia varies with the degree of reduction in pulmonary blood flow. Arterial oxygen saturations of 70 to 85 percent are seen in older children, but in younger children, who may not survive infancy without operation, astonishingly low oxygen saturations are encountered. Saturations of 30 to 35 percent may be seen in patients who can walk only a short distance, and levels of 20 to 25 percent are found in some infants who are unable to walk. Saturations as low as 10 percent have been recorded, usually associated with loss of consciousness from cerebral anoxia. With exercise, there is often a precipitous fall in arterial oxygen saturation, decreasing from a resting level of 70 percent to 20 to 25 percent, clearly indicating the physiologic basis for exertional dyspnea.

Chronic anoxia produces compensatory polycythemia and eventual clubbing of the extremities. Polycythemia is seldom apparent until after 2 years of age, but later hematocrits from 60 to 75 percent are common. Wide variations in hematocrits are found, ranging from normal with mild tetralogies to levels as high as 85 to 90 percent in the most severe forms.

The degree of cyanosis increases significantly in the first few years of life, for visible cyanosis is proportional to the number of grams of unsaturated hemoglobin in the peripheral circulation as well as the actual oxygen concentration. Hence severe cyanosis is visible only after polycythemia has developed. The time of appearance has been used by Nadas for a convenient grouping of the clinical course of the disease. About one-third of patients are cyanotic at birth, another one-third become cyanotic in the first year of life, and one-third develop cyanosis in the next few years. Patients cyanotic at birth from severe anoxia often do not survive infancy unless operation is performed. These patients frequently have significant pulmonary atresia. Patients becoming cyanotic in the first year of life have a milder course but are seriously disabled, while those who develop cyanosis in later years may have little incapacity and little polycythemia—a so-called pink tetralogy. These patients, of course, have only moderate reduction in pulmonary blood flow because of a lesser degree of outflow tract obstruction.

The main threat to life in the first year of life is cerebral infarction, from either thrombosis or anoxia. In severe cases, cyanotic "spells" are seen in which the infant becomes deeply cyanotic and comatose. Spontaneous recovery usually occurs, but death or hemiplegia may ensue. Such infants require emergency operation.

Brain abscess is another serious, often lethal, complication to which patients are peculiarly susceptible. The right-to-left shunt, bypassing the lungs and providing direct access for bacteria in the venous blood to enter the arterial circulation, is the most plausible explanation.

Cardiac failure is rare. Its presence always brings into question the accuracy of the diagnosis. Life expectancy without treatment is short. About 25 percent die in the first year, 40 percent by 3 years, and 70 percent by 10 years. Formerly, only about 10 percent of patients reached 20 years of age.

Clinical Manifestations. ***Symptoms.*** Almost all patients are symptomatic. Dyspnea and cyanosis, markedly aggravated by exertion, are the outstanding features. Two additional characteristics are cyanotic spells and squatting. Cyanotic spells are episodes of sudden increase in intensity of cyanosis, sometimes followed by unconsciousness, usually with spontaneous recovery within a few minutes or hours. Such episodes, representing acute cerebral anoxia, may be fatal or may result in hemiplegia. They are especially frequent between 2 and 6 months of age.

Squatting is an impressive characteristic, for children learn quickly to relieve dyspnea by assuming a squatting position. The physiologic benefit from squatting, apparently a redistribution of blood flow, is probably based on an increase in systemic vascular resistance, which diminishes right-to-left shunting and forces more blood flow into the lungs. Walking for short distances, interrupted by squatting, is a well-recognized hallmark of the tetralogy. Hemoptysis is rare, occurring usually in older children with marked varicosities of the bronchial circulation.

Physical Examination. On physical examination the obvious features are cyanosis of varying severity and clubbing of the digits. The heart usually has a normal size, rate, and rhythm. A systolic murmur of grades II to III intensity is commonly present along the left sternal border at the third or fourth intercostal spaces, accompanied by a thrill in about one-half the patients. With severe pulmonic stenosis or pulmonary atresia, the murmur may be faint or absent because of absence of flow through the pulmonic orifice. The second pulmonic sound is weak or absent, while the aortic second sound is increased.

Diagnosis. The chest radiograph shows a heart of normal size with an unusual contour, termed the *coeur en sabot,* or boot-shaped heart (Fig. 17-31). This unusual appearance results from the combination of a concave pulmonary artery segment, a horizontal ventricular septum produced by the concentric right ventricular hypertrophy, and a left ventricle that is smaller than normal. The lung fields show decreased vascularity.

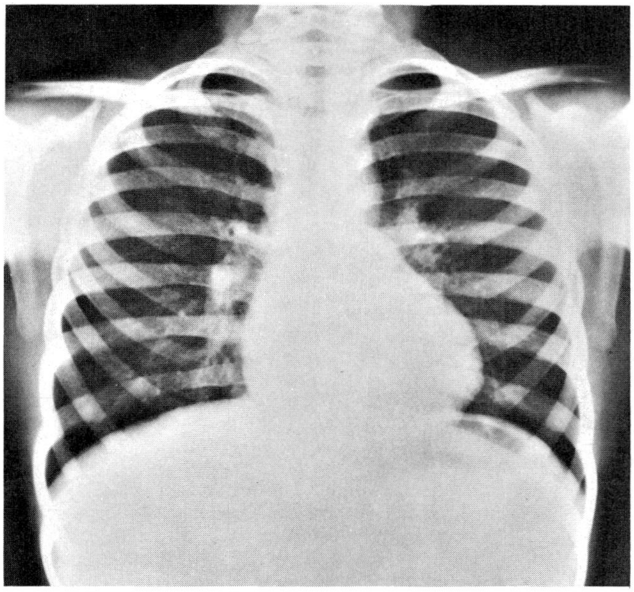

FIG. 17-31. Chest radiograph of child with tetralogy of Fallot, showing typical cardiac silhouette (sabot-shaped heart). Features include heart of normal size with prominent apex from right ventricular hypertrophy. There is increased concavity at base of heart because pulmonic stenosis produces decrease in size or absence of shadow normally seen from pulmonary artery. Vascularity of lung fields may be normal or decreased. *(Courtesy of Dr. Raymond M. Abrams, Department of Radiology, New York University Medical Center.)*

The electrocardiogram is always abnormal, showing right ventricular hypertrophy of varying severity with right axis deviation. The echocardiogram is usually diagnostic. The most important data are obtained by cardiac catheterization and biplane angiography. Abnormalities found at catheterization include the large right-to-left shunt with equal right and left ventricular systolic pressures. Pulmonary artery pressure is decreased, resulting in a large systolic pressure gradient between the right ventricle and pulmonary artery. Calculated pulmonary blood flow is decreased, varying with the severity of the disorder. The degree of decrease will parallel the severity of the arterial hypoxemia. Hematocrit is usually between 60 and 70 percent, ranging from 45 to 90 percent.

The biplane cineangiogram is the most important study, demonstrating all the key morphologic abnormalities when appropriate views are obtained. Essential information includes the type of abnormality in the right ventricular outflow tract, the pulmonary valve annulus, leaflets, main pulmonary artery, and its branches. Care should be taken in studying the size of the main and branch pulmonary arteries because severe hypoplasia of the pulmonary vascular bed may preclude total correction. The typical ventricular septal defect is usually easily seen; additional septal defects, if present, can also be identified. The coronary anatomy should be studied in detail for anomalous origin of the anterior descending from the right coronary.

The diagnosis can usually be made with reasonable certainty from clinical examination combined with radiograph, electrocardiogram, and echocardiogram. The important clinical features are cyanosis with severe exertional dyspnea and squatting. The important physical findings are a heart of normal size with a systolic murmur. Radiographic findings demonstrate a heart of normal size with decreased vascularity of the lung fields, while the electrocardiogram shows right ventricular hypertrophy.

Treatment. ***Indications for Operation.*** Infants with cyanotic spells and significant pulmonary atresia or hypoplastic pulmonary arteries require emergency shunt operation to prevent death or hemiplegia. At present a shunt procedure seems preferable in the first 3 months of life, although a few surgeons use total correction. Although a wide variety of shunts have been used, the safest and most effective is either a standard Blalock-Taussig subclavian pulmonary anastomosis or a modified Blalock-Taussig subclavian-pulmonary Gore-Tex interposition graft. Operative risk with either type of shunt is very small, improvement is usually substantial, and removal of the shunt at the time of a subsequent corrective operation is not complicated. The authors generally prefer the modified Blalock-Taussig Gore-Tex graft in smaller infants or neonates.

Beyond 3 months of age, the increasing tendency is for a primary corrective operation rather than performance of a shunt. Excellent data have been reported from several centers supporting this approach.

Technique of Corrective Operation. A median sternotomy incision is preferred. Extracorporeal circulation with cardioplegia is used. If a previous shunt operation has been performed, the shunt is isolated before extracorporeal circulation is begun and subsequently occluded during bypass before the heart is opened. Once the pericardium has been opened, the outflow tract of the right ventricle is carefully examined for anomalous coronary arteries, choosing an approach that avoids dividing any such arteries.

Five potential zones of obstruction to flow of blood to the lungs should be considered for surgical correction, the location, the severity, and number varying with each patient. These include fusion of the pulmonary valve leaflets; a hypoplastic pulmonic annulus; varying degrees of infundibular stenosis in the right ventricle, either fibrous or muscular; hypoplastic main pulmonary artery; or hypoplastic distal pulmonary arteries. The critical importance of these decisions emphasizes the crucial nature of preoperative selective angiocardiography.

The surgical approach may be through the right atrium or the right ventricle, varying with both the anatomy and the preference of the surgeon. The authors currently approach most cases through the right atrium and perform patch closure of the ventricular septal defect through the tricuspid valve. The main pulmonary artery is then opened and the pulmonary valve and annulus inspected. A short transannular incision is made if the annulus is hypoplastic, extending this incision (Fig. 17-32) beyond the infundibular obstruction. If the pulmonary annulus is of adequate size based on body surface area it is preserved, and a separate small ventriculotomy is used to correct the infundibular stenosis. The ventriculotomy is routinely closed with an appropriate pericardial patch.

A crucial part of the operation is deciding whether the diameter of the pulmonic valve ring is adequate. Sizing of the diameter of the pulmonic ring with Hegar dilators is first done and then evaluated with a nomogram describing normal relationships between body surface area and diameter of the pulmonic annulus. The measurements are particularly useful for smaller children. In larger children a pulmonic valve ring that will accommodate a size 16 Hegar dilator, representing a cross-sectional area slightly less than 2 cm^2, is satisfactory.

Our preference for the prosthetic patch is pericardium (see Fig. 17-32). If the transannular patch is tailored to appropriate size, aneurysmal formation in the patch is rare in the absence of uncorrected branch pulmonary artery stenosis. When the pulmonary arteries are severely hypoplastic a valved pulmonary artery homograft may be used to reconstruct the outflow tract, rather than the standard transannular patch.

Following bypass, intracardiac pressure is measured to confirm that right ventricular obstruction has been corrected. The right ventricular systolic pressure should be reduced to less than 60 to 70 percent of systemic left ventricular systolic pressure. If right ventricular pressure is still elevated above this level, more adequate correction of the ventricular obstruction should be considered, though exact guidelines do not exist. Certainly if the right ventricular pressure remains at systemic levels further intervention is necessary, and a valve conduit or pulmonary homograft should be placed unless obstruction can be better relieved. Otherwise fatal depression of cardiac output from right ventricular failure may occur in the early postoperative course. In most patients following bypass a satisfactory result is obtained, with a systolic pressure near 100 mmHg, a right ventricular systolic pressure between 35 and 50 mmHg, and a pulmonary artery systolic pressure of 20 to 25 mmHg.

Postoperative Course. Following operation, particular attention is required in the first 24 h to intrathoracic bleeding, because older cyanotic patients have an increased hemorrhagic tendency from the longstanding polycythemia. Transfusion of fresh frozen plasma, often combined with platelet transfusions, is the best therapy. Close observation is necessary to detect intrathoracic accumulation of blood with cardiac tamponade.

Adequacy of cardiac output is monitored by direct measurement or indirectly by observing blood pressure, blood-gas concentrations in mixed venous blood, warmth of extremities, and urine output. Left atrial pressure is kept in the range of 10 to 15 mmHg. If perfusion and cardiac output are inadequate small amounts of inotropic drugs (dobutamine, dopamine, epinephrine, or isoproteronol) are infused. Assisted ventilation may be required for 12 to 24 h but seldom for longer.

The risk of operation no longer varies with the age of the patient or the degree of cyanosis. Operative risk is near 2 to 5 percent in most centers. Large clinical series showing low operative mortality have been reported by Kirklin, Malm et al., Shumway et al., and McGoon et al.

Arciniegas et al. reported 209 patients, in whom an outflow patch across the pulmonic annulus was used in nearly 70 percent. Perioperative mortality was 5 percent and delayed mortality was 3

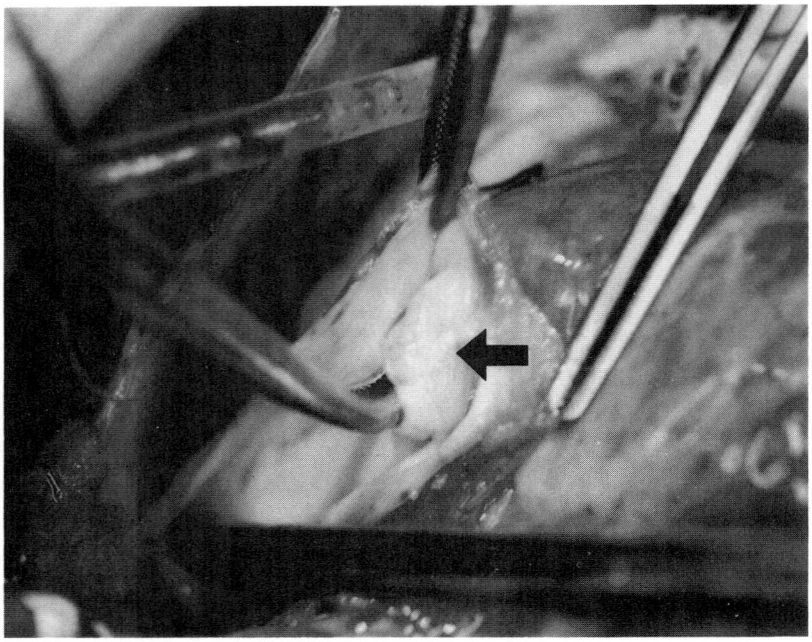

A

FIG. 17-32. Operative photograph of patient with tetralogy of Fallot, with classic combination of valvular, annular, and infundibular right ventricular outflow tract obstruction. *A.* Photograph of open pulmonary artery, demonstrating a domed, monocusp, pulmonary valve and a tightly stenotic 4-mm valve orifice. *B.* Photograph of completed transannular incision demonstrating right and left pulmonary arteries distally (a), open annulus (b), and right ventricular outflow tract incision (c), with 2-cm-thick hypertrophied right ventricular muscle. *C.* Completed pericardial transannular patch reconstruction of right ventricular outflow tract (encircled area). Note ventricular septal defect was repaired through a right atrial incision (Fig. 17-22), minimizing the size of the right ventricular incision. (From: New York University Medical Center.)

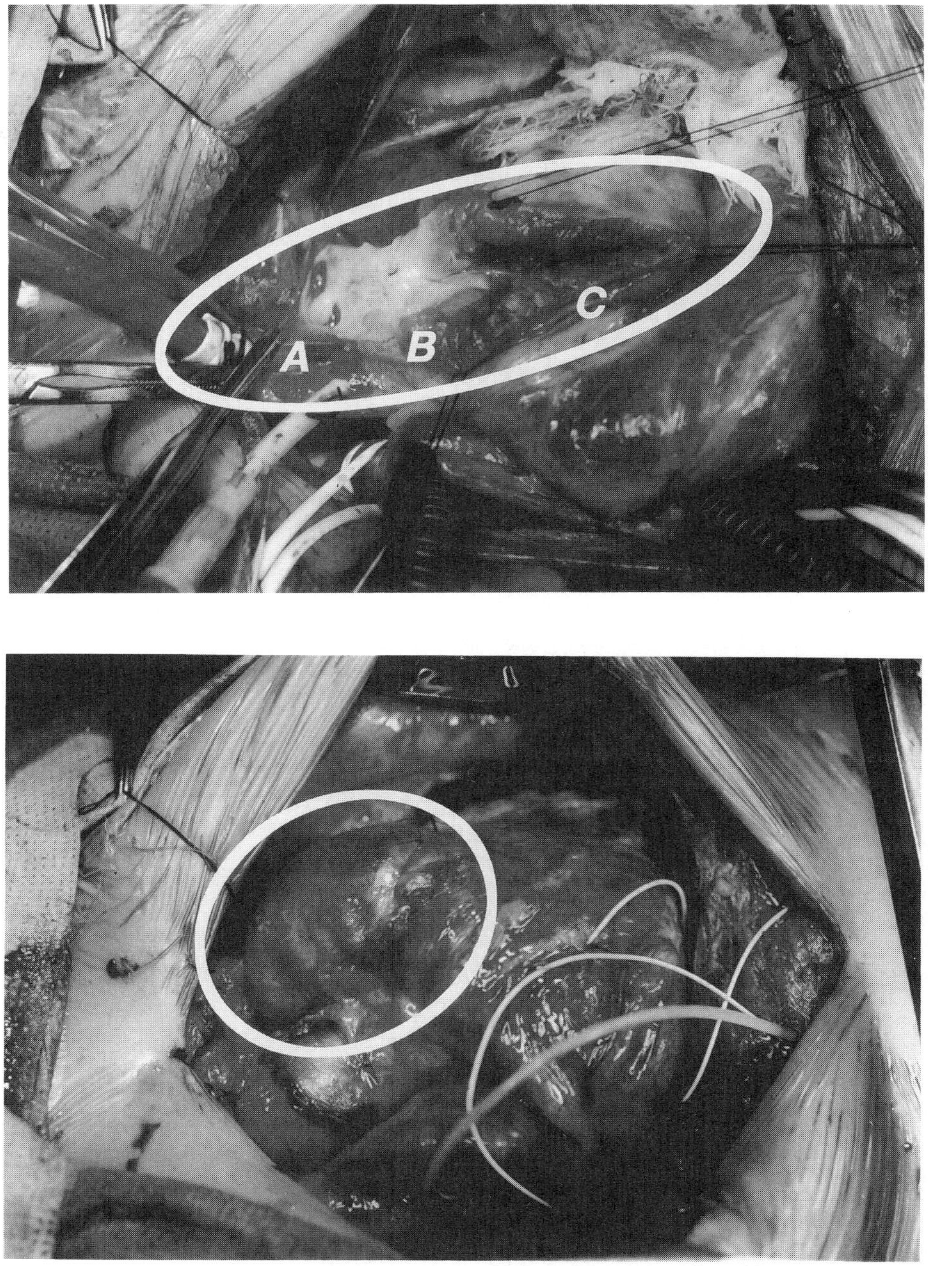

B

C

FIG. 17-32. Continued.

percent. Complete heart block occurred in only one patient. Late results were considered good in 87 percent of the patients.

Following recovery from operation, dramatic improvement is obvious. Cyanosis is, of course, absent, and exercise tolerance within a few months approaches that of a normal individual. If cardiac failure is significant following operation, convalescence may be slow for several weeks. Long-term studies show that most patients have excellent cardiac function.

The tolerance for pulmonic insufficiency after two to three decades is almost unknown, though Lillehei recently reported good long-term results in patients operated upon with a follow-up of more than 30 years. Ebert described repeat operations on 24 patients who had been operated on 1 to 21 years earlier. Several with severe pulmonary valve incompetence and right ventricular dysfunction were treated with insertion of a prosthetic valve. This complication usually occurs secondary to branch pulmonary artery stenosis or hypoplastic peripheral pulmonary arteries, resulting in residual outflow obstruction at the pulmonary artery level, with pulmonary hypertension and progressive valvular insufficiency.

Pulmonary Stenosis-Pulmonary Atresia With Intact Septum

Historical Data. Between 1947 and 1948 Sellers and Brock independently performed the first successful closed valvulotomies for pulmonic valvular stenosis, using a valvulotome through a transventricular approach. Shortly thereafter Blalock reported a series of 19 patients undergoing similar treatment. Open valvulotomy, using hypothermia and venous inflow occlusion, was first done by Swan and Zeavin in 1954. Treatment of pulmonic stenosis with inflow occlusion and open valvulotomy subsequently became the method preferred by many surgeons even after extracorporeal circulation was available. In critically ill infants pulmonary valvulotomy with inflow occlusion is still employed in many centers as the initial treatment for isolated pulmonary stenosis.

Incidence. Pulmonary stenosis is a common defect, constituting 10 percent of all patients with congenital heart disease. Over half of these patients have pure valvular pulmonary stenosis, with the remainder having varying degrees of associated right ventricular outflow tract obstruction. A more severe form of the disease process, pulmonary atresia with intact septum, results in total obstruction of the outflow tract, with atresia of the valve, hypoplasia of the annulus, and differing degrees of hypoplasia and maldevelopment of the right ventricle. Pulmonary atresia with intact septum is less common than pulmonary stenosis, accounting for 1 to 3 percent of congenital heart defects.

Pathologic Anatomy. Pulmonary stenosis and pulmonary atresia with intact septum represent a spectrum of pathologic findings, ranging from isolated valvular stenosis to total valvular atresia with hypoplasia of the body and outflow tract of the right ventricle. With pulmonary stenosis the degree of valvular obstruction may vary from mild, clinically insignificant stenosis to "pinhole" critical stenosis (Fig. 17-33), which produces symptoms during neonatal life similar to pulmonary atresia. The valve is usually tricuspid and domed, with fused commissures, although occasionally valvular dysplasia is present. The annulus may be normal or hypoplastic.

In the majority of cases with pulmonary stenosis the right ventricle is normal, although secondary right ventricular hypertrophy develops in response to the valvular stenosis. Thirty to 40 percent of the cases of pulmonary stenosis will have infundibular obstruction of the right ventricular outflow tract, which is probably acquired as a result of compensatory hypertrophy. Five to 10 percent of the cases will present with isolated infundibular stenosis.

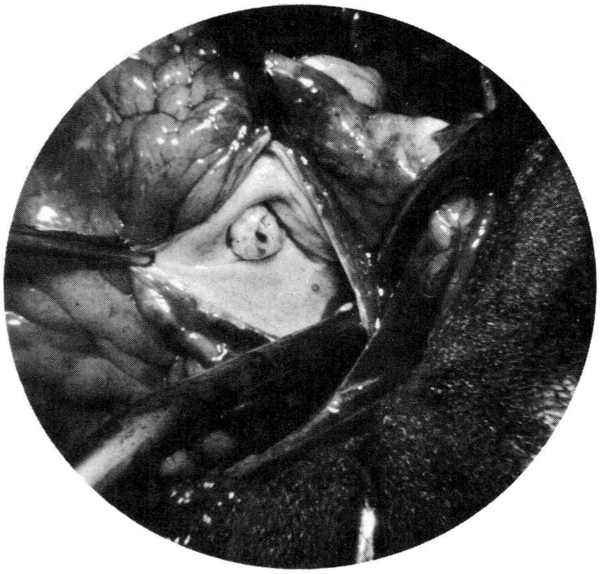

FIG. 17-33. Pulmonic valvular stenosis exposed at operation following incision of pulmonary artery. Dome-shaped structure produced by fusion of valve cusps, with small central opening, is clearly shown. Suction tip has been placed in distal pulmonary artery.

Pulmonary atresia with intact septum is a rare, more severe, disease process. With pulmonary atresia the valve and annulus are atretic, with no forward blood flow. Survival is dependent on right-to-left shunting through a patent foramen ovale and on ductal patency for pulmonary blood flow. The right ventricle is underdeveloped to varying degrees, although the outlet or infundibular portion is usually absent. The body or trabecular portion of the ventricle may also be obliterated and dysfunctional. Cases of pulmonary atresia are at times classified based on the development of the right ventricle as unipartite, bipartite, and tripartite ventricles, depending on the adequacy of the inlet, body, and outlet portions of the ventricle. Knowledge of the right ventricular development is essential, for a minimum of a bipartite ventricle is necessary, and a tripartite ventricle is preferred, if the right heart is to be used in the circulation.

The myocardium exhibits a wide range of pathologic anomalies. Typically the right ventricle is hypertensive, thick-walled, and small, with myocardial muscular disarray. In 25 to 50 percent of the cases with pulmonary atresia sinusoids directly connect the right ventricle with the coronary circulation, at times resulting in a serious condition termed *right ventricular-dependent coronary circulation.*

In patients with pulmonary atresia the tricuspid valve is often regurgitant, but is usually over 75 percent of normal size and the inlet portion of the right ventricle is present. If the tricuspid valve is atretic and the inlet portion of the ventricle is absent the disease becomes part of the tricuspid atresia/hypoplastic right heart syndrome.

Pathophysiology. With severe forms of pulmonary stenosis and with pulmonary atresia forward pulmonary blood flow is minimal or absent. Mixing at the atrial level is necessary to maintain life, with left-to-right shunting across the foramen ovale. If the foramen ovale is of inadequate size it must be stretched shortly after birth with a balloon catheter, a procedure termed *balloon septostomy*. The ductus must be patent to provide pulmonary blood flow. Cyanosis is usually present shortly after birth, and hypoxia and cyanosis progress when the ductus begins to close. Severe acidosis may develop.

With more moderate pulmonary stenosis the physiologic derangements are more insidious. Significant forward pulmonary blood flow is often present and cyanosis is minimal or absent. The obstruction to flow of blood produces elevation in right ventricular systolic pressure with a subsequent secondary hypertrophy of the right ventricle. The severity is determined by the right ventricular outflow gradient, with a 50-mmHg gradient considered mild, and a 80 to 100-mmHg gradient severe. With severe stenosis suprasystemic right ventricular pressures are often present.

As the child grows progressive ventricular hypertrophy may lead to increasing obstruction. If the stenotic valve enlarges with growth, the obstruction may remain moderate or decrease; otherwise a small opening may produce progressively serious obstruction subsequently. Some patients tolerate high levels of right ventricular hypertension for years, while others develop progressive tricuspid insufficiency, right-sided heart failure, and right-to-left shunting across the foramen ovale with resulting hypoxemia and cyanosis.

Clinical Manifestations and Diagnosis. With critical pulmonary stenosis and with pulmonary atresia with intact septum the newborn often looks well except for cyanosis. Cyanosis and hypoxemia markedly worsen over the next 24 hours as the ductus begins to close, with associated metabolic acidosis and respiratory distress. Right-sided heart failure with hepatomegaly is present. A cardiac murmur is frequently absent, although a tricuspid insufficiency murmur may be heard. The second heart sound is single. The electrocardiogram may develop right atrial P waves shortly after birth, but with pulmonary atresia the right ventricular hypertrophy pattern normally seen in the neonate is often absent. The chest radiograph shows decreased pulmonary blood flow and a flat or concave pulmonary artery segment, with a normal or enlarged heart size.

The diagnosis is confirmed by echocardiography, demonstrating either an atretic pulmonary valve and outflow tract or a domed stenotic pulmonary valve. The right ventricle is often thickened and may be hypoplastic. Close attention must be paid to the body and outlet portions of the right ventricle, to the pulmonary valve annular size, to the tricuspid valve size, and to the adequacy of the main pulmonary artery and branch pulmonary arteries. Once the diagnosis is made by echocardiography cardiac catheterization and angiography are indicated to confirm the diagnosis and to demonstrate internal cardiac anatomy prior to operative repair.

With mild or moderate forms of pulmonary stenosis the children are often asymptomatic when first seen. With time dyspnea and easy fatigability occur, and occasionally chest pain or cyanosis develop later in childhood. A harsh systolic ejection murmur is heard best over the second left interspace, and the second heart sound is decreased or absent. The electrocardiogram typically shows progressive right ventricular and right atrial hypertrophy. The chest radiograph shows decreased pulmonary vascular markings and right ventricular cardiac enlargement. Again the diagnosis can be made with accuracy by the echocardiogram. Cardiac catheterization is performed prior to operative repair to measure the pressure gradient across the valve and to outline the details of internal cardiac anatomy.

Treatment. In critically ill neonates urgent operation is required. As soon as the diagnosis is suspected prostaglandin E_1 therapy is begun to maintain ductal patency and acidosis is corrected. For isolated pulmonary stenosis both open and closed valvulotomy are acceptable forms of therapy. The most popular technique is open valvulotomy with venous inflow occlusion, although recently percutaneous closed balloon valvuloplasty has been used with success in selected cases. However, the mortality remains distressingly high with valvulotomy alone, ranging from 10 to 30 percent. This is probably due to a wide spectrum of pathologies that may be present, particularly in terms of right ventricular development. Accordingly many surgeons recommend doing a palliative systemic-to-pulmonary shunt, often with Gore-Tex, in addition to valvulotomy. Both of these approaches usually require further surgery later in life to widely open the outflow tract with a patch. Others have recommended definitive repair with transannular patch in the neonatal period. The therapeutic options and long-term results have been described in detail both for patients with pulmonary stenosis and for patients with pulmonary atresia by Coles et al., but long-term results are clearly better after repair of pulmonary stenosis than with pulmonary atresia. Elective repair performed later in life for pulmonary stenosis has an operative risk of less than 2 to 3 percent with excellent long-term results.

Tricuspid Atresia

Historical Data. Tricuspid atresia was described by Kuhne in 1906, and the clinical features described by Bellet in 1933. Systemic-pulmonary arterial shunts for tricuspid atresia were applied soon after their development between 1945 and 1947 (see Figs. 17-27 and 17-29). There was significant short-term improvement, but long-term results were disappointing. A significant contribution was made by Glenn (see Fig. 17-28), with the development of the superior vena cava-right pulmonary artery anastomosis. The major advance, however, came in 1968 when Fontan successfully separated the right and left circulations in a patient with tricuspid atresia for the first time, a physiologic concept of passive pulmonary blood flow that had seemed feasible in laboratory studies for over a decade but had never been successfully applied in human beings. In the last 15 years, the Fontan procedure has undergone several modifications but has been established clearly as the procedure of choice for this condition.

Pathologic Anatomy. Tricuspid atresia is an important form of congenital heart disease, affecting 2 to 5 percent of children with cyanotic heart disease. The four basic abnormalities are atresia of the tricuspid valve and ventricular inlet, constituting complete obstruction to the flow of blood; a varying degree of hypoplasia of the right ventricle; an atrial septal defect; and frequently a ventricular septal defect. The mitral valve and the left ventricle are usually normal. Blood may enter the rudimentary right ventricle through a ventricular septal defect or may totally mix at the atrial level and enter the lungs only through ductal flow in patients without a ventricular septal defect. Pulmonary atresia or stenosis is seen in 85 percent of the cases with normally located great vessels, further limiting pulmonary blood flow. At times the right heart is totally underdeveloped, without inlet, body, or outlet chambers, a condition that may be referred to as *hypoplastic right heart*.

In about 70 percent of patients, the aorta and pulmonary artery are normally located, while in about 30 percent transposition is present. Hence, there are two major types of tricuspid atresia depending on whether the great vessels are transposed or not. Each of these two major groups has been further subdivided according to whether the pulmonary blood flow is normal, increased, or decreased, or pulmonary atresia is present (Figs. 17-34, 17-35).

In the standard case with normally related great vessels, the majority have a decreased pulmonary blood flow. When the aorta and pulmonary artery are transposed, however, about 70 percent of patients have a normal or increased pulmonary blood flow with overperfusion of the lungs rather than hypoxia.

Pathophysiology. The disability from hypoxia resulting from inadequate pulmonary blood flow is severe. This is most commonly due to the absence of blood flow through the atretic tricuspid valve combined with restriction of flow from the left ventricle through the ventricular septal defect and rudimentary right ventricle into the pulmonary artery. The ventricular septal defect, if present, usually decreases in size in the first year of life, further decreasing pulmonary blood flow. Over 90 percent of patients die before the first year unless operation is performed.

In the minority of patients with an increase in pulmonary blood flow, with either normal or transposed great arteries, congestive heart failure is present with gradual failure of the left ventricle. Only rarely is the pulmonary blood flow near normal.

Clinical Manifestations. Disability is severe, with hypoxia and cyanosis, usually obvious at birth. Over 50 percent of infants are correctly diagnosed during the first day of life. The clinical manifestations are usually those of severe cyanosis and dyspnea, with anoxic spells often terminating in hemiplegia or

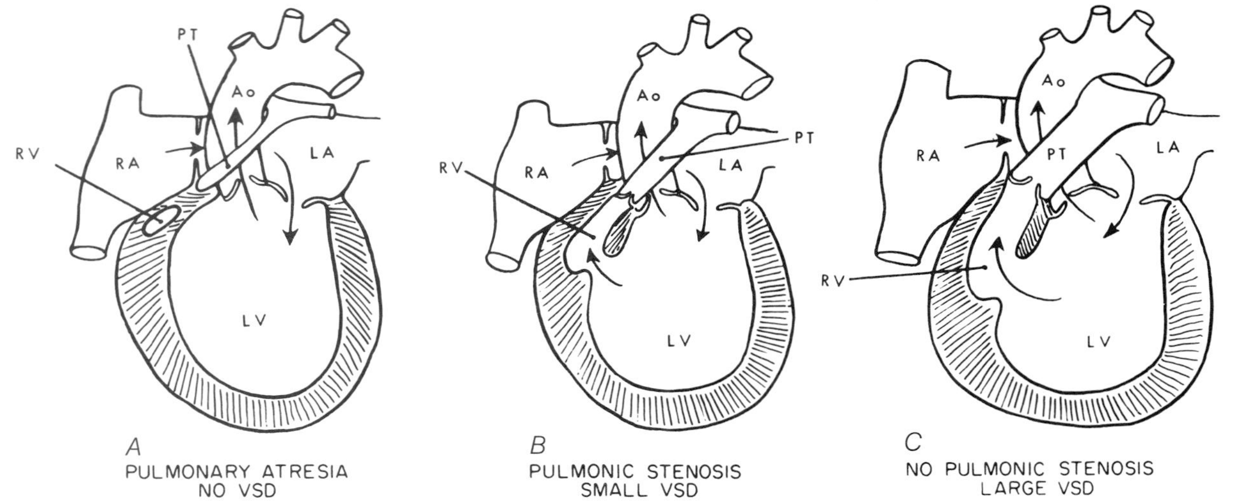

FIG. 17-34. Three basic varieties of tricuspid atresia with normally related great arteries. Proximal to mitral valve, anatomic arrangements are similar, with an interatrial communication providing right atrium (RA) with its only outlet. Beyond mitral valve, anatomic patterns vary (LA, left atrium). *A.* When there is pulmonary atresia, i.e., no interventricular communication, all left ventricular blood enters aorta (Ao). Pulmonary flow depends on a patent ductus arteriosus or systemic arterial collaterals. *B.* When there is pulmonic stenosis, zone of obstruction typically consists of a slitlike ventricular septal defect that represents the only communication between left ventricle (LV) and small right ventricle (RV). Pulmonary trunk (PT) is normal or hypoplastic, and pulmonic valve stenosis may coexist. *C.* Absence of pulmonic stenosis signifies that there is a large ventricular septal defect with unobstructed flow into pulmonary circulation (From: *Perloff JK: The Clinical Recognition of Congenital Heart Disease. Philadelphia, WB Saunders. Ch. 25, p. 555, with permission.*)

death. In the few patients with an increased pulmonary blood flow, signs of pulmonary congestion and heart failure may predominate.

The physical examination is usually not diagnostic, as the systolic murmur present varies widely, depending on the size of the ventricular septal defect and the anatomic relationship of the great vessels. The chest radiograph shows decreased vascularity if pulmonary blood flow is decreased. Both the electrocardiogram and echocardiogram provide the diagnostic clues that establish the diagnosis. The electrocardiogram is strongly suggestive, showing a typical left axis deviation resulting from the underdevelopment of

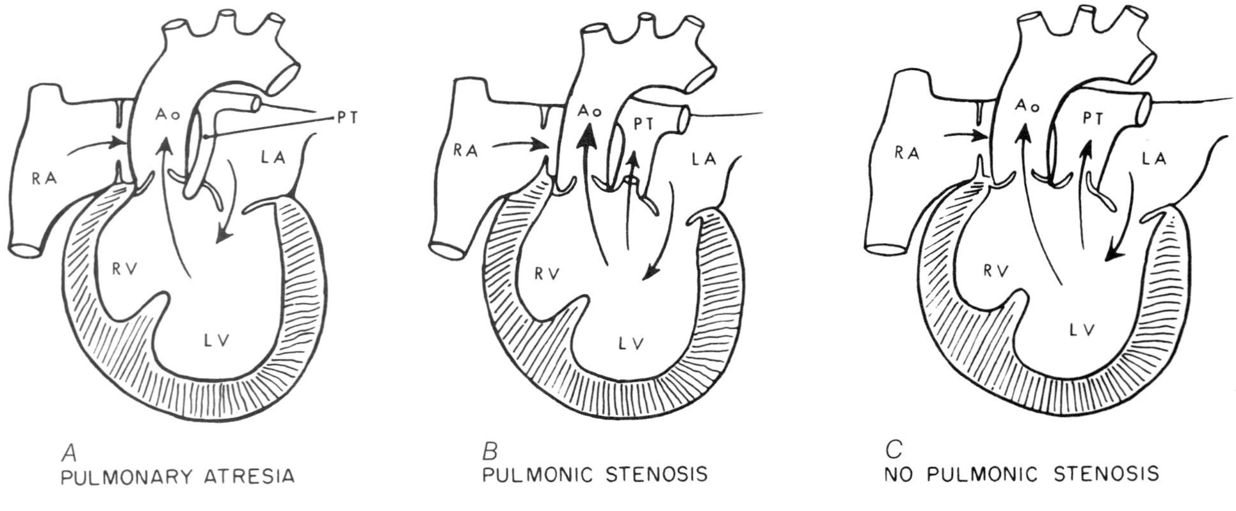

FIG. 17-35. Three basic varieties of tricuspid atresia with complete transposition of great arteries. Proximal to mitral valve, anatomic arrangements are similar, with an interatrial communication providing right atrium (RA) with its only outlet. Ventricular septal defect is characteristically large, so there is no obstruction to flow from left ventricle (LV) into transposed aorta (Ao). Beyond this point anatomic patterns vary. *A.* When there is pulmonary atresia (imperforate pulmonic valve and hypoplastic pulmonary trunk), all left ventricular blood enters aorta. Pulmonary flow depends on a patent ductus arteriosus or systemic arterial collaterals. *B.* When pulmonic stenosis is present obstruction is either valvular or subvalvular. *C.* When there is no pulmonic stenosis, pulmonary vascular resistance determines amount of blood entering the lungs (RV, right ventricle; PT, pulmonary trunk; LA, left atrium). (From: *Perloff JK: The Clinical Recognition of Congenital Heart Disease. Philadelphia, WB Saunders. Ch. 25, p. 555, with permission.*)

the right ventricle. The two-dimensional echocardiogram can often outline the atrial septal defect, the ventricular septal defect, and the relationships of the great arteries. Cardiac catheterization and angiography are required to precisely delineate these abnormalities.

Treatment. An emergency shunt is often necessary in the first few days or weeks of life to prevent death from anoxia. A Gore-Tex interposition shunt, as described in the section on palliative shunts (see Fig. 17-29), is usually the simplest and most satisfactory.

In some patients, a small atrial septal defect (or foramen ovale) may restrict flow of blood from the right atrium to the left atrium. This can be determined at cardiac catheterization, measuring a gradient between the right and left atrium. If a gradient is present, a balloon septostomy can be performed at that time. Surgical enlargement of the atrial septal defect is occasionally required later in life to ensure atrial mixing of blood before more definitive repair (Fig. 17-36). After 6 to 12 months of age, a Fontan procedure can be performed, directing the venous blood into the pulmonary circulation. The procedure is delayed until this time because the pulmonary vascular resistance, normally elevated at birth, must drop to normal levels for a procedure dependent on passive pulmonary blood flow to be effective.

This landmark procedure was first performed by Fontan in France in 1968 and has subsequently been widely used throughout the world with excellent results. Important modifications of the original Fontan concept were made by Kreutzer and by Bjork. At present, two varieties of connections between the right atrium and the pulmonary artery are performed. The simplest is establishment of a large direct communication between the right atrium and the main pulmonary artery, which is divided at its origin, mobilized, and anastomosed directly to a large circular opening in the right atrium. No valve is inserted. Recently some have diminished the size of the right atrium with a tunnel of Dacron or pericardium to decrease the compliance of the atrial chamber. Occasionally a controlled atrial septal defect, made with a 3- or 4-mm punch, is left to allow right-to-left shunting. This is done in high-risk cases, so a sudden rise in pulmonary vascular resistance will not totally stop forward cardiac output.

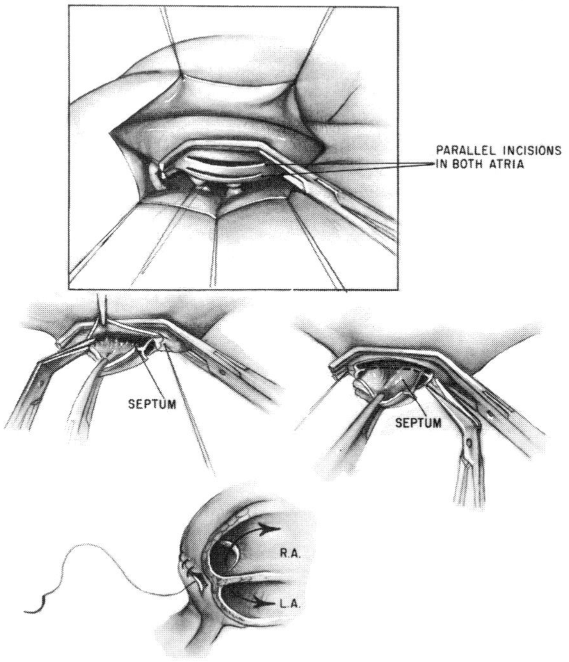

FIG. 17-36. Creation of atrial septal defect (Blalock-Hanlon technique). Right pulmonary veins are mobilized and occluded by traction on ligatures. Pulmonary artery and right main bronchus are also occluded to avoid congestion of lungs during occlusion of pulmonary veins. Tangential occlusion clamp is applied to right and left atria, enclosing atrial septum. Separate incisions are then made in right atrium and left atrium. Exposed atrial septum is then removed, temporarily releasing clamp in order to withdraw more septum from between its jaws and create larger defect. After excision of this septum, incision is sutured, creating large atrial septal defect. (From: *Cooley DA, et al: Arch Surg 93:704, 1966, with permission.*)

Alternately, if the right ventricle is of significant size with a pulmonic valve, a conduit may be established from the right atrium to the right ventricle. In all procedures both the atrial and ventricular septal defects are closed so the two circulations are separated. If an adequate ventricular chamber is present it should be used, otherwise direct atrial-pulmonary connection is used.

The operation physiologically depends on using the venous pressure to perfuse the pulmonary vascular bed resulting in markedly abnormal physiology even after repair. Outcome is usually satisfactory if the right atrial pressure remains below 15 to 18 mmHg. Higher levels result in severe problems such as chylothorax and protein-losing enteropathy. Hence, the Fontan procedure is contraindicated in the presence of an increase in pulmonary vascular resistance, hypoplasia of the pulmonary arteries, or any preexisting condition that results in elevated left ventricular diastolic pressure.

In the minority of patients who are seen with refractory congestive failure from increased pulmonary blood flow in infancy, banding of the pulmonary artery can be done to temporarily decrease pulmonary blood flow and control congestive heart failure, followed 1 to 2 years later by a Fontan procedure and debanding.

The Glenn procedure consists of anastomosis of the superior vena cava to the end of the divided right pulmonary artery (see Fig. 17-28). About 85 percent of patients survive 10 or more years. Arteriovenous fistulas develop in the lung, however, and symptoms tend to gradually recur, probably related to growth of the patient and the basic limitation that only part of systemic venous return has been directed into the pulmonary vascular bed. The Glenn procedure has been largely replaced by the more effective Fontan operation. Recently a bidirectional Glenn or side-to-side caval pulmonary artery anastomosis has been advocated for longer palliation of high-risk cases before a Fontan operation.

While the concept of passive atrial-pulmonary connection with separated circulations introduced by Fontan represents a major breakthrough in the treatment of tricuspid atresia, the corrected patient persists with abnormal, albeit improved, physiology after repair. Because of this long-term results are limited in terms of survival and cardiac functional recovery. Fontan and Kirklin addressed this topic in 1989 in reviewing 334 patients undergoing the Fontan procedure. The variables predicting survival were identified, after which each optimal condition was used to predict outcome after a ''perfect Fontan'' operation. With optimal conditions in each category operative risk was 8 percent, 5-year survival was 86 percent, 10-year survival was 81 percent, and 15-year survival was 73 percent. Of note, the late hazard, or instantaneous risk of death, began to increase after 6 years, and the average NYHA functional status progressively decreased after operation. These data suggest that the late outcome after a Fontan operation is imperfect, presumably because of limitations imposed by the abnormal physiology present. Families of patients undergoing this procedure should be counselled appropriately so that long-term expectations are realistic. However, the procedure still offers the best chance for long-term survival for patients with tricuspid atresia or hypoplastic right heart syndrome.

Transposition of the Great Vessels

Historical Data. The clinical syndrome of transposition of the great vessels was clearly described by Taussig in 1938. The first surgical procedure to achieve significant benefit, creation of an atrial septal defect, was reported in 1948 by Blalock and Hanlon. Because of the excellent results now obtained with balloon septostomy, developed by Rashkind in 1969, surgical creation of an atrial septal defect is now only occasionally necessary to ensure atrial mixing when long-term palliation is necessary (see Fig. 17-36). Another palliative surgical procedure, no longer used, was developed by Baffes around 1957. He transposed the inferior vena cava and the right pulmonary veins. Total correction of transposition by redirecting blood flow at the atrial level was based on work by Arbert in 1955. Senning, in 1957, first completely corrected transposition of the great vessels by repositioning the atrial septum to redirect caval blood through the mitral valve and pulmonary venous blood into the tricuspid valve, but mortality was prohibitively high. Further experience with a modification of the technique was reported by Senning in 1975 with improved results, after which the technique was adopted by several groups as the procedure of choice.

Meanwhile, in 1964 Mustard developed a method of reconstructing the atrial cavity and redirecting vena caval blood into the mitral valve with an intra-atrial baffle. The technique significantly improved the results for correction of transposition of the great vessels and was adopted by most centers as the preferred procedure throughout the 1960s and 1970s. In 1975 Jatene performed the first successful arterial switch procedure for correction of transposition, with coronary artery transfer and reimplantation. This technique had significant long-term advantages in that it used the anatomic left ventricle in the systemic circulation. Although this procedure was initially difficult to duplicate, results improved significantly in the 1980s and the arterial switch operation is now considered the optimal procedure for treatment of transposition.

Incidence and Etiology. Transposition of the great vessels is a frequent disorder, representing 5 to 8 percent of all congenital cardiac malformations and accounting for about 25 percent of deaths in the first year of life. It is the most common cause of cardiac failure in the newborn. It results from abnormal division of the bulbar trunk in embryologic development, occurring between the fifth and seventh uterine week. Etiologic factors are unknown. It is about four times more frequent in males than in females.

Pathologic Anatomy. With transposition of the arteries, the aorta originates from the right ventricle and the pulmonary artery from the left ventricle (Fig. 17-37 and 17-38). As a result, venous blood returning through the venae cavae to the right atrium enters the right ventricle and is then ejected directly into the aorta. Oxygenated blood returning from the lungs through the pulmonary veins to the left atrium enters the left ventricle and is then expelled through the pulmonary artery to the lungs. This dual, parallel circulatory arrangement is obviously incompatible with life without communication between the pulmonary and systemic circulations. Three possible communications exist, a patent ductus arteriosus, an atrial septal defect or foramen ovale, or a ventricular septal defect. One or more of these, of course, must exist for the infant to survive even a few hours after birth. A patent ductus is present for a few weeks after birth in over one-half the patients. A foramen ovale is also frequent, and a ventricular septal defect occurs in 50 to 70 percent of patients.

Associated anomalies are common. One of the most frequent, left ventricular outflow tract obstruction resulting in pulmonic stenosis, occurs frequently enough to constitute a well-defined variant of the syndrome, because the prognosis is unusually favorable. A wide variety of other anomalies may occur, including coarctation of the aorta, pulmonary atresia, and dextrocardia.

Pathophysiology. The two basic physiologic handicaps with transposition are severe anoxia from inability to transport oxygen from the lungs to the tissues of the body and progressive cardiac failure. The severe and rapidly progressive cardiac failure results partly from a high cardiac output into the pulmonary circulation and partly from the fact that the coronary arteries are filled with unoxygenated blood with resulting myocardial anoxia. The relative severity of the anoxia and the cardiac failure varies with

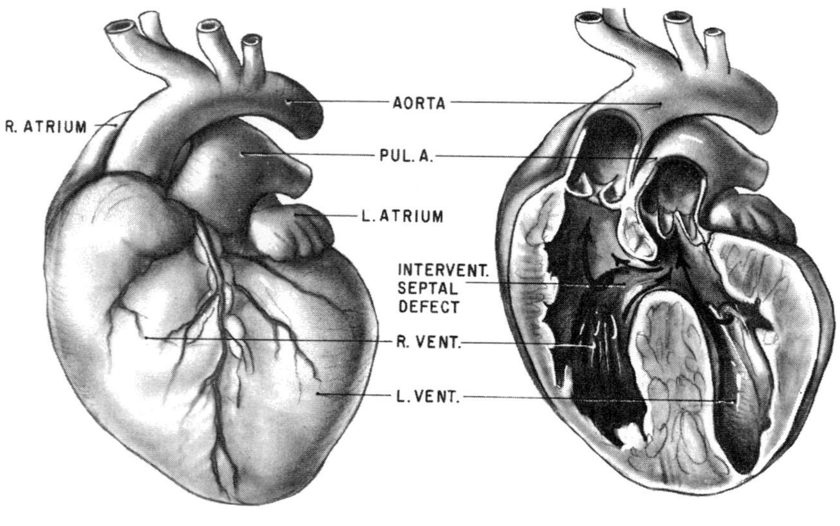

FIG. 17-37. Transposition of great vessels, with aorta arising from right ventricle and pulmonary artery from left ventricle. Ventricular septal defect permits communication between pulmonic and systemic circulations; otherwise condition would be incompatible with life after birth. (From: *Taussig HB: Congenital Malformations of the Heart, 2d ed. Cambridge, Harvard University Press, 1960, p. 149, with permission.*)

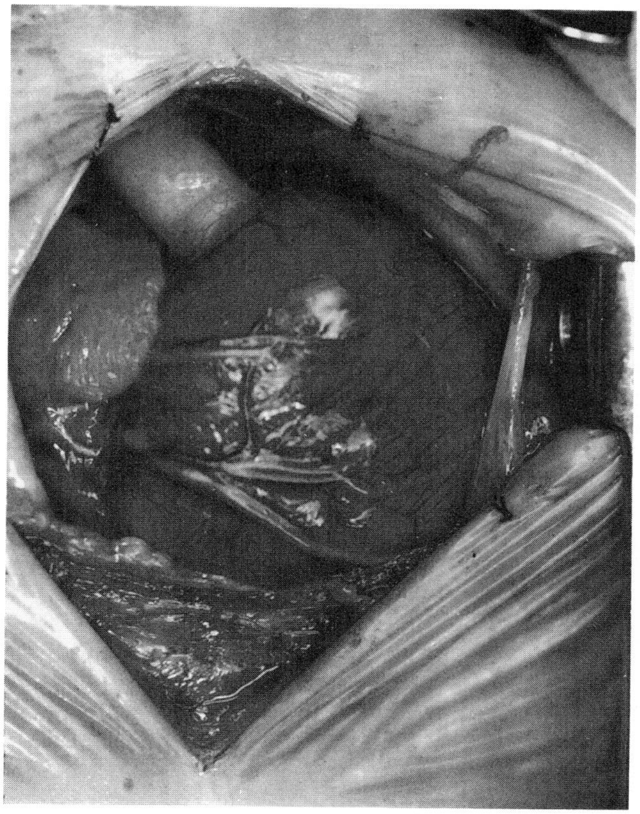

FIG. 17-38. Operative photograph of heart of a child with transposition of great vessels, demonstrating anterior position of aorta. Child underwent successful arterial switch repair. (From: *New York University Medical Center.*)

the nature of the intra-cardiac communications and the adequacy of pulmonary blood flow. Nadas found cardiac failure at birth in 80 percent of live patients.

Transposition is a lethal condition. Patients with an intact ventricular septum, depending on a foramen ovale to communicate between the two circulations, die most rapidly: 30 percent in 1 week, 50 percent in 1 month, and 90 percent by 1 year. Those with a large ventricular septal defect develop pulmonary vascular changes due to increased pulmonary flow at an astonishing rate, often within 6 to 8 weeks, with 80 percent dying within the first year.

Nadas conveniently grouped patients into three clinical categories related to prognosis. Those with an intact ventricular septum do poorly because of inadequate mixing of the pulmonary and systemic circulations. Similarly, those with a large ventricular septal defect do badly because of excessive pulmonary blood flow. Pulmonary vascular resistance rises very rapidly in this group. Patients with the most favorable prognosis have a ventricular septal defect combined with left ventricular outflow obstruction producing pulmonic stenosis. This combination permits mixing of the pulmonary and systemic circulations through the ventricular septal defect, while the outflow tract obstruction prevents excessive pulmonary blood flow with pulmonary congestion and secondary pulmonary hypertension.

Clinical Manifestations. ***Symptoms.*** A high percentage of infants are cyanotic at birth. Over 90 percent are recognized the first day of life. Cardiac failure is similarly frequent. The combination of cardiac failure and cyanosis in a newborn suggests transposition. The most prominent symptoms are cyanosis and dyspnea.

Physical Findings. Cyanosis is usually obvious and is often severe. Signs of congestive failure are almost always found, with cardiac enlargement, hepatomegaly, and pulmonary congestion. A systolic murmur is usually present but is variable and not diagnostic. It can result from any of the different intracardiac communications that may be present. Absence of a murmur, often indicating absence of an intracardiac communication, indicates a particularly unfavorable prognosis.

Diagnosis. The chest radiograph often shows three distinctive abnormalities. The contour of the heart has been described as "egg-shaped," resulting from the prominent right ventricle projecting into the left hemithorax and the dilated right atrium bulging into the right side (Fig. 17-39). The base of the cardiac shadow, termed the *waist,* may be unusually narrow because of the location of the aorta in front of the pulmonary artery, rather than the normal side-to-side relationship. Pulmonary congestion is often marked.

The electrocardiogram consistently shows severe right ventricular hypertrophy. The presence of left ventricular hypertrophy depends on the pulmonary blood flow and the degree of pulmonary valvular stenosis. The echocardiogram is usually diagnostic, outlining the transposed great arteries and the intracardiac communications.

Cardiac catheterization reveals several distinctive features. It may not be possible to enter all four cardiac chambers because of the malformations. The systolic pressure in the right ventricle is

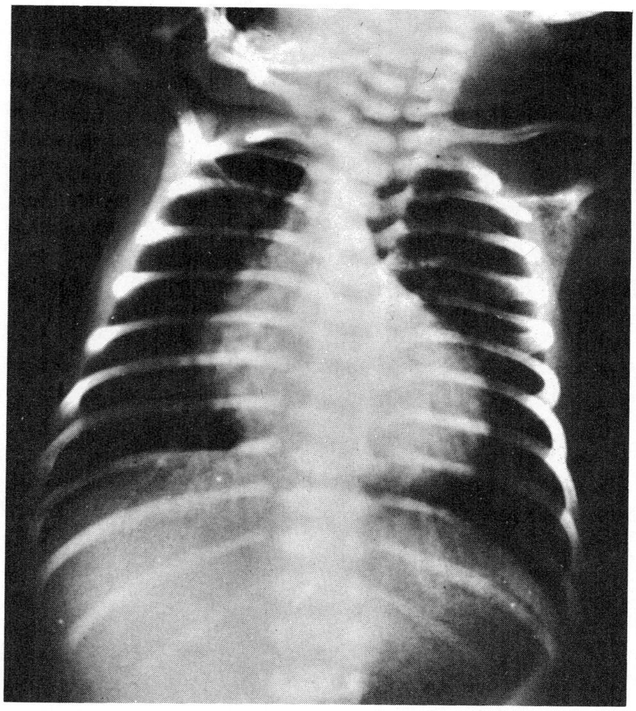

FIG. 17-39. Chest radiograph of child with transposition of great vessels, showing egg-shaped heart with large ventricular silhouette and small "waist," which results from abnormal location of aorta directly anterior to pulmonary artery. *(Courtesy of Dr. Raymond M. Abrams, Department of Radiology, New York University Medical Center.)*

the same as in the aorta, while that in the left ventricle varies with the size of the ventricular septal defect and the presence of outflow tract obstruction. The oxygen saturation in the pulmonary artery is increased. A hallmark of the condition is the fact that oxygen saturation in the pulmonary artery is greater than that in the femoral artery. Varying degrees of arterial oxygen unsaturation are regularly found, ranging from as low as 12 percent to as high as 85 percent. Angiocardiography provides the best means for confirming the diagnosis, for it classically demonstrates the anterior origin of the aorta from the right ventricle, with the more faintly visualized pulmonary artery lying posteriorly.

The diagnosis of transposition should be immediately considered in a seriously ill, cyanotic infant with cardiac enlargement and congestive heart failure. In older children the retardation of physical development is striking. It must be differentiated from tetralogy of Fallot, tricuspid atresia, and total anomaly of venous return. Tetralogy of Fallot is readily identified in many patients by the normal cardiac size, boot-shaped heart, and decreased pulmonary blood flow. Tricuspid atresia is easily recognized by the characteristic of decreased pulmonary blood flow with left axis deviation on the electrocardiogram. Total anomalous drainage of the pulmonary veins may require cardiac catheterization to establish the diagnosis with certainty, although the "snowman"-shaped heart with pulmonary congestion may suggest this diagnosis.

Treatment. In planning therapy transposition may be classified into four broad groups, as follows: (1) intact ventricular septum; (2) ventricular septal defect; (3) ventricular septal defect and left ventricular outflow tract obstruction with decreased pulmonary blood flow; and (4) complex transposition, one of the previous three forms in association with other severe defects such as coarctation of the aorta.

The most critically ill neonates are those with an intact ventricular septum, for the only communication between the pulmonary and systemic circulations is through the foramen ovale. In these patients, a Raskind balloon septostomy provides a dramatic improvement by allowing blood to mix at the atrial level. It should usually be done in the catheterization laboratory at the time the diagnosis is made. Most infants improve dramatically after balloon septostomy, although a few patients do not do well and may require prompt corrective operation.

In previous years operation was delayed after balloon septostomy in stable patients until 3 to 6 months of age, at which time an atrial procedure, either a Senning or a Mustard, was performed. Patients with severe congestive heart failure from a ventricular septal defect received either early atrial repair or palliative pulmonary artery banding with surgical atrial septectomy. Operative risk was 2 to 5 percent with both the Mustard and the Senning operations. However, with this approach 10 to 15 percent of the patients died awaiting operation and the actuarial survival was 80 to 85 percent at 10 years. Both the Senning and the Mustard operations had a significant incidence of late arrhythmias, and systemic tricuspid valve insufficiency often was progressive in those with ventricular septal defects. The Mustard operation also had a significant incidence of late atrial baffle obstruction.

Recently the arterial switch operation (Fig. 17-40) has become the preferred procedure for transposition in most major medical centers. When an intact ventricular septum is present operation should be performed within the first 7 to 10 days of life, before the left ventricle involutes and loses its ability to support the systemic

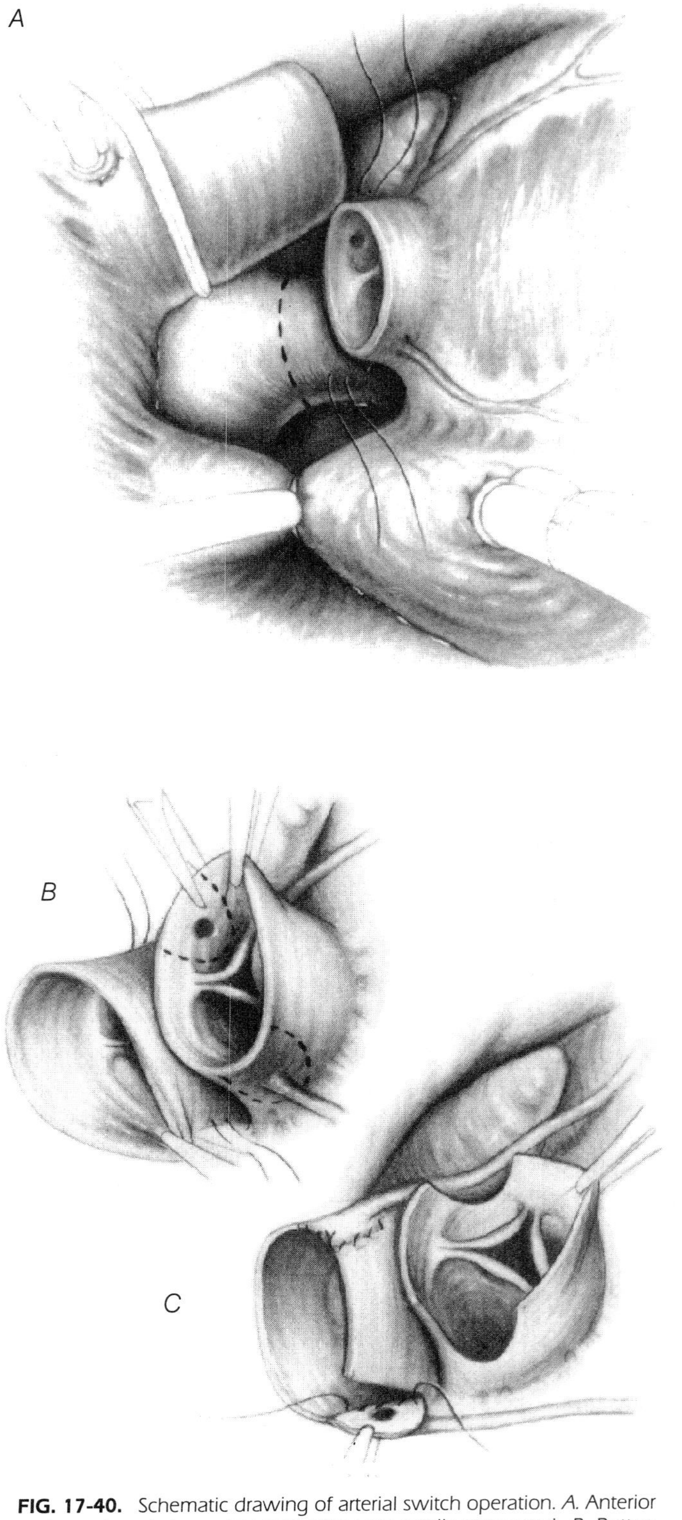

FIG. 17-40. Schematic drawing of arterial switch operation. *A.* Anterior aorta and posterior pulmonary artery are totally transected. *B.* Button containing left coronary artery is excised and transferred to posterior great vessel. *C.* Similar button involving right coronary artery is transferred to posterior great vessel. Subsequently the distal aorta is attached to the posterior great vessel, just beyond the level of the coronary artery transfer (not shown). Pulmonary artery is brought anterior and connected to proximal anterior great vessel (not shown), completing switch operation. (From: *Stark J, de Leval M (eds): Surgery for Congenital Heart Disease, Grune & Stratton. 1983, p. 376, with permission.*)

circulation. Patients with transposition and intact septum who are more than 2 weeks of age may require preliminary banding of the pulmonary artery to induce hypertrophy in the left ventricle and prepare it for the switch operation. This was first proposed by Yacoub, and more recently Jonas reported that only 7 to 10 days of preliminary banding were necessary before proceeding to a rapid two-stage ''switch'' operation. Other surgeons prefer a Senning or Mustard atrial procedure for transposition with intact septum once the child is more than 2 to 3 weeks old.

When a ventricular septal defect is present the arterial switch operation is often done promptly, to avoid congestive heart failure and progressive pulmonary congestion, but operation may be delayed until 2 to 3 months of age if heart failure is not severe. The left ventricle does not usually have a problem supporting the systemic circulation when a ventricular septal defect is present even if the operation is done later, as the ventricle has been working against systemic pressure since birth.

The surgical technique for the arterial switch procedure was described in detail by Jatene, with modifications by Quaegebeur, Castaneda, and others. Deep hypothermia and circulatory arrest is employed routinely. The great vessels are totally transected above the sinuses (see Fig. 17-40A). A small ''button,'' including the ostium of the coronary artery, is resected from the left sinus of the anterior great vessel and transferred to the corresponding sinus of the posterior great vessel (see Fig. 17-40B). A similar transfer is then made with the ''button'' of the right coronary artery, using microvascular technique in both cases to suture the coronary arteries into their new location in the corresponding sinuses of the posterior great vessel (see Fig. 17-40C). The aorta is then relocated, suturing the distal aorta end-to-end to the proximal posterior great vessel, just beyond the coronary artery reimplantation site. The pulmonary artery is brought anteriorly, connecting this to the anterior great vessel, which exits from the right ventricle.

In 1986 Quaegebeur reported results of the arterial switch operation in 66 patients, with a 12 percent operative mortality and no late deaths in the 33 patients followed for 1 to 8 years. In 1991 Castaneda reported results in 505 patients who underwent the arterial switch operation, 326 with intact septum and 179 with ventricular septal defect. Total mortality was 7 percent, with no deaths in the last 150 patients. Arterial switch was successfully carried out in 29 of 30 patients presenting late with intact septum, and undergoing rapid two-stage preliminary banding of the pulmonary artery. Late cardiac catheterization demonstrated excellent hemodynamic results after the operation. Another report in 1991 by Kramer demonstrated a markedly diminished late incidence of cardiac rhythm disturbances in patients undergoing the switch procedure compared to patients receiving the Mustard operation. Thus, the late results after the switch operation are extremely encouraging, and it has emerged as the procedure of choice when feasible.

The subgroup of patients with transposition of the great vessels and ventricular septal defect with left ventricular outflow tract obstruction may not be suitable for atrial repair or arterial switch. This group of patients may require initial palliation with a systemic-to-pulmonary shunt. At 4 to 5 years of age a Rastelli operation is done. This involves use of a prosthetic patch to internally connect the aorta with the left ventricle across the ventricular septal defect. Blood flow is re-established extraanatomically into the pulmonary artery, using a valved conduit or a homograft artery and valve. Operative risk for the Rastelli operation is now less than 10 percent, but late obstruction or degeneration of the extra-anatomic conduit may require reoperation.

Double-Outlet Right Ventricle

This is a congenital malformation in which both great arteries are related to the morphologic right ventricle. It occurs in about 5 percent of all cases of congenital heart disease. Before open heart surgery became possible between 1954 and 1955, a few cases were reported, but modern knowledge of the condition emerged from surgical observations by Kirklin, who, in 1957, first recognized the anatomic problem in the operating room and performed a surgical correction by creation of an intraventricular tunnel, similar to the treatment done today. The term *double-outlet right ventricle* became established as the appropriate designation following a publication by Witham at that time. There are numerous subclassifications of this condition that are beyond the scope of this discussion.

Briefly, four types of relationships of the great arteries at the level of the semilunar valves have been described in this condition, varying with the relationship of the aorta to the pulmonary artery.

In addition, four separate anatomic locations of the ventricular septal defect have been described: subaortic, subpulmonic, beneath both great arteries (''doubly committed''), and beneath neither (''uncommitted''). Theoretically, the existence of two groups of four each creates 16 possible combinations of double-outlet right ventricle. At one extreme the condition is that of classic transposition of the great vessels, while at another extreme the condition merges with tetralogy of Fallot. The classic case report by Taussig and Bing in 1949, leading to the eponym Taussig-Bing syndrome, described a double-outlet right ventricle with a subpulmonic ventricular septal defect, occurring in about 8 percent of cases.

Clinically, three characteristic types of disability occur. Right-to-left shunting occurs to some degree in all types since the aorta arises from the right ventricle. The amount of cyanosis varies, however. With simply a large ventricular septal defect, the presentation is almost identical to that of a large ventricular septal defect because of the high level of pulmonary blood flow present. A high pulmonary vascular resistance develops in infancy with great rapidity. The second familiar clinical syndrome, pulmonic stenosis with a subaortic defect, is virtually identical to that of tetralogy of Fallot. A third variant is the Taussig-Bing syndrome, resembling classic transposition with severe disability in infancy from the combination of pulmonary congestion and hypoxemia.

Echocardiography can usually suggest the diagnosis, but precise biplane angiography is necessary for confirmation and delineation of exact details. With modern surgical techniques, most conditions can be corrected satisfactorily with a precisely constructed intracardiac tunnel to channel blood from the left ventricle through the defect to the aorta. Excellent illustrations of the technique are present in the recent textbook by Kirklin and Barratt-Boyes.

In the Kirklin and Barratt-Boyes book, the combined historic experiences by the authors over a period of 15 years include 98 patients with an overall operative mortality of 30 percent. With the common simpler form, that with a subaortic ventricular septal defect with or without pulmonic stenosis, operative mortality is now less than 5 percent. In the present era most cases of double outlet right ventricle can be repaired with an operative risk of less than 10 percent.

Truncus Arteriosus

Truncus arteriosus is a rare malformation resulting from failure of division of the fetal arterial channel into the aorta and pulmonary arteries and the left and right ventricles. The embryonic origin of the malformation has been analyzed in detail by Rothko.

Pathologic Anatomy. In this condition the entire circulation, including the coronary arteries, the pulmonary arteries, and the systemic arteries, arises from a common arterial trunk (Fig. 17-41). There is always a ventricular septal defect. Only one semilunar valve is present, usually with three or four cusps.

In 80 to 85 percent of patients the pulmonary arteries arise from the truncus, either as a common stem or in close apposition. Infrequently, the origin of the two pulmonary arteries is separated a short distance, complicating the anatomic repair. In most patients the ductus arteriosus is absent; if present, it is usually large with corresponding decrease in size of the aortic isthmus.

Pathophysiology. The disability is a severe one, with about 50 percent of patients dying in the first month of life, and 90 percent within the first year, usually from congestive heart failure. The severe heart failure results from the large left-to-right shunt through the ventricular septal defect. Pulmonary blood flow is significantly increased since the pulmonary arteries arise from the systemic circulation, resulting in extreme degrees of pulmonary congestion. Severe incompetence of the truncal valve, often from nodular myxomatous degeneration, may contribute significantly.

Shunting is both left-to-right and right-to-left, since the aorta receives blood from the right ventricle and the left ventricle. The blood entering the aorta is a mixture of blood from the systemic and pulmonary circulations. Arterial oxygen unsaturation is always present, the degree of cyanosis varying with the volume of pulmonary blood flow. Usually, in infancy, the oxygen saturation is above 80 percent, so cyanosis is minimal. Severe pulmonary vascular disease develops rapidly, often before 6 months of age. As this progresses, arterial oxygen saturation decreases and cyanosis becomes more prominent.

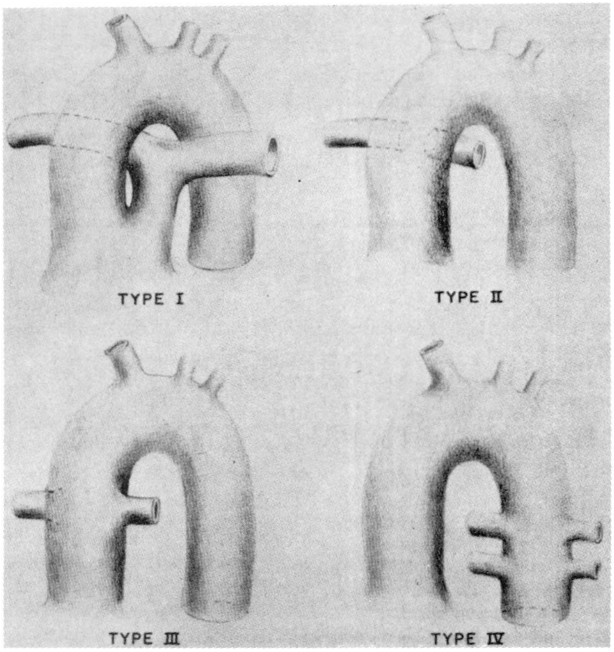

FIG. 17-41. Four anatomic types of truncus arteriosus. (From: *Poirier RA, et al: J Thorac Cardiovasc Surg 69:169, 1987, with permission.*)

The majority of infants are obviously seriously ill, with congestive heart failure and an overactive heart with a wide pulse pressure. Murmurs are variable, not diagnostic, unless a continuous murmur is audible. The chest radiograph shows cardiomegaly and pulmonary congestion. Both right and left ventricular hypertrophy are evident on the electrocardiogram. Two-dimensional echocardiography is diagnostic, outlining the single vascular trunk originating from the base of the heart. Cardiac catheterization and angiography define the anatomy precisely, including the origin of the pulmonary arteries and the presence of insufficiency of the truncal valve. The pulmonary vascular resistance can be determined, indicating the gravity of the problem, and whether operation can be performed or not.

Treatment. Most modern treatment emerged from the excellent work of McGoon, who first successfully used a homograft conduit in 1967. In the procedure developed by McGoon the pulmonary arteries are detached from the truncus, the right ventricle opened, and the ventricular septal defect closed, after which the homograft conduit is inserted between the right ventricle and the distal pulmonary artery.

Most of the early operations were performed on patients over 2 years of age, obviously a selective group as only about 10 percent of patients survive beyond the first year of life.

Current experiences at the Mayo Clinic were summarized in 1985 by DiDonato, who described experiences with 167 patients over a 17-year period. There were 48 hospital deaths (29 percent mortality). Eighty-four percent of 119 surviving patients were alive at 5 years, and 69 percent at 10 years.

In 1985, Sharma reported experiences with 23 patients, 16 of whom were less than 1 year of age. There were only three operative deaths, two of which occurred in critically ill infants operated on under 1 month of age.

As nearly 50 percent of infants die within 1 month, operation must clearly be performed in the neonatal period if heart failure is severe. Otherwise it may be delayed until 3 to 6 months of age, but further delay has the hazard of an irreversible rise in pulmonary vascular resistance.

In 1984, Ebert described experiences with 106 infants. One hundred were corrected by 6 months of age, with 11 operative deaths. Fifteen of the 86 long-term survivors have returned for change of the conduit because of body growth or pseudointimal proliferation in the conduit. There were no mortalities at the time of conduit change.

The long-term course of surviving patients is unknown because to date there are few such patients. A progression in pulmonary vascular resistance has occurred in some patients. Another hazard in surviving patients is the development of insufficiency in the abnormal truncal valve.

Operative mortality has been low in the selective group of patients operated on between 5 and 10 years of age, in whom the pulmonary vascular resistance is less than 0.6 percent of systemic vascular resistance. However, this is a selective group because, as indicated earlier, there is both a high mortality in infancy and also rapid development of irreversible pulmonary vascular disease in many. These considerations were well reviewed in the reports by Poirier in 1975 and by Applebaum in 1976.

Banding of the pulmonary arteries in infancy to protect the pulmonary vascular bed has a surprisingly high mortality, nearly 50 percent from different reports according to Applebaum, and also a significant mortality at the time of attempted correction at a later date. Hence the current recommendation is to perform corrective surgery with a valve conduit at an earlier age, probably between 1 and 3 years, or in the first 6 months of life if symptoms are severe. The current operative risk should be 10 to 15 percent.

OTHER MALFORMATIONS

Cor Triatriatum

Cor triatriatum is a rare maformation. In 1960 a review by Niwayama found only 36 cases. Excellent embryologic and pathologic studies were reported by Van Praagh, and subsequently by Marin-Garcia.

Pathologic Anatomy. The abnormality is best viewed as a variant of total anomalous pulmonary venous drainage except that the unresorbed common venous sinus empties normally into the left atrium through a restricted aperture, rather than through abnormal channels to the right side of the heart. The common venous chamber is superior and posterior to the normal left atrium with a diaphragm separating this chamber from the true left atrium. The left atrial appendage enters the normal small left atrium. A small opening in a thick muscular diaphragm is the only communication between the two chambers.

This abnormality produces severe pulmonary hypertension, identical to mitral stenosis. Gradients as high as 20 mmHg have been recorded between the venous chamber and normal left atrium.

An atrial septal defect, usually a fossa ovalis, is present in about 70 percent of cases, generally entering the common venous chamber and resulting in a left-to-right shunt.

A classic malformation is shown in Fig. 17-42A. The most common variety, with an atrial septal defect between the common venous chamber and the right atrium, is shown in Fig. 17-42B.

Clinical Manifestations. The disability is a severe one from pulmonary congestion, pulmonary hypertension, and heart failure. Without surgical treatment 70 to 75 percent of infants die in the first year of life. The clinical presentation is identical to that of mitral stenosis except that a typical diastolic murmur is often not present.

Diagnostic Considerations. The chest radiograph shows pulmonary congestion with right ventricular enlargement. Right ventricular hypertrophy is evident on the electrocardiogram, varying with the degree of pulmonary hypertension. Two-dimensional echocardiography is diagnostic, outlining the abnormal chambers. Some investigators no longer consider cardiac catheterization necessary, although catheterization and angiography permit measurement of pulmonary artery pressure and more precise delineation of other associated anomalies. The classic physiologic abnormalities at catheterization are an elevated pulmonary artery pressure, an increased wedge pressure, and a *normal* pressure in the left atrium. The differential diagnosis includes the two other conditions that can commonly produce pulmonary venous hypertension: mitral stenosis and stenosis of pulmonary veins, as is often seen with some forms of total anomalous pulmonary venous return or with congenital pulmonary vein stenosis.

Treatment. Operation should be performed promptly when the diagnosis is recognized in infancy because of the high mortality rate. With proper techniques of extracorporeal circulation operative results are usually excellent. Hypothermia and circulatory arrest may be used in very small infants. The abnormal septum between the common venous sinus and the left atrium can be readily excised, eliminating the physiologic abnormality. An accompanying atrial septal defect can be closed at the same time, usually with a patch of pericardium. An approach from the right side of the heart is preferable, though this varies with the precise abnormality present. Results in surviving patients are excellent.

Kirklin and Barratt-Boyes reported excellent results in a group of seven patients operated on over a period of 30 years, emphasizing the rarity of the malformation. Oglietti reported experiences with 25 patients seen over a period of 21 years. The diagnosis was made preoperatively in 14, and established at the time of operation

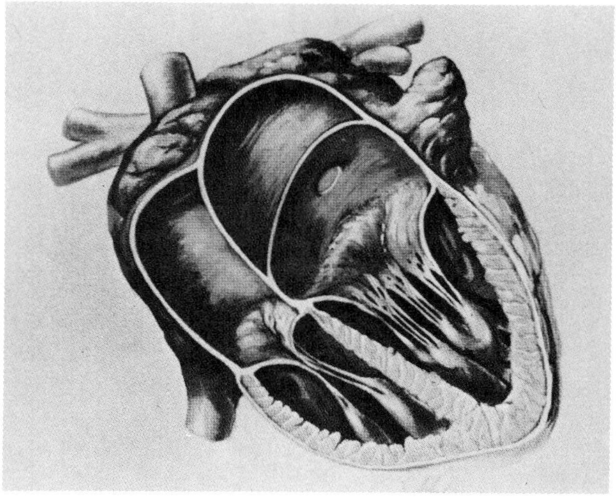
A

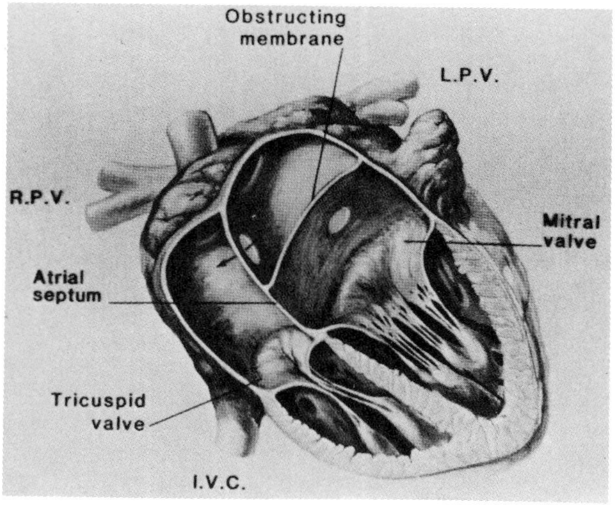

B

FIG. 17-42. *A.* Cor triatriatum with intact atrial septum (Type A). *B.* Cor triatriatum with atrial septal defect between the proximal left atrial chamber and the right atrium (Type A_1). (LPV, left pulmonary vein; RPV, right pulmonary vein; IVC, inferior vena cava.) (From: *Arciniegas E, Hakimi M, et al: 1981, with permission.*)

for other abnormalities in 10. The anomalous membrane was excised in 18 patients, with excellent results in all but 1, who required reoperation because of incomplete excision of the septum. Arciniegas reported on six patients ranging in age from 1.5 to 93 months. There was one postoperative death; the five surviving patients remained in excellent condition 4 years after operation.

Total Anomalous Pulmonary Venous Return

Pathologic Anatomy. A classic pathologic study was reported by Brody in 1942, studying 100 cases of anomalous pulmonary venous drainage, 35 of which were total anomalous drainage. The anomalous veins are supracardiac in about 45 percent of cases, intracardiac in 25 percent, infradiaphragmatic in 25 percent, and mixed in about 5 percent. In almost all cases, the anomalous veins enter a common pulmonary venous sinus, which in turn enters the right side of the heart. With supracardiac drainage, the most common drainage is into a left vertical vein, which in turn enters the left innominate vein. Rarely, the common venous trunk may drain directly into the superior vena cava. With intracardiac drainage, anomalous veins most commonly enter through the coronary sinus. With infracardiac drainage, the common venous trunk traverses the diaphragm and connects with the portal vein or adjacent structures. An atrial septal defect and a patent ductus arteriosus are almost always present.

Pathophysiology. The disability is a severe one, producing death in 50 percent of untreated infants within 3 months, and about 80 percent within the first year. Some degree of obstruction to pulmonary venous drainage is usually present, always so with infradiaphragmatic drainage. This venous obstruction in turn produces severe pulmonary hypertension and pulmonary congestion. The left ventricle often remains small and relatively underdeveloped because of decreased flow, although it develops normally after correction.

In the fortunate 10 to 20 percent of infants without significant venous obstruction and with an adequate atrial septal defect, the patients may do surprisingly well initially. Progressive obstruction with pulmonary congestion can occur, however, although a few patients remain nonobstructed with physiology similar to a large atrial septal defect.

Clinical Manifestations. Severe tachypnea is the dominant system in a seriously ill infant. Infants with severe obstruction often have severe pulmonary congestion and hypoxemia, requiring intubation and respiratory support. Diminished peripheral perfusion from decreased left-sided cardiac output may also be present. The diagnosis is often initially unclear so total anomalous drainage must be considered in any severely tachypneic infant. Cardiac murmurs are not diagnostic. Patients with infracardiac drainage may present earlier with obstructive symptoms. Operation is recommended, however, at the time of diagnosis in all patients since operative risk increases significantly once critical obstruction develops.

The chest radiograph may show definite abnormalities when there is significant dilatation of the common pulmonary vein in adjacent structures. With supracardiac drainage, a well-recognized double contour is visible on the radiograph, termed the *snowman appearance* (Fig. 17-43). This double contour is produced by dilatation of the left innominate vein and right superior vena cava.

Two-dimensional echocardiography can often establish the diagnosis and outline the abnormal channels, but cardiac catheterization and angiography should be done to delineate the abnormal anatomy. At catheterization a classic finding is that blood from the right atrium, pulmonary artery, and femoral artery have a similar oxygen content because of mixing of oxygenated and unoxygenated blood in the right atrium before entering the left atrium through the atrial septal defect.

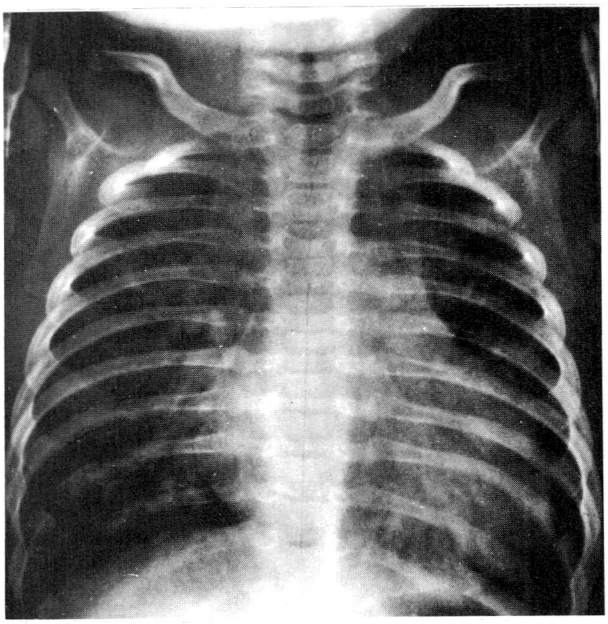

A

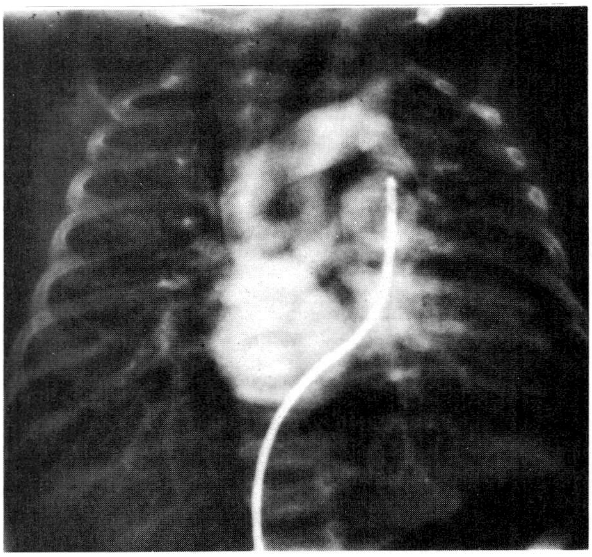

B

FIG. 17-43. *A.* Chest radiograph of child with total anomalous drainage of pulmonary veins through left superior vena cava. Shadow in left upper mediastinum is due to dilated left superior vena cava. *B.* Angiogram demonstrates left superior vena cava emptying into greatly dilated left innominate vein. This radiographic appearance is very suggestive of total anomalous drainage of pulmonary veins into left superior vena cava. *(Courtesy of Dr. Raymond M. Abrams, Department of Radiology, New York University Medical Center.)*

Treatment. Successful total correction was reported by Kirklin in 1956 and also by Cooley. Mortality remained quite high, however, for over a decade but decreased markedly after the introduction of the technique of profound hypothermia and circulatory arrest by Barratt-Boyes around 1969.

Operation must be performed urgently in critically ill infants and should be scheduled promptly in all other patients. The technique of early repair was well described by Clarke and others. It is usually done with the technique of hypothermia and low flow or total circulatory arrest. Surgical correction includes construction of a large (2.5 to 3.0 cm) side-to-side anastomosis between the common venous trunk and the left atrium (Fig. 17-44), followed by closure of the atrial septal defect and ligation of the left vertical vein. Supracardiac drainage is usually approached transatrially, whereas infracardiac drainage may be repaired by lifting the heart and performing part of the atrial-common vein anastomosis from outside of the heart, and part from within the atrium. When anomalous veins enter the coronary sinus, surgical reconstruction is simpler, consisting of creation of a large intracardiac opening between the coronary sinus and the left atrium, with patch closure of the atrial septal defect in a way that directs coronary sinus flow into the left atrium. Operative mortality is now 10 percent in infants. The patients subsequently have almost normal cardiac function. With current techniques late reoperation for recurrent obstruction is rare and late functional results are excellent, as is demonstrated by Clarke's late results.

In the 15 to 20 percent of patients with a large pulmonary blood flow who are operated on after 1 year of age, operative mortality is less than 1 percent.

Single Ventricle (Univentricular Heart)

Single ventricle is a severe malformation that fortunately is quite rare and that represents a variety of complex defects in which there is only a single functioning ventricular chamber. Effective palliative surgery has become possible in a high percentage of cases. The long-term outlook has progressively improved with application of the Fontan procedure to patients with single ventricle complex and to the effective development of cardiac transplantation.

Pathologic Anatomy and Pathophysiology. A wide spectrum of abnormalities exists. The basic abnormality is a single functioning ventricle into which both atrioventricular valves empty. The variations include the type of functioning ventricular chamber (morphologically a "left" or a "right" ventricle), the type of hypoplastic ventricular chamber; different abnormalities in the atrioventricular valves; and the origin of the aorta and pulmonary artery from the normal and hypoplastic ventricular chambers.

The two physiologic abnormalities are hypoxemia from mixture of oxygenated and unoxygenated blood in the single ventricle before entering the aorta, and pulmonary congestion from the high pulmonary blood flow when the origin of the pulmonary artery is from the systemic ventricle. The degree of cyanosis present depends upon the pulmonary blood flow, which depends on which chamber the pulmonary artery arises from and on the degree of obstruction in the outflow tract to the pulmonary artery.

Clinical Manifestations. About one-third of patients do not have significant pulmonic stenosis, so the resulting disability initially resembles that of a large ventricular septal defect with increased pulmonary blood flow and with some cyanosis. At the other extreme, severe cyanosis is present from pulmonic stenosis, requiring an emergency palliative shunt procedure in infancy.

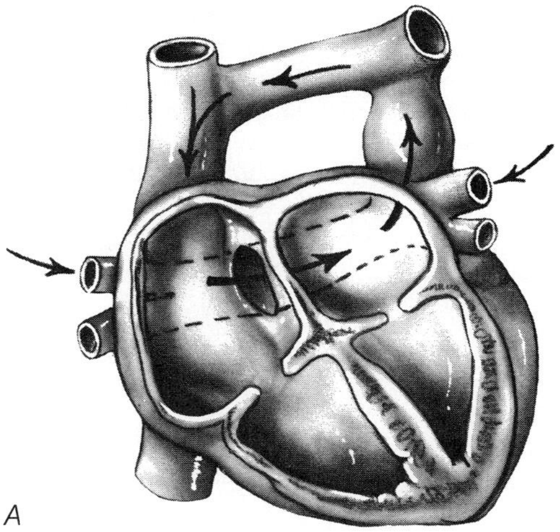

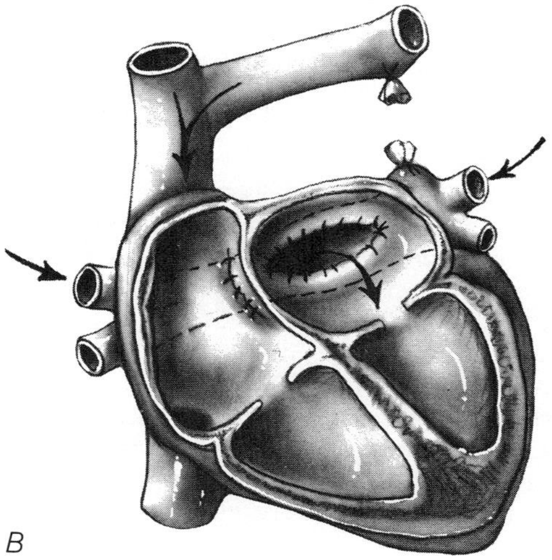

FIG. 17-44. *A.* Abnormal physiology with anomalous drainage of pulmonary veins into left superior vena cava. All pulmonary venous blood flows through left innominate vein into large right superior vena cava and can enter systemic circulation only through atrial septal defect, usually foramen ovale. *B.* At operation, wide opening is made between posteriorly located common pulmonary venous trunk and left atrium, after which opening in atrial septum is closed and left superior vena cava divided. (From: *Benson CD, et al: Pediatric Surgery. Vol. I. Chicago, Year Book Medical Publishers, 1962, p. 446, with permission.*)

In between these two extremes are patients with moderate pulmonic stenosis, often with a pulmonary blood flow about twice normal. Such patients may do reasonably well in the first few years of life because of the balanced nature of their pulmonary blood flow.

In most patients the disability is severe; about 40 percent requiring operation in the first year of life, with only about 50 percent of patients surviving for four years. Excellent morphologic and embryologic studies have been reported by both Van Praagh et al. and by Anderson et al.

Clinical Manifestations and Diagnosis. The clinical picture varies with the pulmonary blood flow. Infants with an increased pulmonary blood flow are acyanotic but disabled from pulmonary congestion and cardiac failure. Such infants have been treated previously with pulmonary artery banding, which unfortunately results in subaortic stenosis in a high percentage of patients within the next 1 to 2 years. At the other extreme, with severely decreased pulmonary blood flow, cyanosis is severe, so a shunt procedure is often required in infancy. The cardiac murmurs, radiograph, and electrocardiogram are usually diagnostic, but a precise diagnosis can be made by two-dimensional echocardiography, noting the absence of the normal ventricular septum. Catheterization with selective angiography can further delineate the precise abnormalities present.

Treatment. Urgent banding or shunting procedures have been used in infants, depending on whether the pulmonary blood flow is increased or decreased. Later in childhood surgically partitioning the ventricle and the Fontan procedure to provide direct atriopulmonary blood flow are the two procedures available. Which procedure is selected depends on the abnormality present and the presence of increased pulmonary vascular resistance. Unfortunately relatively few cases are anatomically suitable for surgical septation of the ventricles because this requires an adequate-sized accessory ventricular chamber and a patent outflow tract leading to the pulmonary artery. Early experiences with partitioning of the ventricle were reported in four cases by Edie and Malm. In 1977, McGoon et al. reported experiences with 23 patients, obtaining satisfactory results in 61 percent. In 1984, Stefanelli et al. described experiences in 166 patients over a period of 15 years with a 10-year actuarial survival rate of 66 percent. Ventricular septation was performed in 36 patients with 15 deaths. The majority of patients developed complete heart block following septation, requiring a pacemaker.

More commonly a Fontan procedure is required for correction of single ventricle. The single ventricle, whether it is morphologically a left ventricle or a right ventricle, is used to support the systemic circulation, while pulmonary blood flow is provided by a Fontan-type direct atrial-pulmonary connection (see Fig. 17-37). Historically, the results of the Fontan procedure are worse when done for single ventricle than when done for tricuspid atresia, with an operative risk of over 20 percent and a 10-year survival of 70 percent or less.

More recently Mayer et al. reported a marked reduction in mortality for patients undergoing the Fontan operation for single ventricle, and the operative risk is now probably less than 10 percent. A good outcome is more likely when the atrioventricular valvular anatomy is favorable and when the child is over 9 years of age, while a poor outcome is more likely when the child is less than 3 years of age, the pulmonary artery pressure is high, or the pulmonary artery anatomy is distorted. Despite recent encouraging reports long-term outlook remains guarded after the Fontan operation, for the reasons cited in the tricuspid atresia section. However, the Fontan operation remains the procedure of choice for many patients with single ventricle, reserving cardiac transplantation or heart-lung transplantation for a limited few with highly distorted anatomy or irreversible pulmonary hypertension.

Corrected Transposition (Ventricular Inversion)

The basic characteristics of this unusual malformation were described by Anderson in 1957, with additional contributions by Schiebler in 1961.

Pathologic Anatomy and Physiology. In this malformation the anatomic right ventricle and the anatomic left ventricle are switched or inverted, hence the name *ventricular inversion*. The tricuspid and mitral valves ''follow'' the ventricles, resulting in a mitral right-sided atrioventricular valve and a tricuspid left-sided atrioventricular valve. The ventricle from which the aorta arises is the morphologic right ventricle, while that from which the pulmonary artery arises is the morphologic left ventricle. The atria and ventricle are also discordant; so blood from the right atrium reaches the pulmonary trunk by traversing a mitral valve and a morphologic left ventricle, while blood from the left atrium reaches the aorta by traversing a tricuspid valve and a morphologic right ventricle. Hence, with the ''double discordance'' the basic circulation is normal. The anatomic relations of the coronary arteries are also altered, with the right coronary artery arising anteriorly, the left coronary posteriorly, and the noncoronary sinus being located at the anterior left border of the heart.

The defect apparently arises from a malrotation of the embryonic heart tube, which bends to the left (L-ventricular loop). The significance of the malformation is primarily from the high incidence of associated abnormalities, for it has been estimated that only 1 to 2 percent of patients do not have an additional malformation. Four separate malformations commonly occur. The most frequent is a disturbance in conduction between the atrium and ventricle, originating from lack of normal continuity from the atrioventricular node to the ventricular septum. Normal atrioventricular conduction is present in less than one-half of patients.

A ventricular septal defect is present in the majority of patients, at least 80 percent. Some degree of pulmonic stenosis frequently occurs, which in some patients is of such severity that shunting must be performed in infancy. The fourth malformation, left-sided atrioventricular valvular insufficiency, gradually develops in older patients, perhaps as a consequence of a tricuspid valve draining into the ventricle from which systemic pressure is generated.

A theoretical question arises from the altered physiology in this condition about whether a morphologic right ventricle can function for a normal lifespan. The systemic morphologic ''right'' ventricle may slowly deteriorate with time, but the long-term data regarding this are unclear. Most patients die before 50 years of age, usually from complications of the associated anomalies or from ventricular deterioration and progressive insufficiency of the left-sided tricuspid atrioventricular valve.

Clinical Manifestations. Conduction defects may cause problems in infancy as 5 to 10 percent of patients are born with a complete heart block, and subsequently heart block appears in about 2 percent of patients each year, with about 30 percent of patients eventually developing complete block.

Even though a large ventricular septal defect is present, some restriction to pulmonary flow may occur and these patients do not develop difficulty as rapidly as others. Eventually severe pulmonary vascular disease develops unless significant pulmonic stenosis is present. In about one-third of patients the pulmonic stenosis is of such severity that a shunt must be surgically corrected in infancy or early childhood.

Physical examination is not diagnostic, though such patients have an unusually loud second sound to the left of the sternum, arising from the aortic valve. The chest radiograph characteristically has a narrow ''waist'' because of the abnormal location of the great arteries.

The electrocardiogram is almost always abnormal, often the first clue to the diagnosis. Characteristic abnormalities include the conduction disturbances and the unusual patterns of ventricular hypertrophy.

Echocardiography is usually diagnostic, but cardiac catheterization and angiography are routinely done to confirm the diagnosis and delineate the severity of associated abnormalities.

Treatment. Closure of the ventricular septal defect is technically difficult because of the uncertainty of the conduction tissue, which tends to course anteriorly and superiorly, on the right side of the superior septal tissue. The preferred approach is the transatrial one through the right atrium. Heart block frequently occurs after operation, with a frequency of at least 10 to 20 percent. Pulmonic stenosis, when severe, is best corrected with an extracardiac conduit placed to the pulmonary trunk because the pathologic anatomy precludes an incision across the stenotic pulmonic valve. When the left-sided tricuspid valve is insufficient, repair or replacement is indicated.

The combined series reported from Kirklin and Barratt-Boyes total almost 100 patients with an operative mortality between 10 and 15 percent and a 10-year survival between 50 and 75 percent. Less favorable long-term results were reported by Metcalfe. Experiences with 19 patients treated over a decade included a high operative mortality, 37 percent, with only one patient asymptomatic 40 months following operation. Thus, the long-term results remain guarded after treatment of corrected transposition.

Ruptured Aneurysm of Sinus of Valsalva

This unusual abnormality produces a distinct syndrome that can be readily diagnosed and effectively treated. Before the development of extracorporeal circulation, it usually caused death from cardiac failure within 1 to 2 years after rupture. The natural history was well described by Sawyer in 1957, reviewing 47 reported patients. Successful operations with extracorporeal circulation were done by Lillehei and by Kirklin in 1956, and other successful care reports soon followed. By 1965 over 90 patients had been operated on.

Pathologic Anatomy. The basic abnormality is a thinning of the aortic media in the wall of the sinus of Valsalva. In embryonic development, the developing ventricular septum inferiorly meets the spiral septum superiorly which separates the aorta and the pulmonary arteries. Incomplete merger of these two structures results in a ventricular septal defect in the membranous septum. An aneurysm of the sinus of Valsalva results from a less severe malformation of a similar type, for the media of the aortic wall does not extend down to the annulus of the aortic valve ring. Hence, there is a spectrum of abnormalities, including ventricular septal defect, aortic valve abnormalities with aortic valve prolapse, and less frequently, pulmonic stenosis.

The right coronary sinus is involved in most patients with rupture into the right ventricle. The noncoronary sinus is involved in about 20 percent of patients, most commonly rupturing into the right atrium. Involvement of the left coronary sinus or rupture into the left atrium or left ventricle is very unusual, probably because of both the differences in anatomy and the high pressures in the left ventricle. The typical aneurysm is usually described as a "windsock" with a wide base at the aortic origin and a nipplelike apex projecting into a cardiac chamber, where rupture eventually occurs.

Clinical Manifestations. Until rupture occurs, there are no abnormalities unless an enlarging aneurysm distorts the aortic leaflets sufficiently to cause aortic insufficiency. The average age at rupture is 31 years. This is usually without known cause, although a few case reports describe the onset during physical exertion.

About one-third of patients develop acute symptoms at the time of rupture, with chest pain, soon followed by dyspnea and palpitation and the appearance of the characteristic murmur. In nearly one-half of patients, however, the onset is more gradual with progressive dyspnea, while a small percentage have very few symptoms when the cardiac abnormalities are detected. Death seldom occurs from right heart failure shortly following rupture, but over the ensuing weeks and months, cardiac failure relentlessly progresses with few patients tolerating the abnormality for more than 1 to 2 years.

On physical examination the classical abnormality is a parasternal murmur, often with a thrill, loudest in the third or fourth interspace. This is often continuous, resembling a patent ductus, but is at a lower location. The usual hemodynamic abnormalities seen with a large patent ductus are present, including a wide pulse pressure, cardiac enlargement, and pulmonary congestion.

The diagnosis can readily be suspected from the history and the physical abnormalities. The chest radiograph shows cardiac enlargement and pulmonary congestion. Cardiac hypertrophy is evident on the electrocardiogram. With two-dimensional echocardiography the diagnosis can be promptly confirmed. Cardiac catheterization and angiography are usually performed to determine the site of origin, the cardiac chamber involved, and the presence of associated lesions, especially ventricular septal defect or aortic insufficiency (Fig. 17-45).

Treatment. Surgical correction, of course, should be performed promptly. The basic objective at operation is to close both the defect and any associated lesions (Fig. 17-46). An approach through both the aorta and the involved cardiac chamber is best, facilitating the correction of associated lesions such as a ventricular septal defect. The aneurysmal sac can be excised back to the aortic origin and closed, preferably with a prosthetic patch. Alternately, the aneurysm can be excised and sutured from within the ventricle, following which a prosthetic patch can be directly sutured over the aortic origin, avoiding any injury to the aortic cusps. The operative risk is small and reported results excellent.

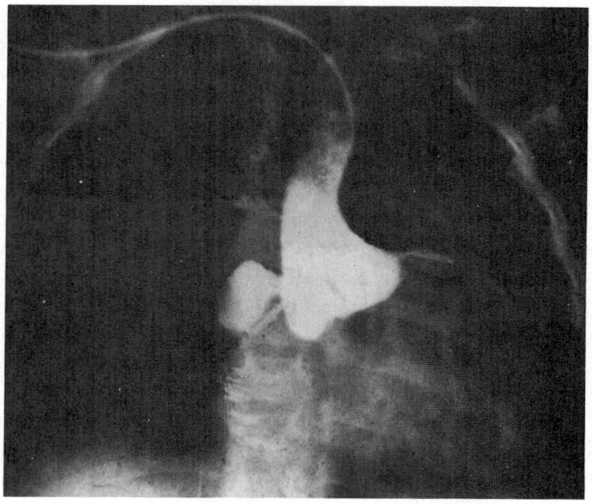

FIG. 17-45. Aortogram confirms diagnosis of ruptured aneurysm of sinus of Valsalva by demonstrating flow of dye from region of aortic sinuses to right atrium. (From: *New York University Medical Center.*)

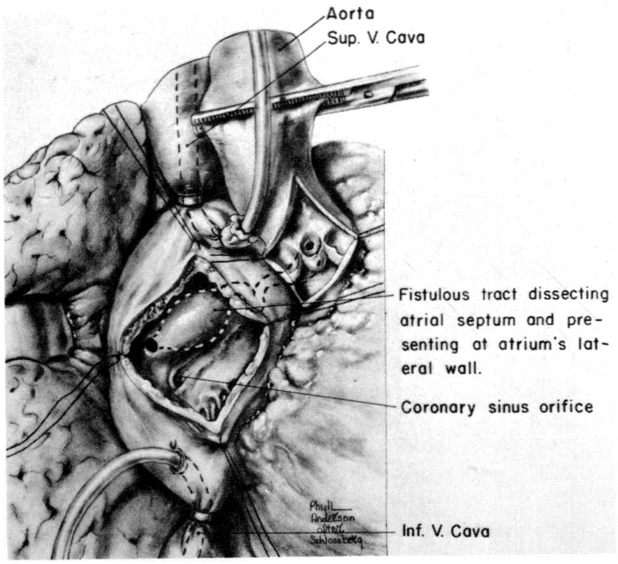

FIG. 17-46. Diagram of unusual type of ruptured aneurysm of sinus of Valsalva. Aneurysm arose from left coronary cusp and developed fistulous tract before rupture into right atrium. Operative closure was performed by opening aorta and closing opening directly. (From: *Ann Surg* 152:965, 1960, with permission.)

Ebstein's Anomaly

This unusual anomaly was described by Wilhelm Ebstein in 1866. The abnormality is uncommon, about 0.5 percent of all cases of congenital heart disease. There is a nearly 400 times increased frequency of Ebstein's malformation when the mother has taken lithium during the pregnancy.

Pathologic Anatomy. The basic abnormality is a malformation of the septal and posterior leaflets of the tricuspid valve. The origin of the leaflets is displaced downward to a variable degree, creating a third chamber on the right side of the heart. Both the leaflet tissue and its chordae are also abnormal. The anterior tricuspid leaflet is usually normal and may be unusually large and prominent, described as "sail-like" (Fig. 17-47). The segment of right ventricular wall between the true annulus of the tricuspid valve and the origin of the displaced leaflets becomes functionally part of the right atrium and has been termed the *atrialized ventricle*. There is a varying degree of hypoplasia of this segment in some patients resembling a true aneurysm that bulges paradoxically. In most patients, the atrialized segment has some muscle fibers with little paradoxical motion. The distal functioning right ventricle is small. Some investigators have believed that there is a true deficiency in the right ventricular fibers as well, contributing to the right ventricular dysfunction in this condition. A foramen ovale or ostium secundum defect is almost always present. The right atrium is usually dilated, often to a huge size in older patients.

The malformation varies widely in severity, ranging from relatively minor valvular abnormalities to virtual atresia of the valve leaflets.

Pathophysiology. The main physiologic disturbance is inadequate cardiac output from the right ventricle, a result of both the tricuspid insufficiency and the dysfunction of the right ventricle. A variety of arrhythmias commonly occur: supraventricular tachycardias occur in over 50 percent of the cases, and Wolff-Parkinson-White syndrome, with an accessory pathway and preexcitation, occurs in 5 percent. Massive dilatation of the right atrium gradually develops in some patients. Cyanosis of moderate degree occurs in at least 50 percent of patients because of a right-to-left shunt through the foramen ovale. It gradually becomes more severe in older patients with progressive right ventricular failure.

Clinical Manifestations. A significant percentage of infants present in the first month of life with tachypnea and cyanosis, probably a manifestation of the elevated pulmonary vascular resistance in the neonatal period. About one-half of patients who are severely symptomatic in the first month of life subsequently die. After the first month, disability decreases, often with loss of cyanosis, so disability during childhood is often small. A mortality of about 15 percent has been estimated to occur between ages one and twenty. The course is a gradual one, so that the average age of diagnosis is in the midteens.

Many adults continue to function reasonably well, depending on the presence of arrhythmias, cyanosis, and cardiac failure. A few patients have lived to beyond 70 years of age, but only about 5 percent of all patients live beyond 50 years.

Diagnostic Considerations. A variety of systolic and diastolic murmurs are present, though Nadas at one time stated that auscultatory findings were highly suggestive, emphasizing a slow cardiac rate with a triple or quadruple rhythm, a systolic murmur of tricuspid regurgitation, and often a low-pitched diastolic murmur.

The chest radiograph may show grotesque cardiac enlargement because of the huge right atrium and the atrialized right ventricle. Vascularity in the lung fields is usually decreased. Electrocardiographic abnormalities are considered typical with conduction disturbances, a prolonged PR interval, and partial right bundle branch block. When Wolff-Parkinson-White syndrome is present the PR interval is short and a delta wave is present.

Two-dimensional echocardiography is virtually diagnostic, outlining the different abnormalities with surprising precision. Cardiac catherization should be done carefully, for fatal arrhythmias have occurred. A right-to-left shunt at the atrial level with arterial hypoxemia is found in 25 to 50 percent of patients. The angiocardiogram is usually diagnostic.

Treatment. Only limited data are available because surgical treatment has only been used frequently in the past decade. Early corrective operations included prosthetic valve replacement by Barnard, and subsequently by Lillehei. Hardy reported a successful valvuloplasty in 1964, based on concepts described by Hunter and Lillehei. Bahnson in 1965 reported successful reconstructive operations in two patients.

The best results have been reported by Danielson at the Mayo Clinic, who described in a 1985 report a total experience with 72 patients. Surgical intervention was recommended for all patients with a class III status, or in those with a cardiothoracic ratio enlarging beyond 0.65. In 81 percent of the group reconstruction of the tricuspid valve was possible, converting the valve to a monocusp valve with the functioning anterior leaflet. Prosthetic valve replacement was used in most of the other patients. There were five hospital and three late deaths. The 39 surviving operated patients were 87 percent class I or II at 5 years. Kirklin and Barratt-

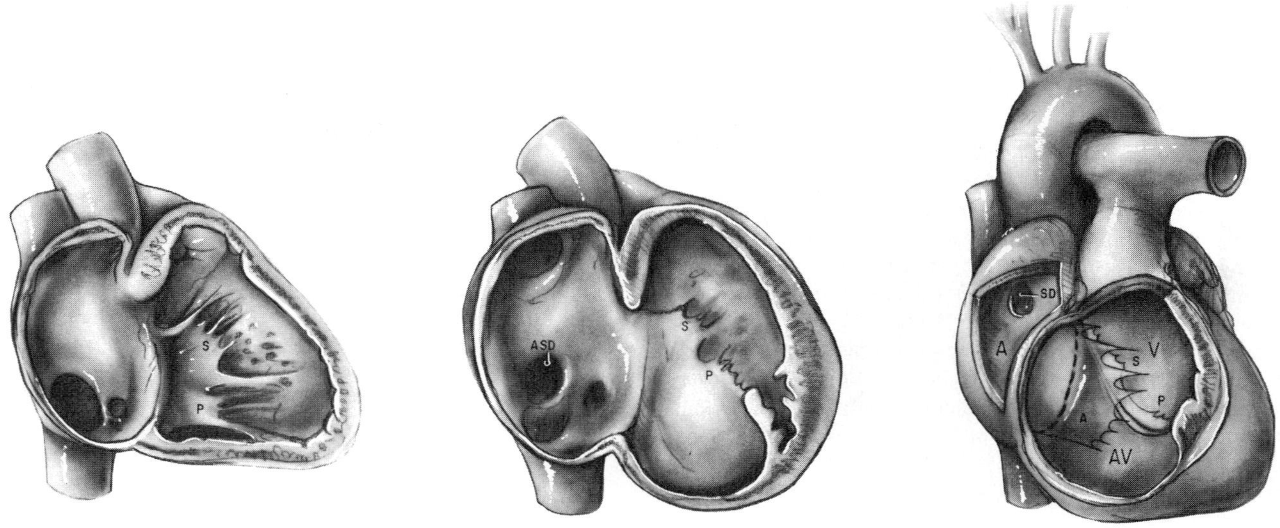

A *B* *C*

FIG. 17-47. *A.* Normal heart showing septal and posterior leaflets of tricuspid valve. *B.* Pathologic anatomy in Ebstein's malformation, with displacement of diminutive septal and posterior leaflets down into normal right ventricular cavity. Large anterior leaflet is not shown. *C.* Abnormal pathologic anatomy in Ebstein's malformation. There is large "sail-like" anterior leaflet with hypoplastic septal and posterior leaflets, which are often displaced downward into ventricle, creating third cardiac chamber interposed between right atrium and functioning right ventricle. (From: *Hardy KL, May IA, et al: 1964, with permission.*)

Boyes, using valve replacement in 20 patients operated on between 1967 and 1980, had an overall mortality of 20 percent. We believe the data of Danielson are quite convincing and most authors would favor attempted valvuloplasty in the majority of patients operated on, but realize that this may prove to be impossible in 10 to 20 percent.

At the time of operation the atrial septal defect is closed. Plication of the atrialized ventricle seems unnecessary in the vast majority of patients, used only when the atrialized segment is extremely thin and contracting paradoxically. Operative risk is now less than 5 percent.

Anomalies of the Coronary Arteries

Anomalous Origin of the Left Coronary Artery

This is a rare malformation, occurring about once in 300,000 live births and representing about 0.25 percent of patients with congenital heart disease. The clinical features were well described by Bland and associates in 1933, emphasizing the similarity of the syndrome to myocardial infarction in adults. A particularly significant contribution was made by Sabiston in 1959, conclusively demonstrating that the flow of blood in the anomalous left coronary artery was *retrograde* into the pulmonary artery. Ligation of the anomalous artery was subsequently performed. Reconstruction was first accomplished by Cooley by detaching the coronary artery and connecting it to the aorta with a saphenous vein graft. Unfortunately, due to late vein graft stenosis, this is no longer considered a satisfactory operation.

Pathologic Anatomy and Physiology. The disability is a severe one, for myocardial infarction and left ventricular failure are commonly present within 3 months after birth. Only about 10 to 20 percent of untreated infants live more than 1 year, apparently because of abundant collateral circulation from the right coronary artery. Symptoms, if present, are usually mild for the first few weeks after birth, probably because of the elevated pulmonary vascular resistance in the neonatal period. Subsequently, symptoms progress with great rapidity. The classic symptom is poor feeding, as attempted feeding produces severe distress. Signs of myocardial infarction or left ventricular failure are soon evident. Initially, only acute episodes occur with feeding, between which the infant may appear normal. During the acute episodes, there is apparently colicky pain, with tachypnea, cyanosis, pallor and sweating, probably angina pectoris, and progressive malnutrition. Subsequently, with chronic congestive failure, tachypnea becomes chronic. On physical examination there may be obvious cardiac enlargement with muffled heart sounds; no characteristic murmurs are found.

The chest radiograph may show extensive enlargement of the left ventricle with pulmonary congestion. Often the electrocardiogram is diagnostic with inverted T waves and prominent Q waves. Transesophageal echocardiography may confirm the diagnosis, demonstrating absence of the normal origin of the left coronary artery from the aorta, and at times actually demonstrating the anomalous origin from the pulmonary artery. Cardiac catheterization and angiography are diagnostic, demonstrating the abnormal origin of the left coronary artery and a small left-to-right shunt at the level of the pulmonary artery. When coronary angiograms are performed in older children, the right coronary is found dilated and tortous, with dye filling the right coronary and subsequently opacifying the left coronary with retrograde flow into the pulmonary artery.

Treatment. Operation should be performed in symptomatic infants to prevent progressive myocardial infarction and death. Though reattachment of the coronary artery to the aorta is clearly the ideal operation, data do not clearly indicate better results with reconstruction as compared with simple ligation and interruption of retrograde flow. A mortality near 50 percent unfortunately is common. The ingenious tunnel operation of Takauchi is the authors' preferred method of reconstruction, creating an intrapulmonary tunnel to connect the anomalous left coronary ostium to the aorta. If the abnormal anatomy is favorable, the left coronary may also be detached from the pulmonary artery and anastomosed directly to the aorta as in the "arterial switch" operation for transposition. In older children a free graft of subclavian artery has been successfully used by several surgeons. A subclavian coronary artery bypass has been successfully performed in a few patients, and internal mammary bypass has been done in older patients.

In patients operated upon after 1 year of age, mortality is low and results excellent. The 18 long-term survivors reported by Kirklin were stated to be in excellent condition. Arciniegas reported experiences with 12 patients with only two deaths, but six seriously ill infants were not operated on, all of whom died. If these six preoperative deaths are included, the total mortality is 40 percent among 20 patients, similar to that reported by other groups.

Coronary Arteriovenous Fistula

Familiarity with this unusual condition grew rapidly with the advent of cardiac angiography and open heart surgery. In 1960 Gasul found 52 cases in a collective review. At this time well over 300 surgical cases have been reported in the literature, and undoubtedly a much larger number have never been reported.

Pathologic Anatomy and Physiology. The right coronary artery is involved in about half of the cases, the left coronary artery in about a third, and both coronaries in only about 5 percent. The artery involved is usually a normal artery with a normal branching pattern. The fistula may be a "side-to-side" one with continuity of the vessel beyond the fistula, or an "end fistula" occurring where the vessel terminates. Over 90 percent of fistulas open into the right heart chambers or its connecting vessels, approximately 25 percent in the right atrium, 40 percent in the right ventricle, 15 to 20 percent in the pulmonary artery, and about 7 percent in the coronary sinus. Fistulas entering the left heart, left ventricle, or left atrium are uncommon. Usually a single fistulous opening is present, in the range of 2 to 5 mm, although occasionally there are several openings or a localized angiomatous network. The involved coronary artery is dilated, aneurysmal, and elongated, at times growing to grotesque serpentine proportions. Actual rupture of an aneurysm, however, is rare.

With fistulas entering the right heart, the resulting shunt is usually small. Only rarely is pulmonary blood flow increased to twice that of systemic flow. As with arteriovenous fistulas elsewhere, the usual course is slow but progressive enlargement over decades, so the volume of the shunt gradually increases with time.

Bacterial endocarditis may develop in a small percentage of cases, about 5 percent.

Clinical Features. The majority of patients are asymptomatic, often evaluated because of the discovery of a continuous murmur. One report found that 80 percent of patients under 20 years of age were asymptomatic, decreasing to less than 50 percent in adults. Rarely, with huge fistulas, symptoms have appeared in the first year of life but are virtually unknown after that during childhood.

In adults the most common symptoms are dyspnea and fatigue from the left-to-right shunt. True angina occurs, probably a "coronary steal," in less than 10 percent. Eventually, congestive heart failure develops in 10 to 15 percent of patients, usually in older life as the shunt gradually enlarges in size.

Treatment involves division of the fistulous tract, either from within the aneurysmal coronary artery or from within the recipient chamber. If the involved coronary artery is extremely aneurysmal, it should be reconstructed in a tapered fashion to avoid excessive stasis, which will result in thrombin formation and late coronary occlusion with myocardial ischemia. Alternately, the involved aneurysmal artery can be divided proximally and distally to fistula. The origin of the fistula is oversewn, and the distal coronary circulation is bypassed with either an internal mammary artery or a saphenous vein graft. Late results are excellent.

Vascular Rings

Incidence and Etiology. Vascular rings are uncommon but are quite significant because surgical therapy is effective with little morbidity or mortality. Embryologically, the vascular rings result from variation in the normal formation of the aorta and pulmonary artery from the six embryonic aortic arches. As six aortic arches exist in the embryo, it is somewhat surprising that such abnormalities are not more frequent. In normal embryonic life, the first two arches disappear, and the fifth never fully develops. The third, fourth, and sixth are significant in normal development. The right common carotid arises from the third arch and the innominate from the right fourth, while the left fourth contributes to the transverse aortic arch. The ductus originates from the sixth.

Pathologic Anatomy. Five types of systemic arterial vascular anomalies of clinical significance have been recognized: (1) double aortic arch; (2) right aortic arch with left ligamentum arteriosum; (3) retroesophageal subclavian artery; (4) anomalous origin of innominate artery; and (5) anomalous origin of left common carotid artery. The last two conditions, anomalous origin of the innominate or the left common carotid, are very rare malformations in which the origin of the artery from the aortic arch is such that the trachea is compressed. Pulmonary artery sling, which is considered separately, is another form of vascular ring that produces tracheal compression. The recommended method of surgical correction of these later conditions consists of mobilizing the anomalous vessel and suturing it into a more normal position. Actually, the mechanism of compression is less precise than in the other three conditions.

A double aortic arch with one limb anterior to the trachea and the other limb posterior to the esophagus (Figs. 17-48 and 17-49) is the most severe of the systemic arterial malformations, producing symptoms in early infancy. Usually one limb is smaller than the other. Often the thoracic aorta descends on the right, rather than on the left. A right aortic arch with a retroesophageal ligamentum arteriosum or left subclavian artery is the other most frequent abnormality (Fig. 17-50). A retroesophageal subclavian artery, consisting of a right subclavian artery originating from the descending aorta beyond the left subclavian artery and coursing posterior to the esophagus to the right upper extremity, is a common anomaly but usually does not cause symptoms (Fig. 17-51).

Clinical Manifestations. Almost all symptoms from vascular rings result from compression of the trachea. Rarely is there difficulty in swallowing from compression of the esophagus.

Symptoms. Infants with a double aortic arch often develop difficulty breathing in the first few months of life and become

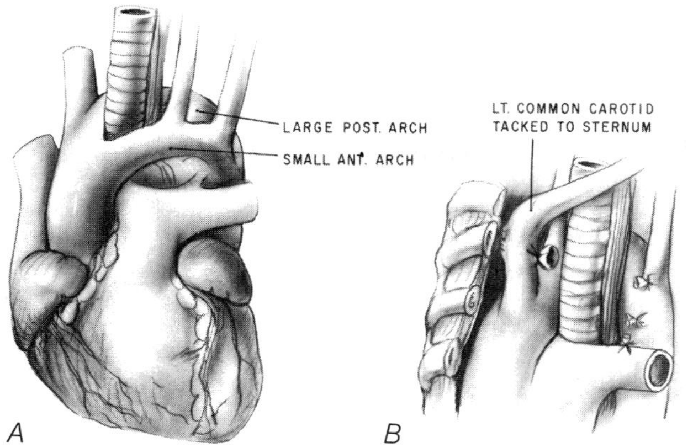

FIG. 17-48. Double aortic arch with small anterior and large posterior limb. *A.* Anterior view of double aortic arch with small anterior limb. *B.* Exposure after division of small anterior arch between left carotid and left subclavian artery, followed by displacement of carotid artery anteriorly toward sternum. (From: *Gross RE: The Surgery of Infancy and Childhood. Philadelphia, Saunders, 1953, p. 917, with permission.*)

critically ill. Stridor is the most frequent prominent symptom. Periodic episodes of serious respiratory distress, with "crowing" respirations, occur. During these attacks, the infant lies in hyperextension, gasping for breath. Feeding often precipitates such episodes, perhaps from flexion of the neck or aspiration. Infants quickly become underweight and malnourished.

Most patients requiring surgical treatment are seen in infancy. Those with mild symptoms developing after 1 year of age may spontaneously recover as they grow older. The most common symptoms are intermittent episodes of respiratory compression, at times with a respiratory infection; difficulty in swallowing, which, if present, is mild; and recurrent episodes of pneumonia, perhaps from aspiration. The mildest clinical picture is produced by the retroesophageal subclavian artery, which may cause mild, intermittent dysphagia. Some patients may be symptomatic in infancy, and spontaneously recover with growth.

Physical Examination. No abnormalities are evident unless respiratory distress is present. If audible stridor is present, the diagnosis should be considered. During episodes of respiratory insufficiency, the infant lies with back arched and neck extended. Attempts to flex the neck may precipitate severe dyspnea and cyanosis.

Laboratory Studies. Both the chest radiograph and electrocardiogram are normal unless aspiration pneumonia is present. Examination of the esophagus with a barium swallow usually establishes the diagnosis, demonstrating a typical area of compression from the retroesophageal artery, usually at the level of the third or fourth thoracic vertebra. This finding virtually confirms the diagnosis.

The precise nature of the obstruction can be defined with further studies. Bronchoscopy may define a discrete area of tracheal narrowing and rule out diffuse tracheomalacia. A tracheogram in the lateral view may provide further evidence of a vascular ring, demonstrating anterior compression of the trachea a short distance above the carina combined with posterior compression of the esophagus. MRI angiography or aortography can precisely delineate the abnormal arteries.

Treatment. Since a vascular ring has no physiologic significance, no treatment is needed in the absence of symptoms. If symptoms are mild, their origin may be uncertain, and a period of observation may be required to be sure that other difficulties are not responsible. If obvious respiratory compression is present,

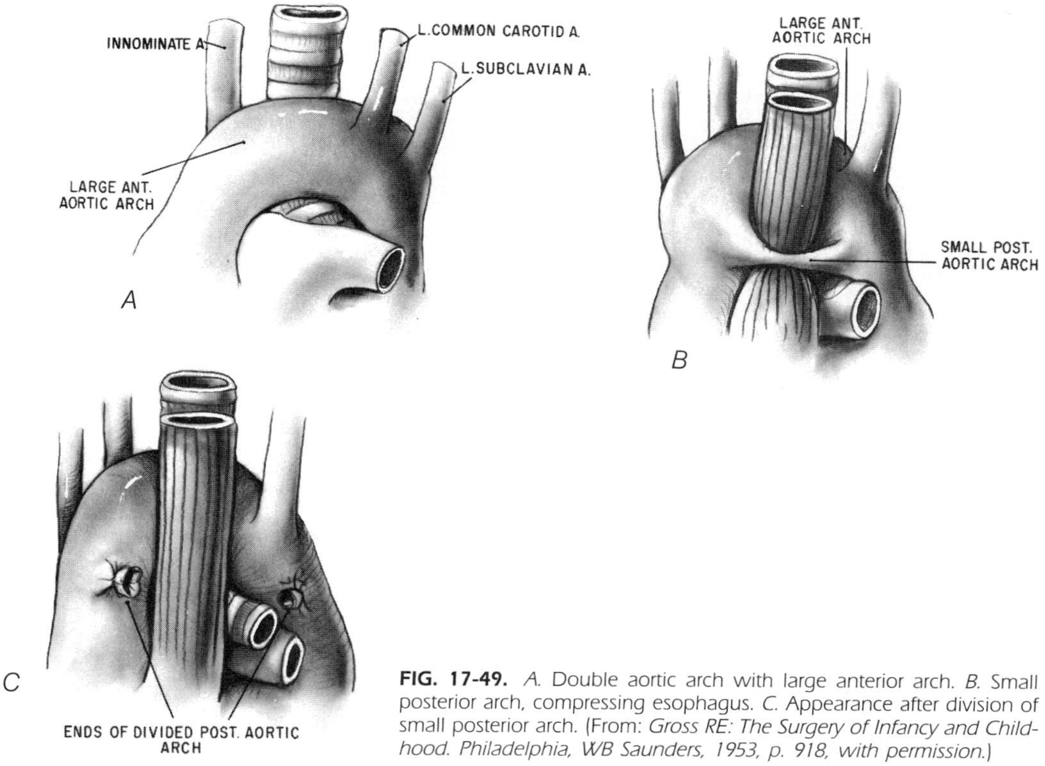

FIG. 17-49. *A.* Double aortic arch with large anterior arch. *B.* Small posterior arch, compressing esophagus. *C.* Appearance after division of small posterior arch. (From: *Gross RE: The Surgery of Infancy and Childhood. Philadelphia, WB Saunders, 1953, p. 918, with permission.*)

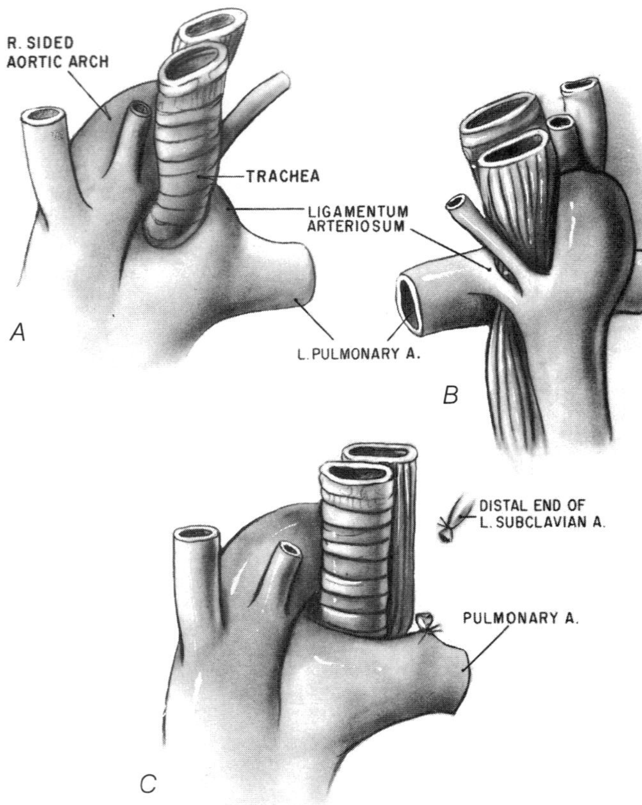

FIG. 17-50. *A.* Right aortic arch with left posterior ligamentum arteriosum. *B.* Posterior view of ligamentum arteriosum extending from right aortic arch to left pulmonary artery, compressing esophagus. Small left subclavian artery arising close to ligamentum arteriosum is also present. *C.* Appearance after division of ligamentum arteriosum and subclavian artery. (From: *Gross RE: The Surgery of Infancy and Childhood. Philadelphia, WB Saunders, 1953, p. 923, with permission.*)

operation should be performed promptly, however, because death from airway obstruction can easily occur.

Operative Technique. If the child is having respiratory distress the airway is secured before the child is fully asleep, and a rigid pediatric bronchoscope should be present in the room. The optimal incision varies with the type of anomaly. Usually an incision through the left four intercostal spaces is selected. An important principle is to dissect the aortic arch completely and identify the innominate artery, the left common carotid artery, and both subclavian arteries. Opening the pericardium facilitates identification of these vessels. The vagus nerve should be traced to the recurrent laryngeal nerve and the ligamentum arteriosum divided. Removal of part of the thymus gland will facilitate exposure. It should be emphasized that operative correction is more than simple division of an abnormal ring, because fibrosis surrounding the adventitia of the abnormal vessel may cause continued compression unless the vessels are widely mobilized and all possible compression is relieved.

With a double aortic arch, the smaller of the two arches should be divided. Usually, with a left descending aorta, the anterior arch is smaller and can be divided between the left common carotid and left subclavian artery, after which the mobilized anterior arch can be sutured to the posterior surface of the anterior chest wall to prevent compression of the trachea. If the posterior arch is smaller, it can be divided behind the esophagus. With a right descending thoracic aorta, almost always the posterior arch is the smaller of the two.

With a right aortic arch and a retroesophageal ligamentum arteriosum, division of the ligamentum arteriosum, combined with mobilization of the abnormal vessels, may be all that is necessary. In some patients the left subclavian artery may be in a retroesophageal location and should also be divided. A nubbin of aorta, constituting an aortic diverticulum, has been found in a retroesophageal location in some patients and may require amputation to relieve compression.

With a retroesophageal subclavian artery as an isolated anomaly, simple division of the artery is all that is necessary. Division of this artery through a cervical incision, followed by reimplantation into the right carotid artery, has been reported.

Postoperative Course. Postoperative care consists primarily of careful attention to respiration, with the infant kept in a highly humidified atmosphere and tracheal secretions aspirated. Tracheostomy is rarely necessary. If tracheal compression was present before operation, serious difficulties may develop afterward, probably from dissection around the trachea, creating postoperative edema. Unusually vigilant care for 24 to 72 h may be necessary. After recovery from operation, symptoms soon disappear. The risk of operation is primarily related to the age of the patient and the severity of compression of the trachea. Excellent results in a group of 70 patients have been reported by Gross, who had only 5 postoperative deaths, all of which occurred in a group of 26 infants

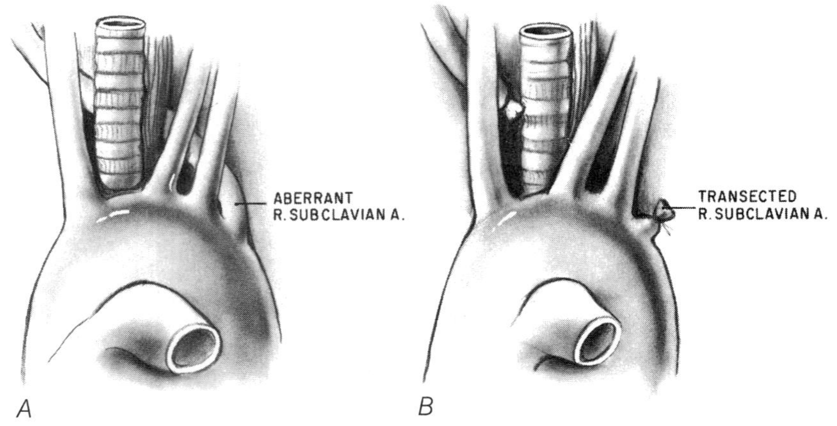

FIG. 17-51. *A.* Retroesophageal right subclavian artery, anomalous vessel arising from aortic arch distal to left subclavian artery. *B.* Appearance after division of anomalous vessel with retraction of distal stump to right of trachea. (From: *Gross RE: The Surgery of Infancy and Childhood. Philadelphia, WB Saunders, 1953, p. 932, with permission.*)

with double aortic arches. Others have subsequently reported excellent results. By contrast, Bertrand et al. noted that 7 of 12 operated patients had residual symptoms. In general most symptoms should resolve with time and long-term results should be excellent.

Pulmonary Artery Sling

Vascular sling is a rare congenital malformation in which the left pulmonary artery arises from the right pulmonary artery and courses to the left between the trachea and esophagus to reach the left lung hilus, thus forming a sling or ring around the trachea (Fig. 17-52). The term originated from a publication by Contro in 1958. Although the first patient was treated surgically by Potts in 1954, total reported surgical experience remains small. A review of Grover in 1975 described experiences with one patient and found a total of 63 patients reported by others. Twenty of 23 unoperated patients died.

The trachea is often narrowed at the site of compression and, in some patients, significant severe tracheal stenosis is present with complete cartilaginous rings. This occurs from abnormal intrauterine development of the trachea, possibly from vascular compromise, and may be fatal when present. Other cardiac anomalies are present in nearly one-half of reported patients.

Clinical Manifestations. Apparently, most infants develop symptoms in the first few months of life, with wheezing, stridor, and choking. The diagnosis may be suspected from abnormalities visible on the chest radiograph, with a density separating the trachea from the esophagus on the lateral view. An esophageal barium swallow is usually diagnostic, showing anterior indentation of the esophagus just above the carina. A tracheogram and bronchoscopy should routinely be performed to evaluate the severity of associated tracheal malformations, one of the most important determinants of postoperative prognosis. A CT scan will also confirm the diagnosis. Catheterization and angiography are routinely performed to confirm the diagnosis and detect additional anomalies.

The major decision before operation is evaluating the extent of inherent diseases in the trachea. Some infants with tracheal stenoses have ultimately died despite division of the sling and attempted correction of the tracheal malformation. Older patients are occasionally seen with minimal or no symptoms. Such patients often require no specific treatment.

Treatment. The operative procedure in the absence of severe tracheal stenosis (Fig. 17-53) is a simple one, dividing the anomalous pulmonary artery at its origin, bringing it from behind the trachea and reanastomosing it to the main pulmonary artery. The ligamentum arteriosum is divided at this time. This has been done through a left lateral thoracotomy and also through a median sternotomy.

When tracheal stenosis is present the procedure becomes more complicated. Isolated tracheal stenosis can be successfully resected at the time of repair. More diffuse stenosis, with complete rings extending the length of the trachea, is a highly fatal condition. The best approach probably involves incision of the length of the trachea and stenting, as advocated by Iddris.

The prognosis following operation is determined principally by the inherent disease present in the trachea. Five patients were recorded by Kirklin and Barratt-Boyes, three of whom died after operation, while the other two remain asymptomatic. Occlusion of the pulmonary artery has been subsequently found in some patients, probably a reflection of the technique of vascular anastomo-

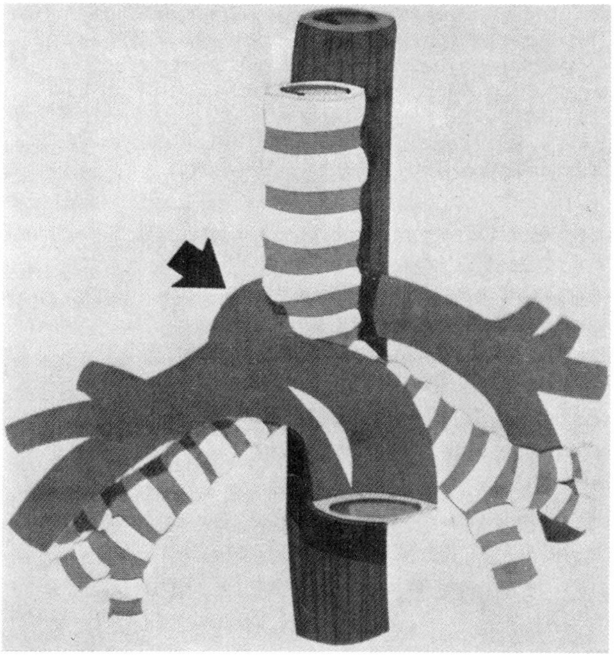

FIG. 17-52. Diagram of anomalous origin of left pulmonary artery from right pulmonary artery. Anatomic relationship of left pulmonary artery to trachea and esophagus is also shown. (From: *Grover FL, Norton JB, et al: 1975, with permission.*)

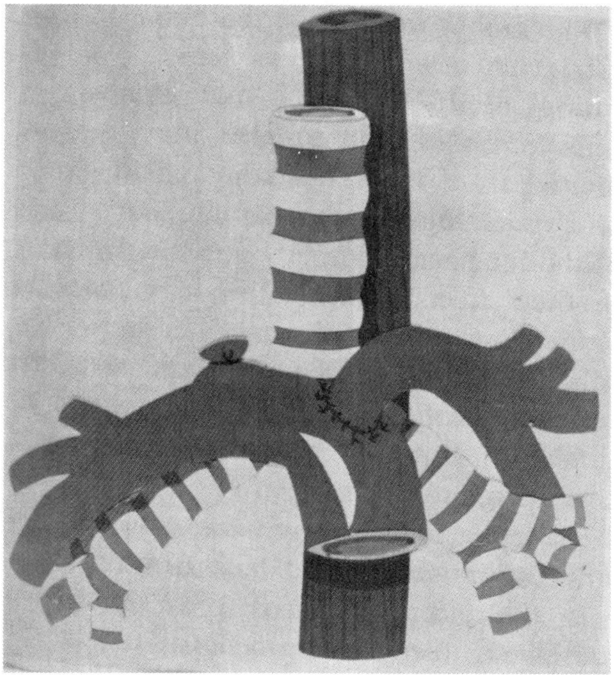

FIG. 17-53. Diagram of anatomy at completion of operation. Note that proximal stump of left pulmonary artery is to right of trachea after having been dissected free. Distal left pulmonary artery has been anastomosed to side of main pulmonary artery. (From: *Grover FL, Norton JB, et al: 1975, with permission.*)

sis. Campbell, in 1983, reported two patients with good surgical results operating through a median sternotomy and also performing an "aortopexy" to minimize postoperative tracheal compression.

Bibliography

Coarctation of the Aorta and Interrupted Aortic Arch

Abbott ME: Coarctation of the aorta of the adult type; statistical study and historical retrospect of 200 recorded cases with autopsy, of stenosis or obliteration of the descending arch in subjects above the age of two years. *Am Heart J* 3:574, 1928.

Brewer LA III, Fosburg RG, et al: Spinal cord complications following surgery for coarctation of the aorta: A study of 66 cases. *J Thorac Cardiovasc Surg* 64:368, 1972.

Brom AG: Narrowing of the aortic isthmus and enlargement of the mind. *J Thorac Cardiovasc Surg* 50:166, 1965.

Campbell DB, Waldhausen JA, et al: Should elective repair of coarctation of the aorta be done in infancy? *J Thorac Cardiovasc Surg* 88:929, 1984.

Crafoord C, Nylin G: Congenital coarctation of the aorta and its surgical treatment. *J Thorac Surg* 14:347, 1945.

Fishman NH, Bronstein MH, et al: Surgical management of severe aortic coarctation and interrupted aortic arch in neonates. *J Thorac Cardiovasc Surg* 71:35, 1976.

Hehrlein FW, et al: Instance and pathogenesis of late aneurysms after patch graft aortoplasty for coarctation. *J Thorac Cardiovasc Surg* 92:226, 1986.

Kirklin JW, Barratt-Boyes BG: *Cardiac Surgery*. New York, Churchill Livingstone, 1993.

Krieger KH, Spencer FC: Is paraplegia after repair of coarctation of the aorta due principally to distal hypotension during aortic cross-clamping? *Surgery* 97:2, 1985.

Lerberg D, Hardesty R, et al: Coarctation of the aorta in infants and children: 25 years of experience. *Ann Thorac Surg* 33:159, 1982.

Momro JL, Bunton RW, et al: Correction of interrupted aortic arch. *J Thorac Cardiovasc Surg* 98:421, 1989.

Perloff JK: *The Clinical Recognition of Congenital Heart Disease,* 3d ed. Philadelphia, WB Saunders, 1987.

Schuster SR, Gross RE: Surgery for coarctation of the aorta: A review of 500 cases. *J Thorac Cardiovasc Surg* 43:54, 1962.

Sealy WC, Harris JS, et al: Paradoxical hypertension following resection of coarctation of the aorta. *Surgery* 42:135, 1957.

Waldhausen, J, Nahrwold D: Repair of coarctation of the aorta with a subclavian flap. *J Thorac Cardiovasc Surg* 51:532, 1966.

Yee ES, Soifer SJ, et al: Infant coarctation: A spectrum in clinical presentation and treatment. *Ann Thorac Surg* 42:488, November 1986.

Congenital Aortic Stenosis (Valvular/Subvalvular)

Bernhard WF, Poirier V, LaFarge CG: Relief of congenital obstruction to left ventricular outflow with ventricular-aortic prosthesis. *J Thorac Cardiovasc Surg* 20:136, 1975.

Brown J, Stevens L: Surgery for discrete subvalvular aortic stenosis: Actuarial survival, hemodynamic results, and acquired aortic regurgitation. *Ann Thorac Surg* 40:151, 1985.

Doty DB, Polansky DB, Jenson CB: Intravalvular aortic stenosis. *J Thorac Cardiovasc Surg* 74:362, 1977.

Frye RL, Kincaid OW, et al: Results of surgical treatment of patients with diffuse subvalvular aortic stenosis. *Circulation* 32:52, 1965.

Hsieh KS, Keane JF: Long-term follow-up of valvotomy before 1968 for congenital aortic stenosis. *Am J Cardiol* 58:338, 1986.

Hunta JC, Carpenter RJ Jr: Prenatal diagnosis and postnatal management of critical aortic stenosis. *Circulation* 75:573, 1987.

Keane JF, Fellows KE, et al: The surgical management of discrete and diffuse supravalvular aortic stenosis. *Circulation* 54:112, 1976.

Kelly DT, Barratt-Boyes BG, Lowe JB: Results of surgery and hemodynamic observations in muscular subaortic stenosis. *J Thorac Cardiovasc Surg* 51:353, 1966.

Koch J, Maron H, et al: Results of operation for obstructive hypertrophic cardiomyopathy in the elderly. Septal myotomy and myectomy in 20 patients 65 years of age or older. *Am J Cardiol* 46:963, 1980.

Konno S, Imai Y, et al: New method for prosthetic valve replacement in congenital aortic stenosis associated with hypoplasia of the aortic valve ring. *J Thorac Cardiovasc Surg* 70:909, 1975.

McKowen RL, Campbell DN, et al: Extended aortic root replacement with aortic allografts. *J Thorac Cardiovasc Surg* 93:366, 1987.

Messina LM, Turley K, et al: Successful aortic valvotomy for severe congenital valvular aortic stenosis in the newborn infant. *J Thorac Cardiovasc Surg* 88:92, 1984.

Misbach G, Turley K, et al: Left ventricular outflow enlargement using the Konno procedure. Paper presented at the American Association for Thoracic Surgery, Phoenix, Arizona, 1982.

Morrow A: Hypertrophic subaortic stenosis. Operative methods utilized to relieve left ventricular outflow obstruction. *J Thorac Cardiovasc Surg* 76:423, 1978.

Peterson TA, Todd DC, Edwards JE: Supravalvular aortic stenosis. *J Thorac Cardiovasc Surg* 50:734, 1965.

Rastelli GC, McGoon DC, et al: Surgical treatment of supravalvular aortic stenosis: Report of 16 cases and review of literature. *J Thorac Cardiovasc Surg* 51:873, 1966.

Schaffer MS, Campbell DN, et al: Aortoventriculoplasty in children. *J Thorac Cardiovasc Surg* 92:391, 1986.

Congenital Mitral Valve Disease

Coles JG, Williams WG, et al: Surgical experience with reparative techniques in patients with congenital mitral valvular anomalies. *Circulation* 76(suppl 3):III-117, 1987.

Grenadier E, Sahn DJ, et al: Two-dimensional echo Doppler study of congenital disorders of the mitral valve. *Am Heart J* 107:319, 1984.

Kadoba KK, Jonas RA, et al: Mitral valve replacement in the first year of life. *J Thorac Cardiovasc Surg* 100:766, 1990.

Ruckman R, Van Praagh R: Anatomic types of congenital mitral stenosis: Report of 49 autopsy cases with consideration of diagnosis and surgical implications. *Am J Cardiol* 42:592, 1978.

Tsuji HK, Shapiro M, et al: Congenital mitral stenosis: Report of two cases and review of the literature. *J Thorac Cardiovasc Surg* 53:850, 1967.

Vitarelli A, Landolina G, et al: Echocardiographic assessment of congenital mitral stenosis. *Am Heart J* 107:319, 1984.

Hypoplastic Left Heart Syndrome

Lang P, Norwood WI: Hemodynamic assessment after palliative surgery for hypoplastic left heart syndrome. *Circulation* 68:101, 1983.

Noonan JA, Nadas AS: The hypoplastic left heart syndrome. An analysis of 101 cases. *Ped Clin North Am* 5:1029, 1958.

Norwood WI, Kirklin JK, et al: Hypoplastic left heart syndrome. Experience with palliative surgery. *Am J Cardiol* 45:87, 1980.

Norwood WI, Lang P, et al: Experiences with operations for hypoplastic left heart syndrome. *J Thorac Cardiovasc Surg* 82:511, 1981.

Atrial Septal Defects/Atrioventricular Canal Defects

Berger T, Blackstone E, et al: Survival and probability of cure without and with operation in complete atrioventricular canal. *Ann Thorac Surg* 27:106, 1979.

Ceithaml EL, Midgley FM, Perry LW: Long term results after repair of incomplete endocardial cushion defects. *Ann Thorac Surg* 48:413, 1989.

Freed MD, Nasas AS, et al: Is routine preoperative cardiac catherization necessary before repair of secundum and sinus venosus atrial septal defects? *J Am Coll Cardiol* 4:333, 1984.

Goldfaden D, Jones M, Morrow A: Long-term results of repair of incomplete persistent atrioventricular canal. *J Thorac Cardiovasc Surg* 82:669, 1981.

King RM, Puga FJ, et al: Prognostic factors and surgical treatment of partial atrioventricular canal. *Circulation* 74:I42, 1986.

McGoon D, Puga F: Atrioventricular canal. *Cardiovasc Clin* 11:311, 1981.

McMullan MH, McGoon DC, et al: Surgical treatment of partial atrioventricular canal. *Arch Surg* 107:705, 1973.

Neill CA: Postoperative hemolytic anemia in endocardial cushion defects. *Circulation* 30:801, 1964.

Paolillo V, Dawkins KD, Miller GA: Atrial septal defect in patients over the age of fifty. *Int J Cardiol* 9:139, 1985.

Ventricular Septal Defects

Barratt-Boyes BG, Neutze JM, et al: Repair of ventricular septal defect in the first two years of life using profound hypothermia-circulatory arrest technics. *Ann Surg* 184:376, 1976.

Danilowicz D, Presti S, et al: Results of urgent or emergent repair of symptomatic infants under one year of age with singular or multiple ventricular septal defects. *Am J Cardiol* 69:699, 1992.

Mattila S, Kostiainen S, et al: Repair of ventricular septal defect in adults. *Scand J Thorac Cardiovasc Surg* 19:29, 1985.

Otterstad JE, Erikssen J, et al: Long term results after operative treatment of isolated ventricular septal defect in adolescents and adults. *Acta Med Scand* 708(suppl):1, 1986.

Richardson J, Schieken R, et al: Repair of large ventricular septal defects in infants and small children. *Ann Surg* 195:318, 1982.

Rizzoli G, Blackstone E, et al: Incremental risk factors in hospital mortality rate after repair of ventricular septal defect. *J Thorac Cardiovasc Surg* 80:494, 1980.

Spencer FC, Doyle EF, et al: Longterm evaluation of aortic valvuloplasty for aortic insufficiency and ventricular septal defect. *J Thorac Cardiovasc Surg* 65:15, 1973.

Walker WJ, Garcia-Gonzalez E, et al: Interventricular septal defect: Analysis of 415 catherterized cases. *Circulation* 31:54, 1965.

Wood P: The Eisenmenger syndrome. *Br Med J* 2:701, 1958.

Yeager SB, Freed MD, et al: Primary surgical closure of ventricular septal defect in the first year of life: Results in 128 infants. *J Am Coll Cardiol* 3:1269, May 1984.

Patent Ductus Arteriosus

Blalock A: Operative closure of the patent ductus arteriosus. *Surg Gynecol Obstet* 82:113, 1946.

Gersony WM, Peckham GJ, et al: Effects of indomethacin in premature infants with patent ductus arteriosus: Results of a national collaborative study. *J Pediatr* 102:895, 1983.

Gold JP, Cohn LH: Operative management of the calcified patent ductus arteriosus. *Ann Thorac Surg* 41:567, 1986.

Gross RE, Hubbard JP: Surgical ligation of a patent ductus arteriosus: Report of first successful case. *JAMA* 112:729, 1939.

Jones JC: Twenty-five years experience with the surgery of patent ductus arteriosus. *J Thorac Cardiovasc Surg* 50:149, 1965.

Kitterman J: Patent ductus arteriosus: Current clinical status. *Arch Dis Child* 55:106, 1980.

Kron IL, Harman PK, et al: The adult ductus surgical results and longterm follow-up. *Am Surg* 49:546, 1983.

Mikhail M, Lee W, et al: Surgical and medical experience with 734 premature infants with patent ductus arteriosus. *J Thorac Cardiovasc Surg* 83:349, 1982.

Aortopulmonary Window

Doty D, Richardson J, et al: Aortopulmonary septal defect: Hemodynamics, angiography, and operation. *Ann Thorac Surg* 32:244, 1981.

Gross RE: Surgical closure of an aortic septal defect. *Circulation* 5:858, 1952.

Jolles PR, Shin MS, Jones WP: Aortopulmonary window lesions: Detection with chest radiography. *Radiology* 159:647, 1986.

Morrow AG, Greenfield LJ, Braunwald E: Congenital aortopulmonary septal defect: Clinical and hemodynamic findings, surgical technique, and results of operative correction. *Circulation* 25:463, 1962.

Scott HW, Sabiston DC: Surgical treatment for congenital aorticopulmonary fistula. *J Thorac Cardiovasc Surg* 25:26, 1953.

Tetralogy of Fallot

Ebert PA: Second operation for pulmonary stenosis or insufficiency after repair of tetralogy of Fallot. *Am J Cardiol* 50:637, 1982.

Hammon JW, Henry CL, et al: Tetralogy of Fallot: Selected surgical management can minimize operative mortality. *Ann Thorac Surg* 40:280, 1985.

Kirklin JW, Blackstone E, et al: Risk factors for early and late failure after repair of tetralogy of Fallot and their neutralization. *J Thorac Cardiovasc Surg* 32:208, 1984.

Lillehei CW, Varco RL, et al: The first open heart repairs of ventricular septal defect, atrioventricular communis, and tetralogy of Fallot using extracorporeal circulation by cross-circulation: A 30-year follow-up. *Ann Thorac Surg* 41:421, 1986.

Roh MS, Hardesty R, et al: Blalock shunt: Procedure of choice in infants. *J Cardiovasc Surg* 25:1, 1984.

Pulmonary Stenosis-Pulmonary Atresia With Intact Septum

Blalock A, Kiefer RF Jr: Valvulotomy for the relief of congenital valvular pulmonary stenosis with intact ventricular septum. Report of 19 operations by the Rock method. *Ann Surg* 32:496, 1950.

Brock RC: Pulmonary valvulotomy for the relief of congenital stenosis: Report of three cases. *Br Med J* 1:112, 1948.

Coles JG, Freedom RM, et al: Surgical management of critical pulmonary stenosis in the neonate. *Ann Thorac Surg* 38:458, 1984.

Coles JG, Freedom RM, et al: Long-term results in neonates with pulmonary atresia and intact ventricular septum. *Ann Thorac Surg* 47:213, 1989.

Griffith B, Hardesty R, et al: Pulmonary valvulotomy alone for pulmonary stenosis: Results in children with and without muscular infundibular hypertrophy. *J Thorac Cardiovasc Surg* 83:577, 1982.

McCaffrey FM, Leatherbury L, et al: Pulmonary atresia and intact ventricular septum. *J Thorac Cardiovasc Surg* 102:617, 1991.

Tricuspid Atresia

Bjork V, Olin C, et al: Right atrial-right ventricular anastomosis for correction of tricuspid atresia. *J Thorac Cardiovasc Surg* 77:452, 1979.

Fontan F, Baudet E: Surgical repair of tricuspid atresia. *Thorax* 26:240, 1971.

Fontan F, Deville C, et al: Repair of tricuspid atresia in 100 patients. *J Thorac Cardiovasc Surg* 85:647, 1983.

Fontan F, Kirklin JW, et al: Outcome after a "perfect" Fontan operation. *Circulation* 81:1520, 1990.

Girod DA, Fontan F, et al: Longterm results after the Fontan operation for tricuspid atresia. *Circulation* 75:605, 1987.

Glenn WW, Patino J: Circulatory bypass of the right heart. In preliminary observations on direct delivery of vena cava blood into pulmonary artery circulation: Azygos vein-pulmonary artery shunt. *Yale J Biol Med* 27:147, 1954.

Glenn WW: Circulatory bypass with the right side of the heart shunt between superior vena cava and distal right pulmonary artery—Report of clinical application. *N Engl J Med* 259:117, 1958.

Kirklin JK, Blackstone EH, et al: The Fontan operation. *J Thorac Cardiovasc Surg* 92:1049, 1986.

Kuhne M: Uber zwefalle Kongenitaler atresia des ostium venosum deytrum. *J Ahrbuch Kinderhekdkunde Physiche Erziehung* 63:235, 1906.

Lee CN, Schaff HB, et al: Comparison of atrial pulmonary vs atrioventricular connections for modified Fontan—Kreutezer repair of tricuspid valve atresia. *J Thorac Cardiovasc Surg* 92:1038, 1986.

Trusler G, Williams G: Long-term results of shunt procedures for tricuspid atresia. *Ann Thorac Surg* 29:312, 1980.

Weinberg P: Anatomy of tricuspid atresia and its relevance to current forms of surgical therapy. *Ann Thorac Surg* 29:306, 1980.

Transposition of the Great Vessels

Albert H: Surgical correction of transposition of the great vessels. *Surg Forum* V:74, 1955.

Ashraf MM, Cotroneo J, et al: Fate of long-term survivors of Mustard procedure (inflow repair) for simple and complex transposition of the great arteries. *Ann Thorac Surg* 42:385, 1986.

Baffes TG, Riker WL, et al: Surgical correction of transposition of the aorta and the pulmonary artery. *J Thorac Cardiovasc Surg* 34:469, 1957.

Bender H, Graham T, et al: Comparative operative results of the Senning and Mustard procedures for transposition of the great arteries. *Circulation* 62(suppl 1):197, 1980.

Castaneda AR, Norwood WI, et al: Transposition of the great arteries and intact ventricular septum: Anatomical repair in the neonate. *Ann Thorac Surg* 38:438, 1984.

Castaneda AR: Arterial switch operation for simple and complex TGA-indication, criterias, and limitations relevant to surgery. *Thorac Cardiovasc Surg* 39(2):151, 1991.

Hanlon CR, Blalock A: Complete transposition of aorta and pulmonary artery: Experimental observations on venous shunts as corrective procedures. *Ann Surg* 127:385, 1948.

Jatene AD, Fontes VF, et al: Successful anatomic correction of transposition of the great vessels: A preliminary report. *Arq Bras Cardiol* 28:461, 1975.

Jatene AD, Fontes VF, et al: Anatomic correction of transposition of the great arteries. *J Thorac Cardiovasc Surg* 83:20, 1982.

Jonas RA, Giglia TM, et al.: Rapid, two-stage arterial switch for transposition of the great arteries and intact ventricular septum beyond the neonatal period. *Circulation* 80(suppl 1):I-203, 1989.

Kramer H, Ramos S, et al.: Cardiac rhythm after Mustard repair and after arterial switch operation for complete transposition. *Int J Cardiol* 32:5, 1991.

Mustard WT, Keith JD, et al: The surgical management of transposition of the great vessels. *J Thorac Cardiovasc Surg* 48:953, 1964.

Piccoli G, Wilkinson J, et al: Appraisal of the Mustard procedure for the physiological correction of ''simple'' transposition of the great arteries. *J Thorac Cardiovasc Surg* 82:436, 1981.

Quaegebeur JM, Rohmer J, et al: The arterial switch operation. An eight-year experience. *J Thorac Cardiovasc Surg* 92:361, 1986.

Senning A: Surgical correction of transposition of the great vessels. *Surgery* 59:334, 1966.

Stewart S, Alexson C, Manning J: Late results of the Mustard procedure in transposition of the great arteries. *Ann Thorac Surg* 42:419, 1986.

Trusler G, Williams W, et al: Current results with the Mustard operation in isolated transposition of the great arteries. *J Thorac Cardiovasc Surg* 80:381, 1980.

Turley K, Wilson J, Ebert P: Atrial repairs of infant complex congenital heart lesions. *Arch Surg* 115:1335, 1980.

Yacoub M, Bernhard A, et al.: Clinical and hemodynamic results of the two-stage anatomic correction of simple transposition of the great arteries. *Circulation* 62:190, 1980.

Double-Outlet Right Ventricle

Anderson RH, Becker AE, et al: Surgical anatomy of double-outlet right ventricle—A reappraisal. *Am J Cardiol* 52:555, 1983.

Judson JP, Danielson GK, et al: Double-outlet right ventricle. *J Thorac Cardiovasc Surg* 85:32, 1983.

Kirklin JW, Barratt-Boyes BG: *Cardiac Surgery,* 2d ed. Churchill Livingstone, New York, 1993, pp. 1469–1500.

Kirklin JW, Pacifico AD, et al: Current risks and protocols for operations for double-outlet right ventricle. Derivation from an 18 year experience. *J Thorac Cardiovasc Surg* 92:913, 1986.

Luber JM, Castaneda AR, et al: Repair of double-outlet right ventricle: Early and late results. *Circulation* 68(suppl 2):II-144, 1983.

Truncus Arteriosus

Ceballos R, Soto B, et al: Truncus arteriosus. An anatomical-angiographic study. *Br Heart J* 49:589, 1983.

DiDonato RM, Fyfe DA, et al: Fifteen-year experience with surgical repair of truncus arteriosus. *J Thorac Cardiovasc Surg* 89:414, 1985.

Ebert PA, Turley K, et al: Surgical treatment of truncus arteriosus in the first 6 months of life. *Ann Surg* 200:451, 1984.

McGoon DC, Wallace RB, Danielson GK: The Rastelli operation: Its indications and results. *J Thorac Cardiovasc Surg* 65:65, 1973.

Rothko K, Moore G, Hutchins G: Truncus arteriosus malformation: A spectrum including fourth and sixth aortic arch interruptions. *Am Heart J* 99:17, 1980.

Sharma AK, Brawn WJ, Mee RB: Truncus arteriosus. Surgical approach. *J Thorac Cardiovasc Surg* 90:45, 1985.

Cor Triatriatum

Arciniegas E, Farooki A, et al: Surgical treatment of cor triatriatum. *Ann Thorac Surg* 32:571, 1981.

Kirklin JW, Barratt-Boyes BG: *Cardiac Surgery,* 2d ed. Churchill Livingstone, New York, 1993, pp. 675–682.

Marin-Garcia J, Tandon R, et al: Cor triatriatum: Study of 20 cases. *Am J Cardiol* 35:59, 1975.

Niwayama G: Cor triatriatum. *Am Heart J* 59:291, 1960.

Oglietti J, Cooley DA, et al: Cor triatriatum: Operative results in 25 patients. *Ann Thorac Surg* 35:415, 1983.

Ostman-Smith I, Silverman NH, et al: Cor triatriatum sinistrum: Diagnostic features on cross sectional echocardiography. *Br Heart J* 51:211, 1984.

Van Praagh R, Corsini I: Cor triatriatum: Pathologic anatomy and a consideration of morphogenesis based on 13 postmortem cases and a study of normal development of the pulmonary vein and atrial septum in 83 human embryos. *Am Heart J* 78:379, 1969.

Total Anomalous Pulmonary Venous Return

Blake HA, Hall RC, Manion WC: Anomalous pulmonary venous return. *Circulation* 32:406, 1965.

Brody H: Drainage of the pulmonary veins into the right side of the heart. *Arch Pathol* 33:221, 1942.

Galloway AC, Campbell D, Clarke D: The value of early repair for total anomalous pulmonary venous drainage. *Pediatr Cardiol* 6:77, 1985.

Turley K, Wilson J, Ebert P: Atrial repairs of infant complex congenital heart lesions. Emphasis on the first three months of life. *Arch Surg* 115:1335, 1980.

Single Ventricle (Univentricular Heart)

Anderson RH, Becker AE, et al: Morphogenesis of univentricular hearts. *Br Heart J* 38:558, 1976.

Anderson RH, Macartney FJ, et al: Univentricular atrioventricular connection: The single ventricle trap unsprung. *Pediatr Cardiol* 4:273, 1983.

Ebert PA: Staged partitioning of single ventricle. *J Thorac Cardiovasc Surg* 88:908, 1984.

Edie RN, Malm JR: Surgical repair of single ventricle. *J Thorac Cardiovasc Surg* 66:350, 1973.

Freedom RM, Benson LN, et al: Subaortic stenosis, the univentricular heart, and banding of the pulmonary artery: An analysis of the courses of 43 patients with univentricular heart palliated by pulmonary artery banding. *Circulation* 73:758, 1986.

McGoon DC, Danielson GK, et al: Correction of the univentricular heart having two atrioventricular valves. *J Thorac Cardiovasc Surg* 74:218, 1977.

Mayer J, Bridges N, et al: Factors associated with marked reduction in mortality for Fontan operations in patients with single ventricle. *J Thorac Cardiovasc Surg* 103:444, 1992.

Stefanelli G, Kirklin JW, et al: Early and intermediate-term (10 year) results of surgery for univentricular atrioventricular connection (''single ventricle''). *Am J Cardiol* 54:811, 1984.

Van Praagh R, Ongley PA, Swan HJC: Anatomic types of single or common ventricle in man. Morphologic and geometric aspects of 60 necropsied cases. *Am J Cardiol* 13:367, 1964.

Van Praagh R, Van Praagh S, et al: Diagnosis of the anatomic types of single or common ventricle. *Am J Cardiol* 15:345, 1965.

Corrected Transposition (Ventricular Inversion)

Guit GL, Kroon HM, et al: Congenitally corrected transposition in the adult: Detection by radionuclide angiocardiography. *Radiology* 157:521, 1985.

de Leval M, Bastos P, et al: Surgical technique to reduce the risks of heart block following closure of ventricular septal defect in atrioventricular discordance. *J Thorac Cardiovasc Surg* 78:515, 1979.

Kirklin JW, Barratt-Boyes BG: *Cardiac Surgery,* 2d ed. Churchill Livingstone, New York, 1993, pp. 1535–1547.

Marcelletti C, Maloney J, et al: Corrected transposition and ventricular septal defect. Surgical experience. *Ann Surg* 191:751, 1980.

Metcalfe J, Somerville J: Surgical repair of lesions associated with corrected transposition. Late results. *Br Heart J* 50:476, 1983.

Schiebler GL, Edwards JE, et al: Congenital corrected transposition of the great vessels: A study of 33 cases. *Pediatrics* 27:851, 1961.

Vargas FJ, Kreutzer GO, et al: Repair of corrected transposition associated with ventricular septal defect and pulmonary stenosis. *Ann Thorac Surg* 40:509, 1985.

Waldo AL, Pacifico AD, et al: Electrophysiological delineation of the specialized A–V conduction system in patients with corrected transposition of the great vessels and ventricular septal defect. *Circulation* 52:435, 1975.

Ruptured Aneurysm of Sinus of Valsalva

Heilman KJ III, Groves BM, et al: Rupture of the left sinus of valsalva aneurysm into the pulmonary artery. *J Am Coll Cardiol* 5:1005, 1985.

Lillehei CW, Stanley P, Varco RL: Surgical treatment of ruptured aneurysms of the sinus of valsalva. *Ann Surg* 146:459, 1957.

Sawyer JL, Adams JE, Scott HW: Surgical treatment for aneurysms of aortic sinuses with aorticoatrial fistula. *Surgery* 41:126, 1957.

Spencer FC, Blake HA, Bahnson HT: Surgical repair of ruptured aneurysm of sinus of valsalva in two patients. *Ann Surg* 162:963, 1960.

Ebstein's Anomaly

Bahnson HT, Bauersfeld SR, Smith JW: Pathological anatomy and surgical correction of Ebstein's anomaly. *Circulation* 31(suppl 1):3, 1965.

Barbero-Marcial M, Verginelli G, et al: Surgical treatment of Ebstein's anomaly. Early and late results in twenty patients subjected to valve replacement. *J Thorac Cardiovasc Surg* 78:416, 1979.

Danielson GK, Fuster V: Surgical repair of Ebstein's anomaly. *Ann Surg* 196:499, 1982.

Hardy KL, May IA, et al: Ebstein's anomaly: A functional concept and successful definitive repair. *J Thorac Cardiovasc Surg* 48:927, 1964.

Kirklin JW, Barratt-Boyes BG: *Cardiac Surgery,* 2d ed. Churchill Livingstone, New York, 1993, pp. 1105–1130.

Mair DD, Seward JB, et al: Surgical repair of Ebstein's anomaly: Selection of patients and early and late operative results. *Circulation* 72:1170, 1985.

Radford DJ, Graff RF, Neilson GH: Diagnosis and natural history of Ebstein's anomaly. *Br Heart J* 54:517, 1985.

Anomalies of the Coronary Arteries

Bland EF, White PD, Garland J: Congenital anomalies of the coronary arteries: Report of an unusual case associated with cardiac hypertrophy. *Am Heart J* 787, 1933.

Donaldson RM, Raphael MJ, et al: Hemodynamically significant anomalies of the coronary arteries. Surgical aspects. *J Thorac Cardiovasc Surg* 30:7, 1982.

Gasul BM, Arcilla RA, et al: Congenital coronary arteriovenous fistula: Clinical, phonocardiographic, angiocardiographic, and hemodynamic studies in five patients. *Pediatrics* 25:531, 1960.

Lowe E, Oldham H, Sabiston D: Surgical management of congenital coronary artery fistulas. *Ann Surg* 194:373, 1981.

Sabiston DC, Neill CA, Taussig HB: The direction of blood flow in anomalous left coronary artery arising from the pulmonary artery. *Circulation* 22:591, 1960.

Takauchi S, Imamura H, et al: New surgical methods for repair of anomalous left coronary artery from the pulmonary artery. *J Thorac Cardiovasc Surg* 78:7, 1979.

Urrutia SCO, Falaschi G, et al: Surgical management of 56 patients with congenital coronary artery fistulas. *Ann Thorac Surg* 35:300, 1983.

Vesterlund T, Thomsen PE, Hansen OK: Anomalous origin of the left coronary artery from the pulmonary artery in an adult. *Br Heart J* 54:110, 1985.

Vascular Rings

Arciniegas E, Hakimi M, et al: Surgical management of congenital vascular rings. *J Thorac Cardiovasc Surg* 77:721, 1979.

Bertrand JM, Chartrand C, et al: Vascular ring: Clinical and physiological assessment of pulmonary function following surgical correction. *Pediatr Pul* 2:378, 1986.

Campbell DN, Lilly JR, et al: The surgery of pulmonary artery ''sling.'' *J Pediatr Surg* 18:855, 1983.

Gross RE: Arterial malformations which cause compression of the trachea or esophagus. *Circulation* 11:124, 1955.

Grover FL, Norton JB, et al: Pulmonary sling: Case report and collective review. *J Thorac Cardiovasc Surg* 69:295, 1975.

Gumbiner C, Mullins C, McNamara D: Pulmonary artery sling. *Am J Cardiol* 45:311, 1980.

Kirklin JW, Barratt-Boyes BG: *Cardiac Surgery,* 2d ed. Churchill Livingstone, New York, 1993, pp. 1365–1382.

Idbeis B, Levinsky L, et al: Vascular rings: Management and a proposed nomenclature. *Ann Thorac Surg* 31:255, 1981.

Idris FS, DeLeon SY, et al: Tracheoplasty with pericardial patch for extensive tracheal stenosis in infants and children. *J Thorac Cardiovasc Surg* 88:527, 1984.

King HA, Walker D: Pulmonary artery sling. *Thorax* 39:462, 1984.

Mahoney EB, Manning JA: Congenital abnormalities of the aortic arch. *Surgery* 55:1, 1964.

Marmon LM, Bye MR, et al: Vascular rings and slings: Long-term follow-up of pulmonary function. *J Pediatr Surg* 19:683, 1984.

Roessler M, De Leval M: Surgical management of vascular ring. *Ann Surg* 197:139, 1983.

CHAPTER 18

Acquired Heart Disease

Aubrey C. Galloway, Stephen B. Colvin, Eugene A. Grossi, and Frank C. Spencer

CLINICAL MANIFESTATIONS

The standard methods for evaluating a patient with heart disease include the history and physical examination; the chest x-ray and electrocardiogram; and special diagnostic studies, especially echocardiography, cardiac catheterization and cineangiography, and special radionuclide studies. Fundamental considerations are discussed in the following sections. More information is described later in the chapter in the specific sections concerning different diseases.

History. The frequent symptoms with cardiac disease include (1) symptoms of left heart failure: dyspnea, other symptoms of pulmonary congestion; (2) symptoms of right heart failure: edema from sodium retention, hepatomegaly and ascites; (3) angina; (4) arrhythmias; (5) syncope; and (6) fatigue. With the exception of angina, symptoms are usually a *late* sign of advanced cardiac disease. The initial change in most cardiac diseases causing heart failure is a rise in intracardiac pressure in the involved cardiac chamber, subsequently followed by cardiac enlargement, usually a combination of dilatation and hypertrophy. This is a manifestation of Starling's law of the heart: an increase in workload can be achieved by an increase in diastolic fiber length. These physiologic and anatomic changes are the early changes from heart disease. Symptoms develop subsequently as different compensatory mechanisms fail. This concept is an important one because abundant data indicate that operation should be considered for many diseases on the basis of physiologic abnormalities, such as a progressive drop in left ventricular ejection fraction or a reduction of cross-sectional area of an aortic or mitral valve below 1.0 cm^2, rather than the presence of symptoms. Delaying operation until symptoms are severe often results in irreversible ventricular injury, which in turn can be a major cause of death in the first few years following operation.

Symptoms of Left Heart Failure. **Dyspnea.** The normal left ventricular end-diastolic pressure is less than 12 mmHg. Pressures in the range of 12 to 20 mmHg represent moderate disease, while pressures of 20 to 30 mmHg represent severe disease. The oncotic pressure of plasma is approximately 25 mmHg. Hence, as left atrial pressure rises, pulmonary congestion develops as left atrial pressure approaches the oncotic pressure of plasma. The tolerance for pulmonary congestion depends on several factors, including the capacity of the pulmonary lymphatics to resorb fluid. *Dyspnea* is one of the cardinal symptoms of left heart failure. It can be graded with the degree of exertion required to initiate dyspnea, as opposed to dyspnea at rest, which represents a severe form of heart disease. With mitral stenosis, dyspnea appears as an early sign because of restriction of flow from the left atrium into the left ventricle. With other forms of heart disease, however, dyspnea is a *late* sign as it develops only after the left ventricle has failed, with the end-diastolic pressure rising above 12 mm. Dyspnea with mitral insufficiency, aortic valvular disease, or coronary disease represents an advanced form of disease, in contrast to mitral stenosis.

A number of other respiratory symptoms represent different degrees of pulmonary congestion. These include orthopnea, paroxysmal nocturnal dyspnea, cough, hemoptysis, and pulmonary edema.

Symptoms of Right Heart Failure. Left-sided heart failure may result in fluid retention and pulmonary congestion, subsequently leading to pulmonary hypertension and progressive right-sided heart failure. Occasionally primary right heart failure may result from right ventricular injury and dysfunction or from primary tricuspid valve disease. Right atrial pressure, normally less than 5 mmHg, may be elevated up to levels of 15 to 30 mmHg or higher. Retention of more than 7 to 10 lb of fluid results in visible edema of the lower extremities. Jugulovenous distention and hepatomegaly develop. With chronic severe right heart failure fluid retention is severe, with marked deformities from accumulation of 20, 30, or more pounds of edema fluid, with ascites and massive hepatomegaly.

Angina. Angina is the hallmark of coronary artery disease, a symptom of myocardial anoxia with subsequent anaerobic metabolism. Classic angina is described as a precordial discomfort appearing with exercise, emotion, or eating, relieved by rest or nitroglycerin. This is discussed in more detail in the section on Coronary Artery Disease. It is present in the classic form in 70 to 75 percent of patients with coronary disease. When this history is elicited, the diagnosis of coronary disease can be made with a high degree of certainty. In perhaps 20 to 25 percent of patients, one of the numerous variations of angina occurs, so-called angina equivalents, with symptoms in the shoulders, arms, jaw, epigastrium, or other areas. Also, in a significant number of patients, the exact frequency of which is unknown, angina apparently does not develop, though ''silent'' ischemia is present.

Angina also is a typical symptom with aortic stenosis, resulting from the combination of decreased cardiac output, left ventricular hypertrophy, and increased ventricular wall tension. It is less common with other forms of heart disease.

With the exception of angina, other forms of pain from heart disease are uncommon; chest pain is usually due to musculoskeletal disorders in the chest wall, pericarditis, or pleural or esophageal disease.

Arrhythmias. Atrial fibrillation is usually one of the first cardiac abnormalities with mitral stenosis, resulting from left atrial hypertrophy evolving from the sustained elevation in left atrial pressure. With other forms of heart disease, arrhythmias are less common, occurring sporadically without any predictable consistency. They are more frequent with older patients, probably from intrinsic disease in the atrioventricular conducting mechanism, and in severe cardiac failure, probably a manifestation of generalized cardiac hypoxia. Severe, life-threatening forms of ventricular tachycardia or ventricular fibrillation may occur in ischemic disease, and areas of scar can serve as a focus of irritability.

Syncope. This is an important symptom with aortic stenosis, apparently from a transient decrease in cerebral blood flow. It is of particular importance because it indicates a severity of aortic stenosis that may unpredictably terminate with sudden death. It must be differentiated from syncope from other causes such as bradycardia, heart block, or sustained ventricular tachycardia.

Fatigue. This is a nonspecific symptom that may arise from many causes. In some patients it probably reflects a generalized decrease in cardiac output. Otherwise, its significance is vague.

Functional Classification. The New York Heart Association developed a classification of patients with heart disease based on symptoms, which has been useful in evaluating clinical course and operative risk.

Class I: No functional limitation. Ordinary physical activity does not cause fatigue, palpation, dyspnea, or angina.
Class II: Slight limitation of physical activity. Such patients are comfortable at rest, but ordinary physical activity results in fatigue, palpitation, dyspnea, or angina.
Class III: Marked limitation of physical activity. These patients are comfortable at rest, but less than ordinary activity will lead to symptoms.
Class IV: Inability to carry on any physical activity without discomfort. Symptoms of congestive heart failure, cardiac insufficiency, or angina are present at rest and symptoms worsen with minimal activity.

Physical Examination. Only a few basic physical abnormalities are discussed in this short section, as abnormal physical findings are best discussed with the specific disease causing them. In some cardiac diseases, physical abnormalities are virtually diagnostic of both the disease and the severity of the problem, while in others, such as coronary disease or aortic stenosis, the paucity or absence of *any* physical abnormality can be seriously misleading.

Cardiac Cachexia. The muscular wasting that occurs from chronic congestive failure, reflected in a weight loss of 10 to 40 lb, is due to the long-standing changes of severe congestive failure in combination with a low cardiac output. In some patients, simply inability to eat may be an important cause, resulting in malnutrition from lack of calories and protein. Such patients are especially susceptible to infection following operation because of a generalized decrease in immunity.

Cardiac Size. When a valvular abnormality produces a significant change in intracardiac pressures, the initial physiologic adaptation is enlargement of the involved cardiac chamber, usually from a combination of dilatation and hypertrophy. A fundamental question in evaluation is, ''Is there cardiac enlargement?'' Accordingly, the finding of a forceful apical impulse in the anterior midaxillary line indicates advanced cardiac disease that usually requires prompt surgical treatment. Less obvious signs of cardiac enlargement may be seen on the chest x-ray, the electrocardiogram, or, most precisely, with the echocardiogram, which can define the exact size of the cardiac chamber and the thickness of the cardiac wall.

Cardiac Murmurs. Diastolic murmurs often establish the diagnosis. The apical diastolic rumble of mitral stenosis is virtually pathognomonic; the parasternal diastolic murmur of aortic insufficiency is also almost equally so.

Systolic murmurs are strongly supportive of the diagnosis of the underlying condition but not to the degree found with diastolic murmurs. These include the basal systolic murmur of aortic stenosis or pulmonic stenosis and the apical systolic murmur of mitral insufficiency.

DIAGNOSTIC STUDIES

Electrocardiography and Radiology. The electrocardiogram and the chest x-ray are the two standard diagnostic studies. The electrocardiogram is used to detect rhythm disturbances, heart block, atrial or ventricular hypertrophy, ventricular strain, myocardial ischemia, and myocardial infarction.

The chest x-ray is excellent for determining cardiac enlargement and pulmonary congestion. A cardiothoracic ratio of over 0.5 represents severe cardiomegaly. Analysis of the pulmonary circulation may show several abnormalities. Pulmonary venous congestion develops when left atrial pressure is chronically elevated above the upper normal limit of 12 mmHg, seen typically with severe mitral stenosis. The signs of pulmonary congestion include engorged pulmonary veins and congestion of pulmonary alveoli. Fluid accumulating in the interlobar planes forms transverse linear opacities perpendicular to the surface of the pleura, termed Kerley "lines." Their presence usually indicates a left atrial pressure exceeding 20 mmHg.

Marked enlargement of the pulmonary arteries may occur from an increase in pulmonary blood flow or an increase in pulmonary vascular resistance with pulmonary hypertension. Normally, the central pulmonary arteries are three to four times larger than the peripheral arteries. With an increase in pulmonary blood flow, as with an atrial septal defect, both central and peripheral arteries are symmetrically enlarged. With pulmonary hypertension, the central pulmonary arteries may become strikingly enlarged while the peripheral arteries are not.

Echocardiography. Noninvasive diagnostic echocardiography incorporates the use of ultrasound and reflected acoustic waves for cardiac imaging. Recently two-dimensional (2-D) echocardiography has largely replaced the older M-mode echocardiographic recording, allowing accurate dynamic imaging of the cardiac chambers and assessment of valvular configuration or mobility. Doppler echocardiography is usually performed with 2-D imaging studies, using Doppler signal velocity and frequency to evaluate the direction and velocity of intracardiac blood flow. Intracardiac pressure, valvular insufficiency, and transvalvular gradients can be estimated from Doppler measurements. Color Doppler information is often superimposed onto the 2-D image, giving a graphic illustration of the directional intracardiac flow pattern and an assessment of valvular insufficiency.

Overall, 2-D color Doppler echocardiography has become an excellent noninvasive method for evaluating myocardial thickness or hypertrophy, cardiac chamber size, cardiac wall motion, intracardiac and pulmonary artery pressures, internal cardiac anatomy, and the degree of valvular stenosis or insufficiency. Corrective operation for valvular disease is now frequently performed on younger patients based on these studies alone. Transesophageal echocardiography, which is done by placement of the 2-D transducer in a flexible endoscope, improves the image quality by minimizing scatter from the chest wall, and is particularly valuable in evaluation of the left atrium, the mitral valve, and the aortic arch.

Radionuclide Studies. Currently, the most widely used myocardial perfusion scan is the thallium scan, which uses the nuclide thallium-201. Initial uptake of thallium-201 into myocardial cells is dependent on myocardial perfusion, while delayed uptake depends on myocardial viability. Thus reversible defects occur in underperfused, ischemic, but viable zones, while fixed defects occur in areas of infarction. The exercise thallium test is used to identify inducible areas of ischemia and is 90 to 95 percent sensitive in detecting multivessel coronary disease. Fixed defects on the thallium scan suggest nonviable myocardium and may be of prognostic value.

Noninvasive assessment of myocardial function is best done by the gated blood pool scan (equilibrium radionuclide angiocardiography) using technetium-99m. This study can detect areas of hypokinesis and measure left ventricular ejection fraction, end-systolic volume, and end-diastolic volume. An exercise-gated blood pool scan is an excellent way to assess a patient's functional response to cardiac stress. Normally the ejection fraction will increase with exercise, but with significant coronary artery disease or valvular disease the ejection fraction may drop. The resting gated blood pool scan is an excellent way to determine the degree of prior cardiac injury, to assess baseline cardiac function, and to assess the functional response to stress.

Positron-emission tomography (PET) scan is a special radionuclide imaging technique used to assess myocardial viability in underperfused areas of the heart. The technique may be more sensitive than the thallium scan for this purpose. The PET scan is based on the myocardial metabolism of glucose or other compounds tagged with positron-emitting isotopes. The PET scan may be most useful in determining whether an area of apparently infarcted myocardium may in fact be "hibernating" and respond to revascularization. These data can be used to determine whether patients with congestive heart failure might improve with operative revascularization.

Cardiac Catheterization. The cardiac catheterization study remains the golden standard for cardiac diagnosis. Complete cardiac catheterization includes the measurement of intracardiac pressures, measurement of cardiac output, localization and quantification of intracardiac shunts, determination of internal cardiac anatomy and ventricular wall motion by cineradiography, and determination of coronary anatomy by coronary angiography (Fig. 18-1).

The cardiac output is usually calculated using the Fick oxygen method, where cardiac index ($1/min/m^2$) = oxygen consumption ($mL/min/m^2$)/arteriovenous oxygen content difference (mL/min). For determining the arteriovenous oxygen difference, the oxygen content is calculated separately in the arterial and venous circulations by the formula: oxygen content (mL oxygen/liter blood) = hemoglobin (g/100 mL) $\times$ % hemoglobin saturation $\times$ 1.36 (mL oxygen/g hemoglobin) $\times$ 10. Calculation of systemic vascular

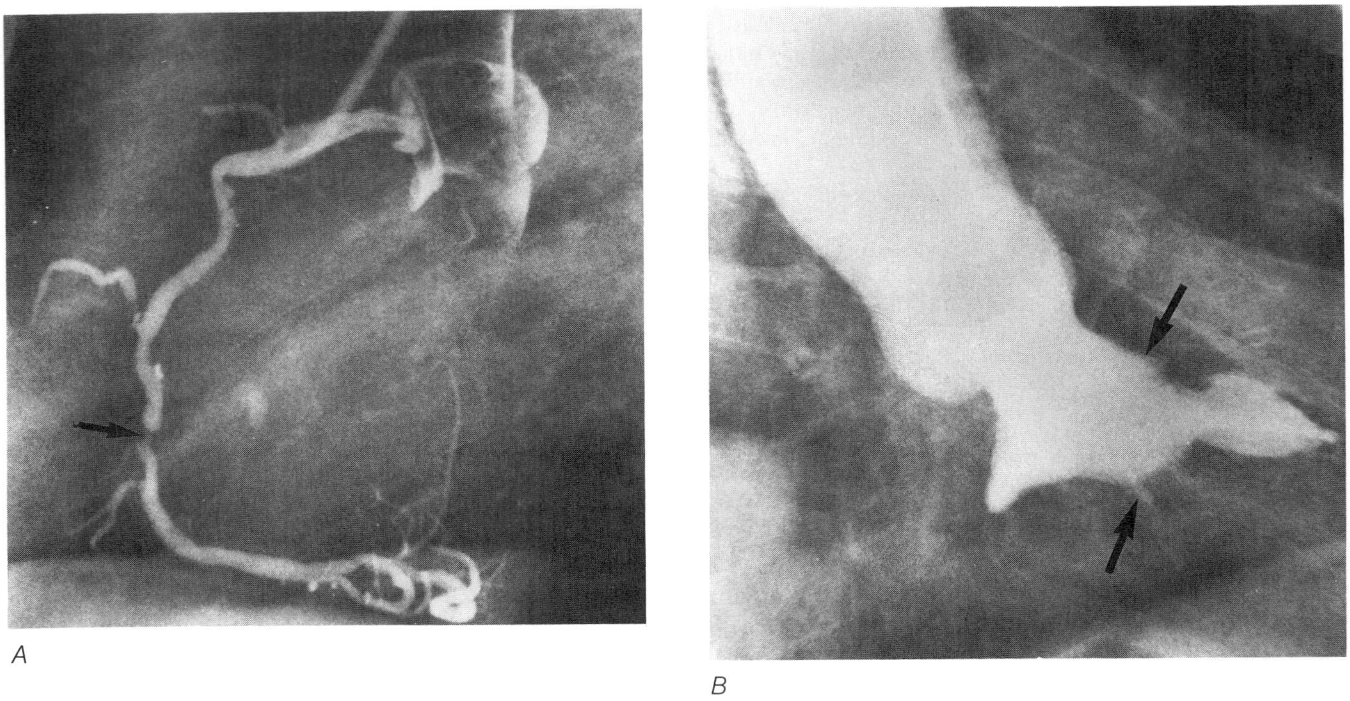

FIG. 18-1. *A.* Coronary angiogram demonstrating a severely stenotic atherosclerotic lesion in the right coronary artery. *B.* A systolic left ventriculogram of a patient with a normal ejection fraction.

resistance (SVR) is by the formula: SVR = (mean systemic arterial pressure minus mean right atrial pressure) × 80/systemic blood flow (cardiac output). The normal SVR is 1200 dynes-sec-cm^{-5}. The pulmonary vascular resistance (PVR) is calculated by the formula: PVR = mean pulmonary artery pressure minus mean left atrial pressure) × 80/pulmonary blood flow (equal to the cardiac output when no shunt is present). The normal PVR is 70 to 80 dynes-sec-cm^{-5}.

The area of a cardiac valve can be determined from measured cardiac output and intracardiac pressures using Gorlin's formula, which relates the valve area to the flow across the valve divided by the square root of the transvalvular pressure gradient (A = f/k × square root of pressure gradient). The Gorlin formula indicates that a small valve area might manifest as a small transvalvular pressure gradient when the cardiac output is low, demonstrating the danger of basing decisions on transvalvular gradient alone. The significance of an obstructing valvular lesion should be based on the calculated valve area, obtained from precise measurements in a cardiac catheterization laboratory. In an adult the normal mitral valve area is 4 to 6 cm^2, and the normal aortic valve area is 2.5 to 3.5 cm^2.

Coronary angiography is essential for the diagnosis of coronary artery disease and is routinely performed before coronary artery bypass operation (see Fig. 18-1). The posterior descending artery and the atrioventricular (AV) nodal artery arise from the right coronary artery in 80 percent of patients, and the right coronary artery is termed dominant in these cases. The left coronary system supplies the major portion of left ventricular myocardium in all cases. In 15 to 20 percent of cases the circumflex branch of the left coronary system also supplies the posterior descending branch and the AV nodal artery and is termed dominant.

Preoperative Assessment of General Surgical Patients. The association of coronary artery disease and peripheral vascular disease is well established in the literature. In one study by Hertzer and associates, 263 patients with abdominal aortic aneurysms had coronary angiography, demonstrating coronary artery disease in 94 percent. Because of the high prevalence of coronary artery disease, patients with peripheral vascular disease require close preoperative evaluation. At New York University these patients undergo screening with history, physical examination, and resting gated blood pool scan, after which they are triaged based on an algorithm established by Pasternack. Patients with significant cardiac symptoms or with a resting ventricular ejection fraction of less than 35 percent undergo cardiac catheterization before surgery, and coronary revascularization is recommended if large areas of myocardium are at risk. Patients with mild or no symptoms and with an ejection fraction of over 35 percent undergo provocative testing with a stress-gated blood pool scan, stress thallium scan, or dipyridamole thallium scan. If significant myocardium is found to be at risk due to inducible ischemia, cardiac catheterization is recommended.

The prevalence of coronary artery disease is less in nonvascular general surgical patients than in vascular patients. For major general surgical procedures preoperative cardiac risk assessment should be established from a detailed history and physical examination. A cardiac risk assessment scale developed by Goldman has been helpful for this purpose, with risk points assigned for age, history of myocardial infarction, congestive heart failure, valvular stenosis, electrocardiogram disturbances, general status (such as renal, hepatic, or respiratory dysfunction), and severity of planned operation. After a thorough preoperative risk assessment is completed, cardiac catheterization is recommended for severely symptomatic patients and for patients with a high cardiac risk profile. Less symptomatic patients with a moderate risk profile should have noninvasive provocative testing as was recommended for vascular patients in the above paragraph. Digital monitoring for silent ischemia may also be helpful in this group of patients. Patients with minimal symptoms and with a low cardiac risk profile need no further workup before surgery.

MEDICAL THERAPY

Coronary Artery Disease. Atherosclerosis is a multifactorial disease resulting in accumulation of lipids, smooth muscle cells, and connective tissue in the vessel wall. This process results in the formation of obstructive lesions in the aorta, the peripheral vessels, and/or the coronary arteries. Atherosclerosis is the leading cause of death in the Western world, and acute myocardial infarction alone accounts for 25 percent of the deaths in the United States each year. Risk factors for coronary artery disease include smoking, obesity, hypertension, diabetes, hypercholesterolemia, hyperlipidemia, sedentary life-style, Type A personality, and male gender. The most important factor in the long-term treatment of coronary disease is the modification of risk factors, including the immediate cessation of smoking, control of hypertension, weight loss, and reduction of serum cholesterol to less than 200 mg/dL.

Angina is the principal manifestation of coronary artery disease. Mild stable angina is sometimes successfully treated with sublingual nitroglycerin for pain. More significant angina is usually treated with a combination of aspirin and beta-blockers. Aspirin presumably works through its antiplatelet affect, while beta-blockers limit ischemia through a reduction in myocardial oxygen consumption and tension-time index. Both agents limit the number of cardiac events and improve survival after myocardial infarction. If angina symptoms are unresponsive to beta-blockers, second-line therapy is begun with either calcium antagonist or long-acting nitrates. For refractory angina "triple therapy" with beta-blockers, calcium antagonists, and nitrates can be used. A progression of angina despite good medical therapy is usually an indication for cardiac catheterization, as is a change in the frequency or severity of angina. Some cardiologists use a stress test evaluation in patients with angina to assess myocardium at risk, and cardiac catheterization is recommended if significant areas of the heart become ischemic at a low work load.

Unstable angina represents a medical-surgical emergency; this condition can progress to acute myocardial infarction and death. Patients with unstable rest angina are admitted to the hospital and treated with aspirin, beta-blockers, and intravenous heparin, with close monitoring for cardiac arrhythmias or recurrent pain. Myocardial oxygen demands should be minimized by obtaining a heart rate of 50 to 60 beats/min and a blood pressure of 100 to 110 mmHg. If angina is not controlled, intravenous nitroglycerin and calcium antagonists may be added. When hypotension or congestive heart failure complicate unstable angina, a Swan-Ganz catheter is placed to optimize preload and an arterial pressure line may be helpful for blood pressure monitoring. Urgent cardiac catheterization is indicated for unstable angina to assess the underlying coronary pathology, and so that revascularization can be planned when appropriate.

Acute myocardial infarction results from acute thrombosis of a coronary artery and accounts for nearly 1.5 million deaths in the United States each year. Patients with acute myocardial infarction should be given oxygen, morphine for pain, and monitored for arrhythmias in an intensive care unit. Arrhythmias occur in more than 75 percent of the cases and may be due to electrical instability, pump failure, or conduction disturbance. Ventricular arrhythmias should be promptly treated with lidocaine, while complete heart block should be treated with a transvenous pacemaker. Recent studies have shown that treatment with thrombolytic therapy (streptokinase, tissue plasminogen activator, anistreplase) within the first 4 to 6 h of an acute infarction may decrease the mortality from 12 to 14 percent to approximately 8 to 9 percent. Thrombolytic therapy is thus indicated whenever feasible. Long-term survival after acute infarction is improved by treatment with beta-blockers and aspirin, both of which are begun within 2 to 4 h after admission to the hospital. Contraindications to thrombolytic therapy are cerebrovascular disease or recent surgery; and contraindications to beta blockade are heart failure, heart block, and bronchospasm.

Postinfarction angina should be treated with intravenous nitroglycerin and urgent cardiac catheterization. Urgent or emergent transluminal coronary angioplasty or coronary bypass might be required for postinfarction angina or for ongoing ischemia after thrombolytic therapy, with an acceptable risk of 1 to 3 percent. Stable postinfarction patients should have a holter monitor to evaluate arrhythmias, and either a modified stress test at 8 to 10 days or a complete stress test at 1 month. If the stress test is positive for significant reversible ischemia, cardiac catheterization is indicated; otherwise, medical therapy is continued.

Cardiogenic shock develops in 10 to 15 percent of patients with acute myocardial infarction but is less frequent after successful thrombolytic therapy. Patients with cardiogenic shock are monitored with a Swan-Ganz catheter and an arterial pressure line. Inotropic support is frequently necessary, and mechanical support with an intraaortic balloon pump is used if hypotension persists. Immediate cardiac catheterization is indicated, and revascularization with angioplasty or coronary bypass operation should be performed if feasible. Operative intervention for cardiogenic shock has a risk of 15 to 25 percent compared with a mortality rate of over 75 percent with medical therapy alone.

Congestive Heart Failure. When congestive heart failure occurs in patients with valvular heart disease, valve replacement is generally indicated. Medical therapy is often necessary, however, while preparations are made for operation. In such cases digitalis and diuretics are used to increase myocardial contractility and control volume overload. Patients with valvular insufficiency or poor cardiac function also benefit from afterload reduction, which increases forward blood flow and relieves pulmonary congestion. Angiotensin converting enzyme inhibitors, such as captopril or enalapril, or intravenous vasodilators, such as sodium nitroprusside, are the agents of choice for afterload reduction. Acutely ill patients in congestive heart failure awaiting valve replacement should be monitored in an intensive care unit with a Swan-Ganz catheter and an arterial pressure line. A combination of short-term inotropic support with dopamine, dobutamine, or amrinone and afterload reduction with intravenous nitroprusside is indicated in these patients.

When chronic congestive heart failure occurs from presumed cardiomyopathy a search for reversible causes, such as ischemia, "hibernating myocardium," or ventricular aneurysm is mandatory. When reversible causes are not found, the cornerstone of current medical therapy for chronic congestive heart failure has become afterload reduction with angiotensin-converting enzyme inhibitors. Afterload reduction minimizes cardiac work, increases forward flow, diminishes pulmonary congestion, improves long-term survival, and may result in beneficial myocardial remodeling. Diuretics are also used to control fluid and salt retention, and digitalis is used to increase the force of cardiac contraction. The beneficial effects of digitalis, however, may not be as widespread as previously believed.

CARDIOPULMONARY BYPASS

Historical Background. The pioneering imagination and efforts of Gibbon were largely responsible for the development of extracorporeal circulation. In 1932, Gibbon initiated laboratory investigations that continued for over 20 years until the first successful open heart operation in human beings was performed by him in 1953. Significant work was also done by Dennis in the late 1940s. Subsequent developments were rapid, with brief use of cross circulation by Lillehei and associates in 1954, followed a short time later by the development of the bubble oxygenator. The disc oxygenator was developed in Sweden by Bjork, Senning, and Crafoord. Kirklin, Donald et al, and Jones et al, all did significant experimental work in the early 1950s, leading to the first large clinical series using the pump oxygenator. For the past decade, membrane and bubble oxygenation have been used almost routinely.

Pumps. The majority of heart-lung machines still use a simple roller pump, originally developed by DeBakey (Fig. 18-2). The resulting flow is almost nonpulsatile, with a pulse pressure of about 15 mmHg. A variety of other pumps have been used, such as centrifugal pumps to minimize trauma to blood elements and pulsatile pumps to improve end organ perfusion. A recurrent physiologic question has been the importance of a pulsatile flow in the normal circulation. Available experimental data indicate that over long periods of time pulsatile flow may be of importance, but for periods up to 4 to 5 h organ perfusion has been equally adequate with pulsatile and nonpulsatile flow. The gradual increase in vasomotor tone that occurs during extracorporeal circulation may be partly due to a physiologic response to nonpulsatile perfusion.

Oxygenators. Since 1970 the disposable membrane and bubble oxygenators have been the most widely used type. Recently hollow-fiber membrane oxygenators have improved the efficiency of gas exchange with minimal trauma to the blood elements. Pump oxygenators in current usage usually require a priming volume in the range of 1500 to 2000 mL. Strenuous efforts are usually made to avoid the use of blood because of the risk of transmission of hepatitis or acquired immunodeficiency syndrome (AIDS); so the pump oxygenator system is usually filled with a crystalloid solution. At NYU a modified Ringer's lactate solution (Plasmalyte) is used that closely approximates the electrolyte composition of blood. The importance of albumin is uncertain, for some institutions seldom use albumin, accepting a much lower oncotic pressure during perfusion, as there are not clear data to indicate what degree of decrease in oncotic pressure is hazardous. A hemodiluted hematocrit of 20 to 25 percent is probably optimal during hypothermic bypass because of viscosity and shear stress, with improved microvascular perfusion. If the hematocrit decreases below 18 to 20 percent, blood is added to the pump oxygenator.

Technique of Perfusion. Sufficient heparin is given to elevate activated clotting time (ACT) well above 600 s, starting with a heparin dose of 4 mg/kg. Venous blood is aspirated by gravity drainage through large cannulae through the right atrium. Oxygenated blood is returned to the arterial circulation, usually through a cannula in the ascending aorta. Initial perfusion is done at a flow rate of about 2.3 to 2.5 L/min/m^2, which is the normal cardiac index. Because oxygen consumption decreases with hypothermia, flow rates may be diminished as the patient is cooled. Safe bypass flow rates for 30°C are 1.8 to 2.2 L/min/m^2, for 25°C are 1.5 to 1.8 L/min/m^2, and for 20°C are 1.2 to 1.5 L/min/m^2. Oxygen flow through the oxygenator is adjusted to produce an arterial oxygen tension above 100 mmHg. Systemic temperature is controlled with a heat exchanger in the circuit; it is usually lowered to 25 to 32°C although colder temperatures are occasionally necessary for some complicated procedures. Spilled intrapericardial or intracardiac blood is aspirated with a suction apparatus, filtered, and returned to the oxygenator. A cell-saving device is routinely used to aspirate spilled blood before and after bypass. Aspirated blood is washed and reinfused in order to avoid blood transfusion.

During perfusion a number of modalities are monitored. Arterial pressure and central venous pressure are monitored through intravascular catheters. A Swan-Ganz catheter can be inserted in adults to monitor pulmonary artery pressures and cardiac output.

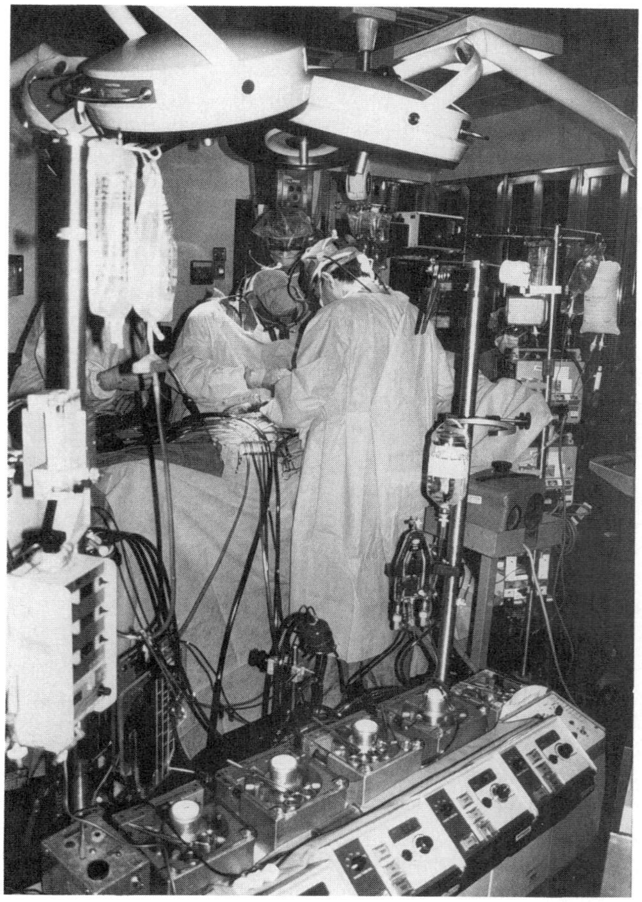

FIG. 18-2. Cardiac surgical operating room at New York University. The cardiopulmonary bypass pump, blood reservoir, and membrane oxygenator are seen in the foreground.

The blood pressure varies widely among different patients during perfusion. It usually decreases sharply with the onset of perfusion, apparently from vasodilatation, and then subsequently rises to above 60 mmHg. The importance of the actual level of mean arterial pressure, as long as flow rate is adequate, is uncertain. As cerebral autoregulation of blood flow becomes ineffective below a mean pressure of 50 to 60 mmHg, perfusion pressure is usually maintained above 50 mmHg, though with moderate hypothermia (25 to 30°C) an arterial pressure of 40 to 50 mmHg seemingly has no harmful physiologic effects. After 15 to 30 min of perfusion, perfusion pressure may gradually rise from progressive vasoconstriction.

Oxygen and carbon dioxide tensions are periodically measured in the venous blood returned to the oxygenator and the oxygenated blood returned to the patient. Preferably the arterial oxygen tension should be above 100 mmHg and the carbon dioxide tension 30 to 35 mmHg. Venous blood returning to the heart-lung machine with the described flow rate will usually have an oxygen saturation greater than 50 percent. With flow rates and oxygen saturations in this range, metabolic acidosis of significant degree does not occur. A drop in venous oxygen saturation or systemic acidosis suggest underperfusion and bypass flow rates should be increased accordingly.

Heparin is gradually metabolized by the body, and so additional heparin is given each hour of perfusion as necessary to keep the ACT above 600 s, usually 1 mg/kg of body weight. During perfusion the lungs are kept stationary in a partially inflated position.

Termination of Perfusion. As perfusion is slowed and stopped, blood is infused from the pump oxygenator to restore normal intracardiac pressures with maintenance of an adequate blood pressure and cardiac output. Close observation of the heart for arrhythmias and adequate contractility is estimated at this phase. Left atrial pressure or pulmonary artery pressure is usually monitored. At NYU an indwelling Swan-Ganz catheter in the pulmonary artery is routinely used to monitor pulmonary artery pressure and cardiac output for 24 to 48 h after operation. In many patients the pulmonary artery diastolic pressure, or wedge pressure, provides a reasonable guide to left atrial pressure. Preload or cardiac filling is optimized with fluids. If cardiac output and systemic blood pressure are inadequate despite an optimal filling pressure, inotropic support is begun, usually with dobutamine, amrinone, epinephrine, or norepinephrine. Peripheral vasodilation is controlled with alpha constrictures.

Heparin is neutralized with protamine, giving sufficient protamine to return the activated clotting time as closely as possible to that existing before bypass. Usually this requires 4 to 5 mg/kg of protamine, given in divided doses. If a coagulopathy is present, the activated clotting time may not return to prebypass levels, indicating the need for infusion of coagulation products, such as fresh frozen plasma, cryoprecipitate, or platelets. This occurs infrequently in routine cases but is more common as the complexity of the procedure and the length of the pump time increases.

Myocardial Preservation. The development of hyperkalemic hypothermic cardiac arrest for myocardial preservation was a major advance in cardiac surgery. This gradually evolved from laboratories throughout the world after 1975–1976. The improved myocardial protection, combined with the increased facility for performing complex cardiac procedures in a dry, quiet field, greatly augmented the safety and effectiveness of virtually all cardiac operations. The results from cardiac operations are now quite different from those obtained before 1980. Many of the complications in earlier years were undoubtedly due to myocardial injury and infarction. Currently protected cross-clamped arrest with multidose cardioplegia can be done for 2 to 3 h duration with near total recovery of cardiac function.

Both crystalloid and blood cardioplegia solutions are widely used, with the exact components of the cardioplegic mixture varying among different institutions. With periods of cardiac arrest for 60 to 90 min, there seems little measurable difference in the two techniques, but with the cold blood technique, regularly used at NYU, the heart can be safely arrested for a surprisingly long period of time, as long as good cardioplegia distribution and uniform myocardial cooling are achieved.

The most widely used blood cardioplegia solution is that developed by Buckberg and associates, with a blood temperature of 7 to 8°C, a potassium concentration near 20 to 30 meq/L, and a low calcium concentration. THAM is used as a buffer against tissue acidosis and the solution is hyperosmolar to minimize myocardial edema.

After the aorta is clamped, blood is infused at a rate sufficient to produce an aortic root pressure initially of 70 to 90 mmHg (200 to 400 mL/min), infusing enough blood to lower myocardial temperature below 10 to 12°C, measured in different zones of the myocardium with a needle thermistor. With normal coronary arteries, this can be achieved with 1000 to 1500 mL of cold blood. When diffuse coronary disease produces maldistribution of blood flow, adequate distribution of cardioplegia and uniform myocardial cooling might be more readily achieved with retrograde delivery of cardioplegia through the coronary sinus, which is now routinely done. Subsequently, while the aorta is clamped, varying amounts of cold blood are reinfused every 20 to 30 min, usually in the range of 300 to 500 mL with a lower potassium concentration of 8 to 12 meq/L. Continuous topical hypothermia, constantly irrigating the pericardium with a 4°C electrolyte solution, is important to keep the heart from being rewarmed. With the combination of periodic infusion of cold blood and topical hypothermia, the myocardial temperature can easily be kept below 10 to 15°C.

Trauma from Perfusion. Extracorporeal circulation inevitably produces some trauma to the blood, primarily from exposure of blood to plastics in the oxygenator and circuits, and from the use of suction to aspirate intracardiac blood. Minimizing the injury to blood during oxygenation is the basis for a membrane oxygenator rather than a bubble oxygenator. Trauma to blood from the pump itself is surprisingly small. At present, tolerance for long periods of perfusion, up to 4 to 5 h, is surprisingly good. Despite this, significant changes in bodily functions occur during cardiopulmonary bypass. These changes most resemble a generalized inflammatory reaction and are probably in part due to the activation of complement and other acute phase inflammatory components by plastics in the pump-oxygenator circuit. The severity of complement activation and the degree of subsequent end organ dysfunction is related to the length of the pump time, with increased capillary permeability occurring throughout the body. Variable organ dysfunction may occur, including confusion, low-grade renal insufficiency, decreased oxygen exchange, and hyperamylasemia. Fortunately, these findings are usually mild and are becoming exceedingly rare as the quality of oxygenators improves.

A low-grade coagulopathy is not uncommon after cardiopulmonary bypass, and, again, this relates to the length of the pump time. Platelet dysfunction may occur due to activation of platelets by artificial surfaces during bypass. Low levels of consumptive coagulopathy and hyperfibrinolysis from plasmin activation may be present. These findings generally do not become clinically relevant for the routine case but may become significant during longer, more complex cases. Recent use of a heparin-bonded bypass tubing has minimized the number of complications related to blood trauma and increased the safety of cardiopulmonary bypass.

Overall, trauma from short-term extracorporeal circulation of up to 3 to 4 h duration is minimal because of the improved design of current pump-oxygenators. By contrast, when the length of cardiopulmonary bypass exceeds 3 to 4 h, the morbidity and mortality of the procedure increases significantly, with severe problems occurring after 6 h.

POSTOPERATIVE CARE AND COMPLICATIONS

General Considerations. Postoperative cardiac surgical care is a prime example of applied cardiovascular physiology. Five key areas are involved: (1) hemodynamic evaluation, (2) electrocardiographic assessment, (3) blood loss, (4) ventilation and pulmonary care, and (5) general care, including nutrition, wound care, renal function, and rehabilitation.

After heart surgery, patients are observed in a specialized recovery room or intensive care unit. The electrocardiogram is monitored continuously, as are the arterial and intracardiac pressures. The Swan-Ganz pulmonary artery catheter is equipped with a thermistor for thermodilution measurement of cardiac output. Accurate hemodynamic profiles can be established on each patient as is outlined below in the section on hemodynamics.

Initial laboratory information should include hemoglobin, hematocrit, electrolytes, BUN, creatinine, PT, PTT, platelet count, amylase, arterial blood gas, mixed venous blood gas, and creatine phosphokinase isoenzyme. The blood gas, hematocrit, and potassium determinations are repeated hourly for 6 h. Flow sheets are used to chart hourly laboratory reports, blood pressure, pulse, hemodynamic data, fluid input and output, and blood loss. Chest x-rays are periodically made to evaluate the mediastinal shadow and the lung fields.

Early postoperative complications include bleeding, tamponade, arrhythmias, myocardial infarction, graft occlusion, coronary spasm, low cardiac output syndrome, cardiac arrest, and stroke. Other complications include delayed bleeding, postpericardiotomy syndrome with pericardial effusion, tamponade, arrhythmias, renal dysfunction, ileus, ischemic bowel, gastrointestinal hemorrhage, pneumothorax, respiratory insufficiency, pneumonia, wound infection, wound dehiscence, and, rarely, chronic cardiac dysfunction. While the incidence of serious complications is relatively low (3 to 8 percent), depending on patient and operative variables, every complication can be potentially life-threatening and associated with significant morbidity.

Our philosophy of postoperative care for cardiac surgical cases differs from others who advocate a diverse multidisciplinary approach. While cardiologists, anesthesiologists, pulmonary consults, and others are important members of the overall team and essential to the long-term care of the patient, one physician should remain responsible for the patient's overall care. For patients undergoing heart surgery, the operating surgeon should remain primarily responsible for all major decisions; the surgeon is best equipped to understand the subtleties of intraoperative physiology, technical problems, myocardial protection, and other similar events that have a profound effect on the patient's clinical course. Similarly, the operating physician's strong commitment to the patient is an essential part of both medical ethics and good patient care and should guide all actions.

Hemodynamic Evaluation. The adequacy of the cardiac function is the key question in any patient following a cardiac operation. Adequacy of cardiac output, of course, is reflected in the blood pressure and the urine output, but exact measurement of cardiac output is far more precise. This can be simply done with a thermodilution technique if a Swan-Ganz catheter has been inserted. This is the mainstay of treatment in any seriously ill patient. A normal cardiac index is 2.5 to 3.0 L/min/m^2. A cardiac index below 1.7 to 1.8 L/min/m^2 is an ominous finding, often resulting in death from inadequate perfusion of peripheral organs unless cardiac output can be increased. The classic clinical findings of low cardiac output with inadequate oxygen transport are the familiar ones of hypotension, vasoconstriction, oliguria, and metabolic acidosis. Untreated low cardiac output is ultimately fatal from either progressive renal failure or arrhythmias.

With treatment of a low cardiac output, the first consideration is to exclude cardiac tamponade or intrathoracic bleeding with hypovolemia. Once these two factors have been excluded, the physiologic causes of low output should be reviewed in terms of *preload, afterload,* and *intrinsic contractility* of the heart. Preload therapy consists of infusion of sufficient fluids to elevate left atrial pressure or pulmonary capillary wedge pressure to an appropriate level; as defined with the Starling concept, cardiac stroke volume rises with a rise in left atrial pressure over a wide range. The cardiac output can be plotted against preload, assuming pulse and afterload are constant, to determine the "optimal" filling pressure of the heart.

Afterload reduction consists of reduction in peripheral vascular resistance with specific drugs to cause vasodilatation. If peripheral vascular resistance is elevated above the normal 1200 dynes/sec/cm^2, afterload reduction should be one of the initial forms of therapy. The most popular drugs for intravenous infusion are nipride or nitroglycerin. Vasodilation, or decreased peripheral resistance, should be treated with vasoconstrictors, as necessary, to maintain an adequate perfusion pressure. In general, afterload should be controlled to keep the systolic blood pressure > 100 mmHg but < 150 mmHg, and the mean arterial blood pressure > 70 mmHg but < 90 to 95 mmHg with a vascular resistance of near normal.

Once bleeding and tamponade are excluded and preload and afterload have been optimized a wide variety of inotropic agents may be used to augment myocardial contractility. Our preference is usually dobutamine or amrinone often augmented with small amounts of norepinephrine, metaraminol, or neosynephrine when the peripheral vascular resistance is low. The latter agents are frequently administered into the left atrium to avoid pulmonary hypertension. Epinephrine can be used if these agents are inadequate.

If cardiac rhythm is not satisfactory, cardiac pacing should be used to maintain both an adequate rate and rhythm. If a sinus mechanism is too slow or not present, atrial pacing or atrial-ventricular pacing is valuable to augment cardiac output. Generally an optimal heart rate to maximize cardiac output without unduly increasing myocardial oxygen consumption is 80 to 90 beats/min.

An intraaortic balloon pump is a valuable form of assisted circulation that can be used when simpler measures fail. The balloon pump (1) decreases afterload and improves forward cardiac flow, (2) decreases preload in the failing heart, (3) provides diastolic counterpulsation to augment both systemic blood pressure and diastolic coronary perfusion, and (4) augments cardiac output about 700 mL/m^2/min. The need for a balloon pump can easily be determined in the operating room by serial measurements of cardiac output following bypass, using an intraaortic balloon pump if cardiac index remains below 1.5 to 1.7 L/min/m^2 despite significant inotropes or pressors. Usually an unexpected fall in cardiac output in the recovery room is due to some specific factor that can be corrected, either in the recovery room or by return of the patient to the operating room. The premature insertion of a balloon pump in this setting, until all other possible causes of a low cardiac output have been eliminated, is a serious error that may have fatal consequences if the basic cause of cardiac decompensation is not recognized. Leg ischemia may be a serious complication of balloon placement. More severe forms of postoperative heart failure may require temporary placement of a left ventricular assist device (see section below).

Electrocardiographic Assessment. The postoperative ECG is important for determining heart block, bundle branch block, infarction (Q waves), ischemia (ST segment elevation, T wave inversion), or other signs of intraoperative injury. The ECG should be followed closely, and patients with signs of ischemia or injury should be monitored carefully in the intensive care unit. Acute ischemia or evolving infarction should be treated initially with nitrates or calcium blockers. If ECG changes do not resolve promptly, a return to the operating room to rule out graft occlusion should be considered. Another important component of postoperative care is constant, 24 h a day, monitoring of the cardiac rhythm on an oscilloscope for at least 2 to 3 days following operation. In an intensive care unit visual monitoring is satisfactory. Otherwise, some form of telemetry with an appropriate alarm mechanism is needed. Only by *constant* monitoring can serious arrhythmias be detected because such arrhythmias may develop unpredictably despite the presence of a normal cardiac output and without any other signs of circulatory failure. Delayed detection of a significant arrhythmia is a major cause of the rare but tragic unexpected death following cardiac operations. The prevalence of bradyarrhythmias is the reason that cardiac pacing wires are routinely left in the right ventricle and right atrium for several days following operation.

Ventricular extrasystoles and ventricular tachycardia are more serious because their appearance may herald the development of ventricular fibrillation. Hypokalemia should always be considered because patients in cardiac failure preoperatively may have significant depletion of body stores of potassium from chronic diuretic therapy. The serum potassium should usually be kept well above 4.0 meq/L.

Intravenous lidocaine, 1 to 3 mg/min, is a valuable form of therapy for temporary control of arrhythmias, as the drug is quickly metabolized. Procainamide is generally used as a second line and bretyllium as a third line agent for serious ventricular arrhythmias. Treatment of more complicated problems should be done in conjunction with a cardiologist.

Methods of treatment of atrial fibrillation, a common arrhythmia, include the use of beta-blocking drugs such as propranolol, a calcium blocking drug such as verapamil, digitalis, procainamide, or quinidine. Unfortunately, virtually all antiarrhythmic agents cause serious side effects in a small percentage of patients; so such patients require careful periodic monitoring. Electric cardioversion is a valuable technique for arrhythmias refractory to simpler forms of therapy. External cardioversion at 400 J should be used for refractory ventricular tachycardia or ventricular fibrillation.

Blood Loss. Management of blood conservation and bleeding associated with cardiac surgery begins preoperatively. Preoperative work-up routinely includes a PT, PTT, and platelet count. Patients with a history of abnormal bleeding and patients with chronic passive congestion of the liver receive full coagulation profiles. In patients taking coumadin the drug is discontinued 3 to 4 days preoperatively so that the PT can return to normal.

Since blood conservation is highly desirable, many patients operated on electively are able to donate autologous blood 1 to 3 weeks before surgery. Donor-directed blood units are solicited of family and friends. Intraoperatively, patients with a large blood volume and an adequate hematocrit may have one unit of fresh whole blood removed before bypass: the unit is saved and reinfused postbypass in order to take advantage of the fresh plasma and noninjured platelets. All blood in the operative field is collected during the procedure, either by suction into the cardiopulmonary bypass pump or into a cell-saver device. Similarly, mediastinal shed blood is collected sterilely and reinfused. By reinfusion of blood from the pump, cell saver, and chest tubes the need for blood transfusion associated with heart surgery has diminished signifcantly, and some patients avoid transfusion altogether.

For most open heart cases, postoperative coagulopathy is nonexistent and postoperative blood loss is insignificant. On completion of the operation, heparin effect is neutralized with protamine. The normal postoperative blood loss should range from a total of 300 to 800 mL. A blood loss in excess of 1 L usually indicates active bleeding and is associated with a high incidence of both early and late cardiac tamponade. For this reason most patients with blood loss of more than 1 L are returned to the operating room to control or rule out active surgical bleeding and to avoid subsequent tamponade.

In some cases the effects of cardiopulmonary bypass can be quite damaging to the blood coagulation system, resulting in severe postoperative coagulopathy. The incidence of coagulopathy relates most strongly to the duration of cardiopulmonary bypass, but coagulopathy is also more frequent when hemodilution is excessive, after severe hypothermia, and in reoperations where ongoing blood loss from scar tissue results in progressive loss of coagulation factors. The diagnosis of coagulopathy is made by the operating surgeon with the observation of abnormal bleeding from the operative field. Laboratory tests can confirm the diagnosis, but treatment should not be delayed until test results return as this might further worsen the coagulation deficit with fatal consequences. Nonsurgical causes of abnormal bleeding after heart surgery include (1) inadequate neutralization of heparin from insufficient protamine, (2) a functional platelet deficit either from aspirin effect or from the activation of platelets by plastics in the cardiopulmonary bypass tubing, (3) a dilutional coagulopathy from the combination of crystalloid priming volume and transfusions, (4) a consumptive coagulopathy from a low-grade activation of the clotting mechanism by the bypass pump oxygenator and tubing, and (5) abnormal fibrinolysis.

Treatment of coagulopathy is urgent. Hypothermia should be corrected and extra protamine should be given until the activated clotting time returns to normal or until no further drop is seen in the activated clotting time. If abnormal bleeding persists, transfusion of platelets, fresh frozen plasma, and cryoprecipitate are given until the clotting deficit is corrected. Epsilon aminocaproic acid (Amicar) may be given to correct fibrinolysis. Recent advances used to minimize coagulopathy in high-risk cases include the use of heparin-bonded pump tubing, preoperative administration of Amicar to prevent fibrinolysis, improved pump oxygenators, less dependence on systemic hypothermia, and possibly the use of aprotinin.

Cardiac tamponade is a serious complication following cardiac surgery. It may occur early postoperatively from the accumulation of intrapericardial blood or less commonly from myocardial edema with pericardial constriction. Later, tamponade can occur from a pericardial effusion. The classic findings of tamponade include (1) elevation of central venous pressure; (2) equalization of central venous pressure, pulmonary artery diastolic pressure, and left atrial pressure; and (3) a pulsus paradoxus of more than 10 mmHg during inspiration. Extreme cases of tamponade may present with life-threatening hypotension, and the diagnosis should be strongly considered in any patient with hypotension and a low cardiac output. A widening of the mediastinal shadow on chest x-ray or a detection of significant pericardial effusion by echocardiography are suggestive of the diagnosis. No single test can exclude tamponade short of surgical exploration. Because of this, any patient with suspected tamponade should be promptly returned to the operating room for definitive diagnosis and treatment.

Ventilatory and Pulmonary Insufficiency. With current pump oxygenators, significant impairment of pulmonary function is uncommon except in patients with severe preexisting pulmonary disease or advanced cardiac failure. The simplest numerical expression of the pulmonary dysfunction is the alveolar-arterial oxygen gradient, representing impaired diffusion of oxygen from the alveoli into the pulmonary venous blood.

Ventilation through an indwelling endotracheal tube for 24 to 72 h is adequate for many patients. If longer periods of ventilation are anticipated, a cricothyroidotomy or tracheostomy should be performed, although some patients may tolerate an indwelling endotracheal tube for several days. Removal of pulmonary secretions, however, a major cause of pulmonary infection, is done much better through a tracheostomy or cricothyroidotomy. Ventilatory support for more than a short time is seldom necessary except in chronically ill elderly patients in whom simple physical weakness may significantly impair the effectiveness of breathing and coughing. Such patients may require ventilatory support for days or even weeks.

While ventilating a patient after heart surgery, the physician should periodically assess the breath sounds, particularly in the posterior bases of the lungs to determine the adequacy of ventilation. Tidal volumes on the respirator are usually set at 10 mL/kg, but occasionally up to 15 mL/kg is necessary in patients with chronic obstructive disease. For most cases, auscultation of the bases and determination of lung compliance (static lung compliance = tidal volume/end inspiratory pressure) are the best ways to determine the optimal tidal volume, with the maxium lung compliance considered optimal compliance for most cases. The adequacy of ventilation and oxygenation is then checked by periodic blood gas determinations. For difficult patients with marginal oxygenation the optimal tidal volume and positive end-expiratory pressure (PEEP) may be better determined on the basis of oxygen delivery, with oxygen delivery equal to cardiac output times arterial oxygen content.

Weaning the patient is done via the intermittent mandatory ventilation (IMV) mode or via progressive continuous positive airway pressure (CPAP) trials. Criteria for extubation include adequate blood gases on CPAP, with an inspired oxygen of less than 50 percent, a respiratory rate of less than 15 to 20 breaths/min, a spontaneous tidal volume of 5 mL/kg, a forced vital capacity of 10 mL/kg, and a negative inspiratory pressure of 15 mL of water as determined by bedside pulmonary function tests. The patient should be awake enough to control the airway.

Postextubation pulmonary care involves use of the incentive spirometer, coughing, and deep breathing. Control of secretions is essential. Difficult cases might require the use of inhaled bronchodilators, such as the β-2-adrenergic agonist albuterol, or use of intravenous aminophylline. Rarely a short course of steroids is beneficial. Tracheobronchitis should be promptly treated with antibiotics. We have found observation of daily sputum specimens to be the bedrock of effective respiratory therapy. Three bottles of sputum specimen should be left at the bedside for daily observation on rounds, serving as a colorimetric test to assess the thickness and quality of sputum. Clearing of secretions by coughing or suctioning is essential if the patient with tracheobronchitis is to recover. Periodic flexible bronchoscopy has been effective in assessing the adequacy of suction and for evaluating the clearance of secretions in the refractory ventilator-dependent patient with tracheobronchitis.

Operation on the patient with a long smoking history and chronic obstructive pulmonary disease poses a special problem. These patients should be strongly counseled on the need to stop smoking preoperatively, with the aid of transdermal nicotine patches if necessary. Evidence suggests that discontinuing smoking for even 1 week is markedly beneficial. Poor pulmonary function, however, usually does not prohibit cardiac surgery. For example, if a patient can function, albeit poorly, with poor pulmonary reserve and critical aortic stenosis, the patient's overall cardiorespiratory function should significantly improve after correction of the valvular pathology. Fortunately, sternotomy has relatively little deleterious effect on pulmonary reserve. A recent study by Bevelaqua and associates noted that heart patients with bad pulmonary function studies had more short-term postoperative pulmonary complications than normal patients, but the hospital mortality was not increased.

General Care. ***Nutrition.*** The need for adequate postoperative nutrition cannot be overemphasized, particularly in elderly or chronically ill patients. The sick postoperative heart patient may require approximately 35 kcal/kg/day. Care should be taken to give adequate protein in patients with normal renal and hepatic function, while special formulas are available for patients with kidney or liver failure. Ill patients who remain intubated in the intensive care unit should have nutritional support started early, either as tube feeding or as intravenous hyperalimentation.

Wound Care. Early postoperative care of the surgical wound consists of the use of a sterile occlusive dressing for the first 24 h. Wounds may be painted twice a day with a povidone-iodine solution or dressed steriley, and examined daily for redness, drainage, or sternal instability. Prophylactic antibiotics are started preoperatively and continued for 24 to 48 h postoperatively, usually until indwelling catheters and chest tubes are removed. The prophylactic antibiotic used should be chosen based on the common organisms causing infection in the hospital.

All fever should be duly recorded and the patient examined for signs of infection. A moderate fever of 100 to 101°F, however, is common in the first 1 to 2 days, usually from inflammatory blood products released during cardiopulmonary bypass and from atelectasis. A fever occurring from 3 to 7 days with a normal white blood cell count might be due to pericardiotomy syndrome. This syndrome is due to irritation of the pericardium from surgical trauma and may be associated with a friction rub, and pericardial or pleural effusions. Postpericardiotomy syndrome can be treated with an anti-inflammatory agent such as ibuprofen, or occasionally prednisone. Significant fevers should be evaluated with a chest x-ray and with blood and urine cultures.

A serious sternal wound infection occurs in 1 to 2 percent of all open heart operations. The incidence is highest in diabetics, especially in diabetics receiving bilateral internal mammary artery grafts. Signs of infection include redness or pain in the wound, purulent drainage, sternal instability, fever, and an elevated white blood cell count. The diagnosis is easily made by sternal aspiration. Early diagnostic sternal aspiration is strongly recommended for any patient with persistent localized sternal pain or unexplained sepsis. Treatment requires prompt operation with either debridement and closure over antibiotic drainage catheters or debridement and open treatment, followed by closure with muscle flaps. The mortality rate from a sternal infection after cardiac surgery is 15 to 25 percent.

Renal Function. Close attention to renal function is necessary. The urine output for most adults should be close to 1 mL/kg/h. The BUN and creatinine are followed for several days postoperatively. Patients with a marginal urine output or with borderline renal function may benefit from low-dose (3 mg/kg/min) dopamine. Some degree of salt and fluid retention is often present during postoperative days 3 to 5, even in patients with normal renal function, and diuretics may be necessary until the patients return to their preoperative weight. In patients with progressive renal dysfunction early dialysis is indicated to control volume overload and to minimize the risk of arrhythmias and infection. Permitting the BUN to rise above 90 to 100 may result in serious cardiac arrhythmias and in immunocompromise. The mortality rate for patients with anuric renal failure after heart surgery exceeds 25 to 50 percent.

Rehabilitation. Since most patients recover uneventfully after heart surgery, a rigorous rehabilitation program is generally unnecessary. Recommendations include daily walking in the halls and a progressive walking schedule of up to 2 mi/day after discharge. The patient should follow normal moderate activities for the first 6 to 8 weeks. More vigorous exercise should be preceded by an exercise stress test, which is recommended after 2 to 3 months, since this amount of time is required before the patient is recovered physically and intellectually. Elderly and debilitated patients should receive a more regimented rehabilitation effort, beginning with physical therapy during the hospital stay and often continuing with a formalized rehabilitation program for the first 2 to 3 weeks after discharge.

CARDIAC ARREST

Cardiac arrest and ventricular fibrillation produce immediate cessation of the circulation. An injury causing generalized cardiac depression, such as anoxia, is more likely to lead to cardiac arrest, while drugs or ischemia that increase myocardial irritability are more likely to produce ventricular fibrillation. Diagnosis and treatment of the two conditions are, however, very similar.

Etiology. Five frequent causes of cardiac arrest of fibrillation that should be routinely considered in the differential diagnosis are coronary occlusion, anoxia, electrolyte abnormalities, drugs, and arrhythmias.

Coronary Occlusion. Coronary disease is present in the majority of patients. An acute myocardial infarction is a common cause of ventricular fibrillation. When chronic coronary disease has produced significant ventricular scarring, cardiac arrhythmias may precipitate ventricular fibrillation in the absence of acute infarction. This is particularly common in patients with ischemic myopathy and in those with ventricular aneurysms.

Anoxia. Sustained anoxia may lead to ventricular fibrillation or bradycardic arrest, both from the low arterial oxygen tension as well as the progressive metabolic acidosis that results. Inadequate ventilation from pneumothorax, from dislodgement of the endotracheal tube, or aspiration of gastric contents or a foreign body are common causes.

Electrolyte Abnormalities. Either a deficiency or an excess of potassium can cause cardiac arrest or fibrillation. A serum potassium below 3.0 meq or above 6.0 meq can be harmful, though the precise influence is determined by the coexisting concentration of calcium ions and the presence of acidosis or alkalosis.

Drugs. Several drugs may induce ventricular fibrillation or cardiac arrest, either from excessive amounts or from an abnormal sensitivity. Digitalis is one of the most frequent of this group because of its widespread usage. The sensitivity of the myocardium to digitalis varies with a number of factors, one of the most important of which is the concentration of potassium. Procainamide and quinidine are examples of drugs with known proarrhythmic effects.

Arrhythmias. A profound bradycardia, with a heart rate below 60 beats/min, may result in ventricular fibrillation or cardiac asystoli. This frequently occurs in patients with complete heart block. Ventricular arrhythmias from any cause may progress to bigeminy, ventricular tachycardia, and fibrillation. This well-known sequence is the reason for constant visual monitoring of the electrocardiogram in a cardiac postoperative unit.

Diagnosis. The cerebral anoxia following circulatory arrest produces brain injury within 3 to 4 min, so the diagnosis must be made and treatment begun rapidly to avoid serious brain injury. Periods of anoxia for 6 to 8 min may produce extensive but reversible brain injury whereas longer periods regularly cause irreversible injury. When the diagnosis of ventricular fibrillation or cardiac arrest is considered, it should either be excluded within 30 to 60 s or treatment should be begun.

In most patients the diagnosis can be simply made. Loss of consciousness occurs within seconds, as well as absence of respiratory activity except for a few agonal gasps. The rapidity of loss of consciousness is awesome. Abruptly, without a sound or any other warning, the patient simply collapses. This is the reason alarm systems are essential in a busy intensive care unit, for otherwise cardiac arrest may not be recognized unless the patient is under direct visual observation. All peripheral pulses are absent, most easily confirmed by palpation of the femoral or carotid arteries. No cardiac sounds can be heard on auscultation of the chest.

Closed-chest massage should be started promptly, within 1 min (Fig. 18-3). The main value of the electrocardiogram is to demonstrate ventricular fibrillation, as opposed to asystole or ventricular tachycardia.

The most common differential diagnosis from cardiac arrest is extreme bradycardia with hypotension, as in someone who has fainted or developed anaphylactic shock from a hypersensitivity syndrome. In such patients, though unconscious, there is slight respiratory activity and cardiac sounds are usually audible.

Treatment. ***Ventilation.*** The immediate first step in treatment is to provide adequate oxygenation. Cardiac massage for more than a few seconds without ventilation of the lungs is futile. Ventilation is most quickly accomplished by mask inflation of the lungs. This can be begun immediately and continued until equipment for an oral airway or endotracheal intubation is obtained. With a laryngoscope, an endotracheal tube can easily be inserted readily by a physician or other trained personnel. In some patients, as in those with a short, thick neck, the anatomy is such that intubation is difficult, at times almost impossible by highly experienced staff. Unless intubation can be accomplished quickly and with certainty, oral insufflation should be continued until a cricothyroidotomy has been performed. In these circumstances a cricothyroidotomy is far simpler than a tracheostomy and equally satisfactory.

An infrequent but serious error can occur when the endotracheal tube is inadvertently placed in the esophagus. Because of this immediate auscultation of the lungs for breath sounds is essential after attempted intubation. If any uncertainty exists after brief auscultation of the lungs, a cricothyroidotomy should be done. A tightly fitting face mask can provide a method of temporary ventilation.

Cardiac Massage. The effectiveness of closed-chest massage probably depends upon intermittent compression of the heart between the sternum and the vertebral column, with lateral motion of the heart limited by the pericardium. The patient must be on a firm surface, usually done by placing a board behind the back. The heel of the hand should be applied over the *lower third* of the sternum with the other hand above it to depress the sternum intermittently for 3 to 4 cm (see Fig. 18-3*A*). The sternal compression should be brisk, depressing the sternum sharply and then releasing it to permit cardiac filling. Mechanical ventilation must be synchronized with massage.

Compression of the sternum near the xiphoid process may injure the liver; compression over the upper sternum or laterally over the chest wall may produce multiple fractures of the ribs. Massage should be at a rate of about 60/min; more than one person is required since the persons performing massage will fatigue quickly.

The amount of force applied should be judged by palpation of a peripheral pulse, usually the femoral. Caution is required to be certain that a regurgitant pulse in the femoral vein is not confused with a pulse in the femoral artery, for a strong retrograde pulse wave may be propagated down the vena cava during massage.

The influence of technique on effectiveness of massage can be easily judged when intraarterial pressure is visually displayed on an oscilloscope. Small adjustments in the technique of massage may change systolic blood pressure 40 to 60 mmHg.

If cerebral function is probably intact, massage should be continued as long as significant cardiac activity is present. Cardiac massage is seldom successful after about 15 min.

Retrospective analyses comparing patients who were and were not successfully resuscitated usually find certain basic differences. Patients successfully resuscitated usually have an electrical failure, such as fibrillation or severe bradycardia, as opposed to a "power" failure from inherent myocardial injury, as with a massive infarction or terminal cardiac failure with anoxia and acidosis. In successfully resuscitated patients, resuscitation is started almost immediately.

Such observations characterize episodes of cardiac arrest from easily reversible causes, as opposed to those secondary to severe myocardial injury. A separate question is whether open-chest massage, mechanically more effective, should be instituted earlier. This is commonly done in the postoperative cardiac patient if closed-chest massage does not produce an adequate blood pressure, because the surgical incision can be quickly reopened and tamponade or intrathoracic hemorrhage recognized. Clearly open cardiac massage is far more effective if instituted promptly. Rarely, open-chest massage may be effectively continued for

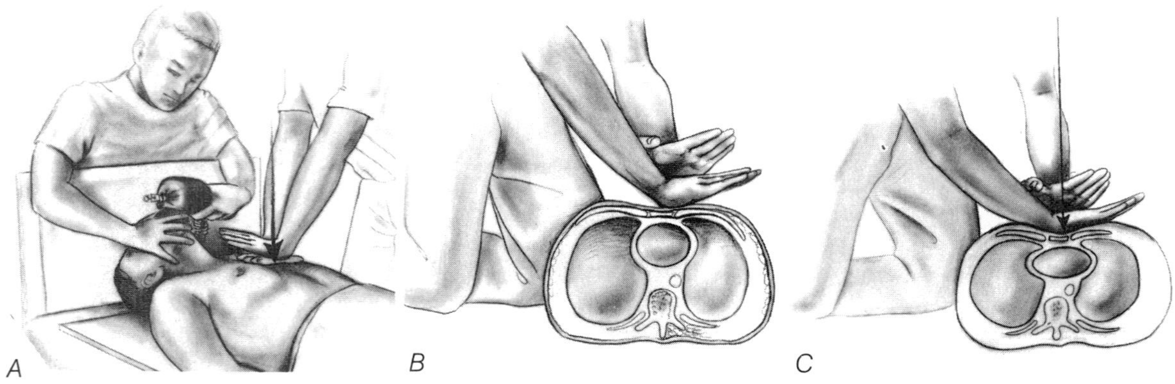

FIG. 18-3. *A.* Close-chest massage. The heel of the hand should be used to compress intermittently the lower portion of the sternum toward the vertebral column. The effectiveness of the compression should be monitored by palpation of a peripheral pulse by another member of the team. Artificial ventilation must be performed at the same time. *B.* Cross-section of the chest showing the anatomic basis for close-chest massage. The heart is seen suspended in the midthorax between the sternum anteriorly and the vertebral column posteriorly. *C.* Compression of the heart as the sternum is depressed downward toward the vertebral column.

hours until the basic condition causing refractory fibrillation or arrest is corrected. The patient is generally returned to the operating room once the chest is opened. If signs of cardiac activity are present, cardiopulmonary bypass is promptly initiated for support.

Drugs and Fluids. Epinephrine, sodium bicarbonate, and calcium are the most useful agents. The protocols suggested by the advanced cardiac life support (ACLS) program are followed. Lidocaine is given primarily for ventricular arrhythmias, followed by procainamide and then bretyllium. Medications are usually ineffective, however, if severe myocardial anoxia is present. Anoxia can be corrected only by the combination of effective cardiac massage and ventilation. Excessive use of drugs before this has been accomplished is probably a futile diversion.

Epinephrine, 1 to 2 mL of 1:10,000 dilution, may be given intravenously or alternately by direct intracardiac injection. Calcium, 3 to 4 mL of a 10% solution, is another powerful stimulant of myocardial contraction. Calcium administration in cardiac arrest may be valuable in some circumstances, harmful in others, and should not be used indiscriminately. Acidosis is usually present and may require intensive therapy to restore a normal pH. Large amounts of sodium bicarbonate may be required. Resuscitation is usually ineffective with a significant acidosis.

Small amounts of fluid should be rapidly infused, for vasodilatation is usually present. An intravenous infusion of a vasoconstrictor, norepinephrine or aramine, is often helpful as well.

Arterial and venous blood gas tension should be serially measured at 5- to 10-min intervals as soon as possible because acidosis invariably recurs with the low cardiac outputs produced by closed-chest massage.

Defibrillation. Ventricular fibrillation can be differentiated from cardiac arrest only by the electrocardiogram or by direct inspection of the myocardium. Initial treatment of cardiac arrest should include a precardial thump, because it is often effective in converting ventricular tachycardia or ventricular fibrillation. If this is not promptly effective and an electrocardiogram is not available, empiric defibrillation may be tried briefly because most resuscitations are effective when defibrillation is promptly done.

Closed-chest defibrillation is usually done by applying electrodes over the base and apex of the heart; an alternate method consists of placing one large electrode posteriorly near the vertebral column and a smaller one anteriorly near the cardiac apex. Defibrillation is best done with a direct current, about 400 J (see Fig. 18-3*B*).

With open-chest defibrillation, the electrodes are applied directly to the heart and an appropriate impulse delivered, usually 20 to 40 J. Unless a serious biochemical abnormality is present, such as hypokalemia or digitalis intoxication, the usual cause of failure to defibrillate is either an anoxic or an acidotic myocardium, or ineffective transmission of an electrical impulse through the myocardium. Vigorous cardiac massage should precede defibrillation to oxygenate the myocardium sufficiently. Perfusion pressure must be maintained to obtain successful defibrillation because ongoing subendocardiac ischemia occurs when the perfusion pressure is inadequate. Correction of acidosis with bicarbonate can be confirmed by blood-gas determinations. Intramyocardial injection of epinephrine may stimulate myocardial tone but should not be done until correction of anoxia and acidosis has been confirmed.

When the electric shock is applied through the electrodes compressing the heart, the myocardium should be observed closely. Adequate transmission of a current through the myocardium will stop all fibrillatory activity, though it may recur within a few seconds. If the fibrillatory activity was not momentarily stopped, enough current was not transmitted, from either inadequate voltage, inadequate electrodes, or inadequate application of the electrodes to the heart. Unless a myocardial infarction has occurred, it should be possible to defibrillate the majority of fibrillating hearts, though the ensuing cardiac arrest may be refractory to therapy. The most significant factor influencing survival is the institution of defibrillation within 1 min of onset of fibrillation or ability to defibrillate with less than five shocks.

Therapy Following Cardiac Resuscitation. Following restoration of an adequate heart beat and blood pressure, the critical question is the extent of injury to the heart and to the central nervous system. Significant brain injury is usually indicated by continuing coma. A detailed neurologic evaluation to elicit specific normal and abnormal reflexes should be done promptly. Permanent brain injury is frequent after more than 5 min of cardiac arrest, even though experimentally cerebral neurons can tolerate nearly 20 min of normothermic ischemic anoxia. Intravenous steroid therapy is usually given for 24 to 48 h to minimize cerebral edema. The efficacy is difficult to measure.

Continuous oscilloscopic monitoring of the cardiac rhythm is essential; arrhythmias are common, and fibrillation may recur. Continuous intravenous infusion of lidocaine or procainamide is useful for suppressing arrhythmias. Adequacy of cardiac function should be promptly determined and ventilation should be monitored by periodic blood-gas determination of arterial and central venous blood. Fluid therapy requires special care, for an adequate blood volume is needed for cardiac and renal function, but excessive fluids may intensify cerebral edema. Underlying causes, such as ischemia, electrolyte imbalance, or graft occlusion, should be promptly treated. Patients should eventually have a 24-h Holter monitor and most should undergo electrophysiologic stimulation (EPS) in the cardiac catheterization laboratory.

Prognosis. If serious cardiac or cerebral injury is not present following resuscitation, prognosis is excellent. This fact is the basis for the enthusiastic development of widespread training in cardiopulmonary resuscitation by all physicians, paramedical personnel, and laypeople, for most effective resuscitation is accomplished when begun within 1 to 2 min after onset of cardiac arrest.

Careful study of patients who survive cardiac arrest subsequently discharged from the hospital has found a sobering recurrence of cardiac arrest within 1 to 3 years, a frequency of 30 to 40 percent or higher. Because of this EPS guided therapy is essential when cardiac arrest occurs secondary to arrhythmias. Survival is significantly greater in patients in whom medical or surgical therapy prevents the induction of a sustained arrhythmia (see sections below on arrhythmia surgery and implantable defibrillators).

CORONARY ARTERY DISEASE

Historical Data. Starting in the late 1930s, different investigators attempted to increase the blood supply of the ischemic heart by developing collateral circulation with vascular adhesions. Beck was the leading investigator, trying different methods for many years, but ultimately all failed.

A separate ingenious concept arose in 1946 when Vineberg developed implantation of the internal mammary artery into a tunnel in the myocardium. This was applied clinically by Vineberg in 1950 and continued for many years. For unknown reasons, the artery remains patent in well over 90 percent of patients, but the amount of flow through the patent artery is distressingly small, often as little as 5 to 10 mL/min. An occasional patient has been reported in whom the implanted artery was of substantial benefit, carrying as much as 50 mL of blood per minute, but these fortunate results were infrequent. For this reason, the procedure has been virtually abandoned.

Attempts at endarterectomy without bypass grafting have been made sporadically since 1956 when this was attempted by Longmire, but late patency rates were prohibitively low, probably from progressive fibrosis in the arterial wall. Similarly Effler and colleagues at the Cleveland Clinic attempted patch graft reconstruction of coronary arteries in the early 1960s, a procedure proposed by Senning in 1961. In recent years some groups have reinvestigated the concept of the combination of endarterectomy with bypass.

Currently over 200,000 bypass procedures are performed annually in the United States. It is estimated that at least 6 million patients in this country have known coronary artery disease.

The development of the bypass operation for coronary occlusive disease between 1967 and 1968 was a dramatic milestone. For the first time it was possible to increase immediately the blood flow to the myocardium. Most of the basic clinical investigations evolved from studies in three centers in the United States during this time. Favalaro and associates from the Cleveland Clinic began using longer and longer segments of saphenous vein to bypass occlusive disease in the right coronary artery, eventually interposing grafts between the aorta proximally and the termination of the right coronary distally. Johnson and associates, in 1969, showed that similar grafts could be effectively used for the left coronary artery. This was a quantum achievement. Previously, direct operative procedures upon the left coronary artery had a prohibitive mortality. Green, following extensive experimental studies by others, anastomosed the left internal mammary artery to the anterior descending, using an operative microscope. The internal mammary was not widely used for over a decade but since 1980 has been widely adopted and is now used in the majority of bypass operations. This change resulted from 10-year angiographic studies that found excellent patency rates of internal mammary grafts, 90 to 95 percent, compared with 10-year patency rates of 50 to 60 percent with saphenous vein grafts. In recent years the trend has been to perform bypass in older patients and in those with more advanced disease, with transluminal angioplasty often used as the initial intervention in patients with less severe disease (see Indications).

Etiology and Pathogenesis. Atherosclerosis is the fundamental cause of coronary artery disease (see above section, Medical Therapy—Coronary Artery Disease). The disease is multifactorial, involving cholesterol metabolism, serum lipids, and possibly local tissue growth factors such as platelet derived growth factor, basic fibroblast growth factor, and others. It is a common disease in the Caucasian male throughout the world, involving males about four times as frequently as females. The frequency varies widely throughout the world, being less common in populations where the average blood cholesterol is less than 200. The frequency is the lowest in Japan, where the average blood cholesterol is near 160 mg/100 mL. The United States has the second highest frequency in the world.

The basic lesion is a segmental atherosclerotic plaque, often localized within the first 5 cm of the origin of the coronary artery from the aorta. Involvement of small distal vessels is usually less extensive; arterioles and intramyocardial vessels are usually free of disease. This segmental localization makes bypass grafts possible. Among the three major coronary arteries, the proximal anterior descending is frequently stenosed or occluded, with the distal half of the artery remaining patent. The right coronary is often stenotic or occluded throughout its course, but almost always the posterior descending and left atrial-ventricular groove branches are patent. The circumflex is often diseased proximally, but one or more distal marginal branches are usually patent.

The popular terminology, single, double, or triple vessel disease, refers, of course, to the number of coronary arteries involved. In over 50 percent of patients, ''triple'' vessel disease is present.

Clinical Manifestations. The myocardial ischemia produced by coronary disease can produce several serious events: angina pectoris, myocardial infarction, congestive heart failure, or sudden death. Angina is the most frequent symptom, but unfortunately myocardial infarction or sudden death may appear without warning. Congestive heart failure usually results as a sequela of myocardial infarction, with significant muscular injury resulting in ischemic myopathy.

Angina pectoris, the most common manifestation, is demonstrated by periodic discomfort, usually substernal, typically appearing with exertion, after eating, or with extreme emotion. Characteristically these symptoms subside within 3 to 5 min or may be dramatically relieved by sublingual nitroglycerin. In about 25 percent of patients, the symptoms are not typical and may radiate to bizarre areas, such as the teeth, the shoulder, or the epigastrium. Establishing a diagnosis of angina in these patients is difficult, perhaps impossible without diagnostic studies. Physical examination is usually normal. Differential diagnosis includes anxiety states, musculoskeletal disorders, and reflux esophagitis or esophageal spasm.

The risk of sudden death varies with the extent of disease and the degree of impairment of ventricular function. It ranges from 2 percent to as high as 10 percent. Death apparently results from ventricular fibrillation in many cases, or from myocardial infarction with acute decompensation.

Myocardial infarction is the most common serious complication. At least 1.5 million infarcts occur in the United States annually as noted in the above section on medical therapy. With modern therapy, mortality is near 7 to 8 percent. Most deaths occur in the first 30 to 60 min after the onset of symptoms, before the patient ever reaches a hospital. With modern treatment in coronary care units, the fatality rate is small.

In a small percentage of patients congestive heart failure eventually develops, resulting from multiple infarctions that ultimately destroy over 40 percent of the left ventricular muscle mass. Often the origin is puzzling. Some patients have had angina for years, with one or more infarctions, but others have been almost asymptomatic for over a decade after a small infarction first established the presence of coronary disease. Despite the paucity of symptoms, ischemic infarction of muscle apparently steadily but ''silently'' progressed. The frequency, diagnosis, and treatment of so-called silent ischemia is currently one of the most active areas in cardiology, where early detection by digital ECG monitoring or stress thallium test is now feasible. Other patients, by contrast, undergo rapid destruction of ventricular function within 2 to 3 years. Multiple small infarctions is the probable mechanism.

With chronic congestive failure, manifested by high intracardiac pressures, the outlook is ominous, for there is insufficient left ventricular muscle to provide adequate cardiac output. Most patients die within 1 to 2 years. Bypass grafting may be futile in such circumstances unless reversible ishemia can be demonstrated on PET scan or thallium scan, or unless there is a large ventricular aneurysm present that can be excised. Cardiac transplantation is now often used in this group of patients with far advanced disease.

Laboratory Studies. The chest x-ray is usually normal, and the electrocardiogram is normal at rest in about 70 percent of patients. Coronary arteriography remains the cornerstone of evaluation, for it outlines both the location and severity of the disease and the degree of impairment of ventricular function. The number of vessels diseased, the location of proximal stenoses, and the ventricular function as measured by ejection fraction are the three most important prognostic indicators of the severity and prognosis with coronary disease.

"Angiographically significant" stenosis is considered present when the diameter is reduced by more than 70 percent, corresponding to a reduction in cross-sectional area greater than 90 percent; some groups use a more liberal indication, considering an angiographic reduction in diameter of 50 percent (equivalent to a 75 percent reduction in cross-sectional area) as significant.

Ventricular function is usually expressed as ejection fraction, considering the range of 0.50 to 0.70 as normal; 0.30 to 0.50 moderately depressed; and below 0.30, especially below 0.20, as severely depressed. An ejection fraction below 0.30 is usually associated with intermittent or chronic congestive heart failure. The long-term course of coronary disease is a balance between two opposing factors, the rate of progression of the atherosclerotic stenoses as balanced by the rate of development of collateral circulation. The ventricular function probably reflects the ability of the heart to develop sufficient collateral circulation to compensate for the arterial stenoses present. Collaterals develop in response to an "ischemic gradient," probably due to a chemical mediator or growth factor that stimulates vessel growth, but this ability varies widely; some patients with extensive triple vessel disease have normal ventricular function with well-developed coronary collaterals, while others with less severe disease have marked impairment in cardiac function and no collaterals.

When a ventriculogram is evaluated, the contraction of individual segments of ventricular wall is separately analyzed, i.e., regional wall motion. Segmental wall motion is classified as normal, hypokinetic (impaired), akinetic (little or no visible contraction), or dyskinetic (paradoxical contraction, as with a left ventricular aneurysm).

Although angiography and ventriculography are the most precise methods for evaluating coronary disease, several limitations of the technique should also be emphasized, for erroneous decisions can easily be made.

An angiogram indicates the severity and complexity of the disease but is seldom, if ever, a reliable guide to state that a patient is "inoperable" because of the diffuse disease present and the small size of the vessels. With the ability to graft vessels as small as 1 mm, combined with endarterectomy when necessary, bypass grafts can virtually always be inserted even though the degree of improvement may be only moderate.

It is also a serious error to conclude from the ventriculogram that a diseased artery supplying an akinetic or dyskinetic area should not be bypassed because that segment of the ventricle is "scar." At operation such areas virtually always contain a significant percentage of viable muscle, estimated to range from 20 to 80 percent. Often improved contractility can be seen following bypass. Newer studies such as the PET scan may be valuable in predicting the response of "apparently nonviable" myocardium to revascularization. The stress thallium test may also be helpful.

The ventriculogram should not be used to conclude that a patient is "inoperable" because of severe impairment of ventricular function, though ejection fraction may be less than 20 percent and end-diastolic pressure above 30 mm. This represents an advanced stage of disease with a grim prognosis, but criteria for operation depend upon the clinical condition of the patient, whether congestive failure is intermittent or chronic, whether angina is present, whether reversible ischemia is demonstrable by other tests, and whether chronic right heart failure is present, reflected by a right atrial pressure near 15 mm or higher, and hepatomegaly.

Coronary Bypass Indications. The clinical status of the patient with coronary disease is usually in one of five groups: asymptomatic—mild angina, chronic moderate—severe angina, unstable angina, acute myocardial infarction, and postinfarction angina.

Asymptomatic-Mild Angina. This includes patients with angiographically significant coronary artery disease but with minimal symptoms and is a common clinical problem. Usually the coronary artery disease was detected because of mild angina or because of a positive stress test. Since angina is not severe, revascularization to improve symptoms or quality of life is not an issue. The key question in these patients is, "Will survival be improved by revascularization?" Three historical randomized studies have attempted to answer this question.

1. *The Veterans Administration Cooperative Study.* This study involved 668 males treated between 1972 and 1974. The study demonstrated improved long-term survival in patients with left main disease treated with surgical therapy. Since this trial, most patients with significant left main disease have been treated with coronary bypass revascularization regardless of their symptoms because of the survival advantage shown.
2. *The European Coronary Surgery Study Group.* This study (1973–1976) randomized men under 65 years of age, 57 percent with mild angina and 42 percent with moderate angina, into medical or surgical therapy. Equal survival was seen in patients with single vessel disease. In patients with double vessel disease in which a proximal anterior descending lesion was present and in patients with triple vessel disease, a long-term survival advantage was seen in patients treated surgically. The study recommended initial surgery for patients with triple vessel coronary disease and for patients with double vessel disease and a proximal anterior descending lesion.
3. *Coronary Artery Surgery Study (CASS).* This multicenter study was done in the United States between 1975 and 1979, randomizing initial treatment for patients with mild angina and operable coronary disease. Patients treated medically could be crossed over to surgery at the discretion of the cardiologist for worsening angina. After 10 years, results suggested that survival was improved by surgery in patients with triple vessel disease when cardiac function was depressed. No survival advantage was demonstrated from early surgery in patients with single, double, or triple vessel disease when ventricular function was normal. Of note, survival was calculated on initial intent for treatment, and a significant number of patients initially treated medically eventually had surgery. For example 38 percent of those with triple vessel disease treated medically eventually required operation. Initial surgical treatment was recommended for patients with triple vessel disease and depressed ventricular function, regardless of symptoms. From these data patients with minimal symptoms and good ventricular function can be safely treated medically, as long as surgery is recommended promptly when symptoms progress.

Other nonrandomized trials and studies involving the overall CASS registry (of both randomized and nonrandomized patients) have suggested that surgical intervention might improve survival and event-free interval in other patients with triple vessel disease. Similarly, studies have suggested that patients with double or triple vessel disease who become ischemic at a low cardiac work load during stress test have a bad prognosis with medical therapy, and these patients might benefit from early surgical intervention.

In summary, most patients with mild angina do well with initial medical therapy. Coronary artery bypass results in improved survival in patients with left main disease and in patients with triple vessel disease and depressed left ventricular function. Bypass operation is recommended in these patients regardless of symptoms. Some patients with triple vessel disease and good ventricular function and some patients with double vessel disease who have a proximal anterior descending lesion may do better with surgical therapy, especially if they have easily inducible ischemia on stress testing. The proper role of angioplasty in the mildly symptomatic patient with single or double vessel disease remains to be determined, but no convincing survival advantage has yet been demonstrated by this procedure. Angioplasty should probably be reserved for symptomatic patients or for those with easily inducible ischemia and isolated, discrete coronary lesions.

Chronic Moderate-Severe Angina. There is uniform agreement that patients with moderate to severe angina, not responding to medical therapy, should undergo revascularization. Currently the mode of revascularization, angioplasty, or surgical coronary bypass depends on the anatomy of the coronary stenosis. Most patients with moderate to severe symptoms and single vessel coronary disease are treated by percutaneous transluminal angioplasty if medical therapy is unsuccessful. Occasionally patients with proximal anterior descending lesions receive bypass grafting with a mammary artery. Most patients with significant symptoms and triple vessel disease undergo coronary artery bypass. Symptomatic patients with double vessel disease and a proximal anterior descending lesion frequently receive surgical therapy, while other combinations of double vessel disease receive angioplasty. The choice of interventional treatment is influenced, of course, by the patient's age and associated risk factors, as well as by the experience of the surgical-interventional teams.

Unstable Angina. "Acute coronary insufficiency" exists when angina is persistent or rapidly progressive and does not respond to therapy with nitroglycerin and other nitrates. It apparently is an acute physiologic state in which the blood flow to a segment of myocardium is seriously jeopardized but necrosis has not yet occurred. It probably arises from a sudden decrease in regional blood flow, usually from thrombus, spasm, or elevation of a plaque. Virtually everyone agrees that the condition is a medical emergency. The patient should be promptly hospitalized in a coronary care unit and managed as outlined earlier under the section on Medical Therapy. If collateral blood flow increases and compensates for the ischemia, manifested by subsidence of the angina, recovery is prompt. Otherwise, acute infarction or death can occur. Cardiac catheterization should be performed promptly in all patients with unstable angina. Patients found to have mild disease can sometimes be managed medically. Most patients require revascularization with angioplasty or coronary bypass based on the anatomy as described above. Untreated patients with unstable angina have a high frequency of infarction or death, hence the term "preinfarction angina."

Acute Infarction. Treatment of myocardial infarction was described in the section on Medical Therapy. Indications for surgical therapy after acute infarction include subendocardial infarction, hemodynamic instability, or postinfarction angina in patients who have left main disease, triple vessel disease, or anatomy unsuitable for angioplasty. Cardiogenic shock after myocardial infarction is usually an indication for emergency angioplasty or coronary bypass since complete revascularization of the noninfarcted zones of the heart is necessary for survival. Mechanical complications of myocardial infarction, such as myocardial rupture, acute ventricular septal defect, and ruptured papillary muscle with acute mitral insufficiency, are indications for surgical intervention since survival is unlikely unless these lesions are promptly repaired. Most stable patients with a myocardial infarction now undergo a stress test either before discharge or at 6 weeks. Cardiac catheterization is done if the stress test is positive. Coronary bypass may be recommended if left main or triple vessel disease is present, and in some cases where proximal anterior descending lesions are found and angioplasty is not advisable.

Congestive Heart Failure. The only absolute contraindication to coronary bypass operation at the author's institution is chronic congestive failure with pulmonary hypertension, a right atrial pressure above 15 mm, hepatomegaly, and no signs of angina or inducible ischemia with the thallium or PET scan. The unfortunate patient in this group usually has already necrosed the majority of the left ventricular muscle, so cardiac transplantation is the only therapy likely to be helpful.

Intermittent congestive failure, manifested by intermittent episodes of pulmonary edema, is not a *contraindication* to operation but actually a strong *indication for immediate operation*. This indicates a serious degree of myocardial ischemia that can easily progress to an irreversible stage or death. The intermittent episodes probably evolve from an acute ischemic episode that elevates end-diastolic pressure sufficiently to produce pulmonary edema. Such patients have been regularly operated on with continuing good long-term results.

A severe depression of ejection fraction to the range of 0.20 to 0.25, or lower, is still erroneously considered a contraindication to bypass, though contrary experiences have been published by several groups. The erroneous concept probably arose from previous experiences with ineffective myocardial preservation that produced some degree of infarction during operation. Jones and associates reported experiences with 188 patients with an ejection fraction below 0.35, about 24 percent of whom had ejection fraction lower than 0.20. Operative mortality was only 2.1 percent.

Pigott and Kouchoukos reported results for 192 patients with an ejection fraction less than 35 percent. Seventy-seven were operated on; 115 were treated medically. Seven-year actuarial survival was 63 percent in the surgical group, 34 percent in the medical group. Recurrent infarction developed in 19 percent of the medical group as compared with 7 percent of the surgical group.

A recent study from our institution reported by Slater and associates evaluated results after bypass operation in 157 patients with severely impaired left ventricular function. Angina was present in 55 percent, but severe congestive heart failure was the predominant symptom in 24 percent. The overall operative mortality rate was 7 percent, and cumulative 4-year survival rate was 67 percent. While congestive heart failure and pulmonary hypertension had a negative impact on long-term survival, 4-year survival was still 49 percent in patients with severe congestive heart failure and pulmonary hypertension, a group that many centers treat by cardiac transplantation.

Operative Technique. At New York University all procedures are performed with extracorporeal circulation and a perfusate temperature of near 30°C. The heart is arrested with the cold blood potassium technique. Cold blood is infused at an aortic root pressure of 70 to 90 mmHg or at a coronary sinus pressure of 20 to 30 mmHg. Retrograde administration of cardioplegia through the coronary sinus venous system has been a big advance in patients with severe disease as this technique avoids maldistribution of cardioplegia due to coronary artery stenosis. Cardioplegia distribution and myocardial cooling are confirmed by measuring regional myocardial temperatures in at least four regions of the myocardium, continuing infusion of cold blood until the ''warmest'' zone has cooled below 10 to 15°C. Topical hypothermia is then employed to prevent rewarming, both by pericardial lavage and by a continuous pericardial infusion of cold electrolyte solution. Blood cardioplegia is reinfused usually after each anastomosis, certainly after every 20 to 30 min. The left heart is decompressed, either by emptying the right heart with a large lumen cannula or with a catheter introduced through a pulmonary vein. Particular attention is given to periodic monitoring of right heart temperatures to be certain that reflux of blood from the cavae does not warm the right ventricle and septum. With this technique, the heart can be arrested for well over 2 to 3 h, even though this is rarely necessary. Experimentally this technique results in complete recovery of cardiac function after 2 h of protected cross clamp. Because of this and other similar techniques of myocardial protection, pump failure is now seldom seen after bypass operation and inotropes are used infrequently for routine cases. There is ample time for grafting all diseased vessels.

Saphenous veins of appropriate size (approximately 4.0 mm) are removed from the lower extremity, using the lesser saphenous or the cephalic veins if adequate greater saphenous veins are not available (Fig. 18-4). The left internal mammary artery is routinely used in the vast majority of patients, usually placed into the left anterior descending artery (Fig. 18-5*A*). In recent years, following the lead of others, bilateral mammary grafting has been employed with increasing frequency, usually in healthy, nondiabetic patients. With the heart arrested and cooled, bypass grafts are attached to all diseased coronary arteries, making a short arteriotomy and attaching the vein end to side with a continuous suture of 7-0 or 8-0 polypropylene. Three- to four-power optical magnification is routinely used. Internal mammary anastomoses are done with 8-0 polypropylene. Cold blood is routinely infused down each graft after it is constructed. When the aorta is unclamped, warm blood is perfused down the grafts until these are attached to the aorta. This is probably superfluous in many patients but seems quite important when serious ischemia is present, especially with left main coronary disease.

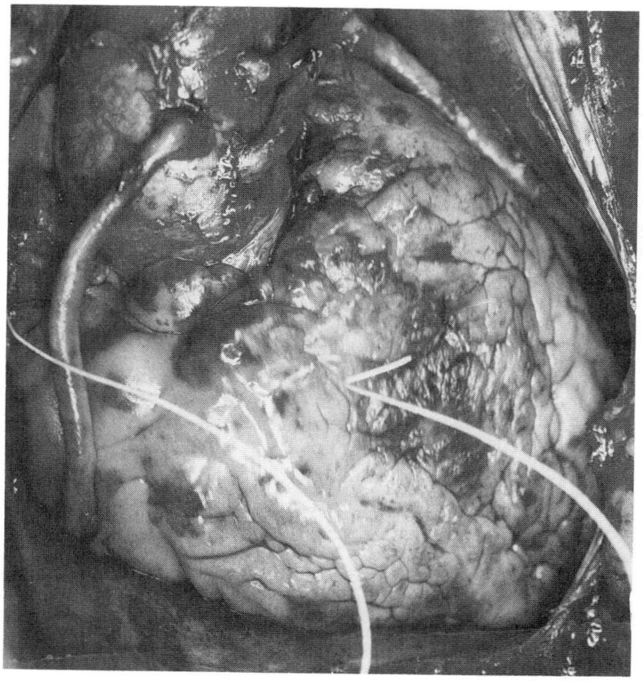

FIG. 18-4. Operative photograph of triple coronary bypass with reverse saphenous vein grafts.

An alternative is to attach several grafts to the aorta proximally before bypass is started and then serially construct the distal anastomoses. This is a simpler and more expeditious method that is used frequently at our institution, though it requires more judgment about the exact length of grafts. This technique allows immediate reperfusion of the heart once the cross clamp is removed. The usual number of anastomoses constructed varies between three and six. As many as nine to ten anastomoses have been constructed in a few patients with no measurable increase in operative mortality. Rarely is coronary endarterectomy necessary. In the authors' experience most patients with diffuse disease are better served with multiple grafts, even if only a part of the vessel has runoff.

Following bypass, flow rates are measured through the grafts with a flowmeter, finding a mean flow between 50 and 100 mL/min in most vessels with an adequate runoff.

Postoperative Management. Postoperative management was covered in detail in the section above. Care is initially given in the recovery room or intensive care unit, with the patient progressing to a monitored intermediate care unit and then to a regular room. Most uncomplicated patients are discharged from the hospital in 7 to 9 days.

Normal sedentary activity is gradually resumed over the next 6 to 8 weeks. After 2 to 3 months have passed, a stress test should be conducted before vigorous physical exercise is permitted. If significant arrhythmias were present preoperatively, these must be carefully monitored indefinitely because these are often not improved with bypass and are a fairly common cause of late death. In patients with normal ventricular function beforehand, after 3 months a full return to normal physical activity, with participation in physically active sports, is usually allowed.

Results. ***Operative Risk and Major Complications.*** Operative risk is very small, near 1 percent for the usual patient. Similar low-risk results have been reported by many experienced cardiac surgical groups throughout the world. Moderate impairment of ventricular function does not increase operative risk, though severe impairment of ventricular function, an ejection fraction less than 0.30, is a significant operative risk factor. Other variables increasing operative risk are cardiogenic shock or hemodynamic instability, emergency operation, preoperative renal failure, congestive heart failure, reoperation, peripheral vascular disease, age, hypertension, diabetes, female gender, left main disease, endarterectomy, and association valvular pathology.

With an uncomplicated operation, electrocardiographic signs of myocardial infarction develop in less than 3 percent of patients. With enzymatic studies, a somewhat higher frequency may be found, though inconsistencies often exist between the electrocardiographic findings and the enzymatic changes. It is rare for enzymatic changes to represent a significant physiologic problem if the patient is asymptomatic without hemodynamic or significant

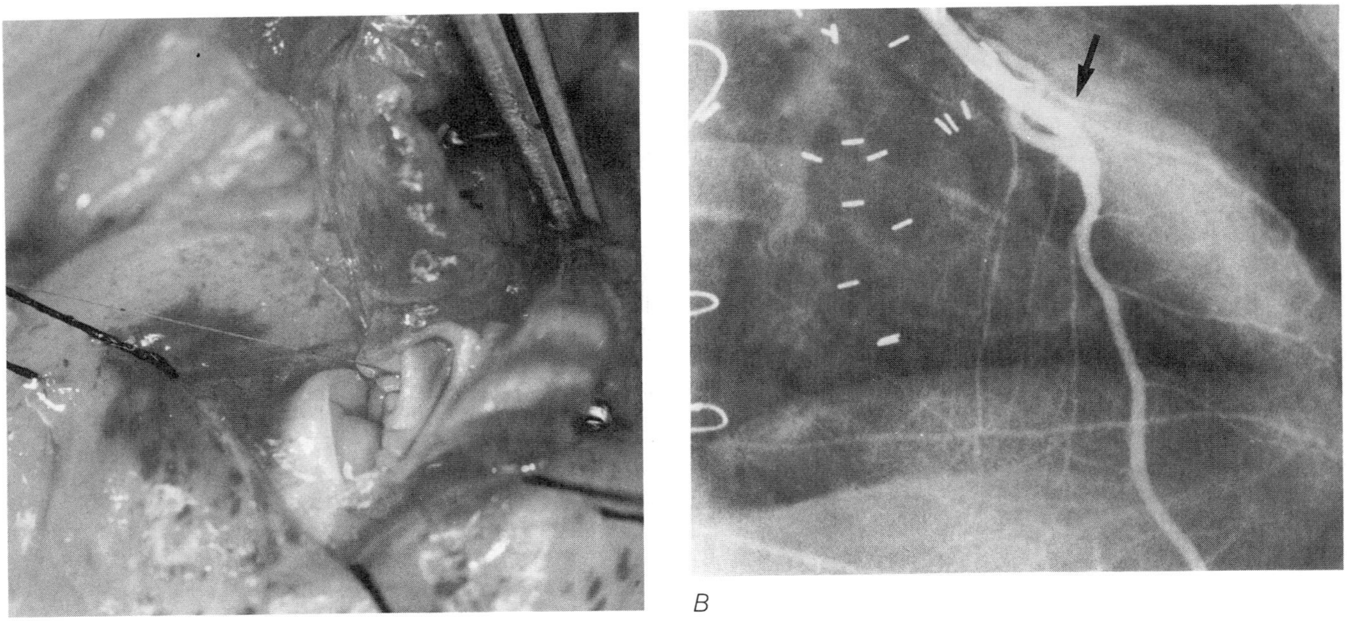

B

A

FIG. 18-5 *A.* Operative photograph of anastomosis between the left internal mammary artery and the left anterior descending artery, using optical magnification, microvascular technique, and continuous 8.0 suture. *B.* Fifteen-year follow-up coronary angiogram demonstrating a widely patent left internal mammary artery–left anterior descending artery bypass graft. The arrow demonstrates the anastomotic site. The mammary artery is virtually free of graft atherosclerosis.

changes on the electrocardiogram. A very minimal elevation of myocardial enzymes indicates the absence of any injury, but moderate elevation is probably related to inadequate myocardial protection. Enzyme elevations are less frequently seen with current myocardial preservation techniques.

The most serious complication with operation is stroke, occurring with a frequency of 1 to 2 percent, more commonly seen in patients in the seventh or eighth decades. The most common cause of stroke is probably embolus of atherosclerotic debris from the aortic arch, although carotid artery disease or emboli from the heart are other causes.

The authors no longer believe that asymptomatic carotid disease is a significant cause of perioperative stroke. Carotid artery disease is surgically treated only in the patient with acute ischemic symptoms such as transient ischemic attacks. If the patient has cerebral symptoms from carotid disease and significant coronary symptoms, the procedures may be done concomitantly. If the coronary symptoms are mild and carotid disease severe, carotid endarectomy is done first, with awake anesthesia and good monitoring. However, unless carotid symptoms are present, we are not aware of any data that show a benefit from performing carotid endarterectomy either before or concurrently with coronary bypass. The only exception is the patient with unilateral total carotid occlusion, with subtotal stenosis of the opposite carotid. Such a patient might benefit from a combined procedure despite the absence of cerebral symptoms.

Considerable attention has been focused on previously unrecognized atherosclerotic disease in the aortic arch as a source of emboli, especially in older patients. Recently, use of intraoperative transesophageal echocardiography has been very helpful in this regard, as this technique can readily detect intraluminal atheroma that are either removed at operation or avoided. In patients over 70 years of age, a special aortic arch cannula is now routinely used, placing the tip beyond the orifice of the left subclavian artery to avoid dislodgment of atherosclerotic material from the transverse arch by the jet of blood emerging from the perfusion cannula. This cannula is routinely used in all patients with any suspected disease in the transverse aortic arch. In patients with palpable disease of the aortic arch or demonstrable intraluminal disease by transesophageal echocardiographic evaluation the aortic arch may be surgically explored, using the technique of circulatory arrest at a perfusate temperature below 18°C. The arch can be readily explored through an appropriately placed 3- to 5-cm aortotomy and any loose atherosclerotic debris removed. Arch exploration generally takes only 5 to 8 min of circulatory arrest time. This has been used in over 100 patients. The exploration is clearly safe, with the strong impression that significant protection from stroke results.

Relief of Angina. The immediate relief of angina is the most dramatic aspect of bypass. Angina is either completely relieved or markedly decreased in at least 90 to 95 percent of patients if complete revascularization is done. Persistent angina almost always indicates that either a graft has become occluded or a significant stenosis was not bypassed. Recurrent angina is unlikely in the first 5 to 7 years, but can occur between 7 and 15 years depending on graft patency and progression of underlying disease. Tight control of risk factors for atherosclerosis minimizes the risk of recurrent angina, as does use of the internal mammary artery.

Improvement in Ventricular Function. With former techniques, significant improvement in impaired ventricular function could not be demonstrated. With present techniques of myocardial preservation, the abnormal responses to exercise existing before operation, principally a fall in ejection fraction, are often abolished following complete revascularization. This is also usually associated with an improvement in regional wall motion abnormalities. Patients with coronary disease undergoing coronary bypass have improved functional results and functional response to exercise compared with patients treated medically. This improvement lasts up to 10 years, and longer in patients receiving mammary grafts.

Vein Graft Patency. With a proper operative technique, combined with the preoperative use of dipyridamole and postoperative use of aspirin, vein graft patency at one month following operation should be about 95 percent. Current data are limited because angiograms are now seldom performed in the immediate postoperative period. Early graft patency is determined by operative technique and by the runoff of the recipient coronary, i.e., vessels with an internal diameter of less than 1 mm are more likely to occlude early. In the first 5 years after operation, patency decreases slowly, about 2 to 3 percent per year, due to intimal hyperplasia in the graft, so 5-year patency is in the range of 80 percent. Intimal hyperplasia can be worsened by trauma to the vein graft at the time of operation, and might be related to local growth factors such as platelet derived growth factor or basic fibroblast growth factor. Intimal hyperplasia is not prevented by antiplatelet therapy.

In the period 5 to 15 years after operation, there is an alarming increase of atherosclerotic disease in the vein grafts, as a result of which vein graft patency at 10 years is only 50 to 60 percent, and significant atherosclerosis is present in many of the grafts remaining patent. Vein graft patency is 30 to 40 percent at 15 years and for unknown reasons, a small number of grafts, near 20 percent, remain in excellent condition more than 15 to 20 years after operation. Late graft patency might be improved with aspirin, and is clearly improved by controlling cardiac risk factors. Cessation of smoking and control of cholesterol are particularly important, as late graft occlusion is 5 to 7 times more frequent when these are not controlled.

In the past few years use of the internal mammary artery has increased markedly including the more frequent use of bilateral and sequential mammary grafts. The 10-year patency rate is 90 to 95 percent for a left internal mammary, and 80 to 90 percent for a right internal mammary graft. Failures are primarily technical, as the mammary develops little late graft atherosclerosis (Fig. 18-5*B*).

Progression of Atherosclerosis. All angiographic studies have reported a serious frequency of progressive atherosclerosis in the coronary arteries, ranging from 5 to 10 percent per year. Progressive disease was observed in between 65 to 70 percent of patients treated either medically or surgically.

The need to control cardiac risk factors cannot be overemphasized. National studies demonstrated that reduction in total plasma cholesterol and low-density lipoprotein cholesterol, often with an elevation in the high-density lipoprotein, resulted in significant improvement and a 2 percent reduction in coronary risk for each 1 percent reduction in plasma cholesterol levels. Discontinuation of smoking can have an even stronger effect. Patients are placed on a low-fat, low-cholesterol diet. Ingestion of meat and foods high in saturated fats should be minimized. Exercise is recommended depending on the cardiac function, and weight loss is strongly encouraged. Attention is given to HDL:LDL cholesterol ratio, but in general if the total cholesterol level remains over 200 to 225 mg/dL, lipid-lowering drugs are begun.

Recurrent Angina. Angina gradually recurs following operation, at a rate of 3 to 5 percent per year after the first 5 years, when angina is infrequent. When significant angina recurs, angiography should be promptly done. In the majority of patients, recurrent angina is due to one of two causes, progressive stenosis or occlusion of a bypass graft or progressive stenosis in a previously ungrafted artery. Either situation can be treated with repeat bypass grafting or occasionally by angioplasty.

Arrhythmias and Sudden Death. Arrhythmias are usually little improved in patients with significant preoperative myocardial scarring. In some patients with good ventricular function, arrhythmias may be improved because ischemia was apparently the basic cause. Effective treatment of arrhythmias associated with ventricular scars remains unsatisfactory. The more frequent use of 24-h electrocardiographic monitoring or EPS may be helpful in developing more effective antiarrhythmic therapy. Patients with recurrent ventricular tachycardia have been effectively treated by electrically locating and then ablating one or more irritable foci. This is now done very effectively in the cardiac catheterization laboratory. Otherwise, various drug regimens are utilized until the EPS-stimulated arrhythmia is suppressed. In refractory cases the implantable defibrillator may be required (see section below).

Sudden death remains a grim possibility in any patient with coronary artery disease. Over 300 patients per year were studied following emergency resuscitation from cardiac arrest on the streets of Seattle. Over 75 percent of the patients had coronary disease, but less than one-half had a significant recent infarction.

The influence of medical and surgical treatment on "sudden death" was reported from results with over 13,000 patients in the CASS. Over a period of 4.6 years, sudden death occurred in 452 patients (3.4 percent of the group). This occurred in 6 percent of the medically treated patients but only 2 percent of the surgically treated patients. These results should be improved further by aggressive 24-h electrocardiographic monitoring and EPS testing as outlined above.

Longevity. The influence of coronary bypass on longevity, of course, depends on the status of the disease process in the patient operated upon. As noted above the CASS data indicate that bypass had little influence on 5-year longevity when performed upon patients with triple vessel disease, little angina, and good ventricular function, although nearly 40 percent of the unusually good risk medically treated group subsequently required operation. Longevity is generally not improved by surgery in patients with single or double vessel disease. For most other categories of patients, which represents a high percentage of all patients with coronary disease, bypass surgery clearly significantly improved longevity. These include patients with left main disease, triple vessel disease with impaired ventricular function, triple vessel disease with severe proximal stenoses or severe angina, patients with easily inducible ischemia and proximal anterior descending disease, and patients with a previous history of severe arrthythmias or "sudden death" with multivessel coronary disease. In our experiences survival for the first 5 to 7 years after bypass is similar to age-sex matched controls. Survival is better than that seen with medical therapy in the groups outlined. This is particularly true because the patients operated on were usually in a high-risk category with severe angina not responding to medical therapy. Loop and associates noted a 5-year survival among different groups of 90 to 93 percent. Kirklin and associates reported a 5-year survival following triple bypass of 89 percent. Most reports show little influence of extent of disease (double or triple vessel disease) on 5-year survival after surgery, in marked contrast to that regularly found in medically treated patients.

A 10-year survival rate of 75 to 88 percent in several thousand patients was reported by Cosgrove and associates. The 10-year survival varied between 84 percent with a normal ventricle and 54 percent with severe impairment. Survival beyond 10 years may be significantly improved by use of the internal mammary artery, with a 10-year survival of nearly 90 percent in those receiving mammary grafts.

Late death, like recurrent angina, is usually found to result from stenosis of a previously inserted bypass graft or progressive disease in an ungrafted vessel. The rare occurrence of death in patients with three functioning grafts, usually from an arrhythmia, also indicates the influence of bypass on longevity. The major factors determining longevity seem to be age, the adequacy of revascularization of all major coronary arteries, the underlying ventricular function before operation (i.e., ejection fraction), and use of the internal mammary artery to graft the anterior descending artery.

Future Considerations. ***Multiple Internal Mammary Anastomoses.*** Since the 1984 report by Grondin documented the alarming deterioration of vein grafts between 5 and 10 years following operation, while mammary arteries remained patent without change in 90 to 95 percent of patients, a wider application of mammary grafting has been reported by several groups. In brief, certain facts are well established with internal mammary grafting.

1. The 10-year patency rate is near 95 percent, with no signs of deterioration after the first few postoperative months. The mammary artery seems to be relatively immune to atherosclerosis.
2. A patent mammary artery can enlarge substantially over a number of years, perhaps responding to a decrease in peripheral resistance in the coronary vascular bed as atherosclerosis occludes adjacent vessels. This striking ability to enlarge with time indicates the possibilities with multiple anastomoses constructed from a single mammary artery.
3. Data now indicate that bilateral mammary grafts can be performed in good-risk patients without significant morbidity. In several significant reports Lytle and associates described experiences with bilateral mammary grafting in 500 patients with little increase in morbidity. Bilateral mammary grafting probably does increase the risk of sternal wound infection, particularly in diabetics. Care should be taken to choose cases appropriately when bilateral mammary grafting is considered, and this procedure may not be indicated in elderly, high-risk, or diabetic patients.

Loop and associates compared longevity in patients who received one mammary graft as compared with those in whom only vein grafts were used. The series included 2306 internal mammary grafts and 3625 vein grafts. There was a statistically significant difference in survival at 10 years, gradually becoming apparent between 5 and 10 years after operation. Results suggest that use of a single mammary bypass can lower the incidence of recurrent symptoms at 10 to 15 years, and these results might be improved even more using double mammary grafts in appropriate patients.

Scanty data are available concerning "free" grafts of mammary artery, in which the artery is divided and reimplanted into the aorta, identical to the method used with a saphenous vein graft. Such "free" grafts no longer function as a pedicle. Loop reported reasonably good results in over 50 such patients operated on under specific circumstances over a period of years, but no series has yet appeared in which such grafts were used routinely. If excellent results similar to those obtained with mammary pedicle grafts can be obtained with "free" grafts, an even wider use of the mammary artery is possible. Similar experiments are now being conducted with use of the inferior epigastric artery and the gastroepiploic artery for coronary bypass, which in combination with mammary grafting could result in total "arterial" revascularization. Results remain to be evaluated, but the procedures may become more widely applicable in the future.

Silent Ischemia. Better therapy is clearly needed to prevent the development of extensive ventricular injury from coronary disease, the so-called "bad" left ventricle with an ejection fraction 0.20 to 0.25 or lower. Such patients are seen too often. The disconcerting fact is that such patients have often had "good" medical management since their coronary disease was first recognized years before and have had neither recurrent major infarctions nor severe angina. Despite periodic medical observation and therapy, the disease has "silently" progressed. Some method other than severity of angina needs to be used to detect such patients and have bypass performed earlier as it is likely that these patients have had ongoing asymptomatic silent ischemia. Some form of periodic stress testing, perhaps at least annually in patients with known coronary disease, seems to be necessary. One of the most definitive studies at present is a measurement of change in ejection fraction with exercise, especially in comparison with studies done in previous years. Similarly, the stress thallium exam may be helpful, and recently 24-h digital ECG monitoring has been highly effective in detecting ongoing silent ischemia. Patients with significant silent ischemia or a positive stress test should undergo cardiac catherization and revascularization if a significant amount of myocardium is at risk.

Ischemic Cardiomyopathy. Patients with ischemic cardiomyopathy and intractable congestive heart failure have been treated by cardiac transplantation in recent years, with roughly a 90 percent 1-year and a 60 percent 5-year survival rate. As noted in the above section on congestive heart failure, these results after transplantation are not markedly different than results seen with bypass operation in patients with low ejection fraction, intractable congestive heart failure, and pulmonary hypertension. The improved outcome noted recently with bypass operation in this group of patients is primarily due to better intraoperative myocardial protection, better detection and treatment of life-threatening arrhythmias, and vigorous medical therapy with afterload reduction after revascularization is completed. Certainly when reversible ischemia is demonstrable in patients with congestive heart failure, standard bypass operation should be considered the procedure of choice. Recently, Carpentier, McGovern, and others have tried to augment left ventricular function in patients with ischemic myopathy by cardiomyoplasty, a procedure that relies on programmed stimulation of the latissimus dorsi muscle for biomechanical cardiac assistance. Cardiomyoplasty has given mixed results thus far, with no demonstrable long-term benefit. As both operative techniques and medical therapy improve, however, a combined multidisciplinary approach to treatment of patients with ischemic cardiomyopathy may be preferable to transplantation in certain patients. This is particularly true in view of the current limitations in organ availability.

LEFT VENTRICULAR ANEURYSM

Historical Data. Safe excision of a ventricular aneurysm was not possible on a routine basis until the development of a pump oxygenator, although Bailey and colleagues reported successful repair of 5 cases between 1954 and 1958. Cooley, in 1958, is credited with one of the first reports of successful excision of an aneurysm with cardiopulmonary bypass. In the next few years, excision became a standard procedure in most cardiac clinics. Effler reported in 1965 that 61 such patients had been operated on at the Cleveland Clinic. Series of more than 100 such aneurysms are now frequently reported. Cooley and colleagues at the Texas Heart Institute have reported more than 4000 ventricular aneurysm repairs over 30 years.

Etiology, Pathology, and Pathogenesis. A left ventricular aneurysm develops over a period of 4 to 8 weeks or longer in 10 to 15 percent of patients following a myocardial infarction. It results when a severe transmural infarction destroys virtually all muscular fibers in the area of the infarction, which are subsequently replaced by fibrous tissue. It probably does not occur more frequently following a transmural infarction because collateral circulation is frequently sufficient to maintain viability of a variable number of muscle fibers in the zone of the infarct.

The classic aneurysm is simply an avascular thin scar, 4 to 6 mm thick, that bulges outward when the remaining left ventricular muscle contracts in systole (Fig. 18-6*A*). Hence, the term, "paradoxical contraction," more commonly termed *dyskinesis,* as opposed to *hypokinesis* (impaired contractility) or *akinesis* (absence of contractility). Mural thrombi are found attached to the ventricular surface of the scar in over one-half of patients, but arterial emboli are rare. The aneurysm usually enlarges a moderate degree and then becomes stationary; progressive enlargement and rupture, as usually occurs with atherosclerotic aortic aneurysms, is rare. Spotty calcification eventually develops in the aneurysmal wall in chronic cases. Over 80 percent of aneurysms are in the anterolateral portion of the left ventricle, evolving after occlusion of the anterior descending coronary. Posterior aneurysms are less common (15 to 20 percent), and lateral aneurysms are rare.

A "false" aneurysm is rare. It is a hematoma that is formed after rupture of a myocardial infarction has been temporarily supported by adjacent fibrous tissue. Excision should be done promptly, for such aneurysms soon expand and rupture.

In 30 to 40 percent of cases, significant coronary disease is limited to the anterior descending coronary, which is either completely occluded or severely stenosed. Multivessel disease is present in the other patients. Small aneurysms (less than 5 cm diameter) have negligible physiologic significance except possibly as a site of arrhythmias. Larger aneurysms decrease ventricular function apparently by dissipating energy of ventricular contraction with the ineffective paradoxical expansion of the wall of the aneurysm during systole. Possibly, the altered geometry of the left ventricular cavity is also significant, though this is difficult to measure. With larger aneurysms, the left ventricular volume is increased and left ventricular hypertrophy develops. The left ventricular end-diastolic pressure is often markedly elevated. The combination of elevated intracavitary pressure and radius results in a significant elevation in wall tension by Laplace's law (tension = pressure × radius). The decrease in effective ventricular contraction eventually results in cardiac failure and angina, though angina may be due to the accompanying coronary disease as well. Arrhythmias are prominent in 15 to 20 percent of patients. Areas of scar tissue around the edge of the aneurysm frequently serve as foci for the origin of ventricular arrhythmias, and patient scar tissue often presents with sustained ventricular tachycardia, syncope, or sudden death.

As the physiologic burden from an aneurysm is related to its size, the magnitude of improvement following operation is somewhat related to the size of the aneurysm. For this reason, it is doubtful that an aneurysm is ever large enough to be truly "inoperable" simply because of size. Improvement is dependent on the amount of functioning myocardium left, and best results are seen when the other walls of the heart contract normally.

As the development of an aneurysm depends upon almost total destruction of muscle fibers, a true aneurysm, composed of dyskinetic scar, must be distinguished from a scar that results from an infarction that may be akinetic but whose wall is composed of varying proportions of fibrous tissue and viable muscle fibers. Excision of such akinetic scars has been investigated in some detail in the past but has not been found clinically beneficial.

Because of the wide spectrum between a ventricular "scar" and a true "aneurysm," accurate data to define natural history are almost impossible to obtain. The natural history of a patient with a ventricular aneurysm will, of course, be determined by at least four factors: the size of the aneurysm, the residual coronary disease, and the function of the remaining viable muscle and the presence of severe arrhythmias. Five-year survival with an untreated aneurysm has ranged from as low as 10 percent to as high as 70 percent among different reports. Brusche and associates reported that 5-year survival in a patient with an akinetic segment was 70 percent; with a dyskinetic segment and good residual ventricular function, 54 percent; with a dyskinetic segment and poor ventricular function, 36 percent.

Clinical Manifestations. Dyspnea or angina, either alone or in combination, are the two most common symptoms. Arrhythmias are prominent in 15 to 20 percent of patients. Abnormalities on physical examination are usually not diagnostic. The apical impulse may be forceful and diffuse with a "double impulse."

The chest x-ray may show a localized enlargement in the anteroapical area of the left ventricle. Electrocardiographic changes usually show only the signs of the previous infarction. Occasionally persistent ST segment elevation in the precordial leads occurs, but this can also be present with a large infarction without aneurysmal disease. A paradoxical area from the aneurysm can be demonstrable by echocardiography or gated blood pool scan. Most diagnostic information comes from the left ventricular angiogram, outlining an akinetic area bulging paradoxically during systole. Often a clear differentiation cannot be made between an akinetic scar and a true aneurysm, with the final decision being made at the time of operation. If a discrete scar is found at operation, containing few or no muscle fibers, resection is indicated. If a diffuse bulging is present without discrete borders and obviously containing a moderate amount of muscle tissue, resection is probably contraindicated. Work-up of arrhythmias is critical. If symptoms suggestive of sustained ventricular tachycardia are present, EPS should be done. If no known arrhythmias exist, a 24-h Holter exam or a signal-averaged ECG should be done to screen for arrhythmias, proceeding with EPS if these studies are positive.

Treatment. Operation is indicated for symptomatic aneurysms larger than 5 to 6 cm. A moderate asymptomatic aneurysm may be simply observed. The operative procedure includes excision of the aneurysm and bypass grafting of the diseased coronary arteries. Grafting of the diseased anterior descending coronary, which often supplies principally ventricular scar, is of questionable value, though at NYU it has usually been grafted because of the possibility the improved blood supply to the ventricular septum might benefit ventricular arrhythmias.

In general, the aneurysm is not manipulated until the heart has been fibrillated or the aorta clamped to prevent dislodgment of mural thrombi. Once the heart is arrested or fibrillated, the heart is

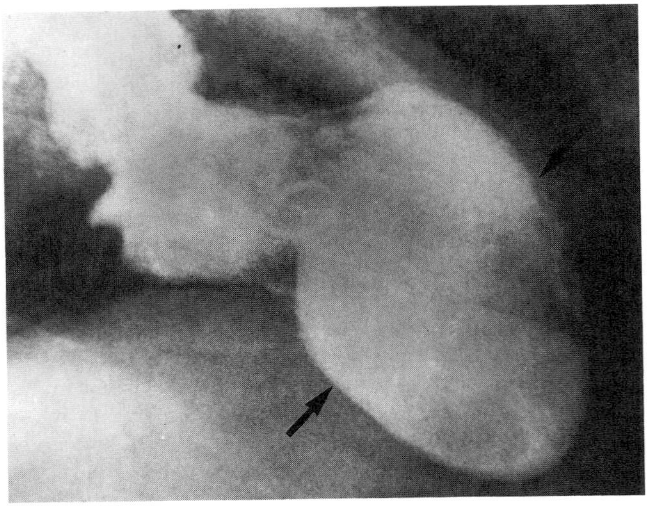

A

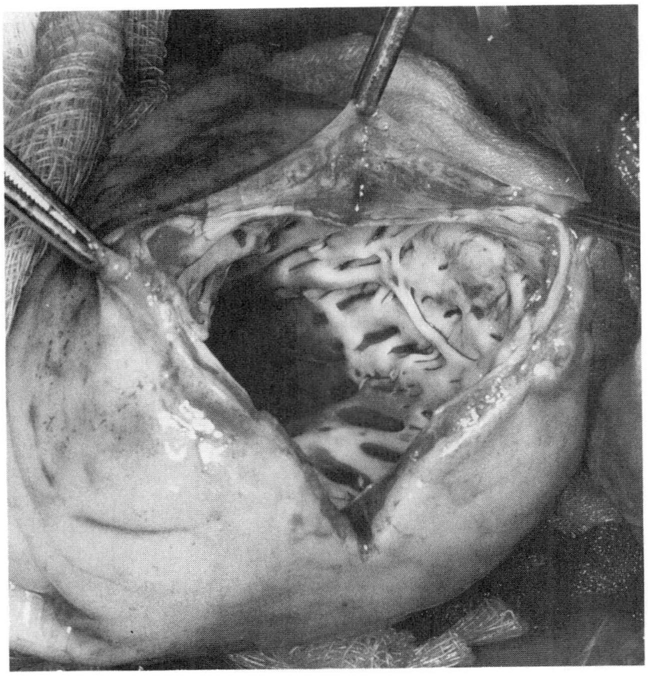

B

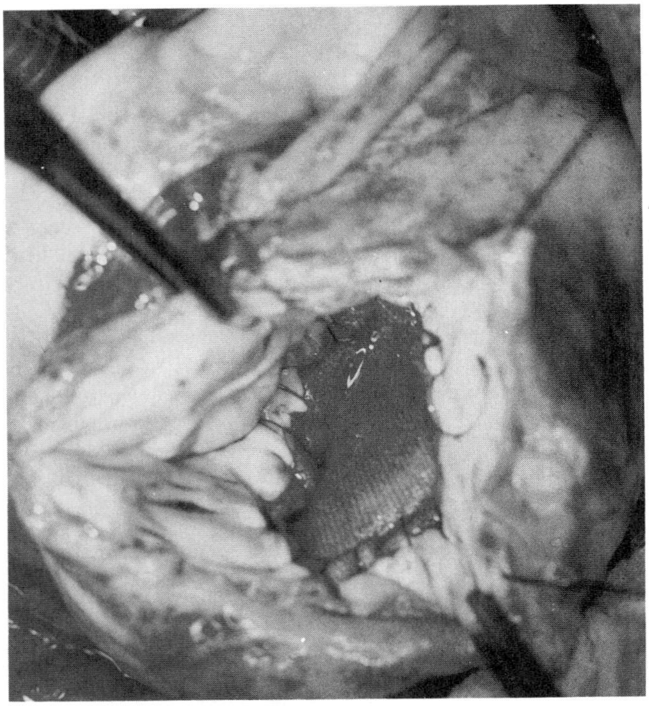

C

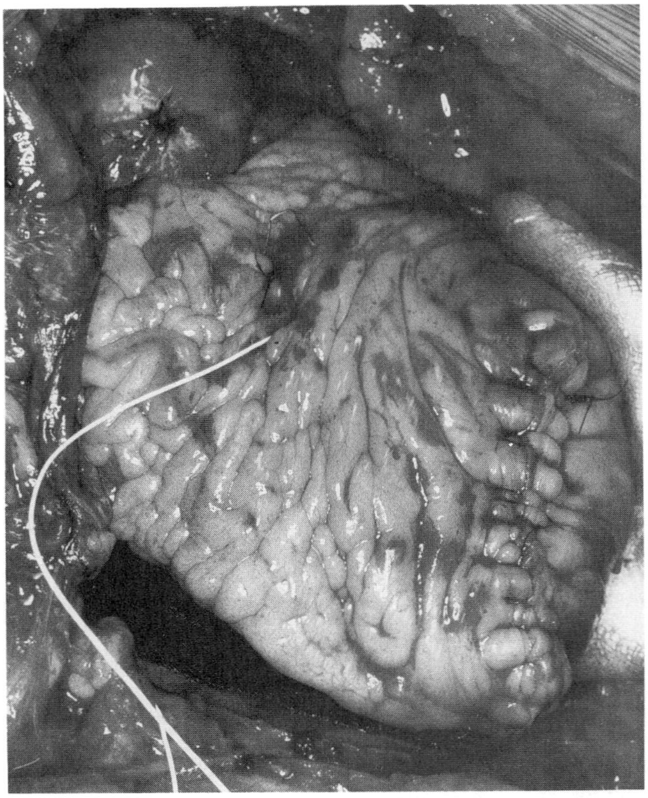

D

FIG. 18-6. *A.* A left ventriculogram demonstrating a large left ventricular aneurysm. Note the contrast to the normal left ventriculogram demonstrated in Fig. 18-1*B*. *B.* Operative photograph of open left ventricular aneurysm. Aneurysmal involvement of the ventricular septum was present, and significant subendocardial scar is seen. *C.* Aneurysm repair using a Dacron patch and the endoaneurysmorrhaphy technique, which excludes the aneurysm and the aneurysmal septum from the normal part of the left ventricular cavity. *D.* The wall of the aneurysm has been closed over the Dacron patch, completing the endoaneurysmorrhaphy technique.

mobilized by freeing the aneurysm from the pericardial adhesions, often by simply incising the wall of the aneurysm and leaving part of the wall attached to the pericardium. For the classic ventricular aneurysm repair a *subtotal* excision of the aneurysm is performed, dividing the wall of the aneurysm about 2 cm from its junction with left ventricular muscle. The *subtotal* concept is a crucial one, as the suture line closing the ventriculotomy is subsequently inserted through scar rather than through viable muscle surrounding the aneurysm. This precaution also avoids any excessive reduction in size of the ventricular cavity. Many operative deaths from excision of huge aneurysms probably have resulted from excessive excision of the wall of the aneurysm with injury of the surrounding viable ventricular muscle.

The classic ventricular aneurysm repair can have a geometrically deforming effect on the remaining left ventricular cavity, due to the linear cardiac closure required after aneurysmal excision. Symptoms often improve after standard repair, although an increase in the ejection fraction does not always occur. A concept of reconstructive intracavitary aneurysm repair has been proposed by Jatene and Cooley. Operative repair involves placement of a Dacron patch to obliterate aneurysmal ventricle and septum, reestablishing a Dacron ''roof'' on the left ventricular cavity (Fig. 18-6*B*, *C*, *D*). The repair results in lowering of diastolic volume without deforming the other walls of the heart. The Dacron patch is sutured circumferentially to the junction of viable and nonviable myocardium and may be combined with subendocardial resection to obliterate conduction of arrhythmias. This technique seems to result in better improvement in cardiac function and control of arrhythmias.

The wall of the aneurysm usually includes the area of the anterior descending coronary, with the scar extending into the ventricular septum. Bypass grafting of the anterior descending in such instances is of uncertain significance, as the muscle supplied by the anterior descending has been infarcted. If significant tributaries to the ventricular septum are patent, the artery should be preserved and a bypass graft attached. Bypass grafts are routinely placed into other areas of viable myocardium if obstructive coronary lesions are present.

Usually, the extent of the endocardial scar is greater than that of the external aneurysm. Because of the hazard of malignant ventricular arrhythmias, an extensive excision of the subendocardial scar for one or more centimeters around the periphery of the aneurysm is important when arrhythmias are present, as this is easily done without significant injury to functioning ventricular muscle. When combined with intracavitary repair and septal obliteration, encircling excision of subendocardial scar provides suprisingly good control of arrhythmias. Electrophysiologic studies have found that trigger zones for arrhythmias are usually located in the scar within 1 to 3 cm of the border of the aneurysm. When severe preoperative ventricular arrhythmias are present, intraoperative electrophysiologic mapping to locate and excise the irritable foci may be necessary.

Results. Prognosis is determined principally by the residual ventricular function, which, in turn, is influenced by the size of the aneurysm and the severity of the coronary disease. In general, if angina was the prominent symptom before operation, 5-year survival is 60 to 70 percent or better, while if congestive heart failure was the principal indication for operation, 5-year survival is around 50 percent.

Most patients are significantly improved following operation, manifested by relief of angina and improvement in ventricular function. With hemodynamic studies, significant improvement in ventricular function can be demonstrated in some patients, while others show very little change. Improvement in ejection fraction may be better after intracavitary repair with reconstructive aneurysmorraphy.

Olearchyk and associates described experiences with 244 cases with a 5-year survival near 70 percent. Dobell and associates in a series of 67 patients found a 5-year survival of 84 percent when angina was the prominent symptom, 53 percent if congestive failure were significant.

Akins and associates in a series of 100 ventricular aneurysms reported a 2 percent operative mortality and a 6-year survival of 77 percent. Jatene reported repair of 508 cases between 1977 and 1983 using reconstructive principles for left ventricular aneurysm repair, with an operative mortality rate of 4 percent. Cooley also reported an operative risk of 4 percent in 100 patients using the intracavitary reconstruction technique, demonstrating a significant improvement in left ventricular ejection fraction after this operation. Sosa and associates reported use of a similar repair in patients with associated sustained ventricular tachycardia, demonstrating an operative risk of 5 percent and freedom from recurrent ventricular tachycardia of 95 percent. Other studies have suggested that aneurysms associated with sustained ventricular tachycardia should be repaired with intraoperative physiologic studies to guide ablation of the arrhythmogenic foci, particularly when sustained ventricular tachycardia is the presenting symptom. Combined aneurysm repair and map-guided ablation can be done with a 5 to 10 percent operative risk.

VALVULAR HEART DISEASE

Pathophysiology: General Principles

With valvular heart disease, ''When should an operation be performed?'' This basic question must be periodically evaluated during the medical therapy of any patient with cardiac valvular disease, because the disease process is usually a progressive one. As a result of several developments, surgical therapy is now being used at a much earlier stage of the disease than in previous years. At present a decision for operation is often made from physiologic abnormalities found with diagnostic studies, such as cardiac catheterization, angiography, echocardiography or radionuclide studies, rather than from the severity and disability from symptoms.

Several developments have combined to indicate that operation should be performed earlier. The safety of operative procedures has increased, with the risk of single valve replacement now being in the range of 1 to 3 percent in good-risk patients. This is principally due to improvements in myocardial preservation with the widespread adoption of hyperkalemic cold cardiac arrest. The virtually indefinite durability of metallic prosthetic valves is now well established, though anticoagulation with warfarin is required. The feasibility of mitral valve reconstruction, which avoids anticoagulation, has made early mitral valve operation even more attractive.

Longevity following cardiac valve replacement is strongly influenced by the myocardial function at the time of operation. Patients with early disability (New York Heart Class II or early III) have a 5-year survival near 90 percent, but only 60 to 70 percent of patients with Class IV disability live 5 years. This striking difference is due to irreversible changes in myocardial function that existed before operation, indicating that operation should not be postponed until symptoms are disabling.

Aortic valve replacement should be seriously considered in asymptomatic patients if the orifice cross-sectional area has decreased to near 1.0 cm^2. This is especially true if left ventricular hypertrophy is developing, or if the left ventricular dimensions are increasing by echocardiographic evaluation. An even more liberal indication should be used with mitral stenosis, considering therapy with an orifice cross-sectional area less than 1.5 cm^2 because a commissurotomy, rather than valve replacement, can usually be performed. The grave hazard always exists of cerebral embolism from thrombi developing in the left atrium, especially when atrial fibrillation has developed.

With aortic and mitral valve insufficiency, selecting the proper time for operation is more difficult, as this depends on the left ventricular function. The demonstration of a fall in left ventricular ejection fraction during exercise is probably the best currently available sign that operation should be done. Similarly, a progressive rise in the left ventricular end-systolic dimension at rest, as measured by echocardiography or by gated blood pool scan, may be a good indication for operative intervention. Postponing operation until serious enlargement of the left ventricle develops or a permanent elevation in left ventricular end-diastolic pressure occurs is clearly a mistake because 5-year prognosis following successful operation is greatly decreased.

A patient with cardiac valvular disease is rarely inoperable. If the basic disease process is cardiac valvular disease, an operation, usually prosthetic valve replacement, can almost always be performed with current techniques of myocardial preservation with an operative risk no greater than 5 to 10 percent regardless of the degree of preoperative disability noted. Patients are still seen with far advanced Class IV failure and cardiac cachexia who simply have postponed operation for years with the concept that operation was "too dangerous." Some benefit, however, will always result from correcting the valvular pathology. For example, the suggestion is wrong that Class IV patients with mitral insufficiency and an ejection fraction of less than 25 to 30 percent will not benefit from operation. The authors have operated on numerous patients in this category with excellent clinical improvement after valve repair or replacement. The magnitude of benefit often cannot be predicted for some months, depending on the unmeasurable irreversible loss of ventricular function. Recent data suggest that valve repair, by preserving the subvalvular apparatus, is especially beneficial in preserving cardiac function in the low ejection fraction ventricle. Most patients improve significantly when severe valvular pathology is corrected. Therefore, except in the unusual case of intrinsic myocardial disease with true "cardiomyopathy," operation should not be denied to patients with advanced valvular heart disease.

Pulmonary hypertension, seen especially with severe aortic or mitral stenosis, less commonly with chronic congestive failure from mitral or aortic insufficiency, almost always improves to a substantial degree following operation. With current techniques, the risk of an operation, even with a pulmonary artery systolic pressure above 100 mmHg, is no more than 5 to 10 percent. This low mortality rate is a result of improvements in myocardial preservation, taking particular care to preserve the hypertrophied right ventricle. Unless massive pulmonary emboli have occurred, intractable right heart failure from pulmonary hypertension, the so-called cor pulmonale, is rare.

Survival following *prosthetic valve replacement* is primarily influenced by the left ventricular function beforehand, i.e., the ejection fraction and the NYHA functional classification. Other risk factors affecting survival are age and the presence of concomitant disease in the coronary arteries or another valve. Late complications from valvular surgery include endocarditis, thromboembolic and anticoagulant-related complications, prosthetic valve failure, and reoperation.

Prosthetic Valves. An ideal prosthetic valve does not exist. The two basic valves available are mechanical prostheses and the tissue prostheses. Both have advantages and disadvantages. The caged ball valve prosthesis, originally used by Starr in 1961 and subsequently undergoing numerous modifications, remains a durable prothesis. "Low profile" disk protheses are now widely used. These may have single or bileaflet disks. The most popular is probably the St. Jude prosthesis, a low-profile bileaflet valve with excellent flow characteristics and durability. The St. Jude valve (Fig. 18-7*A*) has now been used for 15 to 20 years with a very low incidence of mechanical failure and thromboembolic complications. All mechanical prostheses require permanent anticoagulation with warfarin.

Different types of tissue valves have been studied for over two decades because tissue valves have a far lower frequency of thromboembolism. Valves studied include fascia lata valves, dura mater valves, homograft valves, and heterograft valves. The gluteraldehyde-preserved porcine heterograft valve was developed, principally by Carpentier in Paris and Hancock in the United States in the mid-1970s (Fig. 18-7*B*). Unfortunately, late valve failure is significant with all heterograft valves. A pericardial heterograft valve was also developed, primarily by Ionescu in England, and has been widely used, though currently is less popular because of a significant late failure rate. Porcine heterograft prostheses have a very low frequency of thromboembolism if arrhythmias or cardiac enlargement are not present, making anticoagulation unnecessary in a majority of patients, especially those with aortic prostheses. Their principal limitation is durability, currently excellent at 5 years but in the range of 80 to 85 percent near 10 years. As the rate of failure rises sharply per year after 7 or 8 years, the 15-year durability with porcine valves is only 40 to 50 percent. Overall, porcine prostheses have less thromboembolic complications than mechanical prostheses, but they are also less durable.

With mechanical prostheses, the basic problems are thromboembolism and hemorrhage from anticoagulation therapy with warfarin. With proper anticoagulation, keeping the prothrombin time 1½ to 2 times normal (18 to 20 s/control of 12s), thromboembolism is fortunately rare, a range near 1 to 2 percent per patient year. The role of antiplatelet therapy for prevention of thromboembolism is not clearly defined.

Anticoagulant hemorrhage remains a permanent hazard, occurring with a frequency of 1 to 4 percent per year in patients with mechanical prostheses. The frequency of this problem is primarily related to patient compliance and supervision by the physician. With careful supervision based on periodic prothrombin time measurements, significant hemorrhage from warfarin is less common, probably in the range of 1 percent per year. Conversely, anticoagulant hemorrhage can be a serious or lethal problem in a noncompliant patient with inadequate periodic evaluation. Hence, the basic decision in selecting a porcine versus a mechanical prosthesis depends on the patient's understanding and ability to take anticoagulant therapy safely and indefinitely. In general, mechanical prostheses are more durable than porcine prostheses, with a 15-year valve failure rate of only 5 percent, but they may be associ-

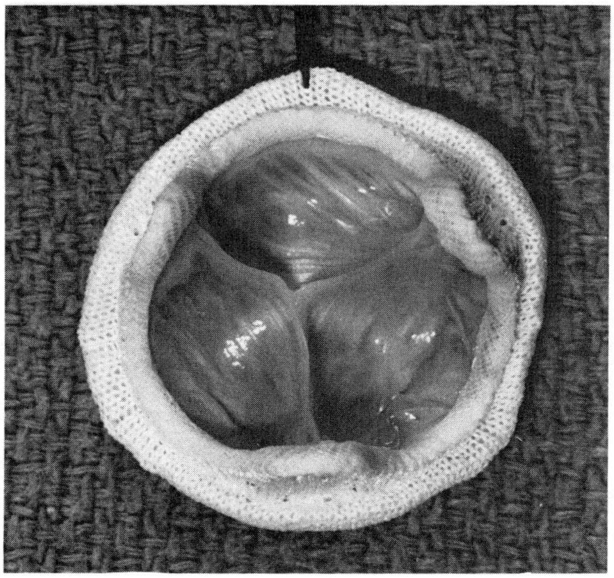

A

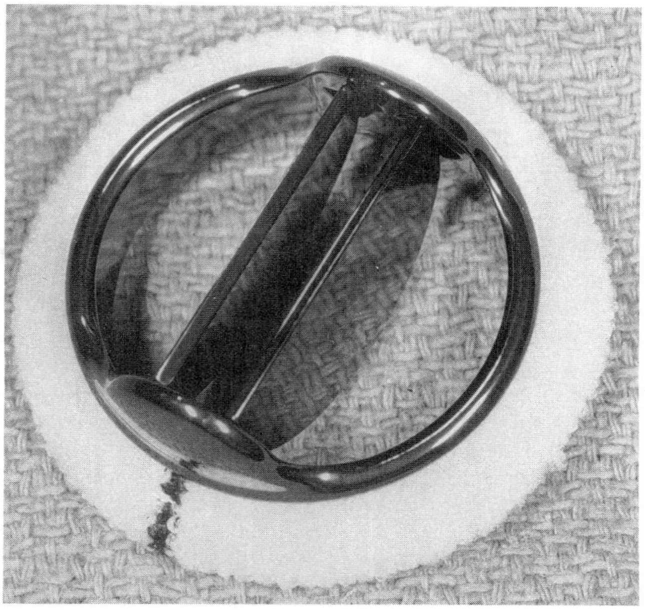

B

FIG. 18-7. *A.* Carpentier-Edwards porcine aortic valve bioprosthesis. *B.* St. Jude bileaflet mechanical mitral valve prosthesis.

ated with a higher incidence of thromboembolic and anticoagulant-related complications. The key question often is whether a patient should have a mechanical valve with permanent anticoagulation but excellent durability, or a porcine valve, which might not require anticoagulation but is likely to fail between 7 and 15 years.

Surgical alternatives to mechanical or porcine prostheses have been developed with attempts to avoid the known complications associated with prosthetic valves. In the 1960s Ross in England and Barrett-Boyes in New Zealand described a procedure for aortic valve replacement using antibiotic-preserved aortic homograft valves. Viable homograft preservation is now possible using cryopreservation techniques, and aortic or pulmonary valve replacement with homograft tissue has gained wider applicability. Similarly, Ross described transplantation of the pulmonary valve into the aortic position, the pulmonary autograft procedure.

In the 1960s McGoon, Kay, and Reed each developed separate plication techniques for reconstruction of the mitral valve for mitral insufficiency, but these methods had limited applicability and were primarily used for treatment of isolated chordal rupture or annular dilation. Renewed interest in surgical reconstruction of the mitral valve resulted from work by Carpentier in Paris in the 1970s. Carpentier's system for valve reconstruction was applicable to a wider range of pathologic findings than prior methods, and the mitral valve reconstruction has proven to be highly reproducible.

Both homograft valve replacement and mitral valve reconstruction are associated with a lower risk of thromboembolism and a lower risk of endocarditis than is noted with prosthetic valve replacement. Neither procedure requires long-term anticoagulation with warfarin. Whether these procedures will be as durable as prosthetic valves remains unknown. Current estimates suggest that the 10- to 15-year durability of aortic homografts may be similar to that noted with porcine valves, with a freedom from reoperation of approximately 50 percent at 15 years, although some reports have suggested better durability than this. The long-term durability of mitral valve reconstruction has been good, over 90 percent at 7 to 10 years, although durability beyond 10 years is less certain. Nevertheless, these procedures offer attractive alternatives to valve replacement for patients who want to avoid long-term anticoagulation.

Recommendations. Before operation, a recommendation should be given by the surgeon to the patient about the appropriate prosthesis or procedure. Some patients are capable of making this decision after the various risks and options are explained and others are not. The surgeon should attempt to learn from the patient whether there is a strong reason to avoid anticoagulation and how the patient feels about the uncertainty of future reoperation. The surgical recommendation is then based on several factors, including the patient's age, intelligence, reliability, and access to follow-up health care. Socioeconomic factors and associated medical conditions are also considered.

In general, for aortic valve replacement a mechanical prosthesis is recommended for most patients under 70 years of age who can take warfarin. A porcine aortic prosthesis is usually recommended for patients older than this because bleeding can be a serious complication in the elderly, and in this population valve failure is unlikely to occur before death from other causes. An aortic homograft or a pulmonary autograft is considered in children and in adults younger than 40 years of age who want to avoid anticoagulation.

For mitral valve disease commissurotomy or valve reconstruction is usually done if feasible. Reconstructive procedures, however, are not recommended unless the likelihood of achieving a durable repair is high. When mitral valve replacement is required, a mechanical prosthesis is recommended in most younger patients and in most patients with atrial fibrillation and a large left atrium, since anticoagulation is already required in this group. Porcine mitral prostheses were frequently used in prior years, but most recently are reserved for elderly patients in whom anticoagulation is considered hazardous.

Mitral Stenosis

Historical Data. A valiant effort to treat mitral stenosis by excising a portion of the valve with a valvulotome was made by Cutler and Levine in 1923, but the resulting mitral insufficiency caused a prohibitive operative mortality. Souttar, in England, performed a digital commissurotomy in one patient in 1925. Thereafter surgical efforts virtually ceased for over 20 years until 1948–1949 when Harken and Bailey independently demonstrated the value of digital commissurotomy. These early commissurotomies, often limited in extent, frequently produced striking clinical improvement, even though mitral stenosis often recurred within 5 years. A transventricular mitral dilator developed around 1957 produced a more extensive commissurotomy and was widely adopted. Subsequently the increasing safety of cardiopulmonary bypass made commissurotomy under direct vision the procedure of choice.

Etiology. All evidence indicates that mitral stenosis is almost always due to rheumatic fever, even though a definite history of rheumatic fever can be obtained in only about 50 percent of patients. Congenital mitral stenosis is very rare, less than 300 cases having been reported. Rarely systemic lupus erythematosus, rheumatoid arthritis, mucopolysaccharide disease, or carcinoid may produce mitral stenosis. In the usual case, after the initial episode of rheumatic fever, symptoms of mitral stenosis may not appear for 10 or more years but may develop as soon as 3 years in some patients and as late as 25 years in others. Selzer and Cohn suggested that scarring of the mitral valve from rheumatic fever produces turbulent flow of blood that in turn causes progressive scarring and contraction over many years. This would explain the appearance of severe mitral stenosis 20 to 30 years after the last known bout of rheumatic fever.

Pathology. Although rheumatic fever produces a pancarditis, involving epicardium, myocardium, and endocardium, serious permanent injury results primarily from the endocarditis. Permanent myocardial injury following recovery from acute myocarditis is uncommon; it is seldom of clinical significance, but an occasional patient is seen with significant myocardial dysfunction. Endocarditis produces ulceration of the endocardium along the edges of the valve leaflets where they normally appose in systole. Tiny, 1- to 2-mm nodules of fibrin and platelets accumulate and may coalesce to fusion of the leaflets at the commissures. A more serious injury evolves from extensive valvulitis with fibrosis and contraction of the body of the leaflets, compounded in subsequent years with calcification and decreasing leaflet mobility. Inflammation of the chordae tendineae similarly leads to fibrosis with contraction, thickening, and fusion. With severe disease the chordae contract and pull the valve leaflets down to fuse with the tips of the papillary muscles.

In many patients mitral stenosis gradually increases in severity over many years, at times more than 20. Previously these progressive changes were considered due to clinically silent episodes of rheumatic fever. The now accepted hypothesis is that the changes are hemodynamic in origin, resulting from turbulent flow of blood with progressive scarring of the mitral orifice.

The possibilities of surgical correction vary greatly with the extent of the valve injury. When simple fusion of the commissures is the only lesion, mitral commissurotomy is highly successful. If the chordae tendineae have contracted and fused to make the leaflets immobile, commissurotomy may be only moderately effective and perhaps impossible. With extensive fibrosis and rigidity of the leaflets, valve replacement is often necessary. How often this is required varies with the type of patient operated on. When operation is performed "early" in the course of the disease (before extensive fibrosis and contraction have occurred), valvular reconstruction, rather than replacement, is possible in the majority of patients, i.e., 85 to 90 percent.

Pathophysiology. A normal mitral valve has a cross-sectional area between 4 and 6 cm^2. Reduction of the cross-sectional area to 2 to 2.5 cm^2 constitutes the mildest form of mitral stenosis. Typical auscultatory findings are present, but the patient is usually asymptomatic (Class I). Further reduction to the range of 1.5 to 2.0 cm^2 produces some symptoms (Class II disability); these are more severe with a cross-sectional area in the range of 1 to 1.5 cm^2. Patients with a cross-sectional area of less than 1 cm^2 are usually seriously disabled (Class IV). A valve area of 0.6 cm^2 or less often results in life-threatening pulmonary edema or death.

Three significant physiologic events result from mitral stenosis—increase in left atrial pressure, decrease in cardiac output, and increase in pulmonary vascular resistance. An increase in left atrial pressure (normally less than 12 mmHg) is the immediate consequence of mitral stenosis. The degree of elevation of left atrial pressure varies with three factors: (1) the cross-sectional area of the mitral orifice, (2) cardiac output, and (3) heart rate. These three factors represent physical laws determining pressure-flow relations through a stenotic orifice, namely, cross-sectional area of orifice, total volume of flow, and duration of time during which flow occurs. When left atrial pressure rises to exceed oncotic pressure of plasma (25 mmHg), transudation of fluid across the pulmonary capillaries will occur. The result of this transudation depends on the capacity of the pulmonary lymphatics to transport the additional fluid. When the fluid load exceeds the capacity of the lymphatic circulation, pulmonary edema results.

Because the normal oncotic pressure of plasma is 25 mmHg, equivalent to a column of blood 12 to 14 in. high, pulmonary congestion in the upright position may be much greater in the lower lobes of the lung than in the upper, for the average thorax is about 20 in. high. A patient with only basilar rales in the upright position may develop extensive pulmonary congestion when supine, with cough, dyspnea, or frank pulmonary edema. This explains paroxysmal nocturnal dyspnea.

The cardiac output is fixed at a low level by the rigid stenotic orifice. With exercise, cardiac output cannot be increased significantly, and dyspnea results. The general fatigue and limitation of physical activity with mitral stenosis is a clinical reflection of this physiologic inability to increase cardiac output.

Chronic pulmonary venous congestion may lead to pulmonary hypertension and increased pulmonary vascular resistance (see Diagnostic Studies). The degree to which pulmonary vascular resistance increases with mitral stenosis varies greatly among different patients. The cause of this variation is unknown. Some, with severe mitral stenosis, have little change, while in others vascular resistance increases to levels 15 to 20 times greater than normal. This increased resistance is primarily a result of congestion and vasoconstriction in the pulmonary arterioles, ultimately intensified by hypertrophy of the media and intima. In far advanced cases recurrent pulmonary emboli may create additional obstruction, but this is uncommon. In the vast majority of patients, the increased vascular resistance either decreases greatly or disappears following surgical correction, a course that is very different from that seen with pulmonary hypertension from congenital heart disease.

Two other serious disabilities that appear with chronic mitral stenosis are atrial fibrillation and systemic embolization. Atrial fibrillation is the ultimate consequence of the atrial hypertrophy produced by chronic left atrial hypertension. Fibrillation produces some decrease in cardiac output and also is often a prelude to more serious arrhythmias. The most serious consequence is the development of thrombi, usually in the ineffectively contracting left atrial appendage. The frequency of thrombi varies with both the duration of mitral stenosis and the presence of atrial fibrillation. Ultimately thrombi develop in 15 to 20 percent of untreated patients, after which episodes of arterial embolism appear with increasing frequency. Before either anticoagulant therapy or operation was possible, cerebral embolism caused death in 20 to 25 percent of patients dying from mitral stenosis.

Clinical Manifestations. ***Symptoms.*** The most important symptom is *dyspnea,* as a result of pulmonary congestion and interstitial edema. This appears whenever mean left atrial pressure exceeds 25 mmHg long enough to produce significant transudation of fluid into the pulmonary capillaries. Characteristically, it first appears with extreme exertion and subsequently, with more severe stenosis, occurs with lesser degrees of exertion. It may also appear with emotion or other circumstances, such as fever or pregnancy, that increase cardiac output.

Several other symptoms subsequently appear, all developing as a result of recurrent pulmonary congestion. A chronic *cough,* worse in the evenings in the recumbent position, is frequent, reflecting basilar congestion. *Orthopnea* and *paroxysmal nocturnal dyspnea* similarly reflect the influence of the upright position on the localization of pulmonary congestion. In the upright position, congestion may be limited to the lower lobes but becomes more diffuse in the supine position. Mobilization of peripheral edema from the lower extremities when the patient is supine intensifies the degree of pulmonary congestion. *Hemoptysis* is a frequent symptom, varying from expectoration of blood-tinged sputum to massive amounts of bright red blood. Such severe hemoptysis, although an alarming symptom, usually subsides spontaneously. Rarely, an emergency mitral valvotomy is required. Episodes of *pulmonary edema* occur when pulmonary congestion greatly exceeds the capacity of the pulmonary lymphatics. In contrast to hemoptysis, pulmonary edema may be fatal unless quickly and effectively treated.

Eventually failure of the right side of the heart appears from the combination of pulmonary hypertension and volume overload, manifested by venous distention, hepatic enlargement, and peripheral edema. This may be intensified by tricuspid insufficiency. Atrial fibrillation develops eventually in most patients. Initially it may be transient, but ultimately in most patients chronic atrial fibrillation is the most common rhythm.

Arterial embolism is a constant threat, especially with atrial fibrillation, although emboli can occur with a sinus rhythm. Emboli evolve from stasis in the dilated left atrium, especially in the atrial appendage. Rarely, large thrombi 5 to 10 cm in diameter may fill much of the left atrium and partly obstruct the ostia of the pulmonary veins.

Angina pectoris develops in about 5 percent of patients. The basic cause is unclear, for it is usually not due to associated coronary atherosclerosis. Possible mechanisms include a low cardiac output, impaired blood flow during diastole because of tachycardia, and recurrent small emboli to the coronary arteries.

Physical Examination. A patient with chronic, severe mitral stenosis may be thin and frail, with the muscular wasting characteristic of a chronic illness. Dilated neck veins are visible if congestive failure is present. Rubor and/or cyanosis are often seen over the fingers or lips. These signs reflect a chronic severe restriction in cardiac output, resulting in blood flowing slowly through peripheral capillary beds. Rales are frequently audible over the lung bases.

Often with pure mitral stenosis, the cardiac size is normal, and the apical impulse is normal or decreased in intensity. A forceful, heaving left ventricular impulse immediately suggests that another disease, such as mitral insufficiency or aortic valvular disease, is present. With increased pulmonary vascular resistance, palpation of the left parasternal area may find a "lift," resulting from contraction of a hypertrophied right ventricle. The pulse rhythm may be regular but is usually irregular atrial fibrillation.

The three significant auscultatory findings with mitral stenosis are the diastolic rumble, an opening snap, and an increased first sound. The apical diastolic rumble, at times sharply localized to an area at the apex only 2 to 3 cm in diameter and heard best with the bell of the stethoscope, is the hallmark of mitral stenosis. It may be of grade I or II intensity in some patients, while in others it is unusually loud with a palpable thrill. The intensity of the murmur, however, does not correlate with the severity of the stenosis. Rarely "silent" mitral stenosis is present without an audible murmur. This results from a calcified, fibrosed valve with little mobility. The increased first sound, the origin of which is not certain, is another distinctive feature and is often the first auscultatory abnormality detected. The opening snap, closely following the second sound, is the third distinctive feature. In many patients careful auscultation can immediately establish the diagnosis of mitral stenosis by finding the triad of an opening snap, followed by a diastolic rumble, and an accentuated first sound.

A short apical systolic murmur may be heard in patients with pure mitral stenosis without any associated mitral insufficiency. Loud pansystolic murmurs, however, which are transmitted to the axilla usually indicate associated mitral insufficiency. A systolic murmur from tricuspid insufficiency may be confused with one arising from mitral insufficiency. The systolic murmur of tricuspid insufficiency, although audible at the apex with hypertrophy of the right ventricle, is usually heard equally well near the sternum and may be accentuated with deep inspiration.

Laboratory Studies. The initial change in mitral stenosis is dilatation of the left atrium. Echocardiography is the simplest and most precise method for making this determination. Once it has been determined that the left atrium is enlarged, there is little correlation between the actual size of the left atrium and the severity of the mitral stenosis. Left atrial enlargement can also be detected with a lateral chest radiograph exposed during oral administration of barium to outline the esophagus. Characteristically, the middle third of the esophagus is displaced backward to form a slight concave curve. With additional degrees of enlargement, the dilated left atrium may be visible as a double shadow in the posteroanterior radiograph, forming a separate dense shadow behind the normal shadow of the right atrium. The left border of the cardiac shadow also shows characteristic changes with mitral stenosis, for the normal concavity between the shadow of the aortic knob and the left ventricle becomes obliterated as both the left atrium and the pulmonary artery enlarge to produce a ''straight'' left heart border. The overall cardiac size may be normal, but lateral views can demonstrate enlargement of the right ventricle when pulmonary vascular resistance has increased. Calcification of the mitral valve is visible with chronic disease in older patients.

Engorged pulmonary veins can be unusually prominent, often with a greater degree of dilatation in the veins to the upper lobes. With pulmonary hypertension the pulmonary arteries are also enlarged. With chronic, severe left atrial hypertension, dilated pulmonary lymphatics become visible as transverse lines across the lower lung fields, ''Kerley lines,'' indicating significant left atrial hypertension.

The electrocardiogram is not diagnostic but often shows T-wave abnormalities characteristic of left atrial enlargement; atrial fibrillation is the most common arrhythmia seen. If pulmonary hypertension is present, right axis deviation and signs of right ventricular hypertrophy are also evident.

2-D echocardiography, however, has been a major advance in noninvasive diagnostic therapy. It can estimate the degree of stenosis and also leaflet mobility. It is of particular value in doubtful cases. Some clinics no longer employ catheterization, simply proceeding from the findings with echocardiography to operation.

Cardiac catheterization can evaluate mitral stenosis precisely, as well as detect the presence of additional valvular disease, such as mitral insufficiency or aortic valvular disease. Left atrial pressure may be estimated from the pulmonary capillary ''wedge'' pressure but this may be falsely elevated in the presence of pulmonary hypertension. The preferred technique is to enter the left atrium directly with a catheter, usually by puncture of the atrial septum. The left atrial pressure in isolated mitral stenosis is increased from the normal range of 5 to 10 mmHg to levels of 20 to 30 mmHg with severe stenosis, producing a diastolic pressure gradient between the left atrium and ventricle of 10 to 20 mmHg. The most precise measurement of the severity of stenosis is done by calculating the cross-sectional area of the mitral valve, determined by the pressure gradient and the cardiac output using Gorlin's formula (see Diagnostic Studies). Angiography may demonstrate rigidity and limited mobility of the valve leaflets but is not of great diagnostic value. It is of particular value, however, in determining the presence of mitral insufficiency by noting the reflux of dye after injection into the left ventricle. Coronary arteriography is an important part of the evaluation of cardiac catheterization, especially in patients older than 40 years of age in whom coronary atherosclerosis may be present.

Treatment. Operation is recommended for all symptomatic patients and should be considered for hemodynamically significant mitral stenosis, even though symptoms are minimal. The operative risk is small, about 1 percent, the possibility of reconstruction rather than replacement very good (over 90 percent). If peripheral embolism has occurred, operation should be performed as soon as the patient has recovered from the embolic episode, for sooner or later emboli almost always recur. Until operation is performed, continuous anticoagulant therapy should be used.

Even though early operation is the preferred approach, it is important to remember that mitral stenosis can almost always be successfully operated on, no matter how far advanced the disease or how severe the pulmonary hypertension. When advanced disease is present, valve replacement is often required due to calcification of the leaflets and fusion of the subvalvular apparatus. The immediate risk of operation is increased with far advanced disease (5 to 7 percent), but surviving patients nearly always show remarkable improvement with a significant decrease, or complete disappearance, of pulmonary hypertension. This improvement is related to the fact that mitral stenosis is a unique condition that keeps blood from entering the left ventricle; so in contrast to other valvular diseases, the left ventricle has not been injured from long-standing hemodynamic stresses.

General Considerations. Since 1971 at New York University virtually all mitral valve operations have been performed with cardiopulmonary bypass and the ''open'' technique. The risk of operation is very small, less than 1 percent. The hazard of emboli from thrombi in the atrium or calcium in the mitral valve is minimal with open technique. Of even greater importance, however, is that effective commissurotomy can usually be performed, although a high percentage of patients require more than simple commissurotomy to totally correct the stenosis. This includes separation of fused chordae, splitting of papillary muscles, debridement of calcium, and often correction of minimal to moderate associated mitral insufficiency with the Carpentier reconstruction techniques.

With the recent interest in catheter balloon valvuloplasty, these considerations are especially pertinent because balloon valvuloplasty has all the limitations of the old ''closed'' commissurotomy methods.

Technique of Open Mitral Commissurotomy. A median sternotomy incision is usually used. This permits ready access to all cardiac structures, including palpation of the tricuspid valve, which is frequently diseased in severely ill patients. The standard cardiopulmonary bypass technique is used, with a perfusate temperature of near 30°C. The heart is arrested with the cold blood hyperkalemic cardioplegia. Topical hypothermia is also used, keeping myocardial temperature below 15°C. The left atrium is incised in the interatrial groove anterior to the point of entry of the right pulmonary veins. By extending the atriotomy beneath the superior vena cava superiorly and the inferior vena cava inferiorly, adequate exposure of the mitral valve can be obtained. The Carpentier self-retraining retractor has been routinely used for the past 5 years and provides far better exposure than that previously obtained with other methods.

Any thrombi in the atrium or atrial appendage are carefully removed. The atrial appendage is subsequently routinely excluded from the atrial cavity by closure of the orifice from within the atrium. This technique has been employed for over a decade without significant injury to other structures, especially the circumflex coronary artery.

The fused commissures of the mitral valve may be exposed by inserting traction sutures into the aortic and mural leaflets or by placing a right angle clamp behind the commissure. As the commissure is incised, the chordae arising from the underlying papillary muscle can be seen and identified. The commissurotomy is carefully performed throughout the length of the fused commissure, stopping where the normal commissural leaflet is found 1 to 2 mm from the mitral annulus.

Division of any chordae is carefully avoided. In at least 30 percent of patients there is significant fusion and contraction of the chordae beneath the commissures, often virtually approximating the fused commissures to the underlying papillary muscles. In such instances the fused chordae papillary muscles are carefully incised for 10 to 15 mm to provide adequate mobility to the mobilized chordae. This greatly increases the efficacy of the commissurotomy by improving mobility of the subvalvular apparatus, and is one of the key advantages of the open procedure.

Opening the fused commissures sufficiently to correct the stenosis without producing significant mitral insufficiency is the key consideration with each operation. After the commissurotomy is completed, the presence of insufficiency can be assessed by a variety of methods. We currently prefer the method popularized by Carpentier, distending the left ventricular cavity with fluid injected through a bulb syringe and noting the apposition of the leaflets. Though subjective, it is simple and has been reasonably reliable. The ability to correct focal insufficiency by a variety of the Carpentier techniques of mitral reconstruction has greatly facilitated the performance of more "radical" commissurotomy.

A final check for mitral insufficiency is performed near the end of bypass with the heart closed, filled with blood, and beating. A finger can be introduced into the left atrium and the functioning mitral valve palpated while the ventricle is ejecting blood with a systolic pressure of 80 to 100 mm.

Following bypass, adequate correction of the mitral stenosis should be routinely confirmed by measuring both left atrial and ventricular pressure by needle puncture, confirming elimination or marked reduction of the end-diastolic pressure gradient. This is an important checkpoint, apparently neglected in many reports of operative technique; with fibrosis and stiff mitral leaflets, an opening that seems anatomically adequate may still be functionally obstructive because of impaired mobility. If a significant residual gradient is present, 5 to 7 mm, a decision must be made as to whether the gradient can be reduced by additional surgical maneuvers, or whether it should be accepted or the valve replaced. A significant residual gradient is usually associated with recurrent symptoms from progressive stenosis within a few years. Intraoperative transesophageal echocardiography is also of value in assessing valvular mobility and the degree of mitral insufficiency.

Following operation, convalescence is usually short and benign. If atrial fibrillation has been present for only a few months, cardioversion may be effective. If atrial fibrillation has been chronic, with significant hypertrophy of left atrial musculature, it is often not successful. The frequency of persistent atrial fibrillation is a strong reason for routine closure of the atrial appendage at the time of operation.

Technique of Mitral Valve Replacement. The initial approach is identical to that used for mitral commissurotomy, described in the preceding section. A sternotomy incision is preferable. Mitral replacement, rather than commissurotomy or reconstruction, is usually necessary if both insufficiency and stenosis are present. The most common pathologic condition requiring replacement is extensive calcification of the valve with stiffening and fibrosis of the valve and the subvalvular structures (Fig. 18-8*A*). Calcification limited to the commissures, however, does not preclude effective commissurotomy.

The valve is excised by incising it a few millimeters from the annulus with a circumferential incision. Underlying papillary muscles are divided near their apices (Fig. 18-8*B*). Usually some chordae can be preserved to the annulus of the mural leaflet, but this may not be possible with advanced disease. The physiologic importance of preserving mural leaflet chordae is uncertain, but the subvalvular chordae and papillary muscles may aid in maintaining cardiac function. The choice of prosthesis was discussed in the preceding section. An identical technique is used for insertion (Fig. 18-8*C*).

The prosthetic valve is inserted with a series of 12 to 18 pledgeted mattress sutures of polyester fabric. How often pledgeted sutures are needed is uncertain as interrupted sutures or a continuous suture have been effectively used by others in some patients; pledgeted mattress sutures have been used at NYU routinely for over 20 years because the technique is simple and significant periprosthetic leak is virtually unknown. Care is taken to insert the sutures in the annulus of the mitral valve but no deeper in order to avoid injury to adjacent structures, especially the circumflex coronary artery or the conduction bundle. Throughout the insertion of the prosthetic valve, care is taken to avoid undue traction on the mitral annulus that may inadvertently tear the annulus from the underlying ventricular muscle and result in subsequent rupture of the left ventricle, discussed in a subsequent section.

Following closure of the atriotomy, fibrillation is induced and the aorta is unclamped. Air is removed by a variety of maneuvers, including aspiration of each cardiac chamber. A left ventricular vent is not used routinely.

Rupture of the left ventricle is a rare but highly lethal complication following insertion. A prospective study of techniques to avoid this complication revealed that routine preservation of a few chordae to the annulus of the mural leaflet, in combination with other techniques, has been associated with absence of this complication for over 10 years, a marked contrast to preceding experiences. Whether preservation of chordae prevents this complication or not cannot be proved, but certainly it is strongly recommended in older high-risk patients until a better explanation is available.

Convalescence is usually benign except in Class IV patients with long-standing congestive failure who are catabolic with the myriads of complications from malnutrition. These patients require intense care for days or weeks, with particular attention to precise caloric and protein intake, recorded on a daily basis. This often entails a combination of tube feeding and hyperalimentation because some chronically ill emaciated patients are simply unable to eat an adequate amount in the first days or weeks following operation.

Antibiotics are routinely given during operation at measured intervals to maintain a bactericidal level of the antibiotic appropriate for the organisms presently existing in the hospital environment. These are stopped 2 to 3 days following operation, usually when intracardiac lines have been removed. Anticoagulation with sodium warfarin is started about 2 days following operation, subsequently maintained with a prothrombin time of 18 to 20 s. We have found maintenance of the prothrombin time at 1.5 to 2 times control a reliable method of following these patients and have no experience using the international ratio (INR) method, although either monitoring technique is acceptable. This has been used for over a decade with satisfactory protection from thromboembolism, but a low frequency of hemorrhage from anticoagulation. Warfarin may be stopped after 3 months in patients with porcine prostheses unless there is chronic atrial fibrillation or a large left atrium. In patients with chronic atrial fibrillation and a large left atrium warfarin should be continued indefinitely. If warfarin is stopped, an antiplatelet agent, usually aspirin, is given for the next year. Warfarin is continued permanently, of course, in patients with mechanical prostheses.

Results Following Open Commissurotomy

Most patients improve promptly after operation, obtaining the full therapeutic benefit within 3 to 6 months. During this time, careful attention to sodium intake and body weight is necessary, for renal excretion of sodium may remain impaired for weeks or months and continued use of diuretics may be necessary.

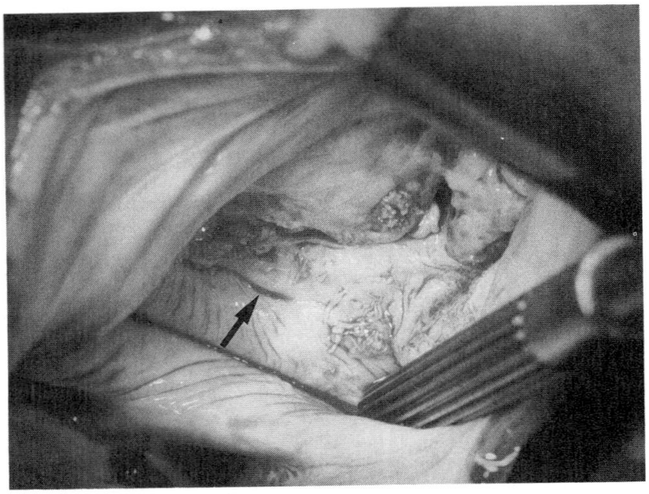

A

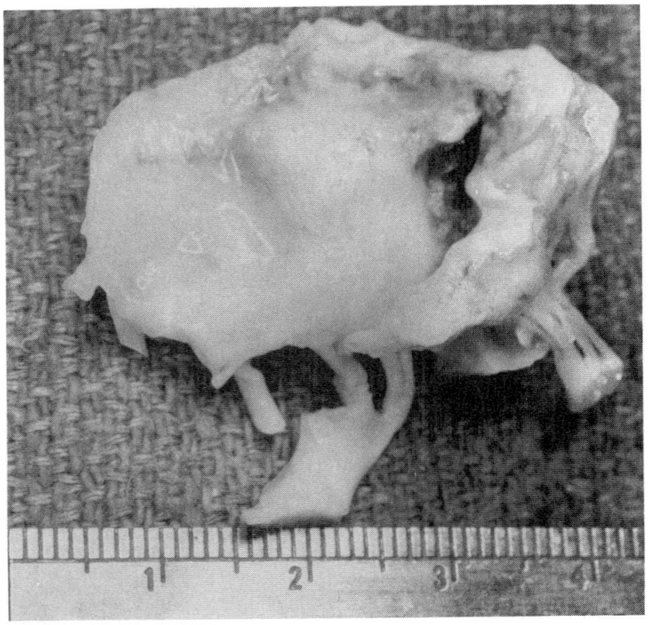

B

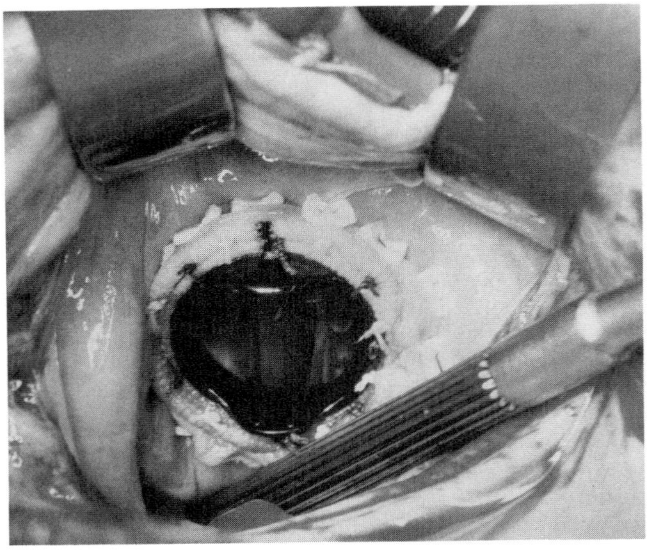

C

FIG. 18-8. *A.* Operative photograph of rheumatic mitral valve with calcific mitral stenosis, viewed through a left atriotomy incision. *B.* Excised calcified mitral valve with fibrotic, shortened chordae tendineae. *C.* St. Jude mechanical mitral valve visualized through the open left atrium. Pledget reinforced sutures were used to secure the valve into the native annulus.

In a report by Halseth and associates, only 11 percent of patients with mitral stenosis required valve replacement at operation. The operative mortality rate was 1.5 percent; the 10-year survival rate was 81 percent. Only 7 percent of the 191 patients required valve replacement in the next several years. In the series reported by Cohn and associates of 120 patients there were no operative deaths and five late deaths from noncardiac causes. Actuarial projections at 10 years found a survival rate near 95 percent, 91 percent freedom from emboli, 84 percent freedom from reoperation. No deaths have occurred at our institution in the last 10 years with open mitral commissurotomy, and late valve function is usually excellent for up to 10 years. After 10 to 15 years, progressive rheumatic disease makes valve replacement increasingly likely.

These experiences are particularly significant because during the 1950s and 1960s a recurrence rate as high as 30 to 40 percent within 5 years after operation was reported following commissurotomy, clearly in retrospect owing to an ineffective commissurotomy with the closed commissurotomy procedure. Pessimism was expressed at that time about the durability of closed commissurotomy, simply because residual stenosis remained following operation.

These considerations are especially pertinent now because of the recent interest in percutaneous balloon mitral valvuloplasty. The effective mitral valve area has been increased from 0.8 to 1.7

cm^2, but some regurgitation occurred in 43 percent of patients. The procedure obviously cannot correct fusion of the chordae and papillary muscles and thus is applicable only to limited pathologic conditions. The noninvasive features make balloon valvuloplasty a serious consideration in patients who are poor candidates for operation because of other diseases such as stroke, cancer, or advanced age. The data do not support, however, that this procedure is more than a palliative one, with results similar to those obtained with digital commissurotomy in the early 1950s. Far better long-term results can be obtained in most patients with an open operative technique.

Results Following Valve Replacement. If valve replacement is necessary, long-term results are excellent. Five-year survival is near 70 to 90 percent, 10 years 60 to 70 percent depending on the functional classification of the patient. A major factor in determining late survival is the severity of congestive heart failure before operation. Patients in Class II or early Class III have a 5-year survival of over 90 percent while those near Class IV are about 60 percent. These data clearly indicate the importance of preventing preoperative irreversible injury and, accordingly, the need for earlier operation. In a comprehensive follow-up study reported from our institution, factors affecting survival after mitral valve operation were age, NYHA Class IV status, previous heart surgery, and concomitant surgical procedures on another valve or on the coronary arteries.

In 1985 Starr summarized his 25 years of experience with over 2000 ball valve prostheses, 34 percent of which were mitral valve replacements. In 1979 Bjork described his experiences with 1800 Bjork-Shiley valves. The 5-year survival after mitral replacement was 66 percent. Frequency of thromboembolism was 4 percent per patient year and frequency of thrombosis of the prosthesis was 1 percent per year. Our experiences have shown that with close medical supervision the incidence of thromboembolic and anticoagulant complications is only 1 percent per year after mechanical mitral valve replacement in selected patients. Edmonds and associates summarized overall reported experiences with thromboembolic complications of different types of valve prostheses, revealing thromboembolic rates of 1 to 4 percent per year.

The major problem with tissue prostheses is durability with an estimated failure rate by 10 years of at least 20 percent, and a failure rate of 50 percent by 15 years. Oyer and associates reported a study of over 1400 patients who received Hancock prostheses. The probability of freedom from tissue failure 5 years following operation was 95 percent. At NYU 976 patients received isolated porcine mitral prosthesis between 1976 and 1987 with a 5-year survival rate of 73 percent and a 5-year freedom from reoperation of 96 percent. While porcine and mechanical prostheses have similar results after 5 years, durability should clearly be better with mechanical prostheses after 10 to 15 years as more porcine valves begin to degenerate.

When either type of prosthetic valve replacement is done, mechanical or porcine, there is a small but permanent risk of endocarditis, ranging between 1 and 2 percent per patient per year. Prophylactic antibiotics should be routinely used when episodes of transient bacteremia can be anticipated, such as with dental extraction, endoscopy, or cystoscopy.

Mitral Insufficiency

Mitral valve replacement has traditionally been the procedure of choice for operative treatment of mitral valve insufficiency, with excellent long-term results reported. The technique for replacement is identical to that described in the section on mitral stenosis. Alternately, over the past 15 years Carpentier has serially reported impressive results using a detailed mitral valve reconstruction technique, a method that has been widely adopted at NYU since 1980. Carpentier's operative techniques for mitral valve reconstruction vary, depending on the valvular pathology. Dilation of the annulus, a frequent finding in most cases of mitral insufficiency, is treated by remodelling ring annuloplasty. Insufficiency due to posterior (mural) leaflet prolapse or chordal rupture is corrected by resection of the diseased mural leaflet, repair of the annulus, and ring annuloplasty (Fig. 18-9). Additional technical maneuvers, applicable to prolapse or ruptured chordae involving the anterior (aortic) leaflet, include shortening of elongated chordae (Fig. 18-10), reimplantation of ruptured chordae onto secondary chordae, or transposition of chordae from the posterior leaflet to the anterior leaflet (Fig. 18-11). Results suggest that mitral valve repair is feasible in most patients with nonrheumatic causes of mitral insufficiency. Ten- to fifteen-year durability has been excellent, and many centers now consider mitral valve reconstruction the preferred treatment for mitral insufficiency due to ruptured chordae, mitral prolapse, or ischemic disease. Late results of valve repair are less certain when mitral insufficiency is due to rheumatic disease.

Etiology. In the United States mitral insufficiency from rheumatic fever has steadily decreased in frequency, now representing only about 30 percent of patients seen. The most common cause of acquired mitral insufficiency is mitral valve prolapse from degenerative disease, often complicated by rupture of chordae tendineae. Degenerative disease accounts for 40 to 50 percent of all mitral insufficiency in this country. Ischemic or infarction of papillary muscle complicating extensive occlusive disease of the coronary arteries has become an increasingly common cause, accounting for 10 to 15 percent. Bacterial endocarditis remains an infrequent but important cause, and rarely congenital mitral disease presents with mitral insufficiency during adulthood.

It is now known that some degree or prolapse of the mitral valve is surprisingly frequent, detectable in as many as 5 percent of the normal population. In the majority of patients, the hemodynamic disturbance is minimal. In chronic cases, however, severe changes evolve with dense extensive calcification, progressive elongation of chordae, and increasing asymmetric dilatation of the annulus of the mitral valve. The mitral valve annulus always dilates posteriorly, as the anterior portion is a fixed part of the fibrous skeleton of the heart.

Pathologic Anatomy. The basic changes with rheumatic fever were described in the preceding section on Mitral Stenosis. Insufficiency develops from fibrosis and contraction of the mitral leaflets, usually combined with calcification restricting mobility. Fibrosis and contraction of chordae tendineae are important contributory factors because they prevent the valve from closing in the proper plane. These changes are usually gradually progressive because of the turbulent flow of blood.

Carpentier, in a study of over 50 rheumatic hearts, carefully delineated the additional pathologic changes that evolve and augment the insufficiency. These are predominantly progressive elongation of chordae and asymmetric dilatation of the mitral annulus, occurring predominantly in the posterior leaflet area. The primary defect in rheumatic mitral insufficiency is from ''restricted leaflet motion.''

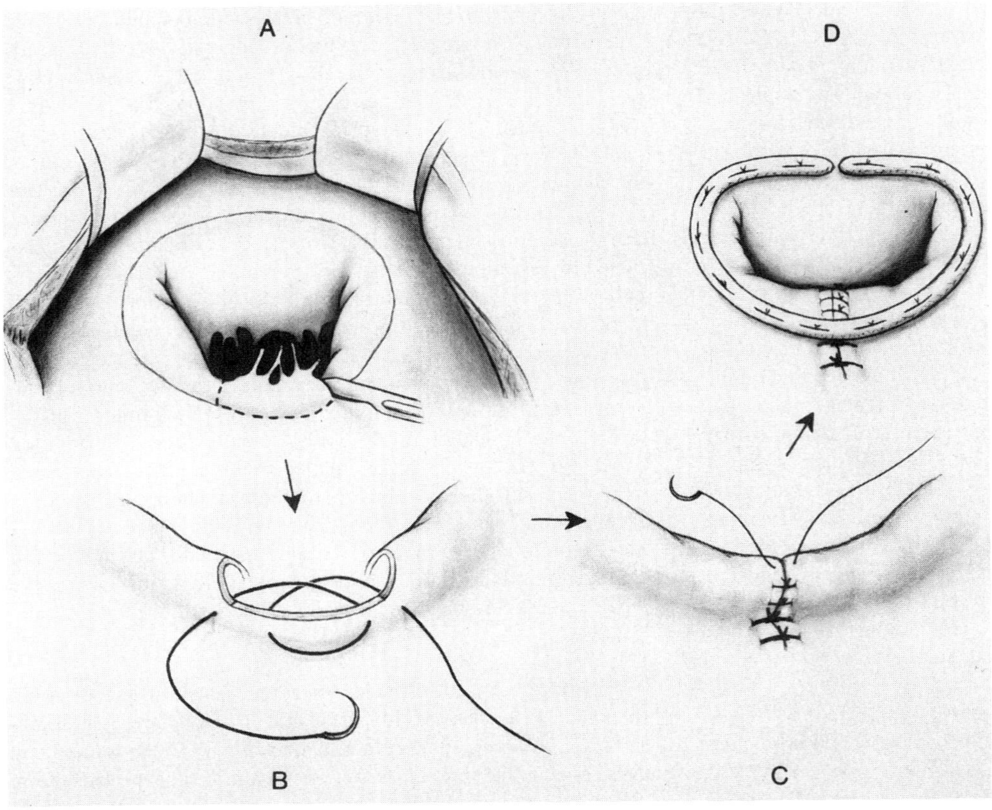

FIG. 18-9. Illustration of Carpentier techniques for posterior leaflet resection and leaflet repair followed by ring annuloplasty. *(Reproduced by permission from Galloway et al, Circulation 78:1087, 1988.)*

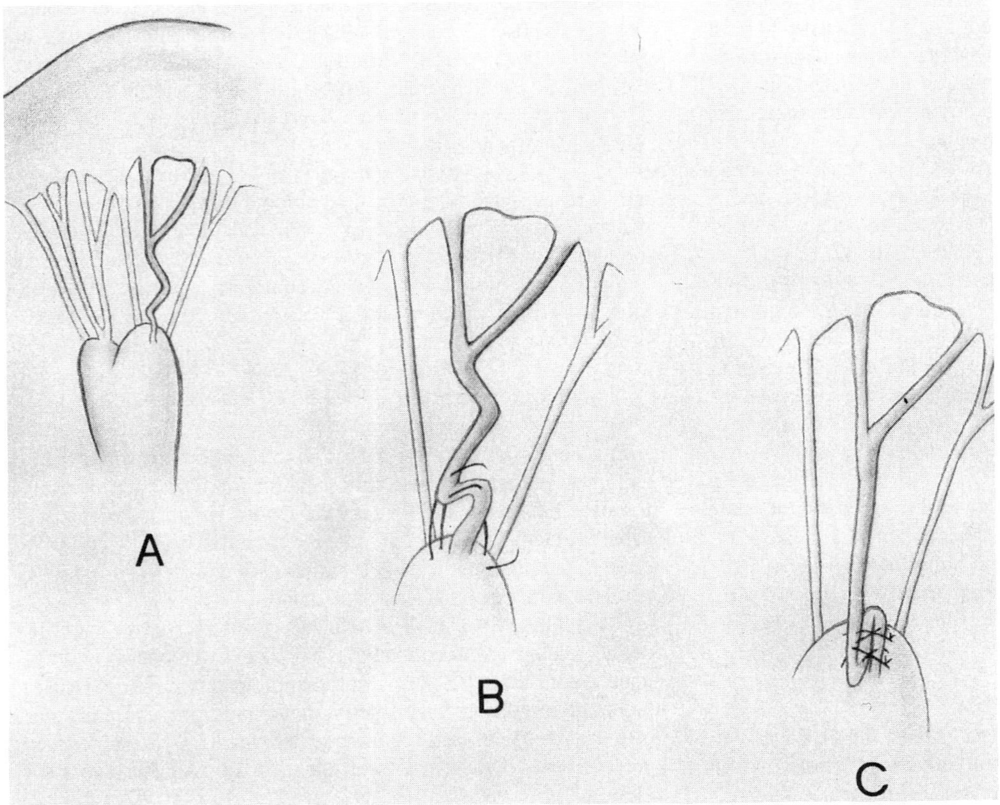

FIG. 18-10. Illustration of Carpentier technique of chordal shortening for anterior mitral valve leaflet prolapse. *(Reproduced by permission from Galloway et al, Circulation 78:1087, 1988.)*

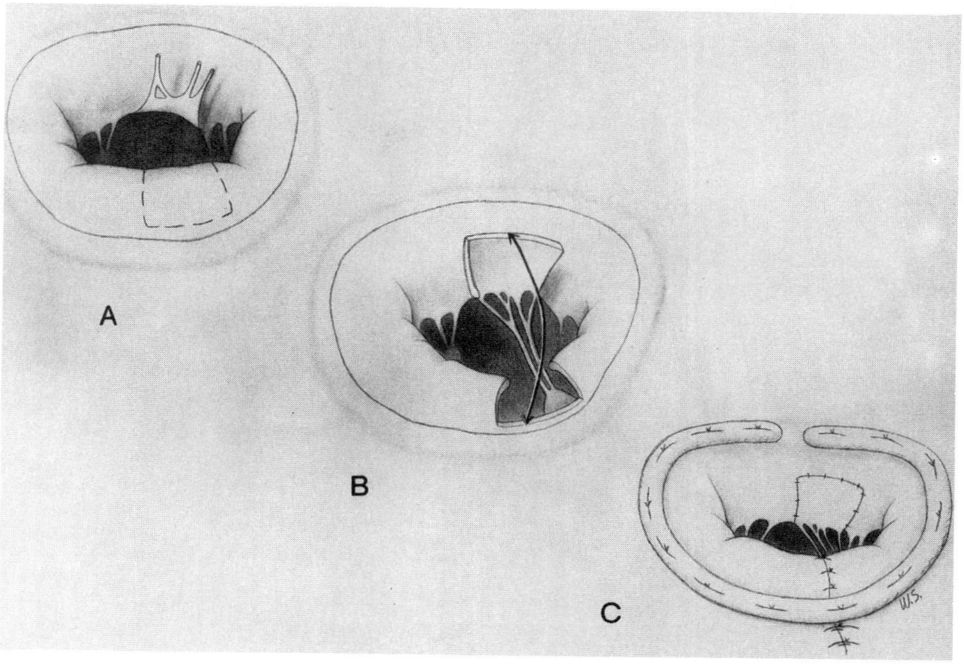

FIG. 18-11. Illustration of Carpentier technique of chordal transposition from the posterior leaflet, used to correct mitral insufficiency due to a flail anterior leaflet. *(Reproduced by permission from Galloway et al, Circulation 78:1087, 1988.)*

By contrast, in mitral insufficiency from degenerative disease, the pathology is primarily a result of ''increased leaflet motion.'' The involved leaflet or leaflets usually prolapse beyond the proper closing plane of the valve, with the leaflets termed ''flail'' when all structural support is loss, as with a ruptured chordae (Fig. 18-12*A*). The chordae are often thinned and elongated, while the leaflet tissue is frequently thinned and increased in size, producing the ''billowing'' mitral valve. Prolapse can occur in the anterior leaflet, the posterior leaflet, or both. Secondary dilation of the posterior portion of the annulus is frequently present.

Several pathologic changes can occur from ischemic disease. At times reversible ischemia of the papillary muscle may be present, and mitral insufficiency may improve after revascularization. In other cases the valve might open and close properly, with mitral insufficiency resulting from annular dilation. This usually occurs when the heart is dilated and the left ventricular end-diastolic pressure is elevated. Finally, the papillary muscle and chordae may be elongated from infarction or be completely ruptured.

Endocarditis can produce discrete leaflet perforation, ruptured chordae, and varying degrees of leaflet destruction. Extensive infection may destroy all viable leaflet tissue or produce a paraannular abscess. Secondary annular dilation occurs if mitral insufficiency is long-standing, as is seen with treated endocarditis and chronic mitral insufficiency. Congenital forms of mitral insufficiency were described in Chap. 17.

Pathophysiology. The basic physiologic change is elevation of the left atrial pressure as blood regurgitates through the incompetent mitral valve during ventricular systole. The ventricular pressure spike is commonly to levels of 30 to 40 mmHg, but levels as high as 80 to 90 mmHg have been recorded. In diastole the left atrial pressure drops sharply to approach the left ventricular diastolic pressure, although a small gradient usually remains because of the large blood flow through the mitral valve during diastole. Mean left atrial pressure is usually 15 to 25 mmHg. The mitral regurgitation produces enlargement of the left atrium, although for unknown reasons the degree of left atrial enlargement varies greatly among different patients and is not proportional to the degree of regurgitation. In some patients with significant regurgitation only slight left atrial enlargement is present, while in others giant left atria evolve, enlarging to contact the right chest wall. In contrast to mitral stenosis, pulmonary vascular changes appear rather late in the course of the disease, perhaps as a result of a large left atrium absorbing much of the kinetic energy of the regurgitating blood without sustained elevation of left atrial pressure. Fortunately, the dilated left ventricle with mitral insufficiency may function adequately for surprisingly long periods of time, maintaining the left ventricular diastolic pressure near the normal range of 8 to 12 mmHg until eventually left ventricular failure appears. This process results in progressive left ventricular dilation and can lead to irreversible changes by the time severe symptoms develop.

As there is little stasis of blood in the left atrium, in contrast to mitral stenosis, left atrial thrombosis and arterial embolism are much less frequent than with mitral stenosis.

Physical Examination. The two characteristic features of mitral insufficiency are the apical systolic murmur and the increased force of the apical impulse. The systolic murmur is heard best at the apex, which is often displaced downward and to the left from enlargement of the left ventricle. It is well transmitted to the axilla. The quality is of a harsh, blowing type. With severe insufficiency, the murmur is pansystolic, appearing immediately after the first sound and continuing until the second sound. The intensity of the murmur does not correlate with the severity of the regurgitation, but the pansystolic characteristic does. Murmurs not extending completely through systole are seen with less serious degrees of regurgitation. The systolic murmur is a highly characteristic feature of mitral insufficiency and is absent only in most unusual circumstances. A diastolic murmur is usually present in addition, resulting from increased flow across the mitral valve as a result of blood regurgitated into the atrium during systole. The absence of an opening snap and the normal quality of the first heart sound

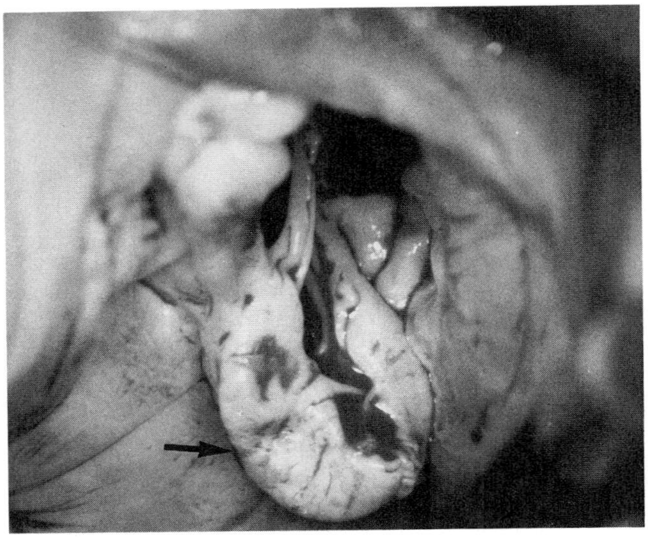

A

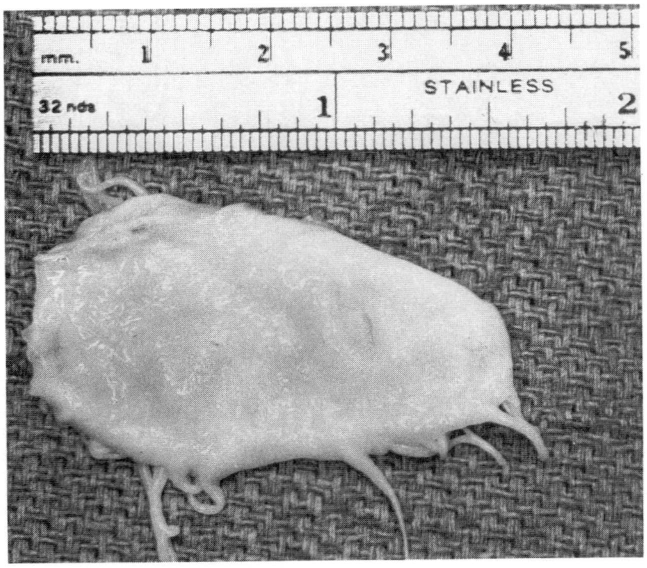

B

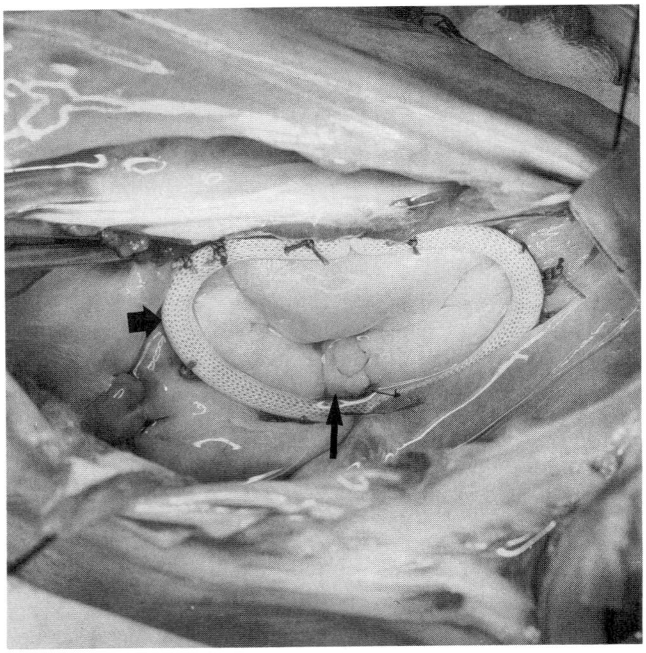

C

FIG. 18-12. *A.* Operative photograph demonstrating massive prolapse of the mitral valve posterior leaflet. *B.* Specimen of resected mitral valve posterior leaflet. *C.* Operative photograph of completed Carpentier-type mitral valve reconstruction. The small arrow indicates the posterior leaflet repair, while the large arrow demonstrates the ring annuloplasty. Note the total correction of leaflet prolapse and annular dilation.

both suggest that the diastolic murmur is due to increased flow of blood rather than anatomic mitral stenosis.

Clinical Manifestations. ***Symptoms.*** Patients with mild mitral insufficiency are usually asymptomatic. The diagnosis is usually made after discovery of an apical systolic murmur. In former years, mitral valve prolapse was confused with rheumatic mitral insufficiency. The development of echocardiography has greatly simplified the differential diagnosis.

With significant mitral insufficiency, the most common symptoms are fatigue, dyspnea on exertion, and palpitation. A most important point is that these symptoms may remain mild despite impressive physical findings of mitral insufficiency with progressive cardiac enlargement. Eventually, left ventricular failure evolves with a rise in end-diastolic pressure and progressive pulmonary congestion. Respiratory symptoms become prominent with exertional dyspnea, cough, and paroxysmal nocturnal dyspnea.

The apical impulse is usually forceful and prolonged, occupying an area of 3 to 4 cm^2. The first heart sound is usually normal, though it may be confused with the early onset of the systolic murmur.

Laboratory Examinations. The chest x-ray shows enlargement of both the left ventricle and the left atrium. In some patients, massive enlargement of the left atrium occurs with the wall of the atrium extending to the right chest wall and producing a grotesque deformity. The electrocardiogram does not contribute materially to the diagnosis. It may be normal with significant disease. In about 50 percent of patients, left ventricular hypertrophy can be recognized. 2-D Doppler echocardiography can approximate the degree of regurgitation. Transesophageal echocardiographic studies have become very accurate, not only in determining the amount of mitral insufficiency, but also in identifying which leaflets are involved. Many patients are now operated on based on this study alone.

The most precise studies are obtained by cardiac catheterization and cineangiography, noting reflux of dye into the left atrium when injected into the left ventricle. With minimal or severe insufficiency the dye studies are quite satisfactory, but with intermediate forms of insufficiency, the method is only reasonably good but thus far the best one available. Left atrial pressure tracings show a prominent V wave from regurgitation of blood during systole.

Treatment. ***Indications for Operation.*** Symptoms of fatigue and dyspnea may remain only moderately severe for a long time despite progressive deterioration in cardiac function, as evidenced by progressive left ventricular enlargement. Selecting the proper time for operation is a combination of physical examination, laboratory studies, and symptoms. A fall in an ejection fraction with exercise, measured with radionuclide studies, is currently a good measurement of early onset of serious impairment in ventricular function. Similarly, a progressive increase in the end-systolic dimension of the heart, measured by echocardiography, suggests significant ventricular deterioration. These changes may well antedate visible enlargement of the left ventricle on the chest x-ray. Operation at this earlier stage will avoid the late onset of cardiac failure 3 to 5 years following valve replacement, apparently from preoperative irreversible ventricular dysfunction. Late cardiac function and long-term survival are both markedly improved when operation is done before the development of NYHA Class IV symptoms. Even with poor cardiac function and debilitating symptoms survival is improved by surgical intervention.

Replacement versus Reconstruction. Up until 1980 to 1985, the majority of patients were treated with mitral valve replacement. Repair was used for some patients with isolated ruptured chordae of the mural leaflet, using the technique developed by McGoon. Kay and Reed successfully used annuloplasty for insufficiency when annular dilatation was prominent. Once Carpentier developed a comprehensive system of repair of mitral insufficiency, mitral valve reconstruction became more widely applicable (Fig. 18-12*B, C*). His overall experiences with over 2000 patients were summarized in 1983. Similarly, since 1980 we have had extensive experience with Carpentier reconstructive techniques at New York University, with excellent results to date in over 700 patients. The operative mortality rate is only 1 to 2 percent. The best results have been in patients with prolapse and ruptured chordae, with a repair durability of 95 percent at 5 to 7 years. Similar encouraging results have been reported by Cosgrove and associates from the Cleveland Clinic. If experiences by others in the future are similar, reconstruction, rather than replacement, may become the most commonly performed operation for nonrheumatic mitral insufficiency.

In 1980 Reed summarized experiences with 198 patients. Results were quite good, with a late mortality of only 9 percent, a low frequency of thromboembolism, and only 8 percent of patients requiring repeat operation. This operation is particularly attractive in children, avoiding the use of the Carpentier rigid annuloplasty ring. Chaval and associates described excellent results with reconstruction in 89 children, 84 of whom had rheumatic valve disease. Ten years following operation 90 percent of patients were alive, 98 percent free from thromboemboli, and 78 percent did not require reoperation.

Late Results. In this country the most extensive late results after mitral valve reconstruction were reported from our institution in 1988, in a report comparing 975 porcine valves, 169 mechanical valves, and 280 Carpentier-type mitral valve reconstructions. Follow-up was 100 percent complete after valve reconstruction, with 82 percent having late echocardiographic studies. Operative mortality was lower and long-term survival was better after valve reconstruction than after valve replacement, but survival was primarily related to the known risk factors such as age, NYHA functional classification, and associated coronary bypass or other cardiac procedures, not to the procedure itself. The incidence of late valve-related complications was less, however, after valve reconstruction than after valve replacement. Furthermore, repair durability was nearly equivalent to that obtained with mechanical prostheses, except in rheumatic patients where reoperation rates were higher. These data suggested that valve reconstruction was associated with less late morbidity than valve replacement (Fig. 18-13). We concluded that mitral valve insufficiency is the procedure of choice for nonrheumatic causes of mitral insufficiency. With rheumatic disease progressive fibrosis results in failure rate of up to 25 percent within 5 to 10 years. Prosthetic mitral valve replacement is often preferable when advanced rheumatic disease is present.

Carpentier has reported excellent durability for 10 to 15 years following valve reconstruction. Again, the incidence of thromboembolic complications was extremely low, less than 1 percent per year without the need for anticoagulation. Other studies have suggested that cardiac function is better maintained after valve repair than after valve replacement, since the chordae tendineae are preserved and the subvalvular apparatus appears to be important in maintaining both global and regional ventricular function.

In summary, mitral valve reconstruction might be the procedure of choice for many patients with mitral insufficiency. Valve reconstruction can be associated with fewer late valve-related complications and may better preserve left ventricular function. Mechanical valve replacement remains the standard in terms of valve durability, and late results are excellent with mechanical valves when the patients are followed closely to avoid anticoagulant-related complications. Consequently, mechanical valves are frequently used in cases with advanced rheumatic disease and when valve repair is unfeasible. Some centers still prefer mechanical valve replacement for most cases. Because of decreased late durability, porcine valves are reserved for the elderly or for the rare case where avoidance of anticoagulation is necessary and valve reconstruction is not feasible.

Aortic Stenosis

Historical Data. Effective surgical treatment of aortic valve disease first became possible in 1960-1961 with the development of satisfactory prosthetic valves by Starr and Edwards and by Harken and associates. Earlier attempts to correct aortic valvular disease by cusp replacement with prosthetic cusps of Teflon cloth or by extensive debridement of calcific material from calcified valve cusps initially gave satisfactory results in some patients, but a high failure rate within 1 to 2 years led to abandonment of these

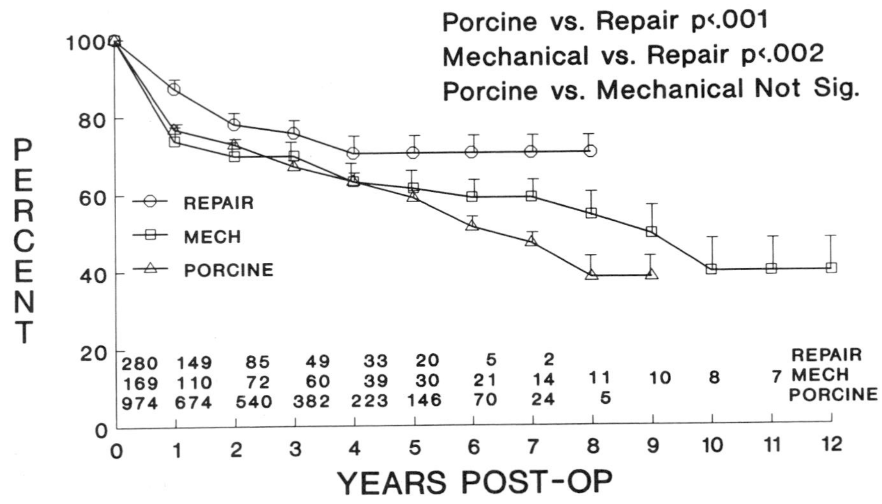

FIG. 18-13. Actuarial freedom from all cardiac-related morbidity and mortality (complication-free survival) after mitral valve reconstruction and mitral valve replacement. Patients with mitral valve reconstruction had significantly fewer late complications or deaths than patients with either mechanical or porcine prostheses. *(Reproduced with permission from Galloway et al, Ann Thorac Surg 47:655, 1989.)*

techniques as soon as a satisfactory prosthetic valve became available.

Several modifications of mechanical prostheses have been evaluated, and three basic designs have proved durable: the original ball valve prosthesis, the tilting disc prosthesis, and the bilateral disk prothesis. Currently, the durability of these prostheses is excellent, but the major limitation of all mechanical prosthetic valves has been thromboembolism, partly controlled with permanent anticoagulation. Despite careful anticoagulation, some thromboembolic events occur with a frequency of 1 to 2 percent per year as noted in the previous sections of this chapter.

With the significant hazard of thromboembolism, there has been a long and continued investigation of tissue prostheses that often do not require permanent anticoagulation and have a much lower frequency of thromboembolism. The aortic homograft, the pulmonary autograft, and the porcine prosthesis are tissue-valve options described earlier in the chapter.

Several other tissues were evaluated and subsequently discarded because of lack of durability, including autologous fascia lata, allograft dura mater valves, and formaldehyde-preserved porcine valves. The glutaraldehyde preserved porcine valve was introduced by Carpentier in 1968 and has subsequently become the most widely used tissue prosthesis. Bovine pericardium, glutaraldehyde treated, was developed by Ionescu but has not been as popular as the porcine valve. At present, 5-year durability with porcine valves is near 95 percent, and decreasing to about 80 percent at 10 years and 50 percent at 15 years.

Etiology. About one-half of patients younger than 70 years of age operated on will be found to have calcification of a congenitally malformed valve, usually a bicuspid valve. Usually, there is a history of negligible disability for decades until calcification has made the valve rigid, with the time interval varying widely from the fourth or even the seventh or eighth decade. In about one-third of patients rheumatic fever is apparently the basic cause. Again calcification eventually makes the valve leaflets progressively rigid, and the degree of stenosis progresses with time (Fig. 18-14*A*).

The third major cause is acquired calcific aortic stenosis, a process of diffuse calcification developing in cusps that are neither congenitally malformed nor show any signs of previous rheumatic inflammation. It is probably similar to calcification that sporadically develops in other soft tissues with aging as this is seen more frequently in patients in their seventh and eighth decades, accounting for one-half of the aortic stenoses seen in patients older than 70 years. Older patients also frequently have associated coronary artery disease.

Pathophysiology. A normal aortic valve has a cross-sectional area of 2.5 to 3.5 cm depending upon body size. Moderately severe stenosis is present when the valve orifice has narrowed to about 1.0 cm; 0.8 cm is an approximate area where operation is usually indicated because of pathophysiologic abnormalities. This is a changing field, however, so operation at an earlier time may be recommended in the future in order to better assure good long-term ventricular function. Cross-sectional areas as low as 0.4 to 0.6 cm^2 may be found in advanced disease, often with a systolic gradient of 100 mm or greater across the valve. Usually, at catheterization a gradient of at least 50 mm is found with significant stenosis. With a low cardiac output the gradient may be misleading, however, and the valve area should always be calculated using the Gorlin formula (see Diagnostic Tests).

The increased workload on the myocardium imposed by the stenosis results in progressive concentric ventricular hypertrophy but little dilatation. For this reason heart size may appear almost normal on the chest x-ray. Despite this, left ventricular hypertrophy results in a stiff, noncompliant ventricle, with diastolic dysfunction. The left ventricular diastolic pressure becomes elevated above the upper limit of normal of 12 mm as the left ventricle gradually fails. Systolic function of the ventricle remains well-preserved early, decreasing later from "afterload mismatch." After systolic function decreases, congestive heart failure progresses.

Myocardial ischemia, manifested as angina pectoris, is a common symptom. This apparently results from the combination of two factors, the increased left ventricular work and myocardial hypertrophy as well as the decreased cardiac output. Such ischemia can also produce arrhythmias. This factor is apparently responsible for the well-known tendency of aortic stenosis to result in "sudden death" with very few premonitory symptoms. Associated coronary artery disease should always be excluded when angina is present.

Clinical Manifestations. ***Symptoms.*** Characteristically, there is a long asymptomatic latent period, sometimes for 10 to 20 years. Classical physical findings may be present with slight dysp-

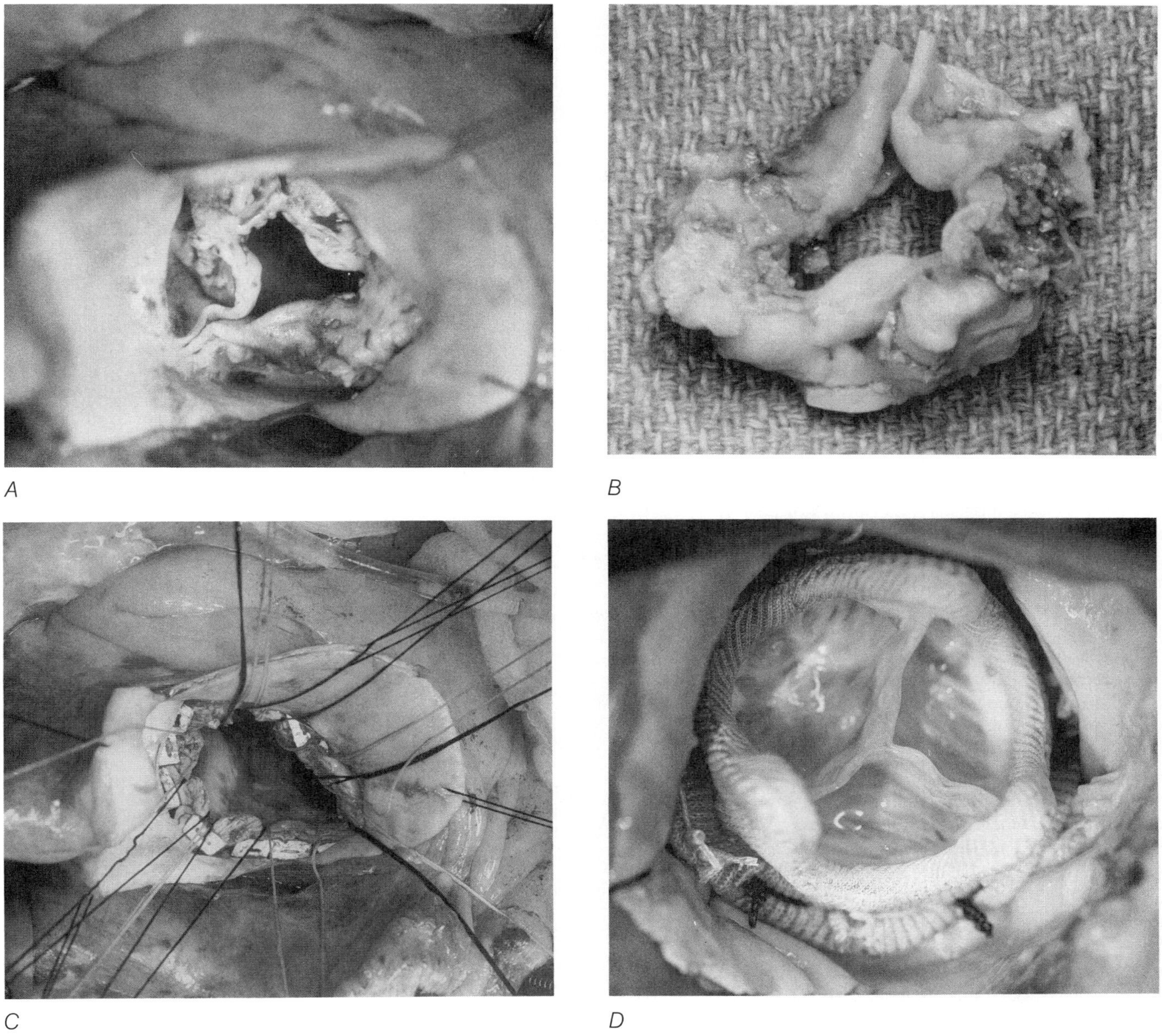

FIG. 18-14. *A.* Operative photograph of calcific aortic stenosis, seen through an oblique aortotomy incision. *B.* Excised aortic valve. The valve leaflets were completely immobile and fixed in the midposition, producing a mixture of aortic stenosis and aortic insufficiency. *C.* After excising the valve, pledget reinforced mattress sutures have been placed into the aortic valve annulus. The sutures will be subsequently placed through the sewing ring of the prosthetic valve. *D.* Porcine valve in the aortic position before closure of the aortotomy incision.

nea on exertion as the only symptom. Three symptoms are characteristic, any or all of which may be present: angina pectoris, syncope, or dyspnea. Sudden death, which accounts for 15 to 20 percent of fatalities from aortic stenosis, becomes much more of a threat once these symptoms are present. Syncope develops in about one-third of patients. This apparently is from decreased cerebral blood flow. In some patients, it may result after minimal effort, with little warning. In a small percentage of patients it may result from a conduction abnormality, apparently an intermittent heart block from involvement of the atrioventricular node by calcium spicules arising from the stenotic valve.

Angina pectoris develops in 30 to 40 percent of patients, a manifestation of myocardial ischemia. Probably these episodes are associated with "silent" episodes of muscle necrosis because some patients with surprisingly few symptoms are found to have large amounts of myocardium replaced by scar tissue.

The average life expectancy once angina or syncope has appeared is about 3 years.

Left ventricular failure is an even more ominous finding, as the life expectancy is slightly more than a year once heart failure is present. Atrial fibrillation, a consequence of prolonged elevation of left atrial pressure, is similarly a grave event, as it indicates an advanced stage of left ventricular failure unless mitral valve disease is present.

The principal change in the left ventricle is concentric hypertrophy, not dilatation. The apical impulse has been described as a ''prolonged heave,'' not a ''forceful thrust,'' as is found with ventricular dilatation from aortic or mitral insufficiency. The peripheral pulse, similarly, is slow and prolonged, well illustrated with a pulse tracing recorded by arterial puncture as a dome-shaped peak in systole, contrasting sharply with the sharp systolic upstroke seen with aortic insufficiency.

Laboratory Studies. The heart size is usually normal on x-ray. Calcification of the aortic valve is usually visible in patients older than 35 years of age.

The electrocardiogram is not reliable because of the wide variation. In some patients left ventricular hypertrophy is evident, but in some seriously ill patients with severe aortic stenosis the electrocardiogram is virtually normal. Conduction abnormalities are frequent, apparently from spicules of calcium projecting into the conduction bundle located just beneath the base of the noncoronary sinus. Some patients develop complete heart block. The 2-D echocardiogram can estimate the peak transvalvular systolic gradient, document ventricular wall thickness, and measure end-systolic and end-diastolic dimensions of the left ventricular cavity.

Cardiac catheterization readily confirms the diagnosis, both measuring the gradient and permitting calculation of the cross-sectional area of the valve. Gradients exceeding 50 mm are usually found with significant stenosis. A cross-sectional area near 0.8 to 1.0 cm^2 is considered the range at which operation should be routinely recommended, though this concept has frequently changed toward more liberal indications for operation as results with aortic valve replacement have improved.

At catheterization coronary arteriography should be routinely done, for associated coronary disease is found in at least 30 to 50 percent of patients studied, the frequency increasing with the age of the patient studied. Other valves should be assessed for concomitant disease, particularly when rheumatic disease is present. Concomitant mitral valve disease and left ventricular function can also be evaluated at catheterization. In some patients with a broad thick chest and distant heart sounds because of emphysematous lungs, the physical findings are deceptively minimal, with a faint unimpressive systolic murmur being the only initial abnormality found on physical examination. In such patients, echocardiography is helpful in deciding whether catheterization should be done, for a benign aortic systolic murmur becomes increasingly common in older age groups.

Treatment. ***Indications for Operation.*** For asymptomatic patients, periodic echocardiographic studies are done to assess the gradient and the end-systolic and end-diastolic dimensions of the heart. A significant gradient with associated left ventricular hypertrophy and a rising end-systolic volume is an indication for catheterization and possible operation. Similarly, a drop in ejection fraction, measured by radionuclide studies, might be an indication for operation. In asymptomatic patients, the finding at catheterization of an aortic cross-sectional area of 0.8 cm is clearly an indication for operation. Sudden death remains a small but definite hazard in such patients, so operation should be clearly urged despite the well-being of the patient. In the presence of any of the classic three symptoms, angina, syncope, or dyspnea, operation should similarly be strongly recommended, especially if catheterization demonstrates an aortic valve area near 1.0 cm^2 or less. The frequency of sudden death increases sharply in symptomatic patients.

Technique of Operation. The operative technique is a standard one, using a median sternotomy, cardiopulmonary bypass with hyperkalemic cardioplegia induced with cold blood. Cardioplegia may be delivered directly into the coronary ostia, or ''retrograde'' through the coronary sinus. Subsequently, topical hypothermia is routinely used with large volumes of a cold electrolyte solution, both filling the pericardium and subsequently wrapping the heart in a laparotomy pad and using a constant infusion of cold fluid. The effectiveness of this method of myocardial preservation is extraordinary because the heart can be safely arrested for 3 h or longer, though this long period of time is seldom necessary.

This form of myocardial preservation provides a dry quiet operative field that has made aortic valve replacement a procedure with a remarkably low mortality and morbidity.

In almost all patients, aortic valve replacement is required. A few elderly patients with a small hypoplastic annulus have been treated by debridement, as long as this does not produce insufficiency. This procedure had a disappointing frequency of recurrence within 1 to 3 years and should be considered a palliative procedure used only when special circumstances indicate prosthetic replacement would be hazardous or unsatisfactory.

After an oblique aortotomy incision is made, the valve is excised totally (Fig. 18-14*B*). Great care is taken at operation to avoid losing any calcific fragments detached during removal of the valve that could subsequently be embolized. A gauze pack is routinely placed in the ventricle before removal of the valve is begun. A number of maneuvers during the procedure (frequent removal of the pack, lavage of the ventricle, and keeping the ventricular cavity dry with a vent) make it possible to avoid emboli in the vast majority of patients.

The choice of a metallic or porcine prosthetic valve was discussed previously emphasizing that the surgeon should make a recommendation based on the specific characteristics of the patient but also emphasizing that the patient should have the final decision. At NYU the St. Jude bileaflet mechanical prosthesis is used for most patients younger than 70 years of age, but other mechanical prostheses are equally efficacious. Flow characteristics are excellent with both single and bileaflet disk prostheses.

With tissue prostheses, the Carpentier porcine prosthesis is currently the most popular. There is flexibility of valve size with porcine prostheses. For valve replacement a pledgeted mattress suture technique is used routinely (Fig. 18-14*C, D*), probably unnecessary in many patients, but it virtually eliminates the hazard of periprosthetic leaks. For homografts and for the pulmonary autograft procedure a ''freehand'' insertion is used, as these grafts have no external sewing ring. A freehand homograft is technically more difficult than the standard prosthetic aortic valve replacement.

The left ventricular-aortic systolic gradient is routinely measured following bypass. Depending on the cardiac output, a gradient is rarely larger than 10 to 20 mm if a prosthesis of adequate size has been chosen.

Associated coronary disease is present in a large percentage of patients and is usually routinely bypassed at the time of operation.

Postoperative Care. Postoperative care is usually uneventful. Arrhythmias are among the more frequent complications, so 24-h monitoring of the cardiac rhythm with an oscilloscope is routinely done for 2 to 3 days. Pacemaker wires are routinely left in the right ventricle and atrium for 4 to 5 days.

Anticoagulant therapy is started 2 to 3 days following mechanical valve replacement, keeping the prothrombin time at 18 to 20 s. Antiplatelet therapy with aspirin is used with porcine aortic valves, and neither anticoagulation nor antiplatelet therapy is required for homograft valves.

Except for patients with serious preoperative ventricular dysfunction, patients become asymptomatic with a normal range of physical activity within 2 to 3 months following operation. Permanent periodic medical supervision, however, should be done for all patients because of the problems inherent with any prosthetic valve. Thromboembolism, anticoagulant hemorrhage, and endocarditis are the three principal complications of any patient with a prosthetic valve that requires periodic monitoring. With current prostheses and good anticoagulant therapy, thromboembolism occurs with a frequency of 1 to 2 percent per year in most reports, but fortunately most of these are small. Bloomfield reported an analysis of 540 patients with a disc or a porcine prosthesis inserted, finding no significant difference in the frequency of thromboembolism in patients with different prostheses. Endocarditis remains a grave hazard in any patient if a transient bacteremia occurs, such as a dental extraction or a cystoscopy. Although thromboemboli occur less with porcine prostheses and with homografts, late valve failure may occur in nearly 50 percent of these patients within 15 years.

Patients with significant cardiac enlargement and decreased ventricular function following operation should be monitored closely. A 24-h electrocardiographic monitor should be used to detect arrhythmias, and, if present, EPS should be performed. Long-term medical treatment with afterload reduction may also be necessary.

Prognosis. The operative mortality from aortic valve replacement is at a remarkably low level, usually between 1 and 2 percent for uncomplicated patients, and seldom exceeding 10 percent, even with far advanced complex problems. Operative risk is only 5 to 10 percent in patients over 70 years of age. Christakis and associates reported an analysis of over 40 variables influencing operative results. Operative death is usually a result of stroke, operative hemorrhage, or subsequent arrhythmias. Heart block has become uncommon.

Five-year survival in the usual patient is now near 85 to 90 percent. With severe impairment of ventricular function before operation, however, 5-year survival is again less, in the range of 60 to 70 percent, emphasizing the need for prompt operation in asymptomatic patients when signs of impaired ventricular function are found with laboratory studies. Reoperation is rare with mechanical prostheses, but reoperation is required with an increasing frequency after 10 years with porcine valves and with homografts.

In the past 1 to 2 years there has been considerable interest in percutaneous balloon valvuloplasty as a palliative procedure. At present, all physiologic data would indicate that balloon valvuloplasty should be restricted to high-risk elderly patients in whom short-term palliation seems the best immediate goal. Its application to good-risk patients, knowing the excellent results with prosthetic replacement, would seem unwarranted. Currently we recommend mechanical aortic valve replacement for most patients younger than 70 years of age, and porcine valve replacement for older patients. Homografts or pulmonary autografts are offered to young patients who want to avoid long-term anticoagulation.

Aortic Insufficiency

Etiology and Pathology. A variety of diseases can produce aortic insufficiency. Inflammatory disease is a frequent cause. At present, perhaps the most common is bacterial endocarditis that has produced destruction or perforation of a valve cusp. Rheumatic fever was formerly the most common inflammatory disease but is steadily declining in frequency in the United States. Syphilis is now a rarity.

Annular ectasia is an unusual type of collagen disease seen with increasing frequency as the average age of the population increases. This is seen in the most extreme form with the classic Marfan's syndrome with extensive cystic medial necrosis in the aorta, most probably in the ascending aorta. The aortic root gradually enlarges, starting in the sinuses of Valsalva and progressing to a discrete aneurysm in the ascending aorta. The pathology is unusual as the dilatation decreases and almost stops at the level of the innominate artery. The size and shape of the aneurysm is quite characteristic, resembling a truncated cone with the narrow apex near the level of the innominate artery. Aortic insufficiency results from dilatation of the aortic ring.

In less severe forms, there is simply a localized aneurysm in the ascending aorta with or without aortic insufficiency and no other signs of connective tissue disease; histologic examination of the excised aneurysm usually finds the characteristic cystic medial necrosis. Atherosclerotic aneurysms produce insufficiency by dilatation of the ring, though the histologic disease in the aorta is principally in the intima and media, contrasting markedly to that with cystic medial necrosis. Both aortoannular ectasia and atherosclerotic aneurysms are discussed in Chap. 19.

Another variant of collagen disease is the so-called floppy valve, a type of myxomatous degeneration of the valve that becomes elongated and sags into the ventricular lumen, often with no other histologic abnormality. The gross appearance suggests a variant of the more common mitral valve prolapse.

A dissecting aneurysm produces insufficiency by dissection of the aortic wall with detachment and prolapse of the valve cusps, usually the noncoronary. This topic was also discussed in Chap. 19. Congenital aortic insufficiency is rarely present at birth but may develop in older patients if stiffening and calcification of the malformed bicuspid valve produces insufficient rather than a stenotic valve.

The cardiac response to blood regurgitating into the left ventricle in diastole is an increase in left ventricular stroke volume, accomplished by dilatation of the heart. This results in gradual dilatation of the left ventricle, producing some of the largest hearts seen in clinical cardiology in neglected cases, with an apex of the left ventricle that extends almost to the chest wall and a cardiac weight approaching 1000 g. This cardiac response is quite different from that with aortic stenosis, where concentric muscular hypertrophy with little dilatation is the predominant change.

Pathophysiology. Surprisingly large volumes of blood regurgitate into the ventricle with severe aortic insufficiency. This results in an increased ventricular end-diastolic volume and a compensatory increase in the left ventricular stroke volume, which may be two or three times greater than the normal stroke volume of 60 to 75 mL. As the ventricular diastolic volume increases (increased preload), dilation and eccentric hypertrophy develop to maintain the wall thickness/cavity radius ratio at normal levels. Diastolic pressure, however, might not increase until later in the clinical course, so symptoms of pulmonary congestion appear only with advanced disease, completely contrasting to their early appearance with mitral stenosis. The process of volume overload, eccentric hypertrophy, and cardiac dilation also contrasts with aortic stenosis, where systolic pressure overload and concentric cardiac hypertrophy occur. As severe cardiac failure progresses, left ventricular end-diastolic pressure rises to 20 to 30 mm. At this time, the clinical findings of insufficiency may actually decrease because the volume of blood regurgitating during diastole is less. Eventually the wall thickness/cavity ratio decreases as cardiac dilation continues, afterload mismatch occurs due to increased systolic wall tension, and systolic function begins to deteriorate.

With marked dilatation of the left ventricle some mitral insufficiency may develop from dilatation of the annulus of the mitral valve. When a rheumatic history is present, it is difficult, or impossible, to determine from angiography whether the mitral insufficiency represents simple dilatation or rheumatic valvulitis. Mitral insufficiency resulting from simple dilatation of the mitral ring usually regresses satisfactorily following replacement of the aortic valve.

Clinical Manifestations. ***Symptoms.*** There is naturally a wide variability in the rate of progression of symptoms, depending on the degree of insufficiency. A symptom-free period of 8 to 10 years is common, but once symptoms appear, death has usually occurred in the past within 4 to 5 years. In general, citing statistics from the presurgical era, about 40 percent of patients died within 10 years, another 50 percent within 20 years. The terminal illness is usually progressive cardiac failure, as sudden death is much less common than with aortic stenosis.

Palpitation is one of the earliest, nonspecific symptoms, apparently arising from forceful contraction of the dilated left ventricle. Angina pectoris is a common symptom with advanced disease, usually with severe aortic incompetence in which the regurgitant flow is more than 50 percent of forward flow. Dyspnea with exertion appears fairly early during the progression of the disease and gradually increases in severity.

Physical Examination. Palpation readily discloses a prominent cardiac impulse, located downward and to the left of the normal location. The hallmark of aortic insufficiency is a high-pitched decrescendo diastolic murmur along the left sternal border, starting immediately after the second sound. The length of the murmur corresponds somewhat with the severity of the insufficiency. If the murmur is loudest to the right of the sternum, dilatation of the aortic ring, as in Marfan's syndrome, is likely. An ejection systolic murmur of moderate intensity is also frequent, and an S_3 gallop may be present. Occasionally a middiastolic rumble is noted, the Austin Flint murmur, which stimulates mitral stenosis.

Examination of the peripheral arterial circulation usually finds several abnormalities. The pulse pressure is increased, partly from an increase in systolic pressure but principally from a decrease in diastolic pressure below the normal range near 80 mm. The diastolic pressure may be as low as 40 mm, but true diastolic pressure, measured by direct arterial puncture, is never less than 30 to 35 mmHg, even though on auscultation a diastolic pressure of 0 may be obtained from dilatation of peripheral arteries. The exact level of diastolic pressure does not closely correlate with the severity of the aortic insufficiency because of the influence of peripheral resistance. With vasodilatation, diastolic pressure may be low without marked regurgitation while conversely, with severe vasoconstriction, diastolic pressure may be elevated but severe regurgitation present.

Peripheral pulses are usually visible, forceful, and bounding. The pulse is described as ''water-hammer,'' or quickly collapsing, the Corrigan's pulse. ''Pistol shot'' sounds are readily heard with the stethoscope over peripheral arteries. A wide variety of other auscultatory phenomena have been described, some over a century ago, all of which indicate vasodilatation and a hyperactive peripheral circulation.

Laboratory Studies and Diagnosis. The chest x-ray shows enlargement of the left ventricle with the apex displaced downward and to the left. As the normal cardiothoracic ratio is 0.5 or less, asymptomatic patients may be periodically followed with biannual x-rays, as long as the heart size is normal. The size of the left ventricle can be evaluated more precisely with 2-D echocardiography, which can demonstrate both the end-systolic and end-diastolic ventricular volume. The electrocardiogram is normal early in the disease, but with cardiac enlargement, signs of left ventricular hypertrophy become prominent. The cardiac rhythm usually remains sinus. Atrial fibrillation is uncommon before advanced disease is present and has an ominous prognosis unless it arises from another cause. Its presence from aortic insufficiency indicates an elevation of left ventricular end-diastolic pressure long enough to produce left atrial hypertrophy. Findings on cardiac catheterization are usually normal except for the visible reflux of dye from the aortic root into the ventricle with angiography. With cardiac failure, left ventricular end-diastolic pressure rises above the normal limit of 12 mm. Values of 15 to 20 are common with early cardiac decompression.

It has long been recognized that postponing operation until symptoms are disabling is not satisfactory, for some patients with early onset of symptoms already have substantial enlargement of the left ventricle and die from cardiac failure in the next 3 to 5 years despite correction of the insufficiency. Hence, clinical investigation for some time has sought a laboratory measurement that would identify the proper time for operation. Simply using changes in the cardiothoracic ratio is also unsatisfactory, for cardiac enlargement to a cardiothoracic ratio of 0.6 or greater indicates advanced disease.

At present, demonstrating a fall in ejection fraction with exercise with radionuclide studies seems one of the best indicators that operation should be performed in asymptomatic patients. Similarly, a rise in the end-systolic dimension of the ventricle, measured by echocardiography, suggests the beginning of systolic dysfunction and may be an indication for operation. The reliability of these ''early warning'' signs is not yet proved by 5- to 10-year postoperative data, but all indications suggest that long-term survival will be improved if operation is done before irreversible systolic dysfunction occurs. Henry assessed echocardiographic findings in this regard and recommended operation when end-systolic dimension had enlarged to 55 mm. A fall in the resting ejection fraction is an indication for operation.

Treatment. The principal decision with treatment is deciding when to operate. If a deterioration in ventricular function is occurring in the presence of severe aortic insufficiency, operation is indicated, preferably before severe, irreversible ventricular dysfunction occurs. The development of dyspnea or other symptoms of congestive heart failure is a clear indication for operation. In some patients who are still alive despite advanced left ventricular dysfunction, with an end-diastolic pressure of 30 mm or above, uncertainty exists about how much improvement can be expected from aortic valve replacement, as it often appears that the principal symptoms are advanced left ventricular dysfunction (or "myopathy"). Available studies do not permit a precise decision in this regard. In even the most advanced cases, valve replacement can usually be performed with an operative risk less than 10 percent. As death is virtually a certainty unless operation is done, operation is rarely contraindicated on the basis of left ventricular dysfunction, carefully explaining to the patient and the family beforehand that the degree of improvement following operation may be limited and cannot be known with any certainty for at least 6 to 12 months following operation. Postoperative medical therapy with digoxin, diuretics, and afterload reduction is beneficial in this group of patients after valve replacement.

The operative technique, choice of valve, postoperative care, and prognosis are very similar to those discussed in the section on Aortic Stenosis. The strongest predictor of late survival is the degree of preoperative left ventricular dysfunction.

Tricuspid Stenosis and Insufficiency

Etiology. Organic disease of the tricuspid valve is almost always due to rheumatic fever. With the exception of septic endocarditis, usually in drug addicts, it virtually never occurs as an isolated lesion, but only in association with extensive disease of the mitral valve. With mitral disease the frequency of associated tricuspid disease is near 10 to 15 percent, although an incidence as high as 30 percent has been reported. Rarely, blunt trauma produces rupture of a papillary muscle or chordae with resulting tricuspid insufficiency.

Tricuspid insufficiency is the more common lesion encountered; pure stenosis is infrequent, as stenotic lesions usually have concomitant insufficiency. Functional tricuspid insufficiency is much more common than insufficiency from organic disease. It develops from dilatation of the tricuspid annulus and right ventricle as a result of pulmonary hypertension and right ventricular failure. These abnormalities, in turn, result from left ventricular failure and chronic elevation of left atrial pressure.

Pathology. With tricuspid stenosis the pathologic changes are similar to those found with the more familiar mitral stenosis. There is fusion of the commissures to form a small central opening 1 to 1.5 cm in diameter. As right atrial pressure is normally only 4 to 5 mmHg, significant tricuspid stenosis may be present with a valve orifice considerably larger than that seen with mitral stenosis. With rheumatic disease combined stenosis and insufficiency or pure insufficiency results from fibrosis and contraction of the valve leaflets, often in association with shortening and fusion of chordae tendineae. Calcification is rare. More commonly functional dilation of the tricuspid annulus results in tricuspid insufficiency. The valve leaflets appear stretched but otherwise are pliable and seemingly normal even though serious regurgitation is present. Apparently the dilatation and deformity of the annulus are irreversible. Valves with severe functional tricuspid insufficiency usually do not regain competency, even though the mitral valve disease is corrected and pulmonary artery systolic pressure returns to normal.

Pathophysiology. With tricuspid stenosis the mean right atrial pressure is elevated to 10 to 20 mmHg. The higher pressures are found with a tricuspid valve orifice smaller than 1.5 cm^2 and a mean diastolic gradient between the atrium and ventricle of 5 to 15 mmHg. A gradient above 5 mm represents significant tricuspid stenosis. When mean right atrial pressure remains above 10 to 15 mmHg, edema and ascites usually appear.

A moderate degree of tricuspid insufficiency may be tolerated, with little adverse influence on the circulation except for a decrease in cardiac output. This is in striking contrast to mitral insufficiency, where the regurgitating blood and elevation of left atrial pressure produces pulmonary congestion. The unusual patient with isolated tricuspid insufficiency produced by a traumatic injury may do well for years, as the only physiologic disturbance is elevation of venous pressure and a decrease in cardiac output. The purest example of the surprising tolerance for tricuspid insufficiency is seen in the drug addict with septic endocarditis who has been treated by total excision of the tricuspid valve. Some, but not all, patients tolerate absence of the tricuspid valve with total tricuspid insufficiency for months or years.

Clinical Manifestations. The symptoms and signs of tricuspid valve disease are similar to those of right heart failure resulting from mitral valve disease. These all result from chronic elevation of right atrial pressure above 15 to 20 mmHg. The most familiar ones are edema, ascites, jugular-venous distention, and hepatomegaly. Characteristic murmurs are present and may be associated with hepatic pulsations. As similar findings result from right heart failure without tricuspid disease, the concomitant presence of tricuspid disease in the patient in heart failure with mitral valve disease may be easily overlooked.

Physical Examination. The characteristic murmur of tricuspid stenosis is best heard as a diastolic murmur at the lower end of the sternum. It is a low-pitched murmur of medium intensity and can easily be overlooked, as it is well localized at the lower end of the sternum. During inspiration the intensity of the murmur increases as the volume of blood returning to the heart is temporarily increased by an increase in intrathoracic negative pressure. Tricuspid insufficiency produces a prominent systolic murmur at the lower end of the sternum and also at the cardiac apex, where it may be confused with the systolic murmur of mitral insufficiency. The murmur is often seen in association with an enlarged pulsating liver and prominent engorged peripheral veins. A prominent jugular pulse, especially when the cardiac rhythm is sinus, may be the best clue to unsuspected tricuspid disease.

Laboratory Studies. The x-ray will show enlargement of the right atrium and right ventricle. Prominent P waves may be visible on the electrocardiogram if a sinus rhythm is present. Echocardiography will confirm enlargement of the right atrium and ventricle and may be helpful with Doppler studies in recognizing tricuspid insufficiency although the echocardiogram often tends to overestimate the degree of tricuspid insufficiency. Cardiac catheterization and angiography are required to confirm the diagnosis. Tricuspid stenosis can be confirmed by demonstrating a diastolic gradient between the atrium and ventricle above 4 to 5 mm. As the gradient is small, precise measurements are essential. Cineangiography is the best method for detecting insufficiency but is not always satisfactory because the catheter through which the dye is injected is lying across the tricuspid orifice and may deform the valve leaflets.

Carpentier has cautioned that palpation at the time of operation may be unreliable. If the blood volume and cardiac output are adequate, intraoperative palpation has been quite useful in our experience. It should be emphasized that the regurgitant jet is quite different from that present with mitral disease, as the pressures are lower. The jet is of lower volume and much more diffuse.

Treatment. Usually the surgical decision about tricuspid insufficiency is a tentative one until the valve is examined at operation. Mild degrees of tricuspid insufficiency are usually left alone, especially in the absence of pulmonary hypertension. The degree of hypertrophy of the right atrial wall is a helpful guide, as the absence of significant right atrial hypertrophy indicates that chronic severe elevation of right atrial pressure has not been present.

With significant tricuspid insufficiency, annuloplasty or tricuspid replacement should usually be done. At times this is necessary as an isolated procedure, often as a reoperation for persistent right heart failure after prior surgery on the other valves. Accordingly, the authors prefer to perform concomitant tricuspid valve repair when severe tricuspid insufficiency accompanies mitral disease or multiple valve disease. Effective tricuspid valve repair in this setting minimizes the risk of late right-sided heart failure and reoperation.

In the majority of patients seen clinically, tricuspid disease is due to dilatation of the annulus, as evidenced not only by the large annulus but also by the absence of fibrotic changes in the leaflets. Usually, the leaflets appear entirely normal. Virtually all such patients can be treated by annuloplasty. For over a decade at NYU a simple posterior leaflet annuloplasty as described by Kay, and by Boyd from our institution in 1974, has been quite satisfactory. The Carpentier ring annuloplasty is a bit more complicated and offers no advantage in our experience. Excellent results with tricuspid repair using the Carpentier technique have been reported by Carpentier and associates and by Kirklin and associates. The DeVega annuloplasty (a purse-string suture technique) has been widely used, but at least two groups have described a significant late failure rate. Data on more than 200 patients from our institution show that the posterior leaflet annuloplasty is simple, safe, and reproducible in the absence of significant intrinsic leaflet disease.

In the minority of patients with tricuspid stenosis from commissural fusion, a commissurotomy may be performed. This may often be combined with annuloplasty. More commonly valve replacement is performed when stenosis is present.

Valve replacement is seldom necessary for pure tricuspid insufficiency, except in patients with significant pulmonary hypertension and leaflet disease precluding annuloplasty. In a 1986 report of experiences with 151 valve replacements and 63 valve repairs, the prosthetic valve subsequently had to be replaced in 20 patients, principally because of progressive thrombosis. These included both ball valves and disc valves. Overall, late thrombosis appears more common with single leaflet disk valves. Excellent late durability and freedom from thrombosis has been noted with mechanical ball valves or bileaflet disk valves. Significant 10-year durability data with porcine prostheses are not yet available, though durability should be higher than the 85 to 90 percent 10-year durability with mitral or aortic porcine prostheses, where higher pressures are present. In our experience, durability of tricuspid valve repair is 98 percent at 5 to 7 years, using the simple posterior lateral annuloplasty technique described earlier.

When the prosthetic valve is inserted, particular care is required along the septal leaflet where the conduction bundle is located between the coronary sinus and the ventricular septum. In this area sutures should be placed through the base of the septal leaflet to avoid injury to the conduction bundle. Nevertheless, a heart block may develop sometime after operation, probably a result of inflammatory reaction stimulated by the prosthetic valve ring.

In the unfortunate patient with septic tricuspid endocarditis, almost always a drug addict, Arbulu demonstrated that total excision of the tricuspid valve *without replacement* could be tolerated. This approach permitted removal of all infected tissue without insertion of a foreign body, increasing the likelihood of cure of the endocarditis with antibiotics. Of the 50 long-term survivors, 11 subsequently required prosthetic replacement. The 15-year survival in this group was near 63 percent, and the majority of late deaths was due to recurrent drug addiction. Stern and Frater questioned this approach, stating that there was little proof that insertion of a prosthetic valve was associated with an immediate high frequency of recurrent endocarditis if the proper antibiotic was given for the infectious organism present. Our experience with similar cases supports the latter conclusion, and we prefer valve replacements with a porcine prosthesis for tricuspid endocarditis.

Operative risk for isolated tricuspid disease is very small, 1 to 2 percent. In previous years, the reported mortality rate for patients undergoing tricuspid surgery in conjunction with aortic or mitral surgery was high, 25 to 40 percent, primarily because the presence of tricuspid disease represented far advanced cardiac failure. An additional cause of high mortality was probably inadequate myocardial preservation of the hypertrophied right ventricle. With present techniques, however, tricuspid surgery seems to add little increased risk to concomitant aortic or mitral surgery. A recent study from our institution, covering 9 years, noted an operative risk of 6.3 percent for mitral valve replacement with associated tricuspid valve surgery.

Prognosis. Starr reported that 5-year survival was 59 percent, 10-year survival 36 percent with mechanical prostheses, and virtually identical with repair techniques, indicating that long-term prognosis is principally determined by residual myocardial function. Current data suggest better results than this, with 5-year survival greater than 70 percent. Prognosis is adversely affected by poor ventricular function, associated coronary disease, and pulmonary hypertension. Tricuspid valve repair procedures have not been associated with undue risk of reoperation.

Multivalvular Disease

Disease involving multiple valves is relatively common. With rheumatic heart disease, more than one valve is frequently involved. Prominent signs in one valve can readily mask disease in others. With aortic valve disease, functional mitral insufficiency can result from a progressive rise in the left ventricular end-diastolic pressure and volume. Similarly, mitral valve disease may result in pulmonary hypertension, right heart failure, and functional tricuspid insufficiency. In general, multiple valve disease is associated with a higher risk of operative repair than single valve disease, since the condition often represents more advanced disease or is associated with significant cardiac dysfunction.

In a 1992 report from our institution 513 patients with multiple valve disease treated surgically between 1976 and 1985 were followed to assess factors influencing operative risk and long-term survival. Three groups accounted for the majority of the cases: 58 percent had aortic and mitral disease (AV + MV), 29 percent had mitral and tricuspid disease (MV + TV), and 12 percent had triple valve disease (AV + MV + TV). Preoperative congestive heart failure was present in 91 percent; 41 percent were NYHA Class III, and 54 percent were NYHA Class IV. The average pulmonary artery systolic pressure was 60 mmHg. Despite chronic symptoms and severe disease the overall operative risk was 12.5 percent and the 5-year survival rate was 67 percent. The variables predicting decreased survival were systolic pulmonary artery pressure, age, triple valve procedure, concomitant coronary disease requiring bypass operation, prior heart surgery, and diabetes. Postoperatively the functional condition of 80 percent improved to NYHA Class I or II, and only 0.6 percent remained NYHA Class IV, suggesting that most patients had significant clinical improvement despite advanced disease. The 5-year freedom from late cardiac related complications or death was 82 percent.

AV + MV. Nine combinations of valvular pathology can produce AV + MV, since each valve can be stenotic, insufficient, or both. Stenosis in both valves may lead to underestimation of the degree of aortic stenosis since return of blood to the left ventricle is limited because of mitral stenosis. Likewise, aortic insufficiency, which produces the Austin Flint murmur, might overshadow and mask true mitral stenosis. With functional mitral insufficiency resulting from severe aortic disease, aortic valve replacement can lead to resolution of insufficiency in some patients, whereas patients with more severe mitral insufficiency may require mitral annuloplasty or valve replacement. Each case should be examined closely for these and other considerations, and cardiac catheterization usually should be performed before operation. The operative risk for isolated AV + MV is 4 to 5 percent.

MV + TV. Nine combinations of valvular pathology are also possible with mitral and tricuspid disease, but mitral disease with functional tricuspid insufficiency is the common scenario, resulting from chronic pulmonary hypertension and right heart failure. This was discussed in the above section on tricuspid disease. The operative risk for isolated MV + TV without prior surgery is approximately 6 percent.

Triple Valve Disease. Trivalvular disease is usually a result of chronic aortic and mitral disease, with pulmonary hypertension and functional tricuspid insufficiency. Occasionally rheumatic disease will affect all three valves, but this is now rare because of the decreasing frequency of rheumatic fever. Clearly the degree of pulmonary hypertension is the most significant predictor of survival with triple valve disease. For example, the overall operative risk for 61 triple valve procedures in the above cited NYU report was 23 percent, whereas the risk of isolated triple valve operation was only 5.6 percent when the pulmonary artery systolic pressure was less than 60 mmHg. As with other forms of valvular heart disease this emphasizes the value of early operation prior to the development of pulmonary hypertension and irreversible ventricular dysfunction. The current results suggest that even the most advanced cases are seldom inoperable.

CARDIAC TRAUMA

Penetrating Trauma

In 1896, Rehn first successfully sutured a stab wound of the heart, but for decades this remained an isolated historic achievement. The hazards of thoracotomy were the principal reason that the 1943 contribution of Blalock and Ravitch, when they introduced pericardial aspiration as a method of treatment for tamponade following penetrating injuries of the heart, was such a significant one. They recognized that many patients survived because the development of tamponade prevented exsanguination. Aspiration remained a definitive and reasonably effective form of therapy for tamponade for over 25 years, but with further advances in therapy has been almost completely replaced for the past two decades with prompt thoracotomy. Aspiration is now used primarily for resuscitation as a lifesaving method of treatment. Removal of as little as 15 to 20 mL of blood by subxyphoid aspiration may abort impending cardiac arrest.

Etiology and Pathology. The two life-threatening problems are tamponade and hemorrhage. Tamponade develops rapidly as the normal pericardium can accommodate only 100 to 250 mL of blood. Small wounds, such as those from an icepick or a knife, often produce tamponade because the laceration in the pericardium is small. Larger wounds, produced by bullets or large knives, threaten immediate death from exsanguination as blood can be expelled through the pericardial laceration into the pleural cavity. The right ventricle, which constitutes most of the anterior portion of the heart, is the cardiac chamber most frequently injured. In patients with penetrating trauma of the chest or upper abdomen a cardiac injury should be suspected. Signs may include hemothorax, hypotension, narrow pulse pressure, tachycardia, jugular venous distention (elevated central venous pressure), blue discoloration of the neck and face, and muffled heart sounds.

Treatment. The dominant problem may be hemorrhage, tamponade, or both. The patient should obviously be taken to the operating room as quickly as possible, which will vary with the circumstances and the hospital environment. As stated by Kirklin and Barratt-Boyes, "No more than 5 min need elapse between admission and the patient's transfer to the operating table." Rapid transfusion of fluids, intubation, emergency pericardiocentesis, and immediate transportation to the operating room are the key principles in treatment.

Initial treatment should include 1 to 2 L of intravenous fluids. Pericardiocentesis can be lifesaving, immediately restoring adequate systolic blood pressure and allowing transport to the operating room. Emergency room thoracotomy is frequently done in some institutions, including Bellevue Hospital. It may be lifesaving in some patients with agonal respirations or impending cardiac arrest but is probably futile with established cardiac arrest in the field and dilated pupils indicating brain injury, as suggested by Moore and associates. After emergency thoracotomy temporary hemostasis may permit restoration of cardiac function long enough for transportation to the operating room. Ivatury reported experiences with emergency room thoracotomy in 22 patients without detectable vital signs in the emergency room. Cardiac function was restored in 16 of these, eight of whom eventually recovered without objective neurologic injury. Thus impending or witnessed cardiac arrest should be treated aggressively.

An emergency unsterile thoracotomy can be quickly done in less than 1 to 2 min by a trained surgeon. With the patient in a slight left anterolateral position, a curved skin incision is made beneath the left nipple to parallel the intercostal spaces. The fourth or fifth intercostal space should be entered, as the pectoralis major arises from the third to the fifth ribs and causes troublesome bleeding with a higher incision. Once the pleural space is entered, the intercostal incision can be quickly completed with scissors, or the fingers separating the ribs, carrying the incision anteriorly beyond the angle of the rib, almost to the sternum. Unless the incision is long enough, exposure is seriously hampered. Subsequent wound infection following an unsterile thoracotomy is surprisingly rare, less than 5 percent.

The key to cardiac tamponade is simply considering the diagnosis in any patient with hypotension and a penetrating thoracic wound. The classic triad emphasized by Beck decades ago was the combination of hypotension, elevated venous pressure, and a small quiet heart. Only a few conditions, such as cardiac failure or pulmonary embolism, produce the combination of hypotension and elevated venous pressure. When the diagnosis is first suspected, fluids are given, and pericardial aspiration or subxyphoid exploration should be promptly done. A most dramatic experience is to remove as little as 20 mL of blood from the pericardium of a moribund patient with an imperceptible blood pressure and be rewarded with a prompt rise in blood pressure to 70 to 80 mmHg and a return of consciousness.

In some patients with severe tamponade, an unusual degree of restlessness is present with the patient wildly rolling about. This contrasts strikingly with the usual quiet apathetic state of patients in hemorrhagic shock. This may be due to severe cerebral anoxia, resulting from the combination of arterial hypotension and venous hypertension.

Operative Therapy. In the operating room a median sternotomy is the preferred incision, as it provides ready access to all chambers of the heart. An anterior thoracotomy can be made more rapidly but does not give good exposure of the right heart.

When circumstances permit, a pump oxygenator, or a simpler apparatus for autotransfusion of blood, should be available. This is not often needed, as most cardiac injuries permitting survival long enough to reach the operating room can be controlled by digital pressure and suturing.

Ventricular lacerations can usually be controlled by digital pressure and then sutured with continuous suture or with interrupted mattress sutures. Occasionally a brief period of inflow occlusion facilitates repair. Atrial lacerations may be initially controlled with tangential application of vascular or wide Allis clamps. With severe injuries, use of cardiopulmonary bypass might be necessary. This is particularly true when mid to proximal anterior descending artery injuries have occurred, as coronary bypass should be done beyond the injured vessel.

Following control of the cardiac laceration, a search should routinely be made for other intrathoracic injuries. Laceration of the internal mammary artery is a common associated injury. Injuries to intracardiac structures, such as a cardiac valve, rarely occur but can be treated at a later time. Injury to the septum, resulting in a ventricular septal defect, should be ruled out in all cases by measuring oxygen saturations in the vena cava and pulmonary artery.

Following successful repair of the cardiac laceration and correction of hypovolemia, recovery is uneventful in most patients. Overall mortality rate is 10 to 20 percent for stab wounds to the heart, and 30 to 60 percent for gunshot wounds. Wound infection, pericarditis, or recurrent bleeding are all uncommon. Late echocardiogram should be done to assess for valvular injury or delayed septal defects. Similarly, a Holter monitor will detect arrhythmias due to ventricular irritability.

Blunt Trauma

Blunt cardiac trauma usually results from automobile accidents, such as a "steering wheel" injury or some similar form of severe blunt injury to the chest wall. Probably 900,000 cases of cardiac trauma occur annually in the United States. Many of these are instantaneously fatal. The direct injury may cause an underlying cardiac contusion. Alternately, when the heart is suddenly compressed, intracardiac pressure apparently becomes high enough to rupture different cardiac structures, such as the ventricular septum, the chordae of the mitral or tricuspid valves, or the free cardiac wall. Injuries of this severity are usually fatal. Only rarely is a patient seen with a laceration of a tricuspid valve or the ventricular septum.

The myocardial contusion varies from simple subepicardial hemorrhage to a full-thickness myocardial contusion, which rarely progresses to an infarction.

The clinical picture is that of pericarditis with a pericardial effusion and chest pain. The classic picture of a myocardial infarction or cardiac failure is uncommon.

The electrocardiogram is a nonspecific diagnostic guide, as false-positive and false-negative results are common. Sinus tachycardia is the most common finding, although ST segment elevation or bundle branch block may be seen. The best diagnostic evaluation is done by a combination of serial measurement of myocardial enzymes, combined with 2-D echocardiography. Frazee and associates summarized experiences with 291 patients with thoracic trauma. Twenty percent of the group (58) had elevated cardiac enzymes (CPK-MB) within 24 h. Of this group, 60 percent were classified as simply "cardiac concussion," as the 2-D echocardiogram was normal. The remaining 40 percent were diagnosed as cardiac contusion, as abnormalities were visible on the echocardiogram. Patients with an abnormal echocardiogram were treated like patients with a subendocardial myocardial infarction, as arrhythmias frequently occurred in this group. The majority recovered within a short period of time. Severe contusion rarely progresses to cardiac necrosis, with myocardial infarction, septal rupture, or ventricular rupture.

Blunt cardiac rarely produces permanent cardiac disability. From a physiologic standpoint, serious cardiac disability does not occur until more than 30 to 50 percent of the myocardium has been lost. An injury severe enough to produce irreversible loss of myocardium of this extent is almost always fatal.

Foreign Bodies

The report by Harken in 1946 is a classic. It describes the successful removal of 56 intramyocardial foreign bodies during World War II without a single death. About two-thirds of the removed foreign bodies had bacteria on culture.

In general, foreign bodies greater than 1 cm usually cause complications, such as pericardial effusion or pericarditis, but smaller foreign bodies are well tolerated. In 1966, Bland and Beebe reported a 20-year follow-up of 40 patients from World War II who had small foreign bodies in the heart. Although major complications did not occur, most patients had a permanent emotional disability, apparently from anxiety associated with the uncertain prognosis of a foreign body in the heart. The difficulty with removing small asymptomatic foreign bodies was emphasized in the report; elective removal was attempted in eight patients, but successfully completed in only three. Recently intraoperative echocardiography has been helpful in locating intracardiac foreign bodies.

The safety of cardiopulmonary bypass, combined with the use of echocardiography, would suggest that all intramyocardial foreign bodies should be surgically removed, usually transatrially. Foreign bodies that are within the cardiac cavities, usually dislodged from a complication of intravascular catheters, may be removed with a percutaneous catheter method, although these occasionally require operation. Uflacker and associates reported the successful percutaneous removal of a foreign body in 20 patients. The authors have operatively removed vena caval umbrellas, vascular sheaths, and other similar devices, as well as numerous bullets.

CARDIAC TUMORS

Primary cardiac neoplasms are rare, occurring with an incidence of 0.001 to 0.3 percent in autopsy series. Benign tumors account for 75 percent of primary neoplasms, while malignant tumors account for 25 percent. The most frequent primary cardiac neoplasm is myxoma, comprising 30 to 50 percent. Other benign neoplasms in decreasing order of occurrence include lipoma, papillary fibroelastoma, rhabdomyoma, fibroma, hemangioma, teratoma, lymphangioma, and others. Most primary malignant neoplasms are sarcomas (angiosarcoma, rhabdomyosarcoma, fibrosarcoma, leiomyosarcoma, liposarcoma), with malignant lymphomas accounting for 1 to 2 percent. Metastatic cardiac neoplasms are more common than primary neoplasms, occurring in 4 to 12 percent of patients dying of cancer.

Symptoms include dyspnea, fever, malaise, weight loss, arthralgias, and dizziness. Clinical findings may include murmurs of mitral stenosis or insufficiency, heart failure, pulmonary hypertension, and systemic embolization.

Diagnosis. The diagnosis is usually readily established by 2-D echocardiography. Transesophageal echocardiography may be useful when transthoracic 2-D findings are equivocal or confusing. Recently MRI has been of value in diagnosis, providing excellent cardiac definition. Cardiac catheterization is not necessary in the majority of cases but may be necessary when other cardiac disease is suspected or if other diagnostic studies are equivocal.

Treatment. Excision is the treatment of choice (Fig. 18-15A, B). This is frequently possible for most benign tumors. Care

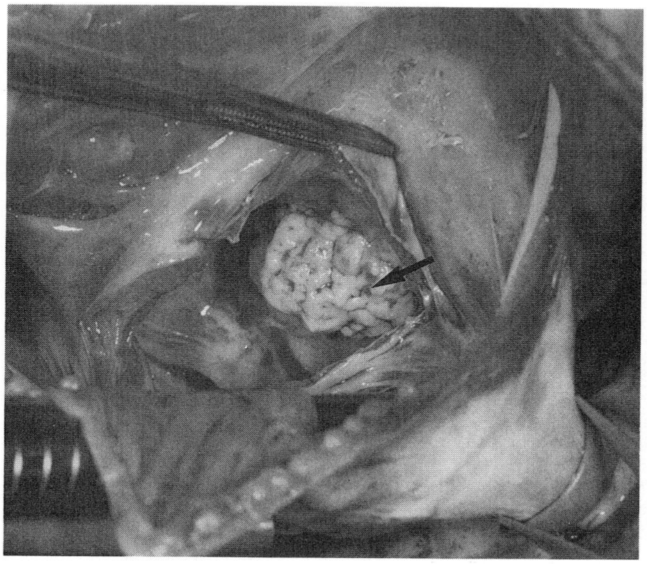

A

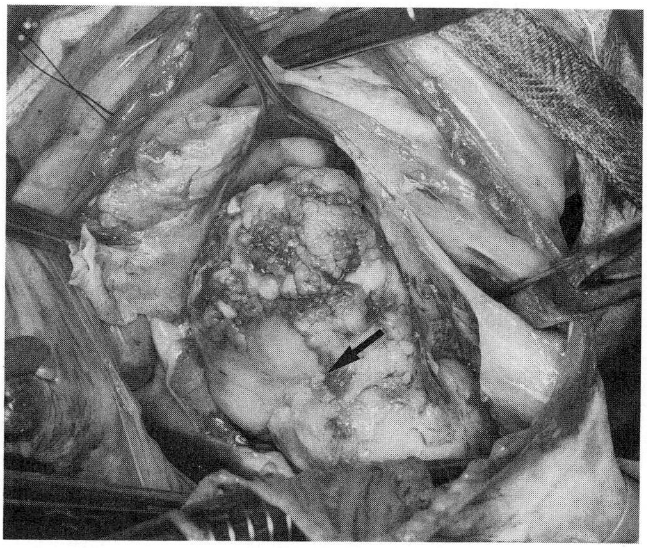

B

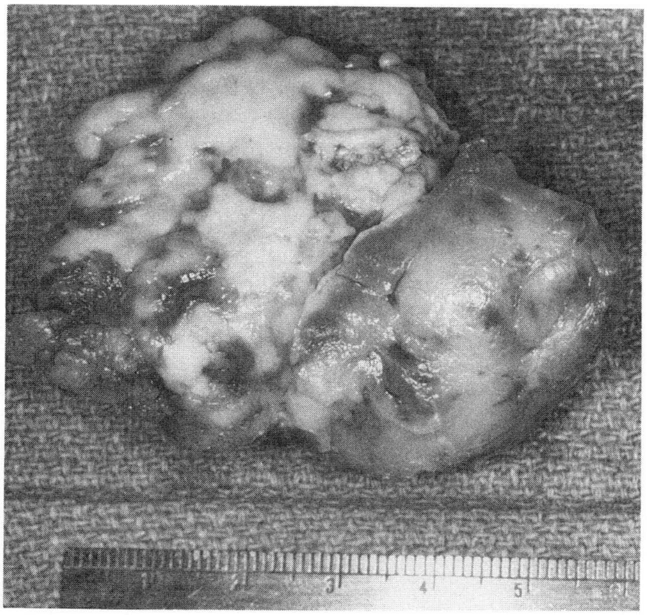

C

FIG. 18-15. *A.* Operative photograph of a patient who presented with nonspecific symptoms and a large left atrial mass, diagnosed preoperatively as a left atrial myxoma. The photograph demonstrates a large left atrial mass *(arrow)* attached to the atrial septum. *B.* The tumor completely fills the left atrial cavity. It was excised by removing a portion of the atrial septum. *C.* The specimen (>6 cm) has none of the classical features of an atrial myxoma. Pathologic examination revealed an extremely rare histiocytoid hemangioendothelioma. The resected portion of the atrial septum was closed with a pericardial patch and the patient recovered uneventfully.

is taken to avoid deformity or destruction of adjacent cardiac structures, and reconstruction of the involved cardiac chamber is occasionally necessary. Total excision of metastatic or primary malignant neoplasms is less frequently possible but should be attempted. Otherwise, incisional diagnostic biopsy is performed. Multimodality therapy, with excision, chemotherapy, and radiotherapy, is indicated for most malignant cardiac neoplasms. Four special cardiac tumor groups will be considered in detail below.

Myxoma

Sixty to seventy-five percent of cardiac myxomas develop in the left atrium, almost always from the atrial septum near the fossa ovalis. Most other myxomas develop in the right atrium. Less than 20 have been found in either the right or left ventricle. The curious predilection for a myxoma to develop from the rim of the fossa ovalis in the left atrium has been studied by several observers, but a satisfactory explanation has not been found.

Myxomas are apparently true neoplasms, although their similarity to an organized atrial thrombus led to considerable debate at one time about whether they represented a true neoplasm or not. Their occurrence in the absence of other organic heart disease, histochemical studies demonstrating mucopolysaccharide and glycoprotein, and a distinct histologic appearance all indicate that myxomas are true neoplasms. The tumors tend to recur locally, but they do not invade or metastasize and are considered benign.

Pathology. The tumors are usually polypoid, projecting into the atrial cavity from a 1- to 2-cm stalk attached to the atrial septum. The maximum size ranges from 0.5 to greater than 10.0 cm. Only the superficial layer of the septum is involved; invasion of the septum does not occur. Over 75 percent of myxomas occur in the left atrium, with the remainder occurring in the right atrium, or rarely in either ventricle. Some myxomas grow slowly, for a few patients have had symptoms for many years. There is no tendency to invade other areas of the heart; distant metastases have rarely been reported. The friable consistency of a myxoma is of particular significance, for fatal emboli have occurred following digital manipulation of the tumor at operation.

Histologically, a myxoma is covered with endothelium and composed of a myxomatous stroma with large stellate cells mixed with fusiform or multinucleated cells. Mitoses are infrequent. Lymphocytes and plasmacytes are regularly found. Hemosiderin, a result of hemorrhage into the tumor, is also common.

Sporadic myxomas usually present in the fifth or sixth decade of life but have been described in younger and older patients. Autosomal dominant genetically transmitted familial myxomas can occur, usually presenting before 30 years of age. Familial "myxoma syndrome" includes myxomas, freckles, pigmented nevi, nodular adrenal cortical disease, mammary myomatous fibroadenomas. Testicular tumors and pituitary adenomas with two or more components are required for diagnosis.

Pathophysiology. A myxoma may cause no difficulty until it grows large enough to obstruct the flow of blood through either the mitral or tricuspid valve, or fragments to produce peripheral emboli. The frequency of embolization, previously estimated to occur in 40 to 50 percent of patients, is not surprising, for an astonishing degree of to-and-fro motion of a myxoma, swinging on a small pedicle with each cardiac contraction, may be seen with echocardiography or angiography. Intermittent acute obstruction of the mitral orifice has been reported to produce syncope or even sudden death. Some myxomas produced generalized symptoms resembling an autoimmune disorder, including fever, weight loss, clubbing, myalgia, and arthralgia. Possibly such patients have an immune reaction to the neoplasm as elevated levels of interleukin 6 and elevated levels of antimyocardial antibodies have been described.

Clinical Manifestations. Symptoms may be those of mitral valve obstruction, resembling mitral stenosis, except for acute exacerbations, presumably due to transient lodging of the myxoma in the mitral orifice; peripheral embolization; or generalized autoimmune symptoms described in the previous section. The diagnosis is made in many patients following an embolic episode, either from histologic examination of the surgically removed embolus or as a result of subsequent diagnostic studies to determine the reason for embolism. The precision and reliability of 2-D echocardiography has greatly simplified diagnosis. Angiography is optional unless additional disease is suspected. Computerized axial tomography has been reported to be helpful with small tumors, but MRI is probably better.

Abnormalities are usually found on examination of the heart and also on the electrocardiogram, but these are not diagnostic.

Treatment. Operation should be performed as soon as possible after the diagnosis has been established because a disabling or fatal cerebral embolus is an ever-present hazard.

A sternotomy incision is used. Once extracorporeal circulation has been established, the aorta is clamped to avoid embolism. Palpation is avoided. The right atrium is opened and the fossa ovalis incised to expose the stalk of the myxoma. The left atrium is then opened in the interatrial groove. With the myxoma visualized, the segment of atrial septum from which the tumor arises is excised, after which the myxoma is removed through the incision in the left atrium (see Fig. 8-15*A*, *B*, *C*). The defect in the atrial septum is closed primarily or with a small patch. The technique is simple and permits exploration of both atria and ventricles.

A few cases of recurrent myxoma have been reported, some of which have been successfully operated on. Initially these were thought to represent inadequate excision of the site of origin, but some have recurred at more remote sites in the atrium, indicating the multipotential source of these unusual neoplasms. Hence, it seems prudent to perform periodic echocardiography routinely for several years following operation.

Larrieu and associates described experiences with 18 myxomas in a series of 25 cardiac tumors over a period of 24 years. Fyke and associates treated 21 patients with mitral myxoma in the first 7 years following the introduction of 2-D echocardiography. The operative risk is currently 1 to 2 percent.

Metastatic Neoplasms

Cardiac metastases have been found in 4 to 12 percent of autopsies performed for neoplastic disease. Although they have occurred from primary neoplasms developing in almost every known site of the body, the most frequent have been carcinoma of the lung or breast, melanoma, and lymphoma. Cardiac metastases involving only the heart are very unusual. Similarly, a solitary cardiac metastasis is infrequent; usually there are multiple areas of involvement. Cardiac involvement is particularly common with leukemia or lymphoma, developing in 25 to 40 percent of patients. All areas of the heart are involved with equal frequency except the cardiac valves, perhaps as a result of the absence of lymphatics in valves.

The diagnosis of a primary cardiac malignant tumor can be suspected in a patient in whom an unexplained hemorrhagic pericardial effusion develops, especially in association with a bizarre cardiac shadow on the radiograph. Echocardiography should confirm the presence of an abnormal cardiac mass. Thoracotomy or sternotomy is usually required to establish the diagnosis. Combined chemotherapy and radiation is indicated, but only rarely is effective therapy possible.

Rhabdomyoma

A cardiac rhabdomyoma is probably not a true tumor but a hamartoma, representing a focal arrest and maturation of cardiac muscle. The nodules have also been termed *nodular glycogenic degeneration,* being interpreted as a manifestation of glycogen storage disease. About one-half of the patients have tuberous sclerosis of the brain. On histologic examination cells with large vacuoles are found in which the nuclei appear suspended by threads of cytoplasm, giving origin to the term ''spider cell.'' Associated adenoma sebaceum and benign kidney tumors are occasionally noted.

Although rhabdomyoma is said to be the most common cardiac tumor in children, it is a rare lesion. Reece and associates indicated that only about 110 cases have been reported in the literature prior to 1984.

The cardiac lesions may be solitary or multiple nodules or may present a diffuse infiltration of the cardiac muscle. The lesions do not grow.

Most cases have been recognized in infancy. The average age was 5 months. The disease is apparently fatal, for older children and adults with such tumors are not seen. Whether the death is from the tumor or from associated disease is uncertain.

Symptoms may result from obstruction of a ventricular chamber or from arrhythmias such as recurrent ventricular tachycardia. Complete excision has been accomplished in a few patients. If tuberous sclerosis of the brain is not present, it appears that a rare infant may be successfully operated on and cured of potentially fatal arrhythmias.

Miscellaneous Tumors

Unusual benign lesions of the heart include fibromas, lipomas, angiomas, teratomas, and cysts. Fewer than 50 examples of each of these types of lesions have been reported. Fibromas have been found most frequently in the left ventricle, often as 2- to 5-cm nodules within the muscle. Sudden death, probably from a cardiac arrhythmia, has been reported with such tumors and may be the reason that only 18 percent of the reported tumors have been found in adults.

Lipomas are rare asymptomatic tumors found projecting from the epicardial or endocardial surface of the heart in older patients. Angiomas are commonly small, focal vascular malformations of no clinical significance, except for four that have been found associated with a heart block. Pericardial teratomas and bronchogenic cysts are rare lesions that may cause symptoms from compression of the right atrium and obstruction of venous return. Most of these occur in children. Some of the larger cysts, up to 10 cm in diameter, may produce grotesque deformities from extensive invagination of the right atrial wall. Myxomas are by far the most common benign tumor in adults, but are seldom found in children except as part of the familial syndrome described in the above section.

PERICARDITIS

Acute Pericarditis

Pericarditis results from acute inflammation of the pericardial space, resulting in substernal chest pain, ECG changes, and a pericardial friction rub. The pain is often inspiratory, worse in the supine position, and relieved by leaning forward. Associated ECG changes frequently occur, most commonly sinus tachycardia, with concave upward ST segment elevation throughout the precordium. The ECG typically progresses to T-wave inversion, followed by the total resolution of all changes. The cause of acute pericarditis is variable, including infection, myocardial infarction, trauma, neoplasm, radiation, autoimmune diseases, drugs, nonspecific causes, and others (Table 18-1). Untreated pericarditis may result in progressive development of a pericardial effusion, with subsequent cardiac tamponade. Alternately, infectious causes may result in septic complications. Chronic constrictive pericarditis may develop after resolution of the acute process.

Diagnosis. The diagnostic work-up should attempt to determine the underlying cause. Blood tests should include sedimentation rate, hematocrit, WBC count, bacterial cultures, viral titers, heterophile antibody, BUN, T_3, T_4, TSH, ANA, rheumatoid fac-

Table 18-1
Causes of Pericarditis

1. Idiopathic (nonspecific)
2. Viral infections: coxsackie A virus, coxsackie B virus, echovirus, adenovirus, mumps virus, infectious mononucleosis, varicella, hepatitis B, AIDS (acquired immunodeficiency syndrome)
3. Tuberculosis
4. Acute bacterial infection: pneumococcus, staphylococcus, streptococcus, gram-negative septicemia, *Neisseria gonorrhoeae,* tularemia, *Legionella pneumophila*
5. Fungal infections: histoplasmosis, coccidioidomycosis, candida, blastomycosis
6. Other infections: toxoplasmosis, amebiasis, mycoplasma, *Nocardia,* actinomycosis, echinococcosis, Lyme disease
7. Acute myocardial infarction
8. Uremia: untreated uremia; in association with hemodialysis
9. Neoplastic disease: lung cancer, breast cancer, leukemia, Hodgkin's disease, lymphoma
10. Radiation
11. Autoimmune disorders: acute rheumatic fever, systemic lupus erythematosus, rheumatoid arthritis, scleroderma, mixed connective tissue disease, Wegener's granulomatosis, polyarteritis nodosa
12. Other inflammatory disorders: sarcoidosis, amyloidosis, inflammatory bowel disease, Whipple disease, temporal arteritis, Behçet disease
13. Drugs: hydralazine, procainamide, diphenylhydantoin, isoniazid, phenylbutazone, dantrolene, doxorubicin, methysergide, penicillin (with hypereosinophilia)
14. Trauma: including chest trauma; hemopericardium following thoracic surgery; pacemaker insertion; cardiac diagnostic procedures; esophageal rupture; pancreatic-pericardial fistula
15. Delayed postmyocardial-pericardial injury syndromes:
    (a) Postmyocardial infarction (Dressler) syndrome
    (b) Postpericardiotomy syndrome
16. Dissecting aortic aneurysm
17. Myxedema
18. Chylopericardium

SOURCE: Reproduced with permission, Lorell BH, Braunwald E: Pericardial disease, in Braunwald E. (ed): *Heart Disease: A Textbook of Cardiovascular Disease,* 4th ed. Philadelphia, WB Saunders, 1992, 1469.

tor, and myocardial enzyme levels. The ECG may be typical or nonspecific. The chest x-ray may be normal or may demonstrate an enlarged cardiac silhouette or a pleural effusion. An echocardiogram to evaluate the degree of pericardial effusion is essential. A pericardiocentesis or pericardial biopsy may be necessary when the diagnosis is uncertain.

Treatment. The preferred treatment obviously depends on the underlying cause. Purulent pyogenic pericarditis requires drainage and prolonged intravenous antibiotic therapy. Postpericardiotomy syndrome, postmyocardial infarction syndrome, viral pericarditis, and idiopathic pericarditis are often self-limiting but can require a short course of treatment with nonsteroidal anti-inflammatory agents. If a significant pericardial effusion is present, surgical drainage is indicated if signs of tamponade are present or if resolution is not prompt with anti-inflammatory agents. Occasionally a 5- to 7-day course of steroids is necessary. Follow-up studies should be done to document resolution of any pericardial effusion or to assess for late constrictive pericarditis.

Chronic Constrictive Pericarditis

Etiology. In the majority of patients, the cause is unknown, probably the end stage of an undiagnosed viral pericarditis. Tuberculosis is a rarity. In recent years, intensive radiation has become a significant cause in some series. Constrictive pericarditis may develop after an open heart operation. In the last 16 years previous cardiac surgery was the cause of 39 percent (13/32) of cases treated surgically for constrictive pericarditis at New York University.

Pathology and Pathophysiology. The pericardial cavity is obliterated by fusion of the parietal pericardium to the epicardium, forming dense scar tissue that encases and constricts the heart. In chronic cases, areas of calcification develop, adding an additional element of constriction.

The physiologic handicap is limitation of diastolic filling of the ventricles. This results in a decrease in cardiac output from a decrease in stroke volume. The right ventricular diastolic pressure is increased with a corresponding increase in right atrial and central venous pressure, ranging from 10 to 30 mmHg. The venous hypertension produces hepatomegaly, ascites, peripheral edema, and a generalized increase in blood volume.

Clinical Manifestations. The disease is a slowly progressive one with increasing ascites and edema. Fatiguability and dyspnea on exertion are common, but dyspnea at rest is unusual. The ascites is often severe, as a result of which the diagnosis is easily confused with cirrhosis.

Hepatomegaly and ascites are often the most prominent physical abnormalities. Peripheral edema is moderate in some patients, severe in others. These findings are manifestations of advanced congestive failure from any form of heart disease. With constrictive pericarditis, however, the usual cardiac findings are a heart of normal size without murmurs or abnormal sounds. Atrial fibrillation is present in about one-third of the patients, and a pleural effusion is common in more severe cases. A paradoxical pulse is found in a small percentage of patients.

Laboratory Findings. Venous pressure is elevated, often to 15 to 20 mmHg or higher. The electrocardiogram, though not diagnostic, is usually abnormal with a low voltage and inverted T waves. The chest x-ray usually shows a heart of normal size, but pericardial calcification may be seen in a significant percentage of cases, often being the first clue to the diagnosis. Echocardiogram, MRI, or CT may demonstrate a thickened pericardium.

Findings on cardiac catheterization are highly characteristic. There is elevation of the right ventricular diastolic pressure with a change in contour, showing an early filling with a subsequent plateau, the ''square root'' sign. Also, there is ''equalization'' of pressures in the different cardiac chambers as right atrial pressure, right ventricular diastolic pressure, pulmonary artery diastolic pressure, pulmonary wedge pressure, and left atrial pressure are similar. The one condition that cannot be excluded with certainty without myocardial biopsy is a restrictive cardiomyopathy.

Treatment. Once the diagnosis has been made, pericardiectomy should be done promptly because the disease relentlessly progresses. Operation can be done through a sternotomy incision or a long left anterolateral thoracotomy. The constricting pericardium should be removed from all surfaces of the ventricle, mobilizing the heart to where it can be held freely upward in the hand. Removal over the atria and the cavae is somewhat optional, although this is usually done as well. The heart-lung machine is usually kept on a standby basis in the event of significant hemorrhage. If this occurs, the patient can be heparinized, the blood aspirated and returned to the patient until the laceration is repaired. The pericardium is removed bilaterally from the pulmonary veins on the right to the pulmonary veins on the left. Both phrenic nerves are mobilized and protected. Particular care is taken to remove pericardium over the pulmonary artery where residual constriction can seriously impair the operative result.

As the constricting scar develops from organization of an exudate between the pericardium and epicardium, the plane of dissection may often be external to the epicardium, which will greatly decrease operative hemorrhage. If the epicardium is thickened, it must be removed from the underlying myocardium, though this is tedious and results in diffuse bleeding.

Intracardiac pressures should be measured by direct needle puncture before and following pericardiectomy. Often with a complete pericardiectomy, the characteristic pressure abnormalities are either eliminated or greatly improved. If significant abnormalities remain, the operative field should be carefully checked for any residual sites of constriction. In all likelihood the slow recovery over many months in the past was simply a result of inadequate pericardiectomy, *not* underlying ''ventricular atrophy.''

Results. Following a radical pericardiectomy that corrects the hemodynamic abnormalities, patients improve promptly with a massive diuresis. The risk of operation varies with the age of the patient and the severity of the disease; it is usually less than 5 percent. A good result can be anticipated, more than 95 percent.

The NYU experience includes 62 patients treated surgically with total pericardiectomy. The majority of patients were NYHA Class III or IV preoperatively. Sixteen percent required cardiopulmonary bypass for treatment of associated pathology, usually tricuspid insufficiency. The operative mortality rate was 3 percent (2/62). After operation, hemodynamic abnormalities promptly corrected, ascites and peripheral edema resolved, and functional status improved dramatically.

ARRHYTHMIA SURGERY

Surgical treatment of cardiac arrhythmias began in 1968 when Sealy first successfully interrupted the bundle of Kent in a patient with Wolff-Parkinson-White (WPW) syndrome. This was possible because of the newly developed EPS and mapping techniques described by Durrer, of Amsterdam, who mapped a patient with WPW syndrome in 1967, demonstrating electrical conduction through an accessory pathway in the area of ventricular preexcitation. Daniel and associates and Kaiser and associates independently reported intraoperative mapping for ischemic ventricular arrhythmias in 1969, but advances in surgical treatment of ventricular tachycardia did not occur until the late 1970s when Guiraudon described the encircling endocardial ventriculotomy and Josephson and associates proposed map-guided subendocardial resection for ablation of recurrent ventricular tachycardia.

Subsequently, surgical methods for treatment of arrhythmias were advanced by Cox and colleagues, and by others. The development of multipoint (160 to 256 channel) computerized cardiac mapping systems greatly improved both the speed and efficiency of arrhythmia mapping, while better operative skills and adjuvant cryoablative techniques similarly improved the efficacy of surgical methods. Recently the development of radiofrequency catheter ablation has allowed treatment of cardiac arrhythmias in the cardiac catheterization laboratory.

Most ablative therapy for arrhythmias, either surgical or nonsurgical, is done for one of four clinical entities: (1) WPW syndrome with preexcitation, (2) paroxysmal supraventricular tachycardia (PSVT) due to (*a*) atrioventricular (AV) node reentry or (*b*) concealed AV pathways, (3) sustained ventricular tachycardia, and (4) chronic atrial fibrillation. Patients with cardiac arrhythmias require EPS before treatment, and further intraoperative mapping is done at the time of surgery. Catheter ablation methods, when appropriate, can be applied in the catheterization laboratory after EPS studies are completed.

Both an epicardial and an endocardial approach have been used for surgical treatment of WPW syndrome and for paroxysmal supraventricular tachycardia, frequently using operative cryoablation as an adjunct. Both operative approaches have been highly successful. The majority of patients with WPW syndrome or PSVT are now treated nonoperatively with less morbidity using radiofrequency catheter ablation techniques. Recent mapping of the slow posterior pathway has even allowed successful catheter treatment of PSVT associated with AV node reentry tachycardia without heart block, and radiofrequency ablation has been near uniformly successful for WPW syndrome.

Arrhythmia surgery has become the preferred method for treatment of sustained ventricular tachycardia which is nonresponsive to medical therapy. These arrhythmias are frequently life-threatening. Typically the ventricular arrhythmia is induced by electrophysiologic studies, and attempts are made to suppress the arrhythmia with pharmacologic agents. If the arrhythmia remains nonsuppressible, surgery is indicated.

Operative map-guided methods have been highly effective for the treatment of sustained ventricular tachycardia associated with left ventricular aneurysms. While results at New York University have been encouraging using ''blind'' (non–map-guided) endocardial resection and remodeling endoaneurysmorraphy for treatment of this combination of diseases (see above section on Left Ventricular Aneurysms), most reports note lower arrhythmia recurrence rates when mapping methods are utilized.

Nonsuppressible ischemic-related sustained ventricular tachycardia without aneurysmal disease may also be treated by definitive map-guided operative ablation, or alternately, by placement of the implantable defibrillator (see section below). Coronary bypass is performed concomitantly if reversible myocardial ischemia is present. While operative mortality rate is less after placement of the implantable defibrillator than with open ablative surgery (3 percent versus 8 to 10 percent), the incidence of late sudden death is lower after operative ablation, and the choice of appropriate treatment remains controversial. However, when ventricular fibrillation is the primary clinical event, and not ventricular tachycardia, the implantable defibrillator becomes the treatment of choice (see section below). Ventricular fibrillation cannot be mapped and electrophysiologic studies cannot be used to follow the response to medications. Nonoperative radiofrequency ablation has not been effective in the treatment of sustained ventricular tachycardia, and neither operative nor radiofrequency ablation methods have been effective for ventricular fibrillation.

A new technique for the treatment of chronic atrial fibrillation, the maze procedure, has been developed by Cox. Initial results with this operation have been encouraging, but long-term results are not yet available. In summary, electrophysiologic studies, catheter ablation techniques, and improved operative methods have given the physician powerful new tools for the treatment of heretofore unmanageable cardiac arrhythmias.

PACEMAKERS/IMPLANTABLE DEFIBRILLATORS/ INTRAAORTIC BALLOON PUMP/ASSIST DEVICES

Pacemakers

Historical Background. Bigelow developed an electric pacemaker that would increase the rate of the hypothermic heart in 1950. In 1952 Zoll demonstrated the clinical possibilities by restarting the hearts of terminal patients with complete heart block using electrical stimulation through the chest wall. A completely implantable permanent pacemaker was described by Chardack in 1960. In 1958 Furman and Robinson found that the heart could be paced by an electrode lead placed on the endocardial surface of the right ventricle, demonstrating that an electrode could be safely left intravenously across the superior vena cava and the tricuspid valve, permanently positioned in the right ventricle. The transvenous method of cardiac pacing quickly became the procedure of choice since the morbidity and mortality were less than with the previously used transthoracic approach.

Indications. Permanent pacemakers were initially used for patients with complete (third-degree) AV heart block, which developed spontaneously in older patients or which occurred secondary to operative trauma. More recently pacemakers have been used for a variety of other arrhythmias including the sick sinus syndrome, with alternating bradycardia and tachycardia, and for any second-degree, bifasicular, or trifasicular heart block associated with intermittent brady-arrhythmias or symptoms. Asymptomatic patients with Mobitz 2 second-degree block or with Mobitz 1 second-degree block at the bundle of His level are also considered to be candidates for a pacemaker by most authorities. The most common indication for permanent pacemaker implantation is sick sinus syndrome, accounting for 50 percent. Temporary pacemakers are used for transient heart block associated with myocardial infarction or cardiac surgery, or in symptomatic patients awaiting a permanent pacemaker.

Pathophysiology of Heart Block. In normal cardiac conduction tissue the cardiac impulse originates in the sinoatrial node near the junction of the superior vena cava with the right atrium.

The impulse is propagated through the right atrium to the AV node, which lies medial to the ostium of the coronary sinus beneath the septal portion of the tricuspid valve, at the apex of the triangle of Koch. From the AV node conduction travels near the annulus of the tricuspid valve, along the bundle of His to pass through the central fibrous body of the ventricular septum, coursing slightly leftward on the crest of the muscular component of the ventricular septum. Here the bundle divides into the left and right bundles, which in turn travel to the respective ventricles.

The most common surgical trauma producing complete heart block occurs during the repair of a ventricular septal defect or an ostium primum atrial septal defect. Complete heart block may rarely follow prosthetic replacement of the aortic, mitral, or tricuspid valves, either from direct injury to conduction tissue or from traction with subsequent fibrosis. Occasionally endocarditis results in complete heart block from an annular abscess. Intrinsic disease may develop in both the SA node and the AV node in the aging population, or may develop as a result of ischemic disease.

Clinical symptoms attributed to first-degree heart block (PR internal > 0.2 s) are rare. With second-degree heart block (intermittent lack of AV conduction) symptoms become apparent if the bradycardia is severe or persistent. Two types of second-degree heart block are described. (1) Mobitz 1 (Wenckeback) typically has progressive prolongation of the PR interval followed by a nonconducted P wave. This is usually benign unless it occurs at the His-Purkinje conduction level. (2) Mobitz 2 second-degree block is more ominous, presenting with normal PR intervals, but with sporadic nonconduction, or third-degree block. Mobitz 2 often progresses to complete third-degree block with associated symptoms.

Third-degree (complete) heart block seriously impairs cardiac output in several ways. The resulting bradycardia varies from 25 to 60 beats/min, which may compromise both the coronary and the cerebral circulation. Refractory congestive failure may exist with heart rates of 45 beats/min or less. Patients with complete heart block frequently have extreme exercise intolerance, and dangerous symptoms of cerebral vascular insufficiency may occur, such as syncope and convulsions (Adams-Stokes syndrome).

Once complete AV disassociation and third-degree heart block occurs, patients often develop a slow ventricular escape rhythm, typically with heart rates of 25 to 60 beats/min. Cardiac arrest and death can occur. Others may develop ventricular tachycardia or ventricular fibrillation instead of a stable ventricular escape mechanism. Although an occasional patient remains asymptomatic with a rate as low as 35 beats/min, most have symptoms once the heart rate is less than 45 beats/min. With Mobitz 2 second-degree block the heart rate may be normal most of the time, but can abruptly change into complete AV disassociation.

Diagnosis. Milder symptoms of light-headedness or near-syncope may be due to intermittent bradycardia or heart block. The differential diagnosis for syncope or near-syncope includes second- or third-degree heart block, sick sinus syndrome, paroxysmal atrial tachycardia, sustained ventricular tachycardia, spontaneous ventricular fibrillation, vasovagal reaction, aortic stenosis, carotid sinus syndrome, occlusive arterial disease of the carotid or cerebral circulation, epilepsy, and idiopathic syncope. The diagnosis of complete heart block can be established with an ECG, whereas the diagnosis of intermittent heart block, sick sinus syndrome (tachy-brady arrhythmias), or paroxysmal atrial tachycardia may require serial ECGs or a 24-h Holter monitor.

Pacemaker Physiology. The efficacy of cardiac pacing depends on the ability of the heart to respond to short bursts (2 ms) of electrical stimulation, ideally with less than 1.5 to 2 mA of current. A direct linear relationship is present between stimulation threshold and the electrode surface area, with more concentrated charge present in smaller electrodes. Characteristics of modern pacemaker generators include a voltage ranging from 2½ to 7½ V, delivering a current of 3.5 to 15 mA. The pulse width of delivered charge can be varied from 0.15 to 2.0 ms. External programming capabilities are usually present.

The pacing threshold determination is particularly important with intravenous implantations to ensure that the pacing lead is in the proper position. With satisfactory location of the intravenous intracardiac electrode, determined by fluoroscopy, an optimal stimulation threshold for pacing is 0.4 to 1.0 mA at 0.2 to 0.5 V, with a pulsewidth 0.5 ms. The resistance of the pacing electrode is calculated from the voltage and current threshold required to achieve cardiac pacing, with 500 to 700 ohms considered acceptable.

Cardiac pacing may be done with either unipolar or bipolar electrodes. In a bipolar system both the positive and negative electrodes are in contact in the heart. When unipolar pacing is used, the tip of the electrode is the stimulating pole and the ground is the metal of the generator. This is the most common method, although sensing is occasionally improved by switching to bipolar leads.

Types of Pacemakers. Demand pacemakers are now almost exclusively used. A more complex and widely used type of pacemaker is the atrial-ventricular pacemaker, or dual-chamber pacemaker, which requires electrodes in both the atrium and the ventricle. Dual-chamber units allow AV sequential pacing (Fig. 18-16) by sensing both chambers and pacing as necessary. Newer pacemakers have rate responsive capabilities, increasing their rate in response to the patient's bodily activity. Almost all pacemakers are now externally programmable.

A standardized code to describe pacemakers has been developed. It usually includes three to five letters which describe the functions of the pacemaker. The first letter describes the chamber paced (V = ventricle, A = atrium, D = dual = chamber pacing). Letter two describes the chamber sensed (V = ventricle, A = atrium, D = dual-chamber sensing, 0 = none). The third letter describes the response of the pacemaker to a sensed beat (T = triggered, I = inhibited, D = dual-chamber inhibition, 0 = not applicable). For example, a DDD pacemaker indicates dual-chamber pacing, sensing, and inhibition. Occasionally a fourth letter is used to indicate either programmability or rate modulation (P = simple programmable, M = multiprogrammability, C = communicating, R = rate modulation), and a fifth letter may be used if antitachycardia or defibrillation function is available (P = antitachycardia pacing, S = shock, D = dual function). These later designs are often combined with the automatic implantable defibrillator (see section below).

Operative Technique. For transient heart block following myocardial infarction a temporary pacing electrode is percutaneously introduced through the subclavian or femoral vein and advanced into the right ventricle. Fluoroscopy may be helpful but is usually not necessary. Temporary pacemaker wires are also commonly placed on the epicardial surface of the heart after cardiac surgical procedures. Temporary transvenous or epicardial pacemaker wires are easily removed prior to hospital discharge.

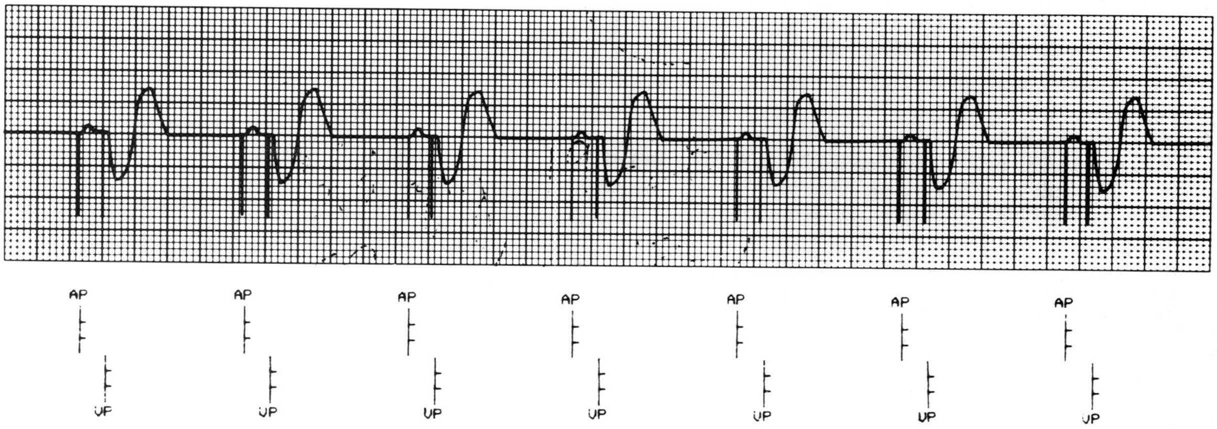

FIG. 18-16. Electrocardiogram of a patient with a functioning AV sequential pacemaker. AP = atrial pace, VP = ventricular pace.

Most permanent pacemakers are now inserted by the transvenous route. The cephalic vein, the external jugular vein, or the internal jugular vein may be used, but more commonly a direct sterile subclavian puncture is used for venous access. Once the needle is in the subclavian vein, a dilator and sheath are passed over a guidewire, and the pacing electrode is advanced through the sheath. The transvenous electrode can be advanced into the appropriate chamber of the heart, guided by fluoroscopic control. Pacing threshold and P wave or R wave sensitivity are then determined. Once the electrode(s) have been positioned, the pacemaker is implanted in a subcutaneous pocket on the anterior chest wall.

Open surgical approaches employ one of three routes: left intercostal, left subcostal, or subxiphoid incisions. Since the morbidity is greater with the direct surgical approach, this method is reserved for special circumstances, i.e., patients with prosthetic tricuspid valves or neonates.

Postoperative Considerations. The morbidity with transvenous pacemaker implantation is small. Migration of the pacing electrode is the most common complication. Perforation of the ventricle can occur, resulting in diaphragmatic pacing or even cardiac tamponade. Infection is surprisingly rare. Recovery following pacemaker placement is usually uneventful. Antibiotics are given for 24 h. Difficulties with the subcutaneous implantation of the generator are rare with the small generators now available.

Following discharge from the hospital, the patient should be seen in 2 to 3 weeks to assess for a rise in the pacing threshold. Telephonic electrocardiographic surveillance has been a significant advance. Data indicate that this type of periodic monitoring is mandatory for good care. As the pulse generator fails, the pacemakers output changes, switching to a fixed mode; this can be determined by telephonic monitoring. When generator failure begins to occur, the pacemaker is electively replaced. Continuous follow-up is essential.

Special problems may occur in pacemaker patients requiring other surgical procedures where the electrocautery is needed. Electromagnetic fields as high as 60 V/m are commonly induced with the electrocautery. This far exceeds the energy level required to activate the sensing circuit in most pacemakers. As a result this electrical signal may inhibit the pulse generator, damage the circuitry, or reset the pacing programs. A variety of arrhythmias have been observed due to subsequent pacemaker malfunction, such as ventricular asystole, multiple premature ventricular contractions, ventricular tachycardia, and ventricular fibrillation. Total destruction of some pacemakers has occurred. In patients for whom use of the electrocautery is necessary brief bursts of cautery should be used, keeping as far away from the generator as possible. A bipolar cautery is probably safest. A pacemaker programming system should be available, and the pacemaker should be interrogated and reprogrammed after use of electrocautery. For patients who are totally pacemaker-dependent a backup transvenous wire and external pacemaker should be available before use of the electrocautery.

Implantable Defibrillators

More than 500,000 deaths occur in the United States each year from sudden cardiac arrest; the majority of these are due to ventricular fibrillation and ventricular tachycardia. Less than 10 percent of these deaths occur in the setting of acute myocardial infarction. The survival for an out-of-hospital cardiac arrest not associated with myocardial infarction is less than 25 percent.

Spontaneous ventricular tachycardia and ventricular fibrillation commonly are a result of underlying structural heart disease such as coronary artery disease, ventricular aneurysm, or cardiomyopathy. Long-term survival in these patients is quite poor, and their risk for sudden death can be stratified by ejection fraction and electrophysiologic studies (see section on Arrhythmia Surgery). For patients with inducible ventricular arrhythmias which are not suppressed with medication, the 2-year survival is less than 40 percent. These patients are candidates for either arrhythmia surgery or for placement of the internal cardioverter defibrillator (ICD).

ICD Devices. The early development of the implantable defibrillator was achieved by Dr. Michael Mirowski with the first human implantation being performed in 1980. In early 1982 a second generation device, the automatic internal cardioverter defibrillator (AICD, CPI, St. Paul, Minnesota) became available. Third- and fourth-generation ICD devices are now in clinical trials. These units allow programmability, backup bradycardia pacing, and antitachycardia pacing as well as standard cardioversion. Up until recently ICD placement required open implantation, but totally transvenous systems are now becoming available.

Indications. The indications for ICD therapy are similar to the indications for arrhythmia surgery:

1. One or more episodes of spontaneous sustained ventricular tachycardia (VT) or ventricular fibrillation (VF) in a patient in whom electrophysiologic testing and/or spontaneous ventricular arrhythmias cannot be used accurately to predict the efficacy of other therapies.
2. Recurrent episodes of spontaneous sustained VT or VF in a patient despite antiarrhythmia drug therapy (guided by electrophysiologic testing or noninvasive methods).
3. Spontaneous sustained VT or VF in a patient in whom antiarrhythmia drug therapy is limited by intolerance or noncompliance.
4. Persistent inducibility of clinically relevant sustained VT or VF on electrophysiologic studies on the best available drug therapy or despite surgical/catheter ablation, in a patient with spontaneous sustained VT or VF.

Results. Several reports have documented the efficacy of ICD therapy. A large series by Winkle documented a 96 percent freedom from sudden death after 5 years with use of the ICD. Although the risk of sudden cardiac death is substantially reduced by ICD therapy, overall survival is still decreased due to congestive heart failure, with a 5-year survival of 70 to 75 percent. Similar results are obtainable with arrhythmia surgery, and the appropriate treatment of these patients remains controversial (see discussion under Arrhythmia Surgery).

Balloon Pump

The intraaortic balloon pump (IABP) is the most common and effective clinical technique for assisted circulation (see above section on Postoperative Care). Approximately 70,000 are inserted annually in this country. The technique was developed by Alstin and associates. A balloon catheter is inserted through the femoral artery and advanced into the thoracic aorta. Insertion of the balloon may either be done by direct arteriotomy or with a percutaneous insertion kit. With electronic synchronization the balloon is alternately inflated during diastole and deflated during systole. Coronary blood flow is increased by improved diastolic perfusion and afterload is reduced. The cardiac index typically improves after insertion and the preload decreases. Total myocardial oxygen consumption is diminished by approximately 15 percent.

The IABP can be used for several days with minimal morbidity. Ischemia of the extremity through which the IABP is inserted is the most serious complication. Viability of the extremity must be confirmed by frequent examination of the extremity. Platelet consumption may also occur.

Ventricular Assist Devices

Temporary assisted circulation is now a valuable clinical modality when transient cardiac injury is present. The most common indication for temporary assisted circulation is cardiac failure after cardiac surgery, manifested by a cardiac index of less than 1.5 L/min/m^2 despite inotropic support. Often an IABP has been used without success. In such instances mechanical cardiac assistance for 24 to 48 h or longer may permit recovery of cardiac function, probably by minimizing reperfusion injury and from resolution of myocardial edema. Similarly, some patients who are dying while awaiting heart transplantation may benefit from circulatory support with a cardiac assist device.

Several types of ventricular assist devices (VAD) are available, including temporary extracorporeal centrifugal pumps, implantable left ventricular assist systems (LVAS), external heterotopic pulsatile ventricular assist devices (VAD), and total artificial hearts (TAH). The most commonly used devices are simple pumps (DeBakey roller pump or Biomedicus centrifugal pump) connected to the left atrium and the aorta. These devices can provide effective support 5 to 7 days, rarely up to 2 weeks. External pulsatile assist devices deliver blood flow in synchrony with the native heart and are used either for short-term support after cardiac surgery or primarily as a bridge to cardiac transplantation. Attempts at total cardiac replacement with an artificial heart, such as the Simbion Jarvik 7 TAH, have been largely unsuccessful due to long-term thromboembolic complications, infection, and trauma to blood elements.

Results. At New York University over 100 temporary ventricular assist devices have been used for postcardiotomy shock in the last 15 years, with an overall survival of approximately 30 percent. Prompt insertion is necessary prior to irreversible myocardial damage. The authors currently use the Biomedicus centrifugal pump with heparin bonded tubing for short-term cardiac assistance (Fig. 18-17). Similar results were reported by Pae and associates, from a combined registry experience of 965 cases, where the hospital survival was 25 percent. Eighty-six percent of the surviving patients were subsequently NYHA functional Class I or II. Survival was equivalent with use of pulsatile pumps or non-

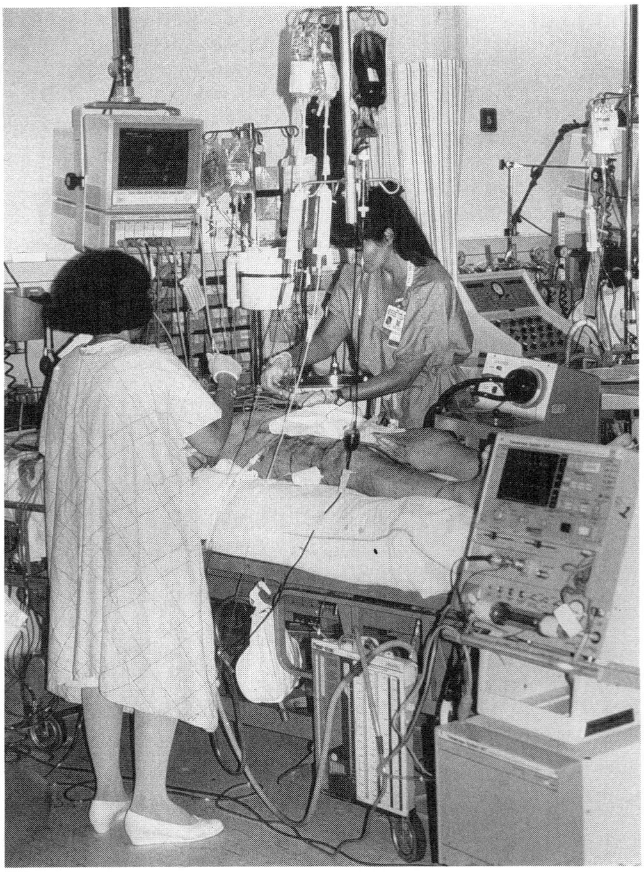

FIG 18-17. Recovery room photograph of a patient requiring ventricular assistance with the intraaortic balloon pump (IABP) and a centrifugal type of ventricular assist device (Biomedicus). The IABP console is in the foreground, and the cardiac assist pump is next to the patient on the bed. This patient was weaned from both devices within 48 h and was discharged from the hospital 3 weeks postoperatively.

pulsatile centrifugal devices. All ventricular assist devices are associated with a significant risk of thromboembolism and infection.

From the registry for the International Society of Heart Transplantation, data exist on the use of ventricular assist devices in 291 patients as a bridge to cardiac transplantation, with 213 patients (73 percent) surviving transplantation. Pretransplant cardiac support ranged from 19 to 159 days. Data from St. Louis University indicate a 48 percent survival when assist devices were used as a bridge to transplantation. However, all patients undergoing cardiac support, either after cardiac surgery or as a bridge to transplantation, would have died had ventricular assist devices not been available. As technology improves long-term cardiac assistance or totally artificial hearts may have an expanded role in the future.

In summary, survival is now possible in patients with end-stage cardiac function or with severe cardiac injury through the use of mechanical cardiac assistance. Artificial cardiac replacement remains to be perfected.

Bibliography

Clinical Manifestations/Diagnostic Studies/Medical Therapy

Braunwald E: *Heart Disease: A Textbook of Cardiovascular Medicine*. Philadelphia, WB Saunders, 1992.

Goldman L, et al: Multifactorial index of cardiac risk in noncardiac surgical procedures. *N Engl J Med* 297:845, 1977.

Goldman L: Multifactorial index of cardiac risk in noncardiac surgery: Ten-year status report. *J Cardiothorac Anesth* 1:237, 1987.

Hertzer NR, et al: Coronary artery disease in peripheral vascular patients: A classification of 1000 coronary angiograms and results of surgical management. *Ann Surg* 199:223, 1984.

Pasternack PF, et al: The value of radionuclide angiography as a predictor of perioperative myocardial infarction in patients undergoing abdominal aortic aneurysm resection. *J Vasc Surg* 1:320, 1984.

Cardiopulmonary Bypass

Bidstrup BP, Royston D, et al: Reduction in blood loss and blood use after cardiopulmonary bypass with high dose aprotinin (Trasylol). *J Thorac Cardiovasc Surg* 97:364, 1989.

Bjork VO: Brain perfusions in dogs with artificially oxygenated blood. *Acta Chir Scand* 96(suppl):137, 1948.

Borowiec J, Thelin S, et al: Heparin-coated circuits reduce activation of granulocytes during cardiopulmonary bypass. A clinical study. *J Thorac Cardiovasc Surg* 104:642, 1992.

Cavarocchi NC, Pluth JR, et al: Complement activation during cardiopulmonary bypass. *J Thorac Cardiovasc Surg* 91:252, 1986.

Cosgrove DM, Loop FD, et al: Determinants of blood utilization during myocardial revascularization. *Ann Thorac Surg* 40:380, 1985.

Crawfoord C, Norberg B, Senning A: Clinical studies in extracorporeal circulation with a heart-lung machine. *Acta Chir Scand* 112:200, 1957.

Dennis C, Spreng DS Jr., et al: Development of a pump-oxygenator to replace the heart and lungs: an example applicable to human patients, and application to one case. *Ann Surg* 134:709, 1951.

Donald DE, Harshbarger HG et al: Experiences with a heart-lung bypass (Gibbon type) in the experimental laboratory: Preliminary report. Proc. staff meet. *Mayo Clin* 30:113, 1955.

Esposito RA, Culliford AT, et al: The role of activated clotting time in heparin administration and neutralization for cardiopulmonary bypass. *J Thorac Cardiovasc Surg* 85:174, 1983.

Esposito R, Culliford A, et al: What is the relationship between plasma heparin concentration and (ACT) activated clotting time? Presented at the 1982 meeting of the American Association for Thoracic Surgery, Phoenix.

Gibbon JH Jr: Application of a mechanical heart and lung apparatus to cardiac surgery. *Minn Med* 37:171, 1954.

Giordano GF, Goldman DS, et al: Intraoperative autotransfusion in cardiac operations—effect on intraoperative and postoperative transfusion requirements. *J Thorac Cardiovasc Surg* 96:382, 1988.

Hackmann T, Gascoyne RD, et al: A trial of desmopressin (1-desamino-8-D-arginine vasopressin) to reduce blood loss in uncomplicated cardiac surgery. *N Engl J Med* 321:1437, 1989.

Harker LA, Malpass TW, et al: Mechanism of abnormal bleeding in patients undergoing cardiopulmonary bypass: Acquired transient platelet dysfunction associated with selective alpha-granule release. *Blood* 56:824, 1980.

Haslam PL, Townsend PJ, Branthwaite MA: Complement activation during cardiopulmonary bypass. *Anaesthesia* 35:22, 1980.

Hisatomi K, Isomura T, et al: Changes in lymphocyte subsets, mitogen responsiveness, and interleukin-2 production after cardiac operations. *J Thorac Cardiovasc Surg* 98:580, 1989.

Jones RE, Donald DE, et al: Apparatus of the Gibbon type of mechanical bypass of the heart and lungs: Preliminary report. Proc. staff meet. *Mayo Clin* 30:105, 1955.

Kirklin JK: The postperfusion syndrome: Inflammation and damaging effects of cardiopulmonary bypass, in Tinker JH (ed): *Cardiopulmonary Bypass: Current Concepts and Controversies*. Philadelphia, WB Saunders, 1989, pp 131–146.

Kirklin JK, Westaby S, et al: Complement and the damaging effects of cardiopulmonary bypass. *J Thorac Cardiovasc Surg* 86:845, 1983.

Krasna MJ, Flancbaum L, Trooskin SZ: Gastrointestinal complications after cardiac surgery. *Surgery* 104:773, 1988.

Lillehei CW, Cohen M, et al: The results of direct vision closure of ventricular septal defects in eight patients by means of control cross circulation. *Surg Gynecol Obstet* 101:446, 1955.

Lillehei CW, Cohen M, et al: Direct vision intracardiac surgical correction of the tetralogy of Fallot, pentalogy of Fallot, and pulmonary atresia defect: A report of first ten cases. *Ann Surg* 142:418, 1955.

Roth JA, Golub SH, et al: Cell mediated immunity is depressed after cardiopulmonary bypass. *Ann Thorac Surg* 31:350, 1980.

Senning A: Ventricular fibrillation during extracorporeal circulation: Use of a method to prevent air-embolisms and to facilitate intracardiac operations. *Acta Chir Scand* 171(suppl):1, 1952.

von Segesser LK, Lachat M, et al: Performance characteristics of centrifugal pumps with end point attached heparin surface coating. *Thorac Cardiovasc Surg* 97:4, 1990.

von Segesser LK, Turino M: Cardiopulmonary bypass without systemic heparinization. Performance of heparin-coated oxygenators in comparison with classic membrane and bubble oxygenators. *J Thorac Cardiovasc Surg* 98:386, 1989.

Postoperative Care and Complications

Bevelaqua F, Garritan S, et al: Complications after cardiac operations in patients with severe pulmonary impairment. *Ann Thorac Surg* 50:602, 1990.

Loop FD (ed), Higgins TL (guest ed): Postoperative care of cardiothoracic surgery patients. *Seminars in Thorac and Cardiovasc Surg* 3, January 1991.

Coronary Artery Disease

Alderman EL, Fisher LD, et al: Results of coronary artery surgery in patients with poor left ventricular function (CASS). *Circulation* 68:785, 1983.

American College of Cardiology/American Heart Association Task Force on Assessment of Diagnostic and Therapeutic Cardiovascular Procedures (Subcommittee on Coronary Artery Bypass Graft Surgery): Guidelines and indications for coronary artery bypass graft surgery. *J Am Coll Cardiol* 17:543, 1991.

Amsterdam EA, Martschinske R, et al: Symptomatic and silent myocardial ischemia during exercise testing in coronary artery disease. *Am J Cardiol* 58:43B, 1986.

Barner HB, Standeven JW, Reese J: Twelve-year experience with internal mammary artery for coronary artery bypass. *J Thorac Cardiovasc Surg* 90:668, 1985.

Bonow RO, Dilsizian V, et al: Identification of viable myocardium in patients with chronic coronary artery disease and left ventricular dysfunction: Comparison of thallium scintigraphy with reinjection and PET imaging with 18F-fluorodeoxyglucose. *Circulation* 83:26, 1991.

Cameron A, Kemp HG Jr, Green GE: Bypass surgery with the internal mammary artery graft: 15 year follow-up. *Circulation* 74:III-30, 1986.

Campeau L, Enjalbert M, et al: Atherosclerosis and late closure of aortocoronary saphenous vein grafts: Sequential angiographic studies at 2 weeks, 1 year, 5 to 7 years, and 10 to 12 years after surgery. *Circulation* 68(suppl II):1, 1983.

Carpentier A, Chachques JC: Clinical dynamic cardiomyoplasty: Method and outcome. *Semin Thorac Cardiovasc Surg* 3:136, 1991.

CASS principal investigators and their associates: Coronary Artery Surgery Study (CASS): A randomized trial of coronary artery bypass surgery. Survival data. *Circulation* 68:939, 1983.

Chaitman BR, David KB, et al: The role of coronary bypass surgery for ''left main equivalent'' coronary disease: The Coronary Artery Surgery Study Registry. *Circulation* 74(suppl III):17, 1986.

Chesebro JH, Clements IP, et al: A platelet-inhibitor drug trial in coronary-artery bypass operations. Benefit of perioperative dipyridamole and aspirin therapy on early postoperative vein-graft patency. *N Engl J Med* 307:73, 1982.

Chesebro JH, Clements IP, et al: A platelet-inhibitor-drug trial in coronary-artery bypass operations. *N Engl J Med* 307:73, 1982.

Chesebro JH, Fuster V, et al: Effect of dipyridamole and aspirin on late vein-graft patency after coronary bypass operations. *N Engl J Med* 310:209, 1984.

Cosgrove DM, Loop FD, et al: Determinants of 10-year survival after primary myocardial revascularization. *Ann Surg* 202:480, 1985.

Crooke GA, Harris LJ, et al: The role of amino acids and enhancement cardioplegia in routine myocardial protection: Experimental results. *J Thorac Cardiovasc Surg*. In press.

Culliford AT, Colvin SB, et al: The atherosclerotic ascending aorta and transverse arch: A new technique to prevent cerebral injury during bypass: Experience with 13 patients. *Ann Thorac Surg* 41:27, 1986.

Detre K, Peduzzi P, et al: Effect of bypass surgery on survival in patients with low- and high-risk groups delineated by the use of simple clinical variables. *Circulation* 63:1329, 1981.

Detre KM, Takaro T, et al: Long-term mortality and morbidity results of the Veterans Administration randomized trial of coronary artery bypass surgery. *Circulation* 72(suppl V):84, 1985.

European Coronary Surgery Study Group: Prospective randomized study of coronary artery bypass surgery in stable angina pectoris. Second interim report. *Lancet* 491, Sept. 6, 1980.

European Coronary Surgery Study Group: Long-term results of prospective randomized study of coronary artery bypass surgery in stable angina pectoris. *Lancet* 2:1173, 1982.

Falcone C, deServi S, et al: Clinical significance of exercise-induced silent myocardial ischemia in patients with coronary artery disease. *J Am Coll Cardiol* 9:295, 1987.

Galbut DL, Traad EA, et al: Twelve-year experience with bilateral internal mammary artery grafts. *Ann Thorac Surg* 40:264, 1985.

Gersh BJ, Califf RM, et al: Coronary bypass surgery in chronic stable angina. *Circulation* 79(suppl I):46, 1989.

Green GE, Spencer FC, et al: Arterial and venous microsurgical bypass grafts for coronary artery disease. *J Thorac Cardiovasc Surg* 60:491, 1970.

Grondin CM, Campeau L, et al: Comparison of late changes in internal mammary artery and saphenous vein grafts in two consecutive series of patients 10 years after operation. *Circulation* 70:1208, 1984.

Grossi EA, Esposito R, et al: Sternal wound infections and use of internal mammary artery grafts. *J Thorac Cardiovasc Surg* 102:342, 1991.

Higgins TL, Estafanous FG, et al: A severity score for cardiac surgery patients. *Crit Care Med* 17:S39, 1989.

Holmes DR Jr, Davis KB, et al: The effect of medical and surgical treatment on subsequent sudden cardiac death in patients with coronary artery disease: A report from the coronary artery surgery study. *Circulation* 73:1254, 1986.

Huddleston CB, Stoney WS, et al: Internal mammary artery grafts: Technical factors influencing patency. *Ann Thorac Surg* 42:543, 1986.

Johnson WD, Brenowitz JB, Gessert R: Long term results of total coronary artery reconstruction. Presented at the American Association for Thoracic Surgery meeting, April 1987.

Kaiser GC, Davis EK, et al: Survival following coronary artery bypass grafting in patients with severe angina pectoris (CASS). *J Thorac Cardiovasc Surg* 89:513, 1985.

Kaiser GC: CABG: Lessons for the randomized trials. *Ann Thorac Surg* 43:3, 1986.

Killip T, Passamani E, et al: Coronary artery surgery study (CASS): A randomized trial of coronary bypass surgery. Eight-year follow-up and survival in patients with reduced ejection fraction. *Circulation* 72(suppl V):102, 1985.

Kirklin JW, Barratt-Boyes BG: Stenotic arteriosclerotic coronary artery disease, in Kirklin JW and Barratt-Boyes BG: *Cardiac Surgery*. New York, Wiley Medical, 1986, p. 207.

Kirklin JW, Naftel DC, et al: Summary of a consensus concerning death and ischemic events after coronary artery bypass grafting. *Circulation* 79(suppl I):81, 1989.

Kirklin JW, Akins CW, et al: ACC/AHA guidelines and indications for coronary artery bypass graft surgery. A report of the American College of Cardiology/American Heart Association Task Force on assessment of diagnostic and therapeutic cardiovascular procedures. *Circulation* 83:1125, 1991.

Klagsbrun M, Edelman ER: Review. Biological and biochemical properties of fibroblast growth factors: Implications for the pathogenesis of atherosclerosis. *Arteriosclerosis* 9:269, 1989.

Kouchoukos NT, Murphy S, et al: Coronary artery bypass grafting for postinfarction angina pectoris. *Circulation* 79(suppl I):68, 1989.

Lee KL, Pryor DB, et al: Prognostic value of radionuclide angiography in medically treated patients with coronary artery disease. A comparison with clinical and catheterization variables. *Circulation* 82:1705, 1990.

Loop FD, Lytle BW, et al: Influence of the internal mammary artery graft on 10-year survival and other cardiac events. *N Engl J Med* 314:1, 1986.

Loop FD, Lytle BW, et al: Free (aorto-coronary) internal mammary artery graft. Late results. *J Thorac Cardiovasc Surg* 92:827, 1986.

Magovern JA, Furnary AP, et al: Indications and risk analysis for clinical cardiomyoplasty. *Semin Thorac Cardiovasc Surg* 3:136, 1991.

Mills NL, Everson CT: Right gastroepiploic artery: A third arterial conduit for coronary artery bypass. *Ann Thorac Surg* 47:706, 1989.

Mock MB, Ringqvist I, et al: The survival of medically treated patients in the coronary artery surgery study (CASS) registry. *Circulation* 66:562, 1982.

Mock MB, Fisher LD, et al: Comparison of effects of medical and surgical therapy on survival in severe angina pectoris and two-vessel coronary artery disease with and without left ventricular dysfunction. A coronary artery surgery study registry. *Am J Cardiol* 61:1198, 1988.

Myers WO, Schaff HV, et al: Improved survival of surgically treated patients with triple vessel coronary artery disease and severe angina pectoris. *J Thorac Cardiovasc Surg* 97:487, 1989.

Orszulak TA, Schaff HV, et al: Initial experience with sequential internal mammary artery bypass grafts to the left anterior descending and left anterior descending diagonal coronary arteries. *Mayo Clin Proc* 61:3, 1986.

Passamani E, Davis KB, et al: A randomized trial of coronary artery bypass surgery. Survival of patients with a low ejection fraction. *N Engl J Med* 312:1665, 1985.

Pigott JD, Kouchoukos NT, et al: Late results of surgical and medical therapy for patients with coronary artery disease and depressed left ventricular function. *J Am Coll Cardiol* 5:1036, 1985.

Rankin JS, Newman GE, et al: Clinical and angiographic assessment of complex mammary artery bypass grafting. *J Thorac Cardiovasc Surg* 92:832, 1986.

Reeder GS, Vlietstra RE, et al: Comparison of angioplasty and bypass surgery in multivessel coronary artery disease. *Int J Cardiol* 10:213, 1986.

Ribakove GH, Katz ES, et al: Surgical implications of transesophageal echocardiography to grade the atheromatous aortic arch. *Ann Thorac Surg* 53:758, 1991.

Ringqvist I, Fisher LD, et al: Prognostic values of angiographic indices of coronary artery disease from the coronary artery surgery study (CASS). *J Clin Invest* 71:1854, 1983.

Rogers WJ, Coggin J, et al: Ten-year follow-up quality of life in patients randomized to receive medical therapy or coronary artery bypass graft surgery. The coronary artery surgery study (CASS). *Circulation* 82:1647, 1990.

Russo P, Orszulak TA, et al: Use of internal mammary artery grafts for multiple coronary artery bypasses. *Circulation* 74:III-48, 1986.

Rutherford JD, Braunwald E: Chronic ischemic heart disease, in Braunwald E (ed): *Heart Disease*. 4th ed. Philadelphia, WB Saunders, 1992, p. 1292.

Ryan TJ, Weiner DA, et al: Exercise testing in the Coronary Artery Surgery Study randomized population. *Circulation* 72(suppl V):31, 1985.

Sauvage LR, Wu HD, et al: Healing basis and surgical techniques for complete revascularization of the left ventricle using only the internal mammary arteries. *Ann Thorac Surg* 42:449, 1986.

Slater J, Chinitz LA, et al: Predictors of operative mortality and long term survival after coronary artery bypass surgery in patients with severely impaired left ventricular function. In press.

Spencer FC: Binocular loupes (microtelescopes) for coronary artery surgery. *J Thorac Cardiovasc Surg* 62:163, 1971.

Spencer FC: The internal mammary artery: The ideal coronary bypass graft? *N Engl J Med* 314:50, 1986.

Spencer FC, Green GE, et al: Surgical therapy for coronary artery disease. *Curr Probl Surg,* September 1970.

Spencer FC, Yong NK, Prachuabmoh K: Internal mammary-coronary artery anastomoses performed during cardiopulmonary bypass. *Cardiovasc Surg* 5:292, 1964.

Stephen Thomas J (ed): *Manual of Cardiac Anesthesia*. New York, Churchill Livingstone, 1984.

Stoney WS, Alford WC Jr, et al: The fate of arm veins used for aorta-coronary bypass grafts. *J Thorac Cardiovasc Surg* 88:522, 1984.

Tector AJ: Fifteen years' experience with the internal mammary artery graft. *Ann Thorac Surg* 42:S22, 1986.

The Veterans Administration Coronary Artery Bypass Surgery Cooperative Study Group: Eleven-year survival in the Veterans Administration randomized trial of coronary bypass surgery for stable angina. *N Engl J Med* 311:1333, 1984.

Tillisch J, Brunken R, et al: Reversibility of cardiac wall-motion abnormalities predicted by positron tomography. *N Engl J Med* 314:884, 1986.

Varnauskas E and the European Coronary Surgery Study Group: Survival, myocardial infarction, and employment status in a prospective randomized study of coronary bypass surgery. *Circulation* 72(suppl V)90, 1985.

Varnauskas E and the European Coronary Surgery Study Group: Twelve-year follow-up of survival in the randomized European Coronary Surgery Study. *N Engl J Med* 319:332, 1988.

Left Ventricular Aneurysm

Akins CW: Resection of left ventricular aneurysm during hypothermic fibrillatory arrest without aortic occlusion. *J Thorac Cardiovasc Surg* 91:610, 1986.

Cooley DA, Frazier OH, et al: Intracavitary repair of ventricular aneurysm and regional dyskinesia. *Ann Surg* 215:417, 1192.

Faxon DP, Myers WO, et al: The influence of surgery on the natural history of angiographically documented left ventricular aneurysm: The coronary artery surgery study. *Circulation* 74:110, 1986.

Jatene AD: Left ventricular aneurysmectomy: Resection or reconstruction. *J Thorac Cardiovasc Surg* 89:321, 1985.

Josephson M, Harken A, Horowitz L: Long-term results of endocardial resection for sustained ventricular tachycardia in coronary disease patients. *Am Heart J* 104:51, 1982.

Kirklin JW, Barratt-Boyes BG: *Cardiac Surgery*. New York, Wiley, 1986.

Novick RJ, Stefaniszyn HJ, et al: Surgery for postinfarction left ventricular aneurysm: Prognosis and long-term follow-up. *Can J Surg* 27:161, 1984.

Olearchyk AS, Lemole GM, Spagna PM: Left ventricular aneurysm. Ten years' experience in surgical treatment of 244 cases. Improved clinical status, hemodynamics, and long-term longevity. *J Thorac Cardiovasc Surg* 88:544, 1986.

Sosa E, Jatene A, et al: Recurrent ventricular tachycardia associated with postinfarction aneurysm: Results of left ventricular reconstruction. *J Thorac Cardiovasc Surg* 103:855, 1992.

Valvular Heart Disease

Mitral Valve Disease

Carpentier A: Cardiac valve surgery—the ''French Correction.'' *J Thorac Cardiovasc Surg* 86:323, 1983.

Carpentier A: Plastic and reconstructive mitral valve surgery, in Jackson JW (ed): *Operative Surgery*. Boston, Butterworths, 1977, p 527.

Carpentier A, Chauvaud S, et al: Reconstructive surgery of mitral valve incompetence: Ten-year appraisal. *J Thorac Cardiovasc Surg* 79:338, 1980.

Carpentier A, Guerinon J, et al: Pathology of the mitral valve, in Jackson JW (ed): *Operative Surgery*. Boston, Butterworths, 1977, p 65.

Cohn LH, Allred EN, et al: Long-term results of open mitral valve reconstruction for mitral stenosis. *Am J Cardiol* 55:731, 1985.

Cosgrove DM, Chavez AM, et al: Results of mitral valve reconstruction. *Circulation* 74(suppl I):I-82, 1986.

David TE, Strauss HD, et al: Is it important to preserve the chordae tendineae and papillary muscles during mitral valve replacement? *Can J Surg* 24:236, 1981.

David TE, Uden DE, Strauss HD: The importance of the mitral apparatus in left ventricular function after correction of a mitral regurgitation. *Circulation* 68(suppl II):II-76, 1983.

Edmunds LH Jr: Thrombotic and bleeding complications of prosthetic heart valves. *Ann Thorac Surg* 44:430, 1987.

Ferrazzi P, McGiffin DC, et al: Have the results of mitral valve replacement improved? *J Thorac Cardiovasc Surg* 92:186, 1986.

Galler M, Kronzon I, et al: Long-term follow-up after mitral valve reconstruction: Incidence of postoperative left ventricular outflow obstruction. *Circulation* 74(suppl I):I-99, 1986.

Galloway AC, Colvin SB, et al: Current concepts of mitral valve reconstruction for mitral insufficiency. *Circulation* 78:1087, 1988.

Galloway AC, Colvin SB, et al: Long-term results of mitral valve reconstruction using Carpentier techniques in 148 patients with mitral insufficiency. *Circulation* 78(suppl I):I-97, 1988.

Galloway AC, Colvin SB, et al: A comparison of mitral valve reconstruction with mitral valve replacement: Intermediate-term results. *Ann Thorac Surg* 47:655, 1989.

Grossi EA, Galloway AC, et al: Experience with twenty-eight cases of systolic anterior motion after mitral valve reconstruction by the Carpentier technique. *J Thorac Cardiovasc Surg* 103:466, 1992.

Halseth W, Elliott D, et al: Open mitral commissurotomy: A modern reevaluation. *J Thorac Cardiovasc Surg* 80:842, 1980.

Hammermeister KE, Henderson WG, et al: Comparison of outcome after valve replacement with a bioprosthesis versus a mechanical prosthesis: Initial 5 year results of a randomized trial. *J Am Coll Cardiol* 10:719, 1987.

Kay GL, Kay JH, et al: Mitral valve repair for mitral regurgitation secondary to coronary artery disease. *Circulation* 74(suppl I):I-88, 1986.

Kay JH, Egerton WS: The repair of mitral insufficiency associated with ruptured chordae tendineae. *Ann Surg* 157:351, 1963.

Kirklin JW: Mitral valve repair for mitral incompetence. *Mod Concept Cardiovasc Dis* 56:7, 1987.

Kirklin JW, Barratt-Boyes BG: *Cardiac Surgery,* New York, Wiley, 1986.

Lillehei CW, Gott VL, et al: Surgical correction of pure mitral insufficiency by annuloplasty under direct vision. *Lancet* 77:446, 1957.

McGoon DC: Repair of mitral insufficiency due to ruptured chordae tendineae. *J Thorac Cardiovasc Surg* 39:357, 1960.

McKay RG, Lock JE, et al: Balloon dilation of mitral stenosis in adult patients: Postmortem and percutaneous mitral valvuloplasty studies. *J Am Coll Cardiol* 9:723, 1987.

Merendino KA, Bruce RA: One hundred seventeen surgically treated cases of valvular rheumatic heart diseases: With preliminary report of two cases of mitral regurgitation treated under direct vision with aid of a pump-oxygenator. *JAMA* 64:749, 1957.

Palacios I, Block PC, et al: Percutaneous balloon valvotomy for patients with severe mitral stenosis. *Circulation* 75:778, 1987.

Perier P, Deloche A, et al: Comparative evaluation of mitral valve repair and replacement with Starr, Bjork, and porcine valve prostheses. *Circulation* 70(suppl I):I-187, 1984.

Reed GE, Pooley RW, Moggio RA: Durability of measured mitral annuloplasty: Seventeen-year study. *J Thorac Cardiovasc Surg* 79:321, 1980.

Reed GE, Tice DA, Clauss RH: Asymmetric exaggerated mitral annuloplasty: Repair of mitral insufficiency with hemodynamic predictability. *J Thorac Cardiovasc Surg* 49:752, 1965.

Sand ME, Naftel DC, et al: A comparison of repair and replacement for mitral valve incompetence. *J Thorac Cardiovasc Surg* 94:208, 1987.

Sarris GE, Fann JI, et al: Global and regional left ventricular systolic performance in the in situ ejecting canine heart: Importance of the mitral apparatus. *Circulation* 80(suppl I):I-24, 1989.

Selzer A, Cohn KE: Natural history of mitral stenosis: A review. *Circulation* 45:878, 1972.

Souttar PW: The surgical treatment of mitral stenosis. *Br Med J* 2:603, 1925.

Spencer FC, Baumann FG, et al: Experiences with 1643 porcine prosthetic valves in 1492 patients. *Ann Surg* 203:691, 1986.

Spencer FC, Colvin SB, et al: Experiences with the Carpentier techniques of mitral valve reconstruction in 103 patients (1980–1985). *J Thorac Cardiovasc Surg* 90:341, 1985.

Spencer FC, Galloway AC, Colvin SB: A clinical evaluation of the hypothesis that rupture of the left ventricle following mitral valve replacement can be prevented by preservation of the chordae of the mural leaflet. *Ann Surg* 202:673, 1985.

Yacoub M, Halim M, et al: Surgical treatment of mitral regurgitation caused by floppy valves: Repair versus replacement. *Circulation* 64(suppl II):II-210, 1981.

Aortic Valve Disease

Arciniegas E: *Pediatric Cardiac Surgery*. Chicago, Year Book Medical, 1985.

Bloomfield P, Kitchin AH, et al: A prospective evaluation of the Bjork-Shiley, Hancock, and Carpentier-Edwards heart valve prostheses. *Circulation* 73:1213, 1986.

Christakis GT, Weisel RD, et al: Can the results of contemporary aortic valve replacement be improved? *J Thorac Cardiovasc Surg* 92:37, 1986.

Galloway AC, Colvin SB, et al: Ten-year experience with aortic valve replacement in 482 patients 70 years of age or older: Operative risk and long-term results. *Ann Thorac Surg* 49:84, 1990.

Isner JM, Salem DN, et al: Treatment of calcific aortic stenosis by balloon valvuloplasty. *Am J Cardiol* 59:313, 1987.

Kirklin JW, Barratt-Boyes BG: *Cardiac Surgery*. New York, Wiley, 1986.

Lombard JT, Selzer A: Valvular aortic stenosis. A clinical and hemodynamic profile of patients. *Ann Intern Med* 106:292, 1987.

Meurs AA, Grundemann AM, et al: Early and 8 year results of aortic valve replacement: A clinical study of 232 patients. *Eur Heart J* 6:870, 1985.

O'Brien MF, Stafford EG, et al: Aortic valve replacement with cryopreserved homograft valves and with antibiotic 4°C stored valves: A comparative follow-up study. Presented at the 67th Annual Meeting of the American Association for Thoracic Surgery, 1987.

Olson LJ, Subramanian R, Edwards WD: Surgical pathology of pure aortic insufficiency: A study of 225 cases. *Mayo Clin Proc* 59:835, 1984.

Perloff JK: *The Clinical Recognition of Congenital Heart Disease,* 3d ed. Philadelphia, WB Saunders, 1987.

Schneider JF, Wilson M, Gallant TE: Percutaneous balloon aortic valvuloplasty for aortic stenosis in elderly patients at high risk for surgery. *Ann Intern Med* 106:696, 1987.

Stark J, de Leval M (eds): *Surgery for Congenital Heart Defects*. London, Grune & Stratton, 1983.

Subramanian R, Olson LJ, Edwards WD: Surgical pathology of pure aortic stenosis: A study of 374 cases. *Mayo Clin Proc* 59:683, 1984.

Tricuspid Valve Disease

Arbulu A, Asfaw I: Tricuspid valvulectomy without prosthetic replacement. Ten years of clinical experience. *J Thorac Cardiovasc Surg* 82:684, 1981.

Baughman KL, Kallman CH, et al: Predictors of survival after tricuspid valve surgery. *Am J Cardiol* 54:137, 1984.

Boyd AD, Engelman RM, et al: Tricuspid annuloplasty. *J Thorac Cardiovasc Surg* 68:344, 1974.

Cobanoglu A, Starr A: Tricuspid valve surgery: Indications, methods, and results. *Cardiovasc Clin* 16:375, 1986.

Galloway AC, Grossi EA, et al: Multiple valve operation for advanced valvular heart disease: Results and risk factors in 513 patients. *J Am Coll Cardiol* 19:725, 1992.

Kay JH, Maselli-Campagna G, Tsuji HK: Surgical treatment of tricuspid insufficiency. *Ann Surg* 162:53, 1965.

Peterffy A: Surgical management of tricuspid valvular disease. Ten years' experience of 141 consecutive patients. *Scand J Thorac Cardiovasc Surg* 26(suppl):1, 1980.

Stern HJ, Sisto DA, et al: Immediate tricuspid valve replacement for endocarditis. Indications and results. *J Thorac Cardiovasc Surg* 91:163, 1986.

Thorburn CW, Morgan JJ, et al: Long-term results of tricuspid valve replacement and the problem of prosthetic valve thrombosis. *Am J Cardiol* 51:1128, 1983.

Wellens F, Jacques G: Tricuspid valve replacement. *Cardiovasc Clin* 17:111, 1987.

Multiple Valve Disease

Bonchek LI, Starr A: Ball valve prostheses: Current appraisal of late results. *Am J Cardiol* 35:843, 1975.

Galloway AC, Grossi EA, et al: Multiple valve operation for advanced valvular heart disease: Results and risk factors in 513 patients. *J Am Coll Cardiol* 19:725, 1992.

Kirklin JW, Barratt-Boyes BG: *Cardiac Surgery*. New York, Wiley, 1986.

Spencer FC, Baumann FG, et al: Experiences with 1643 porcine prosthetic valves in 1492 patients. *Ann Surg* 203:691, 1986.

Cardiac Trauma

Blalock A, Ravitch MM: A consideration of the nonoperative treatment of cardiac tamponade resulting from wounds to the heart. *Surgery* 14:157, 1943.

Bland EF, Beebe GW: Missiles in the heart: A 20-year follow-up report of World War II cases. *N Engl J Med* 274:1039, 1966.

Cogbill TH, Moore EE, et al: Rationale for selective application of emergency department thoracotomy in trauma. *J Trauma* 23:453, 1983.

Estrera AS, Schreiber JT: Management of acute cardiac trauma. *Cardiol Clin* 2:239, 1984.

Evans J, Gray L, et al: Principles for the management of penetrating cardiac wounds *Ann Surg* 189:777, 1979.

Frazee RC, Mucha P Jr, et al: Objective evaluation of blunt cardiac trauma. *J Trauma* 26:510, 1986.

Gay, W: Blunt trauma to the heart and great vessels. *Surgery* 91:507, 1982.

Harken DE: Foreign bodies in and in relation to the heart and thoracic vessels. *Surg Gynecol Obstet* 83:117, 1946.

Harman PK, Trinkle JK: Injury to the heart, in Mattox KL, Moore EE, Feliciano DV (eds): *Trauma*. Norwalk, Appleton & Lange, 1988, p 365.

Holdeger WF, Lyons C, Edwards WS: Indications for removal of intracardiac foreign bodies. *Ann Surg* 163:249, 1966.

Hood RM, Boyd AD, Culliford AT (eds): *Thoracic Trauma*. Philadelphia, WB Saunders, 1989.

Isaacs JP: Sixty penetrating wounds to the heart: Clinical and experimental observations. *Surgery* 45:696, 1959.

Ivatury R, Shah P, et al: Emergency room thoracotomy for the resuscitation of patients with ''fatal'' penetrating injuries of the heart. *Ann Thorac Surg* 32:377, 1981.

Marshall WG Jr, Bell JL, Kouchoukos NT: Penetrating cardiac trauma. *J Trauma* 24:147, 1984.

Mattox KL, Moore EE, Feliciano DV (eds): *Trauma*. Norwalk, CT, Appleton and Lange, 1988.

Moore EE, Moore JB, et al: Postinjury thoracotomy in the emergency department: A critical evaluation. *Surgery* 86:590, 1979.

Reid CL, Kawanishi DT, et al: Chest trauma: Evaluation by two-dimensional echocardiography. *Am Heart J* 113:971, 1987.

Spencer FC, Kennedy JH: War wounds of the heart. *J Thorac Cardiovasc Surg* 33:361, 1957.

Sugg WL, Ecker RR, et al: Penetrating wounds of the heart: An analysis of 459 cases. *J Thorac Cardiovasc Surg* 56:531, 1968.

Tenzer ML: The spectrum of myocardial contusion: A review. *J Trauma* 25:620, 1985.

Cardiac Tumors

Attar S, Lee Y, et al: Cardiac myxoma. *Ann Thorac Surg* 29:397, 1980.

Bahnson HT, Spencer FC, Andrus EC: Diagnosis and treatment of intracavitary myxomas of the heart. *Ann Surg* 145:915, 1957.

Calhoun T, Terry E, et al: Myocardial fibroma or fibrous hamartoma. *Ann Thorac Surg* 32:406, 1981.

Chan HSL, Sonley MJ, et al: Primary and secondary tumors of childhood involving the heart, pericardium, and great vessels. A report of 75 cases and review of the literature. *Cancer* 56:825, 1985.

Fyke FE, Seward JB, et al: Primary cardiac tumors: Experience with 30 consecutive patients since the introduction of two-dimensional echocardiography. *J Am Coll Cardiol* 5(6):1465, 1985.

Larrieu A, Jamieson W, et al: Primary cardiac tumors. Experience with 25 cases. *J Thorac Cardiovasc Surg* 83:339, 1982.

Reece IJ, Cooley DA, et al: Cardiac tumors: Clinical spectrum and prognosis of lesions other than classical benign myxoma in 20 patients. *J Thorac Cardiovasc Surg* 88:439, 1984.

Whorton CM: Primary malignant tumors of the heart. *Cancer* 2:245, 1949.

Pericarditis

Culliford A, Lipton M, Spencer F: Operation for chronic constrictive pericarditis: Do the surgical approach and degree of pericardial resection influence the outcome significantly? *Ann Thorac Surg* 29:146, 1980.

Hier-Madsen K, Saunamaki KI, et al: Purulent pericarditis in children. Review and case report. *Scand J Thorac Cardiovasc Surg* 19:185, 1985.

Kutcher MA, King SB III, et al: Constrictive pericarditis as a complication of cardiac surgery: Recognition of an entity. *Am J Cardiol* 50:742, 1982.

McCaughan BC, Schaff HV, et al: Early and late results of pericardiectomy for constrictive pericarditis. *J Thorac Cardiovasc Surg* 89:340, 1985.

Miller J, Mansour K, Hatcher C: Pericardiectomy: Current indications, concepts, and results in a university center. *Ann Thorac Surg* 34:40, 1982.

Morgan RJ, Stephenson LW, et al: Surgical treatment of purulent pericarditis in children. *J Thorac Cardiovasc Surg* 85:527, 1983.

Nishimura RA, Connolly DC, et al: Constrictive pericarditis: Assessment of current diagnostic procedures. *Mayo Clin Proc* 60:397, 1985.

Seifert FC, Miller DC, et al: Surgical treatment of constrictive pericarditis: Analysis of outcome and diagnostic error. *Circulation* 72(suppl II):II-264, 1985.

Arrhythmia Surgery

Cobb FR, Blumenschein SD, Sealy WC, et al: Successful surgical interruption of the bundle of Kent in a patient with Wolff-Parkinson-White syndrome. *Circulation* 38:1018, 1968.

Cox JL: The surgical management of cardiac arrhythmias, in Sabiston DC Jr, Spencer FC (eds): *Surgery of the Chest,* 5th ed. Philadelphia, WB Saunders, 1990.

Cox JL (guest ed), Loop FD (ed): *Seminars in Thoracic and Cardiovasc Surg* 1(1):1989.

Cox JL, Ferguson TB, et al: Perinodal cryosurgery for atrioventricular node reentry tachycardia in 23 patients. *J Thorac Cardiovasc Surg* 99:440, 1990.

Cox JL, Schuessler RB, et al: The surgical treatment of atrial fibrillation. III. Development of a definitive surgical procedure. *J Thorac Cardiovasc Surg* 101:569, 1991.

Daniel TM, Cox JL, et al: Epicardial and intramural mapping activation of the human heart. A technique for localizing infarction and ischemia of the myocardium. *Circulation* 40(suppl 3):III-66, 1969. Abstract.

Durrer D, Roos JP: Epicardial excitation of the ventricles in a patient with Wolff-Parkinson-White syndrome (type B): Temporary ablation at surgery. *Circulation* 35:15, 1967. Abstract.

Durrer D, Schoo L, et al: The role of premature beats in the initiation and the termination of supraventricular tachycardia in the Wolff-Parkinson-White syndrome. *Circulation* 36:644, 1967.

Guiraudon G, Fontaine G, et al: Encircling endocardial ventriculotomy: A new surgical treatment of life-threatening ventricular tachycardias resistant to medical treatment following myocardial infarction. *Ann Thorac Surg* 26:438, 1978.

Josephson ME, Harken AH, Horowitz LN: Endocardial excision—A new surgical technique for the treatment of recurrent ventricular tachycardia. *Circulation* 60:1430, 1979.

Kaiser GA, Waldo AL, et al: New method to delineate myocardial damage at surgery. *Circulation* 39(suppl 1):83, 1969.

Kehoe R, Zheutlin T, et al: Visually directed endocardial resection for ventricular arrhythmia: Long term outcome and functional status. *J Am Coll Cardiol* 5:497, 1985.

Miller JM, Gottlieb CD, et al: Factors influencing operative mortality in surgery for ventricular tachycardia. *Circulation* 78:44, 1988.

Miller JM, Gottlieb CD, et al: Does ventricular tachycardia mapping influence the success of antiarrhythmic surgery. *J Am Coll Cardiol* 11:112A, 1988.

Sealy WC: The Wolff-Parkinson-White syndrome and the beginnings of direct arrhythmia surgery. *Ann Thorac Surg* 38:176, 1984.

Wolff L, Parkinson J, White PD: Bundle branch block with short PR interval in healthy young people prone to paroxysmal tachycardia. *Am Heart J* 5:685, 1930.

Zobel G, Stein JI, et al: Continuous extracorporeal fluid removal in children with low cardiac output after cardiac operations. *J Thorac Cardiovasc Surg* 101:593, 1991.

Pacemakers/Implantable Defibrillators/Intraaortic Balloon Pump/Assist Devices

Amsterdam E, Awan N, et al: Intra-aortic balloon counterpulsation: Rationale, application and results, in Rackley C (ed): *Critical Care Cardiology*. Philadelphia, FA Davis, 1981.

Axelrod HI, Galloway AC, et al: Percutaneous cardiopulmonary bypass with a synchronous pulsatile pump combines effective unloading with ease of application. *J Thorac Cardiovasc Surg* 93:358, 1987.

Axelrod HI, Galloway AC, et al: A comparison of methods for limiting myocardial infarct expansion during acute reperfusion—primary role of unloading. *Circulation* 76(suppl V):V-28, 1987.

Barold SS, Zipes DP: Cardiac pacemakers and antiarrhythmic devices, in Braunwald E (ed): *Heart Disease*. Philadelphia, WB Saunders, 1992.

Bigelow WG, Callaghan JC, Hoppe JA: General hypothermia for experimental intracardiac surgery: The use of electrophrenic respirations, an artificial pacemaker for cardiac standstill, and radial frequency rewarming in general hypothermia. *Ann Surg* 132:531, 1950.

Bregman D, Casarella W: Percutaneous intraaortic balloon pumping: Initial clinical experience. *Ann Thorac Surg* 29:133, 1980.

Bregman D: Mechanical support of the circulation. *Cleveland Clin Q* 48:181, 1981.

Brodman R, Furman S: Pacemaker implantation through the internal jugular vein. *Ann Thorac Surg* 29:63, 1980.

Carver J, Spitzer S, Mason D: Current concepts in pacing. *Geriatrics* 36:105, 1981.

Chardack WM, Gage AA, et al: The long-term treatment of heart block. *Prog Cardiovasc Dis* 9:105, 1966.

Chardack WM, Gage AA, Greatbatch W: A transistorized, self-contained, implantable pacemaker for the longterm correction of complete heartblock. *Surg* 48:643, 1960.

Culliford A, Isom O, Doyle E: Pacemaker implantation in the extremely young. A safe and cosmetic approach. *J Thorac Cardiovasc Surg* 75:763, 1978.

Furman S, Escher DJ, et al: Implanted transvenous pacemakers: Equipment, technic and clinical experience. *Ann Surg* 164:465, 1966.

Furman S, Robinson G: The use of an intracardiac pacemaker in the correction of total heartblock. *Surg Forum* 9:245, 1958.

Gaines WE, Pierce WS, et al: The Pennsylvania State University paracorporeal ventricular assist pump: Optimal methods of use. *World J Surg* 9:47, 1985.

Glassman E, Engelman RM et al: Method of closed-chest cannulation of left atrium for left atrial-femoral artery bypass. *J Thorac Cardiovasc Surg* 69:283, 1975.

Griffin JC, Mason JW, et al: The treatment of ventricular tachycardia using an automatic tachycardia terminating pacemaker. *PACE* 4:582, 1981.

Griffith BP, Hardesty RL, et al: Temporary use of the Jarvik-7 total artificial heart before transplantation. *N Engl J Med* 316:130, 1987.

Horowitz LN, et al: The automatic implantable cardioverter defibrillator: Review of clinical results 1980–1990. *Pacing and Clinical Electrophysiology* 15(part III):604, 1992.

Joyce LD, DeVries WC, et al: Response of th[illegible] human body to the first permanent implant of the Jarvik-7 total a[illegible] heart. *Trans Am Soc Artif Intern Organs* 29:81, 1983.

Kolff J, Beeb GM: Artificial heart and left [illegible]cular assist devices. *Surg Clin North Am* 65:661, 1985.

Lehmann MH, Saksena S: Naspe Policy Statement: Implantable cardioverter defibrillators in cardiovascular practice: Report of the policy conference of the North American Society of Pacing and Electrophysiology. *PACE* 14:969, 1991.

Levine PA, Balady GJ, et al: Electrocautery and pacemakers: Management of the paced patient subject to electrocautery. *Ann Thorac Surg* 41:313, 1986.

Levinson MM, Smith RG, et al: Thromboembolic complications of the Jarvik-7 total artificial heart: Case report. *Artif Organs* 10:236, 1986.

Macoviak J, Stephenson L, et al: The intraaortic balloon pump: An analysis of five years' experience. *Ann Thorac Surg* 29:451, 1980.

Moses HW, Schneider JA, et al: *A Practical Guide To Cardiac Pacing,* 3d ed. Boston, Little, Brown, 1991.

Pae WE Jr, Pierce WS, et al: Long-term results of ventricular assist pumping in postcardiotomy cardiogenic shock. *J Thorac Cardiovasc Surg* 93:434, 1987.

Pae WE, Miller CA, et al: Ventricular assist devices for postcardiotomy cardiogenic shock: A combined registry experience. *J Thorac Cardiovasc Surg* 104:541, 1992.

Park SB, Liebler GA, et al: Mechanical support of the failing heart. *Ann Thorac Surg* 42:627, 1986.

Pennington DG, Swartz MT: Assisted circulation and mechanical hearts, in Braunwald E (ed): *Heart Disease*. Philadelphia, WB Saunders, 1992.

Pennock JL, Pierce WS, et al: Survival and complications following ventricular assist pumping for cardiogenic shock. *Ann Surg* 198:469, 1983.

Pierce W, Myers J, et al: Approaches to the artificial heart surgery. *Surgery* 90:137, 1981.

Pierce WS: The implantable ventricular assist pump. *J Thorac Cardiovasc Surg* 87:811, 1984.

Pierce WS: The artificial heart—1986: Partial fulfilment of a promise. *ASAIO-Trans* 32:5, 1986.

Reid PR, Griffith LS, et al: Implantable cardioverter-defibrillator: Patient selection and implantation protocol. *PACE* 7(II):1338, 1984.

Rose D, Colvin S, et al: Long-term survival with partial left heart bypass following perioperative myocardial infarction and shock. *J Thorac Cardiovasc Surg* 83:483, 1982.

Rose DM, Colvin SB, et al: Late functional and hemodynamic V status of surviving patients following insertion of the left heart assist device. *J Thorac Cardiovasc Surg* 86:639, 1983.

Saksena S, Camm AJ: Implantable defibrillators for prevention of sudden death—medical and economic cross road. *Circulation* 85:2316, 1992.

Schoen FJ, Palmer DC, et al: Clinical temporary ventricular assist. Pathologic findings and their implications in a multi-institutional study of 41 patients. *J Thorac Cardiovasc Surg* 92:1071, 1986.

Spencer FC, Eiseman B, et al: Assisted circulation for cardiac failure following intracardiac surgery with cardiopulmonary bypass. *J Thorac Cardiovasc Surg* 49:56, 1964.

Sturm J, McGee M, et al: Treatment of postoperative low output syndrome with intraaortic balloon pumping: Experience with 419 patients. *Am J Cardiol* 45:1033, 1980.

Van Citters RL, Bauer CB, et al: Artificial heart and assist devices: Directions, needs, costs, societal and ethical issues. *Artif Organs* 9:375, 1985.

Watkins L, Mirowski M, et al: Automatic defibrillation in man: The initial surgical experience. *J Thorac Cardiovasc Surg* 82:492, 1981.

Zoll PM: Resuscitation of the heart in ventricular standstill by external electric stimulation. *N Engl J Med* 247:768, 1952.

CHAPTER 19

Diseases of Great Vessels

Aubrey C. Galloway, Stephen B. Colvin, and Frank C. Spencer

ANEURYSMS OF THE THORACIC AORTA

Modern treatment of arterial aneurysms was introduced nearly a century ago by Rudolf Matas who described a method of internal repair of aneurysms termed *reconstructive endoaneurysmorrhaphy*. Nearly 50 years later, notable work by Cooley and DeBakey demonstrated the feasibility of successful repair of aneurysms involving the thoracic aorta. Excisional therapy became the mainstay of the modern approach, with resection of the involved aortic segment followed by restoration of blood flow by the placement of an interposition graft, usually made of Dacron. The current method of aneurysm repair often disregards excision of the aneurysmal wall, however, focusing on internal replacement of the involved aortic segment with a graft, which is sewn into normal aorta above and below the area of involvement. The native aortic wall is then closed over the graft; this is termed the *graft inclusion* technique.

Aneurysms of the thoracic aorta may be classified in five groups, varying with the anatomic location: (1) ascending aorta; (2) transverse aortic arch; (3) traumatic, usually occurring distal to the left subclavian artery; (4) descending thoracic aorta; and (5) thoracoabdominal. The etiology, disability, and surgical approach all vary with these different types.

General Considerations. An aortic aneurysm can be defined as a localized or diffuse aortic dilation greater than 5 to 6 cm in diameter, developing from an underlying weakness or defect in the aortic wall. The most frequent causes of thoracic aortic aneurysms are atherosclerosis, aortic dissection, or collagen vascular disease, most frequently Marfan's syndrome. Unusual causes include trauma, infection (syphilitic or other mycotic), autoimmune disease, granulomatous aortitis, and Takayasu arteritis.

Aneurysms are associated with advanced age, hypertension, and smoking. Possible pathogenetic factors include a change in the structure of collagen and elastin within the vessel wall, an increased activity of proteolytic enzymes, and a change in the balance of protease and protease inhibitor activity (Table 19-1), as recently summarized by Griepp.

Separate from etiology, descriptive terms have been helpful in identifying specific areas of aortic involvement. *Aortoannuloectasia* is a descriptive term for a common condition of degenerative dilation of the aortic annulus and the sinuses of Valsalva, producing both aortic insufficiency and a localized aneurysm involving the aortic root and ascending aorta. This lesion is probably a localized form of collagen vascular disease, for it does not develop in vessels in other areas of the body. A traumatic aneurysm generally occurs at a specific location, just distal to the subclavian artery at the site of insertion of the ligamentum arteriosum. The term *dissecting aneurysm* is a misnomer usually meaning aortic dissection resulting from an intimal tear in the aortic wall with subsequent disruption of the media, producing both a true and a false lumen throughout the entire dissected aorta. Aortic dissection is considered separately in a subsequent section, but when a previously dissected aorta chronically dilates to over 5 to 6 cm in diameter, it is appropriately termed chronic aortic dissection or aortic aneurysm secondary to chronic aortic dissection.

Aneurysms of the thoracic aorta are best classified in terms of anatomic location, for both the clinical significance and the surgical approach vary widely. The four major locations are the ascending aorta, transverse aortic arch, descending thoracic aorta, and thoracoabdominal aorta. Aneurysms of the ascending aorta are

Table 19-1
Etiology of Aortic Aneurysms

Deficiency in collagen or elastin in arterial wall
Increased collagenase, elastase, or other proteolytic enzymes
Decreased protease inhibitor activity
Altered protease/antiprotease balance

SOURCE: From Griepp RB, Ergin MA, et al, 1991, with permission.

most frequent, representing over 40 percent of thoracic aneurysms in a large series. Perhaps this is because the ascending aorta is the widest segment; another possibility is that this area is exposed to the high velocity of blood exiting from the heart. The descending aorta is involved in about 35 percent of thoracic aneurysms, and the transverse arch and the thoracoabdominal areas in 10 to 15 percent each. Localizing aneurysms to specific locations may be misleading in some cases, because the entire aorta may be diseased and the most obvious location might be only a portion of a more diffuse disease process.

In all areas of the aorta the natural history of aneurysmal disease is that of progressive enlargement with eventual rupture. This tendency relates primarily to the diameter of the aneurysm, for the lateral wall tension of a vascular tube is related to the radius by Laplace's law (tension = pressure × radius). Thus, the size of the aneurysm is the principal factor determining the risk of rupture. In summarizing data compiled by others, Rutherford outlined the size-related risk of rupture for abdominal aneurysms. For abdominal aneurysms of a 4-cm diameter the risk of rupture at 5 years is 10 to 15 percent, at 6 cm the risk of rupture is 25 to 30 percent at 5 years, but at 8 cm the risk exceeds 75 percent within 5 years. Most data suggest that enlargement and risk of rupture are slightly worse for thoracic aneurysms than for abdominal aneurysms of similar size. In the majority of patients, the aneurysm steadily enlarges until rupture occurs; although rare, sudden leakage or acute rupture has occurred with smaller aneurysms that were not progressively enlarging. In a large series of nonoperated thoracic aneurysms reported by Bikerstaff and associates, 1-year survival was 60 percent, but the 5-year survival was only 13 percent; over 70 percent of the patients died from rupture of the aneurysm. Pressler and McNamara summarized observations in 260 patients with thoracic aneurysms, 126 of whom were treated surgically. Five-year survival in the nonsurgically treated patients was only 21 percent, with high rupture rates noted in both atherosclerotic and dissecting aneurysms. Although chronic traumatic aneurysms progress more slowly than aneurysms from other causes, Finkelmeier demonstrated that 41 percent of patients with chronic traumatic thoracic aneurysms either died or developed symptoms within 5 years. In view of these data, elective treatment for most thoracic aneurysms over 5 to 6 cm in diameter is indicated because of the significant risk of rupture and death.

Clinical Manifestations. The majority of nondissecting aneurysms are asymptomatic until significant enlargement has occurred. Pain may infrequently occur, but the majority are accidentally discovered during a routine chest x-ray. Large aneurysms in the transverse aortic arch create symptoms from compression of adjacent structures such as the trachea or superior vena cava. Syphilitic aneurysms were well known for their tendency to invade bone, producing back pain from erosion of the thoracic spine, but this seldom occurs with other aneurysms. Usually, there are no physical abnormalities or any hemodynamic disturbances, except in aneurysms of the ascending aorta with associated aortic valve insufficiency; in addition, an acute progression in pain or symptoms from an aneurysm is highly significant, as this may indicate leakage or dissection.

Once an abnormal shadow has been recognized on the chest x-ray, diagnosis can be readily established with an aortogram, computed tomography (CT), or magnetic resonance imaging (MRI). Unless the aneurysm is quite small, it should be treated promptly by graft replacement of the involved aortic segment. If serious complicating factors, such as age, previous strokes, or heart disease, significantly increase operative risk, the patient may be observed for a few months or a year, with periodic MRIs or CTs to determine if enlargement is occurring. Once significant enlargement has been demonstrated, operation should be done promptly. Operation should be begun promptly in all cases where the aneurysm is symptomatic.

Treatment. Total excision of the aneurysm is usually unnecessary and often hazardous because of potential injury to adjacent structures. When an aneurysmal segment of aortic wall is excised, the involved area is replaced with an interposition Dacron graft. Some surgeons prefer this technique for aneurysms involving the ascending aorta and aortic arch. A simpler and equally effective method is to replace the involved segment with a prosthetic graft working from within the involved aorta, subsequently wrapping the wall of the aneurysm around the graft. This graft inclusion technique is our preference, as it allows limited dissection, provides coverage of the graft, and minimizes postoperative blood loss.

Aneurysms of the Ascending Aorta

Aneurysms localized to the ascending aorta are often due to a degenerative connective tissue disease of the media of the aortic wall. The origin is usually unknown. This is seen typically as one manifestation of a generalized disorder in Marfan's syndrome or as an isolated disease in Erdheim's cystic medial necrosis. The histologic abnormality described as "cystic medial necrosis" is now recognized as a nonspecific abnormality occurring in several diseases. Atherosclerotic aneurysms occur in the ascending aorta but are seldom limited to this area. Aortic dissection, discussed in the next chapter, frequently involves the ascending aorta. The dissection may stop near the origin of the innominate artery (DeBakey type II) or may extend throughout the entire thoracic aorta (DeBakey type I). Chronic aortic dissection may result in a chronic aneurysm involving the ascending aorta. Syphilis, autoimmune disease, and aortitis are less frequent causes of ascending aneurysms. In a series of 165 ascending and arch aneurysms from this institution, 29 percent were from an aortic dissection, 22 percent from atherosclerosis, 22 percent from cystic medial necrosis, and 29 percent from other causes.

Pathology. An aneurysm in the ascending aorta can be isolated, or it may extend distally and involve the aortic arch (Fig. 19-1). Proximally the aneurysm may involve the aortic root and sinuses of Valsalva. The aortic valve may be normal or may be involved because of aortic stenosis or aortic insufficiency. Valvular involvement may be separate from or continuous with ascending aneurysmal disease. As an aneurysm develops in the proximal ascending aorta, dilatation of the annulus of the aortic valve occurs, stretching the cusps of the aortic valve apart and producing aortic insufficiency. Cardiac failure from the resulting aortic insufficiency is often the significant clinical problem rather than en-

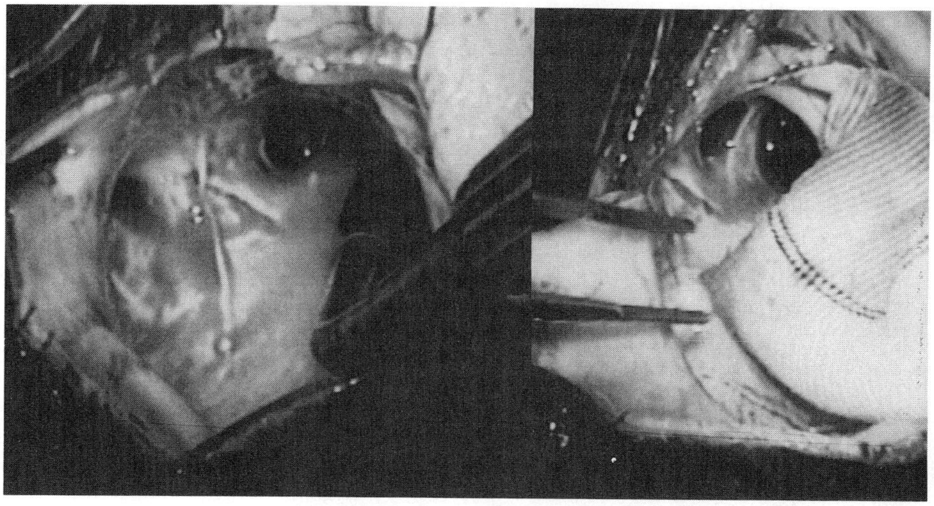

FIG. 19-1. Repair of a large ascending aneurysm with extension into aortic arch. *A*. The aneurysm and aortic arch are opened during hypothermic circulatory arrest. The aortic arch vessels are clearly visualized. *B*. Hemiarch replacement is being performed using a Dacron graft. The inferior portion of the graft extends beneath the arch vessels. The graft results in endoaneurysmorrhaphy, excluding the aneurysmal disease by redirecting blood flow through the graft. The aneurysm wall will be subsequently closed around the graft for coverage.

largement of the aneurysm with compression of adjacent structures or rupture. Once significant aortic insufficiency has developed, progression is rapid, with death from cardiac failure in 1 to 2 years unless operation is performed. Before surgical therapy was available, most patients with Marfan's syndrome died in the third decade from dissecting aneurysms or aortic insufficiency. Gott and associates, based on experience with 50 patients with Marfan's syndrome, concluded that elective operation should be done when the diameter of the aortic root enlarged to 6 cm.

Clinical Manifestations. Patients are often asymptomatic when the diagnosis is made following recognition of dilatation of the ascending aorta on a chest radiograph performed for other purposes. Frequently, the first symptom is due to congestive heart failure from aortic insufficiency. Rarely, expanding saccular aneurysms are seen with symptoms from compression of the superior vena cava or the trachea. Physical examination usually finds no abnormalities except those of aortic insufficiency, the diastolic murmur, and the wide pulse pressure.

Diagnostic Findings. The diagnosis can be suspected from the radiographic findings of dilatation of the ascending aorta. Aortography, MRI, or a CT scan confirms the diagnosis. The aortographic demonstration of a fusiform aneurysm in the proximal ascending aorta, tapering to an aorta of near-normal diameter at the level of the innominate artery, is virtually diagnostic of cystic medial necrosis (Fig. 19-2). Before operative repair, cardiac catheterization is usually recommended to assess aortic valve insufficiency, aortic root disease, and associated coronary artery displacement.

Treatment. Because of the progressive nature of the aortic insufficiency, operation should be performed as soon as possible after the diagnosis is made. As with aortic insufficiency from other causes, postponing operation because of the absence of symptoms while progressive enlargement of the left ventricle occurs is a serious error because the likelihood of sudden death from irreversible ventricular injury is greatly increased in the first few years following operation.

Operation is performed with cardiopulmonary bypass of the ascending aorta with a woven Dacron graft. For isolated disease the ascending aorta is replaced with a graft, beginning just above the coronary ostia and ending just before the innominate artery (Fig. 19-3). Concomitant valve replacement is performed if aortic insufficiency is present.

If aortic valve disease is present but the aortic annulus is not significantly dilated, the aortic valve can be replaced and the prosthetic graft inserted a few millimeters above the site of origin of the coronary arteries, leaving the coronary arteries in their normal anatomic location. However, if the aortic annulus is significantly dilated, this should be replaced also because of the frequency of recurrent aneurysms in this area. This necessitates replantation of the ostia of the coronary arteries. The decision can usually be readily made at operation, for with significant dilatation of the aortic annulus, the ostia of the coronary arteries are displaced more than 1 cm from the aortic ring.

This type of reconstruction is termed the *valve-conduit* operation, consisting of replacement of the aortic valve, replantation of the coronary ostia, and replacement of the ascending aorta with prosthetic graft (Fig. 19-4). Similarly, the valve-conduit operation, or aortic root replacement, can be done using cryopreserved homograft tissue.

The composite operation can be safely performed with excellent results. Kouchoukos and associates reported experiences with 172 patients operated upon over a period of 16 years with an operative mortality of 5 percent. Average follow-up was 81 months with an actuarial survival at 12 years of 48 percent. In 1985, Cabrol and associates reported experiences with 100 patients operated upon over a period of 7 years with an operative mortality of 4 percent and a late mortality of 8 percent during a follow-up period averaging about 3 years. Grey, Ott, and Cooley described experiences with 140 patients, using the composite repair in 89 of the group and a separate graft-valve repair in 51. In the series reported by Moreno-Cabral and associates 85 percent required concomitant aortic valve replacement.

How often the valve-conduit-root replacement operation should be used as opposed to separate graft-valve replacement varies markedly among different institutions. The long-term durability of the composite operation is yet unknown, for pseudoaneurysms have developed at the site of replantation of the coronary ostia in a few patients. At our institution the procedure is reserved for true

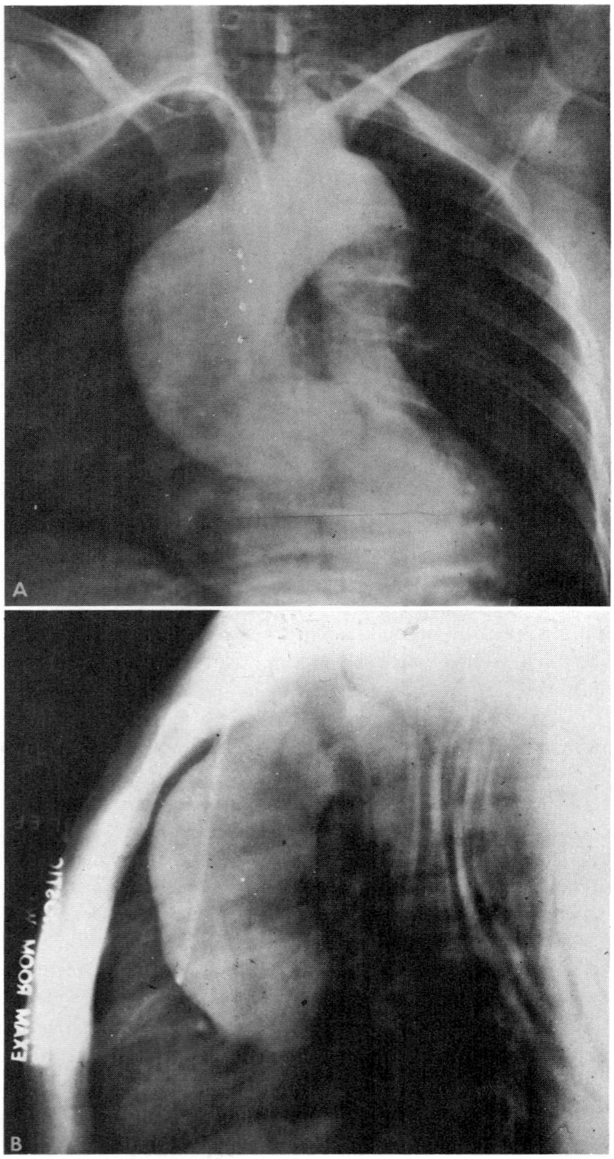

FIG. 19-2. *A.* Posteroanterior view of a thoracic aortogram showing a large aneurysm in the ascending aorta, stopping near the innominate artery. Resection of the aneurysm was successfully performed. The patient was well 15 years following operation. *B.* Lateral view of a thoracic aortogram in the same patient.

aortoannular ectasia, with aneurysmally dilated sinuses of Valsalva and coronary ostial displacement of greater than 2 cm. Most cases with Marfan's syndrome require this procedure.

Aneurysms of the Transverse Aortic Arch

Aneurysms of the transverse aortic arch are due to dissection, atherosclerosis, and other causes, with equal incidence. They may be isolated, or they may represent part of a spectrum involving the ascending aorta, the descending aorta, or both. Diagnosis is usually confirmed with aortography, MRI, or CT to differentiate the aneurysm from a malignant mediastinal tumor. The degree of involvement of the great vessels arising from the aortic arch can also be determined, and both the proximal and distal extent of disease should be clearly defined preoperatively.

Treatment. The operative procedure is a complex one involving both myocardial and cerebral protection, while the circulation is interrupted (Fig. 19-5). Until the concept of combining cardiopulmonary bypass with hypothermia and circulatory arrest was introduced, these aneurysms had the highest operative mortality of any aortic aneurysms, approaching 75 to 80 percent. The demonstration that the brain could tolerate circulatory arrest for up to 1 h if the brain temperature was carefully lowered to 15 to 17°C formed the basis for the modern approach and represents one of the areas of medicine where improved technology has had a dramatic impact. Griepp and associates applied the concept for arch aneurysms, reporting a series of 14 patients with an ischemia time near 42 min. Among 10 patients operated upon electively, only one died.

Crawford and associates described experiences with 129 patients with aortic arch aneurysms, advocating ascending and arch replacement as one procedure, using hypothermic circulatory arrest. Crawford and associates suggested a "staged" distal repair when the descending aorta was also involved. Cooley also pioneered the use of hypothermic circulatory arrest for routine treatment of arch aneurysms. Most groups, including ourselves, have found a brain temperature near 15 to 17°C to be the safest, providing time for a precise reconstruction.

Use of hypothermic circulatory arrest for cerebral protection allows the surgeon to avoid clamping the diseased aorta, thus minimizing the risk of aortic injury or embolization. Brain injury from properly performed circulatory arrest is extremely rare, and the technique may actually diminish the risk of stroke. A recent report from New York University (NYU) described repair of 165 arch aneurysms over 10 years, using hypothermic circulatory arrest in the majority of cases. The operative mortality was 10 to 12 percent, and the frequency of stroke was less than 2 percent. With circulatory arrest the aortic arch can be replaced totally (Fig. 19-5) or partially (Fig. 19-6), tailoring the arch repair with a variation of Cooley's hemiarch replacement.

Frist and associates have proposed reconsidering the old technique of cerebral perfusion, although this technique is cumbersome and appears unnecessary in view of the excellent results obtained with hypothermic circulatory arrest. Circulatory arrest for 45 to 60 min is extremely safe. In the NYU review previously cited 85 percent of the arch repairs had circulatory arrest times less than 45 min, but 15 percent had arrest times greater than 45 min. The risk of stroke was not related to the length of circulatory arrest. In our view the technique is the main advance responsible for successful treatment of complex arch aneurysms in the current era.

Traumatic Thoracic Aneurysms

Etiology and Pathology. Traumatic aneurysms almost invariably arise from transection of the thoracic aorta due to closed-chest trauma. The majority result from horizontal deceleration injuries, typically steering wheel trauma in an automobile accident. McCollum and associates in 1979 described five different forms of trauma. Out of a group of 50 patients, 35 were injured in an automobile accident, 6 were hurt in crushing injuries, and 4 were injured in falls from a height. Traumatic rupture and traumatic thoracic aneurysms have a common etiology but a different clinical course. Traumatic aneurysms evolve in those few patients fortunate enough not to succumb from exsanguinating hemorrhage in the weeks following injury and probably involve only 2 percent of the patients with blunt traumatic aortic disruption. If a patient survives longer than 6 to 8 weeks following injury, the risk of acute rupture is small. In a review of the English and French litera-

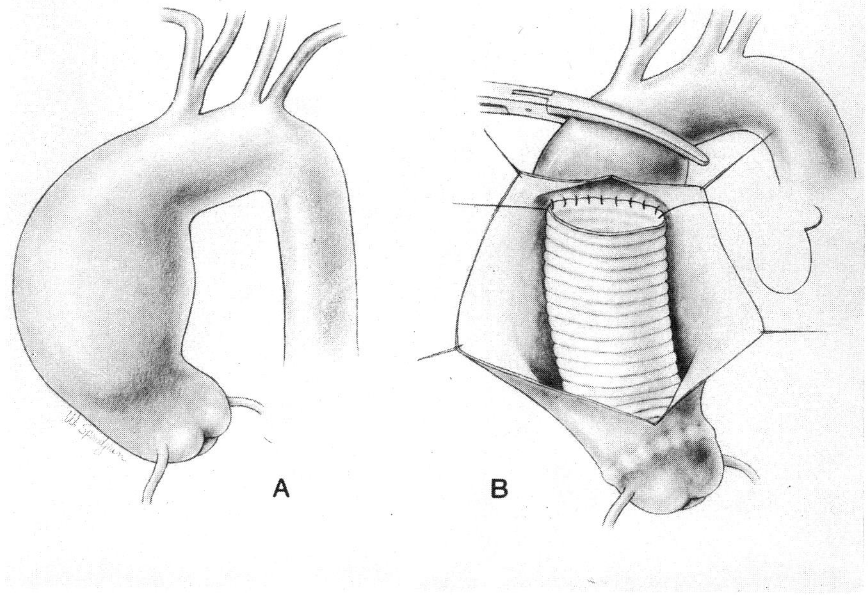

FIG. 19-3. Illustrations of: *A.* Isolated ascending aortic aneurysm. *B.* Repair of ascending aortic aneurysm with a classic supracoronary graft.

ture between 1950 and 1965, Bennett and Cherry found rupture occurring 9 times in a total of 105 aneurysms. The usual course is one of progressive enlargement with compression of adjacent structures.

Most traumatic aneurysms arise just distal to the left subclavian artery, opposite the point of insertion of the ligamentum arteriosum. Fortunately, involvement of the aortic arch or the ascending aorta is rare. Although a huge aneurysm filling most of the hemithorax is occasionally seen, the point of origin is invariably near the ligamentum arteriosum. Reconstruction can usually be done with a short prosthetic graft. Direct anastomosis is seldom possible.

Clinical Manifestions. Unlike most aneurysms from other causes, traumatic thoracic aneurysms enlarge slowly and in some patients remain stationary for 10 to 20 years; the diagnosis is made in retrospect while evaluating an asymptomatic patient with a history of closed-chest trauma 10 to 20 years before. In the series of McCollum and associates, time intervals between trauma and operation varied from 3 months to 32 years, with an average near 12

FIG. 19-4. Illustrations of: *A.* Aorto-annular ectasia, *B.* Valve-conduit procedure with coronary artery reimplantation.

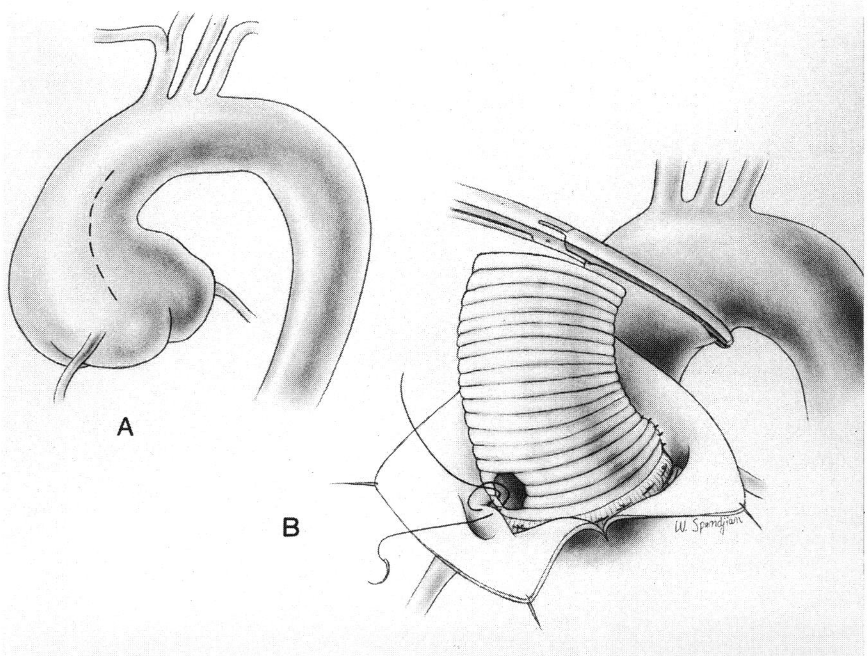

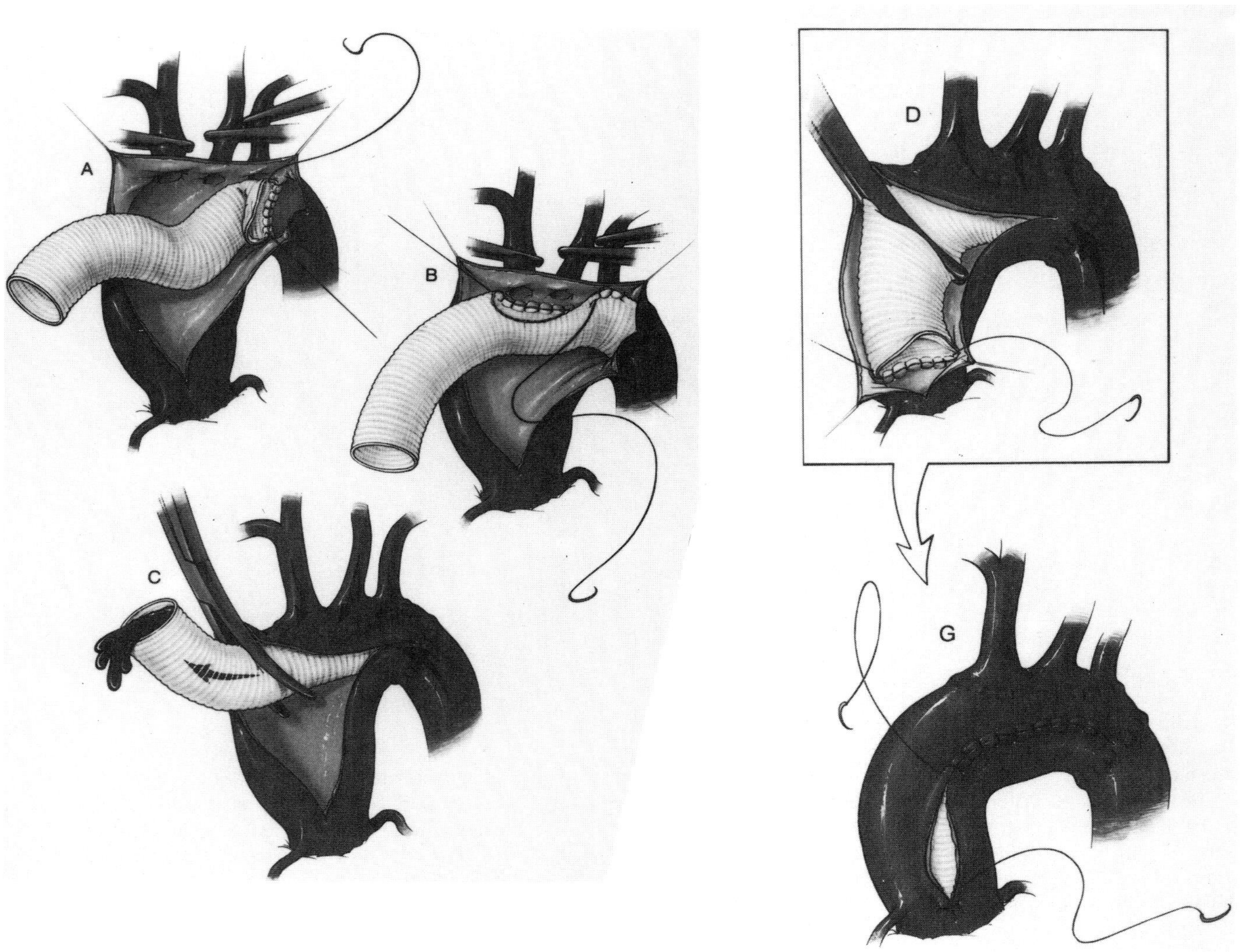

FIG. 19-5. Technique of graft inclusion and total arch replacement. *A.* With the head of the operating table down, the brachiocephalic arteries are clamped. With perfusion just to fill the aorta, the aneurysm is incised. The distal anastomosis is made between the graft and the normal upper descending thoracic aorta using #000 or #0000 prolene sutures. *B.* Anastomatic leakage is checked by clamping the graft and temporarily increasing perfusion. An oval opening is made with the graft under tension and sutured around the brachiocephalic artery origins. *C.* The head is lowered, the free end of the graft is elevated and filled with blood, and the clamps are removed from the brachlocephalic vessels to expel air. *D.* The graft is clamped proximal to the brachiocephalic arteries, full perfusion is resumed, and rewarming is started. Proximal anastomosis is performed depending on the extent of involvement. When uninvolved, the proximal graft is sutured to the ascending aorta. *G.* In either situation, air is removed by filling the heart and graft with blood as the anastomosis is completed and the aneurysmal wall is sutured around the graft. (From: *Crawford ES, Crawford JL: Diseases of the Aorta. Baltimore, Williams & Wilkins, 1984, pp 24–25, with permission.*)

years for the 50 patients. In 25 patients, the interval was greater than 10 years and in 6 greater than 20 years. Finkelmeier and associates, however, reported that 41 percent of patients with traumatic aneurysms died or became symptomatic within 5 years, suggesting that most should be treated surgically.

As the aneurysm enlarges, compression of the left recurrent laryngeal nerve, the left main bronchus, and the esophagus occurs. Symptoms usually announce enlargement well before rupture occurs. This small risk of rupture contrasts with the majority of aneurysms from other causes, where the threat of rupture constitutes the major reason for recommending excision before symptoms develop.

In the McCollum and associates series, pain was the most common symptom, occurring in 24 percent of patients. Hoarseness from recurrent laryngeal involvement was present in 14 percent, dyspnea in 8 percent; 28 percent were asymptomatic. Usually there are no abnormalities on physical examination unless compression of the left main bronchus has occurred. No murmurs can be heard.

Diagnostic Findings. The chest radiograph usually shows an ovoid density near the left subclavian artery. If the aneurysm has been present for several years, calcification is often visible in the wall. Exact dimensions may be outlined by MRI or a CT

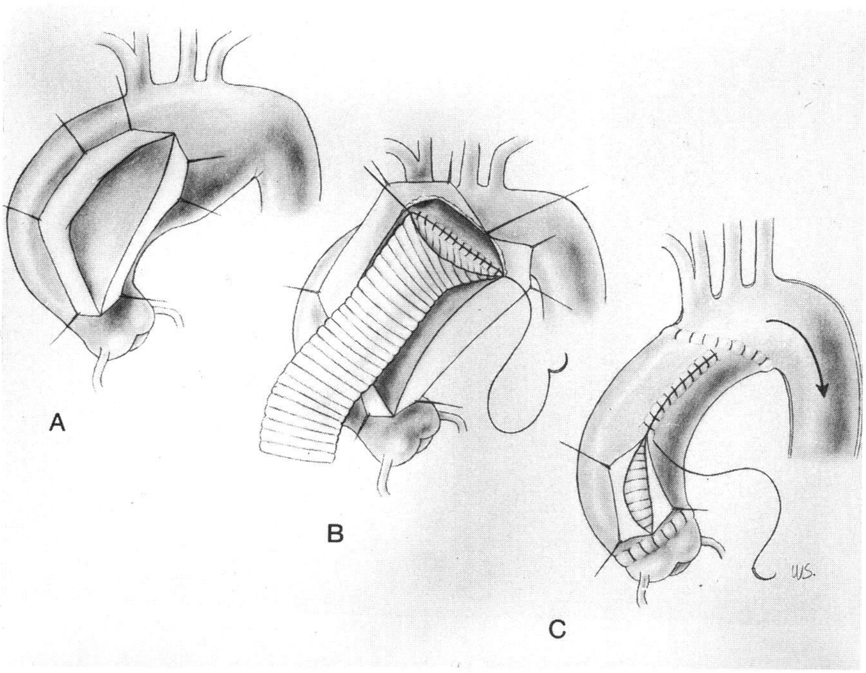

FIG. 19-6. Illustrations of steps (*A* to *C*) in NYU modification of Cooley's hemiarch repair using a graft inclusion technique.

scan. Aortography is occasionally needed to confirm the diagnosis as well as the degree of involvement of adjacent structures (Fig. 19-7).

Treatment. The problem of management of acute traumatic rupture or transection of the thoracic aorta, with the risk of exsanguinating hemorrhage, is discussed in the section Wounds of the Great Vessels. Elective excision is recommended for the majority of patients with chronic traumatic aneurysms. An asymptomatic aneurysm first recognized over a decade after injury presents a choice between periodic observation and elective excision. Operative risk is small (3 to 5 percent) but not insignificant, and so several factors must be evaluated in making a recommendation for an individual patient. Currently elective operation is recommended for most traumatic aneurysms greater than 5.0 cm in diameter. The probability of eventual enlargement requiring operation is the major consideration, as well as the small risk of rupture. We are not aware of an autopsy report of a traumatic aneurysm that remained asymptomatic throughout the patient's lifetime.

Technique of Operation. (See the section Descending Thoracic Aneurysm.)

Aneurysms of the Descending Thoracic Aorta

Etiology and Incidence. Aneurysms in the descending thoracic aorta may result from atherosclerosis, infection, aortitis, trauma, or a dissection of the aortic wall. Most are due to atherosclerosis and are exceeded only by abdominal aneurysms in frequency of occurrence. They are most common in men in the fifth to the seventh decades. Saccular aneurysms from syphilis, once very common, are now rare. Dissecting aneurysms and traumatic aneurysms are considered in the accompanying sections.

The majority of atherosclerotic aneurysms are located in the proximal part of the descending thoracic aorta, beginning distal to the left subclavian artery. They extend for varying distances and often can involve the entire descending thoracic aorta. They are generally fusiform (Fig. 19-8), rather than saccular.

Thoracic aneurysms enlarge and rupture at a rate greater than abdominal aneurysms. Bickerstaff and associates described the natural history of 72 patients observed over a period of 30 years. The descending aorta was involved in 27. In the overall group, rupture occurred in 53 patients (74 percent). Thirty-seven of these had no prior diagnosis of aneurysms; in 16 others the mean interval between diagnosis and rupture was 2 years. Actuarial 5-year survival for all patients was 13 percent, for patients without dissection, 20 percent. Similar statistics have been cited by Pressler and McNamara.

Clinical Manifestations. Most patients are asymptomatic. The diagnosis is made after the accidental finding of an asymptomatic mass on a chest x-ray. In symptomatic patients, most symptoms result from an aneurysm enlarging and compressing the left main bronchus with resulting cough and dyspnea. Erosion into a bronchus or pulmonary parenchyma can produce hemoptysis. Enlarging aneurysms near the left recurrent laryngeal nerve where it encircles the ligamentum arteriosum will paralyze the vocal cord and produce hoarseness.

Physical examination is usually normal. Rarely a bruit is audible in the left paravertebral area. Peripheral pulses are normal unless compression of the origin of the left subclavian artery produces hypotension in the left arm.

Diagnostic Findings. The diagnosis usually can be suspected from the appearance of a mass in the region of the aorta on the chest radiograph. The differential diagnosis includes bronchogenic carcinoma, metastatic carcinoma, or mediastinal tumors. Laminar calcification may be visible in the wall of the aorta.

CT is a valuable noninvasive technique to determine the size of an aneurysm, as is the MRI scan. They are especially useful to periodically evaluate small aneurysms for enlargement. Aortography may be used to confirm the diagnosis and to delineate the precise extent of the aneurysm. Concomitant atherosclerotic disease in the coronary, renal, and carotid arteries frequently occurs.

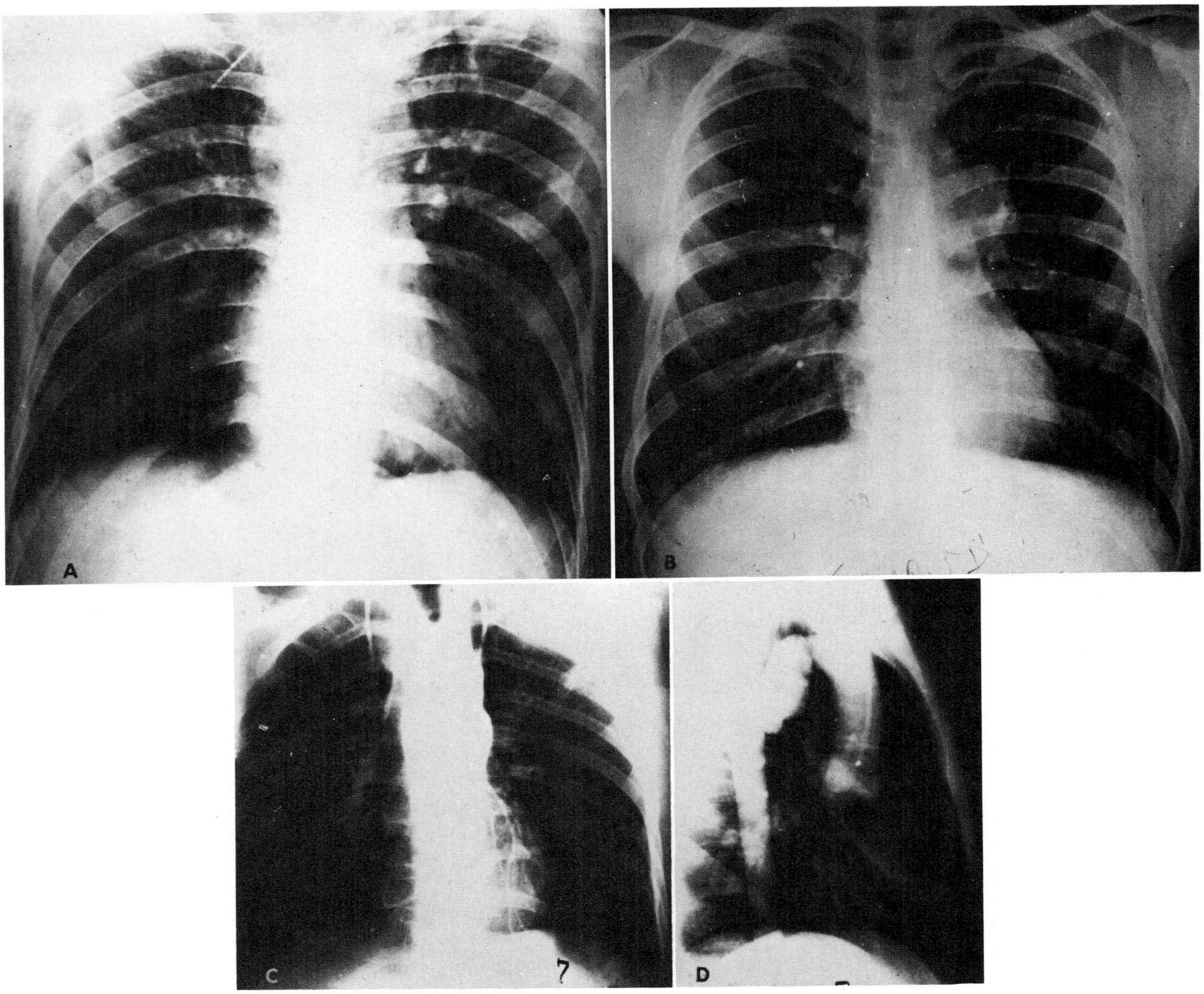

FIG. 19-7. *A.* Chest radiograph following an automobile accident, demonstrating widening of the mediastinum with subcutaneous emphysema. Traumatic rupture of the aorta was not recognized at this time. *B.* Chest radiograph 5 months after the injury demonstrated a left upper mediastinal mass. *C.* Posteroanterior view of an aortogram demonstrating a localized thoracic aneurysm. This lesion was excised successfully. *D.* Lateral view of an aortogram in the same patient. *E.* Chest radiograph in a different patient 2 years after an automobile accident demonstrated an asymptomatic mass in the upper mediastinum. *F.* Aortography demonstrated a saccular thoracic aneurysm, which was subsequently resected successfully. *G.* Aortogram in the same patient as in *F.* This film demonstrated the size and extent of the aneurysm as additional contrast material flowed freely within the lesion.

Hence, preoperative evaluation should carefully investigate these organ systems, often performing a stress test, coronary arteriography, and perhaps carotid arteriography or simpler noninvasive carotid studies.

Treatment. In most patients once the diagnosis of a discrete aneurysm has been made, repair is recommended. Only with small aneurysms associated with significant coronary or cerebral vascular disease is a nonoperative policy of observation with frequent chest radiographs indicated.

The technique of operation is detailed in Fig. 19-9. A left posterolateral thoracotomy through an appropriate interspace, usually the fourth, fifth, or sixth, is made. Initially, the aorta is mobilized and encircled proximal and distal to the aneurysm. With proximal aneurysms involving the left subclavian artery, the aorta is encircled between the left carotid and left subclavian arteries. This is facilitated by opening the pericardium and dissecting the intrapericardial portion of the aortic arch. The vagus nerve and recurrent laryngeal nerve should be mobilized and protected.

Partial bypass is usually used at NYU for repair of isolated descending aneurysms and for chronic traumatic aneurysms in order to protect against paraplegia. A heparinized Gott shunt was used for several years, but this form of shunting is now considered obsolete, as flow rates through the shunt are unpredictable.

Often femoral artery–femoral vein bypass with a pump oxygenator is used; this approach provides excellent distal perfusion and facilitates control of intravascular volume. While partial bypass with a pump oxygenator simplifies hemodynamic manage-

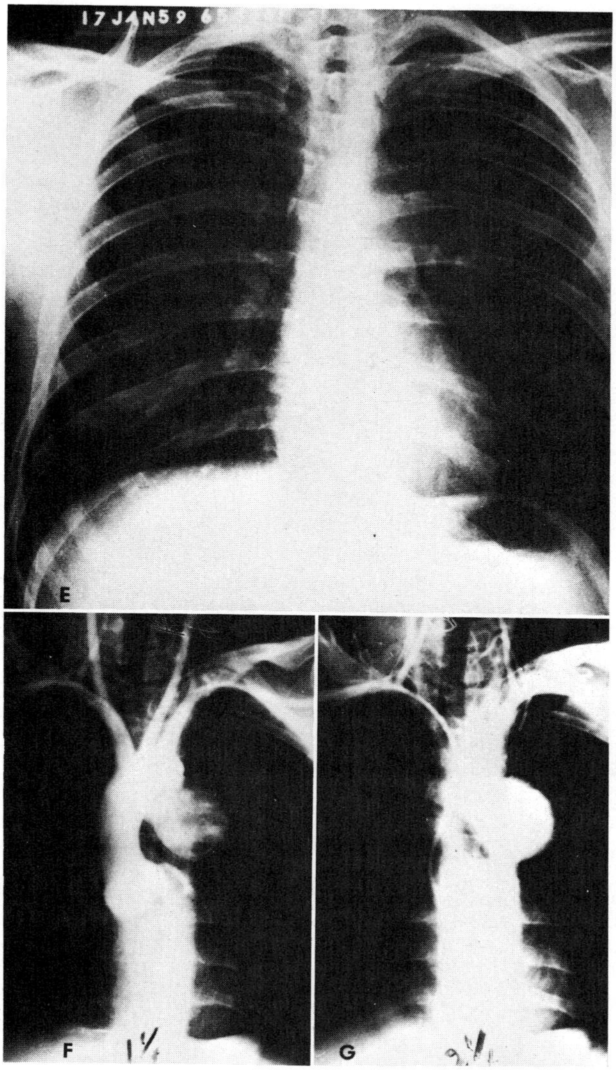

FIG. 19-7. *E, F, G.* Continued.

ment and provides excellent distal perfusion, the technique may be associated with significant bleeding because of the necessity for systemic heparinization. More recently, a partial left atrial–femoral bypass with heparin-bonded tubing and minimal systemic heparin has been used. With this technique alteration of pump flow simultaneously controls proximal hypertension while aiding distal perfusion, and systemic heparinization is minimized or avoided totally. Although we recommend partial bypass and distal perfusion for repair of most isolated descending thoracic aneurysms, others continue to prefer the more standard cross-clamp–and–sew technique of graft placement.

The principal hazards with clamping of the thoracic aorta are paraplegia and renal failure from the distal ischemia produced. Theoretically, this should be preventable by some form of partial bypass, perfusing the distal aorta during this time.

Somatosensory evoked potential (SEP) monitoring to evaluate spinal cord function while the aorta was occluded has been used with the majority of operations performed upon the thoracic aorta at our hospital in recent years. Laboratory and clinical data indicate that paraplegia usually results from spinal cord ischemia from unprotected cross-clamp time and low aortic pressure when thoracic aneurysms do not extend below the diaphragm. With thoracoabdominal aneurysms, direct interruption of critical segmental blood supply to the spinal cord is a major factor. The inability of temporary bypass to protect from paraplegia over the past two decades may have been due to an *inadequate flow through the shunt with inadequate distal perfusion pressure*. In our experience with isolated descending aneurysms, maintaining a distal aortic perfusion pressure above 50 to 60 mmHg using partial bypass has prevented neurologic injury in the majority of cases, even with occlusion of the thoracic aorta for longer than 60 min. The exact flow rate needed cannot be predicted precisely in advance. Flow rates as high as 4 or more L/min have been needed in some patients. Distal aortic pressure, rather than flow rate, is the key requirement in order to perfuse the spinal cord through collateral circulation. Vascular resistance through collateral circulation is greater than the resistance present when spinal cord blood flow is through normal channels. If distal perfusion is adequate and somatosensory potentials remain intact, the risk of paraplegia should be minimal. When somatosensory potentials are lost despite good perfusion, intercostals should be reimplanted promptly to restore segmental blood supply to the cord.

Other published data, however, do not show a significant reduction in the frequency of paraplegia when conventional temporary bypass is used. Livesay and associates reported experiences with 360 thoracic aneurysms employing some form of shunt or bypass in 97 of the group. Paraplegia occurred in 6.5 percent and was not decreased by temporary shunts. Paraplegia occurred principally with extensive aneurysms and with cross-clamp times exceeding 30 min. Crawford and associates suggested that use of evoked-potential monitoring and distal perfusion had no impact on the incidence of paraplegia after repair of 198 descending and thoracoabdominal aneurysms, noting a 7 to 8 percent risk of paraplegia with both clamp-and-sew and bypass-perfusion methods. With thoracoabdominal aneurysms requiring excision of the segment of aorta between T8 and L2, paraplegia occurred in 15 to 20 percent of patients in the series reported by Crawford and associates.

The surgical technique is a standard one. Initial dissection is limited to isolating the aorta proximally and distally sufficiently to permit the application of vascular clamps. The aorta is then opened widely, removing the thrombi from the lumen and any gross areas of calcification or degeneration in the intima. Most of the intima and all the media are carefully preserved. Ostia of bleeding intercostal vessels are directly sutured. A standard woven Dacron graft is then inserted by end-to-end anastomosis, after which the wall of the aneurysmal sac can be sutured around the prosthetic graft to supplement hemostasis and to provide coverage of the graft.

Operative risk is usually less than 5 percent in elective operations unless serious concomitant coronary artery disease is present. Long-term prognosis is principally determined by the concomitant presence of coronary and cerebral atherosclerosis.

Thoracoabdominal Aneurysms

Thoracoabdominal aneurysms are rare, occurring in older patients with extensive atherosclerosis. Excision is a complicated surgical procedure, involving restoration of blood flow to the celiac, superior mesenteric, and renal arteries. The diagnosis is often initially made after a chest x-ray shows enlargement of the aorta near the diaphragm. Even with large thoracoabdominal aneurysms, the abdominal component usually cannot be palpated because it is

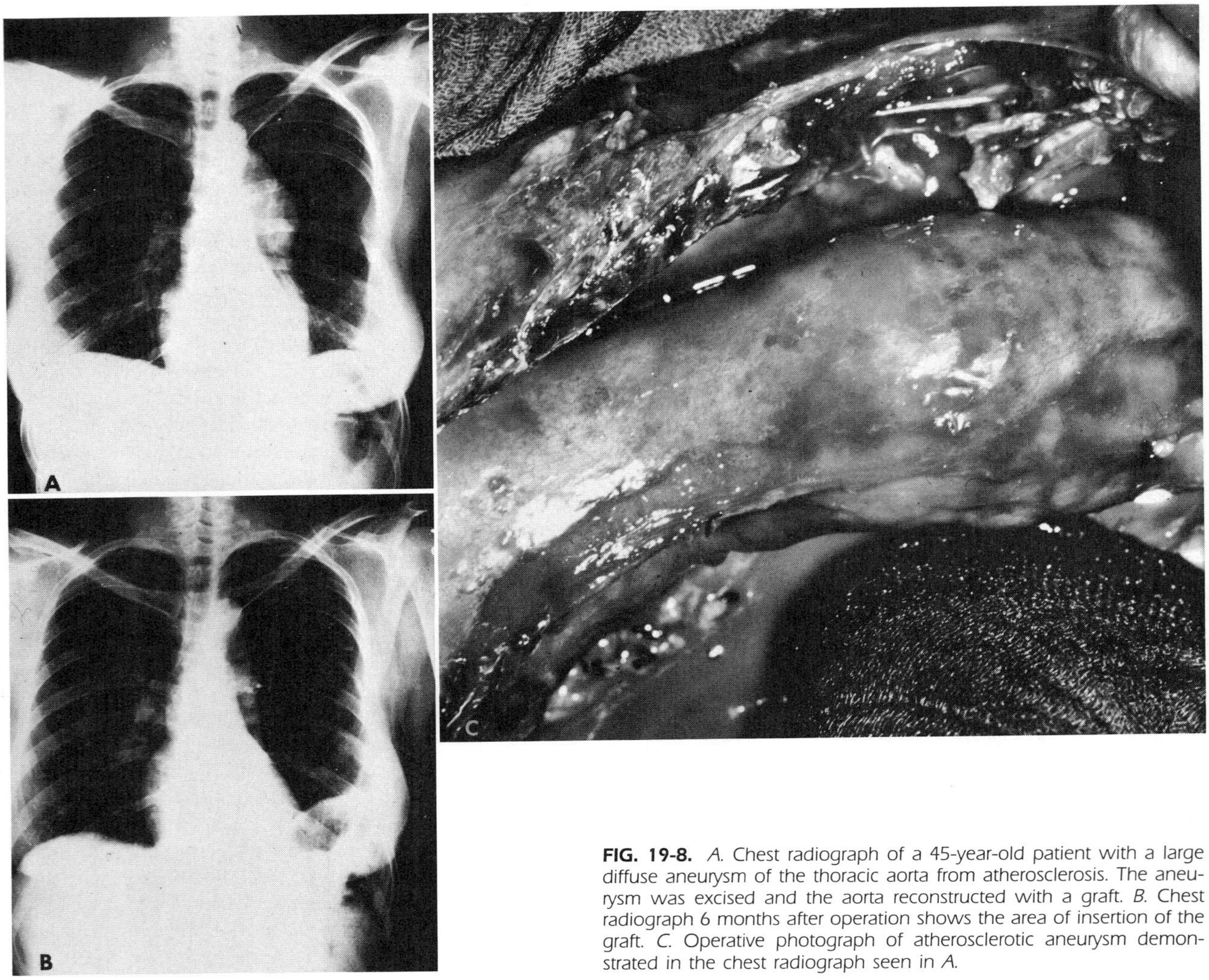

FIG. 19-8. *A.* Chest radiograph of a 45-year-old patient with a large diffuse aneurysm of the thoracic aorta from atherosclerosis. The aneurysm was excised and the aorta reconstructed with a graft. *B.* Chest radiograph 6 months after operation shows the area of insertion of the graft. *C.* Operative photograph of atherosclerotic aneurysm demonstrated in the chest radiograph seen in *A.*

concealed in the upper abdomen by the stomach and pancreas. A diagnosis can be made precisely, however, by aortography, MRI, and CT.

Early experiences with these complex aneurysms were summarized by DeBakey in 1965. A multiple bypass technique was used, attaching a graft from the thoracic aorta above to the abdominal aorta below (Fig. 19-10). From this initial graft, branch grafts were serially attached to the celiac, superior mesenteric, and renal arteries. Operative mortality remained at least 50 percent with this complex procedure.

Subsequently, a major advance was developed by Crawford with the intralumenal technique, simply inserting the graft inside the sac of the aneurysm with appropriate side-to-side anastomoses between the graft and the ostia of the different arteries. In 1978, Crawford and associates summarized experiences with 82 patients, 77 of whom survived operation. In 1986, Crawford and associates summarized their very large experience with 605 such operations. About 70 percent of the patients were symptomatic; rupture had occurred in 4 percent of the group. Operative mortality was about 9 percent.

Crawford and associates also reported significant observations of the natural history of the disease, describing observations upon 94 patients observed over a period of 25 years in whom operation was not performed for a variety of reasons. Only 24 percent of the group were alive 2 years after a decision was made that operation would not be performed; half of the deaths were due to rupture. By contrast, among 604 patients treated surgically, nearly 60 percent were alive 5 years following operation.

Operations upon the segment of aorta between the eighth thoracic and the second lumbar vertebra have the highest associated frequency of paraplegia, ranging between 10 and 40 percent. Crawford has found that the frequency could be significantly decreased by reattaching large lumbar vessels to the aortic graft at the time of operation with a patch graft technique, a technique that Spencer described in laboratory experiments in 1958. The crossclamp is progressively moved down, reimplanted intercostals are reperfused within 20 to 30 min if possible, and the visceral vessels are reperfused as subsequent anastomoses are done. This significantly reduced the frequency of paraplegia to near 10 percent, but to date *no technique* exists that can completely prevent paraplegia

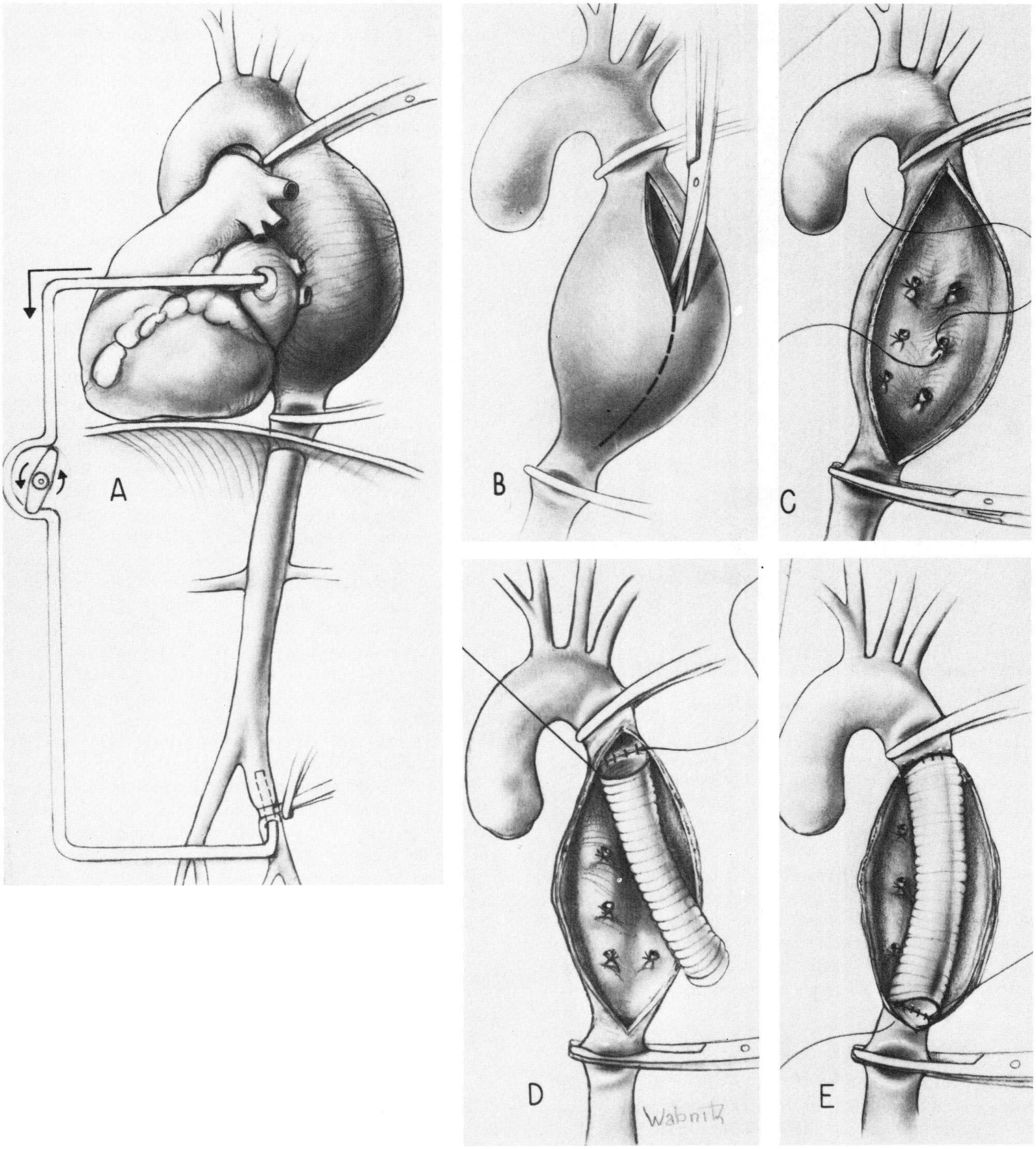

FIG. 19-9. Procedure for excision of an aneurysm of the thoracic aorta. *A.* An aneurysm of the thoracic aorta. Initial dissection is limited to isolation of the aorta proximal and distal to the aneurysm. Left atriofemoral bypass is then instituted at a flow rate of 2 to 4 L/min. (See text for other methods of shunting.) Pressures should be monitored in the aorta and also in the femoral artery to ensure adequacy of perfusion of the arterial circulation proximal and distal to the aneurysm. *B.* Aneurysm is widely opened, removing only the inner lining to avoid excessive bleeding where the aneurysm may be adherent to the vertebral column and lung. *C.* Bleeding intercostal arteries may be oversewed from within the lumen of the aneurysm. *D.* A woven Dacron prosthesis is used for reconstruction of the aorta, employing a continuous suture for the anastomosis. *E.* Following completion of the anastomosis the adventitial sac remaining from the aneurysm can be used to surround the graft (not illustrated).

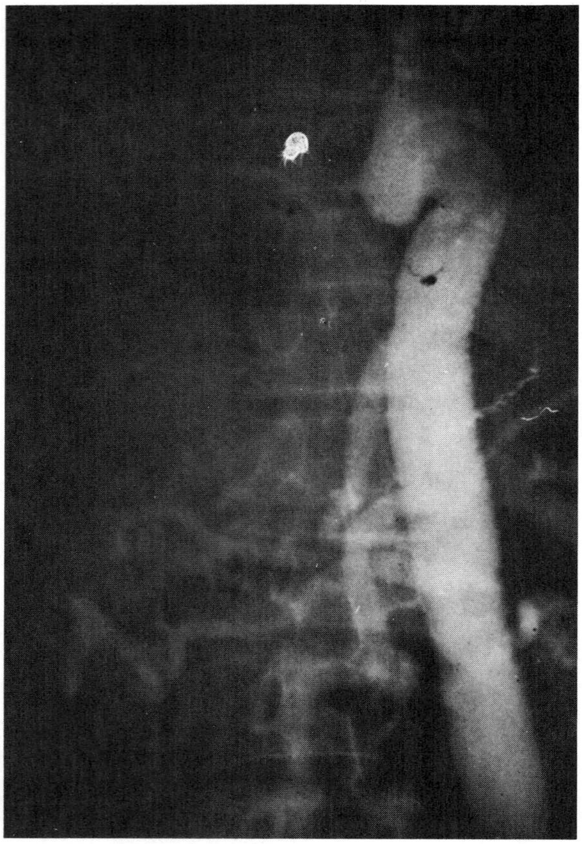

FIG. 19-10. Angiogram of Dacron graft 1 year after excision of thoracoabdominal aneurysm. The graft was inserted between the thoracic aorta, as an end-to-side anastomosis, and the abdominal aorta, not shown in this illustration. Side branches to the superior mesenteric artery, celiac artery, and right and left renal arteries are individually visible.

with this complex problem. Bypass and distal perfusion techniques are not feasible, since the aorta is clamped both above and below the area from which the spinal cord segmental blood supply arises. A technique of cord protection using steroids, cerebral spinal fluid drainage, and intrathecal papaverine was described by Svensson and associates, but its value remains unproven.

AORTIC DISSECTION

Etiology and Incidence. Aortic dissection begins in most cases as a tear in the intima, with entry of blood into and separation of the aortic media for a variable distance, resulting in blood flow down a ''false lumen.'' A localized aneurysm may develop months or years later in an area where the aortic wall has become weakened and enlarged from the original dissection, but a true aneurysm is not present during acute dissection. The disease is three to four times more common in males than in females and occurs predominantly in older patients, those beyond the fifth decade. However, it occurs in every age group, the youngest person being only 14 months of age.

Aortic dissection results from a combination of hypertension and a degenerative disease of the media of the aorta of unknown type. Roberts has emphasized that a history of hypertension may be obtainable in only 60 to 75 percent of patients, but hypertrophy of the left ventricle is present in at least 90 percent. He has found that hypertension is frequently the precipitating factor in patients with Marfan's syndrome who develop dissection, and predicted that proper control of hypertension would virtually eliminate the disease. This prediction well emphasizes the importance of control of hypertension in long-term therapy.

The disease in the media is of unknown cause in most cases but is described histologically as cystic medial necrosis. The prototype of cystic medial necrosis is Marfan's syndrome, in which a genetic defect results in abnormal cross-links in both elastin and collagen, resulting in weakness of the media.

Patients with Marfan's syndrome usually develop a progressive fusiform aneurysm in the ascending aorta, and aortic dissection occurs in 30 to 50 percent if untreated. There is also a greater frequency of dissection in patients with coarctation or congenitally bicuspid aortic valve. Whether this is related to turbulent flow of blood producing these abnormalities or to associated connective tissue defects in the media is uncertain. Disease of the media of the aorta must be a major factor in etiology because there are an estimated 20 million patients with hypertension in the United States, but only about 2000 dissecting aneurysms are reported each year.

It should be emphasized that the disease is *not due* to atherosclerosis. Atherosclerosis is a proliferative disease of the intima and media, occurring most frequently in the abdominal aorta. Aortic dissection is a disease of the media, almost always originating in the thoracic aorta although the dissection often continues distally down to the aortic bifurcation. The frequency of occurrence of aortic dissection in older age groups led to confusion with atherosclerosis. The distinction between the two diseases is most important in evaluating prognosis and planning long-term therapy.

Experimentally, a dissecting aneurysm can be produced in young rats with a diet containing 50 percent sweet peas, which causes a distinct abnormality of connective tissue, known as *lathyrism*. The abnormal chemical agent that weakens the cross-linking of collagen is a beta-amino nitrile. To date, this experimental observation has had little clinical significance except to confirm the probable pathogenesis of aortic dissection.

Wilson and Hutchins reviewed 204 patients undergoing autopsy. The most common associated conditions were hypertension, Marfan's syndrome, and inflammatory injuries of the aortic media. No common pathogenetic mechanism was found.

Pathology. The two major pathologic abnormalities are a transverse tear of the intima and media, usually involving about half the circumference of the aorta, which permits blood to enter the media. The aortic wall then progressively separates (''dissects'') with an inner true lumen and an outer false lumen composed of the outer half of the media and the adventitia. In the detailed analysis published by Roberts, the intimal tear was located in the ascending aorta in about 70 percent of patients, in the aortic arch in 10 percent, in the upper descending thoracic aorta near the ligamentum arteriosum in 20 percent, and in the abdominal aorta in about 2 percent. In the experience of Miller and associates with 175 patients, the intimal tear was in the ascending aorta in 60 percent, in the aortic arch in 10 percent, and in the descending aorta in 30 percent. In a few patients, no tear in the intima can be found at autopsy, a fact that leads to the theory that dissection of the aorta is the primary process with ''rupture of the vasovasorum'' and secondary rupture into the aortic lumen. Almost all clinical data indicate that this hypothesis is unlikely.

Once the dissection begins, it usually extends rapidly through the thoracic and abdominal aorta into the peripheral arteries. Roberts has estimated that the entire aorta will dissect within minutes unless some structural abnormality that has disrupted continuity of the aortic wall, such as atherosclerosis or coarctation, halts the dissection. In over 50 percent of patients, the dissection process extends into a peripheral artery. If this theory is correct, younger patients with less atherosclerosis would more frequently have dissection of the entire aorta. A ''reentry'' tear can be identified in many patients, located in the aorta in about half and in a peripheral artery in the others.

As dissection progresses, branch vessels are sheared off, either becoming obliterated or establishing a communication with the false lumen occluded by the dissection. Proximally, the coronary arteries may be involved. Frequently one or more aortic valve cusps are detached and prolapse into the lumen, creating aortic insufficiency. Usually the noncoronary sinus, or the commissure between the right and noncoronary sinuses, of the aortic valve is involved. Distally, any artery may be involved; carotid artery involvement may produce neurologic injury. Obstruction of the subclavian arteries produces differences in blood pressure between the two arms. Dissection of intercostal arteries may cause spinal cord injury with paraplegia. In one series, 6 of 125 patients had paraplegia on admission. Dissection of renal arteries may produce renal insufficiency. In the extremities, acute obstruction of the iliac or femoral arteries may cause sensory loss, claudication, or even gangrene.

The dissection may terminate fatally at any time by rupture of the false lumen with exsanguination. Rupture into the pericardial cavity is the most common, probably because the adventitia is thin over the intrapericardial ascending aorta and because the velocity of blood flow and diameter are greatest in the ascending aorta. Rupture into the left pleural cavity or the retroperitoneal tissues is less common.

Classification. DeBakey classified aortic dissections into types I, II, and III (Fig. 19-11). In type I the tear site originates in the ascending aorta, usually just above the left main coronary artery, and the dissection continues distally into the descending or abdominal aorta. In type II, the tear site is in a similar location, but the dissection stops distally at the innominate artery. In type III, the tear site is in the upper descending thoracic aorta, just distal to the subclavian artery; in type III-A the dissection is localized in the thoracic aorta, while in type III-B it proceeds into the abdominal aorta.

Based on clinical course and surgical significance, Miller at Stanford reclassified dissections into types A (dissection involves the ascending aorta) or B (dissection only involves the descending aorta). About two-thirds of patients with acute aortic dissection are type A (DeBakey types I and II), while one-third are type B (DeBakey type III). Clinically acute type A dissections have a poor prognosis with medical therapy, with a high incidence of hemodynamic compromise and rupture, and they should be operated on promptly through median sternotomy. For acute type B

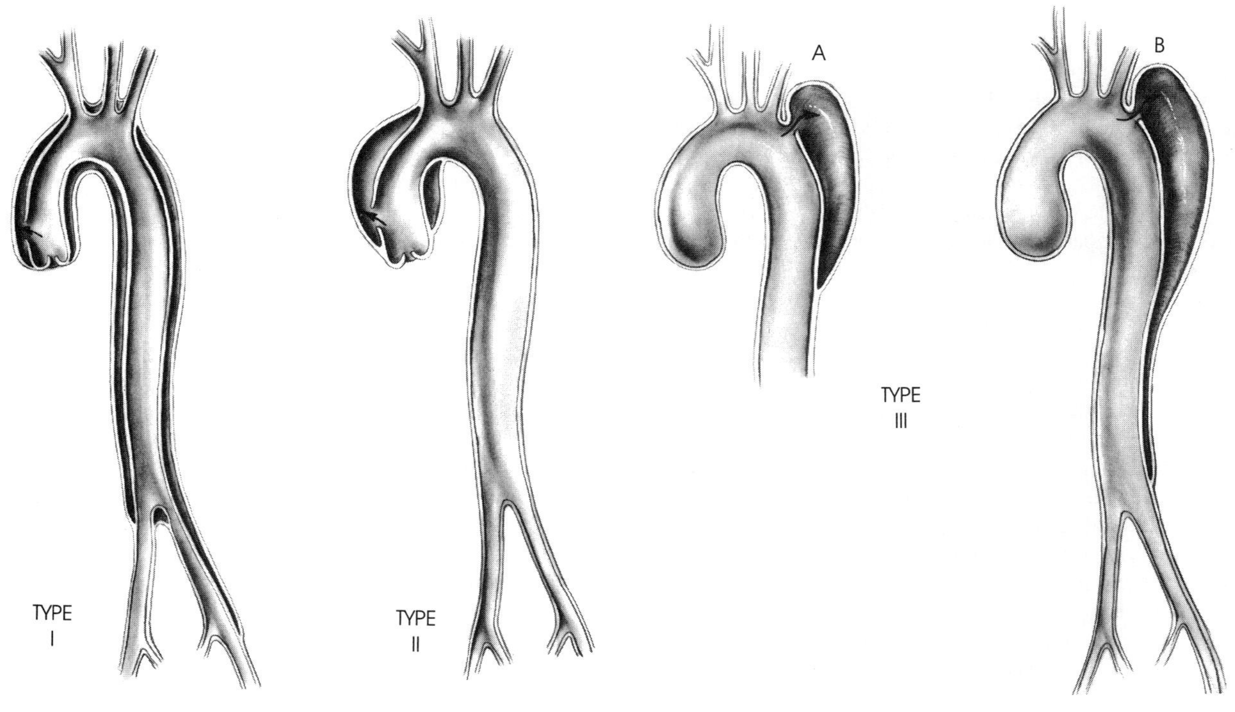

FIG. 19-11. DeBakey classification of aortic dissection. Type I. Dissecting aneurysm that begins in the ascending aorta near the aortic valve and extends throughout the aorta down to the external iliac arteries. Unfortunately, this is a common type of dissecting aneurysm. Type II. Dissecting aneurysm limited to the ascending aorta. This is commonly seen in the Marfan syndrome. Type IIIA. Dissecting aneurysm beginning distal to the left subclavian artery. The localized nature of this aneurysm makes it readily accessible to surgical excision. Type IIIB. Dissecting aneurysm arising distal to the left subclavian artery but extending into the abdominal aorta. Only partial excision of the area of dissection is possible.

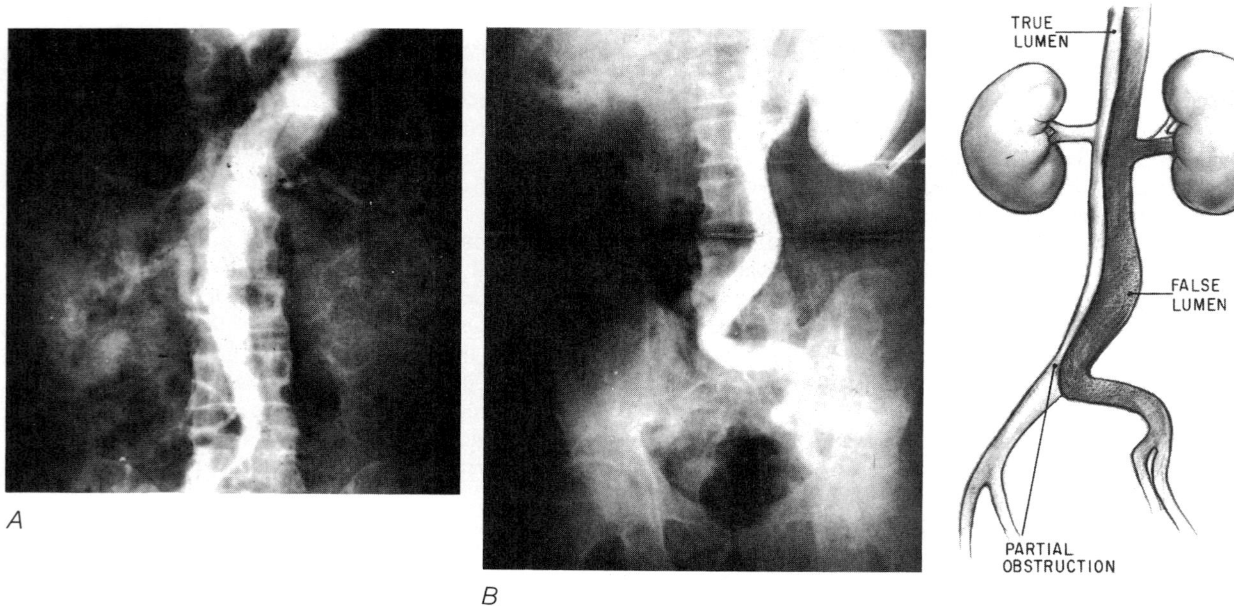

FIG. 19-12. *A.* Aortogram showing an unusual pattern of aortic dissection in which dissection extended from the thoracic aorta into the abdominal aorta, creating two lumens, with the right renal artery arising from one and the left renal artery from the other. Focal stenosis of the right common illiac artery is seen at the lower part of the field producing intermittent claudication, which was the presenting complaint of the patient. *B.* Aortogram performed by a different root opacifies the left kidney and the left common illiac artery. The condition of the dissected aorta is illustrated in the accompanying drawing. Circulation was reestablished by excising the septum between the two channels at the aortic bifurcation. (From: *Gryboski W, Spencer FC: Intermittent claudication caused by a dissecting aneurysm of the aorta. South Med J 58:593, 1965, with permission.*)

dissections the prognosis with immediate medical therapy is good, and early operation is generally done only for complications.

The grim mortality is documented in virtually every report, with 30 to 50 percent of patients dying within 24 h, 50 to 75 percent within 1 to 2 weeks, and 90 percent of untreated patients within 1 to 3 months. In the classic review of 425 cases by Hirst and associates, 74 percent died within 2 weeks and 91 percent within 6 months.

Clearly mortality with acute ascending (Stanford Type B) dissections is much higher with dissection originating in the ascending aorta (DeBakey types I or II, Stanford type A). In a group of 62 patients reported by Lindsay and Hurst, almost all of 40 patients whose dissection began in the ascending aorta died within 3 weeks. Only 8 percent of these patients lived 1 month. This high mortality is the reason emergency operation has been progressively adopted in the last few years for virtually all dissections involving the ascending aorta.

For DeBakey type III (Stanford type B) dissections the initial survival with medical therapy is much better, approaching a 1 month survival of 80 to 90 percent with good in-hospital blood pressure control. Consequently type III dissections are most often treated medically initially, unless a complication such as rupture, visceral ischemia, leg ischemia, or neurologic dysfunction is present.

In the few patients who survive an aortic dissection, endothelial lining of the false lumen develops, termed a *healed dissecting aneurysm*. This occurs in about 20 percent of patients. Such patients have a so-called double-barreled aorta, with a wide variety of bizarre circulatory patterns. For example, one renal artery may arise from the "false" lumen and the other from the true lumen (Fig. 19-12), or alternatively both renal arteries can arise from the false lumen. In other patients, one iliac artery may originate from the false lumen, the other from the true lumen. In most patients the false lumen gradually becomes aneurysmal and ruptures, especially if significant hypertension is present. For patients with chronic dissections, operation is recommended based on the size of the aorta and is usually done once the aorta is more than 5 to 6 cm in diameter.

Clinical Manifestations. The abrupt onset of excruciating pain, almost immediately reaching its peak intensity, is very characteristic of aortic dissection. A myocardial infarction, by contrast, may gradually develop pain of increasing severity over several minutes. Sutton and associates reported that chest pain occurred in nearly 80 percent of 113 patients. Usually this was in the anterior chest. Back pain occurred with dissection of the proximal descending aorta in about a third of patients, indicating that absence of back pain did not exclude the dissection of the thoracic aorta. Another significant characteristic of the pain is its tendency to migrate into different areas as dissection extends distally. As might be predicted from the wide variation in the extent of the dissection process, many pain syndromes may occur. Pain may radiate to the neck, the arm, the epigastrium, or the leg. Seldom is pain completely absent, probably in no more than 10 percent of patients. The pain of acute dissection may mimic myocardial infarction or pulmonary embolus, and the diagnosis of dissection must be considered in order to avoid a fatal treatment error.

Syncope occurs in approximately 10 percent and some neurologic symptoms are present in 10 to 20 percent. These may result from ischemia of the brain, spinal cord, or a peripheral nerve, depending on whether a carotid artery, an intercostal artery, or a peripheral artery has been compromised. Classically, the false lumen obstructs an iliac artery at the aortic bifurcation, resulting in leg ischemia that progresses from decreased sensation, to motor dysfunction, to gangrene. A stroke develops in about 10 percent of patients, paraplegia in 3 to 5 percent.

Hypertension, often of severe degree, is present in 75 to 85 percent of patients. A frequent clinical picture is that of an acutely ill patient who is hypertensive, pale, and sweaty from severe vasoconstriction. An aortic diastolic murmur appears in 20 to 30 percent of patients and is of great diagnostic significance, as it originates from detachment of an aortic valve cusp. Unequal carotid or subclavian pulses may be found, caused by unequal compression of these vessels. A variety of neurologic abnormalities may be detected, the most common being either a monoplegia or paraplegia.

Diagnostic Findings. On the chest radiograph a widened mediastinum or a left pleural effusion from extravasation of blood is frequently seen. In some patients, however, the radiograph may be completely normal. The electrocardiogram is of particular value in distinguishing dissecting aneurysm from myocardial infarction, but there are no characteristic features of aortic dissection. The electrocardiogram can be confused with acute myocardial infarction because of the presence of ST segment elevation secondary to hypertension and ventricular strain. If patients are treated for myocardial infarction with thrombolytic therapy based on this misinterpretation, exsanguination promptly ensues. The most common abnormality is left ventricular hypertrophy from the antecedent hypertension.

Transesophageal echocardiography has recently proven to be extremely accurate in establishing the diagnosis of acute dissection. CT is another valuable noninvasive technique that may establish the diagnosis promptly and quickly in many patients. Aortography has historically been the definitive diagnostic procedure, outlining the double-lumen aorta. In some patients, the diagnosis cannot be made by any other technique, as there are no abnormal physical findings and the only symptom is a history of severe back pain. Transesophageal echocardiography has become the diagnostic test of choice in our institution, and most patients are now treated based on the results of this study alone.

The importance of immediate transesophageal echocardiography, aortography, or CT in any patient with unexplained sustained severe chest pain cannot be overemphasized. The history of pain may be the *only* abnormality detected. Occasionally a patient is seen a few days or weeks after an acute dissection with no symptoms and no abnormality on physical examination, electrocardiogram, or chest x-ray. Such patients often exsanguinate without any preliminary warning symptoms.

Treatment. Modern surgical treatment evolved from the work of DeBakey and Cooley, who reported in 1955 successful excision and grafting of a chronic dissecting aneurysm in the thoracic aorta. Another key concept in treatment, developing from the work of Wheat and colleagues, is the importance of immediate drug therapy both to control the hypertension and to decrease forceful contractility of the left venticle (dP/dt). Drug therapy should be started as soon as the diagnosis is suspected, preferably in the emergency room, because it may stop the dissection process and prevent exsanguination. Wheat and associates discovered the importance of drug therapy following their ingenious evaluation of observations from the poultry industry that the high fatality rate from spontaneous dissecting aneurysm in certain flocks of turkeys could be dramatically reduced by adding a small amount of reserpine to the turkey food. An intravenous infusion of sodium nitroprusside is usually done, preferably combined with immediate administration of a beta-blocking drug. The primary goal of medical therapy is to reduce shear stress by reducing left ventricular dP/dt and to keep the systolic blood pressure less than 110 to 120 mmHg.

Dissections of the ascending aorta are usually operated on emergently because of the high initial mortality with medical therapy. A median sternotomy incision with right atrial–femoral artery bypass and a pump oxygenator is used. The principal surgical objectives are to remove the site of the origination of the tear, replace the ascending aorta and arch as necessary, obliterate the false lumen, redirect blood into the true lumen distally, and correct any associated valvar insufficiency or coronary ischemia. In our experience these goals are best accomplished with the use of deep hypothermia and circulatory arrest, similar to the technique employed for arch aneurysm repair. Routine use of the circulatory arrest technique allows the surgeon to avoid clamping and potentially injuring the diseased aorta and facilitates the distal anastomosis that is done open, under direct vision. At NYU a variation of Cooley's hemiarch replacement (Figs. 19-6 and 19-13) is routinely used for repair of all type A dissections. The NYU method includes internal replacement of the diseased aortic segment with a Dacron graft. The false lumen is obliterated with a continuous 4-0 prolene suture, which approximates intima and adventitia both proximally, adjacent to the aortic valve, and distally in the aortic

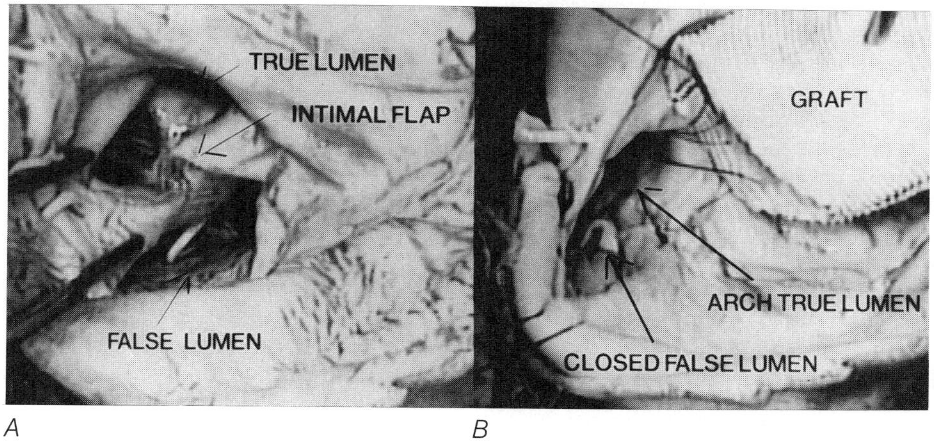

FIG. 19-13. Operative treatment of acute DeBakey type I aortic dissection using circulatory arrest and NYU modification of Cooley's hemiarch repair. *A.* This photo shows the open aortic arch after the torn intima has been removed from the ascending aorta with the intimal flap separating the true lumen from the false lumen. *B.* The false lumen has been obliterated by a continuous suture that circumferentially reapposes the intima to the outer layer of the aorta. The Dacron graft is placed internally into the midarch, serving to remove the torn intima from the circulation and redirect blood flow into the true lumen distally.

arch. The graft is then placed end-to-end internally, and the aortic wall is closed to complete the graft inclusion technique.

Several groups, including ours at NYU, have adopted the technique of performance of the distal aortic hemi-arch anastomosis with the ''open'' technique during a brief period of circulatory arrest (Figs. 19-1 and 19-13). This permits the performance of a more precise anastomosis and also avoids the possible injury of the dissected aorta from application of a vascular clamp. Once the distal anastomosis has been accomplished, the prosthetic graft can be occluded and flow to the brain restored while the proximal anastomosis is performed.

The main cause of operative death is hemorrhage from the suture lines. Performing the distal anastomosis with an ''open'' technique during circulatory arrest permits precise inclusion of all layers of the dissected aorta with less risk of hemorrhage. At NYU the anastomosis is usually performed with a continuous suture of 4-0 prolene, avoiding undue tension on the suture line which can lacerate the friable intima. The graft is wrapped with the native aortic wall. An alternative method is to reconstitute the dissected aorta between two strips of Teflon felt, one placed within the lumen and the other around the adventitia, after which the graft is sutured to this reconstructed aorta.

Other techniques of repair range from internal placement of a sutureless intraluminal graft in the ascending aorta to total excision of the involved aortic segment, followed by aortic replacement with an interposition graft. Some surgeons continue to clamp the aorta and ignore the aortic arch. Clamping the acutely dissected aorta can prove to be extremely hazardous and, in our experience, should be avoided as the intima will tear and redissect distally. Although Miller reported that excision of the tear site does not influence survival, our experience suggests that removal of the tear site from the circulation is a basic principle in the therapy of aortic dissection and should be done whenever possible. Overall, the results of repair of acute type A aortic dissection are excellent, with an operative risk of 10 to 12 percent in most major medical centers.

When the aortic valve is involved with aortic dissection, resulting in aortic insufficiency, resuspension of the valve as described by Spencer in 1962 has been highly effective. Recent reports by Fann and associates have demonstrated satisfactory durability after aortic valve resuspension. In our own experience, complex valve deformities resulting in severe aortic insufficiency are repairable using valve reconstructive techniques borrowed from homograft experience. If a competent valve cannot be assured, however, aortic valve replacement should be performed because the long-term results are excellent after valve replacement in this setting.

With dissections involving the descending thoracic aorta, most groups advocate initial medical therapy. In 10 to 20 percent of patients with acute type B dissection, urgent operation is indicated for complications such as retrograde dissection, recurrent pain, progressive mediastinal hematoma, leakage, acute expansion, visceral organ ischemia, leg ischemia, progressive neurologic injury, and rupture. Operation for type B dissection is performed through a left thoracotomy. Again, the goals of therapy are to exclude the tear site from the circulation, obliterate the false lumen, and redirect flow through a graft distally into the true lumen. Operative mortality for repair for acute type B dissection is 10 to 15 percent even though most such repairs are done emergently. If initial medical treatment is successful in the treatment of type B dissection, the patient is reevaluated in 1 to 2 months, and elective repair is recommended when the late risk of rupture is significant based upon the diameter of the aortic wall, i.e., when a chronic aneurysm greater than 5 to 6 cm is present. In repair of both acute and chronic dissections of the descending aorta, partial bypass techniques have been used to provide distal perfusion, as has been described earlier in the section Repair of Descending Thoracic Aneurysms.

Prognosis. Permanent therapy and close supervision are necessary because aortic dissection is an acute event in a patient with hypertension and a chronic degenerative disease of the media of the aorta. The false lumen remaining beyond the site of aortic reconstruction may gradually enlarge and become aneurysmal in the first few years following operation. Patients over 60 years of age are also in the age group where atherosclerotic disease of the coronary and cerebral circulations is common. In the series of Miller and associates, excluding operative deaths, 5-year survival was 76 percent, 10-year survival 37 percent. Sixty-one percent of late deaths were related to cardiac or cerebral causes. Late rupture in another segment of aorta accounts for 15 to 30 percent of the late deaths of dissection repair.

Control of hypertension is most important, as this lessens the frequency of aneurysmal dilatation of the remaining dissected aorta. More than one fatal aortic rupture has resulted from inadvertent cessation of antihypertensive therapy years after recovery from emergent surgical treatment of aortic dissection. These guidelines are especially important in patients with dissections of the descending thoracic aorta, treated initially with drug therapy. They should be carefully observed at 3- to 6-month intervals for development of an aneurysm, as this occurs in at least 25 to 30 percent of such patients. With the present availability of CT, MRI, and sonography, precise periodic evaluation of the size of the dissected aorta can easily be done and should be performed yearly for the remainder of the patient's life.

WOUNDS OF THE GREAT VESSELS

Penetrating Injuries

With penetrating chest wounds, injuries of the heart or great vessels are a frequent cause of death. The two immediate threats to life are cardiac arrest from exsanguination or tamponade. Tamponade is discussed in Chap. 18.

With injuries of the heart, aorta, or vena cava, only a few patients are alive when first seen in a hospital emergency room. They are usually in profound shock with signs of tamponade or with massive intrathoracic bleeding. Unless an operating room is immediately available, immediate thoracotomy may offer the only chance for survival. ''Slash'' anterolateral thoracotomy or sternotomy with limited aseptic technique has been employed at Bellevue Hospital for several years, occasionally resuscitating a moribund patient. Moore and associates demonstrated that this aggressive technique was justified only when signs of life are present in the field. Infection following such a thoracotomy is surprisingly rare. Once hemorrhage has been controlled, the patient can be transferred to the operating room for definitive surgical exploration and repair.

Most acute aortic wounds can be sutured directly, using 3-0 or 4-0 prolene. Occasionally brief periods of inflow occlusion are extremely helpful so that accurate placement of sutures can be performed. The sutures are then tied with the aid of inflow occlusion to avoid tension and further tearing at the site of injury. The key to success for most cases of penetrating aortic injury is adequate immediate volume resuscitation with fluids and mast trousers. If signs of tamponade are present, pericardiocentesis may temporarily improve hemodynamics while the patient is transported to the operating room. Subxiphoid exploration should not be performed unless the patient is prepped for full sternotomy because subxiphoid drainage alone is often followed by fatal exsanguination.

When threatened exsanguination does not mandate immediate thoracotomy, aortography should be seriously considered in any patient with a possible injury of the great vessels from a penetrating wound of the mediastinum. The development of frequent use of aortography is one of the major advances in therapy of thoracic trauma of the past decade. Indications should be liberal because some grave injuries may not be recognizable by other methods until serious complications develop.

Aortography helps choose between a sternotomy and a thoracotomy. Median sternotomy, combined with extension into the neck if necessary, provides the best combined exposure of the heart and great vessels. Exposure of the left subclavian artery, however, is limited and may require a lateral thoracotomy, converting the sternotomy to a T incision. This extensive incision in the thoracic cage may require ventilatory support for several days afterward, so it should be avoided if a simpler approach is possible. If aortography indicates that injury of the left subclavian artery is the only injury, a left anterior thoracotomy in the third interspace is a better incision.

Richardson and associates described experiences with 76 gunshot wounds of the mediastinum. Immediate operation was performed for 33 patients in *unstable* condition, with 12 deaths. Forty-three patients in *stable* condition had several diagnostic studies, including angiography, after which 27 were operated upon, 11 of whom had injuries to the great vessels. There were three deaths in this group, all from delayed complications (7 percent). In 1985, Zakharia described experiences with nearly 2000 thoracic battle wounds. Over 1400 thoracotomies were performed. Cardiac injuries occurred in 225 patients, great vessel wounds in 54, with an 87 percent survival in those with vessel injuries.

Nonpenetrating Injuries

The possibility of traumatic laceration of the aorta has emerged in the past two decades as one of the most important diagnostic considerations in treating blunt injuries, especially those following an automobile accident. Parmley and associates emphasized that only 10 to 20 percent of patients lived longer than 30 min after injury before exsanguination. The frequency of aortic laceration increases with the severity of the trauma; it is a common finding after severe trauma that produces instant death. In a review by Mattox, 80 to 90 percent of patients with traumatic injuries died before arrival in the hospital. After arrival in the hospital, nonoperated patients had a high mortality of 30 percent by 6 h, 50 percent by 24 h, and 90 percent within 3 months. Liberal use of aortography with *all* severe chest injuries is the best diagnostic approach, because *no single* clinical finding can diagnose or exclude significant vascular injuries and because the mortality from a missed aortic injury is extreme.

Passaro and Pace in 1959 are credited with the first successful repair of a traumatic aortic laceration. In 1961 Spencer and associates reported 15 patients with traumatic injuries and reviewed published experiences of others, finding virtually no successful reports of surgical repairs except the one case reported by Passaro.

Etiology and Pathology. Rupture of the aorta usually results from a deceleration-type injury, typically an automobile accident. In the vast majority of patients, the laceration occurs just distal to the left subclavian artery. Apparently the descending thoracic aorta and the aortic arch decelerate at different rates because of differences in anatomic structure, producing a transverse tear near the site of insertion of the ligamentum arteriosum. The tear may involve part or all of the layers of the aortic wall, varying from laceration of the intima to transection of the aorta with retraction of the two ends (Fig. 19-14). The tear site is usually contained

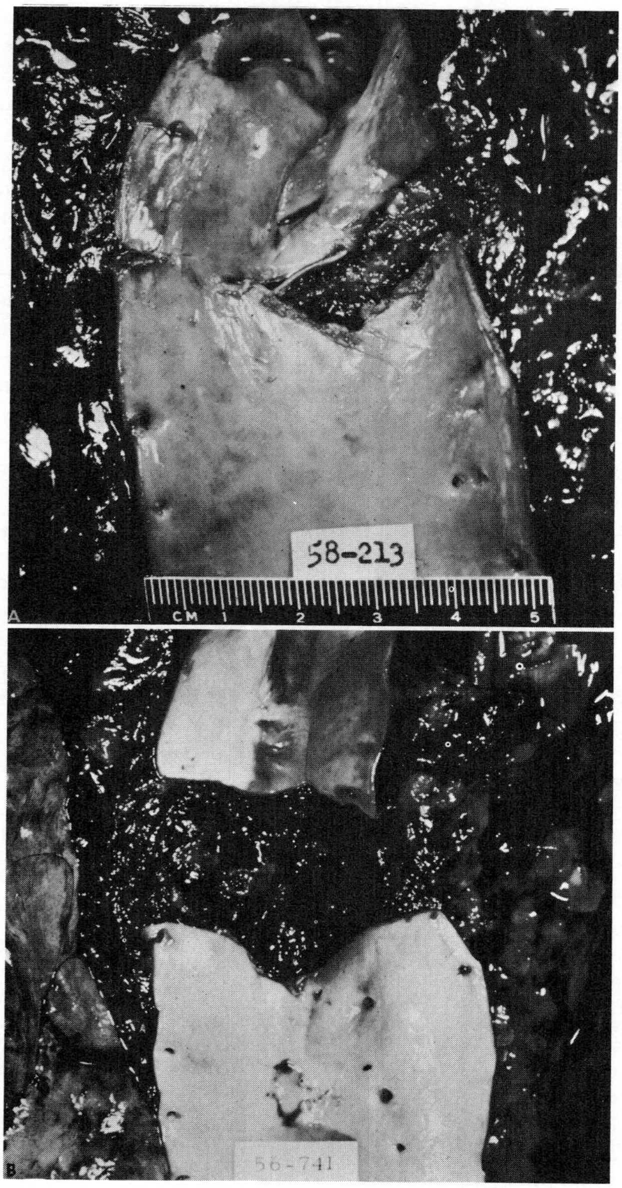

FIG. 19-14. *A.* Transected aorta found at autopsy when the patient exsanguinated 24 h following injury. The patient had only minor chest pain before the terminal event. The sharp, transverse laceration of the aorta is the usual finding, resulting from the deceleration forces at the time of injury. *B.* Partial transection of the aorta found at autopsy when the patient suddenly exsanguinated 3 weeks following an automobile accident. An aortic lesion had not been previously suspected.

by a localized hematoma. Aortic dissection following trauma is rare.

Fatal hemorrhage is prevented in some patients by the adventitia, which has been reported to constitute 60 percent of the tensile strength of the aortic wall. It is quite astonishing at operation to find the transected edges of the intima retracted for 1 to 2 cm, with exsanguination temporarily prevented by the adventitia.

The extensive 1981 review by Fisher and associates summarized available information. They found that aortic and great vessel laceration constituted the most common site of vascular injury after blunt chest trauma, citing 54 cases of their own and 456 cases previously reported by others. The second most common injury was an innominate artery laceration (26 cases). Injuries of the right carotid or right subclavian are virtually unknown; only 4 cases of laceration of the common carotid artery could be found. There were 13 injuries of the subclavian, virtually all of which involved the left subclavian. Multiple vascular lacerations were found in only 3 percent of cases. Lacerations of the aorta in other areas are very rare, with only isolated reports of injury of the ascending aorta or laceration near the diaphragm. Patients with traumatic aortic rupture have a high frequency of associated intracerebral or intraabdominal injuries. Peritoneal lavage should be done to evaluate intraabdominal injuries in most cases. A blown pupil or intraabdominal injury must be addressed in order to prioritize treatment.

In surviving patients, a mediastinal hematoma forms and produces widening of the mediastinal shadow, easily recognized on the chest x-ray. This is the *key to the diagnosis*. Several radiographic abnormalities have been described and are listed in Table 19-2 from a table published by Mattox and associates, but simply recognizing a wide mediastinal shadow is by far the most significant. Several mathematical indices were analyzed, but all were found inferior to the subjective impression of *mediastinal widening*. The critical measurement separating positive from negative cases was a mediastinal width of 8.0 cm.

No single finding either diagnoses or excludes aortic disruption. This can only be done with aortography. A small group of patients, less than 10 percent, has been reported who had aortic transection but did not have significant mediastinal widening.

In surviving patients first seen in the hospital emergency department, there is a grave risk of imminent rupture, as about 50 percent of such patients exsanguinate within the next 24 h. The risk of rupture decreases sharply after 2 weeks. Surviving patients gradually developed a false aneurysm, described earlier in this chapter under Traumatic Thoracic Aneurysms.

Table 19-2
Clues on Plain Chest X-ray Suggestive of Blunt Injury to the Descending Thoracic Aorta

Loss of aortic knob contour
Widened mediastinum (> 8 cm)
Depressed left main stem bronchus (> 140°)
Lateral tracheal deviation
Left pleural apex hematoma (''cap'')
Deviation from midline of nasogastric tube in esophagus
First and/or second rib fracture
Loss of left paraspinal pleural strip
''Calcium layering'' at aortic knob
Massive left hemothorax
Fracture of clavicle or scapula
Fracture or dislocation of thoracic spine
Loss of aortopulmonary window
Anterior displacement of trachea
Fracture of sternum

SOURCE: From Mattox KL, 1991, with permission.

Clinical Manifestations. Usually there are no specific signs to indicate that an aortic injury is present. Dyspnea and chest pain are usually present, but these result from the almost universally present rib fractures. A hemothorax, with varying degrees of shock, is also common. A murmur has seldom been heard. Rarely, signs of acute obstruction of the aorta, apparently from prolapse of a segment of intima into the lumen, are present.

Diagnostic Findings. As the history and the physical examination provide virtually no clues to the diagnosis, the chest x-ray is most important. Widening of the mediastinum (Fig. 19-15) is present in 80 to 90 percent of patients. It may result from causes other than rupture of the aorta; hence, aortography is necessary for the definitive diagnosis (Fig. 19-16). As emphasized earlier, an aortogram should be performed in the majority of patients with severe chest trauma, regardless of clinical findings. The CT scan might also be useful, but aortography has fewer false negative examinations.

Treatment. Thoracotomy should be performed as soon as possible after the diagnosis has been established. Akins and associates provide evidence that prompt operation is indicated in most instances.

Acute aortic rupture is repaired through a left posterolateral thoracotomy done in the fourth intercostal space. The use of partial bypass during operative repair, as opposed to the simpler clamp-and-sew technique, varies widely among institutions. The primary drawback with the use of bypass is the need for systemic heparinization with increased bleeding from associated injuries. In a care-

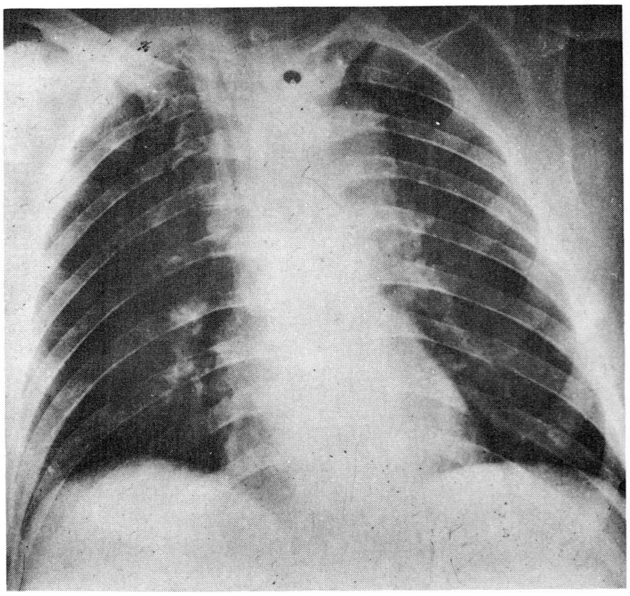

FIG. 19-15. Chest radiograph of a patient with traumatic rupture of the thoracic aorta, illustrating the characteristic widening of the mediastinum. When this is observed following a chest injury, emergency aortography should be performed to establish the diagnosis of rupture of the thoracic aorta.

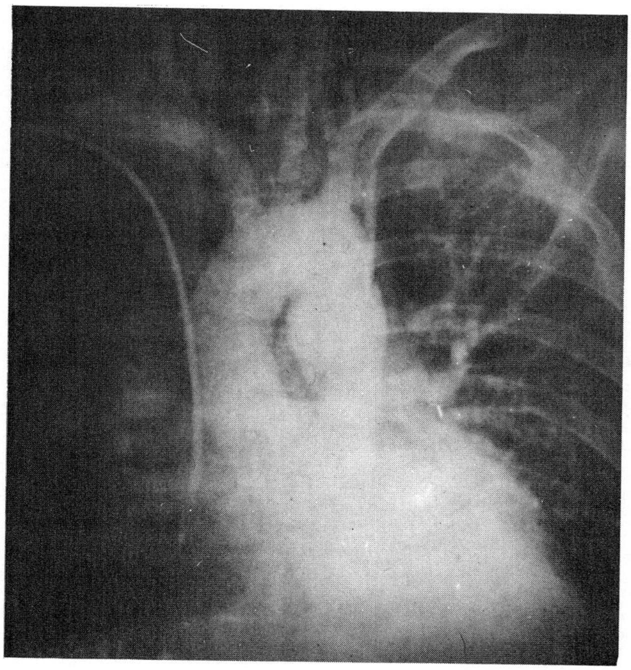

FIG. 19-16. Aortogram demonstrating traumatic rupture of the thoracic aorta distal to the left subclavian artery. The point of rupture can be seen as an irregular border of the thoracic aorta, in association with localized bulging. This angiogram represents the *first* instance in which emergency aortography was employed to establish firmly the diagnosis of traumatic rupture of the aorta. (From: *Spencer FC, Guerin PF, et al: A report of 15 patients with traumatic rupture of the thoracic aorta. J Thorac Cardiovasc Surg 41:1, 1961, with permission.*)

ful review of published reports by others, Payton found that 8 of 30 patients treated by simple clamping and rapid suture repair developed paraplegia (20 percent). Among 68 patients treated with either a shunt or a bypass, only 4 developed paraplegia, for an incidence of 6 percent. Most studies, however, have reported higher mortalities with the use of bypass because of increased bleeding from other injuries. Because of the risk of bleeding from associated injuries, we generally use the clamp-and-sew technique of repair at NYU and have found minimal risk of paraplegia with clamp times of less than 30 min. The goal of operative repair is accurate reconstruction of the aorta on the first attempt, and hurried attempts to achieve a short clamp time should be avoided. Recently a technique using heparin-bonded tubing, the centrifugal pump, and atrial-femoral bypass has been utilized, with total avoidance of systemic heparinization. This technique appears promising, because it provides for safe distal perfusion while avoiding systemic heparinization.

Once the left chest has been opened, the hematoma overlying the thoracic aorta should not be disturbed until proximal aortic control has been obtained. This is best done by opening the pericardium and encircling the aorta between the left carotid and left subclavian and encircling the left subclavian separately. Slight manipulation of the mediastinal hematoma may result in abrupt rupture and massive hemorrhage, and this area should be totally avoided until the cross-clamp is placed. Surgical repair is best done with the insertion of a short Dacron graft, though some groups have reported repair by direct suture or by use of the intraluminal sutureless graft.

Overall mortality with traumatic injuries ranges between 15 and 25 percent, usually because of different associated injuries. In the series of 79 patients reported by Kirklin and Barratt-Boyes, mortality was 24 percent and paraplegia developed in 16 percent.

OBSTRUCTION OF THE SUPERIOR VENA CAVA

Obstruction of the superior vena cava produces an unusual but distinctive clinical syndrome that can be easily recognized once the diagnosis is considered. Diagnostic errors are common, primarily because of the infrequent occurrence of the disease and because of lack of familiarity with the distinctive clinical features. The 1981 report by Parish and associates emphasized that the diagnosis can be made on physical examination in most patients.

Several excellent reviews of this subject have been published in the last three decades, all finding that a malignant tumor is the most frequent cause. Effler and Groves reported 64 patients, 48 of whom had a malignant neoplasm. Banker and Maddison summarized reports totaling 438 cases, only 15 percent of which were from benign causes. Mahajan reviewed published reports of benign causes of superior vena cava obstruction, a total of only 16 cases. Lochridge and associates described 66 cases seen in the previous 10 years; 64 were malignant.

Etiology. Over 90 percent of patients have obstruction from a malignant process. The percentage has apparently risen in recent years, especially since obstruction from expanding aortic aneurysms has decreased. The most common neoplasm is a bronchogenic carcinoma invading the mediastinum. Less frequent lesions are primary mediastinal tumors such as thymoma or lymphoma. Metastatic neoplasms are unusual.

Obstruction from a chronic fibrosing mediastinitis, usually of unknown cause, is infrequent. It is the only condition in which a long-term cure is possible. The etiology in most patients is unknown, although the disorder has been recognized for decades. The Parish and associates report includes three cases resulting from the use of central venous catheters.

Pathophysiology. With obstruction of the superior vena cava there is an increase in venous pressure to levels between 20 and 50 mmHg. The degree of increase in venous pressure varies with both the rate of development of the obstruction and the site of obstruction. Obstruction between the azygos vein and right atrium is less disabling than at other sites because the azygos vein can provide collateral venous decompression. The usual patient will have obstruction of the vena cava above the level of the azygos. Doty, in a 1982 detailed article, cited a venographic report by Dyet, who found that about 40 percent of patients have displacement but incomplete obstruction by tumor, about 20 percent have obstruction between the azygos vein and the heart, and about 40 percent have obstruction of the superior vena cava above the azygos, the usual finding in patients with disabling symptoms.

Acute obstruction of the vena cava, as during a thoracic operation, can produce fatal cerebral edema within a few minutes. This also occurred with early experiences in infants with the Glenn operation of anastomosis of the superior vena cava to the right pulmonary artery. At the opposite extreme are instances where superior vena cava obstruction develops slowly, permitting time for the development of collateral circulation, as a result of which symptoms are mild.

Clinical Manifestations. With mild obstruction, frequent symptoms are headache, swelling of the eyelids, puffiness of the face, or enlargement of the neck. The severity is related to posture. Patients quickly find that symptoms increase if they bend over or lie down. With acute obstruction, resulting from hemorrhage into a rapidly growing neoplasm, more serious symptoms of cerebral congestion appear, including drowsiness and blurring of vision. Edema of the vocal cords produces hoarseness or dyspnea from laryngeal obstruction. As the majority of cases are due to a rapidly growing bronchogenic carcinoma, pulmonary symptoms such as cough and hemoptysis are also often present. In most patients death results within a few months.

In the minority of patients in whom obstruction results from a benign process, usually fibrosing mediastinitis, collateral circulation generally enlarges sufficiently to where little disability is present. Prominent features include dilated veins with edema and cyanosis, the degree varying with the degree of stasis. Venous hypertension is obvious from prominence and distention of veins in the arms and face. Effler and Groves described 16 patients with obstruction from a benign process, all of whom eventually developed sufficient collateral circulation to have minimal symptoms. No fatalities occurred as a result of chronic venous obstruction. We observed one patient over a period of 30 years in whom the superior vena cava became obstructed following an intracardiac operation for correction of anomalous pulmonary veins entering the superior vena cava. Venous hypertension initially was severe, above 35 mmHg, producing a bilateral chylothorax controlled by ligation of the thoracic duct. The child was almost 6 years of age at this time. Within a few months, however, all symptoms subsided, and the patient, now a young married woman with children, has no limitation of physical activities.

Diagnostic Studies. Although the clinical picture is characteristic when fully developed, early manifestations such as swelling of the eyes or headache may be confused with angioneurotic edema, congestive heart failure, or constrictive pericarditis. Elevation of venous pressure, usually between 20 and 50 mmHg, is diagnostic. Venography readily outlines the location and extent of the obstruction, although the elevated venous pressure may result in bleeding. Often venography is omitted if the diagnosis of a malignant process is obvious. The usual consideration is to determine the type of malignancy present by an appropriate biopsy. Thoractomy is usually avoided if malignancy is present. Doty has emphasized that morbidity from a thoracic operation is less if a sternotomy is employed, because venous collateral circulation is interrupted to a lesser degree than with a lateral thoracotomy.

Treatment. With a malignant process, involvement of the superior vena cava almost precludes surgical resection. Isolated exceptions are rare.

The standard therapy is intensive radiation therapy, often in combination with diuretics and chemotherapy. The degree of improvement in symptoms varies with the type of neoplasm, but the majority improve rapidly, within a few weeks, probably from diminution in edema associated with a growing neoplasm. Death from the neoplasm, however, is virtually inevitable within the next several months, with rare survivors to 2 years.

With benign obstructions, as the report of Effler and Groves indicates, there is no urgency in performing an operation if symptoms are mild. In all likelihood these symptoms will improve, or subside completely, as collateral circulation develops. Occasionally, vena caval replacement with a spiral saphenous vein segment, or with a Gore-Tex graft, is indicated.

Little and associates reviewed 42 patients with malignant superior vena cava obstruction. Thirty-three of the patients underwent radiotherapy; in all of these the obstruction clinically resolved within 14 days. Median survival of the entire group was only 5 months, emphasizing again the grim prognosis.

A number of ingenious attempts have been made to reconstruct an obstructed superior vena cava, although the clinical need for superior vena cava reconstruction is uncommon. Prosthetic grafts to date have been almost uniformly unsuccessful although recently better results have been obtained with the use of Gore-Tex material. The most favorable graft is a composite one of autogenous veins. Good results in three patients lasting for several years were reported by Hanlon and Danis. A collective review of surgical approaches was published by Gomes and Hufnagel. The best technique appears to be that reported by Doty that consists of constructing a spiral vein graft by comparing the diameters of the innominate vein and saphenous vein, followed by appropriate mathematical calculations and construction of a composite vein over a stent. Doty summarized his experiences with 10 patients, 4 with benign disease. All grafts remained patent up to 18 months. The 4 patients with benign disease remained asymptomatic 3 months to 6 years after operation, while all with malignancy died within 21 months.

The graft sizes ranged from 9 to 13 mm and could be constructed from a segment of saphenous vein obtained from the thigh within about 30 min. This technique seems clearly superior to prosthetic materials. Unless the saphenous veins are not available, there would seem to be little indication to employ prosthetic materials. The only indication for the operation, however, seems to be the unusual patient with a benign process in whom collateral circulation is inadequate to relieve smptoms.

Rarely, a localized granuloma may compress and thrombose the vena cava. Patency can be restored by opening the vein and removing the thrombus. Three such patients were reported by Pate and Hammon, but the paucity of reports since that time suggests that thrombectomy is not usually feasible.

Bibliography

Aneurysms of the Thoracic Aorta

Bickerstaff LK, Pairolero PC, et al: Thoracic aortic aneurysms: A population-based study. *Surgery* 92:1103, 1982.

Cooley DA, DeBakey ME: Surgical considerations of intrathoracic aneurysms of the aorta and great vessels. *Ann Surg* 135:660, 1952.

Cooley DA, DeBakey ME: Resection of the entire ascending aorta and fusiform aneurysm using cardiac bypass. *JAMA* 162:1158, 1956.

Finkelmeier BA, Mentzer RM, et al: Chronic traumatic thoracic aneurysm: Influence of operative treatment on natural history: An analysis of reported cases, 1950–1980. *J Thorac Cardiovasc Surg* 84:257, 1982.

Griepp RB, Ergin MA, et al: The natural history of thoracic aortic aneurysms. *Seminars in Thoracic Cardiovascular Surgery* 3:258, 1991.

Pressler V, McNamara JJ: Thoracic aortic aneurysm: Natural history and treatment. *J Thorac Cardiovasc Surg* 79:489, 1980.

Rutherford, RB: Infrarenal aortic aneurysms, in Rutherford RB (ed): *Vascular Surgery,* 2d ed. Philadelphia, WB Saunders, 1984, chap 74, p 755.

Aneurysms of the Ascending Aorta

Akins C, Buckley M, et al: Myocardial protection with hypothermia and potassium cardioplegia during operation for ascending aortic aneurysms. *J Thorac Cardiovasc Surg* 79:700, 1980.

Cabrol C, Pavie A, et al: Long-term results with total replacement of the ascending aorta and re-implantation of the coronary arteries. *J Thorac Cardiovasc Surg* 91:17, 1986.

Cooley DA: *Surgical Treatment of Aortic Aneurysms*. Philadelphia, WB Saunders, 1986.

Crawford ES, Crawford JL: *Diseases of the Aorta*. Baltimore, Williams & Wilkins, 1984.

Culliford AT, Cyaliotis B, et al: Aneurysms of the ascending aorta and transverse arch: Surgical experience in 80 patients. *J Thorac Cardiovasc Surg* 83:701, 1982.

Galloway AC, Colvin SB, et al: Ten year operative experience with 165 aneurysms of the ascending aorta and aortic arch. *Circulation* 80(suppl I):I-249, 1989.

Gott VL, Pyeritz RE, et al: Surgical treatment of aneurysms of the ascending aorta in the Marfan syndrome. Results of composite-graft repair in 50 patients. *N Engl J Med* 134:1070, 1986.

Grey DP, Ott DA, Cooley DA: Surgical treatment of aneurysm of the ascending aorta with aortic insufficiency. A selective approach. *J Thorac Cardiovasc Surg* 86:864, 1983.

Kouchoukos NT, Wareing TH, et al: Sixteen-year experience with aortic root replacement: Results of 172 operations. *Ann Surg* 214:308, 1991.

McDonald G, Schaff H, et al: Surgical management of patients with the Marfan syndrome and dilatation of the ascending aorta. *J Thorac Cardiovasc Surg* 81:180, 1981.

Miller D, Stinson E, et al: Concomitant resection of ascending aortic aneurysm and replacement of the aortic valve. Operative and long-term results with "conventional" techniques in ninety patients. *J Thorac Cardiovasc Surg* 79:388, 1980.

Moreno-Cabral CE, Miller DC, et al: Degenerative and atherosclerotic aneurysms of the thoracic aorta. Determinants of early and late surgical outcome. *J Thorac Cardiovasc Surg* 88:1020, 1984.

Pressler V, McNamara JJ: Aneurysm of the thoracic aorta. Review of 260 cases. *J Thorac Cardiovasc Surg* 89:50, 1985.

Aneurysms of the Transverse Aortic Arch

Crawford ES, Crawford JL: *Diseases of the Aorta*. Baltimore, Williams & Wilkins, 1984.

Crawford ES, Snyder DM: Treatment of aneurysms of the aortic arch. A progress report. *J Thorac Cardiovasc Surg* 85:237, 1983.

Crawford ES, Stowe CL, et al: Aortic arch aneurysm: A sentinel of extensive aortic disease requiring subtotal and total aortic replacement. *Ann Aurg* 199:742, 1984.

Ergin M, Griepp R: Progress in treatment of aneurysms of the aortic arch. *World J Surg* 4:535, 1980.

Frist WH, Baldwin JC, et al: A reconsideration of cerebral perfusion in aortic arch replacement. *Ann Thorac Surg* 42:273, 1986.

Galloway AC, Colvin SB, et al: Ten-year operative experience with 165 aneurysms of the ascending aorta and aortic arch. *Circulation* 80(suppl I):I–249, 1989.

Griepp RB, Stinson EB, et al: Prosthetic replacement of the aortic arch. *J Thorac Cardiovasc Surg* 70:1051, 1975.

Kay GL, Cooley DA, et al: Surgical repair of aneurysms involving the distal aortic arch. *J Thorac Cardiovasc Surg* 91:397, 1986.

Livesay JJ, Cooley DA, et al: Open aortic anastomosis: Improved results in the treatment of aneurysms of the aortic arch. *Circulation* 66(suppl I):I–122, 1982.

Livesay JJ, Cooley DA, et al: Surgical experience in descending thoracic aneurysmectomy with and without adjuncts to avoid ischemia. *Ann Thorac Surg* 39:37, 1985.

Ott DA, Frazier OH, et al: Resection of the aortic arch using deep hypothermia and temporary circulatory arrest. *Circulation* 58(suppl I):I–227, 1978.

Sweeney MS, Cooley DA, et al: Hypothermic circulatory arrest for cardiovascular lesions: Technical considerations and results. *Ann Thorac Surg* 40:498, 1985.

Traumatic Thoracic Aneurysms

Bennett DE, Cherry JK: The natural history of traumatic aneurysms of the aorta. *Surgery* 61:516, 1967.

Finkelmeier BA, Mentzer RM, et al: Chronic traumatic thoracic aneurysm: Influence of operative treatment on natural history: An analysis of reported cases, 1950–1980. *J Thorac Cardiovasc Surg* 84:257, 1982.

McCollum C, Graham J, et al: Chronic traumatic aneurysms of the thoracic aorta: An analysis of 50 patients. *J Trauma* 19:248, 1979.

Spencer FC, Guerin PF, et al: A report of fifteen patients with traumatic rupture of the thoracic aorta. *J Thorac Cardiovasc Surg* 41:1, 1961.

Aneurysms of the Descending Thoracic Aorta

Bickerstaff LK, Pairolero PC, et al: Thoracic aortic aneurysms: A population-based study. *Surgery* 92:1103, 1982.

Crawford ES, Crawford JL, et al: Thoracoabdominal aortic aneurysms: Preoperative and intraoperative factors determining immediate and long-term results of operations in 605 patients. *J Vasc Surg* 3:389, 1986.

Crawford ES, Mizrahi EM, et al: The impact of distal aortic perfusion and somatosensory evoked potential monitoring on prevention of paraplegia after aortic aneurysm operation. *J Thorac Cardiovasc Surg* 95:357, 1988.

Culliford A, Ayvaliotis B, et al: Aneurysms of the descending aorta: Surgical experiences in 48 patients. *J Thorac Cardiovasc Surg* 85:98, 1983.

Cunningham JN Jr, Laschinger JC, et al: Measurement of spinal cord ischemia during operations upon the thoracic aorta: Initial clinical experience. *Ann Surg* 196:285, 1982.

Krieger KH, Spencer FC: Is paraplegia after repair of coarctation of the aorta due principally to distal hypotension during aortic cross-clamping? *Surgery* 97:2, 1985.

Laschinger JC, Cunningham JN Jr, et al: Monitoring of somatosensory evoked potentials during surgical procedures on the thoracoabdominal aorta. I. Relationship of aortic crossclamp duration, changes in somatosensory evoked potentials, and incidence of neurologic dysfunction. *J Thorac Cardiovasc Surg* 94:260, 1987.

Laschinger JC, Cunningham JN Jr, et al: Monitoring of somatosensory evoked potentials during surgical procedures on the thoracoabdominal aorta. II. Use of somatosensory evoked potentials to assess adequacy of distal aortic bypass and perfusion after thoracic aortic cross-clamping. *J Thorac Cardiovasc Surg* 94:266, 1987.

Laschinger JC, Cunningham JN Jr, et al: Monitoring of somatosensory evoked potentials during surgical procedures on the thoracoabdominal aorta. III. Intraoperative identification of vessels critical to spinal cord blood supply. *J Thorac Cardiovasc Surg* 94:271, 1987.

Laschinger JC, Cunningham JN Jr, et al: Monitoring of somatosensory evoked potentials during surgical procedures on the thoracoabdominal aorta. IV. Clinical observations and results. *J Thorac Cardiovasc Surg* 94:275, 1987.

Livesay JJ, Cooley DA, et al: Surgical experience in descending thoracic aneurysmectomy with and without adjuncts to avoid ischemia. *Ann Thorac Surg* 39:37, 1985.

Pressler V, McNamara JJ: Aneurysms of the thoracic aorta. Review of 260 cases. *J Thorac Cardiovasc Surg* 89:50, 1985.

Vasko JS, Spencer FC, Bahnson HT: Aneurysm of the aorta treated by excision: Review of 237 cases followed up to seven years. *Am J Surg* 105:793, 1963.

Thoracoabdominal Aneurysms

Crawford ES, Crawford JL, et al: Thoracoabdominal aortic aneurysms: Preoperative and intraoperative factors determining immediate and long-term results of operations in 605 patients. *J Vasc Surg* 3:389, 1986.

Crawford ES, DeNatale RW: Thoracoabdominal aortic aneurysm: Observations regarding the natural course of the disease. *J Vasc Surg* 3:578, 1986.

Crawford ES, Snyder D, et al: Progress in treatment of thoracoabdominal and abdominal aortic aneurysms involving celiac, superior mesenteric, and renal arteries. *Ann Surg* 188:404, 1978.

DeBakey ME, Crawford ES, et al: Surgical considerations in the treatment of aneurysms of the thoraco-abdominal aorta. *Ann Surg* 162:650, 1965.

Spencer FC, Zimmerman JM: The influence of ligation of intercostal arteries on paraplegia in dogs. *Surg Forum* 9:340, 1959.

Svensson LG, Stewart RW, et al: Intrathecal papaverine for the prevention of paraplegia after operation on the thoracic or thoracoabdominal aorta. *J Thorac Cardiovasc Surg* 96:823, 1988.

Aortic Dissection

Crawford ES, Svensson LG, et al: Aortic dissection and dissecting aortic aneurysms. *Ann Surg* 208:254, 1988.

Dalen J, Pape L, et al: Dissection of the aorta: Pathogenesis, diagnostic, and treatment. *Prog Cardiovasc Dis* 23:237, 1980.

Ergin MA, Galla JD, et al: Acute dissections of the aorta. Current surgical treatment. *Surg Clin North Am* 65:721, 1985.

Fann JI, Glower DD, et al: Preservation of aortic valve in type A aortic dissection complicated by aortic regurgitation. *J Thorac Cardiovasc Surg* 102:62, 1991.

Galloway AC, Colvin SB, et al: Experiences with the surgical repair of type A aortic dissection in 66 patients using the circulatory arrest-graft inclusion technique. In press, *J Thorac Cardiovasc Surg*.

Galloway AC, Colvin SB, et al: Ten-year operative experience with 165 aneurysms of the ascending aorta and aortic arch. *Circulation* 80(suppl I):I–249, 1989.

Hirst AE, Johns VJ, Kime SW: Dissecting aneurysm of the aorta: A review of 505 cases. *Medicine (Baltimore)* 37:217, 1958.

Lindsay J, Hurst JW: Clinical features and prognosis in dissecting aneurysm of the aorta. *Circulation* 35:880, 1967.

Miller DC: Surgical management of acute aortic dissection: New data. *Seminars in Thoracic Cardiovascular Surgery* 3:225, 1991.

Miller DC, Mitchell RS, et al: Independent determinants of operative mortality for patients with aortic dissections. *Circulation* 70(suppl I):I–153, 1984.

Roberts W: Aortic dissection: Anatomy, consequences, and causes. *Am Heart J* 101:195, 1981.

Sutton M, Oldershaw P, et al: Dissection of the thoracic aorta. A comparison between medical and surgical treatment. *J Cardiovasc Surg* 22:195, 1981.

Sweeney MS, Cooley DA, et al: Hypothermic circulatory arrest for cardiovascular lesions: Technical considerations and results. *Ann Thorac Surg* 40:498, 1985.

Wheat M: Acute dissecting aneurysms of the aorta: Diagnosis and treatment—1979. *Am Heart J* 99:373, 1980.

Wheat M: Current status of medical therapy of acute dissecting aneurysms of the aorta. *World J Surg* 4:563, 1980.

Wilson SK, Hutchins GM: Aortic dissecting aneurysms: Causative factors in 204 subjects. *Arch Pathol Lab Med* 106:175, 1982.

Wolfe WG, Oldham HN, et al: Surgical treatment of acute ascending aortic dissection. *Ann Surg* 197:738, 1983.

Wounds of the Great Vessels

Akins C, Buckley M, et al: Acute traumatic disruption of the thoracic aorta: A ten-year experience. *Ann Thorac Surg* 31:305, 1981.

Bennett DE, Cherry DK: The natural history of traumatic aneurysms of the aorta. *Surgery* 61:516, 1967.

Burney RE, Gundry SR, et al: Comparison of mediastinal width, mediastinal-thoracic and cardiac ratios, and "mediastinal widening" in detection of traumatic aortic rupture. *Ann Emerg Med* 12:668, 1983.

Fisher RG, Hadlock F: Laceration of the thoracic aorta and brachiocephalic arteries by blunt trauma. Report of 54 cases and review of the literature. *Radiol Clin North Am* 19:91, 1981.

Harman PK, Trinkle JK: Injury to the heart, in Mattox KL, Moore EE, Feliciano DV (eds): *Trauma*. Norwalk, CT, Appleton & Lange, 1988, chap 26, p 365.

Hood RM, Boyd AD, Culliford AT: *Thoracic Trauma*. Philadelphia, WB Saunders, 1989.

Kirklin JW, Barratt-Boyes BG: *Cardiac Surgery*. New York, Wiley, 1986.

Magilligan D, Davila J: Innominate artery disruption due to blunt trauma. *Arch Surg* 114:307, 1979.

Mattox KL: Contemporary issues in thoracic aortic trauma. *Seminars in Thoracic Cardiovascular Surgery* 3:281, 1991.

Mattox KL, O'Gorman RB: Injury to the thoracic great vessels, in Mattox KL, Moore EE, Feliciano DV (eds): *Trauma*. Norwalk, CT, Appleton & Lange, 1988, chap 27, p 385.

Moore EE, Moore JB, et al: Post-injury thoracotomy in the emergency department: A critical evaluation. *Surgery* 86:590, 1979.

Parmley LF, Mattingly TW, Manion WC: Penetrating wounds to the heart and aorta. *Circulation* 17:953, 1958.

Parmley LF, Mattingly TW, et al: Non-penetrating traumatic injury of the aorta. *Circulation* 17:1086, 1958.

Pate JW: Traumatic rupture of the aorta: Emergency operation. *Ann Thorac Surg* 39:531, 1985.

Rich N, Spencer F: *Vascular Trauma*. Philadelphia, WB Saunders, 1978, p 427.

Richardson JD, Flint LM, et al: Management of transmediastinal gunshot wounds. *Surgery* 90:671, 1981.

Robbs J, Baker L, et al: Cervicomediastinal arterial injuries. A surgical challenge. *Arch Surg* 116:663, 1981.

Saylam A, Melo J, et al: Early surgical repair in traumatic rupture of the thoracic aorta. *J Cardiovasc Surg* 21:295, 1980.

Spencer FC, Guerin PF, et al: A report of 15 patients with traumatic rupture of the thoracic aorta. *J Thorac Cardiovasc Surg* 41:1, 1961.

Williams S, Burney RE, et al: Indications for aortography. Radiography after blunt chest trauma: A reassessment of the radiographic findings associated with traumatic rupture of the aorta. *Invest Radiol* 18:230, 1983.

Zakharia AT: Cardiovascular and thoracic battle injuries in the Lebanon war. Analysis of 3,000 personal cases. *J Thorac Cardiovasc Surg* 89:723, 1985.

Obstruction of the Superior Vena Cava

Banker VP, Madison FE: Superior vena cava syndrome secondary to aortic disease. *Dis Chest* 51:656, 1967.

Doty D: Bypass of superior vena cava. Six years' experience with spiral vein graft for obstruction of superior vena cava due to benign and malignant disease. *J Thorac Cardiovasc Surg* 83:326, 1982.

Effler DB, Groves LK: Superior vena caval obstruction. *J Thorac Cardiovasc Surg* 43:574, 1962.

Gomez MN, Hufnagel CA: Superior vena cava obstruction: Review of literature and report of two cases due to benign intrathoracic tumors. *Ann Thorac Surg* 20:344, 1975.

Hanlon CR, Danis RK: Superior vena caval obstruction: Indications for diagnostic thoracotomy. *Ann Surg* 161:771, 1965.

Little AG, Golomb HM, et al: Malignant superior vena cava obstruction reconsidered: The role of diagnostic surgical intervention. *Ann Thorac Surg* 40:285, 1985.

Lochridge S, Knibbe W, Doty D: Obstruction of the superior vena cava. *Surgery* 85:14, 1979.

Mahajan V, Strimlan V, et al: Benign superior vena cava syndrome. *Chest* 68:32, 1975.

Parish J, Marschke R, et al: Etiologic considerations in superior vena cava syndrome. *Mayo Clin Proc* 36:407, 1981.

Pate JW, Hammon J: Superior vena caval syndrome due to histoplasmosis in children. *Ann Surg* 161:778, 1965.

CHAPTER 20

Peripheral Arterial Disease

Richard M. Green and Kenneth Ouriel

The years following World War II have seen a logarithmic increase in the number of patients seeking treatment for diseases of the peripheral arteries. In 1990 almost one million arterial reconstructions were performed in the United States alone. As the geriatric population grows at a disproportionate rate compared to the general population, the incidence of peripheral vascular disease will increase accordingly.

Of necessity, the evolution of vascular surgery awaited the development of arteriography, anesthesia, anticoagulation, blood transfusion, and synthetic graft materials. Nevertheless, Hallowell of England documented the first successful arterial operation in 1759 when he performed a lateral arterial repair of a traumatic wound. Eck is credited with the first formal blood vessel anastomosis when he sutured the portal vein to the inferior vena cava in dogs in 1877. Murphy performed the first end-to-end arterial anastomosis in humans two decades later when he successfully rejoined the femoral artery by invagination of the proximal into the distal end after excision of an arteriovenous fistula of the thigh. Alexis Carrel and Charles Guthrie made remarkable achievements as a result of collaborative efforts beginning in 1904. They pioneered the use of Dorfler's technique of through-and-through sutures of all layers of the vascular wall, and in 1912 Carrel received the Nobel prize in Physiology and Medicine for his work on blood transfusion, vascular suture technique, and organ transplantation in experimental animals.

Rapid advances in vascular surgery began after the second World War, beginning with the treatment of arterial lesions with endarterectomy by dos Santos in 1947 and with bypass using autogenous vein by Kunlin in 1951. Dubost first replaced an abdominal aortic aneurysm with an aortic homograft in 1951, and Voorhees and Blakemore used a synthetic cloth graft the following year. The successful treatment of carotid disease was first reported by Eastcott, Pickering, and Rob in 1954, when a symptomatic carotid bifurcation was resected and reanastomosed, and 2 years later Cooley and his colleagues published a report of carotid endarterectomy for stenotic disease.

PATHOLOGY AND PATHOPHYSIOLOGY

Atherogenesis

Vascular injury and thrombus formation are the major events in the formation and progression of the atherosclerotic lesion. The most widely held view on the genesis of atherosclerosis, the "response-to-injury" hypothesis, was advanced by Ross in 1986. Three categories of vascular injury of increasing severity have been proposed (Table 20-1). In type I injury there is a functional alteration of the endothelial cell without morphologic changes. It has been hypothesized that the injury can occur from flow disturbances in certain parts of the arterial tree. Lipids accumulate in macrophages, and the lipid-laden "foam cells" may represent the earliest sign of atherosclerosis. Type II injuries begin with the release of toxic products from the macrophages. The subsequent adhesion of platelets at sites of injury and the release of a variety of growth factors results in the migration and proliferation of primitive smooth muscle cells and the development of the "fibrointimal" lesion. By the third decade of life some of these lesions become fibrolipid plaques with a cap of smooth muscle cells and collagen surrounding the lipid material. Type III injuries are characterized by fissures and disruption of the plaque with penetration into the media, exposed fibrillar collagen, increased platelet adherence and activation, thrombus formation, and extensive proliferation of smooth muscle cells. This mural thrombus deposited at the site of plaque disruption is important in the progression of the atherosclerotic plaque.

Platelets. Experimental injury models have characterized the time course of the platelet response. Phase I occurs with the immediate deposition of the platelet thrombus after injury and is completed within 24 h. Smooth muscle cells in the media begin to proliferate within 24 h. Phase II begins on day 4 after injury and continues through day 14 and is characterized by migration of the smooth muscle cells into the intima. Phase III lasts from day 14 to 3 months and is marked by the process of intimal thickening and the accumulation of an extracellular matrix. Pigs lacking von Willebrand factor, a protein important in platelet adherence to injured vessel wall, do not develop spontaneous atherosclerosis. Furthermore, rabbits rendered thrombocytopenic do not develop the same degree of intimal thickening when subjected to balloon catheter injury as animals with normal platelet counts.

Macrophages. Macrophages are involved in the earliest stages of atherogenesis. These multipurpose cells facilitate transport and oxidation of cholesterol, secrete a mitogenic growth factor that stimulates the proliferation of smooth muscle cells, and generate toxic products that produce endothelial damage. Most importantly, macrophages release proteases that digest extracellu-

Table 20-1
Response-to-Injury Hypothesis of Atherogenesis

Injury Phase	*Mechanism*	*Result*	*Appearance*
I (1–24 h)	Flow abnormalities, e.g., bifurcations	Deposition of platelet thrombus, accumulation of lipids in macrophages (foam cells)	Functional change in endothelial cells
II (day 4–14)	Toxic products of macrophages, platelet activation	Platelet growth factors, migration and proliferation of smooth muscle cells	"Fibrointimal" lesion
III (day 14 to 3 months)	Plaque disruption with penetration into the media and exposure of collagen	Increased platelet activation and proliferation of smooth muscle cells	Intimal thickening, accumulation of extracellular matrix and mural thrombus

lar matrix, which may be responsible for the plaque disruption that leads to thrombosis.

Plaque Disruption. The intact endothelium is nonreactive to platelets. Recent pathologic data in patients who died of cardiac events suggest that the occluded coronary artery resulted from recurrent episodes of plaque disruption that were sealed by layered thrombus of varying ages in a dynamic and repetitive process. Patients with mild to moderate stenoses may progress rapidly to severe stenosis or total occlusion and sustain a major stroke or an acute myocardial infarction. It has been found, either at operation or postmortem exam, that many of these patients have small to moderate lipid-laden plaques with disruption and that the severe stenosis or occlusion was mainly due to superimposed thrombus. Angiographic studies in patients with acute myocardial infarction who have received thrombolytic therapy have shown that a considerable proportion of these patients have less than a 70 percent stenosis. The soft, lipid-rich plaque of mild to moderate severity is more prone to disruption than the fibrotic, calcified plaque because of the former's high fat content. Once a thrombus forms over an area of vascular injury, further clot deposition occurs. The thrombus encroaches on the vessel lumen and further increases the stenosis, and this increases the shear rate which results in further platelet activation and deposition. Furthermore, residual thrombus itself is one of the most potent thrombogenic surfaces known even in the face of heparin.

Cigarette Effect. Cigarette smoking has a well-documented effect on atherogenesis. The Framingham study shows that the incidence of peripheral vascular disease in smokers is 0.65 percent compared to 0.22 percent for nonsmokers. Other studies have shown that the risk for developing intermittent claudication was 15 times higher in smokers and 7 times higher in female smokers than in nonsmokers. The incidences of abdominal aortic aneurysms, amputations, stroke, and myocardial infarctions are all significantly increased in smokers.

The mechanisms by which cigarettes exert their effect on atherogenesis are complex. Nicotine and carbon monoxide appear to be the most harmful constituents. In addition to the systemic effects of increased heart rate, increased blood pressure, and reduced myocardial oxygen delivery, these compounds exert adverse effects on vascular endothelium. Carbon monoxide causes increased permeability of the vessel wall to lipids. This is important because nicotine produces increased levels of circulating free fatty acids which increase intracellular lipid deposition. Nicotine infused experimentally causes a significant increase in circulating carcasses of endothelial cells. This finding has been reproduced in humans by having them smoke only two cigarettes. Nicotine also decreases cell synthesis of prostacyclin (PGI_2), the most potent inhibitor of platelet aggregation, and promotes the production of thromboxane A_2, which promotes platelet aggregation. Other deleterious effects of smoking include increased blood viscosity and fibrinogen and low-density lipoprotein (LDL) levels and decreased high-density lipoprotein (HDL) levels.

Cessation of smoking reduces the incidence of amputation and increases longevity in patients with peripheral vascular disease, improves walking distances in patients with claudication, and reduces the risk of stroke and myocardial infarction in the general population. The cigarette industry has responded to these data with so-called low-yield cigarettes. These filtered cigarettes do reduce exposure to tar and have been shown to have a lower cancer mortality compared to nonfiltered cigarettes. Unfortunately there has been no reduction in cardiovascular mortality rates associated with filtered cigarettes. Therefore, the most important prophylactic advice that physicians can give patients is to not smoke.

Prevention. Since lipid-rich plaques and subsequent thrombosis play a major role in atherogenesis, strategies for prevention have focused on manipulations in the areas of lipid metabolism and antiplatelet therapy.

Lipid Reduction. Evidence of regression of human atherosclerotic lesions is difficult to obtain because of the lack of reliable methods to quantitate the extent of the process. Angiographic studies of patients with coronary and femoral artery plaques have shown that some regression does occur using lipid-lowering drugs. These studies have shown a small increase in residual lumen size and suggest that the regression is limited to the soft, lipid-rich plaque rather than the extensive calcified fibrotic plaque thereby limiting its clinical usefulness once symptoms from the stenotic or occluded vessel occur. The small effect of lipid-lowering regimens on lumen diameter does not explain the significant reduction of vascular events in the large clinical trials conducted to date. The National Cholesterol Education Program has proposed that persons without vascular disease maintain an LDL cholesterol of 130 mg/dL or less. A patient with a level of greater than 160 mg/dL should be treated with cholesterol-lowering drugs if diet and exercise do not reduce the levels to acceptable ranges.

Antiplatelet Therapy. The interaction between the platelet and the vessel wall is dependent on the balance between thromboxane A_2 and PGI_2. The endothelial cell produces PGI_2 which is responsible for some of the thromboresistant properties of vascular endothelium. In addition, PGI_2 enhances the activity of cholesterol ester hydrolase, suggesting a positive feedback between the prostacyclin system and lipid accumulation in the vessel wall. Prostacyclin generation from atherosclerotic arterial tissue has been shown to be significantly lower than from normal arterial tissue. Platelets in patients with arterial thrombosis produce more thromboxane A_2 than normal.

Aspirin inhibits platelet activation induced by the release of thromboxane A_2 and is the most commonly used antiplatelet drug. Aspirin binds irreversibly to the active site of cyclooxygenase, inhibiting the conversion of arachidonic acid to thromboxane A_2 in the platelet and to PGI_2 in the endothelium. Aspirin has theoretical limits as an antiplatelet agent since platelet aggregation is a complex mechanism that can also be initiated by adenosine diphosphate (ADP) and thrombin in the absence of thromboxane A_2. A single dose of aspirin leads to a platelet defect that lasts 7 days. The effect on the endothelium lasts for a shorter period, presumably because the endothelium can synthesize new enzyme whereas the platelet cannot. Studies on human vascular fragments revealed that aspirin doses of 40 mg/day inhibit both vascular wall PGI_2 and thromboxane A_2 formation with a greater effect on the latter. Less data are available on the efficacy of other antiplatelet agents that work via selective thromboxane A_2 inhibition, phosphodiesterase inhibition (dipyridamole, iloprost, cyprostene), thrombin inhibition (heparin, coumadin, hirudin), calcium channel blockade (ticlopidine), or ACE inhibitors (cilazapril).

Large clinical trials have evaluated the role of antiplatelet drugs in the prophylaxis of myocardial infarction and stroke. Overall, regardless of indication, antiplatelet therapy was most effective in the first year of treatment, there was a smaller but still significant benefit in year 2, and there was no benefit in year 3 and beyond. A cumulative risk reduction of 25 percent was independent of disease categories, age, sex, blood pressure, and type of antiplatelet therapy. A separate analysis of the stroke cohort showed that antiplatelet therapy in high-risk patients resulted in a reduction of occlusive stroke occurrence, a small increase in the number of hemorrhagic strokes, and a substantial and significant net reduction in total stroke occurrence. The effect of antiplatelet therapy on stroke in low-risk patients, i.e., primary prevention, was unclear. In a cardiac cohort, antiplatelet therapy was shown to reduce the incidence of nonfatal myocardial infarction by 33 percent. Unlike the stroke group, the cardiac effect was seen in both primary and secondary prevention.

Thrombogenesis

Thrombogenesis may be conceptualized as the interaction between three pathways: coagulation, platelet deposition, and thrombolysis. Coagulation pathways involve the clotting proteins in the plasma, terminating in the cleavage of fibrinogen and the deposition of fibrin matrix. Platelet pathways involve activating substances in the plasma and, as such, are intimately linked to the coagulation pathway. The end result of these interactions is the activation, attachment, and aggregation of platelets at the site of altered endothelial integrity. Thrombolytic pathways involve the lysis of fibrin by plasmin to maintain luminal patency and tissue perfusion in the event of vessel thrombosis.

Coagulation. The coagulation pathways involve a cascade mechanism, with activation of clotting proteins through two pathways: the intrinsic pathway and the extrinsic pathway. Many of the clotting proteins have been assigned a Roman numeral by the International Committee on Nomenclature of Blood Clotting Factors.

There are two laboratory tests that are widely used to assess the adequacy of anticoagulation. The activated partial thromboplastin time (APTT) reflects the potential activity of the intrinsic coagulation pathway, and the prothrombin time (PT) provides an index of the extrinsic system. The vitamin K-dependent factors II, VII, IX, and X are manufactured in the liver by gamma carboxylation-dependent mechanisms. Warfarin compounds inhibit the production of the vitamin K–dependent factors. The therapeutic control of warfarin anticoagulation is best monitored with the PT. Heparin achieves anticoagulation through its actions on antithrombin III, a potent inhibitor of factor X, and therapeutic control is generally monitored with the APTT.

The intrinsic coagulation pathway is initiated with the activation of Hageman factor (factor XII) by a variety of substances including collagen, trypsin, and endotoxin. Activated factor XII in turn catalyzes the conversion of factor XI to its activated form, and the cascade continues in this fashion through factors IX and X. Activated factor X accelerates the conversion of prothrombin to thrombin, and thrombin cleaves fibrinopeptide A from fibrinogen to form fibrin monomer. Thrombin also activates factor XIII to cross-link the soluble fibrin monomers to form stabilized, insoluble fibrin clot.

The extrinsic pathway is initiated with the release of thromboplastin (tissue factor) from injured endothelial cells, catalyzing the activation of factor X. The coagulation cascade then proceeds through the common pathway to terminate in the formation of insoluble fibrin polymer.

There are several other factors that are important in coagulation mechanisms. Proteins C and S are vitamin K–dependent factors that inactivate factors V and VIII and, as such, function as natural anticoagulants. Calcium (factor IV) is instrumental in the activation of almost all the coagulation reactions, explaining the anticoagulant mechanism of calcium chelators such as ethylenediaminetetraacetate (EDTA) and citrate-phosphate-dextrose compounds. High-molecular-weight kininogen functions with prekallikrein to orient factors XII and XI on negatively charged surfaces to potentiate their activation.

Platelet Deposition. Platelets represent membrane-bound cytoplasmic remnants of bone marrow megakaryocytes. Platelet function is essential in the sealing of vascular defects through the formation of a platelet plug. The intact endothelium normally conceals the adhesive glycoproteins (von Willebrand factor, fibronectin, and collagen) from the blood elements, thereby limiting platelet adhesion to sites of vessel injury. Endothelial damage results in platelet adhesion on the vessel wall, as von Willebrand factor binds to exposed subendothelial collagen and platelet membrane glycoproteins Ib and IIb/IIIa to form a bridge between collagen and the platelet.

Platelet activation follows adhesion, mediated by such agents as ADP, thromboxane A_2, collagen, epinephrine, and thrombin. Platelet arachidonic acid is released from membrane phospholipid and is metabolized by cyclooxygenase to prostaglandins G_2 and H_2, a process blocked by aspirin. These prostaglandin intermediaries are subsequently converted to the potent platelet-aggregating agent thromboxane A_2. Thromboxane A_2 produces platelet activation by interacting with a receptor located on the surface of platelets; thus it must exit from the platelet to bind to the same or a neighboring platelet in order to be effective.

Activated platelets undergo a process known as the *release reaction,* with migration of platelet granules to the cell membrane and release of their contents. The alpha granule contains fibrinogen, platelet factor 4, platelet-derived growth factor, von Willebrand factor, and fibronectin. The secretion of these agents from the platelet amplifies the process of activation, resulting in stimulation of neighboring platelets and initiation of platelet aggregation. It is important to note that the arachidonic acid pathway is not absolutely required for platelet activation. Although aspirin-treated platelets cannot generate thromboxane A_2, two agonists, thrombin and collagen, can cause the release of the contents of platelet storage granules even when the arachidonic acid pathway is blocked.

Platelet aggregation occurs through platelet-platelet cohesive attachment, principally by means of a mechanism involving fibrinogen and platelet glycoprotein IIb/IIIa. Glycoprotein IIb/IIIa is the platelet receptor most densely distributed on the cell membrane, with up to 50,000 molecules present on a stimulated platelet. Glycoprotein IIb/IIIa is unique in its ability to bind multiple ligands, including von Willebrand factor and fibrinogen. The explanation for this finding relates to the presence of a binding site for the tripeptide arginine-glycine-aspartic acid (RGD using the single-letter peptide nomenclature), a sequence that is present in all ligands that bind to the receptor. Through its RDG site, fibrinogen binds to the glycoprotein IIb/IIIa receptors of two platelets and forms a bridge between the two platelets, initiating the process of platelet-to-platelet attachment and formation of a platelet plug.

Thrombolysis. Thrombolysis of formed clot involves the actions of plasmin, a proteolytic enzyme generated by the activation of plasminogen. Activators of plasminogen are present in the endothelium and the plasma [tissue plasminogen activator (TPA)] and can be prepared from bacterial sources (streptokinase) or renal parenchymal cell culture techniques (urokinase). Factor XIIa and prekallikrein also activate plasminogen. Inhibition of plasmin occurs principally through the actions of α_2-antiplasmin. The binding of free plasma plasmin to antiplasmin is critical to the physiologic control of thrombolysis to prevent a systemic fibrinolytic state.

Plasmin lyses both fibrinogen and fibrin to produce proteolytic fragments X, Y, and A through E. Laboratory confirmation of thrombolysis is accomplished by measuring the level of generic fibrin degradation products or of *D dimer,* a unique fragment formed by the covalent binding of two fragment D moieties.

Pathophysiology of Arterial Obstruction

Blood flow in the extremities follows the physical principles of fluid dynamics as described in Bernoulli's principle, which describes the energy changes of liquids flowing in pipes and Poiseuille's law, which describes the effects of viscosity on blood flow. A full explanation of these laws and the impact of the variables in the circulation is beyond the scope of this text. There are, however, a number of concepts that are necessary for understanding the basic pathophysiology of arterial occlusive disease.

Critical Arterial Stenosis. Reductions in pressure and flow (energy loss) do not occur until the cross-sectional area of a vessel is reduced by more than 75 percent. Precise measurements of area reduction due to a stenosis are difficult to obtain, however, because many plaques are irregular. If the lesion is concentric, a 75 percent area reduction corresponds to a diameter reduction of 50 percent. Losses in energy also depend on the velocity of blood flow across the stenosis, so a critical stenosis varies with the resistance of the runoff bed. In the coronary and carotid systems where peripheral resistances are low, a critical stenosis may be reached with less lumenal narrowing than in higher-resistance circuits. This phenomenon explains how an iliac artery lesion that looks insignificant on arteriography can severely restrict a patient during exercise when the resistance in the runoff bed is reduced.

The length of a stenosis is far less important than its diameter. Length effects energy losses related to viscosity. Length enters Poiseuille's equation in the first power whereas radius is elevated to the fourth power. Doubling the length of a stenosis would double the energy loss, but halving the radius would increase the losses by a factor of 16. A considerable energy loss also occurs at the exit from a stenosis where the losses are related to the fourth power of the diameter ratio of the unstenosed to the stenosed vessel. Thus separate stenoses of equal diameter are more significant than a single stenosis of the same diameter whose length equals the sum of the lengths of the two independent lesions.

Collateral Circulation. Flow reduction to the runoff bed distal to a stenosis is dependent on the collateral network, a group of preexisting pathways that enlarge as a stenosis develops in the main arterial supply. Collateral pathways provide flow distal to an occlusion at times sufficient to preserve viability. This perfusion never achieves normal levels because the resistance of the collateral bed always exceeds that of the major artery. The resistance in the collateral bed is fixed because of the smaller diameter of its vessels which negates the vasodilatory effect of exercise, sympathectomy, or vasoactive drugs in the setting of a major arterial occlusion.

Autoregulation. The blood vessels in skeletal muscles are innervated by vasoconstrictor and vasodilator nerve fibers, but these actions are superseded by locally produced metabolites. The term *autoregulation* refers to the ability of vascular beds to provide for a constant blood flow regardless of perfusion pressures. This adaptability is due to a myogenic response of the vessel wall to the local chemical environment. The mechanism fails and flow is not maintained when perfusion pressures fall below 20 to 30 mmHg for skeletal muscle and 50 to 60 mmHg for the brain.

Effect of Exercise. Resting blood flow is decreased in patients with ischemic rest pain. The resting blood flow in patients with intermittent claudication is usually normal because of the collateral circulation and autoregulation. These compensatory mechanisms may even produce an increase in flow during exercise but not one sufficient to meet the local demands of the tissues. As the intramuscular arterioles dilate, resistance falls and flow is maintained or even increased. This results in a fall in pressure distal to the obstructing lesion and explains the finding that palpable pulses may disappear after exercise in some patients with proximal arterial stenoses. The pulse disappears because of the energy loss associated with the increased flow velocities across the high-resistance collateral bed. The mean pressure falls when a stenosis reaches the critical level.

DIAGNOSIS OF OCCLUSIVE ARTERIAL DISEASE

Clinical Manifestations

The patient who presents with symptoms of peripheral vascular disease is likely to have coronary artery disease as well. More than 50 percent of the mortality following arterial reconstruction of any type is due to cardiac disease. Hertzer and colleagues performed coronary arteriograms on 1000 consecutive patients undergoing elective vascular procedures and found that over 90 percent of these patients had evidence of coronary artery disease. Triple-vessel disease was identified in 30 percent of these patients. Despite the high prevalence of coronary disease in the patient with peripheral vascular disease, routine coronary arteriography has not been found to be an efficient method of screening. The risk of perioperative cardiac morbidity can, however, be predicted with the Goldman Cardiac Risk Index, stratifying patients on the basis of age, type and setting of operation, general medical condition, cardiac history and findings on electrocardiogram (ECG). The sensitivity of the Goldman index is not as high as originally suggested, and many patients at high risk for perioperative morbidity will escape detection. Current recommendations for preoperative cardiac evaluation are discussed in the section on aneurysms but apply to all types of elective arterial reconstruction.

Acute Arterial Occlusion. Patients with acute arterial occlusion often seek treatment promptly because of the catastrophic nature of their symptoms. It is essential that the treating physician respond rapidly because the process may quickly become irreversible. There is no fixed time after acute occlusion that ischemia is irreversible and reperfusion no longer indicated. The time interval depends on the preocclusive state, i.e., the status of the collaterals. Examination of the extremity is therefore the single most important determinant of urgency.

The P's of Acute Ischemia. The cardinal features of acute arterial ischemia each begin with the letter "p." They are pulselessness, pallor, poikilothermia, pain, paresthesia, and paralysis.

The diagnosis of acute arterial ischemia is made and the site of occlusion is localized by the absence of pulses on physical examination. Pulses will not be palpable, and they may or may not be detectable with Doppler ultrasound. The degree of collaterial circulation around the occlusion determines whether an audible signal is present and the urgency of revascularization. An embolic occlusion in a previously intact circuit will be poorly collateralized whereas a thrombotic occlusion of a stenotic vessel should be well collateralized. Pallor is associated with decreased skin perfusion and often is accompanied by poikilothermia or a sense of coldness.

Pain is present in the vast majority of patients with acute ischemia. It is not a reliable criterion in an asensate extremity, in a patient on mechanical ventilation, or in an unconscious patient. In these situations the other signs of acute ischemia must be relied upon. The severity of the pain will vary with the degree of collateral circulation.

The tissues in the extremities that are most sensitive to ischemia are the peripheral nerve endings. Therefore, the most important signs for evaluating the degree of ischemia are the neurologic ones, namely paresthesia and paralysis. An extremity that is paralyzed from ischemia will certainly develop gangrene if left untreated. The earliest neurologic findings in the acutely ischemic lower extremity are in the distribution of the peroneal nerve and consist of hypesthesia in the first metatarsal space, inability to dorsiflex the great toe, and eventually a foot drop. Immediate revascularization is indicated when any of these neurologic signs is present.

Chronic Arterial Ischemia. ***Clinical History.*** Chronic arterial ischemia is almost always due to atherosclerotic occlusive disease and can be defined as a state when tissue perfusion is inadequate to meet the metabolic demands of the end organ. This may only occur when the demands are increased, such as during exercise, and produce the symptom of intermittent claudication, the most common complaint of patients with chronic arterial ischemia. Pain is felt during exercise in the region of large muscle groups distal to an arterial occlusion or stenosis and gradually disappears as the activity ceases. Walking tolerance decreases as the degree of arterial insufficiency increases. The symptom of intermittent claudication does not indicate that the extremity is immediately threatened. It does indicate, however, that the patient has a mortality rate from cardiovascular disease of up to 15 times that of persons without peripheral arterial occlusive disease over a 10-year period. This mandates a careful assessment and treatment of any underlying cardiovascular disease including risk factor modification.

When metabolic needs cannot be met at rest, a state of critical ischemia is said to exist and revascularization is indicated to avoid tissue loss. This may take the form of ischemic rest pain, nonhealing ulcerations, or frank gangrene. Ischemic rest pain is a constant burning type of pain that typically involves the distal foot, occurs when the foot is elevated, and is relieved when the foot is dependent. Rest pain can be distinguished from other types of severe foot pain because patients with other causes such as diabetic neuropathy do not have the same positional dependency.

Physical Examination. The diagnosis, site of occlusion, and extent of disease can almost always be determined by physical examination of the patient. A complete vascular exam involves inspection, auscultation, and palpation. Inspection evaluates the skin for color changes and integrity, the status of the nails, and the absence of hair. The stethoscope is used over the neck, abdomen, and groin and the blood pressure is taken in both arms. Upper (brachial, radial, and ulnar) and lower extremity (femoral, popliteal, posterior tibial, and dorsalis pedis) pulses are palpated, and the character and presence are noted. The abdomen is palpated for both the presence and character of the pulse. The legs are elevated for 2 min, and the color of the feet is noted. Normally perfused extremities do not blanch whereas those with significant ischemia will blanch with elevation. The legs are then lowered and the time it takes for capillary filling to occur is noted. Finally, the legs are placed in a dependent position. Severely ischemic feet will exhibit a cherry-red discoloration known as dependent rubor.

Noninvasive Vascular Studies

Noninvasive vascular diagnosis has emerged as an important tool both in the preoperative assessment and postoperative follow-up of patients with peripheral vascular disease. Improvements in instrumentation and techniques have resulted in the development of low-cost, low-risk, reproducible methods of accurately defining the anatomic and physiologic significance of lesions of the peripheral vascular system.

The Doppler ultrasonic flow detector is the most ubiquitous instrument used in vascular diagnosis. This instrument detects the frequency shift of ultrasound from moving particles in the blood and processes them in a variety of ways ranging from an audible sound to a color-flow map as a component of a Duplex scanner. This technique offers the advantages of low cost and simplicity. Its major disadvantage is that it does not detect disease in the absence of hemodynamic alterations. This shortcoming is most relevant in the noninvasive evaluation of the cerebrovascular system where nonstenotic plaques may be clinically important. The combination of real-time B-mode scanning and Doppler spectral analysis is referred to as Duplex scanning and is the most accurate method of detecting and following vascular lesions. In addition to providing an image of vascular lesion, it also allows for the estimation of blood flow. The major disadvantage of Duplex scanning is its high cost.

Plethysmography was once the mainstay of noninvasive diagnosis but has been replaced by the direct imaging modalities. Plethysmography detects changes in volume associated with cardiac contractions. Inferences concerning the vascular status are made from the character of the pulse wave. This modality is most often utilized for measuring segmental limb blood pressures and ophthalmic artery pressures.

Segmental Blood Pressure. A normal patient will have an ankle systolic blood pressure equal to or greater than the arm pressure which can be expressed as a ratio known as the ankle/brachial index (ABI). A reduction in the ABI indicates a hemodynamically significant stenosis or occlusion. Patients with claudication usually have an ABI of 0.5 to 0.7. Patients with critical ischemia have an ABI of less than 0.5 and an absolute ankle pressure of less than 50 mmHg. When the ABI is reduced, segmental pressure measurements are performed by placing blood pressure cuffs on the high thigh, lower thigh, midcalf, and ankle to identify the site of the lesion producing the pressure gradient. Patients with diabetes or end-stage renal disease may have vessels that are not compressible, rendering the test uninterpretable. In this situation, plethysmography is more accurate than pressure measurements. Additional information can be obtained by exercising the patient which exacerbates a pressure gradient in patients with vascular lesions and has no effect on normals.

Duplex Scanning. This state-of-the-art technique evaluates velocity disturbances and provides a real-time image of the blood vessel in question. The velocity information is displayed on an oscilloscope so that the individual frequency components of the signal can be analyzed. By coupling this to the real-time image and using pulsed-Doppler techniques, discrete sample volumes from the midstream of the artery are processed and examined for flow abnormalities that characterize the physiologic disturbance. Recent advances in color-flow imaging depict the flow channel as well as the arterial wall and Doppler spectrum.

Arteriography

Significant advances in contrast media, catheter systems, and imaging techniques provide the essential information about arterial anatomy that makes definitive therapy possible.

Contrast Media. Current ionic contrast agents utilize iodine attached to water-soluble carrier molecules. Many of their adverse side effects are related to a high concentration of sodium or meglumine. Contrast agents are excreted in the kidney, and patients, particularly those with diabetes, with underlying renal dysfunction are at higher risk for complications. Extreme caution must be used when the serum creatinine is greater than 4.5 mg/dL and all patients must be well-hydrated prior to the study. Neurotoxicity with seizures, cortical blindness, or frank stroke can occur particularly with the concentrated (<60 percent weight/volume) sodium-containing agents. Newer agents have osmolalities of 600 to 900 mO/kg as compared to the conventional agents with osmolalities of 2000 mO/kg. The low-osmolality agents have clear advantages but cost considerably more than the conventional agents (25 times). A policy of routine use of low osmolality agents across the United States would add at least 1.5 billion dollars to health care costs per annum.

Idiosyncratic contrast reactions with asthma, laryngeal edema or spasm, and cardiovascular collapse occur infrequently. These reactions are independent of dose. Although there is no reliable sensitivity test for these reactions, it is known that alcoholics, those allergic to iodine, and those with prior serious reactions are more likely to be affected. The absence of a reaction does not ensure that one will not occur with reexposure. Since these reactions appear to be immune-related, prophylactic steroids and antihistamines are administered to high-risk patients. Low-osmolality agents should be used in any patient at high risk for a contrast reaction.

Complications. The common femoral and the axillary arteries are the preferred sites of catheterization. The percutaneous technique described by Seldinger is used by most angiographers. A guide wire is advanced under fluoroscopic control to the appropriate site and a catheter is advanced over the wire. Iatrogenic damage following arterial catheterization may present as hemorrhage, dissection, thrombosis, embolus, false aneurysm, or arteriovenous fistula (Fig. 20-1). The reported incidence of these injuries varies from 1 to 2 percent for diagnostic procedures and up to 44 percent for therapeutic procedures.

Prompt diagnosis and intervention are necessary for successful treatment of these complications which are increasing in incidence as the larger-catheter systems required for endovascular manipulations are used. The critical risk factors are the size of the catheter and sheath, the site and method of puncture, and the duration of the procedure. Large, stiff catheter systems, axillary artery punctures, sheaths left in place for hours and days, and use of anticoagulants or fibrinolytic agents are all associated with a higher incidence of complications. There is an inverse relationship between the number of procedures performed and the complication rate.

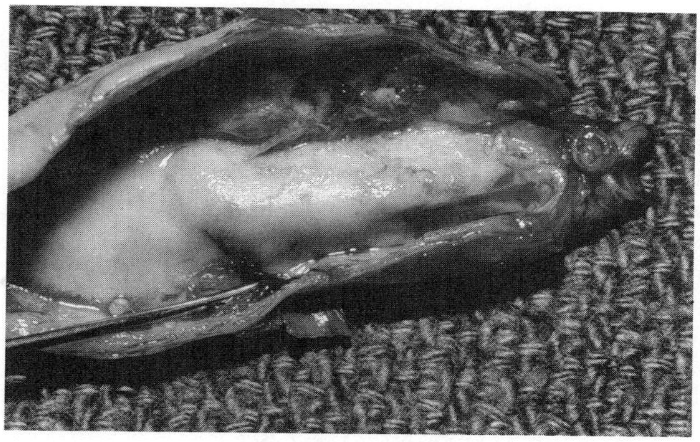

FIG. 20-1. Resected external iliac artery with a probe through a false channel made by a balloon dilatation catheter. The artery was unintentionally dilated in the false channel, and this resulted in acute thrombosis. An emergency operation for correction of the ischemia was required.

The treatment must be tailored to the injury and the general condition of the patient. A large pulsating hematoma in a patient with an acute myocardial infarction who has recently undergone fibrinolytic therapy followed by percutaneous coronary angioplasty presents a different set of challenges than a femoral artery thrombosis following arteriography for claudication in an otherwise healthy patient. The principles of operative repair are discussed in the section on trauma.

Interpretation. Since atherosclerotic plaques typically form at bifurcations, multiple views are necessary to view these bifurcations in profile. This is particularly important in viewing the bifurcations of the common carotid, femoral, and iliac arteries. Simultaneous biplane arteriography minimizes the chance of missing a significant lesion because of vessel overlap but is not always available or possible. Therefore, several injections may be necessary while filming in different obliquities to open up bifurcations. Occasionally vessels will not fill and are considered occluded because the volume of contrast is inadequate or the exposure is too early after injection. If occlusion is diagnosed, contrast must either opacify the distal portion or a branch of the occluded vessel. This may require delayed filming. Digital recording techniques have improved visualization of distal vessels and reduced interpretive errors due to nonvisualization.

ANEURYSMS

Classification

An aneurysm is an irreversible dilatation of an artery to at least one and one-half times its normal diameter. The dangers of pulsatile swellings whose "bright red blood . . . spurted forth with much violence" have been known since the writings of Galen. Aneurysms may involve all layers of the arterial wall (true aneurysm) or only a portion of the vessel wall or surrounding tissue (false aneurysm). Aneurysms can be classified into nonspecific, traumatic, dissecting, mycotic, anastomotic, childhood, and those associated with pregnancy. Whatever the cause, once an aneurysm is formed, it tends to enlarge and may ultimately produce serious if not lethal consequences.

Rupture occurs when the tangential stress at any point exceeds the tensile strength of the wall. Arterial wall strength is dependent on collagen whose tensile strength is ordinarily far in excess of the wall tension. The collagen content of aneurysmal vessels is reduced compared to atherosclerotic and normal vessels, however, placing a greater load on each fiber. Laplace's law, which relates the tensile stress to wall pressure and radius, traditionally has been used to explain why large aneurysms rupture. The stress on the arterial wall is best expressed as a relationship between pressure times radius divided by the wall thickness, a modification of Laplace's law which is only applicable to thin-walled structures where the difference between inside and outside radius is negligible.

Nonspecific Aneurysms. The most common type of aneurysm has been called atherosclerotic, but since the role of atherosclerosis in aneurysmal disease is unclear, the term "nonspecific" is more appropriate. Many consider these aneurysms as degenerative due to an arterial aging process. This view is supported by histologic evidence that demonstrates degeneration of the arterial wall. The intima is usually absent and replaced with compacted fibrin in multiple layers; the media has fragmented and reduced numbers of elastic lamellae; and, most importantly, there is focal loss of elastic tissue. Normal aortic tissue contains 12 percent elastin whereas aneurysmal aortic tissue has only 1 percent elastin. Biochemical data suggest that aneurysm pathogenesis may be related to a systemic connective tissue disorder. An imbalance between the two enzymes important in the metabolism of elastin, elastase (degradation) and α_1-antitrypsin (synthesis), has been identified in patients with aneurysms as compared to occlusive disease. This imbalance becomes even more pronounced in multiple aneurysms and ruptured aneurysm.

Traumatic Aneurysms. Many early descriptions of aneuryms dealt with traumatic or false aneurysms. Currently most traumatic aneurysms are due to arterial catheterization or penetrating injuries. These lesions are characterized by a focal defect in the arterial wall with the hemorrhage controlled by the surrounding tissues. With time a fibrous capsule forms around the hematoma, but a definite risk of rupture is present because the surrounding tissues cannot always withstand arterial pressures and contain the hemorrhage.

True aneurysms can occur following hemodynamic trauma. Aneurysms due to poststenotic dilatation are most often seen in thoracic outlet syndrome distal to a cervical rib, distal to coarctation of the aorta, and distal to aortic or pulmonary valvular stenoses (Fig. 20-2). These aneurysms do not have any preexisting defect but become dilated as a result of the increased lateral wall pressure according to Bernoulli's theorem. Once dilated, these arteries progressively enlarge according to Laplace's law.

Dissecting Aneurysms. The primary pathologic process in a dissecting aneurysm is a longitudinal splitting of the layers of the arterial wall. The entry tear usually extends through the intima and inner two-thirds of the media creating a false channel. External rupture of the outer wall is more common than internal rupture or reentry into the arterial lumen. Hypertension is found in 75 percent of patients with arterial dissections. Other less common causes are pregnancy, Marfan's syndrome, cystic medial necrosis, blunt trauma, cardiopulmonary bypass, and Ehlers-Danlos syndrome.

Mycotic Aneurysms. Infected or mycotic aneurysms can occur anywhere in the body as a consequence of either a blood-borne infection (intravascular) or an infection introduced from outside (extravascular). Blood-borne mycotic aneurysms can be further divided into those preexisting aneurysms that become secondarily infected and those mycotic aneurysms secondary to microbial arteritis. The classic type of this latter entity is the syphylitic aneurysm now rarely seen in the Western world but formerly the cause of over 50 percent of all aneurysms. The only other bacteria with an affinity for arterial walls are *Salmonella* and *Staphylococcus,* which are now the most common organisms cultured from mycotic aneurysms. Infection of a preexisting aneurysm is unusual even though nonspecific aortic aneurysms often grow bacteria from cultured intravascular thrombi.

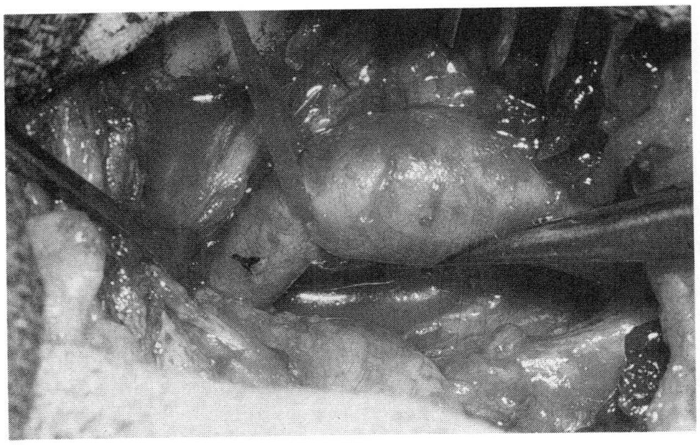

FIG. 20-2. An operative photograph of a fusiform subclavian artery aneurysm secondary to a large bony cervical rib. This exposure was obtained after resection of the medial third of the clavicle. The patient presented with an ischemic hand from embolization. The involved artery was resected and replaced with a segment of saphenous vein. A cervical sympathectomy was also performed because the emboli were irretrievable.

The most common type of extravascular infected aneurysm follows a penetrating injury that contaminates the arterial puncture site and infects the resultant hematoma. Common in the era of bloodletting, the incidence of these aneurysms is increasing again because of our drug culture. Another form of extravascular infected aneurysm is the infected anastomotic aneurysm. Contamination can occur at the time of operation, from erosion of the graft material into the gastrointestinal tract, or from a contiguous hematoma secondarily infected from systemic sepsis.

Mycotic aneurysms should be suspected in patients with sepsis and with inflammatory changes around a pulsatile mass. Intravenous antibiotics are begun based on results of blood cultures and clinical history. Since rupture carries a high morbidity and mortality, emergent operation is indicated after the necessary preparations.

Principles of Operation. The first operative decision is whether revascularization is necessary to prevent tissue loss. If so, a planned two-stage procedure is recommended. The initial stage creates an extraanatomic bypass in a remote operative field through uninfected tissues using autogenous tissue if possible. The second stage consists of resection of the infected arterial segment, debridement of surrounding tissues, and irrigation and drainage with a closed perfusion system of 0.1% betadine solution. If the clinical situation precludes a first-stage remote bypass or the need for revascularization is not certain, the infected aneurysm is approached directly. The same principles of wide excision, debridement, and irrigation are utilized. If revascularization is necessary, it is done so through uninfected tissues immediately after the wounds are closed and all gowns, gloves, drapes, and instruments are changed. Antibiotics are continued for 6 months. Patients with *Salmonella* infections are placed on lifelong treatment.

Anastomotic Aneurysms. Since primary healing of a prosthetic anastomosis never occurs, anastomotic integrity is solely due to the strength of the suture line. Anastomotic aneurysms are the result of a separation between a graft and the host artery that becomes encapsulated with fibrous tissue. These false aneurysms contain no elements of the arterial wall. Most anastomotic aneurysms (80 percent) involve the common femoral artery after aortofemoral bypass.

Etiology. Any suture material that is degradable or easily broken can produce an anastomotic aneurysm. Silk has been abandoned as a vascular suture material because of its high incidence of failure and subsequent anastomotic breakdown. Polypropylene and braided Dacron are currently the most commonly used suture materials in vascular reconstructions and have not been associated with this complication.

In some instances the sutures may remain intact but pull out of the artery. This may occur when the sutures fail to incorporate sufficient amounts of arterial tissue, when there is excessive tension on the anastomosis from a graft that has been cut too short, and when there is degeneration of the artery or a low-grade infection at the anastomosis. An artery that has undergone endarterectomy does not have the same tensile strength as the original artery and care must be taken to take sufficiently large bites of tissue to prevent disruption.

Biologic grafts treated with formaldehyde and more recently gluteraldehyde to prevent rejection are all subject to aneurysmal degeneration. Some of the original prosthetic materials such as Vinyon, nylon, and Orlon quickly lost tensile strength and were abandoned. Dacron has withstood the time test and is the preferred material today. Autogenous grafts are the least apt to develop aneurysms. Saphenous vein has a 4 percent incidence of aneurysm when used in the extremities but a higher incidence when used in the aortorenal position. The conduit least likely to become aneurysmal is autogenous artery.

Diagnosis. Most patients present with a painless pulsatile groin mass. Rupture into surrounding tissues is unusual except when the aortic anastomosis is involved (10 percent). Ultrasonography confirms the diagnosis. Arteriography is necessary to delineate the outflow. Anastomotic aneurysms require repair because they may thrombose, embolize, or rupture.

Treatment. In the case of involvement of the femoral anastomosis, the graft often has retracted into the retroperitoneum. An interposition graft between the old graft limb and the femoral artery is required. This means that control of the graft limb should be obtained under the inguinal ligament. Most of these patients (65 percent) will have associated occlusions of the superficial femoral artery and should have a profundaplasty.

False aneurysms involving an aortic graft usually occur after an end-to-side proximal anastomosis. Rupture into the peritoneal cavity or the duodenum is not unusual. At operation proximal aortic control is best obtained at the supraceliac aorta which is approached through the lesser omentum after division of the crural fibers of the diaphragm (Fig. 20-3). In the absence of infection, the anastomosis is disconnected, the aorta debrided, and an end-to-end anastomosis is created just below the renal arteries using a new interposition graft. A flap of greater omentum is used to cover the new anastomoses. Infection mandates removal of the prosthesis and an extraanatomic bypass.

Aneurysms of Childhood. Aneurysms are rare in children. They are most often attributed to an underlying inherited disorder of connective tissue metabolism but can be acquired as a result of trauma or an arteritis.

Infection. Infectious aneurysms are the most common pediatric aneurysms and usually involve the aorta. Bacterial endocarditis is the most common source of infection, and *Staphylococcus* and *Streptococcus* are the most common bacteria. The aneurysms often develop in the aorta distal to a coarctation. Other predisposing conditions are umbilical artery catheters and bicuspid aortic valves. Prompt resection and reconstruction is indicated because of the high incidence of rupture.

Giant Cell Arteritis. This also affects the aorta and progresses to rupture and death. It is characterized pathologically by immune complex deposition in the vessel wall with complement fixation and neutrophil activation. This produces endothelial injury and transmural arterial ischemia from occlusion of the vasa vasorum. Degeneration and weakening of the vessel wall occur with aneurysm formation and rupture.

Autoimmune Connective Tissue Disease. Children with these aneurysms exhibit the clinical features of an autoimmune process such as polyarteritis nodosa. These aneurysms are less than 3 mm in size and involve the arteries of the kidney, liver, and spleen. Rupture causes symptoms specific to the organ involved but may present as shock from intraperitoneal bleeding. Ligation of the involved artery is indicated.

Kawasaki Disease. This is known as the mucocutaneous lymph node syndrome. The aneurysms occur in the axillobrachial and illofemoral arterial systems. Coronary artery aneurysms occur in 20 to 30 percent of patients and are the most serious manifestation of this disease because of the risk of rupture and sudden death from pericardial tamponade.

Aneurysms Associated with Pregnancy. When aneurysms present during pregnancy, they do so often in the setting of rupture and shock with a mortality rate of 65 percent. Splenic artery aneurysms are the most common followed by aneurysms of the renal and iliac arteries. Pregnancy is also associated with aneurysmal dilatation in the aorta presumably due to weakening of the arterial wall from the hemodynamic stresses of pregnancy and delivery. Matrix and elastic tissue abnormalities in arterial wall have been described during pregnancy which would make the vessel susceptible to rupture.

Abdominal Aortic and Iliac Artery Aneurysms

The infrarenal aorta is the most common site for the development of the nonspecific abdominal aortic aneurysm (AAA), the most common type of aneurysm presenting for treatment. AAAs are normally fusiform in shape and usually arise below the origins of the renal arteries extending a variable distance to and beyond the aortic bifurcation (Fig. 20-4). These aneurysms are found in 2 percent of the elderly population and their incidence is increasing. Males predominate with a ratio of 9:1. There is a definite familial tendency for the development of nonspecific AAAs. The tendency is sex-linked and autosomally inherited. The estimated relative risk for first-degree relatives of affected individuals is 11.6 greater than non–first degree relatives of similar age and sex. Screening with ultrasonography is indicated for relatives of patients with this

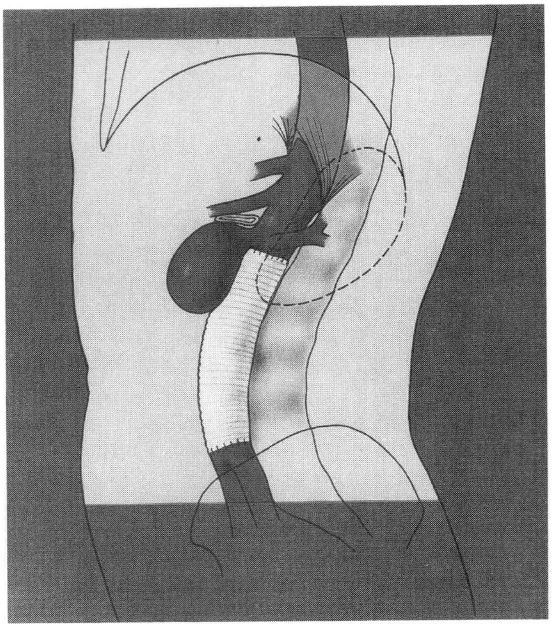

A

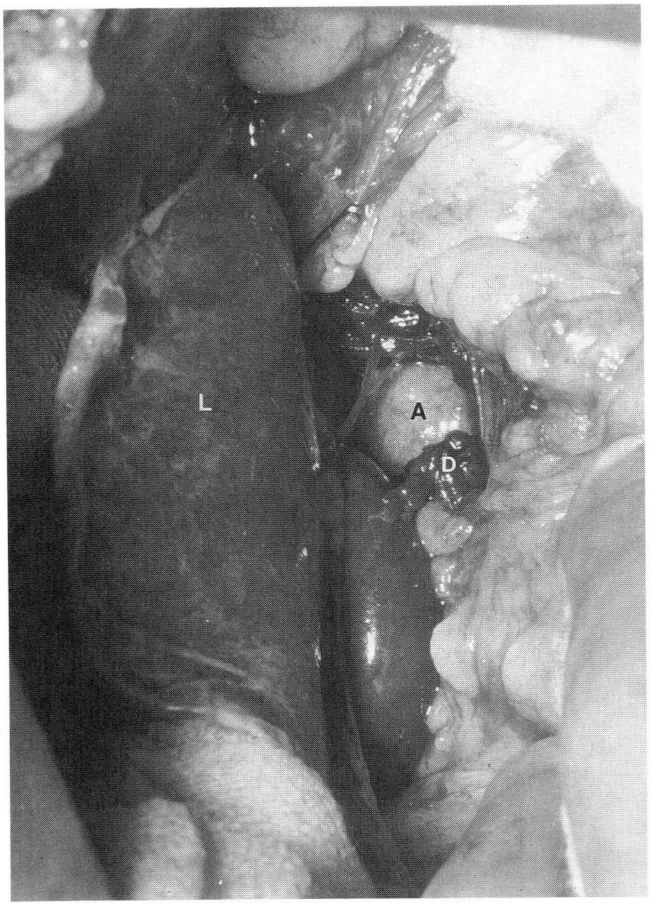

B

FIG. 20-3. *A.* A diagram showing the location of a false aneurysm at the proximal anastomosis of an aortic graft. There is usually no room to control the normal aorta without endangering the renal arteries, left renal vein, or the duodenum. Safe proximal control should be obtained by clamping the supraceliac aorta at the diaphragm *B.* The exposure of the aorta at the diaphragm is done by dividing the triangular liagment, retracting the left lobe of the liver (L) to the right, opening the lesser sac, and dividing the crus of the diaphragm (D). The aorta (A) is mobilized after division of the median arcuate ligament.

lesion. Familial aneurysms tend to occur in individuals at a younger age and affect women more than does the noninherited variety.

Early attempts at repair consisted of wrapping the aneurysm with skin grafts or cellophane, injecting sclerosing agents around the aneurysm, intraluminal wiring, and endoaneurysmorrhaphy, a technique introduced by Matas at the turn of the century. The first successful resection was performed by Dubost in 1951 who restored aortic continuity with a homograft. The modern intrasaccular method of repair was introduced by Creech and DeBakey in 1966. Current indications for operation include prevention of rupture, atheroembolization, associated occlusive disease, or pressure or erosion into contiguous structures.

Risk of Rupture. The decision to recommend resection must balance the immediate risk of operation against the risk of rupture which is directly related to the size of the aneurysm. The natural history of the large aneurysm (>6 cm) was defined by Estes over 30 years ago, and it is generally agreed that these aneurysms should be operated on unless severe comorbid conditions pose unacceptable operative risks or severely limit the patient's life expectancy. The classic study by Szilagyi and coworkers in 1966 clearly demonstrated that the repair of aneurysms greater than 6 cm in diameter prolonged patient survival. Although operations on smaller aneurysms did not prolong survival, in that report the operative mortality was 14 percent, therefore biasing the conclusions toward no operation. Application of current operative mortality rates (2 to 5 percent) would favor resection of even small aneurysms under the proper conditions. Crawford has reported a decline in mortality rates from 19.2 to 1.9 percent over a 25-year period despite a significant increase in operations on high-risk patients.

Less information is available about the natural history of small aneurysms (<6 cm), but there is no question that small aneurysms can rupture. Aneurysms grow an average of 0.45 cm/year, but growth occurs at an uneven rate. In the series by Szilagyi and coworkers, 19.5 percent of aneurysms less than 6 cm ruptured, and these data have been corroborated in more recent series showing a 20 percent risk for rupture in this group over a 5-year period. In a large autopsy study, Darling found that there was a 25 percent rupture rate of aneurysms between 4 and 7 cm and a 9.5 percent rupture rate for aneurysms less than 4 cm.

Raw diameter alone is not a sufficiently accurate predictor of rupture to be used as the sole indication for operation. Cronenwett and coworkers analyzed 30 potential risk factors for a correlation with rupture and found that only diastolic hypertension, initial aneurysm size, and chronic obstructive pulmonary disease were important. The risk of rupture was only 2 percent when the diastolic pressure was less than 75 mmHg, the initial size was less than 3 cm, and there was no reduction in pulmonary function. By contrast, the risk of rupture was 100 percent when the diastolic blood pressure was greater than 105 mmHg, the initial size was greater than 5 cm, and the forced expiratory volume in 1s (FEV_1) was less than 50 percent of the predicted value. Studies have tried

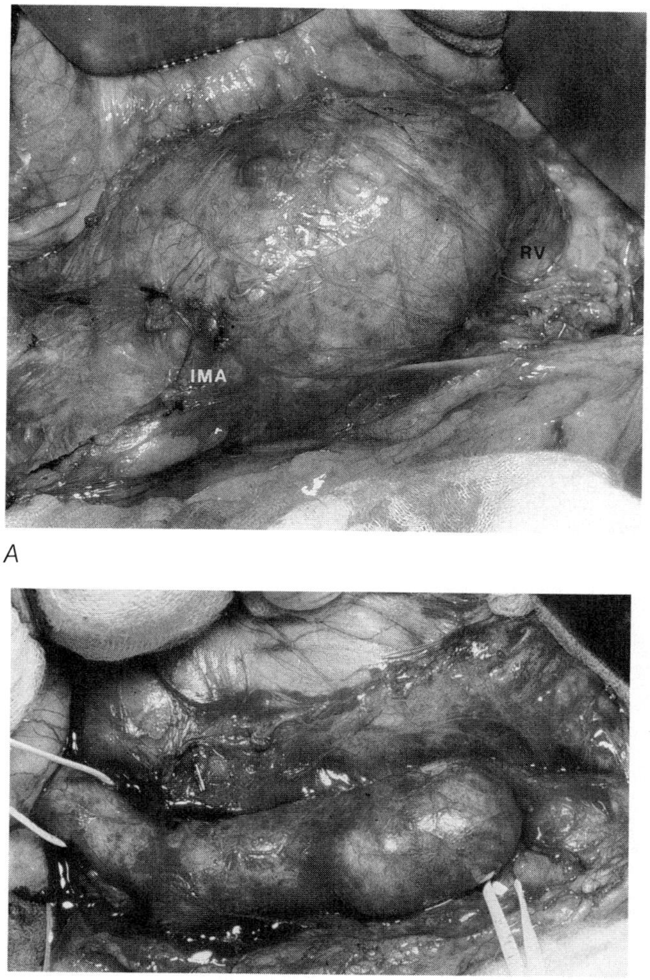

FIG. 20-4. *A.* A large fusiform abdominal aortic aneurysm. The proximal cuff can be seen below the crossing left renal vein (RV). The inferior mesenteric artery (IMA) is isolated. The proximal iliac arteries are ectatic. As these large aneurysms grow the proximal neck angles anteriorly away from the vertebral column facilitating the proximal dissection. *B.* A saccular aortic aneurysm. The aneurysm is confined to the infrarenal aorta below the IMA which is encircled with a vessel loop. Although this process is limited to the anterior surface of the aorta, standard resection and graft replacement are indicated.

to correlate the size of the aorta relative to the size of the patient and the risk for rupture. Ouriel and associates used computed tomography (CT) scanning to measure the transverse diameter of the L-3 vertebral body and calculated a ratio of aortic to vertebral size. Although aneurysms were observed to rupture with diameters as low as 3.5 cm, not one aneurysm ruptured with an aneurysm–to–vertebral-body ratio of less than 1.0. Surgeons should have an elective mortality rate of 1 to 2 percent to justify operation on these small aneurysms since the objective is not only to prevent rupture but also to prolong life.

Diagnostic Evaluation. Most aneurysms (75 percent) are discovered when still asymptomatic, either as a pulsatile mass on physical examination or unexpectedly during the course of an evaluation for an unrelated condition.

Physical Examination. This remains a reliable diagnostic method that is accurate in 88 percent of cases. The infrarenal aorta lies at the level of the umbilicus, so the mass should be felt around the navel. If the lateral borders converge below the costal margins, the aneurysm is probably infrarenal. Thin patients, particularly those with a lordosis have prominent aortas that can be mistaken for aneurysms. An aneurysm can be distinguished from a tortuous aorta because the latter lies to the left and is moveable. An aneurysm can be felt to the right of midline as well as to the left and feels expansile. Size can usually be estimated in a thin patient, and when the diagnosis of aneurysm is made in an obese patient by palpation, the aneurysm is usually larger than 6 cm.

Ultrasonography. The proven accuracy, safety, and low cost of ultrasonography make this the imaging procedure of choice for the diagnosis and follow-up of aneurysms (Fig. 20-5). The variability of the test when performed by the same technician is only 3 mm. Ultrasound can also evaluate blood flow in the renal and visceral arteries. It may not give sufficient information about the juxtarenal aorta or the iliac arteries and may be technically difficult in obese patients and those with excessive intestinal gas.

Computed Tomography. This imaging technique provides an accurate characterization of the entire aorta. New software allows the data to be displayed in a three-dimensional manner (Fig. 20-6). Its accuracy is not influenced by bowel gas or obesity. Furthermore, it provides information about the character and thickness of the aortic wall, the level of the renal arteries relative to the proximal cuff, and the iliac arteries (Fig. 20-7). It is particularly helpful in evaluating patients with symptoms. As little as 10 mL of blood can be detected outside the lumen of the aorta. CT scanning is used in the postoperative period for the evaluation of suspected aortic graft complications.

Magnetic Resonance Imaging. This technique can provide a much more detailed image than that currently available with either ultrasonography or CT scanning. Three-dimensional presentations, showing the aneurysm's lumen and surface anatomy in four separate views, allow the surgeon to visualize the neck, renal arteries, and relationships to other periaortic structures. Unfortunately, progress in vascular imaging with this modality has been limited by lack of appropriate software support, its high cost, and the limitations of scanning obese patients and those with pacemakers.

Arteriography. Although not accurate in determining the size or the presence of an aneurysm, the information provided is helpful in defining associated vascular anatomy, particularly the renal arteries (Fig. 20-8). Many vascular surgeons recommend routine arteriography prior to aneurysm resection, but the issue whether the information learned is worth the cost, discomfort, and potential risk to the patient is unresolved. Arteriographic findings caused a modification of the procedure in 13 to 75 percent of patients usually because of a pathologic condition of the iliac, mesenteric, or renal artery (Fig. 20-9). The data seem to support a selective approach to this diagnostic test with the following indications: (1) suspicion of multiple aneurysms, (2) suspicion of renal or visceral artery involvement, (3) defining upper and lower extent of aneurysm when other tests are inconclusive, (4) hypertension or renal dysfunction, (5) horseshoe kidney, (6) prior colectomy, or (7) peripheral occlusive disease.

Preoperative Cardiac Screening. Cardiac, pulmonary, hepatic, renal, and hematologic screening is essential both in selecting patients for operation, deciding what imaging techniques

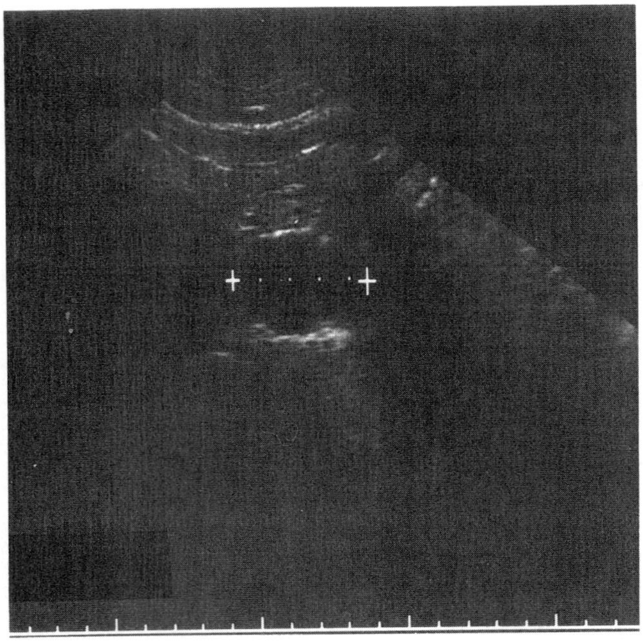

A

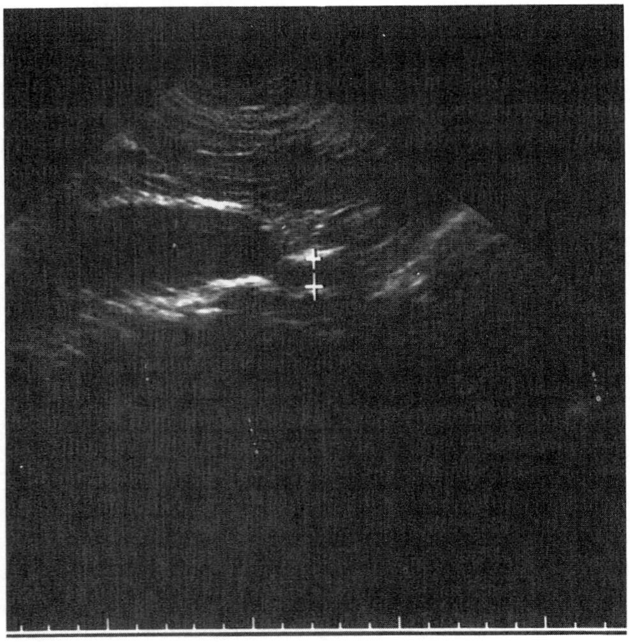

B

FIG. 20-5. Transverse (*A*) and sagittal (*B*) views of an ultrasound of an abdominal aortic aneurysm. Diameters are marked with (+). Ultrasonography is the most cost-effective way to follow the size of the aneurysm. The advantages and limitations of this test are seen. Although the size the aneurysm can be measured, little information is given about the renal or iliac arteries.

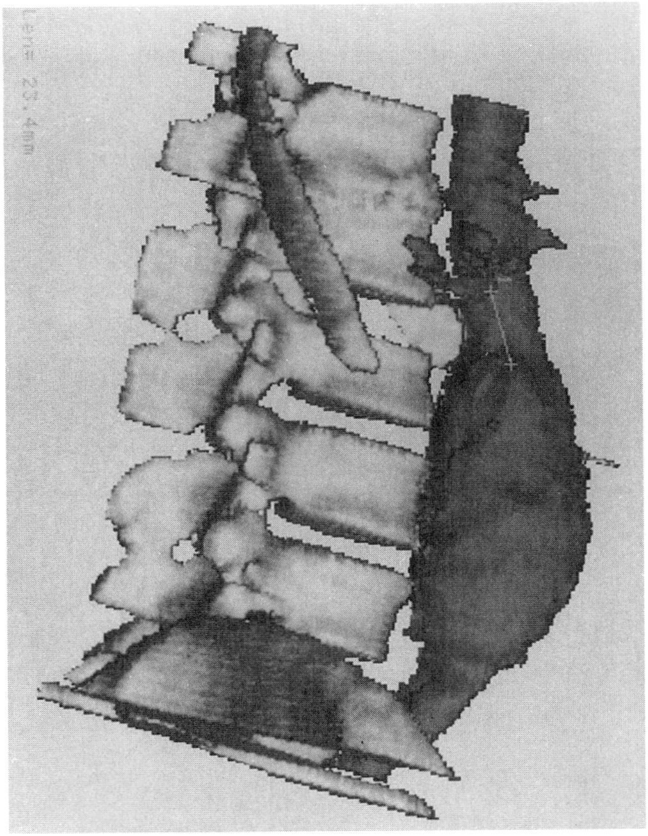

A

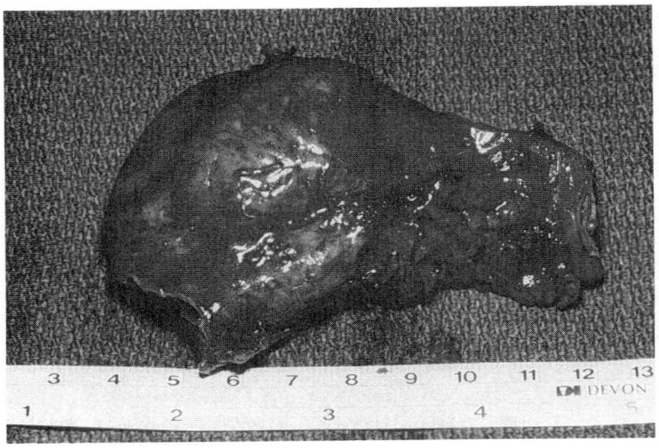

B

FIG. 20-6. *A.* Three-dimensional reconstruction of a CT scan of the abdominal aorta produced on a high-powered video workstation from the digital information obtained on a standard CT scan cut at 5-mm intervals. This technique manipulates the image so that the relationship between the renal arteries and the proximal cuff can be more easily visualized. This technique was originally developed for analyzing intracranial lesions. *B.* This is the resected aneurysm in the same patient showing the accuracy of three-dimensional imaging. The specimen nicely demonstrates the typical anatomy of the infrarenal aortic aneurysm, i.e., a proximal segment of normal aorta below the renal arteries with the aneurysm extending to the aortic bifurcation.

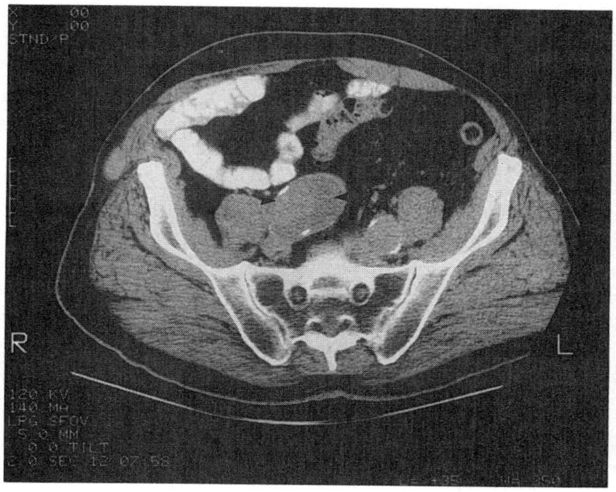

FIG. 20-7. Standard CT scan of the iliac arteries in a patient with an aortic aneurysm diagnosed on ultrasound showing a large and previously unsuspected right iliac artery aneurysm (*arrows*). The oblong shape of this aneurysm is an artifact due to a tangential cut. When an aneurysm is fusiform (which most are), the smaller of the two measurements more accurately defines the true size.

are indicated, and selecting an appropriate incision. Patients with uncorrected coronary artery disease (CAD) undergoing aneurysm resection have an increased risk of myocardial infarction (5 to 10 percent), ischemia-related pulmonary edema (5 to 10 percent), and cardiac death within 30 days (5 to 10 percent). These risks contrast significantly with the 1 to 3 percent cardiac risk in patients without CAD. Preoperative cardiac revascularization has repeatedly been shown to reduce the operative risk in patients with CAD who undergo AAA repair.

Selecting patients at risk for cardiac events has been a difficult task. The Goldman Risk Factor Assessment Index misses up to 50 percent of patients at risk. Exercise-induced ECG ST-segment depression misses a smaller but still significant group. Coronary arteriography is costly and carries some risk and is not appropriate as a screening procedure in an asymptomatic patient. Invasive coronary studies are no longer necessary to discover these high-risk patients because of recent advances in the area of noninvasive cardiac imaging with thallium 201. Patients can be stressed on a treadmill or given dipyridamole, a coronary vasodilator. Interpretation of this test is based on selective regional uptake of isotope as a marker of perfusion. Normally perfused myocardium has a homogeneous uptake, old infarcts do not take up isotope even on delayed scans, and ischemic areas of viable myocardium exhibit delayed uptake, referred to as redistribution. Patients with redistribution are at increased risk (15 to 35 percent) for a postoperative cardiac event. Other markers of increased cardiac risk are angina pectoris, Q waves on ECG, a history of ventricular ectopy, and diabetes mellitus.

The following approach should minimize cardiac risk in patients undergoing aneurysm resection. Patients without a cardiac history and with a normal ECG (30 to 40 percent of AAA patients) can proceed to operation without further work-up. Patients with clinically evident but stable cardiac disease (50 to 60 percent of AAA patients) should have a cardiac perfusion and function (echocardiography) study performed. When two or more clinical factors and significant thallium redistribution are present, the patient

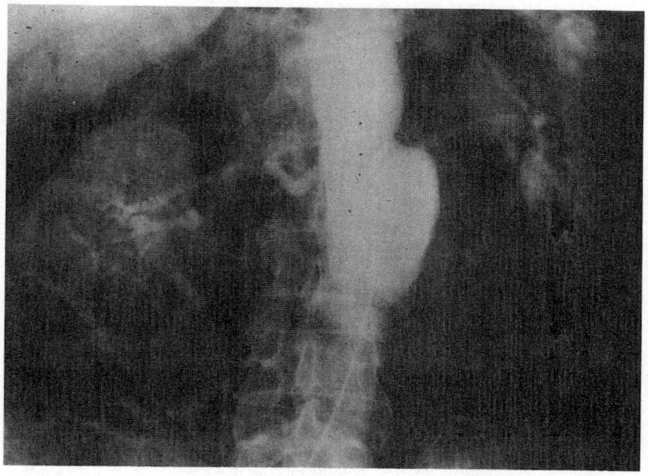

A

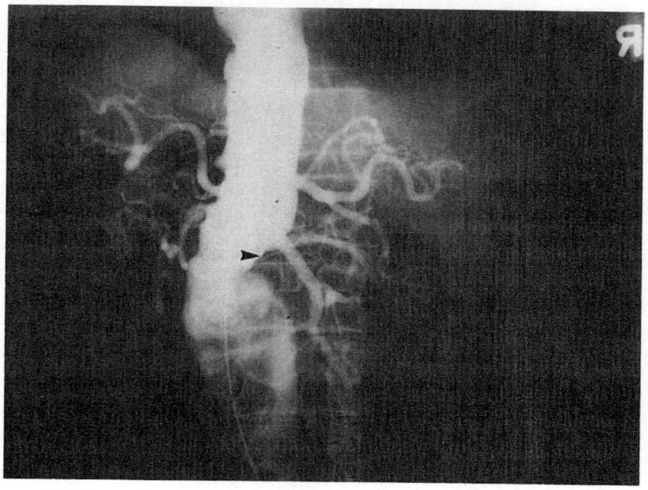

B

FIG. 20-8. *A.* This AP aortogram shows how the anterior angulation of the neck of the aneurysm can obscure the origin of the renal arteries. This view does not provide information about the proximal extent of the aneurysm. *B.* When the relationship between the renal arteries and the proximal extent of the aneurysm is in doubt, a lateral aortogram is necessary. This aortogram shows that a cuff does exist below the renal artery.

should undergo coronary arteriography. Coronary revascularization is indicated prior to AAA repair when there is three-vessel disease or left main stenosis. Patients with mild symptoms, good ventricular function, and normal to mildly abnormal thallium scans can undergo AAA resection with appropriate cardiac monitoring. Patients with clinically severe cardiac disease can bypass noninvasive testing and proceed directly to catheterization and cardiac repair. AAA repair can follow percutaneous coronary dilatation within 10 to 14 days and coronary bypass or valve repair within 6 to 8 weeks. When both the heart and the AAA are symptomatic, combined repair can be performed.

Operation. ***Perioperative Management.*** Significant advances have been made in the anesthetic and medical management of these patients. Patients are volume-loaded beginning at midnight prior to operation. Epidural catheters are used to reduce the amount of anesthetic agent required, to allow for prompt extuba-

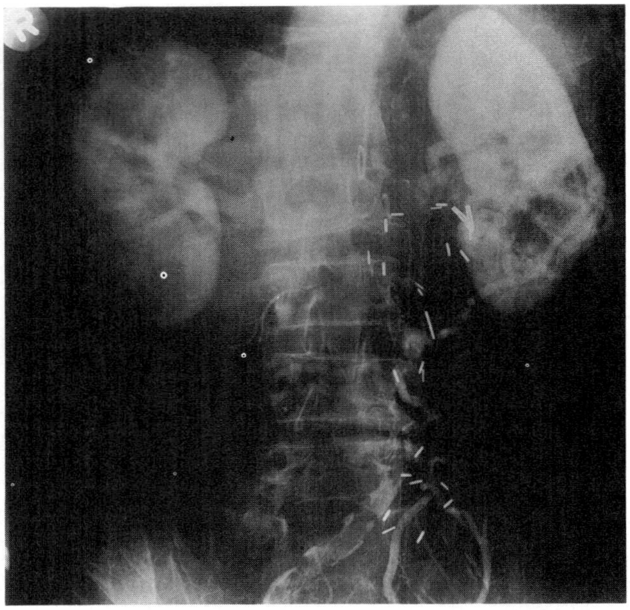

FIG. 20-9. This aortogram shows a meandering mesenteric artery. This may indicate that the inferior mesenteric artery (IMA) is an important vessel and that reimplantation into the body of the aortic graft is necessary. Alternatively, it may indicate that the IMA is occluded and that this represents a large collateral from the superior mesenteric artery. If there is significant backbleeding from the orifice of the IMA when the aneurysm is opened, the latter situation is likely. If little or no backbleeding is noted and the orifice is patent, the IMA should be reimplanted as a Carrel patch.

tion, and to control pain in the postoperative period. Swan-Ganz catheters are used in patients with a cardiac history. Patients are volume-loaded prior to clamping with crystalloid after vasodilatation with nitroglycerin. Blood is returned to the patient with an autotransfusion system to reduce the need for banked blood. Cefazolin or an antibiotic equivalently effective against *Staphylococcus aureus* is administered prior to and for 3 days following operation.

Incision. The choice between a midline transperitoneal or a retroperitoneal approach to the infrarenal abdominal aorta is usually a matter of surgeon preference. Each offers advantages, and the preferable approach varies from patient to patient. The transperitoneal approach is obligatory when access to the right renal artery is required, when there is extensive disease of the right iliac artery, and when access to abdominal contents is necessary. The retroperitoneal approach has advantages when there are extensive intraperitoneal adhesions, marked obesity, gastrointestinal or urinary tract stomata, severe chronic pulmonary disease, or the need to clamp the aorta above the renal arteries.

Exposure. A thorough abdominal exploration is performed. The extent of the aneurysm and the status of the iliac arteries are determined by palpation taking care to avoid extensive manipulation. The intestines are packed off and retracted with a mechanical device fixed to the operating table. An incision is made in the retroperitoneum to the left of the base of the small bowel mesentery and carried proximally around the left margin of the duodenum and distally over the right iliac artery avoiding the ureter (Fig. 20-10). The neck of the aneurysm is exposed below the left renal vein which can be divided if necessary to the right of the adrenal vein to provide additional proximal exposure. Dissection over the aorta is confined to the anterior surface until the neck is clearly identified. Since the aneurysm should not be manipulated at this point, circumferential control is obtained under direct vision only when a normal-appearing aorta is encountered. The anterior and lateral borders of the common iliac arteries are now controlled if the aneurysm ends at the aortic bifurcation. The sympathetic nerves crossing just to the left of the aortic bifurcation are avoided in sexually active men. If iliac artery aneurysms are present, the incision in the retroperitoneum is carried distally on the right and the external and internal iliac arteries are dissected free. The left iliac bifurcation is controlled after lateral mobilization of the sigmoid colon. The inferior mesenteric artery is examined for pulsation and size and is not ligated at this time.

Graft Insertion. The patient is given intravenous heparin by the anesthesiologist and an activated clotting time is checked. The proximal aorta and iliac arteries are clamped and the aneurysm is opened longitudinally. Any intraluminal thrombi are evacuated, and bleeding from lumbar vessels is controlled with 3-0 Prolene sutures. If the inferior mesenteric artery is bleeding briskly, it is ligated at this point. The aortic cuff is examined. When the aneurysm is large, a well-defined sewing ring is present and the graft can be sutured in place without transecting the aorta (Fig. 20-11). A small aneurysm often requires complete transection of the aortic cuff. The distal portion of the aneurysm is inspected and either a bifurcation or a straight tube prosthesis is selected. Anastomoses are sutured with continuous Prolene. The proximal anastomosis is tested before beginning to suture the distal end by removing the aortic clamp once and repositioning it on the graft. Any bleeding areas are reinforced with pledgeted sutures after the aorta is reclamped. The graft limbs must be passed under the ureters if the distal anastomoses are done beyond the iliac bifurcations. Just before the distal clamps are released, the iliac artery clamps and the graft clamp are removed to flush out any residual debris and evacuate air from the system. The anesthesiologist is notified that clamp release is imminent, necessary adjustments in pH are made, and the patient is hyperventilated to blow off CO_2. The proximal clamp is released slowly. Rapid release without adequate fluid and acid-base resuscitation may cause significant hypotension.

Prevention of Colon Ischemia. Visual inspection of the colon is notoriously inaccurate as a predictor of ischemia. If the inferior mesenteric artery is excessively large or the circulation to the sigmoid colon is questionable, Doppler ultrasound can be used to assess flow. If an audible signal is present on the antimesenteric surface, the colon should be viable and no further action is indicated. If no signal is heard, measures must be taken to restore colonic blood flow by reimplanting the inferior mesenteric artery into the body of the graft using the Carrel patch technique. This is an uncommon occurrence particularly when one internal iliac artery is perfused.

Closure. Heparin is reversed with protamine sulfate and the activated clotting time is rechecked. When hemostasis is satisfactory, the walls of the old aneurysm are sutured over the prosthetic graft. The posterior peritoneum is closed to completely isolate the prosthesis. If this cannot be accomplished, a greater omental flap can be brought in a retrocolic fashion and sutured to the surrounding tissues to cover the graft. The abdominal wound is then closed.

Ruptured Aortic Aneurysms

The mortality rates following ruptured AAA range from 15 to 78 percent and are dependent on the status of the patient, the type

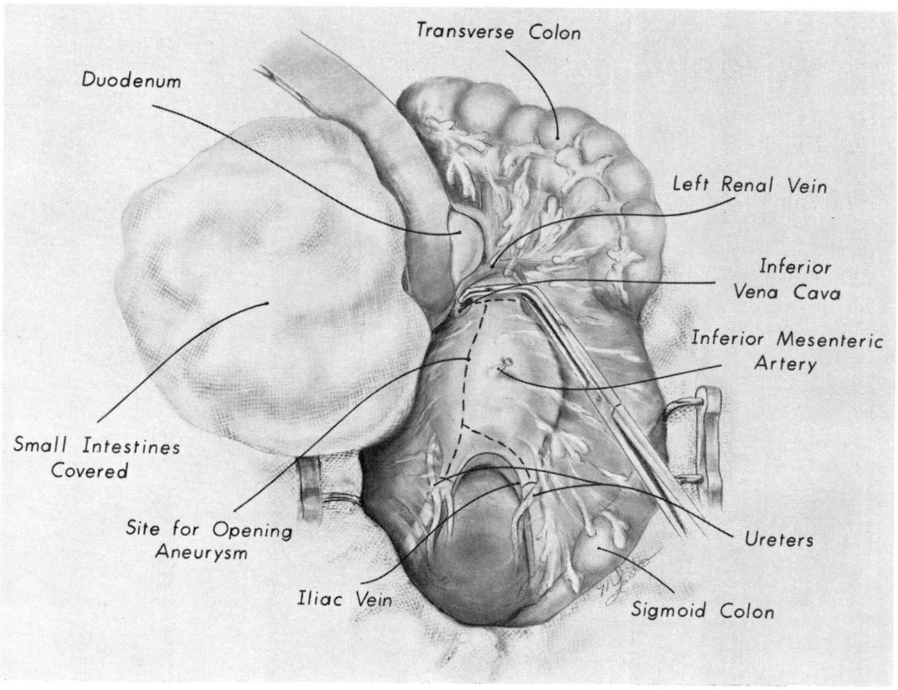

FIG. 20-10. Diagram showing the setup. The duodenum is retracted upward and to the right. The transverse colon is retracted cephalad and the left colon to the left. The staggered line shows the incision in the retroperitoneum to the left of the small-bowel mesentery, avoiding the ureters distally.

of rupture, the experience of the surgical team, and the delay in controlling hemorrhage. Patients present with a variety of dramatic symptoms ranging from generalized abdominal pain, severe back or flank pain, and/or circulatory collapse. Diagnosis may be delayed because this condition may mimic a perforated peptic ulcer, renal or biliary colic, or a ruptured intervertebral disc. The rupture may be contained in the retroperitoneal space, occur freely into the peritoneal cavity, or, in rare instances, into another anatomic structure such as the vena cava or duodenum.

Emergency Room Management. This is a true emergency, and prompt diagnosis, resuscitation, and control of hemorrhage are critical. Factors associated with an increased mortality are a history of cardiac disease or hypertension, hypotension upon arrival, elevated (BUN level (>30 mg/dc), inexperience of the surgical team, duration of operation greater than 400 min, blood transfusions of more than 17 units, and hypotension at the end of the procedure.

The amount of time spent on diagnosis depends on the condition of the patient. When a patient presents in shock with a pulsatile mass and a known history of AAA, no further testing is needed and the patient is taken to the operating room immediately. On the other hand, an obese patient with normal vital signs and severe abdominal, back, or flank pain should undergo an emergency CT scan. If the patient is in shock and the diagnosis is in question, a portable ultrasound exam can be done in the emergency room. Operation should not be delayed in order to resuscitate the patient. Instead, the patient should be brought to the operating room while rapid infusions of fluids are continued and the patient is prepared for exploration.

Operating Room Management. The operating team should be scrubbed and the patient's abdomen prepped prior to the induction of anesthesia. This is a period of significant risk for hypotension due to the vasodilatory effects of the anesthetic agents. If there is free intraperitoneal blood, aortic control is rapidly achieved at the diaphragm using a right-angled retractor to compress the supraceliac aorta against the vertebral column. This maneuver allows the anesthesiologist to resuscitate the patient. The retroperitoneum should not be opened before achieving proximal aortic control if the hematoma is contained. The right-angled retractor can be replaced with a vascular clamp or the retroperitoneal hematoma can be opened while an assistant holds pressure on the supraceliac aorta and the neck of the aneurysm can be clamped below the renal arteries. The aneurysm is opened when iliac control is achieved. We prefer to leave a secure clamp on the supraceliac aorta and suture the proximal anastomosis without a clamp on the infrarenal aorta. This reduces the incidence of left renal vein injury. Heparin is given after the completion of the proximal anastomosis, the iliac arteries are back-bled and reclamped, and the distal end of the graft is sutured to the appropriate outflow artery(s).

Complications. ***Renal Failure.*** Renal failure (rise of BUN and/or creatinine > 20 percent) occurs in roughly 6 percent of elective aneurysm repairs and 75 percent of ruptured AAAs. Acute tubular necrosis can follow prolonged hypotension either from excessive intraoperative blood loss or from declamping hypotension. It is probably the most common form of renal failure after resection of a ruptured AAA but is uncommon in the elective setting. Atheroembolization from the juxtarenal segment during aortic clamping is the most common cause of renal failure in the elective setting. This complication can be avoided by proper selection of a proximal clamp site. In cases where degenerative changes in the cuff are present or the aneurysm is "juxtarenal" the proximal clamp should be placed on the supraceliac aorta to avoid renal damage (Fig. 20-12).

Gastrointestinal Complications. Ischemic colitis involving

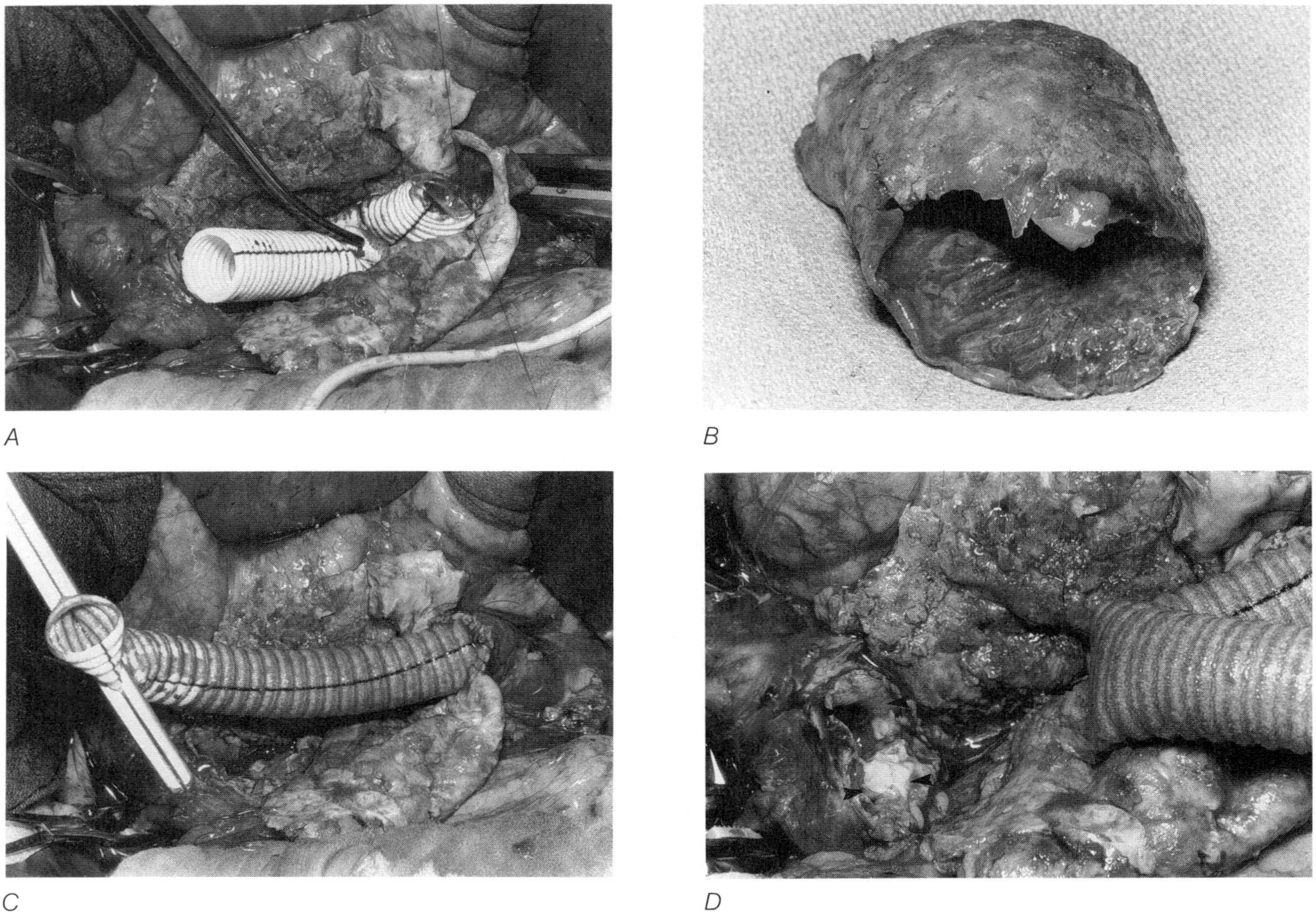

FIG. 20-11. *A.* This operative photograph demonstrates the "inside" suture technique at the proximal anastomosis. A vascular clamp is seen on the proximal cuff. The aneurysm has been opened longitudinally and "T'ed" at the proximal and distal ends, the pannus removed (*B*), and lumbar vessels have been suture-ligated. When large aneurysms are opened, a definite sewing ring can be identified below the renal arteries. The anastomosis is constructed using a continuous suture technique with 3-0 polypropylene. Large bites of tissue are taken posteriorly which incorporate two layers of aortic wall. The suture is continued anteriorly around the sewing ring and tied to the left of midline so that the knot does not irritate the duodenum. *C.* The completed proximal anastomosis with the clamp repositioned on the graft. The old aneurysmal wall will be sewn over the graft after the distal anastomosis is completed. *D.* The distal anastomosis can usually be done at the origins of the common iliac arteries (*arrows*). If the iliac arteries are aneurysmal, a bifurcated graft should be sewn either to the iliac bifurcations or the femoral arteries.

the sigmoid colon is a dreaded complication of operations on the abdominal aorta with an incidence of 1 to 6 percent. The onset of bloody diarrhea, abdominal distention, leukocytosis, and/or signs of peritonitis should prompt immediate sigmoidoscopy. In most instances, the injury is mucosal and the process is self-limited. When the muscularis is involved, a segmental stricture may occur and at a later date might require resection. In cases of full-thickness involvement, immediate resection of the involved intestine prior to contamination of the prosthetic graft is necessary with creation of an end colostomy and mucous fistula.

Spinal Cord Ischemia. Paraplegia that occurs after operations on the infrarenal aorta (0.02 percent) is usually due to pelvic devascularization and occurs with colon ischemia and necrosis of the skin of the buttocks. This is to be differentiated from the paraplegia that occurs after operations on the lower thoracic aorta following interruption of the greater medullary artery of Adamkiewicz (Fig. 20-13). Although the complication is not entirely preventable, its incidence can be reduced by maneuvers that prevent atheroembolization into and ensure perfusion of at least one hypogastric artery and therefore the iliolumbar and lateral sacral arteries. Reimplantation of the inferior mesenteric artery should be considered in patients who have occlusion of both hypogastric arteries.

Iliac Artery Aneurysms

Iliac artery aneurysms are usually dealt with in conjunction with operations for abdominal aneurysms but rarely can occur independently. The common iliac artery is involved in 90 percent of cases with the remaining 10 percent involving the internal iliac arteries. These aneurysms are not often identified on physical examination, and imaging techniques are necessary for diagnosis. An internal iliac artery aneurysm may present as a pulsatile mass

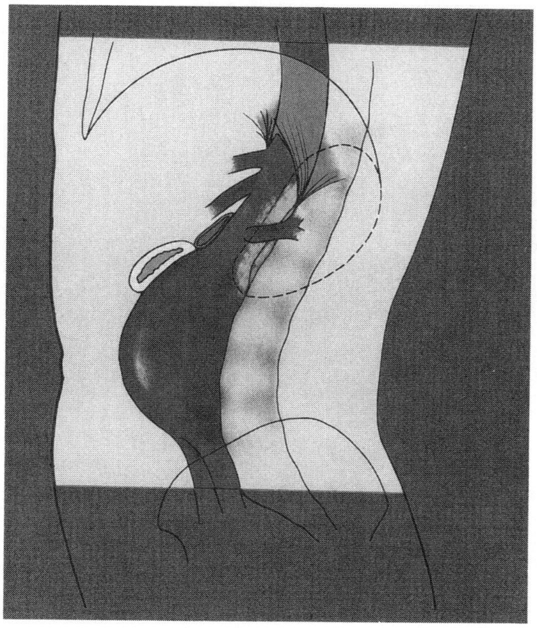

FIG. 20-12. A diagram showing the problem of juxtarenal atherosclerosis. Although the neck of the aneurysm could be clamped below the renal arteries, doing so risks "trashing" the kidneys. Supraceliac clamping is a renal-saving maneuver in this situation. Juxtarenal atherosclerosis should be suspected when one encounters degenerative changes of the aortic cuff on CT scans, lateral aortograms, and/or at operation prior to application of the aortic clamp. It is important that the proximal clamp is initially placed on a normal aortic segment because intraoperative switching from a diseased to a normal segment is usually associated with serious hemorrhagic and atheroembolic complications.

palpable on rectal examination. Isolated iliac aneurysms do rupture, and resection is indicated when the size exceeds 3 cm in diameter. Studies comparing the size of ruptured aortic aneurysms with ruptured iliac artery aneurysms show the latter to be larger at the time of rupture. Follow-up ultrasonography at 6-month intervals is recommended for those patients not undergoing operation.

Isolated unilateral iliac artery aneurysms can be approached through an ipsilateral retroperitoneal flank incision. Common iliac aneurysms are treated with interposition prosthetic grafts. Internal iliac artery aneurysms can usually be ligated proximally, and the outflow vessels can be controlled from within the sac. Bilateral aneurysms are best treated with concomitant replacement of the infrarenal aorta and insertion of a bifurcation graft (Fig. 20-14).

Visceral Artery Aneurysms

Renal Artery Aneurysms. Renal artery aneurysms are uncommon and may present either as a dissection or true aneurysm. The former presents with renal artery thrombosis and often follows blunt abdominal trauma; the latter presents with rupture. Women are more likely to be affected because of the association with fibromuscular dysplasia. The risk of rupture is greatest during pregnancy and for those macroaneurysms greater than 1.5 cm in patients with hypertension. Direct repair with aneurysmorrhaphy or bypass grafting is the procedure of choice for the extraparenchymal lesion. Renal salvage is possible in more than 90 percent of patients. Intraparenchymal lesions often require total or partial nephrectomy especially if rupture has occurred. In some patients an ex vivo repair can be performed for an intraparenchymal lesion prior to rupture.

Splanchnic Artery Aneurysms. See Chap. 33.

Peripheral Aneurysms

Popliteal Artery Aneurysms. Popliteal artery aneurysms are the most common peripheral aneurysm (70 percent), but their incidence is rare. These lesions are often bilateral (50 to 75 percent); are associated with other aneurysms, particularly in the abdominal aorta (50 percent); and occur predominantly in males between the ages of 50 and 70 years. Retrospective studies have shown that roughly 60 percent of untreated patients develop the complications of thrombosis or distal embolization and 20 percent require amputation. Some patients who suddenly develop symptoms present with inoperable situations because of occlusion of the distal arterial tree from embolic material. Early series reported excellent limb salvage rates after ligation which attests to the importance of these embolic events (Fig. 20-15).

Physical examination alone may not distinguish a popliteal from arterial ectasia or a Baker's cyst. Imaging of the popliteal space with B-mode ultrasound, CT scanning, or magnetic reso-

FIG. 20-13. Interruption of the greater medullary artery can result in paraplegia. This is an unavoidable complication of operations on the aorta. Fortunately, this rarely occurs after operations on the infrarenal aorta because this artery is usually located above the renal arteries. Paraplegia following operations on the abdominal aorta is most often due to perfusion abnormalities of the hypogastric circulation either from embolization into or occlusion of the iliolumbar and lateral sacral arteries. Operations that deprive both hypogastric arteries of antegrade inflow carry an increased risk of spinal cord ischemia.

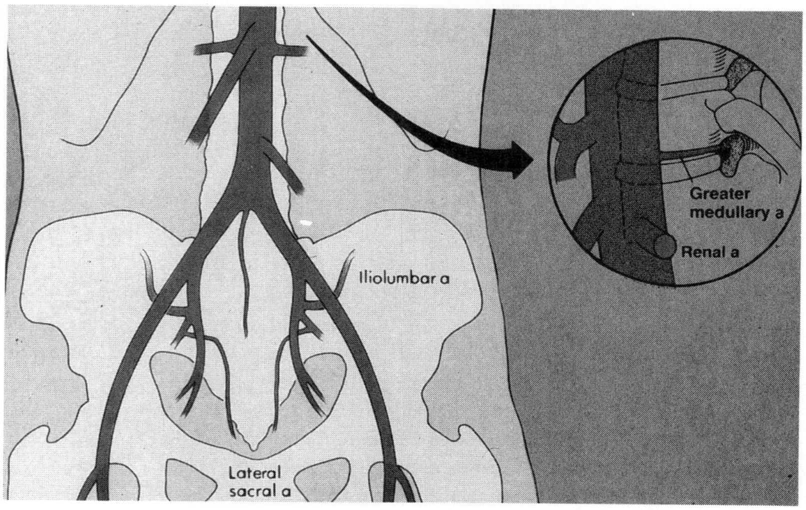

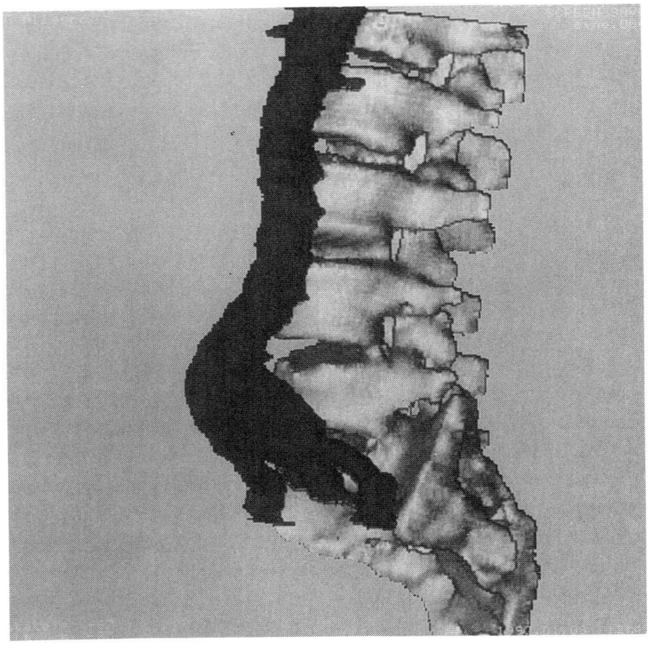

A

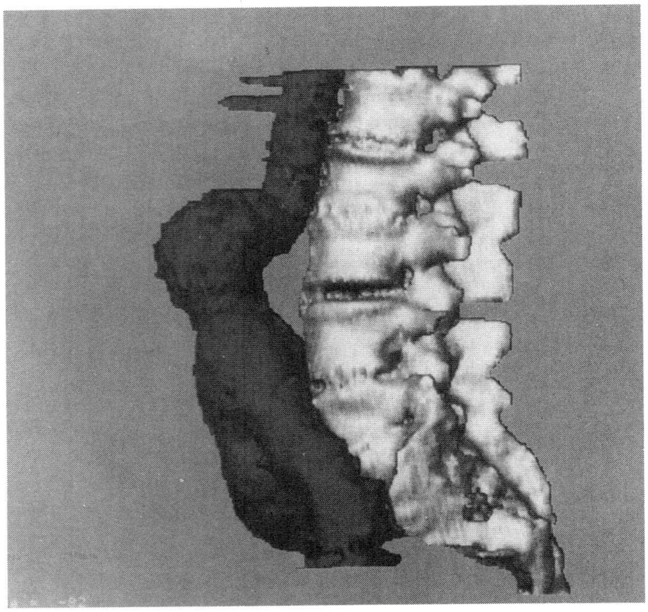

B

FIG. 20-14. Iliac aneurysms can occur independently (*A*) or in association with abdominal aortic aneurysms (*B*). In both cases the treatment is resection and graft replacement in appropriate individuals. Unilateral iliac aneurysms with a suitable proximal cuff can be treated without replacement of the infrarenal aorta.

nance imaging (MRI) is necessary for diagnosis; arteriography should be performed to define the runoff bed (Fig. 20-16).

Indications for operation are debated, but it is clear that long-term results are better when these aneurysms are treated prior to the onset of symptoms. Reports showing that aneurysms greater than 2 cm in diameter were more likely to cause complications than smaller ones have prompted many to advocate repair when

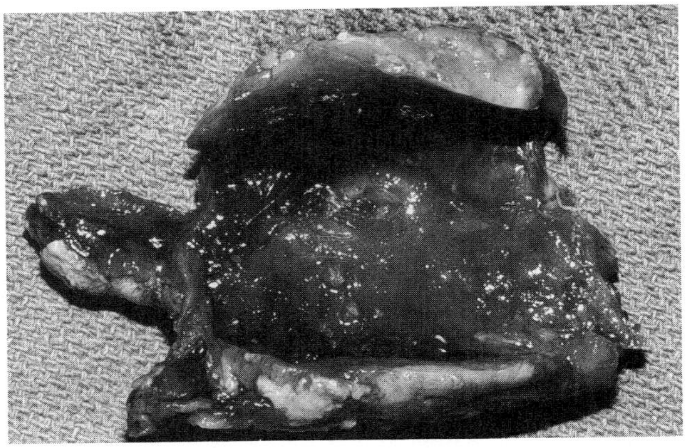

FIG. 20-15. This is a resected popliteal artery aneurysm in a patient who presented with atheroembolic phenomena in the ipsilateral foot. The aneurysm measured 2.5 cm in diameter. The contents were consistent with an organized thrombus similar to that seen in aneurysms of the addominal aorta.

the aneurysm reaches that critical size. By contrast, other claim that thrombosis is more common in the smaller aneurysms. It appears that both statements may be valid, i.e., large aneurysms embolize and small aneurysms thrombose. Repair is therefore indicated in any patient with a popliteal aneurysm without serious comorbidity. Operative management ranges from excision and interposition bypass grafting through a posterior incision and ligation and bypass around the popliteal space through medial incisions. Saphenous vein should be used in most instances.

Femoral Artery Aneurysms. Most of these uncommon aneurysms are found on physical examination. Diagnosis can be verified with ultrasonography. Most are nonspecific in nature, but mycotic and traumatic aneurysms can occur in this site. Most patients develop symptoms of an enlarging groin mass, local pain, venous obstruction, distal embolization, or thrombosis. All symptomatic aneurysms and those asymptomatic aneurysms greater than 2.5 cm in diameter should be repaired. The operation of choice is resection with prosthetic graft replacement.

ACUTE ARTERIAL OCCLUSION

Acute occlusion of the arterial supply to an extremity often represents an emergency. In patients without extensive collateral circulation, or in circumstances in which the occluded artery is the only vessel supplying the end organ, progression to irreversible ischemia may begin 6 h following the event. Prompt diagnosis and treatment in such situations is imperative, both to reestablish flow through the initial site of occlusion, as well as to prevent propagation of the thrombotic process to the distal arterial tree and venous system.

Restoration of perfusion to the threatened limb is the principal objective at the time of initial evaluation. Nevertheless, establishing the nature of the occlusive process is an important secondary goal and should be attempted whenever feasible, since treatment options are affected by the cause. The differential diagnosis of acute arterial occlusion includes embolism, trauma, and thrombosis. Emboli may originate from the heart or from a more proximal artery; in either case there may be no prior or concurrent history of the underlying disorder. Injuries most often associated with arte-

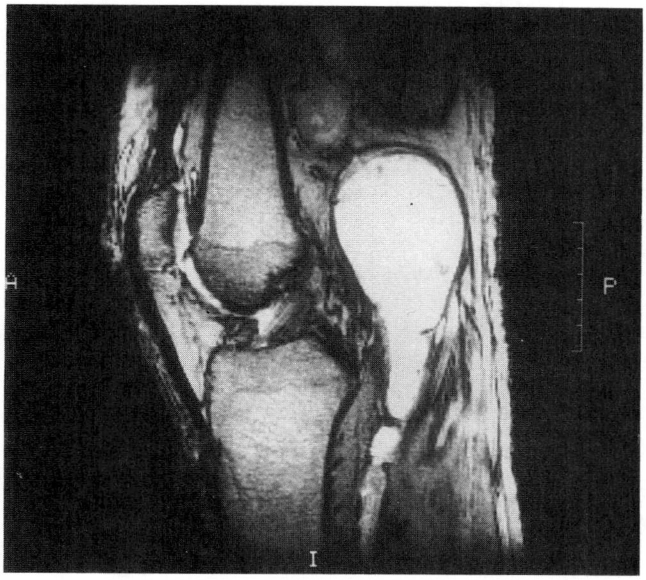

A

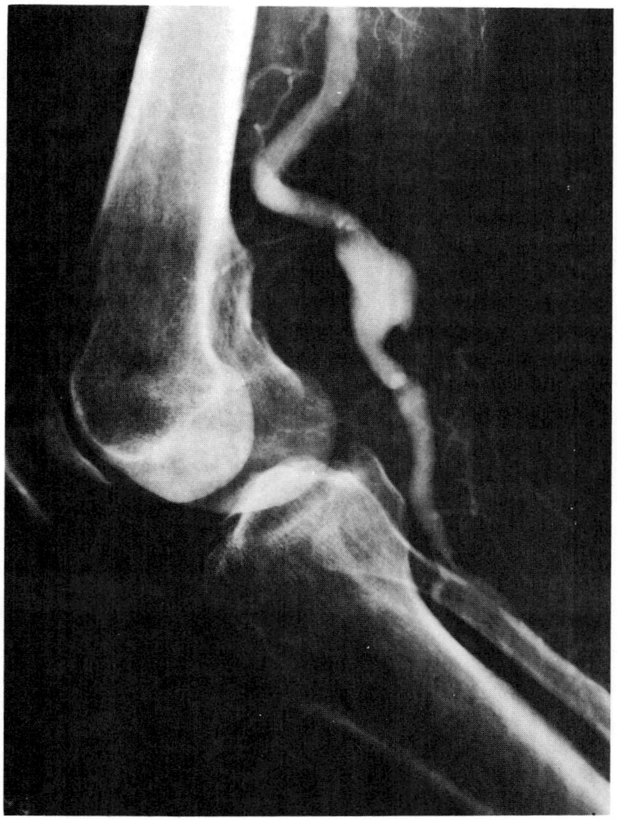

B

FIG. 20-16. *A.* MRI of popliteal space in a patient with a pulsatile mass and a swollen leg. A large popliteal aneurysm is present with compression of the popliteal vein. At operation the popliteal vein was patent but compressed by this large mass. *B.* An arteriogram showing a popliteal aneurysm and runoff. The tortuosity is not an unusual occurrence. This type of aneurysm is best approached posteriorly from the popliteal space, excised, and replaced with a short interposition saphenous vein graft.

rial occlusion are posterior knee dislocation, long bone fractures, penetrating trauma, and catheter-related iatrogenic trauma. Thrombosis may occur in the setting of an atherosclerotic lesion or, less commonly, in the presence of an aneurysm.

Pathophysiology. Acute arterial occlusion results in anoxic ischemia of the tissues supplied by the involved arterial segment. Gangrene will develop in this setting in approximately 50 percent of patients, depending on the site and length of occlusion, and the presence of collaterals. The clinical features of pain, paresthesia, and paralysis relate to the relatively greater susceptibility of nerves to ischemia in comparison to other structures. Striated muscle is only slightly less susceptible to ischemia, and therefore loss of nervous function heralds impending muscle necrosis. Tissue death typically begins 6 to 8 h following the embolic event but may be greatly modified based on the presence of collateral circulation, and in some instances may not occur at all. Thrombus does not propagate beyond branch points when flow through collaterals is sufficiently great, and the clinical findings are less serious. In the presence of stasis, however, thrombosis of the arterial and venous system distal to the initial occlusion does proceed, rendering attempts at operative and pharmacologic therapy futile.

Clinical Manifestations. The most significant features of acute arterial occlusion can be summarized as the five p's: pain, paralysis, paresthesia, pallor, and pulselessness (Table 20-2). Over 75 percent of patients with acute arterial occlusion experience pain as the presenting symptom. Pain may be absent from the clinical syndrome because of diabetic neuropathy, adequate collateral flow resulting in less severe ischemia, or rapid progression to advanced ischemia, with immediate anesthesia. Paresthesia and paralysis are the most critical features to evaluate in the patient with acute arterial occlusion. When present, these findings indicate anoxia of the sensory and motor nerve endings of the extremity, the structures most susceptible to ischemia. Sensory fibers are slightly more sensitive than motor fibers, hence the clinical observation that paresthesia usually precedes paralysis. Paralysis may also be the result of striated muscle necrosis in the setting of more advanced ischemia. The presence of paresthesia and paralysis is an ominous finding, indicating that the limb will almost certainly develop gangrene if the underlying condition is not alleviated within 6 to 8 h, and heralds the need for rapid treatment. By contrast, the patient who does not exhibit these findings is at a much reduced risk of developing ischemic necrosis in the acute setting.

Reduction in blood flow to an extremity results in a pale appearance of the limb and is frequently associated with a sixth p, poikilothermy, or coolness. Discolored, mottled skin that fails to blanch in response to digital pressure is an indicator of irreversible ischemia and is due to extravasation of blood into the dermis from ruptured capillaries. The level at which temperature and color

Table 20-2
Clinical Presentation of Acute Arterial Ischemia: Signs and Symptoms

Pain
Paralysis
Paresthesia
Pallor
Pulselessness
Poikilothermia

changes occur can provide information regarding the level of the arterial occlusion; tissue ischemia usually develops one joint level below the segment of occluded artery. For example, an embolus occluding the origin of the superficial femoral artery produces ischemia distal to the knee joint.

The absence of pulses supports the diagnosis of acute arterial occlusion but does not prove it with certainty, since pulses may be absent chronically in the patient with peripheral vascular disease. The examination of the pulses also assists in locating the level of occlusion. In general, the occlusion can be localized to the segment of the arterial tree immediately proximal to the site of pulselessness. For instance, a patient with a palpable or exaggerated femoral pulse and an absent popliteal pulse can be assumed to have an occlusion of the superficial femoral artery.

In addition to the six p's, evaluation of the muscle turgor in the affected limb yields important information regarding the severity of ischemia and the degree to which the changes are reversible after reperfusion. The muscles are soft immediately following the onset of ischemia. With time, the muscles develop edema, and this is associated with a doughy feeling on physical examination. Necrosis occurs at a more advanced stage, and the muscles feel stiff and hard; when this occurs, the ischemic changes are irreversible, regardless of therapy.

Diagnosis. In some instances, the diagnosis of acute arterial occlusion can be made with relative certainty based on the patient's history and physical examination, and no further work-up is required prior to definitive treatment. An example of this is a patient who presents with the sudden onset of a cold, painful leg, and an absent femoral pulse, and is found to have atrial fibrillation. Groin exploration and femoral embolectomy without preoperative arteriography are appropriate in this case. In the majority of patients, however, either the presence or the precise location of an acute arterial occlusion may be uncertain, and further evaluation is necessary to optimize treatment. Acute arterial occlusion can be confused with nerve root compression, deep venous thrombosis,

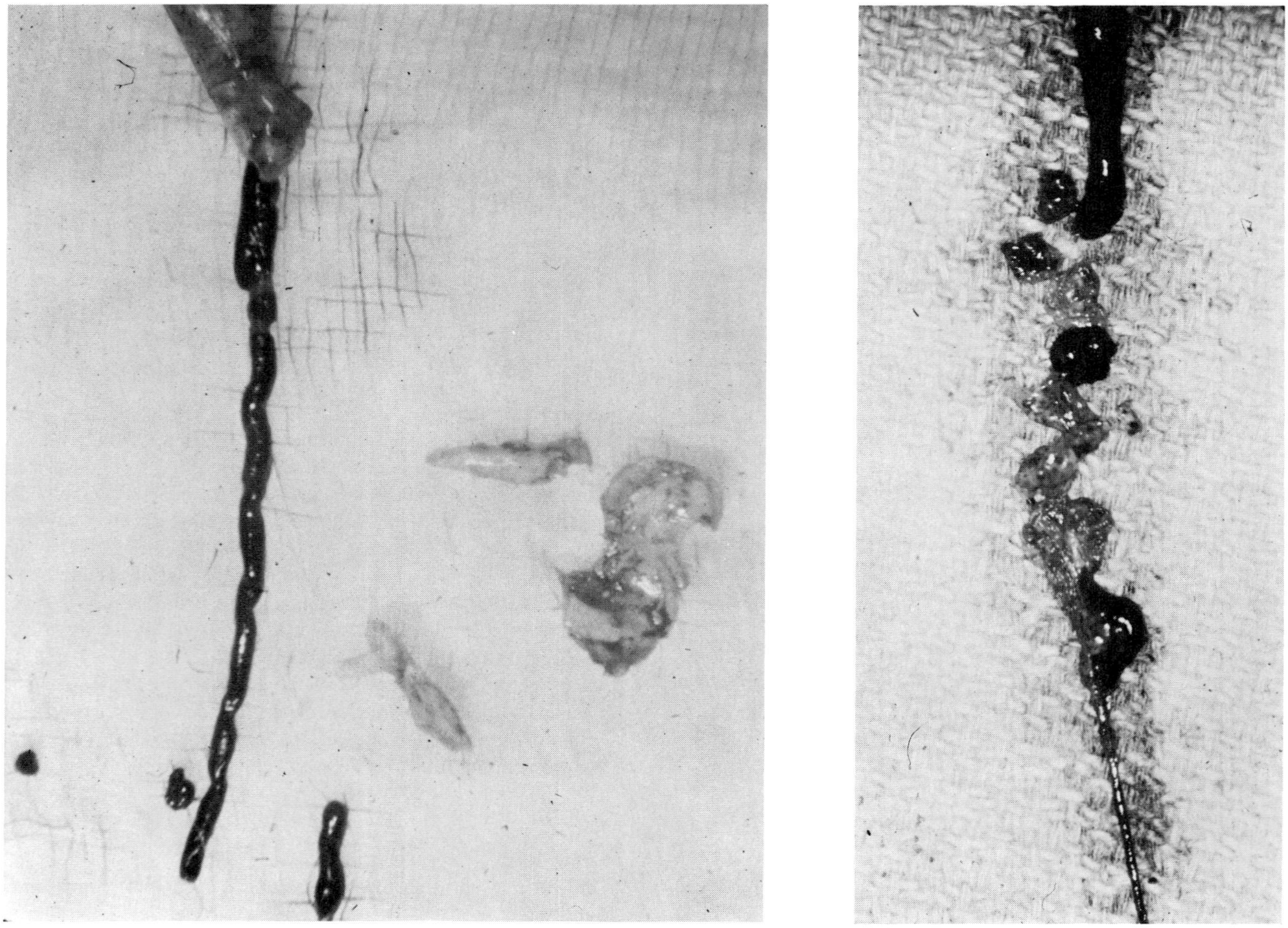

A

FIG. 20-17. *A.* Embolic material and secondary, propagated thrombus. The embolic material formed in the heart overlying an area of injured endocardium, with deposition of platelets and fibrin in excess of red blood cells, producing a salmon-colored thrombus. The propagated clot is composed of a homogenous gelatinous mass containing all the blood elements, which formed when blood flow ceased. As such, the propagated clot is dark red in color. *B.* Frequency of involvement of different peripheral arteries by arterial emboli. In the major of patients, arteries in the lower extremity are involved. (*Redrawn from Haimovici H: Peripheral arterial embolism. Angiology 1:20, 1950, with permission.*)

phlegmasia cerulea dolens, and infectious processes. Rarely, acute dissection of the thoracic aorta may mimic multiple visceral and extremity emboli if these vessels are occluded by the false lumen. Noninvasive studies such as segmental arterial pressures can be helpful in establishing the diagnosis and localizing the site of occlusion in this setting. Arteriography is performed when additional information is required, for instance to determine the appropriate sites of inflow and outflow for a bypass graft. If the ischemia is severe, however, the urgency of revascularization may preclude the advisability of preoperative arteriography.

Arterial Embolism

Arterial emboli can be divided into two categories: emboli that lodge in large-diameter vessels, such as the common femoral artery, the vast majority of which are of cardiac origin; and atheroemboli to smaller vessels, such as branches of the digital arteries, that invariably originate from a plaque or thrombus in a more proximal vessel.

Cardiac Emboli

Etiology. Embolism from the heart may be the first indication of a serious underlying cardiac disorder and may occur in three clinical settings: atrial fibrillation, myocardial infarction, and valvular disease. Appropriate evaluation and treatment of the cardiac disease, when necessary, must be undertaken concurrently with the therapy of the arterial occlusion, and the severity of the underlying cardiac condition must be taken into consideration when deciding on therapy for the arterial occlusion.

Cardiac emboli in the patient with mitral stenosis may result either from valvular vegetations or from mural thrombi that form in a dilated left atrium. Atrial fibrillation, occurring alone or in conjunction with mitral stenosis, predisposes to the formation of mural thrombi, which may then embolize to the peripheral circulation. Similarly, transmural myocardial infarction is associated with the formation of mural thrombus on the subendocardial surface overlying the infarcted ventricle, usually between 2 and 3 weeks following the cardiac event. Rare sources of arterial emboli originating in the heart include bacterial endocarditis, atrial myxoma, prosthetic heart valves, and paradoxical embolization originating in the veins and passing through a patent foramen ovale. A diligent search must be made for the embolic source in all patients, including electrocardiography, echocardiography, and Holter monitoring. Despite a thorough evaluation, however, the source cannot be identified in a significant percentage of patients.

Distribution. The two factors that influence the site in the arterial tree in which an embolus will lodge are patterns of blood flow and changes in vessel diameter. Consequently, 70 percent of cardiac emboli lodge in the arteries of the lower extremities, 13 percent in the arteries of the upper extremities, 10 percent in the cerebral circulation, and 5 to 10 percent in the visceral circulation. In addition, emboli generally lodge at arterial branch points, where the vessel diameter is abruptly reduced. Common sites in the lower extremity include the bifurcation of the abdominal aorta, common iliac artery, common femoral artery, and popliteal artery (Fig. 20-17). A corresponding pattern is seen in the arteries of the upper extremity, with involvement of the brachial artery at its bifurcation into the radial and ulnar arteries or, less commonly, at the takeoff of the profunda brachial artery. The ischemic insult is more severe when the bifurcation of a vessel is occluded, because collateral circulation cannot be supplied by a patent branch vessel.

Evaluation. Once the diagnosis of acute arterial occlusion has been established, it is desirable to differentiate between embolism and thrombosis as the underlying cause, since the treatment options may differ accordingly. A patient with embolic occlusion of an otherwise normal vessel (Fig. 20-18) may only require thromboembolectomy under local anesthesia, whereas a patient with thrombosis of an atherosclerotic artery will likely require a bypass graft around the involved segment, under regional or general anesthesia. Clinical findings suggestive of an embolic cause include the presence of cardiac arrhythmia, myocardial ischemia, and valvular disease; the absence of factors predisposing to atherosclerosis; and the absence of prothrombotic hematologic disorders. The presence of normal pulses on the contralateral side is strongly indicative of an embolic source.

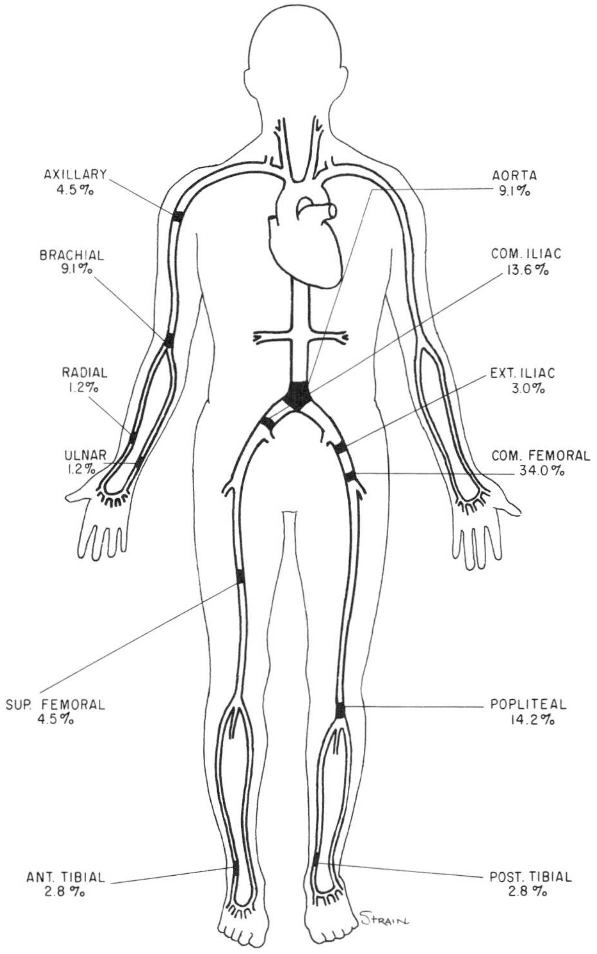

B

FIG. 20-17. *(continued)*

Arterial Atheroemboli

Etiology. The vast majority of emboli that originate in arteries are fragments of an ulcerated atherosclerotic plaque that become dislodged and travel downstream, lodging in a more distal artery. These fragments may be composed of cholesterol crystals, or, alternatively, they may be composed of fibrin-platelet debris that deposit on the surface of the plaque and are then displaced into the circulation. The artery of origin, usually the aorta, iliac, or

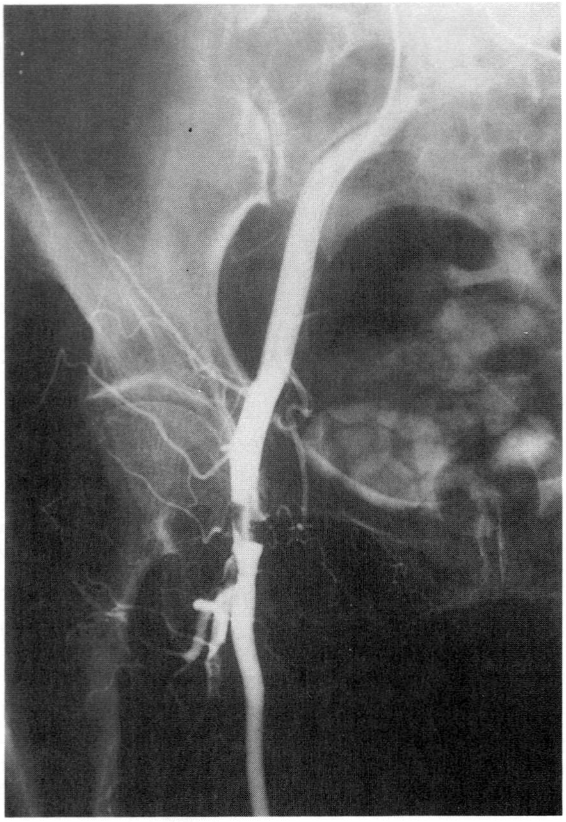

FIG. 20-18. An arteriogram of a patient with a common femoral embolus. The material characteristically occludes the orifices of both the superficial and profunda femoris arteries.

femoral vessels, is often some distance from the artery in which the embolus finally lodges, since these fragments are usually tiny and do not become trapped until they reach a small vessel (Fig. 20-19). It is rare for large vessels such as the common femoral or popliteal arteries to become occluded by atheroemboli, except during operative manipulation of a diseased abdominal aorta. Fragments of intraluminal thrombi, such as those that are seen in association with aneurysms, may also dislodge and occlude distal vessels. This is much less common than atheroemboli but is typically seen in association with popliteal aneurysms. In either case, patients may experience repeated embolic episodes that are individually minor; the additive effects, however, may be quite significant.

Clinical Syndromes. The most common example of atheroemboli is the ''blue-toe'' syndrome. Patients with this syndrome develop severe ischemia of the toes and forefoot in the presence of palpable pulses. The superficial femoral artery, popliteal artery, and at least one tibial vessel are usually patent in order for emboli to travel to the digital arteries; therefore, patients with blue-toe syndrome generally have palpable pedal pulses. This physical finding enables the clinician to differentiate this disorder from lower extremity gangrene resulting from large-vessel atherosclerotic disease. Renal failure or mesenteric ischemia may accompany digital gangrene if the thoracic upper abdominal aorta is the source of emboli. If the digits of the upper extremity are involved, the subclavian artery is usually the source, with disease due either to proximal atherosclerosis or more distal poststenotic aneurysm formation secondary to thoracic outlet obstruction.

Evaluation. Atheroemboli should be suspected when the physical examination reveals digital ischemia in a patient with palpable pulses. The location of the embolic source can be estimated based on the sites where the emboli have lodged; the source must be proximal to the site of the embolus, and bilateral emboli to the feet indicates a source above the aortic bifurcation, while repeated unilateral emboli suggest a more distal source. A thorough arteriographic evaluation is required to confirm the diagnosis and to precisely identify the offending lesion in preparation for operative intervention.

Arterial Thrombosis

Etiology. Spontaneous acute arterial thrombosis occurs most commonly in the presence of an underlying stenosis due to atherosclerotic disease. The thrombotic event may be precipitated by plaque disruption and exposure of the thrombotic core, by hypoperfusion due to inadequate cardiac output, or from a critical reduction in flow across the involved arterial segment. Acute arterial occlusion may also occur in the setting of an aneurysm, commonly popliteal, in which distal embolization of thrombotic material produces occlusion of the outflow tract and ultimately results in thrombosis of the aneurysm itself due to inadequate outflow. Hypercoagulable states, such as the antiphospholipid syndrome, as well as protein C, protein S, and antithrombin III deficiencies may also cause acute arterial occlusion. These disorders should be suspected when the patient lacks the usual risk factors for atherosclerosis (Table 20-3). Rarely, acute arterial thrombosis develops as a result of repeated mild trauma as occurs with a cervical rib compressing the subclavian artery, or from occupational trauma such as the operation of a pneumatic tool, the vibrations of which cause injury to the digital arterial wall. Acute arterial thrombosis may also occur following diagnostic and therapeutic intraarterial procedures, such as cardiac catheterization and peripheral vascular arteriography. An intimal flap can be created by the catheter even with the most careful technique, resulting in thrombosis of the vessel.

Clinical Manifestations. The clinical picture of acute arterial thrombosis may range from severe, limb-threatening ischemia to no symptoms whatsoever, depending on the presence or absence of an adequate collateral network and the size and location of the involved vessel. A patient with a chronic superficial femoral artery stenosis may progress to complete occlusion of the vessel and remain asymptomatic because blood flow is maintained by means of a well-established collateral network. By contrast, a young patient with a coagulation disorder may develop occlusion of the same vessel and have far more severe symptoms due to the absence of collateral circulation. In addition, occlusion of the superficial femoral artery is less serious than occlusion of the popliteal artery, because the profunda femoris artery can provide blood flow to the extremity when the superficial femoral artery is thrombosed, while the popliteal artery is the only major vessel to the foot at the level of the knee.

Diagnosis. The clinical findings in acute arterial thrombosis vary with the severity of ischemia but are essentially the same as those observed with acute arterial embolism and are described by the six p's. In contrast to patients with straightforward peripheral

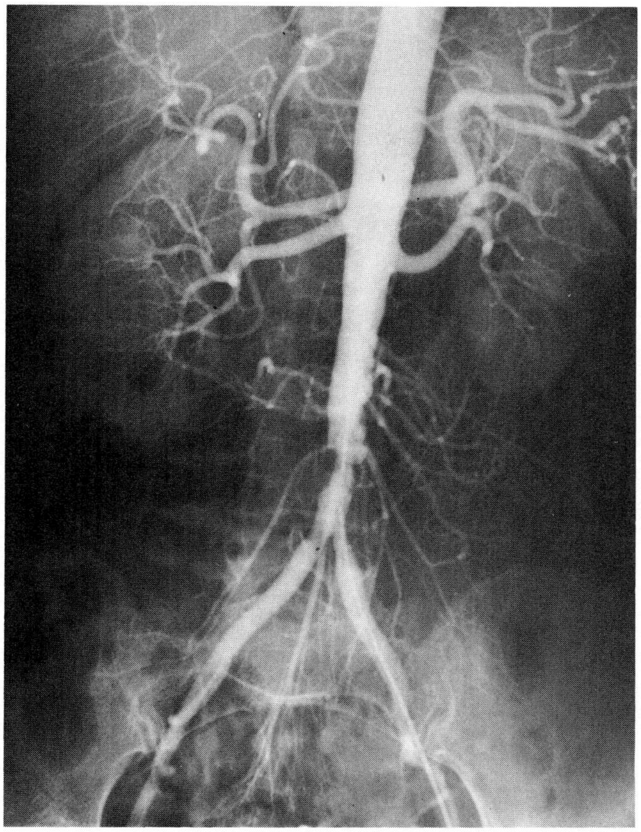

A

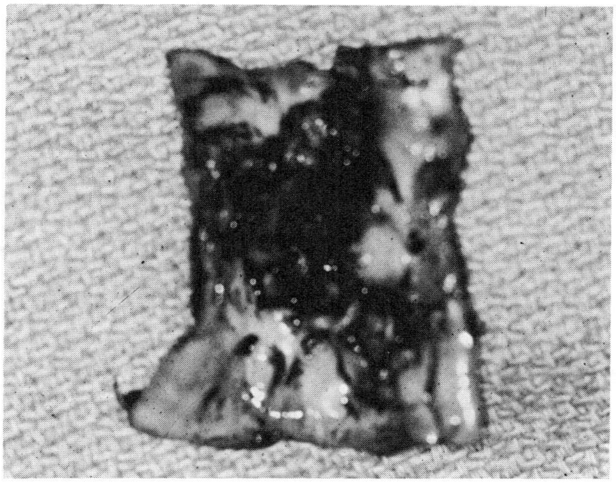

B

FIG. 20-19. Arterioarterial embolization, also known as atheroembolization, in a patient in whom marked ischemia of the toes developed in the presence of palpable pedal pulses. Several attacks occurred with progressive ischemia. *A.* Angiogram showing infrarenal abdominal aortic plaques. Occlusion of small calf arteries without involvement of renal arteries suggested that this infrarenal plaque was the source of emboli. *B.* Aortic plaque removed by endarterectomy. There was no recurrence of embolization at the tenth year follow-up.

embolism, all patients with suspected acute arterial thrombosis should undergo preoperative arteriography unless the degree of ischemia precludes the delay required for the procedure.

The nature of the acute arterial occlusion should be established as either thrombotic or embolic whenever possible. The distinction is often difficult to make, but certain findings on history, physical examination, and arteriography are helpful. A history of peripheral vascular disease (e.g., claudication) in the involved or contralateral limb suggests a thrombotic cause, as does a personal or family history of popliteal or aortic aneurysm. Similarly, physical findings indicative of arterial insufficiency, such as skin and nail changes, or the absence of distal pulses in the uninvolved extremity suggest thrombosis rather than embolus. Conversely, the absence of evidence of peripheral vascular disease on history or physical exam implies an embolic cause. Occasionally, an embolus may be visible arteriographically as a rounded structure at the most proximal site of occlusion. Often, however, this is not seen because of retrograde propagation of the thrombus. Differentiation between these two entities is very important, because although treatment is required for both disorders, the nature of that treatment may be very different. Patients with embolic disease have normal vessels, and operative or pharmacologic treatment is limited to elimination of the thromboembolus. By contrast, the vast majority of patients with thrombotic disease have underlying ath-

Table 20-3
Diagnostic Work-up of Hypercoagulable States

Laboratory Test	*Clinical Entity where Abnormal*
Antithrombin-III level	Congenital antithrombin-III deficiency
Protein C and S levels	Congenital protein C and S deficiency
PTT	Elevated in presence of lupus anticoagulant
Fibrinogen level	Congenital deficiency
Erythrocyte sedimentation rate	Inflammatory and immune disorders
Lupus anticoagulant	Lupus, antiphospholipid syndrome
Anticardiolipin level	Antiphospholipid syndrome
Antinuclear antibody titer	Lupus
Plasminogen level	Congenital or acquired plasminogen deficiency
Platelet count	Benign and malignant thrombocytosis

erosclerotic occlusive disease and will require correction of the lesion responsible for the thrombotic event in addition to removal of the thrombus itself.

Operative Therapy

Operative therapy has been the standard of care for acute arterial thromboembolism for several decades. The introduction and refinement of thrombolytic agents, however, has led to confusion and controversy regarding the indications for use of these two effective therapeutic modalities. In general, thrombolytic therapy is reserved for patients in whom the ischemic event is not so severe that reperfusion cannot be delayed for the time required to perform arteriography and effect clot lysis.

Arterial Embolus. Acute arterial embolism is a disorder that virtually always requires therapy. Most patients with emboli to the peripheral circulation have cardiac disease, and embolectomy can usually be performed through a small incision under local anesthesia. Embolectomy should not be avoided on the basis of its risk to the patient, as the development of extremity gangrene and amputation incurs a far greater physiologic and operative stress. Attempts should not be made to restore blood flow to nonviable limbs, as reperfusion in this setting may result in the return of toxic substances such as potassium, lactic acid, and myoglobin to the circulation. The risk of death in this setting is high, and amputation should be accomplished expeditiously.

The urgency with which blood flow must be restored to the ischemic limb can be estimated based on clinical findings, and when possible, patients should be medically stabilized prior to even the simplest procedure. Systemic heparinization is accomplished as soon the diagnosis is established and is continued throughout the operation. The incision is placed over the presumed site of the embolus. A groin incision is utilized if the thromboembolic process involves the femoral vessels, and a medial incision just below the knee is used for a popliteal embolus. The exception to this rule is embolic occlusion of the aortoiliac segment; in this setting the thromboembolus is removed using bilateral groin incisions. A transverse arteriotomy is performed once the patient has been heparinized and proximal and distal control of the artery has been obtained. The embolus is readily extracted through the arteriotomy, passing an embolectomy catheter proximally and distally to remove all propagated thrombus (Fig. 20-20). Additional incisions may be required to remove thrombus from distal vessels. For example, a below-knee incision would be used to expose the popliteal trifurcation in the case of retained anterior tibial thrombus, since this vessel is often difficult to catheterize from the femoral approach because of the acute angle at which it branches from the popliteal artery. A completion arteriogram should be obtained if there is concern about residual thrombus. Intravascular angioscopy has recently been used to ascertain the effectiveness of thrombectomy. Although usually reserved for trauma, fasciotomies may be performed if compartment swelling is anticipated.

Anticoagulation should be instituted during the early postoperative period. The majority of patients will require long-term oral anticoagulation with warfarin because of cardiac mural thrombi or valvular vegetation. The prognosis for limb salvage is determined by the preoperative condition of the extremity and the success of clot removal. Muscle necrosis and clot propagation are reduced when embolectomy can be accomplished within 6 h of the onset of ischemia. Beyond this time point, the preoperative finding of a soft, pliable calf muscle is predictive of a good outcome. The overall in-hospital mortality in patients with arterial emboli is 25 percent or more, with the majority of deaths occurring as a result of underlying cardiac disease.

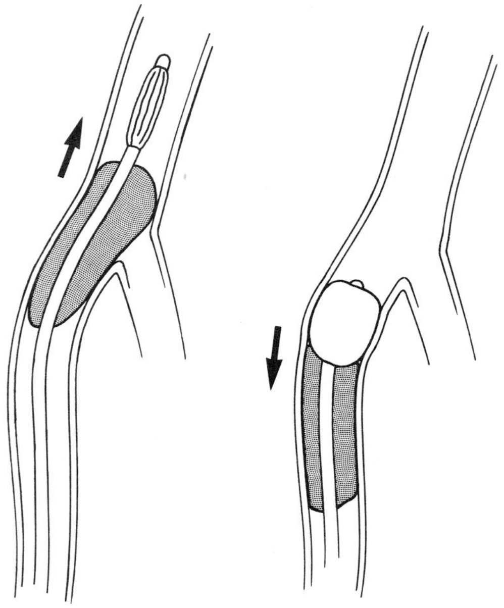

FIG. 20-20. Removal of an embolus from an arterial bifurcation by passing a balloon catheter through a downstream arteriotomy, inflating the balloon, and extracting the embolic material.

Arterial Thrombosis. The operative choices are more complex when acute arterial occlusion develops as a result of thrombosis rather than embolization. Fortunately, time constraints are usually less stringent, as the degree of ischemia is rarely as severe. Operative therapy in this setting is generally a combination of the strategies of thrombus removal established in the section on arterial emboli, and the strategies of bypass grafting established in the section on chronic arterial occlusion.

Thrombolytic Therapy

The introduction of thrombolytic agents in the treatment of acute arterial occlusion by Sherry and associates in 1958 prompted the use of this increasingly popular technique. Many advances and technical refinements have been made since the inception of this therapy, including the use of catheter-directed administration of thrombolytic agents, coaxial catheter systems, and use of safer, more effective agents. Thrombolytic agents are used both instead of and in addition to standard operative techniques, depending on the nature of the occlusion. Thrombolytic agents are unlikely to completely supplant operation in the treatment of acute arterial occlusion in all cases, since many patients have fixed arterial lesions that must be addressed in order to prevent rethrombosis. In addition, some thromboemboli are not susceptible to thrombolysis. In cases of very severe ischemia, the time required to perform a diagnostic arteriogram and achieve pharmacologic clot removal may jeopardize limb salvage.

All thrombolytic agents work by activating the plasmin system, thus effecting lysis of fibrin and dissolution of the clot infrastructure. Streptokinase is a bacterially derived compound that binds plasminogen, and it is this complex that converts plasminogen to form plasmin. Urokinase is derived from renal parenchymal cells, and TPA is derived from vascular endothelial cells; both of these agents activate plasminogen directly. Unlike streptokinase and urokinase, TPA has a greater affinity for plasminogen at the site of the thrombus than for circulating plasminogen but has not been proven to reduce distant bleeding complications associated with either local of systemic administration.

Thrombolytic therapy is indicated in any patient with an acute native arterial or graft occlusion and is most effective when administered within 1 to 2 weeks of thrombosis. There exist a number of important contraindications to the use of lytic therapy, including a history of gastrointestinal or intracerebral lesions, pregnancy, and any contraindication to arteriography. As with catheter thromboembolectomy, blood flow should not be restored to nonviable limbs, since the consequences of reperfusion in this setting may be lethal.

The patient is given an antithrombotic agent such as aspirin or heparin once the decision to administer thrombolytic therapy has been made. This decreases thrombus formation around the catheter itself, reducing the incidence of embolization as the catheter is removed. In addition, platelet activation occurs during thrombolytic therapy and may result in the inhibition of clot lysis or early rethrombosis. Heparin or aspirin may prevent these platelet-associated complications.

Thrombolytic therapy is instituted with catheter placement proximal to the level of the occlusion, followed by the performance of a diagnostic arteriogram. The catheter is then advanced into the clot itself and is used to administer the thrombolytic agent. If the catheter cannot be advanced into the thrombus, attempts at lysis are rarely successful. A high dose of thrombolytic agent is usually administered for the first 4 h, followed by a smaller dose that is continued up to 48 h. Arteriograms are repeated at regular intervals to assess the effectiveness of clot lysis. Therapy is discontinued prior to 48 h if clot lysis is satisfactory, if a complication occurs, if no significant lysis is achieved, or if the rate of lysis is inadequate for limb salvage. There are several treatment options once the thrombolytic agent is discontinued. No further treatment is needed if complete lysis is achieved and there is no arterial lesion, although most of these patients will require evaluation and treatment of the underlying cause of the occlusion. Patients with appropriate arterial or graft lesions may be treated by percutaneous balloon angioplasty. Other patients will require replacement or revision of a bypass graft to correct the underlying lesion.

Thrombolytic therapy has been postulated to be associated with a number of advantages over operative therapy in the treatment of acute arterial occlusion. In the case of thromboembolic disease involving an otherwise normal artery, for example, in a patient with a cardiac embolus or hypercoagulable state, operative intervention may be avoided entirely following successful thrombolysis. Benefit may also be conferred to the patient with an underlying arterial lesion, as the stenosis can be identified arteriographically following clot lysis. As a result, a vein graft may be revised using a patch angioplasty, rather than by replacing it with a new graft, and isolated lesions involving both arteries and grafts can often be treated by percutaneous methods. Finally, thrombolytic agents can lyse thrombi that are inaccessible by operative methods, such as those in the distal tibial vessels, potentially improving the chances of limb salvage.

The risks and complications associated with the use of thrombolytic agents must be weighed against the potential benefits of this therapeutic modality. Administration of any thrombolytic agent may result in a systemic lytic state, which predisposes patients with occult lesions to hemorrhage. The most common site is the gastrointestinal tract, but intracerebral hemorrhage, occurring in 0.5 to 1.0 percent of patients, is by far the most devastating. Bleeding may occur at the catheter site in approximately 15 percent of patients receiving thrombolytic agents, usually in the form of a hematoma that develops following catheter removal. Bleeding complications may be more frequent when the fibrinogen falls below 100 mg/dL, but this has not been demonstrated definitively. The treatment of hemorrhagic complications during thrombolytic therapy involves immediate discontinuation of the agents and appropriate medical or surgical management of the bleeding site. In cases of severe bleeding, particularly intracerebral, epsilon amino caproic acid (AMICAR) should be administered without delay. Streptokinase, derived from beta-hemolytic streptococcus, is antigenic and is associated with an allergic reaction in patients recently exposed to the bacteria or who have recently received streptokinase. The agent should not be given to these individuals. As clot lysis progresses, fragments from the dissolving clot frequently embolize to distal vessels, such as the tibial and digital arteries. When this occurs, the extremity becomes ischemic again, mimicking reocclusion of the vessel. Distal embolization of thrombus responds to continuation of thrombolytic therapy in almost all cases, preferably with advancement of the catheter into the involved segment.

The results of thrombolytic therapy for acute arterial occlusion have been encouraging with most series reporting success rates of 80 to 90 percent, as determined by clot lysis and clinical improvement. Randomized studies comparing the efficacy of operative therapy and thrombolytic therapy have not been completed; hence, it is not known whether thrombolysis actually improves outcome in patients with acute arterial occlusion.

CHRONIC ARTERIAL OCCLUSION

Atherosclerosis is the most common cause of occlusive disease of the arteries supplying the extremities. Although peripheral atherosclerosis is a diffuse process affecting the arterial tree, the most severe lesions tend to occur at discrete sites. Symptomatic peripheral arterial lesions are most frequently located in the infrarenal abdominal aorta, iliac arteries, and the superficial femoral artery at the level of the adductor canal. The presence of arterial stenoses in other locations is usually indicative of coexistent disease processes such as diabetes mellitus (profunda femoris and tibial arteries) or inflammatory arteritides (axillary arteries).

The incidence of symptomatic peripheral atherosclerotic occlusive disease is lower than that of coronary disease, but individuals with significant coronary disease frequently display manifestations of peripheral arterial disease as well. This finding is not surprising, given the common pathogenesis of the two entities. Symptomatic peripheral arterial disease occurs predominantly in males over the age of 50 years. Additional risk factors were documented in the Framingham study and include systolic hypertension, cigarette smoking, hyperlipidemia, and diabetes mellitus (Table 20-4). The pathology observed in affected arteries is usually that of advanced atherosclerosis, with large cholesterol- and calcium-containing plaques encroaching on the lumen. As in all forms of symptomatic atherosclerotic occlusive disease, the pathophysiology is that of gradual plaque enlargement, with eventual thrombosis of the residual lumen. Arterial thrombi are initiated by the deposition of platelets on the plaque surface, attachment and aggregation of ad-

Table 20-4
Risk Factors for Peripheral Atherosclerosis

Male sex
Age
Hypertensive
Tobacco abuse
Hyperlipidemia
Diabetes mellitus

ditional platelets, activation of the coagulation pathways, and deposition of fibrin, terminating in a platelet-fibrin thrombus and occlusion of the vessel. Thrombus formation on the exposed core of an ulcerated plaque can result in acute occlusion of highly stenotic lesions. This luminal thrombus provides the opportunity to recanalize chronic arterial occlusions with fibrinolytic agents, restoring a small channel in an apparently chronically occluded vessel.

Aortoiliac Occlusive Disease

The pathophysiology of the symptoms produced by atherosclerotic occlusive disease of the infrarenal aorta and iliac vessels was first described by Leriche, and the characteristic triad of claudication, impotence, and diminished femoral pulses bears his name. Three patterns of aortoiliac disease have been identified (Fig. 20-21). Localized disease confined to the aorta and common iliac arteries is found in 10 percent of patients (type I). The disease extends into the external iliac arteries in approximately 25 percent of patients (type II). The occlusive process is multisegmental, involving the infrainguinal vessels in the remaining 65 percent of patients (type III).

Clinical Manifestations. Aortoiliac occlusive disease is typically characterized by intermittent claudication involving the thigh, buttock, and calf, and sexual impotence in males. Symptoms may remain stable for years and may even improve as collaterals enlarge with exercise or cessation of smoking. Limb-threatening ischemia is rare with isolated aortoiliac occlusive disease; symptoms are limited to claudication in the absence of concurrent infrainguinal disease. Aortoiliac occlusive disease may also be manifested by atheromatous embolization from ulcerated plaques in the involved arterial segment. The emboli may lodge in the digital arteries of the toes producing gangrene of one or more digits; as previously mentioned, this phenomenon has been termed the blue-toe syndrome. Alternatively, microemboli may travel to dermal vessels, resulting in a blue reticular cutaneous pattern. Biopsy of these lesions reveals cholesterol debris within the terminal arterioles.

Impotence represents a symptom complex of diverse causes. Satisfactory male sexual function requires adequate blood flow to the penis via the hypogastric and internal pudendal arteries, an intact pelvic parasympathetic system, and an appropriate hormonal and psychologic milieu. Impotence can be ascribed to a vascular cause in only a small minority of patients.

Diagnosis. An accurate history and physical examination can establish or exclude the diagnosis of aortoiliac occlusive disease with certainty in the vast majority of instances. The classic findings of thigh claudication and decreased groin pulses may be accompanied by lower abdominal and femoral bruits. The diagnosis may occasionally be confused with that of lumbosacral nerve root compression caused by disc herniation or spinal stenosis. Patients with these disorders can be distinguished from patients with claudication by the fact that their pain is temporally related to changes in position rather than ambulation.

The clinical suspicion of aortoiliac occlusive disease may be difficult to confirm using the noninvasive vascular laboratory. Arterial cuff pressures obtained at the proximal thigh level do not necessarily reflect pressures within the iliac or common femoral systems, since the cuff cannot be positioned high enough to occlude these vessels. A decreased proximal thigh cuff pressure may therefore represent occlusive disease of both the proximal superficial femoral and profunda femoris arteries rather than an inflow lesion of the aortoiliac segment. Common femoral Doppler waveforms have been of some use in the diagnosis of inflow disease. The normal waveform is triphasic, with a negative postsystolic component. Loss of the triphasic waveform and the presence of a blunted, biphasic configuration occurs relatively early in aortoiliac occlusion and is evidence of inflow disease (Fig. 20-22). Percutaneous needle cannulation of the common femoral artery is an invasive, but extremely precise, means of identifying inflow occlusive disease. The presence of a pressure gradient between the brachial and femoral vessels is indicative of significant aortic or iliac stenotic lesions. When a lesion is suspected but no gradient is present, papaverine administration may be helpful in identifying the stenosis. Papaverine is injected intraarterially at the time of cannulation to dilate the distal vasculature, thus reducing peripheral resistance and increasing blood flow across the aortoiliac segment. If a stenosis is present, this will result in a decreased pressure in the femoral artery. A decrease in the femoral to brachial pressure ratio of more than 15 percent after papaverine administration induced hyperemia implies significant occlusive disease involving the aor-

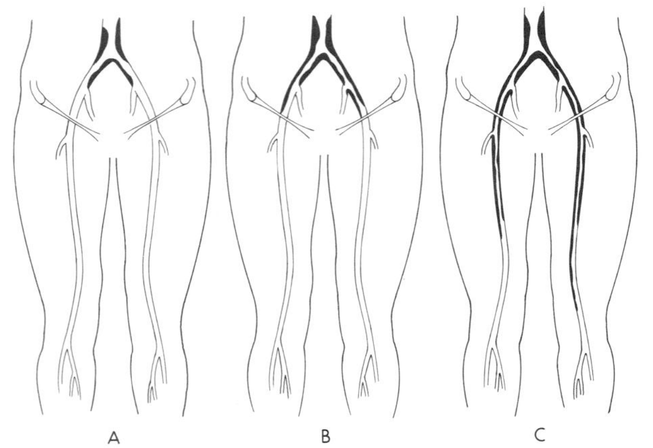

FIG. 20-21. Distribution of stenotic disease in three types of aortoiliac occlusive disease.

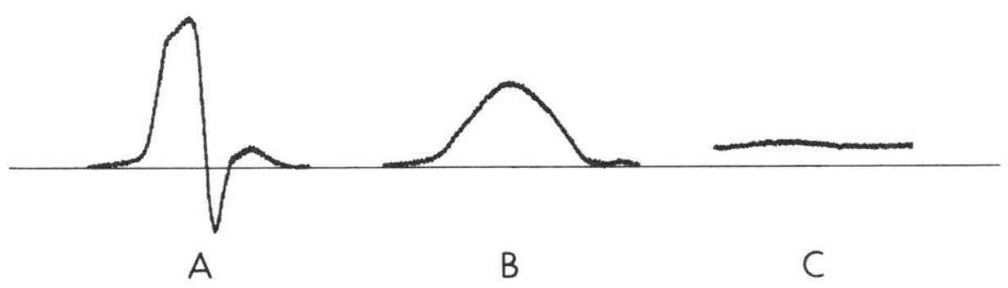

FIG. 20-22. Doppler velocity profile in normal vessels (*A*), vessels with moderate disease proximally (*B*), and vessels with severe proximal disease (*C*).

toiliac segment. It has also been shown to be predictive of symptomatic relief with aortoiliac reconstruction alone, even in the presence of concurrent, uncorrected infrainguinal disease.

Vasculogenic impotence can be differentiated from impotence caused by other disorders using noninvasive laboratory techniques. The penile systolic pressure is measured using a small pneumatic cuff placed around the shaft of the penis and a photoplethysmographic probe on the glans. The penile/brachial index is defined as the penile systolic pressure divided by the brachial systolic pressure, and is approximately 1.0 in potent men. A penile/brachial index of greater than 0.8 confirms the adequacy of penile arterial inflow and virtually excludes the diagnosis of vasculogenic impotence. The converse is not necessarily true; some men are potent despite indices of less than 0.6.

Preoperative standard or digital arteriography is required in patients undergoing elective operation for aortoiliac occlusive disease. The arterial tree should be visualized from the renal arteries to the feet, and the presence of concurrent disease in the inferior mesenteric, hypogastric, and profunda femoris vessels assessed. A transfemoral approach to arteriography is preferable for reasons of ease and safety, but the absence of palpable femoral pulses on either side may necessitate use of a brachial or translumbar route. Intravenous digital studies have been widely used in patients with aortoiliac occlusive disease and absent femoral pulses, but the resolution of this technique is poor because of factors such as bowel gas motion in the abdomen and sluggish blood flow in the extremities.

Treatment. The primary indications for aortoiliac reconstruction are threatened limb loss with rest pain, ulceration, or gangrene and atheroembolic phenomena such as the blue-toe syndrome. Disagreement exists about the advisability of operation for symptoms of claudication alone. In general, claudication of sufficient severity to restrict livelihood or life-style is considered an acceptable indication for aortoiliac reconstruction procedures in medically fit individuals.

Aortoiliac reconstruction can be accomplished using four methods; aortofemoral bypass, aortoiliac endarterectomy, extraanatomic bypass, and balloon catheter dilatation. The durability of aortofemoral bypass and aortoiliac endarterectomy is superior to that of extraanatomic bypass or balloon angioplasty. Extraanatomic procedures, usually in the form of axillofemoral or femorofemoral bypass, are usually reserved for medically unstable patients who are at high risk for perioperative complications in the setting of an intraabdominal procedure. Femorofemoral bypass has a higher patency rate than axillofemoral bypass, but it requires one normal iliac artery for inflow, and so it is not suitable for patients with bilateral disease. Femorofemoral bypass avoids any possibility of pelvic autonomic nerve injury and is therefore frequently employed as a primary reconstructive procedure in young male patients in whom maintenance of normal sexual function is an important issue. Balloon angioplasty is the least invasive method of restoring inflow to the lower extremity, the modality is associated with the success seen with operative bypass in the treatment of isolated common iliac artery lesions only.

Operations on the abdominal aorta are associated with a perioperative mortality of 2 to 10 percent, depending on the presence and severity of associated medical conditions. Complications are most often related to concomitant atherosclerosis involving the coronary and cerebral vasculature. The presence of chronic obstructive lung disease is associated with an increased risk of perioperative pulmonary complications, the most serious of which is the need for prolonged ventilatory support. The preoperative testing for aortoiliac procedures may include pulmonary function tests, dipyridamole-thallium myocardial imaging, dobutamine echocardiography, and coronary angiography, and the evaluation frequently uncovers unsuspected cardiac and pulmonary disease.

The perioperative technical complications of aortoiliac reconstruction are hemorrhage, thrombosis of the reconstruction, and distal embolization of atherosclerotic debris from aortic manipulation. Ischemia of the rectosigmoid colon may be due to interruption of the inferior mesenteric and hypogastric arteries or from atheroembolization to the bowel. Paraplegia is a rare complication that may be secondary to ligation or embolization of a prominent lumbar vessel providing blood flow to the spinal cord through the greater radicular artery of Adamkiewicz (arteria radicularis magna). Damage is usually limited to the anterior two-thirds of the spinal cord in the distribution of the anterior spinal artery, producing a loss of motor function with preservation of sensation. Sexual dysfunction is common after reconstruction of the abdominal aorta; retrograde ejaculation occurs in over 40 percent of patients, and impotence in 25 percent of patients. The frequency of postoperative sexual dysfunction may be decreased by minimizing periaortic dissection, thus preserving the sympathetic and parasympathetic nerves, and by maintaining blood flow through at least one hypogastric artery.

Aortofemoral Bypass. Aortofemoral bypass is currently the treatment of choice for symptomatic aortoiliac occlusive disease. A bifurcated prosthetic graft made of Dacron or, less commonly, polytetrafluoroethylene (PTFE) is utilized to bypass the stenotic lesions. Although there are advantages and disadvantages to each of the prosthetic materials, this is less of a concern in aortofemoral grafting, since patency is excellent with any conduit. The 5- and 10-year patencies of aortoiliac reconstructions are 90 and 75 percent, respectively.

Dacron grafts are constructed in either a knitted or woven configuration. The advantages of the knitted structure are the excellent tissue ingrowth that occurs through the wide interstices of the graft, and the technical ease of handling at the time of operation. Preclotting with the patient's blood is required, however, to avoid massive hemorrhage through the interstices when blood flow through the graft is initially established. Knitted grafts have also been associated with degeneration and aneurysmal dilatation over time. By contrast, preclotting is infrequently required with woven Dacron grafts, and graft dilatation is less common. Dacron grafts have been coated with albumin or collagen, eliminating the need for preclotting, but substantially increasing the cost of the grafts. Using PTFE grafts for aortofemoral bypass also eliminates the need for preclotting, since these grafts are impermeable to blood and aneurysmal degeneration has not yet been reported. Despite these potential advantages, the use of PTFE grafts in the aortofemoral position has not gained widespread acceptance. Currently, the choice of graft material for aortoiliac reconstruction is determined by surgeon preference because there is no difference in patency between the fabrics.

Once the graft has been selected and the patient has been systemically heparinized, the proximal anastomosis between the graft and the infrarenal aorta is created using either an end-to-end or end-to-side technique (Fig. 20-23). The type of anastomosis chosen is determined by the need to maintain antegrade blood flow to the hypogastric vessels. An end-to-side proximal anastomosis is indicated when the external iliac arteries are stenotic or occluded

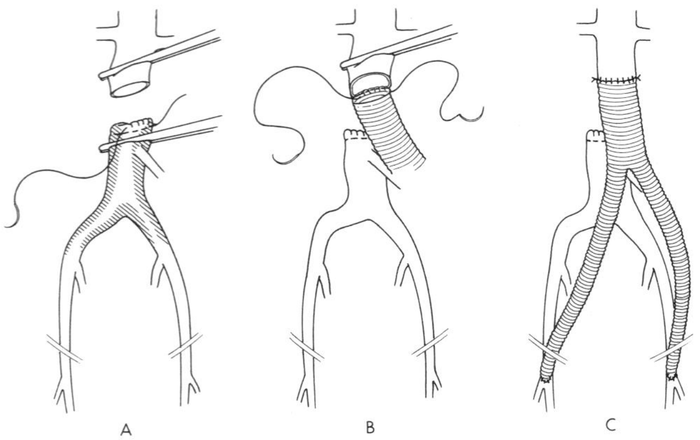

FIG. 20-23. A standard aortobifemoral bypass procedure with *A.* Division of the aorta proximal to the interior mesenteric artery to allow retrograde perfusion of the vessel; *B.* End-to-end proximal anastomosis; *C.* End-to-side distal (common femoral) anastomosis.

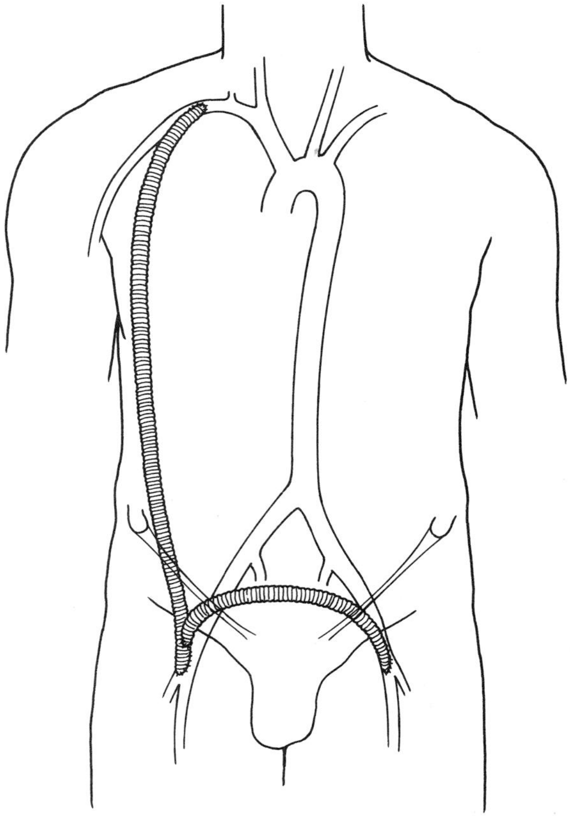

FIG. 20-24. An axillobifemoral bypass with proximal right axillary anastomosis for inflow and bilateral common femoral anastomoses for outflow.

bilaterally, since the arterial flow to the spinal cord and colon in this situation may be dependent on antegrade flow through the distal aorta to the hypogastric and inferior mesenteric arteries. The graft limbs are then delivered to the femoral vessels through tunnels that are created beside the external iliac arteries. The distal anastomoses should be placed at the common femoral level, through bilateral groin incisions. In contrast to patients with aneurysmal aortic disease, bypass to the iliac arteries is unwise in the presence of aortoiliac occlusive disease. Although aortoiliac bypass eliminates the need for groin incisions, the patency rate of this procedure is substantially lower than that of aortofemoral bypass. In addition, bypass to the femoral vessels provides the opportunity to correct proximal profunda femoris artery stenoses by placing the hood of the graft onto the profunda femoris artery beyond the area of narrowing.

Endarterectomy Procedures. Aortoiliac endarterectomy was introduced prior to the advent of prosthetic graft conduits. The aorta and iliac arteries are exposed and all branch vessels are controlled in preparation for clamping. The patient is heparinized and occlusive vascular clamps are placed. The atherosclerotic plaque is removed through one or more arteriotomies, and the arteriotomies are subsequently closed either with or without a patch. Endarterectomy does eliminate the use of prosthetic material, but the procedure is not suitable for patients in whom the atherosclerotic process extends to the external iliac artery. Endarterectomy requires localized atherosclerotic disease with an appropriate ending of the plaque on relatively normal vessel, and early failure of the endarterectomized segment can be predicted in the absence of a suitable end point within 1 or 2 cm of the origin of the external iliac artery. Nevertheless, aortoiliac endarterectomy may be the procedure of choice for young patients with long life expectancies and disease localized to the aorta and common iliac vessels; it achieves excellent patency rates and avoids some of the complications associated with prosthetic graft material.

Extraanatomic Bypass. Extraanatomic revascularization procedures include axillofemoral, femorofemoral, and obturator bypasses (Fig. 20-24). Axillofemoral and femorofemoral procedures are preferred when the patient's medical condition renders the risk of a major intraabdominal operation unacceptable. Other indications include lower extremity ischemia in the presence of an infected aortic graft, reoperation for aortofemoral graft occlusion, and revascularization in a sexually active male to avoid the possibility of postoperative sexual dysfunction. Prosthetic graft materials are almost always employed. The axillary artery provides inflow for an axillofemoral graft; the graft is tunneled subcutaneously along the lateral trunk to the ipsilateral femoral artery in the case of an *axillounifemoral* bypass, or to both femoral arteries in an *axillobifemoral* bypass. The patency of axillounifemoral bypasses is poor, averaging well below 50 percent at 5 years. The flow through axillobifemoral bypasses is twice that of axillounifemoral grafts, resulting in a significantly higher 5-year patency rate. Thus, axillobifemoral bypass is often employed for unilateral leg ischemia in order to improve graft longevity.

The best results of extraanatomic bypass procedures are achieved with femorofemoral bypass grafts; the 5-year patency rate of these grafts is between 50 and 75 percent. The procedure involves exposure of both femoral arteries in the groins and subcutaneous placement of a prosthetic conduit in the suprapubic region. A nonstenotic donor iliac vessel is required; the adequacy of this vessel can be evaluated with femoral arterial pressure measurements made before and after papaverine injection. Concomitant iliac balloon angioplasty has been successfully employed in the presence of iliac stenotic disease to establish adequate inflow to the donor side. The *obturator bypass* is a rarely utilized but extremely effective procedure which is primarily employed to circumvent an infected graft in the groin area. The inflow site is the aorta, iliac artery, or aortofemoral graft limb within the abdomen. The graft is tunneled through the obturator foramen and joins the superficial femoral artery distal to the groin, thus completely avoiding the infected area.

Endovascular Procedures. Percutaneous transluminal angioplasty (PTA) was introduced as a method of reestablishing flow through stenotic vessels by Dotter in 1964. A decade later, Gruntzig further refined the technique of balloon catheter dilatation of arterial stenoses. Currently, the procedure is initiated by the percutaneous cannulation of an accessible vessel, either the common femoral artery or the brachial artery. After a diagnostic arteriogram has been performed and pressure gradients have been measured, a balloon catheter is advanced across the arterial stenosis. The balloon is inflated to several atmospheres of pressure, and completion arteriograms and pressure measurements are obtained. Initially, the mechanism underlying balloon dilatation was believed to be circumferential dilatation of all layers of the arterial wall with compression and remodeling of the plaque. Later studies have suggested that this is not the case; rather, the plaque is cracked, forming fissures and false channels. The media is overstretched, causing destruction of its elastic components. The adventitia remains intact unless the artery has been overdilated. Rupture of the wall with hemorrhage or false aneurysm formation occurs if the artery is excessively overdilated, but this complication is rare.

The results of PTA have been satisfactory in relatively short nonoccluding lesions of the aortoiliac segment, with patency rates (60 to 90 percent at 5 years) approaching those of operative correction. Balloon angioplasty procedures, however, have generally been reserved for patients with less extensive atherosclerosis. Moreover, subjective methods of determining long-term patency rates have been employed to assess the results of PTA rather than the noninvasive laboratory methods routinely utilized to evaluate the results of vascular surgical procedures. These two factors may have resulted in an overestimation of the success of PTA, rendering direct comparisons of patency rates between angioplasty and operative revascularization impossible.

A plethora of new devices designed to relieve arterial stenoses by relatively noninvasive means has been introduced over the last decade. These devices are placed either percutaneously or through femoral arterial cutdowns, and have been collectively termed *endovascular* interventions. The devices have included (1) laser-heated metallic probes designed to remodel plaque as the instrument is advanced through an atherosclerotic lesion, (2) catheters that vaporize atheromata by direct delivery of laser light, (3) "atherectomy" devices that remove plaque with rotational cutting blades, and (4) intraluminal metallic stents designed to maintain the artery in an expanded state and thus decrease the frequency of postprocedural restenosis.

Vascular endoscopes are frequently used to evaluate the results of these interventions, and the instruments have also been helpful in the assessment of operative procedures such as balloon catheter thrombectomy and valve disruption in in situ saphenous vein bypass. Intravascular ultrasound devices have been introduced to provide high-resolution images of atherosclerotic vessels both before and after endovascular manipulation. Unfortunately, the introduction phase of each new device has been associated with unwarranted optimism, prompting premature promotion of the device prior to the demonstration of long-term safety and efficacy. To date, none of new devices has matched the results of standard operative revascularization procedures. It is hoped that the continued development, refinement, and objective long-term evaluation of newer endovascular techniques may someday provide less invasive means of restoring arterial flow to the compromised extremity.

Infrainguinal Occlusive Disease

The infrainguinal vessels are defined as those vessels distal to the inguinal ligament, including the common femoral, superficial and deep femoral, popliteal, and infrapopliteal arteries. The superficial femoral artery is the most common site of atherosclerotic obstruction in the lower extremity. The process is usually first evident at the level of the adductor canal, but recent studies suggest that this is not because the atherosclerotic process begins here. Rather, Zarins and associates have shown that the deposition of atherosclerotic plaque occurs at an equal rate throughout the superficial femoral segment. The normal response to plaque deposition is dilatation of the vessel such that the lumen diameter is maintained. Zarins and associates have suggested that the most severe obliterative process occurs at the level of the adductor canal because this area of the vessel is least likely to display compensatory dilatation in response to plaque deposition.

The risk factors for infrainguinal atherosclerotic arterial disease are the same as those of atherosclerotic disease in general, namely, advanced age, systolic hypertension, cigarette smoking, hyperlipidemia, and diabetes mellitus.

Clinical Manifestations. Stenosis or occlusion limited to only one segment of the arterial tree seldom results in a threatened limb. The most frequent clinical scenario is that of solitary superficial femoral arterial occlusion at the level of the adductor canal, producing symptoms of *calf* claudication following several blocks of ambulation. Critical ischemia manifested by rest pain, ulceration, or gangrene is seen only with the development of multisegmental disease involving the aortoiliac, deep femoral, or tibial vessels in addition to the superficial femoral artery. Rest pain is characteristically located in the forefoot or medial arch and is most severe when the foot is elevated in bed at night. Night-time calf pain is usually the result of benign conditions such as nocturnal cramping and should not be confused with pain from arterial ischemia.

The natural history of infrainguinal arterial occlusive disease is dependent on the severity of the patient's symptoms. Boyd prospectively followed over 1400 patients with intermittent claudication and found that only 7 percent required amputation at 5 years of follow-up. The results of the Framingham study were even more optimistic, with less than 2 percent of patients with claudication losing a limb over a 10-year interval. One must caution, however, that the patients in these studies were not prevented from undergoing arterial reconstructive procedures. Nevertheless, it is clear that symptoms of intermittent claudication alone are not a harbinger of limb loss, and operative procedures designed to relieve claudication must weigh this relatively low risk against the somewhat higher risks of perioperative morbidity and mortality. By contrast to intermittent claudication, symptoms of severe ischemia with pain at rest, ischemic ulceration, and gangrene are associated with a high risk of limb loss unless successful revascularization can be achieved. Over 50 percent of untreated patients with limb-threatening symptoms will required amputation within several months of presentation, and this risk increases as the severity of the ischemic process evolves from rest pain to tissue loss.

The life expectancy of patients with lower extremity occlusive disease must be taken into account when one considers options of operative revascularization. Given the systemic nature of the atherosclerotic process, it is not surprising that the survival of patients with lower extremity occlusive disease is significantly decreased as a result of coexistent coronary disease, cerebrovascular disease, and an increased risk of lung cancer. A consensus of recent studies suggests a 70 percent 5-year and 50 percent 10-year survival rate in patients with chronic lower extremity arterial disease. These rates average 20 to 30 percent below those of age-matched controls.

Diagnosis. The diagnosis of infrainguinal arterial occlusive disease is based on the characteristic clinical findings of intermittent calf claudication, rest pain in the foot, or tissue loss in the form of ischemic ulceration or gangrene. Claudication can be differentiated from other causes of leg pain on the basis of its reproducible relationship to ambulation. Patients with claudication develop pain after walking a distance that is constant for any given patient, and exhibit regression of the pain on cessation of activity, even if the standing position is maintained. By contrast, patients with leg pain secondary to disorders such as nerve root compression exhibit pain that is related to position rather than ambulation.

The physical examination is a most important tool in the diagnosis and localization of lower extremity occlusive disease. Whereas the patient with aortoiliac occlusive disease manifests absent femoral pulses in the groin, patients with infrainguinal disease will have normal femoral pulses and absent popliteal pulses (superficial femoral artery occlusion) or absent pedal pulses (tibial artery occlusive disease). The differential diagnosis of lower extremity ulcerations can frequently be made on the basis of location and appearance. Ulcerations secondary to inadequate arterial blood flow are characteristically found on the lateral aspect of the ankle or on the foot and are pale and devoid of granulation tissue. Ulcerations resulting from venous stasis are located above the medial malleolus, are pink with abundant granulation tissue, and are accompanied by other stigmata of venous disease such as brown discoloration of the pretibial skin.

The noninvasive laboratory examination of the patient with infrainguinal occlusive disease parallels the physical findings. The common femoral Doppler waveforms have the normal triphasic configuration. Proximal thigh Doppler segmental pressures may be normal if either the superficial *or* profunda femoris artery is free of disease, but will be decreased if the proximal portions of *both* vessels are affected. The distal superficial femoral artery is the most frequent site for occlusive disease. The most common Doppler segmental findings, therefore, consist of a proximal thigh cuff pressure equal to or greater than the brachial pressure and a gradient of at least 30 mmHg between the proximal and distal thigh pressures.

Vessel wall calcification, a change characteristically seen in diabetic patients, renders the arterial wall incompressible. Doppler cuff pressures are unobtainable in this situation, since flow through the calcific, rigid vessels cannot be obliterated, even with cuff pressures exceeding 300 mmHg. Pulse volume recordings (PVRs) play an important role in evaluation of the diabetic with incompressible vessels. The PVR does not require compression of the vessels; rather, it relies on volume changes in the leg between systole and diastole. The presence of blunted PVR tracings between two levels in the extremity is indicative of an interval stenosis. Despite the common misperception that diabetic arterial disease is an entity involving the small arteries and arterioles, the larger vessels are actually the most common location of arterial lesions even in diabetics, while the smaller, digital arteries are frequently spared. This feature of diabetic arterial disease makes it possible to use toe pressures to detect arterial insufficiency when the large vessels are incompressible. Toe pressures are obtained by placing a small pneumatic cuff around the base of the digit and a photoplethysmographic sensor distal to the cuff. The systolic pressure at the toe level is normally somewhat less than the brachial pressure, with normal toe indices (toe pressure divided by brachial pressure) averaging 0.70 or more. Patients with claudication usually have toe indices in the range of 0.40, and patients with rest pain, ulceration, or gangrene have toe indices of 0.10 to 0.20.

Arteriography is the most precise method of documenting the location and severity of infrainguinal arterial occlusive disease. Transfemoral standard or intraarterial digital studies offer the highest-quality images. The small caliber and slow flow characteristic of diseased lower extremity vessels diminishes the resolution of intravenous digital studies and renders this form of arteriography inappropriate in most patients with infrainguinal occlusive disease. Recently, Duplex ultrasound has been utilized as a less invasive alternative to contrast arteriography in patients with lower extremity occlusive disease, but the imprecision of the current technique makes it a less adequate method of preoperative evaluation.

Treatment. The indications for infrainguinal arterial reconstruction are comparable to the indications for aortoiliac reconstruction and include severe claudication and limb-threatening ischemia manifested by rest pain, ulceration, or gangrene. Nonoperative management is indicated in patients with mild claudication, and treatment regimens include cessation of tobacco use and institution of a daily program of regular exercise. Vasodilators, including calcium channel blockers have been used with limited success.

Pentoxifylline is an oral agent that reduces blood viscosity, theoretically increasing blood flow through stenotic arteries and small collaterals. Pentoxifylline reduced symptoms of claudication in a randomized, double-blind, multicenter trial. This benefit averaged only 45 percent with the drug, compared to 23 percent with placebo. The therapeutic benefit from pentoxifylline has been unpredictable in actual clinical usage, with many patients experiencing little or no relief of claudication. The documented improvement in microcirculatory flow, however, has led to interest in using pentoxifylline to improve tissue perfusion in patients with limb-threatening ischemia. Encouraging results have been reported in patients with arterial ulcerations, although randomized, blinded studies have yet to be completed.

Three factors are required for successful infrainguinal revascularization: adequate inflow, adequate outflow, and a suitable conduit. As in the case of aortoiliac disease, both endarterectomy and bypass grafting are useful alternatives in the management of arterial insufficiency. For patients requiring infrainguinal reconstruction, however, the concerns of inadequate inflow, inadequate outflow, and type of conduit assume much greater importance. These three issues are rarely of concern in aortoiliac revascularization but are fundamental in more distal reconstructions.

Endarterectomy. Infrainguinal endarterectomy was introduced over four decades ago, prior to the development of adequate bypass conduit materials. The segment of artery containing the atherosclerotic lesion is exposed, the artery is opened, and the atheroma is removed using a spatula or mechanical stripper. The arteriotomy or arteriotomies are then closed primarily or with a venous or prosthetic patch. The long-term success of the procedure appears to be dependent on the size of the artery and the length of the lesion. As with any endarterectomy procedure, the atherosclerotic lesion must terminate distally in an area of normal arterial wall. If care is not taken to ensure that this is the case, dissection of blood beneath the shelf of the atheroma may result in creation of a flap and acute postoperative thrombosis of the reconstruction. Endarterectomy is generally limited to the treatment of short lesions of the superficial femoral artery at the adductor canal and localized stenoses at the origin of the deep femoral artery. Popliteal and tibial artery endarterectomy procedures are rarely successful since the atherosclerotic disease is usually diffuse in these vessels.

Bypass Procedures. Bypass procedure are described by the inflow and outflow sites. Thus, the term *femoropopliteal bypass* indicates that the site of inflow is the femoral artery and the site of outflow is the popliteal artery. The two most commonly performed infrainguinal reconstructions are the femoropopliteal and femorotibial bypasses (Fig. 20-25). Popliteal-to-tibial and popliteal-to-pedal bypasses are important but are performed less commonly, as are more distal reconstructions to the arteries of the foot.

The common femoral artery is the standard site of inflow for infrainguinal bypass procedures. The superficial femoral or popliteal arteries may also be used for inflow in the absence of significant proximal stenoses, and these alternate sources of inflow become particularly important when the length of vein available for the bypass is limited. The choice of inflow and outflow sites is relatively straightforward when a single segment of the arterial tree is involved with an occlusive lesion. For example, a femoropopliteal bypass is appropriate when the occlusive process is limited to the superficial femoral artery between its origin and the knee joint. The presence of multisegmental arterial occlusion, however, requires that a decision be made regarding which levels of occlusion should be bypassed. In general, this decision is based on the magnitude of the ischemic process. The presence of extensive tissue loss in the foot mandates bypassing all levels of occlusion. For example, a patient with a superficial femoral artery occlusion, open popliteal artery, and short proximal occlusions of all three tibial arteries will be well served with a femoropopliteal bypass to the "isolated" popliteal segment if the symptoms are those of claudication or even rest pain. By contrast, a patient with the same arteriographic situation will require bypass to an open distal tibial artery in the presence of a large necrotic ulceration over the dorsum of the foot.

The selection of conduit material is of paramount importance in infrainguinal arterial reconstruction, as the long-term patency rate is highly dependent on two primary factors: the site of outflow and the type of bypass material. The possible graft choices are autogenous vein and prosthetic graft materials (Table 20-5). Presently, PTFE is the most commonly used prosthetic; Dacron is infrequently employed. The use of bovine heterografts has been abandoned because of the propensity for late aneurysm formation, and human umbilical vein biografts have decreased in popularity because they are cumbersome to sew and they too are associated with late aneurysm formation. Saphenous vein is the best infrainguinal bypass conduit material. The patency of saphenous vein grafts is better than that of prosthetic grafts, and problems with postoperative infection are reduced by avoidance of prosthetic material. The difference in patency is of sufficient magnitude that vein should be used for all infrainguinal bypasses, even if this requires use of the lesser saphenous or cephalic veins. Possible exceptions to this rule may occur when the bypass graft does not cross the knee joint as with a femoral-to-supragenicular popliteal artery bypass. In this instance, the patency of venous and prosthetic bypass grafts do not differ substantially, and use of a prosthetic preserves the vein for use in the event of graft failure or for use in a subsequent coronary artery bypass.

There are two general techniques used in autogenous vein bypass procedures, differentiated by the orientation of the vein in relation to the direction of blood flow and the alignment of the venous valves. Advantages and disadvantages have been demonstrated with each method, but most studies have failed to document significant differences in long-term patency rates when pre-

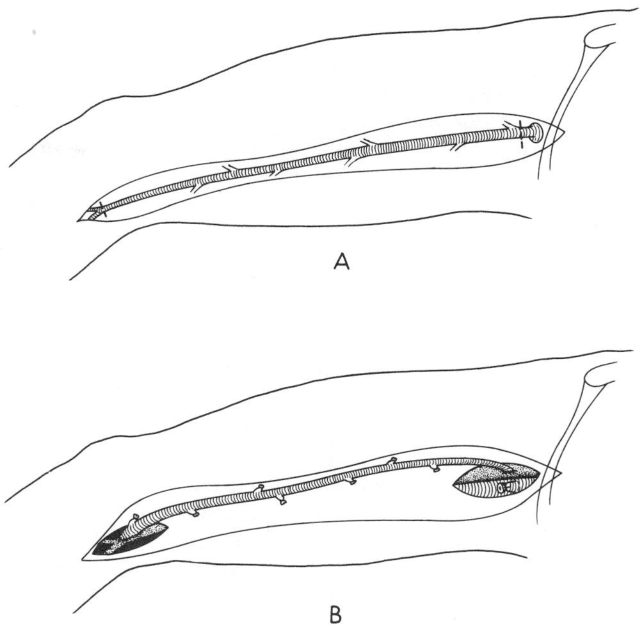

FIG. 20-25. *A.* The greater saphenous vein is exposed from the groin to a distal level appropriate for the required length. The vein may be excised and reversed (reversed vein graft). Alternatively, the vein may be left in its bed and the values rendered incompetent with a valvulotome (in-situ vein graft). *B.* The proximal anastomosis is performed to the side of the common femoral artery, and the distal anastomosis is performed to the side of the infragenicular popliteal artery (femoral below-knee popliteal vein bypass).

Table 20-5
Three-Year Patency Rate of Infrainguinal Bypass Procedures

Bypass Procedure	*Saphenous Vein*	*PTFE*
Femoral popliteal	76 percent	54 percent
Femoral tibial	49 percent	12 percent

cise operative technique has been employed. The *reversed* bypass technique, the first method of infrainguinal vein bypass employed, excises the vein in its entirety and reverses it such that the caudal end is anastomosed proximally and the cranial end distally. The reversed orientation allows blood flow to proceed in the natural direction allowed by the valves, but the small end of the vein is anastomosed to the larger (inflow) artery, and the large end of the vein is anastomosed to the smaller (outflow) artery (Fig. 20-26).

In situ vein bypasses represent a second technique, first performed in the 1960s. The vein is left in its usual orientation, disrupting the venous valves to allow blood to flow from the cranial end of the vein to the caudal end. The large and small ends of the in situ venous conduit are connected to the arterial vessels of corresponding size, and venous vasa vasorum are preserved if the vein is left in its natural bed. A variety of instruments has been devised to assist in the disruption of the valves; some are passed through side branches of the vein and others through the caudal cut end of the conduit. An alternative technique, representing a modification of the in situ method, involves excising the vein, disrupting the valves, and connecting the conduit in an ''excised, nonreversed'' fashion. The excised, nonreversed technique interrupts the potentially advantageous venous vaso vasorum but decreases the risk of vein injury during the valve-cutting process since the vein may be straightened and shortened in an ''accordion'' fashion onto a semirigid valve-cutting instrument.

Endovascular Procedures. Infrainguinal endovascular procedures include percutaneous transluminal balloon angioplasty, laser angioplasty, and catheter atherectomy. None of the devices has matched the success of endovascular procedures in the aortoiliac segment. Balloon angioplasty with or without the use of a stent may have a role in selected patients with superficial femoral disease, but the current results only justify the routine use of this technique for iliac lesions. Currently, laser angioplasty and catheter atherectomy must be considered experimental techniques, and assessment of their safety and efficacy awaits the results of randomized, controlled trials that adhere to uniform reporting standards.

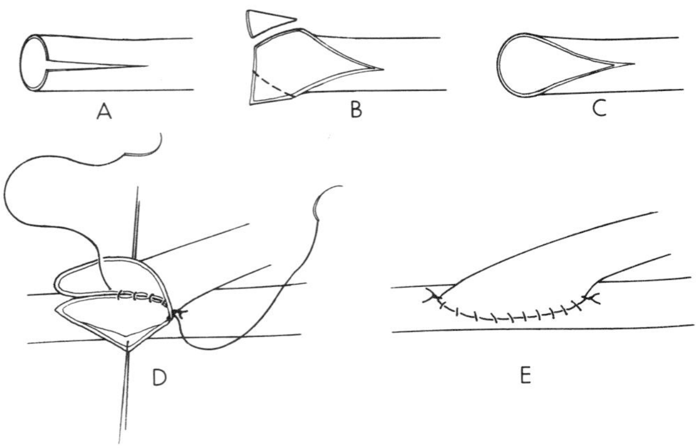

FIG. 20-26. *A.* The graft is spatulated to provide a longer orifice for anastomosis. If necessary, the graft can be tailored to provide a rounded hood. *B, C.* The graft is sewn to the inflow vessel using a continuous suturing technique and an end-of-graft to side-of-artery configuration. *D.* The initial sutures are generally placed at the heel of the anastomosis and the graft is then "parachuted down" onto the artery. *E.* The completed anastomosis with a cobra-head appearance.

The Diabetic Foot

Diabetes mellitus is the risk factor associated with the highest rate of limb-threatening ischemia of the lower extremity; the incidence of gangrene in diabetics is over 50 times greater than in nondiabetics. The anatomic distribution of arterial lesions in diabetics differs from that of the nondiabetic population, but the underlying histopathology is similar. Diabetic arterial disease is more common in the distal profunda femoris artery, the distal popliteal and tibial arteries, and the digital arteries of the foot. The aortoiliac segment is usually spared. The widespread belief that diabetic arterial disease is primarily localized to the small vessels is erroneous. Although diabetics do develop a microangiopathy characterized by thickening of the intima and basement membrane, the primary pathologic process is that of typical large-vessel atherosclerosis. The media of muscular arteries is often heavily calcified in diabetics, rendering the vessels incompressible and difficult to occlude using standard vascular clamps.

Diabetics are predisposed to ulceration and gangrene of the foot, with relatively rapid progression to limb loss. A variety of complex and interrelated factors are responsible for this susceptibility and its rapid progression to limb loss. Diabetic neuropathy produces both motor and sensory deficits in the foot. The loss of efferent motor fibers results in atrophy of the intrinsic muscles, a characteristic high-arched deformity of the foot, and markedly increased pressure on the metatarsal heads. Sensory loss compounds the problem, because the patient is unaware of pressure-induced skin necrosis and minor injuries. Arterial disease accelerates the process, and the presence of apparently trivial external pressure may lead to the development of extensive tissue damage.

The impression that infection is more common in diabetic patients has never been proved, but when infections do occur, they are often very aggressive and are associated with a high incidence of gangrene and limb loss. Infection may develop from seemingly trivial skin defects and can quickly spread along musculofascial planes to involve the tendon sheaths and muscles of the foot and leg. The bacteriology of foot sepsis in the diabetic patient is multimicrobial, with gram-negative, gram-positive, and anaerobic organisms acting in synergy. The bacteria most commonly cultured in diabetic foot ulceration include *Peptococcus* (80 percent), *Proteus* (55 percent), and *Bacteroides* (45 percent), with an average of five or more species per specimen. Organisms cultured from superficial sites differ from the offending organisms deep within the wound in the majority of instances. The inaccuracy of bacterial identification obtained from superficial wound cultures emphasizes the importance of broad-spectrum antibiotic therapy in the treatment of diabetic foot infections. The time-honored approach is to begin treatment with an aminoglycoside, clindamycin, and ampicillin, converting to more specific therapy when deep-wound cultures are obtained at the time of operation. Newer cephalosporins and penicillin derivatives have been used successfully; these agents are of particular importance in the setting of renal insufficiency.

The classic diabetic foot ulcer, the ''mal perforant ulcer,'' is located over the metatarsal heads on the plantar aspect of the foot. This is a *neurotrophic ulceration,* as it results from the sensory neuropathy of the diabetic. The ulcer begins to form beneath a callous and may eventually erode into the bone, producing a secondary osteomyelitis.

Treatment. The treatment of diabetic foot ulcers differs from the treatment of ulcers in nondiabetic patients in a number of ways. The exclusion of significant underlying arterial disease is of primary importance. The presence of calcific, incompressible vessels may falsely elevate Doppler pressure measurements, and normal ankle-brachial indices do not eliminate the possibility of arterial disease in the diabetic patient. Toe pressure determination is an accurate means of evaluating arterial insufficiency in the diabetic patient, since digital artery medial calcinosis is rare. Arterial disease is unlikely when the toe-brachial pressure ratio exceeds 0.70. Arteriography is frequently required to exclude the possibility of reconstructible arterial disease of the infrapopliteal, tibial, and pedal vessels. Revascularization procedures are indicated whenever ulceration occurs in the presence of significant arterial disease. In the absence of arterial disease, local wound care, avoidance of repetitive trauma, and the use of specially fitted shoes are appropriate. Amputation may be necessary when the disease is limited to the most distal vessels or when gangrenous changes have progressed despite apparently adequate arterial supply. Minor resections including digital amputations, transmetatarsal amputations, or creative, unnamed resections involving variable portions of the foot may be appropriate in the diabetic. The presence of a palpable dorsalis pedis or posterior tibial pulse is an excellent predictor of healing, and debridement and amputation should be conservative in this setting. Recently, myocutaneous free-flaps have been of value in covering seemingly insurmountable exposure of subcutaneous tissue and bone. In general, latissimus dorsi or rectus abdominus muscle has been utilized, basing the inflow on a patent tibial artery or vein bypass graft.

Sepsis resulting from diabetic foot infection demands urgent treatment. Control of hyperglycemia, drainage of purulent collections, debridement, and rapid institution of broad-spectrum antibiotic therapy are the important initial interventions. Arterial reconstructive procedures are performed after the septic process has been controlled, minimizing the risk of graft infection by avoidance of prosthetic conduits.

Upper Extremity Occlusive Disease

The causes of chronic upper extremity ischemia are multiple, and although atherosclerosis is the usual cause, nonatherosclerotic causes are also common. Vasospastic and inflammatory arteritides affect the upper extremity more often than the lower extremity, whereas the reverse is true of atherosclerotic disease. The characteristic symptom of chronic upper extremity ischemia is arm claudication. Rest pain and tissue loss are unusual because of the extensive collateral network about the shoulder and elbow. When digital gangrene does occur, it is usually due to microemboli originating from atherosclerotic lesions of the subclavian artery.

Diagnosis. The diagnosis of upper extremity arterial occlusive disease begins with palpation of the axillary, radial, ulnar, and brachial pulses. The most common site of atherosclerotic disease of the upper extremity is the origin of the subclavian arteries proximal to the vertebral artery, a lesion that may produce a supraclavicular bruit. More distal lesions are generally not atherosclerotic in origin, and entities such as giant cell arteritis and thoracic outlet syndrome should be considered in this setting. Proximal subclavian lesions may produce the arteriographic finding of flow reversal in the vertebral artery, since this vessel may serve as a major source of collateral blood flow to the arm. Serial images performed after injection of contrast material into the contralateral nonstenotic subclavian artery will reveal normal antegrade flow in the uninvolved vertebral artery, with retrograde flow in the vertebral artery on the side of the subclavian stenosis. This arteriographic finding is associated with the clinical picture known as the *subclavian steal syndrome* and is characterized by nonhemispheric cerebrovascular symptoms in association with mild arm claudication. This symptom complex develops as a result of a reduction in posterior cerebral arterial flow secondary to the "steal" of blood as it flows in a retrograde direction through the vertebral artery into the subclavian artery. The isolated arteriographic finding of retrograde vertebral flow is rarely associated with cerebral symptoms, since the collateral circulation through the circle of Willis is usually sufficient to compensate for the amount of blood diverted to the arm. The presence of neurologic symptoms in the subclavian steal syndrome should suggest the presence of a coexistant carotid stenosis, limiting the compensatory capacity of the cerebral circulation.

Treatment. The indications for operation in upper extremity arterial occlusive disease include incapacitating arm claudication, emboli to the hand or posterior cerebral circulation, and symptomatic subclavian steal syndrome in the absence of a coexistent carotid lesion. Significant carotid lesions should be corrected first in the subclavian steal syndrome, reserving direct subclavian reconstruction for patients without carotid lesions or in whom carotid endarterectomy fails to alleviate cerebral symptoms.

Endarterectomy of the subclavian artery has decreased in popularity because of the fragility of the subclavian artery and the intrathoracic nature of the procedure. Extrathoracic approaches to the subclavian artery are more commonly utilized, employing a transverse supraclavicular incision to expose the common carotid artery for inflow and the distal subclavian artery for outflow. A carotid-subclavian bypass is generally performed with a Dacron or PTFE conduit; this is one of the few situations where prosthetic material may have a better patency than vein (Fig. 20-27). Other operative alternatives include transposition of the end of the subclavian artery onto the side of the common carotid artery (Fig. 20-28), and axillary-to-axillary artery bypass. Treatment of multiple aortic arch vessel involvement requires a median sternotomy and placement of bypass grafts from the ascending aorta to one or more vessels in the neck. Embolic disease is treated by exclusion of the involved segment of artery from the circulation, usually with a standard carotid-subclavian artery bypass, and ligation of the subclavian artery proximal to the vertebral origin. Lesions of the axillary and brachial arteries are treated with saphenous vein bypass grafts around the occluding lesion; the patency of these grafts is excellent. Cervical sympathectomy has been used in the treatment of nonreconstructible disease such as digital artery occlusion but the results have been discouraging.

MESENTERIC AND RENAL ARTERY OCCLUSIVE DISEASE

Occlusive disease involving the arteries to the viscera and kidneys is associated with the life-threatening complications of intestinal infarction and renal insufficiency. The process may develop suddenly, as in the case of embolization to the vessels. Alternatively, the process can evolve in an insidious fashion, as in the case of progressive encroachment on the arterial lumen by an atherosclerotic plaque. The relative rarity of these disease entities renders the diagnosis elusive, and this diagnostic dilemma is compounded by the inaccessibility of the organs to physical examination.

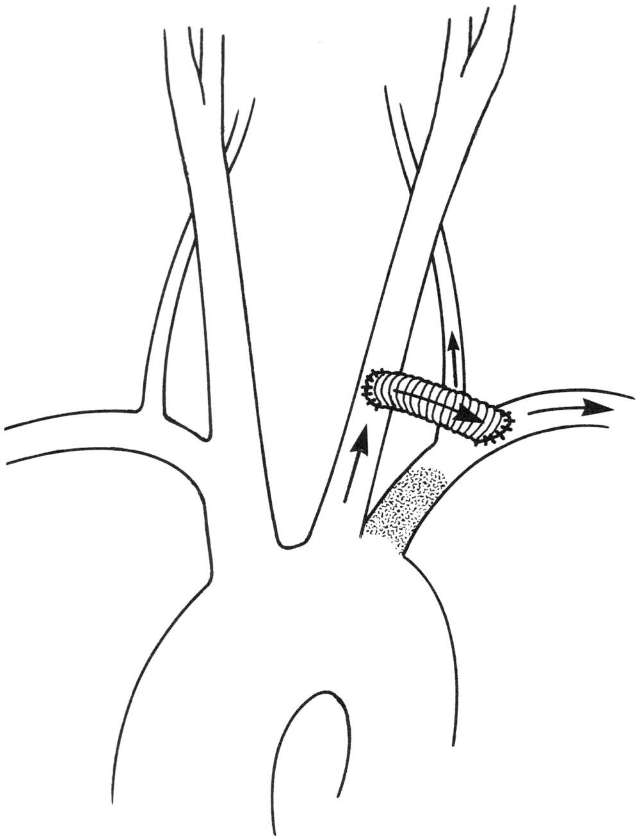

FIG. 20-27. Carotid-subclavian bypass performed for a proximal subclavian occlusion.

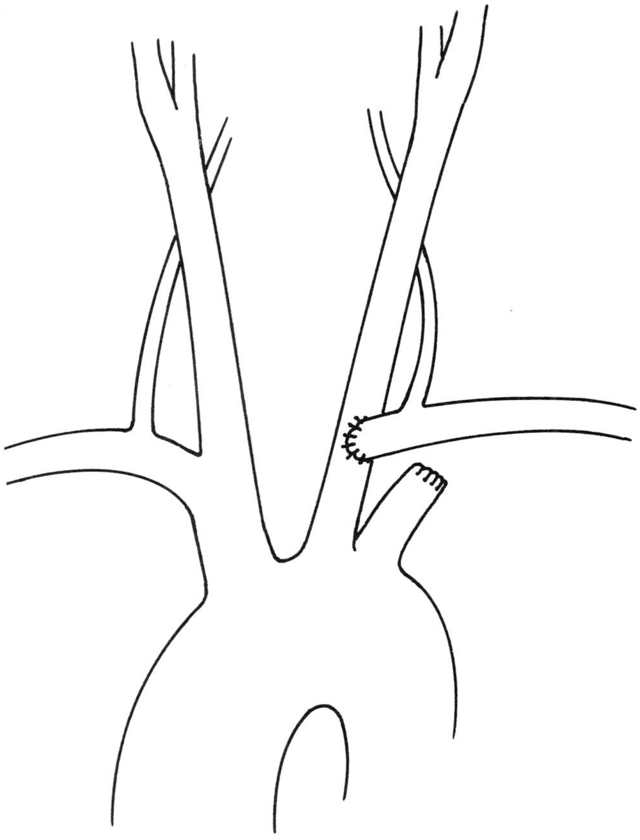

FIG. 20-28. Subclavian-to-carotid transporation performed for proximal subclavian atherosclerotic disease.

Acute Mesenteric Ischemia

Acute mesenteric ischemia is associated with astonishing high mortality rates, approximating 75 percent in most series. The lethality of the entity has not changed substantially over the last few decades, despite advances in operative technique and perioperative management. There are two basic explanations for these dismal results. First, the rarity of the disease renders prompt diagnosis difficult, and an improved outcome can be achieved only through rapid identification of the problem and restoration of blood flow before the onset of irreversible intestinal gangrene. Secondly, acute mesenteric ischemia usually develops in elderly, medically compromised patients who do not tolerate the physiologic insult well.

There are four basic causes of acute mesenteric ischemia; superior mesenteric artery embolization, superior mesenteric artery thrombosis, nonocclusive mesenteric ischemia, and acute mesenteric venous thrombosis. Emboli generally originate from the heart and occur in patients with atrial fibrillation or following myocardial infarction. Thrombosis occurs in the setting of underlying mesenteric atherosclerotic disease, as a critical stenosis progresses to occlusion. Nonocclusive mesenteric ischemia develops in patients with low-cardiac-output states, especially in the presence of digoxin or vasopressors. The pathophysiology of nonocclusive ischemia is that of mesenteric arterial vasoconstriction which is frequently manifest as segmental spasm of the secondary and tertiary branches of the superior mesenteric artery. The precise mechanisms behind nonocclusive ischemia are unclear, but it is probable that the process involves a vicious circle whereby vasoconstriction is induced in the mesenteric arterial bed by a remote stimulus such as cardiogenic shock. Local hypoxia follows, and the resultant bowel ischemia leads to bacterial transudation, worsening shock, and sympathetic stimulation with subsequent perpetuation of the mesenteric vasoconstriction. Venous thrombosis may be secondary to infection or dehydration and will not be considered further.

Electron microscopic changes occur in the intestinal mucosa after only 10 min of ischemia, with light microscopic changes evident after 1 h. Hemorrhagic necrosis develops later, with sloughing of the mucosa, edema of the bowel wall, and hemorrhage into the lumen. The bowel wall becomes permeable to the luminal bacteria once the mucosa is shed. Peritonitis ensues from transudation of microflora across the intestinal wall, and septicemia and bacteremia develop as the organisms enter the portal circulation and overload the filtering capacities of the liver. Massive fluid shifts into the bowel wall and peritoneum follow, resulting in hemoconcentration, oliguria, and hypotension. Serum levels of lactate dehydrogenase (LDH), serum glutamic oxaloacetic transaminase (SGOT), serum glutamic pyruvic transaminase (SGPT), and creatine phosphokinase (CPK) become markedly elevated with the death of intestinal cells.

Diagnosis. The classic presentation of acute mesenteric ischemia is the sudden onset of abdominal pain out of proportion to the physical findings. The patients complain of periumbical pain as a result of the small intestinal ischemia and spasm. The spasm results in gastrointestinal emptying, with emesis and bloody diarrhea. Laboratory changes occur later, with leukocytosis, elevation of the hematocrit, lactate, LDH, SGOT, SGPT, and CPK level elevations, acidosis, and hyperkalemia.

Arteriography has played a crucial role in the early diagnosis of acute intestinal ischemia. Differentiation of the three forms of mesenteric arterial occlusion can be made with lateral views on a transfemoral aortic injection. Mesenteric emboli generally lodge at the orifice of the middle colic artery, generating the characteristic arteriographic picture of a normal-appearing proximal superior mesenteric artery terminating in a ''meniscus sign'' several centimeters from its origin on the aorta. By contrast, mesenteric thromboses occur at the level of the most proximal superior mesenteric artery, prior to the middle colic takeoff. A tapering termination of the superior mesenteric artery is visualized within 1 or 2 cm of its origin, and the development of collateral circulation may be evidence of a long-standing stenotic lesion. Nonocclusive mesenteric ischemia produces the characteristic arteriographic finding of segmental mesenteric vasospasm with a relatively normal appearing main superior mesenteric arterial trunk.

The differentiation of superior mesenteric embolus, thrombosis, and nonocclusive ischemia can frequently be made at the time of laparotomy on the basis of the distribution of the ischemic process. Emboli lodge at the origin of the middle colic artery, distal to the first few jejunal branches of the superior mesenteric artery. Continued perfusion of these jejunal branches spares the proximal jejunum from the gangrenous process. By contrast, thrombotic occlusion occurs at the origin of the superior mesenteric artery, proximal to all the jejunal branches. The gangrenous process runs from the ligament of Treitz to the mid–transverse colon, without sparing of the proximal jejunum. Finally, nonocclusive mesenteric ischemia involves the branches of the superior mesenteric vessel in a segmental fashion and is associated with a patchy appearance of alternating pink and dusky bowel.

Treatment. The treatment of acute mesenteric arterial occlusion is dependent on the cause of the process. It is useful to obtain a preoperative arteriogram so that appropriate management can be planned accordingly. The diagnosis of mesenteric ischemia may not have been made before laparotomy. In addition, some patients may present in a moribund state, and the delay required for arteriography may be ill-advised.

Mesenteric Embolization. The basic goal of operation in superior mesenteric arterial embolus is the rapid restoration of arterial perfusion with removal of the embolus from the vessel. A long midline abdominal incision is usually employed, the transverse colon is lifted superiorly, and the small bowel is reflected toward the right upper quadrant. The superior mesenteric artery is approached at the root of the small-bowel mesentery, usually as it emerges from beneath the pancreas to cross over the junction of the third and fourth portions of the duodenum. A transverse arteriotomy is made in the vessel, and a balloon catheter is inserted proximally and distally to remove the embolus and propagated thrombus. An assessment of intestinal viability must be made after perfusion has been restored, and obviously-nonviable segments must be resected. Numerous technical aids have been employed to predict viable from nonviable bowel, including intraoperative intravenous fluorescein injection and inspection with a Wood's lamp and Doppler assessment of antimesenteric intestinal arterial pulsations. A second-look procedure may be necessary in many patients and is usually scheduled 24 to 48 h following embolectomy. The thesis behind second-look procedures is that the precise extent of intestinal viability may not be evident immediately following reperfusion, and additional resection of ischemic bowel may be necessary. An important tenet of second-look laparotomy is that the decision to proceed with the additional operation must be made at the time of the initial laparotomy. Subsequent analysis of the patient's postoperative course should not alter the decision since the early postoperative status of these patients bears no correlation with the presence or absence of residual nonviable bowel.

Mesenteric Thrombosis. The therapy of mesenteric thrombosis differs from that of embolization as a result of the nature of the superior mesenteric artery. The vessel itself is normal in embolic disease, and simple removal of the thromboembolus is all that is necessary. By contrast, the thrombotic process occurs in a severely atherosclerotic proximal superior mesenteric artery. Therefore, patients with thrombotic disease require placement of a bypass graft to the superior mesenteric artery distal to the occlusive process to restore adequate mesenteric flow. The aorta or iliac artery may be used as the origin of the bypass graft. There exist two advantages of using the supraceliac, infradiaphragmatic aorta rather than the infrarenal aorta as the origin for the graft. First, this segment is usually soft and avoids the problems associated with clamping of the frequently calcific infrarenal aorta. Secondly, the use of the more proximal aorta allows placement of an *antegrade* graft which is less prone to kinking when the small bowel is returned to its normal location after construction of the anastomoses. Saphenous vein is usually the graft material of choice in patients with acute mesenteric ischemia; prosthetic materials should be avoided because of the risk of bacterial seeding from transudation or during intestinal resection.

The principles behind the resection of nonviable bowel are the same for patients with thrombotic and embolic mesenteric ischemia. Doppler and fluorescein techniques can be worthwhile, and a second-look procedure may be advisable. Not infrequently, the length of viable intestine is so short as to be incompatible with life. The treatment of these patients must be individualized on the basis of an understanding of the patient's wishes with respect to permanent intravenous hyperalimentation. Closure of the abdomen without revascularization or resection of bowel may be the most appropriate management in many of these cases.

Thrombolytic therapy is a potential consideration in patients with acute mesenteric ischemia, with intraarterial delivery of the agent into the thrombus at the time of arteriography. Successful lysis of the central core of acute thrombus will return the mesenteric circulation to its chronic, stable state, and subsequent operative revascularization or even balloon angioplasty of the stenotic superior mesenteric artery can be electively undertaken. Percutaneous intraarterial thrombolysis, however, does not provide the opportunity to inspect the potentially nonviable bowel subsequent to reperfusion. In addition, many hours may be lost during the period of time required for clot lysis, and attempts at operative revascularization will be significantly delayed if thrombolysis is unsuccessful. Thus, thrombolytic interventions in acute mesenteric ischemia must be considered investigational at the present time and should be reserved for occasional, selected patients.

Nonocclusive Mesenteric Ischemia. The therapy of nonocclusive mesenteric ischemia is primarily nonoperative. A metabolic cause of the problem should be sought and corrected whenever possible. Intraarterial vasodilating agents such as tolazoline or papaverine can be administered directly into the superior mesenteric artery at the time of arteriography, and the effects of the agents can be objectively documented with serial arteriograms. Resection of nonviable bowel may be required when the patient's condition permits.

Chronic Mesenteric Ischemia

Chronic mesenteric ischemia occurs as the result of atherosclerotic occlusive disease of the superior mesenteric and celiac vessels. Less frequent causes include fibromuscular dysplasia, radiation arteritis, autoimmune arteritides, and a secondary mesenteric arteritis after aortic coarctation repair. An entity known as the "celiac band syndrome" has been described where the celiac axis is compressed by the median arcuate ligament. The significance of this finding as a cause of abdominal symptoms has been argued, but satisfactory results have been achieved after division of the ligament with or without patch angioplasty of the celiac trunk.

The mesenteric atherosclerotic process usually begins with stenotic plaque formation at the origins of the visceral arteries as they exit the aorta. In contrast to acute mesenteric occlusion which produces intestinal infarction with superior mesenteric arterial occlusion alone, the chronic form of the disease is not associated with symptoms until both the celiac axis *and* superior mesenteric arteries are significantly stenosed. The classic symptom complex of postprandial abdominal pain and weight loss is almost uniformly present and is in keeping with the alternate name of "intestinal angina" used to describe the entity.

The anatomy of the collateral arterial circulation is an important feature in chronic mesenteric ischemia (Fig. 20-29). The celiac and superior mesenteric arterial circulations communicate through the gastroduodenal artery and pancreatic branches, respectively. Significant stenotic disease of one system results in dilatation of the gastroduodenal artery to accommodate the increased collateral flow. The inferior mesenteric artery communicates with the superior mesenteric system through two routes. First, a clinically insignificant pathway exists through the left colic artery, marginal artery of Drummond, and middle colic artery. Second, a hemodynamically important pathway may evolve through a "meandering mesenteric artery." This artery is not present in the absence of mesenteric occlusive disease but develops as a tortuous vessel running through the medial aspect of the left mesocolon to provide anastomotic collateral flow between the proximal inferior mesenteric artery and the superior mesenteric artery. A meandering mesenteric artery can be distinguished arteriographically from a normal marginal artery of Drummond by its more medial location, tortuosity, and shorter route between the inferior and superior mesenteric vessels.

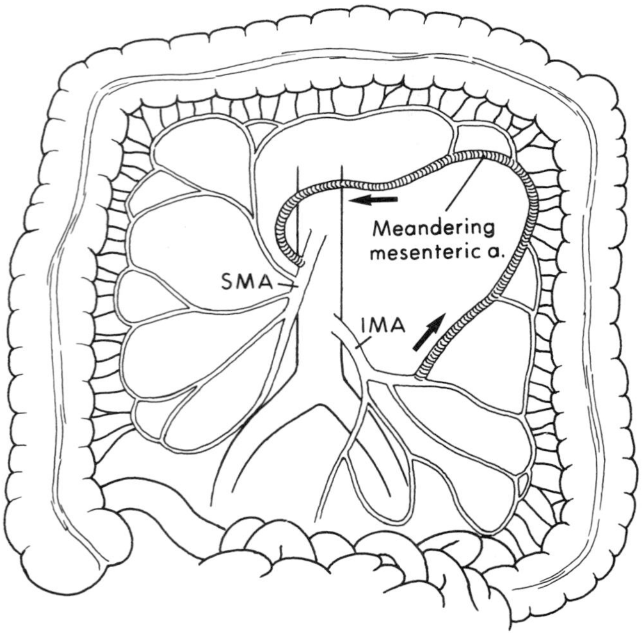

FIG. 20-29. The meandering mesenteric artery represents an important collateral channel between the superior and inferior mesenteric circulation. The artery must be differentiated from the normally present marginal artery of Drummond, which is more lateral, smaller, and of less physiologic significance.

Diagnosis. The most common presentation in patients with chronic mesenteric ischemia is postprandial abdominal pain and weight loss. The pain occurs 20 min to 1 h following a meal, and its intensity correlates with the amount of food ingested. The relationship between food and pain is so striking that patients decrease the size and frequency of meals, giving rise to the term "food fear." This conscious restriction of food intake is the cause of the patients' weight loss, rather than a malabsorption syndrome secondary to ischemic bowel injury.

Physical examination in chronic mesenteric ischemia is remarkable only for the obvious cachectic appearance of the patient and the frequent finding of a midabdominal bruit. Occult blood in the stool is unusual and implies an alternate diagnosis or a more acute ischemic process. Remote stigmata of diffuse atherosclerotic disease are usually present, including carotid and femoral bruits and the absence of palpable lower extremity pulses. Laboratory tests are not generally helpful. Absorption studies such as fecal fat analysis and urinary excretion of orally administered D-xylose are of limited value. Upper and lower gastrointestinal barium contrast studies are usually normal in patients with chronic mesenteric ischemia, although occasional patients will manifest decreased motility and mucosal edema. Duplex scanning of the celiac and superior mesenteric origins has been reported to be a beneficial screening method in patients with suspected mesenteric ischemia, but arteriography is necessary to confirm the diagnosis. Lateral aortography reveals stenosis or occlusion of both the celiac axis and the superior mesenteric artery, frequently in association with a large meandering mesenteric vessel on the anteroposterior views. Mesenteric ischemia so rarely occurs in the presence of a solitary visceral arterial occlusion that the accuracy of the diagnosis is called into question when only one visceral vessel is involved.

Treatment. Revascularization is indicated in all patients with symptomatic mesenteric ischemia in order to prevent the development of catastrophic bowel infarction. Rather impressive visceral artery arteriographic disease may exist in the absence of symptoms. The coexistence of abdominal pain and arteriographic findings does not necessarily imply a causative relationship, and other diagnoses such as occult malignancy or inflammatory bowel disease should be excluded in all patients, irrespective of the arteriographic findings.

A transperitoneal approach to operative revascularization provides the opportunity to thoroughly explore the abdomen to exclude nonvascular causes for the patient's symptoms. Historically, endarterectomy was the first method used in visceral arterial revascularization. Endarterectomy is most easily accomplished through a lateral or posterior aortotomy, removing a plug of atheroma from the celiac trunk and superior mesenteric artery through a "trans-aortic" exposure. The danger in this technique relates to the inability to adequately visualize the termination of the endarterectomy on the visceral vessel, risking inadvertent creation of an intimal flap and early thrombosis of the reconstruction.

Bypass procedures have gained widespread acceptance in visceral arterial reconstruction. As in any arterial reconstructive procedure, the surgeon has three decisions to make; the inflow site, the outflow site, and the type of bypass graft material. The infrarenal aorta, the supraceliac aorta, and the iliac artery all represent satisfactory choices as the site of inflow. The supraceliac aorta has the advantage of a much lower incidence of atherosclerotic change than the more distal sites, thereby decreasing the danger of iatrogenic embolization secondary to the clamping of a diseased vessel. Supraceliac inflow also allows the bypass graft to be placed in an antegrade fashion, avoiding the kinking tendency associated with retrograde grafts from an infrarenal location. Both the celiac and superior mesenteric systems should be revascularized if possible, to provide a margin of safety if one reconstruction fails. In general, anastomosis of one end of the graft to the side of the common hepatic artery will revascularize the celiac system and a similar anastomosis to the superior mesenteric artery will revascularize that arterial bed. Satisfactory results have been achieved with both saphenous vein and prosthetic conduits. The use of a bifurcated Dacron graft from the supraceliac aorta is a commonly performed operation for mesenteric ischemia. This procedure is an antegrade reconstruction that preserves the saphenous vein and reduces the number of vascular anastomoses needed to be performed.

Renovascular Disease

The proximal renal arteries represent a common location for the development of atherosclerotic lesions. Two important disease entities occur as a result of significant renal arterial disease: renovascular hypertension and chronic renal insufficiency. Renovascular hypertension has emerged as the leading cause of surgically correctable hypertension, stimulated by the work of Goldblatt in 1934. In later years, the recognition that renal function improved after renal artery reconstruction fostered interest in the salvage of functioning renal parenchyma irrespective of the presence or absence of hypertension.

Renovascular Hypertension

Hypertension secondary to renal arterial disease is thought to affect 5 to 10 percent of the hypertensive population. Renovascular disease tends to produce a marked elevation in the systolic and diastolic pressures, causing the prevalence of a renovascular etiology to be negligible in the subpopulation of patients with mild to moderate hypertension. Age is also an important correlate of renovascular causes of hypertension. Severe hypertension occurring in young children and elderly adults has the highest probability of a renovascular cause, while hypertension in young and middle-aged adults is usually essential.

Etiology. There are two basic causes of renovascular hypertension; atherosclerosis and fibromuscular dysplasia. The ratio of atherosclerotic to fibromuscular etiologies is roughly 2:1. Atherosclerosis typically occurs at the renal artery ostia, more commonly on the left than the right. Severe atherosclerosis of the abdominal aorta frequently coexists with renal arterial disease.

Fibromuscular dysplasia of the renal artery is an idiopathic entity encompassing a variety of histopathologic subgroups, all producing stenotic lesions of the intima, media, or adventitia. The most common variety consists of medial fibroplasia with alternating stenoses and small aneurysms, producing the characteristic "string of beads" appearance on arteriography (Fig. 20-30). Fibromuscular dysplasia most commonly occurs in young, often multiparous women. In contrast to atherosclerotic disease, the right renal artery is involved more frequently than the left and the lesions frequently occur at the midportion of the renal arteries rather than proximally.

Pathophysiology. Richard Bright was the first to call attention to the relationship between hypertension and renal disease when he observed an association between "hardness of the pulse" and scarred, shrunken kidneys in 1836. Goldblatt defined the cause of the process in his classic canine experiments reported in 1934. Unilateral renal artery constriction produced ipsilateral renal atrophy and systemic hypertension.

The renin-angiotensin-aldosterone system has now been defined as the critical hormonal pathway responsible for the maintenance of the normotensive state. Systemic hypertension may develop as a result of overfilling of the arterial system, arteriolar vasoconstriction, or by a combination of these two factors. Renal arterial stenosis produces a low renal perfusion pressure, a compensatory increase in unilateral renin secretion, increased angiotensin-II formation, and elevated blood pressure secondary to vasoconstriction and hyperaldosteronemic-induced volume overload. A normal contralateral kidney can partially compensate for the hyperrenin state by increasing natriuresis. This compensatory response does not occur in the presence of a diseased or absent contralateral kidney or in the presence of contralateral renal artery stenosis.

Two forms of Goldblatt hypertension provide experimental corollaries to renovascular hypertensives with unilateral versus bilateral renal disease. In the "two kidney, one clip" Goldblatt model a single renal artery is clamped and the opposite kidney is

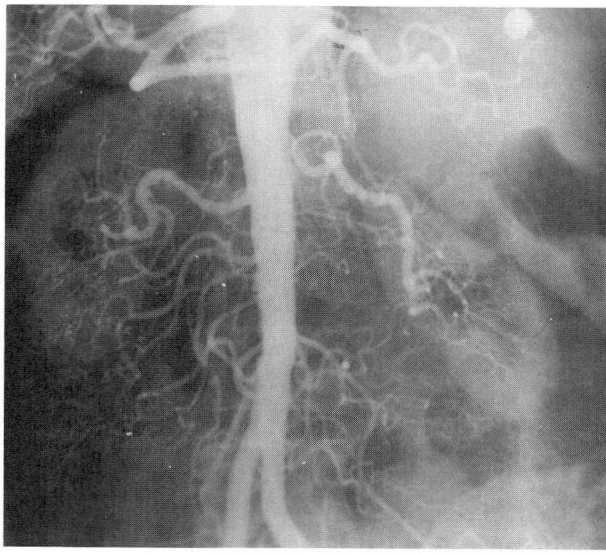

FIG. 20-30. The classic string-of-beads appearance of fibromuscular dysplasia of the renal artery, as seen on intraarterial contrast arteriography.

left undisturbed. In the "one kidney, one clip" model one renal artery is clamped and the contralateral kidney is removed. Renin levels are elevated indefinitely in the two-kidney model, and the administration of angiotensin-II inhibitors results in decreases in blood pressure both initially and in the established phase. By contrast, renin levels are only transiently elevated in the one-kidney model. Elevated renin secretion is soon suppressed by volume expansion from sodium and water retention, and the established phase of hypertension is maintained by volume expansion and not by renin-mediated vasoconstriction. Predictably, angiotensin-II blockade is ineffective in ameliorating the hypertensive state in the established phase of the one-kidney model.

Diagnosis. Although renovascular hypertension is more common when the hypertension is severe, is of recent onset, is associated with an abdominal bruit, and occurs at the extremes of life, none of these characteristics are sufficiently predictive to substantiate or exclude the diagnosis. It is important to rule out such diagnoses as pheochromocytoma or other adrenal tumors with urinary 17-hydroxy ketosteroid and catecholamine levels.

A widely used but highly inaccurate screening test for renovascular hypertension is the intravenous pyelogram. Findings consistent with renovascular cause include a delay in the appearance of contrast on one side, a difference in the length of the two kidneys of 1.5 cm or more, defects in the renal parenchymal outline consistent with segmental infarction, and ureteral notching from compression secondary to dilated collateral vessels. As many as 30 percent of patients with renovascular hypertension will fail to demonstrate abnormal findings on pyelography, with a significantly higher false-negative rate in pediatric patients and patients with bilateral disease.

Radioisotopic renal nuclear scans have been employed in the assessment of renovascular arterial disease using I-131 hippurate as an indirect measure of renal plasma flow and Tc-99 chelated diethylenetriamine pentaacetic acid (DTPA) as an index of glomerular filtration rate. The diagnosis of renal arterial disease is suggested by an asymmetry between appearance and excretion of radiopharmaceutical by the two kidneys. Unfortunately, the nuclear medical techniques are associated with a high incidence of false-negative and false-positive results.

Hypersecretion of renin from a kidney supplied by a stenotic renal artery is the hallmark of surgically curable hypertension. Theoretically, peripheral renin levels should correlate well with renin hypersecretion, since the clearance of renin from the blood remains a constant proportion of the arterial renin concentration. In practice, many patients with curable hypertension exhibit normal peripheral renin determinations. Angiotensin-II blockade provides a means of increasing the sensitivity of peripheral renin determination. The administration of the oral angiotensin-converting enzyme, captopril results in an increase in plasma renin activity to a markedly greater extent in patients with renovascular hypertension than in patients with essential hypertension. The single-dose captopril test accurately discriminates between renovascular and essential hypertension, although the test does not establish which kidney is responsible for the problem.

Split renal function tests were some of the first diagnostic measures used to predict whether patients would benefit from renovascular reconstructive procedures. These evaluations specifically identify which kidney is responsible in the majority of instances. The ureters are individually catheterized and urine is collected. Split function tests are considered suggestive of a renovascular cause for hypertension when one kidney demonstrates a 40 percent reduction in urine volume, a 50 percent increase in creatinine concentration, or a 100 percent increase in para-aminohippuric acid concentration.

Selective renal vein sampling has proved to be a valuable method of determining the presence of a renovascular cause for hypertension. Renal vein renin ratios greater than 1:1.5 between the two kidneys are correlated with a renovascular cause for hypertension and predict a satisfactory response from renovascular reconstruction. Recent appreciation that the kidneys do not remove renin from the arterial blood has fostered the use of subtraction methods for improving the accuracy of renal vein renin testing. Contralateral suppression of renin secretion results in negligible differences between renal arterial and venous renin concentrations on the uninvolved side, and the renin concentration in the inferior vena cava has been shown to approximate the renal arterial renin concentration. In practice, renovascular hypertension should be suspected when the difference between caval and renal vein renin levels is near zero on the uninvolved side and when the renal vein renin increment is 50 percent higher than the caval level on the involved side.

Intravenous digital subtraction angiography has been used as a screening test for the identification of renal artery stenoses. It is a minimally invasive procedure that may be performed on an outpatient basis, injecting dye through an antecubital or femoral vein into the central venous circulation. A computer-subtracted image is obtained as the dye enters the abdominal aorta and renal arteries, and the test is frequently combined with selective renal vein renin sampling. The disadvantages of intravenous digital angiography include its poor resolution, its dependence on adequate cardiac output, and the large amount of dye necessary to obtain adequate images. Intraarterial contrast studies are the most reliable method of delineating renal arterial lesions. Conventional or intraarterial digital techniques provide satisfactory images, and oblique views may be useful to more clearly define proximal stenoses. Intraarterial arteriography is a prerequisite for operative correction of renal arterial disease, and many centers perform this intervention regardless of the results of prior screening tests.

Renal Salvage Procedures. Renal arterial disease may produce significant deterioration in renal excretory function in addition to hypertension. The development of an elevated serum creatinine level implies significant bilateral renal disease. Renal arterial reconstruction can be expected to result in retrieval of function in the azotemic or nonazotemic patient, with objective improvements in glomerular filtration rate and increases in the size of the kidneys following the procedure. A successful surgical outcome is correlated with a preoperative glomerular filtration rate of less than 20 mL/min. Interestingly, the greatest increase in renal size following revascularization occurs with small kidneys.

Treatment. The indications for reconstructive procedures in patients with renovascular disease include all patients with documented renovascular hypertension and patients with chronic renal insufficiency secondary to renal arterial lesions. Operative therapy has been documented as safer than long-term medical management of renovascular hypertension, with significant increases in relief of hypertension and survival, independent of a fibrodysplastic or atherosclerotic cause of the problem. Moreover, long-term therapy with angiotensin-converting enzyme inhibition may be associated with substantial decreases in renal excretory function. Therefore, pharmacologic management of renovascular hypertension is contraindicated in all but the most medically compromised patients. Thrombolytic therapy has been employed in acute renal artery occlusion, such as occurs with emboli to the kidneys. The thrombolytic agent is infused into the renal artery thromboembolus at the time of arteriography. The results of thrombolytic therapy in acute renal ischemia are preliminary, and currently, the procedure must be considered investigative.

There are four choices in the treatment of chronic symptomatic renal artery disease; unilateral nephrectomy, percutaneous transluminal angioplasty, renal artery bypass, and renal endarterectomy. Nephrectomy is indicated in patients with significant renovascular hypertension when the involved kidney is the source of renin production but is so severely damaged from chronic ischemia that the prospects for retrieval of renal function are remote. Renal size and the presence of viable glomeruli on biopsy have been used to predict the likelihood of improving renal function with revascularization, reserving nephrectomy for unilateral renal arterial disease in a small kidney with minimal residual excretory function. Balloon angioplasty has been used with success in renovascular hypertension, but the best results are achieved with lesions distal to the renal ostia. Relative contraindications to balloon angioplasty include lesions involving renal artery bifurcations and bilateral renal artery stenoses. The most favorable results with balloon dilatation occur in patients with fibromuscular dysplasia, and the procedure represents the initial procedure of choice in this patient category, although its long-term benefits remain undefined.

Renal artery bypass and endarterectomy are the two main operative procedures performed to correct renal artery stenoses and occlusions. Exposure of the renal arteries is most easily accomplished by reflecting the left colon medially in the case of left renal arterial reconstructions and by reflecting the right colon and duodenum medially in the case of right renal reconstructions. Alternatively, both renal arteries may be exposed with mobilization of the right colon and ileum and reflection of these structures cranially. The choice of the type of renal reconstruction depends on the status of the abdominal aorta. An aortorenal bypass using autogenous saphenous vein is the procedure of choice when the aorta is relatively spared from atherosclerotic change and clamping will not produce injury or distal embolization. Prosthetic grafts with PTFE or Dacron are acceptable alternatives to saphenous vein. Saphenous vein should be avoided in children, because it is prone to the development of aneurysmal change. Hypogastric artery is the best choice for aortorenal grafting in the pediatric patient. In the presence of aortic atherosclerotic disease, saphenous vein bypass from the hepatic artery to the right renal artery or splenic artery bypass to the left renal artery are the most appropriate alternatives. Both procedures avoid the embolic and hemodynamic consequences of aortic clamping. Splenorenal grafts are performed by transecting the splenic artery and constructing an anastomosis of one end of the splenic artery to one end or side of the left renal artery, and collateral flow from the short gastric vessels obviates the need for splenectomy. Distal renal arterial lesions may be difficult to expose and revascularize with the kidney in situ, and removal of the kidney, ex vivo bench reconstruction, and autotransplantation has provided an excellent alternative in these complex cases.

Renal endarterectomy is appropriate for atherosclerotic lesions but is not applicable in fibrodysplastic disease. The procedure may be accomplished through a transaortic exposure, endarterectomizing the renal orifices through an aortic incision. This procedure is useful in bilateral renal arterial lesions, and a transverse aortotomy across the aorta into both renal arteries avoids the problems associated with a blind ending of the distal extent of the endarterectomy.

EXTRACRANIAL CEREBROVASCULAR DISEASE

The term ''carotid'' originates from the Greek *karotides,* indicating stupor, and was first used by Galen who found that compression of these vessels produced a soporific state. Thomas Willis, a seventeenth century English physician, clearly defined the carotid and vertebral artery supply to the brain in his work *Cebri Anatome*. Despite extensive study of the anatomy of the cerebrovasculature, the relationship between carotid arterial disease and ischemic stroke was not appreciated until the early twentieth century. In 1913, Ramsay Hunt described the relationship between cerebral softening and occlusive lesions involving the main arteries to the brain. He urged that evaluation of the carotid arteries in the neck become a routine part of the physical examination. These early observations were followed by advances in cerebral angiography by Moniz in the 1920s, the elucidation of the pathophysiology of transient neurologic deficits by C. Miller Fisher in 1950, and the first operative carotid reconstruction by Eastcott, Pickering, and Rob in 1953. The first major series describing carotid artery reconstructions was reported by Lyons and Galbraith in 1957, and carotid endarterectomy soon became established as a safe procedure, although its role in improving the natural history of ischemic stroke continues to elicit much controversy.

Nomenclature. Focal cerebral ischemic disease, or stroke, results from insufficient blood flow to the affected portion of the brain. Stroke may be classified in a number of ways, including the anatomic location of the ischemic cerebral insult, the location of the causative arterial lesion, the pathogenesis, and the time sequence. We have found it most helpful to categorize stroke with regard to two of these parameters: (1) location of the cerebral defect, and (2) time course of the event (Table 20-6).

Location. Neurologic deficits may be divided into those that are focal and those that are diffuse. Focal deficits are those that may be specifically localized to a discrete area within the brain. It is useful to classify these deficits into anterior or *hemispheric* symptoms and posterior or *vertebrobasilar* symptoms, since hemispheric symptoms are frequently caused by emboli from the carotid circulation and vertebrobasilar symptoms originate from either flow-limiting or embolic lesions of the aortic arch vessels, the vertebral arteries, or the basilar artery. There has been a recent trend to describe symptoms not referable to the carotid territory as *nonhemispheric* symptoms; these include true vertebrobasilar symptoms as well as the more poorly defined global symptoms of dizziness and syncope. The confluence of both vertebral arteries to form the basilar artery provides a margin of safety with respect to hindbrain ischemia. Disease in one vertebral artery does not produce cerebral hypoperfusion unless the contralateral vertebral artery is diseased or atrophic. Unilateral vertebral lesions can, however, be associated with nonhemispheric symptoms as a result of embolization to either the ipsilateral or contralateral hindbrain.

The *subclavian steal syndrome* is a variant of nonhemispheric ischemia in which a subclavian arterial stenosis proximal to the vertebral origin results in retrograde vertebral perfusion as a source of collateral blood flow to the arm. The arteriographic finding of retrograde vertebral flow is common in the presence of a subclavian lesion, but cerebral symptoms are rare in this setting unless concomitant carotid arterial disease exists. A small percent of ce-

Table 20-6
Classification of Cerebrovascular Events

Description	Duration	Cause: Embolic	Cause: Flow-related
Hemispheric			
TIA	<24 h	Frequent	Rare
RIND	1–21 days	Frequent	Occasional
Completed CVA	>21 days	Frequent	Occasional
Ocular			
Amaurosis fugax	Minutes–hours	Frequent	Rare
Retinal stroke	Permanent	Frequent	Occasional
Ischemic retinopathy	Chronic	Rare	Frequent
Nonhemispheric			
Classic VBI	Variable	Occasional	Frequent
Nonclassic VBI	Variable	Rare	Occasional

RIND = reversible ischemic neurologic defect; CVA = cerebrovascular accident; VBI = vertebrobasilar insufficiency.

rebral infarctions occur as a result of cardiac emboli, and these may travel to the anterior or posterior cerebrum. *Amaurosis fugax* is defined as transient monocular blindness, while persistence of the deficit indicates that the ischemic process has progressed to infarction, and the patient has suffered a *retinal stroke*. The cause of monocular visual symptoms is usually an embolus arising from an atherosclerotic plaque at the carotid bifurcation and traveling through the ophthalmic artery to the terminal arterioles of the retina. The embolus is visible on fundoscopic examination in about 10 percent of patients with amaurosis fugax, appearing as bright intraarteriolar bodies. Although C. Miller Fisher was the first to report this finding in patients with amaurosis fugax, the clinical sign has been given the eponym *Hollenhorst plaque,* after Hollenhorst's report of 27 patients with this finding.

Time Course. Neurologic deficits can be grouped into three categories based on the duration of the signs and symptoms. Transient symptoms resolving completely within 24 h are termed *transient ischemic attacks* (TIAs), although most TIAs actually resolve within minutes rather than hours. When the frequency of TIAs is greater than two or three per day, the term *crescendo TIAs* is applied. Symptoms lasting longer than 24 h but resolving within 3 weeks are known as *reversible ischemic neurologic deficits (RINDs)*. When a deficit lasts longer than 3 weeks, it is considered a *completed stroke*. These definitions are based only on clinical findings. Imaging techniques such as CT and MRI have documented cerebral infarction in a significant percentage of patients with transient symptoms, blurring the distinction between TIA and stroke.

There are two types of stroke that represent an unstable clinical situation; the *stroke-in-evolution* and the *waxing-and-waning neurologic deficit*. In patients with stroke-in-evolution the neurologic deficit worsens through a series of discrete exacerbations. Waxing-and-waning deficits fluctuate between mild and severe neurologic compromise, usually over a period of several hours. Stroke-in-evolution and waxing-and-waning deficits occur in the presence of critical carotid stenoses, usually in excess of 90 percent diameter reduction. The pathophysiology may relate to repeated episodes of embolization or recurrent, borderline cerebral ischemia from low arterial blood flow. In either case, urgent carotid endarterectomy is indicated before irreversible cerebral infarction develops.

Pathophysiology. Carotid and subclavian arterial atherosclerotic lesions usually occur in predictable, focal sites. Atherosclerotic disease involving the carotid artery is almost always limited to the common carotid bifurcation and ends several centimeters distal to the internal carotid origin. This makes it possible to perform endarterectomy procedures rather than bypasses for carotid bifurcation disease, removing all the atherosclerotic plaque and ending the endarterectomy distally on an uninvolved segment of the internal carotid artery. Subclavian atherosclerosis tends to occur at the origin of these vessels, with left-sided stenoses prevailing by a ratio of 4:1.

The particular susceptibility of the carotid bifurcation to atherosclerotic change is most likely due to hemodynamic conditions at this location. Initially, it was assumed that the atherosclerotic propensity of the carotid bifurcation was a result of local turbulence and elevated blood flow rate. These investigators speculated that high wall shear stresses produced endothelial damage, predisposing to atherosclerotic degeneration. Zarins and associates refuted these concepts and offered convincing evidence that plaque formation is accelerated within areas of *low* flow velocity and inhibited in areas with high flow velocity and elevated shear stress. They evaluated transverse light microscopic sections of postmortem human carotid bifurcation specimens. Atherosclerotic plaque was most prominent along the outer, posterior aspect of the proximal internal carotid artery. This finding was correlated with hemodynamic observations within transparent models of human carotid bifurcations. The areas of cadaver artery most susceptible to plaque formation corresponded to regions of low velocity and wall shear stress in the models, while the zones that were relatively free of plaque formation corresponded to regions of high flow and high shear stress.

Mechanism of TIAs. There are two possible mechanisms for the development of TIAs: (1) emboli to the intracranial arteries, and (2) temporary cerebral hypoperfusion. The older literature commonly attributed TIAs to transient decreases in systemic factors such as blood pressure and cardiac output. This theory predicts that TIAs would occur only in patients with hemodynamically significant stenoses. Recent studies, however, have failed to demonstrate a good correlation between the severity of carotid stenosis and prognosis or clinical manifestations of hemispheric, carotid territory TIAs. Further, cardiac disease was less common in patients with carotid TIAs than in the nonhemispheric TIA group. These observations support the concept of an embolic cause for carotid territory TIAs. Nonhemispheric TIAs are likely to be embolic in nature when the symptoms are focal, but global symptoms are more likely to be due to transient hemodynamic compromise in the presence of posterior circulation disease.

Pathologic specimens of carotid lesions from symptomatic patients frequently contain irregular luminal surfaces with exposured subintimal structures. Areas of the vessel lacking the normal intimal layer are termed *ulcers*. Aggregates of platelets and fibrin as well as cholesterol crystals are commonly observed within carotid ulcers (Fig. 20-31).

There are at least three possible causes of embolization from a carotid bifurcation plaque. First, fragments of the cholesterol-calcium plaque may break off and be discharged into the lumen. Second, roughened, thrombogenic subintimal structures may be exposed to the flowing blood, and platelet thrombi may be formed that are easily detached. A third mechanism involves intramural carotid artery hemorrhage. The pathophysiologic mechanisms underlying this process are incompletely understood, but the presence of acute or recent intramural hemorrhage has been reported in over 90 percent of symptomatic patients, compared with less than 30 percent of asymptomatic patients. It is possible that intramural hemorrhage may result in rapid, unpredictable progression of a moderate asymptomatic carotid lesion to a high-grade symptomatic stenosis, with eventual rupture of the intramural process and discharge of the plaque contents into the arterial lumen.

There are several unusual causes of carotid pathologic conditions that may be associated with cerebrovascular symptoms. The artery may be elongated, tortuous, or kinked; these anatomic abnormalities are rarely associated with symptoms. Radiation therapy may induce a symptomatic carotid arterial injury similar in appearance to an atherosclerotic lesion. The internal carotid artery may undergo spontaneous dissection, resulting in neurologic symptoms and thrombosis of the vessel. Treatment of carotid dissection is nonoperative, with anticoagulation and control of hypertension.

Fibromuscular dysplasia is the most common nonatherosclerotic lesion of the carotid artery. The cause of the process is unknown, but it tends to involve long arteries with few branches. The vast majority of affected individuals are females, and the disease is usually bilateral. Four histologic types have been described: intimal fibroplasia, medial hyperplasia, medial fibroplasia, and perimedial dysplasia. Medial hyperplasia is the most frequently encountered variety. Operative intervention is indicated in symptomatic patients, usually in the form of intraluminal dilatation of the involved segment using an open or percutaneous approach. Prophylactic operation in the asymptomatic patient is not recommended, since no objective data exist on the natural history of the process.

Patients with repeated TIAs often experience symptoms in exactly the same anatomic region of the brain with each episode. For example, a patient with crescendo TIAs involving right arm monoplegia will frequently exhibit repeated identical episodes without other deficits such as aphasia or left eye amaurosis fugax. It is reasonable to wonder why the pattern of neurologic dysfunction is frequently reproduced in an identical fashion, since one would expect carotid embolization to occur in a random fashion throughout the distribution supplied by that carotid vessel. This apparent paradox is answered by the fluid dynamics associated with laminar flow. Embolic material originating from a point source in the arterial system tends to travel to the same terminal arterial branch, as illustrated by Millikan. He injected small metallic pellets through a needle placed in the internal carotid artery of monkeys. Subsequent examination of the animals' brains revealed that the pellets stacked up one on the other within the same cortical branch (Fig. 20-32).

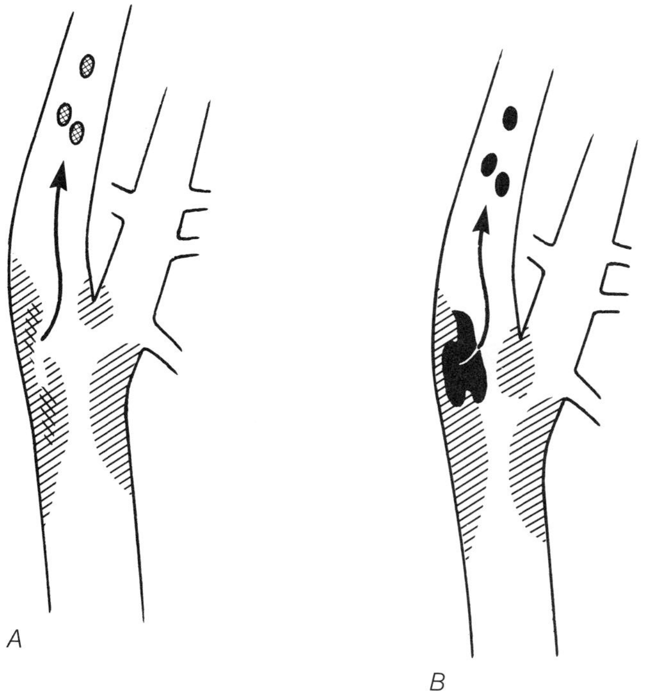

FIG. 20-31. Carotid ulcerations are frequently implicated in the pathogenesis of cerebral events. *A.* Cholesterol debris present within the necrotic core of an atherosclerotic plaque may be discharged into the lumen as the plaque ulcerates. *B.* Platelet-fibrin thrombus may form on the thrombogenic ulcer base and can subsequently be released to embolize distally.

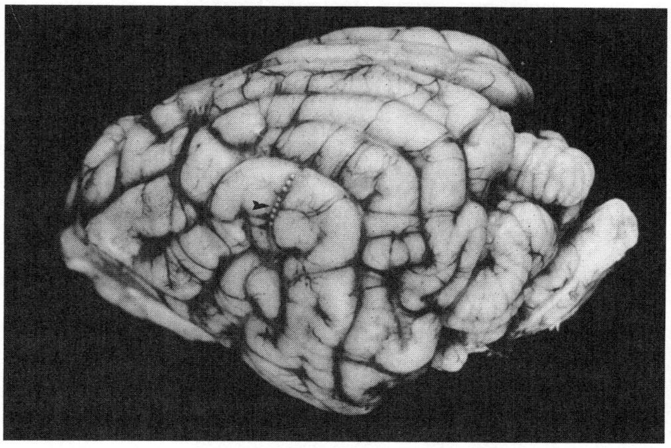

FIG. 20-32. Embolic material originating from a single site in the arterial tree will tend to travel to the same terminal vessel as a result of the presence of consistent flow separation at branch points. This principal is graphically illustrated following the injection of tiny metallic pellets from a single locus in the common carotid artery. Subsequent evaluation of the animal's brain at necropsy revealed consistent embolization to the same branch of the middle cerebral artery.

Diagnosis. The most valuable tool in the diagnosis of carotid artery disease is a careful history and physical examination. A thorough neurologic evaluation is of great importance. The diagnosis of carotid bifurcation disease is facilitated by the relatively superficial location of the vessel, rendering it accessible to study. The cervical carotid pulse is usually normal in patients with carotid bifurcation disease, since the common carotid artery is the only palpable vessel in the neck and is rarely diseased. The superficial temporal artery pulse provides some indication of the status of the external carotid artery, but the internal carotid pulsation is inaccessible to digital palpation. Auscultation has been the most widely employed method of assessing the carotid bifurcation. Carotid bifurcation bruits may be heard just anterior to the sternocleidomastoid muscle near the angle of the mandible. Auscultation in the supraclavicular fossa may reveal bruits originating from stenotic lesions of the subclavian artery. Carotid and subclavian bruits must be differentiated from one another as well as from murmurs due to cardiac lesions such as aortic stenosis, which may be transmitted along the great vessels into the neck. Bruits do not become audible until the stenosis is large enough to reduce the diameter by approximately 50 percent. Bruits may be absent in extremely severe lesions because of the extreme reduction of flow across the stenosis.

The development of noninvasive carotid imaging modalities has provided more precise information regarding the nature and severity of the lesion. Oculoplethysmography (OPG) is a test designed to indirectly measure ophthalmic artery pressure through the use of plastic suction cups applied to the sclera. The ophthalmic artery pressure is a good indicator of internal carotid artery pressure, and abnormalities of this measurement can identify hemodynamically significant carotid artery stenoses. Stenoses of the proximal common carotid artery and the ophthalmic artery must be excluded, as these lesions will produce an abnormal OPG in the absence of significant carotid bifurcation disease. The most useful noninvasive test has been the Duplex ultrasound carotid examination. This test combines pulsed-Doppler measurements with a B-mode ultrasound image to provide data on the velocity of blood flow and the anatomic profile of the carotid bifurcation, respectively. The duplex scan is an extraordinarily accurate noninvasive means of identifying carotid stenoses. The subclavian and vertebral arteries may also be evaluated, but the accuracy in identifying disease is much less in these vessels. The technical difficulty of the test has been largely overcome with the introduction of the color-flow Doppler. This instrument is a modified Duplex scanner that provides a color image in which the velocity and direction of blood flow is keyed to the color of the image at all points within the vessel so that arterial flow can be seen as red and venous as blue. Standard Duplex scans cannot assess the cerebral arterial circulation beyond the first several centimeters of the internal carotid artery. A transcranial Doppler has been developed to evaluate the middle cerebral artery and other intracranial vessels, using a low-frequency Doppler signal to penetrate the thin bone of the temporal and occipital regions. Recently, MRI has been evaluated as a means of imaging the carotid arteries. The resolution of the early MRIs has not been sufficient to accurately define the location and extent of carotid disease, but future technical improvements may provide the vascular specialist with a noninvasive alternative to contrast arteriography.

Arteriography remains the gold standard for the diagnosis of extracranial arterial disease. Intraarterial standard and digital subtraction arteriograms provide the best images and are usually performed by the transfemoral approach, views being obtained in both the anteroposterior and lateral planes (Fig. 20-33). Most images are of sufficient quality to allow precise determination of the severity of the carotid lesion, expressed as the percent diameter reduction in comparison to the normal artery distal to the stenotic process (Fig. 20-34). Intravenous digital images have proved disappointing, with accuracy rates approximating that of noninvasive Duplex ultrasound evaluation. Patients with nonhemispheric symptoms should undergo four-vessel cerebral arteriography (selective injection of both carotid and subclavian arteries) with visualization of the carotid, subclavian, and vertebral vessels.

Treatment. The therapy of cerebrovascular occlusive disease is best considered by dividing patients into two subgroups: those with posterior circulation lesions involving the subclavian or vertebral arteries, and those with anterior circulation lesions involving the carotid arteries.

The indications for operation are relatively straightforward and noncontroversial in patients with subclavian and vertebral disease; operative correction is recommended for symptomatic lesions that are surgically accessible. Proximal subclavian lesions are best treated with a carotid-to-subclavian artery bypass, using end-of-graft to side-of-artery anastomoses at each end. Alternatively, a

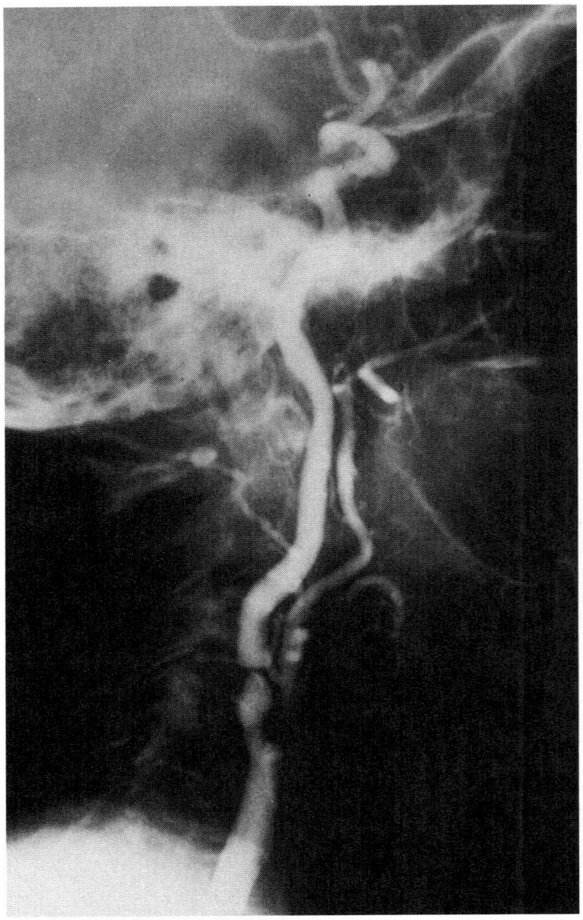

FIG. 20-33. Standard intraarterial contrast arteriographic image of a diseased carotid bifurcation, as viewed in the lateral projection. Note the abrupt termination of atherosclerotic disease within a short distance of the internal carotid origin.

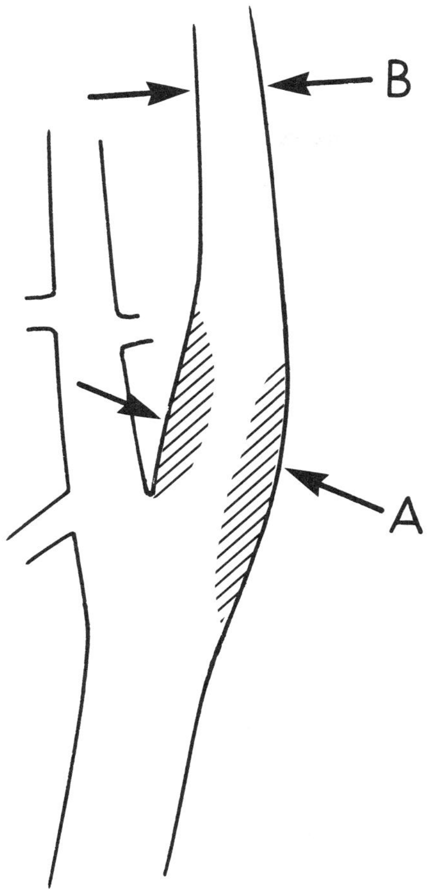

FIG. 20-34. The severity of an internal carotid stenosis is conventionally expressed as the percent diameter reduction compared to the normal internal carotid artery diameter distally. Assuming a circular configuration, the percent reduction in area can be found by the formula 1 − (% diameter reduction/100)^2.

subclavian-to-carotid artery transposition may be performed, with division of the subclavian artery proximal to the vertebral origin and construction of an end-of-subclavian to side-of-carotid anastomosis. Embolic symptoms due to lesions of the subclavian artery require exclusion of the embolic source from the arterial stream. Ligation of the subclavian artery proximal to the vertebral origin is performed in the case of a carotid-to-subclavian artery bypass. Disease involving the vertebral arteries may also be responsible for posterior cerebral symptoms. Vertebral artery lesions usually occur at the origin of the vessel and end within the first centimeter of its course. The stenotic lesion may be endarterectomized and the arteriotomy closed with a patch graft. More commonly, the vertebral artery is transected beyond the stenosis, the stump is ligated, and the distal end is anastomosed to the side of the common carotid artery.

The appropriate treatment of carotid bifurcation disease is currently one of the most controversial topics in vascular surgery. Carotid endarterectomy is the procedure of choice for symptomatic occlusive disease at the carotid bifurcation. The operation is the most frequently performed vascular surgical procedure and reached its zenith of popularity in 1985, when more than 100,000 were carried out. The propriety of this trend as well as the merit of the operation itself has been the topic of much debate.

The medical management of symptomatic carotid disease includes reduction of risk factors such as smoking and hypercholesterolemia, and the use of antiplatelet agents. Current recommendations include a regimen of one to four 325-mg aspirin tablets daily, although recent studies have suggested that doses as low as 30 mg/day produce similar antiplatelet effects. Ticlopidine and other antiplatelet agents have also been used with success. Dipyridamole was once widely employed both solely and in combination with aspirin, but the drug has not been shown to be more effective than aspirin alone. Oral anticoagulation with warfarin has been recommended for patients who continue to experience symptoms on antiplatelet agents.

A myriad of well-designed, randomized trials of antiplatelet therapy for symptomatic carotid disease have been undertaken. Although all the studies revealed a trend toward reduction of the risk of subsequent stroke, none documented a statistically significant benefit of aspirin compared with placebo. It was only when the end points of mortality, myocardial infarction, TIA, and stroke were combined that a significant advantage was achieved with antiplatelet therapy. The effects of aspirin on the incidence of myocardial infarction and on mortality were the most important benefits; the effects on cerebrovascular disease were less striking. Metaanalysis of these results suggested a 15 percent reduction in stroke risk with aspirin, compared to a 40 percent reduction in myocardial infarction and deaths.

The benefit of carotid endarterectomy for patients with symptomatic cerebrovascular disease has recently been established (Table 20-7). The results of the North American Symptomatic Carotid Endarterectomy Trial (NASCET) and the European Carotid Surgery Trial (ECST) have documented a significant reduction in cerebrovascular events following the procedure compared with patients managed medically. The NASCET study randomized patients with symptomatic carotid arterial disease to either carotid endarterectomy or optimal medical care including antiplatelet therapy (generally 1300 mg aspirin daily). In the subset of over 600 patients with stenoses that reduced artery diameter by between 70 and 99 percent, a 26 percent incidence of ipsilateral stroke was observed in the medically managed group at 2 years of follow-up, compared with a 9 percent incidence in the surgical group, a difference which was statistically significant and prompted early termination of the study. On the basis of these results, patients with symptomatic high-grade carotid stenoses should undergo carotid endarterectomy by a surgeon with the low rate of perioperative morbidity that has characterized the centers in the NASCET trial. Patients with minimal stenoses (less than 30 percent diameter reduction) are best managed medically, reserving operative considerations for recurrent symptoms on antiplatelet therapy or for disease progression. The management of the group of patients with moderate stenoses (30 to 69 percent) has not been settled and awaits the results of ongoing randomized trials.

The appropriate treatment of asymptomatic carotid stenosis has not been defined. Several randomized trials are now in progress comparing the results of carotid endarterectomy and antiplatelet therapy. Currently there is no evidence that antiplatelet therapy alters the natural course of the asymptomatic carotid lesion. Several reports have suggested that the use of aspirin in the asymptomatic patient may increase the risk of intraplaque hemorrhage and accelerate the onset of symptoms. Carotid endarterectomy has proven to be a safe procedure in asymptomatic patients, with a low

Table 20-7
Results of Therapy for Severely Stenotic Symptomatic Carotid Stenosis

Mode of Treatment	*Two-year Stroke Risk, %*
None	40*
Aspirin	26†
Carotid endarterectomy	9†

*From metaanalysis of studies in the literature.
†From NASCET study.

incidence of long-term postoperative neurologic sequelae. These observations suggest that carotid endarterectomy may be an appropriate option in the medically uncompromised patient with a high-grade asymptomatic carotid lesion, but objective confirmation of this impression awaits the findings of ongoing clinical trials.

Patients with nonhemispheric cerebral symptoms appear to benefit from correction of carotid lesions, if the patient's symptoms are classic in nature and the stenosis is significant (greater than 60 percent diameter reduction). Patients with nonclassic symptoms such as dizziness or syncope are rarely improved by carotid reconstruction. These patients should be managed as though the lesions were aysmptomatic, reserving operation for the healthy patient with a relatively long life expectancy and a high-grade carotid lesion.

The timing of operation is a critical consideration in the treatment of carotid disease. Patients with unstable neurologic symptoms such as crescendo TIAs or a waxing-and-waning deficit invariably have severe disease and should undergo urgent arteriography and operation. The high risk of cerebral infarction from recurrent embolization or carotid thrombosis in this setting necessitates the administration of systemic anticoagulation at the time of presentation. Patients with a completed stroke should undergo carotid endarterectomy a minimum of 4 weeks following the event, as the risk of perioperative intracerebral bleeding is very great immediately following a stroke. Emergency carotid endarterectomy is indicated for an acute carotid artery thrombosis if the procedure can be performed within a few hours following the event. It is unusual to have the opportunity to restore carotid perfusion so expeditiously, exceptions to this being early postoperative carotid occlusion or carotid occlusion occurring during cerebral arteriography. Operation is contraindicated for an occlusion that is several hours old, since the danger of intracerebral edema and hemorrhage from reperfusion outweighs the potential benefits of revascularization.

Carotid endarterectomy can be performed under local or general anesthesia. The advantage of local anesthesia is that the surgical team can be aware of the patient's mental status at all times, most importantly when the carotid artery is clamped. Changes in level of consciousness or motor deficits at the time of interruption of blood flow signal the need for placement of an intraoperative shunt. General anesthesia confers the advantages of ventilatory support and increased cerebral blood flow with the use of halogenated agents, but alternative methods of assessing the adequacy of cerebral perfusion must be implemented.

The exposure of the carotid bifurcation is accomplished with a vertical incision made along the anterior border of the sternocleidomastoid muscle (Fig. 20-35). The dissection is carried down through the platysma muscle, and the internal jugular vein is mobilized laterally following ligation and division of the facial vein. The carotid bifurcation is exposed along with an adequate length of the common and internal carotid arteries to allow clamping of these structures above and below the plaque. The hypoglossal nerve can be mobilized and reflected craniad for additional exposure. Exposure of the distal internal carotid artery can be achieved by dividing the digastric muscle when needed; further proximal exposure can be accomplished by dividing the omohyoid muscle. The patient is systemically heparinized, the carotid vessels are clamped, and a longitudinal arteriotomy is started on the common carotid artery and carried onto the internal carotid artery, with the distal termination on normal vessel. The plaque is removed using an endarterectomy spatula, and every attempt is made to achieve a smooth tapering distal end point. The termination of the endarterectomy should have a normal adherent intima and media to ensure that the resumption of forward blood flow will not create an occlusive flap. The arteriotomy may be closed primarily with nonabsorbable suture. Alternatively, a vein or prosthetic patch may be employed if the vessel is small.

The collateral cerebral circulation is inadequate to compensate during the period of carotid cross-clamping in a small subset of patients. The use of an indwelling shunt intraoperatively reduces the incidence of intraoperative cerebral infarction in these patients. Some have advocated the routine use of a shunt because it is difficult to predict which patients will not tolerate the period of relative cerebral ischemia. There are disadvantages to the use of a shunt; the shunt can injure the intima at the time of placement and impedes visualization of the end point of the endarterectomy. For these reasons, intraoperative electroencephalographic (EEG) monitoring and internal carotid stump pressure determination have been employed in an effort to identify patients at greatest risk of stroke with temporary carotid interruption. EEG leads are placed on the patient's scalp preoperatively; any slowing of the EEG waveform is indicative of cerebral ischemia and necessitates the insertion of a shunt. Carotid stump pressures of less than 25 mmHg after clamping are also predictive of an increased risk of cerebral infarction during clamping and mandate the placement of a shunt. Use of either EEG or stump pressure determination allows the surgeon to limit the use of indwelling shunts to less than one in five patients undergoing carotid procedures.

The complications of carotid endarterectomy include cranial nerve damage resulting from nerve division, excessive traction, or perineural dissection. The most frequently injured nerves are the vagus, the hypoglossal, the glossopharyngeal, and the marginal mandibular branch of the facial nerve. Revascularization of a severely stenotic carotid artery may result in the "hyperperfusion syndrome," characterized by headache, seizures, and occasionally intracranial bleeding. This phenomenon is felt to result from reperfusion of a chronically ischemic tissue bed in which the arterioles are maximally dilated. With the sudden restoration of blood flow,

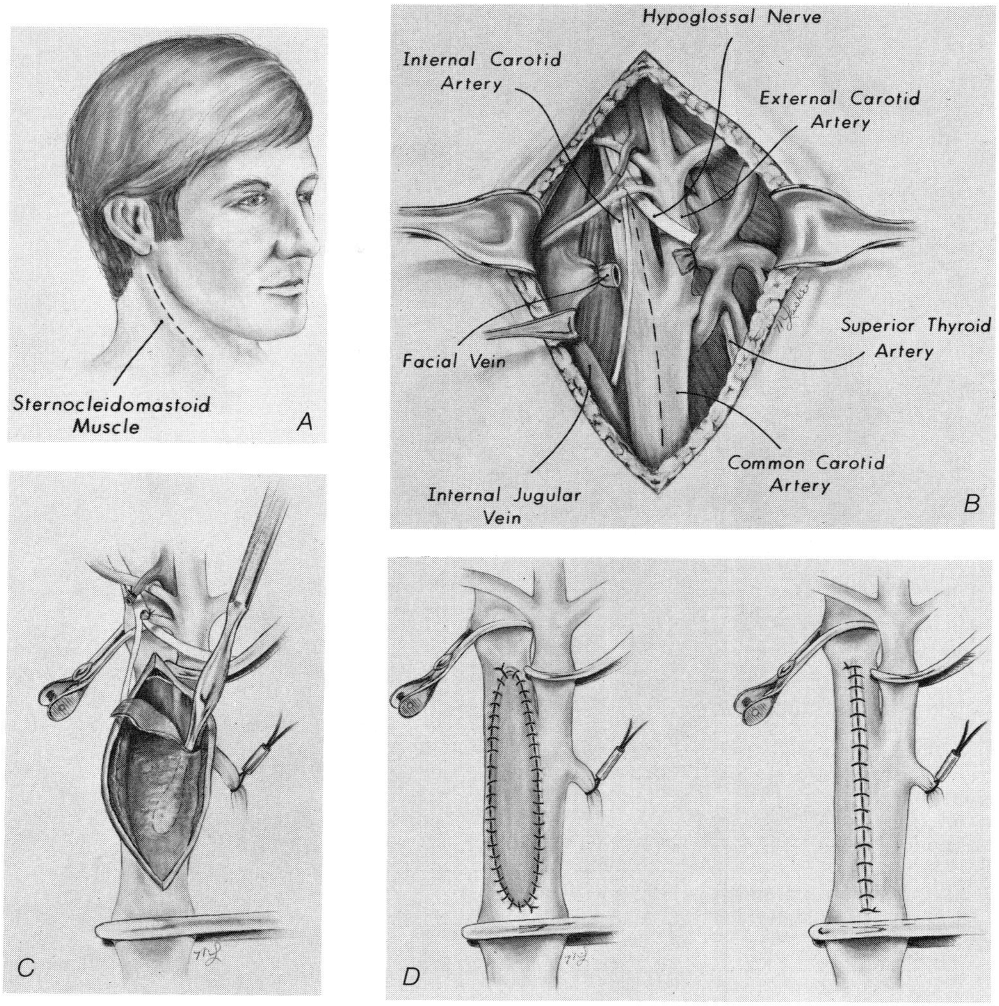

FIG. 20-35. Technique of carotid endarterectomy. *A.* A skin incision is made anterior to the sternocleidomastoid muscle. *B.* The carotid artery branches are widely mobilized. The internal carotid artery is clamped before widely mobilizing the frequently thrombus-containing bulb, thereby protecting the brain from embolization, which may occur during the dissection. The vagus and hypoglossal nerves are carefully protected. Mobilization of the hypoglossal is facilitated by dividing the sternocleidomastoid artery and vein. A longitudinal arteriotomy is made extending above and below the plaque at the carotid bifurcation. *C.* After the intima is divided above the plaque, the plaque can be easily dissected from the underlying media or from the adventitia. The distal intima is carefully inspected and sutured if necessary. *D.* The arteriotomy is either closed primarily with 6-0 prolene, or a vein patch fashioned from autologous saphenous vein is used to avoid producing stenosis. The technique for restoring flow after completion of the closure is crucial to avoid embolization to the brain. The internal carotid clamp is temporarily removed and reapplied. The common and external carotid clamps are removed, and after flushing of the carotid bulb, the internal carotid clamp is removed.

the area becomes markedly edematous and the clinical picture described above develops. Beta-blockers may reduce the severity of symptoms and should be instituted in high-risk patients with the first signs of the syndrome, usually a headache.

The most dreaded complication of carotid endarterectomy is that of perioperative stroke. Perioperative strokes can occur as a result of inadequate cerebral perfusion during the clamp period, embolization of debris from the plaque at the time of operation, or early postoperative thrombosis. Refinements in operative technique have reduced the perioperative stroke rate to less than 5 percent in most institutions and to less than 2 percent in centers with the greatest experience.

The incidence of perioperative myocardial events is distressingly high; they are at least as common as perioperative neurologic events in patients undergoing carotid endarterectomy. Preoperative cardiac screening procedures include myocardial imaging using thallium or echocardiography, often supplemented with exercise, dipyridamole, or dobutamine. In a study performed at the Cleveland Clinic, routine coronary arteriography was used as a screening test in a series of 1000 patients in whom elective vascular procedures were planned; 295 of these patients presented because of pathologic cerebrovascular conditions. Significant coronary lesions were detected in 33 percent of patients with symptoms of cardiac disease and in 17 percent of patients without clinical manifestations of cardiac disease. The 75 percent 5-year survival rate observed in patients who underwent staged cardiac and carotid revascularization procedures was surpassed only by that of the group of patients with normal or minimally diseased coronary arteries (91 percent). Based on the results of this series, it seems reasonable to utilize one of the minimally invasive screening tests, such as dipyridamole-thallium studies, prior to carotid endarterectomy. Coronary arteriography is reserved for patients with overt cardiac symptoms or a positive screening test, and coronary artery bypass is utilized for patients with severe arteriographic coronary artery disease.

NONATHEROSCLEROTIC DISORDERS

Thoracic Outlet Syndrome

The thoracic outlet is the space through which the subclavian artery, vein, and brachial plexus pass from the neck into the upper extremity. Its anatomic boundaries are the chest wall, the scalene muscles, the clavicle, and a variety of anomalous potentially compressive structures such as fibrous bands or cervical ribs (Fig. 20-36). Proper treatment requires a detailed history and physical ex-

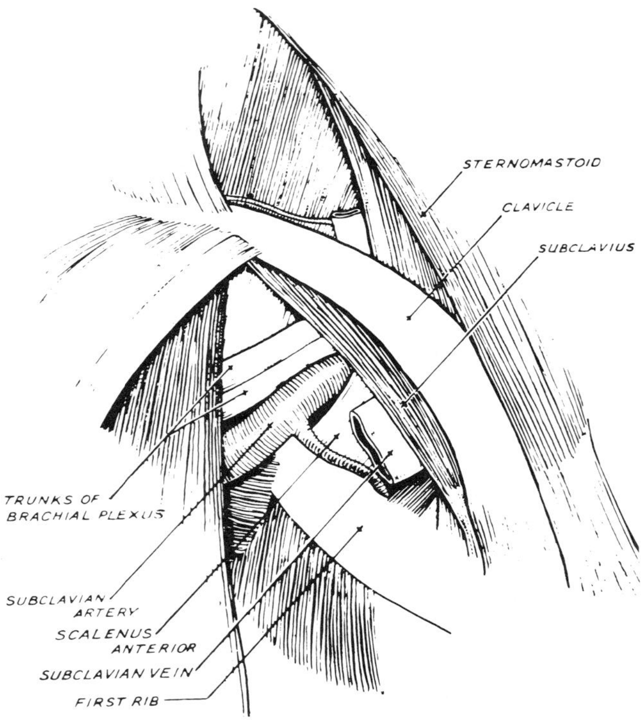

FIG. 20-36. A diagram of the anatomic relationships at the thoracic outlet. This is the space that the subclavian vessels and the trunks of the brachial plexus pass as they leave the neck and enter the upper extremity. The first rib forms the floor of the space, the clavicle the roof, and the scalene muscles the walls which attach to the first rib. The anterior scalene muscle separates the nerves from the artery. Anomalous fibrous bands further subdivide the space and may compress these structures. Treatment of the various compression syndromes involves removal of the first rib, the muscular attachments, and any fibrous bands.

amination, appropriate diagnostic tests, careful patient selection, and understanding of the intricate anatomic relationships in this area.

Arterial Component. The arterial complications of thoracic outlet syndrome (TOS) are due to a bony cervical rib or an anomaly of the first rib. Patients may present with an asymptomatic pulsatile cervical mass, or more often, with upper extremity ischemia ranging from unilateral Raynaud's phenomena to acute ischemia with absent pulses. Symptoms are due to atheroemboli from a poststenotic dilatation or true aneurysm (rarely thrombosis) of the subclavian artery (Fig. 20-37). The evaluation should include cervical x-rays, noninvasive vascular testing, and arteriography when appropriate.

Treatment requires removal of the embolic source, resection of the bony anomaly, and reperfusion, if possible, of the ischemic extremity. The subclavian artery aneurysm is best approached through a supraclavicular incision with or without removal of the medial half of the clavicle. The aneurysm is resected and replaced with an interposition saphenous vein graft. The cervical and first ribs can be excised through this approach, or the patient can be repositioned and the operation completed through the axilla. If the artery is dilated but not aneurysmal, resection is not indicated because bony decompression is sufficient to prevent further atheroemboli in most instances. In this situation the transaxillary approach is preferred because it simplifies removal of the first rib. Any distal embolic material that needs removal should be approached through separate arteriotomies in the arm. Sympathectomy can be a useful adjunct when distal emboli are irretrievable.

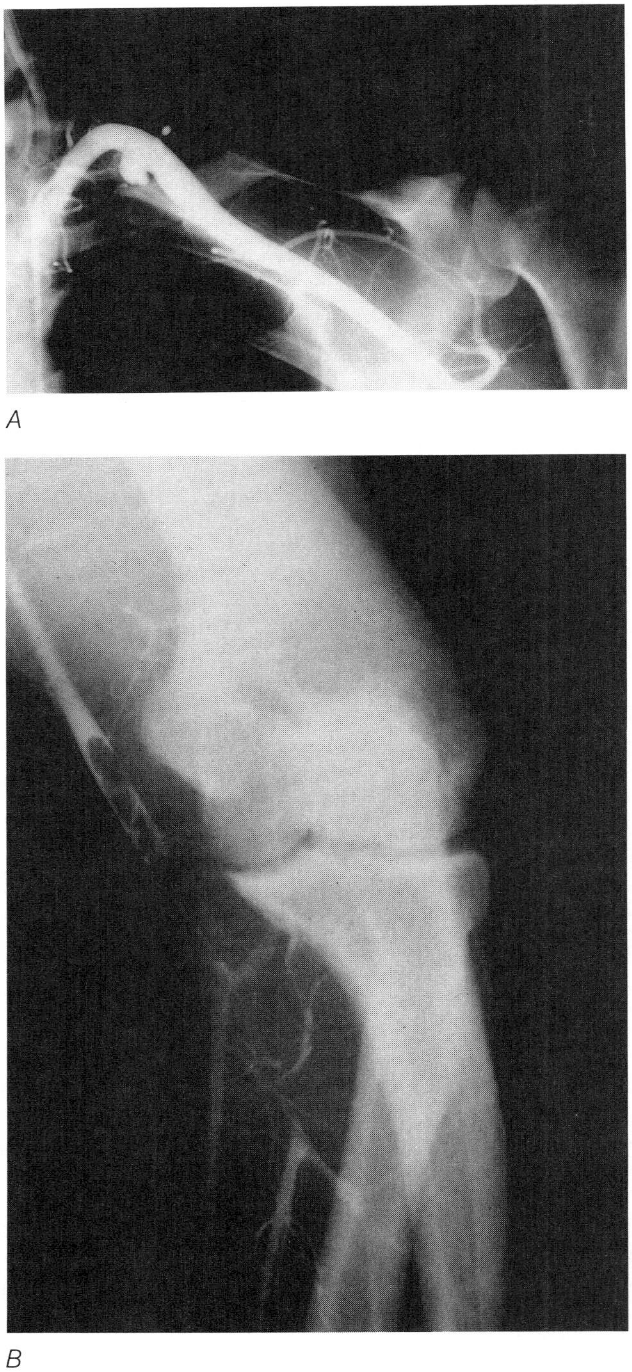

FIG. 20-37. *A.* A subclavian arteriogram in a patient with a bony cervical rib who presented with an ischemic arm due to a brachial artery occlusion. This aneurysm was resected and replaced with a saphenous vein graft. *B.* The brachial arteriogram in this patient revealed an occluding embolus. Fogarty catheter embolectomy is successful in removing this clot and restoring circulation to the arm.

Venous Component. Venous obstruction of the upper extremity is caused by a narrowing of the costoclavicular space between the medial aspect of the first rib and the clavicle. This is the site where the axillary vein passes over the rib and under the clavicle to join the internal jugular vein. Both hyperabduction of the arm and hyperextension of the shoulders can narrow this space causing venous obstruction. Venous obstruction takes one of three forms.

Intermittent Obstruction. These patients present with arm swelling, cyanosis, and pain when the arm is abducted or the shoulders hyperextended. The diagnosis can be made by phlebograms with the arm in both the relaxed and symptomatic positions. A positive exam shows a beaklike appearance to the contrast proximal to the first rib when the arm is stressed and a normal venous anatomy with the arm in a neutral position. Venous pressure measurements can also be made in these same arm positions. Treatment consists of transaxillary first rib resection or medial subtotal claviculectomy.

Acute Thrombosis. Patients are usually young and healthy and present with the sudden onset of arm pain, swelling, and cyanosis. The problem often follows some type of repetitive activity such as throwing a ball, house painting, paper hanging, swimming, rowing a boat, and has been called the "Paget-Schroetter" or "effort thrombosis" syndrome. Phlebograms show a complete obstruction of the subclavian vein often with thrombus distally in the axillary vein.

Treatment options include elevation and heparinization, venous thrombectomy, and local thrombolysis with the latter gaining much support in recent years. Once the diagnosis is confirmed a coaxial catheter is inserted into the basilic vein and placed directly into the thrombus. Urokinase infusion is started with a loading dose of 250,000 IU followed by 4000 IU for the first hour and then 1000 IU for the next 24 h. Heparin is infused into the sheath at a rate of 800 IU/h. If an underlying compressive lesion can be documented, a transluminal balloon venoplasty is performed. The venoplasty does not provide a permanent solution to the underlying compression, and these patients should undergo a transaxillary rib resection. The patient is discharged on coumadin which is continued for 3 months.

Posthrombotic Intermittent Obstruction. Patients with acute obstruction and unsuccessful clot removal, whether chemical or mechanical, have a 50 percent chance of developing residual symptoms of venous obstruction. Phlebograms usually demonstrate an occluded vein with large collaterals around the first rib (Fig. 20-38). Hyperabduction of the arm results in compression of these collateral veins. Either first rib resection or a medial claviculectomy will relieve these symptoms in some patients. Direct repair of the chronically occluded subclavian vein may be preferable and can be achieved by mobilizing the internal jugular vein and turning it down to anastomose into the divided patent axillary vein.

Neurologic Component. The subjective nature of the symptoms and the lack of objective diagnostic criteria make the management of the neurologic component of TOS very difficult. Some would restrict this diagnosis to only those patients with symptoms and signs limited to the T-1 nerve root (ulnar nerve), while others would broaden the entity to include any neurologic symptoms of the neck, upper back, and upper extremity. These symptoms are exacerbated by elevation and abduction of the arm. Trauma may precipitate the symptoms in a susceptible individual.

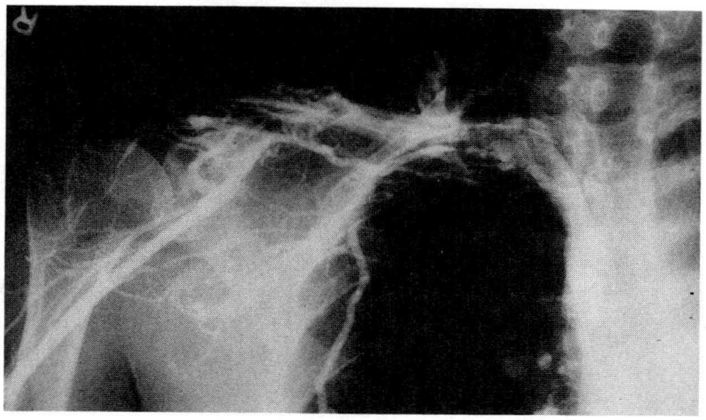

FIG. 20-38. A venogram showing a chronic subclavian vein occlusion with a large venous collateral running along the chest wall. This patient developed arm symptoms of congestion made worse with elevation of the arm. The resting venous pressures were elevated, and a prominent venous pattern was apparent over the chest wall. A transaxillary first-rib resection was performed with significant relief of symptoms particularly with elevation of the arm.

An accurate and complete history is important because the diagnosis is often one of exclusion. Most entities in the differential have reliable diagnostic tests. All these patients should have cervical spine films to identify any bony anomalies and to rule out cervical disc protrusion or spondylitis. Nerve conduction studies are indicated to rule out carpal tunnel syndrome and ulnar nerve compression at the elbow. Orthopaedic and neurologic consultations may be necessary to rule out specific pathologic conditions of the shoulder, multiple sclerosis, and spinal cord tumors. Physical examination includes blood pressure measurements in both arms. The hands are examined for signs of atrophy of the ulnar-innervated interosseus muscles and the median-innervated thenar muscles (Fig. 20-39). Percussion over the median nerve (Tinel's test) and rapid wrist flexion (Phalen's test) are performed to further evaluate the median nerve. A complete neurologic examination of the neck and upper extremity is performed including the application of pressure in the supraclavicular space over the brachial plexus. The traditional Adson's test is totally unreliable in detecting brachial plexus compression and is of no use in making the diagnosis of neurologic TOS. The elevated arm stress test (EAST) described by Roos has the patient raise the arm to 90° and open and close the hands for 3 min. This may reproduce the patient's symptoms but is unfortunately also positive in 90 percent of patients with carpal tunnel syndrome.

When neurologic TOS is the considered diagnosis and treatment is indicated, a conservative approach should always be followed. Patients with severe pain and cervical muscle spasm are initially treated with physical therapy directed at relieving the muscle spasm. Peets' shoulder strengthening exercises are started as the pain subsides. Methods of opening the costoclavicular space by hunching the shoulders upward and forward are used when the patient first feels symptoms recurring. Indications for operation include failed physical therapy, intractable pain, and/or progressive neurologic dysfunction.

Technique of First Rib Resection. Clagett suggested in 1962 that the first rib was the "common denominator" in the various compression syndromes of the thoracic outlet and recommended its resection in appropriate cases. In 1966 Roos described the technique of transaxillary first rib resection which because of its cos-

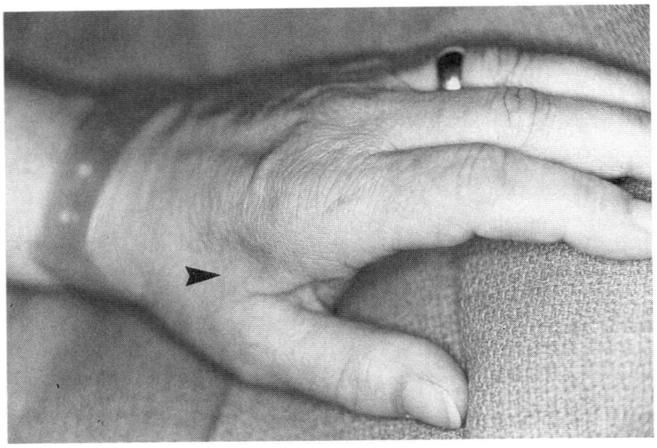

A

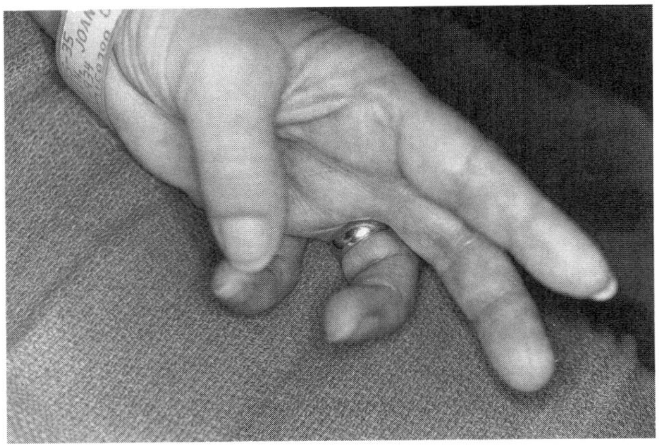

B

FIG. 20-39. *A*. This photograph of the hand in a patient with neurologic thoracic outlet syndrome shows atrophy of the interosseous muscles particularly in the "snuff box" (*arrow*). Nerve conduction studies demonstrated chronic denervation in the distribution of T-1. *B*. The same patient demonstrating the maximum finger flexion possible. A first-rib resection was done which identified a fibrous band extending from the tip of C-7 to the first rib with obvious compression on the T-1 nerve root. There was immediate improvement in function postoperatively but no measurable effect on the muscle atrophy.

metic appeal, simplicity, and alleged safety has become the most frequently performed operation for neurologic TOS.

Using the lateral thoracotomy position with the arm elevated, a skin incision is made in the axillary hair line between the pectoralis major and latissimus dorsi muscles. The first rib is reached by blunt dissection in the axillary tunnel taking care to avoid the intercostobrachial nerve. The subclavian artery and vein are identified and the subclavius muscle tendon divided. The anterior scalene muscle can now be identified and divided at the point where it inserts on the first rib anterior to the artery. At this point a digital search for anomalous bands is performed. These may originate from the C-7 transverse process, from an incomplete cervical rib, from attachment to two places on the first rib, or from the middle scalene muscle. After any bands are divided, the middle scalene muscle and the intercostal muscle attachments are pushed off the first rib. When all muscle fibers are cleared and the T-1 nerve root is visualized and protected, the rib is divided and removed. The wound is irrigated with saline to detect a pneumothorax which if present can be treated by inserting a small chest tube into the pleural space. The tube can be removed in the recovery room if the lung is fully expanded and there is no air leak.

A number of brachial plexus injuries have been reported with this approach, and there are proponents of a supraclavicular approach that avoids any traction on the brachial plexus.

Nonatherosclerotic Popliteal Arterial Disease

There are two causes of nonatherosclerotic popliteal arterial disease that characteristically produce symptoms of calf claudication in young males: popliteal entrapment syndrome and adventitial cystic disease of the popliteal artery.

Popliteal Entrapment Syndrome. Calf claudication in a young male should suggest the diagnosis of popliteal entrapment syndrome. The popliteal artery normally traverses the popliteal fossa between the two heads of the gastrocnemius muscle, but the artery courses medial to the medial head of the gastrocnemius or popliteus muscle in patients with the disorder (Fig. 20-40). The popliteal vein accompanies the artery and is entrapped in just over 10 percent of the cases. Popliteal entrapment is rarely encountered in women, with a male-to-female ratio of 15:1. Bilateral involvement has been observed in one-quarter of the cases.

The findings on physical examination are dependent on whether the popliteal artery is occluded at the time of presentation. The majority of patients present with thrombosis of the vessel and absent pedal pulses. The pedal pulses are present in only one-third of the patients with compressed but nonoccluded vessels. Passive dorsiflexion and active plantar flexion of the foot tense the gastro-

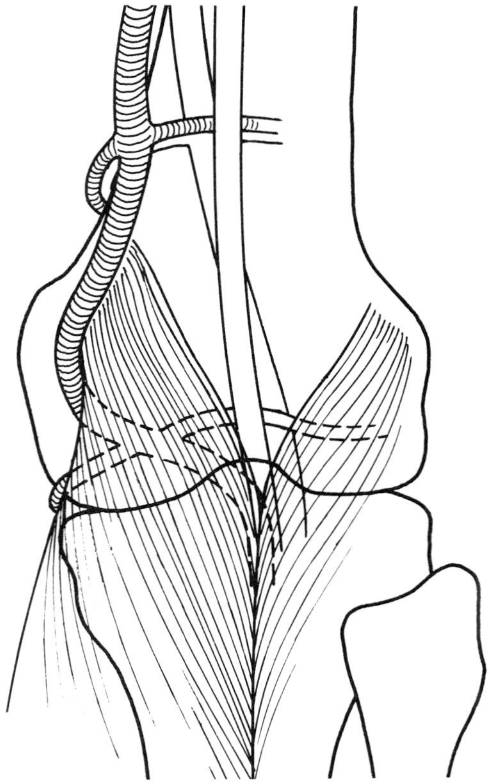

FIG. 20-40. The popliteal entrapment syndrome, with deviation of the popliteal artery around the medial head of the gastrocnemius muscle.

cnemius which compresses the artery, obliterating the pedal pulses. Femoral arteriography with and without plantar flexion of the foot may be instrumental in confirming the diagnosis. Three arteriographic abnormalities of the popliteal artery have been described: medial deviation, occlusion, and post-stenotic dilatation. A computed tomographic scan of the popliteal fossa can be indispensable if the popliteal artery is occluded, defining an abnormal position of the artery with respect to its surrounding muscles.

Operative intervention is indicated in both symptomatic and asymptomatic patients. A posterior approach to the artery is preferred if the artery is patent and extensive proximal and distal exposure is not necessary. Lysis of the constricting gastrocnemius head is all that is required in these instances. Complete resection of the medial head of the gastrocnemius is well tolerated with minimal alteration of function.

Intraarterial thrombolytic agents or balloon catheter thrombectomy are utilized in the recently occluded popliteal artery, followed by lysis of the compressing band if the artery appears otherwise normal. Chronic occlusions necessitate a bypass of the involved segment, with exposure of the proximal popliteal or superficial femoral artery and the distal popliteal or tibial arteries. A medial approach offers advantages in this subgroup, as it facilitates exposure of the inflow and outflow vessels and provides access to the greater saphenous vein.

Adventitial Cystic Disease of the Popliteal Artery. Adventitial cystic disease of the popliteal artery is a rare entity characterized by cystic degeneration of the adventitia of the artery, producing extrinsic compression of the lumen at the level of the knee joint. The cause of the process is unclear, but the two most widely accepted theories invoke a pathogenesis similar to simple ganglia of the wrist, with formation of the cystic cavities as a result of developmental rests of mucin-secreting cells within the adventitia, or abnormal connections between the synovial space of the knee and the wall of the popliteal artery. The cyst contents consist of a viscous material high in proteohyaluronic acid, similar to the fluid found in ganglia. The fluid is colorless in most instances but may take on the appearance of currant jelly if hemorrhage into the cyst has occurred. The cyst may be unilocular or septated.

Popliteal adventitial cystic disease generally produces symptoms of calf claudication in middle-aged men. Arteriography reveals curvilinear stenotic lesions in two-thirds of the patients; popliteal artery occlusions are observed in the remaining one-third of the cases. Ultrasound and computed tomography have been useful in delineating the cyst and its relationship to the arterial lumen.

Although percutaneous cyst aspiration under ultrasound or computed tomographic guidance have been utilized in the treatment of the entity, the long-term results have been discouraging with rapid reaccumulation of the cyst fluid. Operative exploration, incision into the cyst, and evacuation of the contents is the most appropriate treatment if the stenotic process has not progressed to occlusion. Autogenous vein bypass is necessary in the presence of popliteal artery occlusion, with the level of the proximal and distal anastomoses determined by the extent of propagated clot.

Vasospastic Disorders

Arterial vasospasm in the extremities occurs in a variety of clinical situations, including immunologic disorders such as scleroderma and systemic lupus erythematosus, the thoracic outlet syndrome, mechanical (vibratory) or cold-induced small-vessel injury, and the use of drugs such as ergotamine and oral contraceptives.

Raynaud's Syndrome

Raynaud's syndrome represents the prototypic symptom complex associated with peripheral vasospasm. "Raynaud's disease" and "Raynaud's phenomenon" are older terms used to describe a primary benign disorder and a secondary more virulent process, respectively. Improvements in immunologic testing have resulted in a decrease in the frequency of the primary classification, and today over 50 percent of patients with severe Raynaud's symptoms have documented autoimmune disease. Use of the term "Raynaud's syndrome" may be more appropriate than the artificial separation of the entity into primary and secondary forms.

Raynaud's syndrome is characterized by episodic cutaneous color changes consisting of sequential pallor, cyanosis, and rubor. The entity is observed most frequently in the digits of the upper extremities but also may affect the toes. The explanation for the white, blue, and red color changes relates to the pathophysiology of the vasospasm. Initially, cold exposure or emotional stress precipitates intense small-artery vasospasm with digital blanching and numbness. A cyanotic hue develops as partial arterial perfusion is restored and the cutaneous venules become filled with desaturated blood. Finally, the vasospasm resolves and the digits turn bright red as a result of reactive hyperemia.

Between 70 and 90 percent of patients with Raynaud's syndrome are female, almost all younger than age 40. Raynaud symptoms affect the majority of the general population at one time or another, but only a small percentage have symptoms that are severe enough to cause them to seek treatment. Complications include sclerodactylia (atrophy of skin and loss of elasticity, resembling the changes seen in scleroderma), recurrent paronychial infection, and digital ulceration and gangrene. Amputation of the fingers or toes is occasionally necessary, but fortunately the process almost never progresses to involve structures proximal to the digits.

The treatment of Raynaud's syndrome is initially conservative, with avoidance of tobacco, cold exposure, and drugs reported to exacerbate the symptoms such as oral contraceptives, beta-blockers, and ergotamine. Pharmacologic therapy with vasodilating calcium channel blocking agents such as nifedipine has provided partial resolution of symptoms in many patients and represents the mainstay of treatment in the disorder. Cervical sympathectomy has been used in the treatment of severe Raynaud's syndrome, but results have not been gratifying.

Acrocyanosis

Acrocyanosis is a vasospastic disorder occurring almost exclusively in women. The entity is characterized by persistent edema, coolness, and cyanosis of the hands, lower legs, and feet. The pathophysiology is that of cutaneous arteriolar vasospasm. The disease is not as dependent on the temperature of the environment as Raynaud's syndrome, and the process never progresses to tissue loss. Vasodilating agents have been beneficial in acrocyanosis, as has avoidance of cold.

Livedo Reticularis

Livedo reticularis is a condition characterized by constant cyanotic mottling of the skin of the lower legs and feet. The upper extremity is occasionally involved. The changes are always present but become more prominent with exposure to cold. Livedo reticularis occurs as a result of the random spasm of cutaneous arterioles in association with the secondary dilatation of venules to produce a reticulated pattern. The disorder rarely occurs in association with such disease entities as systemic lupus erythematosus and periarteritis nodosa. Most patients have no associated diseases and the process is one of cosmetic concern. Avoidance of cold is the only treatment indicated.

Causalgia

Causalgia, also known as "posttraumatic reflex sympathetic dystrophy," is a painful disorder that develops after incomplete nerve transection. Vasomotor dysfunction is almost always present. The most frequent causes are penetrating missile injuries, fractures, and crush injury. Patients complain of burning pain in the peripheral portions of the extremity, and the symptoms are not limited to the area supplied by the injured nerve. A characteristic feature of the cutaneous dysesthesia is that its intensity is such that the patient cannot tolerate contact of the affected area with clothing or bed sheets. The pain results in limitation of motion and chronic disability. The vasospasm is associated with cyanosis, edema, hyperhydrosis, and coolness of the extremity. Surgical sympathectomy is the treatment of choice and is successful in relieving pain in the vast majority of patients.

Inflammatory Arteritis

The term "inflammatory arteritis" refers to an arterial inflammatory response arising from a group of diseases of unknown or immunologic cause. Many of the arteritides are associated with inflammatory changes in the veins as well, and the term "vasculitides" may be more appropriate when describing these entities. The vasculitides can be classified by the size of the vessels involved and by the coexistent clinical features of the disease process. An immunologic mechanism has been defined in almost all the vasculitides, and most are treated with systemic steroids or cytotoxic agents.

Giant Cell Arteritides. The giant cell arteritides comprise two diseases: temporal arteritis and Takayasu's arteritis. These entities are identical with respect to their histologic appearance and are associated with similar laboratory abnormalities. Anatomically, however, Takayasu's arteritis involves the aorta and its branch vessels near their takeoff, whereas extracranial lesions occur in only 9 percent of patients with temporal arteritis. Takayasu's arteritis occurs almost exclusively in female patients in their teens and twenties. The female predominance is less in temporal arteritis, averaging 3:1, and patients are typically over the age of 50.

Temporal arteritis classically begins with a prodromal phase of malaise, myalgias, headache, and low-grade fever. These symptoms are followed by a second, quiescent phase. A palpable, tender temporal artery may be found in some of the cases. Jaw claudication is a frequent complaint, and an abnormal temporal artery biopsy is found in about 50 percent of patients. The association between polymyalgia rheumatica and temporal arteritis is so striking that some have advocated temporal artery biopsies in all patients with polymyalgia rheumatica to rule out occult arteritis. An elevated erythrocyte sedimentation rate is a uniform finding in temporal arteritis, and the diagnosis should be questioned if the sedimentation rate is normal. Ocular complications in the form of unilateral or bilateral visual loss occur as a result of ischemic optic neuritis. Upper extremity claudication may occur in the unusual patient with extracranial involvement. When extracranial manifestations develop, the characteristic arteriographic finding is that of bilateral smooth tapering or occlusion of the axillary and brachial arteries. The ocular and peripheral arterial complications of temporal arteritis do not generally develop until several months after the onset of symptoms, and the disease is self-limited, with cessation of the process after a period of several years.

Steroid therapy should be initiated early to prevent sudden visual loss from ophthalmic artery thrombosis. Steroids frequently result in remarkable resolution of stenotic lesions over a period of several months, and the erythrocyte sedimentation rate should be followed as an indicator of the efficacy of treatment. Operative revascularization is sometimes necessary for occluded extracranial arterial lesions, but reconstructions tend to thrombose if undertaken during the active phase of the disease and should be delayed until the inflammatory phase of the disease has been adequately suppressed with steroids.

Takayasu's arteritis, also known as "pulseless disease," is a rare disorder associated with stenoses and aneurysms of the aortic branch vessels. Like temporal arteritis, acute and chronic phases are observed. Systemic symptoms and laboratory abnormalities during the acute phase parallel those of temporal arteritis, except for associated findings of erythema nodosum and arthralgias with synovial changes typical of rheumatoid arthritis in some patients. Diagnostic arteriography should include the entire aorta and its branches. Initially, steroid therapy is instituted, following the erythrocyte sedimentation rate as an index of the response to treatment. Cytotoxic agents have been of some benefit. Operative reconstructive procedures are reserved for lesions unresponsive to medical therapy, but when necessary should be delayed beyond the acute disease phase if possible.

Buerger's Disease. Buerger's disease, also known as thromboangiitis obliterans, is an inflammatory vasculopathy occurring in medium-sized and small arteries of young male smokers. The disease is exceedingly rare in females and is not observed in nonsmokers. The lesions occur in the upper and lower extremities and in superficial veins as well as the arteries. The entity was first described by Winiwarter in 1879 and later by Buerger in 1908. Initially Buerger's disease was thought to occur exclusively in the Jewish population, but subsequent studies have shown that this frequency has been exaggerated and the incidence roughly approximates that in other populations.

The cause of Buerger's disease remains obscure. There is evidence for an autoimmune pathogenesis for the disease, with increases in complement factors and anticollagen antibody levels. The disease has also been linked to the presence of certain human lymphocyte antigens (HLAs). Smoking is the most important risk factor in the development and progression of the disease process, although the mechanism behind its effects are undefined.

The histopathologic features of Buerger's disease are those of a panangiitis involving all layers of the vessel wall. Lymphocytes and fibroblasts infiltrate the media and adventitia of the artery in the early stages of the disease. The occluding thrombus is involved with an inflammatory process as well, with multinucleated giant cells and leukocytes giving the appearance of microabscesses within the clot. The late lesion of Buerger's disease is characterized by an occluded, contracted artery with a marked fibrotic reaction in the adventitia, media, and intima. The lesions tend to occur in a localized, segmental fashion, with normal vessel segments interposed between involved segments. The vein and adjacent nerve may be tightly bound to the artery in this dense fibrotic process. The tibial arteries and the vessels of the foot are the predominant sites of involvement in the lower extremity. Approximately 30 percent of patients with Buerger's disease have involvement of the upper extremities, and these lesions occur principally in the vessels of the forearm and hand.

The clinical presentation of patients with Buerger's disease is distinct from that of patients with atherosclerotic disease. Involvement of the smaller arteries may produce symptoms of rest pain and gangrene without antecedent claudication. Necrotic lesions commonly develop at the tips of the fingers and toes. Recurrent superficial thrombophlebitis may develop in the upper or lower extremity. Therapy is directed against the inciting effects of tobacco, with complete arrest of the process once smoking has been abandoned. Vascular reconstructive operations are not frequently feasible as a result of the involvement of the small vessels of the extremity making it difficult to locate suitable outflow sites for bypass grafts. Surgical sympathectomy has been used with some success. Digital amputations are frequently necessary, but major amputations are frequently avoidable because of sparing of the larger vessels.

Periarteritis Nodosa. Periarteritis nodosa is an inflammatory process involving the small and medium-sized arteries of all organs. Uncommonly, digital artery involvement produces Raynaud's symptoms and may progress to ulceration or gangrene. The disease affects males more frequently than females in a ratio of 2:1. Individuals of any age may be affected, but most patients are middle-aged at the time of diagnosis. The pathologic process is that of inflammation progressing to occlusion or aneurysm formation. Renal and gastrointestinal complications occur in the early stages of the disease and include renal failure, intestinal perforation, and intraabdominal hemorrhage. Late mortality occurs as a result of cerebral and cardiovascular events. Steroids have increased the 5-year survival rate to over 50 percent and adjuvant cyclophosphamide therapy has been used with success in severe cases. Operation is reserved for the treatment of hemorrhagic or gangrenous complications.

Hypersensitivity Angiitis. Hypersensitivity angiitis represents a diverse group of disorders involving the smaller arteries, with basement membrane thickening, fragmentation of elastic fibers, and swelling of the collagenous structures, terminating in vascular occlusion. With the exception of scleroderma, all the causative mechanisms involve antigen exposure and the formation of antigen-antibody complexes that damage the small vessels. The antigens include hepatitis-B virus, tumor antigens, and drugs. The primary clinical manifestation of hypersensitivity angiitis is that of digital artery occlusion with digital ischemia, Raynaud's symptoms, ulceration, and gangrene. Vasodilators such as calcium channel blockers and guanethidine have been beneficial despite the lack of demonstrable vasospasm. The results of surgical sympathectomy have been discouraging.

Systemic Lupus Erythematosus. Systemic lupus erythematosus (SLE) is an autoimmune disease with antibodies directed against DNA and other cellular constituents. A prominent component of SLE is an arteritis involving the medium-size vessels of the skin, intestine, kidney, lungs, and heart. Larger arteries and veins are affected with a thrombotic process distinct from the arteritis, secondary to the presence of a circulating substance known as the "lupus anticoagulant." This substance is not specific to SLE and is also found in other vasculitides. Although an elevated partial thromboplastin time is associated with the lupus anticoagulant, a hemorrhagic propensity does not develop. Thrombosis of the arteries of the upper and lower extremity, carotids, and coronaries may occur, as may venous thrombosis involving the inferior vena cava, upper and lower extremity veins, and retinal veins. Steroid and cytotoxic therapy is directed against the arteritis; long-term warfarin anticoagulation is directed against the thrombotic diathesis.

Inherited Connective Tissue Disorders. Marfan's syndrome and Ehlers-Danlos syndromes are two relatively rare autosomal dominant inherited diseases of connective tissue. These disease entities are not vasculitides, as such. The major clinical features are those of aneurysm formation and dissection of the aorta and its major branches. These complications often produce exsanguinating hemorrhage and rapid demise of affected patients in the second through the fifth decade of life.

Marfan's syndrome is characterized by a defect in collagen cross-linking. Mitral valve prolapse, ascending aortic aneurysm, and aortic dissection are the primary cardiovascular manifestations. Therapy is directed at lowering blood pressure with the use of beta-blockers and electively resecting aortic aneurysms when the aortic diameter reaches 6 cm or more.

The Ehlers-Danlos syndromes comprise a group of at least nine disease entities identified by defects in the conversion of procollagen to collagen. Hyperelasticity of the skin, spontaneous rupture of large arteries, aortic aneurysm and aortic dissection are the major clinical manifestations. Arteriography and bypass operations are associated with a substantial risk of hemorrhage, and ligation is the procedure of choice when rupture of a vessel is encountered in Ehlers-Danlos patients.

Antiphospholipid Syndrome

The antiphospholipid syndrome (APS) is a hypercoagulable state characterized by the clinical features of thrombosis, recurrent fetal loss, and thrombocytopenia occurring in association with antiphospholipid antibodies. The two methods currently in use to detect antiphospholipid antibodies are the lupus anticoagulant and anticardiolipin antibody tests, and either or both of these antibodies may be present in patients with APS. Other laboratory abnormalities frequently encountered in patients with APS include thrombocytopenia, elevation of the erythrocyte sedimentation rate, and prolongation of the partial thromboplastin time. The clinical features of APS may be seen in patients with antiphospholipid antibodies and no other concomitant disease process; this is known as primary APS. Alternatively, antiphospholipid antibodies may occur in association with systemic lupus erythematosus or other autoimmune, infectious, malignant, and inflammatory disorders; this is defined as secondary APS. Thrombosis of the venous system is more common than thrombosis of the arterial system in patients with APS, but the latter is far more devastating. In addition, arterial thrombosis due to primary APS may be difficult to distinguish from atherosclerosis, since circulation to the extremities, brain, and myocardium is frequently affected in both disorders, and the resultant ischemic symptoms are identical. Certain clinical features should raise suspicion of the diagnosis, however. In comparison with the atherosclerotic patient population, patients with arterial manifestations of APS are more often female, are significantly younger, and have a higher percentage of upper extremity involvement. Bypass of arterial lesions in patients with APS is associated with a very high incidence of early graft thrombosis (75 to 80 percent), although there is some evidence that preoperative and postoperative treatment with steroids, cytotoxic agents, and coumadin may improve the results of vascular reconstruction.

FROSTBITE

Several forms of cold injury have been described, including acute pernio or chilblains, chronic pernio, trench foot, and frostbite. Acute and chronic pernio represent focal, relatively mild injury of the skin and subcutaneous tissues resulting from cold exposure of moderate severity. The lesions tend to heal rapidly and are seldom a problem for the surgeon. Trench foot is principally a military injury produced by prolonged exposure to a cold, damp environment. Trench foot often occurs with temperatures above freezing, but in the setting of prolonged immobility. Immersion foot is the seagoing counterpart of trench foot.

Frostbite is the cold injury most frequently encountered in civilian practice. Frostbite occurs with exposure of tissues to subfreezing temperatures for a period of several hours. Shorter-term exposure to subzero temperatures results in a different form of frostbite, commonly occurring in airplanes at high altitudes and characterized by the term ''high-altitude'' frostbite. It has been demonstrated experimentally that cold-induced injury to mammalian tissues begins when the temperature reaches 10°C. At −5°C cells lose the ability to recover from the freezing process. Observations in the Korean conflict revealed that frostbite characteristically occurred with exposure to temperatures of −7°C for 7 to 18 h.

Several factors influence the injurious effect of cold exposure, including humidity and wind. Clinical observations have revealed that the most severe cold injuries occur in patients with prolonged contact with moisture or metallic surfaces, both of which function as efficient heat conductors. Wind also accelerates heat loss, presumably through increased evaporation of sweat and disruption of the radiant heat around the body. Coexistent peripheral arterial occlusive disease may contribute to the rapid development of cold-induced tissue injury. Chronic arterial disease should be excluded as a contributing factor anytime severe frostbite is observed in an adult civilian patient.

The pathophysiologic features of frostbite are dependent on the degree of cold-induced injury. Initially, vasoconstriction occurs on exposure to the cold. The histologic findings in mild frostbite consist of a low-grade vasculitis; the process progresses to an intense inflammatory reaction of the intima with severe frostbite. The capillary endothelium becomes permeable, and the resultant extravascular fluid accumulation produces soft tissue edema. Thrombi form in the terminal arterioles and capillaries and irreversible tissue necrosis develops. It is unknown whether the fundamental cold injury occurs as a result of direct freezing with disruption of cell membranes or from ischemic necrosis secondary to widespread thrombosis of the arterioles and capillaries.

Frostbite may be classified into four degrees of severity, analogous to the classification of burn injury. First-degree injury consists of edema and redness without necrosis; blistering becomes evident in second-degree injury; necrosis of skin constitutes third-degree injury; gangrene develops in fourth-degree injury, necessitating amputation of the affected extremity. A simpler subcategorization of frostbite involves division into superficial and deep classifications. Superficial frostbite involves the skin and superficial subcutaneous tissue; deep frostbite involves the deeper subcutaneous tissue, muscle, and even bone.

Treatment. The treatment of frostbite begins with rapid warming of the injured tissue. The involved body part should be immersed in warm water, with a temperature in the range of 40 to 44°C. Complete rewarming generally requires about 20 min. Once warm, the injured extremity should be elevated to minimize the formation of edema, and antibiotic and antitetanus therapy are instituted. The extent of gangrene is difficult to assess early in the course of frostbite. The degree of irreversible injury is often much less than initially feared, because the skin may be involved to a much greater extent than the subcutaneous tissue. For this reason, amputation should be delayed several weeks, until the precise extent of gangrene can be accurately determined.

Experimental and clinical evidence has demonstrated a beneficial effect from early sympathectomy in the treatment of severe frostbite. Operative sympathectomy should be performed within the first few days of injury if the injury is severe enough to produce tissue necrosis. Sympathectomy is also useful in alleviating the late sequelae of cold injury, including hyperhydrosis, cold sensitivity, and pain. Treatment directed against intravascular thrombosis has theoretical advantages; however, no consistent benefit has been achieved with the use of agents such as heparin or dextran.

The late sequelae of frostbite have been well documented in a study by Ervasti of 812 cases followed for 5 to 18 years. Long-term cold sensitivity was present in 82 percent of the patients, color changes of the skin in 73 percent, hyperhydrosis in 59 percent, pain with use of the extremity in 39 percent, and sensory loss in 23 percent. Sympathectomy was associated with improvement in symptomatic residua of frostbite in over 80 percent of patients in whom it was performed.

ARTERIOVENOUS FISTULAE

An arteriovenous fistula is a direct communication between the arterial and venous circulation that bypasses the capillary bed. The congenital variety is present at birth and grows or regresses. Although fistulae rarely cause hemodynamic symptoms, they can produce severe local problems that are often refractory to therapy. Fortunately, most congenital fistulae do not require operative therapy. The acquired arteriovenous fistula is most often the result of penetrating trauma, can produce serious cardiac dysfunction and usually requires repair.

Congenital Fistulae

Classification. Congenital arteriovenous fistulae may be circumscribed or diffuse and are due to abnormal development of the primitive vascular system. Szilagyi and associates have proposed an embryologic classification that divides these malformations into the hemangiomas and the fistulae. Circumscribed fistulae, called cavernous or simple hemangiomas, make up 19 percent of these lesions. There are two forms of this entity: (1) a nonneoplastic lesion that appears at birth and grows with the child and (2) a neoplastic lesion that begins as a small lesion just after birth, grows rapidly, and then usually spontaneously involutes. The distinction is important because of the tendency of the latter form to involute.

The diffuse group makes up 81 percent of these lesions and is characterized by anomalous micro or macro arteriovenous communications. These lesions are complex and have hemangiomatous, fistulous, and aneurysmal elements. Although present at birth, they may not become apparent until the second or third decade of life.

Clinical Manifestations. Many of these lesions are disturbing solely because of their cosmetic appearance which ranges from innocent-looking varicose veins to an ulcerated, bleeding pulsatile mass. The cutaneous changes may be only a small part of the problem, however. CT scanning and more recently MRI provide the most complete diagnostic information about the extent of the malformation and the need for resection. Arteriography and venography have many limitations as a diagnostic procedure because they do not define the extent of muscle and bony involvement and do not visualize the microfistulous connections. Arteriography's principle role is in preoperative localization of the afferent arterial supply and as a portal for embolization prior to resection.

High-output cardiac failure is rare with the congenital arteriovenous malformation. The congenital malformations cause symptoms from mass effect and thrombosis to bleeding from varicosities. Ulceration of the overlying skin with pain and infection is not uncommon because of the accompanying venous hypertension. Progressive growth is the rule because the low resistance on the venous side produces high flows and enlargement of the arterial inflow vessels. Malformations with extensive hemangiomatous changes can be associated with thrombocytopenia and purpura, the Kasabach-Merritt syndrome. One of the more common forms of congenital fistula is the Klippel-Trenaunay syndrome characterized by cutaneous hemangiomas with port-wine staining, varicose veins, and hypertrophy of the involved extremity. Patients with this syndrome may not have a deep venous system, and it is an error to excise the abnormal superficial veins without evidence of an intact deep system.

Treatment. The hemangiomas are more circumscribed and can be completely removed when local symptoms dictate. If changes in consistency or appearance are observed, selected biopsies are indicated because a malignant potential exists. Attempts to control the fistulous malformations are more difficult, and surgery should not be considered unless the lesion is life- or limb-threatening. Simple elastic support may suffice in an extremity lesion with low flow.

Intraarterial embolization and multiple-staged operative procedures for symptomatic lesions have been largely unsuccessful except as a means of short-term palliation (Fig. 20-41). When operative intervention is required as a last resort, a multidisciplinary team of vascular, orthopedic, and plastic surgeons offers a better chance for cure. The major vessels entering and leaving the tumor are initially ligated and the mass is resected with any involved tissue including muscle, bone, subcutaneous tissue, and skin. Reconstruction is then accomplished by the use of appropriate tissue transfers. Lesions in the chest, abdomen, and pelvis may require circulatory support and deep hypothermia.

Acquired Fistulae

Etiology and Diagnosis. These lesions are usually due to penetrating or iatrogenic trauma but can occur spontaneously such as an aortocaval fistula. Although it was once thought the fistula would continue to enlarge, it now seems that spontaneous closure occasionally occurs. On examination, there are usually visible veins surrounding the fistula which may have a palpable thrill and a machinery-type murmur throughout the cardiac cycle. The heart rate may slow with compression of the fistula (Branham's sign). The duplex scanner visualizes the increased flow velocities with the lowered resistance, the dilated outflow vessels, and the often-associated false aneurysm. Arteriography rather than CT or MRI scanning is the essential diagnostic tool for identifying the site of the communication and planning the operative approach.

Pathophysiology. When an arteriovenous connection is suddenly created, there is a decrease in blood flow distal to the lesion and an increase in venous pressure (Fig. 20-42). The peripheral vascular resistance is lowered to that of the venous system, and an increase in cardiac output occurs. As the fistula matures, the collateral circulation increases and the distal perfusion approaches normal and each component dilates. Over the longer term, venous hypertension may develop in the extremity. Growing children may exhibit limb length discrepancies and cardiac failure may occur.

Treatment. Acquired arteriovenous fistulae should be repaired because of the risk of life- or limb-threatening complications. Repair is technically easier when done at an early stage of fistula development. Successful repair requires that all four limbs of the fistula are controlled. An angiographically placed balloon occluding device in the afferent arterial limb can be a helpful adjunct. Once control is obtained, the fistula itself should be exposed and directly divided and sutured. The connection itself may be quite small and can be repaired with several sutures. Larger defects require a patch angioplasty or interposition graft. The long-term prognosis after direct repair is excellent. Early attempts at control by proximal artery ligation were both unsuccessful and dangerous. Ligation of all four vessels without direct exposure of the communication has resulted in a significant incidence of recurrences and distal arterial ischemia. Inaccessible fistulae can be managed angiographically with a variety of coils or plugs of Gelfoam. Recurrences are high with this technique because it requires great skill on the part of the angiographer.

VASCULAR TRAUMA

Major advances have been made in the treatment of arterial injuries based on lessons during wartime and from the management of atherosclerotic disease. The amputation rate following extremity vascular trauma was 50 percent during World War II, 13 percent during the Korean conflict, and is now 2 percent for civilian injuries.

General Considerations

Once the airway has been stabilized and volume replacement begun, patients with major vascular injuries are triaged into one of three groups: (1) those whose injuries are life-threatening and require immediate operation, (2) those whose vascular injuries are obvious but whose vital signs permit an arteriogram, and (3) those whose injuries, while not obvious, require evaluation because of their proximity to vascular structures. The signs of arterial injury include a pulsatile or expanding hematoma, pulsatile bleeding, a bruit or thrill, and/or end-organ ischemia. Suggestive features include unexplained shock, location, a stable hematoma, an injury to an adjacent nerve, or a questionable history of arterial bleeding (Table 20-8). Palpable pulses may be present even in the setting of a significant arterial injury. Arteriography is the gold standard test for the diagnosis of an arterial injury and should be performed whenever possible.

A major priority of treatment is the control of hemorrhage. Direct digital pressure is the most effective maneuver at the scene

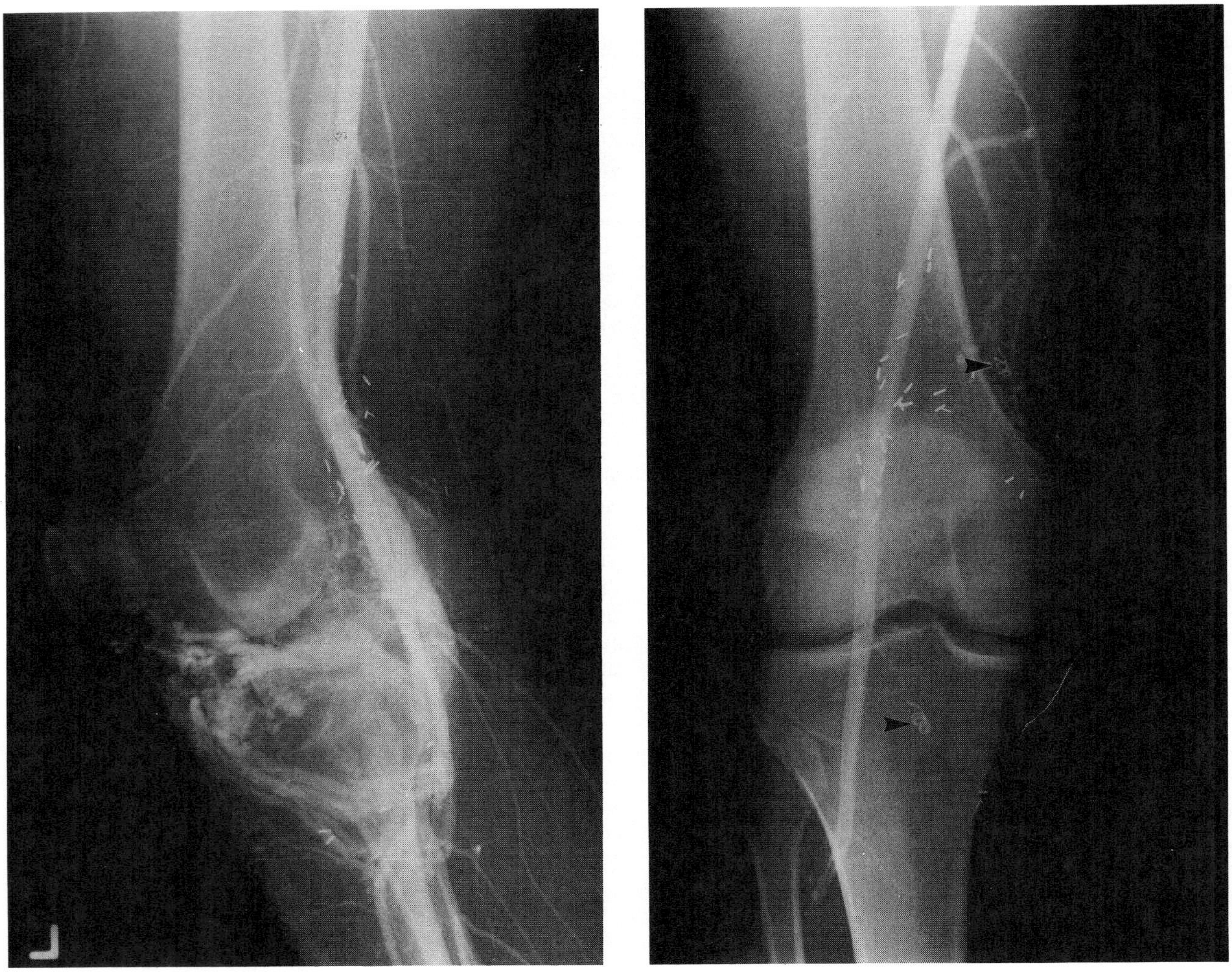

A B

FIG. 20-41. A series of arteriograms in a man with a congenital arteriovenous fistula around his left knee that demonstrate the futility of palliative treatment. *A.* At the time of presentation an attempt at operative control had been done by ligating the feeding vessels only. Hemoclips can be seen around the popliteal artery. The extent of the joint involvement is apparent, and this was confirmed with diagnostic arthroscopy. *B.* Two coils were placed (*arrows*) that occluded inflow to the fistula, and the patient did well for several months until he developed acute pain in his knee with marked swelling and tenderness. A repeat arthroscopy revealed a large hemarthrosis. *C.* A repeat arteriogram revealed the coils (*arrows*) in place but a significant recurrence of the malformation.

of the trauma or in the emergency room. Tourniquets should only be used as a last resort because they can occlude collateral flow and increase tissue damage. Attempts at blind clamping with hemostats should be avoided because this may further damage the injured vessel. Neither an embedded weapon nor a hematoma should be removed until proximal control is achieved because brisk bleeding may ensue.

Table 20-8
Signs of Arterial Injury

Hard signs	*Soft signs*
Pulsatile or expanding hematoma	Unexplained shock
Pulsatile bleeding	Proximity
Bruit or thrill	Stable hematoma
End-organ ischemia	Injury to an adjacent nerve
	Questionable history of arterial bleeding

Since many of these patients are operated on before complete data is available, maximum flexibility is necessary in planning the operative approach. Both legs should be prepped if there is any chance that saphenous vein might be necessary. The chest should be prepped if there is any chance that the arch vessels have been injured or that control of intraabdominal bleeding cannot be achieved transabdominally. Preparations should be made to administer blood with a rapid-infusion device.

Proximal and distal arterial control should be obtained prior to approaching the injury. If an intraluminal thrombus is present, it generally can be removed with a balloon catheter. Systemic heparin is not given to patients with multisystem trauma, and the thrombectomized artery can be flushed with heparinized saline. Once the injury is identified, wide debridement of the vessel is

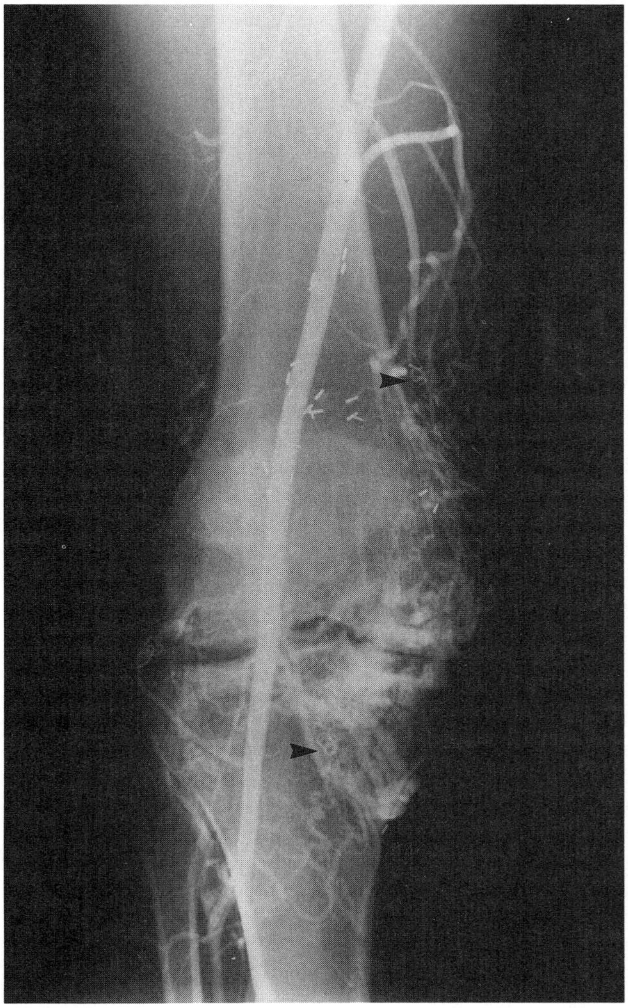

C

FIG. 20-41. *C. (continued)*

necessary. This is especially necessary in high-velocity missile wounds where the damage may extend beyond the obvious injury. The debridement should not be compromised in an attempt to simplify the arterial repair.

The type of arterial repair is ultimately dependent on the nature and extent of the injury. Although some sharp, penetrating wounds can be repaired with lateral arteriorrhaphy or a venous patch angioplasty, most arterial wounds require segmental resection. When an end-to-end anastomosis cannot be performed, an interposition graft using size-matched autogenous vein is used. Contralateral saphenous vein is recommended for extremity repairs to preserve the superficial venous drainage in the affected limb. Use of prosthetic grafts is controversial. Rich and associates reported complications when prosthetic material was used in 20 of 26 patients in the Vietnam Vascular Registry, while a conflicting civilian experience was reported by Mattox and associates from Houston. In their experience 10 percent of vascular repairs became infected when autogenous vein or Dacron was used and no infections were noted using PTFE. Completion arteriography is recommended; distal pulses cannot always be felt even when the repair is satisfactory because of arterial spasm.

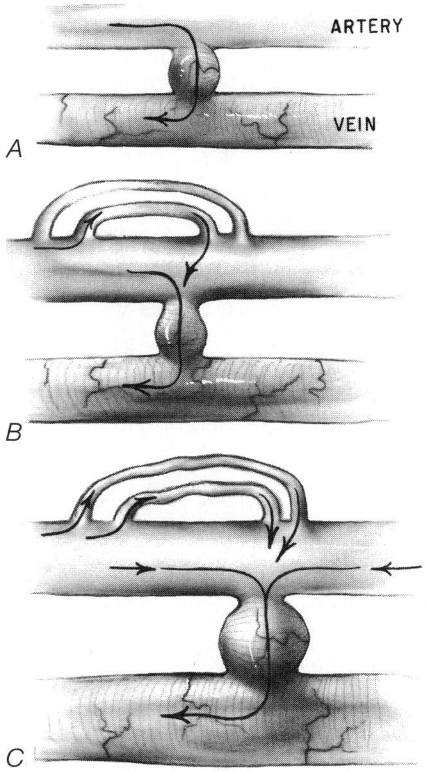

FIG. 20-42. *A.* Immediately following the development of an arteriovenous fistula there is shunting of blood from the artery through the fistula into the vein. The venous pressure rises and blood flow is reduced distal to the fistula. *B.* Collateral circulation develops around the fistula, and the proximal artery and vein dilate as flow through the fistula increases. *C.* Continued development of the collateral circulation and enlargement of the draining veins occurs. Superficial varicosities may occur. In some cases high-output congestive heart failure develops.

Extracranial Vascular Trauma

Carotid Artery. Both penetrating and blunt trauma can injure the carotid artery. The former, by far more common and easier to diagnose, causes either partial or complete transection of the artery. Blunt injuries are the result of hyperextension or a direct blow and are usually diagnosed when neurologic signs appear sometimes hours to days after the insult (Fig. 20-43). This lesion is characterized by intimal or medial tears which lead to dissection, stenosis, or thrombosis of the artery. Carotid arteriography is necessary in any hemodynamically stable patient with a suspected blunt injury.

Patients with penetrating carotid injuries may present with shock or respiratory distress from an expanding cervical hematoma. Pressure may affect cranial nerves IX, X, XI, or XII. Penetrating carotid injuries are anatomically divided into three zones. Zone I is the area below the top of the sternal notch; zone II extends from the sternal notch to the angle of the mandible; zone III is the region above the angle of the mandible. Arteriography is most helpful in zone I for planning the proper incision and in zone III injuries where the specific site and extent of the injury may influence operative strategy.

Preparation must be made for either a left anterior thoracotomy or a median sternotomy to gain control of the proximal carotid artery, if necessary. An oblique incision anterior to the sternomastoid muscle provides exposure of the artery and can be extended

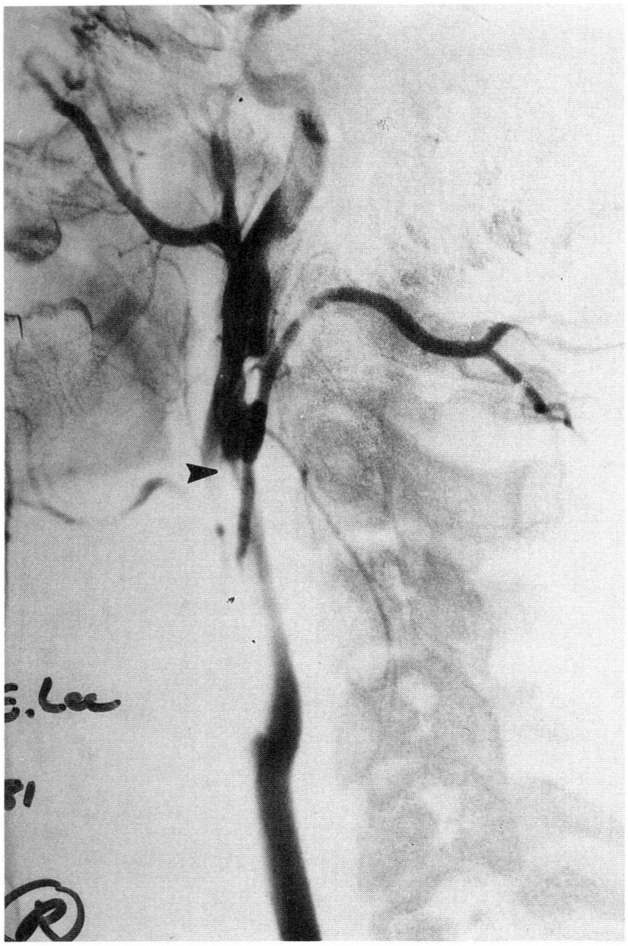

FIG. 20-43. Carotid arteriogram in a high school soccer player who sustained a hyperextension injury to his neck. Shortly after the injury he developed a left hemiparesis which cleared in 10 min. This happened again, and he was brought to the emergency room for evaluation. On arrival his neurologic evaluation was completely normal, but an arteriogram was ordered on the basis of his history. The arrow points to an area of intimal injury at the C-2 level with retrograde clot (poor filling). At operation he had an intimal transection with retrograde thrombosis. The lesion was 1 cm from the base of the skull, and the distal circulation was controlled with a balloon shunt. The intima was debrided and the retrograde thrombus was removed. An autogenous reconstruction was then performed. No further neurologic episodes occured.

caudally into a median sternotomy or craniad behind the ear. Most penetrating carotid injuries can be managed by lateral suture or end-to-end anstomosis. If an interposition graft is needed, either the external carotid artery or the saphenous vein can be used. External carotid artery injuries can be treated with proximal and distal ligation.

There are two areas of controversy in the management of carotid injuries. The first concerns the proper management of the asymptomatic penetrating neck wound. Recommendations vary from obligatory exploration of any wound penetrating the platysma muscle to arteriography and observation. It is reasonable to just follow these patients if they remain asymptomatic and the arteriogram is of sufficient quality to rule out a carotid injury. The second controversy concerns the implications of a neurologic deficit. Although it is accepted that carotid injuries should be repaired in a neurologically intact patient, opinions vary on the indications for operation when deficit exists. The best evidence suggests repair for those patients with mild deficits and those with severe deficits who have prograde flow preoperatively. Ligation is recommended for patients with severe deficits and absence of prograde flow and patients with a distal thrombi that cannot be extracted. Morbidity and mortality rates are lower for all groups of patients, except those in coma, when repair rather than ligation is performed.

Vertebral Arteries. These injuries are usually from penetrating trauma (95 percent). The increased use of arteriography has increased awareness of the problem. Vertebal artery injury rarely causes neurologic symptoms because of the dual blood supply to the basilar artery, but massive hemorrhage can occur. Recent studies have shown most angiographically demonstrated occlusions represent complete transection (52 to 81 percent) which, if left alone, develops into arteriovenous fistula or false aneurysm (5 to 30 percent).

Although there are some proponents of radiologic occlusion of the injured vertebral artery with detachable balloons, this technique does not control the distal vessel and carries the risk of a guide wire being pushed through a false lumen within the bony foramen of the transverse cervical processes. Operative therapy, which consists of proximal and distal ligation of the injured vessel, remains the procedure of choice.

If the proximal artery appears occluded on the arteriogram and there is no pulsatile hematoma present, the proximal artery can be approached at its origin from the subclavian artery through an oblique skin incision in the neck, with retraction of the carotid sheath medially and the anterior scalene muscle laterally. The distal ligation may require control of the interosseous portion of the vessel. This can be achieved by extending the skin incision to the mastoid process, exposing the prevertebral fascia, and gently removing the bone that forms the anterior border of the interosseous canal. If a pulsatile hematoma exists caused by an injury to the proximal vertebral artery, control should be obtained in the chest. Occasionally, repair of the injured vessel is indicated when a proximal transection can be easily transposed onto the common carotid artery or when the contralateral vertebral artery is diseased or absent.

Proximal Brachiocephalic Injuries. Injuries to the innominate, subclavian, and common carotid arteries require immediate diagnosis and control of hemorrhage. The initial presentation may range from an asymptomatic patient with an innocuous-appearing wound to a patient in hypovolemic shock with a massive hemothorax. The wounds should not be explored digitally. Tube thoracostomy is necessary for pneumothorax or hemothorax. Nasogastric tubes should not be placed. Patients in shock require an immediate operation. Arteriography can be performed in a stable patient with a penetrating wound, but a negative result does not replace exploration since sudden hemodynamic collapse is possible (5 percent) and does not rule out a major injury (22 percent). By contrast, arteriography is mandatory in the evaluation of blunt trauma to this region.

The patient is positioned supine with both arms abducted, and the neck, chest, and shoulders are prepped. In hemodynamically unstable patients, lesions on the right side can be controlled with a median sternotomy, and lesions on the left side with an anterolateral thoracotomy. The oblique cervical incision sparing the mediastinum provides exposure for most cervical injuries, but extension to remove the medial portion of the clavicle is sometimes necessary. The chest wall musculoskeletal flap or so-called trap door incision can be used for proximal left subclavian or common carotid injuries. Standard principles of arterial repair follow control of the bleeding. Wound debridement and lateral closure is often possible in these large vessels. Occasionally an autogenous patch is required. Ligation and remote prosthetic bypass is reserved for contaminated cases.

Extremity Injuries

Associated injuries to bones, muscles, veins, and nerves complicate the management of extremity arterial trauma. Signs of arterial involvement may be masked by these associated injuries, and therefore arteriography becomes the most important diagnostic study for establishing the diagnosis and defining the extent of the lesion.

Upper Extremity Injuries. Subclavian artery injuries are the most difficult to manage. They are often associated with injuries to the brachial plexus, either directly or indirectly from the pressure of an accompanying hematoma. Proximal exposure may require a thoracotomy. Results of arterial repair are good, but long-term disability usually follows the nerve injury.

Injuries to the axillary and brachial arteries are handled by incisions directly over the penetrating wound. End-to-end anastomoses are usually possible. The most common upper extremity vascular injury is iatrogenic due to coronary arteriography and transluminal angioplasty and drug abuse. Early repair of these injuries is indicated. Although only one-third of the patients with brachial artery occlusion will develop arm symptoms because of the rich collateral network that exists around the elbow, delayed repair will require a more complicated operation.

Lower Extremity Injuries. Most penetrating injuries of the lower extremity involve the superficial femoral artery; achieving proximal and distal control is similar to performing an elective femoral-popliteal artery bypass. Arteriography should be performed when the diagnosis is questioned. Wounds entering the lateral aspect of the thigh and exiting posteriorly do not need further study unless suggestive signs of arterial injury are present. Medial-entry wounds or those in proximity to a major artery should undergo arteriography.

Limb loss rates from arterial injuries associated with fractures and other soft tissue trauma range as high as 44 percent in civilian practice and higher in military series. Many of the patients with salvaged limbs have decreased function from muscle loss or nerve injury. Long bone fractures may cause arterial damage by acute angulation, laceration, or longitudinal stretching and subsequent thrombosis (Fig. 20-44). The arteries most often involved are the brachial artery just above and below the antecubital fossa, the distal superficial femoral and popliteal arteries, and the proximal tibial arteries around the knee. These lesions may cause immediate or delayed arterial occlusion, and arteriography is indicated in the setting of high-risk fractures in these regions when any evidence of arterial compromise is present.

The sequence of repair of concomitant bony and arterial injuries is controversial regarding fracture stabilization. Initial bone stabilization may correct perfusion abnormalities and protect any subsequent vascular repair from damage due to movement but delays restoration of flow unless a temporary shunt is placed and may impede access to the injured vessel. On the other hand, initial stabilization of the fracture might result in damage to a vascular repair when the latter precedes the former. In general it is preferable to stabilize fractures prior to the vascular repair, but this sequence must be individualized depending on the degree of distal ischemia and the presence of hemorrhage. Important technical considerations in repair of combined injuries are (1) early fasciotomy prior to orthopaedic repair, (2) preferential use of the contralateral saphenous vein, (3) repair of major venous injuries, (4) completion arteriography, and (5) adequate soft tissue coverage using appropriate muscle flaps.

The liberal use of fasciotomy in the injured extremity is important in reducing postoperative edema and the compartmental hypertension that may lead to myonecrosis and nerve damage. Reperfusion injury of ischemic skeletal muscle is related to damage from oxygen-derived free radicals. These compounds increase vascular permeability which permits the loss of intravascular fluid from the capillaries into the interstitial space. Mannitol, a free-radical scavenger, should therefore be given before limb revascularization. Objective measurements of compartment pressures can be made by determining the pressure within a closed system that is required to overcome the pressure in the compartment. Pressures greater than 40 mmHg mandate immediate decompression if clinical signs of elevated compartmental pressures are present. These include sensory loss in the first metatarsal space, inability to dorsiflex the great toe, or a foot drop. Patients with pressures greater than 50 mmHg should have immediate decompression regardless of the clinical findings. Fasciotomy should be performed through limited skin incisions if possible since the fascia is the limiting tissue. Progress in microvascular tissue transfers and improvements in skeletal fixation have increased the number of salvaged extremities. Occasionally early amputation is required because of the magnitude of the injury. Avulsed nerves, extensive soft tissue, and bony destruction may make the limb useless even in the setting of a successful arterial repair. The term "crush syndrome" was applied to the ischemia-induced syndrome of myonecrosis, myoglobinuria, and renal failure during the London Blitz in World War II. Complications in the postoperative period such as metabolic abnormalities from injured skeletal muscle, sepsis, or failure of the arterial repair may also lead to amputation. The principle of life over limb must always be followed when treating these complicated injuries.

Abdominal Vascular Injuries

Most abdominal vascular injuries follow penetrating trauma. Approximately 20 percent of patients with abdominal missile wounds will have a major vascular injury. The aorta, inferior vena cava, and the iliac vessels are most often involved, and the presenting clinical problem is usually exsanguinating hemorrhage. Diagnostic arteriography, although helpful, is rarely indicated. Blunt abdominal trauma is less common and usually involves avulsion of the hepatic veins and visceral arteries. Most of these injuries are associated with trauma to other organ systems, so the surgeon is faced with two problems: (1) control of bleeding and (2) management of solid organ or hollow viscus wounds that may be contaminated.

Principles of Management. Hemostasis is an essential part of the resuscitative effort, so operation must not be delayed for a detailed diagnostic evaluation. The beneficial tamponading effect of the intact abdominal cavity should not be forgotten. In cases of severe hypotension aortic control can be achieved using a left anterolateral thoracotomy through the sixth or seventh interspace. An autotransfusion device should be available, but the salvaged blood should not be reinfused until an intestinal injury is ruled out. The chest, abdomen, and groins are prepped. A midline

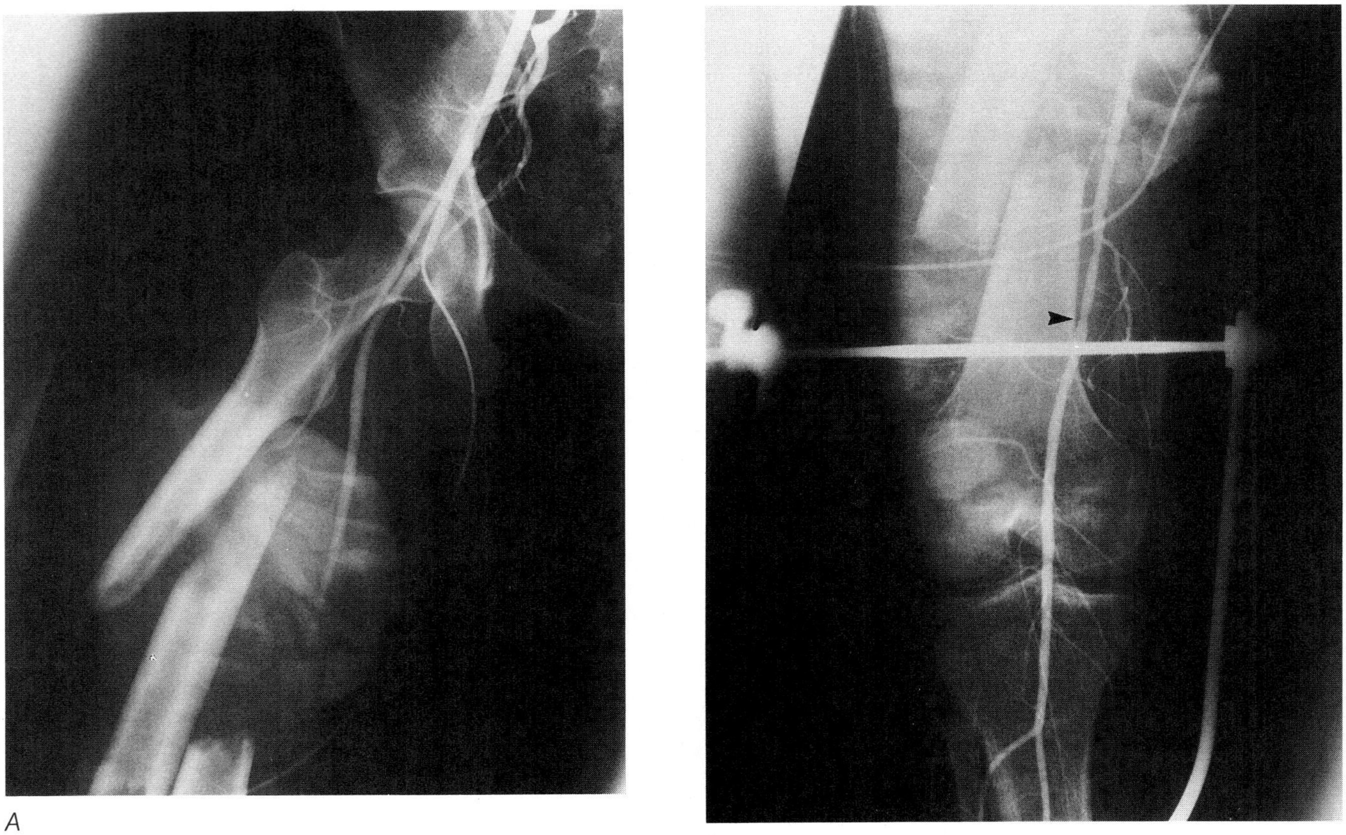

A

B

FIG. 20-44. *A.* An arteriogram taken on the way to the operating room in a 20-year-old woman involved in a motor vehicle accident. She sustained comminuted fractures of her femur and had a cold, pulseless leg. The arteriogram shows an abrupt cutoff of the superficial femoral artery. *B.* The patient was anesthetized and the fracture reduced and stabilized with an external fixator. A repeat arteriogram was done that shows an intimal defect (*arrow*) but a patent system. The foot was examined with Doppler ultrasound, and a biphasic signal was present. The patient was followed with serial noninvasive pressure measurements. The ABI reached 1.0 on the second postreduction day, and as the swelling in the leg subsided a pedal pulse became palpable. This emphasizes the importance of fracture reduction and stabilization in the treatment of combined musculoskeletal and vascular injuries.

abdominal incision should be made for rapid and generous exposure. The aorta is clamped at the diaphragm if arterial bleeding is profuse and cannot be controlled with packing. Blood and clot are rapidly removed, the abdomen packed with large pads, and the blood volume restored. Any intraperitoneal soilage is identified and controlled and then specific injuries are sought out.

Aortic injuries have mortality rates from 50 to 90 percent depending in part on the location of the injury. They are associated with a midline retroperitoneal hematoma and must be approached initially with aortic control at the diaphragm. The hematoma can then be opened and the clamp moved distally. Vena caval and renal artery lesions require mobilization of the right or left colon. Lesions of the suprarenal aorta can be isolated using the technique of medial visceral rotation. Occasionally the incision needs to be extended into the chest for proximal aortic control in the face of uncontrolled hemorrhage. Most patients with aortic injuries who reach the hospital can have the injury repaired with the lateral suture technique. Occasionally a graft is required, and the decision to use one depends on the degree of contamination present. Prosthetic grafts have been used successfully in situations with minimal contamination. Ligation and extraanatomic bypass is preferred, however, in cases where contamination is severe. Iliac artery injuries usually require graft replacement, and the same rules about contamination apply. In this setting a femoral-to-femoral artery bypass usually serves as a satisfactory replacement for the injured iliac artery. The celiac axis and its branches can be ligated in most patients without adverse consequences. Injuries to the proximal superior mesenteric artery and/or vein should be repaired either by lateral suture or saphenous vein bypass. More distal lesions are ligated, and bowel resection may be indicated. These patients require a second-look operation.

Pediatric Injuries. Pediatric arterial injury is uncommon, and a standardized approach is lacking especially in the group of iatrogenic injuries of infancy which make up virtually all of the injuries in children under the age of 2 years. These injuries present special challenges because of the small vessel size and the different implications of nonlimb-threatening ischemia. The manifestations of acute arterial ischemia in a child are similar to those in an adult. Chronic ischemia causes impaired growth in the affected limb rather than claudication or tissue loss. In general, pediatric arterial lesions should be promptly repaired. The only exception may be an iatrogenic femoral artery occlusion in an infant where heparin and observation of an extremity whose viability is not in question may yield better long-term results than early operation.

Bibliography

History of Vascular Surgery

Carrel A, Guthrie CC: Uniterminal and biterminal venous transplantation. *Surg Gynecol Obstet* 2:266, 1906.

Cooley DA, Al-Naaman YD, et al: Surgical treatment of arteriosclerotic occlusion of common carotid artery. *J Neurosurg* 13:500, 1956.

Dubost C, Allary M, et al: Propos de traitement des aneurysmes de l'aorte ablauon de l'aneurysme. Retablissement de la continuité. *Mem Acad Chir* (Paris) 77:381, 1951.

Eastcott HHG: *Arterial Surgery*. Philadelphia, JB Lippincott, 1969, p 235.

Eastcott HHG, Pickering GW, et al: Reconstruction of internal carotid artery in a patient with intermittent attacks of hemiplegia. *Lancet* 2:994, 1954.

Edwards WS, Edwards PD: *Alexis Carrel: Visionary Surgeon*. Springfield, Ill., Charles C Thomas, 1974.

Murphy JB: Resection of arteries and veins injured in continuing end-to-end suture experimental and clinical research. *Med Rec* 51:73, 1897.

Rob CG: The classics of vascular surgery, in Reemtsma K (ed): *The Classics of Surgery Library, Classics in Vascular Surgery*. Medford, NJ, Apollo, 1982.

Voorhees AB, Jaretski A, et al: The use of tubes constructed from vinyon-N cloth in bridging arterial defects. *Ann Surg* 135:322, 1952.

Atherogenesis

Antiplatelet Trialists' Collaboration: Secondary prevention of vascular disease by prolonged antiplatelet treatment. *Br J Med* 296:320, 1988.

Aspirin Myocardial Infarction Study Research Group: A randomized, controlled trial of aspirin in persons recovered from myocardial infarction. *JAMA* 243:661, 1980.

Canadian Cooperative Study Group: Randomized trial of aspirin and sulfinpyrazone in threatened stroke. *N Engl J Med* 299:53, 1978.

Couch NP: On the arterial consequences of smoking. *J Vasc Surg* 3:807, 1986.

Fuster V, Badimon L, et al: The pathogenesis of coronary artery disease and the acute coronary syndromes. *N Engl J Med* 326:242, 1992.

Glagov S, Zarins C, et al: Hemodynamics and atherosclerosis: Insights and perspectives gained from studies of human arteries. *Arch Pathol Lab Med* 112:1018, 1988.

Ip JH, Fuster V, et al: Syndromes of accelerated atherosclerosis: Role of vascular injury and smooth muscle cell proliferation. *J Am Coll Cardiol* 15:1667, 1990.

Lipid Research Clinics Coronary Primary Prevention Trial results. I: Reduction in incidence of coronary heart disease. *JAMA* 251:351, 1984.

Marcus AJ: Recent progress in the role of platelets in occlusive vascular disease. *Stroke* 14:475, 1983.

Report of the National Cholesterol Education Program Expert Panel on Detection, Evaluation and Treatment of High Blood Cholesterol in Adults. The Expert Panel. *Arch Intern Med* 148:36, 1988.

Ross R: The pathogenesis of atherosclerosis—an update. *N Engl J Med* 314:488, 1986.

Stary HC: Evolution and progression of atherosclerotic lesions in coronary arteries of children and young adults. *Arteriosclerosis* 99:(suppl I-19, I-32), 1989.

Thrombogenesis

Badimon L, Badimon JJ, et al: Influence of arterial damage and wall shear rate on platelet deposition. *Arteriosclerosis* 6:312, 1986.

Bennett JS: Integrin structure and function in hemostasis and thrombosis. *Ann N Y Acad Sci* 614:214, 1990.

Francis CW, Marder VJ: Concepts of clot lysis. *Annu Rev Med* 37:187, 1986.

Pathophysiology of Arterial Obstruction

Berguer R, Hwang NHC: Critical arterial stenosis. *Ann Surg* 180:39, 1974.

Conrad MC, Green HD: Hemodynamics of large and small vessels in peripheral vascular disease. *Circulation* 29:847, 1964.

DeWeese JA: Pedal pulses disappearing with exercise: A test for intermittent claudication. *N Engl J Med* 262:1214, 1960.

DeWeese JA, Van deBerg L, et al: Stenoses of arteries of the lower extremity. *Arch Surg* 89:806, 1964.

Flanigan DP, Tullis JP, et al: Multiple subcritical arterial stenoses: Effect on post-stenotic pressure and flow. *Ann Surg* 186:663, 1977.

Fronek A, Johansen KH, et al: Non-invasive physiologic tests in the diagnosis and characterization of peripheral arterial occlusive disease. *Am J Surg* 126:205, 1973.

Hillestad LK: The peripheral blood flow in intermittent claudication. V. Plethysmographic studies. The significance of calf blood flow at rest and in response to timed arrest of the circulation. *Acta Med Scand* 174:23, 1963.

May AG, DeWeese JA, et al: Hemodynamic effects of arterial stenosis. *Surgery* 53:513, 1963.

Moore WS, Malone JM: Effect of flow rate and vessel caliber on critical arterial stenosis. *J Surg Res* 26:1, 1979.

Rutherford RB, Valenta J: Extremity blood flow and distribution: The effects of arterial occlusion, sympathectomy and exercise. *Surgery* 69:332, 1971.

Strandness DE, Bell JW: An evaluation of the hemodynamic response of the claudicating extremity to exercise. *Surg Gynecol Obstet* 119:1237, 1964.

Strandness DE, Sumner DS: *Hemodynamics for Surgeons*. New York, Grune & Stratton, 1975.

Sumner DS: Hemodynamics and pathophysiology of arterial disease, in Rutherford RB (ed): *Vascular Surgery,* 2d ed. Philadelphia, WB Saunders, 1984.

Sumner DS, Strandness DE: The effect of exercise on resistance and blood flow in limbs with an occluded superficial femoral artery. *Vasc Surg* 4:229, 1970.

Yao JST: Hemodynamic studies in peripheral arterial disease. *Br J Surg* 57:761, 1970.

Clinical Manifestations

Boyd AM: The natural course of arteriosclerosis of the lower extremities. *Angiology* 11:10, 1960.

Criqui MH, Langer RD, et al: Mortality over a period of 10 years in patients with peripheral arterial disease. *N Eng J Med* 326:381, 1992.

Cronenwett JL, Warner KG, et al: Intermittent claudication: Current results of nonoperative management. *Arch Surg* 119:430, 1984.

Goldman L: Assessment of the patient with known or suspected ischaemic heart disease for non-cardiac surgery. *Br J Anaesth* 61:38, 1988.

Hertzer NR, Beven EG, et al: Coronary artery disease in peripheral vascular patients. *Ann Surg* 199:223, 1984.

Imparato AM, Kim GE, et al: Intermittent claudication: Its natural course. *Surgery* 78:795, 1975.

Noninvasive Studies

Barnes RW: Noninvasive diagnostic assessment of peripheral vascular disease. *Circulation* 83(suppl I):20, 1991.

Bernstein EF (ed): *Noninvasive Diagnostic Techniques in Vascular Disease*. St. Louis, CV Mosby, 1978.

Gee W, Oller DW, et al: Noninvasive diagnosis of carotid occlusion by ocular pneumoplethysmography. *Stroke* 7:18, 1976.

Strandness DE Jr: Duplex scanning and the vascular surgeon. *J Cardiovasc Surg* 28:235, 1987.

Sumner DS: Presidential address. Noninvasive testing of vascular disease—fact, fancy and future. *Surgery* 93:664, 1983.

Yao JST, Hobbs HT, et al: Ankle systolic pressure measurements in arterial disease affecting the lower extremities. *Br J Surg* 56:676, 1969.

Arteriography

Abrams HL, Adelstein SJ, et al: Optimal radiologic facilities for examination of the chest and the cardiovascular system. Report of the Inter-society Commission for Heart Disease Resources. *Circulation* 43:A135, 1971.

Lang EK, Foreman J, et al: The incidence of contrast medium induced ATN following angiography. *Radiology* 138:203, 1981.

Messina LM: Vascular complications of the lower extremities after percutaneous arterial puncture for diagnosis and therapy, in Ernst CB, Stanley JC (eds): *Current Therapy in Vascular Surgery*. Toronto, B.C. Decker, 1991, p 630.

Seldinger SI: Catheter replacement of the needle in percutaneous arteriography. *Acta Radiol* 39:368, 1953.

Sternberg EP, et al: Safety and cost effectiveness of high-osmolality as compared with low-osmolality contrast material in patients undergoing cardiac angiography. *N Engl J Med* 326:425, 1992.

VanZee BE, Hoy WE, et al: Renal injury associated with intravenous pyelography in nondiabetic and diabetic patients. *Ann Intern Med* 89:51, 1978.

Youkey JR, Clagett GP, et al: Vascular trauma secondary to diagnostic and therapeutic procedures. *Am J Surg* 146:788, 1983.

Aneurysms

Adar R, Rabbi I, et al: Left renal vein division in abdominal aortic aneurysm operations. Effect on renal function. *Arch Surg* 120:1033, 1985.

Bell DD, Gaspar MR: Routine aortography before abdominal aortic aneurysmectomy: A prospective study. *Am J Surg* 144:191, 1982.

Bernstein EF, Dilley RB, et al: Growth rates of small abdominal aortic aneurysms. *Surgery* 80:765, 1986.

Brewster DC, Retana A, et al: Angiography in the management of aneurysms of the abdominal aorta: Its value and safety. *N Engl J Med* 292(16):822, 1975.

Bush HL Jr, Huse JB, et al: Prevention of renal insufficiency after abdominal aortic aneurysm resection by optimal volume loading. *Arch Surg* 116:1517, 1981.

Cambria RP, Brewster DC, et al: Transperitoneal versus retroperitoneal approach for reconstruction of the infrarenal abdominal aorta. *J Vasc Surg* 5:19, 1987.

Crawford ES, DeBakey ME, et al: Surgical considerations of peripheral arterial aneurysms. *Arch Surg* 78:226, 1959.

Crawford ES, Saleh SA, et al: Infrarenal abdominal aortic aneurysm: Factors influencing survival over a 25 year period. *Ann Surg* 193:699, 1981.

Crawford ES, Stowe CL, et al: Inflammatory aneurysms of the aorta. *J Vasc Surg* 2:113, 1985.

Creech O Jr: Endo-aneurysmorrhaphy and treatment of aortic aneurysm. *Ann Surg* 164:935, 1966.

Cronenwett JL, Sargent SK, et al: Variables that affect the expansion rate and outcome of small abdominal aortic aneurysms. *J Vasc Surg* 11:260, 1990.

Darling RC, Messina CR, et al: Autopsy study of unoperated abdominal aortic aneurysms. The case for early resection. *Circulation* 56(suppl 2):161, 1977.

DeBakey ME, Crawford ES, et al: Aneurysm of abdominal aorta: Analysis of results of graft replacement therapy one to eleven years after operation. *Ann Surg* 160:622, 1964.

Dubost C, Allary M, et al: Resection of an aneurysm of the abdominal aorta: Reestablishment of the continuity by a preserved human arterial graft, with result after 5 months. *Arch Surg* 64:405, 1952.

Ernst CB: Prevention of intestinal ischemia following abdominal aortic reconstruction. *Surgery* 93:102, 1982.

Estes JE Jr: Abdominal aortic aneurysm: A study of one hundred and two cases. *Circulation* 2:258, 1950.

Evans WE, Vermillion BD: Popliteal and femoral aneurysms, in Rutherford RB (ed): *Vascular Surgery,* 2d ed. Philadelphia, WB Saunders, 1984, p 814.

Golden MA, Whittemore AD, et al: Selective evaluation and management of coronary artery disease in patients undergoing repair of abdominal aortic aneurysms: A 16 year experience. *Ann Surg* 212:415, 1990.

Graham LM, Zelenock GB, et al: Clinical significance of atherosclerotic femoral aneurysms. *Arch Surg* 115:502, 1980.

Green RM, Ricotta JR, et al: Results of supraceliac aortic clamping in the difficult elective resection of infrarenal abdominal aortic aneurysm. *J Vasc Surg* 9:124, 1989.

Hertzer NR, Beven EG, et al: Coronary artery disease in peripheral vascular patients: A classification of 1000 coronary angiograms and results of surgical management. *Ann Surg* 199:223, 1984.

Hicks G, Eastland MW, et al: Survival improvement following aortic aneurysm resection. *Ann Surg* 181:863, 1975.

Hollier LH, Batson RC, et al: Femoral anastomotic aneurysms. *Ann Surg* 191:715, 1980.

Imparato AM: Abdominal aortic surgery: Prevention of lower limb ischemia. *Surgery* 93:112, 1983.

Johnston KW: Multicenter prospective study of nonruptured abdominal aortic aneurysm. Part II. Variables predicting morbidity and mortality. *J Vasc Surg* 9:437, 1989.

Martin RS, Edwards WH, et al: Ruptured abdominal aortic aneurysm: A 25 year experience and analysis of recent cases. *Am Surg* 54:539,1988.

McCready RA, Pairolero PC, et al: Isolated iliac artery aneurysms. *Surgery* 93:688, 1983.

Ouriel K, Green RM, et al: An evaluation of new methods of expressing aortic aneurysm size: Relationship to rupture. *J Vasc Surg* 15:12, 1992.

Pairolero PC, Gilmore JC, et al: Isolated iliac artery aneurysms. *Surgery* 93:688, 1983.

Peterson LH: Physical factors which influence vascular caliber and blood flow. *Circ Res* 28(suppl 1):3, 1966.

Picone AL, Green RM, et al: Spinal cord ischemia following operations on the abdominal aorta. *J Vasc Surg* 3:94, 1987.

Rapp JH, Pan XM, et al: Angiography by magnetic resonance imaging: Detailed vascular anatomy without ionizing radiation or contrast. *Surgery* 105:662, 1989.

Reilly KM, Abbott WM, et al: Aggressive surgical management of popliteal aneurysms. *Am J Surg* 145:498, 1983.

Reilly LM, Stoney RJ, et al: Improved management of aortic graft infection: The influence of operation sequence and staging. *J Vasc Surg* 5:421, 1987.

Rob CG: Extraperitoneal approach to the abdominal aorta. *Surgery* 53:87, 1963.

Shortell CK, De Weese JA, et al: Popliteal artery aneurysms: A 25 year surgical experience. *J Vasc Surg* 14:771, 992.

Szilagyi DE, Elliott JP, et al: Clinical fate of the patient with asymptomatic abdominal aortic aneurysm and unfit for surgical treatment. *Arch Surg* 104:600, 1972.

Szilagyi DE, Schwartz RL, et al: Popliteal arterial aneurysms. *Arch Surg* 116:724, 1981.

Szilagyi DE, Smith RF, et al: Contribution of abdominal aortic aneurysmectomy to prolongation of life. *Ann Surg* 164:678, 1966.

Thompson JE, Hollier LH, et al: Surgical management of abdominal aortic aneurysms: Factors influencing mortality and morbidity—a 20 year experience. *Ann Surg* 181:654, 1975.

Acute Arterial Occlusion

Belkin M, Belkin B, et al: Intra-arterial fibrinolytic therapy. *Arch Surg* 121:769, 1986.

Billig DM, Hallman GL, et al: Arterial embolism. *Arch Surg* 95:1, 1967.

Cranley JJ, Krause RJ, et al: Peripheral arterial embolism: Changing concepts. *Surgery* 55:57, 1964.

Dale WA: The beginnings of vascular surgery. *Surgery* 76:849, 1974.

Darling RC, Austen WG, et al: Arterial embolism. *Surg Gynecol Obstet* 124:106, 1967.

Dotter CT, Rosch J, et al: Selective clot lysis with low dose streptokinase. *Radiology* 111:31, 1974.

Fisher DR Jr, Clagett GP, et al: Dilemmas in dealing with the blue toe syndrome: Aortic versus peripheral source. *Am J Surg* 148:836, 1984.

Fisher ER, Hellstrom HR, et al: Disseminated atheromatous emboli. *Am J Med* 29:176, 1960.

Fogarty TJ, Cranley JJ, et al: A method for extraction of arterial emboli and thrombi. *Surg Gynecol Obstet* 116:241, 1963.

Gardiner GA Jr, Koltun W, et al: Thrombolysis of occluded femoropoliteal grafts. *AJR* 147:621, 1986.

Haimovici H: Peripheral arterial embolism. *Angiology* 1:20, 1950.

Kassirer JP: Atheroembolic renal disease. *N Engl J Med* 280:817, 1969.

Krupski WC, Feldman RK, et al: Recombinant human tissue-type plasminogen activator is an effective agent for thrombolysis of peripheral arteries and bypass grafts: Preliminary report. *J Vasc Surg* 10:491, 1989.

Marder VJ, Sherry S: Thrombolytic therapy. Current status. *N Engl J Med* 318:1512, 1988.

McNamara TO, Bomberger RA: Intraarterial urokinase as the initial therapy for acutely ischemic lower limbs. *Circulation* 83 (suppl I):I-106, 1991.

Sicard GA, Schier JJ: Thrombolytic therapy for acute arterial occlusion. *J Vasc Surg* 2:65, 1985.

Sullivan KL, Gardiner GA Jr, et al: Efficacy of thrombolysis in infrainguinal bypass grafts. *Circulation* 83 (suppl I):I-99, 1991.

Tawes RL Jr, Harris EJ, et al: Arterial thromboembolism. A 20-year perspective. *Arch Surg* 120:595, 1985.

van Breda A, Katzen BT, et al: Urokinase versus streptokinase in local thrombolysis. *Radiology* 165:109,1987.

Chronic Arterial Occlusion

Blebea J, Ouriel K, et al: Laser angioplasty in peripheral vascular disease—symptomatic versus hemodynamic results. *J Vasc Surg* 13:222, 1991

Dotter CT, Judkins MP: Transluminal treatment of atherosclerotic obstruction: Description of a new technique and a preliminary report of its application. *Circulation* 30:654, 1964.

Gruntzig A, Kumpe DA: Technique of percutaneous angioplasty with Gruntzig balloon catheter. *AJR* 132:547, 1979.

Kannel WB, McGee DL: Update on some epidemiologic features of intermittent claudication: The Framingham study. *J Am Geriatr Soc* 33:15, 1985.

Ouriel K, Fiore WM, et al: Limb threatening ischemia in the medically compromised patient. Amputation or revascularization. *Surgery* 104:667, 1988.

Ouriel K, Green RM, et al: The hemodynamics of thrombus formation in arteries. *J Vasc Surg* 14:757, 1991.

Ouriel K, Smith CR, et al: Endarterectomy for localized lesions of the superficial femoral artery at the adductor canal. *J Vasc Surg* 3:531, 1986.

Ouriel K, Zarins CK: Doppler ankle pressure. An evaluation of three methods of expression. *Arch Surg* 117:1297, 1982.

Porter JM, Cutler BS, et al: Pentoxifylline efficacy in the treatment of intermittent claudication: Multicenter controlled double-blind trial with objective assessment of chronic occlusive arterial disease patients. *Am Heart J* 104:66, 1982.

Ramsey DE, Manke DA, et al: Toe blood pressure—a valuable adjunct to ankle pressure measurement for assessing peripheral arterial disease. *J Cardiovasc Surg* 24:43, 1983.

Veith FJ, Gupta SK, et al: Six-year prospective multicenter randomized comparison of autologous saphenous vein and expanded polytetrafluoroethylene grafts in infrainguinal arterial reconstructions. *J Vasc Surg* 3:104, 1986.

Wilson SE, Sheppard B: Results of percutaneous transluminal angioplasty for peripheral vascular occlusive disease: *Ann Vasc Surg* 4:94, 1990.

Mesenteric and Renal Artery Occlusive Disease

Dean RH, Englund R, et al: Retrieval of renal function by revascularization. Study of preoperative outcome predictors. *Ann Surg* 202:367, 1985.

Dunbar JD, Molnar W, et al: Compression of the celiac trunk and abdominal angina: Preliminary report of 15 cases. *American Journal of Roentgenology, Radium Therapy, and Nuclear Medicine* 95:731, 1965.

Goldblatt H: Studies on experimental hypertension. *J Exp Med* 59:347, 1934.

Hunt JC, Strong CG: Renovascular hypertension. Mechanisms, natural history, and treatment. *Am J Cardiol* 32:562, 1973.

Lawson JD, Boerth RK, et al: Diagnosis and management of renovascular hypertension in children. *Arch Surg* 112:1307, 1977.

Ouriel K, Andrus CH, et al: Acute renal artery occlusion. When is revascularization justified? *J Vasc Surg* 5:348, 1987.

Simon N, Franklin SS, et al: Clinical characteristics of renovascular hypertension. *JAMA* 220:1209, 1972.

Extracranial Cerebrovascular Disease

AbuRahma AF, Boland JP: Antiplatelet therapy in carotid plaque hemorrhage and its clinical implications. *J Cardiovasc Surg* 31:66, 1990.

Antiplatelet Trialists' Collaboration: Secondary prevention of vascular disease by prolonged antiplatelet treatment. *Br Med J* 296:320, 1988.

Carter AB: Clinical aspects of cerebral infarction, in Vinken JP, Bruyn GS (eds): *Handbook of Clinical Neurology: Vascular Disease of the Nervous System,* vol II. New York, North Holland Publishing Company and American Elsevier Publishing Company, 1972.

Eastcott HHG, Pickering GW: Reconstruction of internal carotid artery in a patient with intermittent attacks of hemiplegia. *Lancet* 2:994, 1954.

Ehrenfeld WK, Hoyt WF: Embolization and transient blindness from carotid atheroma. *Arch Surg* 93:787, 1966.

Fisher CM: Observations of the fundus oculi in transient monocular blindness. *Neurology* 9:333, 1959.

Fisher M, Adams RD: Observations on brain embolism with special reference to the mechanism of hemorrhagic infarction. *J Neuropathol Exp Neurol* 10:92, 1951.

Fry DL: Acute vascular endothelial changes associated with increased blood velocity gradients. *Circ Res* 22:165, 1968.

Hollenhorst RW: Significance of bright plaques in the retinal arteriole. *JAMA* 178:23, 1961.

Hertzer NR, Young JR, et al: Coronary artery disease in peripheral vascular patients. A classification of 1000 coronary angiograms and results of surgical management. *Ann Surg* 199:223, 1984.

Lusby RJ, Woodcock JP, et al: The role of intraplaque hemorrhage in the development of cerebro-vascular disease. *Arch Surg* 117:1479, 1982.

Millikan CH: The pathogenesis of transient focal cerebral ischemia. *Circulation* 32:438, 1965.

North American Symptomatic Carotid Endarterectomy Trial collaborators: Beneficial effect of carotid endarterectomy in symptomatic patients with high-grade carotid stenosis. *N Engl J Med* 325:445, 1991.

Ouriel K, DeWeese J: Extracranial cerebral revascularization for nonhemispheric symptoms: Do the results justify the procedures? *Semin Vasc Surg* 2:12, 1989.

Ouriel K, Green RM: Clinical and technical factors influencing carotid restenosis and occlusion after endarterectomy. *J Vasc Surg* 5:702, 1987.

Ouriel K, May AG, et al: Carotid endarterectomy for nonhemispheric symptoms. Predictors of success. *J Vasc Surg* 1:339, 1984.

Ouriel K, Ricotta JJ, et al: Carotid endarterectomy for nonhemispheric cerebral symptoms. Patient selection with ocular pneumoplethysmography. *J Vasc Surg* 4:115, 1986.

Ricotta JJ, Ouriel K, et al: Embolic lesions from the subclavian artery causing transient vertebrobasilar insufficiency. *J Vasc Surg* 4:372, 1986.

Ricotta JJ, Ouriel K, et al: Use of computerized cerebral tomography in selection of patients for elective and urgent carotid endarterectomy. *Ann Surg* 202:783, 1985.

Swanson PD, Calanchini PR, et al: Cooperative study of hospital frequency and character of transient ischemic attacks: II. Performance of angiography among six centers. *JAMA* 237:2202, 1977.

Sze PC, Reitman D, et al: Antiplatelet agents in the secondary prevention of stroke: Metaanalysis of the randomized control trials. *Stroke* 19:436, 1988.

The Dutch TIA Trial Study Group: A comparison of two doses of aspirin (30 mg vs. 283 mg a day) in patients after a transient ischemic attack or minor ischemic stroke. *N Engl J Med* 325:1261, 1991.

Williams II SJ: Chronic upper extremity ischemia: Current concepts in management. *Surg Clin North Am* 66:355, 1986.

Zarins CK, Giddens DP, Glagov S: Atherosclerotic plaque distribution and flow velocity profiles in the carotid bifurcation, in JJ Bergan, Yao JST (eds): *Cerebrovascular Insufficiency,* chap 2. New York, Grune & Stratton, 1983.

Thoracic Outlet Syndrome

Adams JT, DeWeese JA: ''Effort'' thrombosis of the axillary and subclavian veins. *J Trauma* 11:923, 1971.

Claggett OT: Research and prosearch. *J Thorac Cardiovasc Surg* 44:153, 1962.

Cormier JM, Amrane M, et al: Arterial complications of the thoracic outlet syndrome: Fifty-five operative cases. *J Vasc Surg* 9:778, 1989.

Dale WA: Thoracic outlet compression syndrome: Critique in 1982. *Arch Surg* 117:1437, 1982.

DeWeese JA, Green RM: Venous complications of thoracic outlet syndrome and their treatment, in Veith FJ (ed): *Current Critical Problems in Vascular Surgery,* vol 3. St. Louis, Quality Medical Publishing, 1991.

Gilliatt RW: Thoracic outlet compression syndrome. *Br Med J* 1:1274, 1976.

Green RM, McNamara J, et al: Long-term follow-up after thoracic outlet decompression: An analysis of factors determining outcome. *J Vasc Surg* 14:739, 1992.

Haimovici H: Arterial thromboembolism secondary to thoracic outlet compression, in Haimovici H (ed): *Vascular Surgery: Principles and Techniques*. New York, Appleton-Century-Crofts, 1984, p 903.

Lord JW Jr: Critical reappraisal of diagnostic and therapeutic modalities for thoracic outlet syndromes. *Surg Gynecol Obstet* 168:337, 1989.

Machleder HI: Effort thrombosis of the axillosubclavian vein: A disabling vascular disorder. *Compr Ther* 17:18, 1991.

Peet RM, Hendricksen JD, et al: Thoracic outlet syndrome: Evaluation of a therapeutic exercise program. *Proc Mayo Clin* 31:281, 1956.

Rob CG, Standeven A: Arterial occlusion complicating thoracic outlet compression syndrome. *Br J Med* 2:709, 1958.

Roos DB: Thoracic outlet and carpal tunnel syndromes, in Rutherford RB (ed): *Vascular Surgery,* 2d ed. Philadelphia, WB Saunders, 1984.

Roos DB: Transaxillary approach for first rib resection to relieve thoracic outlet syndrome. *Ann Surg* 163:354, 1966.

Roos DB: Congenital anomalies associated with thoracic outlet syndrome: Anatomy, symptoms, diagnosis and treatment. *Am J Surg* 132:771, 1976.

Saunders RRJ, Pearce WH: The treatment of thoracic outlet syndrome: A comparison of three different operations. *J Vasc Surg* 10:626, 1989.

Strange-Vognsen HH, Hauch O, et al: Resection of the first rib, following deep arm vein thrombolysis in patients with thoracic outlet syndrome. *J Cardiovasc Surg* 30:430, 1989.

Wilbourn AJ: Thoracic outlet syndrome is overdiagnosed. *Arch Neurol* 47:328, 1990.

Nonatherosclerotic Popliteal Arterial Disease

Insua JA, Young JR, Humphries AW: Popliteal artery entrapment syndrome. *Arch Surg* 101:771, 1970.

Ishikawa K: Cystic adventitial disease of the popliteal artery and of other stem vessels in the extremities. *Jpn J Surg* 17:221, 1987.

Flanigan DP, Burnham SJ, et al: Summary of cases of adventitial cystic disease of the popliteal artery. *Ann Surg* 189:165, 1979.

Williams LR, Flinn WR, et al: Popliteal artery entrapment: Diagnosis by computed tomography. *J Vasc Surg* 3:360, 1986.

Vasopastic Disorders and Frostbite

Ervasti E: Frostbite of the extremities and their sequelae: A clinical study. *Acta Chir Scand* 299(suppl):1, 1962.

Inflammatory Arteritis

Joyce JW: The giant cell arteritides: Diagnosis and the role of surgery. *J Vasc Surg* 3:8273, 1986.

Klein RG, Hunder GG, et al: Large artery involvement in giant cell (temporal) arteritis. *Ann Intern Med* 83:806, 1975.

Lupi-Herrera E, Sanchez-Torres G, et al: Takayasu's arteritis. Clinical study of 107 cases. *Am Heart J* 43:15, 1977.

Shortell CK, Ouriel K: Involvement of aortic bifurcation and lower extremity vessels in Takayasu's arteritis. *Res Surg* 3:157, 1991.

Shortell CK, Ouriel K: Vascular disease in the antiphospholipid syndrome: A comparison with the patient population with atherosclerosis. *J Vasc Surg* 15:158, 1992.

Congenital Arteriovenous Fistulae

Gloviczki P, Hollier LH, et al: Surgical implications of Klippel-Trenaunay syndrome. *Ann Surg* 197:353, 1983.

Lindenauer SM: The Klippel-Trenaunay syndrome: Varicosity hypertrophy and hemangioma with no arteriovenous fistula. *Ann Surg* 162:303, 1965.

Malan E (ed): *Vascular Malformations (Angiodysplasias)*. Milan, Carlo ERBA Foundation, 1974.

Olcott C IV, Newton TH, et al: Intra-arterial embolization in the management of arteriovenous malformations. *Surgery* 79:3, 1976.

Pearce WH, Rutherford EB, et al: Nuclear magnetic resonance imaging: Its diagnostic value in patients with congenital vascular malformations of the limbs. *J Vasc Surg* 8:64, 1988.

Szilagyi DE, Smith RF, et al: Congenital arteriovenous anomalies of the limbs. *Arch Surg* 111:423, 1976.

Trout HH: Management of patients with hemangiomas and arteriovenous malformations. *Surg Clin North Am* 66:333, 1986.

Acquired Arteriovenous Fistulae

Johansen K: Management of acquired arteriovenous fistulas, in Ernst CB, Stanley JC (eds): *Current Therapy in Vascular Surgery,* 2d ed. Toronto, BC Decker, 1991.

Rich NM, Hobson RW, et al: Traumatic arteriovenous fistulas and false aneurysms: A review of 558 lesions. *Surgery* 78:817, 1975.

Sumner DS: Hemodynamics and pathophysiology of arteriovenous fistulae, in Rutherford RB (ed): *Vascular Surgery,* 2d ed. Philadelphia, WB Saunders, 1984.

Vascular Trauma

Bishara RA, Pasch AR, et al: Improved results in the treatment of civilian vascular injuries associated with fractures and dislocations. *J Vasc Surg* 3:707, 1986.

DeBakey ME, Simeone FA: Battle injuries of the arteries in World War II. *Ann Surg* 123:534, 1946.

Ekbom GA, Towne JB, et al: Intra-abdominal vascular trauma—a need for prompt operation. *J Trauma* 21:1040, 1981.

Flint LM, Snyder WH, et al: Management of vascular injuries in the base of the neck. *Arch Surg* 106:409, 1973.

Graham JM, Feliciano DV, et al: Management of subclavian vascular injuries. *J Trauma* 20:537, 1980.

Holcroft JW, Trunkey DD, et al: Renal trauma and retroperitoneal hematomas—indications for exploration. *J Trauma* 15:1045, 1975.

Mattox KL, McCollum WB, et al: Management of upper abdominal vascular trauma. *Am J Surg* 128:823, 1974.

Meier DE, Brink BE, et al: Vertebral artery injury-recognition and management. *Arch Surg* 116:236, 1978.

Mills JL, Wiedeman JE, et al: Minimizing mortality and morbidity from iatrogenic arterial injuries: The need for early recognition and prompt repair. *J Vasc Surg* 4:22, 1986.

Patman RD: Compartment syndromes in peripheral vascular surgery. *Clin Orthop* 113:103, 1978.

Perry MO: Injuries of the aortic arch and great vessels, in Perry MO (ed.): *The Management of Acute Vascular Injuries*. Baltimore, Williams & Wilkins, 1981, p 55.

Perry MO, Thal ER, et al: Management of arterial injuries. *Ann Surg* 173:403, 1971.

Rich NM: Injuries of the abdominal aorta in vascular trauma, in Rich NB, Spencer FC (eds): *Vascular Trauma*. Philadelphia, WB Saunders, 1978, p 441.

Rich NM, Baugh JH, et al: Popliteal artery injuries in Vietnam. *Am J Surg* 118:531, 1969.

Rich NM, Hobson RW II, et al: Traumatic arteriovenous fistulas and false aneurysms: A review of 558 lesions. *Surgery* 78:817, 1975.

Rich NM, Hughes CW, et al: Management of venous injuries. *Ann Surg* 171:724, 1970.

Smith C, Green RM: Pediatric vascular injuries. *Surgery* 90:20, 1981.

Snyder WH III: Vascular injuries near the knee: An updated series and overview of the problem. *Surgery* 91:502, 1982.

Sumner DS: Aortic thrombus in infants, in Bergan JJ, Yao JST (eds): *Aortic Surgery*. Philadelphia, WB Saunders, 1989 p 453.

Thal ER, Snyder WH III, et al: Management of carotid artery injuries. *Surgery* 76:955, 1974.

Ward RE: Injury to the cervical cerebral vessels, in Blaisdell FW, Trunkey DD (eds): *Trauma Management,* vol III, *Cervicothoracic Trauma*. New York, Thieme, 1986, p 273.

CHAPTER 21

Venous and Lymphatic Disease

Lazar J. Greenfield

VENOUS DISEASE

Functional Anatomy of the Veins

Evolution in human beings to an upright position imposed a significant work load on the venous system. Since the systemic veins contain approximately two-thirds of the circulating blood volume under relatively low pressure, movement from the lower extremities must overcome gravity and intraabdominal pressure to return blood to the right ventricle. The left ventricle provides the initial force called *vis a tergo,* which is reduced through the capillary bed to a pressure of about 15 mmHg in the venules. In addition, the calf muscles provide an important pump function as they compress deep veins within an unyielding fascial compartment. Proximal flow is assured by the presence of the delicate but strong venous valves, which prevent reflux distally. Perforating or communicating veins connect the superficial venous system with the deep and direct flow internally from the superficial veins in all areas of the lower extremity except the foot, where the opposite occurs (Fig. 21-1). Each valve is based within a dilated sinus of the vein, which keeps the valve cusps away from the walls and promotes rapid closure when flow ceases. Numbers of valves increase with distance from the heart while the vena cava and common iliac veins are valveless. Valves are the focal point of most of the pathology of venous thrombosis since their sinuses are where the initial thrombus forms and the loss of valvular function after recanalization of a thrombus produces venous insufficiency.

The structure of veins also is related to their functional requirements, with the unsupported superficial vein walls containing more smooth muscle while the deep veins are thin-walled and lacking in significant smooth muscle. In some areas such as the calf, there are spindle-shaped sinusoids that can become sites of venous stasis when the patient is at bed rest, facilitating the development of venous thrombosis.

The major superficial veins of the lower extremity are the greater and lesser saphenous veins and their tributaries. The deep veins follow the course of the major arteries and share their names. In the lower leg the veins are paired and join at the knee to form

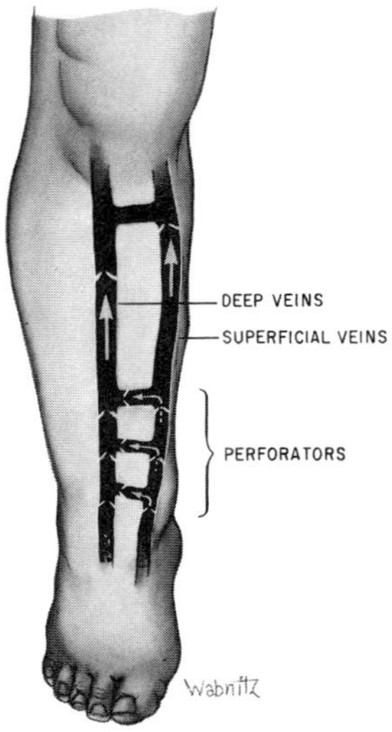

FIG. 21-1. Schematic orientation of venous valves and flow of blood in the superficial, deep, and perforating veins of the lower leg.

the popliteal vein, which continues through the adductor hiatus to become the superficial femoral vein. The latter is joined by the deep femoral vein in the upper thigh to become the common femoral vein, which becomes the external iliac vein as it enters the pelvis beneath the inguinal ligament. The perforating veins are so named because they penetrate the fascia of the lower leg to connect the superficial and deep systems. The perforators adjacent to the medial malleolus are often responsible for the development of stasis ulcers at that level when they become incompetent.

Respiration and exercise have significant effects on normal venous flow. During inspiration, diaphragmatic descent increases intraabdominal pressure, transiently decreasing venous return. During expiration, abdominal pressure falls and the distally trapped blood accelerates flow cephalad. During exercise, the calf muscle pump reduces venous pressure in the deep veins by emptying them, and when the muscle relaxes, the superficial veins drain into the deep system rapidly. The ability to move large volumes of blood during the hyperemia of exercise prevents edema formation by maintaining a normal pressure gradient across the capillary bed.

Etiology of Deep Vein Thrombosis

Development of a thrombus within a vein may be considered functionally as an exaggeration of the normal process of hemostasis. When disruption of normal endothelium occurs, subendothelial structures trigger a reaction in platelets, coagulation proteins, and adjacent endothelial cells that results in a hemostatic plug. Soon fibrin is deposited and within 24 h the platelet plug is replaced by fibrin which allows the vessel to heal. The occurrence of this process in a nontraumatized vein was recognized by Virchow who, in 1856, introduced the term thrombosis and postulated three possible mechanisms: stasis, endothelial damage, and hypercoagulability.

Stasis. In the surgical patient, stasis is the most important factor in the development of deep vein thrombosis (DVT), especially when there is prolonged immobilization in bed. When contrast medium is injected into the veins of the lower extremities of a bedridden patient, it may remain in venous valve sinuses for as long as an hour, confirming the pooling effect in the soleal veins. This is the favored location for the formation of a nidus of thrombus that then promotes successive layering of platelets, fibrin, and leukocytes to produce an organized thrombus. This process can begin under general anesthesia in the operating room but usually requires other contributing factors such as shock, infection, trauma, or congestive heart failure. Aging, obesity, pregnancy, and malignancy are also important added risk factors.

Endothelial Damage. Endothelial injury can occur in collapsed vessels when the intimal walls are in contact, and further injury can be demonstrated after hypoxemia that occurs when there is venous stasis. Similarly, leukocyte adherence to endothelial intracellular junctions can be demonstrated in areas of stasis after trauma at a remote site. In spite of these changes, however, routine histological examination of veins containing thrombus usually fails to show an inflammatory response consistent with vessel wall injury.

Hypercoagulability. Patients who present at an early age with spontaneous venous thrombosis, who have a strong family history of DVT, or who develop recurrent venous thromboembolism are usually considered ''prothrombotic'' or ''hypercoagulable.'' They deserve careful study for associated disorders as described by Shattil and listed in Table 21-1. The lupus anticoagulant listed in Table 21-1 is not a clinical anticoagulant but is associated with an abnormal partial thromboplastin time (PTT) produced by an antiphospholipid antibody. These antibodies, which include anticardiolipin, are being recognized with increased frequency in association with a variety of thrombotic disorders. Their association with unexplained juvenile DVT indicates that screening for antiphospholipid antibodies should be included in the work-up of unexplained DVT.

Table 21-1
Conditions Associated with Recurrent Venous Thromboembolism

Accelerated or inappropriate hemostatic plug formation
Endothelial cell damage
Atherosclerosis and hypercholesterolemia
Homocystinuria
Vasculitis and the lupus anticoagulant
Inappropriate platelet plug formation
Essential thrombocythemia
Paroxysmal nocturnal hemoglobinuria
Heparin-associated thrombocytopenia
Inappropriate fibrin plug formation
Disseminated intravascular coagulation
Infusion of prothrombin complex concentrates
Defects in the mechanism limiting hemostatic plug size
Stasis
Previous deep vein thrombosis
Congestive heart failure
Hyperviscosity syndrome: polycythemia; serum hyperviscosity
Antithrombin III deficiency
Protein C deficiency
Defective lysis of fibrin plugs
Dysfibrinogenemia
Decreased plasminogen activator activity
Decreased plasminogen activity

SOURCE: Shattil SJ: Diagnosis and treatment of recurrent venous thromboembolism. *Med Clin North Am* 68:577–601, 1984.

Idiopathic DVT may also be the first clue to occult malignancy. The association between venous thrombosis and cancer was first suggested by Trousseau and often has been confirmed in postmortem studies. In a series reported by Aderka and associates, 34 percent of otherwise healthy patients with idiopathic DVT were found to have a malignancy diagnosed an average of 24 months later. Increased likelihood of cancer in these patients was associated with age over 65, anemia, and eosinophilia. The earliest onset malignancies were found within 1 year and tended to occur in the pelvic organs and breast. Prolonged follow-up is appropriate, however, since some malignancies did not appear until after 5 years, which also suggests coincidence rather than a direct relationship. There is a direct relationship between the use of oral contraceptive anovulatory agents and thrombotic disorders that occur 3 to 6 times more frequently in those women.

The most common transient hypercoagulable states are associated with recent trauma, major surgical procedures, and sepsis. In addition to the possible roles of stasis and increased circulating procoagulant factors, the fibrinolytic system is inhibited after surgery and trauma and there is less lytic activity in the veins of the lower extremity than in those of the upper extremity.

Pathophysiology

A propagating thrombus may become attached to the opposite wall, causing interruption of flow, retrograde thrombosis, and signs of venous stasis in the extremity (Fig. 21-2). Subsequent formation of edema within the confines of the deep muscular fascia may produce pain and/or limited dorsiflexion of the foot (Homans's sign). The latter sign as originally described by Homans is only an indication of muscular irritability and its use far exceeds its reliability. More commonly, in about 60 percent of patients the thrombus propagates without interrupting flow and develops a long floating "tail" that is more susceptible to breaking loose from its tenuous anchor within the valvular sinus. It is the latter sequence of events that is the most dangerous aspect of the disorder, because major pulmonary embolism can and does occur without premonitory signs or symptoms at its point of origin.

The site of venous obstruction determines the level at which swelling is observed clinically. Swelling at the thigh level always implies obstruction at the level of the iliofemoral system, whereas swelling of the calf or foot suggests obstruction at the femoropopliteal level (Fig. 21-3). Autopsies suggest that it is more common for thrombi to originate in the veins of the soleus and then propagate proximally, but there is evidence that primary thrombosis of the femoral and iliac venous tributaries occurs as well.

Resolution of DVT with recanalization will alter the competence of the valves within the veins and can result in the postthrombotic syndrome, which will be discussed.

Diagnosis

Clinical Manifestations. Major venous thrombosis involving the deep venous system of the thigh and pelvis produces a characteristic clinical picture of pain, extensive pitting edema, and blanching that has been termed *phlegmasia alba dolens* or "milk leg." Association with pregnancy may be related to hormonal effects on blood, relaxation of vessel walls, or mechanical compression of the left iliac vein at the pelvic brim, resulting in the term "milk leg of pregnancy." It was originally believed that the blanching was due to spasm and compromise of arterial flow, but efforts to achieve sympatholysis are ill-advised because it is the

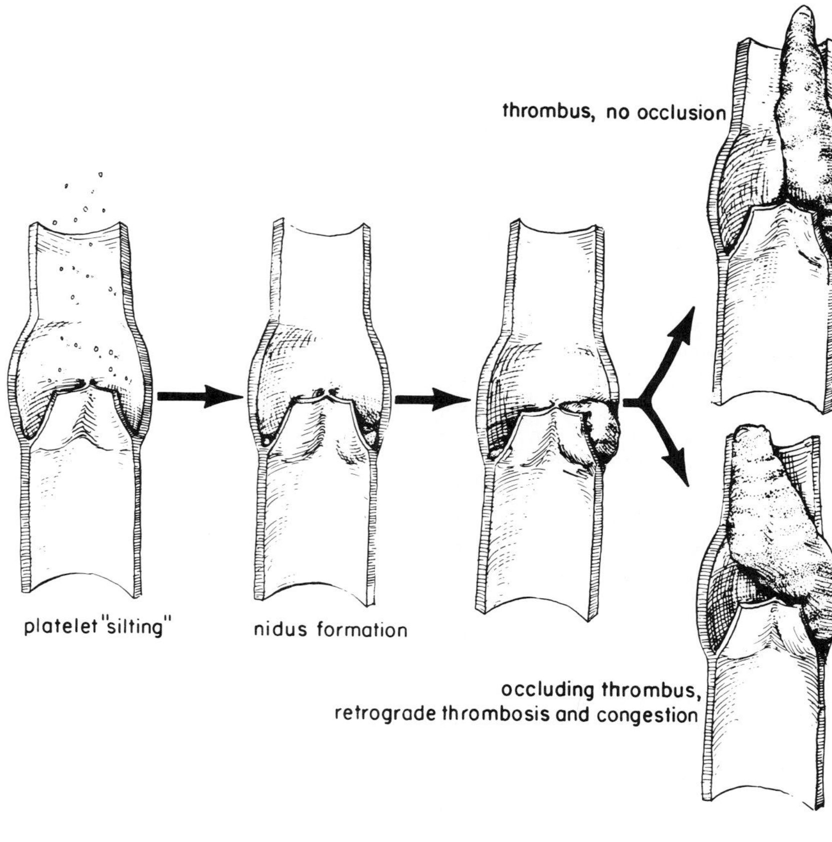

FIG. 21-2. The evolution of venous thrombosis begins with stagnant flow that permits silting of platelets and possibly hypoxemic injury to valvular sinus endothelium. The resulting nidus of thrombus releases thrombin that aggregates more platelets in a cycle of thrombus propagation. As the thrombus grows, it may extend into the lumen without occlusion or may occlude the vein with retrograde thrombosis and venous hypertension. [From: *Greenfield LJ: Acute venous thrombosis and pulmonary embolism, in Hardy JD (ed): Hardy's Textbook of Surgery. Philadelphia, Lippincott, 1983, with permission.*]

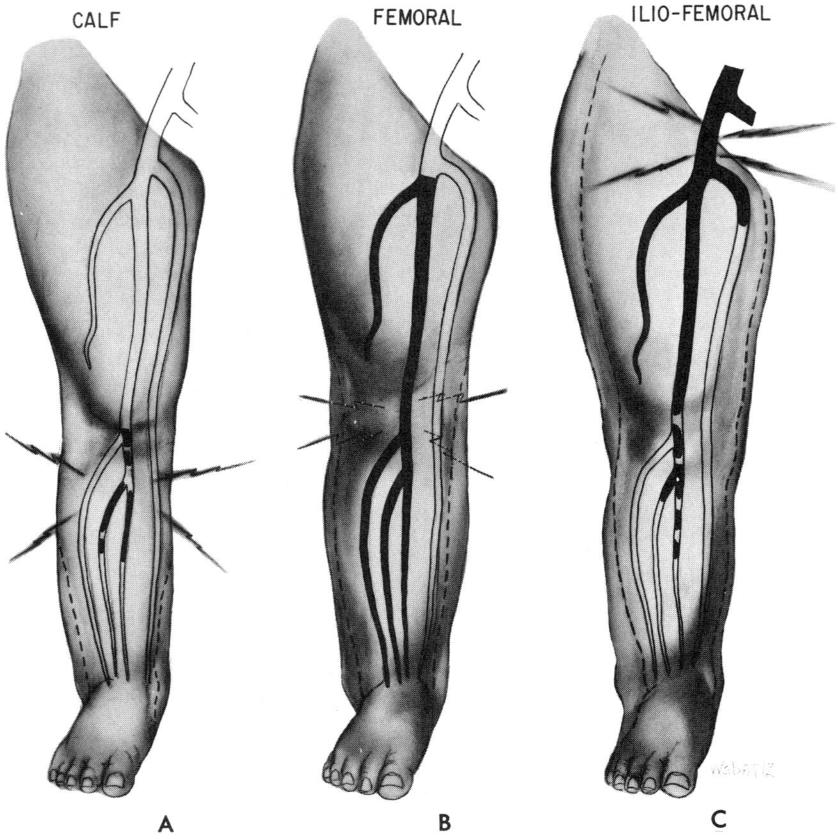

FIG. 21-3. Clinical features of venous thrombosis. *A.* When thrombosis is localized to veins of the calf and the popliteal vein, there is minimal swelling at the level of the ankle. Calf pain and tenderness are usually present. *B.* When there is thrombosis of the femoral vein and associated thrombosis of the calf veins, swelling is usually present and extends to just above the level of the knee. Popliteal tenderness and calf tenderness may be present. *C.* In iliofemoral venous thrombosis, there is thrombosis of the iliac and proximal femoral vein, and frequently the calf veins also are involved. Edema is present from the foot to the inguinal ligament. There is usually tenderness in the groin as well as popliteal and calf tenderness.

subcutaneous edema that is responsible for the blanching. In addition to pregnancy, other mechanical factors that can affect the left iliac vein include compression from the right iliac artery or an overdistended bladder, and congenital webs within the vein. These factors are responsible for the observed 4:1 preponderance of left versus right iliac vein involvement.

As venous thrombosis progresses, impeding most of the venous return from the extremity, there is danger of limb loss from cessation of arterial flow. This clinical picture differs from alba dolens, with more congestion producing *phlegmasia cerulea dolens,* which is characterized by loss of sensory and motor function. Venous gangrene is likely unless an aggressive approach is utilized to remove the thrombus and restore blood flow. A variant of this disorder occurs peripherally in the leg and is associated with concurrent malignant disease and a high mortality rate.

Fortunately, these major complications occur in less than 10 percent of patients with venous thrombosis. Only 40 percent of patients with venous thrombosis have any clinical signs of the disorder. In addition, false-positive clinical signs occur in up to 30 percent of patients studied. Because of this there has been a great deal of interest in the development of screening tests that can reveal thrombi before they become evident clinically. Contrast venography provides direct evidence of both occlusive and nonocclusive thrombi, but it is an invasive procedure and usually requires moving the patient to a radiographic suite. Ideally, the screening test would be accurate, noninvasive, and able to be performed at the bedside. Although the ideal has not yet been achieved, there are a number of tests that have proved useful.

Radioactive-Labeled Fibrinogen. After iodine blockage of the thyroid gland, counts are obtained from marked locations on the lower extremities and expressed as a percentage of the radioactivity measured by counting over the heart. An increase of 20 percent or more in one area indicates the presence of an underlying thrombus. The test permits sequential scanning of the extremities over a period of days and is most sensitive to thrombi forming in the veins of the calves shortly after an operative procedure. It does not permit detection of thrombi in pelvic veins, and it cannot be used in an extremity in which there is a healing wound, fracture, cellulitis, arthritis, edema, ulceration, or superficial thrombophlebitis. These limitations, along with concern for the safety of fibrinogen, have led to abandonment of this test except for selective research studies.

Ultrasound. The Doppler ultrasound probe can be used to advantage to detect major venous thrombi with a high degree of accuracy, but it is a subjective form of testing dependent on the examiner's experience. The principle is based on the change in flow signal produced by intraluminal thrombi. The examination begins at the ankle with identification of the posterior tibial vein signal adjacent to the artery. The flow signal should be altered by distal and proximal compression, producing augmentation and interruption of flow, respectively, which can also be produced by the Valsalva maneuver. The same maneuvers are repeated over the superficial and deep femoral veins and can be done over the popliteal vein as well (Fig. 21-4). Failure of augmentation of flow on compression below the probe or release of interruption of flow

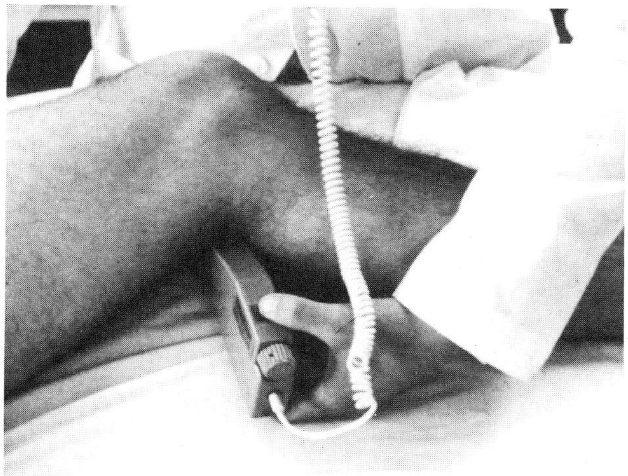

FIG. 21-4. The Doppler probe can be used at the bedside to assess flow in all the venous tributaries of the leg. Distal and proximal compression produce alterations in flow that are attenuated or absent when a thrombus is present.

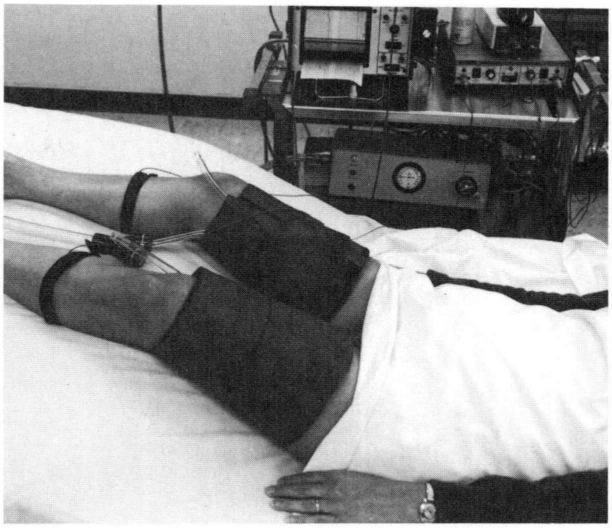

FIG. 21-5. The plethysmograph measures the volume change in the lower extremity following temporary occlusion of venous return by pneumatic cuffs. When the cuff pressure is released, there is rapid outflow of blood and reduction in limb volume unless proximal venous thrombosis is present. Both strain gauge (shown) and impedance sensors may be used for the volume recordings.

above the probe suggests a venous thrombus. The sensitivity of the test exceeds 90 percent, but the specificity is 5 to 10 percent lower because of the possibility of other mechanical problems (e.g., Baker's cyst, hematoma) interfering with venous flow. A negative Doppler ultrasound examination is reassuring, but a positive or equivocal test should be confirmed by imaging. A negative test in the leg is not reassuring when thromboembolism is suspected, because the thrombus may have been evacuated from the extremity.

The addition of real-time B-mode imaging to Doppler measurement in a portable duplex device offers the most useful approach to detection and characterization of venous thrombi. Further refinement with color-flow Doppler facilitates the examination and permits interrogation from calf veins to the iliac system. Increased experience with the duplex study has shown that it has sensitivity, specificity, and accuracy in the range of 90 to 95 percent for detection of lower extremity DVT. More importantly, a negative duplex scan is sufficient to exclude the diagnosis without need for contrast venography. It has become the first-choice diagnostic study for suspected DVT.

Impedance Plethysmography. The impedance method measures the volume of the extremity to temporary occlusion of the venous system. The diagnosis of venous thrombosis depends on the changes in venous capacitance and rate of emptying after release of the occlusion. A proximal thigh cuff is inflated to 50 mmHg or until maximum filling has occurred by plateau of the electrical signal. The cuff is then rapidly deflated, allowing rapid outflow and reduction of volume in a normal limb (Fig. 21-5). Prolongation of the outflow wave suggests major venous thrombosis with 95 percent accuracy. The deficiency of this technique is the lack of detection of calf vein thrombosis or old postthrombotic sequelae. The strain gauge plethysmograph can be used in a similar fashion.

Venography. The injection of contrast material for direct visualization of the venous system of the extremity is the most accurate method of confirming the diagnosis of venous thrombosis and the extent of involvement. Injection is usually made into the foot while the superficial veins are occluded by tourniquet, and a supplemental injection into the femoral veins may be required to visualize the iliofemoral system (Fig. 21-6). Potential false-positive examinations may result from external compression of a vein or washout of the contrast material from venous flow from collateral veins. The procedure can also be performed with isotope injection using a gamma scintillation counter to record flow of the isotope. Delayed imaging of persistent "hot spots" may also reflect isotope retention at the sites of thrombus formation (Fig. 21-7). A perfusion lung scan can also be obtained for baseline comparison and for detection of silent embolism. There is less definition of deep vein thrombi with this technique than with contrast venography, but it is a valuable technique for sequential study of patients and avoids the potential thrombogenesis associated with the injection of contrast medium.

Prophylaxis

Theoretically, it should be possible to prevent formation of venous thrombi either by eliminating or reducing venous stasis or by altering blood coagulability. The belief that early ambulation prevents stasis and reduces the formation of thrombi has been controversial, and studies using tagged fibrinogen have not supported this assumption. One possible explanation for this is that early ambulation often involves having the patient walk to a nearby chair and sit, whereupon the legs are subjected to even more stasis.

There has been more benefit from the prophylactic use of anticoagulant drugs. There are good data to support the use of preoperative oral anticoagulant therapy with warfarin derivatives in high-risk patients. Unfortunately, this procedure increases the risk of hemorrhage, and because of the added difficulties of laboratory control of prothrombin time, there has not been widespread acceptance of this approach. It remains, however, the recommendation

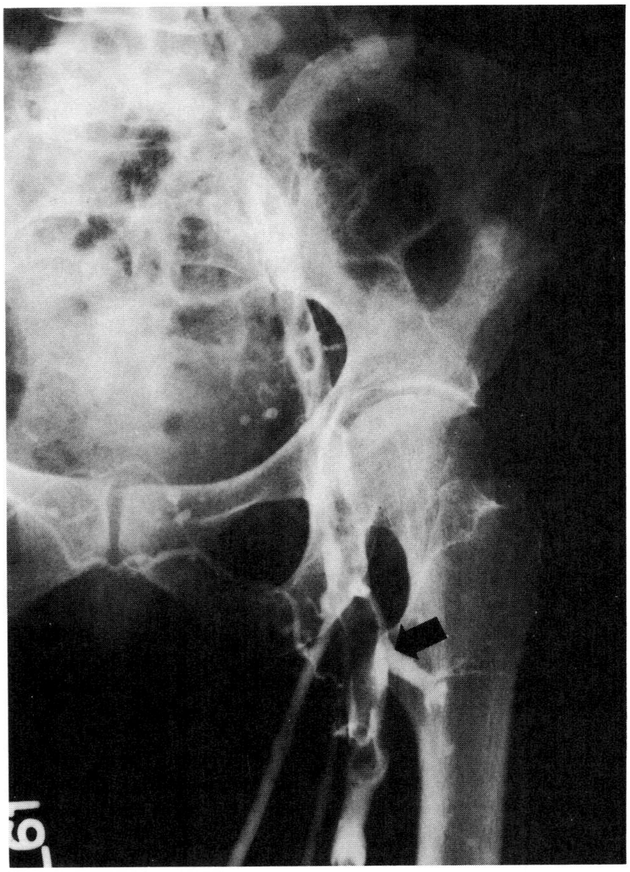

FIG. 21-6. Contrast venogram demonstrating a thrombus within the femoral vein. It is outlined by the contrast material which indicates that it is free-floating at that level. [From: *Greenfield LJ: Complications of venous thrombosis and pulmonary embolism, in Greenfield LJ (ed): Complications in Surgery and Trauma. Philadelphia, Lippincott, 1984, with permission.*]

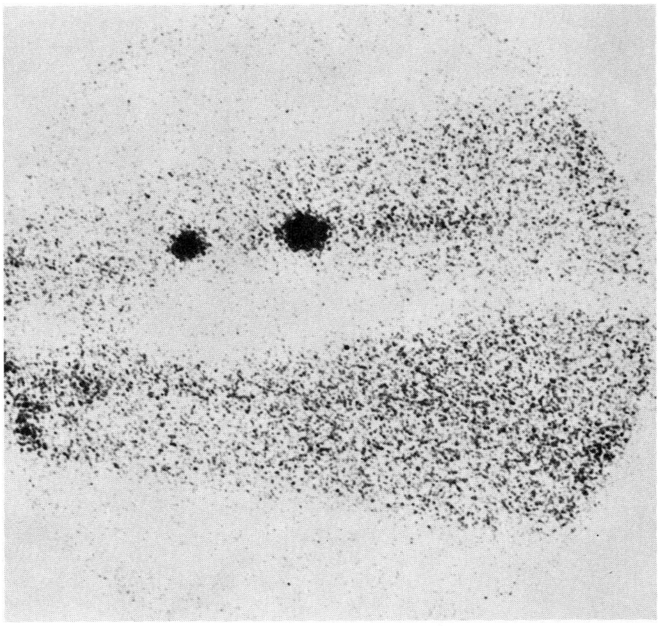

FIG. 21-7. Isotope scan following the injection of macroaggregated albumin ^{131}I showing an acute thrombus in the popliteal vein.

of a national task force on prophylaxis for patients undergoing surgery for fractured hips as reported by Hyers and associates. They also recommend adjusted-dose heparin to prolong the activated partial thromboplastin time (APTT) to the upper normal range for patients having elective hip surgery. The administration of dextran, which produces a variety of effects on platelets and clotting factors, has been demonstrated to reduce the incidence of detectable thrombi. However, it too can produce hemorrhagic problems as well as allergic reactions and, in older patients, congestive heart failure.

There has been much wider acceptance of the administration of heparin before and after surgery in low (''mini'') doses that do not alter the laboratory clotting profile. Generally, a 5000-unit dose is given subcutaneously 2 h preoperatively and then every 12 h postoperatively for 6 days. This provides protection for most high-risk groups with the exception of those undergoing orthopaedic or urologic procedures. The beneficial effect may be due to the enhancement of heparin cofactor (antithrombin III), a natural inhibitor of activated factor X. Although some studies have failed to show a protective effect, Kakkar and associates in a randomized series of 4121 patients showed that heparin protected against fatal pulmonary embolism as well as DVT. Fractionated heparins offer the additional advantage of single daily dose and more anti-Xa activity but are not available in this country.

Intermittent pneumatic leg compression prevents stasis and increases fibrinolytic activity with virtually no side effects. The pneumatic boots can be applied in the operating room to minimize the risk of venous thrombosis beginning under general anesthesia. It is recommended for groups in which low-dose heparin is either contraindicated or ineffective but should not be used in patients with peripheral arterial insufficiency.

Medical Treatment

The approach to management of the patient with DVT is based on three objectives: minimizing the risk of pulmonary embolism, limiting further thrombosis, and facilitating resolution of existing thrombi to avoid the postthrombotic syndrome.

Initially, the patient is anticoagulated and placed at bed rest with the foot of the bed elevated 8 to 10 in. Generally, pain, swelling, and tenderness resolve over a 5- to 7-day period, at which time ambulation can be permitted with elastic stocking support. Standing still and sitting should be prohibited to avoid increased venous pressure and stasis.

Anticoagulation. The foundation of therapy for DVT is adequate anticoagulation, initially with heparin and then with coumarin derivatives for prolonged protection against recurrent thrombosis. Unless there are specific contraindications, heparin should be administered in an initial dose of 100 to 150 units/kg intravenously. Heparin is an acid mucopolysaccharide that neutralizes thrombin, inhibits thromboplastin, and reduces the platelet release reaction. It may be administered by continuous or intermittent intravenous doses regulated by whole blood clotting time or APTT. Bleeding complications can be minimized by doses of heparin that prolong the laboratory clotting determinations by about twice the normal time with no loss of effectiveness. Continuous intravenous infusion regulated by an infusion pump seems to minimize the total dose required for control and is associated with a lower incidence of complications.

Oral administration of anticoagulants is begun shortly after initiation of heparin therapy, because several days are usually required to bring the prothrombin time within the therapeutic range of 1.4 times the control value. The coumarin derivatives block the synthesis of several clotting factors, and prolongation of the prothrombin time beyond the level suggested is associated with a higher incidence of bleeding complications. Fortunately, administration of fresh plasma usually can restore the prothrombin time. After an episode of acute DVT, anticoagulation therapy should be maintained for a minimum of 3 months; some investigators favor 6 months for treatment of thrombi in the larger veins. Many drugs interact with coumarin derivatives (e.g., barbiturates), and therefore it is essential to establish a routine for regular monitoring of prothrombin time after the patient leaves the hospital.

Fibrinolysis. There has been great interest in the use of fibrinolytic agents to activate the intrinsic plasmin system. Both streptokinase and urokinase have been used and found to be effective, although they are associated with a relatively high incidence of hemorrhagic complications as reported by Common and associates. These agents have no advantage over heparin in the treatment of recurrent venous thrombosis or thrombosis that has existed for over 72 h, and they are contraindicated in postoperative or posttraumatic patients.

In a prospective study of 29 patients with major DVT (thrombosis involving the popliteal veins, with or without calf veins), Kakkar and Lawrence compared hemodynamic and clinical results in patients receiving 5-day treatment with heparin or streptokinase, followed by a 6-month course of coumadin. Overall, at 2-year follow-up they found over half of the limbs with evidence of the postthrombotic syndrome. Clinically, 14 percent of patients had no symptoms, 20 percent had severe symptoms, and the remainder demonstrated mild to moderate changes. No difference was seen between patients receiving heparin or streptokinase. Although a drug to restore venous patency and preserve valve function has not yet been found, other thrombolytic drugs such as tissue plasminogen activator (TPA) and single-chain urokinase-type plasminogen activator (SCU-PA) are currently under investigation and may provide better alternatives to treatment.

Surgical Approaches

Operative Thrombectomy. The direct surgical approach to remove thrombi from the deep veins of the leg utilizes the common femoral vein and is facilitated by the use of a Fogarty venous balloon catheter and an elastic wrap for milking the extremity (Fig. 21-8). Although the operative results are impressive, venograms obtained before discharge from the hospital show iliac occlusion in the majority of patients, and there does not seem to be any lesser incidence of the postthrombotic syndrome. Consequently, the procedure is usually reserved for limb salvage in the presence of phlegmasia cerulea dolens and impending venous gangrene.

In considering the reasons why the procedure has not lived up to expectation, there may be an explanation other than rethrombosis. It is customary to assume that the iliac system has been cleared if there is brisk retrograde blood flow after a proximal thrombus has been removed. This can be misleading if the common iliac vein remains obstructed and the retrograde flow is from the internal iliac vein. Conversely, poor retrograde flow may be seen when an iliac vein valve is intact despite removal of all proximal

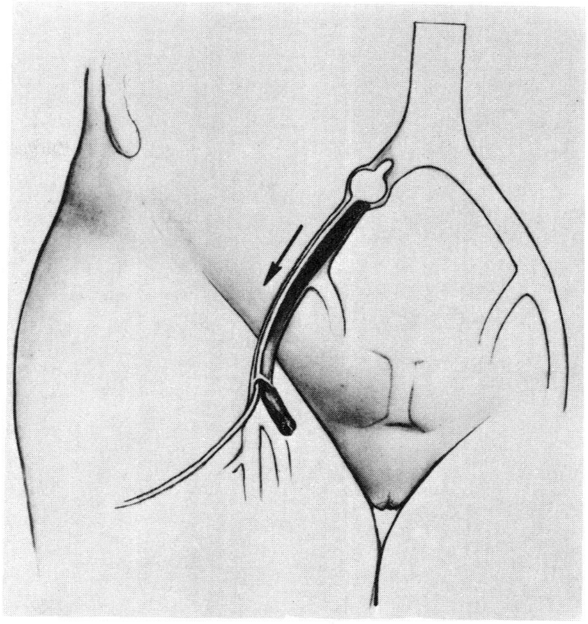

FIG. 21-8. Venous thrombectomy using a Fogarty catheter to extract the proximal thrombus. Increased intraabdominal pressure by the Valsalva maneuver minimizes the risk of embolism. *(Courtesy of C. Rob and R. Smith.)*

thrombi. Therefore, intraoperative venography should be performed in all cases. After completion of the thrombectomy, a small catheter may be left in a branch of the saphenous vein for postoperative regional heparin administration and postoperative venography.

In recent reports, an attempt has also been made to prevent rethrombosis after thrombectomy by creation of a peripheral arteriovenous fistula using the saphenous vein or one of its branches. The fistula is either allowed to close or is occluded surgically or by transcatheter balloon after 2 to 3 months. Early results in 57 patients reported by Einarsson and associates showed patency of the iliofemoral segment by venography in 61 percent, and 75 percent had a good clinical result. Measurement by venous function, however, using plethysmography and foot volumetry showed normal results in only 29 percent.

Vena Caval Interruption. Adequate anticoagulation is usually effective in managing DVT, but if recurrent pulmonary embolism occurs during anticoagulant therapy or if there is a contraindication to anticoagulation, a surgical approach is necessary. Vena caval interruption is also indicated when a complication of anticoagulation forces it to be discontinued, as prophylaxis against recurrence of embolism after pulmonary embolectomy, and in some high-risk patients who could not tolerate even a small embolic recurrence.

Early surgical efforts to prevent recurrence of pulmonary embolism were directed to the common femoral vein, which was ligated bilaterally. This resulted in a high incidence of sequelae due to stasis in the lower extremity and an unacceptable rate of pulmonary embolism. The next approach used was ligation of the inferior vena cava below the renal veins, which added the adverse effect of a sudden reduction in cardiac output under general anesthesia. This effect, coupled with stasis sequelae and recurrent

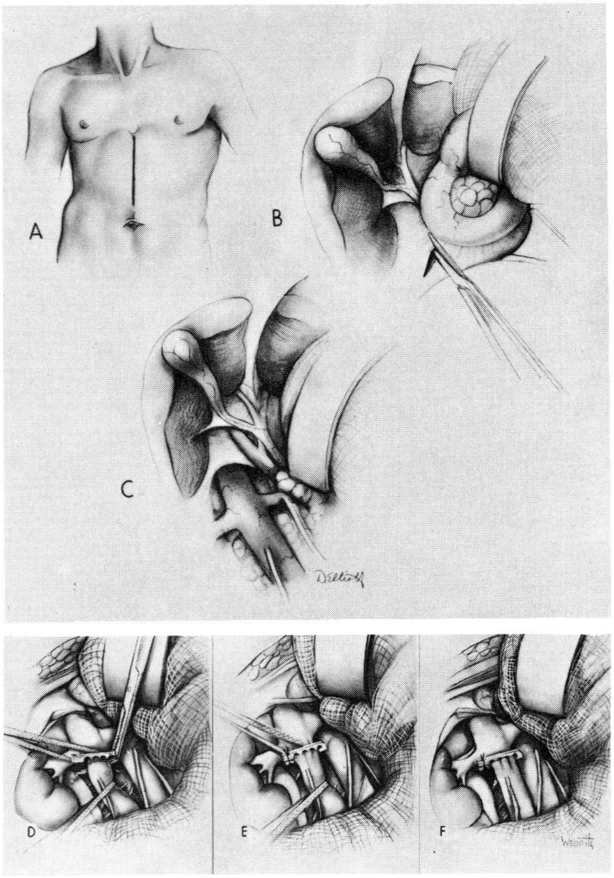

FIG. 21-9. Partial interruption of inferior vena cava using a serrated clip. *A.* Transperitoneal approach is preferred to permit high interruption of vena cava and concomitant ligation of the left spermatic or ovarian veins. *B.* Kocher maneuver. *C.* Vena cava cleared immediately below renal veins. *D.* Clip applied. *E.* Clip closed. *F.* Final position of clip in the immediate infrarenal region to prevent cul-de-sac. (From: *Adams JT, DeWeese JA: Surg Gynecol Obstet 123:1087, 1966, with permission.*)

embolism through dilated collateral veins, led to efforts to compartmentalize the vena cava by means of sutures, staples, and external clips in order to provide filtration without occlusion (Fig. 21-9).

Because these procedures required general anesthesia and laparotomy, the next logical step was to devise a transvenous approach that could be performed under local anesthesia. The Mobin–Uddin ''umbrella'' unit was inserted from the jugular vein and positioned under fluoroscopic control below the renal veins, where it usually produced (in 70 percent of cases) thrombosis of the vena cava and occasionally became detached, resulting in fatal embolism.

The Greenfield cone-shaped filter was developed to maintain patency after trapping emboli. This is possible because of the unique geometry of the cone that collects emboli in its apex and retains perimeter flow. Preservation of flow avoids stasis and facilitates lysis of the embolus (Fig. 21-10). It can be inserted operatively or percutaneously from either the jugular vein or the femoral vein. The rate of recurrent embolism with this device has been 4 percent over 12 years of follow-up. Its long-term patency rate in excess of 95 percent allows it to be placed above the renal veins when necessary for embolism control, such as when there is a thrombus within the renal veins or vena cava.

The indications for insertion of a vena caval filter are listed in Table 21-2 and will be reviewed in the section on pulmonary thromboembolism.

OTHER TYPES OF VENOUS THROMBOSIS

Superficial Thrombophlebitis

The term thrombophlebitis should be restricted to the disorder of the superficial veins characterized by a local inflammatory process that is usually aseptic (Fig. 21-11). The cause of thrombophlebitis in the upper limb is usually acidic fluid infusion or prolonged cannulation. In the lower extremities it is usually associated with varicose veins and may coexist with DVT. Its association with the injection of contrast material can be minimized by washout of the contrast material with heparinized saline.

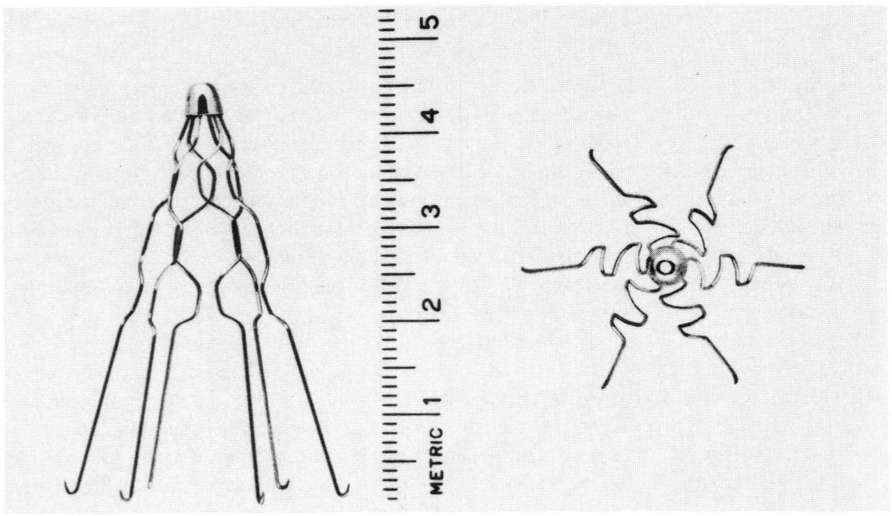

FIG. 21-10. The Greenfield filter is made of stainless steel and shaped in a cone to preserve perimeter flow after an embolus is trapped in its apex. Preservation of flow provides continued filtration, minimizes stasis sequelae, and facilitates lysis of trapped thrombi. The recurved hooks provide secure fixation in the vena cava.

Table 21-2
Indications for Insertion of a Vena Caval Filter

1. Recurrent thromboembolism in spite of adequate anticoagulation
2. Documented thromboembolism in a patient who has a contraindication to anticoagulation
3. Complication of anticoagulation that forces therapy to be discontinued
4. Chronic pulmonary embolism with associated pulmonary hypertension and cor pulmonale
5. Immediately following pulmonary embolectomy
6. Relative indications—patient with more than 50% of the pulmonary vascular bed occluded who cannot tolerate any additional embolism; patient with a large free-floating iliofemoral thrombus on venogram

Thrombophlebitis Migrans

Thrombophlebitis migrans, a condition of recurrent episodes of superficial thrombophlebitis, has been associated with visceral malignancy, systemic collagen vascular disease, and blood dyscrasias. Involvement of the deep veins and the visceral veins has also been described.

Subclavian Vein Thrombosis

Thrombosis of the subclavian vein is most likely to be secondary to an indwelling catheter and can occur in the pediatric age group. It may also occur as a primary event in a young athletic person (effort thrombosis), presumably as a result of injury or compression at the thoracic inlet. If seen within 48 h of onset, it is possible to use thrombolytic drugs followed by a venogram to define a potentially correctable abnormality. If seen later, it usually responds to elevation of the limb and anticoagulation, although some venous insufficiency and discomfort with exercise may persist. A venous bypass procedure using the internal jugular vein can be used to relieve persistent venous hypertension.

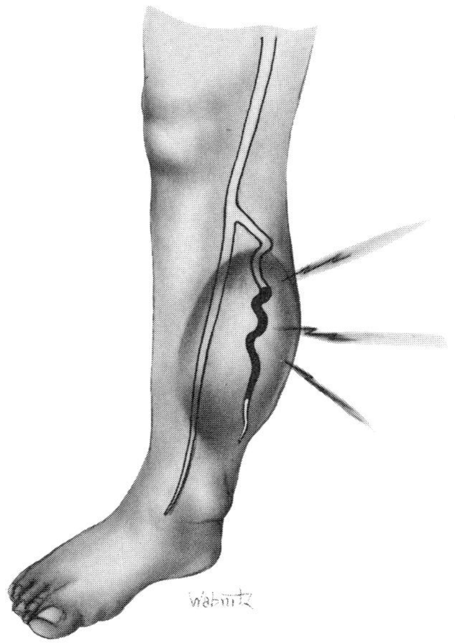

FIG. 21-11. Clinical presentation of superficial venous thrombosis. There is usually redness, tenderness, and swelling surrounding a palpable thrombosed superficial vein.

Inferior Vena Caval Thrombosis

Thrombosis of the inferior vena cava can result from tumor invasion or propagating thrombus from the iliac veins. More commonly, however, it results from ligation, plication, or insertion of partially occluding caval devices. Any caval filtration device can become totally occluded by a trapped massive thrombus, causing sudden reduction in venous return and cardiac output. In the patient with known prior pulmonary embolism it is a grave error to ascribe the resulting hypotension to recurrent pulmonary embolism and treat the patient with vasopressor agents. In this situation the cause of the hypotension is functional hypovolemia which can readily be confirmed by measurement of central venous pressure. Thrombosis of the renal vein can result from extension of vena caval thrombosis but is most likely to occur in association with the nephrotic syndrome. It can be a source of thromboembolism and has been treated successfully by suprarenal placement of the Greenfield filter.

Visceral Venous Thrombosis

Portal vein thrombosis can occur in the neonate, usually secondary to propagating septic thrombophlebitis of the umbilical vein. Collateral development leads to the occurrence of esophageal varices. In the adult, thrombosis of the portal, hepatic, splenic, or superior mesenteric vein can occur spontaneously but usually is associated with hepatic cirrhosis. Thrombosis of mesenteric or omental veins can simulate an acute condition of the abdomen but usually results in prolonged ileus rather than intestinal infarction.

Hepatic vein thrombosis (Budd–Chiari syndrome) usually produces massive hepatomegaly, ascites, and liver failure. It can occur in association with a congenital web, endophlebitis, or polycythemia vera. Although some success has been reported using a direct approach to the congenital webs, the usual treatment is a side-to-side portacaval shunt to allow decompression of the liver.

The development of pelvic sepsis after abortion, tubal infection, or puerperal sepsis can lead to septic thrombophlebitis of the pelvic veins and septic thromboembolism. Ligation of the ovarian vein and vena cava has been the traditional treatment, but the emphasis should be on drainage or excision of the abscesses and appropriate antibiotic therapy. It is also appropriate to use the Greenfield filter in this situation because it is inert stainless steel and avoids the development of an intraluminal abscess that can occur after ligation of the vena cava as demonstrated experimentally by Peyton and associates in 1983.

PULMONARY THROMBOEMBOLISM

The clinical significance of major pulmonary embolism can be appreciated by referring to the annual mortality attributed to it, which has been estimated to be 90,000 deaths in the United States alone. It is estimated that 5 of every 1000 adults undergoing major surgery will die from massive pulmonary embolism. Because it represents the most important complication of DVT, it is of particular concern to surgeons whose patients are prone to develop DVT in the immediate postoperative period.

Just as with DVT, our understanding of the pathophysiology of pulmonary embolism dates back to Virchow, who first recognized the association between the two findings. It also became obvious in the early reports by pathologists that pulmonary embolism could be well tolerated by some patients who then died of other causes.

In fact, the full spectrum of the disorder ranges from asymptomatic minor embolism to sudden death from massive embolism.

Diagnosis

Clinical Manifestations. The signs and symptoms of an embolic episode obviously depend primarily on the quantity of embolus involved and, to a lesser extent, on the cardiopulmonary status of the patient. In the classic presentation, the patient suddenly develops chest pain, cough, dyspnea, tachypnea, and marked anxiety. Although hemoptysis has traditionally been associated with pulmonary embolism, it is actually an uncommon sign, and when present it usually occurs late in the course of the disease and represents pulmonary infarction. Objectively, the patient with major embolism usually shows tachycardia, an increased pulmonary second sound, cyanosis, prominent jugular veins, and varying degrees of collapse. Less commonly, there may be wheezing, a pleural friction rub, splinting of the chest wall, rales, low-grade fever, ventricular gallop, and wide splitting of the pulmonic second sound. The incidence of these findings found in the Urokinase Pulmonary Embolism Trial is shown in Table 21-3.

The differential diagnosis includes esophageal perforation, pneumonia, septic shock, and myocardial infarction. Since all these entities are life-threatening, it is mandatory that an orderly approach be formulated to confirm or reject the working diagnosis. Laboratory studies in general are not very helpful in the differential diagnosis, although a white blood cell count of less than 15,000/mm^3 may be suggestive when a pulmonary infiltrate is present to help rule out pneumonitis. The following examinations are particularly useful in the evaluation of suspected major embolism.

Electrocardiography. The most common electrocardiographic change associated with pulmonary embolism is nonspecific ST and T wave changes (66 percent of patients). More specific signs of right ventricular overload such as the often quoted S_1, Q_3, T_3 pattern are seldom seen. Consequently, the primary value of the electrocardiogram is to exclude the presence of a myocardial infarction. The finding of a myocardial infarction does not exclude the diagnosis of pulmonary embolism, and in some cases a lung scan or pulmonary angiogram may be required to clarify the problem.

Chest Radiography. Although the chest radiograph may suggest the diagnosis of pulmonary embolism because of central vascular enlargement, asymmetry of the vascular markings with segmental or lobar ischemia (Westermark's sign), or pleural effusion, these signs are nonspecific. The chest radiograph then serves to exclude other diagnostic possibilities such as pneumonia, pneumothorax, esophageal perforation, or congestive heart failure. It is also critical in the interpretation of a lung scan, because any radiographic density or evidence of chronic lung disease makes a perfusion defect less likely to represent pulmonary embolism. Any pulmonary vascular or cardiac disease also reduces the applicability of lung scanning to the diagnosis.

Table 21-3
Clinical Manifestations of Major Pulmonary Embolism

Symptoms	*Incidence, %*	*Signs*	*Incidence, %*
Dyspnea	80	Tachypnea	88
Apprehension	60	Tachycardia	63
Pleural pain	60	Accentuated P_2	60
Cough	50	Rales	51
Hemoptysis	27	S_3 or S_4	47
Syncope	22	Pleural rub	17

SOURCE: Data from the Urokinase Pulmonary Embolism Trial: A National Cooperative Study. *Circulation* 2(suppl):47, 1973.

Arterial Blood Gases. The widespread availability of blood gas and pH determinations has improved the assessment of all critically ill patients and provides important support for the diagnosis of pulmonary embolism. Hypoxemia with Pa_{O_2} of less than 60 mmHg is found in the majority of patients and is felt to be due to shunting by overperfusion of nonembolized lung and a widened alveolar-arterial oxygen gradient due to reduced cardiac output. The reduction in arterial P_{CO_2} that follows major embolism is the most discriminating finding, because hypoxemia is present in several disorders likely to be misdiagnosed as massive embolism (e.g., septic shock). If hypoxemia and hypocarbia are not present, the diagnosis of major embolism in the severely ill patient is unlikely, and an alternative diagnosis should be sought.

Central Venous Pressure. In the patient with systemic hypotension, central venous pressure can supply valuable information, and the line provides access for administration of drugs and fluids as well. Low central venous pressure virtually excludes pulmonary embolism as the primary cause of the hypotension because massive embolism almost always is accompanied by right ventricular overload and elevated right atrial pressures. Elevated right ventricular filling pressures may be transient, however, as hemodynamic accommodation occurs, and in subacute or chronic embolism the central venous pressure may be normal.

Lung Scan. The availability and widespread usage of lung photoscanning have led to overemphasis on this test and a tendency to overdiagnose pulmonary embolism. In a nonhypotensive patient with a normal chest radiograph, the lung scan is a valuable screening test that has increasing validity as the size of the perfusion defect approaches lobar distribution (Fig. 21-12). Smaller peripheral perfusion defects are much more difficult to interpret because pneumonitis, atelectasis, or other ventilation abnormalities alter pulmonary perfusion. A normal lung scan, on the other hand, usually excludes the diagnosis of pulmonary embolism. The assumption that the underperfused regions of the lung after embolism will remain normally ventilated, producing the mismatch in the ventilation/perfusion scans, is clouded by the known physiologic effect of bronchoconstriction produced by embolism. The recent multicenter PIOPED study showed that only the high probability scan was sufficiently accurate for the diagnosis of pulmonary embolism, but this reading was found in only 31 percent with confirmed pulmonary embolism. When the additional variable of wide variance in scan interpretation among observers is considered, the diagnosis is much more reliable when it is based on arteriography.

Pulmonary Arteriography. Selective pulmonary arteriography is the most accurate method of confirming the presence, size, and distribution of pulmonary emboli. The procedure is invasive, requiring passage of a cardiac catheter into the pulmonary artery for injection of a bolus of contrast medium. A rapid film changer produces a series of radiographs that outline areas of decreased perfusion and usually show filling defects or the rounded trailing edge of impacted emboli (Fig. 21-13). Straight cutoffs of the smaller pulmonary arteries are more difficult to interpret, par-

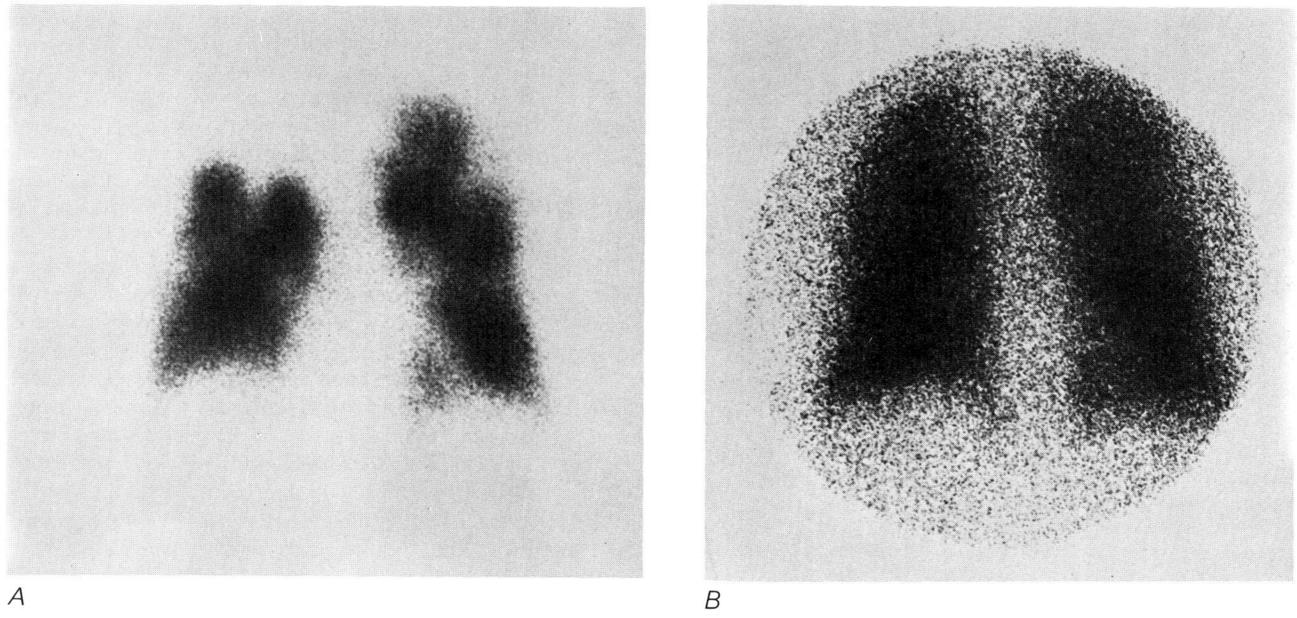

FIG. 21-12. *A.* A radionuclide perfusion scan following intravenous injection of macroaggregated albumin tagged ^{99m}Tc showing filling defects in the right lung. *B.* A ventilation scan performed with ^{133}Xe showing normal ventilation. These findings suggest the diagnosis of pulmonary embolism.

ticularly if there is associated chronic lung disease that tends to obliterate pulmonary vessels. The procedure can be performed with low risk, although pulmonary hypertensive and cardiac patients are at highest risk for this type of study, which usually carries a 0.3 to 0.5 percent mortality rate. Avoidance of injection of contrast medium into the main pulmonary artery minimizes the complications and mortality rates. Additional useful information is obtained before contrast injection by measurement of pulmonary arterial pressures. A normal pulmonary angiogram excludes the diagnosis of pulmonary embolism in acutely ill patients.

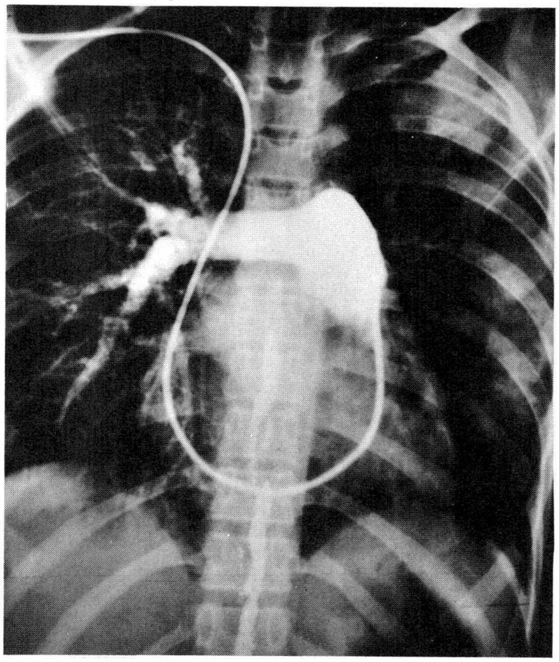

FIG. 21-13. A selective pulmonary angiogram demonstrating absence of filling of left pulmonary arterial branches due to a large embolus obstructing the left main pulmonary artery.

Pathophysiology

Although DVT precedes pulmonary embolism, less than 33 percent of patients with documented pulmonary embolism show clinical signs of venous thrombosis. Despite this, it is estimated that 85 to 90 percent of all pulmonary emboli originate from the veins of the lower extremity, and the remainder arise from the right side of the heart or other veins. In addition, the emboli from a recent thrombus tend to be multiple, fragmenting either in the right side of the heart or during impaction into the pulmonary vascular bed. Older thrombi, however, contain laminated fibrin layers that make them more solid and more difficult to lyse.

Once the embolus has lodged and interrupted pulmonary blood flow, the ratio of regional ventilation to perfusion increases, and the lung responds by bronchoconstriction to reduce wasted ventilation. This response is mediated by a local reduction in CO_2 output, since it can be prevented by ventilation with increased concentration of CO_2. Some experimental studies also suggest a generalized neural reflex vasoconstriction, but even if this occurs in human beings, it is not likely to be as significant a factor in survival as the mechanical effect of major vascular occlusion. Similarly, the effects of vasoactive humoral agents can be demonstrated in animals. There is evidence that serotonin is elaborated from platelets adherent to the embolus, which also contributes to the bronchoconstriction. The ability of heparin to inhibit the release of serotonin adds further justification to the early use of this drug. Other vasoactive agents such as histamine and prostaglandins may play a role in human beings, but the net effect is a reduction in size of peripheral airways, reduced lung volume, and reduced static pulmonary compliance.

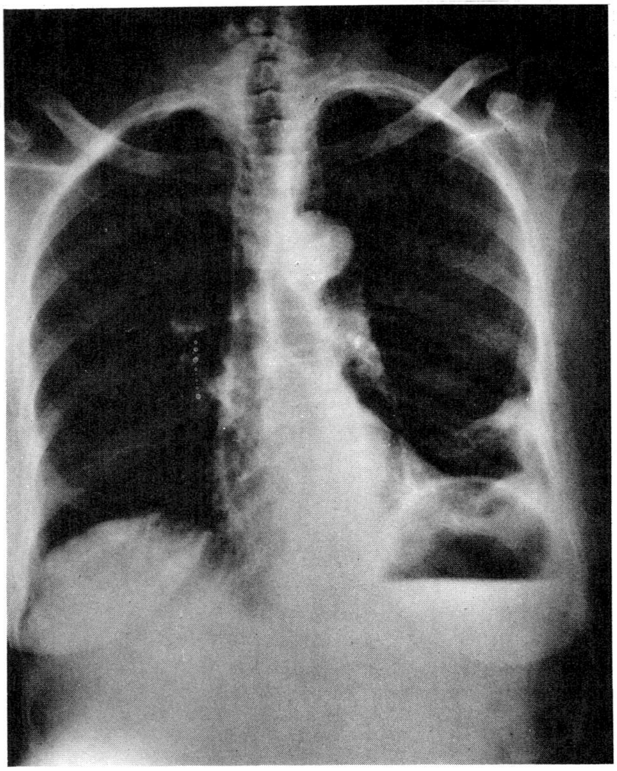

FIG. 21-14. Chest radiograph demonstrating a peripheral wedge-shaped area of infarction on the left side.

The hypoxemia that characterizes major embolism is thought to be due to a ventilation-perfusion imbalance secondary to the ventilation changes described above, although the findings in some patients resemble true arteriovenous shunting. Such shunting is anatomically possible if there is an unobliterated foramen ovale that opens in the presence of elevated right atrial pressures. Such an opening can allow passage of a venous embolus into the systemic circulation; it then is termed *paradoxical embolism*. Although there may be some improvement in Pa_{O_2} after supplemental oxygen is administered, the effects usually are minimal. The return of pulmonary blood flow effected by embolectomy restores respiratory gas exchange, but the ischemia may result in loss of capillary integrity, causing interstitial pulmonary edema or overt pulmonary hemorrhage.

Pulmonary infarction as a consequence of embolism is relatively rare and is associated clinically with problems of poor systemic perfusion such as shock and congestive heart failure. In these patients the symptoms include pleuritic chest pain, dyspnea, cough, and hemoptysis. The signs include fever, tachycardia, splinting, and occasionally friction rub. There is usually prominent leukocytosis, an elevated lactic dehydrogenase level, and bilirubinemia. A wedge-shaped density usually is seen on chest radiography (Fig. 21-14).

The pulmonary vascular and cardiac effects of embolism are a direct consequence of the degree of filling of the pulmonary vascular bed. Occlusion of more than 30 percent of the vascular tree is required to begin to elevate mean pulmonary artery (PA) pressure, and usually more than 50 percent occlusion is required to reduce systemic pressure. The degree of pulmonary hypertension produced is proportional to the extent of angiographic vascular occlusion, but in a previously normal patient the limit of pressure elevation observed is approximately 40 mmHg mean.

The fate of pulmonary emboli in patients is not easy to predict, although a great deal of experimental work in animals has been reported. Injection of autologous thrombi into the pulmonary circulation of dogs is followed by relatively rapid recovery of pulmonary function and objective evidence of lysis over a period of weeks. Activation of plasminogen to plasmin, which is found in high concentration in the pulmonary circulation, promotes this fibrinolytic effect. The resolution of aged thrombi proceeds more slowly and is hampered further by impaction of the embolus and isolation from pulmonary blood flow. Consequently, resolution after massive embolism in patients is unpredictable and often incomplete. It is not unusual to find residual fibrin strands or webs in the pulmonary arteries at autopsy as remnants of prior embolism.

Management

Anticoagulation. The hemodynamic variables mentioned above provide a means of classification of patients that uses four grades of severity and is a useful guide to therapy and prognosis (Table 21-4). The minor degrees of embolism can usually be managed by anticoagulants alone with a satisfactory outcome (Fig. 21-15). Heparin is selected for initial treatment in a dose designed to prolong the partial thromboplastin time to at least twice normal. At this dosage of approximately 150 units/kg, there is adequate protection against further attachment of thrombus and platelets to the embolus. Heparin should be administered intravenously by pump-regulated continuous infusion. Conti and associates have advocated higher doses of heparin to prolong the activated clotting time to 150 to 190 s with no increase in bleeding complications

Table 21-4
Stratification of Pulmonary Thromboembolism

Category	*Signs and Symptoms*	*Gases*	*PA Occlusion (%)*	*Hemodynamics*
Minor	Anxiety Hyperventilation	$Pa_{O_2} < 80$ mmHg $Pa_{CO_2} < 35$ mmHg	20–30	Tachycardia
Major	Dyspnea Collapse	$Pa_{O_2} < 65$ mmHg $Pa_{CO_2} < 30$ mmHg	30–50	CVP elevated, PA > 20 mmHg Responds to resuscitation
Massive	Dyspnea Shock	$Pa_{O_2} < 50$ mmHg $Pa_{CO_2} < 30$ mmHg	>50	CVP elevated, PA > 25 mmHg Requires pressors, inotropes
Chronic	Dyspnea Syncope	$Pa_{O_2} < 70$ mmHg $Pa_{CO_2} <$ 30–40 mmHg	>50	CVP elevated, PA > 40 mmHg Fixed low cardiac output

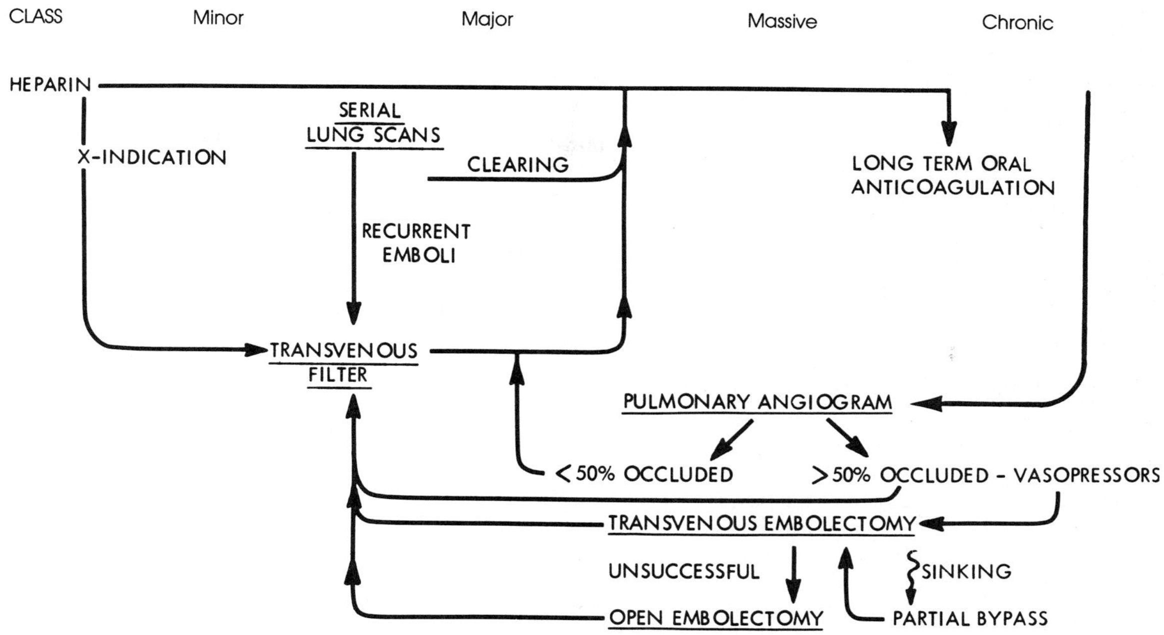

FIG. 21-15. Management algorithm for patients with documented pulmonary embolism stratified by class (see Table 21-4). Treatment is based on anticoagulation as shown for each class. In major embolism, the findings at angiography and hemodynamic status influence the choice of procedures undertaken. [From: *Greenfield LJ: Acute venous thrombosis and pulmonary embolism, in Hardy JD (ed): Hardy's Textbook of Surgery. Philadelphia, Lippincott, 1983, with permission.*]

and improved control of recurrent embolism. Heparin control of recurrent embolism, however, is imperfect, and recurrence was reported in 16 percent of patients by Wilson and associates, with a bleeding complication rate of 27 percent. In spite of this, heparin remains the initial treatment of choice and most clinicians also begin oral anticoagulation therapy to allow several days' overlap of the drugs as prothrombin time is extended into the therapeutic range.

Thrombolytic Therapy. Thrombolytic therapy has been advocated for the treatment of both DVT and pulmonary embolism. Two plasminogen activators, streptokinase and urokinase, are available for this and can be effective as documented in two large clinical trials (Urokinase Pulmonary Embolism Trial). The drugs are administered by intravenous infusion after a loading dose, and beneficial effects in thromboembolism usually can be seen in 12 to 24 h. Present laboratory tests to confirm the presence of a lytic state following streptokinase or urokinase administration have not proved useful in predicting the therapeutic response to these drugs or in preventing hemorrhagic complications. There were hemorrhagic side effects judged to be significant in 30 percent of the patients treated with both drugs, half of whom required transfusion. In addition to bleeding complications, the use of streptokinase for embolism has been associated with allergic reactions, fever, and the adult respiratory distress syndrome as reported by Martin and associates. Also, in the first phase of the study, there was no significant difference between urokinase and heparin treatment in terms of the recurrence rate of embolism or mortality rate at 2 weeks.

More recently, recombinant human tissue–type plasminogen activator (rt-PA) has become available as a relatively clot-specific thrombolytic agent. In a series of 45 patients with documented pulmonary embolism by angiography, peripheral infusion of 100 mg over 2 h improved the angiographic score in 82% of patients as reported by Goldhaber and associates. Since patients with hypotension were excluded, the initial pulmonary arterial pressure was only moderately elevated to 22 mmHg and declined to 17 mmHg after infusion. Significant groin hematomas were seen in five patients, hematuria in two patients, and periodontal oozing in three patients. Two patients had major hemorrhage requiring operative treatment. One patient had recurrent embolism and died for a mortality rate of 3 percent and a morbidity rate of 33 percent in these patients with submassive embolism. In spite of hope that this agent would be specific for thrombus fibrin, plasma fibrinogen declined 55 percent in patients who received 2-chain rt-PA and 34 percent in those who received 1-chain rt-PA. Mitchell and associates reported favorable outcomes for patients in shock.

The advantage of thrombolytic therapy may well be to improve the ultimate resolution of major thromboembolism as demonstrated by Sharma and associates. Their follow-up studies in patients treated with urokinase or streptokinase showed a better restoration of pulmonary-capillary blood volume and diffusing capacity at 2 weeks than in patients treated with heparin and anticoagulants alone. The reason for the continued improvement that was seen at 1 year was not clear but was felt to be related either to more complete early resolution of the embolic condition, allowing more effective natural lytic processes, or to more complete clearance of peripheral venous thrombi, preventing silent recurrent embolism. Therefore, the patient who is not in shock and who has no clear contraindication to the use of thrombolytic therapy would probably benefit from its use.

Vena Caval Interruption. In some patients, anticoagulants cannot be used because of associated problems (e.g., peptic ulcer disease), and management must be directed toward a mechanical means of protection against recurrent embolism as outlined previously (Table 21-2). Other patients, in whom anticoagulation appears to be adequate, sustain recurrent embolism and become candidates for surgical intervention. The third indication is when there has been a complication of anticoagulant therapy forcing it to be discontinued and leaving the patient with untreated DVT. Another indication for a vena caval filter is protection against recurrent embolism in a patient who has sustained massive pulmonary embolism requiring open or catheter embolectomy. In these patients, in spite of a satisfactory embolectomy of the pulmonary circulation, the original focus of venous thrombosis remains untreated, and recurrent embolism is likely.

There are two additional relative indications for a vena caval filter in a patient with active or recent DVT. One is the high-risk patient over 40 years of age who is obese and has a serious associated medical illness (e.g., heart disease), malignant disease, or a history of previous embolism and who undergoes a major abdominal or vascular procedure. The final relative indication is the patient in whom 40 to 50 percent of the vascular bed has been occluded (major) and who would most likely not be able to tolerate additional emboli, particularly if there is associated cardiac or pulmonary disease.

Pulmonary Embolectomy. In patients who sustain massive embolism, management must be a coordinated and rapidly responsive effort, since survival may be only a matter of minutes. As indicated earlier, it is critical to document the diagnosis of massive pulmonary embolism by pulmonary arteriography because the clinical diagnosis, regardless of ''classic'' appearance, often is in error. The initial approach to patients who have either transient collapse or persistent systemic hypotension should include full heparinization and administration of inotropic drugs if necessary to support the circulation while the diagnosis is confirmed. Isoproterenol (4 mg in 1000 mL of 5% dextrose in water) is useful initially because of its bronchodilating and vasodilating effects as well as its positive inotropic cardiac effect. It may provoke arrhythmias, however, and necessitate use of dopamine. In the patient who responds to heparin and does not require vasopressors for systemic pressure or urine output, careful monitoring is essential to determine whether anticoagulation alone will control the disorder (Fig. 21-15). In most circumstances the spontaneous lysis of pulmonary emboli will proceed over a period of days and can be documented by serial lung scans performed at weekly intervals. The rate of clearing may be prolonged for weeks, particularly after a sizable embolism, and may be incomplete, as indicated previously. The latter condition has been observed in association with persistent pulmonary hypertension even after additional lytic drugs (e.g., urokinase) were administered. Lytic agents, however, may become a useful adjunct in management in the future.

The direct surgical approach to pulmonary embolism can be traced back to Trendelenburg (1908), who demonstrated the feasibility of pulmonary embolectomy experimentally but had no successes clinically. It remained for his pupil Kirschner (1924) to confirm the possibility of embolectomy by a successful clinical outcome. Because this procedure was attempted without circulatory support using a direct approach to the pulmonary artery at thoracotomy, the number of survivors was very small, and the first successful case in the United States was not reported until 1958 by Steenburg. The very high mortality rate associated with the Trendelenburg procedure prompted Gibbon to consider the use of extracorporeal circulation to bypass the impacted pulmonary circulation. However, the first successful open embolectomy during cardiopulmonary bypass was not reported by Sharp until 1962.

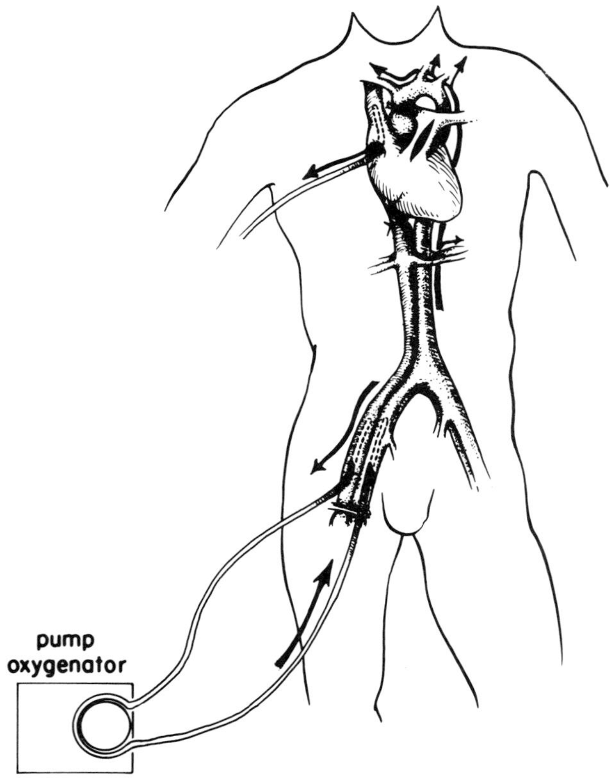

FIG. 21-16. The patient who sustains massive pulmonary embolism with shock and fails to respond to resuscitation must be supported by partial bypass and considered for open pulmonary embolectomy. The femoral artery and vein can be cannulated under local anesthesia as shown. The patient will then tolerate a general anesthetic and sternotomy, at which time a cannula can be inserted into the superior vena cava for total cardiopulmonary bypass. The main pulmonary artery is opened and the emboli are extracted by forceps and suction. [From: *Greenfield LJ: Complications of venous thrombosis and pulmonary embolism, in Greenfield LJ (ed): Complications in Surgery and Trauma. Philadelphia, Lippincott, 1984, with permission.*]

Since then, partial bypass support has also been utilized for the patient in shock. Local anesthesia is used, and the femoral artery and vein are cannulated for venoarterial bypass. The equipment is fully portable (Fig. 21-16), and patients can be supported during pulmonary arteriography and then transported to the operating room, where they can tolerate general anesthesia and sternotomy much better while being maintained on partial cardiopulmonary bypass. Once the mediastinum is opened, the partial bypass can be converted to total bypass by insertion of a superior vena caval catheter; the pulmonary emboli are then removed through a pulmonary arteriotomy.

Open pulmonary embolectomy still carries a mortality rate in the range of 50 percent, however, and uncontrollable pulmonary hemorrhage may follow open restoration of pulmonary perfusion. Consequently, an alternative approach utilizing local anesthesia has been suggested by Greenfield and associates for transvenous removal of pulmonary emboli. A cup device attached to a steerable catheter is inserted in either the jugular or the femoral vein, and the cup is positioned under fluoroscopy adjacent to the embolus seen on arteriography (Fig. 21-17). The position is verified by injection of contrast medium through the catheter. Then syringe suction is applied to aspirate the embolus into the cup, where it is held by suction vacuum as the catheter and captured embolus are with-

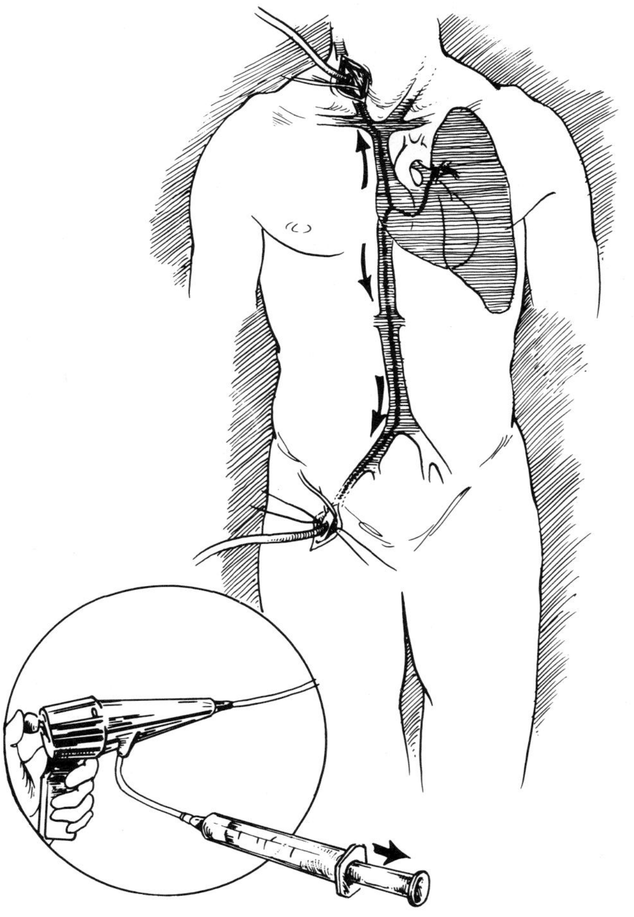

FIG. 21-17. Transvenous pulmonary embolectomy can be performed under local anesthesia via the jugular or femoral vein. The cup-catheter is positioned under fluoroscopy adjacent to the embolus, and syringe suction is applied to capture the embolus within the cup. While suction is maintained, the catheter and trailing embolus are withdrawn through the venotomy. Multiple passages allow clearing of the vascular bed and restoration of cardiac output. [From: *Greenfield LJ: Complications of venous thrombosis and pulmonary embolism, in Greenfield LJ (ed): Complications in Surgery and Trauma. Philadelphia, Lippincott, 1984, with permission.*]

drawn. Clinical experience with the technique in 32 patients showed that emboli could be extracted in 29 of them (91 percent) with an overall survival of 76 percent. Emboli could not be removed when they had been impacted for more than 72 h or if the patient suffered cardiac arrest at the time of angiography, in which case open embolectomy was required. Placement of a Greenfield vena caval filter after removal of sufficient emboli to produce near-normal hemodynamics protected the patients from recurrent embolism.

Pulmonary Hypertension and Thromboembolism

Pulmonary emboli may accumulate gradually over a prolonged period if they fail to undergo lysis and obliterate the pulmonary vascular bed. The clinical picture in this case is one of chronic cor pulmonale because significant pulmonary hypertension results from changes in the pulmonary vascular bed. The presentation may be subtle with only dyspnea or syncope on exertion, but there is a loud P_2 and right-sided strain on the electrocardiogram. The sequence may also occur unaccompanied by significant respiratory symptoms, and this may explain the etiology in some of the patients considered to have primary pulmonary hypertension. When the diagnosis is made, there is very limited life expectancy, but the patient may benefit from a vena caval filter to prevent further embolism even if the disorder is primary pulmonary hypertension as reported by Greenfield and associates. The rationale for this is that they will ultimately develop right heart failure, predisposing to pulmonary embolism that is lethal even if small. When acute cardiopulmonary decompensation occurs in these patients after embolism, they are not good candidates for embolectomy because of fixation of the older thrombi to the pulmonary arterial wall. They should be classified separately (chronic) and managed by long-term anticoagulation therapy, or in some cases should be considered for open pulmonary thromboendarterectomy or heart-lung transplantation.

Recurrent thromboembolic pulmonary hypertension produces exertional dyspnea and signs of right heart strain with cor pulmonale. With further progression of right heart overload, tricuspid insufficiency may develop. This disorder may be difficult to distinguish from primary pulmonary hypertension, although the latter is more likely to be found in women under 20 years of age without a history of DVT. Severe pulmonary hypertension is a serious problem and usually limits the life expectancy to less than 2 years from diagnosis.

Open thrombectomy for chronic occlusion was first performed by Allison and associates in 1958 and remains a possibility for improving pulmonary blood flow. To be eligible for this procedure the occlusion must involve the proximal portion of the pulmonary arterial tree and the distal bed must be patent. The physiologic basis for continued distal patency after proximal occlusion is bronchial arterial collateral flow. The procedure also has a significant mortality, but this has been decreasing with greater experience and identification of risk factors. Daily and associates performed pulmonary thromboendarterectomy on 127 patients under deep hypothermic circulatory arrest with a mortality rate of 12.6 percent. For the majority of patients with severe pulmonary hypertension, however, the outlook is poor unless they receive maximum protection from recurrent embolism, which in our experience has required both anticoagulation therapy and vena caval filter placement.

VARICOSE VEINS

The prevalence of varicose veins in adults increases with age and is generally greater in women. It increases with increasing parity, is directly related to body mass, and has an inconsistent relationship with occupations that require prolonged standing. There is also a striking geographical variation in occurrence that is not well understood, although there appears to be a relationship with low-fiber diets and prolonged sitting as reported by Beaglehole.

Diagnosis

It is important to distinguish between primary varicose veins and the more serious condition of varicosities secondary to underlying deep venous disease. The latter situation is usually associated with stasis dermatitis or ulceration. In primary varicosities there is often a family history and a favorable outcome to medical or surgical treatment. The etiology is unknown, but the more widely accepted hypotheses attribute the disorder to either primary valvular weakness or weakness of the vein walls allowing valvular distraction and incompetence. The theory of arteriovenous communication producing high pressure and flow is less well substantiated. There is rarely an association of varicosities with congenital or acquired

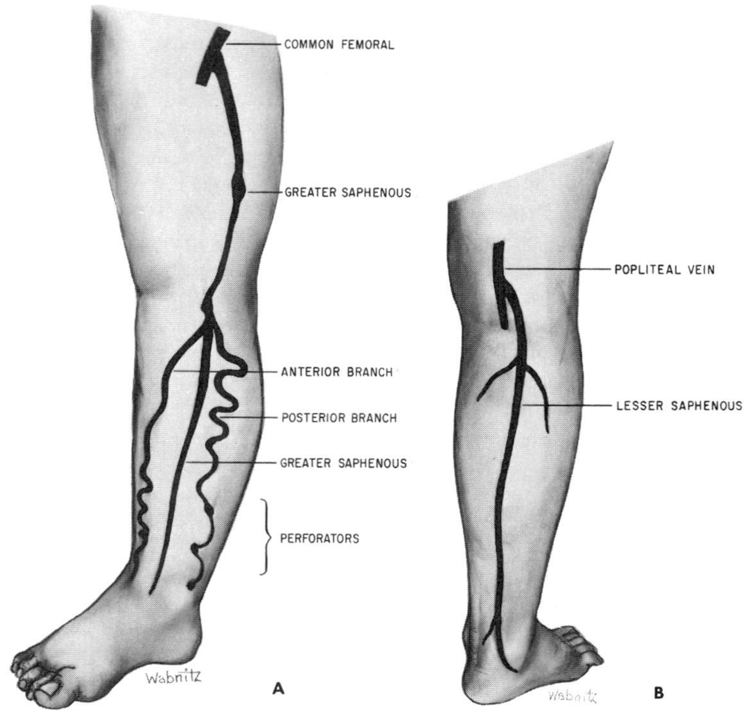

FIG. 21-18. *A.* The usual course of the greater saphenous vein and its major branches in the lower leg, emphasizing the fact that branch varicosities are the ones usually seen. Perforating veins, posterior and superior to medial malleoli, are indicated. *B.* The usual course of the lesser saphenous vein is shown in the lower leg.

arteriovenous fistulas. In the Klippel–Trenaunay syndrome, varicose veins develop in the leg in childhood and there is limb hypertrophy. Pelvic visceral varicosities with hemorrhagic complications also may develop. Servelle advises operative treatment in childhood to avoid limb length abnormality and has occasionally found compressive bands over major veins.

Varicose veins are the most common vascular disorder affecting human beings, who are unique among animals in this susceptibility. The term varicose means dilated and the characteristic enlarged and tortuous superficial veins can be diagnosed by inspection of standing patients. The usual distribution of varices is below the knee in branches of the greater saphenous system (Fig. 21-18). In the absence of postthrombotic sequelae, varicose veins are best evaluated by Doppler ultrasound and venous reflux plethysmography. If the abnormalities found are limited to the superficial veins, the condition is probably primary, whereas the finding of deep or perforator venous disease suggests that the varicosities are secondary and no benefit can be expected from their excision. These patients require lifelong elastic stocking support and may require operative treatment for local complications of their venous insufficiency.

The symptoms associated with varicose veins are nonspecific aching and heaviness of the legs that can be attributed to the congestion and pooling of blood in the enlarged superficial venous system. The symptoms are worsened by prolonged sitting and standing and relieved by elevation of the legs above the level of the heart. The use of calf-length elastic stocking support in the range of 20 to 30 mmHg usually suffices to provide relief. Although mild edema may occur from varicosities alone, it usually reflects additional incompetence of the deep or perforating venous system and may require stronger elastic stocking support. Obviously, the differential diagnosis for any patient presenting with bilateral lower-extremity edema also includes cardiac and renal disease, which should be investigated.

Night cramping of the legs is secondary to muscle spasms and is not usually due to venous disease. Arterial insufficiency should be excluded, but it may not be possible to identify a specific etiology. Some patients obtain relief by performing calf-stretching exercises before retiring and others may be helped by the administration of quinine sulfate, which reduces muscular irritability.

Treatment

The majority of patients can be managed by conservative methods, but if these fail to control symptoms or if additional complications of venous stasis develop, such as dermatitis, bleeding, thrombosis, or superficial ulceration, the patient may become a candidate for more aggressive management. Cosmetic concern or ill-defined pain patterns are less reliably improved by operation.

The two methods of treatment currently employed are ablative surgery and injection sclerotherapy, the latter being more popular in European countries than in this country. The objective of ablation is to redirect venous return through veins with intact valves and to improve appearance by removal or ligation of the varicosities (Fig. 21-19). The traditional procedure includes stripping of the long saphenous vein from ankle to groin by avulsion from its bed. More recently, Ludbrook and others have pointed out that it is advisable to save the normal portion of the saphenous vein below the knee to avoid the complications of its removal at that level and to allow it to be used for arterial bypass at a future time.

Injection sclerotherapy is designed to destroy the endothelium of the vein and promote its obliteration by scar. If pressure is not applied to the vein after injection of the sclerosant, a thrombus will form and later recanalize, leading not only to recurrence but occasionally to worsening of the problem. The technique for injection involves placement of the needle and syringe with the patient standing followed by elevation of the leg, injection of the agent, and bandage compression of the area for 2 to 3 weeks. Efforts are made to sclerose veins in proximity to perforating veins, which

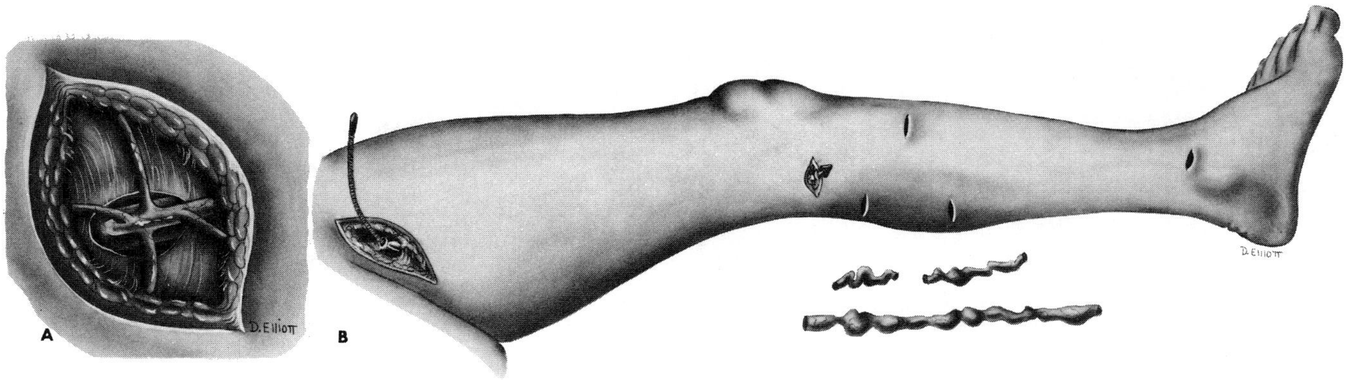

FIG. 21-19. Operative approach for ligation and stripping of the saphenous vein. *A.* The groin incision, showing the junction of the greater saphenous and femoral veins. Note four major branches of the saphenous vein that require ligation and division. *B.* A counterincision at the knee or ankle permits stripping of the saphenous vein. Additional incisions permit removal of branch varicose veins.

can be palpated as fascial defects, in order to reduce the chances of recurrence. Comparison of these techniques has shown that the results are comparable short-term but that surgical treatment clearly produces the best results after 3 to 5 years of observation as reported by Hobbs. Sclerotherapy also can produce allergic reactions, DVT, and inflammatory reaction with possible skin slough if the sclerosant escapes from the vein. It is useful primarily for management of smaller varicose veins and for recurrent or persistent varicosities after operative treatment.

CHRONIC VENOUS INSUFFICIENCY

In spite of optimal anticoagulation and bed rest for patients with acute DVT, approximately 50 percent will develop the postthrombotic syndrome as a reflection of chronic venous insufficiency. The underlying pathology consists of recanalization of the deep veins with persistent deformity and incompetence of the valves. The result is a long column of blood unrestrained by valvular support that transmits pressures of over 100 mmHg to the venules, promoting both fluid and protein loss into the tissues. The perivascular fibrinous deposits remain in place because of inadequate fibrinolysis as demonstrated by Browse and Burnard and interfere with oxygenation and metabolism of the tissues. The result is thickening and liposclerosis of the subcutaneous tissues to produce the characteristic "brawny" edema, which is relatively nonpitting. The loss of red cells results in hemosiderin deposits to produce the characteristic pigmentation. When the distal perforating veins become incompetent, there is additional pressure, with skin atrophy leading ultimately to necrosis and chronic stasis ulceration (Fig. 21-20). There is often an associated dermatitis that may be due to various salves and ointments used to treat the condition. Dryness and scaling with pruritus also occur, and with constant scratching, secondary infection and cellulitis may result.

In contrast to normal patients who reduce their distal venous pressure with exercise, patients with the postthrombotic syndrome gain no benefit from their muscle pump (Fig. 21-21). If there has

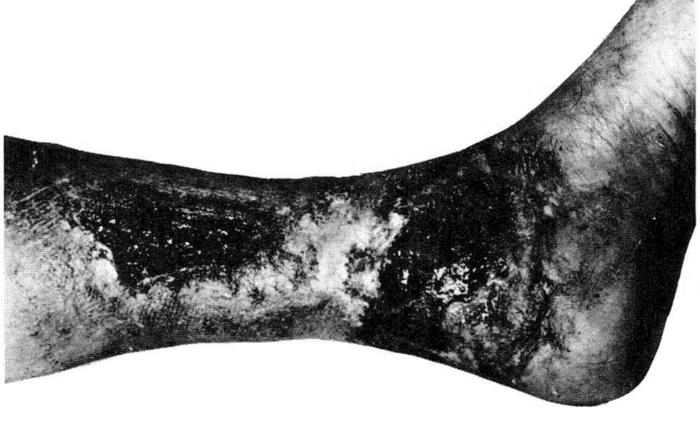

FIG. 21-20. Extensive chronic venous ulcers of the lower leg.

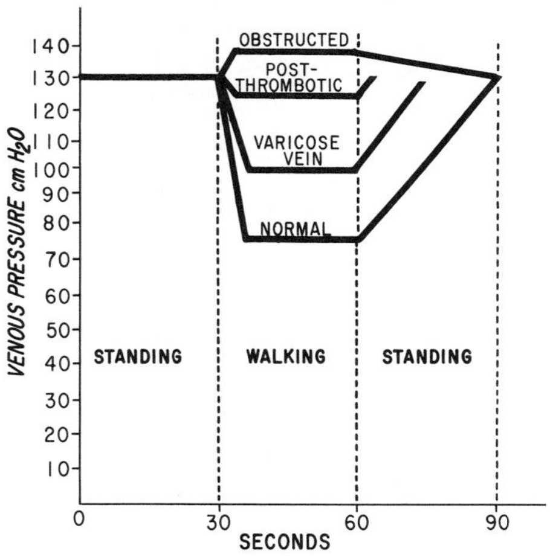

FIG. 21-21. Direct measurement of the responses in venous pressure in the superficial veins at the ankle with exercise. In the standing position, venous pressure is slightly higher than hydrostatic pressure in a column extending from ankle to heart. This pressure is approximately the same for normal persons and for those with venous insufficiency or chronically obstructed veins in which collaterals have formed. With walking, however, normal persons demonstrate a rapid decrease in venous pressure and a slow return to normal when exercise stops; patients with varicose veins show a lesser decrease in pressure with walking but a more prompt return to normal following cessation of exercise; patients with postthrombotic veins demonstrate little if any decrease in venous pressure with walking and a rapid return to normal; patients with obstructed veins show an increase in pressure with walking and a slow return to normal.

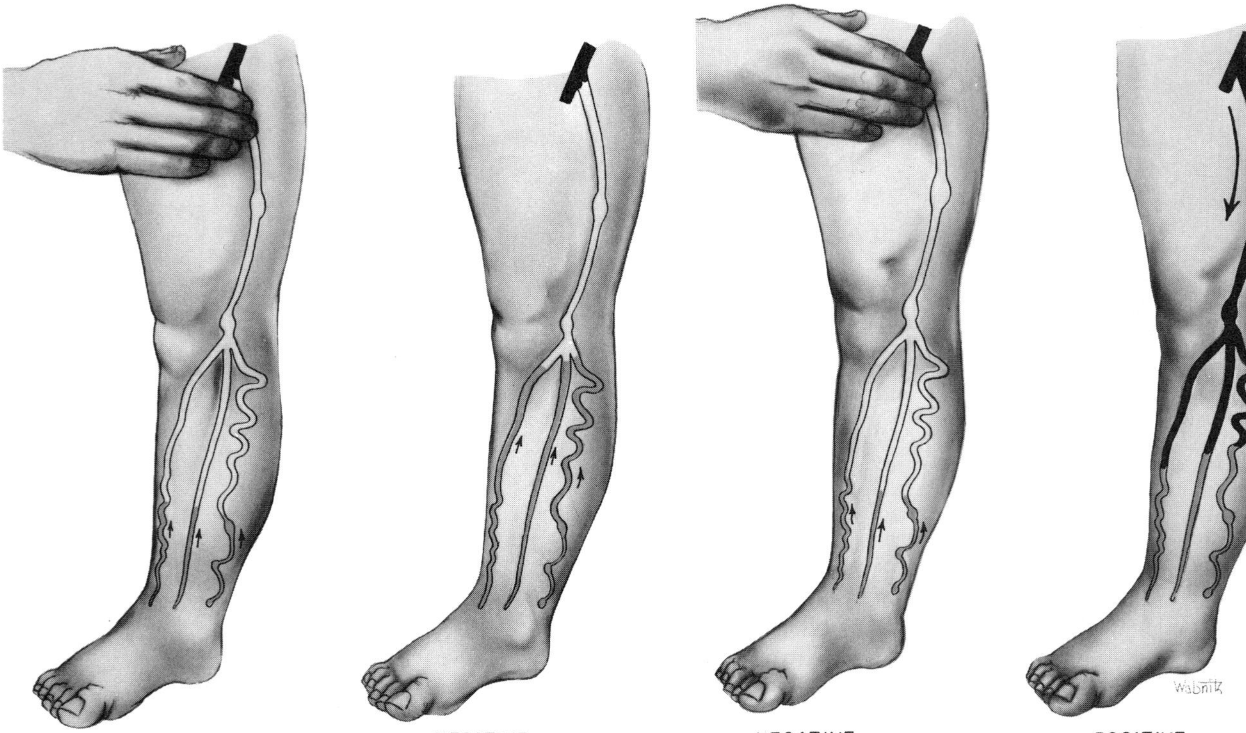

FIG. 21-22. The four possible results of the Trendelenburg compression test. The patient has been lying down with leg elevated; he then stands up with compression over the saphenofemoral junction. *A.* Negative-negative response in which there is gradual filling of veins from below over a 30-s period and there is continued slow filling after release of hand. *B.* Negative-positive response. On standing, there is gradual filling of the distal veins; on release of compression there is rapid retrograde filling of the saphenous vein. *C.* Positive-negative response. With the hand in place, filling of superficial varicosities through incompetent perforators occurs; with release of compression there is further slow filling of the veins. *D.* Positive-positive response. On standing with the hand in place, there is filling of varices through incompetent perforators. On release of compression there is additional rapid filling of the saphenous vein.

been failure of recanalization with persistent obstruction, the increase in blood flow with exercise may increase venous hypertension to produce ischemic pain referred to as ''venous claudication.'' This may become disabling and lead to consideration of venous bypass procedures to be described.

Diagnosis

Before the development of current techniques of noninvasive testing for venous disease, the methods of evaluation depended on physical examination while different sites were compressed. These tests are still useful if a noninvasive vascular laboratory is not available.

Clinical Compression Tests. In the Trendelenburg test the limb is elevated to evacuate the veins; then pressure by hand or tourniquet is applied to the saphenofemoral junction (Fig. 21-22). With the patient standing, the lower leg is observed for the rate of filling of the varicosities. Gradual filling occurs in normal patients when the perforating veins are competent. Rapid filling occurs if the perforators are incompetent. The second phase of the test consists of release of the pressure to see if the upper thigh varices fill rapidly, indicating incompetence of the saphenofemoral valve.

In the Perthes test a tourniquet is placed around the upper leg and the patient is instructed to walk. If the varicose veins disappear, the deep venous system is patent and the perforating veins are competent. If pain occurs with walking, the deep system is obstructed and the superficial system represents the major source of venous outflow. Obviously, it would be a serious error to excise superficial veins under these circumstances. Sequential tourniquets also may be used to define and isolate areas of incompetent perforating veins (Ochsner–Mahorner test).

Laboratory Measurements. Direct measurement of venous pressure by needle and strain gauge provides the most accurate assessment of venous hemodynamics, but it is invasive and cumbersome to use. It has, however, served to validate the noninvasive tests to be described.

Doppler Examination. A directional Doppler can be used at the bedside to determine venous patency and valvular competence. Reflux retrograde flow can be observed at the femoral level during Valsalva maneuver or at the popliteal level with the patient standing and the calf alternately compressed and released (Fig. 21-4). A similar maneuver should be used when listening over perforating veins.

Plethysmography. The strain gauge plethysmograph measures venous capacity and outflow making it more valuable for acute thrombosis than for chronic changes where it may be normal or indicate persistent obstruction. The photoplethysmograph

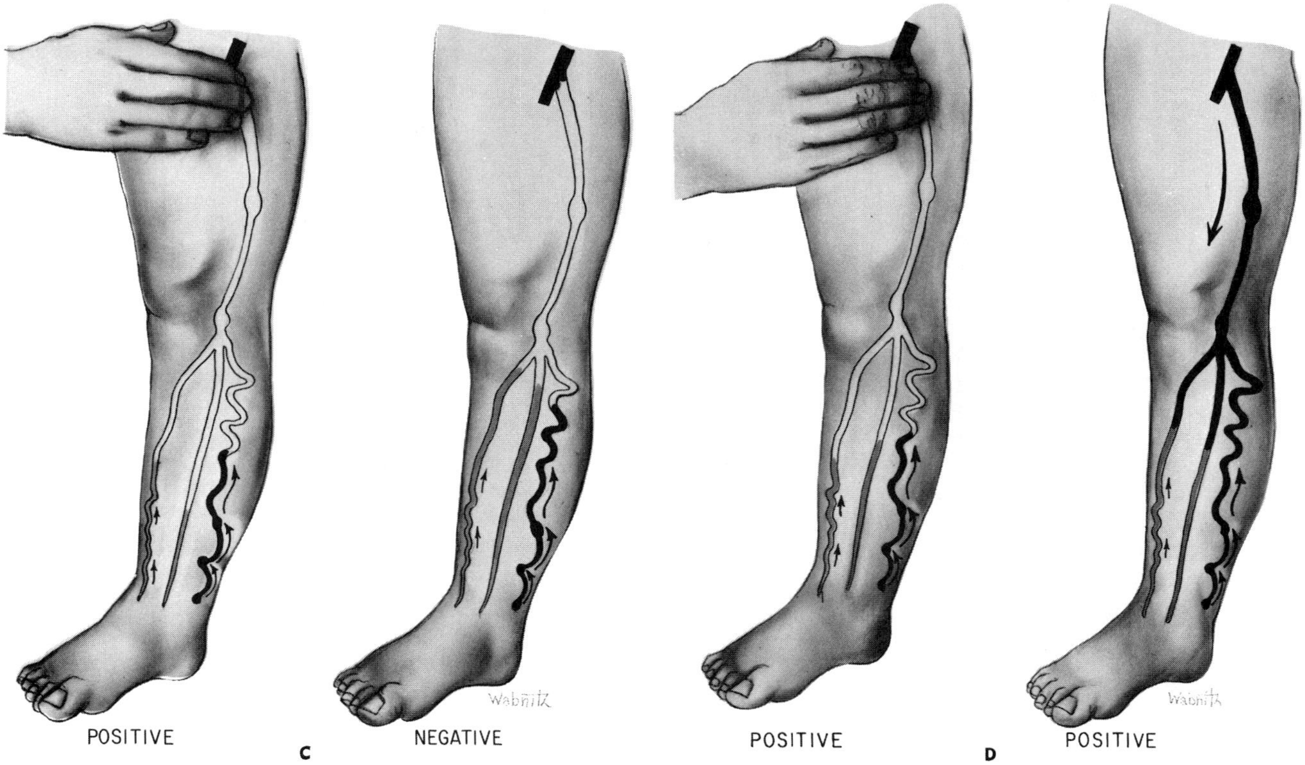

FIG. 21-22. *C,D. Continued.*

(PPG) uses infrared light to measure subcutaneous vascular volume and can provide a reliable index of valvular incompetence. The venous refilling time, after calf muscle exercise empties the veins, will be shortened considerably in the presence of valvular incompetence. Although the technique is primarily qualitative, Norris and associates have developed an in vivo calibration technique to provide quantitative information that correlates well with ambulatory venous pressure measured directly.

Duplex Scanning. The most promising of the newer diagnostic techniques is the combination of ultrasound duplex scanning using a B-mode imager with a pulsed Doppler instrument to provide both imaging and flow patterns. Thrombi can be visualized within the veins and flow observed if the vein remains patent. Normal veins can be compressed by the scanner head over the vessel while thrombosed veins are incompressible. Venous valves can also be visualized and their competence assessed under a variety of flow alterations as demonstrated by Kohler and Strandness.

Supportive Therapy

Perhaps the most important aspect of patient management is the education of the patient to emphasize the importance of elastic stocking support, frequent elevation of the legs above the level of the heart, and the avoidance of prolonged sitting and standing. Frequent follow-up examinations are essential not only to assess compliance with the prescribed regimen but also to detect early recurrent thrombosis. Patient compliance can be improved by including other family members in the discussion and by the use of calf-length elastic stockings, which are easier to manage than full-length hose and less likely to produce a tourniquet effect at the knee. The patient should acquire two sets of pressure gradient stockings so that a clean pair is always available.

Operative Management

The development of a stasis ulcer requires immediate efforts to promote healing by frequent cleansing, bed rest, foot elevation, and the use of paste boots or elastic sealed dressings. The use of local medications should be avoided to minimize allergic reactions. Patients who fail to heal after prolonged outpatient care will require hospitalization and may need skin grafts for larger ulcers.

Perforator Vein Ligation. Permanent healing of chronic stasis ulcers that recur after skin grafting is not likely unless the perforating veins responsible for the ulcer are identified and ligated. The typical location for these is posterior and superior to the medial malleolus. Ligation of the perforator vessels still leads to recurrent ulceration in 15 percent of patients despite vigorous medical therapy, including support stockings, leg elevation, wound care, and patient education. The patients in whom medical and routine surgical therapy fail may be considered for attempted reconstruction of their venous systems.

Venous Reconstruction. The present attitude of most surgeons toward venous reconstruction is critical and pessimistic as reviewed by Bernstein in 1986. The venous system, unlike the arterial system, tends to recanalize, thus making it more difficult to quantitate the obstruction and identify the patient who may benefit from venous reconstruction. Dale estimated that the percentage of patients with chronic venous insufficiency who could benefit from reconstruction was 1 to 2 percent of that population. Surgical reconstruction can be divided into two categories: bypassing obstructive disease and restoring valvular competence. To evaluate patients, it is necessary to obtain both ascending and descending venograms.

The most widely accepted procedure for venous reconstruction is the saphenous vein cross-over graft, first described by Palma and Esperon in 1958. The procedure consists of isolating the normal contralateral saphenous vein and dividing it distally. The vein is then tunneled suprapubically and anastomosed to the contralateral femoral vein, distal to its obstruction. In 1982, Dale described 59 patients who had the Palma bypass with excellent results in 63 percent, good results in 17 percent, and a failure rate of 20 percent. Husni in 1983 and Smith and Trimble in 1977 had reported similar results. The saphenous vein cross-over graft has generally been accepted as useful; however, the natural history of iliac vein occlusion is recanalization, and very few patients with iliofemoral thrombosis became candidates for surgery.

Use of the saphenous vein for popliteal-to-femoral vein bypass was described by Warren and Thayer in 1954, with good clinical results in 10 of 14 patients. The saphenous vein is dissected free below the knee and anastomosed to the popliteal vein, which is obstructed proximally. Husni has popularized this procedure and has reported the outcome in 27 patients, with a good result in 63 percent. Dale reported good results in 10 patients (60 percent), and Smith and Trimble, in a collected series of 59 patients, reported good results in 76 percent. However, with rich collateral veins in the thigh, identifying the patient with an obstructed superficial femoral vein who may benefit from the saphenous-to-popliteal vein bypass is difficult. Kistner and Sparkuhl, on the other hand, recognized that patients with superficial femoral vein incompetence and symptoms of thrombotic syndrome could benefit from superficial femoral vein ligation. They ligated the superficial femoral vein of five patients and had good results in four.

Methods of reconstruction for venous incompetence of the iliofemoral system include valvuloplasty as described by Kistner, venous segment transfer as described by Kistner and Sparkuhl, and valve autotransplantation as described by Taheri and associates.

Valvuloplasty. In 1980, Kistner, after studying 200 limbs with ascending and descending venography, found 28 that could be treated by valve repair, and 72 percent had an excellent result. In this procedure, floppy incompetent valves are tethered against the vein wall or shortened using interrupted 8-0 monofilament suture (Fig. 21-23). After DVT, most patients have scarred and thickened valves that do not lend themselves to this type of reconstruction. Since Kistner routinely combined valvuloplasty with saphenous vein stripping and perforator ligation, the results have been difficult to interpret, but they have found good to excellent results in 80 percent of cases as reported by Ferris and Kistner.

Vein Segment Transfer. In 1979, Kistner and Sparkuhl described six patients who had vein segment transfer. Of these patients, one had venous occlusion and the other five had good results 1 year postoperatively. In this procedure, competent valves are identified in the saphenous vein, superficial femoral vein, and profundus system. The vessel with the incompetent valve identified by descending venography is divided and anastomosed distal to the portion of the system with a competent valve (Fig. 21-24).

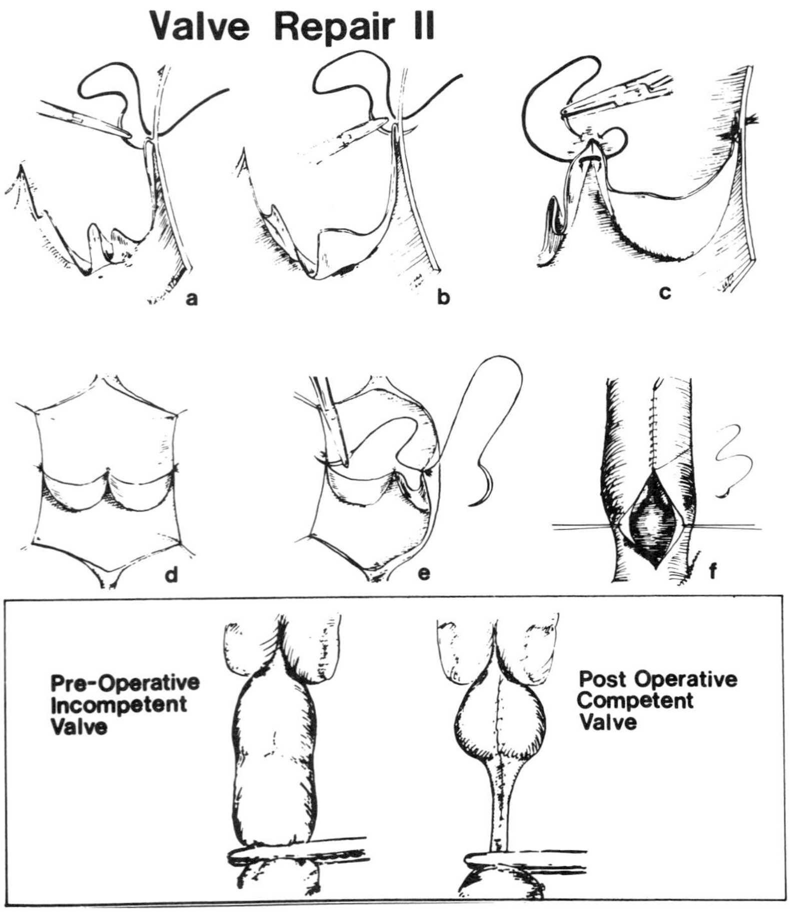

FIG. 21-23. The highest valve in the superficial femoral vein may be eligible for direct repair using the technique proposed by Kistner. A longitudinal venotomy exposes the valve cusps which are repaired by suture plication as shown *(A–E)*. After closure of the vein *(F)*, restored competence of the valve can be demonstrated by milking it proximally. [From: *Bergan J, Yao J (eds): Operative Techniques in Vascular Surgery. Orlando, FL, Grune and Stratton, 1980, with permission.*]

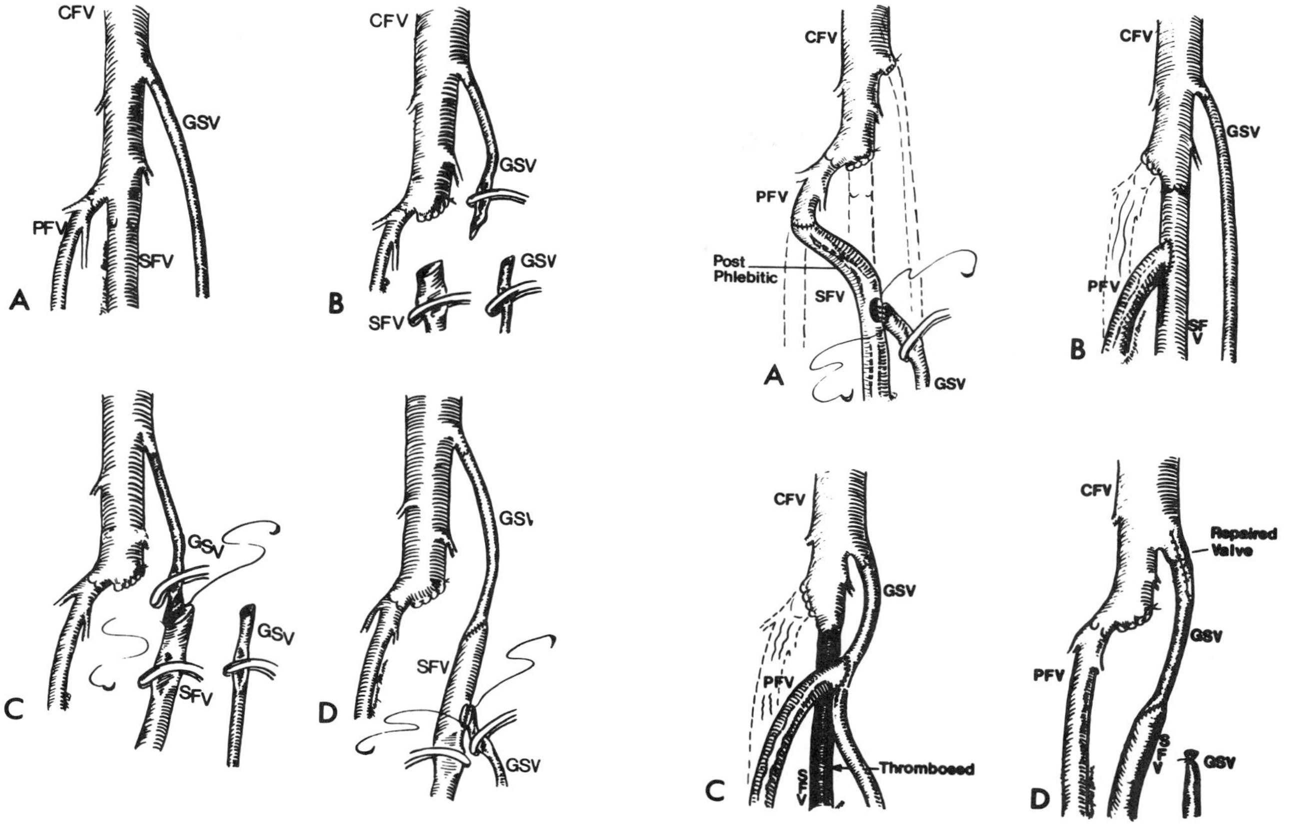

FIG. 21-24. Left. An alternative technique for restoring valvular competence is to use the existing competent greater saphenous vein (GSV) as a new conduit for the incompetent superficial femoral vein (SFV) by dividing the veins at the level of the proposed anastomosis *(A,B)*, connecting the SFV to the GSV *(C)* and then reimplanting the distal GSV into the SFV *(D)*.

Right. Where the SFV shows postphlebitic stenosis, it may be preferable to attach it to a competent profunda femoral vein (PFV) and add the inflow from the GSV *(A)*. Where the PFV is incompetent, it can be connected to a competent SFV *(B)* or to the GSV to bypass an obstructed SFV *(C)*. The transposition procedure can also be used in conjunction with valvuloplasty *(D)* when both techniques are required for restoring valvular competence. [From: *Bergan J, Yao J (eds): Operative Techniques in Vascular Surgery. Orlando, FL, Grune and Stratton, 1980, with permission.*]

This renders the previously incompetent system competent and, when combined with saphenous vein stripping and perforator ligation, improves the clinical and venographic results.

Autologous Vein Transplantation. The third reconstructive procedure for iliofemoral incompetence consists of autologous vein valve transplantation. This was developed by Taheri and coworkers and consists of harvesting a segment of brachial vein with a competent valve from the arm and interposing it into the femoral system just below the origin of the superficial femoral vein or more distally at or above the popliteal vein. In 1986, the investigators described 66 patients, with good results in 78 percent. In this series 31 patients had postoperative venograms, and 28 had valvular competence. This procedure is still considered experimental and is awaiting long-term confirmation. Bergan and colleagues have pointed out that for venous valve surgery to be successful, it usually must be accompanied by saphenous vein stripping and perforator ligation. They reported a series of 12 patients who had only venous valve reconstruction without the more distal stripping and perforator ligation. These patients had good results initially; however, at 1 year, nine of the limbs had reverted to their preoperative condition owing to recurrent symptoms and delayed venous refill time. The difficulty in identifying patients who could benefit from these procedures was put into perspective by Dale who, after 2 years of investigating, failed to identify a group of patients who would benefit from venous valve transplantation or valvuloplasty.

Husni found that venous reconstruction fails in three situations: when the bypass graft is too small in caliber; when venous hypertension is mild to moderate, that is, less than 80 percent of the standing venous pressure; and when a thrombectomy or endophlebectomy has to be performed before anastomosis. In these patients who are at high risk for failure, he has recommended a distal arteriovenous fistula. The use of arteriovenous fistulas after iliofemoral thrombectomy or reconstruction of the venous system is controversial. Most of the experience has been accumulated in Europe where it is believed to reduce the incidence of early rethrombosis. The two most commonly used sites are the femoral triangle and the ankle. After surgery on the iliofemoral system, an H-shaped fistula can be established easily by anastomosing a branch of the saphenous vein end-to-side to the proximal portion of the superficial femoral artery. At the ankle, the posterior tibial artery may be anastomosed to the posterior tibial vein or the greater saphenous vein. Two problems have led to the reluctance of some surgeons to adopt this procedure: the fear of damaging functioning valves distal to the fistula and the requirement for a second operation to close the fistula. Fistulas are usually closed 3 to 4 months postoperatively, and problems with incompetent valves distal to the fistula have not been reported. In 1981, Kroener and Bernstein reported on the effects of arteriovenous fistulas in dogs. They found a marked increase in the success of venous reconstructive procedures when a fistula was used, and no damage to the venous valves was noted when the fistula was taken down after 5 weeks. Two steps during primary venous reconstruction simplify operative closure of the fistula later. The fistula is made distal to the venous reconstruction, thus avoiding damage to this area at reoperation, and a ligature is wrapped around the fistula and left in the subcutaneous tissue where it can be found under local anesthesia. More recently, obliteration of the fistula percutaneously by balloon has been utilized.

It seems reasonable to use the arteriovenous fistula in venous procedures that have been compromised, such as an iliofemoral thrombectomy, when the system has not been effectively cleared, or in a cross-over vein graft where the saphenous vein is of marginal size, since venous dilatation will occur proximal to the fistula. Smith has recommended that the fistula not be used if the ankle-arm index is less than 0.75 to avoid distal arterial problems in the same limb, and that the fistula should not exceed 4 mm in diameter to avoid distal venous hypertension, valvular damage, and significant effects on cardiac hemodynamics.

It has been noted in the past that the majority of iliofemoral thromboses occur on the left side. This is attributed to the right iliac artery compressing the left iliac vein as it crosses the fifth lumbar vertebra. Various autopsy series and operative studies have documented the presence of left iliac vein webs and scarring in patients who have had iliofemoral thrombosis. There was early interest in this problem by Calnan and associates in 1964 and Cockett and Thomas in 1965 who advocated surgical correction of these lesions. Dale reviewed eight such patients identified by venography and subsequently operated on four, trimming out anterior webs or scar tissue and using a venous patch for closure. Two of the patients had excellent results, but edema developed later in one, and a fourth patient had a complicated postoperative course, complaining of excruciating pain and postoperative swelling. Dale recommended operation only for the patient whose symptoms are severe and who will accept the operation knowing that the results are not predictable. Smith and Trimble have followed 30 patients with this problem and have operated on 14, with an 85 percent postoperative improvement rate. Cockett and Thomas, on the other hand, found the results unsatisfactory, and after operating on 30 patients using several different methods, they recommended abandoning the procedure.

VENOUS TRAUMA

Venous injuries of the extremities are usually associated with arterial injuries because of their anatomic proximity. In this situation, application of a tourniquet not only renders the limb ischemic but also can increase blood loss from the venous injury. Since the venous system is under relatively low pressure, direct pressure applied to the wound suffices for control. Direct ligation of injured superficial veins is appropriate treatment except when they are the sole remaining venous drainage of the extremity which mandates their repair.

Treatment of injuries of the deep veins changed dramatically as a result of the military experience in Southeast Asia as reported by Rich and associates. It was well demonstrated that ligation of major extremity veins resulted in higher rates of disability and limb loss than when the veins were repaired or replaced by autogenous vein segments. The concept of primary repair of venous injuries by suture vein patch or vein graft interposition has been extended to civilian injuries by Agarwal and associates with favorable results. These repairs have not been associated with increased complications such as thrombophlebitis or pulmonary embolism as was originally of concern. Although injuries to the inferior vena cava are unusual, the morbidity and mortality rates are high, especially for the retrohepatic vena cava. Kudsk and associates have reported their experience in 70 patients with both penetrating and blunt trauma, resulting in 55 percent survivors. They emphasized the importance of adequate resuscitation and the significance of associated injuries. Malt and associates showed that venous repair is also essential for the success of upper extremity replantation after nearly complete or complete traumatic amputation.

Iatrogenic vascular trauma has increased in frequency with the proliferation of invasive diagnostic and therapeutic puncture and biopsy techniques. The subclavian vein is particularly vulnerable to injury and thrombosis because of its use for venous access and placement of long-term catheters. Placement of these catheters also increases the risk of sepsis and the possibility of catheter breakage with embolism. A technique for retrieval of a catheter fragment in the subclavian vein by Fogarty catheter was reported by Mathur and associates.

Use of a temporary arteriovenous fistula distal to the repair of a traumatic venous injury of the lower extremity in eight patients was reported by Richardson and associates in 1986. The posterior tibial artery and vein were utilized and the external shunt allowed infusion of heparin and access for postoperative venograms. In six patients the shunt functioned for an average of 10 days and all patients with functioning shunts for 72 h or longer had patent venous repairs without subsequent edema.

LYMPHATICS AND LYMPHEDEMA

Developmental Anatomy and Function

The exact origin of lymphatic vessels is a matter of disagreement among embryologists. The original theory of Sabin traced the origin from the venous system while Huntington and McClure suggested that lymphatics form by fusion of mesenchymal spaces or clefts. The latter has been labeled the centripetal theory. By the sixth week of gestation, there are paired lymph sacs in the neck and lumbar areas and at the eighth week, there is a retroperitoneal lymph sac with a developing cisterna chyli. These systems develop communicating channels that ultimately form the thoracic duct by merger of the right lymphatic duct with the left across the fourth to sixth thoracic vertebrae that then drains into the left subclavian vein. Smaller lymphatic ducts persist that drain into the right subclavian vein.

Developmental arrest or abnormalities may result in primary hypoplasia or absence of ducts and lymph nodes. Abnormal growth of jugular lymph sacs can produce unilocular or multilocular lymph cysts termed cystic hygromas. In addition to the neck, these cysts may be found in the axilla, mediastinum, retroperitoneum, or intestinal mesentery. Hyperplastic changes may also occur to produce lymphangiomas with or without other vascular malformations.

The function of the lymphatic system begins with lymphatic capillaries that collect fluid and protein from the extravascular spaces. In addition to the protein that cannot be reabsorbed by the venules, red cells, bacteria, and other larger particles can only be evacuated through the lymphatics. This unique permeability is facilitated by the absence of a basement membrane beneath the lymphatic endothelial cells. The lymphatic capillaries are found beneath the epidermis in the superficial dermis. These vessels drain into valved channels in the deep dermis and subdermal tissues, forming larger channels that follow the vascular pathways superficial to the deep fascia. Although lymphatics can be found in the intermuscular fascia, they are absent in muscles, tendon, cartilage, brain, and cornea.

Lymph is transported by afferent vessels to regional lymph nodes that vary in size according to their function and activity. Within the medullary sinuses of the node, circulating lymphocytes are replaced and initial contact of foreign material with the immune system is made. Efferent lymph leaves the node via hilar channels that are less numerous than the afferent channels that enter the convex side of the node. In addition to direct thoracic duct drainage into the subclavian vein, there are other lymphovenous communications within nodes and in peripheral vessels. Central lymphatic flow is promoted by the lymphatic valves, muscular contractions in larger ducts, respiration, arterial pulsation, and external massage.

Classification of Lymphedema

The original classification of Allen was into two types, one where there was no known cause and one secondary to a known disease or disorder. The primary lymphedemas were called *congenital* when present at birth and *praecox* when there was onset in childhood. When the onset was delayed into later life, Kinmonth added the term *tarda*. With the advent of lymphography it became possible to classify the primary lymphedemas structurally into *hyperplasias* and *hypoplasias*. The present classification as proposed by Kinmonth is as follows:

- I. Primary lymphedema
  - A. Primary hypoplastic
    - (1) Distal hypoplasia or aplasia
    - (2) Proximal hypoplasia
    - (3) Proximal and distal hypoplasia
  - B. Primary hyperplastic
    - (1) Bilateral hyperplasia
    - (2) Megalymphatic
- II. Secondary lymphedema
  - A. Malignancy
  - B. Radiation
  - C. Trauma or surgical excision
  - D. Inflammation or parasitic invasion
  - E. Paralysis

The primary lymphedemas are hypoplastic in 92 percent of cases. Their subgroups are defined by lymphography and behave differently. Those with distal hypoplasia have a mild, nonprogressive form of the disorder provided that their proximal pathways are normal. Most of these patients are women and notice the onset after puberty. In proximal hypoplasia, the lymphedema is more extensive, involving the entire extremity, and it occurs equally among males and females. The combination of proximal and distal hypoplasia shows features of both groups and tends to be progressive.

The primary hyperplastic lymphedemas are uncommon (8 percent), and those with bilateral hyperplasia can usually be recognized by diffuse capillary angiomata on the lateral sides of the feet. Lymphography shows dilated lymphatics with normal valves in contrast to the findings in the megalymphatic group where no valves can be seen. In this latter group, chylous reflux may produce chylometrorrhea, skin vesicles, or chyluria.

The most common cause of secondary lymphedema in this country is malignant disease metastatic to lymph nodes. Surgical removal of nodes, especially when combined with radiation therapy that produces lymphatic fibrosis, is another common cause. In tropical and subtropical countries, filariasis is the most common cause of secondary lymphedema, producing the typical appearance of elephantiasis. Other infective and chemical agents such as silica can enter the lymphatic system via barefoot walking and cause fibrosis of lymphatics and lymph nodes.

Diagnosis

Lymphedema occurs as the result of an abnormality of the lymphatic system, and the term should be restricted to situations where other causes of edema have been excluded or a specific lymphatic abnormality has been demonstrated. The presence of bilateral dependent "pitting" edema usually indicates a renal or cardiac etiology. Other generalized hypoproteinemias may be seen in malnutrition, cirrhosis, and protein-losing enteropathy, or they may be idiopathic. Allergies or hereditary causes are unusual. In unilateral edema, venous disease is the most likely etiology and can be recognized by the examinations described in the previous section.

Clinical Manifestations. The patient with lymphedema complains of swelling and fatigue. Limb size increases during the day and decreases at night but is never normal. It is important to determine whether there is a family history of primary lymphedema and whether the patient has visited any countries where filariasis is endemic. The presence of weight loss and diarrhea suggests small bowel lymphangiectasia. On examination, lymphedema is characteristically firm and rubbery but nonpitting. Lymph vesicles may be present containing fluid of high protein concentration. Complications of lymphedema such as infection, cellulitis, erythema, and hyperkeratosis may be present. It is important to document limb size to identify isolated limb gigantism and the Klippel–Trenaunay syndrome which may have hypoplastic lymphatics in addition to venous abnormalities, capillary nevus, and limb elongation. The patient should be examined for upper extremity and genital lymphedema, hydroceles, and amelogenesis imperfecta.

Lymphatic Visualization. Lymphatics can be visualized by dye injection in the extremities and mesentery, and also by ingestion of cream or milk to visualize intestinal lacteals and major ducts.

Dye Injection. A highly diffusible dye such as patent blue as introduced by Hudack and McMaster or sky blue dye as recommended by Butcher and Hoover can be injected in 0.2-mL amounts subcutaneously into each interdigital web. Massage of the skin and movement of the joints will usually define a network of fine intradermal lymphatics (Fig. 21-25). If the collecting vessels are obstructed or inadequate, the dye will diffuse through the dermal lymphatics to produce a marbled appearance called "dermal backflow."

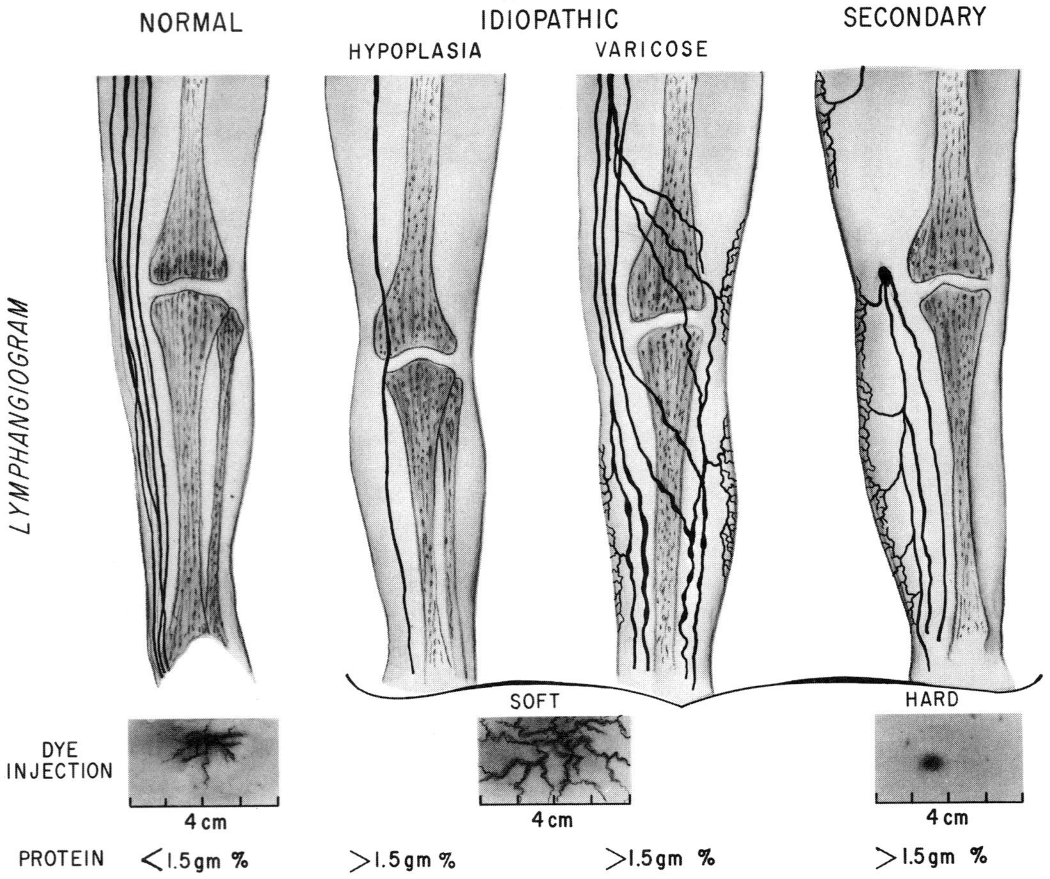

FIG. 21-25. Schematic illustration of the diagnostic procedures for lymphedema: dye injections, lymphangiograms, and protein analysis.

Radiologic Lymphography. The technique of lymphography was developed by Kinmonth, who demonstrated that it was possible to cannulate the lymphatics visualized by dye injection and then inject contrast medium (Lipiodol). This is a meticulous and tedious procedure that may require general anesthesia as originally proposed by Kinmonth. If the lymphatics in the foot are not usable, it is possible either to cannulate lymphatics adjacent to groin nodes or to inject the node directly. With adequate visualization, the lymphatics in the extremity will be identified, often as parallel tracks that are of uniform size and bifurcate as they proceed proximally in contrast to the venous system (Fig. 21-25). Normally, there is some dilatation at the level of the valves.

Radionuclide Lymphatic Clearance. Radionuclide scanning using human serum albumin labeled with radioactive iodine or technetium 99m colloid has been used to monitor lymphatic clearance by serial scanning. Although the technique is simpler than standard lymphography, it has major disadvantages due to haziness of the scan, radiation dosage, and distribution of the radionuclide into the extracellular fluid, making calculations of clearance dependent on leg volume.

Analysis of Tissue Fluid. Tissue fluid or lymph can be aspirated or collected from a tube in the subcutaneous tissues but contributes little to the diagnosis of lymphedema. Characteristically, lymphedema fluid has a protein content of more than 1.5 g/dL in contrast to edema fluid from venous hypertension, which is usually less. Also, the ratio of albumin to globulin is higher in lymphedema fluid than in plasma, which is helpful in the presence of an inflammatory exudate where the protein content is high but the albumin to globulin ratio is normal.

Management

Supportive Treatment. There are significant anatomic and physiologic limitations to the treatment of lymphedema. From the standpoint of physiology, the removal of fluid is not as effective as in edema of other causes because of the residual protein in lymphedema. In addition, from an anatomic standpoint, the development of fibrosis produces irreversible changes in the subcutaneous tissues. Therefore, the options are limited and the primary objectives remain for control of edema, maintenance of healthy skin, and avoidance of the complications of cellulitis and lymphangitis.

The initial objective of control of edema can be approached by elevation and the use of sequential pneumatic compression boots to massage the leg. These treatments can be done at home with equipment rented for this purpose. Once the leg has reached optimal size, the patient should be fitted with firm elastic stockings as described earlier for venous insufficiency. The stockings should be removed at night and the foot of the bed elevated to maintain the pressure gradient from leg to right atrium.

The onset of redness, pain, and swelling usually signifies early cellulitis or lymphangitis which can be recognized by red streaking up the leg. The usual causative organism is either staphylococcus or beta-hemolytic streptococcus which must be treated vigorously, usually with intravenous antibiotics. In the absence of treatment, the infection may obliterate more lymphatics and produce constitutional signs of fever, malaise, nausea, and vomiting. Another frequent complication is eczema, which will usually respond to hydrocortisone cream. Antifungal agents may be necessary, both topically and systemically, for chronic infections, particularly between the toes. In contrast to the stasis edema of venous insufficiency, ulceration is unusual, although fissures and lymph fistulas may develop and require surgical excision.

The secondary lymphedemas may lend themselves to treatment of the underlying disorder such as using diethylcarbamazine for filariasis or appropriate antibiotics for tuberculosis or lymphogranuloma venereum. In rare cases of long-standing secondary lymphedema such as in the arm following radical mastectomy, a lymphangiosarcoma may develop appearing as a raised blue or reddish nodule. Satellite tumors and early metastases may develop if it is not recognized and widely excised.

Operative Treatment. Only 15 percent of patients with primary lymphedema become candidates for operative treatment, which usually is directed to reducing leg size. The indications for operation are related to functional rather than cosmetic improvement since the appearance of the extremity even after a successful procedure will still be abnormal and show extensive scarring. The best results are obtained when the bulk of the extremity has severely impaired movement or when there have been recurrent attacks of cellulitis. Although some efforts have been made to develop techniques to improve lymphatic drainage, most of the established procedures consist of excisional operations.

Three of the excisional procedures were based on the incorrect assumption that the deep fascia acted as a barrier to lymphatic drainage, and the efforts of Kondoleon and associates to excise fascia and/or insert a dermal flap into muscle proved ineffective in improving lymphatic drainage. The original procedure devised by Charles consisting of wide excision of lymphedematous tissue followed by skin grafting is still useful when the overlying skin is in poor condition as in elephantiasis. The procedure used more often, however, is Kinmonth's modification of Homan's procedure where skin flaps are raised to allow excision of the underlying subcutaneous tissues.

The most logical albeit technically demanding approach has been directed to establishing lymphaticovenous anastomoses. Initial efforts in this area were made by Nielubowicz and Olszewski who divided a lymph node, removing the pulp under magnification, and then sutured the node capsule with its afferent lymphatics into a vein. This procedure is more suitable for secondary lymphedema than primary where the disorder lies in the lymphatic channels themselves. Another promising technique of direct lymphovenous connection was developed by Cordeiro and modified by Degni, who used a special needle for insertion of lymphatic vessels directly into veins and fixed them there by a single suture. Using this technique, Fox and associates treated 8 secondary and 12 primary lymphedema patients followed for up to 4 years. Good results were obtained in 2 of 4 postmastectomy lymphedemas with poor results in the 2 patients who had postoperative lymphangitis. Nine of 11 patients with primary lymphedemas had good functional results allowing them to resume normal activity. The authors recommend long-term preoperative anti-inflammatory and antimicrobial therapy to avoid postoperative lymphangitis.

It is obviously difficult to evaluate the results of such procedures when combined with resectional operations and in the absence of postoperative lymphography to demonstrate patency of the anastomoses. However, the deleterious effects of lymphangiographic contrast on lymphatics were well demonstrated by O'Brien and associates, who measured limb volume after lymphangiography in 100 patients and found that 32 percent had a significant increase in leg volume and 19 percent developed lymphangitis. Therefore, it seems advisable to use lymphangiography only for diagnostic studies and not for pre- or postoperative evaluation until safer contrast material becomes available. Further efforts to combine resectional operations with microlymphovenous anastomoses as reported by O'Brien and Shafiroff may offer some brighter prospects for improvement of these debilitating disorders.

Bibliography

Venous Disease

Aderka D, Brown A, et al: Idiopathic deep vein thrombosis in an apparently healthy patient as a premonitory sign of occult cancer. *Cancer* 57:1846, 1986.

Ambrus JS, Ambrus CM, et al: Clinical and experimental studies of fibrinolytic enzymes. *Ann NY Acad Sci* 68:97, 1957.

Common HH, Seaman AJ, et al: Deep vein thrombosis treated with streptokinase or heparin: Follow-up of a randomized study. *Angiology* 27:645, 1976.

Einarsson E, Albrechtsson U, et al: Follow-up evaluation of venous morphologic factors and function after thrombectomy and temporary arteriovenous fistula in thrombosis of iliofemoral vein. *Surg Gynecol Obstet* 163:111, 1986.

Homans J: Diseases of the veins. *N Engl J Med* 231:51, 1944.

Hyers TM, Hull RD, et al: Antithrombotic therapy for venous thromboembolic disease. *Chest* 89(suppl):265, 1986.

Kakkar VV, Carrigan TP, et al: Efficacy of low doses of heparin in prevention of deep vein thrombosis after major surgery: A double blind, randomized trial. *Lancet* 2:101, 1972.

Kakkar VV, Lawrence D: Hemodynamic and clinical assessment after therapy for acute deep vein thrombosis. A prospective study. *Am J Surg* 150:54, 1985.

Lensing AWA, Prandoni P, et al: Detection of deep-vein thrombosis by real-time B-mode ultrasonography. *N Engl J Med* 320:342, 1989.

Palareti G, Legnani C, et al: Prevalence of high levels of antiphospholipid antibodies in otherwise unexplained juvenile venous thromboembolism. *Thromb Haemost* 65:452, 1991.

Peyton JWR, Hylemon MB, et al: Comparison of Greenfield filter and vena caval ligation for experimental septic thromboembolism. *Surgery* 93(4):533, 1983.

Shattil SJ: Diagnosis and treatment of recurrent venous thromboembolism. *Med Clin North Am* 68:577, 1984.

Trousseau A: *Lectures on Clinical Medicine Delivered at the Hôtel-Dieu, Paris.* London, New Syndenham Society, 1985, pp 285–332.

Virchow R: *Gesamelte Abhandlungen zur wissenschaftlichen Medizin.* Frankfurt, Merdinger Sohn, 1856, p 219.

Pulmonary Thromboembolism

Conti S, Daschbach M, et al: Comparison of high-dose versus conventional-dose heparin therapy for deep vein thrombosis. *Surgery* 92:972, 1982.

Daily PO, Dembitsky WP, et al: Risk factors for pulmonary thromboendarterectomy. *J Thorac Cardiovasc Surg* 99:670, 1990.

Goldhaber SZ, Kessler CM, et al: Randomised controlled trial of recombinant tissue plasminogen activator versus urokinase in the treatment of acute pulmonary embolism. *Lancet* 2(8606):293, 1988.

Greenfield LJ: Pulmonary embolism: Diagnosis and management. *Curr Probl Surg* 13:1, 1976.

Greenfield LJ: Intraluminal techniques for vena caval interruption and pulmonary embolectomy. *World J Surg* 3:4559, 1978.

Greenfield LJ, Scher LA, et al: KMA-Greenfield[R] filter placement for chronic pulmonary hypertension. *Ann Surg* 189:560, 1979.

Martin TR, Sandblom RI, et al: Adult respiratory distress syndrome following thrombolytic therapy for pulmonary embolism. *Chest* 1:151, 1973.

Mitchell JP, Trulock: Tissue-plasminogen activator for pulmonary embolism resulting in shock: Two case reports and discussion of the literature. *Am J Med* 90:255, 1991.

PIOPED Investigators: Value of the ventilation/perfusion scan in acute pulmonary embolism. Results of the prospective investigation of pulmonary embolism diagnosis (PIOPED). *JAMA* 263:2753, 1990.

Sharma GVRK, Burleson VA, et al: Effect of thrombolytic therapy on pulmonary capillary blood volume in patients with pulmonary embolism. *N Engl J Med* 303:842, 1980.

Steenburg RW, Warren R, et al: A new look at pulmonary embolectomy. *Surg Gynecol Obstet* 107:214, 1958.

Urokinase Pulmonary Embolism Trial: A National Cooperative Study. *Circulation* 2(suppl):47, 1973.

Wilson JE III, Bynum LJ, et al: Heparin therapy in venous thromboembolism. *Am J Med* 70:808, 1981.

Varicose Veins and Chronic Venous Insufficiency

Beaglehole R: Epidemiology of varicose veins. *World J Surg* 10:898, 1986.

Bergan JJ, Flin WR, et al: Venous reconstruction surgery. *Surg Clin North Am* 62:399, 1982.

Bernstein EF: Future prospects in the treatment of venous disease. *World J Surg* 10:959, 1986.

Browse ML, Burnard KG: The postphlebitic syndrome: A new look, in Bergon JJ, Yao JST (eds): *Venous Problems*. Chicago, Year Book Medical Publications, 1978.

Calnan JS, Kountz S, et al: Venous obstruction in the aetiology of lympyoedema praecox. *Br Med J* 2:221, 1964.

Cockett FB, Thomas ML: The iliac compression syndrome. *Br J Surg* 52:816, 1965.

Dale WA: Reconstructive venous surgery. *Arch Surg* 114:1312, 1979.

Dale WA: Venous bypass surgery. *Surg Clin North Am* 62:391, 1982.

Hobbs JT: Surgery and sclerotherapy in the treatment of varicose veins: A random trial. *Arch Surg* 109:793, 1974.

Husni EA: Reconstruction of veins: The need for objectivity. *J Cardiovasc Surg* 24:525, 1983.

Keister HW, Bowers RF: Results obtained by superficial femoral vein ligation. *Surgery* 47:224, 1960.

Kistner RL: Surgical repair of the incompetent femoral vein valve. *Arch Surg* 110:1336, 1975.

Kistner RL: Primary venous valve incompetence of the leg. *Am J Surg* 140:218, 1980.

Kistner RL, Sparkuhl RD: Surgery in acute and chronic venous disease. *Surgery* 85:31, 1979.

Kohler TR, Strandness DE Jr: Noninvasive testing for the evaluation of chronic venous disease. *World J Surg* 10:903, 1986.

Kroener JM, Bernstein EF: Valve competence following experimental venous valve autotransplantation. *Arch Surg* 110:1467, 1981.

Ludbrook J: Primary great saphenous varicose veins revisited. *World J Surg* 10:954, 1986.

Norris CS, Beyran A, et al: Quantitative photoplethysmography in chronic venous insufficiency: A new method of noninvasive estimation of ambulatory venous pressure. *Surgery* 94:758, 1983.

Palma EC, Esperon R: Vein transplants and grafts in the surgical treatment of the postphlebitic syndrome. *J Cardiovasc Surg* 1:94, 1960.

Servelle M: Klippel and Trenaunay's syndrome: 768 operated cases. *Ann Surg* 201:365, 1985.

Smith DE: Surgical management of obstructive venous disease of the lower extremity, in Rutherford RB (ed): *Vascular Surgery*, 2d ed. Philadelphia, WB Saunders, 1984, pp 1412–1433.

Smith DE, Trimble C: Surgical management of obstructive venous disease of the lower extremity, in Rutherford RB (ed): *Vascular Surgery*. Philadelphia, WB Saunders, 1977, pp 1247–1268.

Taheri SA, Heffener R, et al: Vein valve transplantation. *Contemp Surg* 22:17, 1983.

Taheri SA, Heffener R, et al: Five years' experience with vein valve transplant. *World J Surg* 10:935, 1986.

Taheri SA, Lazar L, et al: Vein valve transplantation. *Surgery* 1:29, 1982.

Warren R, Thayer TR: Transplantation of the saphenous vein for postphlebitic stasis. *Surgery* 35:867, 1954.

Venous Trauma

Agarwal N, Shah PM, et al: Experience with 115 civilian venous injuries. *J Trauma* 22:827, 1982.

Kudsk KA, Bongard F, et al: Determinants of survival after vena caval injury: Analysis of a 14-year experience. *Arch Surg* 119:1009, 1984.

Malt RA, Remonsnyder JP, et al: Long-term utility of replanted arms. *Ann Surg* 176:334, 1972.

Mathur AP, Pochaczevsky R, et al: Fogarty balloon catheter for removal of catheter fragment in subclavian vein. *JAMA* 217:481, 1971.

Rich NM, Hobson RW II, et al: Repair of lower extremity venous trauma: A more aggressive approach required. *J Trauma* 14:639, 1974.

Richardson JB, Jurkovich GJ, et al: A temporary arteriovenous shunt (Scribner) in the management of traumatic venous injuries of the lower extremity. *J Trauma* 26:503, 1986.

Lymphatics and Lymphedema

Allen EV: Lymphedema of the extremities. Classification, etiology and differential diagnosis: Study of 300 cases. *Arch Intern Med* 54:606, 1934.

Cordeiro AK: Novas tecnias de anastomose linfovenoa para tratamento cirurgico de linfedma de membros inferiores e linfedma de membro superior pos mastectomia. *Maternidade Infuncia* 34:211, 1975.

Degni M: New technique of lymphatic-venous anastomosis for the treatment of lymphedema. *Vasa* 3:479, 1974.

Huntington GS, McClure CFW: The anatomy and development of the jugular lymph sacs in the domestic cat. *Am J Anat* 10:177, 1910.

Kinmonth JB: *The Lymphatics. Diseases, Lymphography and Surgery*. London, Arnold, 1972.

Nielubowicz J, Olszewski W: Surgical lymphaticovenous shunts in patients with secondary lymphedema. *Br J Surg* 55:440, 1968.

O'Brien BM, Das SK, et al: Effect of lymphangiography on lymphedema. *Plast Reconstr Surg* 68:922, 1981.

O'Brien BM, Shafiroff BB: Microlymphaticovenous and resectional surgery in obstructive lymphedema. *World J Surg* 3:3, 1979.

Sabin FR: On the origin of the lymphatic system from the veins and the development of lymph hearts and thoracic duct in the pig. *Am J Anat* 1:367, 1902.

CHAPTER 22

Manifestations of Gastrointestinal Disease

David W. McFadden and Michael J. Zinner

INTRODUCTION

Nearly everyone has experienced a gastrointestinal illness. Whether self-limited like gastroenteritis, or imminently life-threatening as in perforated peptic ulcer or colon cancer, the physical and psychosocial impact can be overwhelming. Recent studies demonstrate a prevalence of severe gastrointestinal symptoms in the elderly that approaches 25 percent, with chronic constipation and abdominal pain predominating. Acute and chronic forms of digestive diseases account for approximately 10 percent of the cost of health care in the United States and over 200,000 deaths per year. Approximately 250,000 people miss work each day because of digestive problems. Digestive diseases account for more hospital admissions in the United States than any other disease category.

Symptoms are the subjective manifestations of a disturbance in function and represent pathophysiologic states, not specific diseases. In the gastrointestinal tract numerous alterations in physiologic function can be implicated, affecting secretion, absorption, motility, synthesis, digestion, and transport. The resultant symptoms include abdominal (or extraabdominal) pain, dysphagia or odynophagia, anorexia, weight loss, nausea and vomiting, bloating or distention, constipation, flatulence, and diarrhea. Signs of disease are the objective demonstrations of a pathologic process. These include tenderness, rigidity, masses, altered bowel sounds, bleeding, malnutrition, jaundice, and stigmata of hepatic dysfunction.

The case history remains one of the most useful tools in the diagnosis of digestive diseases. The surgical consultant should review thoroughly every detail of the illness with the patient. The art of physical examination is also of great importance in the diagnosis of digestive diseases. Combining the elicited symptoms from a complete history and the signs from a comprehensive physical examination allows the surgeon to establish a differential diagnosis and formulate a thorough but cost-effective diagnostic evaluation that may require blood tests, radiographs, and histologic confirmation.

PAIN

Pain, from the Latin *poena,* meaning punishment, penalty, or torment, is the singular sensory experience that humans use to identify disease within themselves, and in whose avoidance lies one of the greatest motivational drives known to man. Most diseases of the abdominal viscera are associated with pain sometime during their course (Table 22-1). A brief review of abdominal embryology and pain physiology will assist the clinician in evaluating the patient with acute or chronic abdominal pain.

The gastrointestinal tract comprises a foregut, midgut, and hindgut. Each segment has its own blood supply and innervation, retaining these relationships throughout development and into adulthood. The foregut extends from the oropharynx to the duodenum at the level of the entrance of the common bile duct, and includes the pancreas, liver, biliary tree, and spleen. The midgut is composed of the distal duodenum, jejunum, ileum, appendix, ascending colon, and proximal two-thirds of the transverse colon. The hindgut consists of the remainder of the colon and rectum down to the cloacal bulge, which constitutes the interface between the surface ectoderm and endoderm of the cloaca, corresponding to the dentate line.

The peritoneum is a continuous membrane with visceral and parietal layers. Although both layers are mesodermally derived, they develop separately. Importantly, and for diagnostic reasons, the nerve supply to each layer is separate. The visceral layer, i.e., the layer surrounding all intraabdominal organs, is supplied by autonomic nerves (sympathetic and parasympathetic), and the parietal peritoneum is supplied by somatic innervation (spinal nerves). The pathways relaying the sensation of pain differ for each layer and differ in quality as well. Visceral pain is characteristically dull, crampy, or aching; parietal pain is sharp, severe, and persistent.

Normal embryologic development of the abdominal viscera proceeds with bilateral midline autonomic innervation, which results in visceral pain usually perceived as arising from the midline. The position of pain in the midline is determined by the embryologic origin of the involved viscus. Epigastric pain is typical of foregut origin. Periumbilical pain signifies pain emanating from the midgut. Hypogastric or lower abdominal midline pain indicates a hindgut origin. Pelvic pain is more typical of disease originating in structures derived from the cloaca.

For abdominal pain to be recognized by the patient, nociceptors, or pain receptors, must be noxiously stimulated. Two types of neuronal fibers are involved. A-delta fibers are rapid transmitters and give rise to sharp, well-localized pain sensations. These fibers are distributed to muscle and skin and are involved with the somatic pain transmission through spinal nerves. C fibers are slow transmitters and generate the sensation of dull, poorly localized pain that is more gradual in its onset and of longer duration. These fibers are located intramurally in hollow viscera and in the capsule of solid organs. They are found in muscle, periosteum, and the parietal peritoneum. These fibers are involved in visceral pain transmission through the autonomic nervous system.

Different neural pathways are responsible for pain mediation, depending on whether the source of the pain is the parietal peritoneum or the visceral peritoneum. The anterior and lateral abdominal walls are supplied by nerves arising from spinal segments T7–L1. The posterior abdominal wall is innervated from spinal seg-

Table 22-1
Gastrointestinal and Intraperitoneal Causes of Abdominal Pain

I. Inflammation/Infection
- *A*. Peritoneum
  1. Chemical and nonbacterial peritonitis—perforated peptic ulcer, gallbladder, ruptured ovarian cyst, mitelschmerz
  2. Bacterial peritonitis
     - *a*. Primary peritonitis—pneumococcal, streptococcal, tuberculous
     - *b*. Perforated hollow viscus—stomach, intestine, biliary tract
- *B*. Hollow intestinal organs
  1. Appendicitis
  2. Cholecystitis
  3. Peptic ulceration
  4. Gastroenteritis
  5. Regional enteritis
  6. Meckel's diverticulitis
  7. Colitis—ulcerative, bacterial, amebic
  8. Diverticulitis
- *C*. Solid viscera
  1. Pancreatitis
  2. Hepatitis
  3. Hepatic abscess
  4. Splenic abscess
- *D*. Mesentery
  1. Lymphadenitis
- *E*. Pelvic organs
  1. Pelvic inflammatory disease
  2. Tuboovarian abscess
  3. Endometritis

II. Mechanical (obstruction, acute distention)
- *A*. Hollow intestinal organs
  1. Intestinal obstruction—adhesions, hernia, tumor, volvulus, intussusception
  2. Biliary obstruction—calculi, tumor, choledochal cyst, hematobilia
- *B*. Solid viscera
  1. Acute splenomegaly
  2. Acute hepatomegaly—cardiac failure, Budd-Chiari syndrome
- *C*. Mesentery
  1. Omental torsion
- *D*. Pelvic organs
  1. Ovarian cyst
  2. Torsion or degeneration of fibroid
  3. Ectopic pregnancy

III. Vascular
- *A*. Intraperitoneal bleeding
  1. Ruptured liver
  2. Ruptured spleen
  3. Ruptured mesentery
  4. Ruptured ectopic pregnancy
  5. Ruptured aortic, splenic, or hepatic aneurysm
- *B*. Ischemia
  1. Mesenteric thrombosis
  2. Hepatic infarction—toxemia, purpura
  3. Splenic infarction
  4. Omental ischemia

IV. Miscellaneous
- *A*. Endometriosis

ments L2–L5. Pain arising from the abdominal wall is relayed to the spinal cord through the spinal nerves. Because these pain fibers enter the spinal cord ipsilaterally, pain is perceived as originating from that side. Also, such pain localizes to the area of the abdomen from which it originates. In contrast, pain arising from intraabdominal viscera is perceived to arise in the midline because sensory input from such viscera enters the spinal cord on both sides.

Abdominal pain can be divided into three categories: visceral, somatic, and referred. The aforementioned intramural sensory receptors of the abdominal organs are responsible for visceral pain. A diverse group of destructive stimuli to the abdominal viscera are painless. For example, almost all abdominal organs are insensitive to pinching, burning, stabbing, cutting, and electrical and thermal stimulation. The same is true for the application of acid and alkali to normal mucosa.

There are four general classes of visceral stimulation that result in abdominal pain. These include stretching and contraction; traction, compression, and torsion; stretch; and certain chemicals. The mediating receptors for these responses are located intramurally in hollow organs, on serosal structures such as the visceral peritoneum and capsule of solid organs, intramesenterically (especially associated with large mesenteric vessels and ligaments), and within the mucosa. These receptors are polymodal, or responsive to both mechanical and chemical stimuli. Mucosal receptors respond primarily to chemical stimulation. The major elicitors of visceral pain arise from geometric forces, such as stretching and distention, that result in increased wall tension. Other factors held responsible for visceral pain include ischemia and inflammation. Visceral pain almost always heralds intraabdominal disease but might not indicate the need for surgical therapy. When visceral pain becomes superseded by somatic pain, surgical intervention becomes likely.

Somatic pain arises from irritation of the parietal peritoneum. Mediated mainly by spinal nerve fibers that supply the abdominal wall, somatic pain is localized and perceived as arising from one of the four quadrants of the abdominal wall. In contrast to visceral pain, where geometric changes are responsible for the stimulation of nerve endings, somatic pain arises as a response to acute changes in pH or temperature, as seen in bacterial or chemical inflammation. In addition, somatic pain is felt in response to sudden increases in pressure, as with a surgical incision. Somatic pain is perceived as sharp and pricking and is usually constant. In many clinical situations it is probable that the perception of pain results from multiple stimuli. The pain of pancreatic cancer probably arises from the combination of serosal stretch, vascular and mesenteric compression, and direct neural infiltration. The sensitivity of visceral receptors is also affected by circumstances. Pressure or chemical application to normal gastric mucosa is usually painless, but if the mucosa is inflamed these same stimuli are quite painful.

Referred pain is felt in an area of the body other than the site of its origin, and is one of the characteristic qualities of abdominal pain. Referred pain usually arises from a deep structure, is superficial at its distant presenting location, and frequently is sharp, localized, and persistent at the distant site. It occurs secondary to the existence of shared central pathways for afferent neurons arising from different sites. Two associated features of referred pain are skin hyperalgesia and increased muscle tone of the abdominal wall. A classic example is the ruptured spleen that results in irritation of the left hemidiaphragm, which is innervated by the same cervical nerves; in this setting, referred pain is perceived as arising in the left shoulder (Kehr's sign), also supplied by those nerve roots. A knowledge of referred pain and its patterns can help diagnostically when other evidence of disease is lacking or absent (Table 22-2).

Table 22-2
Possible Origins for Referred Pain

Right Shoulder	**Left Shoulder**
Diaphragm	Diaphragm
Gallbladder	Spleen
Liver Capsule	Tail of pancreas
Right-sided pneumoperitoneum	Stomach
	Splenic flexure (colon)
	Left-sided pneumoperitoneum
Right Scapula	**Left Scapula**
Gallbladder	Spleen
Biliary tree	Tail of pancreas
Groin/Genitalia	
Kidney	
Ureter	
Aorta/iliac artery	
Back-Midline	
Pancreas	
Duodenum	
Aorta	

Acute Abdominal Pain

Acute abdominal pain is loosely defined as pain present for less than 6 hours. The key to the management of the patient with acute abdominal pain is early diagnosis. No aspect of diagnosis is more important than a careful and thorough history. If possible, it is best to allow the patient to give the entire current history before asking specific questions. This should include a past medical history and information concerning associated illnesses. A history of prior similar symptoms is also sought, as well as the presence of any prodromal symptoms.

The character and onset of the pain are important. Colicky pain usually indicates some type of obstructive process, as in bowel obstruction, passing a ureteral calculus, or acute cholecystitis. Colic represents hyperperistalsis of the smooth muscle in an attempt to move fluid or an object past the obstruction. Between attacks, the pain lessens or disappears. During attacks, the pain is persistent and unrelenting. The pain seen with infectious processes such as appendicitis or diverticulitis is sustained and gradually worsens over time. Clues to the underlying cause of pain can be deduced by the type of onset. Pancreatitis is usually gradual in onset and commonly follows an episode of alcohol abuse. In contrast, a perforated hollow viscus produces a sudden onset of pain that the patient may be able to time precisely. The location of the pain is very helpful in establishing the diagnosis. This is especially true with somatic pain that results from an irritation of the parietal peritoneum (Fig. 22-1).

Other factors must also be considered in the evaluation of the patient with abdominal pain. These include any previous history of intraabdominal disease, previous abdominal surgery, and current medications. Familial or concomitant diseases in family members should also be sought. A woman's precise menstrual history should be obtained because this might be the sole clue to the presence of gynecologic disease.

The first and most important step in the physical examination of the patient with an acute abdominal condition is a careful observation of the patient's body habitus and facial expression. The

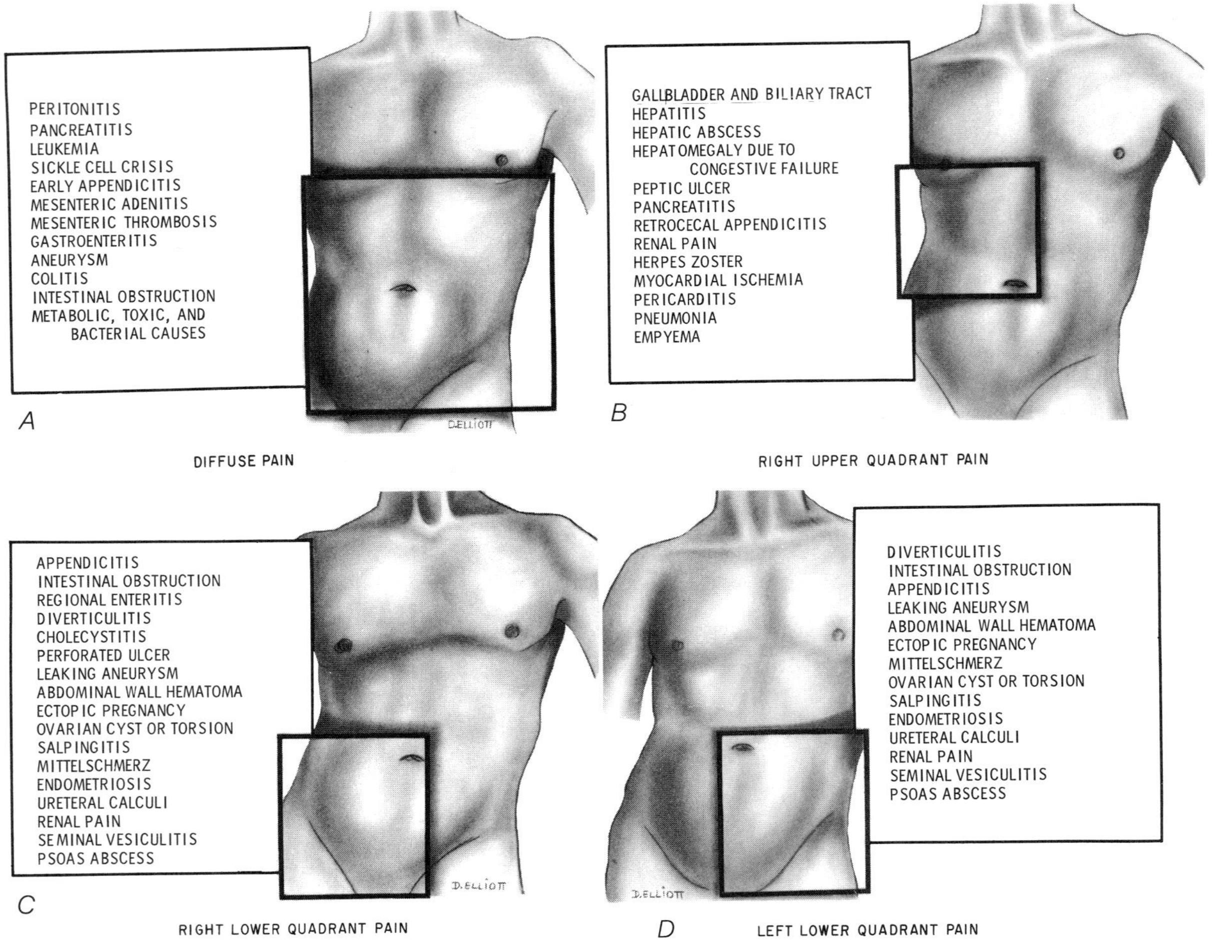

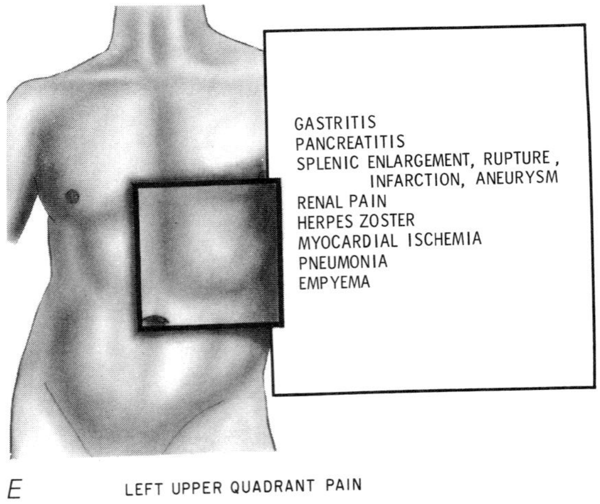

GASTRITIS
PANCREATITIS
SPLENIC ENLARGEMENT, RUPTURE, INFARCTION, ANEURYSM
RENAL PAIN
HERPES ZOSTER
MYOCARDIAL ISCHEMIA
PNEUMONIA
EMPYEMA
E
LEFT UPPER QUADRANT PAIN

FIG. 22-1. Characteristic location of abdominal pain associated with various diseases.

patient's unwillingness to change body position suggests an underlying peritonitis. Hip flexion with the knees drawn up to maintain comfort suggests tension on the abdominal wall and possible peritoneal irritation. Restriction of diaphragmatic excursion with respiration, as noted by shallow breathing and the use of accessory respiratory muscles, is also consistent with peritoneal irritation. By contrast, the presence of colicky pain is frequently manifested by intense movement in an effort to alleviate pain, followed by restful intervals between colicky periods. Inspection of the abdomen for hernial bulges, masses, distention, or areas of inflammation should follow. Careful auscultation of the abdominal cavity for the presence or absence and quality of bowel sounds is performed. The presence and location of bruits should be noted. A careful auscultation of the chest, particularly in the diaphragmatic area, should be undertaken to document diaphragmatic movement and to search for the possibility of a basilar pneumonia that may simulate an acute abdominal condition. Gentle palpation of all quadrants of the abdomen should be performed last. Gentle, rather superficial palpation of the abdomen should be performed initially, proceeding from the quadrant with the least symptomatology to the most painful area. Peritoneal signs or masses, suggested by the superficial exam, can then be confirmed by a deeper, still gentle palpation. Classic rebound tenderness is fraught with examiner error, and a percussion test is kinder and more specific. Having the patient cough, laugh, or maximally distend the abdomen might localize the disease, especially in children. Patients in pain who have been examined by previous unskilled examiners are often quite "sensitized" to the manipulations that are used to elicit rebound. Therefore, a skilled examiner must use diversions to confirm peritonitis. Other techniques, such as using a stethoscope to depress and release the abdomen, the "stethoscope test," are useful. Similarly, shaking the pelvis from side to side may elicit true rebound. Hyperesthesia is uncommonly present but is defined as exquisitely sensitive skin to gentle touch. Hyperesthesia exists because a dermatome is supplied by the same nerve roots as an area of inflamed parietal peritoneum.

Many laboratory tests may offer useful information in the evaluation of the patient with an acute abdominal condition. Minimally, a complete blood count, urinalysis, serum amylase, and, for women with lower abdominal pain, a beta human chorionic gonadotropin or pregnancy test should be requested. Serum electrolytes, blood urea nitrogen, creatinine, and glucose are useful in determining the patient's hydration status, renal function, and basic metabolic state. Liver chemistries are helpful in the patient with upper abdominal pain. In general, laboratory tests should not be performed unless their results could alter the need for additional tests or therapy.

Four radiologic views of the chest and abdomen are essential in the patient without an obvious diagnosis. The physician must be aware of the time and stress of a trip to the radiology suite and assure the stability of the patient's hemodynamic status before this endeavor. An upright and supine film of the abdomen and an upright and lateral radiograph of the chest are then performed. Although only 10 percent of patients with an acute abdominal condition have abnormalities on screening roentgenography, its performance is still suggested unless a clear-cut diagnosis is established. Pneumoperitoneum, gas-fluid levels, fecaliths, gallstones, ascites, and obliteration of the psoas shadows are all helpful diagnostic findings that can be seen on the four screening films. Contrast gastrointestinal studies, ultrasonography, computed axial tomographic scans, and arteriography may all be suggested or required given the findings and clinical suspicions of the evaluating physician.

Numerous surgical causes exist for the patient presenting with acute abdominal pain, and are covered in chapters dealing with the specifics of organ systems. A recent review of over 1100 patients presenting to the emergency ward with abdominal pain revealed that the most common diagnosis was nonspecific abdominal pain, occurring in 35 percent of patients. Appendicitis (17 percent), intestinal obstruction (15 percent), urologic disorders (6 percent), and gallstones (5 percent) were the leading surgical causes. The largest number of admissions occurred in the age groups 10–29 years old (31 percent) and 60–79 years old (29 percent). Surgical procedures were required in 47 percent of patients. The increasing proportion of elderly patients mirrors the rise in the elderly population. Large series of elderly patients presenting with acute abdominal pain have found the leading diagnosis to be cholelithiasis, nonspecific pain, malignancy, incarcerated hernia, ileus, and gastroduodenal ulcer. The presence of comorbid processes, especially cardiovascular disease, stresses the need for rapid diagnosis and timely operation if needed.

Organ systems other than those classically associated within the realm of the alimentary tract must also be considered. Gynecologic causes include pelvic inflammatory disease, ectopic pregnancy, tuboovarian cysts, torsion, hemorrhage, or abscess, and mittelschmerz. Urologic causes include renal, perirenal, or bladder infections, obstructions of the ureter, renal pelvis, or bladder, and acute intrascrotal events. Nonsurgical simulators of acute abdominal conditions include pulmonary, cardiac, neurologic, metabolic, toxic, infectious, and hematologic conditions (Table 22-3).

Acute abdominal pain in the pediatric patient is covered in Chapter 37, but Table 22-4 outlines the differential diagnoses.

Table 22-3
Extraperitoneal Causes of Abdominal Pain

Cardiopulmonary	*Vascular*
Pneumonia	Dissection, rupture, or expansion of aortic aneurysm
Empyema	Periarteritis
Myocardial ischemia	*Metabolic*
Active rheumatic heart disease	Uremia
Blood	Diabetic acidosis
Leukemia	Porphyria
Sickle cell crisis	Addisonian crisis
Neurogenic	*Toxins*
Spinal cord tumors	Bacterial (tetanus)
Osteomyelitis of spine	Insect bites
Tabes dorsalis	Venoms
Herpes zoster	Drugs
Abdominal epilepsy	Lead poisoning
Genitourinary	*Abdominal wall*
Nephritis	Intramuscular hematoma
Pyelitis	*Psychogenic*
Perinephric abscesses	
Ureteral obstruction (calculi, tumors)	
Prostatitis	
Seminal vesiculitis	
Epididymitis	

After cardiac surgery acute abdominal conditions occur in only 1 percent of patients. Abdominal emergencies, however, are responsible for 7 to 10 percent of the total mortality figures in cardiac operations because of their associated 25 to 60 percent mortality figures.

The immunocompromised host comprises a heterogenous group that includes patients receiving allografts, chemotherapy, immunosuppressive drugs for autoimmune disorders, and the patient with the acquired immunodeficiency syndrome (AIDS). Each of these groups has specific abdominal complications that must be appreciated and suspected by the evaluating physician (Table 22-5).

Chronic Abdominal Pain

The patient with chronic abdominal pain remains a common medical and surgical problem. The diagnosis often is elusive despite a variety of investigations. As Hutchinson stated 70 years ago: "In the treatment of the chronic abdomen the most important thing is to catch the patient early. If she has once set her feet on the slippery slope which leads to successive operations she is undone."

The pain pattern in patients with chronic abdominal pain can provide important diagnostic clues. Bouts of pain with entirely normal intervals are usually explained by a discrete intermittent disorder of physiology. Examples include acute intermittent porphyria, internal hernias, endometriosis, and occasionally choledocholithiasis. Chronic abdominal pain that is present most or all of the time is usually due to a clear pathophysiologic abnormality, such as chronic pancreatitis or pancreatic or colonic malignancy. Other cases of chronic abdominal pain may have no specific pathophysiologic abnormality. Nonulcer dyspepsia and irritable bowel syndrome are frequently applied diagnoses—but in reality are diagnoses of exclusion.

Two other sources of chronic abdominal pain should be mentioned. Pain arising from the abdominal wall is frequently misdiagnosed. Specific diagnoses include iatrogenic peripheral nerve injuries, hernias, myofascial pain syndromes, the rib tip syn-

Table 22-4
Differential Diagnoses of Acute Abdominal Conditions in the Pediatric Population

Infants	*Children*	*Adolescents*
Viral enteritis	Meckel's diverticulitis	Pelvic inflammatory disease
Intussusception	Cystitis	Appendicitis
Pyelonephritis	Viral enteritis	Mittelschmerz
Gastroesophageal reflux	Appendicitis	Crohn's disease
Bacterial enterocolitis	Crohn's disease	Pancreatitis
Pneumonitis	Bacterial enterocolitis	Pneumonia
Appendicitis	Pneumonitis	Hematocolpos
Pyloric stenosis	Pancreatitis	Bacterial enterocolitis
Testicular torsion	Ruptured tumors	Viral enteritis
Mesenteric cysts	Poisoning	Peptic ulcer
Ruptured tumors	Pyelonephritis	Poisoning
Pancreatitis	Trauma (child abuse)	Trauma
Meckel's diverticulitis		Ectopic pregnancy
Hirschsprung's disease		Pregnancy
Strangulated hernia		Appendicitis
Poisoning		Cholelithiasis
Trauma (child abuse)		Psychosomatic

drome, abdominal pain of spinal origin, and spontaneous rectus sheath hematoma. Carnett, in 1926, developed a simple test that, when positive, localizes the origin of symptoms to the parietes rather than the viscera. Carnett's test is performed by palpating the abdomen of the supine patient in the usual way. With the palpating fingers located over the tender spot, the patient is asked to contract the abdominal muscles by raising his or her head from the bed. Once the muscles are tensed, pressure is reapplied and the patient is asked if the pain is changed. If the cause of the symptoms is intraabdominal, the tensed muscles should shield the viscera and result in diminished tenderness. On the other hand, if the source resides in the abdominal wall the pain will be worse or no better. Numerous psychiatric disorders are also associated with chronic abdominal pain. Diagnoses include primary affective disorders, somatization disorders, psychogenic (conversion) pain, hypochondriasis, anxiety states, substance abuse disorders, schizophrenia, chronic factitious disorder with physical symptoms (Munchausen syndrome), and malingering.

The control of intractable abdominal pain associated with diseases that cannot be satisfactorily treated is one of the most challenging and frustrating problems the clinician has to face. Examples include unresectable pancreatic carcinoma and chronic pancreatitis. Pharmacologic management, along with behavioral and psychologic therapies, is frequently applied with some success. Neurosurgical and/or chemical ablation techniques may be required in select cases.

Table 22-5
Acute Abdominal Pain in the Immunocompromised Patient

Cytomegalovirus Infection	**Bowel Perforation**
Interstitial pneumonitis	Lymphoma, leukemia (especially after chemotherapy)
Mononucleosis	CMV
Pancreatitis	Colon ulcers
Hepatitis	Kaposi's sarcoma
Cholecystitis	Pseudomembranous Colitis
Gastrointestinal ulceration	Mycobacterial
Neutropenic Enterocolitis	Iatrogenic
Pancreatitis	**Acute Graft vs. Host Disease**
Pentamidine	**Pseudoacute Abdomen**
Steroid	**Fecal Impaction**
Azathioprine	**Standard Abdominal Processes**
CMV	Appendicitis
Hepatitis	Cholecystitis
A, B, C	Diverticulitis
CMV	Bowel obstruction
Epstein-Barr virus	Ulcer disease
Cholecystitis	Pelvic inflammatory disease
CMV	Urinary tract infection
Acalculous	Perirectal abscess
Campylobacter	Lymphadenitis
Hepatosplenic Abscess	
Fungal	
Mycobacterial	
Protozoal	
Splenic rupture	

DYSPHAGIA

Dysphagia, the sensation of swallowed material sticking on its trip from mouth to stomach, is an alarming symptom that demands diagnosis. The symptom of dysphagia originates at either the oropharyngeal or esophageal level. A careful history will supply the diagnosis about 90 percent of the time. Odynophagia, or painful swallowing, is unusual but occurs if esophagitis or diffuse spasm is present. If food becomes impacted above a stricture, pain may result from esophageal contraction.

Normal swallowing is initiated with voluntary pharyngeal contractions pushing food into the hypopharynx, where the upper esophageal sphincter (UES), or cricopharyngeus muscle, relaxes. This permits an involuntary wave of contraction to progress down the normally relaxed esophagus until it reaches the lower esophageal sphincter (LES). The LES relaxes at this juncture, and the contraction wave pushes the bolus into the stomach. In the resting state both the UES and LES are contracted to prevent reflux and aspiration.

The two basic underlying causes of dysphagia are motility disorders and mechanical obstruction. The four basic divisions—mechanical obstruction at the oropharyngeal or esophageal level and motility disorder at the oropharyngeal or esophageal level—have several specific diagnoses (Table 22-6).

Table 22-6
Causes of Esophageal Dysphagia

Cause	*Predominant Sex*	*Age Incidence* 10–45	*Age Incidence* 45 and over	*Salient Historical and Related Characteristics*
Carcinoma	Male	Rare	Common	Duration of symptoms less than 2 years; painful swallowing occurs early, dysphagia later.
Peptic esophagitis	Male	Common	Common	Heartburn for years, often preceding dysphagia; odynophagia later.
Achalasia	Male-female	Common	Common	Liquids, especially cold, cause dysphagia early; regurgitation easy; odynophagia mild and late.
Contractile ring	Male	Rare	Common	Brief, intermittent attacks of dysphagia with no interval symptoms.
Diffuse spasm	Male	Rare	Rare	Affects elderly persons; multiple ringlike contractions along esophageal tube.
Zenker's diverticulum	Male	Rare	Rare	Sticking feeling in neck, gurgling on swallowing; occasional regurgitation of decayed food.
Scleroderma	Female	Common	Rare	Skin changes; Raynaud's disease.
Paraesophageal hiatal hernia	Female	Rare	Rare	Attacks of substernal pressure, pain, dysphagia, and belching during meals.
Extrinsic masses		Common	Rare	Symptoms of primary disorder.

SOURCE: After Ingelfinger, *Med Sci*, Apr. 10, 1960, pp 451–470, with permission.

The basic mechanics of the esophagus were discussed by Edwards more than 20 years ago. A rigid, open tube that passes liquids but not solids suggests early cancer or benign stricture. An elastic tube closed to both solids and liquids that opens with time and the force of gravity suggests achalasia or diffuse spasm. A rigid tube with total obstruction suggests advanced cancer. Pertinent questions to be asked should include the subjective location of where the food sticks. Patients are singularly accurate, and although esophageal dysphagia may be referred proximally, the opposite occurs rarely. The duration of the dysphagia must also be elicited. In general, the longer the duration of dysphagia, the greater the chance of benignancy. The ability to swallow both solids and liquids should be ascertained. At the beginning if dysphagia for both occurred together, a motor disorder is likely; if with solids alone then mechanical obstruction should be suspected. If an initial solids dysphagia progressed to liquids, think malignancy. If the dysphagia is intermittent, consider achalasia, diffuse spasm, or a distal esophageal web (Schatzki's ring). The presence of pain suggests esophagitis, diffuse spasm, or impacted food above a stricture. The association of dysphagia with heartburn or other reflux symptoms should be sought. Difficulty in starting the act of swallowing, or complaint of food refluxing into the nasopharynx, suggests pharyngeal incoordination, which usually arises from neurologic disorders.

Additionally, specific diseases often have specific symptoms. UES dysfunction may present with dysphagia felt in the neck, aspiration, and weight loss if severe. Three percent of patients with gastroesophageal reflux will have UES spasm, which resolves on elimination of the reflux. Zenker's diverticula are suggested by dysphagia, gurgling noises during swallowing, regurgitation of malodorous food, and recurrent aspiration pneumonias. Patients with achalasia frequently drink liquids to push an obstructing food column into the stomach. Nocturnal aspiration and midscapular pain are common. Diffuse esophageal spasm regularly causes pain, which may be located in the lower sternal, epigastric, or midback areas, and is often worsened by stress. Diffuse esophageal spasm may simulate angina pectoris. Schatzki's rings cause intermittent dysphagia, and cold liquids may provoke dysphagia in patients with motor disorders. Dysphagia is also a relatively common manifestation of emotional diseases. Globus hystericus does not cause dysphagia; it is an emotional disorder rendering the constant sensation of a lump in one's throat.

A few tests usually suffice to confirm a working diagnosis. A barium swallow should be the initial step, but cinefluoroscopy should be performed to allow adequate visual documentation of any hypopharyngeal and upper esophageal swallowing abnormalities. A plain chest radiograph can also give clues, as when a large mediastinal air shadow suggests achalasia or hiatal hernia, or irregularities of the air bubble in the upper stomach suggest carcinoma of the cardia. If a stricture is discovered, the next step is esophagoscopy with biopsy. A benign diagnosis with continued clinical suspicion of malignancy mandates repeat biopsy. In most cases the barium radiographs or esophagoscopic results are diagnostic. Motility disorders should be evaluated further by esophageal manometry. Dysphagia lusoria, suggested by a posterior indentation of the upper esophagus, is due to an aberrant origin of the right subclavian or pulmonary artery. Angiography will confirm this rare diagnosis.

Once diagnosed, the dysphagia must be treated. Carcinoma is best treated by resection, benign stricture by dilatation or antireflux procedure. Motility disorders are treated by myotomy and resection of associated diverticula, although achalasia is often amenable to pneumatic dilatation. Schatzki's rings are usually manageable by mercury bougie dilatation. The treatment of the acutely obstructed esophagus is fraught with hazard. Instrumental perforation is common because of the high incidence of associated esophageal disease. A full evaluation of the esophagus must be performed in these patients once the acute obstruction is relieved.

HICCUPS (SINGULTUS)

Hiccups (or singultus) are usually a transient and benign annoyance occasionally experienced by most people but can be quite debilitating if persistent. Hiccups can also be a manifestation of an underlying severe pathologic process. They remain a medical enigma, with no known useful function to the organism. The origin of the word ''singultus'' is believed to be from the Latin *singult,* which means ''the act of attempting to catch one's breath while sobbing.''

The relationship between phrenic nerve irritation and hiccups has been recognized since 1833, and there is now believed to be a hiccup reflex arc. The afferent portion of this arc comprises the phrenic and vagus nerves and the sympathetic chain arising from thoracic segments T6 to T12. The central connection between afferent and efferent limbs of the reflex arc is not ascribable to a specific anatomic location. It appears that the center controlling hiccups is a nonspecific anatomic location between spinal cord segments C3 and C5.

Hiccups have been categorized into those that are benign and self-limited and those causing persistent or intractable episodes; the latter are more likely to result from a serious pathophysiologic process. Benign self-limited hiccups are caused by gastric distention, sudden changes in ambient temperature, alcohol ingestion, and tobacco use. Intractable hiccups are broadly classified as organic, psychogenic, or idiopathic. The organic causes can be divided into central, peripheral, and toxic. The surgeon's interest rests mostly in the peripheral causes arising from either phrenic or vagal nerve stimulation, or direct diaphragmatic stimulation.

Irritation of the vagus nerve anywhere along its course may cause hiccups. In the chest, stimulation may result from trauma, neoplasm, myocardial infarction, pulmonary edema, inflammatory or infectious processes, or intraoperative manipulation of thoracic viscera. Phrenic nerve irritation within the chest caused by intrathoracic inflammation, tumor, infection, or trauma can also lead to hiccups.

A diverse group of abdominal conditions can stimulate the afferent vagal branches. Examples include gastric distention, peptic ulcer disease, pancreatic and biliary disease, bowel obstruction, appendicitis, inflammatory bowel disease, hepatitis, and trauma or intraoperative surgical manipulation. Intraabdominal phrenic nerve stimulation can arise from hiatal hernia, diaphragmatic eventration, subphrenic abscess, perihepatitis, and intraoperative manipulation. Several toxic causes are relevant to the surgeon, including anesthetics and drugs such as intravenous steroids, barbiturates, benzodiazepines, and methyldopa. Metabolic causes include acute alcohol toxicity, uremia, hypocalcemia, and hyponatremia.

The therapies of hiccups are myriad and diverse. Mayo stated in 1932 that ''the amount of knowledge on any subject such as this [hiccups] can be considered as being in inverse proportion to the number of different treatments suggested and tried for it.'' Nonpharmacologic hiccup treatments usually rely on some method of nasopharygeal stimulation and include forcible traction on the tongue, gargling or sipping iced water, swallowing a tablespoon of granulated sugar (the author's favorite), and inhalation of noxious agents (ammonia). Direct pharyngeal stimulation with a rubber catheter is reportedly successful in 90 percent of cases. Pharmacologic treatments include administrating continuous positive-pressure ventilation at 25 to 35 cmH_2O, chlorpromazine, haloperidol, phenytoin, phenobarbital, carbamazepine, and sodium valproate. Other agents sporadically reported in the literature include metoclopramide, amitriptyline, chloral hydrate, and ketamine.

HEARTBURN AND DYSPEPSIA

Heartburn and dyspepsia are very common symptoms that produce considerable irritation and interference in our daily lives. About 10 percent of Americans have daily symptoms referred to as heartburn, and intermittent symptoms are described by one-third of the population. A recent survey revealed the presence of dyspepsia symptoms in 78 percent of the population during the preceding year. Self-medication with over-the-counter antacids is common, of which 80 percent are used for symptoms of heartburn and dyspepsia. The subspecialist in gastroenterology or surgery will see only the minority of patients in whom symptoms have become resistant to nonprescription drugs or in whom complications develop.

Dyspepsia and heartburn are usually manifestations of gastroesophageal reflux or peptic ulcer disease, subjects of separate chapters. Other conditions that have been associated with heartburn and dyspepsia include cholelithiasis, irritable bowel syndrome, and motility disorders or obstructing lesions of the proximal gastrointestinal tract. Almost one-half of affected patients will have dyspeptic symptoms referable to more than one organ system. The link between heartburn and dyspepsia is their postprandial nature and the prosperity of sufferers to seek solace from nonprescription preparations. Another lay description is ''acid indigestion.'' Water brash is occasionally associated with heartburn and dyspepsia. This term, frequently misused, describes the sudden filling of the mouth with clear, slightly salty fluid. The fluid is not regurgitated gastric contents but reflexive salivary gland secretions secondary to acid irritation of the distal esophagus.

Heartburn symptoms are classically offered by the patient as substernal burning sensations that have a tendency to radiate to the mouth. A frequent association with an acid or bitter taste is noted, as well as a tendency to occur within one hour after meals. Aggravation of symptoms by bending over or lying down is common. Regurgitation may occur. Dyspepsia, a more generic term, is a postprandial complaint that includes epigastric distress, nausea, fullness, and bloating.

ANOREXIA

Anorexia is a clinical syndrome characterized by the absence of hunger or appetite. The inappetent state can be secondary to a variety of organic and psychologic disturbances. Since appetite is a central phenomenon, anorexia depends on central effects to produce an appetite loss. Both a feeding center in the lateral hypothalamus and a satiety center in the medial hypothalamus have been demonstrated. Although the stomach plays a minor role, gastric hypofunction, mucosal pallor, and decreases in motility and secretion are described. Numerous gut peptides, colocalized in the central nervous system, have profound effects on feeding and satiety. These peptides, including cholecystokinin, peptide YY, and neuropeptide Y, are currently undergoing extensive evaluation. Nevertheless, the absence of precise pathophysiologic explanations and the variety of disorders associated with anorexia render it of minor diagnostic significance.

Among the organic disorders associated with anorexia are inflammatory processes within the intestinal tract; carcinoma of the stomach, pancreas, liver; hepatitis and alcoholism; advanced liver disease with uremia; congestive heart failure; and various endocrinopathies, including adrenal cortical insufficiency and hyperparathyroidism. Anorexia is virtually always present in cases of acute appendicitis. Although many drugs can cause anorexia, there is no drug that can consistently stimulate an appetite.

Cachexia, defined as anorexia associated with generalized wasting and chronic disease, remains a potentially serious complication, particularly in the cancer patient. A loss of greater than 20 percent of body protein is usually lethal. Supplemental nutrition is not a proven solution as the organism is often unable to utilize the calories effectively. Trials of anabolic β_2-agonists have shown potential in reversing the cancer-induced protein loss in experimental animals.

WEIGHT LOSS

The presenting complaint of unintentional weight loss is a serious one and warrants careful evaluation. Establishing the diagnosis can be a challenge to the physician for several reasons: The patient's complaints may not reflect a true loss of weight; the physician's concern may not be shared by the patient, e.g., eating disorders; the loss may be clinically insignificant; there may be multiple causes; there may be a profound underlying disorder that cannot be found; and the relative roles of biologic and behavioral factors may be difficult to determine. The physician should make several important inquiries. Normal weight variation, which can reach up to 1.5 percent per day, must be assessed. A loss of greater than 5 percent requires investigation. The reported weight loss must be verified, as by change in clothing fit or family corroboration. The time frame of the weight loss and its involuntary nature must be determined. The contributing factors must be sought. Decreased intake, an increased metabolic rate, or catabolic state, incomplete absorption or malabsorption, and psychosocial factors must be clarified.

Studies of patients with weight loss have allowed the formulation of several general conclusions. In most series, the causes of weight loss, usually cancer or gastrointestinal disease, were established within a few months and abnormal signs and laboratory studies were evident on the first visit. Second, a wide variety of gastrointestinal causes were found, too many, in fact, to allow statistical evaluation. Third, about 25 percent of patients remained undiagnosed, despite intensive evaluation. Finally, about 10 percent of all patients were found to have psychologic causes for their weight loss.

Certain medical conditions are associated with chronic weight loss, including endocrine/metabolic disorders (thyrotoxicosis, diabetes mellitus, Addison's disease), chronic infections (tuberculosis, fungal infections, subacute bacterial endocarditis), occult malignancy, and immune disorders. Physiologic changes in weight loss may occur in the elderly, but pathologic causes are common and often multidetermined.

Presumptive gastrointestinal causes can be established from a complete medical history. The relationship of symptoms to meals can be useful, especially as to the presence and location of gastrointestinal obstruction. Obstruction is usually associated with symptomatic worsening after meals. Relief of symptoms after vomiting is also suggestive of an obstructing lesion. Pain from a pancreatic or biliary source often worsens after eating because of the induction of digestive enzyme secretion or muscular contraction. Pancreatic and biliary symptoms are not usually relieved by vomiting. Weight loss associated with ingestion of normal or large quantities of food implies malabsorption, hyperthyroidism, cancer, or diabetes mellitus. The production of voluminous, foul-smelling, oily stools suggests fat malabsorption from pancreatic or intestinal disease. The discriminating value of these symptoms decreases over time as patients decrease their food intake to avoid pain (sitophobia) or diarrhea, or because of associated depressive symptoms. These findings are classically illustrated in the elderly patient with chronic mesenteric ischemia and intestinal angina.

NAUSEA AND VOMITING

Nausea and vomiting are commonly associated complaints that can occur separately. The differential diagnosis is extensive, ranging from addisonian crisis to Zollinger-Ellison syndrome. Nausea usually refers to the feeling of an impending desire to vomit, a formidable sensation with many stimuli and numerous neurologic pathways. Vomiting is defined as the forceful expulsion of gastrointestinal contents through the mouth, usually preceded by nausea. The act of vomiting is complex and involves a series of interactions between the gut and the central nervous system. The latter contains the "vomiting center," located in the reticular formation, the chemoreceptor trigger zone (CTZ) in the area postrema of the fourth ventricle, and various visceral afferent and efferent connections. The vomiting act involves forceful contraction of the abdominal wall musculature, antral and pyloric contraction, elevation of the gastric cardia, decreased lower esophageal sphincter (LES) pressure, and esophageal dilatation. Vomiting is a well-coordinated act that is distinguished from simple regurgitation, which is usually the result of gravity or pressure differences between the abdominal and thoracic cavities. Regurgitation is common in patients with incompetent LES, Zenker's diverticula, and benign peptic stricture. Regurgitation associated with dysphagia mandates a thorough esophageal evaluation.

The relationship of meals to vomiting is of diagnostic significance. Patients with gastric outlet obstruction or gastric atony will usually complain of vomiting several hours postprandially. Patients who vomit from viral gastroenteritis or psychogenic causes are generally symptomatic in the immediate postprandial period. The symptomatic interval can be an important diagnostic point. An acute onset of symptoms in a previously well person usually indicates an infectious or toxin-related agent. Viral gastroenteritis is the most common gastrointestinal disease in the United States, and some viruses, such as the Norwalk and Hawaii viruses, impair gastric motility. Except for nontyphoid salmonellosis, vomiting is rarely associated with bacterial enteric pathogens.

Extragastrointestinal disorders are capable of producing an acute onset of nausea and vomiting. In most cases symptoms are mediated through afferent connections to the central vomiting center. Visceral pain associated with ischemia, colic, or inflammation often stimulates vomiting. Viral hepatitis causes vomiting through an unknown mechanism. Vestibular disturbances cause symptoms via central pathways. A number of metabolic derangements, such as addisonian crisis, uremia, and diabetic ketoacidosis, induce vomiting via the CTZ. Acute small-bowel obstruction due to jejunal volvulus, internal herniation, and intestinal ischemia often stimulates an immediate nausea with vomiting. Surgical patients may have postoperative nausea and vomiting because of the frequent administration of narcotics for pain relief. The acute onset of nausea and vomiting can be elicited by drugs via a local effect on the gut (erythromycin) or via central mechanisms (morphine, cardiac glycosides, chemotherapeutic agents). Erythromycin, possibly acting as an agonist of the hormone motilin, has recently been used as a prokinetic drug in gastric emptying disorders. A careful drug history often identifies the offending agent.

Chronic nausea and vomiting (symptoms longer than one week) are more difficult to diagnose and evaluate. The course of chronically affected patients is often complicated by weight loss, malnutrition, and the metabolic disturbances of hyponatremia, hypokalemia, and metabolic alkalosis. Mechanical obstruction, including benign or malignant causes of gastric outlet obstruction, must be ruled out initially. In this situation, the classic historical finding is the vomiting of undigested food particles up to 12 hours after eating. At times a succussion splash is noted on physical examination. Vomiting associated with bowel obstruction is associated with crampy pain, obstipation, and abdominal distention. Plain abdominal radiographs aid in diagnostic differentiation.

Motility disorders are another major category of diseases that induce chronic nausea and vomiting. Gastroparesis is a motility disorder that complicates several disease states, including diabetes mellitus, gastroesophageal reflux, achlorhydria, and postgastric surgery. In the diabetic patient, the motility disorder called gastroparesis diabeticorum is associated with chronic insulin dependence and peripheral neuropathy and may represent a vagal neuropathy. Upper gastrointestinal tract symptoms can also complicate the course of irritable bowel syndrome (IBS). Idiopathic stasis syndromes are characterized by intractable nausea, vomiting, bloating, early satiety, and bezoar formation. Chronic intestinal pseudoobstruction is another group of disorders that can result in chronic nausea and vomiting. Primary pseudoobstruction may have associated abnormalities in the gut smooth muscle and myenteric plexus. Secondary causes are legion, and include collagen vascular diseases (scleroderma), amyloidosis, primary muscle disease, various endocrine (hypothyroidism) and neurologic disorders, and drugs (amitriptyline, clonidine). Drug-induced gastric stasis can result in chronic nausea and vomiting. Gastric retention has been associated with anticholinergics, β-adrenergic agonists, opiates, tricyclic antidepressants, diphenylhydramine, and aluminum-containing antacids.

Miscellaneous causes of nausea and vomiting include pregnancy (especially the first 14 to 16 weeks of gestation), increased intraabdominal pressure, and psychogenic causes. Hyperemesis gravidarum is a serious vomiting disorder of early pregnancy, frequently requiring hospitalization for intravenous hydration and nutrition. Psychogenic vomiting patients are usually female, with chronic postprandial vomiting without a significant component of nausea. These patients are usually remarkably unconcerned about their disorder and are brought to physicians by concerned families or friends.

Depending on its intensity and duration, vomiting may produce hypovolemia, hypokalemia, acid-base disturbances, and the consequences of starvation. Vomitus, without admixture of ingested food, is isoosmotic with extracellular fluid and contains an elevated concentration of hydrogen ion. The plasma bicarbonate rises along with depletion of total body chloride, potassium, and sodium. With protracted vomiting, the alkalosis becomes profound and there are resultant hypovolemia and malnutrition. Therapy should be instituted early by correcting relatively minor defects, since advanced deficiencies are critical and difficult to reverse. Therapeutic efforts are directed at the underlying pathophysiologic process. Phenothiazines, acting as dopamine antagonists in the CTZ, are commonly used but have frequent extrapyramidal side effects. Metoclopramide, a dopamine antagonist with cholinomimetic effects, has a variety of actions on the central nervous system and the gastrointestinal tract. Other cholinomimetics, such as bethanecol, are occasionally helpful. Cisapride and domperidone are newer experimental agents that act as dopamine or serotonin antagonists and may have therapeutic potential.

GAS AND BLOATING

Excessive gas production is a common presenting complaint for which patients seek medical advice. Cramps, bloating, chest pain, audible bowel sounds, nausea, anorexia, dyspepsia, belching, and flatulence are some of the components. Researchers have documented an increased sensitivity to intestinal stretch and/or the presence of abnormal upper gastrointestinal motility in "gassy" patients rather than an increased gas volume. Abnormal motility of the esophagus, stomach, small intestine, and colon have all been identified, suggesting a generalized motor dysfunction in certain patients.

Abdominal pain and bloating are often attributed to too much gas. Maldigestion (lactase deficiency) may contribute in some cases; in others, the cause is unclear. Other organic causes must be sought, such as regional enteritis, recurrent small bowel obstruction, or giardiasis. Evaluation may require upper gastrointestinal and small bowel barium studies, as well as stool examination for bacterial pathogens and ova and parasites.

Belching is the retrograde passage of esophageal or gastric gas across the upper esophageal sphincter and out the oral cavity. It is initiated by LES relaxation with formation of an esophagogastric chamber of equal pressures. The upper esophageal sphincter then relaxes, allowing reflux of esophageal gas. Involuntary belching, or eructation, following a meal is normal and beneficial due to the swallowed air associated with chewing and eating. Certain foods, such as onions, tomatoes, and mints, facilitate this phenomenon. The majority of upper gastrointestinal air accumulates secondary to aerophagia, especially during eating, drinking, gum chewing, smoking, oral irritation, or nervousness.

Chronic belching is invariably a voluntary phenomenon. Commonly, discomfort from a chronic disorder of the chest or upper abdomen, such as cholelithiasis, peptic ulcer disease, or GER is thought to be partially relieved by eructation. These patients are frequently anxious, and belching becomes habitual and regarded as indicative of digestive problems. The inability to belch may occur in patients who have had fundoplication procedures ("gas-bloat syndrome") for GER. Slow improvement with time is the rule.

The hepatic and splenic flexure syndromes are believed to be caused by the trapping of gas at the colonic flexures with resultant distention of the colonic segment and upper abdominal or thoracic discomfort. Pain can be referred to the chest, shoulder, or neck because of diaphragmatic irritation, and not a few patients have undergone cardiac catheterization for this condition. Many patients are constipated and have emotional disturbances. Symptomatic relief is obtained by defecation or enemas during the attack, and chronic therapy involves relieving the associated constipation.

FLATULENCE

Gas is normally present in the gastrointestinal tract. The complaint of gas has no single connotation, as patients may use it to denote too much belching, abdominal discomfort, or excessive flatulence. The intestines of normal individuals usually contain less than 200 mL of gas at any given time, and the excretion of gas per rectum averages 600 mL per day. Frequent passage of gas per rectum is a disturbing symptom for patients, but rarely is an indicator of serious disease. Studies of young men have found that flatus is passed an average of 14 times per day, with less than 25 being normal. Nitrogen, oxygen, carbon dioxide, and methane compose 99 percent of intestinal gas. Their proportions vary widely, but all four gases are odorless. The characteristic odor of flatus is conferred by a combination of trace gases (ammonia, hydrogen sulfide, volatile amino acids, short-chain fatty acids), which together constitute no more than 1 percent of the total volume of intestinal gas. Swallowed air is the major source of nitrogen and oxygen. Carbon dioxide derives largely from bacterial action on intestinal substrates, which also leads to hydrogen and, in one-third of adults, methane.

Excessive flatulence is difficult to quantitate, but usually results from increased amounts of swallowed air, disorders of intestinal motility, or the altered metabolism of intestinal substrates by intestinal bacteria, of which lactase deficiency is a classic example. A specific search for specific inciting foods should always be performed. Treatments usually involve counseling for air swallowers, elimination of milk, legumes, cabbage, and similar foods, and reassurance. Fiber products may increase flatus because of their propensity for containing nondigestible substrates. If bacterial overgrowth is suspected, a trial of tetracycline or metronidazole for two weeks is usually effective. Several agents have been used to bind or alter intestinal gas, including activated charcoal and simethicone.

CONSTIPATION

Alterations in bowel habits can be related to food ingestion, psychologic disorders, or lesions in the gastrointestinal tract. Intestinal transit is a complicated sequence of neuromuscular and hormonally controlled events. The healthy human stomach is emptied within 3 to 4 hours, and passage through the small intestine occurs at an average rate of 1 inch per minute, or 22 feet in about 4 hours. Ileal effluent is semiliquid, and most colonic water absorption occurs within the cecum and ascending colon. The normal colon absorbs over 1300 mL of the 1500 mL of ileal effluent presented each day, resulting in a stool that remains about 70 percent water. The intensity and frequency of muscular contractions increase aborally, and mass peristalsis carries the bolus from the hepatic flexure onward. Some food products are eliminated within 24 hours, but the majority require several days.

The fecal bolus normally does not pass from the sigmoid into the rectum until defecation is about to occur, brought about by powerful peristaltic waves concurrent with smooth muscle relaxation at the rectosigmoid junction. Distention of the rectum starts afferent nervous impulses conducted via hypogastric and pelvic nerves to the sacral spinal cord where efferent impulses are generated. Defecation can be entirely involuntary, but is usually assisted by voluntary contractions of the abdominal and diaphragmatic muscles, as well as relaxation of the external sphincter. The entire colon, distal to the splenic flexure, is usually emptied. The vagi, splanchnics, and pelvic nerves play a significant role, with the intrinsic myenteric reflexes as the prime movers. Parasympathetic tone augments intestinal motility, whereas sympathetic activity inhibits it, as in the case of reflex ileus.

The external anal sphincter is a voluntary muscle that receives neural input from the gray matter of the conus terminalis, where the defecatory reflex is located. This medullary center has been suggested as a factor in defecatory control, as central nervous system influences can cause either diarrhea or constipation. Chemicals are also capable of influencing defecation, including the cholinergic agents, serotonin, guanethidine, caffeine, nicotine, vasopressin, and potassium, all of which can stimulate intestinal motility. Atropine, morphine, and codeine are capable of inhibiting motility.

Constipation and diarrhea are two of the most frequent manifestations of digestive disorders, and may portend conditions that require surgical intervention. Constipation is much more likely to arise from a surgical condition. The costs of constipation are formidable, especially if one considers the over $400 million spent on laxatives each year in the United States. Data do not exist concerning the additional costs generated by its evaluation, surgery, and time lost from work. Constipation is a difficult term to define, since there is wide diversity in bowel habits. Clinically, a movement that is soft and easy to pass, with a frequency ranging from three per day to one every three days is normal. A patient whose bowel function falls outside these limits, and certainly the patient with a change in bowel habits, deserves evaluation. In the United States, the average daily fiber consumption is 19 grams, and stool weight is between 100 and 200 grams per day. Contrast this to rural Africa, where the average figures are 75 grams and 470 grams, respectively.

The history is important, but often requires a daily record to be kept by the patient for adequate information. The age of onset may suggest congenital causes (Hirschsprung's disease) or an acquired problem. A thorough medical history can identify an associated medical condition, and medications and previous operations must be reviewed. The physical exam must be thorough and focused on the abdomen, perineum, pelvis, and rectum. The presence of fecal soilage should be evaluated by inspecting the patient's undergarments. Resting and contracted anal tone should be evaluated, and perineal descent should be sought for, followed by anal sensitivity and reflex evaluation. Anoscopy and proctosigmoidoscopy are then performed. Constipation can then be classified as in Table 22-7.

Acute constipation is most commonly caused by small or large bowel obstruction. The classic associated findings of distention, nausea and vomiting, and obstipation should alert the examiner to these causes. Colonic pseudoobstruction, or Ogilvie's syndrome, is another important cause. These patients are usually in-hospital, immobile, and many have had recent extraabdominal surgery. Additionally, patients with acute anal disease, such as fissure, abscess, and thrombosed external hemorrhoids, will consciously avoid defecation because of the associated pain. A vicious circle is precipitated by this behavior.

Chronic constipation is a poorly understood, multifactorial complaint frequently seen by the primary care provider, gastroenterologist, and surgeon. Colonic dysmotility, or slow transit constipation, is an idiopathic colonic motility disorder that affects young women. Histologically the colons are normal. The causation has been variously ascribed to deficient rectal sensation (no call to defecate), myenteric plexus abnormalities, laxative abuse, psychosexual pathology, and reduced stool volumes. Bloating and abdominal pain are often worsened by bulk laxatives or fiber. One variety is constipation-predominant irritable bowel syndrome; a history of alternating diarrhea may point to this diagnosis.

Abnormal, or disordered, defecation results from failure of the striated muscles of the pelvic floor to relax on straining (anismus), failure of the internal sphincter to relax on rectal distention (Hirschsprung's disease), pelvic floor laxity (descending perineum syndrome), rectal intussusception (occult rectal prolapse), com-

Table 22-7
Causes of Constipation

Mechanical	
Obstructive	Structural
Neoplasm	Ileus
Hernia	Acute anorectal conditions
Volvulus	Rectal polapse
Adhesive	Endometriosis
Postsurgical abnormalities	Rectocele
Inflammatory bowel disease	Aganglionosis
Enteroliths	Irritable bowel syndrome
Diverticular disease	Chagas' disease
Stricture	Neurofibromatosis
Small bowel obstruction	Inadequate fiber
Abscess	
Ogilvie's syndrome	
Metabolic/Endocrine/Neurologic	
Hypothyroidism	Amyloidosis
Hypercalcemia	Scleroderma
Hypokalemia	Multiple sclerosis
Porphyria	Parkinson's disease
Glucagonoma	Cauda equina tumor
Somatostatinoma	Stroke
Pheochromocytoma	Paraplegia
Pregnancy	Collagen vascular disease
Uremia	Psychologic
MEN IIa	Psychiatric
Panhypopituitarism	Anorexia nervosa
Drug Effects	
Narcotics	Calcium channel blockers
Aluminum (antacids)	Barium sulfate
Psychotropic agents	Diuretics
Ganglionic blockers	Iron supplements
Calcium (antacids, supplements)	Antihypertensives
Sucralfate	Vinca alkaloids
Anticholinergics	Metal intoxication (mercury, lead, arsenic)
Antidepressants	Antispasmodics

plete rectal prolapse (procidentia), anterior rectal herniation (rectocele), posterior rectal herniation, and deficient or ignored rectal sensation. Of these, only Hirschsprung's disease and complete rectal prolapse have well-characterized pathophysiology and defined surgical roles. Specialized evaluative procedures include colon transit studies and pelvic floor evaluation by electromyography, scintigraphic balloon topography, scintigraphy, balloon expulsion, external measurement of perineal descent, and defecating proctography. Treatment options are then discussed on a per diagnosis basis.

DIARRHEA

Diarrhea is defined as an increase in volume, frequency, or fluidity of stool output. The daily stool weight is greater than the average of 200 grams, secondary to an increase in stool water above the normal content of 60 to 75 percent. There may also exist an alteration in stool solids. Diarrhea is a worldwide health problem, as each year more than 5 million people die of acute infectious diarrhea. Of these deaths, 80 percent occur in children under one year of age. The severity of diarrheal illness is primarily due to the enormous secretory capacity of the intestinal tract. All gut segments, from the proximal duodenum to the rectum, are capable of secreting water and electrolytes. Adults infected with cholera can excrete greater than a liter of fluid per hour for several days when adequately rehydrated.

Most people experience diarrheal episodes that last for a few hours to a few days, and whose symptoms resolve spontaneously. Diarrhea acquires greater clinical significance if it persists for more than two weeks, or if a pattern of recurrent, acute episodes becomes established. Of particular surgical importance are episodes of diarrhea that are associated with abdominal pain or gastrointestinal blood loss. Table 22-8 lists some of the causes of diarrhea of interest to the surgeon.

There are four major pathophysiologic mechanisms that lead to an excessive loss of fecal water, or diarrhea: osmotic retention of intraluminal water, luminal secretion of solute and/or water, exudation, and disordered contact between chyme and the absorptive surface. These mechanisms are not mutually exclusive, and more than one mechanism is usually involved. Osmotic diarrhea occurs when poorly absorbed water-soluble moieties are retained, leading to excessive water within the lumen. Examples include lactase deficiency with poorly absorbed sugars, and overusage of saline laxatives or antacids.

Secretory diarrhea results from the stimulation of enteric or colonic mucosa to secrete rather than absorb fluid. This usually occurs at the cellular level where absorptive machinery is turned off and/or secretory mechanisms are turned on. A diverse group of stimuli, or secretagogues, exist and include steatorrhea, wherein fatty acids stimulate the colon and small bowel; ileal resection, by dihydroxy bile acids; islet cell tumors, by vasoactive intestinal peptide as well as other peptides; carcinoid tumors, by serotonin and substance P; medullary thyroid cancer, by calcitonin; toxigenic bacteria (*E. coli, V. cholera,* and others), by enterotoxins; and by laxative abuse, as in anthraquinone cathartics. Whatever the cause, the secretions have a composition similar to extracellular fluid. Infectious diarrheas have been the most studied because of their world health impact.

Enteric organisms cause diarrhea in several ways. Some are noninvasive but secrete toxins that stimulate fluid secretion from intestinal epithelial cells (*V. cholera* species). Others invade and destroy intestinal epithelial cells, thereby altering fluid transport. Selective destruction of enteric villus cells by enteric viruses leaves the secretory crypt portion unopposed. Some enteric organisms are both invasive and toxigenic (*Shigella* species). Others bypass the enterocyte to penetrate the epithelium, and elicit an inflammatory response by interacting with white blood cells in the lamina propria (*Salmonella* species). Others adhere to the luminal surface of the enterocyte, often with cellular membrane fusion, to inject a cytotoxin (*E. coli,* cryptosporidia). Various strains of *E. coli* make use of each of these mechanisms.

Exudative diarrhea results from the copious luminal release of serum proteins, blood, or mucus from sites of inflammation, ulceration, or infiltration. Inflammatory bowel disease, parasitic and bacterial infestations (amebae, salmonellae), and infiltrative disorders (lymphoma, Whipple's disease) can produce diarrhea by this mechanism.

Disordered contact between chyme and the absorptive surface may be secondary to many causes. Abnormal intestinal transit is well described after bowel resection or bypass and in motility disorders. Altered exposure times can impair mixing and shorten contact times necessary for complete digestion. Slowed transit may lead to stasis with bacterial overgrowth, stimulating malabsorption

Table 22-8
Causes of Diarrhea

- Functional enterocolonic disease
    - Mucous colitis
- Organic colonic disease
    - Ulcerative colitis
    - Crohn's colitis
    - Diverticulitis
    - Neoplastic lesions
        - Polyposis
        - Villous adenoma
        - Carcinoma
    - Fecal impaction
    - Lymphogranuloma venereum
    - Endometriosis
    - Toxic colitis
        - Arsenic
        - Mercury
        - Alcohol
- Small intestinal disease
    - Crohn's disease
    - Tuberculous enteritis
    - Malabsorption due to disease
        - Sprue
        - Carcinoid
        - Intestinal lipodystrophy
    - Malabsorption due to mechanical defects
        - Short gut syndrome
        - Blind loop syndrome
        - Fistulas
- Gastric factors
    - Hyperchlorhydria
        - Zollinger-Ellison syndrome
    - Postsurgical problems
        - Dumping syndrome
        - Afferent loop syndrome
        - Gastrojejunocolic fistula
        - Inadvertent gastroileostomy
        - Postvagotomy diarrhea
- Disorders of the solid viscera
    - Pancreatic insufficiency
    - Biliary fistula
    - Watery diarrhea syndrome (VIPoma)
- Enteric infections
    - *Salmonella*
    - *Shigella*
    - Pseudomembranous colitis
- Parasitic infestations
    - Amebiasis
    - Leishmaniasis
    - Ascariasis
    - Liver flukes
    - Schistosomiasis
    - Trichinosis
- Metabolic disorders
    - Thyroid
        - Thyrotoxicosis
        - Medullary carcinoma—calcitonin
    - Hyperparathyroidism
    - Uremia
    - Diabetes mellitus
    - Addison's disease
- Drugs
    - Cathartics
    - Sympatholytic
        - Propranolol
    - Parasympathomimetic
        - Urecholine
        - Neostigmine
        - Acetylcholine

and diarrhea. The so-called nervous diarrhea and irritable bowel syndrome may involve abnormal motility and rapid transit. A complete medication history is essential for the evaluation of the patient with diarrhea, as many drugs can have this symptom as a side effect.

The consequences of diarrhea depend on its severity, cause, and duration. Severe or protracted diarrhea results in fluid and electrolyte loss, hypovolemia, acidosis, and death if there is an inability to replenish the patient. Acidosis may result from the high bicarbonate content in the stool, or it may be related to acid production secondary to starvation or the dehydration compromising renal function.

The evaluation of the patient presenting with diarrhea should include a thorough history to elicit the duration, time of day, description of stool, presence of associated pain and urgency, and the findings of associated symptoms such as fever, nausea, vomiting, and anorexia. A family history of diarrhea, an outbreak in the community of diarrhea, or a history of recent travel points to an infectious cause. Diarrhea that alternates with constipation may occur with colonic lesions such as cancer, diverticulitis, partial obstructions, and chronic laxative abuse. Some variants of irritable bowel syndrome may also have this cyclic bowel activity. Recurrent episodes implicate ulcerative colitis, psychogenic causes, or amebic colitis. Ulcerative colitis can be associated with bloody stools and systemic toxicity. Large, pale, bulky, oily stools suggest pancreatic insufficiency. A pronounced mucous component to the stool suggests ulcerative colitis, colonic carcinoma, or villous adenoma. Pain can be a component with ulcerative colitis, diverticulitis, and occasionally carcinoma. Tenesmus is seen with ulcerative colitis, rectal cancer, and lymphogranuloma venereum. Anorexia, nausea, or vomiting is seen in malignancy, ulcerative colitis, and severe bacillary or amebic dysentery.

The physical exam might be negative and suggestive of a functional origin of the diarrhea. The presence of a mass, ascites, hepatomegaly, or other signs may provide clues to the origin of the diarrhea. Systemic diseases (scleroderma, Addison's disease, hyperthyroidism) may be suspected by specific physical signs. Visual inspection of the anal orifice followed by a digital rectal examination may disclose perianal fistulas (Crohn's disease), reveal a rectal mass, or identify a stricture. Anoscopy is then performed with a careful mucosal inspection for loss of vascularity (chronic ulcerative colitis) or for inflammation, granularity, ulceration, tumors, and hemorrhoids. Stool obtained should be tested for blood, qualitative fat, and leukocytes. Microscopic examination for ova and parasites is particularly pertinent for the diagnosis of infestations. The initial visit should also include proctosigmoidoscopy and blood studies (complete blood count, serum calcium, iron, protein, glucose, electrolytes, and prothrombin time). Depending on the results of these tests, barium enema or full colonoscopy should be performed. Tests for malabsorption, especially fecal fat, should then be chosen if malabsorption remains a significant differential diagnosis.

Specific diarrheas of interest to the surgeon include steatorrhea (pancreatic insufficiency, cystic fibrosis, hepatic disease); inflammatory bowel disease; diarrhea due to medications (chemotherapy, antacids, antibiotics, alcohol); intestinal obstruction; vascular disease; carcinoid syndrome; Zollinger-Ellison syndrome; endocrine tumors, including those that secrete VIP, glucagon, somatostatin, calcitonin, and substance P; and ileostomy diarrhea. The Zollinger-Ellison syndrome produces diarrhea as an initial presenting complaint in 8 percent of cases, and severe diarrhea is a complaint in 20 percent of patients overall. The diarrhea results from the hypersecretion of acid-rich fluid into the small intestine. An easy way to confirm the origin of this diarrhea is by placement of a nasogastric tube, with resultant cessation of the diarrhea.

Numerous antidiarrheal drugs have been tried with variable efficacies. Opiate drugs include codeine, atropine with diphenoxylate, paregoric, and loperamide. Absorbent drugs include Kaopectate and aluminum hydroxide. Bismuth subsalicylate (Pepto-Bismol) blocks the secretory effects of some *V. cholera, E. coli,* and *Shigella* species. Antimicrobials are effective against specific organisms. Newer agents include alpha$_2$-adrenergic agonists (clonidine), somatostatin, prostaglandin synthase inhibitors (indomethacin), calcium channel blockers (verapamil), enkephalins, lithium, and certain weak oral organic acids (nicotinic acid).

OBSTRUCTION

Intestinal obstruction is present when there exists an interference with the normal aboral transit of intestinal contents. Such obstruction can result from extraluminal (adhesions), intraluminal (bezoar, gallstones), or intramural (Crohn's disease) processes. The term *mechanical* bowel obstruction is used to describe an actual physical barrier, whereas *ileus* denotes a functional failure of progressive intestinal transit. Obstruction of the small intestine accounts for 20 percent of all acute surgical admissions and constitutes one of the most common indications for emergency intervention. An estimated 9000 deaths per year occur in the United States from small bowel obstruction.

The classification of intestinal obstruction on clinical and pathologic grounds is required. Simple obstruction refers to an obstructed lumen with an intact blood supply. If the mesenteric vessels are occluded, then strangulated obstruction is present. Finally, closed-loop obstruction results when both limbs of the loop are obstructed. Obstruction is additionally classified as partial or complete, acute or chronic, high or low, and small intestinal versus colonic (Table 22-9).

Table 22-9
Mechanisms of Intestinal Obstructions

- Mechanical obstruction of the lumen
  - Obturation of the lumen
    - Meconium
    - Intussusception
    - Gallstones
    - Impactions—fecal, barium, bezoar, worms
  - Lesions of bowel
    - Congenital
      - Atresia and stenosis
      - Imperforate anus
      - Duplications
      - Meckel's diverticulum
    - Traumatic
    - Inflammatory
      - Regional enteritis
      - Diverticulitis
      - Chronic ulcerative colitis
    - Neoplastic
    - Miscellaneous
      - K^+-induced stricture
      - Radiation stricture
      - Endometriosis
  - Lesions extrinsic to bowel
    - Adhesive band constriction or angulation by adhesion
    - Hernia and wound dehiscence
    - Extrinsic masses
      - Annular pancreas
      - Anomalous vessels
      - Abscesses and hematomas
      - Neoplasms
  - Volvulus
- Inadequate propulsive motility
  - Neuromuscular defects
    - Megacolon
    - Paralytic ileus
      - Abdominal causes
        - Intestinal distention
        - Peritonitis
        - Retroperitoneal lesions
      - Systemic causes
        - Electrolyte imbalance
        - Toxemias
    - Spastic ileus
  - Vascular occlusion
    - Arterial
    - Venous

Obstruction of the small bowel is most commonly due to postoperative adhesions (64 to 79 percent), hernias (15 to 25 percent), and malignant tumors (10 to 15 percent). Intussusception, inflammatory bowel disease, and miscellaneous causes make up the rest. The order of frequency differs for age groups, with hernias more common in the young and previously unoperated on patient. Colonic obstruction usually arises from cancer (60 percent), diverticulitis (15 percent), or volvulus (15 percent). Nearly one-fourth of all patients with colorectal cancer will present with colonic obstruction. In the early part of this century, the mortality from bowel obstruction was greater than 50 percent but is now less than 10 percent, based primarily on a better understanding of fluid and electrolyte therapy, gastrointestinal decompression, and antibiotics.

Simple mechanical obstruction results in an accumulation of succus entericus above the obstruction, deranged motility, and systemic derangements. The volume of fluid that accumulates above the obstruction is striking and inexorable. Fluid accumulates within the lumen, within the bowel wall, and within the peritoneal cavity as transudation. The normal proabsorptive water and electrolyte fluxes of the unobstructed gut become prosecretory, further exacerbating the fluid losses. Vomiting or nasogastric suctioning complicates the fluid losses. In the absence of fluid replacement, progressive hemoconcentration, hypovolemia, renal insufficiency, shock, and death might occur. Intestinal gas also accumulates and accounts for a large proportion of the distention present. Luminal obstruction also increases motility in an attempt to push past the obstruction. After an initial period, regularly recurrent peristaltic bursts are interspersed with quiescent periods. The duration of the quiescent period correlates with the level of the obstruction in the gut—3 to 5 min with proximal small intestine, 10 to 15 min with distal ileal obstruction. These muscular contractions are traumatic to the bowel, with additional edema produced. The bowel distal to the obstruction, after an initial surge, and often with a clinically deceiving bowel movement, becomes progressively quiet due to an inhibitory reflex.

Occlusion of the blood supply to a segment of obstructed bowel is usually referred to as strangulated bowel obstruction. Preoperative recognition of strangulation is essential if patients with small bowel obstruction are to be treated nonoperatively. Interference with the blood supply is the most serious complication of intestinal obstruction. The buildup of fluid and gas within the obstructed segments and the altered motility are rapidly overshadowed by the consequences of venous outflow obstruction, leading to extravasation of bloody, toxin-laden fluid into the bowel, bowel wall, and peritoneal cavity. Mortality from strangulated obstruction still remains prohibitive at 20 to 40 percent.

Closed-loop obstruction, where both the afferent and efferent limbs are obstructed, is an extremely dangerous clinical situation because of the rapid progression to strangulation even before clinical evidence of intestinal obstruction exists. Widespread distention of the intestine and abdominal distention may not occur before strangulation.

Colonic obstruction usually presents less dramatically and with less propensity to strangulate, except with volvulus. Since the colon is essentially a storage organ, systemic derangements are of less magnitude and urgency than those seen with small bowel obstruction. Progressive distention, which may be marked in the presence of a competent ileocecal valve, is the most dangerous aspect of colonic obstruction. If the ileocecal valve is competent, then a closed-loop obstruction is present, with progressive distention and the strong possibility of cecal perforation. The cecum is the location of perforation because of the law of Laplace, which relates pressure to volume.

The four cardinal symptoms and signs of intestinal obstruction are crampy abdominal pain, vomiting, obstipation, and abdominal distention. The findings of localized tenderness, fever, tachycardia, and leukocytosis are supportive of, but not diagnostic for, strangulation obstruction. Crampy abdominal pain coincides with periods of hyperperistalsis and tends to be diffuse and poorly localized. When the obstruction is not relieved, the pain may transform to a steady generalized abdominal discomfort. Steady severe pain without quiescent periods is usually indicative of strangulation. Ileus is usually not painful, except for the generalized discomfort from distention.

Reflexive vomiting occurs almost immediately after the onset of obstruction. A variable quiescent period follows, depending on the level of obstruction. The character and frequency of the vomitus—frequent and bilious with high obstruction or infrequent and feculent with low obstruction—may aid in diagnosis. Reflex vomiting is unusual in colonic obstruction, except in volvulus. When the ileocecal valve is competent, small bowel distention and vomiting may be absent until late in large bowel obstruction.

Obstipation is characteristic, but the patient may spontaneously pass feces and flatus soon after obstruction as part of the bowel's hyperperistaltic surge, thereby evacuating the distal segments. Cramping pain followed by bouts of explosive diarrhea often signifies partial obstruction. Abdominal distention is a late finding, and may be absent in high small-bowel obstruction if vomiting occurs and decompresses the proximal intestine.

The early physical examination may be surprisingly normal. Strangulation is suggested if the patient appears toxic or seriously unwell early in the course or if the patient has pain disproportionate to the physical findings. Palpation during colic demonstrates muscle guarding, and auscultation will reveal loud, high-pitched and metallic rushes of noise. In ileus an occasional high-pitched, cavernous, bowel sound is heard. In strangulated obstruction the intestine is quiet, frequently with evidence of peritonitis. As obstruction progresses, fever, tachycardia, and distention become more apparent.

The serum chemistries may show mild to moderate dehydration early in the course, with hemoconcentration and a decreased output of concentrated urine. The white blood cell count might be modestly elevated in simple obstruction (< 15,000 cells/mL), but elevations above this are suggestive of strangulation. Studies have shown the insensitivity of this measurement, in that 40 percent of patients with strangulation had normal white blood cell counts preoperatively. Very high counts (< 40,000 WBC/mL) are suggestive of primary mesenteric vascular disease. Other blood tests evaluated to differentiate simple obstruction from strangulation include serum amylase, phosphorus, and lactic acid. None of these has been shown sensitive or specific enough to be useful clinically.

Basic abdominal and chest radiographs are perhaps the most important diagnostic maneuver, and should be performed early in the patient's evaluation. Supine and upright, or if the patient is too ill to stand, lateral decubitus, abdominal films with an upright chest radiograph will usually demonstrate gas-fluid levels of diagnostic significance (Fig. 22-2). Gas, although normally present in the stomach and colon of adults, is only occasionally seen in the small bowel, and then only minimal amounts. Gas-fluid levels are highly suggestive of intestinal obstruction, but are also seen in extreme aerophagia, gastroenteritis, severe constipation, sprue, and in infants (Table 22-10).

Contrast radiography has developed as a helpful adjunct in the diagnosis of small and large bowel obstruction. In almost a third of patients, diagnosis is equivocal, based on the aforementioned findings, and contrast exams have been shown to be useful in over 80 percent of patients, without affecting morbidity or mortality. Barium enemas can differentiate colonic obstruction from a distal small bowel lesion if collapsed terminal ileum is seen on barium reflux into the ileum. Colonic volvulus is readily differentiated by this maneuver. The use of barium in either a small bowel series or enteroclysis study can distinguish adynamic ileus from partial or complete small bowel obstruction. In a patient with ileus, barium will take 4 to 6 hours to reach the colon. Mechanical obstruction will produce dilated bowel and progression of the barium to the site of obstruction in one hour or less (Fig. 22-3). Water-soluble contrast studies of the small intestine are extremely limited by their dilution from the fluid present within the lumen. Because they are extremely hypertonic, they may also contribute to the fluid deficits of the patient with small intestinal obstruction.

The differentiation between partial and complete small bowel obstruction is important, as only 12 to 20 percent of patients with the former will require surgical intervention. Nasogastric decompression and metabolic support suffice in the remainder, with most improving within 48 hours. The use of nasoenteric tubes in cases of partial small bowel obstruction belies the evidence of the surgical literature, and most authors now recommend nasogastric tubes. Should resolution not occur with 48 hours of decompression, then contrast radiography or operation should be performed.

Early postoperative bowel obstruction is an infrequent occurrence and is defined as presenting within 30 days of celiotomy. Most cases are secondary to adhesions or inflammatory processes; and in 78 percent of patients in one large study, the obstruction resolved without operation, requiring an average of 6 days of nasogastric decompression. Early postoperative intestinal obstruction occurs an average of 4 days after the procedure. Lower abdominal operations, including colectomy, enterectomy, and

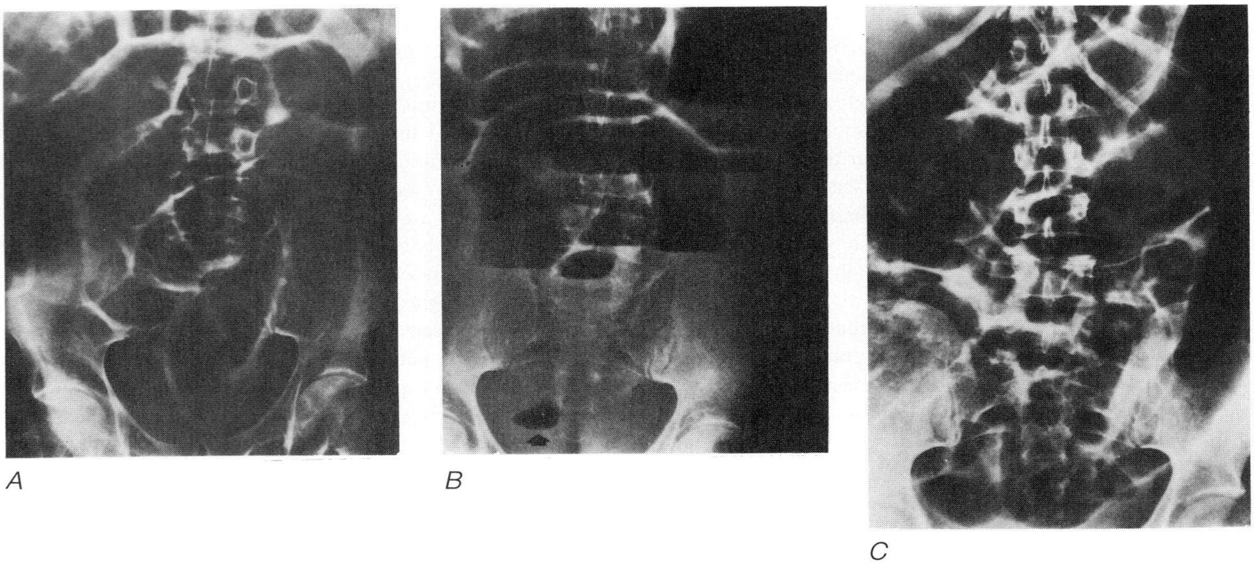

FIG. 22-2. Supine (*A*) and upright (*B*) views demonstrate large amounts of gas in dilated loops of small bowel, but only a single, small collection of gas (*arrow*) in the colon. *C.* Large amounts of gas and fluid are retained in loops of dilated small and large bowel. The entire small and large bowel appear almost uniformly dilated, with no demonstrable point of obstruction. (From: *Eisenberg RL: Gastrointestinal Radiology. Philadelphia, Lippincott, 1983, p 420, Fig 33-10, with permission.*)

exploratory laparotomy, were the most common predisposing procedures. The incidence of strangulation varies from 0 to 12 percent. Once the obstruction is resolved, few patients reobstruct, and if so, less than 15 percent require subsequent exploration.

Small bowel obstruction remains a leading cause of admission to general surgical services. The dilemma is in the patient with a previous cancer who presents with a bowel obstruction, since many will have a benign cause of obstruction. In the reported series, nearly two-thirds of patients with malignant causes of intestinal obstruction had a colorectal primary, and nearly two-thirds of these patients' primaries were in the rectosigmoid. The traditional conservative management with nasogastric or long tube decompression does not appear to facilitate resolution, and its use for over 3 days may be associated with increased morbidity and mortality. Surgical decompression is associated with a 9 to 13 percent mortality and 44 percent morbidity rate, with over 80 percent of patients being discharged home with median survivals of 4.5 months. Operation is recommended in cancer patients with small bowel obstruction who have good performance status. In addition, up to one-third of the patients will be found to have a benign cause of their blockage.

The principles of treatment of intestinal obstruction are fluid and electrolyte therapy, decompression of the gastrointestinal tract, and timely surgical intervention. Except in specific circumstances, most patients will require surgical intervention, and it is the proper timing of operation that is essential. The surgical procedures for the relief of intestinal obstruction may be divided into five categories: (1) procedures not involving opening the bowel, as in adhesiolysis; (2) enterotomy for removal of obturator obstruction, as in bezoars or gallstone ileus; (3) resection of the obstruct-

Table 22-10
Radiologic Signs in Intestinal Obstruction

Sign	*Simple Mechanical Obstruction (See Fig. 22-2A, B)*	*Adynamic Ileus (See Fig. 22-2C)*
Gas in intestine	Large bow-shaped loops in ladder pattern	Copious gas diffusely through intestine
Gas in colon	Less than normal	Increased, scattered through colon
Fluid levels in intestine	Definite	Often very large throughout
Tumor	None	None
Peritoneal exudate	None	Present with peritonitis; otherwise absent
Diaphragm	Somewhat elevated; free motion	Elevated; diminished motion

SOURCE: Eisenberg RL: *Gastrointestinal Radiology*. Philadelphia, Lippincott, 1983, with permission.

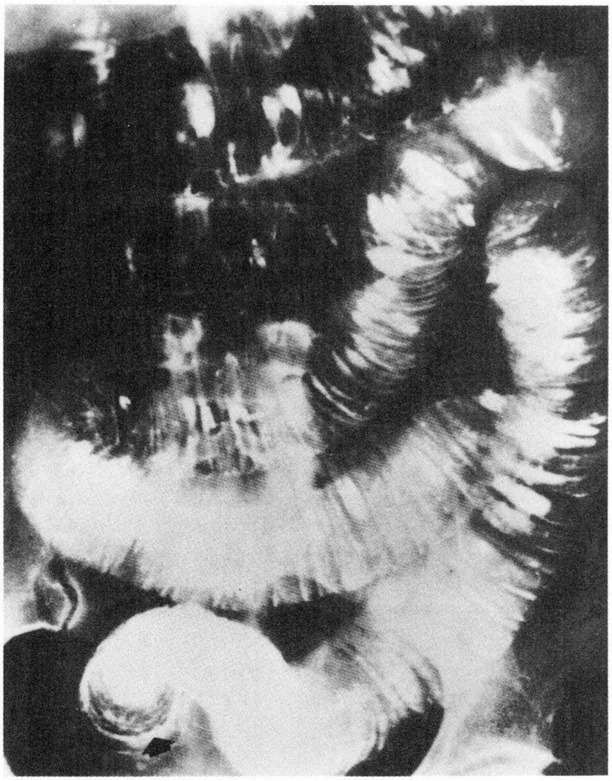

FIG. 22-3. The antegrade administration of barium demonstrates the precise site of small bowel obstruction. A radiolucent gallstone (*arrow*) is causing the distal ileal obstruction. (From: *Eisenberg RL: Gastrointestinal Radiology. Philadelphia, Lippincott, 1983, p 420, Fig 33-13, with permission.*)

ing lesion or strangulated bowel with primary anastomosis; (4) bypass procedures around an obstruction, usually malignant; and (5) formation of a proximal stoma, as in colostomy or cecostomy.

ILEUS

The understanding of the phenomenon of ileus has not advanced substantially in the past few decades. Clearly, the most important advance in the therapy of functional or mechanical bowel obstruction was developed over half a century ago by Wangensteen. He demonstrated that operative management of this problem could be delayed or replaced by nasogastric suction, with greatly improved mortality. Because of the absence of specific therapy, ileus remains a significant clinical problem. Current therapies include nasogastric intubation and intravenous hydration, with resultant increases in hospital stays and costs. In fact, the expense due to ileus has been estimated at $1500 per person, or $750 million a year.

Ileus is divided into three categories: adynamic or inhibition ileus, in which neuromuscular inhibition leads to decreased or absent intestinal motility; spastic ileus, a phenomenon where the intestinal musculature remains tightly contracted without coordinated propulsive motility; and the ileus of vascular occlusion, which is the immobility of the strangulating gut. Spastic ileus is seen in heavy metal poisoning, porphyria, and occasionally in uremia. Its therapy should be directed at the underlying disorder.

Adynamic ileus is extremely common, as it follows every abdominal, many retroperitoneal and thoracic, and some peripheral operations. Irrespective of the mechanism, aboral chyme transit is the final indicator of bowel function, and does not occur during ileus. The presence of bowel sounds, with the subsequent passage of flatus and/or bowel movements, indicates the resumption of normal transit and the end of ileus. Postoperative ileus lasts briefly (< 24 hours) in the small intestine, for 24 to 48 hours in the stomach, and for 48 to 72 hours in the colon.

Occasionally, inhibition of bowel function becomes prolonged, lasting days to weeks, and is referred to as a postoperative paralytic ileus. The paralytic ileus may have a different pathophysiology. Postoperative ileus is thought to arise from temporary inhibition of extrinsic motility regulation and is more severe in the colon. Postoperative paralytic ileus affects all segments of the bowel and may result from further inhibition of local, intrinsic contractile systems. Ileus tends to be more severe after laparotomy, but several studies have shown that the inhibition of bowel activity is independent of both the degree of intraoperative bowel manipulation and the duration of the operation. The return of intestinal activity that signifies the end of ileus is really the resumption of the migrating motor complex activity. The central nervous system, neural reflexes, hormones, medications and anesthetic agents, and local factors all play roles, albeit poorly understood, in the origination and perpetuation of ileus.

The recurrence or prolongation of postoperative ileus may portend intraabdominal inflammation, sepsis, hematoma, or occult wound infection. Metabolic causes include hypokalemia, hyponatremia, and hypomagnesemia. Fractures of the spine or ribs and basal pneumonias may have been overlooked. Drug-induced ileus can result from narcotics, especially morphine, propantheline, antacids, anticoagulants, phenothiazines, and ganglionic blocking agents. The clinical evaluation should include a careful search for occult sepsis, fracture, or bleeding. Metabolic causes, including serum potassium, sodium, magnesium, glucose, and calcium, should be investigated. A current list of medications should be evaluated.

The treatment of ileus involves the treatment of the underlying cause and general support. Treatment has not changed much in the past 100 years. Nasogastric decompression, intravenous hydration and/or nutrition, and correction of existing metabolic abnormalities are essential. No specific drug therapy has been shown effective in double-blind trials. Agents used have included vasopressin, bethanechol, prokinetic agents such as metoclopramide, cisapride, and domperidone, as well as the intraluminal instillation of hyperosmolar or nutritional agents.

FEVER

Fever is a common manifestation of gastrointestinal disease that may herald infection, inflammation, neoplasm, or autoimmune disorders. Fevers of gastrointestinal origin usually result from infection within the abdominal cavity, which are either monomicrobial or polymicrobial. Classic monomicrobial infections include biliary tract infections and spontaneous or primary peritonitis. Most cases of intraabdominal sepsis are polymicrobial, including both aerobic and anaerobic bacteria derived from the normal intestinal flora. Such infections arise from the leakage or perforation of a hollow viscus within the abdominal cavity. Intraabdominal abscesses require drainage, except for most amebic liver abscesses and 70 percent of tuboovarian abscesses.

Fever is also a presenting complaint in 50 percent of patients with Crohn's disease. Such fevers are low grade and usually associated with clinical flares of the disease and its characteristic symptoms of crampy pain, diarrhea, and abdominal masses. Postoperative fevers are common, occurring in 15 to 30 percent of patients after laparotomy. Only 10 to 20 percent of postoperative fevers are due to established infections. Common causes include pulmonary complications, urinary tract infections, wound sepsis, and thrombophlebitis. Acalculous cholecystitis should not be overlooked, and it should be remembered that fever is the presenting symptom in 75 percent of patients with acute hepatitis due to halothane or infectious causes. Occult tumors may also initially present with fever. Twenty percent of fevers of unknown origin are secondary to cancers, either primary or metastatically involved in the abdomen. About 5 percent of fevers in patients with neoplasms are related to the tumor. The most commonly implicated tumors are hypernephroma, liver tumors, lymphomas, and carcinomas of the stomach, colon, and pancreas.

GASTROINTESTINAL BLEEDING

Few events are more frightening to the patient than the expelling of blood from the mouth or anus. Such actions can be the manifestations of a plethora of simple, benign, complex, or malignant disorders. Blood loss may be occult and present late as weakness and orthostasis, or massive, sudden, and fatal. Bleeding may arise along the entire aerodigestive tract, and is the initial symptom of disease in one-third of patients, in whom 70 percent have no prior history of bleeding. Gastrointestinal tract bleeding is usually divided into upper gastrointestinal (UGI) and lower gastrointestinal (LGI) bleeding. UGI bleeding is usually from a source in the esophagus, stomach, or duodenum, where LGI bleeding is usually from the colon, rectum, or terminal ileum.

Hematemesis is the vomiting of blood, and usually represents UGI bleeding proximal to the ligament of Treitz. The presence of blood clots reflects massive bleeding, while "coffee-ground" vomitus usually indicates a slower rate of bleeding with retention of blood in the stomach and alteration of the blood to form hematin. Melena is the passage of black or tarry stool. Only 50 mL of blood is necessary to produce melena, and after a 1000 mL hemorrhage this finding may persist for 5 days. A guaiac-positive stool, indicative of occult blood, may persist for 3 weeks following hematemesis or melena. The conversion of the standard guaiac test to positive requires only 10 mL of blood loss per day. Melena usually reflects a UGI source as well, and melena without hematemesis generally indicates a lesion distal to the pylorus. Hematochezia, or the passage of blood or clots per rectum, usually reflects an LGI source, although massive UGI bleeding may be associated with red or currant jelly stools due to the volume and cathartic effects of the blood. Red or black stools can also result from the ingestion of food dye substances or iron.

Hypotension and shock are the eventual consequences of blood loss, but depend on the rate of bleeding and the patient's response. Hematologic indicators are unreliable until equilibration occurs, which can take up to 48 hours. The clinical development of shock may precipitate myocardial infarction, cerebrovascular accident, renal or hepatic failure. Azotemia occurs in patients with gastrointestinal blood loss. Blood urea nitrogen levels of 30 to 50 mg/dL are common from UGI sources, especially esophageal varices. The BUN to serum creatinine ratio, BUN/Cr, has some diagnostic utility in that if this ratio is greater than 36, the bleeding arises from an UGI source. Average values are 34.8 for UGI and 17.8 for LGI, presumably because of the lack of azotemia seen with colonic bleeding.

Upper Gastrointestinal Bleeding

UGI bleeding continues to be a frequent cause of hospital admission and in-hospital morbidity and mortality. Mortalities are reported between 10 and 20 percent and are dependent on age ($>$ sixty years old), multiorgan system disease, especially hepatic and pulmonary, transfusion requirements ($>$ 5 units), need for operation, and recent stress, as in surgery, trauma, or sepsis. The incidence and causes of UGI bleeding in a given community vary according to the incidence of peptic ulcer disease, alcoholism, use of nonsteroidal anti-inflammatory drugs (NSAIDs), and the elderly. The percentage of patients presenting with UGI bleeding in the over-sixty age group has increased from 10 percent in the 1920s to over 50 percent in the 1970s. Associated with this is the increased mortality of UGI hemorrhage in patients over sixty years old versus those that are younger (20 percent versus 4 percent). Although the incidence of elective surgery for peptic ulcer disease has dramatically decreased over the past 30 years, the need for emergency surgery for bleeding and perforation has not changed appreciably, despite the advent and widespread use of histamine receptor antagonist therapy.

Lesions that present with UGI bleeding include peptic ulceration, acute mucosal lesions, such as gastritis and erosions, esophagogastric varices, reflux esophagitis, Mallory-Weiss tears, and gastric neoplasms. In urban centers, varices and acute mucosal lesions constitute the majority of cases. Surgical intervention is required in only 10 to 20 percent, dependent on the cause, and endoscopic or arteriographic therapies are required in a similar proportion.

Peptic ulceration is a common cause of UGI bleeding. A history of recurrent dyspepsia, especially if nocturnal and ameliorated by antacids or meals, is suggestive, but 10 percent of patients have no previous history of symptoms. Hemorrhage from a duodenal ulcer is four times more common than gastric ulcer bleeding, but duodenal ulcers are four times more common than the gastric variety. Bleeding is the presenting problem in 15 percent of patients, and 10 to 15 percent of all duodenal ulcer patients will have an episode of brisk hemorrhage. Because hemostasis is partially dependent on vessel wall retraction and contraction, chronic ulcers or ulcers in the elderly with atherosclerotic vessels are more likely to bleed persistently. Stomal, or marginal, ulcers should always be considered in the patient with a prior ulcer operation. Incomplete vagotomy is the cause in the majority of cases.

Acute mucosal lesions make up 1 to 33 percent of all UGI bleeding sources. Often multiple, these lesions do not usually extend through the muscularis mucosae, and are therefore erosions rather than true ulcers. Whereas chronic benign gastric ulcers are frequently found on the antrum and lesser curvature, acute mucosal lesions are found in the body and fundus, spare the antrum, and are as frequently on the greater curvature as on the lesser curvature. The term *stress ulceration* is often misapplied, and refers to acute gastroduodenal lesions that arise after or during episodes of shock, sepsis, surgery, trauma, burns (Curling's ulcers), and intracranial pathology or surgery (Cushing's ulcers). Stress ulceration is probably due to decreased gastric blood flow that is secondary to splanchnic vasoconstriction, but sepsis, cytokines, and coagulopathies are also correlated with its presence. UGI bleeding has been described in one-third of patients with septicemia. Eight key risk factors for stress bleeding have been documented, including multiple systems trauma, hypotension, respiratory failure, renal failure, sepsis, jaundice, recent surgery, and burns. The greater the number of risk factors, the more likelihood of stress ulceration and bleeding. Both antacids and histamine receptor antagonists are effective in preventing stress ulcer bleeding.

Curling's ulcers increase in frequency as the percentage of body surface area burned increases. Sepsis, usually burn wound in origin, is frequently present, and bleeding is the presenting symptom in 70 percent of patients. Massive hemorrhage is common, and Curling's ulcers are as often single as multiple, and arise from the gastric mucosa as often as from the duodenum. Cushing's ulcers probably result from the same pathophysiology as stress ulcerations from other surgical trauma, although significant gastric hypersecretion may occur after certain neurosurgical procedures. Ingested substances are often associated with stress ulcerations, including adrenal steroids, NSAIDs, aspirin, cocaine, alcohol, and oral potassium supplements.

Esophagogastric varices constitute a common cause of bleeding in patients with cirrhosis, accounting for 50 to 75 percent of their UGI bleeding. Varices account for about 10 percent of UGI bleeding overall, but 95 percent of all UGI bleeding in the pediatric age group, usually due to extrahepatic portal venous obstruction. A history and physical examination are most helpful in this population, as alcoholism and the physical findings of jaundice, ascites, gynecomastia, palmar erythema, testicular atrophy, and spider angiomata are strongly supportive of a variceal source. Bleeding from varices is often profuse and associated with hematemesis. The precipitating event is believed to be either increased pressure within the varix or ulceration secondary to esophagitis. Treatment is often complicated by the severe malnutrition, hepatic dysfunction, and coagulopathy found in these patients.

Hiatal hernia is a cause of occult chronic blood loss but is the cause of brisk bleeding in only 2 percent of the reported cases. The bleeding is due to reflux peptic esophagitis and is more frequent in patients with paraesophageal hernias. Mallory-Weiss tears of the esophagogastric mucosa are reported to make up 5 to 10 percent of UGI bleeding sources and are preceded by vomiting or retching over 50 percent of the time. More than 90 percent cease spontaneously. Other miscellaneous causes of UGI bleeding, which make up 8 to 18 percent of reported cases, include gastric neoplasms (including adenocarcinoma, leiomyoma, leiomyosarcoma, leukemia, and lymphoma), gastroduodenal polyps, angiomas, aortoenteric fistula, duodenal diverticula with prolapsed mucosa, vasculitic disorders, and hematobilia.

There are three major aspects in managing UGI hemorrhage. The initial priority is to treat the shock and restore blood volume. Second, localization of the source of bleeding is required to perform the third task, that of formulating an interventional plan. The prevention of exsanguination is the initial priority, and the insertion of large-bore intravenous catheters is followed by the rapid infusion of isotonic fluid while blood for laboratory evaluation and cross-matching is obtained. Essential initial laboratory evaluations include a complete blood count, prothrombin and partial thromboplastin times, and an electrolyte profile. Losses of up to 500 mL are frequently well tolerated by the patient, but greater blood loss is heralded by tachycardia, hypotension, and altered mental status. If the patient has stable vital signs in the supine position, a measurement for orthostatic changes after 2 minutes upright is easy, informative, and a good indicator of the need for transfusion. A fall in blood pressure of 20 mmHg or a rise in pulse of 20 beats per minute indicates at least a 20 percent loss of circulating blood volume. A urinary drainage catheter is a rapid and safe way to evaluate the response to resuscitation.

The majority of patients with UGI bleeding will present with melena, so placement of a nasogastric tube is important. A clear bile-stained aspirate generally rules out bleeding proximal to the ligament of Treitz. In the presence of duodenal ulcer bleeding, pylorospasm can occur with the return of bloodless nasogastric aspirate, but this occurs in the minority of cases. If in doubt, the nasogastric tube can be left in place for 24 hours. The tube can also serve to remove a large portion of gastric acid secretions, monitor for rebleeding, and facilitate antacid therapy if necessary.

After initial resuscitation and stabilization, a search for the cause of bleeding should be performed. In most centers this initially consists of esophagogastroduodenoscopy (EGD). Although several large studies have demonstrated no change in overall mortality in patients subjected to early EGD, most believe it to be a required maneuver. The reported complication rate from EGD is less than 0.25 percent, but there is a 30 percent disagreement rate among endoscopists on the findings. Nevertheless, the endoscopic evaluation is especially valuable in disclosing acute gastritis, erosions, ulcers, Mallory-Weiss tears, and varices. The therapeutic options for UGI bleeding lesions have expanded widely over the past decade and are available in most hospitals.

Radiologic studies in acute UGI bleeding are limited to angiography in most cases. Arteriography can localize bleeding points if blood loss exceeds 1 to 2 mL/min, with an accuracy of about 90 percent. Therapeutic advantages include the ability to embolize or infuse vasoconstrictive agents into the responsible vessels. The selective intraarterial infusion of vasopressin for the therapy of bleeding esophageal varices has not been shown to more efficacious than peripheral venous vasopressin infusion. Other treatments for variceal bleeding include balloon tamponade and sclerotherapy. An upper gastrointestinal series, with small bowel follow-through or enteroclysis, is valuable in the more elective setting for occult sources of UGI blood loss. Radionuclide imaging has been highly touted as a valuable tool for localizing sites of gastrointestinal blood loss, with requirements of ongoing blood loss of only 0.1 mL/min reported. Recent studies documented that this test is helpful in less than half of cases, however, and it is often used only as a precursor to arteriographic evaluation.

As previously noted, urgent surgical intervention is uncommonly required for UGI bleeding. Surgical approaches are tailored to the diagnostic entity, and the usual philosophy is to control bleeding first and treat the underlying disorder second if the patient's general condition can tolerate the additional surgical stress.

Lower Gastrointestinal Bleeding

Lesions below the ligament of Treitz that bleed are considered as LGI sources, comprising both midgut and hindgut. The majority of these lesions arise from the colon, and include diverticula, angiodysplastic lesions, cancers, inflammatory bowel disease (IBD), and hemorrhoids. The small intestine, although constituting 90 percent of the gastrointestinal mucosal surface area, is a rare source of bleeding. The small intestinal sources are usually neoplastic, inflammatory, or diverticular. As with UGI bleeding, the source is also a factor of the age of the patient, with Meckel's diverticula, polyps, and IBD being common in the young. Vascular ectasias, cancer, and colonic diverticula predominate in the adult population.

Small Intestinal Bleeding

Small intestinal bleeding, not including the duodenum, can be difficult to investigate and, because of its rarity, may be overlooked in the work-up of patients with chronic gastrointestinal blood loss. Overall, small intestinal sources constitute 10 to 15 percent of all LGI bleeding, with Meckel's diverticulitis, Crohn's disease, and intussusception constituting the most common causes. Meckel's diverticulitis with associated bleeding occurs in the young patient in over 80 percent of cases, and is usually related to ectopic gastric mucosa within the diverticulum. Intussusception is also a characteristic cause of LGI bleeding in the pediatric population, with the passage of currant-jelly stools interspersed with abdominal pain. The cause in pediatric patients is usually undetermined, as nonoperative management suffices in the majority. In adults, intussusception is usually ileocecal and secondary to polyps or tumor.

Regional enteritis, or Crohn's disease, is associated with melena about 5 percent of the time, and some rectal bleeding is noted by approximately 20 percent of patients. Small intestinal tumors, both benign and malignant, occasionally present with brisk LGI bleeding, but more commonly with occult blood loss and anemia, especially for the malignant variety. Overall, almost half of small bowel tumors bleed. The bleeding of aortoenteric fistula is usually seen in patients with prior aortic reconstructive surgery, but primary aortoenteric fistulas are well reported. A sentinel, or herald, bleed is common and warrants immediate evaluation. One must also remember the rare but potentially lethal nonesophageal varices that present with bleeding. Such varices have been reported in the duodenum and jejunum and around cutaneous stomae. They are more common, however, in the colon and rectum. Other rare causes of small intestinal bleeding include blood dyscrasias, non-Meckel's diverticula, mesenteric thrombosis, drug reactions, cytomegalovirus infections, hemangiomas, hereditary telangiectasis, and the polyps of the Peutz-Jeghers syndrome.

Colonic Bleeding

The most common causes of rectal bleeding include carcinoma, diverticula, vascular ectasias, colitis, and polyps. Anorectal lesions, especially hemorrhoids, are a frequent and probably underreported source of rectal bleeding. The evaluating physician must always keep in mind that a frequent source of hematochezia and massive melena is a UGI hemorrhage, and diagnostic nasogastric intubation is recommended. Carcinoma is still the most frequent source of LGI blood loss, but the loss is rarely rapid or profuse. Right-sided cancers classically present with occult blood loss, with the presenting symptoms of fatigue, orthostasis, and heart failure. Only when the anemia is noted does the suspicion of LGI blood loss come to mind. For massive rectal bleeding, diverticulosis and angiodysplasia remain the leading causes.

Angiodysplasia is a common finding in the elderly, and if noted incidentally, rarely becomes bothersome. These lesions are small, usually less than 5 mm in diameter, occur in the cecum and right colon, and are best diagnosed by arteriography or colonoscopy. More than 80 percent of patients with hemorrhaging angiodysplasia will stop bleeding spontaneously. Those patients with bleeding have an unclear risk of rebleeding after cessation. Clinically significant rebleeding occurs in about 50 percent of patients in the subsequent 3 years, and 5 to 30 percent of patients will rebleed after surgery. The risk of bleeding after colonoscopic therapy (electrocoagulation or laser ablation) is more than twice that after surgery, but the risks and benefits of the two procedures must be weighed.

Diverticulosis-related bleeding is thought to arise from erosion of vessels within the neck of the diverticulum. Right-sided diverticula have been recognized as a source of bleeding about 50 percent of the time. The finding of chronic LGI blood loss and diverticulosis should lead to a close look for an associated colonic neoplasm, found in 20 percent of cases. Ulcerative colitis is associated with bloody diarrhea in 95 percent of cases, but massive hemorrhage is seen in only 1 to 2 percent of patients. The mean duration of recognized disease is 2.6 years. Polyps, cecal ulceration, sarcomas, lymphomas, leukemia, hematologic disorders, cytomegalovirus infection, and ischemic syndromes are all rare causes of colonic bleeding. Anorectal sources include hemorrhoids, fistulas, fissures, and proctitis. The presence of these lesions does not rule out a proximal source for the blood loss, and a careful evaluation of the LGI tract is essential.

The evaluation of the patient presenting with LGI bleeding depends on the nature and the volume of the blood loss. For brisk hemorrhage, prompt resuscitation and stabilization of the patient is the initial priority. Passage of a nasogastric tube and aspiration of bloodless, bilious fluid rules out a UGI source in over 90 percent of cases. Since many patients with rectal bleeding have anorectal sites of disease, anoscopy and/or proctosigmoidoscopy is performed as part of the initial evaluation. Colonoscopy is rarely indicated initially because it generally provides no diagnostic information in the face of massive bleeding.

Although 80 percent of patients will stop bleeding spontaneously, any patient who needs more than two units of blood or becomes hypotensive during the hospital course should be considered for urgent radiologic identification of the bleeding site. Radionuclide scans are sensitive for the presence of bleeding, but are diagnostic in less than one-half of patients. Aggressive arteriographic techniques have been shown to be helpful or diagnostic in 65 to 78 percent of cases. Extravasation of contrast or obvious vascular abnormalities are more commonly seen in patients who have required over three units of transfusion and are associated with a greater than 85 percent chance of the need for operation. Arteriographic localization of the bleeding site allows for the therapeutic instillation of vasoconstrictive agents, for methylene blue to assist surgical localization, or for embolization. Localization also facilitates segmental resections of bleeding bowel, which have a lower mortality and morbidity than more global resections. Patients with an arteriographically localized bleeding site in the small bowel are well served by the infusion of methylene blue to localize the bleeding site.

Although the majority of patients with brisk LGI bleeding will have diverticular or arteriovenous sites of origin, recent studies have shown an increasing trend of obscure causes to become less unusual, including cytomegalovirus infections and tumors. Overall mortality figures range from 0 to 21 percent, and improvements have been noted with more liberal use of aggressive arteriographic techniques and precise surgical therapies. The absence of radiologic localization in the face of persistent bleeding and the need for emergency surgery are associated with increased mortalities of 29 to 40 percent.

The evaluation of the patient with chronic LGI blood loss can proceed at a less expedient pace. A thorough history and physical examination will assist in the diagnosis in the majority of cases.

Specific points to be addressed include the presence or absence of pain, weight loss, and family history of gastrointestinal diseases. Physical examination centers on the abdominal, pelvic, and rectal examinations. Colonoscopy has rapidly become the initial diagnostic maneuver of choice and is over 95 percent sensitive and specific for colorectal lesions. Angiodysplastic lesions are identifiable in only 70 percent of patients, but are rarely the source of massive bleeding. In the absence of colonoscopy, proctosigmoidoscopy and a double-contrast barium enema are an acceptable substitute. If angiography is considered either for diagnosis or for treatment, a barium enema should be avoided because residual contrast can obscure small vascular lesions. If these tests are negative, evaluation of the UGI should be performed by esophagogastroduodenoscopy or UGI barium series with small bowel follow-through. If the small bowel is suspected, an enteroclysis study may be performed. Other techniques advocated for chronic occult LGI blood loss include enteroscopy and arteriography with selective infusion of vasodilator or fibrinolytic substances.

JAUNDICE

The word jaundice is derived from the French *jaune,* meaning yellow, and refers to the presence of excess bile pigments in the tissues and serum. The jaundiced patient represents an important diagnostic challenge to the internist and surgeon alike, and the surgeon must decide if the condition requires a surgical procedure. This decision does not require a diffuse diagnostic approach, but rather an understanding of biliary physiology and anatomy. Several studies of jaundiced patients have shown that a diagnostic accuracy of approximately 85 percent can be attained with only a careful history, physical examination, and routine blood chemistries.

The yellowing of the skin and mucous membranes is rarely apparent until total serum bilirubin rises above 2.5 mg/dL. Most of the body's bilirubin is produced in the reticuloendothelial system by the catabolism of heme derived from senescent erythrocytes. Smaller amounts are present from the ineffective erythropoiesis in the bone marrow and the turnover of other heme-containing proteins. Bilirubin, a water-insoluble pigment, has no known physiologic role. Its elimination is dependent on the liver, whose role is to solubilize it and excrete it into the bile and urine.

Bilirubin is bound to plasma albumin, which transports it to the liver, where conjugation occurs by covalent linkage to water-soluble moieties, notably glucuronic acid. The conjugated, or direct, bilirubin is excreted into the bile, where it is poorly absorbed by the gut and, hence, fecally excreted. A small fraction is metabolized by gut flora to urobilinogen and reabsorbed, only to be excreted into the urine or bile. The normal daily fecal excretion of bilirubin is 100 to 200 mg. Normally all conjugated bilirubin is excreted into the bile and does not reflux into the plasma. The minute amounts of conjugated bilirubin reported by most laboratories are artifactually high and assay-related. Almost no conjugated bilirubin is found in the serum or urine. Renal failure can exacerbate jaundice because of the diminished renal excretion of direct bilirubin.

The first step in examining the jaundiced patient is to ascertain if the responsible disease process is hemolytic, hepatocellular, or cholestatic. If cholestatic, then intrahepatic versus extrahepatic obstructions must be distinguished. It is important to reiterate that a complete history and physical exam will answer these preliminary questions almost every time (Table 22-11).

Unconjugated hyperbilirubinemia almost always represents a nonsurgical condition. Hemolytic disorders represent an overload of bilirubin production that may overwhelm the liver's metabolic ability. Rarely will the total serum bilirubin exceed 4 mg/dL, and almost all of the bilirubin is indirect, or unconjugated. If there is concomitant liver disease, or a period of particularly brisk hemolysis, then transiently greater values may appear. The relationship between hemolytic disorders and gallstone formation must always be kept in mind. The second major cause of unconjugated hyperbilirubinemia results from hepatic defects in bilirubin conjugation. An inherited partial deficiency in glucuronyl transferase, or Gilbert's syndrome, affects 3 to 6 percent of the population, and is more common in men. Serum bilirubin fluctuates but is usually below 3 mg/dL. Stress, resulting from surgery, infection, or fasting, can induce higher levels of bilirubin. A lifelong history of mild intermittent jaundice is very suggestive of Gilbert's syndrome. More rare are those patients with Crigler-Najjar syndrome, Types I and II. These conditions represent either a severe deficiency in glucuronyl transferase or its complete absence, respectively. Both present in infancy. Drug-related acquired glucuronyl transferase deficiencies are rarer still. Important points to remember in these patients are that their other liver chemistries are normal, as in patients with hemolytic jaundice. Finally, patients with unconjugated hyperbilirubinemia have minimal to no bilirubinuria because the indirect pigment is water-insoluble.

Conjugated hyperbilirubinemia presents a greater diagnostic challenge to the surgeon, with more potential causes and surgical approaches. They may broadly be classified into three categories: inherited disorders of bilirubin metabolism; hepatocellular, which is frequently subdivided into hepatitic and cholestatic; and mechanical biliary obstruction. Inherited disorders consist of two rare diseases, Dubin-Johnson syndrome and Rotor's syndrome. The former is an inability of hepatocellular excretion of conjugated bile with reflux back into the plasma. Serum bilirubin is usually between 2 and 5 mg/dL. Grossly, the livers are brown or black due to hepatocellular retention of a dark, nonmelanin pigment. Rotor's syndrome represents an impairment of hepatic storage capacity. The liver is grossly normal. Both syndromes are associated with otherwise normal liver function tests.

When jaundice results from hepatocellular damage or dysfunction, surgical intervention is rarely required, and may even be contraindicated. Operative morbidity and mortality are prohibitive in certain situations, such as acute hepatitis and cirrhosis. Hepatic injury can be classified into either hepatocellular or canalicular, although mixed patterns are commonly seen. Jaundice with predominantly conjugated hyperbilirubinemia accompanies both. Prominent increases in the serum transaminases are noted, with lesser degrees of bilirubin and alkaline phosphatase elevation. Other injuries capable of inducing this response include shock, acute viral hepatitis, and drugs. Acutely impacted gallstones in the choledochus can simulate acute hepatitis with transaminase elevations to 600 to 2000 units/L. Their decline is rapid, occurring in less than 72 hours, whereas in acute hepatitis the elevations persist much longer.

Acute alcoholic hepatitis merits special mention. An enlarged, tender liver is usually present, often with marked degrees of fever and leukocytosis. High levels of conjugated bilirubin are seen. Serum transaminases rarely exceed 300 units/L, but the serum glutamic oxaloacetic transaminase to serum glutamic pyruvic

Table 22-11
Analysis of a Case of Hyperbilirubinemia

Fractionate serum bilirubin and measure urine bilirubin and urobilinogen to determine whether:				
I. Unconjugated hyperbilirubinemia Determine mechanism on basis of age, clinical features, and laboratory findings:	*A*. Production of bilirubin beyond excretory capacity. Evidence of:	1. Hemolysis	*a*. Extracorpuscular	(1) Immune body reactions (*a*) Transfusion reactions (*b*) Erythroblastosis (2) Infections and chemicals (3) Physical agents (4) Secondary hemolysis in pregnancy
			b. Intracorpuscular	(1) Congenital hemolytic jaundice (2) Sickle cell anemia (3) Mediterranean anemia
		2. No hemolysis	*a*. Pulmonary infarction *b*. Tranfusion of aged red blood cells *c*. Hematomas *d*. ''Shunt'' hyperbilirubinemia	
	B. Deficient hepatic uptake of bilirubin:	1. ? Gilbert's disease (normal biopsy, low-grade hyperbilirubinemia) 2. ? Acquired liver disease		
	C. Deficient conjugation of bilirubin:	1. Physiologic jaundice of newborn 2. Crigler-Najjar syndrome (transferase deficiency)	*a*. Inadequate bilirubin glucuronide synthesis	
		3. Inhibition of glucuronyl transferase	*a*. Large doses of vitamin K analogs in premature infants *b*. Increased level of pregnanediol *c*. Breast milk containing pregnane $-3\alpha,20\beta$-diol *d*. Novobiocin	
		4. Competitive inhibition	*a*. Drugs detoxified as glucuronides	
		1. Extrahepatic biliary obstruction		

Table 22-11 *(continued)*

II. Conjugated hyperbilirubinemia Determine mechanism on basis of age, clinical features, and laboratory findings:	*A*. Defect in bilirubin excretion Confirm with serum alkaline phosphatase (elevated), cephalin flocculation (normal). In absence of rapid subsidence, exploratory surgery is desirable to differentiate:	Identify by radiologic means and/or direct inspection during surgical intervention.	*a*. Calculus *b*. Stricture *c*. Neoplasm	
		2. Intrahepatic biliary obstruction Confirm absence of extrahepatic biliary obstruction with operative or T-tube cholangiography. Identify localization of lesion by surgical biopsy.	*a*. Lesion of bile canaliculi	(1) Drugs (2) Viruses
			b. Lesion of bile ductules	(1) Drugs (2) Viruses
			c. Lesion of bile ducts	(1) Drugs (2) Viruses
	B. Deficient liver cell secretion of bilirubin May need to differentiate from excretory defect by surgical exploration, cholangiography, or biopsy:	1. Persistence of excretory defect in immature liver after development of adequate glucuronide-synthesizing capacity 2. Dubin-Johnson syndrome (biopsy showing characteristic pigment) 3. Rotor syndrome (absence of characteristic pigment)		
III. Combined unconjugated and conjugated hyperbilirubinemia Determine mechanism on basis of clinical features and laboratory findings:	*A*. Familial defect or immature liver reflected in partial deficiency of glucuronide formation or excretion			
	B. Acquired liver cell damage Confirm with liver function tests and determine primary abnormality:	1. Deficient hepatic uptake of bilirubin 2. Deficient conjugation of bilirubin 3. Deficient secretion or excretion of conjugated bilirubin		
	C. Hemolysis with secondary liver damage Demonstrate presence of hemolysis:	1. Hepatic damage secondary to shock 2. Hepatic damage secondary to hemolysis		
	D. Biliary obstruction with secondary liver damage:	1. Bile stasis with secondary injury 2. Ascending cholangitis		

SOURCE: Leevy CM: *Evaluation of Liver Function in Clinical Practice*. Indianapolis, The Lilly Research Laboratories, 1965, with permission.

transaminase ratio (SGOT/SGPT) is almost always greater than 2:1. The alkaline phosphatase may be two or three times above normal values. The diagnosis can be confirmed in borderline cases by the presence of a nondilated biliary tree on ultrasonography and histologic findings of fatty infiltration, polymorphonuclear inflammation, cellular necrosis, and Mallory's hyalin.

Cholestatic liver injuries differ from hepatic injuries in that they are due to a dysfunction at the level of the bile canaliculi. More pronounced elevations are seen in alkaline phosphatase than in the transaminases. If present, jaundice is usually from the direct, or conjugated, component. Serum bile salts are increased, and pruritus may occur. Intrahepatic cholestasis cannot be reliably distinguished from extrahepatic cholestasis based only on serum chemistries. There are multiple causes of intrahepatic cholestasis, but some commonly seen causes on the surgical service include multiple organ system failure, large transfusion requirements, sepsis, drugs, and total parenteral nutrition. Cholestasis, either intrahepatic or extrahepatic, can result in fat malabsorption and relative vitamin K deficiencies. A prolonged prothrombin time can then be seen with its resultant hemorrhagic complications. Parenteral administration of vitamin K will suffice to correct this problem.

The diagnosis of jaundice caused by extrahepatic biliary obstruction can be made with 90 percent accuracy based on the historical findings, physical exam, and routine laboratory tests, and they are of particular interest to the surgeon. A study by O'Connor et al. compared clinical evaluation, ultrasonography, computed tomography, and radionuclide hepatobiliary scanning in the differential diagnosis of medical versus surgical jaundice. Although clinical evaluation was the least specific (76 percent), it was by far the most sensitive (95 percent), with the best overall accuracy (84 percent). The acute onset of jaundice, right upper quadrant abdominal pain, fever, and nausea and vomiting are typical for choledocholithiasis. A history of classic biliary colic, if present, is helpful. Cholangitis and a history of prior biliary surgery suggest a common duct stone or stricture. An abdominal mass or a palpable nontender gallbladder (Courvoisier's sign) may signify malignant obstruction, especially if the stools contain occult blood and the jaundice is painless. Other signs of malignancy include weight loss, back pain, recent onset of diabetes, and anorexia.

The standard pattern of liver chemistries in extrahepatic biliary obstruction includes an alkaline phosphatase that is two to three times normal and serum aminotransferase levels of less than 300 units/L. An extremely high alkaline phosphatase value is suggestive of an intrahepatic process. Very high aminotransferase levels, simulating acute hepatitis, may also be found in acute extrahepatic obstruction, as in the passage of a gallstone. The increased bilirubin is mainly conjugated, and bilirubinuria may be seen. Serum bile acids and gamma-glutamyl transpeptidase (GGTP) are also elevated. If the obstruction involves only part of the biliary tree, jaundice may be absent despite prominent liver enzyme elevations.

If there is clinical suspicion of extrahepatic bile duct obstruction, then a method of imaging the biliary tree is required. Ultrasonography remains the first test performed by most physicians because of its ease, safety, painlessness, and lack of radiation exposure. Obesity or an abundance of intraabdominal gas makes ultrasound diagnosis difficult, especially for the portal and pancreatic areas. Additionally, ultrasound is considerably more operator-dependent than the other modalities.

Computed tomography (CT) overcomes most of the disadvantages of ultrasound, but its expense and radiation render it a second-line test in the initial evaluation of obstructive jaundice. It is less sensitive in detecting noncalcified gallstones. Associated masses in the porta hepatis and pancreatic head are more reliably detected by CT scanning. Magnetic resonance imaging (MRI) is a newer technique that has a less defined role in evaluating biliary obstruction. It is limited by its expense and lack of availability in many centers. Hepatobiliary scanning with radioactive compounds, usually technetium-iminodiacetic acids, is good for diagnosing complete cystic or common duct obstruction, but offers little anatomic accuracy. It is most useful in the early diagnosis of acute cholecystitis, in identifying postoperative biliary fistulas, and in the pediatric population where direct cholangiography is difficult or impossible. Ultrasonography and CT scanning are anatomic tests whereas hepatobiliary scintography is a functional test.

Direct cholangiography may be needed in the work-up of extrahepatic biliary obstruction. The intrabiliary injection of radiopaque contrast material is justified if surgical intervention is contemplated. The choice of endoscopic retrograde cholangiopancreatography (ERCP) or percutaneous transhepatic cholangiography (PTC) will depend on the suspected cause of the obstruction, local expertise, and consideration of the therapeutic options. Both studies are highly sensitive (99 percent) and specific (99 percent), and either study, if normal, essentially excludes an extrahepatic biliary obstruction. Both techniques can delineate the site and nature of the obstruction in over 90 percent of patients.

PTC can be used when there is intrahepatic ductal dilatation; success rates fall from 90–95 percent to 70 percent in the absence of dilated intrahepatic bile ducts. Minor and major complications occur in 30 percent and 4 to 10 percent, respectively. Contraindications include marked ascites and coagulopathy. ERCP requires more technical skill than PTC but can yield more information and therapeutic options. Successful imaging is possible in over 90 percent of patients, and serious complications, including pancreatitis and cholangitis, occur less than 2 percent of the time. The occurrence of biliary sepsis can be minimized by careful disinfection of instruments, prophylactic antibiotics, and decompression of obstructed ducts by an endoscopically placed nasobiliary tube or stent placement. ERCP should be the procedure of choice in patients who have jaundice after cholecystectomy, as endoscopic sphincterotomy permits stone removal or stricture dilation. ERCP can also be used in patients with suspected malignancy to effect immediate drainage and stent insertion, as well as to obtain material for histologic evaluation.

The complication and success rates for ERCP and PTC are similar. ERCP is currently the initial invasive procedure of choice because of its additional therapeutic and diagnostic possibilities. PTC is usually reserved for situations in which the biliary ducts cannot be visualized by ERCP or if ERCP-placed stent drainage cannot be attained in cases of malignant obstruction. Some authors enjoy the technical facility afforded by the preoperative placement of PTC catheters. Occasionally both procedures are used in particularly difficult cases, in a "push-pull" type of procedure to achieve biliary drainage stent placement.

MULTIPLE ORGAN SYSTEM FAILURE (MOSF)

The gastrointestinal tract was long thought to be inactive or quiescent during periods of critical illness that occurred as a result of infection or trauma. Because laboratory tests are unavailable for the surveillance of the gastrointestinal tract and gut function, the intestine usually ranks low on the problem list of the intensive care unit patient. Recent evidence has supported the growing concept of the contribution of the gut to the development of multiple organ system failure (MOSF) as a manifestation of either occult gastrointestinal disease or deranged gut homeostasis.

The intestine plays a crucial role in the digestion and absorption of nutrients, but it is also essential as a barrier to enteric flora, preventing host invasion by microorganisms or soilage by their toxins. The intestinal barrier may be imperfect during critical illness. Patients in the ICU who are not receiving enteral feedings may contaminate themselves by way of a permeable gastrointestinal tract, possibly resulting in a chronic hypermetabolic state and MOSF.

The intestinal tract consists of smooth muscle, connective tissue, and lymphoid and mucosal cells. The enterocytes and colonocytes cover an extensive surface area and in a normal state are rapidly proliferative. The metabolic demands of the mucosal cells account for the majority of the intestinal nutritional requirements under normal circumstances. Food within the lumen of the gut appears to be the most important stimulus for mucosal growth. When enteral feedings are impossible or inadequate, the intestinal mucosa may atrophy. Recent studies have found that the gut consistently extracts large amounts of the amino acid glutamine as a fuel, while disposing of the majority of its nitrogen as ammonia, alanine, and citrulline. When enteral feedings are inadequate and parenteral nutrition is required, the current therapy is either inadequate or interferes with the production of essential gut nutrients. Since glutamine is absent from current parenteral nutrition formulas, the currently available therapies effectively starve the gut.

MOSF is a disordered hypermetabolic process that arises after 7 to 22 percent of emergency major operations and 30 to 50 percent of laparotomies for sepsis. The mortality figures associated with MOSF are proportional to the number of organ systems involved, but vary between 30 and 100 percent. MOSF is the primary cause for extended stays in surgical intensive care units and accounts for more than 85 percent of deaths in these facilities.

The causes and pathogenesis of MOSF are still unknown. A clinical period of hypermetabolism usually follows the "ebb phase" after injury. This "flow phase" presents 72 to 96 hours after the injury and spontaneously abates within 3 or 4 days. Any complication, such as a wound infection, intraabdominal abscess, or anastomotic leak may potentiate the hypermetabolic flow state but is usually controllable if handled promptly and appropriately. In some patients, however, the crescendo process of MOSF begins, triggered by some unknown physiologic stimuli. Early portents include mental status changes and increases in respiratory rate, pulse, core temperature, and white blood cell count. Later sequelae include hypoxia, hypocarbia, and the radiologic findings of ARDS. Once this cascade is initiated, associated mortality escalates. Worsening encephalopathy accompanies progressive respiratory failure. Serum bilirubin and creatinine rise despite polyuria. The onset of renal failure, typically acute tubular necrosis, is accompanied by staggering rises in mortality. Upper gastrointestinal bleeding, polymicrobial bacteremias, and clinical malnutrition ensue. Finally, coagulopathies and skin and/or wound breakdown develop, presaging the clinical picture of late MOSF dominated by hepatic failure. Most likely, occult liver failure begins much earlier than its clinical recognition, and may well be the final common pathway for MOSF. Although variations of this sequence are the rule rather than the exception, depending upon antecedent disease and physiologic status, most patients with MOSF inexorably succumb to hepatic failure and oliguric renal failure.

It is clear that as the number of organ systems involved in MOSF increasingly fail, the associated mortality rises. In one series of patients with severe pancreatitis, the mean number of organ system failures in survivors was 1.4 versus a mean of 3.2 in nonsurvivors. Once four organ systems are involved, the mortality is virtually 100 percent. In MOSF, respiratory and hepatic failure are reported in over 80 percent of patients, with cardiac, renal, and coagulation failure occurring between 48 and 63 percent of the time.

The failure of multiple organ systems in sequence or simultaneously has fostered much interest and investigation in a common pathophysiologic mechanism. Multiple potential mediators or effectors have been suggested in the pathogenesis of MOSF (Table 22-12). One unifying concept is that MOSF is a biologic summation of numerous humoral mediators, with their trigger being uncontrolled infection. This association of sepsis, in a remote intraabdominal or retroperitoneal focus, and distant organ failure is well documented. However, a large fraction of patients succumbing from MOSF will have no evidence of a septic source either clinically or at autopsy. These findings have led to an increasing amount of attention on the gastrointestinal tract as a reservoir of pathogens that enter the circulation by migrating across the gut mucosal barrier, begin the septic cascade, and perpetuate MOSF.

The transmigration of living bacteria or their endotoxins from the lumen of the gut, through the epithelium, to sites such as the mesenteric lymph nodes, spleen, peritoneal cavity, and blood is called bacterial translocation. The translocation of viable bacteria or their endotoxins has been shown to occur in a number of conditions, including hemorrhagic shock, burns, malnutrition, sepsis, and jaundice. Several factors are acknowledged as promoters of bacterial translocation, including injured tissue, hypotension, protein malnutrition, and altered gut flora. Translocation of indigenous gut pathogens would explain the high incidence of secondary infection by enteric flora. This also might explain the failure of most trials of prophylactic systemic antibiotics, given the failure of most agents to achieve effective levels in gut mucosa or the pancreatic parenchyma.

At least two hypothetical methods of preventing bacterial translocation are clinically intriguing. A therapeutic trial of oral nonabsorbable antibiotics could be done, or some method of stabilizing the gut-blood interface could be attempted. Nonabsorbable antibi-

Table 22-12
Proposed Mediators of MOSF

Mediators	*Effects*
Interleukin-1	Fever, proteolysis
Prostaglandins	Vasodilation
Corticosteroids	Hypermetabolism
Glucagon	Gluconeogenesis
Norepinephrine	Hypermetabolism
Growth, thyroid hormones	Acute catabolism
Complement, anaphylatoxins	Microcirculatory injury
Kinin system, serotonin, histamine	Vasodilation
Oxygen free radicals	Membrane damage
Tumor necrosis factor	Tissue injury, shock
?Myocardial depressant factor	Cardiac dysfunction
Nitric oxide	Vasodilation, hypotension

otics selected to decrease enteric flora have been attempted in "selective decontamination" of the gastrointestinal tract in series of trauma, granulocytopenic, and liver transplantation patients. To date, such studies have demonstrated a decrease in the nosocomial infection rate without overall improvements in patient survival.

It is most likely that the MOSF associated with abdominal inflammatory processes is little different from the MOSF seen with trauma, burns, or other catastrophic illness. The prevention of hypovolemic shock by early resuscitation has decreased the early mortality of patients and presumably decreased the incidence of MOSF. With patients surviving the initial insult, newer techniques to diagnose and treat the late septic complications have also resulted in improved survival. The techniques of early diagnosis, including dynamic computed tomography, percutaneous aspiration of inflammatory masses, and measurement of circulating acute phase reactants have all been used to lessen the morbidity and mortality of sepsis. Furthermore, more aggressive surgical drainage tactics with a tendency toward earlier exploration and frequent reoperation are also decreasing mortality figures.

Current therapy for MOSF consists of a two-pronged attack. First, maximal support of individual organ function (lungs, kidneys, nutrition, etc.) must be aggressively pursued as an initial preventive measure. Second, an aggressive approach to the detection and eradication of occult sepsis must be maintained. The techniques of selective bacterial decontamination and early enteral feeding are both promising and exciting in the eventual goal of the elimination of MOSF-associated death.

Bibliography

Introduction/General References

Abumbad NN, Frexes-Steed M: What getting sick means. *JPEN* 14:157S, 1990.

Balthazar EJ, Chako AC: Computerized tomography in acute gastrointestinal disorders. *Am J Gastroenterol* 85:1445, 1990.

Cutler BS, Dodson TF, et al (eds): *Manual of Clinical Problems in Surgery*. Boston, Little, Brown & Co, 1984.

Eastwood GL, Avanduk C (eds): *Manual of Gastroenterology: Diagnosis and Therapy*. Boston, Little, Brown & Co, 1989.

Moody FG: Surgical consultation in digestive disease, in Moody FG et al (eds): *Surgical Treatment of Digestive Disease,* 2nd ed. Chicago, Year Book Medical Publishers, 1990, pp 53–59.

Schwartz SI: Manifestations of gastrointestinal disease, in Schwartz SI (ed): *Principles of Surgery,* 5th ed. New York, McGraw-Hill, 1989, pp 1061–1101.

Shamburek RD, Farrar JT: Disorders of the digestive system in the elderly. *N Engl J Med* 322:438, 1990.

Spiro HM: Gastrointestinal consultation, in Moody FG et al (eds): *Surgical Treatment of Digestive Disease,* 2nd ed. Chicago, Year Book Medical Publishers, 1990, pp 3–10.

Stellato TA, Shek RR: Gastrointestinal emergencies in the oncology patient. *Semin Oncol* 16:521, 1989.

Pain

Alpers DH: Functional gastrointestinal disorders. *Hosp Pract* 37:139, 1983.

Burnett LS: Gynecologic causes of the acute abdomen. *Surg Clin North Am* 68:385, 1988.

Eisenberg RL, Heineken P, et al: Evaluation of plain abdominal radiographs in the diagnosis of abdominal pain. *Ann Surg* 197:464, 1983.

Fenyo G: Acute abdominal disease in the elderly. *Am J Surg* 143:751, 1982.

Gallegos NC, Hobsley M: Abdominal wall pain: an alternative diagnosis. *Br J Surg* 77:1167, 1990.

Glenn J, Funkhouser WK, et al: Acute illnesses necessitating urgent abdominal surgery in neutropenic cancer patients. *Surgery* 105:778, 1989.

Hatch EI: The acute abdomen in children. *Pediatr Clin North Am* 32:1151, 1985.

Irvin TT: Abdominal pain: a surgical audit of 1190 emergency admissions. *Br J Surg* 76:1121, 1989.

Klein KB, Mellinkoff SM: Approach to the patient with abdominal pain, in Yamada T et al (eds): *Textbook of Gastroenterology*. Philadelphia, Lippincott, 1991, pp 660–679.

Koch MO, McDougal WS: Urologic causes of the acute abdomen. *Surg Clin North Am* 68:399, 1988.

Levine MS: Plain film diagnosis of the acute abdomen. *Emerg Med Clin North Am* 3:541, 1985.

McFadden DW, Zinner MJ: Approach to the patient with acute abdomen and fever of abdominal origin, in Yamada T et al (eds): *Textbook of Gastroenterology*. Philadelphia, Lippincott, 1991, pp 692–707.

Neblett WW, Pietsch JB, et al: Acute abdominal conditions in children and adolescents. *Surg Clin North Am* 68:415, 1988.

Roh JJ, Thompson JS, et al: Value of pneumoperitoneum in the diagnosis of visceral perforation. *Am J Surg* 146:830, 1983.

Schaff MI, Tarr RW, et al: Computed tomography and magnetic resonance imaging of the acute abdomen. *Surg Clin North Am* 68:233, 1988.

Villar HG, Warneke JA, et al: Role of surgical treatment in the management of complications of the gastrointestinal tract in patients with leukemia. *Surg Gynecol Obstet* 165:217, 1987.

Wade DS, Nava HR, et al: Neutropenic colitis. *Cancer* 69:17, 1992.

Weddington WW: Psychiatric aspects of chronic abdominal pain. *Drug Ther Bull* 17:45, 1982.

Dysphagia

Browning TH, et al: Diagnosis of chest pain of esophageal origin. *Dig Dis Sci* 35:289, 1990.

Castell DO: Approach to the patient with dysphagia, in Yamada T et al (eds): *Textbook of Gastroenterology*. Philadelphia, Lippincott, 1991, pp 562–572.

Cattau EL, Castell DO: Symptoms of esophageal dysfunction. *Adv Intern Med* 27:151, 1982.

Edwards DAW: Flow charts, diagnostic keys, and algorithms in the diagnosis of dysphagia. *Scott Med J* 15:378, 1970.

Hiccups (Singultus)

Kolodzik PW, Eilers MA: Hiccups (singultus): review and approach to management. *Ann Emerg Med* 20:565, 1991.

Middleton RK: Drug therapy for hiccups. *Drug Intell Clin Pharm* 21:259, 1987.

Heartburn and Dyspepsia

Castell DO: Medical therapy for reflux esophagitis: 1986 and beyond. *Ann Intern Med* 104:112, 1986.

Castell DO: Clinical approach to the patient with heartburn and dyspepsia, in Moody FG et al (eds): *Surgical Treatment of Digestive Disease,* 2nd ed. Chicago, Year Book Medical Publishers, 1990, pp 11–18.

Graham DY, Smith JL, et al: Why do apparently healthy people use antacid tablets? *Am J Gastroenterol* 78:257, 1983.

Kaul B, Petersen H, et al: Hiatus hernia in gastroesophageal reflux disease. *Scand J Gastroenterol* 21:31, 1986.

Stuart RC, Hennesy TPJ: Primary disorders of esophageal motility. *Br J Surg* 76:1111, 1989.

Talley NJ, Zinsmeister AR, et al: Dyspepsia and dyspepsia subgroups: a population-based study. *Gastroenterology* 102:1259, 1992.

Anorexia

Halmi KA: Anorexia nervosa and bulimia. *Annu Rev Med* 38:373, 1987.
Morley JE, Levine AS: The central control for appetite. *Lancet* 1:398, 1983.
Smith GP, Gibbs J: The effect of gut peptides on hunger, satiety, and food intake in humans. *Ann NY Acad Sci* 499:132, 1987.

Weight Loss

Drossman DA: Approach to the patient with unexplained weight loss, in Yamada T et al (eds): *Textbook of Gastroenterology*. Philadelphia, Lippincott, 1991, pp 634–646.
Huerta G, Viniegra L: Involuntary weight loss as a clinical problem. *Rev Invest Clin* 41:5, 1989.
Leduc D, Rouge PE, et al: Clinical study of 105 cases of isolated weight loss in internal medicine. *Rev Intern Med* 9:480, 1988.
Martin KI, Sox HC, et al: Involuntary weight loss: diagnostic and prognostic significance. *Ann Intern Med* 95:568, 1981.

Nausea and Vomiting

Chaudhuri TK, Fink S: Update: pharmaceuticals and gastric emptying. *Am J Gastroenterol* 85:223, 1990.
Hanson JS, McCallum RW: The diagnosis and management of nausea and vomiting: a review. *Am J Gastroenterol* 80:210, 1985.
Mozwecz H, Pavel D, et al: Erythromycin stearate as prokinetic agent in postvagotomy gastroparesis. *Dig Dis Sci* 35:902, 1990.
Pellegrini C, Ryan T: Management of gastric motility disorders. *Contemp Surg* 22:15, 1983.

Gas and Bloating

Maddock WG, Bell JL: Gastrointestinal gas. *Ann Surg* 130:512, 1949.
Perlman JA, Saltzberg DM: Approach to the patient with gas and bloating, in Yamada T et al (eds): *Textbook of Gastroenterology*. Philadelphia, Lippincott, 1991, pp 681–689.
Roth JA: Gaseousness, in Berk JE (ed): *Gastroenterology*. Philadelphia, Saunders, 1985, p 142.

Flatulence

Lenhard-Jones JE: Functional gastrointestinal disorders. *N Engl J Med* 308:431, 1983.
Levitt MD: Volume and composition of human intestinal gas. *N Engl J Med* 284:1394, 1971.

Constipation

Beck DE: Constipation, in Fazio V (ed): *Current Therapy in Colon and Rectal Surgery*. Toronto, BC Decker, 1990, pp 339–343.
Pemberton JH, Phillips SF: Constipation and diarrhea, in Moody FG et al (eds): *Surgical Treatment of Digestive Disease,* 2nd ed. Chicago, Year Book Medical Publishers, 1990, pp 39–52.
Sander RS, Drossman DA: Bowel habits in apparently healthy young adults. *Dig Dis Sci* 32:841, 1987.
Wald A: Approach to the patient with constipation, in Yamada T et al (eds): *Textbook of Gastroenterology*. Philadelphia, Lippincott, 1991, pp 779–793.
Wexner SD, Dailey T: The diagnosis and surgical treatment of chronic constipation. *Contemp Surg* 32:59, 1988.

Diarrhea

Blacklow NR, Cukor G: Viral gastroenteritis. *N Engl J Med* 304:397, 1981.
Fedorak RN, Field M: Antidiarrheal therapy: prospects for new agents. *Dig Dis Sci* 32:195, 1987.
Field M, Rao MC, et al: Intestinal electrolyte transport and diarrheal disease (parts 1 and 2). *N Engl J Med* 321:800, and 321:879, 1989.
Guerrant RL, Bobak DA: Bacterial and protozoal gastroenteritis. *N Eng J Med* 325:327, 1991.

Obstruction

Brolin RE: Partial small bowel obstruction. *Surgery* 95:145, 1984.
Brolin RE, Rasna MJ, et al: Use of tubes and radiographs in the management of small bowel obstruction. *Ann Surg* 206:126, 1987.
Butler JA, Cameron BL, et al: Small bowel obstruction in patients with a prior history of cancer. *Am J Surg* 162:624, 1991.
Pickleman J, Lee RM: The management of patients with suspected early postoperative small bowel obstruction. *Ann Surg* 210:216, 1989.
Richards WO, Williams LF: Obstruction of the large and small intestine. *Surg Clin North Am* 68:355, 1988.
Riveron FA, Obeid FN, et al: The role of contrast radiography in presumed bowel obstruction. *Surgery* 106:496, 1989.
Sarr MG, Bulkley GB, et al: Preoperative recognition of intestinal strangulation obstruction. *Am J Surg* 145:176, 1983.
Wangensteen OH: Understanding the bowel obstruction problem. *Am J Surg* 135:131, 1978.

Ileus

Graber JN, Schulte WJ, et al: The duration of postoperative ileus related to the extent and site of operative dissection. *Surg Forum* 31:141, 1980.
Livingston EH, Passaro EP: Postoperative ileus. *Dig Dis Sci* 35:121, 1990.
Smith J, Kelly KA, et al: Pathophysiology of postoperative ileus. *Arch Surg* 112:203, 1977.

Fever

Atkins E, Bodel P: Fever. *N Engl J Med* 286:27, 1972.
Freischlag J, Busuttil RW: The value of postoperative fever evaluation. *Surgery* 94:358, 1983.
Galacier C, Richet H: A prospective study of postoperative fever in a general surgery department. *Infect Control* 6:487, 1985.
McFadden DW, Zinner MJ: Approach to the patient with acute abdomen and fever of abdominal origin, in Yamada T et al (eds): *Textbook of Gastroenterology*. Philadelphia, Lippincott, 1991, pp 707–714.
Yeung RSW, Buck JR, et al: The significance of fever following operations in children. *J Pediatr Surg* 17:347, 1982.

Gastrointestinal Bleeding

Christensen A, Bousfield R, et al: Incidence of perforated and bleeding peptic ulcers before and after the introduction of H2-receptor antagonists. *Ann Surg* 207:4, 1988.
Fineberg HV, Pearlman LA: Surgical treatment of peptic ulcer in the United States. *Lancet* 1:1305, 1981.
Greenberger NJ: Gastrointestinal bleeding, in Moody FG et al (eds): *Surgical Treatment of Digestive Disease,* 2nd ed. Chicago, Year Book Medical Publishers, 1990, pp 19–29.
Koval G, Benner KG, et al: Aggressive angiographic diagnosis in acute lower gastrointestinal hemorrhage. *Dig Dis Sci* 32:248, 1987.
Larson DE, Farnell MB: Upper gastrointestinal hemorrhage. *Mayo Clin Proc* 58:371, 1983.
Larson G, Schmidt T, et al: Upper gastrointestinal bleeding: predictors of outcome. *Surgery* 100:765, 1986.
Leitman IM, Paul DE, et al: Evaluation and management of massive lower gastrointestinal hemorrhage. *Ann Surg* 209:175, 1989.

Lewis BS, Waye JD: Chronic gastrointestinal bleeding of obscure origin: role of small bowel enteroscopy. *Gastroenterology* 94:1117, 1988.

McFadden DW, Zinner MJ: Reoperation for recurrent peptic ulcer disease. *Surg Clin North Am* 71:77, 1991.

Peterson WL, Barnett CC, et al: Routine early endoscopy in upper-gastro-intestinal-tract bleeding. *N Engl J Med* 304:925, 1981.

Richards RJ, Donica MB, et al: Can the blood urea nitrogen/creatinine ratio distinguish upper from lower gastrointestinal bleeding? *J Clin Gastroenterol* 12:500, 1990.

Richter JM, Christensen MR, et al: Angiodysplasia. *Dig Dis Sci* 34:1542, 1989.

Robert JH, Sachar DB, et al: Management of severe hemorrhage in ulcerative colitis. *Am J Surg* 159:550, 1990.

Stellato T, Rhodes RS, et al: Azotemia in upper gastrointestinal hemorrhage. *Am J Gastroenterol* 73:486, 1980.

Sugawa C, Steffes CP, et al: Upper GI bleeding in an urban hospital. *Ann Surg* 212:521, 1990.

Uden P, Jiborn H, et al: Influence of selective mesenteric arteriography on the outcome of emergency surgery for massive lower gastrointestinal hemorrhage. *Dis Colon Rectum* 29:561, 1986.

Weber JD, McFadden DW: Carcinoid tumors in Meckel's diverticula. *J Clin Gastroenterol* 1:682, 1989.

Wilson SE, Stone RT, et al: Massive lower gastrointestinal bleeding from intestinal varices. *Arch Surg* 114:1158, 1979.

Zinner MJ, Zuidema GD, et al: The prevention of upper gastrointestinal tract bleeding in patients in an intensive care unit. *Surg Gynecol Obstet* 153:214, 1981.

Jaundice

Foust RT, Schiff ER: Jaundice, in Moody FG et al (eds): *Surgical Treatment of Digestive Disease,* 2nd ed. Chicago, Year Book Medical Publishers, 1990, pp 30–38.

Frank BB: Clinical evaluation of jaundice. *JAMA* 262:3031, 1989.

O'Connor KW, Snodgrass PJ, et al: A blinded prospective study comparing four current noninvasive approaches in the differential diagnosis of medical versus surgical jaundice. *Gastroenterology* 84:1498, 1983.

Traber PG, Gumucio JJ: Approach to the patient with jaundice, in Yamada T et al (eds): *Textbook to Gastroenterology*. Philadelphia, Lippincott, 1991, pp 810–828.

Vennes JA, Bond JA: Approach to the jaundiced patient. *Gastroenterology* 84:1615, 1983.

Multiple Organ System Failure (MOSF)

Alexander JW, Boyce ST, et al: The process of microbial translocation. *Ann Surg* 212:496, 1990.

Fry DE: Multiple system organ failure. *Surg Clin North Am* 68:107, 1988.

McFadden DW: Organ failure and multiple organ system failure in pancreatitis. *Pancreas* 6S:37, 1991.

Page CP: The surgeon and gut maintenance. *Am J Surg* 158:485, 1989.

Saadia R, Schein M, et al: Gut barrier function and the surgeon. *Br J Surg* 77:487, 1990.

Wilmore DW, Smith RJ, et al: The gut: a central organ after surgical stress. *Surgery* 104:917, 1988.

CHAPTER 23

Esophagus and Diaphragmatic Hernia

Jeffrey H. Peters and Tom R. DeMeester

SURGICAL ANATOMY

The esophagus is a muscular tube that starts as the continuation of the pharynx and ends as the cardia of the stomach. When the head is in normal anatomic position, the transition from pharynx to esophagus occurs at the lower border of the sixth cervical vertebra. Topographically this corresponds to the cricoid cartilage anteriorly and the palpable transverse process of the sixth cervical vertebra laterally (Fig. 23-1). The esophagus is firmly attached at its upper end to the cricoid cartilage and at its lower end to the diaphragm; during swallowing, the proximal points of fixation move craniad the distance of one cervical vertebral body.

The esophagus lies in the midline, with a deviation to the left in the lower portion of the neck and upper portion of the thorax, and returns to the midline in the midportion of the thorax near the bifurcation of the trachea (Fig. 23-2). In the lower portion of the thorax, the esophagus again deviates to the left and anterior to pass through the diaphragmatic hiatus.

Three normal areas of esophageal narrowing are evident on the barium esophagogram or during esophagoscopy. The uppermost narrowing is located at the entrance into the esophagus and is caused by the cricopharyngeal muscle. Its luminal diameter is 1.5 cm, and it is the narrowest point of the esophagus. The middle

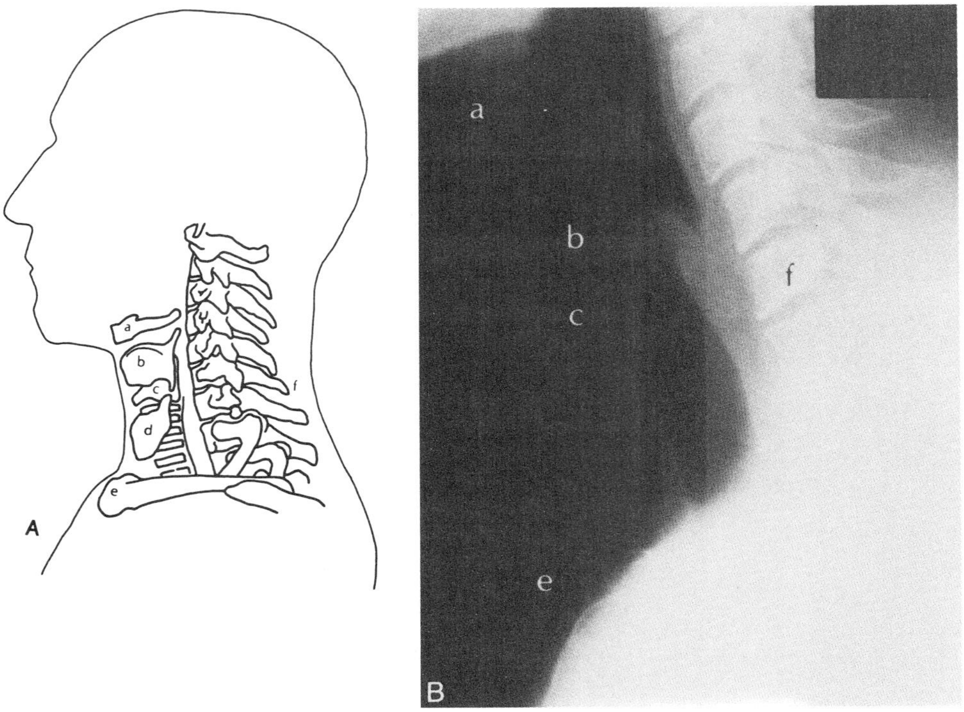

FIG. 23-1. *A.* Topographic relationships of the cervical esophagus: (a) hyoid bone, (b) thyroid cartilage, (c) cricoid cartilage, (d) thyroid gland, (e) sternoclavicular, (f) C6. *B.* Lateral radiographic appearance. (From: *Rothberg M, DeMeester TR: Surgical anatomy of the esophagus, in Shields TW (ed): General Thoracic Surgery, 3rd ed. Philadelphia, Lea & Febiger, 1989, p 77, with permission*).

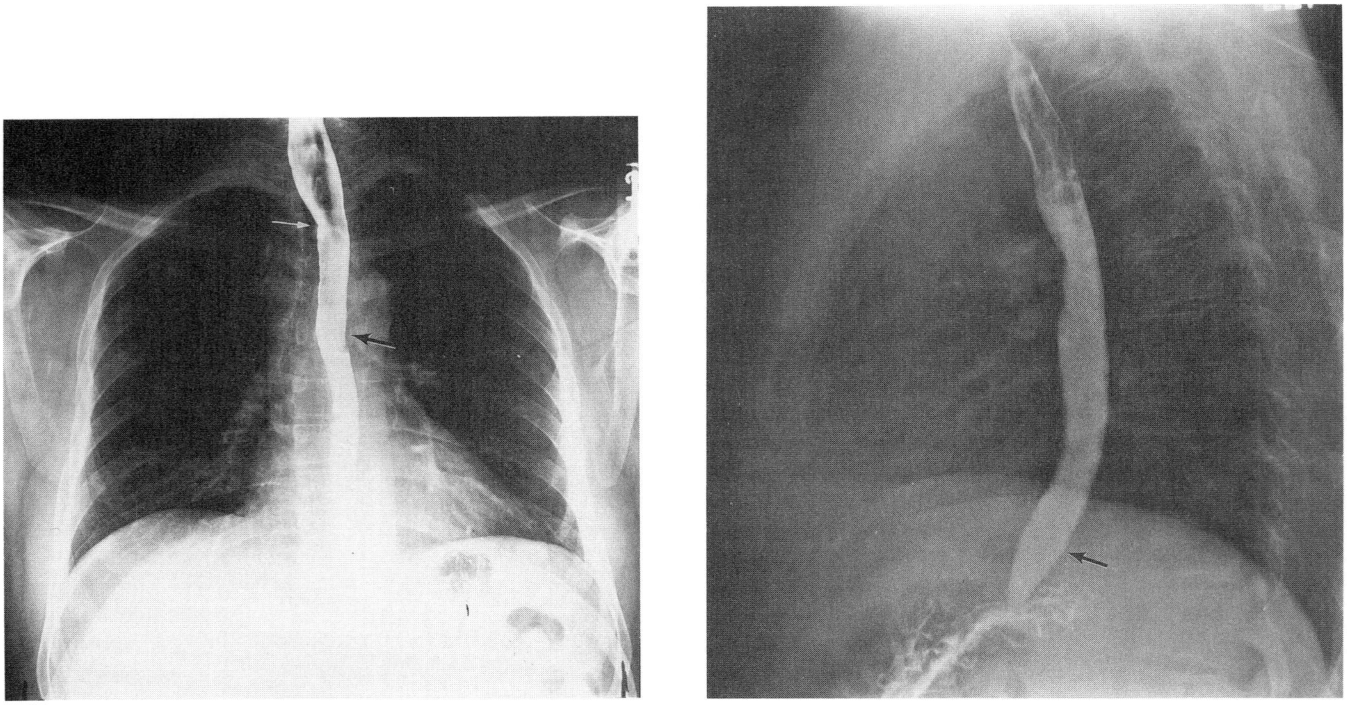

A *B*

FIG. 23-2. Barium esophagogram. *A.* Posterior-anterior view. *B.* Lateral view. White arrow shows deviation to left. Black arrow shows return to midline. Black arrow on lateral view shows anterior deviation. (From: *Rothberg M, DeMeester TR: Surgical anatomy of the esophagus, in Shields TW (ed): General Thoracic Surgery, 3rd ed. Philadelphia, Lea & Febiger, 1989, p 77, with permission.*)

narrowing is due to an indentation of the anterior and left lateral esophageal wall caused by the crossing of the left main stem bronchus and aortic arch. The luminal diameter at this point is 1.6 cm. The lowermost narrowing is at the hiatus of the diaphragm and is caused by the gastroesophageal sphincter mechanism. The luminal diameter at this point varies somewhat depending on the distention of the esophagus by the passage of food, but has been measured at 1.6 to 1.9 cm. These normal constrictions tend to hold up swallowed foreign objects, and the overlying mucosa is subjected to injury by swallowed corrosive liquids due to their slow passage through these areas.

Figure 23-3 shows the average distance in centimeters measured during endoscopic examination between the incisor teeth and the cricopharyngeus, aortic arch, and cardia of the stomach. Manometrically, the length of the esophagus between the lower border of the cricopharyngeus and upper border of the lower sphincter varies according to the height of the individual. Figure 23-4 shows a nomogram for esophageal length based on the height of the subject.

The pharyngeal musculature consists of three overlapping, broad, flat, fan-shaped constrictors (Fig. 23-5). The opening of the esophagus is collared by the cricopharyngeal muscle, which arises from both sides of the cricoid cartilage of the larynx and forms a continuous transverse muscle band without an interruption by a median raphe. The fibers of this muscle blend inseparably with those of the inferior pharyngeal constrictor above and the inner circular muscle fibers of the esophagus below. Some investigators believe that the cricopharyngeus is part of the inferior constrictor; that is, the inferior constrictor has two parts, an upper or retrothyroid portion having diagonal fibers, and a lower or retrocricoid portion having transverse fibers. Keith in 1910 showed that these two parts of the same muscle serve totally different functions. The retrocricoid portion serves as the upper sphincter of the esophagus and relaxes when the retrothyroid portion contracts to force the swallowed bolus from the pharynx into the esophagus.

The cervical portion of the esophagus is approximately 5 cm long and descends between the trachea and the vertebral column from the level of the sixth cervical vertebra to the level of the interspace between the first and second thoracic vertebrae posteriorly or of the suprasternal notch anteriorly. The recurrent laryngeal nerves lie in the right and left grooves between the trachea and the esophagus. The left recurrent nerve lies somewhat closer to the esophagus than the right owing to the slight deviation of the esophagus to the left and the more lateral course of the right recurrent nerve around the right subclavian artery. Laterally, on the left and right sides of the cervical esophagus are the carotid sheaths and the lobes of the thyroid gland.

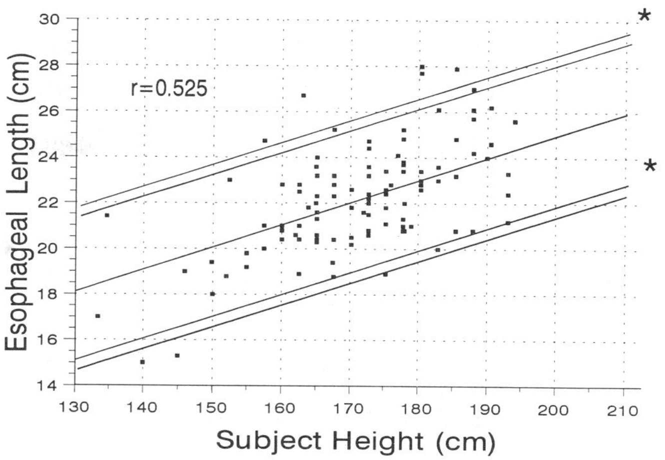

FIG. 23-4. Nomogram for esophageal length based on height of subject. r = coefficient of correlation; * = 2.5, 5, 95, 97.5 percentiles.

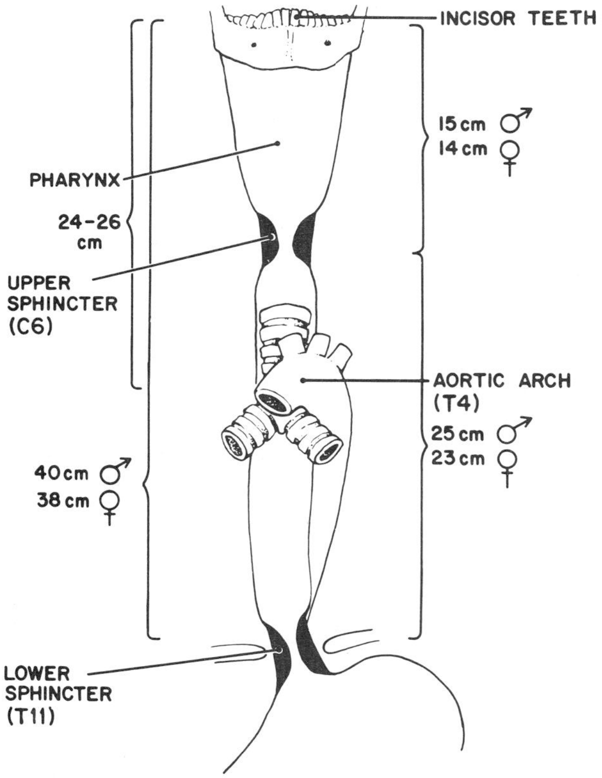

FIG. 23-3. Important clinical endoscopic measurements of the esophagus in adults. (From: *Rothberg M, DeMeester TR: Surgical anatomy of the esophagus, in Shields TW (ed): General Thoracic Surgery, 3rd ed. Philadelphia, Lea & Febiger, 1989, p 78, with permission.*)

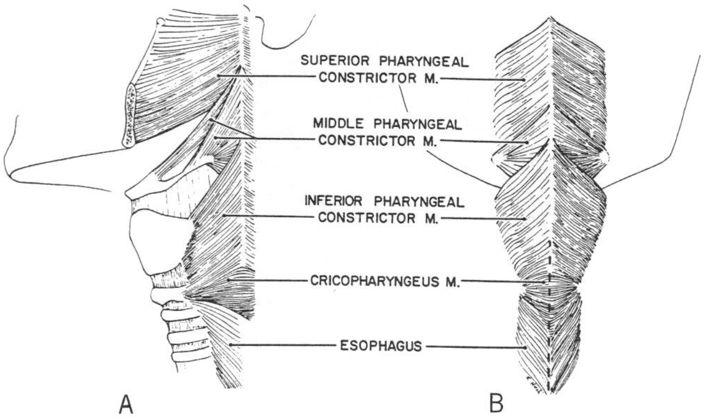

FIG. 23-5. External muscles of the pharynx. *A.* Posterolateral view. *B.* Posterior view. Dotted line represents usual site of myotomy. (From: *Rothberg M, DeMeester TR: Surgical anatomy of the esophagus, in Shields TW (ed): General Thoracic Surgery, 3rd ed. Philadelphia, Lea & Febiger, 1989, p 78, with permission.*)

The thoracic portion of the esophagus is approximately 20 cm long. It starts at the thoracic inlet. In the upper portion of the thorax, it is in intimate relationship with the posterior wall of the trachea and the prevertebral fascia. Just above the tracheal bifurcation, the esophagus passes to the right of the aorta. This anatomic positioning can cause a notch indentation in its left lateral wall on a barium swallow radiogram. Immediately below this notch the esophagus crosses both the bifurcation of the trachea and the left main stem bronchus, owing to the slight deviation of the terminal portion of the trachea to the right by the aorta (Fig. 23-6). From there down the esophagus passes over the posterior surface of the subcarinal lymph nodes, and then descends over the pericardium of the left atrium to reach the diaphragmatic hiatus (Fig. 23-7). From the bifurcation of the trachea downward, both the vagal nerves and the esophageal nerve plexus lie on the muscular wall of the esophagus.

Dorsally, the thoracic esophagus follows the curvature of the spine and remains in close contact with the vertebral bodies. From the eighth thoracic vertebra downward, the esophagus moves vertically away from the spine to pass through the hiatus of the diaphragm. The thoracic duct passes through the hiatus of the diaphragm on the anterior surface of the vertebral column behind the aorta and under the right crus. In the thorax the thoracic duct lies dorsal to the esophagus between the azygos vein on the right and the descending thoracic aorta on the left.

The abdominal portion of the esophagus is approximately 2 cm long. It starts as the esophagus passes through the diaphragmatic hiatus and is surrounded by the phrenoesophageal membrane, a fibroelastic ligament arising from the subdiaphragmatic fascia as a continuation of the transversalis fascia lining the abdomen (Fig. 23-8). The upper leaf of the membrane attaches itself in a circumferential fashion around the esophagus, about 1 to 2 cm above the level of the hiatus. These fibers blend in with the elastic-containing adventitia of the abdominal esophagus and the cardia of the stomach. This portion of the esophagus is subjected to the positive-pressure environment of the abdomen.

The musculature of the esophagus can be divided into an outer longitudinal and an inner circular layer. The upper 2 to 6 cm of the esophagus contains only striated muscle fibers. From there on smooth muscle fibers gradually become more abundant. Most of the clinically significant esophageal motility disorders involve only the smooth muscle in the lower two-thirds of the esophagus. When a surgical esophageal myotomy is indicated, the incision needs to extend only this distance.

The longitudinal muscle fibers originate from a cricoesophageal tendon arising from the dorsal upper edge of the anteriorly located cricoid cartilage. The two bundles of muscle diverge and meet in the midline on the posterior wall of the esophagus about 3 cm below the cricoid (see Fig. 23-5). From this point on, the entire circumference of the esophagus is covered by a layer of longitudinal muscle fibers. This configuration of the longitudinal muscle fibers around the most proximal part of the esophagus leaves a V-shaped area in the posterior wall covered only with circular muscle fibers. Contraction of the longitudinal muscle fibers shortens the esophagus. The circular muscle layer of the esophagus is thicker than the outer longitudinal layer. In situ, the geometry of the circular muscle is helical and makes the peristalsis of the esophagus assume a wormlike drive as opposed to segmental and sequential squeezing. As a consequence, severe motor abnormalities of the esophagus assume a corkscrewlike pattern on the barium swallow radiogram.

The cervical portion of the esophagus receives its main blood supply from the inferior thyroid artery. The thoracic portion receives its blood supply from the bronchial arteries, with 75 percent of individuals having one right-sided and two left-sided branches. Two esophageal branches arise directly from the aorta. The abdominal portion of the esophagus receives its blood supply from the ascending branch of the left gastric artery and from inferior phrenic arteries (Fig. 23-9). On entering the wall of the esophagus, the arteries assume a T-shaped division to form a longitudinal plexus giving rise to an intramural vascular network in the muscular and submucosal layers. As a consequence the esophagus can be mobilized from the stomach to the level of the aortic arch without fear of devascularization and ischemic necrosis. Caution should be exercised as to the extent of esophageal mobilization in patients who have had a previous thyroidectomy with ligation of the infe-

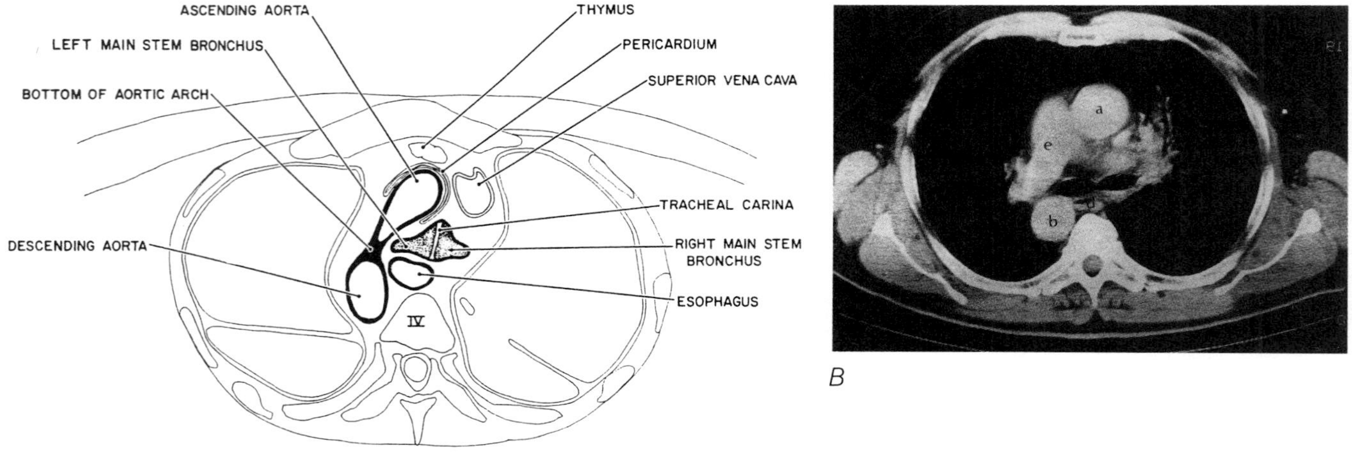

FIG. 23-6. *A.* Cross section of the thorax at the level of the tracheal bifurcation. *B.* CT scan at same level viewed from above: (a) ascending aorta, (b) descending aorta, (c) tracheal carina, (d) esophagus, (e) pulmonary artery. (From: *Rothberg M, DeMeester TR: Surgical anatomy of the esophagus, in Shields TW (ed): General Thoracic Surgery, 3rd ed. Philadelphia, Lea & Febiger, 1989, p 81, with permission.*)

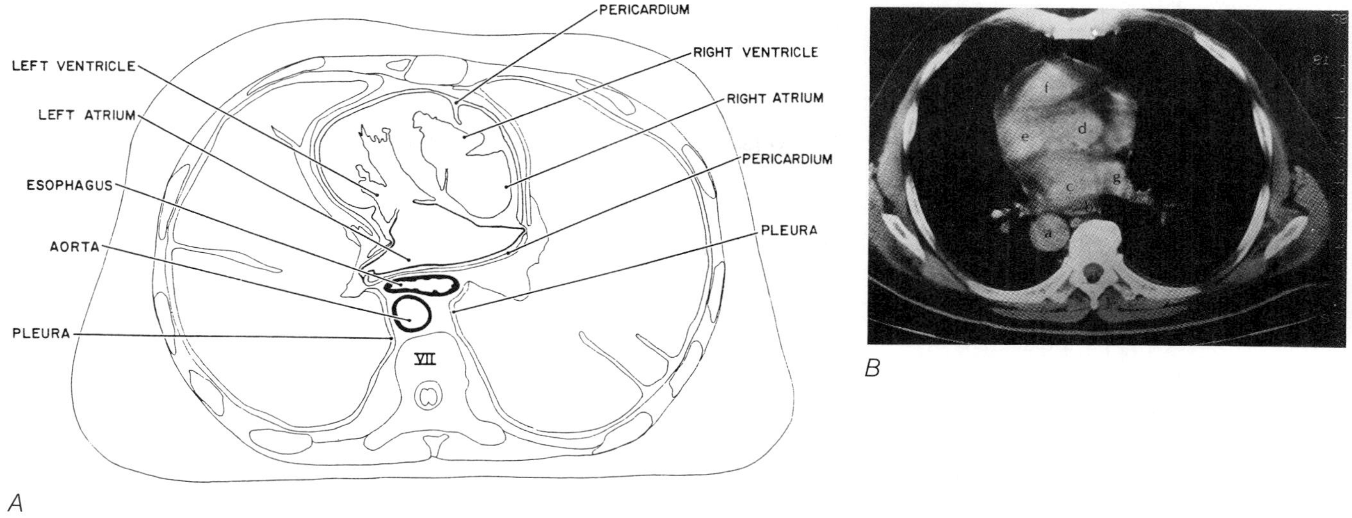

FIG. 23-7. *A.* Cross-section of the thorax at the mid-left atrial level. *B.* CT scan at same level viewed from above: (a) aorta, (b) esophagus, (c) left atrium, (d) right atrium, (e) left ventricle, (f) right ventricle, (g) pulmonary vein. (From: *Rothberg M, DeMeester TR: Surgical anatomy of the esophagus, in Shields TW (ed): General Thoracic Surgery, 3rd ed. Philadelphia, Lea & Febiger, 1989, p 82, with permission.*)

rior thyroid arteries proximal to the origin of the esophageal branches.

Blood from the capillaries of the esophagus flows into a submucosal venous plexus and then into a periesophageal venous plexus from which the esophageal veins originate. In the cervical region, the esophageal veins empty into the inferior thyroid vein; in the thoracic region into the bronchial, azygos, or hemiazygos veins; and in the abdominal region into the coronary vein (Fig. 23-10). The submucosal venous networks of the esophagus and stomach are in continuity with each other, and in patients with portal venous obstruction, this communication functions as a collateral pathway for portal blood to enter the superior vena cava via the azygos vein.

The parasympathetic innervation of the pharynx and esophagus is provided mainly by the vagus nerves. The constrictor muscles of the pharynx receive branches from the pharyngeal plexus, which is on the posterior lateral surface of the middle constrictor muscle and is formed by pharyngeal branches of the vagus nerves with a small contribution from the IXth and XIth cranial nerves (Fig. 23-11). The cricopharyngeal sphincter and the cervical portion of the

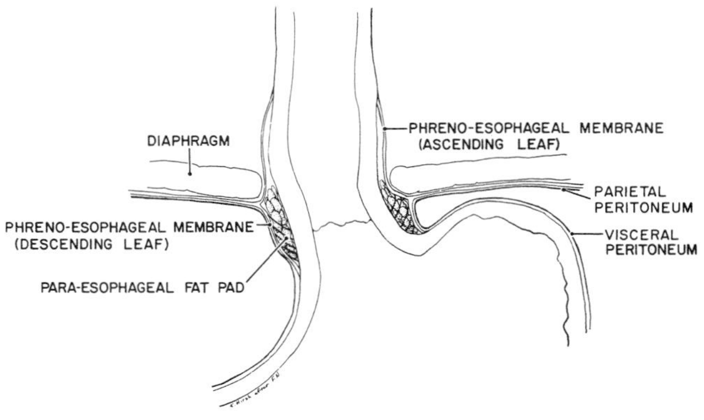

FIG. 23-8. Attachments and structure of the phrenoesophageal membrane. Transversalis fascia lies just above the parietal peritoneum. (From: *Rothberg M, DeMeester TR: Surgical anatomy of the esophagus, in Shields TW (ed): General Thoracic Surgery, 3rd ed. Philadelphia, Lea & Febiger, 1989, p 83, with permission.*)

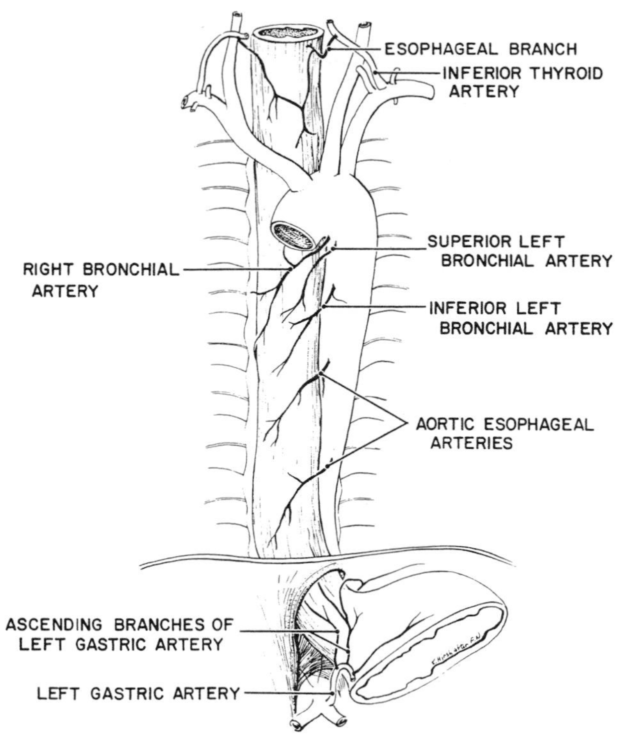

FIG. 23-9. Arterial blood supply of the esophagus. (From: *Rothberg M, DeMeester TR: Surgical anatomy of the esophagus, in Shields TW (ed): General Thoracic Surgery, 3rd ed. Philadelphia, Lea & Febiger, 1989, p 84, with permission.*)

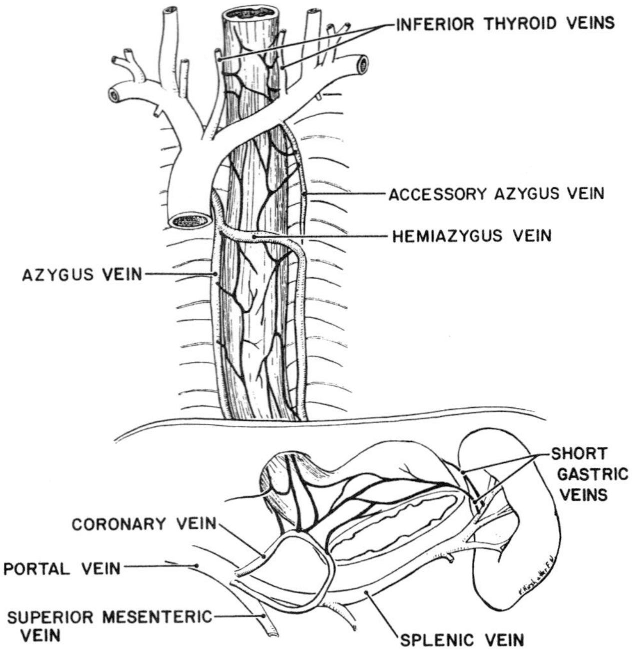

FIG. 23-10. Venous drainage of the esophagus. (From: *Rothberg M, DeMeester TR: Surgical anatomy of the esophagus, in Shields TW (ed): General Thoracic Surgery, 3rd ed. Philadelphia, Lea & Febiger, 1989, p 85, with permission.*)

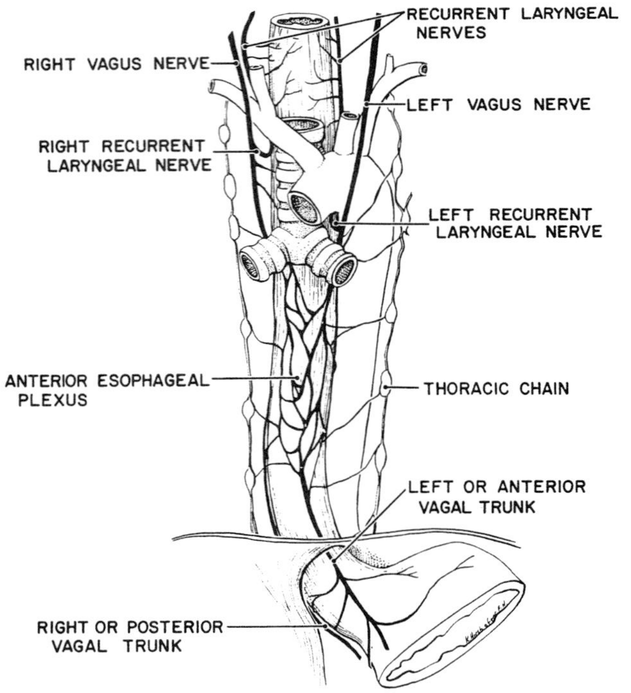

FIG. 23-11. Innervation of the esophagus. (From: *Rothberg M, DeMeester TR: Surgical anatomy of the esophagus, in Shields TW (ed): General Thoracic Surgery, 3rd ed. Philadelphia, Lea & Febiger, 1989, p 85, with permission.*)

esophagus receive branches from both recurrent laryngeal nerves, which originate from the vagus nerves—the right recurrent nerve at the lower margin of the subclavian artery, the left at the lower margin of the aortic arch. They are slung dorsally around these vessels and ascend in the groove between the esophagus and trachea, giving branches to each. Damage to these nerves interferes not only with the function of the vocal cords but also with the function of the cricopharyngeal sphincter and the motility of the cervical esophagus, predisposing the individual to pulmonary aspiration on swallowing.

Afferent visceral sensory pain fibers from the esophagus end without synapse in the first four segments of the thoracic spinal cord, using a combination of sympathetic and vagal pathways. These pathways are also occupied by afferent visceral sensory fibers from the heart; hence, both organs have similar symptomatology.

The lymphatics located in the submucosa of the esophagus are so dense and interconnected that they constitute a single plexus (Fig. 23-12). There are more lymph vessels than blood capillaries in the submucosa. Lymph flow in the submucosal plexus runs in a longitudinal direction, and on injection of a contrast medium the longitudinal spread is seen to be about six times that of the transverse spread. In the upper two-thirds of the esophagus the lymphatic flow is mostly cephalad, and in the lower third caudad. In the thoracic portion of the esophagus, the submucosal lymph plexus extends over a long distance in a longitudinal direction before penetrating the muscle layer to enter lymph vessels in the adventitia. As a consequence of this nonsegmental lymph drainage, a primary tumor can extend for a considerable length superiorly or inferiorly in the submucosal plexus. Consequently, free tumor cells can follow the submucosal lymphatic plexus in either direction for a long distance before they pass through the muscularis and on into the regional lymph nodes. The cervical esophagus has a more direct segmental lymph drainage into the regional

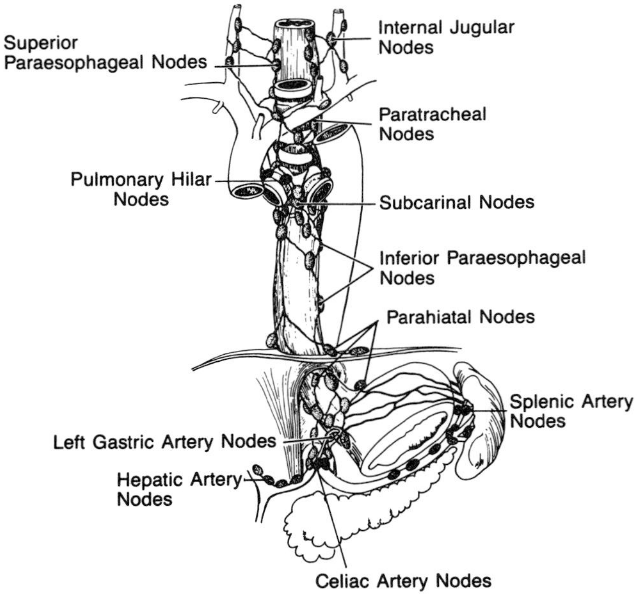

FIG. 23-12. Lymphatic drainage of the esophagus. (From: *DeMeester TR, Barlow AP: Surgery and current management for cancer of the esophagus and cardia: Part I. Curr Probl Surg 25(7):498, 1988, with permission.*)

nodes, and as a result, lesions in this portion of the esophagus have less submucosal extension and a more regionalized lymphatic spread.

The efferent lymphatics from the cervical esophagus drain into the paratracheal and deep cervical lymph nodes, and those from the upper thoracic esophagus empty mainly into the paratracheal lymph nodes. Efferent lymphatics from the lower thoracic esophagus drain into the subcarinal nodes and nodes in the inferior pulmonary ligaments. The superior gastric nodes receive lymph not only from the abdominal portion of the esophagus but also from the adjacent lower thoracic segment.

PHYSIOLOGY

Swallowing Mechanism

The act of alimentation requires the passage of food and drink from the mouth into the stomach. One-third of this distance consists of the mouth and hypopharynx, and two-thirds is made up by the esophagus. To comprehend the mechanics of alimentation, it is useful to visualize the gullet as a mechanical model in which the tongue and pharynx function as a piston pump with three valves, and the body of the esophagus and cardia function as a worm drive pump with a single valve. The three valves in the pharyngeal cylinder are the soft pallet, the epiglottis, and the cricopharyngeus. The valve of the esophageal pump is the lower esophageal sphincter. Failure of the valves or the pumps leads to abnormalities in swallowing—that is, difficulty in food propulsion from mouth to stomach—or regurgitation of gastric contents into the esophagus or pharynx.

Food is taken into the mouth in a variety of bite sizes, where it is broken up, mixed with saliva, and lubricated. Swallowing, once initiated, is entirely a reflex. When food is ready for swallowing, the tongue, acting like a piston, moves the bolus into the posterior oropharynx and forces it into the hypopharynx (Fig. 23-13). Concomitantly with the posterior movement of the tongue, the soft palate is elevated, thereby closing the passage between the oropharynx and nasopharynx. This partitioning prevents pressure generated in the oropharynx from being dissipated through the nose. When the soft palate is paralyzed, as following a cerebral vascular accident, food is commonly regurgitated into the nasopharynx. During swallowing, the hyoid bone moves upward and anteriorly, elevating the larynx and opening the retrolaryngeal space, bringing the epiglottis under the tongue (see Fig. 23-13). The backward tilt of the epiglottis covers the opening of the larynx to prevent aspiration. The whole pharyngeal part of swallowing occurs within 1.5 seconds.

During swallowing, the pressure in the hypopharynx rises abruptly to at least 60 mmHg due to the backward movement of the tongue and contraction of the posterior pharyngeal constrictors. A sizable pressure difference develops between the hypopharyngeal pressure and the less-than-atmospheric midesophageal or intrathoracic pressure (Fig. 23-14). This pressure gradient speeds the movement of food from the hypopharynx into the esophagus when the cricopharyngeus or upper esophageal sphincter relaxes. The bolus is both propelled by peristaltic contraction of the posterior pharyngeal constrictors and sucked into the thoracic esophagus. Critical to receiving the bolus is the compliance of the cervical esophagus; when compliance is lost due to muscle pathology, dysphagia can result. The upper esophageal sphincter closes within 0.5 second of the initiation of the swallow, with the immediate closing pressure reaching approximately twice the resting level of 30 mmHg. The postrelaxation contraction continues down the esophagus as a peristaltic wave (Fig. 23-15). The high closing pressure and the initiation of the peristaltic wave prevents reflux of the bolus from the esophagus back into the pharynx. After the peristaltic wave has passed farther down the esophagus, the pressure in the upper esophageal sphincter returns to its resting level.

Swallowing can be started at will, or it can be reflexly elicited by the stimulation of areas in the mouth and pharynx, among them

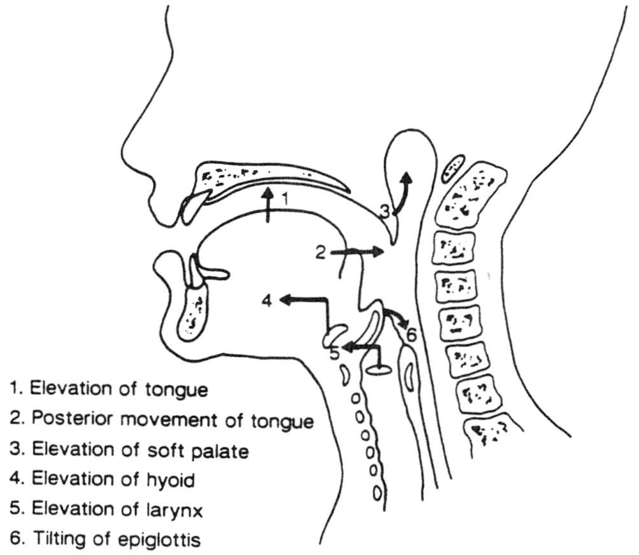

FIG. 23-13. Sequence of events during the oropharyngeal phase of swallowing. (From: *DeMeester TR, Stein HJ, Fuchs KH: Physiologic diagnostic studies, in Zuidema GD, Orringer MB (eds): Shackelford's Surgery of the Alimentary Tract, 3rd ed., Vol I. Philadelphia, Saunders, 1991, p 95, with permission.*)

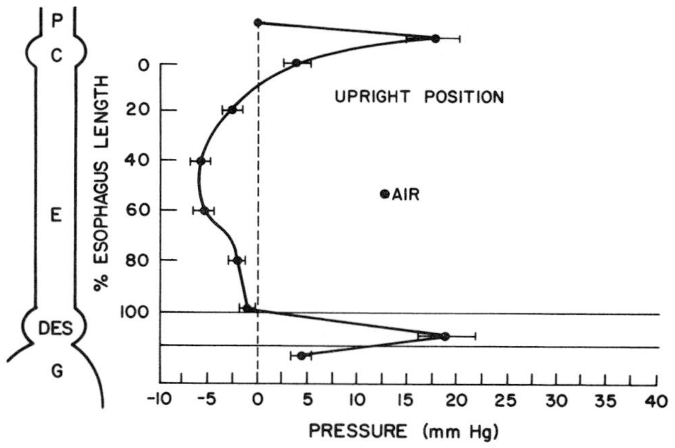

FIG. 23-14. Resting pressure profile of the foregut showing the pressure differential between the atmospheric pharyngeal pressure (P) and the less-than-atmospheric midesophageal pressure (E) and greater-than-atmospheric intragastric pressure (G), with the interposed high-pressure zones of the cricopharyngeus (C) and distal esophageal sphincter (DES). The necessity for relaxation of the cricopharyngeus and DES pressure in order to move a bolus into the stomach is apparent. Esophageal work occurs when a bolus is pushed from the midesophageal area (E), with a pressure less than atmospheric, into the stomach, which has a pressure greater than atmospheric (G). (From: *Waters PF, DeMeester TR: Med Clin North Am 65:1237, 1981, with permission.*)

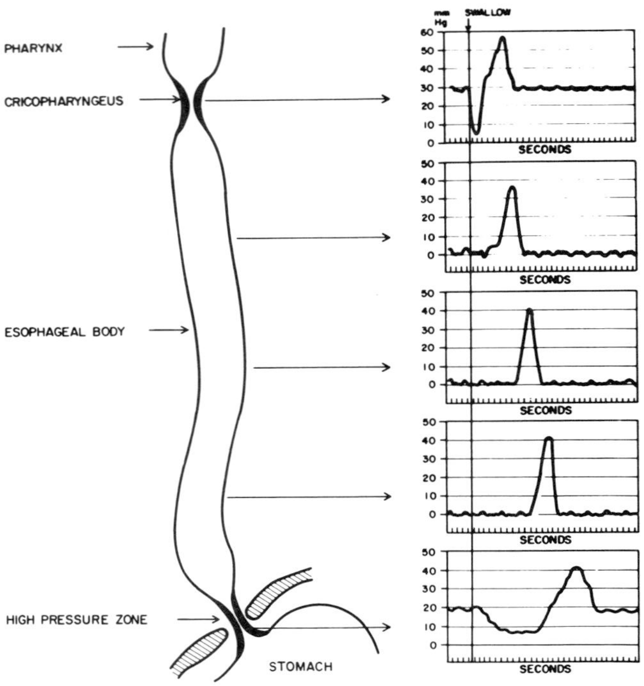

FIG. 23-15. Intraluminal esophageal pressures in response to swallowing. (From: *Waters PF, DeMeester TR: Med Clin North Am 65:1238, 1981, with permission.*)

the anterior and posterior tonsillar pillars or the posterior lateral walls of the hypopharynx. The afferent sensory nerves of the pharynx are the glossopharyngeal nerves and the superior laryngeal branches of the vagus nerves. Once aroused by stimuli entering via these nerves, the swallowing center in the medulla coordinates the complete act of swallowing by discharging impulses through the Vth, VIIth, Xth, XIth, and XIIth cranial nerves, as well as the motor neurons of C1 to C3. Discharges through these nerves occur in a rather specific pattern and last for approximately 0.5 second. Little is known about the organization of the swallowing center except that it can trigger swallowing after a variety of different inputs, but the response is always a rigidly ordered pattern of outflow. Following a cerebral vascular accident, this coordinated outflow may be altered, causing mild-to-severe abnormalitities of swallowing. In more severe injury, swallowing can be grossly disrupted leading to repetitive aspiration.

The striated muscles of the cricopharyngeus and the upper third of the esophagus are activated by efferent motor fibers distributed through the vagus nerve and its recurrent laryngeal branches. The integrity of innervation is required for the cricopharyngeus to relax in coordination with the pharyngeal contraction and resume its resting tone once a bolus has entered the upper esophagus. Operative damage to the innervation can interfere with laryngeal, cricopharyngeal, and upper esophageal function and predispose the patient to aspiration.

The pharyngeal activity in swallowing initiates the esophageal phase. The body of the esophagus functions as a worm drive propulsive pump, due to the helical arrangement of its circular muscles, and is responsible for transmitting a bolus of food into the stomach. The esophageal phase of swallowing represents esophageal work done during alimentation in that food is moved into the stomach from a negative-pressure environment of −6 mmHg intrathoracic pressure to a positive-pressure environment of 6 mmHg intraabdominal pressure or over a gradient of 12 mmHg (see Fig. 23-14). Effective and coordinated smooth muscle function in the lower third of the esophagus is, therefore, important in pumping the food across this gradient.

The peristaltic wave generates an occlusive pressure varying from 30 to 120 mmHg (see Fig. 23-15). The wave rises to a peak in 1 second, lasts at the peak for about 0.5 second, and then subsides in about 1.5 seconds. The whole course of the rise and fall of occlusive pressure may occupy one point in the esophagus for 3 to 5 seconds. The peak of a primary peristaltic contraction initiated by a swallow (primary peristalsis) moves down the esophagus at 2 to 4 cm per second and reaches the distal esophagus about 9 seconds after swallowing starts (see Fig. 23-15). Consecutive swallows produce similar primary peristaltic waves, but when the act of swallowing is rapidly repeated, the esophagus remains relaxed and the peristaltic wave occurs only after the last movement of the pharynx. Progress of the wave in the esophagus is caused by sequential activation of its muscles initiated by efferent vagal nerve fibers arising in the swallowing center.

Continuity of the esophageal muscle is not necessary for sequential activation if the nerves are intact. If the muscles, but not the nerves, are cut across, the pressure wave begins distally below the cut as it dies out at the proximal end above the cut. This allows a sleeve resection of the esophagus to be done without destroying its normal function. Afferent impulses from receptors within the esophageal wall are not essential for progress of the coordinated wave. Afferent nerves, however, do go to the swallowing center from the esophagus, because if the esophagus is distended at any point, a contractual wave begins with a forceful closure of the upper esophageal sphincter and sweeps down the esophagus. This secondary contraction occurs without any movements of the mouth or pharynx. Secondary peristalsis can occur as an independent local reflex to clear the esophagus of ingested material left behind after the passage of the primary wave. Current studies suggest that secondary peristalsis is not as common as once thought.

Despite the rather powerful occlusive pressure, the propulsive force of the esophagus is relatively feeble. If a subject attempts to swallow a bolus attached by a string to a counterweight, the maximum weight that can be overcome is 5 to 10 g. Orderly contractions of the musclar wall and anchoring of the esophagus at its inferior end are necessary for efficient aboral propulsion to occur. Loss of the inferior anchor, as occurs with a large hiatal hernia, can lead to inefficient propulsion.

The lower esophageal sphincter provides a pressure barrier between the esophagus and stomach and acts as the valve on the worm drive pump of the esophageal body. Although an anatomically distinct lower esophageal sphincter has been difficult to identify, microdissection studies show that, in humans, the sphincter-like function is related to the architecture of the muscle fibers at the junction of the esophageal tube with the gastric pouch (Fig. 23-16). The sphincter actively remains closed to prevent reflux of gastric contents into the esophagus and opens by a relaxation that coincides with a pharyngeal swallow (see Fig. 23-15). The lower esophageal sphincter pressure returns to its resting level after the peristaltic wave has passed through the esophagus. Consequently, reflux of gastric juice that may occur through the open valve during a swallow is cleared back into the stomach.

If the pharyngeal swallow does not initiate a peristaltic contraction, then the coincident relaxation of the lower esophageal sphincter is unguarded and reflux of gastric juice can occur. This

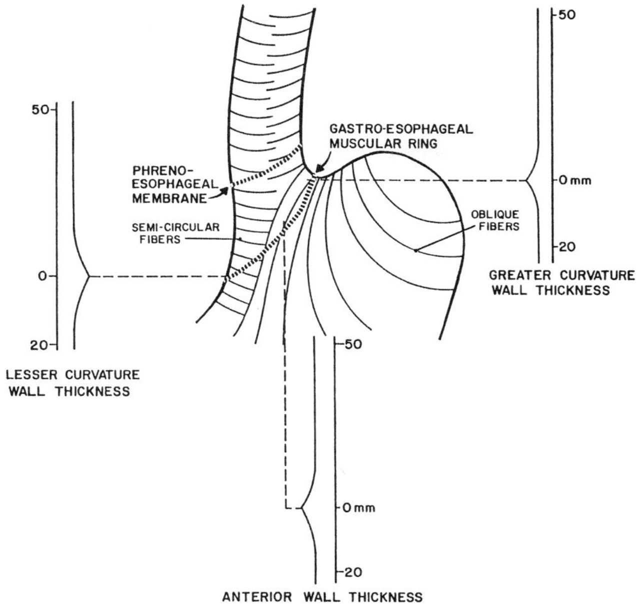

FIG. 23-16. Wall thickness and orientation of fibers on microdissection of the cardia. At the junction of the esophageal tube and gastric pouch, there is an oblique muscular ring composed of an increased muscle mass inside the inner muscular layer. On the lesser curve side of the cardia the muscle fibers of the inner layer are oriented transversely and form semicircular muscle clasps. On the greater curve side of the cardia, these muscle fibers form oblique loops that encircle the distal end of the cardia and gastric fundus. Both the semicircular muscle clasps and the oblique fibers of the fundus contract in a circular manner to close the cardia. (From: *DeMeester TR, Skinner DB: Evaluation of esophageal function and disease, in Glen WWL (ed): Thoracic and Cardiovascular Surgery, 4th ed. Norwalk, Appleton & Lange, 1983, p 461.*)

may be an explanation for the observation of spontaneous lower esophageal relaxation, thought by some to be a causative factor in gastroesophageal reflux disease. The power of the worm drive pump of the esophageal body is insufficient to force open a valve that does not relax. In dogs, a bilateral cervical parasympathetic blockade abolishes the relaxation of the lower esophageal sphincter that occurs with pharyngeal swallowing or distention of the esophagus. Consequently, vagal function appears to be important in coordinating the relaxation of the lower esophageal sphincter with esophageal contraction.

The antireflux mechanism in man is composed of three components: a mechanically effective lower esophageal sphincter, efficient esophageal clearance, and an adequately functioning gastric reservoir. A defect of any one of these three components can lead to increased esophageal exposure to gastric juice and the development of mucosal injury.

Physiologic Reflux

On 24-hour esophageal pH monitoring, healthy individuals have occasional episodes of gastroesophageal reflux. This physiologic reflux is more common when awake and in the upright position than during sleep in the supine position. When reflux of gastric juice occurs, normal subjects rapidly clear the acid gastric juice from the esophagus regardless of their position.

There are several explanations for the observation that physiologic reflux in normal subjects is more common when they are awake and in the upright position than during sleep in the supine position. First, reflux episodes occur in healthy volunteers primarily during transient losses of the gastroesophageal barrier, which may be due to a relaxation of the lower esophageal sphincter or intragastric pressure overcoming sphincter pressure. Gastric juice can also reflux when a swallow-induced relaxation of the lower esophageal sphincter is not protected by an oncoming peristaltic wave. The average frequency of these "unguarded moments" or of transient losses of the gastroesophageal barrier is far less while asleep and in the supine position than while awake and in the upright position. Consequently, there are fewer opportunities for reflux to occur in the supine position. Second, in the upright position there is a 12-mmHg pressure gradient between the resting, positive intraabdominal pressure measured in the stomach, and the most negative intrathoracic pressure measured in the esophagus at midthoracic level. This gradient favors the flow of gastric juice up into the thoracic esophagus when upright. The gradient diminishes in the supine position. Third, the lower esophageal sphincter pressure in normal subjects is significantly higher in the supine position than in the upright position. This is due to the apposition of the hydrostatic pressure of the abdomen to the abdominal portion of the sphincter when supine. In the upright position, the abdominal pressure surrounding the sphincter is negative compared with atmospheric pressure, and, as expected, the abdominal pressure gradually increases the more caudally it is measured. This pressure gradient tends to move the gastric contents toward the cardia and encourages the occurrence of reflux into the esophagus when the individual is upright. By contrast, in the supine position the gastroesophageal pressure gradient diminishes, and the abdominal hydrostatic pressure under the diaphragm increases, causing an increase in sphincter pressure and a more competent cardia.

The lower esophageal sphincter has intrinsic myogenic tone, which is modulated by neural and hormonal mechanisms. Alpha-adrenergic neurotransmitters or beta blockers stimulate the lower esophageal sphincter, and alpha blockers and beta stimulants decrease its pressure. It is not clear to what extent cholinergic nerve activity controls lower esophageal sphincter pressure. The vagus nerve carries both excitatory and inhibitory fibers to the esophagus and sphincter. The hormones gastrin and motilin have been shown to increase lower esophageal sphincter pressure; and cholecystokinin, estrogen, glucagon, progesterone, somatostatin, and secretin decrease lower esophageal sphincter pressure. The peptides bombesin, L-enkephalin, and substance P increase lower esophageal sphincter pressure; and calcitonin gene-related peptide, gastric inhibitory peptide, neuropeptide Y, and vasoactive intestinal polypeptide decrease lower esophageal sphincter pressure. Some pharmacologic agents such as antacids, cholinergics, agonists, domperidone, metoclopramide, and prostaglandin F_2 are known to increase lower esophageal sphincter pressure; and anticholinergics, barbiturates, calcium channel blockers, caffeine, diazepam, dopamine, meperidine, prostaglandin E_1 and E_2, and theophylline decrease lower esophageal sphincter pressure. Peppermint, chocolate, coffee, ethanol, and fat are all associated with decreased lower esophageal sphincter pressure and may be responsible for esophageal symptoms after a sumptuous meal.

ASSESSMENT OF ESOPHAGEAL FUNCTION

A number of tests are currently available for the diagnosis of esophageal disease, but they vary greatly in reliability and appropriate application. The diagnostic tests as presently employed may be divided into five broad groups: (1) tests to detect structural abnormalities of the esophagus; (2) tests to detect functional abnormalities of the esophagus; (3) tests to detect increased esophageal exposure to gastric juice; (4) tests to provoke esophageal symptoms; and (5) tests of duodenogastric function as they relate to esophageal disease.

Tests to Detect Structural Abnormalities. ***Radiographic Evaluation.*** The first diagnostic test in patients with suspected esophageal disease should be a barium swallow followed by full assessment of the stomach and duodenum. Esophageal motility is optimally assessed by observing several individual swallows of barium traversing the entire length of the organ, with the patient in the horizontal position. Hiatal hernias are best demonstrated with the patient prone because the increased intraabdominal pressure produced in this position promotes displacement of the esophagogastric junction above the diaphragm. To detect lower esophageal narrowing, such as rings and strictures, fully distended views of the esophagogastric region are crucial. The density of the barium used to study the esophagus can potentially affect the accuracy of the examination. Esophageal disorders shown well by a full-column technique include circumferential carcinomas, peptic strictures, large esophageal ulcers, and hiatal hernias. A small hiatal hernia is usually not associated with significant symptoms or illness; and its presence is an irrelevant finding unless the hiatal hernia is large (Fig. 23-17), or the hiatal opening is narrow and interrupts the flow of barium into the stomach (Fig. 23-18), or the hernia is of the paraesophageal variety. Lesions extrinsic but adjacent to the esophagus can be reliably detected by the full-column technique if they contact the distended esophageal wall. Conversely, a number of important disorders may go undetected if this is the sole technique used to examine the esophagus. These include small esophageal neoplasms, mild esophagitis, and esophageal varices. Thus, the full-column technique should be supplemented with mucosal relief or double-contrast films to enhance detection of these smaller or more subtle lesions.

Motion-recording techniques greatly aid in evaluating functional disorders of the pharyngoesophageal and esophageal phase of swallowing. The technique and indications for cine-videoradiography will be discussed later, as it is more useful to evaluate function and seldom used to detect structural abnormalities.

The radiographic assessment of the esophagus is not complete unless the entire stomach and duodenum have been examined. A gastric or duodenal ulcer, partially obstructing gastric neoplasm, or scarred duodenum and pylorus may contribute significantly to symptoms otherwise attributable to an esophageal abnormality.

When a patient's complaints include dysphagia and no obstructing lesion is seen on the barium swallow, it is useful to have the patient swallow a barium-impregnated marshmallow, a barium-soaked piece of bread, or a hamburger mixed with barium. This test may bring out a functional disturbance in esophageal transport that can be missed when liquid barium is used.

Endoscopic Evaluation. In any patient complaining of dysphagia, esophagoscopy is indicated, even in the face of a normal radiographic study. A barium study obtained prior to esophagoscopy is helpful to the endoscopist by directing attention to locations of subtle change and alerting the examiner to such potential danger spots as a cervical vertebral osteophyte, esophageal diverticulum, a deeply penetrating ulcer, or a carcinoma. Regardless of the radiologist's interpretation of an abnormal finding, each structural abnormality of the esophagus should be confirmed visually.

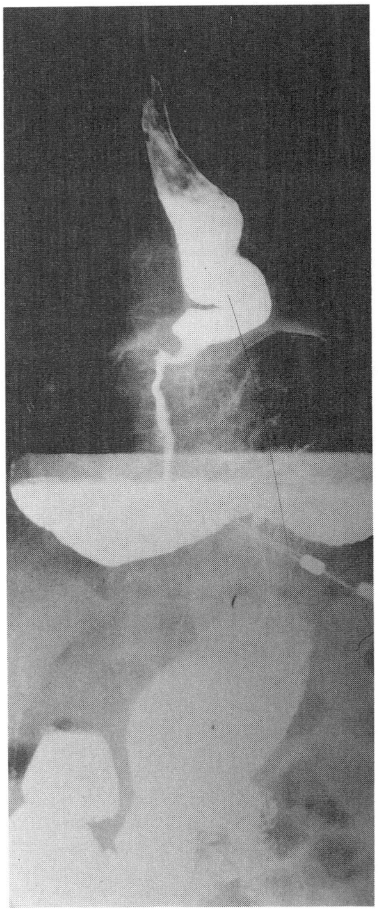

FIG. 23-17. Radiogram of an intrathoracic stomach. This is the end stage of a large hiatal hernia, regardless of its initial classification. (From: *DeMeester TR, Stein HJ, Fuchs KH: Physiologic diagnostic studies, in Zuidema GD, Orringer MB (eds): Shackelford's Surgery of the Alimentary Tract, 3rd ed, Vol I. Philadelphia, Saunders, 1991, p 111, with permission.*)

For the initial endoscopic assessment, the flexible fiberoptic esophagoscope is the instrument of choice because of its technical ease, patient acceptance, and the ability to simultaneously assess the stomach and duodenum. Rigid endoscopy may be required in specific instances and should be part of the armamentarium of the endoscopist. The rigid esophagoscope may be an essential instrument when deeper biopsies are required or the cricopharyngeus and cervical esophagus need closer assessment.

When gastroesophageal reflux disease is the suspected diagnosis, particular attention should be paid to detecting the presence of esophagitis and Barrett's columnar-lined esophagus. When endoscopic esophagitis is seen, severity and the length of esophagus involved are recorded. Grade I esophagitis is defined as reddening of the mucosa without ulceration, and its identification varies depending on the observer. Usually its presence may be confirmed by biopsy. Grade I esophagitis is an unreliable indicator of esophagitis and reflects mainly esophageal mucosal injury secondary to a variety of insults. Grade II esophagitis is defined by the presence of linear erosions lined with granulation tissue that bleeds easily when touched. Grade III esophagitis represents a more advanced stage where the linear ulcerations coalesce, leaving islands of epi-

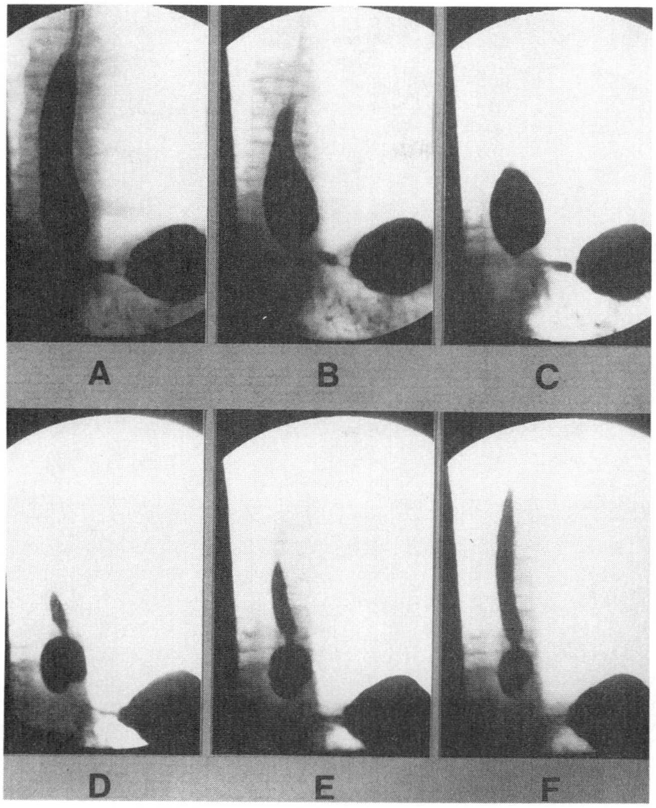

FIG. 23-18. Radiographic barium study showing a primary esophageal wave propelling liquid barium into supradiaphragmatic portion of the stomach in a patient with a hiatal hernia (*A* and *B*). The diaphragmatic impingement on the stomach and the lack of contraction of the supradiaphragmatic stomach prevent passage of the bolus into the distal stomach (*C*). As a consequence, the contents in the supradiaphragmatic portion of the stomach are regurgitated into the thoracic esophagus (*D*, *E*, and *F*). The patient experiences dysphagia and regurgitation. On endoscopy, no anatomic abnormality other than a hiatal hernia was found, and on 24-hour pH monitoring, the patient had normal esophageal acid exposure. Symptoms of dysphagia and regurgitation were relieved by hiatal herniorrhaphy. (From: *Kaul BJ, DeMeester TR: Ann Surg 211:409, 1990, with permission.*)

thelium, which on endoscopy appear as a ''cobblestone'' esophagus. Grade IV esophagitis is the presence of a stricture. Its severity can be assessed by the ease of passing a 36 French endoscope. When a stricture is observed, the severity of the esophagitis above it should be recorded. The absence of esophagitis above a stricture suggests a chemical-induced injury or a neoplasm as a cause. The latter should always be considered and is ruled out only by a tissue biopsy of adequate size.

Barrett's esophagus is a condition where the tubular esophagus is lined with columnar epithelium as opposed to the normal squamous epithelium. It is suspected at endoscopy when there is difficulty in visualizing the squamocolumnar junction at its normal location and by the appearance of a redder, more luxuriant mucosa than is normally seen in the lower esophagus. Its presence is confirmed by biopsy. Multiple biopsies should be taken in a cephalad direction to determine the level at which the junction of Barrett's epithelium with normal squamous mucosa occurs. When this is less than 3 cm above the crura, the diagnosis of Barrett's epithelium is questionable, because of the possibility that the biopsies were taken from a herniated stomach. Barrett's esophagus is susceptible to ulceration, bleeding, stricture formation, and, most important, malignant degeneration. The earliest sign of the latter is severe dysplasia or intramucosal adenocarcinoma (Fig. 23-19). These dysplastic changes have a patchy distribution, so a minimum of five biopsies should be taken from the Barrett's-lined portion of the esophagus. Changes seen in one biopsy are significant. Nishimaki has determined that the tumors occur in an area of specialized columnar epithelium near the squamocolumnar junction in 85 percent of the patients and within 2 cm of the squamocolumnar junction in virtually all patients. Particular attention should be focused in this area in patients suspected of harboring a carcinoma.

A hiatal hernia is endoscopically confirmed by finding a pouch lined with gastric rugal folds lying 2 cm or more above the margins of the diaphragmatic crura, identified by having the patient sniff. A prominent sliding hiatal hernia frequently is associated with increased esophageal exposure to gastric juice. When a paraesophageal hernia is observed, particular attention is taken to exclude a gastric ulcer or gastritis within the pouch. The intragastric retroflex or ''J'' maneuver is important in evaluating the full circumference of the mucosal lining of the herniated stomach.

When an esophageal diverticulum is seen, it should be carefully explored with the flexible scope to exclude ulceration or neoplasia. When a submucosal mass is identified, biopsies are usually not taken. Normally a submucosal leiomyoma or reduplication cyst can be easily dissected away from the intact mucosa, but if a biopsy is taken, the mucosa may become fixed to the underlying abnormality. This complicates the surgical dissection by increasing the risk of mucosal perforation.

Tests to Detect Functional Abnormalities. In many patients with symptoms of an esophageal disorder, standard radiographic and endoscopic evaluation fails to demonstrate a structural abnormality. In these situations, esophageal function tests are necessary to identify a functional disorder.

Stationary Manometry. Esophageal manometry is a widely used technique to examine the motor function of the esophagus and its sphincters. Manometry is indicated whenever a motor abnormality of the esophagus is suspected by the complaints of dysphagia, odynophagia, or noncardiac chest pain, and the barium swallow or endoscopy does not show a clear structural abnormality. Esophageal manometry is particularly necessary to confirm the diagnosis of specific primary esophageal motility disorders, i.e., achalasia, diffuse esophageal spasm, nutcracker esophagus, and hypertensive lower esophageal sphincter. It also identifies nonspecific esophageal motility abnormalities and motility disorders secondary to systemic disease such as scleroderma, dermatomyositis, polymyositis, or mixed connective tissue disease. In patients with symptomatic gastroesophageal reflux disease, manometry of the esophageal body can identify a mechanically defective lower esophageal sphincter and evaluate the adequacy of esophageal peristalsis and contraction amplitude.

Esophageal manometry is performed using electronic pressure-sensitive transducers located within the catheter or water-perfused catheters with lateral side holes attached to transducers outside the body. The catheter usually consists of a train of five pressure transducers or five or more water-perfused tubes bound together. The transducers or lateral openings are placed at 5-cm intervals from the tip and oriented radially at 72° from each other around the

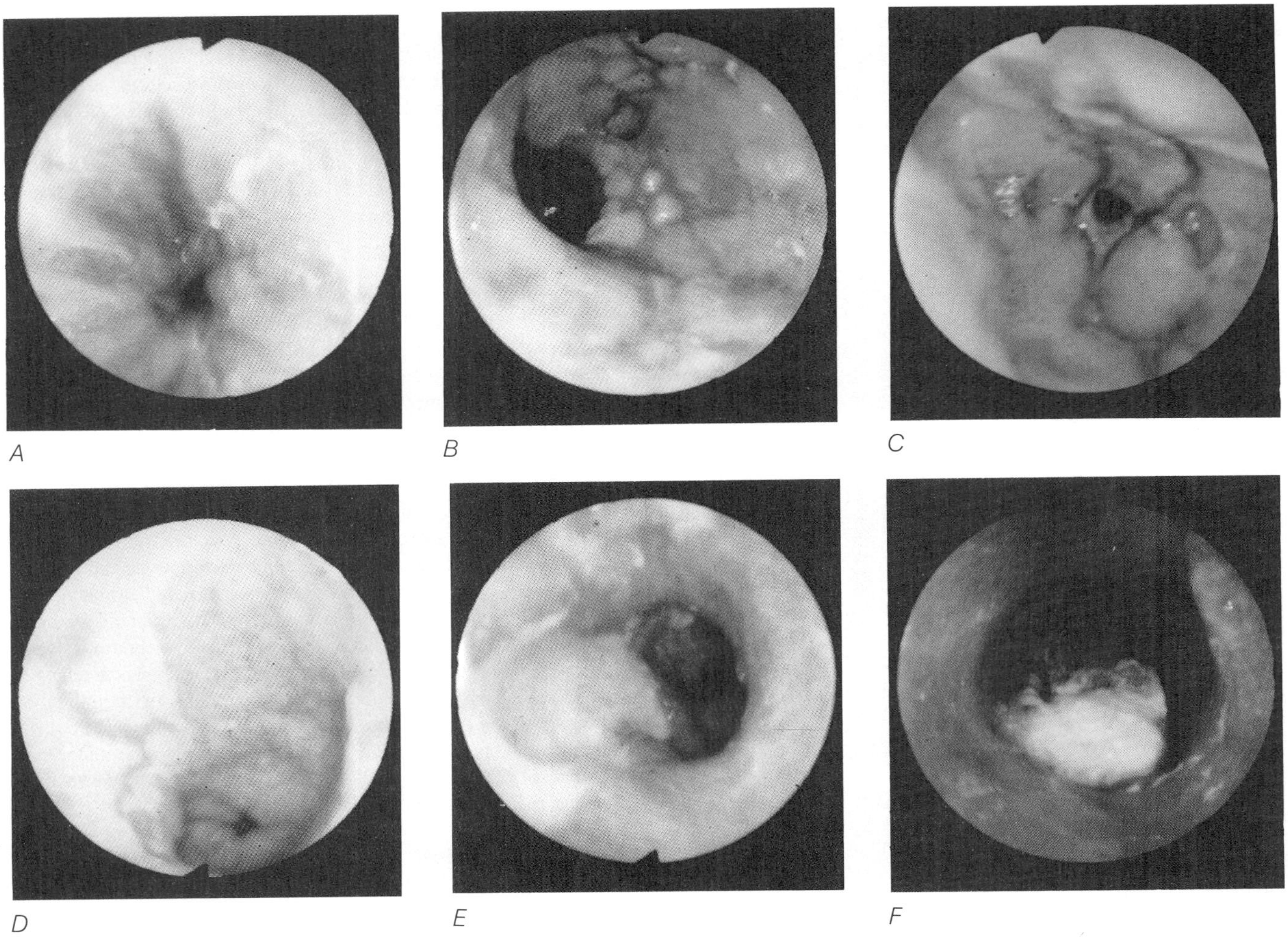

FIG. 23-19. Complications of reflux disease as seen on endoscopy. *A.* Linear erosion of grade II esophagitis. *B.* Cobblestone mucosa of grade III esophagitis. *C.* Stricture associated with grade III esophagitis. *D.* Uncomplicated Barrett's mucosa. *E.* Large ulcer in Barrett's mucosa. *F.* Adenocarcinoma arising in Barrett's mucosa.

circumference of the catheter. A special catheter assembly consisting of four lateral openings at the same level, oriented at 90° to each other, is of special use in measuring the three-dimensional vector volume of the lower esophageal sphincter. Other specially designed catheters can be used to assess the upper sphincter.

As the pressure-sensitive station is brought across the gastroesophageal junction, a rise in pressure above the gastric baseline signals the beginning of the lower esophageal sphincter. The respiratory inversion point is identified when the positive excursions that occur in the abdominal cavity with breathing change to negative deflections in the thorax. The respiratory inversion point serves as a reference point at which the amplitude of lower esophageal sphincter pressure and the length of the sphincter exposed to abdominal pressure are measured. As the pressure-sensitive station is withdrawn into the body of the esophagus, the upper border of the lower esophageal sphincter is identified by the drop in pressure to the esophageal baseline. From these measurements the pressure, abdominal length, and overall length of the sphincter are determined (Fig. 23-20). To account for the asymmetry of the sphincter (Fig. 23-21), the pressure profile is repeated with each of the five radially oriented transducers, and the average values for sphincter pressure above gastric baseline, overall sphincter length, and abdominal length of the sphincter are calculated.

Table 23-1 shows the values for these parameters in 50 normal volunteers without subjective or objective evidence of a foregut disorder. The level at which a deficiency in the mechanics of the lower esophageal sphincter occurs was defined by comparing the frequency distribution of these values in the 50 healthy volunteers with a population of similarly studied patients with symptoms of gastroesophageal reflux disease. The presence of increased esophageal exposure to gastric juice was documented by 24-hour esophageal pH monitoring. Based on these studies, a mechanically defective sphincter is identified by having one or more of the following characteristics: an average lower esophageal sphincter pressure of less than 6 mmHg, an average length exposed to the positive-pressure environment in the abdomen of 1 cm or less, and an average overall sphincter length of 2 cm or less. Compared with the normal volunteers, these values are below the 2.5 percentile for sphincter pressure and overall length, and abdominal length. More recently it has been shown that the resistance of the sphincter to reflux of gastric juice is determined by the integrated effects of radial pressures extended over the entire length, resulting in three-

Table 23-1
Normal Manometric Values of the Distal Esophageal Sphincter, n = 50

		Percentile	
	Median	*2.5*	*97.5*
Pressure (mmHg)	13	5.8	27.7
Overall length (cm)	3.6	2.1	5.6
Abdominal length (cm)	2	0.9	4.7
	Mean	*Mean −2 SD*	*Mean +2 SD*
Pressure (mmHg)	13.8 ± 4.6	4.6	23.0
Overall length (cm)	3.7 ± 0.8	2.1	5.3
Abdominal length (cm)	2.2 ± 0.8	0.6	3.8

SOURCE: DeMeester TR, Stein HJ: Gastroesophageal reflux disease, in Moody FG, Carey LC, et al (eds): *Surgical Treatment of Digestive Disease,* 2nd ed. Chicago, Year Book Medical Publishers, 1989, p 89, with permission.

dimensional computerized imaging of sphincter pressures. Calculating the volume of this image reflects the sphincter's resistance and is called the sphincter pressure vector volume (Fig. 23-22). A calculated SPVV less than the 5th percentile is an indication of a mechanically defective sphincter.

In a study of 50 normal volunteers and 150 patients with increased esophageal exposure to gastric juice and various degrees of esophageal mucosal injury, the calculation of the sphincter pressure vector volume increased the ability of manometry to identify a mechanically defective sphincter compared with standard techniques (Fig. 23-23). This was particularly so in patients without mucosal injury and borderline sphincter abnormalities. Three-dimensional lower esophageal sphincter manometry and calculation of the vector volume should, therefore, become the standard technique to assess the barrier function of the lower esophageal sphincter in patients with gastroesophageal reflux disease. Patients with gastroesophageal reflux disease and an SPVV below the 5th percentile of normal or a deficiency of one, two, or all three mechanical components of a lower esophageal sphincter on standard manometry have a mechanical defect of their antireflux barrier that a surgical antireflux procedure is designed to correct.

To assess the relaxation and postrelaxation contraction of the lower esophageal sphincter, a pressure transducer is positioned within the high-pressure zone, with a distal transducer located in

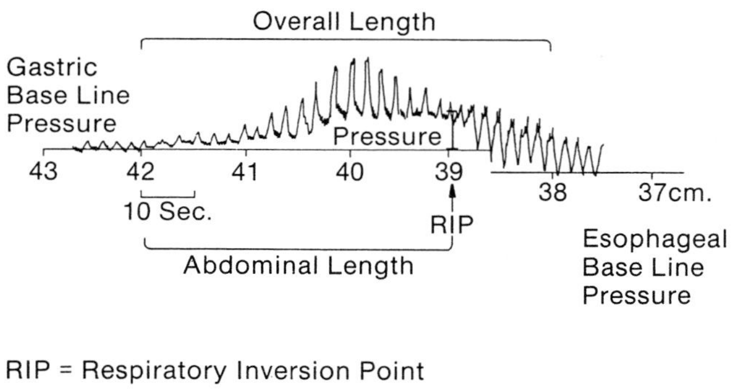

FIG. 23-20. Manometric pressure profile of the lower esophageal sphincter. The distances are measured from the nares. (From: *Zaninotto G, DeMeester TR, et al: Am J Surg 155:105, 1988, with permission.*)

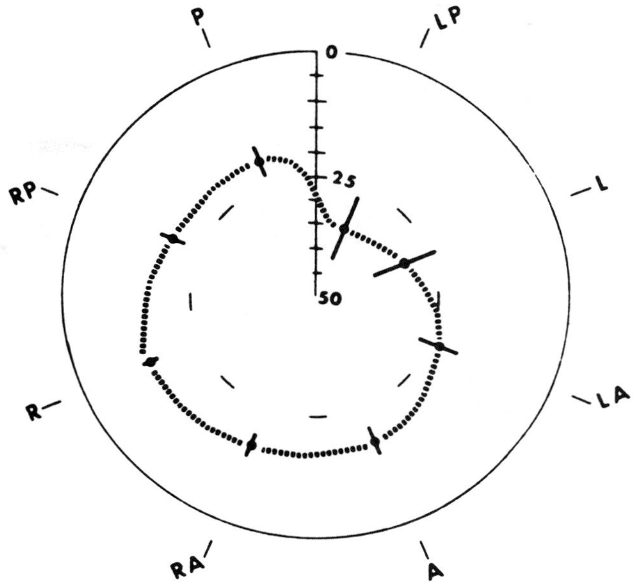

FIG. 23-21. Radial configuration of the lower esophageal sphincter. A = anterior; L = left; LA = left anterior; LP = left posterior; P = posterior; R = right; RA = right anterior; RP = right posterior. (From: *Winans CS: Dig Dis 22:348, 1977, with permission.*)

the stomach and the proximal transducer within the esophageal body. Ten wet swallows (5 mL water each) are performed. The normal pressure of the lower esophageal sphincter should drop to the level of gastric pressure during each wet swallow.

The function of the esophageal body is assessed with the five pressure transducers located in the esophagus. To standardize the procedure the most proximal pressure transducer is located 1 cm below the well-defined cricopharyngeal sphincter. By this method

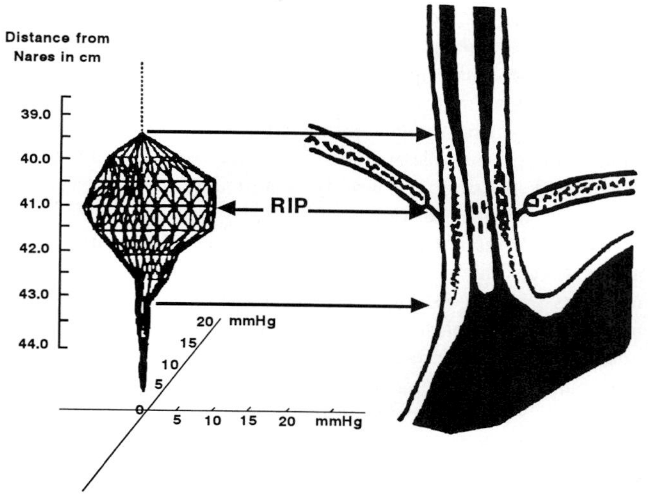

FIG. 23-22. Computerized three-dimensional imaging of lower esophageal sphincter. A catheter with four to eight radial side holes is withdrawn through the gastroesophageal junction. For each level of the pullback, the radially measured pressures are plotted around an axis representing gastric baseline pressure. When a stepwise pullback technique is used, the respiratory inversion point (RIP) can be identified. (From: *Stein HJ, DeMeester TR, et al: Ann Surg 214:377, 1991, with permission.*)

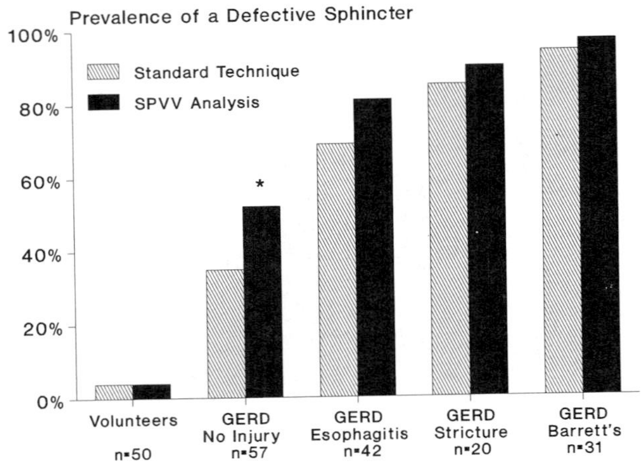

FIG. 23-23. Comparison of standard manometric techniques and SPVV analysis in the identification of a mechanically defective lower esophageal sphincter. *: $p < 0.05$ versus standard manometry. (From: *Stein HJ, DeMeester TR, et al: Ann Surg 214:380, 1991, with permission.*)

a pressure response throughout the whole esophagus can be obtained on one swallow. The study consists of recording ten wet swallows. Amplitude, duration, and morphology of contractions following each swallow are calculated at all recorded levels of the esophageal body. The delay between the onset or peak of esophageal contractions at the various levels of the esophagus is used to calculate the speed of wave propagation. The relationship of the esophageal contractions following a swallow is classified as peristaltic or simultaneous. From this information, motor disorders of the esophagus are identified.

The position, length, and pressure of the cricopharyngeal sphincter are assessed with a stationary pull-through technique similar to the lower esophageal sphincter. The manometric catheter is withdrawn in 0.5-cm intervals from the upper esophagus through the upper esophageal sphincter region into the pharynx. The relaxation of the upper esophageal sphincter is studied by straddling the eight pressure transducers across the sphincter so that some are in the pharynx and some in the upper esophagus. High-speed graphic recordings (50 mm/sec) are necessary to obtain an assessment of the coordination of cricopharyngeal relaxation with hypopharyngeal contraction. It has been difficult to consistently demonstrate a motility abnormality in patients with pharyngoesophageal disorders.

24-Hour Ambulatory Manometry. The development of miniaturized electronic pressure transducers and portable digital data recorders with large storage capacity has made ambulatory monitoring of esophageal motor function over an entire circadian cycle possible. The broad clinical application of this new technology in a large number of asymptomatic normal volunteers and patients with primary esophageal motor disorders or gastroesophageal reflux disease provides new insights into esophageal motor function in health and disease under a variety of physiologic conditions. In both normal volunteers and symptomatic patients, esophageal motor activity increases with the state of consciousness and focus on eating activity, i.e., from the supine, to the upright, to meal periods. In the normal situation there is a higher prevalence of nonperistaltic contractions then appreciated on stationary manometry.

Compared with standard manometry, ambulatory esophageal manometry provides a more than 100 times larger database for the classification and quantification of abnormal esophageal motor function and leads to a change in the diagnosis in a substantial portion of patients with symptoms suggestive of a primary esophageal motor disorder (Fig. 23-24). In patients with nonobstructive dysphagia, the circadian esophageal motor pattern is characterized by an inability to organize the motor activity into peristaltic contraction during a meal period (Fig. 23-25). This finding can be used to provide a new classification of motility disorders in regards to when they may give rise to dysphagia (Fig. 23-26). In patients with noncardiac chest pain, ambulatory motility monitoring can document a direct correlation of abnormal esophageal motor activity with the symptom and shows that the abnormal motor activity immediately preceding the pain episodes is characterized by an increased frequency of simultaneous, double- and triple-peaked, high-amplitude, and long contractions. In patients with gastroesophageal reflux disease, ambulatory motility monitoring shows that the contractility of the esophageal body deteriorates with increasing severity of esophageal mucosal injury, compromising the clearance function of the esophageal body. Ambulatory esophageal manometry will replace standard manometry in the assessment of esophageal body function and has the potential to improve the diagnosis and management of patients with esophageal motor abnormalities. The combination of ambulatory 24-hour esophageal manometry with esophageal and gastric pH monitoring is currently the most physiologic way to assess patients with foregut motility disorders.

Esophageal Transit Scintigraphy. Esophageal transit scintigraphy is a recently described technique for the evaluation of esophageal function. The esophageal transit of a 10-mL water bolus containing technetium 99m sulfur colloid is recorded with a gamma camera. The transit time is measured separately in the proximal and distal esophagus. Using this technique, delayed bolus transit has been shown in patients with a variety of esophageal motor disorders, including achalasia, scleroderma, diffuse esophageal spasm, and nutcracker esophagus. It appears that transit scintigraphy is a reliable technique to quantify and document esophageal transit abnormalities. The test lacks specificity since it

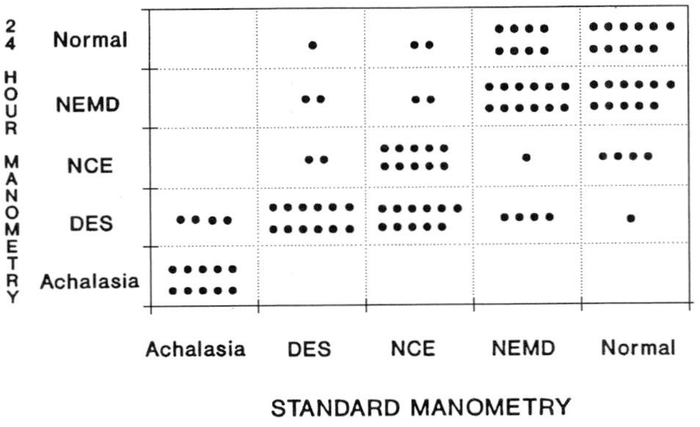

FIG. 23-24. Classification of esophageal motility disorders on standard and ambulatory 24-hour manometry in 78 patients. NEMD = nonspecific esophageal motility disorders; NCE = nutcracker esophagus; DES = diffuse esophageal spasm. (From: *DeMeester TR, Stein HJ: Surgery for esophageal motor disorders, in Castell DO (ed): The Esophagus. Boston, Little, Brown, 1992, p 412, with permission.*)

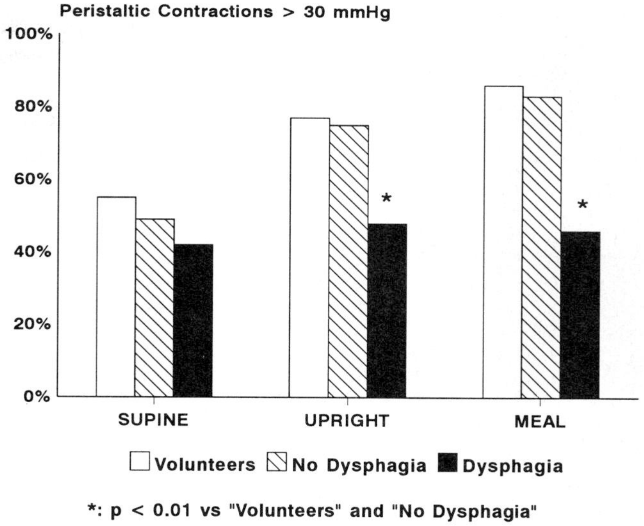

FIG. 23-25. Frequency of peristaltic contractions with an amplitude >30 mmHg during supine, upright, and meal periods, showing that patients with nonobstructive dysphagia are unable to organize their esophageal contractions with increasing states of awareness, from sleep (supine) to alertness (upright) to focus on eating (meals). (From: *Stein HJ, DeMeester TR: Indications, technique, and clinical use of ambulatory 24-hour esophageal motility monitoring in a surgical practice. Ann Surg 217(2):128, 1993, with permission.*)

cannot define the precise nature of a swallowing abnormality. Its best use is to quantify the effect of an esophageal motility disorder by measuring esophageal emptying time.

Video/Cineradiography. High-speed cine or video recording of radiographic studies allows reevaluation by reviewing the studies at various speeds. This technique is more useful than manometry in the evaluation of the pharyngeal phase of swallowing. Observations suggesting oropharyngeal or cricopharyngeal dysfunction include misdirection of barium into the trachea or nasopharynx, prominence of the cricopharyngeal muscle (Fig. 23-27), a Zenker's diverticulum, a narrow pharyngoesophageal segment, and stasis of the contrast medium in the valleculae or hypopharyngeal recesses (Fig. 23-28). These findings are usually not specific, but rather common manifestations of neuromuscular disorders affecting the pharyngoesophageal area. Studies using liquid barium, barium-impregnated solids, or radiopaque pills aid the evaluation of normal and abnormal motility in the esophageal body. Loss of the normal stripping wave or segmentation of the barium column with the patient in the recumbent position correlates with abnormal motility of the esophageal body. In addition, structural abnormalities such as small diverticula, webs, and minimal extrinsic impressions of the esophagus may be recognized only with motion-recording techniques.

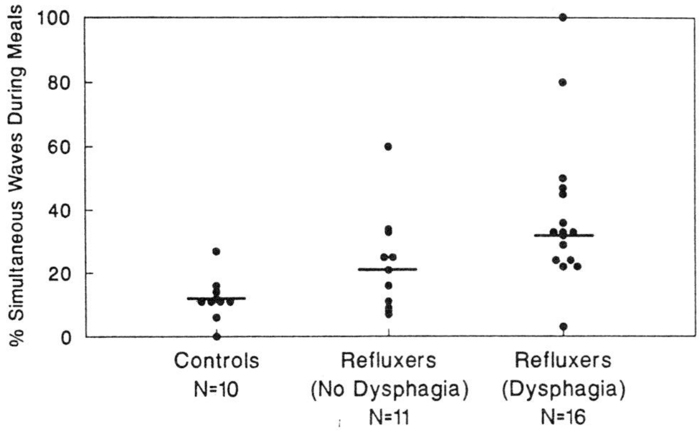

FIG. 23-26. Scattergram showing individual patient data for percentage of simultaneous waves during the meal periods in normal subjects and in patients. The bar denotes median value for each group, with a significant difference between patients with reflux and dysphagia and the other groups, $p < 0.05$. (From: *Singh S, Stein HJ, et al: Am J Gastroenterol 87(5):562, 1992, with permission.*)

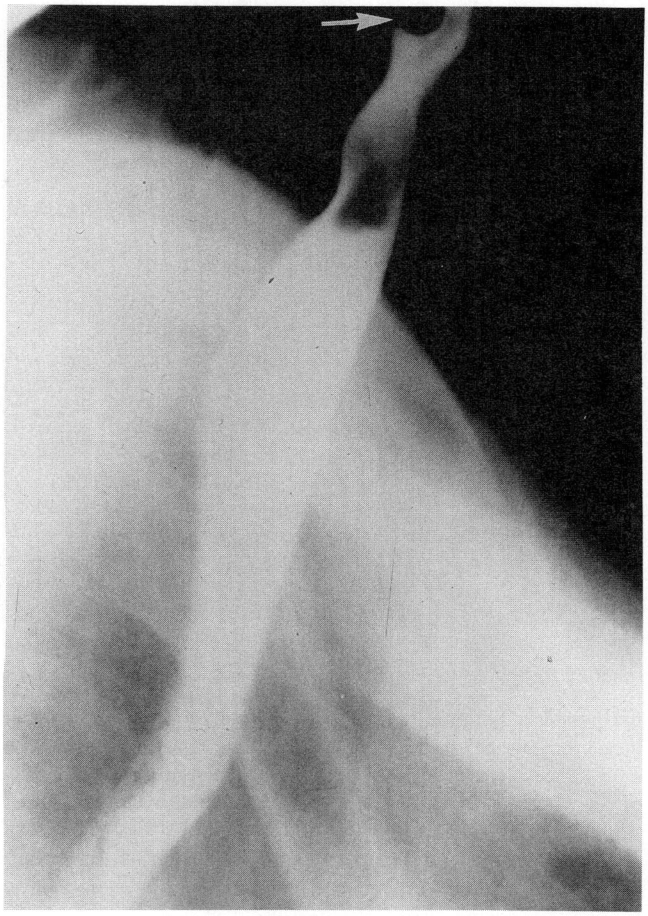

FIG. 23-27. Barium contrast radiogram of pharyngeal swallowing activity showing prominent cricopharyngeal indentation *(arrowhead)* in a patient who presented with dysphagia resulting from bulbar poliomyelitis. (From: *Bonavina L, Khan NA, DeMeester TR: Arch Surg 120:543, 1985, with permission.*)

Tests to Detect Increased Exposure to Gastric Juice.

24-Hour Ambulatory pH Monitoring. The most direct method of measuring increased esophageal exposure to gastric juice is by an indwelling pH electrode. Prolonged monitoring of esophageal pH is performed by placing a pH probe 5 cm above the manometrically measured upper border of the distal sphincter for 24 hours. It quantifies the actual time the esophageal mucosa is exposed to gastric juice, measures the ability of the esophagus to clear refluxed acid, and correlates esophageal acid exposure with

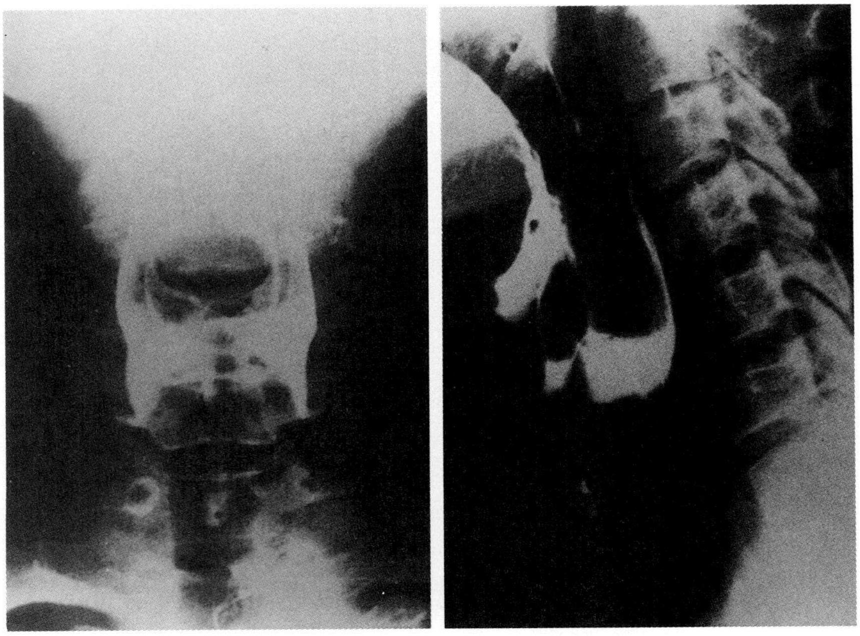

A B

FIG. 23-28. Esophagograms from a patient with cricopharyngeal achalasia. *A.* Anteroposterior film showing retention of the contrast medium at the level of the vallecula and piriform recesses, with no barium passing into the esophagus. *B.* Lateral film, taken opposite the C5–C6 vertebrae, showing posterior indentation of the cricopharyngeus, retention in the hypopharynx, and tracheal aspiration. (From: *Lafontaine E: Pharyngeal dysphagia, in DeMeester TR, Matthews H (eds): International Trends in General Thoracic Surgery, Vol 3, Benign Esophageal Disease. St Louis, CV Mosby, p 345, 1987, with permission.*)

the patient's symptoms. A 24-hour period is necessary so that measurements are made over one complete circadian cycle. This allows measuring the effect of physiologic activity, such as eating or sleeping, on the reflux of gastric juice into the esophagus (Fig. 23-29).

The 24-hour esophageal pH monitoring should not be considered a test for reflux, but rather a measurement of the esophageal exposure to gastric juice. The measurement is expressed by the time the esophageal pH was below a given threshold during the 24-hour period. This single assessment, although concise, does not reflect how the exposure has occurred: that is, did it occur in a few long episodes or several short episodes? Consequently, two other assessments are necessary: the frequency of the reflux episodes and their duration.

The units used to express esophageal exposure to gastric juice are (1) cumulative time the esophageal pH is below a chosen threshold, expressed as the percent of the total, upright, and supine monitored time; (2) frequency of reflux episodes below a chosen threshold, expressed as number of episodes per 24 hours; and (3) duration of the episodes, expressed as the number of episodes greater than 5 minutes per 24 hours and the time in minutes of the longest episode recorded. Table 23-2 shows the normal values for these components of the 24-hour record at the whole number pH threshold derived from 50 normal asymptomatic subjects. The upper limits of normal were established at the 95th percentile. Most centers use pH 4 as the threshold.

To combine the result of the six components into one expression of the overall esophageal acid exposure below a pH threshold, a pH score was calculated by using the standard deviation of the mean of each of the six components measured in the 50 normal subjects as a weighing factor. By accepting an abstract zero level two standard deviations below the mean, the data measured in normal subjects could be treated as though they had a normal distribution. Thus, any measured patient value could be referenced to this zero point and, in turn, be awarded points based on whether it was below or above the normal mean value for that component.

$$\text{Component score} = \frac{\text{Pt Value} - \text{Mean}}{\text{SD}} + 1$$

The upper limits of normal for the composite score for each whole number pH threshold is shown in Table 23-3.

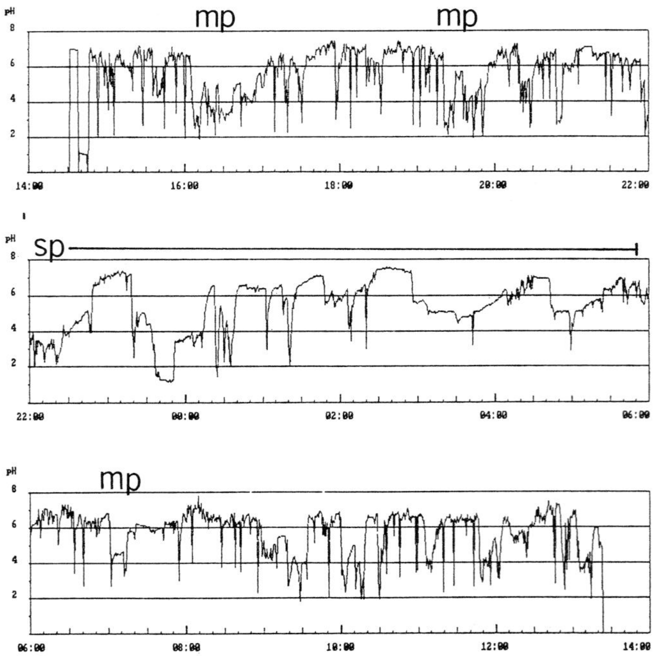

FIG. 23-29. Strip chart display of a 24-hour esophageal pH monitoring study in a patient with increased esophageal acid exposure. mp = meal period; sp = supine period. (From: *DeMeester TR, Stein HJ, Fuchs KH: Physiologic diagnostic studies, in Zuidema GD, Orringer MB (eds): Shackelford's Surgery of the Alimentary Tract, 3rd ed, Vol I. Philadelphia, Saunders, 1991, p 119, with permission.*)

Table 23-2
Normal Values for Esophageal Exposure to pH < 4 (n = 50)

Component	*Mean*	*SD*	*95%*
Total time	1.51	1.36	4.45
Upright time	2.34	2.34	8.42
Supine time	0.63	1.0	3.45
No. of episodes	19.00	12.76	46.90
No. > 5 minutes	0.84	1.18	3.45
Longest episode	6.74	7.85	19.80

SOURCE: DeMeester TR, Stein HJ: Gastroesophageal reflux disease, in Moody FG, Carey LC, et al (eds): *Surgical Treatment of Digestive Disease,* 2nd ed. Chicago, Year Book Medical Publishers, 1989, p 68, with permission.

The detection of increased esophageal exposure to acid gastric juice is more dependable than the detection of increased exposure to alkaline gastric juice. The latter is suggested by an increased alkaline exposure time above pH 7 or 8. Increased exposure in this pH range can be caused by abnormal calibration of the pH recorder, dental infection which increases salivary pH, esophageal obstruction which results in static pools of saliva with an increase in pH secondary to bacterial overgrowth, or regurgitation of alkaline gastric juice into the esophagus. Using a properly calibrated probe, in the absence of dental infections or esophageal obstruction, the percentage of time the pH is measured above 7 correlates with the concentration of bile acids continuously aspirated over a 24-hour period.

When done in a test population with an equal distribution of normal healthy subjects and patients with the classical reflux symptoms and a defective sphincter, 24-hour esophageal pH monitoring had a sensitivity and specificity of 96 percent. This gave a predictive value of a positive and a negative test of 96 percent and an overall accuracy of 96 percent. Based on these studies and extensive clinical experience, 24-hour esophageal pH monitoring has emerged as a gold standard for the diagnosis of gastroesophageal reflux disease.

Standard Acid Reflux Test (SART). The development of powerful acid reduction agents such as omeprazole has created difficulties in the measurement of esophageal acid exposure. Many patients are placed on the medications prior to study, altering normal physiology and thus complicating interpretation of ambulatory pH monitoring. The acid-reducing effects of omeprazole have been noted to be present as long as 40 days following cessation of the drug, making a prolonged period without the medication necessary before study. Standard acid reflux testing can be used to provide additional information when it is suspected that the results of ambulatory monitoring may have been altered by medications.

Table 23-3
Normal Composite Score for Various pH Thresholds

pH threshold	*Upper level of normal value (95th percentile)*
< 1	14.2
< 2	17.37
< 3	14.10
< 4	14.72
< 5	15.76
< 6	12.76
> 7	14.90
> 8	8.50

SOURCE: DeMeester TR, Stein HJ: Gastroesophageal reflux disease, in Moody FG, Carey LC, et al (eds): *Surgical Treatment of Digestive Disease,* 2nd ed. Chicago, Year Book Medical Publishers, 1989, p 69, with permission.

The SART was popularized by Skinner et al. as a diagnostic test for increased esophageal acid exposure. The test is performed following manometry by placing a pH electrode 5 cm above the upper border of the lower esophageal sphincter. The manometry catheter is then advanced temporarily into the stomach, and 300 mL of 0.1 N HCl is infused. In children the gastric acid load is reduced accordingly. The manometry catheter is flushed and then pulled back into the body of the esophagus. The pH of the esophagus is monitored while the patient rests quietly in the supine position and then while he or she performs four maneuvers: deep breathing, Valsalva, Mueller (inspiration against a closed glottis), and cough. These maneuvers are repeated in the right and left lateral decubitus position and with the head down 20°, giving 16 possibilities for acid reflux to occur. A decrease in esophageal pH to less than 4 is considered evidence of reflux. At the beginning of the test, before the patient is placed in the supine position, the distal esophagus must have a pH greater than 4. In some patients this necessitates their standing erect and swallowing repeatedly in order to clear the esophagus of acid.

Patients who fail to clear the esophagus in the erect position after 20 effective swallows monitored on a motility tracing are considered to be abnormal in all positions and maneuvers and are scored as 16. Among 90 healthy volunteers, only 2 individuals had more than two reflux episodes. Accordingly, one or two drops in pH during these challenges to the cardia are considered normal, and three or more drops in pH are taken as evidence of a mechanical incompetence of the cardia. Patients with severe reflux may be unable to clear acid from the esophagus after reflux has been documented.

When used in a test population with an equal distribution of normal healthy subjects and patients with classic symptoms of gastroesophageal reflux disease, the SART had a sensitivity, i.e., the ability to detect the disease when known to be present, of 59 percent, and a specificity, i.e., the ability to exclude the disease when known to be absent, of 98 percent. This gave a predictive value of a positive test of 96 percent and a negative test of 75 percent, with an overall accuracy of 81 percent.

Radiographic Detection of Gastroesophageal Reflux. The definition of radiographic gastroesophageal reflux varies depending on whether reflux is spontaneous or induced by various maneuvers. In only about 40 percent of patients with classic symptoms of gastroesophageal reflux disease is spontaneous reflux observed by the radiologist, i.e., reflux of barium from the stomach into the esophagus with the patient in the upright position. In most patients who show spontaneous reflux on radiography, the diagnosis of increased esophageal acid exposure is confirmed by 24-hour esophageal pH monitoring. Therefore, the radiographic demonstration of spontaneous regurgitation of barium into the esophagus in the upright position is a reliable indicator that reflux is present. Failure to see this does not indicate the absence of disease.

Scintigraphic Detection of Gastroesophageal Reflux. A scintigraphic test for the detection of gastroesophageal reflux disease was introduced in 1976 by Fisher et al. For this test 100 Ci of ^{99m}Tc sulfur colloid is mixed with 300 mL of physiologic saline and drunk by the patient or instilled into the stomach via a nasogastric tube. The patient is placed in a supine position, and abdominal pressure is raised using an abdominal binder. Gastroesophageal reflux can be quantified with a gamma camera. A major disadvantage of the test is the short duration of the monitoring period and the unphysiologic means by which reflux is induced.

Tests to Provoke Esophageal Symptoms. The spontaneous occurrence of symptoms during a standard esophageal motility study is rare, especially in patients with noncardiac chest pain. Consequently, a number of provocative tests have been designed to identify the esophagus as the cause of these symptoms. Of these, intraesophageal acid perfusion (Bernstein) test, edrophonium (Tensilon) test, and intraesophageal balloon distention are the most common.

Acid Perfusion Test. Since its introduction in 1958 by Bernstein and Baker, the esophageal acid perfusion test has been widely used to determine whether a patient's symptoms can be reproduced by the infusion of acid into the esophagus. If positive, the test indicates that the esophagus is sensitive to acid. Increased esophageal exposure to acid is assumed. In the original technique the distal esophagus is perfused with 0.1 N HCl at 6 to 8 mL/min with the patient sitting upright. Ideally, a placebo is also infused, i.e., acid is perfused in alteration with physiologic saline without the patient knowing the identity of the perfusate. The patient is asked to report any symptom that develops during infusion. Consistent reproduction of the patient's usual symptoms only during acid perfusion and rapid abatement during saline perfusion or after antacid administration indicate a positive test. Development of symptoms during both the saline and acid perfusion or development of symptoms foreign to the patient's usual experience represents an equivocal test. Failure to develop any symptoms during a 30-minute acid perfusion indicates a normal status.

Various investigators have reported that 34 to 100 percent of patients with typical symptoms of gastroesophageal reflux disease have a positive acid perfusion test. Failure to include other components of gastric juice, such as pepsin, bile, and pancreatic enzymes, in the perfusate may account for some of the normal results. A false-negative result can also occur in patients who have an insensitive esophagus and has been noted in patients who have severe hemorrhagic esophagitis without pain and patients with Barrett's esophagus. False-positive results are seen in 15 percent of asymptomatic subjects. Of concern is that symptomatic subjects whose pain is not due to reflux may have a similar incidence of false-positive tests, resulting in an erroneous diagnosis. Patients with duodenal ulcer may have heartburn as well and often develop symptoms during esophageal acid perfusion. Consequently the test can lead to diagnostic confusion.

Edrophonium (Tensilon) Test. The edrophonium test is used to identify the esophageal origin of chest pain in patients in whom cardiac disease has been excluded. The cholinesterase inhibitor edrophonium hydrochloride (Tensilon) is injected intravenously at a dose of 80 μg/kg. A syringe with 1 mg of the antidote atropine should always be at hand when performing the test. The test is ideally placebo-controlled. The end point of the test is the patient's chest pain and the similarity of the pain to that which is experienced spontaneously. A positive test is defined as replication of the patient's chest pain within 5 minutes of edrophonium but not placebo injection. The test is positive in 20 to 30 percent of patients with noncardiac chest pain, but not in asymptomatic volunteers. In both, edrophonium causes a marked increase in amplitude and duration of esophageal contractions, but the end point of the test is the reproduction of the patient's typical chest pain rather than a specific change in esophageal motility. The disadvantages of the test are its risk of side effects, that it reproduces symptoms with an unphysiologic stimulus, and that it is helpful in only a small portion of patients with chest pain. The test should not be performed in patients with asthma, chronic obstructive airway disease, or cardiac arrhythmias.

Balloon Distention Test. Balloon distention of the esophagus was described in 1955 as a diagnostic test to distinguish esophageal from cardiac chest pain. An inflatable balloon is positioned 10 cm above the lower esophageal sphincter and gradually inflated with air in 1-mL increments. Esophageal motility is simultaneously monitored. The test is considered positive when typical symptoms are reproduced with gradual distention of the balloon. Recent studies indicate that the procedure induces spastic esophageal motor activity and reproduces chest pain episodes in up to 48 percent of patients with noncardiac chest pain but not in volunteers. Although the test has a greater diagnostic yield than provocative drug studies, it is relatively invasive and provides no information on spontaneously occurring symptoms.

Tests of Duodenogastric Function. Esophageal disorders are frequently associated with abnormalities of duodenogastric function. Abnormalities of the gastric reservoir or increased gastric acid secretion can be responsible for increased esophageal exposure to gastric juice. Reflux of alkaline duodenal juice, including bile salts, pancreatic enzymes, and bicarbonate, is thought to have a role in the pathogenesis of esophagitis and complicated Barrett's esophagus. Furthermore, functional disorders of the esophagus are often not confined to the esophagus alone, but are associated with functional disorders of the rest of the foregut, i.e., stomach and duodenum. Tests of duodenogastric function that are helpful to investigate esophageal symptoms include gastric emptying studies, gastric acid analysis, and cholescintigraphy (for the diagnosis of pathologic duodenogastric reflux). The single test of 24-hour gastric pH monitoring can be used to identify gastric hypersecretion and imply the presence of duodenogastric reflux and delayed gastric emptying.

Gastric Emptying. Gastric emptying studies are performed with radionuclide-labeled meals. Emptying of solids and liquids can be assessed simultaneously when both phases are marked with different tracers. After ingestion of a labeled standard meal, gamma camera images of the stomach are obtained at 5- to 15-minute intervals for 1.5 to 2 hours. After correction for decay, the counts in the gastric area are plotted as percentage of total counts at the start of the imaging. The resulting emptying curve can be compared with data obtained in normal volunteers. In general, normal subjects will empty 59 percent of a meal within 90 minutes.

Gastric Acid Analysis. The gastric secretory state is usually evaluated by determination of the titratable gastric acid in aspirated gastric juice. Interdigestive or basal gastric acid secretion (BAO) is measured in the fasting state and varies between 0 and 5 mmol/h in normal volunteers. The maximal secretory capacity (MAO) of the stomach, which reflects the available parietal cell mass, is calculated following stimulation of gastric acid secretion with pentagastrin or histamine. Acid hypersecretors have a BAO $>$ 5 mmol/h and an MAO $>$ 30 mmol/h.

Cholescintigraphy. Scintigraphic hepatobiliary imaging is performed after intravenous injection of 5 μCi of technetium 99m iminodiacetic acid derivates such as disofenin (DISIDA). Gamma camera images of the upper abdomen including the gallbladder and stomach are obtained at 5-minute intervals for 60 minutes. Imaging is continued for an additional 30 minutes after stimulation of gallbladder contraction with 20 mg/kg of synthetic C-terminal octapeptide of cholecystokinin (CCK). Duodenogastric reflux is demonstrated as an increase of radioactivity in the stomach in the sequential images. The clinical value of this test is limited due to its short duration and a relatively high false-positive rate in normal volunteers.

24-Hour Gastric pH Monitoring. Monitoring is performed over a complete circadian cycle with a pH electrode placed 5 cm below the manometrically located lower esophageal sphincter. The patient is fully ambulatory during the test and is encouraged to perform normal daily activity. The gastric pH profile is assessed separately for the meal, postprandial period, and fasting period. The latter is divided into the time spent upright and supine.

The interpretation of continuous gastric pH recordings is more difficult than that of esophageal pH recordings. This is because the gastric pH environment is determined by a complex interplay of acid secretion; mucous secretion; ingested food; swallowed saliva; regurgitated duodenal, pancreatic, and biliary secretions; and the effectiveness of the mixing and evacuation of the chyme. Using 24-hour gastric pH monitoring to evaluate the gastric secretory state is based on studies that have shown that a good correlation exists between increased basal acid output on standard gastric acid analysis and a left shift on the frequency distribution graph of gastric pH recordings during the supine fasting period. The evaluation of gastric emptying by 24-hour gastric pH monitoring is based on studies demonstrating a good correlation between the emptying of a solid meal and the duration of the postprandial plateau and decline phase of the gastric pH record.

Using 24-hour gastric pH monitoring to evaluate duodenogastric reflux is based on the observation that reflux of alkaline duodenal juice into the stomach can alkalinize the gastric pH environment. The measurement is not straightforward because of the effect of meals, and reduction in acid secretion can result in changes in gastric pH that mimic alkaline reflux episodes. To overcome this problem, computerized measurements of the number and height of alkalinizing peaks, the baseline pH, the postprandial pH plateau, and the pattern of pH decline from the plateau can be used to identify the probability of duodenogastric reflux. The results are presented as an overall score that indicates the likelihood of pathologic duodenogastric reflux. Initial data indicate that this approach has a higher sensitivity and specificity for the diagnosis of pathologic duodenogastric reflux than scintigraphic methods do.

Combined 24-hour esophageal and gastric pH monitoring has been recently introduced. Using this technique, excessive alkaline duodenogastric and alkaline gastroesophageal reflux can be identified in symptomatic patients. The combined tracings can often identify simultaneous gastric and esophageal alkalinization, suggesting a duodenal origin for the esophageal alkaline exposure (Fig. 23-30).

Integrated Ambulatory Foregut Monitoring. Integrated ambulatory foregut monitoring, consisting of 24-hour esophageal and gastric pH monitoring and ambulatory motility monitoring, has been introduced. This allows an evaluation of the foregut function during one 24-hour period in a physiologic outpatient environment with only minor discomfort to the patient. This technology may replace the series of laboratory tests currently required to thoroughly evaluate foregut function and give surgeons the ability to evaluate complex foregut problems in their own offices. Integrated monitoring of foregut function therefore has potential to give surgical therapy for functional abnormalities of the foregut a more scientific basis than was previously possible (Fig. 23-31).

GASTROESOPHAGEAL REFLUX DISEASE

Definition. Gastroesophageal reflux is a common disease that accounts for approximately 75 percent of esophageal pathology. Despite its common prevalence, it can be one of the most challenging diagnostic and therapeutic problems in benign esophageal disease. A contributing factor to this is the lack of a universally accepted definition of the disease.

The simplest approach is to define the disease by its symptoms. However, symptoms thought to be indicative of gastroesophageal reflux disease, such as heartburn or acid regurgitation, are very common in the general population, and many individuals consider them to be normal and do not seek medical attention. Even when excessive, these symptoms are not specific for gastroesophageal reflux and can be caused by other diseases such as achalasia, diffuse spasm, esophageal carcinoma, pyloric stenosis, cholelithiasis, gastritis, gastric or duodenal ulcer, and coronary artery disease. On the other hand, gastroesophageal reflux can present with atypical symptoms, such as nausea, vomiting, postprandial fullness, chest pain, choking, chronic cough, wheezing, and hoarseness. Furthermore, bronchiolitis, recurrent pneumonia, idiopathic pulmonary fibrosis, and asthma can be primarily due to gastroesophageal reflux disease. To confuse the issue further, gastroesophageal reflux disease can coexist with cardiac and pulmonary disease. Thus, using symptoms to define gastroesophageal reflux disease lacks sensitivity and specificity.

An alternative definition for gastroesophageal reflux disease is the presence of endoscopic esophagitis. Using this criterion for diagnosis assumes that all patients who have esophagitis have excessive regurgitation of gastric juice into their esophagus. This is true in 90 percent of patients, but in 10 percent the esophagitis has other causes, the most common being unrecognized chemical injury from drug ingestion. In addition, the definition leaves undiagnosed those patients who have symptoms of gastroesophageal reflux but do not have endoscopic esophagitis.

A third approach to define gastroesophageal reflux disease is to measure the basic pathophysiologic abnormality of the disease, that is, increased exposure of the esophagus to gastric juice. In the past this was inferred by the presence of a hiatal hernia, later by endoscopic esophagitis, and more recently by a hypotensive lower esophageal sphincter pressure. The recent development of a miniaturized pH electrode and data recorder allowed measurement of esophageal exposure to gastric juice by calculating the percentage of time the pH was less than 4 over a 24-hour period. This provided an opportunity to objectively identify the presence of the disease and stimulated a rational stepwise approach to determining the cause for the abnormal esophageal exposure to gastric juice.

Etiology. Having established that the patient has abnormal exposure to acid or alkaline juice, it is necessary to determine which mechanism is responsible for the abnormality. There are three known causes of increased esophageal exposure to gastric juice in patients with gastroesophageal reflux disease. The first is a

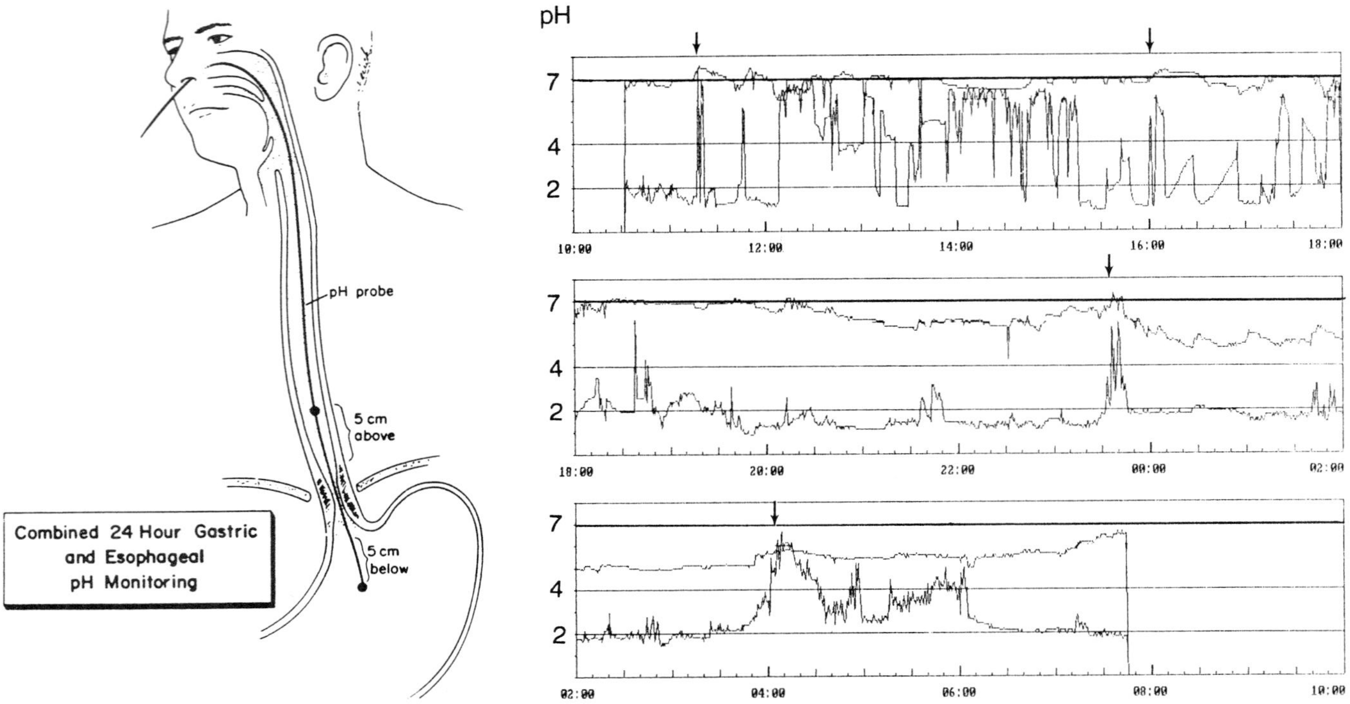

A B

FIG. 23-30. *A.* Combined esophageal and gastric pH monitoring showing position of probes in relation to the lower esophageal sphincter. *B.* Combined ambulatory esophageal *(upper tracing)* and gastric *(lower tracing)* pH monitoring showing duodenogastric reflux *(arrows)* with propagation of the alkaline juice into the esophagus of a patient with complicated Barrett's esophagus. The gastric tracing *(lower)* is taken from a probe lying 5 cm below the upper esophageal sphincter. The esophageal tracing *(upper)* is taken from a probe lying 5 cm above the lower esophageal sphincter. Note that in only a small proportion of time does duodenogastric reflux move the pH of the esophagus above the threshold of 7, causing the iceberg effect. (From: *DeMeester TR, Stein HJ, Fuchs KH: Physiologic diagnostic studies, in Zuidema GD, Orringer MB (eds): Shackelford's Surgery of the Alimentary Tract, 3rd ed, Vol I. Philadelphia, Saunders, 1991, p 123, with permission.*)

mechanically incompetent lower esophageal sphincter. This accounts for about 60 to 70 percent of gastroesophageal reflux disease. The identification of this cause is important, since it is the one that antireflux surgery is designed to correct. The other two causes are inefficient esophageal clearance of refluxed gastric juice and abnormalities of the gastric reservoir that augment physiologic reflux. Conceptually, these three main causes of gastroesophageal reflux can be thought of as a valve, a pump, and a reservoir. As alluded to above, because antireflux surgery is directed principally at restoring the function of the valve, the relative contributions of each of these components in general can be, and should be, determined prior to undertaking surgical therapy.

Lower Esophageal Sphincter. Failure of the lower esophageal sphincter is caused by inadequate pressure, inadequate overall length, or abnormal position, i.e., the portion exposed to the positive-pressure environment of the abdomen as measured by manometry (see Fig. 23-20). The probability of increased exposure to gastric juice is 69 to 76 percent if one component of the sphincter is abnormal, 65 to 88 percent if two components are abnormal, and 92 percent if all three are abnormal. This indicates that the failure of one or two of the components of the sphincter may be compensated for by the clearance of the esophageal body. Failure of all three sphincter components inevitably leads to increased esophageal exposure to gastric juice.

The most common cause of a mechanically defective lower esophageal sphincter is inadequate sphincter pressure. The reduced pressure is most likely due to an abnormality of myogenic function. This is supported by two observations. First, the location of the lower esophageal sphincter, in either the abdomen or the chest, is not a major factor in the genesis of the sphincter pressure, since it can still be measured when the chest and abdomen are surgically opened and the distal esophagus is held freely in the surgeon's hand. Second, Biancani and coworkers have shown that the distal esophageal sphincter's muscle response to stretch is reduced in patients with an incompetent cardia. This suggests that sphincter pressure depends on the length and tension properties of the sphincter's smooth muscle. Surgical fundoplication has been shown to restore the mechanical efficiency of the sphincter to normal by correcting the abnormal length-tension characteristics.

Although an inadequate pressure is the most common cause of a mechanically defective sphincter, the efficiency of a sphincter with normal pressure can be nullified by an inadequate abdominal length or an abnormally short overall resting length. An adequate abdominal length is important in preventing reflux caused by increases in intraabdominal pressure, and an adequate overall length is important in providing the resistance to reflux caused by increases in intragastric pressure independent of intraabdominal pressure. Therefore, patients with a low sphincter pressure or

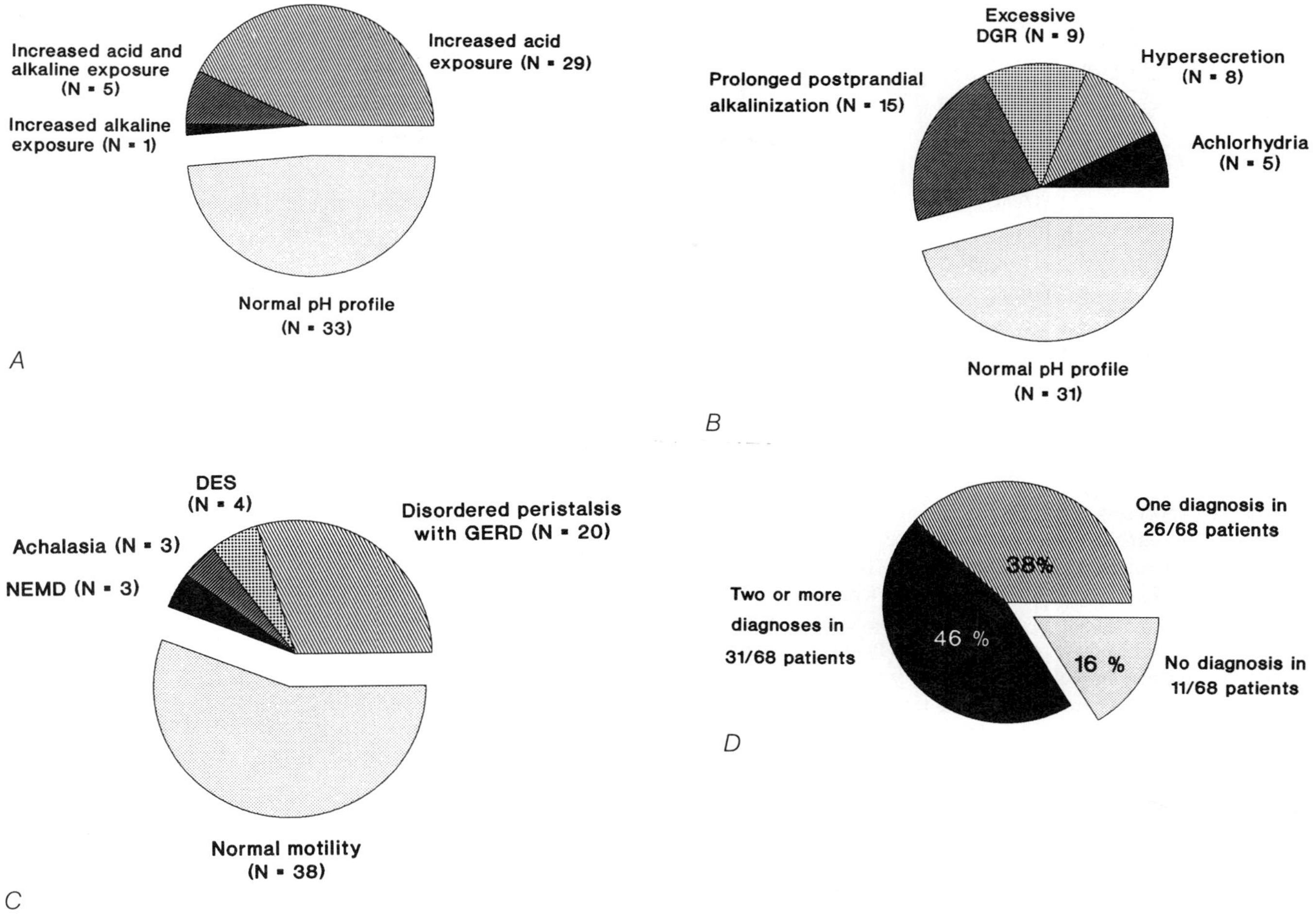

FIG. 23-31. Results of outpatient integrated monitoring of *(A)* esophageal pH, *(B)* gastric pH, and *(C)* esophageal motility in 68 patients with complex foregut pathology. The ability to make a diagnosis in these patients is shown in *D*. (From: *Stein HJ, DeMeester TR: Integrated ambulatory foregut monitoring in patients with functional foregut disorders, in Nyhus LM (ed): 1992 Surgery Annual, Part 1, Vol 24. Norwalk, CT, and San Mateo, CA, Appleton & Lange, 1992, pp 171–175, with permission.*)

those with a normal pressure but a short abdominal length are unable to protect against reflux caused by fluctuations of intraabdominal pressure that occur with daily activities or changes in body position. Patients with a low sphincter pressure or those with a normal pressure but short overall length are unable to protect against reflux related to independent increases in gastric pressure caused by outlet obstruction, aerophagia, gluttony, or altered pressure-volume relationship of the stomach as occurs in various gastropathies. In this situation, reflux can occur whenever an increase in gastric pressure exceeds the sphincter pressure that is necessary to provide competency for the overall length of sphincter. Persons who have a short overall length on a resting motility study are at a disadvantage in protecting against normal fluctuations in gastric pressure secondary to eating, and suffer postprandial reflux. This is because with normal dilatation of the stomach sphincter, length becomes shorter, and if short in the resting state, there is very little tolerance for further shortening before incompetency occurs.

The combined effects of pressure, overall length, and abdominal length on the resistance of the sphincter to the reflux of gastric juice can be determined by integrating the effects of radial pressures extended over the entire length of the sphincter. This can be quantified by three-dimensional computerized imaging of pressures throughout the sphincter length and calculating the volume of this image. This is referred to as the sphincter pressure vector volume. Figure 23-32 shows the three-dimensional sphincter representations for a normal volunteer and a patient with Barrett's esophagus before and after Nissen fundoplication. The marked improvement in the sphincter is apparent.

Esophageal Clearance. A second portion of the human antireflux mechanism is effective esophageal clearance. Ineffective esophageal clearance can result in an abnormal esophageal exposure to gastric juice in individuals who have a mechanically effective lower esophageal sphincter and normal gastric function but fail to clear physiologic reflux episodes. This situation is relatively rare, and ineffectual clearance is more apt to be seen in association with a mechanically defective sphincter, which augments the esophageal exposure to gastric juice by prolonging the duration of each reflux episode.

Four factors important in esophageal clearance are gravity, esophageal motor activity, salivation, and anchoring of the distal esophagus in the abdomen. The loss of any one can augment

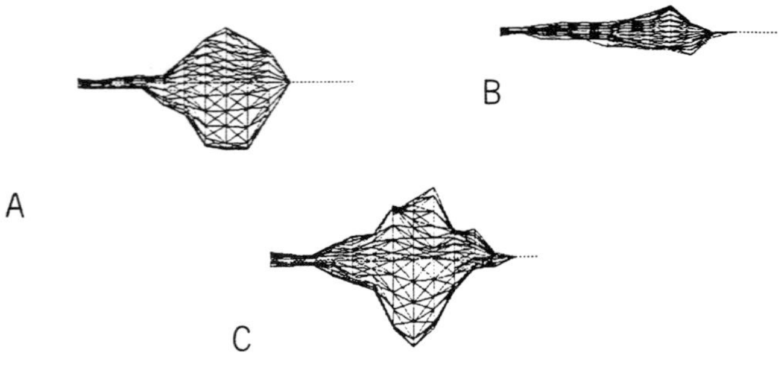

FIG. 23-32. The three-dimensional lower esophageal sphincter pressure profile in (A) a normal volunteer, (B) a patient with a mechanically defective sphincter, and (C) the same patient 1 year after Nissen fundoplication. (From: *DeMeester TR, Stein HJ: Surgical treatment of gastroesophageal reflux disease, in Castell DO (ed): The Esophagus. Boston, Little, Brown & Company, 1992, p 619, with permission.*)

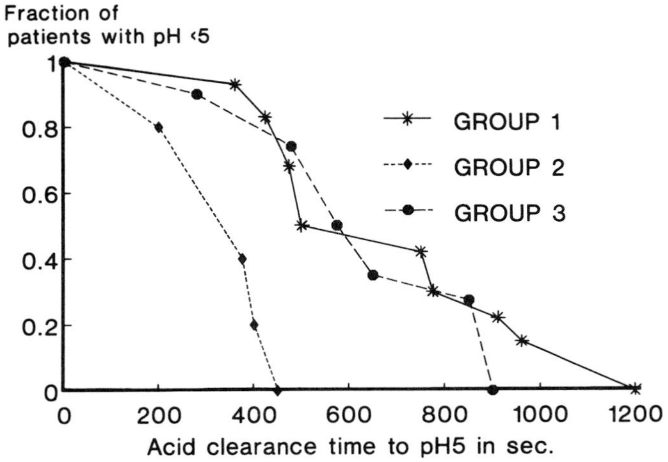

FIG. 23-33. Acid clearance in subjects with hiatal hernia and symptoms of gastroesophageal reflux disease (group 1), subjects with no hiatal hernia but symptoms of gastroesophageal reflux disease (group 2), and subjects with hiatal hernia but no symptoms of gastroesophageal reflux disease (group 3). The *y* axis shows the number of patients who persist with esophageal pH less than 5. The acid clearance time to pH 5 or greater is significantly faster in group 2 (symptomatic, no hiatal hernia) compared with group 1 (symptomatic, hiatal hernia) and group 3 (asymptomatic, hiatal hernia). Groups 1 and 3 have similar acid clearance times. (From: *Mittal RK, Lange RC, McCallum RW: Identification and mechanisms of delayed esophageal clearance in subjects with hiatus hernia. Gastroenterology 92:132, 1987, with permission.*)

esophageal exposure to gastric juice by contributing to ineffective clearance. This explains why, in the absence of peristalsis, reflux episodes are prolonged in the supine position. The bulk of refluxed gastric juice is cleared from the esophagus by a primary peristaltic wave initiated by a pharyngeal swallow. Secondary peristaltic waves are initiated by either distention of the lower esophagus or a drop in the intraesophageal pH. Ambulatory motility studies indicate that secondary waves are less common and play less of a role in clearance than previously thought. The esophageal contractions initiated by a drop in esophageal pH rarely have a normal peristaltic pattern and usually have a broad-based, powerful and synchronous pattern, which reduces the efficiency of esophageal clearance and encourages the regurgitation of refluxed material into the pharynx, predisposing the patient to aspiration.

Manometry of the esophageal body can detect failure of esophageal clearance by analysis of the pressure amplitude and speed of wave progression through the esophagus. The work of Kahrilas and Dodds has shown that the amplitude of an esophageal contraction required to clear the esophagus of barium varies according to the level. Lower segments require a greater amplitude than upper segments. Inadequate amplitude results in ineffective clearance.

Salivation contributes to esophageal clearance by neutralizing the minute amount of acid that is left following a peristaltic wave. Return of esophageal pH to normal takes significantly longer if salivary flow is reduced, such as after radiotherapy, and is shorter if saliva is stimulated by sucking lozenges. Saliva production may also be increased by the presence of acid in the lower esophagus. The patient experiences excessive mucus in the throat. Clinically, this is referred to as "water brash."

A hiatal hernia can also contribute to an esophageal propulsion defect due to loss of anchorage of the esophagus in the abdomen. This results in a reduction in the efficiency of acid clearance (Fig. 23-33). Kahrilas has shown that complete esophageal emptying without retrograde flow was achieved in 86 percent of test swallows in control subjects without a hiatal hernia, 66 percent in patients with a reducing hiatal hernia, and only 32 percent of patients with a nonreducing hiatal hernia. Impaired clearance in patients with nonreducing hiatal hernias suggests that the presence of a hiatal hernia contributes to the pathogenesis of gastroesophageal reflux disease.

Gastric Reservoir. Abnormalities of the gastric reservoir that increase esophageal exposure to gastric juice include gastric dilatation, increased intragastric pressure, persistent gastric reservoir, and increased gastric acid secretion. The effect of gastric dilatation is to shorten the overall length of the lower esophageal sphincter, resulting in a decrease in the sphincter resistance to reflux. This is analogous to the shortening of a balloon neck on inflation. Excessive gastric dilatation in patients with gastroesophageal reflux disease commonly results from aerophagia due to an unconscious increase in pharyngeal swallowing in an effort to improve esophageal clearance and accounts for the symptom of bloating often seen in these patients. Each pharyngeal swallow results in the propulsion of 1 to 2 mL of air into the stomach. This occurs in chronic gum chewers, in patients with decreased saliva from Sjögren's syndrome or previous head and neck radiation, and in patients who are unable to initiate secondary peristalsis and require multiple pharyngeal swallows to propel food into the stomach.

Increased intragastric pressure occurs from the outlet obstruction of a scarred pylorus or duodenum, from a vagotomy, and in the diabetic patient with gastroparesis. The latter two conditions are secondary to abnormalities of the normal active relaxation of the stomach. The increase in intragastric pressure due to alteration in the pressure-volume relationship in these abnormalities can overcome the sphincter resistance and results in reflux.

A persistent gastric reservoir results from delayed gastric emptying and increases the exposure of the esophagus to gastric juice by accentuating physiologic reflux. It is caused by myogenic abnormalities such as gastric atony in advanced diabetes, diffuse neuromuscular disorders, anticholinergic medications, and postviral infections. Nonmyogenic causes are vagotomy, antropyloric dysfunction, and duodenal dysmotility. Delayed gastric emptying can result in increased exposure of the gastric mucosa to bile and pancreatic juice refluxed from the duodenum into the stomach, with the development of gastritis.

Gastric hypersecretion can increase esophageal exposure to gastric acid juice by the physiologic reflux of concentrated gastric acid. Barlow has shown that 28 percent of patients with increased esophageal exposure to gastric juice measured by 24-hour pH monitoring have gastric hypersecretion. A mechanically defective sphincter was more important than gastric hypersecretion in the development of complications of reflux disease. In this respect, gastroesophageal reflux disease differs from duodenal ulcer disease, as the latter is specifically related to gastric hypersecretion.

Complications of Gastroesophageal Reflux. The complications of gastroesophageal reflux result from the damage inflicted by gastric juice on the esophageal mucosa or respiratory epithelium and changes caused by their subsequent repair and fibrosis. Complications due to repetitive reflux are esophagitis, stricture, and Barrett's esophagus, and to repetitive aspiration, progressive pulmonary fibrosis. The severity of the complications is directly related to the prevalence of a mechanically defective sphincter (Table 23-4). The observation that a mechanically defective sphincter occurs in 42 percent of the patients without complications suggests that the mechanical defect of the sphincter is primary and not the result of inflammation or tissue damage. The presence of a mechanically defective sphincter allows unrestricted reflux of gastric juice into the esophagus and overwhelms its normal clearance mechanisms. This leads to mucosal injury with progressive deterioration of esophageal contractility, particularly in patients with strictures and Barrett's esophagus, and regurgitation into the pharynx with aspiration.

The observation that complications of gastroesophageal reflux can occur in patients with a mechanically normal sphincter, and that some patients who have a mechanically defective sphincter can be free of complications, indicates that factors other than a mechanically defective sphincter, such as the composition of the refluxed gastric juice, are important in the development of the complications. Refluxed acid gastric juice has been generally regarded as the major damaging agent in gastroesophageal reflux disease. But recent studies have shown that the presence and severity of reflux complications, i.e., esophagitis, stricture, and Barrett's esophagus, are related to the presence of a mechanically defective sphincter and an increased esophageal exposure to *both* acidity and alkalinity (Fig. 23-34). Combined esophageal and gastric pH monitoring shows that the alkaline component is due to

Table 23-4
Complications of Gastroesophageal Reflux Disease: 150 Consecutive Cases with Proven Gastroesophageal Reflux Disease (24-Hour Esophageal pH Monitoring, Endoscopy, and Motility)

Complication	*No.*	*Normal sphincter*	*Defective sphincter*
None	59	58%	42%
Esophagitis	47	23%	77%*
Stricture	19	11%	89%
Barrett's esophagus	25	0%	100%
Total	150		

*Grade more severe with defective cardia

SOURCE: DeMeester TR, Stein HJ: Gastroesophageal reflux disease, in Moody FG, Carey LC, et al (eds): *Surgical Treatment of Digestive Disease*, 2nd ed. Chicago, Year Book Medical Publishers, 1989, p 81, with permission.

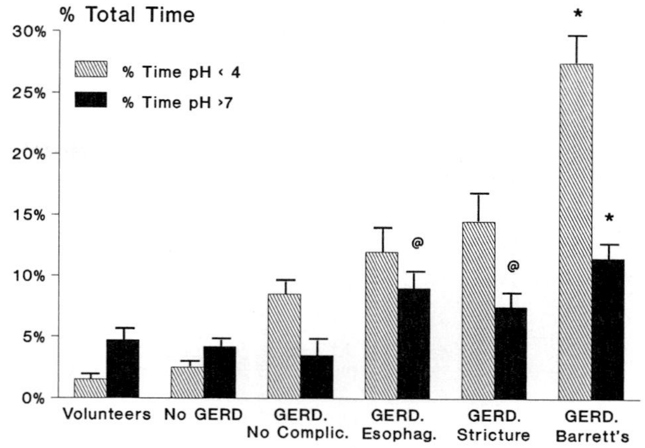

FIG. 23-34. Esophageal acid and alkaline exposure expressed as percentage of total time pH < 4 and pH > 7. *: $p < 0.01$ vs. GERD patients with no complication. @: $p < 0.05$ vs. GERD patients with no complications. (From: *Stein HJ, Barlow AP, et al: Ann Surg 216:39, 1992, with permission.*)

excessive reflux of duodenal contents through the stomach and into the distal esophagus (see Fig. 23-30). In support of this observation is that the prevalence of complications of gastroesophageal reflux disease is significantly higher in patients with acid/alkaline reflux as compared with those with only acid reflux. In patients who have acid reflux only, complications are unusual if there is a mechanically normal sphincter and somewhat more frequent in those who have a mechanically defective sphincter. By contrast, complications are almost always present in patients who have a mechanically defective sphincter and an alkaline component to their acid reflux. In addition to the prevalence of complications, the severity of the complications progressively increases from patients with a normal lower esophageal sphincter and only acid reflux to patients with a defective sphincter and acid/alkaline reflux. Patients with a normal lower esophageal sphincter and acid reflux were more apt to have esophagitis or no complications, whereas those with a mechanically defective sphincter and acid/alkaline reflux were more likely to have a stricture or Barrett's esophagus.

Our current understanding of the role of the various ingredients in gastric juice in the development of reflux complications is based on the elegant studies of Johnson and Harmon and is graphically illustrated in Fig. 23-35. Hydrogen ion injury to the esophageal squamous mucosa occurs only at a pH below 2. In acid refluxate, the enzyme pepsin appears to be the major injurious agent. Reflux of bile and pancreatic enzymes into the stomach can either protect against or augment esophageal mucosal injury. For instance, the reflux of duodenal contents into the stomach may prevent the development of peptic esophagitis in a patient whose gastric acid secretion maintained an acid environment because the bile salts would attenuate the injurious effect of pepsin and the acid would inactivate the trypsin. Such a patient would have bile-containing acid gastric juice that, when refluxed, would irritate the esophageal mucosa but cause less esophagitis than if it were acid gastric juice containing pepsin. By contrast, the reflux of duodenal contents into the stomach of a patient with limited gastric acid secretion can result in esophagitis, because the alkaline intragastric environment would support optimal trypsin activity and the soluble bile salts with a high pK_a would potentiate the enzyme's effect. Hence, duodenal-gastric reflux and the acid secretory capacity of

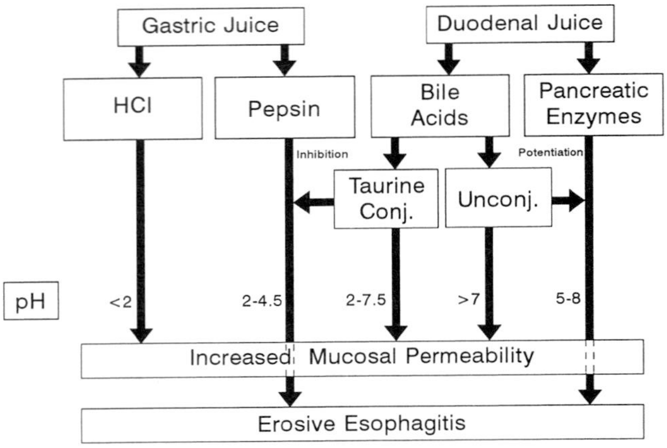

FIG. 23-35. Schematic diagram of the interaction of injurious agents refluxed into the esophagus of patients with gastroesophageal reflux disease related to the pH of the refluxed gastric juice. (From: *DeMeester TR: Definition, detection, and pathophysiology of gastroesophageal reflux disease, in DeMeester TR, Matthews H (eds): International Trends in General Thoracic Surgery, Vol III: Benign Esophageal Disease. St. Louis, CV Mosby, 1987, p 122, with permission.*)

the stomach interrelate by altering the pH and enzymatic activity of the refluxed gastric juice to modulate the injurious effects of enzymes on the esophageal mucosa.

Similarly, the disparity in injury—i.e., mucosal barrier abnormalities caused by acid and bile alone as opposed to gross esophagitis caused by pepsin and trypsin—provides an explanation for the poor correlation between the symptom of heartburn and endoscopic esophagitis. The reflux of acid gastric juice contaminated with duodenal contents could break the esophageal mucosal barrier, irritate nerve endings in the papillae close to the luminal surface, and cause severe heartburn. Despite the presence of intense heartburn, the bile salts present can inhibit pepsin, the acid pH would inactivate trypsin, and the patient would have little or no gross evidence of esophagitis. By contrast, the patient who refluxed alkaline gastric juice may have minimal heartburn because of the absence of hydrogen ions in the refluxate, but have endoscopic esophagitis because of the bile salt potentiation of trypsin activity on the esophageal mucosa. Consequently, changing the pH of refluxed duodenogastric juice from acid to alkaline, by the administration of H_2 blockers or proton pump inhibitors, may intensify the mucosal injury, while at the same time giving the patient a sense of security by alleviating the symptom of heartburn. This is supported by recent clinical studies that indicate that the presence of alkaline reflux is associated with the development of reflux complications (Table 23-5). This suggests that the combination of duodenogastric reflux and gastroesophageal reflux may be more detrimental than gastroesophageal reflux alone.

When the composition of the refluxed gastric juice is such that sustained or repetitive esophageal injury occurs, two sequelae can result. First, a luminal stricture can develop from submucosal and eventually intramural fibrosis. Second, a Barrett's esophagus can develop by replacement of repetitively destroyed squamous mucosa with columnar epithelium. The columnar epithelium is resistant to acid and is associated with the alleviation of the complaint of heartburn. Endoscopically the Barrett's changes can be quiescent or associated with complications of esophagitis, stricture, Barrett's ulceration, and dysplasia. Clinical evidence suggests that

Table 23-5
Alkaline Esophageal Exposure

	No.	*% Time pH > 7*
Normal subjects	50	2.8
Esophagitis	53	8.7*
Barrett's esophagus	23	11.8*

*$p < 0.05$

SOURCE: DeMeester TR, Stein HJ: Gastroesophageal reflux disease, in Moody FG, Carey LC, et al (eds): *Surgical Treatment of Digestive Disease,* 2nd ed. Chicago, Year Book Medical Publishers, 1989, p 85, with permission.

the complications associated with Barrett's may be due to the continuous irritation from refluxed alkalinized duodenogastric juice. Most important is that the metaplastic Barrett's epithelium may become dysplastic and progress to adenocarcinoma with an incidence that is yet to be determined but is predicted to be between 0.5 and 10 percent.

An esophageal stricture can be associated with severe esophagitis or Barrett's esophagus. In the latter situation, it occurs at the site of maximal inflammatory injury, i.e., the columnar-squamous epithelial interface. As the columnar epithelium advances into the area of inflammation, the inflammation extends higher into the proximal esophagus, and the site of the stricture moves progressively up the esophagus. Patients who have a stricture in the absence of Barrett's esophagus should have the presence of gastroesophageal reflux documented before the causation of the stricture is ascribed to reflux esophagitis. In patients with normal acid exposure, the stricture may be due to a drug-induced chemical injury resulting from the lodgment of a capsule or tablet in the distal esophagus. In such patients, dilatation usually corrects the problem of dysphagia. Heartburn, which may have occurred only because of the chemical injury, need not be treated. It is also possible for drug-induced injuries to occur in patients who have underlying esophagitis and a distal esophageal stricture secondary to gastroesophageal reflux. In this situation, a long stringlike stricture progressively develops as a result of repetitive caustic injury from capsule or tablet lodgment on top of an initial reflux stricture. These strictures are often resistant to dilatation.

When the refluxed gastric juice is of sufficient quantity, it can reach the pharynx, with the potential for pharyngeal tracheal aspiration, causing symptoms of repetitive cough, choking, hoarseness, and recurrent pneumonia. This is often an unrecognized complication of gastroesophageal reflux disease, since either the pulmonary or the gastrointestinal symptoms may predominate in the clinical situation and focus the physician's attention on one to the exclusion of the other. Clinical studies have identified three factors that are important in these patients: First, the loss of respiratory epithelium secondary to the aspiration of gastric contents can take up to 7 days to recover and may give rise to a chronic cough between episodes of aspiration. When studied during this time the cough may not be related to a reflux episode. Second, the presence of an esophageal motility disorder is observed in 75 percent of patients with reflux-induced aspiration and is believed to promote the aboral movement of the refluxate toward the pharynx. Third, if in patients with increased esophageal acid exposure, the pH is below 4 for 3 percent of the time in the cervical esophagus, the respiratory symptoms have a high probability of being caused by aspiration.

Medical Therapy

Gastroesophageal reflux disease is such a common condition that most patients with mild symptoms carry out self-medication. Patients when first seen with symptoms of heartburn without obvious complications can reasonably be placed on 8 to 12 weeks of simple antacids before extensive investigations are carried out. In many situations, this successfully aborts the attacks. Patients should be advised to elevate the head of the bed, avoid tight clothing, eat small frequent meals, avoid eating their nighttime meal shortly before retiring, lose weight, and avoid alcohol, coffee, and peppermints, which may aggravate the symptoms.

Alginic acid, used in combination with simple antacids, may augment symptomatic relief by creating a physical barrier to reflux as well as by acid reduction. Alginic acid reacts with sodium bicarbonate in the presence of saliva to form a highly viscous solution that floats like a raft on the surface of the gastric contents. When reflux occurs, this protective layer is refluxed into the esophagus and acts as a protective barrier against the noxious gastric contents. Medications to promote gastric emptying such as metoclopramide, domperidone, or cisapride have been of little value.

The second phase of medical therapy is acid suppression. This is achieved in patients with persistent symptoms by administering H_2-blocker therapy. In high doses, it can cause 70 to 80 percent reduction in gastric acidity. This treatment, however, achieves healing of esophagitis in only about 50 percent of patients after an 8-week course of therapy. The new hydrogen potassium proton pump inhibitor, omeprazole, which can totally shut off gastric acid secretion, causes an almost complete disappearance of symptoms and results in a more than 75 percent healing rate of mild esophagitis and a 50 percent healing rate of severe esophagitis after a 12-week course of therapy. The problem with these medications is that they should not be continued long-term because of the cost and the danger of developing complications secondary to the alkaline component of the reflux gastric juice while symptoms are being masked with therapy. Unfortunately, within 6 months of discontinuation of any form of medical therapy for gastroesophageal reflux disease, 80 percent of patients have a recurrence of symptoms. This is because a mechanically defective sphincter is not corrected or repaired by acid suppression therapy.

A reasonable protocol for managing patients with gastroesophageal reflux disease is shown in Fig. 23-36. All patients whose symptoms persist despite simple antacid therapy should undergo endoscopy to determine if the complications of reflux disease such as esophagitis, stricture, or Barrett's esophagus are present. All are then placed on H_2-blocker or omeprazole therapy. If their symptoms disappear completely after 12 weeks of therapy, the medication should be discontinued and the patient observed. If their symptoms recur within 4 weeks, they should be studied with manometry and 24-hour foregut pH monitoring. Patients who on repeat endoscopy show persisting complications of the disease should also be studied. Depending on the results of the tests, further intensive medical therapy may be instituted, or the patient may be considered for surgical therapy if the criteria are met. Patients whose symptoms do not reoccur within 4 weeks and are free of complications of the disease should be monitored and treated intermittently when symptoms occur.

Surgical Therapy

Historical Background. From a historical perspective, gastroesophageal reflux disease was not recognized as a significant clinical problem until the mid 1930s and was not identified as a precipitating cause for esophagitis until after World War II. Initially, the symptoms of gastroesophageal reflux were associated with a hiatal hernia. This led to the conclusion that the hernia itself was the cause of the symptoms. It seemed reasonable to attempt to correct these symptoms by surgically reducing the hernia with simple closure of the crura. The result of this first surgical effort was uniform failure. For a period, the reasons for the failures did not become evident, because of the inability to understand the relationship between hiatal hernia and reflux. This was due to the lack of esophageal function studies and the difficulty of performing rigid endoscopy. Consequently, a hiatal hernia became an indication for operation, and many patients had dissatisfying results.

Phillip Allison was the first to link the symptomatology of hiatal hernia to the occurrence of gastroesophageal reflux. This con-

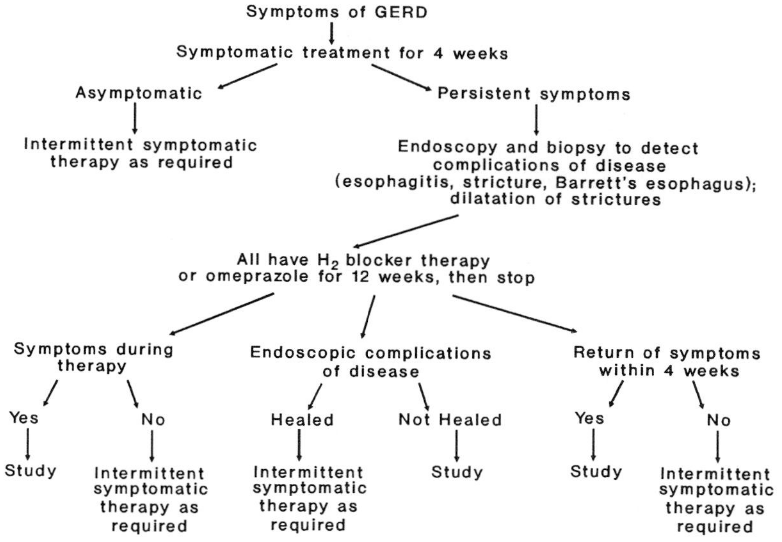

FIG. 23-36. Algorithm showing medical management and indications for functional studies (i.e., 24-hour pH monitoring and manometry) in patients with symptoms of gastroesophageal reflux disease (GERD). (From: *Hinder RA, DeMeester TR: Gastroesophageal reflux disease and hiatal hernia in adults, in Scott WH Jr, Sawyers JL (eds): Surgery of the Stomach, Duodenum, and Small Intestine, 2nd ed. Boston, Blackwell Scientific Publications, 1992, p 422, with permission.*)

tribution encouraged surgeons to improve the function of the cardia rather than simply reducing the hernia. The Allison repair, introduced in 1951, represented the first effort in this direction. He emphasized the need to place the gastroesophageal junction in its normal intraabdominal position in order to improve its function. Although the repair was associated with a high incidence of recurrence, Allison justly received the credit for initiating the modern era of antireflux surgery.

The experience with the Allison repair demonstrated that relief from the symptoms of reflux occurred in those patients whose gastroesophageal junction remained in the intraabdominal position. Consequently, surgeons were stimulated to develop procedures designed to place and anchor the lower esophagus more effectively in the intraabdominal position. Initially, these operations consisted of various forms of gastropexy in which an intraabdominal esophagus was achieved by pulling the stomach down in the abdomen, whether it was herniated or not, and attaching it to the anterior abdominal wall or to any posterior peritoneal structure that seemed strong enough to maintain it there. The design of the gastropexy operation placed the stomach and esophagus on a great deal of continual tension, which was further stressed by the normal respiratory and swallowing movements. Consequently, dislodgement of the gastropexies occurred with the return of reflux symptoms. The most popular of these operations was the Hill procedure, which anchors the gastroesophageal junction posteriorly to the median arcuate ligament.

With the exception of the Hill procedure, these operations did not stand the test of time and were gradually abandoned as more durable methods were sought to achieve an intraabdominal esophagus. One of these was the Belsey Mark IV repair and another the Nissen fundoplication. Both procedures incorporate a portion of the distal esophagus into the stomach to assure that it will be affected by changes in intraabdominal pressure transmitted by the gastric conduit. The Belsey Mark IV procedure is, in essence, a partial fundoplication, or an enveloping of the distal esophagus with the gastric fundus over 280°, while the Nissen is a complete fundoplication, or a 360° enveloping of the distal esophagus by the gastric fundus.

With wider application of the Nissen procedure, it became evident that a successful Nissen fundoplication is not simply a matter of wrapping the stomach around the lower esophagus and sewing it in place. Rather, a good deal of judgment and experience is required to determine how tight and how long to make the fundoplication, what portion of the stomach should be used, and what conditions preclude the use of the operation. Consequently, Nissen fundoplications have contributed to a number of severe postoperative complications. Most can be attributed to surgical technique and inaccurate selection of patients for operation. If the fundoplication is constructed too long or performed as a wrap rather than an enveloping of the esophagus by the fundus, permanent dysphagia or odynophagia may result. Such a fundoplication precludes physiologic belching and vomiting. Instead of performing the operation properly, surgeons began to introduce a variety of partial fundoplications to avoid these problems. They are usually constructed by covering either the anterior or the posterior wall of the distal esophagus with the stomach. This necessitates suturing the fundus of the stomach to the esophagus as the primary and most important portion of the procedure. This suture line is subject to a great deal of stress and, as a consequence, has a limited durability. Although the partial fundoplication operations are successful in preventing reflux and permitting physiologic belching when they remain intact, they disrupt with a distressing frequency.

The most durable of the partial fundoplication procedures is the Belsey Mark IV operation. In this procedure the attachment of the esophagus to the stomach is more extensive than that advocated for the other partial fundoplications, and the procedure is performed transthoracically, so that the esophagus can be adequately mobilized to construct the repair without undue tension. The main drawback of the Belsey Mark IV procedure is that, when universally applied by surgeons with varied skills, the antireflux protection achieved is not as predictable as with a complete Nissen fundoplication. This is because the Belsey procedure is difficult to teach and communicate and has less margin for error. In experienced hands the success of the Belsey operation appears similar to that of the Nissen.

More recently, it has become recognized that as reflux disease progresses, the esophagus becomes shorter. This is particularly so in patients with a stricture or Barrett's esophagus. Under these conditions, it is difficult to get an adequate length of abdominal esophagus for a proper repair without undue tension on the repair or without placing the fundoplication around the stomach which has been deformed into a tube from chronic traction through the esophageal hiatus. Both of these errors result in a high incidence of recurrence and a bad reputation for surgical therapy.

Indications for Antireflux Surgery. Before proceeding with an antireflux procedure, it is necessary to confirm that the patients' symptoms are caused by increased esophageal exposure to gastric juice secondary to a mechanically defective lower esophageal sphincter. This requires performing esophageal function studies, i.e., 24-hour esophageal pH monitoring and esophageal manometry. As outlined in the algorithm in Fig. 23-36, esophageal function studies should be done if the patient has persistent symptoms or unimproved esophageal mucosal injury after 8 to 12 weeks of acid suppression therapy. Patients who respond to a course of medical therapy but have recurrence of symptoms within 4 weeks after cessation of therapy should also be studied, since they are prone to drug dependency.

The requirements to proceed with an antireflux procedure in such patients are listed in Table 23-6.

If 24-hour esophageal pH monitoring is normal in a patient with unequivocal endoscopic esophagitis, the possibilities of alkaline, drug-induced, or retention esophagitis should be considered. Patients with increased esophageal exposure to gastric juice in whom the sphincter is manometrically normal should be evaluated for a gastric or esophageal cause of reflux. Approximately 40 percent of these patients will have gastric acid hypersecretion and respond to more aggressive antisecretory therapy. Patients with increased esophageal acid exposure, a mechanically defective sphincter, and no complications of the disease should be given the

Table 23-6
Requirements to Proceed with Antireflux Procedure

1. Increased esophageal exposure to gastric juice on 24-hour esophageal pH monitoring
2. Documentation of a mechanically defective lower esophageal sphincter
3. Adequate esophageal contractility on manometry

option of surgery if they are drug-dependent to control their symptoms.

If the patient responds symptomatically to medical therapy but endoscopic esophagitis persists, surgery should be performed. Without surgery, these patients can progress to develop a stricture or Barrett's esophagus while on therapy and lose esophageal body function while on therapy because reflux of alkalized gastric contents continues through the mechanically defective sphincter. In this situation, an antireflux procedure corrects the mechanically defective sphincter, prevents the formation of a stricture or Barrett's esophagus and heals the esophagitis.

Preoperative Evaluation. Before proceeding with an antireflux operation, several factors should be evaluated. First, the propulsive force of the body of the esophagus should be evaluated by esophageal manometry to determine if it has sufficient power to propel a bolus of food through a newly reconstructed valve. Patients with normal peristaltic contractions do well with a 360° Nissen fundoplication. When peristalsis is absent, severely disordered, or the amplitude of the contraction is below 20 mmHg, the Belsey two-thirds partial fundoplication is the procedure of choice.

Second, anatomic shortening of the esophagus can compromise the ability to do an adequate repair without tension and lead to an increased incidence of breakdown or thoracic displacement of the repair. Esophageal shortening is identified radiographically by a sliding hiatal hernia that will not reduce in the upright position or that measures larger than 5 cm between the diaphragmatic crura and gastroesophageal junction on endoscopy. When an esophageal shortening is present, the motility of the esophageal body must be carefully evaluated and, if adequate, a gastroplasty should be performed. In patients who have a motility study that shows the absence of contractility or more than 50 percent interrupted or dropped contractions or a history of several failed previous antireflux procedures, esophageal resection should be considered as an alternative.

Third, the surgeon should specifically query the patient for complaints of epigastric pain, nausea, vomiting, and loss of appetite. In the past, these symptoms were accepted as part of the reflux syndrome, but we now realize that they can be due to excessive duodenogastric reflux, which occurs in about one-third of patients with gastroesophageal reflux disease. This problem is most pronounced in patients who have had previous upper gastrointestinal surgery, particularly cholecystectomy, although this is not always the case. In such patients, the correction of only the incompetent cardia may result in a disgruntled individual who continues to complain of nausea and epigastric pain on eating. In these patients, 24-hour pH monitoring of the stomach may help to detect and quantitate duodenogastric reflux. The abnormality can also be documented with a ^{99m}Tc-HIDA scan if excessive reflux of radionucleotide from the duodenum into the stomach can be demonstrated. Antireflux surgery may reduce duodenogastric reflux by improving the efficiency of gastric emptying. If the symptoms of duodenogastric reflux persist after antireflux surgery, the administration of sucralfate may relieve the persistent complaint of nausea and epigastric pain. In a few patients this may give inadequate relief, and eventually a bile diversion procedure may be necessary.

Fourth, approximately 30 percent of patients with proven gastroesophageal reflux on 24-hour pH monitoring will have hypersecretion on gastric analysis; 2 percent to 3 percent of patients who have an antireflux operation will develop a gastric or duodenal ulcer. These factors may modify the proposed antireflux procedure in patients with active ulcer disease or documentation of previous ulceration, by the addition of a highly selective vagotomy.

Fifth, delayed gastric emptying is found in approximately 40 percent of patients with gastroesophageal reflux disease and can contribute to symptoms after an antireflux repair. Usually, however, mild degrees of delayed gastric emptying are corrected by the antireflux procedure and only in patients with severe emptying disorders is there a need for an additional gastric procedure.

Principles of Surgical Therapy. The primary goal of antireflux surgery is to safely reestablish the competency of the cardia by mechanically improving its function while preserving the patient's ability to swallow normally, to belch to relieve gaseous distention, and to vomit when necessary. Regardless of the choice of the procedure, this goal can be achieved if attention is paid to five principles in reconstructing the cardia. First, the operation should restore the pressure of the distal esophageal sphincter to a level twice resting gastric pressure—i.e., 12 mmHg for a gastric pressure of 6 mmHg—and its length to at least 3 cm. This can be achieved by buttressing the distal esophagus with the fundus of the stomach. Preoperative and postoperative esophageal manometry measurements have shown that the resting sphincter pressure and the overall sphincter length can be surgically augmented over preoperative values, and that the change in the former is a function of the degree of gastric wrap around the esophagus (Fig. 23-37).

Second, the operation should place an adequate length of the distal esophageal sphincter in the positive-pressure environment of the abdomen by a method that ensures its response to changes in intraabdominal pressure. The permanent restoration of 1.5 to 2 cm of abdominal esophagus in a patient whose sphincter pressure has been augmented to twice resting gastric pressure will maintain the competency of the cardia over various challenges of intraabdominal pressure. All three of the popular antireflux procedures increase the length of the sphincter exposed to abdominal pressure by an average of 1 cm. When poorly performed, however, an operation may result in a reduction of the length of abdominal sphincter. Increasing the length of sphincter exposed to abdominal pressure will improve competency only if it is acted on by challenges of intraabdominal pressure. Thus, the creation of a conduit

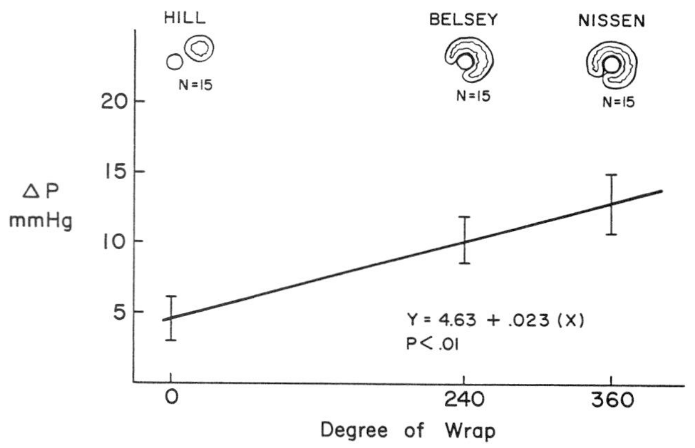

FIG. 23-37. The relationship between the augmentation of sphincter pressure over preoperative pressure (ΔP) and the degree of gastric fundic wrap in three popular antireflux procedures. (From: *O'Sullivan GC et al: Am J Surg 143:43, 1982, with permission.*)

that will ensure the transmission of intraabdominal pressure changes around the abdominal portion of the sphincter is a necessary aspect of surgical repair. The fundoplication in the Nissen and Belsey repairs serves this purpose.

Third, the operation should allow the reconstructed cardia to relax on deglutition. In normal swallowing a vagally mediated relaxation of the distal esophageal sphincter and the gastric fundus occurs. The relaxation lasts for approximately 10 seconds and is followed by a rapid recovery to the former tonicity. To ensure relaxation of the sphincter, three factors are important: (*a*) only the fundus of the stomach should be used to buttress the sphincter, since it is known to relax in concert with the sphincter; (*b*) the gastric wrap should be properly placed around the sphincter and not incorporate a portion of the stomach or be placed around the stomach itself, since the body of the stomach does not relax with swallowing; and (*c*) damage to the vagal nerves during dissection of the thoracic esophagus should be avoided because it may result in failure of the sphincter to relax.

Fourth, the fundoplication should not increase the resistance of the relaxed sphincter to a level that exceeds the peristaltic power of the body of the esophagus. The resistance of the relaxed sphincter depends on the degree, length, and diameter of the gastric fundic wrap and on the variation in intraabdominal pressure. A 360° gastric wrap should be no longer than 2 cm and constructed over a 60 French bougie. This will ensure that the relaxed sphincter will have an adequate diameter with minimal resistance. This is not necessary when constructing a partial wrap.

Fifth, the operation should ensure that the fundoplication can be placed in the abdomen without undue tension and maintained there by approximating the crura of the diaphragm above the repair. Leaving the fundoplication in the thorax converts a sliding hernia into a paraesophageal hernia with all the complications associated with that condition. Maintaining the repair in the abdomen under tension predisposes to an increased incidence of recurrence. This occurs in patients who have a stricture or Barrett's esophagus and is probably due to shortening of the esophagus from the inflammatory process. This problem can be resolved by lengthening the esophagus by gastroplasty and constructing a partial fundoplication.

Primary Antireflux Repairs

The most common antireflux procedure is the Nissen fundoplication (Fig. 23-38). The procedure can be performed through the abdomen or the chest. Rudolph Nissen described the procedure as a 360° gastric wrap around the lower esophagus for a distance of 4 to 5 cm. Although this provided good control of reflux, it was associated with a number of side effects, which have encouraged several modifications of the originally described procedure. These include using only the gastric fundus to envelope the esophagus in performing the fundoplication, sizing the fundoplication with a 60 French bougie, and limiting the length of the fundoplication to 1 to 2 cm.

In the presence of altered esophageal motility, where the propulsive force of the esophagus is not sufficient to overcome the outflow obstruction of a complete fundoplication, a partial fundoplication may be indicated. The Belsey Mark IV repair is the prototype of such a partial fundoplication and consists of a 270° gastric wrap generally performed through the chest. The dissections of the Belsey Mark IV and the transthoracic Nissen operations are the same, differing only in the technique of constructing the gastric fundoplication (Fig. 23-39).

In patients with a short esophagus due to stricture, Barrett's esophagus, or a large hiatal hernia, a Collis gastroplasty (Fig. 23-40) is performed as an esophageal lengthening procedure. The gastroplasty will lengthen the tubular esophagus by constructing a gastric tube, allowing tension-free construction of a Belsey Mark IV or Nissen fundoplication around the gastric tube, with placement of the repair in the abdomen. Because of the absence of peristalsis in the gastric tube, most surgeons prefer to combine the gastroplasty with a 280° Belsey Mark IV fundoplication rather than a 360° Nissen fundoplication.

Indications for performing an antireflux procedure by the transthoracic approach are

1. A patient who has had a previous antireflux procedure.
2. A patient who requires a concomitant esophageal myotomy for achalasia or diffuse spasm.
3. A patient who has an esophageal stricture or Barrett's esophagus. In this situation, the thoracic approach is preferred in order to obtain maximum mobilization of the shortened esophagus and, if necessary, perform a gastroplasty to place the repair without tension below the diaphragm.
4. A patient with a sliding hiatal hernia that does not reduce below the diaphragm during a radiographic barium study in the upright position. This can indicate esophageal shortening and, again, a thoracic approach is preferred for the reasons stated.
5. A patient who has associated pulmonary pathology. In this situation, the nature of the pulmonary pathology can be evaluated and the proper pulmonary surgery in addition to the antireflux repair can be performed.
6. An obese patient. In this situation, the abdominal repair is difficult because of poor exposure, whereas the thoracic approach gives better exposure and allows a more precise repair.

Antireflux surgery is different from an operation to extirpate a diseased organ whose function is of no concern, since it will be destroyed with its removal. Rather, antireflux surgery is designed to improve the function of an organ that will remain in the patient, i.e., to provide complete and permanent relief of all symptoms and complications of gastroesophageal reflux secondary to an incompetent cardia. Currently the Nissen fundoplication, the Belsey Mark IV repair, and the Hill posterior gastropexy are the most widely used antireflux repairs. Table 23-7 shows that each of the procedures, based on the reported experience in the literature, provides good to excellent relief of reflux symptoms in 84 to 89 percent of patients. Each of these procedures has different strengths and weaknesses and may be more applicable in certain situations, as shown in Table 23-8.

Experience and randomized studies have shown that the Nissen fundoplication is an effective and durable antireflux repair with minimal side effects while providing relief of reflux symptoms in 91 percent of patients over 10 years. This is accomplished by restoring normal mechanical characteristics to a defective lower esophageal sphincter. In patients with good esophageal contractility and normal esophageal length the Nissen fundoplication is the procedure of choice for a primary antireflux repair. The Nissen repair has been criticized for not being applicable to the broad spectrum of patients or to those with advanced disease. A recent cooperative study that prospectively randomized medical and surgical therapy for complicated reflux disease, however, showed that immediate Nissen fundoplication was the best therapy for control of symptoms and healing of complications in addition to providing the best patient satisfaction.

The explosion of laparoscopic general surgical procedures in the early 1990s included laparoscopic antireflux surgery. Laparo-

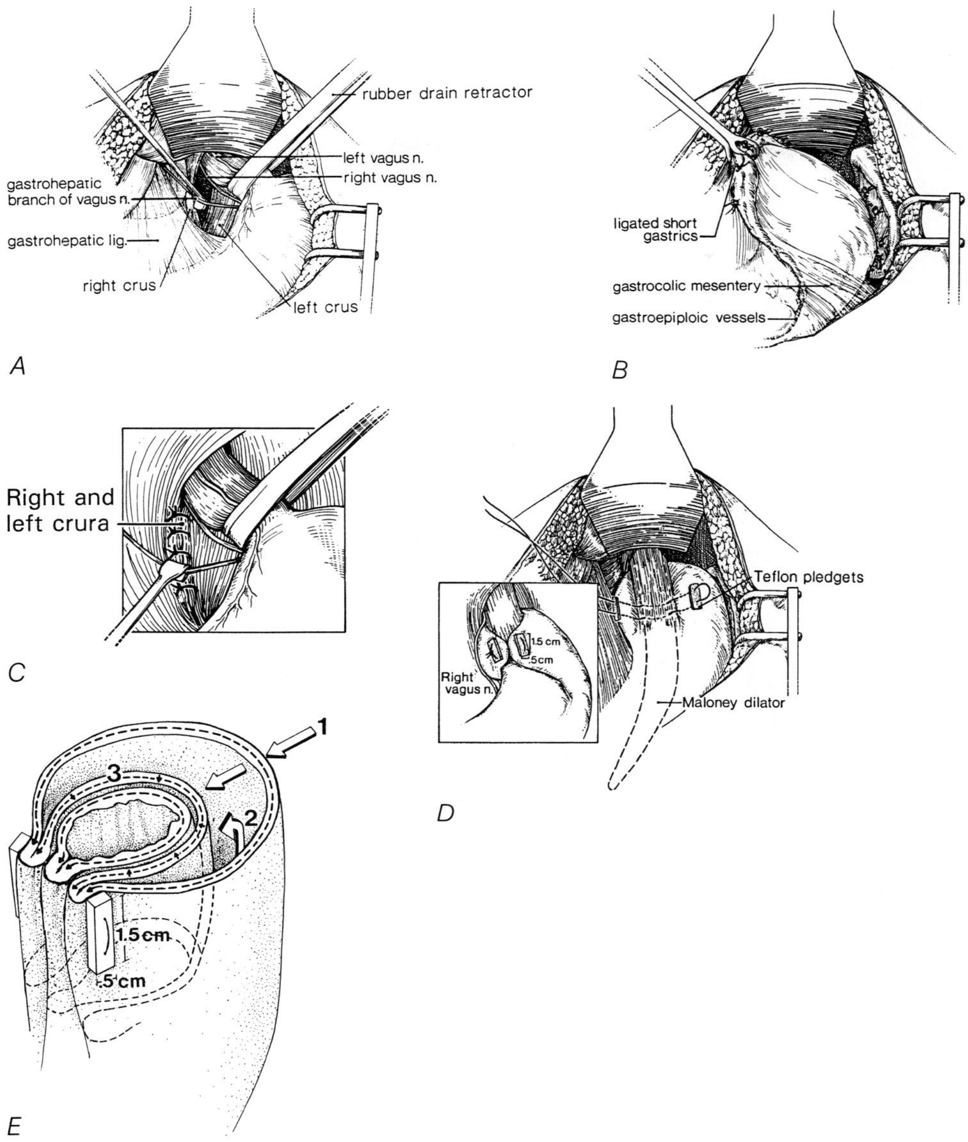

FIG. 23-38. *A.* Completed hiatal dissection done through the transabdominal approach showing the vagal nerves, position of the rubber drain around the esophagus, and the right and left crus. *B.* The mobilized gastric fundus after division of the short gastric vessels. Some of these vessels can take a retroperitoneal course, tethering the fundus of the stomach posteriorly. *C.* The closed esophageal hiatus. Notice that the esophageal body has been displaced anteriorly by the approximation of the right and left crura. *D.* Construction of the fundoplication by the transabdominal approach illustrating the placement of the horizontal mattress stitch and the positions of the pledgets. The wrap is formed over a 60 F bougie with enough space left over to allow the passage of an index finger through the wrap adjacent to the bougie. *Inset,* the completed fundoplication. *E.* Schematic cross section of a Nissen fundoplication done with 1.5 × 0.5 cm pledgets illustrating how the pledgets compress the stomach and esophagus together and how intragastric pressure *(1)*, intraabdominal pressure *(2)*, and gastric fundic muscle tone *(3)* are transmitted to the sphincter. (From: *DeMeester TR: Surgical management of gastroesophageal reflux, in Castell DO, Wu WC, Oh DJ (eds): Gastroesophageal Reflux Disease: Pathogenesis, Diagnosis, Therapy. Mount Kisco, NY, Futura Publishing Company, 1985, p 266, with permission.*)

Table 23-7
Results of Primary Surgical Antireflux Repairs for Gastroesophageal Reflux Disease

Repair	*Authors*	*Number of patients*	*Follow-up period*	*% Good results*	*% Reflux recurrence*	*% Dysphagia*	*% Gas bloat*	*Mortality*
Belsey	Skinner	632	1–5 years	85	7.0	—	—	1.2
Mark IV	Orringer	892	3–15 years	84	11.0	—	—	1.0
Hill	Hill 1967	149			4.8	2		
posterior	Hill 1983							
gastopexy	(1) No intraoperative motility	541			4.8		—	0
	Intraoperative motility	191			1.5			
	(2) No intraoperative motility	72	92.6 months	65	4.1	0		0
	Intraoperative motility	83	47 months	89	0	0		0
	Maher 1978	65		82	9			4.6
Nissen	5 reports	1141	1–12 years	87	7	8(4/48)	8(97/1115)	1.0

SOURCE: DeMeester TR, Stein HJ: Surgical treatment of gastroesophageal reflux disease, in Castell DO (ed): *The Esophagus*. Boston, Little, Brown & Company, 1992, p 615, with permission.

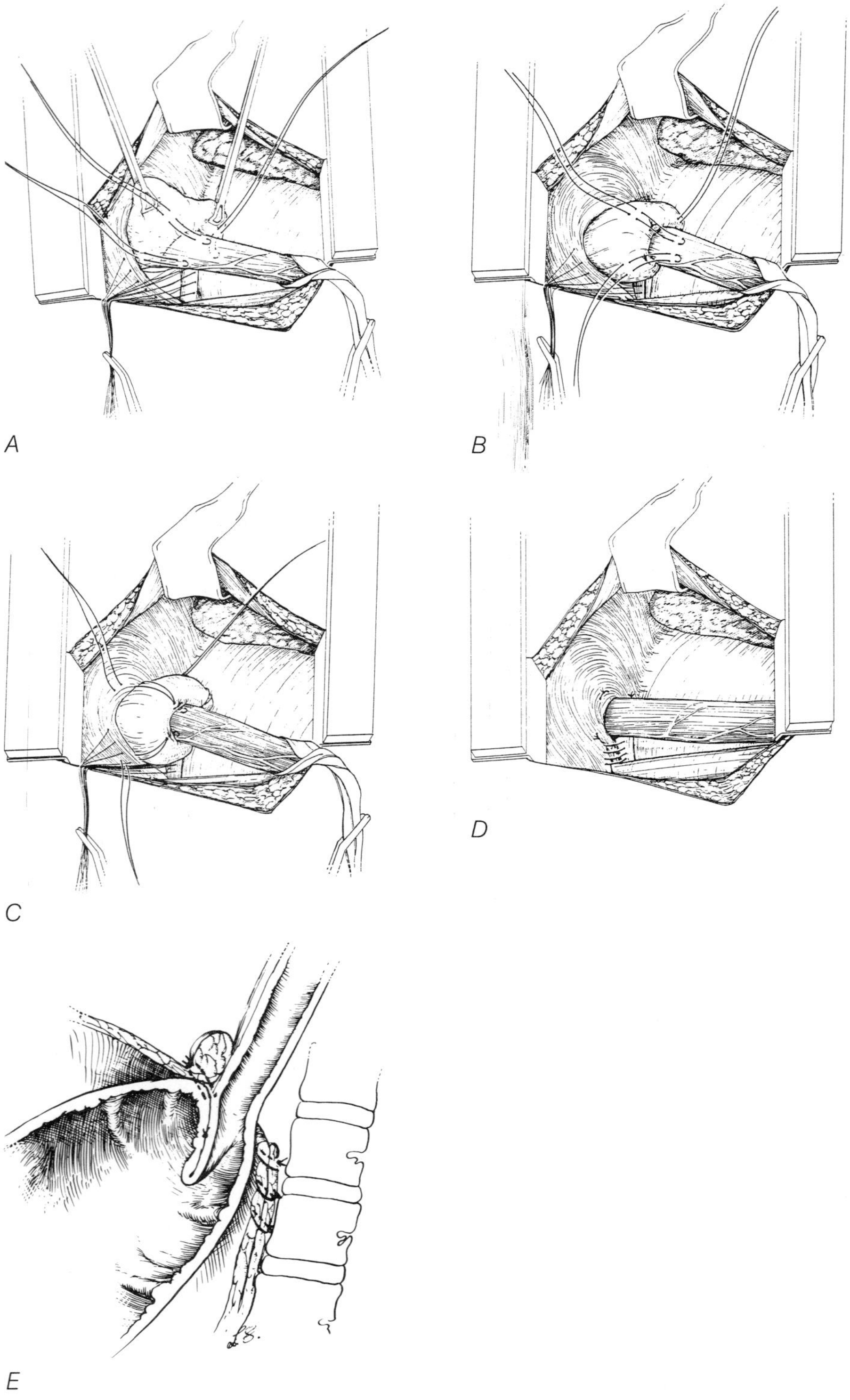

FIG. 23-39. *A.* Construction of a Belsey 240° gastric fundic wrap showing placement of the first row of sutures 1.5 cm above the gastroesophageal junction. Particular attention must be given to placement of the right lateral suture. *B.* Continued construction of the Belsey 240° gastric fundic wrap showing placement of the second row of sutures 1.5 to 2.0 cm above the previously tied sutures of the first row. *C.* Continued construction of the Belsey 240° gastric fundic wrap showing placement of the tails of the previously tied second row of sutures through the diaphragm, 0.5 cm apart and 1.0 to 1.5 cm from the edge of the hiatus. Note the placement of the sutures at the 4, 8, and 12 o'clock positions on an imaginary clock face oriented with the 6 o'clock position posterior in the hiatus between the right and left crura just anterior to the aorta. *D.* The completed Belsey 240° gastric fundic wrap showing the right and left crura approximated by tying the previously placed sutures. *E.* Sagittal section of the complete repair showing posterior sutures in the crus and first and second row of sutures used to hold the partial fundoplication. Note the second row of sutures joins diaphragm, stomach, and esophagus. The position of the tied holding sutures is also shown. (From: *DeMeester TR: Transthoracic antireflux procedures, in Nyhus LM, Baker RJ (eds): Mastery of Surgery. Boston, Little Brown, & Company, 1984, p 388, with permission.*)

scopic Nissen fundoplication has been shown to be a safe procedure, although data regarding its long-term efficacy have yet to be produced. The requirements for laparoscopic antireflux surgery are identical with its open counterparts. Patients selected for laparoscopic antireflux surgery should undergo the same preoperative evaluation as candidates for an open procedure. Patients with early, uncomplicated gastroesophageal reflux are the best candidates for a laparoscopic approach. A short esophagus, often present in patients with severe disease, with strictures, or with Barrett's esophagus, is of concern. From a laparoscopic viewpoint, a short intraabdominal esophagus poses a formidable challenge which may result in fundoplication placed at the level of the cardia

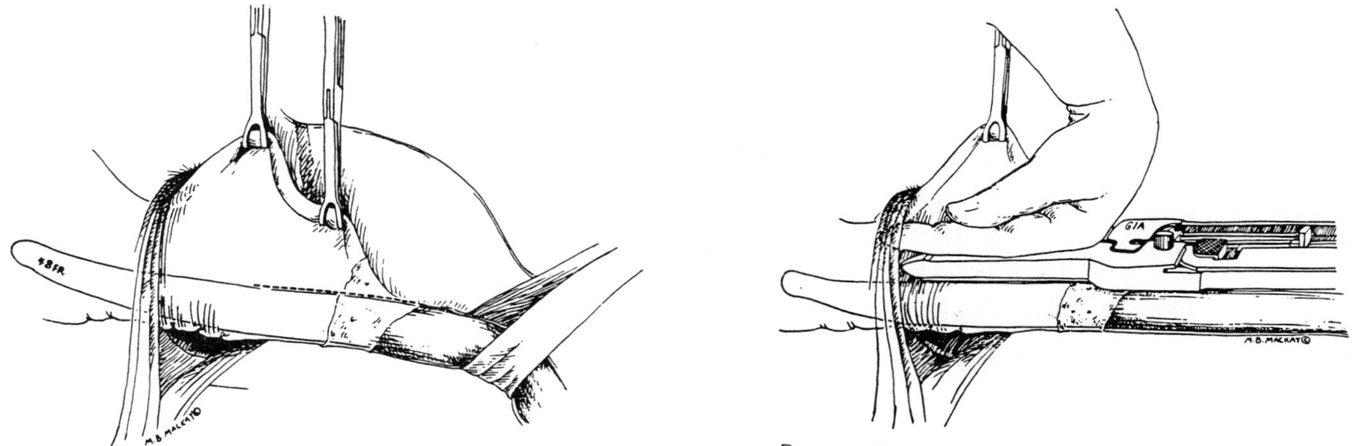

A

B

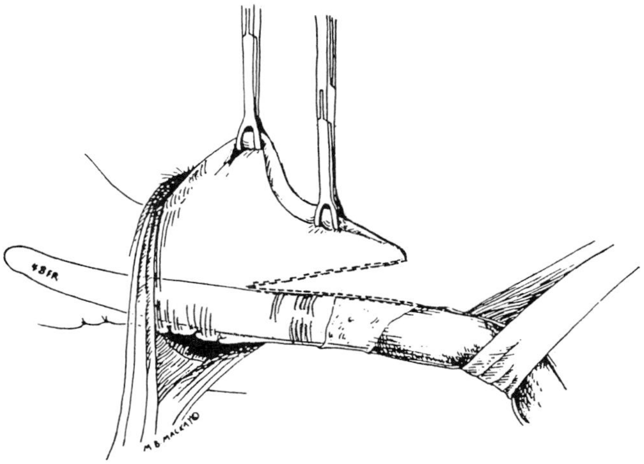

C

FIG. 23-40. *A.* Construction of a Collis gastroplasty. A 48 French bougie is passed into the stomach. The dotted line indicates the site of division of the gastric wall for construction of the gastric tube in continuity with the esophagus. *B.* Continued construction of the Collis gastroplasty. The stomach is divided with a GIA stapler. Traction is exerted on the greater curvature side of the fundus before closing the jaws of the stapler. This ensures that the gastric tube closely approximates the diameter of the indwelling 48 French bougie throughout its length. *C.* After stapling and division of the stomach, a 5-cm gastric tube is formed along the proximal portion of the lesser curvature. This effectively lengthens the esophagus and allows the construction of a Belsey partial fundoplication which can be placed below the diaphragm without tension. (From: *Pearson FG, Cooper JD, et al: Ann Surg 206:475, 1982, with permission.*)

Table 23-8
Comparison of Current Antireflux Procedures

Operation	*Concept of function*	*Ease of instruction*	*Effectiveness of the value*	*Outflow resistance*	*Toleration of tension*	*Best use*
Hill posterior gastropexy	Complex	Difficult	Dependent on intraoperative manometrics	Dependent on degree of imbrication of cardia	Good	Previous gastric resection
Belsey partial fundoplication	Simple	Most difficult	Effective—patient usually able to belch	Lowest	Poor	Poor esophageal pump
Nissen fundoplication	Simple	Average	Most effective—patient unable to belch	Highest; long and tight wrap can cause permanent dysphagia	Fair	Standard antireflux procedure
Collis-Belsey (Pearson procedure)	Simple	Difficult	Effective—patient unable to belch	Low	Best	Poor esophageal pump and short esophagus

SOURCE: DeMeester TR, Stein HJ: Surgical treatment of gastroesophageal reflux disease, in Castell DO (ed): *The Esophagus*. Boston, Little, Brown & Company, 1992, p 614, with permission.

and not around the esophagus itself. This situation will result in uniformly unsatisfactory results. Obesity and extensive adhesions secondary to previous upper abdominal surgery may, at present, represent relative contraindications to laparoscopic antireflux repair.

It is important to stress that, when utilizing a laparoscopic approach, the technical elements are the same as those of an open abdominal procedure. A Nissen fundoplication is the laparoscopic procedure of choice (Fig. 23-41). Five 10-mm ports are utilized. A fan retractor, placed into the lateral right-sided port, holds the left lateral segment of the liver toward the anterior abdominal wall. The stomach is retracted with a Babcock clamp toward the patient's feet. The phrenoesophageal ligament is grasped and incised to expose the right and left crura of the diaphragm. A blunt-tipped grasper is placed within the esophageal hiatus laterally or anteriorly to facilitate exposure. The posterior or right vagus is identified and dissected away from the esophagus. The anterior or left vagus is left in place. The crura are approximated with three to four interrupted 0 silk sutures, staying above the aortic decussation and working anteriorly. The fundus is mobilized by ligating several short gastric vessels and passed behind the esophagus. A 60 French bougie is passed to properly size the fundoplication. The fundoplication is then sutured as described for an open procedure.

Complicated Reflux Disease

Barrett's Esophagus. The condition whereby the tubular esophagus is lined with columnar epithelium rather than squamous epithelium was first described by Norman Barrett in 1950. He incorrectly believed it to be congenital in origin. It is now realized that it is an acquired abnormality, occurs in 7 to 10 percent of patients with gastroesophageal reflux disease, and represents the end stage of the natural history of this disease. It is also understood to be distinctly different from the congenital condition in which islands of mature gastric columnar epithelium are found in the upper half of the esophagus.

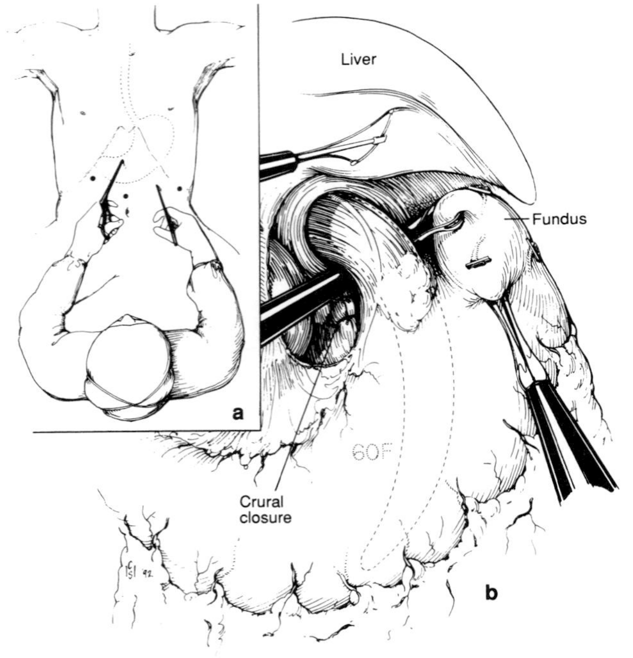

FIG. 23-41. Laparoscopic construction of a Nissen fundoplication illustrating the exposure obtained with video-assisted technology. This allows the traditional components of the open procedure, i.e., crural closure, fundic mobilization, and construction of a short fundoplication over a 60 F bougie, to be done without a laparotomy.

In the spectrum of gastroesophageal reflux disease, Barrett's esophagus stands out as being associated with profound mechanical deficiency of the lower esophageal sphincter (LES), severe impairment of esophageal body function, and the most marked esophageal acid exposure. Gastric hypersecretion occurs in 44 percent of patients.

The typical complications in Barrett's esophagus include ulceration in the columnar-lined segment, stricture formation, and a dysplasia-cancer sequence. Ulceration is unlike the erosive ulceration of reflux esophagitis, in that it more closely resembles peptic ulceration in the stomach or duodenum and has the same propensity to bleed, penetrate, or perforate. The strictures found in Barrett's esophagus occur at the squamocolumnar junction, and are typically higher than peptic strictures in the absence of Barrett's. The risk of adenocarcinoma developing in Barrett's mucosa is variously estimated at 1 in 50 patient-years to 1 in 400 patient-years, but even the most conservative estimates still represent a risk forty times that of the general population. Most cases of adenocarcinoma of the esophagus have arisen in Barrett's esophagus (Fig. 23-42). Conversely, about one-third of all patients with Barrett's present with malignancy.

The development of complications is related to the nature of the refluxed gastric juice, particularly when containing an alkaline component due to the concomitant excessive duodenogastric reflux. Nearly 60 percent of patients with complications of Barrett's esophagus had abnormal esophageal alkaline exposure compared with 6 percent of patients without complications. The columnar mucosal insensitivity that results from repetitive injury may be important in allowing severe tissue damage to progress without worsening of the patient's symptoms.

The approach to the patient with suspected Barrett's esophagus starts with a barium radiogram and upper GI endoscopy. The esophagogram may show a hiatus hernia, which if it fails to reduce in the upright posture may indicate a shortened esophagus. It may also show a high esophageal stricture or a penetrating ulcer. Endoscopically, Barrett's esophagus is recognized by the appearance of gastric-type mucosa extending 2 cm or more into the tubular esophagus. Smaller segments of Barrett's mucosa have been discovered by biopsy and are prone to the same risks. The columnar mucosa may be in the form of a tongue, and need not be circumferential. The endoscopic diagnosis must be confirmed histologically. To avoid sampling errors, we recommend performing at least two biopsies for every 1-cm interval along the length of the Barrett's segment. The most important feature to identify is the presence of intestinalization of the mucosa and whether dysplasia has occurred and, if so, whether of high or low grade.

Patients with a low risk of developing complications and whose symptoms are readily controlled by medication are suitable for medical therapy. H_2 blockers and omeprazole often brings symptomatic improvement, especially if hypersecretion of acid is an etiologic factor. Objective healing of ulcers and stabilization of strictures are not as reliably achieved. The value of prokinetic agents such as bethanechol or cisapride is usually minimal because of the loss of esophageal body function. The chief problem with medical treatment is that acid reduction therapy does nothing to correct the underlying defective sphincter and, therefore, does

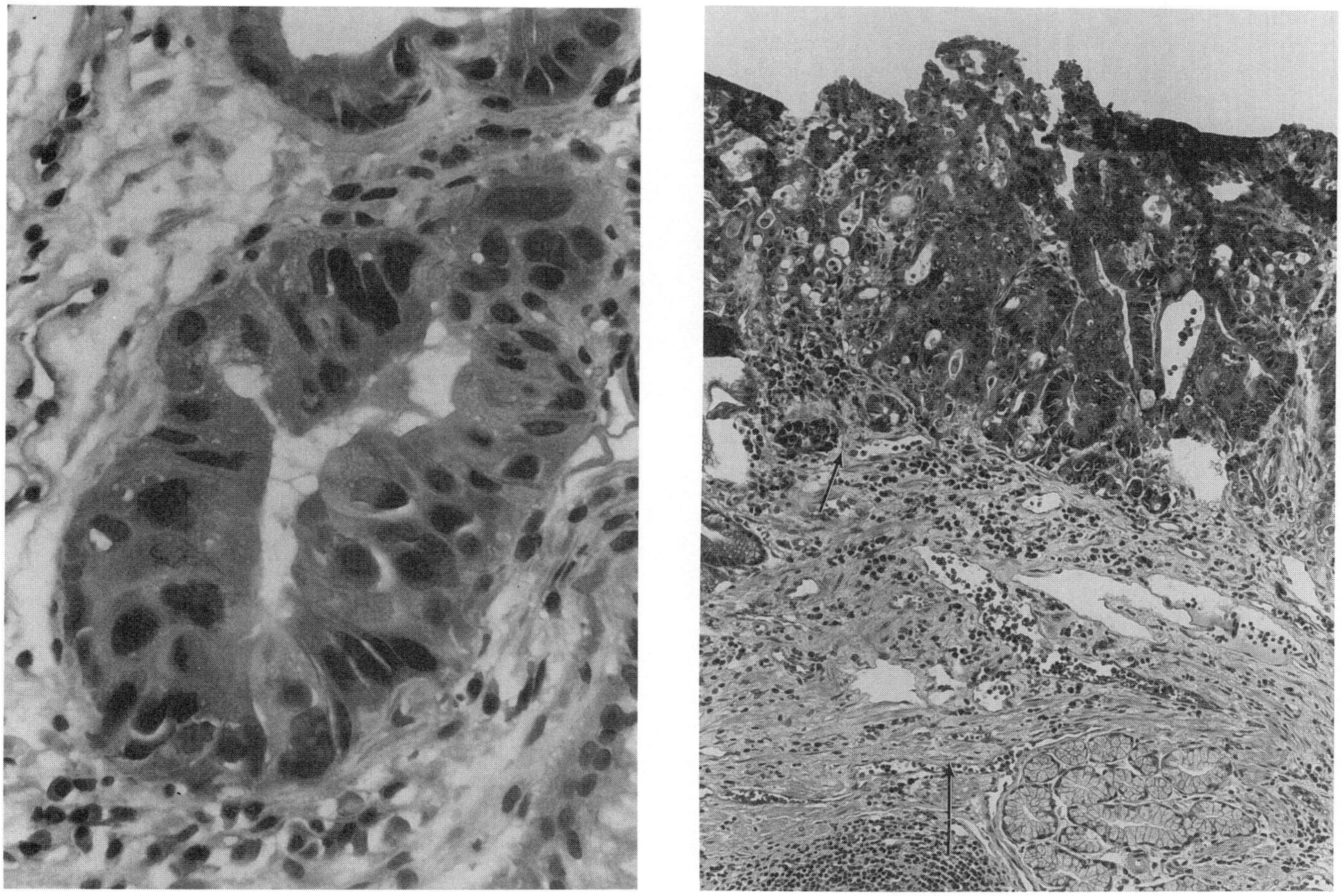

A B

FIG. 23-42. Photomicrographs. *A.* Barrett's epithelium with severe dysplasia. (×200.) Note nuclear irregularity, stratification, and loss of polarity. *B.* Barrett's epithelium with intramucosal carcinoma. (×66.) Note malignant cells in the mucosa (*upper arrow*), but not invading the muscularis mucosae (*bottom arrow*). (From: *DeMeester TR, Stein HJ, Fuchs KH: Physiologic diagnostic studies, in Zuidema GD, Orringer MB (eds): Shackelford's Surgery of the Alimentary Tract, 3rd ed, Vol I. Philadelphia, Saunders, 1991, p 113, with permission.*)

nothing to reduce the reflux of alkalized gastric juice or prevent aspiration. The symptomatic relief may allow tissue damage to progress unnoticed, so that advancement of the disease continues to occur. For this reason, surgery may be appropriate earlier in the course of the disease.

In uncomplicated Barrett's esophagus, the loss of esophageal body function can still occur but the patients are less often referred for surgery. More often, patients with complicated Barrett's esophagus are referred for surgery; and the problems of esophageal damage render it necessary to modify the operative strategy. These include esophageal body shortening, loss of peristaltic propulsive force, stricture formation, and a large ulcer.

In these circumstances it is wiser to use a transthoracic approach, as it allows thorough mobilization of the infraaortic esophagus and provides the option of performing a Collis gastroplasty if shortening of the esophagus persists despite full mobilization. It also puts the surgeon in the best position to deal with mediastinal inflammation secondary to a penetrating ulcer, where there is a risk of creating a full-thickness defect in the esophagus after mobilization. If this occurs, esophageal replacement is usually necessary.

Since Barrett's esophagus is a premalignant condition, there are strong theoretical grounds for reversing the underlying cause before malignancy develops, by performing antireflux surgery. The goal of antireflux surgery is to prevent progression of the disease rather than produce regression of the Barrett's epithelium. Regression of Barrett's epithelium after surgery has not often been reported, and when it is reported the cause may have been an artifact related to surgical relocation of the esophagogastric junction. Despite the lack of regression, there is a growing body of evidence to attest to the ability of fundoplication to protect against dysplasia and invasive malignancy. Although some cancers have developed after antireflux surgery, the absence of preexistent dysplasia or the efficacy of the particular operative procedure in reducing 24-hour esophageal acid exposure to normal has not been documented. A long-term registry maintained on patients with Barrett's free of dysplasia on entry recently reported that the development of dysplasia and cancer in patients healed medically was 19.7 percent and 1.3 percent, respectively, whereas in those treated by fundoplication, dysplasia emerged in only 3.4 percent and no cancers developed. This evidence has been used to recommend surgery as a prophylactic measure in patients with a segment of Barrett's mucosa free of dysplasia. It is unknown what effect antireflux surgery has on low-grade dysplasia. The situation is more clear when high-grade dysplasia is discovered at biopsy. If this is confirmed by two knowledgeable pathologists, an esophagectomy is recommended, as 50 percent of such specimens will show early invasive carcinoma.

Stricture. The development of a stricture while on acid suppression therapy, in a patient with a mechanically defective sphincter, represents a failure of medical therapy, and is an indication for a surgical antireflux procedure. Before surgery, a malignant cause of the stricture should be excluded and the stricture progressively dilated up to a 60 French bougie. Three factors become important in the management of these patients: (1) the response to dilatation, (2) an assessment of esophageal length by endoscopy or barium swallow, and (3) adequacy of esophageal contractility on motility studies.

If dysphagia is relieved and the amplitude of esophageal contractions and the length of the esophagus are adequate, a total fundoplication can be performed. In a patient with adequate esophageal length in whom dysphagia persists or esophageal contractility is compromised, a partial fundoplication should be done. If in either of these situations the esophagus is shortened by the disease process, a gastroplasty and partial fundoplication should be performed. When esophageal acid exposure is normal in a patient with a stricture, the cause is most likely a drug-induced injury, and dilatation is commonly all that is necessary. It should be remembered, however, that in patients with peptic strictures, medications can lodge in the narrowed area and add a superimposed chemical injury onto the existing reflux injury. This can give rise to long strictures that are difficult to dilate. Such patients should limit their medications to those available in the liquid form.

Atypical Reflux Symptoms. Chronic respiratory symptoms, such as chronic cough, recurrent pneumonias, episodes of nocturnal choking, waking up with gastric contents in the mouth, or soilage of the bed pillow, may also indicate the need for surgical therapy. The chest radiogram in patients suffering from repetitive pulmonary aspiration secondary to gastroesophageal reflux often shows signs of pleural thickening, bronchiectasis, and chronic interstitial pulmonary fibrosis. If 24-hour pH monitoring confirms the presence of increased esophageal acid exposure and manometry shows a mechanical defect of the lower esophageal sphincter and normal esophageal body motility, an antireflux procedure can be done with an expected good result. Usually these patients have, however, a nonspecific motor abnormality of the esophageal body which tends to propel the refluxed material toward the pharynx. In some of these patients the motor abnormality will disappear following a surgical antireflux procedure. In others, the motor disorder will persist and contribute to postoperative aspiration of swallowed saliva and food. Consequently the results of an antireflux procedure in patients with a motor disorder of the esophageal body are variable.

Chest pain may be an atypical symptom of gastroesophageal reflux and is often confused with coronary artery disease. Fifty percent of patients in whom a cardiac cause of the chest pain has been excluded will have increased esophageal acid exposure as a cause of the episode of pain. An antireflux procedure provides relief of the chest pain with greater constancy than will occur with medical therapy.

Dysphagia, regurgitation, and/or chest pain on eating in a patient with normal endoscopy and esophageal function studies can be an indication for an antireflux procedure. These symptoms are usually related to the presence of a large paraesophageal hernia, intrathoracic stomach, or a small hiatal hernia with a narrow diaphragmatic hiatus. A Schatzki ring may be present with the latter. All these conditions are easily identified with an upper gastrointestinal radiographic barium examination done by a knowledgeable radiologist. These patients may have no heartburn, since the lower esophageal sphincter is usually normal and reflux of gastric acid into the esophagus does not occur. The surgical repair of the hernia usually includes an antireflux procedure because of the potential of destroying the competency of the cardia during the surgical dissection. If a Schatzki ring is identified in a patient with dysphagia, a hiatal hernia, a normal size of hiatus, and normal esophageal acid exposure, dilatation with a 60 F dilator is usually effective therapy and surgery is not required.

Scleroderma. Gastroesophageal reflux in association with scleroderma is a particularly difficult situation due to the complete absence of the lower esophageal sphincter and contractility in the distal esophagus. Intensive medical therapy should be used initially until symptoms of severe esophagitis can no longer be controlled. When this occurs, a Belsey Mark IV partial fundoplication in association with a gastroplasty can be done with the expectation that this will reduce esophageal acid exposure but not return it to normal. The gastroplasty is added because of the shortening of the esophagus that occurs as a consequence of the disease. About 50 percent of the patients receive excellent to good results with this approach.

Previous Gastric Surgery. The presence of a mechanically defective sphincter after vagotomy and gastric resection or pyloroplasty can allow reflux of gastric and pancreaticobiliary secretions into the esophagus. This problem is usually manifested by symptoms of regurgitation and pulmonary aspiration. Heartburn may be present. Endoscopic esophagitis can occur and is usually mild. Medical therapy designed to control both acid and alkaline reflux usually fails; and a bile-diverting procedure, without reconstruction of the cardia, is of little benefit in preventing the symptoms of aspiration and may contribute to delayed gastric emptying. A simple antireflux procedure may be difficult when a resection has been done. In this situation, the proper surgical therapy usually requires a gastric resection with a Roux-en-Y esophagojejunostomy and a Hunt-Lawrence pouch.

Reoperation for Failed Antireflux Repairs

Failure of an antireflux procedure occurs when the patient, after the repair, is unable to swallow normally, experiences upper abdominal discomfort during and after meals, and has recurrence or persistence of reflux symptoms. The assessment of these symptoms and the selection of patients who need further surgery are challenging problems. Functional assessment of patients who have recurrent, persistent, or emergent new symptoms following a primary antireflux repair is critical to identify the cause of failure. A retrospective analysis of patients requiring reoperation after a previous antireflux procedure showed that placement of the wrap around the stomach is the most frequent cause for failure. This is followed by partial or complete breakdown of the wrap, herniation of the repair into the chest, and construction of a too tight or too long wrap (Table 23-9). Attention to the technical details during construction of the primary procedure will avoid these failures in most instances. The critical role of preoperative esophageal function tests, before the initial procedure, is emphasized in that 10

Table 23-9
Reasons for Failure of the Primary Antireflux Repair in 63 Patients Requiring Surgery

Reason for failed repair	*No. of patients*	*(%)*
1. Placement of wrap around the stomach	17	(77)
2. Partial or complete breakdown of repair	11	(17)
3. Herniation of the repair into the chest	11	(17)
4. Too tight or too long a wrap	5	(8)
5. Disordered motility of the body	6	(10)
6. Necrosis or fistulization of lower esophagus	2	(3)
7. Extraesophageal symptoms	11	(17)

SOURCE: DeMeester TR, Stein HJ: Surgical treatment of gastroesophageal reflux disease, in Castell DO (ed): *The Esophagus*. Boston, Little, Brown & Company, 1992, p 620, with permission.

percent of these patients had antireflux procedure for a misdiagnosed underlying esophageal motor disorder.

The preferred surgical approach to a patient who has had a previously failed antireflux procedure is through a left thoracotomy with a peripheral circumferential incision in the diaphragm to provide for simultaneous exposure of the upper abdomen and safe dissection of the previous repair from both abdominal and thoracic sides of the diaphragm. Patients who have recurrence of heartburn and regurgitation without dysphagia and have good esophageal motility are most amenable to reoperation and can be expected to have an excellent outcome. When dysphagia is the cause of failure, the situation is more difficult to manage. If the dysphagia occurred immediately following the repair, it is usually due to a technical failure, most commonly a misplaced fundoplication around the upper stomach, and rerepair is usually satisfactory. When dysphagia is associated with poor motility and multiple pervious repairs, serious consideration should be given to esophageal resection and replacement. It should be kept in mind that with each reoperation the esophagus is damaged further and the chances of preserving function become less. Also, blood supply is reduced and ischemic necrosis of the esophagus can occur after several previous mobilizations.

Gastroesophageal Reflux in Children

In children with gastroesophageal reflux disease, esophagitis can progress to a stricture in a matter of weeks, even while on medical therapy. Consequently, once increased esophageal exposure to gastric juice has been confirmed in a child with esophagitis, the need for a surgical antireflux procedure becomes urgent. In infants, failure to thrive, anemia, and aspiration pneumonia may be the only evidence that reflux is present. Esophageal pH monitoring may be normal in this age group because gastric acid production does not reach adult levels until six months of age. A surgical antireflux procedure should only be performed in infants in the presence of well-documented complications of gastroesophageal reflux disease, i.e., esophagitis, stricture, and pulmonary aspiration.

The presence of reflux esophagitis after balloon dilatation for achalasia that persists despite medical therapy is an indication for early surgical intervention, since esophagitis in the presence of a severe motility disorder progresses rapidly to stricture formation. A Belsey Mark IV partial fundoplication should be done in this situation because its low outflow resistance makes it particularly suitable to an esophageal body that has no propulsive activity. Once a stricture has developed under these conditions, esophageal resection and a colon interposition are usually necessary to reestablish alimentation.

MOTILITY DISORDERS OF THE PHARYNX AND ESOPHAGUS

Clinical Manifestations. Dysphagia, i.e., difficulty in swallowing, is the primary symptom of esophageal motor disorders. Its perception by the patient is a balance between the severity of the underlying abnormality causing the dysphagia and the adjustment made by the patient in altering eating habits. Consequently, any complaint of dysphagia must include an assessment of the patient's dietary history. It must be known whether the patient experiences pain, choking, or vomits with eating; whether the patient requires liquids with the meal, is the last to finish, or has interrupted a social meal; or whether he or she has been admitted to the hospital for food impaction. These assessments, in addition to the ability to maintain nutrition, help to quantify the dysphagia, and are important in determining the indications for surgical therapy.

Based on the underlying cause of nonobstructive dysphagia the surgeon has a number of operations designed to improve the patient's swallowing ability. The results can profoundly improve the patient's ability to ingest food, but rarely return the function of the foregut to normal. In most situations, the principle of the operation is to make a defect in order to correct a defect, resulting in an improvement in the patient's ability to swallow.

To apply surgical therapy to the problem of dysphagia, the surgeon needs to know the precise functional abnormality causing the symptom. This usually entails a complete esophageal motility evaluation. A clear understanding of the physiologic mechanism of swallowing and determination of the motility abnormality giving rise to the dysphagia are essential for the choice of operation. Endoscopy is necessary only to exclude the presence of tumor or inflammatory changes as the cause of dysphagia.

Motility Disorders of the Pharyngoesophageal Segment

Disorders of the pharyngoesophageal phase of swallowing result from a discoordination of the neuromuscular events involved in chewing, initiation of swallowing, and propulsion of the material from the oropharynx into the cervical esophagus. They can be categorized into one or a combination of the following abnormalities: (1) inadequate oropharyngeal bolus transport; (2) inability to pressurize the pharynx; (3) inability to elevate the larynx; (4) discoordination of pharyngeal contraction and cricopharyngeal relaxation; and (5) decreased compliance of the pharyngoesophageal segment secondary to muscle pathology. The latter results in incomplete anatomic relaxation of the cricopharyngeus and cervical esophagus.

The causation of pharyngoesophageal swallowing disorders is usually congenital or acquired disease involving the central and peripheral nervous system, which includes cerebrovascular accidents, brainstem tumors, poliomyelitis, multiple sclerosis, Parkinson's disease, pseudobulbar palsy, peripheral neuropathy, or operative damage to the cranial nerves involved in swallowing. Muscular diseases such as radiation-induced myopathy, dermatomyositis, myotonic dystrophy, and myasthenia gravis are less common causes. Occasionally extrinsic compression by thyromegaly, cervical lymphadenopathy, or hyperostosis of the cervical spine can cause pharyngoesophageal dysphagia.

Abnormalities of pharyngoesophageal swallowing are difficult to assess with manometric techniques because of the rapidity of the oropharyngeal phase of swallowing, the movement of the gullet, and the asymmetry of the cricopharyngeus. Video/cineradiography is currently the most objective test to evaluate oropharyngeal bolus transport, pharyngeal compression, relaxation of the pharyngoesophageal segment, and the dynamics of airway protection during swallowing. It readily identifies a diverticulum (Fig. 23-43), stasis of the contrast medium in the valleculae, a cricopharyngeal bar, and/or narrowing of the pharyngoesophageal segment. These are anatomic manifestations of neuromuscular disease, and result from the loss of muscle compliance in portions of the pharynx and esophagus composed of skeletal muscle.

Careful analysis of video/cineradiographic studies combined with manometry using specially designed catheters can identify the cause of a pharyngoesophageal dysfunction in most situations. Motility studies may demonstrate inadequate pharyngeal pressurization (Fig. 23-44), insufficient or lack of cricopharyngeal relaxation (Fig. 23-45), marked discoordination of pharyngeal pressurization, cricopharyngeal relaxation and cervical esophageal contraction (Fig. 23-46), or a hypopharyngeal bolus pressure suggesting decreased compliance of the skeletal portion of the cervical esophagus (Fig. 23-47).

In patients with a Zenker's diverticulum it has been difficult to consistently demonstrate a motility abnormality of discoordination of pharyngeal/esophageal events. The abnormality most apt to be present is a loss of compliance in the pharyngoesophageal segment manifested by an increased bolus pressure. Esophageal muscle biopsies in patients with Zenker's diverticulum have shown histologic evidence of a restrictive myopathy in the pharyngoesophageal segment. These findings correlate well with the observation of a decreased compliance of the upper esophagus on videoradiographic and detailed manometric studies in these patients. They suggest that the diverticulum develops as a consequence of the repetitive stress of bolus transport through a noncompliant muscle of the pharyngoesophageal segment.

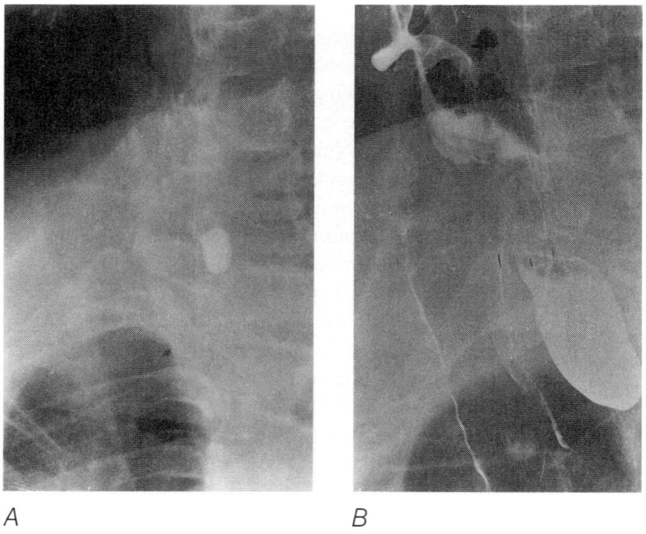

FIG. 23-43. *A.* Zenker's diverticulum, initially discovered 15 years ago and left untreated. *B.* Note its marked enlargement and evidence of laryngeal inlet aspiration on recent esophagogram. (From: *Waters PF, DeMeester TR: Med Clin North Am 65:1257, 1981, with permission.*)

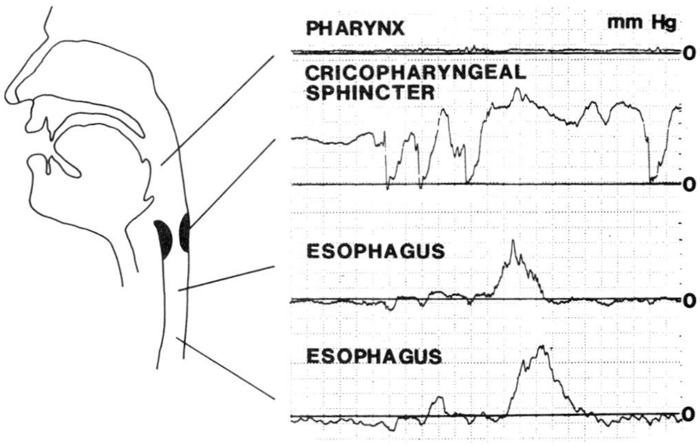

FIG. 23-44. Manometric record showing absence of a pharyngeal pressure wave in pharynx during swallowing. Cricopharyngeal sphincter relaxation is complete but brief and initiates a normal cervical esophageal pressure wave. (From: *Bonavina L, Khan NA, DeMeester TR: Arch Surg 120:546,' 1985, with permission.*)

Other manifestations of this noncompliant segment may be a cricopharyngeal bar or a more extended segment of narrowing seen in the upper esophagus. Increasing the diameter of this noncompliant segment by an esophageal myotomy reduces the resistance it imposes to a swallowed bolus. Consequently, patients unable to pressurize the pharynx or those who have an increased bolus pressure as a result of a noncompliant pharyngoesophageal segment can be improved by a cricopharyngeal myotomy.

The requirements for the successful pharyngoesophageal myotomy are (1) adequate oropharyngeal bolus transport; (2) the presence of an intact swallowing reflux; (3) reasonable coordination of pharyngeal pressurization with cricopharyngeal relaxation; (4) a cricopharyngeal bar, Zenker's diverticulum, or a narrowed pharyngoesophageal segment on videoesophagogram and/or the presence of excessive pharyngoesophageal shoulder pressure on motility study.

Zenker's Diverticulum

In the past, the most common recognized sign of the pharyngoesophageal dysfunction was the presence of a Zenker's diverticulum, originally described by Ludlow in 1769. The eponym resulted from Zenker's classic clinicopathologic descriptions of 34 cases published in 1878. Pharyngoesophageal diverticula have been reported to occur in 0.1 percent of 20,000 routine barium examinations and classically occur in elderly white males. Zenker's diverticula tend to enlarge progressively with time due to the decreased compliance of the skeletal portion of the cervical esophagus.

Presenting symptoms include dysphagia, associated with the spontaneous regurgitation of undigested, bland material, often interrupting eating or drinking. The symptom of dysphagia initially is due to the loss of muscle compliance in the pharyngoesophageal segment, later augmented by the presence of an enlarging diverticulum. On occasion, the dysphagia can be severe enough to cause debilitation and severe weight loss. Chronic aspiration and repetitive respiratory infection are common associated complaints. The diagnosis, once suspected, is established by a barium swallow. Endoscopy is usually difficult in the presence of a cricopharyngeal diverticulum, and potentially dangerous, owing to obstruction of

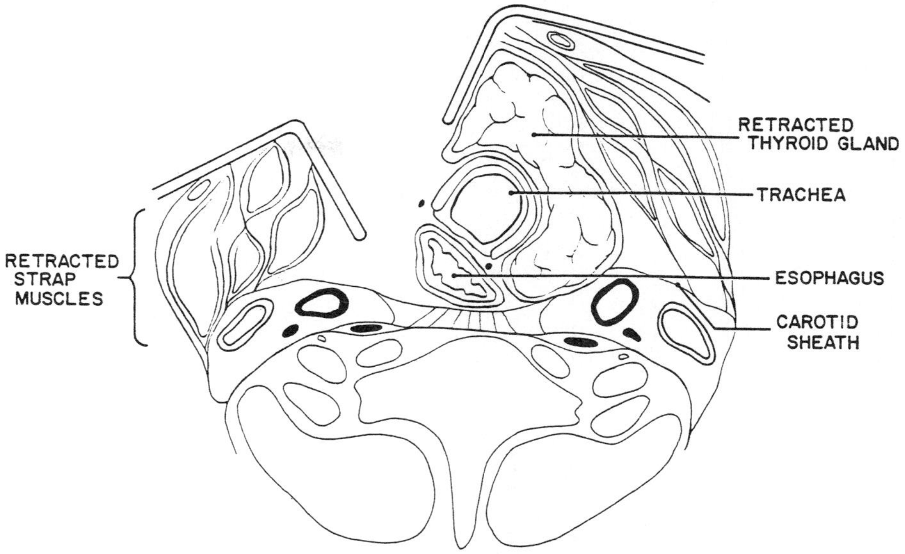

FIG. 23-45. Manometric record from a patient after a cerebrovascular accident showing lack of cricopharyngeal sphincter relaxation in response to pharyngeal contraction. (From: *Waters PF, DeMeester TR: Med Clin North Am 65:1259, 1981, with permission.*)

the true esophageal lumen by the diverticulum and the attendant risk of diverticular perforation.

Pharyngocricoesophageal Myotomy

The low morbidity and mortality of a cricopharyngeal and upper esophageal myotomy has encouraged a liberal approach toward its use for almost any problem in the oropharyngeal phase of swallowing. This attitude has resulted in an overall success rate in the relief of symptoms of only 64 percent. When patients are selected using radiographic or motility markers of disease as outlined above, it is unusual for patients not to be benefited.

The myotomy can be performed under local or general anesthesia through an incision along the anterior border of the left sternocleidomastoid muscle. The pharynx and cervical esophagus are exposed by retracting the sternocleidomastoid muscle and carotid sheath laterally and the trachea and larynx medially (Fig. 23-48). When a pharyngoesophageal diverticulum is present, localization of the pharyngoesophageal segment is easy. The diverticulum is carefully freed from the overlying areolar tissue to expose its neck, just below the inferior pharyngeal constrictor and above the cricopharyngeus muscle. It can be difficult to identify the cricopharyngeus muscle in the absence of a diverticulum. A benefit of local anesthesia is that the patient can swallow and demonstrate an area of persistent narrowing at the pharyngoesophageal junction. Further, before closing the patient, gelatin can be fed to ascertain whether the symptoms have been relieved and to inspect the opening of the previously narrowed pharyngoesophageal segment.

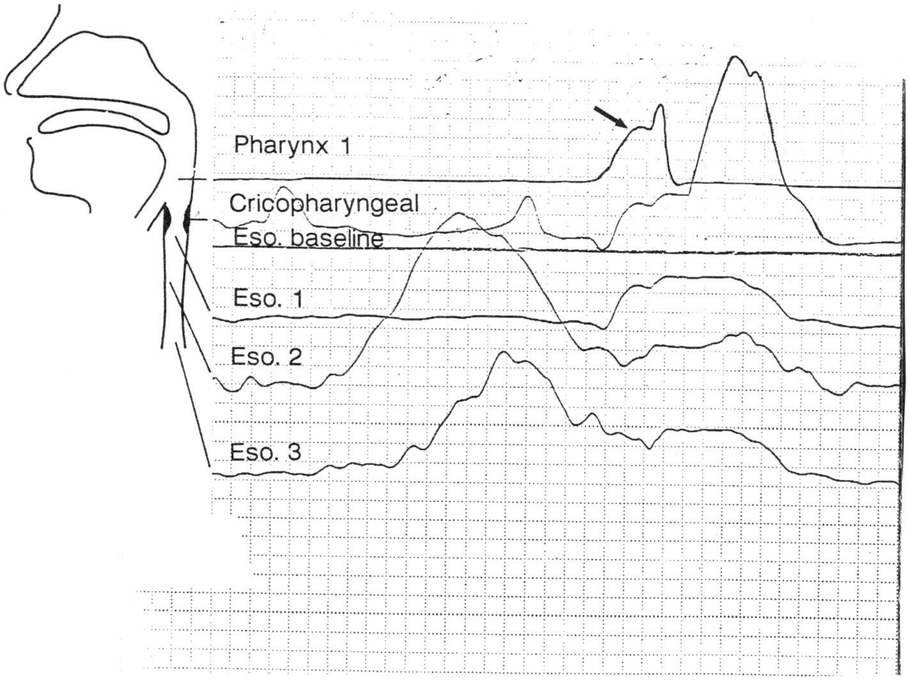

FIG. 23-46. Manometric record showing severe pharyngocricopharyngeal discoordination. Pharyngeal contraction with large shoulder pressure (*arrow*) occurs at the time of cricopharyngeal closure. There is incomplete relaxation of the cricopharyngeus. The upper esophageal port is located just below the cricopharyngeus and with movement during swallowing records cricopharyngeal closure. Lower esophageal ports show early contraction of the cervical esophagus, reducing its compliance to receive a bolus.

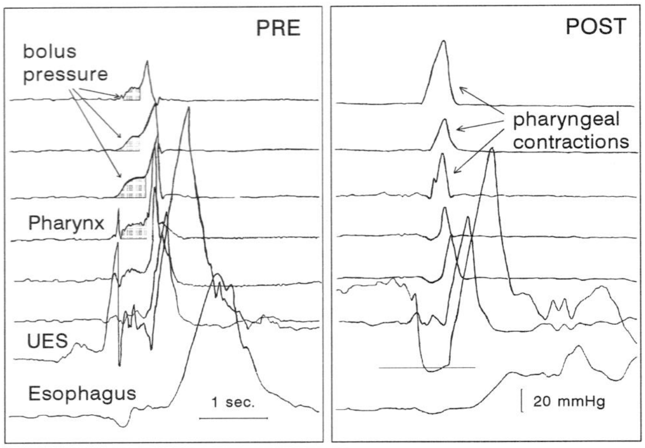

FIG. 23-47. Pharyngoesophageal manometric tracing in a patient with Zenker's diverticulum before and after diverticulectomy and myotomy. A nonrelaxing upper esophageal sphincter (UES) and a prominent bolus pressure are evident in the preoperative recording. Myotomy increased the compliance of the pharyngoesophageal segment, with complete disappearance of the bolus pressure in the pharyngeal contractions.

Under general anesthesia, placement of a nasogastric tube to the level of the manometrically determined cricopharyngeal sphincter helps in localization of the structures. The myotomy is extended cephalad by dividing 1 to 2 cm of inferior constrictor muscle of the pharynx and caudally by dividing the cricopharyngeal muscle and the cervical esophagus for a length of 4 to 5 cm. The cervical wound is then closed without drainage, and oral alimentation is started the following day. The patient is usually discharged on the first or second postoperative day.

If a diverticulum is present and is large enough to persist after a myotomy, it may be sutured in the inverted position to the prevertebral fascia using a permanent suture, i.e., diverticulopexy (Fig. 23-49). If the diverticulum is excessively large so that it would be redundant if suspended, or its walls are thickened, a diverticulectomy should be performed.

Postoperative complications consist of fistula formation, abscess, hematoma, recurrent nerve paralysis, difficulties in phonation, and Horner's syndrome. The incidence of the first two are reduced with myotomy and diverticulopexy. Recurrence of a Zenker's diverticulum occurs late, and is more common after diverticulectomy without myotomy, presumably due to persistence of the underlying loss of compliance of the cervical esophagus when a myotomy is not performed.

Postoperative motility studies have shown that the peak pharyngeal pressure generated on swallowing is not affected, the resting pressure is reduced but not eliminated and the cricopharyngeal sphincter is shortened. Consequently, after myotomy some protection against pharyngoesophageal regurgitation persists.

Motility Disorders of the Esophageal Body and Lower Esophageal Sphincter

Disorders of the esophageal phase of swallowing result from abnormalities in the propulsive pump action of the esophageal body or the relaxation of the lower esophageal sphincter. These disorders result from either primary esophageal abnormalities or from generalized neural, muscular, or collagen vascular disease (Table 23-10). With the introduction of standard esophageal manometry, specific primary esophageal motility disorders have been recognized, out of a pool of nonspecific motility abnormalities. These include achalasia, diffuse esophageal spasm, the so-called nutcracker esophagus, and the hypertensive lower esophageal sphincter. The manometric characteristics of these disorders are shown in Table 23-11.

The boundaries between the primary esophageal motor disorders are, however, vague, and intermediate types exist. This is because their diagnosis usually is based on the analysis of 10 wet swallows performed in a laboratory setting. The recently introduced technique of ambulatory 24-hour monitoring of esophageal motor activity allows the classification of esophageal motor disorders to be performed on the basis of more than 1000 contractions recorded during different physiologic states, i.e., normal daily activity, eating, and sleeping. Application of this technique has shown that there are significant differences in the classification of esophageal motor disorders when based on standard manometry or ambulatory monitoring (see Fig. 23-24). The degree of reclassification that occurs when analysis of esophageal motor function is done on the basis of ambulatory manometry indicates that the classic categories of esophageal motor disorders are inappropriate. These findings indicate that esophageal motility disorders should be looked at as a spectrum of abnormalities which reflects various stages of destruction of esophageal motor function.

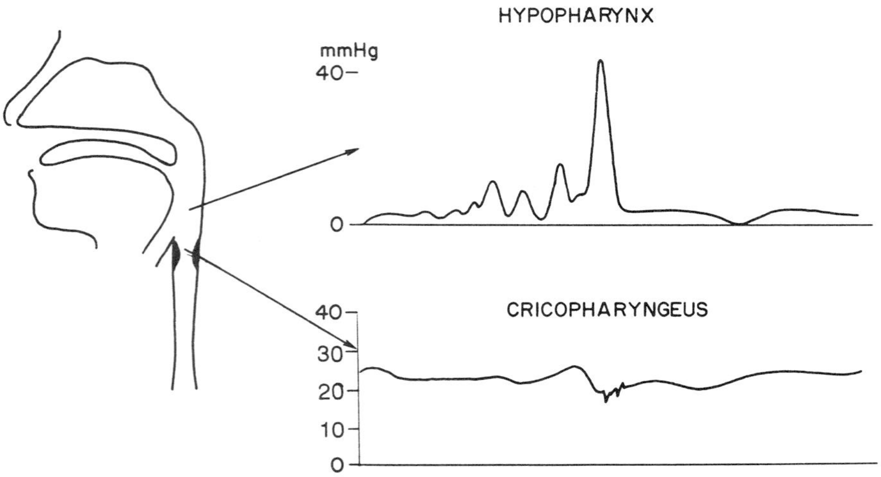

FIG. 23-48. Cross section of the neck at the level of the thyroid isthmus that shows the surgical approach to the hypopharynx and cervical esophagus. (From: *DeMeester TR, Stein HJ: Surgery for esophageal motor disorders, in Castell DO (ed): The Esophagus. Boston, Little, Brown & Company, 1992, p 418, with permission.*)

Table 23-10
Esophageal Motility Disorders

1. *Primary Esophageal Motility Disorders:*
   —Achalasia, "vigorous" achalasia
   —Diffuse and segmental esophageal spasm
   —Nutcracker esophagus
   —Hypertensive lower esophageal sphincter
   —Nonspecific esophageal motility disorders
2. *Secondary Esophageal Motility Disorders:*
   —Collagen vascular diseases: progressive systemic sclerosis, polymyositis and dermatomyositis, mixed connective tissue disease, systemic lupus erythematosus, et al.
   —Chronic idiopathic intestinal pseudoobstruction
   —Neuromuscular diseases
   —Endocrine and metastatic disorders

Achalasia

The best known and understood primary motility disorder of the esophagus is achalasia, with an incidence of 6 per 100,000 population per year. Although complete absence of peristalsis in the esophageal body has been proposed as the major abnormality, present evidence indicates achalasia is a primary disorder of the lower esophageal sphincter. This is based on 24-hour outpatient esophageal motility monitoring which shows that even in advanced disease up to 5 percent of contractions can be peristaltic. Abnormal esophageal peristalsis develops as a result of the increased resistance provided by the nonrelaxing lower esophageal sphincter. This is supported by experimental studies in which a Gore-Tex band loosely placed around the gastroesophageal junction in cats did not change sphincter pressures, but resulted in impaired relaxation of the lower esophageal sphincter and led to a markedly increased frequency of simultaneous contractions and a decrease of contraction amplitude in the esophageal body. This was associated with radiographic dilatation of the esophagus and was reversible after removal of the band. Clinical observations in patients with pseudoachalasia due to tumor infiltration, a tight stricture in the distal esophagus, or an antireflux procedure that is too tight also indicate that dysfunction of the esophageal body can be caused by the increased outflow obstruction of a nonrelaxing lower esophageal sphincter. The observation that esophageal peristalsis can return in patients with classic achalasia following dilatation or myotomy provides further support for a primary disease of the lower esophageal sphincter.

Table 23-11
Manometric Characteristics of the Primary Esophageal Motility Disorders

Achalasia:
—Incomplete lower esophageal sphincter (LES) relaxation ($< 75\%$ relaxation)
—Aperistalsis in the esophageal body
—Elevated LES pressure ≥ 26 mmHg
—Increased intraesophageal baseline pressures relative to gastric baseline
Diffuse Esophageal Spasm (DES):
—Simultaneous (nonperistaltic contractions) ($> 10\%$ of wet swallows)
—Repetitive and multipeaked contractions
—Spontaneous contractions
—Intermittent normal peristalsis
—Contractions may be of increased amplitude and duration
Nutcracker Esophagus:
—Mean peristaltic amplitude (10 wet swallows) in distal esophagus ≥ 180 mmHg
—Increased mean duration of contractions (> 7.0 seconds)
—Normal peristaltic sequence
Hypertensive Lower Esophageal Sphincter:
—Elevated LES pressure (≥ 26 mmHg)
—Normal LES relaxation
—Normal peristalsis in the esophageal body
Nonspecific Esophageal Motility Disorders:
—Decreased or absent amplitude of esophageal peristalsis
—Increased number of nontransmitted contractions
—Abnormal wave forms
—Normal mean LES pressure and relaxation

LES = lower esophageal sphincter

SOURCE: DeMeester TR, Stein HJ, Fuchs KH: Physiologic diagnostic studies, in Zuidema GD, Orringer MB (eds): *Shackelford's Surgery of the Alimentary Tract,* 3rd ed, Vol I. Philadelphia, Saunders, 1991, p 115, with permission.

The pathogenesis of achalasia is presumed to be a neurogenic degeneration, which is either idiopathic or due to infection. In experimental animals, the disease has been reproduced by destruction of the nucleus ambiguus and the dorsal motor nucleus of the vagus nerve. In patients with the disease, degenerative changes have been shown in the vagus nerve and in the ganglia in the Auerbach plexus of the esophagus itself. This degeneration results in hypertension of the lower esophageal sphincter, a failure of the sphincter to relax on deglutition, elevation of intraluminal esophageal pressure, and a subsequent loss of progressive peristalsis in the body of the esophagus. The combination of a nonrelaxing

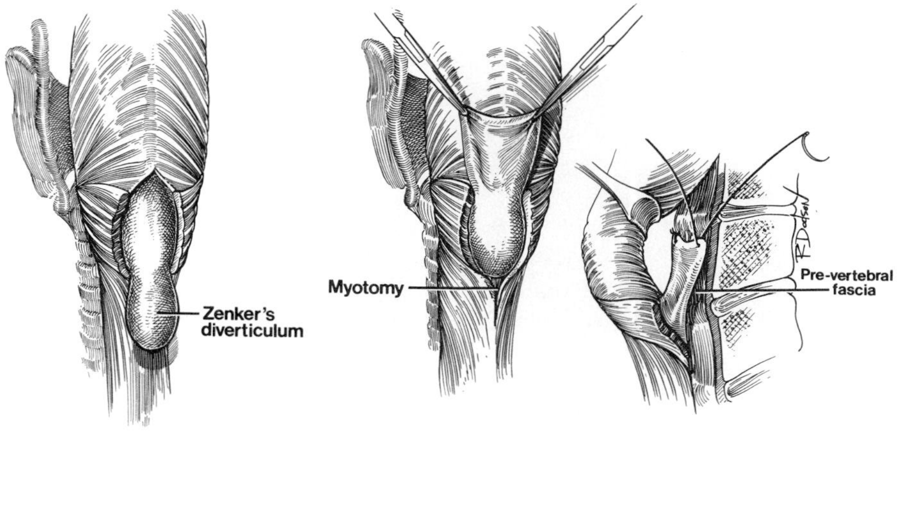

FIG. 23-49. Posterior of the anatomy of the pharynx and cervical esophagus showing pharyngoesophageal myotomy and pexing of the diverticulum to the prevertebral fascia.

sphincter, which causes a functional holdup of ingested material in the esophagus, and elevation of intraluminal pressure from repetitive pharyngeal air swallowing results in dilatation of the esophageal body. With time, the functional disorder results in anatomic alterations seen on radiographic studies as a dilated esophagus with a tapering, beaklike narrowing of the distal end (Fig. 23-50). There is usually an air-fluid level in the esophagus that reflects the degree of resistance imposed by the nonrelaxing sphincter. As the disease progresses, the esophagus becomes massively dilated and tortuous.

A subgroup of patients with otherwise typical features of classic achalasia have simultaneous contractions of their esophageal body which can be of high amplitude. This manometric pattern has been termed ''vigorous achalasia,'' and chest pain episodes are a common finding in these patients. Differentiation of vigorous achalasia from diffuse esophageal spasm can be difficult. In both diseases videoradiographic exam can show a corkscrew deformity of the esophagus and diverticulum formation.

Diffuse and Segmental Esophageal Spasm

This esophageal motor disorder is characterized clinically by substernal chest pain and/or dysphagia. Diffuse esophageal spasm differs from classic achalasia in that it is primarily a disease of the esophageal body, produces a lesser degree of dysphagia, causes more chest pain, and has less effect on the patient's general condition. True symptomatic diffuse esophageal spasm is a rare condition, occurring about five times less frequently than achalasia.

The causation and neuromuscular pathophysiology of diffuse esophageal spasm are unclear. The basic motor abnormality is

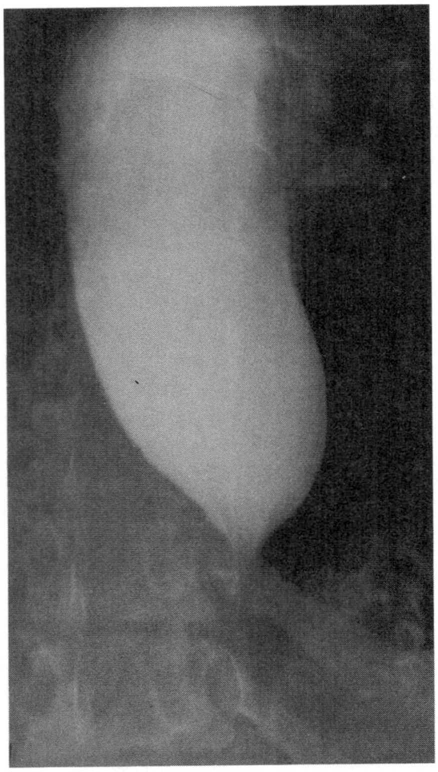

FIG. 23-50. Barium esophagogram showing a markedly dilated esophagus and characteristic "bird's beak" in achalasia. (From: *Waters PF, DeMeester TR: Med Clin North Am 65:1244, 1981, with permission.*)

rapid progression of contractions down the esophagus secondary to an abnormality in the latency gradient. Hypertrophy of the muscular layer of the esophageal wall and degeneration of the esophageal branches of the vagus nerve have been observed in this disease, although these are not constant findings. Manometric abnormalities in diffuse esophageal spasm may be present over the total length of the esophageal body, but are usually confined to the distal two-thirds. In segmental esophageal spasm the manometric abnormalities are confined to a short segment of the esophagus.

The classic manometric finding in these patients is characterized by the frequent occurrence of simultaneous and repetitive esophageal contractions which may be of abnormally high amplitude or long duration. Key to the diagnosis of diffuse esophageal spasm is that the esophagus retains a degree of peristaltic performance in excess of that seen in achalasia. A criterion of 20 percent or more simultaneous contractions in 10 wet swallows has been used to diagnose diffuse esophageal spasm. This figure is, however, arbitrary and often debated. Discriminate analysis has identified a series of abnormalities on the ambulatory motility record of patients with classic diffuse esophageal spasm. A composite score based on these parameters of the ambulatory motility record has allowed diagnosis of the disease with a sensitivity of 90 percent and a specificity of 100 percent. When applied prospectively this scoring system identified severely deteriorated esophageal motor function in symptomatic patients despite the absence of the classic motility abnormalities of diffuse spasm on standard manometry.

The lower esophageal sphincter in patients with the disease usually shows normal resting pressure and relaxation on deglutition. A hypertensive sphincter with poor relaxation may also be present. In patients with advanced disease the radiographic appearance of tertiary contractions appears helical and has been termed *corkscrew esophagus* or *pseudodiverticulosis* (Fig. 23-51). Patients with segmental or diffuse esophageal spasm can compartmentalize the esophagus and develop an epiphrenic or midesophageal diverticulum (Fig. 23-52).

Nutcracker Esophagus

The disorder termed *nutcracker* or *supersqueezer esophagus* was recognized in the late 1970s. Other terms used to describe this entity are ''hypertensive peristalsis'' or ''high-amplitude peristaltic contractions.'' It is the most frequent of the primary esophageal motility disorders. By definition the so-called nutcracker esophagus is a manometric abnormality in patients with chest pain characterized by peristaltic esophageal contractions with peak amplitudes greater than 2 standard deviations above the normal values in individual laboratories. Contraction amplitudes in these patients can easily be above 400 mmHg. Ambulatory 24-hour monitoring of esophageal motor function in patients classified as ''nutcracker esophagus'' has identified a subgroup of patients with a motor pattern characteristic of diffuse esophageal spasm. These patients usually complain of dysphagia in addition to chest pain and probably are misclassified by standard manometry. The identification of these patients is important, since esophageal myotomy is a therapeutic option for patients with dysphagia and diffuse esophageal spasm but is of questionable value in patients with chest pain thought secondary to nutcracker esophagus.

Hypertensive Lower Esophageal Sphincter

This abnormality was first described as a separate entity by Code et al. in patients with chest pain or dysphagia. This disorder

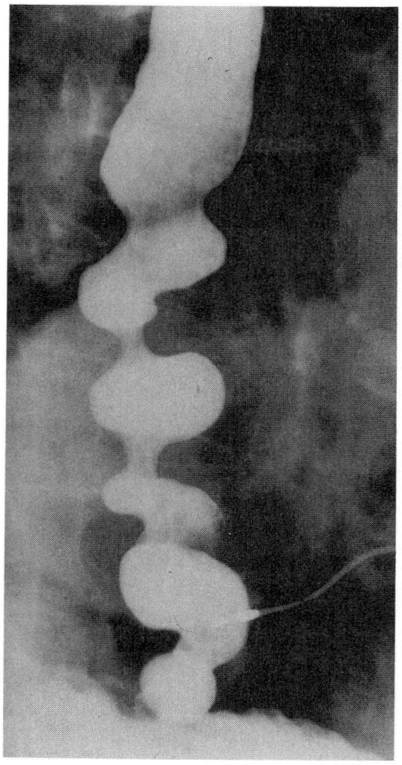

FIG. 23-51. Barium esophagogram of patient with diffuse spasm showing the "corkscrew" deformity.

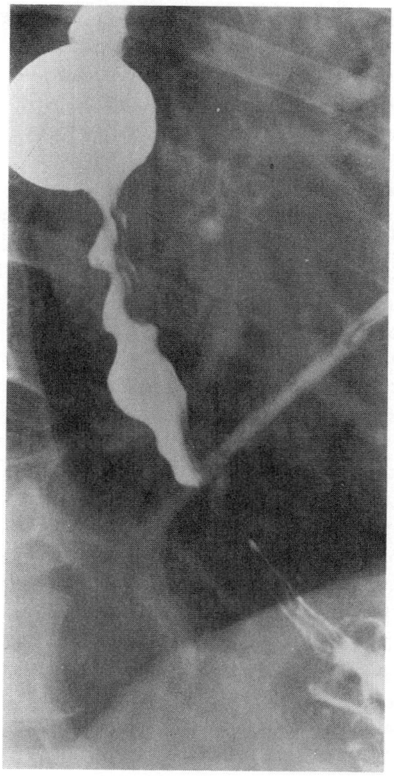

FIG. 23-52. Barium esophagogram showing a high epiphrenic diverticulum in a patient with diffuse esophageal spasm. (From: *DeMeester TR, Stein HJ: Surgery for esophageal motor disorders, in Castell DO (ed): The Esophagus. Boston, Little, Brown & Company, 1992, p 415, with permission.*)

is characterized by an elevated basal pressure of the lower esophageal sphincter with normal relaxation and normal propulsion in the esophageal body. About half of these patients, however, have associated motility disorders of the esophageal body, particularly hypertensive peristalsis and simultaneous contractions. In the remainder, the disorder exists as an isolated abnormality. Dysphagia in these patients may be caused by a lack of compliance of the sphincter even in its relaxed state. Myotomy of the lower esophageal sphincter may be indicated in patients not responding to medical therapy or dilatation.

Nonspecific Esophageal Motor Disorders

Many patients complaining of dysphagia or chest pain of noncardiac origin demonstrate a variety of contraction patterns on esophageal manometry that are clearly out of the normal range but do not meet the criteria of a primary esophageal motility disorder. Esophageal manometry in these patients frequently shows an increased number of multipeaked or repetitive contractions, contractions of prolonged duration, nontransmitted contractions, an interruption of a peristaltic sequence at various levels of the esophagus, or contractions of low amplitude. These motility abnormalities have been termed *nonspecific esophageal motility disorders*. The significance of these abnormal contractions in the causation of chest pain or dysphagia is still unclear. Surgery plays no role in the treatment of these disorders unless there is an associated diverticulum.

A clear distinction between primary esophageal motility disorders and nonspecific esophageal motility disorders is often not possible. Patients diagnosed as having nonspecific esophageal motility abnormalities on repeated studies will occasionally show abnormalities consistent with nutcracker esophagus. Similarly, progression from a nonspecific esophageal motility disorder to classic diffuse esophageal spasm has been demonstrated. The finding of a nonspecific esophageal motility disorder, therefore, may represent only a manometric marker of an intermittent more severe esophageal motor abnormality. Furthermore, combined ambulatory 24-hour esophageal pH and motility monitoring has shown that an increased esophageal exposure to gastric juice is common in patients diagnosed as having a nonspecific esophageal motility disorder. In some situations the motor abnormalities may be induced by the irritation of refluxed gastric juice; in other situations it may be a primary event unrelated to the presence of reflux.

Diverticula of the Esophageal Body

Radiographic abnormalities such as segmental spasm, corkscrewing, compartmentalization, and diverticulum are the anatomic results of disordered motility function. Of these the most persistent and easiest to demonstrate is an esophageal diverticulum. Diverticula most commonly occur with nonspecific motility disorders but can occur with all of the primary motility disorders. In the latter situation the motility disorder is usually diagnosed prior to the development of the diverticulum. When present, a diverticulum may temporarily alleviate the symptom of dysphagia by becoming a receptacle for the food, and replace it with postprandial symptoms of pain and regurgitation of undigested food. If an abnormality of the function of the esophageal body or lower esophageal sphincter cannot be identified manometrically, a traction or congenital cause for the diverticulum should be considered. Historically, since radiographic studies preceded manometric studies, diverticula of the esophagus were considered to be the primary abnormality rather than the consequence of motility disorders. Consequently earlier texts focused on them as specific entities based upon their location.

Epiphrenic diverticula arise from the terminal third of the thoracic esophagus and are usually found adjacent to the diaphragm (see Fig. 23-52). They have been associated with distal esophageal muscular hypertrophy, esophageal motility abnormalities, and increased luminal pressure. They are classicially ''pulsion'' diverticula, and have been associated with diffuse spasm, achalasia, or nonspecific motor abnormalities in the body of the esophagus.

Whether the diverticulum should be surgically resected or suspended depends upon its size and proximity to the vertebral body. When diverticula are associated with esophageal motility disorders, esophageal myotomy from the distal extent of the diverticulum to the stomach is indicated; otherwise one can expect a high incidence of suture line rupture due to the same intraluminal pressure that gave rise to the diverticulum initially. If the diverticulum is suspended to the prevertebral fascia of the thoracic vertebra, a myotomy is begun at the neck of the diverticulum and extended across the lower esophageal sphincter. If the diverticulum is excised by dividing the neck, the muscle is closed over the excision site and a myotomy is performed on the opposite esophageal wall, starting at the level of diverticulum. When a large diverticulum is associated with a hiatal hernia, the diverticulum is excised, a myotomy is performed if there is an associated esophageal motility abnormality, and the hernia is repaired because of the high incidence of postoperative reflux when it is omitted.

Midesophageal or traction diverticula were first described in the nineteenth century (Fig. 23-53). At that time they were frequently noted in patients who had mediastinal lymph node involvement with tuberculosis. It was theorized that adhesions form between the inflamed mediastinal nodes and the esophagus. By contraction, the adhesions exerted ''traction'' on the esophageal wall and led to a localized diverticulum (Fig. 23-54). This theory was based on the findings of early dissections, where adhesions between diverticula and lymph nodes were commonly found. It is now believed that some diverticula in the midesophagus may also be caused by motility abnormalities.

Most midesophageal diverticula are asymptomatic and incidentally discovered during investigation for nonesophageal complaints. In such patients, the radiologic abnormality may be ignored. Patients with symptoms of dysphagia, regurgitation, chest pain, or aspiration in whom a diverticulum is discovered should be thoroughly investigated for an esophageal motor abnormality and treated appropriately. An occasional patient will present with a bronchoesophageal fistula manifested by a chronic cough on ingestion of meals. Such patients are most likely to have an inflammatory etiology.

The indication for surgical intervention is the degree of their symptomatic disability. Usually midesophageal diverticula can be suspended due to their proximity to the spine. If motor abnormality is documented, a myotomy should be performed similar to that described for an epiphrenic diverticulum.

Operations

Long Esophageal Myotomy for Motor Disorders of the Esophageal Body. A long esophageal myotomy is indicated for dysphagia caused by any motor disorder characterized by

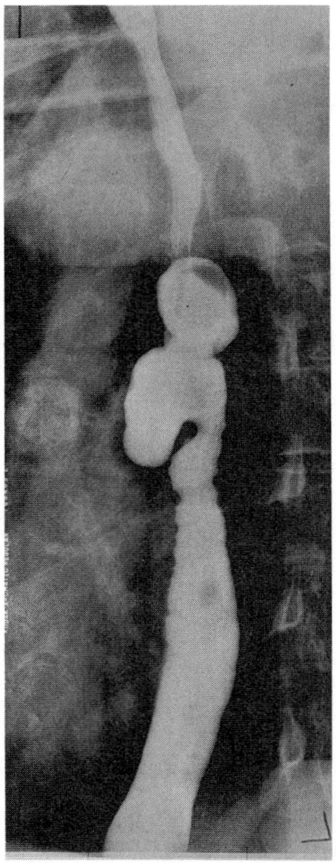

FIG. 23-53. Barium esophagogram showing a midesophageal diverticulum. Despite the anatomic distortion, the patient was asymptomatic. (From: *Waters PF, DeMeester TR: Med Clin North Am 65:1255, 1981, with permission.*)

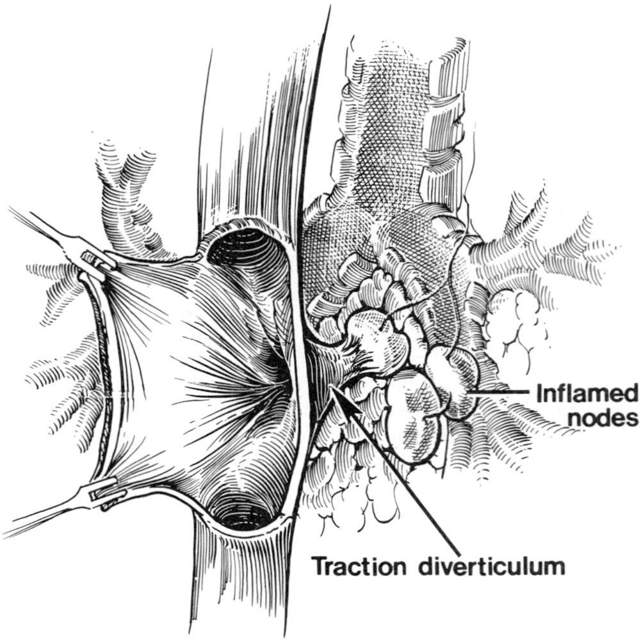

FIG. 23-54. Illustration of the pathophysiology of midesophageal diverticulum showing traction on the esophageal wall from adhesions to inflamed subcarinal lymph nodes.

segmental or generalized simultaneous contractions in a patient whose symptoms are not relieved by medical therapy. Such disorders include diffuse and segmental esophageal spasm, vigorous achalasia, and nonspecific motility disorders associated with a mid or epiphrenic esophageal diverticulum. The recent introduction of 24-hour ambulatory motility monitoring has greatly aided in the identification of patients with symptoms of dysphagia and chest pain who might benefit from a surgical myotomy.

The decision to operate rests on a balance of the patient's symptoms, diet, life-style adjustments, and nutritional status, with the driving force being the opportunity to improve patient's swallowing disability. The symptom of chest pain alone is not an indication for a surgical procedure.

In patients selected for myotomy of the esophageal body, preoperative manometry is essential to determine the proximal extent. Most surgeons extended the myotomy distally across the lower esophageal sphincter to reduce outflow resistance. Consequently, some form of antireflux protection is needed to avoid gastroesophageal reflux if there has been extensive dissection of the cardia. In this situation most authors prefer a partial fundoplication in order not to add resistance that will further interfere with the ability of the myotomized esophagus to empty. If the symptoms of reflux are present preoperatively, 24-hour pH monitoring is required to confirm its presence.

The procedure is performed through a left thoracotomy in the sixth intercostal space (Fig. 23-55). An incision is made in the posterior mediastinal pleura over the esophagus, and the left lateral wall of the esophagus is exposed. The esophagus is not circumferentially dissected unless necessary. A 2-cm incision is made into the abdomen through the parietal peritoneum at the midportion of the left crus. A flap of gastric fundus is pulled into the chest. This exposes the gastroesophageal junction and its associated fat pad. The latter is excised to give a clear view of the junction. A myotomy is performed through all muscle layers, extending distally over the stomach 1 to 2 cm below the gastroesophageal junction and proximally on the esophagus over the distance of the manometric abnormality. The muscle layer is dissected from the mucosa laterally for a distance of 1 cm. Care is taken to divide all minute muscle bands, particularly in the area of the junction. The gastric fundic flap is sutured to the margins of the myotomy over the distal 4 cm and replaced into the abdomen. This maintains separation of the muscle and acts as a partial fundoplication to prevent reflux.

If an epiphrenic diverticulum is present it is excised by dividing the neck and closing the muscle. The myotomy is then performed on the opposite esophageal wall. If a midesophageal diverticulum is present, the myotomy is made so that it includes the muscle around the neck, and the diverticulum is inverted and suspended by attaching it to the paravertebral fascia of the thoracic vertebra.

The results of myotomy for motor disorders of the esophageal body have improved in parallel with the improved preoperative diagnosis afforded by manometry. Previous published series report between 40 and 92 percent symptomatic improvement, but interpretation is difficult due to the small number of patients involved and the varying criteria for diagnosis of the primary motor abnormality. When myotomy is accurately done, 93 percent of the patients had effective palliation of dysphagia after a mean follow-up of 5 years, and 89 percent would have the procedure again if it was necessary. Most patients gain or maintain their weight after the operation. Postoperative motility studies show that myotomy reduces the amplitude of esophageal contractions to near zero, eliminating both simultaneous and peristaltic waves. The dysphagia of the patient, therefore, is likely to be improved by the procedure only if the benefit of reducing the prevalence of simultaneous waves, and as a consequence their adverse effect on bolus propulsion, exceeds the adverse effect on bolus propulsion caused by the loss of peristaltic wave amplitude. If not, the patient is likely to continue to complain of dysphagia and to have little improvement from the operation. Thus, a delicate balance exists between success and failure of a long esophageal myotomy and emphasizes the importance of preoperative motility studies.

Myotomy of the Lower Esophageal Sphincter. Secondary to reflux disease, achalasia is the most common functional disorder of the esophagus to require surgical intervention. Relief of the functional obstruction of a nonrelaxing sphincter can be achieved by an uncontrolled instrumental rupture of the sphincter muscle or by a controlled surgical myotomy. Pneumatic dilation has been suggested as adequate treatment but only relieves dysphagia and pharyngeal regurgitation in 70 percent of patients. It becomes clear that patients, when questioned carefully, tend to overemphasize the benefit they receive from pneumatic dilation, and are slow to accept failure of the procedure. Consequently, adequate treatment with a surgical myotomy is delayed, leading to progressive esophageal dilatation and the resulting tortuosity. Whether to treat newly diagnosed esophageal achalasia by forceful dilation or by operative cardiomyotomy remains controversial. Both large retrospective reviews and prospective randomized studies comparing the two modes of therapy indicate that surgical myotomy is associated with low morbidity and gives better long-term results (Table 23-12). Consequently, the data support surgical myotomy as the procedure of choice; however, in practice most patients are dilated. An inherent risk of pneumatic dilation is rupture of the esophagus. This is reported to occur in 2 percent of patients, but in carefully monitored studies can be as high as 15 percent. Although it has been reported that a myotomy after previous balloon dilation is more difficult, this has not been a universal experience unless the cardia has been ruptured. In this situation, operative intervention either immediately or after healing has occurred can be difficult.

In performing a surgical myotomy of the lower esophageal sphincter, there are four important principles: (1) minimal dissection of the cardia, (2) adequate distal myotomy to reduce outflow resistance, (3) prevention of postoperative reflux, and (4) preventing rehealing of the myotomy site. The use of a partial fundoplication after a myotomy to prevent reflux has been debated, but when the experience is tallied regarding the postoperative symptoms of reflux, it supports the addition of the antireflux procedure. The development of a reflux-induced stricture due to the loss of competency after a myotomy is a serious problem that usually necessitates esophagectomy for relief and further encourages the need for reflux protection.

A modified Heller myotomy is performed through a left thoracotomy in the sixth intercostal space along the upper border of the seventh rib. The esophagus is exposed as described for a long myotomy. A myotomy through all muscle layers is performed, extending distally over the stomach to 1 to 2 cm below the junction and proximally on the esophagus for 4 to 5 cm. The cardia is reconstructed by suturing the gastric fundic flap to the margins of the myotomy to prevent rehealing of the mytomy site and to provide reflux protection in the area of the divided sphincter. If an extensive dissection of the cardia has been done, a more formal Belsey repair is performed. The gastric fundic flap is allowed to

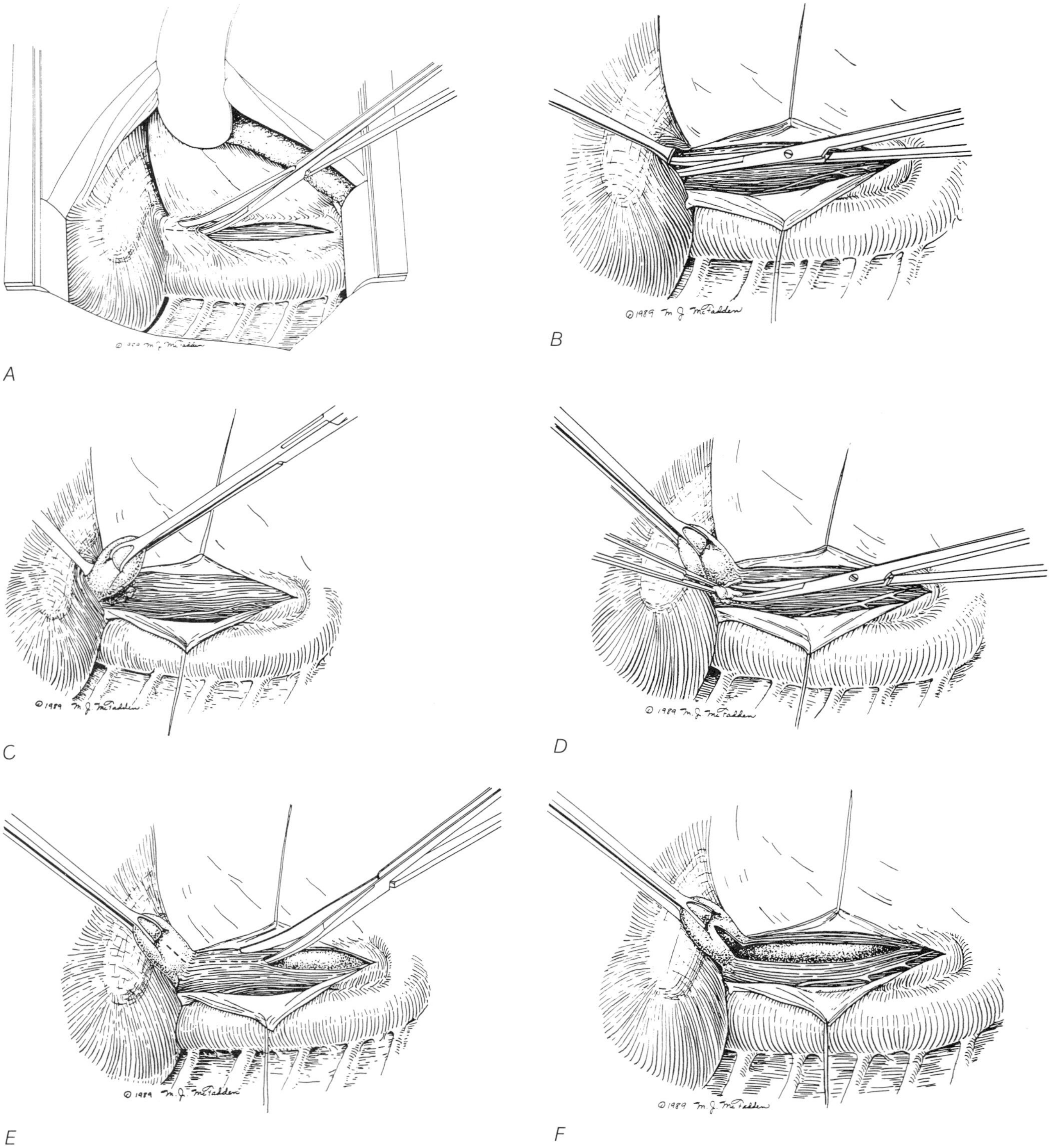

FIG. 23-55. Technique of long myotomy: *A.* Exposure of the lower esophagus through the left sixth intercostal space and incision of the mediastinal pleura in preparation for surgical myotomy. *B.* Location of a 2-cm incision made through the phrenoesophageal membrane into the abdomen along the midlateral border of the left crus. *C.* Retraction of tongue of gastric fundus into the chest through the previously made incision. *D.* Removal of the gastroesophageal fat pad to expose the gastroesophageal junction. *E.* A myotomy down to the mucosa is started on the esophageal body. *F.* Completed myotomy extending over the stomach for 1 cm. *G.* Reconstruction of the cardia after a myotomy, illustrating the position of the sutures used to stitch the gastric fundic flap to the margins of the myotomy. *H.* Reconstruction of the cardia after a myotomy, illustrating the intraabdominal position of the gastric tongue covering the distal 4 cm of the myotomy.

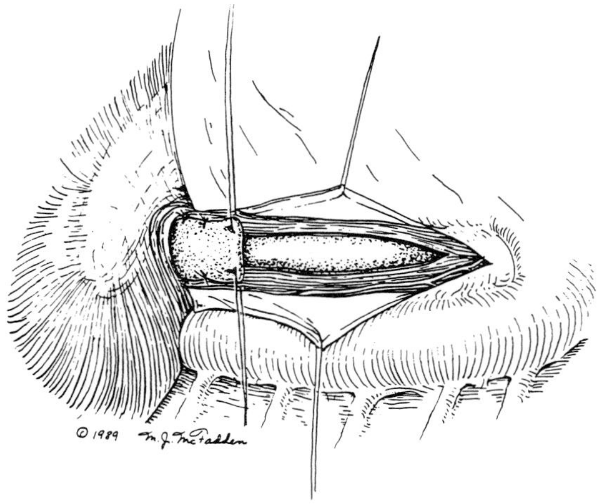

G

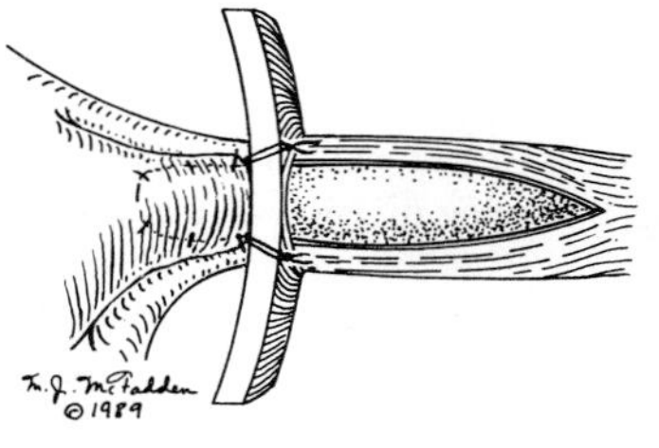

H

FIG. 23-55. *(continued)*

retract into the abdomen. Postoperatively, nasogastric drainage is maintained for 6 days to prevent distention of the stomach during healing. An oral diet is resumed on the seventh day, after a barium swallow study shows unobstructed passage of the bolus into the stomach without extravasation.

Csendes et al. (1981) reported the long-term follow-up of 81 patients randomized between forceful dilation and surgical myotomy for achalasia. They showed that myotomy was associated with a significant increase in the diameter at the gastroesophageal junction and a decrease at the middle third of the esophagus on follow-up radiographic studies. Further there was a greater reduction in sphincter pressure and improvement in the amplitude of esophageal contractions following myotomy. Thirteen percent of patients regained peristalsis after dilation compared with 28 percent after surgery. These findings were shown to persist over 5 years of follow-up, at which time 95 percent of those treated with surgical myotomy were doing well. Of those who received dilation, only 54 percent were doing well, while 16 percent required redilation and 22 percent eventually required surgical myotomy to obtain relief.

If simultaneous esophageal contractions are associated with the sphincter abnormality, the so-called vigorous achalasia, then the myotomy should extend over the distance of the motility abnormality as mapped by the preoperative motility study. Failure to do this will result in continuing dysphagia and a dissatisfied patient. The best objective evaluation of improvement in the patient following either balloon dilation or myotomy is a scintigraphic measurement of esophageal emptying time. A good therapeutic response improves esophageal emptying toward normal. Some degree of dysphagia may, however, persist despite improved esophageal emptying due to disturbances in esophageal body function. Recent studies have shown that when an antireflux procedure is added to the myotomy it should be a partial fundoplication. A 360° fundoplication is associated with progressive retention of swallowed food, regurgitation and aspiration to a degree that exceeds the patient's preoperative symptoms.

Endosurgical Esophageal Myotomy. It has been shown that video-assisted endosurgical myotomy can be accomplished safely either laparoscopically or thoracoscopically. A thoracic

Table 23-12
Recent Series with > 100 Patients Giving Follow-up Results of Myotomy or Balloon Dilation for Achalasia

Author	*Year*	*No. of patients*	*Mortality*	*Follow-up years*	*Response good-excellent*
		SURGICAL MYOTOMY			
Black, et al	1976	108	0	4	65%
Menzies Gow	1978	102	0	8	98%
Okike, et al	1979	456	1	1–17	85%
Ellis, et al	1984	113	0	3.5	91%
Csendes, et al	1988	100	0	6.8	92%
		BALLOON DILATION			
Sanderson, et al	1970	408			81%
Vantrappen, et al	1979	403	17	7.8	76%
Okike, et al	1979	431	2	1–18	65%

SOURCE: DeMeester TR, Stein HJ: Surgery for esophageal motor disorders, in Castell DO (ed): *The Esophagus*. Boston, Little, Brown & Company, 1992, p 424, with permission.

approach is preferable as it entails minimal dissection of the esophageal hiatus and thereby is less disruptive to antireflux mechanisms.

The procedure is performed with the patient in the left lateral decubitus position. A double-lumen endotracheal tube is used to allow selective ventilation of the right lung. A four-port technique is employed in addition to a small (1-inch) incision along the left costal margin for placement of retracting instruments. With selective ventilation of the right lung, it is not necessary to insufflate the left hemithorax. Angled-viewing laparoscopes/thoracoscopes are preferable to the zero-degree scopes. Occasionally a fifth port may be necessary to retract the lung following division of the inferior pulmonary ligament.

Identification and dissection of the esophagus are aided by the concomitant use of an endoscope within the esophageal lumen. The mediastinal pleura overlying the terminal esophagus is divided sharply with scissors. The myotomy is performed with a hook-type electrocautery probe (Fig. 23-56). Having an endoscope within the esophagus helps prevent mucosal injury. Once the esophageal mucosa is clearly identified, the myotomy is carried distally with either the electrocautery probe or scissors. The inferior extent of the myotomy is judged utilizing the endoscope. The myotomy is ended when it has reached the endoscopic gastroesophageal junction, and the spasm of the valve commonly associated with achalasia is alleviated.

The laparoscopic approach is similar to the Nissen fundoplication in terms of the trocar placement, exposure and dissection of the esophageal hiatus. Once the esophagus is mobilized, the myotomy is performed in a fashion analogous to the thoracoscopic approach.

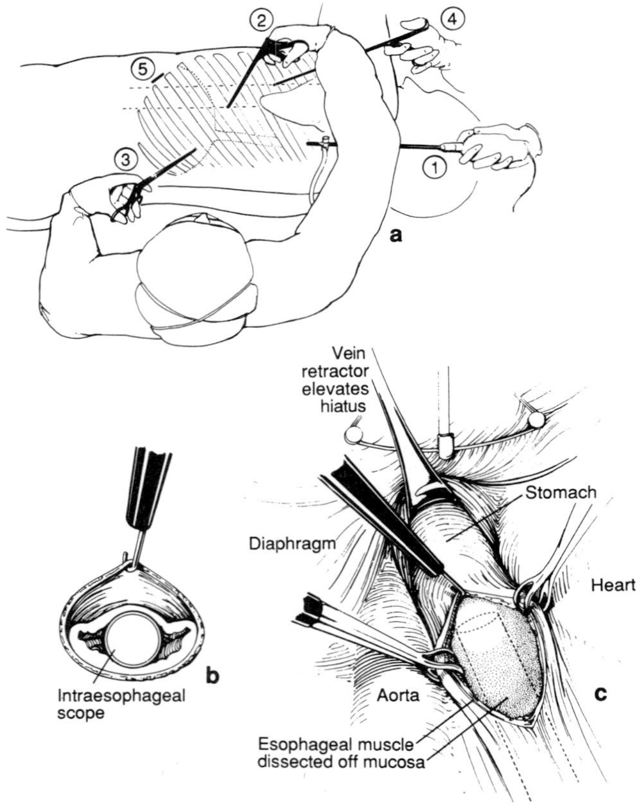

FIG. 23-56. Thoracoscopic esophageal myotomy illustrating the exposure obtained with video-assisted technology. This allows the traditional myotomy of the esophageal lower sphincter or body to be done without a thoracotomy.

Esophageal Resection for End-Stage Motor Disorders of the Esophagus. Patients with dysphagia and long-standing benign disease, whose esophageal function has been destroyed by the disease process or multiple previous surgical procedures, are best managed by esophagectomy. Fibrosis of the esophagus and cardia can result in weak contractions and failure of the distal esophageal sphincter to relax. Another sign of fibrosis is the loss of the secondary peristaltic reflex, which propels into the stomach a bolus of food that has failed to reach that destination with the primary peristaltic wave. The presence of these abnormalities signals end-stage motor disease. In these situations esophageal replacement is usually required to establish normal alimentation.

Before proceeding with esophageal resection for patients with end-stage benign disease, the choice of the organ to substitute for the esophagus, i.e., stomach, jejunum, or colon, should be considered. The choice of replacement is affected by a number of factors, as described later in the section on techniques of esophageal reconstruction.

CARCINOMA OF THE ESOPHAGUS

Squamous carcinoma accounts for the majority of esophageal carcinomas. Its incidence is highly variable, ranging from approximately 20 per 100,000 in the United States and Britain to 160 per 100,000 in certain parts of South Africa and the Honan province of China, and even 540 per 100,000 in the Guriev district of Kazakhstan. The environmental factors responsible for these sharply localized high incidences have not been conclusively identified, though additives to local foodstuffs (nitroso compounds in pickled vegetables and smoked meats) and deficiencies (zinc and molybdenum) have been suggested. In Western societies, smoking and alcohol consumption are strongly linked with squamous carcinoma. Other definite associations link squamous carcinoma with long-standing achalasia, lye strictures, tylosis (an autosomal dominant disorder characterized by hyperkeratosis of the palms and soles), and human papilloma virus.

Adenocarcinoma of the esophagus, once an unusual malignancy, is diagnosed with increasing frequency (Fig. 23-57) and now accounts for over 40 percent of esophageal cancer in some Western countries. The gross appearance resembles that of squamous cell carcinoma. Microscopically, when it originates in metaplastic mucosa, it resembles gastric cancer. When it arises in the submucosal glands, it forms intramural growths which resemble the mucoepidermal and adenoid cystic carcinomas of the salivary glands. The most important etiologic factor in the development of primary adenocarcinoma of the esophagus is a metaplastic columnar-lined or Barrett's esophagus, which occurs as a complication in approximately 10 percent of patients with gastroesophageal reflux disease. The incidence of adenocarcinoma in a patient with Barrett's esophagus has been estimated between 1/56 to 1/441 patient years. Although this risk appears to be small, it is at least thirty to forty times that expected for a similar population without Barrett's esophagus. This risk is similar to the risk for developing cancer of the lung in a person with a 20 pack-year history of smoking. Endoscopic surveillance for patients with Barrett's esophagus is recommended for two reasons: (1) at present there is no reliable evidence that medical therapy or an antireflux procedure removes

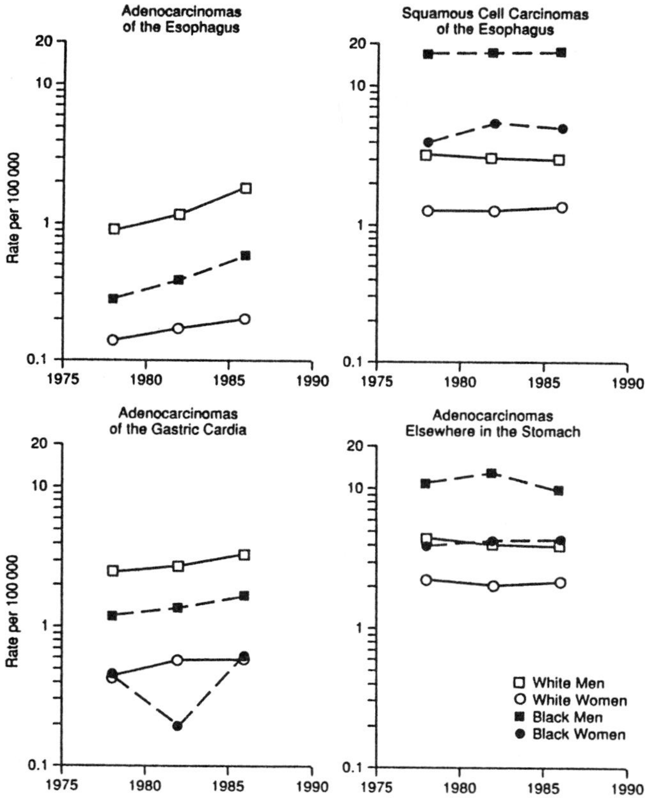

FIG. 23-57. Trends in age-adjusted incidence rates of esophageal and stomach cancers by histology and anatomic site, sex and race showing a rise in the incidence of both adenocarcinoma of the esophagus and gastric cardia, suggesting that factors responsible for the development of these concerns may be similar. (From: *Blot WJ, Devesa SS, et al: JAMA 265:1288, 1991, with permission.*)

the risk of neoplastic transformation; and (2) malignancy in Barrett's esophagus is curable if detected at an early stage.

Clinical Manifestations. Esophageal cancer is a disease affecting patients of advancing age, with dysphagia and weight loss being by far the most common symptoms at the time of diagnosis. In a few patients, dysphagia does not occur and symptoms arise from invasion of the primary tumor into adjacent structures or from metastases. Extension of the primary tumor into the tracheobronchial tree can cause stridor, and if a tracheoesophageal fistula develops, coughing, choking, and aspiration pneumonia result. Severe bleeding from erosion into the aorta or pulmonary vessels occurs on rare occasion. Vocal cord paralysis may result from the invasion of either recurrent laryngeal nerve. Metastases are usually manifested by jaundice or bone pain. The situation is different in high-incidence areas where screening is practiced. In these communities, the most prominent early symptom is pain on swallowing rough or dry food.

Dysphagia usually presents late in the natural history of the disease because the lack of a serosal layer to the esophagus allows the smooth muscle to dilate with ease. As a result, the dysphagia becomes severe enough to motivate the patient to seek medical advice only when more than 60 percent of the esophageal circumference is infiltrated with cancer. Thus, the disease is usually far advanced at the time of diagnosis. Tracheoesophageal fistula may be present in some patients on their first visit to the hospital, and more than 40 percent will have evidence of distant metastases. With tumors of the cardia, anorexia and weight loss usually precede the onset of dysphagia. The physical signs of esophageal tumors are those of distant metastases, as discussed earlier.

Staging. The stage of the disease is determined by the depth of penetration of the primary tumor (Fig. 23-58) and the presence of lymph node and distant organ metastasis. Classification of these factors for tumors in the thoracic esophagus usually is not clinically possible and currently is based on imaging techniques (Table 23-13 *A* and *B*). CT scans are of little value in the staging of early tumors of the thoracic esophagus or cardia, and generally only confirm clinical findings when extensive disease is present. Their use in the evaluation of tumors of the cervical esophagus is no better than clinical examination. The technology of nuclear magnetic resonance imaging has so far not been shown to be superior to CT scans for the classification of esophageal carcinomas. Consequently, preoperative staging shows only minor differences in long-term survival between various stages of the disease (Table 23-14).

In an analysis of patients with early disease, who underwent a potentially curative en bloc resection that included the regional lymph nodes, it was observed that only metastasis to lymph nodes and tumor penetration of the esophageal wall had a significant and independent influence on prognosis (Table 23-15). Further, it was shown that the effect of having fewer than four to six peritumoral nodes involved, particularly if the ratio of involved to uninvolved nodes is less than 1 in 5, is the same as having no nodes involved.

Other factors such as tumor size, cell type, degree of cellular differentiation, and location of the tumor within the esophagus had no effect on survival of these relatively early lesions. This indicated that resectable esophageal tumors, which met the criteria of no wall penetration and/or fewer than four regional lymph node

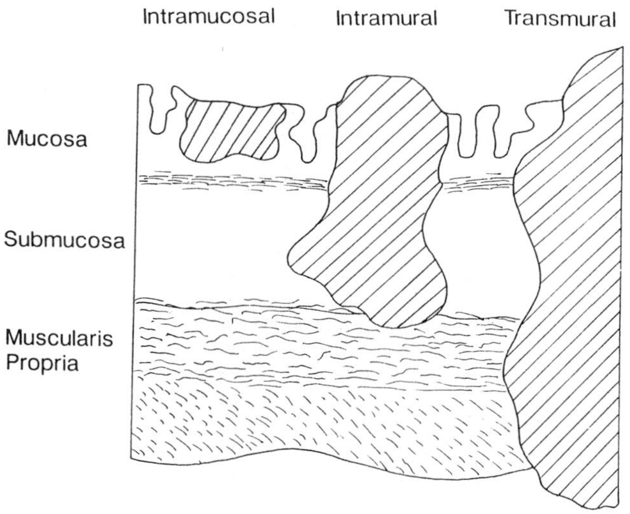

FIG. 23-58. Staging of the primary tumor according to the depth of invasion using standard anatomic landmarks: intramucosal carcinoma if through the basement membrane but limited by the muscularis mucosae, intramural carcinoma if through the muscularis mucosae but not the muscularis propria, and transmural if through the muscularis propria. (From: *DeMeester TR, Attwood SEA, et al: Ann Surg 212:530, 1990, with permission.*)

Table 23-13A
TNM Staging Criteria for Esophageal Cancer

Clinical		*Postsurgical resection*
	Primary Tumor (T)	
Tumor <5 cm long, no obstruction, not circumferential, no extraesophageal spread	T1	Tumor limited to mucosa and submucosa
Tumor without extension beyond muscularis propria, but >5 cm long, circumferential or obstructing	T2	Tumor invading into but not through muscularis propria
Any tumor with evidence of extraesophageal spread	T3	Tumor invading beyond muscularis propria
	Nodal Involvement (N)	
Regional nodes not involved	N0	Regional nodes not involved
Regional nodes not accessible for clinical evaluation	NX*	—
Movable unilateral palpable nodes†	N1	Regional nodes involved (for cervical tumors, unilateral involvement only)
Movable bilateral palpable nodes†	N2	—
Fixed nodes†	N3	Extensive regional node involvement (cervical tumors only)
	Distant Metastases (M)	
No distant metastases	M0	No distant metastases
Distant metastatic involvement	M1	Distant metastatic improvement

*Usually applied to tumors of the thoracic esophagus and cardia.

†Applies only to tumors of the cervical esophagus.

SOURCE: Ferguson MK, Little AG, Skinner DB: Cancer of the esophagus, in Roth JA, Ruckdeschel JC, Weisenburger TH (eds): *Thoracic Oncology*. Philadelphia, Saunders, 1989, p 374, with permission.

metastases, could be defined as potentially curable regardless of their size, histologic grade, cell type, and location. The problem is to determine this preoperatively.

The important goal of clinical staging of esophageal carcinoma is to determine if the end point of a surgical procedure is cure or palliation. Properly defined, a curable resection is an adequate en bloc resection of a tumor in a patient whose pre-resection physical condition and tumor characteristics have the potential of long-term survival. This requires selection of the physically fit patient and the curable lesion. Making the selection for cure or palliation prior to resection has several benefits. It identifies the mission of the operation and emphasizes adequate surgery for cure and sufficient surgery for palliation. It does not conceal the curative benefits of surgery by reporting the survival of patients in whom the procedure was done only for palliation. It also emphasizes the use of a more durable reconstruction of the gastrointestinal tract in patients operated on for cure and identifies patients for multimodal therapy if surgical cure is not possible.

Table 23-13B
The Japanese and UICC* TNM Staging System

Primary Tumor (T)	
T1	Tumor invades into but not beyond submucosa
T2	Tumor invades into but not beyond muscularis propria
T3	Tumor invades adventitia
T4	Tumor invades contiguous structures
Regional Lymph Nodes (N)	
N0	No lymph node involvement
N1	Involvement of mediastinal and perigastric nodes
Metastases (M)	
M0	No distant metastases
M1	Metastases to other viscera or nonregional lymph nodes

*UICC = Union Internationale Contre le Cancer

SOURCE: Ferguson MK, Little AG, Skinner DB: Cancer of the esophagus, in Roth JA, Ruckdeschel JC, Weisenburger TH (ed): *Thoracic Oncology*. Philadelphia, Saunders, 1989, p 374, with permission.

Clinical Approach to Carcinoma of the Esophagus and Cardia. The selection of a curative versus a palliative operation for cancer of the esophagus is based on the location of the tumor, the patient's age, physiologic fitness, the extent of the disease, and intraoperative staging. Figure 23-59 shows an algorithm of the clinical decisions important in the selection for curative or palliative therapy.

Tumor Location. The selection of surgical therapy for patients with carcinoma of the esophagus depends not only on the anatomic stage of the disease and an assessment of the swallowing capacity of the patient, but also on the location of the primary tumor.

It is estimated that 8 percent of the primary malignant tumors of the esophagus occur in the cervical portion (Fig. 23-60). These tumors, particularly those in the postcricoid area, represent a separate pathologic entity for a number of reasons: (1) they are more common in females and appear to be a unique entity in this regard; and (2) the efferent lymphatics from the cervical esophagus drain completely differently from those of the thoracic esophagus. The latter drain directly into the paratracheal and deep cervical or internal jugular lymph nodes with minimal flow in a longitudinal direction. Except in advanced disease, it is unusual for intrathoracic

Table 23-14
Five-Year Survival from Esophageal Cancer by Pathologic Stage

System		*Stage*	*Five-year survival (%)*
American Joint Committee on Cancer Staging (AJCCS) TNM	I	(T1N0M0)	50.0
	II	(T2N0M0)	44.9
	III	(T3N0M0; any T, N1–3, M0)	24.8
	IV	(Any T, any N, M1)	6.7
Japanese, UICC TNM	I	(T1N0M0)	60.8
	IIa	(T2–3, N0M0)	39.7
	IIb	(T1–2, N1M0)	24.8
	III	(T3N1M0; T4N0–1M0)	15.5
	IV	(Any T, any N, M1)	4.9
WNM	I	(W1N0M0)	55.0
	II	(W1N1M0)	27.0
	III	(W2N0M0)	15.0
	IV	(W2N1–2M0; any W, any N, M1)	8.0

SOURCE: Ferguson MK, Little AG, Skinner DB: Cancer of the esophagus, in Roth JA, Ruckdeschel JC, Weisenburger TH (eds): *Thoracic Oncology*. Philadelphia, Saunders, 1989, p 374, with permission.

lymph nodes to be involved. For all practical purposes the tumor is managed as though it were a head and neck tumor. Lesions that are not fixed to the spine, do not invade the vessels, and do not have fixed cervical lymph node metastases should be resected. If lymph node metastases are present, the resection should be considered palliative, since cure at this stage of disease is rare.

Low cervical lesions that reach the level of the thoracic inlet are usually unresectable due to early invasion of the great vessels and trachea. The length of the esophagus below the cricopharyngeus is insufficient to allow intubation or construction of a proximal anastomosis for a bypass procedure. Consequently palliation of these tumors is very difficult, and patients inflicted with disease at this location have a poor prognosis. Upper airway obstruction or the development of tracheoesophageal fistulas in such tumors may demand surgical intervention on a palliation basis.

Tumors that arise within the middle or upper third of the thoracic esophagus lie too close to the trachea and aorta to allow an en bloc resection without removal of these vital structures. Consequently, in this location only tumors that have not penetrated through the esophageal wall and have not metastasized to the regional lymph nodes are potentially curable. In essence, the resection for a tumor at this level is done similarly whether for palliation or cure, and long-term survival is a chance phenomenon. This does not mean that efforts to remove the adjacent lymph nodes, when resecting such tumors, should be abandoned. To do so may inadvertently leave unrecognized metastatic disease behind and hamper the patient's overall survival by recurrent local disease and compression of the trachea.

Tumors of the lower esophagus and cardia are usually adenocarcinomas. Squamous cell carcinoma of the lower esophagus, however, does occur. Both types of tumor are amenable to en bloc resection. Unless preoperative and intraoperative staging clearly demonstrate an incurable lesion, an en bloc resection in continuity with a lymph node dissection should be performed. The principles of a curative resection as applied elsewhere in the gastrointestinal tract require that tumors be resected on all sides by a layer of normal tissue. Because of the propensity of gastrointestinal tumors to spread for long distances submucosally, long lengths of grossly normal gastrointestinal tract should be resected. The longitudinal lymph flow in the esophagus can result in skip areas, with small foci of tumor above the primary lesion, which underscores the importance of a wide resection of esophageal tumors. Wong has shown that local recurrence at the anastomosis can be prevented by obtaining a 10-cm margin of normal esophagus above the tumor. Anatomic studies have also shown that there is no submucosal lymphatic barrier between the esophagus and the stomach at the cardia, and Wong has shown that 50 percent of the local recurrences in patients with esophageal cancer who are resected for cure occur in the intrathoracic stomach along the line of the gastric resection. Considering that the length of the esophagus ranges from 17 to 25 cm, and the length of the lesser curve of the stomach is approximately 12 cm, a curative resection requires a cervical division of the esophagus and a greater than 50 percent proximal gastrectomy in most patients with carcinoma of the distal esopha-

Table 23-15
Postsurgical Staging Criteria Based on Specific Prognostic Factors

Wall Penetration (W)
- W0 Carcinoma in situ
- W1 Penetration into but not through muscularis propria
- W2 Transmural extension of primary tumor through muscularis propria

Regional Lymph Node Involvement (N)
- N0 No lymph nodes involved
- N1 1 to 5 regional lymph nodes involved
- N2 Greater than 5 regional nodes involved

Metastases (M)
- M0 No distant metastases
- M1 Visceral or distant lymph node metastases

SOURCE: Ferguson MK, Little AG, Skinner DB: Cancer of the esophagus, in Roth JA, Ruckdeschel JC, Weisenburger TH (eds): *Thoracic Oncology*. Philadelphia, Saunders, 1989, p 375, with permission.

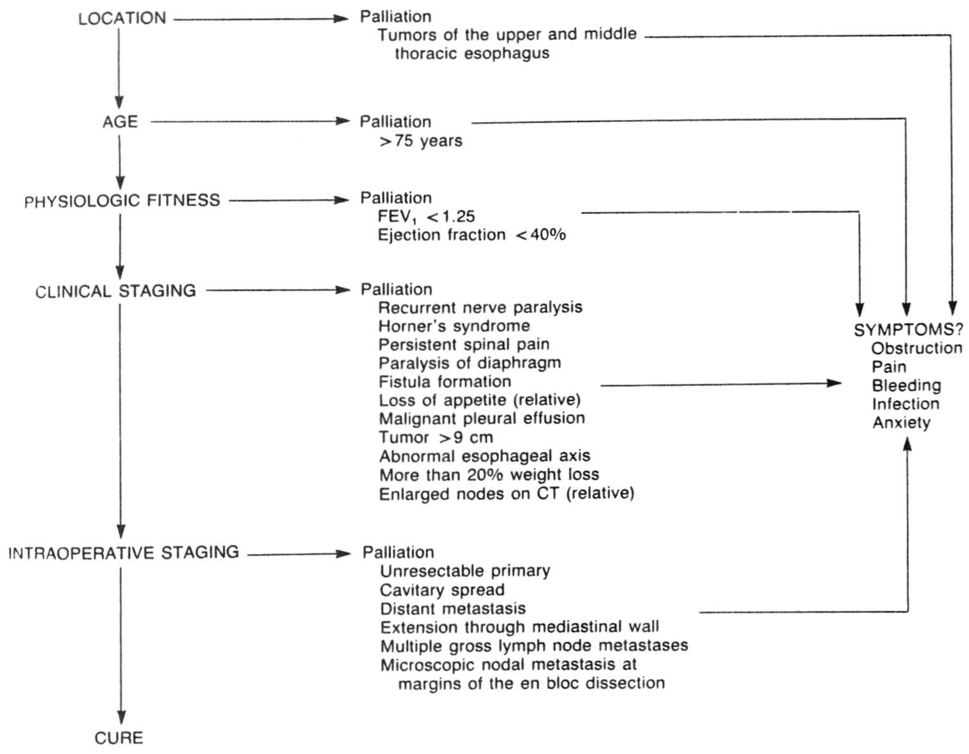

FIG. 23-59. Algorithm of decisions of patients with carcinoma of the esophagus and cardia for curative resection or palliation. (From: *DeMeester TR, Stein HJ: Cancer of the esophagus, in Bayless TM (ed): Current Therapy in Gastroenterology and Liver Disease, 3rd ed. Burlington, Ontario, BC Decker Inc, 1990, p 53, with permission.*)

gus or cardia. This compromises the length of the stomach and esophagus remaining to reestablish gastrointestinal continuity and necessitates a colon interposition.

Age. An en bloc resection for cure of carcinoma of the esophagus is unwise in patients older than seventy-five years because of the additional operative risk in face of a short life expectancy.

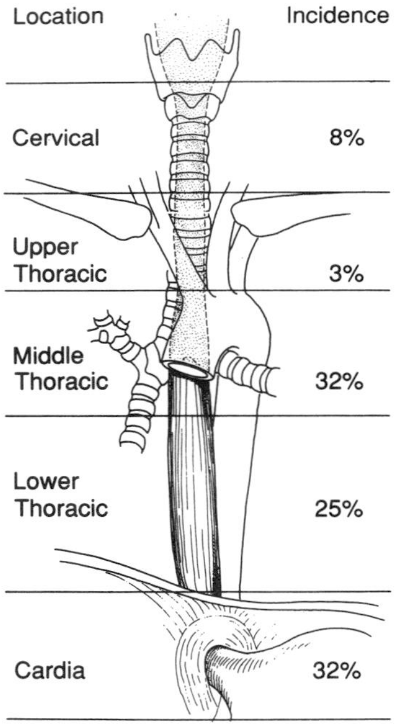

FIG. 23-60. Incidence of carcinoma of the esophagus and cardia based on tumor location.

Regardless of how favorable their pathology appears, a palliative resection is performed in these patients. This approach provides relief of symptoms with less surgery, and cure is still a chance possibility.

Physiologic Status. Patients undergoing esophageal resection should have sufficient cardiopulmonary reserve to tolerate the operation. Consequently, the physiologic status of the patient will affect the decision regarding the extent of surgery. The respiratory function is best assessed with the FEV_1, which ideally should be 2 L or more. Any patient with an FEV_1 of less than 1.25 L is a poor surgical candidate because he or she carries a 40 percent risk of dying from respiratory insufficiency within 4 years. In such a patient the chances of long-term survival, even if cured from the disease, do not justify an extensive en bloc resection. Clinical evaluation and electrocardiogram are not sufficient indicators of cardiac reserve. Echocardiography and dipyridamole thallium imaging provides accurate information on wall motion, ejection fraction, and myocardial blood flow. A defect on thallium imaging may require further evaluation with preoperative coronary angiography. A resting ejection fraction of less than 40 percent, particularly if there is no increase with exercise, is an ominous sign. We prefer to perform a palliative resection in such a patient, regardless of how favorable the pathology appears.

Clinical Stage. Clinical factors that indicate an advanced stage of carcinoma and exclude surgical cure are recurrent nerve paralysis, Horner's syndrome, persistent spinal pain, paralysis of the diaphragm, fistula formation, and malignant pleural effusion. Factors that make surgical cure unlikely include a tumor greater than 8 cm in length, abnormal axis of the esophagus on a barium radiogram, enlarged lymph nodes on CT, a weight loss of greater than 20 percent, and loss of appetite. In patients where these findings are not present, staging depends primarily on the length of the tumor measured with endoscopy and the degree of wall penetration and lymph node metastasis seen with endoscopic ultrasound. A high incidence of favorable parameters was present for tumors less than 4 cm in length, a lower incidence was found for tumors between 4 and 8 cm, and favorable criteria were absent for tumors greater than 8 cm in length. Consequently, a tumor greater than 8 cm in length should exclude curative resection, the finding of a smaller tumor should encourage an aggressive approach, and the smaller the tumor the more aggressive the approach should be. Endoscopic ultrasound imaging of esophageal tumors has recently become available, and provides further information regarding the size, wall penetration, and lymph node status of the lesion (Fig. 23-61*A*, *B*).

Intraoperative Staging. Intraoperative staging is designed for intraoperative selection of favorable candidates for a curative en bloc resection. It is based on the observation that patients with a tumor that penetrates through the esophageal wall, or has multiple or distant lymph node metastasis, have a poor survival. It requires an operative approach that allows switching from a curative to a palliative resection. If during the course of an operation an incurable situation is identified, the surgeon should change to a palliative procedure. Figure 23-62 shows an algorithm of intraoperative decision making. A curative en bloc dissection is abandoned if intraoperative staging reveals an unresectable primary tumor, cavitary spread of the tumor, distant organ metastasis, extension of the tumor through the mediastinal pleura, multiple gross lymph node metastases, or microscopic evidence of lymph node involvement at the margins of an en bloc resection, i.e., low paratracheal, portal triad, or subpancreatic periaortic lymph nodes. Experience has shown that for cancers of the distal esophagus and cardia, patients with a favorable stage of disease can be identified by a combination of preoperative and intraoperative assessment with an 86 percent accuracy. The overall five-year survival of these selected patients after a curative en bloc resection is between 40 and 55 percent. If the tumor does not extend through the esophageal wall and there are less than 6 lymph nodes positive the five-year survival is 75 percent. These results support a clinical approach in which an en bloc resection of the esophagus and stomach is advocated for patients most apt to benefit.

Management of Patients Excluded from Curative Resection. If the patient is considered incurable on preoperative or intraoperative evaluation, the severity of dysphagia or other incapacitating symptoms is assessed. Dysphagia of grade IV or higher (Table 23-16) is an indication for a palliative resection. If the patient is physiologically fit, a simple esophageal resection and reconstruction with esophagogastrostomy offers the best palliation. It allows the patient to eat without dysphagia and prevents the local complications of perforation, hemorrhage, fistula formation, and incapacitating pain. Occasionally a patient will be cured by a palliative resection, but this should not be used as justification for a palliative resection in the absence of dysphagia. The presence of a malignant pleural effusion, obvious mediastinal spread, or distant organ metastases usually discourages a palliative resection. In this setting, if dysphagia is not a problem, nothing more need be done.

If an obstructing tumor cannot be resected due to invasion of the trachea, aorta or heart, or when the patient's general condition precludes an operative procedure, relief of dysphagia by reestablishing the esophageal lumen is the focus of therapy. In this situation, the objective is to provide relief of dysphagia with the lowest mortality and the shortest hospital stay. A variety of techniques including bouginage, intubation, laser ablation, and electrical coagulation are available and can be used alone or in combination. Most centers prefer intubation of the esophagus.

Surgical Treatment

The nutritional status of the patient is of paramount importance for the outcome of an esophageal resection. Low serum protein levels have a deleterious effect on the cardiovascular system, and a poor nutritional status affects the host resistance to infection and the rate of anastomotic and wound healing. A serum albumin level of less than 3.4 g/dL on admission indicates poor caloric intake and an increased risk of surgical complications, including anastomotic breakdown. A feeding jejunostomy tube provides the most reliable and safest method for nutritional support in patients who cannot consume an oral diet and have a functionally normal small bowel. In severely malnourished patients, the jejunostomy is performed as a separate procedure to allow for preoperative nutritional support. In these patients the abdomen is entered through a small supraumbilical midline incision. Otherwise, the jejunostomy tube is placed

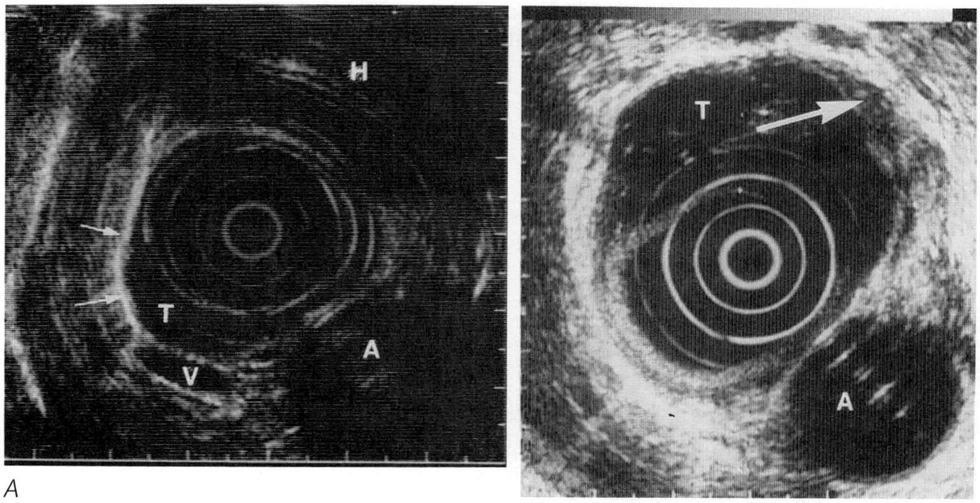

A

B

FIG. 23-61. *A.* Endoscopic ultrasound image of a tumor confined to the esophageal wall. T = tumor; V = azygos vein; H = heart; A = aorta; *arrows* = intact adventitia. *B.* Endoscopic ultrasound image of an advanced esophageal carcinoma with tumor penetrating through all layers of the esophagus. T = tumor, A = aorta; *arrow* shows tumor penetrating through the adventitia into periesophageal tissues. (From: *Bremner RM, DeMeester TR: Surgical treatment of esophageal carcinoma, in Wong RKH (ed): Gastroenterology Clinics of North America, Vol 20, No 4. Philadelphia, Saunders, 1991, p 748, with permission.*)

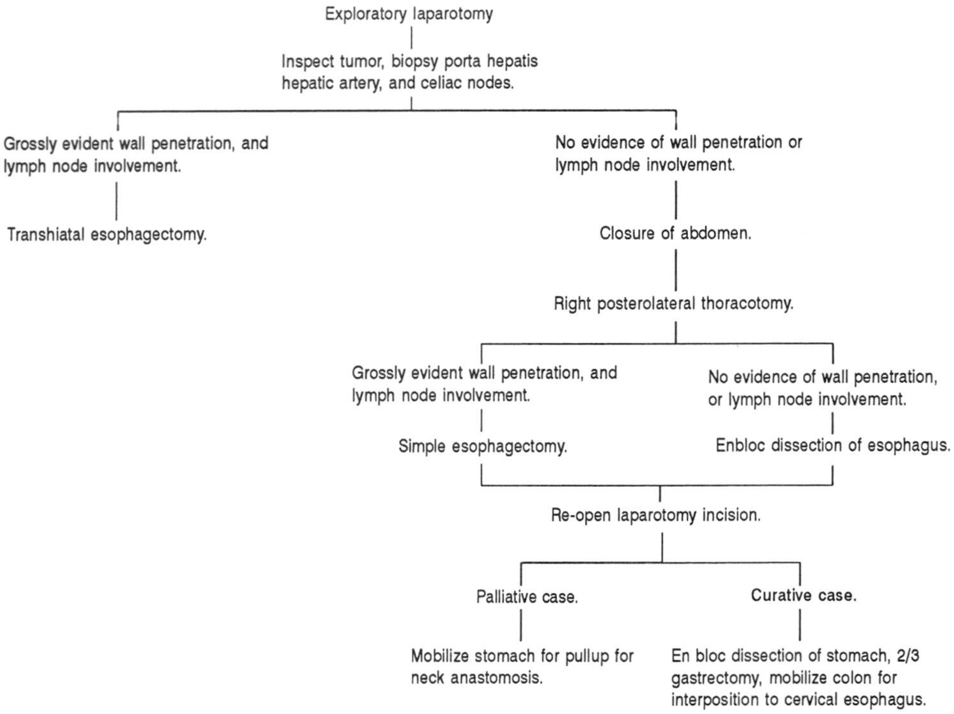

FIG. 23-62. Algorithm of intraoperative decision making for cancer of the lower esophagus and cardia.

at the time of esophageal resection, and feeding is begun on the third postoperative day.

Cervical Esophageal Cancer. Czerny reported the first successful resection of a carcinoma of the cervical esophagus in 1877. Initially it was hoped that the prognosis for patients with this disease might be better than for those with carcinoma of the thoracic esophagus. Unfortunately, this has not been proven to be true. Early experience with resection of the cervical esophagus resulted in a high mortality rate, and reconstruction by neck flaps often required multiple operations. Because of these complexities and the generally disappointing results, radiotherapy frequently was elected. Immediate mortality decreased, but control of the tumor was not satisfactory. The difference between the two forms of therapy is in the manner in which the disease recurs. Tumors treated with radiation therapy initially tend to recur locally as well as systemically, and cause unmanageable local disease with eventual erosion into neck vessels and trachea, causing hemorrhage and dyspnea. Patients who undergo surgical therapy have few local recurrences of the tumor provided total excision was possible, but they succumb to metastatic disease. Colin has reported a local failure rate of 80 percent after definitive radiation therapy, and 20 percent of these patients required palliative surgery in order to control the disease locally. Improvements in the techniques of immediate esophageal reconstruction have reduced the complications of the surgical treatment of this disease and encouraged a more aggressive surgical approach. The data reported by Colin suggest that an initial aggressive surgical resection yields longer survival than radiation therapy (Fig. 23-63). However, positive surgical margins, tracheal invasion that cannot be removed, and vocal cord paralysis correlate with a significantly shorter survival following surgery. His data also indicate that palliation was better achieved in patients who underwent esophagectomy with immedi-

Table 23-16
Functional Grades of Dysphagia

Grade	*Definition*	*Incidence at Dx (%)*
I	Eating normally	11
II	Requires liquids with meals	
III	Able to take semisolids but unable to take any solid food	30
IV	Able to take liquids only	40
V	Unable to take liquids, but able to swallow saliva	7
VI	Unable to swallow saliva	12

SOURCE: Modified from Takita H, Vincent RG, et al: Squamous cell carcinoma of the esophagus: a study of 153 cases. *J Surg Oncol* 9:547, 1977, with permission.

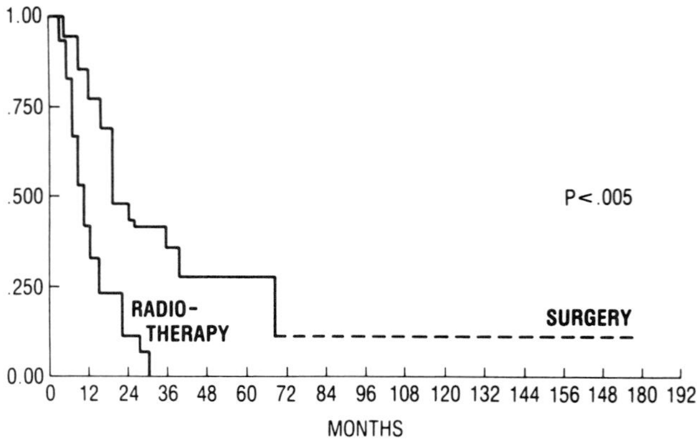

FIG. 23-63. Actuarial survival of patients with carcinoma of the cervical esophagus treated by surgery or 5000+ rads of radiotherapy. (From: *Colin CF, Spiro RH: Am J Surg 148:460, 1984, with permission.*)

ate gastric pull-up than in those who underwent primary radiation therapy or chemotherapy.

In general, lesions of the cervical esophagus that are not fixed to the spine, do not invade the vessels, and do not have fixed cervical lymph node metastasis should be resected. If nonfixed lymph node metastases are present, the resection should be considered palliative, since cure at this stage of disease is rare. The larynx is often invaded with microscopic tumor, and 94 percent of the time, a total laryngectomy in combination with esophagectomy is necessary. Most authors feel that the trachea should be removed even if gross tumor cannot be visualized. A simultaneous en bloc bilateral neck lymph node dissection is done, sparing the jugular veins on both sides.

The thoracic esophagus is removed by blunt dissection through a cervical and upper abdominal incision, and the continuity of the gastrointestinal tract is reestablished by pulling the stomach up through the esophageal bed. A permanent tracheostomy stoma is constructed in the lower flap of the cervical incision. The division of the trachea in some patients may preclude the possibility of a permanent cervical standard tracheostomy, since the remaining tracheal stump distal to the tumor will not reach the suprasternal notch. Removal of the medial head of the clavicles and the manubrium down to the sternal angle of Louis provides excellent exposure and allows the construction of a mediastinal tracheostomy. A bipedicle skin flap over the pectoralis muscle can be advanced upward, or a single-pedicle musculocutaneous flap including the pectoralis muscle and its overlying skin can be rotated to cover the defect. A circular incision in the flap can be used as a port through which the tracheal remnant is brought out to the skin. The overall operative mortality for this procedure is approximately 7 percent, and the 5-year survival rate is 20 to 25 percent.

Tumors of the Thoracic Esophagus and Cardia. A combined transthoracic and transhiatal approach is used to remove tumors in the middle or upper third of the thoracic esophagus because of their tendency to adhere to hilar structures. The procedure is performed through a combined right anterior thoracotomy and an upper midline abdominal incision. As many regional lymph nodes as possible are taken out with the specimen. Through a left neck incision the esophagus is divided and the previously dissected thoracic esophagus is removed transhiatally. Gastrointestinal continuity is reestablished by pulling up the previously prepared stomach through the posterior mediastinum and anastomosing it to the esophagus in the neck (Fig. 23-64). The 5-year survival of these lesions is largely dependent on the penetration of the tumor through the wall of the esophagus. In patients with an early lesion, some surgeons prefer a posterolateral thoracotomy with an en bloc removal of the lower esophagus and all available lymph nodes above the carina. The patient is then repositioned for a laparotomy and neck incision, and gastrointestinal continuity is reestablished with the stomach in the substernal position.

To remove tumors in the lower third of the thoracic esophagus and cardia, we prefer either an en bloc resection for cure or a transhiatal removal for palliation. A curative procedure is performed according to the principles of an en bloc resection in continuity with the regional lymph nodes (Fig. 23-65). It is attempted in a patient whose pre-resection physical condition and tumor characteristics have the potential for long-term survival. The en bloc resection is done through three incisions in the following order: right posterolateral thoracotomy, en bloc dissection of the distal esophagus, and mobilization of the esophagus above the aortic arch, closure of the thoracotomy, repositioning of the patient in the recumbent position; upper midline abdominal incision, en bloc dissection of the stomach and associated lymph nodes; left neck incision, proximal division of the esophagus, transhiatal removal of the previously en bloc-dissected distal esophagus and mobilized proximal esophagus, and distal division of the stomach at the angulus. Gastrointestinal continuity is reestablished with a left colon interposition. During the thoracic and abdominal dissection, intraoperative staging is done. If during the course of the operation an incurable situation is identified, the en bloc resection is abandoned and a palliative resection is performed in a manner similar to that described for tumors of the middle and upper thoracic esophagus. The hospital mortality for the group undergoing a curative en bloc resection was 7 percent. If preoperative staging has shown that the patient is a candidate for palliative resection, a transhiatal esophagectomy as popularized by Orringer is performed (Fig. 23-66). A standard left thoracotomy with intrathoracic anastomosis for lower lesions or an Ivor Lewis combined approach for higher lesions is not advocated because of (1) the proven need to resect long lengths of the esophagus to eradicate submucosal spread, (2) the higher morbidity of a thoracic anastomotic leak, and (3) the high incidence of esophagitis secondary to reflux following an intrathoracic anastomosis.

The conceptual aspects of the procedure for cardial carcinoma outlined above are based upon traditional Halstedian concepts of cancer spread, which have yet to be disproven for tumors arising within the thorax. It is clearly more of an en bloc procedure than most surgeons choose to undertake. There is little evidence that simply removing the esophagus and a portion of the stomach offers the patient the best chance for cure. Removing a 10-cm cuff of normal stomach and long lengths of apparently normal esophagus

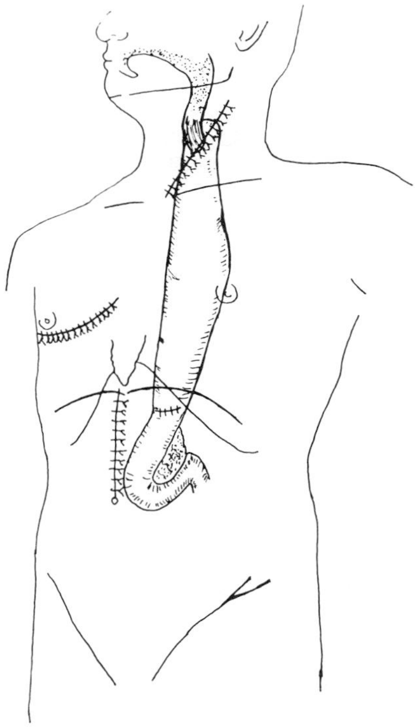

FIG. 23-64. Reconstruction of the gastrointestinal tract following resection of a middle or upper third esophageal cancer. A combined laparotomy and anterior thoracotomy is used to remove the tumor.

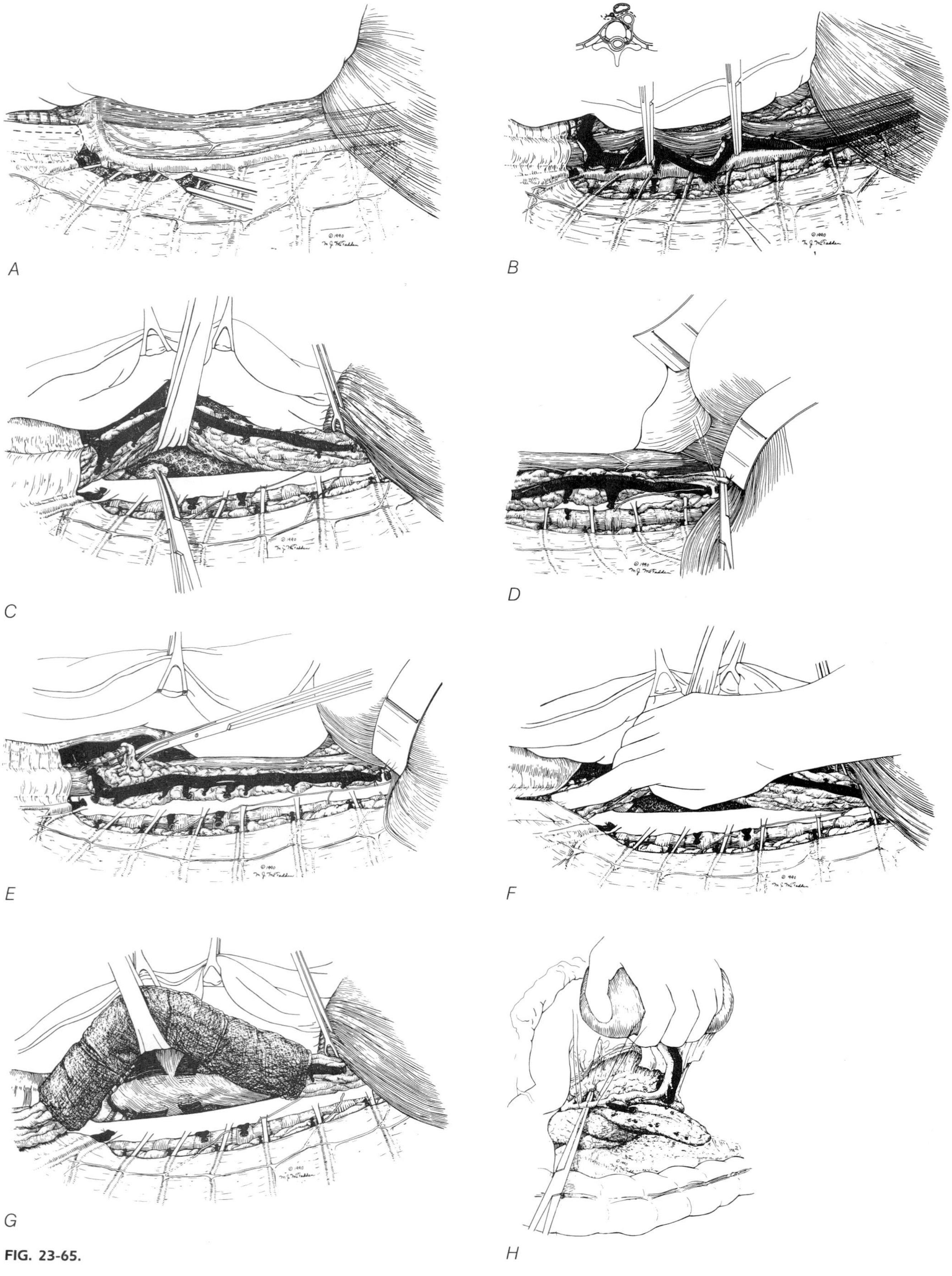

FIG. 23-65.

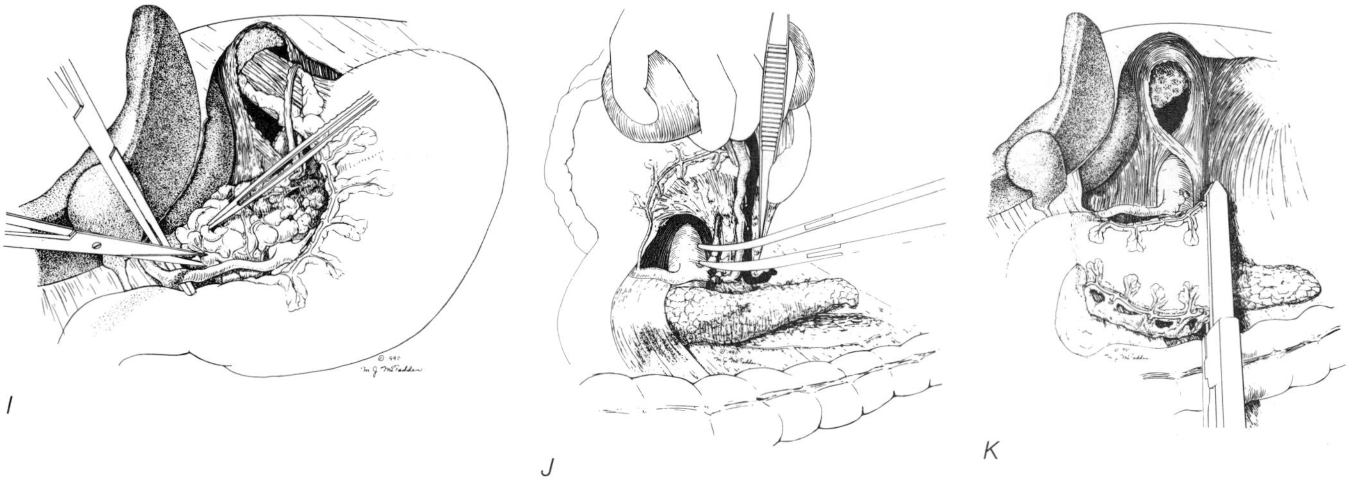

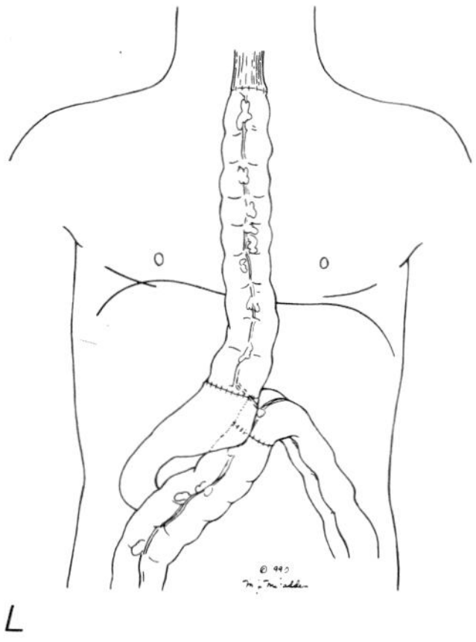

FIG. 23-65. Technique of en bloc esophagogastrectomy. The procedure is performed through a right posterolateral thoracotomy followed by repositioning the patient and an upper abdominal laparotomy and left neck incision. The steps in the procedure are: *A.* Division of the intercostal veins over the course of the azygos vein. *B.* Division of the hemiazygos veins (*insert* shows plane of dissection). *C.* Dissection along the intercostal arteries and over the anterior surface of the aorta into the left chest. *D.* Ligation of the thoracic duct and terminal end of the azygos. *E.* Dissection of the subcarinal lymph nodes. *F.* Blunt finger dissection of the proximal esophagus. *G.* Specimen wrapped, and left in chest while thoracotomy is closed and patient is repositioned for the abdominal portion of the procedure. *H.* Dissection of splenic artery in the beginning of the celiac and splenic lymphadenectomy. *I.* Opening of the gastrohepatic ligament and continuation of the lymphadenectomy along the common hepatic artery. *J.* Completion of the celiac and splenic lymphadenectomy with division of the left gastric artery. *K.* Transection of the stomach and removal of the specimen through the hiatus after division of the esophagus in the neck. *L.* Completed procedure with reconstruction of the gastrointestinal tract with left colon interposition.

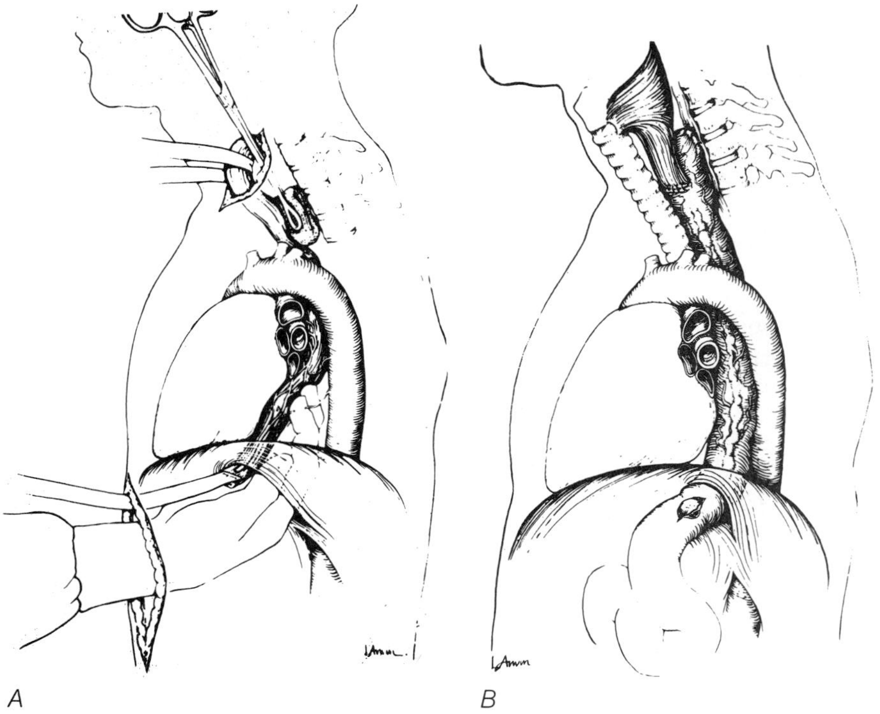

FIG. 23-66. Transhiatal esophagectomy. *A.* Illustration of blunt dissection of the thoracic esophagus through combined abdominal and neck incisions without thoracotomy. *B.* Reestablishment of gastrointestinal continuity using the stomach brought through the posterior mediastinum and cervical esophagogastrostomy.

to prevent recurrence is supported by evidence suggesting submucosal lymphatic spread of esophageal cancers. Most surgeons obtain more modest margins of the stomach and do not perform a true en bloc dissection in patients with potentially curable disease. The consequence of leaving potentially involved lymphatic disease behind is of concern, given the Japanese experience that patients with esophageal carcinoma and limited lymph node metastases can be cured. Consequently, some surgeons advocate that if the morbidity of the procedure is acceptable, aggressive surgical attempts at cure with an en bloc dissection are justified.

Alternative Therapies

Primary treatment with radiation therapy does not produce results comparable with those obtained with surgery. Currently, the use of radiotherapy is restricted to patients who are not candidates for surgery. Palliation of dysphagia is short term, generally lasting only 2 to 3 months. Furthermore, the length and course of treatment are difficult to justify in patients with a limited life expectancy. Consequently there is a reluctance to treat patients with advanced disease.

The use of chemotherapy to treat a disease with a high degree of systemic dissemination, as in advanced esophageal cancer, is appealing. A complete remission after single chemotherapeutic agents occurs occasionally, but the duration of the response is brief. Combination chemotherapy has been more promising. Most regimens involve cisplatin in combination with one or more drugs, usually 5-fluorouracil. Response rates are 40 to 50 percent, with a duration of about 7 months, at which time dysphagia returns. Unfortunately, a response is usually seen in patients with a Karnowski score higher than 50, while response is poor and toxicity increased in those with a score lower than 50.

Despite advances obtained by curative en bloc resection of early esophageal carcinoma, the results of surgery alone in advanced disease remain undeniably disappointing. Many hope that cytoreduction or debulking of tumors by surgery in combination with irradiation and chemotherapy will offer a promising new approach for long-term survival in patients with esophageal carcinoma.

Preoperative irradiation is most commonly applied in divided fractions over a 4-week period adding up to 40 Gy, with surgery to follow in 4 to 6 weeks when the acute inflammatory response has subsided and before tissue fibrosis occurs. This protocol does not appear to affect operative mortality, but does increase resectability rates by reducing the tumor size. Disagreement exists regarding the effect of preoperative radiation therapy on the incidence of lymph node metastases and the degree of tumor penetration. There is no evidence that preoperative radiation therapy improves the 5-year survival rate.

Postoperative irradiation is attractive because it can be selectively offered to the patients who, in light of the knowledge gained at the operation, might benefit from it and it can be targeted to a particular area. It is now clear that postoperative radiotherapy does not prolong survival and may be detrimental to the gastric or colonic reconstruction.

The use of combined chemotherapy prior to surgery has shown encouraging initial results in terms of tumor destruction. Combinations of cisplatin with 5-fluorouracil have resulted in downstaging of squamous cell tumors in 30 to 50 percent of patients before the operation. A major drawback with preoperative chemotherapy regimens is the inability to obtain precise staging of the patient prior to the institution of therapy. This removes the most important prognostic determinant, in regard to both patient management and interpretation of subsequent survival data. Disappointingly the most common cause of failure in patients treated with preoperative chemotherapy is the emergence of systemic disease. This may suggest that its major effect is on the primary tumor. The synergistic effect of chemotherapy and surgery on long-term survival remains to be established.

The theoretical advantage of combining chemotherapy and radiation is that the drugs may act as radiation sensitizers. Several trials are currently under way to evaluate the effect of combined modality treatment consisting of chemotherapy, radiation, and surgery. To date, the most impressive conclusion is that concurrent radiation therapy and chemotherapy increase the number of patients who achieve a complete response prior to surgery, i.e., no microscopic evidence of tumor in the resected specimen. The significance of this is not clear with regard to long-term survival. The results of combination therapy, although exciting in single patients, are not sufficiently predictable to consider it as standard therapy, particularly in patients with early lesions. More work needs to be focused on the selection of those patients apt to receive benefit. Concerns regarding the ability to control systemic disease remain.

SARCOMAS OF THE ESOPHAGUS

Sarcomas and carcinosarcomas are rare neoplasms, accounting for approximately 0.1 to 1.5 percent of all esophageal tumors. Despite their infrequent occurrence these neoplasms exhibit several significant behavior patterns that are important in their management. Clinically, they present with the symptom of dysphagia, which does not differ from the dysphagia associated with the more common epithelial carcinoma. Tumors located within the cervical or high thoracic esophagus can cause symptoms of pulmonary aspiration secondary to esophageal obstruction. Large tumors originating at the level of the tracheal bifurcation can produce symptoms of airway obstruction and syncope by direct compression of the tracheobronchial tree and heart (Fig. 23-67). The duration of dysphagia and age of the patients affected with these tumors are similar to those with carcinoma of the esophagus.

A barium swallow usually shows a large polypoid intraluminal esophageal mass, causing partial obstruction and dilatation of the esophagus proximal to the tumor. The smooth polypoid nature of the lesion, although not itself diagnostic, is distinctive enough to suggest the presence of a sarcoma rather than the more common ulcerating, stenosing carcinoma.

Esophagoscopy commonly shows an intraluminal necrotic mass. When biopsy is attempted, it is important to remove the necrotic tissue until bleeding is seen on the tumor's surface. When this is not done, the biopsy shows only tissue necrosis. Even when viable tumor is obtained on biopsy, it has been our experience that it cannot be identified as either carcinoma, sarcoma, or carcinosarcoma, depending on the histology of the portion biopsied. Therefore, one cannot rely totally on the biopsy results to identify the presence of sarcoma and must depend on the polypoid nature of the lesion to arouse suspicion that it may be something other than carcinoma.

Polypoid sarcomas of the esophagus, in contrast to infiltrating carcinomas, remain superficial to the muscularis propria and are less likely to metastasize to regional lymph nodes. This growth characteristic was dramatically demonstrated in 14 patients who

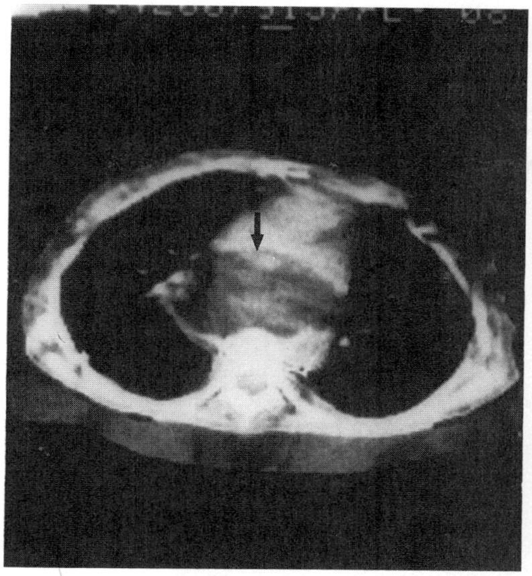

A

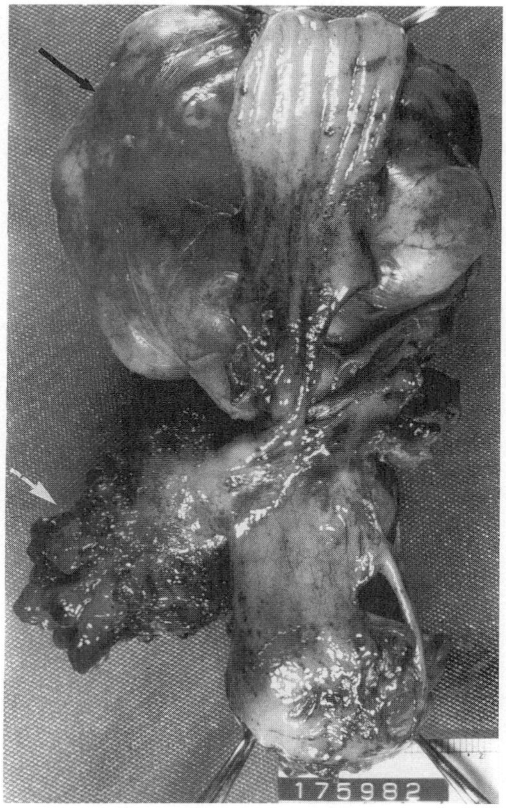

B

FIG. 23-67. *A.* CT scan of a leiomyosarcoma (*black arrow*) that caused compression of the heart and symptoms of syncope. *B.* Surgical specimen of above with a pedunculated luminal lesion (*white arrow*) and a large extraesophageal component (*black arrow*). There was no evidence of lymph node metastasis at the time of operation.

were diagnosed postmortem. In only 5 of the 14 patients would local extension or tumor metastasis have prevented a potentially curative resection. Thus the presence of a large polypoid tumor should not deter the surgeon from resecting the lesion.

Sarcomatous lesions of the esophagus can be divided into epidermoid carcinomas with spindle cell features, such as carcinosarcoma, and true sarcomas that arise from mesenchymal tissue, such as leiomyosarcoma, fibrosarcoma, and rhabdomyosarcoma. Based on current histologic criteria for diagnosis, fibrosarcoma and rhabdomyosarcoma of the esophagus are extremely rare lesions of doubtful existence.

Surgical resection of polypoid sarcoma of the esophagus is the treatment of choice, since radiation therapy has little success and the tumors remain superficial, with local invasion or distant metastases occurring late in the course of the disease. As with carcinoma, the absence of both wall penetration and lymph node metastases is necessary for curability, and surgical resection is consequently responsible for the majority of the reported 5-year survivals. Resection also provides an excellent means of palliating the patient's symptoms. The surgical technique for resection and the subsequent restoration of the gastrointestinal continuity is similar to that described for carcinoma.

In a review of the literature we were able to find eight patients with carcinosarcoma who survived resection for cure and who either died from recurrent disease during their follow-up period or lived longer than 5 years. Patients who had not reached the 5-year mark but who were reported alive and well during the follow-up period were excluded. Four of the eight patients survived for 5 years or longer—one for 5 years, one for 13 years, and two for 10 years. Even though this number is small, it suggests that resection produces better results in epithelial carcinoma with spindle cell features than in squamous cell carcinoma of the esophagus.

Similarly, with leiomyosarcoma of the esophagus, the same scattered reports exist with little information on survival. We were able to find seven patients who had surgical resection for cure and who either died from their disease within the follow-up period or survived 5 years or longer. Of the seven patients, two died from their disease—one in 3 months and the other 4 years and 7 months after resection. The other five patients were reported to have survived 12, 7, 7, 6, and 5 years, respectively. Turnbull et al. reported on three patients who received radiotherapy for leiomyosarcoma of the esophagus. Two died 2 and 17 months after radiation, and the third survived 11 years before dying of recurrent widespread disease.

It is difficult to evaluate the benefits of resection for leiomyoblastoma (Fig. 23-68) of the esophagus, due to the small number of reported patients with tumors in this location. Most leiomyoblastomas occur in the stomach, and 38 percent of these patients succumb from the cancer in 3 years. Fifty-five percent of patients with extragastric leiomyoblastoma also died from the disease at an average of 3 years. Consequently, leiomyoblastoma should be considered a malignant lesion and apt to behave like a leiomyosarcoma. In general, the presence of nuclear hyperchromatism, increased mitotic figures (more than 1 per high-power field), tumor size larger than 10 cm, and clinical symptoms of longer than 6 months duration are signs of poor prognosis.

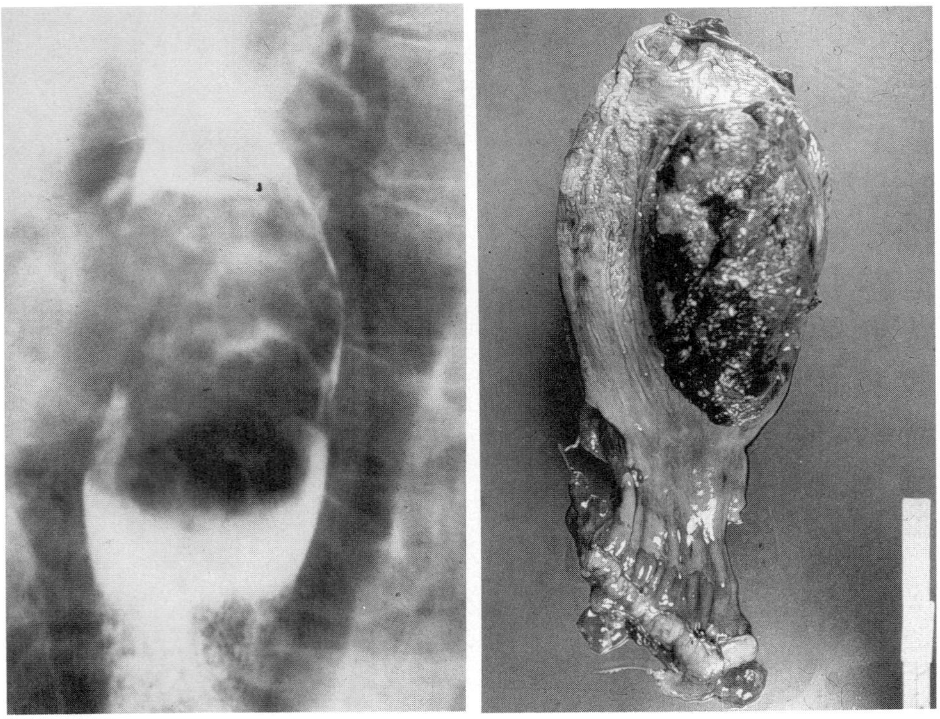

A B

FIG. 23-68. *A.* Barium esophagogram showing a classical polypoid lesion of the esophagus suggesting a sarcoma. *B.* Surgical specimen of above showing a large polypoid tumor which on histologic examination was a leiomyoblastoma.

BENIGN TUMORS AND CYSTS

Benign tumors and cysts of the esophagus are relatively uncommon. Leiomyoblastomas are, by far, the most common benign esophageal tumors. From both the clinical and pathologic perspective, benign tumors may be divided into those that are within the muscular wall and those that are within the lumen of the esophagus.

The intramural lesions are either solid tumors or cysts. The vast majority of intramural tumors are leiomyomas. They are made up of varying portions of smooth muscle and fibrous tissue. Fibromas, myomas, fibromyomas, and lipomyomas are closely related and occur rarely. Other histologic types of solid intramural tumors have been described such as lipomas, neurofibromas, hemangiomas, osteochondromas, granular cell myoblastomas, and glomus tumors and are medical curiosities.

Intraluminal lesions are polypoid or pedunculated growths which usually originate in the submucosa, develop mainly into the lumen, and are covered with normal stratified squamous epithelium. The majority of these tumors are composed of fibrous tissue of varying degrees of compactness with a rich vascular supply. Some are quite loose and myxoid such as myxoma and myxofibroma, others more collagenous such as fibroma, and some contain adipose tissue such as a fibrolipoma. These different types of tumor are frequently collectively designated as fibrovascular polyps or simply as polyps. Pedunculated intraluminal tumors should be removed. If the lesion is not too large, endoscopic removal with a snare is feasible.

Leiomyomas

Leiomyomas constitute more than 50 percent of benign esophageal tumors. Along with cysts they can be considered the prototype of benign intramural tumors. The average age at presentation is thirty-eight years, which is in sharp contrast to that seen with esophageal carcinoma. Leiomyomas are twice as common in males. Because they originate in smooth muscle, 90 percent are located in the lower two-thirds of the esophagus. They are usually solitary, but multiple tumors have been found on occasion. They vary greatly in size and shape. Tumors as small as 1 cm in diameter or as large as 10 lb have been removed.

Typically, leiomyomas are oval. During their growth, they remain intramural, having the bulk of their mass protruding toward the outer wall of the esophagus. The overlying mucosa is freely movable and normal in appearance. Neither their size nor location correlates with the degree of symptoms. Dysphagia and pain are the most common complaints, the two symptoms occurring more frequently together than separately. Bleeding directly related to the tumor is rare, and when hematemesis or melena occurs in a patient with an esophageal leiomyoma, other causes should be investigated.

A barium swallow is the most useful method to demonstrate a leiomyoma of the esophagus (Fig. 23-69). In profile the tumor appears as a smooth, semilunar or crescent-shaped filling defect which moves with swallowing, is sharply demarcated, and is covered and surrounded by normal mucosa. Esophagoscopy should be performed to exclude the reported observation of a coexistence with carcinoma. The freely movable mass, which bulges into the lumen, should not be biopsied because of an increased chance of mucosal perforation at the time of surgical enucleation.

Despite their slow growth and limited potential for malignant degeneration, leiomyomas should be removed surgically unless there are specific contraindications. The majority can be removed by simple enucleation. If during removal the mucosa is inadvertently entered, the defect can be repaired primarily. Following

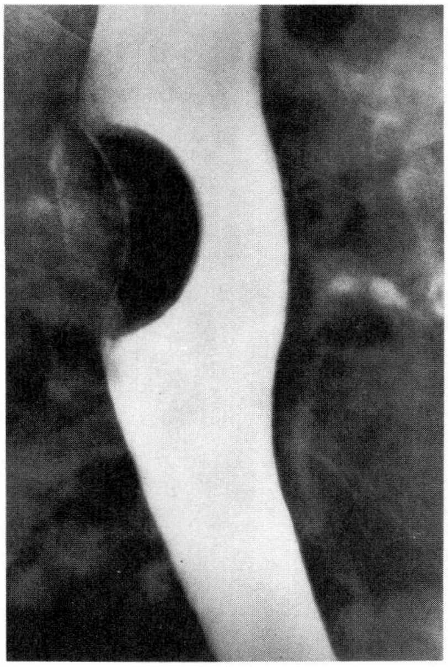

FIG. 23-69. Barium esophagogram showing the typical smooth contour punched-out defect of a leiomyoma.

tumor removal the outer esophageal wall should be reconstructed by closure of the muscle layer. The location of the lesion and the extent of surgery required will dictate the approach. Lesions of the proximal and middle esophagus require a right thoracotomy, whereas distal esophageal lesions require a left thoracotomy. Recently videothoracoscopic approaches have been reported. The mortality of enucleation is less than 2 percent, and success in relieving the dysphagia is universal. Large lesions or those involving the gastroesophageal junction may require esophageal resection.

Esophageal Cysts

Cysts may be congenital or acquired. Congenital cysts are lined wholly or partly by columnar ciliated epithelium of the respiratory type, by glandular epithelium of the gastric type, by squamous epithelium, or by transitional epithelium. In some, epithelial lining cells may be absent. Confusion over the embryologic origin of congenital cysts has led to a variety of names, such as enteric, bronchogenic, and mediastinal cysts. Acquired retention cysts also occur, probably from obstruction of the excretory ducts of the esophageal glands.

Enteric and bronchogenic cysts are the most common and arise as a result of developmental abnormalities during the formation and differentiation of the lower respiratory tract, esophagus, and stomach from the foregut. During its embryologic development, the esophagus is lined successively with simple columnar, pseudostratified ciliated columnar, and finally stratified squamous epithelium. This sequence probably accounts for the fact that the lining epithelium may be any or a combination of these. Consequently the presence of cilia does not necessarily indicate a respiratory origin.

Cysts vary in size from small to very large and are usually located intramurally in the middle to lower third of the esophagus. Their symptoms are similar to those of a leiomyoma. The diagnosis similarly depends on radiographic and endoscopic findings. Surgical excision is the preferred treatment, with most able to be enucleated without damage to the mucosa. During removal, a fistulous tract connecting the cysts to the airways should be looked for, particularly in patients who have had repetitive bronchopulmonary infections.

ESOPHAGEAL PERFORATION

Perforation of the esophagus constitutes a true emergency. It most commonly occurs following diagnostic or therapeutic procedures. Spontaneous perforation, referred to as Boerhaave's syndrome, is the cause for only 15 percent of such patients, foreign bodies for 14 percent, and trauma 10 percent. Pain is a striking and consistent symptom and strongly suggests that an esophageal rupture has occurred, particularly if located in the cervical area following instrumentation of the esophagus or substernally in a patient with a history of resisting vomiting. If subcutaneous emphysema is present, the diagnosis is almost certain.

Spontaneous rupture of the esophagus has a poor survival because of the delay in recognition and treatment. Although there usually is a history of resisting vomiting in a small number of patients, the injury occurs silently without any antecedent history. When the condition presents with a chest radiogram showing air or an effusion in the pleural space, it is often misdiagnosed as a pneumothorax or pancreatitis. An elevated serum amylase caused by the extrusion of saliva through the perforation may fix the diagnosis of pancreatitis in the mind of an unwary physician. If the chest radiogram is normal, the diagnosis is often confused with a myocardial infarction or dissecting aneurysm.

Spontaneous rupture usually occurs into the left pleural cavity or just above the gastroesophageal junction. Fifty percent of patients have concomitant gastroesophageal reflux disease, suggesting that minimal resistance to the transmission of abdominal pressure into the thoracic esophagus is a factor in the pathophysiology of the lesion. During vomiting, remarkably high peaks of intragastric pressure can be recorded, frequently exceeding 200 mmHg, but since extragastric pressure remains almost equal to intragastric pressure, stretching of the gastric wall is minimal. The amount of pressure transmitted to the esophagus varies considerably depending on the position of the gastroesophageal junction. When it is in the abdomen and exposed to intraabdominal pressure, the pressure transmitted to the esophagus is must less than when it is exposed to the negative thoracic pressure. In the latter situation, the pressure in the lower esophagus will frequently equal intragastric pressure if the glottis remains closed. Cadaver studies have shown that when this pressure exceeds 150 mmHg, rupture of the esophagus is apt to occur. When a hiatal hernia is present and the sphincter remains exposed to abdominal pressure, the lesion produced is usually a Mallory-Weiss mucosal tear, and bleeding rather than perforation is the problem. This is due to the stretching of the supradiaphragmatic portion of the gastric wall. In this situation the hernia sac represent an extension of the abdominal cavity, and the gastroesophageal junction remains exposed to abdominal pressure.

Diagnosis. Abnormalities on the chest radiogram can be variable and should not be depended upon to make the diagnosis. This is because the abnormalities are dependent on three factors: (1) the time interval between the perforation and the radiographic examination, (2) the site of perforation, and (3) the integrity of the mediastinal pleura. Mediastinal emphysema, a strong indicator of perforation, takes at least one hour to be demonstrated and is present in only 40 percent of patients. Mediastinal widening secondary to edema may not occur for several hours. The site of perforation can also influence the radiographic findings. In cervical perforation, cervical emphysema is common and mediastinal emphysema rare; the converse is true for thoracic perforations. Frequently, air will be visible in the erector spinae muscles on a neck radiogram before it can be palpated or seen on a chest radiogram (Fig. 23-70). The integrity of the mediastinal pleura influences the radiographic abnormality in that rupture of the pleura results in a pneumothorax. This finding occurs in 77 percent of patients. In two-thirds the perforation is on the left side, 20 percent right-sided, and 10 percent bilateral. If pleural integrity is maintained, mediastinal emphysema (rather than a pneumothorax) appears rapidly. A pleural effusion secondary to inflammation of the mediastinum occurs late. In 9 percent of patients the chest radiogram will remain normal.

The diagnosis is confirmed with a contrast esophagogram which will demonstrate extravasation in 90 percent of patients. The use of a water-soluble medium such as Gastrografin is preferred. Of concern is that there is a 10 percent false-negative rate. This may be due to obtaining the radiographic study with the patient in the upright position. When the patient is upright, the passage of water-soluble contrast material can be too rapid to demonstrate a small perforation. The studies should be done with the patient in the right lateral decubitus position (Fig. 23-71). In this position the contrast material fills the whole length of the esophagus, thereby allowing the actual site of perforation and its interconnecting cavities to be shown in almost all patients.

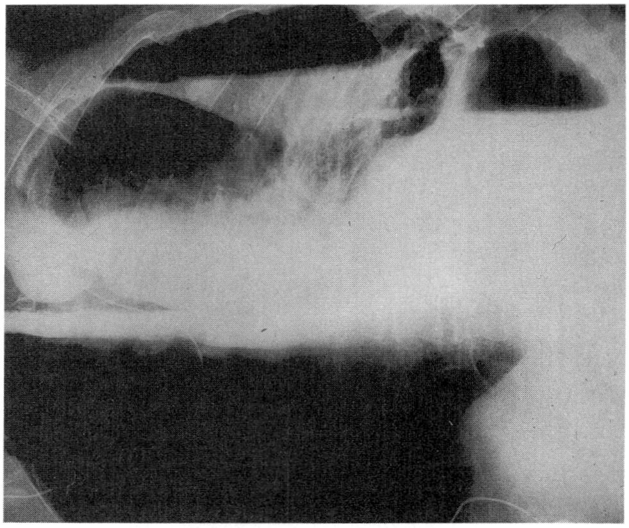

FIG. 23-71. Radiographic study of a patient with a perforation of the esophagus using water-soluble contrast material. The patient is placed in the lateral decubitus position with the left side up to allow complete filling of the esophagus and demonstration of the defect.

Management. The key to optimum management is in early diagnosis. The most favorable outcome is obtained following primary closure of the perforation within 24 hours, resulting in 80 to 90 percent survival. Figure 23-72 is an operative photograph taken through a left thoracotomy of an esophageal rupture following a pneumatic dilation for achalasia. The most common location for the injury is the left lateral wall of the esophagus just above the gastroesophageal junction. To get adequate exposure of the injury a dissection similar to that described for esophageal myotomy is performed. A flap of stomach is pulled up and the soiled fat pad at the gastroesophageal junction is removed. The edges of the injury

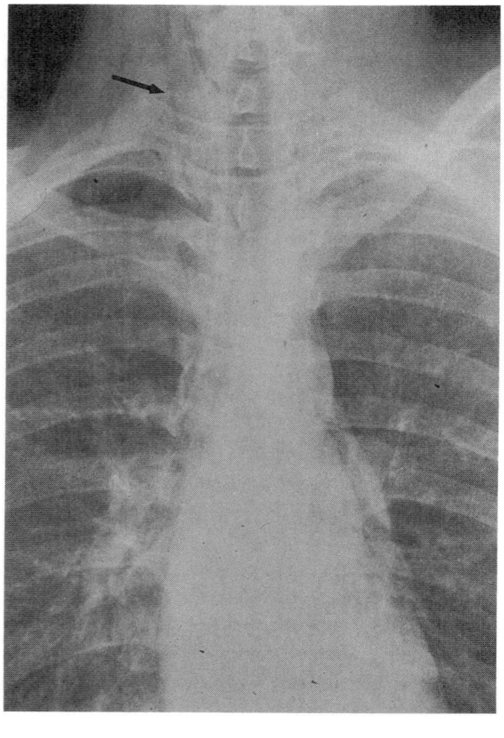

FIG. 23-70. Chest radiogram showing air in the deep muscles of the neck following perforation of the esophagus (*arrow*). This is often the earliest sign of perforation and can be present without evidence of air in the mediastinum.

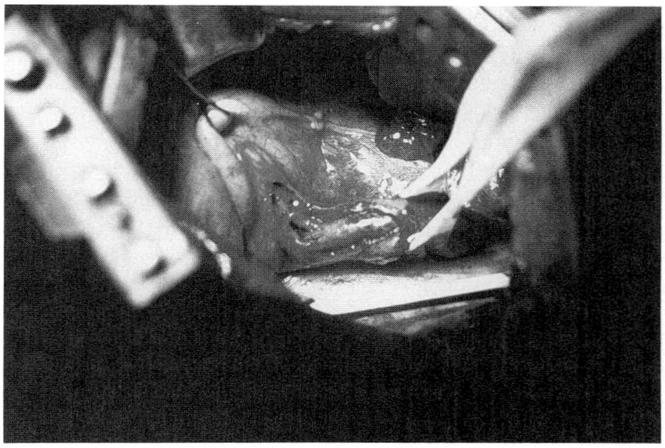

FIG. 23-72. Left thoracotomy in a patient with an esophageal rupture at the gastroesophageal junction following forceful dilation of the lower esophagus for achalasia (the surgical clamp is on the stomach, and the Penrose drain encircles the esophagus). The injury consists of a mucosal perforation and extensive splitting of the esophageal muscle from just below the Penrose drain on to the stomach.

are trimmed and closed using a modified Gambi stitch (Fig. 23-73*A*). The closure is reinforced by the use of a pleural patch or construction of a Nissen fundoplication (Fig. 23-73*B*).

Mortality of immediate closure varies between 8 and 20 percent. After 24 hours survival decreases to less than 50 percent and is not influenced by the type of operative therapy, that is, drainage alone or drainage plus closure of the perforation. If the time delay prior to closing a perforation approaches 24 hours and the tissues are inflamed, division of the cardia and resection of the diseased portion of the esophagus is recommended. The remainder of the esophagus is mobilized and as much normal esophagus as possible is saved and is brought out as an end cervical esophagostomy. In some situations the retained esophagus may be so long that it loops down into the chest. The contaminated mediastinum is drained and a feeding jejunostomy tube is inserted. The recovery from sepsis is often immediate, dramatic, and reflected by a marked change in the patient's course in 24 hours. On recovery from the sepsis the patient is discharged and returns on a subsequent date for reconstruction with a substernal colon interposition. Failure to apply this aggressive therapy can result in a mortality in excess of 50 percent in patients in whom the diagnosis has been delayed.

Nonoperative management of esophageal perforation has been advocated in select situations. The choice of conservative therapy requires skillful judgment and necessitates careful radiographic examination of the esophagus. This course of management usually follows an injury occurring during dilation of esophageal strictures or pneumatic dilations of achalasia. Conservative management should not be used in patients who have free perforations into the pleural space. Cameron proposed three criteria for the nonoperative management of esophageal perforation: (1) the barium swallow must show the perforation to be contained within the mediastinum and drain well back into the esophagus (Fig. 23-74); (2) mild symptoms should be present; and (3) there should be minimal evidence of clinical sepsis. If these conditions are met, it is reasonable to treat the patient with hyperalimentation, antibiotics, and cimetidine to decrease acid secretion and diminish pepsin activity. Oral intake is resumed in 7 to 14 days, dependent on subsequent radiographic examinations.

CAUSTIC INJURY

Accidental caustic lesions occur mainly in children and, in general, rather small quantities are taken. In adults or teenagers, the swallowing of caustic liquids is usually deliberate during suicide attempts. Consequently, greater quantities are swallowed. Alka-

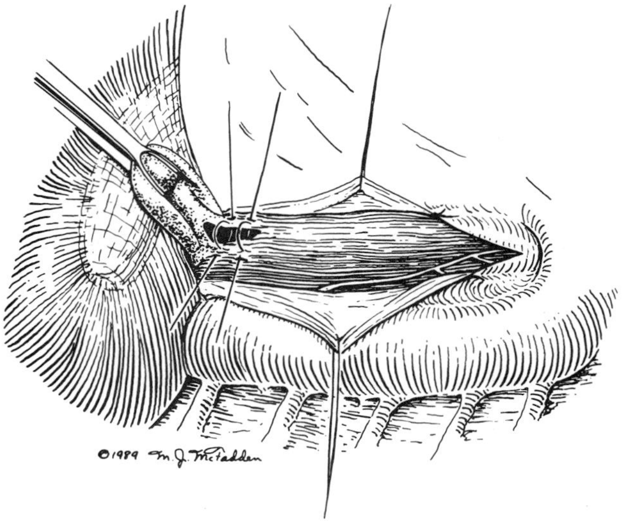

A

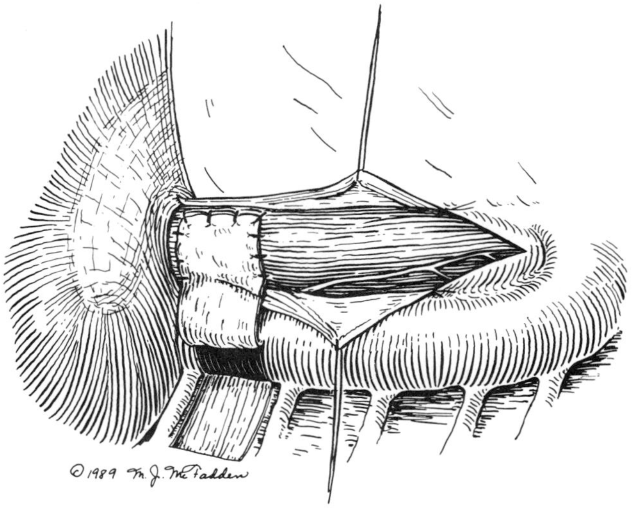

B

FIG. 23-73. The technique of closure of an esophageal perforation through a left thoracotomy. *A.* A tongue of stomach is pulled up through the esophageal hiatus and the gastroesophageal fat pad is removed; the edges of the mucosal injury are trimmed and closed using interrupted modified Gambi stitches. *B.* Reinforcement of the closure with a parietal pleural patch.

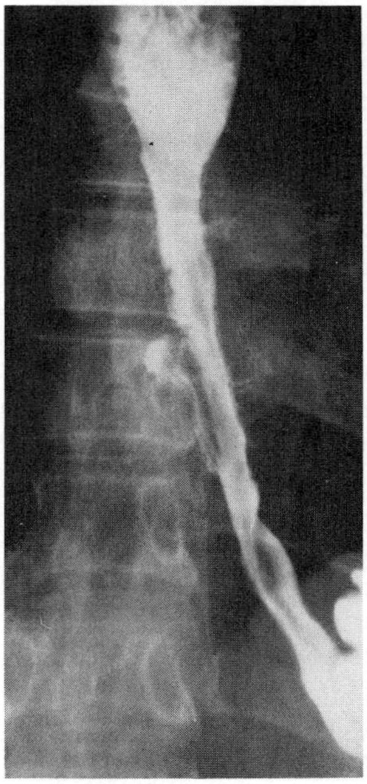

FIG. 23-74. Barium esophagogram showing a stricture and a contained perforation following dilation. The injury meets Cameron criteria: it is contained within the mediastinum and drawn back into the esophagus; the patient had mild symptoms with no evidence of clinical sepsis. Nonoperative management was successful.

lies are more frequently swallowed accidentally than acids because strong acids cause an immediate burning pain in the mouth.

Pathology. The swallowing of caustic substances causes both an acute and a chronic injury. Care focuses during the acute phase on controlling the immediate tissue injury and the potential for perforation; during the chronic phase on strictures and disturbances in pharyngeal swallowing. In the acute phase the degree and extent of the lesion are dependent on several factors: the nature of the caustic substance, its concentration, the quantity swallowed, and the time the substance is in contact with the tissues. Acids and alkalies affect tissue in a different manner. Alkalies dissolve tissue and, therefore, penetrate more deeply, while acids cause a coagulative necrosis which limits their penetration. Animal experiments have shown that there is a correlation between the depth of lesion and the concentration of sodium hydroxide solution. When a solution of 3.8 percent comes into contact with the esophagus for 10 seconds, it causes a necrosis of the mucosa and the submucosa but spares the mucsular layer. A concentration of 22.5 percent penetrates the whole esophageal wall and into the periesophageal tissues. The pertinence of these data is obvious if one remembers that cleansing products can contain up to 90 percent NaOH. The strength of esophageal contractions varies according ot the level of the esophagus, being weakest at the striated-smooth muscle interface. Consequently, clearance from this area may be somewhat slower, so caustic substances are in contact longer with the mucosa. This can explain why the esophagus is preferentially and more severely affected at this level than in the lower portions.

The lesions caused by lye injury occur in three phases. First is the acute necrotic phase, lasting 1 to 4 days after injury. During this period coagulation of intracellular proteins results in cell necrosis, and the living tissue surrounding the area of necrosis develops an intense inflammatory reaction. Second is the ulceration and granulation phase, starting 3 to 5 days after injury. During this period the superficial necrotic tissue sloughs, leaving an ulcerated, acutely inflamed base, and granulation tissue fills the defect left by the sloughed mucosa. This phase lasts 10 to 12 days, and it is during this period that the esophagus is the weakest. Third is the phase of cicatrization and scarring, which begins the third week following injury. During this period the previously formed connective tissue begins to contract, resulting in narrowing of the esophagus. Adhesions between granulating areas occurs, resulting in pockets and bands. It is during this period that efforts must be made to reduce stricture formation.

Clinical Manifestations. The clinical picture of an esophageal burn is determined by the degree and extent of the lesion. In the initial phase, complaints consist of pain in the mouth and substernal region, hypersalivation, pain on swallowing, and dysphagia. Fever correlates best with the presence of an esophageal lesion. Bleeding can occur, and frequently the patient vomits. These initial complaints disappear during the quiescent period of ulceration and granulation. During the cicatrization and scarring phase the complaint of dysphagia reappears and is due to fibrosis and retraction resulting in narrowing of the esophagus. Of the patients who develop strictures, 60 percent do so within 1 month, and 80 percent within 2 months. If dysphagia does not develop within 8 months it is unlikely that a stricture will occur. Serious systemic reactions such as hypovolemia and acidosis resulting in renal damage can occur in burns caused by strong acids. Respiratory complications such as laryngospasm, laryngedema, and occasionally pulmonary edema can occur, especially when strong acids are aspirated.

Inspection of the oral cavity and pharynx can indicate that caustic substances were swallowed, but does not mean that the esophagus has been burned. The reverse situation also occurs, i.e., esophageal burns can be present without apparent oral injuries. Because of this poor correlation, early esophagoscopy is advocated to establish the presence of an esophageal injury. The scope should not be introduced beyond the proximal esophageal lesion, in order to lessen the possibility of perforation. The degree of injury can be graded according to Table 23-17. Even if the esophagoscopy is normal, strictures may appear later. Radiographic examination is not a reliable means to identify the presence of early esophageal injury but is important in later follow-up to identify strictures. The most common locations of caustic injuries are shown in Table 23-18.

Treatment. Treatment of a caustic lesion of the esophagus attempts to cope with both the immediate and late consequences of the injury. The immediate treatment consists of limiting the burn by swallowing neutralizing agents. To be effective, this must be done within the first hour. Lye or other alkali can be neutralized with half-strength vinegar, lemon or orange juice. Acid can be neutralized with milk, egg white, or antacids. Sodium bicarbonate is not used because it generates CO_2, which might increase the danger of perforation. Emetics are contraindicated, since vomiting renews the contact of the caustic substance with the esophagus and can contribute to perforation if too forceful. Hypovolemia is corrected and broad-spectrum antibiotics are administered to lessen the inflammatory reaction and prevent infectious complications. If necessary a feeding jejunostomy tube is inserted to provide nutrition. Oral feeding can be started when the dysphagia of the initial phase has regressed.

In the past, surgeons waited until the appearance of a stricture before starting treatment. More recently dilations are started the first day after the injury, with the aim of preserving the esophageal lumen by removing the adhesions that occurred in the injured segments. This approach, however, is controversial in that dilations can traumatize the esophagus, causing bleeding and perforation, and there are data indicating that excessive dilations cause increased fibrosis secondary to the added trauma. The use of steroids to limit fibrosis has been shown to be effective in animals, but their effectiveness in man is debatable.

Extensive necrosis of the esophagus frequently leads to perforation and is best managed by resection. When there is extensive gastric involvement, the esophagus is nearly always necrotic or severely burned, and total gastrectomy and near-total esophagectomy are necessary. The presence of air in the esophageal wall is an indication of muscle necrosis and impending perforation and should encourage esophagectomy.

Table 23-17
Endoscopic Grading of Corrosive Esophageal and Gastric Burns

1° =	Mucosal hyperemia and edema
2° =	Limited hemorrhage, exudate, ulceration and pseudomembrane formation
3° =	Sloughing of mucosa, deep ulcers, massive hemorrhage, complete obstruction of lumen by edema, charring, and perforation

Table 23-18
Location of Caustic Injury (n = 62)

Pharynx		10%
Esophagus		70%
Upper	15%	
Middle	65%	
Lower	2%	
Whole	18%	
Stomach		20%
Antral	91%	
Whole	9%	
Both stomach and esophagus		14%

Management of acute injury is summarized in the algorithm in Fig. 23-75. Some authors have advocated the use of an intraluminal esophageal stent (Fig. 23-76) in patients who are operated upon and found not to have evidence of extensive esophagogastric necrosis. In these patients, a biopsy of the posterior gastric wall should be performed in order to exclude occult injury. If histologically there is a question of viability, a second-look operation should be done within 36 hours. If a stent is inserted it should be kept in position for 21 days, and removed after a satisfactory barium esophagogram. Esophagoscopy should be done and if strictures are present, dilations initiated.

Once the acute phase has passed, attention is turned to the preventon and management of strictures. Both antegrade dilation with a Hurst or Maloney bougie and retrograde dilation with a Tucker bougie have been satisfactory. Occasionally, particularly with severe strictures, the patient is instructed to swallow a string, over which metal Sippy dilators are passed until an adequate lumen can be obtained for passage of a mercury bougie. Reported experience with early dilations started during the acute phase in 1079 patients gave excellent results in 78 percent, good in 13 percent, and poor in 2 percent. Fifty-five patients died during the treatment. By contrast, the experience with 333 patients whose stricture were dilated when they became symptomatic, showed that only 21 percent had excellent results, 46 percent good, and 6 percent poor, with 3 dying during the process. The length of time the surgeon should persist with dilation before consideration of esophageal resection is problematic. An adequate lumen should be reestablished within 6 months to 1 year, with progressively longer intervals between dilations. If during the course of treatment an adequate lumen cannot be established or maintained, i.e., smaller bougies must be used, operative intervention should be considered. Surgical intervention is indicated when there is (1) complete stenosis in which all attempts from above and below have failed to establish a lumen, (2) marked irregularity and pocketing on barium swallow, (3) the development of a severe periesophageal reaction or mediastinitis with dilatation, (4) a fistula, (5) the inability to dilate or maintain the lumen above a 40 French bougie, or (6) a patient who is unwilling or unable to undergo prolonged periods of dilation.

The choice of operation cannot be stated dogmatically. The variety of abnormalities seen requires that creativity be used when considering esophageal reconstruction. Skin tube esophagoplasties are used much less frequently in recent years and are mainly of historic interest. Currently the stomach, jejunum, and colon are the organs used to replace the esophagus through either the posterior mediastinum or the retrosternal route. A retrosternal route is chosen when there has been a previous esophagectomy or there is extensive fibrosis in the posterior mediastinum. When all factors are considered, the order of preference for an esophageal substitute is (1) colon, (2) stomach, and (3) jejunum. Free jejunal grafts

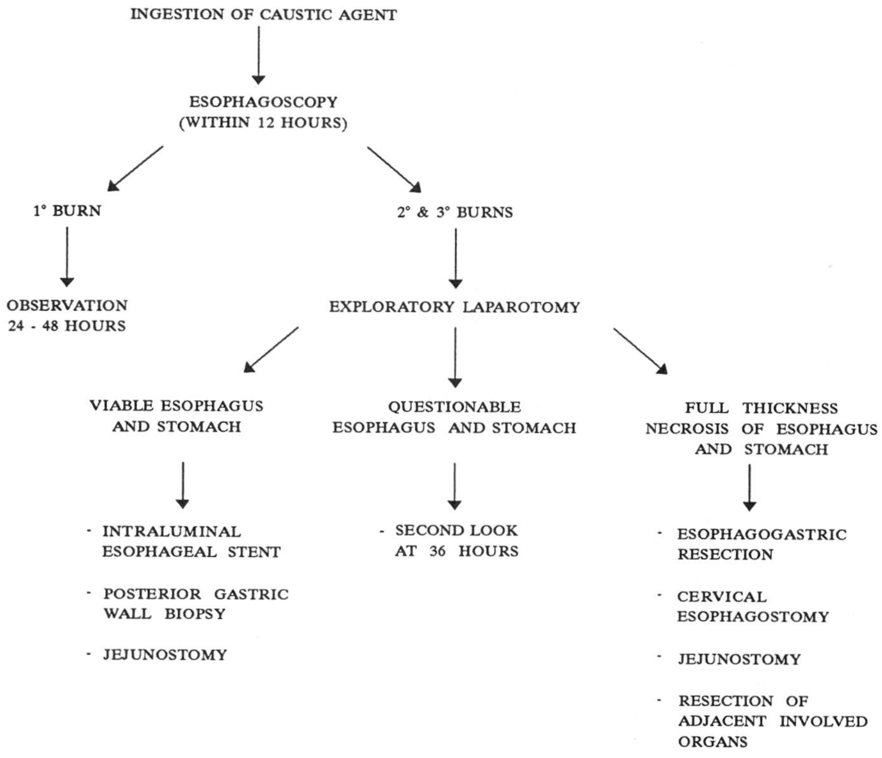

FIG. 23-75. Algorithm summarizing the management of acute caustic injury.

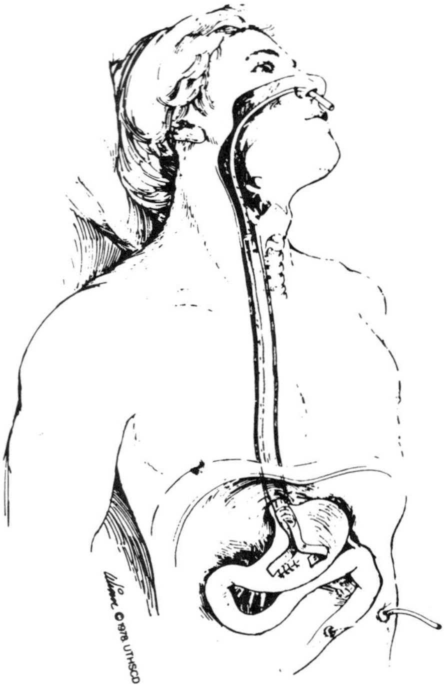

FIG. 23-76. The use of an esophageal stent to prevent stricture. The stent is constructed from a chest tube and placed in the esophagus at the time of an exploratory laparotomy. A Penrose drain is placed over the distal end as a flap valve to prevent reflux. The stent is supported at its upper end by attaching it to a suction catheter which is secured to the nares. Continuous suction removes saliva and mucus trapped in the pharynx and upper esophagus.

based on the superior thyroid artery have provided excellent results. Whatever method is selected, it must be emphasized that these procedures cannot be taken lightly, minor errors of judgment or technique may lead to serious or even fatal complications.

Critical in the planning of the operation is the selection of the site for proximal anastomosis, whether cervical esophagus, pyriform sinus, or posterior pharynx. The site of the upper anastomosis depends on the extent of the pharyngeal and cervical esophageal damage encountered. When the cervical esophagus is destroyed and a pyriform sinus remains open, the anastomosis can be made to the hypopharynx (Fig. 23-77). When the pyriform sinuses are completely stenosed, a transglottic approach is used to perform an anastomosis to the posterior oropharyngeal wall (Fig. 23-78). This allows excision of supraglottic strictures and elevation and anterior tilting of the larynx. In both of these situations the patient must relearn to swallow. Recovery is long and difficult and may require several endoscopic dilations and often reoperations. Sleeve resections of short strictures are not successful because the extent of damage to the wall of the esophagus can be greater than realized, and almost invariably the anastomosis is carried out in a diseased area.

The management of a bypassed damaged esophagus after injury is problematic. If the esophagus is left in place, ulceration from gastroesophageal reflux or the development of carcinoma must be considered. However, the extensive dissection necessary to remove the esophagus, particularly in the presence of marked periesophagitis, has a significant morbidity. Further, leaving the esophagus in place preserves the function of the vagus nerves, and

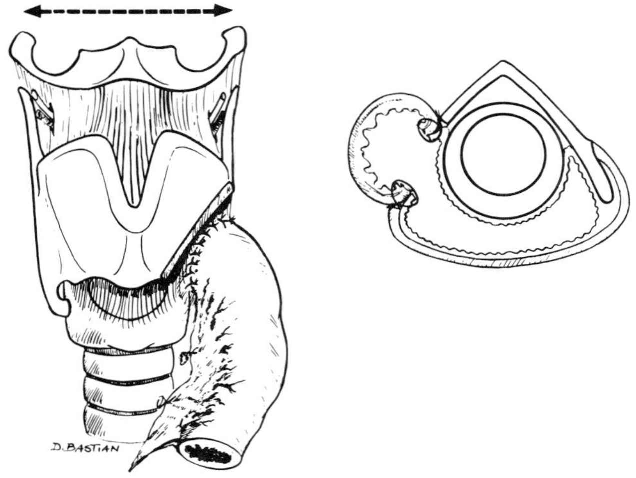

FIG. 23-77. Anastomosis of the bowel to a preserved pyriform sinus. To identify the site, a finger is inserted into the free pyriform sinus through a suprahyoid incision (*dotted line*). This requires removing the lateral inferior portion of the thyroid cartilage as shown in cross section. (From: *Huy PTB, Celerier M: Ann Surg 207:442, 1988, with permission.*)

in turn the function of the stomach. On the other hand, leaving a damaged esophagus in place can result in multiple blind sacs and subsequent development of mediastinal abscesses years later. In general, most experienced surgeons recommend that the esophagus should be removed unless the operative risk is unduly high.

DIAPHRAGMATIC HERNIAS

With the advent of clinical radiology, it became evident that a diaphragmatic hernia was a relatively common abnormality and was not always accompanied by symptoms. Three types of esophageal hiatal hernia were identified: (1) the sliding hernia, Type I, characterized by an upward dislocation of the cardia in the poste-

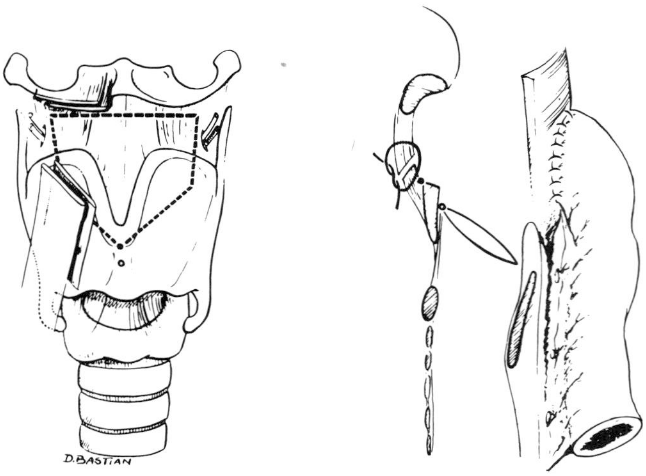

FIG. 23-78. Anastomosis of the bowel to the posterior oropharynx. The anastomosis is done through an inverted trapezoid incision above the thyroid cartilage (*dotted line*). A triangle-shaped piece of the upper half of the cartilage is resected. Closure of the oropharynx is done so that the larynx is pulled up (sagittal section). (From: *Huy PTB, Celerier M: Ann Surg 207:442, 1988, with permission.*)

rior mediastinum (Fig. 23-79*A*); (2) the rolling or paraesophageal hernia, Type II, characterized by an upward dislocation of the gastric fundus alongside a normally positioned cardia (Fig. 23-79*B*); and (3) the combined sliding-rolling or mixed hernia, Type III, characterized by an upward dislocation of both the cardia and the gastric fundus (Fig. 23-79*C*). The end stage of a Type I and II hernia occurs when the whole stomach migrates up into the chest by rotating 180° around its longitudinal axis, with the cardia and pylorus as fixed points. In this situation the abnormality is usually referred to as an intrathoracic stomach (Fig. 23-79*D*).

Incidence and Etiology. The true incidence of a hiatal hernia in the overall population is difficult to determine because of the absence of symptoms in a large number of patients who are subsequently shown to have a hernia. When radiographic examinations are done in response to gastrointestinal symptoms, the incidence of a sliding hiatal hernia is seven times higher than that of a paraesophageal hernia. The age distribution of patients with paraesophageal hernias is significantly different from that observed in sliding hiatal hernias. The median age of the former is sixty-one, whereas the latter is forty-eight years. Paraesophageal hernias are more likely to occur in women by a ratio of 4 to 1.

Structural deterioration of the phrenoesophageal membrane over time may explain the higher incidence of hiatal hernias in the older age group. These changes involve thinning of the upper fascial layer of the phrenoesophageal membrane (i.e., the supradiaphragmatic continuation of the endothoracic fascia) and loss of elasticity in the lower fascial layer (i.e., the infradiaphragmatic continuation of the transversalis fascia). Consequently, the phrenoesophageal membrane yields to stretching in the cranial direction due to the persistent intraabdominal pressure and the tug of esophageal shortening on swallowing. The upper fascial layer is formed only by loose connective tissue and is of little importance. The lower fascial layer is thick, stronger, and more important. It divides into an upper and lower leaf about 1 cm before attaching intimately with the esophageal adventitia. Due to stretching in the cranial direction, the attachment of the lower leaf protrudes upward and can frequently be identified in the thoracic cavity (Fig. 23-80).

These observations suggest that the development of a hiatal hernia appears to be a phenomenon related to age and is secondary to repetitive upward stretching of the phrenoesophageal membrane. A paraesophageal hernia rather than a sliding hernia develops when there is a defect, perhaps congenital, in the esophageal hiatus anterior to the esophagus. The persistent posterior fixation of the cardia to the preaortic fascia and the median arcuate ligament is the only essential difference between a sliding and paraesophageal hernia. When an anterior defect in the hiatus occurs in association with a loss of fixation of the cardia, a mixed or Type III hernia develops.

Clinical Manifestations. The clinical presentation of a paraesophageal hiatal hernia differs from that of a sliding hernia. There is usually a higher prevalence of symptoms of dysphagia and postprandial fullness with paraesophageal hernias, but the typical symptoms of heartburn and regurgitation present in sliding hiatal hernias can also occur. Both are caused by gastroesophageal reflux secondary to an underlying mechanical deficiency of the cardia. The symptoms of dysphagia and postprandial fullness in patients with a paraesophageal hernia are explained by the compression of the adjacent esophagus by a distended cardia, or twisting of the gastroesophageal junction by the torsion of the stomach that occurs as it becomes progressively displaced in the chest.

About one-third of patients with a paraesophageal hernia complain of hematemesis due to recurrent bleeding from ulceration of the gastric mucosa in the herniated portion of the stomach. Respiratory complications are frequently associated with a paraesophageal hernia and consist of dyspnea from mechanical compression and recurrent pneumonia from aspiration. With time the stomach migrates into the chest and can cause intermittent obstruction due to the rotation that has occurred. Conversely, many patients with paraesophageal hiatal hernia are asymptomatic or complain of very minor symptoms. On the other hand, the presence of a paraesophageal hernia is life-threatening in one-fifth of patients in that the hernia can lead to sudden catastrophic events, such as excessive bleeding or volvulus with acute gastric obstruction or infarction. With mild dilatation of the stomach, the gastric blood supply can be markedly reduced, causing gastric ischemia, ulceration, perforation, and sepsis.

The symptoms of sliding hiatal hernias are usually due to functional abnormalities associated with gastroesophageal reflux and include heartburn, regurgitation, and dysphagia. These patients have a mechanically defective lower esophageal sphincter, giving rise to the reflux of gastric juice into the esophagus and the symptoms of heartburn and regurgitation. The symptom of dysphagia occurs from the presence of mucosal edema, Schatzki's ring, stricture, or the inability to organize peristaltic activity in the body of the esophagus as a consequence of the disease.

There are a group of patients with sliding hiatal hernias not associated with reflux disease who have dysphagia without any obvious endoscopic or manometric explanation. Video barium radiograms have shown that the cause of dysphagia in these patients is an obstruction of the swallowed bolus by diaphragmatic impingement on the herniated stomach. Manometrically, this is reflected by a double-humped high-pressure zone at the gastroesophageal junction (Fig. 23-81). The first pressure rise is due to diaphragmatic impingement on the herniated stomach and the second to the true distal esophageal sphincter. These patients usually have a mechanically competent sphincter, but the impingement of the diaphragm on the stomach can result in propelling the contents of the supradiaphragmatic portion of the stomach up into the esophagus and pharynx, resulting in complaints of pharyngeal regurgitation and aspiration. Consequently this abnormality is often confused with typical gastroesophageal reflux disease. Surgical reduction of the hernia results in relief of the dysphagia in 91 percent of patients.

Diagnosis. A radiogram of the chest with the patient in the upright position can diagnose a hiatal hernia if it shows an air-fluid level behind the cardiac shadow (Fig. 23-82). This is usually caused by a paraesophageal hernia or an intrathoracic stomach. The accuracy of the upper gastrointestinal barium study in detecting a paraesophageal hiatal hernia is greater than for a sliding hernia, since the latter can often spontaneously reduce. The paraesophageal hiatal hernia is a permanent herniation of the stomach into the thoracic cavity, so that a barium swallow provides the diagnosis in virtually every case. Attention should be focused on the position of the gastroesophageal junction, when seen, to differentiate it from a Type II hernia (see Fig. 23-79*B,C*).

Fiberoptic esophagoscopy is very useful in the diagnosis and classification of a hiatal hernia because of the ability to retroflex the scope. In this position, a sliding hiatal hernia can be identified

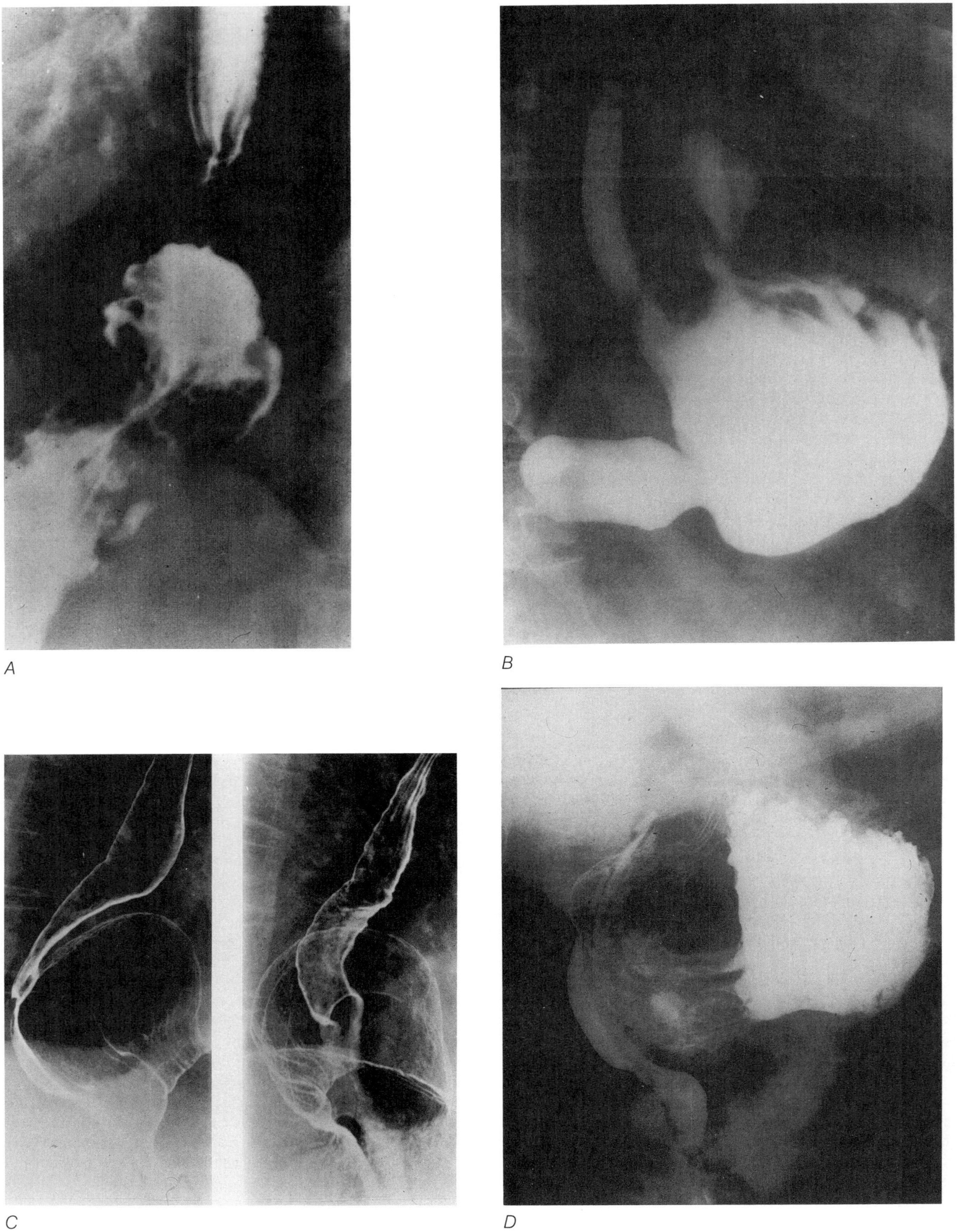

FIG. 23-79. *A.* Radiogram of a Type I sliding hiatal hernia. *B.* Radiogram of a Type II rolling or paraesophageal hernia. *C.* Radiogram of a Type III combined sliding-rolling or mixed hernia. *D.* Radiogram of an intrathoracic stomach. This is the end stage of a large hiatal hernia regardless of its initial classification. Note that the stomach has rotated 180° around its longitudinal axis, with the cardia and pylorus as fixed points. (From: *DeMeester TR, Bonavina L: Paraesophageal hiatal hernia, in Nyhus LM, Condon RE (eds): Hernia, 3rd ed. Philadelphia, Lippincott, 1989, pp 684, 685, 686, with permission.*)

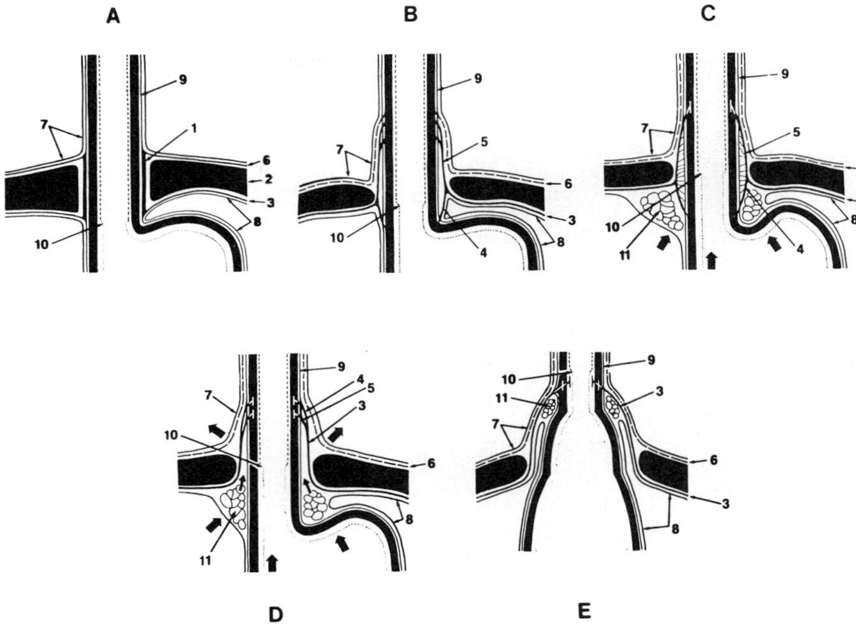

FIG. 23-80. Changes in the anatomy of the phrenoesophageal membrane over time based on the dissection of 163 human cadavers from the fetal period to age seventy-five years. *A.* Fetus. *B.* Newborn and small infants and young adults twenty to thirty years of age. *C.* Old adults fifty-five to seventy years of age. *D.* Old adults in transition to a hiatal hernia. *E.* Old adults with hiatal hernia. (From: *DeMeester TR, Bonavina L: Paraesophageal hiatal hernia, in Nyhus LM, Condon RE (eds): Hernia, 3rd ed. Philadelphia, Lippincott, 1989, p 687, with permission.*)

by noting a gastric pouch lined with rugal folds extending above the impression caused by the crura of the diaphragm (Fig. 23-83), or measuring at least 2 cm between the crura, identified by having the patient sniff, and the squamous-columnar junction on withdrawal of the scope (Fig. 23-84). A paraesophageal hernia is identified on retroversion of the scope by noting a separate orifice adjacent to the gastroesophageal junction into which gastric rugal folds ascend (Fig. 23-85). A sliding-rolling or mixed hernia can be identified by noting a gastric pouch lined with rugal folds above the diaphragm, with the gastroesophageal junction entering about midway up the side of the pouch (Fig. 23-86).

Pathophysiology. It has been assumed for a long time that a sliding hiatal hernia is associated with an incompetent distal esophageal sphincter, whereas a paraesophageal hiatal hernia constitutes a pure anatomic entity and is not associated with an incompetent cardia. Accordingly, surgical therapy has been directed toward restoration of the physiology of the cardia in patients with a sliding hernia, and simply reducing the stomach into the abdominal cavity and closing the crura for a paraesophageal hernia.

Over the past three decades there has been an increased interest in the physiology of the gastroesophageal junction and its relationship to the various types of hiatal hernias. Physiologic testing with 24-hour esophageal pH monitoring has shown increased esophageal exposure to acid gastric juice in 60 percent of the patients with a paraesophageal hiatal hernia compared with the observed 71 percent incidence in patients with a sliding hiatal hernia. Thus, it is now recognized that paraesophageal hiatal hernia can be associated with pathologic gastroesophageal reflux.

Physiologic studies have shown that the competency of the cardia depends on an interrelationship of distal esophageal sphincter pressure, the sphincter's length exposed to the positive-pressure

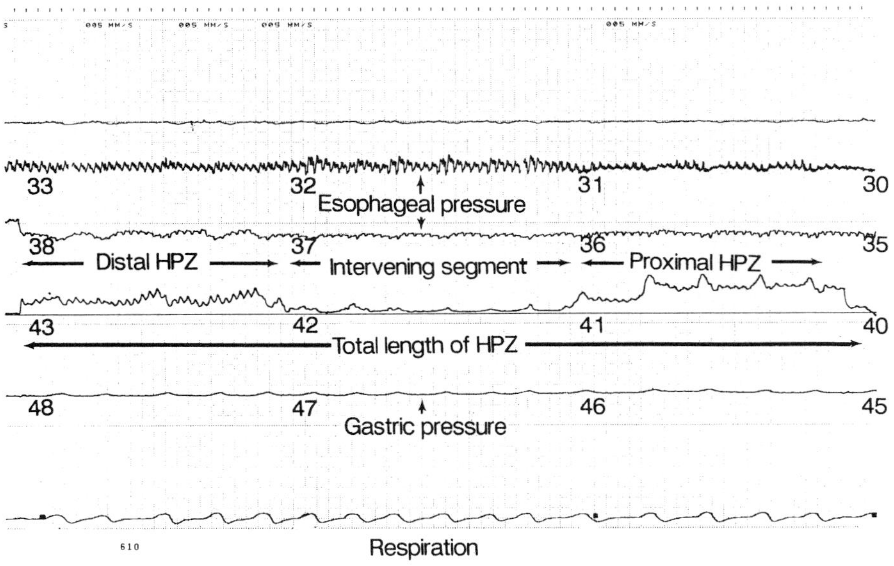

FIG. 23-81. The double-hump phenomenon seen on esophageal manometry showing various divisions of the double-hump segment. HPZ = high pressure zone. (From: *Kaul BK, DeMeester TR, et al: Ann Surg 211:407, 1990, with permission.*)

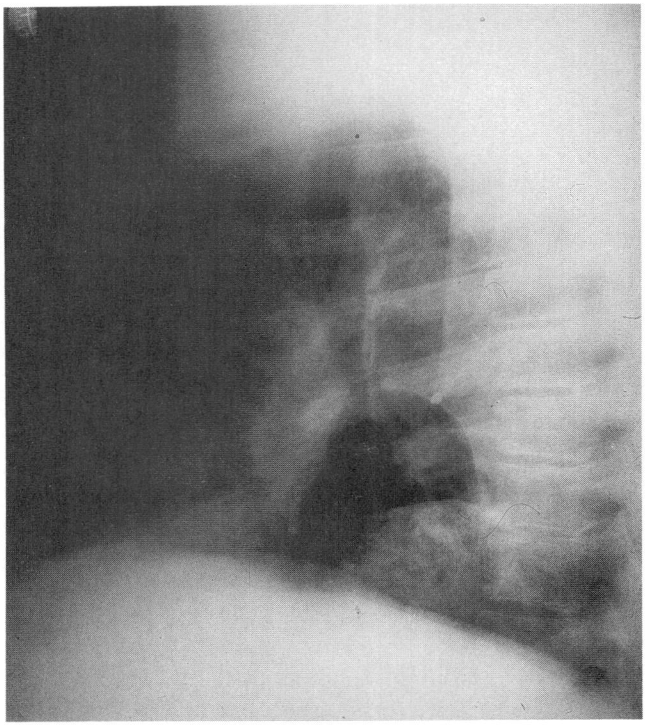

FIG. 23-82. Lateral chest radiogram showing a posterior mediastinal air-fluid level in a gas bubble, indicating the presence of a paraesophageal hernia. (From: *DeMeester TR, Bonavina L: Paraesophageal hiatal hernia, in Nyhus LM, Condon RE (eds): Hernia, 3rd ed. Philadelphia, Lippincott, 1989, p 688, with permission.*)

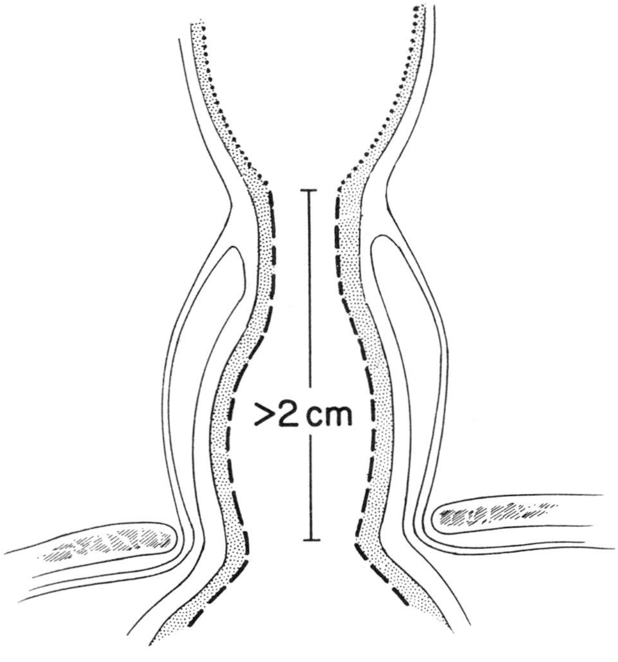

FIG. 23-84. Schematic diagram of the endoscopic criteria for diagnosing a sliding hiatal hernia: a gastric pouch above the crural impression measuring at least 2 cm between the crura, identified by having the patient sniff, and the squamocolumnar junction with the patient resting in the left lateral position and breathing quietly. (From: *DeMeester TR, Bonavina L: Paraesophageal hiatal hernia, in Nyhus LM, Condon RE (eds): Hernia, 3rd ed. Philadelphia, Lippincott, 1989, p 689, with permission.*)

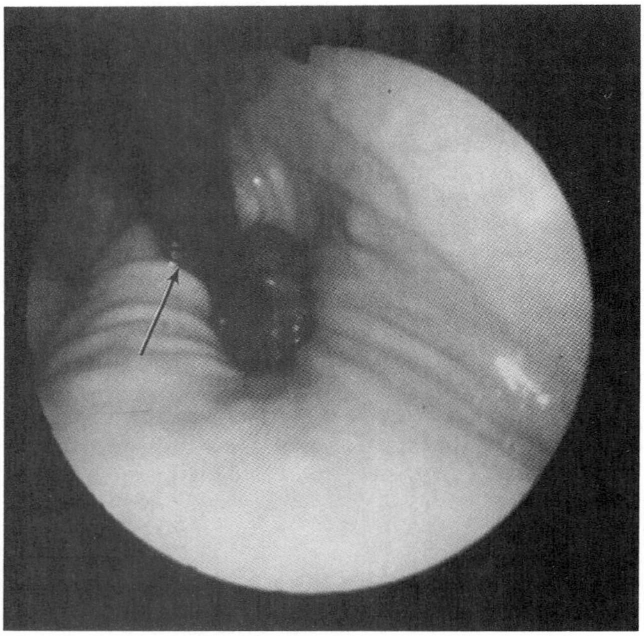

FIG. 23-83. Endoscopic view through a retroflexed fiberoptic gastroscope showing the shaft of the scope (*arrow*) coming down through a sliding hernia. Note the gastric rugal folds extending above the impression caused by the crura of the diaphragm. (From: *DeMeester TR, Bonavina L: Paraesophageal hiatal hernia, in Nyhus LM, Condon RE (eds): Hernia, 3rd ed. Philadelphia, Lippincott, 1989, p 689, with permission.*)

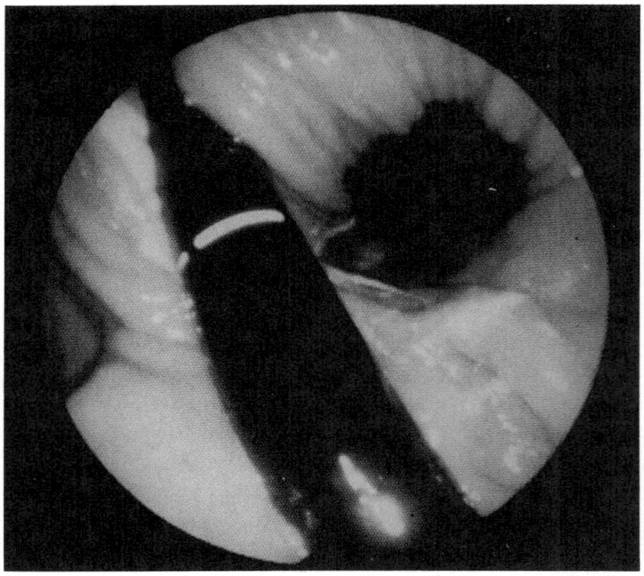

FIG. 23-85. Endoscopic view through a retroflexed fiberoptic gastroscope showing the shaft of the scope coming down through the gastroesophageal junction adjacent to a separate orifice of the paraesophageal hernia into which the gastric rugal folds ascend. (From: *DeMeester TR, Bonavina L: Paraesophageal hiatal hernia, in Nyhus LM, Condon RE (eds): Hernia, 3rd ed. Philadelphia, Lippincott, 1989, p 689, with permission.*)

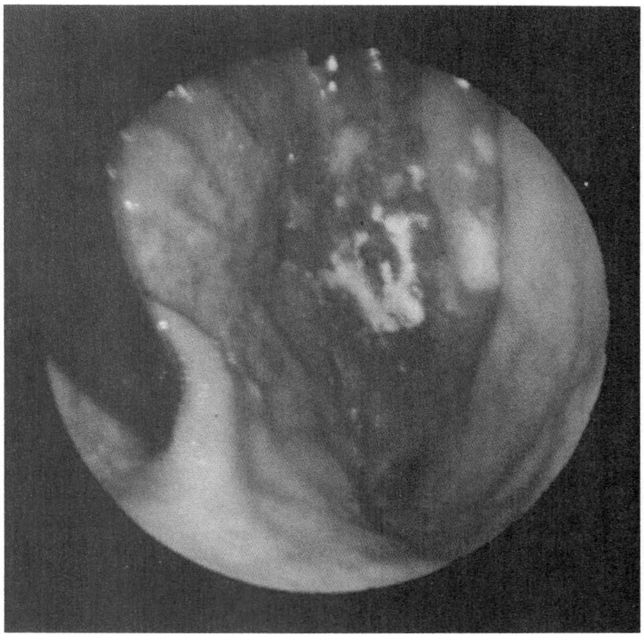

FIG. 23-86. Endoscopic view through a retroflexed fiberoptic gastroscope showing the shaft of the scope entering a hernia about midway up the side of a mixed hiatal hernial pouch that extends high into the thorax. (From: *DeMeester TR, Bonavina L: Paraesophageal hiatal hernia, in Nyhus LM, Condon RE (eds): Hernia, 3rd ed. Philadelphia, Lippincott, 1989, p 689, with permission.*)

environment of the abdomen, and its overall length. A deficiency in any one of these manometric characteristics of the sphincter is associated with incompetency of the cardia regardless of whether a hernia is present. Patients with a paraesophageal hernia who have incompetent cardias have been shown to have a distal esophageal sphincter with normal pressure but a shortened overall length and displacement outside the positive-pressure environment of the abdomen (Fig. 23-87). In a sliding hernia, even though the sphincter appears to be within the chest on a radiographic barium study, it still can be exposed to abdominal pressure because of the surrounding hernial sac which functions as an extension of the abdominal cavity. A high insertion of the phrenoesophageal membrane into the esophagus gives adequate length of the distal esophageal sphincter exposed to abdominal pressure. A low insertion gives inadequate length (Fig. 23-88). The importance of the anatomic length of esophagus within the hernial sac has been emphasized by Bombeck, Dillard, and Nyhus in their careful dissections of the hiatus. They showed that in 55 patients who underwent postmortem dissection, there were 8 who had a hiatal hernia, 5 of whom had no evidence of esophagitis and, therefore, a competent cardia. In these 5 patients, the phrenoesophageal membrane inserted 2 to 5 cm (with a mean of 3.6 cm) above the gastroesophageal junction. The other 3 patients had evidence of esophagitis and therefore an incompetent cardia. In these patients the membrane inserted 1 cm or less with a mean of 0.5 cm) above the gastroesophageal junction. This difference was significant and emphasized the importance of an adequate length of intraabdominal esophagus in maintaining competency of the cardia even in the presence of a hiatal hernia.

In contrast to a paraesophageal hernia, where the sphincter remains fixed in the abdomen, in a mixed Type III hernia the sphincter moves extraperitoneally into the thorax through the widened hiatus along with a portion of the lesser curvature of the stomach and cardia and forms part of the wall of the hernial sac. Consequently, the lower esophageal sphincter lies outside the abdominal cavity and is unaffected by its environmental pressures. The loss of normal esophageal fixation that occurs in a Type I sliding hernia or a Type III mixed hernia results in the body of the esophagus being less able to carry out its propulsive function. This contributes to a greater exposure of the distal esophagus to refluxed gastric juice when components of an incompetent cardia are present. In summary, the causes for a mechanical incompetency of the cardia are similar regardless of the type of hernia and are identical with those in patients who have an incompetent cardia and no hiatal hernia.

Therapy. The presence of a paraesophageal hiatal hernia is an indication for surgical repair. The catastrophic, life-threatening complications of bleeding, infarction, and perforation that are part of the natural history of the hernia in about 25 percent of patients drive its surgical correction even in the elderly with a shorter life expectancy.

In the report of Skinner and Belsey, 6 of 21 patients with a paraesophageal hernia treated medically died from the complications of strangulation, perforation, or exsanguinating hemorrhage secondary to acute dilatation of the herniated intrathoracic stomach. These catastrophes occurred for the most part without warning. With this in mind, patients with a paraesophageal hernia are counseled to have elective repair of their hernia regardless of the severity of their symptoms or the size of the hernia. If surgery is delayed and repair is done on an emergency basis, there is a 19 percent operative mortality, compared with less than 1 percent for an elective repair.

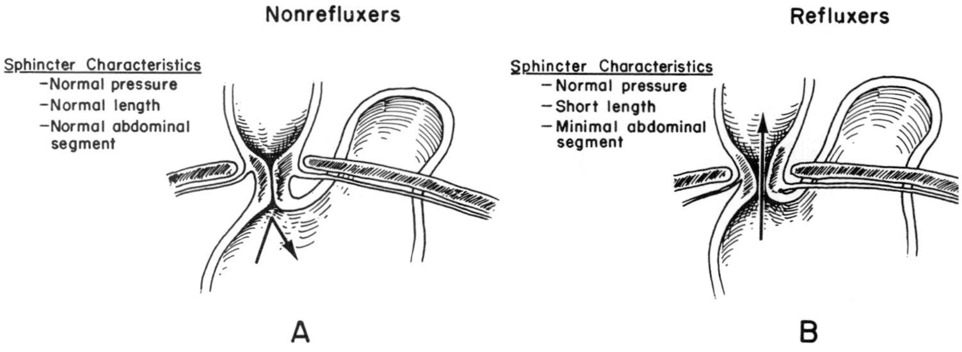

FIG. 23-87. Schematic diagram of the anatomic and manometric difference between patients with a paraesophageal hiatal hernia with reflux and those without reflux, based on 24-hour esophageal pH monitoring. (From: *DeMeester TR, Bonavina L: Paraesophageal hiatal hernia, in Nyhus LM, Condon RE (eds): Hernia, 3rd ed. Philadelphia, Lippincott, 1989, p 690, with permission.*)

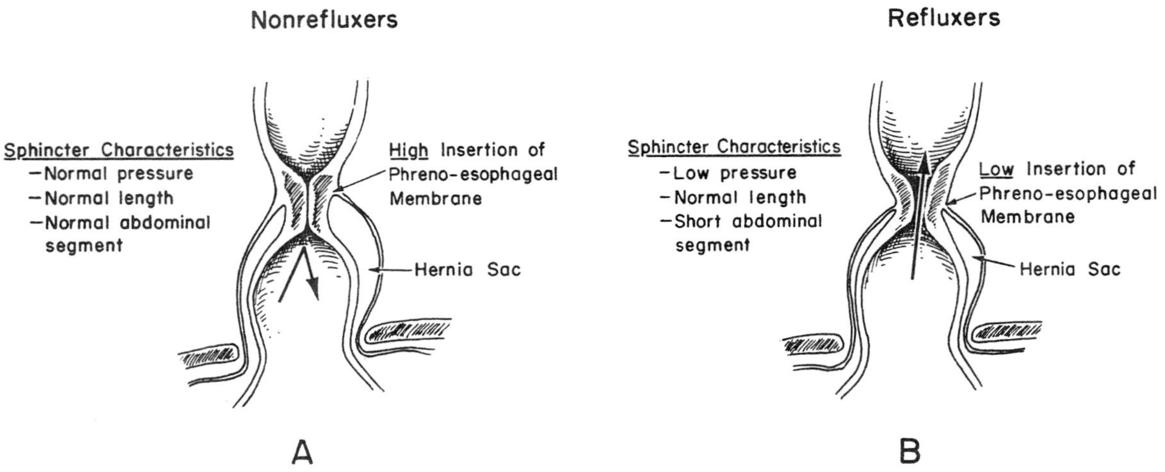

FIG. 23-88. Schematic diagram of the anatomic and manometric difference between patients with a sliding hiatal hernia with reflux and those without reflux, based on 24-hour esophageal pH monitoring. (From: *DeMeester TR, Bonavina L: Paraesophageal hiatal hernia, in Nyhus LM, Condon RE (eds): Hernia, 3rd ed. Philadelphia, Lippincott, 1989, p 691, with permission.*)

Based on pathophysiologic studies on patients with a paraesophageal hiatal hernia, the repair of a paraesophageal hernia should include an antireflux procedure to correct the sphincter characteristics associated with a mechanically incompetent cardia. This is particularly necessary when the operation is performed on an urgent basis without preoperative studies. If time permits, preoperative evaluation with 24-hour esophageal pH monitoring and esophageal manometry allows the identification of patients with competent cardias. Such patients are candidates for a simple anatomic repair, provided it can be done without surgical dissection of the cardia. If dissection of the cardia is necessary, an antireflux procedure should be added to the repair. Operative repair of sliding hiatal hernias is driven by symptoms of or complications of gastroesophageal reflux disease, unless it is determined that the patient has impingement of the stomach by the diaphragm as a cause of symptoms as discussed above.

MISCELLANEOUS ESOPHAGEAL LESIONS

Plummer-Vinson Syndrome

This uncommon clinical syndrome is characterized by dysphagia associated with atrophic oral mucosa, spoon-shaped fingers with brittle nails, and chronic anemia. It characteristically occurs in middle-aged edentulous women. Iron-deficiency anemia is a common finding; thus the synonym sideropenic dysphagia has been advocated by some. The syndrome is more common in the Scandinavian countries than in the United States, and its presentation is variable. Not all patients exhibit the classic syndrome, some lacking iron-deficiency anemia and others with the typical clinical stigmata but lacking dysphagia or the presence of an esophageal web.

Videoradiographic study as well as endoscopic findings have demonstrated a fibrous web just below the cricopharyngeus muscle as the cause of dysphagia in these patients. Treatment consists of dilation of the web and iron therapy to correct the nutritional deficiency.

Clinical observation suggests that the esophageal web may actually be a drug-induced lesion. Since these patients have an iron-deficiency anemia, it would be logical for physicians to prescribe ferrous sulfate, a drug known to cause esophageal injury. It is reasonable to suspect that a number of such patients may have had a drug-induced esophageal injury develop at the site where the web is commonly observed. Not knowing the cause of the esophageal abnormality, the early observers reported the web as part of the syndrome.

Malignant lesions of the oral mucosa, hypopharynx, and esophagus have been noted to occur in up to 100 percent of patients when followed long-term.

Schatzki's Ring

Schatzki's ring is a thin submucosal circumferential ring in the lower esophagus at the squamocolumnar junction, often associated with a hiatal hernia. Its significance and pathogenesis are unclear (Fig. 23-89). The ring was first noted by Templeton, but Schatzki and Gary defined it as a distinct entity in 1953. Its prevalence varies from 0.2 to 14 percent in the general population, depending on the technique of diagnosis and the criteria used. Stiennon believed the ring to be a pleat of mucosa formed by infolding of redundant esophageal mucosa due to shortening of the esophagus. Others believe the ring to be congenital, and still others suggest it is an early stricture resulting from inflammation of the esophageal mucosa caused by chronic reflux.

Schatzki's ring is a distinct clinical entity having different symptoms, upper gastrointestinal function studies, and response to treatment when compared with patients with a hiatal hernia but without a ring. Twenty-four-hour esophageal pH monitoring showed that patients with a Schatzki's ring have a lower incidence of reflux than hiatal hernia controls. They also have better lower esophageal sphincter function. This, together with the presence of a ring, could represent a protective role to prevent gastroesophageal reflux.

Clinical symptoms associated with Schatzki's ring are episodes of short-lasting dysphagia during hurried ingestion of solid foods. Its treatment has varied from dilation alone to dilation with antireflux measures, antireflux procedure alone, incision, and even excision of the ring. Little is known about the natural progression of Schatzki's rings. Radiologically, Chen et al. showed progressive

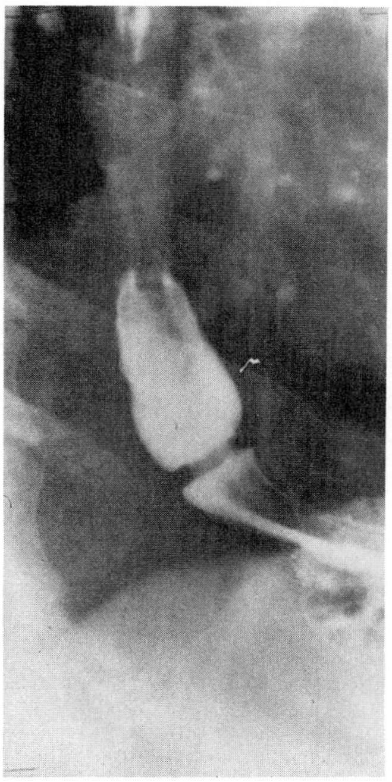

FIG. 23-89. Barium esophagogram showing Schatzki's ring, i.e., a thin circumferential ring in the distal esophagus at the squamocolumnar junction. Below the ring is a hiatal hernia.

stenosis of rings in 59 percent of patients, whereas Schatzki found the rings to decrease in diameter in 29 percent of patients and to remain unchanged in the remainder.

Symptoms in patients with a ring are caused more by the presence of the ring than by gastroesophageal reflux. Furthermore most patients with a ring but without proven reflux respond to one dilation, while most patients with proven reflux require repeated dilations. In this regard, the majority of Schatzki's ring patients without proven reflux have a history of ingestion of drugs known to be damaging to the esophageal mucosa. Bonavina et al. have suggested drug-induced injury as the cause of stenosis in patients with a ring but without a history of reflux. Since rings also occur in patients with proven reflux, it is likely that gastroesophageal reflux also plays a part. This is further supported by the fact that these patients have less drug ingestion. Thus Schatzki's ring is probably an acquired lesion that can lead to stenosis from chemical-induced injury by pill lodgment in the distal esophagus or from reflux-induced injury to the lower esophageal mucosa.

The best form of treatment of a symptomatic Schatzki's ring in patients who do not have reflux consists of esophageal dilation for relief of the obstructive symptoms. In patients with a ring who have proven reflux and a mechanically defective sphincter, an antireflux procedure is necessary to obtain relief and avoid repeated dilation.

Mallory-Weiss Syndrome

In 1929 Mallory and Weiss described four patients with acute upper gastrointestinal bleeding who were found at autopsy to have mucosal tears at the gastroesophageal junction. This syndrome, characterized by acute upper gastrointestinal bleeding following repeated vomiting, is considered to be the cause of up to 15 percent of all severe upper GI bleeds. The mechanism is similar to spontaneous esophageal perforation, i.e., an acute increase in intraabdominal pressure against a closed glottis in a patient with a hiatal hernia.

Mallory-Weiss tears are characterized by arterial bleeding which may be massive. Vomiting is not an obligatory factor, as there may be other causes of an acute increase in intraabdominal pressure, such as paroxysmal coughing, seizures, and retching. The diagnosis requires a high index of suspicion, particularly in the patient who develops upper gastrointestinal bleeding following prolonged vomiting or retching. Upper endoscopy confirms the suspicion, by identifying one or more longitudinal fissures in the mucosa of the herniated stomach as the source of bleeding.

In the majority of patients the bleeding will stop spontaneously with nonoperative management. In addition to blood replacement, the stomach should be decompressed and antiemetics administered, as a distended stomach and continued vomiting aggravate further bleeding. A Sengstaken-Blakemore tube will not stop the bleeding, as the pressure in the balloon is not sufficient to overcome arterial pressure. Only occasionally will surgery be required to stop blood loss. The procedure consists of laparotomy and high gastrotomy with oversewing of the linear tear. Mortality is uncommon and recurrence is rare.

Scleroderma

Scleroderma is a systemic disease wherein esophageal abnormalities occur in approximately 80 percent of patients. In most, the disease follows a prolonged course. Renal involvement occurs in a small percentage of patients and signals a poor prognosis. The onset of the disease is usually in the third or fourth decade of life, occurring twice as frequently in women as in men.

Small vessel inflammation appears to be an initiating event, with subsequent perivascular deposition of normal collagen which may lead to vascular compromise. In the gastrointestinal tract, the predominant feature is smooth muscle atrophy. Whether the atrophy in the esophageal musculature is a primary effect or occurs secondary to a neurogenic disorder is unknown. The results of pharmacologic and hormonal manipulation, with agents that act either indirectly via neural mechanisms or directly on the muscle, suggest that scleroderma is a primary neurogenic disorder. Methacholine, which acts directly on smooth muscle receptors, causes a similar increase in lower esophageal sphincter pressure in normal controls and in patients with scleroderma. Edrophonium, a cholinesterase inhibitor which enhances the effect of acetylcholine when given to patients with scleroderma, causes an increase in lower esophageal sphincter pressure that is less marked in these patients than in normal controls, suggesting the neurogenic rather than myogenic nature of the disorder. Muscle ischemia due to perivascular compression has been suggested as a possible mechanism for the motility abnormality in scleroderma. Others have observed that, in the early stage of the disease, the manometric abnormalities may be reversed by reserpine, an agent that depletes catecholamines from the adrenergic system. This suggests that an adrenergic overactivity may be present in early scleroderma which causes a parasympathetic inhibition and supports a neurogenic mechanism of the disease. In advanced disease manifested by smooth muscle atrophy and collagen deposition, reserpine no longer produces this reversal. Consequently, from a gastrointestinal perspective, we have a patient with a poor esophageal pump and a poor valve.

The diagnosis of scleroderma can be made manometrically by the observation of normal peristalsis in the proximal striated esophagus, with absent peristalsis in the distal smooth muscle portion (Fig. 23-90). The lower esophageal sphincter pressure is progressively weakened as the disease advances. Because many of the systemic sequelae of the disease may be nondiagnostic, the motility pattern is frequently used as a specific diagnostic indicator. Gastroesophageal reflux commonly occurs in patients with scleroderma, since they have both hypotensive sphincters and poor esophageal clearance. This combined defect can lead to severe esophagitis and stricture formation. The typical barium swallow shows a dilated, barium-filled esophagus, stomach, and duodenum, or a hiatal hernia with distal esophageal stricture and proximal dilatation (Fig. 23-91).

Traditionally, esophageal symptoms have been treated with H_2 blockers, antacids, elevation of the head of the bed, and multiple dilations for strictures, with generally unsatisfactory results. The degree of esophagitis is usually severe and leads to marked esophageal shortening. Consequently a Collis gastroplasty in combination with a Belsey antireflux repair is the usual procedure for the surgical management of this problem. Surgery reduces esophageal acid exposure but does not return it to normal because of the poor clearance function of the body of the esophagus. Consequently only 50 percent of the patients have a good to excellent result. If the esophagitis is severe or there has been a previous failed antireflux procedure and the disease is associated with delayed gastric emptying, a gastric resection with Roux-en-Y esophagojejunostomy and a Hunt-Lawrence pouch has proved the best option.

Acquired Fistula

The esophagus lies in immediate contact with the membranous portion of the trachea and left bronchus, predisposing to the formation of fistula to these structures. Most acquired esophageal fistulas are to the tracheobronchial tree and secondary to either esophageal or pulmonary malignancy. Traumatic fistulas and those associated with esophageal diverticula account for the remainder. Fistulas associated with traction diverticula are usually due to mediastinal inflammatory disease, and traumatic fistula usually occur secondary to penetrating wounds, lye ingestion, or iatrogenic injury.

Clinically these fistulas are characterized by paroxysmal coughing following the ingestion of liquids and by recurrent or chronic pulmonary infections. The onset of cough immediately after swallowing suggests aspiration, whereas a brief delay (30 to 60 seconds) suggests a fistula.

Spontaneous closure is rare, owing to the presence of malignancy or a recurrent infectious process. Surgical treatment of benign fistula consists of division of the fistulous tract, resection of irreversibly damaged lung tissue, and closure of the esophageal defect. To prevent recurrence, a pleural flap should be interposed. Treatment of malignant fistulas is difficult, particularly in the presence of prior irradiation. Generally only palliative treatment is indicated. This can be best done by using a specially designed esophageal endoprosthesis that bridges and occludes the fistula, allowing the patient to eat. Rarely esophageal diversion, coupled with placement of a feeding jejunostomy, can be used as a last resort.

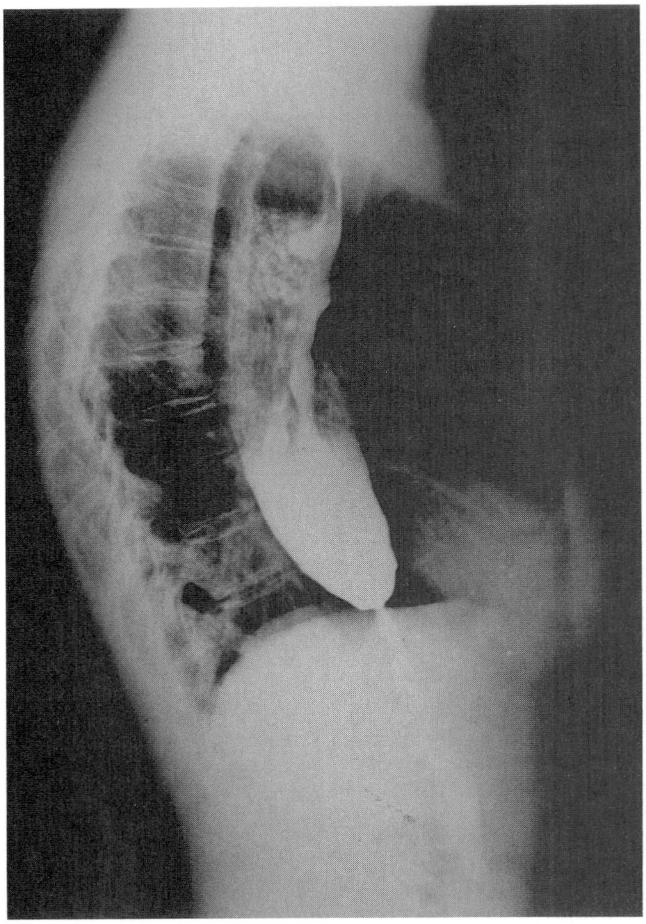

FIG. 23-91. Barium esophagogram of a patient with scleroderma and stricture. Note the markedly dilated esophagus and retained food material. (From: *Waters PF, DeMeester TR: Med Clin North Am 65:1253, 1981, with permission.*)

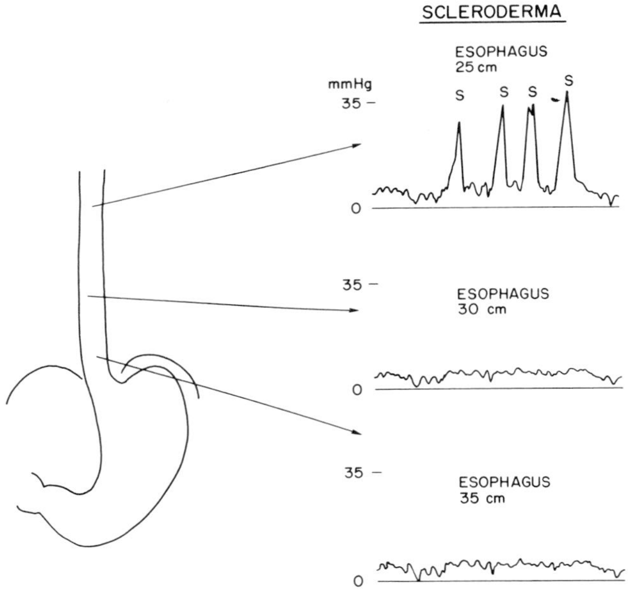

FIG. 23-90. Esophageal motility record in a patient with scleroderma showing aperistalsis in the distal two-thirds of the esophageal body with peristalsis in the proximal portion. (From: *Waters PF, DeMeester TR: Med Clin North Am 65:1252, 1981, with permission.*)

TECHNIQUES OF ESOPHAGEAL RECONSTRUCTION

Options for esophageal substitution include gastric advancement, colonic interposition, and either jejunal free transfer or advancement into the chest. Rarely combinations of these grafts will be the only possible option. The indications for esophageal resection and substitution include malignant and end-stage benign disease. The latter includes reflux- or drug-induced stricture formation that cannot be dilated without damage to the esophagus, a dilated and tortuous esophagus secondary to severe motility disorders, lye strictures, and multiple previous antireflux procedures. The choice of esophageal substitution has significant impact upon the technical difficulty of the procedure and influences the long-term outcome.

Partial Esophageal Resection. Low-lying benign lesions, with preserved proximal esophageal function, are best treated with the interposition of a segment of proximal jejunum into the chest and primary anastomosis. A jejunal interposition can reach to the inferior border of the pulmonary hilum with ease, but the architecture of its blood supply rarely allows the use of the jejunum above this point. Because the anastomosis is within the chest, a thoracotomy is necessary.

The jejunum is a dynamic graft and contributes to bolus transport, whereas the stomach and colon function more as a conduit. The stomach is a poor choice in this circumstance because of the propensity for the reflux of gastric contents into the upper esophagus following an intrathoracic esophagogastrostomy. It is now well recognized that this occurs, and can lead to incapacitating symptoms and esophageal destruction in some patients. Short segments of colon, on the other hand, lack significant motility and have a propensity for the development of esophagitis above the anastomosis.

Replacement of the cervical portion of the esophagus while preserving the distal portion is occasionally indicated in cervical esophageal or head and neck malignancy and following the ingestion of lye. Free transfer of a portion of jejunum to the neck has become a viable option and is successful the majority of the time. Revascularization is achieved via use of the internal mammary artery and the internal mammary or innominate vein. Removal of the sternoclavicular joint aids in performing the vascular and distal esophageal anastomosis (Fig. 23-92).

Reconstruction Following Total Esophagectomy. No pretense should be made that the intrathoracic stomach or colon functions as well as the native esophagus after an esophagogastrectomy. The choice between these organs will be influenced by several factors, such as the adequacy of their blood supply and the length of resected esophagus that they are capable of bridging. If the stomach is involved with pathology, or has been contracted or reduced by previous gastric surgery, the length available for esophageal replacement may not be adequate. The presence of diverticular disease, unrecognized carcinoma, or colitis prohibits the use of the colon. The blood supply of the colon is more affected than the stomach's by vascular disease, which may prevent its use. Of the two, the colon provides the longest graft. The stomach can usually reach to the neck if the amount of lesser curve resected does not interfere with the blood supply to the fundus. Gastric interposition has the advantage that only one anastomosis is required. On the other hand, there is greater potential for aspiration of gastric juice or stricturing of the cervical anastomosis from chronic reflux when stomach is used for replacement.

Patients following an esophagogastrectomy may have discomfort during or shortly after eating. The most common symptom is a postprandial pressure sensation or a feeling of being stuffed, which probably results from the loss of the gastric reservoir. This symptom is less common when the colon is used as an esophageal

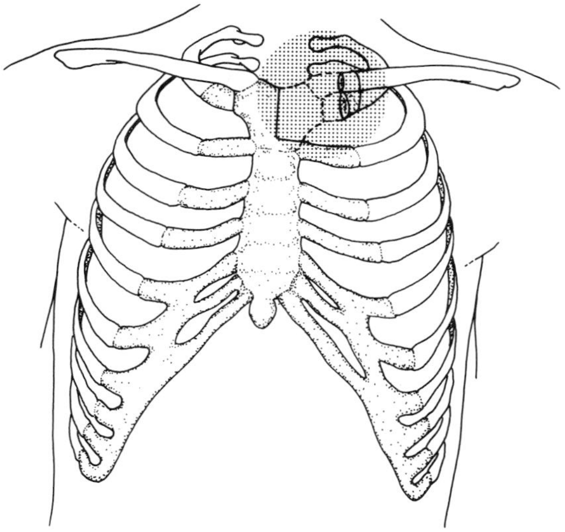

A

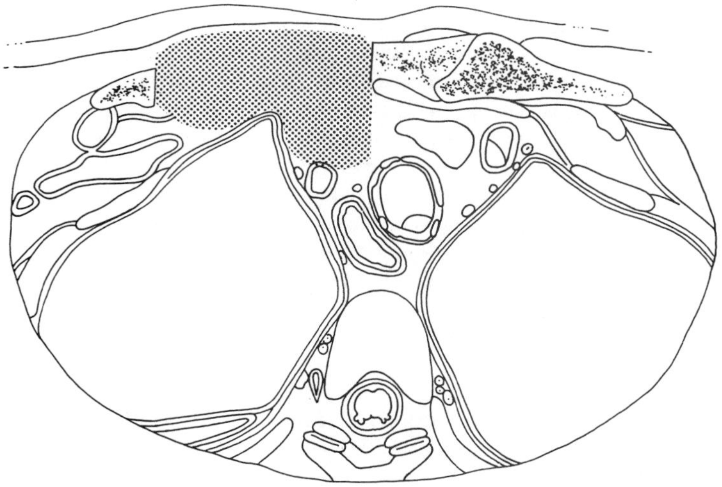

B

FIG. 23-92. *A.* The portion of the thoracic inlet to be resected in order to provide space for a free jejunal graft and access to the internal mammary artery. *B.* Cross section showing the space available after resection of the sternoclavicular joint and half of the manubrium. (From: *Rothberg M, DeMeester TR: Exposure of the cervical esophagus, in Shields TW (ed): General Thoracic Surgery, 3rd ed. Philadelphia, Lea & Febiger, 1989, p 419, with permission.*)

substitute, probably because the distal third of the stomach is retained in the abdomen and the interposed colon provides an additional reservoir function.

King and Hölscher have reported a 40 percent and 50 percent incidence of dysphagia after reestablishing gastrointestinal continuity with the stomach following esophagogastrectomy. This incidence is similar to Orringer's results after using the stomach to replace the esophagus in patients with benign disease. More than half of the patients experienced dysphagia postoperatively, two-thirds of whom required postoperative dilation and one-fourth of whom have persistent dysphagia and require home dilation. By contrast, dysphagia is uncommon and the need for dilation is rare following a colonic interposition. Isolauri reported on 248 patients with colonic interpositions and noted a 24 percent incidence of dysphagia 12 months after the operation. When it occurred, the most common cause was recurrent mediastinal tumor. The high incidence of dysphagia with the use of the stomach is probably related to the esophagogastric anastomosis in the neck and the difficulty this imposes on the passage of a swallowed bolus.

Another consequence of the transposition of the stomach into the chest is the development of postoperative duodenogastric reflux. It may be explained by pyloric denervation. Adding a pyloroplasty may worsen this problem. Following gastric advancement, the pylorus lies at the level of the esophageal hiatus, and a distinct pressure differential develops between the intrathoracic gastric and intraabdominal duodenal lumina. Unless the pyloric valve is extremely efficient, the pressure differential will encourage reflux of duodenal contents into the stomach. Duodenogastric reflux is less likely to occur following colonic interposition, because there is sufficient intraabdominal colon to be compressed by the abdominal pressure and the pylorus and duodenum remain in their normal intraabdominal position.

Although there is general acceptance of the concept that an esophagogastric anastomosis in the neck results in less postoperative esophagitis and stricture than one at a lower level, reflux esophagitis following a cervical anastomosis does occur, albeit at a slower rate than when the anastomosis is at a lower level. Most patients undergo cervical esophagogastrostomy for malignancy; thus the long-term sequelae of an esophagogastric anastomosis in the neck are not of concern. Patients who have had a cervical esophagogastrostomy for benign disease, however, may develop problems associated with the anastomosis in the fourth or fifth postoperative year severe enough to require anastomotic revision. This is less likely in patients who have had a colonic interposition for esophageal replacement. Consequently, in patients who have a benign process or a potentially curable carcinoma of the esophagus or cardia, a colonic interposition is used to obviate the late problems associated with a cervical esophagogastrostomy. Colonic interposition for esophageal substitution is a more complex procedure than gastric advancement, with the potential for greater perioperative morbidity, particularly in inexperienced hands.

Composite Reconstruction. Occasionally a combination of colon, jejunum and stomach is the only reconstructive option available. This situation may arise because of previous gastric or colonic resection, because of recurrence of dysphagia after a previous esophageal resection, or following postoperative complications such as ischemia of an esophageal substitute. Although not ideal, combinations of colon, jejunum, and stomach used to restore gastrointestinal continuity function surprisingly well. This recognition may allow alimentary reconstruction in an otherwise impossible situation.

Bibliography

General References

Castell DO (ed): *The Esophagus*. Boston, Little, Brown & Company, 1992.

DeMeester TR, Barlow AP: Surgery and current management for cancer of the esophagus and cardia: Part I. *Curr Probl Surg* 25(7):477, 1988.

DeMeester TR, Barlow AP: Surgery and current management for cancer of the esophagus and cardia: Part II. *Curr Probl Surg* 25(8):535, 1988.

Moody FG, Carey LC, et al (eds): *Surgical Treatment of Digestive Disease*, 2nd ed. Chicago, Year Book Medical Publishers, 1989.

Roth JA, Ruckdeschel JC, Weisenburger TH (eds): *Thoracic Oncology*. Philadelphia, Saunders, 1989.

Scott WH Jr., Sawyers JL (eds): *Surgery of the Stomach, Duodenum, and Small Intestine*, 2nd ed. Boston, Blackwell Scientific Publications, 1992.

Shields TW (ed): *General Thoracic Surgery*, 3rd ed. Philadelphia, Lea & Febiger, 1989.

Stein HJ, DeMeester TR, Hinder RA: Outpatient physiologic testing and surgical management of functional foregut disorders. *Curr Probl Surg* 24(7):418, 1992.

Zuidema GD, Orringer MB (eds): *Shackelford's Surgery of the Alimentary Tract*, 3rd ed, Vol I. Philadelphia, Saunders, 1991.

Surgical Anatomy

Gray SW, Rowe JS Jr, Skandalakis JE: Surgical anatomy of the gastroesophageal junction. *Am Surg* 45(9):575, 1979.

Halber MD, Daffner RH, Thompson WM: CT of the esophagus (carcinoma). *AJR* 133:1051, 1979.

Hurwitz A, Duranceau A, Haddad J: Disorders of esophageal motility. *Major Problems in Internal Medicine*, Vol XVI, Chap VII, 1979.

Johnson JB, Clagett OT, McDonald JR: Smooth-muscle tumors of the esophagus. *Thorax* 8:251, 1953.

Klinkhamer AC: *Esophagography in Anomalies of Aortic Arch System*. Amsterdam, Excerpta Medica Foundation, 1969.

Phillips MM, Hendrix TR: Dysphagia. *Postgrad Med* 50:81, 1977.

Physiology

Barlow AP, DeMeester TR, et al: The significance of the gastric secretory state in gastroesophageal reflux disease. *Arch Surg* 124:937, 1989.

Biancani P, Zabinski MP, Behar J: Pressure, tension, and force of closure of the human lower esophageal sphincter and esophagus. *J Clin Invest* 56:476, 1975.

Bonavina L, Evander A, et al: Length of the distal esophageal sphincter and competency of the cardia. *Am J Surg* 151:25, 1986.

Davenport HW: *Physiology of the Digestive Tract*, 5th ed. Chicago, Year Book Medical Publishers, 1982, pp 52–69.

DeMeester TR: What is the role of intraoperative manometry? *Ann Thorac Surg* 30:1, 1980.

DeMeester TR, Lafontaine E, et al: The relationship of a hiatal hernia to the function of the body of the esophagus and the gastroesophageal junction. *J Thorac Cardiovasc Surg* 82:547, 1981.

DeMeester TR, Stein HJ, Fuchs KH: Physiologic Diagnostic Studies, in Zuidema GD, Orringer MB (eds): *Shackelford's Surgery of the Alimentary Tract*, 3rd ed, Vol I. Philadelphia, Saunders, 1991, pp 94–126.

Helm JF, Dodds WJ, et al: Acid neutralizing capacity of human saliva. *Gastroenterology* 83:69, 1982.

Helm JF, Dodds WJ, et al: Effect of esophageal emptying and saliva on clearance of acid from the esophagus. *N Engl J Med* 310:284, 1984.

Helm JF, Dodds WJ, Hogan WJ: Salivary responses to esophageal acid in normal subjects and patients with reflux esophagitis. *Gastroenterology* 93:1393, 1982.

Helm JF, Riedel DR, et al: Determinants of esophageal acid clearance in normal subjects. *Gastroenterology* 85:607, 1983.

Joelsson BE, DeMeester TR, et al: The role of the esophageal body in the antireflux mechanism. *Surgery* 92:417, 1982.

Johnson LF, DeMeester TR: Evaluation of elevation of the head of the bed, bethanechol, and antacid foam tablets on gastroesophageal reflux. *Dig Dis Sci* 26:673, 1981.

Kahrilas PJ, Dodds WJ, Hogan WJ: Effect of peristaltic dysfunction on esophageal volume clearance. *Gastroenterology* 94:73, 1988.

Kaye MD, Showalter JP: Pyloric incompetence in patients with symptomatic gastroesophageal reflux. *J Lab Clin Med* 83:198, 1974.

Lieberman-Meffert D, Allgower M, et al: Muscular equivalent of the esophageal sphincter. *Gastroenterology* 76:31, 1979.

McCallum RW, Berkowitz DM, Lerner E: Gastric emptying in patients with gastroesophageal reflux. *Gastroenterology* 80:285, 1981.

Mittal RK, Lange RC, McCallum RW: Identification and mechanism of delayed esophageal acid clearance in subjects with hiatus hernia. *Gastroenterology* 92:130, 1987.

Price IM, El-Sharkawy, et al: Effects of bilateral cervical vagotomy on balloon-induced lower esophageal sphincter relaxation in the dog. *Gastroenterology* 77:324, 1979.

Zaninotto G, DeMeester TR, et al: The lower esophageal sphincter in health and disease. *Am J Surg* 155:104, 1988.

Assessment of Esophageal Function

Akberg O, Wahlgren L: Dysfunction of pharyngeal swallowing: a cineradiographic investigation in 854 dysphagial patients. *Acta Radiol Diagn* 26:389, 1985.

Barish CF, Castell DO, Richter JE: Graded esophageal balloon distention: a new provocative test for non-cardiac chest pain. *Dig Dis Sci* 31:1292, 1986.

Battle WS, Nyhus LM, Bombeck CT: Gastroesophageal reflux: diagnosis and treatment. *Ann Surg* 177:560, 1973.

Behar J, Biancani P, Sheahan DG: Evaluation of esophageal tests in the diagnosis of reflux esophagitis. *Gastroenterology* 71:9, 1976.

Benjamin SM, Richter JE, et al: Prospective manometric evaluation with pharmacologic provocation of patients with suspected esophageal motility dysfunction. *Gastroenterology* 84:893, 1983.

Bennett JR, Atkinson M: Oesophageal acid-perfusion in the diagnosis of precordial pain. *Lancet* 2:1150, 1966.

Benz LJ, Hootkin LA, et al: A comparison of clinical measurements of gastroesophageal reflux. *Gastroenterology* 62:1, 1972.

Bernstein IM, Baker CA: A clinical test for esophagitis. *Gastroenterology* 34:760, 1958.

Breen KJ, Whelan G: The diagnosis of reflux oesophagitis: an evaluation of five investigative procedures. *Aust NZ J Surg* 46:156, 1978.

Cade CF, Creamer B, et al: *An Atlas of Esophageal Motility in Health and Disease*. Springfield, IL, Charles C Thomas, 1981.

Castell DO, Richter JE, Dalton CB (eds): *Esophageal Motility Testing*. New York, Elsevier, 1987.

DeMeester TR, Johnson LF, et al: Patterns of gastroesophageal reflux in health and disease. *Ann Surg* 184:459, 1976.

DeMeester TR, Stein HJ, Fuchs KH: Physiologic diagnostic studies, in Zuidema GD, Orringer MB (eds): *Shackelford's Surgery of the Alimentary Tract*, 3rd ed, Vol I. Philadelphia, Saunders, 1991, pp 94–126.

DeMeester TR, Wang CI, et al: Technique, indications and clinical use of 24-hour esophageal pH monitoring. *J Thorac Cardiovasc Surg* 79:656, 1980.

DeMoraes-Filho JPP, Bettarello A: Lack of specificity of the acid perfusion test in duodenal ulcer patients. *Am J Dig Dis* 19:785, 1974.

Dent J: A new technique for continuous sphincter pressure measurement. *Gastroenterology* 71:263, 1976.

Dodds WJ: Current concepts of esophageal motor function: clinical implications for radiology. *AJR* 128:549, 1977.

Donner MW: Swallowing mechanism and neuromuscular disorders. *Semin Roentgenol* 9:273, 1974.

Emde C, Armstrong F, et al: Reproducibility of long-term ambulatory esophageal combined pH/manometry. *Gastroenterology* 100:1630, 1991.

Emde C, Garner A, Blum A: Technical aspects of intraluminal pH-metry in man: current status and recommendations. *Gut* 23:1177, 1987.

Fisher RS, Malmud LS, et al: Gastroesophageal (GE) scintiscanning to detect and quantitate GE reflux. *Gastroenterology* 70:301, 1976.

Fuchs KH, DeMeester TR, Albertucci M: Specificity and sensitivity of objective diagnosis of gastroesophageal reflux disease. *Surgery* 102:575, 1987.

Fuchs KH, DeMeester TR, et al: Concomitant duodenogastric and gastroesophageal reflux: the role of twenty-four-hour gastric pH monitoring, in Siewert JR, Holscher AH (eds): *Diseases of the Esophagus*. New York, Springer-Verlag, 1988, pp 1073–1076.

Iascone C, DeMeester TR, et al: Barrett's esophagus: functional assessment, proposed pathogenesis and surgical therapy. *Arch Surg* 118(5):543, 1983.

Johnson LF, DeMeester TR: Twenty-four-hour pH monitoring of the distal esophagus: a quantitative measure of gastroesophageal reflux. *Am J Gastroenterol* 62:325, 1974.

Johnson LF, DeMeester TR: Development of 24-hour intraesophageal pH monitoring composite scoring. *J Clin Gastroenterol* 8:52, 1986.

Johnson LF, DeMeester TR, Haggitt RC: Endoscopic signs for gastroesophageal reflux objectively evaluated. *Gastrointest Endosc* 22:151, 1976.

Kramer P, Hollander W: Comparison of experimental esophageal pain with clinical pain of angina pectoris and esophageal disease. *Gastroenterology* 29:719, 1955.

Landon RL, Ouyang A, et al: Provocation of esophageal chest pain by ergonovine or edrophonium. *Gastroenterology* 81:10, 1981.

Mittal RK, Stewart WR, Schirmer BD: Effect of a catheter in the pharynx on the frequency of transient lower esophageal sphincter relaxations. *Gastroenterology* 103:1236, 1992.

Reid BJ, Weinstein WM, et al: Endoscopic biopsy can detect high-grade dysplasia or early adenocarcinoma in Barrett's esophagus without grossly recognizable neoplastic lesions. *Gastroenterology* 94:81, 1988.

Richter JE, Hackshaw BT, Wu WC: Edrophonium: a useful provocative test for esophageal chest pain. *Ann Intern Med* 103:14, 1985.

Russell COH, Hill LD, et al: Radionuclide transit: a sensitive screening test for esophageal dysfunction. *Gastroenterology* 80:887, 1981.

Schwesinger WH: Endoscopic diagnosis and treatment of mucosal lesions of the esophagus. *Surg Clin North Am* 69(6):1185, 1989.

Schwizer W, Hinder RA, DeMeester TR: Does delayed gastric emptying contribute to gastroesophageal reflux disease? *Am J Surg* 157:74, 1989.

Seaman WB: Roentgenology of pharyngeal disorders, in Margulis AR, Burhenne JH (eds): *Alimentary Tract Roentgenology*, 2nd ed, Vol I. St Louis, CV Mosby, 1973, pp 305–336.

Smout AJPM: Ambulatory manometry of the oesophagus—the method and the message. *Gullet* 1:155, 1991.

Stein HJ, DeMeester TR, et al: Three-dimensional imaging of the lower esophageal sphincter in gastroesophageal reflux disease. *Ann Surg* 214:374, 1991.

Tolin RD, Malmud LS, et al: Esophageal scintigraphy to quantitate esophageal transit (quantitation of esophageal transit). *Gastroenterology* 76:1402, 1979.

Welch RW, Lickmann K, et al: Manometry of the normal upper esophageal sphincter and its alteration in laryngectomy. *J Clin Invest* 63:1036, 1979.

Wickremesinghe PC, Bayrit PQ, et al: Quantitative evaluation of bile diversion surgery utilizing ^{99m}Tc HIDA scintigraphy. *Gastroenterology* 84:354, 1983.

Winans CS: Manometric asymmetry of the lower esophageal high pressure zone. *Dig Dis Sci* 22:348, 1977.

Gastroesophageal Reflux Disease

Allison PR: Peptic ulcer of the esophagus. *J Thorac Surg* 15:308, 1946.

Allison PR: Reflux esophagitis, sliding hiatus hernia and the anatomy of repair. *Surg Gynecol Obstet* 92:419, 1951.

Allison PR: Hiatus hernia: a 20 year retrospective survey. *Ann Surg* 178:273, 1973.

Altorki NK, Sunagawa M, et al: High-grade dysplasia in the columnar-lined esophagus. *Am J Surg* 161:97, 1991.
Barlow AP, DeMeester TR, et al: The significance of the gastric secretory state in gastroesophageal reflux disease. *Arch Surg* 124:937, 1989.
Bonavina L, DeMeester TR, et al: Drug-induced esophageal strictures. *Ann Surg* 206:173, 1987.
Bremner CG: Barrett's esophagus. *Br J Surg* 76:995, 1989.
Cameron AJ, Lomboy CT: Barrett's esophagus: age, prevalence, and extent of columnar epithelium. *Gastroenterology* 103:1241, 1992.
Chen MF, Wang CS: A prospective study of the effect of cholecystectomy on duodenogastric reflux in humans using 24-hour gastric hydrogen monitoring. *Surg Gynecol Obstet* 175:52, 1992.
Collard J-M, DeMeester TR: Correction of failed antireflux procedures based on preoperative functional assessment and intraoperative findings. (In preparation.)
Cuschieri A, Shimi S, Nathanson LK: Laparoscopic reduction, crural repair, and fundoplication of large hiatal hernia. *Laparoscopy* 163:425, 1992.
Dallemagne B, Weerts JM, et al: Laparoscopic Nissen fundoplication: Preliminary report. *Surg Laparosc Endosc* 1(3):138, 1991.
DeMeester TR: Management of benign esophageal strictures, in Stipa S, Belsey RHR, Moraldi A (eds): *Medical and Surgical Problems of the Esophagus*. New York, Academic Press, 1981, pp 173–176.
DeMeester TR, Bonavina L, Albertucci M: Nissen fundoplication for gastroesophageal reflux disease—evaluation of primary repair in 100 consecutive patients. *Ann Surg* 204:9, 1986.
DeMeester TR, Bonavina L, et al: Chronic respiratory symptoms and occult gastroesophageal reflux. *Ann Surg* 211:337, 1990.
DeMeester TR, Fuchs KH, et al: Experimental and clinical results with proximal end-to-end duodenojejunostomy for pathologic duodenogastric reflux. *Ann Surg* 206:414, 1987.
DeMeester TR, Johansson KE, et al: Indications, surgical technique, and long-term functional results of colon interposition or bypass. *Ann Surg* 208(4):460, 1988.
DeMeester TR, Stein HJ: Gastroesophageal reflux disease, in Moody FG, Carey LC, et al (eds): *Surgical Treatment of Digestive Disease*, 2nd ed. Chicago, Year Book Medical Publishers, 1989, pp 65–108.
DeMeester TR, Stein HJ: Surgical treatment of gastroesophageal reflux disease, in Castell DO (ed): *The Esophagus*. Boston, Little, Brown & Company, 1992, pp 579–625.
Donahue PE, Samelson S, et al: The floppy Nissen fundoplication: effective long-term control of pathologic reflux. *Arch Surg* 120:663, 1985.
Feussner H, Petri A, et al: The modified AFT score: an attempt to make the results of anti-reflux surgery comparable. *Br J Surg* 78:942, 1991.
Fiorucci S, Santucci L, et al: Gastric acidity and gastroesophageal reflux patterns in patients with esophagitis. *Gastroenterology* 103(3):855, 1992.
Fuchs KH, DeMeester TR: Cost benefit aspects in the management of gastroesophageal reflux disease, in Siewert JR, Holscher AH (eds): *Diseases of the Esophagus*. New York, Springer-Verlag, 1988, pp 857–861.
Fuchs KH, DeMeester TR, et al: Computerized identification of pathologic duodenogastric reflux using 24-hour gastric pH monitoring. *Ann Surg* 213:13, 1991.
Geagea T: Laparoscopic Nissen's fundoplication: preliminary report on ten cases. *Surg Endosc* 5:170, 1991.
Gillen P, Keeling P, et al: Implication of duodenogastric reflux in the pathogenesis of Barrett's oesophagus. *Br J Surg* 75(6):540, 1988.
Gotley DC, Ball DE, Owen RW, et al: Evaluation and surgical correction of esophagitis after partial gastrectomy. *Surgery* 111:29, 1992.
Henderson RD, Henderson RF, Marryatt GV: Surgical management of 100 consecutive esophageal strictures. *J Thorac Cardiovasc Surg* 99(1):1, 1990.
Hinder RA, et al: Relationship of a satisfactory outcome to normalization of delayed gastric emptying after Nissen fundoplication. *Ann Surg* 210:458, 1989.
Hinder RA, Filipi CJ: The technique of laparoscopic Nissen fundoplication. *Surg Laparosc Endosc* 2(3):265, 1992.
Jacob P, Kahrilas PJ, Herzon G: Proximal esophageal pH-metry in patients with "reflux laryngitis." *Gastroenterology* 100:305, 1991.
Jamieson JR, Hinder RA, et al: Analysis of 32 patients with Schatzki's ring. *Am J Surg* 158:563, 1989.
Kahrilas PJ, Dodds WP, Hogan WJ: Effect of peristaltic dysfunction on esophageal volume clearance. *Gastroenterology* 94:73, 1988.
Kaul BK, DeMeester TR, et al: The cause of dysphagia in uncomplicated sliding hiatal hernia and its relief by hiatal herniorrhaphy: a roentgenographic, manometric, and clinical study. *Ann Surg* 211:406, 1990.
Lin KM, Ueda RK, et al: Etiology and importance of alkaline esophageal reflux. *Am J Surg* 162:553, 1991.
Lind JF, et al: Motility of the gastric fundus. *Am J Physiol* 201:197, 1961.
Little AG, et al: Duodenogastric reflux and reflux esophagitis. *Surgery* 96:447, 1984.
Little AG, Ferguson MK, Skinner DB: Reoperation for failed antireflux operations. *J Thorac Cardiovasc Surg* 91:511, 1986.
Nissen R: Eine einfache Operation zur Beeinflussung der Refluxoesophagitis. *Schweiz Med Wochenschr* 86:590, 1956.
Nissen R: Gastropexy and fundoplication in surgical treatment of hiatus hernia. *Am J Dig Dis* 6:954, 1961.
Orringer MB, Skinner DB, Belsey RHR: Long-term results of the Mark IV operation for hiatal hernia and analyses of recurrences and their treatment. *J Thorac Cardiovasc Surg* 63:25, 1972.
O'Sullivan GC, DeMeester TR, et al: Twenty-four-hour pH monitoring of esophageal function: its use in evaluation in symptomatic patients after truncal vagotomy and gastric resection or drainage. *Arch Surg* 116:581, 1981.
Patti MG, Debas HT, et al: Esophageal manometry and 24-hour pH monitoring in the diagnosis of pulmonary aspiration secondary to gastroesophageal reflux. *Am J Surg* 163:401, 1992.
Pearson FG, Cooper JD, et al: Gastroplasty and fundoplication for complex reflux problems. *Ann Surg* 206(4):473, 1987.
Pelligrini CA, DeMeester TR, et al: Gastroesophageal reflux and pulmonary aspiration: incidence, functional abnormality, and results of surgical therapy. *Surgery* 86:110, 1979.
Richardson JD, Larson GM, Polk HC: Intrathoracic fundoplication for shortened esophagus: treacherous solution to a challenging position. *Am J Surg* 143:29, 1982.
Richter JE, Castell DO: Gastroesophageal reflux: pathogenesis, diagnosis and therapy. *Ann Intern Med* 97:93, 1982.
Salama FD, Lamont G: Long-term results of the Belsey Mark IV antireflux operation in relation to the severity of esophagitis. *J Thorac Cardiovasc Surg* 100:17, 1990.
Salzman M, Barwick K, McCallum RW: Progression of cimetidine-treated reflux esophagitis to a Barrett's stricture. *Dig Dis Sci* 27(2):181, 1982.
Schindlpeck NE, Klauser AG, et al: Three year follow up of patients with gastroesophageal reflux disease. *Gut* 33:1016, 1992.
Schwizer W, Hinder RA, DeMeester TR: Does delayed gastric emptying contribute to gastroesophageal reflux disease? *Am J Surg* 157:74, 1989.
Siewert JR, Isolauri J, Feussuer M: Reoperation following failed fundoplication. *World J Surg* 13:791, 1989.
Sontag SJ: The medical management of reflux esophagitis: role of antacids and acid inhibition. *Gastroenterol Clin North Am* 19(3):683, 1990.
Spechler SJ, Department of Veterans Affairs Gastroesophageal Reflux Disease Study Group: Comparison of medical and surgical therapy for complicated gastroesophageal reflux disease in veterans. *N Engl J Med* 326(12):786, 1992.
Stein HJ: The development of complications in gastroesophageal sphincter, esophageal acid and acid/alkaline exposure, and duodenogastric reflux. *Arch Surg* (in press).
Stein HJ, et al: Clinical use of 24-hour gastric pH monitoring vs. *O*-diisopropyl iminodiacetic acid (DISIDA) scanning in the diagnosis of pathologic duodenogastric reflux. *Arch Surg* 125:966, 1990.

Stein HJ, Barlow AP, et al: Complications of gastroesophageal reflux disease: role of the lower esophageal sphincter, esophageal acid and acid/alkaline exposure, and duodenogastric reflux. *Ann Surg* 216(1):35, 1992.

Stein HJ, Bremner RM, et al: Effect of Nissen fundoplication on esophageal motor function. *Arch Surg* 127:788, 1992.

Stein HJ, Smyrk TC, et al: Clinical value of endoscopy and histology in the diagnosis of duodenogastric reflux disease. *Surgery* 112:796, 1992.

Stirling MC, Orringer MB: Surgical treatment after the failed antireflux operation. *J Thorac Cardiovasc Surg* 92:667, 1986.

Tolin RD, et al: Enterogastric reflux in normal subjects and patients with Billroth II gastroenterostomy: measurement of enterogastric reflux. *Gastroenterology* 77:1027, 1979.

Walther BS, Courtney JV, et al: The effect of paraesophageal hernia on sphincter function and its implication on surgical therapy. *Am J Surg* 147:111, 1984.

Wattchow DA, Jamieson GG, et al: Distribution of peptide-containing nerve fibers in the gastric musculature of patients undergoing surgery for gastroesophageal reflux. *Ann Surg* 290(2):153, 1992.

Welch NT, Yasui A, et al: Effect of duodenal switch procedure on gastric acid production, intragastric pH, gastric emptying, and gastrointestinal hormones. *Am J Surg* 163:37, 1992.

Williamson WA, Ellis FH Jr, et al: Effect of antireflux operation on Barrett's mucosa. *Ann Thorac Surg* 49:537, 1990.

Zaninotto G, DeMeester TR, et al: Esophageal function in patients with reflux-induced strictures and its relevance to surgical treatment. *Ann Thorac Surg* 47:362, 1989.

Motility Disorders of the Pharynx and Esophagus

Achem SR, Crittenden J, et al: Long-term clinical and manometric follow-up of patients with nonspecific esophageal motor disorders. *Am J Gastroenterol* 87(7):825, 1992.

Andreollo NA, Earlam RJ: Heller's myotomy for achalasia: is an added antireflux procedure necessary? *Br J Surg* 74:765, 1987.

Bianco A, Cagossi M, et al: Appearance of esophageal peristalsis in treated idiopathic achalasia. *Dig Dis Sci* 90:978, 1986.

Bonavina L, Khan NA, DeMeester TR: Pharyngoesophageal dysfunctions: the role of cricopharyngeal myotomy. *Arch Surg* 120:541, 1985.

Bonavina L, Nosadinia A, et al: Primary treatment of esophageal achalasia: long-term results of myotomy and Dor fundoplication. *Arch Surg* 127:222, 1992.

Browning TH, et al: Diagnosis of chest pain of esophageal origin. *Dig Dis Sci* 35(3):289, 1990.

Cassella RR, Brown AL, Jr, et al: Achalasia of the esophagus: pathologic and etiologic considerations. *Ann Surg* 160:474, 1964.

Castell DO, Richter JE, Dalton CB (eds): *Esophageal Motility Testing*. New York, Elsevier, 1987.

Chakkaphak S, Chakkaphak K, et al: Disorders of esophageal motility. *Surg Gynecol Obstet* 172:325, 1991.

Code CF, Schlegel JF, et al: Hypertensive gastroesophageal sphincter. *Mayo Clin Proc* 35:391, 1960.

Cook IJ, Blumbergs P, et al: Structural abnormalities of the cricopharyngeus muscle in patients with pharyngeal (Zenker's) diverticulum. *J Gastroenterol Hepatol* 7(6):556, 1992.

Cook IJ, Gabb M, et al: Pharyngeal (Zenker's) diverticulum is a disorder of upper esophageal sphincter opening. *Gastroenterology* 103(4):1229, 1992.

Csendes A, Braghetto I, et al: Late subjective and objective evaluation of the results of esophagomyotomy in 100 patients with achalasia of the esophagus. *Surgery* 104:469, 1988.

Csendes A, Braghetto I, et al: Late results of a prospective randomized study comparing forceful dilatation and oesophagomyotomy in patients with achalasia. *Gut* 30:299, 1989.

Csendes A, Velasco N, et al: A prospective randomized study comparing forceful dilatation and esophagomyotomy in patients with achalasia of the esophagus. *Gastroenterology* 80:789, 1981.

Dalton CB, Castell DO, Richter JE: The changing faces of the nutcracker esophagus. *Am J Gastroenterol* 83:623, 1988.

DeMeester TR, Johansson KE, et al: Indications, surgical technique and long-term functional results of colon interposition or bypass. *Ann Surg* 208:460, 1988.

DeMeester TR, Lafontaine E, et al: The relationship of a hiatal hernia to the function of the body of the esophagus and the gastroesophageal junction. *J Thorac Cardiovasc Surg* 82:547, 1981.

DeMeester TR, Stein HJ: Surgery for esophageal motor disorders, in Castell DO (ed): *The Esophagus*. Boston, Little, Brown & Company, 1992, pp 401–439.

Donner MW: Swallowing mechanism and neuromuscular disorders. *Semin Roentgenol* 9:273, 1974.

Ekberg O, Wahlgren L: Dysfunction of pharyngeal swallowing: A cineradiographic investigation in 854 dysphagial patients. *Acta Radiol Diagn* 26:389, 1985.

Ellis FH Jr, Crozier RE: Cervical esophageal dysphagia: indications for and results for cricopharyngeal myotomy. *Ann Surg* 194:279, 1981.

Evander A, Little AG, et al: Diverticula of the mid and lower esophagus. *World J Surg* 10:820, 1986.

Eypasch EP, Stein HJ, et al: A new technique to define and clarify esophageal motor disorders. *Am J Surg* 159:144, 1990.

Ferguson MK: Achalasia: current evaluation and therapy. *Ann Thorac Surg* 52:336, 1991.

Ferguson MK, Skinner DB (eds): *Diseases of the Esophagus, Vol 2, Benign Diseases*. Mount Kisco, NY, Futura Publishing, 1990.

Ferguson TB, Woodbury JD, Roper CL: Giant muscular hypertrophy of the esophagus. *Ann Thorac Surg* 8:209, 1969.

Foker JE, Ring WE, Varco RL: Technique of jejunal interposition for esophageal replacement. *J Thorac Cardiovasc Surg* 83:928, 1982.

Gillies M, Nicks R, Skyring A: Clinical, manometric, and pathologic studies in diffuse oesophageal spasm. *Br Med J* 2:527, 1967.

Kahrilas PJ, Logemann JA, et al: Pharyngeal clearance during swallowing: a combined manometric and videofluoroscopic study. *Gastroenterology* 103(1):128, 1992.

Lafontaine E: Pharyngeal dysphagia, in DeMeester TR, Matthews HR (eds): *International Trends in General Thoracic Surgery, Vol 3, Benign Esophageal Disease*. St Louis, CV Mosby, 1987.

Lam HGT, Dekker W, et al: Acute noncardiac chest pain in a coronary care unit. *Gastroenterology* 102:453, 1992.

Lang IM, Dantas, Cook IJ, et al: Videographic, manometric, and electromyographic analysis of canine esophageal sphincter. *Am J Physiol* 260:G911, 1991.

Lerut J, Elgariani A, et al: Zenker's diverticulum. Surgical experience in a series of 25 patients. *Acta Gastroenterol Belg* 46:189, 1983.

Lerut T, VanRaemdonck D, et al: Pharyngo-oesophageal diverticulum (Zenker's). Clinical, therapeutic and morphologic aspects. *Acta Gastroenterol Belg* 53:330, 1990.

Little AG, Correnti FS, et al: Effect of incomplete obstruction on feline esophageal function with a clinical correlation. *Surgery* 100:430, 1986.

Mellow MH: Return of esophageal peristalsis in idiopathic achalasia. *Gastroenterology* 70:1148, 1976.

Moser G, Vacariu-Granser GV, et al: High incidence of esophageal motor disorders in consecutive patients with globus sensation. *Gastroenterology* 101(6):1512, 1991.

Pellegrini C, Wetter LA, et al: Thoracoscopic esophagomyotomy: initial experience with a new approach for the treatment of achalasia. *Ann Surg* 216(3):291, 1992.

Richter JE: Surgery or pneumatic dilation for achalasia: A head-to-head comparison. *Gastroenterology* 97:1340, 1989.

Shimi SM, Nathanson LK, Cuschieri A: Thoracoscopic long oesophageal myotomy for nutcracker oesophagus: initial experience of a new surgical approach. *Br J Surg* 79:533, 1992.

Stein HJ, DeMeester TR, Eypasch EP: Ambulatory 24-hour esophageal manometry in the evaluation of esophageal motor disorders and noncardiac chest pain. *Surgery* 110:753, 1991.

Stein HJ, Eypasch EP, DeMeester TR: Circadian esophageal motility pattern in patients with classic diffuse esophageal spasm and nutcracker esophagus. *Gastroenterology* 96:491, 1989.

Streitz JM Jr, Glick ME, Ellis FH Jr: Selective use of myotomy for treatment of epiphrenic diverticula: manometric and clinical analysis. *Arch Surg* 127:585, 1992.

Vantrappen G, Janssens J: To dilate or to operate? That is the question. *Gut* 24:1013, 1983.

Waters PF, DeMeester TR: Foregut motor disorders and their surgical management. *Med Clin North Am* 54:1235, 1981.

Carcinoma of the Esophagus

Akiyama H: Surgery for carcinoma of the esophagus. *Curr Probl Surg* 27(2):, 1980.

Akiyama H, Hiyama M, Miyazono H: Total esophageal reconstruction after extraction of the esophagus. *Ann Surg* 182:547, 1975.

Akiyama H, Kogure T, Itai Y: The esophageal axis and its relationship to the resectability of carcinoma of the esophagus. *Ann Surg* 176:30, 1971.

Akiyama J, Tsurumaru M, et al: Principles of surgical treatment for carcinoma of the esophagus: analysis of lymph node involvement. *Ann Surg* 194:438, 1981.

Baker JW Jr, Schechter GL: Management of paraesophageal cancer by blunt resection without thoracotomy and reconstruction with stomach. *Ann Surg* 203:491, 1986.

Beatty JD, DeBoer G, Rider WD: Carcinoma of the esophagus: pretreatment assessment, correlation of radiation treatment parameters with survival, and identification and management of radiation treatment failure. *Cancer* 43:2254, 1979.

Borrie J: Sarcoma of esophagus: surgical treatment. *J Thorac Surg* 37:413, 1959.

Bremner CG: Barrett's esophagus, in DeMeester TR, Matthews HR (eds): *International Trends in General Thoracic Surgery, Vol III: Benign Esophageal Disease*. St Louis, CV Mosby, 1987.

Cameron AJ, Ott BJ, Payne WS: The incidence of adenocarcinoma in columnar-lined (Barrett's) esophagus. *N Engl J Med* 313:857, 1985.

Carey JS, Plested WG, Hughues RK: Esophagogastrectomy—how to do it. *Ann Thorac Surg* 14:59, 1972.

Castrini G, Pappalardo G: Carcinoma of the cardia. Tactical problem. *J Thorac Cardiovasc Surg* 82:190, 1981.

Clinical staging system for carcinoma of the esophagus. The American Joint Committee for Cancer Staging and End Results Reporting, October 1973.

Colin CF, Spiro RH: Carcinoma of the cervical esophagus: changing therapeutic trends. *Am J Surg* 148:460, 1984.

DeMeester TR: Surgical anatomy of the esophagus, in Shields TW (ed): *General Thoracic Surgery*, 2nd ed. Philadelphia, Lea & Febiger, 1983, pp 82–91.

DeMeester TR, Attwood SEA, et al: Surgical therapy in Barrett's esophagus. *Ann Surg* 212:528, 1990.

DeMeester TR, Barlow AP: Surgery and current management for cancer of the esophagus and cardia: Part II. *Curr Probl Surg* 25(8):535, 1988.

DeMeester TR, Skinner DB: Polypoid sarcomas of the esophagus. *Ann Thorac Surg* 20:405, 1975.

DeMeester TR, Stein HJ: Surgical therapy for cancer of the esophagus and cardia, in Castell DO (ed): *The Esophagus*. Boston, Little, Brown & Company, 1992, pp 299–341.

DeMeester TR, Zaninotto G, Johansson KE: Selective therapeutic approach to cancer of the lower esophagus and cardia. *J Thorac Cardiovasc Surg* 95:42, 1988.

Duhaylongsod FG, Wolfe WG: Barrett's esophagus and adenocarcinoma of the esophagus and gastroesophageal junction. *J Thorac Cardiovasc Surg* 102:36, 1991.

Fisher DR, Brawley RK, Kielfer RF: Esophagogastrostomy in the treatment of carcinoma of the distal two-thirds of the esophagus. *Ann Thorac Surg* 14:658, 1972.

Fleming JAC: Carcinoma of thoracic esophagus: some notes on its pathology and spread in relation to treatment. *Br J Radiol* 16:212, 1943.

Gomes MN, Kroll S, Spear SL: Mediastinal tracheostomy. *Ann Thorac Surg* 43:539, 1987.

Goodner JT: Treatment and survival in cancer of the cervical esophagus. *Am J Surg* 20:405, 1975.

Grummy AB, Wegner GP, et al: Azygos venography. An aid in the evaluation of esophageal carcinoma. *Ann Thorac Surg* 6:522, 1968.

Guernsey JM, Knudsen DF: Abdominal exploration in the evaluation of patients with carcinoma of the thoracic esophagus. *J Thorac Cardiovasc Surg* 59:62, 1970.

Hawley PR, Westerholm P, Morson BC: *Br J Surg* 57:877, 1970.

Heatley RV, Lewis MH, Williams RHP: Preoperative intravenous feeding—a controlled trial. *Postgrad Med J* 55:541, 1979.

Heimlich HJ: Carcinoma of the cervical esophagus. *J Thorac Cardiovasc Surg* 59:309, 1970.

Holub E, Simecek C: Pneumomediastinography in carcinoma of the esophagus. *Thorax* 23:77, 1968.

Kron IL, Joob AW, et al: Blunt esophagectomy and gastric interposition for tumors of the cervical esophagus and hypopharynx. *Am Surg* 52:140, 1986.

Lavin P, Hajdu SI, Foote FW Jr: Gastric and extragastric leiomyoblastomas. *Cancer* 29:305, 1972.

Law SYK, Fok M, et al: A comparison of outcomes after resection for squamous cell carcinomas and adenocarcinomas of the esophagus and cardia. *Surg Gynecol Obstet* 175:107, 1992.

Levine DS, Reid BJ: Endoscopic diagnosis of esophageal neoplasms. *Gastrointest Clin North Am* 2(3):395, 1992.

Lewis I: The surgical treatment of carcinoma of the esophagus with special reference to a new operation for the growths of the middle third. *Br J Surg* 34:18, 1946.

Logan A: The surgical treatment of carcinoma of the esophagus and cardia. *J Thorac Cardiovasc Surg* 46:150, 1963.

Lund O, Hasenkam JM, et al: Time related changes in characteristics of prognostic significance of carcinomas of the esophagus and cardia. *Br J Surg* 76:1301, 1989.

McCort JJ: Esophageal carcinosarcoma and pseudosarcoma. *Radiology* 102:519, 1972.

Moore TC, Battersby JS, et al: Carcinosarcoma of the esophagus. *J Thorac Cardiovasc Surg* 45:281, 1963.

Mori S, Kasai M, et al: Preoperative assessment of resectability for carcinoma of the thoracic esophagus. *Ann Surg* 190:100, 1979.

Murray GF, Wilcox BR, Starek P: The assessment of operability of esophageal carcinoma. *Ann Thorac Surg* 23:393, 1977.

Naunheim KS, Petruska PJ, et al: Preoperative chemotherapy and radiotherapy for esophageal carcinoma. *J Thorac Cardiovasc Surg* 103:887, 1992.

Nicks R: Colonic replacement of the esophagus. *Br J Surg* 54:124, 1967.

Orringer MB: Transhiatal esophagectomy without thoracotomy for carcinoma of the thoracic esophagus. *Ann Surg* 200(3):282, 1984.

Orringer MB, Forastiere AA, et al: Chemotherapy and radiation therapy before transhiatal esophagectomy for esophageal carcinoma. *Ann Thorac Surg* 49:348, 1990.

Orringer MB, Skinner DB: Unusual presentations of primary and secondary esophageal malignancies. *Ann Thorac Surg* 11:305, 1971.

Papachristou DN, Fortner JG: Adenocarcinoma of the gastric cardia. *Ann Surg* 192:58, 1980.

Payne SW, Bernatz PE: One stage resection and reconstruction of carcinoma of the esophagogastric junction, in Varco AL, Delaney JP (eds): *Controversy in Surgery*. Philadelphia, Saunders, 1976, Chap 26, p 591.

Pera M, Trastek VF, et al: Barrett's esophagus with high-grade dysplasia: an indication for esophagectomy? *Ann Thorac Surg* 54:199, 1992.

Piccone VA, Ahmed N, et al: Esophagogastrectomy for carcinoma of the middle third of the esophagus. *Ann Thorac Surg* 28:369, 1979.

Postlethwait RW: Carcinoma of the esophagus. *Curr Probl Cancer*, Vol II, No 8, 1978.

Ravitch M: *A Century of Surgery*. Philadelphia, Lippincott, 1981, p 56.

Reid BJ, Weinstein WM, et al: Endoscopic biopsy can detect high-grade dysplasia or early adenocarcinoma in Barrett's esophagus without grossly recognizable neoplastic lesions. *Gastroenterology* 94:81, 1988.

Resano JH: Treatment of cancer of the esophagus. *Bull Soc Int Chir* 6:311, 1957.

Rice TW, Boyce GA, et al: Esophageal ultrasound and the preoperative staging of carcinoma of the esophagus. *J Thorac Cardiovasc Surg* 101:536, 1991.

Robertson CS, Mayberry JF, Nicholson JA: Value of endoscopic surveillance in the detection of neoplastic changes in Barrett's esophagus. *Br J Surg* 75:760, 1988.

Rösch T, Lorenz R, et al: Endosonographic diagnosis of submucosal upper gastrointestinal tract tumors. *Scand J Gastroenterol* 27:1–8, 1992.

Rosenberg JC, Budev H, et al: Analysis of adenocarcinoma in Barrett's esophagus utilizing a staging system. *Cancer* 55:1353, 1985.

Rosenberg JC, Franklin R, Steiger Z: Squamous cell carcinoma of the thoracic esophagus: an interdisciplinary approach. *Curr Probl Cancer* 5, 1981.

Saidi F, Abbassi A, et al: Endothoracic endoesophageal pull-through operation: a new approach to cancers of the esophagus and proximal stomach. *J Thorac Cardiovasc Surg* 102:43, 1991.

San Segaua M, Curto Cardus J: The value of azygography in carcinoma of the esophagus. *Surg Gynecol Obstet* 141:248, 1975.

Sarr MG, Hamilton SR, et al: Barrett's esophagus: its prevalence and association with adenocarcinoma in patients with symptoms of gastroesophageal reflux. *Am J Surg* 149:187, 1985.

Silver CE: Surgical management of neoplasms of the larynx, hypopharynx and cervical esophagus. *Curr Probl Surg* 14(9):2, 1977.

Skinner DB, Dowlatshahi KD, DeMeester TR: Potentially curable carcinoma of the esophagus. *Cancer* 50:2571, 1982.

Skinner DB, Ferguson MK, Little AG: Selection of operation for esophageal cancer based on staging. *Ann Surg* 204:391, 1986.

Smith R, Gowing WFC: Carcinoma of the esophagus with histological appearances simulating a carcinosarcoma. *Br J Surg* 40:487, 1953.

Soga J, Kobayashi K, et al: The role of lymphadenectomy in curative surgery for gastric cancer. *World J Surg* 3:701, 1979.

Spechler SJ: Endoscopic surveillance for patients with Barrett's esophagus: does the cancer risk justify the practice? *Ann Intern Med* 106:902, 1987.

Stout AP, Humphreys GH, Rottenberg LA: A case of carcinosarcoma of the esophagus. *AJR Radium Ther Nucl Med* 61:461, 1949.

Streitz JM Jr, Ellis FH Jr, et al: Adenocarcinoma in Barrett's esophagus. *Ann Surg* 213(2):122, 1991.

Sunderland DA, McNeer G, et al: *Cancer* 6:987, 1953.

Thomas PA: Physiologic sufficiency of regenerated lung lymphatics. *Ann Surg* 192:162, 1980.

Talbert JL, Cantrell JR: Clinical and pathologic characteristics of carcinosarcoma of the esophagus. *J Thorac Cardiovasc Surg* 45:1, 1963.

Turnbull AD, Rosen P, et al: Primary malignant tumors of the esophagus other than typical epidermoid carcinoma. *Ann Thorac Surg* 15:463, 1973.

Watson WL, Goodner JT: Carcinoma of the esophagus. *Am J Surg* 93:259, 1957.

Watson WP, Pool L: Cancer of the cervical esophagus. *Surgery* 23:893, 1948.

Wolfel DA, Lindborg EJ, Light JP: The abnormal azygogram: an index of inoperability. *AJR* 97:933, 1966.

Benign Tumors and Cysts

Bardini R, Segalin A, et al: Videothoracoscopic enucleation of esophageal leiomyoma. *Ann Thorac Surg* 54:576, 1992.

Esophageal Perforation

Brewer LA III, Carter R, et al: Options in the management of perforations of the esophagus. *Ann J Surg* 152:62, 1986.

Chang C-H, Lin PJ, et al: One-stage operation for treatment after delayed diagnosis of thoracic esophageal perforation. *Ann Thorac Surg* 53:617, 1992.

Gouge TH, Depan HJ, Spencer FC: Experience with the Grillo pleural wrap procedure in 18 patients with perforation of the thoracic esophagus. *Ann Surg* 209(5):612, 1989.

Jones WG II, Ginsberg RJ: Esophageal perforation: a continuing challenge. *Ann Thorac Surg* 53:534, 1992.

Pate JW, Walker WA, et al: Spontaneous rupture of the esophagus: a 30-year experience. *Ann Thorac Surg* 47:689, 1989.

Caustic Injury

Anderson KD, Rouse TM, Randolph JG: A controlled trial of corticosteroids in children with corrosive injury of the esophagus. *N Engl J Med* 323(10):637, 1990.

Ferguson MK, Migliore M, et al: Early evaluation and therapy for caustic esophageal injury. *Am J Surg* 157:116, 1989.

Sugawa C, Lucas CE: Caustic injury of the upper gastrointestinal tract in adults: a clinical and endoscopic study. *Surgery* 106:802, 1989.

Zargar SA, Kochhar R, et al: The role of fiberoptic endoscopy in the management of corrosive ingestion and modified endoscopic classification of burns. *Gastrointest Endosc* 37(2):165, 1991.

Diaphragmatic Hernias

Bombeck TC, Dillard DH, Nyhus LM: Muscular anatomy of the gastroesophageal junction and role of the phrenoesophageal ligament. *Ann Surg* 164:643, 1966.

Bonavina L, Evander A, et al: Length of the distal esophageal sphincter and competency of the cardia. *Am J Surg* 151:25, 1986.

Dalgaard JB: Volvulus of the stomach. *Acta Chir Scand* 103:131, 1952.

DeMeester TR, Bonavina L: Paraesophageal hiatal hernia, in Nyhus LM, Condon RE (eds): *Hernia*, 3rd ed. Philadelphia, Lippincott, 1989, pp 684–693.

DeMeester TR, Lafontaine E, et al: The relationship of a hiatal hernia to the function of the body of the esophagus and the gastroesophageal junction. *J Thorac Cardiovasc Surg* 82:547, 1981.

Eliska O: Phreno-oesophageal membrane and its role in the development of hiatal hernia. *Acta Anat* 86:137, 1973.

Kleitsch WP: Embryology of congenital diaphragmatic hernia. I. Esophageal hiatus hernia. *Arch Surg* 76:868, 1958.

Menguy R: Surgical management of large paraesophageal hernia with complete intrathoracic stomach. *World J Surg* 12:415, 1988.

Postlethwait RW: *Surgery of the Esophagus*. New York, Appleton-Century Crofts, 1979, pp 195–255.

Skinner DB, Belsey RHR: Surgical management of esophageal reflux and hiatus hernia: long-term results with 1030 patients. *J Thorac Cardiovasc Surg* 53:33, 1967.

Walther B, DeMeester TR, et al: The effect of paraesophageal hernia on sphincter function and its implication on surgical therapy. *Am J Surg* 147:111, 1984.

Miscellaneous Esophageal Lesions

Burt M, Diehl W, et al: Malignant esophagorespiratory fistula: management options and survival. *Ann Thorac Surg* 52:1222, 1991.

Mathisen DJ, Grillo HC, et al: Management of acquired nonmalignant tracheoesophageal fistula. *Ann Thorac Surg* 52:759, 1991.

Techniques of Esophageal Reconstruction

Bonavina L, Anselmino M, et al: Functional evaluation of the intrathoracic stomach as an oesophageal substitute. *Br J Surg* 79(6):529, 1992.
Curet-Scott MJ, Ferguson MK, et al: Colon interposition for benign esophageal disease. *Surgery* 102:568, 1987.
DeMeester TR, Johansson K-E, et al: Indications, surgical technique, and long-term functional results of colon interposition or bypass. *Ann Surg* 208(4):460, 1988.
Ellis FH Jr, Gibb SP: Esophageal reconstruction for complex benign esophageal disease. *J Thorac Cardiovasc Surg* 99(2):192, 1990.
Fok M, Cheng SWK, Wong J: Pyloroplasty versus no drainage in gastric replacement of the esophagus. *Am J Surg* 162:447, 1991.
Heitmiller RF, Jones B: Transient diminished airway protection after transhiatal esophagectomy. *Am J Surg* 162:442, 1991.
Wu M-H, Lai W-W: Esophageal reconstruction for esophageal strictures or resection after corrosive injury. *Ann Thorac Surg* 53:798, 1992.

CHAPTER 24

Stomach

Frank G. Moody and Thomas A. Miller

ANATOMY

Functional Relationships. The stomach is an expanded segment of the foregut responsible for the initial breakdown and predigestion of a meal. Its location in the upper abdomen beneath the left hemidiaphragm allows for free expansion of its thin-walled distensible fundus, which receives and stores solid foods that pass into it from the esophagus above. The thicker-walled, more muscular distal portion of the stomach, the antrum, grinds and mixes the food and then forces it back into the fundus for further reduction in size and predigestion. Small particles move forward into the duodenum where they are further processed by intestinal secretions. The distal stomach is delineated by a thick band of circular smooth muscle, the pyloric sphincter. This sphincter prevents duodenogastric reflux and assists in gastric emptying by relaxing during antral propulsive contractions.

The fundus is lined by a highly specialized epithelium that secretes hydrochloric acid, pepsin, and intrinsic factor. The mucosa of the antrum participates in the process of gastric acid secretion by releasing the secretagogue, gastrin, into the circulation. This event is mediated by vagal release of acetylcholine and is modulated by the pH of the antral lumen. The stomach, therefore, can be considered as two organs: its proximal portion is designed for storage and digestion, and its distal part is adapted to the role of mixing and evacuation. Although older textbooks divided the stomach into three sections, namely a fundus, cardia, and antrum, physiologically it comprises only two, a fundus and antrum. Thus, in further discussion throughout this chapter, only these two functional parts will be recognized.

Of importance to the functional activity of the stomach in disease is its relationship to other intraabdominal organs. The most important adjacent organs are the pancreas and the liver, which lie dorsad and ventrad, respectively, and the spleen, which lies directly to the left of the stomach's greater curve (Fig. 24-1). Inflammation of the pancreas may delay gastric emptying, while enlargement by neoplasm may cause a sense of fullness or even obstruction to the gastric outlet. Liver or splenic enlargement may also interfere with the storage capacity of the stomach by infringing on its lumen. The transverse colon, which lies caudad, may also interfere with gastric function by direct neoplastic extension. More commonly, however, the stomach affects adjacent organs by penetration from peptic ulceration of either the stomach or duodenum. Another closely related structure is the biliary tree. It runs posterior to the first part of the duodenum only a few centimeters from the gastric outlet and is vulnerable to injury not only from peptic ulcer of the duodenum but from attempts at treatment by gastrectomy.

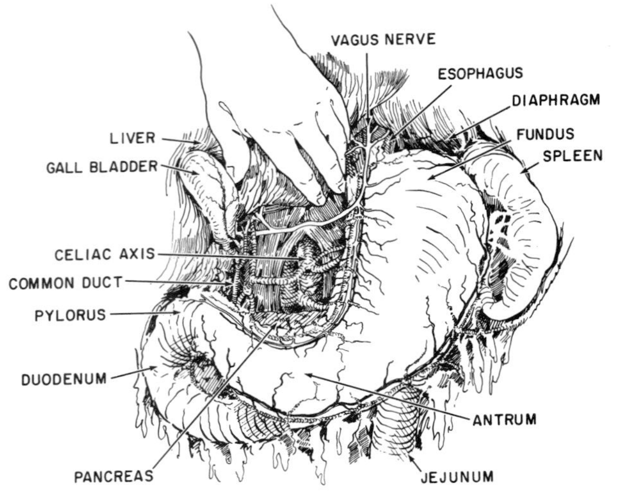

FIG. 24-1. Position of the stomach relative to the other principal organs of the upper abdomen.

Blood Supply and Lymphatics. The stomach has a blood supply so extensive and interconnected that three of its four major nutrient arteries can be ablated without incurring necrosis or even significant dysfunction. A submucosal plexus of arterioles provides for rapid healing of wounds and a low incidence of anastomotic disruption after operative manipulation. Because of this vascular anatomy, mucosal lesions may bleed extensively, even when small or superficial. The major arterial supply to the stomach is shown in Fig. 24-2. The lesser curve of the stomach is supplied primarily by the left gastric artery, which arises from the celiac axis. The right gastric artery, arising from the ascending hepatic artery, is usually a small vessel that provides branches to the first part of the duodenum and the pylorus. Right and left gastroepiploic arteries arise from the gastroduodenal and splenic arteries, respectively. They form an arcade along the greater curve, the right providing blood to the antrum and the left supplying the lower portion of the fundus. The short gastric arteries arising from the splenic artery are small and relatively insignificant in terms of the amount of blood that they deliver to the most proximal portion of the body of the stomach.

The lymphatic drainage of the stomach follows the distribution of the blood supply. An understanding of lymphatic channels and their nodal communications is important to the assessment of tumor spread from gastric cancer (see Fig. 24-3). Lymph from the upper lesser curvature of the stomach drains into the left gastric and paracardial nodes. The antral segment on the lesser curve drains into the right suprapancreatic nodes. Lesions high on the greater curvature flow into the left gastroepiploic and splenic nodes, while the distribution of flow along the right gastroepiploic

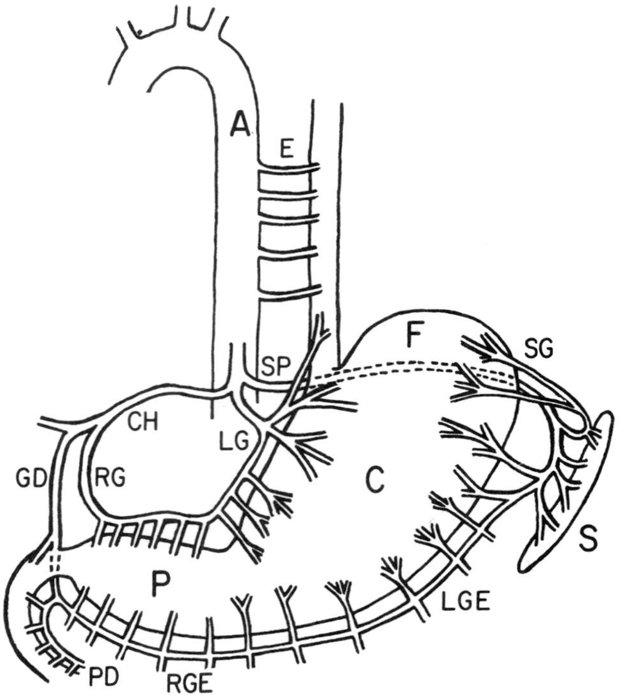

FIG. 24-2. Blood supply to the stomach. Legend: F—fundus; C—cardia; P—pylorus; S—spleen; A—aorta; E—esophageal arteries; SP—splenic artery; LG—left gastric artery; CH—common hepatic artery; RG—right gastric artery; GD—gastroduodenal artery; PD—pancreaticoduodenal artery; RGE—right gastroepiploic artery; LGE—left gastroepiploic artery; SG—short gastric arteries. (*Courtesy of KR Larsen, PhD.*)

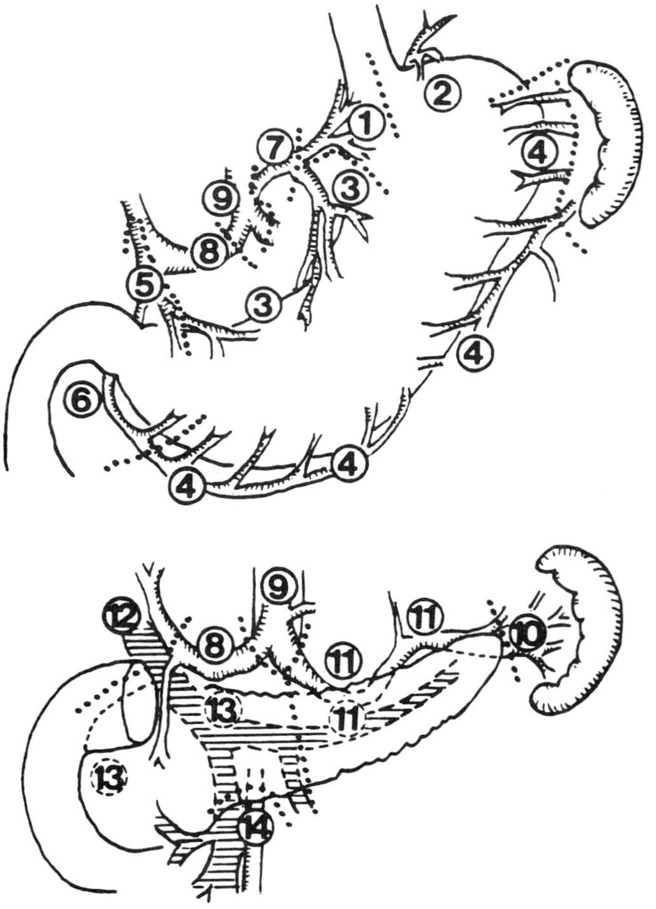

FIG. 24-3. Lymphatic drainage of the stomach with numerical designation of major regional lymph nodes. (From: *Iehiyoshi Y, et al: Surgery 107:490, 1990, with permission.*)

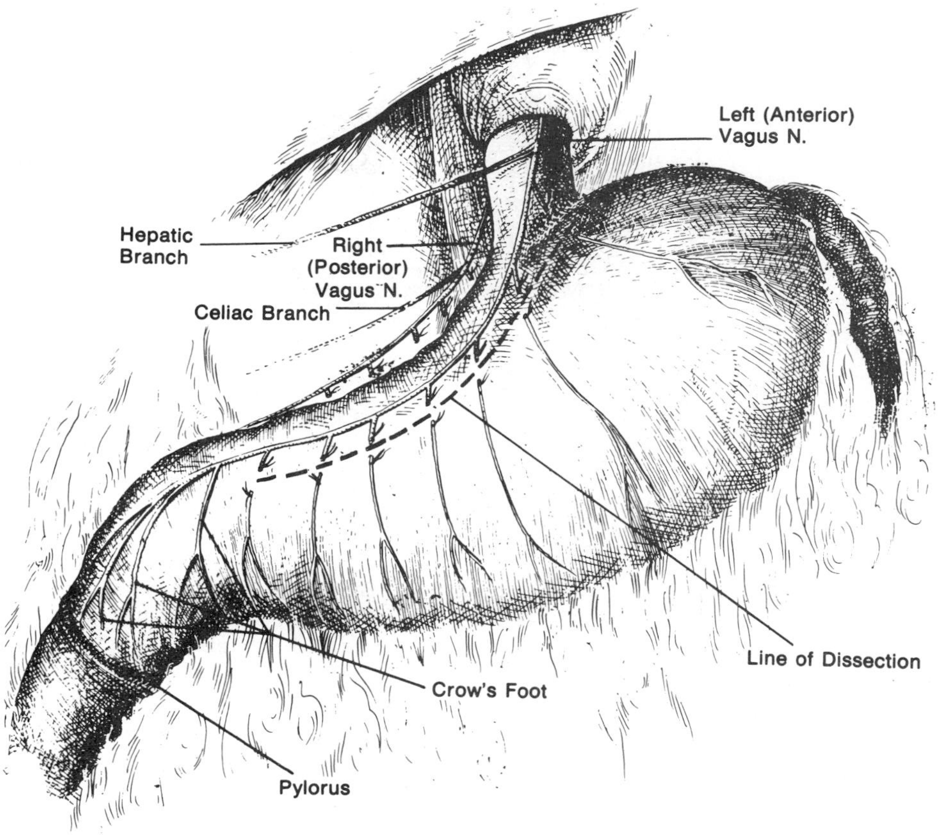

FIG. 24-4. Diagram of the distribution of the vagus nerve within the abdomen. It also shows where the branches of the nerve of Laterjet are divided for a parietal cell vagotomy. (From: *Moody FG: Mt Kisco, NY: Futura, 1:1–15, 1980.*)

enters nodes at the base of the vascular pedicle serving this area. Knowledge of these patterns of lymph flow is of practical importance when operating for cure of gastric cancer. Unfortunately, the routes of metastatic spread in this disease are unpredictable. Removal of lymph nodes until recently was thought to be more important for ascertaining prognosis than for gaining a cure. Important results of long-term survival after extensive removal of all lymph nodes within the potential lymphatic drainage of the tumor have led to a more detailed consideration of specific lymph nodes within each region (see Fig. 24-3).

Innervation. Motor aspects as well as secretory aspects of gastric function are controlled by the autonomic nervous system. The vagus nerves provide a predominant part of this innervation. The major branches of the vagi are shown schematically in Fig. 24-4. Each vagus has a single branch within the abdomen: the hepatic arising from the left anterior vagus, and the celiac from the right posterior vagus. The axial orientation of the vagi relates to the rotation of the stomach to the left as the lengthened foregut returns to the celomic cavity from the yolk sac during gestation. Each vagus terminates in the anterior and posterior nerves of Laterjet, respectively. Small branches course along the smaller blood vessels as they enter the gastric wall along its lesser curve. Knowledge of the anatomy of these nerves has resulted in a new technique, highly selective vagotomy, for treatment of peptic ulcer. In this procedure, the antral branches called the ''crow's-foot'' are preserved, while the more proximal branches are divided as they enter the stomach. The left anterior vagus will often divide into two or three branches before passing through the esophageal hiatus. The right posterior vagus may occasionally give off a small branch that courses to the left behind the esophagus to join the cardia. This branch has been termed the ''criminal nerve of Grassi'' in recognition of its important role in the etiology of recurrent ulcer when it is left undivided.

The splanchnic innervation to the stomach is less distinct than that of vagal origin. It has been demonstrated that some of the vagal fibers are adrenergic as well as cholinergic. The majority of sympathetic innervations, however, appear to be adrenergic. They accompany the gastrosplenic artery and its branches, which is appropriate for their function of control of blood flow and muscular function rather than secretory events within the mucosa. There is, in general, a paucity of knowledge about the precise role that local sympathetic nerves play in gastric function.

Morphology. The gastric wall consists of an external serosa that covers an inner oblique, a middle circular, and an outer longitudinal layer of smooth muscle. The submucosa and mucosa provide a continuous inner integument that is separated by a thin sheet of smooth muscle, the muscularis mucosa (Fig. 24-5). A prominent characteristic of the mucosa is a rich mucosal capillary network that is derived from small arteries that originate in the submucosa. Arteriovenous shunts are rarely seen within the gastric wall.

The mucosal lining of the gastric antrum (distal one-third) is distinctly different from that of the gastric fundus (proximal two-thirds). The latter has an elaborate network of deep glands, four or five of which join an indentation within the mucosal surface called a *pit* or *foveolus*. Individual pits are seen along with the cells that line the interfoveolar area in a scanning electron micrograph in Fig. 24-6. The gastric glands consist of six major cell types: sur-

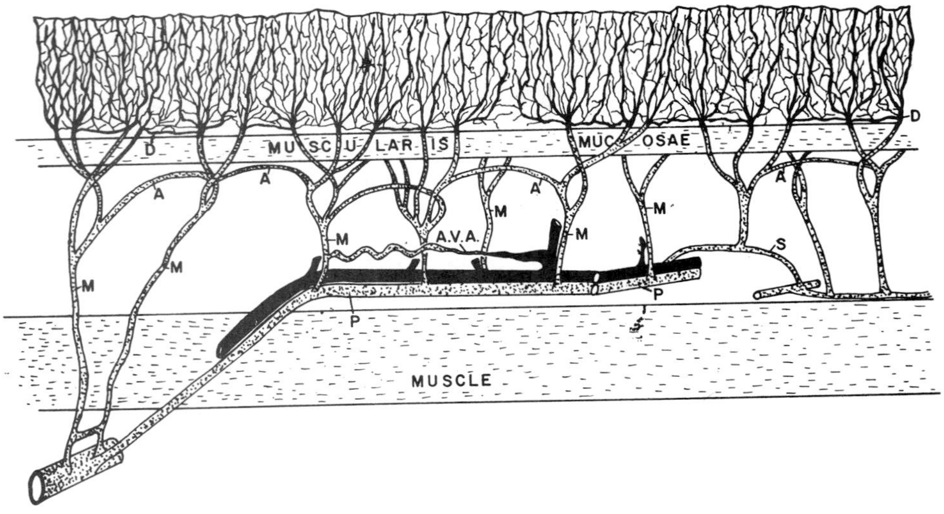

FIG. 24-5. Diagram of the lush mucosal capillary network of the stomach and the network of relatively large caliber arterioles that exist in the submucosa. Legend: D—anastomosing channels; A—anastomosis; M—mucosal arteries; AVA—arteriovenous anastomosis; P—submucous plexus; S—subsidiary anastomosing channels. (From: *Barlow TE, et al: Surg Gynecol Obstet 93:668, 1951, with permission.*)

face, mucous neck, progenitor, chief, parietal, and endocrine cells. (Fig. 24-7). The surface epithelial cells are distinguished by abundant mucous granules within their apical surface. These cells are designed to protect the epithelium from ingestants and the injurious effects of gastric acid. They are also the likely source of a sodium-rich alkaline secretion. The mucous neck cells line the entrance to gastric glands. They may serve the purpose of partially buffering nascent acid as it enters the gastric pits. Cells at the base of the gastric pits serve as stem or progenitor cells for the development of new surface cells and also the cells of the gastric glands. Knowledge of the function of the parietal cells distributed within the gastric glands is more secure than that of surface cells, for it has been proved that they are the site of secretion of hydrochloric acid. The characteristics of a resting and secreting cell are shown in Fig. 24-8*A* and *B*. Chief cells are the source of pepsinogen, a proteolytic enzyme that is converted to its active form, pepsin, at a pH below 2.5. A variety of endocrine cells exist within the gastric gland. Some secrete gastrin or serotonin, while the function of the others has not as yet been elucidated.

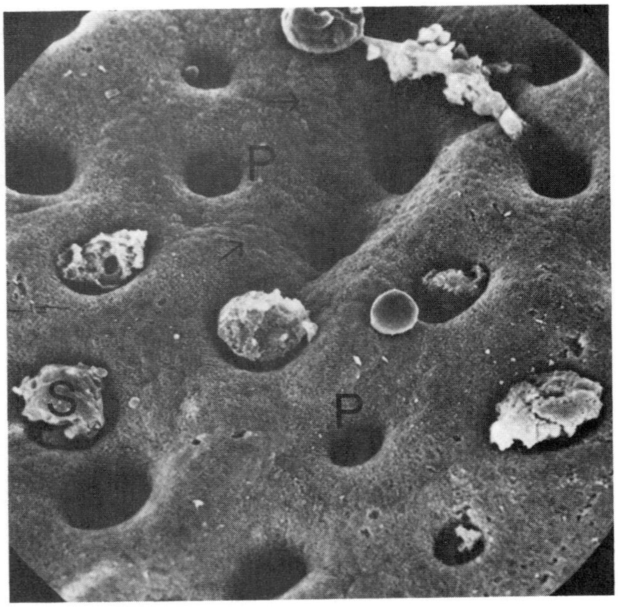

FIG. 24-6. Fundic gastric mucosa illustrating multiple gastric pits (P), some of which are filled with secretion (S). "Cobblestone" appearance of the epithelium is suggested (*arrows*) (×400). (*Courtesy of CA Zalewsky, PhD.*)

The antral mucosa is less specialized than that within the fundic area. In fact, by light microscopy, one can only identify surface epithelial cells and mucous neck cells. There are no parietal or chief cells. Gastrin-producing cells (G-cells), however, can be identified by radioimmunofluorescence.

Sphincters. The entrance of ingestants into the stomach is controlled by a highly specialized 5-cm area of smooth muscle, termed the *lower esophageal sphincter*. This sphincter, which presents a high-pressure zone between the esophagus and stomach, relaxes to allow the passage of foodstuffs. It then contracts to prevent the regurgitation of gastric contents into the esophagus. This sphincter is important because it protects the esophageal mucosa from corrosion by gastric acid.

The lower esophageal sphincter does not have an anatomic correlate, i.e., an identifiable mound of smooth muscle that can be easily felt and even seen when cut in cross section. By contrast, the pyloric sphincter, which prevents (or minimizes) duodenogastric reflux, is both anatomic and physiologic. It also serves as a metering point for the movement of food particles into the duodenum. Particles that are more than 2 mm in size are rejected and forced back into the body of the stomach for further trituration and preliminary digestion.

PHYSIOLOGY

Storage. The major function of the stomach is to prepare ingested food for digestion and absorption as it descends through the small intestine. The process of early digestion requires that solid foodstuffs be stored for a prolonged period of time (4 hours) as they undergo reduction in size and preliminary breakdown into basic metabolic constituents. Once the meal has been processed to an appropriate particulate size and chemical composition, it is delivered intermittently to the duodenum for further digestion.

The storage function of the stomach is greatly enhanced by the process of receptive relaxation. This is an event whereby the upper

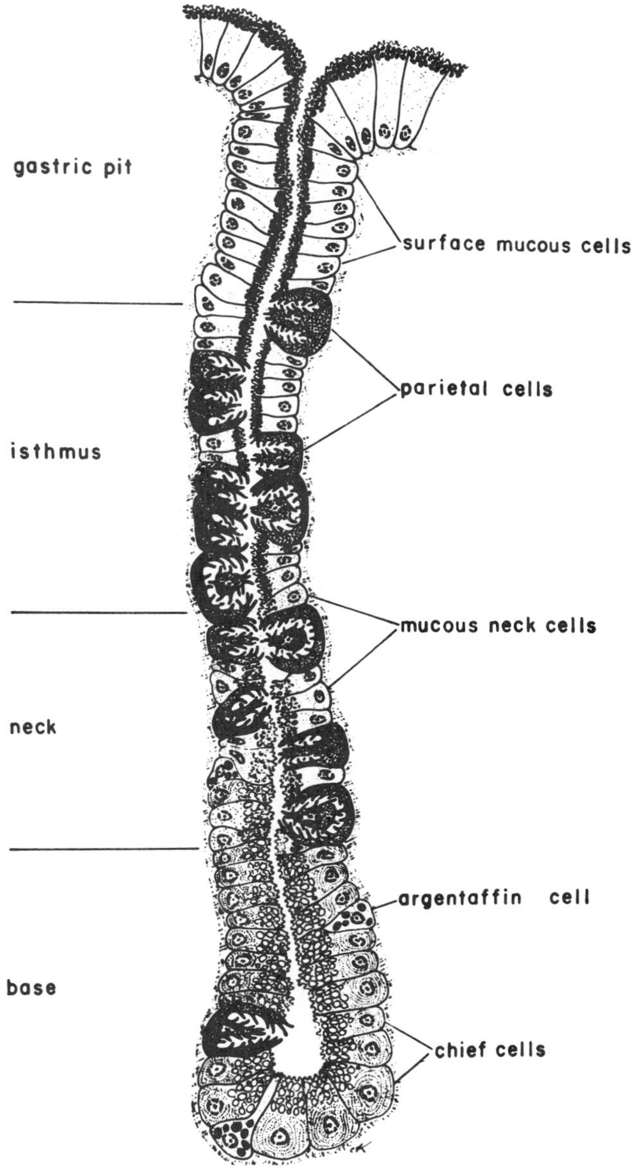

FIG. 24-7. Diagram of a single gastric gland of the bat. Between five and seven of these units open into the base of a single gastric pit (foveolus). (From: *Ito S, et al: J Cell Biol 16:543, 1963, with permission.*)

portion of the stomach relaxes as the intake of food is anticipated. Solid food settles and layers within the greater curvature of the fundic area of the stomach. Liquids pass rapidly from the stomach along its lesser curve (the magenstrasse), thereby leaving the solid mass quite undisturbed. Processing of the food mass is initiated by a skimming from the outermost layers of the gastric bolus. Salivary digestion occurs within its middle and gastric digestion at its periphery. Food particles are reduced in size by a grinding action of the antrum as well as digestion and dilution by the gastric secretions. The storage function of the stomach is enhanced by the antrum and pylorus, which constantly return material to the proximal stomach until it is ready for delivery to the duodenum. A surprising aspect of this very active mechanical process is that it proceeds for several hours after a solid meal without sensation of its occurrence.

Satiety is a feeling of gratification after eating. Morbidly obese individuals do not experience this feeling until they have consumed more food (calories) than they need. Appetite control is based on genetic, cultural, psychological, environmental, and physical factors, all of which play a role in how much one eats. The pathophysiologic consequence of abnormalities of this appetite control mechanism is obesity more often than malnutrition.

Digestion. Gastric digestion involves the breakdown of foodstuffs into fine particles. Starches undergo enzymatic breakdown as long as the pH within the center of the gastric bolus remains favorable for the activity of salivary alpha-amylase ($pH > 5$). Peptic digestion within the stomach is primarily designed to reduce the size of meat particles and initiate the dispersion of fats, proteins, and carbohydrates by breaking down cells walls. The gastric mucosa also secretes a lipase that assists in the early phase of fat digestion. The majority of digestion occurs within the duodenum and upper small bowel. The stomach is merely responsible for improving the efficiency of the process.

Gastric Acid Secretion. Acid-peptic disease of the esophagus, stomach, and duodenum represents one of the most common pathologic entities of the foregut. While gastric acid is usually not the single or even the predominant causative factor in peptic diseases, it is a critical component in their genesis. The dictum ''no acid, no ulcer'' has gained general support since the discovery by Beaumont (1833) that the stomach could secrete hydrochloric acid. Furthermore, all therapies for gastric and duodenal ulcer are based on control of intraluminal pH by either neutralization or inhibition of acid secretion.

It is convenient to consider the secretion of gastric acid in terms of its neurohumoral control. There is only a low rate of acid secretion during the interdigestive period when the stomach is at rest (2 to 3 meq/h). The sight and smell of food and its ingestion lead to a brisk secretion of hydrochloric acid. This activity is initiated by stimuli that pass from the cerebral cortex to the vagal centers within the hypothalamus. Action potentials descend the vagi and release acetylcholine within the enteric plexuses and their nerve endings in the gastric wall. Acetylcholine in turn leads to the release of gastrin from the antral mucosa and the secretion of acid and pepsinogen from the fundic mucosa. Gastrin is also a stimulant of acid secretion, and its action is greatly enhanced by the vagal release of acetylcholine. Histamine also participates in the acid secretory event and may, in fact, be a critical modulator of the process.

The gastrointestinal hormone, gastrin, is a polypeptide that has been well studied during the past decade since its isolation and purification by Gregory and Tracy. Numerous clinicians and scientists have made important contributions to our understanding of how this hormone might carry out its important activities within the gastrointestinal tract. Foremost among these is the late Morton Grossman who, over a 30-year period, stimulated numerous collaborators to find out how gastrin might contribute to acid secretion in the normal state and in disease. Unfortunately, the answer is still not known. It is to the credit of Yalow and Berson, and their collaborators, that the technique of radioimmunoassay has allowed a reasonably full description of its biologic function.

The vagal release of gastrin is enhanced by antral distention and contact of its mucosa with proteins. The ingestion of a meal is associated with a cumulative release of gastrin that provides for a

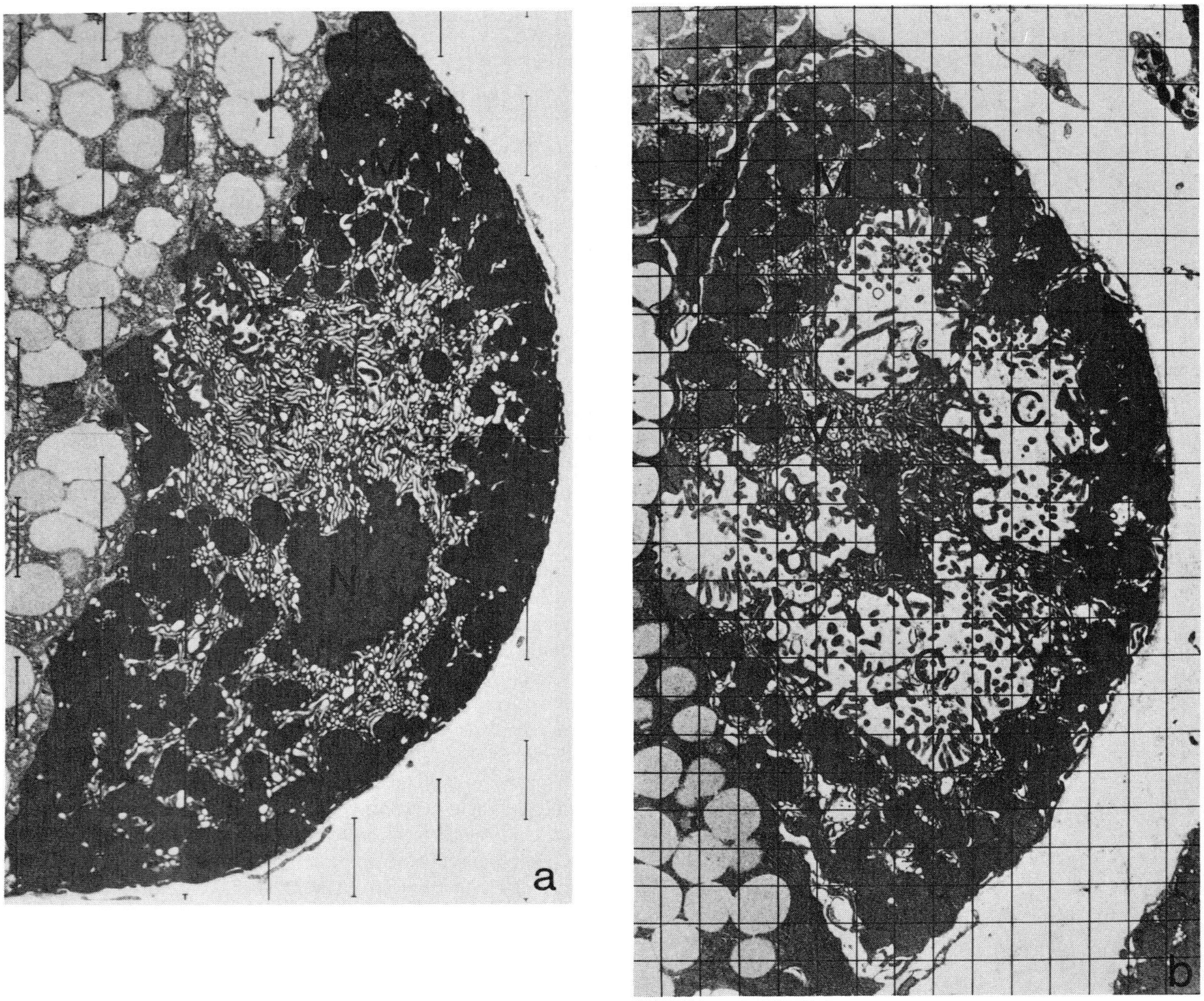

FIG. 24-8. *A.* Resting, unstimulated parietal cell in which the cytoplasm is occupied primarily by tubulovesicles (V) and peripheral mitochondria (M). Apical canaliculi (C) and nucleus (N) are present. A stereometric grid to measure membrane density covers the cell (×9500). *B.* Histamine-stimulated parietal cell with extensive development of canaliculi (C). Remaining tubulovesicles (V) surround the nucleus (N), and mitochondria (M) occupy the periphery. A stereometric grid to measure membrane density covers the cell (×9000). *(Courtesy of CA Zalewsky, PhD.)*

constant flow of acid secretion during gastric digestion. This gastrin release is facilitated as long as the intraluminal pH is high. Conversely, gastrin release is attenuated by a low pH on the antral mucosal surface. This negative feedback mechanism provides the principal control for the rate of acid secretion. Furthermore, it offers a check on the indiscriminate secretion of acid during the interdigestive period. The process described above is called the ''cephalogastric'' phase of acid secretion.

The duodenum and intestines also play a role in controlling acid secretion. Acidification of the duodenum leads to the release of secretin. Secretin inhibits both gastrin release and the secretion of gastric acid. Gastrin, which is also present within the mucosa of the duodenum and upper intestine, may be the source of the small stimulus for acid secretion that occurs as the products of a meal move through the intestinal tract. The intestinal phase of gastric secretion accounts for about 5 percent of the cumulative acid secretory response during the ingestion of a meal.

Parietal Cell Function. The parietal cell (Fig. 24-8*A* and *B*) is the established site of hydrochloric acid secretion. In the resting state, its cytoplasm consists of numerous mitochondria and tubulovesicles. With stimulation, there is a remarkable elaboration of membrane into an intracellular canaliculus. This is the presumed site of the transfer of hydrogen ions (H^+) to the luminal side of the plasma membrane into the tubule of the gastric gland. How this occurs is not completely known. A current scheme involves the translocation of a proton (H^+) at some site on the membrane in exchange for a potassium ion (K^+). This H^+ for K^+ exchange requires energy provided by oxidative phosphorylation (Fig. 24-9). The hydrolysis of ATP derived from this process is facilitated by a specific enzyme, adenosine triphosphatase

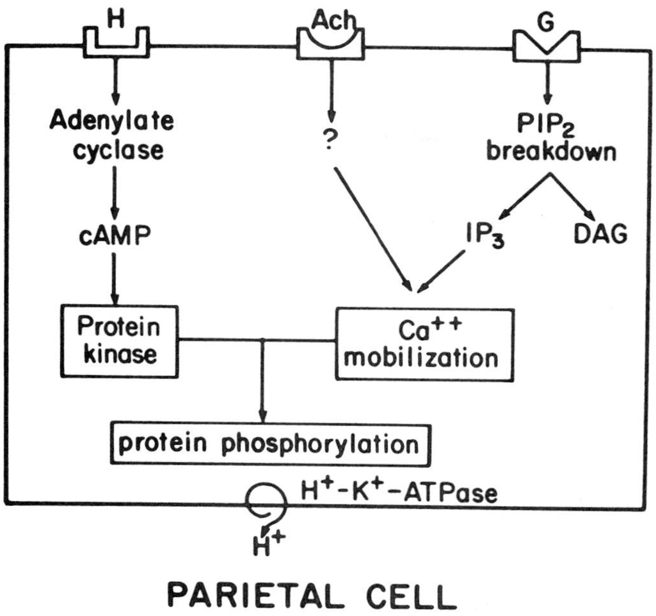

FIG. 24-9. Cellular mechanism of acid secretion. Legend: H—histamine; G—gastrin; DAG—diacylglycerol. (From: *Debas HT, Mulholland MW: Curr Probl Surg 26:14, 1989, with permission.*)

(ATPase). There is speculation that the Cl^- in this process is provided by its own translocation process. The extraordinary aspect of gastric acid secretion is that it moves H^+ against a millionfold chemical gradient (10^{-7} in the blood to 10^{-1} in gastric juice).

The parietal cell will secrete acid in response to acetylcholine, gastrin, and histamine. Acid secretion can be inhibited by a class of agents that block histamine receptors on the parietal cell (H_2, as opposed to the heart and lung histamine receptors called H_1). Because of this unique ability of these agents to block the H_2 receptor, they are commonly called H_2-receptor antagonists. Clinically available H_2 blockers include cimetidine (Tagamet), ranitidine (Zantac), famotidine (Pepcid), and nizatidine (Azid). Recently, an inhibitor of the hydrogen-potassium ATPase has been discovered. Because of its specificity, this inhibitor, omeprazole (Prilosec), has already been found to have clinical value in the treatment of various acid-peptic disorders, particularly acid reflux esophagitis. Prostaglandins are also potent inhibitors of acid secretion that are being evaluated for their clinical usefulness. The only prostaglandin currently available for clinical use is misoprostol (Cytotec), which has its greatest efficacy in the treatment and prevention of gastric injury from consumption of nonsteroidal anti-inflammatory compounds such as aspirin, indomethacin, and ibuprofen. Anticholinergics in high doses are partial antagonists of the secretory process, but their pronounced delaying effects on gastric emptying preclude their value as antisecretory agents. A new anticholinergic drug, pirenzepine, which appears to inhibit acid secretion without inducing other side effects, may prove to be of value in various acid-peptic disorders, but additional studies are needed to validate this notion. Vagotomy profoundly diminishes the response of the parietal cell to gastrin and histamine, an effect that has contributed to its effectiveness as a therapy for peptic ulcer.

Surface Cell Function. The surface epithelial cells line the outermost layer of the gastric epithelium and thereby are exposed to the contents of the gastric lumen. They are relatively impervious to H^+ ions and are protected from mechanical injury by a thin layer of mucus. This mucus layer is renewed constantly by a large number of mucus granules stored beneath the apical plasma membrane. Surface cells also produce a sodium-rich alkaline (bicarbonate) secretion. Numerous studies over the past decade strongly suggest that these mucous and bicarbonate secretions act in tandem to form a mucus-bicarbonate barrier that plays an important role under physiologic conditions as a gastric mucosal defense mechanism. As currently conceived, mucus sets up a pH gradient between the lumenal contents and the surface epithelium such that the pH on the lumenal side of mucus is acidic and that on the mucosal surface approaches neutrality. As hydrogen ions in the lumenal contents diffuse across this mucus-gel, they are not only slowed by the mucus itself, but bicarbonate secreted by the surface cells into this mucus neutralizes the diffusing hydrogen ions, giving rise to water and carbon dioxide. The net results of mucus and bicarbonate working together are maintenance of the pH gradient and protection of the surface epithelium from acid injury. Although much more needs to be learned about the physiology of this barrier and the conditions under which it is perturbed, current knowledge strongly implicates its importance as a major defense mechanism.

Gastric Analysis. There are a variety of ways to assess the acid secretory capacity of the stomach. The most accurate is to aspirate gastric contents under controlled conditions through a nasogastric tube. It is best to have the patient lying in a semirecumbent position on the left side. The study is commenced by aspirating the stomach of its contents and then instilling and immediately recovering 50 mL of normal saline. Complete recovery reveals appropriate tube placement. Aspirations are then done by hand syringe every 5 min for 1 h. The aspirates are pooled in 15-min aliquots. At the end of the final aspirate, the stomach is stimulated to secrete by the intravenous administration of histalog in a dose of 2 μg/kg, or pentagastrin in a dose of 6 μg/kg. Aspiration is continued as described above, with four 15-min collections obtained over a 1-h period. The volume of the collections is measured, and an aliquot is titrated electrometrically to determine its content of H^+. The rate of secretion is then expressed as the number of milliequivalents produced per hour during the basal or prestimulatory phase and during maximal and peak output. Maximal acid output (MAO) is obtained by averaging the output of the two final 15-min periods. Peak output is the highest rate of secretion obtained during a 15-min period after stimulation. Basal acid output (BAO) is normally 2 to 3 meq/h; secretory output (MAO) is in the range of 10 to 15 meq/h. Patients with duodenal ulcer generally have higher values, while those with gastric ulcer may have lower values. However, there is remarkable overlap between either condition and the normal, so identifying patients with peptic ulcer disease using purely acid secretory data alone is usually not possible. For this reason, most clinicians have found routine use of gastric analysis to be of little value in the workup of patients suspected of having gastric or duodenal ulcers. One situation in which gastric analysis may be of benefit is its use as a screen for the Zollinger-Ellison (ZE) syndrome. In this illness characterized by flagrant ulcer disease, basal acid outputs may be in excess of 50 meq/h.

Pepsinogen. The role of pepsinogen in gastroduodenal disease has not been well defined. Pepsinogen, a proenzyme, does not assume its proteolytic activity until activated by a pH below 2.5. Pepsin, the activated enzyme, can digest food as well as devitalized tissue but has virtually no effect on healthy, well-nourished cells. Its role in the pathogenesis of peptic ulcer is uncertain, but its ability to digest devitalized cells probably contributes to the formation of the ulcer crater. Thus, the well-circumscribed, clean nature of a peptic ulcer bed is likely a consequence of its activity. Pepsinogen is stored within chief cells in the form of granules whose release is under vagal control. It is interesting that so little is known about a substance that assumes illusionary importance by the terms ''peptic ulcer'' and ''dyspepsia.''

Gastric Emptying. ***Control Mechanisms.*** Gastric emptying is modulated by a highly integrated process that includes mechanical, chemical, and neurohumoral mechanisms. Solids are preprocessed in the stomach over a period of hours during which they are reduced in size and dispersed within the gastric juice for efficient digestion. In addition, the osmolality of the chyme is reduced by dilution. The latter function is important in the prevention of the dumping syndrome. Dumping occurs when an osmotic load is delivered to the intestine, causing an influx of water, intestinal distention, and rapid transit of the predigested meal. This leads to light-headedness, sweating, tachycardia, crampy abdominal pain, and diarrhea. It is, therefore, logical that one of the important control mechanisms should include osmoreceptors within the duodenum.

An understanding of the neurohumoral control of gastric emptying is currently incomplete. The observation that truncal vagotomy does not predictably lead to delayed gastric emptying has led to ambiguity about the role of the autonomic nervous system. In fact, vagotomy may hasten the transit of liquids when a pyloroplasty or gastroenterostomy has been performed. The antrum appears to be the key component in propulsion from the stomach, and its activity is clearly under vagal control. Apparently the myenteric plexuses that are a component of the enteric nervous system can continue to function in response to intraluminal stimulation of food even in the absence of central vagal innervation. Furthermore, denervation causes an increase in serum gastrin as a consequence of loss of antral acidification. Possibly the law of Cannon, in which denervated receptors become more sensitive to chemical stimuli, is at work in this situation, whereby the gastrin receptors that stimulate gastric smooth muscle contractions may be rendered supersensitive to a point of compensating for the loss of centrally mediated vagal release of acetylcholine.

What is known is as follows: Anticipation of a meal leads to vagally mediated gastrin release, gastric acid secretion, receptive relaxation of the proximal stomach, rhythmic antral contractions, and coordinated relaxation of the pyloric sphincter. Ingestion of the meal accentuates all of these responses. Emptying of liquids is continuous and relatively rapid, depending on the osmolarity. Solids must be reduced to a few millimeters in diameter before antral discharge occurs.

Gastric motor function is related in some way to the electromyographic activity within its smooth muscle. The stomach has a pacemaker high on the greater curve that likely initiates contractions in the area by phasic spike potentials that entrain a series of action potentials toward the pylorus (Fig. 24-10). The precise role of the myoelectric entrainment is not understood, nor is it a critical phenomenon since division of the stomach does not interfere with aborad electrical activity or gastric emptying.

Fats delay gastric emptying by an unknown mechanism. Gastric lipase may be responsible in that it is slow to reduce the droplet size of fats. It is also possible that the antral or duodenal mucosa may have a chemical sensor for specific fatty acids. Finally, lipid-related cholecystokinin release may affect gastric emptying by retarding emptying.

Gastric Emptying Studies. There are a variety of ways to assess gastric emptying. The simplest is to instill a known volume of saline into the stomach and attempt to recover it at a fixed time. Lewis recommends instillation of 750 mL into the unoperated

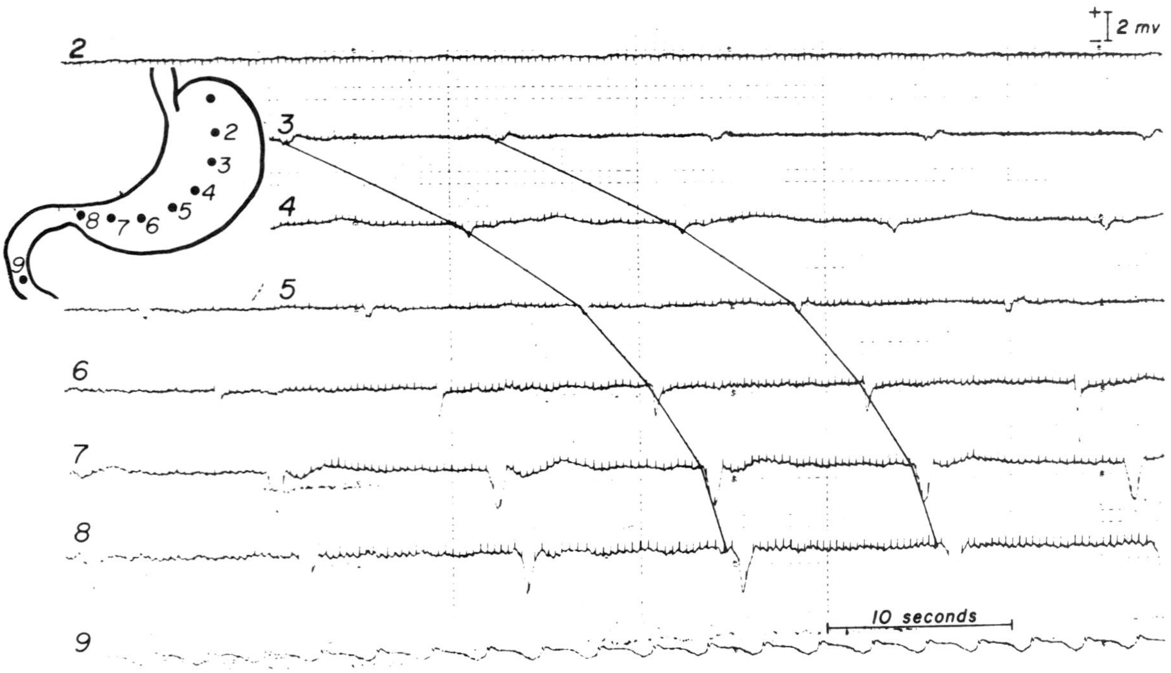

FIG. 24-10. Illustration of electrical activity measured at different sites on the stomach. The recordings demonstrate the distal migration of myoelectric complexes from the gastric pacemaker. (From: *Kelly KA, et al: Am J Physiol 217:465, 1969, with permission.*)

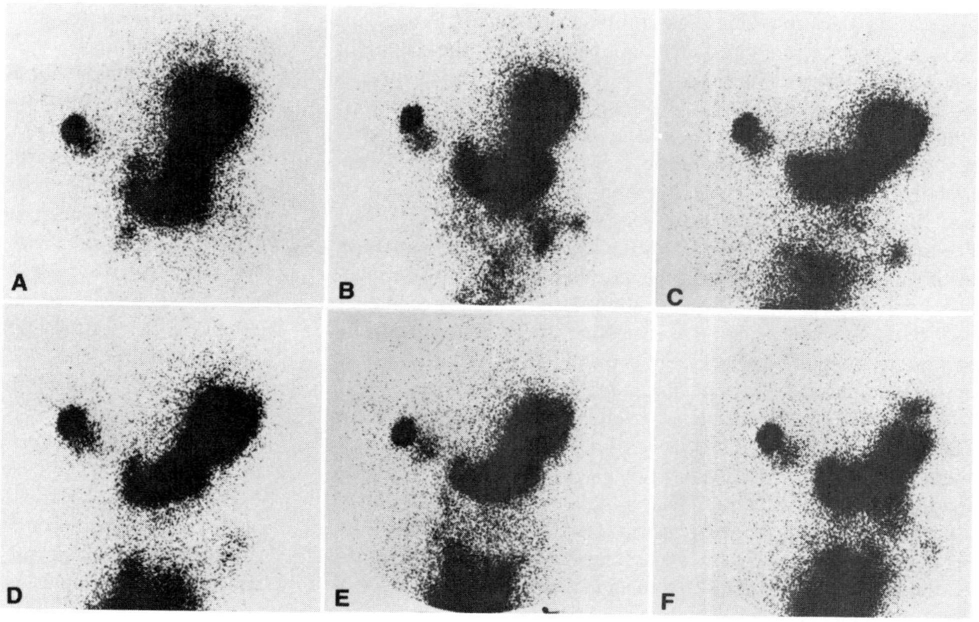

FIG. 24-11. A normal solid-phase gastric emptying study using 100 μC technetium sulfur colloid. Gamma camera images were made at *A*, immediately after ingestion of the radioactive meal; *B*, after 15 min; *C*, after 30 min; *D*, after 45 min; *E*, after 60 min; and *F*, after 90 min. The sequential pictures show more activity in the small bowel and less in the stomach. (*Courtesy of P Christian.*)

stomach. Gastric aspiration at 30 min with returns of less than 200 mL indicates normal pyloric function. Pyloric dysfunction or obstruction usually yields a volume greater than 400 mL. This saline load test can provide a qualitative view of the stomach's capacity to empty a liquid meal. A barium radiograph can also provide some information on adequacy of emptying and may reveal pathology that might contribute to a delay such as pyloric obstruction. Computerized radionuclide scans have provided a quantitative way to measure the emptying rate of liquids as well as solids. Radiolabeled technetium is used to monitor the rate of liquid emptying. The solid phase is measured with radioactive chicken livers. An example of the appearance of such a study is shown in Fig. 24-11. These studies are particularly helpful in patients who have gastric atony from vagal denervation, diabetes, or other associated illness.

Other Gastric Functions. The stomach plays an important role in hematopoiesis through its production of intrinsic factor by the parietal cell. Intrinsic factor is essential for the ileal absorption of vitamin B_{12}. Of added, but not critical, importance is a relationship between acid secretion and iron absorption by the duodenum, a relationship that involves the important role of acid in proteolysis and breakdown of animal cells. Additionally, iron absorption takes place in the duodenum and proximal jejunum where it is best enhanced because of the ferrous state (Fe^{2+}) which is facilitated by ascorbic acid and other reducing substances that are commonly present in this region of the gut.

Gastric acidification is also important in maintaining sterility of the foregut. Only a few unusual fusiform bacillae can withstand the challenges of a low gastric pH. It is known that the upper gastrointestinal tract is rapidly colonized by enteric bacteria when the stomach is rendered achlorhydric by medical or surgical means.

Immunologic Sensing. It is reasonable to assume that the gastric mucosa is involved in the detection of harmful ingestants. It is well suited for this purpose with its ability to protect its surface by rapid mucus release, creating an unstirred layer that may form a first line of defense against harmful macromolecules. If potentially dangerous substances (with chemical or oncological portent) should permeate the mucosa, they immediately encounter the lamina propria and its army of mast cells and free-floating macrophages and lymphocytes. The role of the gastric mucosa in immunosurveillance has not yet been elucidated.

Heat Exchange. The stomach with its lush mucosal microcirculation is an excellent heat exchanger. This is an important function, for it ensures the intraluminal contents a relatively stable thermal environment for their enzymatic digestion. Furthermore, the mechanism offers protection against cooling of adjacent viscera or significant changes in core temperature.

GASTRIC DYSFUNCTION

Symptoms. ***Anorexia.*** Lack of appetite, or anorexia, is a common symptom that everyone has from time to time, especially during a viral illness. In fact, it is so frequently associated with psychologic stress that it may initially be overlooked as an early sign of a serious illness. For example, most patients with cancer of the gastrointestinal tract will recall that they were anorectic during the early phase of their illness. Anorexia is usually the reason for weight loss in neoplastic as well as other diseases within the gastrointestinal tract.

Nausea and Vomiting. The gastrointestinal tract is capable of protecting itself from harmful ingestants by a forceful evacuation of its contents through the mouth, known as *vomiting*. Vomiting is a complex process. After a deep breath, the glottis is closed. The stomach then evacuates its contents by retropulsion. The reversed movement of gastrointestinal contents is assisted by a tightening of the muscles of the abdomen and thorax, a decrease in acid secretion, and an autonomic response that includes sweating, pallor, and tachycardia. Nausea is a sensation of impending emesis and may be of central or peripheral origin. It is not always accompanied by vomiting. In fact, many patients with vaguely defined gastrointestinal disease will complain of nausea. It is a symptom that accompanies low-grade visceral pain such as might occur in gallstone disease, mild pancreatitis, peptic ulcer, or the early phase of acute appendicitis.

The vomiting of "intestinal origin" is often associated with other signs such as abdominal distention or emesis of blood (varices, gastritis, or peptic ulcer) or intestinal contents. The character of the vomitus may be helpful in establishing a diagnosis. Lack of bile suggests a point of obstruction above the papilla of Vater. Feculent vomiting is associated with low small bowel obstruction, its brown color and foul odor being a result of bacterial overgrowth by enteric organisms. Obstruction at this level is usually accompanied by generalized abdominal distention, in contrast to chronic pyloric obstruction in which there is distention of the mid and left upper abdomen from a fluid- and air-filled stomach.

Pain. The mucosa of the stomach is devoid of pain endings. This explains in part the relatively painless nature of erosive gastritis, gastric cancer, and even peptic ulcer disease of the stomach. Acute gastric distention may also be a relatively pain-free event, especially in the postoperative period. Acid-peptic disease of the duodenum, however, has a very characteristic pain pattern depending on the depth of ulceration. Early superficial ulceration is usually associated with a gnawing sensation within the midepigastrium. When acid is unbuffered, such as might occur in the early morning hours, the pain is sharp and more intense. A characteristic of duodenal ulcer pain is that it disappears as soon as an antacid or other neutralizing substance is ingested. Gastric ulcer pain is more subtle and diffuse in nature, often coming on during or after eating, rather than before. The sudden onset of severe, unrelenting, generalized abdominal pain is a sign of ulcer perforation. This, of course, is a catastrophic event that requires immediate surgical attention.

Regurgitation. The reflux of gastric contents into the esophagus may be associated with three complaints: (1) heartburn, (2) expectoration of gastric chyme, and (3) cough from aspiration. Heartburn is a sensation of mild to moderate substernal discomfort. It is an annoying, diffuse, burning pain that is usually well tolerated by the patient. Not only acid but also alkaline regurgitation can cause this symptom, which may be associated with inflammation within the esophageal mucosa. A severe subxiphoid or substernal pain exacerbated by feeding (odynophagia) is a sign of esophageal ulceration. Difficulty in swallowing (dysphagia) accompanies esophageal obstruction from peptic stricture, esophagogastric cancer, or a primary motor disturbance such as achalasia or esophageal spasm.

Regurgitation is a sign of loss of the high-pressure zone that normally exists between the stomach and esophagus. Recall that the pressure within the body of the esophagus reflects intrathoracic pressure, and therefore is subatmospheric (-5 to -10 mmHg). Gastric pressures are positive, 5 to 10 mmHg. The pressures within the lower esophageal segment (LES) must, therefore, be in excess of 15 mmHg in order to prevent reflux. Factors that control the pressure within the LES are not completely known, but they include vagal release of acetylcholine, intraabdominal pressure, intragastric pressure, and ill-defined humoral mechanisms, which may include cyclic nucleotides and prostaglandins. Pharmacologic doses of acetylcholine, metoclopramide, gastrin, and calcium blocking agents can reconstitute low esophageal sphincter pressures. The LES can also be repaired operatively by wrapping the upper part of the stomach around the lower end of the esophagus (Nissen fundoplication).

Signs. ***Bleeding.*** Upper gastrointestinal bleeding demands a thorough evaluation of the alimentary tract. Hematemesis (vomiting of blood) may be a dramatic, exsanguinating event, or it may be a manifestation of a minor bleed from gastritis or peptic ulcer. The nature of the vomitus may provide a clue to the rate and site of bleeding. Coffee-ground emesis (acid-hematin) is usually a sign of peptic ulcer. Bright-red emesis may be from an esophageal varix, a gastric mucosal tear, gastritis, or a peptic ulcer. Gastric or duodenal bleeding can occur without hematemesis. In this instance the stool is usually black. More rapid bleeding, however, can result in bright-red stools. Newer technology now permits rapid identification and control of the offending lesion. This is accomplished by upper gastrointestinal endoscopy whereby the esophagus, stomach, and duodenum can be safely and quickly inspected. Bleeding sites can be controlled by electrocoagulation or photocoagulation, and biopsies of suspicious lesions can be obtained for histologic examination.

Weight Loss. Gastric disease, especially neoplasia, is usually accompanied by gradual loss of weight. Benign gastric ulcer is associated with weight loss as a consequence of the avoidance of food which might induce abdominal pain. Duodenal ulcer is usually accompanied by weight gain in response to pain control by the ingestion of milk and other alkalinizing foods.

Gastric Distention. Acute gastric dilatation provokes an intense autonomic response that includes pallor, rapid respirations, bradycardia, and hypotension. This is a dramatic and serious complication that may follow any operation within the abdomen. It can easily be diagnosed by inspection and percussion of the abdomen which reveals a markedly distended stomach. Once recognized, the problem is easily remedied, by the passage of a nasogastric tube and gastric aspiration.

Abdominal Tenderness. Peptic ulcer disease may be accompanied by tenderness on deep palpation within the midepigastrium. This is a common sign when an active ulcer is present within the duodenum; gastric ulcers, except when they penetrate through the gastric wall, are usually nontender. Gastric neoplasms are also not associated with discomfort on palpation. Perforated ulcers are usually accompanied by marked, generalized tenderness in response to the intense chemical peritonitis that accompanies the leak of gastric acid into the abdominal cavity. Because of the intense abdominal rigidity that results from the peritoneal irritation, "a boardlike abdomen" has been the description assigned to this finding.

Palpable Tumor. Gastric neoplasms of the distal stomach may present as a palpable mass within the epigastrium or left upper abdomen. Gastric tumors can usually be distinguished from mass lesions that arise within the pancreas, since they are more anterior and often movable. Liver tumors are even more superficial and usually will descend with deep inspiration. Neoplasms of the proximal stomach are hidden from detection by physical examination by the left hemithorax.

Diagnosis. ***Radiography.*** Visualization of the upper gastrointestinal tract by barium radiography has provided a safe, convenient, reliable way to detect gastric and duodenal disease. Unfortunately, over half of the acute lesions of the duodenum and almost all superficial erosions of the stomach go undetected by this type of examination. It still remains, however, a starting point for patients with chronic symptoms of upper gastrointestinal disease. A normal upper gastrointestinal barium series is shown in Fig. 24-

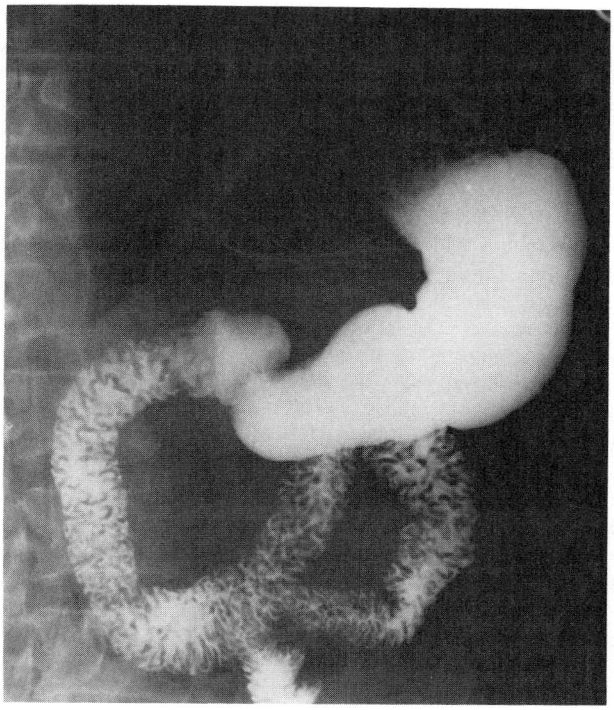

FIG. 24-12. Normal upper gastrointestinal barium radiograph.

12. Multiple views are required to gain a full view of the stomach and duodenal bulb.

Endoscopy. Patients who present with the signs and symptoms of upper gastrointestinal hemorrhage are usually subjected to endoscopy early in their hospital course, especially when the bleeding is massive or persistent. Endoscopy for chronic symptoms is also a routine procedure that can be done on an ambulatory basis with high yield and little risk or discomfort to the patient. Most gastroenterologists, and an increasing number of general surgeons, are proficient at the technique of upper gastrointestinal endoscopy. An advantage of the technique is the opportunity it provides to obtain photographs and biopsies of suspicious lesions.

Postgastrectomy Syndromes. Operations on the stomach that include resection, pyloric ablation (pyloroplasty) or bypass (gastroenterostomy), and total gastric vagotomy may be accompanied by unpleasant side effects. For convenience, they have been termed ''postgastrectomy syndromes'' (Table 24-1). They occur to varying degrees in about 20 percent of patients in the early months after stomach surgery. With time and attention to diet, the symptoms disappear in the majority of patients. About 5 percent of patients, however, remain symptomatic for the remainder of their lives, and 1 percent become permanently disabled to a point of being considered ''gastric cripples.'' It is for this reason that lesser procedures such as proximal gastric vagotomy without drainage have replaced the more extensive 75 percent gastric resection and truncal vagotomy and varying degrees of partial gastric resection for the treatment of acid-peptic disease of the duodenum.

Table 24-1
Postgastrectomy Syndromes

Small capacity
Dumping
Bile gastritis
Afferent loop
Efferent loop
Postvagotomy diarrhea
Anemia
Metabolic bone disease

Surprisingly, total gastrectomy with esophagojejunal reconstruction is fairly well tolerated by patients who require it for gastric cancer or the Zollinger-Ellison syndrome. They usually remain on the slender side but have few gastrointestinal complaints if they eat several small meals a day. It is essential that they receive injections of vitamin B_{12} on a monthly basis, since they cannot absorb it from the gut in the absence of intrinsic factor that formerly came from the parietal cells.

The dumping syndrome, characterized by light-headedness, diaphoresis, palpitations, crampy abdominal pain, and diarrhea, is a consequence of the rapid movement of gastric contents into the upper intestinal tract. It usually is related to the ingestion of a high-carbohydrate meal. Pyloric bypass or ablation appears to be the main contributor to this syndrome. Vagotomy and the type of gastric reconstruction do not appear to be important variables in its frequency. The mystery is why it occurs as a chronic symptom so infrequently. Management of patients with dumping can usually be accomplished with modifications in diet, particularly carbohydrate content, and altering the volume of a given meal and instead instituting six smaller feedings spaced evenly throughout the day rather than the usual three regular feedings. In the event that these measures do not work, treatment with octreotide, a synthetic somatostatin analogue, has proved effective in selected individuals.

Extensive gastrectomy is accompanied by early satiety, a symptom called the *small-capacity syndrome*. This is a serious problem, since it can lead to profound weight loss and malnutrition.

Truncal vagotomy requires an accompanying drainage procedure (pyloroplasty or gastroenterostomy); otherwise gastric stasis may lead to nausea, vomiting, or gastric ulceration. The extragastric vagal denervation associated with this procedure may also contribute to gallstone formation and incapacitating, explosive diarrhea.

Bile gastritis has been recognized as a consequence of gastrectomy in recent years. It is an entity that is characterized by vague symptoms of low-grade epigastric pain, chronic nausea, and bilious vomiting. Barium examination of the stomach is usually nonrevealing. Erosive gastritis may be seen during endoscopic examination of the gastric mucosa. Biopsy often reveals round cell infiltration and edema, especially at the site of mucosal lesions. Unfortunately, patients without gastrointestinal complaints may have similar findings. The strongest evidence that bile may be involved in the syndrome relates to the observation that approximately half of individuals who undergo biliary diversion by Roux en Y gastrojejunostomy will gain symptomatic relief.

The afferent loop syndrome is a clearly defined entity that is characterized by bilious vomiting after distal gastric resection and gastrojejunal anastomosis (Billroth II). The patient will complain of a severe midepigastric pain after eating which is relieved by the emesis of a large volume of bile. Its pathogenesis relates to an obstruction at the junction of the afferent limb coming from the duodenum to the gastric remnant. Food usually has already passed from the stomach into the efferent limb; therefore, it is not mixed with the emesis, as is the case when the efferent loop is obstructed. These conditions are mechanical in nature, as a consequence of either recurrent ulcer or a technical error at the time of reconstruction. Their correction requires reoperation.

Acid-reducing procedures of all types can be accompanied by an iron deficiency or even macrocytic anemia. Bile gastritis and duodenal bypass may increase the frequency and severity of hematologic disturbances. Also of concern is the possibility of an increased incidence of cancer in the gastric remnant after acid reduction procedures for duodenal ulcer, although opinion on this eventuality is by no means uniform.

Diarrhea is one of the most common and distressing complaints after gastric surgery. In a small number of patients it contributes to profound, life-threatening malnutrition. In most patients, however, avoidance of foods that contribute to dumping provides a return to a normal bowel habit. Postvagotomy diarrhea is explosive and unpredictable, a most undesirable sequela. Until recently the only therapy for this condition has been the use of antimotility drugs without consistent success. With the development of the somatostatin analogue, octreotide, initial trials with this drug suggest that it can effectively manage postvagotomy diarrhea as it does dumping. Occasionally, gastric surgery will unmask nontropical sprue or a lactase deficiency. These conditions can be diagnosed by small bowel mucosal biopsy, with specific histochemical staining for the presence or absence of lactase.

Recurrent ulcer is a disappointing postgastrectomy sequela. Some patients may present with multiple symptoms including dumping, bilious vomiting, and pain from recurrent ulcer. This presents a quandary in diagnosis and management. Most students of the postgastrectomy syndromes are ultraconservative in offering patients further reconstructive surgery, since the results are modest even in the hands of those skilled in the management of such complex problems.

GASTRIC DISEASE

Peptic Ulcer—Duodenum

Peptic ulcer disease of the duodenum is one of the most common illnesses of the foregut. The stomach's complicity relates to the presumed role of gastric acid secretion in ulcerogenesis. While it is true that achlorhydric patients rarely develop peptic ulcers and that most patients with hyperchlorhydria from gastrinoma (Zollinger-Ellison syndrome) have severe ulcer disease, patients with more common forms of duodenal ulcer may not have hypersecretion of acid. It is for this reason that the role of acid in ulcerogenesis is ambiguous and to this day subject to challenge.

Pathophysiology. Chronic duodenal ulceration is almost never of neoplastic origin except in rare instances of duodenal cancer. Acute ulcers may occur in a setting of extreme psychological or physical stress. The etiology of acute and chronic ulceration is multivariate. It involves aggressive factors, such as gastric acid and pepsin, and protective factors, which include the alkaline duodenal secretions (bile, pancreatic juice, and duodenal secretion from Brunner's glands) and the duodenal epithelium (hydrogen for sodium exchange, bicarbonate secretion, blood flow, and release of antisecretory hormones such as secretin).

Several observations suggest that duodenal ulcer disease in many patients is a consequence of the secretion of acid in excess of the amount that can be efficiently disposed of by the duodenum. Such patients have an increased basal and stimulated acid secretory output. In addition, they have an augmented cumulative gastrin response to an ingested meal. They also have acidification of the duodenum for prolonged periods ($pH < 2$), an event rarely seen in normal patients. That hypersecretion of acid can cause duodenal ulceration has been well established in experimental animal models. Furthermore, as mentioned above, patients with hypersecretion of acid on the basis of hypergastrinemia from a pancreatic tumor have a severe ulcer diathesis that subsides when acid secretion is controlled by antisecretory agents. The usual forms of duodenal ulcer also heal when gastric acid is either neutralized by ingestion of antacids or inhibited by antisecretory agents.

There is abundant evidence that reduction of duodenal buffers contributes to ulceration. An example is the removal of bile from the duodenum by biliary diversion into a limb of jejunum. Another is the reduction in the flow of pancreatic juice in chronic pancreatitis or following extensive pancreatic resection. Transposition of the bile and pancreatic secretions into the small intestine at a point where they cannot reflux into the duodenum in experimental animals uniformly leads to chronic duodenal ulceration.

The surgical treatment of peptic ulcer (particularly duodenal ulcer) has as its rationale the reduction of acid secretory output to a point that will provide permanent cure for peptic ulcer. There has been a gradual evolution of how this can best be accomplished. Initial efforts were directed toward diversion of acid from the duodenum (gastroenterostomy) and reduction of the acid secretory mass by extensive resection. Knowledge that acid secretion is under vagal control has led to vagotomy as a simpler operative approach with less immediate and late morbidity.

Clinical Manifestations. Chronic duodenal ulcer disease can present in a number of ways. It usually has its onset in early or midadult life and occurs more frequently in males than in females (4 to 1). The clinical stereotype of an intense, compulsive, cigarette-smoking, alcohol-drinking executive has not been well established in careful epidemiologic studies, but such individuals do represent a high-risk group. There may also be genetic factors other than those that relate to families with gastrinoma or hyperparathyroidism as a component of a multiple endocrine neoplasia syndrome (MEN).

Abdominal Pain. The most common feature of duodenal ulcer is a gnawing, sometimes sharp, well-localized midepigastric pain. The pain is tolerable and usually relieved by alkali or milk. It is for this reason that many patients do not seek medical advice until they have had the disease for many years. In addition, the pain is episodic, coming and going over periods of months for unknown reasons. There appears to be a spring and fall seasonal occurrence and a relapse during periods of extreme stress. The development of constant pain is a sign of deep penetration. Referral of pain to the back is often associated with penetration into the pancreas. Generalized severe abdominal pain is a sign of free perforation.

Bleeding. Gastrointestinal bleeding is a common manifestation of duodenal ulcer. This is not surprising, since the duodenal wall has an abundant blood supply, and there are several large blood vessels posterior to the duodenal bulb. In fact, most cases of massive upper gastrointestinal hemorrhage are secondary to a posterior ulcer that has penetrated into the gastroduodenal artery or one of its branches. Most ulcers are more superficial or are located on the duodenal wall that is not adjacent to large blood vessels.

This is the reason why most duodenal ulcers present with only minor bleeding episodes, usually detected by melenic (black) or guaiac-positive feces.

Obstruction. Duodenal ulcer during a period when the disease is active is often associated with delayed gastric emptying characterized by anorexia, or nausea, or vomiting. These symptoms may be a consequence of pylorospasm or obstruction to the gastric outlet by an inflammatory mass. In cases of protracted vomiting, patients may become dehydrated and develop a hypokalemic, hypochlorhydric alkalosis from the loss of large amounts of gastric juice that is rich in hydrogen, chloride, and potassium ions. To correct for the volume losses that occur from vomiting, the kidneys initially attempt to correct the acid-base imbalance by excreting excess bicarbonate in the urine to compensate for the developing alkalosis. If vomiting continues, maintenance of intravascular volume and osmolality become more important priorities. To address these problems, the kidneys respond by enhancing sodium reabsorption via the distal tubule in exchange for potassium. Compounding this excessive potassium excretion is increased bicarbonate reabsorption with further aggravation of the existing alkalosis. With continued gastric losses, the potassium in the extracellular space moves intracellularly in exchange for hydrogen ion in a further attempt to reestablish acid-base balance. As the extracellular potassium depletion continues, the kidneys now reabsorb sodium in exchange for hydrogen ion. The net effect of these aberrations is an increase in the alkalotic state that results in a paradoxically acid urine commonly seen in states of prolonged metabolic alkalosis. It is for these reasons that therapy must include intravenous restitution of these losses and nasogastric suction for control and assessment of replacement needs. Until the chloride and potassium deficits have been replaced, the kidney is unable to correct the metabolic alkalosis. Therapy, therefore, includes intravenous restitution of these losses and nasogastric suction for control and assessment of replacement needs.

Long-standing duodenal ulcer, with recurrent episodes of healing and repair, may lead to cicatricial stenosis of the lumen of the duodenum. Patients with pyloric obstruction on this basis usually have painless vomiting of large volumes of undigested food once or twice a day. The stomach in this condition is usually massively dilated and has lost its muscular tone. This form of obstruction may be associated with marked weight loss and malnutrition. Treatment is always surgical after appropriate metabolic and nutritional preparation that may include a period of parenteral hyperalimentation.

Perforation. Penetration of an ulcer through the duodenal wall is usually accompanied by an effort at containment by the greater omentum or adjacent viscera. Occasionally (about 5 percent of the time), a penetrating ulcer will perforate into the free peritoneal cavity. This is a dramatic clinical event, characterized by severe generalized abdominal pain, fever, tachycardia, dehydration, and ileus. This complication represents a surgical emergency. The diagnosis is easily made by palpation of the abdomen, which almost always reveals exquisite tenderness, rigidity, and rebound. Percussion demonstrates loss of liver dullness. An upright radiograph of the chest will usually demonstrate free air beneath the diaphragm. Operation to close the perforation and clean the peritoneal cavity should be carried out within a few hours after the patient enters the emergency department. Operation should be delayed only for appropriate fluid resuscitation. Early intervention will usually reveal sterile exudate within the abdomen; delay will most certainly be associated with a subsequent septic complication. A prompt operation may also provide an opportunity for performing an acid-reducing procedure if indicated.

Zollinger-Ellison Syndrome. The description of an association between a pancreatic tumor and severe ulcer disease by Zollinger and Ellison in 1955 initiated a new era in the study and treatment of acid-peptic disease of the duodenum. Their observation was made before the isolation and characterization of gastrin and the ability to measure its presence in the bloodstream by radioimmunoassay. Gastrointestinal endoscopy was in its early phase of development, and medical treatment for ulcer disease centered on antacids. A great deal of knowledge about peptic ulcer has derived from the study of the Zollinger-Ellison syndrome, a disease characterized clinically by flagrant duodenal ulcer disease, high basal acid secretory outputs, and a pancreatic tumor. Serum gastrin levels are usually in excess of 1000 pg/mL, but in some cases, the serum gastrin may be only mildly elevated for reasons not yet known. In the latter cases, serum gastrin levels can be increased by provocation with the intravenous administration of calcium or secretin. Increase in serum gastrin to above 350 pg/mL when calcium is infused at a rate of 4 $\mu g/(kg \cdot h)$ is indicative of a gastrinoma. An increase of serum gastrin in excess of 150 pg/mL in response to a bolus dose of 2 $\mu g/kg$ of secretin is also considered to be a positive response. The value of these tests has been established.

The pancreatic tumor of Zollinger-Ellison disease is a true neoplasm. In fact, approximately half of the patients have metastases to adjacent pancreatic nodes or the liver at the time of the discovery of the disease. Fortunately, the neoplasm has a slow growth pattern, and survival, even with proved metastases, is in the range of decades rather than months or years, as is true of most gastrointestinal malignancies.

Diagnosis. Active ulcer disease of the duodenum can usually be detected by a directed history and careful physical examination. When epigastric pain and tenderness are the only findings, a clinical trial of antacid or antisecretory therapy may be sufficient to provide symptomatic relief, healing, and in some instances a cure. This is especially true when symptoms are of an acute nature and related to environmental stress. In most cases, however, there is a history of chronic dyspepsia, and activity is manifested by bleeding or incapacitating pain. These symptoms require endoscopic examination of the duodenum to determine the precise nature of the lesion. Examination of the upper gastrointestinal tract by barium radiography is also a useful study to determine the location and depth of penetration of the ulcer, as well as the extent of deformation from chronic fibrosis (Fig. 24-13). Unfortunately, superficial ulceration will not be detected by this technique. False-negatives in the range of 50 percent have been documented by follow-up endoscopy when ulcer symptoms are present and barium radiographs are negative. Pyloric obstruction is easily diagnosed by an upright radiograph of the abdomen; perforation is best detected by a chest x-ray also performed in the upright position (Fig. 24-14*A* and *B*).

Treatment. ***Medical.*** The medical therapy of duodenal ulcer is based upon the premise that it is a chronic, incurable disease. Treatment, therefore, is directed toward symptomatic relief during periods of acute exacerbation. This is best accomplished by a 6- to 8-week course of H_2-receptor antagonist therapy. Cur-

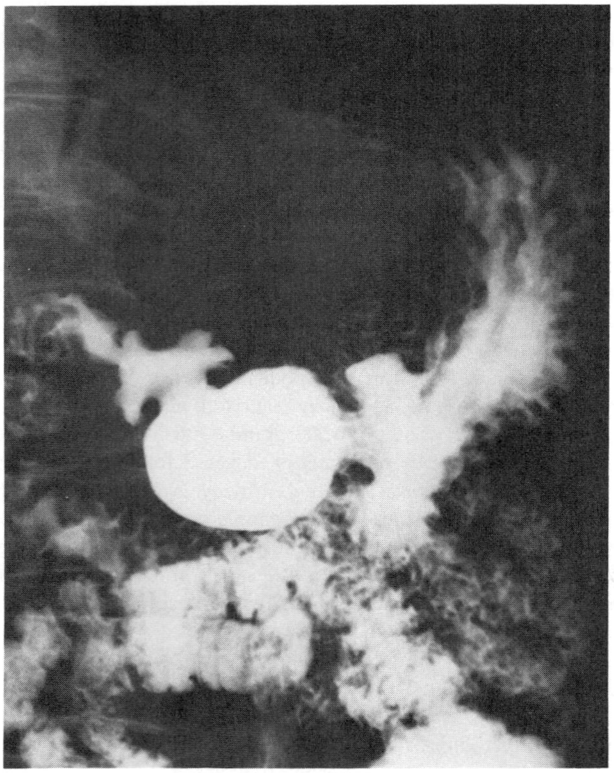

FIG. 24-13. Barium radiograph demonstrating the classic cloverleaf appearance of a deformed duodenal bulb due to the scarring of chronic ulcer disease. (*Courtesy of FA Mann, MD.*)

rently, four H_2 blockers are available for clinical use. These include cimetidine (Tagamet), ranitidine (Zantac), famotidine (Pepcid), and nizatidine (Azid). For the most part, the efficacy of these drugs is equivalent. Their differences mainly center around the frequency of dosing, side effects (most of which are minimal), and relative costs. Of these agents, famotidine is especially attractive because it only requires two doses daily (i.e., 20 mg orally every 12 h), has virtually no side effects, and from a cost standpoint is generally less expensive. The frequent ingestion of antacids (7 times daily: before meals, after meals, and at bedtime) is as effective as antisecretory therapy for symptomatic relief, but the H_2 blockers shorten the period of complete healing. Furthermore, patient compliance appears to be better with H_2 blockers in view of the ease of taking a pill and the avoidance of the undesirable intestinal symptoms (diarrhea or constipation) associated with most antacid ingestion. Tranquilizers and diets have not proved to be efficacious, although both are used on an empiric basis by most clinicians. A six-feeding bland diet may help to reduce the gastric phase of acid secretion, but evidence that it enhances ulcer healing is lacking. Tranquilizers themselves have a modest antisecretory effect. A highly specific inhibitor of acid secretion that acts by inhibiting the proton pump is omeprazole (Prilosec). As with the four H_2 blockers, this agent has been approved by the Federal Drug Administration (FDA) for duodenal ulcer management. Early trials with omeprazole have demonstrated its ability to heal duodenal ulcer. Whether it will prove to be superior to the H_2 blockers remains to be seen. The aforementioned advances in duodenal ulcer therapy not only offer the possibility of providing symptomatic relief during activity but also the possibility of protection against recurrences. Knowledge derived from their mecha-

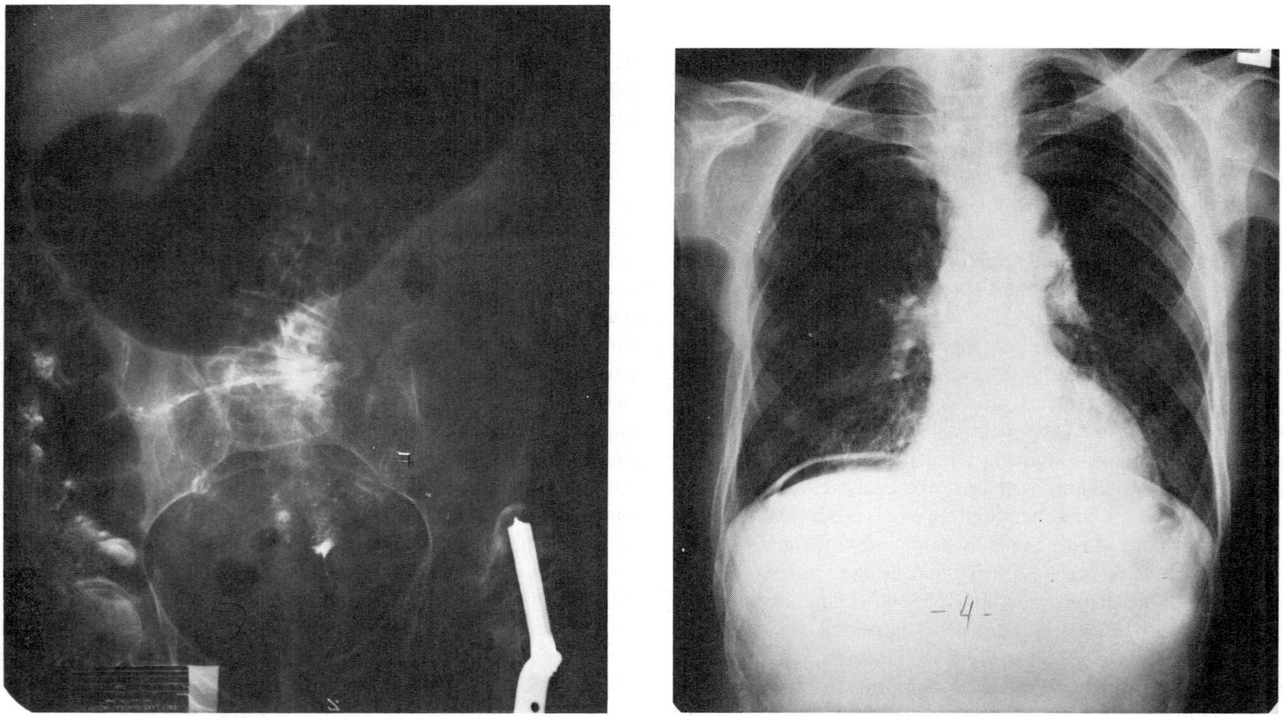

A B

FIG. 24-14. *A.* Plain abdominal film demonstrating massive gastric distention. *B.* Erect chest film demonstrating free air under the right hemidiaphragm.

nisms of action may also lead to an understanding of the pathogenesis of the disease and its ultimate prevention. There is no question that acid antisecretory agents have made a profound impact on the treatment of this common disease.

Surgical. Surgical therapy for chronic duodenal ulcer has two purposes: (1) to salvage patients from the life-threatening complications of perforation, massive hemorrhage, and gastric outlet obstruction and (2) to provide cure for the disease in the form of protection from recurrence and the pain and discomfort associated with this disorder. The indications for surgery, therefore, include perforation, obstruction, massive bleeding, and intractable abdominal pain.

The objective of therapy for perforation is early recognition of the complication and prompt closure of the opening in the duodenum. This procedure, termed "plication," is accomplished through an upper midline incision. Usually placement of three or four silk (00) sutures in seromuscular fashion across the site of perforation is sufficient for secure closure. It is customary to tie in a tag of omentum with these sutures to provide a biologic buttress, a procedure termed a "Graham patch." Thorough cleansing of the peritoneal cavity by irrigation is an essential part of the operation. A major decision relates to whether an acid-reducing procedure should be performed as part of the therapy. The criteria for this approach include long-standing ulcer symptoms, a perforation of less than 6 h duration, and a patient whose condition is conducive to a longer operation than is associated with simple plication. In our opinion, the procedure of choice is a truncal vagotomy and Heineke-Mikulicz pyloroplasty (Fig. 24-15) with excision of the ulcer that is almost always on the anterior surface of the first part of the duodenum. Others have recommended proximal vagotomy with a Graham patch for the treatment of duodenal ulcer perforation as the preferred therapy.

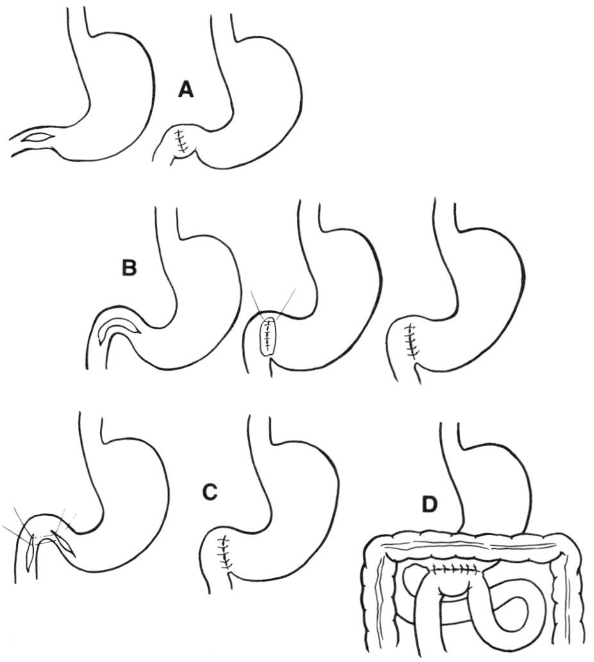

FIG. 24-15. Diagram of the most frequently used drainage procedures: *A.* Heineke-Mikulicz pyloroplasty. *B.* Finney pyloroplasty. *C.* Jaboulay pyloroplasty. *D.* Gastroenterostomy.

Pyloric obstruction can be treated by either a partial gastrectomy or vagotomy and drainage procedure. The former is preferred when the stomach is massively dilated. By this approach, the potentially deleterious effects of vagotomy on gastric emptying are avoided. Truncal vagotomy with pyloroplasty or gastroenterostomy, however, conserves the gastric reservoir and can be done with a lower risk in these patients who may have incompletely corrected fluid and electrolyte imbalance or malnutrition. A newer and more rational approach is the performance of a proximal gastric vagotomy with either a pyloroplasty or gastroenterostomy (Fig. 24-15). This operation allows for preservation of the antral pump, thereby reducing the incidence of dumping, gastric stasis, and bile reflux gastritis.

Rapid, uncontrolled bleeding from a duodenal ulcer (usually posterior) requires surgical intervention once the intravascular volume has been reconstituted. Debate continues, however, concerning the definition of uncontrolled bleeding. In our judgment, the recommendations of Enquist and associates should be followed. Thus, if the patient's original blood volume is not adequately restored with three units of whole blood or its equivalent, or if greater than 500 mL of whole blood or its equivalent is required in any subsequent 8-h period, the patient should be subjected to operation. The allowance of excessive numbers of blood transfusions in the hope that hemorrhage will eventually cease can be disastrous, not only because of the dilution of clotting factors that commonly occurs with multiple transfusions, but also because of the continued stress on the cardiovascular system to maintain hemodynamic stability.

Once the decision to operate has been made, a generous upper midline laparotomy is performed. Immediately on entering the abdomen, the surgeon incises through the midanterior aspect of the distal 3 cm of stomach and the proximal 2 cm of duodenum. This incision provides direct visualization of the posterior wall of the duodenum, the ulcer crater, and the spurting vessel within its base. Bleeding can be controlled by compression with the left index finger, and the open vessel can then be easily secured by undersewing the finger with 00 silk on a stout needle. Sutures should be placed above and below this point in order to ensure complete encirclement of the gastroduodenal artery in this area. It may be necessary to place sutures deep at all four quadrants of the lesion. Some surgeons prefer a horizontal mattress stitch to encompass the bleeding vessel. Careful suture ligature of the vessel is essential if rebleeding is to be avoided. The operation is completed by a truncal vagotomy and pyloroplasty. A gastric resection should not be attempted because of the possibilities of pancreatic injury, anastomotic leak, or blown duodenal stump, complications that account for the majority of deaths in ulcer surgery.

The management of a medically controlled major bleed, or recurrent minor bleed, is controversial. Availability of effective antisecretory agents has introduced an element of uncertainty in these complications that were considered to be indications for operation in the recent past. Proximal gastric vagotomy is the preferred approach for reasons that will be discussed below.

Intractable pain is no longer a common indication for ulcer surgery. It has been reasonably well demonstrated that patients with intractable pain are usually poorly compliant in their antacid therapy. Antisecretory therapy has improved compliance of medical therapy and may account for the remarkable decrease in the number of patients with intractable pain referred for surgical therapy during the past 5 to 10 years. An operative approach is necessary in truly noncompliant patients or in those who cannot bear the

Table 24-2
Results of Operations for Duodenal Ulcer

	Mortality	*Morbidity*	*Recurrence*
Partial gastrectomy	3%	10%	5%
Vagotomy and antrectomy	2%	12%	1%
Vagotomy and drainage	1%	15%	10%
Proximal gastric vagotomy	0.5%	5%	15%

expense or inconvenience of prolonged or repeated courses of H_2 blockage. These individuals should have a proximal gastric vagotomy as the next step in the treatment of their disease.

The relative advantages of the various operations for duodenal ulcer are shown in Table 24-2. Notice that proximal gastric vagotomy has a remarkably low morbidity and mortality but has a recurrence rate that is comparable with or even higher than truncal vagotomy and drainage. Antrectomy and vagotomy provide the best assurance of a low recurrence rate but at a mortality and morbidity that would be unacceptable for patients with easily controllable ulcer symptoms, which represents the majority. Candidates for vagotomy and antrectomy include patients who are to undergo an elective operation for a major complication of their ulcer and who are at high risk for recurrence. These would include individuals in high-stress situations, heavy smokers, chronic alcoholics, and patients who have known high acid secretory rates unrelated to hypergastrinemia. Such patients are usually middle-aged, heavy-set, aggressive, reasonably successful males.

There is some evidence that females do not tolerate truncal vagotomy as well as males. The availability of proximal gastric vagotomy offers an excellent alternative to partial gastrectomy for use in females needing surgery for peptic ulcer. The surgical therapy for duodenal ulcer, other than Zollinger-Ellison syndrome and the exceptions listed above, is based on the reduction of the acid secretory response by vagotomy. This can be accomplished by division of the vagi above their major abdominal branches, thereby incurring a complete vagal denervation of the intraabdominal viscera. Selective vagotomy, whereby the major trunks are divided below the hepatic and celiac branches to include transection of the nerves of Laterjet, provides for total gastric denervation. Proximal gastric vagotomy, wherein the small branches of the nerves of Laterjet to the fundus are divided close to the gastric wall, leaves the vagal innervation undisturbed to the antrum and other intraabdominal viscera. Truncal vagotomy is currently the most popular method of gastric denervation because of its simplicity. Selective vagotomy is the best way to denervate the gastric remnant following antrectomy, but it does not reduce the incidence of postgastrectomy sequelae. Because of its low early and late morbidity, proximal gastric vagotomy has emerged as the preferred operation for duodenal ulcer when drainage is not required.

Truncal and selective vagotomy may lead to gastric stasis and therefore must be accompanied by a drainage procedure. Three types of pyloroplasty (Heineke-Mikulicz, Finney, and Jaboulay) are recommended for this purpose. They differ in the way in which the pylorus is reconstructed or bypassed, as shown in Fig. 24-15. A gastroenterostomy is also an acceptable way to prevent stasis following truncal gastric vagotomy, but it is more complex than pyloroplasty and therefore used when the latter cannot be easily performed.

Gastric resections are described by the amount of stomach removed: antrectomy (one-third), hemigastrectomy (one-half), partial gastrectomy (two-thirds), subtotal gastrectomy (three-fourths), and total gastrectomy. Except as described below for gastric cancer and the Zollinger-Ellison syndrome, attempts are made to preserve antral function and the gastric reservoir. When resection is required for benign ulcer of the duodenum or stomach, the gastric remnant is usually anastomosed to the duodenum (Billroth I), whereas resection for neoplasm is usually followed by a gastrojejunostomy (Billroth II) in order to avoid obstruction from tumor recurrence at the anastomosis (Fig. 24-16).

The surgical treatment of the Zollinger-Ellison syndrome has undergone dramatic change in recent years since the introduction of the H_2 blockers and, more recently, omeprazole. When H_2 blockers are used, doses in excess of what is usually required for duodenal ulcer are needed. As an example, generally dosages of cimetidine in the range of 600 mg four times a day have been needed to effectively control the severe ulcer diathesis associated with the syndrome. When omeprazole has been used to control the hypersecretory state in Zollinger-Ellison patients, a starting dose of 60 mg/day is usually required. In unusual situations, doses up to 120 mg three times a day have been needed. Unfortunately, medical control precludes staging of the extent of the neoplastic process within the pancreas and adjacent lymph nodes and viscera. In addition, there are increasing numbers of reports documenting that many patients with a gastrinoma gradually become refractory to H_2 blockers and require total gastrectomy for control of ulcer disease. Whether a similar situation will occur with omeprazole therapy remains to be determined. More recently it has been observed that proximal gastric vagotomy serves as a useful adjunct to medical therapy by rendering the acid secretory cells more sensitive to lower doses of the antisecretory drug employed. Another advantage to utilizing proximal gastric vagotomy as a component of initial pharmacologic therapy is the opportunity it provides for assessing the extent of tumor. Occasionally (<5 percent of the time), the gastrinoma consists of a single tumor mass located within the distal pancreas that is readily accessible to excision leading to permanent cure. It is generally agreed that Zollinger-Ellison patients should not have partial gastric resections, since recurrences in this situation can be catastrophic. Total gastrectomy with esophagojejunostomy in Roux en Y fashion (Fig. 24-17) is a safe operation that is well tolerated in the Zollinger-Ellison patient.

Peptic Ulcer—Stomach

Acute Erosive Gastritis

The gastric epithelium is constantly at risk of injury from ingestants in combination with its own secretions. Acute mucosal injury, called *erosive gastritis,* is the most common cause of upper gastrointestinal bleeding and by far the most frequent pathologic process within the stomach. The clinical problem is compounded by its relatively frequent occurrence in the setting of severe illness, or following physical or thermal injury, sepsis, or shock. Stress erosive gastritis has been of particular interest to the surgeon since it may require a surgical intervention in an already critically ill patient. Fortunately, advances in the understanding of the pathogenesis of the disease have led to a variety of ways to prevent its occurrence or progression.

Mechanisms. The pathogenesis of erosive gastritis involves five variables: (1) acid secretion, (2) rate of back-diffusion of H^+ ions (the gastric barrier), (3) gastric mucosal blood flow, (4) mucus and alkaline secretion, and (5) submucosal buffers. Obviously, many other factors are involved in maintaining normal

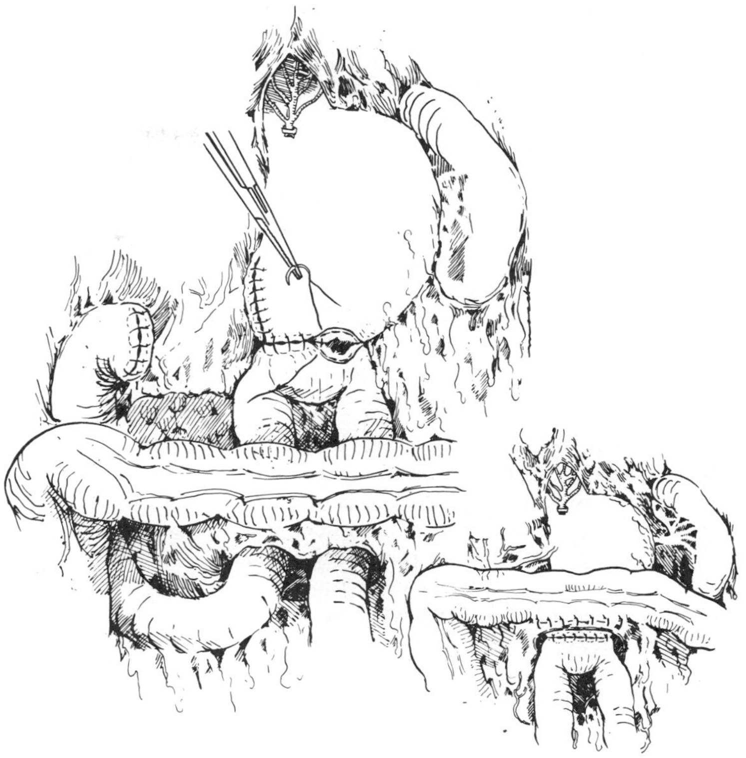

FIG. 24-16. Diagram of a Billroth II gastrojejunostomy placed behind the transverse colon. For cancer, the anastomosis is usually done in front of the colon away from areas of possible recurrence.

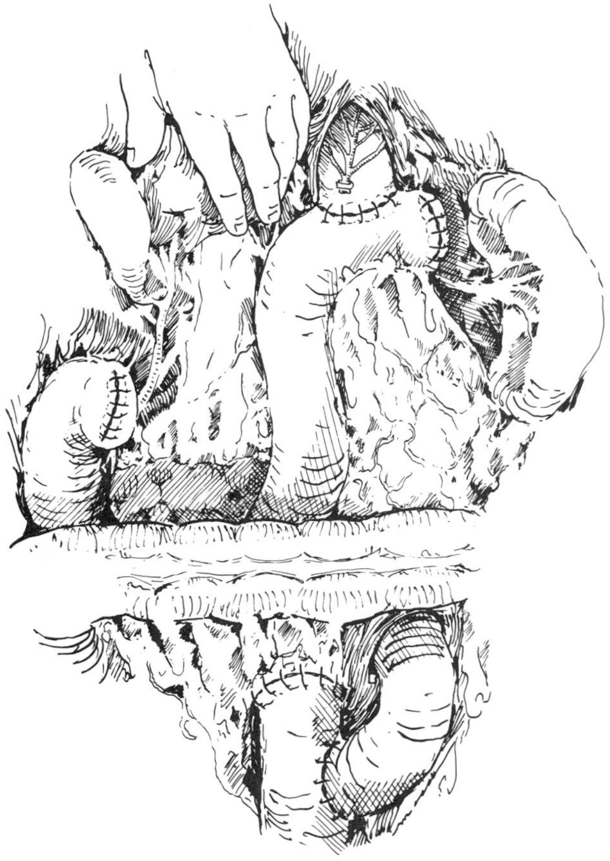

FIG. 24-17. Roux en Y reconstruction after total gastrectomy.

epithelial function, but their role in the pathogenesis of erosive gastritis has not yet been identified.

The dictum "no acid, no ulcer" clearly applies to erosive gastritis. This has been well established in experimental models and in the clinical situation. In fact, it represents the basis for modern therapy of the disease.

The precise role of H^+ ions in ulcerogenesis is not known. It has been well established, however, that the gastric epithelium is relatively impervious to H^+ ions, thereby accounting for their millionfold gradient from blood to gastric lumen. A disruption of this cation barrier leads to an influx of H^+ ions and an efflux of Na^+ ions, bicarbonate, and water. Breaking of the barrier by noxious agents such as aspirin, alcohol, or bile salts may lead to acute erosions within the superficial layers of the gastric epithelium. A variety of protective mechanisms attempt to counteract this possibility. Mucus and an alkaline secretion are produced by the surface epithelial cells in an attempt to wash away and neutralize the effects of the barrier breaker and H^+ ions by dilution and alkalinization. These functions of the surface cell represent the first line of defense against external injury.

Gastric mucosal blood flow maintains the epithelial integrity by delivery of buffers and nutrients to the gastric cells. Substrates for oxidative metabolism such as oxygen play a key role in this regard. Curiously, even prolonged intervals of hypoxia or hypoperfusion do not induce injury in the absence of H^+ ions and chemical disruption of the barrier. A critical relationship exists between the rate of hydrogen ion back diffusion, gastric mucosal blood flow, and extent of mucosal injury.

The role of mucus and buffer secretion by surface cells is only now being studied in a comprehensive way. Knowledge of these events is much too new to make a clear statement of their importance in the pathogenesis of acute lesions. It is possible that thickening of the mucus coat on the luminal side of the surface cell may provide an unstirred layer that allows entrapment and a titration sink for H^+ ions. Several laboratories are actively involved in attempting to define more clearly the role of mucus and bicarbonate in gastric mucosal defense.

Another area of intense inquiry relates to the fate of H^+ ions once they permeate the surface cell layer. It has been well established that acidification of the lamina propria can lead to surface cell injury, and that neutralization of this process by parenteral alkalinization can prevent cell loss. For example, the secreting stomach is less prone to experimental injury, possibly as a consequence of the delivery of alkali to the lamina propria following its discharge into the gastric venous effluent after the secretion of an H^+ ion into the stomach. The importance of this concept to the clinical problem has yet to be defined.

Diagnosis. Upper gastrointestinal bleeding is the clinical hallmark of erosive gastritis. It may be characterized by hematemesis, bloody nasogastric aspirate, melena, or anemia associated with the detection of occult blood in the stool. Pain is uncommon and, when present, is a sign of a penetrating ulcer. Small amounts of blood in the nasogastric aspirate of patients in a critical care setting are so common that they provide enough evidence for making a presumptive working diagnosis without further work-up. Massive hematemesis requires gastric lavage for cleansing and endoscopic examination to determine the anatomic lesion. Superficial erosions rarely bleed rapidly; vomiting of large volumes of blood is an indication of penetration of an erosion into a large blood vessel within the submucosa or the presence of a chronic gastric or duodenal ulcer. Barium studies are not useful in this disease.

Treatment. The therapy of erosive gastritis is directed toward intravascular volume replacement and early control of hemorrhage by nonsurgical means. Gastric lavage with room temperature solutions such as water or saline is an important first step in therapy. The stomach must be completely evacuated of its blood contents in order to reduce fibrinolysis at bleeding sites. In addition, the stomach will be stimulated to secrete acid if the antrum is distended by clots. More than 80 percent of patients stop bleeding with this simple maneuver.

The third step in management is to provide for intragastric neutralization. This may be accomplished by inhibiting acid secretion with an H_2 blocker such as cimetidine (300 mg I.V. every 6 h), or the instillation of antacids (30 to 60 mL/h) into the stomach, checking its effectiveness by assessing gastric neutrality ($pH > 5$) by pH-sensitive paper at the end of each hour. The latter process must be pursued diligently if further penetration of erosions with rebleeding is to be avoided.

If bleeding persists or recurs, the patient should be treated by transendoscopic bipolar electrocautery or by laser photocoagulation. Pharmacologic control by the selective infusion of pitressin into the left gastric artery is also effective, since it induces spasm and thrombosis of the bleeding artery. The associated decrease in mucosal perfusion does not lead to further ulceration if the gastric contents are carefully alkalinized during therapy. Transluminal occlusion of the left gastric artery by a gel forms a clot, or a coil is also an effective way to control bleeding from a branch of this vessel.

Bleeding that recurs or persists is an indication for operation. The criteria we use to determine when an operation should be performed for bleeding have been discussed in the section on duodenal ulcer disease. Since most erosions occur in the fundus of the stomach, a long anterior gastrotomy is made in this area. The gastric lumen is cleared of blood, and the mucosal surface is inspected for bleeding points in deeply penetrating lesions. These are secured with silk (00) by a figure-of-eight stitch taken deep within the gastric wall. Each actively bleeding site should be secured in this way. The majority of superficial erosions will not be actively bleeding and do not require ligature unless a blood vessel can be felt or seen at its base. The operation is completed by closure of the anterior gastrotomy and the performance of a truncal vagotomy and pyloroplasty. The incidence of rebleeding is less than 5 percent if bleeding points are carefully looked for and secured.

Some surgeons prefer a liberal partial gastrectomy and vagotomy. In fact, near-total gastrectomy even has its advocates because of concern over the possibilities of rebleeding. In our opinion, this radical surgical approach has no justification except in the rare instance in which suture ligature with vagotomy and pyloroplasty fails.

Prevention. An understanding of the importance of intragastric acidity in the pathogenesis of erosive gastritis has provided a rationale for the prevention of the disease in critically ill patients. The efficacy of alkalinization of intraluminal acid by topical antacids as well as by inhibition of acid production by various antisecretory substances in preventing hemorrhage from erosive gastritis has been clearly established by randomized controlled trials. Numerous studies over the past decade have clearly shown that H_2 blockers are equal to antacids in accomplishing this goal and are easier to use. The three H_2 blockers that have found efficacy in this situation include cimetidine, ranitidine, and famotidine; they all can be administered intravenously, which is the route required in these critically ill individuals. As with other acid-peptic disorders treated with these agents, the differences to be considered among these three H_2 blockers include dosing schemes, drug side effects, and relative costs. In our experience, famotidine has proved to be especially useful as it can effectively prevent bleeding from acute gastritis with virtually no side effects and at a reasonable cost when given twice daily (10 mg I.V. every 12 h).

Prostaglandins of the E series have emerged as a potentially important group of compounds that may in themselves offer protection to the gastric epithelium. Their mechanism of action is not precisely known, but they may work through stimulation of mucus and alkaline secretion, enhancement of mucosal blood flow, or inhibition of acid secretion. The importance of the latter biologic property of prostaglandins has been challenged, since prostaglandins provide cytoprotection at dosages below those that inhibit acid secretion, and noninhibitory prostaglandins can also prevent experimentally induced gastritis. The only prostaglandin currently available clinically is misoprostol (Cytotec), which has not proved useful in the management of erosive gastritis because of its diarrheal side effect.

Chronic Gastric Ulcer

Differential Diagnosis. Chronic gastric ulceration presents a unique challenge in diagnosis since malignant and benign lesions share many clinical and pathologic features. The advent of endoscopic biopsy and brush cytology has reduced uncertainty in this area, but a significant false-negative rate (about 5 percent), i.e., the lesion is neoplastic but the biopsies are benign, still exists. It is for this reason that patients with gastric ulcer require careful follow-up by radiographs and repeat endoscopy with biopsy if the ulcer persists. It is also for this reason that multiple biopsies (i.e., 7 to 9) rather than the previously recommended 4-quadrant biopsy of the lesion in question should be undertaken. Gastric analysis can also be helpful since achlorhydria to maximal histamine stimulation excludes the possibility of a peptic ulcer.

The pathogenesis of a benign gastric ulcer remains unknown. Several prominent contributing factors are age (>40), sex (female/male, 2/1), ingestion of barrier-breaking drugs such as aspirin, and malnutrition. Numerous attempts have been made to implicate chronic gastric ischemia, but with little success. The occurrence of the lesions on the lesser curvature at the junction of the antral and fundic mucosa suggests the possibility of a breakdown of mucosal protective factors at that site, but there is no evidence to support this speculation. It has been well demonstrated, however, that patients with gastric ulcer have an epithelium that is "leaky" to H^+ ions. This observation has suggested that regurgitation of bile acids and other barrier breakers within the duodenal succus may play an important role in the disease. Against this possibility is the fact that the experimental rerouting of bile through the stomach by a cholecystogastrostomy does not cause ulceration. Furthermore, chronic gastric ulceration is uncommon in patients with a gastroenterostomy, a situation in which bile is constantly bathing the mucosa of the gastric antrum. The most compelling evidence that the disease is acid-peptic in origin relates to the rapid healing that follows antacid therapy or vagotomy, even when the lesion-bearing portion of the stomach is left intact.

Ulceration within a gastric cancer is somewhat easier to explain. This lesion is most likely a consequence of local ischemia and malnourishment of the tissues within the center of the neoplastic process. It is easy to visualize how this might occur as the younger cells at the advancing edge of the penetrating neoplasm deprive the older cells within its center of nutrients and oxygen. The bulk lesion and infiltration of the gastric wall as revealed by barium radiographs provide the major diagnostic clues of the neoplastic nature of malignant ulcers. Furthermore, achlorhydria precludes peptic digestion of devitalized cells within the ulcer bed, resulting in an irregular, shaggy appearance in contrast to the clean, well-demarcated base of a benign peptic ulcer.

Symptoms. Lack of appetite with vague upper abdominal distress following a meal is a common presenting complaint of patients with a benign gastric ulcer. This form of dyspepsia usually is accompanied by a gradual loss of weight as a consequence of a decrease in the intake of food. Severe pain is an unusual manifestation of the disease, except when the ulcer is located within the distal stomach or pyloric channel. Ulcers in this location assume the characteristics of a duodenal ulcer in that they are associated with increased rates of acid secretion, epigastric pain during the interdigestive period, and prompt relief with antacid ingestion. Gastric ulcers in the proximal stomach have less dramatic symptomatology and consequently may assume a large size and extensive depth of penetration before their detection.

Massive hemorrhage is an unusual event in chronic gastric ulceration; melena, or the detection of occult blood in the stool, is common. Gastric outlet obstruction as manifested by nausea and vomiting is also a rare finding, unless the ulcer is within the pyloric channel or near the gastric outlet, while delayed gastric emptying is frequent and the likely source of the vague "indigestion" experienced by this patient population.

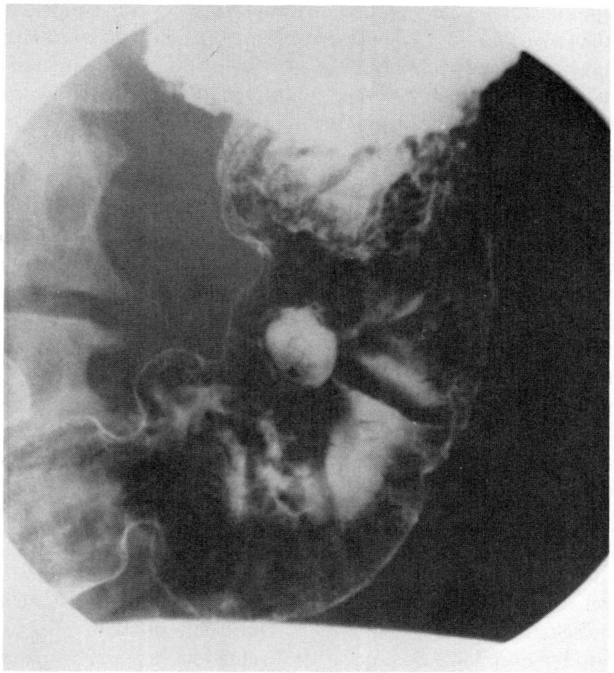

FIG. 24-18. This air contrast barium radiograph shows an ulcer with smooth margins. The rugal folds radiate toward the ulcer crater. This is the typical appearance of a benign ulcer. (*Courtesy of FA Mann, MD.*)

Diagnosis. ***Radiography.*** The upper gastrointestinal barium radiograph is the first step in diagnosis after a careful history and physical examination have focused attention on the stomach as the likely source of the patient's complaints. This is a simple, safe, convenient study that provides a great deal of diagnostic information in the hands of a well-trained radiologist. The radiographic characteristics of a benign gastric ulcer are shown in Fig. 24-18. A common mistake in the diagnostic approach is the utilization of endoscopic visualization of the lesion without obtaining a barium study. The two procedures complement each other. Their order of performance is obvious; barium examination performed first serves to identify the presence and location of a lesion and the probability of its benign or malignant nature; subsequent endoscopy with biopsy provides a histologic diagnosis.

Endoscopy. The endoscopic appearance of a gastric ulcer offers information about its pathologic identity. Benign lesions usually have a well-demarcated, "punched-out" appearance, with a smooth base and a sharp, flat margin. Malignant ulcers usually have an irregular, "heaped-up" margin and a rough, necrotic-appearing base. Unfortunately, there is overlap, especially between benign ulcers and ulcerating cancers early in their genesis. This is why careful endoscopic biopsy at multiple sites at the margin of all gastric ulcers is a mandatory diagnostic procedure. It should not be omitted even when the radiograph and the eye suggest that the lesion is benign in appearance.

Treatment. ***Medical.*** The initial therapy for a benign gastric ulcer is a so-called medical trial. Unfortunately, there is no specific therapy for a gastric ulcer, since its etiology is unknown. The empiric use of antacid therapy appears to hasten the rate of ulcer healing. H_2 blockers have also been shown to promote healing of gastric ulcers, but their efficacy in this regard is only about half that noted when they are used for duodenal ulcer management. There has been a great deal of interest in diet manipulation that includes abstention from alcohol, spicy foods, and large meals that might aggravate symptoms associated with delayed gastric emptying. A six-feeding bland gastric diet is usually recommended for this reason. Aspirin and other barrier-breaking drugs (nonsteroidal anti-inflammatory agents) must be stopped during the period of therapy, and elimination of smoking has also been shown to be quite beneficial in enhancing gastric ulcer healing. Sulfated glycoproteins (sucralfate), a new generation of antiulcer agents, appear to hasten the healing rate of gastric ulcer by binding to the devitalized tissues within the ulcer bed and thereby protecting it from further peptic digestion. Cytoprotective agents such as the prostaglandins of the E series may also play a role in the future of patients who must take barrier-threatening drugs on a chronic basis. This is currently an active area of investigation. Misoprostol (a PGE analogue) has been shown to effectively prevent gastric injury in patients requiring treatment with nonsteroidal anti-inflammatory compounds.

Unfortunately, some gastric ulcers, even when benign, fail to heal at a satisfactory rate (6 weeks) to provide symptomatic relief or assurance that they are not neoplastic. This situation requires a period of hospitalization for further evaluation and careful supervision of medical therapy. Since gastric ulcers are notorious for their tendency to recur even after a successful course of medical therapy, an operative approach should be considered early in patients with recalcitrant or recurrent benign gastric ulcers or when malignancy is even a remote possibility.

Surgical. The indications for surgical management of benign gastric ulcer are fairly clear-cut and include persistent bleeding, perforation, obstruction, failure to heal, recurrence, and suspicion of malignancy. Combined gastric and duodenal ulcer is also best treated by an acid-reducing procedure such as truncal vagotomy and antrectomy to include resection of the gastric ulcer. In fact, it is important to keep in mind that the surgical treatment of gastric ulcer must include a consideration of the presence of duodenal ulcer disease, since the rate of anastomotic ulcer is high (50 percent) if only a distal gastrectomy is used for this purpose.

The most popular operation for a benign lesser curvature gastric ulcer is a distal gastrectomy (antrectomy) without vagotomy to include the ulcer. Gastroduodenostomy is preferred since it reduces the risk of bile gastritis, iron deficiency, and afferent loop syndrome. The recurrence rate and incidence of undesirable side effects are low with this approach in the absence of duodenal ulcer disease or an overlooked cancer. If a concomitant duodenal ulcer is present, vagotomy should be included as a component of therapy.

High-lying gastric ulcers near the esophagogastric junction present a special challenge in management. These can be locally excised or left in place in conjunction with a concomitant antrectomy. Giant (>4 cm) benign ulcers are also a problem, since they may require an extensive gastric resection. Usually they occur in a malnourished, elderly patient who may have an underlying chronic disease. These patients are best managed by a period of hospitalization, parenteral hyperalimentation, and interval surgery (4 to 6 weeks) if inability to eat persists. Usually the ulcer reduces to a small size or heals during this period. Distal gastric and pyloric channel ulcers should be treated as a duodenal ulcer, since they usually are similar in their clinical presentation and relationship to acid hypersecretion.

Gastric Neoplasia

Malignant Tumors

The vast majority of gastric tumors are malignant, and of these, adenocarcinoma of the stomach is by far the most common (95 percent). Lymphomas (4 percent) and leiomyosarcomas (1 percent) constitute the rest, except for rare lesions such as squamous cell carcinoma, angiosarcoma, carcinosarcoma, and metastasis from adjacent or distant primary sites.

Cancer. ***Epidemiology.*** Gastric cancer is a biologically aggressive disease that is virtually incurable when discovered in its symptomatic phase. While it is worldwide in occurrence, its frequency varies greatly. Chile, Japan, and Iceland have the highest incidence. The disease is rarely encountered in Malaysia. The United States has experienced a rapid decline in stomach cancer deaths from a rate of 30 per 100,000 in 1930 to 8 per 100,000 today. The reason for this favorable trend is not known. Nor is the high incidence in some geographic areas understood, although a high consumption of smoked fish appears to be a characteristic common to these high-risk populations. Patients with pernicious anemia and blood group A also have an increased incidence of the disease, suggesting that genetic as well as environmental factors play a role.

Symptoms and Signs. Anorexia with weight loss is the most common sign of gastric cancer (>95 percent). Unfortunately, patients are relatively asymptomatic until there is extensive involvement of the gastric wall and adjacent viscera, or widespread metastases. Massive hematemesis occurs in less than 5 percent of patients, although the finding of occult blood in the stool is common. Nausea and vomiting may occur when distal lesions encroach upon the pylorus. Dysphagia is a dominant symptom when cancer arises within the cardia of the stomach. Pain is a late and uncommon complaint. While abdominal tenderness is a rare finding, a palpable abdominal mass is common (50 percent). Hepatomegaly is also a frequent finding and must arouse suspicion of liver metastases. Peritoneal seeding may cause massive ascites or involvement of the ovaries (Krukenberg tumor) or pelvic cul-de-sac (Bloomer's shelf) by gravitational metastases. These manifestations of advanced gastric cancer may lead to pelvic pain and constipation. A palpable lymph node in the left supraclavicular space (Virchow's node) is also a sign of advanced malignancy.

Pathologic Features. Gastric cancer may involve the stomach in a variety of ways (Table 24-3), even though each type usually originates from the progenitor cells at the base of the gastric pits. The most favorable form of the disease is superficial spreading carcinoma. In that condition, the neoplastic process does not penetrate through the muscularis mucosa, nor is it associated with a breakdown of the epithelium and chronic ulceration. Early detection by endoscopic biopsy and gastrectomy is associated with a good prognosis (75 percent with 10-year survival). Lesions of this type are usually detected by mass screening of high-risk populations by endoscopic visualization or photography.

Table 24-3
Types of Gastric Cancer

Superficial spreading
Polypoid
Ulcerative
Scirrhous-linitis plastica

Most symptomatic gastric cancers are infiltrating lesions that penetrate deep into the gastric wall. The luminal portion of the neoplastic process may be represented by a bulky tumor mass, a polypoid excrescence, or a flat, ulcerating lesion. Large cancers of this type are easily detected by radiography or endoscopy. Linitis plastica is an extensive infiltration of the gastric wall without tumor or ulceration. This form of gastric cancer produces a peculiar ''leather-bottle'' appearance to the gastric radiograph because of the rigid, nondistensible stomach.

Gastric cancer may spread in four ways: (1) lymphatics, (2) bloodstream, (3) peritoneal seeding, and (4) direct extension. More than half of the patients already have tumor spread at the time they seek medical therapy. It, therefore, is important to recognize high-risk groups. A family history of gastric cancer, detection of pernicious anemia, unexplained weight loss, and gastric symptoms that have their onset many years after gastrectomy require careful medical evaluation. There is concern that chronic hypochlorhydria, even when obtained by H_2 blockers, may present a high-risk situation since bacterial overgrowth within the stomach may allow a buildup of oncogenic substances such as nitrosoureas.

Natural History. The tendency for gastric cancer to be advanced at the time of its detection has led to considerable therapeutic nihilism. This is not entirely justified, since gastric resection can provide excellent palliation in most patients and an occasional cure when the cancer is confined to the gastric epithelium. The latter form of the disease mimics chronic gastric ulcer. Even when such neoplastic ulcers are neglected, patients with them may survive for prolonged periods of time.

Chronic wasting and progressive weakness and cachexia constitute the usual mode of death. Liver and pulmonary metastases are common. Metastases to bone are uncommon; therefore, pain is usually not a major problem in management. Nutrition becomes the rate-limiting step in maintaining function due to mechanical or functional gastric obstruction caused by the cancer.

Therapeutic Alternatives. The therapy of gastric cancer is primarily surgical. Radiation and chemotherapy have little to offer even in the way of palliation. Except in advanced cases of carcinomatosis, a palliative subtotal gastrectomy should be done to provide a route for oral alimentation. When there is no evidence of distal spread, a radical subtotal gastrectomy should be performed for cure. This operation includes resection of the gastrocolic omentum and ligation of the right gastric, right gastroepiploic, and left gastric arteries at their origin. Approximately 4 cm of the proximal duodenum is included in the resection. More than 85 percent of the stomach is removed, and gastrointestinal continuity is reestablished by a gastrojejunostomy. Splenectomy and even total gastrectomy may be required when the lesion is large or within the proximal portion of the stomach.

Gastric resection usually provides a symptom-free interval of 1 or 2 years. Recurrences may respond to chemotherapy, although such responses are usually of short duration. The reported 5-year survival rate when gastric resection is performed for cure is less than 10 percent. Clearly, efforts must be directed toward early detection and prevention if survival statistics are to be improved. Mass screening in Japan by gastroscopy has established the validity of an aggressive public health approach. Cure rates are reported in the range of 85 percent at 5 years when gastric cancer is discovered in an early stage, when it is still confined to the epithelial surface of the stomach. The results of surgery on over 6000 cases of gastric cancer have been reported by Kim and associates. The average 5-year survival rates for stages I and II were good, 98 percent and 72 percent, respectively. By contrast, the results for stages III and IV were poor, 31 percent and 0.7 percent, respectively. In an attempt to improve these results, immunochemosurgery was initiated in 1975.

Lymphoma (Lymphosarcoma). Gastric lymphoma may occur as an isolated neoplasm confined to the stomach, or it may be a manifestation of widespread infiltrative disease. The lesion may present as a tumor mass or, more commonly, as a thickening of the rugal epithelial folds secondary to lymphocytic infiltration within the submucosa. Anorexia and weight loss are the most common presenting complaints. Early satiety may also be a prominent symptom as the gastric wall becomes thickened, and the lumen is progressively compromised by the neoplastic infiltrate. Bleeding is uncommon. Definitive diagnosis is made by endoscopic biopsy. Bulky lesions, with associated gastric outlet obstruction, are best treated by subtotal gastric resection and postoperative irradiation. Radiation therapy alone, however, provides a long-standing remission that is equal to that obtained by gastric resection in most cases. Radiation, in fact, has emerged as the treatment of choice because of its low morbidity. A combined approach is associated with an 85 percent, 5-year survival when the process is limited to the stomach. Involvement of the stomach by generalized lymphosarcoma is usually treated by radiation or chemotherapy. Gastrectomy in such cases is undertaken only when complications ensue or when the stomach is the major source of disabling symptoms, e.g., obstruction.

Leiomyosarcoma. This tumor of smooth muscle origin is the least common of gastric malignancies. Unfortunately, it usually grows to a very large size before detection because of its outward growth away from the gastric lumen. Distal spread, however, is late, and even massive tumors that become adherent to the liver or pancreas can be resected with prolonged survival. Leiomyosarcomas are not responsive to radiation or chemotherapy. They usually are detected following a gastrointestinal hemorrhage from a breakdown of overlying epithelium or as a consequence of malnutrition secondary to compromise of gastric storage capacity. They often are palpable on abdominal examination when they present in this way. Preoperative assessment can be enhanced by visceral angiography in order to determine mesenteric or hepatic vascular interrelationships to the tumor. Cleansing and chemical preparation of the large intestine are also useful, since resection of its transverse portion or splenic flexure may be required in order to encompass the tumor. Resection is the preferred treatment, even when all the tumor cannot be safely removed, since long-term survival is usual even in this incurable situation.

Benign Tumors

Polyps. Papillary excrescences of the gastric epithelium (polyps) are the most common benign tumors of the stomach of clinical significance. They are of two types—inflammatory and adenomatous. While the latter are less common, they represent the more important lesion, since they are true neoplasms and may have a malignant potential. They can be distinguished from inflammatory polyps because of their long stalk and tendency to occur in the atrophic mucosa of patients with pernicious anemia. Occasionally, adenomatous polyps will arise in the stomach in conjunction with the multiple small bowel polyposis of the Peutz-Jeghers syndrome or the familial polyposis of Gardner's syndrome.

Inflammatory polyps are usually sessile excrescences within the antrum or fundus of the stomach. They are asymptomatic, except when they are adjacent to and prolapse through the pylorus. Hypertrophic gastritis (Menetrier's disease) may also be associated with multiple inflammatory polypoid lesions within the fundic area of the stomach. These lesions can be distinguished from multiple gastric adenomatous polyposis by biopsy and histologic examination. They do not require surgical extirpation.

Gastric polyps should be biopsied and excised by ensnarement through the endoscope when their adenomatous nature has been determined. Malignant polyps should be treated as a gastric cancer by a partial gastrectomy. Patients with pernicious anemia require careful monitoring by gastric barium radiograph or endoscopy in order to detect neoplastic polyps early in their genesis.

Leiomyoma. Small, benign leiomyomas are commonly found within the smooth muscle of the gastric wall at autopsy or during palpation of the stomach at laparotomy. They are of little clinical significance until they enlarge to greater than 4 cm in diameter. At this point, they begin to compromise the blood supply to the overlying gastric epithelium. This leads to ulceration and proteolytic digestion of the core of the neoplasm that itself may have undergone central necrosis. This process culminates in a massive upper gastrointestinal hemorrhage that may require emergency gastric resection for control. Such lesions when large cannot be distinguished from their malignant counterparts and therefore should be treated by distal gastrectomy with a liberal margin (4 cm) proximally. Smaller lesions (<4 cm) can be shelled out of the gastric wall or removed by a wedge resection.

Lipoma. Lipomas of the stomach are asymptomatic submucosal lesions that are a radiographic curiosity, distinguished by their smooth contour. Endoscopy will reveal their submucosal position. They need not be biopsied or excised.

Ectopic Pancreas. Rarely, a pancreatic rest will reside within the antrum of the stomach. While this lesion is usually submucosal, it often will present within the gastric lumen as an umbilicated dimple. It may require excision if there is a question about its nature or when patients present with unremitting dyspeptic symptoms that are refractory to antiulcer therapy.

Other Gastric Lesions

Hypertrophic Gastritis (Menetrier's Disease)

Menetrier's disease is a rare inflammatory disease of the gastric epithelium that is characterized by massive gastric folds within the proximal stomach. In advanced stages, the epithelium assumes the appearance of large multiple polypoid excrescences as shown in Fig. 24-19. Histologic examination reveals that the thickened folds consist of a hypertrophy of the gastric glandular epithelium as well as a remarkable increase in the size of the submucosa that is edematous and contains a large number of small round cells. The latter finding has suggested that the disease may have an autoimmune component.

Menetrier's disease is characterized clinically by the massive amount of plasma proteins that can be lost through an epithelium that ordinarily is extremely tight to large molecules. The reason for this extraordinary event is not known. The immunologic aspects of the disease have not yet been clarified.

Most cases of hypertrophic gastritis can be managed nonoperatively with treatment directed toward maintaining good nutrition and symptomatic relief of the vague gastric complaints offered by these patients. Rarely, loss of plasma proteins is so persistent and rapid that hypoproteinemia ensues. If left unrecognized, a state of severe protein deprivation may develop (kwashiorkor), with its attendant hepatic dysfunction, ascites, and peripheral edema. Cases with massive protein loss should have a total gastrectomy following a period of parenteral hyperalimentation. Individuals with less severe forms of the disease should be followed carefully by barium or endoscopic examination in view of the high incidence of gastric cancer reported in some series.

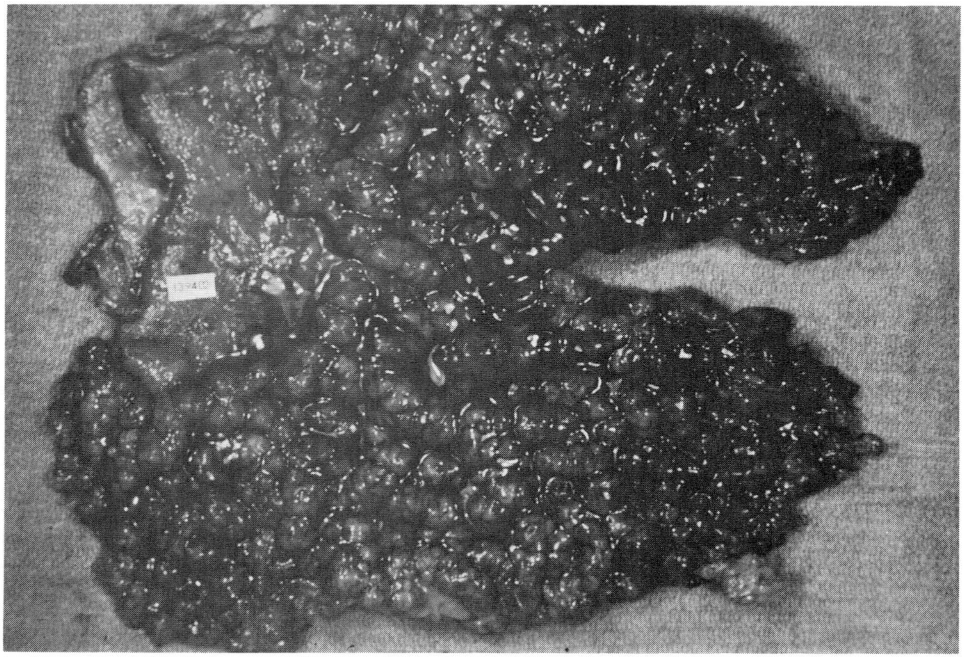

FIG. 24-19. Gross appearance of hypertrophic gastritis (Menetrier's disease).

Mallory-Weiss Tear

Violent retching can lead to a disruption of the gastric mucosa high on its lesser curve at the esophagogastric junction. The usual story is that of retching after ingestion of solid food, which is followed shortly thereafter by bright red hematemesis. The mucosal tear often extends deep into the submucosa where a large arteriole is encountered as the source of bleeding. However, this lesion is associated with massive upper gastrointestinal bleeding in only 10 percent of cases. Alcoholics with portal hypertension may have as their source of bleeding a submucosal gastric or esophageal varix.

The diagnosis is suspected by history and confirmed by esophagogastroscopy. Rapidly bleeding lesions require immediate operation following reconstitution of intravascular volume. Nonactively bleeding tears can be safely observed and usually proceed to complete healing without symptoms or further evidence of bleeding.

The operation for persistent bleeding from a Mallory-Weiss tear is carried out through an upper midline incision. The lesion at the esophagogastric junction is approached through a long anterior gastrotomy. This provides a full view of the bleeding site which is secured by several deep 2-0 silk ligatures placed in such a way that the mucosal edges are reapproximated in an anatomic fashion. A supplemental antisecretory operation is not necessary. Extension of the tear into the lower end of the esophagus may require mobilization of the esophagogastric junction in order to approximate the margins of the esophageal component of tear. The operation is completed by a fundoplication whereby the upper part of the stomach is wrapped around the lower end of the esophagus. Lesions of this type occur in association with reflux esophagitis and direct hiatal hernia.

Gastric Mucosal Prolapse

There is uncertainty about whether the prolapse of antral gastric mucosa through the pylorus can lead to gastrointestinal symptoms. Unfortunately, it is observed as a radiologic finding in some patients with symptoms of acid-peptic disease who otherwise have no other findings to explain them. It is unlikely that the nonspecific complaints offered by such patients are a consequence of this radiographic curiosity. Accordingly, no specific treatment is recommended when this finding is identified.

Acute Gastric Dilatation

Sudden rapid distention of the stomach is associated with a vagovagal response characterized by pallor, sweating, bradycardia, hypotension, and abdominal pain in the nonsedated patient. Unfortunately, many patients develop this problem early after an operative procedure when they are under the influence of anesthetics and analgesics. If left unrecognized, gastric dilatation may lead to vomiting with aspiration, tissue decompensation from hypoxia, or bleeding from stress erosive gastritis. Treatment consists of nasogastric aspiration which can be dramatic in providing relief of associated symptoms. The stomach often requires a period of 24 to 48 h to regain normal emptying. Nasogastric aspiration should be maintained throughout this period of recovery.

Gastric Volvulus

Torsion of the stomach is an uncommon, serious complication that occurs in association with a paraesophageal hiatal hernia. In this condition, the stomach, which is located within the mediastinum in an orad-caudad reversal (upside-down stomach), can rotate in a clockwise manner, thereby entrapping ingestants, air, and gastric juice. The associated distention and venous obstruction lead to ischemic gangrene of the gastric wall and subsequent perforation. It is for this reason that patients with the otherwise relatively asymptomatic condition of paraesophageal hiatal hernia are advised to have an operative repair. The procedure usually involves returning the stomach to the abdominal cavity and closure of the large opening within the diaphragm adjacent to the right crus.

Foreign Bodies and Bezoars

The stomach becomes a repository for objects other than food that are taken into the mouth. Infants and those who are mentally deranged represent those most vulnerable to this complication. Children most commonly swallow coins, small parts of toys, or their diaper pins when they are very young. As a rule of thumb, blunt objects that enter the stomach will usually pass on through the intestinal tract. Sharp objects should be retrieved by endoscopy. If this cannot be easily accomplished, the progress of the object should be followed radiographically while carefully observing the patient for signs of perforation. Adults may ingest numerous large objects that make endoscopic retrieval both time-consuming and difficult. These cases usually require operative evacuation. Bulky, solid, nondigestible objects, retained for prolonged periods of time, may, even when single, require operative extraction.

Bezoars are conglomerates of nondigestible materials usually of vegetable origin. Persimmon peels or pits, orange or grapefruit pulp, or fruit pits are the usual offenders, especially in the postgastrectomy stomach. Patients of this type must be advised to avoid foodstuffs that have a great deal of cellulose or other vegetable fiber. Bezoars are associated with vague upper abdominal discomfort, nausea, and vomiting. A barium radiograph will reveal a mass lesion within the lumen of the stomach. Treatment consists of dissolution of the undigested bolus by ingestion of proteolytic enzymes such as papain or by mechanical fragmentation via the endoscope. Recurrence can be prevented by dietary management.

Atrophic Gastritis

Pernicious anemia is associated with a gradual thinning of the gastric epithelium of the proximal stomach and a complete loss of parietal cells. This results in achlorhydria and a loss of the secretion of intrinsic factor which is responsible for the absorption of vitamin B_{12}. A deficiency of this vitamin will develop within 3 or 4 years if it is not provided by monthly replacement (1000 μg I.M.). Atrophic gastritis itself does not produce symptoms. Its major significance is a high risk for gastric malignancy.

Eosinophilic Antritis

Rarely, eosinophils may infiltrate beneath the submucosa of the antrum, producing a nodular deformity. Patients with this lesion usually present with ill-defined complaints. The diagnosis can be confirmed by endoscopic biopsy. The pathogenesis and natural history of these lesions are unknown. Careful follow-up and observation are therefore essential if for no other reason than to learn what the clinical significance of this lesion might be.

Corrosive Gastritis

The ingestion of strong alkali or acid may lead to gastric as well as esophageal injury. Lye remains a principal cause of this problem even though alterations in packaging of caustic materials have decreased the frequency of accidental ingestion. Suicide attempts by ingestion of large volumes of liquid lye lead to severe erosive esophagitis and gastritis. The subsequent healing process may be associated with gastric outlet obstruction as well as esophageal stricture. Gastric perforation, however, is unusual.

The ingestion of strong acid (sulfuric or hydrochloric) may lead to a full-thickness perforation of the stomach. History of this form of caustic injury requires endoscopic visualization of the gastric epithelium. The identification of large areas of epithelial necrosis should lead to immediate exploration and resection of the involved stomach.

GASTRIC PROCEDURES FOR MORBID OBESITY

Rationale. Excessive fat accumulation in relationship to other constituents of the body mass is a condition termed ''morbid obesity.'' Patients with this problem manifest excessive weight gain at puberty or in their early adult years. In spite of dieting and strenuous exercise, they frequently exceed twice their ideal weight. There is usually a strong family history associated with the disorder. Morbid obesity is usually not associated with symptoms or disease in early life. By midlife, however, the morbidly obese may develop hypertension, carbohydrate intolerance (adult-onset diabetes), degenerative arthritis, cardiopulmonary dysfunction, or gallstones. Possibly of equal importance is the fact that afflicted individuals are forced to live a suboptimum life since our culture is designed for slim people.

The pathogenesis of morbid obesity is poorly understood. Of the many factors involved, probably the most dominant is a combination of a genetic predisposition and an affluent society where there is an abundance of food. Childhood or teenage onset obesity appears to have this background. However, obesity that starts in midlife does not usually reach massive proportions. Obesity has been presumed to be an inequality of energy intake versus expenditure. Recent results from both animal and human studies suggest that body weight is not always directly related to the amount of food one eats. Some obesity may result from an inability to burn off excess calories as heat, leading to storage of these calories as fat. It is speculated that this disturbance in thermogenesis is due to a decreased amount of brown adipose tissue.

It is generally agreed that morbid obesity is refractory to medical therapy. Jejuno-ileal bypass, wherein the length of the small bowel is shortened, has been an effective way to induce weight loss in the morbidly obese. Its efficacy has been based on the malabsorption of excess food. Diarrhea associated with overeating also contributes to a reduction in food intake. Unfortunately, the operation which involves anastomosis of the jejunum 14 in. beyond the ligament of Treitz to the ileum, 4 in. from the ileocecal valve, requires bypass of the majority of the small bowel. The bypassed segment in some way contributes to the development of liver disease in 5 to 10 percent of patients. Malabsorption is associated with fluid and electrolyte abnormalities in an additional 5 percent. Over 50 percent of jejuno-ileal bypass patients develop oxalate kidney stones. Bloating with crampy abdominal pain is also a common complaint. These side effects have led to an abandonment of the procedure.

Operations. Gastric operations for morbid obesity are designed to reduce the daily intake of food to less than 800 cal until weight reduction has been achieved. Two operations depicted in

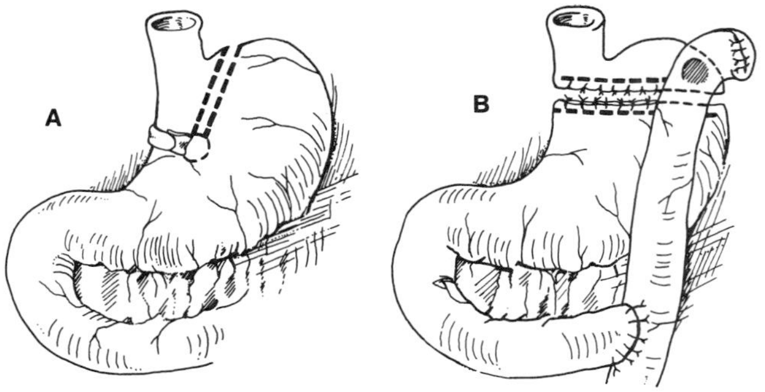

FIG. 24-20. Most common procedures designed to reduce gastric capacity and induce weight loss. *A.* Vertical banded gastroplasty. *B.* Small pouch gastric bypass.

Fig. 24-20, the Mason vertical banded gastroplasty and the Greenville small pouch gastric bypass with Roux en Y limb reconstruction, have been shown to be safe and effective. They received general acceptance by the medical community at a recent National Institutes of Health (NIH) consensus conference. Both operations provide for early satiety by the formation of a proximal gastric pouch that will hold less than 15 mL of ingesta. They differ in that the gastric bypass does not allow food to enter the distal stomach, thereby introducing an element of maldigestion. Furthermore, the ingestion of carbohydrates after this operation will lead to a rapid transit through the intestine and produce the symptomatology of the dumping syndrome. Possibly this is why the small pouch gastric bypass has emerged as the superior operation with regard to weight loss and long-term weight containment. Furthermore, the procedure appears to be associated with less unpleasant side effects such as chronic vomiting, a prominent symptom for some patients following a vertical banded gastroplasty. Following a small pouch gastric bypass patients usually lose 75 percent of their excess weight by 2 years and sustain this weight loss with only a 5 to 10 percent increment in weight in subsequent years. An important component to a successful outcome is a close and ongoing relationship between the surgeon and the patient in the early and late postoperative period. While the complication rate is low for either procedure, and the morbidity nil in the hands of those expert in this type of surgery, problems can arise quickly in the postoperative period. Pulmonary emboli represent the most serious complication, while atelectasis is the most common. Wound complications such as fluid accumulation, infection, or wound dehiscence are relatively uncommon (1 to 3 percent), considering the size of the wound in most patients.

It is now known that patients must remain on a low caloric intake (about 1000 or less kcal) for the remainder of their lives. They must take multivitamin supplements on a daily basis. The patients must be carefully monitored for adequacy of their nutrition and for problems such as iron or vitamin B_{12} deficiency anemias.

The surgical treatment of morbid obesity has been slowly evolving over the past 30 years toward an acceptable treatment for the complications associated with extreme obesity. The gastric restrictive procedures are not only associated with weight reduction but also lead to an increase in mobility, a decrease in blood pressure, an amelioration of glucose intolerance, and a reduction in pain within the joints of the lower extremities. While it is known that obesity is associated with a shortened life span, it is not yet known whether successful weight containment will prolong life. It is clear, however, that patients who have a successful outcome are very satisfied with the opportunities provided to them by their lower body mass.

The superobese (over 300 lb) continue to present a challenge in that they require in addition to a small gastric pouch an added element of malabsorption that is gained by making a long nondigestive jejunal limb. In this operation, the limb that carries the gastric succus, bile, and pancreatic juice is attached to the limb that carries the food from the gastric pouch at varying levels between the midgut and the ileocecal valve. The results of these procedures that combine an element of restricted intake with varying degrees of malabsorption are currently being assessed. It is clear that the superobese represent an extraordinary expression of the gene (or lack thereof) that has led to their obesity.

Bibliography

History

Beaumont W: *Experiments and Observations on the Gastric Juice and the Physiology of Digestion*. New York, Dover, 1959.

Blalock JB Jr: History and evolution of peptic ulcer surgery. *Am J Surg* 141:317, 1981.

Jordan PH Jr: Duodenal ulcers and their surgical treatment: Where did they come from? *Am J Surg* 149:2, 1985.

Wagensteen OH, Wagensteen SD: Gastric surgery, in *The Rise of Surgery*. Minneapolis, University of Minnesota Press, 1978.

Zollinger RM: Reflections on gastric surgery. *Am J Surg* 139:10, 1980.

Anatomy

Bentley FH, Barlow TE: Stomach: Vascular supply in relation to gastric ulcer, in *Surgery Progress 1952*. London, Butterworth, 1953.

Griffith CA: Anatomy, in Harkins HN, Nyhus LM (eds): *Surgery of the Stomach and Duodenum*. Boston, Little, Brown, 1969, p 25.

Lillibridge CB: The fine structure of normal human gastric mucosa. *Gastroenterology* 47:269, 1964.

McGuigan JE: Gastric mucosal intracellular localization of gastrin by immunofluorescence. *Gastroenterology* 55:315, 1968.

Michels NA: Blood supply of the stomach and the esophagus, in *Blood Supply and Anatomy of the Upper Abdominal Organs*. Philadelphia, Lippincott, 1955, p 248.

Schofield GC: Anatomy of muscular and neural tissues in the alimentary canal, in Code CF (ed): *Handbook of Physiology*. Washington, DC, American Physiological Society, 1968, sec 6, p 1579.

Physiology

Bukhave K, Rask-Madsen J, et al: Proximal duodenal prostaglandin E_2 release and mucosal bicarbonate secretion are altered in patients with duodenal ulcer. *Gastroenterology* 99:951, 1990.

Card WI, Marks IN: The relationship between the acid ouput of the stomach following "maximal" histamine stimulation and the parietal cell mass. *Clin Sci* 19:147, 1960.

Cooke AR: Control of gastric emptying and motility. *Gastroenterology* 68:804, 1975.

Davenport HW: Gastric secretion, in *Physiology of the Digestive Tract*. Chicago, Year Book Medical Publishers, 1971, p 95.

Davenport HW: Why the stomach does not digest itself. *Sci Am* 226:86, 1972.

Davenport HW, et al: Functional significance of gastric mucosal barrier to sodium. *Gastroenterology* 57:142, 1964.

Debas HT, Hollinshead J, et al: Vagal control of gastrin release in the dog: Pathways for stimulation and inhibition. *Surgery* 95:34, 1984.

Dragstedt LR: The physiology of the gastric antrum. *Arch Surg* 75:552, 1957.

Edkins JS: The chemical mechanism of gastric secretion. *J Physiol* 34:183, 1906.

Flemstrom G: Gastroduodenal mucosal secretion of bicarbonate and mucus. Physiologic control and stimulation by prostaglandins. *Am J Med* 81:18, 1986.

Fordtran JS, Walsh JH: Gastric acid secretion rate and buffer control of the stomach after eating: Results in normal subjects and in patients with duodenal ulcer. *J Clin Invest* 52:645, 1973.

Gregory RA: Memorial lecture: The isolation and chemistry of gastrin. *Gastroenterology* 51:953, 1966.

Gregory RA, Tracy HJ: The constitution and properties of two gastrins extracted from hog antral mucosa. *Gut* 5:103, 1964.

Grossman MI: Neural and hormonal stimulation of gastric secretion of acid, in Code CF (ed): *Handbook of Physiology*. Washington, DC, American Physiological Society, 1967, sec 6, vol II, p 835.

Grossman MI, et al: Candidate hormones of the gut. *Gastroenterology* 67:730, 1974.

Heading RC, et al: Gastric emptying rate measurement in man. A double isotope scanning technique for simultaneous study of liquid and solid components of a meal. *Gastroenterology* 71:45, 1976.

Hunt JN, Knox MT: Regulation of gastric emptying, in Code CF (ed): *Handbook of Physiology*. Washington, DC, American Physiological Society, 1968, sec 6, vol IV, p 1917.

Hunt JN, Stubbs DF: The volume and energy content of meals as determinants of gastric emptying. *J Physiol* (*London*) 245:209, 1975.

Ippoliti AF, et al: Demonstration of the intestinal phase of gastric acid secretion in man. *Gastroenterology* 70:896, 1976.

Jeffries GH: Gastric secretion in intrinsic factor, in Code CF (ed): *Handbook of Physiology*. Washington, DC, American Physiological Society, 1967, sec 6, vol II, p 919.

Johnson LR: Progress in gastroenterology: The trophic action of gastrointestinal hormones. *Gastroenterology* 70:278, 1976.

Kelly KA, Code CF: Canine gastric pacemaker. *Am J Physiol* 220:112, 1971.

Kleibeuker JH, Eysselein VE, et al: Role of endogenous secretin in acid-induced inhibition of human gastric function. *J Clin Invest* 73:526, 1984.

Makhlouf GM, et al: A quantitative statement of the two component hypothesis of gastric secretion. *Gastroenterology* 51:149, 1966.

Malagelada JR, et al: Measurement of gastric function during digestion of ordinary solid meals in man. *Gastroenterology* 70:203, 1976.

Meyer JH, Mayer EA, et al: Gastric processing and emptying of fat. *Gastroenterology* 90:1176, 1986.

Nyhus LM, et al: The control of gastric release: An experimental study illustrating a new concept. *Gastroenterology* 39:582, 1960.

Richardson CT, et al: Studies on the role of cephalic-vagal stimulation in the acid secretory response to eating in normal human subjects. *J Clin Invest* 60:435, 1977.

Samloff IM: Pepsinogens, pepsins and pepsin inhibitors. *Gastroenterology* 69:586, 1971.

Sircus W: The intestinal phase of gastric secretion. *Q J Exp Physiol* 38:91, 1953.

Thompson JC: Gastrointestinal hormones—introduction to symposium on gastrointestinal hormones. *World J Surg* 3:389, 1979.

Uvnas B: Role of duodenum in inhibition of gastric acid secretion. *Scand J Gastroenterol* 6:113, 1971.

Walsh JH, Grossman MI: Gastrin. *N Engl J Med* 292:1324, 1975.

White CM, Poxon V, et al: The importance of the distal stomach in gastric emptying of liquids in man. *Surg Gastroenterol* 3:13, 1984.

Wolf S, Wolff HG: *Human Gastric Function*. London, Oxford University Press, 1943.

Woodward ER: The role of the gastric antrum in the regulation of gastric secretion. *Gastroenterology* 38:7, 1960.

Gastric Dysfunction

Alexander-Williams J: Alkaline reflux gastritis: A myth or a disease? *Am J Surg* 143:17, 1982.

Barnes AD, Cox AG: Diarrhea, in Williams JA, Cox AG (eds): *After Vagotomy*. London, Butterworth, 1969, p 211.

Baron JH: The clinical use of gastric function tests. *Scand J Gastroenterol Suppl* 6:9, 1970.

Becker JM, Sava P, et al: Intestinal pacing for canine postgastrectomy dumping. *Gastroenterology* 84:383, 1983.

Camilleri M, Malageleda JR, et al: Effect of six weeks of treatment with cisapride in gastroparesis and intestinal pseudoobstruction. *Gastroenterology* 96:704, 1989.

Condon JR, et al: The cause and treatment of postvagotomy diarrhea. *Br J Surg* 62:309, 1975.

Ferguson GH, MacLennon I, et al: Outcome of revisional gastric surgery using a Roux-en-Y biliary diversion. *Br J Surg* 77:551, 1990.

Fiore AC, et al: Surgical management of alkaline reflux gastritis. *Arch Surg* 117:689, 1982.

Geer RJ, Richards WO, et al: Efficacy of octreotide acetate in treatment of severe postgastrectomy dumping syndrome. *Ann Surg* 212:678, 1990.

Goldberg J, et al: A clinical evaluation of the maximal histalog test. *Am J Dig Dis* 12:468, 1967.

Greene FL: Gastroscopic screening of the post-gastrectomy stomach: Relationship of dysplasia to remnant cancer. *Am Surg* 55:12, 1989.

Grundy A, Belli A: Balloon dilation of upper gastrointestinal tract strictures. *Clin Radiol* 39:229, 1988.

Gustavsson S, et al: Scintigraphic assessment of biliary reflux into the residual stomach after subtotal gastrectomy and gastrojejunostomy. *Acta Radiol [Diagn] (Stockh)* 21:639, 1980.

Halpern NB, et al: Failure to achieve success with remedial gastric surgery. *Am J Surg* 125:108, 1973.

Herrington JL Jr, Sawyers JL: Surgical management of alkaline reflux gastritis and esophagitis. *Surg Annu* 13:341, 1981.

Herrington JL Jr, et al: Surgical management of reflux gastritis. *Ann Surg* 180:526, 1974.

Hirschowitz BI, et al: Demonstration of a new gastroscope, the "Fiberscope." *Gastroenterology* 35:50, 1958.

Isenberg JI, et al: Pentagastrin vs betazole as stimulant of gastric secretion. *JAMA* 206:2897, 1968.

Janssens J, Peeters TL, et al: Improvement of gastric emptying in diabetic gastroparesis by erythromycin: Preliminary studies. *N Engl J Med* 322:1028, 1990.

Johnston GW, Spencer EF, et al: Proximal gastric vagotomy: Follow-up at 10–20 years. *Br J Surg* 78:20, 1991.

Johnstone FR, et al: Postgastrectomy problems in patients with personality defects: The "albatross" syndrome. *Can Med Assoc J* 96:1559, 1967.

Jordon GL: Surgical management of postgastrectomy problems. *Arch Surg* 102:251, 1971.

Kelly KA: Gastric motility in health and after gastric surgery. *Viewpoints, Dig Dis* 8:1, 1976.

Kennedy T: The failures of gastric surgery. *Br J Surg* 68:677, 1981.

Laufer I: A simple method for routine double contrast study of the upper gastrointestinal tract. *Radiology* 117:513, 1975.

Laufer I, et al: The diagnostic accuracy of barium studies of the stomach and duodenum—correlation with endoscopy. *Radiology* 115:569, 1975.

LeQuesne LP, et al: The dumping syndrome—1. Factors responsible for the symptoms. *Br Med J* 1:141, 1960.

Lundh G: Intestinal digestion and absorption after gastrectomy. *Acta Chir Scand Suppl* 231:1, 1958.

Macintyre IMC, Miller A: Highly selective vagotomy—A safe operation for duodenal ulcer: Immediate and long-term complications and sequelae in 500 patients. *Eur J Surg* 157:261, 1991.

Martin LF, Larson GM, et al: Bleeding from stress gastritis. Has prophylactic pH control made a difference? *Am Surg* 5:189, 1985.

Mathias JR, Fernandez A, et al: Nausea, vomiting, and abdominal pain after Roux en Y anastomosis: Motility of the jejunal limb. *Gastroenterology* 88:101–107, 1985.

Metzger WH, et al: Effect of metoclopramide in chronic gastric retention after gastric surgery. *Gastroenterology* 71:30, 1976.

Miller TA: Derangements in gastric function secondary to previous surgery, in Miller TA (ed): *Physiologic Basis of Modern Surgical Care*. St. Louis, CV Mosby, 1988, p 320.

Phillips JC, et al: Gastric leiomyosarcoma; Roentgenologic and clinical findings. *Am J Dig Dis* 15:239, 1970.

Reasbeck PG, Van Rij AM: The effect of somatostatin on dumping after gastric surgery: A preliminary report. *Surgery* 99:462, 1986.

Reber HA, Way LW: Surgical treatment of late postgastrectomy syndromes. *Am J Surg* 129:71, 1975.

Sakita T, Oguro Y: Endoscopic diagnosis of early gastric cancer, in Berry LH (ed): *Gastrointestinal Pan-Endoscopy*. Springfield, IL, Charles C Thomas, 1974, p 278.

Sawyers JL, et al: Remedial operation for alkaline reflux gastritis and associated postgastrectomy syndromes. *Arch Surg* 115:519, 1980.

Seaman WB: Non-neoplastic diseases of the stomach, in Margulis AR, Burhenne HJ (eds): *Alimentary Tract Roentgenology*. St Louis, CV Mosby, 1973, vol 1, p 607.

Shaffer EA: The effect of vagotomy on gallbladder function and bile composition in man. *Ann Surg* 195:413, 1982.

Sheiner HJ, et al: Gastric motility and emptying in normal and post-vagotomy subjects. *Gut* 21:753, 1980.

Shirakabe H, et al: *Atlas of X-ray Diagnosis of Early Gastric Cancer*. Philadelphia, Lippincott, 1966.

Tovey FI, Clark CG: Anaemia after partial gastrectomy: A neglected curable condition. *Lancet* 1:956, 1980.

van Heerden JA, et al: Postoperative reflux gastritis. *Am J Surg* 129:82, 1975.

Vogel SB, Vair DB, et al: Alterations in gastrointestinal emptying of 99m-technetium-labeled solids following sequential antrectomy, truncal vagotomy and Roux Y gastroenterostomy. *Ann Surg* 198:506, 1983.

Vogel SB, Woodward ER: The surgical treatment of chronic gastric atony following Roux-Y diversion for alkaline reflux gastritis. *Ann Surg* 209:756, 1989.

Wormsley KG, Grossman MI: Maximal histalog test in control subjects and patients with peptic ulcer. *Gut* 6:427, 1965.

Yalow RS, Berson SA: Radioimmunoassay of gastrin. *Gastroenterology* 58:1, 1970.

Zboralske FF: Gastric ulcer, in Margulis AR, Burhenne HJ (eds): *Alimentary Tract Roentgenology*. St Louis, CV Mosby, 1967, vol 1, p 475.

Gastric and Duodenal Disease

Adami H, Enander L, et al: Recurrences one to ten years after highly selective vagotomy in prepyloric and duodenal ulcer. *Ann Surg* 199:393, 1984.

Adkins RB Jr, DeLozier JB III, et al: The management of gastric ulcers: A current review. *Ann Surg* 201:741, 1985.

Amdrup E: Recurrent ulcer. *Br J Surg* 68:679, 1981.

Amdrup E, Jensen HE: Selective vagotomy of the parietal cell mass preserving innervation of the undrained antrum. *Gastroenterology* 59:522, 1970.

Amdrup E, et al: Clinical results of parietal cell vagotomy (highly selective vagotomy) two to four years after operation. *Ann Surg* 180:279, 1974.

Amdrup E, et al: Parietal cell (highly selective or proximal gastric) vagotomy for peptic ulcer disease. *World J Surg* 1:19, 1977.

Anderson JR, et al: Cholelithiasis following peptic ulcer surgery: A prospective controlled study. *Br J Surg* 67:618, 1980.

Asbaugh D, et al: Gastroscopy in corrosive burn of the stomach. *JAMA* 216:1638, 1971.

Bader JP: The surgical treatment of peptic ulcer disease. A physician's view. *Dig Dis Sci* 30(11 suppl):52S, 1985.

Bardhan DD: Refractory duodenal ulcer. *Gut* 25:711, 1984.

Barragry TP, Blatchford JW, et al: Giant gastric ulcers, a review of 49 cases. *Ann Surg* 203:255, 1986.

Bergegardh S, et al: Gastric acid responses to graded I.V. infusion of pentagastrin and histalog in peptic ulcer patients before and after antrum-bulb resection. *Scand J Gastroenterol* 11:337, 1976.

Berne CJ, Rosoff L: Peptic ulcer perforation of the gastroduodenal artery complex. *Ann Surg* 169:141, 1969.

Binder HJ, et al: Cimetidine in the treatment of duodenal ulcer: A multicenter double-blind study. *Gastroenterology* 74:380, 1978.

Bittner R, Schirrow H, et al: Total gastrectomy: A 15-year experience with particular reference to the patient over 70 years of age. *Arch Surg* 120:1120, 1985.

Blumenthal IS: Digestive disease as a national problem. III. Social cost of peptic ulcer. *Gastroenterology* 54:86, 1968.

Bonfils S, et al: Cimetidine treatment of acute and chronic Zollinger-Ellison syndrome. *World J Surg* 3:597, 1979.

Bringaze WL III, Chappuis CW, et al: Early gastric cancer. *Ann Surg* 204:103, 1986.

Burgess JN, et al: Sarcomatous lesions of the stomach. *Ann Surg* 173:758, 1971.

Burhenne HJ: The postoperative stomach, in Margulis AR, Burhenne HJ (eds): *Alimentary Tract Roentgenology*. St Louis, CV Mosby, 1973, vol 1, p 740.

Castrini G, Pappalardo G: Carcinoma of the cardia: Tactical problem. *J Thorac Cardiovasc Surg* 82:190, 1981.

Cathcart PM, et al: Tumors of gastric smooth muscle. *South Med J* 73:18, 1980.

Cello JP, Grendell JH: Endoscopic laser treatment for gastrointestinal vascular ectasias. *Ann Intern Med* 104:352, 1986.

Christiansen J, et al: Prospective controlled vagotomy trial for duodenal ulcer: Primary results, sequelae, acid secretion, and recurrence rates two to five years after operation. *Ann Surg* 193:49, 1981.

Chung R, DenBesten L: Fiberoptic endoscopy in treatment of corrosive injury of the stomach. *Arch Surg* 110:725, 1975.

Collen MJ, Howard JM, et al: Comparison of ranitidine and cimetidine in the treatment of gastric hypersecretion. *Ann Intern Med* 100:52, 1984.

Conn HO, et al: Intra-arterial vasopressin in the treatment of upper gastrointestinal hemorrhage. A prospective, controlled clinical trial. *Gastroenterology* 68:211, 1975.

Cooke AR: The role of the mucosal barrier in drug-induced gastric ulceration and erosions. *Am J Dig Dis* 21:155, 1976.

Cooperative Study Group: Omeprazole in duodenal ulceration: Acid inhibition, symptom relief, endoscopic healing, and recurrence. *Br Med J* 289:525, September 1984.

Cowley DJ, et al: Acid secretion in relation to recurrence of duodenal ulcer after vagotomy and drainage. *Br J Surg* 60:517, 1973.

Cox AJ Jr: Pathology, in Harkins HN, Nyhus LM (eds): *Surgery of the Stomach and Duodenum,* 2d ed. Boston, Little, Brown, 1969.

Crofts TJ, Park KGM: A randomized trial of nonoperative treatment for perforated peptic ulcer. *N Engl J Med* 320:970, 1989.

Cross S, et al: Carbenoxolone: Its protective action on gastric mucosa, in *Biologie et Gastroenterologie*. 9th International Congress of Gastroenterology, Paris, 5:568C, 1972.

Csendes A, Braghetto L, et al: Surgical treatment of high gastric ulcer. *Am J Surg* 149:765, 1985.

Czaja AJ, et al: Gastric acid secretion and acute gastroduodenal disease after burns. *Arch Surg* 111:243, 1976.

DeBakey M, Ochsner A: Bezoars and concretions. *Surgery* 4:934, 1938.

Debas HT, Mulholland MW: Drug therapy in peptic ulcer disease. *Curr Probl Surg* 26:9, 1989.

Diggory RT, Cuschieri A: R2/3 gastrectomy for gastric carcinoma: An audited experience of a consecutive series. *Br J Surg* 72:146, 1985.

Donahue PE, Yoshida J: Proximal gastric vagotomy with drainage for obstructing duodenal ulcer. *Surgery* 104:757, 1988.

Donovan AJ, et al: Selective treatment of duodenal ulcer with perforation. *Ann Surg* 189:627, 1979.

Dougherty SH, et al: Stomach cancer following gastric surgery for benign disease. *Arch Surg* 117:294, 1982.

Dragstedt LR, Owens FM Jr: Supradiaphragmatic secretion of vagus nerves in treatment of duodenal ulcer. *Proc Soc Exp Biol Med* 53:152, 1943.

DuPlessis DJ: Pathogenesis of gastric ulceration. *Lancet* 1:974, 1965.

Duthie HL, et al: Surgical treatment of gastric ulcers. Controlled comparison of billroth-I gastrectomy and vagotomy and pyloroplasty. *Br J Surg* 57:784, 1970.

Elashoff JD, Van Deventer G, et al: Long-term follow-up of duodenal ulcer patients. *J Clin Gastroenterol* 5:509, 1983.

Ellis FH Jr: Esophagogastrectomy for carcinoma: Technical considerations based on anatomic location of lesion. *Surg Clin North Am* 60:265, 1980.

Emas S, Aly A: Acid and pepsin responses to graded doses of pentagastrin in duodenal and corporeal gastric ulcer patients before and after selective proximal vagotomy. *Am J Surg* 150:543, 1985.

Emas S, Fernstrom M: Prospective, randomized trial of selective vagotomy with pyloroplasty and selective proximal vagotomy with and without pyloroplasty in the treatment of duodenal, pyloric, and prepyloric ulcers. *Am J Surg* 149:236, 1985.

Engstrom PF, Lavin PT, et al: Postoperative adjuvant 5-fluorouracil plus methyl-CCNU therapy for gastric cancer patients: Eastern Cooperative Oncology Group Study (EST 3275). *Cancer* 55:1863, 1985.

Enquist IF, Karlson KE, et al: Statistically valid ten-year comparative evaluation of three methods of management of massive gastroduodenal hemorrhage. *Ann Surg* 162:550, 1965.

Fakhry SM, Herbst CA Jr, et al: Complications requiring intervention after gastric bariatric surgery. *South Med J* 78:536, 1985.

Farris JM, Smith GK: Vagotomy and pyloroplasty: A solution to the management of bleeding duodenal ulcer. *Ann Surg* 152:416, 1960.

Feczko PJ, Halpert RD: Gastric polyps: Radiological evaluation and clinical significance. *Radiology* 155:581, 1985.

Finsberg HV, Pearlman LA: Surgical treatment of peptic ulcer in the United States. Trends before and after the introduction of cimetidine. *Lancet* 1:1305, 1981.

Fleischer D: Endoscopic laser therapy for gastrointestinal neoplasms. *Surg Clin North Am* 64:947, 1984.

Fleming ID, et al: The role of surgery in the management of gastric lymphoma. *Cancer* 49:1135, 1982.

Fordtran JS, et al: In vivo and in vitro evaluation of liquid antacids. *N Engl J Med* 288:293, 1973.

Foster JH, et al: Factors influencing mortality following emergency operation for massive upper gastrointestinal hemorrhage. *Surg Gynecol Obstet* 117:257, 1963.

Fraser AG, Brunt PW, et al: Comparison of highly selective vagotomy with truncal vagotomy and pyloroplasty: One surgeon's results after 5 years. *Br J Surg* 70:485, 1983.

Fraser GM, Earnshaw PM: Double-contrast barium meal: Correlation with endoscopy. *Clin Radiol* 34:121, 1983.

Friedman GD, et al: Cigarettes, alcohol, coffee and peptic ulcer. *N Engl J Med* 290:469, 1974.

Gall FP, Hermanek P: New aspects in the surgical treatment of gastric carcinoma—a comparative study of 1636 patients operated on between 1969 and 1982. *Eur J Surg Oncol* 11:19, 1985.

Gentsch HH, et al: Results of surgical treatment of early gastric cancer in 113 patients. *World J Surg* 5:103, 1981.

Gilbert DA, Surawicz CM, et al: Prevention of acute aspirin-induced gastric mucosal injury by 15-R-15 methyl prostaglandin E_2: Endoscopic study. *Gastroenterology* 86:339, 1984.

Gledhill T, Buck M, et al: Cimetidine or vagotomy? Comparison of the effects of proximal gastric vagotomy, cimetidine, and placebo on nocturnal intragastric acidity and acid secretion in patients with cimetidine-resistant duodenal ulcer. *Br J Surg* 70:7043, 1983.

Goldstein F, Kline TS, et al: Early gastric cancer in a United States hospital. *Am J Gastroenterol* 78:715, 1983.

Goligher JC: A technique for highly selective (parietal cell or proximal gastric) vagotomy for duodenal ulcer. *Br J Surg* 61:337, 1974.

Goligher JC, et al: Controlled trial of vagotomy and gastroenterostomy, vagotomy and antrectomy and subtotal gastrectomy in elective treatment of duodenal ulcer: Interim report. *Br Med J* 1:455, 1964.

Goligher JC, et al: Five to eight year results of truncal vagotomy and pyloroplasty for duodenal ulcer. *Br Med J* 1:7, 1972.

Gough KR, Korman MG, et al: Ranitidine and cimetidine in prevention of duodenal ulcer relapse: Double-blind, randomized, multicenter, comparative trial. *Lancet* 2:659, 1984.

Gouzi JL, Huguier M, et al: Total versus subtotal gastrectomy: Analysis of an Amsterdam cohort. *Int J Cancer* 46:792, 1990.

Graffner HO, Liedberg GF, et al: Parietal cell vagotomy in the surgical treatment of chronic duodenal, pyloric and prepyloric ulcer disease. *Int Surg* 70:139, 1985.

Graffner HO, Liedberg GF, et al: Recurrence after parietal cell vagotomy for peptic ulcer disease. *Am J Surg* 150:336, 1985.

Grant CS, Kim CH, et al: Gastric leiomyosarcoma: Prognostic factors and surgical management. *Arch Surg* 126:985, 1991.

Greenall MJ, Lehnert T: Vagotomy or gastrectomy for elective treatment of benign gastric ulceration? *Dig Dis Sci* 30:353, 1985.

Greenall MJ, et al: Long term effect of highly selective vagotomy on basal and maximal acid output in man. *Gastroenterology* 68:1421, 1975.

Gregory RA, et al: Extraction of gastrin-like substance from pancreatic tumor in case of Zollinger-Ellison syndrome. *Lancet* 1:1045, 1960.

Griffith CA, Harkins HN: Partial gastric vagotomy. An experimental study. *Gastroenterology* 32:96, 1957.

Grossman MI: Some minor heresies about vagotomy. *Gastroenterology* 67:1016, 1974.

Grossman MI, et al: A new look at peptic ulcer. *Ann Intern Med* 84:57, 1976.

Grossman MI, et al: Peptic ulcer: New therapies, new diseases. *Ann Intern Med* 95:609, 1981.

Gunvén P, Maruyama K: Non-ominous micrometastases of gastric cancer. *Br J Surg* 78:351, 1991.

Hallenbeck GA, et al: Proximal gastric vagotomy: Effects of two operative techniques on clinical and gastric secretory results. *Ann Surg* 184:435, 1976.

Hastings PR, et al: Mallory-Weiss syndrome, review of 69 cases. *Am J Surg* 142:560, 1981.

Herrington JL, et al: A twenty-five year experience with vagotomy-antrectomy. *Arch Surg* 106:469, 1973.

Hirschowitz BI, Luketic GC: Endoscopy in the post-gastrectomy patient: An analysis of 580 patients. *Gastrointest Endosc* 18:27, 1971.

Hoffmann J, Olesen A, et al: Prospective 14- to 18-year follow-up study after parietal cell vagotomy. *Br J Surg* 74:1056, 1987.

Howard TJ, Zinner MJ, et al: Gastrinoma excision for cure: A prospective analysis. *Ann Surg* 211:9, 1990.

Hunt PS: Surgical management of bleeding chronic peptic ulcer: A 10-year prospective study. *Ann Surg* 199:44, 1984.

Hunt PS, et al: The management of bleeding gastric ulcer: A prospective study. *Aust NZ J Surg* 50:41, 1980.

Iishi H, Tatsuta M, et al: Endoscopic diagnosis of minute gastric cancer of less than 5 mm in diameter. *Cancer* 56:655, 1985.

Inberg MV, et al: Total and proximal gastrectomy in the treatment of gastric carcinoma: A series of 305 cases. *World J Surg* 5:249, 1981.

Ippoliti AF, et al: Cimetidine versus intensive antacid therapy for duodenal ulcer: A multicenter trial. *Gastroenterology* 74:393, 1978.

Isenberg JI, Peterson WL, et al: Healing of benign gastric ulcer with low-dose antacid or cimetidine: A double-blind randomized, placebo-controlled trial. *N Engl J Med* 308:1319, 1983.

Ivy AC, et al: *Peptic Ulcer*. Philadelphia, Blakiston, 1950.

Jaffin BW, Kaye MD: The prognosis of gastric outlet obstruction. *Ann Surg* 201:176, 1985.

Johnston D, Wilkinson AR: Highly selective vagotomy without a drainage procedure in the treatment of duodenal ulcer. *Br J Surg* 57:289, 1970.

Jordan PH Jr: Surgery for peptic ulcer disease. *Curr Probl Surg* 28:271, 1991.

Jordan PH Jr, Condon RE: A prospective evaluation of vagotomy-pyloroplasty and vagotomy-antrectomy for treatment of duodenal ulcer. *Ann Surg* 172:547, 1970.

Kim JP, Kwon OJ, et al: Results of surgery on 6589 gastric cancer patients and immunochemosurgery as the best treatment of advanced gastric cancer. *Ann Surg* 216:269, 1992.

Klein TS, Goldstein F: Malignant lymphoma involving the stomach. *Cancer* 32:961, 1973.

Knauer CM: Mallory-Weiss syndrome. Characterization of 75 Mallory-Weiss lacerations in 528 patients with upper gastrointestinal hemorrhage. *Gastroenterology* 71:5, 1976.

Koga S, et al: Results of total gastrectomy for gastric cancer. *Am J Surg* 140:636, 1980.

Koo J, Lam SK, et al: Proximal gastric vagotomy, truncal vagotomy with drainage, and truncal vagotomy with antrectomy for chronic duodenal ulcer: A prospective, randomized controlled trial. *Ann Surg* 197:265, 1983.

Kuster GGR, et al: Gastric cancer in pernicious anemia and in patients with and without achlorhydria. *Ann Surg* 175:783, 1972.

Laine L, Winstein WM: Histology of alcoholic hemorrhage "gastritis": A prospective evaluation. *Gastroenterology* 94:1254, 1988.

Lamers CBHW, Lind T, et al: Omeprazole in Zollinger-Ellison syndrome: Effects of a single dose and of long-term treatment in patients resistant to histamine H_2-receptor antagonists. *N Engl J Med* 310:758, 1984.

Lamothe PH, Rao E, et al: Comparative efficacy of cimetidine, famotidine, ranitidine, and Mylanta in post-operative stress ulcers: Gastric pH control and ulcer prevention in patients undergoing coronary artery bypass graft surgery. *Gastroenterology* 100:1515, 1991.

Laurence BH, et al: Endoscopic laser photocoagulation for bleeding peptic ulcers. *Lancet* 1:124, 1980.

Lieberman DA, Keller FS, et al: Arterial embolization for massive upper gastrointestinal tract bleeding in poor surgical candidates. *Gastroenterology* 86:376, 1984.

Lind T, Cederberg C: 24-hour intragastric acidity and plasma gastrin after omeprazole treatment and after proximal gastric vagotomy in duodenal ulcer patients. *Gastroenterology* 99:1593, 1990.

Littman A (ed): The Veterans Administration cooperative study on gastric ulcer. *Gastroenterology* 61:567, 1971.

Longmire WP Jr: Gastric carcinoma: Is radical gastrectomy worthwhile? *Ann R Coll Surg Engl* 62:25, 1980.

Lucas CE, et al: Natural history and surgical dilemma of "stress" gastric bleeding. *Arch Surg* 102:266, 1971.

Lunde OC, Liavag I, et al: Proximal gastric vagotomy and pyloroplasty for duodenal ulcer with pyloric stenosis: A thirteen-year experience. *World J Surg* 9:165, 1985.

Lygidakis NJ: Gastric stump carcinoma after surgery for gastroduodenal ulcer. *Ann R Coll Surg Engl* 63:203, 1981.

Lygidakis NJ: Total gastrectomy for gastric carcinoma: A retrospective study of different procedures and assessment of a new technique of gastric reconstruction. *Br J Surg* 68:649, 1981.

McCarthy DM: Report of the United States experience with cimetidine in the Zollinger-Ellison syndrome and other hypersecretory states. *Gastroenterology* 74:453, 1978.

McCarthy E, et al: H_2-histamine receptor blocking agents in the Zollinger-Ellison syndrome. *Ann Intern Med* 87:668, 1977.

MacLeod LA, Mills PR, et al: Neodymium-yttrium-aluminum-garnet laser photocoagulation for a major hemorrhage from peptic ulcers and single vessels: A single-blind controlled study. *Br Med J* 286:345, 1983.

Madsen P, Kronborg O: Recurrent ulcer $5\frac{1}{2}$–8 years after highly selective vagotomy without drainage and selective vagotomy with pyloroplasty. *Scand J Gastroenterol* 15:193, 1980.

Malagelada JR: Medical versus surgical therapy for duodenal ulcer: Making the right choices. *Mayo Clin Proc* 55:25, 1980.

Malagelada JR, Ahlquist DA, et al: Defects in prostaglandin synthesis and metabolism in ulcer disease. *Dig Dis Sci* 31(suppl 2):20S, 1986.

Malagelada J, Edis AJ, et al: Medical and surgical options in the management of patients with gastrinoma. *Gastroenterology* 84:1524, 1983.

Malagelada J, Phillips SF, et al: Postoperative reflux gastritis: Pathophysiology and long-term outcome after Roux en Y diversion. *Ann Intern Med* 103:178, 1985.

Mallory GK, Weiss S: Hemorrhages from lacerations of cardiac orifice of the stomach due to vomiting. *Am J Med Sci* 178:506, 1929.

Marshak RH, Lindner AE: The Zollinger-Ellison syndrome, in *Radiology of the Small Intestine*. Philadelphia, WB Saunders, 1970, p 88.

Maton PN, Frucht H, et al: Medical management of patients with Zollinger-Ellison syndrome who have had previous gastric surgery: A prospective study. *Gastroenterology* 94:294, 1988.

Maton PN, Vinayek R, et al: Long-term efficacy and safety of omeprazole in patients with Zollinger-Ellison syndrome: A prospective study. *Gastroenterology* 97:827, 1989.

Mekelvey STD: Gastric incontinence and postvagotomy diarrhea. *Br J Surg* 57:741, 1970.

Mendeloff AI: What has been happening to duodenal ulcer? *Gastroenterology* 67:1020, 1974.

Menetrier P: Des polyadenomes gastriques et de leurs rapports avec le cancer de l'estomac. *Arch Physiol Norm Path* 1:32, 226, 1888.

Menguy R: Pathophysiology of peptic ulcer. *Am J Surg* 120: 282, 1970.

Menguy R, et al: Mechanism of stress ulcer: Influence of hypovolemic shock on energy metabolism in the gastric mucosa. *Gastroenterology* 66:46, 1974.

Menguy R, et al: The surgical management of acute gastric mucosal bleeding. Stress ulcer, acute erosive gastritis, and acute hemorrhagic gastritis. *Arch Surg* 99:198, 1969.

Messer J, Reitman D, et al: Association of adrenocorticosteroid therapy and peptic ulcer disease. *N Engl J Med* 309:21, 1983.

Miller TA: Gastroduodenal mucosal defense: Factors responsible for the ability of the stomach and duodenum to resist injury. *Surgery* 103:389, 1988.

Miller TA: Emergencies in acid-peptic disease. In Merrell RL (ed): *Gastroenterological Emergencies*. Philadelphia, WB Saunders, 1988, p 303.

Miller TA: Gastric neoplasia. In Miller TA (ed): *Physiologic Basis of Modern Surgical Care*. St. Louis, CV Mosby, 1988, p 310.

Miller TA, Reed RL, et al: Gastrointestinal hemorrhage. In Barie PS, Shires GT (eds): *Surgical Intensive Care*. Boston, Little, Brown, 1992, in press.

Miller TA, Smith GS, et al: Gastroduodenal defense: Role of epithelial factors. In Goldie R (ed): *Immunopharmacology of Epithelial Barriers*. London, Academic Press, 1992, p 743.

Miller TA, Tornwall MS, et al: Stress erosive gastritis. *Curr Probl Surg* 28:459, 1991.

Miller TA, Victor BE: Gastritis and gastric ulcer. In Moody FG (ed): *Surgical Treatment of Digestive Disease*. Chicago, Year Book Medical Publishers, 1990, p 174.

Mizuno H, et al: Endoscopic followup of gastric polyps. *Gastrointest Endosc* 21:112, 1975.

Moertel CG, et al: Sequential and combination chemotherapy of advanced gastric cancer. *Cancer* 38:678, 1976.

Monaco AP, et al: Adenomatous polyps of the stomach. A clinical and pathological study of 153 cases. *Cancer* 15:456, 1962.

Moody FG: Role of mucosal blood flow in the pathogenesis of gastric ulcers, in Holton P (ed): *International Encyclopedia of Pharmacology and Therapeutics*. Oxford, Pergamon, 1973, sec 39A, vol 1.

Moody FG, et al: Stress and the acute gastric mucosal lesion. *Am J Dig Dis* 21:148, 1976.

Mozell E, Stenzel P, et al: Functional endocrine tumors of the pancreas: Clinical presentation, diagnosis, and treatment. *Curr Probl Surg* 27:309, 1990.

Newman PL, Wadden C, et al: Gastrointestinal stromal tumours: Correlation of immunophenotype with clinicopathological features. *J Pathol* 164:107, 1991.

Nicosia J, et al: Surgical management of corrosive gastric injuries. *Ann Surg* 180:139, 1974.

Norton JA, Doppman JL, et al: Aggressive resection of metastatic disease in selected patients with malignant gastrinoma. *Ann Surg* 203:352, 1986.

Nyhus LM: Gastric ulcer, in Harkins HN, Nyhus LM (eds): *Surgery of the Stomach and Duodenum,* 2d ed. Boston, Little, Brown, 1969, p 203.

O'Brien JJ, Burakoff R, et al: Early gastric cancer: Clinicopathologic study. *Am J Med* 78:195, 1985.

Ochsner A, et al: Cancer of the stomach. *Am J Surg* 141:10, 1981.

O'Connor HJ, Newbold KM: Effect of Roux-en-Y diversion of *Campylobacter pylori*. *Gastroenterology* 97:958, 1989.

Oi M, et al: The location of gastric ulcer. *Gastroenterology* 36:45, 1959.

O'Neill JA, et al: Studies related to the pathogenesis of Curling's ulcer. *J Trauma* 7:275, 1967.

Orlando R III, Welch JP: Carcinoma of the stomach after gastric operation. *Am J Surg* 141:487, 1981.

O'Rourke IC: Elective surgery for peptic ulcer: A five-year review. *Med J Aust* 143:13, 1985.

Overholt BF, Jeffries GH: Hypertrophic, hypersecretory protein-losing gastropathy. *Gastroenterology* 58:80, 1970.

Paimela H, Tuompo PK, et al: Peptic ulcer surgery during the H_2-receptor antagonist era: A population-based epidemiological study of ulcer surgery in Helsinki from 1972 to 1987. *Br J Surg* 78:28, 1991.

Palmer ED: The vigorous diagnostic approach to upper gastrointestinal tract hemorrhage. *JAMA* 207:1477, 1969.

Pellegrini CA, Patti MG, et al: Alkaline reflux gastritis and the effect of biliary diversion on gastric emptying of solid food. *Am J Surg* 150:166, 1985.

Pipeleers-Marichal M, Somers G, et al: Gastrinomas in the duodenums of patients with multiple endocrine neoplasia type 1 and the Zollinger-Ellison syndrome. *N Engl J Med* 322:723, 1990.

Primrose JN, Ratcliffe JG, et al: Differences between peptic ulcer and control patients on the basis of the response to secretion. *Digestion* 32:249, 1985.

Rackner VL, Thirlby RC, et al: Role of surgery in multimodality therapy for gastrointestinal lymphoma. *Am J Surg* 161:570, 1991.

Rauws EAJ, Tytgat GNJ: Cure of duodenal ulcer associated with eradication of *Helicobacter pylori*. *Lancet* 335:1233, 1990.

Richardson CT, Peters MN, et al: Treatment of Zollinger-Ellison syndrome with exploratory laparotomy, proximal gastric vagotomy, and H_2-receptor antagonists: A prospective study. *Gastroenterology* 89:357, 1985.

Richardson CT, Walsh JH: The value of a histamine H_2-receptor antagonist in the management of patients with the Zollinger-Ellison syndrome. *N Engl J Med* 294:133, 1976.

Ritchie WJ Jr: Alkaline reflux gastritis, late results on a controlled trial of diagnosis and treatment. *Ann Surg* 203:537, 1986.

Romanus ME, Neal JA, et al: Comparison of four provocative tests for the diagnosis of gastrinoma. *Ann Surg* 198:608, 1983.

Rossi RL, et al: Parietal cell vagotomy for intractable and obstructing duodenal ulcer. *Am J Surg* 141:482, 1981.

Rotter JL, et al: Genetics of peptic ulcer disease: Segregation of serum group I pepsinogen concentrations in families with peptic ulcer disease. *Clin Res* 25:114A, 1977.

Rutledge PL, Warshaw AL: Diagnosis of symptomatic alkaline reflux gastritis and prediction of response to bile diversion operation by intragastric alkali provocation. *Am J Surg* 155:82, 1988.

Sakita T, et al: Observations on the healing of ulcerations in early gastric cancer. The life cycle of the malignant ulcer. *Gastroenterology* 60:835, 1971.

Sawyers JL, Scott HW Jr: Selective gastric vagotomy with antrectomy or pyloroplasty. *Ann Surg* 174:541, 1971.

Schafer LW, Larson DE, et al: Risk of development of gastric carcinoma in patients with pernicious anemia: A population-based study in Rochester, Minnesota. *Mayo Clinic Proc* 60:444, 1985.

Scott HW Jr, Adkins RB Jr, et al: Results of an aggressive surgical approach to gastric carcinoma during a twenty-three-year period. *Surgery* 97:55, 1985.

Shepherd AF, Allan RN, et al: The surgical treatment of gastroduodenal Crohn's disease. *Ann R Coll Surg Engl* 67:382, 1985.

Shimm DS, Dosoretz DE, et al: Primary gastric lymphoma: An analysis with emphasis on prognostic factors and radiation therapy. *Cancer* 52:2044, 1983.

Sirinek KR, et al: Simple closure of perforated peptic ulcer. Still an effective procedure for patients with delay in treatment. *Arch Surg* 116:591, 1981.

Sonnenberg A: Costs of medical and surgical treatment of duodenal ulcer. *Gastroenterology* 96:1445, 1989.

Stabile BE, Passaro E Jr: Recurrent peptic ulcer. *Gastroenterology* 70:124, 1976.

Stanten A, Peters H Jr: Enzymatic dissolution of phytobezoars. *Am J Surg* 130:259, 1975.

Stempien SJ, et al: Hypertrophic hypersecretory gastropathy. *Am J Dig Dis* 9:471, 1964.

Swain CP, Storey DW, et al: Nature of the bleeding vessel in recurrently bleeding gastric ulcers. *Gastroenterology* 90:595, 1986.

Tanphiphat C, Tanprayoon T, et al: Surgical treatment of perforated duodenal ulcer: A prospective trial between simple closure and definitive surgery. *Br J Surg* 72:370, 1985.

Tersmette AC, Offerhaus GJA, et al: Occurrence of non-gastric cancer in the digestive tract after remote partial gastrectomy: Analysis of an Amsterdam cohort. *Int J Cancer* 46:792, 1990.

Thomas WE, et al: The long-term outcome of billroth I partial gastrectomy for benign gastric ulcer. *Ann Surg* 195:189, 1982.

Thompson NW, Vinik AI, et al: Microgastrinomas of the duodenum: A cause of failed operations for the Zollinger-Ellison syndrome. *Ann Surg* 209:396, 1989.

Thomsen F, et al: Cimetidine treatment of recurrent ulcer after vagotomy. *Acta Chir Scand* 146:35, 1980.

Vallon AG, et al: Randomized trial of endoscopic argon laser photocoagulation in bleeding peptic ulcers. *Gut* 22:228, 1981.

Walan A, Bader JP, et al: Effect of omeprazole and ranitidine on ulcer healing and relapse rates in patients with benign gastric ulcer. *N Engl J Med* 320:69, 1989.

Wara P: Endoscopic management of the bleeding ulcer. *Danish Med Bull* 33:1, 1986.

Wastell C, Ellis H: Volvulus of the stomach. *Br J Surg* 58:557, 1971.

Weaver RM, Temple JG: Proximal gastric vagotomy in patients resistant to cimetidine. *Br J Surg* 72:177, 1985.

Weiland D, et al: Gastric outlet obstruction in peptic ulcer disease: An indication for surgery. *Am J Surg* 143:90, 1982.

Weinberg JA: Treatment of the massively bleeding duodenal ulcer by ligation. Pyloroplasty and vagotomy. *Am J Surg* 102:158, 1961.

Wermer P: Multiple endocrine adenomatosis: Multiple hormone producing tumors, a familial syndrome. In Bonfils S (ed): *Endocrine-Secreting Tumours of the Gastrointestinal Tract*. Philadelphia, WB Saunders, 1974, p 671.

Wilson SD, Ellison EH: Survival in patients with Zollinger-Ellison syndrome treated with total gastrectomy. *Am J Surg* 111:787, 1966.

Wilson WS, et al: Superficial gastric erosions. Response to surgical treatment. *Am J Surg* 126:133, 1973.

Wyllie JH, et al: Effect of cimetidine on surgery for duodenal ulcer. *Lancet* 1:1307, 1981.

Yalow RS, Berson SA: Size and charge distinctions between endogenous human plasma gastrin in peripheral blood and heptadecapeptide gastrins. *Gastroenterology* 58:609, 1970.

Yamazaki H, Oshima A: A long-term follow-up study of patients with gastric cancer detected by mass screening. *Cancer* 63:613, 1989.

Yan CJ, Brooks JR: Surgical management of gastric adenocarcinoma. *Am J Surg* 149:771, 1985.

Zollinger RM: Gastrinoma: Factors influencing prognosis. *Surgery* 97:49, 1985.

Zollinger RM, Ellison RH: Primary peptic ulcerations of the jejunum associated with islet cell tumors of the pancreas. *Ann Surg* 142:709, 1955.

Gastric Procedures for Morbid Obesity

Agha FP, Eckhauser FE, et al: Mason's vertical banded gastroplasty for morbid obesity: Surgical procedure and radiographic evaluation. *Radiology* 150:825, 1984.

Brolin RE, Kenler HA, et al: Long-limb gastric bypass in the superobese: A prospective randomized study. *Ann Surg* 215:387, 1992.

Buckwalter JA: Clinical trial of jejunoileal and gastric bypass for the treatment of morbid obesity: Four-year progress report. *Ann Surg* 46:377, 1980.

Flickinger EG, Pories WJ, et al: The Greenville gastric bypass: Progress report at 3 years. *Ann Surg* 199:555, 1984.

Flickinger EG, Sinar DR, et al: The bypassed stomach. *Am J Surg* 149:151, 1985.

Freeman JB, Burchett HJ: A comparison of gastric bypass and gastroplasty for morbid obesity. *Surgery* 88:433, 1980.

Gannon MX, Pears DJ, et al: The effect of gastric partitioning on gastric emptying in morbidly obese patients. *Br J Surg* 72:952, 1985.

Gentry K, Halverson JD, et al: Psychologic assessment of morbidly obese patients undergoing gastric bypass: A comparison of preoperative and postoperative adjustment. *Surgery* 95:215, 1984.

Griffen WO Jr, et al: Experiences with conversion of jejunoileal bypass to gastric bypass: Its use for maintenance of weight loss. *Arch Surg* 116:320, 1981.

Hall JC, Watts JM, et al: Gastric surgery for morbid obesity: The Adelaide study. *Ann Surg* 211:419, 1990.

Halverson JD, et al: Gastric bypass for morbid obesity: A medical-surgical assessment. *Ann Surg* 194:152, 1981.

Halverson JD, Koehler RE: Assessment of patients with failed gastric operations for morbid obesity. *Am J Surg* 145:357, 1983.

Krol JA, Strodel WD, et al: Critical appraisal of horizontal gastroplasty. *Am J Surg* 153:256, 1987.

MacLean LD, Rhode BM, et al: Late results of vertical banded gastroplasty for morbid and super obesity. *Surgery* 107:20, 1990.

Makarewicz PA, Freeman JB, et al: Vertical banded gastroplasty: Assessment of efficacy. *Surgery* 98:700, 1985.

Mason EE: Vertical banded gastroplasty for obesity. *Arch Surg* 117:701, 1982.

Miller DK, Goodman GN: Gastric bypass procedures. In Deitel M (ed): *Surgery for the Morbidly Obese Patient*. Philadelphia, Lea & Febiger, 1989, p 113.

Nightengale ML, Sarr MG, et al: Prospective evaluation of vertical banded gastroplasty as the primary operation for morbid obesity. *Mayo Clin Proc* 66:773, 1991.

Stunkard AJ, Harris JR, et al: The body-mass index of twins who have been reared apart. *N Engl J Med* 322:1483, 1990.

Sugarman HJ, Fairman RP, et al: Gastric surgery for respiratory insufficiency of obesity. *Chest* 90:81, 1986.

Sugarman HJ, Starkey JV, et al: A randomized prospective trial of gastric bypass versus vertical banded gastroplasty for morbid obesity and their effects on sweets versus non-sweets eaters. *Ann Surg* 205:613, 1987.

Waters GS, Pories WJ, et al: Long-term studies of mental health after the Greenville gastric bypass operation for morbid obesity. *Am J Surg* 161:154, 1991.

Index

Page numbers in italics refer to figures; page numbers followed by t indicate tables.